MW01630032

SECTION 9 Problems of Ingestion, Digestion, Absorption, and Elimination

SECTION 10 Problems of Urinary Function

SECTION 11 Problems Related to Regulatory and Reproductive Mechanisms

SECTION 12 Problems Related to Movement and Coordination

ABBREVIATIONS

ABG	arterial blood gas
ACE	angiotensin-converting enzyme
ACLS	advanced cardiac life support
ACS	acute coronary syndrome
ACTH	adrenocorticotropic hormone
ADH	antidiuretic hormone
AED	automatic external defibrillator
AIDS	acquired immunodeficiency syndrome
AKA	above-knee amputation
AKI	acute kidney injury
ALI	acute lung injury
ALL	acute lymphocytic leukemia
ALS	amyotrophic lateral sclerosis
AMI	acute myocardial infarction
ANA	antinuclear antibody
ANS	autonomic nervous system
AORN	Association of periOperative Room Nurses
APD	automated peritoneal dialysis
aPTT	activated partial thromboplastin time
ARDS	acute respiratory distress syndrome
ATN	acute tubular necrosis
BCLS	basic cardiac life support
BKA	below-knee amputation
BMI	body mass index
BMR	basal metabolic rate
BMT	bone marrow transplantation
BPH	benign prostatic hyperplasia
BSE	breast self-examination
BUN	blood urea nitrogen
CABG	coronary artery bypass graft
CAD	coronary artery disease; circulatory assist device
CAPD	continuous ambulatory peritoneal dialysis
CAVH	continuous arteriovenous hemofiltration
CBC	complete blood count
CCU	coronary care unit; critical care unit
CDC	Centers for Disease Control and Prevention
CIS	carcinoma in situ
CKD	chronic kidney disease
CLL	chronic lymphocytic leukemia
CML	chronic myelocytic leukemia
CMP	cardiomyopathy
CN	cranial nerve
CNS	central nervous system
CO	cardiac output
COPD	chronic obstructive pulmonary disease
CPAP	continuous positive airway pressure
CPR	cardiopulmonary resuscitation
CRRT	continuous renal replacement therapy
CRNA	certified registered nurse anesthetist
CSF	cerebrospinal fluid
CT	computed tomography
CVA	cerebrovascular accident; costovertebral angle
CVAD	central venous access device
CVI	chronic venous insufficiency
CVP	central venous pressure
D&C	dilation and curettage
DDD	degenerative disk disease
DI	diabetes insipidus
DIC	disseminated intravascular coagulation
DJD	degenerative joint disease
DKA	diabetic ketoacidosis
DM	diabetes mellitus; diastolic murmur
DRE	digital rectal examination
DVT	deep vein thrombosis
ECF	extracellular fluid
ECG	electrocardiogram
ED	emergency department; erectile dysfunction
EEG	electroencephalogram
EMG	electromyogram
EMS	emergency medical services
ENT	ear, nose, and throat
ERCP	endoscopic retrograde cholangiopancreatography
ERT	estrogen replacement therapy
ESKD	end-stage kidney disease
ESR	erythrocyte sedimentation rate
ET	endotracheal
FEV	forced expiratory volume
FRC	functional residual capacity
FUO	fever of unknown origin
GCS	Glasgow Coma Scale
GERD	gastroesophageal reflux disease
GFR	glomerular filtration rate
GH	growth hormone
GI	glycemic index
GTT	glucose tolerance test
GU	genitourinary
GYN, Gyn	gynecologic
HAI	health care—associated infection
HAV	hepatitis A virus
Hb, Hgb	hemoglobin
HBV	hepatitis B virus
Hct	hematocrit
HCV	hepatitis C virus
HD	hemodialysis, Huntington disease
HDL	high-density lipoprotein
HF	heart failure
HIV	human immunodeficiency virus
H&P	history and physical examination
HPV	human papillomavirus
HSCT	hematopoietic stem cell transplantation
IABP	intraaortic balloon pump
IBS	irritable bowel syndrome
ICP	intracranial pressure
I&D	incision and drainage
IE	infective endocarditis
IFG	impaired fasting glucose
IGT	impaired glucose tolerance
INR	international normalized ratio
IOP	intraocular pressure
IPPB	intermittent positive-pressure breathing
ITP	idiopathic thrombocytopenic purpura
IUD	intrauterine device
IV	intravenous
IVP	intravenous push; intravenous pyelogram
JVD	jugular venous distention
KS	Kaposi sarcoma
KUB	kidney, ureters, and bladder (x-ray)
KVO	keep vein open
LAD	left anterior descending
LDL	low-density lipoprotein

LEWIS'S

Medical-Surgical Nursing

ASSESSMENT AND MANAGEMENT OF CLINICAL PROBLEMS

LEWIS'S

Medical-Surgical Nursing

13TH EDITION

ASSESSMENT AND MANAGEMENT OF CLINICAL PROBLEMS

Mariann M. Harding,
PhD, RN, CNE, FAADN
Nursing Program Administrator
College of Applied and Technical Studies
Kent State University Tuscarawas
New Philadelphia, Ohio

SECTION EDITORS

Jeffrey Kwong,
DNP, MPH, RN, ANP-BC, FAANP, FAAN
Nurse Practitioner
NYU Langone Health
New York, New York

Debra Hagler,
PhD, RN, ACNS-BC, CNE, CHSE, ANEF, FAAN
Clinical Professor
Edson College of Nursing and Health Innovation
Arizona State University
Phoenix, Arizona

Courtney Reinisch,
DNP, RN, FNP-BC
Professor
School of Nursing
Montclair State University
Montclair, New Jersey

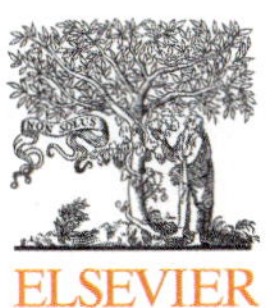

ELSEVIER

Elsevier
3251 Riverport Lane
St. Louis, Missouri 63043

LEWIS'S MEDICAL-SURGICAL NURSING: ASSESSMENT
AND MANAGEMENT OF CLINICAL PROBLEMS, THIRTEENTH EDITION ISBN: 978-0-443-12179-1

Notice

Practitioners and researchers must always rely on their own experience and knowledge in evaluating and using any information, methods, compounds or experiments described herein. Because of rapid advances in the medical sciences, in particular, independent verification of diagnoses and drug dosages should be made. To the fullest extent of the law, no responsibility is assumed by Elsevier, authors, editors or contributors for any injury and/or damage to persons or property as a matter of products liability, negligence or otherwise, or from any use or operation of any methods, products, instructions, or ideas contained in the material herein.

Previous editions copyrighted 2023, 2020, 2017, 2014, 2011, 2007, 2004, 2000, 1996, 1992, 1987, and 1983.

Executive Content Strategist: Lee Henderson
Senior Content Development Specialist: Rebecca Leenhouts
Publishing Services Manager: Catherine Jackson
Senior Project Manager: Jodi Willard
Design Direction: Brian Salisbury

Printed in India

Last digit is the print number: 9 8 7 6 5 4 3 2 1

ABOUT THE AUTHORS

MARIANN M. HARDING, PhD, RN, CNE, FAADN

Mariann Harding is a professor of nursing and nursing program director at Kent State University Tuscarawas, New Philadelphia, Ohio, where she has been a member of the faculty since 2005. She received her diploma in nursing from Mt. Carmel School of Nursing, her bachelor of science in nursing from Ohio University, her master of science in nursing as an adult nurse practitioner from the Catholic University of America, and her doctorate in nursing from West Virginia University. Dr. Harding's nursing experience has primarily been in critical care nursing and teaching in licensed practical, associate, and baccalaureate nursing programs. Her research has focused on pedagogy for promoting student success and health promotion. Dr. Harding is coauthor of *Clinical Reasoning Cases in Nursing* and *Conceptual Nursing Care Planning.* She is a fellow in the Academy of Associate Degree Nursing.

DEBRA HAGLER, PhD, RN, ACNS-BC, CNE, CHSE, ANEF, FAAN

Debbie Hagler is a clinical professor in the Edson College of Nursing and Health Innovation at Arizona State University in Phoenix. Dr. Hagler earned a practical certificate in nursing, associate degree, and bachelor of science in nursing from New Mexico State University. She earned a master of science in nursing from the University of Arizona and a doctorate in learning and instructional technology from Arizona State University. Dr. Hagler is a clinical nurse specialist with experience in adult health and critical care nursing. Currently, she teaches students in the undergraduate honors, master's, and doctoral programs. For many years, she has led writing groups to support nurses and health professionals in becoming published authors. Dr. Hagler is the senior editor of *Innovative Teaching Strategies in Nursing,* associate editor for credentialing at *The Journal of Continuing Education in Nursing,* and coauthor of *Conceptual Nursing Care Planning.* She is a fellow in the American Academy of Nursing and the National League for Nursing Academy of Nursing Education.

JEFFREY KWONG, DNP, MPH, RN, ANP-BC, FAANP, FAAN

Jeffrey Kwong is a nurse practitioner at NYU Langone Health in New York City, where provides primary care for the LGBTQ+ community and persons living with HIV. He has over 16 years of academic nursing experience and most recently was a member of the faculty at Rutgers, the State University of New Jersey. There he was a professor in the Division of Advanced Nursing Practice. Dr. Kwong received his undergraduate degree from the University of California—Berkeley, received his nurse practitioner degree from the University of California—San Francisco and completed his doctoral training at the University of Colorado—Denver. He has a master of public health degree from the University of California—Los Angeles. He is a fellow in the American Association of Nurse Practitioners and the American Academy of Nursing.

COURTNEY REINISCH, DNP, RN, FNP-BC

Courtney Reinisch is a professor in the School of Nursing at Montclair State University, Montclair campus, in New Jersey. She served as the founding undergraduate program director when the school opened in 2016. Dr. Reinisch earned her undergraduate degree from Immaculata College and her nursing degree and master's in nursing from the University of Delaware. Dr. Reinisch has worked as a primary care and urgent care family nurse practitioner with a special interest in underserved communities for over 25 years. She earned her doctorate in nursing practice from Columbia University and has been involved in both undergraduate and graduate nursing education for 18 years. Dr. Reinisch provides primary care in a volunteer medical clinic.

CONTRIBUTORS

Maura Abbott, PhD, AOCNP, CPNP-PC and AC
Associate Professor of Nursing
Columbia University School of Nursing;
Nurse Practitioner
Hematology/Oncology
Columbia University Medical Center
New York, New York

Cynthia Bernat Amerson, MSN, MS, RN, CNE
Discipline Lead
Division of Nursing
Collin College
McKinney, Texas

Vera Barton-Maxwell, PhD, APRN, FNP-BC
Associate Professor, Program Director
Family Nurse Practitioner Program
Georgetown University
Washington, DC;
Nurse Practitioner
Wheeling Health Right
Wheeling, West Virginia

Samantha J. Bonaduce, DNP, RN, CNE
Associate Professor
Nursing
Kent State University Tuscarawas
New Philadelphia, Ohio

Diana Taibi Buchanan, PhD, RN
Affiliate Associate Professor
Biobehavioral Nursing and Health Informatics
University of Washington
Seattle, Washington

Mary M. Cameron, MSN, RN
Associate Lecturer
Nursing Technology
Kent State University Tuscarawas
New Philadelphia, Ohio

Lori Cogan, DNP, DCC, ACNP-BC, ANP-BC, CCTC, WCC
Nurse Practitioner
Center For Liver Disease and Transplantation
NewYork-Presbyterian/Weill Cornell Medical Center
New York, New York

Julia B. Corbo, MSN, CRNP, AGACNP-BC, FNP-BC
Nurse Practitioner
Cardiology
Jefferson Hospital
Philadelphia, Pennsylvania

Ann H. Crawford, PhD, MSN, RN, CNS, CEN, CPEN
Professor
Scott & White School of Nursing
University of Mary Hardin-Baylor
Belton, Texas;
Relief Charge/Staff Nurse
Emergency Department
Baylor Scott & White Health McLane Children's Medical Center
Temple, Texas

Sylvia Dao, MSN, MPA, RN, NE-BC
Patient Care Director
8W Burn Center
NewYork-Presbyterian/Weill Cornell Medical Center
New York, New York

Kimberly Day, DNP, MSN-Ed, RN, CNE, CHSE
Clinical Professor
Edson College of Nursing and Health Innovation
Arizona State University
Phoenix, Arizona

Hazel A. Dennison, DNP, RN, FNP-BC, CHCP, CPHQ, CNE
Nursing Faculty
College of Nursing
Virtua Our Lady of Lourdes Hospital
Stratford, New Jersey;
Faculty
College of Nursing
Walden University
Minneapolis, Minnesota

Jane K. Dickinson, RN, PhD, CDCES
Program Director/Senior Lecturer
Health & Behavior Studies
Teachers College
Columbia University
New York, New York

Susan Doyle-Lindrud, DNP, ANP
Assistant Dean of Academic Affairs
Columbia University School of Nursing
New York, New York

Marybeth Duffy, DNP-DCC, RN, FNP-BC, ACNP-BC, PMHNP
Associate Professor
School of Nursing
Montclair State University
Montclair, New Jersey

Rebekah O. Filson, DNP, RN, ACNS-BC, ANP-BC
Founder, Healthcare Consultant
Neurosciences, Orthopedics and Spine
NOS Healthcare Consulting
Wetumpka, Alabama

Jessica I. Goldberg, PhD, RN, AGPCNP-BC, ACHPN
Nurse Practitioner and Nurse Scientist
Supportive Care Service
Memorial Sloan Kettering Cancer Center
New York, New York

Sherry A. Greenberg, PhD, RN, GNP-BC, FGSA, FNAP, AGSF, FAANP, FAAN
Evelyn Lauder Chair in Adult Gerontology;
Professor; Specialty Director, Adult-Gerontology Primary Care Nurse Practitioner Program
Nursing
Hunter-Bellevue School of Nursing, Hunter College, The City University of New York
New York, New York

Debra Hagler, PhD, RN, ACNS-BC, CNE, CHSE, ANEF, FAAN
Clinical Professor
Edson College of Nursing and Health Innovation
Arizona State University
Phoenix, Arizona

Diana Rabbani Hagler, MSN-Ed, RN
Registered Nurse
Intensive Care Unit
Banner Health
Gilbert, Arizona;
Adjunct Faculty
Nursing
Grand Canyon University
Phoenix, Arizona;
Adjunct Faculty
Nursing
Maricopa Community College
Phoenix, Arizona

Mariann M. Harding, PhD, RN, CNE, FAADN
Nursing Program Administrator
College of Applied and Technical Studies
Kent State University Tuscarawas
New Philadelphia, Ohio

Julia A. Hitch, MS, FNP, CDCES
Nurse Practitioner
Diabetes
Level2
Eden Prairie, Minnesota

Haley Hoy, PhD, NP
Associate Professor
Nursing
University of Alabama in Huntsville
Huntsville, Alabama;
Nurse Practitioner
Vanderbilt Lung Transplantation
Vanderbilt Medical Center
Nashville, Tennessee

Patricia Keegan, DNP, NP-C, FACC
Medical Science Liaison
Heart Recovery
Johnson and Johnson MedTech
Danvers, Massachusetts

Kristen J. Keller, DNP, ACNP-BC, PMHNP-BC, RNFA
Nurse Practitioner
Trauma and Acute Care Surgery
Banner Thunderbird Medical Center
Glendale, Arizona

Jeffrey Kwong, DNP, MPH, RN, ANP-BC, FAANP, FAAN
Nurse Practitioner
NYU Langone Health
New York, New York

Anthony Richard Lutz, MSN, NP-C, CUNP
Urology Nurse Practitioner
Atlantic Medical Group Urology
Atlantic Health System
Summit, New Jersey

Ruthie R. Mangino, DNP, APRN, ACNS-BC, ANP-C
Clinical Nurse Specialist
Department of Nursing—Professional Practice and Quality
Mayo Clinic
Phoenix, Arizona

Helen Miley, PhD
Program Director, Online
Nursing
Herzing University
St. Louis Park, Minnesota;
Adjunct Faculty
School of Nursing
Montclair State University
Montclair, New Jersey;
Adult-Gerontology Acute Care Nurse Practitioner
Critical Care
Robert Wood Johnson Hospital
New Brunswick, New Jersey

Eugene E. Mondor, MN, RN, BScN, CNCC(C)
Clinical Nurse Specialist
Department of Critical Care
Royal Alexandra Hospital
Edmonton, Alberta, Canada

Tracie Clark Morgan, DNP, CRNP
Clinical Assistant Professor
Nursing
University of Alabama in Huntsville
Huntsville, Alabama

Brenda C. Morris, EdD, MS, BSN, RN, CNE
Clinical Professor
Edson College of Nursing and Health Innovation
Arizona State University
Phoenix, Arizona

Yeow Chye Ng, PhD, CRNP, CPC, AAHIVE, FAANP, FAAN
Professor
College of Nursing
University of Alabama in Huntsville
Huntsville, Alabama

Leslie Ogburn, MSN, NP-C
Nurse Practitioner
Cardiology
Emory Healthcare
Atlanta, Georgia

Shila Pandey, DNP, AGPCNP-BC, ACHPN
Nurse Practitioner
Supportive Care Service
Memorial Sloan Kettering Cancer Center
New York, New York

Amisha Parekh de Campos, PhD, MPH, RN, CHPN
Quality and Education Coordinator
Hospice Care at Home
Middlesex Health
Middletown, Connecticut;
Assistant Clinical Professor
School of Nursing
University of Connecticut
Storrs, Connecticut

LaToya Patterson, PhD, CRNP
Clinical Nursing Instructor
College of Nursing
University of Alabama in Huntsville
Huntsville, Alabama

Lillian A. Pryor, DNP, RN, CNN
VANAP-U Co-Director
Nursing Education
VA Atlanta Health Care
Decatur, Georgia

Margaret R. Rateau, PhD, RN, CNE
Associate Professor (Retired)
Nursing
Robert Morris University
Moon Township, Pennsylvania

Catherine R. Ratliff, PhD, GNP-BC, CWOCN, CFCN, FAAN
Clinical Associate Professor/Nurse Practitioner
School of Nursing/Department of Surgery/Vascular Surgery
UVA Health
Charlottesville, Virginia

Courtney Reinisch, DNP, RN, FNP-BC
Professor
School of Nursing
Montclair State University
Montclair, New Jersey

Sandra Irene Rome, MN, RN, AOCN
Clinical Nurse Specialist
Oncology/Hematology/Cellular Therapy
Cedars-Sinai Medical Center
Los Angeles, California;
Volunteer Assistant Clinical Professor
UCLA School of Nursing
Los Angeles, California

William E. Rosa, PhD, MBE, NP-BC, FAANP, FAAN
Assistant Attending Behavioral Scientist
Department of Psychiatry and Behavioral Sciences
Memorial Sloan Kettering Cancer Center
New York, New York

Diane M. Rudolphi, MSN
Senior Instructor
Nursing
University of Delaware
Newark, Delaware

Amanda Sanders, MSN, APRN-CNP
Nurse Practitioner
Urology
Aultman Urology
Canton, Ohio;
Clinical Adjunct Faculty
Associate Nursing
Kent State University Tuscarawas
New Philadelphia, Ohio

Janice A. Sarasnick, PhD, MSN, RN
Professor of Nursing
Nursing
Robert Morris University
Coraopolis, Pennsylvania

Michelle L. Sauve, MSN, RN, CPAN
Nursing Supervisor
MOR, PACU, Extended Recovery, Perianesthesia Resource Pool
Mayo Clinic Arizona
Phoenix, Arizona

Andrew Scanlon, PhD, DNP, MN, MNS, RN, FACN, FACNP
Adjunct Senior Lecturer
School of Nursing and Midwifery
La Trobe University
Bundoora, Victoria, Australia;
Nurse Practitioner
Neurosurgery
Austin Health
Heidelberg, Victoria, Australia

Robyn Schafer, PhD, CNM, FACNM
Assistant Professor
Division of Advanced Nursing Practice
Rutgers School of Nursing
Newark, New Jersey;
Assistant Professor
Department of Obstetrics, Gynecology, and Reproductive Sciences
Robert Wood Johnson Medical School
New Brunswick, New Jersey

Aaron M. Sebach, PhD, DNP, MBA, AGACNP-BC, FNP-BC, NRP, CP-C, CEN, CPEN, CGNC, CLNC, CNE, CNEcl, SFHM, FNAP, FAANP
Dean and Professor
College of Health Professions and Natural Sciences
Wilmington University
New Castle, Delaware;
Nurse Practitioner
Mobile Integrated Health
TidalHealth
Salisbury, Maryland

Rose B. Shaffer, MSN, RN, ACNP-BC, CCRN, FAHA
Nurse Practitioner
Cardiology
Thomas Jefferson University Hospital
Philadelphia, Pennsylvania

Janice Smolowitz, PhD, DNP, EDD
Dean and Professor
Nursing
Montclair State University
Montclair, New York

Kara Ann Ventura, DNP, PNP, FNP
Clinical Program Director
Abdominal Transplant
Yale New Haven Hospital
Fairfield, Connecticut

Lori Ann Wenz, MSN, AGNP-C, BC-ADM, FOMA
Nurse Practitioner
Owner/Founder
Western Colorado Weight Care
Colorado Springs, Colorado

Rita Wermers, DNP, ANP-BC
Nurse Practitioner and Clinic Manager
Health Services
Arizona State University
Phoenix, Arizona

Daniel P. Worrall, MSN, ANP-BC
Nurse Practitioner
Sexual Health Clinic
Massachusetts General Hospital
Boston, Massachusetts

AUTHORS OF TEACHING AND LEARNING RESOURCES

Test Bank

Debra Hagler, PhD, RN, ACNS-BC, CNE, CHSE, ANEF, FAAN
Clinical Professor
Edson College of Nursing and Health Innovation
Arizona State University
Phoenix, Arizona

Case Studies (Interactive and Applying Clinical Judgment With Multiple Patients)

Mariann M. Harding, PhD, RN, CNE, FAADN
Nursing Program Administrator
College of Applied and Technical Studies
Kent State University Tuscarawas
New Philadelphia, Ohio

Brenda C. Morris, EdD, MS, RN, CNE
Clinical Professor
Edson College of Nursing and Health Innovation
Arizona State University
Phoenix, Arizona

PowerPoint Presentations

Jane Grages, MS, RN
Associate Professor of Nursing (Retired)
Pennsylvania College of Technology
Williamsport, Pennsylvania

TEACH for Nurses

Margaret R. Rateau, PhD, RN, CNE
Associate Professor (Retired)
Nursing
Robert Morris University
Moon Township, Pennsylvania

NCLEX® Examination Review Questions

Shelly Stefka, MSN, RN
Senior Lecturer
Nursing
Kent State University Tuscarawas
New Philadelphia, Ohio

Study Guide

Collin Bowman-Woodall, MS, RN
Assistant Professor
San Francisco Peninsula Campus
Samuel Merritt University
San Mateo, California

Clinical Companion

Debra A. Hagler, PhD, RN, ACNS-BC, CNE, CHSE, ANEF, FAAN
Clinical Professor
Edson College of Nursing and Health Innovation
Arizona State University
Phoenix, Arizona

Evidence-Based Practice Boxes

Margaret R. Rateau, PhD, RN, CNE
Associate Professor (Retired)
Nursing
Robert Morris University
Moon Township, Pennsylvania

Nursing Care Plans

Mariann M. Harding, PhD, RN, CNE, FAADN
Nursing Program Administrator
College of Applied and Technical Studies
Kent State University Tuscarawas
New Philadelphia, Ohio

PREFACE

The thirteenth edition of *Lewis's Medical-Surgical Nursing: Assessment and Management of Clinical Problems* contains the most current medical-surgical nursing information in an easy-to-use format. This textbook is a comprehensive resource describing standards of nursing clinical practice for providing safe and comprehensive patient care. The text and accompanying resources include many features to help students learn key medical-surgical nursing content, including patient and caregiver teaching, gerontology, interprofessional care, patient safety, nutrition and drug therapy, evidence-based practice, and much more, that will prepare them to deliver compassionate, inclusive care across diverse populations.

This edition incorporates the AACN 4 Spheres of Clinical Care to help students learn to apply nursing knowledge to improve patient outcomes across the continuum of care. Here's a brief overview of each:

1. **Health Promotion** — Focuses on disease prevention, wellness strategies, and patient education to support long-term health.
2. **Acute and Rehabilitative Care** — Aims to return patients to their highest level of function after illness or injury.
3. **Chronic Care** — Involves managing long-term conditions such as diabetes, heart disease, or chronic obstructive pulmonary disease (COPD), often requiring coordinating care and teaching patient self-management strategies.
4. **Palliative Care** — Emphasizes comfort, symptom management, and quality of life for patients with serious, life-limiting illnesses.

Special content has been enhanced to assist with NCLEX® preparation and the development of clinical judgment based on NCSBN's Clinical Judgment Measurement Model (CJMM). At the end of each unit, the reader will find Applying Clinical Judgment With Multiple Patients, featuring traditional and Next-Generation NCLEX® (NGN)—style questions. Discussion questions in the management chapters' Case Studies focus on the 6 cognitive skills identified in the CJMM: Recognize Cues (Recognize), Analyze Cues (Analyze), Prioritize Hypotheses (Prioritize), Generate Solutions (Plan), Take Actions (Act), and Evaluate Outcomes (Evaluate).

This edition features updated visuals that reflect the rich diversity of today's patients and health care professionals, bringing inclusivity to the forefront of nursing education. The authentic imagery combined with content on promoting health equity reinforces the textbook's commitment to fair and inclusive health care.

Great effort has been put into continuing to improve readability and lower the reading level. Readers will find clear and easier-to-read language, with an engaging, conversational style. The narrative addresses the reader directly, helping make the text more personal and an active learning tool.

ORGANIZATION

Content is organized into 2 major divisions. The first division, Sections 1 through 3 (Chapters 1 through 17), discusses general concepts related to the care of adult patients. The second division, Sections 4 through 13 (Chapters 18 through 68), presents nursing assessment and nursing management of medical-surgical problems. At the beginning of each chapter, the Conceptual Focus helps students focus on the key concepts and integrate concepts, with exemplars affecting different body systems. Learning Outcomes and Key Terms assist students in identifying the key content for that chapter.

The various body systems are grouped to reflect their interrelated functions. Each section is organized around 2 central themes: assessment and management. Chapters dealing with assessment of a body system include a discussion of the following:

1. A brief review of anatomy and physiology, focusing on information that will promote understanding of nursing care
2. Health history and noninvasive physical assessment skills to expand the knowledge base on which treatment decisions are made
3. Common diagnostic studies, expected results, and related nursing responsibilities to provide easily accessible information

Management chapters focus on the pathophysiology, clinical manifestations, diagnostic studies, interprofessional care, and nursing management of various problems. The conceptual focus at the beginning of each chapter helps students focus on the key concepts and integrate concepts, with exemplars affecting different body systems. The nursing management sections are organized into assessment, clinical problem, planning, implementation, and evaluation.

SPECIAL FEATURES

- Features that are focused on developing clinical judgment include:
  - Applying Clinical Judgment With Multiple Patients, featuring traditional and Next-Generation NCLEX® (NGN)—style questions at the end of each unit.
  - Prioritization questions in case studies and Bridge to NCLEX® Examination Questions.
  - ***Enhanced!* Case Studies** help students learn how to prioritize care and manage patients in the clinical setting. Discussion questions focus on the 6 cognitive skills identified in the CJMM: Recognize Cues (Recognize), Analyze Cues (Analyze), Prioritize Hypotheses (Prioritize), Generate Solutions (Plan), Take Actions (Act), and Evaluate Outcomes (Evaluate), with a special focus on patient

safety. Answer guidelines are provided on the Evolve website.

- ***Expanded!* Nursing Management** tables focus on the actions nurses need to take to deliver safe, quality, effective patient care. New tables throughout the text focus on problems such as pancreatitis, acute respiratory failure, and hemodialysis.
- ***Expanded!* Drug Therapy** tables provide more detailed information on drug therapy and associated nursing considerations. Concise **Drug Alerts** highlight important safety considerations for key drugs.
- ***Enhanced!* Evidence-Based Practice** boxes use a case study approach to help students learn to use evidence in making decisions at the patient and systems levels.
- Interprofessional care delivered by physicians, nurses, and other health care team members is highlighted in **Interprofessional Care** tables throughout the text.
- **Safety Alert** boxes highlight important patient safety issues and focus on the National Patient Safety Goals.
- **Bridge to NCLEX® Examination Questions** at the end of each chapter match the Learning Outcomes and help students learn the important points in the chapter. Answers are provided just below the questions for immediate feedback, and rationales are provided on the Evolve website.
- Teaching is an ongoing theme and highlighted in **Patient and Caregiver Teaching** tables.
- Gerontology is addressed throughout the text under Gerontologic Considerations headings and in **Gerontologic Differences in Assessment** tables.
- Nutrition is highlighted throughout the textbook. **Nutrition Therapy** tables summarize nutrition interventions and promote healthy lifestyles.
- **Promoting Population Health** boxes address strategies to improve health outcomes as they relate to specific disorders, such as diabetes and cancer, and to health promotion, such as preserving hearing and maintaining a healthy weight.
- **Check Your Practice** boxes challenge students to think critically, analyze patient assessment data, and implement the appropriate intervention. Scenarios and discussion questions are provided to promote active learning.
- **Ethical/Legal Dilemma** boxes promote critical thinking for timely and sensitive issues that nursing students may deal with in clinical practice—topics such as informed consent, advance directives, and confidentiality.
- **Emergency Management** tables outline the emergency treatment of health problems most likely to require emergency intervention.
- **Nursing Care Plans** on the Evolve website focus on common problems. These care plans incorporate clinical problems, interventions, and outcomes in a way that the student can translate them readily to clinical nursing practice.
- **Nursing Assessment** and **Health History** tables summarize key subjective and objective data related to common problems. Subjective data are organized by functional health patterns.
- **Assessment Abnormalities** tables in assessment chapters alert the nurse to commonly encountered abnormalities and their possible etiologies.
- **Focused Assessment** boxes in all assessment chapters provide brief checklists that help students do a more practical "assessment on the run" or bedside approach to assessment. They can be used to evaluate the status of previously identified health problems and monitor for signs of new problems.
- Genetics content includes:
  - **Genetics in Clinical Practice** boxes that summarize the genetic basis, genetic testing, and clinical implications for genetic disorders that affect adults.
  - **Genetic Link** headings in the management chapters, which highlight the specific genetic bases of many disorders.

LEARNING SUPPLEMENTS FOR STUDENTS

- The **Clinical Companion** presents more than 200 common medical-surgical problems and procedures in a concise, alphabetical format for quick clinical reference. Designed for portability, this popular reference includes the essential, need-to-know information for treatments and procedures in which nurses play a major role. An attractive and functional full-color design highlights key information for quick, easy reference.
- The revised **Study Guide** contains more than 500 pages of review material that reflects the content found in the textbook. It features a wide variety of clinically relevant exercises and activities, including NCLEX®-format multiple-choice and alternate-format questions, anatomy review, critical thinking activities, and much more. The revised case studies mirror the NCLEX® Examination, with NGN Examination–style case studies and questions reflecting phases of the CJMM. It features an attractive full-color design and many alternate-item format questions to better prepare students for the NCLEX® Examination. An answer key is included to provide students with immediate feedback as they study.
- The **Evolve Student Resources** are available online at http://evolve.elsevier.com/Lewis/medsurg. They include the following valuable learning aids organized by chapter:
  - Printable **Key Points** summaries for each chapter.
  - 1000 NCLEX® Examination **Review Questions.**
  - **Answer Guidelines** to the Case Studies in the textbook.
  - Rationales for the Bridge to NCLEX® Examination Questions in the textbook.
  - 55 **Interactive Case Studies** with state-of-the-art animations and a variety of learning activities, which provide students with immediate feedback. Ten of the Case Studies are enhanced with photos and narration of the clinical scenarios.
  - Customizable **Nursing Care Plans** for more than 60 common patient problems.
  - Conceptual Care Map Creator.

- **Audio Glossary** of key terms, available as a comprehensive alphabetical glossary and organized by chapter.
- Content Updates.

TEACHING SUPPLEMENTS FOR INSTRUCTORS

- The **Evolve Instructor Resources** (available online at http://evolve.elsevier.com/Lewis/medsurg) remain the most comprehensive set of instructor's materials available, containing the following:
  - **TEACH for Nurses Lesson Plans** with electronic resources organized by chapter help instructors develop and manage the course curriculum. This exciting resource includes:
    - Objectives
    - Preclass activities
    - Nursing curriculum standards
    - Student and instructor chapter resource listings
    - Teaching strategies, with learning activities and assessment methods tied to learning outcomes
    - Case studies with answer guidelines
  - The **Test Bank** features more than 2000 NCLEX®–style test questions with text page references and answers coded for NCLEX® Client Needs category, nursing process, and cognitive level. The test bank includes hundreds of prioritization, delegation, and multiple patient questions. Alternate-item format questions are included.
  - Unfolding and standalone **Next-Generation NCLEX® (NGN) Examination–Style Case Studies** can be used to help strengthen students' clinical judgment and prepare them for NGN success.
  - The **Image Collection** contains more than 800 full-color images for use in lectures.
  - The **PowerPoint Presentations** include more than 125 different presentations focused on the most common patient problems. They feature unfolding case studies and NCLEX® Examination–style questions for use with classroom response media.

ACKNOWLEDGMENTS

The editors are especially grateful to many people at Elsevier who assisted with this revision effort. In particular, we wish to thank the team of Lee Henderson, Rebecca Leenhouts, and Jodi Willard. We also thank our contributors and reviewers for their assistance with the revision process.

We hope that this book will assist both students and clinicians in practicing professional nursing and providing safe, quality patient care to all.

Mariann M. Harding
Debra Hagler
Jeffrey Kwong
Courtney Reinisch

CONTENTS

CONCEPT EXEMPLARS

Acid–Base Balance
Chronic Kidney Disease
Chronic Respiratory Disease
Diabetic Ketoacidosis
Metabolic Acidosis
Metabolic Alkalosis
Respiratory Acidosis
Respiratory Alkalosis

Cellular Regulation
Anemia
Breast Cancer
Cervical Cancer
Colon Cancer
Endometrial Cancer
Head and Neck Cancer
Leukemia
Liver Cancer
Lung Cancer
Lymphoma
Melanoma
Prostate Cancer

Clotting
Disseminated Intravascular Coagulopathy
Pulmonary Embolism
Thrombocytopenia
Venous Thromboembolism

Cognition
Alcohol Withdraw
Alzheimer Disease
Delirium

Elimination
Benign Prostatic Hypertrophy
Chronic Kidney Disease
Constipation
Diarrhea
Intestinal Obstruction
Pyelonephritis
Prostatitis
Renal Calculi

Fluids and Electrolytes
Burns
Hyperkalemia
Hypernatremia
Hypokalemia
Hyponatremia

Gas Exchange
Acute Respiratory Failure
Acute Respiratory Distress Syndrome
Asthma
Chronic Obstructive Pulmonary Disease
Cystic Fibrosis
Lung Cancer
Pulmonary Embolism
Tuberculosis

Glucose Regulation
Cushing Syndrome
Diabetes

Hormonal Regulation
Addison Disease
Hyperthyroidism
Hypothyroidism

Immunity
Allergic Rhinitis
Anaphylaxis
HIV Infection
Organ Transplantation
Psoriasis

Infection
Antimicrobial Resistant Infections
COVID-19
Health Care–Associated Infections
Hepatitis
Pneumonia
Tuberculosis
Urinary Tract Infection

Inflammation
Appendicitis
Cholecystitis
Glomerulonephritis
Pancreatitis
Pelvic Inflammatory Disease
Peritonitis
Rheumatoid Arthritis

Intracranial Regulation
Brain Tumor
Head Injury
Meningitis
Seizure Disorder
Stroke

Mobility
Fractures
Low Back Pain
Multiple Sclerosis
Osteoarthritis
Parkinson Disease
Spinal Cord Injury

Nutrition
Gastroesophageal Reflux Disease
Inflammatory Bowel Disease
Metabolic Syndrome
Malnutrition
Obesity
Peptic Ulcer Disease

Pain
Burns
Palliative Care
Postoperative Care
Sickle Cell Disease

Perfusion
Acute Coronary Syndrome
Atrial Fibrillation
Cardiogenic Shock
Coronary Artery Disease
Endocarditis
Heart Failure
Hyperlipidemia
Hypertension
Hypovolemic Shock
Mitral Valve Prolapse
Peripheral Artery Disease
Septic Shock
Sickle Cell Disease

Reproduction
Early Pregnancy Loss
Ectopic Pregnancy
Infertility

Sensory Perception
Cataracts
Glaucoma
Hearing Loss
Macular Degeneration
Otitis Media

Sexuality
Erectile Dysfunction
Leiomyomas
Menopause
Sexually Transmitted Infection

Sleep
Insomnia
Sleep Apnea

Thermoregulation
Fever
Frostbite
Heat Stroke
Hyperthyroidism

Tissue Integrity
Burns
Pressure Injuries
Wound Healing

LEWIS'S

Medical-Surgical Nursing

ASSESSMENT AND MANAGEMENT OF CLINICAL PROBLEMS

1

Professional Nursing

Mariann M. Harding

http://evolve.elsevier.com/Lewis/medsurg/

CONCEPTUAL FOCUS

Care Coordination
Clinical Judgment
Collaboration
Communication
Evidence
Person-Centered Care
Professional Identity
Safety

LEARNING OUTCOMES

1. Describe the definition and domains of professional nursing practice.
2. Compare the different scopes of practice available to professional nurses.
3. Describe the role of clinical judgment skills and clinical practice frameworks in providing patient-centered care.
4. Apply the SBAR procedure and effective communication techniques in the clinical setting.
5. Explore the role of the professional nurse in delegating care to licensed practical/vocational nurses and assistive personnel.
6. Discuss the role of integrating safety and quality improvement into nursing practice.
7. Evaluate the role of informatics and health care technologies in nursing practice.
8. Apply concepts of evidence-based practice to nursing practice.

KEY TERMS

advanced practice registered nurse (APRN)
clinical judgment
clinical pathway
delegation
electronic health records (EHRs)
evidence-based practice (EBP)
failure to rescue (FTR)
interprofessional team
nursing
nursing process
patient handoff
SBAR (Situation-Background-Assessment-Recommendation)
serious reportable event (SRE)
spheres of care
telehealth

This chapter presents an overview of professional nursing practice, discussing the wide variety of roles and responsibilities nurses fulfill to meet health care needs. This overview includes the core competencies that are part of registered nursing practice. These include providing safe, patient-centered care and collaborating with others.

PROFESSIONAL NURSING PRACTICE

You have never been more important to health care than you are today. As a nurse, you are at the forefront of patient care (Fig. 1.1). Beyond nursing's reputation for compassion and dedication lies a highly specialized profession.[1] Nursing continues to evolve to meet society's health care needs.

As a nurse, you (1) offer skilled care to those recovering from illness or injury, (2) advocate for patients' rights, (3) teach patients to manage their health, (4) support patients and their caregivers at critical times, and (5) help them navigate the complex health care system. You can practice in virtually all health care settings and communities. Wherever you practice, recipients of your care include individuals, families, groups, or communities. Nurses work collaboratively with other health care providers to manage the needs of persons and groups.

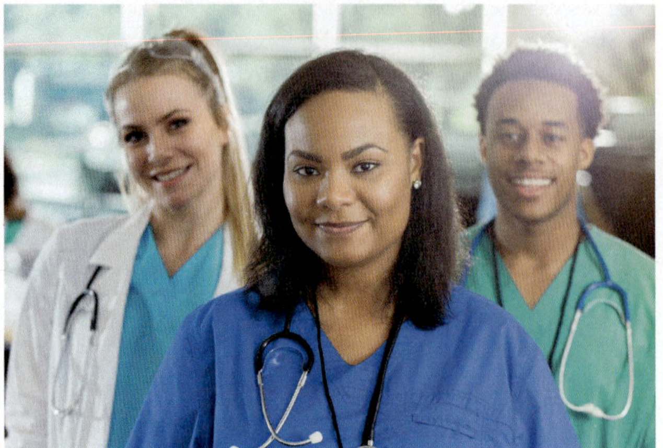

Fig. 1.1 Nurses are frontline professionals of health care. (© SDI Productions/iStock.com.)

PROFESSIONALISM

What Is Nursing?

Nursing is described as both an art and a science; a heart and a mind.[1] Well-known definitions of nursing show that the basic themes of caring, health, and illness have existed since Florence Nightingale first described nursing. The current definition of nursing by the American Nursing Association (ANA) reflects the ongoing evolution of nursing practice:

"**Nursing** integrates the art and science of caring and focuses on the protection, promotion and optimization of health and human functioning; prevention of illness and injury; facilitation of healing; and alleviation of suffering through compassionate presence. Nursing is the diagnosis and treatment of human responses, and advocacy in the care of individuals, families, groups, communities, and in recognition of the connection of all humanity."[2]

Your professional identity as a nurse will begin to develop in nursing school as you embrace the values of nursing. Through interactions in clinical and with your peers and faculty, you will begin to think, act, and feel like a nurse.

Professional Licensure

Professional licensure is established to protect public safety and authorize practice. A registered nurse is granted a professional license by a specific state, commonwealth, or territory to practice nursing.[2] The nurse's scope of practice is defined by their license. The extent that the nurse engages in their scope of practice depends on their education, experience, role, and state law.

To enter practice, a nurse must complete an accredited program and pass the NCLEX-RN, a test that verifies the nurse has the basic knowledge needed to provide safe care. Entry-level nurses with associate or baccalaureate degrees are prepared to function as generalists. At this level, nurses provide direct health care to patients across the lifespan in a variety of settings.

Experienced nurses may specialize in a specific practice area. Certification is a formal way for nurses to obtain professional recognition for having expertise in a specialty area. Many nursing organizations offer certification in specialty practice. Certification requires a certain amount of clinical experience and successfully passing a test. Recertification usually requires ongoing clinical experience and ongoing education. Common nursing specialties include critical care, women's health, geriatric, medical-surgical, perinatal, emergency, mental health, and community health nursing.

A nurse may pursue graduate-level education to be in advanced practice. Education requirements vary by specialty and education program. Besides managing and delivering expert direct patient care, nurses with graduate-level education have roles in patient and staff education, leadership, quality improvement, research, and consulting. Examples include clinical nurse leader (CNL), informatics, education, and administration. Nurses with a research-focused doctorate (PhD) typically work as nurse faculty, clinical experts, researchers, and health care executives.

You may choose to become an **advanced practice registered nurse (APRN).** An APRN is educated at the master's or doctoral level. APRNs include 4 roles: clinical nurse specialists, nurse practitioners, nurse midwives, and nurse anesthetists. They have advanced education in pathophysiology, pharmacology, and health assessment. APRNs play a vital role in the health care delivery system.

Standards of Professional Nursing Practice

You are accountable for the quality of care you deliver. To guide nurses in how to perform professionally, the ANA defines Standards of Professional Nursing Practice. These standards describe the actions and behaviors that all nurses are expected to perform competently. When you follow them, patients receive better care, and the clinical environment is more positive. There are 2 parts, Standards of Practice and Standards of Professional Performance.[2] The Standards of Practice describe a competent level of nursing care based on the nursing process. The Standards of Professional Performance describe a nurse's professional behavior. You are following the performance standards when you practice ethically and use evidence-based practice. Communicating effectively and staying competent in practice are essential. You must be able to work in collaboration with other health care team members, patients, and caregivers.

INFLUENCES ON NURSING

Expanding Knowledge and Technology

Ever-changing technology and rapidly expanding clinical knowledge add to the complexity of health care. The increased treatment, diagnostic, and care options available change care delivery and extend patients' lives. People are living longer. The number of people with chronic illnesses and multiple comorbidities is increasing. Patients with chronic illnesses have complex needs. They see different health care providers over an extended period and often move among health care settings. You need to be able to manage and coordinate care when patients transition among different settings.

Patient Population

The population is more diverse than ever. Diversity stems from race, ethnicity, age, gender identity, sexual orientation, socioeconomic status, religious beliefs, or other ways people perceive themselves. You must consider patients' and caregivers' beliefs and values when delivering care. Bias, prejudice, and stereotyping can lead to disparities in health care. Health care disparities occur across illnesses and in delivery services. You will need to effectively coordinate resources to provide safe, quality, equitable care.

Patients today are often engaged in their health care. They are very knowledgeable about their health and use technology to gather information about health problems and health care. Many want to have a voice in making decisions about their health and want to know their options for health care services. They expect high-quality, coordinated, and financially reasonable care. As a nurse, you must be able to help patients access, interpret, and use safe health care information (Fig. 1.2).

Health Care Environment

The work environment directly influences health care delivery and nursing practice. In some health care systems, staff shortages contribute to increased nursing workload. Staff shortages affect how care is provided and how well it meets standards. Other aspects of the work environment, such as workplace violence, feeling unsupported, and administrative burdens, negatively affect nursing.[3]

Nurses' health and well-being are affected by the demands of their workplace. Increased workplace demands are associated with burnout. Burnout is a threat to health care. Among nurses, burnout is associated with increased patient mortality and hospital-transmitted infections. As a nurse, you must take a leadership role in creating health care systems that promote safe, positive work environments.

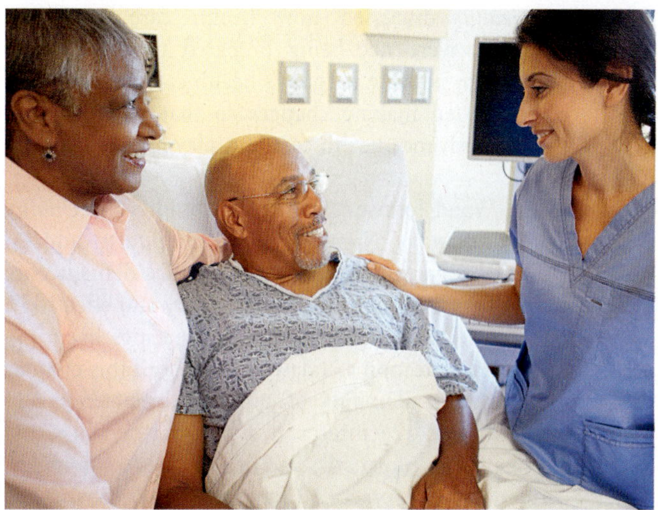

Fig. 1.2 The patient, caregiver, and nurse collaborate as part of coordinating care. (© monkeybusinessimages/iStock/.)

Professional Nursing Organizations

The ANA is the primary professional nursing organization. There are many professional specialty organizations, such as the American Association of Critical-Care Nurses (AACN), National Association of Orthopedic Nurses (NAON), and Oncology Nursing Society (ONS). Professional organizations play a role in promoting quality patient care and professional nursing practice. These roles include developing standards of practice and codes of ethics, supporting research, and lobbying for legislation and regulations. Major nursing organizations research the causes of errors, develop strategies to prevent errors, and address nursing issues that affect the nurse's ability to deliver patient care safely. Nurses join a professional organization to keep current in their practice and network with others interested in a specific practice area.

A program that supports nurses is the American Nurses Credentialing Center's Magnet Recognition Program. Health care agencies that have Magnet designation have created environments in which high-quality nursing care is provided.[4] Magnet agencies provide a positive practice environment for nurses. Nurses who work in Magnet agencies have low turnover and burnout rates and more professional and personal growth opportunities. This leads to better patient outcomes and greater career satisfaction.

Domains of Nursing Competence

Several reports have highlighted problems with health care quality. One report, *The Future of Nursing: Leading Change,*

Advancing Health, discussed how health care providers, including nurses, were not being prepared to provide the highest quality care possible in today's health care systems. The report recommended making changes so that nurses would have the skills to advance health care and play leadership roles in health care.[5]

The Robert Wood Johnson Foundation funded the *Quality and Safety Education for Nurses (QSEN) Institute* to address nursing's role in solving these problems. QSEN defined core competencies that nurses need to practice safely and effectively. These competencies have since been integrated into licensing, accreditation, and education standards. The rest of this chapter describes 5 common domains of nursing competence: (1) patient-centered care, (2) interprofessional partnerships, (3) quality and safety, (4) informatics and health care technologies, and (5) evidence-based practice (Table 1.1).[6] When you are licensed as a registered nurse, you accept responsibility to base your practice on these domains.

PATIENT-CENTERED CARE

Nurses have long shown that they deliver compassionate and coordinated care based on each person's unique needs and respect for their preferences and values. We build relationships that make patients a full partner in their care. Patients and caregivers are involved in making decisions and coordinating care. Patient-centered care is interrelated with quality and safety. With patient-centered care, patients and caregivers seek and receive care from competent and knowledgeable health care providers.

Clinical Judgment

Complex health care environments require that you use clinical judgment to make decisions that lead to the best patient outcomes. **Clinical judgment** is your ability to make decisions and solve problems by making sense of information in a situation. It

TABLE 1.1 Domains of Nursing Competency

Domain	Examples of Competencies
Patient-Centered Care Provide holistic, compassionate, and coordinated care based on respect for person's preferences, values, and needs and guided by a scientific body of knowledge	• Provide care with sensitivity and respect • Consider the person's perspectives, beliefs, and culture • Communicate effectively • Engage in relationship-centered care that promotes health, well-being, and self-care management • Use assessment skills, diagnose health problems, and develop and deliver a plan of care
Interprofessional Partnerships Function effectively within nursing and interprofessional teams	• Value the expertise of each team member • Delegate work to team members based on their roles and competency • Initiate appropriate referrals • Follow communication practices that minimize risks associated with hand-offs and care transitions • Take part in interprofessional rounds • Manage conflict among team members
Safety and Quality Minimize risk of harm to patients and providers and use data to monitor outcomes of care to improve quality and safety	• Follow national safety recommendations • Communicate concerns about hazards and errors • Contribute to designing systems to improve safety • Be accountable for reporting unsafe conditions and near misses • Recognize how to prevent workplace violence • Take part in implementing practice changes
Informatics and Health Care Technologies Use information and technology to manage care, gather data, communicate, reduce errors, and support decision making	• Protect confidentiality of protected health information • Document appropriately in electronic health records • Use technology to coordinate patient care • Respond correctly to clinical decision-making alerts
Evidence-Based Practice Integrate best evidence with clinical expertise and patient preferences and values in making patient care decisions	• Read research, clinical practice guidelines, and evidence reports related to area of practice • Base patient care on patient's values, clinical expertise, and evidence • Use new knowledge in clinical practice • Develop or revise policies based on new evidence

Data from QSEN competencies. Retrieved from www.qsen.org/competencies. The Essentials. Retrieved from https://www.aacnnursing.org/Portals/0/PDFs/Publications/Essentials-2021.pdf.

is not memorizing a list of facts or the steps of a procedure. Instead, you use nursing knowledge to assess situations, identify priority problems, and generate the best possible solutions to deliver safe patient care.[7] It involves understanding the medical and nursing implications of a patient's situation when making decisions about patient care. You use clinical judgment when you identify a change in a patient's status, consider the context and patient and caregiver concerns, and decide what to do.

Because of the diversity and complexity of patient care, there may not be a right solution in each situation. Therefore you need to learn and implement clinical judgment skills through experience. Various experiences in nursing school help you to learn to make decisions about patient care. Learning activities, including unfolding case studies and simulation, help you practice using clinical judgment. Throughout this book, case studies and practice questions promote your use of clinical judgment.

Clinical Practice Frameworks

Depending on the situation, nurses use different scientific models when providing patient care. Many use the nursing process. The **nursing process** is a problem-solving approach to the identification and treatment of patient problems. It is the foundation of nursing practice. The nursing process framework provides a structure for delivering nursing care and the knowledge, judgments, and actions that nurses use to achieve the best patient outcomes.

The nursing process consists of 5 phases: assessment, diagnosis, planning, implementation, and evaluation (ADPIE) (Fig. 1.3). The nursing process begins with assessment. *Assessment* is the collection of subjective and objective patient information on which you will base your care plan. *Diagnosing* is the act of analyzing the assessment data and making conclusions. During *planning,* you develop patient outcomes or goals and identify nursing interventions to accomplish the outcomes. The right expected outcomes provide criteria you can use to measure and evaluate the impact of the interventions you provide. *Implementation* is the action phase of the plan with the use of nursing interventions. *Evaluation* is a continual activity of deciding whether patient outcomes were met. If the outcomes were not met, a review of the process helps to figure out why. You may need to obtain more assessments and revise diagnoses, outcomes, and interventions. Once started, the nursing process is continuous and cyclic.

There are other clinical practice frameworks. These include Tanner's Clinical Judgment Model (with the phases of Noticing, Interpreting, Responding, and Reflecting) and the National Council of State Boards of Nursing's Clinical Judgment Measurement Model (NCJMM) (Fig. 1.4).[7] The NCJMM was designed to test your clinical judgment on the NCLEX-RN. All 3 models emphasize assessment, making decisions, taking action, and evaluating outcomes. Some clinical agencies use a "shortened version" of the nursing process—Assess, Act, Reassess.

In this book, we use an ADPIE format to help you learn how to care for patients with certain health problems. We use the term "clinical problem" for the diagnostic naming phase of nursing clinical practice (see Appendix A). It is intended to be a synonym for nursing diagnoses, nursing problems, patient problems, or any label that describes patient problems, conditions, or diagnoses requiring health care.[8] Clinical problems can be diagnosed based on a single clinical finding, such as pain or anxiety, or result from a decision about a particular focus, such as impaired nutrition or musculoskeletal problem. Clinical problems are the basis for selecting nursing interventions to achieve patient outcomes for which nursing is accountable.

A nursing intervention is "a single nursing action, treatment, procedure, activity, or service designed to achieve an outcome of a nursing or medical diagnosis for which the nurse is accountable."[9] This includes treatments that you perform and direct or indirect care. When planning care for a patient, choose specific interventions for the patient based on the clinical problem and desired patient outcomes. You collaborate with patients to decide when and which interventions to use for the specific situation.

In the clinical setting, you will be responsible for developing a plan of care that includes problems, outcomes, and interventions. In clinical practice, electronic care plans often

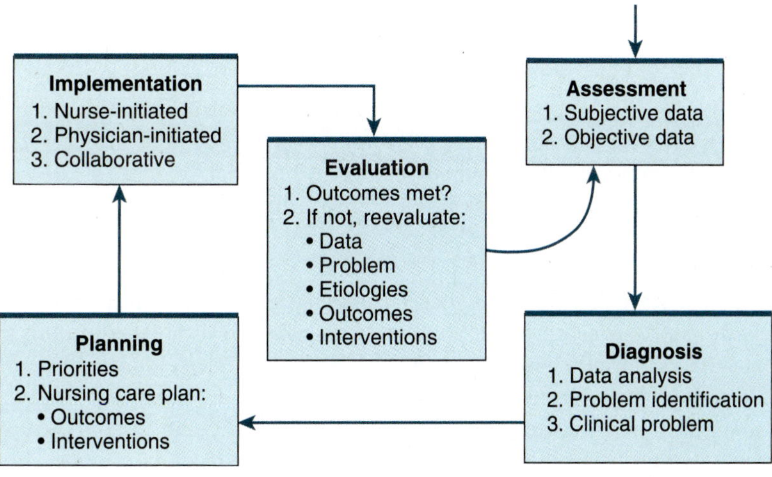

Fig. 1.3 Nursing process.

Model/theory	Components					
NCSBN clinical judgment model	Recognize cues	Analyze cues	Prioritize hypotheses	Generate solutions	Take action	Evaluate outcomes
Nursing process (ADPIE or AAPIE)	Assessment	Diagnosis or analysis		Planning	Implementation	Evaluation
Tanner model	Noticing	Interpreting		Responding		Reflecting

Fig. 1.4 Comparison of the phases of clinical practice frameworks. (From https://evolve.elsevier.com/education/next-generation-nclex/resources/continuing-nursing-education/.)

follow a standard format that has been adapted for that specific setting. These plans are guides for routine nursing care. You customize each to your patient's unique needs and problems.

In nursing education, you will likely document the nursing process differently from clinical practice. The nursing process is often recorded in nursing care plans like those found on the website for this book (http://evolve.elsevier.com/Lewis/medsurg). These nursing care plans are teaching and learning tools. When you use one of the nursing care plans, you will need to customize the plan for your patient. You must use clinical judgment to evaluate the situation and revise the clinical problems, outcomes, and interventions to fit each patient's unique care needs. You usually must give rationales for the interventions you choose.

A *concept map* is another way to record a nursing care plan. A concept map records the nursing process in a visual diagram. The map shows patient problems and interventions and relationships among clinical data. Nurse educators use concept mapping to teach nursing processes and care planning. Concept maps have various formats.

Conceptual care maps blend a concept map and a nursing care plan. On a conceptual care map, assessment data used to identify the primary health concern are in the center. Diagnostic test data, treatments, and medications surround the assessment data. Positioned below are the clinical problems that represent the patient's responses to their health state. Listed with those are the supporting assessment data, outcomes, nursing interventions with rationales, and evaluation. After completing the map, you draw connections between identified relationships and concepts. A conceptual care map creator is available online on the website for this book. Concept maps for select case studies at the end of management chapters are available on the website at http://evolve.elsevier.com/Lewis/medsurg.

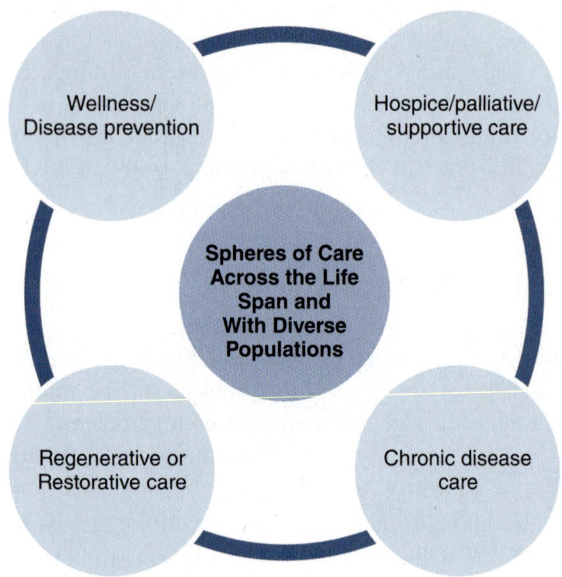

Fig. 1.5 Spheres of care.

Spheres of Care

Spheres of care describe the health care needs of individuals, families, and populations and the care and services required to address these needs and promote health.[10] The 4 spheres of care (Fig. 1.5) represent the scope of a persons' health status and the reason people seek health care. Nurses deliver care to meet people's needs across the lifespan in all 4 spheres.

Most people use health care services within the wellness and disease prevention sphere. The care goals are centered around keeping people healthy and managing minor acute and intermittent care needs. Nursing care within this sphere includes care for minor injuries and illness and health promotion interventions, such as vaccinations, screenings, prenatal care, and patient education.[11]

Chronic disease care represents the health care needs of people with one or more chronic health conditions that need ongoing management.[11] This includes persons with heart, lung, or kidney disease and diabetes. Care goals for chronic disease care include optimal disease management, preventing complications, and maximizing quality of life. Chapter 5 addresses the key role you play in helping patients manage chronic illness.

Persons who have an unexpected serious health event, major illness, or a serious injury that requires a higher level of care need regenerative or restorative care.[11] This includes a person who has an acute exacerbation of a chronic condition that needs acute, complex care.[10] There are many examples of problems that require acute care. These include stroke, myocardial infarction, traumatic injury, heart failure, and sepsis. Nurses providing care to patients with complex needs often need special skills. For example, the nurse in a cardiac intensive care unit must know how to manage a mechanical ventilator and titrate medications that affect blood pressure and heart rhythm.

The fourth sphere is hospice/palliative/supportive care. Palliative care occurs across the trajectory of serious illness and includes hospice and end-of-life care. End-of-life care is provided to patients and their families in the days leading up to and just after the death of the patient.[12] This sphere also includes rehabilitative and extended care for persons with complex chronic problems.[11] Chapter 10 discusses the nurses' role in providing palliative care.

Care Settings

Although the hospital is the mainstay for acute care, community-based settings offer patients the opportunity to live or recover in settings that maximize their independence and preserve human dignity. Decisions about the best setting for obtaining health care often depend on the cost of care and the patient's health insurance plan and personal finances.

Community-based health care settings include ambulatory care, transitional care, and long-term care. *Transitional care* settings provide care in between the acute care and the home or long-term care setting. Patients may receive transitional care at an acute rehabilitation facility after head trauma or a spinal cord injury. *Long-term care* refers to the care of patients for a period longer than 30 days. It may be needed for those who have severe development disabilities, cognitive issues, or physical problems requiring continuous medical and nursing care. These include patients who are ventilator dependent or have Alzheimer disease. Long-term care facilities include skilled nursing facilities, assisted living facilities, and residential care facilities.

Care coordination is important when patients transition between care settings. *Transition of care* refers to patients moving among health care practitioners, settings, and home as their condition and care needs change.[13] As a nurse, you are an essential part of care coordination by stressing actions that meet patients' needs and facilitate safe, quality care. Collaborating with other members of the health care team is critical. A lack of communication can result in an ineffective care transition, leading to drug errors and higher hospital readmission rates. For example, you are a nurse in acute care admitting a long-term care patient who has been receiving propranolol 20 mg/5 mL twice a day. The admitting orders read, "propranolol 20 mg/mL, give 5 mL twice a day." The patient could have received 100 mg instead of the 20 mg dose ordered. Using communication to reconcile the difference averts a drug error.

Nursing Care Delivery

Nurses deliver patient-centered care in collaboration with the interprofessional health care team and within the framework of a care delivery model. A care delivery model outlines how responsibilities and authority are structured to carry out patient care. Better outcomes occur when the number and type of care providers match patient needs and there is a designated care coordinator.

In acute care settings, 2 basic models are used: team care and total patient care. *Team care* models involve a group of providers who work together to deliver care. A professional nurse is usually the team leader. As the team leader, you manage and coordinate care with others, such as licensed practical/vocational nurses (LPN/VNs) and assistive personnel (AP). You have accountability for the quality of care delivered by team members during a work period. In total patient care models, you are responsible for planning and providing all care.

Case management involves managing the patient's care with other health care team members and available resources across multiple care settings and levels of care to meet their health needs. It is thought to promote quality, cost-effective outcomes. In nursing case management, a registered nurse assumes the role of case manager. In this role, the nurse assesses the needs of patients and/or caregivers, coordinates services for them, makes referrals, and evaluates the progress toward meeting care goals.

For example, a nurse case manager in an outpatient clinic has been working for 3 months with an older male patient with multiple comorbidities, including coronary artery disease, diabetes, and osteoarthritis. After the patient is scheduled for a coronary artery bypass, the nurse manager coordinates care with other health care team members. The nurse arranges the patient's preoperative appointments and informs the other team members so that everyone understands the patient's unique needs. After surgery, the patient develops a deep venous thrombosis in the leg. The case manager then works with the health care team to evaluate the patient's discharge needs and decide whether rehabilitation or home health care is necessary for the patient. With the patient and caregiver, the team decides to discharge the patient to a rehabilitation facility. The case manager helps with the transition, again coordinating care so that the providers at the rehabilitation facility are aware of the patient's needs.

Telehealth provides health care and information using telehealth technologies in virtual environments. These include smartphones and watches, kiosks, and web or digital platforms. The type of telehealth visit depends on the setting and patient need.[14] Among the many uses are triaging patients, monitoring patients with chronic or critical conditions, helping patients manage symptoms, providing patient and caregiver education and support, and providing follow-up care. Telehealth can increase access to care. The nurse engaged in telehealth can assess the patient's health status, deliver interventions, and evaluate the outcomes of nursing care while separated geographically from the patient (Fig. 1.6).

Supporting Caregivers

Caregivers play a valuable role in the patient's health and are members of the health care team. They contribute to the patient's well-being by (1) linking the patient to news from the outside world; (2) facilitating decision making and advising the patient; (3) helping with activities of daily living; (4) acting as liaisons to advise the health care team of the patient's wishes for care; and (5) providing safe, caring, familiar relationships for the patient.

When someone is ill, care extends beyond the patient to the patient's caregivers. Caregivers need your guidance and support. Anxiety and concerns about the patient's condition, prognosis, and pain are common. Caregivers may have a

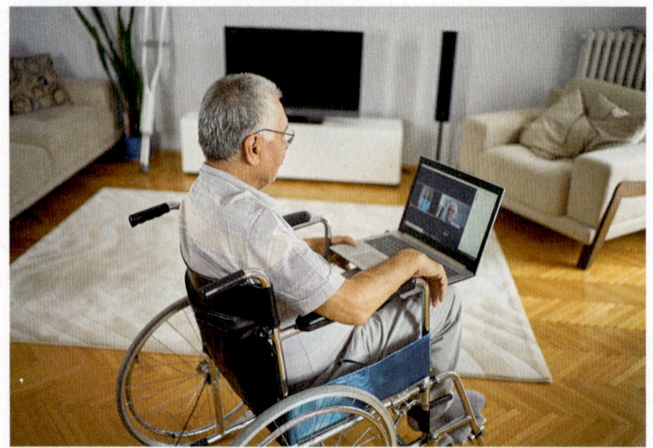

Fig. 1.6 Patient at home videoconferencing with the nurse and physician. (© Phynart Studio/iStock.com.)

concern about financial issues related to a hospital stay. They often disrupt their daily routines to support the patient. Conduct a family assessment and intervene as needed. Recognize the caregivers' feelings, listen to them openly and without being judgmental, and acknowledge their decisions. Consult other team members, such as a chaplain or social worker, as needed to help caregivers cope.

The key needs of caregivers include information, communication, and access. Lack of information is a major source of anxiety. Assess their understanding of the patient's status, treatment plan, and prognosis and provide them with information. Identify a spokesperson to help coordinate information exchange between the health care team and caregivers. Have them meet team members. Include caregivers in rounds and patient care conferences. It helps caregivers cope when they see that the team is caring and competent, decisions are deliberate, and their input is valued. Invite the caregivers to take part in patient care if they want.

Caregivers need access to the patient. Assess patients' and caregivers' needs and preferences and include these in the plan of care. Caregivers should have the choice to be present at the bedside when patients are undergoing invasive procedures (central line insertion) or cardiopulmonary resuscitation (CPR). Even when the outcomes are not favorable, being present helps caregivers to (1) overcome doubts about the patient's condition, (2) reduce their anxiety and fear, (3) meet their need to be together with and to support their loved one, and (4) begin the grief process if death occurs.

INTERPROFESSIONAL PARTNERSHIPS

Interprofessional Team

To deliver high-quality care, you need to have effective working relationships with other health care team members. The **interprofessional team** is made up of providers from various disciplines, working together and sharing their expertise to provide customized care. It may consist of physicians, nurses, pharmacists, occupational and physical therapists, and others (Table 1.2). To be competent in interprofessional practice, you must collaborate in many ways by exchanging knowledge, sharing responsibility for problem solving, and making patient care decisions. You may be responsible for coordinating care among the team members, taking part in interprofessional team meetings or rounds, and making referrals when you need expertise in specialized areas to help the patient. To do so, you must be aware of the knowledge and skills of other team members and be able to communicate effectively with them.

To help you develop the competencies necessary to practice within an interprofessional clinical environment, you may take part in activities with students from other disciplines. Throughout this book, case studies and review questions discuss the roles others have in managing patient care.

Communication

Effective communication is key to fostering teamwork and coordinating care. To provide safe, effective care, team members must exchange information clearly and accurately. Everyone involved in a patient's care should understand the patient's condition and needs. Unfortunately, many issues result from a breakdown in communication.

One model used to improve communication is the **SBAR (Situation-Background-Assessment-Recommendation)** technique (Table 1.3). SBAR offers a structured way to discuss a patient's condition between team members. It allows you to communicate vital patient information that needs immediate attention and action. There will be times when you will be alarmed about a patient situation and need to alert team members. At those times, you can use another model: Concerned, Uncomfortable, Safety (CUS) (Table 1.4). With CUS you state that you are concerned, feel uncomfortable, or perceive a safety issue to stress important or critical information.

A **patient handoff** is the transfer of patient information and care responsibility to another team member during a care transition.[15] The handoff should include information about the patient's condition and any recent or anticipated changes. There should be an opportunity to ask questions and a way to confirm information, such as check-back. Examples of handoffs include shift changes and unit or facility transfers. Good communication is important during handoffs.

Huddles and rounds promote effective communication among team members. A huddle is a short, daily meeting that often happens at the start of each day.[16] Huddles let team members discuss patient concerns, safety concerns, and updates. They improve care quality by helping to solve problems that are affecting patient care (Box 1.1). Interprofessional rounds allow team members to discuss patient care and discharge plans. Rounding at the bedside involves the patient in planning care.

Clinical Pathways

Clinical pathways or care protocols are interprofessional plans that outline the care and desired outcomes for patients

TABLE 1.2 Interprofessional Health Care Team Members

Team Member	Services Provided
Dentist	Provides preventive and restorative treatments for problems affecting the teeth and mouth
Dietitian	Provides general nutrition services, including dietary consultation about health promotion or specialized diets
Occupational therapist (OT)	Aids patient with fine motor coordination, performing activities of daily living, cognitive-perceptual skills, sensory testing, and the use of assistive or adaptive equipment
Pastoral care	Offers spiritual support and guidance to patients and caregivers
Pharmacist	Prepares medications and infusion products
Physical therapist (PT)	Works with patients to improve strength and endurance, gait training, transfer training, and developing a patient education program
Physician (medical doctor [MD])	Practices medicine and treats illness and injury by prescribing medication, performing diagnostic tests and evaluations, performing surgery, and providing other medical services and advice
Physician assistant	Conducts physical exams, diagnoses and treats illnesses, and counsels on preventive health care in collaboration with a physician
Respiratory therapist	Provides therapies to maintain or improve lung function by assessing respiratory problems, conducting diagnostic tests, and administering respiratory treatments
Social worker	Assists patients with developing coping skills, meeting caregiver concerns, securing adequate financial resources or housing, or making referrals to social service or volunteer agencies
Speech pathologist	Focuses on treating speech defects and disorders, especially by using physical exercises to strengthen muscles used in speech, speech drills, and audiovisual aids that develop new speech habits

TABLE 1.3 Guidelines for Communicating Using SBAR

Purpose: SBAR is a model for effective transfer of information by providing a standard structure for concise factual communication from nurse-to-nurse, nurse-to-physician, or nurse-to—other health professionals.

Steps to Use: Before speaking with a physician or other health care professional about a patient problem, assess the patient yourself, read the most recent progress notes, and have the patient's health record available.

S Situation	• What is the situation you want to discuss? What is happening right now? • Identify self, unit. State: I am calling about: *patient, room number.* • Briefly state the problem: what it is, when it happened or started, and how severe it is. State: I have just assessed the patient and am concerned about: *describe why you are concerned.*
B Background	• What is the background or circumstances leading up to the situation? State pertinent background information related to the situation that may include: • Admitting diagnosis and date of admission • List of current medications, allergies, IV fluids • Most recent vital signs • Date and time of any laboratory testing and results of previous tests for comparison • Synopsis of treatment to date • Code status
A Assessment	• What do you think the problem is? What is your assessment of the situation? State what you think the problem is: • Changes from prior assessments • Patient condition unstable or worsening
R Recommendation/Request	• What should we do to correct the problem? What is your recommendation or request? State your request. • Specific treatments • Tests needed • Patient needs to be seen now

Data from Institute for Health Care Improvement: SBAR technique for communication: A situational briefing model. Retrieved from www.ihi.org/resources/Pages/Tools/SBARTechniqueforCommunicationASituationalBriefingModel.aspx.

with a specific problem. Think of a clinical pathway as a road map the patient and health care team should follow. As the patient progresses along the road, the patient should receive specific care and meet specific goals. If a patient's progress differs from the planned path, a variance has occurred. A negative variance occurs when specific goals are not met. The nurse usually identifies when a negative variance is present and works with team members to create a plan to address the issue.

The exact content and format of clinical pathways vary among agencies and settings. Each agency usually has its own pathways based on evidence-based practice guidelines. Common components include assessment guidelines, laboratory and diagnostic testing, medications, activity, diet, and teaching.

In acute care, clinical pathways often describe which patient care components are needed at specific times (Fig. 1.7). The case types that have pathways are usually high volume or high risk and predictable, such as myocardial infarction and surgical procedures, like laparoscopy or cataract surgery.

Delegation and Assignment

As a registered nurse (RN), you will delegate nursing care and supervise those who are qualified to deliver care. **Delegation** allows a care provider to perform a specific nursing activity, skill, or procedure beyond their usual role.[17] Delegating and assigning nursing activities is a process that, when used appropriately, results in safe, effective, and efficient patient care. Delegating can allow you more time to focus on complex patient care needs. Delegating care and supervising others will be one of your essential roles as a professional nurse.

Delegation usually involves tasks and procedures that licensed LPN/VNs and AP perform. Nursing interventions that require independent nursing knowledge, skill, or judgment (initial assessment, patient teaching, evaluating care) are your responsibility and cannot be delegated. State nurse practice acts and agency policies identify what you can delegate to LPN/VNs and AP. You will use professional judgment to select which activities to delegate. Your decision will be based on the patient's needs, the LPN/VN's and AP's education and training, and the amount of supervision needed. Commonly delegated nursing actions involve aspects of direct patient care. For example, you can delegate measuring oral intake and urine output to AP, but you use your nursing judgment to decide if the intake and output are adequate.

The general guideline for LPN/VN practice is that they can function independently in a stable, routine situation. However, they must work under the direct supervision of a professional nurse in acute, unstable situations in which a patient's condition can rapidly change. In most states, LPN/VNs may give medications, perform sterile procedures, and perform a wide variety of interventions planned by the RN. The procedure itself is not the issue when an RN is determining what to delegate. Instead, the patient's stability determines whether an RN should delegate a procedure to an LPN/VN. For example, the LPN/VN can change an abdominal surgical wound dressing, but the RN should do the first dressing change and wound assessment.

AP have many titles, including nurse aides, certified medication aides, nursing assistants, patient care assistants, or

TABLE 1.4 Communicating Using CUS

CUS: Concerned, Uncomfortable, Safety	
"I am **C**oncerned that…"	State your concern about the patient or situation.
"I am **U**ncomfortable because…!"	State why you feel uncomfortable with what is occurring.
"This is a **S**afety issue because…"	Describe why there is a safety issue and state what actions you think should be taken.
Example: "I'm concerned that the patient is more confused and having difficulty breathing. I am uncomfortable because of the sudden onset of these symptoms. I believe the patient is not safe; there may be something serious going on, and we need to call the rapid response team."	

BOX 1.1 EVIDENCE-BASED PRACTICE

Participating in Post-Fall Huddles

You are caring for J.R., a 76-year-old female admitted for acute kidney injury. She has a history of falls at home, none of which resulted in serious injury. Despite correct identification of her fall risk and implementation of the fall prevention bundle, J.R. fell trying to get up to the bedside commode without calling for help. Based on unit policy, there is a post-fall huddle after any patient fall to evaluate contributing circumstances and any unidentified patient risk factors. You are taking part in the fall huddle as J.R.'s assigned nurse. J.R. and her daughter are joining the huddle.

Making Clinical Decisions

Synthesis of Best Available Evidence

After-action reviews, also called huddles or debriefs, are implemented after a key event (e.g., a patient fall) to discuss contributing factors, identify lessons learned, and determine how those lessons can be implemented to avoid future incidents. Debriefing increases knowledge and improves patient outcomes. Debriefing is widely used as part of an evidence-based fall prevention program. The team members convened after a patient fall often include the assigned nurse, any AP, and the charge nurse, as well as physical therapists, respiratory therapists, and pharmacists. A family member may be included. Nursing staff and the family provide information about what the patient was doing at the time of the fall, the location of the fall, how it was discovered, the severity of any patient injury, interventions intended to be placed, and changes in the plan of care needed to decrease the risk of another fall.

Clinician Expertise

Although the research is limited and has not shown that post-fall huddles decrease fall occurrence, you know that the huddle is part of a unit culture of reflection and open communication. You review J.R.'s current medications and discuss with the pharmacist the potential impact on fall risk. The physical therapist and you discuss the potential value of a balance and core strengthening exercise plan for J.R.

Patient Preferences and Values

J.R. and her daughter express concern about the risk of injury with future falls, but they also want to preserve J.R.'s independence.

Implications for Nursing Practice

1. How does taking part in post-fall huddles encourage teamwork and a culture of patient safety?
2. How can the results of post-fall huddles be shared for wider learning by all staff?

Reference for Evidence

Parekh A, Hill KD, Guerbaai RA: Exploring post-fall management interventions in long-term care facilities and hospitals for older adults: A scoping review. *J Clin Nurs* 34:408, 2025.

Outcome	0–6 hours	6–24 hours	Day 2
Respiratory	Extubate within 4–6 hours	• O_2 therapy to maintain saturation greater than 94% • Incentive spirometry (10 times/h)	• O_2 therapy to maintain saturation greater than 94% • Incentive spirometry (10 times/h)
Pain Control	IV sedation	IV Morphine	Oral pain medication
Diet	NPO	Clear liquids within 6–8 hours	Diet as tolerated
Activity	• Head of bed at 30° • Turn every 2 hours	Sit at bedside	• Sit in chair twice daily • Walk to bathroom with assistance
Bowel Motility	Remove NG tube before extubation	GI assessment	• GI assessment • Begin stool softeners
Education	Unit orientation for patient and caregivers	• Respiratory care measures • Cardiac rehabilitation	• PT, social work, diet referrals

Fig. 1.7 Clinical pathway for heart surgery.

technicians. The activities AP perform typically include obtaining routine vital signs on stable patients, feeding and helping patients at mealtimes, ambulating stable patients, and helping patients with bathing and hygiene.

Delegation can occur among professional nurses. For example, if one RN has accountability for an outcome and asks another RN to perform a specific intervention related to that outcome, that is delegation. This type of delegation typically occurs when one RN leaves the unit/work area for a meal break.

Assignment is different from delegation. The term *assign* is used when you direct an LPN/VN or AP to do an activity or procedure that is part of their everyday job.[17] An assignment must be within the authorized scope of practice of the LPN/VN or part of the routine function of the AP. For example, you can assign an LPN/VN to give medications to a patient because this is within the LPN/VN's scope of practice. You cannot assign an LPN/VN to a patient who needs an admission assessment because an RN must perform the initial patient assessment.

Whether you delegate or assign staff tasks, you are responsible for the patient's total care during your work period. You need to decide what patient care tasks must be carried out during the given period, identify who will do them, and prioritize the order in which the tasks must be completed. You are responsible for supervising AP and LPN/VNs. Clearly communicate the tasks that need to be completed and give necessary guidance. Because you are accountable for ensuring that delegated tasks are completed competently, evaluate the care provided, follow up as needed, and make sure no care was missed.

You need to use clinical judgment to ensure that you follow the 5 Rights of Delegation (Table 1.5). This is a skill that is learned, and you must practice it to be proficient in managing patient care. To help you learn to delegate, there is information on delegation in nursing management tables and case study questions at the end of the management chapters.

CHECK YOUR PRACTICE

A float AP is assigned for the first time to your unit today. The nurse manager shares with you that the AP is a new employee and just finished orientation. How would you determine what tasks you would assign to the AP?

SAFETY AND QUALITY

Quality care and safety are related: the higher the culture of safety, the better the quality of care. A safe environment minimizes risks to patients and health care providers. Preventable medical errors are a serious problem and a leading cause of death in the United States. Several groups address this issue by outlining safety goals for health care organizations and identifying safety competencies for health professionals. Implementing procedures and systems that improve safety minimizes the risk of harm. These systems should address how errors and near misses are reported and analyzed when they occur.

Serious Reportable Events

The National Quality Forum (NQF) uses the term **serious reportable event** (SRE), also called a *never event,* to describe serious, largely preventable, and harmful clinical events.[18] The current list of SREs consists of 29 events. These events include a patient acquiring a stage 3 or greater pressure injury after admission and death or injury from a fall or hypoglycemia. The health care agency may not receive reimbursement for care if a patient experiences an SRE.

To reduce the occurrence of SREs, the NQF has a list of effective *Safe Practices* that health care settings should use to provide safe patient care (www.qualityforum.org). You are implementing NQF practices when you perform a time-out before a surgical procedure; reconcile medication records; and implement interventions to prevent hospital-acquired infections, pressure injuries, and falls.

National Patient Safety Goals

The Joint Commission (TJC), an accrediting agency for health care organizations, gathers and reports data on serious errors they call sentinel events. A *sentinel event* is a patient safety event unrelated to the patient's illness or underlying condition that results in death, permanent harm, or severe, temporary harm.[19] Events are "sentinel" because they signal the need for immediate investigation and response. Many sentinel events are also

TABLE 1.5 Rights of Delegation

The 5 Rights of Delegation

The registered nurse uses clinical judgment to be sure that the delegation or assignment is:

1. The right task
2. Under the right circumstances
3. To the right person
4. With the right directions and communication
5. Under the right supervision and evaluation

Rights of Delegation	Description	Questions to Ask
Right Task	One that can be delegated to a specific person	Is it appropriate to delegate based on agency policy or their job description? Is the person able and willing to do the specific activity?
Right Circumstances	Health condition of the patient must be stable	What are the patient's needs right now? Has the patient's condition changed? Are the patient needs a "fit" with the delegatee?
Right Person	Delegatee has the right knowledge and skills to perform the activity	Is the delegatee willing and able? Has the person been trained and evaluated in performing the activity?
Right Directions and Communication	Clear, concise description of activity, including instructions and information pertinent to the situation	Have you given clear communication? With directions, limits, and expected outcomes? Does the delegatee understand what needs to be done? Does the delegatee know what and when to report?
Right Supervision and Evaluation	Appropriate monitoring, evaluation, and feedback	How and when you will evaluate the outcome? How often do you need to directly observe? Will you be able to give feedback if needed?

Data from National Council of State Boards of Nursing: Delegation. Retrieved from https://www.ncsbn.org/nursing-regulation/practice/delegation.page.

serious reportable events. If the patient has a wrong-site or wrong-procedure surgery, is assaulted in the health care setting, or receives an incompatible blood product, the occurrence is both a sentinel event, reportable to TJC, and a serious reportable event, reportable to NQF.

To address specific patient safety concerns, TJC issues National Patient Safety Goals (NPSGs).[20] NPSGs promote patient safety by giving evidence-based solutions to common safety problems. Table 1.6 lists the current NPSGs.

The safety goal focusing on using clinical alarm systems safely greatly affects nursing. Patient monitoring systems give us vital information. Alarms that work well improve patient safety and care by telling you when a patient needs your attention. However, so many alarms can go off that *alarm fatigue* occurs, and you can become less sensitive to the sounds. By better managing alarm settings, we reduce alarm fatigue and improve patient safety.

Failure to rescue (FTR) occurs when there is failure or delay in recognizing a patient has developed complications. As a result, the patient worsens and has an adverse outcome. FTR often involves subtle signs and symptoms that are thought to be of no concern or are missed entirely. You can prevent FTR by recognizing changes in a patient's condition, taking the right actions based on the problem, and activating a response team when needed.

Because you have the most interaction with patients, you play a key role in promoting safety. Many describe nurses as the patient's last line of defense. Every nurse has the responsibility to ensure the patient receives care in a manner that prevents errors and promotes patient safety. Throughout this book, safety alerts highlighting patient care issues and NPSGs will help you learn to apply safety principles.

Quality Improvement Programs

Quality improvement (QI) is a process that uses data to monitor and improve patient care and enhance safety. Health care systems focused on quality outcomes use practice standards and protocols based on reliable knowledge and evidence. QI is an interprofessional team effort that accrediting agencies require.

As part of your nursing practice, you will coordinate the complex aspects of patient care, including monitoring the care delivered by others and looking for and correcting issues associated with poor quality or unsafe care. You need to be able to collect data using QI tools, implement interventions to improve patient care, and monitor patient outcomes. Think to yourself, "How can I do my job better?" Identify where changes can be made and be part of making them.

Patient outcomes are an important indicator of health care quality. Several public and private groups focusing on improving health care quality have developed standard QI measures. These performance measures assess how well the health care team cares for a patient with a certain condition or receives a specific treatment. They describe what data the team must collect and monitor. Fig. 1.8 shows an example of a QI system for patients with heart failure (HF). In this example, you would review records from patients newly diagnosed with HF to decide if HF

TABLE 1.6 National Patient Safety Goals

Safety Goal	Examples
Identify patients correctly	• Use at least 2 ways to identify patients (have them state full name and date of birth).
Improve communication among the health care team	• Get critical test results to the right person on time.
Use medicines safely	• Before a procedure, label all medicines. Discard any found unlabeled. • Use proper precautions with patients who take anticoagulants. • Find out what medicines each patient is taking. Make certain that it is safe for the patient to take any new medicines with their current ones. • Give a medication list to the patient and the caregiver before discharge. Explain the list.
Use alarm systems safely	• Respond to alarms promptly. • Do not turn alarms off.
Prevent health care–associated infections	• Follow hand hygiene guidelines. • Use evidence-based practices to prevent infections related to central lines, indwelling urinary catheters, and multidrug-resistant organisms
Identify patient safety risks	• Assess patients at risk for suicide. • Assess any risks, such as fires, for patients who are getting home oxygen therapy. • Use measures to reduce fall risk. • Prevent pressure injuries.
Improve health care equity	• Have the personal skills and competencies to advance health equity.
Prevent mistakes in surgery	• Conduct a time-out before the start of any surgery. • Confirm correct patient, procedure, and site.

Adapted from The Joint Commission (TJC): *National patient safety goals*. Retrieved from www.jointcommission.org/standards_information/npsgs.aspx.

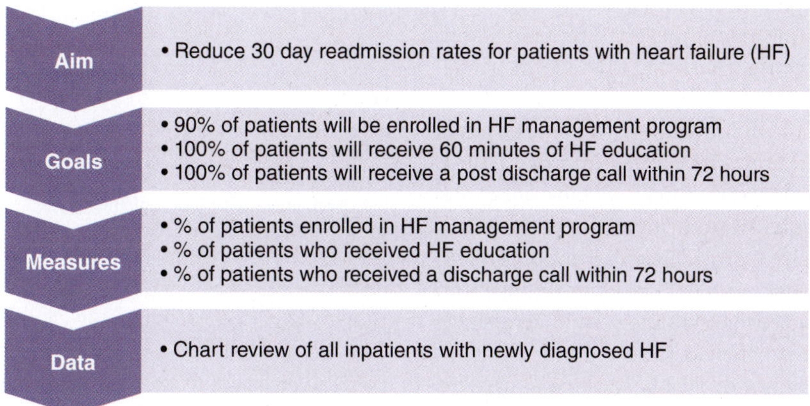

Fig. 1.8 Quality improvement system.

education rates are 100%. You would share the results with the team and work as a team to implement measures to correct the problem if the standard was not met.

The National Database of Nursing Quality Indicators (NDNQI) provides data on nursing-sensitive measures to evaluate the impact of nursing care on patient outcomes. Patient outcomes are nursing sensitive if they improve with a greater quantity or quality of nursing care. NDNQI outcomes are unique because they identify how nursing workforce factors, including nurse staffing and skill mix, directly influence patient outcomes. NDNQI data show the incidence of falls and health care–associated pressure injuries and infections decreases with adequate staffing and increased nurse education and satisfaction with the work environment. Table 1.7 lists the current NDNQI.

INFORMATICS AND HEALTH CARE TECHNOLOGY

Nursing is an information-intense profession. Technology has changed the way nurses plan, deliver, document, and evaluate care. All nurses, regardless of their setting or role, use informatics and technology every day in practice. You will use informatics to obtain and review diagnostic information, make clinical decisions, communicate with patients and health care team members, document, and provide care.

Technology advances have increased the efficiency of nursing care, improving the work environment and the care nurses provide. Computers and mobile devices allow you to document when you deliver care and give you quick and easy access to information, such as clinical decision-making tools, patient

TABLE 1.7 National Database of Nursing Quality Indicators

NDNQI include information from 3 main indicator groups:

- Structure indicators
    - Nurse turnover
    - Patient volume, flow, and contacts
    - RN education and certification
    - Staff and skill mix: RNs, LPN/VNs, AP, agency staff
- Process indicators
    - Advance care planning
    - BMI screening and follow-up
    - Care coordination
    - Depression screening and follow-up
    - Diabetes care
    - Hypertension screening and follow-up
    - Patient falls
    - Pressure injuries
    - Restraint use
- Outcome indicators
    - Assaults on nursing personnel
    - Health care–associated infection rate
    - Perioperative care

Data from National Database of Nursing Quality Indicators. Retrieved from https://www.pressganey.com/platform/ndnqi/.

education materials, and references. Texting, video chat, and e-mail enhance communication among health care team members and help you deliver the right message to the right person at the right time.

Technology plays a key role in providing safe, quality patient care. Medication administration applications improve patient safety by flagging potential errors, such as look-alike and sound-alike medications and adverse drug interactions, before they can occur. Computerized provider order entry (CPOE) systems can reduce errors caused by misreading or misinterpreting handwritten orders. Sensor technology can decrease the number of falls in high-risk patients. Care reminder systems give cues that decrease the amount of missed nursing care.

Using technology skills to communicate and access information is an essential part of nursing practice. You must be able to use word processing software, communicate by e-mail and messaging, access information, and follow security and confidentiality rules. You need to have the ability to use patient care technologies and electronic documentation systems safely.

Protected health information (PHI) is highly sensitive. *The Health Insurance Portability and Accountability Act (HIPAA)* is part of federal legislation that addresses actions for how we use and disclose PHI. With the increased use of informatics and technology are concerns on how to follow HIPAA regulations and maintain a patient's privacy. Wireless technologies, increased use of e-mail and computer networking, and the ongoing threat of computer viruses increase the need for properly protecting a patient's privacy. We must assure patients of their privacy and that only those with a right to know are accessing protected information.

As a nurse, you have an obligation to ensure the privacy of your patient's health information. To do so, you need to understand your agency's policies about the use of technology. You need to know the rules about accessing patient records and releasing PHI, what to do if information is released accidentally or intentionally, and how to protect all your passwords. If you are using social networking, you must not place PHI online (Box 1.2).

BOX 1.2 ETHICAL/LEGAL DILEMMAS

Social Networking: HIPAA Violation

Situation

You log into a closed group on a social networking site and read a post from a fellow nursing student. The post describes in detail the complex care the student gave to a patient in a local hospital the previous day. The student says how stressful the day was and asks for advice on dealing with similar patients in the future.

Ethical/Legal Points for Consideration

- Protecting and maintaining patient privacy and confidentiality are basic obligations defined in the Code of Ethics for Nurses, which nurses and nursing students should uphold.[1]
- As outlined in the Health Insurance Portability and Accountability Act (HIPAA), a patient's private health information is any information that relates to the person's past, present, or future physical or mental health. This includes not only specific details such as a patient's name or picture but also information that gives enough details that someone may be able to identify that person.
- You may unintentionally breach privacy or confidentiality by posting patient information (diagnosis, condition, situation) on a social networking site. Using privacy settings or being in a closed group does not guarantee the secrecy of posted information. Others can copy and share any post without your knowledge.
- Potential consequences for not using social networking properly vary based on the situation. These may include (1) disciplinary action by the state board of nursing; (2) being disciplined, suspended, or fired by your employer; (3) dismissal from a nursing program; and (4) civil and/or criminal charges.
- A student nurse who had a stressful day and is looking for advice and support from peers (e.g., "Today my patient died. It made me cry.") could share by clearly limiting the post to the student's perspective and not sharing any identifying information.

Discussion Questions

1. How would you deal with the situation involving the fellow nursing student?
2. How would you handle a situation if you saw a staff member who violated HIPAA?

Reference

1. Code of Ethics for Nurses. Retrieved from www.nursingworld.org/DocumentVault/Ethics-1/Code-of-Ethics-for-Nurses.html.

Electronic Health Records

The largest use of informatics is **electronic health records (EHRs)**, also called *electronic medical records*. An EHR is a computerized record of patient information. It is shared among all health care team members involved in a patient's care and moves with the patient—to other providers and across care

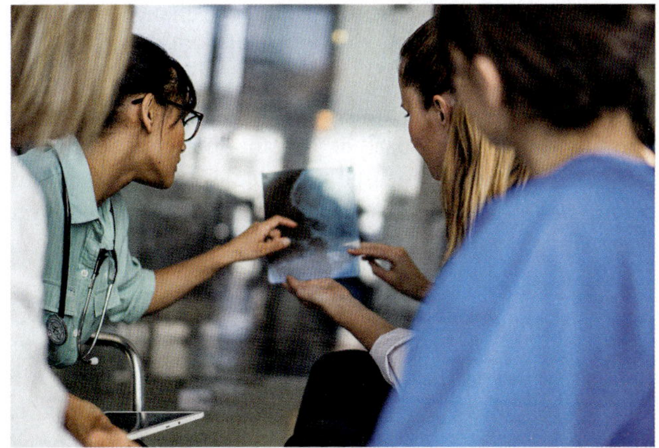

Fig. 1.9 Members of the interprofessional team review a patient's electronic health record. (© Portra/iStock.)

settings. The ideal EHR is a single place for team members to review and update a patient's health record, document care given, and enter patient care orders, including medications, procedures, diets, and diagnostic and laboratory tests (Fig. 1.9).

Several obstacles are still in the way of fully implementing EHRs. EHRs are expensive and technologically complex. They require many resources and training to implement and maintain. Communication is still lacking among computer systems and software applications. Finally, challenges in the use of EHRs, including increased workload and the need for workarounds, affect implementation.

EVIDENCE-BASED PRACTICE

Evidence-based practice (EBP) is a problem-solving approach to clinical decision making. Using the best available evidence (e.g., research findings, QI data) combined with your expertise and the patient's values, beliefs, and preferences leads to better clinical decisions and improved patient outcomes. EBP closes the gap between research and practice, providing more reliable and predictable care than that based on tradition, opinion, and trial and error.

EBP does not mean that you conduct a research study. Instead, EBP means you take an active role in using the best available evidence when delivering care. You need to have an ongoing curiosity about the best nursing practices. Routinely ask questions about your patient's care. Know when you need more information. When you base your practice on valid evidence, you are solving problems and supporting best patient outcomes.

Steps of the Evidence-Based Practice Process

The EBP process has 6 steps (Table 1.8).

TABLE 1.8 Steps of the Evidence-Based Practice Process

1. Ask the clinical question using the **PICOT** format:
   Patients/population
   Intervention
   Comparison or comparison group
   Outcome(s)
   Time (as applicable)
2. Search for the best evidence based on the clinical question.
3. Critically appraise and synthesize the evidence.
4. Implement the evidence in practice.
5. Evaluate the practice decision or change.
6. Share the outcomes of the decision or change.

Step 1

Step 1 is asking a clinical question about a practice issue or concern. Developing the clinical question is the key step in the EBP process. A good clinical question sets the context for integrating evidence, clinical judgment, and patient preferences. The question guides the literature search for the best evidence to influence practice.

You may ask the clinical question using the PICOT format. An example is, "In adult abdominal surgery patients (**P** = patients/population) is splinting with an elasticized abdominal binder (**I** = intervention) or a pillow (**C** = comparison) more effective in reducing pain associated with ambulation (**O** = outcome) on the first postoperative day (**T** = time period)?" A clinical question may not have all components of PICOT. Some only have 4 components. The (T) timing and (C) comparison components are not appropriate for every question. The (C) component may include a comparison with a specific intervention, the usual standard of care, or no intervention at all.

Step 2

Step 2 is searching for the best evidence that applies to the clinical question. Technology provides you with ready access to data. You can easily search online resources and collect information and evidence. It is important to evaluate the data sources for their credibility and reliability. Not all evidence is equal. Fig. 1.10 presents the hierarchy of evidence. As you go up the pyramid, the evidence is stronger. Systematic reviews and evidence-based clinical practice guidelines save time and effort in the EBP process. However, they are available for only a limited number of clinical topics and may not suit all types of clinical questions. When insufficient research exists to guide practice, recommendations from expert panels and authority figures may be the best evidence available.

Step 3

Step 3 is to critically appraise the evidence you found. A successful critical appraisal process focuses on 3 essential questions: (1) What are the results? (2) Are the results reliable and valid? and (3) Will the results help me in caring for my patients? You appraise the strength of the evidence and synthesize the findings related to the clinical question to conclude what the best practice is. For example, you find strong evidence

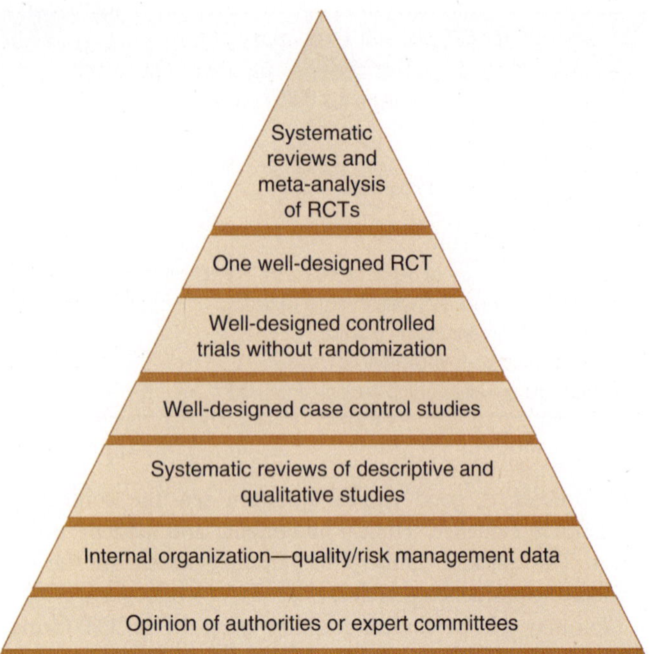

Fig. 1.10 Hierarchy of evidence. (Modified from Melnyk BM, Fineout-Overholt E: *Evidence-based practice in nursing and healthcare: A guide to best practice,* ed 3, Philadelphia, 2014, Lippincott Williams & Wilkins.)

supporting the effectiveness of elasticized binders and pillows in reducing pain associated with ambulation. However, binders appear to be most effective if the patient is obese or had prior abdominal surgery.

Step 4

Step 4 involves implementing the evidence in practice. The decision to implement change is made by considering the evidence, clinical judgment, and preferences and values of patients and caregivers. You may be part of an interprofessional team charged with implementing a practice change or applying evidence in a specific patient care situation. This may include developing clinical practice guidelines, policies, and procedures, or new assessment, teaching, or documentation tools. For example, you may be part of a team implementing a new postoperative protocol focused on using elasticized abdominal binders with patients who are obese or had prior abdominal surgery.

Step 5

Step 5 is evaluating the outcome of the practice change. After implementing the change for a specific period, you should monitor outcomes to decide whether the change has improved patient outcomes. Accrediting bodies require documentation of outcome measures to show that the organization is using evidence to improve patient care.

Step 6

Step 6 is sharing the results of the EBP change. If you do not share the outcomes of EBP, then other health care providers and patients cannot benefit from what you learned from your experience. You can share information locally using media, newsletters, and posters and regionally and nationally through journal publications and presentations at conferences.

Implementing EBP

To implement EBP, you must seek and incorporate into practice scientific evidence that supports best patient outcomes. Throughout this book, Evidence-Based Practice boxes allow you to practice applying EBP to patient scenarios. To help you identify the use of evidence in this book, an asterisk (*) in the reference list at the end of each chapter indicates evidence-based information for clinical practice.

BRIDGE TO NCLEX EXAMINATION

The number of the question corresponds to the same-numbered outcome at the beginning of the chapter.

1. An example of a nursing activity that best reflects the American Nurses Association's definition of nursing is
   - **a.** treating dysrhythmias that occur in a patient in the coronary care unit.
   - **b.** diagnosing a patient with a feeding tube as being at risk for aspiration.
   - **c.** setting up protocols for treating patients in the emergency department.
   - **d.** prescribing antianxiety drugs to a patient with a disturbed sleep pattern.
2. A nurse working in the critical care unit at an urban hospital would like to become certified in critical care nursing. The nurse knows that this process would most likely require
   - **a.** a bachelor's degree in nursing.
   - **b.** formal education as an advanced practice nurse.
   - **c.** experience for a specific period in critical care nursing.
   - **d.** membership in a critical care nursing specialty organization.

3. The nurse is assigned to care for a newly admitted patient. Number in order the steps for using the nursing process to prioritize care. (Number 1 is the first step, and number 5 is the last step.)
   ___ Determine whether the plan was effective.
   ___ Identify any clinical problems.
   ___ Collect patient information.
   ___ Carry out the plan.
   ___ Decide on a plan of action.
4. Using the SBAR format, number in order the steps for how the nurse would communicate information with the provider. (Number 1 is the first step, and number 4 is the last step.)
   ____ "I would like you to order an IV medication and come evaluate the patient as soon as possible."
   ____ "This is Nurse M.H. I am calling from the unit because your patient, D.R., has a new onset of atrial fibrillation."
   ____ "The atrial fibrillation started about 10 minutes ago. The heart rate is 124; BP 90/60. The patient is reporting dizziness."
   ____ "D.R., who is 2 days postoperative for a bowel resection for an obstruction, has a history of mitral valve disease."
5. The nurse is caring for a patient with diabetes who had a wound debridement. Which task is appropriate for the nurse to delegate to AP?
   a. Check the patient's vital signs.
   b. Assess the patient's pain level.
   c. Palpate the patient's pedal pulses.
   d. Monitor the patient's IV catheter site.
6. The nurse's role in addressing the National Patient Safety Goals includes (**Select all that apply.**)
   a. answering all patient monitoring alarms promptly.
   b. obtaining a correct list of patient medications on admission.
   c. memorizing all the rules published by The Joint Commission.
   d. encouraging patients to be actively involved in their health care.
   e. using side rails and alarm systems as necessary to prevent patient falls.
7. Advantages of using informatics in health care delivery are (**Select all that apply.**)
   a. reduced need for nurses in acute care.
   b. increased patient anonymity and confidentiality.
   c. the ability to deliver high standards of safe, quality care.
   d. access to decision-making tools for health care team members.
   e. improved communication of the patient's health status to the health care team.
8. When using evidence-based practice, the nurse
   a. must use clinical practice guidelines developed by national health agencies.
   b. should use findings from randomized controlled trials to plan care for all patient problems.
   c. uses clinical decision making and judgment to decide what evidence is appropriate for a specific clinical situation.
   d. analyzes the relationship of nursing interventions to patient outcomes to discover evidence for patient interventions.

1. b; 2. c; 3. 5, 2, 1, 4, 3; 4. 4, 1, 3, 2; 5. a;
6. a, b, e; 7. c, d, e; 8. c.

For rationales to these answers and even more NCLEX review questions, visit http://evolve.elsevier.com/Lewis/medsurg.

REFERENCES

To access the References for this chapter, please scan the QR code with a mobile device.

2

Social Determinants of Health

Andrew Scanlon and Courtney Reinisch

http://evolve.elsevier.com/Lewis/medsurg/

CONCEPTUAL FOCUS

Culture
Health Disparities and Health Equity
Diversity, Equity, and Inclusion

LEARNING OUTCOMES

1. Identify the social determinants of health.
2. Explain how social determinants may affect health.
3. Describe factors that contribute to health disparities and health equity.
4. Define cultural competence and related terminology.
5. Discuss how cultural factors affect health and health care.
6. Examine ways to identify health disparities.
7. Describe nursing interventions to promote health equity.

KEY TERMS

acculturation
cultural competence
culture
ethnicity
ethnocentrism
health disparities
health equity
place
race
racism
social determinants of health
stereotyping
structural barriers
structural competency

SOCIAL DETERMINANTS OF HEALTH

Why are there differences in people's health status? How do these differences occur? The social determinants of health (SDH) are nonmedical factors that (1) influence the health of persons and groups and (2) explain why some people have poorer health than others.[1] The SDH can be broken down into 5 groups. These are neighborhood, economic stability, education, health care access, and community context (Fig. 2.1). Where people are born, grow up, live, work, and age helps to determine their health status, behaviors, and care.

Health status is a holistic concept that is more than the presence or absence of disease. It encompasses life expectancy and self-assessment of health. Many measures make up the concept of health status. For a person, this means the sum of their current health problems plus their coping resources (e.g., family, financial resources). For a community, health status is the combination of health measures for all people living in the community. Community health measures include birth and death rates, life expectancy, access to care, and morbidity and mortality rates related to disease and injury.

Factors in a person's social and physical environment, including personal relationships, workplace, housing, transportation, and neighborhood violence, contribute to health status.[1] For example, the risk of youth homicide is much higher in neighborhoods with gang activity and high crime rates. The physical environment in which one lives, works, and plays may expose a person to risks such as environment hazards (workplace injuries), toxic agents (industrial pollution), or unsafe traffic patterns (lack of sidewalks). There may be a lack of fresh, healthy food choices.

Social determinants of health

Economic stability	Neighborhood	Education	Community context	Health care
Employment Income Expenses Debt Medical bills Support	Housing Transportation Safety Recreation Walkability Zip code/ geography Food	Literacy Language Early childhood education Vocational training Higher education	Social integration Support systems Community engagement Discrimination Stress	Health coverage HCP availability Linguistic and cultural competency Quality of care

Health outcomes
Mortality, morbidity, life expectancy, health status, functional limitations

Fig. 2.1 Social determinants of health.

Neighborhood

Place refers to the geographic and environment location where a person is born, grows, lives, works, and ages. Your neighborhood affects the use of health services, health status, and health behaviors.

Housing is a basic need. It protects us from environmental harm. Housing can contribute to poor health outcomes. Unsafe or poor-quality housing is associated with exposure to lead, indoor air pollution, and asthma triggers (dust, mold, rodents). Overcrowded living conditions can contribute to the spread of infectious disease. Living close to hazards can affect pregnancy outcomes. It increases the risk of cancer and neurologic problems.

Health behaviors affected by place are physical activity and nutrition. Safe, walkable neighborhoods with playgrounds promote physical activity. Source and price of healthy foods affect diet intake and weight. Social support positively affects coping with illness. Social networks are more likely in communities where neighbors interact and rely on one another.

Differences in access to health care services between rural and urban settings create geographic health disparities.[2] People in rural areas may need to travel long distances to receive health care. This can result in inadequate or less frequent access to health care services. Some parts of the rural United States are "medically underserved" because of low numbers of HCPs. Rural populations tend to be older than urban populations. They are more likely to have cancer, heart disease, diabetes, depression, obesity, and injury-related deaths than people in urban areas.

Living in urban centers may predispose a person to other health disparities. People in high-crime areas may not visit HCPs. High rates of chronic health problems and premature deaths occur in neighborhoods with social inequalities. These include high poverty rates, high crime rates, and residential segregation.

Structural barriers, such as zoning laws and economic policies, play a role in access to health care and overall health outcomes. Zoning laws can restrict where health care facilities, grocery stores, and recreation areas are located. This may make it harder for some communities to have services. Economic policies affecting employment, wages, and housing affordability affect economic stability. People living in poor or poorly zoned areas experience worse health outcomes than more affluent communities.[3]

Structural competency is essential for understanding and addressing how systemic factors like zoning, economic policies, and resource distribution affect health. It encourages us as health care team members to look beyond individual behaviors and recognize how broader community structures affect health. By understanding these influences, we can advocate for policy changes and interventions that address the root causes of health disparities, promoting more equitable outcomes.[3]

Economic Stability

The main nonmedical factor affecting health is socioeconomic status. Socioeconomic status is related to wealth, education, and occupation. Those living in poverty cannot afford healthy food, health care, and safe housing. People of lower income report worse health and die at a younger age. Hazardous work environments and high-risk occupations increase health risk and contribute to higher rates of illness, injury, and death.

Health Care

Access to health care contributes to a person's health. Many people do not have access to quality health care. Health care coverage is a key factor that contributes to health disparities. People who are underinsured, have no insurance, or lack financial resources to pay for treatment of diseases may forgo health care visits, screenings, and treatments. This affects both individual and community health. Patients who lack the knowledge and/or access to apply for government aid programs (e.g., Medicaid) are also at risk.

The health care system may contribute to health disparities. For example, a clinic located in an area with a large population of non–English-speaking immigrants that does not provide interpreters or educational materials and financial forms in languages other than English may limit these families' ability to understand how to access health care.

Discrimination and *bias* based on a patient's race, ethnicity, gender, age, body size, sexual orientation, or ability to pay are likely to result in less aggressive or negative treatment practices. Discrimination can result in the delay of a diagnosis because of assumptions made about the patient. Sometimes discrimination is hard to recognize, especially when it occurs at the institutional level. Even well-intentioned HCPs who try to eliminate bias in their care can show their prior beliefs or prejudices through nonverbal communication. Many policies are in place to eliminate discrimination, but it still exists.

Poorer health outcomes for minorities are linked to the shortage of culturally and ethnically diverse HCPs, who are underrepresented in the health professions. A diversity gap exists between the ethnic composition of the health care team and the overall population in the United States (Fig. 2.2). For example, the diversity of nurses in the United States is increasing but still lags that of the overall population. People who are Black, Hispanic/Latino, and Native American make up more than 35% of the population but only 16% of the nation's nurses.[4] Biased behaviors against nurses of diverse cultural and ethnic backgrounds by patients and health care professionals may contribute to their underrepresentation.

Cultural differences affect how well patients think they can communicate with their HCP. In the United States, minority patients may have difficulty understanding and communicating with their HCP. Communication issues include not understanding the HCP, feeling that they are not listened to, and having questions but not asking them.

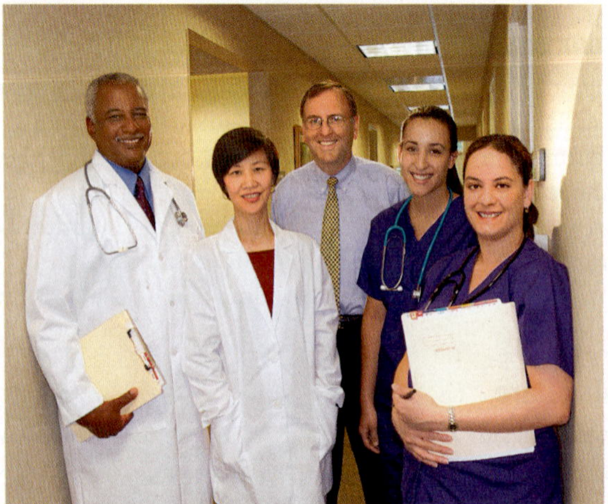

Fig. 2.2 Interprofessional team working together in a multicultural health care environment. (© Thinkstock/Stockbyte/Thinkstock.)

Education

Where you live influences your access to quality education. Some communities have better schools than others. People with higher levels of education tend to be healthier. Adults without a high school diploma or equivalent are 3 times more likely to die before age 65 than those with a college degree.

Health literacy is the degree to which a person has the capacity to obtain, process, and understand basic health information and services needed to make health decisions. This includes the ability to (1) read, understand, and analyze information; (2) understand instructions; (3) weigh risks and benefits; and (4) make decisions and act. Low health literacy is related to more hospitalizations, greater use of emergency department care, decreased use of cancer screening and influenza vaccine, decreased ability to use medications correctly, and higher mortality rates among older adults. See Chapter 4 for more about health literacy.

Community

Our sense of connection with family, friends, coworkers, and community members affects our health and well-being. Positive relationships can improve health. Persons who are bullied may not get the support they need. Nurses can help people get social support in the community to reduce health disparities.

HEALTH DISPARITIES AND HEALTH EQUITY

Health disparities are differences in the incidence, prevalence, mortality rate, and burden of diseases that exist among specific population groups. Many factors can lead to health disparities (Table 2.1). In the United States, health disparities occur because of social, economic, or environmental disadvantages. They can affect population groups based on gender, age, ethnicity, socioeconomic status, education, location, sexual orientation, or disability status (Box 2.1).[5] **Health equity** is achieved when every person can attain their health potential and no one is disadvantaged. Social and cultural factors

TABLE 2.1 Factors and Conditions Leading to Health Disparities

- Age
- Disability status
- Education
- Ethnicity and race
- Food insecurity
- HCP attitudes/biases
- Health literacy
- Income status
- Lack of health care services access
- Language barrier
- Occupation or unemployment
- Place
- Sexual orientation
- Unemployment
- Unstable housing

BOX 2.1 ETHICAL/LEGAL DILEMMAS

Health Disparities

Situation

E.M., a 47-year-old Latino female living with type 2 diabetes, comes to the clinic to have her blood glucose measured. It has been 12 months since her last visit. At that time, the nurse asked that she bring along her glucometer and strips to show how she checks her blood glucose because her glucose values were high at her previous visits.

When you check E.M.'s equipment and glucose strips, you find the strips are for a different machine and expired 2 years ago. When you inquire about the situation, E.M. says that she cannot afford to come to the clinic or to buy new equipment and supplies to check her blood glucose level. During the day, E.M. cares for her 3 grandchildren so her daughter can work. E.M. spends most of her income on food for her family, so she has little money left for her health care.

Ethical/Legal Points for Consideration

- Ethnic minorities and other vulnerable or disadvantaged groups have higher rates of certain chronic illnesses. Limited access to high-quality, accessible, and affordable health care services is related to an increased incidence of complications and a reduced life span.
- People with certain health problems such as diabetes may have difficulty obtaining health care insurance. Consider these issues in the broader context of social justice.
- The legal definition of the role of the professional nurse includes patient advocacy. Advocacy includes the obligation to provide adequate follow-up care for all patients, regardless of race, gender, or ability to pay.
- A nurse who sees disparities must consider the possibility of discrimination. Professional nurses are legally and ethically responsible for patient advocacy. The nurse may incur legal liability if failure to fulfill this obligation results in patient harm.

Discussion Questions

1. How would you work with E.M. to help her obtain the necessary resources and knowledge to care for her diabetes?
2. What can you do to begin working on the problems of health disparities in your community?

influence equity in health care. Awareness of these factors will help you to provide optimal patient care.

Ethnicity and Race

The terms ethnicity and race are subjective and based on self-report. We often use these terms interchangeably. They are not defined by genetic markers. Social context and lived experiences influence people's decision about the ethnic and race category with which they identify or are assigned. Ethnic and race categories may differ on a person's birth certificate and death certificate.

People often identify their own ethnicity and race for health data collection (e.g., health plans, birth certificates). Collection of health data based on self-reported ethnic and race categories is important for research, to inform policy, and to understand and eliminate disparities. People identify their race using 1 or more categories. Law requires federal agencies to list a minimum of 5 race categories: White, Black, American Indian or Alaska Native, Asian, and Native Hawaiian or another Pacific Islander. Federal agencies must also list a minimum of 2 ethnicities for people who self-identify as either *Hispanic or Latino* and *Not Hispanic or Latino.* A Hispanic or Latino is typically a person of Cuban, Mexican, Puerto Rican, South or Central American, or other Spanish descent, regardless of race. In the United States, minority groups include Hispanic/Latino (20%), Black (14%), and Asian (6%).[5] Native Hawaiian and other Pacific Islander, Native American and Native Alaskan, and 2 or more races make up 4% of the population.[5] The number for most of these groups is expected to increase in the coming decades.

Although treatment advances have prolonged and improved quality of life for many, racial and ethnic minorities have received less benefit from these advances. Obesity and chronic illness rates for diabetes, hypertension, chronic obstructive pulmonary diseases, cancer, and stroke are higher among minorities. Racial, ethnic, and cultural differences exist in health services, treatments provided, and access to HCPs. Race and ethnicity also influence health outcomes. For example, after myocardial infarction, minority patients are at greater risk of rehospitalization and death. They are less likely to receive potentially beneficial treatments.[6]

Racism affects health outcomes. **Racism** is the structures, policies, practices, beliefs, and behaviors in a society that create an unfair advantage for some people and unfair or harmful treatment of others based on their race or ethnic group.[7] Racism affects the physical, social, and economic conditions of where people live, learn, work, and play, including access to health care services.

Gender

Health disparities exist between males and females. Adult females use health care services more than males. Females may not receive the same quality of care. When we combine gender with racial and ethnic differences, the disparities are even greater.

Age

Biases toward older adults that affect their care, or ageism, are discussed in Chapter 5. Older adults are at risk for experiencing health disparities in the number of diagnostic tests done and aggressiveness of treatments used. Older adults of low socioeconomic status have greater disability, more limitations in activities of daily living, and more frequent and rapid cognitive decline. Black and Latino older adults are disproportionately affected by chronic illnesses, disability, depression, and substandard quality of life.[8]

CULTURE

Culture is a way of life for a group of people. It includes the behaviors, beliefs, values, traditions, and symbols that the group accepts, generally without thinking about them. This way of life is passed along by communication and imitation from 1 generation to the next. You can also think of culture as behavior that one acquires through social learning. It is the totality of a

TABLE 2.2 Basic Characteristics of Culture

- Dynamic and ever-changing
- Not always shared by all members of a cultural group
- Adapted to specific conditions such as environmental factors
- Learned through oral and written histories in addition to socialization

person's learned, accumulated experience that is socially transmitted. The basic characteristics of culture are described in Table 2.2.

Values are the sets of rules by which persons, families, groups, and communities live. They are the principles and standards that serve as the basis for beliefs, attitudes, and behaviors. All cultures have values. The types and expressions of those values differ among cultures. These cultural values develop over time, guide decision making and actions, and may affect a person's self-esteem. Cultural values often unconsciously develop early in life as a child learns about acceptable and unacceptable behaviors. The extent to which a person's cultural values are internalized influences that person's tendency toward judging other cultures. We usually use our own culture as the accepted standard.

Although persons within a cultural group may have many similarities through their shared values, beliefs, and practices, there is also diversity within groups. Each person is culturally unique. Such diversity may result from different perspectives and interpretations of situations (Fig. 2.3). These differences may be based on age, gender, marital status, family structure, income, education level, religious views, and life experiences. Within any cultural group, there are smaller groups that may not hold all the values of the dominant culture. These smaller cultural groups have experiences that differ from those of the dominant group. These differences may be related to ethnic background, residence, religion, occupation, health, age, gender, education, or other factors that unite the group. Members of a subculture share certain aspects of culture that are different from those of the overall cultural group. For example, people from a cultural group seek professional health care right away when symptoms appear. Others from the same culture rely first on folk healers. A third group may seek the opinion of family and friends before seeking formal health care.

Cultural beliefs about symptom tolerance and health care–seeking behavior can contribute to health disparities. Some cultures consider pain something to endure or ignore. As a result, patients may not seek help. Some cultures may view diseases or problems fatalistically. This means there is no reason to seek treatment because they believe there is no hope. Some cultures view the signs and symptoms of an illness as "God's will" or as a punishment for some prior behavior. In some cultures, it may not be acceptable to see an HCP who is not of the same gender or ethnic group. Such beliefs can result in delays in seeking health care or inadequate treatment.

Acculturation is the lifelong process of incorporating cultural aspects in which a person grows, lives, works, and ages. It is often bidirectional. In other words, the context changes as a person's culture influences it. Change may be in attitudes, behaviors, and values. For example, a sedentary person who loves to cook may change their attitude toward exercise when living with athletic roommates. Their roommates may also change as they begin to appreciate cooking. Behaviors change when an immigrant child learns the local language while influencing the conduct of classmates. A deeply held value such as self-sufficiency may change for a person exposed to a culture in which reliance on others dominates.

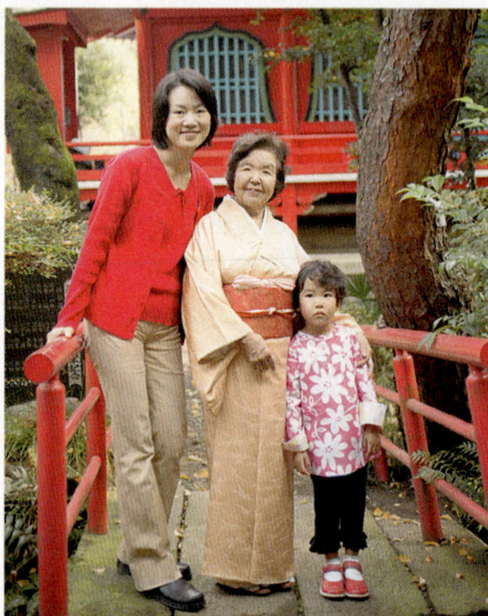

Fig. 2.3 Each person is culturally unique. (© Jupiterimages/Photos.com/Thinkstock.)

Newcomers may adopt both the strengths and limitations of the dominant culture. This is relevant when considering health behaviors and the quality of health care delivered by professionals. For example, an immigrant may be negatively influenced by a dominant cultural context in which unhealthy eating habits prevail.[9]

The result of acculturation may be new cultural variations in attitudes, behaviors, and values. People who move to a new community or country are more aware of the acculturation experience than people who are not exposed to new experiences. Exposure to new cultural contexts increases a nurse's cultural competency.

Stereotyping refers to an overgeneralized viewpoint that members of a specific culture, race, or ethnic group are alike and share the same values and beliefs. This oversimplified approach does not consider the individual differences that exist within a culture. Being a member of a particular cultural, ethnic, or racial group does not make the person an expert on other members of that same group. Such stereotyping can lead to false assumptions and affect a patient's care. For example, it would be inappropriate for you to assume that just because a nurse is of a particular culture, they would know how a person of the same culture's beliefs may affect that patient's health care practices. As another example, a young Latino nurse born and raised in a large city experienced a different culture than the older patient who was born and raised in a rural area of the same country of origin.

Ethnocentrism refers to the belief that one's own culture and worldview are superior to those of others from different cultural, ethnic, or racial backgrounds.[9] Comparing others' ways to your own can lead to seeing others as different or inferior. HCPs' ethnocentrism can result in poor communication, patient alienation, and potentially inadequate treatment. To avoid ethnocentrism, you need to remain open to a variety of perspectives and maintain a nonjudgmental view of the values, beliefs, and practices of others. Failure to do this can result in ethnic stereotyping or cultural imposition.

Cultural imposition occurs when we impose our own cultural beliefs and practices on another person or group of people. In health care, it can result in disregarding a patient's health care beliefs or practices. Cultural imposition may happen when an HCP is unaware of the patient's cultural beliefs and plans and implements care without taking them into account.

Cultural safety describes care and advocacy for a person of another culture determined by that person or family. Care that is culturally safe prevents cultural imposition. Culturally safe care requires cultural competency and action to ensure that cultural histories, experiences, and traditions of patients, their families, and communities are valued and shape health care approaches and policies.

CULTURAL COMPETENCE

Cultural competence is the ability to understand, appreciate, and work with people from cultures other than your own. It involves an awareness and acceptance of cultural differences, self-awareness, knowledge of the patient's culture, and adaptation of skills to meet the patient's needs. The 4 components of cultural competence are (1) cultural awareness, (2) cultural knowledge, (3) cultural skill, and (4) cultural encounter (Table 2.3). *Cultural humility* is the next step beyond cultural competence. It is a lifelong process of learning and examining one's own personal bias. It is the evaluation of a person of a certain culture as an individual. You avoid assigning stereotypes or assumptions to people of a particular race or ethnicity.

Providing culturally competent care may increase patient satisfaction, promote health equity, increase patient safety, and prevent misunderstandings between you and your patients. It also involves integrating cultural practices into Western medicine. For example, before some diagnostic procedures and interventions, it is typical to have patients remove personal objects they are wearing on the body. Ask patients whether they wear personal objects and the significance of their removal, because they may have cultural or spiritual significance. Know

TABLE 2.3 How to Develop Cultural Competence

Description	Role of Nurse
Cultural Awareness	
• Ability to understand patients' unique cultural needs	• Understand your own cultural background, values, and beliefs, especially as related to health and health care. • Examine your own cultural biases toward people whose cultures differ from your own.
Cultural Knowledge	
• Process of learning key aspects of a group's culture, especially as it relates to health and health care practices • Patients are best source of information about their culture	• Learn basic general information about predominant cultural groups in your geographic area. Cultural guides are a good resource. • Assess patients for presence or absence of cultural traits based on an understanding of generalizations about a cultural group. • Do not make assumptions based on cultural background because the degree of acculturation varies among persons. • Read research studies that describe cultural differences. • Read ethnic newspaper articles and books. • View documentaries about cultural groups.
Cultural Skill	
• Ability to collect relevant cultural data • Perform a cultural assessment	• Be alert for unexpected responses with patients, especially as related to cultural issues. • Become aware of cultural differences in predominant ethnic groups. • Develop assessment skills to do a competent cultural assessment for any patient (Table 2.7). • Learn assessment skills for different cultural groups, including cultural beliefs and practices.
Cultural Encounter	
• Direct cross-cultural interactions between people from culturally diverse backgrounds • Extended contact with a cultural group to enhance understanding of its values and beliefs	• Create opportunities to interact with predominant cultural groups. • Attend cultural events, such as religious ceremonies, significant life passage rituals, social events, and demonstrations of cultural practices. • Visit markets and restaurants in ethnic neighborhoods. • Explore ethnic neighborhoods, listen to different types of ethnic music, and learn games of various ethnic groups. • Visit or volunteer at health fairs in local ethnic neighborhoods. • Learn about prominent cultural beliefs and practices and include this knowledge when planning nursing care.

whether wearing these objects will affect patient safety, test results, or outcomes of the intervention.

When HCPs from different cultures work together as members of the health care team, opportunities for miscommunication and conflict can occur. We call this *cultural conflict.* The cultural origins of miscommunication and conflict in the workplace are often connected with cultural beliefs, values, and etiquette. Seeking clarification is a communication strategy to foster effective teamwork among a multicultural health care team.

CULTURAL FACTORS AFFECTING HEALTH AND HEALTH CARE

Culture greatly affects health and health care. It affects our perceptions of health, illness, and death; ideas about causes of disease; ways of promoting health; how we experience and express illness and pain; where we seek care; and preferred treatments. Potential factors are outlined in Table 2.4. It may be helpful to review general characteristics associated with a cultural group when preparing to care for a patient. However, remember that patients may not identify with the assumed cultural group, and our biases and stereotypes may affect the patient and result in more patient-provider barriers.

Folk Healers and Traditions

Many cultures have folk healers, also known as *traditional healers.* Most folk healers speak the person's native language and cost less than conventional HCPs. Among the many folk healers found worldwide, patients from regions in Mexico and Central and South America may choose to use a *curandero* (or *curandera*). Some cultures employ lay midwives (e.g., *parteras* for Latino females) in the care of pregnant females.

Folk medicine and traditions are culturally based forms of prevention and treatment. They traditionally rely on oral transmission of healing techniques from 1 generation to the next. Patients may not use the term *folk medicine* but think of these as cultural home remedies or treatment practices. Patients can practice folk medicine at home without using a folk healer. It is important to assess whether patients are practicing traditional or folk healing. Some herb remedies could pose potential interactions with medications.

Some traditions practiced as a rite of passage in some cultures are considered harmful in the dominant culture in the United States. For example, female genital cutting is a tradition that is illegal in most countries yet still practiced in many countries in Africa and the Middle East. It results in physical and emotional trauma and may affect childbirth.

Spirituality and Religion

Spirituality refers to a person's effort to find purpose and meaning in life. It is influenced by a person's unique life experiences and reflects one's personal understanding of life's mysteries. Spirituality relates to the soul or spirit more than to the body. It may provide hope and strength for a person during

TABLE 2.4 Cultural Factors Affecting Health and Health Care

Beliefs and Practices
- Care provided in established health care programs may not be perceived as culturally relevant.
- Religious reasons, beliefs, or practices may affect a person's decision to seek or not seek health care.
- Patients may delay seeking health care because of fear or dependence on folk medicine and herbal remedies.
- Patients may stop treatment or visits for health care because the symptoms are no longer present, and they think that further care is not needed.
- Some patients associate hospitals and extended care facilities with death.
- Patients may have had a previous negative experience with culturally incompetent HCPs or discriminatory practices.
- Some people mistrust the majority population and institutions dominated by them.
- Some patients may feel apprehensive about unfamiliar diagnostic procedures and treatment options.

Communication and Language
- Patients may not speak English and may not be able to communicate with the HCP.
- It may be hard to communicate, even with interpreters.

Economic Factors
- Patients may not get health care because they cannot pay for it or because of the costs of travel for health care.
- Refugee or undocumented immigrant status may deter some patients from using the health care system.
- Immigrant women who are heads of households or single mothers may not seek health care for themselves because of childcare costs.
- Patients may lack health insurance.

Health Care System
- Patients may not make or keep appointments because of the time lag between the onset of an illness and an available appointment.
- Hours of operation of health care facilities may not accommodate patients' need to work or use public transportation.
- Requirements to access some types of care may discourage some patients from taking the steps to qualify for health care or health care payment assistance.
- Some patients have a general distrust of HCPs and health care systems.
- Lack of ethnic-specific health care programs may deter some people from seeking health care.
- Transportation may be a problem for patients who must travel long distances for health care.
- Adequate interpreter services may be unavailable.
- Patients may not have a primary HCP. They may use emergency departments or urgent care centers for health care.
- Shortages of HCPs from specific ethnic groups may deter some people from seeking health care.
- Patients may lack knowledge about the availability of existing health care resources.
- Agency policies may not be culturally competent (e.g., hospital policy may limit the number of visitors, which is problematic for cultures that value having many family members present).

Time Orientation
- For some cultures, it is more important to deal with a social role than to arrive on time for an appointment with an HCP.
- Some cultures are future oriented; others are past or present oriented.

an illness. *Religion* is a more formal and organized system of beliefs, including belief in or worship of God or gods. Religious beliefs include the cause, nature, and purpose of the universe and involve prayer and rituals. Religion is based on beliefs about life, death, good, and evil.

Spirituality and religion are aspects of culture that may affect a person's beliefs about health, illness, and end-of-life care (Table 2.5). They may also play a role in nutrition and decisions related to health, wellness, and how to respond to or treat an illness. Interventions to meet patients' religious and spiritual

TABLE 2.5 Health-Related Beliefs and Practices of Selected Religious Groups

Amish
- Prohibit drinking alcohol.
- Prohibit abortion, artificial insemination, and stem cell use.
- Seldom buy commercial health insurance.
- Prohibit drugs unless prescribed by HCPs.

Buddhism
- Prohibit drinking alcohol and using illicit drugs.
- Practice moderation in diet and avoidance of extremes.
- Central tenets are maintaining right views, intentions, speech, actions, livelihood, effort, mindfulness, and concentration.

Catholicism
- Fast and abstain from meat and meat products on Ash Wednesday and the Fridays of Lent.
- Prohibit artificial contraception and direct abortion.
- Indirect abortion (e.g., treatment of uterine cancer in a pregnant female) may be morally justified.
- Sacrament of the Sick includes anointing of sick with oil, blessing by a priest, and communion (unleavened wafer made of flour and water).

Church of Jesus Christ of Latter-Day Saints (Mormons)
- Strict diet code called Word of Wisdom prohibits all alcohol, hot drinks (nonherbal teas and coffee), tobacco, and recreational drugs.
- Fast for a 24-hour period each month on "Fast Sunday."
- During hospitalization or serious illness, an elder anoints the ill person with oil while a second elder seals the anointing with a prayer and blessing (laying on of hands).
- Prohibit abortion except when the mother's life is in danger.

Hinduism
- Prohibit eating meat because it involves harming a living creature.
- Cremation is the usual form of body disposal, but fetuses or newborns are sometimes buried.

Islam
- Fasting during daytime hours occurs during a month-long period called Ramadan.
- Perform a ritual cleansing with water before eating and before prayer.
- Prohibit eating pork or taking medicines with pork derivatives.
- Prohibit drinking alcohol.
- Artificial insemination is permissible only if from the husband to his own wife.

Jehovah's Witness
- Prohibit blood transfusions in any form or agents in which blood is an ingredient.
- Blood volume expanders are acceptable if they are not derivatives of blood.
- Prohibit transplants that involve bodily mutilation.
- Prohibit artificial insemination and therapeutic and on-demand abortions.

Judaism
- Prohibit eating pork, shellfish, or predatory fowl or mixing milk dishes and meat dishes when preparing foods.
- Certain foods and drinks are designated as kosher, which means "proper." All animals must be ritually slaughtered.
- On the 8th day after birth, boys are circumcised in a ritual called *brit milah.* Girls are given a dedication ceremony involving prayers and blessings.
- Prohibit abortion except when the mother's life is in danger.
- Organized support system for the sick includes a visit from the rabbi. The rabbi may pray with the sick person alone or in a minyan, a group of 10 adults older than age 13.
- If an autopsy is done, all body parts must be returned for burial.

Seventh-Day Adventism
- Encourage a vegetarian diet.
- Nonvegetarian members do not eat foods derived from any animal having a cloven hoof that chews its cud (e.g., pigs, goats).
- Prohibit eating shellfish; eating fish with fins and scales is acceptable.
- Prohibit drinking alcohol.
- Some church members practice voluntary fasting.

From Andrews MM, Boyle JS: *Transcultural concepts in nursing care,* ed 7, Philadelphia, 2016, Lippincott Williams & Wilkins.

needs include prayer, scripture reading, listening, and referral to a chaplain, rabbi, or religious leader.

Many patients find that rituals help them during times of illness. Rituals help a person make sense of life experiences. They may take the form of prayer, meditation, or other rituals that patients may create. Include spiritual questions in your patient assessment and plan care accordingly. Table 10.2 has a spiritual assessment guide you can use with patients.

Cross-Cultural Communication

Communication refers to an organized, patterned system of behavior that may be verbal or nonverbal (Fig. 2.4). Verbal communication includes not only one's language or dialect but also voice tone, volume, timing, and ability to share thoughts and feelings. More than 60 million people in the United States speak a language other than English in their home. Spanish is the most common. Hispanic people who do not speak English at home are less likely to receive a variety of health care services even if they are comfortable speaking English.

Nonverbal communication may take the form of writing, gestures, body movements, posture, facial expressions, and personal dress in some cultures. It includes eye contact, use of touch, body language, style of greeting, and spatial distancing. Eye contact varies among cultural groups. Other variables to consider include the role of gender, age, acculturation, and status. For example, Muslim-Arab women exhibit modesty when avoiding eye contact with men other than their husbands and when in public situations.

Silence has many meanings. It is important to understand and clarify what silence means in a patient interaction. Some people are comfortable with silence. They use silence for thinking and carefully considering a response. In these interactions, silence shows respect for the other person and the importance of the remarks. The speaker may stop talking and leave a period of silence for the listener to think about what was said before continuing. Sometimes the person may interpret silence as meaning agreement. Patients sometimes nod their head or say "yes" as if agreeing with you or to show they understand. They may be doing this because it is a culturally acceptable manner of showing respect, not because they understand or agree. Others become uncomfortable and may speak to decrease the amount of silent time.

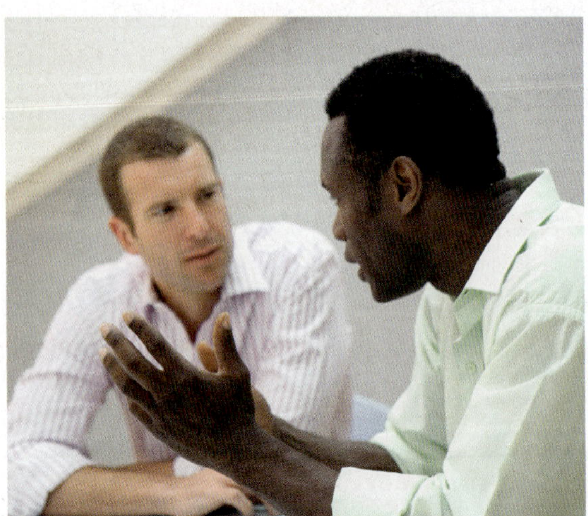

Fig. 2.4 Coworkers from different cultures communicate with verbal and nonverbal cues. (© BananaStock/Thinkstock.)

Racism and Microaggression Affect Communication

Microaggressions are social exchanges in which a person says or does something that can either intentionally or unintentionally belittle or alienate a person, especially someone of a different racial/ethnic group. It is important that we seek to understand racism and microaggression through education, self-awareness, and open dialogue with peers.

Family Roles and Relationships

Family roles differ from one culture to another. It is important to determine who should be involved in communication and decision making related to health care. Some groups emphasize interdependence rather than independence. In the United States, many in the mainstream culture have strong beliefs related to autonomy. We expect a patient to sign consent forms when receiving health care. In some cultural groups, patients may expect a family member to make health care decisions. The health care system may have difficulty with how a patient makes decisions. We may have to delay treatment while the patient waits for family members to arrive before giving consent for a procedure or treatment. In other instances, patients may make a decision that is best for the family despite adverse outcomes for themselves. Being aware of such values will better prepare you to be a patient advocate.

Some cultural differences relate to expectations of family members in providing care. In some cultures, family members expect to provide care for the patient even in the hospital. Others may expect that family, along with the HCPs, will provide all care. This view is the opposite of the predominant Western expectation that patients will assume self-care as quickly as possible.

Ask about culturally relevant gender relationships. For example, in some cultures, it is not appropriate for a man to be alone with a woman other than his wife. Nor is it appropriate for a woman other than a man's wife to provide physical care for him. The clinical implication of this cultural belief is that nurses cannot provide direct physical care for patients of the opposite gender. In some instances, patients may receive procedures or treatments only from providers of the opposite gender if a third party is present.

Personal Space

Personal space zones are the variable and subjective distance at which 1 person feels comfortable talking to another. As a nurse, you often interact with patients at the intimate or personal distance, which may be uncomfortable for the patient.

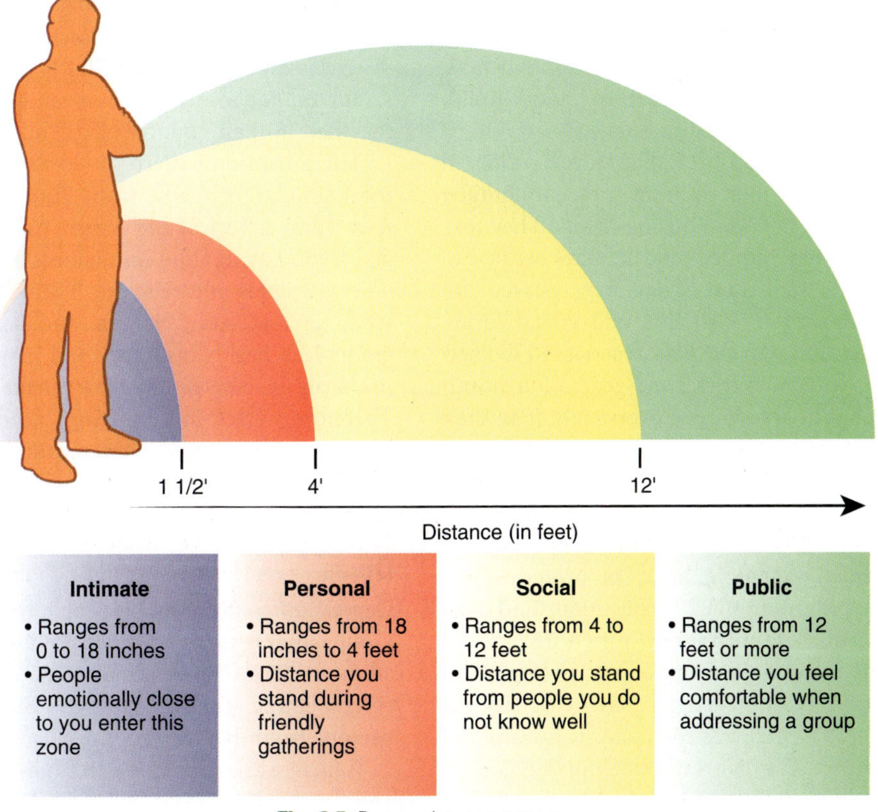

Fig. 2.5 Personal space zones.

Personal space distances vary from culture to culture and within a culture. An American nurse of European descent may be comfortable with a certain distance. A representative example of personal space zones for European Americans is shown in Fig. 2.5. A person from a Hispanic or Middle Eastern background may believe that the distance is too far and will move closer. This may make you feel uncomfortable. If you then move away to a more comfortable distance, this may cause the other person to think that you are unfriendly, or the person may be offended.

Touch

Physical contact with patients conveys various meanings depending on the culture. Performing a physical assessment requires touching a patient. Many people of Asian and Hispanic heritage believe that touching a person's head is a sign of disrespect because the head is the source of one's strength and/or soul. Many people in the world believe in the evil eye, or *mal ojo.* In this culture-bound syndrome, illness—usually in a child or a woman—results from excess admiration by another person. In some cultures, the way to ward off the evil eye is to touch the area of admiration. For example, if the person admires the hair, the top of the head may be touched. It is important for you to ask permission before touching anyone, particularly if it is necessary to touch the person's head.

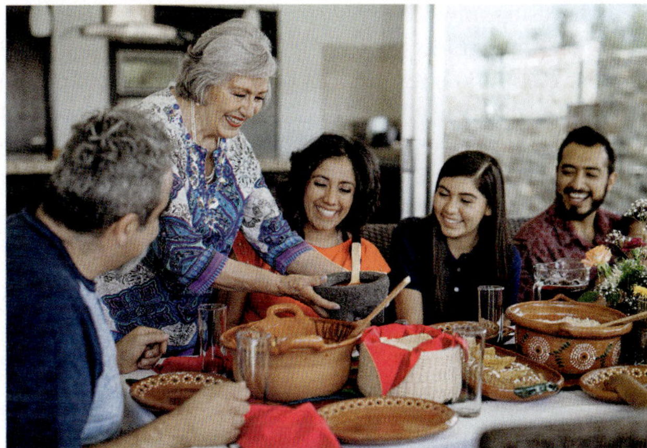

Fig. 2.6 Members of this family share a common heritage. (© Drazen/iStock.com.)

Nutrition

An important part of cultural practices is food, including both the foods that one eats and rituals and practices associated with food (Fig. 2.6). We should consider food-related cultural beliefs, practices, and habits when discussing nutrition with patients and planning their diets.

Patients may need to make major changes in their diets because of health problems. Muslims fast during the daytime during the Islamic month of Ramadan. Such practices may affect when and how patients take medications. A person may use food to cope with life changes such as homesickness. Specific foods may be considered essential to good health during pregnancy or other life stages.

When people immigrate to an area that is very different from their country of origin, they may encounter unfamiliar foods, food storage systems, and food buying habits. They may come from countries that have limited food supplies because of poverty, wars, and poor sanitation. They may arrive with conditions such as malnutrition, diarrhea, and dental caries. Other problems may develop after the person arrives in the new country. For example, with obesity, second-generation immigrants have a greater chance of becoming overweight than their first-generation counterparts.[9]

Immigration

Several conditions drive migration, such as overcrowding, natural disasters, geopolitical conflict, persecution, and economic forces. Because of these migrations, a rich diversity of cultures exists in many communities and countries (Fig. 2.7).

Immigrants who have recently arrived may be at risk for physical and mental health problems for many reasons. Conditions in their countries of origin (e.g., malnutrition, poor sanitation, civil war) may have resulted in chronic health problems. For example, most cases of tuberculosis in the United States occur in persons born outside the United States.[10] Relocation is associated with many losses and can cause economic hardship, physical stress, and mental distress.

As new immigrants go through the acculturation process, many have cultural stress as they adjust to their new environment, especially if they have left relatives behind or are unable to return to their home country. Older immigrants are especially affected by changes in role and social position. This may result in depression. People who have survived wars and violence may have posttraumatic stress disorder. Immigrants may face barriers to social acceptance, such as prejudice or discrimination. There may be a lack of ethnic and cultural resources. For some, it may mean loss of the social status that they had in their country of origin.

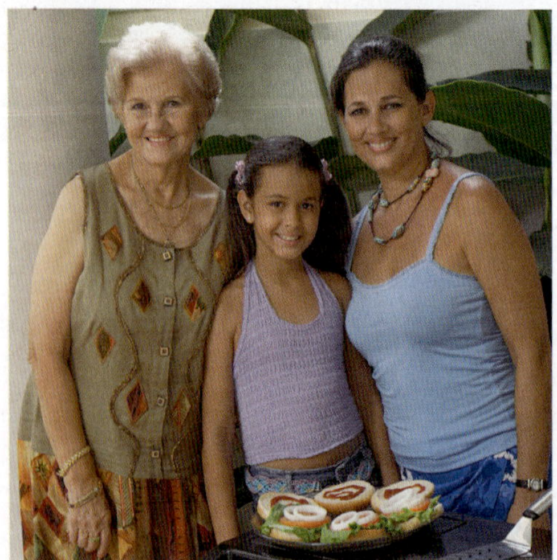

Fig. 2.7 Recently arrived immigrants join a neighbor for a barbecue, a common American tradition. (© Jack Hollingsworth/Photodisc/Thinkstock.)

The migration pattern of North America has shifted. Once, most immigrants came from Europe. Now, most come from Asia, Latin America, and Africa. An increased number of first- and second-generation immigrants enter the United States after visiting friends and relatives. They have a higher risk for malaria, typhoid fever, cholera, and hepatitis A.[11] Many immigrants lack health insurance and may obtain their health care primarily in emergency departments and urgent care clinics. Therefore nurses in all settings need to be aware of refugee health screening, treatment recommendations, and resources for access to health care and social services.

Drugs

Genetic differences among people from diverse ethnic or racial groups may explain differences in drug choice, dosage, or administration. For example, some drugs are more effective in certain ethnic groups than others. Side effects may vary among persons from diverse backgrounds.

Genetic variations can affect how the body processes a drug and the overall effect of selected drugs on the body. Although race and ethnicity are imprecise indicators of genetic differences, they can be helpful in predicting variations in drug response. For example, in treating hypertension, some populations respond better to angiotensin-converting enzyme (ACE) inhibitors and β-blockers. Others respond to diuretics. Genetics and drug metabolism are discussed in Chapter 13.

Problems can result from interactions between cultural remedies and prescription drugs. Some people may self-treat their depression with St. John's wort. This can result in adverse effects if taken with prescription antidepressants. Others may avoid standard Western medicine until herbs and other remedies become ineffective or the illness becomes acute. The challenge for us is to try to accommodate patients' desires for traditional aspects of care while using evidence-based approaches that are appropriate and acceptable to patients. Evaluate the safety and appropriateness of traditional cultural healing therapies.

Develop a collaborative, trusting relationship with patients and encourage them to discuss their traditional approaches to healing. Seek out information on potential drug and herb product interactions from the pharmacist. Honor patient choices if safe and effective. This will enhance collaboration and may have a positive impact on health outcomes.

Psychologic Factors

Symptoms are interpreted through a person's cultural norms and may vary from the recognized interpretations of Western medicine. All symptoms have meaning. The meanings may vary from one culture to another. For example, cultural views can affect the degree of depression after a cardiac diagnosis. It is important to ask patients what their illness means to them, what they believe is the cause, and what they think is the best treatment.

❖ NURSING MANAGEMENT: SOCIAL DETERMINANTS OF HEALTH AND CULTURALLY COMPETENT CARE

Self-Assessment

The first step in promoting health equity and providing culturally competent care is for you to assess your own cultural background, values, and beliefs, especially those that are related to health and health care. Many tools are available to help you with this process. One is available through the Georgetown University National Center for Cultural Competence (http://nccc.georgetown.edu).

Table 2.3 suggests ways for you to improve your cultural competence. Culturally competent care requires continual learning and self-reflection.[12] It is important to understand that cultures evolve and change over time. This will help you to better understand patients and provide culturally competent care.

In today's increasingly multicultural environment, you will meet patients, families, significant others, and members of the health care team from many different cultures. You will find yourself in care situations that require an understanding of the patient's cultural beliefs and practices. Even when you provide care for patients from your own cultural background, you may be from a different subculture than the patient. For example, there are more than 574 federally recognized Native American tribes in the United States.[13] It would be inappropriate for you to assume that a Native American nurse can give culturally appropriate care to all Native American patients. A nurse from an urban upbringing may find cultural differences with a patient from a rural community.

◆ Assessment

We play a key role in promoting health equity. The causes of health disparities are not always easy to identify. Administer an SDH screening tool, such as the Protocol for Responding to and Assessing Patient's Assets, Risks, and Experiences (PRAPARE) (Table 2.6). Assess patients for risk of reduced health care services because of limited access, inadequate resources, age, or low health literacy. Review patients' eligibility for various resources, such as insurance, food assistance, and unemployment,

Perform a cultural assessment.[12] Table 2.7 lists key components of the assessment. Assess patients' (1) health beliefs and health care practices and (2) perspective of the meaning, cause, and preferred treatment of illness. How can you be aware of the differences among ethnic groups? Using guides for cultural assessment will promote optimal care when working with patients, families, or other groups who are from different cultures. Although guides can help you, be careful not to stereotype or assume that common cultural characteristics pertain to each patient. Use guides to explore the degree to which patients share commonalities with the traits attributed to their cultural group. You need to know about traditional characteristics of cultural groups while recognizing that culture is constantly evolving and unique for each person.

TABLE 2.6 Protocol for Responding to and Assessing Patient's Assets, Risks, and Experiences (PRAPARE)

Category	Question
Personal characteristics	Are you Hispanic or Latino?
	Which race(s) are you?
	At any point in the past 2 years, has seasonal or migrant farm work been your or your family's main source of income?
	Have you been discharged from the armed forces of the United States?
	What language are you most comfortable speaking?
Family and home	How many family members, including yourself, do you currently live with?
	What is your housing situation today?
	Are you worried about losing your housing?
	What is your address?
Money and resources	What is the highest level of school that you have finished?
	What is your current work situation?
	What is your main insurance?
	During the past year, what was the total combined income for you and your family members you live with?
	In the past year, have you or any family members you live with been unable to get food, clothing, utilities, childcare, phone, medicine, or health care when it was really needed?
	Has lack of transportation kept you from medical appointments, meetings, work, or getting things needed for daily living?
Social and emotional health	How often do you see or talk to people who you care about and feel close to?
	How stressed are you?

Adapted from the National PRAPARE® Social Determinants of Health Protocol developed by the National Association of Community Health Centers, Association of Asian Pacific Community Health Organizations, and Oregon Primary Care Organization and their development partners. www.nachc.org/prapare. © National Association of Community Health Centers. All rights reserved. Retrieved from http://www.nachc.org/wp-content/uploads/2019/04/NACHC_PRAPARE_Full-Toolkit.pdf.

◆ Implementation

Although the issues associated with health disparities can seem overwhelming, several strategies are available to reduce and eliminate health disparities. Table 2.8 presents nursing interventions to promote health equity.

Advocacy

Strategies to increase health care access and insurance are critical for making sure more people get important health care services. The solutions to reduce health disparities often rest with the policymakers. Economic issues often determine health care delivery. Access and public policy decisions determine who

TABLE 2.7 Cultural Assessment

A cultural assessment should include these areas:

- Communication
  - Languages spoken; skill in speaking, reading, and writing in English
  - Eye contact, interpersonal space
  - Preferred way to communicate with patient and family
- Cultural group person identifies with
- Cultural restrictions and taboos
- Decision making within the family
- Diet practices
- Organizations providing cultural support
- Personal beliefs about health and illness
  - Meaning and beliefs about cause of illness
  - Practices or rituals used to improve health
  - Use of alternative medicine
  - Acceptability of direct care by gender
- Presence of social network
- Religious affiliation, practices, and rituals
- Socioeconomic considerations
- Spiritual beliefs
- Place of birth; if outside the United States, length of time in the United States and circumstances

TABLE 2.8 NURSING MANAGEMENT

Interventions to Promote Health Equity

- Treat all patients equally.
- Be aware of your own biases or prejudices and work toward eliminating them.
- Learn about services and programs that focus on specific cultural/ethnic groups.
- Inform patients about health care services available for their specific cultural/ethnic group.
- Follow the same standards of care for all patients regardless of culture or ethnicity.
- Recognize health care practices and cultural practices that are important to cultural and ethnic identity.
- Take part in research focused on understanding and improving care to culturally and ethnically diverse populations.
- Identify stereotypic attitudes toward a culture/ethnic group that may interfere with getting health care.
- Support patients who are fearful about traveling outside the accepted neighborhood for health care services.
- Advocate for patients of specific cultural/ethnic groups to receive health care services that pay special attention to English-language limitations and cultural health practices.
- Learn advocacy and interpersonal strategies from leaders of specific cultural/ethnic groups. For example, some cultures emphasize themes such as "do it for your loved ones."
- Ensure availability of culturally appropriate patient educational resources.

is eligible for federal and state health insurance coverage. You play an important role in improving health care access.

You, along with the social worker, can help by identifying key resources in the community, including transportation services, reduced-fee screening programs, and federal and state offices for Medicaid and Medicare. Be an advocate in your health care setting by helping to create a community advisory group. Such a group can be helpful when setting up health programs within a community. This can increase the distribution of culturally sensitive information. Another powerful strategy is to increase the number of underrepresented populations in the health care professions (Fig. 2.8).

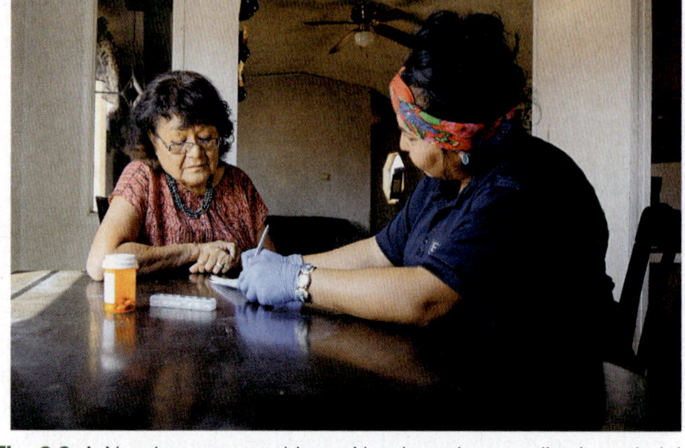

Fig. 2.8 A Navajo nurse teaching a Navajo patient medication administration in the home. (© RichLegg/iStock.com.)

Standard Guidelines

The use of standard, evidence-based care guidelines can reduce racial or cultural disparities in treatment and outcome. For example, the management of hypertension should be based on guidelines and the patient's BP, symptoms, history, and laboratory values rather than characteristics such as gender, age, or culture. In addition, recommendations related to cultural competency will guide you in your learning and practice.

The National Standards for Culturally and Linguistically Appropriate Services in Health Care (CLAS standards) are guidelines that improve the quality of health care.[14] The CLAS standards provide practical guidance for care of people with limited English proficiency and of diverse cultural backgrounds.

Communication

Improving interpersonal skills is an important first step in providing culturally competent care. To show respect for patients, consider their usual communication style. For instance, conduct a health history in an unhurried manner and in a way that is appropriate for the culture. In some cultures, it is best to start with general rather than direct questions. For some cultures, it is most effective to engage in "small talk," with the discussion including answers that may seem to be unrelated to the questions. If you appear to be "too busy," communication may be impaired.

When meeting patients or family members, introduce yourself and indicate how you would like them to address you—whether they should use first names; Mr., Ms., or Mrs.; or a title, such as Doctor or Pastor. Ask patients how they prefer to be addressed. This shows respect and will help you begin the relationship in a culturally appropriate manner.

If you need to gather personal information, it is important to understand the most effective approach to use. For instance, when talking with people from some cultural groups, you must

TABLE 2.9 Using a Medical Interpreter

Choosing an Interpreter
- Use an agency interpreter if possible.
- Use a trained medical interpreter who knows how to interpret, has a health care background, understands patients' rights, and can help with advice about the cultural relevance or appropriateness of the health care plan and instructions.
- Use a family member only if necessary. Be aware of limitations if the family member does not understand medical terms, is younger or a different gender from the patient, or is not aware of the health care procedures or medical ethics.
- Interpreter should be able to do the following:
    - Interpret the patient's nonverbal and verbal communication.
    - Translate the message into understandable terms.
    - Act as a patient advocate to represent the patient's needs to the health care team.
    - Be culturally competent and understand how to give teaching instructions.

Strategies for Working With an Interpreter
- If possible, have the interpreter meet with the patient ahead of time to establish rapport before the interpreting begins.
- Speak slowly.
- Maintain eye contact with the patient.
- Talk to the patient, not the interpreter.
- Use simple language with as few medical terms as possible.
- Speak 1 or 2 sentences at a time to allow for easier interpretation.
- Avoid raising your voice during the interaction.
- Obtain feedback to be certain the patient understands.
- Plan to take twice as long to complete the interaction.

take time to establish trust and listen to the patient's responses to questions. There may be long silences as the person thinks about the question, showing respect by giving the question consideration before answering. Take time to listen and help establish trust. Consider how the age may affect their views and

TABLE 2.10 Tips for Overcoming Language Barriers

- Speak slowly and clearly.
- Use simple words and avoid medical jargon.
- Keep sentences short and to the point.
- Discuss 1 topic at a time.
- Do not use slang.
- Use drawings, pictures, or even props to illustrate concepts.
- If appropriate, demonstrate with gestures.
- Use a HIPAA-compliant translation application.
- Pay attention to the patient's body language and facial expressions.
- Maintain appropriate eye contact.
- Encourage the patient to ask questions, and use the teach-back method to ensure they understand.

communication. For example, older adults with mental health concerns may struggle with shame, uncertainty, and lack of trust.

Do not try to serve as an interpreter if your patient does not understand English, because this could lead to misunderstandings. Get the help of a person who is qualified to do medical interpretation when you cannot speak the patient's primary language (Table 2.9). Interpreters are available by phone or video communication anywhere in the United States through a fee-based service. Use the service rather than a family member. Table 2.10 offers guidelines for communicating when no interpreter is available.

Many websites and applications can translate spoken words and documents from one language into another. Patients may find it helpful if you have a prepared list of questions and potential answers in several languages. Be careful because some applications may not accurately reflect your intended question or statement. It is helpful to have resources for people from cultural groups who often use your agency. This is especially beneficial when a qualified medical interpreter is not readily available.

CASE STUDY

Health Disparities

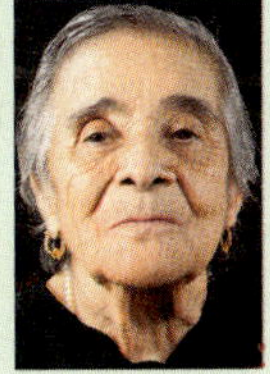

©Luevanos/iStock.

Patient Profile

M.S. is an 81-year-old female who came to the United States from India 4 years ago with her son and daughter-in-law and their 4 children. She has several health problems, including coronary artery disease, hypertension, osteoarthritis in her right hip, and diabetes. Her daughter-in-law is the primary caregiver. She often brings her to the urban health clinic for health-related problems. Recently M.S. has been having memory problems.

The entire family comes to the health clinic with M.S. Because English is a second language (Hindustani is their first language) for all the adult family members, the staff relies on the oldest granddaughter to interpret.

At this clinic visit, M.S. has shortness of breath. Through her granddaughter's interpretation, she tells the nurse that she is having trouble walking up the stairs in the apartment building. The nurse does a history and assessment, checks her glucose (which is within normal limits), and tells M.S. that she should get more exercise. Given M.S.'s memory problems and limited English, the nurse does not complete a 24-hour diet recall or teach her or the family about diabetes management. M.S. is scheduled for an appointment with the cardiologist for an evaluation of her hypertension and heart disease. Two weeks later, when she sees the cardiologist, her shortness of breath is much worse, and she is having chest pain. She is hospitalized immediately.

Meanwhile, the clinic supervisor is completing a chart audit for the clinic's quality review program. She is reviewing M.S.'s chart and notices that, although she has been a patient in the clinic for 3 years, she has never received instructions on blood glucose monitoring or diabetes management. The clinic manager reviews these findings with the nurse and asks why M.S. did not receive diabetes education. The nurse states that with M.S.'s memory problems and the language barrier, she assumed that M.S. and her family would not benefit.

Discussion Questions

1. ***Recognize:*** What type of health disparity has M.S. experienced?
2. ***Analyze:*** What factors led to her not receiving the standard of care?
3. ***Analyze:*** What other assessment should have been done at the initial visit?
4. ***Act:*** What strategies may have worked to enhance patient education?
5. ***Act:*** How would you consider M.S.'s religious and spiritual needs?
6. ***Evaluate:*** If you were the clinic manager, how would you recommend that the nurse improve her practice?

Answers available at http://evolve.elsevier.com/Lewis/medsurg.

BRIDGE TO NCLEX EXAMINATION

The number of the question corresponds to the same-numbered outcome at the beginning of the chapter.

1. Which factors are part of the social determinants of health? **(Select all that apply.)**
   - **a.** Genetics
   - **b.** Economic status
   - **c.** Family history of disease
   - **d.** Social and physical environment
   - **e.** Type and quality of health care received
2. What are structural barriers in health care?
   - **a.** Genetic predispositions that affect disease risk
   - **b.** Psychologic factors affecting patient compliance
   - **c.** Personal health behaviors that affect individual health outcomes
   - **d.** Community factors that influence access to care and health outcomes
3. In identifying patients at the *greatest* risk for health disparities, the nurse would note that
   - **a.** patients who live in urban areas have readily available access to health care services.
   - **b.** cultural differences may exist in patients' ability to communicate with the health care provider.
   - **c.** a patient receiving care from a health care provider of a different culture will have decreased quality of care.
   - **d.** persons who immigrate to the United States are less likely to have health problems once they establish residency.
4. Forcing one's own cultural beliefs and practices on another person is an example of
   - **a.** stereotyping.
   - **b.** ethnocentrism.
   - **c.** cultural relativity.
   - **d.** cultural imposition.
5. Which statement *most* accurately describes cultural factors that may affect health?
   - **a.** Diabetes and cancer rates differ by cultural/ethnic groups.
   - **b.** There are limited ethnic variations in physiologic responses to drugs.
   - **c.** Most patients find that religious rituals help them during times of illness.
   - **d.** Silence after providing patient education means the patient understands the instructions.
6. As part of the nursing process, cultural assessment is *best* accomplished by
   - **a.** judging the patient's cultural values based on observations.
   - **b.** using a cultural assessment guide as part of the nursing process.
   - **c.** seeking guidance from a nurse from the patient's cultural background.
   - **d.** relying on the nurse's previous experience with patients from that cultural group.
7. An important intervention in promoting health equity is to
   - **a.** discourage use of evidence-based practice guidelines.
   - **b.** insist that patients adhere to established clinical guidelines.
   - **c.** teach patients to use the Internet to find resources related to their health.
   - **d.** engage in active listening and establish relationships with patients and families.

1. b, d, e; 2. b; 3. d; 4. d; 5. a; 6. b; 7. d

For rationales to these answers and even more NCLEX review questions, visit http://evolve.elsevier.com/Lewis/medsurg.

REFERENCES

To access the References for this chapter, please scan the QR code with a mobile device.

3

Health History and Physical Examination

Courtney Reinisch

http//evolve.elsevier.com/Lewis/medsurg/

CONCEPTUAL FOCUS

Clinical Judgment
Communication
Patient-Centered Care

LEARNING OUTCOMES

1. Explain the purpose, components, and techniques of a health history and physical examination.
2. Obtain a nursing history using a functional health pattern format.
3. Select appropriate techniques of inspection, palpation, percussion, and auscultation for the physical examination.
4. Distinguish among emergency, comprehensive, and focused assessments in terms of indications, purposes, and components.
5. Promote health equity and respect by awareness of bias and using adept communication skills to conduct an assessment.

KEY TERMS

auscultation
clinical manifestations
database
functional health patterns
inspection
nursing history
objective data
palpation
subjective data

During an assessment, you will obtain a patient's health history and perform a physical examination. This is part of the interprofessional team's patient evaluation. The findings of your nursing assessment (1) contribute to data that identifies the patient's current and past health status and (2) provide a baseline against which we evaluate future changes. Assessment is the first step of the nursing process. The purpose of the nursing assessment is to enable you to make clinical judgments about your patient's health status.[1] Assessment is performed continually throughout the nursing process to evaluate nursing interventions and progress toward patient outcomes.

DATA COLLECTION

The **database** is all the health information about a patient. It includes (1) nursing history and physical examination, (2) the medical history and physical examination, and (3) laboratory and diagnostic test results. A nurse and HCP perform an assessment using formats and data based on each discipline's focus. The goal is to have a complete database based on findings and assessments. All the findings related to a specific problem are the **clinical manifestations** of that problem.

Medical Assessment

A *medical history* is used by the HCP to determine risk for disease and diagnose medical conditions. The medical history is usually collected by a physician, advanced practice nurse (APN), resident, physician's assistant, or medical student. The HCP's physical examination and diagnostic tests aid in establishing medical diagnoses and implementing and monitoring the medical treatment plan. The information the HCP collects and reports is used by nurses and other health care team

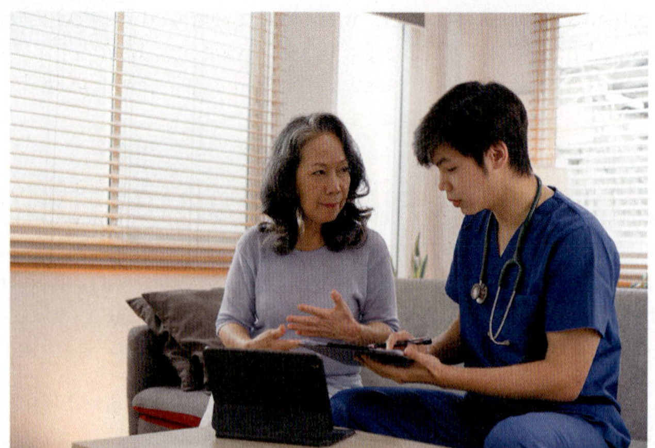

Fig. 3.1 Conducting a nursing focused interview. (© Korrawin/iStock.com.)

members (e.g., pharmacist, physical therapist, dietitian) based on the focus of their care. For example, the abnormal results of a neurologic examination by an APN may help diagnose a stroke. You use the same results to identify fall risk in a patient. A physical therapist uses the information to plan therapy involving range-of-motion exercises.

Nursing Assessment

The purpose of the **nursing history** is to obtain information about the patient's past and present health state (Fig. 3.1). We use the information from the nursing assessment to determine the patient's strengths and responses to a health problem. For example, a patient with diabetes may respond with anxiety or lack knowledge about managing the condition. This patient may have the physical response of the abnormal fluid loss caused by hyperglycemia. These human responses to the condition of diabetes are diagnosed and treated by nurses. With your assessment, you obtain and record the data to support decisions about nursing care (Table 3.1).

The amount of time you need to complete an assessment varies with the format and your experience. It may be completed in 1 or several sessions, depending on the setting and patient. An older adult patient with a low energy level may need a few brief sessions to allow time to give the needed information. You must judge the amount of information to collect on initial contact with the patient. In taking a health history with patients with chronic disease, patients in pain, and patients in emergency situations, ask only those questions that are pertinent to a specific problem. You can complete the health history at a more appropriate time.

It is important for you to determine the patient's priority concerns and expectations. Your priorities may be different from the patient's. For example, your priority may be to complete the assessment, while the patient is interested only in pain relief. Until the patient's priority need is met, you will probably be unsuccessful in obtaining a complete and accurate assessment.

TABLE 3.1 NURSING MANAGEMENT

Assessment and Data Collection

- On admission, complete a comprehensive assessment (Table 3.4).
- Obtain a health history by interviewing patient and/or caregiver.
- Perform physical examination using inspection, palpation, percussion, and auscultation as appropriate.
- Record findings from the assessment in the medical record.
- Organize patient data into functional health patterns (Table 3.3).
- Develop and prioritize nursing problems.
- Throughout hospitalization, perform focused assessments based on the health history or clinical manifestations (Table 3.8).
- Refer patients to the proper community-based services.
- Supervise aspects of data collection by AP:
  - Vital signs
  - Height and weight, oral intake, and output
  - Per agency policy, point-of-care testing, such as glucose

Rate the patient's reliability as a historian. The complexity and duration of health problems may make it hard for the patient to be an accurate historian. An older adult may give a false impression about their mental status because of a prolonged response time or vision and hearing problems.

Types of Data

The database includes subjective and objective data. **Subjective data**, or *symptoms,* are collected by interviewing the patient and/or caregiver. This type of data includes information that can be described or verified only by the patient or caregiver. It is what the person tells you, either spontaneously or in response to a direct question.

Objective data, or *signs,* are data that we can observe or measure. You obtain objective data using inspection, palpation, percussion, and auscultation. Objective data are also obtained by diagnostic testing. Patients often provide subjective data while you are performing their physical assessment. You will see objective signs while interviewing patients.

Promoting Health Equity in Assessment

Creating a climate of trust and respect is critical to establishing a therapeutic relationship during your assessment.[2] You need to communicate acceptance of the patient as a person by using an open, responsive, and nonjudgmental approach. You communicate through spoken language and actions, including your manner of dress, gestures, and body language.

The process of obtaining an assessment is an intimate experience for you and the patient. The ease of asking questions, particularly those related to sensitive areas such as sexual function, comes with training and experience. Be sensitive to issues of eye contact, space, modesty, and touching. Determine whether the patient would like to have someone present or someone of a preferred gender to perform the assessment. You may feel uncomfortable obtaining information related to sexuality, identity, and preferences. However, it is important to take a history in a nonjudgmental way. Refer the patient to a more experienced HCP if needed.

Promote health equity in your assessment. Remember that bias exists. Some biases are surface, and others are hidden. As nurses, we must avoid harm caused by implicit or unconscious bias. Structural racism leads to negative health status. Be aware of your personal conscious and unconscious beliefs. It is easier to identify your conscious beliefs. Pay attention to the language that you use when you document. Guard against contributing to bias when you write notes.

Culture influences the words, gestures, and postures we use and the information we share with others (see Chapter 2). Ask patients about cultural values to avoid bias related to cultural practices. Knowing cultural norms related to male-female relationships is especially important during the physical assessment.

Symptom Investigation

At any time during the assessment, the patient may report a symptom such as pain, fatigue, or weakness. Because we do not observe symptoms patients experience, we need to ask further questions. Table 3.2 shows a mnemonic (PQRST) to help you remember the areas to explore when a symptom is reported. The information you receive may help determine the cause of the symptom. A common symptom that you will assess is pain (see Chapter 9). If a patient says they have "pain in their leg," you would assess and record the data using PQRST.

Patient has right midcalf pain that occurs at work when climbing stairs after lunch (P). Pain is alleviated by stopping and resting for 2 to 3 minutes. States they have been "eating a banana every day for extra potassium" but "it hasn't helped" (P). Describes pain as "stabbing" and nonradiating (Q, R). Pain is so severe (rating 9 on a 0–10 scale) that patient cannot continue activity (S). Onset is abrupt, occurring once or twice daily. It last occurred yesterday while cutting the lawn (T).

Data Organization

You must systematically organize the assessment so you can readily analyze the patient's health status and any health problems. Some assessment forms are organized by body system. Although helpful, these types of forms may be incomplete because they may omit areas, such as health promotion behaviors, sleep, coping, and values.

Functional health patterns, developed by Gordon, provide the framework used throughout this book for obtaining a nursing history.[3] This format includes an initial collection of important health information followed by assessment of 11 areas of health status or function (Table 3.3). Data organized in this format allow for the identification of areas of wellness (or positive function) and health problems.[2]

NURSING HISTORY: SUBJECTIVE DATA

Health Information

Having key health information offers an overview of past and present medical problems and treatments. Include the health history, medications, allergies, and surgery or other treatments.

Health History

The history provides information about the patient's prior state of health. Ask about major childhood and adult illnesses, injuries, hospitalizations, and surgeries. Specific questions are more effective than asking whether the patient has had any illness or health problems in the past. For example, asking "Do you have a history of diabetes?" elicits better information than asking "Do you have any chronic health problems?"

Medications

Take a thorough medication history. Ask for specific details related to past and current medications, including prescription and illicit drugs, over-the-counter (OTC) drugs, and vitamins. Record the dose (if known), frequency, length of time taken, any side effects, and the reason for taking the medication. Encourage patients to bring all medication bottles and any inhalers to each visit with an HCP. Ask about use of herbs and supplements. These products can interact adversely with prescribed medications.

TABLE 3.2 Investigation of Patient-Reported Symptom

	Factor	Questions for Patient and Caregiver	Record
P	Precipitating and Palliative	Were there any events that came before the symptom? What makes it better? Worse? What have you done for the symptom? Did this help?	Influence of physical and emotional activities. Patient's attempts to alleviate or treat the symptom
Q	Quality	Tell me what the symptom feels like (e.g., aching, dull, pressure, burning, stabbing).	Patient's own words, such as "Like a pinch or stabbing feeling"
R	Radiation	Where do you feel the symptom? Does it move to other areas?	Region of body. Local or radiating, superficial or deep
S	Severity	On a scale of 0–10, with 0 meaning no pain and 10 being the worst pain you could imagine, what number would you give your symptom?	Pain rating number (e.g., 5/10)
T	Timing	When did the symptom start? Was it sudden or gradual? Any particular time of day, week, month, or year? Has the symptom changed over time? Has the symptom happened before? What are you doing when the symptom occurs?	Time of onset, duration, periodicity, and frequency. Course of symptoms. Where patient is and what patient is doing when the symptom occurs

TABLE 3.3 HEALTH HISTORY

Functional Health Pattern Format

Demographic Data

Name, preferred name, preferred pronouns, address, age, occupation, gender assigned at birth, gender identity

Race, ethnicity, culture, spirituality

Health Information

Health history

Medications, supplements

Allergies

Surgery or other treatments

Immunizations such as tetanus, hepatitis, COVID, flu vaccines

Health Perception—Health Management

1. Reason for visit?
2. History of present problem. Cause? Action taken? Results?
3. Describe your general health.
4. Things done to keep healthy? Self-examinations? Colorectal cancer, hypertension, and diabetes screening? Papanicolaou (Pap) test?
5. Who are your HCPs? Primary?
6. Health adherence problems?
7. Things important to you while here?
8. Family history (e.g., cardiovascular disease, hypertension, cancer, diabetes, psychiatric illness, genetic disorders)?
9. Injury risk factors (e.g., sexual abuse, intimate partner abuse, violence)?
10. Personal health habits (e.g., smoking, alcohol use)?
11. Exposure to environment hazards (e.g., lead)?

Nutritional-Metabolic

1. Typical daily food intake (describe)? Supplements?
2. Typical daily fluid intake (describe)?
3. Weight loss or gain (amount, time span, intentional)?
4. Desired weight?
5. Appetite?
6. Gastrointestinal symptoms: Discomfort? Nausea? Diet restrictions?
7. Change in appetite with stress?
8. Diet restrictions? Food preferences?
9. Food allergies?
10. Dentition: Dental problems? Well-fitting dentures?
11. Difficulty obtaining food?

Elimination

1. Bowel elimination pattern (describe): Frequency? Character? Discomfort? Laxatives? Enemas?
2. Urinary elimination pattern (describe): Frequency? Problem in control? Diuretics?
3. Any external devices?
4. Excess perspiration? Odor problems? Itching?

Activity-Exercise

1. Ability to take part in desired or required activities?
2. Exercise pattern? Type? Regularity?
3. Spare time (leisure) activities?
4. Dyspnea? Chest pain? Palpitations? Stiffness? Aching? At rest? With activity?
5. Perceived ability for (rate Functional Level 0—III for each): Eating __ Cooking __ Grooming __ Transfer (e.g., bed to chair) __ Toileting __ Bathing __ Dressing __ Shopping __ General mobility __

   Functional Levels

   Level 0: Full self-care

   Level I: Requires use of equipment or device

   Level II: Needs help or supervision from another person

   Level III: Dependent and does not participate

Sleep-Rest

1. Generally rested and ready for daily activities after sleep?
2. Sleep onset problems? Aids (drugs, CPAP)? Dreams (nightmares)? Early awakening?
3. Usual sleep rituals?
4. Usual sleep pattern?

Cognitive-Perceptual

1. Impaired hearing? Hearing aids?
2. Vision? Wear glasses? Wear contact lenses? Last checked?
3. Any change in taste? Any change in smell?
4. Any recent change in memory?
5. Easiest way to learn things?
6. Any discomfort? Pain (rating on scale of 0—10)? How managed?
7. Ability to communicate (e.g., primary language)?
8. Understanding of illness? Treatments?

Self-Perception—Self-Concept

1. Self-description? Self-perception?
2. Effect of illness on self-image?

Role-Relationship

1. Live alone? Family/caregiver? Family structure?
2. Family problems?
3. Family problem solving?
4. Family dependence on you for things? How managing?
5. Family's and others' feelings about illness or hospitalization?[a]
6. Problems with children? Hard to handle?[a]
7. Belong to social groups? Have close friends? Feel lonely (frequency)?
8. Work (school) satisfaction? Income sufficient for needs?[a]
9. Feel part of or isolated from neighborhood where living?

Sexual-Reproductive

1. Any changes or problems in sexual relations?[a]
2. Effect of illness?
3. Use of contraceptives? Problems?
4. When menstruation started? Last menstrual period? Menstrual problems? Gravida? Para?[b]
5. Effect of present condition or treatment on sexuality?
6. Sexually transmitted infections?
7. Safety?

Coping—Stress Tolerance

1. Tense a lot of the time? What helps? Use any drugs, alcohol?
2. Have someone to confide in? Available to you now?
3. Recent life changes?
4. Problem-solving techniques? Effective?
5. Efforts to promote mental health or wellness?

Value-Belief

1. Satisfied with life?
2. Religion important in your life?
3. Conflict between treatment and beliefs?
4. Religious practices we need to be aware of?

[a]If appropriate.

[b]For females.

CPAP, Continuous positive airway pressure.

Modified from Gordon M: *Manual of nursing diagnosis,* ed 13, Boston, 2016, Jones & Bartlett.

Ask about medication routines. Patients may not take medications as prescribed because of cost, difficulty swallowing, or not understanding the directions or reason for the drug. Look for issues related to medication cost and polypharmacy. Changes in absorption, metabolism, and elimination of drugs can potentially pose serious problems.[4]

Allergies

Assess for a history of allergies to drugs, latex, contrast media, food, and the environment (e.g., pollen). Include a detailed description of any allergic reaction(s).

Surgery and Other Treatments

Record all surgeries. Note the date, reason for the surgery, and outcome. Was the problem resolved? Are there any residual effects? Ask about and record any blood products the patient has received.

Functional Health Patterns

Assess the patient's functional health patterns to identify effective, dysfunctional, and potential dysfunctional health patterns. *Dysfunctional health patterns* occur with disease. *Potential dysfunctional patterns* identify risk conditions for problems. You may identify patients with effective health function who want a higher level of wellness. Table 3.3 gives examples of possible questions to ask related to functional health patterns.

Health Perception–Health Management

This pattern focuses on the patient's perceived level of health, well-being, and personal practices for maintaining health. Ask the patient to describe their personal health and any concerns or questions about it. Explore with the patient what they feel helps or hinders their sense of well-being. Ask the patient to rate their health as excellent, good, fair, or poor. Record this information in the patient's words if possible.

Have the patient describe their understanding of the current health problem, including its onset, course, and treatment. These questions yield information about a patient's knowledge of the health problem and ability to use resources to manage the problem. Ask about all HCPs the patient uses. Does the hospitalized patient have expectations for their experience?

Obtain a thorough family history. Seek to identify risk factors by exploring personal health habits (e.g., tobacco, alcohol use) and any exposure to environment hazards.

Nutritional-Metabolic

This pattern assesses the processes of ingestion, digestion, absorption, and metabolism. A 24-hour diet recall can evaluate the quantity and quality of foods and fluids consumed. If there is a concern, ask patients to keep a 3-day food diary for a more careful analysis of diet intake. Assess the impact of psychologic factors such as depression, anxiety, stress, and self-concept on nutrition. Evaluate socioeconomic factors, such as food budget. What are their food preferences? Who prepares the meals? Determine whether the patient's present condition has interfered with eating and appetite by exploring any symptoms of nausea, intestinal gas, or pain. Note any food allergies and food intolerances, such as lactose or gluten intolerance. Consider oral health, which may affect the ability to eat or drink.

Elimination

The elimination pattern involves bowel, bladder, and skin function. Ask about the frequency of bowel and bladder activity. Do they have urgency, incontinence, and diuretic use? Inquire about stool consistency, stool color, and laxative use. Assess the skin here in terms of its excretory function.

Activity-Exercise

This pattern assesses the patient's usual pattern of exercise, work activity, leisure, and recreation. Ask about the ability to perform activities of daily living (ADLs) and note any specific problems. Table 3.3 includes a scale for rating the functional levels of common activities.

Sleep-Rest

The sleep-rest pattern describes the patient's perception of their pattern of sleep, rest, and relaxation in a 24-hour period. Ask "Do you feel rested when you wake up?" Assess the use of sleep aides. Review their sleep-wake patterns. Include napping.

Cognitive-Perceptual

This pattern involves describing senses and cognitive function. Assess pain as a sensory perception (see pain assessment in Chapter 9). Ask about any sensory deficits that affect the ability to perform ADLs. Record how patients compensate for any sensory-perceptual problems. Ask how they learn best and in what language. Assess what they understand about the illness and treatment plan. Begin to plan patient teaching according to identified needs and preferences. See Chapter 4 for details on patient teaching.

Self-Perception–Self-Concept

The patient's self-concept influences how they interact with others. Assess their attitudes about self, perception of personal abilities, body image, identity, and general sense of worth. Ask patients for a self-description and about how their health condition affects self-concept. Hopelessness or loss of control can reflect an inability to care for oneself.

Role-Relationship

This pattern reveals the patient's roles and relationships, including major responsibilities. Ask patients to describe family, social and work roles, and relationships. Have them rate their performance of the expected behaviors. Determine whether these roles and relationships are satisfactory. Is any strain present? Note the patient's feelings about how the health condition affects their roles and relationships.

Sexuality-Reproductive

This pattern describes satisfaction with personal sexuality, sexual preference, identity, and reproductive issues. This is important because many illnesses, surgeries, and drugs affect sexual function. Patients may express sexual and reproductive concerns.

Coping—Stress Tolerance

Coping-stress describes the patient's general coping and the effectiveness of coping mechanisms. Assessment here involves analyzing the specific stressors or problems that confront the patient. Ask about their perception of stressors. What is their response to their stressors? Review any major losses or stressors experienced in the previous year. Note strategies used to deal with stressors and relieve tension. What persons and groups make up the patient's social support networks? Ask about efforts to promote mental health and wellness.

Value-Belief

This pattern describes the values, goals, and beliefs (including spiritual) that guide health-related choices. Review the effects of culture and beliefs on health practices. Note and respect patients' wishes about continuing religious or spiritual practices and the use of religious articles.

PHYSICAL EXAMINATION: OBJECTIVE DATA

General Survey

Begin with making a general survey statement. This is your general impression of a patient, including behavior observations. The initial survey begins with your first encounter with the patient and continues during the entire assessment.

The major areas included in the general survey statement are (1) body features, (2) mental state, (3) speech, (4) body movements, (5) obvious physical signs, (6) nutrition status, and (7) behavior. Vital signs, body mass index (BMI) (calculated from height and weight [kg/m^2]), and waist circumference may be included. The following is a sample of a general survey statement:

A.H. is a 34-year-old female, BP 120/78, P 88, R 18. No distinguishing body features. Alert, anxious. Speech is rapid with trailing thoughts. Wringing hands and shuffling feet during interview. Skin appears flushed; hands clammy. BMI = 28.3 kg/m^2 meets overweight criteria. Waist measures 88.9 cm (35 in). Sits with eyes downcast, shoulders slumped, and avoids eye contact.

Physical Examination

The *physical examination* is the systematic assessment of a patient's physical status. Explore positive findings using the same criteria used when investigating a symptom in the nursing history (Table 3.2). A *positive finding* shows that the patient has or had a problem or condition. For example, if the patient with jaundice has an enlarged liver, it is a positive finding. You then need to gather relevant information about this problem.

Negative findings may be significant. A pertinent *negative finding* is the absence of a sign or symptom usually associated with a problem. For example, peripheral edema is common with advanced liver disease. If edema is not present in a patient with advanced liver disease, specifically note this as "no peripheral edema."

Techniques

Four major techniques are used in assessment: inspection, palpation, percussion, and auscultation. The techniques are usually performed in the same sequence—inspection, palpation, percussion, and auscultation. The abdominal examination is an exception. Inspection is first, followed by auscultation, percussion, and palpation. Performing percussion and palpation before auscultation can alter bowel sounds and produce false findings. Not every assessment area requires the use of all 4 assessment techniques. The musculoskeletal system requires only inspection and palpation.

Inspection. **Inspection** is the visual assessment of a part or region of the body to rate normal conditions or deviations. Inspection is more than just looking. This technique is deliberate, systematic, and focused. Compare what is seen with the known, generally visible characteristics of the body part that you are inspecting. For example, most 30-year-old males have hair on their legs. Absence of hair may indicate a vascular problem and the need for further investigation, or it may be normal for the patient. Always compare each side of the body to the other to assess for any abnormal findings.

Palpation. **Palpation** is the assessment of the body using touch. Using light and deep palpation can yield information about masses, pulsations, organ enlargement, tenderness or pain, swelling, muscular spasm or rigidity, elasticity, vibration of voice sounds, crepitus, moisture, and texture. Different parts of the hand are more sensitive for specific assessments. For example, use the dorsa (backs) of your hands and fingers to assess skin temperature and tips of your fingers to palpate pulses (Fig. 3.2).[1]

Percussion. *Percussion* is a technique that produces a sound and vibration to obtain information about the underlying area (Fig. 3.3). The sounds and vibrations are relative to the underlying structures. Normally lung tissue is resonant; dense organs like the liver are dull. A change from an expected sound may indicate a problem. For example, you would need further assessment if you heard dullness in the right lower quadrant instead of the normal tympany. Specific percussion sounds of various body parts and regions are discussed in the appropriate assessment chapters.

Auscultation. **Auscultation** involves listening to sounds produced by the body with a stethoscope to assess normal and abnormal conditions. It is useful in evaluating sounds from the heart, lungs, abdomen, and vascular system (Fig. 3.4). The bell of the stethoscope is more sensitive to low-pitched sounds

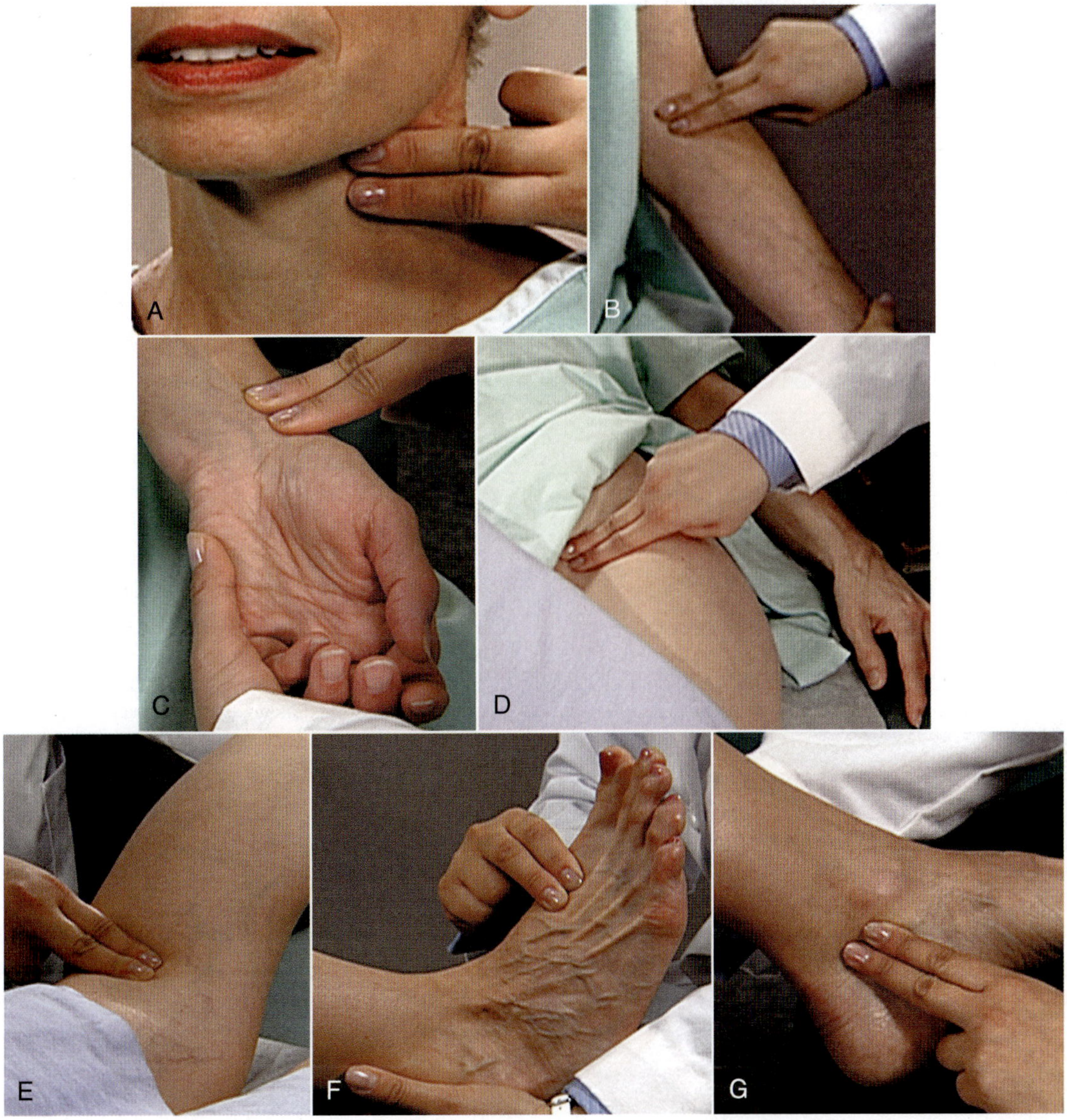

Fig. 3.2 Palpating peripheral pulses. (A) carotid, (B) brachial, (C) radial, (D) femoral, (E) popliteal, (F) dorsalis pedis, (G) posterior tibial. (From Ball JW, Dains JE, Flynn JA, et al: *Seidel's guide to physical examination,* ed 9, St. Louis, 2018, Elsevier.)

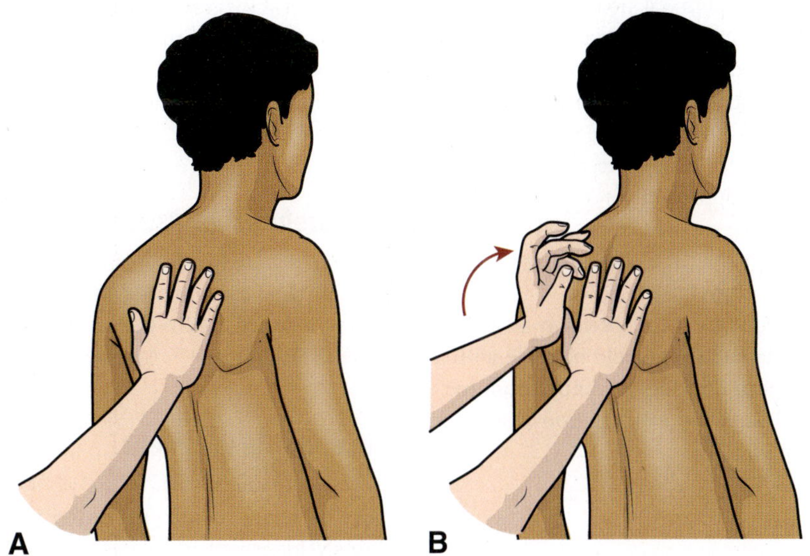

Fig. 3.3 (A) To perform percussion, place the nondominant hand with the fingers slightly separated directly on the area you are assessing. (B) Use the fingers of the dominant hand to strike the joint of the middle finger of the nondominant hand to produce a sound vibration.

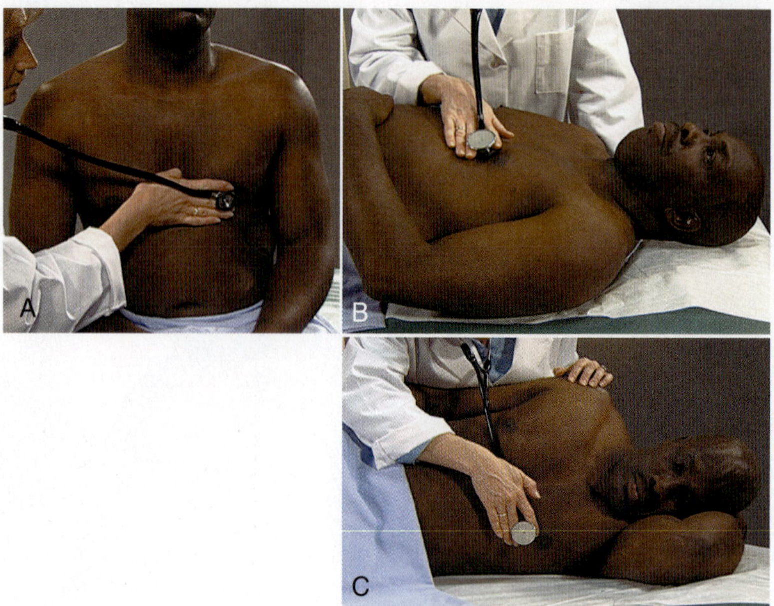

Fig. 3.4 Patient positions for auscultating heart sounds. (A) Sitting, (B) supine, and (C) left lateral. (From Ball JW, Dains JE, Flynn JA, et al: *Seidel's guide to physical examination,* ed 9, St. Louis, 2018, Elsevier.)

(e.g., heart murmurs). The diaphragm of the stethoscope is more sensitive to high-pitched sounds (e.g., bowel sounds). Some stethoscopes have only a diaphragm that can transmit low- and high-pitched sounds. To listen for low-pitched sounds, hold the diaphragm lightly on the skin. For high-pitched sounds, press the diaphragm firmly on the skin.[1] Specific sounds and auscultation techniques are discussed in the appropriate assessment chapters.

Organizing the Examination

Perform the physical examination systematically and efficiently. Give explanations to the patient as you proceed. Consider the patient's comfort, safety, and privacy. Follow the same sequence every time to avoid omitting a procedure, a step in the sequence, or a part of the body. Table 3.4 presents a comprehensive, organized physical examination outline.

Collect the equipment you need before you begin (Table 3.5). This saves time and energy for you and the patient. It promotes trust by showing a level of professionalism. The use of specific equipment is discussed in the appropriate assessment chapters.

You may need to adapt your approach for the older adult patient, who may have problems, such as decreased mobility, limited energy, and perceptual changes.[5] An outline listing some useful adaptations is found in Table 3.6.

A nurse with appropriate education can perform advanced techniques. A dilated retinal examination would be done with a complete eye examination. Speculum and bimanual examination of females and the prostate gland examination would be done after inspecting the genitalia.

Documentation

At the end of the examination, record the normal and abnormal findings in the health record. Table 3.7 shows an example of how to record findings of a normal physical examination of a healthy adult. See Table 5.4 to find age-related assessment findings in the book.

TYPES OF ASSESSMENT

We use different types of assessment to obtain patient information. There are 3 approaches: emergency, comprehensive, and focused (Table 3.8). The type of assessment to perform is based on the clinical situation. Sometimes the health care agency provides guidelines. Other times it is your nursing judgment.

Emergency Assessment

An *emergency assessment* may be done in an emergency or life-threatening situation. This involves a rapid health history and physical examination to identify life- or limb-threatening conditions that can be stabilized promptly, ensuring better patient outcomes.[6]

Comprehensive Assessment

A *comprehensive assessment* includes a detailed health history and physical examination of all body systems. This is typically done on admission to the hospital or onset of care in a primary care setting.

Focused Assessment

A *focused assessment* is an abbreviated health history and physical examination. It is used to evaluate the status of previously identified problems and monitor for signs and symptoms of new problems. It can be done when a specific problem (e.g., pneumonia) is identified. The patient's clinical cues guide

TABLE 3.4 Physical Examination Outline

1. General Survey

Observe general state of health (with patient seated):

- Body features
- Mental state and level of orientation
- Speech
- Body movements
- Physical appearance
- Nutrition status
- Behavior

2. Vital Signs

Obtain vital signs:

- Blood pressure—both arms for comparison
- Apical/radial pulse
- Respiration
- Temperature
- Oxygen saturation

Record height and weight; calculate body mass index (BMI).

3. Skin

Assess skin, noting:

- Color
- Integrity (e.g., lacerations, lesions, breakdown)
- Scars, tattoos, piercings
- Bruises, rash
- Edema
- Moisture
- Texture
- Temperature
- Turgor
- Vascularity

Assess nails, noting:

- Color
- Lesions
- Size
- Shape
- Angle
- Capillary refill time

4. Head and Neck

Assess head:

- Shape and symmetry of skull
- Masses
- Tenderness
- Condition of hair and scalp
- Temporal arteries
- Temporomandibular joint

Test cranial nerves (CNs):

- Sensory (CN V, light touch, pain)
- Motor (CN VII, shows teeth, purses lips, raises eyebrows)
- Looks up, wrinkles forehead (CN VII)
- Raises shoulders against resistance (CN XI)

Assess neck:

- Skin (vascularity and visible pulsations)
- Symmetry
- Range of motion
- Pulses and bruits (carotid)
- Midline structure (trachea, thyroid gland, cartilage)
- Venous distention, pulsations, waves
- Lymph nodes (preauricular, postauricular, occipital, mandibular, tonsillar, submental, anterior, and posterior cervical, infraclavicular, supraclavicular)

Test visual acuity.

Assess eyes and vision, noting:

- Position and movement of eyelids (CN VII)
- Visual fields (CN II)
- Extraocular movements (CN III, IV, VI)
- Cornea, sclera, conjunctiva
- Pupillary response (CN III)
- Red reflex

Assess nose and sinuses, noting:

- External nose: Shape, blockage
- Internal nose: Patency of nasal passages, shape, turbinates or polyps, discharge
- Frontal and maxillary sinuses

Assess ears and hearing:

- Placement
- Pinna
- Auditory acuity (whispered voice, ticking watch) (CN VIII)
- Mastoid process
- Auditory canal
- Tympanic membrane

Assess mouth:

- Lips (symmetry, lesions, color)
- Buccal mucosa (Stensen's and Wharton's ducts)
- Teeth (absence, state of repair, color)
- Gums (color, receding from teeth)
- Tongue for strength (asymmetry, ability to stick out tongue, side to side, fasciculations) (CN XII)
- Palates
- Tonsils and pillars
- Uvular elevation (CN IX)
- Posterior pharynx
- Gag reflex (CN IX and X)
- Jaw strength (CN V)
- Moisture
- Color
- Floor of mouth

5. Extremities

Observe size and shape, symmetry and deformity, involuntary movements.

Assess arms, fingers, wrists, elbows, shoulders:

- Strength
- Range of motion
- Joint pain
- Swelling
- Pulses (radial, brachial)
- Sensation (light touch, pain, temperature)
- Test reflexes: Triceps, biceps, brachioradialis

Assess legs:

- Strength
- Range of motion
- Joint pain
- Swelling, edema
- Hair distribution
- Sensation (light touch, pain, temperature)
- Pulses (dorsalis pedis, posterior tibialis)
- Test reflexes: Patellar, Achilles, plantar

6. Posterior Thorax

Inspect for muscular development, scoliosis, respiratory movement, anteroposterior (AP) diameter.

Palpate symmetry of respiratory movement.

Assess CVA tenderness, spinous processes, tumors or swelling, tactile fremitus.

Auscultate lungs for breath sounds. Assess egophony, bronchophony, whispered pectoriloquy.

Continued

TABLE 3.4 Physical Examination Outline—cont'd

7. Anterior Thorax

Assess breasts:

- Configuration, symmetry, dimpling of skin
- Assess nipples for rash, direction, inversion, retraction

Assess apical impulse and precordium for thrills, lifts, heaves, tenderness

Auscultate heart sounds for rate and rhythm; character of S_1 and S_2 in the aortic, pulmonic, Erb's point, tricuspid, mitral areas; bruits at carotid, epigastrium

8. Abdomen

Inspect for scars, shape, symmetry, bulging, muscular position and condition of umbilicus, movements (respiratory, pulsations, presence of peristaltic waves)

Auscultate for peristalsis (i.e., bowel sounds), bruits

Percuss then palpate to confirm positive findings; check liver (size, tenderness), spleen, kidney (size, tenderness), urinary bladder (distention)

Palpate femoral pulses, inguinofemoral nodes, abdominal aorta

9. Neurologic

Observe motor status:

- Gait
- Toe walk
- Heel walk
- Drift

Observe coordination and proprioception:

- Finger to nose
- Romberg sign
- Heel to opposite shin
- Proprioception (position sense of great toe)

10. Genitalia

Male External Genitalia

- Inspect penis, noting hair distribution, prepuce, glans, urethral meatus, scars, ulcers, eruptions, structural changes, discharge
- Inspect epidermis of perineum, rectum
- Inspect skin of scrotum; palpate for descended testes, masses, pain

Female External Genitalia

- Inspect hair distribution; mons pubis, labia (minora and majora); urethral meatus; Bartholin's, urethral, Skene's glands (palpate, if indicated); introitus; any discharge
- Assess for presence of cystocele, prolapse
- Inspect perineum, rectum

TABLE 3.5 Common Physical Examination Equipment

- Alcohol swabs
- Blood pressure cuff
- Cotton balls
- Examining table or bed
- Eye chart (e.g., Snellen eye chart)
- Paper cup with water
- Patient gown
- Penlight
- Reflex hammer
- Stethoscope (with bell and diaphragm or a dual-purpose diaphragm; tubing 15–18 inches [38–46 cm])
- Tongue blade
- Watch (with second hand or digital)

a focused assessment. For example, abdominal pain signals the need for a focused assessment of the abdomen. Some problems need a focused assessment of more than one body system. A patient with a headache may need musculoskeletal, neurologic, and head and neck examinations. Examples of focused assessments are found in every assessment chapter of this book.

Using Assessment Approaches

Assessment in an inpatient, acute care hospital setting is different from assessment in other settings. Focused assessment of the hospitalized patient is done more often and by many different HCPs. A team approach demands a high degree of consistency among HCPs from a variety of disciplines.

TABLE 3.6 GERONTOLOGIC ASSESSMENT DIFFERENCES

Adaptations in Physical Assessment Techniques

General Approach

Keep patients warm and comfortable because loss of subcutaneous fat decreases ability to stay warm. Adapt positioning to physical limitations. Avoid unnecessary changes in position. Perform as many activities as possible in the position of comfort for the patient.

Skin

Handle with care because of fragility and loss of subcutaneous fat.

Head and Neck

Provide a quiet environment free from distraction because of possible sensory impairments (e.g., decreased vision, hearing).

Extremities

Use gentle movements and reinforcement techniques. Avoid having patient hop on one foot or perform deep knee bends if patient has limited range of motion of the extremities, decreased reflexes, or diminished sense of balance.

Thorax

Adapt examination for changes related to decreased force of expiration, weakened cough reflex, and shortness of breath.

Abdomen

Use caution in palpating patient's liver as it is readily accessible because of a thinner, softer abdominal wall. The older adult patient may have diminished pain perception in the abdominal wall.

TABLE 3.7 Example of Findings From a Healthy Adult Physical Examination

General Status
- Well-nourished, well-hydrated, well-developed female (or male) in no acute distress, appears stated age, speech clear and evenly paced. Alert and oriented ×3; cooperative, calm. BMI 23.8

Skin
- Skin clear s̄ lesions, warm and dry, trunk warmer than extremities, normal skin turgor, no ↑ vascularity, no varicose veins
- Nails well-groomed round 160-degree angle s̄ lesions, nail beds pink, capillary refill <2 seconds
- Hair thick, brown, shiny, normal (male, female) distribution

Head
- Normocephalic, nontender

Eyes
- Visual fields intact on gross confrontation

Visual acuity s̄ glasses: Right eye 20/20
Left eye 20/20
Both eyes 20/20
- EOM: Intact on all gazes s̄ nystagmus
- Pupils: PERRLA, negative cover and uncover tests

Ears
- Pinna intact, in proper alignment; external canal patent; small amount of cerumen present bilaterally; TMs intact; pearly gray, light reflex visible, not bulging; whisper heard at 3 ft bilaterally

Nose
- Patent bilaterally; turbinates pink, no swelling
- Sinuses nontender

Mouth
- Moist and pink, soft, and hard palates intact, uvula rises midline on "ahh," 24 teeth present and in good repair
- Tonsils surgically removed, no redness
- Tongue moist, pink, size appropriate for mouth, no lesions

Neck
- Supple, no masses or bruits, lymph nodes nonpalpable and nontender
- Thyroid: Palpable, smooth, not enlarged
- ROM: Full, intact, strong
- Trachea: Midline, nontender

Breasts
- Soft, nonpendulous, no dimpling or puckering
- Nipples: Inversion, point in same direction, areola dark and symmetric, no discharge, no masses, nontender

Axilla
- Hair present, no lesions, no palpable lymph nodes

Thorax and Lungs
- Respiratory rate 18, regular rhythm, oxygen saturation 98% on room air; AP < transverse diameter, no ↑ in tactile fremitus, no tenderness, lungs resonant throughout, diaphragmatic excursion 4 cm bilaterally, chest expansion symmetric, lung fields clear throughout

Heart
- Rate 82, regular rate, and rhythm; BP: right arm: 122/76, left arm: 120/78; no lifts, heaves
- Apical impulse: 5th ICS at MCL; no palpable thrills; S_1, S_2 present; no S_3, S_4; no murmurs, rubs, clicks
- Carotid, femoral, pedal, and radial pulses present; equal, 2+ bilaterally

Abdomen
- No pulsations visible, rounded, positive bowel sounds in 4 quadrants, no bruits or CVA tenderness, no palpable masses
- Liver lower border percussed at costal margin, smooth, nontender; approx. 9-cm span
- Spleen nonpalpable nontender

Neurologic System
- Cranial nerves I—XII intact
- Motor (drift, toe stand) intact
- Sensation (touch, vibration, proprioception) normal bilaterally, upper and lower extremities
- Coordination (finger to nose, Romberg) intact
- Reflexes: See diagram

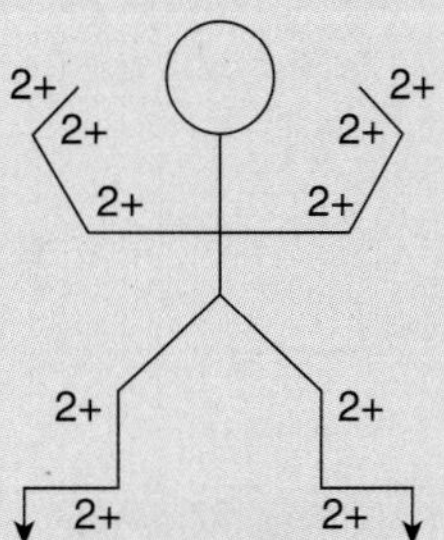

Grading Scale
- 0: No response
- 1+: Diminished
- 2+: Normal
- 3+: Increased
- 4+: Hyperactive

Musculoskeletal System
- Well developed, no muscle wasting, crepitus, nodules, or swelling, no scoliosis
- ROM: Full and equal bilaterally, upper and lower extremities
- Strength: Equal, strong 5/5 bilaterally, upper and lower extremities
- Gait: Walks erect 2-foot steps, arms swinging at side s̄ staggering

Female Genitalia[a]
- External genitalia: No swelling, redness, tenderness; normal hair distribution, no cysts
- Vagina: No lesions, discharge; bulging, pink
- Cervix: Os closed; pink, no lesions, erosions, nontender
- Uterus: Small, firm, nontender
- Adnexa: No enlargement; nontender
- Rectovaginal: Sphincter intact; confirms above findings

Male Genitalia[a]
- Normal male hair distribution, negative inguinal hernia
- Penis: Urethral opening patent; no redness, swelling, discharge; no lesions, structural changes
- Scrotum: Testes descended; no redness, masses, tenderness
- Rectal: No lesions, redness; sphincter intact; prostate small, nontender

[a]Some data would be obtained only if the nurse has the appropriate education.
AP, Anterior-posterior; *CVA*, costovertebral angle; *EOM*, extraocular movements; *ICS*, intercostal space; *MCL*, midclavicular line; *PERRLA*, pupils equal, round, reactive to light and accommodation; *ROM*, range of motion; *TM*, tympanic membrane.

TABLE 3.8 Types of Assessment

Description	When and Where Performed	Where to Find in Book
Emergency		
• Limited to assessing life-threatening conditions (e.g., inhalation injuries, anaphylaxis, myocardial infarction, shock, stroke) • Done to ensure survival. Focuses on elements in primary survey (e.g., airway, breathing, circulation, disability) • After life-saving interventions are started, perform brief systematic assessment to identify other injuries or problems	• Done in any setting when signs or symptoms of a life-threatening condition appear (e.g., emergency department, critical care unit, surgical setting)	• Chapter 21, Table 21.3, Table 21.5 • Emergency Management tables throughout the book and listed in Table 21.1
Comprehensive		
• Detailed assessment of all body systems (head-to-toe assessment) • Data are used to plan and deliver individualized patient care	• Initial visit in primary or ambulatory care setting • Admission to hospital, rehabilitation, or long-term care setting • Initial home care visit • Admission to hospice care	• Assessment chapters for each body system • Physical examination outline (Table 3.4) • Findings from physical examination of a healthy adult (Table 3.7)
Focused		
• Brief assessment that focuses on one or more body systems that are the focus of care • Includes assessment related to a specific problem (e.g., pneumonia, specific abnormal laboratory findings) • Monitors for signs and symptoms of new problems	• Throughout hospital admission—at beginning of a shift and as needed throughout shift • Revisit in ambulatory care setting or home care setting	• Focused assessment tables in each assessment chapter • Tables on nursing assessment of specific diseases throughout book

TABLE 3.9 Clinical Applications for Types of Assessment

This is an example of how different types of assessment would be used as a patient progresses from the emergency department to a clinical unit of a hospital.

Timeline	Type of Assessment
Emergency Department	
• Patient arrives in acute respiratory distress • Problem is found, and critical interventions are performed • Patient stabilizes	• Perform emergency assessment (see Table 21.3) • Conduct a focused assessment of the respiratory and related body systems (e.g., cardiovascular) • May begin comprehensive assessment of all body systems
Clinical Unit	
• Patient is admitted to a monitored clinical unit • Beginning of each shift: Reassess per orders and more often as determined by the nurse	• Complete comprehensive assessment of all body systems within proper timeframe • Perform focused assessment of respiratory system and other related body systems per agency protocol • Perform focused assessment of appropriate body system(s) if new symptoms are reported

As you gain experience, you will be able to form a mental image of a patient's status from a few basic details, such as "85-year-old female admitted for COPD exacerbation." Details from a complete verbal report, including length of stay, laboratory results, physical findings, and vital signs, will help you have a clear picture. Next, perform your own assessment using a focused approach. During your assessment, you will confirm or revise the findings that you read in the medical record and what you heard from other HCPs.

Remember, the process does not end once you have done your first assessment on a patient during rounds. Continue to gather information about your patients throughout your shift. You consider everything you learned previously about each patient considering new information. For example, when you are doing a respiratory assessment on your patient with COPD, you now hear crackles in the lungs. This leads you to do a cardiovascular assessment because heart problems can cause crackles. As you gain experience, the importance of new findings will become more clear. Case studies in the assessment chapters will help you develop your assessment skills.

Table 3.9 shows how you perform different types of assessments based on a patient's progress through a given hospital stay. When a patient arrives at the emergency department with a life-threatening condition, you will perform an emergency assessment based on the elements of a primary survey (e.g., airway, breathing, circulation, disability) (see Table 21.3). Once the patient is stable, you can begin a focused assessment of related body systems. After the patient is admitted, you perform a comprehensive assessment of all body systems.

BRIDGE TO NCLEX EXAMINATION

The number of the question corresponds to the same-numbered outcome at the beginning of the chapter.

1. The nursing health history and physical examination provide the nurse with information primarily to
   - **a.** diagnose a medical problem.
   - **b.** investigate a patient's signs and symptoms.
   - **c.** classify subjective and objective patient data.
   - **d.** make clinical judgments about the patient's health.
2. The nurse would place information about a patient's concern that an illness is threatening job security in which functional health pattern?
   - **a.** Role-relationship
   - **b.** Cognitive-perceptual
   - **c.** Coping–stress tolerance
   - **d.** Health perception–health management
3. The nurse is preparing to examine a patient's abdomen. Place in order the proper steps for an abdominal assessment, using the numbers 1 to 4, with 1 = the first technique and 4 = the last technique:
   - **a.** ___ Inspection
   - **b.** ___ Palpation
   - **c.** ___ Percussion
   - **d.** ___ Auscultation
4. Which situation would require the nurse to obtain a focused assessment? **(Select all that apply.)**
   - **a.** A patient seeking care with a new primary provider.
   - **b.** A patient who reports a new symptom during rounds.
   - **c.** A previously identified problem needs reassessment.
   - **d.** An admission assessment for a patient in long-term care.
   - **e.** A patient with an emergent problem needing immediate care.
5. A nurse needs to be aware of personal bias to be able to:
   - **a.** promote health equity and respect for all patients.
   - **b.** determine which patient health beliefs are important.
   - **c.** recognize similarities in patients from a cultural group.
   - **d.** use personal beliefs to evaluate a patient care situation.

1. d; 2. a; 3. 1, 4, 3, 2; 4. b, c; 5. a.

For rationales to these answers and even more NCLEX review questions, visit http://evolve.elsevier.com/Lewis/medsurg.

REFERENCES

To access the References for this chapter, please scan the QR code with a mobile device.

4

Patient and Caregiver Teaching

Brenda C. Morris

http//evolve.elsevier.com/Lewis/medsurg/

CONCEPTUAL FOCUS

Communication
Health Promotion
Patient Education
Self-Management

LEARNING OUTCOMES

1. Apply the teaching-learning process to diverse patient populations.
2. Select strategies to support patient learning.
3. Evaluate the role of the caregiver in patient teaching.
4. Relate the physical, psychologic, and sociocultural characteristics of the patient and caregiver to the teaching-learning process.
5. Prioritize patient teaching goals for patients and caregivers.
6. Choose appropriate teaching strategies for patients and caregivers.
7. Choose appropriate methods to evaluate patient and caregiver learning.

KEY TERMS

caregivers
health literacy
learning
learning needs
motivational interviewing
self-efficacy
teaching
teaching plan
teaching process

This chapter describes the process of patient and caregiver teaching and strategies that contribute to successful teaching and learning. The concept of patient and caregiver (family member or significant other) teaching is central to delivering quality patient care. It is a dynamic, interactive process that involves a change in a patient's knowledge, behavior, and/or attitude to maintain or improve health. You will find that teaching is a challenging and rewarding role. Teaching patients and caregivers is a key nursing intervention that makes a difference in their lives.

ROLE OF PATIENT AND CAREGIVER TEACHING

The general goals of patient teaching include health promotion, disease prevention, illness management, and appropriate choice and use of treatment options. In patients with acute and chronic health problems, your teaching can prevent complications and promote recovery, self-care, and independence. In the United States 6 in 10 adults have a chronic health problem.[1] How patients manage their health problems and maintain quality of life depends on what they learn about their conditions and how they use this knowledge. Patients with the knowledge, skills, and desire to manage their health are more likely to follow medication and treatment plans.[2] Patients who receive education before surgery are more likely to have a reduced length of hospital stay and less likely to have complications after surgery.[3]

Teaching may be needed wherever you work as a nurse. Although agencies may have advanced practice nurses or patient educators provide patient teaching programs, you are always responsible for teaching patients and caregivers.[4] You cannot delegate teaching to AP.

In patient teaching, the teaching-learning process involves the patient, the patient's caregiver(s), and you. Every interaction with a patient and a caregiver is a potential *teachable moment.* On any given day, more informal opportunities to teach occur than formal opportunities. For example, when you teach a patient with asthma how to use a peak flow meter, you do not need a formal teaching plan. However, when your patient has a specific learning need about health promotion or managing a health problem, you should develop a teaching plan. A teaching plan includes (1) assessing the patient's ability and readiness to learn, (2) identifying teaching needs, (3) developing learning goals with the patient, (4) implementing plans for the teaching, and (5) evaluating learning.

TEACHING-LEARNING PROCESS

Teaching is the act of conveying information to facilitate learning. Nurses often teach patients using methods such as direct instruction, coaching, counseling, and behavior modification. Teaching may be formal, such as giving a planned presentation to a group of patients, or informal, such as teaching a patient about medications before giving them.

Learning is the act of acquiring knowledge or skills that may produce a change in behavior. Observation of this change is a sign that learning has occurred. However, learning may not result in any observable change. A patient who understood what was taught can choose not to change behavior.

Adult Learning Principles

Understanding how and why adults learn is important for you to effectively teach patients and caregivers. Knowles identified 6 principles of *andragogy* (adult learning) that are important for you to consider when teaching adults (Table 4.1).[5]

Models to Promote Health

Patients and caregivers may progress through a series of steps before they are willing or able to change their health behaviors. Prochaska and Velicer proposed 6 stages of change in their *Transtheoretical Model of Health Behavior Change* (Table 4.2).[6] This model is often used for planning to help patients stop smoking, manage diabetes, and lose weight.

Motivational interviewing is a nonconfrontational communication method to motivate patients to change behavior.[7] This strategy includes interventions that enhance the patient's

TABLE 4.1 Adult Learning Principles Applied to Patient and Caregiver Teaching

Principles	Teaching Implications for Nurse	Examples
Need to know	• Patients need to know why they should learn something, what they need to learn, and how it will help them. • Ask the patient questions such as, "What do you think you need to learn about this topic?"	Your patient and their caregiver ask what they need to know about exercise guidelines after a heart attack.
Readiness to learn	• Readiness and motivation to learn are high when facing new tasks. • Health crises provide opportunities for patients to learn and change behavior. • Stress and anxiety may interfere with learning, thus requiring frequent reinforcement of content.	While recovering from a transient ischemic attack, your patient tells you that they are ready to learn about the changes they need to take to reduce their risk for stroke.
Prior experiences	• Motivation is increased when one already knows something about the subject from past experiences. • Identification of knowledge and experiences can help find familiar ground to increase patients' confidence.	Your patient needs to begin injections of enoxaparin. They tell you that they give their father insulin injections and are ready to learn how to give this medication.
Motivation to learn	• Patients prefer to apply learning at once. • Long-term goals may have less appeal than short-term goals. • Focus teaching on information that the patient views as needed right now.	Your patient is scheduled for discharge in the morning. Both the patient and their caregiver have received instruction on wound care and have watched the procedure. The caregiver tells you that they want to perform the wound care today.
Orientation to learning	• Patients seek out various resources for specific learning and prefer choices. • When the patient does not recognize the relevancy of the teaching, offer explanations of the value of the learning. • Teaching should target the specific problem or circumstance.	Your patient, who is newly diagnosed with diabetes, tells you that they are worried about the diet changes they will need to make. Share several options with them to learn about diet changes (e.g., cooking classes, online tutorials, mobile applications, sessions with the dietitian, brochures).
Self-concept	• Patients need control and self-direction (sense of autonomy) to maintain their sense of self-worth. • Patients do not learn when we treat them like children and tell them what they must do.	The patient with a temporary colostomy says they are not ready to look at the stoma. Work out a schedule with them for learning colostomy care that meets their need for control and prepares them for self-care.

TABLE 4.2 Stages of Change in Transtheoretical Model

Stage	Patient Behavior	Nursing Implications
1. Precontemplation	Is not considering a change. Is not ready to learn.	Provide support, increase awareness of condition. Describe benefits of change and risks of not changing.
2. Contemplation	Thinks about a change. May recognize need to change. Says "I know I should," but identifies barriers.	Introduce what is involved in changing the behavior. Reinforce the stated need to change.
3. Preparation	Starts planning the change, gathers information, sets a date to start change, shares decision to change with others.	Reinforce the positive outcomes of change, give information and encouragement, develop a plan, help set priorities, and identify sources of support.
4. Action	Begins to change behavior through practice. Tentative and may experience relapses.	Reinforce behavior with reward, encourage self-reward, discuss choices to help minimize relapses and regain focus. Help patient plan to deal with potential relapses.
5. Maintenance	Practices the behavior regularly. Able to sustain the change.	Continue to reinforce behavior. Provide more teaching on the need to maintain change.
6. Termination	Change has become part of lifestyle. Behavior no longer considered a change.	Evaluate effectiveness of the new behavior. No further intervention needed.

Adapted from Prochaska J, Velicer W: The transtheoretical model of health behavior change, *Am J Health Promot* 12:38, 1997 (Classic).

TABLE 4.3 Key Aspects of Motivational Interviewing

- Listen rather than tell.
- Adjust to, rather than oppose, patient resistance.
- Express empathy through reflective listening.
- Focus on the positive. Do not criticize the patient.
- Gently persuade with the understanding that change is up to the patient.
- Focus on the patient's strengths to support the hope needed to make changes.
- Avoid argument and direct confrontation. They can cause defensiveness and a power struggle.
- Help the patient recognize the "gap" between where they are and where they hope to be.

motivation for change (Table 4.3). The techniques used in motivational interviewing are linked to the stages of change identified by Prochaska and Velicer.[6]

During the process of change, relapse and recycling through the stages are expected. Sometimes patients do not change behaviors. Some return to previous behaviors after a period of change. This may mean that the interventions used did not consider the patient's stage of change. Identify the patient's current stage of readiness for change and the stage to which they are moving. Patients who are in the early stages of change need and use different kinds of motivational support than patients at later stages of change.

For example, a hospitalized patient who smokes cigarettes may be in the *precontemplation* or *contemplation* stage of change. In the precontemplation stage, the patient is not concerned about their smoking and not considering quitting. During this stage, it is important to help the patient increase awareness of risks and problems related to smoking. Ask them what they think could happen if they continued smoking. Give evidence of the problem (e.g., x-ray changes). Share facts about the risks of smoking. Although they may not be ready to change behavior now, the idea for a future change may be in their mind. In other cases, such as when a patient has a life-threatening condition (e.g., heart attack), there may be an immediate awareness of the problem and motivation to change.

A patient in the *contemplation* stage of change often is ambivalent. The patient understands the behavior is a problem and that change is necessary. However, they believe that change is too hard or that the behavior is worth the risks. This is seen in the patient who says, "I know that I have to stop smoking. This heart attack really scared me. I know I need to lose weight and start exercising, but I can't change everything all at once. Smoking helps me control my eating. I can't stop until I lose some weight." During this stage, help the patient consider the positive and negative aspects of their behavior (e.g., tobacco use). Helping the patient discover internal motivators in addition to those external motivators (e.g., second heart attack, lung disease) that push the patient toward change can move the patient from contemplating change to preparation and action. Throughout this process, emphasize the patient's personal choices and responsibilities for change.

As the patient moves from contemplation to *preparation,* we can help strengthen the commitment to change by helping the patient develop **self-efficacy**.[7] This is the belief that one can succeed in a given situation. In this example, it is the patient's belief that they can change their tobacco use. Support even the smallest effort to change. Movement through action and maintenance stages of change requires continued support for the patient's involvement and participation in treatment. You can find strategies for using motivational interviewing to create a plan for change at https://www.niaaa.nih.gov/health-professionals-communities/core-resource-on-alcohol/conduct-brief-intervention-build-motivation-and-plan-change.

The resolution of acute health problems or discharge from the hospital often occurs before the patient moves to the preparation and action stages of change. As the patient develops readiness in the contemplative stage of change, provide referrals to community and outpatient resources.

Teaching Competencies

Knowledge of Subject Matter

Develop confidence as a teacher by becoming knowledgeable about the topic. For example, if you are teaching patients about managing hypertension, you must be able to explain what hypertension is and why treating it is important. Teach patients what they need to know about exercise, diet, medications, BP monitoring, and situations to report to the HCP. Provide patients with resources such as credible websites, brochures, and information about support organizations (e.g., American Heart Association [AHA]).

Do not expect to be an expert in all subject areas. Sometimes you will not be able to answer patients' or caregivers' questions. Clarify the questions to be sure of what they are asking. When you do not know the answer, tell them that you will find out an answer. Seek help from co-workers, patient educators, and other reliable sources to answer the question.

Communication Skills

Patient teaching depends on effective communication between you and the patient or caregiver. Medical jargon can be intimidating and frightening. Introduce medical words and define their meanings. Limit the use of acronyms (e.g., CABG for coronary artery bypass graft) and abbreviations (e.g., IV). Have the patient and caregiver clarify their understandings of the disease process. Ask them to explain what they know in their own words. For example, if a patient has leukopenia, define this term. Explain that *leuko-* refers to a leukocyte, a white blood cell that fights infections, and that *penia* refers to a shortage. Use a brief explanation such as, "You do not have enough white blood cells. They are cells that fight infection."

Nonverbal communication is critical when teaching. Cultural practices often guide nonverbal communication. For example, in Western culture, sitting in an open, relaxed position facing the patient with eyes at the same level delivers a positive nonverbal message (Fig. 4.1). Sit in a chair at the bedside and use open body gestures to communicate interest and a willingness to share. Patients from some cultures may prefer that you avoid direct eye contact and give health information to a family spokesperson rather than directly to the patient.

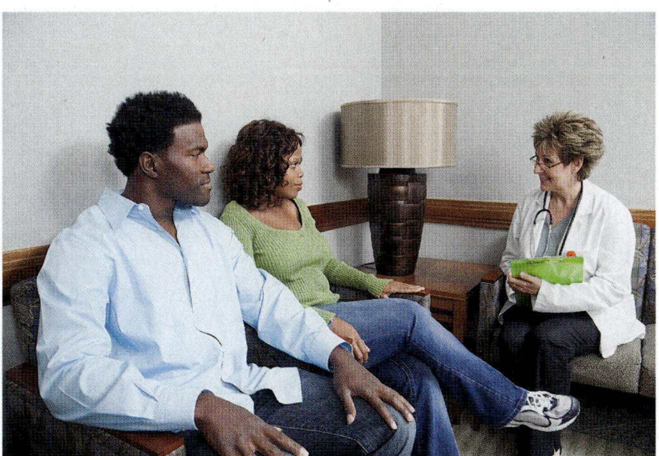

Fig. 4.1 Open, relaxed positioning of patient, spouse, and nurse at eye level promotes communication in teaching and learning. (© Jupiterimages/Photos.com/Thinkstock.)

Develop the art of active listening. Pay attention to what the patient says, listen to understand, and observe nonverbal cues. Do not interrupt. Nod in response to the patient's statements. Restate what is said to help clarify communication.

Empathy is the courage to enter the world of another in a manner that does not judge or correct but tries to understand. Empathy means putting aside your own self and stepping into the patient's shoes. Active listening, combined with empathy, is a powerful way to communicate caring and prepare patients to learn.

Challenges to Nurse-Teacher Effectiveness

Teaching patients and caregivers has many challenges. These include (1) lack of time, (2) your own feelings as a teacher, (3) nurse-patient differences in learning goals, and (4) rapid or early discharge from the health care system.

Lack of time can be a barrier to effective teaching. For example, the patient's physical needs may compete for time that you could use for teaching. To make the most of limited time, set learning priorities with the patient. Tell the patient at the beginning of the interaction how much time you can devote to the session. Deliver or reinforce teaching during every contact with the patient or caregiver. For example, when giving a medication, explain the purpose and side effects. Reinforcing small pieces of information over time is an effective teaching strategy, especially if information is new or complex.

Other potential barriers are your own feelings as a teacher and insecurity about your knowledge and skill. Teaching is a skill that takes time to master. Consult with nurse educators or experienced co-workers for further help with developing your teaching skills. Become familiar with the resources for patient teaching available at your agency.

Sometimes disagreements arise among the patient, the caregiver, and you about the expectations or outcomes of teaching. Realistic discussions about discharge plans, timelines, and home care options can emphasize the need for learning. For example, after emergent valve surgery, the patient and caregiver may reject teaching efforts until they accept the seriousness of the patient's health problem.

Another challenge is early and quick patient discharges from the health care facility. Shorter lengths of stays have resulted in patients receiving only basic teaching. This makes it important to begin teaching patients soon after admission to the health care system and continue throughout their stay.

Caregiver Support in Patient Teaching

The teaching and learning process applies to the caregiver. **Caregivers** are people who care for those who cannot care for themselves. Most caregivers are family members or significant others who (1) give or help with direct patient care; (2) provide emotional, social, spiritual, and possibly financial support for the patient; and (3) manage and coordinate health care services.

About 1 in 4 American adults serves as a caregiver to a person with a long-term disability or illness.[8] The most common caregivers are spouses, adult children, parents, grandparents, and life partners. Identify the key caregiver(s). Assess their roles and relationships to the patient. Because the patient's health problem affects family roles and functions, identify the needs of caregivers. Caregivers with unmet needs may be unable to assist the patient (Table 4.4).

Consider cultural differences when assessing the caregiver. In some cultures, a male family member may be the designated spokesperson to receive and communicate information among family members and the patient. Ensure that the family spokesperson and caregivers who will provide care for the patient are included in discharge planning. See Chapter 2 for more information on culturally sensitive care.

When possible, teach the patient and the caregiver together. Explain the goals of the teaching plan. Caregivers may need help when learning the physical and technical requirements of care, finding resources for home care, finding equipment and supplies, and rearranging the home to accommodate the patient. Sources of support for the transition from hospital to home include community-based agencies, social workers, and case managers at the hospital and insurance companies.

Patients and caregivers may have different teaching needs. For example, the priority of an older patient with a leg ulcer may be to learn how to transfer from a bed to a chair in the least painful manner. On the other hand, the caregiver may be most concerned about learning the technique for dressing changes. Both the patient's and caregiver's learning needs are important.

The patient and caregiver may have different or conflicting views of the illness and treatment options. Developing a successful teaching plan requires you to view the patient's needs within the context of the caregiver's needs. For instance, you may teach a patient with right-sided weakness self-feeding techniques with special tools. Then, at a home visit you find the caregiver feeding the patient. On questioning, the caregiver reveals that it is too hard to watch the patient struggle with feeding, it takes too long, and it is messy. As a result, the caregiver decided that it is easier to feed the patient. This is an example of a situation in which the patient and caregiver need more discussion and teaching about goals for self-care.

Discuss potential resources provided by support groups, family and friends, and community organizations. Support groups help by sharing experiences and information, offering understanding and acceptance, and suggesting solutions to common problems and concerns.

TABLE 4.4 Assessing Caregiver Needs

Ask caregivers the following questions:

1. How are you coping with your caregiver role?
2. Do you have any problems performing your caregiver responsibilities?
3. How much support do you get from outside sources (e.g., other family members, friends)?
4. Are you aware of and do you use community resources (e.g., disease-specific professional organizations [such as Alzheimer's Association, AHA, ACS], adult day care centers, religious/spiritual organizations)?
5. Do you know about resources that are available for respite (someone caring for your loved one while you have time to yourself)?
6. What kind of help or services do you need now and in the near future?
7. How can I or other health care providers help you in your caregiving role?

Regulatory Mandates for Patient Teaching

Several important agencies have specific mandates related to teaching hospitalized patients. The Joint Commission's (TJC's) accreditation standards, National Patient Safety Goals,[9] and the American Hospital Association's Patient Care Partnership[10] state that patients have a fundamental right to receive information about their care. This information includes their diagnosis, treatment, and prognosis in terms that they can understand. For example, written materials must be at the patient's reading level. One program started by TJC, SpeakUp™, was developed to encourage patients to become more involved and informed about their plan of care.[11] The SpeakUp™ program offers infographics and videos for patients. Another program is Ask Me 3.[12] Both programs encourage patients to ask specific questions about their care.

PATIENT TEACHING PROCESS

We use many different approaches in patient teaching. The approach used most often by nurses parallels the nursing process. The **teaching process** includes assessment, goal setting, implementation, and evaluation. The teaching process, like the nursing process, may not always flow in linear order, but the steps serve as checkpoints.

Assessment

During the general nursing assessment, determine whether the patient has learning needs. For example, what does the patient know about the health problem? How do they perceive the problem? If you identify a learning need, conduct a more detailed assessment, and address that problem with a teaching plan. Include caregivers as you assess their role and ability to care for the patient at home. Key questions to use are outlined in Table 4.5.

Physical Factors

The patient's age and experience affect the plan for teaching. An older adult may have experience related to learning health self-management. A young adult who has never thought about

TABLE 4.5 Assessing Factors Affecting Patient Teaching

Physical
- What is the patient's age?
- Is the patient acutely ill?
- Is the patient fatigued or in pain?
- What is the primary diagnosis?
- Are there other medical problems?
- What is the patient's current mental status?
- What is the patient's hearing ability? Visual ability? Motor ability?
- What drugs does the patient take that may affect learning?

Psychologic
- Does the patient appear anxious, afraid, depressed, defensive?
- Is the patient in a state of denial?
- What is the patient's level of motivation? Self-efficacy?

Sociocultural
- What are the patient's beliefs about their illness or treatment?
- Is the proposed teaching consistent with the patient's cultural values?
- What is the patient's educational experience, reading ability, primary language?
- What is the patient's present or past occupation?
- How does the patient describe their financial status?
- What is the patient's living arrangement?
- Does the patient have family or close friends?

Learner
- What does the patient already know about the health problem?
- What does the patient think is most important to learn?
- What prior learning experiences could be a frame of reference for current learning needs?
- Is the patient ready to learn? Change behavior?
- How does the patient learn best (e.g., reading, listening, looking at pictures, doing, playing games)?
- In what type of environment does the patient learn best? Formal classroom? Computer/online setting? Informal setting, such as home? Alone or in a group?
- In what way should the caregiver(s) be involved in patient teaching?

mortality may struggle to accept the long-term health implications of diabetes and the needed areas of learning.

Sensory problems (e.g., hearing or vision loss) that decrease sensory input can alter learning. Nervous system problems (e.g., stroke, head trauma) and other diseases (e.g., liver problems, heart failure) can affect cognition. Patients with altered cognition may have a hard time learning and need more caregiver involvement in the teaching process. Manual dexterity is needed to perform skills such as giving injections or BP monitoring.

Pain, fatigue, and certain drugs influence the ability to learn. No one can learn effectively when in severe pain. Provide teaching after the patient's pain is controlled. A tired, weak patient may be unable to concentrate. Sleep problems are common during hospitalization. Patients are often sleep deprived at the time of discharge. Drugs that cause central nervous system depression, such as opioids and sedatives, decrease mental alertness and can affect the patient's ability to learn new information. Adjust the teaching plan by setting high-priority goals based on need-to-know information and realistic expectations. Patients often need a referral for follow-up care so that teaching can continue after discharge.

Psychologic Factors

Psychologic factors have a major influence on the patient's ability to learn. Anxiety and depression are common reactions to illness. Although mild anxiety increases perceptual and learning abilities, moderate or severe anxiety limits learning. Anxiety and depression can negatively affect motivation and readiness to learn. For instance, the patient newly diagnosed with diabetes who is depressed about the diagnosis may not listen or respond to instructions about glucose testing. Discussions with the patient about these concerns or referrals to a support group may help the patient learn that managing diabetes is possible.

Patients respond to the stress of illness with a variety of defense mechanisms, such as denial, rationalization, or even humor. A patient who denies having cancer will not be receptive to information related to treatment options. A person may have a hard time accepting a terminal diagnosis. A patient using rationalization could produce many reasons for avoiding change or for rejecting teaching. For example, a patient with heart disease who does not want to change diet habits will relate stories of people who have eaten bacon and eggs every day and lived to be 100 years old. Some patients use humor to filter reality or decrease anxiety. They may use laughter to escape from the experience of facing threatening situations. Humor in the teaching process is important and useful unless the humor is used to avoid reality.

One key factor in successful adoption of new behaviors is the patient's sense of self-efficacy. There is a strong relationship between self-efficacy and outcomes of illness management (Box 4.1). Self-efficacy increases when a person gains new skills in managing a threatening situation. It decreases if the person has repeated failure. Plan easily achievable goals early in the teaching sessions. Proceed from simple to more complex content to support a feeling of success.

Sociocultural Factors

Health literacy. Health literacy is the degree to which a person can obtain, understand, and use basic health information to inform health decisions.[13] Almost 90% of U.S. adults have limited health literacy skills.[14] Currently, only 57% of adults report being involved in health care decisions as much as they wanted.[15] Only 26% report that an HCP asked them to describe how they will follow the instructions provided.[15]

Patients with low levels of health literacy have trouble understanding and acting on health information. Even patients with high levels of health literacy may have a hard time understanding complex health information if they are sick or stressed. Interventions for improving health literacy in patients improve self-efficacy and the ability to manage chronic disease, leading to improved health outcomes.[16]

BOX 4.1 EVIDENCE-BASED PRACTICE

You are a nurse at a general GI postsurgical clinic. Following the first 3 months after surgery, you note a decrease in patient compliance and an increase in complications. The health care team recognizes that these complications may partly be due to patients' lack of motivation for continuing healthy lifestyle recommendations after surgery.

Making Clinical Decisions

Synthesis of Best Available Evidence

As the nurse, you believe an individual approach to patient teaching may help improve self-efficacy, thus decreasing complications. Self-efficacy is the belief that one can succeed in a particular situation or perform a certain behavior. The empowerment approach provides patient-centered education aimed at promoting self-efficacy.

Clinician Expertise

You and your colleagues design and implement an individual education program. The program includes interactive sessions between the nurse and small patient groups for the first 6 weeks followed by video call follow-ups for 3 months. All sessions will allow for face-to-face interaction and the opportunity for patients to ask questions about their care.

Patient Preferences and Values

After a 6-month period, the nursing staff noted an increase in attendance in the 3-month video sessions. On average, 65% of patients attending the sessions asked questions about lifestyle changes to help maintain control of their conditions and improve their overall health status.

Implications for Nursing Practice

1. What influencing factors should you consider when designing an interactive nurse-patient education program designed to improve patient outcomes?
2. As the nurse, how would you recognize improved self-efficacy in the patient?

Reference for Evidence

Guo L, Li L, Lu Y, et al: Effects of empowerment education on the self-management and self-efficacy of liver transplant patients: A randomized control trial, *BMC Nurs* 22:146, 2023.

It is challenging to assess health literacy. Patients may be embarrassed to admit that they are having trouble understanding health information. Health professionals often overestimate patients' health literacy, so it is important to routinely assess health literacy level. Easy-to-use assessment tools are available. The Single-Item Literacy Screener (SILS) uses one question to identify adults who need help with reading.[17] The question is, "How often do you need to have someone help you when you read instructions, pamphlets, or other written material from your doctor or pharmacy?"

Another approach is to implement health literacy universal precautions. These are the steps to take when we assume that all patients may have difficulty understanding important health information and accessing health services. These include using simple communications about health information and verifying patient understanding.[14]

TJC states that we must tailor teaching to the patient's literacy needs. For example, teach patients and give them

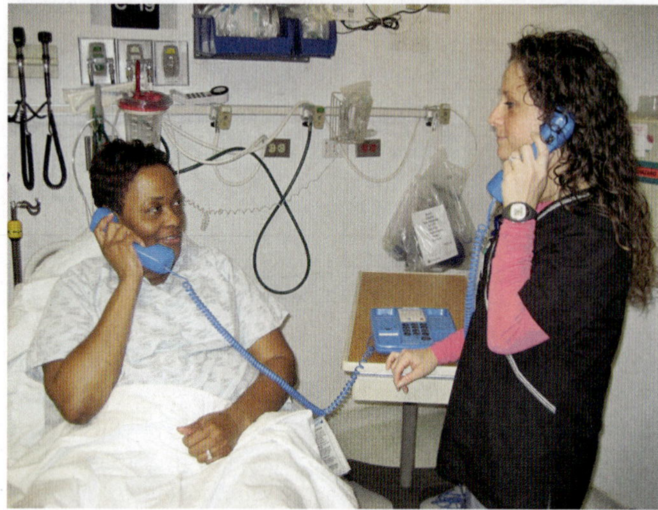

Fig. 4.2 Nurse communicating with a non–English-speaking patient using a translation phone service. (Courtesy Linda Bucher, RN, PhD, CEN, CNE, Staff Nurse, Virtua Memorial Hospital, Mt. Holly, NJ.)

written materials in their primary language. It is best to use medical interpreters instead of family members or friends to protect patient privacy (Fig. 4.2). Medical interpreters are discussed in Table 2.9. Choose patient teaching materials written at the 5th grade or lower reading level. Other interventions to help patients with low levels of health literacy include using the teach-back method, providing visual aids, highlighting key text, offering videos, and teaching content in small increments.

Culture. Cultural traditions influence our health practices, beliefs, and behavior. These traditions, which can affect patient teaching, can be identified in a cultural assessment (see Table 2.5). Ask patients to describe their beliefs about health and illness. TJC requires that we tailor patient teaching to the patient's cultural needs.[18]

Assess the patient's use of cultural remedies and healing practices. Consider how the cultural remedies may support or conflict with the treatment plan. One cultural element that affects the teaching-learning process is a conflict between cultural beliefs and values and the behaviors promoted by the health care team.

Last, determine who has authority in the patient's culture. Patients may defer to the authority, such as an elder or a spiritual leader, for decisions. In this case identify and work with the patient and the decision makers in the patient's cultural group. See Chapter 2 for more information on cultural competence.

Socioeconomic. Consider a variety of socioeconomic factors when preparing to teach patients. Knowing the patient's occupation may help you decide the vocabulary to use during teaching. For example, an auto mechanic may understand the volume overload from heart failure as flooding an engine. An engineer may understand the principles of physics associated with gravity and pressures when discussing vascular problems.

Ask about living arrangements. Whether the patient lives alone, with friends, or with family influences who you include in the teaching process. If the patient has unmet learning needs at the time of discharge, arrange for further teaching.

Learner Factors

Learning needs. Learning needs are the new knowledge and skills that a person must have to meet a goal. Assess what the patient already knows and any past experiences with health problems. Patients with long-standing health problems may have different learning needs from those patients with newly diagnosed health problems.

What patients should learn about managing health and illness may seem obvious to you. However, what you think is important may be different from what patients want to know. Remember, adults learn best when given information that they view as being needed at once (Table 4.1). Having patients prioritize their own learning needs lets you begin with the patient's most important needs. Ask what they see as the most critical "need to know" information. Give them a list of the recommended topics and then ask them to identify other topics not on the list.

Readiness to learn. Motivation and readiness to learn depend on multiple factors, such as perceived need, attitudes, and beliefs. When teaching adults, identify what information the person values. Readiness to learn increases when the patient perceives a need for information, has a belief that a behavior change has value, or perceives the learning activities as new and engaging.[5]

Assess where the patient is in the stages of change (Table 4.2). If the patient is in the precontemplation stage, provide support and increase the patient's awareness of the problem until they are ready to consider a behavior change. Nurses in outpatient settings and home health care can continue to assess the patient's readiness to learn and implement the teaching plan as the patient moves through the stages of change. Reinforcement throughout the change process is a strong motivational factor for achieving a desired behavior. *Positive reinforcement* involves rewarding the expected behavior with positive feedback or other rewards to maintain the behavior.[6]

Learning style. Each person has preferred styles of learning. The 3 general learning styles are (1) *visual* (reading, pictures), (2) *auditory* (listening), and (3) *physical* (doing things). People often use several learning styles to gain new knowledge or skills. Ask how the patient likes to learn and has learned effectively in the past. Identify those who have low health literacy or do not read. The patient may tell you that they like to learn from television. Assess *ehealth literacy.* This is the degree that patients use digital information (e.g., webinars, online health tools) and communication technologies (e.g., online communication with HCP, online support groups) to improve their health (Fig. 4.3).[19] When possible, use the patient's and caregiver's preferred learning style in developing teaching plans.

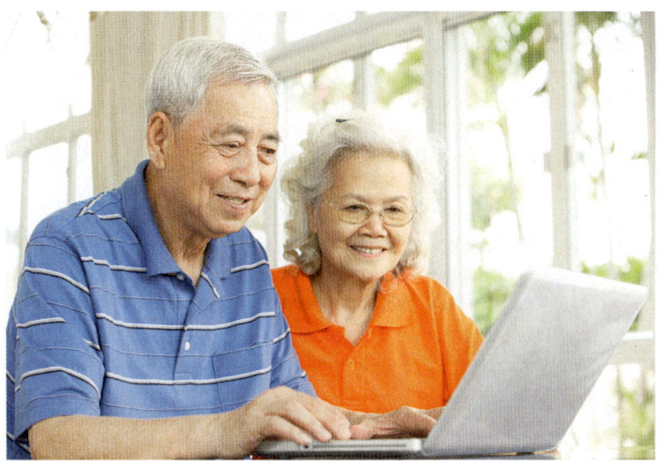

Fig. 4.3 Older couple accessing online health information. (© monkeybusinessimages/iStock/Thinkstock.)

Clinical Problems

Clinical problems for the patient and caregiver related to teaching include:

- Deficient knowledge
- Literacy problem

Planning

Prioritize the patient's learning needs and agree on learning goals. If the patient is not able to take part, then involve caregiver(s) in planning.

Setting Goals

Set clear and measurable learning goals (Table 4.6). Learning goals relate to the intended outcome of the learning process, guide the choice of teaching strategies, and help evaluate the patient's progress. Learning goals are parallel to patient outcomes in the nursing care plan (NCP). Most settings have standardized NCPs with preset goals and interventions for specific learning needs. Modify standard NCPs based on the patient's unique sociocultural and learner characteristics.

Choosing Teaching Strategies

Factors that influence the choice of teaching strategies are (1) patient characteristics (e.g., learning style, education background, culture, language skills), (2) subject matter, and (3) available resources. Table 4.7 summarizes learner characteristics and recommended teaching approaches based on the generation of the patient or caregiver.

Consider various strategies (Table 4.8) in the teaching plan. We often use multiple teaching strategies to improve learning (Fig. 4.4). Discussion is the most common type of interaction used in teaching patients and caregivers. A type of group teaching involves *peer teaching,* as occurs in support groups. Patients dealing with common problems such as cancer,

TABLE 4.6 Writing Learning Goals

Elements of Learning Goals

Learning goals are written statements that define exactly how patients demonstrate their knowledge of the content. Goals address the following questions:

1. ***Who will perform the activity or acquire the desired behavior?***
   Examples:
   - I (the patient) will
   - I (the caregiver) will
   - We (patient's family/caregivers) will
2. ***What is the behavior the learner will exhibit to show mastery of the goal?***
   Examples:
   - List the symptoms.
   - Self-administer an insulin injection.
   - Choose from a hospital menu.
3. ***What are the conditions under which the behavior will be demonstrated?***
   Examples:
   - In front of the nurse
   - From a random list
   - Using sterile technique
4. ***What are the specific criteria that will be used to measure success, such as time and degree of accuracy?***
   Examples:
   - With 100% accuracy
   - Over the next week
   - Before discharge

Verbs in Learning Goals

Avoid vague, ambiguous verbs that are hard to measure:	*Use verbs that have precise descriptions with few interpretations:*
• Appreciate	• Choose
• Enjoy	• Describe
• Feel	• Demonstrate
• Learn	• Identify
• Know	• List
• Understand	• Perform
• Value	

Poorly and Well-Written Learning Goals

Example of Poorly Written Learning Goal	**Examples of Well-Written Learning Goals**
• The patient will understand the importance of managing their own colostomy. *Analysis:* It is not clear how the patient will show that they "understand" the importance of managing their colostomy, when and to whom they will demonstrate this behavior, or what criteria will be used to determine whether the goal has been met.	• The patient will describe to the nurse the basic steps for changing the colostomy pouch and skin barrier by 2/14/25. • Using correct technique, the patient will empty their colostomy pouch when one-third full. • The caregiver will perform colostomy care, including changing the pouch and skin barrier. • Given a list of signs and symptoms related to complications of a colostomy, the patient and caregiver will identify signs and symptoms to report to a health care provider before discharge. *Analysis:* When learning goals are clear and specific and documented in the patient's record, all members of the health care team can work together to achieve the same outcomes.

alcoholism, and eating disorders can receive help from peer teaching.

Adapt your methods when teaching patients with a disability. Plan to modify teaching methods to meet the needs of patients with cognitive impairment, hearing loss, limited manual dexterity, or vision loss. Magnifying glasses, bright lighting, and materials printed in a large font may help those with impaired vision read teaching materials. Providing more visual information can help people with hearing loss. Using adaptive equipment may help those with problems performing manual skills. Table 4.9 presents strategies for teaching patients who have disabilities.

Learning materials. Use learning materials in multiple formats. Learn what resources are available in your agency and from support services and professional groups. Videos are helpful, particularly when teaching visual content such as the steps of a procedure (e.g., giving an injection). The health care agency's television system may show patient teaching programs on demand or on a rotating schedule (Fig. 4.4).

Printed materials are useful, especially for those whose preferred learning style is reading. Some health organizations, such as the American Cancer Society (ACS) and the AHA, provide free, high-quality patient education materials. Some government organizations, such as the National Institutes of Health and the Centers for Disease Control and Prevention, have free learning materials for patients and caregivers. These materials can be used with other teaching strategies. For instance, after a discussion on the health effects of smoking, material from the ACS can reinforce the information.

When writing new teaching materials, use techniques to keep the text at a 5th-grade reading level. These include (1) organize the content logically; (2) highlight or place key information in bold or italics; (3) use short, common words of 1 or 2 syllables; (4) define medical words in simple language; (5) keep sentences short, between 10 and 15 words; (6) use pictures or drawings; and (7) use active voice as you would normally speak.[13] You can check written materials for readability level using word processing (e.g., Microsoft Word) or other online (e.g., www.wordscount.info) programs.

Using technology. Patients may use the Internet and other digital technology (e.g., smartphones) to obtain information and manage their health. Patients can quickly do an online search or open a software application for access to information about diseases, drugs, treatments, and surgeries. Help patients sift through the information and determine whether it is valid, reliable, and usable. Encourage patients to use websites maintained by the government, universities, or reputable health organizations (e.g., American Diabetes Association, AHA, ACS, National Institutes of Health). Teach patients to search for valid health information. Organizations dedicated to improving the quality of life for older adults publish guides to help evaluate online health information (e.g., www.mlanet.org/resources/userguide.html).

The quantity and complexity of digital health care technology available to you and your patients will continue to increase.

TABLE 4.7 Learner Characteristics and Teaching Strategies by Generation

Birth Year	Learner Characteristics	Recommended Teaching Strategies
Generation Z, iGen Late 1990s to mid-2010s	• Digital natives • Social learners or independent learners • Socially conscious • Hands-on or applied learning • Technology focused • Connected to the virtual world • Prefers instant feedback	• Use personal stories to engage learners • Integrate technology and social media in teaching • Use self-paced learning activities • Provide hands-on learning experiences • Facilitate digital engagement with learning
Millennials (Generation Y) 1981–2000	• Digital natives • Prefer interactive and virtual environments • Technologically focused • Prefer structured learning • Accustomed to learning whatever, wherever, whenever • Prefers frequent feedback	• Integrate technology and social media in teaching • Incorporate health-related mobile apps and websites in teaching • Use active or group teaching approaches
Generation X (Xers, Digital Natives) 1965–1980	• Self-motivated to meet personal learning goals • Prefers regular, ongoing feedback	• Incorporate technology and social media in teaching • Engage in active learning • Integrate health-related mobile applications and websites in teaching
Baby Boomers 1946–1964	• Digital immigrants • Views teacher as authority • Prefers comprehensive feedback	• Assess health literacy and consider strategies as appropriate • Consider lecture or lecture-discussion (e.g., PowerPoint presentation) • Use patient education TV channels • Provide printed materials

Compiled from Oermann ME, DeGagne JC, Phillips BC: *Teaching in nursing and role of the educator: the complete guide to best practice in teaching, evaluation, and curriculum development,* ed 3, New York, 2022, Springer; and Chunta K, Shellenbarger T, Chicca J: Generation Z students in the online environment, *Nurse Educ* 46:87, 2021.

Telehealth, a broad term that refers to the delivery of health-related services and information via telecommunications technologies, allows for (1) remote HCP-patient consultations *(telemedicine);* (2) monitoring physical parameters, such as vital signs, weight, heart rhythm, and glucose; and (3) ongoing patient teaching.

There are disparities in access to digital health information for those with lower income, with some types of disabilities, and in some geographic locations. These patients may benefit from community or government programs that provide Internet access and education on how to use digital health care technologies, such as video-conferencing services for telehealth, patient portals for scheduling appointments and accessing health information, and health tracking applications.

Implementation

During the implementation phase, use the planned strategies to present information and teach new skills. Determine how the patient can participate based on the assessment of the physical, psychologic, sociocultural, and learner characteristics. Whenever possible and appropriate, involve the caregiver(s) in the teaching-learning process.

Evaluation

Evaluation, the last step in the learning process, is a measure of the degree to which the patient has achieved the learning goals. You can use various evaluation techniques (Table 4.10). Use techniques such as "teach back" to determine the knowledge and skill levels of the patient and/or caregiver throughout the teaching and learning process (Fig. 4.5). If goals are not reached, reassess the patient and revise the teaching plan as needed.

Avoid assumptions about a patient's knowledge and skills. Confirm prior knowledge while you are teaching and evaluating new skills.

Long-term evaluation of learning goals often requires follow-up after discharge. Provide a written schedule of visits and referrals before the patient leaves the hospital or clinic. Share this information with the caregiver(s) so that everyone involved in the patient's long-term progress has the same information.

TABLE 4.8 Teaching Strategies

Description	Advantages	Limitations
Discussion ("Teach Back")		
• Purpose is to exchange points of view about a topic or to arrive at a decision or conclusion • Can be done with patient, with patient and caregiver, or with group • *Example:* Weight loss	• Allows for an active exchange of information and experiences among participants • Good when patients have experience with subject and have information to share • Nonthreatening format • Can use peers (patients with common problems) to teach	• May need more time depending on topic and number of participants
Lecture-Discussion		
• Useful when group of patients and caregivers can benefit from basic information • Lecture part is short (i.e., 15–20 min) • Discussion ("teach back") follows lecture • *Example:* Basic principles of cardiac rehabilitation (e.g., exercise, nutrition)	• Combines short lecture to present basic information with time for discussion • Provision of printed material related to lecture content is useful and recommended	• Need to limit number of lecture topics to 3–5 • May need more time depending on topic and number of participants
Demonstration/Return Demonstration ("Show Back")		
• Purpose is to teach patient and caregiver to perform a skill • Return demonstration ("show back") can show patient's ability to perform skill (see Fig. 4.5) • *Examples:* Dressing change, injection	• Provides for learning and practice of physical skills • Dividing skill into series of smaller steps helps mastery and provides reinforcement	• May need more time for practice to master skill • Patients with limited manual dexterity may have difficulty
Use of Teaching Resources		
• Audiovisual aids to supplement teaching • Printed materials (e.g., brochures) • CDs/DVDs • Hospital-based TV (see Fig. 4.4) • Digital and communication technologies (e.g., mobile applications, online patient education programs, game-based education, online support groups) • Telehealth	• Enhances the presentation through visual and/or auditory stimulation • Best used in combination with other teaching strategies • Use of digital and communication technologies for health information is the preferred choice for many • Internet access in patient rooms is standard in most health care agencies • Health information can be given and reinforced to patients remotely	• Review materials for accuracy, reading level, completeness, before using • Evaluate websites, games, applications, programs, for validity of information • May not be appropriate for all learners (e.g., lack of interest, decreased mental capacity) • Finances (e.g., equipment purchase, Internet service) may be a limiting factor to using digital technology

Documentation is an essential part in the teaching-learning process. Record the teaching goals, strategies, and evaluation results so that the information is clear, complete, and available to the team members.

CHECK YOUR PRACTICE

Your patient is a 53-year-old male with type 1 diabetes who entered the hospital with a glucose level of 550 mg/dL (30.53 mmol/L). He is now stable and soon will be discharged.

You prepare his insulin and plan to give him the syringe to let him do his own injection. Before you go to his room, your preceptor suggests that you watch him prepare the insulin and give the injection. This puzzles you because he has had diabetes for 32 years and should know how to do it.

When you go to his room, you ask him to prepare the insulin injection ("show back"). You notice that he filled the syringe with 30 units of insulin and 10 units of air instead of 40 units of insulin. After correcting the dose and questioning the patient more fully ("teach back"), you wonder what happened.

What are possible reasons that he did not draw up the correct amount of insulin?

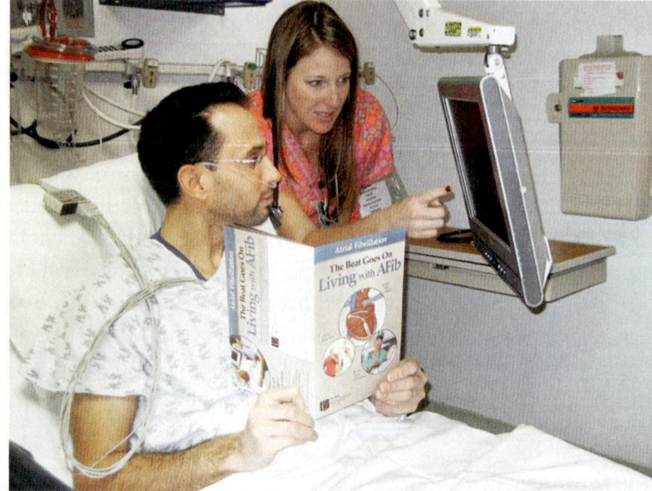

Fig. 4.4 Effective teaching using a variety of strategies (written materials, computer-based patient education programs). (Courtesy Linda Bucher, RN, PhD, CEN, CNE, Staff Nurse, Virtua Memorial Hospital, Mt. Holly, NJ.)

TABLE 4.9 Teaching Patients Who Have Disabilities

Hearing Loss[20]

- Sit in front of the patient at eye level with the light shining on your face
- Use assistive listening devices to amplify sound
- Speak slowly and clearly, using short, simple sentences
- Create a quiet environment that eliminates or minimizes background noises
- Assess patient's preferred communication method (sign language or lip reading)
- If patient prefers to use sign language:
  - Leave as much freedom as possible for their dominant hand to allow for signing
  - Use a sign language interpreter to preserve patient privacy and confidentiality
  - If using a sign language interpreter, speak to the patient, not the interpreter
- If the patient prefers lipreading:
  - Make sure the patient can see your lips
  - Face the patient and maintain eye contact
  - Ensure there is good lighting on your lips
  - Speak in a normal rhythm and tone
  - Use facial expressions to help convey meaning

Limited Manual Dexterity

- Provide assistive (ease of use) devices to help the patient perform necessary tasks to perform a skill

Mild Cognitive Impairment[21]

- Explain what you will be doing
- Use simple wording
- Present one instruction at a time
- Ask yes/no questions
- Avoid open-ended questions
- Be patient
- Answer repeated questions as if it were the first time the question was asked
- Reinforce instructions often
- Create a quiet environment and minimize distractions

Vision Loss[22,23]

- Use low-vision aids, such as magnifiers, high-power reading glasses, or handheld or mounted telescopes
- Use technology, such as screen readers that read text on the computer screen using a speech synthesizer or convert text to braille
- Use electronic tablets or smartphones with adjustable text size
- Use large-print publications
- Ensure that there is good lighting in the environment
- Minimize distractions and eliminate background noise
- Give educational materials available in braille
- Provide verbal or tactile instruction instead of written instruction

TABLE 4.10 Evaluating Patient and Caregiver Learning

Technique	Strategy and Examples

Observe patient or caregiver directly	• Ask person to show you how to change the dressing
	• Return demonstration ("show back") determines whether:
	  • Skill has been mastered
	  • Further instruction is needed
	  • Patient and caregiver are ready for new or more content

Observe verbal and nonverbal cues	• Teaching may have to be delayed, more teaching needed, or different strategy used if patient or caregiver:
	  • Asks you to repeat instructions
	  • Loses eye contact
	  • Begins to doze in chair or bed
	  • Becomes restless or fidgety
	  • Does not speak English

Ask open-ended questions ("teach back")	• Open-ended questions provide more information about understanding than closed-ended questions, which need only a "yes" or "no"
	• Ask questions such as:
	  • "How often do you need to change the dressing?"
	  • "What will you do if you develop chest pain at home?"

Talk with caregiver ("teach back")	• Involve caregiver in the evaluation process
	• Ask questions such as:
	  • "What medications are they taking?"
	  • "When do they use their oxygen?"

Seek the patient's self-evaluation of progress	• Ask patient's opinion about their progress • Assess what evidence the patient has that the goals are being met • Assess if the patient is ready to learn new material

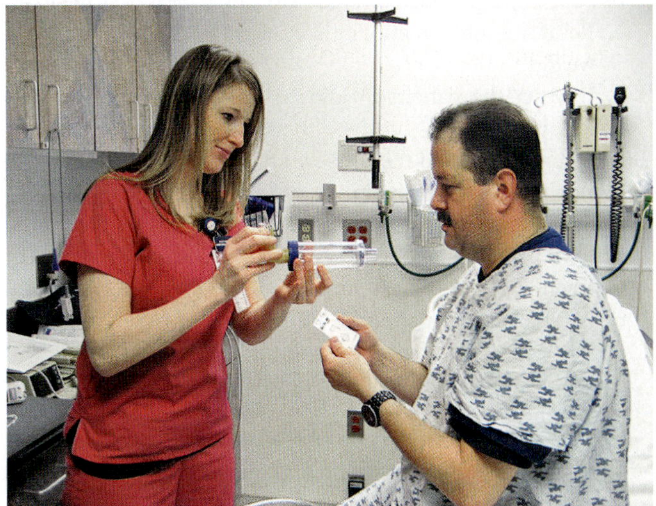

Fig. 4.5 Teaching using discussion ("teach back") and demonstration/return demonstration ("show back") increases successful learning. (Courtesy Linda Bucher, RN, PhD, CEN, CNE, Staff Nurse, Virtua Memorial Hospital, Mt. Holly, NJ.)

CASE STUDY

Patient and Caregiver Teaching

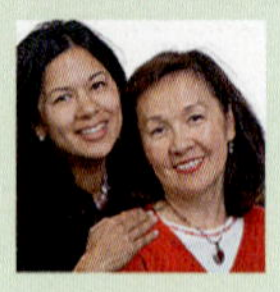
(© azndc/iStock.)

Patient Profile

M.L., a 60-year-old Asian female, is admitted to the hospital with a diagnosis of exacerbation of chronic obstructive pulmonary disease (COPD).

Subjective Data

- History of COPD for 10 years. Admitted twice in the past 8 months for COPD exacerbations. Reports a chronic cough. Denies any recent change in sputum color. States: "I stopped smoking last year, but my son-in-law smokes in the house."
- Medical history: Gastroesophageal reflux disease; macular degeneration in right eye.
- Social history: Widowed 5 years ago. Lives with daughter and son-in-law, who work full time. Cares for 2 young grandchildren after school. English is M.L.'s second language.

Objective Data

Physical Assessment

- Alert, oriented, anxious, thin female with dyspnea on minimal exertion. Speaks in short phrases. States: "I have no energy."
- Oxygen via nasal cannula at 2 L/min
- Weight 100 lb, height 5 ft 2 in

Diagnostic Studies

- Chest x-ray negative for acute infection
- O_2 saturation via pulse oximetry during 6-min walk test on room air = 83%

Interprofessional Care

- Medications: bronchodilator therapy (inpatient nebulizer therapy, inhalers at home), oral corticosteroids
- Continuous home O_2 therapy 2 L/min via nasal cannula
- Pulmonary rehabilitation: inpatient and outpatient

Discussion Questions

1. ***Recognize:*** What potential challenges might you expect when planning to teach M.L.? How would you manage them?
2. ***Analyze:*** What factors (e.g., sociocultural, physical, psychologic) noted in the assessment may influence M.L.'s response to teaching?
3. ***Plan/Prioritize:*** Choose 2 of M.L.'s priority learning needs. Develop a teaching plan for each of these needs.
4. ***Evaluate:*** What assessment data would you collect to decide if teaching was effective?

Answers available at http://evolve.elsevier.com/Lewis/medsurg.

BRIDGE TO NCLEX EXAMINATION

The number of the question corresponds to the same-numbered outcome at the beginning of the chapter.

1. A patient who is overweight tells the nurse that they know they should lose weight. Which nursing action would match this patient's readiness for change?
   a. Confirm that the patient is serious about losing weight.
   b. Assess the patient's awareness of their dietary behaviors.
   c. Reinforce information that supports a need to lose weight.
   d. Instruct the patient to join an organized group weight-loss program.

2. Which action would the nurse *prioritize* when limited time is available for patient teaching?
   a. Setting realistic goals that are important to the patient
   b. Referring the patient to a nurse educator for patient teaching
   c. Asking more experienced nurses how to teach faster and more efficiently
   d. Providing reading materials for the patient instead of discussing the information

3. Which rationale supports including caregivers in patient teaching? (**Select all that apply.**)
   a. Caregivers provide all the care for patients after discharge.
   b. They might feel rejected if they are not included in the teaching.
   c. Patients have better outcomes when their caregivers are involved.
   d. The patient may be too ill or too stressed to fully understand the teaching.
   e. Caregivers are responsible for the overall management of the patient's care.

4. Which patient characteristic enhances learning outcomes?
   a. Feeling moderate anxiety
   b. Developing high self-efficacy
   c. Laughing about the current health problem
   d. Being in the precontemplation stage of change

5. Which goal applies when planning to teach a female patient about ways to relieve symptoms of menopause?
   a. Prevent the development of future disease.
   b. Provide information on possible treatments.
   c. Maintain the patient's current state of health.
   d. Change the patient's beliefs about herbal supplements.

6. A patient tells the nurse that they enjoy talking with others and sharing experiences but often falls asleep when reading. Which teaching strategy would the nurse plan for this patient?
   a. Formal lecture
   b. Journal writing
   c. Digital technology
   d. Small-group discussion

7. The nurse taught a caregiver how to administer insulin. Which action would the nurse take to evaluate the caregiver's learning?
   a. Monitor the patient's glucose readings.
   b. Arrange for follow-up with a home care nurse.
   c. Ask the caregiver to "show back" the ability to administer insulin.
   d. Assess what the caregiver thought was effective about the teaching.

1. c; 2. a; 3. c, d; 4. b; 5. b; 6. d; 7. c.

For rationales to these answers and even more NCLEX review questions, visit http://evolve.elsevier.com/Lewis/medsurg.

REFERENCES

To access the References for this chapter, please scan the QR code with a mobile device.

5

Chronic Illness and Older Adults

Sherry A. Greenberg

http://evolve.elsevier.com/Lewis/medsurg/

CONCEPTUAL FOCUS

Cognition
Family Dynamics
Functional Ability
Mobility
Nutrition
Sensory Perception

LEARNING OUTCOMES

1. Explain the characteristics of a chronic illness.
2. Describe the prevention and major causes of chronic illness.
3. Describe the demographics of aging.
4. Explain the needs of special populations of older adults.
5. Describe types of elder mistreatment and appropriate nursing interventions.
6. Distinguish among care alternatives and ways to create systems of care to meet older adults' needs.
7. Describe common problems of older adults related to hospitalization and acute illness and the nurse's role in assisting them.
8. Describe the nurse's role in health promotion and managing the special needs of older adults.

KEY TERMS

ageism
elder mistreatment (EM)
ethnogeriatrics
frail older adult
gerontologic nursing
Medicaid
Medicare
old-old adult
young-old adult

This chapter discusses issues related to chronic illness and aging. The number of older adults is growing rapidly. You need to consider their multiple complex health care conditions and needs when planning and providing patient care. Functional ability in older adults with chronic illness is interrelated with several concepts. These include mobility, perfusion, nutrition, cognition, and sensory perception. Managing a chronic illness greatly affects the lives of older adults, families, and caregivers. Family dynamics and caregiving shape the care provided to those who need help meeting their needs.

CHRONIC ILLNESS

Illness can be categorized as either acute or chronic (Table 5.1). The US health care system faces a growing burden of chronic illness as the population ages. Chronic illnesses account for 70% of all deaths in the United States. Chronic illness results in limitations in physical functioning, work productivity, and quality of life for nearly 1 out of 10 Americans (Fig. 5.1). Many older adults live with at least 1 chronic illness. Many live with multiple chronic conditions. In 2020, 20% of older adults age 65 to 74 assessed their health as fair or poor, compared with 27% of those age 75 and older.[1] A large portion of health care dollars goes toward treating chronic illnesses.

Societal changes and social determinants of health contribute to the increase in chronic illnesses. These include lack of physical activity, poor nutrition, and tobacco and alcohol use.[2]

Trajectory of Chronic Illness

The person with a chronic illness can move from a level of optimum functioning, with the illness well controlled, to a period of physical instability. Corbin and Strauss proposed a view of chronic illness as a trajectory (Fig. 5.2) with overlapping phases (Table 5.2).[3] This trajectory depicts the common course of most chronic conditions. Corbin and Strauss also identified the 7 tasks of those who are chronically ill (Table 5.3). We discuss these tasks next.

Preventing and Managing a Crisis

Most chronic illnesses have the potential for an acute exacerbation of symptoms. This may result in further disability or death. Examples include patients with heart disease who have another myocardial infarction or patients with asthma who have a severe attack. A major task for patients and caregivers is to learn to prevent or manage the crisis. First, they need to understand the potential for the crisis to occur. Second, they need to know ways to prevent or modify the threat. This often involves adhering to a prescribed medical and overall health plan. Patients need to know the signs and symptoms of the onset of a crisis or exacerbation. Depending on the chronic illness, signs and symptoms may occur suddenly (e.g., bleeding in patients with inflammatory bowel disease) or slowly (e.g., heart failure in persons with untreated hypertension). It is important for patients and caregivers to have a plan to manage a crisis that is likely to occur.

TABLE 5.1 Characteristics of Acute and Chronic Illness

Description	Characteristics
Acute Illness	
Diseases that have a rapid onset and short duration *Examples:* colds, influenza, acute gastroenteritis	• Usually self-limiting • Responds readily to treatment • Infrequent complications • After illness, return to previous level of functioning
Chronic Illness	
Diseases that are prolonged, do not resolve spontaneously, rarely cured completely *Examples:* Cancer, COPD, diabetes, heart disease, stroke	• Permanent impairments or deviations from normal • Irreversible pathologic changes • Residual disability • Special rehabilitation needed • Need for long-term medical and/or nursing management

COPD, Chronic obstructive pulmonary disease.

Carrying Out the Prescribed Treatment Plan

Treatment plans vary in the degree of difficulty and the impact they have on the person's lifestyle. Some plans may be perceived as challenging or time consuming, such as changing a dressing multiple times a day or following a toileting program. However, they generally save time, prevent complications, and improve outcomes.

Controlling Symptoms

An important task for those with chronic illnesses is to learn to control symptoms so that they can continue to do what matters to them. Some change their lifestyle by learning to plan. Persons with heart failure adjust the time they take diuretics when going out for the day to avoid needing to rush to a bathroom. Encourage independence in decision making and collaborating with the HCP about treatment plans Others may change their living space. Patients and their families need to learn about the pattern of symptoms, such as typical onset, duration, and

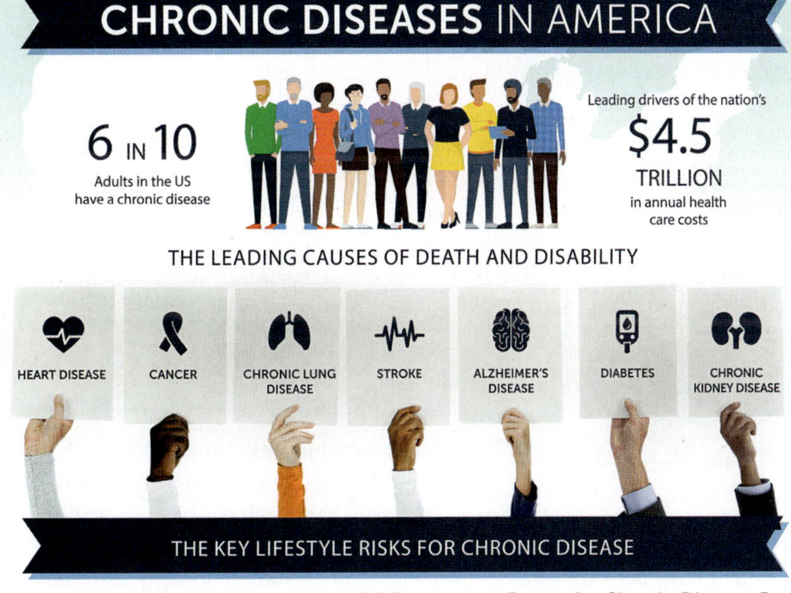

Fig. 5.1 Demographics of chronic illness. (From CDC's National Center for Chronic Disease Prevention and Health Promotion [NCCDPHP].)

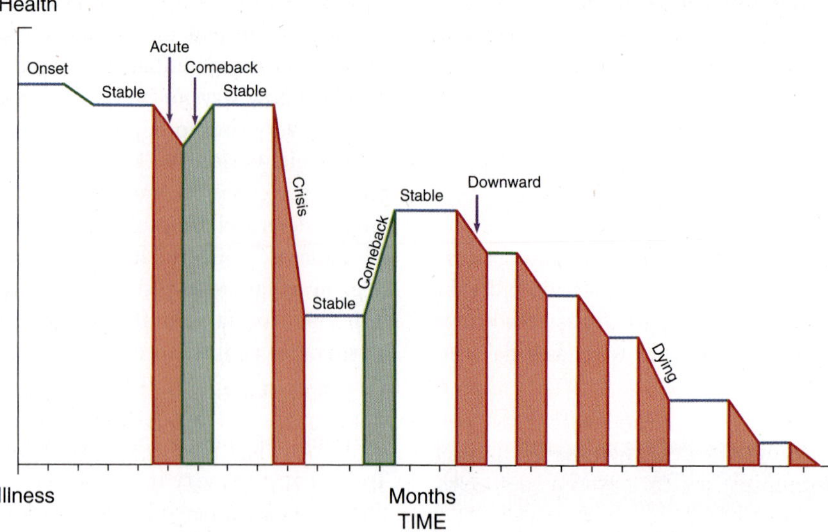

Fig. 5.2 The chronic illness trajectory is a theoretical model of chronic illness. The trajectory model of chronic illness recognizes that chronic illness will have many phases (Table 5.3). (From Woog P: *The chronic illness trajectory framework: the Corbin and Strauss nursing model*, New York, 1992, Springer.)

TABLE 5.2 Chronic Illness Trajectory

Phases	Description
Onset	• Signs and symptoms are present • Disease diagnosed
Stable	• Illness course and symptoms controlled by treatment plan • Maintains daily activities
Acute	• Active illness with severe and unrelieved symptoms or complications • Hospitalization may be needed for management
Comeback	• Gradual return to an acceptable way of life
Crisis	• Life-threatening situation occurs • Emergency services are necessary
Unstable	• Unable to keep symptoms or disease course under control • Life disrupted while patient works to regain stability • Hospitalization not required
Downward	• Gradual and progressive deterioration in physical or mental status • Accompanied by increasing disability and symptoms • Continuous changes in daily life activities
Dying	• Patient has to relinquish life interests and activities, let go, and die peacefully • Immediate weeks, days, hours preceding death

From Woog P: *The chronic illness trajectory framework: The Corbin and Strauss nursing model*, New York, 1992, Springer.

severity, so that they can make lifestyle changes and maintain safety.

Reordering Time

Persons with chronic illness often report having too much or too little time. Treatment plans that take large amounts of time may require changing schedules or eliminating other activities. For example, patients with a new ileostomy need to plan for increased time in the bathroom to change the drainage bag.

TABLE 5.3 Tasks of People With Chronic Illnesses

- Prevent and manage a crisis
- Carry out prescribed treatment plan
- Control symptoms
- Reorder time
- Adjust to changes in course of disease
- Prevent social isolation
- Attempt to normalize interactions with others

From Corbin JM, Strauss A: A nursing model for chronic illness management based upon the trajectory framework, *Sch Inq Nurs Pract* 5:155, 1991.

Adjusting to Changes in the Course of Disease

Some diseases have unpredictable courses that make planning activities difficult. Part of the person's task is to develop a personal identity that includes the chronic illness and to adjust to the necessary lifestyle changes. For example, a person with a mechanical heart valve taking warfarin may need to avoid sports that have a high risk for injury.

Preventing Social Isolation

Social isolation may occur with chronic illness. The person may choose to withdraw from social activities. For example, a person with aphasia after a stroke may not want to take part in social activities because they are embarrassed about communication issues. Sometimes others withdraw from the ill person.

Attempting to Normalize Interactions With Others

Some persons with chronic illness try to manage symptoms so that they can hide their disabilities or disfigurement. This may involve wearing a prosthesis. They may want to show they can function the same as a person without a disability or chronic illness. An example is a person with heart failure who stops walking to catch their breath but appears to be looking at a store display.

NURSING MANAGEMENT: CHRONIC ILLNESS

Health Promotion

Chronic illnesses are often preventable. *Primary prevention* refers to measures such as eating a healthy diet, getting proper exercise, and receiving immunizations that prevent a specific disease. Immunizations include influenza, pneumococcal, herpes zoster, COVID-19, tetanus/diphtheria/pertussis (Td/Tdap), and hepatitis A and B. *Secondary prevention* refers to actions aimed at health screening and early detection of disease. Examples include colon cancer and breast cancer screening. *Tertiary prevention* refers to activities that limit disease progression. These include rehabilitation and chronic disease self-management programs.

Chronic Care

Diagnosis and treatment of the acute phase or acute exacerbations of a chronic illness sometimes take place in a hospital. Other phases of a chronic illness are regularly assessed and managed in an ambulatory care setting, at home, in an assisted living facility, or in a skilled nursing facility.

An assessment of health status, at least annually, includes a person's level of daily function and their perception of relative health, function, and illness. This assessment includes activities of daily living (ADLs), such as bathing, dressing, eating, and toileting, and instrumental ADLs (IADLs). These include activities such as shopping, preparing food, housekeeping, doing laundry, taking medications, and handling finances.

Because most chronic illnesses are treated in an ambulatory care setting, it is important for patients and caregivers to understand and manage their own health. The term *self-management* refers to the person's ability to manage their health, especially in response to living with a chronic illness. It includes the ability to manage symptoms, treatment plans, physical and psychosocial consequences, and lifestyle changes. Self-management is done in conjunction with the family and HCP.

You play a key role in managing patients with chronic illness. This includes conducting a complete history and physical assessment, teaching patients and caregivers about the treatment plan, implementing symptom management plans, and evaluating patient outcomes.

Family caregivers (e.g., spouses, partners, adult children) often have important roles. The ideal situation is when family caregivers work together with the patient to manage any chronic problems. This collaboration begins under the direction of the health care team at the time of diagnosis. When the caregiver is a spouse or partner who is also older, they may have a chronic illness or multiple chronic conditions as well. This may add complexity to the coordination of care.

OLDER ADULTS

DEMOGRAPHICS OF AGING

The growth of the older adult population continues to outpace the rest of the population. More than 1 in 6 US residents, or 16.8% of the population, was age 65 or older in 2020.[4] This is projected to reach 95 million in 2060. The 65 to 74 age group represented over half of the 65 and over population in 2020. This group had the largest growth of an older adult age group since 2010 (Fig. 5.3).

We predict life expectancy to continue to increase. By 2060, life expectancy is projected to be 83.9 years for males and 87.3 years for females.[4] We do not know the reason for this difference. The increase in life span is the result of new therapies and a greater emphasis on health promotion, early detection, and better care management. Interesting to note is that in 2020, people reaching age 65 had an average life expectancy of another 18.5 years, a decrease from 19.6 years in 2019. We think this is because of mortality from COVID-19, unintentional injuries, heart disease, homicide, and diabetes.[1]

The number of persons age 65 and older from racial and ethnically diverse populations continues to grow. People of Hispanic ethnicity, who may be of any race, represented 9% of the older population in 2020.[1] By 2050, we estimate that this number will increase to 19.5% of the population. Asians are expected to increase to 8.4% and Blacks to increase to 11.8%.[5] Overall, the number of older adults of racial or ethnicity populations in the United States is projected to be 27.7 million by 2040 (34% of older adults), an increase from 13.5 million in 2020 (24% of older adults).[1]

The terms **young-old adult** (65 to 74 years of age) and **old-old adult** (85 years of age and older) describe 2 groups of older adults with distinct characteristics, needs, and living arrangements. Young-old adults typically are healthier and independent and maintain good cognitive function. The old-old adult is often a widowed, divorced, or single female dependent on family for support or care. Many old-old adults have outlived children, spouses or partners, and siblings.

The **frail older adult** is usually over age 75 with multiple physical, cognitive, and/or mental health conditions. These often interfere with self-management and the ability to perform daily activities independently.

ATTITUDES TOWARD AGING

Who is old? The answer often depends on your age and attitude. Your "real" age is set by a date in time. Many factors influence how "old" you feel. These include emotional and physical health, development stage, socioeconomic status, and culture. We all age. As we do, we have different life experiences.

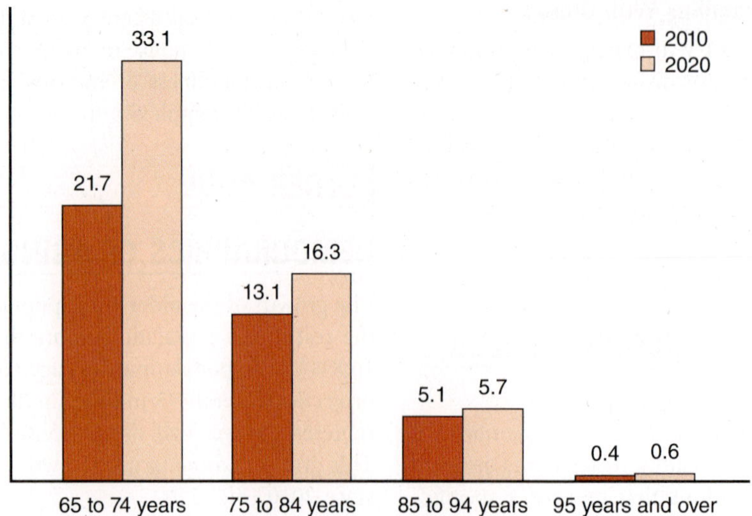

Source: U.S. Census Bureau, 2020 Census Demographic and Housing Characteristics File (DHC).

Fig. 5.3 Population size of older age groups, 2010 and 2020. (Data from U.S. Census Bureau, 2020 Census Demographic and Housing Characteristics [DHC].)

The accumulation of these differences makes older adults more diverse than any other age group.

As you assess older adults, consider and value their diversity and life history. Assess their feelings of what it means to be an older adult. Most older adults report having good-to-excellent health despite having a chronic condition. However, those with poor health often report a higher perceived age and lower sense of well-being. Age is important, but it may not be the most relevant factor in determining the appropriate care of an individual older adult.

Ageism is a negative attitude based on age. Ageism leads to discrimination and disparities in the care given to older adults. The media often supports myths and stereotypes about aging. If you have negative attitudes, it may be because you fear your own aging process. Or you may not be knowledgeable about aging and the health care needs of the older adult. Consider taking time to self-reflect about your own feelings about aging.

BIOLOGIC AGING

From a biologic view, *aging* reflects the changes that occur over time. Biologic aging is a multifactorial process involving genetics, diet, and environment. In part, we view biologic aging as a balance of positive and negative factors (Fig. 5.4). Research is directed at increasing older adults' average life span, functional status, and quality of life. The hope is that we can develop new antiaging therapies to slow down or reverse age-related changes that result in chronic illness and disability.

Age-related changes affect every body system. These changes are normal, common, and occur as people age. The age at which specific changes occur differs from person to person and within the same person. For instance, a person who has gray hair at age 55 may have fairly unwrinkled skin at age 80. As a nurse, you will assess for age-related changes. Table 5.4 shows where to find tables outlining age-related assessment findings.

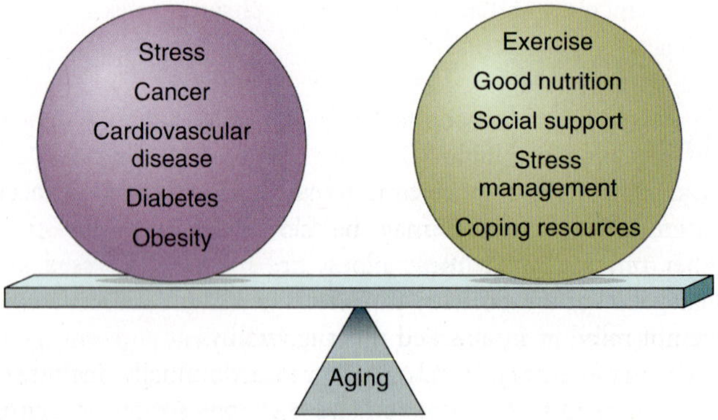

Fig. 5.4 The aging process can be viewed as a balance between negative and positive factors.

SPECIAL OLDER ADULT POPULATIONS

Chronically Ill Older Adults

Living with chronic illness is a reality for many older adults. The incidence of chronic illness triples after age 45. Most people 65 years of age and older have at least 1 chronic condition. Many have multiple conditions. Leading chronic conditions among adults age 65 and older include arthritis, heart disease, hypertension, cancer, chronic obstructive pulmonary disease, and diabetes.[1] In 2020, 30% of older adults age 65 and over were obese.[1] Other common chronic conditions include Alzheimer disease, vision and hearing deficits, osteoporosis, Parkinson disease, and depression.

TABLE 5.4 GERONTOLOGIC ASSESSMENT DIFFERENCES

Tables Throughout the Book

Title	Chapter
Adaptations in Physical Assessment Techniques	3
Auditory System	23
Cardiovascular System	35
Cognitive Function	5
Hematologic Studies	33
Immune System	14
Endocrine System	52
Gastrointestinal System	43
Integumentary System	24
Musculoskeletal System	66
Nervous System	60
Reproductive Systems	55
Respiratory System	27
Urinary System	49
Visual System	22

TABLE 5.5 GERONTOLOGIC ASSESSMENT DIFFERENCES

Cognitive Function

Effect of Aging	Cognitive Function
Improves with aging	• Vocabulary and verbal reasoning • Crystallized intelligence (ability to use skills, knowledge, experience)
Declines during middle age	• Mental performance speed • Synthesis of new information • Fluid intelligence (ability to think logically and solve problems in new situations)
Declines during old age	• Short-term recall memory
Constant (no change with aging)	• Long-term recall memory

Cognitively Impaired Older Adults

Most healthy older adults have no noticeable decline in cognitive abilities (Table 5.5). They may have a mild decline in memory and need more time to recall events or new information. New learning may be slower. This differs from cognitive impairment. Refer older adults with memory loss to their HCP for an evaluation. Teach them to use memory aids, attempt recall in a calm and quiet environment, and engage in enhancing memory. Memory aids include clocks, calendars, notes, marked pillboxes, safety alarms, and wearable technology. Memory techniques include word association, mental imaging, and mnemonics.

Dementia, delirium, and depression can occur and may coexist in older adults. Declining physical health and acute illness influence cognition. For example, an older adult who has surgery may have an acute change in mental status called *delirium.*[6] Delirium superimposed on dementia may signify an acute condition such as heart failure, electrolyte imbalance, or infection. Hence, it is important to distinguish the signs and symptoms of each. Cognitive impairment, delirium, and dementia are discussed in Chapter 64.

Rural Older Adults

Key barriers to health care access for rural older adults are transportation, limited supply of health care, lack of quality health care, social isolation, and financial limitations. Particularly vulnerable are older adults of racial or ethnic minorities living in rural areas, who have even less access to HCPs. Older adults who live in rural areas may be less likely to engage in health-promoting activities.

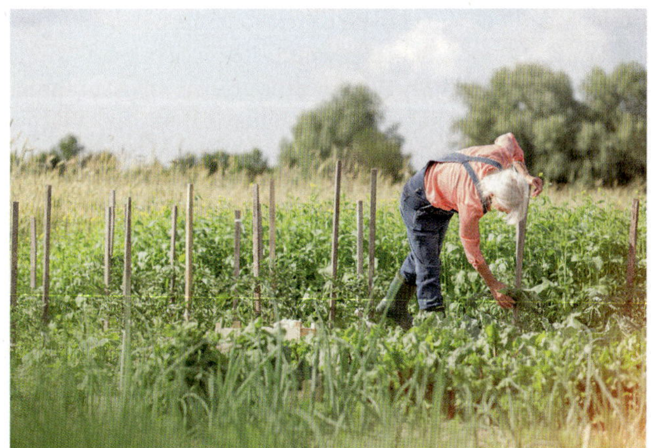

Fig. 5.5 Older adults living in rural areas often enjoy outside activities, such as gardening. (© Caiaimage/Agnieszka Wozniak/iStock.com.)

When you work with older adults in rural areas, recognize lifestyle values and practices of rural life (Fig. 5.5). In planning care, be aware that transportation is the top barrier to health care for rural older adults. Alternative service approaches such as DVDs, radio, community centers, and church events may be used to promote healthy practices or to conduct health screenings (Fig. 5.6). Older adults are increasingly using technology in their daily lives. Most older adults use the Internet and cell phones. Telehealth has enhanced the ability to provide care to those who are more isolated.[7]

Homeless Older Adults

The number of older adults who are homeless is increasing. Key factors associated with homelessness include (1) having a low income, (2) having reduced cognitive capacity, (3) living alone, and (4) living in a community that lacks affordable housing. Homeless older adults may be chronically homeless or recently homeless because of a crisis in either health, economic, or social status.

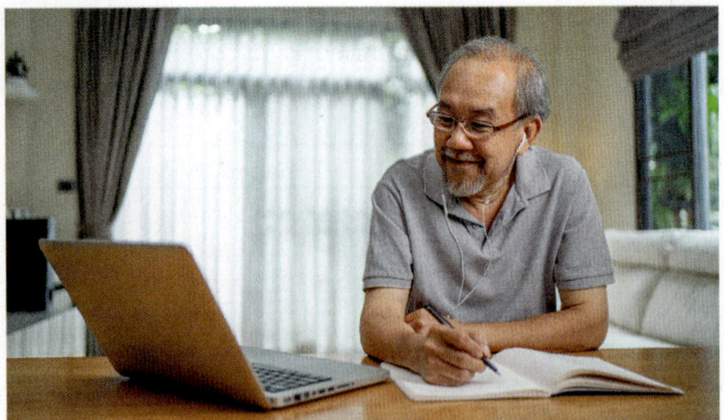

Fig. 5.6 Older adults are using computers more often and accessing health care information on the Internet. (© Kiwis/iStock.com.)

Mortality rates for homeless older adults are higher than those who have housing. Older homeless adults are at higher risk for more health problems because many aging network services are not designed to reach out to homeless people. They are less likely to use shelters or meal site services than younger homeless people. This may be because of fear of institutionalization. Care for homeless older adults requires an interprofessional approach (including nurses, physicians, social workers, clerical workers, and transporters) that links shelters with primary care, Medicare and Medicaid offices, pharmacies, senior centers, and Area Agencies on Aging. Long-term care placement is often an alternative to homelessness, especially when the person is cognitively impaired.

Frail Older Adults

Frailty is a common clinical syndrome seen in older adults. The Fried phenotype considers a person with 3 or more of these criteria as frail: (1) unintentional weight loss (10 pounds or more in a year), (2) self-reported exhaustion, (3) weakness (measured by grip strength), (4) slow walking speed, and (5) low level of physical activity.[8] Risk factors include disability, multiple chronic conditions, and dementia. People are more likely to become frail if they smoke, have a history of depression or long-term medical health problems, or are underweight. The old-old adult is most at risk for frailty, although many in this age group are healthy and robust.

Older frail adults often have declining function and decreasing daily energy. When stressful life events (e.g., death of a close friend) and daily strain (e.g., caring for an ill spouse) occur, frail older adults may have ineffective coping mechanisms. As a result, they may become ill themselves. Common health problems of frail older adults include limited mobility, sensory impairment, cognitive decline, and falls.

Frail older adults may tire easily and have little physical reserve. They are at risk for malnutrition, physical dependence, and institutionalization. Monitor frail older adults for adequate calorie, protein, iron, calcium, vitamin D, and fluid intake. Use the SCALES tool to assess the risk factors for poor nutrition status in older adults (Table 5.6). Consider how to meet an older adult's nutrition needs. Common interventions include home-delivered meals, dietary supplements, Supplemental Nutrition Assistance Program (SNAP), dental referrals, and vitamin supplements. Because some drugs affect appetite or interact with nutrients, obtain a thorough medication history. Nutrition is discussed in Chapter 44.

TABLE 5.6 SCALES: Nutrition Assessment of Older Adults

The acronym SCALES can remind you to assess important nutrition indicators:

Sadness, or mood change
Cholesterol, high
Albumin, low
Loss or gain of weight
Eating problems (e.g., mechanical problems, such as impaired swallowing, poor dentition)
Shopping and food preparation problems

Culturally Diverse Older Adults

The term **ethnogeriatrics** describes the specialty area of providing culturally competent care to older adults.[9] Support for older adults of racial or ethnic minority is most often found in the family, religious practices, and isolated geographic or community ethnic clusters. As American society changes, ethnic institutions and neighborhoods may also change. For a person with strong ethnic and cultural roots, there may be a loss of friends who speak the native language, a loss of the religious institution that supports social and ethnic activities, and a loss of stores that carry desired ethnic foods. This sense of loss is increased when children and others deny or ignore ethnic and cultural practices.

Older adults may live in neighborhoods where physical security and personal safety related to crime may be a concern. Those who identify with specific ethnic groups often have disproportionately lower incomes. They may not be able to afford Medicare deductibles or drugs needed to treat illnesses. Older adults from minority populations may use health care services less often compared with nonminority groups.[10]

Assess each older adult's ethnic and cultural background. Assume that ethnicity and culture are important and of value to them unless they tell you otherwise. A sense of respect and clear communication are critical for you to provide high-quality care. Culturally competent care is discussed in Chapter 2.

ELDER CARE

A network of services supports older adults in the community and health care agencies. In the United States most older adults are the beneficiaries of at least 1 social or governmental service. To understand the older adult's situation, learn about government structures that fund and regulate programs for older adults.

Family Caregivers

Many older adults need caregiving from family members. This includes those with multiple chronic conditions, those who need help with ADLs and IADLs, and persons with dementia. The most common caregivers are spouses, adult children, parents, grandparents, and life partners. Older adult females, age 65 or older, are the most common family caregivers. Many family caregivers care for themselves, their aging parents, and their children and grandchildren.

The caregiver usually takes on responsibilities gradually. For example, a caregiver may initially need only to adjust work schedules to accommodate a patient's health care appointments. Later, as the patient's needs become greater, the caregiver has to reduce work hours and provide more help with ADLs.

Caregiving is an experience for which most people are not prepared. It is common for caregivers to become physically, emotionally, and economically overwhelmed by the responsibilities and demands of caring for a loved one. The stress of caregiving may lead to emotional problems such as depression, anger, and resentment. Signs of caregiver stress include irritability, inability to concentrate, fatigue, and sleeplessness. The caregiver often experiences decreased social interactions and is at risk for social isolation. Multiple commitments, fatigue, and, at times, the patient's socially inappropriate behaviors contribute to the caregiver's social isolation. Stress can progress to burnout and result in patient negligence and abuse by the caregiver. Consider collaborating with a social worker if caregiver stress or strain is present and caregivers need respite.

Encourage caregivers to take care of themselves. Suggest journaling or joining a support group to help them share feelings. Remind caregivers that getting regular exercise and sleep and eating balanced meals will enhance their well-being. Encourage contact with others to give emotional support. Finally, humor is important. Sometimes its use by caregivers can provide distraction and relieve stress-filled situations.

Elder Mistreatment

Elder mistreatment (EM) describes intentional acts of omission or commission by a caregiver or "trusted other" that cause harm or serious risk for harm to a vulnerable older adult. EM may occur in community (home, assisted living facility) or long-term care (institutional) settings.

Between 2% and 10% of community-dwelling older adults in the United States are abused, neglected, or exploited by trusted others.[11] Although EM rates are similar in females and males, most victims are female because of the larger number of older females. Victims of EM have a mortality risk that is 3 times higher than those who are not mistreated. This higher risk may be the result of stress-related illnesses associated with prolonged mistreatment.

EM is a hidden problem. For every reported case in the community setting, more than 5 cases go unreported. Underreporting may be higher based on immigration status, ethnic background, or sexual orientation. Victims are unlikely to report mistreatment by "trusted others" because of isolation; impaired cognitive or physical function; feelings of shame, guilt, or self-blame; fear of reprisal; pressure from family members; fear of long-term care; or cultural norms. HCPs also underreport EM, possibly from a failure to suspect or recognize it, perceived inability to successfully intervene, desire to avoid responsibility for further action, or ageism.

Family members commit up to 90% of domestic EM. Adult children who abuse, neglect, or exploit their parents are usually dependent on them for housing and financial support, have a history of violence, are unemployed, and/or are disabled from substance use or mental illness. Abusive spouses or partners may either begin intimate partner violence at an older age or continue a lifelong pattern of abuse.

Many factors put community-dwelling older adults at risk for domestic EM. These include (1) physical or cognitive problems that lead to an inability to perform ADLs (and thus depend on others for care); (2) any psychiatric diagnoses, including dementia; (3) alcohol use; (4) decreased social support; (5) living with several household members other than a spouse; and (6) low income. In long-term care settings, the same factors that lead to institutionalization are risk factors for mistreatment by staff, visitors, and others. These include dependence on others for care because of physical or cognitive limitations.

Types of EM, characteristics, and manifestations are shown in Table 5.7. In institutional settings, EM also includes failure to follow the plan of care, unauthorized use of physical or chemical restraints, overuse or underuse of medication, or isolation as punishment.

Follow your agency's protocols for EM screening and interventions. Screen for mistreatment as part of the history and physical assessment. It is important that you interview people alone. If mistreatment is occurring, they may not disclose it in the presence of the person who is with them, especially if that person is the abuser. Be especially attentive to explanations about injuries that are not consistent with what you observe, contradictory explanations between the patient and caregiver, or behavior clues that suggest the patient is being threatened or intimidated. Other assessments and interventions are listed in Table 5.8. In most states, health care workers are among those mandated to report suspected or actual EM to adult protective services (APS) and/or law enforcement. Know your legal responsibilities by checking the laws in your state.

Self-Neglect

Most referrals made to APS are for self-neglect. Older adults who self-neglect are often unable to meet their basic needs and refuse help, have multiple untreated medical or psychiatric conditions, and live alone and often in squalor.[12] Older community-dwelling adults who self-neglect face a higher risk for mortality than peers who do not self-neglect. Nursing

TABLE 5.7 Types of Elder Mistreatment

Characteristic	Manifestations
Abandonment	
Desertion of an older person by a person who has assumed responsibility for providing care or by a person with physical custody.	Older adult reports of being abandoned; deserting an older adult at a hospital or skilled nursing facility, shopping center, or other public place.
Financial Abuse	
Denying access to personal resources, stealing money or possessions. Coercing to sign contracts or durable power of attorney. Making changes in will or trust.	Living situation below level of personal resources. Sudden change in personal finances, sudden transfer of assets.
Neglect	
Failure or refusal to provide basic life needs, including food, water, medications, clothing, and hygiene. Failure to provide physical aids such as dentures, eyeglasses, and hearing aid. Failure to ensure safety.	Older adult reports of being neglected. Untreated or infected pressure injuries on sacral area or heels. Weight loss, malnutrition. Laboratory values showing dehydration. Poor personal hygiene. Lack of adherence with treatment.
Failure to provide social stimulation. Leaving alone for long periods. Failure to provide companionship.	Depression, withdrawn behavior, agitation. Ambivalent attitude toward caregiver or family member.
Physical Abuse	
Slapping, striking, restraining, incorrect positioning. Oversedation with medications.	Bruises, bilateral injuries (upper arms, ankles, wrists), repeated injuries in various stages of healing, burn marks, oversedation. Use of several emergency departments.
Psychologic Abuse	
Berating verbally, harassment, intimidation, threats of punishment, or deprivation. Childlike treatment, isolation.	Depression, withdrawn behavior, agitation. Ambivalent attitude toward caregiver or family member.
Sexual Abuse	
Nonconsensual sexual contact, including inappropriate touching. Forced sexual contact.	Older adult reports sexual abuse. Unexplained vaginal or anal bleeding, bruised breasts. Unexplained sexually transmitted or genital infections.
Violation of Personal Rights	
Denying right to privacy or right to make decisions about health care or living environment. Forcible eviction.	Sudden inexplicable changes in living situation, confusion.

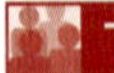

TABLE 5.8 NURSING MANAGEMENT

Elder Mistreatment

When elder mistreatment is suspected, it is important to do the following:

- Screen for possible elder mistreatment, including domestic violence.
- Conduct a thorough history and physical assessment.
- Record your findings. Include statements made by the patient and accompanying persons.
- If the patient is in immediate danger, implement a safety plan in collaboration with the health care team members involved in the patient's care.
- Identify, collect, and preserve physical evidence (e.g., dirty or bloody clothing).
- After obtaining consent, take photographs to document physical findings of suspected abuse or neglect. If possible, do this before treating or bathing the patient.
- If you suspect that mistreatment is occurring, report your findings to the state agency and/or law enforcement as mandated by state law.
- Initiate needed consultations with social work, forensic nursing, and adult protective services.

interventions include assessing for possible self-neglect and referring to long-term case management and APS as needed.

Medicare and Medicaid

Medicare is a federally funded health insurance program for people ages 65 years or older.[13] It also covers people under age 65 with certain disabilities and those of any age with end-stage renal disease requiring dialysis or a kidney transplant.

Medicare has 4 options for coverage: A, B, C, and D (Fig. 5.7). Part A covers inpatient hospital care and partially covers skilled nursing facility care, hospice, and home health care (HHC). Part A coverage is supported through Medicare through payroll taxes. Part B partially covers outpatient care, physicians' or primary care providers' services, and HHC. It also covers some preventive services, such as mammograms. Part B is voluntary and has a monthly premium. There is an annual deductible before payment begins. Medicare Advantage Plans, sometimes called "Part C" or "MA Plans," are offered by private companies approved by Medicare to provide Part A and

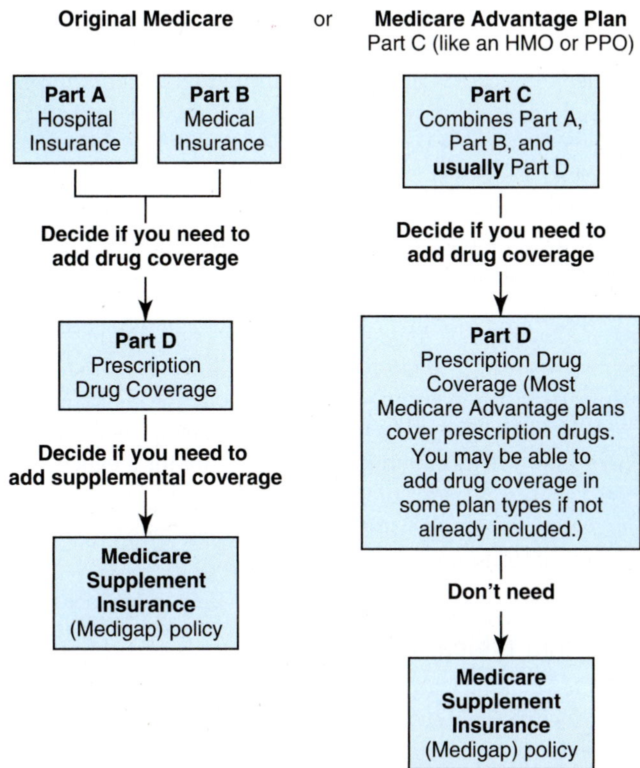

Fig. 5.7 The 2 main ways in which beneficiaries can get Medicare coverage. (Modified from U.S. Department of Health and Human Services, Centers for Medicare and Medicaid Services, Baltimore, MD.)

Part B benefits. Part D is available to Medicare enrollees and provides a prescription drug benefit. Members pay a yearly deductible, monthly premium, and copayment. People with lower incomes and limited assets may qualify for extra help to pay for prescriptions.

Medicare does not cover long-term care, custodial ADLs or IADLs care, dental care or dentures, hearing aids, or eyeglasses. More information is available at www.medicare.gov. Out-of-pocket expenditures for people on Medicare continue to rise. The costs increase with age, functional disabilities, number of chronic conditions, and number of hospitalizations.[13]

Medicaid is a state-administered, needs-based program to help eligible low-income people, including Medicare beneficiaries, with certain medical expenses. Those who qualify for both Medicare and Medicaid are referred to as *dual-eligible.* Eligibility and coverage vary by state. For qualified Medicare beneficiaries, Medicaid pays Medicare premiums, deductibles, coinsurance, and long-term care and home health expenses. In the United States most long-term care is paid for by Medicaid or private pay. More information is available at www.medicaid.gov.

Care Alternatives for Older Adults

Older adults with special care needs include people who are homeless, in need of help with ADLs, cognitively impaired, homebound, or no longer able to live at home. Older adults may be served by adult day care, adult day health care, HHC, and long-term care. Continuing-care retirement communities, congregate housing, and assisted living facilities are housing options for older adults.

Adult Day Care and Adult Day Health Care

Adult day care centers provide social, recreation, and health-related services to people in a safe, community-based environment. This includes daily supervision, social activities, opportunities for social interaction, and help with ADLs. They serve 2 groups of adults: (1) those who are cognitively impaired and (2) those who have problems performing ADLs. Adult day care programs provide services based on need. Programs for adults who are cognitively impaired offer therapeutic recreation, support for families, family counseling, and social involvement.

Adult day health care centers are like adult day care but provide care to meet the needs of older adults and people with disabilities who need a higher level of care. This might include health monitoring, therapeutic activities, 1-on-1 ADLs training, and personal services. Both may offer respite to allow continued employment for the caregiver and delay institutionalization.

States set standards and regulate centers. Medicare does not cover costs. Adult day health care is tax deductible as dependent care. Placement in an adult care program that matches the person's needs is important. You can help by knowing the available centers in your area and assessing the needs of older adults and their families. You will then be able to help them make good decisions about their care.

Home Health Care

HHC can be a cost-effective care alternative for older adults who are homebound, have health needs that are intermittent or acute, and have supportive caregiver involvement. HHC is not an alternative for adults in need of 24-hour help with ADLs or continuous safety supervision. Private-duty care may be an alternative in these situations. HHC services require HCP orders and skilled nursing care for Medicare reimbursement. Unless one meets these requirements, Medicare will not pay for home health aides for ADLs management or a homemaker for IADLs management. In addition to HHC, caregivers often seek homemaker services and respite and personal care through organizations that provide nonmedical assistance. These services help older adults stay at home.

Long-Term Care Facilities

Three factors appear to lead to placement in a long-term care facility: (1) rapid patient deterioration, (2) caregiver inability to continue care because of stress and burnout, and (3) a change in or loss of the family support system. Progressive dementia, urinary incontinence, or a major health event (e.g., stroke) can hasten long-term care placement.

The conflicts and fears faced by older adults and their families make placement a difficult transition. Common caregiver concerns include: (1) Will the older adult resist admission? (2) Will the level of care given by staff be sufficient? (3) Will the resident be lonely? (4) Will care be affordable?

Physical relocation may lead to adverse health effects. *Relocation stress syndrome* is associated with the disruption, confusion, and challenges that older adults face when moving to a new environment. Older adults may have anxiety, depression, and disorientation. Appropriate interventions can reduce the effects of relocation. Whenever possible, involve older adults in the decision to move and fully inform them about the location. Caregivers can share information, pictures, or a video recording of the new location. Staff members can send a welcome message. On arrival, they can greet new residents and provide orientation. To bridge the relocation, new residents can be "buddied" with seasoned residents.

Programs for All-Inclusive Care for the Elderly

Programs for All-Inclusive Care for the Elderly (PACE) provide care for adults age 55 and older. PACE services include primary care, including prescription medications and wound care; physical, occupational, recreational, and speech therapy; adult day care; dental care; podiatry; social services; and HHC. Respite care, hospitalization, short-term rehabilitation, and long-term care are provided as needed.[14]

A person who has Medicaid will not have to pay a monthly premium for the long-term portion of the PACE benefit. A person who does not qualify for Medicaid but has Medicare must pay a monthly premium to cover the long-term care portion.

Age-Friendly Health Systems

To address the challenges that older adults face as they age, especially the complexity of care, we have developed a new care model called the Age-Friendly Health System's Model of Care.[15] The aim of this initiative is to build a social movement so that all older adult care is age friendly. This means care is guided by a set of evidence-based practices, causes no harm, and is consistent with what matters to the older adult and their family caregivers. The key components are the 4Ms: (1) *What Matters* to the older adult—considering what is most important to the patient, family, and caregivers, including care goals and preferences; (2) *Medication*—making sure all medications have a clear indication and are prescribed at the lowest effective dose and frequency; (3) *Mentation*—assessing and managing dementia, delirium, and/or depression; and (4) *Mobility*—maintaining or improving mobility and function (Fig. 5.8). Use the 4Ms model to guide the care you provide older adults. Oftentimes, when using the 4Ms to plan care for a patient, it is necessary to work with other health care team members. This allows for a comprehensive, age-friendly assessment and plan for each older adult in your care.

Legal and Ethical Issues

Many older adults need legal guidance and assistance. Legal issues include advance directives, estate planning, tax issues, appeals for denied services (e.g., disability), financial decisions, or exploitation by strangers or "trusted others."

Advance directives are written statements of a person's wishes about medical care. A health care proxy may be appointed to make medical decisions if a person is unable to make their own medical decisions. These documents allow people to direct their own care at end of life. Advance directives are discussed in detail in Chapter 10 and Table 10.3.

When working with older adults, you may find ethical issues that influence practice, such as the assessment of older adults' ability to make decisions. Other ethical issues relate to end-of-life care. These include decisions about resuscitation, nutrition and hydration, and transfer to more intensive treatment units

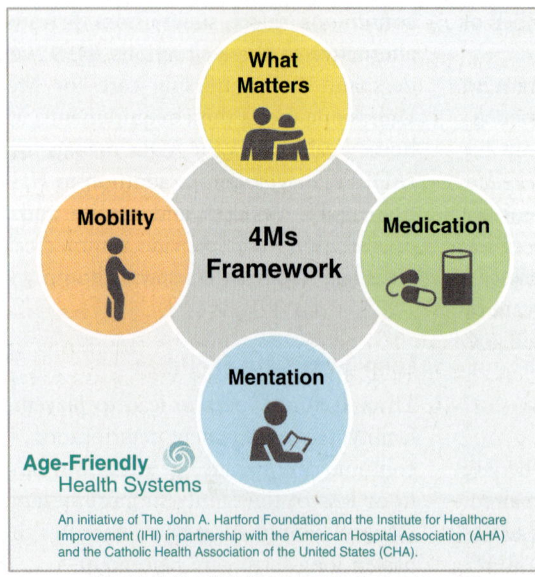

What Matters
Know and align care with each older adult's specific health outcome goals and care preferences including, but not limited to, end-of-life care, and across settings of care.

Medication
If medication is necessary, use Age-Friendly medication that does not interfere with What Matters to the older adult, Mobility, or Mentation across settings of care.

Mentation
Prevent, identify, treat, and manage dementia, depression, and delirium across settings of care.

Mobility
Ensure that older adults move safely every day in order to maintain function and do What Matters.

Fig. 5.8 The 4Ms framework of age-friendly health systems. (© Institute for Healthcare Improvement, http://www.ihi.org/Engage/Initiatives/Age-Friendly-Health-Systems/Pages/default.aspx.)

and the hospital. These situations are often complex, especially during emotionally stressful times. You can assist the older adult, family, and other health care workers by (1) keeping current on the ethical issues, (2) acknowledging when an ethical dilemma is present, and (3) advocating for an institutional ethics committee to help provide guidance in making decisions and assist when differences of opinion occur.

NURSING MANAGEMENT: OLDER ADULTS

Gerontologic nursing is the care of older adults based on the specialty body of knowledge of gerontology and nursing. These specialty nurses provide care for older adults using a whole-person (e.g., physical, psychologic, functional, developmental, socioeconomic, cultural) perspective. Care of older adults is complex and presents challenges that require skilled assessment and interventions tailored to this population.

For older adults, the stress of an illness may lead to fear and anxiety. They may view health care personnel as helpful but perceive institutions as negative and potentially harmful places. Communicate a sense of concern and care by use of direct and simple statements, eye contact, direct touch, and gentle humor. These actions help the older adult relax in this stressful situation.

Assessment

Diseases and conditions in older adults may be hard to accurately assess and diagnose. Older adults may underreport symptoms and try to manage them by changing their functional status. For example, a patient with loss of feeling in the feet from neuropathy may start using a walker but not report the symptom to the HCP. The older adult may attribute a new symptom to "aging" and ignore it. Or someone may eat less, sleep more, or "wait it out."

In older adults, disease symptoms are often atypical. The most common atypical presentations are "delirium" or "acute change in mental status" and change in functional status. For example, confusion may be a sign of a urinary tract infection. A caregiver may say that a relative "is acting differently," "is not their self," or is no longer taking part in usual activities or self-care. Conditions with similar symptoms can be confused. For example, depression may be misdiagnosed and treated as dementia.

In older adults, a *cascade disease pattern* may occur. For example, a person who has insomnia treats the condition with sleeping medication. They become lethargic and delirious and fall, sustaining a hip fracture. This decreases activity and mobility, leading to pneumonia and/or pressure injuries. Nurses play a vital role in preventing this downward trajectory.

The focus of a geriatric assessment is to determine interventions needed to support and enhance the health, quality of life, function, and independence of older adults. At a minimum, it includes the medical history, functional assessment, medication review, cognitive and mood evaluation, social resources, and physical assessment followed by recommended diagnostic tests. Several providers may be involved. These often include a nurse, an HCP such as a physician or advanced practice nurse, and a social worker. It may also include a physical and/or occupational therapist, dietitian, podiatrist, ophthalmologist, dentist, and pastoral care.

Specific elements in a complete nursing assessment include a thorough history, mood assessment, functional assessment including ADLs and IADLs, mental status evaluation, social-environment assessment, and physical assessment. Although the health history may be lengthy, it is important to obtain. Review medical records and determine what information is most relevant or needs more detail.

Before an assessment, address the person's primary needs. For example, ensure that older adults are comfortable and ask if they need to use the bathroom. If they normally use eyeglasses and hearing aids, ask them to use these during the assessment. Place all assistive devices, such as walkers, within reach. Assess your patient's level of fatigue and pause the assessment if necessary. Allow adequate time to offer information and time for the person to respond to questions. Interview the older adult and their family or caregivers. You can do this separately unless the patient is cognitively impaired or specifically requests the caregiver's presence.

Evaluation of mental status is important because these results often determine the potential for independent living. SPICES is an effective tool for obtaining assessment data in older adults. It may be used as an initial nursing assessment in any setting (Fig. 5.9). Multiple evidence-based geriatric assessment tools and best practice approaches to nursing care for older adults are available from the *Try This:* Series at the Hartford Institute for Geriatric Nursing (HIGN) (available at https://hign.org/consultgeri/try-this).

Assess for fall risk. Those at increased risk for falls have a history of falls or a fear of falling. Other factors that increase fall risk include use of certain drugs; infection; orthostatic hypotension; dehydration; electrolyte imbalance; arthritis; changes in gait, balance, and mobility; neurologic problems (e.g., stroke, Parkinson disease); decreased muscle strength; and decreased visual acuity. Assess for symptoms of dizziness or lightheadedness upon standing. Other risk factors include hazards in the environment, foot problems, poor footwear, incorrect use of an assistive device such as a cane, or bed in an incorrect position, such as too high.

Patient name:	Date:	
	EVIDENCE	
SPICES	Yes	No
Sleep disorders		
Problems with eating or feeding		
Incontinence		
Confusion		
Evidence of falls		
Skin breakdown		

Fig. 5.9 SPICES. (Adapted from Fulmer T: The geriatric nurse specialist role: a new model, *Nurs Manag* 22:91, 1991.)

Evaluation of the results of the assessment helps determine needed services and potential long-term placement needs. Collect data about community resources that will help older adults and their caregivers in supporting maximal function. The goal is to plan and implement actions that help older adults stay as functionally independent as possible and promote their quality of life.

◆ Planning

When setting goals with older adults, identify their strengths and abilities. Include caregivers in planning. Priority goals may include gaining a sense of control, feeling safe, and reducing stress.

◆ Implementation

When carrying out a plan of action for older adults, adjust your approach and actions based on their physical, functional, and mental status. The small body size of a frail older adult may require the use of pediatric equipment (e.g., BP cuff). Safety is a primary concern when caring for an older adult. Those with bone and joint changes often need transfer assistance, altered positioning, and the use of gait belts and lift devices. Older adults with declining energy reserves may need extra time to complete tasks. A slower approach and the use of other adaptive equipment may be needed. Cognitive impairment, if present, requires that you have a calm approach to avoid producing anxiety and resistance. Depression can result in apathy and poor cooperation with the treatment plan.

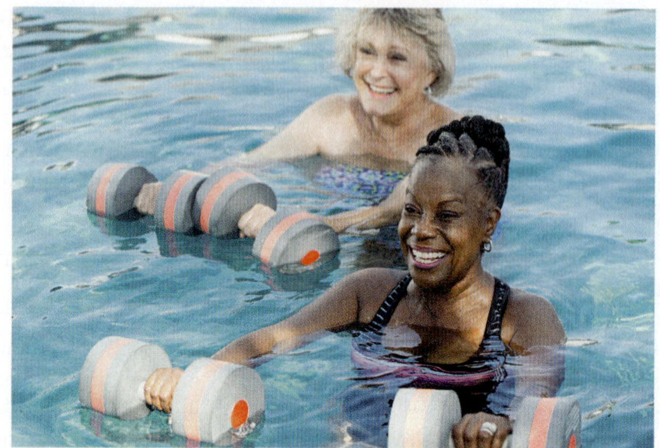

Fig. 5.10 Water aerobics is an example of a health promotion activity for older adults. (© kali9/iStock.com.)

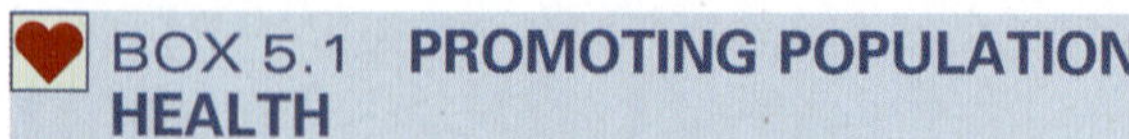

BOX 5.1 PROMOTING POPULATION HEALTH

Promoting Health in Older Adults

- Get recommended vaccines.
- Create an environment free of hazards to reduce the risk of falling.
- Drink plenty of liquids. Limit drinks with lots of added sugar or salt.
- Obtain at least 150 min of moderate-intensity exercise each week.
- Maintain an appropriate weight based on a nutrient-rich diet.
- Use medications, herbs, and supplements according to the HCP's direction.

Health Promotion

Health promotion and prevention of health problems for older adults focus on 3 areas: (1) increased participation in health promotion and disease prevention activities (Fig. 5.10), (2) reduction in diseases and health-related issues, and (3) increased use of services that reduce health hazards. Programs exist for screening for chronic health conditions, tobacco cessation, geriatric foot care, vision and hearing screening, stress reduction, exercise programs, fall prevention programs, drug use, crime prevention, elder mistreatment, and home safety assessment. Teach older adults about the need for preventive services and available programs (Box 5.1).

Include health promotion and disease prevention in nursing interventions and plans at any setting or level of care in which nurses and older adults interact. You can use health promotion activities to increase personal responsibility for health and independent functioning. Teaching and reinforcement are important tools for you to use to enhance self-care practices in older adults. Patient teaching is discussed in Chapter 4.

Acute Care

The hospital may be the first point of contact for older adults with the health care system. Conditions that often result in hospitalization include falls, dysrhythmias, heart failure, stroke, fluid and electrolyte imbalances, pneumonia, urosepsis, and hip fractures. Hospitalized older adults often have multiple problems, acute and chronic.

When older adults are being cared for in the acute care setting, both patients and caregivers need help with a variety of functions (Table 5.9). The outcome of hospitalization for older adults varies. Of special concern are patients having high-risk surgeries (e.g., hip replacement) and those who have delirium while hospitalized.

Care transitions. The time of a care transition to another setting (e.g., acute care hospital to rehabilitation) is challenging for many older adults. While in the hospital, patients and caregivers are counseled on how to prepare for posthospital care. Those with multiple health conditions have a higher risk for rehospitalization.

Medicare regulations require a registered nurse, social worker, or qualified person to develop a care transition plan for patient discharge. Safe and effective care transitions are most likely to occur when health care team members work together with the patient and family to coordinate care.

The Transitional Care Model (TCM) is an evidence-based, innovative approach to care coordination and management of patients with complex needs. In the TCM, a transitional care nurse delivers and coordinates care by nurses and other team members throughout potential and acute episodes of illness.

TABLE 5.9 NURSING MANAGEMENT

Care of the Hospitalized Older Adult

Give special consideration to the following interventions when caring for hospitalized older adults:

- Identify older adults at risk for consequences of medical and/or surgical treatments.
- Consider discharge and postacute needs early in the hospital stay, especially help with activities of daily living and medications.
- Encourage the development and use of health care teams, special care units, and providers who focus on the special needs of older patients.
- Implement standard protocols to screen for at-risk conditions common in the hospitalized older adult, such as urinary tract infections and delirium.
- Implement mobility and exercise programs to prevent functional decline.
- Monitor for and prevent skin integrity changes.
- Implement measures focused on safety (e.g., fall prevention).
- Refer patients to community-based services.

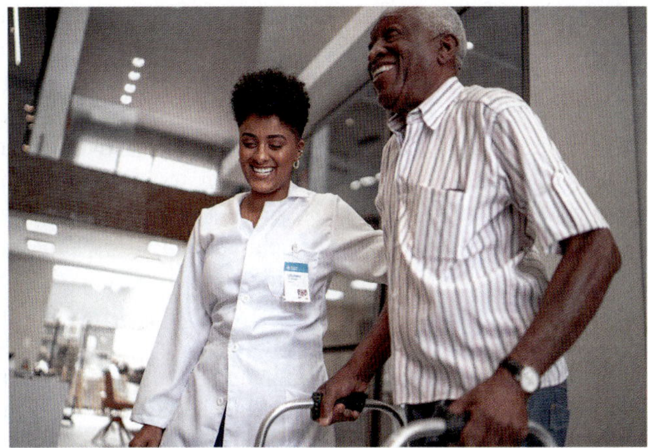

Fig. 5.11 The nurse assists a patient in a geriatric rehabilitation facility. (© FG Trade/iStock.com.)

Those most likely to benefit from transitional care nursing include older adults and those with functional deficits, behavior or psychiatric issues, multiple chronic conditions, polypharmacy, a recent hospitalization, lack of a support system, low health literacy, and history of nonadherence to treatment.[16]

Chronic Care

Rehabilitation. Rehabilitation helps older adults adapt to or recover from disability or an acute functional decline. The goal is to strive for maximal function and physical capabilities considering the person's current health and functional status. Rehabilitation may occur in acute inpatient rehabilitation, subacute rehabilitation, or long-term care settings. With proper training, assistive equipment, and attendant personal care, people with functional deficits may live independently. Older adults, primarily through Medicare reimbursement, can receive rehabilitative care through acute inpatient rehabilitation (limited days) and HHC programs (Fig. 5.11).

Older adults with chronic conditions, such as arthritis, have an increased risk for functional decline. Decreased function or disabilities lead to increased self-care deficits, increased rates of institutionalization, decreased quality of life, and higher mortality rates.

Several factors influence rehabilitation. First, preexisting conditions associated with decreased reaction time, visual acuity, fine motor ability, physical strength, and cognitive function affect the short- and long-term rehabilitation potential. Older adults may have anxiety, fear, or concern about falling. Poor nutrition and financial issues may limit the rehabilitation process. Encouragement, support, and acceptance from the health care team members and caregivers can help older adults remain motivated for potentially physically challenging rehabilitation.

Second, older adults often lose function because of inactivity and immobility. This deconditioning can occur because of unstable acute medical conditions, lack of assistive devices, and a lack of motivation to stay fit. The effect of inactivity leads to "use it or lose it" consequences. Older adults can improve flexibility, strength, and aerobic capacity even into very old age. Passive and active range-of-motion exercises are done to preserve muscle tone and strength and prevent deconditioning and subsequent functional decline.

Assistive devices. Consider the use of assistive devices as interventions for older adults. Using assistive devices such as dentures, glasses, hearing aids, walkers, wheelchairs, adaptive utensils, elevated toilet seats, and skin protective devices can increase function. Include these tools and devices in the older adult's care plan when needed and teach the use of the devices. For example, using a cane correctly may decrease fall risk.

Technology can help with rehabilitation and living with functional impairments. For example, we can use electronic monitoring equipment to monitor heart rhythm and BP. Monitoring can find a person with dementia who has wandered away from home. Computer devices may help patients with speech problems after a stroke. Small electronic devices can serve as memory aids.

Social support. Social support for older adults occurs at 3 levels. First, family members are the primary and preferred providers of social support. Second, semiformal support is found in clubs, religious (faith-based) organizations, neighborhoods, adult day care, and senior centers. Third, older adults may be linked to formal systems of social welfare agencies, health agencies, and government support. Generally, you, as a nurse, are part of the formal support system.

Safety. Safety is crucial in maintaining an older adult's health. Older adults are at higher risk for accidents because of normal sensory changes, slowed reaction time, decreased thermal and pain sensitivity, changes in gait and balance, and drug effects. Most accidents occur in or around the home. Falls, motor vehicle accidents, and fires are common causes of accidental death. Declining thermoregulation impairs the older person's ability to adapt to extremes in environment temperatures. An older adult's body can neither conserve nor dissipate heat as efficiently, increasing risk for hypothermia and hyperthermia. The older adult age group accounts for most deaths during severe cold spells and heat waves. Fear of falling can affect the older adults' decisions about the activities that they engage in and how active they remain.

Review the environment for needed changes that can improve safety. Measures such as colored step strips, tub and toilet grab bars, and stairway handrails can be effective in "safety-proofing" living spaces. Uncluttered floor space (e.g., removing throw rugs), railings, and increased lighting and nightlights are some of the easiest and most practical adaptations. Advocate for home fire and security alarms. Other interventions to decrease fall risk include exercise, physical therapy, and management of foot and footwear issues. Encourage the use of glasses and hearing aids as needed. Advocate for home fire and security alarms.

Older adults who are new to inpatient or long-term care settings need a thorough orientation to the environment. Reassure them that they are safe. Answer all questions and refer to team members and specialists as needed. Foster orientation by displaying large-print clocks, keeping wall designs simple, clearly designating doors and exits, and using simple bed and nurse or family-call controls. Provide diffuse lighting while avoiding glare.

Medication use. Medication use in older adults requires thorough and regular assessment, care planning, and evaluation. Nonadherence to medication plans by older adults may occur because of inability to read prescription drug labels and/or understand the health information that we provide them.

Age-related changes alter drug pharmacodynamics and pharmacokinetics. Drug-drug, drug-nutrient, and drug-disease interactions influence the absorption, distribution, metabolism, and excretion of drugs. The most dramatic changes with aging are related to drug metabolism (Fig. 5.12). Hepatic blood flow and the enzymes responsible for drug metabolism decrease markedly with aging. These increase drug half-life in older adults and lead to greater risk for drug toxicity and adverse drug events. With age comes a decline in the renal clearance of drugs. Older adults with altered renal function may need a lower dose and/or decreased frequency of a drug excreted by the kidney. When drug-level monitoring is available (e.g., digoxin), identify toxic levels by serum monitoring at regular intervals, especially when there is a change of dose and/or frequency.

Older adults may have difficulty managing drug therapy because of cognitive impairment, altered sensory perception, and limited hand mobility or dexterity. Table 5.10 lists common reasons for drug errors made by older adults.

Polypharmacy (the use of multiple medications by a person who has more than 1 health problem), overdose, dependence,

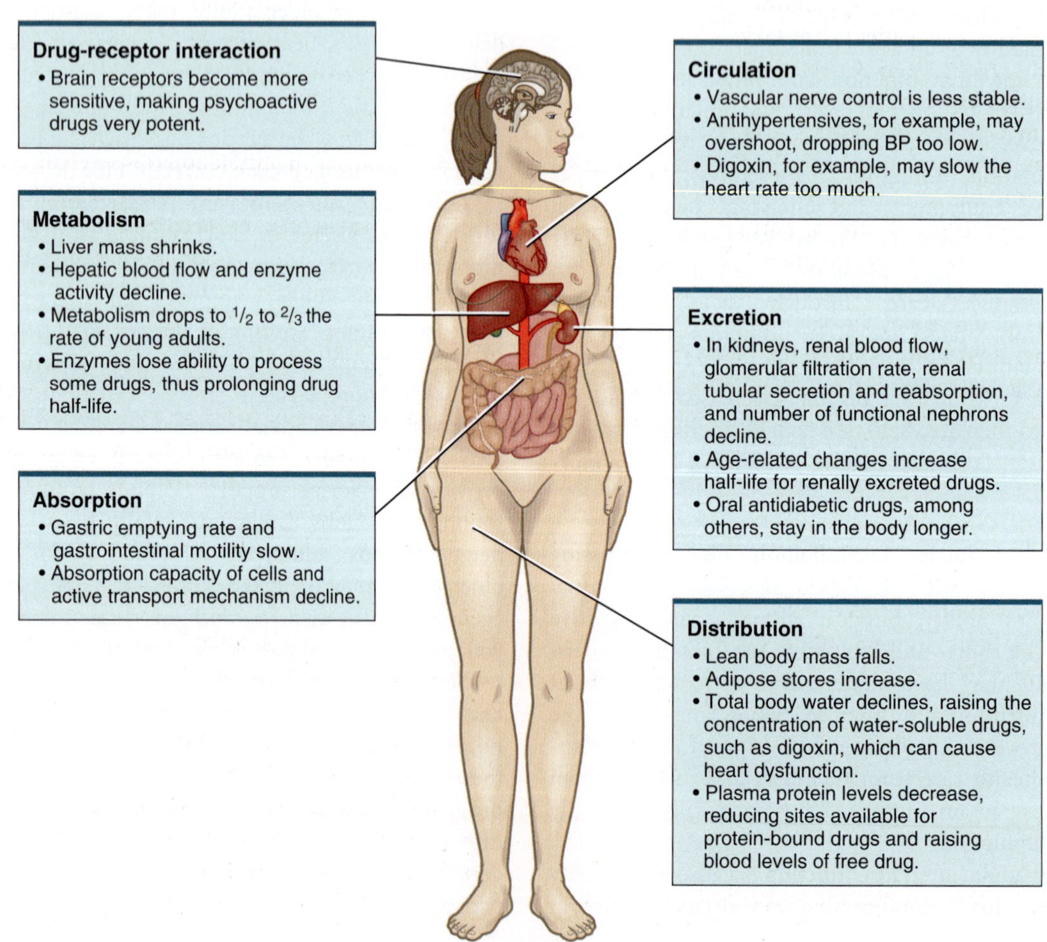

Fig. 5.12 The effects of aging on drug metabolism.

TABLE 5.10 Drug Therapy

Causes of Medication Errors by Older Adults

- Decreased vision
- Forgetting to take drugs
- Taking drugs incorrectly
- Use of drugs prescribed for someone else
- Lack of financial resources to obtain prescription drugs
- Refusal to take a drug because of undesirable side effects
- Failure to understand instructions or importance of drug treatment

TABLE 5.11 Drug Therapy

Safe Medication Use by Older Adults

When older adults are using medications, it is important to take the following measures to prevent medication errors:

- Assess cognitive function and monitor for changes.
- Assess their ability to self-administer medication.
- Obtain and maintain a complete medication record.
- Assess for alcohol and illicit drug use.
- Encourage the use of written or electronic medication-reminder systems.
- Encourage the use of 1 pharmacy.
- Work with HCPs and pharmacists to set up routine drug profiles on all older adult patients.
- Try to reduce drug use that is not essential by consulting the HCP and pharmacist.
- Advocate for low-income prescription support services.

and addiction to prescription drugs are major causes of illness in older adults. Potential medication errors include (1) taking both brand-name and generic medications, (2) taking medications incorrectly, and (3) drug-drug interactions. These errors can be prevented by having a pharmacist review medications regularly. Suggest the use of 1 pharmacy for filling all prescription medications.

The effects of medications in patients with multiple health problems are particularly challenging to assess and manage. As 1 disease is treated, another may be affected. For example, the use of oxybutynin to treat overactive bladder may cause confusion. To assess medication knowledge and use, ask older adults to bring all medications that they take regularly or occasionally to their health care appointments. You can then assess all medications that patients are taking. The American Geriatrics Society (AGS) Beers Criteria for Potentially Inappropriate Medication Use in Older Adults is designed to reduce problems with medications in older adults.[17] Table 5.11 describes other nursing interventions to help older adults follow a safe medication routine.

Depression. Depression is not a normal part of aging. However, it is often an underrecognized problem in older adults. Around 15% of older adults living in their homes have depression. Rates of depression in older adults in institutional settings are higher. Older adults make up 18% of suicides.[18]

Depression is associated with female gender, being divorced or separated, low socioeconomic status, poor social support, and a recent adverse and unexpected event. Depression tends to arise from a loss of self-esteem and may be related to life situations, such as retirement or loss of a spouse or partner. Problems such as pain, insomnia, lethargy, agitation, weight loss, and dementia are associated with depression.

Late-life depression often occurs together with medical conditions, such as heart disease, stroke, diabetes, and cancer. Depression can worsen medical conditions by affecting adherence to diet, exercise, or drug regimens. Be alert in your assessment for problems that may have symptoms similar to those of depression (e.g., thyroid disorders, vitamin deficiencies).

Encourage older adults with depressive symptoms to seek treatment. Because older adults with depression may feel unworthy, withdrawn, and isolated, the support of the family or others in encouraging older adults to seek treatment is important. Assist an older adult caregiver with depressive symptoms to seek medical care. Help them to secure respite services and support for their caregiving role.

Disruptive behavior. Behavior symptoms, such as crying and shouting, may arise from comorbidities, pain, medication effects, unmet needs, and/or environment factors. Evaluate whether disruptive behaviors signal unmet physiologic or psychosocial needs. For example, a patient who tries to get out of bed without help may be trying to reach the toilet. A toileting schedule will help curtail such attempts and prevent incontinence.

When behavior manifestations are present, ask questions to better understand the patient's behavior: Is the person able to say what they need or want? People with dementia may respond by speaking, gesturing, nodding, or making eye contact. Questions that use "yes" or "no" answers are better than open-ended questions. Ask family, friends, or staff members from previous care settings about the patient's (1) history; (2) usual communication style and cues to indicate pain, fatigue, hunger, or a need to urinate or defecate; (3) abilities in ADLs; and (4) daily routines (e.g., "Are they often awake at night or an early riser?" "Do they eat breakfast before dressing? Take an afternoon nap? Have a routine for bedtime?").

Physical restraints are devices, materials, and equipment that physically prevent persons from moving freely, such as walking, standing, lying, transferring, or sitting. *Chemical restraints* are drugs used to restrict a patient's freedom of movement or, in some cases, to sedate a patient. The current standard is to provide safe care without using restraints of any form, whether physical or chemical. Restraints are a last resort. Only use restraints to ensure the person's safety or the safety of others.[19] Before considering the use of any restraint, assess the perceived need for it and document the assessment.

Long-term care regulations and The Joint Commission set standards for restraint use. These include a time limit, observation, care, mandating the use of least restrictive measures (e.g., mittens), and alternatives to restraint use. Restraint alternatives include low beds, body props, and electronic devices (such as bed and chair alarm signaling). Such approaches support the development of a restraint-free, safe environment.

TABLE 5.12 Evaluating Nursing Care for Older Adults

Use the following questions to evaluate the effectiveness of care for older adults:

- Is there an identifiable change in function, mental status, or signs and symptoms of exacerbation of chronic conditions?
- Does the person consider their health state to be improved?
- Does the person think the plan is helpful?
- Do the person and caregiver think the care is worth the time and cost?
- Can you document positive changes that support the interventions?

Alternatives to restraints require vigilant, creative, and sensitive nursing care.

All restraints require an order from an HCP. Document restraint use and the reason for use. It is not appropriate to use restraints to prevent falls, avoid interference with medical devices, or reduce irritating behaviors, such as calling out. Frequent scheduled reviews of the ongoing need for the restraint are done with consideration of when to discontinue them.

◆ Evaluation

Your evaluation of nursing care is similar for all patients. The results of the evaluation direct you to continue the plan of care or revise as needed. When evaluating nursing care with older adults, focus on functional improvement and quality of life. Useful questions to consider when evaluating the plan of care for older adults are outlined in Table 5.12.

CASE STUDY

Older Adults

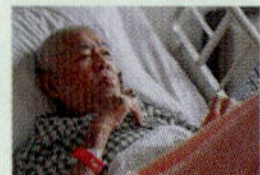

(©Edwin Tan/ iStock.com)

Patient Profile

H.W., an 81-year-old Chinese male, was admitted with confusion and found to have community-acquired pneumonia. His medical history includes hypertension, diabetes, prostate cancer, stage 3b chronic kidney disease, depression, Parkinson disease, and significant hearing loss.

Subjective Data

- Decreased upper extremity strength and persistent tremors from Parkinson disease
- Unplanned weight loss of 15 pounds in the past year
- Spends his days either in bed or in a recliner watching television
- Confusion, cough, and shortness of breath for the past 2 days

Psychosocial Data

- Came to the United States 35 years ago from Hong Kong.
- Speaks Cantonese with limited English proficiency.
- Lives with his adult daughter, who is unemployed, and her husband who was recently laid off from his job. His daughter provides help with ADLs and IADLs.
- Has a younger son who lives out of state, about 10 hours away.
- Limited financial resources but has Medicare and Medicaid benefits.
- Son raises concerns about his father's care and safety at home, given his brother-in-law's history of anger issues and alcohol use disorder.
- When the son asks his sister how she and her husband care for their father, she says, "We're doing the best we can. You don't live with him, so you don't know what it's like. He's stubborn and doesn't want to go to any appointments or take his medications. We do everything for him. He doesn't seem to know what is going on. I don't know how much longer we can do this . . . sometimes I wish it would end!"
- Daughter states their father does not want to go to a nursing home.

Objective Data

Physical Assessment

- Unwashed, matted hair; poor oral hygiene; overgrown toenails
- 2 stage 3 sacral pressure injuries
- Unstageable right heel pressure injury
- Multiple small bruises on his forearms and shins
- 5 × 10 cm bruise in the middle of his back

Diagnostic Tests

- Albumin 2.4 g/dL
- Creatinine 1.8 mg/dL
- Estimated glomerular filtration (eGFR) 36 mL/min/1.73 m^2
- Chest x-ray shows right lower lobe consolidation

Discussion Questions

1. ***Recognize:*** What additional history do you need to assess H.W.'s condition? What issues would you be most concerned about?
2. ***Recognize:*** What risk factors does H.W. have for developing frailty?
3. ***Analyze:*** Define ageism and explain how it may be manifested in this case.
4. ***Analyze:*** What are important findings regarding H.W.'s ability to manage his chronic illnesses?
5. ***Plan:*** Identify the stage of Corbin and Strauss's chronic illness trajectory that describes H.W.'s status. Which stage is the goal of your nursing care?
6. ***Plan:*** Based on your assessment of H.W., what will you include in your care planning to optimize his self-care ability?
7. ***Plan:*** Because he has an expressed desire to return home, what referrals would be indicated if this were the plan?
8. ***Prioritize:*** What are the interprofessional team's priorities for H.W.?
9. ***Act:*** To ensure H.W.'s safety, what interventions are necessary during his hospitalization?
10. ***Safety:*** What risk factors does H.W. have for becoming a victim of elder mistreatment? List and provide the rationale for nursing interventions and legal and ethical responsibilities in this case.
11. ***Evaluate:*** What care setting would be best for H.W. upon hospital discharge?

Answers available at http://evolve.elsevier.com/Lewis/medsurg.

BRIDGE TO NCLEX EXAMINATION

The number of the question corresponds to the same-numbered outcome at the beginning of the chapter.

1. Characteristics that differentiate chronic illness from acute illness include (**Select all that apply.**)
   a. resolve with antibiotics.
   b. requires specialty referral.
   c. infrequent complications.
   d. may have residual disability.
   e. irreversible pathologic changes.
2. A patient is ordered medication and diet therapy to manage type 2 diabetes. The nurse recognizes this as
   a. primary prevention for hyperglycemia.
   b. secondary prevention for hypoglycemia.
   c. tertiary prevention to reduce progression of diabetes.
   d. a recommended treatment to prevent nephrotoxicity.
3. Demographic trends among older Americans in the United States suggest
   a. a decrease in people living past age 85.
   b. females having the same life expectancy as males.
   c. increased frailty in persons between 65 and 75 years.
   d. an increase in older adults of racial or ethnic populations.
4. A nurse is discharging an older adult patient who lives in a rural farming community 40 miles from the nearest hospital. Which actions show the nurse understands the patient's needs? (**Select all that apply.**)
   a. Asks the patient if they have ever done a telehealth visit
   b. Inquires if the patient has a mail order pharmacy service
   c. Asks the social worker if there are any online support groups
   d. Teaches the patient to return weekly for a blood pressure check
   e. Asks the patient who can go to their home in case they need assistance
5. Which situation poses the highest risk for elder mistreatment?
   a. Older adult with recurrent syncopal episodes
   b. Adult living at home with chronic kidney disease
   c. Patient with dementia attending an adult day care program
   d. Adult children with financial dependency on an older adult family member
6. Which action is aligned with the 4Ms model of an age-friendly health system?
   a. Working with the patient to set a daily mobility goal
   b. Telling the patient that they need to live on their own
   c. Asking for a sleeping medication for a patient with insomnia
   d. Telling the patient that medical issues need addressing before functional issues
7. Which action is a *priority* for a newly admitted patient?
   a. Applying a pressure injury dressing
   b. Assessing the patient's mental status
   c. Administering a pneumococcal vaccine
   d. Assessing the patient's ability to do ADLs
8. Which nursing intervention is focused on health promotion for community-dwelling older adults?
   a. Assessing for delirium
   b. Helping complete legal documents
   c. Asking if the patient uses the Internet
   d. Assessing if recommended vaccines have been received

1. d, e; 2. c; 3. d; 4. a, b, c, e; 5. d; 6. a; 7. b; 8. d.

For rationales to these answers and even more NCLEX review questions, visit http://evolve.elsevier.com/Lewis/medsurg.

REFERENCES

To access the References for this chapter, please scan the QR code with a mobile device.

6

Caring for Lesbian, Gay, Bisexual, Transgender, Queer or Questioning, and Gender Diverse Patients

Jeffrey Kwong

http://evolve.elsevier.com/Lewis/medsurg/

CONCEPTUAL FOCUS

Health Disparities

Sexuality

LEARNING OUTCOMES

1. Describe the difference between biologic sex, sexual orientation, and gender identity.
2. Explain how health disparities affect lesbian, gay, bisexual, transgender, queer or questioning, and gender diverse (LGBTQ+) populations.
3. Explain strategies to create an LGBTQ+ inclusive environment.
4. Discuss options for gender-affirming hormone therapy.
5. Discuss interprofessional management for persons undergoing gender-affirming surgery.

KEY TERMS

biologic sex
cisgender
gender-affirming hormone therapy (GAHT)
gender-affirming surgery
gender dysphoria
gender identity
minority stress model
sexual orientation
transgender

This chapter provides an overview of care considerations for persons who identify as lesbian, gay, bisexual, transgender, queer, questioning, or gender diverse (LGBTQ+). There is a growing recognition of the health disparities and needs of the LGBTQ+ community. Nurses need to be aware of best practices to provide care that is unconditional, inclusive, and respectful.

BIOLOGIC SEX, GENDER IDENTITY, AND SEXUAL ORIENTATION

Biologic sex, also called *sex assigned at birth,* is determined by a person's external genitalia, internal reproductive organs, and chromosomes. Persons born with a penis and testicles and who have XY chromosomes are biologically male. Their sex assigned at birth is male. Sometimes the term *assigned male at birth (AMAB)* is used. Persons born with a vagina, uterus, and ovaries and who have XX chromosomes are biologically female. Their sex assigned at birth is female. Sometimes the term *assigned female at birth (AFAB)* is used. Some persons may have genitalia that we cannot categorize as either male or female or have a chromosomal makeup that we cannot clearly categorize as one or the other sex. In these situations, we sometimes use the term *intersex.*[1]

Gender identity refers to a person's self-perceived gender. It may be the same as or different from their sex assigned at birth. The term **cisgender** refers to persons whose gender identity aligns with their sex assigned at birth. **Transgender** refers to someone whose gender identity or gender expression is different from their sex assigned at birth. Someone whose sex assigned at birth is male but feels or identifies as a female would be considered a transgender female. Someone whose sex assigned at birth is female but feels and identifies as a male would be considered a transgender male. Some believe the term *transgender* to be an umbrella term that includes many different forms of gender identity and expression.[2] The term *transexual* is an old term that refers to persons who use medical interventions to change their bodies. Many transgender persons do not identify as transexual. We should not use this term when identifying a person. It is best to ask a person how they identify.

Gender is a socially constructed idea based on cultural standards. In traditional Western culture, there are 2 primary options for gender selection: male and female. However, this is beginning to change. In many cultures there is a recognition of genders beyond a binary (male/female) construct. People may take on more blended characteristics. For example, in the indigenous American culture, the term *two-spirit* is used to describe those who are born of one gender but who take on roles or identities of the opposite gender.[3] In India, *hijras* is a feminine gender identity that is taken on by persons whose sex assigned at birth was male or intersex. Within the Albanian culture, *burrnesha* are females who take a vow of celibacy and live their lives as males.

Gender expression refers to how someone expresses their gender in an outward appearance. It is a combination of behavior, mannerisms, interests, and appearance associated with gender. An example is the use of clothing or accessories. We traditionally considered gender a binary category, meaning either male or female. Now, there is growing acceptance that gender can be considered along a continuum that may change over time. *Nonbinary,* also termed *gender fluid* or *gender queer,* are terms that we use to describe someone who does not define themselves as completely one gender or the other. This term differs from *cross-dressing.* Cross-dressing typically refers to males (usually heterosexual) who wear women's clothing for pleasure or performance in specific settings and in a manner that may not lead to permanent changes to their appearance. They do not choose to live full-time in the opposite gender.

Gender dysphoria is a diagnostic classification that describes the distress that occurs when there is conflict between a person's gender identity and their sex assigned at birth.[4] There are defined diagnostic criteria for gender dysphoria, with specific criteria for children, adolescents, and adults. Gender dysphoria is typically diagnosed by a psychologist or other mental health professional. Gender dysphoria differs from *gender nonconformity.* Gender nonconformity is the extent that a person's gender identity, role, or expression differs from expected cultural norms.[5] Gender nonconformity is not a mental health disorder.

Sexual orientation refers to how one identifies based on their sexual or romantic attraction to others. When thinking about sexual orientation, it is helpful to consider 3 different aspects: behavior, attraction, and identity. These 3 aspects are not always tied together. For instance, some men may have sex with other men but may not identify as gay. Sexual orientation and sexual behavior can be considered across a continuum. They can be influenced by social and cultural norms. Remember that having a gender identity as transgender is separate from sexual orientation. Transgender persons may identify as gay, lesbian, bisexual, or heterosexual.

The term *heterosexual,* or "straight," implies a person who has sex with or is attracted to persons of the opposite gender. The term *homosexual* is considered offensive by some because of the stigma and derogatory use of this word. The preferred terms used to describe persons who have sex with or are attracted to persons of the same gender include *gay man* or *lesbian.* Bisexual (or "bi") describes those who are sexually attracted to or have sex with persons of more than one gender. Besides the commonly accepted terms *lesbian, gay,* and *bi,* several other terms are used to describe sexual orientation (Table 6.1).

LGBTQ+ HEALTH INEQUITIES

The LGBTQ+ population experiences various health inequities compared with non-LGBTQ+ populations. Many of the inequities stem from stigma and discrimination. These issues are based on cultural, political, legal, and historic contexts. Researchers describe this phenomenon as the **minority stress model**. This model assumes that a large part of the **health disparities** experienced by the LGBTQ+ community stems from stressors associated with a culture that is hostile. It results in a lifetime of harassment and victimization.[6] For example, up until 1973 the American Psychiatric Association considered homosexuality a mental illness. This had far-reaching impact by making people who identified as gay or lesbian believe they had a mental illness or that there was something "wrong with them."

Certain societal and cultural beliefs further perpetuate discrimination and stigma. Some religions do not acknowledge or accept same-sex behaviors or feelings. People who do not identify as heterosexual may be excluded, shamed, or become targets of fear and hatred. Some laws and regulations have institutionalized these inequalities and stigma.

In some parts of the country, a person can be subject to criminal actions or denied certain privileges because of their sexual orientation or gender identity. Some states restrict gender-affirming care to persons over 18 years of age.[7] In 2015 the U.S. Supreme Court legalized same-sex marriage. Federal recognition of same-sex marriage represented a major milestone, not only in terms of recognition of same-sex unions, but the legal right of marriage has implications that can affect the provision of health care.[8] This includes who has legal visitation rights during a patient's hospitalization, who can make health care decisions, and the ability to provide spousal coverage on a health insurance plan. Surveys of LGBTQ+ persons found that 53% experienced discrimination because of their sexual orientation and 1 in 3 transgender persons reported being refused health care because of their gender identity.[9]

Poverty stems from stigma and discrimination. Research shows that there are inequities in the socioeconomic status of LGBTQ+ persons compared with non-LGBTQ+ persons. An analysis found that 17% of LGBTQ+ people live in poverty in

TABLE 6.1 Terms Used to Describe Gender and Sexual Identity[a]

Term	Meaning or Significance
AFAB	Assigned female at birth
AMAB	Assigned male at birth
Asexual	Not feeling sexual attraction or desire for partnered sexuality
Bi, bisexual	Person who is emotionally, sexually, or affectionally attracted to more than one gender
Cis, cisgender	Term to describe persons whose gender identity matches their physical sex assigned at birth
Gay male	Male who is sexually, romantically, or relationally attracted to other males
Gender queer/ gender nonconforming	Person whose gender identity or expression falls outside the traditional male/female binary
Intersex	Person who has biologic or secondary sex traits that are inconsistent with what is typically considered male or female
Lesbian	Female who is sexually, romantically, or relationally attracted to other females
LGBTQ+, LGBTQI+, LGBTQIA+	Abbreviations for lesbian, gay, bisexual, queer/ questioning (LGBTQ), intersex (LGBTQI), and ally/asexual (LGBTIA) The plus (+) acknowledges that more identities exist
MSM	Men who have sex with men
Nonbinary	Refers to a spectrum of gender and not being in 1 of 2 categories Typically, the 2 gender categories are male and female
Omnigender	Term that describes possessing all genders
Poly (polyamorous)	Having more than 1 romantic relationship at the same time
Queer	Term that can mean people who identify as lesbian, gay, bisexual, or transgender or who identify outside of the traditional societal definitions of gender or sexual orientation Some consider the term offensive, as it was previously used as a slur Members of the LGBTQ+ community have taken back this term as a form of empowerment
Questioning	Persons who are in the process of examining or understanding their gender identity or sexual orientation
Same-gender loving	Term to describe persons who are attracted physically, romantically, or relationally to persons of the same gender
Trans, transgender	An umbrella term for people whose gender identity differs from their sex assigned at birth
Two spirit	A term used by Native American and Canadian First Nation people to describe persons who identify with a third gender that has both masculine and feminine qualities
WSW	Women who have sex with women

[a]This table is not meant to be an exhaustive list of terms or definitions.
Adapted from University of California San Francisco Lesbian Gay Bisexual and Transgender Resource Center. Retrieved from https://lgbt.ucsf.edu/glossary-terms.

the United States compared with 12% of cisgender straight people.[10] The rate of poverty is higher among LGBTQ+ persons of color. Poverty is associated with lack of access to health insurance and a lower likelihood of engaging in wellness behaviors. Both affect health outcomes.

Other health inequities and disparities that occur within the LGBTQ+ population include higher rates of substance use, tobacco use, depression, anxiety, violence, and victimization. We estimate that rates of substance use, including alcohol and tobacco use, are nearly twice as high among LGBTQ+ persons compared with non-LGBTQ+ persons.[11] Similarly, mental health issues, such as depression and anxiety, are more prevalent among people who identify as LGBTQ+. A national survey found the rates of depression and anxiety were nearly twice as common in LGBTQ+ people.[12]

Rates of mental health disorders are high among LGBTQ+ youth (Fig. 6.1). A 2023 report of LGBTQ+ youth found that 67% reported experiencing anxiety, 54% reported experiencing depression, and 41% considered attempting suicide.[13] These rates are higher compared with non-LGBTQ+ youth.

Rates of violence and victimization are higher among LGBTQ+ populations compared with heterosexual populations. Hate crimes and intimate partner violence rates greatly affect LGBTQ+ persons. The rates of violence among transgender persons are much higher compared with their cisgender counterparts. A disproportionate number of violent crimes are committed against transgender and gender nonconforming persons of color. Recent data found that 63% of fatal violence against transgender persons occurred in Black transgender women.[14]

Certain cancers occur at a high rate within the LGBTQ+ community.[15] We believe that lesbians have a higher incidence of breast cancer. Risk factors associated with these higher rates include tobacco use, obesity, and nulliparity. The rates of anal cancer from human papillomavirus infection in men who have sex with men (MSM) without HIV is estimated to be 20 times higher than non-MSM. In MSM with HIV, the rate is nearly 40

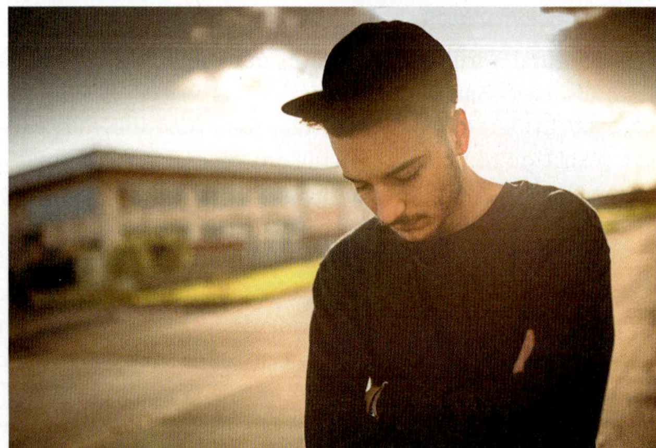

Fig. 6.1 Rates of mental health disorders are higher among LGBTQ+ youth. (© ©franckreporter/iStock.com.)

times higher. Lung cancer rates are higher. This is in part because of higher rates of tobacco use.

Lesbian and bisexual females have higher rates of being overweight or obese compared with heterosexual women.[16] Obesity itself is a risk factor for other chronic conditions. These include diabetes, heart disease, hypertension, and osteoarthritis.

HIV and sexually transmitted infections (STIs), such as syphilis, are disproportionately higher, especially among MSM and transgender women. In the United States most new HIV infections occur among MSM. Among Black communities, the rates are even more staggering. The Centers for Disease Control and Prevention (CDC) estimates that in 2021 among the 36,189 new diagnoses of HIV, Black MSM accounted for 37% of new diagnoses, Hispanic/Latino males accounted for 34%, and White MSM accounted for 24%.[17]

One of the structural barriers that contributes to health disparities is the limited amount of training that health professionals receive in how to provide LGBTQ+ culturally appropriate care. Studies estimate that medical providers receive less than 5 hours of clinical training in LGBTQ+ health. Lack of knowledge about care considerations and a lack of preparation in how to communicate with such patients contribute to the challenges and barriers LGBTQ+ people experience.

GERONTOLOGIC CONSIDERATIONS

Older LGBTQ+ adults (those age 65 years or older) experience different challenges with their health and caregiving. Many older LGBTQ+ adults do not have children to help support them as they age. Thus more than half of older LGBTQ+ adults rely on a partner or friend to help or care for them (Fig. 6.2). The aging population lived through the early years of the HIV epidemic. Many people lost their friends, partners, and social networks. This has implications for higher rates of isolation as that generation reaches older adulthood. Some who need to receive care at a long-term care facility go "back in the closet" and again hide their sexual orientation or gender identity because of negative and sometimes violent reactions from other residents or care staff.[18] These issues add to the physical and mental health disparities between LGBTQ+ and non-LGBTQ+ persons.

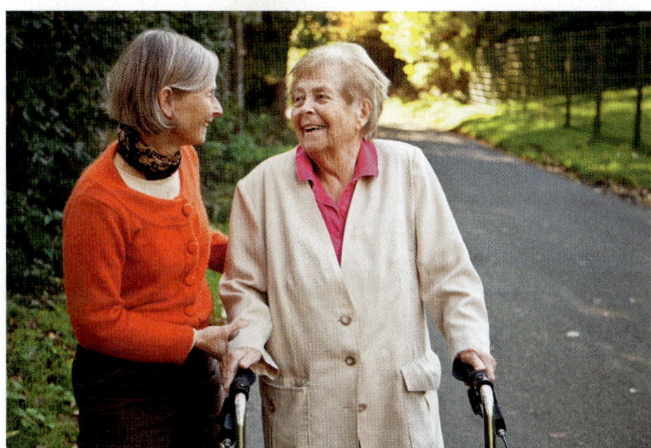

Fig. 6.2 Older LGBTQ+ adults tend to rely on partners or friends for caregiving. (© ©SilviaJansen/iStock.com.)

ESTABLISHING INCLUSIVE ENVIRONMENTS

The Joint Commission developed guidelines that are part of accreditation to improve the health care experience of LGBTQ+ patients. Examples include having nondiscrimination visitation policies, having unisex or single-stall bathrooms, and using patient intake forms that collect information on sexual and gender identity.[19]

Establishing a Welcoming Environment

Creating a welcoming environment starts the moment a patient enters a health care agency or makes contact with a facility (Table 6.2). For instance, when patients enter a building or a hospital unit, displaying an inclusive patient bill of rights is important. Have signs or symbols that indicate a safe space for LGBTQ+ persons. This can be in the form of signage or visual cues that have the rainbow flag (a universal symbol of LGBTQ+ pride), advertisements or posters that include same-sex couples or transgender persons, all-inclusive or nongender-specific restrooms, or having LGBTQ+ literature or magazines in the waiting areas. Staff can incorporate visual cues on ID badges. These strategies help establish a welcoming environment before having any direct interaction with patients or their caregivers.

TABLE 6.2 Promoting an Inclusive Environment

- Post the agency's nondiscrimination policy and patient bill of rights.
- Have waiting rooms and common areas that are inclusive of LGBTQ+ patients and caregivers.
- Create or designate unisex or single-stall restrooms.
- Allow patients to identify a support person of their choice.
- Implement visitation policies in a fair and nondiscriminatory manner.
- Honor and respect the patient's decision and pacing in providing information.
- Make sure forms use inclusive, gender-neutral language that allows for self-identification.
- Provide information and guidance for the specific health concerns facing LGBTQ+ people.
- Ensure that the disclosure of sexual orientation and gender identity information is voluntary.
- Make sure that strong privacy protections for all patient data are in place.

From The Joint Commission: *Advancing effective communication, cultural competence, and patient-and-family centered care for the LGBT community: a field guide.* Retrieved from https://www.jointcommission.org/-/media/tjc/documents/resources/patient-safety-topics/health-equity/lgbtfieldguide_web_linked_verpdf.pdf?db=web&-hash=FD725DC02CFE6E4F21A35EBD839BBE97&-hash=FD725DC02CFE6E4F21A35EBD839BBE97.

CHECK YOUR PRACTICE

You are working on a medical unit caring for a 42-year-old transgender woman admitted for appendicitis. Your patient prefers the name Sara Smith. You hear the surgical team during their rounds discussing Sara's case. A member of the team refers to the patient as Mr. Smith. You correct them and say the patient uses the name Sara and identifies as female. The surgical team member says, "He still has a penis, so he is Mr. Smith."

How would you respond?

Health History and the Intake Process

As part of taking a health history, establish the patient's identity. Introduce yourself. Ask the patient their preferred name, gender identity, and pronouns. Using a patient's chosen name is important, as it shows recognition for the person's identity. This is true for all persons, not just LGBTQ+ persons. For example, some people may have the legal name Jennifer, but they prefer you call them Jen or Jenny. Some people may go by their middle name or a nickname.

For transgender persons, they may still have their legal name on their insurance cards but no longer wish to use this name. They sometimes refer to that name as their "dead name." Having legal documents with a given name (which may be a different gendered name) poses a challenge for transgender persons as they begin the transition process or even years after. Some agencies now include a preferred name on the electronic health record. Verify this before starting the health history. The easiest way to obtain the name a person wishes to use is to ask, "Is there a name you would like for us to use for you while you are here with us?" This will include those whose legal name is William and use Bill and those whose legal name is William but use the name Jennifer. The crucial element is that the question is asked of everyone.

Asking about gender identity is important. Some agencies include this information on an intake form, and patients can complete the information directly. If the information is pre-entered into the electronic health record, verify that the information is correct before proceeding. If this information is not preentered into the medical record system, use a 2-step process for asking about gender identity. Ask the patient their sex assigned at birth and their current gender identity. Ask if the patient has any gender-specific pronouns (e.g., he/him, she/her, they/them). Make note to use these pronouns when talking about the patient. If you make a mistake and misgender a person or address them by the wrong name, acknowledge your error right away. Apologize to the patient. Table 6.3 describes other ways to be more inclusive in your communication.

TABLE 6.3 Inclusive Communication Strategies

Use these strategies to be more inclusive and welcoming when communicating with patients.

Do

Use a 2-step gender question:

- "What was your sex assigned at birth?"
- "What is your current gender?"

Ask and use a patient's preferred name and pronoun:

- "Do you have a preferred name that you would like me to use?"
- "What pronouns do you use?"

Avoid using gender terms with new patients until all information is known:

- Instead of "How may I help you, sir?" ask "How may I help you?"
- Use the patient's preferred first and last name instead of "Mr." or "Ms."
- Instead of saying "He is here for his appointment" say "The patient is here."
- Do not ask a transgender person for their "real" name. This may offend people who no longer identify with their given name.

Use the term "transition" to accurately reflect the process and continuum of change that transgender persons experience.

Do not ask unnecessary questions. Focus on why the patient is being seen or evaluated. Remember not every problem or issue is related to sexual orientation or gender identity.

Terms to Avoid

- "Sexual preference"—Alludes to the concept that sexual orientation is a choice.
- "Transgendered"—Transgender is an adjective, not a noun. Avoid referring to someone as "a transgender," just like you would not call someone "a straight."
- Do not add "-ed" at the end of transgender. This makes it sound like a condition.
- Do not use these terms "preop" or "postop sex change" when referring to a transgender person. These terms are outdated and considered offensive.

Adapted from Centers for Disease Control and Prevention: *Patient-centered care for transgender people: recommended practices for health care settings.* Retrieved from https://www.cdc.gov/hiv/clinicians/transforming-health/health-care-providers/affirmative-care.html#strategies; GLAAD: *An ally's guide to terminology: talking about LGBT people and equality.* Retrieved from https://www.glaad.org/sites/default/files/allys-guide-to-terminology_1.pdf.

Social History

As part of the social history, use gender-neutral terms when asking about a patient's relationship status or living situation. For example, when asking about a patient's partner or spouse, do not assume that a male patient will have a wife or a girlfriend. Rather, you can either wait for the patient to disclose the gender of their partner or if you are unclear or they do not specify, then you can ask the patient to clarify for you. It is better to ask for clarification versus making an automatic assumption. If you make a mistake, acknowledge the error and apologize.

In the absence of people to rely on from their families of origin, LGBTQ+ persons often have a family of choice, often made up of friends, partners, and perhaps a few relatives. Ask the patient who is part of their family of choice and if they have any advance directives. LGBTQ+ patients are especially vulnerable if they do not have advance directives in place.

Without an advance directive naming a surrogate decision maker, LGBTQ+ patients who are single or not legally married are at risk of having someone from their family of origin rather than their family of choice make health care decisions if they cannot make decisions for themselves (Box 6.1).

Sexual and Reproductive History

Taking an inclusive sexual history is an important aspect of providing holistic care. The most important element to taking a sexual history is to understand, before asking questions, what you need to know to provide care to that person. A sexual history may not be done in all clinical settings. When obtaining a sexual history use nonjudgmental language. Be sensitive to the range of sexual practices for *all* patients, not just the LGBTQ+ community.[20] You need to feel comfortable asking these questions. If you appear uncomfortable, patients will sense your uneasiness. They may choose not to disclose information. Consider asking questions that speak specifically to pregnancy (prevention, family planning) or STI risk and prevention. This will help guide your conversation to the sexual practices and away from questions that seem probing or unnecessary.

Questions about fertility and family planning are important to ask regardless of sexual orientation or practices. LGBTQ+ persons may have children or have an interest in parenting children (Fig. 6.3). You can find more information on sexual history taking in Chapter 55.

BOX 6.1 ETHICAL/LEGAL DILEMMAS

Durable Power of Attorney for Health Care

Situation

B.R., a 59-year-old gay male, has been in a vegetative state for 3 weeks after a hemorrhagic stroke. He has minimal brain activity on his electroencephalogram (EEG). He has a feeding tube providing nutrition. The HCP indicated that B.R. has a limited chance of recovery and the feeding tube is the only intervention keeping him alive. B.R.'s parents are deceased. He has 1 sister, but they have not spoken in 20 years because she could not accept the fact that he was gay. However, after B.R.'s stroke, the sister decided to come to the hospital and has been with him for the last 3 weeks. B.R. has a life partner of 15 years whom he chose as his proxy in his signed durable power of attorney. B.R. has said many times that he would never want to be kept alive if he were to live his life in a comatose or vegetative state. B.R.'s partner asks the HCP to remove the feeding tube, but his sister refuses and asks the HCP to keep the feeding tube in. The HCP refuses to recognize B.R.'s partner as proxy because he is not a blood relative.

Ethical/Legal Points for Consideration

The Patient Self-Determination Act (1990) requires all health care agencies receiving Medicare and Medicaid funding to make available advance directives allowing persons to state their preferences or refusals of health care if they are incapable of consenting for themselves. Durable power of attorney for health care is one type of advance directive in which people, when they are competent, identify someone else to make decisions for them should they lose their decision-making ability in the future (see Table 10.3).

You need to know the decision-making laws and regulations in your state. Teach patients and families about advance directives. You need to (1) make sure that HCPs are aware of and follow advance directives, (2) assist the patient and family in communicating with the HCPs when a "No Code" order is requested, and (3) assist a conflicted family in obtaining counseling whenever needed.

Many HCPs mistakenly think that proxies must be family members or blood relatives. LGBTQ+ persons often have difficulty having their partnership recognized as valid, especially if the patient's family disputes their rights. Counsel LGBTQ+ patients on the importance of having a health care proxy and a will to legally protect their end-of-life choices.

Discussion Questions

1. How can you assess the patient and family's understanding of durable power of attorney and assist them in understanding their role in decision making?
2. What should you do when an HCP declines to remove a feeding tube when you know that this goes against the patient's advance directive?

PREVENTIVE HEALTH

Preventive health is an important part of providing care (Box 6.2). In addition to standard guidelines for preventive health screenings and vaccinations, offer MSM vaccinations for hepatitis A and B if they have not previously received them. Rates of these preventable forms of viral hepatitis are higher among MSM because of sexual practices. Although not a vaccine-preventable form of hepatitis, the rate of hepatitis C

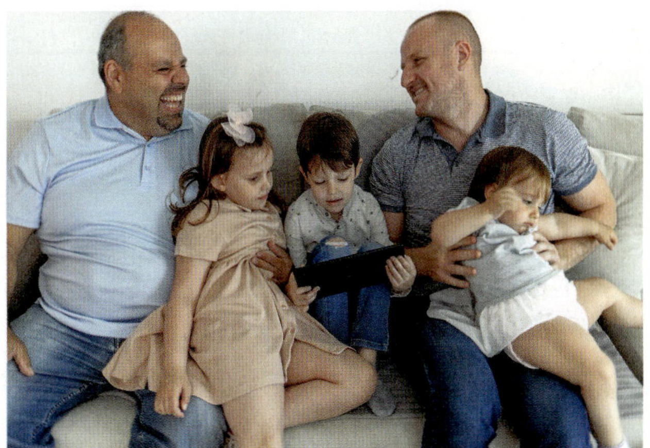

Fig. 6.3 A growing number of LGBTQ+ persons are having and raising families. (©© Jelena Stanojkovic/iStock.com.)

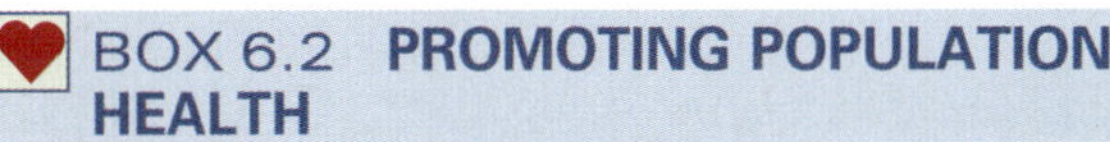

BOX 6.2 PROMOTING POPULATION HEALTH

Improving the Health and Well-Being of LGBTQ+ Persons

- Provide supportive social services to reduce suicide among LGBTQ+ persons.
- Implement antibullying policies in schools and the workplace.
- Provide health care professionals with knowledge of the health needs of the LGBTQ+ community and training on related mental health issues.
- Continue efforts to expand domestic partner health insurance coverage.
- Establish community advisory boards and LGBTQ+ health centers.
- Disseminate effective HIV and sexually transmitted infection interventions.

infection among MSM and transgender women, especially those living with HIV, is higher than for heterosexual males. Screening for hepatitis C virus (HCV) antibodies is recommended for those at risk. Vaccines for Mpox and meningitis are recommended for MSM who have additional risk factors.[21,22]

Given the higher rates of HIV infection and STIs among MSM and transgender women, assess the patient's awareness of their HIV and STI status. Teach those without HIV about strategies to prevent it. Include preexposure prophylaxis (PrEP) and postexposure prophylaxis (PEP) (see Chapter 15).

Breast and cervical cancer screenings are important for lesbian and bisexual females. Ensuring that females receive appropriate preventive screening and early detection can help reduce the complications associated with these cancers.

Remember that not all transgender people undergo surgical transition. In fact, many choose not to undergo surgical transition for a variety of reasons. Thus a transgender woman may still have a prostate and be at risk for prostate cancer. Similarly, a transgender man with a cervix should have a screening for cervical cancer. Do not assume that a transgender patient has had gender-affirming surgery.

Tobacco use is thought to be 2 to 3 times higher among LGBTQ+ persons. Tobacco use increases the risk for conditions such as pulmonary and cardiovascular problems. Screen for tobacco use as part of routine care. For those who report using tobacco, provide education and assistance by referring them to a tobacco cessation program or specialist. See more about cessation in Chapter 11.

GENDER-AFFIRMING CARE

Gender-Affirming Hormone Therapy

Testosterone and estrogen are both naturally occurring hormones in those assigned male and female at birth. Testosterone is responsible for physical attributes such as increased muscle mass, facial hair, and a lower voice. Estrogen produces female characteristics. These include softer skin, breast development, and changes in the distribution of body fat.

Gender-affirming hormone therapy (GAHT) provides transgender persons the opportunity to transition from their sex assigned at birth to the gender that aligns with their sense of being. Table 6.4 provides a summary of GAHT options for transgender persons. For a person whose sex assigned at birth was female but who identifies as male, testosterone therapy is used. A person who was assigned male sex at birth but whose

TABLE 6.4 Gender-Affirming Hormone Therapy

Masculinizing Hormone Therapy Options

Hormone	Anticipated Effects	Nursing Considerations
Testosterone *Available formulations:* • Injectable testosterone • Topical testosterone	• ↑ Abdominal fat • Acne • Amenorrhea • Clitoromegaly • Deepening voice • ↑ Facial hair • ↑ Hemoglobin and hematocrit • ↑ Muscle mass • Vaginal dryness • Oily skin	When given IM or subcutaneously, teach injection techniques. Review importance of rotating injection sites. For topical therapy, apply daily. Avoid skin contact with others until testosterone has dried to avoid unintentional transfer of testosterone. Contraindications include pregnancy, unstable coronary artery disease, and untreated polycythemia with a hematocrit of 55% or higher. Patients with history of breast or estrogen-dependent cancers should consult with oncologist before hormone use. Although menses may cease, persons at risk for pregnancy should consider another method of birth control.

Feminizing Hormone Therapy Options

Hormone	Anticipated Effects	Considerations for Care
Estradiol *Available formulations:* • Oral or sublingual estradiol • Injectable estradiol valerate • Transdermal estradiol patch	• Breast growth • Erectile dysfunction • Fat redistribution from the abdomen to the hips • ↓ Libido • ↓ Prostate and testicular size • Skin softens • Slowing of androgenetic hair loss	Bioidentical forms are preferred. Take oral/sublingual formulations daily. ↑ Risk of venous thromboembolic (VTE) events. Contraindicated in persons with previous VTE related to an underlying hypercoagulable condition, history of estrogen-sensitive cancers, or end-stage liver disease. For persons using injectable therapy, teach injection techniques. Some patients on estrogen therapy are at risk of prolactinomas. Refer for evaluation patients with new-onset galactorrhea, vision changes, or headaches. May worsen migraines, so patients with preexisting migraines should start on lower doses and titrate upwards as needed.
Antiandrogen *Available formulations:*		
• Spironolactone		Monitor potassium levels, especially for patients with renal disease or who are on ACEs or ARBs.
• Finasteride/dutasteride		Preferred for patients unable to tolerate or with contraindications to spironolactone.

ACE, Angiotensin-converting enzyme; *ARB*, angiotensin receptor blocker.

Data from Hembree WC, Cohen-Kettenis PT, Gooren L, et al: Endocrine treatment of gender-dysphoric/gender-incongruent persons: an Endocrine Society clinical practice guideline, *J Clin Endocrinol Met* 102:3869, 2017; Fenway Health: *Medical care of trans and gender diverse adults.* Retrieved from https://fenwayhealth.org/wp-content/uploads/Medical-Care-of-Trans-and-Gender-Diverse-Adults-Spring-2021-1.pdf.

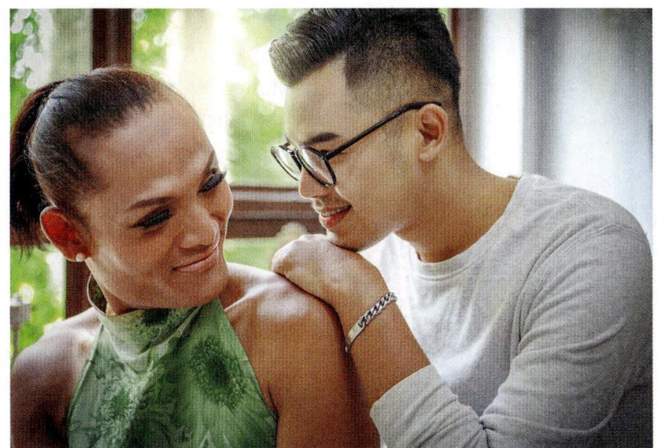

Fig. 6.4 The goal of gender-affirming hormone therapy is to align a person's hormones and physical appearance with their identified gender. (©TwilightShow/iStock.com.)

gender is female is prescribed feminizing hormone therapy with estrogen and an antiandrogen.[23] The goal of GAHT is to align a person's hormones and physical attributes with their affirmed gender (Fig. 6.4).

The physical changes of GAHT occur over an extended period, much like puberty. Transgender men who start testosterone therapy will typically experience cessation of menses and increased body hair within the first few months of starting therapy. Transgender women who are starting feminizing hormones with estrogen and an antiandrogen agent may develop breast buds after several months of therapy. For many people, the maximum effects of hormone therapy can take several years.

Several guidelines for the care and management of transgender persons exist. The World Professional Association for Transgender Health (WPATH) is an international organization of health professionals who have developed standards of care for transgender persons.[23] The Endocrine Society and TransLine (a collaborative of transgender medicine specialists) have published guidelines on the use of GAHT and gender-affirming surgery.[24,25]

As part of an initial assessment before GAHT, ask patients about their desires for future fertility and reproductive health. Hormone or medical therapy may affect future fertility. We should have a conversation and provide resources about sperm or egg preservation for those who are interested.

Counsel patients starting GAHT about possible side effects and the importance of adherence to hormone therapy. Teach those receiving injectable therapy how to properly inject hormones if they are going to be doing self-injections. If someone on GAHT is hospitalized, maintain their hormone therapy during their hospitalization if there are no contraindications.

Nonsurgical Gender-Affirming Interventions

Some transgender persons may begin their transition process by including nonsurgical or nonhormonal interventions to help align their physical appearance with their gender identity.[26] Examples include chest binding of the breasts for transgender men who wish to have a more masculine-appearing chest. Transgender women with a penis may "tuck" their penis to flatten the front part of their genital area. Those who do chest binding or tucking may develop skin irritation in these areas. Assess if they have any issues with skin infections, rashes, or irritations and intervene as needed.

Other nonsurgical interventions include laser hair removal or dermal fillers.[27] Transgender women can use these fillers to feminize facial features; transgender men can use fillers to make facial features more masculine. When implanted correctly, fillers are a safe and effective way to create wanted changes to the appearance of the body in a similar manner to non-transgender people. Some transgender women may get silicone or other substances injected illicitly in nonmedical settings (sometimes referred to as "pumping parties"). Use of these substances can lead to serious complications.

Vocal therapy is an intervention used by transgender women to help feminize their voices.[28] A speech pathologist who is trained in working with transgender patients can help them achieve a higher pitch to their voice. In some cases, the person may have vocal surgery.

Gender-Affirming Surgery

Gender-affirming surgery (sometimes called *gender reconstructive surgery*) refers to surgical procedures performed to create either more masculinizing features in a transgender man or feminizing features in a transgender woman.[23] There are a number of gender-affirming surgical options for transgender persons. The range and type of surgery depend on several factors. The main one is patient desires and goals. Not all transgender persons wish to have gender-affirming surgery. Table 6.5 outlines the types of gender-affirming surgeries and procedures. Depending on the type of procedure done, a person may need to have several procedures over time to achieve the desired outcome.

More hospitals are performing gender-affirming surgery. Nurses caring for patients having gender-affirming surgery need to be familiar with providing appropriate and supportive care before surgery and through the recovery period. For patients who need wound care after surgery, home care nurses and office-based primary care nurses may need to provide wound care teaching.

Chest Masculinization Surgery

Chest masculinization surgery is a surgical intervention for transgender men. As part of this procedure, breast tissue is removed and the chest is reshaped to have a more masculine appearance. The nipples may be repositioned to provide a more masculine-appearing chest. There are several surgical approaches and techniques based on the patient's anatomy and surgical preference. These include variation in incision site, incision size, and preservation of nerve sensation in the nipples. Previous hormone therapy with testosterone is not a requirement.

TABLE 6.5 Gender-Affirming Surgical Procedures

Feminizing Surgical Procedures	
Breast augmentation/ feminizing augmentation mammoplasty	• Implants (saline or silicone) are placed under the breast muscle to enhance breast size. • May be done using fat transferred from another part of the body.
Facial feminization surgery	• Surgical procedures done to make the face softer and more feminine in appearance. • Includes brow lifts, hairline adjustment, nose reshaping, cheek implants, blepharoplasty, mandibular angle reduction, chin width reduction, lip reshaping, tracheal shave (thyroid chondroplasty).
Orchiectomy	• Removal of the testicles.
Vaginoplasty	• Creates a vagina. • Penis, testicles, and scrotum are removed. The tissue is then reshaped to create a neo-vagina. May have skin grafting from the abdomen or thigh. • Dilators used afterward to help keep the graft from contracting and to improve elasticity of the vagina.
Masculinizing Surgical Procedures	
Hysterectomy and oophorectomy	• Removal of the uterus and ovaries.
Masculinizing chest reconstruction (mastectomy)	• Breast tissue is removed and reshaped to have a more masculine appearance.
Metoidioplasty (meta)	• Creation of a penis from existing genital tissue, including the clitoris.
Pectoral implants	• Implants used to create a more masculine chest.
Phalloplasty	• Multistage procedure that creates a penis. • Several techniques exist. • Typically involves lengthening the urethra, creating a scrotum, removing the vagina, placing erectile and testicular implants, and grafting additional skin and muscle from the forearm, thigh, or latissimus dorsi.
Scrotoplasty	• Creation of a scrotum. • Typically includes testicular implants.

From Li VY, Demzik A, Snyder L, et al: Genital gender affirming surgery. *Am Surg* 88:2817, 2022.

Feminizing Breast Augmentation

Feminizing breast surgery provides transgender women an opportunity to augment their breasts with implants to create a more feminine appearance. Although GAHT can cause breast development in transgender women, in some people, hormone therapy alone does not produce the desired results for breast development. Some surgical centers require a person to be on hormone therapy for at least 12 months to allow for maximal breast growth before surgery. Options for breast implants include gel or saline implants and fat transfer. With fat transfer, body fat is removed from one part of the body and injected or placed around the breast to enhance or augment the shape.

NURSING MANAGEMENT: GENDER-AFFIRMING SURGERY

Assessment

Current guidelines for transgender care recommend that patients undergoing either chest masculinization or breast augmentation surgery have persistent and well-documented gender dysphoria, the capacity and ability to provide informed consent, be the age of majority, and have any medical or mental health concerns well controlled.[23] The surgical team should work closely with the patient's hormone therapy and mental health providers to make sure that the patient is a good candidate for surgery and prepared for the procedure and postsurgical recovery period.

Implementation

Acute Care

After surgery, provide general postoperative care as described in Chapter 20. Some patients having chest masculinization or breast augmentation surgery may have surgical drains. If drains are present, assess the amount and type of drainage. A chest binder or other supportive dressings are in place until the surgical wounds are healed. Assess the dressing for signs of excess bleeding.

Pain management during the recovery period is important for patients having either chest masculinization or breast augmentation surgery. Assess pain level. Give analgesics as ordered to keep patients comfortable.

Postprocedure complications include seromas, hematomas, and infection. Teach and monitor patients for signs or symptoms of infection. Patients will often have limited range of motion for several weeks afterward. Teach patients how to minimize movement. Have patients avoid activities such as heavy lifting or reaching. They may need help with certain activities or must make modifications in the home or work environment. For example, moving items from a high shelf to a lower shelf or countertop will help avoid stretching.

Chronic Care

Although breast tissue is removed with chest masculinization surgery, there is still a potential for breast cancer development. Counsel those with a history of breast cancer or a high risk for breast cancer on the importance of regular screening. There are limited data on breast cancer prevalence in persons who have had feminizing breast augmentation surgery. Some guidelines recommend that breast cancer screening in transgender women at average risk begin at age 40 if the person has been on estrogen therapy for at least 5 years.[29] The length of exposure to feminizing hormones influences the risk of breast cancer.

CASE STUDY

Breast Cancer

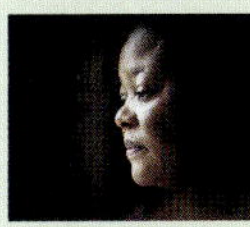

(©ands456/ iStock.com)

Patient Profile

M.P. is a 57-year-old cisgender female who identifies as a lesbian. She was diagnosed with stage IIB breast cancer and had a mastectomy. She is admitted to your unit after surgery.

Subjective Data

- Diagnosed with stage IIB breast cancer last month
- Noted a mass in her right breast earlier in the year after having some discomfort
- Avoided getting a mammogram for several years
- Has a female partner of 7 years

Objective Data

- Temperature: 98.2°F, BP: 118/78 mm Hg, heart rate 78 beats/min, respiratory rate is 16 breaths/min and unlabored
- Reports 4/10 pain in her right breast
- Surgical dressing is dry and intact
- 2 Jackson-Pratt drains with a minimal amount of blood-tinged drainage
- Has a flattened affect and is tearful

Discussion Questions

1. ***Recognize:*** What do you know about the rates of cancer in the LGBTQ+ community?
2. ***Recognize:*** What factors may have caused M.P. to delay seeking care?
3. ***Plan:*** What other interprofessional team members might be useful to involve?
4. ***Prioritize:*** Based on the information provided, what are the priority nursing interventions?
5. ***Act:*** M.P. tells you that she is concerned about how her surgery will affect her sexual relationship with her partner. How would you respond?

Answers available at http://evolve.elsevier.com/Lewis/medsurg.

BRIDGE TO NCLEX EXAMINATION

The number of the question corresponds to the same-numbered outcome at the beginning of the chapter.

1. The nurse caring for a patient who was assigned male at birth but identifies as female understands that the
   - **a.** patient is gay.
   - **b.** patient's gender is female.
   - **c.** patient is a cisgender female.
   - **d.** patient requires testosterone therapy.
2. A nurse is caring for a cisgender female patient who underwent a bilateral mastectomy for breast cancer. The patient discloses that she identifies as a lesbian. Which statement demonstrates an understanding of health disparities and the LGBTQ+ community?
   - **a.** "When was your last eye exam?"
   - **b.** "Have you been screened for arthritis?"
   - **c.** "Has anyone ever tried to hurt or harm you?"
   - **d.** "Do you need a referral to a hormone therapy specialist?"
3. Strategies for creating an LGBTQ+ inclusive environment include
   - **a.** Limiting use of single-stall bathrooms to those in wheelchairs.
   - **b.** Referring to patients only by the name on their insurance card.
   - **c.** Assigning a transgender patient to a private room, when possible.
   - **d.** Only allowing a patient's immediate biologic family visiting rights.
4. A patient is starting feminizing gender-affirming hormone therapy with oral estrogen. What would the nurse include as part of patient teaching? **(Select all that apply.)**
   - **a.** Educate about changes in libido
   - **b.** Educate about the cessation of menses
   - **c.** Discuss the rate of increased hair growth
   - **d.** Review the symptoms of a pulmonary embolism and stroke
   - **e.** Educate on the need to seek medical attention if they have increased headaches
5. You are caring for a transgender man who underwent chest masculinization surgery. What information would be part of the discharge instructions?
   - **a.** "You can stop testosterone therapy."
   - **b.** "You will need regular prostate cancer screening."
   - **c.** "Talk with your surgeon about your need for mammograms."
   - **d.** "Discuss with your hormone therapy provider about resuming estrogen."

1. b; 2. c; 3. c; 4. a, d, e; 5. c.

For rationales to these answers and even more NCLEX review questions, visit http://evolve.elsevier.com/Lewis/medsurg.

REFERENCES

To access the References for this chapter, please scan the QR code with a mobile device.

7

Stress Management

Margaret R. Rateau

http://evolve.elsevier.com/Lewis/medsurg/

CONCEPTUAL FOCUS

Risk for Disease

Stress and Coping

LEARNING OUTCOMES

1. Explain the nature of stress and stressors.
2. Describe the role of the nervous and endocrine systems in the stress process.
3. Describe the effects of stress on the immune system.
4. Discuss the effects of stress on health.
5. Explain the role of coping in managing stress.
6. Select coping and relaxation strategies that a person experiencing stress can use.
7. Describe the assessment and management of a patient experiencing stress.

KEY TERMS

biofeedback
coping
emotion-focused coping
imagery
massage
meditation
problem-focused coping
relaxation breathing
stress
stressors

All people have stress. Stress has a powerful effect on the mind and a significant effect on health and well-being. Chronic stress is a major factor in causing and worsening chronic health conditions. This in turn is a major driver of soaring health care costs.

High levels of stress are common among patients and caregivers. How they deal with their stress is critical to their well-being. As a nurse, you play a key role in helping them recognize stress and manage stressful events. This chapter focuses on how stress can affect the mind, body, and spirit and how a person can effectively cope with stress.

WHAT IS STRESS?

Stress is a state of worry or mental tension created by a demanding life situation. Stress is a natural human response. We all experience stress at some point in time.[1] Stress is more prevalent in women. Increased stress levels are associated with unemployment for both males and females.[2]

Many different things can be **stressors**. They can be physical, like illness and pain; mental, like death of a loved one or fear; or situational, like the loss of a home through fire (Fig. 7.1). Mental and situational stressors can be positive or negative. For example, the birth of a baby is usually a positive stressor. Marital discord is a negative stressor.

Perception of the potential stressor influences the way a person responds to that stressor. Responses to the same stressor vary greatly. What one person perceives as stressful may not be perceived as stressful to someone else. This is shown in the following examples:

- B.J., a 37-year-old female, seems depressed after a laparoscopic hysterectomy for cervical cancer. She is unwilling to take part in normal self-care activities. You think she had

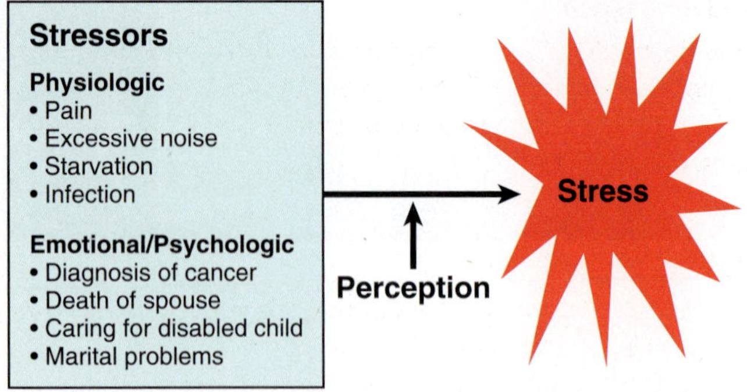

Fig. 7.1 Stressors can be physiologic or emotional/psychologic. Events or circumstances become stressful when you perceive them to be.

a simple surgery and should be recovering more quickly. After further assessment, you discover that removing her uterus is a great stressor because she was considering having another baby.

- K.R., a 59-year-old female, has just been told by her HCP of a new diagnosis of type 2 diabetes. You were prepared to provide emotional support because of the stress of this new diagnosis. However, you are puzzled when she is smiling and feeling relieved. K.R. tells you that she is so relieved because for weeks she was worried that her symptoms were caused by cancer.

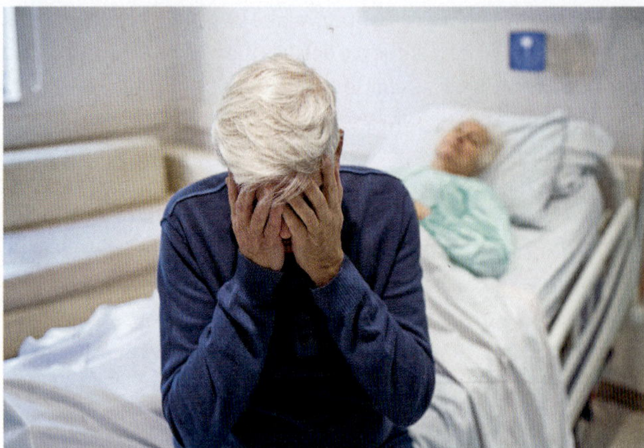

Fig. 7.2 During stressful situations, demands may exceed resources. (© izusek/iStock.com.)

Is Stress Bad or Good?

Any event or situation that is out of the ordinary can be a stressor. We tend to think of stress as bad or a threat because too much can be harmful (Fig. 7.2). Things that we normally consider happy or enjoy, such as getting married or going on vacation, can be a stressor. Stress can be helpful. A little stress can motivate you. Stress can inspire you to achieve a goal or become more confident.

The body responds to the stressor with the same stress response. The stress response is the way our bodies react both physically and emotionally to any change. The body cannot tell between bad and good or real or imagined stress. It responds to the stressor with the same stress response.

As a nursing student, a test can be a stressful situation. A little bit of stress related to an upcoming test makes you study and become better prepared. If you feel mildly stressed during the test, it may help your test performance. A little stress heightens your awareness and increases your mental acuity. However, if you are too stressed, it causes mental blocks, lack of concentration, and inability to remember things.

TABLE 7.1 Factors Affecting Response to Stress

Internal
• Age
• Attitude
• Experience with stressors
• Genetic background
• Hardiness
• Health status
• Nutrition status
• Optimistic outlook
• Personality characteristics
• Resilience
• Sleep status
External
• Cultural and ethnic influences
• Number of stressors present
• Religious or spiritual influences
• Socioeconomic status
• Social support
• Timing of stressors

Factors Affecting Response to Stress

Why do people respond so differently to stress? Why do some people cope better with stress than others? Some people experience significant adverse life events but do not succumb to the effects of stress. Your mind is the most powerful weapon that you have to deal with and conquer stress. You have a choice in how you respond to a crisis or a difficult time. Even if the outcome of the situation is not what you wanted, you can emerge with a winning attitude.

Internal and external factors play a role in the ability to cope with stress (Table 7.1). Being surrounded by a strong social support system and receiving positive support from friends and family have a large impact on your ability to cope with stress (Fig. 7.2).

Key personal characteristics that buffer the effects of stress are attitude, hardiness, being optimistic, and resilience. *Resilience* is being resourceful and flexible and having good problem-solving skills. People who have a high degree of resilience are not as likely to perceive an event as stressful.

Hardiness is a combination of 3 characteristics: commitment, control, and openness to change. Together they give the courage and motivation needed to turn stressful circumstances from potential calamities into opportunities for personal growth.

Attitude can influence the effect of stress on a person. People with positive attitudes view situations differently from those with negative attitudes. Attitude also influences how they manage stress. To some extent, positive attitudes can prevent disease and prolong life.[3]

Being optimistic can help you cope better with stress.[3] Optimism also reduces the chance of developing stress-related illnesses. When optimistic people do become ill, they tend to recover more quickly.

PHYSIOLOGIC RESPONSE TO STRESS

The nervous, endocrine, and immune systems are involved in the stress response. These systems are interrelated. This interrelationship is reflected in the physiologic response to stress (Fig. 7.3). Stress activation of these systems affects other body systems, such as the cardiovascular, respiratory, gastrointestinal (GI), renal, and endocrine systems. A person's response to a stressor determines the impact that stress will have on the body.

Nervous System

Cerebral Cortex

The areas of the cerebral cortex, or cerebrum, involved in the control of cognition, affect, and movement influence how we perceive stressors. We evaluate the stressor in light of past experiences and future consequences. This gives us some control over our response to stress. The motor areas send signals to the adrenal medulla that directly relate to how stressors are managed.

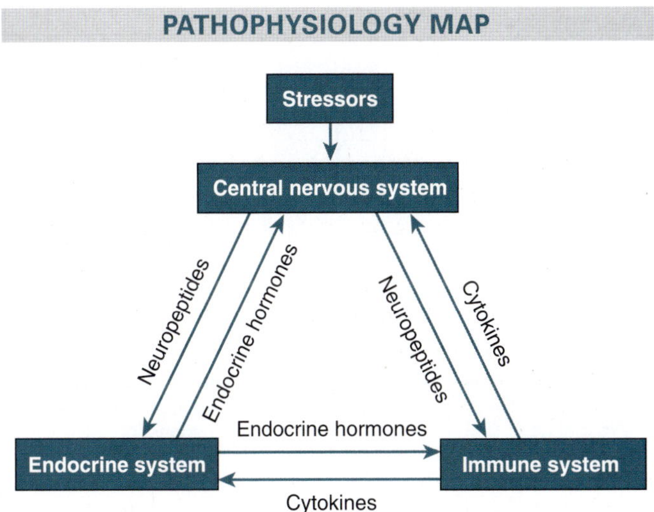

Fig. 7.3 Neurochemical links among the nervous, endocrine, and immune systems. The communication among the systems is bidirectional.

Limbic System

The limbic system is an important mediator of emotions and behavior. When the limbic system is stimulated, emotions, feelings, and behaviors can occur that ensure survival and self-preservation.

Reticular Formation

The reticular formation contains the reticular activating system (RAS), which sends impulses contributing to alertness to the limbic system and cerebral cortex. When the RAS is stimulated, it increases its output of impulses, leading to wakefulness. Stress usually increases the degree of wakefulness and can lead to sleep problems.

Hypothalamus

The hypothalamus has many functions that aid in adapting to stress. Stress activates the limbic system, which in turn stimulates the hypothalamus. Because the hypothalamus secretes neuropeptides that regulate the release of hormones by the anterior pituitary, it is central to the connection between the nervous and endocrine systems in responding to stress (Fig. 7.4).

The hypothalamus plays a key role in the stress response by regulating the function of both the sympathetic and parasympathetic branches of the autonomic nervous system. When a person perceives a stressor, the hypothalamus sends signals that initiate both the nervous and endocrine responses to the stressor. It does this mainly by sending signals via nerve fibers to stimulate the sympathetic nervous system (SNS) and by

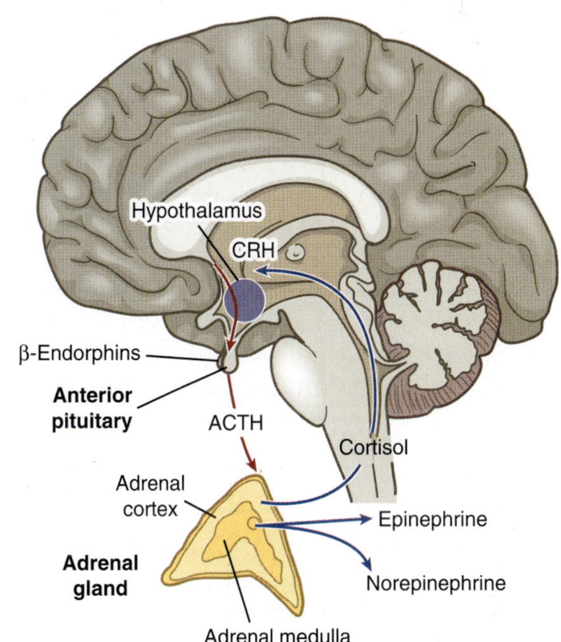

Fig. 7.4 Hypothalamic-pituitary-adrenal axis. *ACTH,* Adrenocorticotropic hormone; *CRH,* corticotropin-releasing hormone.

releasing corticotropin-releasing hormone (CRH). CRH stimulates the pituitary to release adrenocorticotropic hormone (ACTH) (see Chapter 52).

Endocrine System

Once the hypothalamus is activated in response to stress, the endocrine system becomes involved. The SNS stimulates the adrenal medulla to release epinephrine and norepinephrine (catecholamines). The effect of catecholamines and the activation of the SNS, including the response of the adrenal medulla, is referred to as the *sympathoadrenal response.* Epinephrine and norepinephrine prepare the body for the *fight-or-flight response* (Fig. 7.5).

Stress activates the hypothalamic-pituitary-adrenal (HPA) axis. In response to stress, the hypothalamus releases CRH, which stimulates the anterior pituitary to release proopiomelanocortin (POMC). Both ACTH (a hormone) and β-endorphin (a neuropeptide) are derived from POMC. Endorphins have analgesic-like effects and blunt pain perception during stress situations involving pain stimuli. ACTH in turn stimulates the adrenal cortex to synthesize and secrete corticosteroids (e.g., cortisol) and, to a lesser degree, aldosterone.

Corticosteroids are essential for the stress response. Cortisol produces several physiologic effects, such as increasing glucose levels, increasing the action of catecholamines on blood vessels, and inhibiting the inflammatory response. Corticosteroids play an important role in "turning off" or blunting the stress response, which, if uncontrolled, can become self-destructive. This is shown by their ability to suppress the release of proinflammatory mediators, such as the cytokines tumor necrosis factor (TNF) and interleukin-1 (IL-1). The persistent release of these mediators is thought to initiate organ dysfunction in conditions such as sepsis or autoimmune disease. Thus corticosteroids act not only to support the body's adaptive response to a stressor but also to suppress an overzealous and potentially self-destructive response.

The stress response involves increases in (1) cardiac output (from the increased heart rate and increased stroke volume), (2) glucose levels, (3) oxygen consumption, and (4) metabolic rate (Fig. 7.5). Dilation of skeletal muscle blood vessels increases blood supply to the large muscles and supports quick movement. Increased cerebral blood flow increases mental alertness. Increased blood volume from increased extracellular fluid and the shunting of blood away from the GI system helps to maintain adequate circulation to vital organs.

Summary of Stress Response

In summary, the fight-or-flight response is an important and necessary adaptive mechanism of the body to acute stress. We activate this response to stressors whether they are physiologic or emotional/psychologic. Acute stress leads to physiologic changes that are important to a person's survival. This is your "alarm system." It puts you on high alert. The acute stress response is a state of physiologic and psychologic arousal characterized by increased SNS activity that leads to increased heart and respiratory rate, increased BP, and decreased skin temperature (Fig. 7.6).

Immune System

Stress affects the immune system. Because neuroanatomic and neuroendocrine pathways connect the brain to the immune system, stressors have the potential to lead to changes in immune function (Fig. 7.7).

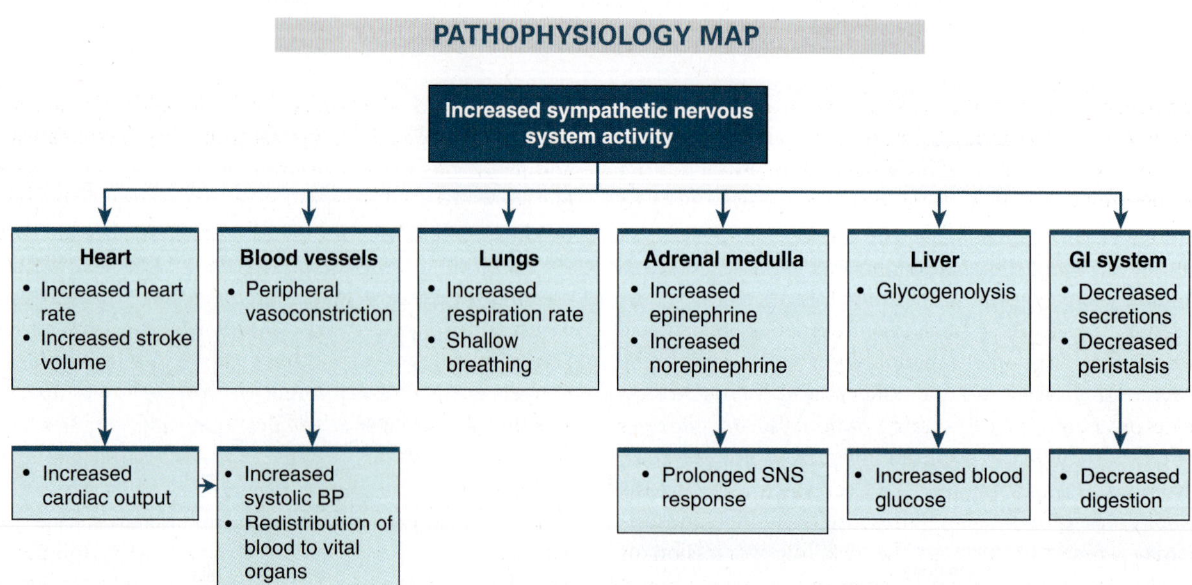

Fig. 7.5 "Fight-or-flight" reaction. Alarm reaction responses resulting from increased sympathetic nervous system *(SNS)* activity.

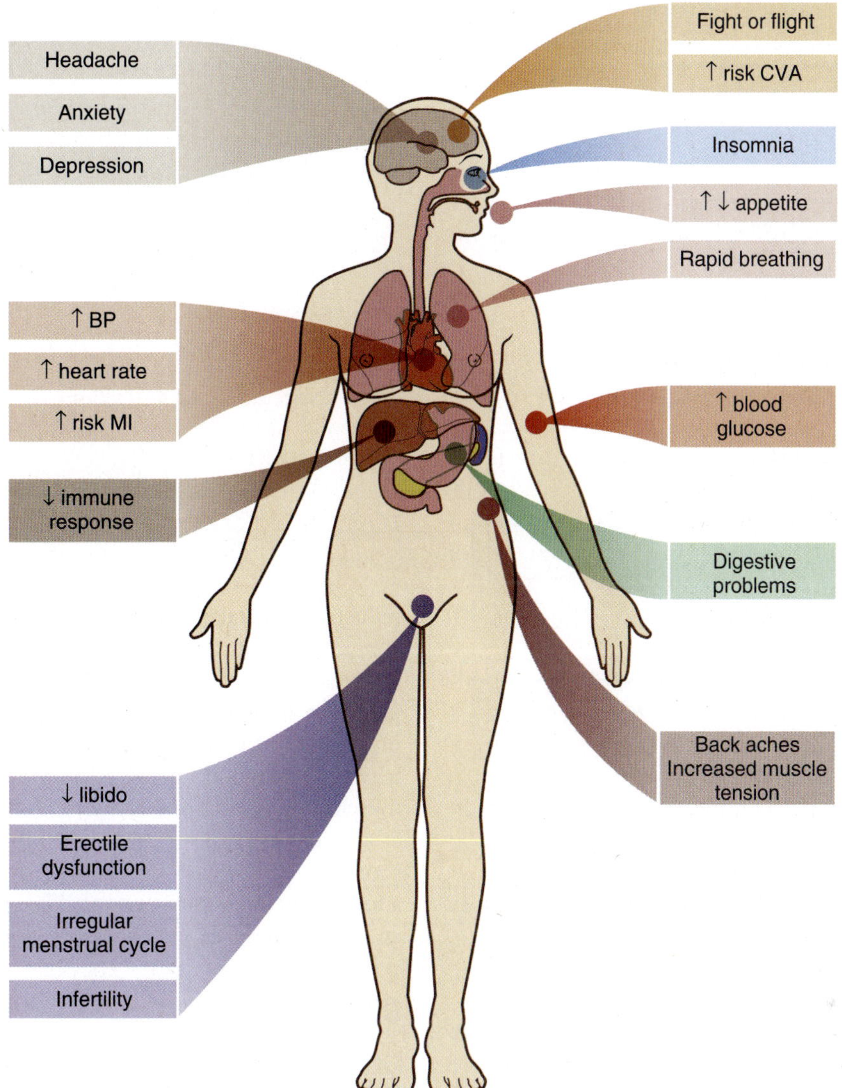

Fig. 7.6 Effects of stress on the body. (From Halter MJ: *Varcarolis' foundations of psychiatric mental health nursing*, ed 9, Philadelphia, 2022, Saunders.)

Nerve fibers extend from the nervous system and synapse on cells and tissues of the immune system (i.e., spleen, lymph nodes). In turn, the cells of the immune system have receptors for many neuropeptides and hormones. This allows them to respond to nervous and neuroendocrine signals. As a result, the mediation of stress by the central nervous system leads to corresponding changes in immune cell activity.

Both acute and chronic stress can cause immunosuppression. Stress affects immune function by (1) decreasing the number and function of natural killer cells; (2) decreasing lymphocyte proliferation; (3) altering production of *cytokines* (soluble factors secreted by white blood cells and other cells, e.g., interferon, interleukins); and (4) decreasing phagocytosis by neutrophils and monocytes. Stress-induced immunosuppression may worsen or increase the risk for progression of immune-related diseases such as asthma, inflammatory bowel syndrome, and diabetes.[4]

The network that links the brain and immune system is bidirectional (Fig. 7.3). Signals from these systems travel back and forth, allowing for communication between these systems. Not only do emotions influence the immune response, but products of immune cells send signals back to the brain and alter its activity. Many of the communication signals sent from the immune system to the brain are mediated by cytokines, which are central to the coordination of the immune response. For example, IL-1 (a cytokine made by monocytes) acts on the temperature regulatory center of the hypothalamus and initiates the febrile response to infectious pathogens (see Fig. 12.4).

EFFECTS OF STRESS ON HEALTH

The acute stress response is your alarm system and puts you on alert. However, your body was not meant to be on high alert all the time. If stress is excessive or prolonged, these same

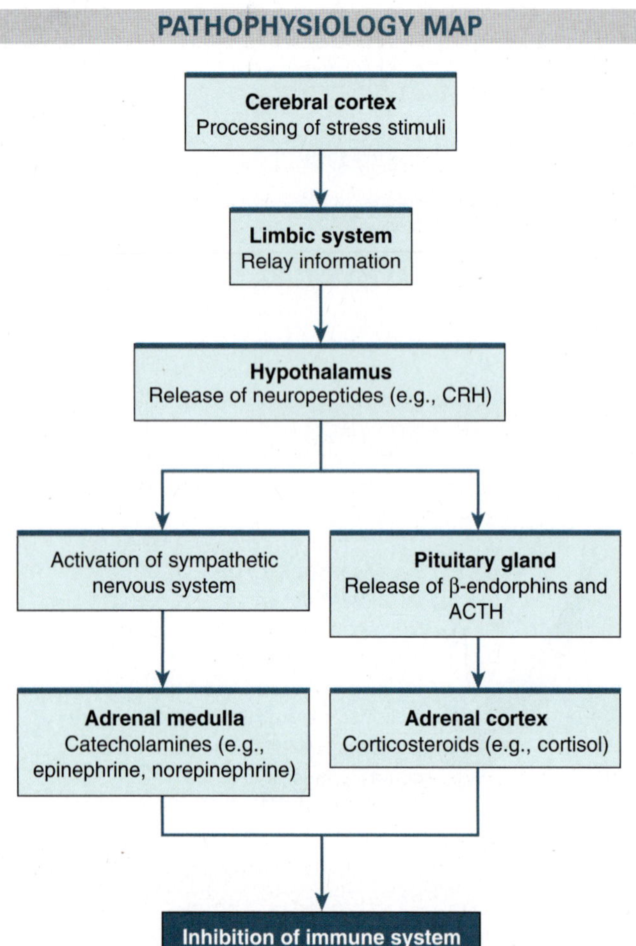

Fig. 7.7 The cerebral cortex processes stressful stimuli and relays the information via the limbic system to the hypothalamus. Corticotropin-releasing hormone *(CRH)* stimulates the release of adrenocorticotropic hormone *(ACTH)* from the pituitary gland. ACTH stimulates the adrenal cortex to release corticosteroids. Sympathetic nervous system stimulation causes the release of epinephrine and norepinephrine. The result is immune system inhibition.

"helpful" physiologic responses can lead to harm and disease. When a person has chronic, unrelieved stress, the body's defenses cannot keep up with the demands. This is how stress plays a role in the development and/or progression of stress-related illness (Table 7.2). This is why it is important for you and your patients to learn to cope effectively with stress.

Stress can have effects on cognitive function, including poor concentration, memory problems, distressing dreams, sleep problems, and impaired decision making. It can cause a wide variety of changes in behavior. These include withdrawing from others, decreased interest in physical appearance, changing eating habits, drinking excess alcohol, or being irritable.[5] Stress is linked to accidents and suicides. Long-term exposure to catecholamines from SNS activation may increase the risk for cardiovascular diseases such as heart attack, hypertension, and stroke.[6] Problems that are worsened by stress include diabetes, asthma, and anxiety. Behavior interventions aimed at stress reduction and relaxation have helped manage these diseases in conjunction with standard medical treatment.[7]

TABLE 7.2 Common Health Problems With a Stress Component

- Cancer
- Depression
- Dyspepsia
- Eating disorders
- Erectile dysfunction
- Fatigue
- Fibromyalgia
- Headaches
- Hypertension
- Insomnia
- Irritable bowel syndrome
- Low back pain
- Menstrual irregularities
- Peptic ulcer disease
- Sexual problems

Stress can make a person more susceptible to infection, including the common cold.[8] At the cellular level, stress may promote earlier onset of age-related diseases. There is a link between stress and telomere length. Telomeres are the protective end caps on chromosomes. Their diminishing size is a sign of age. Telomeres are highly susceptible to stress. Telomeres are shorter in people who are stressed. Thus chronic stress can have a long-term effect on our overall health by changing our DNA and accelerating the rate at which our cells age.[9]

COPING STRATEGIES

Coping is a person's efforts to manage stressors. *Coping strategies* are what you do (your behaviors and actions) to help deal with stress. Coping can be either positive or negative. Positive coping includes activities such as exercise and spending time with friends and family. Healthy coping helps you handle your stressors so that they do not overwhelm you. Negative coping may include substance use and denial.

Some coping strategies make the stress worse. Sometimes coping strategies temporarily relieve the stress, but in the long run they increase the stress. For example, you may really enjoy watching a favorite TV show as a form of coping. However, if you become fixated on several reality shows, then TV becomes an addiction and an escape from dealing with your real stressors.

We can use a number of coping strategies. Table 7.3 has examples of coping strategies that you can use in your life and teach to your patients and their caregivers. Coping strategies can be divided into 2 broad categories: emotion-focused coping and problem-focused coping. **Emotion-focused coping** involves managing the emotions that you feel when a stressful event occurs. When a situation is unchangeable or uncontrollable, emotion-focused coping may predominate. Emotion-focused coping helps decrease negative emotions and create a

TABLE 7.3 Coping Strategies

Strategy	Description	How to Implement
Aromatherapy	• Use of essential oils (fragrant molecules from plants) for inhalation or topical application • Variety of essential oils, including lavender, peppermint, rosemary, eucalyptus, tea tree	• Place 5–8 drops in a full bath and agitate water before bathing • Place a few drops on a tissue or in diffuser or vaporizer • Apply diluted with an oil and massage
Art Therapy	• Allows a person to nonverbally express and communicate feelings, emotions, and thoughts • Can reduce stress, promote relaxation, and help process experiences • Based on the belief that the creative process is healing and life enhancing	• Paint or draw • Get a piece of paper and doodle • Get a coloring book and crayons and just start coloring • Do knitting or crochet work • Make a themed collage or scrapbook
Exercise	• Any form of movement, especially aerobic movement • Can be viewed as meditation in motion	• Walk, swim, garden, bicycle, dance, climb stairs, take part in group exercises
Humor	• Can take the form of laughter, cartoons, funny movies, videos, riddles, comic books, and joke books	• Keep a "tickler" scrapbook with funny photos, cartoons • Humor carts can be set up in the clinical setting for patient and family use
Journaling	• Allows a person to express self in writing • Enhances personal development and awareness through self-reflection	• Use a journaling notebook or computer to write down thoughts, feelings, memories, and perceptions
Pet Therapy (Animal-Assisted Therapy) (Fig. 7.8)	• Use of animals as a form of treatment • Improves social, emotional, or cognitive functioning	• Pet therapist or family member or friend brings a pet with which patient can socialize
Social Support	• Relationships with family and friends • Self-help groups and professional help	• Get together with family and friends on a regular basis • Join a support group that specifically helps to meet needs (e.g., grief support group)

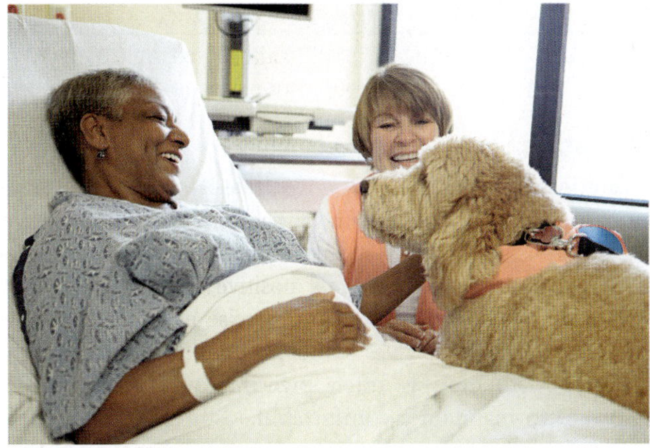

Fig. 7.8 Pet therapy can be used in a variety of settings including stress management counseling. (© monkeybusinessimages/iStock.com.)

feeling of well-being. Examples include discussing feelings with a friend or taking a hot bath.

Problem-focused coping involves attempts to resolve the problems causing the stress. If you can change or control a problem, this strategy is the most helpful. Problem-focused coping allows a person to reduce stress by actively addressing the problem. Setting priorities, collecting information, and seeking advice are examples of problem-focused coping.

We often use a combination of strategies to cope with the same stressor. Table 7.4 gives examples of emotion- and problem-focused coping applied to the same stressful situation.

TABLE 7.4 Problem- and Emotion-Focused Coping Examples

Stressor	Problem-Focused Coping	Emotion-Focused Coping
Failing an examination	Obtaining a tutor	Going for a run
Being diagnosed with diabetes	Attending education classes about diabetes	Getting a massage
Receiving questionable mammogram results	Scheduling follow-up testing for ultrasound	Expressing feelings of anxiety to friends and nurse

RELAXATION STRATEGIES

The *relaxation response* is a state of physiologic and psychologic rest. It is opposite of the stress response. The relaxation response is characterized by decreased SNS activity. This leads to decreased heart and respiratory rate, decreased BP, decreased muscle tension, decreased brain activity, and increased skin temperature.

We can use various relaxation strategies to elicit the relaxation response (Table 7.5). Regularly eliciting the relaxation response is an effective treatment for a wide range of stress-related disorders, including chronic pain, insomnia, and hypertension. People who regularly use relaxation strategies cope better with everyday life and can decrease their stress levels in their bodies and minds.[10]

TABLE 7.5 Common Relaxation Strategies

- Biofeedback
- Imagery
- Massage
- Meditation
- Muscle relaxation
- Music
- Qigong
- Relaxing breathing
- Tai Chi
- Yoga

Relaxation Breathing

The way you breathe affects every aspect of life. When you are stressed, muscles tense and breathing becomes shallow and rapid. So, a simple and effective way to stop the stress response is to breathe deeply and slowly. It is hard to stay tense when breathing in a slow, deep, and relaxed pattern. **Relaxation breathing** forms the basis for most relaxation strategies (Table 7.6). It is especially useful during a stressful or anxious situation to reduce stress. You can do relaxation breathing while sitting, standing, or lying down. It is natural for newborns and sleeping adults.

We often use chest breathing, which involves the upper chest and shoulders, during times of anxiety and distress. Relaxation breathing is a more efficient type of breathing. It involves the primary use of the diaphragm and less use of the upper chest and shoulders to help in each breath. In this type of breathing, the abdomen gently moves in and out during exhalation and inhalation. The breaths should be slow, steady, and deep.

A basic technique for relaxation breathing is as follows: (1) Inhale slowly and deeply, pushing the abdomen out. Think about breathing in peace. (2) Exhale slowly, letting the abdomen come in and all the muscles relax. Think about breathing out tension. (3) Repeat these deep breaths 10 times without interruption. As with any breathing exercise, if a light-headed feeling arises, stop for 30 seconds and then start again. Other methods used to teach relaxation breathing are the 4 × 4 technique and relaxation sigh.

At first, relaxation breathing may feel strange. With practice it becomes easier, and its relaxing benefits are soon obvious. You should personally learn to use relaxation breathing before teaching it to patients and their caregivers. Once learned, you can easily teach relaxation breathing to patients in a variety of settings, particularly when they are undergoing stressful and painful procedures.

Biofeedback

Biofeedback helps you become more aware of involuntary body responses such as breathing, heart rate, and muscle activity. Electrodes attached to the skin, or in some cases, hand-held sensors measure these processes and display them on a monitor. This feedback allows the person to learn to control their responses. This gives a person the power to use thoughts to control the body, often to improve a health condition or improve activities of daily living.[11]

TABLE 7.6 Relaxation Breathing Techniques

Breathing Assessment

1. Place one hand gently on your abdomen below your waistline.
2. Place the other hand on the center of your chest on the sternum.
3. Without changing the normal breathing pattern, take several breaths. During inhalation notice which hand rises the most.
4. When relaxation breathing is done properly, the hand on the abdomen should rise more than the hand on the chest.

4 × 4 Technique

1. Sit up straight with your back flush to the support of the chair and your feet flat on the floor.
2. Rest your arms on your lap, thighs, or arms of the chair.
3. Take in a deep breath through your nose to a count of 4 (1 … 2 … 3 … 4).
4. Hold your breath to a count of 4 (1 … 2 … 3 … 4).
5. Release your breath through your mouth to a count of 4 (1 … 2 … 3 … 4).
6. Rest for a count of 4 (1 … 2 … 3 … 4).
7. Repeat the cycle 4 times.

Relaxing Sigh

1. Sit up straight with your back against the support of the chair and your feet flat on floor.
2. Inhale a natural breath and then sigh deeply. Let out a sound of relief as the air rushes out of your lungs.
3. Do not think about inhaling at the end of the sigh; just let the air come in naturally as you breathe deeply.
4. Repeat this sigh about 4–6 times very slowly.
5. You can repeat this exercise whenever you need it.

Meditation

Meditation is a practice of concentrated focus on a sound, object, visualization, the breath, or movement. The purpose of meditation is to increase awareness, reduce stress, promote relaxation, and enhance personal and spiritual growth.

It is best to practice meditation in a quiet place, free of distractions. Table 7.7 gives some basic guidelines on how to meditate. Meditation is often practiced while seated. It is important to maintain a comfortable posture. Meditation can be done while walking and focusing on a single action such as the movement of the feet. In the beginning, you typically start with just 5 to 10 minutes of meditation at a time. Increase the time as the practice becomes more comfortable.

Imagery

Imagery is the use of your mind to generate images that have a calming effect on the body. It involves focusing the mind and incorporates all the senses to create physiologic and emotional changes. It is a simple technique that needs no equipment other than your imagination. *Guided imagery* is a variation of imagery in which another person (either live or through technology) suggests the images to you.

You can use imagery in your own life or use guided imagery with your patients. One use of imagery is to create a special place

TABLE 7.7 Guide to Meditation

You can teach yourself the basics of meditation by following a few simple steps:

1. Find a quiet place.
2. Make sure there are no distractions.
3. Sit in a comfortable position.
4. Close your eyes.
5. Shut out the world so that your brain can stop processing information coming from your senses.
6. Pick a focus word, short phrase, song verse (melody), or prayer that is firmly rooted in your belief system, such as *one, peace, The Lord is my shepherd, Hail Mary full of grace,* or *shalom.*
7. Breathe slowly and practice relaxation breathing. Say your focus word, short phrase, song verse, or prayer silently to yourself as you exhale.
8. Say the word or phrase again and again.
9. Try saying the word or phrase silently to yourself with every exhalation. The monotony will help you focus.
10. Relax your muscles, progressing from your feet to your calves, thighs, abdomen, shoulders, head, and neck.
11. Do not be concerned when other thoughts come to mind. Just acknowledge them and return calmly to your word or phrase.
12. Continue for 10–20 min, but even 5 min can leave you feeling calm and refreshed. Rise slowly.
13. Practice once or twice daily.

TABLE 7.8 Imagery

Creating Your Special Place

1. Begin by closing your eyes and taking several slow, deep breaths.
2. Imagine a place where you feel completely comfortable and peaceful. It may be a real place or one you imagine. Use a place from your past or a place you have always wanted to go.
3. Allow this special place to take form, slowly. As it takes form, look around to your left, to your right. Enjoy the scenery: the colors, the texture, the shapes.
4. Listen carefully to the sounds of your place. What do you hear?
5. Is there a gentle breeze or sunshine warming your face? Pick up or touch some favorite objects from your special place.
6. Take in a deep breath through your nose and notice the rich smells around you. Perhaps your favorite flower is in bloom, or you smell the scents of the ocean.
7. Take another deep breath and relax. Enjoy the peace, comfort, and safety of your special place.
8. This is your special place. You relax and feel thankful that you are here, in your special place.
9. You can return to this place any time that you wish.

for a mental retreat. Table 7.8 describes the steps involved in creating a special place. It is best to perform imagery in a comfortable position. Take slow, deep breaths. Focus should involve all senses (sight, hearing, touch, smell). For example, you can use an image, such as Fig. 7.9, engaging all the senses as you focus on the image.

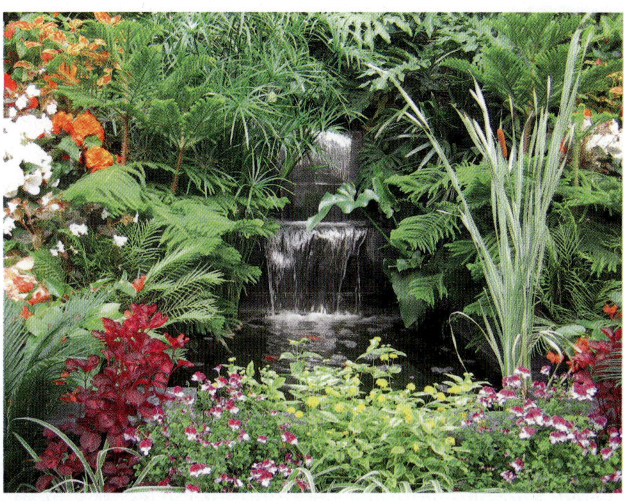

Fig. 7.9 In imagery, special places are created involving all the senses, such as a place where you can hear flowing water, smell flowers, feel the wind, and see a colorful landscape. (© LanaCanada/iStock.com.)

TABLE 7.9 Examples of Imagery for Specific Health Problems

Problem	Images
Arthritis	• Cells working as carpenters to rebuild their bones, tendons, and ligaments
Asthma	• Tiny elastic rubber bands that constrict the airways pop open
Cancer	• Shark gobbles up cancer cells • Radiation or chemotherapy treatments enter the body like healing rays of light; they destroy cancer cells
Depression	• Attach troubles and feelings of sadness to big colorful helium balloons that float off into a clear blue sky
Infection	• White blood cells are warriors who are attacking invaders
Pain	• Place painful sensations on a raft and watch them float away on a river

Imagery can be used in many settings for stress reduction and pain relief. Benefits include reduced anxiety, decreased muscle tension, improved comfort during procedures, enhanced immune function, decreased recovery time after surgery, and fewer sleeping problems. Special images can be created to ease symptoms or treat specific health problems. The image should be strong and vivid for the person, using many senses to create the image. Table 7.9 describes some suggestions for using imagery in specific diseases or disorders.

You can use imagery to enhance performance or process stressful or difficult tasks. For example, an athlete or musician can use imagery to achieve greater success. Imagery allows you to mentally rehearse a difficult or challenging situation. Imagery can help you start an IV line or perform a difficult procedure. It can be used with patients who are afraid of having a stressful or painful procedure, such as a bone marrow biopsy.

Massage

Massage includes a range of techniques that manipulate the soft tissues and joints of the body through touch and movement. It is typically delivered with the hands. Massage reduces muscle tension and positively affects mental and emotional states.

Massage is an important form of touch. It is a form of caring, communication, and comfort. Your role related to massage differs from that of the registered massage therapist. A massage therapist can provide more comprehensive massage therapies. As a nurse, you can use specific massage techniques as part of nursing care. For example, you can give a back massage to help promote sleep. For a bedridden patient, gentle massage can stimulate circulation and help prevent skin breakdown. A simple hand massage can have a calming and relaxing effect, especially for patients who are anxious or agitated. During end-of-life care, hospice nurses may include massage in their nursing care as massaging touch can lessen pain and restlessness.

When you believe that massage may be useful, first assess the patient's preference about touch and massage. Consider cultural and social beliefs and discuss potential benefits with the patient. You can teach family members to massage their loved one, giving a way for family members to take part in patient care. This can be therapeutic for the patient and family, even when the loved one is cognitively impaired or unresponsive.

Music

Music can help achieve relaxation and bring about healthy changes in emotional or physical states. Listening to relaxing music can divert one's focus from a stressful situation. Music can be used in many settings. It is noninvasive, safe, inexpensive, and easy to use. Music decreases anxiety and elicits the relaxation response. It helps people with insomnia to sleep, manage pain from health problems, and relieve depression.[12]

Each person considers different types of music to be relaxing. Music that has 60 to 80 beats/min is considered soothing. Many find low-pitched tones and music without words best for relaxation. Mozart's music is popular for relaxation. On the other hand, fast-tempo music can stimulate and uplift a person. Assess each patient's interest and preference in music. Find music that best matches the person's needs and circumstances. Create a listening environment by helping the patient find a comfortable position and minimizing interruptions. Evaluate patients' responses to the music, asking them how it sounds and how it makes them feel.

Prayer

Prayer can be a form of meditation. It is a spiritual communion with God or an object of worship. Many people find deep comfort in their faith. Religious services, conversations with clergy, and personal worship and prayer may help ease stress and give greater perspective, strength, and inspiration.

NURSING MANAGEMENT: STRESS

Assessment

Patients and caregivers face many potential stressors that can have health consequences. Be aware of situations that are likely to result in stress. As a nurse, you are in a key position to (1) assess stress in patients and caregivers, (2) help them identify high-risk periods for stress, and (3) implement stress management strategies that can prevent the negative consequences of stress on their health.

The first step in managing stress is to become aware of its presence. Assess what the stressors are and the person's response to them. Consider the type and number of stressors and their intensity (mild, moderate, or severe). Assess the duration (acute or chronic) of stress. Ask if they have experienced this stressor before. How did they handle it? What worked well and what did not? Assess the personal and cultural meaning attached to the stressful situation to provide useful insight for planning stress management strategies.

Assess patients for the signs and symptoms of the stress response. These include an increased heart rate and BP, hyperventilation, sweating, headache, musculoskeletal pain, GI upset, loss of appetite, insomnia, and fatigue. Patients may show stress-related illness (Table 7.2).

Behavior manifestations of stress may include an inability to concentrate, accident proneness, impaired speech, anxiety, crying, frustration, and irritability. Work-related responses to stress may include absenteeism or tardiness at work, decreased productivity, and job dissatisfaction. Cognitive responses include self-reports about the inability to make decisions and forgetfulness. Some of these responses may be apparent to others.

Consider the caregivers' responses to the stressors. A patient's illness often causes stress for the caregiver and other family members. Assess what aspects of the illness are the most stressful for the patient and caregiver. These may include the patient's physical health, job responsibilities, finances, and children. This information helps you to understand their perspective of the stressors. Knowledge of stressors, the feelings these stressors evoke, and the psychologic effects they can produce will help you recognize potential and actual sources of stress and their effect on the patient.

Clinical Problems

Clinical problems for patients with stress include:

- Caregiver role strain
- Difficulty coping
- Spiritual problem

Planning

The overall goals are that patients with stress will (1) report decreased levels of stress, (2) use positive coping strategies, and (3) be free from complications resulting from stress.

◆ Implementation

Nursing care focuses on helping persons recognize stress and implementing measures to help manage stress. Keep in mind that you may want to include other health care team members such as mental health professionals, social work health professionals, and clergy or other religious professionals. Recognize when you need to refer a patient or caregiver to a professional with advanced training in counseling.

The interventions you choose depend on the severity of the stress experience. For example, a patient with multiple trauma expends energy to physically survive. As a nurse, you direct efforts toward life-supporting interventions and approaches aimed at reducing added stressors for the patient. The patient is much less likely to adapt or recover if faced with more stressors, such as sleep deprivation or an infection. You can assume a primary role in implementing stress management strategies.

Ideas for how to include stress management strategies in nursing practice are described in Table 7.10. Although some require special training, many stress management strategies are within the scope of nursing practice. These include relaxation breathing, imagery, music, exercise, massage, meditation, art therapy, and journaling.

Coping strategies used should be helpful and not a source of added stress for patients. You can teach most coping and relaxation strategies to patients in 10 to 15 minutes. Choose a coping or relaxation strategy to best suit the patient and situation. Effective stress management provides a sense of control of stressful situations. As stress management practices become part of daily activities, the person can increase their confidence and self-reliance and limit the emotional response to the stressful circumstances. Having a sense of control can prevent the harmful effects of a stress response.

NURSING AND SELF-CARE

As a nurse, stress can have a significant effect on you. A primary source of stress for a nurse can be the work environment. This includes challenging patient care situations, time constraints when providing care, and tensions among co-workers and supervisors.[13] Your stress level influences your ability to provide nursing care. Your ability to manage stress is important in providing proper care to your patients and in maintaining a healthy and meaningful life for yourself.

You must care for yourself. Self-care is a way to reduce the stress that comes with nursing. It replenishes your ability to provide compassionate, quality care. Assess where you are with your self-care. What stress are you experiencing? How are you managing your stress? Develop a personal plan for your self-care. Some tips for nursing self-care are shown in Table 7.11. These tips will help you personally and enhance your own level of health and wellness. Many professional organizations, such as the American Nurses Association, offer resources to help you manage stress (www.nursingworld.org). Once you include these strategies in your life, you can share them with patients and caregivers.

TABLE 7.10 How to Implement Stress Management in Practice

1. Learn relaxation breathing. It is the easiest method of relaxation to use.
2. Pick coping strategies (Table 7.3) and relaxation strategies that are appropriate for your clinical area.
3. Practice using the strategy yourself. It becomes easier with time.
4. Take advantage of opportunities to teach coping and relaxation strategies to patients.
5. Continue learning. Study and attend workshops on stress management.

TABLE 7.11 Tips for Nursing Self-Care

Physical
- Exercise
- Eat a well-balanced diet
- Get adequate sleep

Mental
- Listen to audiobooks or podcasts
- Do puzzles or play games
- Be creative—journal, build, make
- Read
- Engage in a favorite hobby, like cooking

Social
- Spend quality time with loved ones and friends
- Share your feelings
- Keep a sense of humor; laugh often
- Work to resolve conflicts with other people
- Volunteer for something you are passionate about

Spiritual
- Meditate or pray
- Spend time in nature
- Attend religious service

Emotional
- Work with a therapist or life coach
- Learn to "let go" of things that are outside of your control
- Use relaxation breathing and imagery
- Use positive affirmations

Professional
- Socialize with your colleagues
- Do something you enjoy on breaks
- Take a mental health day without feeling guilty
- Have a boundary between work and personal time

CASE STUDY

Stress-Induced Illness

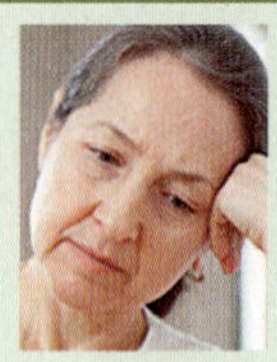
(© JackF/iStock.)

Patient Profile

K.F., a 48-year-old female, recently moved to the United States from Romania with her 2 teenage children. She has no family in the country and was recently divorced. She works as a server in a hectic restaurant and as a seamstress out of her home in the evenings. K.F. must maintain these 2 jobs so that she can provide for her rent and other financial responsibilities. K.F.'s family remains in Romania, and she is unable to visit them.

She has come to see the nurse practitioner at a community clinic. Although she says that she was in good health when she left Romania, she now presents with fatigue, inability to sleep, and aches all over her body. Even when she gets some extra sleep, she still feels exhausted. Her co-worker told her she has fibromyalgia.

Discussion Questions

1. ***Recognize:*** Considering K.F.'s situation, what history and assessment data should you obtain from the patient and why? Describe how this information influences the plan of care being developed for K.F.
2. ***Plan:*** How would you involve other members of the interdisciplinary health care team?
3. ***Prioritize:*** What are the priority coping strategies should you include in K.F.'s plan of care?
4. ***Act:*** What cultural considerations should you include when delivering care?
5. ***Evaluate:*** Identify 2 outcomes that would indicate the interprofessional plan of care delivered was effective.

Answers available at http://evolve.elsevier.com/Lewis/medsurg.

BRIDGE TO NCLEX EXAMINATION

The number of the question corresponds to the same-numbered outcome at the beginning of the chapter.

1. Determining whether an event is a stressor is based on a person's:
   a. tolerance.
   b. perception.
   c. adaptation.
   d. stubbornness.
2. The nurse would expect which finding in a patient due to the physiologic effect of stress on the reticular formation?
   a. An episode of diarrhea while awaiting painful dressing changes
   b. Refusal to communicate with nurses while awaiting a cardiac catheterization
   c. Inability to sleep the night before beginning to self-administer insulin injections
   d. Increased blood pressure, decreased urine output, and hyperglycemia after a car accident
3. The nurse uses the knowledge of stress on the immune system through the understanding of which process?
   a. Infection risk increases with prolonged exposure to stress.
   b. The body's stress response does not affect cytokine production.
   c. Phagocytosis by neutrophils and monocytes is stronger when illness occurs.
   d. Natural killer cells remain constant during both relaxation and stress periods.
4. The nurse understands that a person who has chronic stress could be at higher risk for (**Select all that apply.**)
   a. asthma.
   b. osteoporosis.
   c. fibromyalgia.
   d. colds and influenza.
   e. high blood pressure.
5. The nurse recognizes that a patient with newly diagnosed breast cancer is using an emotion-focused coping process when she
   a. joins a support group for women with breast cancer.
   b. considers the pros and cons of the various treatment options.
   c. delays treatment until her family can take a weekend trip together.
   d. tells the nurse that she has a good prognosis because the tumor is small.
6. During a stressful circumstance that is unchangeable, which type of coping strategy is the *most* effective?
   a. Avoidance
   b. Coping flexibility
   c. Emotion-focused coping
   d. Problem-focused coping

7. An appropriate nursing intervention for a hospitalized patient who says she cannot cope with her illness is
   - **a.** controlling the environment to prevent sensory overload and promote sleep.
   - **b.** encouraging the patient's family to offer emotional support by frequent visiting.
   - **c.** arranging for the patient to phone family and friends to maintain emotional bonds.
   - **d.** asking the patient to describe previous stressful situations and how she managed to resolve them.

1. b; 2. c; 3. a; 4. a, d, e; 5. a; 6. c; 7. d.

For rationales to these answers and even more NCLEX review questions, visit http://evolve.elsevier.com/Lewis/medsurg.

REFERENCES

To access the References for this chapter, please scan the QR code with a mobile device.

8

Sleep and Sleep Disorders

Diana Taibi Buchanan

http://evolve.elsevier.com/Lewis/medsurg/

CONCEPTUAL FOCUS

Functional Ability
Mood and Affect
Sleep

LEARNING OUTCOMES

1. Define sleep.
2. Describe the stages of sleep.
3. Explain the relationship of various health problems and sleep disorders.
4. Describe the etiology, clinical manifestations, and interprofessional and nursing management of insomnia.
5. Describe the etiology, clinical manifestations, and interprofessional and nursing management of obstructive sleep apnea.
6. Describe clinical manifestations and interprofessional management of narcolepsy, parasomnias, and circadian rhythm disorders.
7. Select strategies for managing sleep problems associated with shift work sleep disorder.

KEY TERMS

circadian rhythms
continuous positive airway pressure (CPAP)
insomnia
jet lag disorder
narcolepsy
obstructive sleep apnea (OSA)
parasomnias
periodic limb movement disorder (PLMD)
shift work sleep disorder
sleep
sleep-disordered breathing (SDB)
sleep disorders
sleep disturbance
sleep hygiene
wake behavior

SLEEP

Sleep is a state in which a person lacks conscious awareness of their surroundings but can be easily aroused. Sleep is distinct from unconscious states such as coma, in which the person cannot be aroused. Sleep is a basic, dynamic, highly organized, and complex behavior that is essential for healthy functioning and survival. Sleep influences mood, behavior, memory, physical functioning, hormone secretion, glucose metabolism, immune function, and temperature.

Most adults need 7 to 8 hours of sleep within a 24-hour period.[1] *Sleep insufficiency* is sleep that does not support optimal alertness, functioning, and health. It may be caused by sleep deprivation or sleep fragmentation. *Sleep deprivation* is too little sleep to meet the person's needs. *Sleep fragmentation* means a person frequently wakes up or almost wakes (called an arousal), interrupting continuous sleep. Sleep fragmentation can have negative outcomes even when a person gets the right amount of sleep.[2]

Sleep disturbance is a broad term that refers to poor sleep quality from various causes. Sleep disturbance may be related to environment factors such as noise or light. It can be caused by health-related factors such as pain or by sleep disorders. Sleep disorders include insomnia, obstructive sleep apnea syndrome, periodic limb movement disorder, circadian sleep disorders, narcolepsy, and parasomnias.

Sleep disturbances and sleep disorders can result in sleep insufficiency. Many people are not in bed long enough to allow for an adequate amount of sleep. Data for Healthy People 2030 show 32.5% of U.S. adults report insufficient sleep (Fig. 8.1).[3] We estimated 50 to 70 million people in the United States have a sleep disorder.[1] Many are unaware that they have a problem. People with chronic illnesses have the greatest risk for sleep disturbances. COVID-19 intensified the public health impact of poor sleep health not only from direct effects of the disease, but also due to social impacts of the pandemic such as isolation, stress, and financial strain.[1]

A 2021 position statement from the American Academy of Sleep Medicine (AASM) emphasized the importance of sleep health. The AASM proposed greater emphasis on sleep in primary and health professional education, and attention to sleep health by health professionals and workplaces.[3]

Sleep problems cause health, safety, and economic consequences. Severe daytime sleepiness can interfere with work and social functioning. Driving while drowsy is thought to contribute to 6000 fatal crashes each year.[4] Sleep problems and daytime sleepiness cost billions of dollars each year in health care, work-related accidents, and lost productivity.[1]

Physiologic Sleep Mechanisms

Sleep-Wake Cycle

The brain controls the cyclic changes between sleep and waking. Complex networks in areas of the forebrain (cerebral cortex, hypothalamus, thalamus) and brainstem interact to regulate the sleep-wake cycle.

Wake behavior. Wake behavior is maintained by an integrated network of arousal systems from the brainstem to the forebrain. A cluster of neuron structures in the brainstem, called the *ascending reticular activating system (ARAS)*, promotes general activation of the cerebral cortex, which is responsible for higher brain functions. This activation gives rise to typical wake behaviors such as alertness and attention. Various neurotransmitters (glutamate, acetylcholine, norepinephrine, dopamine, histamine, serotonin) promote wake behavior. Adenosine inhibits wake-promoting mechanisms.[5] The popular stimulant, caffeine, is an adenosine antagonist.

People with Alzheimer disease lose cholinergic neurons in the forebrain, which results in sleep problems. In Parkinson disease, wake-promoting dopamine neurons in the ARAS degenerate. This causes daytime sleepiness. Histamine neurons in the hypothalamus stimulate cortical activation and wake behavior.[6] The sedating properties of certain sleep medications result from inhibiting histamine-related arousal.

Orexin (hypocretin) is a neuropeptide found in the hypothalamus. Orexin is involved in regulating the sleep-wake cycle. It has a key role in keeping people awake. Orexin inhibitors, a newer class of prescription sleep medication, block the wake-promoting effects of orexin. Decreased levels of orexin or its receptors lead to problems staying awake, a syndrome called *narcolepsy*.[5]

Sleep behavior. An area in the hypothalamus just above the optic chiasm contains many sleep-promoting neurons. These neurons inhibit the ARAS and promote sleep via several neurotransmitters and peptides. The primary sleep-promoting neurotransmitter is γ-aminobutyric acid (GABA).[5] The immune system can also affect sleep-wake regulation. When a person has an infection, proinflammatory cytokines (interleukin-1, tumor necrosis factor, interleukin-6) contribute to sleepiness and lethargy.

Melatonin is a hormone made by the pineal gland. Melatonin secretion is linked to the environment light-dark cycle. Its release signals the time for sleep by "turning off" the mechanisms that promote wakefulness. Under normal day-night conditions, we release melatonin in the evening, as it gets dark. Light exposure at night can suppress melatonin secretion.[5]

Circadian rhythms. Many biologic rhythms of behavior and physiology fluctuate within a 24-hour period. These 24-hour patterns are called circadian rhythms.[7] The suprachiasmatic

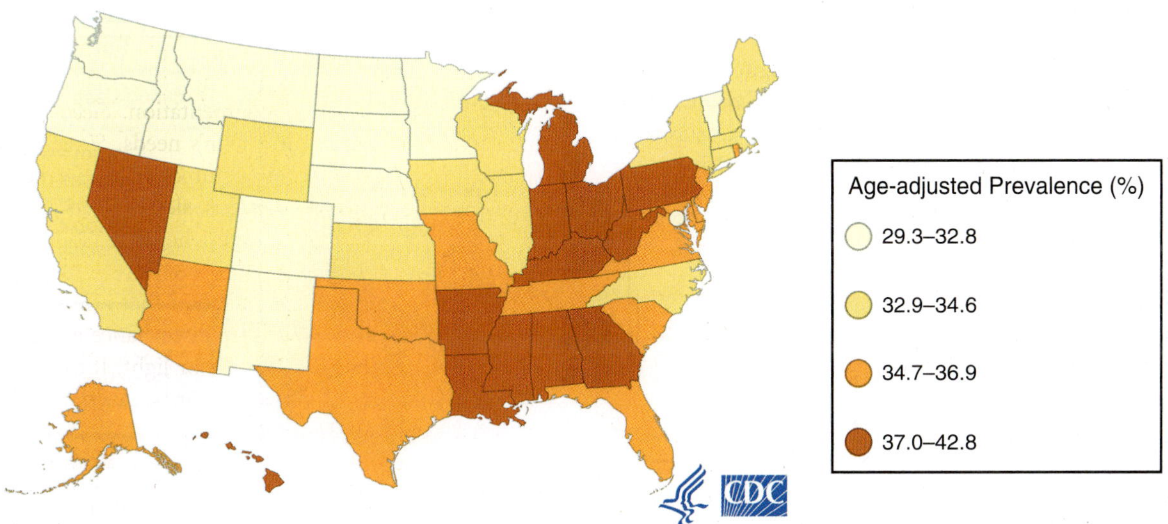

Fig. 8.1 U.S. adults that obtain less than 7 hours of sleep each night. (Modified from https://www.cdc.gov/sleep/data-and-statistics/Adults.html.)

nucleus (SCN) in the hypothalamus is the master clock of the body. The SCN synchronizes the genetic clocks within individual body cells and regulates the 24-hour sleep-wake cycle. Circadian rhythm timing is synchronized to environment light and dark periods through specific light detectors in the retina. Pathways from the retina reach the SCN, and pathways from the SCN innervate brain regions controlling wake and sleep behavior. When sleep timing is misaligned with a person's internal rhythms, the person may experience a circadian sleep disorder.[7] This may occur for social reasons, such as staying up late on weekends, or occupational reasons, such as shift work.

Light is the strongest cue for the sleep-wake rhythm. Thus we can use light as a therapy to shift the timing of the sleep-wake rhythm. For example, bright light used early in the morning will cause the sleep-wake rhythm to move to an earlier time. Bright light used in the evening will cause the sleep-wake rhythm to move to a later time. For some people, being outside in daylight without sunglasses may be helpful. Others use a light therapy device that provides very bright light.

Sleep Architecture

Sleep architecture refers to the pattern of nighttime sleep recorded from physiologic measures using *polysomnography* (PSG). PSG measures we record include (1) muscle tone with an electromyogram (EMG), (2) eye movements with an electrooculogram (EOG), and (3) brain activity recorded through an electroencephalograph (EEG).[8]

Sleep consists of 2 basic states: *rapid eye movement (REM) sleep* and *non–rapid eye movement (NREM) sleep.* During sleep, the body cycles between NREM and REM sleep. Once asleep, a person goes through 4 to 6 NREM and REM sleep cycles, each cycle lasting 60 to 110 minutes (Fig. 8.2).

NREM sleep. Healthy adults spend about 75% to 80% of sleep time in NREM sleep. NREM sleep has 3 stages.[5]

- *N1* is the stage that occurs at the beginning of sleep. It is characterized by slow eye movements. N1 is a transition phase from wakefulness to sleep. During N1 the person can be easily awakened.
- *N2* is the stage that takes up most of the night's sleep. The heart rate slows down and body temperature drops. N2 is associated with specific brain wave forms measured by EEG that represent sleep-maintaining neural activity.
- *N3* is the deepest stage of sleep. We call N3 slow-wave sleep (SWS) because of the characteristic large, low-frequency EEG waves. These delta waves are a measure of sleep intensity. SWS declines as people age. Most adults over 60 years of age have little N3 sleep.

REM sleep. REM sleep accounts for 20% to 25% of sleep. REM sleep follows NREM sleep in a sleep cycle. In this stage, brain waves resemble wakefulness. Postural muscles are inhibited, leading to greatly reduced skeletal muscle tone. During REM sleep a person cannot initiate muscle movement (e.g., cannot stand up). REM sleep is the period when most vivid dreaming occurs.

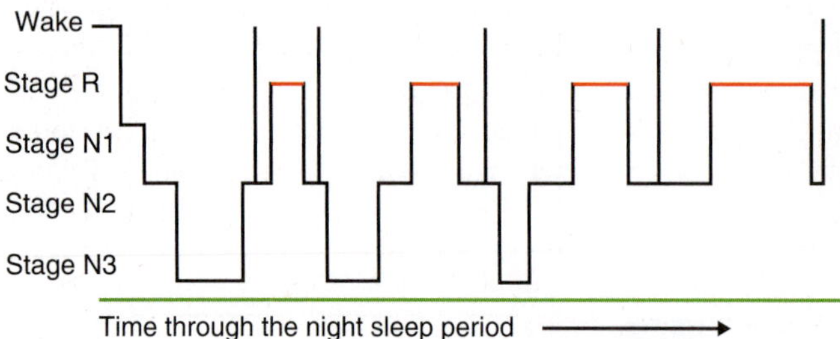

Fig. 8.2 Sleep stages graphed across a complete sleep cycle. (From Goldman L, Cooney KA: *Goldman-Cecil medicine,* ed 27, Philadelphia, 2024, Elsevier.)

EFFECTS OF INSUFFICIENT SLEEP

Insufficient sleep is associated with changes in body function (Fig. 8.3) and health problems (Table 8.1). Impaired cognitive function and impaired performance on simple behavior tasks occur within 24 hours of sleep loss. The effects of sleep loss are cumulative. Those who report less than 6 hours of sleep a night are at increased risk for heart disease, diabetes, obesity, and all-cause mortality.[9] Chronic sleep loss places people at risk for depression, impaired daytime functioning, social isolation, and overall decreased quality of life.[9]

Sleep Disturbances in the Hospital

Hospitalized patients, especially in the intensive care unit (ICU), may have decreased total sleep time, disrupted normal sleep stages, and altered circadian rhythms.[9] In the hospital, a

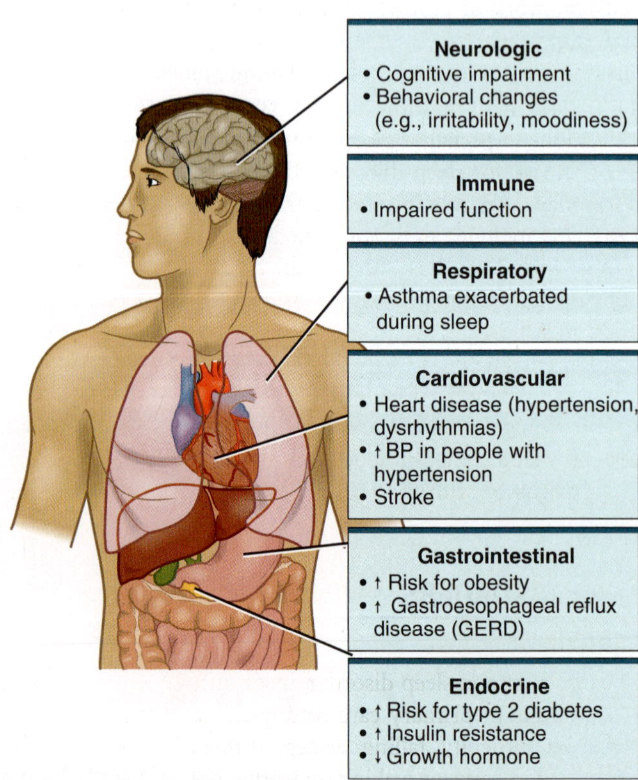

Fig. 8.3 Effects of sleep deprivation and sleep disorders on the body.

TABLE 8.1 Common Effects of Sleep on Health

Health Condition	Related Sleep Problems/Effects
Cancer	• Insufficient sleep is associated with breast and colorectal cancers.
Cardiovascular (CV) Disease	• People with sleep apnea or sleep disorders are at increased risk for CV disorders, including hypertension, dysrhythmias, and coronary artery disease. • Effects of sleep disruption on CV health likely are due to sympathetic activation, impaired glucose metabolism, and inflammation.
Immune Response	• Long-term sleep deficiency can suppress the immune response to infection. • Sleep deficiency can increase inflammation, which contributes to CV disease, metabolic syndrome, and other conditions associated with sleep loss.
Mental Health	• Sleep disturbance can worsen depression and anxiety.
Metabolic Disorders	• Insufficient sleep is linked to increased risk for type 2 diabetes. • Short sleep duration may result in metabolic changes that are linked to obesity. • Sleep deprivation in healthy people increases insulin resistance and leads to increased food intake.

disruptive environment, psychoactive medications, and acute and critical illness contribute to poor sleep. Environment factors include around-the-clock noise, light, and patient care activities. Hospital and ICU noise often persists day and night from sources such as ventilator alarms, bedside monitors, infusion alarms, and staff conversations. Bright lights during the night disrupt sleep and reduce melatonin levels. Patient care activities, like blood draws, vital sign monitoring, and medication administration, often disrupt patients' and their roommates' ability to get sound, continuous sleep. Inactivity, boredom, and napping during the day and evening can affect nighttime sleep. Symptoms, including pain, dyspnea, and nausea, can contribute to sleep loss in acutely ill patients. Preexisting sleep disorders may worsen or be triggered in hospitalized patients.

Sleep problems can cause delirium and delayed recovery. Decreased sleep duration and sleep loss cause patients to be more sensitive to pain and less able to tolerate pain.[9] Adequate pain management may improve total sleep time. But many pain medications, especially opioids, alter sleep quality and place a person at risk for sleep-disordered breathing.

You play a key role in creating an environment conducive to sleep. This includes how you schedule medications and procedures, including those performed by other team members. Reducing light and noise levels at night can promote sleep. Other measures include scheduling rest periods, obtaining measurements without disturbing the patient, opening curtains during the daytime, providing eye masks/ear plugs for sleep, and providing comfort measures (e.g., massage). Hypnotic sleep-aid medications may be given on an as-needed basis or can be discussed with the HCP.

SLEEP DISORDERS

Insomnia

The most common sleep disorder, insomnia, affects about 50% of U.S. adults in primary care settings.[10] **Insomnia** is characterized by difficulty falling asleep, difficulty staying asleep, waking up too early, or waking up feeling unrefreshed.[10] People with insomnia report overall dissatisfaction with sleep quality and quantity.

Short-term insomnia disorder refers to problems falling or remaining asleep at least 3 nights per week for less than 3 months. *Chronic insomnia disorder* is defined by the same symptoms and a daytime problem related to poor sleep (e.g., fatigue, poor concentration, interference with social or family activities) that persist for 3 months or longer. It is more common in females and those who are divorced, widowed, and separated. It is more prevalent in people with low socioeconomic status and less education.[11]

Etiology and Pathophysiology

Behaviors, lifestyle, diet, physical and mental conditions, and medications may contribute to insomnia. Insomnia is worsened by behaviors such as varying bedtime and rise time, taking long naps in the afternoon, spending time awake in bed trying to sleep, sleeping late in the morning, and exercising near bedtime.

Lifestyle factors can contribute to insomnia. Although the sedative effects of alcohol help people fall asleep, it suppresses REM sleep and causes restlessness and awakenings later in the night. Stimulants, including nicotine in tobacco and nicotine replacement products, caffeine, or cough and cold medications, especially those containing pseudoephedrine, can worsen insomnia. Insomnia is a common side effect of many medications (e.g., antidepressants, antihypertensives, corticosteroids, psychostimulants, analgesics).

Chronic insomnia may be related to various factors. Often people report that the insomnia symptoms started after a stressful life event, such as losing a job or the death of a loved one. Patients with psychiatric or medical conditions are more likely to have insomnia than those without these conditions. Once insomnia becomes chronic, symptoms are likely to persist.

Clinical Manifestations

Manifestations of insomnia include 1 or more of the following symptoms: (1) difficulty falling asleep (long sleep latency),

(2) prolonged nighttime awakenings or awakening too early and not being able to fall back to sleep (difficulty maintaining sleep), (3) awakening earlier than desired, (4) avoidance or resistance to a scheduled bedtime, and (5) inability to sleep without intervention.[10] Daytime or functional consequences include fatigue, trouble concentrating at work or school, impaired functional performance, and having an altered mood. Behavior manifestations include irritability, sleepiness during the day, heightened states of arousal (e.g., aggression or hyperactivity), and reduced energy.

Diagnostic Studies

Self-report. The diagnosis of insomnia is made based on subjective reports and an evaluation of a 1- or 2-week sleep diary completed by the patient. A diary or log usually includes the number and times of naps; times of going to bed, awakening, and getting up; number of awakenings; and overall sleep quality ratings.

In ambulatory care settings, the evaluation of insomnia requires a comprehensive sleep history. This establishes the type of insomnia and screens for possible psychiatric, medical, or other sleep disorders requiring specific treatment. We often use questionnaires to assess sleep quality and negative daytime symptoms related to insomnia. Examples include the Pittsburgh Quality Sleep Index, Insomnia Severity Index, and Epworth Daytime Sleepiness.

Actigraphy. *Actigraphy* is a method of monitoring rest and activity cycles. An actigraph is a device worn on the wrist that measures overall motor activity. The unit continuously records the patient's movements. These data are downloaded to a computer and analyzed. Activity corresponds to time spent awake. Continuous inactivity corresponds to time spent asleep. Actigraphy is not necessary for diagnosing insomnia. It is useful for confirming patients' sleep self-reports and monitoring the effects of treatments.

Interprofessional Care

Insomnia treatments are directed toward changing behaviors that perpetuate insomnia and managing symptoms (Table 8.2). The goal is to (1) prevent short-term insomnia from becoming chronic and (2) treat chronic insomnia. An important first step is teaching about sleep and behavior strategies. **Sleep hygiene** is a variety of practices that are important to normal, quality nighttime sleep and daytime alertness (Table 8.3). Patients are often familiar with some sleep hygiene principles. They may benefit from coaching on using the principles effectively.

Cognitive-behavioral therapy for insomnia. *Cognitive-behavioral therapy for insomnia* (CBT-I) is the first-line treatment for chronic insomnia.[10] CBT-I is based on structured treatment plans that include cognitive and behavioral components. The cognitive part may include stress management techniques (e.g., relaxation breathing, imagery) or strategies to address misconceptions about sleep. The specific approach used varies based on the patient. The behavior part includes focused teaching and coaching on how to effectively use sleep hygiene practices (Table 8.3). CBT-I requires behavior change, which can be hard.

TABLE 8.2 Interprofessional Care

Insomnia

Diagnostic Assessment

- Self-report sleep log or diary
- Sleep assessment (Table 8.5)
- Pittsburgh Sleep Quality Index
- Insomnia Severity Index
- Epworth Sleepiness Scale

Management

Nondrug Therapy

- Sleep hygiene (Table 8.3)
- Cognitive-behavioral therapies for insomnia (CBT-I)

Drug Therapy (Table 8.4)

- Antidepressants
- Benzodiazepines
- Benzodiazepine-receptor—like agents
- Dual orexin-receptor antagonists
- Melatonin-receptor agonists

TABLE 8.3 PATIENT & CAREGIVER TEACHING

Sleep Hygiene

Include the following instructions when teaching patients ways to promote sleep:

- Do not go to bed if you are not tired.
- If you are not asleep after 20 min, get out of bed and do a nonstimulating activity. Return to bed only when you are sleepy.
- Have a regular time to go to bed and to get up.
- Set a bedtime that allows for 7 to 8 hours of uninterrupted sleep.
- Practice the same sleep routine every night in the same order.
- Sleep in a quiet, dark, and cool room.
- Use a fan or white noise machine to reduce excess noise.
- Do not read, write, eat, watch TV, talk on the phone, or use technologies such as smartphones and tablet computers in bed.
- Avoid caffeine, nicotine, and alcohol 4 to 6 hours before bedtime.
- Do not go to bed hungry, but do not eat a big meal or spicy food 2 to 4 hours before bedtime.
- Do not exercise or take a hot bath or shower right before bedtime.
- Limit the use of sleeping pills or use them cautiously.
- Practice relaxation techniques (e.g., relaxation breathing) to help cope with stress.

Adapted from American Academy of Sleep Medicine: *Healthy sleep habits.* Retrieved from www.sleepeducation.org/treatment-therapy/healthy-sleep-habits/.

A trained HCP should deliver CBT-I treatment. CBT-I has become more accessible to patients through health technologies. It can be offered via telehealth. There are also several online interactive programs developed by sleep experts. Nox Health (http://noxhealth.com) provides the first Food and Drug Administration (FDA)—approved prescription digital online therapeutic program for insomnia.

You can apply many CBT-I principles to help patients. Teach the person with insomnia to avoid naps. Older adults may have difficulty fully avoiding naps. You can teach them that naps are less likely to affect nighttime sleep if they are less than 15 to 20 minutes, once per day, and occur within 7 to 9 hours after waking in the morning. Regular exercise may enhance sleep quality but should not be done within several hours of bedtime.

Drug therapy. Drug therapy is useful in treating insomnia in certain situations.[10] Most drugs for insomnia work by producing sleepiness to promote the onset or maintenance of sleep. Based on the characteristics (onset, half-life, mechanism of action), certain medications may be used for specific patterns of insomnia but not for others. They can treat problems falling asleep (sleep onset), waking during the night and having trouble falling back asleep (sleep maintenance), or both. Medications that treat insomnia can cause next-day drowsiness and impair driving and other activities that require alertness. People can be impaired even when they feel fully awake. Many people who take over-the-counter (OTC) or prescription medications to treat insomnia risk becoming psychologically and physically dependent on them. *Rebound insomnia* is worsening of sleep problems that may occur when one abruptly stops certain sleep medications.

Medications are generally recommended for short-term treatment of insomnia. There is little evidence to support the use of medications for chronic insomnia.[10,12] Initial drug classes used to treat insomnia are benzodiazepine-receptor agonists, followed by a dual orexin-receptor antagonist (DORA), melatonin receptor agonists, or antidepressants. Benzodiazepines, antihistamines, and antipsychotics require special considerations and may be less effective (Table 8.4).[10]

Benzodiazepine-receptor agonists. Benzodiazepine-receptor agonists have long been the mainstay of drug treatment of insomnia. They act at GABA receptors more selectively than benzodiazepines, resulting in better safety. Zaleplon (Sonata) is used for sleep onset insomnia. Zolpidem (Ambien) and eszopiclone (Lunesta) are used for sleep onset and sleep maintenance insomnia.[10] There is some evidence that these drugs may be safe for prolonged use, but intermittent (rather than daily) use is still recommended. These agents have a short duration of action that reduces the risk for daytime sedation. Newer formulations have improved specific therapeutic uses. A controlled-release formulation of zolpidem (Ambien CR) lengthens the action of the medication, improving its use for sleep maintenance insomnia. A dissolvable tablet form of zolpidem (Edluar) and an oral spray formulation (ZolpiMist) may be used with those who have trouble swallowing pills or are on restricted oral fluid intake.

DRUG ALERT

- Sleepwalking, sleep driving, and engaging in other activities while not fully awake may occur after taking a benzodiazepine-receptor agonist.
- Tell patients to stop taking the drug at once if they have such an episode.

Dual orexin-receptor antagonists (DORAs). Suvorexant, lemborexant, and daridorexant promote sleep by blocking the wake-promoting effects of orexin. They should be taken once per night, within 30 minutes of going to bed, with at least 7 hours remaining before the planned time of waking. Use is best for sleep onset or sleep maintenance insomnia. The most common side effect is drowsiness.[10]

Melatonin-receptor agonist. Ramelteon (Rozerem) is a prescription melatonin-receptor agonist. It has a rapid onset. Ramelteon is recommended for insomnia with difficulty falling asleep, not for insomnia due to waking up during the night. Ramelteon does not cause tolerance, but it is not always effective in improving sleep quality.[12]

Antidepressants. Certain tricyclic antidepressants (e.g., doxepin, amitriptyline) are used as sleep aids due to their side effect of sedation. The insomnia dose is much lower than the antidepressant dose. Doxepin is used for sleep maintenance insomnia.[12] It improves sleep without next-day drowsiness in adults with chronic primary insomnia.

Trazodone, an atypical antidepressant, is the most commonly prescribed agent for insomnia, even though the drug is not FDA approved for such use.[10] Giving this drug to older adults is controversial. Daytime sleepiness is common. Tolerance can develop within a few weeks. Trazodone is not recommended because there is not enough research to determine whether the benefit outweighs risks for side effects.[12]

TABLE 8.4 Drug Therapy

Insomnia

Antidepressants
- Amitriptyline (Elavil)
- Doxepin (Silenor)
- Mirtazapine (Remeron)
- Nortriptyline (Pamelor)
- Trazodone

Antihistamines
- Diphenhydramine
- Doxylamine (Unisom)

Benzodiazepines
- Alprazolam
- Temazepam (Restoril)
- Triazolam (Halcion)

Benzodiazepine-Receptor–Like Agents
- Eszopiclone (Lunesta)
- Zaleplon (Sonata)
- Zolpidem (Ambien, Ambien CR, Edluar, ZolpiMist)

Melatonin-Receptor Agonists
- Melatonin (controlled release)
- Ramelteon (Rozerem)
- Tasimelteon (Hetlioz)

Orexin-Receptor Antagonists
- Daridorexant
- Lemborexant (Dayvigo)
- Suvorexant (Belsomra)

Benzodiazepine hypnotics. Benzodiazepines activate GABA receptors to promote sleep. Triazolam (Halcion) is recommended for sleep onset insomnia. Temazepam (Restoril) is used for both sleep onset and sleep maintenance insomnia.[12] Some benzodiazepines are not recommended for treating insomnia (e.g., diazepam, alprazolam). However, you may still see patients who are prescribed these drugs for insomnia. Other benzodiazepines (flurazepam, oxazepam) lack enough research to support clinical recommendations. The prolonged half-life of some of these drugs can result in daytime sleepiness, amnesia, dizziness, and rebound insomnia. Tolerance develops. There is a risk of dependence and the potential for misuse. These drugs should be used for only 2 to 3 weeks. In addition, they can cause dangerous levels of sedation if used with alcohol and other central nervous system (CNS) depressants.

Antihistamines. Many people use OTC sleep aids such as doxylamine (Unisom) and diphenhydramine. Any OTC medication labeled "PM" may have diphenhydramine. Research does not show that diphenhydramine improves sleep. It should be used cautiously in older adults. Antihistamines have anticholinergic side effects, including daytime sleepiness, impaired cognitive function, blurred vision, urinary retention, constipation, and risk for increased intraocular pressure.[12]

Complementary and alternative therapy. People use many types of complementary and alternative therapies as sleep aids. Melatonin may be effective for circadian rhythm disorders (e.g., jet lag).[13] It can help night shift workers sleep during the daytime. Melatonin can allow for slight decreases in time-to-sleep and increase the amount of sleep. It is not a recommended treatment for insomnia. Issues with OTC melatonin products include a lack of FDA regulation and purity concerns in many products.

Some patients use herbal remedies that they believe will improve sleep. Common supplements include valerian, melatonin, hops, passion flower, kava, and skullcap. Tell patients that many of these products do not have FDA approval or oversight. Patients may have adverse effects or herb-drug interactions. While we now better understand the mechanisms behind many herbal remedies, further testing in clinical trials is needed to guide clinical use.[14] The legalization of cannabis in many states has led patients to use these products for sleep, but we know little about the clinical efficacy or risks.[10]

Nursing Management: Insomnia

Assessment

As a nurse, you are in a key position to assess for sleep problems. Sleep assessment is important in helping patients identify personal habits and environment factors that contribute to poor sleep. Family caregivers may have sleep disruptions from the need to provide care to patients in the home. These sleep disruptions can increase the burden of caregiving.

We use self-report and objective data to assess sleep. Ask patients about their sleep and problems with sleep. Use the following questions to screen for insomnia in primary care patients: (1) Do you have trouble getting to sleep or staying asleep? and (2) Do you feel well rested during the day?[10] Obtain a sleep history. Include sleep duration, the pattern of sleep, and daytime alertness (Table 8.5). Occasional difficulty getting to sleep or awakening during the night is not unusual. However, sleep disturbances longer than 1 month are problematic. Assess diet and caffeine intake.

Ask patients about sleep aids including OTC and prescription medications. Note the drug dose, frequency of use, and any side effects (e.g., daytime drowsiness, dry mouth). Ask about alcohol use and whether it is used as a sleep aid. Do they use any herbal supplements?

Encourage patients to keep a sleep diary for 1 to 2 weeks. Free sleep diaries are available from the National Sleep Foundation (http://thensf.org/nsf-sleep-diary/) and the National Institutes of Health (https://www.nhlbi.nih.gov/resources/sleep-diary). You can help patients choose a sleep diary smartphone application that tracks sleep information. Activity monitors to track sleep vary in accuracy. Encourage people with sleep problems to share this information with their HCP to help identify sleep patterns.

The medical history can provide important information about factors related to poor sleep. For example, a male with benign prostatic hyperplasia may report frequent awakenings during the night for voiding. Mental health problems (e.g., depression, anxiety, posttraumatic stress disorder [PTSD], drug use) are associated with sleep problems. Disturbed sleep often develops as a result or complication of a chronic or terminal illness (e.g., heart disease, dementia, cancer). Painful conditions such as arthritis may contribute to nighttime awakenings.

TABLE 8.5 NURSING ASSESSMENT

Sleep

Use the following questions to do an initial sleep assessment:

1. What time do you normally go to bed at night? What time do you normally wake up in the morning?
2. Do you often have trouble falling asleep at night?
3. About how many times do you wake up at night?
4. If you do wake up during the night, do you usually have trouble falling back asleep?
5. Does your bed partner say or are you aware that you frequently snore, gasp for air, or stop breathing?
6. Does your bed partner say or are you aware that you kick or thrash about while asleep?
7. Are you aware that you ever walk, eat, punch, kick, or scream during sleep?
8. Are you sleepy or tired during much of the day?
9. Do you usually take 1 or more naps during the day?
10. Do you usually doze off without planning to during the day?
11. How much sleep do you need to feel alert and function well?
12. Are you currently taking any type of medication or other preparation to help you sleep?

Shift work contributes to reduced or poor-quality sleep. Ask about work schedules and cross-country and international travel. Work-related behaviors resulting from poor sleep may include poor performance, decreased productivity, and job absenteeism.

◆ Clinical Problems

Clinical problems related to sleep include:

- Impaired sleep
- Fatigue

◆ Implementation

Care depends on the severity and duration of the sleep problem. Although teaching about sleep hygiene practices (Table 8.3) is beneficial, patients with chronic insomnia need more in-depth intervention using CBT-I strategies. An important part of sleep hygiene is reducing intake of caffeine-containing substances (Table 8.6). Caffeine has a half-life of about 6 hours and as long as 9 hours in older adults. Patients should avoid caffeinated beverages starting 6 to 9 hours before bedtime.

Suggest and implement changes in home and agency environments to enhance sleep. Reducing light and noise levels enhances sleep. Some people sleep better when they do not look at the clock during the night. Awareness of time passing and watching the clock adds to anxiety about not falling asleep or returning to sleep. Keeping the bedroom dark and cool is conducive to good sleep.

Teach patients about sleep medications. Sleep agents should be taken right before bedtime and when the patient is prepared to sleep at least 6 to 8 hours. Tell patients not to plan activities the next morning that require highly skilled psychomotor coordination. Teach patients not to take these medications with high-fat food (delays absorption), alcohol, or other CNS depressants. Follow-up is important. Ask patients about daytime sleepiness, nightmares, and any problems with activities of daily living.

Obstructive Sleep Apnea

Sleep-disordered breathing (SDB) describes abnormal respiratory patterns associated with sleep. These include snoring, apnea, and hypopnea. *Apnea* is the cessation of respiratory airflow (90% or greater decrease) lasting longer than 10 seconds. *Hypopnea* is a condition characterized by shallow respirations with a 30% to 90% decrease in airflow. SDB results in frequent sleep disruptions and changes in sleep stages.

Obstructive sleep apnea (OSA), also called *obstructive sleep apnea–hypopnea syndrome* (OSAHS), is characterized by partial or complete upper airway obstruction during sleep. Obstructive sleep apnea is the most diagnosed SDB problem.[15] Airflow obstruction in OSA occurs because of (1) narrowing of the air passages with relaxation of muscle tone during sleep and/or (2) the tongue and soft palate falling backward and partially or completely obstructing the pharynx (Fig. 8.4).[16]

TABLE 8.6 Caffeine Content of Select Beverages

Beverage	Caffeine (mg)
Coffee, brewed (8 oz)	96
Coffee, instant (8 oz)	62
Coffee, espresso (1 oz)	64
Coffee, decaffeinated	2
Cola (8 oz)	22
Energy drink (8 oz)	72
Energy shot (1 oz)	215
Tea, black (8 oz)	47
Tea, green (8 oz)	28

Used with permission of the Mayo Foundation for Medical Education and Research, all rights reserved. From Mayo Clinic: *Caffeine content for coffee, tea, soda, and more*, 2022. Retrieved from www.mayoclinic.org/healthy-lifestyle/nutrition-and-healthy-eating/in-depth/caffeine/art-20049372.

Each obstruction may last from 10 to 90 seconds. During the apneic period, the patient can have *hypoxemia* (decreased Pa_{O_2} or Sp_{O_2}) and *hypercapnia* (increased Pa_{CO_2}). These changes stimulate ventilation and cause brief arousals, which end the apnea or hypopnea episode. Arousals are often under the threshold of awakening. Therefore persons with OSA might not remember these events the next day.

When an arousal occurs, the person with OSA resumes regular ventilation with a generalized startle response. This event includes snorts and gasps, which cause the tongue and soft palate to move forward and the airway to open. Apnea and arousal cycles occur repeatedly throughout the night. Apneic episodes occur most often during REM sleep, when airway muscle tone is lowest.

There is no single cause for OSA. The condition is related to multiple factors that influence airway patency and airway muscle tone. Risk factors include obesity (body mass index [BMI] greater than 30 kg/m^2), age older than 65 years, neck circumference 16 inches or larger, male sex, and post-menopausal status in women.[16]

Clinical Manifestations

Manifestations include frequent arousals during sleep, insomnia, excess daytime sleepiness, and witnessed apneic episodes. The patient's bed partner may complain about the patient's loud snoring. Morning headaches are common. They are caused by hypercapnia or increased blood pressure that causes vasodilation of cerebral blood vessels. Persons with OSA may have personality changes or irritability.

Untreated OSA can lead to serious health problems. Apnea during sleep causes hypoxia, nocturnal arousals, and increased pressure in the thoracic cavity. These events can lead to negative physiologic patterns, including overactivation of the sympathetic nervous system, increased vascular resistance, and reduced oxygenation of the heart muscle. Long-term effects include hypertension, type 2 diabetes, dysrhythmias, coronary heart

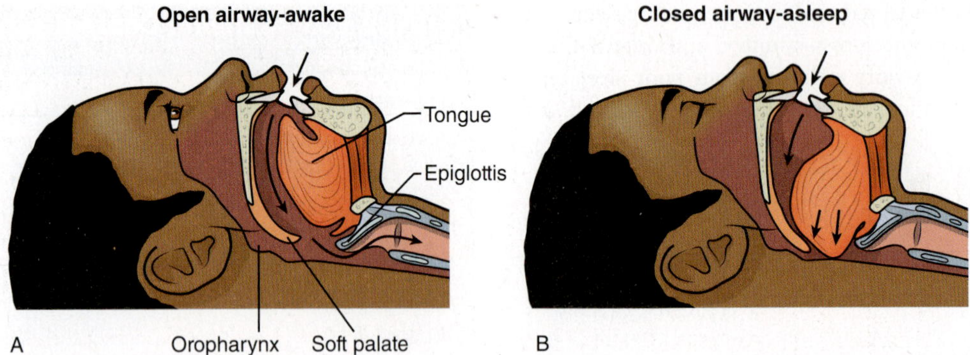

Fig. 8.4 How sleep apnea occurs. (A) The patient predisposed to obstructive sleep apnea (OSA) has a small pharyngeal airway. (B) During sleep, the pharyngeal muscles relax, allowing the airway to close. Lack of airflow results in repeated apneic episodes.

disease, arteriosclerosis, heart failure, and cardiovascular-related mortality.[16]

Chronic sleep loss predisposes the person to diminished ability to concentrate, impaired memory, failure to complete daily tasks, and interpersonal problems. Males may have impotence. Hypercapnia and arousals contribute to daytime sleepiness. Driving accidents may occur due to excessive daytime sleepiness. Family life and the patient's ability to maintain employment may be compromised. As a result, the patient may become depressed. The bed partner's awareness of apnea episodes is usually a source of anxiety because of fear that breathing may not resume.

Diagnostic Studies

Assessment of patients with OSA includes a thorough sleep and medical history. Tools used to screen for OSA are the Berlin and STOP-BANG questionnaires.[16] Each assesses for manifestations of OSA, including snoring, known apneic episodes, sleepiness/fatigue, hypertension, obesity, older age, neck size, and sex. The Epworth Sleepiness Scale may be used to check for sleepiness associated with OSA.[16]

PSG is the gold standard for OSA diagnosis but is expensive and often impractical.[16] Home testing may be done for patients with high likelihood of OSA based on our assessment. In a PSG study, electrodes simultaneously record physiologic measures (muscle tone, eye movement, and brain activity) that define the main stages of sleep and wakefulness. In laboratory and home testing, key measurements include chest and abdominal movement, oral and nasal airflow, and Spo_2. In the laboratory, additional measures include limb movements, EEG, and heart rate.

A diagnosis of sleep apnea is based on calculation of the apnea-hypopnea index (AHI). This is an hourly average of apneic events or hypopneas of at least 10 seconds' duration. OSA is defined as an AHI greater than 5 events per hour with a 3% to 4% decrease in oxygen saturation. Severe apnea can be associated with more than 30 to 50 apneic events per hour of sleep.[16]

Interprofessional and Nursing Management

Behavior treatment. Mild sleep apnea (AHI of 5 to 10) may respond to simple behavior measures. Sleeping on one's side rather than on the back (called *positional therapy*) can be effective in some cases by reducing the effects of gravity on the airway. Elevating the head of the bed may eliminate OSA in some patients.

Behavior treatment may involve weight loss and avoiding medications or substances that make apnea worse. Excess body weight worsens sleep apnea. The pressure of adipose tissue in the neck and on the chest restricts ventilation. Referral to a weight loss program may be needed. Substances that relax airway muscle tone often make OSA worse. Teach patients to avoid taking sedatives or drinking alcoholic beverages for 3 to 4 hours before sleep. Sleep medications often make OSA worse.

Teach patients the dangers of driving or using heavy equipment due to the profound sleepiness that is common in people with OSA. Some find a support group helpful to express concerns and feelings and discuss strategies for resolving problems. Insomnia is common in people with OSA. They may need specific treatment for insomnia (such as CBT-I).

Medical devices. Medical devices are key to managing OSA. For persons with more severe symptoms (>15 apnea/hypopnea events/hour), treatment guidelines recommend the use of devices that deliver positive airway pressure.[16] The most common device is a **continuous positive airway pressure (CPAP)** machine. With CPAP, the patient applies a nasal or oral-nasal mask that is attached to a high-flow blower (Fig. 8.5). The blower is adjusted to maintain enough positive pressure (5 to 25 cm H_2O) in the airway during inspiration and expiration to prevent airway collapse.

Some patients cannot adjust to wearing a mask over the nose or mouth or to exhaling against the high pressure. A more sophisticated therapy, bilevel positive airway pressure (BiPAP), can deliver a higher inspiration pressure and a lower expiration pressure. The lower mean pressure of BiPAP can relieve apnea symptoms. It may be better tolerated.

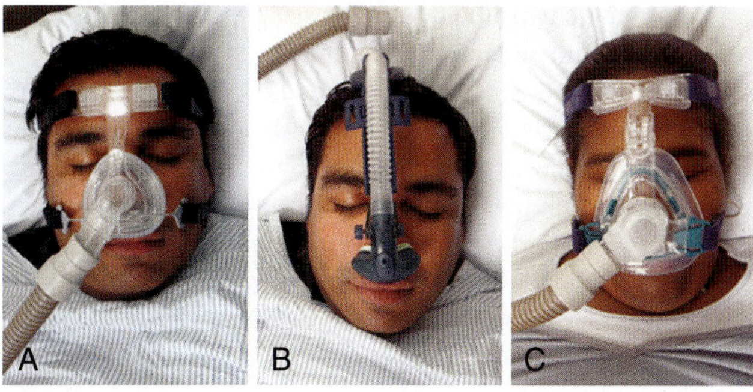

Fig. 8.5 Examples of positive airway pressure devices for sleep apnea. (A) Patient wearing a nasal mask and headgear (positive pressure only through nose). (B) Patient wearing nasal pillows (positive pressure only through nose). (C) Patient wearing a full face mask (positive pressure to nose and mouth). (From Goldman L, Cooney KA: *Goldman-Cecil medicine,* ed 27, Philadelphia, 2024, Elsevier.)

Regular CPAP use reduces apnea episodes, daytime sleepiness, and fatigue. It improves quality of life and returns cognitive functioning to normal. Benefits of CPAP are dose-dependent based on how long the patient uses CPAP during the night. CPAP adherence is defined as use of the device more than 4 hours per night on at least 70% of nights.[16] Many patients have problems using CPAP every day. Many report side effects such as nasal stuffiness.

Assess the patient's knowledge about OSA and CPAP. Involve the bed partner in teaching. Assess the patient for nasal resistance. To ensure successful adherence to CPAP treatment, involve patients in choosing the mask and device. Patient-centered care may improve patient outcomes given that OSA treatment requires behavior and lifestyle changes. Facilitate goal-setting discussions between patients and HCPs to arrive at feasible and mutually agreed upon treatment plans.

When patients with a history of OSA are hospitalized, receiving opioid analgesics and sedating medications that depress respiration may worsen OSA symptoms. A patient who uses home CPAP or BiPAP may need to continue this therapy in the hospital when resting or sleeping. Many patients can use their own equipment if allowed by agency policy.

For patients with mild to moderate OSA, oral appliances might be preferable to positive airway pressure. Oral appliances bring the mandible and tongue forward to enlarge the airway space, thereby preventing airway occlusion.

Surgical treatment. If other measures fail, OSA can be managed surgically. The goal of OSA surgery is to reduce collapsibility and increase patency of the upper airway, including oral, nasal, and pharyngeal passages. The most common procedures are uvulopalatopharyngoplasty (UPPP or UP3) and genioglossal advancement and hyoid myotomy (GAHM). UPPP involves removal of obstructing tissue from the tonsillar pillars, uvula, and posterior soft palate. GAHM involves advancing the attachment of the muscular part of the tongue on the mandible. When GAHM is done, UPPP is often done as well. Depending on the site of the obstruction, symptoms are relieved in up to 80% of patients.

Radiofrequency ablation (RFA) is the least invasive surgical intervention. RFA of obstructive tissues is used alone or in combination with other surgical techniques.

Complications of airway obstruction or hemorrhage occur most often in the immediate postoperative period. Patients are usually discharged home within 1 day after surgery. Teach patients what to expect during the postoperative recovery period. Tell patients to expect a sore throat. A foul breath odor may be reduced by rinsing with diluted mouthwash and then salt water for several days. Snoring may persist until the inflammation has subsided. Follow-up care after surgery is important, including a repeat PSG in 3 to 4 months.

Surgically implanted neurostimulators increase the tone of airway muscles. We are still testing this treatment for effectiveness and safety. It tends to be more expensive than other treatment options.

Periodic Limb Movement Disorder

Periodic limb movement disorder (PLMD) is characterized by *periodic limb movements in sleep* (PLMS): involuntary, repetitive movement of the limbs that affects people only during sleep.[17] PLMD usually involves the legs and rarely involves the arms. Sometimes abdominal, oral, and nasal movement accompanies PLMD. Movements typically occur for 0.5 to 10 seconds, in intervals separated by 5 to 90 seconds. PLMD causes poor-quality sleep and excessive daytime sleepiness.

We do not know the cause of PLMD. Iron deficiency and dopamine dysfunction in the CNS might contribute.[17] PLMS can occur with sleep disorders (e.g., sleep apnea, narcolepsy) and certain medications (e.g., antidepressants). For a diagnosis of PLMD, the occurrence of PLMS must not be due to another disorder. PLMS affects many people with restless legs syndrome (RLS). RLS is discussed in Chapter 63.

PLMD is diagnosed using a detailed history from the patient and/or bed partner and doing PSG. It is treated by medications aimed at reducing or eliminating the limb movements or the arousals. The benzodiazepine clonazepam is used to treat PLMD. It likely helps patients by improving sleep quality rather than reducing limb movements. Other medications used are valproic acid, an antiseizure drug that reduces muscle activity, and selegiline, a dopaminergic agent. Dopamine agonists (pramipexole, ropinirole) are used to treat RLS, but there is little research on their efficacy for PLMD. However, HCPs commonly prescribe these drugs to treat PLMD.

Circadian Rhythm Disorders

Circadian rhythm disorders can occur when the circadian time-keeping system loses alignment with the time cues from the environment such as light/dark phases indicating day and night. We call this loss of synchrony. Lack of synchrony between the circadian time-keeping system and environment disrupts the sleep-wake cycle and affects the ability to have quality sleep. Common symptoms are insomnia and excessive sleepiness. Jet lag disorder and shift work sleep disorder (see the

Special Sleep Needs of Nurses section) are the most common types of circadian rhythm disorders.[7]

Jet lag disorder occurs when a person travels across multiple time zones. The result is the body's time and the environment time are not synchronized. Most people crossing at least 3 time zones have jet lag. The number of time zones crossed affects the symptom severity and the recovery time. Resynchronization of the body's clock occurs at a rate of about 1 h/day when traveling eastward and 1.5 h/day when traveling westward. Melatonin and exposure to daylight help synchronize the body's rhythm.

Several strategies may help reduce the risk for developing jet lag. Before travel, the person can begin harmonizing with the time schedule of the destination. When time at the destination is brief (2 days or less), keeping home-based sleep hours rather than adopting destination sleep hours may reduce sleepiness and jet lag symptoms.

Narcolepsy

Narcolepsy is a chronic neurologic disorder caused by the brain's inability to regulate sleep-wake cycles normally. At various times throughout the day, people with narcolepsy have uncontrollable urges to sleep. Patients with narcolepsy often go directly into REM sleep from wakefulness.[18] This unique feature of narcolepsy does not occur in normal sleep. Patients with narcolepsy also have fragmented and disturbed nighttime sleep. There are 2 types of narcolepsy: with cataplexy *(type 1)* and without cataplexy *(type 2)*.[18] Cataplexy is a brief and sudden loss of skeletal muscle tone. It can manifest as a brief episode of muscle weakness or complete postural collapse and falling. Laughter, anger, or surprise often triggers episodes.

The onset of narcolepsy typically occurs in adolescence or early in the patient's 20s. Head trauma, a sudden change in sleep-wake habits, and infection may trigger the onset. The cause of narcolepsy is unknown. It is associated with destruction of neurons that make orexin, thought to be due to an autoimmune process.[5,18] The resulting deficiency of orexin causes transitions from wake to sleep that occur unpredictably.

Narcolepsy is diagnosed based on a history of sleepiness, PSG, and daytime *multiple sleep latency tests* (MSLTs).[18] For the MSLT, patients undergo an overnight PSG evaluation followed by 4 or 5 naps scheduled every 2 hours during the next day. Short sleep latencies and onset of REM sleep in more than 2 MSLTs are diagnostic signs of narcolepsy.

Narcolepsy cannot be cured. Management focuses on common symptoms: excessive daytime sleepiness, nighttime sleep disturbance, and cataplexy. Provide teaching about sleep and sleep hygiene (Table 8.3). Teach patients to take 2 to 3 short (15- to 20-minute) naps throughout the day. You can play a key role in ensuring patient safety by teaching safety behaviors and encouraging adherence to the prescribed medication plan. Safety precautions, especially when driving, are critically important for patients with narcolepsy. The behavior therapies for insomnia are used to address the sleep problems. Stimulants are used to counter daytime sleepiness.

Modafinil (Provigil) and armodafinil (Nuvigil) are non-amphetamine wake-promotion drugs that are part of first-line drug therapy. Newer drugs include pitolisant (Wakix), which exerts effects at the histamine receptor, and solriamfetol (Sunosi). It is thought to inhibit norepinephrine and dopamine reuptake.[19] Sodium oxybate (Xyrem), a metabolite of GABA, is another wake-promoting drug that is effective for treating both daytime sleepiness and cataplexy. Antidepressants, including tricyclics and selective serotonin reuptake inhibitors (SSRIs), are used to treat cataplexy.[18]

Parasomnias

Parasomnias are unusual and often undesirable behaviors that occur while falling asleep, transitioning between sleep stages, or arousing from sleep.[19] They are due to CNS activation and often involve complex behaviors. The parasomnia is generally goal directed, although the person is not aware or conscious of the act. Parasomnias may result in fragmented sleep and fatigue.

Sleepwalking and sleep terrors are arousal parasomnias that occur during NREM sleep. *Sleepwalking* behaviors can range from sitting up in bed, moving objects, and walking around the room to driving a car. While sleepwalking, the person may not speak and may have limited or no awareness of the event. On awakening, the person does not remember the event. In the ICU, a parasomnia may be misinterpreted as ICU psychosis. Sedated ICU patients can have manifestations of a parasomnia.

Sleep terrors (night terrors) are characterized by a sudden awakening from sleep along with a loud cry and signs of panic. The person has marked increases in heart rate and respiration and diaphoresis. Factors in the ICU such as sleep disruption and deprivation, fever, stress, and exposure to noise and light can contribute to sleep terrors.

Nightmares are a parasomnia characterized by recurrent awakening with recall of a frightful or disturbing dream. These normally occur during REM sleep during the final third of sleep. In critically ill patients, nightmares are common and likely due to medications. Drug classes most likely to cause nightmares are sedative-hypnotics, β-adrenergic antagonists, dopamine agonists, and amphetamines.

Gerontologic Considerations: Sleep

Older age is associated with overall shorter total sleep time, decreased sleep efficiency, and more awakenings (Fig. 8.6). A common misconception is that older people need less sleep than younger people. In fact, the amount of sleep needed as a person ages stays relatively constant. Other sleep disorders (e.g., sleep-disordered breathing) increase with age and may manifest with symptoms of insomnia. Some older adults have a

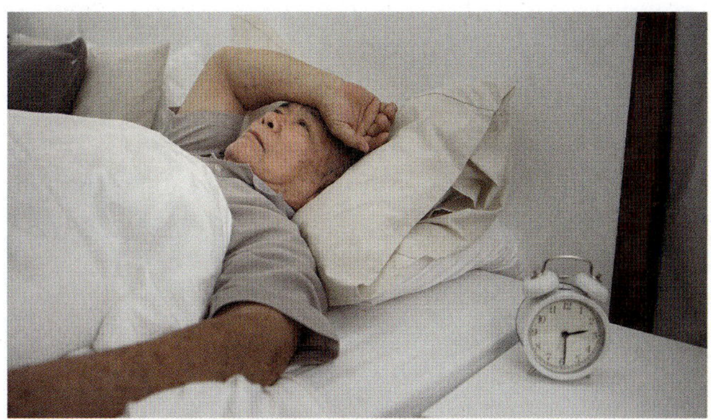

Fig. 8.6 Many older people have sleep problems. (© Nattakorn Maneerat/iStock.com.)

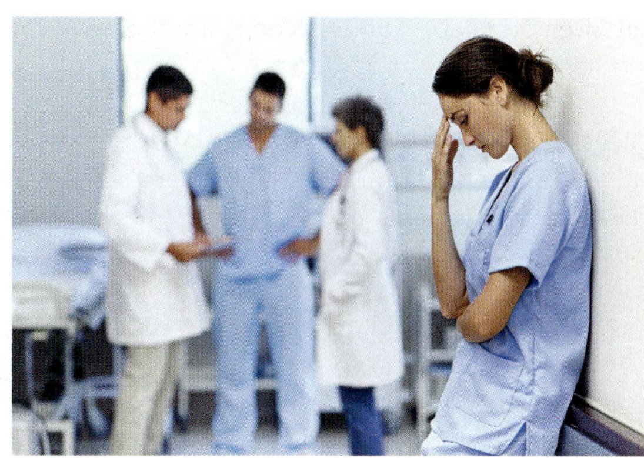

Fig. 8.7 Sleep problems are common among nurses. (© iStock.com/kupicoo.)

shift in their circadian sleep timing so that they get sleepy earlier in the evening and awaken early in the morning.

Many factors impair older adults' ability to obtain quality sleep. Chronic conditions that are common in older adults (chronic obstructive pulmonary disease [COPD], diabetes, dementia, chronic pain, cancer) can affect sleep quality.[20] Medications used to treat these conditions and OTC medications can contribute to sleep problems.

Awakening and getting out of bed during the night (e.g., to use the bathroom) increases the risk of falls. Older adults' use of OTC medications or alcohol as sleep aids further increases the risk for falls at night. Chronic, disturbed sleep in older adults can result in disorientation, delirium, impaired intellect, disturbed cognition, and an increased risk for accidents and injury.

Because older adults may attribute their disturbed sleep to normal aging, they may not report sleep problems to their HCPs. Alternatively, providers may overlook sleep disorders by attributing symptoms to other health issues.[20]

Sleep medications should be used with great caution in older adults. Metabolism of most hypnotic drugs decreases with aging. Thus drugs given for sleep disturbances are started at lower doses and monitored carefully.[20] Whenever possible, long-acting benzodiazepines should be avoided. Older adults receiving benzodiazepines are at increased risk of daytime sedation, falls, and cognitive and psychomotor impairment. Diphenhydramine should be used cautiously by older adults.

Special Sleep Needs of Nurses

In many settings, nurses work alternating and rotating day and night shifts. Unfortunately, nurses who work these shifts often report less job satisfaction, less social engagement, and more job-related stress.

Nurses on permanent night or rapidly rotating shifts are at increased risk for **shift work sleep disorder**. It is characterized by insomnia, sleepiness, and fatigue. Nurses on rotating shifts get the least amount of sleep. With repeated periods of inadequate sleep, the sleep debt grows. Chronic fatigue in nurses doing shift work poses challenges for the individual nurse's health and for patient safety (Fig. 8.7).

Shift work alters the synchrony between circadian rhythms and the environment, leading to sleep disruption. Nurses working the night shift are often too sleepy to be fully alert at work and too alert to sleep soundly the next day. Sustained changes in circadian rhythms such as rotating shift work are linked to increased morbidity and mortality risks from cardiovascular problems. Rates of mood disorders such as anxiety are higher in nurses who work rotating shifts.

From a safety perspective, disturbed sleep and subsequent fatigue can result in errors and accidents that affect nurses and their patients. Fatigue diminishes or distorts perceptual skills, judgment, and decision-making capabilities. Lack of sleep reduces the ability to cope and handle stress, which may result in physical, mental, and emotional exhaustion.

The problem of sleep disruption is important to nursing. Several strategies may help reduce the problems with rotating shift work. These include brief periods of on-site napping. Maintaining a consistent sleep-wake schedule even on days off is best but hard to do. For night shift work, scheduling the sleep period just before going to work increases alertness and vigilance, improves reaction times, and decreases accidents during night shift work. Nurses who have control over their work schedules appear to have less sleep disruption. As a nurse, you need to manage the impact of sleep disruption by using sleep hygiene practices.

CASE STUDY

Insomnia

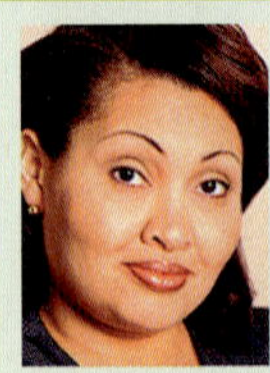

(© JackF/ iStock.)

Patient Profile

G.P. is a 49-year-old female who is being seen in the primary care clinic for chronic fatigue and disturbed sleep. She says she is healthy except for problems related to her sleep. Currently she is taking OTC diphenhydramine each night at bedtime to help her sleep. Her partner, who is with her, states that her snoring has gotten worse over the past year. It is interfering with his sleep.

Subjective Data

- Does not report any other health problems. Takes a multivitamin.
- States she was a sound sleeper before the menopausal transition but now awakens 5 or more times during the night.
- Attributes her awakenings to hot flashes.
- Has difficulty falling asleep, usually taking 30 to 60 minutes, and has trouble falling back asleep after waking during the night.
- Says she is very sleepy during the day. Falls asleep in the evening when watching television and has occasionally fallen asleep at work.
- Her partner states she stops breathing for around 30 seconds.
- Has difficulty concentrating on her work at times due to fatigue.
- On a usual workday drinks 2 cups of hot tea in the morning and a can of diet cola in the late afternoon.

Objective Data

Physical Assessment

- Alert and oriented but appears tired
- Height is 5′6″; weight 190 lb (BMI 30.7)
- Vital signs: BP 140/88 mm Hg, HR 80/min, respiratory rate 18/min, temp 36.8°C, SpO_2 97% on room air

Diagnostic Studies

- Nighttime PSG study revealed an apnea-hypopnea index of 24 with reduced pulse O_2 readings. This indicates moderate obstructive sleep apnea.

Interprofessional Care

- Prescription of CPAP nightly
- Referral for weight reduction counseling and teaching about sleep hygiene

Discussion Questions

1. ***Recognize:*** What are G.P.'s risk factors for sleep apnea?
2. ***Analyze:*** What are the major health risks for G.P. from sleep apnea?
3. ***Plan:*** What referrals may be indicated for G.P.?
4. ***Prioritize:*** Based on the assessment data provided, what are the priority clinical problems?
5. ***Act:*** What teaching will you provide so G.P. can successfully self-manage care and improve her sleep quality?
6. ***Evaluate:*** What assessment data would you need to collect to decide if care was effective?
7. ***Safety:*** What safety concerns should you address with the patient?

Answers available at http://evolve.elsevier.com/Lewis/medsurg.

BRIDGE TO NCLEX EXAMINATION

The number of the question corresponds to the same-numbered outcome at the beginning of the chapter.

1. Which statement *best* describes sleep?
  a. A loosely organized state similar to coma
  b. A quiet state in which there is little brain activity
  c. A state in which a person has reduced sensitivity to pain
  d. A state lacking conscious awareness of the environment

2. Which statements are true about rapid eye movement (REM) sleep? **(Select all that apply.)**
  a. The EEG pattern is quiescent.
  b. Muscle tone is greatly reduced.
  c. It occurs only once in the night.
  d. It is physiologically similar to NREM sleep.
  e. The most vivid dreaming occurs during this phase.

3. Which factors does the nurse associate with insufficient sleep? **(Select all that apply.)**
  a. Increased body mass index
  b. Increased insulin resistance
  c. Impaired cognitive functioning
  d. Increased daytime temperature
  e. Enhanced immune responsiveness

4. When teaching a patient with insomnia about sleep hygiene, which information would the nurse emphasize?
  a. The importance of daytime naps
  b. The need for long-term use of hypnotics
  c. Recommending vigorous exercise 1 hour before bedtime
  d. Planning to avoid caffeine for 6 to 9 hours before bedtime

5. An overweight patient with sleep apnea would like to avoid using a nasal CPAP device. Which recommendation would the nurse make to help the patient manage sleep apnea without using CPAP?
  a. Lose excess weight
  b. Take a nap each afternoon
  c. Eat a high-protein snack at bedtime
  d. Use mild sedatives or alcohol at bedtime

6. While caring for a patient with a history of narcolepsy with cataplexy, which activity can the nurse delegate to assistive personnel (AP)?
  a. Teaching about the timing of medications
  b. Walking the patient to and from the bathroom
  c. Developing a plan of care with a family member
  d. Planning a diet that avoids caffeine-containing foods

7. Which strategy reduces drowsiness on the job for night shift workers?
   a. Exercising before going to work
   b. Taking melatonin before working the night shift
   c. Sleeping for at least 2 hours immediately before work time
   d. Walking for 10 minutes every 4 hours during the night shift

1. d; 2. b, e; 3. a, b, c; 4. d; 5. a; 6. b; 7. c.

For rationales to these answers and even more NCLEX review questions, visit http://evolve.elsevier.com/Lewis/medsurg.

REFERENCES

To access the References for this chapter, please scan the QR code with a mobile device.

9

Pain

William E. Rosa and Jessica I. Goldberg

http://evolve.elsevier.com/Lewis/medsurg/

CONCEPTUAL FOCUS

Coping
Functional Ability
Pain

LEARNING OUTCOMES

1. Define pain.
2. Describe the neural mechanisms of pain and pain modulation.
3. Distinguish between nociceptive and neuropathic types of pain.
4. Explain the physical and psychologic effects of unrelieved pain.
5. Interpret data from a comprehensive pain assessment.
6. Apply principles of effective pain management.
7. Describe drug and nondrug methods of pain relief.
8. Explain your role and responsibility in pain management.
9. Discuss ethical and legal issues related to pain and pain management.
10. Evaluate the influence of one's own knowledge, beliefs, and attitudes about pain assessment and management.

KEY TERMS

analgesic ceiling
breakthrough pain (BTP)
central sensitization
complex regional pain syndrome (CRPS)
equianalgesic dose
modulation
multimodal analgesia
neuropathic pain
nociception
nociceptive pain
pain
patient-controlled analgesia (PCA)
patient-controlled epidural analgesia (PCEA)
peripheral sensitization
transduction
transmission
trigger point

PAIN

Pain is a complex, multidimensional experience that is closely related to suffering and decreased quality of life. Pain is a major reason that people seek health care. To effectively assess and manage patients with pain, you need to understand the physiologic and psychosocial dimensions of pain. Pain is interrelated with many concepts. Culture and spirituality influence the expression of pain. Acute pain adversely affects mobility and sleep, leading to fatigue. Having pain is a stressor that can lead to depression. Those with severe or chronic pain are more likely to describe their health as poor and may have increased mortality. This chapter presents information to help you assess and safely manage pain in collaboration with other interprofessional team members.

Millions of people suffer from pain. Each year in the United States, at least 25 million people have acute pain from an injury or surgery. Common chronic pain conditions, such as arthritis, migraine headache, and back pain, affect more than 1 million American adults. Pain is a common symptom experienced by

TABLE 9.1 **Negative Consequences of Unrelieved Acute Pain**

Response	Possible Consequences
Cardiovascular	
↑ Cardiac output	Deep vein thrombosis
↑ Coagulation	Hypertension
↑ Heart rate	Myocardial infarction
↑ Myocardial O_2 consumption	Unstable angina
↑ Peripheral vascular resistance	
Endocrine and Metabolic	
↑ Adrenocorticotropic hormone (ACTH)	↑ BP
↑ Aldosterone	Fluid overload
↑ Antidiuretic hormone (ADH)	↑ Heart rate
↑ Cortisol	Hyperglycemia
↑ Epinephrine and norepinephrine	↑ Respiratory rate
Gluconeogenesis	Shock
Glycogenolysis	Urinary retention, ↓ urine output
↓ Insulin	Weight loss (from ↑ catabolism)
Muscle protein catabolism	
Gastrointestinal	
↓ Gastric and intestinal motility	Anorexia
	Constipation
	Paralytic ileus
Immune	
↓ Immune response	Infection
Musculoskeletal	
Impaired muscle function	Immobility
Muscle spasm	Weakness and fatigue
Neurologic	
Impaired cognitive function	Confusion
	Impaired ability to think, reason, make decisions
Renal	
↓ Urine output	Electrolyte imbalance
Urinary retention	Fluid imbalance
Respiratory	
↓ Cough with sputum retention	Atelectasis
Hypoxemia	Pneumonia
↓ Tidal volume	

patients with cancer.[1] Many people experience inadequate pain management. Consequences of unrelieved acute pain are shown in Table 9.1.

DEFINITIONS AND DIMENSIONS OF PAIN

The International Association for the Study of Pain (IASP) defines **pain** as "an unpleasant sensory and emotional experience associated with actual or potential tissue damage." This definition emphasizes the subjective nature of pain, in which the patient's self-report is the most valid means of assessment. Although understanding the patient's experience and relying on self-report is essential, this view is problematic for many patients. For example, patients who are comatose or who have dementia, who are mentally disabled or challenged, or who have expressive aphasia have varying abilities to report pain. In these instances, you must include nonverbal information, such as observed behaviors, in your pain assessment.

TABLE 9.2 **Dimensions of Pain**

Dimension	Description
Affective	• Emotional responses to pain include anger, fear, depression, anxiety • Negative emotions impair patient's quality of life
Behavior	• Observable actions (e.g., grimacing, irritability, coping skills) are used to express or control pain • People unable to communicate may have behavior changes (e.g., agitation, combativeness)
Cognitive	• Beliefs, attitudes, memories, and meaning attributed to pain influence the ways in which a person responds to pain
Physiologic	• Genetic, anatomic, and physical determinants of pain influence how we process, recognize, and describe painful stimuli
Sociocultural	• Age and gender influence nociceptive processes and responses to opioids • Families and caregivers influence patient's response to pain through their beliefs, behaviors, and support • Culture affects pain expression, medication use, pain-related beliefs, and coping methods

The emotional distress of pain can cause suffering, especially when the pain is unrecognized or undertreated.[2] Suffering can result in a sense of insecurity, lack of control, and spiritual distress. It is important to assess the ways in which a person's spirituality influences and is influenced by pain.

The biopsychosocial model of pain includes the physiologic, affective, cognitive, behavior, and sociocultural dimensions of pain (Table 9.2). Each person understands and conceptualizes their pain in their own way. This influences how a person responds to pain. Some people cope with pain by distracting themselves. Others convince themselves that the pain is permanent and untreatable. People who believe their pain is uncontrollable and overwhelming are more likely to have poor outcomes.

For example, a female in labor will have pain. She may choose to manage it without analgesics because she associates it with a joyful event. She may feel control over her pain because of the training she received in prenatal classes and the knowledge that the pain is time limited. In contrast, a female with chronic, undefined musculoskeletal pain may be stressed by thoughts that others think that her pain is "not real." She may feel her pain is uncontrollable and have difficulty coping.

Families and caregivers influence the patient's response to pain through their beliefs and behaviors. For example, families may discourage the patient from taking opioids because they fear that the patient may become addicted. Understanding these beliefs helps you address them through patient and family teaching.

Pain Mechanisms

Nociception is the physiologic process by which we communicate information about tissue damage to the central nervous system (CNS). It involves 4 processes: (1) transduction, (2) transmission, (3) perception, and (4) modulation (Fig. 9.1).

Transduction

Transduction involves the conversion of a noxious (tissue-damaging) stimulus into an electrical signal called an action potential. Noxious stimuli can be thermal (e.g., sunburn), mechanical (e.g., surgical incision), or chemical (e.g., toxic substances). They cause the release of chemicals, such as substance P and adenosine triphosphate (ATP), into the damaged tissues. Other chemicals are released by mast cells (e.g., serotonin, histamine, prostaglandins) and macrophages (e.g., cytokines). These chemicals activate nociceptors (specialized receptors), or free nerve endings, which respond to painful stimuli. Activating the nociceptors results in an action potential. The action potential is then carried to the spinal cord by small, rapidly conducting, myelinated A-delta fibers and slowly conducting unmyelinated C fibers.

Inflammation and the subsequent release of chemical mediators lower nociceptor thresholds. As a result, nociceptors may fire in response to stimuli that previously were insufficient to elicit a response. They may also fire in response to noxious stimuli, such as light touch. We call this increased susceptibility to nociceptor activation **peripheral sensitization**. Leukotrienes, prostaglandins, cytokines, and substance P are involved in peripheral sensitization. Cyclooxygenase (COX), produced in the inflammatory response, plays a key role in peripheral sensitization. An example of this process is sunburn. Thermal injury causes inflammation that results in pain when the affected skin is lightly touched. Peripheral sensitization amplifies signal transmission. This contributes to central sensitization (discussed under Dorsal Horn Processing). The pain from activation of peripheral nociceptors is called nociceptive pain.

Therapies that change either the local environment or sensitivity of the peripheral nociceptors can prevent transduction and initiation of an action potential. Decreasing the effects of chemicals released at the periphery is the basis of several drug approaches to pain relief. For example, nonsteroidal antiinflammatory drugs (NSAIDs) exert their analgesic effects by blocking the action of COX-2 enzymes.

Transmission

Transmission is the process by which we relay pain signals from the periphery to the spinal cord and then to the brain. Nerves that carry pain impulses from the periphery to the spinal cord are called *primary afferent fibers.* These include A-delta and C fibers. Each is responsible for a different pain sensation. A-delta fibers conduct pain rapidly. They are

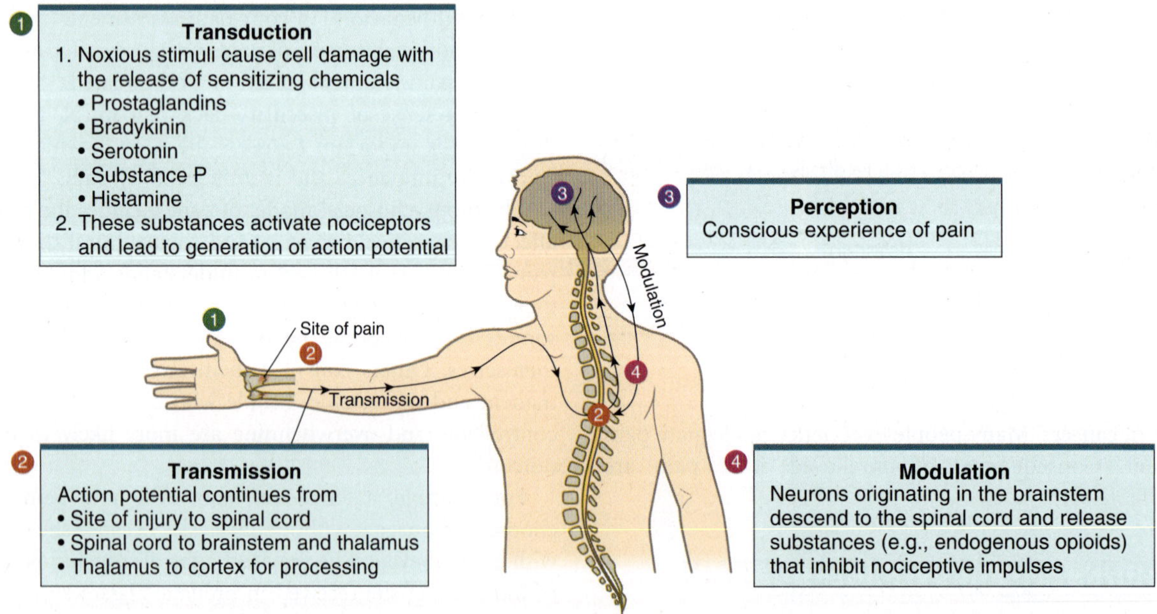

Fig. 9.1 Nociceptive pain originates when tissue is injured. (1) Transduction occurs when there is release of chemical mediators. (2) Transmission involves the conduct of the action potential from the periphery (injury site) to the spinal cord and then to the brainstem, thalamus, and cerebral cortex. (3) Perception is the conscious awareness of pain. (4) Modulation involves signals from the brain going back down the spinal cord to modify incoming impulses.

responsible for the initial, sharp pain that accompanies tissue injury. C fibers transmit painful stimuli more slowly. They produce pain that is typically aching or throbbing. Primary afferent fibers end in the dorsal horn of the spinal cord. Activity in the dorsal horn integrates and modulates pain inputs from the periphery.

Drugs that stabilize the neuronal membrane act on peripheral sodium channels to inhibit movement of nerve impulses. These drugs include local anesthetics (e.g., injectable or topical lidocaine, bupivacaine) and antiseizure drugs (e.g., gabapentin).

Fig. 9.1 shows the movement of pain impulses from the site of transduction to the brain. Three segments are involved in nociceptive signal transmission: (1) transmission along the peripheral nerve fibers to the spinal cord, (2) dorsal horn processing, and (3) transmission to the thalamus and cerebral cortex.

Transmission to spinal cord. The *first-order neuron* extends the entire distance from the periphery to the dorsal horn with no synapses. For example, an afferent fiber travels from the great toe through the 5th lumbar nerve root into the spinal cord. It is a single cell. Once generated, an action potential travels all the way to the spinal cord unless it is blocked by a sodium channel inhibitor (e.g., local anesthetic) or disrupted by a lesion, such as a dorsal root entry zone lesion.

Dorsal horn processing. Once a nociceptive signal arrives in the spinal cord, it is processed within the dorsal horn. Neurotransmitters released from the afferent fiber bind to receptors on nearby cells. Some of these neurotransmitters (e.g., glutamate, substance P) cause activation. Others (e.g., γ-aminobutyric acid [GABA], serotonin) inhibit activation. In this area, exogenous and endogenous opioids (e.g., encephalin, β-endorphin) play a vital role by binding to opioid receptors and blocking the release of neurotransmitters, especially substance P. They produce analgesic effects like those of exogenous opioids, such as morphine. We call the neurons that project to the thalamus *second-order neurons.*

Increased sensitivity and hyperexcitability of neurons in the CNS is called **central sensitization**. With central sensitization, the central processing circuits are altered. Peripheral tissue damage or nerve injury can cause central sensitization. Continued nociceptive input from the periphery maintains it (Fig. 9.2). In some cases, central sensitization can be long lasting due to multiple changes that occur in the periphery and CNS.

Because of the increased excitability of CNS neurons, normal sensory inputs cause abnormal sensing and responses to painful and other stimuli. This explains why some people have significant pain from touch or tactile stimulation that is not typically painful. We call this *allodynia.* It also explains why some people have *hyperalgesia,* an exaggerated or increased pain response to noxious stimuli.

With ongoing stimulation of slowly conducting unmyelinated C-fiber nociceptors, firing of specialized dorsal horn neurons gradually increases. These inputs can lead to the sprouting of wide dynamic range (WDR) neuron dendrites and the induction of glutamate-dependent *N*-methyl-D-aspartate (NMDA) receptors. This results in an increased capacity to transmit a broader range of stimuli-producing signals, which we then pass up the spinal cord and to the brain. This process is known as *wind-up.* Activation of NMDA receptors plays a role in wind-up. NMDA receptor antagonists, such as ketamine, potentially interrupt or block mechanisms that lead to or sustain central sensitization. Wind-up is like central sensitization and hyperalgesia in that it occurs in response to C-fiber inputs. Wind-up is different in that it can be short-lasting. Central sensitization and hyperalgesia persist over time.

It is important to understand that acute, unrelieved pain leads to chronic pain through central sensitization. Even brief intervals of acute pain can induce long-term neuronal remodeling and sensitization *(plasticity),* chronic pain, and lasting psychologic distress.

Neuroplasticity refers to processes that allow neurons in the brain to compensate for injury and adjust their responses to new situations or changes in their environment. Neuroplasticity contributes to adaptive mechanisms for reducing pain. It can also result in maladaptive mechanisms that enhance pain sensitivity.

Transmission to thalamus and cortex. From the dorsal horn, nociceptive stimuli are communicated to the *third-order neuron,* primarily in the thalamus. Fibers of dorsal horn projection cells enter the brain through several pathways, including the spinothalamic tract and spinoreticular tract. Distinct thalamic nuclei receive nociceptive input from the spinal cord and have projections to several regions in the cerebral cortex. This is where we think that pain perception occurs.

Therapeutic approaches that target pain transmission include opioid analgesics. They bind to opioid receptors on primary afferent and dorsal horn neurons. These agents mimic the inhibitory effects of endogenous opioids. Baclofen inhibits pain transmission by binding to GABA receptors, thus mimicking the inhibitory effects of GABA.

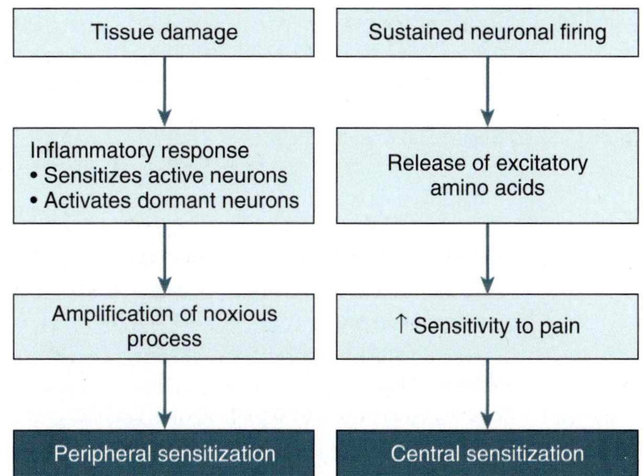

Fig. 9.2 Sequence of mechanisms leading to peripheral and central sensitization. Increased susceptibility to nociceptor activation is called *peripheral sensitization.* Increased sensitivity and hyperexcitability of neurons in the CNS is called *central sensitization.*

Perception

Perception occurs when pain is recognized, defined, and assigned meaning by the person experiencing the pain. In the brain, nociceptive input is perceived as pain. Pain perception involves several brain structures. We think that the reticular activating system warns the person to address the pain stimulus. The somatosensory system is responsible for localization and characterization of pain. Our emotional and behavior responses may originate in the limbic system.

Cortical structures are crucial to constructing the meaning of the pain.[3] This makes behavior strategies, such as distraction and relaxation, effective pain-reducing therapies for many people. Meditation and imagery can affect pain perception. By directing attention away from the pain sensation, patients can reduce the sensory and affective components of pain.

Modulation

Modulation involves the activation of descending pathways that exert inhibitory or facilitatory effects on pain transmission (Fig. 9.1). Depending on the type and degree of modulation, we may or may not perceive nociceptive stimuli as pain. Modulation of pain signals can occur at the level of the periphery, spinal cord, brainstem, and cerebral cortex. Descending modulatory fibers release chemicals, such as serotonin, norepinephrine, GABA, and endogenous opioids, which can inhibit pain transmission.

Several antidepressants exert their effects through modulation. For example, tricyclic antidepressants (TCAs) (e.g., amitriptyline) and serotonin norepinephrine reuptake inhibitors (SNRIs) (e.g., venlafaxine) are used to manage chronic noncancer and cancer pain. These agents interfere with the reuptake of serotonin and norepinephrine. This increases their availability to inhibit noxious stimuli.

CLASSIFYING PAIN

We classify pain in several ways. Most often, we classify pain as nociceptive or neuropathic based on underlying pathology (Table 9.3). Another way is to classify pain as acute or chronic (Table 9.4).

Nociceptive Pain

Nociceptive pain is caused by damage to somatic or visceral tissue. *Somatic pain* often is further described as superficial or deep. *Superficial pain* arises from skin, mucous membranes, and subcutaneous tissues. It is often described as sharp, burning, or prickly. *Deep pain* is often described as aching or throbbing. It originates in bone, joint, muscle, skin, or connective tissue.

Visceral pain results from the activation of nociceptors in the internal organs and lining of the body cavities, such as the thoracic and abdominal cavities. Visceral nociceptors respond to inflammation, stretching, and ischemia. Stretching of hollow viscera in the intestines and bladder that occurs from tumor involvement or obstruction can cause intense cramping pain. Examples of visceral nociceptive pain include pain from a surgical incision, pancreatitis, and inflammatory bowel disease.

Neuropathic Pain

Neuropathic pain is caused by damage to peripheral nerves or structures in the CNS. It is typically described as numbing, hot, burning, shooting, stabbing, sharp, or electric shock–like.

TABLE 9.3 Comparison of Nociceptive and Neuropathic Pain

	Nociceptive Pain	Neuropathic Pain
Definition	Normal processing of stimulus that damages normal tissue or has the potential to do so if prolonged	Abnormal processing of sensory input by the peripheral nervous system or CNS
Treatment	Usually responsive to nonopioid and/or opioid drugs	Usually treated with adjuvant analgesics May be responsive to opioid drugs
Types	**Superficial Somatic Pain** Pain arising from skin, mucous membranes, subcutaneous tissue. Tends to be localized *Examples:* Sunburn, skin contusions **Deep Somatic Pain** Pain arising from muscles, fascia, bones, tendons. Local or diffuse and radiating *Examples:* Arthritis, tendonitis, myofascial pain **Visceral Pain** Pain arising from visceral organs, such as the GI tract and bladder. Well or poorly localized. Often referred to cutaneous sites *Examples:* Appendicitis, pancreatitis, cancer affecting internal organs, irritable bowel and bladder syndromes	**Central Pain** Caused by primary lesion or CNS problems *Examples:* Poststroke pain, pain associated with multiple sclerosis **Peripheral Neuropathies** Pain felt along the distribution of 1 or many peripheral nerves caused by damage to the nerve *Examples:* Diabetic neuropathy, alcohol-nutrition neuropathy, trigeminal neuralgia, postherpetic neuralgia **Deafferentation Pain** Pain resulting from a loss of or altered afferent input *Examples:* Phantom limb pain, postmastectomy pain, spinal cord injury pain **Sympathetically Maintained Pain** Pain that persists due to autonomic nervous system dysfunction *Examples:* Phantom limb pain, complex regional pain syndrome

TABLE 9.4 Differences Between Acute and Chronic Pain

	Acute Pain	Chronic Pain
Onset	Sudden	Gradual or sudden
Duration	<3 mo or as long as it takes for normal healing to occur	>3 mo. May start as acute injury or event but continues past the normal time for recovery
Severity	Mild to severe	Mild to severe
Cause of pain	Usually can identify a precipitating event (e.g., illness, surgery)	May not be known Original cause of pain may differ from mechanisms that maintain the pain
Course of pain	Decreases over time and goes away as recovery occurs	Typically pain does not go away Characterized by periods of increasing and decreasing pain
Typical physical and behavior manifestations	Manifestations vary but can reflect sympathetic nervous system activation: • ↑ Heart rate, respiratory rate, BP • Confusion, anxiety, agitation • Diaphoresis, pallor • Urine retention	Common behavior manifestations: • Fatigue • Flat affect • ↓ Physical activity • Withdrawal from social interaction
Usual goals of treatment	Pain control with ability to take part in recovery activities Minimize side effects of treatment	Pain control to the extent possible Focus on enhancing function and quality of life Minimize side effects of treatment

Neuropathic pain can be sudden, intense, short lived, or lingering. Paroxysmal firing of injured nerves is responsible for shooting and electric shock—like sensations. It is often associated with diabetic neuropathy and other neuropathic pain syndromes, like phantom limb sensation and trigeminal neuralgia. Other causes include trauma, inflammation, metabolic diseases, alcohol use disorder, nervous system infections (e.g., herpes zoster), tumors, toxins, some chemotherapy agents, and neurologic diseases (e.g., multiple sclerosis). Some types of neuropathic pain (e.g., postherpetic neuralgia) are caused by more than 1 neuropathologic mechanism.

CNS lesions or dysfunction cause *central pain. Deafferentation pain* results from loss of or altered afferent input from either peripheral nerve injury (e.g., amputation) or CNS damage, including a spinal cord injury. Painful peripheral polyneuropathies (pain felt along the distribution of multiple peripheral nerves) and painful mononeuropathies (pain felt along the distribution of a damaged nerve) arise from damage to peripheral nerves. They generate pain that people may describe as burning, paroxysmal, or shocklike. Patients may have positive or negative motor and sensory signs, including numbness, allodynia, or change in reflexes and motor strength.

Sympathetically maintained pain is associated with a group of conditions that have a degree of change in autonomic nervous system. One especially debilitating type is **complex regional pain syndrome (CRPS)**.[4] Typical features include changes in the color and temperature of the skin over the affected limb or body part, with intense burning pain, skin sensitivity, sweating, and swelling. Triggers for CRPS type I include tissue injury, surgery, or a vascular event, such as stroke. CRPS type II includes all these features and a peripheral nerve lesion.

Opioid analgesics alone are often not effective in treating neuropathic pain. Treatment often requires a multimodal approach combining various adjuvant analgesics from different drug classes. These include TCAs (e.g., amitriptyline), SNRIs (e.g., bupropion [Wellbutrin]), antiseizure drugs (e.g., pregabalin [Lyrica]), transdermal lidocaine, and α_2-adrenergic agonists (e.g., clonidine). NMDA receptor antagonists, such as ketamine, have shown promise in alleviating neuropathic pain refractory to other drugs.[5]

Acute and Chronic Pain

Acute pain and chronic pain differ in their cause, course, manifestations, and treatment (Table 9.4). Acute pain functions as a signal, warning the person of potential or actual tissue damage. Examples include postoperative pain, labor pain, trauma (e.g., lacerations, fractures, sprains), infection (e.g., dysuria from cystitis), and acute ischemia. For acute pain, treatment includes analgesics and treatment of the underlying cause (e.g., splinting for a fracture, antibiotic therapy for an infection). Normally, acute pain decreases over time as healing occurs. Sometimes acute pain can persist and lead to a disabling chronic pain state. For example, pain from herpes zoster subsides as the acute infection resolves, usually within a month. Sometimes the pain persists and develops into a chronic pain state called *postherpetic neuralgia.* Because of the connection between inadequately treated acute pain and chronic pain, it is important to treat acute pain aggressively.

Chronic pain, or *persistent pain,* lasts for longer periods. We often define this as longer than 3 months or past the time when an expected acute pain or acute injury should subside. The severity and functional impact of chronic pain are often disproportionate to objective findings because of changes in the nervous system that are not detectable with standard tests. Chronic pain does not appear to have an adaptive role. It can be disabling. Patients may have anxiety and depression.

INTERPROFESSIONAL AND NURSING MANAGEMENT: PAIN

You are an important member of the interprofessional pain management team. You provide input into the assessment and reassessment of pain (Table 9.5). You help in planning and implementing treatments, including teaching, advocacy, and support of the patient, caregiver, and family. Because patients in any care setting can have pain, you must be knowledgeable about current therapies and flexible in approaches to pain management.

PAIN ASSESSMENT

Assessment is an essential step in pain management. It is important to regularly screen all patients for pain. When present, perform a more thorough pain assessment. The key to accurate and effective pain assessment is to consider the principles of pain assessment (Table 9.6).

The goals of a pain assessment are to (1) describe the patient's pain experience in order to implement pain management techniques and (2) identify the patient's goal for therapy and resources for self-management.

Most components of a pain assessment involve direct interview or patient observation. Diagnostic studies and physical assessment findings complete the initial assessment. The assessment differs with the clinical setting, patient population, and point of care (e.g., whether the assessment is part of an initial workup or a reassessment of pain following therapy). Your evaluation of pain should always be multidimensional (Table 9.7).

Before beginning any assessment, recognize that patients may use words other than "pain."[6] For example, some patients may deny that they have pain but respond positively when asked if they have soreness or aching. Record the specific words that the patient uses to describe pain. Then consistently ask the patient about pain using their words.

Document the pain assessment. This is critical to ensure safe, effective communication among interprofessional team members. Many health care agencies have specific tools to record an initial pain assessment, treatment, and reassessment. There also are many multidimensional pain assessment tools, such as the Brief Pain Inventory, the McGill Pain Questionnaire, and the Neuropathic Pain Scale.

Pain Pattern

Assessing pain *onset* involves determining when the pain started. Patients with acute pain resulting from injury, acute illness, or treatment (e.g., surgery) often know exactly when their pain began. Those with chronic pain may be less able to relate when the pain started. Establish the *duration* of the pain (how long it has lasted). This helps to determine whether the pain is acute or chronic and helps identify the cause of the pain. For example, a patient with advanced cancer who has chronic low back pain from spinal stenosis reports a sudden, severe pain in the back that began a week ago. Knowing the onset and duration leads to a diagnostic workup that reveals new metastatic disease in the spine.

The pain pattern gives clues about the cause of the pain and directs its treatment. Many types of chronic pain (e.g., arthritis pain) can increase and decrease over time. A patient may have pain all the time (around-the-clock pain), as well as periods of intermittent pain.

Breakthrough pain (BTP) is transient, moderate to severe pain that occurs in patients with stable chronic pain. The average peak of BTP can be 3 to 5 minutes. It can last up to 30 minutes or even longer. BTP can be either predictable or unpredictable. Patients can have 1 to many episodes per day. Short-acting analgesics (e.g., hydromorphone) can be effective to treat BTP.

End-of-dose failure is pain that occurs before the expected duration of a specific analgesic. It should not be confused with BTP. Pain that occurs at the end of the duration of an analgesic often leads to a prolonged increase in the baseline persistent pain. For example, in a patient on transdermal fentanyl (Duragesic patches), the typical duration of action is

TABLE 9.5 NURSING MANAGEMENT

Pain Management

- Assess pain characteristics (pattern and onset, area or location, intensity, quality, associated symptoms, and management strategies) (Table 9.7).
- Collaborate with the patient, caregivers, and interprofessional team members to develop a pain management plan.
- Give ordered analgesia. Base the decision on administering range orders on a thorough pain assessment and knowledge of the medication being given.
- Adhere to system safeguards that minimize the potential for misuse of controlled substances.
- Implement measures to reduce or eliminate common side effects of drug therapy.
- Give pretreatment analgesia and/or nonpharmacologic strategies before painful procedures.
- Collaborate with the patient, caregiver, and other health professionals to select and implement nondrug pain relief measures (Tables 9.14 and 9.15).
- Evaluate whether treatment plan is effective through ongoing assessment.
- Implement measures to address problems that precipitate or increase the pain experience, such as depression.
- Help patients develop strategies to help with participation in activities of daily living in the home, at work, and socially.
- Promote adequate periods of rest and sleep and institute measures to address impaired sleep if present.
- Help patients and caregivers cope with the pain experience by using positive coping and stress management behaviors.
- Teach patients and caregivers about treatment plan (Tables 9.16 and 9.17).
- Implement discharge teaching about pain management.
- Provide effective supervision of AP:
  - Help with screening for pain, and notify RN if the patient expresses pain.
  - Take and report vital signs before and after pain medications are given.
  - Note and report if the patient is refusing to take part in ordered activities, such as ambulation (may indicate inadequate pain management).

TABLE 9.6 Principles of Pain Assessment

Principle	Nursing Implications
1. Patients have the right to assessment and management of pain.	• Assess pain in *all* patients.
2. Pain is always subjective.	• Patient's self-report of pain is the single most reliable indicator of pain. • Accept and respect this self-report unless there are clear reasons for doubt.
3. Physiologic and behavior signs of pain are not reliable or specific for pain.	• Do not rely on observations and objective signs of pain unless the patient is unable to self-report pain.
4. Pain is an unpleasant sensory and emotional experience.	• Address physical and psychologic aspects of pain when assessing pain.
5. Assessment approaches, including tools, must be appropriate for the patient.	• Special considerations are needed for assessing pain in patients with difficulty communicating. • Include family members in the assessment process when appropriate.
6. Pain can exist even when no physical cause can be found.	• Do not attribute pain that does not have an identifiable cause to psychologic causes.
7. Different patients have different levels of pain in response to comparable stimuli.	• A uniform pain threshold does not exist.
8. Patients with chronic pain may be more sensitive to pain and other stimuli.	• Pain tolerance varies depending on several factors, such as genetics, energy level, coping skills, and experience with pain.
9. Unrelieved pain has adverse consequences. Acute pain that is not adequately controlled can result in physiologic changes that increase the chance of developing persistent pain.	• Encourage patients to report pain, especially patients who are reluctant to discuss pain, deny pain when it is probably present, or fail to follow through on prescribed treatments.

72 hours. An increase in pain after 48 hours on the drug would be an end-of-dose failure. End-of-dose failure signals the need for changes in the dose or scheduling of the analgesic.

Episodic, procedural, or *incident pain* is a transient increase in pain caused by a specific activity or event. Examples include dressing changes, movement, position changes, and procedures, such as catheterization.

Location

The *location* of pain helps us identify possible causes and treatment. Ask the patient to (1) describe the site(s) of pain, (2) point to painful areas on the body, or (3) mark painful areas on

TABLE 9.7 NURSING ASSESSMENT

Pain

Subjective Data

Important Health Information

Health history: Pain history includes onset, location, intensity, quality, patterns, aggravating and alleviating factors, and expression of pain. Coping strategies. Past treatments and their effectiveness. Health care use related to the pain problem (e.g., emergency department visits, treatment at pain clinics, visits to primary HCPs and specialists)

Medications: Use of any prescription or OTC, illicit, or herbal products for pain relief. Alcohol and marijuana use

Nondrug measures: Use of therapies, such as massage, heat or ice, aromatherapy, acupuncture, hypnosis, yoga, meditation

Functional Health Patterns

Health perception–health management: Social and work history, mental health history, smoking history. Effects of pain on emotions, relationships, sleep, and activities. Interviews with family members. Records from psychologic treatment related to the pain. Knowledge and beliefs about pain and expectations about pain management.

Elimination: Constipation related to opioid drug use, other medication use, or pain related to elimination

Activity-exercise: Fatigue, effect of pain on activities of daily living (ADLs), pain related to use of muscles

Sexuality-reproductive: Decreased libido

Coping–stress tolerance: Current and past use of stress management and coping strategies

Objective Data

Physical assessment, including evaluation of functional limitations

Psychosocial evaluation, including measures to assess depression, anxiety

a pain map. Some patients may be able to specify the precise location(s) of their pain. Others may describe general areas or comment that they "hurt all over." Because many patients have more than 1 site of pain, make sure that the patient describes every location.

Consider the possibility of referred pain when interpreting the location of pain reported by the person with an injury or a disease involving visceral organs. The origin of the pain may be distant from where the patient reports (Fig. 9.3). For example, the patient often reports pain from liver disease in the right upper abdominal quadrant. It can be referred to the anterior and posterior neck region, shoulder area, and posterior flank area. If we do not consider referred pain when evaluating a pain location report, diagnostic tests and therapy could be misdirected.

Intensity

Assessing the severity, or *intensity,* of pain provides a reliable measure to determine the type of treatment and its effectiveness. Pain scales help patients communicate pain intensity. Base your choice of a scale on a patient's development needs and cognitive status (Fig. 9.4). Many adults can rate their pain intensity using a numeric rating scale (e.g., 0 = no pain, 10 = the worst pain). Patients who wish to have word choices to quantify pain may prefer a verbal descriptor scale (e.g., none, mild, moderate, severe). For those oriented to vertical representations, the Pain Thermometer Scale is an option. Other visual pain measures, such as the Wong-Baker FACES pain tool, are useful for patients with cognitive or language barriers to describe their pain. Pain assessment measures for cognitively impaired adults and nonverbal adults are addressed later in this chapter.

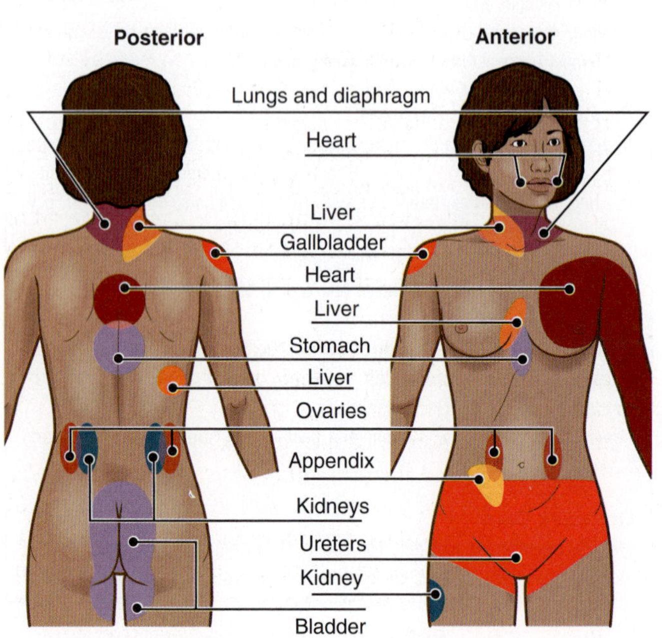

Fig. 9.3 Typical areas of referred pain.

Quality

Quality refers to the nature or characteristics of the pain. For example, patients often describe neuropathic pain as burning, numbing, shooting, stabbing, or electric shock–like. Nociceptive pain may be described as sharp, aching, throbbing, dull, and cramping. Since the quality of pain relates to a degree to the classification of pain (e.g., neuropathic, nociceptive), these descriptors help guide treatment options that best address the specific pain mechanism.

Associated Symptoms

Pain may worsen associated symptoms, such as anxiety, fatigue, and depression. Patients often report poor sleep and subsequent daytime sleepiness. Poor sleep can further increase pain perception. Ask about aggravating factors that increase pain and activities and situations that alleviate pain. For example, musculoskeletal pain may increase or decrease with movement and ambulation. Resting can decrease pain. Knowing what makes pain better or worse can help characterize the type of pain and be helpful in selecting treatments.

Management

As people experience and live with pain, they may cope differently and have varying levels of willingness to try pain management strategies. To maximize the effectiveness of the pain treatment plan, ask patients what they are using now to control pain, what they have used in the past, and whether the methods work. Strategies include prescription and nonprescription drugs and nondrug therapies, such as hot and cold applications, and complementary and alternative

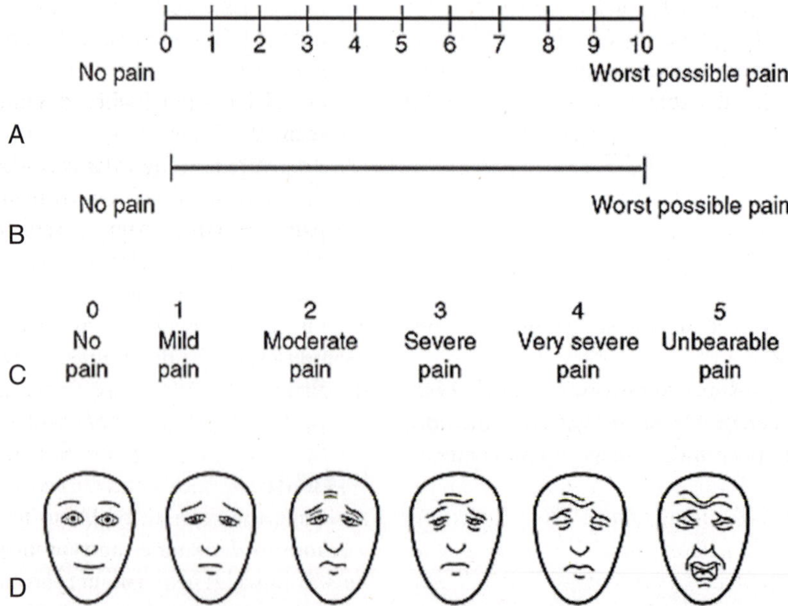

Fig. 9.4 Pain intensity scales. (A) 0 to 10 numeric scale. (B) Visual analog scale. (C) Descriptive scale. (D) Faces Pain Scale. (Modified from Baird M: *Manual of critical care nursing: nursing interventions and collaborative management*, ed 7, St Louis, 2016, Elsevier.)

therapies (e.g., acupuncture). Some people cope by distracting themselves and using relaxation strategies (e.g., imagery).

Impact of Pain

Pain can have a profound influence on quality of life and functioning. Assess the effect of the pain on the ability to sleep, enjoy life, interact with others, perform work and household duties, and engage in physical and social activities. Assess the impact of pain on the patient's mood.

In an acute care setting, time limits may dictate a shortened assessment. At a minimum, assess the effects of the pain on sleep and daily activities, relationships with others, physical activity, and emotional well-being. Include the ways in which the patient describes the pain and strategies used to cope with and control the pain.

Patient's Beliefs, Expectations, and Goals

Patient and family beliefs, attitudes, and expectations influence responses to pain and pain treatment. Assess for attitudes and beliefs that may hinder effective treatment (e.g., belief that opioid use will result in addiction). Ask about expectations and goals for pain management.

Reassessment

It is critical for you to reassess pain at appropriate intervals. Reassessment provides real-time evaluation data on the efficacy of pain management interventions. The frequency and scope of reassessment are guided by factors such as pain severity, physical and psychosocial condition, type of intervention, risks for adverse effects, and agency policy. For example, we frequently reassess postoperative patients for the effectiveness of each analgesic dose. In a long-term care facility, residents with chronic pain are reassessed at least quarterly or with a change in condition or functional status.

PAIN MANAGEMENT

Basic Principles

All pain treatment plans are based on the following 10 principles and practice standards:

1. *Follow the principles of pain assessment* (Table 9.6). Remember that pain is a subjective experience. The patient is the best judge of their pain and the expert on the effectiveness of pain treatment.
2. *Use a holistic approach to pain management.* The pain experience affects all aspects of a person's life. Thus it requires a holistic approach to assessment, treatment, and evaluation.
3. *Every patient deserves adequate pain management.* Many patient populations, including those with impaired cognition and people with substance use problems, are at risk for inadequate pain management. Be aware of your own biases and ensure that we treat all patients respectfully.
4. *Base the treatment plan on the patient's goals.* Discuss with patients realistic goals for pain relief during the initial pain assessment. We can describe some goals in terms of pain intensity (e.g., the desire for average pain to decrease from "8/10" to "3/10"). With chronic pain, encourage functional goal setting (e.g., a goal of performing certain daily activities, such as socializing and recreational activities). Encourage functional activities for patients with acute pain as well. For example, the pain must be at a level that allows the patient to use the incentive spirometer, get out of bed, and ambulate. Over time, reassess these goals and progress made toward meeting them. The patient, in collaboration with the health care team, determines new goals. If the patient has unrealistic goals for therapy, such as wanting to be completely rid of all chronic arthritis pain or be completely pain free after a major surgery, work with the patient to establish a more realistic goal.
5. *Use both drug and nondrug therapies.* Although we consider analgesics the mainstay of therapy, include self-care and nondrug therapies to increase the overall effectiveness of therapy and minimize adverse drug effects.
6. *When appropriate, use a multimodal approach to analgesic therapy.* **Multimodal analgesia** uses 2 or more classes of analgesic agents to take advantage of the various mechanisms of action. The goal is to combine analgesics from different classes to achieve maximum pain relief with minimal adverse effects. For acute, postoperative pain, a multimodal approach may include the use of an opioid (morphine), NSAID, and/or antiseizure drug (e.g., gabapentin). Regional anesthesia and continuous peripheral neural blockade used with local anesthetics are part of multimodal regimens. Age, organ function, type of surgery, risk for developing chronic pain, and coexisting conditions are all considered when designing a multimodal analgesic regimen.
7. *Address pain using an interprofessional approach.* The expertise of an interprofessional team is often necessary to provide effective pain assessment and therapies. For hospitalized patients or those with complex acute or chronic pain issues, anesthesiology-based pain services may be available to manage patients with technology-supported pain care (e.g., patient-controlled analgesia [PCA]). Palliative care teams may help manage complex pain symptoms in those with serious illness. Team members may include pain management nurses, nurse practitioners, clinical nurse specialists, anesthesiologists, and clinical pharmacists. These teams help establish realistic goals with patients and families to facilitate recovery and discharge. Many patients have access to outpatient pain management centers or clinics. Some provide comprehensive pain care and employ multiple providers, including

anesthesiologists, rehabilitation physicians, nurses, psychologists, physical and occupational therapists, and social workers. Services may focus on medication management, interventional pain therapies, counseling, cognitive and behavior therapies, physical and occupational therapy, and social services. Specialized pain treatment centers may offer more holistic therapies, such as massage, music and art therapy, and acupuncture.

8. *Evaluate the effectiveness of all therapies to ensure that they are meeting the patient's goals.* Achieving an effective treatment plan often requires trial and error. Adjustments in drug, dosage, or route are common to achieve maximal benefits while minimizing adverse effects. This trial-and-error process can become frustrating for patients and caregivers. Reassure them that pain relief, if not pain cessation, is usually possible and that the health care team will continue to work with them to achieve adequate pain relief.
9. *Prevent and/or manage medication side effects.* Side effects or adverse events are a major reason for treatment failure and nonadherence. Side effects are managed in several ways (Table 9.8). You play a key role in monitoring for and treating side effects and in teaching patients and caregivers how to minimize these effects.
10. *Include patient and caregiver teaching throughout assessment and treatment.* Develop a pain management plan with the patient. Teach the patient and caregiver about the causes of the pain, pain assessment, treatment goals and options, expectations of pain management, safe use of drugs, side effect management, and nondrug and self-help pain relief measures.

TABLE 9.8 Drug Therapy

Managing Side Effects of Pain Medications

Effect	Management Considerations
General	• Decrease the dose of analgesic by 10%–15%. • Change to a different agent in the same class. • Use an administration route that minimizes drug concentrations.

Constipation	• Start a bowel regimen at the beginning of opioid therapy; continue for as long as the person takes opioids.
	  • Most should use a gentle stimulant laxative.
	  • Add a stool softener if the patient has hard stools.
	  • Encourage diet fiber, fluids, and exercise.
	• Administer a peripheral opioid receptor antagonist as needed.

Nausea	• Administer as needed antiemetics. • Decrease environment stimuli.
Respiratory Depression and Sedation	• Monitor respiratory rate and sedation level using a sedation scale. • Providing interventions based on the level of sedation (Table 9.11). • Administer psychostimulants as needed with persistent sedation.

Drug Therapy

We generally divide pain medications into 3 categories: nonopioids, opioids, and adjuvant drugs. Patient-centered treatment plans may include medications from 1 or more of these groups. Mild pain often can be relieved using nonopioids alone. Moderate to severe pain usually requires an opioid. Some types of pain, such as neuropathic pain, typically require adjuvant drug therapy alone or in combination with an opioid or another class of analgesics. We may treat pain caused by cancer with analgesics, as well as chemotherapy or radiation therapy.

Nonopioids

Nonopioid analgesics include acetaminophen, aspirin and other salicylates, and NSAIDs (Table 9.9).[7] As a group, these drugs do not produce tolerance or physical dependence. Many are available without a prescription. To provide safe care, monitor over-the-counter (OTC) analgesic use to avoid serious problems related to drug interactions, side effects, and overdose.

Nonopioids are effective for mild to moderate pain. They are often used in conjunction with opioids because they allow for effective pain relief using lower opioid doses (thereby causing fewer opioid side effects). This is called the *opioid-sparing effect.* They have an **analgesic ceiling**. This means that increasing the dose beyond an upper limit provides no greater analgesia.

Aspirin is effective for mild pain. Its use is limited by its common side effects, including increased risk for bleeding, especially gastrointestinal (GI) bleeding. Acetaminophen (Tylenol) has analgesic and antipyretic effects.[8] Unlike aspirin, it has no antiplatelet or antiinflammatory effects. Acetaminophen is often well tolerated. It is metabolized by the liver. Liver toxicity may result from chronic dosing of more than 3 g/day, acute overdose, or use by patients with severe liver disease. Adding acetaminophen to opioid therapy produces an opioid-sparing effect, lower pain scores, and fewer side effects. This is the reason for opioid-acetaminophen combinations.

IV acetaminophen is used alone to treat acute mild to moderate pain, as an adjunct to opioid analgesics, or part of a multimodal analgesic regimen for moderate to severe pain. It has a short duration of action.

NSAIDs represent a broad class of drugs with varying efficacy and side effects. All NSAIDs inhibit COX. It is the enzyme that converts arachidonic acid into prostaglandins and related compounds. The enzyme has 2 forms: COX-1 and COX-2. COX-1 is found in almost all tissues. It is responsible for several protective physiologic functions. In contrast, COX-2 is made mainly at the sites of tissue injury, where it mediates inflammation (Fig. 9.5). Inhibiting COX-1 causes many of the untoward effects of NSAIDs, such as renal problems, bleeding tendencies, GI irritation, and ulceration. COX-2 inhibition is

TABLE 9.9 **Drug Therapy**

Select Nonopioid Analgesics

Drug	Nursing Considerations
Nonsalicylates	
acetaminophen (Tylenol)	• Antipyretic; not antiinflammatory • Sustained release, rectal suppository, and IV forms • Maximum daily dose of 3 g/day for adults ≥50 kg • Oral doses of >3 g may cause liver toxicity • Acute overdose: Acute liver failure • Give IV form over 15 min
Nonsteroidal Antiinflammatory Drugs (NSAIDs)	
celecoxib (Celebrex)	• Causes fewer GI side effects (e.g., bleeding) than other NSAIDs, but risk still present • More costly than other NSAIDs • May increase risk for serious cardiovascular thrombotic events, myocardial infarction, and stroke • Risks may increase with duration of use, preexisting cardiovascular disease, or risk factors for cardiovascular disease
diclofenac K	• Use lowest effective dose for shortest possible duration • Available in oral, ophthalmic, topical preparations
ibuprofen (Advil, Motrin)	• Use lowest effective dose for shortest possible duration • Increased risk for serious GI adverse events (bleeding, ulceration, perforation), especially in older adults • May increase risk for serious cardiovascular thrombotic events, myocardial infarction, and stroke • May increase risk for hypertension and renal insufficiency
ketorolac	• Limit treatment to 5 days • May cause renal failure in dehydrated patients
naproxen (Naprosyn, Aleve)	• Use lowest effective dose for shortest possible duration • Increased risk for serious GI adverse events (bleeding, ulceration, perforation), especially in older adults • Contraindicated for treating pain after coronary artery bypass graft (CABG) surgery
Salicylates	
aspirin	• Rectal suppository and sustained-release preparations available • Chance of upper GI bleeding • Used more often in low doses as a cardioprotective measure than for its analgesic properties

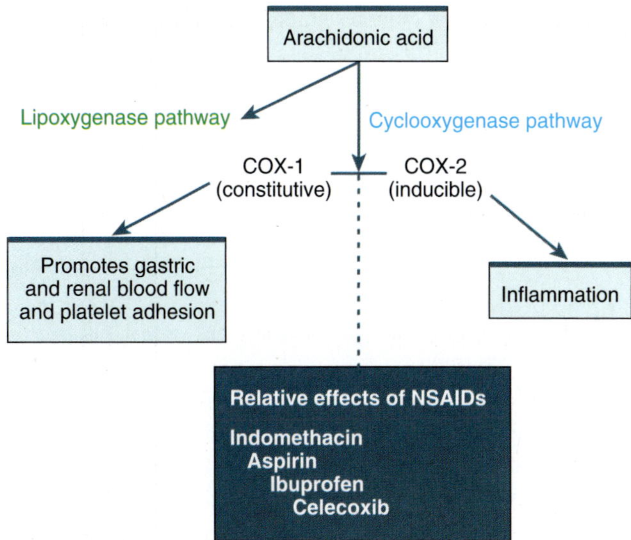

Fig. 9.5 Arachidonic acid is oxidized by 2 pathways: lipoxygenase and cyclooxygenase. The cyclooxygenase *(COX)* pathway leads to 2 forms of the enzyme COX: COX-1 and COX-2. COX-1 is *constitutive* (always present). COX-2 is *inducible* (its expression varies markedly depending on the stimulus). NSAIDs differ in their actions, with some having more effects on COX-1 and others more on COX-2. Indomethacin acts primarily on COX-1. Ibuprofen is equipotent on COX-1 and COX-2. Celecoxib primarily inhibits COX-2.

associated with the therapeutic, antiinflammatory effects of NSAIDs. Celecoxib (Celebrex) is a COX-2 inhibitor. Older NSAIDs, such as ibuprofen, inhibit both forms of COX. We call these nonselective NSAIDs.

Patient response to a specific NSAID varies greatly. We should suggest another NSAID if the first one does not provide relief. NSAIDs have many side effects. They can cause cognitive problems and hypersensitivity reactions with asthma-like symptoms.

NSAID-associated GI toxicity ranges from dyspepsia to life-threatening ulceration and hemorrhage. Patients at risk include those who have a recent history of peptic ulcer disease, patients who are older than 65, and those also using corticosteroids or anticoagulants. When patients at risk for GI bleeding use NSAIDs, they should also receive misoprostol (Cytotec) or a proton pump inhibitor, such as omeprazole. NSAIDs should not be given with aspirin because this increases the risk for GI bleeding.

DRUG ALERT

NSAIDs

- NSAIDs, except aspirin, are linked to a higher risk for cardiovascular events, such as myocardial infarction, stroke, and heart failure.
- Patients who have just had heart surgery should not take NSAIDs.

Opioids

Opioids (Table 9.10) produce their effects by binding to receptors in the CNS. This results in (1) inhibition of the transmission of nociceptive input from the periphery to the spinal cord, (2) altered limbic system activity, and (3) activation of the descending inhibitory pathways that modulate transmission in the spinal cord. Thus opioids act on several nociceptive processes.

TABLE 9.10 Drug Therapy

Opioid Analgesics

Drug	Routes	Nursing Considerations
Mu Agonists		
codeine oral (with acetaminophen [Tylenol #3]), codeine injectable	Oral, subcutaneous	• Associated with higher incidence of nausea and constipation than other mu agonists • Many codeine preparations are combined with acetaminophen • 5%–10% of European Americans lack the enzyme to metabolize codeine to morphine
fentanyl (Sublimaze [IV]), (Actiq [transmucosal]), (Fentora [buccal tablet])	IV, epidural, intrathecal, transmucosal, transdermal	• Immediate onset after IV route, 7–8 min after IM route, 5–15 min after transmucosal route, up to 6 h after transdermal route • For procedures, IV fentanyl often combined with benzodiazepines for analgesia and sedation • Very potent; dosage is in micrograms (mcg) • Transdermal fentanyl used only for chronic pain and should not be given to opioid-naive patients
hydrocodone with acetaminophen, hydrocodone with bitartrate (Hysingla ER), hydrocodone with ibuprofen	Oral (short-acting, long-acting)	• Used for moderate or moderately severe pain • For short-term management of acute pain (e.g., trauma, musculoskeletal)
hydromorphone (Dilaudid)	Oral (short-acting, long-acting), rectal, IV, subcutaneous, epidural, intrathecal	• Slightly shorter duration than morphine • For moderate to severe pain • Sustained-release tablets should be swallowed whole and must not be broken, chewed, dissolved, or crushed • Preparations for neuraxial administration are preservative free
levorphanol	Oral, IV, IM, subcutaneous	• Accumulates with repeated dosing
methadone	Oral, IV, IM	• High oral and rectal bioavailability • Accumulates with repeated dosing • Use with caution in older adults • Risk for QT interval prolongation and hypoglycemia with high doses
morphine (MS Contin, Duramorph)	Oral (short-acting, sustained-release), rectal, IV, subcutaneous, epidural, intrathecal, sublingual, intranasal	• Standard of comparison for opioid analgesics (Table 9.13) • For moderate to severe pain • Can stimulate histamine release, leading to pruritus, with systemic administration • Sustained-release tablets are to be swallowed whole and must not be broken, chewed, dissolved, or crushed • Preparations for neuraxial administration must be preservative free
oxycodone (Roxicodone) oxycodone extended release (OxyContin) oxycodone plus acetaminophen (Percocet) oxycodone plus aspirin (Percodan)	Oral (short-acting, extended-release)	• Available as single agent and in combination with a nonopioid • Used for moderate to severe pain • Often combined with a nonopioid for acute, moderate pain • Extended release indicated for chronic pain
tapentadol (Nucynta)	Oral (short-acting, extended release)	• Dual mechanism of action: Mu opioid agonist and blocks reuptake of norepinephrine and serotonin
tramadol	Oral (short-acting, extended release)	• Dual mechanism of action: Mu opioid agonist and blocks reuptake of norepinephrine and serotonin • Used for moderate pain
Mu Mixed Agonist-Antagonists		
butorphanol	Nasal spray, injectable form	• Psychotomimetic effects lower than with pentazocine • May precipitate withdrawal in opioid-dependent patients • Injectable used for acute pain • Nasal spray given for migraine headaches
Partial Agonists		
buprenorphine	Sublingual, injectable, implant	• Sublingual form should not be chewed or swallowed • Lower abuse potential than morphine • May precipitate withdrawal in opioid-dependent patients. Not readily reversed by naloxone • Buprenorphine plus naloxone used as a sublingual preparation to treat opioid dependence for easier withdrawal when necessary to taper from opioids
buprenorphine plus naloxone sublingual (Suboxone)	Sublingual	

Types of opioids. We categorize opioids by their physiologic action (e.g., agonist, antagonist) and binding at specific opioid receptors (e.g., mu, kappa, delta). The most common subclass of opioids is the pure opioid agonists, or morphine-like opioids. They bind to mu receptors.

Opioids are used for acute and chronic pain. Although nociceptive pain seems to be more responsive to opioids than neuropathic pain, opioids may be used to treat both types of pain. Pure opioid agonists include morphine, oxycodone (OxyContin), hydrocodone, codeine, methadone, hydromorphone (Dilaudid), and levorphanol. These drugs are effective for moderate to severe pain because they are potent, theoretically have no analgesic ceiling, and can be given by several routes. When opioids are prescribed for moderate pain, they are usually combined with a nonopioid analgesic, such as acetaminophen or ibuprofen.

Methadone has a unique mechanism of action as an NMDA receptor antagonist and mu opioid receptor agonist.[9] It is most often a treatment for chronic pain but can be used for acute pain. It produces analgesic effects independent of its action as an opioid.

Mixed agonist-antagonists (e.g., butorphanol) bind as agonists on kappa receptors and as weak antagonists or partial agonists on mu receptors. Because of this difference in binding, they cause less respiratory depression than drugs that act only at mu receptors. However, these drugs cause more dysphoria and agitation. Opioid agonist-antagonists have an analgesic ceiling. They can precipitate withdrawal if used by a patient who is physically dependent on mu agonist drugs. Partial opioid agonists (e.g., buprenorphine) can produce some pain relief but bind tightly to mu receptors and block the effect of other drugs. Agonist-antagonists and partial agonists currently have limited clinical application in pain management.

Dual-mechanism agents. Some opioid analgesics have 2 distinct actions, or dual mechanisms. Tramadol is a weak mu agonist and inhibits the reuptake of norepinephrine and serotonin.[10] It can be effective in treating low back pain, osteoarthritis, fibromyalgia, diabetic peripheral neuropathic pain, polyneuropathy, and postherpetic neuralgia. The common side effects are like those of other opioids, including nausea, constipation, dizziness, and sedation. As with other drugs that increase serotonin and norepinephrine, patients with a history of seizures should avoid this drug because it lowers the seizure threshold.

Tapentadol (Nucynta) is a centrally acting opioid analgesic that works at mu receptors and inhibits norepinephrine reuptake.[11] It is approved for managing moderate to severe acute pain. For chronic moderate to severe pain, an extended-release formula is available. The side effects are similar to those of conventional opioids except that this drug causes less nausea and constipation.

Opioids to avoid. Some opioids should be avoided for pain relief because of limited efficacy and/or toxicities. The American Pain Society does not recommend the use of meperidine (Demerol) as an analgesic. It can cause neurotoxicity (e.g., seizures) from the accumulation of its metabolite, normeperidine. When given, use is limited to the very short-term (less than 48 hours) treatment of acute pain when other opioid agonists are contraindicated.

Opioid side effects. Common side effects include constipation, nausea and vomiting, sedation, and respiratory depression (Table 9.8).[12] With continued use, many side effects diminish. The exception is constipation. Less common side effects include itching, urinary retention, myoclonus, dizziness, confusion, and hallucinations.

Constipation is the most common side effect. Left untreated, it may increase the person's pain and lead to fecal impaction, bowel obstruction, and paralytic ileus. A bowel regimen should be started at the beginning of opioid therapy and continued for as long as the person takes opioids.[13] Although diet fiber, fluids, and exercise should be encouraged, these may not be enough. Most patients should use a gentle stimulant laxative. A stool softener (e.g., docusate sodium) may be added if the patient has hard stools. Be aware that a stool softener will not increase the number of bowel movements. Other agents (e.g., bisacodyl, lactulose) can be added if needed. Methylnaltrexone (Relistor), naldemedine (Symproic), and naloxegol (Movantik) are peripheral opioid receptor antagonists used for opioid-induced constipation when the response to laxative and stool softener therapy is insufficient.

Nausea is often a problem in opioid-naive patients. The use of an antiemetic, such as ondansetron (Zofran), metoclopramide, transdermal scopolamine, or hydroxyzine, can prevent or minimize nausea and vomiting until tolerance develops. This usually occurs within 1 week. Opioids delay gastric emptying. Patients may report gastric fullness. Metoclopramide can reduce this effect. If nausea and vomiting are severe and persistent, changing to a different opioid may be needed.

Sedation usually occurs in opioid-naive patients being treated for acute pain. Regularly monitor patients receiving opioid analgesics, especially in the first few days after starting therapy (e.g., after surgery). Be aware that the risk for unintended sedation in postoperative patients is greatest within 4 hours after leaving the postanesthesia care unit. Opioid-induced sedation resolves as tolerance develops. Persistent sedation with chronic opioid use can often be treated with psychostimulants, such as caffeine, dextroamphetamine (Dexedrine), methylphenidate (Ritalin), or the anticataleptic drug modafinil (Provigil).

The risk for *respiratory depression* is higher in opioid-naive, hospitalized patients being treated for acute pain. Clinically significant respiratory depression is rare in opioid-tolerant patients and when opioids are titrated to analgesic effect. Patients most at risk for respiratory depression include those who are age 65 or older, have a history of snoring or witnessed apneic episodes, report excess daytime sleepiness, have underlying heart or lung disease, are obese, have a 20+ pack-year history of smoking, or are receiving other CNS depressants (e.g., sedatives, benzodiazepines). For postoperative patients, the greatest risk for opioid-related respiratory adverse events is in the first 24 hours after surgery.

Frequently monitor both the sedation level and respiratory rate in patients receiving opioid analgesics. Use a sedation scale to monitor and provide interventions based on the level of sedation (Table 9.11).

! SAFETY ALERT

Sedation and Respiratory Depression

- If the patient's respiratory rate falls below 8 or 10 breaths/min and the sedation level is 3 or greater, vigorously stimulate the patient and try to keep them awake.
- If the patient becomes oversedated (respiratory rate less than 8–10 breaths/min or obtunded), follow agency protocol and prepare to administer naloxone.

For patients who are sedated or unresponsive, we can give naloxone, an opioid antagonist that rapidly reverses the effects of opioids. It can be given by IV, subcutaneous, or intranasal routes. A hand-held autoinjector containing naloxone (Evzio) can be used by a caregiver or family member to treat a person known or suspected to have had an opioid overdose. Since naloxone is an opioid antagonist, its use can precipitate severe, agonizing pain, profound withdrawal symptoms, hypertension, and pulmonary edema. Because naloxone's half-life is shorter than that of most opioids, frequently monitor the patient. You may need to give repeated doses.

A rare but concerning problem with long-term and sometimes short-term use of high-dose opioids is *opioid-induced hyperalgesia* (OIH).[14] OIH is a state of nociceptive sensitization caused by opioid exposure. It is a paradoxical response in which patients become more sensitive to certain painful stimuli and report increased pain with opioid use. We do not understand the exact cause of OIH.

CHECK YOUR PRACTICE

A 73-year-old patient returns to the unit after abdominal surgery with a PCA pump. His husband tells you that the patient seems difficult to arouse. You note that the O_2 saturation monitor became disconnected. When you reconnect it, you see that the patient's O_2 saturation is 89% and his respiratory rate ranges from 8 to 10 breaths/min.

- What should you do?

Adjuvant Analgesic Therapy

Analgesic adjuvant drugs are used alone or in conjunction with opioid and nonopioid analgesics (Table 9.12). Most of these drugs were developed for other purposes (e.g., antiseizure drugs, antidepressants) and found to be effective for treating pain. Antidepressants and antiseizure drugs are the recommended first-line agents for treating neuropathic pain.[15]

α_2-Adrenergic agonists. Clonidine and tizanidine (Zanaflex) are the most widely used α_2-adrenergic agonists. They likely work on the central inhibitory α-adrenergic receptors. These agents may also decrease norepinephrine release peripherally. They are helpful in treating chronic headache and neuropathic pain.

TABLE 9.11 Pasero Opioid-Induced Sedation Scale (POSS) With Interventions

Level of Sedation	Nursing Intervention
S = Sleep, easy to arouse	• Acceptable • No action necessary • May increase opioid dose if needed
1. Awake and alert	• Acceptable • No action necessary • May increase opioid dose if needed
2. Slightly drowsy, easily aroused	• Acceptable • No action necessary • May increase opioid dose if needed
3. Frequently drowsy, arousable, drifts off to sleep during conversation	• Unacceptable • Monitor respiratory status and sedation level closely until sedation level is stable at <3 and respiratory status is satisfactory • Decrease opioid dose 25%–50% or notify HCP or anesthesiologist for orders • Consider giving a nonsedating, opioid-sparing nonopioid, such as acetaminophen or an NSAID, if not contraindicated
4. Somnolent, minimal or no response to verbal or physical stimulation	• Unacceptable • Stop opioid • Consider giving naloxone • Notify HCP or anesthesiologist • Monitor respiratory status and sedation level closely until sedation level is stable at <3 and respiratory status is satisfactory

Adapted from Pasero C: Assessment of sedation during opioid administration for pain management, *J PeriAnesthesia Nurs* 24:186, 2009.

Antidepressants. TCAs enhance the descending inhibitory system by preventing the cellular reuptake of serotonin and norepinephrine. Higher levels of serotonin and norepinephrine in the synapse inhibit the transmission of nociceptive signals in the CNS. Other beneficial actions include sodium channel modulation, α_1-adrenergic antagonist effects, and weak NMDA receptor modulation. They are effective for a variety of pain syndromes, especially neuropathic pain syndromes. Side effects, such as sedation, dry mouth, blurred vision, and weight gain, limit their use. Antidepressants that selectively inhibit reuptake of serotonin and norepinephrine (SNRIs) are effective for many neuropathic pain syndromes and have fewer side effects than TCAs. These agents include venlafaxine, desvenlafaxine (Pristiq), milnacipran (Savella), and bupropion.

Antiseizure drugs. Antiseizure drugs affect peripheral nerves and the CNS in several ways. These include sodium channel modulation, central calcium channel modulation, and changes in excitatory amino acids and other receptors. Agents such as gabapentin (Neurontin), lamotrigine (Lamictal), and pregabalin (Lyrica) are valuable adjuvant agents in chronic pain therapy. We are using them more for treating acute pain.

GABA-receptor agonist. Baclofen, an agonist at GABA receptors, can interfere with the transmission of nociceptive

TABLE 9.12 Drug Therapy

Adjuvant Drugs Used for Pain

Drug	Specific Indication	Nursing Considerations
α_2-Adrenergic Agonists		
clonidine (Duraclon) tizanidine (Zanaflex)	Especially useful for neuropathic pain when given intrathecally	• Side effects: Sedation, orthostatic hypotension, dry mouth • Often combined with anesthetics (e.g., bupivacaine)
Anesthetics: Local		
capsaicin (active compound of chili peppers)	Pain associated with arthritis, postherpetic neuralgia, diabetic neuropathy	• Apply sparingly onto affected area • Use gloves or wash hands with soap and water after application • Side effects: Skin irritation (burning, stinging) at application site • May cause cough when inhaled
lidocaine (L-M-X)	Topical local anesthetic cream applied to intact skin before venipuncture or lumbar puncture. May be effective for postherpetic neuralgia	• Apply bubble layer to intact skin and wait at least 20–30 min before wiping and performing painful procedure • Duration is around 60 min after wiped from skin • Available without prescription
lidocaine 2.5% + prilocaine 2.5% (topical eutectic mixture of local anesthetics)	Longer time to take effect than L-M-X	• Apply under an occlusive dressing (e.g., Tegaderm, DuoDERM) or on an anesthetic disk • Side effects: Mild redness, edema, skin blanching
Anesthetics: Oral or Systemic		
5% lidocaine-impregnated transdermal patch (Lidoderm patch)	Postherpetic neuralgia	• Local skin reactions (e.g., change in color, colored spots, irritation, itching, rash, burning) occur at the site of application; typically mild
mexiletine	Diabetic neuropathy Neuropathic pain	• Side effects: Nausea, dizziness, perioral numbness, paresthesia, tremor, seizures (at high doses), dysrhythmias, myocardial depression • Avoid in patients with heart disease
Antidepressants		
Tricyclic Antidepressants (TCAs)		
amitriptyline desipramine (Norpramin) doxepin imipramine (Tofranil) nortriptyline (Pamelor)	Neuropathic pain	• Side-effect profile differs for each agent and is often dose-dependent • Side effects: Anticholinergic effects (e.g., dry mouth), sedation • Titrate slowly over days to weeks to reach optimal therapeutic doses
Serotonin Norepinephrine Reuptake Inhibitor (SNRI) Antidepressants		
duloxetine (Cymbalta) milnacipran (Savella) venlafaxine (Effexor ER)	Neuropathic pain Multimodal therapy for acute pain (venlafaxine) Fibromyalgia (duloxetine, milnacipran)	• Side effects vary with each agent • Decreased arousal and desire for sex
Other Antidepressants		
bupropion (Wellbutrin)	Neuropathic pain Headaches	• Distinguished from TCAs and SNRIs as an inhibitor of norepinephrine and dopamine uptake
Antiseizure Drugs (see Table 63.7)		
carbamazepine (Tegretol), gabapentin (Neurontin), lamotrigine (Lamictal), phenytoin (Dilantin), pregabalin (Lyrica)	Neuropathic pain Multimodal therapy for acute pain (gabapentin, pregabalin) Fibromyalgia (pregabalin)	• Start with low doses, increase slowly • Side effects vary with each agent
Cannabinoids		
dronabinol (Marinol)	Neuropathic pain Certain pain syndromes	• May relieve nausea and increase appetite • May have opioid-sparing effects, possibly reducing opioid tolerance and symptoms of opioid withdrawal
Corticosteroids		
dexamethasone	Inflammation	• Avoid high doses for long-term use
γ-Aminobutyric Acid (GABA)–Receptor Agonist		
baclofen (Lioresal)	Neuropathic pain Muscle spasms	• Monitor for weakness, urinary problems • Avoid abrupt discontinuation because of CNS irritability

impulses. It helps manage muscle spasms and neuropathic pain. It crosses the blood-brain barrier poorly and is much more effective for spasticity when delivered intrathecally.

Corticosteroids. Corticosteroids include dexamethasone, prednisone, and methylprednisolone. They are used for managing acute and chronic cancer pain, pain from spinal cord compression, and inflammatory joint pain syndromes. Mechanisms of action may be related to the ability of corticosteroids to decrease edema and inflammation. Because they act through the same final pathway as NSAIDs, do not give corticosteroids with NSAIDs.

Local anesthetics. Local anesthetics, such as bupivacaine and ropivacaine, can be given epidurally by continuous infusion or by intermittent or continuous infusion with regional nerve blocks to manage acute pain from surgery or trauma. A systemic lidocaine IV infusion is sometimes used for neuropathic and postoperative visceral pain. Topical applications interrupt transmission of pain signals to the brain. For example, 5% lidocaine patch (Lidoderm) is a first-line agent for treating several types of neuropathic pain. Oral therapy with mexiletine may be an option for treating chronic severe neuropathic pain that is refractory to other analgesics.

Cannabinoids. Cannabinoid-derived medications show promise in treating neuropathic pain, certain pain syndromes, and some symptoms.[16] Synthetic cannabinoids (e.g., dronabinol [Marinol]) have been approved for medical use. Smoking marijuana or cannabis rapidly increases plasma levels of tetrahydrocannabinol (THC). The increase depends on composition of the marijuana cigarette and inhalation technique. As a result, this form has variable pain relief. With commercially available oral preparations, absorption and bioavailability are more reliable and predictable.

Cannabinoids exert their analgesic effects primarily through the cannabinoid-l (CB1) and CB2 receptors. Activation of these receptors modulates neurotransmission in the serotoninergic, dopaminergic, and glutamatergic systems, as well as other systems. Cannabinoids also enhance the endogenous opioid system. Other beneficial effects include alleviating nausea and increased appetite. They may have opioid-sparing effects, possibly reducing opioid tolerance and symptoms of opioid withdrawal.

Administration

Scheduling. Appropriate analgesic scheduling focuses on preventing or controlling pain rather than providing analgesics only after pain has become severe. An example is premedicating a patient before a procedure or activity that will likely cause pain. Similarly, a patient with constant pain should receive analgesics around the clock rather than on an "as needed" (PRN) basis. These strategies control pain before it starts and usually result in lower analgesic requirements.

Titration. *Analgesic titration* is dose adjustment based on assessment of the adequacy of analgesic effect versus the side effects produced. The amount of analgesic needed to manage pain varies widely. Titration is an important strategy in addressing this variability. An analgesic can be titrated upward or downward, depending on the situation. For example, in a postoperative patient the dose of analgesic decreases over time as the acute pain resolves. On the other hand, opioids for chronic, severe cancer pain may be titrated upward many times over the course of the disease to maintain adequate pain control. The goal of titration is to use the smallest dose of analgesic that provides effective pain control with the fewest side effects.

Do not dose patients with opioids solely based on reported pain scores. Opioid "dosing by numbers" can lead to unsafe practices and serious adverse events. We can achieve safe analgesic administration by balancing pain relief with analgesic side effects and using a multimodal approach. We can adjust therapy to promote better pain control and minimize adverse outcomes.

Equianalgesic dosing. The term **equianalgesic dose** refers to a dose of one analgesic that is equivalent in pain-relieving effects to a given dose of another analgesic (Table 9.13). This equivalence helps guide opioid dosing when changing routes or opioids when a specific drug is ineffective or causes intolerable side effects. Equianalgesic charts and conversion programs are available in clinical guidelines, in agency pain protocols, and on the Internet. They are useful tools, but you need to understand their limitations because these doses are estimates. The amounts can be affected by many factors, including patient variability, type of pain, and tolerance. To ensure safety, carefully monitor patients with all changes in opioid therapy and adjust the dose as needed.

Administration routes. We can deliver opioids and other analgesic agents by many routes. This flexibility allows the HCP to (1) target the source of the pain, (2) achieve therapeutic blood levels rapidly, when necessary, (3) avoid certain side effects through local administration, and (4) provide analgesia when patients are unable to swallow.

Oral. Oral administration is the route of choice for the person with a functioning GI system. Most pain medications are available in oral preparations, such as liquid and tablet. For opioids, larger oral doses are needed to achieve the equivalent analgesia of doses given IM or IV (Table 9.12). For example, 5 mg of IV morphine is equivalent to around 15 mg of oral morphine. The reason larger doses are needed is related to the *first-pass effect* of

TABLE 9.13 Opioid Equianalgesic Doses[a]

	DOSE EQUAL TO PARENTERAL MORPHINE 10 mg	
Drug	**Oral (mg)**	**Parenteral (IM, IV, Subcutaneous) (mg)**
Codeine	200	120–130
Fentanyl	NA	0.1 (100 mcg)
Hydrocodone	30	NA
Hydromorphone	7.5	1.5
Levorphanol	4	2
Morphine	30	10
Oxycodone	20	NA

[a]All equivalencies are approximate.

hepatic metabolism. This means that oral opioids are absorbed from the GI tract into the portal circulation and shunted to the liver. Partial metabolism in the liver occurs before the drug enters the systemic circulation and becomes available to peripheral receptors or can cross the blood-brain barrier and access CNS opioid receptors, which is needed to produce analgesia. Oral opioids are as effective as parenteral opioids if the dose is large enough to compensate for the first-pass metabolism.

Many opioids are available in short-acting (immediate-release) and long-acting (sustained-release or extended-release) oral preparations. Immediate-release products are effective in providing rapid, short-term pain relief. Sustained-release or extended-release preparations are often given every 8 to 12 hours. Some preparations may be dosed every 24 hours.

! SAFETY ALERT

Sustained-Release or Extended-Release Preparations

- These drugs should be swallowed whole. They are not to be crushed, broken, dissolved, or chewed.
- If all the drug is released into a person at once, serious side effects can occur, including death from overdose.

Transmucosal and buccal. Transmucosal absorption allows the drug to enter the bloodstream and travel directly to the CNS. Pain relief typically occurs 5 to 7 minutes after administration. Several transmucosal fentanyl products are options in treating BTP. Oral transmucosal fentanyl citrate (Actiq) contains fentanyl in a flavored lozenge on a stick. The lozenge is rubbed against the buccal surface (not sucked as a lollipop), allowing the buccal mucosa to absorb the fentanyl. Fentanyl buccal tablet (Fentora) is a quickly dissolving buccal tablet. These agents should be used only for patients who are already receiving and are tolerant to opioid therapy.

Although we can give morphine sublingually to people with cancer pain who have problems swallowing, little of the drug is absorbed from the sublingual tissue. Most of the drug dissolves in saliva and is swallowed, making its absorption like that of oral morphine.

Intranasal. Intranasal administration allows delivery of medication to highly vascular mucosa and avoids the first-pass effect. Butorphanol is given for acute headache and other intense, recurrent types of pain.

Rectal. We often overlook the rectal route. It is especially useful for patients who cannot take an analgesic by mouth, such as with severe nausea and vomiting or at end of life. Analgesics that are available as rectal suppositories include hydromorphone, oxymorphone, morphine, and acetaminophen. If rectal preparations are not available, many oral agents can be given rectally.

Transdermal. Transdermal patches offer systemic or local delivery. Fentanyl is useful for patients who cannot tolerate oral analgesic drugs. Absorption from the patch is slow. It takes 12 to 17 hours to reach full effect with the first application. Therefore transdermal fentanyl is not suitable for rapid dose titration but is better if the patient's pain is stable and the dose needed to control it is known. Patches may have to be changed every 48 hours rather than the recommended 72 hours based on the response. Remove a fentanyl patch if the patient has a fever. The elevated body heat can cause increased absorption of the medication and lead to increased side effects. Teach patients to avoid heat application over the patch for extended periods of time (e.g., heating pad, long hot showers). A transdermal PCA system (iontophoretic transdermal system [ITS]) is available.

A 5% lidocaine-impregnated transdermal patch (Lidoderm patch) can be used for local delivery of pain medication. The patch is left in place for up to 12 hours. There are few systemic side effects, even with chronic use.

Creams and lotions containing 10% trolamine salicylate (e.g., Aspercreme) are available for joint and muscle pain. This aspirin-like substance is absorbed locally. This route avoids GI irritation but not the other side effects of high-dose salicylates. Topical diclofenac solution or a diclofenac patch (Flector) can be effective in treating local pain, such as osteoarthritic knee pain.

Other topical analgesic agents, such as capsaicin (e.g., Zostrix) and lidocaine (L-M-X cream), can provide analgesia. Derived from red chili pepper, capsaicin acts on C-fiber heat receptors. If used 3 or 4 times a day for 4 to 6 weeks, it will cause the C nociceptor fibers to become inactive. The result is neuronal resistance to painful stimuli. Capsaicin may control pain from diabetic neuropathy, arthritis, and postherpetic neuralgia. We can apply L-M-X cream to control pain from venipunctures. Cover the targeted area of intact skin with a layer of L-M-X for at least 20 to 30 minutes, then wipe it off before beginning.

Parenteral. Parenteral routes include IV and subcutaneous administration. Single, repeated, or continuous dosing is possible with parenteral routes. IV administration is the best route when immediate analgesia and rapid titration are needed. Continuous IV infusions provide excellent steady-state analgesia through stable blood levels.

Onset of analgesia after subcutaneous administration is slow. Thus we rarely use the subcutaneous route for acute pain management. Continuous subcutaneous infusions are effective for pain management at the end of life. This route is especially helpful for people with abnormal GI function and limited venous access.

The IM route is not recommended. Injections cause significant pain and result in unreliable absorption. With chronic use, IM injections can result in abscesses and fibrosis.

Intraspinal. Intraspinal or neuraxial opioid therapy involves inserting a catheter into the subarachnoid space *(intrathecal delivery)* or the epidural space *(epidural delivery)* (Fig. 9.6). Analgesics are injected either by intermittent bolus doses or continuous infusion.

Percutaneously placed temporary catheters are used for short-term therapy (2 to 4 days). Epidural catheters may be placed at any point along the spinal column (cervical, thoracic, lumbar, or caudal). The lumbar region is the most common

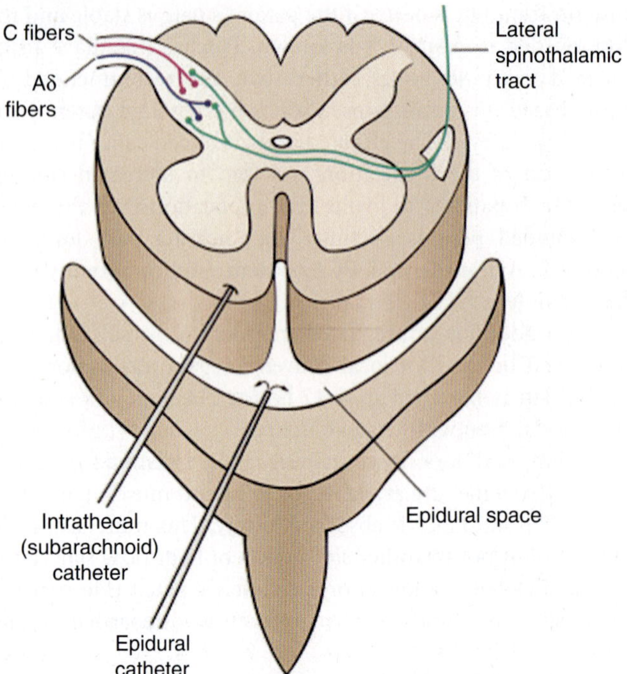

Fig. 9.6 Cross section of spinal cord with placement of catheters into the subarachnoid space (intrathecal delivery) and the epidural space (epidural delivery). (From Urden LD, Stacy KM, Lough ME: *Critical care nursing: diagnosis and management,* ed 8, St Louis, 2018, Elsevier.)

site. The tip of the epidural catheter is placed as close to the nerve supplying the painful dermatome as possible. For example, a thoracic catheter is placed for upper abdominal surgery, and a high lumbar catheter is used for lower abdominal surgery. Fluoroscopy ensures correct placement of the catheter.

Intraspinal analgesics are highly potent because they are delivered close to the receptors in the spinal cord dorsal horn. Smaller doses of analgesics are needed than with other routes. For example, 1 mg of intrathecal morphine equals 10 mg of epidural morphine and 100 mg of IV morphine. Intraspinal analgesics include morphine, fentanyl, sufentanil (Sufenta), alfentanil (Alfenta), hydromorphone, clonidine, and ziconotide. Ziconotide is a calcium channel receptor modulator for treating neuropathic pain syndromes. Nausea, itching, and urinary retention are common side effects of intraspinal opioids.

Complications of intraspinal analgesia include catheter displacement and migration, accidental infusions of neurotoxic agents, epidural hematomas, and infection. Manifestations of catheter displacement or migration depend on catheter location and the drug. A catheter that migrates out of the intrathecal or epidural space causes a decrease in pain relief with no improvement with more boluses or increases in the infusion rate. If an epidural catheter migrates into the subarachnoid space, increased side effects become quickly apparent. Somnolence, confusion, and increased anesthesia (if the infusion contains an anesthetic) may occur. Follow agency policy for aspirating cerebrospinal fluid to determine intrathecal catheter placement. Migration of a catheter into a blood vessel may cause an increase in side effects because of systemic drug distribution.

Many drugs and chemicals are highly neurotoxic when given intraspinally. These include antibiotics, chemotherapy agents, potassium, parenteral nutrition, and many preservatives, such as alcohol and phenol. To avoid accidental injection of IV drugs into an intraspinal catheter, clearly mark the catheter as an intraspinal access device.

Infection is a rare but serious complication of intraspinal analgesia. Assess the skin around the exit site for inflammation, drainage, or pain. Manifestations of an intraspinal infection include diffuse back pain, pain or paresthesia during bolus injection, and unexplained sensory or motor deficits in the lower limbs. Fever may or may not be present. Acute bacterial infection (meningitis) is manifested by photophobia, neck stiffness, fever, headache, and altered mental status. Regular, meticulous wound care and using sterile technique when caring for the catheter and injecting drugs reduces infection risk.

Long-term epidural catheters may be placed for terminal cancer patients or patients with certain pain syndromes that are unresponsive to other treatments. If a long-term indwelling epidural catheter is used, bacterial filters are recommended.

Implantable pumps. Intraspinal catheters are used for long-term pain relief. The surgical placement of an intrathecal catheter to a subcutaneously placed pump and reservoir allows for the delivery of drugs directly into the intrathecal space. The pump is normally placed in a pocket made in the subcutaneous tissue of the abdomen. It may be programmable or fixed. Pumps are refilled every 30 to 90 days, depending on flow rate, mixture, and reservoir size.

Patient-controlled analgesia. **Patient-controlled analgesia (PCA)** (demand analgesia) is a method that allows patients to self-administer preset doses of an analgesic within a prescribed time period by activating an infusion pump. Routes of administration include IV and epidural (**patient-controlled epidural analgesia [PCEA]**). PCA also can be adapted for oral administration. With PCA/PCEA, a dose of opioid is delivered when the patient decides a dose is needed. PCA/PCEA uses an infusion system in which patients push a button to receive a bolus infusion of an analgesic. PCA/PCEA is used widely for the management of acute pain, including postoperative and cancer pain.

Opioids, such as morphine and hydromorphone, are often given via PCA therapy. Sometimes IV PCA is given with a continuous or background infusion called a *basal rate,* depending on the patient's opioid requirement. Adding a basal rate in opioid-naive patients and those at risk for adverse respiratory outcomes (e.g., older age, obstructive sleep apnea, lung disease) may lead to serious respiratory events.

PCEA often combines an opioid and local anesthetic. Basal rates are often used with PCEA. Because the medication is delivered directly into the epidural space, the amount of opioid is 10 times less than is needed by IV route. This lessens the risk for respiratory depression but does not eliminate it.

Patient teaching is important with the use of PCA/PCEA. Help patients understand the mechanics of the machine. Teach them to self-administer the analgesic before pain is severe. Assure patients that they cannot "overdose" because the pump is programmed to deliver a maximum number of doses per hour. They will not receive more analgesic once they reach the maximum dose. If the maximum dose is inadequate to relieve pain, we can reprogram the pump to increase the amount or frequency of dosing. You can give bolus doses if they are part of the HCP's orders. To make a smooth transition from infusion PCA to oral drugs, patients should receive increasing doses of oral drug while we taper the PCA analgesic.

Patient-controlled delivery systems are intended for use by the patient. An *authorized agent-controlled analgesia (AACA)* is a method of delivery performed by a consistently available and competent person for patients who are unable to independently activate PCA devices. This authorized agent must be carefully selected, taught the principles of PCA, and capable of recognizing pain and the appropriate times to give medication via the PCA device. Understand your agency's policies about PCA and AACA.

Interventional Therapy

Therapeutic Nerve Blocks

Nerve blocks involve injecting local anesthetics into an area to produce pain relief. We also call these techniques *regional anesthesia.* Nerve blocks interrupt all afferent and efferent transmission to the area and are not specific to nociceptive pathways. They include local infiltration of anesthetics into a surgical area (e.g., chest incisions, inguinal hernia) and injection of anesthetic into a specific nerve (e.g., occipital, pudendal nerve) or nerve plexus (e.g., brachial, celiac plexus). Nerve blocks can be used during and after surgery to manage pain. For longer-term relief of chronic pain syndromes, we can give local anesthetics by a continuous infusion.

Adverse effects of nerve blocks are like those for local anesthetics delivered by other systemic routes. Effects include systemic toxicity resulting in dysrhythmias, confusion, nausea and vomiting, blurred vision, tinnitus, and metallic taste. Temporary nerve blocks affect motor function and sensation and typically last 2 to 24 hours, depending on the agent and the site of injection. Motor ability generally returns before sensation.

Neuroablative techniques. *Neuroablative interventions* are done for severe pain that is unresponsive to all other therapies. They involve destroying nerves, thereby interrupting pain transmission. Destruction is by surgical resection or thermocoagulation, including radiofrequency coagulation. Neuroablative interventions that destroy the sensory division of a peripheral or spinal nerve are classified as *neurectomies, rhizotomies,* and *sympathectomies.* Neurosurgical procedures that ablate the lateral spinothalamic tract are classified as *cordotomies* if the tract is interrupted in the spinal cord or *tractotomies* if the interruption is in the medulla or midbrain of the brainstem (Fig. 9.7).

Neuroaugmentation

Neuroaugmentation involves electrical stimulation of the brain and spinal cord. The most common use is for chronic back pain caused by nerve damage that is unresponsive to other therapies. Other uses include CRPS, spinal cord injury pain, and interstitial cystitis. Potential complications include those related to the surgery (bleeding, infection), migration of the generator (which usually is implanted in the subcutaneous tissues of the upper gluteal or pectoralis area), and nerve damage.

Nondrug Therapies

Nondrug strategies have a key role in pain management (Table 9.14). They can reduce the dose of an analgesic needed to relieve pain and thereby minimize side effects of drug therapy. They increase the patient's sense of personal control about managing pain and increase coping skills. We think some strategies alter ascending nociceptive input or stimulate descending pain modulation mechanisms. These nondrug therapies are useful for both acute and chronic pain.

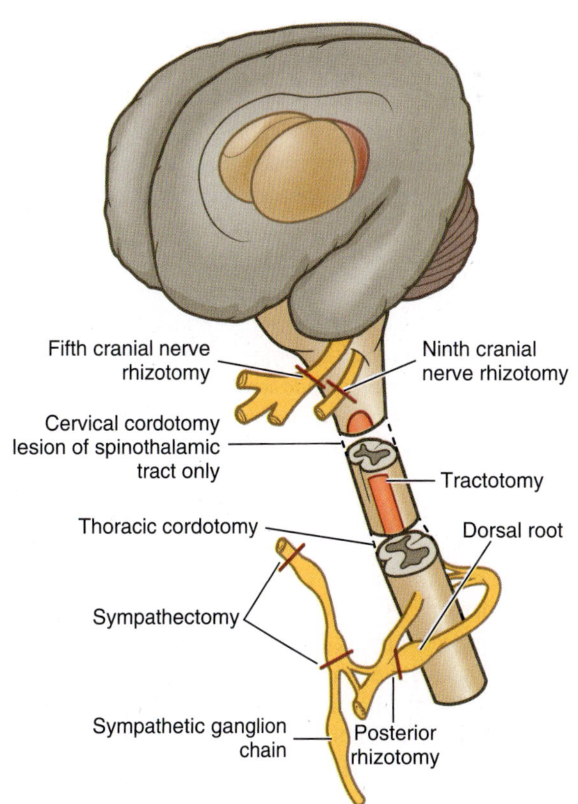

Fig. 9.7 Sites of neurosurgical procedures for pain relief.

TABLE 9.14 Nondrug Therapies for Pain

Physical Therapies
- Acupuncture
- Application of heat and cold (Table 9.15)
- Exercise
- Massage
- Transcutaneous electrical nerve stimulation (TENS)

Cognitive Therapies
- Distraction
- Hypnosis
- Imagery
- Relaxation strategies (see Chapter 7)
  - Art therapy
  - Imagery
  - Meditation
  - Music therapy
  - Relaxation breathing

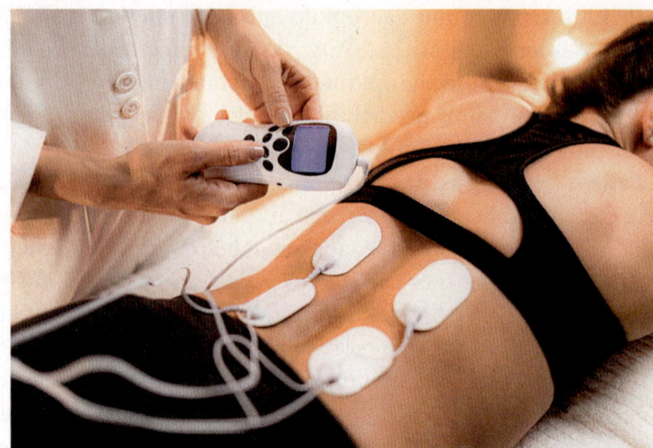

Fig. 9.8 TENS treatment for a patient with low back pain. (© microgen/iStock.com.)

Physical Pain Relief Strategies

Massage. Massage may be useful to alleviate certain types of acute and chronic pain.[17] Many different massage techniques exist. These include moving the hands or fingers over the skin slowly or briskly with long strokes or in circles (superficial massage) or applying firm pressure to the skin to maintain contact while massaging the underlying tissues (deep massage). Another type is trigger point massage. A **trigger point** is a circumscribed hypersensitive area within a tight band of muscle. It is caused by acute or chronic muscle strain. It feels like a tight knot under the skin. Trigger point massage is done by applying strong, sustained digital pressure; deep massage; or gentler massage with ice followed by muscle heating. See more about massage in Chapter 7.

Exercise. Exercise is an essential part of the treatment plan for patients with chronic pain, especially those with musculoskeletal pain.[18] Many patients become physically deconditioned from their pain, which in turn leads to more pain. Exercise acts via many mechanisms to relieve pain. It enhances circulation and cardiovascular fitness, reduces edema, increases muscle strength and flexibility, and enhances physical and psychosocial function. It is important to tailor an exercise program to the patient's physical needs and lifestyle. It may include aerobic exercise, stretching, and strengthening exercises. Trained personnel (e.g., physical therapist) should supervise the program.

Transcutaneous electrical nerve stimulation. *Transcutaneous electrical nerve stimulation* (TENS) involves the delivery of an electric current through electrodes applied to the skin surface over the painful region, at trigger points, or over a peripheral nerve.[19] A TENS system consists of 2 or more electrodes connected by lead wires to a small, battery-operated stimulator (Fig. 9.8). A physical therapist is often responsible for delivering TENS therapy, although nurses can be trained in the technique. TENS may be used for acute pain, including postoperative pain and pain from physical trauma. The effects of TENS on chronic pain are less clear, but it may be effective in these cases.

Acupuncture. Acupuncture is a technique of traditional Chinese medicine in which very thin needles are inserted into the body at designated points.[20] It is used for many kinds of pain. Acupuncture is described in Chapter 7.

Heat therapy. Heat therapy is the application of either moist or dry heat to the skin. Heat therapy can be either superficial or deep. We can apply heat using an electric heating pad (dry or moist), a hot pack, hot moist compresses, warm wax (paraffin), or a hot water bottle. To expose large areas of the body, patients can immerse themselves in a hot bath, shower, or whirlpool. Physical therapy departments provide deep-heat therapy through techniques such as short-wave diathermy, microwave diathermy, and ultrasound therapy. Patient and caregiver teaching about heat therapy is described in Table 9.15.

Cold therapy. Cold therapy involves the application of either moist or dry cold to the skin. Dry cold can be applied by using an ice bag. Moist cold can be applied by using towels soaked in ice water, cold hydrocollator packs, or immersion in a bath or under running cold water. Icing with ice cubes or blocks of ice made to resemble popsicles is another technique used for pain relief. Patient and caregiver teaching about cold therapy is described in Table 9.15.

Cognitive Therapies

Techniques to alter the affective, cognitive, and behavior components of pain include a variety of cognitive strategies and behavior approaches.[21] For example, patients can identify and challenge negative pain-related thoughts and replace them with more positive coping thoughts. Some techniques need little training. Patients may adopt them independently. For others, a trained therapist is needed.

Distraction. Distraction involves redirection of attention away from the pain and onto something.[22] It is a simple but powerful strategy to relieve pain. Distraction involves engaging patients in any activity that can hold their attention (e.g., watching TV or a movie, conversing, listening to music). It is important to match the activity with the patient's energy level and ability to concentrate.

Hypnosis. Hypnotherapy is a structured technique that allows patients to achieve a state of heightened awareness and focused concentration that can be used to alter pain

TABLE 9.15 PATIENT & CAREGIVER TEACHING

Heat and Cold Therapy

Include the following instructions when teaching the patient and caregiver about superficial heat or cold techniques:

Heat Therapy
- Do not use heat on an area that is being treated with radiation therapy, is bleeding, has decreased sensation, or has been injured in the past 24 hours.
- Do not use any menthol-containing products (e.g., Ben-Gay, Icy Hot) with heat applications because this may cause burns.
- Cover the heat source with a towel or cloth before applying to the skin to prevent burns.

Cold Therapy
- Cover the cold source with a cloth or towel before applying to the skin to prevent tissue damage.
- Do not apply cold to areas that are being treated with radiation therapy, have open wounds, or have poor circulation.
- If it is not possible to apply the cold directly to the painful site, try applying it right above or below the painful site or on the opposite side of the body on the corresponding site (e.g., left elbow if the right elbow hurts).

TABLE 9.16 PATIENT & CAREGIVER TEACHING

Pain Management

Include the following information in the teaching plan for the patient with pain and caregiver:
- Cause of the pain, if known, and how long it may last
- Factors that may be contributing to pain
- Pain assessment methods and reason for frequent monitoring of pain
- Expectations about pain management
- Self-management techniques
- Realistic goals for pain control
- Negative consequences of unrelieved pain
- Need to maintain a record of pain level and effectiveness of treatment
- Safe use of analgesia
- Treat pain with drugs and/or nondrug therapies before it becomes severe
- Medication may stop working after it is taken for a time period. Dosages may need to be adjusted
- Potential side effects and complications associated with pain therapies can include nausea and vomiting, constipation, sedation and drowsiness, itching, urinary retention, and sweating
- Need to report when pain is not relieved to tolerable levels

perception.[23] Hypnosis should be delivered and monitored only by specially trained clinicians.

Relaxation strategies. Relaxation strategies reduce stress, decrease anxiety, distract from pain, ease muscle tension, combat fatigue, promote sleep, and enhance the effectiveness of other pain relief measures. Relaxation strategies include relaxation breathing, music, imagery, meditation, muscle relaxation, and art (see Chapter 7).

Challenges to Effective Pain Management

Communication Barriers

Because pain is subjective, patients need to feel confident that their reporting of pain will be believed and will not be perceived as "complaining." The patient and caregiver need to know that you consider the pain significant and understand that pain may profoundly disrupt a person's life. Communicate concern and commit to helping the patient obtain pain relief and cope with any unrelieved pain. Support the patient and caregiver through the period of trial and error that may be necessary to implement an effective therapeutic plan. It is important to clarify responsibilities in pain relief. Help the patient understand the role of the interprofessional team members, as well as the patient's roles and expectations.

Evaluate the impact that the pain has on the lives of the patient and caregiver. Table 9.16 addresses teaching needs of patients and caregivers related to pain management.

Fear of Addiction

Common challenges to effective pain management include misunderstandings about tolerance, physical dependence, and addiction. It is important for you to understand and be able to explain these concepts. Table 9.17 lists barriers to pain management and strategies to address them.

Tolerance. *Tolerance* occurs with chronic exposure to a variety of drugs. In the case of opioids, tolerance to analgesia is characterized by the need for an increased opioid dose to maintain the same degree of analgesia. The incidence of clinically significant analgesic opioid tolerance in chronic pain patients is unknown, because dosage needs may increase as the disease (e.g., cancer) progresses. It is essential to assess for increased analgesic needs in patients on long-term therapy. The interprofessional team must evaluate and rule out other causes of increased analgesic needs, such as disease progression or infection.

If significant tolerance to opioids develops and the opioid is losing its effectiveness or if intolerable side effects occur with dose escalation, the practice of *opioid rotation* may be considered. This involves switching from one opioid to another, assuming that the new opioid will be more effective at lower equianalgesic doses. However, very high opioid doses can result in OIH rather than pain relief. This means that increases in the dose can lead to higher pain levels.

Physical dependence. Like tolerance, physical dependence is a normal physiologic response to ongoing exposure to drugs. It is manifested by a withdrawal syndrome when the drug is abruptly decreased. When opioids are no longer needed to provide pain relief, a tapering schedule should be used with careful monitoring. A typical tapering schedule may involve reducing the dose by 20% to 50% per day. The goal is to reduce the amount of medication and at the same time minimize adverse and withdrawal effects.

Addiction. *Addiction* is a complex neurobiologic condition characterized by aberrant behaviors arising from a drive to obtain and take substances for reasons other than the

TABLE 9.17 **PATIENT & CAREGIVER TEACHING**

Reducing Barriers to Pain Management

When teaching patients and caregivers about pain management discuss the following barriers:

Barrier	Nursing Considerations
Fear of addiction	• Acknowledge and normalize fears. • Reinforce that health care team members will be monitoring for signs of addiction.
Fear of tolerance	• Teach that tolerance is a normal physiologic response to chronic opioid therapy. If tolerance does develop, the drug may have to be changed (e.g., morphine in place of oxycodone). • Teach that there is no absolute upper limit to pure opioid agonists (e.g., morphine). Dosages can be increased, and patient should not save drugs for when the pain is worse. • Teach that tolerance develops more slowly to analgesic effects of opioids than to side effects (e.g., sedation, respiratory depression).
Concern about side effects	• Teach ways to prevent and to treat common side effects. • Stress that some side effects, such as sedation and nausea, decrease with time. • Explain that different drugs have unique side effects. Other pain drugs can be tried to reduce the specific side effect.
Fear of injections	• Explain that oral medicines are preferred. • Stress that even if oral route becomes unusable, transdermal or indwelling parenteral routes can be used rather than injections.
Desire to be "good" patient	• Discuss that patients are partners in their care. That partnership requires open communication by both patient and nurse. • Stress to patients that they have a responsibility to keep you informed about their pain.
Desire to be stoic	• Explain that although stoicism may be a valued behavior in some circumstances, failure to report pain can result in undertreatment and severe, unrelieved pain.
Forgetting to take analgesic	• Discuss using reminders, such as pill containers. • Recruit caregivers to help with the analgesic regimen.
Concern that pain indicates disease progression	• Explain that increased pain or the need for analgesics may reflect tolerance. • Stress that new pain may come from a non–life-threatening source (e.g., muscle spasm, urinary tract infection). • Use drug and nondrug strategies to reduce anxiety. • Ensure that patient and caregivers have current, accurate information about the disease and prognosis. • Provide psychologic support.
Sense of fatalism	• Explain that pain can be managed in most patients. • Explain that most therapies require a period of trial and error. • Stress that side effects can be managed.
Ineffective medication	• Teach that there are multiple options within each category of medication (e.g., opioids, NSAIDs), and another medication from the same category may provide better relief. • Discuss that finding the best treatment regimen may require trial and error. • Include nondrug approaches in treatment plan.

prescribed therapeutic value (see Chapter 11). Tolerance and physical dependence are not indicators of addiction. Rather, they are normal physiologic responses to chronic exposure to certain drugs, including opioids. If we suspect addiction, it must be investigated and appropriately diagnosed. The hallmarks of addiction include (1) compulsive use, (2) loss of control of use, and (3) continued use despite risk of harm.

Pseudoaddiction. Inadequate treatment of pain can lead to a phenomenon called *pseudoaddiction.* This occurs when patients show behaviors associated with addiction (e.g., frequent requests for analgesic refills or higher dosages), but the behaviors resolve with adequate treatment of the patient's pain. These patients are often labeled as drug seeking. This can result in mistrust between the patient and HCP. Effective communication strategies and optimal pain management can help avoid this problem.

Inadequate Education

Other barriers to effective and safe pain management include inadequate HCP education and lack of agency support. Traditionally, medical and nursing school curricula spent little time teaching future physicians and nurses about pain and symptom management. We have made progress in this area. Medical and nursing schools devote more time to addressing pain. Numerous professional organizations have published evidence-based guidelines for assessing and managing pain in many patient populations and clinical settings.

Agency commitment and practices are changing clinical practice. One major step is the development and adoption of The Joint Commission (TJC) guideline on pain. Under these standards, health care agencies are required to (1) recognize the patient's right to assessment and management of pain; (2) identify pain in patients during their initial assessment and as needed, during ongoing, periodic reassessments; (3) teach HCPs about pain assessment and management and ensure competency; and (4) teach patients and their families about pain management.

A common concern of health care professionals and caregivers is that giving enough drug to relieve pain will hasten or precipitate death of a terminally ill person. However, there is no scientific evidence that opioids can hasten death, even among patients at the very end of life. Moreover, you have a moral obligation to provide comfort and pain relief at the end of life. Even if there is a concern about the possibility of hastening death, the rule of double effect provides ethical justification. This rule states that if an unwanted consequence (i.e., hastened death) occurs because of an action taken to achieve a moral good (i.e., pain relief), the action is justified if the nurse's intent is to relieve pain and not to hasten death.

MANAGING PAIN IN SPECIAL POPULATIONS

Older Adults

Persistent pain is a common problem in older adults. It is often associated with physical disability and psychosocial problems. The prevalence of chronic pain among community-dwelling older adults exceeds 50%. Among older nursing home patients, it is around 80%. The most common painful conditions among older adults are musculoskeletal conditions, such as osteoarthritis and low back pain. Chronic pain often results in depression, sleep problems, decreased mobility, increased health care use, and physical and social role problems. Despite its high prevalence, pain in older adults is often inadequately assessed and treated.

Several barriers to pain assessment in older patients exist. Older adults and their HCPs often believe that pain is a normal, inevitable part of aging and that nothing can be done to relieve the pain. Older adults may not report pain for fear of being a "burden" or a "complainer." They may fear taking opioids. Older patients are more likely to use words such as "aching," "soreness," or "discomfort" rather than "pain." Be persistent in asking older adults about pain. Perform your assessment in an unhurried, supportive manner.

Another barrier is the increased prevalence of cognitive, sensory-perceptual, and motor problems that interfere with a person's ability to process information and communicate. Examples include dementia, delirium, and poststroke aphasia. Hearing and vision problems may complicate assessment. Pain assessment tools may have to be adapted for older adults. For example, you may need to use a large-print pain intensity scale. Most older adults, even those with mild to moderate cognitive impairment, can use quantitative scales accurately and reliably.

In older patients with chronic pain, perform a thorough physical assessment and history to identify causes of pain, possible therapies, and potential problems. Assess for depression and functional impairments. They are common among older adults with pain.

Treatment of pain in older adults is complicated by several factors. First, older adults metabolize drugs more slowly than younger people. Thus they are at greater risk for higher blood levels and adverse effects. Apply the adage "start low and go slow" to analgesic therapy in this age group. Second, the use of NSAIDs in older adults is associated with a high frequency of GI bleeding. Third, older adults often are taking many drugs for 1 or more chronic conditions. The addition of analgesics can result in dangerous drug interactions and increased side effects. Last, analgesics, such as opioids, antidepressants, and antiseizure drugs, can worsen cognitive problems and ataxia. This requires that HCPs titrate drugs slowly and monitor carefully for side effects.

Treatment plans for older adults must include nondrug modalities. Exercise and patient teaching are important nondrug interventions for older adults with chronic pain. Include family and caregivers in the treatment plan (Tables 9.16 and 9.17).

Patients Unable to Self-Report Pain

Although self-report is the gold standard of pain assessment, many illnesses and conditions affect a patient's ability to report pain. These diagnoses and conditions include dementia and delirium. For these people, behavior and physiologic changes may be the only indicators of pain. You must be astute at recognizing behavior symptoms of pain.

A guide for assessing pain in nonverbal patients is outlined in Table 9.18. Several scales are available to assess pain-related behaviors in nonverbal patients, especially those with advanced dementia and the critically ill. Links to several pain assessment tools are available at the City of Hope Pain and Palliative Care Resource Center website (http://prc.coh.org).

Patients in the Critical Care Unit

Unrelieved pain is common among critical care patients and can lead to poor outcomes. Inadequate pain control is linked

TABLE 9.18 Assessing Pain in Nonverbal Patients

The following assessment techniques are recommended:

- Obtain a self-report when possible.
- Never assume a nonverbal person is unable to communicate pain; blinking, writing, hand gestures, or nodding can be ways to express pain or the absence of pain.
- Assess potential causes of pain.
- Observe patient behaviors that indicate pain (e.g., grimacing, frowning, rubbing a painful area, groaning, restlessness).
- Obtain reports of pain from professional and family caregivers.
- Try to use analgesics and reassess the patient for a decrease in pain-related behaviors.

Modified from Herr K, Coyne PJ, Ely E, et al: Pain assessment in the patient unable to self-report: clinical practice recommendations in support of the ASPMN 2019 position statement, *Pain Manag Nurs* 20:404, 2019.

with agitation, fear, and anxiety and adds to the stress response. Patients at high risk for pain include those who (1) have medical conditions that include ischemic, infectious, or inflammatory processes; (2) are immobilized; (3) have invasive monitoring devices, including endotracheal tubes (ETs); and (4) undergo procedures.

For many critically ill patients (e.g., those intubated), continuous IV sedation (e.g., propofol [Diprivan]) and an analgesic agent (e.g., fentanyl) provide sedation and pain control. However, patients getting deep sedation are often unresponsive. This prevents us from fully assessing neurologic status. To address this issue, all patients who can safely tolerate an interruption in sedation usually receive a daily, scheduled interruption of sedation, or "sedation holiday." These allow you to awaken the patient to conduct a neurologic examination.

Patients With Substance Use Problems

The American Society for Pain Management Nursing has established guidelines for pain management in patients with addiction. These guidelines reflect a team approach in which patients with addictive disease and pain have the right to be treated with dignity, respect, and the same quality of pain assessment and management as all other patients.

HCPs are often reluctant to give opioids to patients at risk for addiction or those with substance use problems for fear of promoting or worsening addictions. However, there is no evidence that providing opioid analgesia to these patients in any way worsens their addictive disease. In fact, the stress of unrelieved pain may contribute to relapse in the recovering patient or increased drug use in the patient who actively misuses drugs.

CHECK YOUR PRACTICE

A 27-year-old female patient is admitted for IV antibiotics to treat an abscess in her arm that developed from using injection drugs. She received 2 mg of IV hydromorphone 1 hour ago. She tells you that her pain level is 8 out of 10 and she appears irritable and anxious because she is not getting enough pain medication. She yells at you and says that you are treating her unfairly.

- What should you do?

Several opioid risk assessments are available to help us assess patients for misuse and addiction. Other tools assess the risk of addiction with opioid analgesia. These include the Opioid Risk Tool (www.drugabuse.gov/sites/default/files/files/OpioidRiskTool.pdf) and the Screener and Opioid Assessment for Patient Pain (https://www.mcstap.com/docs/SOAPP-5.pdf) We may use a controlled substance agreement for those at risk. Patient monitoring with urine drug screens and access to state prescription monitoring programs to track prescriptions are effective in detecting misuse of drugs.

If the patient acknowledges substance use, determine the types and amounts of drugs used. Avoid exposing the patient to the misused drug. Effective equianalgesic doses of other opioids may be determined if daily drug doses are known. If a history of drug use is unknown or if the patient does not acknowledge substance use, be suspicious when normal doses of analgesics do not relieve pain.

Aggressive behavior patterns and signs of withdrawal may occur. Withdrawal symptoms can worsen pain and lead to drug-seeking behavior or illicit drug use. Toxicology screens may be helpful in determining recently used drugs. Discussing these findings with the patient may help gain their cooperation in pain control.

Severe pain should be treated with opioids. They will likely need to be at much higher doses than those used with drug-naive patients. The use of a single opioid is best. Avoid using a mixed opioid agonist-antagonist (e.g., butorphanol) or a partial agonist (e.g., buprenorphine), because these drugs may precipitate withdrawal symptoms. Nonopioid and adjuvant analgesics and nondrug pain relief measures may be used as needed. To maintain opioid blood levels and prevent withdrawal symptoms, provide analgesics around the clock. Use supplemental doses to treat BTP. IV or PCA infusions may be an option for acute pain management.

Pain management for people with addiction is challenging and needs an interprofessional team approach. When possible, the team includes pain management and addiction specialists. Team members need to be aware of their own attitudes about people with substance use problems, which may result in undertreatment of pain.

CASE STUDY

Pain

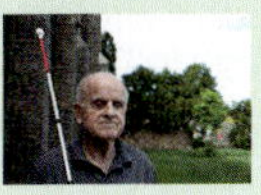

(© Johnrob/ iStock.com.)

Patient Profile

S.W. is a 135-lb (61-kg) 68-year-old male with diabetes, hypertension, and cervical radiculopathy. He has diabetic retinopathy with a visual acuity of 20/200, which makes him legally blind. S.W. was admitted for anterior cervical discectomy with fusion to help relieve the pain he was experiencing from his cervical radiculopathy. He is being discharged on his second postoperative day.

Subjective Data

- Lives alone
- Desires 0 pain but will accept 1 or 2 on a scale of 0 to 10
- Reports incision area pain in his neck as a 3 or 4; pain as high as 7 in both of his arms when he changes position or tries to raise his arms to do things like feed himself or brush his teeth
- Describes the pain in his arms as a burning and shooting sensation that originates in his neck and radiates to his hands
- In the hospital his pain has been treated with gabapentin and oxycodone
- He tells you he does not like taking pain medications

Objective Data

- Needs to wear neck brace until his next follow-up appointment
- For discharge, prescribed oral oxycodone 1 tablet every 4 h as needed for pain and gabapentin 300 mg 3 times daily

Discussion Questions

1. ***Recognize:*** Describe the assessment data that are important for determining whether S.W. has adequate pain management.
2. ***Analyze:*** What can you do to respect S.W.'s beliefs about using pain medication?
3. ***Plan:*** How would you involve other interprofessional team members in S.W.'s care?
4. ***Prioritize:*** Based on the data presented, what are the priority clinical problems?
5. ***Prioritize:*** What are the priority nursing interventions for S.W.?
6. ***Safety:*** What side effects might he have because of his pain medication? How can these be safely managed?
7. ***Act:*** What teaching will you provide so S.W. can successfully self-manage care at home?

Answers available at www.evolve.elsevier.com/Lewis/medsurg.

BRIDGE TO NCLEX EXAMINATION

The number of the question corresponds to the same-numbered outcome at the beginning of the chapter.

1. The nurse provides comprehensive pain management based on which principles? **(Select all that apply.)**
   a. Older patients rarely report pain.
   b. Pain has an emotional component.
   c. Pain consists of an unpleasant sensory experience.
   d. Families and caregivers do not play a role in pain response.
   e. Observed behaviors are used to assess pain in nonverbal patients.
2. A patient is receiving a patient-controlled analgesia (PCA) infusion after spinal surgery. They are sleeping soundly, awaken when the nurse speaks to them in a normal tone of voice, and reports their pain as "mild and tolerable." Their respirations are 8 breaths/min. The *most* appropriate nursing action is to
   a. stop the PCA infusion.
   b. continue to closely monitor the patient.
   c. assess surgical dressing for signs of bleeding.
   d. call the rapid response team and administer naloxone.
3. A patient with a below-the-knee amputation of the right leg reports right foot pain. The nurse knows that this type of pain
   a. originates from the skin.
   b. is best treated with steroids.
   c. arises from damage to peripheral nerves.
   d. is associated with visceral nociceptive pain.
4. Unrelieved pain is
   a. inevitable in persons in hospice.
   b. expected in a person with peripheral neuropathy.
   c. a source of suffering and can cause difficulty sleeping.
   d. something to expect because of the opioid addiction epidemic.
5. The nurse is assessing a postoperative patient for pain. The best way to approach this assessment is to
   a. obtain a blood pressure.
   b. ask the patient to rate their pain on a 0 to 10 scale.
   c. determine the amount of pain medication that has been used.
   d. have the patient point to the area that is causing them discomfort.
6. Which statement by the nurse shows an understanding of the basic principles of treating pain?
   a. "Tell me what level of pain is acceptable to you."
   b. "If you take too much of this medication you will become addicted."
   c. "Do not push the PCA button more than once an hour or you could overdose."
   d. "I am only allowed to give you the medication when your pain is a 9 out of 10."
7. A patient with cancer reports constant, moderate pain with short periods of severe pain during dressing changes. The best approach in managing this patient's pain is
   a. intermittent heat and cold therapy.
   b. deep breathing, acupuncture, and meditation.
   c. as needed long-acting opioids and topical lidocaine.
   d. a combination of a long-acting and a short-acting opioid.

8. Nursing responsibilities related to pain management include (**Select all that apply.**)
   a. reassess the effect of analgesia.
   b. trust the patient's subjective pain report.
   c. assume nonverbal patients do not experience pain.
   d. teach patient and caregiver about the treatment plan.
   e. withhold pain medication for patients with addiction.
9. Giving opioids to an actively dying patient who is reporting severe pain
   a. will hasten the person's death.
   b. is ineffective unless given in an IV formulation.
   c. is an appropriate and ethically justified nursing action.
   d. will not be helpful as they need a higher dose than what the nurse can give.
10. A nurse believes that all patients recovering from laparoscopic surgery should not need more than acetaminophen for pain. This statement reflects
   a. a belief that results in effective pain management.
   b. a belief based on the nurse's own personal experience with pain
   c. a lack of knowledge about factors affecting pain, leading to poor pain management.
   d. a belief that will not have any effect on the type of care provided to patients in pain.

1. b, c, e; 2. b; 3. c; 4. c; 5. b; 6. a; 7. d;
8. a, b, d; 9. c; 10. c.

For rationales to these answers and even more NCLEX review questions, visit http://evolve.elsevier.com/Lewis/medsurg.

REFERENCES

To access the References for this chapter, please scan the QR code with a mobile device.

10

Palliative and End-of-Life Care

Amisha Parekh de Campos, Shila Pandey, and William E. Rosa

http://evolve.elsevier.com/Lewis/medsurg/

CONCEPTUAL FOCUS

Stress and Coping
Ethics
Family Dynamics
Health Care Organizations
Palliative Care
Spirituality

LEARNING OUTCOMES

1. Distinguish the purpose of palliative care and hospice care.
2. Describe the physical and psychologic manifestations at the end of life.
3. Discuss ethical and legal issues related to palliative care.
4. Describe the nursing management of the dying patient.
5. Explore the special needs of family caregivers in palliative care.
6. Explain the process of grief and bereavement at the end of life.
7. Discuss the special needs of the nurse who cares for dying patients and their families.
8. Examine cultural and spiritual issues related to palliative care.

KEY TERMS

advance care planning
advance directives
anticipatory grief
bereavement
brain death
death
do-not-resuscitate (DNR) order
end of life
grief
hospice
palliative care
spirituality

PALLIATIVE CARE

Palliative care is the active holistic care of persons with serious health-related suffering from severe illness.[1] The severe illness may be acute or chronic, with a high mortality rate. Patients with serious illnesses experience a significant burden of suffering. The illness may affect quality of life and role function and create increased burden related to symptoms, treatment, or caregiver stress. Health care has a role in the care of the dying, but interventions at end of life are often excessive, exclude contributions from families and friends, and increase suffering.[2]

Although palliative care can be started at any time, optimal benefits occur when it begins after the diagnosis of a serious illness. These illnesses include neurodegenerative diseases, cancer, heart failure, chronic obstructive pulmonary disease (COPD), dementia, or end-stage kidney disease.[3] The growing number of people with problems such as diabetes and heart disease contributes to the increased need for and use of palliative care.[4]

Palliative care is considered supportive care. It involves assessing and managing pain and other symptoms, supporting caregiver needs, and coordinating care. The approach is patient and family centered. The goal is to reduce the burden of health-related suffering while improving quality of life (Fig. 10.1). Palliative care (1) improves quality of life for those with chronic illness, (2) decreases health care costs, and (3) eases caregiver burden.[5]

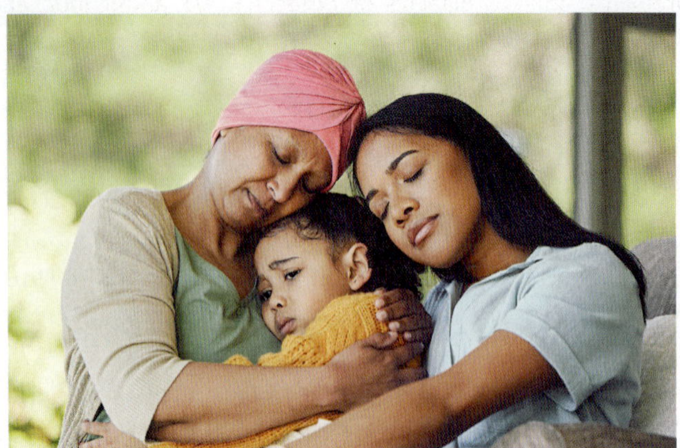

Fig. 10.1 One goal of palliative care is to improve the quality of the patient's remaining life. (©Jacob Wackerhausen/iStock.com.)

TABLE 10.1 Goals of Palliative Care

- Provide relief from pain and other physical symptoms
- Maximize quality of life
- Provide psychosocial and spiritual care
- Provide support to the family and the caregivers during the patient's illness and in bereavement

The International Association for Hospice and Palliative Care. Retrieved from https://hospicecare.com/what-we-do/publications/getting-started/what-is-palliative-care/.

Palliative care can be provided as the primary focus of care or concurrently with medical/curative treatment (Table 10.1). Ideally, all patients receiving curative or restorative care should receive palliative care at the same time. Palliative care extends into the period of end-of-life (EOL) care and offers patient and family support while planning for EOL needs.[5] Grief and bereavement care follow the patient's death (Fig. 10.2).

The American Nurses Association (ANA) and the Hospice and Palliative Nurses Association suggest that every nurse should deliver primary palliative care, regardless of setting. In other words, all who care for seriously ill patients should provide basic palliative care interventions.[6] Hospice nurses focus on pain control and symptom management, spiritual assessment, and assessment and management of family needs. To meet patient and family needs, the hospice nurse needs excellent teaching skills, compassion, flexibility, cultural competence, and adaptability.

Primary palliative care includes basic symptom management, routine discussions about care goals, and assessment of psychologic, social, cultural, and spiritual care needs.[7] Specialist palliative care clinicians offer complex symptom management, have difficult discussions and clarify care goals, and help with accessing care.

The palliative care team is an interprofessional collaboration. The interprofessional team (IPT) often includes nurses, advanced practice nurses, social workers, pharmacists, physicians, chaplains, and other health care professionals.[8] Empathetic, respectful, and reflective communication among the patient, family, and IPT is vital to ensuring patient- and family-centered care. Patients receive palliative care services in multiple settings. These include the home, long-term and acute care, mental health agencies, rehabilitation centers, and prisons. Many agencies have established palliative care teams.

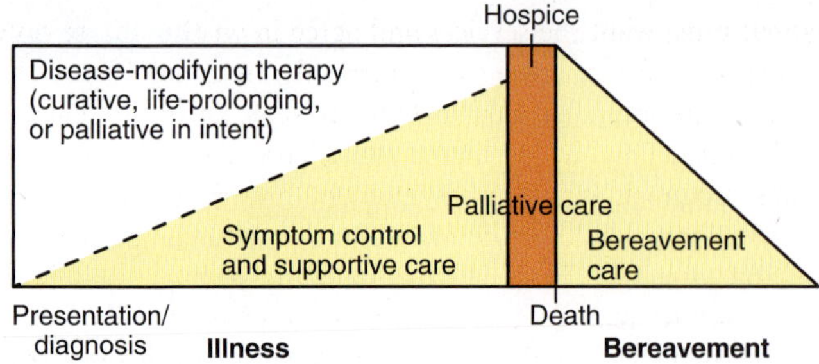

Fig. 10.2 Continuum-of-care model showing integration of curative care, palliative and end-of-life/hospice care, and bereavement care. (Redrawn from Robert Wood Johnson Foundation: *The EPEC Project: Elements and models of end-of-life care*, Chicago, 1999, American Medical Association.)

HOSPICE CARE

Hospice care is a subcategory of palliative care. **Hospice** is a concept of EOL care with an emphasis on symptom management, advance care planning, spiritual care, and family support.[9] Hospice clinicians provide compassion, concern, and support for patients in the last phases of a serious illness. The main goal of hospice care is to help the patient live as fully and comfortably as possible while dying with dignity.

Hospice care is an option when a patient has a limited life expectancy—specifically 6 months or less. Hospice is often underused. Many wrongly assume patients must be actively dying. On the contrary, it is important that patients be referred to hospice as early as possible to ease the physical, emotional, and spiritual distress so common at the EOL. Almost half of the Medicare patients who die in the United States are in hospice care. More than 75% of patients in hospice are over the age of 65 years. Most patients have cancer, dementia, stroke, or heart or respiratory conditions.[9]

Discussions about hospice should be started early so that patients can understand the philosophy, services, benefits, and limitations. The decision to begin hospice care is hard for several reasons. Many patients, families, and HCPs lack information about hospice care. Some people may not use hospice because of a lack of awareness of hospice services, a desire to continue with potentially curative treatment, and concerns about lack of minority hospice workers. HCPs may be reluctant to give referrals if they view a patient's functional decline as their personal failure. Some patients or family members see hospice care as "giving up" or receiving second-rate care. Openly discuss this concern and provide reassurance in the quality of hospice care.

In the United States Medicare, Medicaid, and many private insurance agencies cover hospice services. Admission to a hospice program has 2 criteria. The first criterion is that the patient must want the services and agree in writing to use only hospice care, not curative care, to treat the terminal illness. The second criterion is that the patient must be medically eligible for hospice. This means that 2 physicians certify that the patient's prognosis is terminal, with less than 6 months to live. After this initial certification, only 1 physician (e.g., the hospice medical director) is needed to recertify the patient. It is important to realize that the physician who certifies that a hospice patient is terminal does not "guarantee" death within 6 months.

Hospice patients can receive care for other health problems that are not related to the terminal illness. However, the hospice, Medicare, Medicaid, or insurance company may not cover those services. If a patient in hospice survives beyond 6 months, Medicare and other organizations will continue to reimburse if the patient still meets enrollment criteria. Occasionally, a patient's condition stabilizes. A patient may be discharged from hospice care after review of the treatment plan and input from the hospice team. Patients can voluntarily withdraw from hospice at any time.

It is important to consider potential barriers to hospice care for vulnerable populations. These may include veterans, immigrants, and persons who are impoverished, uninsured, disabled, institutionalized, or incarcerated. The hospice team may need to collaborate with community partners to facilitate support services.

DOMAINS OF PALLIATIVE CARE

The National Consensus Project for Quality Palliative Care Guidelines outline 8 key domains for quality palliative care: (1) care structure and processes; (2) physical aspects of care; (3) psychologic and psychiatric aspects; (4) social aspects of care; (5) spiritual, religious, and existential aspects of care; (6) culture care; (7) care of the patient nearing EOL; and (8) ethical and legal aspects (Fig. 10.3).[5]

Care Structure and Processes

Palliative care is coordinated and provided holistically. The IPT works together to support the patient and family across all settings throughout the illness trajectory. Nurses serve as advocates, provide direct care, coordinate additional care, teach, and continually reevaluate patient and family needs. The IPT establishes a plan of care and continually refines it based on the goals of the patient and communication with IPT members.

The initial patient assessment includes a history, assessment, and discussions with the patient and family. Assess their understanding of the serious illness. Discuss advance care planning, including care goals and treatment preferences, and review advance directives. Obtain the patient's medical history, medication record, and laboratory and diagnostic results. Note the specific event or change that brought the patient into the health care setting. Do a brief review of systems. Note any current symptoms. Assess for discomfort, pain, nausea, and dyspnea. Evaluate for comorbidities or acute episodes of problems, such as diabetes or headache. Ask about food and fluid intake, sleep patterns, and responses to the stress of illness. Consider factors related to the social determinants of health, caregiver support, and emotional and spiritual concerns.

Physical Aspects of Care

Symptom management can improve patients' physical well-being and function. We can anticipate and prevent some symptoms with assessment and continued monitoring. Symptom management considers physical, emotional, spiritual, and cultural factors that can contribute to the burden of pain and suffering related to serious illness.

Pay close attention to the onset, quality, and severity of symptoms. Note factors that worsen or relieve the symptom and prior treatments such as medications or interventions. Consider the impact of symptoms on function and quality of life (Box 10.1). Timely reassessment is needed to determine whether treatments are effective, if new symptoms arise, and if the patient and family can manage the plan of care.

Psychologic and Psychiatric Aspects

A diagnosis of serious illness can affect the mental health of a patient and family. Anxiety, depression, delirium, post-traumatic stress disorder, and substance use may be a factor in the progression of the patient's illness. The IPT can support, provide treatment, and coordinate care to manage psychosocial distress.

The nurse's role is to ensure support for the patient and family during their journey with serious illness. A social worker

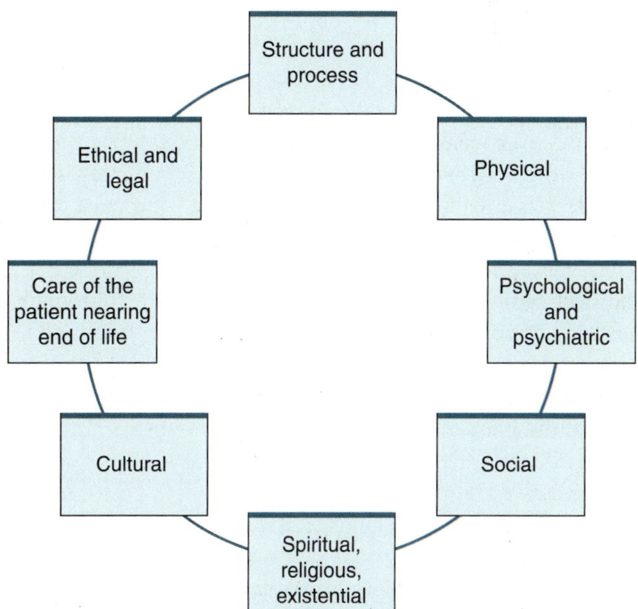

Fig. 10.3 Domains of palliative care. (Created from National Consensus Project for Quality Palliative Care: *Clinical practice guidelines for quality palliative care,* ed 4, Richmond, 2018, National Coalition for Hospice and Palliative Care. Retrieved from https://www.nationalcoalitionhpc.org/ncp.)

BOX 10.1 EVIDENCE-BASED PRACTICE

Nonpharmacologic Pain Management

You are caring for an 82-year-old patient who had an ischemic stroke. The patient is intermittently awake, responds to simple questions, and is paralyzed on the left side. Based on behavior cues, you believe the patient is experiencing pain. She is moaning softly, appears tense, and shifts restlessly in the bed. BP and heart rate are elevated since the previous assessment 4 hours ago. A request for palliative care is made after a team conference with the family.

Making Clinical Decisions

Synthesis of Best Available Evidence

Pain is a common experience for patients receiving palliative care. Proper pain management often includes drug and nonpharmacologic interventions (NPIs). NPIs can be a beneficial addition to the pain management plan. They can reduce the dose of analgesia needed to relieve pain and minimize side effects of drug therapy. NPIs are associated with general relaxation and greater comfort.

Clinician Expertise

Six weeks ago, the unit educator and manager began working with the EBP Committee to start a standard NPI pain protocol for all palliative care patients. The protocol includes a 10-minute back and leg massage in the morning and evening using a recommended lavender lotion. The protocol was implemented 6 days ago. You begin to note that patients are less restless and sleeping for longer periods at night.

Patient Preferences and Values

The patient's daughter comments to you, "My mother seems much calmer and more comfortable. I was really concerned to see her so restless and unsettled." She asks how she can continue this care after discharge.

Implications for Nursing Practice

1. How often would pain be assessed in patients using NPI?
2. How would you involve patients and family members in using NPI for pain management?

Reference for Evidence

van Veen S, Drenth H, Hobbelen H, et al: Non-pharmacological interventions feasible in the nursing scope of practice for pain relief in palliative care patients: A systematic review. *Palliat Care Soc Pract* 18, 2024.

can help manage psychologic symptoms. Refer to counseling if needed. Discuss any sign of suicidal ideation or a serious and/or persistent mental illness immediately with the IPT. Treatment of psychologic or mental health issues can include behavior, therapeutic, and pharmacologic interventions. Cultural or complementary therapies may be used.

Social Aspects of Care

Social aspects include environment and social factors that affect the quality of life. Issues we address include access to medication and treatment, transportation to appointments, and financial constraints. Assess social factors that surround

TABLE 10.2 Spiritual Assessment

Obtain basic spiritual-related information. Include:
• Religious preference
• If the patient is part of a spiritual or religious community
• If religion is significant to them
• Whether the patient would like a chaplain or other person involved
• Whom the patient turns to when they need help
• Use of spiritual-related coping strategies
• Any religious or spiritual practices the patient wants to take part in
• Presence of any concerns or conflicts between spiritual or religious beliefs and health care
• Sources of hope, strength, comfort, and peace

persons who are uninsured, underinsured, homeless, or undocumented.

Assess the patient and family's social support and care environment. Do they have access to reliable food, housing, and transportation? This assessment should reflect their culture, values, goals, and preferences. These may change over time, so continued reassessment is important. Identify specific roles and contributions of caregivers, along with resources and community services.

Spiritual, Religious, and Existential Aspects of Care

Spiritual care is fundamental to addressing the suffering associated with serious illness.[10] **Spirituality** is a broad concept that encompasses beliefs, values, and purpose related to the search for existential meaning and purpose. Some define spirituality as a relationship with a supreme being that directs beliefs and practices. Spiritual needs do not necessarily equate to religious beliefs in a higher power. A patient may not practice a specific religion but have a deep spirituality. The IPT should care for patients and families in a manner that respects their spiritual beliefs and practices. We should respect when patients and families decline to discuss their beliefs or accept spiritual support.

Assess spiritual needs (Table 10.2). What are the preferences related to spiritual guidance or pastoral care services? Spiritual distress is a state of suffering related to meaning of connectedness to self, others, or a higher power. Patients may question their beliefs about their journey through life, religion, and an afterlife (Fig. 10.4). *Existential distress* may occur as the person reexamines their lives and questions their prior understandings of meaning.[10] Make needed referrals. Professional chaplains are trained to address spiritual issues.

Cultural Care

Cultural beliefs affect a patient's values and traditions related to health, illness, family caregiving roles, and decision making. Acknowledge and respect a patient and family's culture and provide care that is sensitive to these needs.

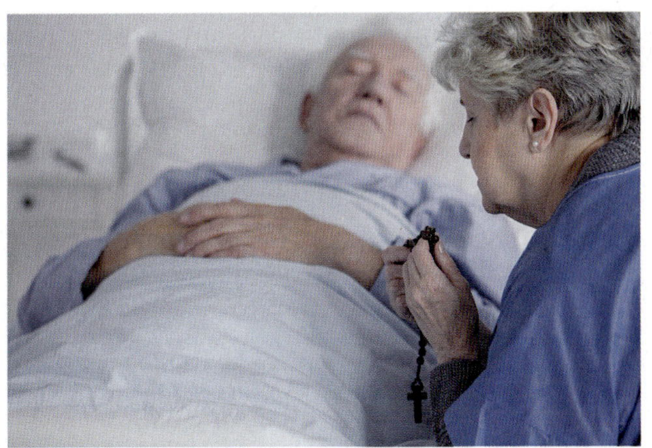

Fig. 10.4 Spiritual needs are an important consideration in end-of-life care. (© KatarzynaBialasiewicz/iStock.com.)

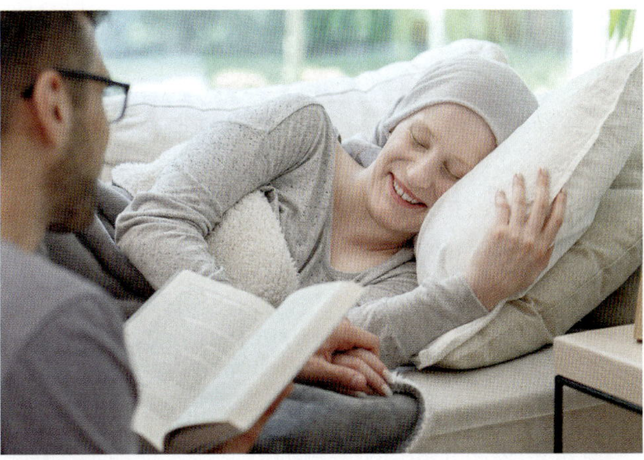

Fig. 10.5 Inpatient hospice settings are designed to make the atmosphere as relaxed and homelike as possible. (© KatarzynaBialasiewicz/iStock.com.)

Cultural variations exist in symptom expression (e.g., pain expression), communication, and use of health care services. Consider a patient's language, cognitive capacity, disabilities, and developmental stage. Assess nonverbal cues, such as grimaces, body position, and decreased or guarded movements. Communicate with attention to verbal, nonverbal, and symbolic details. Use medical interpreter services when communicating with those who do not understand English and sign language interpreters for patients who are hearing impaired.

Care of the Patient Nearing the End of Life

End of life is the period during which patients cope with declining health from a terminal illness or from the frailties associated with advanced age, even if death is not clearly imminent.[11] In some cases it is obvious to HCPs that the patient is at the EOL. In other cases, they may be uncertain if the EOL is near. This uncertainty adds to the challenge of answering the common question asked by the patient and family, "How much time is left?"

End-of-life care (EOL care) is the term used for issues and services related to death and dying. The goals for EOL care are to (1) provide comfort and supportive care during the dying process, (2) improve the quality of the patient's remaining life, (3) help ensure a dignified death, and (4) provide emotional support to the family. Some patients are at home. Hospice services are available 24 hours a day, 7 days a week to help patients and families with home care. Inpatient hospice settings often have a relaxed and homelike atmosphere (Fig. 10.5).

Ethical and Legal Aspects of Care

Patients and families struggle with many decisions associated with a serious illness or EOL experience. Palliative care focuses on honoring patient preferences. Decisions may involve the choice for (1) advance directives (e.g., living wills), (2) specific treatments (e.g., chemotherapy, surgery), (3) cardiopulmonary resuscitation (CPR), (4) organ and tissue donations, and (5) feeding tube placement. Provide information to help patients with these decisions.

Advance Care Planning and Advance Directives

Advance care planning is a process of having patients (1) think through their values and goals for treatment, (2) talk about their values and goals with others, and (3) document their preferences. **Advance directives** are the written documents that provide information about the patient's wishes and designated spokesperson (Table 10.3). Under the 1990 Patient Self-Determination Act (PSDA), patients must receive information on advance directives from health care agencies.

Each state has specific advance directive forms. A *living will* details a person's wishes to avoid, limit, or withhold interventions. These forms are often combined with a *durable power of attorney for health care* (DPAHC), *medical power of attorney* (MPOA), and *power of attorney for health care* (POAH) or *health care proxy.* If the patient is unable to communicate or is incapacitated, the DPAHC allows the agent to make all health care decisions. Patients may change their minds about desired treatments as their disease state progresses, so it is important to reassess the advance directives. For cognitively impaired older adults who lack decision-making capacity, consider the patient's values, collaborate with the IPT, and engage the surrogates in medical decisions.

In addition to state-specific advance directive forms, documents such as the Five Wishes help people discuss their care preferences with their loved ones and HCP.[12] Verbal directives can be given to the attending physician in the presence of 2 witnesses. To improve communication of advance directives, the Physician Order for Life-Sustaining Treatment (POLST) or Medical Order for Life-Sustaining Treatment (MOLST) outlines the patient's desire for treatment (Table 10.3).

The patient should keep a copy of all advance directives and let family know where the copy is kept. In the absence of advance directives and if the patient is not capable of communicating, the surrogate decision maker (most often

TABLE 10.3 Common Advance Care Planning Legal Documents

Term	Description	Special Considerations
Advance directive	Written documents that state information about the patient's future health care decisions or choices. Guide for families, caregivers, health care team on the patients' goals and wishes for care.	• Document has various forms • Should adhere to guidelines in the state of residence
Allow natural death (AND)	Acknowledges the patient's wish to avoid aggressive measures. May be associated with care focusing on dignity and comfort.	• Preferred term for a do-not-resuscitate order • May be called do not attempt resuscitation (DNAR)
Combined directives	Includes more than 1 form. Contains directives about health care, values/goals, and/or appointed health care proxy. Example includes the "Five Wishes" advance directive.	• Not a legal document in all states • May be used to start discussion about advance directives between patient, family, and health care team
Do not resuscitate (DNR)	Written order reflecting a patient's wish to avoid or not attempt CPR.	• Signed by a physician or nurse practitioner (varies by state) • Record that discussion was held
Durable power of attorney for health care (DPAHC)	Defines who will serve as the surrogate decision maker when the patient loses decision-making capacity.	• Also called medical power of attorney, health care proxy, appointment of a health care agent or surrogate • Does not include financial decisions
Living will	Lay term for a written legal document that describes the patient's preferences about future health care decisions or choices.	• Must identify specific treatments that a person wants or does not want at EOL
Physician/practitioner order for life-sustaining treatment (POLST)	Legal form completed by the patient and HCP listing treatments wanted, not wanted, or limited. Guides current treatment and acts as medical orders across health care settings.	• State-specific form • May be signed by a physician and/or nurse practitioner (varies by state) and patient or patient surrogate • Also called medical order for life-sustaining treatment (MOLST)

family or significant other) will be asked to make decisions. Surrogates rely on information from the IPT to make crucial decisions. Record discussions and decisions in the medical record to keep the IPT informed and assure appropriate care.

CPR is an important topic of discussion. HCPs sometimes avoid discussing CPR, which can lead to inappropriate or unwanted use of resuscitation methods. Patients and families may have unrealistic expectations about survival potential after CPR. The patient with no preferred limits on life support has a *full code* status. This choice allows for resuscitation attempts with chest compressions, defibrillation, intubation, vasopressors, and other life-sustaining interventions.

After considering health problems, prognosis, and personal values, some patients may request a **do-not-resuscitate (DNR) order**. A DNR order is a written medical order that documents a patient's wishes about resuscitation and the patient's desire to avoid CPR.[13] Use language cautiously. Terms such as *do not attempt resuscitation (DNAR)* or *allow natural death (AND)* may more accurately reflect the meaning of this intervention.

Some hospitals may define a DNR order as only cardiac resuscitation attempts and use a *do not intubate (DNI)* order for patients who decline intubation or mechanical ventilation efforts. A *chemical code* may involve the use of drugs for resuscitation, such as vasopressors, without the use of CPR. Some health care settings may have a *comfort measures only* (CMO) order, or an EOL order set that assists with selecting only interventions that will provide comfort and limit invasive measures. Some states have implemented a form called *out-of-hospital DNR* for use by terminally ill patients who wish to have no heroic measures used to prolong life after they leave an acute care agency.

Do not hospitalize (DNH) is a status used by skilled nursing agencies if a patient does not want to go to the hospital for treatment. These terms never mean that care is withheld; rather, care is focused to relieve suffering and promote dignity at the EOL.

An advance directive may include withholding or withdrawing treatments such as a ventilator, artificial hydration, and nutrition. The ANA states that the decision to withhold artificial nutrition and hydration should be made by the patient or surrogate together with the IPT. The nurse continues to provide expert care for patients who are withdrawing treatments.

Organ and Tissue Donation

Patients may choose organ donation of a body part or the entire body. Advance directives and organ donor information should be in the medical record and identified on the patient's care plan. The decision to donate organs may be made by immediate family after the patient's death. Next-of-kin permission must be obtained at the time of donation.[14] Organ and tissue donations follow specific legal guidelines and agency policies. Prompt notification to the right personnel when organ donation is intended is important because some tissues must be used within hours after death.

Euthanasia and Physician-Assisted Suicide

Euthanasia is the deliberate act of hastening death. It is not legal in the United States. The ANA statement on requests for medical aid in dying clearly states euthanasia is inconsistent with the core commitments of the nursing profession. Nurses are ethically prohibited from giving aid-in-dying medication.[15] *Physician-assisted suicide,* or *aid-in-dying laws,* are offered in some states. In this case the physician provides the means and/or information for a terminally ill patient to self-administer medication to hasten death.

Nurses have the obligation to support patients at the EOL by understanding these laws and providing prompt, humane, and comprehensive EOL care. *Palliative sedation* refers to giving medications to intentionally produce sedation to relieve distressing symptoms in a patient who is imminently dying. The intent of palliative sedation is to relieve unmanageable pain and suffering. It is not to shorten life or to hasten death.

The use of opioids for symptom management at the EOL is often misunderstood and feared by patients, families, and HCPs. Many patients refuse opioids for pain, which leads to physical and emotional suffering. However, opioids for pain management and shortness of breath are the gold standard in EOL care. Relieving patient suffering includes giving medications such as opioids that have the potential to produce harm (Box 10.2). Teach the patient and family about addiction, tolerance, and dependence. Opioids should not be withheld at the EOL, even for those with a history of addiction. Pain management is discussed in Chapter 9.

DEATH

Death occurs when all vital organs and body systems cease to function. It is the irreversible cessation of cardiovascular, respiratory, and brain function. In some states and under specific circumstances, a registered nurse is legally allowed to pronounce death. Policies and procedures vary by state and among health care agencies.

Brain death is an irreversible loss of all brain functions. Brain death is a clinical diagnosis. It occurs when the cerebral cortex stops functioning or is irreversibly destroyed. The diagnostic criteria for clinical diagnosis of brain death include coma or unresponsiveness, absence of brainstem reflexes, and apnea.[16] Physicians perform specific assessments to confirm each criterion. Current legal and medical standards require that all brain function cease to be able to pronounce brain death. Diagnosing brain death is of special importance when organ donation is an option.

BOX 10.2 ETHICAL/LEGAL DILEMMAS

Pain Management at End of Life

Situation

A.P. is a terminally ill 50-year-old female with metastatic breast cancer who is hospitalized with severe bone pain. She has had multiple complications including respiratory failure, infections, and difficult-to-manage pain. Goals-of-care discussions led to decisions to focus exclusively on comfort measures. She continues to moan at rest and shows signs of severe pain with any movement. The team recently increased the doses of pain medications. She is intermittently awake, and her family is at the bedside. Some of the nurses do not feel comfortable giving the high doses of opioid for fear they will hasten death.

Ethical/Legal Points for Consideration

- Adequate pain relief at end of life (EOL) is fundamental to the quality of life of the patient and experience of family caregivers.
- The *Code of Ethics for Nurses* and position statement from the American Nurses Association (ANA) address the ethical responsibility of the nurse to relieve pain and the suffering it causes, along with counseling patients and families about pain and symptom management.[1,2]
- The goal of adequate pain control in seriously ill or terminally ill patients is based on the *principle of nonmaleficence to ease suffering* (preventing or reducing harm to the patient). Access to adequate pain and symptom management at EOL follows the *principle of beneficence,* which includes promoting good. Because the intent of this action is to ease suffering, not hasten death, it is ethically justified by the principle of *double effect.* Though administering opioids and sedatives at the EOL may cause sedation, it is justified to relieve suffering.
- Nurses are responsible for providing comprehensive and compassionate EOL care. Legally, the *standard of care* is used to define the nursing acts required for safe and competent nursing practice. Nursing care that is below the standard is considered negligent and unsafe.
- In A.P.'s situation the standard of care includes access to opioids for relief of pain at the EOL. Failure of the nurse to act assertively to achieve pain relief for the patient and failure to effectively use resources to obtain that pain relief will be considered below the standard of care and unsafe and incompetent practice. Nurses should seek counsel from mentors and the interprofessional team (IPT) to gain comfort with providing this care.

Discussion Questions

1. What types of discussions should occur among the IPT, patient, and family as this patient approaches EOL?
2. How can nurses reduce moral distress when managing pain at the EOL?
3. What training is needed for nurses to safely give opioids at the EOL?

References

1. American Nurses Association: *The code of ethics for nurses with interpretive statements.* Retrieved from https://codeofethics.ana.org/provision-1-3.
2. American Nurses Association: *Position statement: The ethical responsibility to manage pain and the suffering it causes.* Retrieved from https://www.nursingworld.org/practice-policy/nursing-excellence/official-position-statements/id/the-ethical-responsibility-to-manage-pain-and-the-suffering-it-causes/.

Physical Manifestations at End of Life

As death approaches, the body gradually slows down until all functions end. Respiratory changes are common. Respirations may be rapid or slow, shallow, and irregular. Breath sounds may become wet and noisy, both audibly and on auscultation. Mouth breathing and mucus accumulation in the airways cause noisy, wet-sounding respirations. We call these *terminal secretions*, or *the death rattle.* Cheyne-Stokes respiration is a pattern of breathing with alternating periods of apnea and deep, rapid breathing. When respirations cease, the heart stops beating within a few minutes. The physical manifestations of approaching death are listed in Table 10.4.

Psychosocial Manifestations at End of Life

A variety of feelings and emotions can affect the patient and family at the EOL (Table 10.5). The patient and family may feel overwhelmed, fearful, powerless, and fatigued. They may also feel at peace with death and feel gratitude for a "life well lived." The family's response depends in part on the type and length of the illness and their relationship with the patient.

Respect the patient's needs and wishes. Patients need time to express their feelings. Response time to questions may be sluggish from fatigue, weakness, and confusion.

TABLE 10.4 Physical Manifestations at End of Life

System	Manifestations
Cardiovascular	• ↑ Heart rate; later slowing and weakening of pulse • Irregular rhythm • ↓ BP • Delayed absorption of drugs given IM or subcutaneous
Gastrointestinal	• Hypoactive bowel sounds, constipation, abdominal distention • Anorexia, no oral intake • Loss of sphincter control with incontinence • Bowel movement before imminent death or at time of death
Musculoskeletal	• Gradual immobility • Sagging of jaw resulting from loss of facial muscle tone • Difficulty speaking • Swallowing becoming more difficult • Difficulty maintaining body posture and alignment • Loss of gag reflex • Jerking seen in patients on high doses of opioids
Nervous	• ↑ Confusion or delirium, hallucinations, impaired cognition • Temperature swings: hypothermia and fever • Possible seizures, nonreactive pupils
Respiratory	• ↑ Respiratory rate • Irregular breathing, Cheyne-Stokes respiration, periods of apnea, episodic deep, rapid breaths • Inability to cough or clear secretions resulting in grunting, gurgling, or noisy congested breathing (death rattle or terminal secretions)
Sensory	• Hearing is usually last to disappear • ↓ Taste and smell • ↓ Sensation • ↓ Response to tactile stimuli • Blurred vision • Sinking and glazing of eyes • Blink reflex absent • Inability to close eyelids
Skin	• Mottling on hands, feet, coccyx, arms, and legs • Skin breakdown, especially in pressure areas • Peripheral cyanosis of nose, nail beds, knees • Cold, clammy skin or "waxlike" skin when death is imminent
Urinary system	• Gradual decrease in urine output • Incontinence • Inability to urinate

Bereavement and Grief

Bereavement is the period after the death of a loved one during which we experience grief and mourning occurs. The time spent in bereavement depends on several factors. These include how attached one was to the person who died and how much time one spent expecting the loss.

Grief is a normal reaction in response to the real loss of a loved one and the loss of what might have been. Psychologic responses include anger, guilt, anxiety, sadness, depression, and despair. Physiologic reactions include sleeping problems, changes in appetite, physical problems, and illness.

Grief is a complex and intense emotional experience. Many describe grief in phases (Table 10.6).[17] Common feelings are associated with each phase. There is no typical way to move through grief. Some people do not experience all the phases, and the phases are not always progressive. It is common to be in a phase and then go backward. For example, a person may be in the bargaining phase and then revert to anger.

TABLE 10.5 Psychosocial Concerns at End of Life

Dimension	Manifestations
Social	• Ability to say goodbye or give/receive forgiveness • Ability to express love to significant persons • May seek to strengthen bonds with family and friends, ensure their legacy, or find meaning in their relationships. • May feel isolated from their loved ones, especially if family and friends are struggling to cope with their emotions or if they feel uncomfortable with death • Worry about burdening others
Distress	• Grief over their impending loss and the loss of relationships and future possibilities • Anger from the unfairness of the situation or from feelings of powerlessness
Uncertainty	• Fear of the unknown, the pain of death, or the burden on loved ones can be overwhelming • Uncertainty about what comes after death can contribute to anxiety • Acceptance of mortality, engagement in planning for one's death, experiencing peacefulness
Reflection	• Legacy work and life review • Regret about missed opportunities or unresolved issues • Enhanced meaning of life, ability to talk about death • Questions about the nature of existence and the prospect of death can lead to feelings of despair, confusion, and a search for meaning

TABLE 10.6 Phases of Grief

Phase	What Person May Say	Characteristics
Shock	I can't believe this. This isn't happening.	React to the learning of a loss with numbness. Shock may provide an emotional buffer and protect the person from being overwhelmed.
Denial	I'm doing fine. The results are wrong.	Denies the loss has taken place. Feelings of defensiveness may be present. May act withdrawn. Temporary response may last minutes to months.
Anger	Why me? This is not fair. Why could this happen? Who is to blame?	Emotional response as the realization of severity of illness increases. Feelings of anger may be directed at inanimate objects, friends, family, or health care team. May be angry at the person who inflicted the hurt (even after death) or at the world for letting it happen. May be angry with self for letting an event (e.g., car accident) take place, even if nothing could have stopped it. Loved ones may be angry at the dying or deceased patient.
Bargaining	If I could trade their life for mine.... I promise to quit smoking. If only I had seen the oncologist sooner....	Normal reaction to feeling helpless and vulnerable. Statements made out of sense to regain control. Attempts to rationalize current state. Associated with feelings of guilt. May make bargains with God.
Depression	I'm dying, so what's the point? I'm so sad, so why bother with anything?	Feelings of sadness, despair, and regret as one recognizes mortality. Patients and families may be quiet, seek isolation, or appear mournful.
Acceptance	I'm okay with it all. It's going to be okay.	Embracing of mortality and inevitable death. Able to engage in life review and feel at peace with one's death or death of a loved one.

Adapted from Oates JR, Maan-Fogelman PA: *Nursing grief and loss*. Retrieved from https://www.ncbi.nlm.nih.gov/books/NBK518989/.

Another model of grief is seen in the grief wheel (Fig. 10.6). After a loss, the person feels *shock* (numbness, denial, inability to think straight). Next is the *protest* stage, in which a person may have anger, guilt, sadness, fear, and searching. Then comes the *disorganization* stage, with despair, apathy, anxiety, and confusion. In the *reorganization* stage, a person gradually returns to normal functioning but feels different. The last stage is the *new normal*. Eventually the destabilization experienced in grief resolves and the challenge is to accept the new normal. Trying to go back to the "old" normal (which is not there anymore) causes a great deal of anxiety and stress.

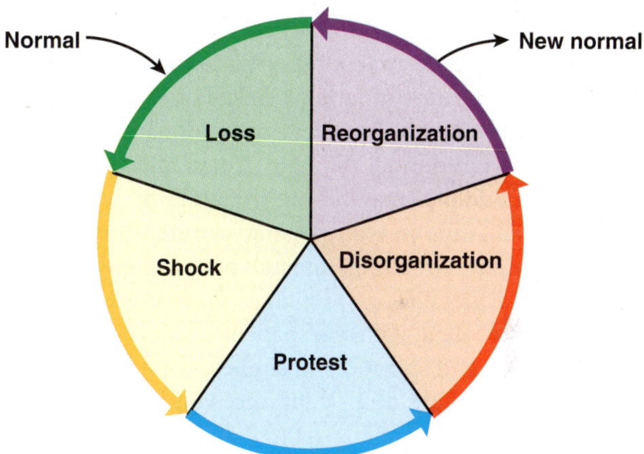

Fig. 10.6 The grief wheel model begins with the normal state at the bottom. After a person goes through the grief process, eventually the grief will resolve. Because of the loss, the normal state is different from before. The challenge is to accept the "new normal."

The way a person grieves depends on factors such as the relationship with the person who has died (e.g., spouse, parent), physical and emotional coping resources, other life stresses, cultural beliefs, and personality. Other factors that affect the grief response include mental and physical health, economic resources, religious or spiritual beliefs, family relationships, social support, and time spent preparing for the death. Conflict may affect the grief response.[18]

The grief experience for the caregiver or family of the patient with a severe illness often begins long before the actual death. We call this **anticipatory grief.** Patients at the EOL can have anticipatory grief.

Working in a positive way through the grief process helps to adapt to the loss. Grief that helps the person accept the reality of death is a healthy response called *adaptive grief.* It may be grieving before death occurs or when the death is expected. Signs of adaptive grief include the ability to see some good resulting from the death and positive memories of the deceased person.

Dysfunctional reactions to loss can occur. The physical and psychologic impact of the loved one's death may persist for years. *Prolonged grief disorder,* formerly called *complicated grief,* is a term for lengthy and intense mourning. Prolonged grief disorder can include recurrent and severe distressing emotions and intrusive thoughts related to the loss of a loved one, self-neglect, and denial of the loss for longer than 6 months. About 1 in 5 bereaved people have grief disorder. They have a higher risk for illness and may have impaired work and social role function.

Bereavement and grief counseling are core parts of palliative care. The goal of a bereavement program is to provide support and to help survivors transition to a life without the deceased person. Include grief support into the plan of care for the family and significant others during the patient's illness and after the death.

Priority interventions for grief focus on providing an environment that allows the patient and family to express their feelings, such as anger, fear, and guilt. Discussing feelings helps them work toward resolution of the grief process. Respect the patient's privacy and need to talk or remain silent. Be honest in answering questions and giving information.

Spirituality and religion offer meaning to many and are associated with decreased despair in patients at EOL.[19] Some dying patients are secure in their faith about the future. Religion may offer a sense of peace and recognition in the broader cosmic context.[19] It is common for patients to give away material possessions and focus on values that they believe will lead them on to another place.

Culturally Competent Care: End of Life

Culture and ethnicity are important considerations for patients receiving palliative and EOL care and their families. Cultural beliefs affect a person's understanding of and reaction to death or loss. They affect decision making about life support, withholding and withdrawing treatments, and using palliative or hospice care.[20] Perform a cultural assessment and tailor care to the patient and family.

Rituals associated with dying are part of all cultures. Many differences exist among cultural beliefs and values in relation to death and dying. Being aware of specific cultural traditions may help anticipate patient and family needs. For example, some in the Jewish faith may not engage in organ donation. They may keep constant vigil during EOL and 7 days after burial. Some Hindus and Buddhists may believe in karma or reincarnation and prefer cremation. In many Islamic cultures, the traditional rites of washing, shrouding, funeral prayers, and burial are done as soon as possible.

Plan care to align with the patient's language, diet, and cultural beliefs and practices. Families with non–English-speaking members are at risk for receiving less information about their family member's critical illness and prognosis.[20] Access medical interpreter services, if needed, so that the patient's wishes are known. Culturally competent care is discussed in Chapter 2.

NURSING MANAGEMENT: END OF LIFE

Nurses spend more time with patients near the EOL than any other health care professionals. Respect, dignity, and comfort are important for the patient and family. The treatment plan still consists of assessment, planning, implementation, and evaluation. The main difference is that the focus of care is on symptom management.

Assessment

Be sensitive and do not perform repeated, unnecessary assessments. When possible, use health history data available in the medical record rather than tiring the patient with an interview. Assess functional status, intake, patterns of sleep and rest, and response to the stress of terminal illness. Review their ability to cope with the diagnosis and prognosis. Assess the family's ability to manage the needed care and to cope with the illness and its consequences.

The physical assessment focuses on changes that accompany terminal illness and the specific disease process (Table 10.4). The frequency depends on the patient's stability. Assessment is done at least every 8 hours in the agency setting. For patients cared for in their homes by hospice programs, assessment may occur weekly. Pay attention to patients who are nonverbal for subtle changes in their condition. As changes occur, you may assess and document more often.

Key elements of a social assessment include the relationships and patterns of communication among the family. Listen to concerns. Evaluate the goals of the patient and family. Differences in expectations and interpersonal conflict can cause disruptions during the dying process and after the death of the loved one.

Monitor the patient for multiple systems failing with attention to subtle physical changes. Neurologic assessment is especially important and includes level of consciousness, reflexes, and pupil responses. Vital signs, skin color, and temperature show changes in circulation. Monitor respiratory status, character and pattern of respirations, and breath sounds. Assess nutrition and fluid intake, urine output, and bowel function to obtain data about renal and gastrointestinal functioning. Assess the skin on an ongoing basis because fragile skin may easily break down.

In the last hours of life, limit assessments to those that determine patient comfort. Assessment of pain and respiratory status may be the most important during this time. It may be more peaceful and comforting to the patient and family if you refrain from measuring BP or checking for pupil response. As death approaches, provide emotional and psychosocial support to the patient and family. Limit tasks that will not affect the comfort or outcome for the patient.

Clinical Problems

Clinical problems for patients who are dying and their families include grief and the dying process.

Planning

The overall goals are that the patient who is dying will (1) make decisions about EOL care and (2) experience a peaceful death. Involve the patient and family in planning and coordinating EOL care. Develop a comprehensive plan to support, teach, and evaluate patients and families. Care goals during the last stages of life involve comfort and safety measures and care of patients' emotional and physical needs. These may include determining where patients would like to die and whether this is possible. For example, a patient may want to die at home, but the family may object or be unable to manage the physical care.

◆Implementation

Advocate for the patient's wishes to be met where possible. Patients and families need ongoing information on the disease, the dying process, the care you will be providing, and how to cope. Denial and grieving may be barriers for both the patient and family.

Psychosocial Care

As death approaches, respond appropriately to the patient's psychosocial manifestations at the EOL (Table 10.7). Patients and family members may have difficulties expressing themselves. Allow time for them to express their feelings and thoughts. Empathy and active listening are essential. Listen and interact in a sensitive way to enhance the relationship among you, the patient, and the family. Often silence is related to the overwhelming feelings experienced at the EOL. Silence can also allow time to gather thoughts. Listening to the silence sends a message of acceptance and comfort.

Most terminally ill and dying people do not want to be alone. Many dying patients are afraid that loved ones will not be able to cope with their imminent death and will abandon them. Simply being present offers support and comfort (Fig. 10.7). Holding hands, touching, and listening are important nursing interventions. Providing companionship allows the patient a sense of security.

Prepare family members for changes in the patient's emotional and cognitive function as death nears. The patient's speech may become confused, disoriented, or garbled. Patients may speak to or about family members or others who have predeceased them or give instructions to those who will survive them.

Anxiety and depression. Patients often show signs of anxiety and depression during the EOL period. Causes of anxiety and depression may include uncontrolled pain and dyspnea, psychosocial factors related to the disease process or impending death, altered physiologic states, and drugs used in high dosages. Anxiety is often related to fear. Encouragement, support, and teaching may help. Management may include both medications and nonpharmacologic interventions. Relaxation strategies, such as relaxation breathing, muscle relaxation, music, and imagery, may be useful (see Chapter 7).

Anger. Anger is a common and normal response to grief. A grieving person cannot be forced to accept the loss. The surviving family members may be angry with the dying loved one who is leaving them. Encourage the expression of feelings, but it is hard to come to terms with loss. As a nurse, you may be the target of the anger. Understand the anger response and avoid reacting on a personal level.

Hopelessness and powerlessness. Hopelessness and powerlessness are common during the EOL period. Encourage realistic hope within the limits of the situation. Support the patient's involvement in decision making about care to foster a sense of control and autonomy. Allow the patient and family to deal with what is within their control. Help them recognize what is beyond their control.

TABLE 10.7 NURSING MANAGEMENT

Psychosocial Care at End of Life

Dimensions	Nursing Management
Preparing for Death	
Serious illness can create strain on relationships. Facilitate meaningful discussions for the patient and family to prepare for death. They may reconcile the past to find meaning in the present.	Encourage the patient and family to share their feelings of love, sadness, loss, forgiveness. Saying goodbye can be therapeutic. Encourage physical touch (e.g., hand holding, hugging) and expressions such as crying. Allow the patient and family privacy to express their feelings and comfort one another.
Spiritual Needs	
Religion, faith, and spirituality may be sources of strength for patients and families. Patients and family members may experience spiritual longing.	Assess spiritual needs, cultural norms, hopes, values, and fears. Address the needs of the family and caregivers. Allow patient to express concerns about quality of life, fear of death or dying, spiritual practices, and significant relationships. Recognize the presence of spiritual or existential distress. Promote visits by spiritual care service provider, chaplain, family member.
Unusual Communication	
May indicate altered coping that may prevent the patient from resolving issues and letting go. Comorbid psychiatric conditions may worsen. Patients may become restless and agitated, which may be a manifestation of terminal delirium.	Assess for depression, anxiety, and/or delirium. Encourage the family to talk with and reassure the patient. Coordinate referrals for counseling.
End-of-Life Dreams and Visions	
Patients talk to persons who are not there or see places and objects not visible. They may report dreams of living or deceased loved ones. These experiences may comfort the patient in coming to terms with meaning in life and transitioning from it.	Assess for the presence, distress, or comfort from these visions. Affirm the patient's experience as a part of transition from this life. Teach families and caregivers about the patient's experiences.
Withdrawal	
May be an emotional response or part of grieving. Patients near death may seem withdrawn from the physical environment, maintaining the ability to hear but unable to respond.	Allow the patient to sleep and rest. Converse as though the patient were alert, using a soft voice and gentle touch. Encourage meaningful tasks and discussions during periods of wakefulness.

Fear. Fear is a typical feeling associated with dying. Specific fears include fear of pain, shortness of breath, loneliness, abandonment, and meaninglessness. Fear of meaninglessness leads people to review their lives. Assist patients with *life review* to help them recognize the value of their lives. Practical

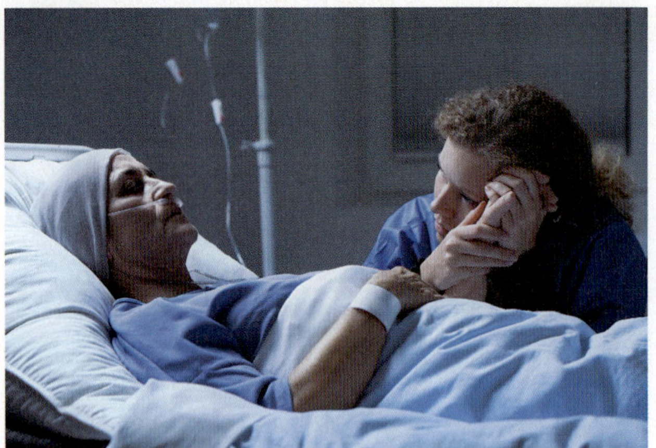

Fig. 10.7 Dying patients often want someone who they know and trust to stay with them. (© KatarzynaBialasiewicz/iStock.com.)

ways of helping may include looking at photo albums or collections of important mementos while sharing thoughts and feelings.

Many people assume that pain accompanies death. There is no evidence that death is always painful. Most patients want their pain relieved without the side effects of grogginess or sleepiness. Pain relief measures do not have to deprive the patient of the ability to interact with others. Assure the patient and family that drugs will be given promptly when needed and that any side effects will be managed. As many EOL patients are unable to swallow, other routes, such as patches, sublingual, and rectal routes, may be used. Consider alternative methods like massage, music, aromatherapy, and mindfulness.

Physical Care

Physical care at the EOL focuses on symptom management and comfort (Table 10.8). The priority is meeting the patient's physiologic and safety needs. Physical care focuses on the needs for oxygen, nutrition, pain relief, mobility, elimination, and skin care. People who are dying deserve and require the same physical care as people who are expected to recover. Discuss the goals of care with the patient and family before treatment begins.

Respiratory distress and dyspnea are common near the EOL. The sensation of air hunger results in anxiety for the patient and family. Current treatments include opioids, bronchodilators, and oxygen, depending on the cause of the dyspnea. Anxiety-reducing agents (e.g., anxiolytics) may help the patient relax.

Postmortem care. After a patient is pronounced dead, you will need to prepare or delegate preparing the patient's body for immediate viewing by the family. Consider cultural customs and follow your agency policy for postmortem care (Table 10.9). In some cultures, such as Hinduism and Judaism, it may be important to allow the family to prepare or help in caring for the patient's body.[21] When the death is unexpected, preparing the patient's body for viewing or release to a funeral home depends on state law and agency policy.

Care of and discussion related to the patient should continue to be respectful even after death. Allow the family privacy and as much time as they need with the deceased patient. Never refer to the deceased patient as "the body."

SPECIAL NEEDS OF CAREGIVERS AND NURSES

Family Caregivers

Family caregivers are important in meeting the patient's physical and psychosocial needs. Their role includes working and communicating with the patient and other family members, supporting the patient's concerns, and helping the patient resolve any unfinished business. Families often face emotional, physical, and economic consequences from caring for a family member who is dying. The caregiver's responsibilities do not end when the patient is admitted to an acute care, inpatient hospice, or long-term care agency.[22]

Being present during a family member's dying process can be highly stressful. Recognize signs and behaviors of abnormal grief reactions among family members. Warning signs may include dependency and negative feelings about the dying patient, inability to express feelings, sleep problems, a history of depression, difficult reactions to previous losses, perceived lack of social or family support, low self-esteem, multiple previous bereavements, or alcohol or substance use. Caregivers with concurrent life crises (e.g., divorce) are especially at risk.

Encourage caregivers to continue their usual activities where possible to maintain some control over their lives. Inform them about resources for support, including respite care, community counseling, and local support in working through grief. Encourage caregivers to build a support system of extended family, friends, faith community, and clergy to call on to express any feelings they are experiencing.

Special Needs of Nurses

Nurses who care for the dying need to recognize their own needs when dealing with grief and dying. Caring for patients and their families at the EOL is challenging and rewarding but also intense and emotionally charged. A bond or connection may develop between you and the patient or family. When you provide care for terminally ill or dying patients, you are not immune to feelings of loss. Be aware of how grief personally affects you. It is common to feel helpless and powerless when dealing with death. Be aware of what you can and cannot control. Express feelings of sorrow, guilt, and frustration. Recognize your own values, attitudes, and feelings about death. Realizing that it is okay to cry with the patient or family during the EOL may be important for your well-being.

To meet your personal needs, focus on interventions to decrease your stress. Get involved in hobbies or other interests, schedule time for yourself, ensure time for sleep, maintain a peer support system, and develop a support system beyond the workplace. Many hospice agencies offer support groups and discussion sessions that can help you cope.

TABLE 10.8 NURSING MANAGEMENT

Physical Care at End of Life

Manifestation	Nursing Management
Anorexia, Dehydration, Nausea, and Vomiting • May be caused by complications of disease process • Hunger and thirst significantly decrease in the last days of life • Dehydration is common • Medications contribute to nausea • Constipation, impaction, and bowel obstruction can cause anorexia, nausea, vomiting	• Assess the patient for nausea or vomiting and possible contributing causes • Provide antiemetics as needed and before meals if ordered • Offer and provide frequent meals with small portions of favorite foods; offer culturally appropriate foods • Do not force the patient to eat or drink • Provide frequent mouth care • Encourage consumption of ice chips and sips of fluids or use moist cloths to moisten the mouth • Use moist cloths and swabs for unconscious patients to avoid aspiration • Apply lubricant to the lips and oral mucous membranes as needed • Ensure uninterrupted mealtimes • Teach family that hunger and thirst naturally decrease at end of life
Bowel Patterns • Immobility, opioid use, depression, lack of diet fiber, dehydration, obstructive cancer can cause constipation • Diarrhea may occur from laxative use, obstruction, fecal impaction, infection, medications, chemotherapy	• Assess bowel function and associated symptoms • Assess for and remove fecal impactions • Encourage movement and physical activities as tolerated • Encourage diet fiber if appropriate; discuss the role of IV fluids in context of goals of care • Use suppositories, stool softeners, laxatives, and/or enemas as ordered, especially if on opioids • Assess for confusion, agitation, restlessness, and pain, which may be signs of constipation • Encourage the intake of simple carbohydrates, if appropriate, and use of antidiarrheals as needed
Oral Conditions • Candidiasis may be present with chemotherapy, immunosuppression • Xerostomia or dry mouth is common; this may be the result of comorbidities, medication, radiation, dehydration	• Assess oral cavity and cause of problem • If ordered, give oral antifungal • Clean dentures and other dental appliances to prevent reinfection • Provide oral hygiene and use soft toothbrush or sponge
Delirium and Restlessness • Develops over a short period with severity fluctuating through the day • Confusion, disorientation, restlessness, clouding of consciousness, incoherence, fear, anxiety, excitement, hallucinations • May be misidentified as depression, psychosis, anger, anxiety • Contributing factors include medications, underlying disease, environment, sensory impairment, metabolic problems • Associated with adverse outcomes • Considered reversible • Common in final days of life	• Perform a thorough assessment for delirium using a validated tool • Assess for risk factors for delirium, including pain, constipation, and urinary retention, and treat as needed • Include appropriate nonpharmacologic interventions • Provide a room that is quiet, well lit, and familiar to reduce the effects of delirium • Reorient the patient to person, place, and time with each encounter • Give ordered antipsychotics, benzodiazepines, and sedatives as needed • Stay physically close to frightened patient; reassure in a calm, soft voice with touch and slow strokes of the skin • Avoid physical restraints whenever possible • Provide family with emotional support and encouragement in their efforts to cope with the behaviors associated with delirium
Difficulty Swallowing • May occur because of cancer, neurologic problems, weakness • Common at EOL • May lead to aspiration of liquids and/or solids, pneumonia, malnutrition, dehydration, death • Drooling/inability to swallow secretions may be present	• Assess level of alertness and safety of oral intake • Collaborate referral for evaluation based on goals of care; refer to speech-language pathologist • If needed, use alternative routes for (rectal, buccal, transdermal, IV) drug administration for symptom management • Modify diet to focus on comfort or pleasure, as tolerable by patient • Teach family on safety and risk for aspiration • Review medications and stop nonessential • Hand-feed small meals • Elevate the head for meals and at least 30 minutes after

TABLE 10.8 NURSING MANAGEMENT—cont'd

Physical Care at End of Life

Manifestation	Nursing Management
Dyspnea, Terminal Secretions, and Cough • Can significantly impair quality of life • Dyspnea is often accompanied by chest tightness, fear of suffocation, anxiety • Terminal secretions, or death rattle, is noisy breathing from secretion accumulation; very common in the hours before death • Presence of terminal secretions can be distressing to family members • Cough is a reaction to an irritation of the respiratory tract and can be debilitating	• Assess respiratory status regularly • Assess for anxiety and other associated symptoms including pain and fatigue • Elevate the head and/or position patient on side to improve chest expansion • Use a fan or air conditioner to help movement of cool air • Teach and encourage the use of pursed-lip breathing • Teach relaxation and guided imagery techniques for relaxation • Administer opioids as ordered for dyspnea • Administer benzodiazepines for anxiety • Administer anticholinergic medications for secretion management • Administer antitussives, expectorants, mucolytics, opioids, or inhaled anesthetics for cough • O_2 use should be based on the goals of care • Avoid deep suctioning; gentle oral suctioning may be used • Teach the patient and family on these symptoms and treatments; provide emotional support for caregivers
Myoclonus • Mild to severe abnormal movement that may be a brief jerking, twitching, or movement of the extremities • Can be caused by medications, metabolic imbalances, central nervous system damage	• Assess for onset, duration, any discomfort or distress • Review potential causes, including medications • Treat symptoms with benzodiazepines • Provide teaching and emotional support to patient and family
Pain (see also Chapter 9) • Major symptom at EOL, can contribute to suffering, and the most feared • Often associated with other symptoms and sources of distress • Often requires opioids for management • Physical and emotional stressors can worsen pain	• Assess pain thoroughly and regularly to determine the onset, duration, quality, intensity, location, and aggravating and alleviating factors • Assess for associated symptoms including anxiety, social or spiritual distress • Give medications around the clock, in a timely manner, and on a regular basis to provide constant relief • Provide nonpharmacologic interventions, such as guided imagery, massage, and relaxation techniques as needed (see Chapter 7) • Frequently evaluate effectiveness of pain relief measures • Ensure that the patient is on a correct, adequate drug regimen • Monitor for side effects of opioids, such as nausea or constipation, and treat as appropriate • Teach the patient and family on all interventions and medications • Do not delay or deny pain relief measures to a terminally ill patient
Skin Breakdown • Skin integrity is hard to maintain at the end of life • Immobility, urinary and bowel incontinence, dry skin, malnutrition, anemia, friction, and shearing forces lead to a high risk for skin breakdown • Disease and other processes may impair skin integrity • In the last days of life, circulation to the extremities decreases and they become cool, mottled, cyanotic	• Assess skin for signs of breakdown or injury • Assess risk factors for skin breakdown and implement protocols to prevent • Perform wound assessments as needed • Follow protocols for dressing wounds • Premedicate if turning, repositioning, or wound care causes discomfort • Follow protocols to prevent skin irritation and breakdown from urinary and bowel incontinence • Use blankets to cover for warmth • Use lotions to prevent dryness
Urinary and Bowel Incontinence • May result from disease progression or changes in the level of consciousness, medications, decreased mobility • As death becomes imminent, the perineal muscles relax, causing incontinence of bowel and bladder	• Assess urinary and bowel function • Use absorbent pads for incontinence and barrier creams to prevent irritation • Follow protocols for the use and management of indwelling or external catheters • Implement measures to prevent skin irritation and breakdown from urinary and bowel incontinence
Weakness and Fatigue • Decline in mental status and energy is expected • Causes include metabolic demands related to disease, underlying chronic condition, cancer, malnutrition, insomnia, infection	• Assess the patient's tolerance for physical and mental activities • Help the patient identify and complete valued or desired activities • Modify and time nursing interventions to conserve energy • Refer to physical and occupational therapy for safe movement • Review nutrition and hydration based on goals of care • Give frequent rest periods and adjust environment to allow for quiet surroundings

TABLE 10.9 NURSING MANAGEMENT

Postmortem Care

- Provide privacy throughout the process. Teach family and caregivers on process if present.
- Assess cultural and/or religious preferences or rituals about this process from family or caregivers before starting.
- Obtain supplies needed before starting. This may include a kit or individual items. Ask for help if needed.
- Wash hands, and use protective equipment as needed.
- Close the patient's eyes and jaw.
- Replace dentures; if unable, place in labeled cup.
- Remove jewelry, eyeglasses, and other personal belongings.
- Remove tubes and dressings (per policy).
- Wash the body as needed, then apply clothes selected by the patient or family (home) or a clean gown (agency). Comb and arrange the hair neatly.
- Place a waterproof pad or incontinence brief to absorb urine and feces.
- Straighten the body, placing the arms at their sides or across the abdomen with palms down.
- Follow instructions per policy in home or agency setting.

CASE STUDY

Spiritual Distress at End of Life

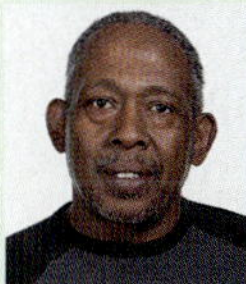
((©XiXinXing/iStock.com))

Patient Profile

G.M. is a 42-year-old male with end-stage liver disease and recently diagnosed liver cancer. He could not receive any therapy and is now in hospice. He has a history of excess alcohol use. He reports increased abdominal pain, nausea, vomiting, and anorexia. Current medications include fentanyl transdermal patch and hydromorphone for pain, ondansetron for nausea and vomiting, sertraline for depression, and mirtazapine for appetite. He is divorced with 2 children, age 10 and 8. He was raised Christian but says faith is not important to his care.

Subjective Data

- Reports pain at 7 (0- to 10-point scale) not relieved by medication
- Reports feeling that he is being punished for his previous lifestyle and getting divorced
- Asks why God would leave his children without a father and questions if there "is a God"
- States he is worried about losing his health benefits and what will happen to his children

Objective Data

Assessment

- Dry skin with scratch marks
- Weight 145 lb, height 5 ft 10 in
- Yellow sclera

Interprofessional Care

- Review pain medication usage and assess for dosage adjustment
- Consult chaplaincy and review ways to address distress
- Social work consult to review medical benefits and disability application
- Psychology consult for counseling and promoting discussions with ex-wife and children
- Ensure that advance directives are in place

Discussion Questions

1. ***Recognize:*** What are G.M.'s risk factors for spiritual and existential distress?
2. ***Analyze:*** Based on the data given, what are the major health problems for G.M.?
3. ***Plan:*** What cultural considerations should be included when planning care?
4. ***Prioritize:*** Based on your assessment of G.M., what are the top 3 priority nursing interventions?
5. ***Act:*** What teaching will be important so the patient can self-manage symptoms and care?
6. ***Evaluate:*** What outcomes would indicate interprofessional care was effective?
7. ***Safety:*** Describe specific nursing actions you would take to promote patient safety.

Answers available at http://evolve.elsevier.com/Lewis/medsurg.

BRIDGE TO NCLEX EXAMINATION

The number of the question corresponds to the same-numbered outcome at the beginning of the chapter.

1. An older adult with emphysema is receiving palliative care along with pulmonary management. Which statements provide accurate information for planning this patient's care? **(Select all that apply.)**
   - **a.** This patient does not need palliative care.
   - **b.** The pulmonologist can provide primary palliative care.
   - **c.** Palliative care can help improve coping and quality of life.
   - **d.** Palliative care can help with symptom burden, such as dyspnea.
   - **e.** The patient is at end of life because palliative care is only for those who are dying.
2. Which clinical manifestations are common in a patient who is actively dying? **(Select all that apply.)**
   - **a.** Noisy secretions
   - **b.** Increased sensation
   - **c.** Mottling of hands and feet
   - **d.** Cheyne-Stokes respirations
   - **e.** Increased response to tactile stimuli

3. A nurse is completing the admission assessment for a patient admitted with heart failure. The nurse asks about advance directives, and the patient does not know what this means. Which response would accurately describe advance directives?
   - **a.** "These are forms that tell your doctor when you want to withdraw care."
   - **b.** "These forms will tell your loved ones where your money goes after you die."
   - **c.** "These are forms, such as a living will, where you detail your treatment preferences."
   - **d.** "You cannot fill out any advance directives right now because you are in the hospital."
4. A 35-year-old female with sarcoma arrives to the clinic for chemotherapy. She reports severe pain at a level of 7 (0- to 10-point scale) in her right lower extremity. Which action would the nurse take before starting the chemotherapy?
   - **a.** Auscultate for bowel sounds.
   - **b.** Ask about advance directives.
   - **c.** Hold any medications that may cause sedation.
   - **d.** Review orders and give prescribed pain medications.
5. A female has been widowed for 2 years after her husband died from cancer. She stopped working, does not leave the house often, and cries daily. The nurse notes that she has not removed her husband's items from the home. The nurse would describe this grieving as
   - **a.** adaptive
   - **b.** disruptive
   - **c.** anticipatory
   - **d.** prolonged
6. A patient on home hospice tells the nurse, "I can't believe God would do this to me. I've always been healthy until this cancer. I don't understand!" Which states is the patient exhibiting? **(Select all that apply.)**
   - **a.** Denial
   - **b.** Loneliness
   - **c.** Fear of death
   - **d.** Spiritual distress
   - **e.** Existential distress
7. A nurse who often works with patients at the end of life reports feeling sad and exhausted. Which actions could help support the nurse? **(Select all that apply.)**
   - **a.** Plan for adequate sleep each day.
   - **b.** It is okay to cry about the patient situation.
   - **c.** Schedule time for your hobbies and interests.
   - **d.** Avoid bonding with families to decrease stress.
   - **e.** Express your feelings to a trusted colleague or friend.
8. The nurse is assigned a patient with breast cancer who speaks only Cantonese. Several family members are at the bedside. Which action would the nurse take first?
   - **a.** Assess the patient's language preferences and beliefs.
   - **b.** Call a pastor or priest for the family to help them cope.
   - **c.** Avoid using a translator for fear of offending the family.
   - **d.** Ask for a different nurse to have this patient assignment.

1. b, c, d; 2. a, c, d; 3. c; 4. d; 5. d; 6. a, d; 7. a, b, c, e; 8. a.

For rationales to these answers and even more NCLEX review questions, visit http://evolve.elsevier.com/Lewis/medsurg.

REFERENCES

To access the References for this chapter, please scan the QR code with a mobile device

11

Substance Use Disorders in Acute Care

Mariann M. Harding

http://evolve.elsevier.com/Lewis/medsurg/

CONCEPTUAL FOCUS

Addiction
Cognition
Stress and Coping

LEARNING OUTCOMES

1. Relate the effects of substance use to its resulting health complications.
2. Discern the effects of using stimulants, depressants, and cannabis.
3. Explain your role in promoting tobacco use cessation.
4. Review the nursing and interprofessional management of patients with overdose or withdrawal from stimulants and depressants.
5. Apply the Screening, Brief Intervention, and Referral to Treatment approach in nursing practice.
6. Describe the effects of substance use in an older adult.

KEY TERMS

acute alcohol toxicity
alcohol use disorder (AUD)
alcohol withdrawal syndrome (AWS)
binge drinking
Screening, Brief Intervention, and Referral to Treatment (SBIRT)
substance use disorder (SUD)
tobacco use disorder (TUD)
vaping

Substance use is a serious problem. Substance-related disorders involve several types of substances. These range from widely used and accepted tobacco and alcohol to illegal, brain-altering drugs such as heroin and cocaine. **Substance use disorders (SUDs)** are defined as the chronic use of drugs and/or alcohol that causes physical and/or mental impairment leading to health issues and the inability to function in daily life (Table 11.1).[1]

Many patients with SUDs receive acute care for associated problems—and there are many. Every drug associated with SUD harms some tissue or organ. Substance use causes specific health problems, such as liver damage related to alcohol use or lung cancer related to smoking. Other problems result from injuries associated with substance use, such as falls or motor vehicle accidents. Common health problems related to substance use are outlined in Table 11.2.

There is a high incidence of overlap between SUD and mental health disorders. Mental health disorders associated with SUD include anxiety disorders, depression, bipolar disorder, attention deficit hyperactivity disorder (ADHD), and personality disorders. Patients with chronic pain have an increased risk for SUD.[2]

This chapter focuses on the nurse's role in identifying and managing patients with SUD in the acute care setting. Hospitalized patients who use substances can develop withdrawal when substance use abruptly stops. You need to be able to recognize substance use and its effects on health problems and manage withdrawal. The health care setting offers an

TABLE 11.1 Diagnostic Criteria

Substance Use Disorder

These general criteria can be used to identify the presence of SUD.

Impaired Control
- Taking more or for longer than intended
- Not quitting use despite multiple times of trying
- Spending a great deal of time obtaining, using, or recovering from use
- Urge or craving to use the substance

Social Impairment
- Missing school, work, or other responsibilities because of use
- Continuing use despite problems caused or worsened by use
- Giving up or reducing important activities because of use
- Use takes precedence over other interests or enjoyments, daily activities, or health or personal care
- Use takes a key role in the person's life

Dependence
- Physical tolerance to effects of the substance
- Presence of withdrawal symptoms when not using or using less
- Repeated use to prevent or alleviate withdrawal symptoms

From Saunders JB, Latt NC: Diagnosis and classification of substance use disorders. In Johnson B, editor: *Addiction medicine: science and practice,* ed 2, Philadelphia, 2020, Elsevier.

TABLE 11.2 Health Problems Related to Substance Use

	Health Problems[a]
Substance	
Amphetamines	• Dysrhythmias, myocardial ischemia, hypertension • Liver, lung, kidney damage • Mood changes, violent behavior, psychoses
Cannabis	• Chronic cough, lung infections • Impaired memory • Mental health problems
Cocaine	• Dysrhythmias, myocardial ischemia and infarction • Psychosis, panic attacks • Seizures, stroke
Inhalants	• Kidney and liver damage • Cognitive and motor impairment
Opioids	• Impaired cognition • Psychosis • Sexual problems
Sedative-hypnotics	• Impaired memory • Personality changes, depression
Behaviors	
Injecting drugs	• Blood clots, phlebitis, skin infections • Hepatitis C • HIV • Other infections: endocarditis, cellulitis, pneumonia, meningitis, tetanus, bone and joint infections, lung abscesses
Personal neglect	• Accident injuries • Malnutrition
Risky sexual behavior	• Hepatitis B and C • HIV • Sexually transmitted infections
Snorting drugs	• Chronic sinusitis • Nasal sores, nasal damage • Loss of smell

[a]Health problems related to substance use disorder are discussed in the chapters where they are risk factors for a specific problem.
Adapted from National Institute on Drug Abuse: *Medical consequence of drug abuse.* Retrieved from www.drugabuse.gov/related-topics/medical-consequences-drug-abuse.

opportunity for screening and teaching about substance use. It is your responsibility to motivate patients to change behavior and refer them to treatment programs.

TOBACCO USE

You are most likely to encounter people with **tobacco use disorder (TUD)**. People with TUD are dependent on the drug nicotine from using tobacco products. Products that contain nicotine include smoked tobacco (cigarettes, cigars, pipes), smokeless tobacco (chew, snuff, dip), and some electronic cigarettes. Cigarette smoking is the main form of tobacco use in the United States.

Effects of Use

Nicotine is a central nervous system stimulant. Within seconds of entering the body, nicotine reaches the brain, causing the release of adrenaline and creating feelings of a "high" or a "buzz." The effects last about 1 to 2 hours before withdrawal symptoms occur, leaving the person feeling tired, irritable, and anxious. The need to have the "high" or "buzz" feelings again makes the person crave more nicotine, leading to addiction.

Smoked tobacco is the most harmful method of nicotine use. Smoking harms nearly every organ in the body and reduces the person's general health.[3] Smoking causes lung disease, lung and other cancers, and heart disease. It is a major factor in many health problems (Fig. 11.1).

Although using smokeless tobacco has less risk for lung disease, it can cause serious health problems. Holding tobacco in the mouth is associated with periodontal disease and cancer of the mouth, cheek, tongue, throat, and esophagus. The nicotine in smokeless tobacco affects the cardiovascular system. This increases the risk for high blood pressure, heart attack, and stroke.

Vaping is the use of electronic cigarettes, or e-cigs. These battery-operated devices turn nicotine and other chemicals into an inhaled vapor. The vapor that users breathe can contain harmful substances, including nicotine, heavy metals, and cancer-causing chemicals. Vaping is associated with health risks. It can cause e-cig vaping–associated lung injury (EVALI) and other lung and heart problems. It can harm adolescent brain development and negatively influence pregnancy outcomes.[4] Although some think e-cigs aid in smoking

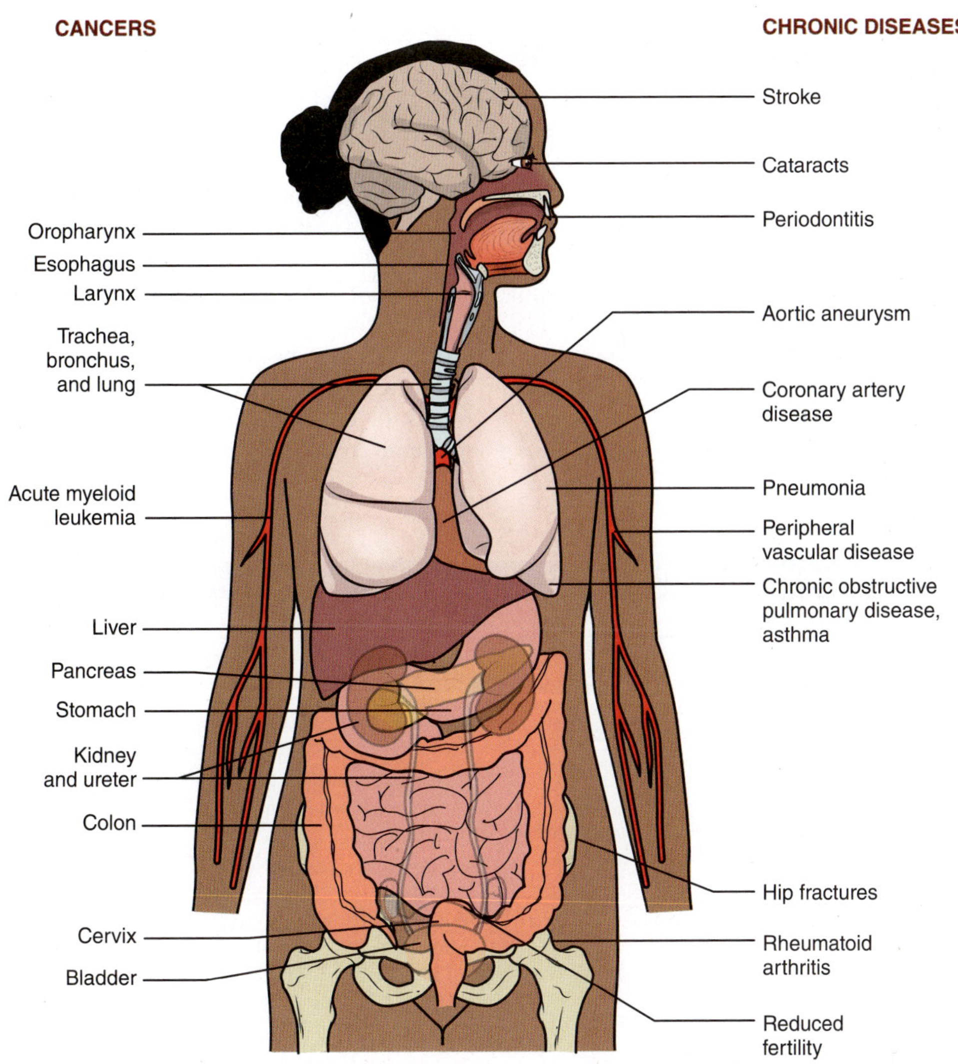

Fig. 11.1 Health effects of smoking.

cessation, the FDA has not found e-cigs to be safe or effective in helping smokers quit. Instead, you should encourage those who vape to use the same cessation strategies recommended for TUD.

Interprofessional and Nursing Management

As a nurse, you have a professional responsibility to help people stop smoking or using tobacco. Ask all patients about tobacco use and whether risk factors for use are present. When smoking is identified, encourage the patient to quit. Offer specific information on ways to stop using tobacco. Patients who receive even brief advice and intervention from you are more likely to quit than those who receive no intervention.

There are several tools we can use to encourage users to quit (Tables 11.3 and 11.4).[5,6] Use the "5 *As* and 5 *Rs*" with each patient encounter. It will help you identify tobacco users, determine their willingness to quit, assist them in quitting, and arrange for follow-up. A patient teaching guide (Table 11.5) expands on the fourth strategy, *Assist,* to help you when the

TABLE 11.3 5 *As* and 5 *Rs*

Brief TUD Intervention

The 5 *As* for Users Who Want to Quit	The 5 *Rs* for Users Unwilling to Quit
1. **Ask:** Identify all tobacco users at every contact. 2. **Advise:** Strongly urge all tobacco users to quit. 3. **Assess:** Determine willingness to make a quit attempt. 4. **Assist:** Develop a plan with the patient to help the patient quit (e.g., counseling, medication). 5. **Arrange:** Schedule follow-up contact.	1. **Relevance:** Ask the patient to say why quitting is personally relevant (e.g., health). 2. **Risks:** Ask the patient to identify their potential risks/ consequences of tobacco use. 3. **Rewards:** Ask the patient to relate potential benefits of stopping tobacco use. 4. **Roadblocks:** Ask patient to identify barriers or impediments to quitting. 5. **Repetition:** Repeat process every clinic visit.

From Agency for Healthcare Research and Quality: *AHCPR supported clinical practice guideline: treating tobacco use and dependence—2008 update,* Washington, DC, 2008, U.S. Public Health Service.

TABLE 11.4 NURSING MANAGEMENT

Inpatient Tobacco Cessation Interventions

- Ask each patient if they use tobacco, and document tobacco use status.
- For current tobacco users, list tobacco use status on the problem list and as a discharge diagnosis.
- Offer nicotine-replacement therapy or medication to help the tobacco user stay abstinent and treat withdrawal symptoms.
- Provide counseling on how to stay abstinent after discharge.
- Arrange for follow-up care. Provide supportive contact for at least a month after discharge.

From Rojewski AM, Palmer AM, Toll BA: Treatment of tobacco dependence in the inpatient setting. In Eakin MN, Kathuria H, editors: *Tobacco dependence: a comprehensive guide to prevention and treatment,* Cham, 2023, Humana, pp 149–162.

user is willing to quit. If a tobacco user is not willing to quit, using the "5 *Rs*" may encourage them to quit in the future.

A variety of products are available to help support users in quitting. Nicotine replacement products include skin patches, lozenges, and gum. They are helpful because they reduce the craving and withdrawal symptoms of cessation by supplying the body with smaller amounts of nicotine (Table 11.6).

Because most health care agencies are tobacco-free, admitted patients addicted to nicotine may have withdrawal symptoms because they are unable to smoke. These symptoms are the same as for the person who stops using tobacco "cold turkey." Offering nicotine replacement therapy to every patient who wants to quit will help control withdrawal symptoms and promote continued cessation after discharge.

TABLE 11.5 PATIENT & CAREGIVER TEACHING

Smoking and Tobacco Use Cessation

The following interventions are methods that work for quitting tobacco use. Tobacco users have the best chance of quitting if they use more than 1 method.

Develop a Quit Plan

- Set a quit date, ideally within 2 weeks.
- Talk to your HCP about getting help to quit.
- Tell family, friends, and coworkers about quitting and request understanding and support.
- Expect withdrawal symptoms and challenges when quitting.
- Before quitting, avoid smoking in places where you spend a lot of time (work, car, home).
- Throw away all tobacco products from your home, car, and work.
- Have support options in place by your quit date.

Use Approved Nicotine Replacement Systems

- Use a nicotine replacement agent unless you are a pregnant or nursing female (Table 11.6).
- Do not use other forms of tobacco when using nicotine replacement systems.

Support and Encouragement

- Joining a quit-tobacco support group will increase your chances of stopping permanently.
- If you get the urge for tobacco, call someone to help talk you out of it—preferably an ex-user.
- Be proud every time you reach a quit milestone and reward yourself.
- Do not be afraid to talk about how you feel while quitting, especially fears of not being able to quit for good. Ask your spouse or partner, friends, and coworkers to support you. Self-help materials, mobile phone applications, and hotlines are available:
  - American Lung Association: 800-LUNGUSA; www.lung.org
  - American Cancer Society: 800-227-2345; www.cancer.org
  - National Cancer Institute: LiveHelp; www.smokefree.gov

Dealing With Urges to Use Tobacco

- Identify situations that may cause you to want to smoke or use other tobacco, such as being around other smokers, being under time pressure, feeling sad or frustrated, and drinking alcohol.
- Avoid difficult situations while you are trying to quit. Try to lower your stress level.
- Exercise can help, such as walking, jogging, or bicycling.
- Distract yourself from thoughts of smoking and the urge to use tobacco by talking to someone, going to a movie, getting busy with a task, or having a game night with friends.
- Drink a lot of water.
- Keep your hands busy with a pen or toothpick.

Avoiding Relapse

Most relapses occur within the first 3 months after quitting. Do not be discouraged if you start using tobacco again. Remember, most people try several times before they finally quit. Explore different ways to break habits. You may need to deal with triggers that cause relapse.

- *Change your environment.* Get rid of cigarettes, tobacco (in any form), and ashtrays in your home, car, and place of work. Get rid of the smell of cigarettes in your car and home.
- *Alcohol.* Consider limiting or stopping alcohol use while you are quitting tobacco.
- *Other smokers at home.* Encourage housemates to quit with you. Work out a plan to cope with others who smoke and avoid being around them.
- *Weight gain.* Tackle 1 problem at a time. Work on quitting tobacco first. You will not necessarily gain weight, and increased appetite is often temporary. Eat healthy and exercise.
- *Negative mood or depression.* If these symptoms persist, talk to your HCP. You may need treatment for depression.
- *Withdrawal symptoms.* Your body will go through many changes when you quit tobacco. You may have a dry mouth, cough, or scratchy throat, and you may feel irritable. The nicotine patch or gum may help with cravings (Table 11.6).
- *Focus on the benefits of quitting:*
  - Your blood pressure and heart rate will lower almost at once.
  - Your risk for a heart attack declines within 24 hours. The blood will become less likely to clot, making dangerous blood clots less likely.
  - Within a few weeks, you will be less short of breath, cough less, and have more energy. Your ability to smell and taste should improve.
  - Your immune system will be stronger, so you will be less likely to be sick.
  - Quitting will improve your night vision and help preserve your overall vision.

Adapted from National Cancer Institute: *Quit smoking.* Retrieved from https://smokefree.gov/quit-smoking.

TABLE 11.6 **Drug Therapy**

Smoking Cessation

Agents	Side Effects	Considerations
Nicotine Replacement Agents		
Nicotine gum (OTC) • 2-mg, 4-mg strengths • Use for 12 wk • Use 1 piece q1–2h for 6 wk then q2–4h for 3 wk • Maximum dose: 24 pieces/day	Hiccups, mouth/jaw pain, mouth ulcers, heartburn, throat irritation, nausea	Use "chew and park," alternating chewing with periods of holding the gum between cheek and teeth. Repeat for 30 min then discard gum. Do not eat or drink 15 min before and during use. Dose depends on how much user smokes each day.
Nicotine lozenge (OTC) • 2 sizes (regular, mini) each comes in 2-mg and 4-mg strengths • Use 8–12 wk • Use 1 lozenge q1–2h for 6 wk, tapering to 1 lozenge q4–8h by 12 wk	Insomnia, nausea, sore throat, mouth ulcers, cough, heartburn, headache	Dissolves in mouth in 20–30 min. Do not chew or swallow. Do not eat or drink 15 min before and during use. Occasionally rotate around the mouth. Do not eat or drink 15 min before and during use.
Nicotine patch (OTC) • 3 strengths: 7 mg, 14 mg, 21 mg • 1 patch applied daily and worn for 24 h	Local skin irritation, insomnia, nausea, headache	Provides steady level of nicotine. Rotate sites to decrease skin irritation. Users who smoke more than 10 cigarettes/day should start with a 21 mg/day patch.
Nicotine nasal spray • 1–2 doses (2 sprays)/h • Use ≥6 mo	Nose and throat irritation, sneezing, rhinitis, headache, cough	Requires a prescription. Quick-acting. Do not sniff, swallow, or inhale while spraying. Tilt head back slightly for best results.
Nicotine inhaler • Use 6 cartridges/day for first 3–6 wk • Limit 16 cartridges/day	Cough, mouth and throat irritation, headache, nausea, hiccups	Requires a prescription. Mouthpiece simulates smoking, which satisfies oral urges. Do not eat or drink 15 min before and during use.
Nonnicotine Agents		
Bupropion • 150 mg/day for 2 days, then 150 mg bid • Use 12 wk; can use up to 6 mo	Insomnia, dry mouth, irritability, rash, tremors, anorexia	Increases risk for seizures or eating disorders. Limit or avoid alcohol use. Take doses at least 8 h apart. Start taking 1–2 wk before quit date.
Varenicline • 0.5 mg/day for 3 days, 0.5 mg bid for 4 days, then 1 mg bid • Use 12 wk; additional 12 wk may be used in select patients	Nausea, insomnia, kidney stones, flatulence, vivid dreams, headache	Start taking at least 1 wk before quit date. Monitor kidney function tests. Take with food or full glass of water.

Nonnicotine products play a role in helping users quit. Varenicline is one drug used to aid smoking cessation. Varenicline has agonist and antagonist actions. The agonist activity at one type of nicotinic receptor provides some nicotine effects to ease withdrawal symptoms. If the person does resume smoking, the antagonist action blocks the effects of nicotine at another type of nicotinic receptor, making smoking less enjoyable. Bupropion, an antidepressant drug, reduces the urge to smoke, reduces some withdrawal symptoms, and helps prevent weight gain from smoking cessation.

DRUG ALERT

Varenicline and Bupropion

- Behavior changes, hostility, aggression, depression, anxiety, suicidal thoughts, attempted suicide, and delusions may occur.
- Tell patients to stop taking these drugs and contact the HCP at once if any of these occur.

Along with using a smoking cessation product, users who wish to quit are most likely to succeed if they take part in a tobacco cessation program.[6] You should be aware of available community resources. Cessation programs may involve behavior counseling, aversion therapy, group support, individual therapy, and self-help options. Many programs teach users to avoid high-risk situations for smoking relapse, such as those that promote cue-induced craving. They help them develop coping skills, such as cigarette refusal skills, assertiveness, alternative activities, and peer support systems.

ALCOHOL USE

Of Americans ages 18 and older, 67% consume alcohol. Most people use alcohol in moderation.[7] *Moderate drinking* is up to 1 drink per day for females and up to 2 drinks per day for males (Fig. 11.2). **Alcohol use disorder (AUD)**, or alcoholism, affects about 11.3% of U.S. adults.[7] More people engage in periodic

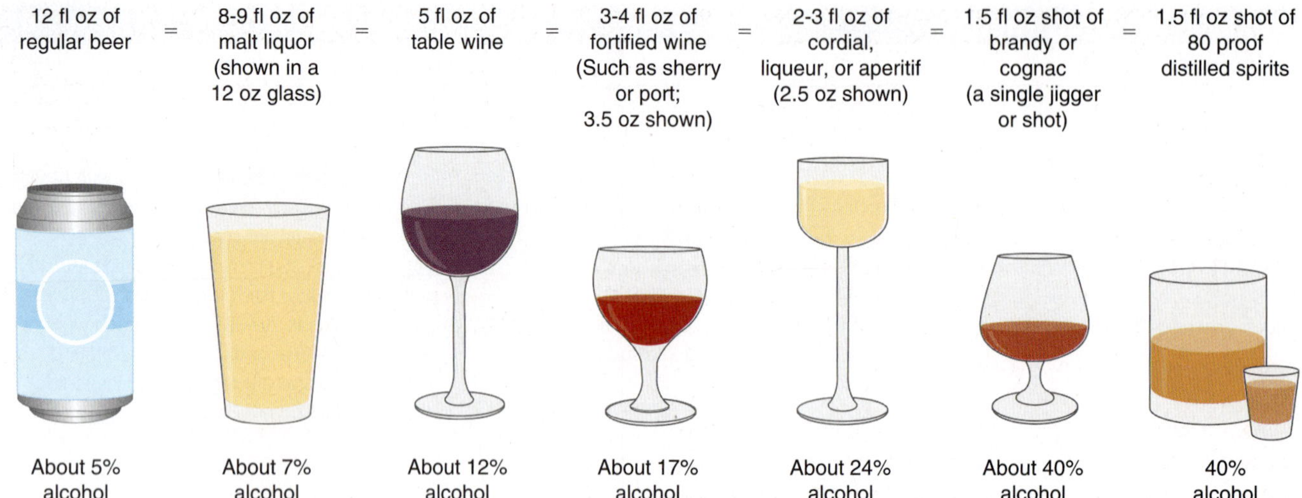

Fig. 11.2 U.S. standard drink equivalents. Each beverage represents 1 alcoholic drink equivalent, defined in the United States as any beverage containing 0.6 fl oz or 14 g of pure alcohol. (Adapted from NIAAA: *What's a standard drink?* Retrieved from https://www.niaaa.nih.gov/what-standard-drink.)

excess alcohol use. **Binge drinking** is consuming 5 or more alcoholic drinks for males or 4 or more alcoholic drinks for females on the same occasion at least once per month. AUD and binge drinking can have harmful physical, emotional, and social consequences.

Effects of Use

Alcohol affects almost all cells of the body. It changes neurotransmitter levels in the central nervous system (CNS), affecting all areas and functions of the CNS. These include centers that control our impulses, mood, and behavior; coordinate motor activity; and promote respiratory and cardiac function. The immediate effects of alcohol depend on a person's susceptibility to alcohol and the blood alcohol concentration (BAC).

For the person who is not dependent on alcohol, the BAC generally predicts alcohol's effects. The relationship between BAC and behavior is different in a person who has developed tolerance to alcohol and its effects. The *tolerant person* can usually drink large amounts without obvious impairment and perform complex tasks at BAC levels much higher than levels that would produce obvious impairment in the *nontolerant drinker.* Females have higher blood alcohol levels than males do after the same amount of alcohol intake.

Alcohol use causes many health problems (Table 11.7). These problems are often the reason that people seek health care. Long-term alcohol use can lead to hypertension, heart disease, stroke, liver disease, and digestive problems. Short-term excess alcohol use increases the risk for injury to self and others from motor vehicle crashes, falls, firearms, assault, drowning, and burns. Patients with AUD having surgery have increased in-hospital death rates and longer lengths of stay.

TABLE 11.7 Effects of Chronic Alcohol Use

Body System	Effects
Cardiac	Hypertension, heart failure, cardiomyopathy, stroke, coronary artery disease, dysrhythmias
Gastrointestinal (GI)	Gastritis, gastroesophageal reflux disease (GERD), ulcers, esophagitis, esophageal varices, GI bleeding, pancreatitis, GI cancers
Hematologic	Bone marrow depression, anemia, leukopenia, thrombocytopenia, blood clotting problems
Hepatic	Alcoholic hepatitis, cirrhosis, liver cancer
Musculoskeletal	Myopathy, osteoporosis, gout
Neurologic	Alcoholic dementia, Wernicke-Korsakoff syndrome; impaired cognition, psychomotor skills, abstract thinking, and memory; depression, anxiety, attention deficit, labile moods, seizures, insomnia, peripheral neuropathy, chronic headache
Nutrition	Diabetes, anorexia, malnutrition, vitamin deficiencies (especially thiamine)
Reproductive	Breast cancer, decreased beard growth, decreased libido, infertility, gynecomastia, impaired sexual function
Skin	Palmar erythema, spider angiomas, rosacea, rhinophyma
Urinary	Diuretic effect from inhibition of antidiuretic hormone

Complications may arise from the interaction of alcohol with commonly prescribed or over-the-counter (OTC) medications. Those that interact with alcohol in an additive manner include antihypertensives, antihistamines, and antianginals. Alcohol taken with aspirin may cause or worsen gastrointestinal (GI) bleeding. Alcohol taken with acetaminophen may increase the risk of liver damage. Taking a CNS depressant with alcohol can increase, or potentiate, the effect of both. An alcohol-dependent person may have cross-tolerance, needing higher doses of CNS depressants to achieve the desired effect.

Alcohol Toxicity

Acute alcohol toxicity occurs when a person has a high blood alcohol level, generally after ingesting a large amount of alcohol. This leads to behavior changes and impaired neurologic function, resulting in respiratory and circulatory failure. Unconsciousness, coma, and death can occur. Other common effects include hypokalemia, hypomagnesemia, and hypoglycemia.

Obtain a health history as able and assess for injuries, diseases, and hypoglycemia. No antidote for alcohol is available. Implement supportive care measures to maintain airway, breathing, and circulation (the ABCs) until the alcohol metabolizes. Frequently monitor vital signs and level of consciousness. Maintain IV access and administer IV fluids for hypotension.

Patients with hypoglycemia need glucose. Give IV thiamine before or with IV glucose to prevent *Wernicke-Korsakoff syndrome,* which can cause seizures and brain damage.[8] Administer electrolyte solutions with magnesium and potassium as ordered. Place patients with nausea or vomiting in a lateral position and give antiemetic drugs.[8]

Agitation and anxiety are common. Stay with the patient as much as possible, orienting as necessary. Assess the patient for increasing anger and the potential for violence. Use protective measures because the patient is at risk for injury as a result of lack of coordination and impaired judgment.

Alcohol Withdrawal Syndrome

Alcohol withdrawal syndrome (AWS) can develop in a patient when the use of alcohol abruptly stops. The onset of AWS depends on the quantity, frequency, pattern, and duration of alcohol use. The early signs often develop within a few hours after the last drink. They peak after 24 to 48 hours and then disappear unless withdrawal progresses to alcohol withdrawal delirium.

Alcohol withdrawal delirium is a serious complication that can occur from 2 to 3 days after the last drink and last 2 to 3 days—the greater the patient's dependence on alcohol, the greater the risk for alcohol withdrawal delirium. Death may result from multiorgan failure, dysrhythmias, or peripheral vascular collapse.

Management begins with identifying at-risk persons. Use a symptom assessment tool, such as the Clinical Institute Withdrawal Assessment of Alcohol Scale, Revised (CIWA-Ar), to determine treatment (Table 11.8).[9] Table 11.9 outlines the clinical manifestations and treatment for AWS. A nursing care plan (see eNursing Care Plan 11.1) for patients with AWS is available on the website at http://evolve.elsevier.com/Lewis/medsurg.

TABLE 11.8 Clinical Institute Withdrawal Assessment of Alcohol Scale, Revised (CIWA-Ar)

CIWA-Ar Categories	Score Range in Each Category
Agitation	0–7
Anxiety	0–7
Auditory disturbances	0–7
Headache	0–7
Clouding of sensorium	0–4
Paroxysmal sweats	0–7
Tactile disturbances	0–7
Tremor	0–7
Visual disturbances	0–7

Score:
<10: Very mild withdrawal
10–15: Mild withdrawal
16–20: Modest withdrawal
>20: Severe withdrawal

From University of Maryland School of Medicine. Available at www.umem.org/files/uploads/1104212257_CIWA-Ar.pdf.

CHECK YOUR PRACTICE

A 34-year-old patient was admitted with multiple trauma after a car accident. Her boyfriend tells you that she drinks too much, and he knew she would "get in trouble" someday.

- What signs and symptoms would alert you to the presence of AWS?
- What measures would you use to promote her safety?
- How would you involve members of the health care team in planning patient care?

STIMULANT USE

Frequently used stimulants include cocaine, amphetamines, and methamphetamines. Although using cocaine and methamphetamine is illegal, amphetamines have a role in treating narcolepsy, obesity, and attention deficit disorder. Though most people responsibly use prescribed stimulants, some people do misuse them. Stimulants increase cardiac activity and excite the CNS by increasing norepinephrine, serotonin, and dopamine levels. People use these drugs to produce feelings of euphoria, increase alertness, and boost their energy. They are highly addictive. Health problems associated with using stimulants are outlined in Table 11.2.

Stimulant Overdose

Patients with stimulant overdose present with *sympathetic overdrive,* or increased stimulation of the sympathetic nervous system. The patient has restlessness, agitation, impaired judgment, and paranoia with psychotic symptoms. Physical effects include hypertension, tachycardia, fever, seizures, and confusion. Death may occur from stroke, dysrhythmias, or

TABLE 11.9 Manifestations and Treatment of Alcohol Withdrawal

Manifestations	Interprofessional Care	Nursing Management
Alcohol Withdrawal Syndrome		
• Agitation • Anxiety • ↑ BP • Fever • Headache • ↑ HR • Hyperactivity • Insomnia • Nausea and vomiting • Slurred speech • Sweating • Tactile disturbances (numbness, itching, burning, "bugs under the skin" • Tremors	• Benzodiazepines (lorazepam, diazepam) to lessen symptoms • Thiamine to prevent Wernicke-Korsakoff syndrome • Multivitamins (folate, B vitamins) • Magnesium sulfate to treat low magnesium • IV dextrose solution to treat hypoglycemia • β-Blockers (atenolol) or α_2-agonists (clonidine) to stabilize vital signs • Respiratory support as needed	• Monitor vital signs and neurologic status. • Infuse thiamine before IV solutions that contain dextrose. • Maintain NPO status. • Implement seizure precautions. • Calculate CIWA-Ar score q4h until it is less than 8 for 24 h. • Use measures to manage any fever and pain. • Provide a quiet, low-stimulating, well-lit environment. • Maintain adequate nutrition and fluid intake.
Alcohol Withdrawal Delirium		
• Delusions • Disorientation • Hallucinations • Seizures	• Continued use of benzodiazepines • Antiseizure agents (e.g., gabapentin) • Antipsychotic agents (haloperidol) • Chlordiazepoxide if psychosis persists after receiving benzodiazepines	• Orient the patient as needed. • Provide a safe environment. • Implement measures to address any hallucinations.

TABLE 11.10 EMERGENCY MANAGEMENT

Stimulant Overdose

Assessment Findings	Interventions
Cardiovascular • ↑ BP • Chest pain • Diaphoresis • Dysrhythmias • ↑ HR • Myocardial ischemia • Palpitations **Central Nervous System** • Agitation • Confusion • Fever • Hallucinations • Insomnia • Psychosis • Pupil dilation • Seizures	• Ensure patent airway. • Establish IV access and start fluid replacement. • Obtain a 12-lead ECG and start ECG monitoring. • Treat dysrhythmias as needed. • Treat hypertension and chest pain with nitrates. • Give IV diazepam or lorazepam for seizures and sedation. • Give IV antipsychotic drugs for psychosis and hallucinations. • Monitor vital signs and level of consciousness. • Use cooling measures for fever. • Implement measures to treat insomnia. • Start gastric lavage in cases of recent ingestion.

myocardial infarction. Emergency management depends on the manifestations at the time of treatment (Table 11.10). There is no specific antidote. Treatment focuses on supportive care.

Stimulant Withdrawal

Stimulant withdrawal is usually not an emergency. Abrupt cessation can lead to a "crash." The patient may be depressed and have fatigue, disturbed sleep, vivid dreams, general aching, irritability, increased appetite, and mood swings. Craving for the drug is intense during the first hours to days of drug cessation and may continue for weeks. Treatment focuses on supportive care. Provide a safe, quiet environment, and allow the patient to sleep and eat as desired.[10] If a patient has severe depression, implement suicide precautions and refer for further treatment.

OPIOID USE

Opioids include substances directly derived from the opium poppy (morphine), semisynthetics (heroin, hydromorphone), and synthetic compounds (fentanyl). Opioid use disorder (OUD) is a major threat to health. Most overdose deaths involve an opioid.[11] Common health problems resulting from OUD are outlined in Table 11.2.

Opioids act on opiate receptors and neurotransmitter systems in the CNS, causing sedation and analgesia. The person taking an opioid has euphoria, mood changes, mental clouding, drowsiness, and pain reduction. Although this makes prescription opioids useful in treating some medical problems, their pleasurable effects promote misuse. Opioids have rapid development of tolerance and dependence. People with OUD include those who use illegal drugs and those who misuse prescription opioids. Those who misuse prescription opioids take them in a way not directed by a provider, including without a prescription, or use in greater amounts, more often, or longer than told. Inappropriate access to prescription opioids by a person at risk of addiction and HCP prescribing patterns are other factors.

TABLE 11.11 EMERGENCY MANAGEMENT

Opioid and Sedative-Hypnotic Overdose

Assessment Findings	Interventions
• Agitation • ↓ BP • Confusion • Decreased level of consciousness • ECG changes • Hallucinations • Lethargy • ↓ O_2 saturation • Pinpoint pupils • Respiratory or cardiac arrest • Seizures • Slow, shallow respirations • Slurred speech • Seizures	• Ensure patent airway. • Expect intubation if respiratory distress is present. • Establish IV access. • Give the right antidotes (e.g., naloxone for opioid overdose). • Monitor vital signs, level of consciousness, and O_2 saturation. • Obtain 12-lead ECG and start continuous ECG monitoring. • Obtain information about substance (name, route, when taken, amount). • Obtain drug levels or comprehensive toxicology screen. • Obtain a health history, including drug use and allergies. • Perform gastric lavage if necessary. • Give activated charcoal and cathartics if ordered.

Opioid Overdose

Opioid overdose can cause death from CNS and respiratory depression. The priority of care is the ABCs and giving the opioid antagonist naloxone (Table 11.11). Naloxone reverses respiratory depression and other manifestations of an overdose.[12] Monitor the patient closely because naloxone has a shorter duration of action than most opioids. Repeated doses or IV infusion of naloxone may be needed until the opioid is metabolized. In many areas, naloxone is publicly available. This allows police, first responders, family members, and friends to give someone naloxone in emergencies, thus reversing the effects of an overdose sooner. As a result, you may have patients who need postreversal care.

Opioid Withdrawal

Opioid withdrawal symptoms depend on the opioid used, route of use, and duration of use. It is usually not life threatening but can be quite uncomfortable. With short-acting drugs, withdrawal begins 6 to 12 hours after the last dose. With longer-acting drugs, manifestations may begin 24 to 48 hours after the last dose and may last 3 weeks or more. Classic symptoms include craving, runny nose, sweating, and watery eyes. Other symptoms include anxiety, fever, nausea and vomiting, muscle aches, tachycardia, increased respirations and blood pressure, tremor, insomnia, and irritability. Most symptoms subside over 5 to 7 days. Craving and irritability can last for months.

Treatment focuses on relieving symptoms and often requires drug therapy. Giving a long-acting opioid (methadone, buprenorphine) at low doses or α_2-adrenergic agonists (e.g., clonidine) decreases withdrawal symptoms. Other therapies include medications for GI distress (loperamide, ondansetron), acetaminophen or nonsteroidal antiinflammatory agents for muscle aches and fever, and antihistamines for anxiety and insomnia.

SEDATIVE-HYPNOTIC USE

Common sedative-hypnotic agents include barbiturates and benzodiazepines. This class includes all prescription sleeping agents and almost all antianxiety agents. These drugs depress the CNS, causing sedation at low doses and sleep at high doses. Their use produces euphoria and intoxication that resemble that of alcohol. Tolerance develops rapidly to the effects of these drugs, requiring higher doses to achieve euphoria. However, tolerance may not develop to the brainstem-depressant effects. As a result, an increased dose may trigger hypotension and respiratory depression, resulting in death.

Sedative-Hypnotic Overdose

An overdose can cause death from respiratory and CNS depression. The priority of care is the ABCs. Supporting respiratory and cardiovascular function and continuous monitoring of neurologic status is critical until the patient is stable. The patient receives hydration, vasopressors, and treatments to promote drug elimination. Some may receive activated charcoal if their airway can be maintained. Dialysis is used in some situations. Emergency management depends on the substance used and the clinical manifestations (Table 11.11).

On occasion, a patient with a benzodiazepine overdose may receive flumazenil, a specific benzodiazepine antagonist. Because flumazenil may have a shorter duration of action than some benzodiazepines, repeated doses may be needed until the benzodiazepine is metabolized. Place the patient on safety precautions, as flumazenil can cause seizures. There are no antagonists for barbiturates or other sedative-hypnotic drugs.

Sedative-Hypnotic Withdrawal

Withdrawal can be life threatening. The body responds with rebound hyperactivity with cessation of use. Early, the patient may have tremors, anxiety, insomnia, fever, and disorientation. Delirium, seizures, and respiratory and cardiac arrest may occur within 24 hours after the last dose. Treatment consists of tapering doses of a long-acting benzodiazepine. IV diazepam is an option for severe manifestations. Closely monitor the patient. Frequently assess neurologic status and vital signs. Supportive care includes implementing patient safety and comfort measures and providing reassurance and orientation.

INHALANT USE

Persons with inhalant use disorder inhale hydrocarbon-based fumes, such as those found in glues or paints, to change their mental state.[1] Inhalants are rapidly absorbed and reach the

CNS quickly. Most are depressants. They cause a brief period of euphoria and disinhibition, followed by drowsiness and lightheadedness. Long-term use can result in neurologic problems, including damage to parts of the brain that control cognition, movement, vision, and hearing (Table 11.2).

Patients with inhalant toxicity may have lethargy, dizziness, slurred speech, blurry vision, tremors, and impaired coordination.[1] The effects usually resolve within minutes to a few hours. Inhalant toxicity is managed with supportive care. In rare cases, users need emergency treatment for dysrhythmias, bronchospasms, or seizures. Using some inhalants, like toluene, can result in kidney damage, so monitor renal function. Withdrawal is rare, as most inhaled substances have a very short duration.

CANNABIS USE

The use of cannabis, or marijuana, continues to increase in the United States. Cannabis is available in forms that can be smoked, vaporized, or ingested. The main ingredient is tetrahydrocannabinol (THC). At low to moderate doses, THC produces euphoria, relaxation, and sleepiness. Adverse effects include impaired memory, impaired coordination, altered judgment, and, in high doses, paranoia and psychosis. Long-term use is associated with a wide range of effects, particularly on cardiopulmonary and mental health (Table 11.2).

The legal use of cannabis for specific medical reasons continues to grow. Pain, sleep problems, cancer, posttraumatic stress disorder, seizure disorders, and nausea are some of the most common conditions for which cannabis can be authorized medically.[13] The synthetic THC-based medications dronabinol (Marinol) and nabilone (Cesamet) are used for chemotherapy-induced nausea and to boost appetite in those with AIDS. Epidiolex (cannabidiol, CBD) is approved to treat rare forms of epilepsy. CBD is a chemical found in the cannabis plant. It does not cause the euphoria that comes from THC.

There are many synthetic cannabinoid drugs (e.g., K2, spice). They act on the same receptors as THC but affect the brain differently. Many are illegal. They contain varying amounts of different ingredients. The result is that these products have unpredictable effects and are more toxic. Sometimes, death has occurred with 1 use.

Patients with cannabis toxicity may have acute psychotic episodes, especially if the patient used a synthetic derivative. Tachycardia and hypertension can trigger dysrhythmias and myocardial infarction. Support the patient's ABCs. Panic and flashbacks are managed by maintaining a quiet environment and reassuring the patient. Benzodiazepines give symptom relief.

Withdrawal symptoms occur within 24 to 48 hours after cessation and peak at 2 to 6 days. Symptoms last a few weeks. The patient may have irritability, insomnia, anorexia, anger, anxiety, and restlessness. There is no specific drug therapy for treating withdrawal. Supportive care includes measures to promote sleep, safety, and patient comfort, including analgesics and hydration.[14]

CAFFEINE USE

Caffeine is the most widely used substance in the world. It is very weak compared with the other stimulants. Most people use it to promote wakefulness. Other uses include promoting motor activity and treating headaches. Its use is safe for most people. Problems from high doses of caffeine have occurred from "energy" drinks. A large caffeine intake can cause dysrhythmias, hypertension, disturbed sleep, seizures, and anxiety. Treatment consists of supportive care. The patient may need IV hydration, β-blockers for tachycardia, and antiseizure medications. Patients with caffeine withdrawal during restriction on usual intake may have muscle pain, drowsiness, irritability, and headaches.

❖ NURSING MANAGEMENT: SUBSTANCE USE

◆ Assessment

You need to be able to determine whether patients use substances in a way that places them at risk or if SUD is present. Screening is a simple, effective way to identify patients who need further assessment. Use the **Screening, Brief Intervention, and Referral to Treatment (SBIRT)** approach (Fig. 11.3). SBIRT consists of 3 parts: (1) screening to quickly identify and assess the severity of any substance use problems, (2) providing a brief intervention or teaching patients about the consequences of substance use, and (3) referring those who screen positive for further treatment.[15]

Screening is the first step of SBIRT. As a baseline, ask every patient about the use of all substances, including medications, caffeine, tobacco, and recreational drugs. Record why a patient is taking a prescribed agent that places them at risk. Use simple screening tests to detect alcohol, tobacco, and other substance use problems (Table 11.12).

If a patient has a positive screen, follow up with a detailed assessment to identify specific problems. Two tools, the Alcohol Use Disorders Identification Text (AUDIT) and CAGE

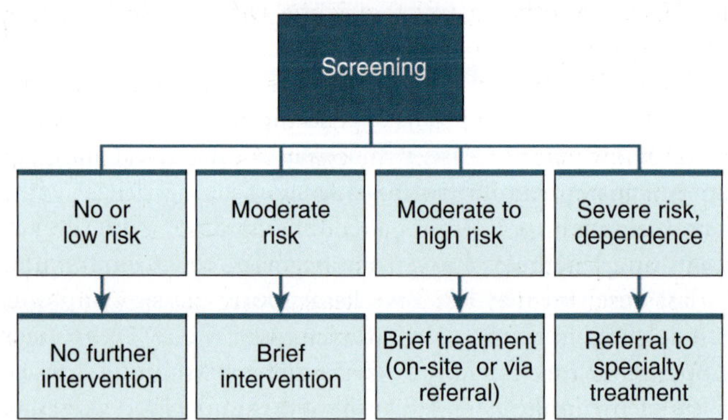

Fig. 11.3 Screening, brief intervention, and referral to treatment approach. (From Substance Abuse and Mental Health Services Administration [SAMHSA]: *Systems-level implementation of screening, brief intervention, and referral to treatment, Technical Assistance Publication [TAP] Series 33.* HHS Publication No. 13-4741, Rockville, 2013, SAMHSA.)

TABLE 11.12 Brief Screening Tools for Substance Use

Single-Question Tests

Use 1 of these questions to screen for the presence of alcohol, drug, or tobacco use:

- In the past year, on how many days did you have more than a few sips of beer, wine, or other drink containing alcohol?
- How many times in the past year did you use marijuana or prescription medications for nonmedical reasons?
- In the past year, how many days did you use tobacco products?

Two-Question Tests

Use the following 2 questions to screen for alcohol or drug use:

- In the past year, have you ever drunk or used drugs more than you meant to?
- Have you felt you wanted or needed to cut down on your drinking or drug use in the past year?

TABLE 11.13 CAGE Questions

C: Cut	Have you ever felt you should cut down on your drinking?
A: Annoyed	Have people annoyed you by criticizing your drinking?
G: Guilty	Have you ever felt bad or guilty about your drinking?
E: Eye	Eye opener: Have you ever had a drink first thing in the morning to steady your nerves or to get rid of a hangover?

Scoring: Score item responses on the CAGE questions as 0 for "no" and 1 for "yes." A total score of 2 or greater is considered significant.

From National Institute on Drug Abuse. Retrieved from https://nida.nih.gov/nidamed-medical-health-professionals/screening-tools-resources/chart-screening-tools.

TABLE 11.14 Drug Abuse Screening Test (DAST-10)

In the last 12 months:

1. Have you used drugs other than those required for medical reasons?	No	Yes
2. Do you use more than 1 drug at a time?	No	Yes
3. Are you always able to stop using drugs when you want to?	No	Yes
4. Have you had "blackouts" or "flashbacks" as a result of drug use?	No	Yes
5. Do you ever feel bad or guilty about your drug use?	No	Yes
6. Does your spouse (or parents) ever complain about your involvement with drugs?	No	Yes
7. Have you neglected your family because of your use of drugs?	No	Yes
8. Have you engaged in illegal activities in order to obtain drugs?	No	Yes
9. Have you ever had withdrawal symptoms or felt sick when you stopped taking drugs?	No	Yes
10. Have you had medical problems because of your drug use?	No	Yes

Score 1 point for each question answered "Yes," except for question 3, for which a "No" receives 1 point.

Score	Degree of Problem	Suggested Action
0	None	None at this time
1–2	Low	Monitor, reassess later
3–5	Moderate	Investigate further
6–8	Substantial	Intensive assessment
9–10	Severe	Intensive assessment

Retrieved from https://cde.drugabuse.gov/sites/nida_cde/files/DrugAbuseScreeningTest_2014Mar24.pdf.

(Table 11.13), measure the extent of alcohol use. The AUDIT is a 10-question survey. Questions include how often and how much the person drinks, if they feel guilty or remorse about their drinking, and if a relative or friend has been concerned about their drinking. The range of scores is 0 to 40. Scores of 1 to 7 indicate low risk; 8 to 14, potentially harmful use; and 15 and above, a strong chance of moderate to severe alcohol use and AUD.[16] Another useful tool is the Drug Abuse Screening Test (DAST-10), shown in Table 11.14.

If there is any sign of substance use, determine when the patient last used the substance. Knowing this information will let you know when to expect the onset of withdrawal and help you anticipate drug interactions. Assess for other factors that influence withdrawal. These include the dose taken, method of intake, and length of time the patient has used the substance. You may find that the patient is dealing with *polysubstance use*, or the use of more than 1 substance. Alert the HCP, as these patients need care tailored to all the substances used.

Assess for health problems related to substance use. Assess the patient's general appearance and nutrition status. Examine the abdomen, skin, and cardiovascular and respiratory systems. Assess level of consciousness, speech, and memory. Is there a mental health disorder, such as anxiety or depression, which increases the risk for SUD? Serum and urine drug screens can identify the type and amounts of drugs present. A complete blood count, serum electrolytes, blood urea nitrogen, creatinine, and liver function tests may show electrolyte imbalances and heart, kidney, or liver problems.

During your assessment, look for patient behaviors such as denial, avoidance, underreporting or minimizing substance use, or giving inaccurate information. Behaviors and physical manifestations suggesting substance use are outlined in Table 11.15. Remember, these behaviors are not all inclusive (Box 11.1).

◆ Clinical Problems

Clinical problems for patients with SUD include:

- Substance use
- Risk for injury
- Impaired cognition

◆ Planning

The overall goals are that patients with a substance use problem will (1) have normal physiologic functioning, (2) be free from

TABLE 11.15 Findings Suggesting Substance Use

Physiologic
- Fatigue
- Insomnia
- Headaches
- Changes in mood
- Anorexia, weight loss
- Vague physical problems
- Appearing older than age, unkempt appearance
- Sexual problems, decreased libido, erectile dysfunction
- Standard doses of sedatives do not have a therapeutic effect

Behavior
- Mouthwash or toiletries overuse
- Trauma from falls, auto accidents, fights, or burns
- Citations for driving while intoxicated or impaired
- Leisure activities that involve alcohol or other drugs
- Financial problems, including those related to spending on substances
- Defensive or evasive answers to questions about substance use and its importance in the person's life
- Problems in areas of life function, such as frequent job changes; marital problems; work-related accidents, tardiness, or absenteeism; legal problems; social isolation, estranged from friends or family

complications resulting from withdrawal, (3) admit to a substance use problem, and (4) commit to abstaining from substance use.

◆ Implementation

The immediate result of overconsumption is acute toxicity or overdose. Overdoses occur for several reasons. Overdose in the community setting can occur when a person deliberately misuses an illegal or prescription opioid or takes an opioid prescribed for someone else. A person may misunderstand dosing instructions. Unintentional overdose often occurs, especially when depressants are used with alcohol or other drugs.[12] Overdose in the inpatient setting may occur when patients receive an incorrect or high dose, when patients with impaired kidney or liver function receive the drug, or when we give drugs that enhance respiratory depression.

The priority of care is supporting the patient's ABCs, especially respiratory status. The patient may present with trauma or injuries. In addition to treating injuries, provide supportive care until detoxification can occur. Nursing care includes frequently assessing neurologic status and vital signs, giving IV fluids to prevent dehydration, orienting to time and place, and implementing patient safety measures.

Sometimes, uncertainty exists as to what substances are involved. If the patient used multiple substances, a complex clinical picture could result. For example, a patient presents with an overdose, and we do not know what substances are involved. Although blood and urine tests will help identify the substances, treatment is started while waiting for the test results. The patient in this situation would usually receive naloxone. If the substance used is a barbiturate or another CNS depressant, naloxone will not help the patient, but it will not hurt the patient either. If the patient does not respond to a total dose of 10 mg of naloxone, opioids are likely not involved.

Once acute health issues are resolved, you are in a unique position to empower behavior change. When patients seek care for health problems related to substance use or when being hospitalized interferes with the use, their awareness of any substance use problem increases. Intervention at this time can promote behavior change. Take an active role in performing motivational interviewing and providing counseling aimed at cessation. Motivational interviewing is discussed in Chapter 4.

BOX 11.1 ETHICAL/LEGAL DILEMMAS

Board of Nursing Disciplinary Action

Situation

The state board of nursing has received multiple complaints about J.R., an RN who works in a long-term care agency. J.R. has signed off on 3 controlled substances counts that have been inaccurate. The investigation revealed that a few members of the nursing staff knew about J.R.'s reported behavior. They did not report their observations to the unit administrator because the administrator is J.R.'s aunt. After the investigation, the board of nursing subpoenas J.R. to a meeting to discuss charges in preparation for a disciplinary hearing.

Ethical/Legal Points for Consideration
- Regulation of nursing practice is the right of each state. Most have regulatory agencies charged with writing regulations and rules to implement the State Nurse Practice Act. The regulations approved by these agencies carry the weight of the law. Failure to behave accordingly places a nurse at risk for disciplinary action.
- The RN charged with unprofessional behavior is entitled to the same legal rights as any other person. This includes a fair and timely hearing, opportunity to confront the accusers, right to be represented by an attorney, and right to prepare a defense.
- Possible disciplinary actions include temporary suspension or revocation of the nursing license, mandatory rehabilitation for substance use, and mandated supervision and evaluation of practice. Sometimes disciplinary action includes fines and requires reeducation. The state board of nursing may report the action to the state attorney general if evidence suggests the person committed a crime. The RN who is found guilty of unprofessional practice must report this action on all applications for nursing positions.
- All RNs should be familiar with their state's nurse practice act and regulations and the composition and actions of the state board of nursing. Nurses should pay attention to the examples of actionable behavior and disciplinary actions sanctioned by the state.
- RNs have a legal and ethical obligation to report suspected illegal behavior to their administrators and to continue reporting until the situation is resolved. By failing to report, the RN may be charged as an accessory to the act or with unprofessional behavior. The RN risks losing their nursing license.

Discussion Questions
1. What would you do if you suspected a coworker of substance use?
2. How would you handle a situation where retaliation for reporting unprofessional behavior may occur?

Help the patient understand the problem. Discuss the risks associated with substance use and provide counseling. Gauge their level of motivation to access treatment. If the patient agrees, help them access care through referral to treatment.

Gerontologic Considerations: Substance Use

Substance use in older adults is a growing health problem. SUD among older adults is expected to increase as they use more prescription medications and those with a history of unhealthy use from a younger age grow older.[17] Some use alcohol or drugs to cope with grief and loss, such as the death of a spouse.

Because of age-related changes and the higher rate of chronic medical problems, older adults are at greater risk for issues related to substance use. Common problems include liver damage and cardiovascular, GI, and endocrine problems. Substance use may cause confusion, delirium, memory loss, and neuromuscular impairment. Physiologic changes may lead to serum levels that may not have been a problem at a younger age. Withdrawal symptoms may be more severe.

It is important to screen older adults for substance use. The effects of alcohol and drugs can be mistaken for medical conditions common among older adults, such as dementia. So, we may attribute substance use problems to another cause and not offer treatment. Common screening tools may not identify an older adult with a substance use problem. The Short Michigan Alcoholism Screening Test—Geriatric version (SMAST-G) is a short-form alcohol use screening tool for older adults that can identify potential AUD. Family members are important sources of information. Other potential sources include friends, home health aides, meal delivery personnel, and staff members at senior citizen centers and long-term care agencies.

Smoking and other tobacco use is another issue. Those who have smoked for decades may feel unable to stop or believe there is no benefit to stopping at an advanced age. However, smoking contributes to and worsens many chronic illnesses found in older adults. Smoking cessation at any age is beneficial. The information about smoking cessation discussed earlier can help older adults with smoking cessation (Tables 11.3 to 11.6).

Teach the older adult about the desired effects, possible side effects, and proper use of prescribed and OTC drugs. When you suspect alcohol or substance use, refer the patient for treatment. It is a mistaken belief that older people have little to gain from alcohol and drug dependence treatment. The rewards of treatment can lead to greater quality and quantity of life for older adults.

CASE STUDY

Substance Use Disorder

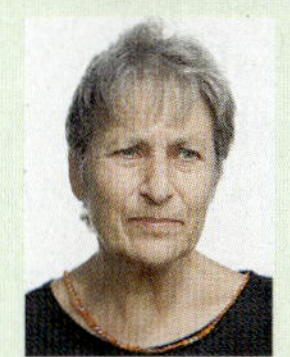

(©XiXinXing/iStock.com)

Patient Profile

C.M., a 78-year-old female, is in the emergency department after falling at home and fracturing her right hip. She has been widowed for 4 years and lives alone. Recently her best friend died. Her only family is a daughter who lives out of state. When contacted by phone, the daughter tells the nurse that her mother has appeared more disoriented and confused over the past few months when she has talked to her on the phone. The patient will be admitted to the medical unit and scheduled for surgical repair.

Subjective Data

- Describing severe pain in her right hip
- Admits she had some wine in the late afternoon to stimulate her appetite
- Has had several falls in the past 2 months
- Reports that she fell after taking a prescribed sleeping pill because she does not sleep well
- Speech is hesitant and slurred
- Says she smokes about a half-pack of cigarettes a day

Objective Data

Physical Assessment

- Oriented to person and place but not time
- BP 162/94, pulse 92, respirations 24
- Severe pain and tenderness in the right hip region
- Bilateral hand tremors

Diagnostic Tests

- X-ray reveals a subtrochanteric fracture of the right femur
- Blood alcohol concentration (BAC) 120 mg/dL (0.12%)
- Complete blood count: Hemoglobin 10.6 g/dL, hematocrit 33%

Discussion Questions

1. ***Recognize:*** What other information do you need to assess C.M.'s condition?
2. ***Recognize:*** What risk factors for substance use are present?
3. ***Analyze:*** What complications and injury risks may occur during C.M.'s postoperative recovery?
4. ***Plan:*** What treatment will C.M. need for substance use?
5. ***Plan:*** What referrals are indicated?
6. ***Prioritize:*** Based on the assessment data given, what are the priority clinical problems?
7. ***Prioritize:*** What are the priority nursing interventions during C.M.'s preoperative period?
8. ***Act:*** How would you use the AP on the postoperative unit to carry out the interventions you identified in question 6?
9. ***Safety:*** To ensure C.M.'s safety, what nursing interventions are necessary after surgery?

Answers available at http://evolve.elsevier.com/Lewis/medsurg.

BRIDGE TO NCLEX EXAMINATION

The number of the question corresponds to the same-numbered outcome at the beginning of the chapter.

1. Which patient is *most* likely to have substance use disorder (SUD) as a contributing factor?
   - **a.** A young adult with multiple sclerosis
   - **b.** An older adult in myasthenic crisis
   - **c.** A middle-aged adult with end-stage liver disease
   - **d.** A middle-aged adult with early onset Alzheimer disease
2. The nurse would suspect cocaine overdose in the patient who is experiencing
   - **a.** agitation, confusion, and seizures.
   - **b.** diarrhea, nausea and vomiting, and confusion.
   - **c.** blurred vision, constricted pupils, and paranoia.
   - **d.** slow, shallow respirations; bradycardia; and hypotension.
3. The *most* appropriate nursing intervention for a patient who is being treated for an exacerbation of emphysema and is not interested in quitting smoking is to
   - **a.** accept the patient's decision and not intervene until the patient expresses a desire to quit.
   - **b.** realize that some smokers never quit and trying to assist them increases the patient's frustration.
   - **c.** ask the patient to identify the risks and benefits of quitting and what barriers to quitting are present.
   - **d.** motivate the patient to quit by describing how continued smoking will worsen the breathing problems.
4. While caring for a patient with alcohol withdrawal, the nurse would **(Select all that apply.)**
   - **a.** monitor neurologic status on a routine basis.
   - **b.** provide a quiet, nonstimulating, dimly lit environment.
   - **c.** pad the side rails and place suction equipment at the bedside.
   - **d.** orient the patient to the environment and person with each contact.
   - **e.** give antiseizure drugs and sedatives to relieve withdrawal symptoms.
5. A patient admitted for scheduled surgery has a positive brief screening test for alcohol use disorder. Which initial action is *most* appropriate?
   - **a.** Notify the health care provider.
   - **b.** Complete a detailed alcohol use assessment.
   - **c.** Initiate a referral to a specialty treatment center.
   - **d.** Provide patient teaching on postoperative health risks.
6. What point would the nurse include in a community presentation about substance use in older adults?
   - **a.** The use of drugs is declining as the population ages.
   - **b.** Older adults who use tobacco do not benefit from cessation.
   - **c.** There is a lower risk of medical problems from substance use.
   - **d.** The effects of drug use may be mistaken for another health problem.

1. c; 2. a; 3. c; 4. a, c, d, e; 5. b; 6. d.

For rationales to these answers and even more NCLEX review questions, visit http://evolve.elsevier.com/Lewis/medsurg.

REFERENCES

To access the References for this chapter, please scan the QR code with a mobile device.

CASE STUDY

Applying Clinical Judgment With Multiple Patients

It is 0715. The following 3 patients are among the 6 you are assigned to care for today on the medical unit. You have an experienced AP assigned to assist you. A float RN can be paged if needed.

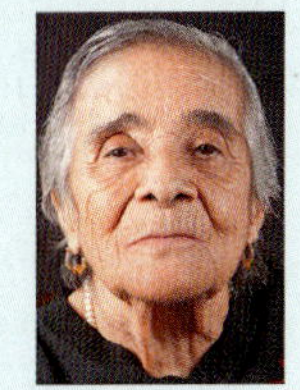 ©Luevanos/iStock	M.S., an 81-year-old female, was admitted yesterday with heart failure. She came to the United States from India 4 years ago. She speaks minimal English, relying on her oldest granddaughter to translate. M.S. has type 2 diabetes and, recently, some memory problems. Vital signs: BP 152/78, pulse 96, RR 24, and O_2 saturation 96% on 2 L/min via nasal cannula.
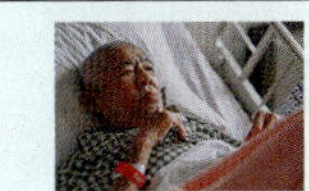 ©Edwin Tan/iStock.com	H.W., an 81-year-old Chinese male, was admitted with confusion and pneumonia. He is receiving IV antibiotics. The next dose is due at 1000. His history includes hypertension, diabetes, prostate cancer, stage 3b chronic kidney disease, Parkinson disease, and significant hearing loss. Lives with his daughter and son-in-law. They are asking when they can take H.W. home.
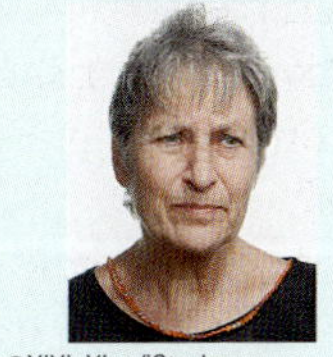 ©XiXinXing/iStock.com	C.M. is a 78-year-old female admitted the previous evening with a right hip fracture. She is in Buck traction. Surgery is scheduled later this morning. She has a history of substance use. Her blood alcohol content (BAC) was 120 mg/dL (0.12%) on admission. The nurse reports she has been confused and restless overnight. She is receiving IV morphine as needed for pain. The last dose was at 0530.

1. Highlight all the findings that require your follow-up.
2. Which patient would you see first? Why?
3. The AP tells you that you need to see M.S. immediately. You enter M.S.'s room and find her sitting up in bed with labored respirations. Although you cannot understand what she is saying, you note that she is unable to say more than a few words without stopping for a breath. Use an X for the nursing actions listed that are indicated (appropriate or necessary) or contraindicated (could be harmful) for M.S. at this time.

Nursing Action	Indicated	Contraindicated
Perform a respiratory assessment.		
Direct the AP to stay with M.S. while you contact the HCP.		
Obtain an order for cardiac biomarkers.		
Access the hospital's translation services.		
Place the head of the bed flat.		
Obtain vital signs with O_2 saturation.		
Prepare for emergency intubation.		

Case Study Progression

M.S.'s assessment reveals bibasilar crackles, 2+ dependent pitting edema, BP 175/84, pulse 116, RR 32, temp 98.2°F (36.8°C), and pulse oximetry 90% on 2 L/min via nasal cannula. You increase the O_2 to 4 L/min per protocol and obtain an order from M.S.'s HCP for furosemide 40 mg IV stat. After giving the diuretic, M.S.'s granddaughter arrives, and you discuss her grandmother's condition. She tells you that her grandmother asked her to bring in potato chips and soda yesterday. She did not think her grandmother should be eating salt, but M.S. insisted that the dietitian said that she could eat them.

4. On further investigation, the dietitian tells you that a translator was not available when she saw M.S. yesterday. Because the dietitian did not understand what M.S. was saying, she could not respond to her questions. She planned to visit M.S. today when the granddaughter is present. Being a culturally competent nurse, you realize that M.S. likely interpreted the dietitian's silence as:
   a. agreement with what M.S. was asking.
   b. demonstrating a lack of respect for M.S.'s wishes.
   c. a lack of understanding by the dietitian as to what M.S. was asking.
   d. a need for the dietitian to get more information before answering questions.

Case Study Progression

Knowing that C.M.'s confusion and restlessness may indicate acute alcohol withdrawal, you go to perform her assessment. You find C.M. trying to pull out the IV line and remove the Buck traction.

5. What action would you take *first*?
   a. Have the AP stay with C.M.
   b. Ask C.M.'s daughter to stay with her.
   c. Obtain a restraint order from the HCP.
   d. Move C.M. to a room closer to the nurse's station.
6. Your assessment reveals a score of 11 on the CIWA-Ar Scale. Choose the *best* option for the information missing from the statement that follows by selecting from the options provided.

*Based on C.M.'s condition, the priority need will be prevention of ______**1**______. To reduce this risk, you would plan to give _____**2**_____ per the HCP's order.*

Options for 1	Options for 2
alcohol withdrawal delirium	enoxaparin
deep vein thrombosis	lorazepam
respiratory depression	naloxone

Case Study Progression

You find yourself falling behind in the care you need to provide for your assigned patients. The charge nurse tells you that the float RN is free to assist you for an hour.

7. Insert an X in each row to indicate which interventions you would include delegate to the AP and which interventions to the float RN.

Intervention	AP	RN
Reapply M.S.'s external urinary incontinence device.		
Titrate M.S.'s O_2 to maintain a pulse oximetry reading of 95%.		
Reassess M.S. after having administered furosemide.		
Move C.M. to a room closer to the nurse's station.		
Reinforce diet teaching for M.S. and her granddaughter.		
Assess H.W.'s IV site for signs of phlebitis.		
Assist H.W. with morning care.		

8. As you assess H.W. you are concerned about the possibility of elder abuse. Which assessment findings would suggest mistreatment? **(Select 5 correct options.)**
   a. Two stage 1 sacral pressure injuries
   b. Asking when his family is coming to visit
   c. Appears to have symptoms of depression
   d. Multiple small bruises on the forearms and shins
   e. Matted hair, poor oral hygiene, overgrown toenails
   f. H.W. becomes silent when his family comes to visit
9. The float RN informs you that the AP is not following H.W.'s fall risk protocol. What is the *most* appropriate action?
   a. Notify the unit manager as soon as possible.
   b. Ask the float RN to explain hospital protocol to the AP.
   c. Write up the AP's actions so they will be included in her evaluation.
   d. Talk to the AP about the importance of following protocol to prevent C.L. from sustaining a fall-related injury.

Answers available at http://evolve.elsevier.com/Lewis/medsurg.

12

Inflammation and Healing

Catherine R. Ratliff

http//evolve.elsevier.com/Lewis/medsurg/

CONCEPTUAL FOCUS

Health Promotion
Inflammation
Nutrition
Pain
Perfusion
Sensory Perception
Tissue Integrity

LEARNING OUTCOMES

1. Describe the inflammatory response, including vascular and cellular responses and exudate formation.
2. Explain local and systemic manifestations of inflammation and their physiologic bases.
3. Describe the drug therapy, nutrition therapy, and nursing management of inflammation.
4. Distinguish among healing by primary, secondary, and tertiary intention.
5. Describe the factors that delay wound healing and common complications of wound healing.
6. Describe the nursing and interprofessional management of wound healing.
7. Explain the etiology and clinical manifestations of pressure injuries.
8. Apply a patient risk assessment to measures used to prevent the development of pressure injuries.
9. Discuss nursing and interprofessional management of patients with pressure injuries.

KEY TERMS

dehiscence, Table 12.9
evisceration, Table 12.9
fibroblasts
inflammatory response
pressure injury
regeneration
repair
shear

This chapter focuses on inflammation, wound healing, and preventing and managing pressure injuries. Maintaining skin and tissue integrity is a key nursing role. Multiple concepts are closely related to tissue integrity. Adequate nutrition and perfusion promote healing when an injury occurs. Impaired mobility and sensory perception increase the risk for injury. When an injury occurs, pain and problems regulating temperature and fluid and electrolyte balance are common.

INFLAMMATION

The **inflammatory response** is a sequential reaction to cell injury. It neutralizes and dilutes the inflammatory agent, removes necrotic materials, and sets up an environment suitable for healing and repair. The term *inflammation* is not a synonym for *infection*. Inflammation is always present with infection, but infection is not always present with inflammation. An infection

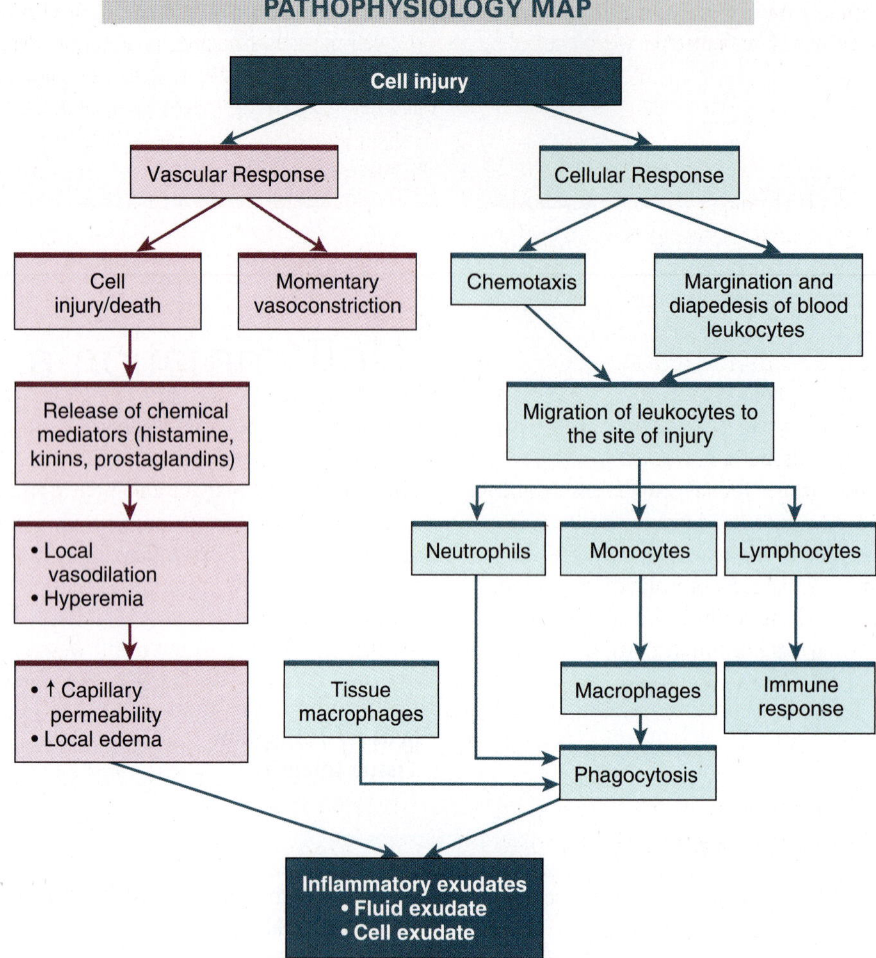

Fig. 12.1 Vascular and cellular responses to tissue injury.

involves the invasion of tissues or cells by microorganisms, such as bacteria, fungi, and viruses. In contrast, heat, radiation, trauma, chemicals, allergens, and an autoimmune reaction can cause inflammation. A person who is neutropenic may have an infection without an inflammatory response.

The intensity of the inflammatory response depends on the extent and severity of the injury and the person's reactive capacity. The inflammatory response is divided into a vascular response, cellular response, exudate formation, and healing. Fig. 12.1 shows the vascular and cellular response to injury. Healing is discussed later in this chapter.

Vascular Response

After cell injury, local arterioles constrict briefly. After release of histamine and other chemicals by the injured cells, the vessels dilate. Chemical mediators increase capillary permeability and promote fluid movement from capillaries into tissue spaces. At first, this inflammatory exudate is made up of serous fluid. Later, it contains plasma proteins, primarily albumin. These proteins exert oncotic pressure that further draws fluid from blood vessels into the area of injury. Both vasodilation and increased capillary permeability are responsible for redness, heat, and swelling around the site of injury.

As the plasma protein fibrinogen leaves the blood, it is activated to fibrin by the products of the injured cells. Fibrin strengthens a blood clot formed by platelets. In tissues, the clot functions to trap bacteria, preventing their spread, and serves as a framework for the healing process. Platelets release growth factors that start the healing process.

Cellular Response

Neutrophils and monocytes move from circulation to the site of injury (Fig. 12.1). *Chemotaxis* is the directional migration of these white blood cells (WBCs) accumulating at the site of injury.

Neutrophils

Neutrophils are the first WBCs to arrive at the injury site (usually within 6 to 12 hours). They phagocytize (engulf) bacteria, other foreign material, and damaged cells. With their short lifespan (24 to 48 hours), dead neutrophils soon accumulate. In time, a mix of dead neutrophils, digested bacteria, and other cell debris accumulate as a creamy substance called *pus.*

To keep up with the demand for neutrophils, the bone marrow releases more neutrophils into circulation. This results in a high WBC count, especially the neutrophil count. Mature neutrophils are called *segmented neutrophils.* Sometimes the demand for neutrophils increases to the extent that the bone marrow releases immature neutrophils *(bands)* into circulation.

We call an increased number of band neutrophils in circulation a *shift to the left.* This is common in patients with acute bacterial infections.

Monocytes

Monocytes are the second type of phagocytic cells that migrate from circulating blood. They usually arrive at the site within 3 to 7 days after the onset of inflammation. On entering the tissue spaces, monocytes transform into macrophages. Together with the tissue macrophages, these new macrophages help with phagocytosis of the inflammatory debris. Because the area must be clean so it can heal, they play a key role in the healing process. Macrophages have a long lifespan. They can multiply and may stay in the damaged tissues for weeks.

When particles are too large for a single macrophage, macrophages accumulate and fuse to form a *multinucleated giant cell.* Collagen encapsulates this giant cell, leading to the formation of a granuloma. A classic example of this process occurs in tuberculosis of the lung. While the *Mycobacterium* bacillus is walled off, a chronic state of inflammation exists. The granuloma formed is a cavity of necrotic tissue.

Lymphocytes

Lymphocytes arrive later at the site of injury. Their primary role is related to humoral and cell-mediated immunity (see Chapter 14).

Chemical Mediators

Table 12.1 describes inflammatory response mediators.

Complement System

The complement system is an enzyme cascade (C1 to C9) consisting of pathways to mediate inflammation and destroy invading pathogens. Major functions of the complement system are enhanced phagocytosis, increased vascular permeability, chemotaxis, and cellular lysis. These activities are important in the inflammatory response and healing.

Cell lysis occurs when the final components create holes in the cell membranes and cause targeted cell death by membrane rupture. In autoimmune disorders, complement activation and the resulting inflammatory response can damage healthy tissue. Examples of this include rheumatoid arthritis and systemic lupus erythematosus.

Prostaglandins and Leukotrienes

With cell injury, the arachidonic acid in the cell membrane is rapidly converted to produce prostaglandins (PGs), thromboxane, and leukotrienes (Fig. 12.2). PGs are considered proinflammatory. They are potent vasodilators contributing to increased blood flow and edema formation.

Some subtypes of PGs form when platelets are activated. They can inhibit platelet and neutrophil aggregation. PGs have a significant role in sensitizing pain receptors to arousal by stimuli that would normally be painless. PGs stimulate the temperature-regulating area of the hypothalamus, producing a febrile response.

Thromboxane is a powerful vasoconstrictor and platelet-aggregating agent. It causes brief vasoconstriction and skin pallor at the injury site and promotes clot formation. It has a short half-life. The pallor soon gives way to vasodilation and redness, which is caused by PGs and histamine.

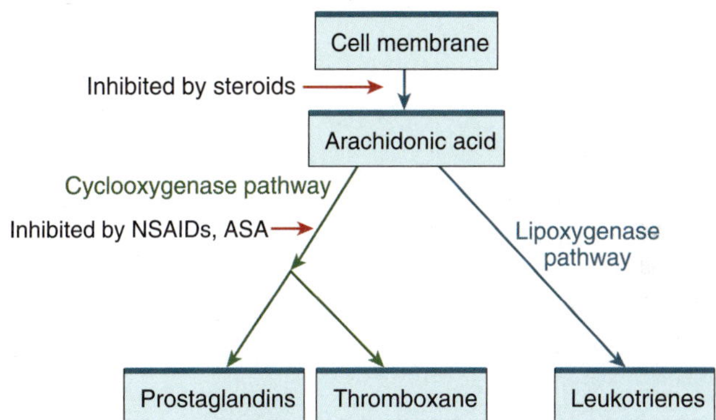

Fig. 12.2 Pathway of generation of prostaglandins, thromboxane, and leukotrienes. Corticosteroids, *NSAIDs,* and acetylsalicylic acid *(ASA)* act to inhibit various steps in this pathway.

TABLE 12.1 Mediators of Inflammation

Mediator	Source	Mechanisms of Action
Complement components (C3a, C4a, C5a)	Anaphylatoxins generated from complement pathway activation	Stimulate histamine release and chemotaxis
Cytokines (see Table 14.3)	Mainly produced by macrophages and lymphocytes	Act as intercellular and intracellular messengers
Histamine	Stored in granules of basophils, mast cells, platelets	Cause vasodilation and increased capillary permeability
Kinins (e.g., bradykinin)	Produced from precursor factor kininogen because of activation of Hageman factor (XII) of clotting system	Cause contraction of smooth muscle and vasodilation. Result in stimulation of pain
Prostaglandins (PGs) **and leukotrienes** (LTs)	Produced from arachidonic acid (Fig. 12.2)	PGs cause vasodilation. LTs stimulate chemotaxis
Serotonin	Stored in platelets, mast cells, enterochromaffin cells of GI tract	Same as histamine. Stimulate smooth muscle contraction

TABLE 12.2 **Types of Inflammatory Exudate**

Type	Description	Examples
Catarrhal	Found in tissues where cells produce mucus Inflammatory response accelerates mucus production	Runny nose from an upper respiratory tract infection
Fibrinous	Occurs with increasing vascular permeability and fibrinogen leakage into interstitial spaces Excess amounts of fibrin that coats tissue surfaces may cause them to adhere	Adhesions, gelatinous ribbons seen in surgical drain tubing Often covers fluid-exuding wounds, such as venous injuries
Hemorrhagic	Results from rupture or necrosis of blood vessel walls	Hematoma, bleeding after surgery, tissue trauma
Purulent (pus)	Consists of WBCs, microorganisms (dead and alive), liquefied dead cells, and other debris	Furuncle (boil), abscess, cellulitis (diffuse inflammation in connective tissue)
Serosanguineous	Found during the midpoint in healing after surgery or tissue injury Composed of RBCs and serous fluid, which is semiclear pink and may have red streaks	Surgical drain fluid
Serous	Results from outpouring of fluid. Seen in early stages of inflammation or when injury is mild	Skin blisters, pleural effusion

Leukotrienes form the slow-reacting substance of anaphylaxis (SRS-A). SRS-A constricts smooth muscles of the bronchi, causing narrowing of the airway, and increases capillary permeability. This leads to airway edema.

Exudate Formation

Exudate consists of fluid and WBCs that move from the circulation to the site of injury. The nature and quantity of exudate depend on the type and severity of the injury and tissues involved (Table 12.2).

Types of Inflammation

The basic types of inflammation are acute, subacute, and chronic. In *acute inflammation,* the healing occurs in 2 to 3 weeks and usually leaves no residual damage. Neutrophils are the main cell type at the site of inflammation. *Subacute inflammation* has the features of the acute process but lasts longer. For example, subacute infective endocarditis has acute inflammation, but it can last for weeks (see Chapter 40).

Chronic inflammation lasts for weeks, months, or even years. The injurious agent persists or repeatedly injures tissue. The main cell types present at the site of inflammation are lymphocytes and macrophages. Examples include rheumatoid arthritis and osteomyelitis. Chronic inflammation may result from an altered immune response (e.g., autoimmune disease) and can lead to physical decline.

Clinical Manifestations

Local manifestations of inflammation include redness, heat, pain, swelling, and loss of function (Table 12.3 and Fig. 12.3). Systemic manifestations include an increased WBC count with a shift to the left, fatigue, nausea, anorexia, increased pulse and respiratory rate, and fever.

TABLE 12.3 **Local Manifestations of Inflammation**

Manifestations	Cause
Heat	Increased metabolism at inflammatory site
Loss of function	Swelling and pain
Pain	Change in pH. Nerve stimulation by chemicals (e.g., histamine, prostaglandins). Pressure from fluid exudate
Redness	Hyperemia from vasodilation
Swelling	Fluid shift to interstitial spaces. Fluid exudate accumulation

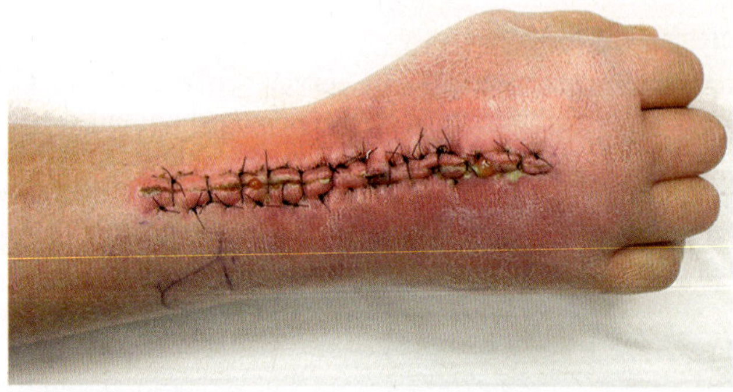

Fig. 12.3 Inflammation with a deep wound infection after wrist surgery. (From Hayden RJ, Jebson PJL: Wrist arthrodesis, *Hand Clin* 21[4]:631, 2005.)

Leukocytosis results from the increased release of WBCs from the bone marrow. The causes of other systemic manifestations may be related to complement activation and the release of cytokines. Some cytokines (e.g., interleukins [ILs], tumor necrosis factor [TNF]) are important in causing fever and other systemic manifestations of inflammation. An increase in pulse and respiration follows the rise in metabolism because of an increase in temperature.

Fever

Cytokine release triggers the onset of fever. Cytokines cause fever by initiating metabolic changes in the temperature-regulating center in the hypothalamus (Fig. 12.4). PG synthesis is the most critical metabolic change. PGs act directly to increase the thermostatic set point. The hypothalamus then activates the autonomic nervous system to stimulate increased muscle tone and shivering and decrease perspiration and peripheral blood flow. Epinephrine released from the adrenal medulla increases the metabolic rate. The net result is fever.

With the physiologic thermostat raised to a higher-than-normal temperature, the body increases heat production and conservation until the temperature reaches that new set point. At this point, the person feels chilled and shivers. The shivering response is the body's way of raising the body's temperature to the new set point. This seeming paradox is dramatic. The body is hot, yet the person piles on blankets and may go to bed to get warm. When the temperature reaches the setpoint, the chills and warmth-seeking behavior cease.

The released cytokines and the fever that they trigger activate the body's defense mechanisms. Benefits of fever include increased killing of microorganisms, increased phagocytosis by neutrophils, and increased proliferation of T cells.[1] Fever may enhance the activity of interferon, the body's natural virus-fighting substance (see Chapter 14).

PATHOPHYSIOLOGY MAP

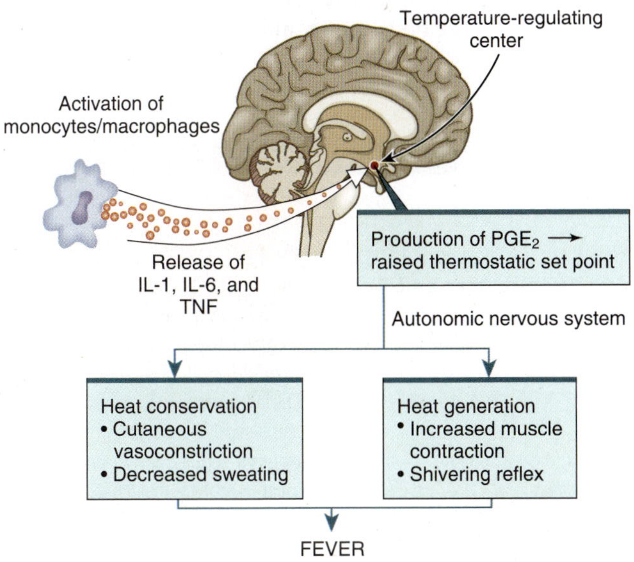

Fig. 12.4 Fever production. When monocytes/macrophages are activated, they secrete cytokines such as interleukin-1 *(IL-1)*, interleukin-6 *(IL-6)*, and tumor necrosis factor *(TNF)*, which reach the hypothalamic temperature-regulating center. These cytokines promote the synthesis and secretion of prostaglandin E_2 *(PGE_2)* in the anterior hypothalamus. PGE_2 increases the thermostatic setpoint. This stimulates the autonomic nervous system, resulting in shivering, muscle contraction, and peripheral vasoconstriction.

NURSING MANAGEMENT: INFLAMMATION

Assessment

Early recognition of inflammation is important so that proper treatment can begin. Assess for the cause of the inflammation (Table 12.4). Are there any risk factors that may limit the patient's ability to respond to inflammation? In the immunosuppressed person (e.g., taking corticosteroids, receiving chemotherapy), the classic manifestations of inflammation may be masked. The only early symptoms may be malaise or "just not feeling well."

Note the patient's vital signs with any inflammation. When infection is present, the temperature, pulse, and respiratory rate may increase.

Clinical Problems

Clinical problems for patients with inflammation include:

- Inflammation
- Altered temperature
- Impaired tissue integrity

A nursing care plan for patients with a fever (eNursing Care Plan 12.1) is available on the website for this chapter at http://evolve.elsevier.com/Lewis/medsurg.

Implementation

Most treatment of inflammation depends on the cause. The care of patients with acute inflammation is directed at mediating the inflammatory process to promote tissue healing. This may include rest, drug therapy, or specific treatment of the injured site. Immediate treatment may prevent the extension and complications of inflammation. Interventions for those with chronic inflammation aim to prevent or slow tissue damage.

TABLE 12.4 Common Causes of Inflammation

Acute Inflammation	Chronic Inflammation
• Allergic reaction	• Asthma
• Anaphylaxis	• Chronic obstructive pulmonary disease (COPD)
• Appendicitis	• Cirrhosis
• Burn injury	• Diverticulitis
• Cholecystitis	• Fibromyalgia
• Foreign-body injury	• Inflammatory bowel disease
• Infection	• Multiple sclerosis
• Insect bite or sting	• Myasthenia gravis
• Joint strain or sprain	• Osteoarthritis
• Nephritis	• Psoriasis
• Septic shock	• Rheumatoid arthritis
• Trauma	• Systemic lupus erythematosus
• Upper respiratory infection	• Tuberculosis

Adequate nutrition provides the necessary factors to promote healing after injury. A high fluid intake will replace fluid loss from perspiration. There is a 7% increase in metabolism for every 1°F increase in temperature above 100°F (37.8°C), or a 13% increase for every 1°C increase. The increased metabolic rate increases a patient's need for calories.

Fever

The nursing management of patients with a fever is outlined in Table 12.5. Because mild to moderate fever usually does little harm, imposes no great discomfort, and may help host defense mechanisms, antipyretic drugs are rarely essential. Moderate fevers (up to 103°F [39.4°C]) cause few problems in most patients.[1] However, if the patient is very young or very old, is very uncomfortable, or has a significant medical problem (e.g., severe heart or lung disease, brain injury), antipyretic use should be considered. Fever in immunosuppressed patients should be treated immediately with antibiotic therapy because infections can rapidly progress to septicemia. Neutropenia is discussed in Chapter 34.

High fever, especially if greater than 104°F (40°C), can damage body cells, including those in the brain. Delirium and seizures can occur. At temperatures greater than 105.8°F (41°C), the hypothalamic temperature control center becomes impaired. Older adults have a blunted febrile response to infection. The temperature may not rise to the level expected for a younger adult, or there may be a delay in the onset of the rise. The blunted response can delay diagnosis and treatment. By the time fever (as defined for younger adults) is present, the illness may be more severe. Patients who are taking nonsteroidal antiinflammatory drugs (NSAIDs) on a regular basis may have a blunted febrile response.

TABLE 12.5 NURSING MANAGEMENT
Patient With a Fever

- Notify the HCP of a fever per agency policy.
- Monitor the patient with a temperature up to 103°F (39.4°C) without trying to lower it. Focus interventions on patient comfort.
- Give medications as prescribed, including antibiotics, and antipyretics or antiinflammatories (Table 12.6).
- Ensure adequate fluid intake through oral or IV fluid therapy as prescribed.
- Assess for fluid volume deficit.
- Implement needed measures to decrease temperature, such as:
  - Applying cooling blankets
  - Providing a tepid bath
  - Applying cold packs
  - Using a fan to cool the environment
- Keep linens and clothing clean and dry.
- Initiate fall and seizure precautions for the patient with neurologic or neuromuscular manifestations.
- Provide optimal skin and oral care.

Drug Therapy

Drugs can decrease the inflammatory response and lower the temperature (Table 12.6). Some NSAIDs (e.g., ibuprofen) have antipyretic effects. Corticosteroids are antipyretic through preventing cytokine production and PG synthesis. This results in dilation of superficial blood vessels, increased skin temperature, and sweating.

CHECK YOUR PRACTICE

A 76-year-old female patient has acute osteomyelitis after a fractured femur. You check her temperature every 2 hours and giving acetaminophen when it is higher than 102°F. However, you notice that her temperature fluctuates from 96°F to 103°F.

- What should you do?

Antipyretics cause a sharp decrease in temperature. They should be given regularly at 2- to 4-hour intervals to prevent acute swings in temperature. Given intermittently, they can induce or perpetuate chills. When the antipyretic wears off, the body may initiate a compensatory involuntary muscular contraction (i.e., chill) to raise the body temperature back up to its previous level.

RICE

Rest, **I**ce, **C**ompression, **E**levation (RICE) is a key treatment for soft tissue injuries and related inflammation.

Rest. Rest, or immobilization, prevents further injury and gives the body time to heal. It decreases the tissues' metabolic needs and helps the body use its nutrients and O_2 for healing. The repair process is facilitated by allowing fibrin and collagen

TABLE 12.6 Drug Therapy
Inflammation

Drug	Mechanism of Action
Antiinflammatory and Antipyretic	
Corticosteroids	Inhibit accumulation of inflammatory cells at site, tissue granulation, lysosome release, prostaglandin (PG) synthesis, and cytokine release and induce immunosuppressive effects (decreased lymphocyte synthesis)
NSAIDs (e.g., ibuprofen, piroxicam)	Inhibit PG synthesis (Fig. 12.2). Act on heat-regulating center in hypothalamus to lower temperature.
Salicylates (aspirin)	Inhibit PG synthesis (Fig. 12.2). Lower temperature by action on heat-regulating center in hypothalamus, resulting in peripheral vasodilation and heat loss. Reduce capillary permeability.
Antipyretic	
Acetaminophen	Lowers temperature by action on heat-regulating center in hypothalamus.

to form across the wound edges with little disruption. Applying a cast or splint supports fractured bones and prevents further tissue injury from sharp bone fragments that could sever nerves or blood vessels, causing bleeding (see Chapter 67).

Ice (thermal therapy). Cold application is usually best at the time of the initial trauma. Cold promotes vasoconstriction and decreases swelling, pain, and congestion from increased metabolism in the area of inflammation. Heat may be used later (e.g., after 24 to 48 hours) to promote healing by increasing circulation to the inflamed site. This promotes the removal of debris. Heat can localize inflammatory agents. Warm, moist heat may help debride the wound if necrotic material is present.

Compression. Compression counters the vasodilation effects and development of edema. Compression by direct pressure over a laceration occludes blood vessels and stops bleeding. Compression bandages support injured joints when tendons and muscles are unable to provide support. Assess distal pulses and capillary refill before and after applying compression to make sure the compression does not compromise circulation (e.g., pale color of skin, loss of feeling).

Elevation. Elevating the injured extremity above the level of the heart reduces edema at the inflammatory site by increasing venous and lymphatic return. It helps reduce pain from blood engorgement at the injury site. Elevation may be contraindicated in patients with reduced arterial circulation.

HEALING PROCESS

The last phase of the inflammatory response is healing. Healing includes 2 major components: regeneration and repair.

Regeneration

Regeneration is the replacement of lost cells and tissues with cells of the same type. The ability of cells to regenerate depends on the cell type (Table 12.7).

Repair

Repair is the more common type of healing, with connective tissue replacing lost cells. Repair is a more complex process than regeneration. Repair healing occurs by primary, secondary, or tertiary intention and usually results in scar formation (Fig. 12.5).

Primary Intention

Primary intention healing takes place when wound margins are neatly approximated, as in a surgical incision or a paper cut. A continuum of processes is associated with primary healing (Table 12.8). These include 4 phases: hemostasis, inflammatory, proliferation, and remodeling.

Hemostasis phase. In hemostasis, the edges of the incision are aligned and sutured (or stapled) in place. The incision area fills with blood from the cut blood vessels. Blood clots form, and platelets release growth factors to begin the healing process. This forms a matrix for WBC migration.

TABLE 12.7 Regenerative Ability of Different Types of Tissues

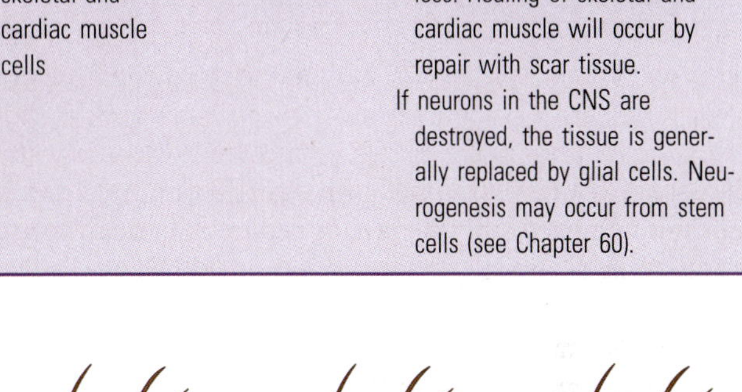

Tissues	Cell Type	Description
Skin, lymphoid organs, bone marrow, mucous membranes	Labile cells	Cells divide constantly. Injury to these organs is followed by rapid regeneration.
Liver, pancreas, kidney, bone cells	Stable cells	Retain their ability to regenerate but do so only if the organ is injured. Regeneration is slow.
Neurons of the central nervous system (CNS), skeletal and cardiac muscle cells	Permanent cells	Do not divide. Damage to CNS neurons or skeletal or heart muscle can lead to permanent loss. Healing of skeletal and cardiac muscle will occur by repair with scar tissue. If neurons in the CNS are destroyed, the tissue is generally replaced by glial cells. Neurogenesis may occur from stem cells (see Chapter 60).

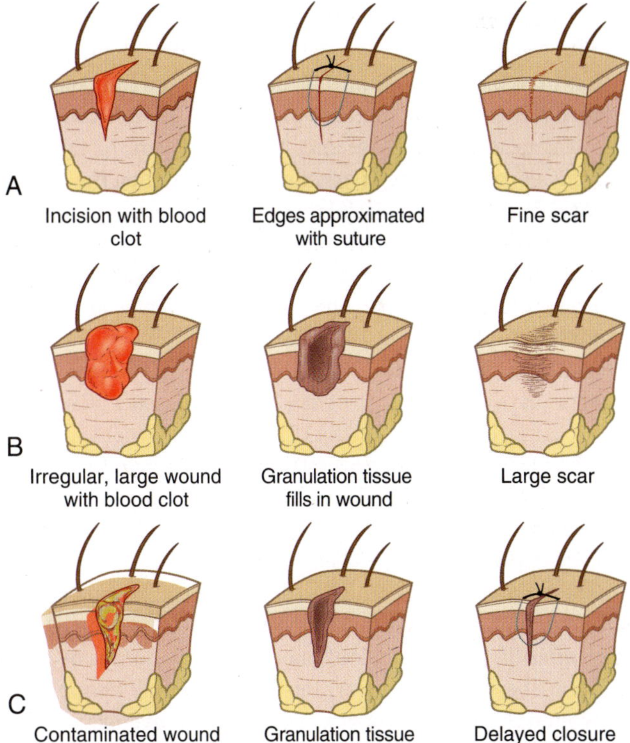

Fig. 12.5 Types of wound healing. (A) Primary intention. (B) Secondary intention. (C) Tertiary intention.

Inflammatory phase. An acute inflammatory reaction occurs with WBC migration. Fibrin clots, red blood cells (RBCs), neutrophils (dead and dying), and other debris are in the area of injury. Macrophages ingest and digest cellular debris, fibrin fragments, and RBCs. Extracellular enzymes derived from

TABLE 12.8 **Phases in Primary Intention Healing**

Phase	Duration	Description
Hemostasis	Up to 2 days	Approximation of incision edges. Clot serving as meshwork for starting capillary growth
Inflammatory	3–5 days	Macrophages ingest and digest cellular debris, fibrin fragments, and RBCs
Proliferative	5 days to 4 weeks	Migration of fibroblasts. Secretion of collagen. Abundance of capillary buds. Wound fragile
Remodeling	7 days to several months	Remodeling of collagen. Strengthening of scar

macrophages and neutrophils help digest fibrin. As the wound debris is removed, the fibrin clot serves as a meshwork for future capillary growth and migration of epithelial cells.

Proliferation phase. Cytokines drive the proliferation of fibroblasts and formation of granulation tissue. Granulation tissue includes proliferating fibroblasts, proliferating capillary sprouts *(angioblasts)*, various WBCs, exudate, extracellular matrix, proteoglycans, hyaluronic acid, collagen, and elastin.

Fibroblasts are immature connective tissue cells that migrate into the healing site and secrete collagen. In time, the collagen is organized and restructured to strengthen the healing site. At this stage, we call it *fibrous* or *scar tissue.*

During the granulation phase, the wound is pink and vascular. Numerous red granules (young budding capillaries) are present. At this point, the wound is friable, at risk for **dehiscence**, and resistant to infection.

Surface epithelium at the wound edges begins to regenerate. In a few days, a thin layer of epithelium migrates across the wound surface in a 1-cell-thick layer until it contacts cells spreading from the opposite direction. The epithelium thickens and begins to mature, and the wound now closely resembles the adjacent skin. In a superficial wound, reepithelialization may take 3 to 5 days.

Remodeling phase. Remodeling, during which scar contraction occurs, overlaps with granulation. It may begin 7 days after the injury and continue for several months or years. Collagen fibers are further organized. Fibroblasts disappear as the wound becomes stronger. The active movement of the myofibroblasts causes contraction of the healing area, helping to close the defect and bring the skin edges closer together. A mature scar is then formed. A mature scar is virtually avascular and pale. The scar may be more painful at this phase than in the granulation phase.

Secondary Intention

Wounds that occur from trauma, injury, and infection have large amounts of exudate and wide, irregular wound margins with extensive tissue loss. These wounds may have edges that cannot be approximated or brought together. The inflammatory reaction may be greater than in primary healing. This results in more debris, cells, and exudate. We may have to clear the debris away *(debride)* before healing can take place.

Healing by secondary intention is basically the same as healing by primary intention. The major differences are the greater defect and the gaping wound edges. Healing and granulation take place from the edges inward and from the bottom of the wound upward until the wound is filled. There is more granulation tissue. The result is a much larger scar.

Tertiary Intention

Tertiary intention (delayed primary intention) healing occurs with delayed suturing of a wound in which 2 layers of granulation tissue are sutured together. This occurs when a contaminated wound is left open and sutured closed after the infection is controlled. It also occurs when a primary wound becomes infected, is opened, allowed to granulate, and then sutured. Tertiary intention usually results in a larger and deeper scar than primary or secondary intention.

Wound Classification

A *wound* is a break or opening into the skin. Wounds often occur because of surgery, accidents, or injuries. Types of wounds can range from minor scrapes to deep wounds involving bones, blood vessels, and nerves.

We classify wounds by their cause (surgical or nonsurgical; acute or chronic) and the depth of tissue affected (superficial, partial thickness, or full thickness) (Fig. 12.6). A *superficial wound* involves only the epidermis. *Partial-thickness* wounds extend into the dermis. *Full-thickness* wounds have the deepest layer of tissue destruction. They involve the subcutaneous tissue and sometimes extend into the fascia and underlying structures, including muscle, tendon, or bone.

A *skin tear* is a wound caused by shear, friction, and/or blunt force resulting in the separation of skin layers. A skin tear can be partial thickness or full thickness. This type of wound is common, especially in older adults and critically or chronically ill adults.[2]

Complications of Healing

Factors that can impede wound healing and lead to complications are described in Table 12.9.

NURSING MANAGEMENT: WOUND HEALING

Assessment

In general, you are responsible for assessing wounds and managing wound care (Table 12.10). You may work with a Wound, Ostomy, and Continence Nurse (WOCN) or HCP

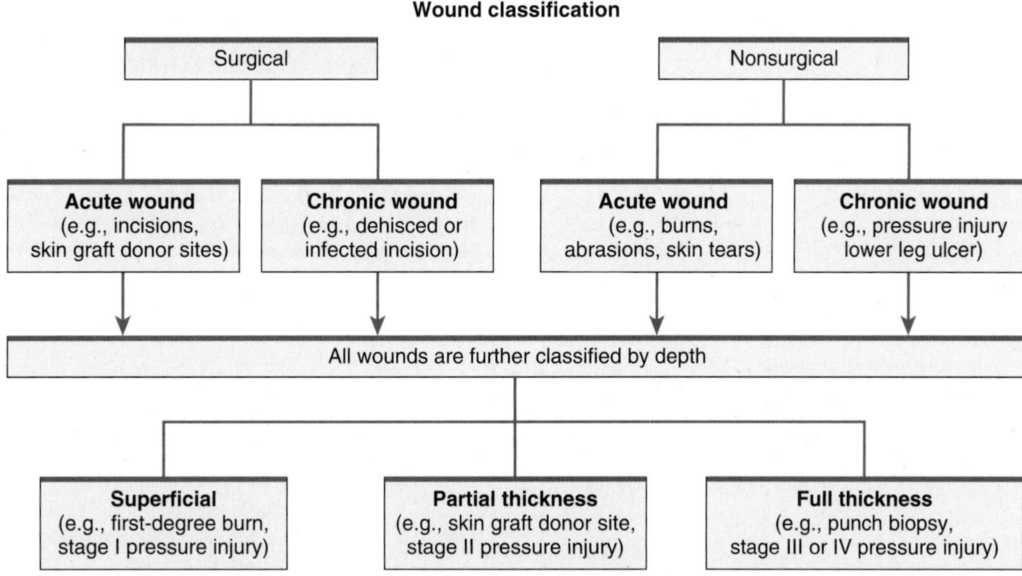

Fig. 12.6 Classification of wounds by their cause and the depth of tissue affected.

TABLE 12.9 Complications of Wound Healing

Adhesions
- Bands of scar tissue that form between or around organs
- May occur in the abdominal cavity or between the lungs and the pleura
- In the abdomen may cause an intestinal obstruction

Contractions
- Wound contraction is a normal part of healing
- Complications occur when excessive contraction results in deformity
- Shortening of muscle or scar tissue, especially over joints, results from excessive fibrous tissue formation

Dehiscence
- Separation and disruption of previously joined wound edges
- Usually occurs when a primary healing site bursts open
- May be caused by:
  - Infection causing inflammation
  - Granulation tissue not strong enough to withstand forces imposed on wound
  - Obesity, because adipose tissue has less blood supply and may slow healing
  - Pocket of fluid (seroma, hematoma) developing between tissue layers and preventing the edges of the wound from coming together

Evisceration
- Occurs when wound edges separate to the extent that intestines protrude through wound
- Usually needs immediate surgical treatment

Excess Granulation Tissue
- Excess granulation tissue protrudes above surface of healing wound
- If the tissue is cauterized or cut off, healing continues in normal manner

Fistula Formation
- An abnormal passage between organs or a hollow organ and skin (abdominal or perianal fistula)

Infection (Fig. 12.3)
- Risk increases when wound contains necrotic tissue, or with impaired blood supply, impaired immune function (e.g., from immunosuppressive drugs), undernutrition, multiple stressors, hyperglycemia

Hemorrhage
- Causes include suture failure, clotting problems, dislodged clot, infection, erosion of a blood vessel by a foreign object (tubing, drains), infection

Hypertrophic Scars
- Inappropriately large, raised red and hard scars
- Occur when an overabundance of collagen is made during healing

Keloid Formation
- Great protrusion of scar tissue that extends beyond wound edges and may form tumor-like masses of scar tissue
- Permanent without any tendency to subside
- May be tenderness, pain, and paresthesia, especially in early stages
- Occurs most often in persons with dark skin

specializing in wound management to treat and manage chronic wounds, traumatic or draining wounds, pressure injuries, and fistulas.

Assess the wound on admission or first clinic visit and then on a regular basis. Begin by obtaining a history of the wound. What is the cause of the wound? If it is a chronic wound, how long has it been present? In healthy people, wounds heal at a normal, predictable rate. Assess for factors that may delay wound healing or contribute to a wound not healing as expected (Table 12.11). Continually assess for complications

TABLE 12.10 NURSING MANAGEMENT

Wound Care

- Assess patient for factors that may delay wound healing and develop a plan of care to address these factors (see Table 12.11).
- Assess and document initial wound appearance, including wound size, depth, color, and drainage (see Table 12.12).
- Provide proper wound care, choosing dressings and therapies for wound treatment in conjunction with the HCP or WOCN (see Table 12.14).
- Implement measures to promote wound healing and prevent further injury, including positioning devices to reduce shear and pressure, moisture management, and nutrition care.
- Implement needed infection control measures.
- Assist the patient with managing any body image concerns and fears.
- Provide effective pain management.
- Evaluate whether wound care is effective in promoting wound healing.
- Teach patient and caregivers about wound care and pressure injury prevention.
- Supervise LPN/VN:
  - Perform dressing changes.
  - Apply ordered topical agents to wounds.
  - Apply prescribed medications for wound debridement.
  - Collect and record wound assessment data.
- Collaborate with dietitian to:
  - Assess and monitor patient's nutrition status.
  - Outline diet to support proper wound healing.

(e.g., infection) associated with healing (Table 12.9). If wound deterioration occurs, assess and document changes more often.

Perform a thorough wound assessment (Table 12.12). Determine the type of wound and its involvement (Table 12.13).[3] Note the location and size. There are several ways to measure a wound. One way is shown in Fig. 12.7. Assess the wound margin and wound bed. Record the consistency, color, approximate amount, and odor of any drainage. Report if abnormal for the situation. *Staphylococcus* and *Pseudomonas* are common organisms that cause purulent, draining wounds.

Implementation

The type of wound management and dressings needed depend on the type, extent, and characteristics of the wound and the phase of healing.[4] The purposes of wound management include (1) protecting a clean wound from trauma so that it can heal normally, (2) cleaning a wound to remove any dirt and debris from the wound bed, and (3) preventing and treating infection.[5] There are many wound products (Table 12.14).

Clean Wounds

Superficial skin injuries may only need cleansing. Materials used to close wounds include adhesive strips (e.g., Steri-Strips), sutures (stitches), staples, and tissue adhesives (fibrin sealants). We use adhesive strips for some injuries because they decrease scarring and are easy to care for. Sutures are used when wounds need mechanical support to

TABLE 12.11 Factors Delaying Wound Healing

Factor	Effect on Wound Healing
Advanced Age	Slows collagen synthesis by fibroblasts, impairs circulation, needs longer time for epithelialization of skin, alters phagocytic and immune responses
Anemia	Supplies less O_2 at tissue level
Corticosteroid Drugs	Impair phagocytosis by WBCs, inhibit fibroblast proliferation and function, depress formation of granulation tissue, inhibit wound contraction
Diabetes	Decreases collagen synthesis, delays capillary growth, impairs phagocytosis (result of hyperglycemia), reduces supply of O_2 and nutrients due to vascular disease
Impaired Perfusion	Decreases supply of nutrients to injured area, decreases removal of exudative debris, inhibits inflammatory response
Infection	Increases inflammatory response and tissue destruction
Mechanical Friction on Wound	Destroys granulation tissue, prevents apposition of wound edges
Nutrition Deficiencies	
Vitamin C	Delays formation of collagen fibers and capillary development
Protein	Decreases supply of amino acids for tissue repair
Zinc	Impairs epithelialization
Obesity	Decreases blood supply in fatty tissue
Poor General Health	Causes general absence of factors necessary to promote wound healing
Smoking	Nicotine, a potent vasoconstrictor, impedes blood flow to healing areas

TABLE 12.12 NURSING ASSESSMENT

Wound Assessment

Include the following when performing a wound assessment and monitoring for wound healing:

- Location of the wound
- Type of wound
- Measure the depth, length (head to toe), and width of the wound (see Fig. 12.7)
- Wound bed tissue type (e.g., granulation tissue, eschar, slough)
- Wound margins for tunneling, undermining, rolling (epibole), fibrotic changes, not attached
- Presence, type, and amount of drainage:
  - Serous, serosanguineous, sanguineous, purulent
  - None, scant, minimal, moderate, large
- Presence of odor after cleansing the wound
- Perfusion to the wound and surrounding tissue
- Condition of tissue around the wound
- Signs and symptoms of infection
- Associated symptoms, including pain, loss of function

Adapted from Nagle SM, Stevens KA, Wilbraham SC: *Wound assessment*. Retrieved from https://www.ncbi.nlm.nih.gov/books/NBK482198/.

TABLE 12.13 **Wound Classifications by Degree of Tissue Involvement**

Involved Tissues	Types of Wounds
Epidermis	Grade 0 diabetic foot ulcer Partial thickness, superficial burn Stage 1 pressure injury Superficial injury, abrasions Type 1a skin tear
Epidermis, dermis	Grade 1 diabetic foot ulcer Partial thickness, deep burn Skin graft donor site Stage 2 pressure injury Type 1b, 2, and 3 skin tears
Epidermis, dermis, subcutaneous tissue, and fascia	Grade 2 diabetic foot ulcer Full-thickness burn Punch biopsy Stage 3 pressure injury
Epidermis, dermis, subcutaneous tissue and fascia, deep fascia, underlying structures (muscle, bone, tendon)	Dehisced surgical wound Full-thickness burn Grade 3 diabetic foot ulcer Stage 4 pressure injury

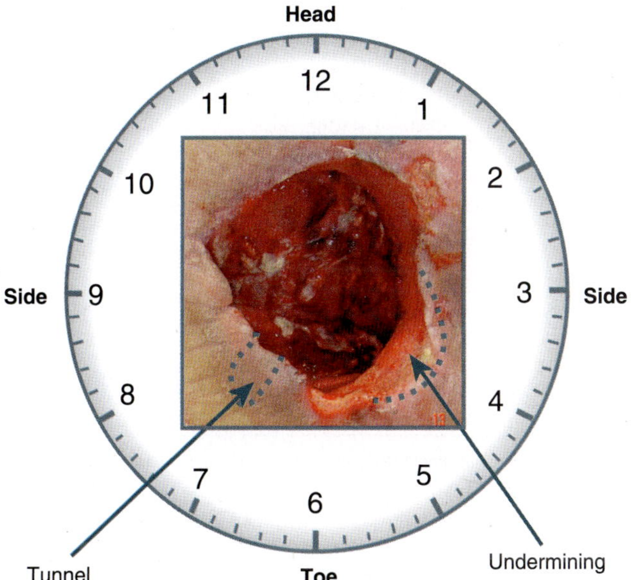

Fig. 12.7 Wound measurements are made in centimeters. The first measurement is oriented from head to toe, the second is from side to side, and the third is the depth (if any). Chart any tunneling or undermining in respect to a clock, with 12 o'clock being toward the patient's head. You would chart this wound as a full-thickness, red wound, 7 × 5 × 3 cm, with a 3-cm tunnel at 7 o'clock and 2 cm undermining from 3 o'clock to 5 o'clock. (Courtesy Robert B. Babiak, RN, BSN, CWOCN, San Antonio, TX.)

sustain closure. A wide variety of suturing materials are available. Tissue adhesives are biologic adhesives that are applied alone or with sutures or tape. Topical skin adhesive is a liquid that holds surgical incisions and laceration wound edges together instead of sutures or staples.

A dressing material that keeps the wound surface clean and slightly moist promotes epithelialization. For wounds that heal by primary intention, we often cover the wound or incision with a dry dressing. It is removed when the drainage stops or in 2 to 3 days. Transparent film or adhesive semipermeable dressings are common choices. Sometimes an HCP will leave a surgical wound uncovered or remove the dressing within 48 hours after surgery. Medicated sprays that form a transparent film on the skin may be used as a dressing on a clean incision or injury. Keep clean wounds that are granulating and reepithelializing slightly moist and protected from further trauma until they heal naturally. Do not let a wound that has the potential to heal dry out. Wounds need a moist environment to heal.[6] Unnecessary manipulation during dressing changes may destroy new granulation tissue and break down fibrin formation.

Sometimes drains are inserted into the wound to help remove fluid. The Jackson-Pratt (JP) drain is a suction drainage device consisting of a flexible plastic bulb connected to an internal plastic drainage tube (Fig. 12.8).

Contaminated Wounds

A contaminated wound must be converted into a clean wound before healing can occur normally. Debridement of a wound that has debris or dead tissue may be needed. The debridement method used depends on the type of wound, amount of debris, and the condition of the wound tissue (Table 12.15).

One option is absorptive dressings. They can absorb exudate and draw excess drainage from the wound surface. The amount of wound drainage and type of dressing dictate the frequency of dressing changes.

In hydrocolloid dressings, the inner part of the dressing interacts with the exudate, forming a hydrated gel over the wound. When we remove the dressing, the gel separates and stays over the wound. Clean the wound gently to prevent damage to newly formed tissue. These dressings can stay in place for up to 7 days or until leakage occurs around the dressing.

Negative-Pressure Wound Therapy

Negative-pressure wound therapy (NPWT) is used to treat acute and chronic wounds (Box 12.1). A vacuum source creates continuous or intermittent negative pressure inside the wound to remove fluid, exudates, and infectious materials. We do not know exactly how NPWT promotes tissue granulation. We think that it pulls excess fluid from the wound, reduces bacterial load, and increases blood flow into the wound base.[7]

NPWT systems consist of a vacuum pump, drainage tubing, a foam dressing, and an adhesive film dressing that covers and seals the wound.[7] In NPWT, we cleanse the wound, then cut a foam dressing to fit the dimensions of the wound. A larger occlusive dressing is applied, with a small hole made over the foam dressing where the tubing is attached (Fig. 12.9). The tubing connects to the vacuum pump, which creates the negative pressure. The vacuum pump may be an electrical or a disposable battery-operated device.

TABLE 12.14 Types of Wound Dressing

Type of Dressing	Description	Uses	Considerations
Alginates			
Examples: Algisite, CalciCare, Kalginate, Melgisorb	Derived from processed seaweed or kelp. Form a nonstick gel on contact with draining wound. Highly absorbent. Hemostatic.	Wounds with moderate to heavy exudates.	Easy to use over irregular-shaped wounds. Require a secondary dressing. Nonadherent. Changed every 1–7 days. Do not use in dry wounds or wounds with minimal drainage.
Antimicrobials			
Examples: Aquacel AG, Exufiber AG, Acticoat, SilverSorb, Silvercel	Antimicrobial action. Include silver, iodine, honey, or polyhexamethylene biguanide (PHMB). Available as sponges, impregnated woven gauzes, film dressings, absorptive products, nylon fabric, nonadherent barriers, or a combination of materials.	Locally infected or colonized wounds. May be used prophylactically in nonhealing wounds to prevent or treat wound infection.	Absorbent ability varies. Must come into direct contact with wound bed to be effective.
Foams			
Examples: Allevyn, Cutimed, Hydrocell, Lyofoam, Mepilex, Permafoam, Aquacel Foam	Film-coated gel or polyurethane, multilayer absorbent dressing.	Primary dressing for absorption, secondary dressing for wounds with packing. Used to prevent sacral pressure injuries.	Nonadherent. May need a secondary dressing. Can absorb large amount exudate. Some cause a foul-smelling discharge.
Gauze (Impregnated and Nonimpregnated)			
Examples: Curity, Kerlix	Made of woven or nonwoven material.	Can be a primary dressing on almost any wound. Cleanse and pack a wound, usually moistened. Often combined with another kind of dressing.	Absorbs exudate. If dry, gauze can adhere and damage wound base. Dressings changed often because gauze tends to dry out quickly.
Hydrocolloids			
Examples: Bursamed, Comfeel, DuoDerm, Hydrocoll, PrimaCol	Gelatin, pectin, or carboxymethylcellulose bonded to a film or sheet. Produce a flat occlusive dressing that forms a gel on wound surface. Occlusion does not interfere with wound healing. Autolytic debridement. Prevents secondary infections.	Wounds with light to moderate drainage, such as small abrasions, superficial burns, pressure injuries	Avoid with wound infection. Some leave a foul-smelling residue on the wound surface. Change every 3–5 days. Comfortable.
Hydrogels			
Examples: Aquasite, Curasol, IntraSite, Purilon, Solosite	Available in gels, gel-covered gauze, or sheets. Give moisture to a dry wound and maintain a moist environment. Can rehydrate wound tissue. Autolytic debridement from moisturizing effects.	Dry wounds. Wounds with minimal drainage. Necrotic wounds.	May have a soothing effect in a painful wound. Dressings often changed daily. Do not apply the gel to the surrounding skin as maceration can occur. Requires a secondary dressing.
Nonadherent			
Examples: Adaptic, Vaseline gauze, Xeroform	Woven or nonwoven dressings. May be impregnated with saline, petrolatum, or antimicrobials.	Applied over skin tears, open wounds, minor wounds, or as a second dressing.	Dressing changes every 24–48 h to prevent product from drying and adhering to wound bed. Minimally absorbent. Does not harm intact skin.
Transparent Films			
Examples: Bioclusive, Biofilm, OpSite, Tegaderm, Transeal	Generally composed of polyurethane. Transparency allows wound visualization. Enhance autolytic debridement. Varying degrees of permeability.	Dry, uninfected wounds or wounds with minimal drainage. Often used as a secondary dressing to secure other dressing materials, such as foams.	Can result in further tissue loss in fragile wounds (e.g., skin tears) when removed. Can draw in moisture, increasing risk for infection. Minimally absorbent. Easy to apply, flexible.

Data from Hess CT: *Product guide to skin and wound care,* 2020, Philadelphia, Wolters Kluwer; Jaszarowski K, Murphree RW: Wound cleansing and dressing selection. In *Core curriculum wound management,* 2022, Philadelphia, Wolters Kluwer.

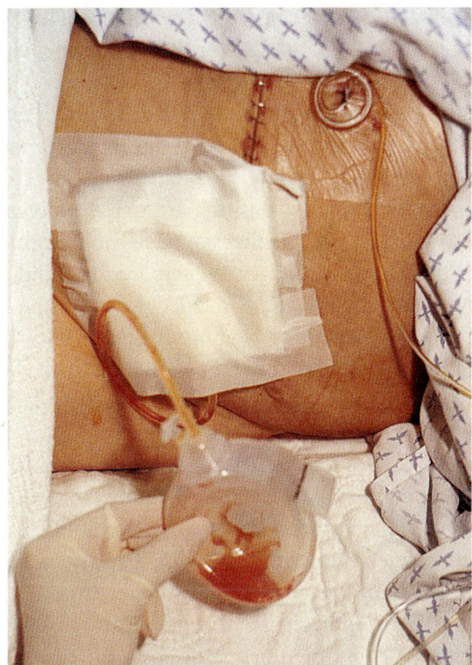

Fig. 12.8 Jackson-Pratt drainage device. (From Perry AG, Potter PA, Elkin MK: *Nursing interventions and clinical skills,* ed 5, St. Louis, 2012, Mosby.)

Another type of NPWT uses fluid instillation with NPWT. Saline or antibiotic-containing solution is instilled into the wound bed and allowed to remain for 10 to 20 minutes to distribute the solution across the wound. Negative pressure is applied at 125 mm Hg for up to 6 hours, then the fluid instillation reoccurs. NPWT has also been adapted for the adjunctive treatment of closed wounds, such as closed surgical incisions.

Hyperbaric Oxygen Therapy

Hyperbaric O_2 therapy (HBOT) delivers O_2 at increased atmospheric pressures. It can be given topically by creating a chamber around the injured limb. It also can be given systemically with the patient in an enclosed chamber, receiving 100% O_2 at 1.5 to 3 times the normal atmospheric pressure. Most systemic treatments last from 90 to 120 minutes. The number of treatments is highly variable (from 10 to 60), depending on the condition being treated.

HBOT allows O_2 to diffuse into the serum and be transported to the tissues. By increasing O_2 content in the serum, HBOT moves the O_2 past narrowed arteries and capillaries where RBCs cannot go. The high O_2 levels stimulate angiogenesis, kill anaerobic bacteria, and increase the killing power of WBCs and certain antibiotics (e.g., fluoroquinolones, aminoglycosides). HBOT accelerates granulation tissue formation and wound healing.[8]

Drug Therapy

Platelet-derived growth factor is released from the platelets. It stimulates cell proliferation and migration. Becaplermin (Regranex), a recombinant human platelet-derived growth factor gel, actively stimulates wound healing. It is used to treat patients with lower extremity diabetic neuropathic ulcers. Becaplermin should be used only when the wound is free of dead tissue and infection. It is contraindicated at wound sites with known cancer.

TABLE 12.15 Types of Debridement

Type	Description
Noninstrumental Debridement	
Autolytic	• Slow debridement that occurs naturally • Can be aided by using topical agents and moisture-retentive semiocclusive or occlusive dressings (e.g., hydrocolloids, transparent films, hydrogels) (see Table 12.14) that soften dry eschar by autolysis • Need a moist wound environment. Assess area around wound for maceration
Biologic (larval therapy)	• Use of living organisms, such as maggots, to remove necrotic or dead tissue from a wound • Applied either free range (direct contact method) or via a biobag (indirect contact method) dressing
Enzymatic/chemical	• Drug applied topically to dissolve necrotic tissue and then covered with moist dressing (e.g., saline-moistened gauze) • Process can be slow. Thick eschar may have to be scored with scalpel
Mechanical	• *Wet-to-dry dressings,* in which open-mesh gauze is moistened with normal saline, lightly packed into wound surface, and outer layer allowed to dry. Wound debris adheres to dressing, and then dressing is removed • *Wound irrigation.* Make certain bacteria are not driven into wound with high irrigation pressure • Noncontact low-frequency ultrasound and ultrasonic mist
Instrumental Debridement	
Conservative sharp	• May be done at the bedside • Use of scalpels, curettes, scissors to remove nonviable tissue • Ensure adequate vascular blood supply
Surgical	• Done in the operating room • Quick method of debridement to prevent, control, or remove infection • Used when large amounts of nonviable tissue are present • Prepares wound bed for healing, skin grafting, or flaps

Nutrition Therapy

Special nutrition can promote wound healing. A high fluid intake is needed to replace fluid loss from perspiration and exudate formation. An increased metabolic rate intensifies water loss. Persons at risk for wound healing problems are those with malabsorption problems (e.g., Crohn disease,

BOX 12.1 EVIDENCE-BASED PRACTICE

Negative Pressure Wound Therapy (NPWT)

A.C. is a 64-year-old male admitted to the hospital with unhealed diabetic foot ulcers (DFUs). He has had type 2 diabetes since age 38. He has retinopathy and moderate vision loss from microvascular complications of the disease. You find that A.C. has difficulty preparing food due to vision loss. He often eats frozen foods. He has mobility problems because of pain from the DFUs. The HCP has ordered NPWT to treat the DFUs. Because of your membership on the unit's Evidence-Based Practice (EBP) Committee, you are interested in reviewing the evidence related to this use of NPWT.

Making Clinical Decisions

Synthesis of Best Available Evidence

Traditionally, we use wet gauze dressings to treat DFUs. You take the question of NPWT effectiveness in treating DFUs to the EBP Committee and work with a peer to do a literature search. Although you find several studies addressing NPWT with and without irrigation, most are small cohort studies. Many studies had methodologic problems, including premature end or treatment changes. Few studies address NPWT as a treatment for DFUs.

Clinician Expertise

You learn that some research findings were clinically important. Compared with standard wet-to-dry dressings, some studies have found NPWT decreases costs and treatment time. Patients have reported greater satisfaction with NPWT wound treatment. The EBP Committee discusses the concept of clinical importance, including implications for current practice.

Patient Preferences and Values

A.C. expresses concern about past failed treatments and shares his hopes that the NPWT will speed healing of the ulcers.

Implications for Nursing Practice

1. How should you consider research findings for patients such as A.C.?
2. How can you use the evidence to maximize A.C.'s treatment?
3. What could committee members do with the results of the evidence review?

Reference for Evidence

Yang L, Zhao N, Yang M, et al: Diabetic foot wound ulcers management by vacuum sealing drainage: a meta-analysis, *International Wound Journal,* Sep 13, 2023.

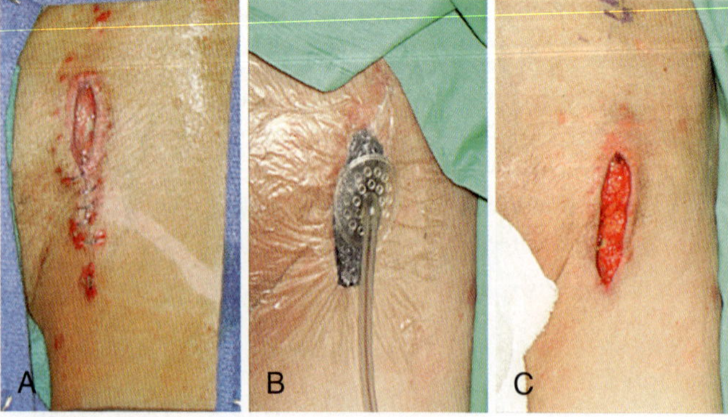

Fig. 12.9 Negative-pressure wound therapy. (A) Femoral wound that is not healing. (B) NPWT in place. (C) Granulation tissue formation after therapy. (From Abai B, Zickler RW, Pappas PJ, et al: Lymphorrhea responds to negative pressure wound therapy, *J Vascular Surg* 45 [3]:610–613, 2007.)

gastrointestinal [GI] surgery, liver disease), deficient intake or high energy demands (e.g., cancer, major trauma or surgery, sepsis, fever), and diabetes.

Undernutrition puts a person at risk for poor healing. A diet high in protein, carbohydrates, and vitamins with moderate fat intake is needed for healing. Protein helps to correct the negative nitrogen balance resulting from the increased metabolic rate. It is needed for the synthesis of immune factors, WBCs, fibroblasts, and collagen, which are the building blocks for healing. Carbohydrates are needed to meet the increased metabolic energy needed for healing. If there is a carbohydrate deficit, the body will break down protein for the needed energy. Fats help in the synthesis of fatty acids and triglycerides, which are part of the cell membrane.

Vitamin C is needed for capillary synthesis and collagen production by fibroblasts. The B-complex vitamins are necessary as coenzymes for many metabolic reactions. Vitamin B deficiency disrupts protein, fat, and carbohydrate metabolism. Vitamin A aids in epithelialization. It increases collagen synthesis and tensile strength of the healing wound.

If the patient is unable to eat but has a functional GI tract, enteral nutrition (EN) and oral supplements should be the first choice. Parenteral nutrition (PN) is used when EN is contraindicated or not tolerated. EN and PN are discussed in Chapter 44.

Infection Prevention and Control

You and the patient must follow aseptic procedures, including handwashing, to keep the wound free from infection. Do not allow the patient to touch a recently injured area. The patient's environment should be as free as possible from contamination from items introduced by roommates and visitors. Some patients may receive prophylactic antibiotics.

If an infection develops, a culture and sensitivity test can determine the organism and the most effective antibiotic for that specific organism. Obtain the culture before giving the first dose of antibiotic. We can obtain wound cultures by needle aspiration, tissue culture, or swab technique. HCPs perform needle and tissue punch biopsies.

To obtain cultures using the swab technique, rotate a culture swab over a cleansed 1-cm^2 area near the center of the wound. Use enough pressure to extract wound fluid from deep tissue layers. Take a culture of the clean tissue because exudate and necrotic tissue will not provide an accurate sample. Send the sample to the laboratory within 30 minutes.

Psychologic Care

The patient may be distressed at the sight of an incision or wound and fear scarring or disfigurement. Drainage and odor from a wound often cause alarm. The patient needs to understand the healing process and normal changes that occur as the wound heals.

When changing a dressing, avoid inappropriate facial expressions that may alert the patient to problems with the wound or raise doubts about your ability to provide wound care. Wrinkling your nose may convey disgust to the patient. Treat the patient as a total person rather than focusing only on the wound.

Patient Teaching

Patients and caregivers must know how to care for the wound and perform dressing changes. Wound healing may take 4 to 6 weeks or longer. Emphasize the importance of adequate rest and good nutrition throughout this time. Physical and emotional stress should be minimized. Observing the wound for complications, such as contractures, adhesions, and secondary infection, is important. Teach patients and caregivers the signs and symptoms of infection. Have them note changes in the wound color and amount of drainage. Teach them to notify the HCP of any signs of abnormal wound healing.

Review drug-specific side effects and adverse effects with patients and caregivers and ways to prevent side effects (e.g., taking with food). Teach patients to contact the HCP if any of these effects occur. Discuss the need to complete the entire course of therapy. This will help prevent a more severe, drug-resistant infection.

PRESSURE INJURIES

Etiology and Pathophysiology

A **pressure injury** is localized damage to the skin and/or underlying soft tissue. It usually occurs over a bony prominence or is related to a medical or other device. The injury occurs because of intense and/or prolonged pressure or pressure in combination with shear. The most common site for pressure injuries is the sacrum, with the heels being second.

Factors that influence the development of pressure injuries include the amount of pressure (intensity), length of time the pressure is exerted on the skin (duration), and ability of the patient's tissue to tolerate the pressure. Other contributing factors include *excessive moisture* (increases risk for skin breakdown) and **shear**. Shear is the pressure exerted on the skin when it adheres to the bed, and the skin layers slide with body movement. This may occur when pulling the patient up in bed. The tolerance of soft tissue for pressure and shear is affected by microclimate, nutrition, perfusion, comorbidities, and condition of the soft tissue.[9]

Factors that put patients at risk for developing a pressure injury are outlined in Table 12.16. Patients at risk include those who are older, incontinent, unable to reposition or unaware of the need to reposition (e.g., spinal cord injury), and bed- or wheelchair-bound.

TABLE 12.16 Risk Factors for Pressure Injuries

- Advanced age
- Anemia
- Cognitive impairment, unconsciousness
- Critically ill, cared for in critical care setting
- Debilitation
- Decreased body weight (15% less than ideal body weight)
- Diabetes
- Fever
- Friction (rubbing of surfaces together)
- Hip fracture
- History of pressure injury
- Immobility; inability to turn and position body
- Impaired immune function
- Incontinence of feces, urine, or both
- Long and/or extensive surgical procedure
- Low diastolic blood pressure (<60 mm Hg)
- Major trauma
- Malnutrition
- Musculoskeletal problems, contractures, weakness
- Neurologic problems; stroke, altered sensation
- Obesity
- Peripheral vascular disease
- Spinal cord injury

Clinical Manifestations

The manifestations of pressure injuries depend on the extent of the tissue involved. The injury can present as intact skin or an open injury and may be painful. We stage pressure injuries based on the visible or palpable tissue in the wound bed. Table 12.17 shows the stages of pressure injury.

A medical device–related pressure injury results from the use of devices designed and applied for diagnostic or therapeutic purposes.[10] The resulting injury generally conforms to the pattern or shape of the device. The most implicated devices include splints, braces, indwelling lines, and respiratory devices. The most common site is the ears, from O_2 tubing and masks. Another common site is the foot, from casts and splints. A mucosal membrane pressure injury (MMPI) can occur on mucous membranes that contact a medical device such as an endotracheal tube or nasogastric tube.

If the pressure injury becomes infected, the patient may have signs of infection (e.g., leukocytosis, fever). The pressure injury may increase in size, odor, and drainage; have necrotic tissue; and be indurated, warm, and painful. Untreated pressure injuries may lead to *cellulitis*, chronic infection, and sepsis. The most common complication of a pressure injury is recurrence. It is important to note the location of previously healed pressure injuries on a patient's admission assessment.

! SAFETY ALERT

Pressure Injuries

A Stage 3 or 4 (full skin–thickness injury) pressure injury acquired after admission to a health care setting (hospital-acquired pressure injury [HAPI]) is a serious reportable event (SRE) (see Chapter 1).

TABLE 12.17 Diagnostic Criteria

Pressure Injury Staging

Stage 1: Nonblanchable Erythema of Intact Skin

Intact skin with nonblanchable redness of a localized area, usually over a bony prominence. Blanchable redness or changes in sensation, temperature, or firmness may precede visual changes. May be hard to detect in persons with dark skin tones.

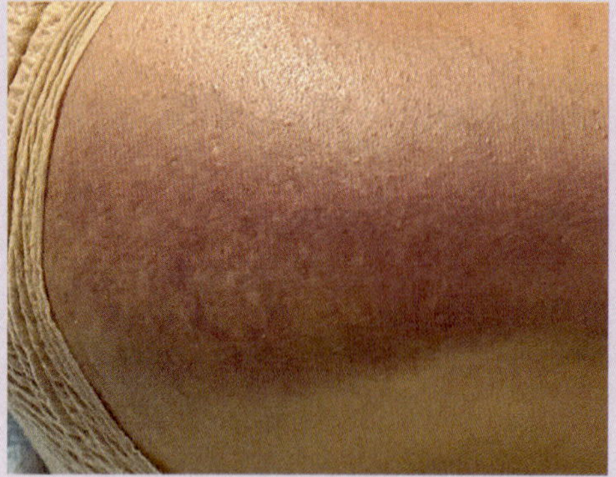

Stage 2: Partial-Thickness Skin Loss With Exposed Dermis

Blister or partial thickness loss of skin with exposed dermis. Wound bed is viable, pink or red, and moist. No slough, eschar, or granulation tissue.

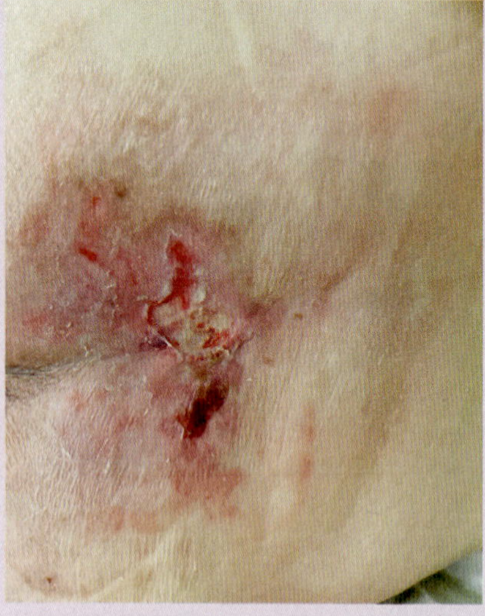

Stage 3: Full-Thickness Tissue Loss

Full-thickness tissue loss. Subcutaneous fat may be visible. Granulation tissue and rolled wound edges are often present. Slough and/or eschar may be present. Depth varies by location. Undermining and tunneling may occur.

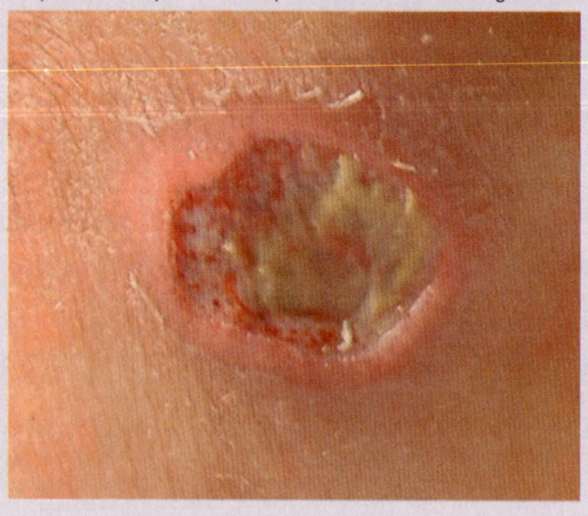

Stage 4: Full-Thickness Skin and Tissue Loss

Full-thickness skin and tissue loss with muscle, tendon, ligament, cartilage, or bone involvement. Slough and/or eschar may be present. Often includes undermining and/or tunneling. Depth varies by location.

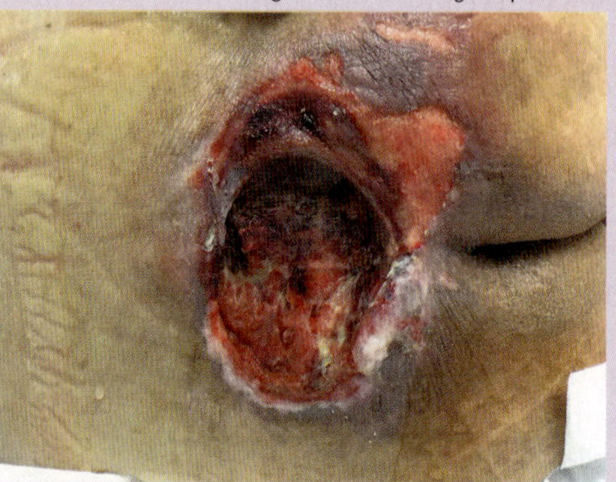

Unstageable: Obscured Full-Thickness Skin and Tissue Loss

Full-thickness skin and tissue loss in which the extent of the injury cannot be determined because the base of the injury is covered by slough or eschar. Stage 3 or Stage 4 pressure injury is present after removing slough or eschar. Stable eschar (i.e., dry, adherent, intact without redness) on the heel or ischemic limb should not be removed.

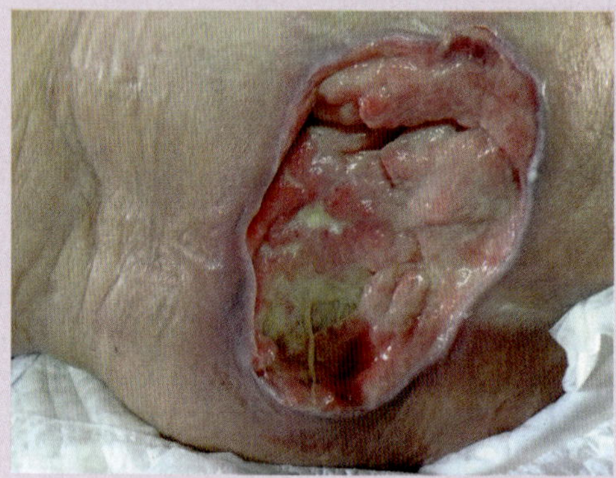

Deep Tissue Pressure Injury (DTPI): Persistent Nonblanchable Deep Red, Maroon, or Purple Discoloration

Intact or nonintact skin with local area of persistent nonblanchable deep red, maroon, purple discoloration, or epidermal separation revealing a dark wound bed or blood-filled blister. Pain and temperature changes often precede skin color changes. May be hard to detect in persons with dark skin. May evolve to reveal the actual extent of tissue injury or resolve without tissue loss.

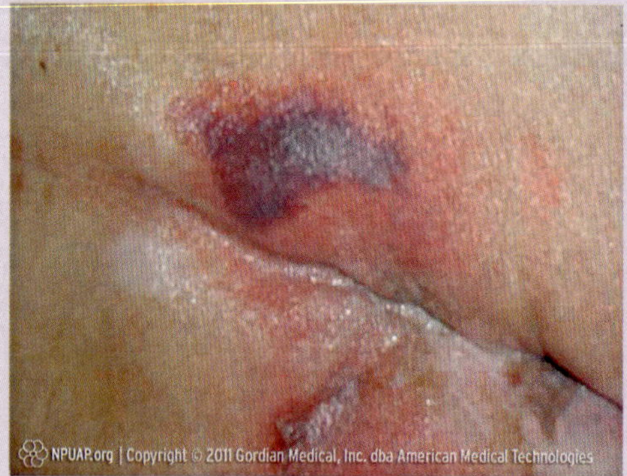

Stage 1. © iStock.com/Jodi Jacobson.
Stage 2. © C5C/iStock.com.
Stage 3. From MNHHS RBWH.
Stage 4. © Boonyarit/iStock.com.
Unstageable. © Suphanni Chongmithorn/iStock.com.
Deep Tissue Pressure Injury. Used with permission of the European Pressure Ulcer Advisory Panel, National Pressure Injury Advisory Panel, and Pan Pacific Pressure Injury Alliance; Haesler E, editor: *Prevention and treatment of pressure ulcers/injuries: quick reference guide,* ed 3, 2019. https://www.internationalguideline.com/static/pdfs/Quick_Reference_Guide-10Mar2019.pdf. © NPUAP.

NURSING MANAGEMENT: PRESSURE INJURIES

You play a key role in preventing and treating pressure injuries. Other members of the health team, such as the wound care specialist, plastic surgeon, WOCN, dietitian, and physical therapist, can provide input into the complex management needed to prevent and treat pressure injuries. The eNursing Care Plan 12.2 (available on the website for this chapter at http://evolve.elsevier.com/Lewis/medsurg) outlines the care for patients with a pressure injury.

Assessment

Assess patients for pressure injury risk within the first 24 hours of admission and/or home visit and at periodic intervals based on the patient's condition (Table 12.16). Use a validated assessment tool, such as the Braden Scale (available at www.bradenscale.com). Knowing the level of risk can help determine how aggressive preventive measures should be. Conduct a thorough head-to-toe assessment on admission to identify and document any pressure injuries. After admission, conduct periodic reassessments of the skin and wounds.

! SAFETY ALERT

Assessing for Pressure Injuries

- In acute care, reassess patients for pressure injuries every 24 hours.
- In long-term care, reassess residents weekly for the first 4 weeks after admission and then at least monthly or quarterly.
- In home care, reassess patients at every nurse visit.

Implementation

Health Promotion

The main nursing responsibilities are (1) identifying patients at risk for developing pressure injuries (Table 12.16) and (2) implementing pressure injury prevention strategies for those at risk (Table 12.18). Prevention is the best treatment for pressure injuries. Implementing evidence-based pressure injury prevention programs can reduce the occurrence of health care–acquired pressure injuries.[11]

In the past, standard care was to turn and reposition patients every 2 hours. However, this practice is not evidence-based. Individualize time schedules and frequency based on risk factors, patient's overall condition, and type of mattress and support surface. For example, we may need to turn and reposition some high-risk patients every hour, while we may turn and reposition others at lower risk only every 3 to 4 hours.[12]

TABLE 12.18 Preventing Pressure Injuries

The plan of care for patients who are at risk for pressure injury should include:

- Skin assessment
- Skin cleansing, care for dry skin, use of moisture barriers
- Nutrition support based on an individualized nutrition assessment
- A plan to maintain and, when appropriate, increase mobility
- Positioning, repositioning, transferring, and turning techniques that reduce friction and shear
- Devices to reduce pressure and shear (e.g., low-air-loss mattresses, foam mattresses, wheelchair cushions, padded commode seats, boots [foam, air], lift sheets) as needed.
- Ways to reduce exposure to excess moisture

Acute Care

Care of patients with a pressure injury requires wound care and support of the whole person, including adequate nutrition, pain management, control of other medical conditions, and redistributing pressure. Both conservative and surgical strategies are used in treating a pressure injury, depending on the stage and condition of the injury.

We base our interventions on the injury characteristics (e.g., stage, size, location, amount of exudate, type of wound, presence of infection or pain) and the patient's general status (e.g., nutrition state, age, cardiovascular status, level of mobility). Document the size of the pressure injury. Document the healing wound using one of several available pressure injury healing tools, such as the NPIAP Pressure Ulcer Scale for Healing (PUSH) tool (available at https://npiap.com/page/PUSHTool). Some agencies require taking pictures of the pressure injury initially and at regular intervals during treatment.

Pressure injuries generally heal by secondary intention. Care may involve debridement, wound cleaning, applying a dressing, and offloading pressure. It is important to choose the right pressure-redistributing techniques (e.g., mattress replacement, mattress overlay, integrated bed system, seat cushion, seat cushion overlay) to move pressure off areas of injury. Whenever possible, do not turn the patient onto a body surface that has blanchable redness. Massage is contraindicated in acute inflammation and where there is the possibility of damaged blood vessels or fragile skin.

A pressure injury with necrotic tissue or eschar (except for dry, stable necrotic feet or heels) should have the tissue removed by surgical, mechanical, enzymatic, or autolytic debridement methods (Table 12.15). Once the pressure injury has been debrided and has a clean granulating base, plan to support moist wound healing and prevent disruption of the newly formed granulation tissue. Reconstruction of the pressure injury site by surgical repair, including skin grafting, skin flaps, musculocutaneous flaps, or free flaps, may be necessary.

Clean pressure injuries with noncytotoxic solutions (e.g., normal saline) that do not kill or damage cells, especially fibroblasts. Use enough irrigation pressure (4 to 15 psi) to clean the wound without causing trauma or damage. You can achieve this pressure using a 30-mL syringe and a 19-gauge needle.

After cleansing the pressure injury, cover it with a proper dressing. Keep a pressure injury slightly moist rather than dry to enhance reepithelialization. Some factors to consider when choosing a dressing are maintaining a moist environment, preventing the wound from drying out, absorbing the wound drainage, location of the wound, amount of caregiver time needed to change the dressing, cost of the dressing, presence of infection, clean versus sterile dressings, and care delivery setting. Dressings are described in Table 12.14.

Stages 2 through 4 pressure injuries are considered contaminated or colonized with bacteria. Remember that in people who have chronic wounds or are immunocompromised, the signs and symptoms of infection (purulent exudate, odor, redness, warmth, tenderness, edema, pain, fever, high WBC count) may not be present even when the pressure injury is infected.

Maintaining adequate nutrition is an important nursing responsibility for patients with a pressure injury. Often patients are debilitated and have a poor appetite from inactivity. Oral feedings must be adequate to meet the patient's nutrition requirements. The caloric intake needed to correct and maintain nutrient balance may be 30 to 35 calories/kg/day and 1.25 to 1.50 g of protein/kg/day.[13] EN can supplement oral feedings. When oral feedings and EN are inadequate, PN with amino acid and glucose solutions is given. PN and EN are discussed in Chapter 44.

Pressure injuries affect the quality of life of patients and their caregivers. Because pressure injuries often recur, teach prevention techniques to patients and caregivers (Table 12.19).

TABLE 12.19 PATIENT & CAREGIVER TEACHING

Pressure Injury

When teaching the patient and caregiver to prevent and care for pressure injuries, do the following:

1. Identify and explain risk factors and cause of pressure injuries.
2. Discuss ways to manage incontinence. If incontinence occurs, cleanse skin at time of soiling and use absorbent pads or briefs.
3. Review correct positioning to decrease risk for skin breakdown. NEVER position the patient directly on the pressure injury, if possible.
4. Teach caregiver to reposition a bed-bound patient at least every 2 hours and a chair-bound patient every hour.
5. Review the available resources (i.e., caregiver's availability and skill, finances, equipment) of patients who need pressure injury care at home.
6. Teach patient and/or caregiver how to change dressings. Review the disposal of contaminated dressings.
7. Teach patient and caregiver to inspect skin daily. Tell them to report any significant changes to the HCP.
8. Review the importance of good nutrition to enhance injury healing.

Caregivers need to know the cause of pressure injuries, prevention techniques, early signs, nutrition support, and care techniques for actual pressure injuries. Because patients with a pressure injury often need extensive care for other health problems, it is important that the nurse support caregivers who have an added responsibility for pressure injury treatment.

CASE STUDY

Pressure Injury

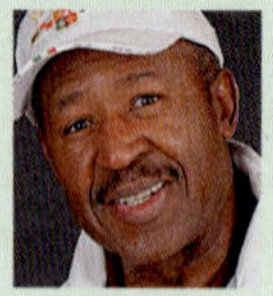

(© iStockphoto/ Thinkstock.)

Patient Profile

G.N., a 62-year-old male, is admitted to the medical unit with a urinary tract infection. He has multiple sclerosis, which has led to the loss of feeling and mobility in his lower extremities. During the admission assessment, you note a Stage 2 sacral pressure injury. His wife, who has been caring for him at home, is with him.

Subjective Data

- Wheelchair-bound for 8 years
- Requires 1 person to assist with transferring
- Reports a decreased appetite and problems swallowing
- Drinks 2 oral nutrition supplements daily
- Had been using a trapeze to help with repositioning in bed, but states that its use has become harder lately due to feeling weaker

Objective Data

Physical Assessment

- Vital signs: 118/62, 88 and regular, 18, 100.4°F (38°C)
- Wound dimensions: 2.8 × 2.0 × 1.0 cm
- Continent of urine and stool

Laboratory Studies

- WBC count 16,400/μL (26.4 × 10^9/L) with 80% neutrophils (10% bands)

Discussion Questions

1. ***Recognize:*** What risk factors contributed to his developing a pressure injury?
2. ***Recognize:*** Describe the assessment you need to obtain in relation to his pressure injury.
3. ***Analyze:*** What would you expect a Stage 2 pressure injury to look like?
4. ***Analyze:*** Why does he have a fever?
5. ***Analyze:*** What is the significance of his WBC count and differential?
6. ***Plan:*** What are your options for dressing G.N.'s wound?
7. ***Prioritize:*** What are the priority clinical problems?
8. ***Act:*** What referrals could you initiate?
9. ***Act:*** What interventions would you implement to promote wound healing?
10. ***Evaluate:*** What outcomes would indicate that interprofessional care was effective?

Answers available at http://evolve.elsevier.com/Lewis/medsurg.

BRIDGE TO NCLEX EXAMINATION

The number of the question corresponds to the same-numbered outcome at the beginning of the chapter.

1. A patient 1 day postoperative after abdominal surgery has incisional pain, 99.5°F temperature, slight redness at the incision margins, and 30 mL serosanguineous drainage in the Jackson-Pratt drain. Based on this assessment, what conclusion would the nurse make?
   - **a.** The patient has a normal inflammatory response.
   - **b.** The abdominal incision shows signs of an infection.
   - **c.** The abdominal incision shows signs of impending dehiscence.
   - **d.** The patient's health care provider must be notified about their condition.
2. The nurse assessing a patient with a chronic leg wound finds redness and edema. The patient reports pain at the wound site. Which test would the nurse expect to be prescribed to assess the patient's systemic response?
   - **a.** Serum protein analysis
   - **b.** WBC count and differential
   - **c.** Punch biopsy of the center of the wound
   - **d.** Culture and sensitivity of the wound
3. A patient in the unit has a 103.7°F temperature. Which intervention would be *most* effective in restoring normal body temperature?
   - **a.** Using a cooling blanket while the patient is febrile
   - **b.** Giving antipyretics on an around-the-clock schedule
   - **c.** Providing increased fluids and having the AP give sponge baths
   - **d.** Giving prescribed antibiotics and placing warm blankets for comfort
4. A nurse is caring for a patient who has a pressure injury that is treated with debridement, irrigations, and moist gauze dressings. How would the nurse expect healing to occur?
   - **a.** Cell regeneration
   - **b.** Tertiary intention
   - **c.** Secondary intention
   - **d.** Remodeling of tissues
5. Which patient has the *greatest* risk for delayed wound healing?
   - **a.** 65-year-old female who has stress incontinence
   - **b.** 78-year-old male who has a history of hypertension
   - **c.** 52-year-old female who has obesity and type 2 diabetes
   - **d.** 30-year-old male who drinks 2 alcoholic beverages per day
6. Which prescribed action should a nurse question in the plan of care for an older adult, immobile stroke patient who has a pink, clean Stage 3 pressure injury?
   - **a.** Turn and position the patient every hour.
   - **b.** Clean the wound daily with a cytotoxic solution.
   - **c.** Pack the wound with an absorbent foam dressing.
   - **d.** Assess for pain and medicate before dressing change.
7. Which patients are at *most* risk for pressure injuries? **(Select all that apply.)**
   - **a.** A patient with right sided-paralysis and fecal incontinence
   - **b.** An older adult who is alert and needs assistance to ambulate
   - **c.** A young adult patient with paraplegia after a gunshot wound
   - **d.** An ambulatory patient who has occasional stress incontinence
   - **e.** A young adult with a tibial fracture from a motor vehicle accident
   - **f.** A patient who is morbidly obese and has an open abdominal wound
8. An 85-year-old patient has a score of 16 on the Braden Scale. Which action should the nurse include in the plan of care?
   - **a.** Implementing a 1-hour turning schedule with skin assessment.
   - **b.** Elevating the head of the bed 90 degrees when the patient is supine.
   - **c.** Continuing with weekly skin assessments with no special precautions.
   - **d.** Placing a silicone foam dressing on the patient's sacrum to prevent breakdown.
9. An 82-year-old male is being cared for at home by his family. A pressure injury on his right buttock measures 1 × 2 × 0.8 cm, and pink subcutaneous tissue is visible on the wound bed. Which stage would the nurse document on the wound assessment form?
   - **a.** Stage 1
   - **b.** Stage 2
   - **c.** Stage 3
   - **d.** Stage 4

1. a; 2. b; 3. b; 4. c; 5. c; 6. b; 7. a, c, f; 8. a; 9. c.

For rationales to these answers and even more NCLEX review questions, visit http://evolve.elsevier.com/Lewis/medsurg.

REFERENCES

To access the References for this chapter, please scan the QR code with a mobile device.

13

Genetics

Janice Smolowitz and Marybeth Duffy

http://evolve.elsevier.com/Lewis/medsurg/

CONCEPTUAL FOCUS

Cellular Regulation

Ethics

LEARNING OUTCOMES

1. Describe common terms related to genetics and genetic disorders.
2. Distinguish between the 2 common causes of genetic mutations.
3. Compare and contrast the 3 common inheritance patterns of genetic disorders.
4. Describe common classifications of genetic disorders.
5. Explore the ethical and social implications of genetic testing.
6. Analyze the role of pharmacogenomics and pharmacogenetics in drug therapy.
7. Discuss your role in assisting the patient and family in dealing with genetic and genomic issues.

KEY TERMS

epigenetics
genes
genetics
genome
genomics
hereditary, Table 13.1
heterozygous, Table 13.1
homozygous, Table 13.1
mutation
pharmacogenetics
pharmacogenomics

GENETICS AND GENOMICS

Genes are the basic units of heredity. They are composed of sequences of deoxyribonucleic acid (DNA) that are arranged along a person's chromosomes. Genes are passed from one generation to the next. The **genome** is the complete set of DNA. It includes all the organism's genes. An organism's genome has all the information it needs to build and maintain itself.[1]

Genetics is the study of genes and their role in inheritance. Genetics determines the way that certain traits or conditions are passed down through genes. A person's genes can have a profound impact on health and disease. We think more than 10,000 diseases are related to altered genes.[2]

Genomics is the study of all a person's genes (the *genome*), including interactions of these genes with each other and with the person's environment. Genomics includes the study of complex diseases, such as heart disease, diabetes, and cancer. These diseases are typically caused by a combination of genetic and environment factors rather than by a single gene. Genomics may help us understand why some people who eat healthy diets and exercise die at a young age of heart disease, while others eat unhealthy diets and never exercise and live to old age.[2] Table 13.1 presents common terms used in genetics and genomics.

Advances in genetic and genomic research and technology affect health care delivery. In response, nursing organizations have established practice standards that provide a framework for caring for persons with genetic and genomic concerns. Other standards outline competencies and education in relation to professional practice and genetics.[3]

Identifying a genetic basis for many diseases has the potential to influence the care of patients at risk for or diagnosed

TABLE 13.1 **Glossary of Genetic and Genomic Terms**

Term	Definition
Allele	One of a series of alternative forms (genotypes) at a specific region (locus) of a chromosome
Autosome	A chromosome other than X or Y. The human genome has 44 autosomes (22 pairs of autosomes)
Carrier	Person who is heterozygous for a gene variant that causes autosomal recessive or X-linked recessive disease. Used to describe heterozygotes for risk alleles of complex traits with variable penetrance, regardless of inheritance type
Carrier testing	Method to identify at-risk family members of populations who are usually asymptomatic but may have a pathogenic variant for an autosomal recessive or X-linked disorder
Chromosome	Microscopic structures in the cell nucleus composed of chromatin, which contain genetic information. Each cell normally has 46 chromosomes in 23 pairs (22 autosome pairs and 2 sex chromosomes)
Codominance	Expression of each pair of alleles when present in the heterozygous state (e.g., AB blood type)
Consanguineous	Reproduction between 2 persons from the same bloodline, such as 1st or 2nd cousins. Consanguineous parentage increases the chance of a rare recessive disease
Dominant allele	Gene that is expressed in the phenotype of a heterozygous person
Familial disorder	A trait that appears with higher frequency among close relatives than in the general population
Gene	Functional unit of heredity. A gene is a unit of DNA sequence that encodes for a specific functional product, such as RNA
Genetic risk	Probability that a trait will occur or recur in a family, based on knowledge of its genetic pattern of transmission
Genetics	Study of genes and their role in inheritance
Genome	All the DNA contained in a person. A person's genetic constitution
Genomics	Study of how genes interact and influence people's biologic and physical characteristics
Genotype	Genetic identity of a person, comprised of the entire complex of genes inherited from both parents
Haploid	Cells or organisms that have 1 copy of each autosomal chromosome and 1 copy of each sex chromosome. Ova and sperm are haploid. Fertilization results in an embryo with 1 set of chromosomes from each parent (diploid embryo)
Hereditary	Transmission of a disease, condition, or trait from parent to children
Heterozygous	Having 2 different alleles for 1 given gene, 1 inherited from each parent
Homozygous	Having 2 identical alleles for 1 given gene, 1 inherited from each parent
Locus	Position of a gene on a chromosome
Mutation	A change in a gene that affects function. Types include nonsense, missense silent, and frameshift. A *pathogenic variant* is a mutation associated with a disease. Sometimes parents pass mutations to children.
Oncogene	Gene that contributes to the conversion of normal cells to cancer cells. Usually dominant
Pedigree	A graphic representation that shows family relationships, gender, age, and presence of diseases for each family member
Pharmacogenetics	Study of variability of drug metabolism related to variations in single genes
Pharmacogenomics	Study of variability of drug metabolism in relation to variations in and interactions of multiple genes or the person's genome
Phenotype	Observable characteristics of a person. Measured categorically or quantitatively
Protooncogene	Genes that can be turned into oncogenes by a dominant activating mutation. Oncogenes produce structurally altered proteins that result in cancer
Recessive allele	Allele that has no noticeable effect on the phenotype in a heterozygous person
Trait	Physical characteristics a person inherits, such as hair or eye color
X-linked gene	Gene found on the X chromosome rather than an autosome. In general, sex-linked disorders occur in males

with a disease that has a genetic link. You need to know basic genetic principles, be familiar with the impact that genetics has on health and disease, and be prepared to aid the patient and family with genetic issues.

Basic Principles of Genetics

Chromosomes

Chromosomes are found in the cell nucleus. They occur in pairs. Humans have 23 pairs of chromosomes. Twenty-two of the 23 pairs of chromosomes are *homologous autosomes.* This means the pair of chromosomes has corresponding DNA sequences. Autosomes are the same in both males and females. The sex chromosomes make up the 23rd pair. A female has 2 X chromosomes, and a male has 1 X and 1 Y chromosome. One chromosome of each pair is inherited from the mother and one from the father. Half of each child's chromosomes (and thus their genetic makeup) comes from their father and half from their mother.

Genes

Genes carry the instructions for making proteins that direct the activities of cells. Genes control how a cell functions, including how quickly it grows, how often it divides, and how long it lives. To control these functions, genes make proteins that perform specific tasks and act as messengers for the cell. Each gene must have the correct instructions, or "code," for making its protein so that the protein can perform the proper function for the cell.

Genes are arranged in a specific linear formation along a chromosome (Fig. 13.1). Each gene has a specific location on a chromosome, called the *locus.* An *allele* is 1 of 2 or more alternative forms of a gene that occupy corresponding loci on

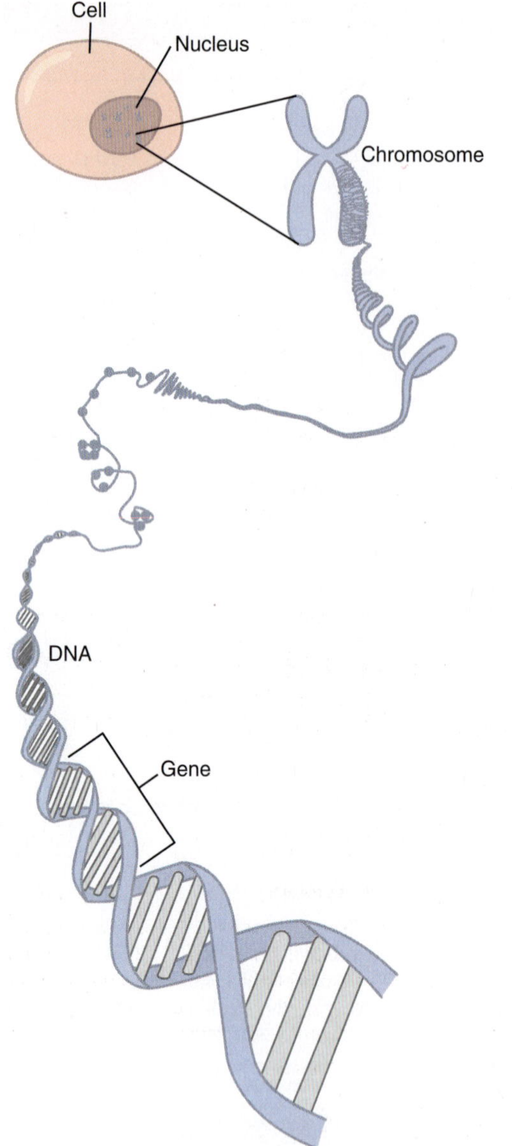

Fig. 13.1 Long, stringy DNA that makes up genes is spooled within chromosomes inside the nucleus of a cell. Note: A gene would be a much longer stretch of DNA than what we show here.

homologous chromosomes. Each allele codes for a specific inherited characteristic.

When the alleles are different, the allele that is fully expressed is the *dominant allele.* The allele that cannot express itself in the presence of a dominant allele is the *recessive allele.* The actual genetic makeup of the person is the *genotype.* Physical traits expressed by a person are the *phenotype.*

DNA

Genes are made up of a nucleic acid called DNA. DNA stores genetic information and encodes the instructions for producing specific proteins needed to maintain life. It dictates the rate at which proteins are made. Every somatic cell in a person's body has the same DNA.

The information in DNA is stored as a code made up of 4 nitrogenous bases: adenine (A), guanine (G), cytosine (C), and thymine (T). Human DNA consists of about 3 billion bases. More than 99% of those bases are the same in all people. The order, or sequence, of these bases determines the information for building and maintaining an organism. This is similar to how we use letters of the alphabet to create words and sentences.

DNA bases pair up with each other, A with T and C with G, to form units called *base pairs.* Each base is attached to a sugar molecule and a phosphate molecule (Fig. 13.2). Together, a base, sugar, and phosphate form a *nucleotide.* Nucleotides are arranged in 2 long strands that form a spiral called a *double helix.* The structure of the double helix is like a ladder. The base pairs form the ladder's rungs. The sugar and phosphate molecules form the ladder's vertical sidepieces.

DNA can *replicate* or make copies of itself. Each DNA strand in the double helix can serve as a pattern for duplicating the sequence of bases. When cells divide, each new cell must have an exact copy of the DNA that was in the parent (original) cell.

RNA

Ribonucleic acid (RNA) is similar to DNA but with some major differences. RNA contains the nitrogenous bases adenine, guanine, and cytosine, but it contains uracil instead of thymine. RNA is single, not double, stranded. It contains ribose instead of deoxyribose sugar. RNA transfers the genetic information obtained from DNA to the proper location for protein synthesis.

Protein Synthesis

Protein synthesis, or the making of proteins, occurs in 2 steps: *transcription* and *translation.* Transcription is the process by which messenger RNA (mRNA) is made from single-stranded DNA. The mRNA attaches to a ribosome, where translation occurs. At this point, another specialized type of RNA, transfer RNA (tRNA), arranges the amino acids in the correct sequence to assemble the protein. Once the protein is complete, the ribosome releases the protein. It can perform its specific function in the cell.

Mitosis

Mitosis is a type of cell division that results in the formation of genetically identical daughter cells. Before cell division, the chromosomes duplicate, and each new cell (called *daughter cells*) receives an exact replica of the chromosomes from the original cell (called the *parent cell*).

Meiosis

Meiosis occurs only in germline or sexual reproductive cells. Two consecutive nuclear divisions, meiosis I and meiosis II, occur without chromosomes replicating in between. This process results in the production of 4 haploid sex cells. Each has 1 copy of each chromosome.

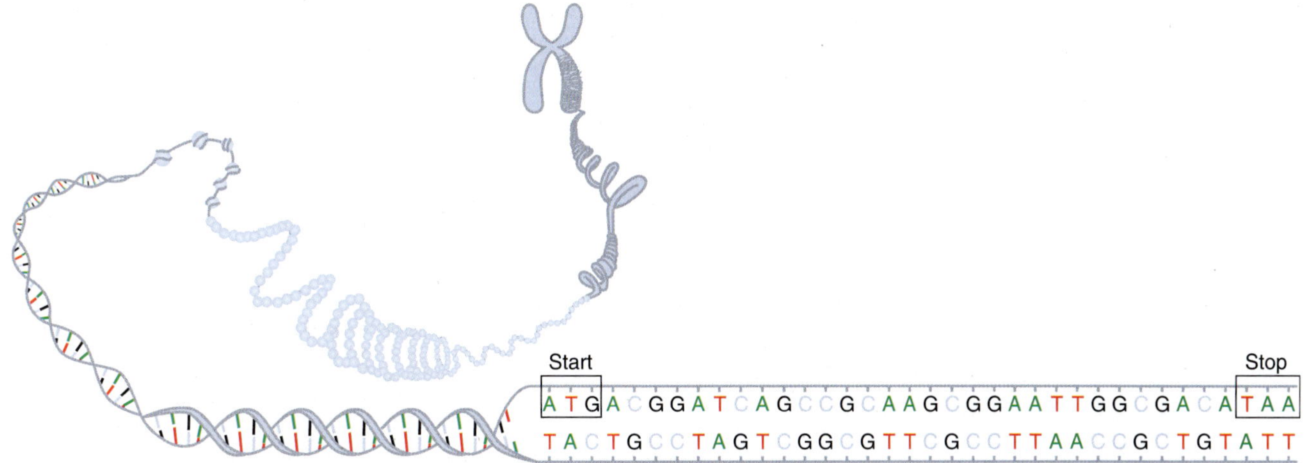

Fig. 13.2 DNA consists of 2 long, twisted chains made up of nucleotides. Each nucleotide contains a base, a phosphate molecule (P), and the sugar molecule deoxyribose (S). The bases in DNA nucleotides are adenine *(A)*, thymine *(T)*, cytosine *(C)*, and guanine *(G)*.

Genetic Mutations

A **mutation** is any change in the usual DNA sequence. Mutations range in size from a single DNA base (building block) to a large segment of a chromosome. The change in gene structure may change the type and/or amount of protein made. The protein may not work at all, or it may work incorrectly. In some cases, genetic mutations do not have a visible effect on the people who have them. Some gene variations result in a disease or an increased risk for the disease. For example, in people with sickle cell disease, a substitution of a single base (thymine replaces adenine) in a single gene (β-globin gene) causes the disease (Fig. 13.3).

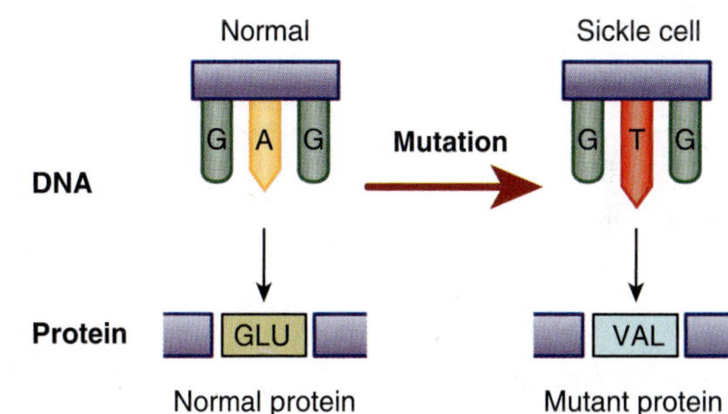

Fig. 13.3 In sickle cell disease, a single gene mutation leads to mutant (incorrect) protein. The substitution of valine *(VAL)* for glutamic acid on the β-globin chain of hemoglobin produces abnormal hemoglobin, hemoglobin S (Hb S). In response to low O_2 levels, erythrocytes with Hb S stiffen and elongate, taking on a sickle shape.

Types of Mutations

Genetic mutations occur in 2 ways. *Germline mutations* pass from parent to child. These mutations are present in the oocyte and sperm cells. This type of mutation is present throughout a person's life in almost every cell in the body.

Acquired (somatic) mutations occur in the DNA of a cell at some time during a person's life. An acquired mutation passes on to all cells that develop from that single cell. These mutations in somatic cells cannot be passed on to the next generation. Acquired mutations can occur if (1) a mistake occurs as DNA replicates during cell division or (2) environment factors alter the DNA.

Mutations can occur when a cell is dividing. Sometimes mistakes, such as deletions, insertions, or duplication of DNA material, occur during replication. Although DNA repair enzymes can correct replication errors, mistakes can go uncorrected.

DNA damage can occur from environment factors. For example, ultraviolet (UV) radiation can cause DNA damage, leading to skin cancer. Toxins in cigarettes can lead to lung cancer. Many chemotherapy drugs used to treat cancer target the DNA of cancer cells and healthy cells. In the process, these drugs increase a person's risk for developing secondary cancers (see Chapter 16).

Cells have built-in mechanisms that catch and repair most of the changes that happen during DNA replication or from environment damage. However, as we age, our DNA repair does not work as effectively. Thus we accumulate changes in our DNA.

Inheritance Patterns

We can inherit genetic conditions in several ways. These include autosomal dominant, autosomal recessive, X-linked, and Y-linked disorders (Table 13.2). If the mutant gene is on an autosome, the genetic disorder is called *autosomal.* If the mutant gene is on the X chromosome, it is an *X-linked* genetic disorder. These 3 patterns are mendelian patterns of inheritance. They occur less often than multifactorial or complex traits and disorders. Family pedigrees for autosomal recessive and dominant disorders and X-linked recessive disorders are shown in Figs. 13.4 and 13.5. These diagrams are discussed later in this chapter in the context of recording a pedigree and family history.

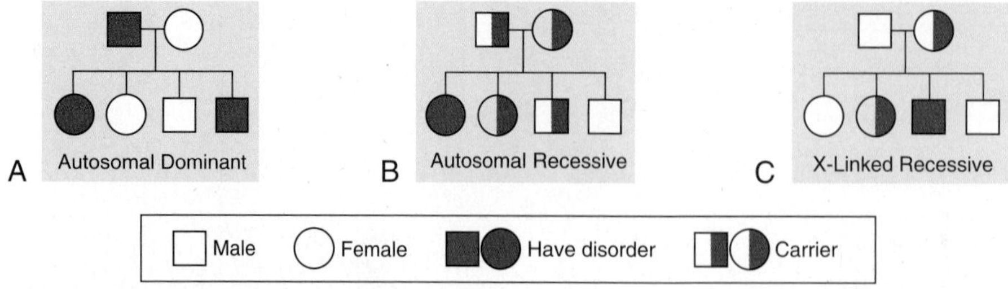

Fig. 13.4 Family pedigrees showing inheritance of (A) autosomal dominant, (B) autosomal recessive, and (C) X-linked recessive disorders.

TABLE 13.2 Comparison of Genetic Disorders

Characteristics	Examples
Autosomal Dominant	
• Males and females are affected or have the disease equally • Affected persons show variable expression • Affected persons may have an affected parent • Children of a heterozygous (affected) parent have a 50% chance of being affected • Affects persons in successive generations	• Breast and ovarian cancer related to *BRCA* genes • Familial hypercholesterolemia • Hereditary nonpolyposis colorectal cancer • Huntington disease • Neurofibromatosis • Marfan syndrome
Autosomal Recessive	
• Affects males and females equally • Heterozygotes are carriers and usually asymptomatic • Affected persons may have unaffected parents who are heterozygous for trait • Children of 2 heterozygous parents have a 25% chance of being affected and a 50% chance of being carriers (see Fig. 13.9) • Often no family history of disease	• Cystic fibrosis • Phenylketonuria • Sickle cell disease • Tay-Sachs disease • Thalassemia
X-Linked Recessive	
• Most affected persons have unaffected parents • Affected persons are usually male • Daughters of affected males are carriers • Sons of affected males are unaffected (unless mother is a carrier)	• Duchenne muscular dystrophy • Hemophilia • Wiskott-Aldrich syndrome

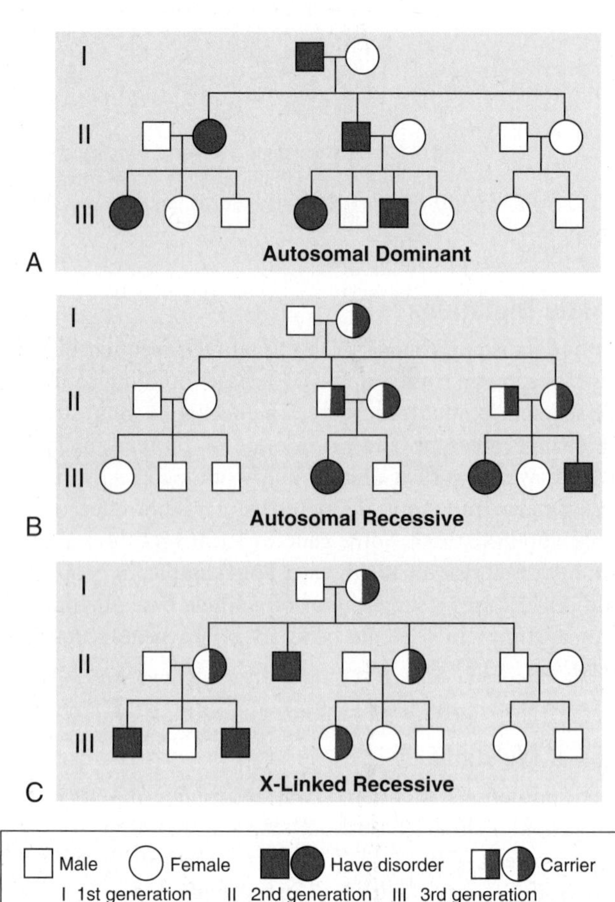

Fig. 13.5 Family pedigrees showing 3 generations. (A) Family pedigree suggesting an autosomal dominant disorder. (B) Family pedigree suggesting an autosomal recessive disorder. (C) Family pedigree suggesting an X-linked recessive disorder.

Autosomal dominant disorders are caused by a mutation of a single gene pair (heterozygous) on a chromosome. A dominant allele prevails over a normal allele. *Penetrance* describes the chance that a carrier of a dominant mutation will show signs of the disorder. *Incomplete penetrance* occurs when a person with a genetic mutation does not have signs of the disorder. It explains why a parent who has a genetic disorder may not have signs of the disorder, but the child does. Autosomal dominant disorders show variable expressivity. *Expressivity* describes the way the phenotype manifests. This accounts for how symptoms of a disorder vary from person to person, even though they have the same mutated gene. Symptoms are also influenced by other, usually unknown, genetic factors, gene-environment interactions, and chance events.

Autosomal recessive disorders are caused by mutations of 2 gene pairs (homozygous) on a chromosome. A person who inherits 1 copy of the recessive allele does not develop the disease because the normal allele predominates. However, this person is a *carrier.* A couple who are carriers may have affected children. These disorders occur in 1 generation and more often among children of parents who are blood relatives, such as 1st cousins. Disorders affect males and females with equal frequency and severity.

X-linked recessive disorders are caused by a mutation on the X chromosome. They can severely affect males because they have only 1 X chromosome. Females who carry the mutated gene on 1 X chromosome have another X chromosome to compensate for the mutation. Females who carry the mutated gene can transmit it to their offspring.

Y chromosomal inheritance occurs for genes that are only on the Y chromosome. They only affect males. An affected father transmits the disorder to all his sons.[4,5]

Human Genome Project

The Human Genome Project (HGP), completed in 2003, mapped 92% of the human genome.[6] In 2022, the Telomere to Telomere (T2T) consortium team continued this work and identified the remaining 8% of the human genome. The knowledge gained through the HGP and T2T consortium (1) helps improve the diagnosis of diseases, (2) allows for earlier detection of genetic predisposition to diseases, and (3) plays a key role in determining risk assessment for genetic-related diseases. The results of the HGP help match organ donors with transplant recipients.

GENETIC DISORDERS

A *genetic disorder* is caused in whole or in part by a change in the DNA sequence. They can be inherited (person born with altered genetic code) or acquired (e.g., replication errors, toxic damage to DNA).[4] Genetic disorders can be caused by (1) a mutation in 1 gene (single gene disorder); (2) mutations in multiple genes (multifactorial inheritance disorder), which are often related to environment factors; or (3) damage to chromosomes (changes in the number or structure of chromosomes).

Classification of Genetic Disorders

Single Gene Disorders

Some genetic disorders result from a single gene mutation (Fig. 13.6A). Examples include cystic fibrosis, sickle cell disease, and polycystic kidney disease. The pattern of inheritance for single gene disorders can be autosomal dominant, autosomal recessive, or X-linked. Single gene disorders are relatively rare compared with more common multifactorial genetic disorders.

Multifactorial Inherited Conditions

Multifactorial inherited conditions are complex diseases that result from inherited variations in genes acting together with environment factors (Fig. 13.6B). These disorders run in families but do not show the same inherited characteristics as the single gene mutation conditions. Examples include heart disease, diabetes, and some cancers.[5]

Rare hereditary mutations in a single gene can cause disease. In these cases, genetic mutations that cause or strongly predispose a person to these diseases run in a family. These mutations can significantly increase each family member's risk of developing the disease. One example is breast cancer. Inheriting a mutated *BRCA1* or *BRCA2* gene confers a significant risk for developing breast cancer.

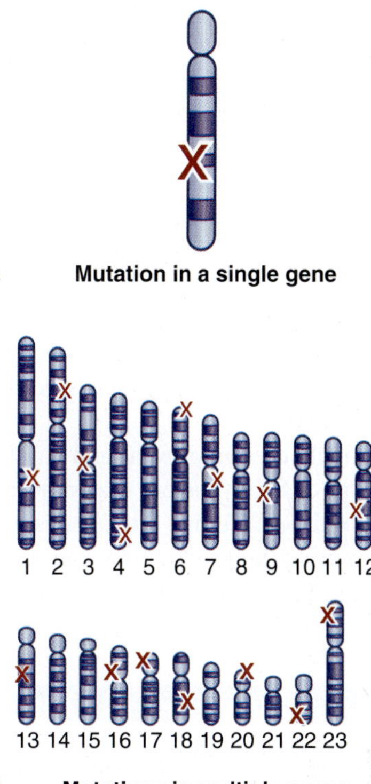

Fig. 13.6 (A) Genetic disorders can be caused by a mutation in a single gene (e.g., sickle cell disease, cystic fibrosis). (B) Most genetic disorders are multifactorial genetic disorders caused by a combination of mutations in multiple genes, often interacting with environment factors. Examples include cancer, diabetes, and hypertension.

Epigenetics. **Epigenetics** is the study of inheritable changes in gene expression that do not involve changes in the DNA sequence. There is a change in phenotype without a change in genotype. Epigenetic modifications define how the information in genes is expressed and used by cells.

Epigenetics influences the way cells terminally differentiate to become distinct types of cells (e.g., skin, liver) or result in disease. Epigenetic changes occur regularly. They can be influenced by age, the environment, exercise, diet, and disease. Identical twins, who have the same genetic makeup, do not always develop the same diseases or at the same rate. Twins share the same genes, but their environments become different as they age. This unique aspect of twins makes them an excellent model for understanding how genes and the environment contribute to certain traits, especially complex behaviors and diseases.

Chromosome Disorders

Chromosome disorders are caused by structural changes within chromosomes or by an excess or deficiency of the genes on chromosomes. For example, an extra copy of chromosome 21 causes Down syndrome (called *trisomy 21*). There are 3 copies of this chromosome instead of 2. In Down syndrome, there is no individual abnormal gene on the chromosome. Chromosomal translocation, in which portions of 2 chromosomes (chromosomes 9 and 22) are switched, can cause chronic myelocytic leukemia. This translocation is called the *Philadelphia chromosome.*[5]

GENETIC SCREENING AND TESTING

Genetic screening is the first level of detection. It is offered to general or targeted populations who are at risk for a disorder but do not have symptoms or have a family history of the disorder. An example is α-fetoprotein screening, which can detect fetal anomalies.

Genetic testing focuses on persons and families for a specific reason. Symptoms or family history may show an increased risk for a specific condition. Testing procedures analyze chromosomes, genes, or any gene product that can determine whether a mutation or predisposition to a condition exists. We can obtain samples for genetic testing from a person's blood, skin, hair, or saliva. We can also obtain tissues and cells prenatally. Insurance companies may not cover the cost of genetic testing.

Genetic testing has become important in health care (Table 13.3). Genetic tests are available for more than 2000 diseases. Most tests assess single genes. They can help diagnose genetic disorders, such as cystic fibrosis or Duchenne muscular dystrophy.[5] Some genetic tests look at rare inherited mutations of otherwise protective genes, such as *BRCA1* and *BRCA2.* They are responsible for some types of hereditary breast and ovarian cancers.[5]

Test results are used to assess risk or diagnose a disorder, a key step in providing ongoing care for the person and family. They help us to identify people at high risk for conditions that may be preventable. For example, persons who have inherited a gene for familial adenomatous polyposis (FAP) need ongoing monitoring.[5]

TABLE 13.3 Use of Genetic Tests

Type of Test	Description	Examples
Carrier screening	• Used to identify unaffected persons who carry 1 copy of a gene • Offered to persons who have a family history of a genetic disorder and to those in ethnic groups with an increased risk for specific genetic conditions • If both parents are tested, the test can provide information about a couple's risk for having a child with a genetic condition	• Cystic fibrosis • Sickle cell disease • Hemophilia
Diagnostic testing	• Used to diagnose, exclude, or confirm a specific genetic or chromosomal condition • Used to confirm findings when signs and symptoms suggest a genetic disorder • Can be done at any time • Not available for all genes or all genetic conditions	• Cystic fibrosis • Sickle cell disease • Polycystic kidney disease • Hemophilia • Familial hypercholesterolemia
Forensic testing	• Done to identify a person for legal purposes	• Identify crime or victims in catastrophic situations • Exclude or implicate a crime suspect
Newborn screening	• Most widespread use of genetic testing • Early intervention to treat a disorder can eliminate or reduce symptoms that may otherwise cause a lifetime of disability	• Phenylketonuria • Congenital hypothyroidism • Cystic fibrosis
Parental testing	• Establish biologic relationships between people	• Paternity testing
Pharmacogenomic testing	• Identifies genetic variations that influence a person's response to drugs • Results provide information to select drug therapy that is best for the person	• Warfarin dose
Predictive testing	• Can identify mutations that increase a person's risk for developing disorders • If results are positive, person can have prophylactic measures (e.g., mastectomy, oophorectomy) to prevent development of cancer	• Breast cancer • Ovarian cancer
Preimplantation genetic diagnosis (PGD)	• Fertilized embryos tested before implantation and pregnancy • Allows embryos free of a specific disorder can be placed into the uterus	• For persons known to have or be a carrier for a genetic mutation (e.g., Huntington disease)
Prenatal diagnostic testing	• Fluid obtained from amniocentesis or tissue from chorionic villus used to obtain fetal cells. Can obtain fetal samples from mother's blood • Detect changes in genes or chromosomes of fetus before birth • Testing offered to a couple with an increased risk for having a baby with a genetic or chromosomal disorder	• Down syndrome • Genetic alterations in fetuses
Presymptomatic testing	• Detects genetic mutations associated with disorders that appear later in life • Can be helpful to people who have a family member with a genetic disorder but who have no features of the disorder themselves at the time of testing • Results can provide information about a person's risk for developing a specific disorder and help with making decisions about treatment	• Huntington disease • Adult polycystic kidney disease • Hemochromatosis • Familial adenomatous polyposis • Hereditary nonpolyposis colorectal cancer syndrome

Genetic testing may raise ethical questions. People considering genetic testing should receive counseling about the various issues. They should be aware that test results in their medical records might not be private, and there is the potential for discrimination by employers and insurance companies. To protect people from this discrimination, the federal government passed the Genetic Information Nondiscrimination Act (GINA) in 2008 (Box 13.1).[7]

If a person has genetic testing, it may uncover information that may affect a family member who was not tested. These persons may not have taken part in the decision-making process to have testing. Similarly, if a whole family is tested, the results may show that a biologic relationship is not what the family believed it to be.

Interpreting Genetic Test Results

The results of genetic tests are not always straightforward. This often makes them challenging to interpret and explain. When interpreting test results, we need to consider the reason for the test, pretest counseling provided, the person's medical history, the family history, and the type of genetic test.

A *positive test* result means that the laboratory found a change in a particular gene, chromosome, or protein that was being tested. Depending on the purpose of the test, this result may confirm a diagnosis (e.g., Huntington disease). It may show that a person is a carrier of a specific genetic mutation (e.g., cystic fibrosis). A positive test can identify an increased risk for developing a disease (e.g., breast cancer) or suggest a need for further testing. A positive result of a predictive or presymptomatic genetic test usually cannot establish the absolute risk for developing a disorder. A positive test cannot predict the course or severity of a condition.

It is hard to interpret a positive result in some situations because some people who have the genetic mutation never develop the disease. For example, having the *apolipoprotein E-4 (Apo E-4)* allele increases the risk of developing Alzheimer disease. However, many people who test positive for *Apo E-4* never develop Alzheimer disease (see Chapter 64).

A *negative test* result means that the laboratory did not find an altered form of the gene, chromosome, or protein under consideration. This result means a person is not affected by a specific disorder, is not a carrier of a specific genetic mutation, or does not have an increased risk for developing a certain disease. It is possible that the test missed a disease-causing genetic alteration. Many tests cannot detect all the genetic changes that cause a specific disorder. The person may need more testing to confirm a negative result.

BOX 13.1 GENETICS IN CLINICAL PRACTICE

Genetic Information Nondiscrimination Act (GINA)

The GINA is a federal law prohibiting discrimination in health care coverage and employment based on genetic information. Genetic information is any data about a person's genetic tests, family members' genetic tests, and family history of a genetic disease.

- Addresses concerns about discrimination that might prevent people from seeking genetic tests
- Enables people to take part in research studies without fear that their DNA information may be used against them in the workplace or prevent them from getting health insurance
- Prevents health insurers from denying health insurance coverage and discriminating against a person based on genetic or family history information
- Prevents health insurers from asking that a person have a genetic test
- Prohibits most employers from using genetic information for hiring, firing, or promotion decisions and any decisions about terms of employment
- Protection does not extend to life insurance, disability insurance, or long-term care insurance

Courtesy National Human Genome Research Institute, https://www.genome.gov/about-genomics/policy-issues/Genetic-Discrimination.

Direct-to-Consumer Genetic Tests

Direct-to-consumer genetic tests are marketed directly to people via television, print advertisements, or the Internet. The person receives the test kit directly rather than having a specimen collected in an HCP's office. The test typically involves collecting a DNA sample at home, often by swabbing the inside of the cheek, and mailing the sample back to the laboratory. In some cases, the person must visit a health clinic to have blood drawn. People receive their results by mail, over the telephone, or online. In some cases, a genetics counselor or other HCP is available to explain the results and answer questions.[8]

Direct-to-consumer genetic tests have risks and limitations. People may want their genetic information, but they may not understand what it means. They may be misled by unproven or invalid test results. Without guidance from an HCP, they may make important decisions about disease treatment or prevention based on inaccurate, incomplete, or misunderstood information about their health. People may experience an invasion of genetic privacy if testing companies use their genetic information in an unauthorized way. When people are considering using these kinds of genetic tests, nurses should provide education and suggest they discuss the issue with their HCP or a genetic counselor. Teaching related to genetic testing is outlined in Table 13.4.

Genetic Technology

DNA Fingerprinting

DNA (genetic) fingerprinting begins by extracting DNA from the cells in a sample of blood, saliva, semen, or other appropriate fluid or tissue. *Polymerase chain reaction (PCR)* is a quick, easy method to provide unlimited copies of a DNA or RNA sequence using only a small sample. PCR involves the artificial replication of a DNA or RNA sequence. The DNA or RNA strands can be separated to form new templates that are used for replication.

TABLE 13.4 PATIENT & CAREGIVER TEACHING

Genetic Testing

General Information

Provide the following general information when teaching patients and caregivers about genetic testing:

- Genetics counseling can help you understand the purpose of genetic testing, considerations before testing, and the emotional and medical impact of the test results.
- A genetic test will only tell you whether there is a specific genetic variant or mutation. Positive tests do not always mean you will develop that disease. Neither can the results tell you when you will develop the disease.
- If a genetic test shows a genetic predisposition to an inherited disease, the news can be depressing.
- Knowledge of a genetic predisposition to a disease may motivate you to take preventive measures (e.g., taking drugs for high cholesterol) or make lifestyle changes to lower the risk for a disease (e.g., exercising to decrease the risk for type 2 diabetes).
- If a genetic test reveals you are at risk for a specific genetic disease, there is the chance that other family members may be at risk.
- If a genetic test reveals you are at risk for developing an inherited disease, whether you decide to share that information with family members is a personal and ethical decision that you will have to make.
- Genetic testing may provide important information that you can use when making decisions about having children.
- Genetic testing can be expensive. Your health insurance may not cover the cost.

PCR is a key element in *genetic fingerprinting*. It is an essential technique for finding mutations in genes. We use it in forensic medicine to identify the DNA of criminal suspects by using samples from blood, hair, saliva, and semen. Results have freed persons who are wrongly incarcerated. PCR is used in paternity testing and as a confirmatory test in HIV testing. This is especially important when an infant of a mother who is HIV-antibody positive tests HIV positive. PCR can determine whether the baby is infected with HIV or if the antibodies are from the mother.

DNA Microarray (DNA Chip)

Although all a person's somatic cells have identical genetic material, the same genes are not active in every cell. Studying which genes are active and inactive in different cell types helps to understand (1) how these cells function normally and (2) how they are affected when various genes do not perform properly.

Gene expression profiling uses a technology called *DNA microarrays* (DNA chips). The chip is a small glass plate enclosed in plastic. The surface of each chip has thousands of short, synthetic, single-stranded DNA sequences. Together they represent the normal gene, as well as known variations of the gene.[9] DNA chips can identify changes in gene sequences or if certain genes are turned off in cells and tissues. It can serve as a diagnostic test or determine whether certain medications might have a better therapeutic effect for certain people.

Genome-Wide Association Study (GWAS)

Genome-wide association study (GWAS) is an approach that involves rapidly scanning complete sets of DNA, or genomes, of many people to find genetic variations associated with the development or progression of a specific disease.

With GWAS, researchers can study large numbers of genes and proteins, including how they act and interact. This gives us a more complete picture of what goes on in a person. We may learn how to stop or jump-start genes on demand, change the course of a disease, or prevent it from ever happening. GWAS is useful in finding genetic variations that contribute to multifactorial inherited disorders, such as cancer and heart disease. The information can help us tailor prevention programs.[10]

PHARMACOGENOMICS AND PHARMACOGENETICS

Patients vary widely in their response to drugs. Although the reasons for this are complex, genetic factors may account for a percentage of individual variability. **Pharmacogenomics** looks at how drugs affect and interact with the genome and output expression. Pharmacogenomics allows for the identification of variations in multiple genes that affect drug response. **Pharmacogenetics** is the study of variable drug responses, including adverse events from differences in inheritable genes. These terms have been used interchangeably when describing the relationship between pharmacology and genetic variability in determining a person's response to drugs. Pharmacogenetics has a narrower focus than pharmacogenomics.

Pharmacogenetic and pharmacogenomic studies could lead to the development of drugs that can be tailor-made or adapted to each person's genetic makeup. This will make it possible to have personal medicine by choosing the right drug and the right dose for the right person. HCPs are starting to use pharmacogenomic information to prescribe drugs. Table 13.5 shows a few examples.

One area of study has focused on the hepatic cytochrome P450 (CYP450) enzyme system. It is responsible for oxidizing many drugs and chemicals. The enzymes in this system share certain amino acid sequences. Each is coded by a separate gene. People with a less active form of the enzyme (who metabolize the drug slowly) may get too much of the drug. People with a

TABLE 13.5 Examples of Pharmacogenomics

Drug	Role of Pharmacogenetics
abacavir (Ziagen)	• Some people are at greater risk for serious allergic reactions when first starting treatment with this drug. • Genetic testing for *HLA-B*5701* before taking the drug can identify those who carry a genetic marker associated with life-threatening hypersensitivity reactions.
clopidogrel (Plavix)	• For clopidogrel to work, cytochrome P450 enzymes in the liver (particularly CYP2C19) must convert the drug to its active form. • About 2%–14% of the population are poor metabolizers of the drug. These patients may not receive the full benefits of the drug. • Genetic tests can identify genetic differences in CYP2C19 function.
crizotinib (Xalkori)	• Used to treat patients with late-stage, non–small cell lung cancers (NSCLCs) who express the abnormal anaplastic lymphoma kinase *(ALK)* gene. • *ALK* gene abnormality causes cancer development and growth. • Blocks certain proteins called *kinases,* including the protein made by the abnormal *ALK* gene. • Genetic test can determine whether a patient with NSCLC has the abnormal *ALK* gene.
trastuzumab (Herceptin)	• In breast cancer, drug works only for women whose tumors have genes that lead to the overproduction of a protein called HER-2. • Drug is a monoclonal antibody to HER-2. After the antibody attaches to the antigen, it kills the cells. • Genetic testing provides information on good candidates for treatment with drug.
vemurafenib (Zelboraf)	• Approved for patients with late-stage (metastatic) or unresectable melanoma whose tumors express a gene mutation called *BRAF V600E.*
warfarin (see Fig. 13.7)	• Genetic variants in the genes *VKORC1* and cytochrome P450 2C9 *(CYP2C9)* affect people's sensitivity to warfarin (Fig. 13.7). These variations explain about 50% of the required dose difference between persons. • Persons with specific variations in these genes need a lower warfarin dose to maintain therapeutic levels of anticoagulation. • Persons with other variations need higher doses. • Testing for *CYP2C9* and *VKORC1* genotype information can assist in choosing the starting dose.

more active form of the enzyme (who metabolize the drug quickly) may get too little of the drug. It may appear that the medication is not effective. These persons may need more frequent dosing. Pharmacogenomic testing can help HCPs in prescribing the right dose based on a patient's genetic makeup (Fig. 13.7).

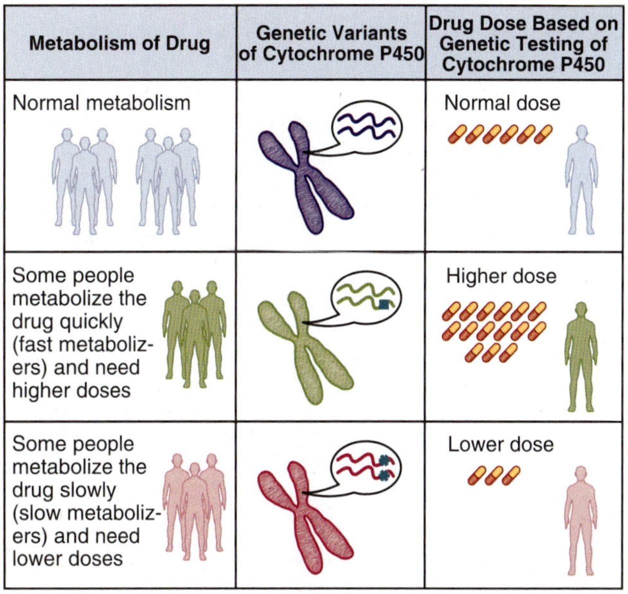

Metabolism of Drug	Genetic Variants of Cytochrome P450	Drug Dose Based on Genetic Testing of Cytochrome P450
Normal metabolism		Normal dose
Some people metabolize the drug quickly (fast metabolizers) and need higher doses		Higher dose
Some people metabolize the drug slowly (slow metabolizers) and need lower doses		Lower dose

Fig. 13.7 People respond differently to the drug warfarin. This is partially due to genetic variants in 1 of the cytochrome P450 genes.

GENE THERAPY

Gene therapy is used to treat the underlying cause of a disease. Gene therapy may be able to supply a missing gene, provide the missing gene's role, or enhance the treatment of a disease. The goal is to provide a normally functioning gene to a person with a pathogenic gene variant.

A carrier molecule called a *vector* is used to deliver the therapeutic gene to the target cells. Currently, one of the most common vectors is a genetically altered virus to carry normal human DNA. The vector is given IV or directly injected into tissue. The vector unloads its genetic material containing the therapeutic human gene into the target cell. If the treatment is successful, the new gene will make a functional protein and restore the target cell to normal. A diagram of gene therapy is shown in Fig. 13.8.[5] Gene therapy is a promising treatment for several diseases, including inherited disorders, some types of cancer, and certain viral infections.[11]

STEM CELL THERAPY

Stem cells are unspecialized cells in the body that have the ability to (1) remain in their unspecialized state and divide or (2) differentiate and develop into specialized cells. The use of stem cells may allow for the regeneration of lost tissue and restoration of function in various diseases. Stem cells can be derived from human embryos or adult somatic tissues. Stem cells can be totipotent, pluripotent, multipotent, or unipotent. Totipotent cells can produce all the cell types of the developing organism. Pluripotent cells can make any body cell because they make all cells of the embryo. Multipotent cells only make cells within a specific germ layer. Unipotent cells make a single cell type.[12]

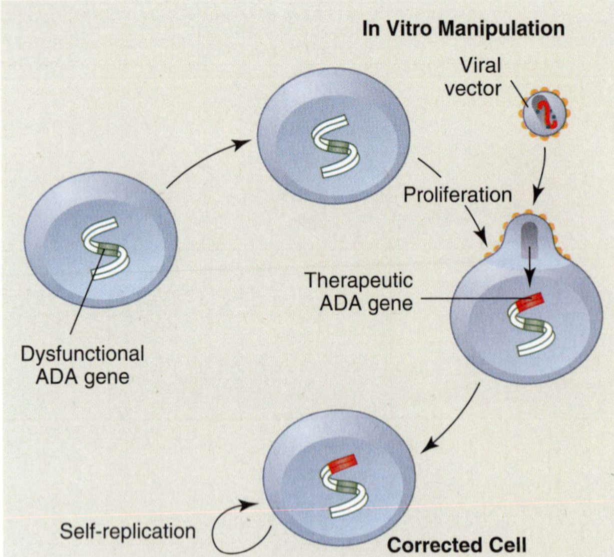

Fig. 13.8 Gene therapy for adenosine deaminase *(ADA)* deficiency. The viral vector containing the therapeutic ADA gene is inserted into the patient's lymphocytes. These cells can then make the ADA enzyme.

Adult stem cells are undifferentiated cells that exist in small numbers in many organs and tissues. These include the brain, bone marrow, peripheral blood, blood vessels, skeletal muscle, skin, teeth, heart, GI tract, liver, ovarian epithelium, and testes. The primary roles of adult stem cells are to maintain and repair the tissues in which they are found. They are generally multipotent cells, giving rise to a closely related family of cells within the tissue. For example, skin stem cells produce new skin cells. Hematopoietic stem cells in the bone marrow can form all the various blood cells. These cells are prolific by design.[12]

We use stem cells to treat people with many different disorders, including severe burns and orthopedic conditions requiring bone grafting. Hematopoietic stem cell transplantation is a standard treatment for hematologic cancers and bone marrow failure (see Chapter 16).[12]

NURSING MANAGEMENT: GENETICS AND GENOMICS

You need to understand genetics and genomics to assist persons and families seeking information and making decisions related to genetic issues.[3] By understanding the influence that genetics has on health and illness, you can aid the patient and family in making critical decisions related to genetic issues, such as genetic testing. You can facilitate access to resources and provide education.

You will collaborate with other health care team members, including genetic counselors and nurses. A genetic nurse is a nurse with special education and training in genetics. Nurses with *GCN* after their names are baccalaureate-prepared RNs who have specialty credentialing as a Genetic Clinical Nurse (GCN). Nurses with *APNG* after their names are RNs with a master's degree who have specialty credentialing as an Advanced Practice Nurse in Genetics (APNG).

People considering genetic testing should meet with a genetics nurse or counselor who is specially trained in medical genetics and counseling. The special knowledge and counseling skills they have are often important in genetic testing, which may raise many emotional issues. Knowledge of the carrier status of a genetic disorder may influence a person's career, marriage, and childbearing decisions. It may affect family members as they contemplate potentially serious life and health care issues.

Genetic testing raises ethical questions. Who should know the results of a genetic test? Who should protect the privacy of test results and prevent persons from discrimination? People may not want to share or disclose information about family history or genetic test results. They may fear they are vulnerable to discrimination based on their DNA. As a nurse, you need to understand how different health care policies relate to genetic testing. It is important to explain how the GINA protects persons from discrimination by employers and health care insurance companies (Box 13.2).[7]

BOX 13.2 ETHICAL/LEGAL DILEMMAS

Genetic Testing

Situation

A 30-year-old patient tells you she is 3 months pregnant. She and her husband have 2 biologic children. This pregnancy was unplanned, and their youngest child has cystic fibrosis (CF). They express concern about the chance of having another child with CF and would like to have genetic testing on their fetus. The husband asks you what the chance is of having another child with CF.

Ethical/Legal Points for Consideration

- With genetic testing, the couple can find out whether their child will have CF.
- Genetic counseling is recommended before and after genetic testing because of the complexity of the information and the emotional issues involved with implications and options.
- Knowing that CF is an autosomal recessive condition, you can use Punnett squares (Fig. 13.9) or a family pedigree (Figs. 13.4 and 13.5) to show them the chance of having another child with CF.

Discussion Questions

1. What information would you give the couple about genetic testing so they can make an informed decision?
2. How would you help the couple if the genetic test results reveal that the fetus has CF?

Family History

It is important that you ask patients about their family history and identify and assess inheritance patterns. The family health history is a written or graphic record of the health problems in one's family (see Chapter 3). You may construct a family pedigree (Figs. 13.4 and 13.5). A pedigree is a graphic representation of the family health history. The family health history and pedigree should include a minimum of 3 generations.[5]

To help people record information about their family history, federal agencies developed a Web-based tool called My Family Health Portrait (https://phgkb.cdc.gov/FHH/html/index.html). Other web-based programs are available to help create pedigree diagrams based on the information entered.

When constructing the pedigree, start with the proband or person being interviewed. For each family member, record date of birth, health problems, and the age when diagnosed. Include age and cause of death for deceased relatives. Note racial and ethnic information and information that is unknown. Note any shared ancestors. Review the information to identify key features that may increase a person's risk for genetic-related diseases. These include:

- Disease in more than 1 close relative
- Disease that does not usually affect a certain gender (e.g., breast cancer in a male)
- Disease that occurs at an earlier age than expected (e.g., myocardial infarction before age 35)
- Certain combinations of diseases within a family (e.g., breast and ovarian cancer, heart disease and diabetes)

If we identify 1 or more of these features, the family history may hold important clues about a person's risk for a genetic disease. These persons may benefit from further clinical investigation, screening, and diagnostic testing. As a nurse, you may refer these persons to a specialist for information about the benefits and risks of genetic screening and testing. Throughout the book, Genetics in Clinical Practice boxes describe risks related to genetic disorders. You can use that information to assess family history.

As a nurse, you can support the person and family by providing education and reinforcing the information they receive throughout the process. Use the family history, pedigree, and Punnett squares (Fig. 13.9) to explain the risk for inheritable disease. When a diagnosis is confirmed, you can discuss health promotion activities. People with multifactorial disorders may benefit from lifestyle modification that addresses risky behaviors (e.g., smoking, unhealthy eating habits). You can help the person and family understand how we use evidence-based guidelines for monitoring, screening, and ongoing follow-up. For example, it is important to monitor cholesterol levels in a person with a family history of high cholesterol.

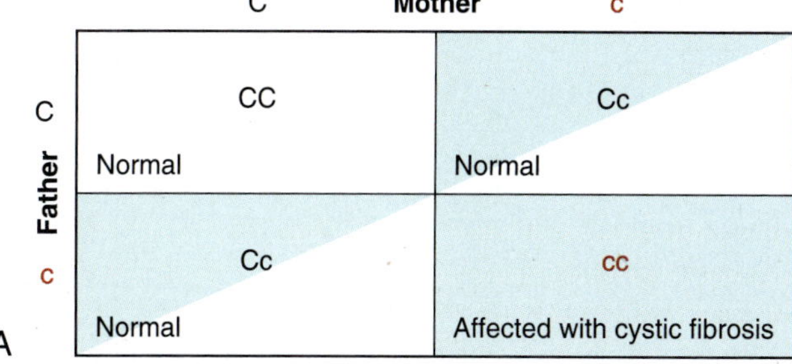

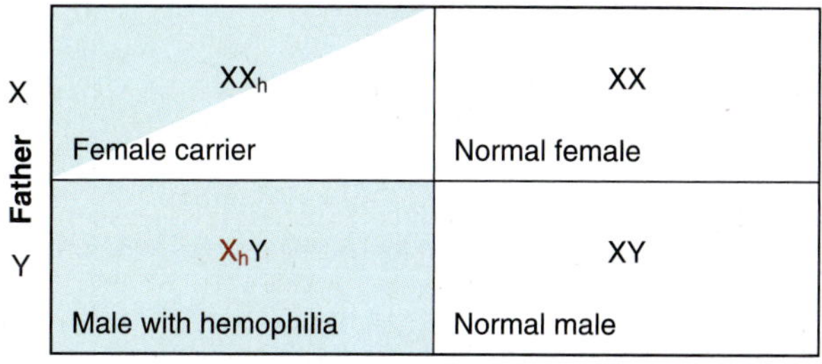

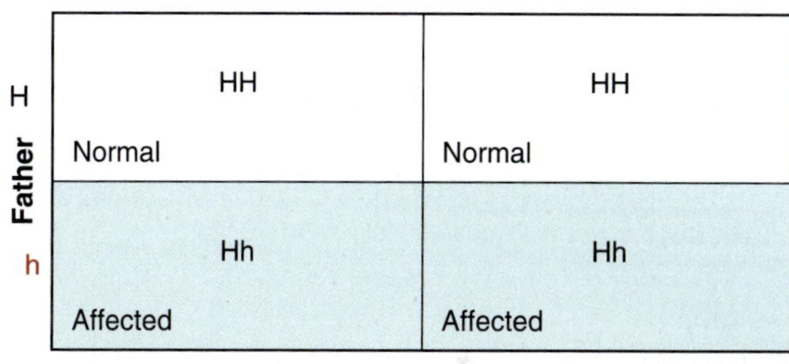

Fig. 13.9 Punnett squares show inheritance possibilities. (A) If the mother and father are both carriers of cystic fibrosis, there is a 25% chance that offspring will have cystic fibrosis. (B) If the mother is a carrier for the hemophilia gene and the father has a normal genotype, there is a 50% chance that any male offspring will have hemophilia. There is a 50% chance that any female offspring will be a carrier. (C) If the mother has a normal genotype and the father has Huntington disease, there is a 50% chance that offspring will have the disease.

BRIDGE TO NCLEX EXAMINATION

The number of the question corresponds to the same-numbered outcome at the beginning of the chapter.

1. If a person is heterozygous for a given gene, it means that the person
   a. is a carrier for a genetic disorder.
   b. is affected by the genetic disorder.
   c. has 2 identical alleles for the gene.
   d. has 2 different alleles for the gene.

2. Common causes of genetic mutations include (**Select all that apply.**)
   a. DNA damage from toxins.
   b. DNA damage from UV radiation.
   c. inheritance of altered genes from father.
   d. inheritance of altered genes from mother.
   e. inheritance of somatic mutations from either parent.

3. A father who has an X-linked recessive disorder and a wife with a normal genotype will
   a. pass the carrier state to all his children.
   b. pass the carrier state to his male children.
   c. pass the carrier state to his female children.
   d. not pass on the genetic mutation to any of his children.

4. What characterizes multifactorial genetic disorders?
   a. Often caused by single-gene alterations
   b. Genetic testing available for most disorders
   c. Many family members report having the disorder
   d. Caused by complex interactions of genetic and environment factors

5. If a person tests positive for a genetic mutation, it means (**Select all that apply.**)
   a. the laboratory found an alteration in a gene.
   b. the person is predisposed to develop a genetic disease.
   c. there is the chance other family members may be at risk.
   d. the person will definitely develop the disease at some point.
   e. the person should not have any children or any more children.

6. What role does pharmacogenomics have in health care?
   a. It can assess individual variability to many drugs.
   b. Information can assess the effectiveness of a drug.
   c. It provides important assessment data for gene therapy.
   d. It can assess the variability of drug responses due to single genes.

7. A couple who recently had a son with hemophilia A is consulting with a nurse. They want to know if their next child will have hemophilia A. The nurse can tell the parents that if their child is a
   a. male, he will have hemophilia A.
   b. male, he will be a carrier of hemophilia A.
   c. female, she will be a carrier of hemophilia A.
   d. female, there is a 50% chance she will be a carrier of hemophilia A.

1. d; 2. a, b, c, d; 3. c; 4. d; 5. a, c; 6. d; 7. d.

For rationales to these answers and even more NCLEX review questions, visit http://evolve.elsevier.com/Lewis/medsurg.

REFERENCES

To access the References for this chapter, please scan the QR code with a mobile device.

14

Immune Responses and Transplantation

Tracie Clark Morgan, LaToya Patterson, Yeow Chye Ng, and Haley Hoy

http://evolve.elsevier.com/Lewis/medsurg/

CONCEPTUAL FOCUS

Immunity
Infection
Inflammation
Tissue Integrity

LEARNING OUTCOMES

1. Describe the components and functions of the immune system.
2. Characterize the 5 types of immunoglobulins.
3. Distinguish among the 4 types of hypersensitivity reactions in terms of immunologic mechanisms and resulting alterations.
4. Outline the clinical manifestations and emergency management of an anaphylactic reaction.
5. Describe the assessment and interprofessional care of patients with chronic allergies.
6. Describe the etiologic factors, clinical manifestations, and treatment of autoimmune diseases.
7. Discern the categories of immunodeficiency.
8. Distinguish among the types of rejections after transplantation.
9. Identify the types and side effects of immunosuppressive therapy.
10. Describe interprofessional care of patients receiving biologic response modifiers.

KEY TERMS

anergy
antigen
autoimmunity
biologic response modifiers (BRMs)
cell-mediated immunity
human leukocyte antigen (HLA)
humoral immunity
hypersensitivity reactions
immunocompetence

One of our most complex defense mechanisms is the immune response. Immune processes must function properly for the body to defend itself against the presence of foreign substances. Many problems occur when the immune response is altered. These problems are closely related to the concepts of inflammation, infection, and tissue integrity. You will find that the care of patients with immune disorders discussed in this chapter is similar to the care of patients with inflammation (see Chapter 12), neutropenia (see Chapter 34), and general infection (see Chapter 15).

IMMUNE RESPONSE

Immunity is the body's ability to resist disease. Immune responses serve the following 3 functions:

1. *Defense:* The body protects against invasion by microorganisms and prevents the development of infection by attacking foreign antigens and pathogens.
2. *Homeostasis:* Damaged cellular substances are digested and removed. Through this mechanism, the body's different cell types stay uniform and unchanged.

3. *Surveillance:* Mutations continually arise. They are recognized as foreign cells and destroyed.

Immunocompetence exists when the body's immune system can identify and inactivate or destroy foreign substances. When the immune system is incompetent or underresponsive, severe infections, cancers, and immunodeficiency diseases may occur. When the immune system overreacts, hypersensitivity disorders such as allergies and autoimmune diseases may develop.

An **antigen** is a substance that elicits an immune response. Most antigens are made up of protein. However, other substances such as large polysaccharides, lipoproteins, and nucleic acids can act as antigens. All the body's cells have antigens on their surface. They are unique to that person and enable the body to recognize itself. The immune system normally becomes "tolerant" to our own molecules. This makes us nonresponsive to "self" antigens.

Types of Immunity

We classify immunity as innate or acquired.

Innate Immunity

Innate immunity is present at birth. Its primary role is first-line defense against pathogens. This type of immunity involves a nonspecific response. Neutrophils and monocytes are the primary white blood cells (WBCs) involved. Innate immunity is not antigen specific. So, it can respond within minutes to an invading pathogen without prior exposure to that organism.

Acquired Immunity

Acquired immunity is the development of either active or passive immunity (Table 14.1).

Active acquired immunity. *Active acquired immunity* results from the invasion of the body by foreign substances such as microorganisms and the subsequent development of antibodies and sensitized lymphocytes. With each reinvasion of the microorganism, the body responds more rapidly and vigorously to fight the invader. Active acquired immunity may result naturally from a disease or artificially through immunization.

TABLE 14.1 Types of Acquired Specific Immunity

Type	Natural	Artificial
Active	Natural contact with antigen through actual infection (e.g., chickenpox, measles, mumps)	Immunization with antigen (e.g., vaccines for chickenpox, measles, mumps)
Passive	Transplacental and colostrum transfer from mother to child (e.g., maternal immunoglobulins passed to baby)	Injection of serum with antibodies from 1 person (e.g., injection of hepatitis B immune globulin) to another person who does not have antibodies

Because the body makes antibodies, immunity takes time to develop but is long lasting.

Passive acquired immunity. In *passive acquired immunity,* the person receives antibodies to an antigen rather than making them. This may take place naturally through the transfer of immunoglobulins across the placental membrane from mother to fetus. Artificial passive acquired immunity occurs through injection with gamma globulin (serum antibodies). The benefit of this immunity is its immediate effect. Unfortunately, passive immunity is short lived because the person does not make the antibodies and memory cells for the antigen.

Lymphoid Organs

The lymphoid system is composed of central (or primary) and peripheral lymphoid organs. The *central lymphoid organs* are the bone marrow and thymus. We make lymphocytes in the bone marrow. They eventually migrate to the peripheral organs. The thymus is involved in T-lymphocyte differentiation and maturation. This makes it essential for a cell-mediated immune response. The thymus is its largest during childhood. After puberty, the thymus starts to slowly shrink and become replaced by fat. By age 75, the thymus is little more than fatty tissue and makes few T lymphocytes.

The *peripheral lymphoid organs* are the lymph nodes; tonsils; spleen; and gut-, genital-, bronchial-, and skin-associated lymphoid tissues (Fig. 14.1). The spleen is the primary site for filtering foreign antigens from the blood. The lymphoid tissue in the GI submucosa (gut-associated), genitourinary (genital-associated), and respiratory (bronchial-associated) tracts protect the body from external microorganisms.

When antigens enter the body, they may be carried by the bloodstream or lymph channels to regional lymph nodes. The

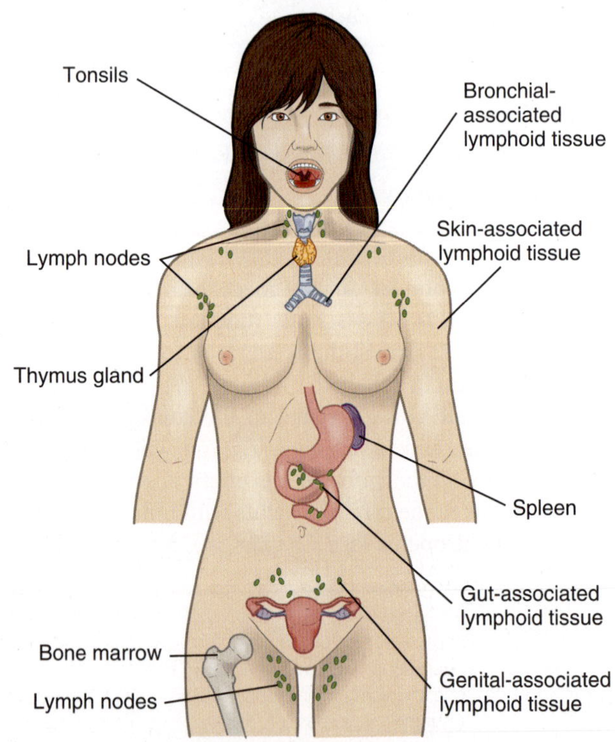

Fig. 14.1 Organs of the immune system.

antigens interact with B and T lymphocytes and macrophages in the lymph nodes. The 2 major functions of lymph nodes are (1) filtration of foreign material brought to the site and (2) circulation of lymphocytes.

The skin-associated lymph tissue consists mainly of lymphocytes and Langerhans cells (type of dendritic cell) found in the epidermis of skin. When Langerhans cells are depleted, the skin cannot initiate an immune response. Therefore a delayed hypersensitivity reaction (as determined by skin testing with injected antigens) does not occur.

Cells Involved in Immune Response

Mononuclear Phagocytes

The *mononuclear phagocyte system* includes monocytes in the blood and macrophages found throughout the body. Mononuclear phagocytes have a critical role in the immune system. They are responsible for capturing, processing, and presenting the antigen to the lymphocytes. This stimulates a humoral or cell-mediated immune response. Capturing is accomplished through phagocytosis. The macrophage-bound antigen, which is highly immunogenic, is presented to circulating T or B lymphocytes and thus triggers an immune response (Fig. 14.2).

Lymphocytes

We make lymphocytes in the bone marrow (Fig. 14.3). They then differentiate into B and T lymphocytes.

B lymphocytes. B cells differentiate into *plasma cells* when activated. Plasma cells make antibodies (immunoglobulins) (Table 14.2).

T lymphocytes. Cells that migrate from the bone marrow to the thymus differentiate into *T lymphocytes* (thymus-dependent cells). The thymus secretes hormones, including thymosin, that stimulate the maturation and differentiation of T lymphocytes.

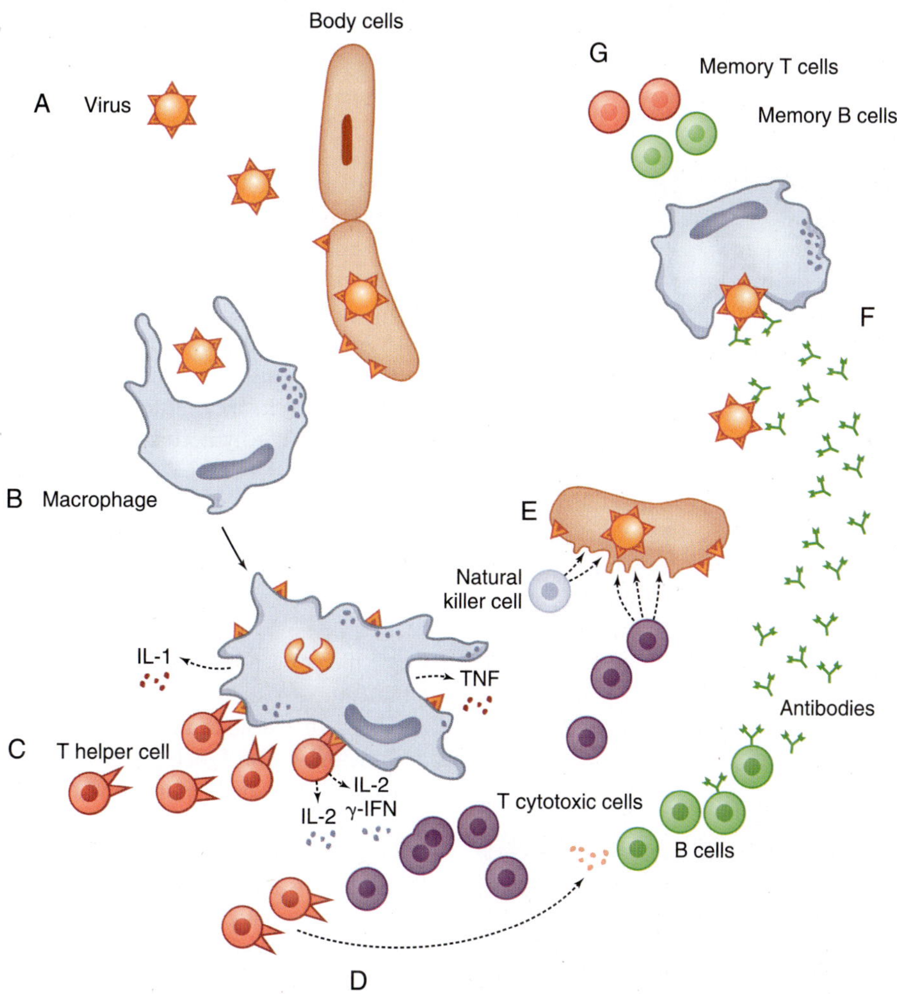

Fig. 14.2 The immune response to a virus. (A) A virus invades the body through a break in the skin or another portal of entry. The virus must make its way inside a cell to replicate itself. (B) A macrophage recognizes the antigens on the surface of the virus. The macrophage digests the virus and displays pieces of the virus (antigens) on its surface. (C) T helper cell recognizes the antigen displayed and binds to the macrophage. This binding stimulates the production of cytokines such as interleukin (IL)-1 and tumor necrosis factor (TNF) by the macrophage and IL-2 and γ-interferon *(γ-IFN)* by the T cell. These cytokines are intracellular messengers that provide communication among the cells. (D) IL-2 instructs other T helper cells and T cytotoxic cells to proliferate (multiply). T helper cells release cytokines, causing B cells to multiply and make antibodies. (E) T cytotoxic cells and natural killer cells destroy infected body cells. (F) The antibodies bind to the virus and mark it for macrophage destruction. (G) Memory B and T cells stay behind to respond quickly if the same virus attacks again.

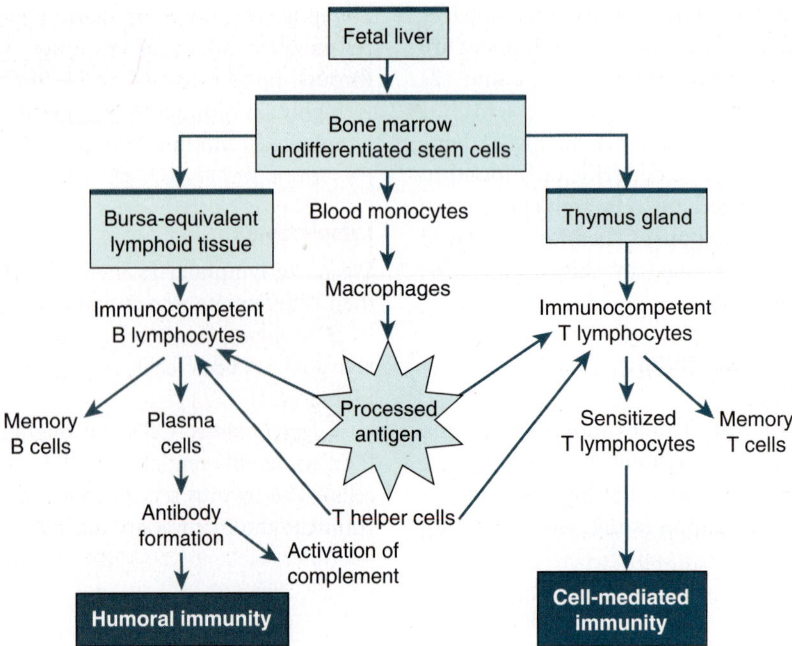

Fig. 14.3 Relationships and functions of macrophages, B lymphocytes, and T lymphocytes in an immune response.

TABLE 14.2 Characteristics of Immunoglobulins

Class	Serum Concentration (%)	Location	Characteristics
IgG	76	Plasma, interstitial fluid	Only immunoglobulin that crosses placenta Responsible for secondary immune response
IgA	15	Body secretions, including tears, saliva, breast milk, colostrum	Lines mucous membranes and protects body surfaces
IgM	8	Plasma	Responsible for primary immune response Forms antibodies to ABO blood antigens
IgD	1	Plasma	Present on lymphocyte surface Aids in the differentiation of B lymphocytes
IgE	0.002	Plasma, interstitial fluids	Causes symptoms of allergic reactions Fixes to mast cells and basophils Aids in defense against parasitic infections

T cells make up 70% to 80% of the circulating lymphocytes. They are mainly responsible for immunity to intracellular viruses, tumor cells, and fungi. T cells can live from a few months to the life span of a person. They account for long-term immunity.

We categorize T lymphocytes as T cytotoxic and T helper cells. Antigenic characteristics of WBCs can be classified using monoclonal antibodies. These antigens are classified as *clusters of differentiation,* or *CD antigens.* We refer to many types of WBCs, especially lymphocytes, by their CD designations. All mature T cells have the CD3 antigen.

T cytotoxic cells. T cytotoxic (CD8) cells are involved in attacking antigens on the cell membrane of foreign pathogens and releasing cytolytic substances that destroy the pathogen. These cells have antigen specificity and are sensitized by exposure to the antigen. Much like B cells, some sensitized T cells do not attack the antigen but remain as memory T cells. As in the humoral immune response, a second exposure to the antigen results in a more intense and rapid cell-mediated immune response.

T helper cells. T helper (CD4) cells are involved in regulating cell-mediated immunity and the humoral antibody response. T helper cells differentiate into subsets of cells that make distinct types of cytokines (discussed in a later section). These subsets are T_H1 cells and T_H2 cells. T_H1 cells stimulate phagocyte-mediated ingestion and killing of microbes, the key component of cell-mediated immunity. T_H2 cells stimulate eosinophil-mediated immunity. It is effective against parasites and involved in allergic responses.

Natural killer cells. Natural killer (NK) cells are involved in cell-mediated immunity. These cells do not need prior sensitization for their generation. These cells engage in recognition and killing of virus-infected cells, tumor cells, and transplanted grafts. They have a vital role in immune surveillance for malignant cell changes. We do not fully understand the mechanism of recognition.

Dendritic Cells

Dendritic cells make up a system of cells that is important to the immune system, especially the cell-mediated immune response. They have an atypical shape with extensive dendritic processes that form and retract. They are found in many places in the body, including the skin (where they are called *Langerhans cells*) and the lining of the nose, lungs, stomach, and intestine. There are many immature dendritic cells in the blood.[1]

Dendritic cells capture antigens at sites of contact with the external environment (e.g., skin, mucous membranes) and then transport the antigen until it meets a T cell with specificity for that antigen. In this role, they have an important function in activating the immune response.

Cytokines

The complex interactions of T cells, B cells, monocytes, and neutrophils depend on *cytokines* (soluble factors secreted by WBCs and a variety of other cells in the body). Cytokines act as messengers among the cell types. Cytokines instruct cells to alter their proliferation, differentiation, secretion, or activity.

Currently, we know of more than 100 different cytokines. They are classified into distinct categories. Table 14.3 lists some of these cytokines. Cytokines have a beneficial role in hematopoiesis and immune function. They can have detrimental effects such as those seen in chronic inflammation, autoimmune diseases, and sepsis. Cytokines such as colony-stimulating factors (CSFs), interferons, and interleukin (IL)-2 have clinical uses (Table 14.4). CSFs act as growth-regulating factors for hematopoietic cells. In general, ILs are immunomodulatory and antiviral factors.

Interferon helps the body's natural defenses attack tumors and viruses. We know of 3 types of interferon (Table 14.3). Interferon is not directly antiviral. It produces an antiviral effect in cells by reacting with them and inducing the formation of a second protein termed *antiviral protein* (Fig. 14.4). This protein mediates the antiviral action of interferon by changing the cell's protein synthesis and preventing new viruses from becoming assembled.

TABLE 14.3 Types and Functions of Common Cytokines

Type	Primary Functions
Colony-Stimulating Factors (CSFs)	
Erythropoietin	Stimulates erythroid progenitor cells in bone marrow to make red blood cells.
Granulocyte colony-stimulating factor (G-CSF)	Stimulates proliferation and differentiation of neutrophils, enhances functional activity of mature polymorphonuclear neutrophils (PMNs).
Granulocyte-macrophage colony-stimulating factor (GM-CSF)	Stimulates proliferation and differentiation of PMNs and monocytes.
Macrophage colony-stimulating factor (M-CSF)	Promotes proliferation, differentiation, and activation of monocytes and macrophages.
Interferons (IFNs)	
α-IFN β-IFN	Inhibits viral replication, activates natural killer (NK) cells and macrophages, antiproliferative effects on tumor cells.
γ-IFN	Proinflammatory mediator. Activates macrophages, neutrophils, and NK cells. Promotes B-cell differentiation. Inhibits viral replication.
Interleukins (ILs)	
IL-1	Proinflammatory mediator. Promotes proliferation of B cells. Activates T cells, NK cells, and macrophages.
IL-2	Activates T cells, NK cells, and macrophages. Stimulates release of other cytokines (α-IFN, TNF, IL-1, IL-6).
IL-3	Hematopoietic growth factor for hematopoietic precursor cells.
IL-4	Antiinflammatory mediator. B-cell growth and differentiation. Induces differentiation into T_H2 cells. Stimulates mast cell growth.
IL-5	B-cell growth and differentiation. Promotes growth and differentiation of eosinophils.
IL-6	Proinflammatory mediator. T- and B-cell growth factor promotes differentiation of B cells into plasma cells and stimulates antibody secretion. Induces fever. Synergistic effects with IL-1 and TNF.
Tumor necrosis factor (TNF)	Proinflammatory mediator. Activates macrophages and granulocytes. Promotes immune and inflammatory responses. Kills tumor cells. Responsible for weight loss with chronic inflammation, cancer.

Humoral and Cell-Mediated Immunity

We need both humoral and cell-mediated immunity to remain healthy. Each type of immunity has unique properties, different methods of action, and reactions against particular antigens. Table 14.5 compares humoral and cell-mediated immunity.

Humoral Immunity

Humoral immunity consists of antibody-mediated immunity. The term *humoral* comes from the Greek word *humor*, which means body fluid. Because antibodies are made by plasma cells (differentiated B cells) and found in plasma, we use the term *humoral immunity*. Antibody production is an essential part of the humoral immune response. Each of the 5 classes of immunoglobulins (IgG, IgA, IgM, IgD, IgE) has specific characteristics (Table 14.2).

When a pathogen (especially bacteria) enters the body, it may encounter a B cell that is specific for antigens found on that bacterial cell wall. In addition, a monocyte or macrophage may phagocytize the bacteria and present its antigens to a B cell. The B cell recognizes the antigen because it has receptors

TABLE 14.4 Clinical Uses of Common Cytokines

Cytokine	Clinical Uses
Colony-Stimulating Factors	
Erythropoietin epoetin alfa (Epogen, Procrit) Darbepoetin alfa (Aranesp)	Anemia related to chronic kidney disease, cancer, chemotherapy
G-CSF filgrastim (Neupogen), pegfilgrastim (Neulasta)	Chemotherapy-induced neutropenia
GM-CSF sargramostim (Leukine)	Neutropenia, myeloid recovery after bone marrow transplantation
Interferons	
α-Interferon (Roferon-A, Intron A)	Hairy cell leukemia, chronic myelogenous leukemia, melanoma, renal cell cancer, ovarian cancer, multiple myeloma, Kaposi sarcoma, hepatitis B and C
β-Interferon (Betaseron, Avonex, Rebif)	Multiple sclerosis
Interleukins	
IL-2 aldesleukin (Proleukin)	Metastatic renal cell cancer, metastatic melanoma
IL-11 (platelet growth factor) oprelvekin (Neumega)	Thrombocytopenia related to chemotherapy

G-CSF, Granulocyte colony-stimulating factor; *GM-CSF,* granulocyte-macrophage colony-stimulating factor.

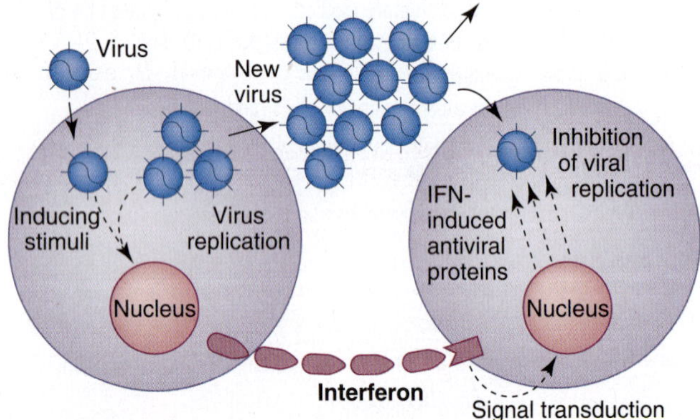

Fig. 14.4 Mechanism of action of interferon *(IFN).* When a virus attacks a cell, the cell begins to make viral DNA and IFN. IFN serves as an intercellular messenger and induces the production of antiviral proteins. Then the virus is not able to replicate in the cell.

on its cell surface specific for that antigen. When the antigen comes in contact with the cell surface receptor, the B cell becomes activated, and most B cells differentiate into plasma cells (Fig. 14.3). The mature plasma cell secretes immunoglobulins. Some stimulated B cells remain memory cells.

The primary immune response becomes evident 4 to 8 days after the first exposure to the antigen (Fig. 14.5). IgM is the first type of antibody formed. Because of its large size, the IgM molecule is confined to the intravascular space. As the immune response progresses, we make IgG. IgG can move from intravascular to extravascular spaces.

When a person is exposed to the antigen the second time, a secondary antibody response occurs. This response occurs

TABLE 14.5 Comparison of Humoral and Cell-Mediated Immunity

Characteristics	Humoral Immunity	Cell-Mediated Immunity
Cells involved	B lymphocytes	T lymphocytes, macrophages
Products	Antibodies	Sensitized T cells, cytokines
Memory cells	Present	Present
Protection	Bacteria Respiratory and GI pathogens Viruses (extracellular)	Chronic infectious agents Fungi Tumor cells Viruses (intracellular)
Examples	Anaphylactic shock Atopic diseases Bacterial infection Transfusion reaction	Contact dermatitis Destruction of cancer cells Fungal infection Graft rejection Tuberculosis

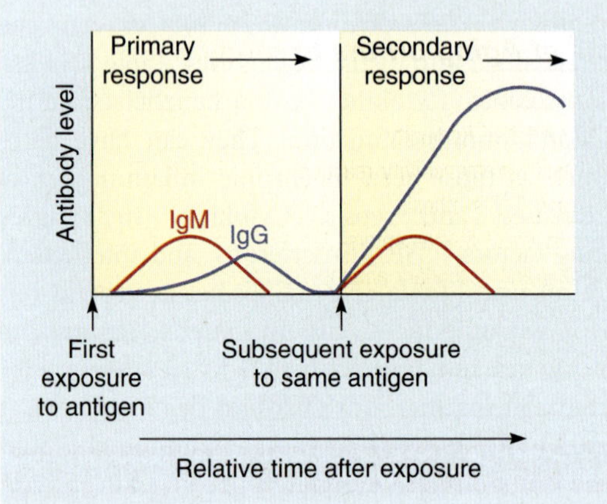

Fig. 14.5 Primary and secondary immune responses. The introduction of antigen induces a response dominated by 2 classes of immunoglobulins: IgM and IgG. IgM dominates in the primary response, with some IgG appearing later. After the host's immune system is primed, another challenge with the same antigen induces the secondary response, in which some IgM and large amounts of IgG are made.

faster (1–3 days), is stronger, and lasts for a longer time than a primary response. Memory cells account for the memory of the first exposure to the antigen and the more rapid production of antibodies. IgG is the primary antibody found in a secondary immune response.

IgG crosses the placental membrane. It provides the newborn with passive acquired immunity for at least 3 months. Infants may get some passive immunity from IgA in breast milk and colostrum.

Cell-Mediated Immunity

Immune responses that we initiate through specific antigen recognition by T cells are termed **cell-mediated immunity**. Several cell types and factors are involved in cell-mediated immunity. These include T cells, macrophages, and NK cells. Cell-mediated immunity is important in (1) immunity against pathogens that survive inside of cells, including viruses and some bacteria (e.g., mycobacteria); (2) fungal infections; (3) transplant tissue rejection; (4) contact hypersensitivity reactions; and (5) tumor immunity.

Gerontologic Considerations: Effects of Aging on the Immune System

With advancing age, there is a decline in the function of the immune response (Table 14.6). The main evidence of *immunosenescence* is the high incidence of cancer in older adults. Older people are also more susceptible to infections (e.g., influenza, pneumonia) from pathogens that they were more immunocompetent against earlier in life. Bacterial pneumonia is the leading cause of death from infections in older adults. The antibody response to immunizations (e.g., flu vaccine) in older adults is much lower than in younger adults.[1]

The bone marrow is unaffected by increasing age. Immunoglobulin levels decrease with age, leading to a suppressed humoral immune response in older adults. The thymus shrinks with age, along with decreased numbers of T cells. These changes in the thymus gland are a primary cause of immunosenescence. Both T and B cells show deficiencies in activation, transit time through the cell cycle, and differentiation. However, the most significant changes involve T cells. As thymic output of T cells diminishes, the differentiation of T cells increases. Consequently, there is an accumulation of memory cells rather than new precursor cells responsive to previously unencountered antigens.

The delayed hypersensitivity reaction, as determined by skin testing with injected antigens, is often decreased or absent in older adults. This altered response reflects **anergy** (an immunodeficient condition characterized by lack of or diminished reaction to an antigen or a group of antigens).

TABLE 14.6 GERONTOLOGIC ASSESSMENT DIFFERENCES

Effects of Aging on the Immune System

- ↑ Autoantibodies
- ↓ Cell-mediated immunity
- ↓ Delayed hypersensitivity reaction
- ↓ IL-1 and IL-2 synthesis
- ↓ Expression of IL-2 receptors
- ↓ Primary and secondary antibody responses
- ↓ Proliferative response of T and B cells
- Thymus shrinks

ALTERED IMMUNE RESPONSES

Hypersensitivity Reactions

Sometimes the immune response is overreactive against foreign antigens or reacts against its own tissue, resulting in tissue damage. These responses are termed **hypersensitivity reactions**. *Autoimmune disease,* a type of hypersensitivity response, occurs when the body does not recognize self-proteins and reacts against self-antigens.

We can classify hypersensitivity reactions by the source of the antigen, time sequence (immediate or delayed), or immunologic mechanisms causing the injury. Four types of hypersensitivity reactions exist (Table 14.7). Types I, II, and III are

TABLE 14.7 Types of Hypersensitivity Reactions

Type I: IgE-Mediated	Type II: Cytotoxic	Type III: Immune-Complex	Type IV: Delayed Hypersensitivity
Antigen			
Pollen, food, drugs, dust	Cell surface of RBCs Cell basement membrane	Extracellular fungal, viral, bacterial	Intracellular or extracellular
Rate of Development			
Immediate	Minutes to hours	Hours to days	Several days
Complement Involved			
No	Yes	Yes	No
Mediators of Injury			
Histamine Leukotrienes Mast cells Prostaglandins	Complement lysis Macrophages in tissues	Complement lysis Lysosomal enzymes Monocytes, macrophages Neutrophils	Cytokines T cytotoxic cells
Examples			
Allergic rhinitis Angioedema Asthma Atopic dermatitis Hives	Goodpasture syndrome Grave disease Immune thrombocytopenic purpura Transfusion reaction	Acute glomerulonephritis Rheumatoid arthritis Systemic lupus erythematosus (SLE)	Contact dermatitis (e.g., to poison ivy)
Skin Test			
Wheal and flare	None	Erythema and edema in 3–8 h	Erythema and edema in 24–48 h

RBC, Red blood cell.

immediate and are examples of humoral immunity. Type IV is a delayed hypersensitivity reaction and is related to cell-mediated immunity.

Type I: IgE-Mediated Reactions

Anaphylactic reactions are type I reactions that occur only in susceptible people who are highly sensitized to specific allergens. IgE antibodies, made in response to the allergen, have a characteristic property of attaching to mast cells and basophils (Fig. 14.6). Within these cells are granules that contain potent chemical mediators (histamine, serotonin, leukotrienes, eosinophil chemotactic factor of anaphylaxis [ECF-A], kinins, bradykinin). Chemical mediators of inflammation are discussed in Chapter 12 and Table 12.1.

On the first exposure to the allergen, IgE antibodies are made and bind to mast cells and basophils. On any subsequent exposures, the allergen links with the IgE bound to mast cells or basophils and triggers degranulation of the cells and the release of chemical mediators from the granules. In this process, the mediators that are released attack target tissues, causing clinical symptoms of an allergic response. These effects include smooth muscle contraction, increased vascular permeability, vasodilation, hypotension, increased mucus secretion, and itching. Fortunately, mediators are short acting and their effects are reversible. Table 14.8 lists these mediators.

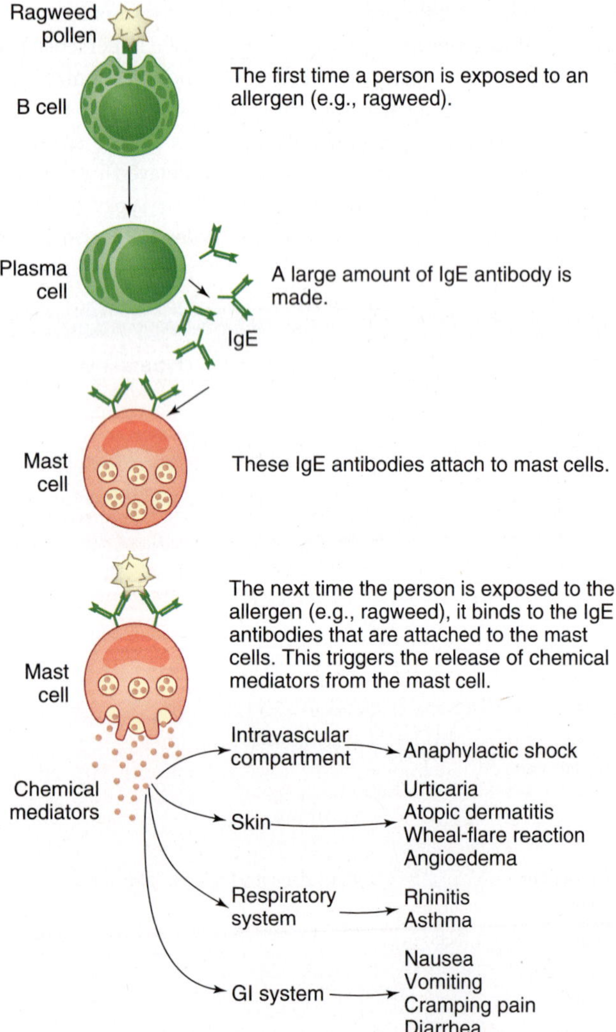

Fig. 14.6 Steps in a type I allergic reaction.

The manifestations of an anaphylactic reaction depend on whether the mediators stay local or become systemic and whether they affect specific organs. When the mediators are local, a skin response called a *wheal-and-flare reaction* occurs. This reaction is characterized by a pale wheal containing edematous fluid surrounded by a red flare from the hyperemia. The reaction occurs in minutes or hours. It is usually not dangerous. An example of a wheal-and-flare reaction is a mosquito bite. The wheal-and-flare reaction has a diagnostic purpose by showing allergic reactions to specific allergens during skin tests.

Common allergic reactions include anaphylaxis and atopic reactions.

Anaphylaxis. *Anaphylaxis* can occur when mediators are released systemically (e.g., after injection of a drug, after an insect sting). The reaction commonly occurs within minutes but can be delayed. It can be life threatening because of bronchial constriction and subsequent airway obstruction and vascular collapse. The target organs affected are shown in Fig. 14.7. Initial symptoms include edema and itching at the site of exposure to the allergen. Shock can occur rapidly. It is manifested by rapid, weak pulse; hypotension; dilated pupils; dyspnea; and possibly cyanosis. Bronchial edema and angioedema can compound shock. Death will occur without emergency treatment. Table 14.9 lists some common allergens that can cause anaphylactic shock in hypersensitive people. Insect stings and drugs, especially antibiotics, are common triggers.[2]

Atopic reactions. Around 20% of people are *atopic*. This means they have an inherited tendency to become sensitive to environment allergens. Atopic diseases that can result are allergic rhinitis, asthma, atopic dermatitis, hives, and angioedema.

Allergic rhinitis, or hay fever, is the most common type I hypersensitivity reaction. It may occur year-round (perennial allergic rhinitis) or be seasonal (seasonal allergic rhinitis). Airborne substances such as pollens, dust, and molds are the primary causes of allergic rhinitis. Dust, molds, and animal dander often cause perennial allergic rhinitis. Pollen from trees, weeds, or grasses often causes seasonal allergic rhinitis. The target areas affected are the conjunctiva and the mucosa of the upper respiratory tract. Symptoms include nasal discharge; sneezing; tearing; mucosal swelling with airway obstruction;

TABLE 14.8 Allergic Response Mediators

- Anaphylatoxins (C3a, C4a, C5a from complement activation)
- Histamine
- Kinins
- Leukotrienes
- Platelet-activating factor
- Prostaglandins
- Serotonin

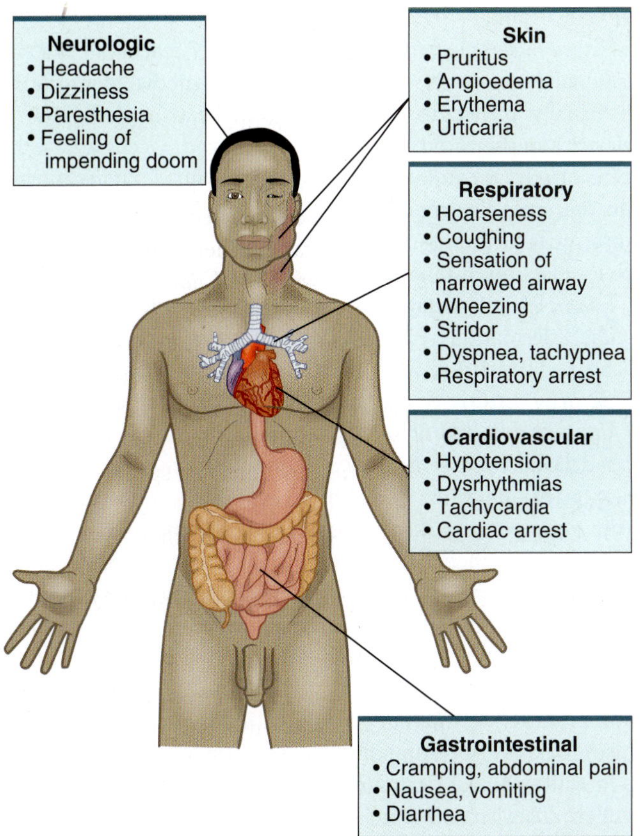

Fig. 14.7 Manifestations of a systemic anaphylactic reaction.

TABLE 14.9 Allergens Causing Anaphylactic Shock

Animal Sera
- Diphtheria antitoxin
- Rabies antitoxin
- Snake venom antitoxin
- Tetanus antitoxin

Drugs
- Aspirin
- Cephalosporins
- Chemotherapy drugs
- Insulins
- Local anesthetics
- Nonsteroidal antiinflammatory drugs
- Penicillins
- Sulfonamides
- Tetracycline

Foods
- Eggs, milk, nuts, peanuts, shellfish, fish, chocolate, strawberries

Insect Venoms
- Wasps, hornets, yellow jackets, bumblebees, ants

Treatments
- Allergy extracts used in immunotherapy
- Blood products (whole blood and components)
- Iodine-contrast media for CT scan or other radiologic procedures

and itching of the eyes, nose, throat, and mouth. Treatment of allergic rhinitis is discussed in Chapter 29.

Many patients with *asthma* have an allergic component to their disease. These patients often have a history of atopic disorders (e.g., infantile eczema, allergic rhinitis, food intolerances). Inflammatory mediators cause bronchial smooth muscle constriction, excess secretion of thick mucus, edema of the mucous membranes of the bronchi, and decreased lung compliance. These changes cause dyspnea, wheezing, coughing, tightness in the chest, and thick sputum. Asthma is discussed in depth in Chapter 31.

Atopic dermatitis is a chronic, inherited skin disorder characterized by exacerbations and remissions. It is caused by environment allergens. These allergens are often hard to identify. The features are not the typical, local wheal-and-flare type I reactions. The skin lesions are more general and involve blood vessel vasodilation. This causes interstitial edema with vesicle formation. Dermatitis is discussed in Chapter 25.

Urticaria (hives) is a skin reaction against systemic allergens occurring in atopic people. Transient wheals (pink, raised, edematous, itchy areas) that vary in size and shape occur. They may be all over the body. Hives develop rapidly after exposure to an allergen. They may last minutes or hours. Histamine causes local vasodilation (erythema), transudation of fluid (wheal), and flaring. Flaring is the result of dilated blood vessels on the edge of the wheal. Histamine causes the associated itching.

Angioedema is a local lesion similar to hives but involving deeper layers of the skin and submucosa. The principal areas involved include the eyelids, lips, tongue, larynx, hands, feet, GI tract, and genitalia (Fig. 14.8). Swelling usually begins in the face and then progresses to the airways and other parts of the body. Dilation and engorgement of the capillaries from the release of histamine causes the diffuse swelling. Welts are not present as in hives. The outer skin appears normal or has a reddish hue. The lesions may burn, sting, or itch. It can cause acute abdominal pain if in the GI tract. The swelling may occur suddenly or over several hours. It usually lasts for 24 hours.

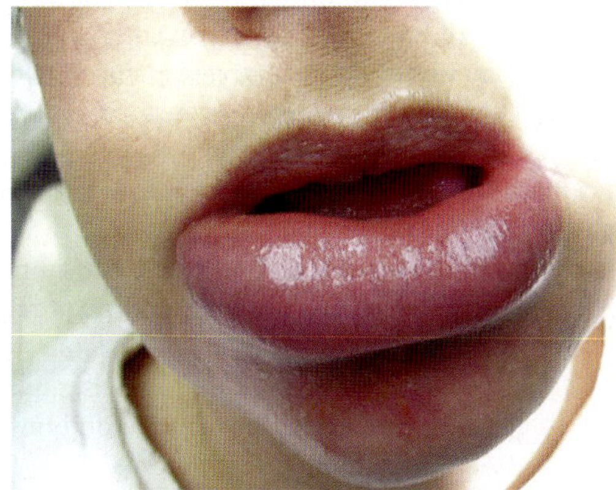

Fig. 14.8 Allergic reaction with angioedema of the lip. (From Soto AP, Meyer SL: Oral implications of polypharmacy in older adults, *Clin Geriatr Med* 39:273, 2023.)

Type II: Cytotoxic and Cytolytic Reactions

Cytotoxic and cytolytic reactions are type II hypersensitivity reactions involving the direct binding of IgG or IgM antibodies to an antigen on the cell surface. Antigen-antibody complexes activate the complement system, which mediates the reaction. Cell tissue is destroyed by either (1) activation of the complement system resulting in cytolysis or (2) enhanced phagocytosis.

Target cells often destroyed in type II reactions are red blood cells (RBCs), platelets, and leukocytes. The tissue damage usually occurs rapidly. Some of the antigens involved are the ABO blood group, Rh factor, and drugs. Pathophysiologic disorders characteristic of type II reactions include ABO incompatibility transfusion reaction, Rh incompatibility transfusion reaction, autoimmune and drug-related hemolytic anemias, leukopenia, thrombocytopenia, erythroblastosis fetalis (hemolytic disease of the newborn), and Goodpasture syndrome.

Hemolytic transfusion reactions. A classic type II reaction occurs when a recipient receives ABO-incompatible blood from a donor. Naturally acquired antibodies to antigens of the ABO blood group are in the recipient's serum but are not present on the RBC membranes. For example, a person with type A blood has anti-B antibodies, a person with type B blood has anti-A antibodies, a person with type AB blood has no antibodies, and a person with type O blood has anti-A and anti-B antibodies.

If the recipient is transfused with incompatible blood, antibodies immediately coat the foreign RBCs, causing *agglutination* (clumping). The clumping of cells blocks small blood vessels in the body, uses existing clotting factors, and depletes them. This leads to bleeding. Within hours, neutrophils and macrophages phagocytize the agglutinated cells. The complement system is activated. Cell lysis occurs, which causes the release of hemoglobin into the urine and plasma. Acute kidney injury can result from hemoglobinuria. See Chapter 34 for more about blood transfusions.

Type III: Immune-Complex Reactions

Tissue damage in immune-complex reactions, which are type III reactions, results from antigen-antibody complexes. Soluble antigens combine with IgG and IgM to form complexes that are too small for the mononuclear phagocyte system to effectively remove them. Therefore the complexes deposit in tissue or small blood vessels. They cause activation of the complement system and release of chemotactic factors that lead to inflammation and destruction of the involved tissue.

Type III reactions may be local or systemic and immediate or delayed. The manifestations depend on the number of complexes and the location in the body. Common sites for deposit are the kidneys, skin, joints, blood vessels, and lungs. Severe type III reactions are associated with autoimmune disorders such as systemic lupus erythematosus (SLE), acute glomerulonephritis, and rheumatoid arthritis. See more about SLE and rheumatoid arthritis in Chapter 69. Acute glomerulonephritis is discussed in Chapter 50.

Type IV: Delayed Hypersensitivity Reactions

A *delayed hypersensitivity reaction*—a type IV reaction—is a *cell-mediated immune response.* Although cell-mediated responses are usually protective mechanisms, tissue damage occurs in delayed hypersensitivity reactions. Sensitized T cells attack antigens or release cytokines. Some cytokines attract macrophages into the area. The macrophages and the enzymes they release cause most of the tissue destruction. In the delayed hypersensitivity reaction, it takes 24 to 48 hours for a response to occur.

Examples of delayed hypersensitivity reactions include contact dermatitis (Fig. 14.9); hypersensitivity reactions to bacterial, fungal, and viral infections; and transplant rejections. Some drug sensitivity reactions also fit this category.

Contact dermatitis. *Allergic contact dermatitis* is an example of a delayed hypersensitivity reaction involving the skin. The reaction occurs when the skin is exposed to substances that easily penetrate the skin to combine with epidermal proteins. The substance then becomes antigenic. Over a period of 7 to 14 days, memory cells form to the antigen. On subsequent exposure to the substance, a sensitized person develops eczematous skin lesions within 48 hours. The most common antigenic substances are metal compounds (e.g., those containing nickel or mercury); rubber compounds; poison ivy, poison oak, and poison sumac; cosmetics; and some dyes.

In acute contact dermatitis, the skin lesions appear red and swollen. They are covered with papules, vesicles, and bullae. The involved area itches. It may burn or sting. When contact dermatitis becomes chronic, the lesions resemble atopic dermatitis because they are thickened, scaly, and lichenified. The main difference between contact dermatitis and atopic dermatitis is that contact dermatitis is local and restricted to the area exposed to the allergens. Atopic dermatitis is usually widespread.

Microbial hypersensitivity reactions. The classic example of a microbial cell-mediated immune reaction is the body's defense against the tubercle bacillus. Tuberculosis (TB) results from

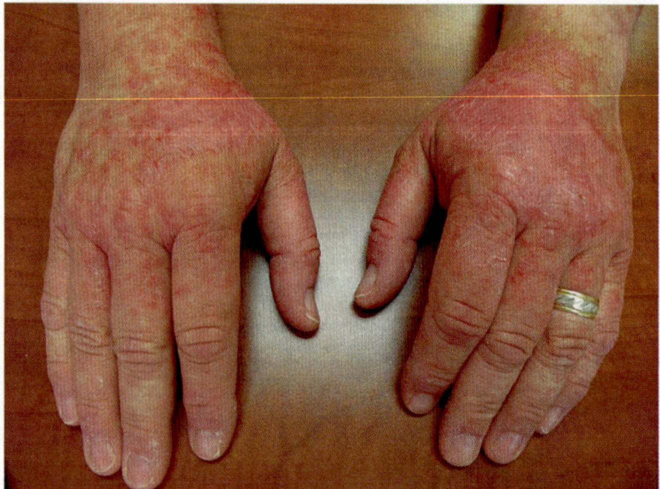

Fig. 14.9 Contact dermatitis to rubber. (From Rich R, Fleisher AT, Shearer WT, et al: *Clinical immunology: principles and practice,* ed 5, St. Louis, 2019, Elsevier.)

invasion of lung tissue by the highly resistant tubercle bacillus. The organism itself does not directly damage the lung tissue. Antigenic material released from the tubercle bacilli reacts with T cells, initiating a cell-mediated immune response. The resulting response causes extensive necrosis of the lung.

After the first cell-mediated reaction, memory cells persist. Subsequent contact with the tubercle bacillus or an extract of purified protein from the organism causes a delayed hypersensitivity reaction. This is the basis for the purified protein derivative (PPD) TB skin test. See Chapter 30 for more about a TB skin test.

INTERPROFESSIONAL AND NURSING MANAGEMENT: ALLERGIC DISORDERS

Assessment

Obtain a complete history and physical assessment, diagnostic workup, and skin testing for allergens. Take a history of past and present allergies (Table 14.10). Family history, including information about atopic reactions in relatives, is especially important in identifying at-risk patients. Obtain information about the manifestations and course of allergic reaction. The time of year when an allergic reaction occurs can be a clue to a seasonal allergen. Ask about all medications used to treat allergies. Note any reactions to medication.

Social and environment factors, especially the physical environment, are important. Ask about pets, trees and plants on the property, pollutants in the air, floor coverings, houseplants, and cooling and heating systems in the home and workplace. A daily or weekly food diary with a description of any untoward reactions may be useful.[3] Ask about the patient's lifestyle and stress level in connection with the allergic symptoms.

List all allergies on the chart, nursing care plan, and medication record. During the physical assessment, focus attention on the site of the allergic manifestations (Table 14.10).

TABLE 14.10 NURSING ASSESSMENT

Allergies

Subjective Data

Important Health Information

Health history: Details about past and present allergies, including associated symptoms and their severity, age symptoms started, speed of symptom onset after contact with allergen, duration of symptoms, frequency of occurrence, reproducibility of symptoms with further exposure, seasonal exacerbations. Details of any previous treatment, including any medications to treat allergies. Recurrent respiratory problems. Unusual reactions to insect bites or stings.

Medications: Unusual reactions to any medications.

Functional Health Patterns

Health perception—health management: Family history of allergies or atopic disease; malaise.

Nutritional-metabolic: Food intolerances, vomiting.

Elimination: Abdominal cramps, diarrhea.

Activity-exercise: Fatigue; hoarseness, cough, dyspnea.

Cognitive-perceptual: Itching, burning, stinging of eyes, nose, throat, or skin; chest tightness.

Role-relationship: Altered home and work environment, presence of pets.

Objective Data

Eyes, Ears, Nose, and Throat

Eyes: Conjunctivitis, lacrimation, rubbing or excessive blinking, dark circles under the eyes ("allergic shiner")

Ears: Diminished hearing, immobile or scarred tympanic membranes, recurrent ear infections

Nose: Nasal polyps, nasal voice, nose twitching, itchy nose, rhinitis; pale, boggy mucous membranes; sniffling, repeated sneezing; swollen nasal passages; recurrent, unexplained nosebleeds; crease across the bridge of nose ("allergic salute")

Throat: Continual throat clearing, swollen lips or tongue, red throat, palpable neck lymph nodes

Respiratory

Wheezing, stridor; thick sputum

Skin

Rashes, including hives, wheal and flare, papules, vesicles, bullae; dryness, scaliness, scratches, irritation

Possible Diagnostic Findings

Eosinophilia of serum, sputum, or nasal and bronchial secretions; increased serum IgE levels; positive skin tests; abnormal chest and sinus x-rays

Diagnostic Studies

We use various immunologic techniques to detect abnormalities of lymphocytes, eosinophils, and immunoglobulins. A complete blood count (CBC) with WBC differential is done, with an absolute lymphocyte count and eosinophil count. Immunodeficiency is diagnosed if the lymphocyte count is below 1200/μL (1.2×10^9/L). T-cell and B-cell quantification can diagnose specific immunodeficiency syndromes. The eosinophil count and serum IgE level are high in type I hypersensitivity reactions. Serum IgE level serves as a diagnostic indicator of atopic diseases.

We can test sputum and nasal and bronchial secretions for the presence of eosinophils. Pulmonary function tests are helpful for patients with asthma. Serum tryptase, which reflects basophil and mast cell degranulation, diagnoses IgE-mediated anaphylaxis.

We need to identify the offending allergen. Sometimes we can do this with skin testing. With food allergies an elimination diet is an option. If an allergic reaction occurs, the patient should stop all foods eaten shortly before the reaction and gradually reintroduce them 1 at a time until the offending food is detected.

Skin tests. Skin testing can identify the specific allergens that are causing the allergy symptoms. With the use of empiric allergy medications as the treatment of choice for most allergic rhinitis, it has become more common to omit skin testing for specific allergens. However, diagnosing a specific allergy allows patients to avoid an allergen and makes them a candidate for immunotherapy.

Unfortunately, we cannot do skin testing on patients who cannot stop taking drugs that suppress the histamine response or patients with food allergies. In these instances, blood allergy testing is used. Blood testing may be done if a person cannot tolerate the many needle scratches needed for skin testing or has a skin disorder (e.g., severe eczema, dermatitis, psoriasis).

We can do skin testing by 3 different methods: (1) a scratch or prick test, (2) an intradermal test, or (3) a patch test. The areas of the body usually used in skin testing are the arms and back. Allergen extracts are applied to the skin in rows with a corresponding control site opposite the test site. Saline or another diluent is applied to the control site. In the *scratch test* a drop of allergen is placed on the skin, and then a pricking device is used so that the allergen can enter the skin. In the *intradermal test* the allergen extract is injected under the skin, similar to a PPD test for TB. In the patch test an allergen is applied to a patch that is placed on the skin.

In the scratch and intradermal tests, the reaction occurs in 5 to 10 minutes. In the patch test the patches must be worn for 48 to 72 hours. If the person is hypersensitive to the allergen, a positive reaction will occur within minutes after insertion in the skin. It may last for 8 to 12 hours. We will see a local wheal-and-flare response with a positive reaction.

The size of the positive reaction does not always correlate with the severity of allergy symptoms. False-positive and false-negative results may occur. Negative results from skin testing do not always mean the person does not have an allergic disorder. Positive results do not always mean that the allergen was causing the manifestations. Positive results imply that the person is sensitized to that allergen. Correlating skin test results with the health history is important.

A highly sensitive person is always at risk for developing an anaphylactic reaction to skin tests. Therefore never leave a patient during the testing period. If a severe reaction does occur with a skin test, immediately remove the extract. Apply an antiinflammatory topical cream to the site. For intradermal testing, the arm is best so that a tourniquet can be applied during a severe reaction. The patient may need a subcutaneous epinephrine injection.

Interventions

Anaphylaxis

The key principle in managing anaphylaxis is speed in (1) recognizing signs and symptoms of an anaphylactic reaction, (2) maintaining a patent airway, (3) giving drugs, and (4) treating for shock. Table 14.11 outlines the emergency treatment of anaphylactic shock.

Epinephrine is the drug of choice to treat an anaphylactic reaction. It is given IV or IM. Patients taking β-blockers may be resistant to epinephrine. They can develop refractory hypotension and bradycardia. These patients should receive glucagon. Its inotropic and chronotropic effects are not mediated through β-receptors. Severe anaphylaxis may result in hypovolemic shock. Increased capillary permeability causes intravascular fluid to move into the interstitial spaces.[4]

TABLE 14.11 EMERGENCY MANAGEMENT

Anaphylactic Shock

Cause

- Injection of, inhalation of, ingestion of, or topical exposure to substance that produces profound allergic response (Table 14.9)

Assessment Findings

- Detailed in Fig. 14.7

Interventions

Initial

- Ensure patent airway. Intubation if evidence of impending obstruction.
- Remove insect stinger if present.
- Establish IV access.
- Give epinephrine, options include:
  - 0.3 to 0.5 mg (0.3–0.5 mL) subcutaneous or IM, preferably in the mid-outer thigh. Repeat every 5 to 10 min.
  - 0.1 to 0.25 mg (1–2.5 mL) IV over 5 min or continuous infusion at 5 to 15 mcg/min.
- Give high-flow O_2 (8–10 L/min) via face mask. Can give up to 100% as needed.
- Nebulized albuterol for bronchospasm resistant to epinephrine.
- IV diphenhydramine for hives.
- IV corticosteroids.

Hypotension

- Place recumbent and elevate legs
- IV normal saline rapid bolus of 1 to 2 L
- Maintain BP with fluids, volume expanders, vasopressors (e.g., dopamine)

Ongoing Monitoring

- Monitor vital signs, respiratory effort, O_2 saturation, level of consciousness, heart rhythm, urine output
- Anticipate intubation with severe respiratory distress
- Anticipate cricothyrotomy or tracheostomy with severe laryngeal edema

Peripheral vasoconstriction and stimulation of the sympathetic nervous system occur to compensate for the fluid shift. However, unless shock is treated early, the body will no longer be able to compensate and irreversible tissue damage will occur, leading to death.

CHECK YOUR PRACTICE

You are caring for a patient who has been receiving IV antibiotic therapy for 2 days. Several minutes after starting the latest infusion, the patient states that his chest feels tight and begins coughing. You take his BP, and it is 100/64 and his pulse is 124.

- What would you do?

Chronic Allergies

Most allergic reactions are chronic. Periods of remissions and exacerbations of symptoms occur. Treatment is aimed at reducing exposure to the offending allergen, treating symptoms with drug therapy, and, if needed, desensitizing the person through immunotherapy.

Allergen recognition and control. You play a key role in helping patients make lifestyle adjustments so there is minimal exposure to offending allergens. Reinforce that even with drug therapy and immunotherapy the patient will never be totally desensitized or completely symptom free. Help patients use various preventive measures to control symptoms.

Many allergic reactions, especially asthma and hives, may worsen with fatigue and stress. Help patients plan a stress management program. Have patients practice relaxation techniques when coming in for immunotherapy.

Sometimes control of symptoms requires environment control. This might include changing an occupation, moving to a different climate, or giving up a favorite pet. With airborne allergens, sleeping in an air-conditioned room, damp dusting daily, covering mattresses and pillows with hypoallergenic covers, and wearing a mask outdoors may be helpful.

If the allergen is a drug, have the patient avoid the drug. Patients have the responsibility to make any drug allergies known to all health care team members. Patients should wear a medical alert bracelet listing the drug allergy and have the drug allergy listed on all medical and dental records.

For patients allergic to insect stings, commercial kits containing automatic injectable epinephrine are available. Teach the patient and family how to use the injector and have them practice assembling and using the training device (Table 14.12). This patient should wear a medical alert bracelet and carry an insect-sting kit whenever going outdoors.

TABLE 14.12 PATIENT & CAREGIVER TEACHING

Automatic Epinephrine Injectors

Include the following information when teaching the patient and caregiver how to use an automatic epinephrine injector:

1. Fill the prescription at once and keep at least 2 doses available.
2. Always keep at least 1 autoinjector with you.
3. Keep an autoinjector in a place where others can easily find it in case of an emergency. Tell family and friends where it is stored.
4. Keep the autoinjector in the original case, at room temperature, away from extremes of cold and heat.
5. Mark your calendar when the autoinjector expires, although you can use an expired autoinjector if there is no alternative. Replace solutions that are discolored or contain particles.
6. Use the device if you have any sign of anaphylaxis, such as trouble breathing or feeling tightness in the throat or lightheaded.
7. When needed:
   - Inject the drug into the top of the thigh, slightly to the outside, at a 90-degree angle. Hold in place for at least 2 to 3 sec.
   - You can inject the drug through clothes. Avoid pockets and seams where the fabric is thick.
   - After use, call 911 and get to the nearest hospital for monitoring. Take the autoinjector with you.

Drug Therapy

The major categories of drugs used for symptomatic relief include antihistamines, sympathomimetic/decongestant drugs, corticosteroids, antipruritic drugs, and mast cell–stabilizing drugs. Many of these drugs are available over the counter (OTC).

Antihistamines. Antihistamines are the best drugs for treating allergic rhinitis, itching, and hives (see Table 29.2). They are less effective for severe allergic reactions and do not prevent bronchoconstriction. They act by competing with histamine for H_1-receptor sites, thus blocking the effect of histamine. Results are best if they are taken as soon as allergy symptoms appear. With seasonal rhinitis, antihistamines should be taken during peak pollen seasons.

Sympathomimetic/decongestant drugs. The major sympathomimetic drug is epinephrine. Epinephrine is made by the adrenal medulla and stimulates α- and β-adrenergic receptors. Stimulation of the α-adrenergic receptors causes vasoconstriction of peripheral blood vessels. β-Receptor stimulation relaxes bronchial smooth muscles. Epinephrine acts directly on mast cells to stabilize them against further degranulation. The action of epinephrine lasts only a few minutes.

Minor sympathomimetic agents include drugs containing phenylephrine and pseudoephedrine. They differ from epinephrine because they are taken orally or nasally. Their effects last several hours. These drugs are mainly used to treat allergic rhinitis (see Table 29.2).

Corticosteroids. Nasal corticosteroid sprays are effective in relieving the symptoms of allergic rhinitis. Sometimes a brief course of oral corticosteroids can be used for severe symptoms.

Antipruritic drugs. Antipruritic drugs provide relief from itching and protect the skin. They are most effective when applied topically to intact skin. Common OTC drugs include calamine lotion, coal tar solutions, and camphor. Menthol and phenol may be added to other lotions to relieve itching.

Mast cell–stabilizing drugs. Cromolyn is a mast cell–stabilizing agent that inhibits the release of histamines, leukotrienes, and other agents from the mast cell after antigen-IgE interaction. It is available as an inhalant nebulizer solution or a nasal spray. Cromolyn is used to manage allergic rhinitis (see Table 29.2).

Leukotriene receptor antagonists. Leukotriene receptor antagonists (LTRAs) block leukotriene, a major mediator of the allergic inflammatory process. These medications can be taken orally. They are used to treat allergic rhinitis and asthma.

Immunotherapy

Immunotherapy is the recommended treatment for control of allergic symptoms when the allergen cannot be avoided and drug therapy is not effective. It involves giving small titers of an allergen extract in increasing strengths until hyposensitivity to the specific allergen is achieved. The incremental increases cause the immune system to become less sensitive to the substance, probably by causing production of a "blocking" antibody, which reduces the symptoms of allergy when the substance is encountered in the future. The allergens included are based on the results of skin testing. Immunotherapy is indicated for those with anaphylactic reactions to insect venom. Unfortunately, not all allergy-related conditions respond to immunotherapy. Peanut allergy is the only food allergy treatment available.

Method of administration. *Subcutaneous immunotherapy (SCIT)* involves the subcutaneous injection of titrated amounts of allergen extracts biweekly or weekly. The dose is small at first, then increased slowly until a maintenance dosage is reached. It often takes 1 to 2 years of immunotherapy to reach the maximal therapeutic effect. Therapy may continue for about 5 years. After that, some patients may stop therapy. Many have a sustained decrease in symptoms after the treatment is stopped. Those with severe allergies or sensitivity to insect stings may continue maintenance therapy indefinitely.

Sublingual immunotherapy (SLIT) involves allergen extracts taken under the tongue. Sublingual products include a 5-grass pollen tablet (Oralair), a single-grass pollen tablet (Grastek), and a ragweed pollen tablet (Ragwitek).[5]

Patients usually take SLIT once daily at home. The first dose is usually given under medical supervision. Some patients have local site reactions (e.g., oral pruritus, throat irritation, tongue swelling). Local reactions subside in many patients within a few days to a week. Systemic reactions are markedly fewer than with SCIT. SLIT has the advantage of being a convenient, self-administered oral therapy. Its main disadvantage is that the patient must consistently adhere to the therapy.[6]

NURSING MANAGEMENT: IMMUNOTHERAPY

You will often be the person responsible for giving SCIT. Immunotherapy always carries the risk for a severe anaphylactic reaction. Therefore an HCP, emergency equipment, and essential drugs should be available whenever injections are given. Always anticipate adverse reactions, especially when using a new dose strength, after a previous reaction, or after a missed dose. Early manifestations of a systemic reaction include itching, hives, sneezing, laryngeal edema, and hypotension. If these occur, begin emergency measures for anaphylactic shock at once.

Describe any local reaction according to the degree of redness and swelling at the injection site. If the area is greater than the size of a quarter in an adult, report the reaction to the HCP. The allergen dosage may need decreased.

Accurate record keeping can help prevent an adverse reaction to the allergen extract. Before giving an injection, check the patient's name against the name on the vial. Next, review the strength, amount of last dose, date of last dose, and any reaction information.

Always give the allergen extract in an extremity away from a joint so you can apply a tourniquet for a severe reaction. Rotate the site for each injection. After giving the injection, observe the patient for 20 to 30 minutes, because systemic reactions are most likely to occur immediately. However, teach the patient that a delayed reaction can occur up to 24 hours later.

For best results, teach patients to avoid the offending allergen whenever possible because complete desensitization is impossible.

Latex Allergies

Allergies to latex products have become an increasing problem for patients and health care workers. The increase coincides with the sharp increase in glove use. The more frequent and prolonged the exposure to latex, the greater the risk for developing a latex allergy.[7]

Besides gloves, we use many other latex-containing products in health care. These include BP cuffs, stethoscopes, tourniquets, IV tubing, syringes, electrode pads, O_2 masks, tracheal tubes, colostomy and ileostomy pouches, urinary catheters, anesthetic masks, and adhesive tape. Latex proteins can become aerosolized through powder on gloves and can result in serious reactions when inhaled by sensitized persons. All health care agencies should use powder-free gloves to avoid respiratory exposure to latex proteins.[8]

Types of Latex Allergies

Two types of latex allergies can occur: type IV allergic contact dermatitis and type I allergic reactions. *Type IV contact dermatitis* is caused by the chemicals used in making latex gloves. It is a delayed reaction that occurs within 6 to 48 hours. Typically, the person first has dryness, itching, fissuring, and cracking of the skin, followed by redness, swelling, and crusting at 24 to 48 hours. Chronic exposure can lead to lichenification, scaling, and hyperpigmentation. Dermatitis may extend beyond the area of physical contact with the allergen.

A *type I allergic reaction* is a response to the natural rubber latex proteins. It occurs within minutes of contact with the proteins. The manifestations can vary from skin redness, hives, rhinitis, conjunctivitis, or asthma to full-blown anaphylactic shock. Systemic reactions to latex may result from exposure to latex protein via various routes, including the skin, mucous membranes, inhalation, and blood.

Latex-Food Syndrome

Because some proteins in rubber are similar to food proteins, some foods may cause an allergic reaction in people who are allergic to latex. We call this *latex-food syndrome.* The most common of these foods are banana, avocado, chestnut, kiwi, tomato, water chestnut, guava, hazelnut, potato, peach, grape, and apricot. Most people with latex allergy have a positive allergy test to at least 1 related food.

NURSING MANAGEMENT: LATEX ALLERGIES

Identifying people sensitive to latex is crucial to prevent adverse reactions. Obtain a health history and history of any allergies, especially for patients with a history of latex contact symptoms. The greatest risk factor is long-term multiple exposures to latex products (e.g., health care personnel, those who have had multiple surgeries, rubber industry workers). Other risk factors include a history of allergic rhinitis, asthma, and allergies to latex-related foods.

Use latex precaution protocols for those patients with a positive latex allergy test or a history of signs and symptoms related to latex exposure. Many health care agencies have created latex-free product carts to use with patients with latex allergies. Because we cannot identify all latex-sensitive people, even with a thorough history, follow general recommendations for preventing allergic reactions to latex (Table 14.13).

Because of the potential for severe symptoms of food allergy, teach patients to avoid those foods. Other recommendations for people with latex and food allergies include wearing a medical alert bracelet or necklace and carrying an injectable epinephrine pen.

Multiple Chemical Sensitivity

Multiple chemical sensitivity (MCS) is marked by recurrent, vague, nonspecific symptoms associated with low-dose chemical exposure. Common associated substances include smoke, pesticides, plastics, synthetic fabrics, scented products, petroleum products, and paint fumes. Females between the ages of 30 and 50 are more likely to develop symptoms.

People have a wide range of nonspecific symptoms. These include runny nose, shortness of breath, palpitations, headache, burning eyes, sore throat, dizziness, confusion, fatigue, irritability, nausea, and muscle and joint pain. CNS symptoms include short-term memory loss, confusion, and depression.[9]

Diagnosis is usually made based on the health history. There are no tests to diagnose MCS. The most effective treatment is to avoid the chemicals that may trigger symptoms and create a chemical-free and odor-free home and workplace. Psychotherapy is recommended. Antidepressants, including selective serotonin reuptake inhibitors (SSRIs; e.g., citalopram), are options. Drugs for anxiety and sleep also have been used.

TABLE 14.13 Guidelines for Preventing Allergic Latex Reactions

- Use nonlatex gloves for activities that are not likely to involve contact with infectious materials (e.g., food preparation, housekeeping).
- If you choose latex gloves, use powder-free gloves.
- Do not use oil-based hand creams or lotions when wearing latex gloves.
- Wash hands with soap and water after wearing gloves.
- Frequently clean work areas that are contaminated with latex-containing dust (e.g., carpets, ventilation ducts).
- Frequently change the ventilation filters and vacuum bags used in latex-contaminated areas.
- Learn to recognize the symptoms of latex allergy: skin rash; hives; flushing; itching; nasal, eye, or sinus symptoms; asthma.
- If symptoms of latex allergy develop, avoid direct contact with latex gloves and products.
- Wear a medical alert bracelet and carry an epinephrine pen.

AUTOIMMUNITY

Autoimmunity is an immune response against self in which the immune system no longer differentiates self from nonself. For some unknown reason, immune cells that are normally unresponsive (tolerant to self-antigens) are activated. In autoimmunity, autoantibodies and autosensitized T cells cause tissue damage.

The cause of autoimmune diseases is unknown. Age may play some role because the number of circulating autoantibodies increases in people over age 50. We think the main factors in the development of autoimmunity are (1) the inheritance of susceptibility genes, which contribute to the failure of self-tolerance, and (2) initiation of autoreactivity by triggers, such as infections, which activate self-reactive lymphocytes.

Autoimmune diseases tend to cluster. A given person may have more than 1 autoimmune disease (e.g., rheumatoid arthritis, Addison disease). We often group autoimmune diseases according to organ-specific and systemic diseases (Table 14.14).

Family members may have the same or related autoimmune diseases. This observation has led to the concept of genetic predisposition to autoimmune disease. Most of the genetic research correlates certain human leukocyte antigen (HLA) types with an autoimmune condition.

Even in a genetically predisposed person, some trigger is needed to initiate autoreactivity. This may include infectious agents such as a virus. Viral infections can change cells or tissues that are not normally antigenic. The virally induced changes make the cells or tissues antigenic. Viruses may be involved in the development of diseases such as type 1 diabetes. Rheumatic fever and rheumatic heart disease are autoimmune

TABLE 14.14 Examples of Autoimmune Diseases

- Addison disease
- Autoimmune hemolytic anemia
- Autoimmune hepatitis
- Celiac disease
- Diabetes, type 1
- Glomerulonephritis
- Goodpasture syndrome
- Grave disease
- Guillain-Barré syndrome
- Hemochromatosis
- Hypothyroidism
- Immune thrombocytopenic purpura (ITP)
- Inflammatory bowel disease
- Multiple sclerosis
- Myasthenia gravis
- Pernicious anemia
- Primary biliary cirrhosis
- Rheumatic heart disease
- Rheumatoid arthritis
- Scleroderma (systemic sclerosis)
- Systemic lupus erythematosus
- Thyroiditis

responses triggered by streptococcal infection. Antibodies against group A β-hemolytic streptococci cross-react with heart muscles, heart valves, and synovial membranes.

Drugs can be precipitating factors. Hemolytic anemia can result from methyldopa administration. Procainamide can induce the formation of antinuclear antibodies and cause a lupus-like syndrome.

Sex and hormones have a role. More females have autoimmune disease. During pregnancy, many autoimmune diseases get better. After delivery, females with an autoimmune disease often have an exacerbation.

Apheresis

Apheresis is a procedure to separate components of the blood followed by the removal of 1 or more of these components. It is an effective treatment for several autoimmune diseases and other diseases and disorders. Compound words are often used to describe a specific apheresis procedure, depending on the blood components being collected. *Plateletpheresis* is the removal of platelets. It often involves collecting platelets from normal persons to infuse into patients with low platelet counts (e.g., patients taking chemotherapy who develop thrombocytopenia). *Leukocytapheresis* is a general term describing the removal of WBCs. It is used in chronic myelogenous leukemia to remove high numbers of leukemic cells.

Apheresis is used in hematopoietic stem cell transplantation to collect stem cells from peripheral blood. These stem cells can then be used to repopulate a person's bone marrow after high-dose chemotherapy. See Chapter 16 for more on hematopoietic stem cell transplants.

Plasmapheresis

Plasmapheresis is the removal of plasma containing components causing or thought to cause disease. It can be used to get plasma from healthy donors to give to patients as replacement therapy.

Plasmapheresis involves removing whole blood through an IV device, then circulating the blood through an apheresis machine. Inside the machine the blood is divided into plasma and its cellular components by centrifugation or membrane filtration. The plasma is replaced with normal saline, lactated Ringer's solution, fresh-frozen plasma, plasma protein fractions, or albumin. When we manually remove blood, we can only take 500 mL at 1 time. However, with the use of apheresis procedures, more than 4 L of plasma can be pheresed in 2 to 3 hours.

Plasmapheresis is used to treat autoimmune diseases such as SLE, glomerulonephritis, Goodpasture syndrome, myasthenia gravis, rheumatoid arthritis, and Guillain-Barré syndrome. Many of these disorders have circulating autoantibodies (usually of the IgG class) and antigen-antibody complexes. Performing therapeutic plasmapheresis in autoimmune disorders can remove pathologic substances and inflammatory mediators present in plasma that cause tissue damage. Immunosuppressive therapy can prevent recovery of IgG production, and plasmapheresis can prevent antibody rebound.

The most common complications are hypotension and citrate toxicity. Hypotension is usually the result of a vasovagal reaction or transient volume changes. Citrate, used as an anticoagulant, may cause hypocalcemia. The patient may have a headache, paresthesias, and dizziness.

IMMUNODEFICIENCY

When the immune system does not adequately protect the body, *immunodeficiency* exists. Immunodeficiency disorders involve an impairment of 1 or more immune mechanisms, which include (1) phagocytosis, (2) humoral response, (3) cell-mediated response, (4) complement, and (5) a combined humoral and cell-mediated deficiency. Immunodeficiency is primary if the immune cells are improperly developed or absent and *secondary* if an illness or treatment causes the deficiency. Primary immunodeficiency is rare and often serious. Secondary disorders are more common and less severe.

Primary Immunodeficiency

The basic categories of primary immunodeficiency disorders are (1) phagocytic defects, (2) B-cell deficiency, (3) T-cell deficiency, and (4) a combined B-cell and T-cell deficiency (Table 14.15).

Secondary Immunodeficiency Disorders

Key factors that may cause secondary immunodeficiency disorders are shown in Table 14.16. Drug-induced immunosuppression is the most common. Immunosuppressive therapy is prescribed for patients to treat autoimmune disorders

TABLE 14.15 Primary Immunodeficiency Disorders

Disorder	Affected Cells	Genetic Basis
Ataxia-telangiectasia	B, T	Autosomal recessive
Bruton X-linked agammaglobulinemia	B	X-linked
Chronic granulomatous disease	PMNs, monocytes	X-linked
Common variable hypogammaglobulinemia	B	—
DiGeorge syndrome (thymic hypoplasia	T	—
Graft-versus-host disease	B, T	—
Job syndrome	PMNs, monocytes	—
Severe combined immunodeficiency disease	Stem, B, T	X-linked or autosomal recessive
Selective IgA, IgM, or IgG deficiency	B	Some X-linked
Wiskott-Aldrich syndrome	B, T	X-linked

Ig, Immunoglobulin; *PMNs,* polymorphonuclear neutrophils.

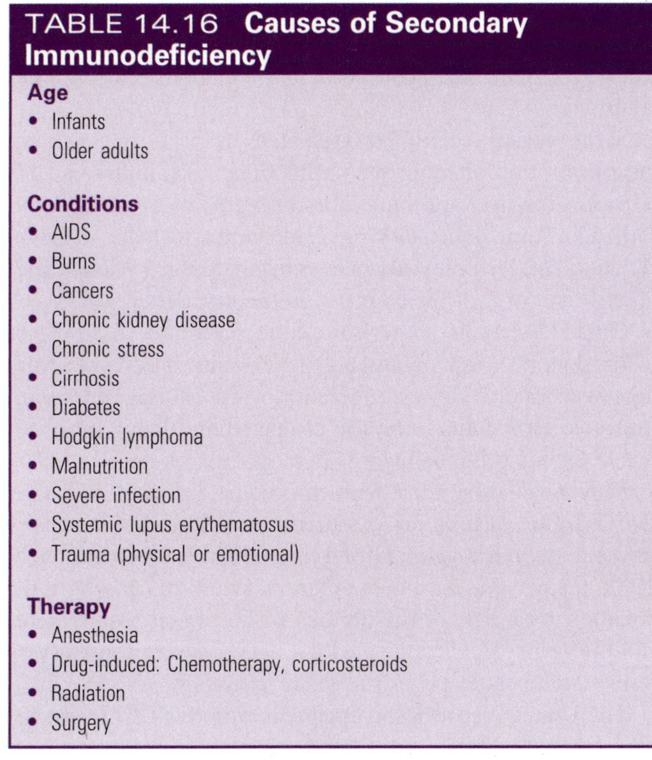

TABLE 14.16 Causes of Secondary Immunodeficiency

Age
- Infants
- Older adults

Conditions
- AIDS
- Burns
- Cancers
- Chronic kidney disease
- Chronic stress
- Cirrhosis
- Diabetes
- Hodgkin lymphoma
- Malnutrition
- Severe infection
- Systemic lupus erythematosus
- Trauma (physical or emotional)

Therapy
- Anesthesia
- Drug-induced: Chemotherapy, corticosteroids
- Radiation
- Surgery

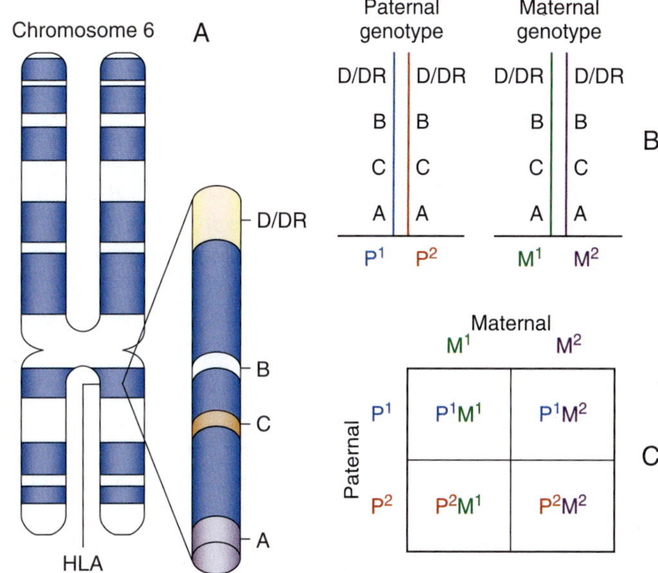

Fig. 14.10 Patterns of human leukocyte antigen (HLA) inheritance. (A) HLA genes are found on chromosome 6. (B) The 2 haplotypes of the father are labeled P^1 and P^2, and the haplotypes of the mother are labeled M^1 and M^2. Each child inherits 2 haplotypes, 1 from each parent. (C) Only 4 combinations—P^1M^1, P^1M^2, P^2M^1, and P^2M^2—are possible, and 25% of the offspring will have identical HLA haplotypes.

and prevent transplant rejection. Immunosuppression is a serious side effect of chemotherapy. General leukopenia often results, leading to a decreased humoral and cell-mediated response. This makes secondary infections common in immunosuppressed patients.

Malnutrition alters cell-mediated immune responses. When protein is deficient over a prolonged period, the thymus gland atrophies and lymphoid tissue decreases. An increased susceptibility to infections always exists.

Hodgkin lymphoma impairs the cell-mediated immune response, and patients may die of severe viral or fungal infections (see Chapter 34). Viruses, especially rubella, may cause immunodeficiency by direct cytotoxic damage to lymphoid cells. Systemic infections can place such a demand on the immune system that resistance to a secondary or another infection is impaired.

Radiation can destroy lymphocytes either directly or through depletion of stem cells. As the radiation dose is increased, more bone marrow atrophies. This leads to severe pancytopenia and suppression of immune function. Splenectomy in children is especially dangerous. They may develop sepsis from a simple respiratory tract infection.

Stress may alter the immune response. This response involves interrelationships among the nervous, endocrine, and immune systems (see Chapter 7).

HUMAN LEUKOCYTE ANTIGEN SYSTEM

The antigens responsible for rejection of genetically unlike tissues are called the *major histocompatibility antigens.* These antigens are products of histocompatibility genes. In humans, they are called the **human leukocyte antigen (HLA)** system. The genes for the HLA antigens are linked and occur together on the sixth chromosome. HLAs are present on all nucleated cells and platelets. We use the HLA system in matching organs and tissues for transplantation.

An important characteristic of HLA genes is that they are highly *polymorphic* (variable). Each HLA locus can have many possible alleles, so many combinations exist. Each person has 2 alleles for each locus, 1 inherited from each parent. Both alleles of a locus are expressed independently, meaning they are codominant.

The entire set of A, B, C, D, and DR genes (the HLA genes) on 1 chromosome is a *haplotype.* This complete set is inherited as a unit. One haplotype is inherited from each parent (Fig. 14.10). This means that a person has HLA genes that are half identical to those of each parent. The HLA genes of 1 person have a 25% chance of being identical to the HLA genes of a sibling. In organ transplantation we mainly use A, B, and DR for compatibility matching. The specific allele at each locus is identified by a number. For example, a person could have an HLA of A2, A6, B7, B27, DR4, and DR7. Currently more than 8000 HLA alleles have been identified for the various HLA genes.

Several diseases show significant associations with specific HLA alleles. People who have these alleles are much more likely to develop the associated disease than those who do not have the alleles. However, having a particular HLA allele does not mean that the person will necessarily develop the associated disease—only that the risk is greater than in the general population. Most people who inherit a specific HLA type that is associated with a disease will never develop that disease.

Many HLA-associated diseases are autoimmune disorders. Examples of HLA types and disease associations include (1) HLA-B27 and ankylosing spondylitis; (2) HLA-DR2, HLA-DR3, and SLE; and (3) HLA-DR3, HLA-DR4, and diabetes.

Currently the relationship between HLAs and certain diseases is of minimal practical clinical importance. Research is promising for the development of clinical applications. For example, with some autoimmune diseases, it may be possible to identify family members at risk for developing the same or a related autoimmune disease. These people would need preventive care (if possible) and early diagnosis and treatment to prevent chronic complications.

ORGAN TRANSPLANTS

Transplant success has improved with advances in surgical technique and histocompatibility testing and more effective immunosuppressant drugs. Common transplants include corneas, skin, bone marrow, heart valves, kidneys, and livers (Fig. 14.11).[10] Corneal transplants can prevent or correct blindness. Skin grafts are used in managing burn patients. Donated bone marrow can help patients with leukemias and other cancers.

Transplanted organs come from many different body systems. These organs include the heart, lung, liver, kidney, pancreas, and intestine. Multiple organs can be transplanted together, such as kidney and pancreas, kidney and liver, kidney and heart, or the complete intestinal tract. For example, some patients with diabetes who receive a pancreas transplant also receive a kidney transplant because the diabetes led to kidney failure.

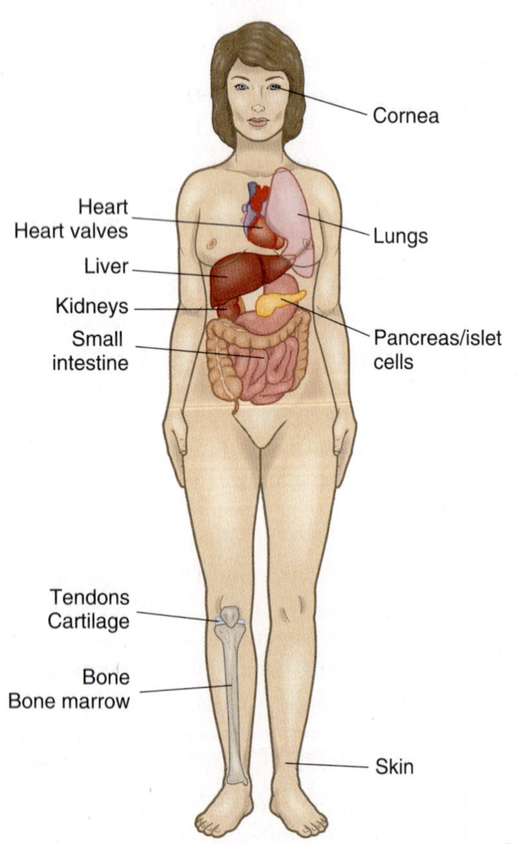

Fig. 14.11 Tissues and organs that can be transplanted.

Some organs can be transplanted in parts or segments instead of transplanting an entire organ. Examples include transplanting liver and lung lobes or segments of an intestine. This allows for 1 person's organ donation to help many recipients. This technique also allows living donors to donate part of an organ or 1 of their organs, in the case of kidneys.

Organ donations come from either deceased (cadaver) or living donors. Most organs and tissues currently come from deceased donors. However, because of the shortage of organs from deceased donors, the use of related and living unrelated donor organs is increasing.

People can show their wish to become a donor when they sign a donor card or driver's license or join a donor registry (depending on the state). However, on their death or imminent death, the person's legal next of kin may need to consent to the donation regardless of the donor's wishes. Legal requirements and the agency's policy for the legal next of kin to consent vary from state to state and from agency to agency.

The United Network for Organ Sharing (UNOS) maintains the national waiting list. Fewer people receive transplants annually than need them. The Uniform Anatomical Gift Act regulates organ and tissue donations to allow for fair and consistent transplantation laws among all states.[11] Patients are matched to available donors based on several factors: ABO blood and HLA typing, medical urgency, time on the waiting list, and geographic location. Transporting and storing donated organs can take time. The "best" match may live many miles from the "ideal" recipient. The need to have the "best" matches must be balanced against the time it takes to obtain and transport a donated organ and then transplant it.

Tissue Typing

The recipient usually receives a transplant from an ABO blood group–compatible donor. The donor and recipient do not need to share the same Rh factor.

HLA Typing

HLA typing is done on potential donors and recipients. Currently we think only the A, B, and DR antigens are significant for transplants. We try to match as many antigens as possible between the HLA-A, HLA-B, and HLA-DR loci. Antigen matches of 5 and 6 antigens and some 4-antigen matches have better clinical outcomes. This means the patient is less likely to reject the transplanted organ. A perfect match is nearly impossible unless the tissue is from an identical twin or, in some cases, a sibling.

The degree of HLA matching needed or suitable for successful transplantation depends on the type of organ and degree of acceptable risk. Certain organ and tissue transplants need a closer histocompatibility match than other organs. For example, nearly anyone can accept a cornea transplant. Corneas are avascular, so no antibodies can reach the cornea and cause rejection. In kidney and bone marrow transplants, HLA matching is very important, because these transplants are at high risk for graft rejection. HLA mismatches have little impact on graft survival for liver transplants. Heart and lung transplants fall somewhere in between, but minimizing HLA mismatches significantly improves survival. For liver, lung, and heart transplants, few donors are available, and it is hard to get good HLA matches.

Panel of Reactive Antibodies

A panel of reactive antibodies (PRA) shows the recipient's sensitivity to various HLAs before receiving a transplant. PRA allows us to decide whether a recipient is of high or low reactivity to potential donors. To detect preformed antibodies to HLA, the recipient's serum is mixed with a randomly selected panel of donor lymphocytes to assess reactivity. Patients awaiting a transplant usually have a PRA panel done on a regular basis.

We calculate PRA results in percentages. A high PRA means that the person has many cytotoxic antibodies and is highly sensitized. There will be a poor chance of finding a crossmatch-negative donor. They may have been exposed to HLA antigens by previous blood transfusions, pregnancy, or a previous organ transplant. In highly sensitized patients (high PRA), plasmapheresis and IV immunoglobulin (IVIG) are options to lower the number of antibodies.

Crossmatch

A crossmatch is done to determine the existence of antibodies against the potential donor. A crossmatch uses serum from the recipient mixed with donor lymphocytes to test for any preformed anti-HLA antibodies to the potential donor organ. The crossmatch can be used as a screening test when living donors are being considered or once a cadaver donor is chosen.

A negative crossmatch means that no preformed antibodies are present and it is safe to go ahead with transplantation. A positive crossmatch means that the recipient has cytotoxic antibodies to the donor. This is an absolute contraindication in living donor transplants. Live donor transplants may be done for patients with a positive crossmatch if no other live donors with a negative crossmatch exist. In this situation, plasmapheresis or IVIG can remove antibodies.

It is not always possible to complete a crossmatch before a transplant. If a crossmatch is done after, the results will affect the immunosuppression protocols after the transplant. A prospective crossmatch is especially important for kidney transplants. It is not an option for lung, liver, and heart transplants.

Transplant Rejection

Rejection is a major problem after an organ transplant. Organ rejection occurs as a normal immune response to foreign tissue. Immunosuppression therapy, performing ABO and HLA matching, and ensuring that the crossmatch is negative reduce the risk for rejection. Rejection can be hyperacute, acute, or chronic. Prevention, early diagnosis, and treatment of rejection are essential for long-term graft function.

Hyperacute Rejection

Hyperacute rejection occurs within 24 hours after a transplant. It occurs because the person had preexisting antibodies against the transplanted tissue or organ. There is no treatment for hyperacute rejection. We must remove the transplanted organ. Fortunately, hyperacute rejection is a rare event. This is because of improved immunosuppressive drugs, and the final testing before surgery usually determines whether the recipient is sensitized to any donor HLAs.

Acute Rejection

Acute rejection most often occurs in the first 6 months after a transplant. This type of rejection is usually a cell-mediated immune response by the recipient's lymphocytes, which are activated against the donated (foreign) tissue or organ (Fig. 14.12). Another type of acute rejection occurs when the recipient develops antibodies to the transplanted organ (humoral rejection).

It is common to have at least one rejection episode, especially with organs from deceased donors. These episodes are usually reversible with more immunosuppressive therapy. This may include increased corticosteroid doses or polyclonal or monoclonal antibodies. Unfortunately, immunosuppressants

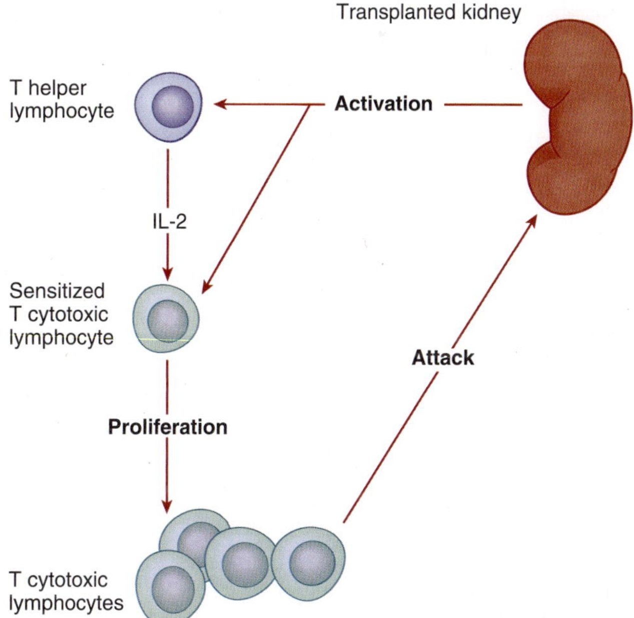

Fig. 14.12 Mechanism of action of T cytotoxic lymphocyte activation and attack of transplanted tissue. The transplanted organ (e.g., kidney) is recognized as foreign and activates the immune system. T helper cells are activated to make interleukin-2 *(IL-2)*, and T cytotoxic lymphocytes are sensitized. After the T cytotoxic cells proliferate, they attack the transplanted organ.

increase the risk for infection. To combat acute rejection, all patients with transplants need long-term use of immunosuppressants, putting them at high risk for infection, especially in the first few months after transplant when the immunosuppressive doses are highest.

Chronic Rejection

Chronic rejection is a process that occurs over months or years. It is irreversible. Chronic rejection can occur for unknown reasons or from repeated episodes of acute rejection. Large numbers of T and B cells infiltrate the transplanted organ, with ongoing, low-grade, immune-mediated injury. Chronic rejection results in fibrosis and scarring. In heart transplants it manifests as accelerated coronary artery disease. In lung transplants it manifests as bronchiolitis obliterans. In liver transplants we see a loss of bile ducts. In kidney transplants it manifests as fibrosis and glomerulopathy. Treatment is supportive. Chronic rejection is hard to manage and does not have the optimistic prognosis of acute rejection.

Immunosuppressive Therapy

Immunosuppressive therapy requires a lifelong balance between rejection and infection. The immune response must be suppressed to prevent rejection of the transplanted organ. On the other hand, an adequate immune response must be maintained to prevent overwhelming infection and the development of cancers.[12]

Many drugs used to achieve immunosuppression have significant side effects. Because transplant recipients must take immunosuppressants for life, the risk for toxicity continues for the rest of their lives.

Immunosuppressant drugs are listed in Table 14.17.[13] With the use of a combination of agents that work during different phases of the immune response (Fig. 14.12), we can give lower doses of each drug to produce effective immunosuppression while minimizing side effects.

The major immunosuppressive agents are (1) calcineurin inhibitors; (2) corticosteroids (prednisone, methylprednisolone); (3) purine synthesis antagonists, including mycophenolate mofetil (CellCept, Myfortic) and azathioprine (Imuran); and (4) sirolimus. IV muromonab-CD3 and either horse antithymocyte globulin (Atgam) or rabbit antithymocyte globulin (ATG) are used for short periods to prevent early rejection or reverse acute rejection.

Immunosuppression protocols vary among transplant centers, with different drug combinations being used. Most patients are initially on triple therapy. The standard triple therapy usually includes a calcineurin inhibitor, a corticosteroid, and mycophenolate mofetil.

The doses of immunosuppressant drugs are reduced over time after the transplant. The trend in many transplant centers is to follow an immunosuppression protocol that uses minimal corticosteroids because of their many side effects. Patients taking corticosteroids may be weaned off after a few years.

Calcineurin Inhibitors

This group of drugs includes tacrolimus (Prograf, Envarsus XR) and cyclosporine (Sandimmune). They are the most effective agents and serve as the foundation of most immunosuppression regimens. Calcineurin inhibitors work by preventing a cell-mediated attack against the transplanted organ (Fig. 14.13). They are usually used in combination with corticosteroids, mycophenolate mofetil, and sirolimus. Tacrolimus is the most widely used. Envarsus XR is an extended-release, long-acting formulation of tacrolimus that is dosed once daily. Cyclosporine is being used less often as a first-line drug choice.

DRUG ALERT

Tacrolimus and Cyclosporine

- A substance in grapefruit and grapefruit juice prevents metabolism of these drugs.
- Consuming grapefruit or grapefruit juice while using these drugs can increase their toxicity.

Mycophenolate Mofetil

Mycophenolate mofetil inhibits purine synthesis with suppressive effects on T and B cells. The major limitation of this drug is GI toxicity, including nausea, vomiting, and diarrhea. In many cases the side effects can be lessened by lowering the dose or giving smaller doses more often.

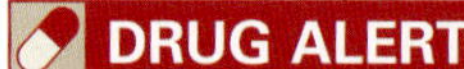

Mycophenolate Mofetil

- When given IV, it can only be reconstituted in D_5W.
- Do not give as IV bolus. Give over 2 or more hours.

Sirolimus

Sirolimus suppresses T-cell activation and proliferation. It is used in combination with corticosteroids, cyclosporine, and/or tacrolimus.

Monoclonal Antibodies

Monoclonal antibodies are used to prevent and treat acute rejection episodes. Muromonab-CD3 is a mouse monoclonal antibody that binds with the CD3 antigen found on the surface of human thymocytes and mature T cells. It interferes with the function of all T cells, the pivotal cells involved in rejection. It is given by IV bolus. Within minutes after the first infusion, the number of circulating T cells decreases significantly.

A flulike syndrome occurs during the first few days of treatment because of cytokine release. Side effects include fever, chills, headache, myalgias, and various GI problems. To reduce the expected side effects, give patients acetaminophen, diphenhydramine, and IV methylprednisolone beforehand.

TABLE 14.17 **Drug Therapy**

Immunosuppressive Therapy

Agent	Route	Mechanism of Action	Side Effects
Calcineurin Inhibitors			
cyclosporine (Gengraf, Neoral, Sandimmune)	Oral, IV	Acts on T helper cells to prevent production and release of IL-2 T- and B-cell proliferation	Kidney toxicity, ↑ infection risk, neurotoxicity (tremors, seizures), liver toxicity, lymphoma, ↑ BP, tremors, hirsutism, leukopenia, gingival hyperplasia
tacrolimus (Astagraf XL, Envarsus XR, Prograf)	Oral, IV	Same as cyclosporine but more effective	Same as cyclosporine
Corticosteroids			
prednisone, methylprednisolone	Oral, IV	Suppress inflammatory response Inhibit cytokine production (IL-1, IL-6, TNF) and T-cell activation and proliferation	Peptic ulcers, ↑ BP, osteoporosis, Na^+ and H_2O retention, muscle weakness, easy bruising, delayed healing, hyperglycemia, ↑ infection risk
Cytotoxic (Antiproliferative) Drugs			
azathioprine (Imuran)	Oral, IV	Inhibits purine synthesis Suppresses proliferation of T and B cells	Bone marrow suppression (neutropenia, anemia, thrombocytopenia)
cyclophosphamide	Oral, IV	Cross-links DNA, leading to cell injury and death ↓ in number and activity of T and B cells	Neutropenia, hemorrhagic cystitis
everolimus (Afinitor, Zortress)	Oral	Binds to mechanistic target of rapamycin (mTOR), thereby suppressing T-cell activation and proliferation	Peripheral edema, constipation, ↑ BP, nausea, anemia, urinary tract infection, hyperlipidemia
mycophenolate mofetil (CellCept, Myfortic)	Oral, IV	Inhibits purine synthesis Suppresses T- and B-cell proliferation	Diarrhea, nausea and vomiting, neutropenia, thrombocytopenia, ↑ infection risk, ↑ cancer risk
sirolimus (Rapamune, Torisel)	Oral	Same as everolimus	↑ Infection risk, leukopenia, anemia, thrombocytopenia, hyperlipidemia, hypercholesterolemia, arthralgias, diarrhea; ↑ cancer risk
Monoclonal Antibodies			
alemtuzumab (Campath, Lemtrada)	IV	Monoclonal antibody that targets the CD52 antigen on T and B cells, monocytes, and macrophages Causes prolonged T-cell depletion	Fever, chills, dyspnea, chest pain, nausea, vomiting; neutropenia, anemia, thrombocytopenia ↑ Risk for opportunistic infections
basiliximab (Simulect)	IV	Monoclonal antibody that targets IL-2 receptor and inhibits T-cell activation and proliferation	Can cause acute hypersensitivity reaction, including anaphylaxis
Other			
belatacept (Nulojix)	IV	Prevents T-cell activation	Anemia, diarrhea, constipation, urinary tract infection, peripheral edema
Polyclonal Antibodies			
Horse antithymocyte globulin (ATG), eATG (Atgam)	IV	Prepared by immunizing horse or rabbit with human thymocytes or T cells	Fever, chills, dyspnea, myalgia, chest pain, nausea and vomiting, anaphylaxis, leukopenia,
Rabbit ATG, rATG (Thymoglobulin)	IV	Polyclonal antibodies directed against T cells, thus depleting them	thrombocytopenia, rash, ↑ infection risk

IL, Interleukin; *TNF,* tumor necrosis factor.

Newer-generation monoclonal antibodies are a hybrid of mouse and human antibodies. They have fewer side effects because they have been "humanized." Agents include basiliximab, which targets the IL-2 receptor and impairs lymphocyte proliferation. Another monoclonal antibody is alemtuzumab. It targets the CD52 antigen found on T and B cells, monocytes, and macrophages. Prolonged T-cell depletion can result.

Polyclonal Antibodies

Antithymocyte globulin (ATG) is an infusion of horse- or rabbit-derived polyclonal antibodies against T cells and their precursors (thymocytes). These agents are derived by injecting the animals with human lymphoid cells, then obtaining and purifying the resultant antibody. They are often used for inducing immunosuppression and treating acute rejection. The 2 ATG agents are rabbit ATG or rATG (Thymoglobulin) and equine (horse) ATG or eATG (Atgam).

Allergic reactions to the foreign proteins from the animal are common but usually not severe enough to prevent use. Manifestations include fever, arthralgias, and tachycardia. These effects can be decreased by giving the preparation slowly, over 4 to 6 hours, and premedicating patients with acetaminophen, diphenhydramine, and methylprednisolone. The main toxicities are leukopenia and thrombocytopenia. They are caused by antibody contaminants that are not completely removed during preparation of the antibodies.

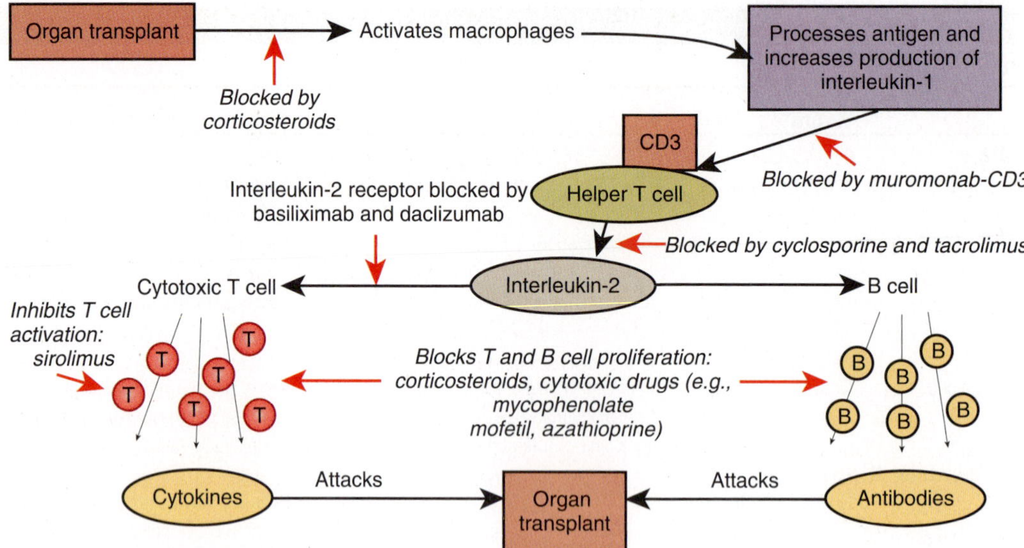

Fig. 14.13 Sites of action for immunosuppressive agents. (Adapted from McKenry L, Tessier E, Hogan M: *Mosby's pharmacology in nursing*, St Louis, 2006, Mosby.)

GRAFT-VERSUS-HOST DISEASE

Graft-versus-host disease (GVHD) occurs when an immunodeficient patient receives immunocompetent cells. In most transplantation situations, the biggest concern is the patient's (host's) rejection of the organ or transplant. However, in GVHD, the graft (donated tissue) rejects the host (recipient) tissue.[13] A GVHD response is most common in hematopoietic stem cell transplants.

The GVHD response may begin 7 to 30 days after transplantation. Once the reaction is started, little can be done to change its course. We do not understand the exact mechanisms involved. It does involve donor T cells attacking and destroying vulnerable host (recipient) cells.

The target organs for the GVHD phenomenon are the skin, liver, and GI tract. The skin disease may be a maculopapular rash, which may be itchy or painful. It initially involves the palms and soles of the feet. It can progress to a generalized erythema with bullous formation and desquamation (shedding of the outer layer of skin). Liver disease may range from mild jaundice with high liver enzymes to hepatic coma. GI manifestations may include mild to severe diarrhea, severe abdominal pain, GI bleeding, and malabsorption.

The biggest problem with GVHD is infection, with different types of infections seen in different periods. Bacterial and fungal infections can occur right after transplantation when granulocytopenia exists. Interstitial pneumonitis is the primary concern later.

High-dose corticosteroids are the first-line treatment.[13] Immunosuppressive agents (e.g., methotrexate, cyclosporine) are more effective as a preventive rather than treatment measure. Radiating blood products before they are given is another way to prevent T-cell replication. Ibrutinib (Imbruvica), a kinase inhibitor that is used to treat several forms of leukemia and lymphoma, is an option for some patients with chronic GVHD.

BIOLOGIC RESPONSE MODIFIERS

Biologic response modifiers (BRMs), or *biologics* or *immunotherapy*, are a class of antibody- or protein-based drugs that can modify the body's immune response. We classify BRMs by their mechanism of action (Table 14.18). They play a key role in treating various conditions, including transplants, autoimmune diseases, and cancer. BRMs are contraindicated in patients who have active infections, immunodeficiency syndromes, and diseases of demyelination.

Mechanism of Action

BRMs have complex interactions within the immune system and targeted pathways. The specific mechanism of action varies among BRMs, which is reflective of the diverse diseases they are used to treat. BRMs can either enhance or suppress an immune response, depending on the mechanism of action needed for the specific target. With autoimmune diseases such as inflammatory bowel disease or rheumatoid arthritis, BRMs often target proinflammatory cytokines like tumor necrosis factor-alpha (TNF-α), IL-1, or IL-6. With cancer treatment, BRMs often target immune checkpoint inhibitors. Some BRMs deplete specific cell populations (e.g., rituximab targets B cells). Others alter the activation state or the function of the immune cells. For example, pembrolizumab keeps T cells from attacking other cells.

Side Effects

Side effects vary depending on the BRM and the underlying disease. Common side effects include flulike symptoms, such as nausea, weakness, and muscle aches. These are generally self-limiting or treatable. More serious complications include infusion reactions, risk for bleeding, and infections. Serious infections are the most feared complications and require screening before initiation and monitoring while patients are taking the medications.[14] Reactivation of hepatitis and TB;

TABLE 14.18 Drug Therapy

Biologic Response Modifiers (BRMs)

Class	Agents	Indications	Considerations
Alpha 4-integrin inhibitors Block α_4-integrin, an adhesion molecule Prevent migration of leukocytes from bloodstream to inflamed tissue	natalizumab (Tysabri)	Crohn disease, relapsing-remitting multiple sclerosis (RRMS)	IV infusion. Monitor for infection and liver problems. Side effects: GI distress, rashes, headache, fever, dizziness, allergic reactions. Because of the risk for progressive multifocal leukoencephalopathy, natalizumab is available only through a restricted program.
	vedolizumab (Entyvio)	Crohn disease, ulcerative colitis	IV infusion, subcutaneous. Monitor for infection and liver problems. Side effects: GI distress, fatigue, headache, joint pain.
CD20-targeted monoclonal antibody Binds to CD20, an antigen on B cells, destroying B cells and suppressing immune response	rituximab (Rituxan)	Non-Hodgkin lymphoma, rheumatoid arthritis	IV infusion, subcutaneous. Monitor for infection and bleeding. Side effects: Fever, chills, GI distress, headache, joint pain, fatigue. No live virus vaccines during treatment. Monitor for low BP if taking BP medication.
IL-1 inhibitor Blocks the action of IL-1, ↓ inflammatory response	anakinra (Kineret)	Rheumatoid arthritis	Do not use with TNF inhibitors. Injection site reaction generally occurs in first month of treatment and decreases with continued therapy. Monitor for infection and kidney problems.
IL-6 inhibitor Blocks action of IL-6, thus ↓ inflammatory response	sarilumab (Kevzara)	Rheumatoid arthritis, juvenile idiopathic arthritis, giant cell arteritis, cytokine release syndrome	Subcutaneous injection. Monitor for infection, bleeding, liver problems. Side effects: Chills, cough, fever, mouth sores, injection site reactions. Monitor cholesterol levels every 4 wk.
	tocilizumab (Actemra)	Juvenile idiopathic arthritis, polymyalgia rheumatica, rheumatoid arthritis	IV infusion. Side effects: GI distress, fatigue, headache, joint pain. Monitor for infection, liver and heart problems, mood changes.
IL-12/IL-23 inhibitor Binds IL-12 and IL-23, preventing the activation of T-helper and natural killer cells	risankizumab (Skyrizi) ustekinumab (Stelara)	Crohn disease, psoriasis, psoriatic arthritis, ulcerative colitis	IV infusion, subcutaneous. Monitor for infection, bleeding, liver problems. Side effects: Chills, cough, dizziness, fever, joint and muscle pain, rashes, stuffiness. Warm medicine to room temperature before injecting.
IL-17 inhibitor	secukinumab (Cosentyx)	Psoriasis, psoriatic arthritis, ankylosing spondylitis	Subcutaneous injection. Side effects: Cough, GI distress, headache, mouth sores, injection site reactions.
JAK inhibitors Block JAK enzyme, preventing it from activating immune cells that cause inflammation	baricitinib (Olumiant) tofacitinib (Xeljanz) upadacitinib (Rinvoq)	Crohn disease, rheumatoid arthritis, ulcerative colitis	Oral agents taken daily. Should not be given with other biologics. Monitor for infection, liver problems. Avoid pregnancy. Side effects: GI distress, headache, mouth sores, rash.
PD-1 inhibitors	atezolizumab (Tecentriq)	Various cancers, including liver, lung, and skin cancers	IV infusion. Side effects: Fatigue, GI distress, rash. Monitor thyroid and lung function.
	pembrolizumab (Keytruda)	Various cancers, including melanoma, lung, cervical, breast, kidney, head and neck, and stomach cancers	IV infusion. Monitor thyroid and heart function. Side effects: Fatigue, GI distress, rash, vision changes.
T-cell costimulation inhibitor Inhibits T-cell activation, thus suppressing immune response	abatacept (Orencia)	Rheumatoid arthritis, juvenile idiopathic arthritis	IV infusion, subcutaneous. Do not give with TNF inhibitors. Monitor for infection. Side effects: GI distress, headache, fatigue, injection site reactions. Avoid pregnancy.

Continued

TABLE 14.18 Drug Therapy—cont'd

Biologic Response Modifiers (BRMs)

Class	Agents	Indications	Considerations
TNF inhibitors Inhibit the cytokine tumor necrosis factor (TNF)	adalimumab (Humira), certolizumab pegol (Cimzia) etanercept (Enbrel) golimumab (Simponi) infliximab (Remicade)	Crohn disease, psoriatic arthritis, psoriasis, rheumatoid arthritis, ulcerative colitis	↑ Risk for tuberculosis. Do yearly testing. Monitor for infection, bleeding, cancers. Side effects: Cold symptoms, headache, rash, injection site reactions. For infliximab: Monitor for infusion reaction. For other agents: Subcutaneous injection site reaction generally occurs in first month of treatment and ↓ with continued therapy.

IL, Interleukin.

opportunistic infections; and cancers, especially lymphoma, may occur. Some develop liver and pancreas problems.

DRUG ALERT

Biologic Therapies

- Perform TB test and chest x-ray before starting therapy.
- Monitor for signs of infection. Notify HCP if acute infection develops, as therapy may be stopped temporarily.
- Report bruising or bleeding.

NURSING MANAGEMENT: BRMS

Nursing care of patients receiving BRMs involves a comprehensive approach to ensure safe and effective care. Care includes patient education, monitoring and assessment, and infusion management. Review the purpose of the drug, mechanism of action, administration route, and potential side effects. Include how to prevent and recognize early signs and symptoms of infection, including fever, cough, malaise, and dyspnea. Discuss the significance of reporting any unusual or worsening symptoms promptly. BRMs require regular CBC monitoring because they can suppress the bone marrow and lead to infections and bleeding. Cardiac function testing is recommended every 3 to 6 months for many BRMs.

Patients need to know the risks before starting biologic therapy. The agents may cause allergic reactions. They are immunogenic, meaning that patients receiving them often make antibodies against them. Immunogenicity leads to acute infusion reactions and delayed hypersensitivity-type reactions. The drugs are most effective when given at regular intervals. Infusion reactions are more likely if a drug is stopped and then restarted.

Before starting therapy, patients are tested for latent TB and hepatitis B. Age-appropriate screening for cancer and pregnancy should be done. Therapy must be delayed if an active infection is present. Vaccines should be updated. Live vaccines should be given 4 weeks before starting treatment.

BRMs are mainly given IV or subcutaneous. Administration can be done in a clinical setting or in the home. When given in a clinical setting we perform frequent vital sign checks and neurologic assessment. Observe for infusion and local reactions. Infusion reactions often manifest as fever, chills, rash, itching, shortness of breath, or hypotension. Reactions can be immediate or delayed. Severe reactions may lead to anaphylaxis. Premedication and a slower infusion rate may be used to mitigate these reactions. Home administration requires teaching about self-administration and treating allergic reactions.

CASE STUDY

Anaphylaxis

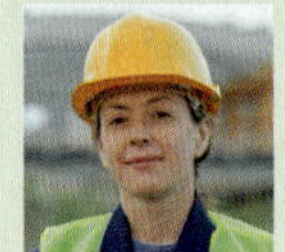

(© shironosov/iStock.com.)

Patient Profile

J.S., a 43-year-old female, presents to the emergency department with an anaphylaxis reaction. Her symptoms started while she was wearing latex gloves at work.

Subject Data

- Works as a construction site manager
- Reports tightness in the vocal cord, dizziness
- States she is having difficulty breathing
- Both hands are "itchy" with burning sensations

Objective Data

Physical Assessment

- BP 80/40 mm Hg, temp 100.1°F (37.8°C), O_2 saturation 94% on room air
- Wheezing noted throughout all lung fields
- Heart rate is 110 and regular
- Both upper hands have erythema, with irregular-shaped wheals that are warm to touch

Interprofessional Care

- Epinephrine (1 mg/mL preparation). 0.5 mg IM in vastus lateralis. Repeat q5 to 15 minutes.
- Cetirizine 10 mg IV now
- 1 L IV normal saline by rapid bolus
- Place patient in a recumbent position and elevate legs
- Monitor vital signs and O_2 saturation

Discussion Questions

1. ***Recognize:*** What clinical manifestations of anaphylaxis does J.S. have?
2. ***Analyze:*** How would IgE antibody immunoassays be beneficial in the diagnose of latex sensitivity?
3. ***Plan:*** Provide the rationale for each HCP order.
4. ***Prioritize:*** What are your priority nursing interventions for J.S.?
5. ***Act:*** Which interventions can you delegate to AP or other members of the health care team?
6. ***Evaluate:*** What outcomes would indicate nursing interventions were successful?

Answers available at http://evolve.elsevier.com/Lewis/medsurg.

BRIDGE TO NCLEX EXAMINATION

The number of the question corresponds to the same-numbered outcome at the beginning of the chapter.

1. A patient with a low number of monocytes would have a decreased ability to
   a. stimulate the production of T and B lymphocytes.
   b. make antibodies after exposure to foreign substances.
   c. bind antigens and stimulate natural killer cell activation.
   d. capture antigens by phagocytosis and present them to lymphocytes.
2. Newborns are protected for the first 3 months of life from bacterial infections because of the maternal transmission of
   a. IgA.
   b. IgE.
   c. IgG.
   d. IgM.
3. In a type I hypersensitivity reaction the primary immunologic disorder appears to be
   a. binding of IgG to an antigen on a cell surface.
   b. deposit of antigen-antibody complexes in small vessels.
   c. release of cytokines used to interact with specific antigens.
   d. release of chemical mediators from IgE-bound mast cells and basophils.
4. The nurse would be alerted to possible anaphylaxis after a patient has received IV penicillin by the development of
   a. edema and itching at the injection site.
   b. sneezing and itching of the nose and eyes.
   c. a wheal-and-flare reaction at the injection site.
   d. chest tightness and production of thick sputum.
5. The nurse tells a friend who asks him to administer his allergy shots that
   a. it can be done if the friend has injectable epinephrine available.
   b. avoiding allergens is a more effective treatment than allergy shots.
   c. it is illegal for nurses to give injections outside of a medical setting.
   d. immunotherapy should be given in a setting where emergency equipment is available.
6. A patient is undergoing plasmapheresis for treatment of systemic lupus erythematosus. The nurse explains that the purpose of plasmapheresis is to
   a. remove T lymphocytes in her blood that are producing antinuclear antibodies.
   b. remove normal particles in her blood that are being damaged by autoantibodies.
   c. exchange her plasma that contains antinuclear antibodies with a substitute fluid.
   d. replace viral-damaged cellular components of her blood with replacement whole blood.
7. The *most* common cause of secondary immunodeficiency is
   a. drugs.
   b. stress.
   c. malnutrition.
   d. human immunodeficiency virus.
8. What accurately describes rejection after transplantation?
   a. Hyperacute rejection can be treated with antimetabolites.
   b. Acute rejection can be treated with sirolimus or tacrolimus.
   c. Chronic rejection can be treated with tacrolimus or cyclosporine.
   d. Hyperacute reaction can be avoided if crossmatching is done before transplantation.
9. The nurse is giving cyclosporine to a patient after a transplant. The nurse would assess for primary adverse effects relating to which system?
   a. Lung
   b. Kidney
   c. Immune
   d. GI tract
10. Which points would be included in a teaching plan for a patient starting biologic response modifier therapy? (**Select all that apply.**)
    a. Possibility of local injection site reactions
    b. Symptoms to report to the health care provider
    c. How to self-administer subcutaneous injections
    d. Importance of receiving necessary vaccinations
    e. Need to undergo monthly TB and hepatitis B testing

1. d; 2. c; 3. d; 4. a; 5. d; 6. c; 7. a; 8. d; 9. c; 10. a, b, c, d.

For rationales to these answers and even more NCLEX review questions, visit http://evolve.elsevier.com/Lewis/medsurg.

REFERENCES

To access the References for this chapter, please scan the QR code with a mobile device.

15

Infection

Jeffrey Kwong

http://evolve.elsevier.com/Lewis/medsurg/

CONCEPTUAL FOCUS

Adherence
Coping
Immunity
Infection
Inflammation
Nutrition

LEARNING OUTCOMES

1. Discuss principles of epidemiology related to infectious disease.
2. Describe the impact of emerging and reemerging infections on health care.
3. Identify interventions to reduce health care–associated infections.
4. Evaluate methods health care workers can take to protect themselves from infection.
5. Describe the manifestations, management, and prevention of COVID-19.
6. Describe methods used to diagnose and monitor HIV infection.
7. Discuss the management of HIV infection.
8. Summarize the characteristics of opportunistic diseases associated with HIV infection.
9. Describe the nursing management of patients with HIV and those at risk for HIV infection.

KEY TERMS

acquired immunodeficiency syndrome (AIDS)
emerging infection
health care–associated infections (HAIs)
human immunodeficiency virus (HIV)
incidence
nonoccupational postexposure prophylaxis (nPEP)
opportunistic diseases
personal protective equipment (PPE)
postexposure prophylaxis (PEP)
preexposure prophylaxis (PrEP)
prevalence
standard precautions
transmission-based precautions
viral load
window period

This chapter presents a brief overview of the concept of emerging and health care–associated infections (HAIs). This includes identifying persons most at risk, recognizing signs and symptoms of infection, and understanding ways to treat or manage infection. Infection, immunity, and inflammation are closely related. The chapter closes with a discussion of human immunodeficiency virus (HIV) infection.

INFECTIONS

Infections such as pneumonia, COVID-19, malaria, HIV, and tuberculosis (TB) are responsible for many deaths worldwide. Infection occurs when a *pathogen* (microorganism that causes disease) invades the body, multiplies, and causes disease, usually causing harm to the host. The signs and symptoms of infection are a result of specific pathogen activity, which triggers inflammation and other immune responses.

We categorize infections as local, disseminated, or systemic. A *local* infection is limited to a small area. A *disseminated* infection has spread to areas of the body beyond the initial site of infection. *Systemic* infections have spread extensively throughout the body, often via the blood.

EPIDEMIOLOGY CONCEPTS

Epidemiology is the study of the distribution and determinants of health conditions, such as infections or diseases.[1] Important concepts include incidence and prevalence. **Incidence** is the number of new cases of a health-related issue or problem that occur during a specific period. For example, the annual incidence of new HIV cases in the United States is around 36,400 cases per year. This means that each year, about 36,400 people are diagnosed with HIV. **Prevalence** is the total number of people who have a specific health-related issue, problem, disease, or illness at any given time. For example, we think the prevalence, or total number of people living with HIV in the United States, is 1.2 million.

Endemic describes the baseline level of disease in a particular area. *Epidemic* refers to a rise or increase of a disease or condition within a certain community or area. For example, the 2022 mpox outbreak is an example of an epidemic. *Pandemic* is a type of epidemic that has significant geographic spread and affects entire countries or the world. COVID-19 in 2020 is an example of a pandemic.

TYPES OF PATHOGENS

Pathogens include bacteria, viruses, fungi, protozoa, and prions. *Bacteria* are one-celled organisms that are common throughout nature. Many bacteria are normal flora. They live harmoniously in or on the human body without causing disease under normal circumstances. Normal flora protect the human body by preventing the overgrowth of other microorganisms. For example, *Escherichia coli* is part of the normal flora in the large intestine.

Bacteria cause disease in 2 ways: by entering the body and growing inside human cells (e.g., TB) or by secreting toxins that damage cells (e.g., *Staphylococcus aureus*). Bacteria are classified based on their shape. *Cocci,* such as streptococci and staphylococci, are round. *Bacilli* are rod shaped. They include tetanus and TB. *Curved rods* include *Vibrio* bacteria, one of which causes cholera. *Spirochetes* are spiral shaped. They include pathogens that cause leprosy and syphilis. Table 15.1 lists common bacteria that cause disease.

Viruses do not have a cell structure. They are simple particles that consist of a small amount of genetic material (either ribonucleic acid [RNA] or deoxyribonucleic acid [DNA]) and a protein envelope. Viruses can reproduce only after releasing their genetic material into the cell of another living organism. Table 15.2 shows some infectious diseases that are caused by viruses.

Fungi are organisms similar to plants, but they lack chlorophyll. *Mycosis* is any disease caused by a fungus. Pathogenic fungi cause infections that are usually local. Tinea pedis (athlete's foot) and tinea corporis (ringworm) are common examples. Systemic infections occur much less often but are much more dangerous. This can happen in an immunocompromised person. Some fungi are normal flora in the body, but when overgrowth occurs, disease can result. For example, overgrowth of *Candida albicans* can cause candidiasis in the mouth (thrush), esophagus, intestines, and vagina. Table 15.3 lists other fungi and the infections they cause.

TABLE 15.1 Disease-Causing Bacteria

Bacteria	Diseases Caused
Chlamydia trachomatis	Chlamydia, lymphogranuloma venereum
Clostridia	
• *Clostridium botulinum*	Food poisoning with progressive muscle paralysis
• *Clostridium tetani*	Tetanus (lockjaw)
Corynebacterium diphtheriae	Diphtheria
Escherichia coli	UTIs, peritonitis, hemolytic-uremic syndrome
Haemophilus	
• *Haemophilus influenzae*	Nasopharyngitis, meningitis, pneumonia
• *Haemophilus pertussis*	Pertussis (whooping cough)
Helicobacter pylori	Peptic ulcers, gastritis
Klebsiella-Enterobacter organisms	UTIs, peritonitis, pneumonia
Legionella pneumophila	Pneumonia (Legionnaires disease)
Mycobacteria	
• *Mycobacterium leprae*	Hansen disease (leprosy)
• *Mycobacterium tuberculosis*	TB
Neisseriae	
• *Neisseria gonorrhoeae*	Gonorrhea, pelvic inflammatory disease, proctitis
• *Neisseria meningitidis*	Meningococcemia, meningitis
Proteus species	UTIs, peritonitis
Pseudomonas aeruginosa	UTIs, meningitis
Salmonella	
• *Salmonella typhi*	Typhoid fever
• Other *Salmonella* organisms	Food poisoning, gastroenteritis
Shigella	Shigellosis; diarrhea, abdominal pain, and fever (dysentery)
Staphylococcus aureus	Skin infections, pneumonia, UTIs, acute osteomyelitis, toxic shock syndrome
Streptococci	
• *Streptococcus faecalis*	Genitourinary infection, surgical wound infections
• *Streptococcus pneumoniae*	Pneumococcal pneumonia
• *Streptococcus pyogenes* (group A β-hemolytic streptococci)	Pharyngitis, scarlet fever, rheumatic fever, acute glomerulonephritis, erysipelas, pneumonia
• *S. pyogenes* (group B β-hemolytic streptococci)	UTIs
• *Streptococcus viridans*	Bacterial endocarditis
Treponema pallidum	Syphilis

UTI, Urinary tract infection.

TABLE 15.2 Disease-Causing Viruses

Virus	Diseases Caused
Adenoviruses	Upper respiratory tract infection (URI), pneumonia
Arbovirus	Syndrome of fever, malaise, headache, myalgia; aseptic meningitis; encephalitis
Coronavirus	Respiratory tract infection
• SARS-CoV-2	COVID-19
• SARS	Severe acute respiratory syndrome (SARS) Middle Eastern respiratory syndrome (MERS)
Coxsackieviruses A and B	URI, gastroenteritis, acute myocarditis, aseptic meningitis
Ebola	Hemorrhagic fever
Echoviruses	URI, gastroenteritis, aseptic meningitis
Hepatitis A, B, C	Viral hepatitis
Herpesviruses	
• Cytomegalovirus (CMV)	Gastroenteritis; pneumonia and retinal damage in immunosuppressed persons, infectious mononucleosis-like syndrome
• Epstein-Barr	Mononucleosis, Burkitt lymphoma (possibly)
• Herpes simplex type 1	Herpes labialis ("fever blisters"), genital herpes infection
• Herpes simplex type 2	Genital herpes infection
• Varicella-zoster	Chickenpox, shingles
HIV	HIV infection, AIDS
Influenza A and B	URI, H1N1 (swine) flu, H5N1 avian (bird) flu
Mumps	Parotitis, orchitis in postpubertal males
Papillomavirus	Genital warts, cervical and anal cancer
Parainfluenza 1–4	URI
Parvovirus	Gastroenteritis
Poliovirus	Poliomyelitis
Pox viruses	Smallpox, molluscum contagiosum, mpox
Reoviruses 1, 2, 3	URI
Respiratory syncytial virus	Gastroenteritis, respiratory tract infection
Rhabdovirus	Rabies
Rhinovirus	URI, pneumonia
Rotaviruses	Gastroenteritis
Rubella	German measles
Rubeola	Measles
West Nile virus	Flulike symptoms, meningitis, encephalitis
Zika virus	Flulike symptoms, fetal microcephaly

TABLE 15.3 Disease-Causing Fungi

Fungi	Diseases Caused	Organs Affected
Aspergillus fumigatus	Aspergillosis	Lungs[a]
	Otomycosis	Ears
Blastomyces dermatitidis	Blastomycosis	Lungs,[a] various organs
Candida albicans	Candidiasis	Intestines
	Vaginitis	Vagina
	Thrush	Skin,[b] mouth
Coccidioides immitis	Coccidioidomycosis	Lungs[a]
Epidermophyton	Tinea corporis	Skin[b]
Microsporum	Tinea capitis	Skin[b]
Pneumocystis jirovecii	Pneumocystis pneumonia (PCP)	Lungs[a]
Sporothrix schenckii	Sporotrichosis	Skin, lymph vessels
Trichophyton	Tinea pedis	Skin[b]

[a]See Table 30.15: Fungal Infections of the Lungs.
[b]See Table 25.7: Common Fungal Infections of the Skin and Nails.

Protozoa are single-cell, animal-like microorganisms. Protozoa normally live in soil and bodies of water. If they enter the body, they can cause infection. Protozoal parasites cause amoebic dysentery and giardiasis. A sporozoan called *Plasmodium malariae* causes malaria.

Prions are infectious particles that have abnormally shaped proteins. Not all prions cause disease. Those that do often affect the nervous system. They can cause a group of illnesses called *transmissible spongiform encephalopathies (TSEs).* Examples of TSEs are Creutzfeldt-Jakob disease and bovine spongiform encephalopathy in cattle (mad cow disease).

TYPES OF INFECTIONS

Emerging Infections

An **emerging infection** is an infectious disease that has recently increased in incidence or that threatens to increase in the immediate future.[2] They can originate from unknown sources, from contact with animals, changes or mutations of a known infectious agent, or biologic warfare. Table 15.4 lists examples of emerging infections. COVID-19 (caused by SARS-CoV-2) and mpox virus are examples. Other emerging infections occur when a previously treatable organism develops resistance to antibiotics, such as carbapenem-resistant Enterobacteriaceae (CRE).

TABLE 15.4 Emerging Infections

Microorganism	Related Disease
Bacteria	
Borrelia burgdorferi	Lyme disease
Campylobacter jejuni	Diarrhea
Escherichia coli 0157:H7	Hemorrhagic colitis, hemolytic-uremic syndrome
Helicobacter pylori	Peptic ulcer disease
Legionella pneumophila	Pneumonia (Legionnaires disease)
Vibrio cholerae 0139	New strain of epidemic cholera
Virus	
Chikungunya	Fever, muscle aches, rash
Ebola virus	Ebola hemorrhagic fever
H1N1	H1N1 (swine) flu
Hantavirus	Hemorrhagic fever with severe pulmonary syndrome
Hepatitis C virus	Parenterally transmitted hepatitis
Hepatitis E virus	Enterically transmitted hepatitis
HIV	HIV infection, AIDS
Human herpesvirus 6 (HHV-6)	Roseola subitem
Human herpesvirus 8 (HHV-8)	Kaposi sarcoma in immunosuppressed patients, including people with HIV infection
Mpox virus	Cutaneous pox lesions, mucosal ulcerations
SARS-Cov-2	COVID-19
West Nile virus	West Nile fever
Zika virus	Fever, rash, muscle aches; microcephaly in children born to infected mothers
Parasite	
Cryptosporidium parvum	Acute and chronic diarrhea

Studies in *zoonosis* (science of transmission of diseases from animals to humans) have shown that many infectious diseases come from animal and insect vectors. Rabies, Lyme disease, mpox, West Nile virus, Ebola virus, and severe acute respiratory syndrome (SARS) are examples of zoonotic infections.

Ebola virus has been an ongoing public health challenge since we first saw it in 1976. In 2014 rates of Ebola increased significantly in East Africa and the first cases of Ebola occurred in the United States. These first cases were from travelers or medical aid workers who were working in Africa. Ebola virus can cause severe hemorrhagic fever. It is usually lethal. Treatments are limited. The natural reservoir and path of transmission are unknown, which makes it impossible to effectively combat Ebola virus and the disease it causes.

Mpox is a viral illness that was first identified in monkeys in 1958. The first human case was identified in 1970 in the Democratic Republic of Congo. In July 2022, there was a global rise in mpox infections resulting in the World Health Organization (WHO) declaring mpox a public health emergency of international concern. Mpox is thought to be transmitted from an infected animal or human. Person-to-person transmission can occur from close contact with infectious materials or respiratory droplets in prolonged face-to-face exposure.

Influenza viruses are another example of how disease can spread between animals and humans. Variants of influenza A viruses are responsible for many influenza epidemics. We traced the 2009 influenza A (H1N1) outbreak to pigs, hence the name *swine flu.* In 1997 and 2003, outbreaks of the influenza A (H5N1) strain of avian flu resulted from transmission of influenza virus from chickens to humans.

Coronaviruses are a group of viruses that can circulate between animals and humans. These viruses get their name because of their crownlike structure. Most coronaviruses cause respiratory illnesses in humans, including pneumonia. The most notable coronavirus is SARS-CoV-2. It is the virus that causes COVID-19.

Unlike other recent infectious disease outbreaks, the COVID-19 pandemic was unique. The rapid spread of the infection, high mortality rate, strain on the health care system, massive quarantine initiatives, and global response had not been seen with other infectious disease outbreaks. Major issues at the beginning of the pandemic included the limited amount of information about how the virus was transmitted and how to treat and prevent infection. Researchers and clinicians worked rapidly to develop and deploy diagnostic tests, effective treatments, and preventive vaccines.

Reemerging Infections

Although vaccines and treatments have led to the near eradication of some infections (e.g., smallpox, polio), infective agents can reemerge under the right conditions. Factors such as population density, inadequate sanitation, antibiotic misuse, climate change, bioterrorism, and other social determinants have increased the risk for widespread distribution of these infections. Domestic outbreaks have typically occurred in areas with low vaccination rates or access to medical care. For example, infections such as measles, diphtheria, polio, and pertussis have had sporadic resurgences. This is in part because of people not receiving recommended vaccines. More recently, there has been a rise in congenital syphilis. We think this is associated with lack of routine syphilis screening during pregnancy and access to prenatal care.

International travel is an obstacle for the eradication of some diseases. For example, measles is no longer endemic in the United States but is still a leading cause of death in developing countries. Some cases occurred in people who have recently traveled to measles-endemic areas outside the United States.

Antimicrobial-Resistant Infections

Resistance occurs when pathogenic organisms change in ways that decrease the ability of a drug (or a family of drugs) to treat disease.[3] Any organism (virus, fungi, parasite) can develop drug resistance to agents typically used to treat them. This is why we use the term *antimicrobial resistance* to describe resistance across different classes of organisms.

Microorganisms can become resistant to classic treatments (e.g., penicillin) and to newer antimicrobial agents. Microorganisms are highly adaptable. They have evolved genetic and biochemical mechanisms to defend against antimicrobials. Genetic mechanisms include mutation and acquisition of new DNA or RNA. Biochemically, bacteria can make enzymes that destroy or inactivate the drugs. Drug target sites are then altered so that the antibiotic cannot bind to or enter the bacteria. If the drug cannot enter the cell, it cannot kill the bacteria. Table 15.5 describes common antibiotic-resistant bacteria.

Drug-resistant bacteria are becoming more prevalent in the community. For example, we initially considered methicillin-resistant *S. aureus* (MRSA), a form of *S. aureus* that does not respond to methicillin- or penicillin-based therapies, a health care–associated infection (HA-MRSA). A variant strain of MRSA that is mainly acquired in the community (community-acquired MRSA [CA-MRSA]) has emerged.[4] This strain of

TABLE 15.5 Common Antibiotic-Resistant Organisms and Treatment

Bacteria	Resistant to	Preferred Treatment
Enterococcus faecalis	vancomycin streptomycin gentamicin	daptomycin linezolid (Zyvox) oritavancin (Orbactiv) tigecycline (Tygacil)
Enterococcus faecium	vancomycin streptomycin gentamicin	daptomycin linezolid (Zyvox) tigecycline (Tygacil)
Klebsiella pneumoniae	Carbapenems (e.g., imipenem, meropenem)	ceftazidime and avibactam (Avycaz)
Streptococcus pneumoniae	penicillin G	ceftriaxone cefotaxime

MRSA is more *virulent* (able to cause disease or infection) compared with HA-MRSA. CA-MRSA can cause rapidly forming skin infections and systemic diseases, including pneumonia and sepsis. Vancomycin-resistant enterococci (VRE) infection is another concern. VRE are more virulent than MRSA and can survive on environment surfaces for weeks. Hospital patients and those with a suppressed immune system are more likely to be exposed and develop infection.

HCPs contribute to the development of drug-resistant microorganisms by (1) giving antibiotics for viral infections, (2) prescribing unnecessary antibiotic therapy, (3) using inadequate drug regimens to treat infections, or (4) using broad-spectrum or combination agents for infections that should be treated with first-line agents. Patients contribute to resistance development by skipping doses and not taking antibiotics for the full duration of prescribed therapy. Limited resources and access to care make it hard for some patients to get adequate treatment for infections. Many health care organizations campaign for the proper use of antibiotics to address these problems.

Health Care–Associated Infections

Health care–associated infections (HAIs) are infections that are acquired because of exposure to microorganisms in a health care setting. Every day, nearly 1 in every 31 hospital patients and 1 in every 43 nursing home residents acquires at least 1 HAI.[5] Around one-third of HAIs are preventable. HCPs often transmit HAIs from patient to patient through direct contact. Improvements in infection control have resulted in fewer infections in recent years. We have seen decreases in several major types of HAIs. These include central line–associated bloodstream infections (CLABSIs), catheter-associated urinary tract infections (CAUTIs), surgical site infections (SSIs), and *C. difficile* infection.

Any organism can cause HAIs, but certain bacteria, including *E. coli, S. aureus, Enterobacter aerogenes,* and various types of streptococci, are most common. Some bacteria that do not normally cause disease can cause infections in high-risk patients because of illness or treatment of illness. Surgical and immunocompromised patients are at highest risk.

NURSING MANAGEMENT: INFECTION

You play a key role in reducing the risk of infection by prioritizing infection control in practice. Assess the patient's risk for infection. Note factors that increase risk (Table 15.6). Monitor for signs and symptoms of infection on an ongoing basis. Create a safe environment that addresses the patient's risks (Table 15.7). Teach patients and caregivers ways to reduce infection risk.

Infections vary by severity, location, the patient's response to treatment, and the potential for harm. Managing infections requires both treating the infection and providing supportive care. The main treatment goal is to eradicate the infection.

Many nursing interventions are supportive. Provide measures to manage pain, fatigue, and fever (see Table 12.5). Monitor for problems with fluid and electrolyte balance. Give antimicrobials and IV fluids as prescribed. Help patients maintain adequate nutrition and rest.

TABLE 15.6 Risk Factors for Infection

- Age
- Autoimmune disease
- Being unimmunized
- Burns
- Cancer and its treatment
- Chronic kidney disease
- Chronic obstructive pulmonary disease (COPD)
- Crowded or unsanitary living conditions
- Debilitation
- Diabetes
- High-risk sexual behavior
- Impaired immune function
- Impaired nutrition
- Indwelling urinary catheter
- Invasive lines and mechanical ventilation
- IV drug use
- Lack of preventive health care
- Liver disease
- Low socioeconomic status
- Medications: Antimicrobials, biologic response modifiers, corticosteroids
- Poor hand hygiene
- Recent surgery
- Recent travel, especially outside the United States or to an underdeveloped area
- Recurrent infections
- Trauma (physical, emotional)

TABLE 15.7 NURSING MANAGEMENT

Infection Prevention

- Perform screening and assess for signs and symptoms of infection, implementing appropriate actions as needed.
- Perform hand washing or use an alcohol-based hand sanitizer before and after patient contact or procedures.
- Change gloves and wash hands when moving between tasks, even when working with the same patient.
- Implement appropriate transmission-based precautions and use PPE.
- Ensure reusable equipment is properly cleaned before use with a new patient.
- Avoid or limit use of invasive interventions when possible.
- Give antimicrobial therapy as prescribed (Table 15.8).
- Use proper aseptic technique when performing procedures.
- Ensure all environment surfaces are properly cleaned, disinfected, and maintained.
- Implement specific care bundles to prevent CAUTI, SSI, CLABSI, and VAP.
- Properly dispose of patient-care equipment contaminated with blood, body fluid, secretions, and excretions.
- Maintain closed catheter systems, such as hemodynamic monitoring, chest tubes, urinary catheters, and IV infusions, when possible.

CAUTI, Catheter-associated urinary tract infection; *CLABSI,* central line–associated bloodstream infection; *PPE,* personal protective equipment; *SSI,* surgical site infection; *VAP,* ventilator-associated pneumonia.

Antimicrobial Therapy

Antimicrobial therapy is the main treatment for many infections. Laboratory testing helps to determine the right antimicrobial. Common classes of antibiotics are shown in Table 15.8. Antibiotics within a class tend to have similar effectiveness, side effects, and allergic potential.

TABLE 15.8 Drug Therapy

Antibiotics

Drug	Action	Side Effects	Considerations
Aminoglycosides			
amikacin gentamycin neomycin tobramycin	Bactericidal Inhibits protein synthesis of many gram-negative bacteria	GI distress Kidney toxicity Ototoxicity	Encourage fluids Monitor kidney function and hearing Give IM dose by deep injection
Cephalosporins			
1st-generation: cefazolin, cephalexin 2nd-generation: cefaclor, cefoxitin, cefuroxime 3rd-generation: cefdinir, ceftriaxone 4th-generation: cefepime 5th-generation: ceftaroline (Teflaro)	Bactericidal Inhibits bacterial cell wall synthesis	Allergic reactions Bleeding GI distress Rash	Take with food Avoid alcohol while taking Monitor kidney function Cross allergy with penicillin Monitor CBC and assess for bleeding Have vitamin K available if bleeding occurs
Fluoroquinolones			
ciprofloxacin (Cipro) levofloxacin moxifloxacin (Avelox) ofloxacin	Bactericidal Interferes with DNA replication in gram-negative bacteria	GI distress Headache Kidney toxicity Photosensitivity Rash Tendonitis	Monitor kidney function tests Take 1 h before or 2 h after meals or antacids Encourage fluids Minimize sun exposure
Lincosamides			
clindamycin	Bacteriostatic and bactericidal Inhibits bacterial protein synthesis	Allergic reactions Colitis GI distress Liver toxicity Rash	Monitor liver function tests Take with a full glass of water Give IM dose by deep injection
Macrolides			
azithromycin erythromycin	Bacteriostatic and bactericidal Inhibits bacterial protein and cell wall synthesis	GI distress Liver toxicity Mental status changes	Take 1 h before or 2 h after meals Take with a full glass of water, avoiding juice Monitor liver function tests
Nitroimidazoles			
metronidazole (Flagyl) secnidazole (Solosec) tinidazole (Tindamax)	Bactericidal Used for anaerobic bacterial and parasitic infections Commonly used for GI and reproductive tract infections	Bitter taste Dizziness GI distress Headache Rash	Avoid alcohol Take with food Encourage fluids May turn urine reddish-brown
Penicillins			
amoxicillin ampicillin nafcillin penicillin G penicillin V	Bactericidal Inhibits bacterial cell wall synthesis	Allergic reactions GI distress Rash	Give IM dose by deep injection, rotating sites Take with a full glass of water, avoid juice Monitor IV site
Sulfonamides			
trimethoprim/sulfamethoxazole	Bacteriostatic Prevents bacterial synthesis of folic acid	Allergic reactions GI distress Liver toxicity Kidney toxicity Peripheral neuropathy Photosensitivity Stomatitis	Take with food and a full glass of water Minimize sun exposure Monitor liver and kidney function tests
Tetracyclines			
doxycycline minocycline tetracycline	Bacteriostatic Inhibits bacterial protein synthesis	GI distress Photosensitivity Rash	Avoid use in pregnancy Minimize sun exposure Take 1 h before or 2 h after meals Avoid dairy products, antacids, iron
Vancomycin	Bactericidal Inhibits bacterial cell wall synthesis	Kidney toxicity Ototoxicity Rash Thrombophlebitis	Monitor kidney function and hearing Monitor IV site

Spectrum refers to the number of organisms affected by an antibiotic (broad or narrow spectrum). *Activity* refers to how an antibiotic kills bacteria. Bactericidal agents attack and kill the bacteria directly. Bacteriostatic agents interfere with bacterial replication.

Before giving any antibiotic, obtain a history of any allergic reactions. Have you collected needed cultures? Perform baseline and infection-specific assessments. Ensure baseline laboratory results, such as liver function tests, are done. Set up an around-the-clock dosing schedule to maintain effective blood levels. Review all drugs the patient is taking to make sure oral agents are not given at the same time as antacids and products containing calcium, iron, or magnesium.

During therapy, monitor for adverse effects, including allergic reactions and superinfections. Superinfections can occur when antibiotics reduce or eliminate the normal bacterial flora. This allows other bacteria or fungi to take over and cause infection. Teaching patients and caregivers the proper use of antibiotics (Table 15.9) is crucial to treatment success and preventing drug-resistant pathogens.

Currently, antiviral therapy is available for a small number of viral infections. These drugs target viruses that cause conditions such as herpes, hepatitis, varicella, HIV, COVID-19, and some influenza infections. Most antiviral drugs work by suppressing viral replication. Table 15.10 shows some common drugs used to treat herpes and cytomegalovirus infections. See Table 48.7 for the drug therapy for hepatitis infection and Chapter 29 for information about influenza treatment.

Antifungals fall into 2 main groups: drugs for systemic infections and drugs for local infections (Table 15.11). A few drugs treat both. Systemic fungal infections and some localized ones are treated with oral or IV drugs. Fungi are often very difficult to kill, and resistance is common. Many drugs have potential toxicity problems.

TABLE 15.9 PATIENT & CAREGIVER TEACHING

Decreasing the Risk for Antibiotic-Resistant Infection

Include the following instructions when teaching patients or their caregivers how to decrease the risk for antibiotic-resistant infection:

1. Only take antibiotics prescribed for you.
2. Wash your hands frequently. Hand washing is the most important thing you can do to prevent infection.
3. Follow the directions for taking antibiotics. Not taking your antibiotic as prescribed or skipping doses can allow antibiotic-resistant bacteria to develop.
4. If your HCP says that you do not need an antibiotic, chances are you do not. Antibiotics are not effective against viruses, which cause colds and flu.
5. Finish your antibiotic. Do not stop taking your antibiotic when you feel better. If you stop taking your antibiotic early, the hardiest bacteria survive and multiply. Eventually you could develop an infection resistant to any antibiotics. You should never have leftover antibiotics.
6. Do not use leftover drugs from other people. This is dangerous because the leftover antibiotic may not be appropriate for you and your illness may not be a bacterial infection. Old antibiotics can lose their effectiveness and, in some cases, can be fatal.

Occupational Safety and Health Administration Guidelines

The Occupational Safety and Health Administration (OSHA) is a federal agency that protects workers from injury and illness in places of employment and supports activities that minimize or eliminate exposure to infectious materials in the workplace. OSHA mandates that any employer whose employees could be exposed to potentially infectious materials implement standard policies and procedures to protect those employees. Employees must be provided with appropriate **personal protective equipment (PPE)**, which are items that prevent infection or injury to the wearer.[6] PPE includes gloves, gowns, facial protection, and disposal systems for sharps (Table 15.12). PPE must be provided in the right sizes. Hypoallergenic gloves or

TABLE 15.10 Drug Therapy

Antivirals for Herpes and Cytomegalovirus Infections

Drug	Indications	Side Effects	Considerations
acyclovir (Zovirax)	CMV HSV VZV	Diarrhea Headache Irritation (topical)	Given oral, IV, topical. Encourage fluids. Monitor kidney function. Monitor IV site. Give IV dose over at least 1 h.
cidofovir	CMV	GI distress Kidney toxicity	Given IV. Monitor kidney function.
famciclovir	HSV VZV	Fatigue Fever GI distress Headache	Given oral. Encourage fluids. Monitor CBC and kidney function.
foscarnet (Foscavir)	CMV HSV VZV	Electrolyte imbalances GI distress Headache Liver toxicity Kidney toxicity Seizures	Given IV. Monitor kidney and liver function. Monitor electrolytes.
ganciclovir	CMV	Bleeding Neutropenia Sore throat	Given IV, oral, ocular. Monitor CBC. Avoid use in pregnancy. Monitor IV site.
valacyclovir (Valtrex)	HSV VZV	GI distress Headache	Given oral. Encourage fluids. Monitor CBC and kidney function.
valganciclovir (Valcyte)	CMV	Anemia GI distress	Given oral. Monitor CBC. Do not crush; avoid contact with powder. Avoid use in pregnancy. Encourage fluids.

CMV, Cytomegalovirus; *HSV*, herpes simplex virus; *VZV*, varicella-zoster virus.

TABLE 15.11 Drug Therapy

Antifungals

Drug	Route	Side Effects	Considerations
Echinocandins			
anidulafungin (Eraxis)	IV	GI distress Hypokalemia Liver toxicity Peripheral edema	Encourage fluid intake. Monitor CBC, electrolytes, and liver function tests. Avoid use in pregnancy.
caspofungin (Cancidas)	IV	GI distress Infusion-related reaction Liver toxicity	Monitor CBC and liver function tests. Monitor for problems during IV infusion. Avoid use in pregnancy.
micafungin (Mycamine)	IV	Cognitive changes GI distress Liver toxicity Kidney toxicity	Monitor kidney and liver function tests. Infuse over at least 1 h. Avoid use in pregnancy.
Imidazoles			
ketoconazole (Extina)	Oral, topical	GI distress Rash, burning (topical)	Do not take orally within 2 h of drugs that affect stomach acid.
Polyenes			
amphotericin B (Abelcet, Ambisome)	IV	Bone marrow suppression Dysrhythmias Electrolyte imbalances Infusion-related reaction Kidney toxicity	Monitor CBC, electrolytes, and kidney function. Pretreat before IV dose with antipyretics, antihistamines, antiemetics, and/or corticosteroids as ordered. Monitor vital signs and IV site during infusion.
nystatin	Oral, topical	GI distress Rash, burning	Do not eat or drink 30 min after oral treatment. Remove dentures before oral treatment. Do not use while breastfeeding.
Triazoles			
fluconazole (Diflucan)	IV, oral	Bone marrow suppression Dysrhythmias GI distress Liver toxicity	Monitor CBC and liver function tests.
isavuconazonium (Cresemba)	IV, oral	Cognitive changes GI distress Liver toxicity Infusion-related reaction Kidney toxicity Peripheral edema	Monitor kidney and liver function tests. Monitor I & O, daily weights. Avoid use in pregnancy.
itraconazole (Sporanox, Tolsura)	Oral	GI distress Hepatitis	Take tablets with food. Take solution on an empty stomach. Monitor liver function tests. Avoid use in pregnancy.
posaconazole (Noxafil)	IV, oral	BP changes Cough Dysrhythmias Edema Fatigue GI distress Musculoskeletal pain	Monitor vital signs and ECG. May need antiemetic agent. Give with food. Avoid use in pregnancy.
voriconazole (Vfend)	IV, oral	Dysrhythmias GI distress Hallucinations Liver toxicity Kidney toxicity Photophobia, vision changes	Monitor kidney and liver function tests. Monitor vision function with long-term therapy. Take on empty stomach. Avoid use in pregnancy.

TABLE 15.12 PPE Requirements

The following equipment minimizes exposure to blood-borne pathogens.

Equipment	Indications for Use
Gloves	• Must be used when employee can reasonably expect having contact with blood or other potentially infectious materials, when performing vascular access procedures, and when handling or touching contaminated items or surfaces. • Gloves must be replaced if torn, punctured, or contaminated or their ability to function as a barrier is compromised.
Clothing (gowns, aprons, caps, boots)	• Must be used when occupational exposure is expected. • Type depends on the task and degree of exposure expected.
Face protection (mask and glasses with solid side shields or a chin-length face shield)	• Must be used when splashes, sprays, spatters, or droplets of blood or other potentially infectious materials pose a hazard to the eyes, nose, or mouth.

From Occupational Safety and Health Administration (OSHA): *Blood-borne pathogens and needlestick prevention.* Retrieved from www.osha.gov/SLTC/bloodbornepathogens.

similar alternatives must be made available to those who have an allergic sensitivity to gloves.

Appropriate PPE varies depending on the situation. You need to use sound judgment when deciding when and how to use PPE. Knowing how to properly put on and take off PPE is important for the health and safety of you and your patients. Isolated infections can be caused when bacteria that normally stay in one area of the body are introduced into another area. Therefore you must take care to change gloves and wash hands when moving from one task to another, even when working with the same patient.

Infection Precautions

There are 2 levels of precautions to help reduce infections: (1) **standard precautions**, designed for the care of all patients in hospitals and health care facilities, and (2) **transmission-based precautions**, designed for specific diseases.[7] The purpose of precautions is to prevent the transmission of organisms from patients to HCPs, from HCPs to patients, from patients to other patients, and from health care personnel and patients to people outside of the hospital (Table 15.13).

Standard precautions apply to (1) blood; (2) all body fluids, secretions, and excretions; (3) nonintact skin; and (4) mucous membranes. Standard precautions are designed to reduce the risk for transmission of microorganisms in hospitals. They should be applied to *all* patients regardless of diagnosis or presumed infection status. Standard precautions include all the OSHA blood-borne pathogens standard requirements.

TABLE 15.13 Isolation Precautions Used in Health Care Settings

Type	Examples
Standard Precautions	
• Used for care of all patients, regardless of diagnosis or presumed infection status	Includes hand washing and PPE use.
Transmission-Based Precautions	
• Provides additional precautions beyond standard precautions to prevent transmission of pathogens • Used for patients known or suspected to be infected or colonized with pathogens that can be transmitted by airborne or droplet transmission or by contact with dry skin or contaminated surfaces • Used in addition to standard precautions	**Airborne precautions:** Health care personnel should wear fit-tested N-95 mask or higher-level respirators. Used for infections spread in small particles in the air, such as chickenpox (varicella), measles, and TB. **Droplet precautions:** Health care personnel should use facial protection (mask and eye protection). Used for infections spread in large droplets by coughing, talking, or sneezing, such as influenza and bacterial meningitis. **Contact precautions:** Health care personnel should use gowns and gloves. Used for infections spread by skin-to-skin contact or contact with other surfaces, such as *C. difficile,* MRSA, VRE.

MRSA, Methicillin-resistant *Staphylococcus aureus; PPE,* personal protective equipment; *TB,* tuberculosis; *VRE,* vancomycin-resistant enterococci.

Transmission-based precautions are used for patients known to be or suspected of being infected with highly transmissible pathogens that require additional precautions to interrupt transmission and prevent infection. Transmission-based precautions include airborne, droplet, and contact precautions. *Airborne precautions* are used if the organism can cause infection over long distances when suspended in the air (e.g., TB, rubeola). *Droplet precautions* minimize contact with pathogens that spread through the air at close contact and that affect the respiratory system or mucous membranes (e.g., influenza, pertussis). *Contact precautions* minimize the spread of pathogens that are acquired from direct or indirect contact, especially multidrug-resistant organisms (e.g., MRSA, VRE, CRE). Precautions may be combined for diseases with multiple routes of transmission. Transmission-based precautions should always be used in conjunction with standard precautions.

CHECK YOUR PRACTICE

While providing care to a patient on contact precautions, you ask the AP to obtain vital signs for you on the patient in the next room. The AP leaves the room only to return a few minutes later. The AP tells you that the BP cuff is not working in the other room, then proceeds to take the BP cuff from the patient on contact precautions and walk into the other patient's room without disinfecting it.

What would you do?

Gerontologic Considerations: Infections in Older Adults

The rate of HAIs is 2 to 3 times higher in older adults. This risk is higher for persons in long-term care facilities. Age-related changes (e.g., impaired immune function) and comorbidities, such as diabetes and physical disabilities, contribute to the higher infection rates.

Infections common in older adults include pneumonia, urinary tract infections (UTIs), skin infections, and TB. UTIs are more common in those who live in long-term care facilities. Patients with indwelling catheters are at particular risk.

Infections in older adults often have atypical manifestations, such as cognitive and behavior changes, before they develop fever, pain, or changes in laboratory values. Do not rely on the presence of fever to indicate infection in older adults. Many have lower core body temperatures and decreased immune responses. We should suspect a problem if a patient shows changes in the ability to perform daily activities or in cognitive function. Underlying diseases and increased frequency of drug reactions can complicate the treatment of an older adult with infection.

COVID-19

The COVID-19 pandemic forever affected communities worldwide. Since the infection was first recognized in 2019, it has caused significant morbidity and mortality globally. During the first year of the pandemic, we estimate 2.33 million people died from COVID-19 infection. COVID-19 mainly spreads through respiratory droplets. Once infected, the incubation period can be up to 14 days. During this period, persons with COVID-19 may not show any symptoms but can transmit the infection to others.

Pathophysiology

Like other coronaviruses, *SARS-CoV-2* is an RNA virus that is surrounded by a protein envelope that has "spikes" on the outer surface.[8] These spikes give the virus a crownlike appearance (hence the name "corona," which means crown). The spikes from the virus's outer envelope bind with angiotensin-converting enzyme 2 (ACE2) receptors, which allow entry of virus into cells. The virus tends to infect cells within the upper respiratory tract. Research suggests that cells within the conjunctiva and gastrointestinal tract can be sites of entry. Once infected, cell-mediated and humoral immune responses occur. These immune responses lead to a release of cytokines and disruption of cell integrity.

The time from infection to initial symptoms is about 5 days. For mild cases of COVID-19, symptoms and immune response peak within the first week. In more severe cases, a significant inflammatory cascade is triggered, leading to acute respiratory distress syndrome (ARDS) and multiple organ dysfunction syndrome (MODS) (Fig. 15.1). See Chapter 32 for more about ARDS and Chapter 42 about MODS.

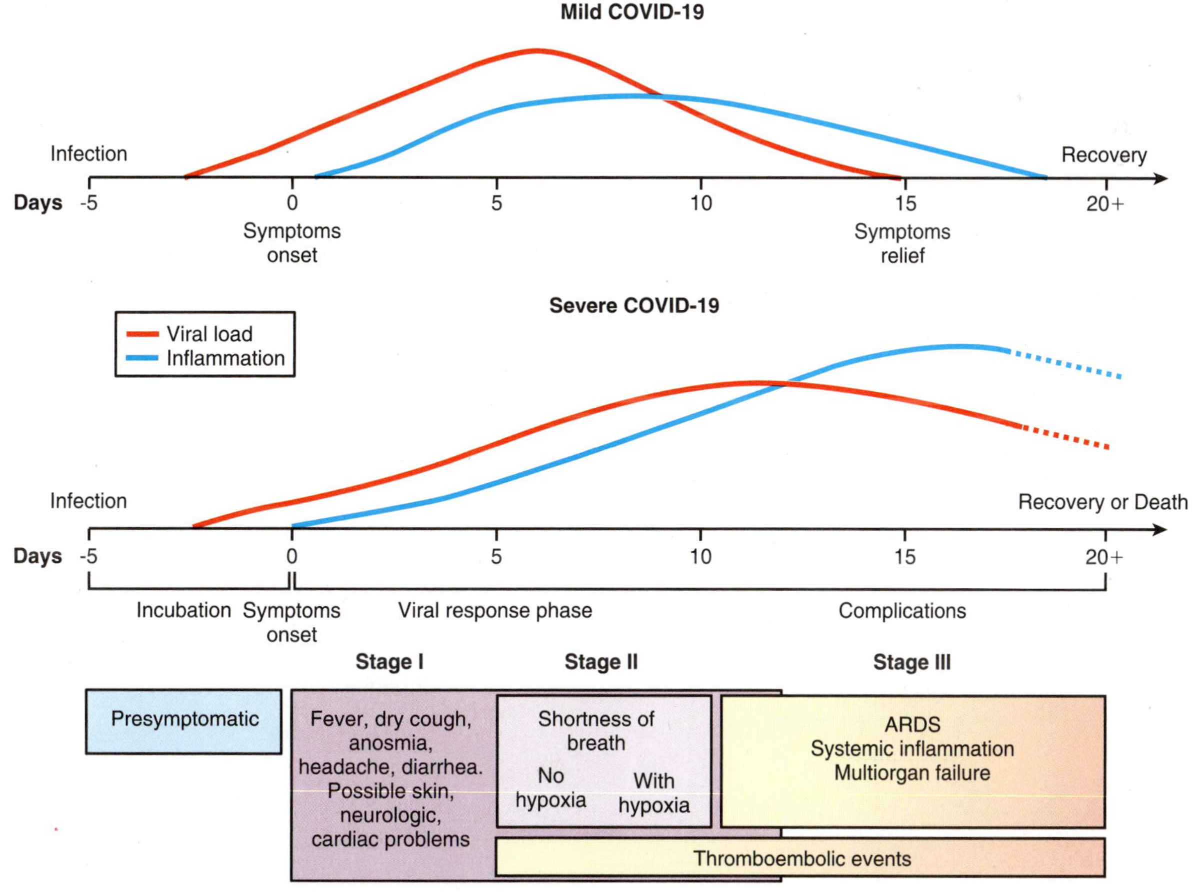

Fig. 15.1 The time course of the immune response in COVID-19 infection.

One challenge in battling COVID-19 is the appearance of variants. Variants occur when the virus mutates. This can result in a variety of different outcomes, including a virus that is more infectious or one that may not respond to established treatments or vaccines. There is ongoing monitoring of viral variants across the globe.[9]

TABLE 15.14 Manifestations of COVID-19

- Cough
- Diarrhea
- Dyspnea
- Fatigue
- Fever
- Headache
- Muscle or body aches
- Nausea and vomiting
- New loss of taste or smell
- Sore throat
- Runny nose, congestion

Other symptoms may include:

- Malaise
- Mental status changes
- Respiratory distress
- Sputum production

Adapted from Centers for Disease Control and Prevention. Retrieved from https://www.cdc.gov/coronavirus/2019-ncov/hcp/clinical-guidance-management-patients.html.

Clinical Manifestations and Complications

The clinical spectrum of COVID-19 varies widely (Table 15.14). Some patients have a mild flulike illness. Others develop serious pneumonia and respiratory failure (Fig. 15.2). It is most severe in older persons and those with preexisting conditions (Table 15.15). The range of illness has been classified into 5 categories[10]:

- Asymptomatic or presymptomatic infection. This occurs when someone has evidence of infection on a viral test for COVID-19 but has no symptoms.
- Mild illness. People with mild illness may have cough, fever, loss of taste or smell, general malaise, sore throat, or diarrhea. Most people with mild illness can be managed at home.
- Moderate illness. People have similar symptoms as those with mild illness, but they usually have more significant signs of respiratory illness, including signs of pneumonia.
- Severe illness. Patients with severe illness typically have decreased oxygenation (SpO_2 <94% on room air, respiratory rate >30 breaths/min, lung infiltrates >50%). They may have signs of sepsis.
- Critical illness. This stage is characterized by ARDS; septic shock; and cardiac, liver, renal, central nervous system (CNS), or thrombotic problems. These patients need intensive care unit (ICU) care and mechanical ventilation.

Most people recover from their symptoms in a few weeks. Some people, though, have persistent symptoms or complications that continue for months. *Post-COVID conditions* is the term used to describe the range of symptoms that people have

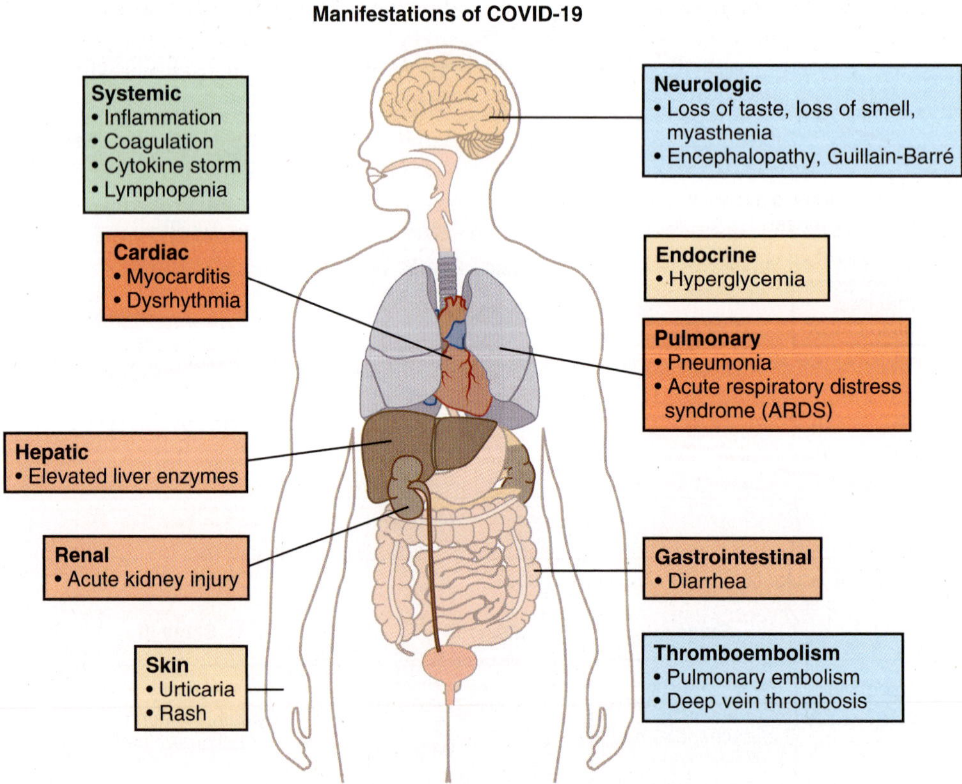

Fig. 15.2 Manifestations of COVID-19 infection.

TABLE 15.15 Risk Factors Associated With Severe COVID-19

Age (≥65 yr)
Cancer
Cerebrovascular disease
Chronic kidney disease
Cystic fibrosis
Diabetes
Down syndrome
Heart conditions (heart failure, coronary artery disease, cardiomyopathies)
Immune deficiencies, including HIV
Immunosuppressive drugs
Liver problems (cirrhosis, autoimmune hepatitis)
Lung disease (asthma, COPD, pulmonary fibrosis, pulmonary hypertension)
Neurologic conditions, including dementia
Obesity, overweight
Pregnancy and recent pregnancy
Smoking (current and former)
Sickle cell disease
Solid organ or blood stem cell transplantation
Substance use disorders
Thalassemia
Tuberculosis

COPD, Chronic obstructive pulmonary disease.
Adapted from CDC. Retrieved from https://www.cdc.gov/coronavirus/2019-ncov/hcp/clinical-care/underlyingconditions.html.

that persist beyond 4 weeks from the onset of initial infection.[11] These persons (sometimes called "long haulers") can have lingering problems. These include prolonged loss of taste or smell, dyspnea, heart problems, fatigue, cognitive changes, and psychologic issues.

Diagnostic Tests

Testing respiratory or oral-pharyngeal samples for COVID-19 is the standard for diagnosis. Antibody testing detects antibodies to COVID-19. It is used to determine past infection or can be seen in vaccinated persons.

Laboratory findings include lymphopenia, increased liver enzymes, low albumin, low platelets, high inflammatory markers (C-reactive protein, ferritin, sedimentation rate), increased D-dimer, and increased lactate dehydrogenase. Chest CT imaging may show diffuse opacities.[10]

Interprofessional and Nursing Management

Most patients with asymptomatic, mild, or moderate COVID-19 can be treated on an outpatient basis. Advise them to follow quarantine restrictions. Keep up to date with your agency and local health department's recommendations on quarantining, as these policies may change regularly. Teach patients good hand washing. Discuss when to contact the HCP. Some patients may need therapy for specific symptoms.

Hospitalization may be needed for severely ill or debilitated patients. In the acute care setting, follow agency policies for isolation and transmission-based precautions. Nursing care focuses on monitoring respiratory status and hemodynamics. Patients may decline rapidly and need transition to the ICU. Provide measures to decrease symptoms, such as acetaminophen for fever.

Disease-specific treatments include antiviral agents and immune-based therapies (Table 15.16). Immune-based therapies include monoclonal antibodies. They are laboratory-made proteins that mimic the immune system and attack infectious agents, like COVID-19. Other immune-based therapies include Janus kinase inhibitors (JAK inhibitors), which can help limit inflammatory responses. Oral antivirals are recommended for most people who can be treated as an outpatient or do not need supplemental O_2. Some treatments for people with more severe disease require IV administration.

Vaccines

Several types of vaccines are available for preventing COVID-19. These vaccine mechanisms include messenger RNA (mRNA) vaccines, protein subunit vaccines, and viral vector vaccines.[12] *mRNA vaccines* use a technology that provides instructions to the hosts' immune cells to create one of the "spike proteins" found on the outer coating of COVID-19. This helps the body create antibodies to the protein. The vaccines do not change your genes (they never get inside the nucleus). The mRNA is destroyed soon after it completes giving instructions to the immune system.

Viral vector vaccines use a harmless version of adenovirus to act as a transport mechanism to deliver genetic material to the cells. The viral vector vaccine contains a small piece of DNA that triggers the body's immune system to create antibodies to the spike protein found on COVID-19. The DNA does not change or interact with the host's DNA in any other way.

Protein subunit vaccines contain a small amount of the protein found on the outer surface of the virus, known as a "spike" protein. Similar to viral vector vaccines, subunit vaccines stimulate the immune system to produce antibodies against the virus. If the immune system is exposed to the actual virus, the antibodies will prevent the virus from reproducing. Protein subunit vaccines are not able to cause COVID-19 infection.

Common vaccine side effects are similar. They include injection site reactions, fatigue, tiredness, fever, and muscle pain. Teaching patients about vaccination and potential side effects is important.

TABLE 15.16 Select Therapies for Treatment of COVID-19

Agent	Considerations
Antiviral	
molnupiravir	• Molnupiravir considered second-line for those unable to take ritonavir-boosted nirmatrelvir
remdesivir (Veklury)	• Hospital patients who need conventional O_2 • IV infusion • Side effects: Nausea, increased liver function tests
ritonavir-boosted nirmatrelvir (Paxlovid)	• Recommended as first-line therapy for patients with mild to moderate COVID-19 who do not need supplemental O_2 and those who are hospitalized for reasons other than COVID-19 • Give PO twice daily for 5 days • Start within 5 days of symptom onset • Available in 2 dosages based on estimated glomerular filtrate rate (eGFR); do not use in persons with eGFR <30 mL/min • Multiple drug-drug interactions
Corticosteroids	
dexamethasone	• Recommended for hospital patients who need high-flow nasal cannula O_2 (HFNC), mechanical ventilation, extracorporeal membrane oxygenation (ECMO)
Recombinant Humanized Anti–Interleukin-6 Receptor Monoclonal Antibody	
tocilizumab (Actemra)	• Used for patients receiving dexamethasone therapy who have rapid respiratory decompensation or who need HFNC, mechanical ventilation, or ECMO • IV infusion
Janus Kinase (JAK) Inhibitor	
baricitinib	• Used for patients receiving dexamethasone therapy who have rapid respiratory decompensation or who need HFNC, mechanical ventilation, ECMO • Given PO • Dose adjusted for patients with renal impairment

Adapted from National Institutes of Health: *COVID-19 treatment guidelines*. Retrieved from https://www.covid19treatmentguidelines.nih.gov/therapeutic-management.

HUMAN IMMUNODEFICIENCY VIRUS

Human immunodeficiency virus (HIV) is a retrovirus that causes immunosuppression. More than 1.2 million people are living with HIV in the United States. About 36,400 new infections occur annually.[13] In North America, men who have sex with men (MSM) account for the largest group of persons living with HIV. With effective treatment, HIV is considered a chronic condition.

HIV Transmission

HIV can only be transmitted through contact with infected blood, semen, vaginal secretions, or breast milk. Health care personnel have a low risk of acquiring HIV at work, even after a needlestick injury.

Sexual Transmission

The most common mode of transmission is unprotected sexual contact with a person who has a high HIV viral load. It is not possible to transmit HIV sexually if the person with HIV has an undetectable viral load.[14] This concept of not being able to sexually transmit HIV with an undetectable viral load is known as "U = U," or undetectable equals untransmittable. Sexual activity involves contact with semen, vaginal secretions, and/or blood, all of which have lymphocytes that may contain HIV. Sexual activities that cause trauma to local tissues increase the risk for transmission. Genital lesions from other sexually transmitted infections (STIs), such as herpes or syphilis, increase the chance of transmission.

Contact With Blood and Blood Products

HIV can be transmitted from exposure to blood when sharing drug-using paraphernalia. Needles, syringes, straws, and other equipment may be contaminated with HIV or other bloodborne organisms.

Routine screening of blood donors to identify at-risk persons and testing donated blood for the presence of HIV have improved the safety of the blood supply. In countries that routinely test donated blood, HIV infection because of blood transfusions or hemophilia clotting factors is unlikely.

Puncture wounds are the most common means of work-related HIV transmission. The risk for infection after a needlestick exposure to HIV-infected blood is less than 1%.[15] The risk is higher if the exposure involves blood from a patient with a high level of circulating HIV, a deep puncture wound, a needle with a hollow bore and visible blood, or a device used for venous or arterial access. Splash exposures of blood on skin with an open lesion present some risk, but it is much lower than from a puncture wound.

Perinatal Transmission

Perinatal transmission from mother to child can occur during pregnancy, delivery, or breastfeeding. Fortunately, the early use of HIV antiretroviral therapy (ART) during pregnancy has decreased the risk of perinatal transmission to less than 1% in the United States.

Pathophysiology

HIV is an RNA virus. RNA viruses are called *retroviruses* because they replicate in a "backward" manner (going from RNA to DNA). Like all viruses, HIV cannot replicate unless it is inside a living cell. The *$CD4^+$ T cell (CD4 cell),* a type of lymphocyte, is the target cell for HIV. HIV enters the CD4 cell by binding to protein receptors on the outside of the cell (Fig. 15.3). This process is known as *fusion* (Fig. 15.4).

Once HIV is attached and fused with the CD4 cell, HIV RNA enters the CD4 cell. This triggers the release of *reverse transcriptase,* an enzyme that transforms HIV RNA into a single strand of DNA. This strand copies itself, becoming double-stranded viral DNA. Another enzyme, called *integrase,* allows the newly formed double-stranded DNA to integrate itself into the host's genetic structure. This action has 2 consequences: (1) because all genetic material is replicated during cell division, all daughter cells are infected and (2) viral DNA in the genome directs the cell to make new HIV.

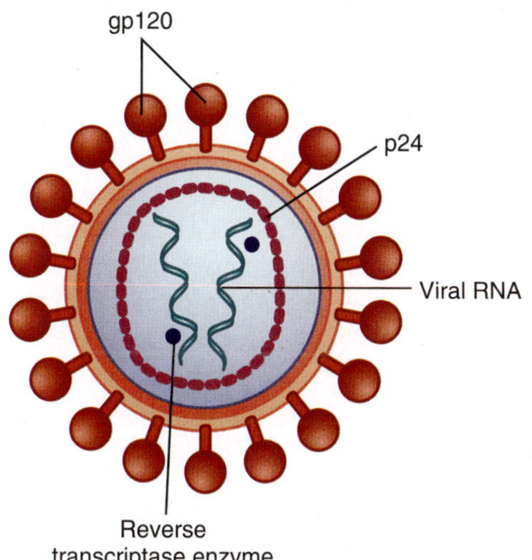

Fig. 15.3 HIV is surrounded by an envelope made up of proteins (including gp120) and a core of viral RNA and proteins.

Protease, another enzyme involved in the replication process, cleaves the newly formed strands of HIV genetic material into smaller pieces. New HIV virions are then formed and released and then the CD4 cell is destroyed.

HIV destroys about 1 billion CD4 cells every day. For many years, the body can make new CD4 cells to replace the destroyed ones. However, over time HIV destroys more CD4 cells than the body can replace. The decline in the CD4 cell count impairs immune function. In general, the immune system remains healthy with more than 500 CD4 cells/μL. Immune problems begin to occur when the count drops below 500 CD4 cells/μL. Severe problems develop with fewer than 200 CD4 cells/μL.

With HIV, a point is eventually reached at which so many CD4 cells have been destroyed that not enough are left to regulate immune responses (Fig. 15.5). This allows **opportunistic diseases** (infections and cancers that occur in immunosuppressed patients) to develop. Opportunistic diseases are the main cause of disease, disability, and death in patients with HIV infection.

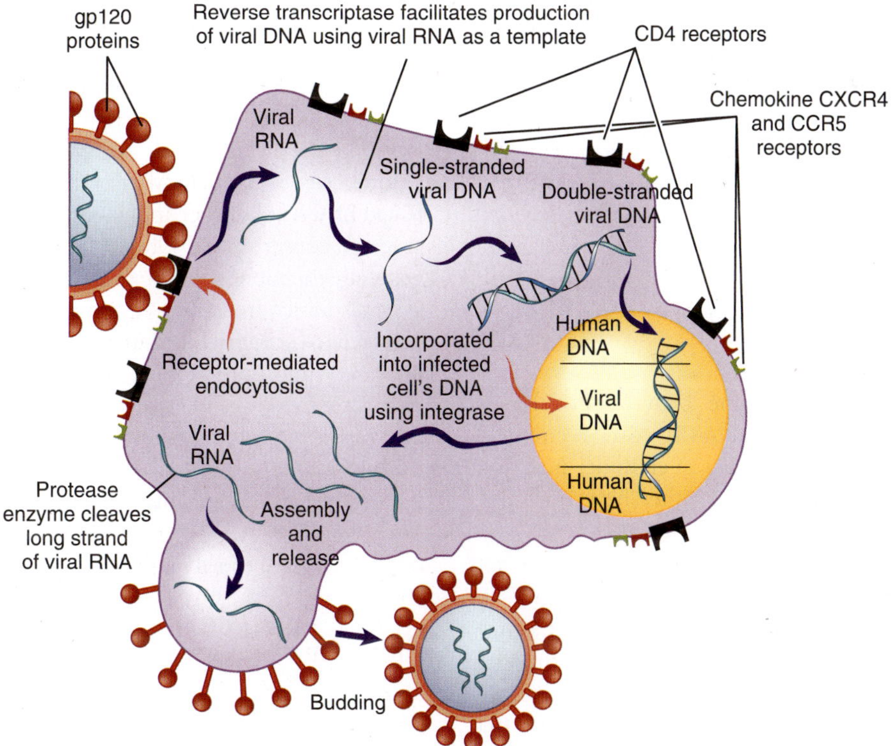

Fig. 15.4 HIV has gp120 glycoproteins that attach to CD4 and chemokine CXCR4 and CCR5 receptors on the surface of CD4 cells. Viral RNA then enters the cell and makes viral DNA in the presence of reverse transcriptase. It incorporates itself into the cell genome in the presence of integrase, causing permanent cell infection and the production of new virions. New viral RNA develops initially in long strands that are cut in the presence of protease and leave the cell through a budding process that contributes to cell destruction.

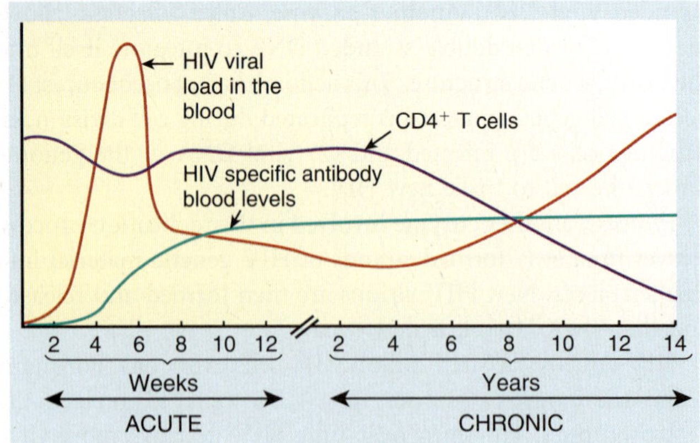

Fig. 15.5 Viral load in the blood in relationship to number of CD4 cells over the spectrum of untreated HIV infection.

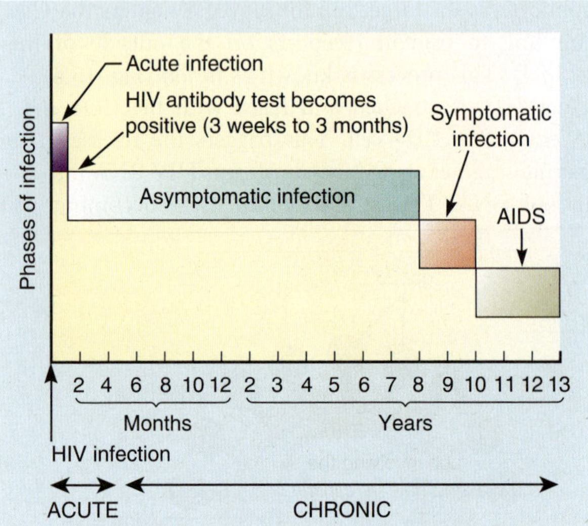

Fig. 15.6 Timeline for the spectrum of untreated HIV infection. The timeline represents the course of untreated illness from the time of infection to clinical manifestations of disease.

Clinical Manifestations and Complications

The typical course of untreated HIV infection follows the pattern shown in Fig. 15.6.[16] Remember that (1) disease progression is highly individualized, (2) treatment can significantly alter this pattern, and (3) prognosis is unpredictable.

Acute Infection

About 2 to 4 weeks after someone becomes newly infected with HIV, they typically develop *acute HIV infection.* During this period, a person can have a mononucleosis-like syndrome of fever, swollen lymph nodes, sore throat, headache, malaise, nausea, muscle and joint pain, diarrhea, and/or a diffuse rash. Many people, including HCPs, mistake these symptoms for the flu. Some people have neurologic problems, such as aseptic meningitis, peripheral neuropathy, facial palsy, or Guillain-Barré syndrome. During acute infection, there is a high **viral load**, the amount of HIV circulating in the blood. This is why people are most infectious during this stage. CD4 cell counts fall temporarily but quickly return to baseline or near-baseline levels (Fig. 15.5).

Chronic HIV Infection

Asymptomatic infection. The time between initial HIV infection and a diagnosis of AIDS is about 10 years in untreated infection. During the first several years after initial infection, people are typically asymptomatic and either have no symptoms or limited signs of infection.

Because symptoms during early infection are vague and nonspecific for HIV, people may not be aware that they are infected. They continue their usual activities, which may include sexual and drug-using behaviors that can transmit HIV to others even though they have no symptoms. Their personal health is affected because they are not receiving treatment that could improve the quality and length of their lives.

Symptomatic infection. As the CD4 cell count declines closer to 200 cells/μL and the viral load increases, HIV advances to a more active stage. Symptoms such as persistent fever, night sweats, chronic diarrhea, recurrent headaches, and severe fatigue may develop.

A common infection during this phase is oropharyngeal candidiasis (thrush) (Fig. 15.7). Other infections that can occur at this time include shingles (caused by the varicella-zoster virus); persistent vaginal candidal infections; outbreaks of oral or genital herpes; bacterial infections; and Kaposi sarcoma (KS), caused by human herpesvirus 8 (Fig. 15.8). *Oral hairy leukoplakia,* an Epstein-Barr virus infection that causes painless, white, raised lesions on the lateral aspect of the tongue (Fig. 15.9), is a sign of disease progression.

AIDS. A diagnosis of **acquired immunodeficiency syndrome (AIDS)** is made when a person with HIV meets established criteria. This occurs when the immune system becomes severely compromised (Table 15.17). Opportunistic diseases generally do not occur in the presence of a functioning immune system. Many infections, a variety of cancers, wasting, and HIV-related cognitive changes can occur in patients with impaired immunity (Table 15.18). Organisms that do not cause severe disease in people with functioning immune systems can cause debilitating, life-threatening infections during this stage. Several opportunistic diseases may occur at the same time, making diagnosis and treatment more difficult. Advances in HIV treatment have decreased the occurrence of opportunistic diseases.

Diagnostic Studies

Diagnosis of HIV infection is made by testing for HIV antibodies and/or antigens. Screening tests can be done using blood or saliva. It can take several weeks after infection before a screening test can detect evidence of HIV (Fig. 15.5). This delay is the **window period**. The typical window period is about 3 weeks (Table 15.19). If a newly infected person is tested

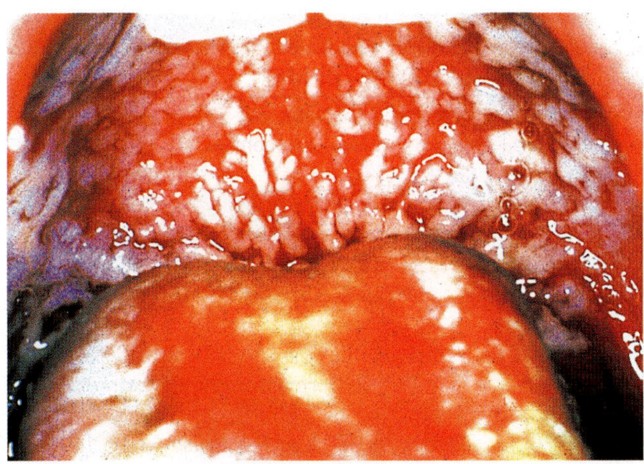

Fig. 15.7 Oral thrush involving the tongue and mucosa. (From Cross SS: *Underwood's pathology: a clinical approach*, ed 8, St. Louis, 2025, Elsevier.)

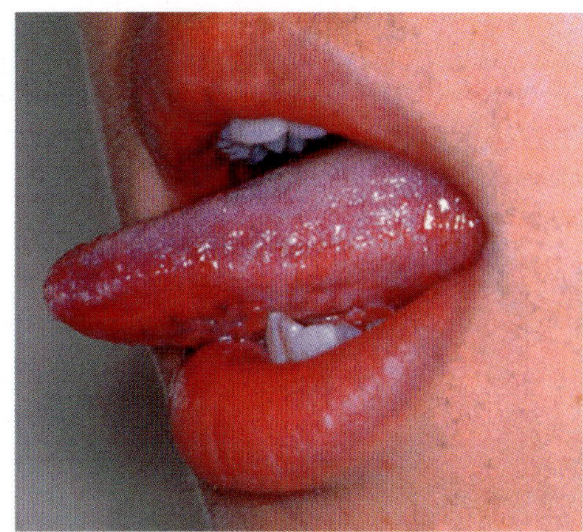

Fig. 15.9 Oral hairy leukoplakia on the lateral aspect of the tongue. (From Chan R, Chio M, Koh HY: Cutaneous manifestations of HIV infection, *Dermatology* 78:1364, 2018.)

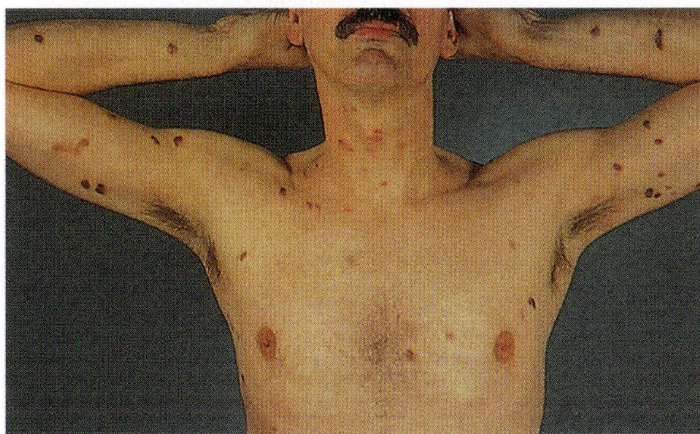

Fig. 15.8 Kaposi sarcoma (KS). KS lesions can appear anywhere on the skin surface or on internal organs. Lesions vary in size from pinpoint to large. They may appear in a variety of shades. (Courtesy Jeffrey Kwong.)

during the window period, the test may not be able to detect infection and there will be a false-negative result.

We monitor HIV progression by assessing CD4 cell count and viral load.[17] The CD4 cell count reflects immune function. The normal range for CD4 cells is 800 to 1200 cells/μL. As the disease progresses, the number of CD4 cells usually decreases (Fig. 15.5). Viral levels provide an assessment of disease progression. The lower the viral load, the less active the disease. In HIV, viral loads are reported as real numbers (e.g., 1260 copies/μL). The goal of treatment is to suppress the viral load to the lowest level possible, which is below the level of detection on a commercial assay. This is referred to as "undetectable." "Undetectable" does *not* mean that the virus has been eliminated from the body or that the person is cured of HIV. Rather, it means that the amount of circulating HIV in the blood is below the level of detection of the test.

Abnormal blood test results are common. They may be caused by HIV, opportunistic diseases, or complications of therapy. Decreased platelet and white blood cell (WBC) counts, with lymphopenia and neutropenia, often occur. Anemia occurs from the chronic disease process and adverse effects of ART. Altered liver function, caused by HIV infection, drug therapy, or coinfection with a hepatitis virus, may be seen. Early identification of coinfection with hepatitis B or hepatitis C virus

TABLE 15.17 Diagnostic Criteria

AIDS

AIDS is diagnosed when a person with HIV develops at least one of the following conditions:

1. $CD4^+$ T-cell count drops below 200 cells/μL
2. One of the following opportunistic infections (OIs):
   - *Bacterial:* Tuberculosis (TB; any site); any disseminated or extrapulmonary mycobacteria, including *Mycobacterium avium* complex (MAC) or *Mycobacterium kansasii;* recurrent pneumonia; recurrent *Salmonella* septicemia
   - *Fungal:* Candidiasis of bronchi, trachea, lungs, or esophagus; *Pneumocystis jirovecii* pneumonia (PCP); disseminated or extrapulmonary coccidioidomycosis; disseminated or extrapulmonary histoplasmosis
   - *Protozoal:* Toxoplasmosis of the brain, chronic intestinal isosporiasis, chronic intestinal cryptosporidiosis
   - *Viral:* Cytomegalovirus (CMV) disease other than liver, spleen, or nodes; CMV retinitis (with loss of vision); herpes simplex with chronic ulcer(s) or bronchitis, pneumonitis, or esophagitis; progressive multifocal leukoencephalopathy (PML); extrapulmonary cryptococcosis
3. One of the following opportunistic cancers:
   - Burkitt lymphoma
   - Immunoblastic lymphoma
   - Invasive cervical cancer
   - Kaposi sarcoma
   - Primary lymphoma of the brain
4. Wasting syndrome (*wasting* is defined as a loss of 10% or more of ideal body mass)

Modified from Centers for Disease Control and Prevention: *Revised surveillance case definition for HIV infection—United States, 2014.* Retrieved from https://www.cdc.gov/mmwr/preview/mmwrhtml/rr6303a1.htm#Tab.

TABLE 15.18 Common Opportunistic Diseases Associated With HIV Infection

Organism or Disease	Clinical Manifestations
Candida albicans	Thrush (Fig. 15.7), esophagitis, vaginitis; whitish yellow patches in mouth, esophagus, GI tract, vagina
Coccidioides immitis	Pneumonia and fever, weight loss, cough
CNS lymphoma	Cognitive problems, motor impairment, aphasia, seizures, personality changes, headache
Cryptococcus neoformans	Meningitis, impaired cognition, motor impairment, fever, seizures, headache
Cryptosporidium muris	Gastroenteritis, watery diarrhea, abdominal pain, weight loss
Cytomegalovirus (CMV)	Retinitis: retinal lesions, blurred vision, vision loss Esophagitis, stomatitis: difficulty swallowing, colitis or gastritis: bloody diarrhea, pain, weight loss Pneumonitis: respiratory symptoms Neurologic disease: CNS manifestations
Herpes simplex virus (HSV)	HSV-1 (type 1): orolabial and mucocutaneous vesicular and ulcerative lesions; keratitis, vision changes, encephalitis, CNS manifestations HSV-2 (type 2): genital and perianal vesicular and ulcerative lesions
Histoplasma capsulatum	Pneumonia: fever, cough, weight loss Meningitis: CNS manifestations, disseminated disease
JC papovavirus	Progressive multifocal leukoencephalopathy (PML), CNS manifestations, mental and motor declines
Kaposi sarcoma (KS) caused by human herpesvirus 8 (HHV-8)	Vascular lesions on the skin (Fig. 15.6), mucous membranes, and viscera with wide range of presentation: firm, flat, raised, or nodular; pinpoint to several cm in size; hyperpigmented, multicentric Can cause lymphedema and disfigurement Usually not serious unless it occurs in the respiratory or GI system
Mycobacterium avium complex (MAC)	Gastroenteritis, watery diarrhea, weight loss
***Mycobacterium tuberculosis* (MTB, TB)**	Respiratory and disseminated disease; productive cough, fever, night sweats, weight loss
***Pneumocystis jirovecii* pneumonia (PCP)**	Pneumonia, nonproductive cough, hypoxemia, progressive shortness of breath, fever, night sweats, fatigue
Toxoplasma gondii	Encephalitis, cognitive problems, motor impairment, fever, headache, seizures, sensory problems
Varicella-zoster virus (VZV)	Shingles: red, maculopapular rash along dermatomal planes, pain, pruritus Ocular: progressive outer retinal necrosis (PORN)

TABLE 15.19 HIV Testing

HIV Antibody/Antigen Testing

- A highly sensitive test detects antibodies and antigens associated with HIV. Blood samples that are negative for HIV infection are reported as negative. The antigen/antibody testing algorithm includes confirmation with HIV viral load testing for any indeterminate results.
- If the patient has a negative HIV antibody/antigen test but reports recent risky behaviors, encourage retesting in 4 to 6 wk. Assess persons at ongoing risk and teach risk reduction interventions, including PrEP.
- If the results are positive and consistent with HIV infection, aid the patient in getting counseling, support, and follow-up HIV primary care.
- Rapid HIV antibody testing
  - Rapid testing results are highly accurate. It can be done in a variety of settings (mobile health units, HCP offices, privacy of a person's home). Results are typically available within 20 min.
  - In-home HIV test kits are available. Testing is done on saliva.
  - Follow a negative rapid test with a risk assessment to determine the need for repeat tests.
  - Positive rapid tests can be disclosed to the patient but must be confirmed with a standard HIV assay. This requires a blood draw and a return appointment to get results.

PrEP, Preexposure prophylaxis.

is important. These infections have a more serious course in patients with HIV, may limit options for ART, and can cause liver-related morbidity and mortality.[18]

Resistance tests can determine whether a patient's HIV is resistant to drugs used for ART. *Genotype* and *phenotype* assays help HCPs to know which drugs can best control a patient's infection. These tests are similar to culture and sensitivity testing used for antibiotic selection.

Interprofessional Care

HIV is a chronic condition. Care focuses on (1) monitoring HIV disease progression and immune function, (2) starting and monitoring ART, (3) preventing opportunistic diseases, (4) detecting and treating opportunistic diseases, (5) managing symptoms, (6) preventing or decreasing treatment complications, and (7) preventing further HIV transmission.

Drug Therapy

ART is a combination of medications used to control and suppress HIV replication. The goals of ART are to (1) decrease the viral load, (2) maintain or increase CD4 cell counts, (3) prevent HIV-related symptoms and opportunistic diseases, (4) delay disease progression, (5) improve quality of life, and (6) prevent HIV transmission.[19] When taken consistently and correctly, ART can reduce viral loads by 90% to 99%. This makes adherence to treatment very important.

A major principle of treating HIV is to use combination therapy with drugs from different classes. Drugs used to treat HIV work at various points in the HIV replication cycle

TABLE 15.20 Drug Therapy

HIV Infection

Drug Classification	Mechanism of Action	Considerations
Attachment Inhibitors		
fostemsavir (Rukobia) ibalizumab-uiyk (Trogarzo)	Interrupts the ability of HIV to attach to the CD4 cell	Fostemsavir taken twice daily orally. May cause heart and liver problems. Ibalizumab-uiyk given IV. An initial loading dose followed by 15- to 30-min infusion every 14 days. May ↑ glucose.
Capsid Inhibitors		
lenacapavir (Sunleca)	Alters capsid, a protein that encapsulates HIV RNA Prevents viral entry, formation, and development of new viruses	Starting therapy involves taking a combination of oral tablets and injectable forms. After initial dosing period, given as 2 subcutaneous injections every 6 mo.
Entry Inhibitors		
enfuvirtide (Fuzeon) maraviroc (Selzentry)	Prevents binding of HIV to cells, thus preventing entry of HIV into cells where replication would occur	Enfuvirtide given subcutaneously twice daily. May cause peripheral neuropathy. Maraviroc may cause heart and liver problems. Taken orally.
Integrase Inhibitors		
bictegravir cabotegravir (Vocabria, Apretude) dolutegravir (Tivicay) elvitegravir raltegravir (Isentress)	Binds with integrase enzyme and prevents HIV from incorporating its genetic material into the host cell	Elvitegravir and bictegravir are available only in fixed-dose combinations with tenofovir and emtricitabine (Table 15.15). Cabotegravir available orally or long-acting injectable. Can cause severe skin reactions, widespread inflammation.
Protease Inhibitors (PIs)		
atazanavir (Reyataz) darunavir (Prezista) fosamprenavir (Lexiva) lopinavir/ritonavir (Kaletra) nelfinavir (Viracept) ritonavir (Norvir) tipranavir (Aptivus)	Prevents the protease enzyme from cutting HIV proteins into the proper lengths needed to allow viable virions to assemble and bud out from the cell membrane	Taken orally as tablets. All part of therapy with other HIV agents, either separately or in a fixed-dose agent. May cause liver problems, ↑ glucose, ↑ cholesterol. Should not take with most statins (e.g., lovastatin). Ritonavir often used in low doses with other PIs to boost effect.
Reverse Transcriptase Inhibitors		
Nonnucleoside Reverse Transcriptase Inhibitors (NNRTIs)		
doravirine (Pifeltro) efavirenz etravirine (Intelence) nevirapine (Viramune, Viramune XR) rilpivirine (Edurant)	Inhibits the action of reverse transcriptase	Taken orally. May cause liver problems and neuropsychiatric symptoms, such as nightmares, hallucinations, suicidal thoughts.
Nucleoside Reverse Transcriptase Inhibitors (NRTIs)		
abacavir (Ziagen) emtricitabine (Emtriva) lamivudine (Epivir) zidovudine (Retrovir)	Inserts a piece of DNA into the developing HIV DNA chain, blocking further development of the chain and leaving the production of the new strand of HIV DNA incomplete	Can cause rashes and skin problems, liver problems, peripheral neuropathy, lactic acidosis. Taken orally as tablet or solution.
Nucleotide Reverse Transcriptase Inhibitor (NtRTI)		
tenofovir (Viread)	Combines with reverse transcriptase enzyme to block the process needed to convert HIV RNA into HIV DNA	Oral powder must be added to 2 to 4 ounces of soft food such as applesauce, baby food, or yogurt. Do not mix with liquid. May cause liver or kidney problems, lactic acidosis.

(Tables 15.20 and 15.21). The major advantage of combination therapy is it inhibits viral replication in different ways. This makes it more difficult for the virus to recover and decreases the chance of drug resistance. Resistance can develop rapidly when drugs are used alone or taken in inadequate doses. Improvements in ART have simplified therapy. Many persons now take combination therapy in a single tablet. Disadvantages of ART include drug side effects and expense.

! SAFETY ALERT

Antiretroviral Therapy Drug Interactions

- Many ARTs have interactions with other drugs and herbal therapies.
- Significant interactions occur with over-the-counter (OTC) drugs, including antacids and proton pump inhibitors, in addition to certain supplements, such as St. John's wort.
- Ask patients about prescribed and OTC drugs in addition to herbal products and supplements.

TABLE 15.21 Fixed-Dose Drug Combination Products

HIV Infection

Mechanism of Action

More than 1 drug combined into a single tablet or administered concurrently as a complete regimen. Drugs may be from the same or different classes.

Examples

Atripla (tenofovir DF + emtricitabine + efavirenz)
Biktarvy (tenofovir AF + emtricitabine + bictegravir)
Cabenuva (cabotegravir + rilpivirine)[a]
Combivir (lamivudine + zidovudine)
Complera (tenofovir DF + emtricitabine + rilpivirine)
Delstrigo (tenofovir DF + lamivudine + doravirine)
Descovy (tenofovir AF + emtricitabine)
Dovato (lamivudine + dolutegravir)
Epzicom (abacavir + lamivudine)
Evotaz (atazanavir + cobicistat[b])
Genvoya (tenofovir AF + emtricitabine + elvitegravir + cobicistat[b])
Juluca (dolutegravir + rilpivirine)
Odefsey (tenofovir AF + emtricitabine + rilpivirine)
Prezcobix (darunavir + cobicistat[b])
Temixys (tenofovir DF + lamivudine)
Triumeq (abacavir + lamivudine + dolutegravir)
Truvada (tenofovir DF + emtricitabine)
Stribild (tenofovir DF + emtricitabine + elvitegravir + cobicistat[b])
Symfi, Symfi Lo (tenofovir DF + lamivudine + efavirenz)
Symtuza (tenofovir AF + emtricitabine + darunavir + cobicistat[b])

[a]Injectable formulations must be given concurrently.
[b]Cobicistat is a pharmacologic booster that enhances the potency of some HIV antiretrovirals. It has no direct effects against HIV.
AF, Alafenamide; *DF,* disoproxil fumarate.

Drug Therapy for Opportunistic Diseases

Management of HIV is complicated by the many opportunistic diseases that can develop as the immune system deteriorates (Table 15.18). Prevention is the preferred approach to opportunistic diseases. Several opportunistic diseases associated with HIV can be delayed or prevented with ART, vaccines (including hepatitis A, hepatitis B, meningococcal, and pneumococcal), and disease-specific prevention measures.[20] Although we usually cannot eliminate opportunistic diseases once they occur, prophylactic therapy can increase life expectancy.

BOX 15.1 ETHICAL/LEGAL DILEMMAS

Individual vs. Public Health Protection

Situation

A nurse in the emergency department is assessing M.T., a 22-year-old male who is being seen today for facial injury that he said happened after "tripping on the sidewalk." M.T. was diagnosed with HIV infection 2 weeks ago. He discloses that his partner verbally and physically abuses him. M.T. says he had not yet told his partner about the HIV diagnosis because he is afraid that he will hurt him. He has not used any protection during sex with his partner since learning of his test results because he thinks his partner infected him.

Ethical/Legal Points for Consideration

- You face a conflict between preventing further harm to M.T. (risk of intimate partner violence), providing care to his partner (his need for an HIV test), and protecting the public health (potential spread of HIV infection to his partner or from his partner to others in the community). Patient teaching and support are essential because your primary obligation is to the patient.
- Because relevant laws vary, be familiar with your state law concerning mandated reporting for domestic partner abuse and infectious diseases.
- Federal laws about protection of privacy in HIV testing apply everywhere.
- In many states, reporting domestic abuse is mandatory only when the reporter witnesses the abuse or the immediate effects of the abuse (e.g., wounds, contusions, broken bones).[1]
- Be familiar with local crisis counseling services.

Discussion Questions

1. How can you protect the patient's confidentiality to prevent further intimate partner violence?
2. What services does your state offer to notify a partner without disclosing the source patient's name? How would M.T. access those services in your state?
3. How can you protect the partner from possible infection while protecting M.T. from further violence?
4. What advice would you give M.T. to address intimate partner violence? What resources would M.T. have in your community?

Reference

1. National Domestic Violence Hotline. Retrieved from https://www.thehotline.org/.

NURSING MANAGEMENT: HIV INFECTION

Assessment

Assessment of people without HIV infection should focus on behaviors that put the person at risk for HIV and other STIs and blood-borne infections. Assess risk by asking basic questions: (1) Have you ever had a blood transfusion or used clotting factors? If so, was it before 1985? (2) Have you ever shared drug-using equipment with another person? (3) Have you ever had a sexual experience in which your penis, vagina, rectum, or mouth came into contact with another person's penis, vagina, rectum, or mouth? (4) Have you ever had an STI? (5) Have you ever had sexual contact with someone known to have HIV? Follow up a positive response to any question with an in-depth exploration of issues related to the identified risk (Box 15.1).

The first patient visit for a patient with HIV provides an opportunity to gather baseline data and start establishing rapport. Obtain a complete history and physical assessment, including an immunization history and psychosocial and diet evaluations (Table 15.22). Repeated assessments are essential so we can identify and address problems quickly.

Planning

Nursing care can help patients to (1) adhere to ART; (2) adopt a healthy lifestyle that includes avoiding exposure to other STIs

TABLE 15.22 NURSING ASSESSMENT

Patients With HIV

Subjective Data

Important Health Information

Health history: Route of infection. Hepatitis, other STIs, tuberculosis. Frequent viral, fungal, and/or bacterial infections.

Medications: Immunosuppressive drugs.

Functional Health Patterns

Health perception—health management: Perception of illness. Alcohol and drug use. Malaise.

Nutritional—metabolic: Weight loss, anorexia, nausea, vomiting. Lesions, bleeding, or ulcerations of lips, mouth, gums, tongue, or throat. Sensitivity to acidic, salty, or spicy foods. Difficulty swallowing, abdominal cramping. Skin rashes, lesions, or color changes.

Elimination: Persistent diarrhea, change in character of stools. Painful urination, low back pain.

Activity—exercise: Chronic fatigue, muscle weakness, difficulty walking. Cough, shortness of breath.

Sleep—rest: Insomnia, night sweats, fatigue.

Cognitive—perceptual: Headaches, stiff neck, chest pain, rectal pain, retrosternal pain. Blurred vision, photophobia, diplopia, loss of vision. Impaired hearing. Confusion, forgetfulness, attention deficit, changes in mental status, memory loss, personality changes. Paresthesias, hypersensitivity in feet, pruritus.

Role—relationship: Support system(s), career or job, financial resources.

Sexuality—reproductive: Lesions on genitalia or anus (internal or external), pruritus or burning in vagina, penis, or anus. Painful sexual intercourse, rectal pain or bleeding, changes in menstruation, vaginal or penile discharge. Use of birth control measures, pregnancies, desire for future children.

Coping—stress tolerance: Stress level, previous losses, coping patterns, self-concept; social withdrawal.

Objective Data

Cardiovascular

Pericardial friction rub, murmur, bradycardia, tachycardia

Eyes

Presence of exudates, retinal lesions or hemorrhage, papilledema

GI

Mouth lesions, including blisters (HSV), white-gray patches (*Candida* infection), painless white lesions on the side of the tongue (hairy leukoplakia), discolorations (Kaposi sarcoma). Gingivitis, tooth decay, or loosening. Redness or white patchy lesions of throat. Vomiting, diarrhea, incontinence, rectal lesions, hyperactive bowel sounds, abdominal masses, hepatosplenomegaly.

General

Lethargy, persistent fever, lymphadenopathy, peripheral wasting, fat deposits in truncal areas and upper back.

Musculoskeletal

Muscle wasting, weakness.

Neurologic

Ataxia, tremors, lack of coordination. Sensory loss, slurred speech, aphasia. Memory loss, peripheral neuropathy, apathy, agitation, depression, inappropriate behavior. Decreasing levels of consciousness, seizures, paralysis, coma.

Respiratory

Tachypnea, dyspnea, intercostal retractions. Crackles, wheezing, productive or nonproductive cough.

Reproductive

Genital lesions or discharge, abdominal tenderness secondary to pelvic inflammatory disease.

Skin

Dry skin, diaphoresis. Pallor, cyanosis. Lesions, eruptions, discolorations, bruising of skin or mucous membranes. Vaginal or perianal excoriation. Alopecia. Delayed wound healing.

Possible Diagnostic Findings

Positive HIV antibody/antigen assay. Detectable viral load. ↓ CD4 cell count, ↓ WBC count, lymphopenia, anemia, thrombocytopenia. Electrolyte imbalances. ↑ Liver function tests. ↑ Cholesterol, ↑ triglycerides, ↑ glucose.

HSV, Herpes simplex infection; *STI,* sexually transmitted infection.

and blood-borne diseases; (3) protect others from HIV; (4) have supportive relationships; (5) maintain activities and productivity; (6) explore spiritual issues; (7) come to terms with issues related to disease, disability, and death; and (8) cope with symptoms caused by HIV and its treatments.

◆ Implementation

Health Promotion

HIV infection is preventable. The goal is to develop safer, healthier, and less risky behaviors (Box 15.2). The more consistently and correctly one uses prevention methods, the more effective they are in preventing HIV infection. Measures to prevent HIV transmission are based on an assessment of the person's risk behaviors. Provide culturally sensitive, language-appropriate, and age-specific teaching and behavior change counseling. Nurses who are comfortable with and know how to talk about sensitive topics such as sexuality and drug use are best prepared to provide prevention education.

Biomedical prevention. Preexposure prophylaxis (PrEP) is a prevention method in which people who do not have HIV take HIV medicine to reduce their risk for acquiring HIV sexually or through IV drug use.[21] PrEP should be used before exposure to HIV and combined with other prevention actions such as condoms, risk reduction counseling, and regular HIV testing. There are various forms of PrEP, including oral and injectable agents. Although the agents used for PrEP are the same as those taken by persons to treat HIV infection, a PrEP option only contains drugs from 1 class of antiretrovirals. The oral PrEP option consists of 2 HIV antiretroviral drugs combined into 1 tablet. Both oral tablets contain emtricitabine. They are combined with either tenofovir disoproxil fumarate

BOX 15.2 PROMOTING POPULATION HEALTH

Prevention and Early Detection of HIV

- Increase safer sexual practices, including condom use
- Decrease equipment sharing among IV drug users
- Increase clinician skills to assess for risk factors for HIV infection, recommend HIV testing, and provide counseling for behavior change
- Make HIV testing a routine part of health care
- Increase access to new HIV testing technologies, especially rapid testing
- Increase access to HIV testing in alternative care settings, such as drug and alcohol treatment facilities and community-based organizations
- Increase behavior change messages to people with HIV to prevent new infections
- Discuss and offer PrEP to persons at risk for HIV infection
- Discuss the option of nPEP for persons at risk for HIV who had an unanticipated exposure
- Decrease perinatal HIV infection by offering HIV testing as a part of routine prenatal care
- Counsel and support those with HIV to take ART as prescribed

ART, Antiretroviral therapy, *nPEP,* nonoccupational postexposure prophylaxis; *PrEP,* preexposure prophylaxis.

(Truvada) or tenofovir alafenamide (Descovy). Another option is the integrase inhibitor cabotegravir (Apretude) given as an intramuscular injection every 8 weeks. If someone on PrEP becomes infected with HIV, they will need to be placed on additional classes of ART.

Nonoccupational postexposure prophylaxis (nPEP) is another prevention option to reduce the risk of HIV infection.[22] With nPEP, combination HIV ART is given to someone within 72 hours after a potential exposure (e.g., sex, needlestick). Treatment is typically given for 28 days. We monitor patients after the incident with repeat HIV testing.

Behavior modification. Many activities can reduce the risk for HIV infection. Help people choose the methods that best fit their needs and circumstances. We consider prevention techniques as *safer activities* (those that have minimal risk) or *risk-reducing activities* (those that decrease, but do not eliminate, risk). A combination of prevention methods (e.g., PrEP, using protective barriers, limiting the number of sex partners) increases the prevention effect.

Decreasing risks related to sexual intercourse. *Safe sexual activities* eliminate the risk for exposure to HIV in semen and vaginal secretions. Abstaining from all sexual activity is an effective way to achieve this goal. There are safe options for those who cannot or do not wish to abstain. Limiting sexual behavior to activities in which the mouth, penis, vagina, or rectum does not come into contact with a partner's mouth, penis, vagina, or rectum eliminates contact with blood, semen, or vaginal secretions. Safe activities include masturbation, mutual masturbation ("hand job"), and other activities that meet the "no contact" requirements.

Risk-reducing sexual activities decrease the risk of contact with HIV. Protective barriers can be used when engaging in insertive sexual activity (oral, vaginal, anal) with a partner who has HIV or whose HIV status is not known. The most-used barrier is the male condom (Box 15.3). They offer protection during anal, vaginal, and oral intercourse. Female condoms are an alternative to male condoms. Squares of latex (dental dams) can be used as a barrier during oral sexual activity.

Decreasing risks related to drug use. The major risk for HIV related to using drugs involves sharing equipment or having unsafe sexual experiences while under the influence of drugs. Basic risk reduction rules are (1) do not use drugs; (2) if you use drugs, do not share equipment; and (3) do not have sexual intercourse when under the influence of any drug, including alcohol, which impairs decision making.

The safest method is to abstain from drugs. This may not be a practical option for users who are not prepared to quit or have no access to drug treatment services. The risk for HIV infection for these persons is eliminated if they do not share injecting equipment. Blood can contaminate equipment used to snort (straws) or smoke (pipes) drugs and should not be shared.

BOX 15.3 EVIDENCE-BASED PRACTICE

Condom Use and HIV

As a nurse in an HIV clinic, you are counseling M.J., a 27-year-old male, and his male partner. M.J. is on antiretroviral therapy (ART). His viral load is very low, and his CD4 cell count is normal. He tells you that because the drugs are working, he and his partner (who is HIV negative) are considering not using condoms in the future.

Making Clinical Decisions

Best Available Evidence

One of the best ways to prevent HIV transmission continues to be the consistent and correct use of latex condoms. Those with HIV who take ART and have an undetectable viral load (<200 copies/mL) have no risk for transmitting HIV to their sexual partners. Behavior change programs provided by HCPs, peers, and others can reduce risk behaviors among those with HIV.

Clinician Expertise

Risk-reducing sexual activities in this situation include the continued use of condoms. You know that although an undetectable viral load decreases the risk for HIV transmission, the risk of transmission of other sexually transmitted infections (STIs) is not completely eliminated.

Patient Preferences and Values

M.J. and his partner tell you that they are in a committed relationship and have no other partners. They do not like using condoms.

Implications for Practice

1. What information would you discuss related to HIV transmission, ART and viral load, and the risks of unprotected sexual activity?
2. What measures besides condom use would you discuss with them to reduce the risk for HIV transmission?

References for Evidence

CDC: *Evidence of HIV treatment and viral suppression in preventing the sexual transmission of HIV.* Retrieved from www.cdc.gov/hiv/pdf/risk/art/cdc-hiv-art-viral-suppression.pdf.

CDC: *Proven HIV prevention methods.* Retrieved from www.cdc.gov/nchhstp/newsroom/docs/factsheets/hiv-proven-prevention-methods-508.pdf.

Access to sterile equipment is an important risk elimination tactic. Some communities have syringe service programs (SSPs) that provide sterile equipment in exchange for used equipment. In communities with SSPs, drug use does not increase, and rates of HIV and other blood-borne infections are controlled.[23] Proper cleaning of equipment can reduce risk by decreasing the chance of blood contact.

Decreasing perinatal transmission. ART treatment during pregnancy decreases the rate of perinatal transmission from 25% to less than 1%.[24] Ask persons with HIV who can become pregnant about their reproductive desires. Discuss family planning methods. Someone who is contemplating pregnancy should receive HIV counseling, be offered access to voluntary HIV testing, and, if they have HIV, be offered optimal ART.[24]

Decreasing risks at work. The risk for infection from occupational exposure to HIV is small but real. OSHA requires employers to protect workers from exposure to blood and other potentially infectious materials (Table 15.12). Precautions and safety devices decrease the risk for direct contact with blood and body fluids. Should exposure to HIV-infected fluids occur, **postexposure prophylaxis (PEP)** with combination ART can significantly decrease the risk for infection.[15] The need for timely treatment and counseling makes it critical for nurses to report all blood exposures.

HIV testing. Around 14% of people with HIV in the United States do not know they are infected. They are more likely to transmit the infection to others. Current guidelines recommend universal, voluntary testing as part of routine medical care.[25] The goal is to normalize the test, decrease the stigma related to HIV testing, find hidden cases, get infected persons into care, and prevent new cases of infection.

Acute Care

Table 15.23 shows a summary of nursing goals, assessments, and interventions throughout the course of HIV infection.

TABLE 15.23 NURSING MANAGEMENT

HIV Infection

Nursing Goals	Assessment	Interventions
Acute Care		
Promote health and limit disability	*Physical health:* Is the patient having problems? *Mental health:* How is the patient coping? *Resources:* Does the patient have family or social support? Is the patient accessing community services? Is money or insurance a problem? Does the patient have access to spiritual support as desired?	• Provide case management or referrals such as social work. • Teach about HIV, the spectrum of infection, options for care, signs and symptoms to report, treatment options, immune enhancement, risk reduction, and ways to adhere to treatment. • Establish trusting relationships with patient, family, and significant others. • Provide emotional and spiritual support. • Develop resources for legal needs: discrimination prevention, wills, advance directives, childcare wishes. • Empower the patient to identify needs, direct care, and seek services.
Manage problems caused by HIV infection	*Physical health:* Has the patient had an acute exacerbation of problems related to immunodeficiency, opportunistic disease, or risk factors (e.g., substance use)? *Mental health status:* Has the patient's ability to cope with psychosocial issues deteriorated?	• Provide care during acute exacerbations: recognition of life-threatening developments, life support, rapid intervention with treatments and drugs, comfort, and hygiene needs. • Support patient and family during crisis. • Assist the patient with mental health issues. Provide referral to mental health specialist as needed.
Chronic Care		
Maintain optimal health	*Physical health:* Are new symptoms developing? Are there drug side effects or interactions?	• Continue physical care for chronic disease process: treatments, drugs, comfort, and hygiene needs. • Continue case management. • Teach about changing treatment options and continued adherence.
Maximize quality of life	*Mental health:* How is the patient coping? What adjustments have been made? *Finances:* Can the patient maintain health care and basic standards of living? *Family, social, and community support:* Are these available? Is the patient using support in an effective manner? Do family or significant others need teaching, encouragement, or stress relief? *Spirituality issues:* Does the patient desire support from a religious organization or spiritual counselor?	• Refer the patient to resources to support finances. • Support patient and family or significant others in a trusting relationship. • Assist with end-of-life issues, including resuscitation orders, comfort measures, funeral plans, estate planning, childcare. • Assess desires and refer to resources that will help in meeting spiritual needs. • Empower patient to continue to direct care and to make desires known to family and significant others.

Early intervention. Early intervention after detection of HIV infection can promote health and limit disability. Findings from the history, assessment, and laboratory tests help determine patient needs. Ongoing assessment should focus on early detection of symptoms, opportunistic diseases, and psychosocial problems (Table 15.22). Begin teaching about HIV disease, prevention of transmission to others, health promotion, and family planning. Use patient input to develop a plan of care and determine the need for referrals. Remember that newly diagnosed patients may not be able to retain or understand information. Be prepared to repeat and clarify information over the course of several months.

Table 15.24 outlines patient and caregiver teaching on HIV treatment and initial follow-up. One of the most important components of successful treatment is adherence to ART. Taking drugs as prescribed is important. Missing even a few doses can lead to drug resistance. Provide teaching about ART (Table 15.25). Include (1) advantages and disadvantages of treatments, (2) dangers of poor adherence, (3) how and when to take each drug, (4) drug interactions to avoid, and (5) side effects to report to the HCP.

CHECK YOUR PRACTICE

You are caring for a patient living with HIV. When you ask them about their HIV treatment, they tell you, "I heard that HIV drugs are hard on the liver. I'm afraid to take anything that will make me feel sick, so I don't always take my HIV pills." How would you respond?

Reactions to an HIV diagnosis are similar to the reactions of people who are diagnosed with any life-threatening, debilitating, or chronic illness. These reactions include anxiety, panic, fear, depression, denial, hopelessness, anger, and guilt. Unfortunately, all these emotions are overlaid with the stigma and discrimination that continue to infuse societal reactions to HIV. The patient's family, friends, and caregivers have many of the same reactions.

Acute exacerbations. Nursing care becomes more complex as a patient's immune system declines and new problems arise to compound existing problems. Nursing care can help prevent many opportunistic diseases. We can ensure that the patient is adhering to the ART regimen and, if appropriate, taking prophylactic therapy for opportunistic infections.

When opportunistic diseases or treatment side effects develop, provide symptom management and specific treatment. For example, a patient with *Pneumocystis jirovecii* pneumonia (PCP) needs care to ensure adequate oxygenation. If the patient with meningitis is confused, maintain a safe environment.

Chronic Care

HIV infection affects the entire range of a person's life. As a nurse, you are often the person who works with patients who are coping with living with HIV.

Psychosocial care. As time passes, patients and their loved ones will be confronted with complex treatment decisions; feelings of loss, anger, powerlessness, depression, and grief; social isolation; and the possibility of death. Infections, cancers, debility, and psychosocial or economic issues may interact to overwhelm a patient's ability to cope. Review coping and stress management strategies. Refer patients to counseling as needed. Encourage them to get involved in support groups and counseling.

Persons with HIV share problems experienced by those with chronic diseases, but these problems are worsened by negative social attitudes and beliefs surrounding HIV. Some people conclude that people with HIV brought the disease on themselves and deserve to be sick. Some view behaviors related to HIV infection as immoral (e.g., same-sex activity, promiscuity). Other behaviors are sometimes illegal (e.g., using drugs, sex work). The fact that people with HIV can transmit the virus to others creates fear, which leads to stigma and discrimination.[26] Although the Americans with Disabilities Act (ADA) prohibits many forms of discrimination, people with HIV have lost jobs, homes, and insurance. Discrimination can lead to social isolation, dependence, frustration, low self-image, loss of control, and economic pressures.

TABLE 15.24 PATIENT & CAREGIVER TEACHING

Antiretroviral Drugs

To decrease the risk for developing resistance, include the following instructions when teaching the patient and/or caregiver about ART:

1. Discuss options with your HCP to find the best regimen for you.
2. Know the drugs you are taking and how to take them (some must be taken with food, some must be taken on an empty stomach, some cannot be taken together). If you do not understand, ask. Have your nurse write the instructions for you.
3. Take the full dose prescribed and take it on schedule.
4. Tell the HCP if you cannot take the drug because of side effects or other problems. Do not quit taking one drug while continuing the others. If you cannot tolerate any of your drugs, talk to your HCP, who will recommend a way to deal with the side effects or a new set of drugs.
5. Many antiretroviral drugs interact with other drugs, including many common drugs you can buy without a prescription. Be sure your HCP and pharmacist know all the drugs that you are taking. Do not take any new drugs without checking for possible interactions.
6. The goals of ART are to decrease the amount of virus in your blood (your viral load) and to keep your CD4 cell count high. Most HCPs do laboratory work every 3 to 6 months.
7. At 2 to 4 weeks after you start on drug therapy or change your therapy, your HCP will test your viral load to find out how the drugs are working.
   a. Your viral load is reported in absolute numbers. You want to see the viral load drop.
   b. Your CD4 cell count is reported in absolute numbers or percentages. It is best for your CD4 cell count to be above 500 cells/μL. If reported in percentages, you would like your CD4 cell value to be above 14%.
8. An undetectable viral load means that the amount of virus is extremely low. HIV cannot be found in the blood using current testing technology. It does not mean that the virus is gone. The virus can be in lymph nodes and organs that blood tests cannot detect. HIV cannot be transmitted through sexual contact if you have an undetectable viral load.

ART, Antiretroviral therapy.

TABLE 15.25 PATIENT & CAREGIVER TEACHING

Improving Adherence to Antiretroviral Therapy

The following are strategies that you can use to improve a patient's adherence to antiretroviral therapy (ART):

1. Determine whether the patient understands the importance of adherence and is ready to start therapy.
2. Provide teaching on ART dosing.
3. Review potential ART side effects. Assure the patient that side effects can be treated. If not, ART regimens can be changed.
4. Use memory aids, including smartphone apps, pillboxes, and calendars.
5. Engage family and friends in the teaching process. Solicit their support to help the patient take treatment.
6. Simplify regimens, dosing, and food requirements as much as possible.
7. Use a team of nurses, HCPs, pharmacists, case managers, and mental health and peer counselors to support the patient.
8. Help the patient integrate the ART regimen into their typical life activities and work schedules.

Modified from Panel on Antiretroviral Guidelines for Adults and Adolescents: *Guidelines for the use of antiretroviral agents in adults and adolescents living with HIV.* Retrieved from https://clinicalinfo.hiv.gov/en/guidelines/adult-and-adolescent-arv/whats-new-guidelines.

CHECK YOUR PRACTICE

You are receiving report on a patient newly admitted to the oncology unit. She is a 62-year-old female patient who is being treated for lung cancer. The nurse giving report casually mentions, "Oh, by the way, I'd be careful—she has AIDS. I bet she's a drug user."

- How would you respond?

Disease and drug side effects. Teach patients to recognize symptoms that may indicate disease progression and drug side effects so that prompt medical care can be started. Table 15.26 gives an overview of symptoms that patients should report. Teach about hand hygiene and ways to avoid exposure to new infectious agents.

Promoting a healthy immune system may delay the progression of HIV disease. Nutrition support can help maintain lean body mass and ensure optimal nutrition. Encourage moderating or eliminating alcohol, tobacco, and drug use. Keep patients up to date with recommended vaccines. Adequate rest provides the body with the energy needed for optimal immune function. Taking part in safe exercise and activities helps maintain physical and pulmonary function.

Physical problems related to HIV or its treatment can interfere with patients' ability to maintain a desired lifestyle. Persons with HIV can suffer from anxiety, fear, depression, diarrhea, peripheral neuropathy, pain, nausea, vomiting, and fatigue. Implement nursing measures to manage symptoms. For example, management of diarrhea includes recommending diet changes, encouraging fluid and electrolyte replacement, teaching about skin care, and managing perianal skin breakdown. Approaches for fatigue include teaching patients to assess fatigue patterns; determine contributing factors; set activity priorities; conserve energy; schedule rest periods; and exercise regularly.

TABLE 15.26 PATIENT & CAREGIVER TEACHING

Signs and Symptoms Patients With HIV Need to Report

Teach the patient with HIV infection and the caregiver to report the following signs and symptoms:

Report Immediately

- Any change in level of consciousness: lethargic, hard to arouse, unable to arouse, unresponsive
- Headache with nausea and vomiting, changes in vision, changes in ability to perform coordinated activities, or after any head trauma
- Vision changes: blurry or black areas in vision field, new floaters, double vision
- Persistent dyspnea with activity not relieved by a short rest period
- Nausea and vomiting with abdominal pain
- Vomiting blood
- Dehydration: unable to eat or drink because of nausea or mouth lesions; severe diarrhea or vomiting; dizziness when standing
- Yellow skin discoloration
- Any rectal bleeding unrelated to hemorrhoids or trauma (e.g., from anal sexual intercourse)
- Pain in the flank with fever and inability to urinate for more than 6 h
- Blood in the urine, dysuria
- New onset of weakness, numbness, or difficulty speaking
- Chest pain not related to a cough
- Seizures
- New rash or oral lesions with a fever
- Severe depression, anxiety, hallucinations, delusions, or thoughts of causing danger to self or others

Report the Following Signs and Symptoms Within 24 Hours

- New or different headache; constant headache not relieved by pain medication
- Headache with fever, nasal congestion, or cough
- Burning, itching, or discharge from the eyes
- New or productive cough
- New, significant, or watery diarrhea (more than 6 times a day)
- Significant new rash (widespread; painful; or following a path down the leg or arm, around the chest, or on the face)
- Problems eating or drinking because of mouth lesions
- Vaginal discharge, pain, or itching

End-of-life care. Despite new HIV treatments, many patients eventually have disease progression, disability, and death. Sometimes these occur because treatments do not work for the patient. Sometimes the HIV becomes resistant to all available drug therapies. ART is now allowing people with HIV to live longer and to develop diseases of aging, such as cardiovascular and endocrine problems, that lead to death.

Nursing care during the terminal phase focuses on keeping the patient comfortable, facilitating emotional and spiritual acceptance, helping significant others deal with grief and loss, and maintaining a safe environment. End-of-life care is discussed in Chapter 10.

 Gerontologic Considerations: HIV Infection

The number of older adults who have HIV disease is increasing because (1) HIV treatment has been effective in reducing the number of deaths from HIV-related opportunistic infections and (2) people 60 and older are being infected at increasing rates. Older adults may be ashamed and hesitate to tell anyone that they have HIV infection. This may make it hard for them to get health care and support. As a nurse, you need to recognize that HIV will affect an increasing number of older adults and be prepared to help the older person with HIV.

Older adults with HIV are susceptible to the same diseases as older adults without HIV. These include heart disease, cancer, diabetes, bone disease, arthritis, hypertension, kidney disease, and cognitive problems. People with HIV infection may develop these diseases at an earlier age and be at higher risk for comorbidities related to ART.[27] We do not know why this happens. It is likely a combination of factors including genetic predisposition, chronic stress, long-term infection with HIV, and side effects of ART. Management of these other chronic conditions focuses on detecting problems early, managing risk factors, and helping patients cope with emerging problems and changes to treatment plans.

In general, older adults take multiple medications to manage various chronic diseases. Some agents may interact with or be potentiated by ART. Careful monitoring and assessment of possible drug interactions are important when providing care.

CASE STUDY

HIV Infection

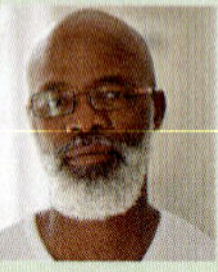

(© iStock.com/ Cecilie_Arcurs.)

Patient Profile

J.N. is a 66-year-old male with HIV, type 2 diabetes, chronic obstructive pulmonary disease (COPD), and hypertension. He was admitted 2 days ago with acute diverticulitis.

Subjective Data

- Diagnosed with HIV infection at age 47 after developing *Mycobacterium avium* complex infection.
- Has had issues taking ART consistently, "I have too many pills to keep track of."
- Has fatigue and frequent oral candidiasis outbreaks.
- Identifies as bisexual. Has a history of sex with both males and females; no partner currently.
- Reports 6 out of 10 left lower quadrant pain.
- Expresses concern about his future, "I don't know who will take care of me. I don't have any family around."

Objective Data

Physical Assessment

- 5 ft 10 in tall, 150 lb, temperature 100.4°F (38°C), O_2 saturation 98% on room air
- + Bowel sounds in all 4 quadrants, tenderness to palpation in left lower quadrant

Laboratory Studies

- CD4 cell count 210 cells/μL
- Viral load 4520 copies/μL
- Abdominal CT scan: Local bowel wall thickening without abscess, perforation, or obstruction
- White blood cell count 16.1 × 10^3/μL

Interprofessional Care

- Levofloxacin IV and metronidazole IV
- Morphine sulfate IV every 2 h as needed for pain
- Combination ART: tenofovir alafenamide, emtricitabine, bictegravir
- Complete bowel rest, NPO

Discussion Questions

1. ***Recognize:*** Why were levofloxacin and metronidazole ordered, and what are common side effects?
2. ***Analyze:*** What teaching needs should be covered before J.N. is discharged from the hospital to return home?
3. ***Plan:*** Older LGBT adults often lack familial social support as they age. What barriers could this cause for J.N.'s treatment? How could the interprofessional team assist in addressing these issues? What referrals may be made?
4. ***Prioritize:*** What are the priority nursing interventions? What nursing care will he need after discharge?
5. ***Act:*** How can we help J.N. adhere to his ART schedule?
6. ***Evaluate:*** What assessment data would you need to collect to decide if care was effective?
7. ***Safety:*** The nurse needs to start an IV to administer the antibiotic. What type of PPE is recommended in this situation?

Answers available at http://evolve.elsevier.com/Lewis/medsurg.

BRIDGE TO NCLEX EXAMINATION

The number of the question corresponds to the same-numbered outcome at the beginning of the chapter.

1. A surgical unit's quality improvement committee notes the incidence of surgical site infections (SSIs) decreased over the past 6 months. The nurse understands that this means:
   a. there is an epidemic of SSIs on the unit.
   b. the prevalence of vancomycin resistance is increasing.
   c. there has been improvement in infection control practices.
   d. there has been a decrease in adherence with aseptic technique.
2. Emerging infections have been associated with **(Select all that apply.)**
   a. bioterrorism.
   b. international travel.
   c. mutation of viruses or bacteria.
   d. completing full courses of antibiotics.
   e. transmission of disease from animal sources.

3. Interventions to prevent health care–associated infections include (**Select all that apply.**)
   a. always wearing a face mask.
   b. administering antibiotics as ordered.
   c. limiting visitors to persons over age 18.
   d. washing hands before and after patient contact.
   e. decontaminating equipment used for patient care.
4. When working with a patient who has bacterial meningitis, the nurse would
   a. use sterile gloves.
   b. wear face and eye protection.
   c. have the patient wear an N-95 mask.
   d. put the patient on airborne precautions.
5. Preferred treatment options for COVID-19 include the use of
   a. miconazoles
   b. cephalosporins
   c. fluoroquinolones
   d. immune modulators
6. Diagnosing HIV is best done using
   a. a CD4 cell count.
   b. an antigen/antibody test.
   c. a complete blood cell count.
   d. a culture and sensitivity test.
7. Goals of starting HIV antiretrovirals include (**Select all that apply.**)
   a. reducing the viral load.
   b. increasing life expectancy.
   c. decreasing the CD4 cell count.
   d. preventing transmission to others.
   e. eliminating the desire to use injection drugs.
8. A patient with HIV is being treated for *Pneumocystis jirovecii* pneumonia. The nurse recognizes that this
   a. is seen more in advanced disease.
   b. occurs in patients with high CD4 counts.
   c. should be treated with an immune modulator.
   d. requires stopping HIV ART until the condition is cured.
9. When teaching a patient about preexposure prophylaxis (PrEP), the nurse should inform the patient about
   a. taking PrEP for a total of 28 days.
   b. the importance of regular HIV testing.
   c. getting a CD4 cell count every 3 to 6 months.
   d. the need to take PrEP within 72 hours after an exposure.

1. c; 2. a, b, c, e; 3. b, d, e; 4. b; 5. d; 6. b; 7. a, b, d; 8. a; 9. b.

For rationales to these answers and even more NCLEX review questions, visit http://evolve.elsevier.com/Lewis/medsurg.

REFERENCES

To access the References for this chapter, please scan the QR code with a mobile device.

16

Cancer

Susan Doyle-Lindrud

http://evolve.elsevier.com/Lewis/medsurg/

CONCEPTUAL FOCUS

Cellular Regulation
Coping
Health Promotion

LEARNING OUTCOMES

1. Describe the epidemiology of cancer in the United States.
2. Discuss the pathophysiology of cancer.
3. Outline the stages of cancer development.
4. Discuss the role of the nurse in the prevention, detection, and diagnosis of cancer.
5. Explain the use of surgery, chemotherapy, radiation therapy, immunotherapy, targeted therapy, and hormone therapy in treating cancer.
6. Identify the classifications of chemotherapy drugs and methods of administration.
7. Distinguish between external beam radiation and brachytherapy.
8. Describe the effects of radiation therapy and chemotherapy on normal tissues.
9. Identify the types and effects of immunotherapy and targeted therapy.
10. Describe the nursing management of patients receiving chemotherapy, radiation therapy, immunotherapy, and targeted therapy.
11. Describe nutrition therapy for patients with cancer.
12. Identify complications associated with cancer.
13. Describe support interventions for cancer patients, survivors, and their caregivers.

KEY TERMS

angiogenesis
brachytherapy
cancer
carcinogens
carcinoma in situ (CIS)
chemotherapy
external beam radiation
hematopoietic stem cell transplantation (HSCT)
histologic grading
immunologic surveillance
immunotherapy
metastasis
oncogenes
peripheral stem cell transplantation (PSCT)
protooncogenes
staging
targeted therapy
vesicants

Cancer is a group of diseases characterized by uncontrolled and unregulated cell growth. The resulting problems may be directly related to the cancer, a consequence of cancer treatment, or a combination of both. The shared physiologic, psychologic, and social impact of cancer on patients and their caregivers is considerable. A lot of anxiety and fear are associated with a cancer diagnosis.

Educating HCPs and the public is essential to promote realistic attitudes about cancer and cancer treatment. You are in a key position to lead efforts to change attitudes about cancer. You can help people decrease their risk for cancer and take part in cancer screening. You need to know about types of cancer, treatments, managing side effects of therapy, and supportive therapies. By supporting patients and caregivers as they cope with the effects of cancer and treatment, you are helping them adhere to cancer management plans and improve quality of life.

EPIDEMIOLOGY

Around 1.9 million people in the United States are diagnosed each year with cancer. This number excludes basal and squamous cell skin cancers and carcinoma in situ of any site except the bladder.[1] The incidence of many cancers, such as colorectal, lung, and bladder cancers, has declined largely because of preventive efforts. The incidence of other cancers, such as kidney, pancreas, liver, endometrial, and oropharyngeal, is increasing.[2]

The incidence and death rates for specific cancers are shown in Tables 16.1 and 16.2. Although mortality rates from all cancers combined are on the decline, it is still the second most common cause of death in the United States. Cancer is the leading cause of death in people 40 to 79 years of age. Each year about 600,000 Americans die of cancer. This is more than 1600 deaths per day.[1,2] Overall cancer incidence and mortality rates are higher in males.

Cancer incidence is disproportionately higher in Black and other minority persons. Although overall racial disparities in cancer death rates have been declining, death rates continue to be higher among Black persons. Black persons are more likely to have later-stage disease at the time of diagnosis.[1]

We have made great progress in controlling cancer for long periods. More than 18 million Americans with a history of cancer are alive today. This includes those who have cancer and are undergoing treatment, are disease free, or are in remission.[2]

We attribute differences in survival rates to a combination of factors. These include poverty, difficult access to and poorer quality of health care, and more comorbid conditions. Disparities in cancer care exist throughout the continuum, from prevention and screening to end-of-life care and survivorship. The disparity in prevention and screening results in cancer being in advanced stages at the time of diagnosis.[1,2]

TABLE 16.1 Cancer Incidence by Site and Sex (Male/Female)[a]

MALE		FEMALE	
Type	**%**	**Type**	**%**
Prostate	9	Breast	31
Lung	12	Lung	13
Colon/rectum	8	Colon/rectum	8
Urinary bladder	6	Uterus	7
Melanoma	6	Melanoma	4
Kidney and renal pelvis	5	Non-Hodgkin lymphoma	4
Non-Hodgkin lymphoma	4	Thyroid	3
Oral cavity and pharynx	4	Kidney and renal pelvis	3
Leukemia	4	Pancreas	3
Pancreas	3	Leukemia	3

[a]Numbers are estimates and exclude basal and squamous cell skin cancers and carcinoma in situ.
From National Cancer Institute: Cancer stat facts. Retrieved from https://seer.cancer.gov/statfacts.

A concern is that cancer incidence and mortality will be affected by the impact of the COVID-19 pandemic on missed or postponed HCP appointments for cancer screening and delays in cancer treatment. This may result in an increase in advanced stage disease at the time of diagnosis and an increase in cancer mortality rates over the next few years.[2]

BIOLOGY OF CANCER

Defect in Cell Proliferation

Defective cell proliferation, or growth, is a key factor in cancer development. All cells are controlled by an intracellular mechanism that determines when cell proliferation is necessary. A state of equilibrium is present under normal conditions. This means cell proliferation equals cell degeneration or death. Normally, cell division and proliferation are activated only in the presence of cell degeneration or death *(apoptosis).* Cell proliferation also occurs if the body has a physiologic need for more cells. For example, a normal increase in white blood cell (WBC) count occurs with infection.

Another means of proliferation control in normal cells is *contact inhibition.* Normal cells respect the boundaries and territory of the cells around them. They will not invade an area that is not their own. We think the neighboring cells inhibit cell growth through the physical contact of their cell membranes. Cancer cells have a loss of contact inhibition. They have no regard for cell boundaries. They grow on top of one another and on top of or between normal cells.

The rate of cell proliferation from cell birth to cell death differs in each body tissue. In some tissues, such as bone marrow, hair follicles, and epithelial lining of the gastrointestinal (GI) tract, the rate of cell proliferation is rapid. In other tissues, such as myocardium and cartilage, cell proliferation does not occur or is slow.

Cancer cells proliferate at the same rate as the normal cells of the tissue from which they arise. However, cancer cells respond differently to the intracellular signals that regulate cell proliferation. The result is that cancer cell proliferation is

TABLE 16.2 Cancer Deaths by Site and Sex (Male/Female)

MALE		FEMALE	
Type	**%**	**Type**	**%**
Lung and bronchus	21	Lung and bronchus	21
Prostate	11	Breast	15
Colon/rectum	9	Colon/rectum	8
Pancreas	8	Pancreas	8
Liver and bile ducts	6	Ovary	5
Leukemia	4	Uterus	5
Esophagus	4	Liver and bile ducts	4
Urinary bladder	4	Leukemia	3
Non-Hodgkin lymphoma	4	Non-Hodgkin lymphoma	3
Brain and other nervous system	3	Brain and other nervous system	3

From National Cancer Institute: Cancer stat facts. Retrieved from https://seer.cancer.gov/statfacts.

indiscriminate and continuous. Sometimes they produce more than 2 cells at the time of mitosis. In this way, there is continuous growth of a tumor mass: 1 × 2 × 4 × 8 × 16 and so on. We call this the *pyramid effect.* The time needed for a tumor mass to double in size is known as its *doubling time.*

Defect in Cell Differentiation

Cell differentiation describes the processes by which immature cells with less specificity become mature cells with a specific function. Most tissues have a population of undifferentiated cells known as stem cells. These stem cells ultimately differentiate and become mature, functioning cells of a specific tissue. This is normally an orderly process. Since all body cells are derived from the fertilized ova, all cells initially have the potential to perform all body functions. As cells differentiate, this potential is repressed. The mature cell can perform only specific functions. Normally, this differentiated cell is stable and will not *dedifferentiate* or return to its previous undifferentiated state. Cancer cells can lose the special properties of the mature cell and dedifferentiate.

Cancer Genomics

Cancer involves the malfunction of genes that control differentiation and proliferation. Two types of normal genes that can be affected by mutation are *protooncogenes* and *tumor suppressor genes.* **Protooncogenes** are normal cell genes that are important regulators of normal cell processes. Protooncogenes promote growth. Mutations that change the expression of protooncogenes can cause them to function as **oncogenes** (tumor-inducing genes).

Think of the protooncogene as the genetic lock that keeps the cell in its mature functioning state. When this lock is "unlocked," which can occur through exposure to carcinogens or oncogenic viruses, genetic alterations and mutations occur. Thus oncogenes can change a normal cell to a cancer cell. The cancer cell regains a fetal appearance and function. For example, some cancer cells make new proteins characteristic of the embryonic and fetal periods of life. These proteins, found on the cell membrane, include carcinoembryonic antigen (CEA) and α-fetoprotein (AFP). They can be found in the blood by laboratory studies. Other cancer cells, such as small cell lung cancer, make hormones that are usually made by cells arising from the same embryonic cells as the tumor cells.

Tumor suppressor genes suppress growth. They prevent cells from going through the cell cycle. Mutations can change tumor suppressor genes and make them inactive. This results in a loss of their tumor-suppressing action. Examples of tumor suppressor genes are *BRCA1* and *BRCA2.* Changes in these genes increase the risk for breast and ovarian cancer. Another tumor suppressor gene is the *APC* gene. *APC* mutations increase the risk for familial adenomatous polyposis, a precursor for colorectal cancer (see Chapter 47). Mutations in the *p53* tumor suppressor gene have been found in many cancers. These include bladder, breast, colorectal, esophageal, liver, lung, and ovarian cancers.

Immune Surveillance

The immune system has the potential to tell normal (self) cells from abnormal (nonself) cells. Cancer cells can be perceived as nonself. This can elicit an immune response, resulting in their rejection and destruction. However, cancer cells arise from normal human cells and, although they are mutated and thus different, the immune response that is mounted against cancer cells may be inadequate to effectively kill them.

Cancer cells may have altered cell-surface antigens. These antigens are termed *tumor-associated antigens (TAAs)* (Fig. 16.1). We think that the immune system responds to TAAs through a process called **immunologic surveillance.** In this process, lymphocytes continuously check cell-surface antigens. They detect and destroy cells with abnormal or altered cell-surface antigens. Under most circumstances, immune surveillance prevents transformed cells from developing into detectable tumors.

Immune response to cancer cells involves B cells, cytotoxic T cells, natural killer (NK) cells, and macrophages. B cells can make specific antibodies that bind to tumor cells. These antibodies are often detectable in serum and saliva.

Cytotoxic T cells play a key role in resisting tumor growth. These cells can kill tumor cells. T cells are important in cytokine production (e.g., interleukin-2 [IL-2], γ-interferon), which stimulate T cells, NK cells, B cells, and macrophages. NK cells can directly kill tumor cells without any prior sensitization. γ-Interferon (made by T cells) and IL-2 (released from T cells) stimulate NK cells, resulting in increased cytotoxic activity.

Monocytes and macrophages have several important roles in tumor immunity. γ-Interferon can activate macrophages to become nonspecifically lytic for tumor cells. Macrophages secrete cytokines, including IL-1, tumor necrosis factor (TNF), and colony-stimulating factors (CSFs). The release of IL-1, coupled with the presentation of the processed antigen, stimulates T-cell activation and production. α-Interferon augments the killing ability of NK cells. TNF causes hemorrhagic necrosis of tumors and exerts cytocidal or cytostatic actions against tumor cells. CSFs regulate the production of various blood cells in the bone marrow and stimulate the function of various WBCs.

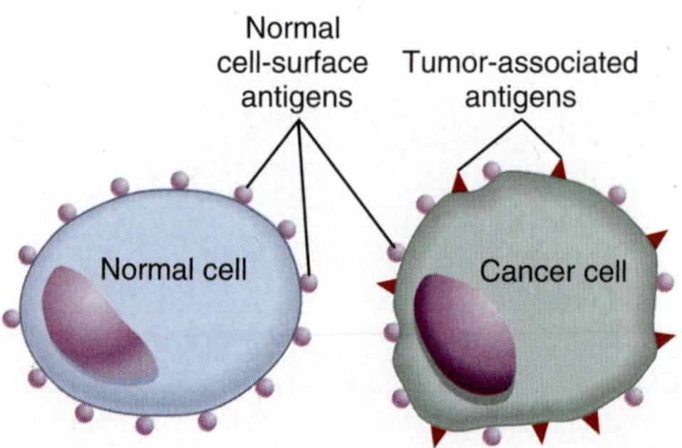

Fig. 16.1 Tumor-associated antigens appear on the cell surface of cancer cells.

Immunologic escape is the process by which cancer cells evade the immune system. Possible mechanisms for immunologic escape include (1) suppression of factors that stimulate T cells to react to cancer cells; (2) weak surface antigens allowing cancer cells to "sneak through" immunologic surveillance; (3) development of tolerance of the immune system to some tumor antigens; (4) suppression of the immune response by products secreted by cancer cells; (5) induction of suppressor T cells by the tumor; and (6) blocking antibodies that bind TAAs, thus preventing their recognition by T cells (Fig. 16.2).

Oncofetal Antigens and Tumor Markers

Oncofetal antigens are a type of tumor antigen. They are on the surfaces and the inside of cancer cells and fetal cells. These antigens are an expression of the shift of cancerous cells to a more immature metabolic pathway. This expression is usually associated with embryonic or fetal periods of life. We think the reappearance of fetal antigens is the result of the cell regaining its embryonic capability to differentiate into many different cell types.

Examples of oncofetal antigens are CEA and AFP. CEA is found on the surfaces of cancer cells from the GI tract and normal cells from the fetal gut, liver, and pancreas. Normally, CEA disappears during the last 3 months of fetal life. High CEA levels often occur with colorectal cancer. However, high CEA levels can occur in nonmalignant conditions (e.g., cirrhosis, ulcerative colitis, heavy smoking).

Oncofetal antigens can be used as *tumor markers* that may be useful to monitor the effect of therapy and indicate tumor recurrence. However, they are not 100% specific for tumor recurrence. Various factors affect tumor markers. We must consider these factors when reviewing results. For example, high CEA titers that persist after surgery means that some cancer is still present. A rise in CEA levels after chemotherapy may mean recurrence or spread of the cancer, or it may be due to chronic lung disease and smoking.

AFP is made by liver cancer cells, metastatic liver growth, and fetal liver cells. AFP has diagnostic value in primary liver cancer. This makes AFP valuable in tumor detection and evaluating tumor progression. AFP levels are also high in some cases of testicular cancer and viral hepatitis.

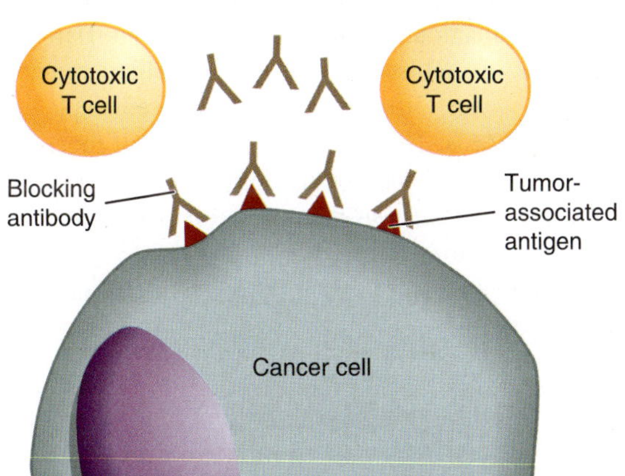

Fig. 16.2 Blocking antibodies prevent T cells from interacting with tumor-associated antigens and from destroying the cancer cell.

Other examples of oncofetal antigens are CA-125 (ovarian cancer), CA-19-9 (pancreatic and gallbladder cancer), prostate-specific antigen (PSA) (prostate cancer), and CA-15.3 and CA-27-29 (breast cancer). Molecular markers for specific tumors include KRAS (an oncogene in colon cancer), epidermal growth factor receptor (EGFR) in lung cancer, and human epidermal growth factor receptor-2 (HER-2) expression in breast cancer.

Cancer Development

The following is a theoretical model of cancer development. The cause and development of each type of cancer are likely to be multifactorial. A common misbelief is that cancer development is a rapid, haphazard event. However, cancer is usually an orderly process that occurs over time. The 3-stage theory of cancer development is initiation, promotion, and progression (Fig. 16.3).

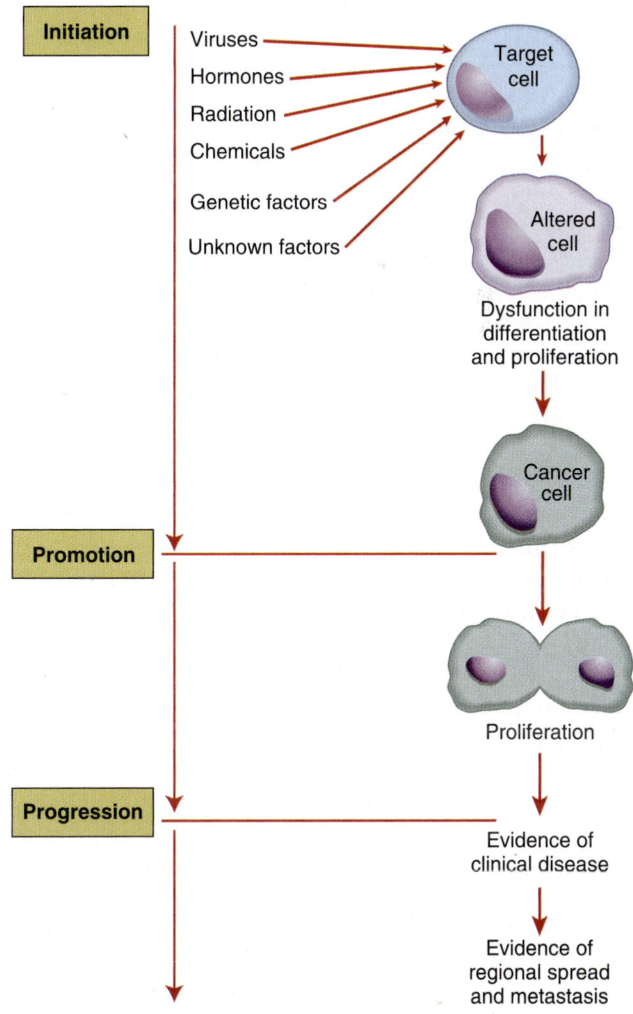

Fig. 16.3 Process of cancer development.

Initiation

Cancer cells arise from normal cells because of changes in genes. The first stage, *initiation,* involves a mutation in the cell's genetic structure.[3] A *mutation* is any change in the usual DNA sequence. Gene mutations can occur in 2 ways: *inherited* from a parent (passed from one generation to the next) or *acquired* during a person's lifetime.

We think that 5% to 10% of all cancers are due to an inherited gene mutation. These genetic changes can lead to a high risk for developing a specific type of cancer. However, most cancers do not result from inherited genes. They are acquired from damage to your genes. The damaged cell may die or repair itself. However, if cell death or repair does not occur before cell division, the cell will replicate into daughter cells, each with the same genetic alteration. Thus an acquired mutation is passed on to all cells that develop from that single cell.

Carcinogens. **Carcinogens** are cancer-causing agents capable of producing cell alterations. Many are detoxified by protective enzymes and harmlessly excreted. If this protective mechanism fails, carcinogens can enter the cell's nucleus and change deoxyribonucleic acid (DNA). Carcinogens may be chemical, radiation, or viral.

Chemical. Many chemicals are carcinogens (e.g., benzene, arsenic, formaldehyde). People exposed to these chemicals over time have a greater incidence of certain cancers. The long latency period from the time of exposure to cancer development makes it hard to identify cancer-causing chemicals.

Radiation. Radiation can cause cancer in almost any body tissue. When cells are exposed to a source of radiation, damage occurs to DNA. A higher incidence of cancer occurs in people exposed to radiation in certain occupations, such as radiologists, radiation chemists, aircrews, and uranium miners.

Ultraviolet (UV) radiation is associated with melanoma and squamous and basal cell skin cancers. Skin cancer is the most common type of cancer in the United States. Sunlight exposure is the main source of UV exposure. UV radiation from tanning beds causes skin cancer.[4]

Viral. Certain DNA and ribonucleic acid (RNA) viruses, termed *oncogenic,* can alter the cells they infect and induce malignant transformation. Burkitt lymphoma is associated with Epstein-Barr virus (EBV).[5] People with AIDS, caused by HIV, have a high incidence of Kaposi sarcoma (see Chapter 15). Other viruses linked to cancer include hepatitis B and C virus, which is associated with primary liver cancer. Human papillomavirus (HPV) can cause lesions that progress to squamous cell cancers, such as cervical, anal, and head and neck cancers.[5]

Promotion

A single change in a cell's genetic structure is not enough to cause cancer. The odds of cancer development increase with the presence of promoting agents. *Promotion* is characterized by the reversible proliferation of the altered cells. An increase in the altered cell population increases the likelihood of more mutations.

An important distinction between initiation and promotion is that the activity of promoters is reversible. This is a key concept in cancer prevention. Promoting factors include obesity, tobacco use, and alcohol use. Changing a person's lifestyle to modify these risk factors can reduce the chance of developing cancer. Around 40% of newly diagnosed cancers in the United States are potentially avoidable. These include cancers caused by obesity, alcohol use, unhealthy diet, smoking, and physical inactivity.[1]

Several promoting agents have activity against specific body tissues. These agents tend to promote specific kinds of cancer. For example, cigarette smoke is a promoting agent in lung cancer. Alcohol use is a promoter of esophageal and bladder cancers.

Some carcinogens, termed *complete carcinogens,* are capable of both initiating and promoting cancer development. Cigarette smoke is an example of a complete carcinogen.

The time between the first genetic alteration and clinical evidence of cancer is the *latent* period. It includes the initiation and promotion stages. The variation in the length of time that elapses before the cancer becomes clinically evident is related to the mitotic rate of the tissue of origin and environment factors. In most cancers, this process is years or even decades long. For cancer to be clinically evident, the cells must reach a critical mass. A tumor that is 1.0 cm (0.4 inch), the size usually detectable by palpation, has 1 billion cancer cells.

Progression

Progression is the last stage. Here, we see increased growth rate of the tumor, increased invasiveness, and **metastasis** (spread of the cancer to a distant site). As the tumor increases in size, developing its own blood supply is critical to its survival and growth. The process of forming blood vessels within the tumor itself is termed tumor **angiogenesis**. It is facilitated by tumor angiogenesis factors made by the cancer cells.

Metastasis is a multistep process. It begins with the rapid growth of the primary tumor (Fig. 16.4). Tumor cells can detach from the primary tumor, invade the tissue surrounding the tumor, and penetrate the walls of lymph or vascular vessels for metastasis to a distant site. Once free, metastatic tumor cells often travel to distant sites by hematogenous or lymphatic routes. Some cancers have an affinity for a particular tissue or organ as a site of metastasis. For example, colon cancer often spreads to the liver. Other cancers are unpredictable in their pattern of metastasis. The most common sites of metastasis are lungs, liver, bone, and brain (Fig. 16.5).

Hematogenous metastasis involves several steps. It begins with primary tumor cells penetrating blood vessels. These tumor cells then enter the circulation, travel through the body, and adhere to and penetrate small blood vessels of distant organs. Most tumor cells do not survive this process. They are destroyed by mechanical mechanisms (e.g., turbulence of blood flow) and cells of the immune system. The formation of a combination of tumor cells, platelets, and fibrin deposits may protect some tumor cells from destruction in blood vessels.

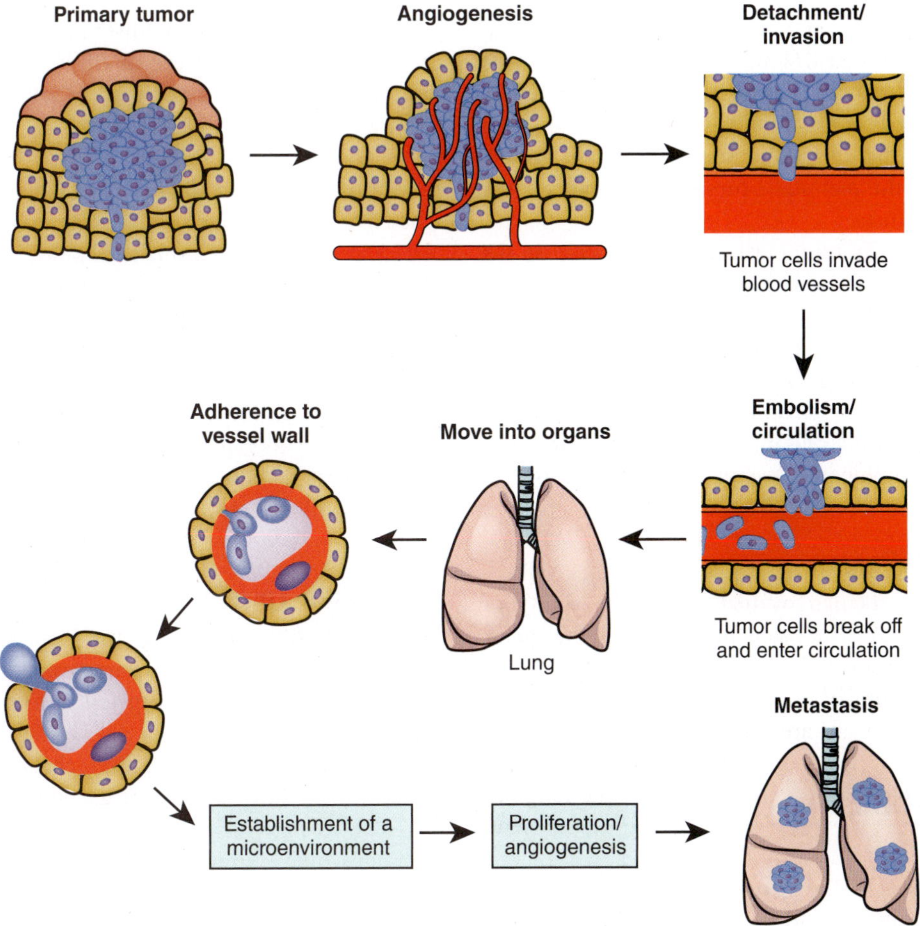

Fig. 16.4 The pathogenesis of cancer metastasis. To produce metastases, tumor cells must detach from the primary tumor and enter the circulation, survive in the circulation to rest in the capillary bed, adhere to capillary basement membrane, gain entrance into the organ parenchyma, respond to growth factors, proliferate, induce angiogenesis, and evade host defenses.

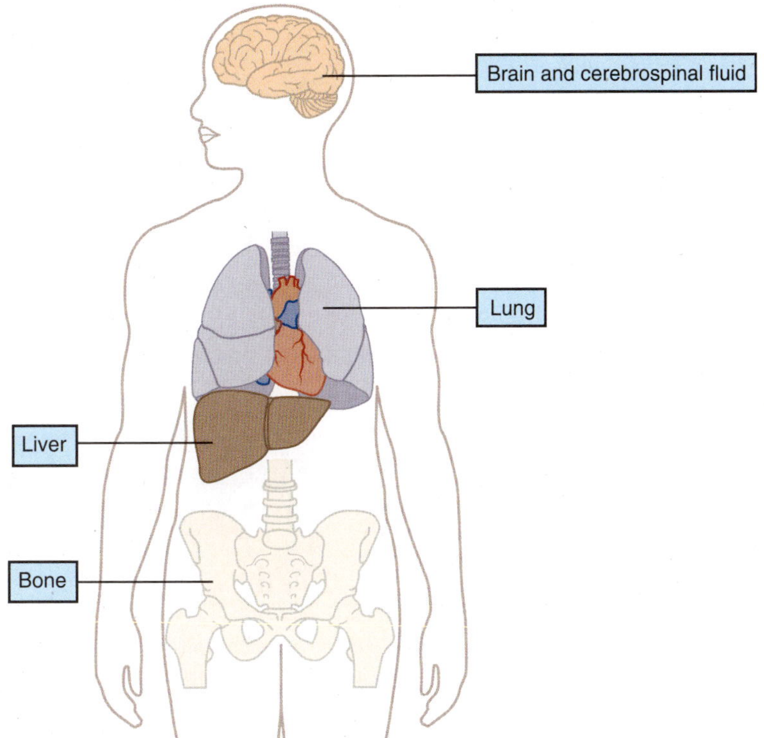

Fig. 16.5 Main sites of metastasis.

Tumor cells that survive the process of metastasis must create an environment in the distant organ site that promotes their growth and development. This is facilitated by the tumor cells' ability to evade cells of the immune system and produce a blood supply within the metastatic site. This blood supply provides nutrients to the metastatic tumor and allows for the removal of waste products.

In the lymphatic system, tumor cells can be "trapped" in the first lymph node to which cancer cells are most likely to spread from a tumor. This lymph node is the *sentinel lymph node.* A sentinel lymph node biopsy (SLNB) can help determine the extent of the cancer. A positive SLNB means cancer is present in the sentinel node and may have spread to other lymph nodes and organs. Sometimes, the tumor cells may bypass local lymph nodes and travel to distant lymph nodes. We call this *skip metastasis.*

Benign Versus Malignant

We classify tumors as benign or malignant. The ability of malignant tumor cells to invade and metastasize is the major difference between benign and malignant neoplasms. Other differences are outlined in Table 16.3.

DIAGNOSTIC STUDIES

Biopsy

A *biopsy* is the removal of a tissue sample for pathologic analysis. This pathologic evaluation is the only definitive way to diagnose cancer. The pathologist examines the tissue to determine (1) whether it is benign or malignant, (2) the anatomic tissue from which the tumor arises *(histology),* and (3) the degree of cell differentiation *(histologic grade).* Other information that we can obtain includes the size of tumor and depth, evidence of invasiveness, adequacy of surgical excision (positive or negative surgical margins), and mitotic rate. Special staining techniques may give insight into responsiveness of the tumor to treatment or disease behavior (receptor status, tumor markers).

The method used to obtain a biopsy depends on the location and size of the suspected tumor. *Percutaneous biopsy* is often done for tissue that can be safely reached through the skin. *Endoscopic biopsy* may be used for lung or other intraluminal lesions (esophageal, colon, bladder). When a tumor is not easily accessible, surgery (laparotomy, thoracotomy, craniotomy) may be done to obtain a piece of the tumor tissue. Many radiographic techniques may be used to improve tissue localization with a biopsy. These include CT, MRI, ultrasound-guided biopsy, and stereotactic biopsy.

Various types and sizes of biopsy needles are available. The choice depends on the type of tissue to be sampled. *Fine-needle aspiration* (FNA) uses a small-gauge aspiration needle to obtain some cells from the mass for cytologic examination. *Large-core biopsy* cutting needles deliver an actual piece of tissue (core) for analysis. An advantage is that it preserves the histologic architecture of the tissue specimen. *Excisional biopsy* involves the surgical removal of the entire lesion, lymph node, nodule, or mass. So, it is therapeutic as well as diagnostic. If an excisional biopsy is not feasible, an *incisional biopsy* (partial excision) may be done with a scalpel or dermal punch.

TABLE 16.3 Comparison of Benign and Malignant Neoplasms

Characteristic	Benign	Malignant
Encapsulated	Usually	Rarely
Differentiated	Normally	Poorly
Metastasis	Absent	Capable
Recurrence	Rare	Possible
Vascularity	Slight	Moderate to marked
Mode of growth	Expansive	Infiltrative and expansive
Cell characteristics	Fairly normal, like parent cells	Cells abnormal, become more unlike parent cells

Diagnostic Tests

Other tests done depend on the suspected primary or metastatic site(s) of the cancer. Examples include:

- Cytology studies (e.g., Pap test, bronchial washings)
- Chest x-ray
- Complete blood count (CBC), chemistry profile
- Liver function studies (e.g., aspartate aminotransferase [AST])
- Endoscopic examination: upper GI, sigmoidoscopy, or colonoscopy (including guaiac test for occult blood)
- Radiographic studies (e.g., mammography, ultrasound)
- Radioisotope scans (e.g., bone, lung, liver, brain)
- Positron emission tomography (PET) scan (Fig. 16.6)

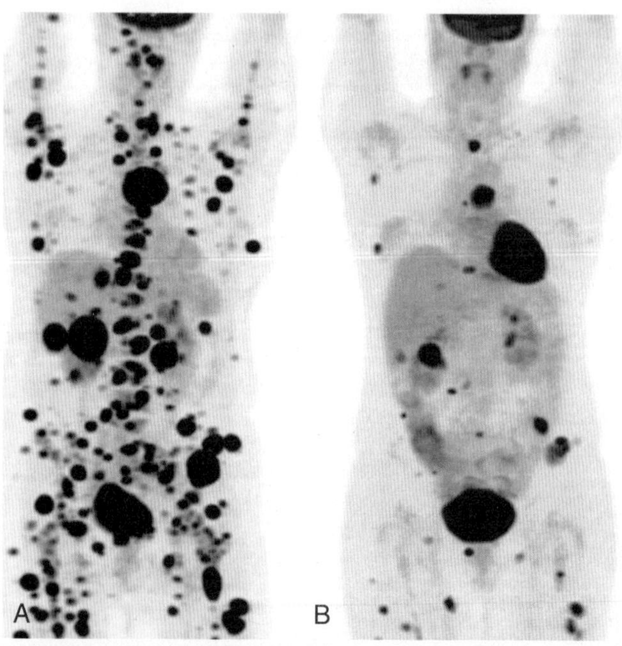

Fig. 16.6 PET scan before treatment (A) showing multiples metastases in the skeleton, soft tissues, muscles, mediastinum, lymph nodes, liver, kidneys, and thyroid gland. PET scan after treatment (B) shows the effects of therapy. (From Faria S, Devine C, Viswanathan C, et al: FDG-PET assessment of other gynecologic cancers, *PET Clinics* 13:203, 2017.)

- Tumor markers (e.g., CEA, AFP, PSA, CA-125)
- Genetic markers (e.g., *BRCA1, BRCA2*)
- Molecular receptor status (e.g., estrogen, progesterone, HER-2)
- Bone marrow examination

We use other rating scales to describe the patient's health status at the time of diagnosis, treatment, retreatment, and at each follow-up appointment. For example, the Karnofsky Performance Scale and Katz Index of Independence in Activities of Daily Living describe functional performance.

CANCER CLASSIFICATION

Tumors can be classified by anatomic site, histology (grading), and extent of disease (staging). Tumor classification systems provide a standard way to (1) communicate the status of the cancer to all members of the health care team, (2) assist in determining the most effective treatment plan, (3) evaluate the treatment plan, (4) predict prognosis, and (5) compare groups for statistical purposes.

Anatomic

In the *anatomic classification,* the tumor is identified by the tissue of origin, anatomic site, and behavior of the tumor (benign or malignant) (Table 16.4). *Carcinomas* originate from embryonal *ectoderm* (skin and glands) and *endoderm* (mucous membrane linings of the respiratory tract, GI tract, and genitourinary [GU] tract). *Sarcomas* originate from embryonal *mesoderm* (connective tissue, muscle, bone, fat). Lymphomas and leukemias originate from the hematopoietic system.

TABLE 16.4 Anatomic Classification of Tumors

Site	Benign	Malignant
Epithelial Tissue Tumors	**-oma**	**-carcinoma**
Surface epithelium	Papilloma	Carcinoma
Glandular epithelium	Adenoma	Adenocarcinoma
Connective Tissue Tumors	**-oma**	**-sarcoma**
Fibrous tissue	Fibroma	Fibrosarcoma
Cartilage	Chondroma	Chondrosarcoma
Striated muscle	Rhabdomyoma	Rhabdomyosarcoma
Bone	Osteoma	Osteosarcoma
Nervous Tissue Tumors	**-oma**	**-oma**
Meninges	Meningioma	Meningeal sarcoma
Nerve cells	Ganglioneuroma	Neuroblastoma
Hematopoietic Tissue Tumors		
Lymphoid tissue	—	Hodgkin lymphoma, non-Hodgkin lymphoma
Plasma cells	—	Multiple myeloma
Bone marrow	—	Lymphocytic and myelogenous leukemia

Histologic

In **histologic grading**, the appearance of cells and degree of differentiation are evaluated pathologically. Grading is based on the degree to which the cells resemble the tissue of origin. Poorly differentiated (undifferentiated) tumors have a poorer prognosis than those that are closer in appearance to the normal tissue of origin (well-differentiated). We use 4 grades for many tumor types:

Grade I: Cells differ slightly from normal cells (mild dysplasia) and are well-differentiated (low grade).

Grade II: Cells are more abnormal (moderate dysplasia) and moderately differentiated (intermediate grade).

Grade III: Cells are very abnormal (severe dysplasia) and poorly differentiated (high grade).

Grade IV: Cells are immature, primitive *(anaplasia),* and undifferentiated. Cell origin is hard to determine (high grade).

Grade X: Grade cannot be assessed.

Staging

Classifying the extent and spread of disease is termed **staging**. Staging is based on the anatomic extent of disease. Although there are similarities in the staging of various cancers, there are many differences for specific types of cancer. Staging can be done initially and at several points. Clinical staging is done at the completion of the diagnostic workup to guide treatment selection.

Clinical

The clinical staging classification system determines the anatomic extent of the cancer by stages:

Stage 0: Cancer in situ

Stage I: Tumor limited to the tissue of origin; local tumor growth

Stage II: Limited local spread

Stage III: Extensive local and regional spread

Stage IV: Metastasis

Clinical staging is used as a basis for staging a variety of tumor types. Look at the examples for colorectal cancer (see Table 47.33) and Hodgkin lymphoma (see Fig. 34.15). Other cancers (e.g., leukemia) do not use this staging approach. **Carcinoma in situ (CIS)** refers to a cancer whose cells are local and show no tendency to invade or metastasize to other tissues.

TNM Classification

For many types of cancer, we use the *TNM classification system* (Table 16.5) to determine the anatomic extent of cancer involvement. There are 3 parameters: tumor size and invasiveness (T), presence or absence of regional spread to the lymph nodes (N), and metastasis to distant organ sites (M). An example of the TNM classification system is shown in Table 47.22. We do not use TNM staging with all cancers. For example, we do not stage leukemia with TNM because they are not solid tumors. CIS has its own designation in the system

TABLE 16.5 TNM Classification System

Primary Tumor (T)	
T_0	No evidence of primary tumor
T_{is}	Carcinoma in situ
T_{1-4}	Ascending degrees of increase in tumor size and involvement
T_x	Tumor cannot be measured or found
Regional Lymph Nodes (N)	
N_0	No evidence of disease in lymph nodes
N_{1-4}	Ascending degrees of nodal involvement
N_x	Regional lymph nodes unable to be assessed clinically
Distant Metastases (M)	
M_0	No metastases
M_{1-4}	Metastases present
M_x	Cannot be determined

(T_{is}). CIS has all the histologic characteristics of cancer except invasion, a key feature of the TNM staging.

Cancer staging guidelines for some cancers add nonanatomic factors when making the final determination of stage. Staging is still based on the TNM classification, but it adds grade and hormone receptor expression. When appropriate, it includes genomic profile results (e.g., Oncotype DX, Mammaprint). This information allows for a more accurate determination of prognosis and can better guide therapy.

Surgical staging (pathologic stage) refers to the extent of disease as determined by surgical excision, exploration, and/or lymph node sampling. Surgical staging results may differ from clinical staging results because of what is found on the pathology sample. For example, surgery may find more spread of tumor than had been seen by imaging. Exploratory surgical staging is used less often as noninvasive diagnostic technology becomes more advanced.

After the extent of the disease is determined, the stage classification is set. If the patient needs more treatment, or if treatment fails, retreatment staging is done to determine the extent of the disease before retreatment. "Restaging" classification (rTNM) is distinguished from the stage at diagnosis because the clinical significance may be different. Staging cannot decrease, but the stage can increase. For example, a patient may initially be a stage 3. After treatment failure, the tumor metastasizes, and now the patient is a stage 4.

NURSING MANAGEMENT: CANCER PREVENTION AND DETECTION

We can reduce the incidence of cancer through a stronger emphasis on prevention by promoting healthy lifestyles (Box 16.1). As a nurse, you have an essential role in the prevention and early detection of cancer. Reducing risk factors reduces the incidence of cancer. For example, smoking-related cancers (e.g., lung and bladder cancer) have declined with a reduction in smoking rates.[1]

BOX 16.1 PROMOTING POPULATION HEALTH

Prevention and Early Detection of Cancer

Teach patients and the public about cancer prevention and early detection. Points include:

- Limit alcohol use.
- Get regular physical activity (e.g., 30 min or more of moderate physical activity 5 times weekly).
- Maintain a normal weight.
- Have regular physical examinations.
- Obtain regular colorectal screenings.
- Avoid cigarette smoking and other tobacco use.
- Get regular mammography screening and Pap tests.
- Be familiar with your own family history and risk factors for cancer.
- Obtain adequate rest of at least 6–8 hours per night.
- Use sunscreen with a sun protection factor of 15 or higher. Avoid tanning beds.
- Eliminate, reduce, or change the perception of stressors and enhance the ability to effectively cope with stress (see Chapter 7).
- Eat a balanced diet that includes vegetables and fresh fruits, whole grains, and fiber. Reduce dietary fat and preservatives. Limit smoked and salt-cured meats with high nitrite concentrations.

TABLE 16.6 Warning Signs of Cancer

Change in bowel or bladder habits
A sore that does not heal
Unusual bleeding or discharge from any orifice
Thickening or a lump in the breast or elsewhere
Indigestion or difficulty in swallowing
Obvious change in a wart or mole
Nagging cough or hoarseness

Early detection and prompt treatment are responsible for increased survival rates. Colonoscopy is important in reducing colon cancer mortality both by early detection of colon cancer and prevention (e.g., excision of adenomatous polyps).

The goals of public education are to (1) motivate people to recognize behaviors that may negatively affect health and (2) encourage awareness of and participation in health-promoting behaviors. When you teach about cancer, try to lessen the fear that surrounds the diagnosis.

Teach people to be familiar with their bodies and how to perform self-examinations. Review the 7 warning signs of cancer (Table 16.6). Encourage them to seek immediate medical care if they notice a change in what is normal for them or if cancer is suspected. Following recommended cancer screening guidelines for breast, colorectal, cervical, and prostate cancer from the American Cancer Society (ACS) is important.[6]

Diagnosis of Cancer

Facing a possible diagnosis of cancer is a stressful time for patients and caregivers. Patients may undergo several days to weeks of diagnostic studies. During this time, fear of the unknown may be more stressful than the actual diagnosis of cancer. Patients may feel overwhelmed or confused by the need for multiple diagnostic studies and consultations. Help coordinate care among specialists and explain the purpose of required tests and any special preparation needed.

Some agencies have oncology teams and services housed in the same building. This helps to coordinate care among cancer specialists. These centers combine appointments to make the experience convenient and comfortable for patients and caregivers.

While patients are waiting for the results of diagnostic studies, actively listen to their concerns. Anxiety may arise from myths and misconceptions about cancer (e.g., cancer is a "death sentence," cancer treatment is "horrible"). Correcting misconceptions can help lessen their anxiety.

Learn to have difficult conversations. Avoid communication that hinders exploration of feelings and meaning. These include providing false reassurances (e.g., "It's probably nothing"), redirecting the discussion (e.g., "Let's discuss that later"), and generalizing (e.g., "Everyone feels this way"). These strategies deny patients the opportunity to share the meaning of their experience. They can jeopardize your ability to build a trusting relationship with your patients.

During this time of high anxiety, patients may need repeated explanations of the diagnostic plan. Include as much information as needed for patients and caregivers. Give clear, understandable explanations. Avoid overly technical language. Reinforce teaching as needed. Written information is helpful to reinforce verbal information.

A diagnostic plan for the person suspected of having cancer includes the health history, identifying risk factors, the physical assessment, and specific diagnostic studies. Many people receive a cancer diagnosis after an abnormal screening test (e.g., mass on mammogram). Others are alerted to the presence of cancer by a presenting symptom or cluster of symptoms (e.g., cough and hemoptysis, anorexia with weight loss).

Review their risk factors for cancer. Obtain information about a family and personal history of cancer. Is there any exposure to or use of known carcinogens (e.g., cigarette smoking, occupational pollutants or chemicals, radiation exposure)? Do they have a history of diseases characterized by chronic inflammation or immunosuppression (e.g., ulcerative colitis) and treatments (e.g., hormone therapy, previous anticancer therapies)? Assess factors that may call for additional supportive care during therapy, including alcohol or drug use, living situation, social support, and coping strategies for perceived stressors.

INTERPROFESSIONAL CARE

TREATMENT GOALS

The goals of cancer treatment are cure, control, and palliation (Fig. 16.7). Knowing the treatment goals will help you communicate with, teach, and support patients. The main factors that determine the therapy plan are tumor histology and staging outcomes. Other crucial factors are patients' physiologic

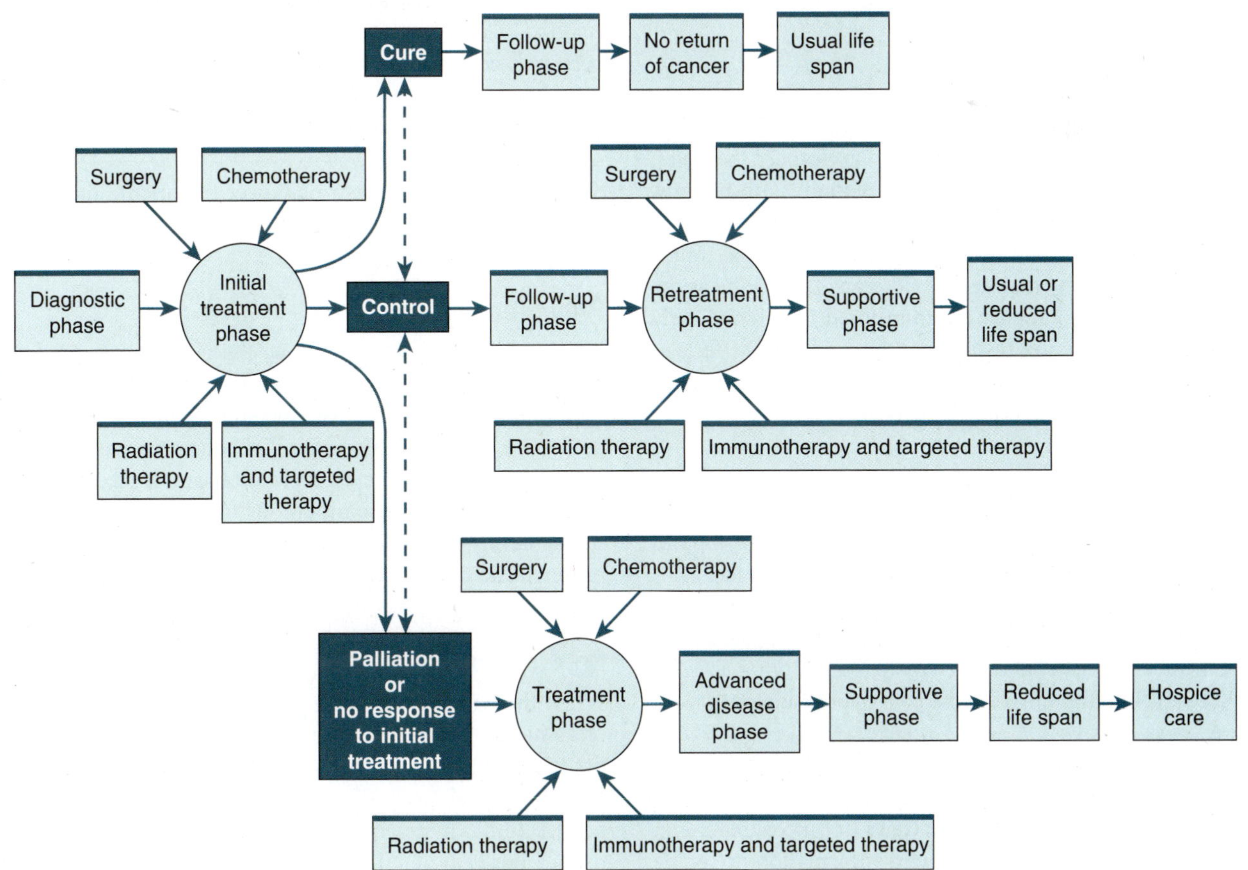

Fig. 16.7 Goals of cancer treatment.

status (e.g., presence of comorbid illnesses), psychologic status, and personal desires (e.g., active treatment versus palliation).

These factors influence (1) the treatment modalities (e.g., surgery, radiation therapy, chemotherapy), (2) how therapies are sequenced, and (3) the length of time of treatment. A therapy can be used alone or in any combination during initial treatment, as maintenance therapy, and in retreatment if the disease does not respond or recurs after remission.

Many patients receive 2 or more treatment modalities (known as *multimodality therapy* or *combined modality therapy*) to achieve the goal of cure or long-term control. Multimodality therapy is more effective because it takes advantage of more than one mechanism of action, although it does come with a risk of greater toxicity.

Cure

When *cure* is the goal, we expect treatment to have the greatest chance of eradicating the cancer. Curative cancer therapy differs by the type of cancer. It may involve local therapies (e.g., surgery or radiation) alone or in combination, with or without adjunctive systemic therapy (e.g., chemotherapy, immunotherapy, targeted therapy).

The time frame to consider a person "cured" differs depending on the tumor and its characteristics. In general, the risk for recurrent disease gradually decreases the longer the patient is cancer free after treatment. Cancers with a higher mitotic rate, a measure of how fast cancer cells are dividing, are more likely to recur than cancers with slower mitotic rates.

Control

Control is the goal of treatment for cancers that we cannot completely eradicate but are responsive to anticancer therapies. Some cancers can be controlled for long periods with therapy. Examples include multiple myeloma and chronic lymphocytic leukemia (see Chapter 34). Patients may receive an initial course of treatment followed by maintenance therapy for as long as the disease is responding. Patients are monitored closely for early signs and symptoms of progression and the cumulative effects of therapy. Evidence of tumor resistance (e.g., disease progression) may call for changing to a different therapy.

Palliation

Palliation is the goal of treatment when the goals are symptom control or relief and maintaining a satisfactory quality of life. Palliative care and treatment are not mutually exclusive and can take place concurrently. An example of treatment in which palliation is the goal includes using radiation therapy to reduce tumor size and relieve subsequent symptoms, like the pain of bone metastasis.

PERSONALIZED MEDICINE

Personalized medicine is an emerging trend in cancer treatment. It involves using the patient's genetic information to guide decisions about cancer prevention, diagnosis, and treatment. Many studies (tumor markers, genetic markers) are useful in determining treatment.

Before personalized medicine, most patients with a specific type and stage of cancer received the same treatment. However, some treatments worked well for some patients and not as well for others. Research has found that genetic differences in people and their tumors explain some of the different treatment responses. By performing genetic tests and analysis, we can personalize some treatments.[7]

Next-generation sequencing, or massive parallel sequencing, can sequence millions of DNA fragments. This technology can determine whether a patient's cancer is caused by a hereditary cancer syndrome or whether it is sporadic. Results guide which specific drugs target a patient's mutation and help identify clinical trials specific to the genetic mutation.[8]

Targeted therapy targets a cancer's specific genes or proteins that contribute to cancer growth and survival. Treatment with a targeted therapy depends on assessing whether the tumor has the specific target. This is usually done by testing a sample of the tumor obtained through a biopsy.

Pharmacogenomics and *pharmacogenetics* are the study of genomic variation in drug responses.[9] Examples of how the results of genetic testing can be applied to cancer drug therapy are shown in Table 13.5. For example, vemurafenib is a treatment for patients with metastatic melanoma. It is indicated only for those with tumors that express a gene mutation called *BRAF V600E.*

Not all types of cancer have personalized treatment options. Genetic testing may be costly and time consuming. Many insurance plans do not cover the costs of these tests. Some personalized treatments can be expensive.[7]

SURGICAL THERAPY

Surgery is the oldest form of cancer treatment. Today surgery can meet a variety of goals (Fig. 16.8).

Prevention

Surgery can eliminate or reduce the risk for cancer development. Prophylactic removal of nonvital organs has been successful in reducing the risk for some cancers. For example, patients with adenomatous familial polyposis may benefit from a total colectomy to prevent colorectal cancer (see Chapter 47). Those who have genetic mutations of *BRCA1* or *BRCA2* and a strong family history of early-onset breast cancer may consider prophylactic mastectomy (see Chapter 56).

Cure or Control

When the goal is cure or control, the objective is to remove all or as much resectable tumor as possible while sparing normal tissue. Examples of surgeries used for cure or control of cancer include radical neck dissection, mastectomy, thyroidectomy, nephrectomy, hysterectomy, and oophorectomy. The trend is toward less radical surgeries.

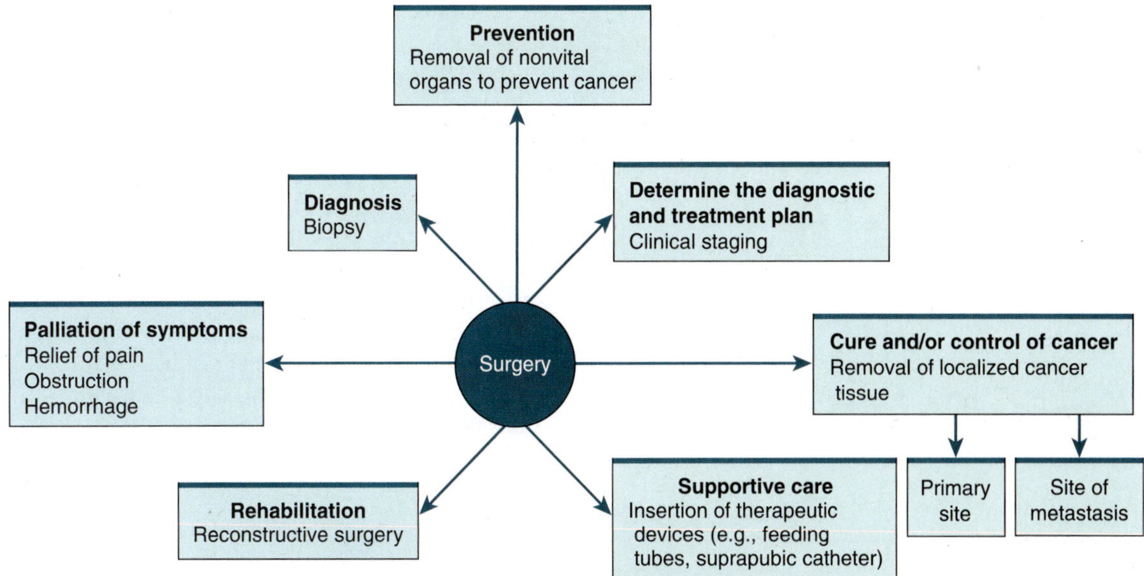

Fig. 16.8 Role of surgery in treating cancer.

A patient may undergo a *debulking* or *cytoreductive procedure* if the tumor cannot be completely removed (e.g., a tumor attached to a vital organ). With debulking, as much tumor as possible is removed. The patient then receives chemotherapy and/or radiation therapy. This type of surgery can make chemotherapy or radiation therapy more effective, since the tumor mass is reduced before treatment is started. At other times, a patient may need to receive *neoadjuvant* (treatment before surgery) chemotherapy or radiation therapy to reduce tumor size and improve the surgical outcome.

Supportive and Palliative Care

Procedures can be part of supportive care that maximizes bodily function or facilitates cancer treatment. Examples of supportive surgeries include:

- Inserting a feeding tube to maintain nutrition during head and neck cancer treatment
- Placing a central venous access device to deliver chemotherapy
- Prophylactic surgical fixation of bones at risk for pathologic fracture

Effects of treatment or symptoms may require surgical intervention for palliation. Examples include (1) tumor debulking to relieve pain or pressure, (2) colostomy for the relief of a bowel obstruction (see Chapter 47), and (3) laminectomy for the relief of a spinal cord compression (see Chapter 65).

CHEMOTHERAPY

Chemotherapy is the use of chemicals as a systemic therapy for cancer. The goal of chemotherapy is to eliminate or reduce the number of cancer cells in the primary and metastatic tumor site(s). It is a mainstay of treatment for most solid tumors and hematologic cancers (e.g., leukemias, lymphomas). Chemotherapy can offer cure for some cancers, control other cancers for long periods, and in some cases, offer palliative relief of symptoms when cure or control is no longer possible (Fig. 16.9).

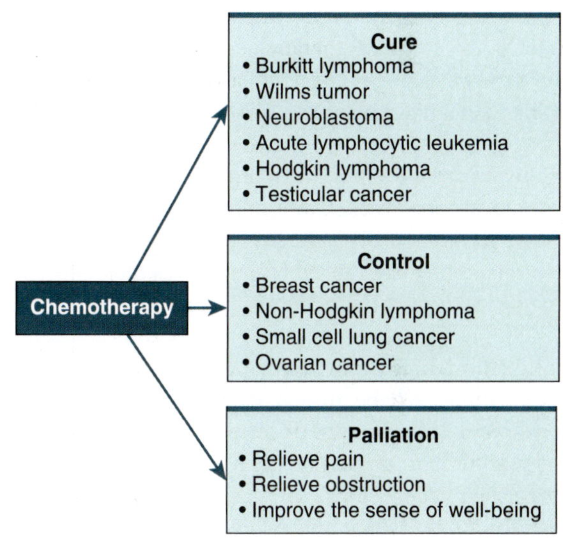

Fig. 16.9 Goals of chemotherapy.

Effect on Cells

All cells (cancer cells and normal cells) enter the cell cycle for replication and proliferation. We describe the effects of chemotherapy in relation to the cell cycle. The 2 major categories of chemotherapy are cell cycle phase–nonspecific and cell cycle phase–specific drugs (Fig. 16.10). *Cell cycle phase–nonspecific chemotherapy drugs* have their effect on the cells during all phases of the cell cycle. This includes the process of

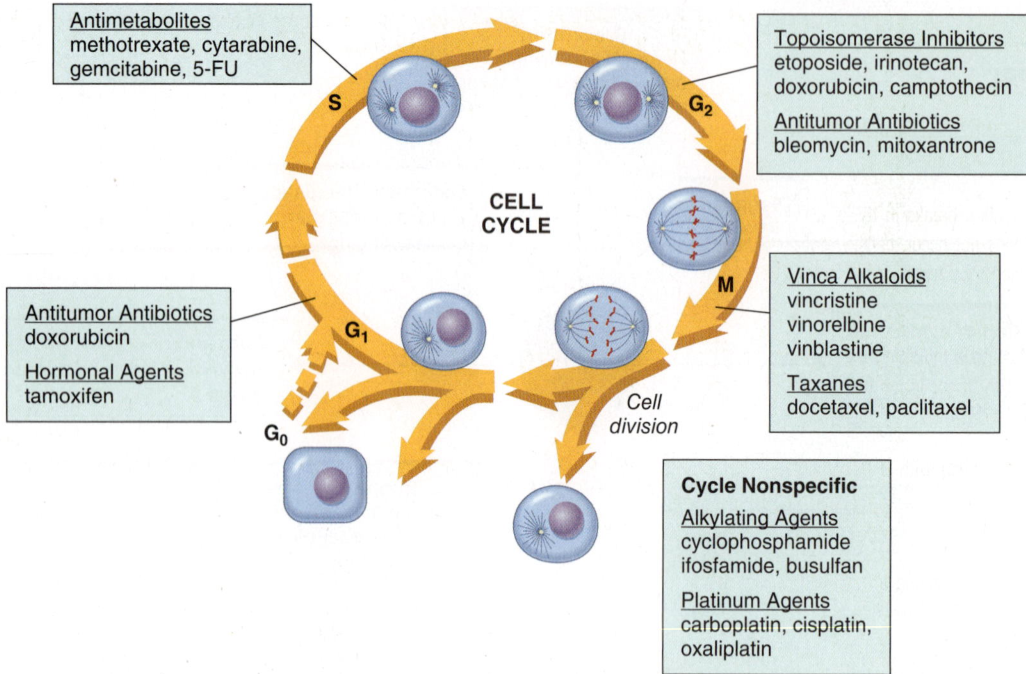

Fig. 16.10 Cell life cycle and chemotherapeutic agents.

cell replication and proliferation and the resting phase (G_0). *Cell cycle phase–specific chemotherapy drugs* have their greatest effects during specific phases of the cell cycle (e.g., when cells are in the process of replication or proliferation during G_1, S, G_2, or M). Giving cell cycle phase–specific and cell cycle phase–nonspecific drugs together maximizes their effectiveness by using drugs that act in different ways and throughout the cell cycle.

When cancer first begins to develop, most of the cells are actively dividing. As the tumor increases in size, more cells become inactive and convert to a resting state (G_0). Because most chemotherapy drugs are only effective against dividing cells, cells can escape death by staying in the G_0 phase. A challenge is to overcome the effect of resistant resting and noncycling cells.

Classification

Chemotherapy drugs are classified in general groups by their molecular structure and mechanisms of action (Table 16.7). Each drug in a particular class has many similarities. However, there are differences in how the drugs work and the unique side effects associated with drugs in each class.

Chemotherapy Preparation

Only persons specifically trained in chemotherapy handling techniques should be involved with the preparation and administration of cancer drugs.[10] Cancer drugs may pose a hazard to health care persons who do not follow safe handling guidelines. A person preparing, transporting, or giving chemotherapy may absorb the drug through inhalation of particles when reconstituting a powder or through skin contact from exposure to droplets or powder. There may be some risk in handling the body fluids and excretions of people during the first 48 hours after they receive chemotherapy.

Methods of Administration

Chemotherapy is given by multiple routes. The IV route is the most common. Major concerns associated with IV chemotherapy administration include venous access problems, device or catheter-related infection, and *extravasation.*[11] It is the infiltration of drugs into tissues surrounding the infusion site, causing local tissue damage (Fig. 16.11).

Many chemotherapy drugs are either irritants or vesicants. *Irritants* damage the intima of the vein, causing phlebitis and sclerosis and limiting future peripheral venous access. They will not cause tissue damage if infiltrated. **Vesicants**, if inadvertently infiltrated into the skin, may cause severe local tissue breakdown and necrosis. It is important to monitor for and take prompt action if extravasation of a vesicant occurs. To lessen discomfort and risks of infection and infiltration, IV chemotherapy can be given through a *central venous access device* (CVAD). CVADs are placed in large blood vessels. They allow frequent, continuous, or intermittent administration of chemotherapy, immunotherapy, targeted therapy, and other products. This avoids multiple venipunctures for vascular access. See more about CVADs in Chapter 17.

With advances in drug formulation techniques, more oral chemotherapy drugs are available. An advantage to oral drugs is that patients take them at home. This makes it easier for patients, although adherence to oral medication regimen may become an issue.

TABLE 16.7 Drug Therapy

Chemotherapy

Mechanisms of Action	Examples
Cell Cycle Phase—Nonspecific	
Alkylating	
Damage DNA by causing breaks in the double-stranded helix. If repair does not occur, cells will die immediately (cytocidal) or when they try to divide (cytostatic).	bendamustine (Treanda), busulfan (Myleran), chlorambucil (Leukeran), cyclophosphamide, dacarbazine, ifosfamide (Ifex), melphalan, temozolomide (Temodar), thiotepa
Antitumor Antibiotics	
Bind directly to DNA, thus inhibiting the synthesis of DNA and interfering with transcription of RNA.	bleomycin, dactinomycin, daunorubicin, doxorubicin (Doxil), epirubicin (Ellence), idarubicin, mitomycin, mitoxantrone, valrubicin (Valstar)
Nitrosoureas	
Break DNA helix, interfering with DNA replication. Cross blood-brain barrier.	carmustine (BiCNU, Gliadel), lomustine (Gleostine), streptozocin (Zanosar)
Platinum Drugs	
Bind to DNA and RNA, miscoding information and/or inhibiting DNA replication, and cells die.	carboplatin, cisplatin, oxaliplatin
Cell Cycle Phase—Specific	
Antimetabolites	
Mimic naturally occurring substances, thus interfering with enzyme function or DNA synthesis. Primarily act during S phase. Purine and pyrimidine are building blocks of nucleic acids needed for DNA and RNA synthesis.	
• Interfere with purine metabolism	cladribine, clofarabine (Clolar), fludarabine, mercaptopurine (Purixan), nelarabine (Arranon), pentostatin (Nipent), thioguanine
• Interfere with pyrimidine metabolism	capecitabine (Xeloda); cytarabine, floxuridine, fluorouracil, gemcitabine
• Interfere with folic acid metabolism	methotrexate (Trexall), pemetrexed (Alimta)
• Interfere with DNA synthesis	hydroxyurea (Hydrea, Droxia)
Mitotic Inhibitors	
Taxanes	
Antimicrotubule agents that interfere with mitosis. Act during the late G_2 phase and mitosis to stabilize microtubules, thus inhibiting cell division.	albumin-bound paclitaxel (Abraxane), docetaxel (Taxotere)
Vinca Alkaloids	
Act in M phase to inhibit mitosis.	vinblastine, vincristine, vinorelbine
Microtubular Inhibitors	
Disrupt the function of microtubules, which stops or slows down cell division.	ixabepilone (Ixempra), eribulin (Halaven)
Topoisomerase Inhibitors	
Inhibit topoisomerases (normal enzymes) that function to make reversible breaks and repairs in DNA that allow for flexibility of DNA in replication.	etoposide, irinotecan (Camptosar), topotecan (Hycamtin)

Regional Chemotherapy

Regional treatment with chemotherapy involves delivery of the drug directly to the tumor site. The advantage of this method is that we can deliver higher concentrations of the drug to the tumor with less systemic toxicity. Examples include intra-arterial, intraperitoneal, intrathecal, intraventricular, and intravesical chemotherapy.

Intraarterial

Intraarterial chemotherapy delivers the drug to the tumor through the arteries supplying the tumor. This method is used to treat osteogenic sarcoma, head and neck cancer, primary liver cancer, and retinoblastoma. We can also deliver chemotherapy through a surgically placed catheter that is connected to an external or implanted infusion pump.

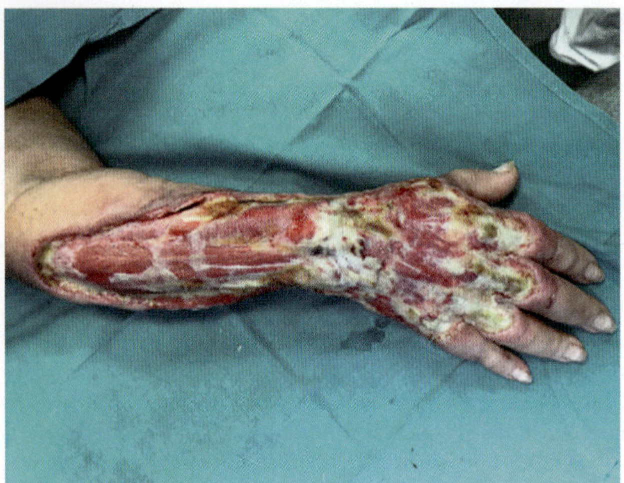

Fig. 16.11 Extravasation injury from infiltration of chemotherapy drug. (From Faenza M, Ferraro GA, Fonzone Caccese FP, et al: Combined approach with negative pressure wound therapy and dermal substitute for extravasation injury, *JPRAS Open* 25:62, 2020.)

Intraperitoneal

Intraperitoneal chemotherapy involves the delivery of chemotherapy to the peritoneal cavity. It is a treatment for peritoneal metastases from primary colorectal and ovarian cancers and malignant ascites. For short-term administration, we can place an imported port or temporary Silastic catheter (Tenckhoff, Hickman, Groshong) percutaneously or surgically into the peritoneal cavity. Chemotherapy is generally infused into the peritoneum in 1 to 2 L of fluid and allowed to *dwell* in the peritoneum for 1 to 4 hours. After the *dwell time*, the fluid is drained from the peritoneum.

Intrathecal or Intraventricular

Cancers that metastasize to the central nervous system (CNS) are hard to treat because the blood-brain barrier often prevents distribution of chemotherapy to this area. One method used to treat metastasis to the CNS is intrathecal chemotherapy. This involves a lumbar puncture and injection of chemotherapy into the subarachnoid space. To reduce the need for repeated lumbar punctures, patients may have an Ommaya reservoir inserted. An Ommaya reservoir is a soft, plastic, dome-shaped disk with an extension catheter. It is surgically implanted through the cranium into a lateral ventricle.

Intravesical Bladder

Intravesical bladder chemotherapy involves instilling chemotherapy into the bladder. This is done through a urinary catheter. The solution is retained for 1 to 3 hours.

Effects of Chemotherapy on Normal Tissues

Chemotherapy drugs cannot selectively distinguish between normal cells and cancer cells. Chemotherapy-induced side effects result from the destruction of normal cells, especially those that are rapidly proliferating. These include cells in the bone marrow, lining of the GI tract, and integument (skin, hair, nails) (Table 16.8). We classify the general and drug-specific adverse effects as acute, delayed, or chronic. Some side effects fall into more than one category. For example, nausea, vomiting, and diarrhea can be both acute and delayed.

TABLE 16.8 Cells With a Rapid Rate of Proliferation

Cells	Generation Time	Effect of Cell Destruction
Bone marrow stem cell	6–24 h	Myelosuppression (infection, bleeding, anemia)
Epithelial cells lining the GI tract	12–24 h	Anorexia, mucositis (including stomatitis, esophagitis), nausea, vomiting, diarrhea
Hair follicle cells	24 h	Alopecia
Neutrophils	12 h	Leukopenia, infection
Ova and testes	24–36 h	Reproductive problems

Acute toxicity occurs during and right after drug administration. It includes anaphylactic and hypersensitivity reactions, extravasation or flare reactions, anticipatory nausea and vomiting, and dysrhythmias.

Delayed effects are numerous. They include delayed nausea and vomiting, mucositis, alopecia, skin rashes, bone marrow suppression, altered bowel function (diarrhea, constipation), and various cumulative neurotoxicities.

Chronic toxicities involve damage to organs, such as the heart, liver, kidneys, and lungs. Chronic toxicities can be either long-term effects that develop during or right after treatment and persist or late effects that are absent during treatment and manifest later.

Treatment Plan

The most common treatment plans combine drugs in multidrug regimens. Multidrug plans target more than one signaling pathway. They are more effective in managing most cancers. The plans involve drugs with different mechanisms of action and varying toxicity profiles. However, combination chemotherapy can increase toxicities.

Drug regimens are based on evidence supporting their use in specific cancers. Sometimes they are customized to meet specific patient needs. Chemotherapy is most effective when the tumor burden is low, therapy is not interrupted, and the patient receives the intended dose. Drug doses are based on the person's weight and height using the body surface area calculation.

Mutation of cancer cells within the tumor can result in cells that are resistant to chemotherapy. With multiple drugs working at different times in the cell cycle, cancer cells can be more effectively killed. This decreases mutation and resistance.

RADIATION THERAPY

Radiation therapy is used to treat a carefully defined area of the body. Many cancer patients receive radiation at some point in their treatment. Radiation may be used by itself, in combination with systemic therapy or surgery to treat primary tumors, or for palliation of metastatic lesions.

Radiation therapy uses high-energy particles or waves, such as electron beams, x-rays, or protons. Radiation breaks the chemical bonds in DNA. The damaged DNA causes cells to stop growing and dividing. Over time, this causes cell death. Technologic advances have expanded and refined the sources and methods of delivering radiation therapy. This allows for more accurate and less invasive treatments.

Principles of Radiobiology

As the radiation beam passes through the treatment field, energy is deposited. *Low-energy beams* (e.g., electrons) expend energy quickly on impact with matter, so they penetrate only a short distance. They are useful in treating cancers that affect the skin, such as cutaneous T-cell lymphoma. *High-energy beams* (e.g., photons) are more widely used due to their greater depth of penetration. This makes them suitable for delivering optimal doses to internal organs.

Some cancers are more responsive to the effects of radiation than others (Table 16.9). Radiosensitivity is the relative responsiveness of cells and tissues to the effects of radiation. In highly responsive tumors (such as lymphomas), radiation therapy can affect even a large tumor. In less responsive tumors, there may be a slower or incomplete response. Local prostate cancer responds very slowly to radiation (several months after treatment is complete).

TABLE 16.9 Tumor Radiosensitivity

High Radiosensitivity
- Hodgkin lymphoma
- Neuroblastoma
- Non-Hodgkin lymphoma
- Ovarian dysgerminoma
- Testicular seminoma
- Wilms tumor

Moderate Radiosensitivity
- Bladder carcinoma
- Breast adenocarcinoma
- Esophageal carcinoma
- Oropharyngeal carcinoma
- Prostate carcinoma
- Uterine and cervical carcinoma

Mild Radiosensitivity
- Colon adenocarcinoma
- Gastric adenocarcinoma
- Renal adenocarcinoma
- Soft tissue sarcomas (e.g., chondrosarcoma)

Poor Radiosensitivity
- Osteosarcoma
- Malignant glioma
- Melanoma
- Testicular nonseminoma

When planning radiation treatment, we must establish a balance between the likelihood of radiation-induced toxicity and control of the tumor. This is the *therapeutic ratio.* The ratio is most beneficial when the dose is minimized to normal tissue and maximized to the tumor. There is a lifetime dose limit to the amount of radiation an area of the body can receive.

Radiation doses are expressed in units called *gray* (Gy) or centigray (cGy). A *centigray* is equal to 1 rad; 100 centigray equals 1 gray. Once the total dose to be delivered is determined, that dose is divided into daily *fractions.* Doses between 180 and 200 cGy/day are considered *standard fractionation.* Hypofractionated radiotherapy is a shortened treatment duration with a higher dose of radiation per day. This type of treatment is currently being used in breast and prostate cancer treatments.

Simulation and Treatment Planning

Simulation is a process by which the radiation treatment fields are defined, filmed, and marked on the skin. The target is defined using a variety of imaging techniques (e.g., CT, MRI, PET scans), physical assessment, and surgical reports. The radiation oncologist specifies the dose and volume of area to be treated. Treatment volumes include the (1) *gross target volume* (GTV), which is the gross extent of the tumor; (2) the *clinical target volume* (CTV), which is the GTV plus additional margin to encompass any potential microscopic or subclinical disease; and (3) the *planning target volume* (PTV). PTV is the GTV/CTV plus additional margin to allow for organ motion or variance in daily set-up position.

During the simulation, the patient is positioned on a simulator. A diagnostic imaging machine re-creates the actions of the linear accelerator. The radiation fields are marked on the patient's skin. Immobilization devices (e.g., casts, bite blocks, thermoplastic face masks) are often used to help the patient stay in a stable position (Fig. 16.12). Temporary tattoos may be placed to ensure the position is precisely reproduced with each treatment.

External Radiation

External beam radiation is the most common form of radiation treatment. With this technique, the patient is exposed to radiation from a megavoltage treatment machine. The beam passes through the external tissues to reach the internal target. A linear accelerator is the most commonly used machine for delivering external beam radiation (Fig. 16.13). *Gamma knife technology* uses highly accurate gamma rays to deliver stereotactic treatment to a local area. It is often used for brain tumors.

Internal Radiation

Brachytherapy, or internal radiation, consists of the implantation or insertion of radioactive materials directly into the tumor

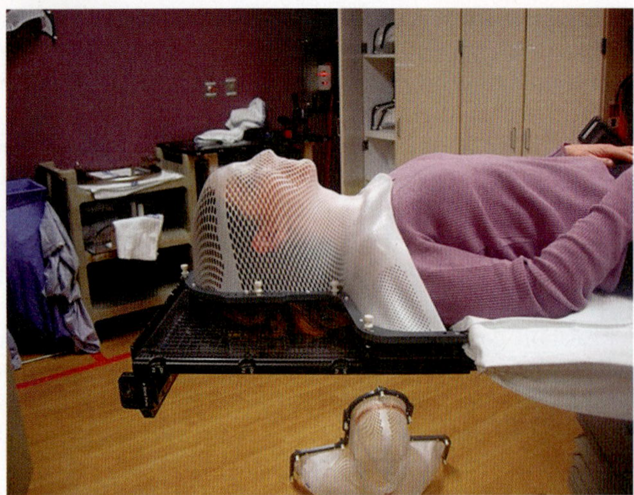

Fig. 16.12 Immobilization device. A head holder and an immobilization mask ensure accurate positioning for daily treatment of head and neck cancer. (Courtesy Jormain Cady, Virginia Mason Medical Center, Seattle, WA.)

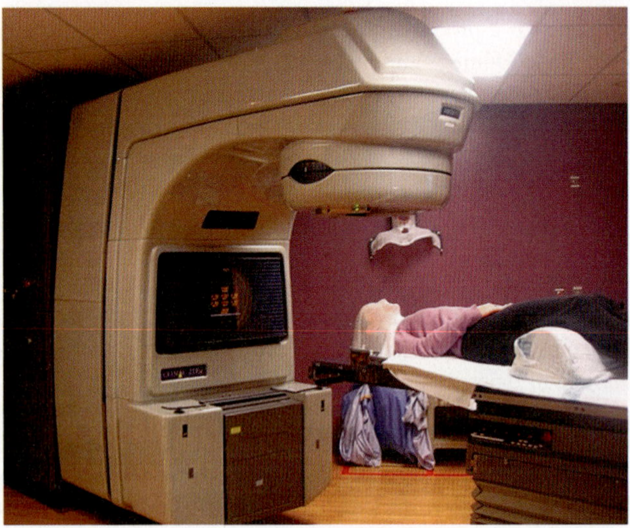

Fig. 16.13 Linear accelerator used to deliver radiation therapy. Patient is positioned on radiation treatment table for treatment of head and neck cancer. (Courtesy Jormain Cady, Virginia Mason Medical Center, Seattle, WA.)

(interstitial) or near the tumor (intracavitary or intraluminal). This allows for direct delivery of radiation to the target with minimal exposure to surrounding healthy tissues. It may be a primary or adjuvant therapy. It is often used in combination with external radiation as a supplemental "boost" treatment. The most common cancers treated with brachytherapy are uterine, cervical, breast, head and neck, and prostate.

The isotopes used include high–dose rate sources (e.g., iridium-192) and low–dose rate sources (e.g., iodine-125, palladium-103, cesium-131). Brachytherapy implants are permanent or temporary. Permanent brachytherapy delivers a low dose rate via pellets or seeds that are inserted into the tumor with thin hollow needles. These seeds are left in place after treatment is complete. Temporary brachytherapy can be either high or low dose. Using hollow needles, catheters or fluid-filled balloons are inserted through hollow needles near the cancer for a period of time. They are removed after treatment has ended.

Radioactive drugs, or radiopharmaceuticals, are used to treat some cancers systemically. They may be given orally as a capsule or drink (e.g., iodine-131 for thyroid cancer). IV examples include yttrium-90 for liver cancer and radium-223 for bone metastases in prostate cancer. The drug is sometimes bound to monoclonal antibodies. The antibodies attach to the cancer cell, directly delivering the radiation. This may minimize the effects of the radiation on healthy cells.

Care of the person undergoing brachytherapy or receiving radioactive drugs requires you to be aware when the patient is emitting radioactivity. Patients with temporary implants are radioactive only while the source is in place. In those with permanent implants, because the sources have short half-lives and are weak emitters, the radioactive exposure to the outside and to others is low.

Since interstitial seeds emit low energy with limited tissue penetration, patients are not considered radioactive. However, some initial radiation precautions may be recommended because of the small risk of seed dislodgement. Over time, the isotopes decay and are no longer radioactive. We can predict the time frame for treatment side effects based on the rate of decay for the isotope used.

The principles of *ALARA (as low as reasonably achievable)* and *time, distance,* and *shielding* are vital to our safety when caring for the person with a source of internal radiation. The radiation safety officer will say how much time at a specific distance one can spend with the patient. This is determined by the dose delivered by the implant. Small differences in distance are critical. Organize care to limit the time spent in direct contact with the patient. Only care that must be delivered near the source, such as checking placement of the implant, is done in proximity. Use shielding, if available. Do not deliver care without wearing a film badge (dosimeter) showing cumulative radiation exposure. Do not share the film badge. To lessen anxiety and confusion, tell the patient the reason for time and distance limitations before the treatment.

When the patient is to be discharged, we perform a radiation survey to verify that radiation levels surrounding the patient are sufficiently low. We give the patient a card with information about their treatment and radiation oncology contact information. In most circumstances, the patient is advised to maintain a safe distance from pregnant females and young children for a specified period of time based on the isotope used.

NURSING MANAGEMENT: CHEMOTHERAPY AND RADIATION THERAPY

You play a key role in helping patients deal with the side effects of chemotherapy and radiation therapy. Before starting teaching, assess the patient's ability to process information. Tailor teaching to meet the patient's and caregiver's learning needs.

Table 16.10 outlines the common side effects of chemotherapy and radiation. Bone marrow suppression, fatigue, GI problems, skin and mucosal problems, and pulmonary and reproductive effects are discussed here.

Bone Marrow Suppression

Treatment-induced myelosuppression can result in life-threatening and distressing effects. These include infection, hemorrhage, and overwhelming fatigue. Myelosuppression is one of the most common effects of chemotherapy. To a lesser extent, it can occur with radiation. The major difference between them is that radiation (a local therapy) only affects bone marrow within the treatment field. Chemotherapy (a systemic therapy) affects bone marrow function throughout the body. When the therapies are combined, the risk for myelosuppression increases.

In general, the onset of bone marrow suppression is related to the life span of the type of blood cell. WBCs (especially neutrophils) are affected first (within 1 to 2 weeks), platelets in 2 to 3 weeks, and red blood cells (RBCs), with a longer life span of 120 days, later. The severity of myelosuppression depends on the drugs used, drug dosages, and the radiation treatment field. Radiation to large marrow-containing regions of the body causes more clinically significant myelosuppression. In adults, most active marrow is in the pelvis and thoracic and lumbar vertebrae.

Monitor the CBC. Patients often have the lowest blood cell counts (called the *nadir*) between 7 and 10 days after starting therapy. However, the exact onset depends on the drug regimen.

Neutropenia is more common in patients receiving chemotherapy. It is a serious risk factor for life-threatening infection and sepsis. Significant neutropenia will prompt treatment delay or adjustments (e.g., lower dosages). Take every measure to

TABLE 16.10 NURSING MANAGEMENT

Problems Caused by Chemotherapy and Radiation Therapy

Etiology	Nursing Management
Biochemical	
Hyperuricemia	
↑ Uric acid levels due to chemotherapy-induced cell destruction. Can cause secondary gout and obstructive uropathy.	• Monitor uric acid levels. • Give prescribed allopurinol. • Maintain increased fluid intake. • Monitor intake and output.
Cardiovascular	
Cardiotoxicity	
Some chemotherapy drugs (e.g., anthracyclines, taxanes) can cause ECG changes and rapidly progressive heart failure.	• Monitor heart with ECG and cardiac ejection fractions. • Drug therapy may need to be changed for symptoms or deteriorating cardiac function studies. • Administer antidysrhythmic drugs as ordered.
Pericarditis and Myocarditis	
Inflammation from radiation injury. Complication from chest wall radiation. May occur up to 1 year after treatment. Side effect of some chemotherapy.	• Monitor for manifestations of these problems (e.g., dyspnea). • Give prescribed cardiac medications. • Encourage adequate rest.
Comfort	
Fatigue	
Anabolic processes result in accumulation of metabolites from cell breakdown.	• Assess for reversible causes of fatigue and address them as indicated. • Reassure patient that fatigue is a common side effect of therapy. • Encourage patient to rest when fatigued, to maintain usual lifestyle patterns, as much as possible, and to pace activities in accordance with energy level. • Encourage moderate exercise as tolerated.
Gastrointestinal System	
Anorexia	
Release of TNF and IL-1 from macrophages has appetite-suppressant effect. Therapy-induced GI effects (mucositis, nausea, vomiting, bowel problems) and anxiety reduce appetite.	• Monitor weight. • Encourage patient to eat small, frequent meals of high-protein, high-calorie foods. • Gently encourage patient to eat, but do not nag. • Recommend keeping a food diary to track daily calories and fluids. • Serve food in pleasant environment.

Continued

TABLE 16.10 NURSING MANAGEMENT—cont'd

Problems Caused by Chemotherapy and Radiation Therapy

Etiology	Nursing Management
Constipation	
Autonomic nervous system dysfunction decreases intestinal motility. Caused by neurotoxic effects of plant alkaloids (vincristine, vinblastine).	• Teach patients to take stool softeners as needed, eat high-fiber foods, and increase fluid intake. • Increase activity (e.g., walking) if tolerated.
Diarrhea	
From denuding of epithelial lining of intestines. Side effect of chemotherapy. Follows radiation to abdomen, pelvis, lumbosacral areas.	• Give antidiarrheal drugs as needed. • Encourage fluid intake of at least 3 L/day. • Encourage low-fiber, low-residue diet. • Other foods to avoid include fried, fatty, or highly seasoned foods and foods that are gas producing.
Hepatotoxicity	
Toxic effects from chemotherapy (usually transient and resolve when drug is stopped).	• Monitor liver function tests.
Nausea and Vomiting	
Release of intracellular breakdown products stimulates vomiting center in brain. Drugs stimulate vomiting center in brain. Radiation and chemotherapy destroy lining of GI tract.	• Encourage patient to eat and drink when not nauseated. • Give prophylactic antiemetics before chemotherapy and on as-needed basis (see Table 46.1). • Teach patients to take antiemetics on a scheduled basis for 2–3 days after chemotherapy. • Use appropriate diversional activities.
Stomatitis, Mucositis, and Esophagitis	
Chemotherapy or radiation treatment destroy epithelial cells located in field (e.g., head and neck, stomach, esophagus). Rapid cell destruction causes inflammation and ulceration.	Assess oral mucosa daily and teach patient to do the following: • Use nutrition supplements (e.g., Ensure, Boost) if intake is decreasing. • Be aware that eating, swallowing, and talking may be difficult and patient may need analgesics. • Teach avoidance of irritating spicy or acidic foods or too hot or too cold food (extremes in temperature). • Teach how to choose moist, bland, and softer foods. • Keep oral cavity clean and moist by frequent oral rinses with saline or salt and soda solution. • Use artificial saliva to manage dryness (radiation). • Discourage use of irritants, such as tobacco and alcohol. • Apply topical anesthetics (e.g., viscous lidocaine).
Genitourinary Tract	
Hemorrhagic Cystitis	
Chemotherapy destroys cells lining the bladder. Side effect of radiation when in the treatment field.	• Increase fluid intake 24–72 h after treatment as tolerated. • Monitor for urgency, frequency, and hematuria. • Give cytoprotectants (mesna [Mesnex]) and hydration. • Provide supportive care to manage symptoms (e.g., flavoxate).
Nephrotoxicity	
Exposure to nephrotoxic drugs (cisplatin and high-dose methotrexate) directly damages renal cells. Precipitation of metabolites of cell breakdown (tumor lysis syndrome [TLS]).	• Monitor BUN and creatinine levels. • Avoid potentiating drugs. • Alkalinize the urine by adding sodium bicarbonate to IV infusion • Give allopurinol or rasburicase for TLS prevention.
Reproductive Problems	
Therapy damages cells of testes or ova.	• Discuss risk with patients before starting treatment. • Offer opportunity for sperm and ova banking before treatment for patients of childbearing age.

TABLE 16.10 NURSING MANAGEMENT—cont'd

Problems Caused by Chemotherapy and Radiation Therapy

Problem	Nursing Management
Hematologic System	
Anemia	
Therapy causes bone marrow depression. Cancer cells infiltrate bone marrow.	• Monitor hemoglobin and hematocrit levels. • Give iron supplements and erythropoietin. • Encourage intake of foods that promote RBC production (see Table 34.5).
Leukopenia	
Chemotherapy or radiation therapy causes bone marrow depression. Infection is the most frequent cause of death in cancer patients. Respiratory and genitourinary systems are usual sites of infection.	• Monitor WBC count, especially neutrophils. • Tell patient to report fever and manifestations of infection. • Teach patient good handwashing (see Table 34.24). • Give WBC growth factors as indicated (Table 16.14).
Thrombocytopenia	
Chemotherapy causes bone marrow depression. Cancer cells infiltrate bone marrow. Spontaneous bleeding can occur with platelet counts $\leq$20,000/μL.	• Observe for signs of bleeding (e.g., petechiae, bruising). • Monitor platelet counts. • For patient teaching, see Table 34.15.
Nervous System	
Cognitive Changes ("chemo brain")	

Occur during and after treatment (especially with chemotherapy).
Problems with concentration, memory lapses, trouble remembering details, taking longer to finish tasks.
May happen quickly and last a short time. Some people have mild long-term effects.
	• Teach patients to
	  • Use detailed daily planner.
	  • Get enough sleep and rest.
	  • Exercise brain (learn something new, do word puzzles).
	  • Focus on one thing (no multitasking).

Intracranial Pressure	
May result from radiation edema in central nervous system.	• Monitor neurologic status. • May be controlled with corticosteroids.
Peripheral Neuropathy	
Paresthesias, areflexia, skeletal muscle weakness, and smooth muscle dysfunction can occur as a side effect of plant alkaloids, taxanes, and cisplatin.	• Monitor for manifestations in patients on these drugs. • Consider temporary chemotherapy dose interruption or reduction until symptoms improve. • Antiseizure drugs (e.g., gabapentin) may be given.
Respiratory System	
Pneumonitis	
Radiation pneumonitis develops 2–3 mo after start of treatment. After 6–12 mo, fibrosis occurs and is evident on x-ray. Side effect of some chemotherapy and immunotherapy drugs.	• Monitor for dry, hacking cough; fever; and dyspnea with exertion. • Encourage activity and respiratory exercises.
Skin	
Alopecia	
Chemotherapy or radiation to scalp destroys hair follicles. Hair loss usually is temporary with chemotherapy, may be permanent with radiation.	• Suggest ways to cope with hair loss (e.g., hair pieces, scarves, wigs). • Cut long hair before therapy. • Avoid excess shampooing and grooming. • Implement scalp cooling. • Avoid use of electric styling products. • Discuss effect of hair loss on self-image.
Chemotherapy-Induced Skin Changes	
Acneiform eruptions Acral erythema Hyperpigmentation Photosensitivity Telangiectasia	• Alert patient to potential skin changes. • Encourage patient to avoid sun exposure. • Implement symptomatic management as needed depending on specific skin effect (e.g., application of lotions, corticosteroid creams).
Radiation Skin Changes (dry to moist desquamation)	
Radiation damages skin	Table 16.11 describes patient management.

prevent infections. Hand hygiene is the mainstay of patient safety. Patients and their contacts, including health care team members, should follow handwashing guidelines.

Monitor temperature. Any sign of infection should be treated promptly. Fever in the presence of neutropenia is a medical emergency. WBC growth factors (e.g., filgrastim [Neupogen]) are often used to reduce the duration of chemotherapy-induced neutropenia. They are used as a prophylactic measure to prevent neutropenia from myelosuppressive chemotherapy.[12] Neutropenia is discussed in Chapter 34. See the patient teaching guide in Table 34.24.

Thrombocytopenia can result in spontaneous bleeding or major hemorrhage. The risk for serious bleeding is generally not present until the platelet count falls below 20,000/μL. When the count drops that low, we often give platelet transfusions. Implement measures to reduce risk of bleeding (see Chapter 34). Teach patients to avoid activities that place them at risk for injury or bleeding. See the patient teaching guide in Table 34.15.

Anemia is common in patients undergoing either radiation therapy or chemotherapy. It generally has a later onset (about 3 to 4 months after starting treatment). Patients with low hemoglobin levels may receive RBC growth factors (e.g., darbepoetin, epoetin [Procrit]). Patients who are symptomatic may need RBC transfusions.

Fatigue

Fatigue is a nearly universal symptom affecting most patients with cancer. Many describe fatigue as the most disturbing treatment-related side effect. Fatigue may persist long after treatment has ended.

Anemia is one cause of fatigue. Other causes may be related to the (1) toxic substances left in the body from cells killed by cancer treatment, (2) need for extra energy to repair and heal body tissue damaged by treatment, and (3) lack of sleep caused by some chemotherapy drugs or steroids. Assess for reversible causes of fatigue. These include anemia, hypothyroidism, depression, insomnia, dehydration, or infection.

Use guidelines to manage cancer-related fatigue.[13] Stress that fatigue is common. Teach patients energy conservation measures. Help them identify days or times during the day when they typically feel better. Encourage them to be more active during those periods.

Patients may need to rest before activity. Others can help patients with work or home tasks. Ignoring fatigue or overstressing the body when fatigue is tolerable may lead to an increase in symptoms. Maintaining exercise and activity within tolerable limits is often helpful in managing fatigue. Walking programs are a way for most patients to keep active without overtaxing themselves. Staying active helps improve mood and avoid the debilitating cycle of fatigue-depression-fatigue that can occur in patients with cancer. Use guidelines to manage cancer-related fatigue.[13]

GI Effects

The intestinal mucosa is one of the most sensitive tissues to radiation and chemotherapy. GI problems include nausea and vomiting, diarrhea, mucositis, and anorexia. These problems can significantly affect hydration, nutrition, and sense of well-being.

There are several reasons GI problems occur. These include (1) the release of serotonin from the GI tract, which stimulates the chemoreceptor trigger zone (CTZ) and the vomiting center in the brain, and (2) cell death and resulting damage to GI mucosa. Radiation to treatment fields that contain GI structures (e.g., abdominopelvic, lumbosacral, lower thoracic areas) and select chemotherapy drugs cause direct injury to GI epithelial cells.

Nausea and Vomiting

Nausea and vomiting are common side effects of chemotherapy and sometimes radiation therapy. Chemotherapy-induced nausea and vomiting (CINV) may occur within 1 hour of chemotherapy administration. Vomiting may start a few hours after radiation therapy to the chest or abdomen. It may persist for 24 hours or more.

Anticipatory nausea and vomiting can develop if a patient had poorly controlled nausea and vomiting with prior chemotherapy administration. In this phenomenon, encountering the cues even without receiving treatment may precipitate nausea and vomiting. Preventing nausea and vomiting with the first cycle lowers the risk. If it does occur, we initiate control measures. This includes giving prophylactic antiemetic and antianxiety medication 1 hour before treatment. The patient may find that eating a light meal of nonirritating food before treatment is helpful. *Delayed nausea and vomiting* can develop 24 hours to a week after treatment.

Assess patients with nausea and vomiting for signs and symptoms of dehydration. Treatment includes antiemetic drugs, diet, and nondrug interventions (e.g., relaxation breathing). Several antiemetic drugs are used (see Table 46.1). Serotonin (5-HT_3) receptor antagonists (ondansetron, palonosetron) and neurokinin-1 receptor antagonists (NK_1RA) (e.g., aprepitant [Emend], rolapitant [Varubi]) can reduce CINV. Dexamethasone given with other antiemetics helps manage CINV.

Diarrhea

Diarrhea is a reaction of the bowel mucosa to radiation and some chemotherapy. Patients can have an increase in frequency and liquidity of stool. The small bowel is very sensitive and does not tolerate significant radiation doses. With pelvic radiation, patients may receive treatment with a full bladder. This moves the small bowel out of the treatment field. Radiation and chemotherapy-induced diarrhea are best managed with diet, antidiarrheals, antimotility drugs, and antispasmodics (see Table 47.2).

Recommend a diet low in fiber and residue before chemotherapy known to cause diarrhea. This includes limiting foods high in roughage (e.g., fresh fruits, vegetables, seeds, nuts). Bowel mucosal injury from radiation may cause temporary lactose intolerance. Avoiding milk products is helpful for some patients during and right after treatment. Depending on the severity, patients may need hydration and electrolyte supplements.

The rectal area must be clean and dry to maintain skin integrity. Inspect the perianal area for skin breakdown. Lukewarm sitz baths may ease discomfort and cleanse the rectal area if irritation develops. Systemic analgesia may be used for painful skin irritations. Note the number, volume, consistency, and character of stools per day. Have patients keep a diary or log to record episodes and aggravating and alleviating factors.

Mucositis

Mucositis is irritation, inflammation, and/or ulceration of the mucosa. The mucosal linings of the oral cavity, oropharynx, and esophagus are very sensitive to the effects of radiation and chemotherapy. Patients with head and neck cancer who receive radiation are at high risk.

Certain factors can compound the problem. For example, patients undergoing head and neck radiation may face the added challenge of radiation-induced parotid gland dysfunction. This may result in decreased salivary flow, causing acute or chronic *xerostomia* (dry mouth). Dryness or thick saliva compromises the protective salivary functions of assisting with cleansing teeth, moistening food, and swallowing. Good oral care during and for a long time after treatment reduces the risk for cavities, which may occur due to decreased saliva. Teach patients to continue regular dental follow-up every 6 months. They should use fluoride supplements as recommended by their dentist. Saliva substitutes or sucking sugar-free candy may help patients with dry mouth. Many patients find that drinking small amounts of water frequently has a similar effect.

Dysphagia and dysgeusia (taste loss) may develop. By the end of treatment, patients often report that all food has lost its flavor. Patients may report feeling that they have a "lump" as they swallow and that "foods get stuck." Those with *odynophagia* (painful swallowing) caused by oropharyngeal or esophageal irritation and ulceration may need analgesics before meals.

Oral assessment and careful intervention to keep the oral cavity moist, clean, and free of debris is essential to prevent infection and promote nutrition intake. Implement oral care protocols that address prevention and management of mucositis.

Routinely assess the oral cavity, mucous membranes, characteristics of saliva, and ability to swallow. Referral to a dentist for all necessary dental work is common before starting treatment. Teach patients to self-examine the oral cavity and how to perform oral care. They should perform oral care before and after each meal, at bedtime, and as needed throughout the day. A saline solution of 1 tsp of salt in an 8-ounce glass of water is an effective cleansing agent. Adding 1 tsp of sodium bicarbonate to the oral care solution can decrease odor, ease pain, and dissolve mucin. Have patients use a soft-bristled toothbrush.

Treat mucositis or pain in the throat with systemic and topical analgesics and antibiotics if infection is present. Monitor and get prompt treatment for oral candidiasis (which often occurs with mucositis). Frequently cleanse with saline and water and apply topical anesthetic gels directly to the lesions.

Anorexia

Anorexia (loss of appetite) is common. It is a side effect of cancer and cancer treatment. Anorexia may be related to an inflamed mouth or esophagus, which creates difficulty chewing or swallowing, or to emotions, such as anxiety or depression. It is important to have a dietitian involved in patient care before cancer treatment starts.

Patients with nausea and vomiting, bowel problems, mucositis, and taste changes typically have little desire to eat. Anorexia seems to peak at about 4 weeks of treatment. It resolves more quickly than fatigue when treatment ends.

Monitor patients during and after treatment to ensure that weight loss does not become excess. Observe for dehydration. Most tolerate small, frequent meals of high-protein, high-calorie foods best. Nutrition supplements can be helpful. Patients may need enteral nutrition (EN) or parenteral nutrition (PN) if they are severely malnourished, if symptoms will interfere with nutrition for a time, or if the bowel needs rest. Monitor for and manage other symptoms that interfere with appetite (e.g., nausea, vomiting, pain, depression).

CHECK YOUR PRACTICE

Your 67-year-old female patient with heart failure and Stage III colorectal cancer has just completed chemotherapy. At her clinic visit, she reports being so nauseated that she "can barely keep anything down." She reports mucositis and ongoing weakness. The patient says to you, "Is this treatment worth it?"

- How would you respond?

Skin Reactions

Radiation Skin Changes

With radiation therapy, skin effects are local, occurring only in the treatment field. Radiation-induced skin changes can be acute or chronic depending on the area irradiated, the dosage, and technique. The skin-sparing ability of modern radiation equipment limits the severity of these reactions.

Redness may develop 1 to 24 hours after a single treatment. It generally occurs progressively as the treatment dose accumulates. It is an acute response followed by dry desquamation (Fig. 16.14). If the rate of cell sloughing is faster than the ability of the new epidermal cells to replace dead cells, a wet desquamation occurs with exposure of the dermis and weeping of serous fluid (Fig. 16.15). Skin reactions are especially evident in areas of skinfolds or where skin is subjected to pressure. This includes behind the ear; in gluteal folds; on the perineum, breast, or collar line; and bony prominences.

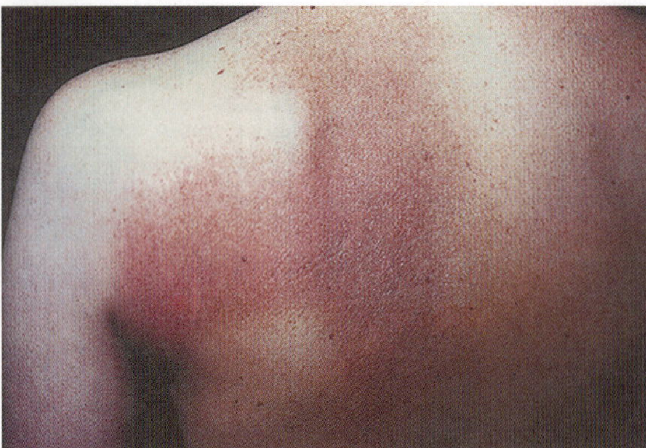

Fig. 16.14 Dry desquamation.

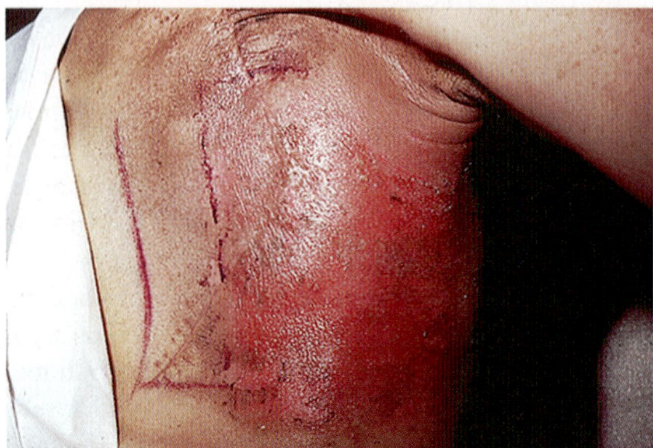

Fig. 16.15 Wet desquamation.

The goal of skin care is to prevent infection and promote wound healing. Although protocols vary, some basic principles apply. Protect radiated skin from temperature extremes. Do not use heating pads, ice packs, and hot water bottles in the treatment field. Avoid constricting garments, rubbing, harsh chemicals, and deodorants because they may traumatize the skin. Dry reactions are uncomfortable and cause pruritus. Lubricate dry skin with a nonirritating lotion emollient that contains no metal, alcohol, perfume, or additives. These can be irritating. Calendula ointment and topical hyaluronic acid cream are effective for managing radiation dermatitis. Aloe vera gel is useful for preventing skin problems.

Wet desquamation generally causes pain, drainage, and increased risk for infection. Skin care includes keeping tissues clean with normal saline compresses or 0.5% chlorhexidine solution. Protect the skin from further damage with soft, absorbent, silicone foam bandages. Reassess and clean the area every 24 to 48 hours. Because protocols vary widely, verify the guidelines in Table 16.11 with your agency's radiation oncology department.

Chemotherapy Skin Changes

Chemotherapy causes a wide range of skin problems. These can range from mild redness and hyperpigmentation to more serious acral erythema and *erythrodysesthesia syndrome* (hand-foot syndrome). Hand-foot syndrome causes mild redness and tingling of the palms of the hands and soles of the feet. It may also cause painful moist desquamation, ulceration, blistering, and pain.

Alopecia is an easily recognizable effect of cancer treatment.[14] Hair loss from radiation is local. Chemotherapy affects hair throughout the body. The degree and duration of hair loss depends on the type and dose of the chemotherapy agent. Alopecia from chemotherapy is usually reversible. Usually, the hair does not grow back until 3 to 4 weeks after the end of therapy. Sometimes the new hair is a different color and texture.

Scalp cooling may be used for certain chemotherapies to reduce alopecia. Cold caps are placed on the head before, during, and after a treatment. Common side effects are headache and cold sensation.

TABLE 16.11 PATIENT & CAREGIVER TEACHING

Radiation Skin Reactions

Include the following instructions when teaching the patient and caregiver to clean and protect the skin in a radiation treatment area:

1. Gently cleanse the skin in the treatment field using a mild soap (Dove, Basis), tepid water, a soft cloth, and a gentle patting motion. Rinse thoroughly and pat dry.
2. Apply nonmedicated, nonperfumed, moisturizing lotion or cream, such as calendula ointment, aloe gel, Aquaphor, or Eucerin cream, to alleviate dry skin. Some substances must be gently cleansed from the treatment field before each treatment and reapplied. Over-the-counter hydrocortisone cream 1% may reduce itching.
3. Avoid antiperspirants as these can increase the amount of radiation received. Deodorant may be used but should be discontinued if redness, swelling, or soreness develop.
4. Observe the area daily for signs of infection.
5. Avoid wearing tight-fitting clothing, including brassieres and belts, over the treatment field.
6. Avoid wearing harsh fabrics, such as wool and corduroy. A lightweight cotton garment is best. If possible, expose the treatment field to air.
7. Use gentle detergents (e.g., Tide Free and Gentle) to wash clothing that will come in contact with the treatment field.
8. Avoid direct exposure to the sun. If the treatment field is in an area that is exposed to the sun, wear protective clothing, such as a wide-brimmed hat, when out in the sun and apply sunscreen lotion.
9. Avoid all sources of excess heat (hot water bottles, heating pads, sunlamps) on the treatment field.
10. Avoid exposing the treatment field to cold temperatures (ice bags, cold weather).
11. Avoid swimming in salt water or in chlorinated pools while in treatment.
12. Avoid using potential irritants (e.g., perfumes, powders, or cosmetics) on the skin in the treatment field. Use other topical medications or lotions as directed by the HCP. Avoid tape, dressings, and adhesive bandages unless allowed by the radiation therapist.
13. Continue to protect sensitive skin after the treatment is completed. Do the following:
    - Avoid direct exposure to the sun. A sunscreen agent and protective clothing must be worn if the potential of exposure to the sun is present.
    - Use an electric razor if shaving is needed in the treatment field.

Patients have a range of emotions at the prospect of losing their hair and when hair loss occurs. They may have anger, grief, or embarrassment. Hair loss is a visible reminder of their cancer and the challenges of treatment. For some people, hair loss is one of the most stressful events experienced during treatment. The ACS's "Look Good, Feel Better" program is an excellent resource for people with hair loss and body image changes.

Lung Effects

Chemotherapy and radiation have the potential to cause irreversible and progressive lung damage. Distinguishing between the complications of treatment and those related to the disease can be challenging. There are acute and late effects of radiation on the lung. Acute effects can mimic symptoms (e.g., cough, dyspnea) that may have led to the cancer diagnosis.

Pneumonitis is a delayed acute inflammatory reaction that may occur within 1 to 6 months after completing thoracic radiation. Symptoms include cough, fever, chest congestion, dyspnea, and chest pain. Some patients may develop pulmonary fibrosis, a late effect of therapy.

Other common effects of chemotherapy include pulmonary edema (noncardiogenic) related to capillary leak syndrome or fluid retention, interstitial fibrosis, and pneumonitis due to an inflammatory reaction or destruction of alveolar-capillary endothelium.

Cardiovascular Effects

Radiation to the thorax can damage the pericardium, myocardium, valves, and coronary blood vessels. The pericardium is most often involved. Pericardial effusion and pericarditis are key problems. Patients with preexisting coronary artery disease are especially at risk.

Anthracyclines (e.g., doxorubicin, daunorubicin) cause cardiotoxicity. Acute cardiotoxicities may cause ECG changes. Late effects cause left ventricular dysfunction and heart failure. Baseline and periodic echocardiograms to monitor left ventricular function during treatment are usually done.

Cognitive Effects

Cognitive effects can happen at any time during cancer, especially after treatment. Patients describe this change in mental function, often called *chemo brain,* as mental cloudiness or fog. Patients can have altered short-term memory. Speech and learning ability can be affected. These effects can last a short time or for years. They can be so severe that patients may not be able to perform activities that require mental effort, including school, work, or social activities.[15]

Reproductive Effects

Reproductive problems from radiation and chemotherapy depend on the radiation treatment field and dosage, the chemotherapy drugs and dosage, and the patient (e.g., age). Treatment can cause temporary or permanent gonadal failure. Problems occur most often when reproductive organs are part of the radiation field or with alkylating drug treatment.

The testes are highly sensitive to radiation. We protect them with a testicular shield whenever possible. Combined modality treatment or prior chemotherapy with alkylating drugs enhances and prolongs the effects of radiation on the testes. When radiation is used alone with conventional doses and shielding, testicular recovery often occurs. Erectile dysfunction may occur after pelvic radiation.

The radiation dose that induces ovarian failure changes with age. With radiation therapy, we shield the ovaries whenever possible. The cervix and endometrium tissues can withstand a high radiation dose with minimal sequelae. This accounts for the ability to treat endometrial and cervical cancer with high external and brachytherapy doses. Acute reactions, such as tenderness, irritation, and loss of lubrication, can compromise sexual activity. Late effects of combined internal and external radiation therapy include vaginal shortening related to fibrosis and loss of elasticity and lubrication. After pelvic radiation, specific suggestions include using a water-soluble vaginal lubricant and a vaginal dilator.

Provide the patient and partner with information about the expected effects of treatment. Encourage discussion of issues related to reproduction and sexuality. Potential infertility can be a significant consequence. Counseling may be needed. We should address fertility preservation before starting cancer treatment. Pretreatment harvesting of sperm, ova, or ovarian tissue may be an option.[16]

Late Effects of Radiation and Chemotherapy

Radiation therapy and chemotherapy may cause long-term effects *(late effects)* that occur months to years after therapy.[17] They can affect every body system to some extent.

Late radiation effects occur most often in postmitotic cells (e.g., liver, kidney, lung, heart, muscle, bone, connective tissues). Once they occur, the late effects may be progressive and generally are permanent. Examples range from skin telangiectasias to strictures, fistulas, or radiation necrosis. Alteration of the lymphatic channels (e.g., axillary lymph node dissection) may contribute to lymphedema.

Long-term effects of chemotherapy include cardiac toxicity, cataracts, arthralgia, endocrine problems, renal insufficiency, hepatitis, osteoporosis, and neurocognitive problems. The additive effects of multiagent chemotherapy before, during, or after a course of radiation therapy can significantly increase the resulting late effects.

Cancer survivors may be at risk for secondary cancers, including leukemia, angiosarcoma, and skin cancer. Patients treated with alkylating drugs and those treated with high-dose radiation have an increased risk. The potential risk for developing secondary cancer does not contraindicate having cancer treatment.

IMMUNOTHERAPY AND TARGETED THERAPY

Immunotherapy uses the immune system, the body's main defense against infection and disease, to fight cancer. Immunotherapy can (1) boost or manipulate the immune system and create an environment that is not conducive for cancer cells to grow or (2) attack cancer cells directly. Immunotherapies are outlined in Table 16.12. Some types of immunotherapy are called *biologic response modifiers (BRMs)* or *biologics.* BRMs are discussed in Table 14.18.

Checkpoint inhibitors are one type of immunotherapy. T-cells have proteins that turn on an immune response when we have an infection and proteins that turn off the immune response when it is no longer needed. These proteins are called checkpoint proteins. Immune checkpoint inhibitors work by blocking the function of checkpoint proteins by preventing the

TABLE 16.12 Drug Therapy

Immunotherapy and Targeted Therapy

Type and Mechanism of Action	Examples
Angiogenesis Inhibitors	
Bind vascular endothelial growth factor (VEGF), thereby inhibiting angiogenesis.	bevacizumab (Avastin) pazopanib (Votrient) ramucirumab (Cyramza) cabozantinib (Cometriq) lenvatinib mesylate (Lenvima)
CD20 Monoclonal Antibodies	
Bind CD20 antigen, causing cytotoxicity and radiation injury.	ibritumomab tiuxetan/yttrium-90 (Zevalin)
Bind CD20 antigen, causing cytotoxicity.	ofatumumab (Arzerra) rituximab (Rituxan) ocrelizumab (Ocrevus)
CD52 Monoclonal Antibody	
Bind CD52 antigen (found on T and B cells, monocytes, natural killer [NK] cells, neutrophils).	alemtuzumab (Campath)
Cytokines (see Table 14.3)	
Inhibit DNA and protein synthesis. Suppress cell proliferation. ↑ Cytotoxic effects of NK cells.	α-interferon (Intron A)
Stimulate proliferation of T and B cells. Activate NK cells.	interleukin-2 (aldesleukin [Proleukin])
Human Epidermal Growth Factor Receptor-2 (HER-2)	
Monoclonal antibody to HER-2 that attaches to the antigen. It is taken into the cells and eventually kills them.	pertuzumab (Perjeta) trastuzumab (Herceptin)
Trastuzumab with the chemotherapy drug DM1.	ado-trastuzumab emtansine (Kadcyla)
Immunomodulatory Drugs (IMiDs)	
Inhibit production of tumor necrosis factor (TNF), IL-6, and VEGF, leading to antiangiogenic effects. Stimulate T and NK cells. ↑ γ-interferon and IL-2 production.	apremilast (Otezla) lenalidomide (Revlimid) pomalidomide (Pomalyst) thalidomide (Thalomid)
Kinase Inhibitors	
Anaplastic Lymphoma Kinase (ALK) Inhibitors	
Inhibit ALK.	ceritinib (Zykadia) crizotinib (Xalkori) entrectinib (Rozlytrek)
BCR-ABL Tyrosine Kinase Inhibitors	
Inhibit BCR-ABL TK. Primarily used in chronic myeloid leukemia.	bosutinib (Bosulif) dasatinib (Sprycel) imatinib (Gleevec) nilotinib (Tasigna)
BRAF Kinase Inhibitors	
Inhibit BRAF enzymes.	dabrafenib (Tafinlar) vemurafenib (Zelboraf) encorafenib (Braftovi)
Inhibit MEK enzymes.	trametinib (Mekinist) cobimetinib (Cotellic) binimetinib (Mektovi)
EGFR Tyrosine Kinase (TK) Inhibitors	
Inhibit epidermal growth factor receptor (EGFR) TK.	cetuximab (Erbitux) erlotinib gefitinib (Iressa) panitumumab (Vectibix)
Inhibit EGFR-TK and bind HER-2.	lapatinib (Tykerb)
Multi-Tyrosine Kinase Inhibitors	
Inhibit multiple TKs.	axitinib (Inlyta) cabozantinib (Cometriq) pazopanib (Votrient) regorafenib (Stivarga) sorafenib (Nexavar) sunitinib (Sutent) vandetanib (Caprelsa)
mTOR Kinase Inhibitors	
Inhibit the mechanistic target of rapamycin (mTOR) protein.	everolimus (Afinitor) temsirolimus (Torisel)
Programmed Death Receptor (PD)-1 Blockers	
Block PD-1, a protein on T cells that normally helps keep T cells from attacking other cells. This boosts immune response against cancer cells.	nivolumab (Opdivo) pembrolizumab (Keytruda) dostarlimab (Jemperli)
Proteasome Inhibitors	
Inhibit proteasome activity, which functions to regulate cell growth.	bortezomib (Velcade) carfilzomib (Kyprolis)
Vaccines	
Live attenuated strain of *Mycobacterium bovis* induces immune response. Used intravesically to treat bladder cancer (see Chapter 50).	Bacille Calmette-Guérin (BCG) vaccine
Stimulates the immune system against prostate cancer (see Chapter 59).	sipuleucel-T (Provenge)

"off" switch from being sent. This allows an increased immune response.[18]

Chimeric antigen (CAR) T-cell therapy uses T cells taken from the patient's blood. They are changed in a lab by adding a gene receptor that fights a specific cancer antigen. These cells are then given back to the patient to fight their cancer. This treatment is approved for some types of lymphoma and leukemia.

Targeted therapy interferes with cancer growth by targeting specific cell receptors and pathways that are important in tumor growth.[18,19] Targeted therapies work at sites that are on the cell surface, at the intracellular level, or in the extracellular domain (Fig. 16.16 and Table 16.12). We classify targeted therapies as small or large molecule drugs. Small molecule drugs are small enough to enter a cancer cell and work inside the cell. A large molecule drug usually cannot enter a cell. They work by attaching to targets on the cell. Because targeted therapies are selective for specific molecular targets, an advantage is that they do less damage to normal cells than chemotherapy.

A key class of targeted therapy is tyrosine kinase inhibitors. Tyrosine kinases are enzymes responsible for activating many proteins by signal transduction cascades. EGFR is a transmembrane molecule that activates intracellular tyrosine kinase (TK). Overexpression of EGFR is associated with unregulated cell growth and a poor prognosis. Drugs that inhibit EGFR suppress cell proliferation and promote *apoptosis* (programmed cell death).

EGFRs belong to the same receptor family as HER-2. HER-2 is overexpressed in certain cancers (especially breast cancers). It is associated with more aggressive disease and decreased survival. Trastuzumab (Herceptin) is a drug mainly used to treat breast cancer. It binds to HER-2 and inhibits the growth of breast cancer cells that overexpress HER-2.

Chronic myeloid leukemia (CML) cells make an abnormal active enzyme called BCR-ABL tyrosine kinase. Drugs, such as imatinib (Gleevec), that inhibit this enzyme suppress proliferation of CML cells and promote cell death.

Antibodies are proteins made by the immune system that bind to a target antigen on the cell surface. Because each antibody is specific to an antigen, that mechanism is used to develop specific drugs to treat cancer. Monoclonal antibodies (MoAb) work in this manner.

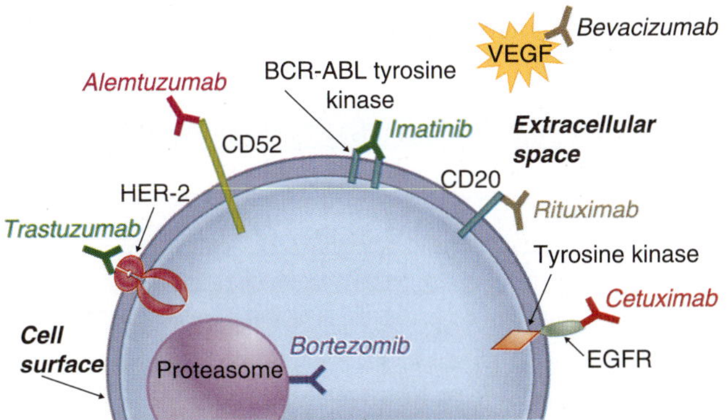

Fig. 16.16 Sites of action of targeted therapy. Examples of targeted therapy drugs that work at the specific site of action are shown in colored, italicized font. *EGFR*, Epidermal growth factor receptor; *HER-2*, human epidermal growth factor receptor-2; *VEGF*, vascular endothelial growth factor.

Angiogenesis inhibitors prevent the mechanisms and pathways necessary for tumor vascularization. Bevacizumab (Avastin), a recombinant human MoAb, binds with vascular endothelial growth factor (VEGF), a compound that stimulates blood vessel growth. When this occurs, VEGF cannot bind with its receptors on vascular endothelial cells and promote new vessel formation. This inhibits further tumor growth.

Proteasomes are intracellular multienzyme complexes that degrade proteins. In cancer cells, proteasome inhibitors (e.g., bortezomib [Velcade]) promote the accumulation of proteins, leading to cell death.

Cancer cells can become resistant to targeted therapies. This can occur because (1) the target changes through mutation and the therapy no longer interacts with it, and (2) the tumor finds a new growth pathway and no longer depends on the target. Because of the risk of resistance, targeted therapies work best in combination treatments such as with a chemotherapy drug.

Side Effects

The administration of immunotherapy usually induces the endogenous release of other agents. The release and action of these agents result in systemic immune and inflammatory responses. The toxicities and side effects are related to dose and schedule.

Common side effects are flu-like symptoms, including headache, fever, chills, myalgias, fatigue, malaise, weakness, photosensitivity, anorexia, and nausea. Those receiving interferon therapy almost always have flu-like symptoms. The severity generally decreases over time. Bone marrow depression is generally more transient and less severe than that with chemotherapy.

Tachycardia and orthostatic hypotension are common. IL-2 and MoAbs can cause *capillary leak syndrome*, which can result in pulmonary edema. A wide range of neurologic problems can occur with interferon and IL-2. Other side effects involve the renal, hepatic, and cardiovascular systems.

MoAbs are given IV. Patients may have infusion-related symptoms, including fever, chills, hives, mucosal congestion, nausea, diarrhea, and myalgias. Hypertension and liver toxicity can occur.

Skin rashes are common in patients receiving EGFR inhibitors. They generally manifest as redness and acneiform-like rash that can cover a large part of the upper body. Angiogenesis inhibitors can cause arterial thrombi, hemorrhage, hypertension, impaired wound healing, and proteinuria.

❖ NURSING MANAGEMENT: IMMUNOTHERAPY AND TARGETED THERAPY

Some problems experienced by patients receiving immunotherapy and targeted therapy occur more acutely and are dose limited (e.g., effects resolve when therapy is over). Combining these agents with chemotherapy expands the spectrum of treatment-related effects. Assess the patient's side effects and tolerance. Proactive nursing care can prevent some problems. Interventions to manage side effects can improve quality of life.

Capillary leak syndrome and pulmonary edema often require critical care nursing. Nursing interventions for flu-like syndrome include giving acetaminophen before treatment and every 6 hours after treatment. Large amounts of fluids reduce symptom severity. IV meperidine (Demerol) can help control severe chills or rigors.

Other care includes monitoring vital signs and temperature, planning for rest periods, assisting with activities of daily living (ADLs), and monitoring for adequate oral intake. Teach patients and caregivers to observe for neurologic problems (e.g., confusion, memory loss, difficulty making decisions, insomnia), report their occurrence, and institute safety and support measures.

HORMONE THERAPY

The hormones estrogen and progesterone can enhance the growth of some breast cancers. Androgen (testosterone) can enhance the growth of some prostate cancers. When given as a cancer treatment, hormone therapy drugs can block the effects of the hormone and stop the growth of cancer cells (Table 16.13). Surgery (oophorectomy, orchiectomy) can be done to remove the effects of the hormone on cancer growth.

TABLE 16.13 Drug Therapy

Hormone Therapy

Type and Mechanism of Action	Examples
Androgen Receptor Blockers	
Selectively attach to androgen receptors, blocking androgen from binding. Inhibits tumor growth.	bicalutamide (Casodex), enzalutamide (Xtandi), apalutamide (Erleada), darolutamide (Nubeqa)
Aromatase Inhibitors	
Inhibit aromatase, thus preventing estrogen production.	anastrozole (Arimidex), exemestane (Aromasin), letrozole (Femara)
Estrogens	
Interfere with the effect of testosterone.	estradiol, estramustine (Emcyt), estrogen (Menest)
Estrogen Receptor Blockers	
Selectively attach to estrogen receptors, blocking estrogen from binding. Inhibits tumor growth.	fulvestrant (Faslodex), tamoxifen, toremifene (Fareston)
Estrogen Receptor Modulator	
Has both estrogen-agonistic effects on bone and estrogen-antagonistic effects on breast tissue.	raloxifene (Evista)

HEMATOPOIETIC GROWTH FACTORS

Hematopoietic growth factors are used to support patients through their cancer treatment (Table 16.14). Colony-stimulating factors (CSFs) are a family of glycoproteins made by various cells. CSFs stimulate production, maturation, regulation, and activation of cells of the hematologic system. The name of the CSF is based on the specific cell line it affects.

Erythropoiesis-stimulating agents (ESAs) can be used to treat anemia from chemotherapy that is not intended to cure. ESA use has safety concerns when the target hemoglobin is greater than 12 g/dL. They can cause thromboembolic and cardiovascular events and increase the risk of death. Therefore we give the lowest dose that will gradually increase hemoglobin to the lowest level sufficient to avoid the need for blood transfusion. Monitor the hemoglobin level regularly.

HEMATOPOIETIC STEM CELL TRANSPLANTATION

Hematopoietic stem cell transplantation (HSCT) and **peripheral stem cell transplantation (PSCT)** are effective, life-saving treatments for several malignant and nonmalignant diseases (Table 16.15). Both allow for the safe use of very high doses of chemotherapy and/or radiation therapy in patients whose tumors have developed resistance (refractory) or did not respond to standard doses of chemotherapy and radiation. Overall, cure rates are steadily increasing. Even when a cure is not achieved, a transplant can result in a period of remission. The drawback is that patients may have long-term or delayed complications that can affect quality of life.

Many call either procedure a "bone marrow transplant." This is because when it was first developed, bone marrow was the source of stem cells. However, advances in harvesting and cryopreservation have opened new pathways to collecting stem

TABLE 16.14 Drug Therapy

Hematopoietic Growth Factors

Growth Factor	Drug Name	Indications	Side Effects
Erythropoietin	epoetin alfa (Epogen, Procrit)	Anemia of chronic cancer	↑ BP, thrombosis, headache
	darbepoetin alfa (Aranesp)	Anemia related to chemotherapy	↑ BP, thrombosis, headache
Granulocyte colony-stimulating factor (G-CSF)	filgrastim (Neupogen) filgrastim-sndz (Zarxio) pegfilgrastim (Neulasta) tbo-filgrastim (Granix)	Chemotherapy-induced neutropenia	Bone pain, nausea, vomiting
Granulocyte-macrophage colony-stimulating factor (GM-CSF)	sargramostim (Leukine)	Myeloid cell recovery after bone marrow transplant	Nausea, vomiting, diarrhea, fever, chills, myalgia, headache, fatigue
Interleukin-11 (platelet growth factor)	oprelvekin (Neumega)	Thrombocytopenia related to chemotherapy	Fluid retention, peripheral edema, dyspnea, ↑ HR, nausea, mouth sores

TABLE 16.15 Indications for Hematopoietic Stem Cell Transplant

Malignant Diseases
- Acute and chronic lymphocytic leukemia
- Acute and chronic myelogenous leukemia
- Hodgkin lymphoma
- Multiple myeloma
- Myelodysplastic syndrome
- Non-Hodgkin lymphoma

Nonmalignant Diseases
- Aplastic anemia
- Chronic granulomatous disease
- Fanconi anemia
- Hematologic diseases
- Immunodeficiency diseases
- Severe combined immunodeficiency disease (SCID)
- Sickle cell disease (severe)
- Thalassemia
- Wiskott-Aldrich syndrome

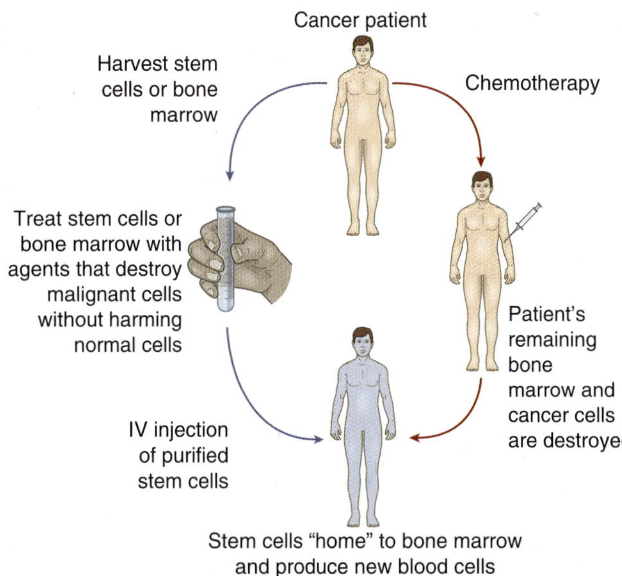

Fig. 16.17 Autologous stem cell transplant.

cells from the peripheral blood.[20] Therefore the terminology has changed.

The approach in HSCT is to eradicate diseased tumor cells and/or clear the bone marrow of its components to make way for engraftment of the transplanted, healthy stem cells. This is done by giving higher than usual dosages of chemotherapy with or without radiation therapy. Life-threatening consequences from pancytopenia and other adverse effects can result. After chemotherapy and radiation therapy are over, healthy stem cells are infused. These healthy stem cells "rescue" the damaged bone marrow through subsequent proliferation and differentiation of the donated stem cells in the recipient.

HSCT is an intensive procedure with many risks. Some patients die of treatment-related complications or from recurrence of the original disease. Because it is a highly toxic therapy, patients must weigh the significant risks for treatment-related death or treatment failure (relapse) against the hope of a cure.

Types of Hematopoietic Stem Cell Transplants

We categorize HSCTs as allogeneic, syngeneic, or autologous. The sources of stem cells include bone marrow, peripheral blood, and umbilical cord blood. In an *allogeneic transplant,* stem cells are acquired from a donor (graft) who, through human leukocyte antigen (HLA) tissue typing, has been HLA matched to the recipient (host). HLA typing involves testing WBCs to identify genetically inherited antigens common to both donor and recipient that are important in the compatibility of transplanted tissue. HLA tissue typing is discussed in Chapter 14. The donor is often a family member. It may be an unrelated donor found through a national or international bone marrow registry. These are known as matched unrelated donor (MUD) transplants. Increased risks and toxicities may be associated with an MUD. Common indications for allogeneic transplant are certain leukemias, multiple myeloma, and lymphoma.

A *syngeneic transplant* is a type of allogeneic transplant that involves obtaining stem cells from one identical twin and infusing them into the other. Identical twins have identical HLA types and are a perfect match.

In *autologous transplants,* patients receive their own stem cells back after *myeloablative* (destroying bone marrow) chemotherapy (Fig. 16.17). The aim of this approach is "rescue." It allows patients to receive intensive chemotherapy and radiation by supporting them with their previously harvested stem cells until their marrow generates blood cells again on its own. Restoration usually takes about 4 to 6 weeks.

Procedures

Harvest Procedures

Hematopoietic stem cells are *harvested* from a donor (allogeneic transplant) or the recipient (autologous transplant) via 2 methods. Harvesting stem cells from bone marrow is done in the operating room using general or spinal anesthesia. Multiple bone marrow aspirations (usually from the iliac crest, sometimes the sternum) are carried out to obtain stem cells. The harvested marrow is processed to strain out bone fragments. The entire bone marrow harvest procedure takes about 1 to 2 hours. The patient can be discharged after recovery. Postharvest, the donor may have pain at the collection site that lasts up to 7 days. It can be treated with mild analgesics. The donor's body will replenish the removed bone marrow in a few weeks.

Peripheral stem cell transplants are obtained from the peripheral blood in an outpatient procedure. Cell separator equipment automatically separates the stem cells from the blood circulating through the machine and returns the remaining blood components to the donor. The process takes about 2 to 4 hours. Sometimes it takes longer depending on donor factors and the quality of the venous access. Often it takes more than 1 procedure to obtain enough stem cells. Because blood has fewer stem cells than bone marrow, "mobilizing" stem cells from the bone marrow into the peripheral blood can be achieved with chemotherapy and/or hematopoietic growth factors.

Growth factors, such as granulocyte-macrophage colony-stimulating factor (GM-CSF) and granulocyte colony-stimulating factor (G-CSF), may be given to increase stem cell production for collection (Table 16.14). When patients receive growth factors for mobilization, stem cells are harvested 4 or 5 days after growth factor injections.

After collection, the marrow or peripheral stem cells are used immediately or bagged with preservatives for cryopreservation and stored until they are needed. Because they come from the patient, autologous stem cells are sometimes treated (purged) to remove undetected cancer cells. Many different pharmacologic, immunologic, physical, and chemical agents are used for this purpose.

Umbilical cord blood is rich in hematopoietic stem cells. Successful allogeneic transplants have been done using this source. Cord blood can be HLA-typed and cryopreserved. A disadvantage of cord blood is the risk of insufficient numbers of stem cells to allow a transplant to adults. Considerable research is currently ongoing to define the optimal use of this technology.

Preparative Regimens and Stem Cell Infusions

Patients receive myeloablative dosages of chemotherapy with or without adjunctive radiation to treat the underlying disease. Total-body irradiation (TBI) can be used for immunosuppression or to treat the disease. These preparative therapies are known as the *conditioning regimen.*

Stem cell infusions are given IV. They can be injected via the slow bolus method or infused, much like a blood transfusion (using tubing without a filter). The infused stem cells reconstitute the bone marrow elements, "rescuing" the recipient's hematopoietic system. It usually takes 2 to 4 weeks for the transplanted marrow to start making hematopoietic blood cells. During this period, the patient has pancytopenia. The patient must be protected from exposure to infection and supported with electrolyte supplements, nutrition, and blood component transfusions (as needed) to maintain adequate levels of circulating RBCs and platelets.

Complications

Bacterial, viral, and fungal infections are common after HSCT. Prophylactic therapies are used to reduce their incidence. A potentially serious complication of allogeneic transplant is graft-versus-host disease. This occurs when the T cells from the donated marrow (graft) recognize the recipient (host) as foreign and begin to attack certain organs, such as the skin, liver, and GI tract. Graft-versus-host disease is discussed in Chapter 14.

The occurrence and severity of posttransplant complications depend on the drugs used (some are more toxic than others) and the stem cell source. Because stem cells in the peripheral blood are more mature than those harvested from the marrow, the hematologic recovery period in PSCT is shorter, and fewer, less severe complications occur.

CANCER COMPLICATIONS

Patients may develop complications related to the cancer growing into normal tissue or to the side effects of treatment.

NUTRITION PROBLEMS

Malnutrition

Patients may have protein and calorie malnutrition with fat and muscle depletion. Promoting optimal nutrition is discussed in Chapter 44. If malnutrition cannot be treated with diet intake, it may be necessary to use enteral or parenteral nutrition.

Soft, nonirritating, high-protein, and high-calorie foods should be eaten throughout the day. Teach patients to avoid extremes of temperature, tobacco, alcohol, spicy or rough foods, and other irritants. Encourage nutrition supplements (e.g., Ensure) as an adjunct to meals and fluid intake. Nutrition supplements can be used in place of milk when cooking or baking. Foods to which supplements can be easily added include scrambled eggs, pudding, custard, mashed potatoes, cereal, and cream sauces. Instant supplements can be used as indicated or sprinkled on cereals and other foods. Caregivers may need to help the patient with eating.

Weigh the patient at least twice each week to monitor for weight loss. Suggest a referral for diet counseling to the patient or HCP as soon as a 5% weight loss is noted or if the patient has impaired nutrition. Monitor albumin and prealbumin levels. Once a 10-lb (4.5-kg) weight loss occurs, it may be hard to maintain nutrition status.

Altered Taste (Dysgeusia)

Cancer cells may release substances that stimulate the bitter taste buds. Patients may have changes in the sweet, sour, and salty taste sensations. Meat may taste bitter or bland. We do not know the cause of these taste changes.

Teach patients with taste problems to avoid foods that they dislike. Often, patients may feel compelled to eat certain foods they believe are beneficial. Tell patients to try different ways to mask the taste changes. Some find stronger seasonings and spices effective. Others find it better to avoid strong flavors and eat more bland foods. Avoiding strong smells, drinking more water with food, oral care before eating, eating smaller amounts more often, and using plastic utensils may help.[21]

Cancer Cachexia

Cancer cachexia (wasting syndrome) is a complex, multifactorial syndrome characterized by anorexia and/or unintended loss of weight and appetite. It is accompanied by general tissue wasting, skeletal muscle atrophy, immune dysfunction, and metabolic problems. Nutrition therapy cannot reverse weight loss. Patients with upper GI and pancreatic cancers are prone to cachexia. As cancer progresses, cachexia can affect many cancer patients. It is associated with increased morbidity.[22]

The best way to manage cancer cachexia is to treat the cancer. Unfortunately, this is not a realistic goal for patients with advanced cancer. A second option is to increase intake, but this does not completely reverse the wasting. A third option is to use megestrol acetate. It is a synthetic form of the hormone progesterone, which stimulates appetite in patients with cachexia.

INFECTION

Infection is a leading cause of death in patients with cancer. Common sites of infection include the lungs, GU system, mouth, rectum, peritoneal cavity, and blood (septicemia). Infection occurs because of the ulceration and necrosis caused by the tumor, the tumor compressing vital organs, and neutropenia from the cancer or cancer treatment.

Teach patients at risk for neutropenia to call their HCP if they have a temperature of 100.4°F (38°C) or greater. Assessment often includes signs and symptoms of fever, determining the possible cause (e.g., sinuses, mucous membranes, respiratory, GI, urinary, sites of any tubes or lines), and CBC.

Many patients are neutropenic when an infection develops. In these persons, infection may cause significant morbidity. It may be rapidly fatal if not treated promptly. The classic manifestations of infection are often subtle or absent in patients with neutropenia and a depressed immune system. Neutropenia is discussed in Chapter 34.

ONCOLOGIC EMERGENCIES

Oncologic emergencies are life-threatening emergencies that occur because of cancer or cancer treatment. Emergencies can be obstructive, metabolic, or infiltrative (Table 16.16).

Tumor obstruction of an organ or blood vessel causes most obstructive emergencies. Problems include superior vena cava syndrome (Fig. 16.18), spinal cord compression syndrome, third space syndrome, and intestinal obstruction. Infiltrative emergencies occur when cancer infiltrates major organs or from cancer treatment. The most common infiltrative emergencies are cardiac tamponade and carotid artery rupture.

Metabolic emergencies are caused by the production of ectopic hormones directly from the tumor or from metabolic problems caused by the cancer or cancer treatment. Ectopic hormones arise from tissues that do not normally make these hormones. Cancer cells return to a more embryonic form, thus allowing the cells' stored potential to become evident.

Metabolic emergencies include syndrome of inappropriate antidiuresis (see Chapter 54), hypercalcemia (see Chapter 17), tumor lysis syndrome, septic shock (see Chapter 44), and disseminated intravascular coagulation (see Chapter 34).

CANCER PAIN

Moderate to severe pain occurs in around 59% of patients who are receiving active treatment for cancer and 64% of patients with advanced cancer.[23] Pain is a cancer symptom that patients fear, and unfortunately, undertreatment of cancer pain is common. Ineffective pain management causes needless suffering, decreases quality of life, and increases caregiver burden.

Pain Assessment

Inadequate pain assessment is the single greatest barrier to effective pain management. Data, such as vital signs and patient behaviors, are not reliable indicators of pain, especially long-standing, chronic pain. Determine whether pain is persistent or episodic, positional, or breakthrough pain. Obtain a comprehensive pain assessment (Table 16.17). Include the quality, location, intensity, duration, and precipitating and alleviating factors. Distinguishing between types of pain (e.g., visceral, somatic, neuropathic) is important in developing an effective pain management plan.

Assess pain on an ongoing basis to determine the effectiveness of the treatment plan. Obtain data and document at regular intervals the location and intensity of the pain, what it feels like, and how it is relieved. Assess change in pain (e.g., a change in the intensity, character, worsening, or location) to determine the cause (e.g., disease progression). Having patients keep a pain management diary may help.[23]

Pain Management

Pain management must address both persistent and breakthrough components of pain if they are present. Adjuvant therapies need to be delivered specific to the type or nature of the pain.

Drug therapy, including NSAIDs (e.g., ibuprofen), opioids (e.g., morphine), and adjuvant pain medications, should be used and selected based on the character and cause of the pain. Opioids normally are prescribed for the treatment of moderate to severe cancer pain. Corticosteroids are part of many drug regimens. They are antiinflammatory, reducing swelling and inflammation, which may contribute to cancer pain.

Drug dosages are adjusted to control pain with the fewest side effects. Analgesic medications (e.g., morphine, fentanyl) should be given on a regular schedule (around the clock) with more doses available as needed for breakthrough pain. In general, oral administration is preferred. Other routes (e.g., transdermal, transmucosal) are options.

Treatment plans should be developed that balance analgesia and side effects to maintain optimal functional status. It is important for you to pay attention to common side effects of pain medications (e.g., constipation) to ensure the patient's well-being and adherence to the pain management program. NSAIDs often serve as helpful adjuncts to opioid therapy, especially for bone pain. Antidepressant and antiseizure drugs may be helpful in managing neuropathic pain, which is often resistant to opioids.

Radioactive drugs (e.g., radium 223) may help patients with symptomatic diffuse bone metastases. Nerve blocks or epidural or intrathecal analgesia may help patients with unrelieved pain or to minimize opioid use.

TABLE 16.16 Oncologic Emergencies

Description	Manifestations	Management
Obstructive Emergencies		
Spinal Cord Compression		
• Neurologic emergency caused by cancer in epidural space of spinal cord. • Common causes are breast, lung, prostate, GI, renal cancers, melanoma. • Lymphomas can invade epidural space.	• Intense, local, and persistent back pain with vertebral tenderness. • Motor weakness, sensory paresthesia, and loss. • Autonomic dysfunction (e.g., change in bowel or bladder function).	• Radiation therapy, corticosteroids. • Surgical decompressive laminectomy. • Activity limitations and pain management.
Superior Vena Cava Syndrome (SVCS)		
• Results from obstruction of superior vena cava by tumor or thrombosis. • Common causes are lung cancer, non-Hodgkin lymphoma, metastatic breast cancer. • Presence of central venous catheter and previous mediastinal radiation increase risk.	• Facial edema, periorbital edema. • Distention of veins of head, neck, and chest. • Headache, seizures. • Mediastinal mass on chest x-ray.	• Serious medical problem. • Radiation therapy to site of obstruction. • Chemotherapy for tumors more sensitive to this therapy.
Third Space Syndrome		
• Shifting of fluid from vascular space to interstitial space. • Occurs due to extensive surgical procedures, immunotherapy, septic shock.	• Signs of hypovolemia: ↓ BP, ↑ HR, ↓ central venous pressure, ↓ urine output.	• Fluid, electrolyte, plasma protein replacement. • During recovery hypervolemia can occur, causing ↑ BP, ↑ central venous pressure, weight gain, shortness of breath.
Metabolic Emergencies		
Hypercalcemia		
• Occurs in metastatic bone disease, multiple myeloma, or when cancer cells secrete a parathyroid hormone–like substance. • Immobility and dehydration can contribute to or worsen hypercalcemia.	• Serum calcium higher than 12 mg/dL (3 mmol/L) often produces symptoms. • Apathy, depression, fatigue, muscle weakness, ECG changes, polyuria and nocturia, anorexia, nausea, vomiting. • High calcium elevations can be life threatening. • Chronic hypercalcemia can result in renal failure.	• Treat primary disease. • Hydration (3 L/day) • Diuretics (especially loop diuretics) used to prevent heart failure or edema. • Infusion of bisphosphonate zoledronate or pamidronate (Aredia). • RANKL inhibitor injection, denosumab (Xgeva)
Syndrome of Inappropriate Antidiuresis (SIAD)		
• Tumor cells can produce abnormal or sustained production of antidiuretic hormone (ADH). • Many chemotherapy drugs may contribute to ectopic ADH production or potentiate ADH effects.	• Water retention and hyponatremia (hypotonic hyponatremia) (see Chapter 49). • Weight gain without edema, weakness, anorexia, nausea, vomiting, personality changes, seizures, oliguria, ↓ in reflexes, coma.	• Treat underlying cancer. • Take measures to correct sodium-water imbalance, including fluid restriction, oral salt tablets or isotonic (0.9%) saline administration, and IV 3% sodium chloride solution (severe cases). • Furosemide used in early phases. • Monitor sodium level. Correcting SIAD quickly may cause seizures or death.
Tumor Lysis Syndrome (TLS)		
• Metabolic complication characterized by rapid release of intracellular components in response to chemotherapy and radiation therapy (less often). • Massive cell destruction releases intracellular components (potassium, phosphate, DNA, RNA) that are metabolized to uric acid by liver.	• *Hallmark signs:* hyperuricemia, hyperphosphatemia, hyperkalemia, hypocalcemia. • Weakness, muscle cramps, diarrhea, nausea, vomiting, cardiac dysrhythmia, seizure, syncope. • Occurs within 24–48 h after starting chemotherapy. • May last 5–7 days. • Metabolic abnormalities and concentrated uric acid (which crystallizes in distal tubules of kidneys) can lead to acute kidney injury.	• Identify patients at risk. • Monitor for and address abnormal electrolyte values. • Maintain high urine output with hydration therapy. • Decrease uric acid concentration with allopurinol. • Implement safety precautions.

Continued

TABLE 16.16 Oncologic Emergencies—cont'd

Description	Manifestations	Management
Infiltrative Emergencies		
Cardiac Tamponade		
• Fluid accumulation in pericardium. • Caused by constriction of pericardium by tumor or pericarditis from radiation therapy to the chest.	• Heavy feeling over chest, shortness of breath, ↑ HR, cough, dysphagia, hiccups, hoarseness. • Nausea, vomiting, excess perspiration. • ↓ Level of consciousness, distant or muted heart sounds. • Extreme anxiety.	• Decrease fluid around heart using (1) surgery to create a pericardial window or (2) an indwelling pericardial catheter. • Administer O_2 therapy, IV hydration, vasopressor therapy.
Carotid Artery Rupture		
• Invasion of arterial wall by tumor or erosion following surgery or radiation therapy. • Occurs most often in patients with head and neck cancer.	• Bleeding: ranges from minor oozing to spurting of blood in the case of a "blowout" of artery.	• Give IV fluids and blood products. • Surgery: ligation of carotid artery above and below rupture site and reduction of local tumor.

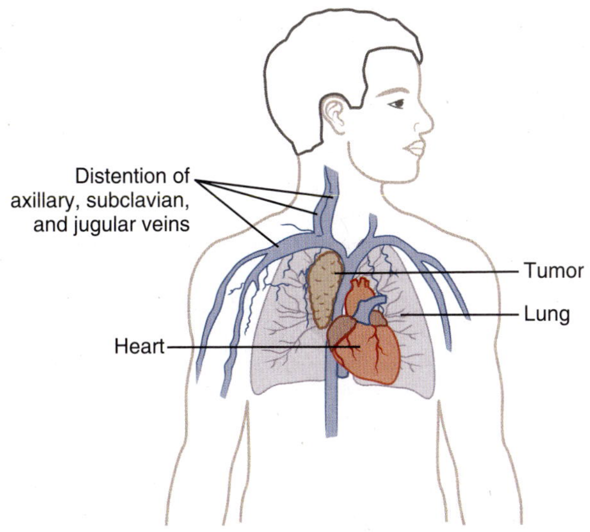

Fig. 16.18 Superior vena cava obstruction in bronchial cancer.

TABLE 16.17 Pain Assessment in Cancer Patients

Characteristic	Questions to Ask
Location	• Where is the pain? • Is the pain in more than one place? Is the pain in a new location? • Does location of pain correlate with known diagnosis?
Intensity	• How bad is the pain? • Rate the pain on a scale of 0–10.
Quality	• What does the pain feel like—sharp, dull, burning, shooting, aching, or other?
Pattern	• Has the pain changed? • Is the pain getting better, worse, or unchanged? • What makes the pain better or worse?
Relief measures	• What do you do to control your pain? • Do you use medications? • Do the relief measures help much? How much?

Discuss pain management goals with patients, especially those needing large or chronic doses of opioids. Assess for risk factors for opioid misuse. Clarify myths and misconceptions. Reassure patients and caregivers that cancer pain can be effectively relieved. Address any fear of addiction. It is a significant barrier in pain management. Nondrug interventions, including relaxation therapy and imagery, are part of pain management (see Chapter 7). Other measures to relieve pain are discussed in Chapter 9.

COPING WITH CANCER

You play a key role in helping patients and caregivers cope with the psychosocial issues associated with cancer and cancer treatment. They may have a variety of concerns, including fears of dependency, loss of control, family and relationship stress, financial burden, and fear of death. Anxiety and fear may occur throughout the continuum, including at diagnosis, during or after treatment, and in association with long-term follow-up.

Repetitive office visits or hospitalizations, continuing medications, and frequent laboratory testing force patients to confront their cancer every day. Treatment-related uncertainties and fears are often most evident at the beginning of therapy. However, anxiety and fear may be present throughout treatment and when therapy is completed (e.g., fear of recurrence, less available support).

Several factors influence adaptation and coping with a cancer diagnosis. These include demographics, prior coping skills and strategies, social support, and religious and spiritual beliefs (Table 16.18). You are in a key position to assess the patient's and caregiver's responses and support positive coping

TABLE 16.18 Factors Affecting How Patients Cope With Cancer

Factor	Description
Ability to cope with past stressful events	How patients coped with previous stressful events (e.g., loss of job, major disappointment, significant traumatic event) affects how they cope with diagnosis of cancer.
Ability to express feelings and concerns	Patients who express feelings and needs and ask for help cope better than those who internalize feelings and needs.
Age at the time of diagnosis	Age determines coping strategies to a great degree. For example, a young mother and a 70-year-old female with cancer may have different concerns.
Attitude associated with the cancer	Patients who feel in control and have a positive outlook about cancer and cancer treatment cope better with the diagnosis and treatment of cancer than those who feel hopeless, helpless, and out of control.
Availability of significant others	Patients who have effective support systems cope better than those who do not.
Negative body image	Negative body image (e.g., deformity, ostomy, mastectomy) may intensify the psychologic impact of cancer.
Extent of disease	Cure or control of the disease process is usually easier to cope with than the reality of terminal illness.
Experience with cancer	Negative experiences with cancer (personal or with others) influence perceptions about the current situation.
Symptoms	Symptoms such as fatigue, nausea, diarrhea, and pain may intensify the psychologic impact of cancer.

strategies. To promote effective coping and to support them during the various stages of cancer, you should

- Be available and continue to be available, especially during difficult times.
- Be open, honest, and caring.
- Listen actively to fears and concerns.
- Help provide relief from distressing symptoms.
- Provide accurate, essential information about cancer and cancer care.
- Help establish realistic expectations about what the patient will experience.
- Maintain a relationship based on trust and confidence.
- Help the patient in setting realistic, reachable short-term and long-term goals.
- Help the patient maintain usual lifestyle patterns.
- Maintain hope, which is the key to effective cancer care.

Hope varies, depending on the patient's status—hope that the symptoms are not serious, hope that the treatment is curative, hope for independence, hope for relief of pain, hope for longer life, hope to achieve meaningful goals, or hope for a peaceful death. Hope provides control over what is occurring. It is the basis of a positive attitude toward cancer and cancer care.

Patients and caregivers need ongoing education and support. Give information and support to help minimize the negative impact of cancer treatment on quality of life. Teaching and symptom management help patients to self-manage their illness (e.g., adjusting treatment schedules to allow patients to work when possible, making referrals to support groups). Work with the oncology nurse navigators, who serve as the liaison between the patient and the health care team.

Arrange for patients to meet with people who have successfully completed therapy. This can increase their hopefulness and confidence. Make regular supportive telephone contacts between office visits. Assist with planning for transportation, nutrition, and emotional support.

Patients and caregivers may benefit from a variety of psychosocial interventions. These include supportive listening, stress management techniques, individual or group counseling, and cognitive-behavioral therapy. Assess psychosocial concerns and emotional responses so that you can connect them with supportive care resources. Use the available resources in the community, such as the ACS, Cancer Lifeline, churches, and other community resources.

Gerontologic Considerations: Cancer

Cancer is usually a disease of aging. Approximately 88% of cancers occur in people 50 years or older.[1] The percent of cancer deaths is highest in ages 65 to 74. This is especially important since the proportion of the population that is older than 65 years is increasing.

Manifestations of cancer in older adults may be mistakenly attributed to age-related changes and ignored by the person. Older adults are especially at risk for complications of both cancer and cancer treatment. This is due to a decline in physiologic functioning, social and emotional resources, and cognitive function.

Age alone is not a good predictor of tolerance or response to treatment. Advances in cancer treatment are making cancer therapies beneficial to more older adults, including those with suboptimal health. Use the cancer-specific geriatric assessment to predict treatment-related toxicities. It is a multidimensional assessment that includes comorbidity, functional status, nutritional status, social support, cognition, and psychologic status.[24]

Some important questions to consider when an older adult is diagnosed with cancer include: Will the treatment provide more benefits than harm? Will they be able to tolerate the treatment safely? Is there a need to treat comorbidities or nutrition or functional status before starting treatment? What are the patient's preferences and wishes (Box 16.2)?

BOX 16.2 ETHICAL/LEGAL DILEMMAS

Medical Futility

Situation

D.M., a 65-year-old female, has breast cancer with metastasis to the liver and bone. The family asks you why their mother is not receiving chemotherapy. They want to make sure that she will be resuscitated should her heart stop. They are aware of her diagnosis and that she only has a few weeks to live. In morning rounds, you hear that D.M. does not want any more treatment that would prolong her life.

Ethical/Legal Points for Consideration

- Although court decisions have varied, legally there is substantial consensus about the right to privacy (a constitutional right), right to informed consent and refusal of treatment, and rights about end-of-life decision making. The *Code of Ethics for Nurses* addresses the key components in the informed consent process that nurses must address.[1]
- An adult patient who is competent (defined as capable of understanding and interpreting information, making choices, and communicating those choices) solely retains the right to make personal health care decisions.
- The Patient Self-Determination Act requires that we ask patients on admission whether they have an advance directive. If available, place it in the medical record. Document if a patient does not have an advance directive.
- The National POLST Paradigm is an approach to end-of-life planning that emphasizes patients' wishes about the care they receive. It emphasizes medical orders and includes coverage regardless of location (e.g., hospital, home, assisted living).[2]
- Families may have difficulty accepting a terminal diagnosis.
- Sometimes family members have conflicting interests (e.g., finances, property, inheritance rights) that influence their decision-making abilities.

Discussion Questions

1. How can you help D.M. communicate her wishes to her family?
2. How can you help the family in planning end-of-life care that considers their mother's wishes?
3. Are there cultural issues that should be considered in D.M.'s case and if so, what would they be?

References

1. Code of Ethics for Nurses. Retrieved from www.nursingworld.org/practice-policy/nursing-excellence/ethics/code-of-ethics-for-nurses/.
2. Physician Orders for Life Sustaining Treatment (POLST) Paradigm. Retrieved from www.polst.org.

SURVIVORSHIP

As the overall death rate from cancer decreases, the number of cancer survivors continues to increase. There are currently more than 18 million cancer survivors in the United States. Some of these persons are cancer free. Others still have evidence of cancer and may be receiving treatment. The increase in survivorship is attributed to the aging and growth of the population and improvements in early detection and treatment. Survival statistics vary by the type and stage of cancer.[1,2]

We are developing a greater awareness of the long-term health and quality-of-life issues that a cancer diagnosis

TABLE 16.19 PATIENT & CAREGIVER TEACHING

Survivorship

You can help cancer survivors by doing the following:

1. Provide all cancer patients with a treatment summary and care plan outlining treatment exposures, risk for late effects, preventive care recommendations, and follow-up surveillance plan after completion of treatment.
   - Identify all members of the interprofessional team and their responsibilities for follow-up care.
   - Include referrals to supportive care and community resources that would help the patient in recovery or ongoing care.
2. Coordinate care among the oncology team, primary HCP, and other specialists.
3. Teach cancer survivors to look for and report any ongoing symptoms resulting from treatment, including late effects of radiation therapy and chemotherapy.
4. Teach cancer survivors healthy behaviors:
   - *Prevention:* good nutrition, exercise, smoking avoidance, maintaining proper weight, cardiac risk reduction, bone health.
   - *Early detection:* routine health screenings (e.g., breast, colon), cholesterol, diabetes, osteoporosis screening as recommended.
5. Encourage cancer survivors to have regular follow-up examinations with their HCP.
6. Assess for psychologic, financial, health insurance, or employment problems related to cancer. Assist patients in getting help if necessary.

TABLE 16.20 Resources for Cancer Survivors

Organization	Purpose
ACS Cancer Survivors Network	Provides survivorship information and resources and online forum for connecting with others affected by cancer. (https://csn.cancer.org/)
CancerCare	Provides a variety of free support services delivered by professional oncology social workers for patients and anyone else affected by cancer. (www.cancercare.org)
Cancer.Net	American Society of Clinical Oncology (ASCO) patient support site that includes extensive information and resources for cancer survivors. (www.cancer.net)
National Cancer Institute Office of Cancer Survivorship	Supports research into the short- and long-term physical, social, emotional, and economic effects of cancer survivorship. Offers educational and support resources for cancer survivors, caregivers, and advocates. (www.cancercontrol.cancer.gov/ocs/)
National Coalition for Cancer Survivorship	Advocates for quality cancer care. Seeks to teach patients and advocates about issues that affect the quality of life of cancer survivors. (www.canceradvocacy.org)
National Comprehensive Cancer Network	An alliance of leading cancer centers has developed patient and caregiver resources, including information to assist cancer survivors and their families with issues post treatment. (https://www.nccn.org/patientresources/patient-resources)

imposes. Cancer survivors have a variety of long-term and late effects after treatment. You need to be aware of the effects of the various treatments so that you can teach patients and their caregivers.

The impact of cancer and its treatment confers greater risk for non–cancer-related death and comorbidities (e.g., heart disease, diabetes, osteoporosis) among survivors. They may continue to have symptoms or impaired function related to treatment for years after treatment. Emotional issues can play a profound role in a patient's life after cancer. Many find living in uncertainty challenging. Cancer survivors often report financial, vocational, marital, and spiritual concerns long after treatment is over.

Some patients may wish to return to their normal lives as soon as possible. They may not go to scheduled follow-up appointments. Others become cancer advocates or active members of a support group. Still others allow their lives to revolve around cancer and may even resist giving up the illness role.

Tips to help cancer survivors are described in Table 16.19. Connecting cancer survivors to online support and resources can enhance positive health outcomes (Table 16.20).

BRIDGE TO NCLEX EXAMINATION

The number of the question corresponds to the same-numbered outcome at the beginning of the chapter.

1. When planning education for patients about early detection and cancer screening, the nurse is aware that:
   a. prostate cancer is the leading cause of death in males.
   b. breast cancer is the leading cause of cancer death in females.
   c. lung cancer is a leading cause of death among males and females.
   d. the incidence of thyroid cancer is higher in males compared with females.
2. The patient asks how cancer cells differ from normal cells. The response to this question is based on the knowledge that:
   a. Cancer cells mature faster and more rapidly.
   b. Normal cells do not exhibit contact inhibition.
   c. Cancer cells may regain a fetal appearance and function.
   d. Cancer cells only proliferate when there is a need for more cells.
3. Modifying alcohol use or smoking affects which stage of cancer development?
   a. Initiation
   b. Promotion
   c. Progression
   d. Maturation
4. The nurse is caring for a male who is preparing for surgery for lung cancer. He is withdrawn and tearful. He says that he is scared to die and leave his wife alone. The *most* effective nursing intervention is to use this opportunity to
   a. redirect the conversation.
   b. ask if he completed an advanced directive.
   c. let him communicate about the meaning of this experience.
   d. tell him about a grief support group for families of cancer patients.
5. The role of chemotherapy is to (**Select all that apply.**)
   a. cure cancer.
   b. control cancer.
   c. prevent cancer.
   d. provide palliation.
   e. stimulate oncogenes.
6. The *most* effective method of administering a chemotherapy agent that is a vesicant is to
   a. give it orally.
   b. give it intraarterially.
   c. use a central venous access device.
   d. use the smallest gauge needle through a peripheral line.
7. Teaching for a patient who is being treated with brachytherapy seeds for prostate cancer would include
   a. how to cope with hair loss.
   b. the risk of exposing others to radiation is low.
   c. the need to return monthly to have the seeds replaced.
   d. the need to avoid being around others due to the risk of radiation.
8. A patient on chemotherapy and pelvic radiation for metastatic prostate cancer has hematuria and a temperature of 100.8°F. What finding on the CBC would be the most serious?
   a. Hgb of 11.2 g/dL
   b. WBC count of 1.9×10^9/L
   c. Neutrophil count of 0.8×10/L
   d. Platelet count of 100,000 per microliter
9. The nurse is managing a patient on immunotherapy who develops flu-like symptoms, including headache, fatigue, and myalgias. What would the nurse include in the plan of care?
   a. Decrease fluid intake.
   b. Increase activity level.
   c. Administer dexamethasone.
   d. Give scheduled acetaminophen.
10. The nurse determines the patient understands how to manage diarrhea associated with chemotherapy when the patient states
    a. "I will only drink two glasses of liquid a day."
    b. "I should eat more fresh fruits and vegetables."
    c. "I will decrease fried and fatty foods in my diet."
    d. "Increasing the fiber in my diet will bulk up my stools."
11. What teaching would the nurse provide to a patient receiving cancer treatment who is having problems maintaining their weight?
    a. Counsel them to eat foods low in fiber.
    b. Recommend high-fat foods that are spicy.
    c. Stress the need for three large meals daily.
    d. Discuss the use of oral nutrition supplements.

12. A patient who recently started chemotherapy has uncontrollable nausea, diarrhea, muscle cramps, and dizziness. Which complication of cancer is this *most* likely caused by?
    a. Tumor lysis syndrome
    b. Third space syndrome
    c. Spinal cord compression
    d. Superior vena cava syndrome

13. A male who recently completed treatment for testicular cancer is having a hard time adjusting to the end of his active treatments. What can the nurse discuss as possible next steps? **(Select all that apply.)**
    a. Join a support group.
    b. Family counseling to discuss expectations.
    c. Encourage regular follow-up with his HCP.
    d. Teach about potential late effects of treatment.
    d. Provide the patient with a cancer survivorship care plan.

1. c; 2. c; 3. b; 4. c; 5. a, b, d; 6. c; 7. b; 8. c; 9. d; 10. c; 11. d; 12. a; 13. a, b, c, d, e.

For rationales to these answers and even more NCLEX review questions, visit http://evolve.elsevier.com/Lewis/medsurg.

REFERENCES

To access the References for this chapter, please scan the QR code with a mobile device.

17

Fluid, Electrolyte, and Acid-Base Imbalances

Margaret R. Rateau

http://evolve.elsevier.com/Lewis/medsurg/

CONCEPTUAL FOCUS

Acid-Base Balance
Fluid and Electrolytes
Perfusion
Safety

LEARNING OUTCOMES

1. Describe the composition of the major body fluid compartments.
2. Define processes involved in maintaining fluid and electrolyte balance.
3. Describe the etiology, manifestations, and interprofessional management of:
   a. Fluid imbalance: fluid volume deficit and fluid volume excess
   b. Sodium imbalance: hypernatremia and hyponatremia
   c. Potassium imbalance: hyperkalemia and hypokalemia
   d. Magnesium imbalance: hypermagnesemia and hypomagnesemia
   e. Calcium imbalance: hypercalcemia and hypocalcemia
   f. Phosphate imbalance: hyperphosphatemia and hypophosphatemia
4. Identify the processes involved in maintaining acid-base balance.
5. Discuss the etiology, manifestations, and nursing and interprofessional management of acid-base imbalances.
6. Describe the composition of and indications for common IV fluid solutions.
7. Discuss the types and nursing management of common central venous access devices.

KEY TERMS

acidosis
alkalosis
buffers
central venous access devices (CVADs)
electrolytes
hydrostatic pressure
hypercalcemia
hyperkalemia
hypernatremia
hypertonic
hypocalcemia
hypokalemia
hyponatremia
hypotonic
isotonic
osmolality

Fluids and electrolytes play an important role in maintaining *homeostasis,* the body's stable internal environment. Body fluids are in constant motion transporting nutrients, electrolytes, and oxygen to cells and carrying waste products away from cells. The body uses many adaptive processes to keep the composition and volume of fluids and electrolytes within narrow limits to maintain homeostasis and promote health.

Fluid and electrolyte imbalances occur in most patients with a major illness or injury because illness disrupts normal homeostatic processes. Illness or disease directly causes some fluid and electrolyte imbalances, like burns or heart failure (HF). Other times, therapeutic measures (e.g., nasogastric [NG] suction, diuretics) cause or contribute to imbalances. Perioperative patients are at risk for developing fluid and electrolyte imbalances because of fluid restrictions, blood or fluid loss, and the stress of surgery.

Imbalances are often reflected by changes in perfusion, gas exchange, mobility, and cognition. For example, a patient with metastatic cancer may develop hypercalcemia because of bone destruction from tumor invasion. They have severe muscle weakness and confusion. Chemotherapy used to treat cancer may result in nausea and vomiting, causing dehydration and hypotension. When correcting dehydration with IV fluids, the patient needs close monitoring to prevent fluid overload.

We classify fluid and electrolyte imbalances as *deficits* or *excesses.* Fluid volume deficit *(hypovolemia)* and volume excess *(hypervolemia)* are common clinical conditions. Volume imbalances are usually accompanied by one or more electrolyte imbalances, especially changes in the sodium level.

It is common for more than one imbalance to occur in the same patient. For example, a patient with prolonged NG suction will lose sodium, potassium, hydrogen, and chloride. This may result in low sodium and potassium levels, fluid volume deficit, and metabolic alkalosis from the loss of HCl acid.

It is important to anticipate the potential for fluid and electrolyte imbalances associated with certain disorders and medical therapies, recognize the signs and symptoms of imbalances, and intervene with the appropriate action. This chapter describes the (1) normal control of fluids, electrolytes, and acid-base balance; (2) conditions that disrupt these processes and their manifestations; and (3) actions that the HCP and you can take to manage fluid, electrolyte, and acid-base imbalances and restore homeostasis.

HOMEOSTASIS PROCESSES

BODY WATER CONTENT

The body is mainly composed of water. It accounts for about 50% to 60% of body weight in adults. Water content varies with body mass, gender, and age (Fig. 17.1). Lean body mass has a higher percentage of water, and fat tissue has a lesser percentage of water. So, the more fat present in the body, the less the total water content. Females and older adults generally have a lower percentage of body water because they tend to have less lean body mass. In older adults, body water content averages 45% to 50% of body weight. This places them at a higher risk for fluid-related problems.

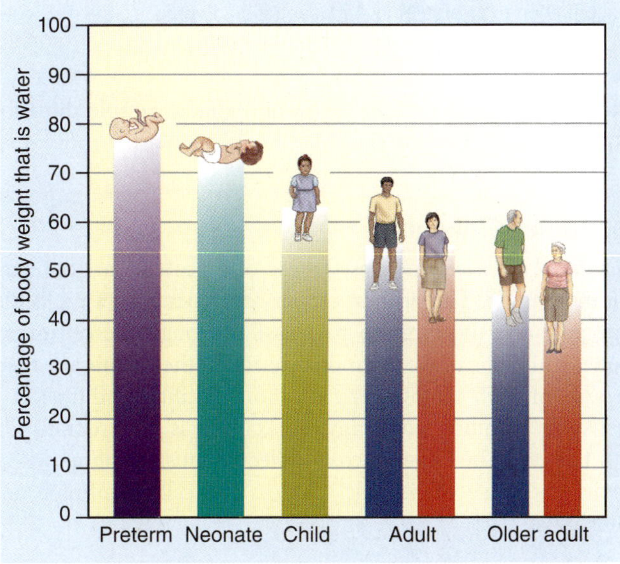

Fig. 17.1 Body water over the life span.

Fluid Compartments

The 2 fluid compartments in the body are the *intracellular space* (inside the cells) and the *extracellular space* (outside the cells) (Fig. 17.2). About two-thirds of body water is found within cells. It is the *intracellular fluid* (ICF). ICF makes up about 40% of body weight of an adult. This means a 70-kg person would have about 42 L of water, with about 28 L of that water within their cells.

The fluid in the extracellular space is *extracellular fluid* (ECF). The 2 main compartments containing ECF are the *interstitial fluid,* the fluid in the spaces between cells, and the intravascular fluid or *plasma,* the liquid part of blood. Other ECF compartments include lymph and *transcellular fluids.* Transcellular fluids include cerebrospinal fluid; fluid in the gastrointestinal (GI) tract and joint spaces; and pleural, peritoneal, intraocular, and pericardial fluid. ECF makes up about one-third of the body water. This amounts to about 14 L in a 70-kg person. About one-third of ECF is in the intravascular space as plasma (3 L in a 70-kg person). Two-thirds are in the interstitial space, or about 10 L in a 70-kg person. The fluid in the transcellular spaces totals about 1 L at any given time.

Calculating Fluid Gain or Loss

One liter of water weighs 2.2 lb (1 kg). Body weight change, especially a sudden change, is a key indicator of overall fluid volume loss or gain. For example, if a patient drinks 240 mL (8 oz) of fluid, weight gain will be 0.5 lb (0.23 kg). A patient receiving diuretic therapy who loses 4.4 lb (2 kg) in 24 hours has a fluid loss of about 2 L. An adult patient who is fasting may lose 1 to 2 lb/day. Weight loss exceeding this is likely the result of loss of body fluid.

ELECTROLYTES

Electrolytes are substances whose molecules dissociate, or split, into ions when placed in water. *Ions* are electrically charged particles. *Cations* are positively charged ions. Examples include sodium (Na^+), potassium (K^+), calcium (Ca^{2+}), and magnesium (Mg^{2+}) ions. *Anions* are negatively charged ions.

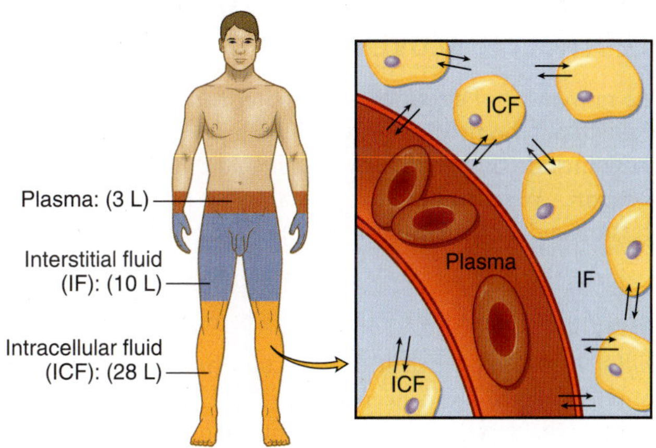

Fig. 17.2 Relative volumes of 3 body fluids. Values represent fluid distribution in a young male adult.

TABLE 17.1 Normal Serum Electrolyte Values

Electrolyte	Reference Interval
Anions	
Bicarbonate (HCO_3^-)	22 to 26 mEq/L (22 to 26 mmol/L)
Chloride (Cl^-)	98 to 106 mEq/L (98 to 106 mmol/L)
Phosphate (PO_4^{3-})	3.0 to 4.5 mg/dL (0.97 to 1.45 mmol/L)
Cations	
Calcium (Ca^{2+}) (total)	9.0 to 10.5 mg/dL (2.25 to 2.62 mmol/L)
Calcium (ionized)	4.5 to 5.6 mg/dL (1.05 to 1.3 mmol/L)
Magnesium (Mg^{2+})	1.3 to 2.1 mEq/L (0.65 to 1.05 mmol/L)
Potassium (K^+)	3.5 to 5.0 mEq/L (3.5 to 5.0 mmol/L)
Sodium (Na^+)	136 to 145 mEq/L (136 to 145 mmol/L)

Examples include bicarbonate (HCO_3^-), chloride (Cl^-), and phosphate (PO_4^{3-}) ions. Most proteins bear a negative charge and thus are anions.

We express electrolyte concentration in body fluids as milliequivalents (mEq) per liter. Because electrolytes are active chemicals, we express their concentration according to their chemical activity or the number of electrolytes able to combine chemically. Ions combine milliequivalent for milliequivalent. For example, 1 mEq (1 mmol) of sodium combines with 1 mEq (1 mmol) of chloride. Table 17.1 lists normal serum electrolyte values. These values reflect the electrolyte's concentration in the plasma.

Electrolyte Composition of Fluid Compartments

Electrolyte composition varies between ECF and ICF. While the overall concentration of electrolytes is nearly the same in the ECF and ICF, the concentrations of specific ions differ greatly (Fig. 17.3). In ECF, the main cation is sodium, with small amounts of potassium, calcium, and magnesium. The primary ECF anion is chloride, with small amounts of bicarbonate, sulfate, and phosphate anions. In ICF, the main cation is potassium, with small amounts of magnesium and sodium. The main ICF anion is phosphate, with some protein and a small amount of bicarbonate.

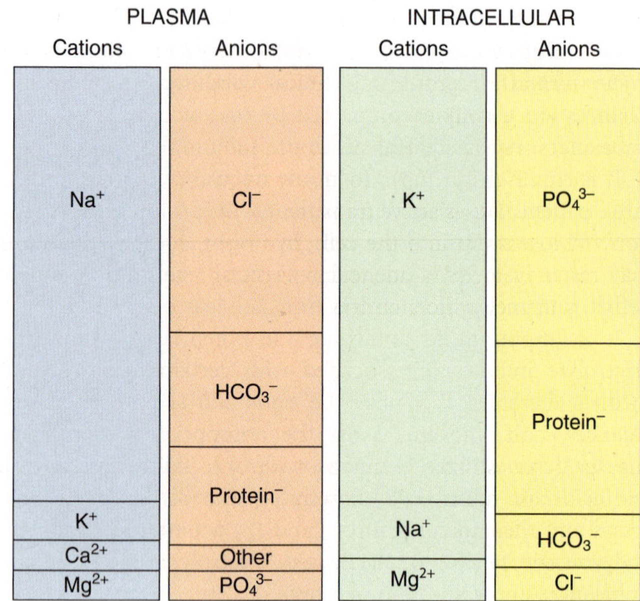

Fig. 17.3 Concentrations of the major cations and anions in the intracellular space and the plasma.

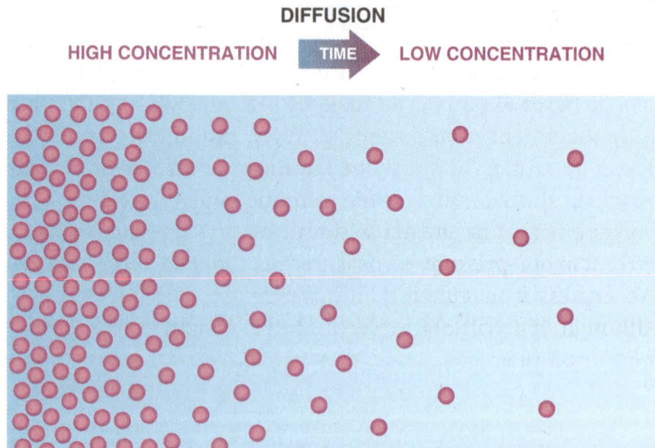

Fig. 17.4 Diffusion is the movement of molecules from an area of high concentration to an area of low concentration. Eventually, the molecules are evenly distributed. (© petrroudny/iStock.com.)

PROCESSES CONTROLLING FLUID AND ELECTROLYTE MOVEMENT

The movement of electrolytes and water between ICF and ECF to maintain homeostasis involves many different processes. These include simple diffusion, facilitated diffusion, and active transport. Water moves as driven by 2 forces: hydrostatic pressure and osmotic pressure.

Diffusion

Diffusion is the movement of molecules from an area of high concentration to low concentration (Fig. 17.4). Net movement of molecules stops when the concentrations are equal in both areas. It occurs in liquids, gases, and solids. Simple diffusion requires no external energy.

Facilitated Diffusion

Facilitated diffusion involves the use of a protein carrier in the cell membrane. The protein carrier combines with a molecule, especially one too large to pass easily through the cell membrane, and helps move the molecule across the membrane from an area of high to low concentration. Facilitated diffusion is passive and requires no energy. An example is glucose transport into the cell. The large glucose molecule must combine with a carrier molecule to be able to cross the cell membrane and enter most cells.

Active Transport

Active transport is a process in which molecules move against the concentration gradient. External energy is needed for this process. An example is the sodium-potassium pump. The concentrations of sodium and potassium differ between the ICF and ECF (Fig. 17.3). To maintain this concentration difference, the cell uses active transport to move sodium out of the cell and potassium into the cell (Fig. 17.5). The energy source for this movement is adenosine triphosphate (ATP). ATP is made in the cell mitochondria.

Osmosis

Osmosis is the movement of water "down" a concentration gradient, that is, from a region of low solute concentration to one of high solute concentration, across a semipermeable membrane. Osmosis requires no outside energy sources. It stops when the concentration differences disappear or when hydrostatic pressure builds and opposes any further movement of water. Imagine a chamber with 2 compartments separated by a membrane that only allows the movement of water (Fig. 17.6). If you add albumin to one side, water will move from the less concentrated side (has more water) to the more concentrated side of the chamber (has less water) until the concentrations are equal.

Whenever dissolved substances are contained in a space with a semipermeable membrane, they can pull water into the space by osmosis. The concentration of the solution determines the strength of the osmotic pull. The higher the concentration, the greater a solution's pull or osmotic pressure. *Osmotic pressure* is measured in milliosmoles (mOsm). We express it as either fluid osmolarity or fluid osmolality. Although you will often see the terms *osmolarity* and *osmolality* used interchangeably, they are different measurements.

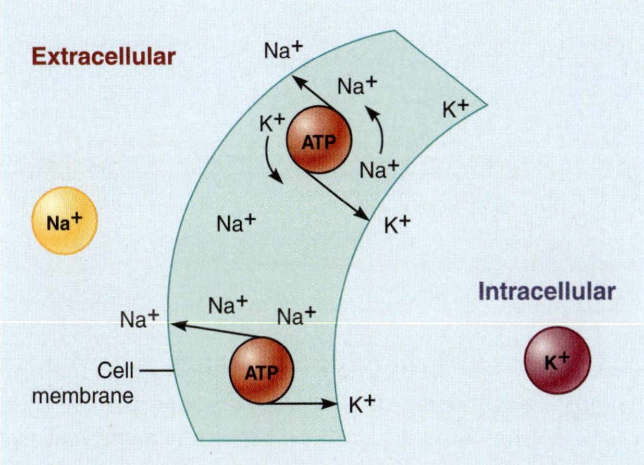

Fig. 17.5 Sodium-potassium pump. As sodium *(Na⁺)* diffuses into the cell and potassium *(K⁺)* diffuses out of the cell, an active transport system supplied with energy delivers Na^+ back to the extracellular compartment and K^+ to the intracellular compartment. *ATP,* Adenosine triphosphate.

Osmolarity measures the total milliosmoles per liter of solution, or the concentration of molecules per volume of solution (mOsm/L). **Osmolality** measures the number of milliosmoles per kilogram of water, or the concentration of molecules per weight of water. Osmolality is the preferred measure to evaluate the concentration of plasma, urine, and other body fluids. Changes in the ECF osmolality can cause significant changes in the ICF osmolality. These changes can affect normal cell function and volume.[1]

Measurement of Osmolality

Osmolality is nearly the same in the body fluid spaces. Measuring or estimating plasma osmolality is a good way to assess the state of the body's water balance. Calculate the estimated plasma osmolality using the following formula:[2]

$$\text{Plasma Osmolality} = (1.86 \times \text{Na}) + (\text{Glucose}/18) + (\text{BUN}/2.8)$$

Normal plasma osmolality is between 280 and 295 mOsm/kg. A value greater than 295 mOsm/kg means that either the concentration of solute is too great or the water content is too little. This condition is called *water deficit.* A value less than 280 mOsm/kg means there is either too little solute for the amount of water or too much water for the amount of solute. This is called *water excess.* Both conditions are clinically significant.

Urine osmolality can range from 100 to 1300 mOsm/kg. It depends on fluid intake, the amount of antidiuretic hormone (ADH) in circulation, and the renal response to ADH.

Osmotic Movement of Fluids

The osmolality of the fluid surrounding cells affects them. Fluids with the same osmolality as the cell interior are **isotonic**. Normally, ECF and ICF are isotonic to one another, so no net movement of water occurs.

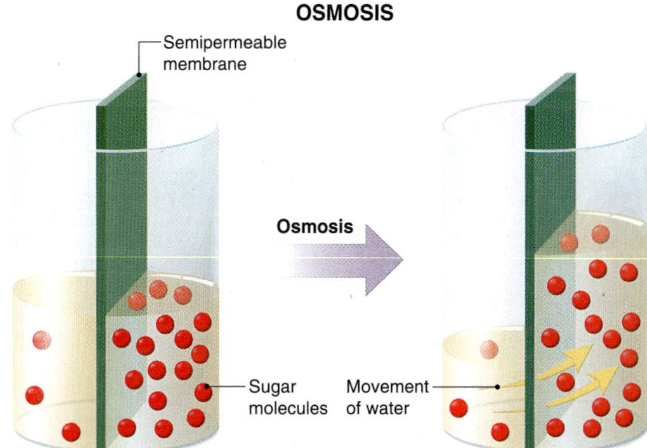

Fig. 17.6 Osmosis is the process of water movement through a semipermeable membrane from an area of low solute concentration to an area of high solute concentration. (© ttsz/iStock.com.)

Changes in the osmolality of ECF change the volume of cells. Solutions in which the solutes are less concentrated than in the cells are **hypotonic** (hypoosmolar). If a cell is surrounded by hypotonic fluid, water moves into the cell, causing it to swell and possibly burst. Fluids with solutes more concentrated than in cells, or an increased osmolality, are **hypertonic** (hyperosmolar). If hypertonic fluid surrounds a cell, water leaves the cell to dilute ECF. The cell shrinks and may eventually die (Fig. 17.7).

Hydrostatic Pressure

Hydrostatic pressure is the force of fluid in a compartment pushing against a cell membrane or vessel wall. In the blood vessels, hydrostatic pressure is the BP generated by the heart's contraction. Hydrostatic pressure in the vascular system gradually decreases as the blood moves through the arteries until it is about 30 mm Hg in the capillary bed. At the capillary level, hydrostatic pressure is the major force that pushes water out of the vascular system and into the interstitial space.

Oncotic Pressure

Oncotic pressure (colloidal osmotic pressure) is the osmotic pressure caused by plasma colloids (large molecules) in solution. The major colloids in the vascular system contributing to osmotic pressure are proteins, such as albumin. We have large amounts of protein in plasma and little amounts in the interstitial space. Plasma protein molecules attract water, pulling fluid from the tissue space to the vascular space. Under normal conditions, plasma oncotic pressure is about 25 mm Hg. The small amount of protein found in the interstitial space has an oncotic pressure of about 1 mm Hg.

FLUID MOVEMENT IN CAPILLARIES

As plasma flows through the capillary bed, 4 factors determine whether fluid moves out of the capillary and into the interstitial space or if fluid moves back into the capillary from the interstitial space. The amount and direction of movement are determined by the interaction of (1) capillary hydrostatic pressure, (2) plasma oncotic pressure, (3) interstitial hydrostatic pressure, and (4) interstitial oncotic pressure.

Capillary hydrostatic pressure and interstitial oncotic pressure move water out of the capillaries. Plasma oncotic pressure and interstitial hydrostatic pressure move fluid into the capillaries. At the arterial end of the capillary, capillary hydrostatic pressure exceeds plasma oncotic pressure, and fluid moves into the interstitial space. At the venous end of the capillary, the capillary hydrostatic pressure is lower than plasma oncotic pressure. The oncotic pressure created by plasma proteins draws fluid back into the capillary (Fig. 17.8).

Fluid Shifts

If capillary or interstitial pressures change, fluid may abnormally shift from one compartment to another. An increase in the plasma osmotic or oncotic pressure draws fluid into the plasma from the interstitial space. This could happen when we give colloids, dextran, mannitol, or hypertonic solutions. Increasing the tissue hydrostatic pressure is another way of causing a shift of fluid into plasma. Wearing elastic compression gradient stockings or hose to decrease peripheral edema is a therapeutic application of this effect.

Edema is an accumulation of fluid in the interstitial space. It occurs if plasma oncotic pressure decreases, interstitial oncotic pressure increases, or venous hydrostatic pressure increases, which inhibits fluid movement back into the capillary. Causes of increased venous pressure include fluid overload, HF, liver failure, obstruction of venous return to the heart (e.g., tourniquets, restrictive clothing, venous thrombosis), and venous insufficiency (e.g., varicose veins). Edema may also develop if an obstruction of lymphatic outflow causes a decrease in the removal of interstitial fluid.

Red blood cells

A Hypotonic solution B Isotonic solution C Hypertonic solution

Fig. 17.7 Effects of water status on red blood cells. (A) Hypotonic solution (H_2O excess) results in cell swelling. (B) Isotonic solution (normal H_2O balance) results in no change. (C) Hypertonic solution (H_2O deficit) results in cell shrinking.

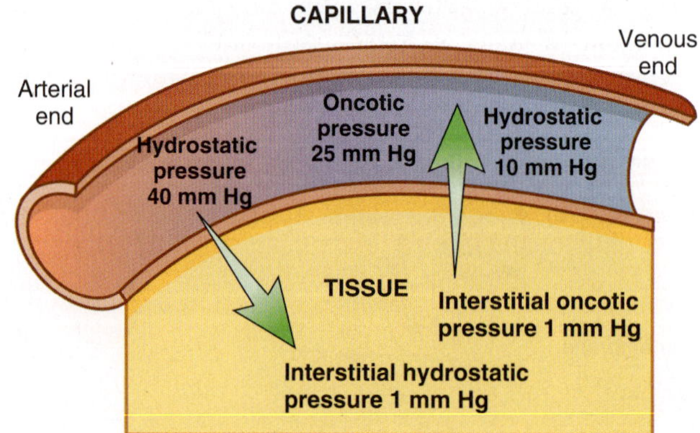

Fig. 17.8 Dynamics of fluid exchange between a capillary and tissue. An equilibrium exists between forces filtering fluid out of the capillary and forces absorbing fluid back into the capillary. Note that the hydrostatic pressure is greater at the arterial end of the capillary than at the venous end. The net effect of pressures at the arterial end of the capillary causes a movement of fluid into the tissue. At the venous end of the capillary, there is net movement of fluid back into the capillary.

Fluid stays in the interstitial space if the plasma oncotic pressure is too low to draw fluid back into the capillary. Low plasma protein content decreases oncotic pressure. This can result from excess protein loss (renal problems), decreased protein synthesis (liver disease), and decreased protein intake (malnutrition). Trauma, burns, and inflammation can damage capillary walls and allow plasma proteins to accumulate in the interstitial space. This increases interstitial oncotic pressure, draws fluid into the interstitial space, and holds it there.

FLUID SPACING

Fluid spacing is a term used to describe the distribution of body water. *First spacing* describes the normal distribution of fluid in ICF and ECF compartments. *Second spacing* refers to an abnormal accumulation of interstitial fluid (i.e., edema). *Third spacing* occurs when excess fluid collects in the nonfunctional area between cells. This fluid is trapped where it is difficult or impossible for it to move back into the cells or blood vessels. Third spacing occurs with ascites; fluid leaking into the abdominal cavity with peritonitis or pancreatitis; and edema from burns, trauma, or sepsis.

REGULATION OF WATER BALANCE

Many factors are involved in maintaining the finely tuned balance among water intake, use, and excretion. For proper fluid balance, an average healthy adult needs a daily water intake of between 2000 and 3000 mL (Table 17.2). This amount replaces what the body loses in urinary output and insensible losses. Oral fluid intake accounts for most of the water intake. Water intake also includes water from food metabolism and water present in solid foods.

Insensible water loss occurs with the invisible vaporization from the lungs and skin. It helps regulate body temperature. Accelerated body metabolism, which occurs with increased body temperature and exercise, increases the amount of water lost and may result in the need for more water replacement.

Do not confuse water loss through the skin with the vaporization of water excreted by sweat glands. Insensible perspiration causes only water loss. Excess sweating *(sensible perspiration)* caused by exercise, fever, or high environment temperatures may lead to large losses of water and electrolytes.

TABLE 17.2 Normal Fluid Balance in the Adult

Intake	
Fluids	1200 mL
Solid food	1000 mL
Water from oxidation	300 mL
Total	2500 mL
Output	
Insensible loss (skin and lungs)	900 mL
In feces	100 mL
Urine	1500 mL
Total	2500 mL

Hypothalamic-Pituitary Regulation

Water ingestion equals water loss in the person who has free access to water, intact thirst and ADH mechanisms, and normally functioning kidneys. A body fluid deficit or increase in plasma osmolality activates osmoreceptors in the hypothalamus. This stimulates thirst and the release of ADH from the posterior pituitary gland. ADH acts on the distal tubules and collecting ducts in the kidney by making them more permeable to water. The result is increased water reabsorption from the tubular filtrate into the blood and decreased excretion in the urine. Because ADH is only able to regulate how much water the body holds onto, thirst is our main protection against developing dehydration or hyperosmolality. Thirst causes us to increase the amount of water we drink. Together these result in increased free water in the body, decreasing plasma osmolality and restoring fluid volume.

Many factors influence ADH secretion and thirst. Decreased BP, nausea, pain, hypoglycemia, and hypoxemia stimulate ADH release. In postoperative patients, the stress response to surgery and receiving analgesics and anesthesia cause ADH release and decreased osmolality. Unconscious or cognitively impaired patients are at increased risk for fluid deficit and hyperosmolality because of an inability to express thirst and act on it. A dry mouth will cause a person to drink, even when there is no body water deficit.

Renal Regulation

The kidney's main function is to regulate fluid and electrolyte balance by adjusting urine volume and the excretion of most electrolytes (see Chapter 49). The kidneys filter the total plasma volume many times each day. In the average adult, the kidneys reabsorb 99% of this filtrate, producing around 1.5 L of urine per day. Under the influence of ADH, aldosterone, and other hormones, selective reabsorption and secretion of water and electrolytes in the renal tubules result in urine that is different in composition and concentration from plasma. This process helps maintain normal plasma osmolality, electrolyte balance, blood volume, and acid-base balance.

With severely impaired renal function, the kidneys cannot maintain fluid and electrolyte balance. This results in edema, potassium and phosphate retention, acidosis, and other electrolyte imbalances (see Chapter 51).

Adrenal Cortical Regulation

Glucocorticoids and mineralocorticoids secreted by the adrenal cortex help regulate water and electrolyte balance. Mineralocorticoids enhance sodium retention and potassium excretion (Fig. 17.9). Aldosterone is the main mineralocorticoid. Decreased renal perfusion or decreased sodium in the distal renal tubule activates the renin-angiotensin-aldosterone system

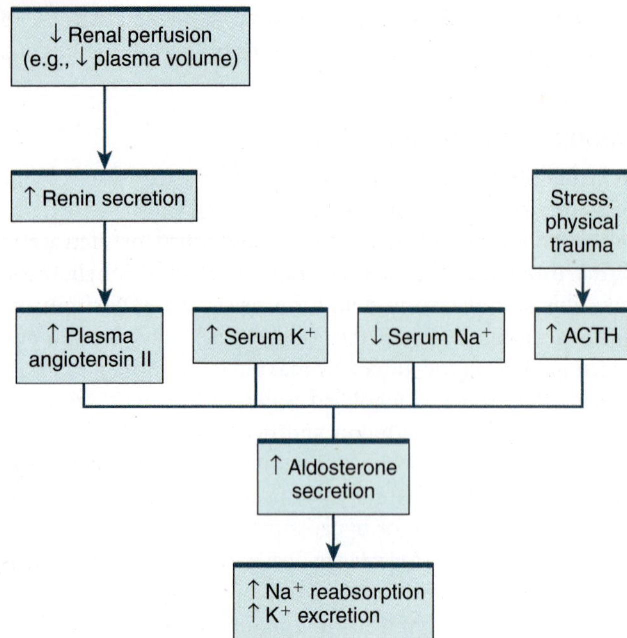

Fig. 17.9 Factors affecting aldosterone secretion. *ACTH,* Adrenocorticotropic hormone.

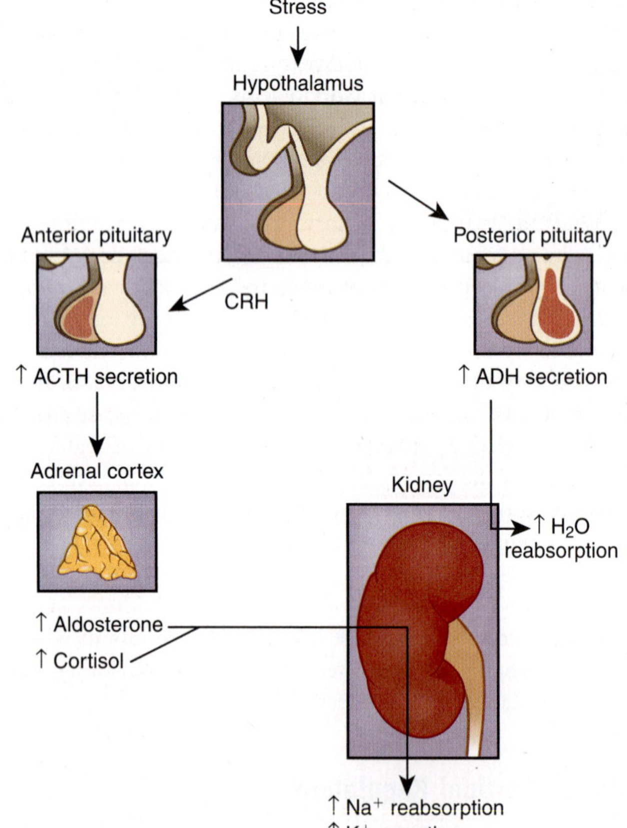

Fig. 17.10 Effects of stress on fluid and electrolyte balance. *ACTH,* Adrenocorticotropic hormone; *ADH,* antidiuretic hormone; *CRH,* corticotropin-releasing hormone.

(RAAS), resulting in aldosterone secretion. Increased potassium, decreased sodium, and increased adrenocorticotropic hormone (ACTH) stimulate aldosterone secretion. Aldosterone increases sodium and water reabsorption in the renal distal tubules, decreasing plasma osmolality and restoring fluid volume.

Glucocorticoids mainly have an antiinflammatory effect and increase glucose levels. Cortisol is the most abundant glucocorticoid. In large doses, cortisol has both glucocorticoid (glucose-elevating, antiinflammatory) and mineralocorticoid (sodium retention) effects. Increased cortisol secretion occurs in response to stress. This affects many body functions, including fluid and electrolyte balance (Fig. 17.10).

Cardiac Regulation

Natriuretic peptides, including atrial natriuretic peptide (ANP) and b-type natriuretic peptide (BNP), are hormones made by cardiomyocytes in response to increased atrial pressure (increased volume, such as in HF) and high sodium levels. They are natural antagonists to the RAAS and suppress secretion of aldosterone, renin, and ADH and the action of angiotensin II. In the renal tubules, peptides promote excretion of sodium and water, decreasing blood volume and BP.

Gastrointestinal Regulation

In addition to oral intake, the GI tract normally secretes around 8000 mL of digestive fluids each day. It normally reabsorbs most of this fluid, with only a small amount eliminated in feces. This is why diarrhea and vomiting, which prevent GI reabsorption of the secreted fluid, can lead to significant fluid and electrolyte loss.

Gerontologic Considerations: Fluid and Electrolytes

Normal physiologic changes with aging increase susceptibility to fluid and electrolyte imbalances. Structural changes to the kidneys and a decrease in renal blood flow lead to decreased glomerular filtration rate and loss of the ability to concentrate urine and conserve water. Hormonal changes include a decrease in renin and aldosterone and an increase in ADH and ANP. Subcutaneous tissue loss and thinning of the dermis lead to increased moisture lost through the skin.

FLUID IMBALANCES

FLUID VOLUME DEFICIT

Fluid volume deficit can occur with abnormal body fluid loss (e.g., diarrhea, vomiting, hemorrhage, polyuria), inadequate fluid intake, or a shift from plasma to interstitial fluid. Though often used interchangeably, *fluid volume deficit* and *dehydration* are not the same. *Dehydration* refers to loss of pure water alone without the loss of sodium. Table 17.3 lists causes and manifestations of fluid volume deficit.

Interprofessional Care

We manage fluid volume deficit by correcting the underlying cause and replacing both water and any needed electrolytes. Replacement therapy depends on the severity and type of volume loss. In mild losses, we can use oral rehydration. If the deficit is more severe, we may replace volume with blood products or isotonic IV solutions. The choice of fluid depends on the cause and the patient's electrolyte status. For rapid volume replacement, 0.9% sodium chloride is preferred. Blood is given when volume loss is the result of blood loss.

FLUID VOLUME EXCESS

Fluid volume excess may result from excess fluid intake, abnormal fluid retention (e.g., HF, renal failure), or a shift of fluid from interstitial fluid into plasma fluid. Weight gain is the most consistent manifestation of fluid volume excess. Table 17.3 lists additional causes and manifestations of fluid volume excess.

Interprofessional Care

We manage fluid volume excess by treating the underlying cause and removing fluid without causing abnormal changes in the electrolyte composition or osmolality of ECF. Diuretics and fluid restriction are the main therapies. Some patients also need sodium restrictions. If the fluid excess leads to ascites or pleural effusion, an abdominal paracentesis or thoracentesis may be done.

TABLE 17.3 Extracellular Fluid Imbalances

Causes and Manifestations

ECF Volume Deficit	ECF Volume Excess
Causes	
• Arginine vasopressin disorder	• Corticosteroid use long-term
• GI losses: vomiting, NG suction, diarrhea, fistula drainage	• Cushing syndrome
• Hemorrhage	• Heart failure
• Inadequate fluid intake	• Primary polydipsia
• ↑ Insensible water loss or perspiration (high fever, heatstroke)	• Renal failure
• Osmotic diuresis	• Syndrome of inappropriate antidiuresis
• Overuse of diuretics	
• Third-space fluid shifts: burns, pancreatitis	
Manifestations	
• ↓ Capillary refill	• Bounding pulse, ↑ BP, ↑ CVP
• Confusion, restlessness, drowsiness, lethargy	• Confusion, headache, lethargy
• Cold clammy skin	• Dyspnea, crackles, pulmonary edema
• Postural hypotension, ↑ HR, ↓ CVP	• Edema
• ↑ Respiratory rate	• Jugular vein distension
• Seizures, coma	• Muscle spasms
• Thirst, dry mucous membranes	• Polyuria (with normal renal function)
• ↓ Urine output, concentrated urine	• S_3 heart sound
• Weakness, dizziness	• Seizures, coma
• Weight loss	• Weight gain

CVP, Central venous pressure; *ECF*, extracellular fluid; *NG*, nasogastric.

NURSING MANAGEMENT: FLUID IMBALANCES

Assessment

Careful assessment and management of fluid volume changes is a key nursing role (Table 17.4).

Does the patient have a history of kidney, heart, GI, or lung problems that could affect the present fluid balance? Ask about specific diseases such as diabetes, arginine vasopressin disorder (AVP disorder), renal failure, HF, and liver disease. Assess for any prior fluid balance problems. Ask the patient about any recent changes in body weight.

Ask about the patient's exercise pattern and any excess perspiration. Is the patient exposed to extremely high temperatures during leisure or work activity? Ask the patient what they do to replace fluid and electrolytes lost through excess perspiration. Assess the patient's activity level for any functional problems that could affect food and fluid intake.

Obtain a medication history. Many drugs, including diuretics and corticosteroids, can cause fluid imbalance. Ask the patient about past or present renal dialysis, kidney surgery, or

TABLE 17.4 NURSING MANAGEMENT

Fluid Volume Changes

- Assess for manifestations of fluid imbalances.
- Assess for risk factors for a fluid imbalance, including the patient's ability to self-manage hydration.
- Give IV fluids and medications as ordered.
- Monitor pulse oximetry and give O_2 therapy as ordered.
- Evaluate intake and output and weight trends.
- Implement fall precautions.
- Provide diet appropriate for the specific fluid imbalance.
- Initiate referrals, such as dietitian, as needed.
- Supervise AP:
  - Obtain daily weights and vital signs.
  - Record accurate intake and output.
  - Perform skin care and frequent oral care.
  - Assist with frequent position changes and toileting as needed.
  - Elevate edematous extremities.
  - Encourage oral fluids as appropriate.
- Monitor for effectiveness of therapy.

bowel surgery. Does the patient have an external collecting system, such as an ileostomy?

Perform a complete physical assessment because fluid imbalances can affect all body systems. As you assess each system, check for manifestations that you would expect with an imbalance (Table 17.3).

Monitor available laboratory results and calculate plasma osmolality. Patients with a fluid volume deficit often have increased blood urea nitrogen (BUN), sodium, and hematocrit levels with increased plasma and urine osmolality. With fluid volume excess, patients will have decreased BUN, sodium, and hematocrit levels, with decreased plasma and urine osmolality.

◆ Clinical Problems

Clinical problems for patients with a fluid imbalance include:

- Fluid imbalance
- Impaired tissue perfusion
- Altered blood pressure
- Impaired respiratory system function
- Impaired urinary elimination

◆ Planning

The overall goals are that patients with a fluid imbalance (1) achieve and maintain fluid balance, (2) be free from complications from abnormal fluid levels, (3) adhere to the prescribed care plan, and (4) recognize factors that can lead to a fluid imbalance and take preventive action.

◆ Implementation

Daily Weights

Daily weights are the most accurate measure of volume status. An increase of 1 kg (2.2 lb) is equal to 1000 mL (1 L) of fluid retention, provided the person has maintained usual diet and oral intake. Obtain the weight under standard conditions. Weigh the patient at the same time every day, wearing the same clothes and on the same calibrated scale. Remove excess bedding and empty all drainage bags before weighing the patient. If items are present that are not there every day, such as bulky dressings or tubes, note this with the weight.

Intake and Output

Intake and output records give valuable information about fluid and electrolyte balance. An accurate intake and output will identify sources of excess intake or fluid losses. Intake should include oral and IV fluids, enteral nutrition (EN) or tube feedings, and retained irrigation solutions. Output includes urine, excess perspiration, wound or tube drainage, vomitus, and diarrhea. Estimate fluid loss from wounds and perspiration. Note the amount and color of the urine. Measure the urine specific gravity. Readings greater than 1.025 mean urine is concentrated, while readings less than 1.010 mean urine is dilute.

Cardiovascular Care

Monitor vital signs and perform a cardiovascular assessment as needed. Changes in BP, central venous pressure (CVP), pulse force, and jugular venous distention (JVD) reflect ECF volume imbalances. In fluid volume excess, the pulse is full, bounding, and not easily obliterated. Increased volume causes distended neck veins (JVD), increased CVP, and high BP. Auscultate heart sounds, being alert for the presence of an S_3.

In mild to moderate fluid volume deficit, sympathetic nervous system compensation increases the heart rate and results in peripheral vasoconstriction to try to keep BP within normal limits. Pulses may be weak and thready. Assess for orthostatic changes. A change in position from lying to sitting or standing may decrease BP or further increase the heart rate (orthostatic hypotension). In more severe deficits, hypotension may be present.

Respiratory Care

Monitor pulse oximetry and auscultate lung sounds as needed. ECF excess can cause pulmonary congestion and pulmonary edema, as increased hydrostatic pressure in the pulmonary vessels forces fluid into the alveoli. The patient will have shortness of breath and moist crackles on auscultation. Patients with ECF deficit will have an increased respiratory rate because of decreased tissue perfusion and resultant hypoxia. Give O_2 as ordered.

Patient Safety

Patients with fluid volume deficit are at risk for falls because of orthostatic hypotension, muscle weakness, and impaired cognition. Assess level of consciousness, gait, and muscle strength. Implement fall precautions. If orthostatic hypotension is present, teach the patient to change positions slowly when rising from a bed or chair.

Skin Care

Assess the skin for turgor and mobility. Normally, a fold of skin, when pinched, will readily move and, on release, rapidly return to its former position. In ECF volume deficit, there is diminished skin turgor with tenting or a lag in the pinched skinfold's return to its original state. Skin areas over the sternum, abdomen, and anterior forearm are the usual sites we use to assess turgor (Fig. 17.11). In older people, decreased skin turgor is less predictive of fluid deficit because of the loss of tissue elasticity.

In mild fluid deficits, the skin may appear warm, dry, and wrinkled. These signs may be hard to assess in the older adult

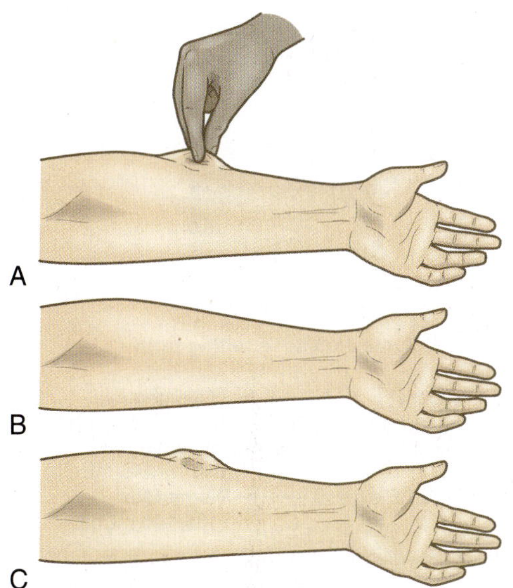

Fig. 17.11 Assessment of skin turgor. (A and B) When normal skin is pinched, it resumes shape in seconds. (C) If the skin stays wrinkled for 20 to 30 seconds, the patient has poor skin turgor.

because the person's skin may be normally dry, wrinkled, and nonelastic. In more severe deficits, the skin may be cool and moist if there is vasoconstriction to compensate for the decreased fluid volume. Oral mucous membranes will be dry, and the tongue may be furrowed. The person often is thirsty. Oral care is important for the comfort of a patient who is dehydrated or on a fluid restriction.

Edematous skin may feel cool because of fluid accumulation and a decrease in blood flow from the pressure of the fluid. The fluid can stretch the skin, causing it to feel taut and hard. Assess edema by pressing with a thumb or forefinger over the edematous area. Use a grading scale to standardize the description if an indentation (ranging from 1+ [slight edema; 2-mm indentation] to 4+ [pitting edema; 8-mm indentation]) remains when pressure is released. Assess for edema in areas where soft tissues overlie a bone, especially the tibia, fibula, and sacrum.

Skin care is important. Protect tissues from extremes of heat and cold, prolonged pressure, and trauma. Frequent skin care and changes in position will prevent skin breakdown. Elevate edematous extremities to promote venous return and fluid reabsorption. Dehydrated skin needs frequent care without the use of soap. Applying moisturizing creams or oils increases moisture retention and stimulates circulation.

Fluid Therapy

Give IV fluids as ordered. Monitor the rates of IV infusions, especially when you are giving large volumes of fluid. This is especially true in patients with heart, renal, or neurologic problems.

With fluid volume deficit, you can use several interventions to maintain adequate oral intake. Assess the patient's ability to obtain adequate fluids independently, express thirst, and swallow effectively. Fluids should be easily accessible. Provide an assortment of fluids that are appealing to the patient. Serve fluids at a temperature preferred by the patient. Offer fluids every 1 to 2 hours and at select times, such as when giving medications. Remind the patient to finish all drinks.

If the patient is choosing to limit intake to decrease nocturia or incontinence, make it easier for the patient to reach the toilet when needed. Help those with physical limitations, such as arthritis, to open and hold containers. Involve the dietitian, speech therapist, or occupational therapist for help with patients with dysphagia or physical limitations.

ELECTROLYTE IMBALANCES

SODIUM

Sodium is the main cation of ECF. It plays a major role in maintaining the concentration and volume of ECF and influencing water distribution between ECF and ICF. Sodium is important in generating and transmitting nerve impulses, muscle contractility, and regulating acid-base balance.

The sodium level reflects the ratio of sodium to water, not necessarily the amount of sodium in the body. Changes in the sodium level can reflect a primary water imbalance, primary sodium imbalance, or combination of the two. Sodium imbalances are typically associated with imbalances in ECF volume (Figs. 17.12 and 17.13). Because sodium is the main determinant of ECF osmolality, sodium imbalances have parallel changes in osmolality.

The GI tract absorbs sodium from foods. Typically, daily intake of sodium far exceeds the body's daily requirements. Sodium leaves the body through urine, sweat, and feces. The kidneys mainly regulate sodium balance. The kidneys control ECF sodium concentration by excreting or retaining water under the influence of ADH. Aldosterone plays a smaller role in sodium regulation by promoting sodium reabsorption from the renal tubules.

Hypernatremia

Hypernatremia (high serum sodium) may occur with inadequate water intake, excess water loss, or, rarely, sodium gain. Because sodium is the main determinant of ECF osmolality, hypernatremia causes hyperosmolality. ECF hyperosmolality causes water to move out of the cells to restore equilibrium, leading to cell dehydration. As discussed earlier, the main protection against developing hyperosmolality is thirst. Hypernatremia is not a problem in an alert person who has

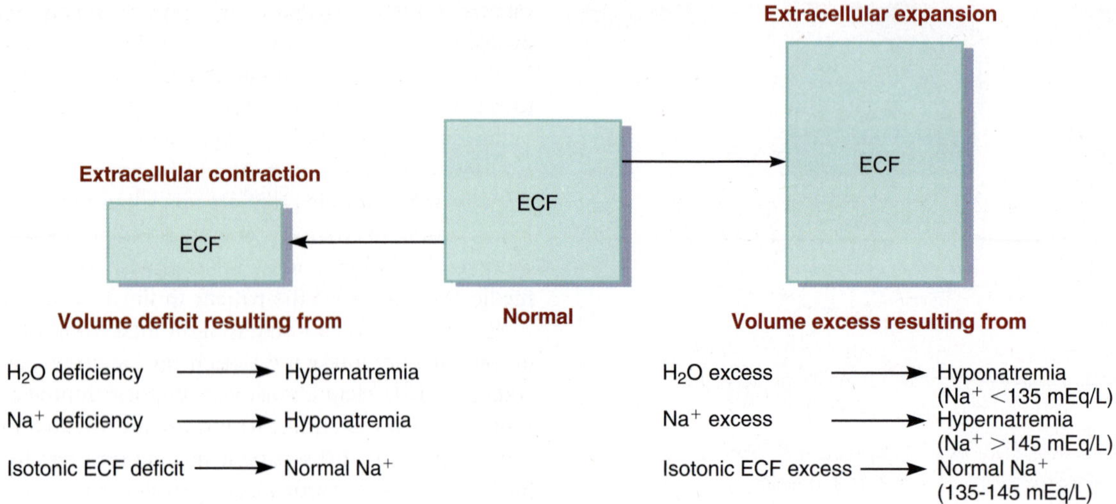

Fig. 17.12 Assessment of extracellular fluid *(ECF)* volume.

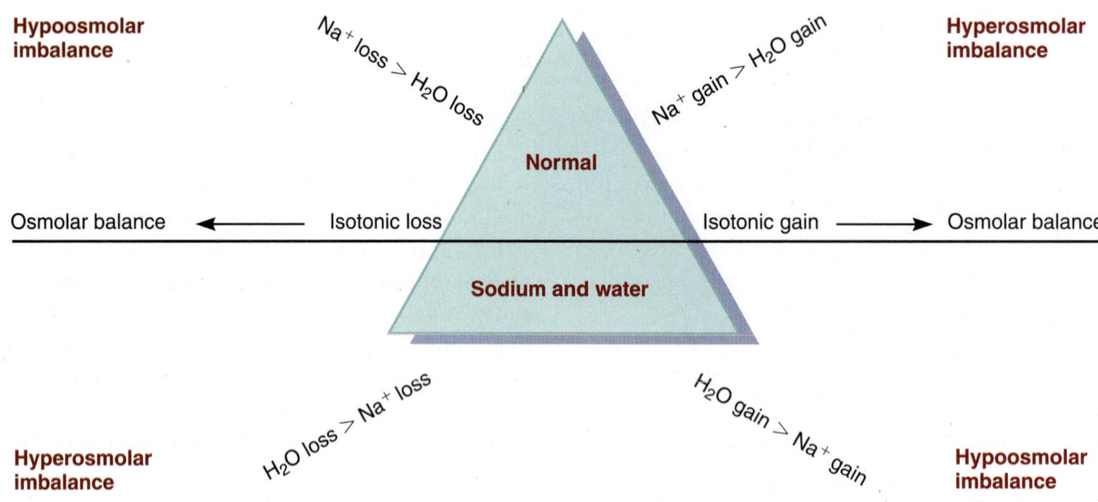

Fig. 17.13 Isotonic gains and losses affect mainly the extracellular fluid (ECF) compartment, with little or no water movement into the cells. Hypertonic imbalances cause water to move from inside the cell into the ECF to dilute the concentrated sodium, causing cell shrinkage. Hypotonic imbalances cause water to move into the cell, causing cell swelling.

access to water, can sense thirst, and is able to swallow. Hypernatremia from water deficiency can happen with an impaired level of consciousness or inability to obtain fluids.

Several clinical states can cause hypernatremia from water loss (Table 17.5). Problems with the synthesis or release of ADH from the posterior pituitary gland (arginine vasopressin disorder-deficiency [AVP-D]) or a decrease in kidney responsiveness to ADH (arginine vasopressin disorder-resistance [AVP-R]) can result in profound diuresis, causing a water deficit and hypernatremia. Hyperosmolality with osmotic diuresis can result from hyperglycemia associated with uncontrolled diabetes or giving concentrated hyperosmolar EN.

Excess sodium intake with inadequate water intake can lead to hypernatremia. Examples include IV administration of hypertonic saline or sodium bicarbonate, use of sodium-containing drugs, and excess oral intake of sodium (e.g., ingesting seawater). *Primary aldosteronism* from an adrenal gland tumor causes excess aldosterone secretion, increasing sodium reabsorption.

TABLE 17.5 Sodium Imbalances

Causes and Manifestations

Hypernatremia (Na^+ >145 mEq/L [mmol/L])	Hyponatremia (Na^+ <136 mEq/L [mmol/L])
Causes	
Excess Sodium Intake	***Excess Sodium Loss***
• Hypertonic enteral nutrition without water supplements • IV fluids: hypertonic NaCl, excess isotonic NaCl, IV sodium bicarbonate • Near-drowning in salt water	• *GI losses:* diarrhea, vomiting, fistulas, NG suction • *Renal losses:* diuretics, adrenal insufficiency, Na^+ wasting renal disease • *Skin losses:* burns, wound drainage
Inadequate Water Intake	***Inadequate Sodium Intake***
• Unconscious or impaired cognition	• Fasting diets
Excess Water Loss (↑ Sodium Concentration)	***Excess Water Gain (↓ Sodium Dilution)***
• Diarrhea • ↑ Insensible water loss (high fever, heatstroke, prolonged hyperventilation) • Osmotic diuretic therapy	• Excess hypotonic IV fluids • Primary polydipsia
Diseases	***Diseases***
• Arginine vasopressin disorder • Cushing syndrome • Primary hyperaldosteronism • Uncontrolled diabetes	• Cirrhosis • Heart failure • Primary hypoaldosteronism • Syndrome of inappropriate antidiuresis
Manifestations	
With Decreased ECF Volume	***With Decreased ECF Volume***
• Agitations, restlessness, lethargy, seizures, coma • Dry swollen tongue, intense thirst, sticky mucous membranes • Postural hypotension, ↓ CVP, weight loss, ↑ HR • Weakness, muscle cramps	• Apprehension, irritability, confusion, dizziness, personality changes, tremors, seizures, coma • Cold and clammy skin • Dry mucous membranes • Postural hypotension, ↓ CVP, ↓ jugular venous filling, ↑ HR, thready pulse
With Normal or Increased ECF Volume	***With Normal or Increased ECF Volume***
• Agitations, restlessness, twitching, seizures, coma • Edema, peripheral and pulmonary • Intense thirst, flushed skin • Weight gain, ↑ BP, ↑ CVP	• Apathy, headache, confusion, muscle spasms, seizures, coma • Nausea, vomiting, diarrhea, abdominal cramps • Weight gain, ↑ BP, ↑ CVP

CVP, Central venous pressure; *NG*, nasogastric.

Clinical Manifestations

The manifestations are mainly the result of water shifting out of cells into ECF with resultant dehydration and shrinkage of cells (Table 17.5). Dehydration of brain cells results in changes in mental status, ranging from fatigue, mood changes, and confusion to seizures and coma.[3] If there is an accompanying ECF volume deficit, manifestations such as postural hypotension, tachycardia, and weakness occur.

Interprofessional and Nursing Management

Managing hypernatremia depends on the underlying cause and the patient's volume status. In primary water deficit, fluid replacement is given either orally or IV with isotonic solutions such as 0.9% sodium chloride.[4] If the problem is sodium excess, expect diluting the high sodium concentration with sodium-free IV fluids, such as 5% dextrose in water, and promoting sodium excretion with diuretics. Diet sodium intake is often restricted. If the patient has altered consciousness or is having seizures, initiate seizure precautions.

Monitor sodium levels, plasma osmolality, and the patient's response to therapy. The sodium level should not decrease by more than 12 mEq/L in a 24-hour period.[4] Quickly reducing levels can cause a rapid shift of water back into the cells, causing cerebral edema and neurologic complications. This risk is greatest in patients who develop hypernatremia over several days or longer.

Hyponatremia

Hyponatremia (low serum sodium) may result from a loss of sodium-containing fluids, water excess in relation to the amount of sodium (dilutional hyponatremia), or a combination of both (Table 17.5). Hyponatremia is usually associated with ECF hypoosmolality from the excess water. To restore balance, fluid shifts out of the ECF and into the cells, leading to cell edema.

Common causes of hyponatremia from loss of sodium-rich body fluids include draining wounds, diarrhea, vomiting, and primary adrenal insufficiency. Inappropriate use of sodium-free or hypotonic IV fluids causes hyponatremia from water excess. This may occur in patients after surgery or major trauma or if we give fluids to patients with renal failure. Patients with psychiatric disorders may have an excess water intake. Syndrome of inappropriate diuresis (SIAD) results in dilutional hyponatremia caused by abnormal retention of water (see Chapter 54).

Clinical Manifestations

The manifestations are the result of cell swelling and first appear in the central nervous system (CNS). Mild hyponatremia has minor, nonspecific neurologic symptoms. These include headache, irritability, and difficulty concentrating. More severe hyponatremia can cause confusion, vomiting, seizures, and even coma. If hyponatremia is severe and develops rapidly, irreversible neurologic damage or death from brain herniation can occur.

Interprofessional and Nursing Management

We manage hyponatremia from fluid loss by replacing fluid using isotonic sodium-containing solutions, encouraging oral intake, and withholding all diuretics.[5] In mild hyponatremia caused by water excess, fluid restriction may be the only treatment. Loop diuretics and demeclocycline may be given. If hyponatremia is acute or more serious, small amounts of IV hypertonic saline solution (3% sodium chloride) can restore the sodium level while the body is returning to a normal water balance.

Selective vasopressin 2 receptor antagonists increase water excretion from the kidneys without affecting sodium excretion. They are used to treat patients who cannot tolerate fluid restrictions or have excess fluid volume.[5] These drugs include conivaptan (Vaprisol) and tolvaptan (Samsca). Conivaptan, which inhibits both V1a and V2 vasopressin receptors, is given IV to hospitalized patients with severe hyponatremia from water excess. Tolvaptan is given orally to treat hyponatremia from HF or SIAD.

Monitor sodium levels and the patient's response to therapy. Avoid rapid correction or overcorrection. The level should not increase by more than 10 to 12 mEq/L in 24 hours.[5] Quickly increasing sodium can cause osmotic demyelination syndrome with permanent damage to nerve cells in the brain. An accurate urine output record is essential. The patient may need a urinary catheter placed if unable to help with monitoring output. If the patient has an altered consciousness or is having seizures, initiate seizure precautions.

POTASSIUM

Potassium is the major ICF cation, with 98% of the body potassium being in cells. Potassium concentration in ECF is 3.5 to 5.0 mEq/L. The sodium-potassium pump in cell membranes maintains this concentration difference by pumping potassium into the cell and sodium out. Insulin helps by stimulating the sodium-potassium pump.

Because the ratio of ECF to ICF potassium is the major factor in the resting membrane potential of nerve and muscle cells, potassium imbalances often affect neuromuscular and cardiac function. Potassium is involved with regulating intracellular osmolality and promoting cell growth. It is required for glycogen to be deposited in muscle and liver cells. It plays a role in acid-base balance.

Diet is the main source for potassium. The typical Western diet contains around 50 to 100 mEq of potassium daily. This mainly comes from protein-rich foods and various fruits and vegetables. Many salt substitutes used in low-sodium diets have substantial potassium. Patients may receive potassium from IV sources, including IV fluids; transfusions of stored, hemolyzed blood; and some medications (e.g., potassium penicillin).

The kidneys eliminate about 90% of the daily potassium intake. Potassium excretion depends on the potassium level, urine output, and renal function. When potassium is high, urine potassium excretion increases. When levels are low, excretion decreases. Large urine output can cause excess potassium loss. Impaired kidney function can cause potassium retention. An inverse relationship exists between sodium and potassium reabsorption in the kidneys. Factors that cause sodium retention (e.g., low blood volume, hyponatremia, aldosterone secretion) cause potassium excretion.

Hyperkalemia

Hyperkalemia (high serum potassium) may result from impaired renal excretion, a shift of potassium from ICF to ECF, a massive potassium intake, or a combination of these factors (Table 17.6). The most common cause is renal failure. Adrenal

TABLE 17.6 Potassium Imbalances

Causes and Manifestations

Hyperkalemia (K^+ >5.0 mEq/L [mmol/L])	Hypokalemia (K^+ <3.5 mEq/L [mmol/L])
Causes	
Excess Potassium Intake	***Potassium Loss***
• Excess or rapid IV administration • Potassium-containing drugs (e.g., potassium penicillin) • Potassium-containing salt substitute	• Dialysis • Diaphoresis • *GI losses:* diarrhea, vomiting, fistulas, NG suction, ileostomy drainage • *Renal losses:* diuretics, hyperaldosteronism, magnesium depletion
Shift of Potassium Out of Cells	***Shift of Potassium Into Cells***
• Acidosis • Intense exercise • Tissue catabolism (e.g., fever, crush injury, sepsis, burns) • Tumor lysis syndrome	• Alkalosis • ↑ Epinephrine (e.g., stress) • ↑ Insulin release (e.g., IV dextrose load) • Insulin therapy (e.g., with diabetic ketoacidosis)
Failure to Eliminate Potassium	***Lack of Potassium Intake***
• Adrenal insufficiency • *Medications:* Angiotensin II receptor blockers, ACE inhibitors, heparin, potassium-sparing diuretics, NSAIDs • Renal disease	• Diet low in potassium • Failure to include potassium in IV fluids if NPO • Starvation
Clinical Manifestations	
• Abdominal cramping, diarrhea, vomiting • Confusion • Fatigue, irritability • Irregular pulse • Loss of muscle tone • Muscle weakness, cramps • Paresthesias, ↓ reflexes • Tetany	• Constipation, nausea, paralytic ileus • Fatigue • ↑ Glucose • Irregular, weak pulse • Muscles soft, flabby • Muscle weakness, leg cramps • Paresthesias, ↓ reflexes • Shallow respirations
ECG Changes	***ECG Changes***
• Loss of P wave • Prolonged PR interval • ST segment depression • Widening QRS • Tall, peaked T wave • Ventricular fibrillation • Ventricular standstill	• Peaked P wave • Prolonged QRS • ST segment depression • Flattened T wave • Presence of U wave • Ventricular dysrhythmias • First- and second-degree heart block

ACE, Angiotensin-converting enzyme; *NSAID,* nonsteroidal antiinflammatory drug.

insufficiency with subsequent aldosterone deficiency leads to potassium retention. Factors that cause potassium to move from ICF to ECF include acidosis, massive cell destruction (as in burn or crush injury, tumor lysis, severe infections), and intense exercise. In metabolic acidosis, potassium ions shift from ICF to ECF in exchange for hydrogen ions moving into the cell.

Digoxin-like drugs and β-adrenergic blockers (e.g., propranolol) can impair entry of potassium into cells, resulting in higher ECF potassium concentrations. Several drugs, such as NSAIDs, potassium-sparing diuretics, angiotensin II receptor blockers (e.g., losartan), and angiotensin-converting enzyme (ACE) inhibitors (e.g., lisinopril), can contribute to hyperkalemia by reducing the kidney's ability to excrete potassium.[6]

Clinical Manifestations

Increased potassium concentration outside the cell changes the normal ECF and ICF ratio. This results in increased cell excitability and changes in impulse transmission to the nerves and muscles. The most significant problem is changes in cardiac conduction. The initial finding is tall, peaked T waves. As potassium increases, cardiac depolarization decreases. This leads to loss of P waves, a prolonged PR interval, ST segment depression, and widening QRS complex (Fig. 17.14). Life-threatening dysrhythmias may occur.[6]

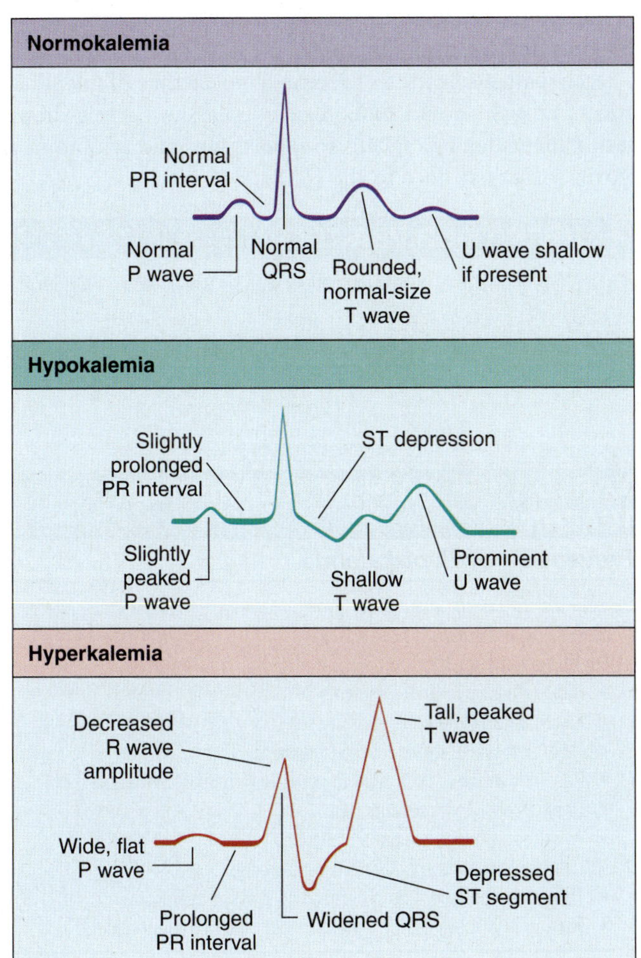

Fig. 17.14 ECG changes associated with changes in potassium levels.

The patient may have fatigue, confusion, tetany, and paresthesias. As potassium increases, loss of muscle tone and weakness or paralysis of other skeletal muscles, including the respiratory muscles, can occur, leading to respiratory arrest. Abdominal cramping, vomiting, and diarrhea occur from hyperactivity of GI smooth muscles.

Interprofessional and Nursing Management

Therapies to manage hyperkalemia include:

1. Stop oral and IV potassium intake.
2. Increase potassium excretion. This may be done with loop or thiazide diuretics, hemodialysis, and GI agents (e.g., patiromer, sodium zirconium cyclosilicate, sodium polystyrene sulfonate [Kayexalate]). Kayexalate, given orally or rectally, binds potassium in the bowel. Each gram removes roughly 1 mEq of potassium and frees 1 to 2 mEq of sodium.[6] Patiromer, given orally, exchanges calcium for potassium in the lower GI tract. It may take up to 7 hours to take initial effect and 2 days to see maximal results. It is best for patients with hyperkalemia caused by chronic renal failure. Sodium zirconium cyclosilicate (ZS-9, Lokelma) traps potassium in the GI lumen, increasing fecal excretion. Onset occurs within 1 hour.[6] The risk of toxicity is low because the drug is not absorbed systemically.
3. Force potassium from ECF to ICF. A combination of IV regular insulin with dextrose and a β-adrenergic agonist stimulates the sodium-potassium pump, shifting potassium into cells. Using these drugs together is more effective than using either alone. Metered-dose inhalers and nebulized β-adrenergic agonists (e.g., nebulized albuterol) are equally effective. IV sodium bicarbonate is an option if the patient is acidotic.[6]
4. Stabilize cardiac membranes. IV calcium chloride or calcium gluconate does not lower potassium but serves as an antagonist to reverse the toxic effects on the cardiac cell membrane. This protects the patient from life-threatening dysrhythmias.[6]

When the potassium elevation is mild and the kidneys are functioning, it may be enough to (1) withhold potassium from the diet and IV sources and (2) increase renal potassium excretion by giving loop or thiazide diuretics and fluids. Patients with severe hyperkalemia or symptomatic patients should receive treatment to force potassium into cells.

Use continuous ECG monitoring for all patients with clinically significant hyperkalemia to detect dysrhythmias and monitor the effects of therapy. Patients with dangerous dysrhythmias should receive IV calcium. Monitor BP because giving calcium rapidly can cause hypotension. When giving insulin, monitor for hypoglycemia and give glucose as needed. Monitor potassium levels.

Hypokalemia

Hypokalemia (low serum potassium) can result from an increased loss of potassium, an increased shift of potassium from ECF to ICF, or, rarely, decreased potassium intake. The most common causes are abnormal losses from either the kidneys or GI tract. GI tract losses occur with diarrhea, laxative misuse, vomiting, and ileostomy drainage. Renal losses occur when a patient has increased urinary output, is using loop or other potassium-depleting diuretics, or has a low magnesium level. Low magnesium levels stimulate renin and aldosterone release, resulting in potassium excretion.

Factors causing potassium to move from ECF to ICF are insulin therapy, especially in conjunction with diabetic ketoacidosis, and β-adrenergic stimulation (catecholamine release in stress, coronary ischemia). Alkalosis can cause a shift of potassium into cells in exchange for hydrogen, which lowers potassium in ECF.

Clinical Manifestations

Hypokalemia alters the resting membrane potential, resulting in hyperpolarization (an increased negative charge within the cell) and impaired muscle contraction. Therefore the manifestations of hypokalemia involve changes in cardiac and muscle function (Table 17.6).

The most serious clinical problem is cardiac changes. These include impaired repolarization, resulting in a flattened T wave, depressed ST segment, and the presence of a U wave. The P waves peak and the QRS complex is prolonged (Fig. 17.14). There is an increased incidence of heart block and potentially lethal ventricular dysrhythmias.

As with hyperkalemia, skeletal muscle weakness and paresthesia may occur. Severe hypokalemia can cause paralysis. This usually involves the extremities but can involve the respiratory muscles, leading to shallow respirations and respiratory arrest. Changes in smooth muscle function may lead to decreased GI motility (e.g., constipation, paralytic ileus). Finally, hypokalemia impairs insulin secretion, leading to glucose intolerance and hyperglycemia.

Interprofessional and Nursing Management

We manage hypokalemia by giving oral or IV potassium chloride (KCl) supplements and increasing potassium intake in the diet. Consuming potassium-rich foods can usually correct mild hypokalemia. See Table 17.7 for foods that are high in potassium. Clinically significant hypokalemia requires giving oral or IV KCl.

SAFETY ALERT

IV KCl

- Always dilute IV KCl, and do not give in concentrated amounts.
- Never give KCl as an IV push or bolus.
- Invert IV bags with KCl several times to ensure even distribution in the bag.
- Do not add KCl to a hanging IV bag to prevent giving a bolus dose.

IV KCl infusion rates should not exceed 10 mEq/h unless the patient is in a critical care setting with continuous ECG monitoring and central line access for administration.[7] IV KCl must be given by infusion pump to ensure the correct administration rate. Because KCl is irritating to the vein, assess IV sites at least hourly for phlebitis and infiltration. Infiltration can cause necrosis and sloughing of the surrounding tissue.

Patients who are critically ill and those at risk for hypokalemia should have continuous ECG monitoring to detect cardiac changes. Monitor potassium levels and urine output as appropriate. KCl is usually given only if the urine output is at least 0.5 mL/kg of body weight per hour. Because patients on digoxin therapy have an increased risk for toxicity if their potassium level is low, monitor the patient for digitalis toxicity. Manifestations include confusion, lethargy, anorexia, vision problems, nausea, and vomiting.[8]

Teach patients ways to prevent hypokalemia (Table 17.8). Patients at risk should have regular potassium levels drawn. Teach patients taking digitalis to report signs and symptoms of digoxin toxicity at once to the HCP.

CHECK YOUR PRACTICE

You are taking care of a 78-year-old patient with HF who is taking furosemide and digitalis.

- What would you be alert for in a patient who takes both drugs?

TABLE 17.7 NUTRITION THERAPY

High-Potassium Foods

Fruits	Vegetables	Other Foods
• Apricot, raw (medium)	• Baked beans	• Bran or bran products
• Avocado (¼ whole)	• Butternut squash	• Chocolate (1.5 to 2 oz)
• Banana (¼ whole)	• Refried beans	• Granola
• Cantaloupe	• Black beans	• Milk, all types (1 cup)
• Dried fruits	• Broccoli, cooked	• Nuts and seeds (1 oz)
• Grapefruit juice	• Carrots, raw	• Peanut butter (2 Tbsp)
• Honeydew	• Greens, except kale	• Salt substitutes, Lite Salt
• Orange (medium)	• Mushrooms, canned	• Salt-free broth
• Orange juice	• Potatoes, white and sweet	• Yogurt
• Prunes	• Spinach, cooked	
• Raisins	• Tomatoes, tomato products	
	• Vegetable juices	

TABLE 17.8 PATIENT & CAREGIVER TEACHING

Prevention of Hypokalemia

Include the following instructions when teaching at-risk patients how to prevent hypokalemia:

1. For all patients at risk:
   - Report the signs and symptoms of hypokalemia (Table 17.5) to your health care provider.
   - Have potassium levels checked regularly.
   - Regularly include foods high in potassium in your diet (Table 17.6).
   - Drink alcohol in moderation.
   - Avoid eating large amounts of licorice.
2. For patients taking oral potassium supplements:
   - Take the supplement as prescribed to prevent overdosing.
   - Take with a full glass of water. Do not crush or chew tablets.

CALCIUM

Calcium has a role in many metabolic processes. It is the main cation in bones and teeth. Calcium plays a role in blood clotting, nerve impulse transmission, myocardial contractions, and muscle contractions. The major source for calcium is diet intake. Calcium absorption requires the active form of vitamin D. Vitamin D is obtained from foods or made in the skin by the action of sunlight on cholesterol.

The total body content of calcium is about 1200 g. The bones contain 99% of the body's calcium; the rest is in plasma and body cells. Of the calcium in plasma, 50% is bound to plasma proteins, mainly albumin. Around 40% is in a free or ionized form. The rest is found bound with phosphate, citrate, or carbonate. The ionized or free calcium is biologically active. The serum pH influences how much calcium is ionized or bound to albumin. A decreased plasma pH (acidosis) decreases calcium binding to albumin, leading to more ionized calcium. An increased plasma pH (alkalosis) increases calcium binding, leading to decreased ionized calcium.

Calcium levels reflect the total level of all forms of calcium. Albumin levels affect total calcium levels. Calcium levels increase or decrease directly with albumin levels. Ionized calcium levels are measured using special laboratory techniques or calculated using a formula. Albumin levels do not affect ionized calcium levels.

Parathyroid hormone (PTH) and calcitonin regulate calcium levels. Because the bones serve as a readily available store of calcium, the body can usually keep calcium levels normal by regulating the movement of calcium into or out of the bone. Low calcium levels stimulate the parathyroid glands to make and release PTH. PTH increases bone resorption (movement of calcium out of bones), increases GI absorption of calcium, and increases renal calcium reabsorption. High calcium levels stimulate calcitonin release. Calcitonin has the opposite effect of PTH. It lowers the calcium level by increasing calcium deposition into bone, increasing renal calcium excretion, and decreasing GI absorption.

Hypercalcemia

Hypercalcemia (high serum calcium) is caused by hyperparathyroidism in about two-thirds of persons. Cancers, especially kidney, breast, prostate, ovarian, hematologic, and lung cancers, cause the remaining third. Cancers lead to hypercalcemia through tumor-producing factors that prompt osteoclastic activity and bone resorption.[9] Rare causes include thiazide diuretic use, prolonged immobilization, and increased calcium intake (e.g., calcium-containing antacids).

Excess calcium acts like a sedative, leading to reduced excitability of muscles and nerves. Neurologic manifestations begin with fatigue, lethargy, weakness, and confusion and progress to hallucinations, seizures, and coma. Changes in cardiac conduction can lead to dysrhythmias, including heart block and ventricular tachycardia. Table 17.9 lists the causes and manifestations of hypercalcemia.

Interprofessional and Nursing Management

Management depends on the degree of hypercalcemia, patient's condition, and underlying cause. Patients with mild hypercalcemia should stop any medications related to hypercalcemia, start a diet low in calcium, and increase weight-bearing activity. The patient must drink 3000 to 4000 mL of fluid daily to promote the renal excretion of calcium and decrease the chance of kidney stones. Fluids that promote urine acidity (cranberry or prune juice) will help prevent stone formation.

We manage severe hypercalcemia by giving IV isotonic saline, a bisphosphonate, and calcitonin. IV saline therapy requires careful monitoring. Fluid overload can occur in patients who cannot excrete the excess sodium because of impaired

TABLE 17.9 Calcium Imbalances

Causes and Manifestations

Hypercalcemia (Ca^{2+} >10.5 mg/dL [2.62 mmol/L])	Hypocalcemia (Ca^{2+} <9.0 mg/dL [2.25 mmol/L])
Causes	
Increased Total Calcium	***Decreased Total Calcium***
• Hyperparathyroidism • Adrenal insufficiency • Cancers with bone metastasis • Excess dairy intake • Hematologic cancer • *Medications:* Thiazide diuretics, calcium-containing antacids, vitamin A or D • *Mycobacterium* infection • Paget disease • Prolonged immobilization • Thyrotoxicosis	• Acute pancreatitis • Chronic alcohol use • Diarrhea • Malnutrition, vitamin D deficiency • ↓ Magnesium level • *Medications:* Bisphosphonates, loop diuretics • ↑ Phosphate level • Primary hypoparathyroidism • Renal insufficiency • ↓ Serum albumin • Tumor lysis syndrome
Increased Ionized Calcium	***Decreased Ionized Calcium***
• Acidosis	• Alkalosis • Receiving excess citrated blood
Manifestations	
• ↑ BP • Bone pain, fractures • Confusion, psychosis • Fatigue, lethargy, weakness • ↓ Reflexes • Impaired memory • Kidney stones • Nausea, vomiting, anorexia • Polyuria, dehydration • Seizures, coma	• ↓ BP • Chvostek sign • Confusion, depression, irritability • Fatigue, weakness • ↑ Reflexes, muscle cramps • Laryngeal and bronchial spasms • Numbness and tingling in extremities and around mouth • Tetany, seizures • Trousseau sign
ECG Changes	***ECG Changes***
• Short ST segment • Short QT interval • Ventricular dysrhythmias • Increased digitalis effect	• Prolonged ST segment • Prolonged QT interval • Ventricular tachycardia

renal function. Bisphosphonates (e.g., pamidronate, zoledronic acid) are the gold standard in treating hypercalcemia, especially when caused by cancer. They interfere with the activity of osteoclasts, cells that break down bone. Because it takes 2 to 4 days for them to achieve maximum effect, patients receive calcitonin injections for an immediate effect. Calcitonin rapidly increases renal calcium excretion. However, therapy is effective for only a few days and may cause tachycardia. For patients who do not respond to bisphosphonates or have cancer-induced hypercalcemia, denosumab (Prolia) is an alternative.[10] Dialysis is an option in life-threatening situations.

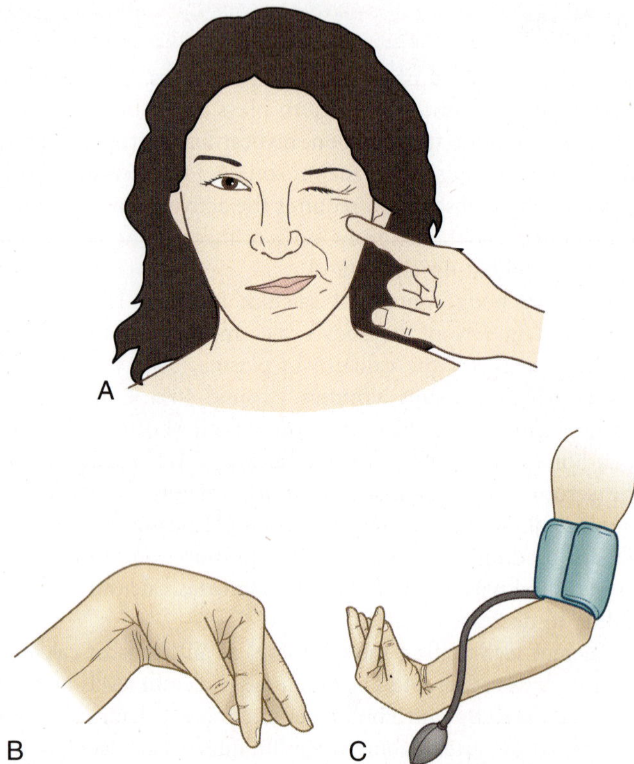

Fig. 17.15 Tests for hypocalcemia. (A) Chvostek sign is contraction of facial muscles in response to a light tap over the facial nerve in front of the ear. (B) Trousseau sign is a carpal spasm induced by (C) inflating a BP cuff above the systolic pressure for a few minutes.

Hypocalcemia

Hypocalcemia (low serum calcium) can result from any condition associated with PTH deficiency. This may occur with surgical removal of part of or injury to the parathyroid glands during thyroid or neck surgery or with neck radiation. Patients who receive multiple blood transfusions can develop hypocalcemia. This is because citrate, used as an anticoagulant in blood bags, binds with calcium, decreasing ionized calcium levels. Sudden alkalosis may result in symptomatic hypocalcemia despite a normal total calcium level. The high pH increases calcium binding to protein, decreasing the amount of ionized calcium. Table 17.9 lists causes and manifestations of hypocalcemia.

Low ionized calcium levels decrease the threshold for activating the sodium channels that cause cell membrane depolarization. This results in increased nerve excitability and sustained muscle contraction, or *tetany.* Signs of tetany include Chvostek sign and Trousseau sign. *Chvostek sign* is contraction of facial muscles in response to a tap over the facial nerve in front of the ear (Fig. 17.15A). *Trousseau sign* refers to carpal spasms induced by inflating a BP cuff on the arm (Fig. 17.15B and C). When you inflate the cuff above the systolic pressure, carpal spasms occur within 3 minutes if hypocalcemia is present. Other manifestations of tetany are laryngeal stridor, dysphagia, paresthesia, and numbness and tingling around the mouth (circumoral) or in the extremities. Cardiac effects include decreased cardiac contractility and ECG changes. A prolonged QT interval may develop into ventricular tachycardia.

Interprofessional and Nursing Management

Managing hypocalcemia depends on the underlying cause and the presence of symptoms. We treat mild or asymptomatic hypocalcemia with a diet high in calcium-rich foods and calcium and vitamin D supplementation. Symptomatic hypocalcemia, including the presence of tetany and significant ECG changes, is treated with IV calcium gluconate.[11] Measures to promote CO_2 retention, such as breathing into a paper bag or sedating the patient, can control muscle spasms and other symptoms of tetany until the calcium level is corrected. Patients taking loop diuretics may need to change to thiazide diuretics to decrease urinary calcium excretion. Assess any patient who had thyroid or neck surgery in the immediate postoperative period for hypocalcemia because of the proximity of the surgery to the parathyroid glands. Adequately treat pain and anxiety because hyperventilation-induced respiratory alkalosis can precipitate hypocalcemic symptoms.

PHOSPHORUS

Phosphorus is the primary anion in ICF and the second most abundant element in the body after calcium. Most phosphorus is in bones and teeth as calcium phosphate. The remaining phosphorus is metabolically active in the form of phosphate salts. Thus we use the terms *phosphorus* and *phosphate* interchangeably here. Phosphate is essential to the function of muscle, red blood cells (RBCs), and the nervous system. It is involved in the acid-base buffering system; the mitochondrial formation of ATP; cell uptake and use of glucose; and carbohydrate, protein, and fat metabolism.

PTH maintains phosphate levels and balance. Phosphate balance requires adequate renal functioning because the kidneys are the main route of phosphate excretion. When the phosphate level in the glomerular filtrate falls below normal or PTH levels are low, the kidneys reabsorb more phosphate. A reciprocal relationship exists between phosphate and calcium. This means a low calcium level will result in a high phosphate level and vice versa.

Hyperphosphatemia

Hyperphosphatemia (high serum phosphate) is common in patients with acute kidney injury or chronic kidney disease because both alter the kidney's ability to excrete phosphate.

TABLE 17.10 Phosphate Imbalances

Causes and Manifestations

Hyperphosphatemia (PO_4^{3-} >4.5 mg/dL [1.45 mmol/L])	Hypophosphatemia (PO_4^{3-} <3.0 mg/dL [0.97 mmol/L])
Causes	
• Excess ingestion (e.g., phosphate-containing laxatives) • Hyperthermia • Hypoparathyroidism • Phosphate enemas (e.g., Fleet Enema) • Renal failure • Rhabdomyolysis • Sickle cell anemia, hemolytic anemia • Tumor lysis syndrome • Thyrotoxicosis	• Chronic alcohol use • Chronic diarrhea • Diabetic ketoacidosis • Malabsorption syndromes • Malnutrition, vitamin D deficiency • Hyperparathyroidism • Parenteral nutrition • Phosphate-binding antacids • Refeeding syndrome • Respiratory alkalosis
Manifestations	
• ↑ Reflexes, muscle cramps • ↓ Calcium • Numbness and tingling in extremities and around mouth • Tetany, seizures • Calcium-phosphate precipitates in skin, soft tissue, cornea, viscera, blood vessels	• CNS depression (confusion, coma) • Heart problems (dysrhythmias, heart failure) • Muscle weakness, including respiratory muscle weakness • Polyneuropathy, seizures • Rhabdomyolysis • Rickets, osteomalacia

Other causes include excess phosphate intake from the use of phosphate-containing laxatives or enemas or a shift of phosphate from ICF to ECF. This may occur in patients with tumor lysis syndrome or rhabdomyolysis. Hypoparathyroidism and vitamin D intoxication cause increased kidney phosphate reabsorption. Table 17.10 describes causes and manifestations of hyperphosphatemia.

High phosphate levels can be asymptomatic unless calcium binds with phosphate, leading to manifestations of hypocalcemia. These include tetany, muscle cramps, paresthesias, hypotension, dysrhythmias, and seizures.[12] Long-term increased phosphate levels result in the development of calcified deposits outside of the bones. These calcium deposits can be found in soft tissues, such as joints, arteries, skin, corneas, and kidneys, and cause organ dysfunction, notably renal failure.

Management involves identifying and treating the underlying cause. Restrict the intake of foods and fluids high in phosphorus (e.g., dairy products). Oral phosphate-binding agents (e.g., calcium carbonate) limit intestinal phosphate absorption and increase phosphate secretion in the intestine. With severe hyperphosphatemia, hemodialysis may be used to rapidly decrease levels. Volume expansion and forced diuresis with a loop diuretic may increase phosphate excretion. If hypocalcemia is present, institute measures to correct calcium levels. See Chapter 51 for more information about treating high phosphate from kidney disease.

Hypophosphatemia

Hypophosphatemia (low serum phosphate) can result from decreased intestinal absorption, increased urinary excretion, or ECF-to-ICF shifts. Malabsorption, diarrhea, and phosphate-binding antacids lead to decreased absorption. Phosphate shifts occur in respiratory alkalosis, treatment of diabetic ketoacidosis, and refeeding syndrome (reinstitution of nutrition to patients who are severely malnourished). Low phosphate levels may occur in those who are malnourished or receive parenteral nutrition (PN) with inadequate phosphorus replacement. Table 17.10 lists causes and manifestations of hypophosphatemia.

Most of the manifestations result from impaired cell energy and O_2 delivery because of low levels of cell ATP and 2,3-diphosphoglycerate (2,3-DPG). It is an enzyme in RBCs that facilitates O_2 delivery to the tissues. Mild to moderate hypophosphatemia is often asymptomatic. Severely low phosphate may be fatal because of decreased cell function. Acute manifestations include CNS depression, muscle weakness and pain, HF, and respiratory failure. Chronically low phosphate levels alter bone metabolism, causing rickets and osteomalacia.

Symptomatic hypophosphatemia usually requires IV sodium phosphate or potassium phosphate. During IV replacement, monitor calcium and phosphate levels every 6 hours and perform frequent assessments.[13] Complications include hypocalcemia, hyperkalemia, hypotension, and dysrhythmias. We treat mild phosphate deficiency with phosphate supplements or by increasing oral intake of food rich in phosphorus like dairy products, meats, and beans. Dairy products may be better tolerated because phosphate supplements often cause adverse GI effects, including diarrhea.[13]

MAGNESIUM

Magnesium, the second most abundant intracellular cation, plays a key role in essential cell processes. It is a cofactor in many enzyme systems, including those responsible for carbohydrate metabolism, DNA and protein synthesis, blood glucose control, and BP regulation. Magnesium is needed for the production and use of ATP, the energy source for the sodium-potassium pump. Muscle contraction and relaxation, normal neurologic function, and neurotransmitter release depend on magnesium.

We store about 50% to 60% of our magnesium in muscle and bone. About 30% is in cells, with only 1% in ECF. The kidneys and GI system regulate magnesium by controlling the amount of magnesium reabsorbed in the ascending loop of Henle and distal tubules and absorbed in the small intestine. GI absorption and renal reabsorption increase when magnesium levels are low.

Hypermagnesemia

Hypermagnesemia (high serum magnesium level) usually occurs only with increased magnesium intake accompanied by renal insufficiency or failure. Patients with chronic kidney disease who ingest products containing magnesium (e.g., Maalox, Milk of Magnesia) will have a problem with excess magnesium. Magnesium excess could develop in pregnant females receiving magnesium sulfate for the treatment of eclampsia or in patients taking laxatives and antacids that contain magnesium. Table 17.11 lists the causes and manifestations of hypermagnesemia.

Excess magnesium inhibits acetylcholine release at the myoneural junction and calcium movement into cells. This impairs nerve and muscle function. Initial manifestations include hypotension, facial flushing, lethargy, urinary retention, nausea, and vomiting. As magnesium levels increase, deep tendon reflexes are lost, followed by muscle paralysis and coma. Respiratory and cardiac arrest can occur.

Management begins with stopping magnesium-containing drugs and limiting intake of magnesium-containing foods (e.g., green vegetables, nuts, bananas, oranges, peanut butter, chocolate). If renal function is adequate, increased fluids and diuretics promote urinary excretion of magnesium. Patients with impaired renal function may need dialysis. If the patient is symptomatic, giving IV calcium gluconate will oppose the effects of the excess magnesium on cardiac muscle.[14]

Hypomagnesemia

Hypomagnesemia (low serum magnesium level) occurs in patients with limited magnesium intake or increased GI or renal losses. Causes from insufficient food intake include prolonged fasting or starvation and chronic alcohol use. Another potential cause is prolonged PN without magnesium supplementation. Fluid loss from the GI tract, acute pancreatitis, and poorly controlled diabetes may contribute to low magnesium. Diuretics, proton pump inhibitors, and some antibiotics may lead to magnesium loss.[15] Table 17.11 lists the causes and manifestations of hypomagnesemia.

Clinically, hypomagnesemia resembles hypocalcemia. Neuromuscular manifestations are common. These include muscle cramps, tremors, hyperactive deep tendon reflexes, Chvostek sign, and Trousseau sign. Neurologic manifestations include confusion, vertigo, and seizures. Dysrhythmias, such as torsades de pointes and ventricular fibrillation, can occur.

Management depends on the underlying cause and the patient's symptoms. We treat mild magnesium deficiency with oral supplements and increased intake of foods high in magnesium. We give IV magnesium (e.g., magnesium sulfate) if the deficiency is severe or if hypocalcemia is present.

TABLE 17.11 Magnesium Imbalances

Causes and Manifestations

Hypermagnesemia (Mg^+ >2.1 mEq/L [1.05 mmol/L])	Hypomagnesemia (Mg^+ <1.3 mEq/L [0.65 mmol/L])
Causes	
• Adrenal insufficiency • Antacids, laxatives • Hypothyroidism • IV administration of magnesium, especially for treatment of eclampsia • Metastatic bone disease • Renal failure • Tumor lysis syndrome	• Acute pancreatitis • Chronic alcohol use • GI tract fluid losses (e.g., diarrhea, NG suction) • Hyperglycemia • Malabsorption syndromes • Prolonged malnutrition • Proton pump inhibitor therapy • ↑ Urine output
Manifestations	
• ↓ Deep tendon reflexes • Flushed, warm skin, especially facial • Lethargy, drowsiness • Nausea, vomiting • Muscle weakness • ↓ HR, ↓ BP • Urinary retention	• Chvostek and Trousseau signs • Confusion • Hyperactive deep tendon reflexes • Muscle cramps • ↑ HR, ↑ BP, dysrhythmias • Tremors, seizures • Vertigo

! SAFETY ALERT

IV Magnesium

- Always give using an infusion pump.
- Monitor vital signs, level of consciousness, and reflexes.
- Rapid administration can lead to hypotension and cardiac or respiratory arrest.
- Keep IV calcium gluconate on hand.

ACID-BASE BALANCE

ACID-BASE REGULATION

The body normally maintains a steady balance between the acids continually produced during normal metabolism and the bases that neutralize and promote acid excretion. Because these acids alter the body's internal environment, their regulation is necessary to maintain homeostasis and acid-base balance (Table 17.12). An acid-base imbalance is not a disease, but a symptom of an underlying health problem. Many health problems may lead to acid-base imbalances. Patients with diabetes, chronic obstructive pulmonary disease (COPD), and kidney disease often develop acid-base imbalances.

pH and Hydrogen Ion Concentration

The acidity or alkalinity of a solution depends on its hydrogen ion (H^+) concentration. We express H^+ concentration as a negative logarithm (symbolized as *pH*). An increase in H^+ concentration leads to acidity. The higher the H^+ concentration, the lower the pH. A decrease in H^+ concentration leads to alkalinity. The lower the H^+ concentration, the higher the pH. A decrease leads to alkalinity.

The pH of a chemical solution may range from 1 to 14. A solution with a pH of 7 is considered neutral. An acid solution

TABLE 17.12 Acid-Base Imbalances

Causes	Pathophysiology	Laboratory Findings
Respiratory Acidosis		

• Atelectasis
• Chest wall abnormality
• Chronic respiratory disease (e.g., COPD)
• Mechanical hypoventilation
• Pneumonia (severe)
• Pulmonary edema
• Respiratory muscle weakness
• Sedative overdose
	• ↑ CO_2 retention from hypoventilation
	• Compensatory response is ↑ HCO_3^- retention by kidney
		• ↓ Plasma pH
		• ↑ $Paco_2$, HCO_3^- normal (uncompensated)
		• ↑ HCO_3^- (compensated)
		• *Sample ABG (uncompensated):*
		  • pH 7.31
		  • $Paco_2$ 54 mm Hg
		  • HCO_3^- 25 mEq/L

Respiratory Alkalosis		

• Hyperventilation (e.g., hypoxia, anxiety, fear, pain, exercise, fever)
• Liver failure
• Mechanical hyperventilation
• Stimulated respiratory center (e.g., septicemia, stroke, meningitis, encephalitis, brain injury, salicylate poisoning)
	• ↑ CO_2 excretion from hyperventilation
	• Compensatory response is ↑ HCO_3^- excretion by kidney
		• ↑ Plasma pH
		• ↓ $Paco_2$, HCO_3^- normal (uncompensated)
		• ↓ HCO_3^- (compensated)
		• *Sample ABG (uncompensated):*
		  • pH 7.52
		  • $Paco_2$ 27 mm Hg
		  • HCO_3^- 25 mEq/L

Metabolic Acidosis		

• Diabetic ketoacidosis
• Diarrhea
• GI fistulas
• Lactic acidosis
• Renal failure
• Renal tubular acidosis
• Shock
• Starvation
	• Gain of fixed acid, inability to excrete acid or loss of base
	• Compensatory response is ↑ CO_2 excretion by lungs
		• ↓ Plasma pH
		• $Paco_2$ normal (uncompensated)
		• ↓ $Paco_2$ (compensated)
		• ↓ HCO_3^-
		• *Sample ABG (uncompensated):*
		  • pH 7.29
		  • $Paco_2$ 38 mm Hg
		  • HCO_3^- 18 mEq/L

Metabolic Alkalosis		

• Diuretic therapy
• Excess $NaHCO_3$ intake
• Hypokalemia
• Mineralocorticoid use
• NG suctioning
• Vomiting
	• Loss of strong acid or gain of base
	• Compensatory response is ↑ CO_2 retention by lungs
		• ↑ Plasma pH
		• $Paco_2$ normal (uncompensated)
		• ↑ $Paco_2$ (compensated)
		• ↑ HCO_3^-
		• *Sample ABG (uncompensated):*
		  • pH 7.50
		  • $Paco_2$ 40 mm Hg
		  • HCO_3^- 34 mEq/L

ABG, Arterial blood gas; *COPD,* chronic obstructive pulmonary disease.

has a pH less than 7, and an alkaline solution has a pH greater than 7. Blood is slightly alkaline and has a normal arterial pH of 7.35 to 7.45. Medically, if the pH drops below 7.35, a person has **acidosis**. If the blood pH is greater than 7.45, the person has **alkalosis** (Fig. 17.16).

The body uses 3 processes to regulate acid-base balance and keep the pH between 7.35 and 7.45. These are the buffer systems, respiratory system, and renal system. Each process reacts at different speeds. Buffers are the fastest, reacting immediately. The respiratory system responds in minutes and reaches maximum effectiveness in hours. The renal response occurs hours to days after a change in pH. The kidneys can maintain balance indefinitely in patients with chronic imbalances. But if the person has impaired kidney function, the kidneys will not be effective in maintaining acid-base balance.

Buffer System

Buffering is the primary regulator of acid-base balance. **Buffers** act chemically to change strong acids into weaker ones or bind acids to neutralize them. This minimizes the effect of acids on blood pH until they can be excreted from the body. Buffers can maintain pH only if the respiratory and renal systems function adequately.

All body fluids contain buffers. The major buffer in ECF is the carbonic acid–bicarbonate system (H_2CO_3/HCO_3^-). Other

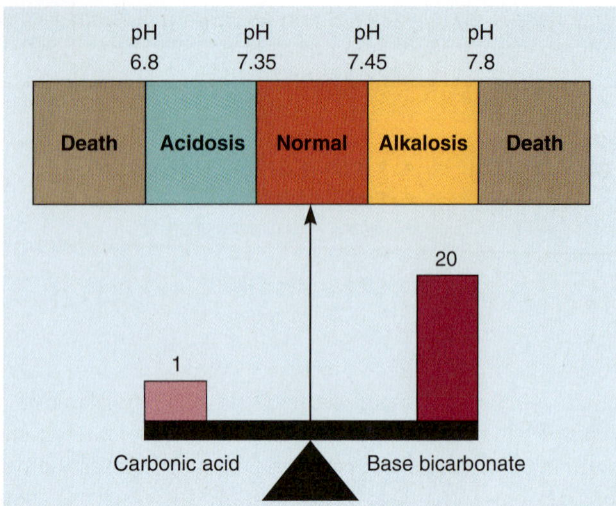

Fig. 17.16 The normal range of plasma pH is 7.35 to 7.45. A normal pH is maintained by a ratio of 1 part carbonic acid to 20 parts bicarbonate.

buffer systems include phosphate, protein, and hemoglobin. The cell can act as a buffer by shifting H^+ in and out of the cell. When ECF levels of H^+ are increased, H^+ enters the cell in exchange for potassium. This may result in hyperkalemia as potassium moves into the ECF. Conversely, with decreased H^+ levels, H^+ enters plasma in exchange for potassium. This is why a patient with alkalosis can develop hypokalemia.

A buffer consists of a weak acid, which releases H^+ when fluid is too alkaline, or a base and its salt, which takes up H^+ when fluid is too acidic. The carbonic acid–bicarbonate buffer system neutralizes hydrochloric acid (HCl), a strong acid, by combining it with a strong base. This prevents the acid from making a large decrease in pH.

$$\underset{\text{Strong Acid}}{HCl} + \underset{\text{Strong Base}}{Na_2CO_3} \rightarrow \underset{\text{Salt}}{NaCl} + \underset{\text{Weak Acid}}{H_2CO_3}$$

Carbonic acid is broken down into H_2O and CO_2. The lungs excrete CO_2, either combined with insensible H_2O as carbonic acid or alone as CO_2.

The phosphate, protein, and hemoglobin buffer systems act in the same way as the bicarbonate system. The main components of the phosphate system are monohydrogen phosphate and dihydrogen phosphate ($H_2PO_4^-$). A phosphate combined with sodium can neutralize a strong acid, such as HCl, by forming sodium chloride (NaCl) and sodium biphosphate (NaH_2PO_4), a weak acid. If a strong base, such as sodium hydroxide (NaOH), is present, sodium biphosphate (NaH_2PO_4) neutralizes it to a weaker base (Na_2HPO_4) and H_2O.

Intracellular and extracellular proteins can act as an acid or base. Because the chemical structure of amino acids has an acid and a base, they can either accept H^+ if pH decreases or release H^+ if fluid is too alkaline. Some amino acids have basic radicals (NH_3OH [ammonium hydroxide]) that can dissociate into NH_3^+ (ammonia) and OH^- (hydroxide). The OH^- can combine with H^+ to form H_2O.

Hemoglobin can bind with both H^+, forming a weak acid, and CO_2, forming carbaminohemoglobin ($HbCO_2$). $HbCO_2$ dissociates in the lungs, releasing CO_2 for exhalation. Because H^+ can combine only with hemoglobin that has released its O_2, venous blood is a better buffer than arterial blood, which contains saturated hemoglobin. Hemoglobin also aids in controlling pH by shifting chloride in and out of RBCs in exchange for bicarbonate.

The buffer system maintains a 20:1 ratio between HCO_3^- and carbonic acid in ECF. The body's ability to keep this ratio is important in controlling pH. For example, excess carbonic acid increases the ratio and decreases pH, resulting in acidosis. In response, the body can increase HCO_3^- levels to keep the ratio 20:1 and keep the pH near normal—a state called *compensation.* For example, a ratio of 40:2 is present in compensated acid-base balance.

Respiratory System

The lungs help maintain a normal pH by excreting CO_2 and water, which are by-products of cell metabolism. When released into the circulation, CO_2 enters RBCs and combines with H_2O to form H_2CO_3. Carbonic acid dissociates into H^+ and HCO_3^-. Hemoglobin buffers the free H^+, and the HCO_3^- diffuses into the plasma. This process is reversed in the pulmonary capillaries, forming CO_2 that is excreted by the lungs.

The amount of CO_2 in the blood directly relates to carbonic acid and H^+ concentration. With increased respirations, the lungs expel more CO_2, so less stays in the blood. This leads to less carbonic acid and less H^+. With decreased respirations, more CO_2 stays in the blood. This leads to increased carbonic acid and more H^+.

The respiratory center in the medulla controls the rate of excretion of CO_2. If increased amounts of CO_2 or H^+ are present, the respiratory center stimulates an increased rate and depth of breathing to "blow off" CO_2 through hyperventilation. If the center senses low H^+ or CO_2 levels, respirations are reduced and CO_2 is retained. The older adult has an impaired compensatory ability because of decreased respiratory function.

Renal System

Under normal conditions, the body depends on the kidneys to reabsorb and conserve all the HCO_3^- they filter and excrete some of the acid produced by cell metabolism. The 3 processes of acid excretion include (1) secreting small amounts of free hydrogen into the renal tubule, (2) combining H^+ with ammonia (NH_3) to form ammonium (NH_4^+), and (3) excreting weak acids.

The kidneys normally excrete acidic urine (average pH is 6). As a compensatory process, the urine pH can decrease to 4 or increase to 8. To compensate for acidosis, the kidneys can reabsorb more HCO_3^- and excrete excess H^+. This increases the blood pH and decreases the urine pH. In the older adult, the kidneys are less able to compensate for acid load.

Acid-Base Imbalance

An acid-base imbalance results when there is a change in the ratio of 20:1 between base and acid content. This occurs when a disease or process alters one side of the ratio (e.g., CO_2 retention in pulmonary disease) and the compensatory processes that maintain the other side of the ratio (e.g., increased renal HCO_3^- reabsorption) either fail or are inadequate. The compensatory process may be inadequate because either the pathophysiologic activity is overwhelming or there is not enough time for the compensatory process to work.

Acid-base imbalances are classified as respiratory or metabolic. *Respiratory imbalances* result from changes in carbonic acid concentration. *Metabolic imbalances* affect the base HCO_3^-. Acidosis occurs with an increase in carbonic acid (respiratory acidosis) or decrease in HCO_3^- (metabolic acidosis). Alkalosis occurs with a decrease in carbonic acid (respiratory alkalosis) or an increase in HCO_3^- (metabolic alkalosis). We further classify imbalances as acute or chronic. Chronic imbalances allow greater time for compensatory changes.

Respiratory Acidosis

Respiratory acidosis (carbonic acid excess) occurs when a person has hypoventilation (Table 17.12). Hypoventilation leads to a buildup of CO_2, resulting in an accumulation of carbonic acid in the blood. Carbonic acid dissociates, releasing H^+ and decreasing pH. If CO_2 is not eliminated from the blood, acidosis results from the accumulation of carbonic acid (Fig. 17.17A).

During acute respiratory acidosis, the renal compensatory processes begin to work within 24 hours. The kidneys conserve HCO_3^- and secrete increased H^+ into the urine. Until the renal processes have an effect, the HCO_3^- level will usually be normal and then increase.

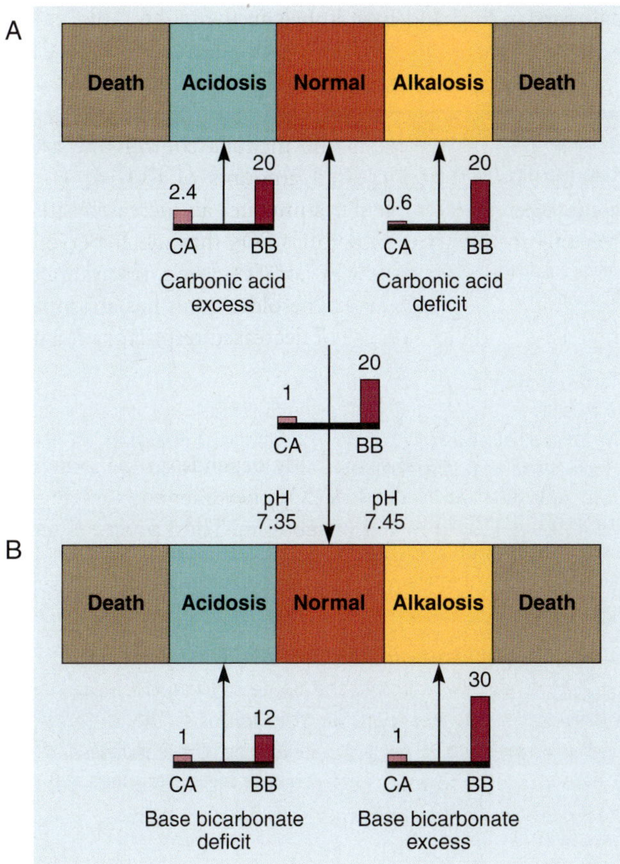

Fig. 17.17 Types of acid-base imbalances. (A) Respiratory imbalances caused by carbonic acid *(CA)* excess and carbonic acid deficit. (B) Metabolic imbalances caused by base bicarbonate *(BB)* deficit and base bicarbonate excess.

Respiratory Alkalosis

Respiratory alkalosis (carbonic acid deficit) occurs with hyperventilation or an increase in respiratory rate or volume (Table 17.12). The main cause of respiratory alkalosis is hypoxemia from acute pulmonary disorders (e.g., pneumonia, pulmonary embolus). Hyperventilation can occur as a physiologic response to metabolic acidosis and increased metabolic demands (e.g., fever). Pain, anxiety, and some CNS disorders can increase respirations without a physiologic need. The decrease in the arterial CO_2 level leads to decreased carbonic acid concentration in the blood and an increased pH (Fig. 17.17A).

Compensated respiratory alkalosis is rare. In acute respiratory alkalosis, aggressive treatment of the cause of hypoxemia is essential. This usually does not allow time for compensation to occur. If the respiratory alkalosis is caused by significant pain, anxiety, or panic, breathing into a closed system to rebreathe eliminated CO_2 can aid in the compensatory process. Some buffering may occur with the shifting of HCO_3^- into cells in exchange for chloride ions (Cl^-). In chronic respiratory alkalosis that occurs with pulmonary fibrosis or CNS disorders, compensation may include renal excretion of HCO_3^-.

Metabolic Acidosis

Metabolic acidosis (base bicarbonate deficit) occurs when an acid other than carbonic acid accumulates in the body or when bicarbonate is lost in body fluids (Table 17.12 and Fig. 17.17B). Ketoacid accumulation in diabetic ketoacidosis and lactic acid accumulation with shock are examples of acid accumulation. Severe diarrhea resulting in loss of HCO_3^- is an example of a base deficit. In renal disease, the kidneys lose their ability to reabsorb HCO_3^- and secrete H^+. To compensate for metabolic acidosis, the kidneys try to excrete extra acid and the lungs increase CO_2 excretion. The patient often develops *Kussmaul respirations* (deep, rapid breathing) when trying to compensate for metabolic acidosis.

If metabolic acidosis is present, calculating the anion gap helps you figure out the source of the acidosis. The *anion gap* is the difference between the measured cations and anions in ECF:

$$\text{Anion gap} = Na^+ - (HCO_3^- + Cl^-)$$

A normal anion gap is 8 to 12 mmol/L. The anion gap increases in metabolic acidosis from acid gain (e.g., lactic acidosis, diabetic ketoacidosis). It is normal in metabolic acidosis caused by bicarbonate loss (e.g., diarrhea).

Metabolic Alkalosis

Metabolic alkalosis (base bicarbonate excess) occurs when a loss of acid (e.g., from prolonged vomiting or gastric suction) or a gain in HCO_3^- (e.g., from ingestion of baking soda) occurs (Table 17.12 and Fig. 17.17B). Renal excretion of HCO_3^- occurs in response to metabolic alkalosis. The lung's compensatory response is limited. The respiratory rate decreases to retain plasma CO_2. However, once hypoxemia occurs or plasma CO_2 reaches a certain level, stimulation of chemoreceptors will increase respirations.

Mixed Acid-Base Disorders

A mixed acid-base disorder occurs when 2 or more disorders are present at the same time. The pH depends on the type, severity, and acuity of each disorder involved and any compensatory processes at work. Respiratory acidosis combined with metabolic alkalosis (e.g., a patient with atelectasis and NG suction) may result in a near-normal pH. Respiratory acidosis combined with metabolic acidosis causes a greater decrease in pH than either disorder alone. An example of a mixed acidosis is a patient in severe shock with poor perfusion and hypoventilation. Mixed alkalosis can occur in a patient hyperventilating because of postoperative pain who is losing acid from NG suctioning.

Clinical Manifestations

Manifestations of acidosis and alkalosis are outlined in Tables 17.13 and 17.14. In both respiratory and metabolic acidosis, the CNS is depressed. Headache, lethargy, weakness, and confusion develop, leading eventually to coma and death. Compensation also produces specific manifestations. For example, the deep, rapid (Kussmaul) respirations of a patient with metabolic acidosis occur with respiratory compensation.

In both types of alkalosis, symptoms usually result from an accompanying electrolyte abnormality rather than the alkalosis. Hypocalcemia occurs because of increased calcium binding with albumin, lowering the amount of ionized, active calcium. Therefore muscle cramping and symptoms of CNS excitability, including tingling and numbness of the fingers and tetany, occur. Although respiratory alkalosis itself is not usually life-threatening, the underlying cause may be.[16]

Blood Gas Values

Arterial blood gas (ABG) values give objective information about acid-base status, the underlying cause of an imbalance, and the body's ability to regulate pH. Knowing the patient's clinical situation and the extent of renal and respiratory compensation allows you to identify acid-base disorders and the patient's ability to compensate. ABG analysis also shows the partial pressure of arterial O_2 (PaO_2) and O_2 saturation. Table 17.15 lists normal ABG values. These values help you evaluate the patient's overall oxygenation status and identify hypoxemia. Table 17.16 shows *ROME,* a quick memory device for understanding acid-base imbalances.

TABLE 17.13 Manifestations of Acidosis

Respiratory (↑ $PaCO_2$)	Metabolic (↓ HCO_3^-)
Neurologic	
Lethargy	Lethargy
Confusion	Confusion
Dizziness	Dizziness
Headache	Headache
Coma	Coma
Cardiovascular	
↓ BP	↓ BP
Ventricular fibrillation (related to hyperkalemia from compensation)	Dysrhythmias (related to hyperkalemia from compensation)
Warm, flushed skin	Cold, clammy skin
Gastrointestinal	
No significant findings	Nausea, vomiting, diarrhea, abdominal pain
Neuromuscular	
Seizures	Muscle weakness
Respiratory	
Hypoventilation with hypoxia	Deep, rapid respirations

TABLE 17.14 Manifestations of Alkalosis

Respiratory (↓ $PaCO_2$)	Metabolic (↑ HCO_3^-)
Neurologic	
Dizziness	Irritability
Lightheadedness	Lethargy
Confusion	Confusion
Headache	Headache
Cardiovascular	
Tachycardia	Tachycardia
Dysrhythmias (related to hypokalemia from compensation)	Dysrhythmias (related to hypokalemia from compensation)
Gastrointestinal	
Nausea, vomiting, diarrhea	Nausea, vomiting
Epigastric pain	Anorexia
Neuromuscular	
Tetany	Tetany
Numbness	Tremors
Tingling of extremities	Tingling of fingers and toes
↑ Reflexes	Muscle cramps, hypertonic muscles
Seizures	Seizures
Respiratory	
Hyperventilation (lungs are unable to compensate if there is a respiratory problem)	Hypoventilation (compensatory action by lungs)

TABLE 17.15 Normal Arterial Blood Gas Values

Parameter	Reference Interval
pH	7.35 to 7.45
$Paco_2$	35 to 45 mm Hg
Bicarbonate (HCO_3^-)	22 to 26 mEq/L (mmol/L)
Pao_2[a]	80 to 100 mm Hg
Sao_2	>95%
Base excess	±2.0 mEq/L

[a]Decreases above sea level and with increasing age.

TABLE 17.16 ROME

Memory Device for Acid-Base Imbalances

For acid-base imbalances, use this quick memory device (mnemonic):

In ***Respiratory*** conditions, the pH and the $Paco_2$ go in ***Opposite*** directions.

- In respiratory alkalosis, the pH is ↑ and the $Paco_2$ is ↓.
- In respiratory acidosis, the pH is ↓ and the $Paco_2$ is ↑.

In ***Metabolic*** conditions, the pH and the HCO_3^- go in the same direction ***(Equal)***.

- In metabolic alkalosis, pH and HCO_3^- are ↑.
- In metabolic acidosis, pH and HCO_3^- are ↓.

To interpret the results of an ABG, perform the following 5 steps:

1. Look at each value. If the pH is between 7.35 and 7.45 and the CO_2 and Pao_2 are within normal limits, the ABGs are normal. If any value is out of normal, then continue.
2. Look at the pH first. Values less than 7.35 indicate acidosis. Values greater than 7.45 indicate alkalosis. A normal pH means there is normal acid-base status, compensation is occurring, or a mixed disorder is present.
3. Use ROME (Table 17.16) to figure out if the origin is respiratory or metabolic. Remember "respiratory opposite and metabolic equal."
4. Once the metabolic or respiratory origin is determined, look at the remaining value, either the CO_2 or HCO_3^-, to figure the level of compensation. If the value is moving in the opposite direction, the body is trying to compensate. If the remaining value moving to compensate is abnormal and the pH is higher or lower than normal, *partial compensation* has occurred. If the pH is within normal limits, *full compensation* has occurred.
5. Assess the Pao_2 and O_2 saturation. If these values are abnormal, hypoxemia is present.

Table 17.17 explains how to analyze ABG results. The laboratory findings section of Table 17.12 shows ABG findings of the 4 major acid-base imbalances. See Chapter 27 for further discussion of ABGs.

ASSESSMENT OF ELECTROLYTE AND ACID-BASE IMBALANCES

Assessing patients for electrolyte and acid-base imbalances is an important part of your nursing practice. In addition to assessing for the manifestations discussed earlier in this chapter, obtain subjective and objective data from any patient with suspected electrolyte or acid-base imbalances.

TABLE 17.17 Applying Arterial Blood Gas (ABG) Analysis

Sample ABG Values	Analysis
pH 7.32 $Paco_2$ 30 HCO_3^- 16 Pao_2 95	1. Look at each of the values. If the pH is between 7.35 and 7.45 and the CO_2, HCO_3^-, and Pao_2 are within normal limits, the ABGs are normal. If any value is out of normal, then continue. *The pH, CO_2, HCO_3^- are all abnormally low. Continue with analysis.* 2. Look at the pH first. Values less than 7.35 indicate acidosis and values greater than 7.45 indicate alkalosis. *The pH is below 7.35, indicating acidosis.* 3. Use ROME to figure out if the origin is respiratory or metabolic. Remember "respiratory opposite and metabolic equal." *Using ROME, the pH and CO_2 are not going in the opposite direction (the disorder is not respiratory in origin). The pH and HCO_3^- are moving in the same or equal direction, so the disorder is metabolic in origin.* 4. Once the metabolic or respiratory origin is determined, look at the remaining laboratory value (either CO_2 or HCO_3^-) to determine the level of compensation. *Because the disorder is metabolic in origin, review the remaining laboratory value (in this case the CO_2). CO_2 is low, meaning the lungs are trying to compensate by lowering acid levels.* 5. Assess the Pao_2 and O_2 saturation. If these values are abnormal, hypoxemia is present. *The Pao_2 is normal and does not indicate hypoxemia.*

Interpretation

This ABG shows metabolic acidosis with partial compensation. Partial compensation is occurring because the pH remains abnormal. Full compensation would occur after the pH returns within normal limits.

Subjective Data

Important Health Information

Health history. If the patient has a problem related to electrolyte and acid-base balance, obtain a detailed description of the illness, including onset, course, and treatment. Ask about any history of problems involving the kidneys, heart, GI system, or lungs that could affect the present electrolyte and acid-base balance. Determine whether they have problems such as diabetes, endocrine problems, COPD, renal failure, liver disease, GI problems, or cancer. Ask the patient about past or present renal dialysis, kidney surgery, or bowel surgery.

Medications. Assess the patient's current and past use of medications. Many drugs, especially over-the-counter drugs, are hidden sources of sodium, potassium, calcium, magnesium, and other electrolytes. Other drugs, including diuretics, corticosteroids, and electrolyte supplements, can cause electrolyte imbalances.

Functional Health Patterns

Nutritional-metabolic. Ask the patient about their usual diet and any special diet practices. Weight reduction diets, fad diets, or any eating disorders, such as anorexia or bulimia, can lead to electrolyte problems. If the patient is on a special diet, such as low sodium or high potassium, assess the ability to adhere to the prescribed diet. Ask if they add salt to their food.

Elimination. Make note of the patient's usual bowel and bladder habits. Explore any problems, such as diarrhea, oliguria, polyuria, or incontinence. Do they have a temporary or permanent external collecting system, such as an ileostomy?

Activity-exercise. Ask the patient about exercise and any excess perspiration. Is the patient exposed to extremely high temperatures during leisure or work activity? Ask the patient what they do to replace fluid and electrolytes lost through excess perspiration.

Cognitive-perceptual. Ask about any changes in sensations, such as numbness, tingling, or muscle weakness, which could signal an electrolyte problem. Ask the patient and caregiver if there have been any changes in cognition, such as confusion, memory impairment, or lethargy.

Objective Data

Physical Assessment

Perform a complete physical assessment because electrolyte and acid-base balance affects all body systems. Identify patients in need of emergency management so that they can be stabilized. As you assess each system, check for manifestations that you would expect with an imbalance. Common abnormal assessment findings of major body systems offer clues to possible imbalances (Table 17.18).

TABLE 17.18 ASSESSMENT ABNORMALITIES

Fluid and Electrolyte Imbalances

Finding	Possible Cause
Blood Pressure	
Hypotension	Fluid volume deficit, low Ca^{2+}, high Mg^{2+}
Hypertension	Fluid volume excess, high Ca^{2+}, low Mg^{2+}
Muscular	
Chvostek sign	Low Ca^{2+}, high PO_4^{3-}, low Mg^{2+}
Muscle cramping	High K^+, low Ca^{2+}, high PO_4^{3-}, low Mg^{2+}
Muscle weakness	High or low K^+, high Ca^{2+}, low PO_4^{3-}, high Mg^{2+}
Trousseau sign	Low Ca^{2+}, low Mg^{2+}
Neurologic	
Confusion	Fluid volume excess, high or low Na^+, high or low K^+, low Ca^{2+}, high or low Mg^{2+}, low PO_4^{3-}
Decreased level of consciousness	Fluid volume deficit or excess, high or low Na^+, low PO_4^{3-}
Fatigue	Fluid volume deficit, low K^+, high Ca^{2+}
Irritability	Low Na^+, high K^+, low Ca^{2+}, high PO_4^{3-}
Tremors, seizures	High Na^+, low K^+, low Ca^{2+}, high PO_4^{3-}, low Mg^{2+}
Respirations	
Crackles	Fluid volume excess
Dyspnea	Fluid volume excess
Rapid respirations	Fluid volume deficit
Restricted airway	Low Ca^{2+}, high PO_4^{3-}
Pulse	
Bounding pulse	Fluid volume excess
Rapid, weak, thready pulse	Fluid volume deficit
Weak, irregular, rapid pulse	Severe low K^+, low Mg^{2+}
Weak, irregular, slow pulse	Severe high K^+, high Mg^{2+}
Skin	
Cold, clammy skin	Fluid volume deficit, low Na^+
Flushed, dry skin	High Na^+, high Mg^{2+}
Pitting edema	Fluid volume excess

Laboratory Values

Assessing serum electrolyte values is a good starting point for evaluating fluid and electrolyte balance (Table 17.1). Electrolytes can provide vital information about acid-base balance. Changes in HCO_3^- occur with metabolic acidosis (low HCO_3^-) or alkalosis (high HCO_3^-).

! SAFETY ALERT

Managing Critical Test Results

- Promptly report critical laboratory values to the HCP.
- Assess the patient and take appropriate actions (e.g., ECG monitoring).

Remember that electrolyte values often provide limited information. They reflect the concentration of that electrolyte in ECF but not necessarily in ICF. For example, most potassium is found in the cells. Changes in potassium values may be the result of a true deficit or excess of potassium or reflect the movement of potassium into or out of the cell during acid-base imbalances. An abnormal sodium level may reflect a sodium problem or, more likely, a water problem.

Other laboratory tests include plasma osmolality, glucose, BUN, creatinine, and ABGs. Urine tests include measures of osmolality, specific gravity, and electrolytes.

Clinical Problems

Clinical problems for patients with an electrolyte or acid-base imbalance include:

- Electrolyte imbalance
- Acid-base imbalance
- Impaired cardiac function
- Impaired cognition
- Impaired respiratory function
- Risk for injury
- Health care–associated complication

TABLE 17.19 NURSING MANAGEMENT

Electrolyte and Acid-Base Imbalances

- Assess for manifestations of electrolyte and acid-base imbalances.
- Determine risk factors and assess for the potential cause of an imbalance.
- Be prepared to institute resuscitation protocols and respiratory support.
- Give IV fluids and medications as prescribed.
- Treat dysrhythmias according to agency policy.
- Provide prescribed diet appropriate for specific electrolyte imbalance.
- Properly obtain laboratory specimens for electrolyte levels and ABG analysis.
- Provide a safe environment for the patient with neurologic or neuromuscular manifestations by instituting fall and seizure precautions.
- Monitor for complications from or measures to correct the balance.
- Implement measures to orient the patient as needed.
- Help the patient prioritize activities and alternate rest and activity periods.
- Implement measures to reduce side effects from electrolyte supplements.
- Evaluate response to therapies addressing the electrolyte or acid-base imbalance.

Planning

The overall goals are that patients will (1) achieve and maintain electrolyte and acid-base balance, (2) be free from any complications, and (3) adhere to the prescribed therapies.

Implementation

The general nursing care of patients with electrolyte or acid-base imbalances is outlined in Table 17.19.

FLUID AND ELECTROLYTE REPLACEMENT

ORAL FLUID AND ELECTROLYTE THERAPIES

Oral rehydration solutions may be used to correct mild fluid and electrolyte deficits. They generally contain water, potassium, sodium, and glucose. Glucose provides calories and promotes sodium and water absorption in the small intestine. Commercial oral rehydration solutions are now available for home use. Avoid cola drinks because they do not contain adequate electrolyte replacement, and the sugar content may lead to osmotic diuresis.

! SAFETY ALERT

Using Smart Infusion Pumps

- Smart infusion pumps can calculate IV drug dose and delivery rates.
- If you make an error and enter incorrect data, you will get incorrect results.
- Have a second RN confirm the settings for high-risk drugs.
- Use your best judgment when using smart infusion pumps and follow agency policy.

IV FLUID AND ELECTROLYTE THERAPIES

IV fluid and electrolyte therapy is necessary to treat many different fluid and electrolyte imbalances. Many patients need maintenance IV fluid therapy when they cannot take oral fluids (e.g., during and after surgery). Other patients need corrective or replacement therapy for losses that are ongoing or have already occurred. The amount and type of solution are determined by the normal daily maintenance requirements and by imbalances identified by laboratory results. We classify IV replacement solutions by their concentration or tonicity (Table 17.20). Tonicity is a key factor in determining the appropriate solution to correct imbalances.

Solutions

Hypotonic

A hypotonic solution has a lower osmolality compared with plasma. Infusing a hypotonic solution dilutes ECF, lowering plasma osmolality. Osmosis then produces a movement of water from ECF to interstitial spaces and cells, causing cells to swell. After achieving equilibrium, ICF and ECF have the same osmolality. Hypotonic solutions (e.g., 0.45% NaCl) are useful in treating patients with hypernatremia. They are a good maintenance fluid because normal daily losses are hypotonic. They are not good for replacement because they can deplete ECF and lower BP. Because hypotonic solutions have the potential to cause cell swelling, monitor patients for changes in mentation that may signal cerebral edema.

Although 5% dextrose in water is technically an isotonic solution, the dextrose quickly metabolizes. The net result is the administration of hypotonic-free water with equal expansion of ECF and ICF. One liter of a 5% dextrose solution provides 50 g of dextrose or 170 calories. Although this amount of dextrose is not enough to meet caloric requirements, it helps prevent ketosis associated with starvation.

Isotonic

An isotonic solution has an osmolality similar to plasma. Because of this similarity, giving an isotonic solution expands only ECF, and the fluid does not move into cells. This makes isotonic solutions the ideal fluid replacement for patients with ECF volume deficits. Examples of isotonic solutions include 0.9% NaCl and lactated Ringer's solution.

Isotonic saline (0.9% NaCl), or *normal saline,* has a sodium concentration (154 mEq/L) slightly higher than that of plasma (135 to 145 mEq/L) and a chloride concentration (154 mEq/L) significantly higher than the plasma chloride level (96 to 106 mEq/L). Therefore giving too much isotonic saline has the potential to increase sodium and chloride levels. Isotonic saline is used when a patient has had both fluid and sodium losses (e.g., diarrhea, vomiting).

Lactated Ringer's solution contains sodium, potassium, chloride, calcium, and lactate (the precursor of bicarbonate) in about the same concentrations as ECF. This makes it the ideal fluid in certain situations, such as surgery, burns, or GI fluid losses. Patients with liver problems, hyperkalemia, and severe hypovolemia should not receive lactated Ringer's because they have a decreased ability to convert the lactate to bicarbonate.

TABLE 17.20 Common Crystalloid Solutions

Solution	Tonicity	mOsm/kg	Contents	Indications and Considerations
Dextrose in Water				
5%	Isotonic, but physiologically hypotonic	278	50 g/L dextrose	• Contains free water only, no electrolytes • Provides 170 cal/L • Used to replace water losses and treat hypernatremia
10%	Hypertonic	556	100 g/L dextrose	• Contains free water only, no electrolytes • Provides 340 cal/L • Used with parenteral nutrition
Saline				
0.45%	Hypotonic	154	77 mEq/L Na^+ 77 mEq/L Cl^-	• Contains free water, Na^+, and Cl^-, no calories • Used to treat hypernatremia and uncontrolled hyperglycemia • Used as a maintenance solution
0.9%	Isotonic	308	154 mEq/L Na^+ 154 mEq/L Cl^-	• Contains Na^+ and Cl^- in excess of plasma levels • Does not contain free water or calories • Used to expand intravascular volume and replace extracellular fluid losses • Only solution given with blood products • May cause volume overload in patients with heart or kidney disease
3.0%	Hypertonic	1026	513 mEq/L Na^+ 513 mEq/L Cl^-	• Contains more Na^+ and Cl^- than plasma • Used to treat symptomatic hyponatremia and trauma patients with head injury • Give slowly because it may cause volume overload and pulmonary edema
Dextrose in Saline				
5% in 0.225%	Isotonic	355	50 g/L dextrose 34 mEq/L Na^+ 34 mEq/L Cl^-	• Provides Na^+, Cl^-, and free water • Used to replace hypotonic losses and treat hypernatremia • Provides 170 cal/L
5% in 0.45%	Hypertonic	432	50 g/L dextrose 77 mEq/L Na^+ 77 mEq/L Cl^-	• Provides Na^+, Cl^-, and free water because of rapid metabolism of the dextrose • Used as a maintenance solution
5% in 0.9%	Hypertonic	586	50 g/L dextrose 154 mEq/L Na^+ 154 mEq/L Cl^-	• Contains more Na^+ and Cl^- than plasma • Used to treat metabolic alkalosis and volume deficits in patients with hyponatremia
Multiple Electrolyte Solutions				
Ringer's solution	Isotonic	309	147 mEq/L Na^+ 156 mEq/L Cl^- 4 mEq/L K^+ 4 mEq/L Ca^{2+}	• Similar to plasma except that it has excess Cl^-, no Mg^{2+}, no HCO_3^- • Does not provide free water or calories • Used to expand the intravascular volume and replace extracellular fluid losses
Lactated Ringer's (Hartmann's) solution	Isotonic	273	130 mEq/L Na^+ 109 mEq/L Cl^- 4 mEq/L K^+ 3 mEq/L Ca^{2+} 28 mmol/L lactate	• Similar in composition to normal plasma except does not contain Mg^{2+} • Does not provide free water or calories • Used to treat hypovolemia, burns, and GI fluid losses • Cannot be used in patients with alkalosis or lactic acidosis

Hypertonic

A hypertonic solution has a higher osmolality than plasma. The higher osmotic pressure draws water out of the cells into ECF. It is useful in the treatment of hyponatremia and trauma patients with head injuries. Those receiving hypertonic solutions need frequent monitoring of BP, lung sounds, and sodium levels because of the risk for intravascular fluid volume excess.

Although concentrated dextrose and water solutions (10% dextrose or greater) are hypertonic solutions, once the dextrose is metabolized, the net result is the administration of water. This free water ultimately expands ECF and ICF. The primary use of these solutions is providing calories as part of PN (see Chapter 44). You may give solutions containing 10% dextrose or less through a peripheral line. You must use a central line to give solutions with dextrose concentrations greater than 10%.

IV Additives

Additives in basic IV solutions replace specific losses. KCl, calcium, magnesium, and HCO_3^- mEq/L are common additives. The use of each was described earlier in the discussion of the specific electrolyte deficiencies. Many premixed IV solutions containing specific additives are available. Using these solutions reduces error, as the solution contains the correct amount of the electrolyte in the right volume and type of IV solution.

Colloids

Colloid solutions contain large molecules that increase oncotic pressure and pull fluid into the blood vessels. Because this action restores blood volume, we also call colloids *volume expanders* or *plasma expanders*. Colloids include human plasma products (albumin, fresh frozen plasma, blood) and semisynthetic solutions (dextran, starches).

Albumin is available in 5% and 25% solutions. The 5% solution has an albumin concentration similar to that of plasma. Use results in plasma volume expansion equal to the volume infused. This makes it ideal for treating hypovolemic patients. In contrast, 25% albumin solution is hypertonic and draws fluid from the interstitial space. This makes it useful in treating patients with burns, liver failure, and ascites.

Dextran solutions are synthetic complex sugar solutions. There are 2 types: low-molecular-weight dextran (dextran 40) and high-molecular-weight dextran (dextran 70). Because dextran metabolizes slowly, it stays in the vascular system for a prolonged period. It pulls fluid into the intravascular space, expanding it by more volume than what is infused. Hydroxyethyl starches (e.g., Hespan) are synthetic colloids that work similarly to dextran to expand plasma volume.

Colloids can lead to circulatory overload because they pull fluid into ECF. Monitor vital signs and urine output. Assess for signs and symptoms of fluid volume excess. Colloids affect blood coagulation by interfering with coagulation factor VII.[17] Monitor coagulation times and implement any necessary precautions. Fatal anaphylactic reactions have occurred with Hespan and dextran. Monitor the patient for a hypersensitivity reaction and stop an infusion at once if a reaction occurs.

If the patient has lost blood, whole blood or packed RBCs are given. Packed RBCs have the advantage of giving the patient mostly RBCs rather than RBCs and fluid volume. Although packed RBCs have a decreased plasma volume, they increase the oncotic pressure and pull fluid into the intravascular space. The use of whole blood, with its added fluid volume, may cause circulatory overload, especially in patients who are susceptible to complications from excess circulating volume (e.g., HF). To prevent fluid volume excess, loop diuretics may be given with blood and colloids. See Chapter 34 for more about giving blood and blood products. See Table 17.21 for nursing management of IV therapy.

CENTRAL VENOUS ACCESS DEVICES

Central venous access devices (CVADs) are catheters placed in large blood vessels (e.g., subclavian vein, jugular vein) of people who need frequent or special access to the vascular system.

TABLE 17.21 NURSING MANAGEMENT

IV Therapy

- Assess for manifestations of fluid and electrolyte imbalances.
- Know if the indications for prescribed therapies are appropriate.
- Choose and insert appropriate IV catheters and infusion devices.
- Give IV fluids and medications.
- Monitor for adverse reactions to IV fluids or medications.
- Assess for fluid and electrolyte imbalance and initiate appropriate changes in IV fluids.
- Adhere to agency policy and evidence-based infection prevention practices.
- Evaluate if IV therapies are addressing patient's fluid and electrolyte needs.
- Provide patient and caregiver education about IV therapies.
- Collaborate with the pharmacist to:
  - Determine appropriateness of IV therapies and need for dose adjustments.
  - Prepare IV infusions and medications.
  - Screen for potential problems, such as compatibility issues.
  - Monitor response to therapy.

There are 3 main types of CVADs: centrally inserted catheters, peripherally inserted central catheters (PICCs), and implanted ports.

Advantages of CVADs include immediate access to the central venous system, a reduced need for multiple venipunctures, and decreased risk for extravasation injury. CVADs permit frequent, continuous, rapid, or intermittent administration of fluids and medications. They allow us to administer more safely drugs that are potential *vesicants* (agents that can cause tissue damage), blood and blood products, and PN. CVADs can provide a means to perform hemodynamic monitoring and obtain venous blood samples. They are useful with patients who have limited peripheral vascular access or who have a projected need for long-term vascular access. Table 17.22 gives examples of when we use CVADs.

The major disadvantages are an increased risk for systemic infection and the invasiveness of the procedure. Extravasation (leakage of fluid) can still occur if there is displacement of or damage to the device.

Centrally Inserted Catheters

The tip of centrally inserted catheters (also called *central venous catheters [CVCs]*) rests in the distal end of the superior vena cava near its junction with the right atrium (Fig. 17.18). The other end of the catheter exits through a separate incision on the chest or abdominal wall. *Nontunneled catheters* are usually placed in the subclavian or internal jugular vein, more rarely in the femoral vein. They are best for patients with short-term needs in an acute care setting. *Surgically placed tunneled catheters* (e.g., Hickman, Broviac, Groshong) are suitable for long-term needs. Tunneling of the catheter through the subcutaneous tissue and the synthetic cuff used to anchor the catheter provide stability and decrease infection risk. After the site heals, the catheter does not need a dressing, making it easier for the patient to maintain the site at home.

TABLE 17.22 Common Indications for Central Venous Access Devices (CVADs)

Condition	Indications for Use
Autoimmune disorders	Perform plasmapheresis
Blood sampling	Multiple blood draws for diagnostic tests over time
Blood transfusions	Infusion of blood or blood products
Heart failure	Perform ultrafiltration
Hemodynamic monitoring	Used to measure CVP and assess fluid balance
Medication administration	
• Cancer	Chemotherapy, infusion of irritating or vesicant medications
• Contrast media	Inject radiopaque contrast media for diagnostic testing
• Infection	Long-term administration of antibiotics
• Pain	Long-term administration of pain medication
• Drugs at risk for causing phlebitis	Epoprostenol Calcium chloride Potassium chloride Amiodarone
Nutrition replacement	Parenteral nutrition IV high percentage dextrose solutions
Renal failure	Perform hemodialysis (especially on an acute basis) or continuous renal replacement therapy
Shock, burns	Infusion of high volumes of fluid and electrolyte replacement

CVP, Central venous pressure.

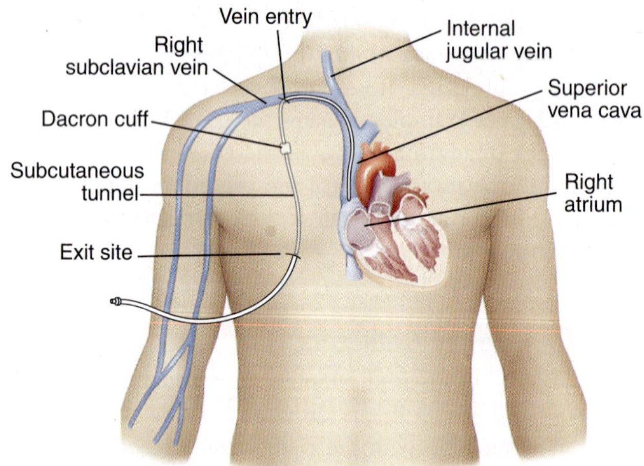

Fig. 17.18 Tunneled central venous catheter. Note tip of the catheter in the superior vena cava.

CVCs are available with single, double, or triple lumens. Multilumen catheters are used in critically ill patients because each lumen can be used simultaneously to provide a different therapy. For example, incompatible drugs infuse in separate lumens without mixing, while a third lumen gives access for blood sampling.

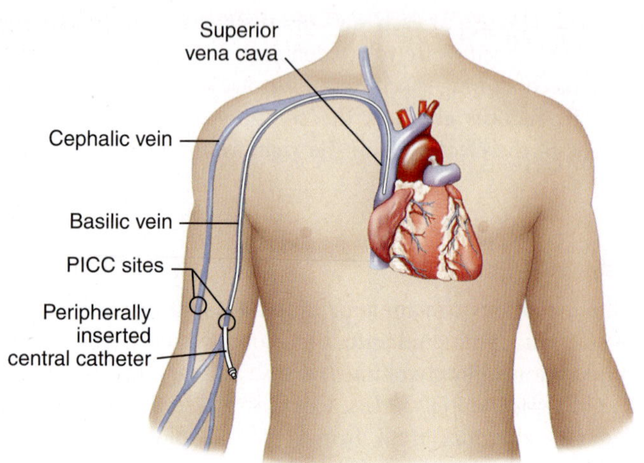

Fig. 17.19 Peripherally inserted central catheter *(PICC)* can be inserted using the basilic or cephalic vein.

Peripherally Inserted Central Catheters

PICCs are CVCs inserted into a vein in the arm. The basilic vein is best because of its large diameter (Fig. 17.19). The cephalic, median cubital, or brachial veins are other options. Single, double, or triple lumens are available. Double lumens are preferred because they allow for simultaneous use. PICCs are used with patients who need vascular access for 1 week to 6 months, but they can be in place for longer periods.

Advantages of a PICC over a CVC are lower infection rate, fewer insertion-related complications, decreased cost, and ability to insert at the bedside or in an outpatient area. PICCs, however, have an increased risk for deep vein thrombosis and phlebitis (Table 17.23). If phlebitis occurs, it usually happens within 7 to 10 days after insertion. Do not use the arm with the PICC to take a BP reading or draw blood. When the BP cuff is inflated, the PICC can touch the vein wall, increasing the risk for vein damage and thrombosis.

Implanted Infusion Ports

An implanted infusion port consists of a surgically implanted CVC connected to a reservoir or port (Fig. 17.20A). The catheter tip lies in the desired vein. The port lies in a surgically created subcutaneous pocket on the upper chest or arm. It consists of a titanium or plastic reservoir covered with a self-sealing silicone septum. You access the port by using a special noncoring needle with a deflected tip. This prevents damage to the septum that could make the port useless (Fig. 17.20B).

We place drugs in the reservoir by a direct injection or through injection into an established IV line. The reservoir then slowly releases the medicine into the bloodstream. Implanted ports are good for long-term therapy and have a low risk for infection. The hidden port offers the patient cosmetic advantages and overall has less maintenance than other types of CVADs. Monitor accessed ports for infiltration that can occur if the needle is not in place or dislodges.

TABLE 17.23 Complications of Central Venous Access Devices (CVADs)

Possible Cause	Manifestations	Management
Catheter Migration		
• Improper suturing • Insertion site trauma • Changes in intrathoracic pressure • Forceful catheter flushing • Spontaneous	• Sluggish infusion or aspiration • Edema of chest or neck during infusion • Patient reports gurgling sound in ear • Dysrhythmias • Increased external catheter length	• Prepare for fluoroscopy to confirm position • Assist with removal and new CVAD placement
Catheter-Related Infection (Local or Systemic)		

• Contamination during insertion or use
• Migration of organisms along catheter
• Immunosuppressed patient
	• *Local:* redness, tenderness, purulent drainage, warmth, edema
	• *Systemic:* fever, chills, malaise
		• *Local:*
		  • Culture drainage from site
		  • Apply warm, moist compresses
		  • Remove catheter if needed
		• *Systemic:*
		  • Take blood cultures
		  • Give antibiotic therapy
		  • Give antipyretic therapy
		  • Remove catheter if needed

Catheter Occlusion		
• Clamped or kinked catheter • Tip against wall of vessel • Thrombosis • Precipitate buildup in lumen	• Sluggish infusion or aspiration • Inability to infuse and/or aspirate	• Have patient change position, raise arm, and cough • Assess and alleviate any clamping or kinking • Flush with normal saline using a 10-mL syringe; do not force flush • Instill anticoagulant or thrombolytic agent
Embolism		
• Catheter breaking • Dislodgment of thrombus • Entry of air into circulation	• Chest pain • Respiratory distress (dyspnea, tachypnea, hypoxia, cyanosis) • ↓ BP • ↑ HR	• Apply O_2 • Clamp catheter • Place patient on left side with head down (air emboli) • Notify provider
Pneumothorax		
• Perforation of visceral pleura during insertion	• Decreased or absent breath sounds • Respiratory distress (cyanosis, dyspnea, tachypnea) • Chest pain • Distended unilateral chest	• Apply O_2 • Place in semi-Fowler's position • Prepare for chest tube insertion

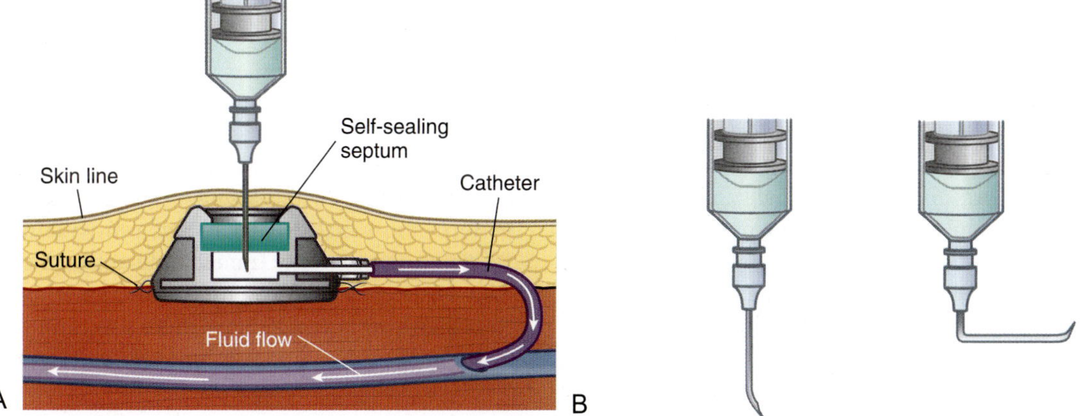

Fig. 17.20 (A) Cross section of implantable port displaying access of the port with the Huber-point needle. Note the deflected point of the Huber-point needle, which prevents coring of the port's septum. (B) Huber-point needles used to enter the implanted port. The 90-degree needle is used for top-entry ports for continuous infusion.

Midline Catheters

Midline catheters technically are peripheral catheters because they do not enter a central vein. However, their use and care are similar to a PICC. A specially trained nurse can insert a midline catheter. A catheter can be from 3 to 8 inches long and have single or double lumens. They are inserted in the antecubital area through either the basilic or cephalic vein, often under ultrasound guidance. The basilic vein is best because it has a larger diameter. The tip rests right below the axilla, staying below the shoulder joint to reduce the risk for vein irritation from moving the shoulder. These lines can stay in place for up to 4 weeks.

Complications

CVADs always have a potential for complications. Monitoring and assessment will help you to identify potential complications early. Table 17.23 lists common complications, potential causes, manifestations, and interventions.

NURSING MANAGEMENT: CENTRAL VENOUS ACCESS DEVICES

Nursing management includes assessment, dressing changes and cleansing, injection cap changes, and maintaining catheter patency. The frequency and procedures for these requirements vary by type of CVAD and agency, so it is important to follow your agency's policies. The following section discusses some general guidelines.

Catheter and insertion site assessment includes inspecting the site for redness, edema, warmth, drainage, tenderness, or pain. Observe the catheter for misplacement or slippage. Perform a pain assessment. Note any reports of chest or neck discomfort, arm pain, or pain at the insertion site. Do not use a newly placed CVAD until the tip position is verified with a chest x-ray.

> **CHECK YOUR PRACTICE**
>
> You are taking care of a 74-year-old patient with a left triple-lumen subclavian catheter. When you are changing the dressing, you note some redness at the site with a small amount of yellow, foul-smelling drainage.
>
> - What should you do?

Before manipulating a catheter, perform hand hygiene. Perform dressing changes and cleanse the catheter insertion site using strict sterile technique. Typical dressings include transparent semipermeable dressings or gauze and tape. If the site is bleeding, a gauze dressing may be preferable. Otherwise, transparent dressings are best. They allow observation of the site without having to remove the dressing. Transparent dressings may be in place for up to 1 week. Change any dressing at once if it becomes damp, loose, or soiled.

Cleanse the skin around the catheter insertion site according to agency policy. A chlorhexidine-based preparation is the cleansing agent of choice.[18] When using chlorhexidine, cleansing the skin with friction is critical to preventing infection. When applying a new dressing, allow the area to air dry completely. Secure the lumen ports to the skin above the dressing site. Document the date and time of the dressing change and initial the dressing.

Disinfect catheter hubs, needleless connectors, and injection ports before accessing the catheter. Use an alcohol chlorhexidine preparation, 70% alcohol, or povidone-iodine per agency policy. Change injection caps at regular intervals according to policy or if they have damage from excess punctures. Use strict sterile technique. Teach the patient to turn the head to the opposite side of the insertion site during cap change. If you cannot clamp the catheter, have the patient lie flat in bed and perform the Valsalva maneuver whenever the catheter is open to air to prevent an air embolism.

Flushing is one of the most effective ways to maintain catheter patency. It also keeps incompatible drugs or fluids from mixing. Use a normal saline solution in a syringe that has a barrel capacity of 10 mL or more to avoid excess pressure on the catheter. If you feel resistance, do not apply force. This could result in a ruptured catheter or create an embolism if a thrombus is present. Because of the risk for contamination and infection, use solution from prefilled syringes or single-dose vials rather than multiple-dose vials when flushing catheters. If you are not using a positive-pressure valve cap, clamp any unused lines after flushing.

Use the push-pause technique when flushing all catheters. Push-pause creates turbulence within the catheter lumen, promoting the removal of debris that adheres to the catheter lumen and decreasing the chance of occlusion. This technique involves injecting saline with a rapid alternating push-pause motion, instilling 1 to 2 mL with each push on the syringe plunger. If you are using a negative-pressure cap or neutral-pressure cap, clamp the catheter while maintaining positive pressure while instilling the last 1 mL of saline. This prevents reflux of blood back into the catheter. If a positive-pressure valve cap is present, it works to prevent the reflux of blood and resultant catheter lumen occlusion. Remove the syringe before clamping the catheter to allow the positive pressure valve to work correctly.

CVAD Removal

Remove a CVAD according to agency policy. In many agencies, nurses with proven competency can remove PICCs and nontunneled CVCs. The procedure involves removing any sutures and then gently withdrawing the catheter. Have the patient perform the Valsalva maneuver as you withdraw the last 5 to 10 cm of the catheter. Immediately apply pressure to the site with sterile gauze to prevent air from entering and to control bleeding. Inspect the catheter tip to determine that it is intact. After bleeding has stopped, apply an antiseptic ointment and sterile dressing to the site.

CASE STUDY

Fluid and Electrolyte Imbalance

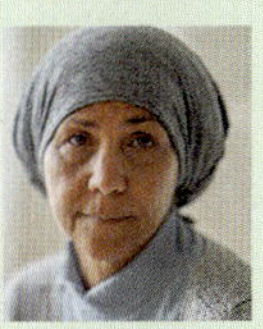
(© FatCamera/ Stock.com.)

Patient Profile

S.S., a 63-year-old female with acute lymphocytic leukemia, has been receiving chemotherapy on an outpatient basis. She completed her 3rd treatment 5 days ago and has had nausea and vomiting for 2 days despite using ondansetron. S.S.'s daughter brings her to the hospital, where she is admitted to the medical unit. As the admitting nurse, you perform an admission assessment.

Subjective Data

- Reports lethargy, weakness, dizziness, and dry mouth
- States she has been too nauseated to eat or drink anything for 2 days
- Reports "little urination" over the previous 24 h

Objective Data

- Heart rate 110 beats/min, pulse thready
- BP 100/65
- Weight loss of 5 lb since she received her chemotherapy treatment 5 days ago
- Dry oral mucous membranes

Discussion Questions

1. ***Recognize:*** What are her risk factors for fluid and electrolyte imbalances?
2. ***Recognize:*** What additional assessment data should you obtain?
3. ***Analyze:*** Based on her manifestations, what fluid imbalance does S.S. have?
4. ***Analyze:*** You draw blood for a chemistry evaluation. What electrolyte imbalances are likely and why?
5. ***Analyze:*** S.S. is at risk for which acid-base imbalance? Describe the changes that would occur in S.S.'s ABGs with this acid-base imbalance. How would the body compensate?
6. ***Plan:*** What priority nursing interventions would be in the plan of care?
7. ***Prioritize:*** What is the interprofessional team's priority at this time for S.S.?
8. ***Act:*** The provider orders dextrose 5% in 0.45% saline to infuse at 100 mL/h. How will it help S.S.'s fluid imbalance?
9. ***Act:*** S.S. has a double-lumen PICC in her left arm. One lumen is connected to the IV infusion; the other is unused. What is the recommended practice for maintaining the patency of the unused lumen?
10. ***Evaluate:*** What outcomes will indicate that interprofessional care was effective?

Answers available at http://evolve.elsevier.com/Lewis/medsurg.

BRIDGE TO NCLEX EXAMINATION

The number of the question corresponds to the same-numbered outcome at the beginning of the chapter.

1. During the postoperative care of a 76-year-old patient, the nurse monitors the patient's intake and output, knowing that the patient is at risk for fluid and electrolyte imbalances because

a. older adults have impaired thirst and need reminders to drink fluids.
b. older adults are more likely than younger adults to lose extracellular fluid during surgeries.
c. water accounts for a greater percentage of body weight in the older adult than in younger adults.
d. small losses of fluid are significant because body fluids account for 45% to 50% of body weight in older adults.

2. The process involved in equalizing the fluid concentration between ECF and the cells in a patient receiving hypertonic IV solution is:

a. osmosis.
b. diffusion.
c. active transport.
d. facilitated diffusion.

3a. Assessment findings that would lead the nurse to suspect fluid volume deficit in a patient with GI bleeding include **(Select all that apply.)**

a. weight loss.
b. dry oral mucosa.
c. full bounding pulse.
d. engorged neck veins.
e. orthostatic hypotension.
f. increased central venous pressure.

3b. Nursing care for a patient with hyponatremia and fluid volume excess includes

a. fluid restriction.
b. administration of hypotonic IV fluids.
c. administration of a cation-exchange resin.
d. placement of an indwelling urinary catheter.

3c. The nurse would be alert for which manifestations in a patient receiving a loop diuretic?

a. Restlessness and agitation
b. Paresthesias and irritability
c. Weak, irregular pulse and poor muscle tone
d. Increased blood pressure and muscle spasms

3d. Which patient is at *greatest* risk for developing hypermagnesemia?

a. An 83-year-old male with lung cancer and hypertension
b. A 65-year-old female with hypertension taking β-adrenergic blockers
c. A 42-year-old female with systemic lupus erythematosus and renal failure
d. A 50-year-old male with benign prostatic hyperplasia and a urinary tract infection

3e. The nurse would assess for which manifestation(s) in a patient who has just undergone a total thyroidectomy? **(Select all that apply.)**

a. Confusion
b. Weight gain
c. Depressed reflexes
d. Circumoral numbness
e. Positive Chvostek sign

3f. The long-term treatment of a patient with hyperphosphatemia from renal failure will include
- **a.** fluid restriction.
- **b.** calcium supplements.
- **c.** magnesium supplements.
- **d.** increased intake of dairy products.

4. The lungs act as an acid-base buffer by
- **a.** increasing respiratory rate and depth when CO_2 levels in the blood are high, reducing acid load.
- **b.** increasing respiratory rate and depth when CO_2 levels in the blood are low, reducing base load.
- **c.** decreasing respiratory rate and depth when CO_2 levels in the blood are high, reducing acid load.
- **d.** decreasing respiratory rate and depth when CO_2 levels in the blood are low, increasing acid load.

5. A patient has the following arterial blood gas results: pH 7.52, $Paco_2$ 30 mm Hg, HCO_3^- 24 mEq/L. These results indicate
- **a.** metabolic acidosis.
- **b.** metabolic alkalosis.
- **c.** respiratory acidosis.
- **d.** respiratory alkalosis.

6. The typical fluid replacement for the patient with a fluid volume deficit is
- **a.** dextran.
- **b.** 0.45% saline.
- **c.** lactated Ringer's solution.
- **d.** 5% dextrose in 0.45% saline.

7. The nurse is unable to flush a central venous access device and suspects occlusion. The *best* nursing action would be to
- **a.** apply warm moist compresses to the insertion site.
- **b.** try to force 10 mL of normal saline into the device.
- **c.** place the patient on the left side with the head down.
- **d.** have the patient change positions, raise arm, and cough.

1. d; 2. a; 3a. a, b, e; 3b. a; 3c. c; 3d. c; 3e. a, d, e; 3f. b; 4. a; 5. d; 6. c; 7. d.

For rationales to these answers and even more NCLEX review questions, visit http://evolve.elsevier.com/Lewis/medsurg.

REFERENCES

To access the References for this chapter, please scan the QR code with a mobile device.

CASE STUDY

Applying Clinical Judgment With Multiple Patients

It is 0715 and you are assigned to care for the following 3 patients in the stepdown unit. You have an AP to assist you. You have just finished receiving shift report.

 © Stockphoto/Thinkstock.	G.N., a 62-year-old male, was admitted with a urinary tract infection. He has multiple sclerosis and a stage 2 sacral pressure injury. He is receiving O_2 at 4 L/min via nasal cannula. Vital signs: 118/62, 88 and regular, RR 18, 100.4°F (38°C), and O_2 saturation 93%. His WBC count is 26,400/μL (26.4 × 109/L) with 80% neutrophils (10% bands). The wound dressing needs changed.
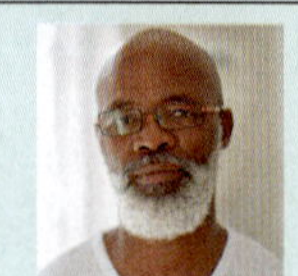 © iStock.com/ Cecilie_Arcurs.	J.N. is a 66-year-old male with HIV, type 2 diabetes, COPD, and hypertension. He was admitted 2 days ago with acute diverticulitis. He is to receive his next doses of IV levofloxacin and metronidazole at 0800. Vital signs: 124/72, 98 and regular, RR 20, 100.4°F (38°C), O_2 saturation 98%.
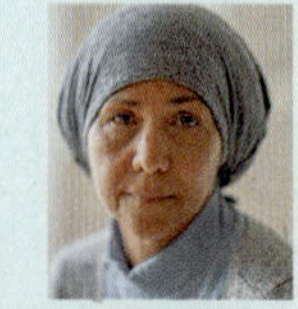 © FatCamera/iStock.com	S.S., a 63-year-old female with acute lymphocytic leukemia, completed her 3rd chemotherapy treatment 5 days ago. She was admitted with dehydration after having nausea and vomiting for 2 days despite taking ondansetron. Vital signs: BP 90/50, 112 and regular, RR 22, O_2 saturation 95% on 2 L/via nasal cannula. Her last emesis was 3 hours ago.

1. Highlight all the findings that require your follow-up.
2. Which patient would you see first? Why?
3. Which nursing actions would you include in S.S.'s plan of care right now? Use an X for the nursing actions listed that are indicated (appropriate or necessary) or contraindicated (could be harmful).

Nursing Actions	Indicated	Contraindicated
Place S.S. on strict NPO status.		
Suggest a referral to the dietitian for enteral nutrition.		
Provide oral care after episodes of emesis.		
Administer as-needed antiemetics.		
Administer prescribed IV fluid replacement therapy.		
Initiate daily weights and intake and output.		
Monitor electrolyte levels as ordered.		

CASE STUDY—cont'd

Applying Clinical Judgment With Multiple Patients

4. Which morning tasks would you delegate to the AP? **(Select all that apply.)**
   a. Provide oral care for G.N.
   b. Change G.N.'s sacral dressing.
   c. Calculate intake and output on S.S.
   d. Take J.N. to radiology for a chest x-ray.
   e. Perform a respiratory assessment on G.N.

Case Study Progression

When preparing J.N.'s AM medications, you note that he is scheduled to receive 2 IV medications at 0800: metronidazole 500 mg/100 mL normal saline over 30 minutes every 8 hours and levofloxacin 500 mg/100 mL over 60 minutes daily. He has 1 IV site in the left arm.

5. Which action is your *best* option right now?
   a. Call the HCP to change the administration times.
   b. Obtain a second peripheral IV site in the right arm.
   c. Check with pharmacy to see if they can mix the drugs in the same bag.
   d. Administer the metronidazole first because it takes less time to infuse.

After you start J.N.'s IV antibiotic therapy, you ask the AP to obtain vital signs on your other patients while you begin a more thorough assessment of J.N. During your assessment of J.N., you note gray-white patches on the inside of his mouth.

6. You recognize these as *most* likely caused by
   a. *Candida albicans.*
   b. poor oral hygiene.
   c. *Coccidioides immitis.*
   d. irritation from recent mouth care.
7. Choose the *best* option for the information missing from the statement that follows by selecting from the lists of options provided.
   You receive notification that morning laboratory results are available. S.S.'s chemistry panel results show a potassium level of 2.5 mEq/L. Based on this result, the priority need will be prevention of ______1______. To detect this complication, you will prioritize the assessment of S.S.'s ______2______.

Options for 1	Options for 2
Diarrhea	Bowel function
Dysrhythmias	Cardiac rhythm
Respiratory depression	Muscle strength

8. Which medication would you administer first?
   a. Daily subcutaneous enoxaparin to J.N.
   b. IV Bactrim, ordered twice daily, to G.N.
   c. IV proton pump inhibitor, ordered twice daily, to S.S.
   d. As-needed IV morphine to J.N., who reports pain at a level 5 (1 to 10 scale)
9. As the day continues, you find that you are getting busy. Which nursing task should be your priority?
   a. Changing G.N.'s sacral wound dressing
   b. Reviewing new antibiotic orders from the HCP for J.N.
   c. Starting a 500-mL fluid bolus to S.S., whose most recent BP is 76/42
   d. Calling the hospital chaplain to speak with S.S., who is upset over her condition
10. By late morning, you are able to change G.N.'s dressing and perform his assessment. For each assessment finding, use an X to indicate whether the interventions were effective (helped to meet expected outcomes) or ineffective (did not help meet expected outcomes).

Assessment Finding	Effective	Ineffective
Urine output clear yellow		
Alert and oriented to person only		
Afebrile		
WBC count 14,600/μL (14.6 × 10^9/L)		
O_2 saturation 96% with O_2 at 2 L per nasal cannula		
Small amount of purulent drainage on wound dressing.		

11. While sitting at the computer charting your shift assessments, you overhear the AP state that J.N. deserves what he got because "HIV is a punishment for being LGBTQ+." Your *most* appropriate response would be to
    a. report the AP's actions to the supervisor.
    b. ask the AP to keep her opinions to herself.
    c. ignore the conversation because it does not affect patient care.
    d. talk to the AP about keeping personal feelings separate from patient care.

Answers available at http://evolve.elsevier.com/Lewis/medsurg.

18 Preoperative Care

Michelle L. Sauve and Ruthie R. Mangino

http://evolve.elsevier.com/Lewis/medsurg/

CONCEPTUAL FOCUS

Anxiety
Patient Education
Safety

LEARNING OUTCOMES

1. Distinguish the common purposes, settings, and phases of perioperative care.
2. Describe the purpose and components of a preoperative nursing assessment.
3. Interpret the significance of data related to the preoperative patient's health status and operative risk.
4. Analyze the components and purpose of informed consent for a procedure.
5. Examine the nursing role in the preparation of the surgical patient.
6. Prioritize the nursing responsibilities related to day-of-procedure preparation for the surgical patient.
7. Discern the purposes and types of common preoperative drugs.
8. Plan care to include special considerations of preoperative preparation for the older adult surgical patient.

KEY TERMS

ambulatory surgery
elective surgery
emergency surgery
informed consent
perianesthesia
perioperative
preoperative care
same-day admission
surgery

SURGICAL PROCEDURES

Surgery is the art and science of treating diseases, injuries, and deformities by operation and instrumentation. The **perioperative** period includes the time before surgery (preoperative period), the time spent during the actual surgical procedure (intraoperative period), and the period after the surgery is over (postoperative or recovery period). We refer to the preoperative period (preanesthesia phase) and postoperative period (post-anesthesia phase) as **perianesthesia** phases of care. Perianesthesia nursing encompasses the special nursing care required for patients undergoing a procedure who receive sedation, analgesia, and/or anesthesia. We use the term **preoperative care** to describe any type of preprocedural care and care planning.

The surgical experience involves an interprofessional health care team, including the patient, surgeon, anesthesia care provider (ACP), nurse, and others. Preparing patients for surgery or a procedure is an important nursing role. Preprocedural care is provided before interventional radiology, cardiac catheterization, surgery, endoscopy procedures, and other procedures. The procedure and routines of the surgery setting guide the patient's preparation. The Association of periOperative Registered Nurses (AORN) and American Society of

TABLE 18.1 Suffixes Describing Surgical Procedures

Suffix	Meaning	Example
-ectomy	Excision or removal of	Appendectomy
-orrhaphy	Repair or suture of	Herniorrhaphy
-oscopy	Looking into	Endoscopy
-ostomy	Creation of opening into	Colostomy
-otomy	Cutting into or incision of	Tracheotomy
-plasty	Repair or reconstruction of	Mammoplasty

PeriAnesthesia Nurses (ASPAN) provide standards and recommended practices to guide nursing interventions in all perioperative settings.[1]

This chapter discusses the preanesthesia phase for patients having surgery or other procedures. Preparation measures for specific surgeries (abdominal, thoracic, orthopedic surgery) are discussed in other chapters of this book.

Patients have surgery or procedures for many reasons. These include:

- *Diagnosis:* Determine the presence and extent of a condition (e.g., lymph node biopsy, bronchoscopy).
- *Cure:* Eliminate or repair a pathologic condition (e.g., remove a ruptured appendix).
- *Palliation:* Alleviate symptoms without cure (e.g., cutting a nerve root to reduce pain, creating a colostomy to bypass an inoperable bowel obstruction).
- *Prevention:* Reduce the risk of developing a condition (e.g., removal of a mole before it becomes malignant).
- *Cosmetic improvement:* Alter physical appearance (e.g., repairing a burn scar, breast reconstruction after a mastectomy).
- *Exploration:* Determine the nature or extent of a disease (e.g., laparotomy). Exploration is becoming less common because we can identify many problems noninvasively through diagnostic imaging tests.

Surgical procedures are usually described by combining specific suffixes with a body part or organ (Table 18.1).

SURGICAL SETTINGS

Surgery may be a carefully planned event (**elective surgery**) or may arise with unexpected urgency (**emergency surgery**). Elective and emergency procedures are done in a variety of settings. The type of procedure, potential complications, the patient's health status, and the patient's ability for self-care afterward influence the choice of setting.

Some surgeries require postoperative admission (**same-day admission**) for specific inpatient care and teaching. Patients may also have surgery during a hospital admission. Patients who are in the hospital before surgery are usually there because of acute or chronic health problems and return to the inpatient setting for ongoing recovery and management.

Many elective surgeries and procedures are done on an outpatient basis (also called ambulatory or *same-day procedures*). Some use minimally invasive methods such as laparoscopy or endoscopy. Outpatient procedures take place in endoscopy clinics, HCP offices, surgical clinics, hospital outpatient surgery units, or interventional suites. These procedures can include general, regional, or local anesthesia, and/or sedation. Patients require less than a 24-hour stay after the procedure. Many go home with a caregiver soon after meeting specific discharge criteria. These less invasive procedures require less time under anesthesia than traditional surgery thus have a shorter recovery.

Patients and HCPs often prefer outpatient procedures. There is a lower risk for health care–associated infections. Patients like the convenience of recovering at home. HCPs prefer the flexible scheduling. The costs are usually less for the patient and the insurer. Other benefits include earlier mobility, quicker return to self-care, and less sedation/anesthesia time with reduced postoperative complications.[2]

PREOPERATIVE ASSESSMENT

You play a vital role in preparing patients for a procedure. Start with identifying the type of procedure and specific procedure information. The goal of the preoperative history and physical assessment (H&P) is to identify risk factors and plan care to ensure patient safety and optimize patient outcomes (Fig. 18.1). To achieve this, you will need to:

- Establish rapport with the patient and obtain patient preferences for how to be addressed (preferred name, pronouns).
- Establish baseline data for comparison in the intraoperative and postoperative periods.
- Determine the patient's psychologic status to reinforce the use of coping strategies.
- Determine physiologic factors related to the planned procedure that may contribute to operative risk factors.
- Participate in the identification and marking of the surgical site according to agency policy.
- Identify drugs and supplements the patient takes that may affect the surgical outcome.
- Review the results of preoperative diagnostic studies and share this information with the appropriate HCPs.
- Identify cultural and ethnic factors that may affect the surgical experience.
- Determine whether the patient received adequate information from the surgeon to make an informed decision to have surgery. Verify that the consent form is signed and witnessed.
- Assess previous anesthesia history including any adverse outcomes, such as postoperative nausea or vomiting.
- Begin appropriate and safe discharge planning per agency policy.

Patient Interview

Preoperative interviews are an important nursing responsibility. The nurse who works in the HCP's office, ambulatory surgery center, or hospital may do the interview. It can occur in advance or on the day of surgery.

The main purposes of the interview are to (1) obtain health information, (2) provide and clarify information about the

Perioperative Care Impacted by the Preoperative Assessment	Examples
Communication	• Important updates on clinical condition • Ensuring alignment of team regarding risks
Perioperative care	• Information about previous difficult intubation • Anticoagulation/antiplatelet plans
Day of surgery	• Requirements for specific operating room equipment • Pretreatment for specific conditions • Orders for needed day-of-surgery labs
Postoperative care	• Need for ICU bed based on comorbidities • Wound care consultation
Patient safety	• VRE, MRSA planning • Allergies/sensitivities (e.g., antibiotics, latex, metal)
Patient requests	• Documentation of advance directives • Begin discharge planning

Fig. 18.1 The health care team uses preoperative assessment information in many ways to ensure safe patient outcomes.

TABLE 18.2 Psychosocial Assessment of Preoperative Patient

Situational Changes	Concerns With the Unknown	Concerns With Body Image	Experiences	Need for Information
• Define degree of personal control, decision making, and independence • Assess for presence of hope and anticipation of positive results • Consider the impact of surgery and hospitalization and effects on lifestyle • Identify support systems, including family, other caregivers, and religious and spiritual groups	• Identify degree of anxiety and fears related to the surgery (e.g., pain) • Identify expectations of surgery, changes in health status, effects on daily living, and sexual activity (if appropriate)	• Identify current roles or relationships and view of self • Determine perceived or potential changes in roles or relationships and their impact on body image	• Review previous surgical experiences, hospitalizations, and treatments • Determine responses to those experiences (positive and/or negative) • Identify perceptions of the planned procedure in relation to the above and information from others (e.g., a friend's view of their surgical experience)	• Determine the amount and type of information the patient wants • Assess understanding of surgical procedure, including preparation, care, interventions, preoperative activities, restrictions, and expected outcomes • Review the accuracy of information the patient has received from others, including health care team, family, friends, and media

planned procedure, (3) assess the patient's emotional state and readiness for the procedure, and (4) begin the discharge plan. The interview gives the patient and caregiver an opportunity to ask questions about the anesthesia plan and postprocedure care. Often patients ask about taking their routine drugs, such as insulin, anticoagulants, or heart medications, and if they will have pain.

When speaking with patients, assess their response to stress related to the procedure or aftercare. You can provide the information and support needed to reduce anxiety and provide reassurance.

Psychosocial Assessment

Surgery is a stressful event, even for a minor procedure. Reactions to surgery may elicit the stress response with sympathetic nervous system activation (e.g., BP and heart rate). The stress response enables the body to meet the perioperative demands, but excess stressors or responses may affect recovery. Many factors influence the patient's reaction to stress, including age, experiences with illness and pain, current health, and socioeconomic status. Avoid medical jargon. Use common words and language familiar to the patient.

Your role in psychologically preparing patients for surgery is to assess them for potential or actual stressors that could negatively affect outcomes (Table 18.2). Communicate concerns to the appropriate surgical team member and during the hand-off of care if the concern may require intervention later. The most common psychologic reactions that patients express are anxiety, fear, and hope.

Anxiety. Most people are anxious when facing surgery because of the unknown. This is a normal survival mechanism. However, a high anxiety level can impair cognition, decision making, and coping mechanisms and affect the ability to learn or follow instructions.

Anxiety can arise from a lack of knowledge. This can range from not knowing what to expect to uncertainty about the outcome. Past experiences and stories from friends or the media can contribute. You can decrease some anxiety by giving information about what to expect. This is often done before surgery through videos or Internet-based/printed teaching materials. Inform the surgeon if the patient needs more information or has excess anxiety.

The patient may receive drugs that provide an amnesic effect, so they will not remember what occurs during surgery. Telling the patient this helps decrease anxiety.

Patients may have anxiety when surgery conflicts with their religious or cultural beliefs. For example, patients who are Jehovah's Witnesses may decline to receive blood or blood products.[3] Identify, record, and communicate patient decisions about the possibility of blood transfusions.

Common fears. Patients fear surgery for many reasons. The most common fear is the risk of death or permanent disability. Sometimes the fear comes after hearing or reading about the risks during the informed consent process. Other fears are related to pain, change in body image, or results of diagnostic procedures.

Fear of death can influence the surgical outcome through the patient's emotional state and stress response. Notify the HCP if the patient has a strong feeling of impending death. The HCP may delay the surgery.

Fear of pain during and after surgery is common. If the fear is extreme, notify the ACP or HCP. Reassure patients that drugs and other therapeutic interventions such as repositioning and splinting are often used to help with pain control. Pain is an expected part of the process and improves with healing. Setting a pain goal with realistic expectations provides patients with a sense of control. Tell patients to communicate with the care team to achieve a tolerable level of pain after the procedure. Teach them how to use a pain intensity scale (e.g., 0 to 10, FACES). See Chapter 9 for more on pain scales.

Fear of mutilation or *altered body image* can occur whether the surgery is radical, such as amputation, or minor, such as breast biopsy. Even a small scar on the body can be upsetting. Fear of keloid development (overgrowth of a scar) may be a concern. Listen to and assess the patient's concern with an accepting attitude.

Fear of anesthesia may arise from the unknown, personal experience, or tales of others' bad experiences. These concerns can also result from information about anesthesia risks (e.g., brain damage, paralysis). Many patients fear losing control while under anesthesia. Patients with a history of post-traumatic stress disorder may have a higher risk of being triggered by anesthesia. If you identify any of these fears or risks, include this information in the hand-off and/or ask the ACP to talk with the patient.

Fear of disruption of life functioning may range from fear of permanent disability to concern about limiting usual activities for a few weeks. You may find concerns about loss of role function, separation from family, and how the family will manage. Financial concerns include dealing with an expected loss of income and the costs of surgery and recovery.

Consulting with the caregiver, a social worker, a spiritual advisor, or a psychologist may be appropriate. Financial advisors at the hospital may provide information about financial options and support.

CHECK YOUR PRACTICE

Your 19-year-old male patient is in the holding area. He is scheduled for an orchiectomy for testicular cancer. He is visibly sweating and agitated. When you ask him how he is doing, he responds, "I am scared. Wouldn't you be?"

- What can you do to reduce his fear?

Hope. Hope may be the patient's strongest way of coping. To deny or minimize hope may negate the positive mental attitude necessary for a quick and full recovery. Some patients hopefully anticipate surgery to repair (e.g., plastic surgery for burn scars), rebuild (e.g., total joint replacement to reduce pain), or save and extend life (e.g., remove a tumor). Assess and support the presence of hope and the patient's anticipation of positive results.

Health History

Ask about current and past health problems and procedures. Record the reason for any hospitalizations and the dates. Identify any problems with previous surgeries and anesthesia. For example, the patient may have had a wound infection, nausea and/or vomiting, or a drug reaction. Does the patient have any implanted devices? Identify any home use of medical equipment, such as O_2. Assess whether the patient understands the reasons for surgery.

Does the patient have an acute infection (e.g., influenza, COVID-19)? Elective surgery may be canceled if the patient has an acute infection. Ask about recent travel that may have exposed them to infection. Patients with active chronic infections such as hepatitis B or C, AIDS, or tuberculosis may have surgery if needed. We will need to make sure that we take appropriate infection control precautions to protect the patient and health care team. Infection control guidelines are discussed in Chapter 15.

Screen for risk of pregnancy. Ask about menstrual and obstetric history, date of the last menstrual period, number of pregnancies, and history of cesarean section as appropriate. Immediately tell the HCP if the patient may be pregnant or tests positive. Maternal and fetal exposure to anesthetics should be avoided during the first trimester.

Ask about blood relatives with any traits that may affect the surgical outcome. Record family history of heart and endocrine problems. For example, if a patient reports a parent with hypertension, sudden cardiac death, or myocardial infarction (MI), this should alert you that the patient may have a similar predisposition or condition. Is there a family history of adverse reactions to or problems with anesthesia? For example, malignant hyperthermia has a genetic predisposition. If present, measures will be taken to decrease complications associated with this condition (see Chapter 19).

Medications

Record all current medications, including over-the-counter drugs and supplements. Share this with the perioperative health care team. The ACP will decide the best schedule and dose of the patient's routine drugs before and after surgery. Ensure that you identify all the patient's drugs and implement any changes in the medication plan. Monitor the patient for potential interactions and complications.

The interaction of the patient's current drugs and anesthetics can alter anesthesia effects (Table 18.3). For example, some antidepressants potentiate the effect of opioid agents used for anesthesia or pain control. Antihypertensive drugs may predispose the patient to hypotension or shock from the combined effect of the drug and the vasodilator effect of some anesthetics. Most patients taking beta-blockers for hypertension, coronary artery disease, or dysrhythmias should continue taking them on the day of surgery.[1]

Insulin and hypoglycemic agents may need adjustments during the perioperative period because of decreased oral intake, stress, and anesthesia. Antiplatelet agents (e.g., aspirin, clopidogrel) inhibit platelet aggregation and may contribute to bleeding. Drugs taken for chronic pain may be continued to help manage pain after surgery and prevent acute opioid withdrawal.

HCPs may ask patients to withhold some drugs before surgery. Specific time frames for withholding drugs depend on the drug and the patient. Patients on long-term anticoagulation therapy (e.g., warfarin, rivaroxaban, apixaban) present a unique challenge. Options include (1) continuing therapy, (2) withholding therapy for a time before and after surgery, or (3) withholding the therapy and starting subcutaneous or IV heparin therapy during the perioperative period. We often call this "bridge therapy." The strategy selected is based on the patient and the procedure.[4]

TABLE 18.3 Common Drugs Requiring Preoperative Adjustment

- Angiotensin-converting enzyme (ACE) inhibitors
- Angiotensin II receptor blocker (ARB)
- Angiotensin receptor-neprilysin inhibitor (ARNi)
- Anticoagulants
- Antiplatelets
- Aspirin
- Corticosteroids
- Diuretics
- Glucagon-like peptide-1 (GLP-1) agonists
- Hypoglycemic medication
- Insulin
- Monoamine oxidase (MAO) inhibitors
- Nonsteroidal antiinflammatory drugs (NSAIDs)
- Oral contraceptive therapy
- Phosphodiesterase inhibitors
- Sodium-glucose cotransporter-2 (SGLT2) inhibitors
- Triptans
- Weight loss drugs

Ask about the use of supplements. Many patients do not include them on their medication list. Supplements taken with anticoagulants or antiplatelet drugs can cause excess postoperative bleeding that may require a return to the operating room (OR).[5]

Ask about substance use. This includes tobacco, alcohol, opioids, marijuana, cocaine, and amphetamines. Screen for alcohol and opioid use disorders using validated screening tools. Chronic alcohol and opioid use can place the patient at risk because of lung, gastrointestinal (GI), or liver damage. Decreased liver function prolongs the metabolism of anesthetic agents, alters nutrition status, and increases the risk for complications. Alcohol and opioid withdrawal can occur during lengthy surgery or recovery. Proper planning and management help prevent this life-threatening condition (see Chapter 11).

Allergies

Ask about drug intolerances and drug allergies. Drug intolerance usually results in side effects that are unpleasant but not life threatening. Common intolerances include nausea, constipation, and diarrhea. A true drug allergy or hypersensitivity reaction activates the immune system. Allergies are discussed in Chapter 14.

Ask specifically about allergies to antibiotics. Prophylactic antibiotics are given before most surgeries to prevent surgical site infections. Ask about reactions to metal or skin cleansers such as chlorohexidine and/or povidone-iodine as these products may be used on the skin.

! SAFETY ALERT

Allergies

- Some local anesthetic agents contain bisulfite preservatives.
- Notify the ACP if the patient has an allergy to sulfur-containing drugs.

Ask about food and environment (e.g., latex, pollen, animals) allergies. Patients with a history of any allergic reactions have a greater potential for hypersensitivity reactions to drugs given during anesthesia. Though many agencies are latex-free environments, we still need to screen for latex allergies. Risk factors for latex allergy include long-term, multiple exposures to latex products, such as those experienced by health care and rubber industry workers. Other risk factors include hay fever, contact dermatitis, asthma, and allergies to certain foods (e.g., eggs, avocados, bananas).[6]

Review of Systems

The last part of the history is the body systems review. Ask specific questions to confirm the presence or absence of health problems (Table 18.4). This alerts you to areas that you will need to assess in the preoperative physical

TABLE 18.4 Preoperative Patient Assessment[a]

System	Risk Factor for Complications	Assessment
Cardiovascular	• Blood clotting disorder • Coronary artery disease • Heart failure • Hypertension • Hypovolemia • MI • Prosthetic valve • VTE	• Identify any medication (e.g., aspirin) or herbs (e.g., ginkgo) that may affect coagulation. • Identify presence of prosthetic heart valves, pacemakers, or implantable cardioverter-defibrillators. • Assess for edema (including dependent areas), noting location and severity. • Inspect neck veins for distention. • Obtain bilateral baseline BPs. • Assess capillary refill, skin color and temperature, and pulses for rate, rhythm, and quality.
Endocrine	• Diabetes • Adrenal problems • Thyroid problems	• Assess glucose and electrolyte levels. • Assess for use of corticosteroids and thyroid replacement therapy.
Gastrointestinal	• Liver problems • Malnutrition • Obesity • Substance use disorder	• Determine patterns of food and fluid intake. • Weigh patient and note any recent changes. • Review usual pattern of bowel movements, including date of last bowel movement. • Assess for presence of dentures and bridges (loose dentures or teeth may be dislodged during intubation). • Auscultate abdomen for presence of bowel sounds. • Review liver function and electrolyte tests. • Inspect skin color and sclera for jaundice.
Genitourinary	• Kidney disease	• Determine ability to void. • Note color, amount, and characteristics of urine. • Determine pregnancy status. • Review kidney function tests.
Immune	• Immunodeficiency	• Note any immunodeficiency.
Musculoskeletal	• Limited mobility	• Assess for limitations in joint range of motion and muscle strength. • Assess for joint or muscle pain. • Assess mobility, gait, and balance.
Neurologic	• Impaired cognition • Stroke	• Determine orientation to person, place, and time. • Assess baseline mental status. Note any confusion, disorderly thinking, or inability to follow commands. • Identify a history of stroke, transient ischemic attacks, neurologic problem (e.g., Parkinson disease, multiple sclerosis), or sensory deficit.
Respiratory	• Asthma • COPD • Current infection • Sleep apnea • Smoking; vaping	• Note use of CPAP machine, O_2 therapy. • Assess for vaping and tobacco use, include date/time of last use. • Determine baseline O_2 saturation and respiratory rate and rhythm. • Observe for cough, dyspnea, and use of accessory muscles. • Auscultate breath sounds.
Skin	• History of pressure injury	• Note any current or previous skin problems (e.g., eczema, bruising). • Inspect skin for rashes, breakdown, or infection, especially around the planned surgical site. • Examine skin around bone pressure points. • Inspect mucous membranes and skin moisture for signs of dehydration.

[a]See specific body system chapters for more detailed assessments and related laboratory studies.

examination. The combined review of systems and history provides essential data to determine the preoperative tests that the patient needs.

Cardiovascular system. Evaluate cardiovascular (CV) function to see if there are any problems. Is there a history of hypertension, angina, dysrhythmias, heart failure, or MI? Ask about the current treatment for any CV problem and the level of functioning. The goal is to optimize the medical management (e.g., BP, cardiac rhythm control) to reduce potential harm during and after the procedure.[7]

Patients scheduled for a noncardiac procedure are screened for risk of a perioperative adverse cardiac event by the HCP. If indicated, the patient should have a 12-lead ECG and coagulation studies, and the results should be on the chart before surgery. A cardiology consultation is often obtained if the patient has a significant CV history (e.g., recent MI, valve disease, implantable cardiac device, heart failure). The CV assessment provides data on what other measures the patient needs. For example, the patient on diuretic therapy may need to have a serum potassium level drawn before surgery.

Immobility and operative positioning increase the risk of venous thromboembolism (VTE). Patients at high risk for VTE include those with previous thrombosis, blood-clotting problems, cancer, varicosities, obesity, tobacco use, heart failure, or chronic obstructive pulmonary disease (COPD).[8] Prophylactic anticoagulants may be given before the procedure based on the patient's VTE risk.[9]

Respiratory system. Ask about recent or chronic respiratory problems or infections. COVID-19 can have long-term effects such as fatigue and dyspnea.[10] Elective surgery may be postponed if the person has an upper respiratory tract infection. Upper airway infections increase the risk for bronchospasm, decreased O_2 saturation, and problems with respiratory secretions. Report any dyspnea at rest or with exertion, coughing (dry or productive), or hemoptysis (coughing blood) to the ACP and HCP. Depending on the H&P, baseline pulmonary function tests and arterial blood gases may be done before surgery.

If a patient has asthma, ask about the use of inhaled or oral corticosteroids and bronchodilators, and the frequency and triggers of asthma attacks. The patient with COPD is at high risk for pulmonary complications, including hypoxemia and atelectasis. When was the last time the patient brushed their teeth? Tooth brushing within 4 hours of beginning sedation reduces the risk of pneumonia.[11]

Gather information about tobacco use, including vaping. The HCP and you should encourage the patient to stop smoking at least 6 weeks before surgery. Smoking increases the risk for pulmonary and vascular complications during and after surgery.

Screen for sleep apnea and sleep-disordered breathing.[1] Identify any home use of medical equipment, such as O_2 or continuous positive airway pressure (CPAP). Report conditions likely to affect respiratory function such as sleep apnea, obesity, and spinal, chest, or airway deformities. Patients are often asked to bring their sleep apnea devices with them to the hospital or surgical center.

Neurologic system. Baseline cognitive function is important for comparison during and after surgery. Assess the patient's ability to respond to questions, follow commands, and maintain orderly thought patterns. Record their ability to pay attention, concentrate, and respond appropriately.

If you note deficits in cognitive function, determine the extent of the problems and whether they can be corrected before surgery. If the problems cannot be corrected, it is important to involve a legal guardian or person with durable power of attorney for health care to aid the patient and provide informed consent for surgery.

Changes in hearing and vision may affect responses and the ability to follow directions. Make sure the patient has access to their eyewear and auditory aids. Obtain information about a history of strokes, transient ischemic attacks, or spinal cord injury. Ask about neurologic problems, such as Parkinson disease or multiple sclerosis and any treatments used. Do they have an implantable device such as a cochlear implant, nerve stimulator, or intrathecal pump?

The older adult may have intact mental abilities before surgery but is more prone to adverse outcomes during and after surgery. This is due to the added stressors of surgery, anesthesia, and adjunctive drugs, as well as the unfamiliar environment. These factors contribute to *postoperative delirium,* a condition that may be falsely labeled as senility or dementia.

Gastrointestinal system. Anesthesia and procedures can affect the GI system. These effects include nausea, vomiting, and constipation because of the neuromuscular blockade during anesthesia. Assess baseline GI function as it may affect the anesthesia plan of care. For example, chronic nausea may require additional antiemetics. Ask about gastroesophageal reflux disease and gastric motility disorders. Disruptions in the GI tract can affect drug absorption. Assess bowel habits. Constipation is common after surgery.

The liver detoxifies many anesthetics and adjunctive drugs. Patients with liver problems have an increased risk for clotting abnormalities and adverse drug responses. Consider the presence of liver disease with jaundice, hepatitis, alcohol and/or drug misuse, or obesity.

Genitourinary system. Assess for renal or urinary tract problems, such as chronic kidney disease or repeated urinary tract infections. Renal problems are associated with fluid and electrolyte imbalances, blood clotting problems, infection, and impaired wound healing. The kidneys metabolize and excrete many drugs. Many patients have renal function tests (e.g., serum creatinine, estimated glomerular filtration rate [eGFR], blood urea nitrogen [BUN]) before surgery.

Record and share with the perioperative team if the patient has problems voiding (e.g., incontinence, hesitancy). Older male patients may have an enlarged prostate that can interfere with the insertion of a bladder catheter or impair voiding after surgery.

Skin. Ask about any skin problems. Plan for special attention to padding areas to prevent pressure injuries. Patients with a history of pressure injuries may need extra protection during surgery.

Body art such as tattoos and piercings are common. When possible, select pigment-free areas for injections, IV sites, and laboratory draws. Piercings may put the patient at risk for burns at the piercing site during the procedure when the electrosurgical cautery is activated. Ensure all metal piercings and jewelry are removed before the procedure. If jewelry cannot be removed, notify the HCP and surgical team to plan for patient safety.

Musculoskeletal system. Note any musculoskeletal and mobility problems, especially in older adults. Identify any joints affected by arthritis. Mobility restrictions may influence intraoperative and postoperative positioning and ambulation. Spinal anesthesia may be difficult if the patient cannot flex the lumbar spine enough to allow easy needle insertion. If the neck is affected, intubation and airway management may be difficult. Any mobility aids (e.g., cane, walker) should be with the patient on the day of surgery.

Endocrine system. Patients with diabetes are especially at risk for adverse effects of anesthesia and surgery. Hypoglycemia, hyperglycemia, delayed wound healing, and infection are common perioperative complications of diabetes. Most agencies have protocols for managing preprocedural insulin and hypoglycemic agents. Assess glucose and notify the HCP if the glucose is outside normal parameters. Reassess glucose according to agency protocol.

Ask about chronic steroid use, such as in Addison disease. Chronic steroid use affects the ability to heal. Patients who take maintenance steroids may need additional steroid doses to manage the physiologic stress of the perioperative period.

Immune system. Note if the patient has a compromised immune system or takes immunosuppressive drugs. This includes patients on chemotherapy or those who have received organ or tissue transplants. An impaired immune system can lead to delayed wound healing and an increased risk for infection.[12]

Fluid and electrolyte balance. Ask about any recent conditions that increase the risk for fluid and electrolyte imbalances, such as vomiting, diarrhea, or completing a bowel prep. Note the time of last food and fluid intake as this can affect gastric emptying and increase risk for intraprocedural aspiration and/or postprocedural pneumonia. Identify drugs that change fluid and electrolyte status, such as diuretics. We often assess electrolyte levels before surgery. Patients who have fluids restricted before surgery may develop dehydration if surgery is delayed. Patients with dehydration may need more fluids and electrolytes before or during surgery.

Nutrition. Knowing that a patient has a nutrition problem can help the health care team provide more customized care. For example, if the patient has little subcutaneous tissue, additional positioning support on the OR table can prevent pressure injuries. Notify the team if a patient has body mass index (BMI) greater than 35 kg/m^2 (morbid obesity) to allow time to obtain special equipment needed (e.g., longer instruments for abdominal surgery, weight limits on procedural equipment).

Obesity stresses the heart and lungs and makes access to the surgical site and anesthesia administration more difficult.[13] The decreased perfusion of fat tissue predisposes the patient to wound dehiscence, wound infection, and incisional herniation after surgery. The patient may be slower to recover from anesthesia because fat tissue absorbs and stores inhalation agents and some opioids (e.g., fentanyl). See Chapter 45 for the special perioperative needs of patients who are obese.

Nutrition problems impair surgical recovery. If the nutrition problem is severe, surgery may be postponed. Protein and vitamin A, vitamin C, and vitamin B complex deficiencies are particularly important because these substances are essential for wound healing. The older adult is often at risk for malnutrition and fluid volume deficits. Patients who are malnourished may need supplemental nutrition during the perioperative period.

Identify patients who drink large quantities of coffee, caffeinated drinks, or "energy" drinks. Withholding caffeinated beverages can lead to severe withdrawal headaches.[14] These headaches can be confused with spinal headaches. Giving caffeinated beverages after surgery, when possible, may prevent these headaches.

Physical Examination

The Joint Commission requires that all patients admitted to the OR have an H&P in their chart that was done in the last 30 days. There must be an addendum with any changes on the day of procedure.[15] HCPs qualified to perform the H&P include advanced practice nurses, physicians, physician assistants, and ACPs. Findings from the H&P enable the ACP to assign the patient a physical status rating for anesthesia administration (Table 18.5). This rating indicates the patient's perioperative risk and may influence perioperative decisions. The scale is P1 to P6 or ASA I to VI. Patients having surgery in ambulatory or outpatient settings generally have ratings of P1, P2, or P3. Other designations to the ASA status, such as an "E," designate an "emergent" procedure.

Complete a physical assessment of the patient before surgery (Table 18.4). Review the documentation in the chart, including the H&P. Record all findings and share any relevant findings at once with the surgeon or ACP.

Diagnostic Studies

Obtain and assess the results of diagnostic tests that were done before surgery. Ensure that all laboratory and diagnostic reports are in the chart. Missing reports may result in a delay or cancellation of the surgery. Common tests are listed in Table 18.6.

Ideally, these are ordered based on the H&P. For example, patients taking an antiplatelet drug (e.g., aspirin) may have a coagulation profile done. Patients on diuretic therapy may need a potassium level. An ECG may be done based on risk factors, such as taking medication for dysrhythmias or having high BP.[16] Some settings test specific patient populations (cardiac surgery, joint replacement) for methicillin-resistant *Staphylococcus aureus.* Those with positive results are prescribed antibiotics for several days before surgery.[17]

During periods of widespread communicable infections such as pandemics, patients may be tested for a specific organism before surgery. Those who test positive for infection may have nonemergent procedures rescheduled.

TABLE 18.5 Diagnostic Criteria

American Society of Anesthesiologists' (ASA) Physical Classification System

Rating	Definition
P1 (ASA I)	Normal healthy person
P2 (ASA II)	Patient with mild systemic disease
P3 (ASA III)	Patient with severe systemic disease
P4 (ASA IV)	Patient with severe systemic disease that is a constant threat to life
P5 (ASA V)	Moribund patient who is not expected to survive without surgery
P6 (ASA VI)	Declared brain-dead patient whose organs are being removed for donor purposes

Used with Permission from American Society of Anesthesiologists: Statement on *ASA Physical Status Classification System,* 2020. Available at: https://www.asahq.org/standards-and-practice-parameters/statement-on-asa-physical-status-classification-system

TABLE 18.6 Common Preoperative Diagnostic Studies

Test	Assessment
Albumin	Nutrition status
Arterial blood gases (ABGs), pulse oximetry	Respiratory and metabolic function, oxygenation status
Blood urea nitrogen (BUN), creatinine	Renal function
Chest x-ray	Lung problems, cardiac enlargement, heart failure
Complete blood count (CBC): red blood cells (RBCs), hemoglobin (Hgb), hematocrit (Hct), white blood cells (WBCs)	Anemia, immune status, infection
ECG	Heart disease, dysrhythmias
Electrolytes	Metabolic status, renal function, diuretic side effects
Glucose	Metabolic status, diabetes
Human chorionic gonadotropin (hCG)	Pregnancy status
Liver function tests	Liver status
Prothrombin time (PT), partial thromboplastin time (PTT), international normalized ratio (INR), platelet count	Coagulation status
Pulmonary function studies	Pulmonary status
Type and crossmatch	Blood available for replacement (elective surgery patients may have own blood available)
Urinalysis	Renal status, hydration, urinary tract infection
Test or culture for communicable disease	Presence of communicable disease

Culturally Competent Care: Preoperative Patient

Consider culture when assessing and implementing preoperative patient care. For example, culture often determines one's expression of pain and ability to verbally express needs. One's culture may require that the family be included in any decision making. Ask about specific cultural considerations that may affect care. Respect these patient preferences. If the patient or caregiver does not speak English, use a qualified interpreter or translator. This can be completed via video, by phone, or in person. See more on culturally competent care in Chapter 2.

PREOPERATIVE TEACHING

Base preoperative nursing interventions and patient teaching on the assessment of the patient's specific needs. In most settings, patients arrive a short time before surgery. Preoperative teaching for these patients generally occurs in the HCP's office, a preadmission surgical clinic, or by video or phone call. We reinforce information on the day of surgery. Patients have a right to know what to expect and how to take part in their care during the experience. Teaching increases patient satisfaction and can reduce fear, anxiety, and stress.[18] It may decrease the incidence of complications, length of hospitalization, and recovery time after discharge.

Assess what the patient wants to know and give priority to those concerns. Patients with varying cultures, backgrounds, and experiences may want different types of information. See Table 4.5 for factors affecting patient teaching.

Find a balance between explaining so much that the patient is overwhelmed and telling so little that the patient is unprepared. Observe and listen carefully to the patient to determine how much information is enough. Remember that anxiety and fear may limit learning ability.

Generally, preoperative teaching includes 3 types of information: sensory, process, and procedural.[19] With *sensory information,* patients find out what they will see, hear, smell, and feel during the surgery. For example, you may tell them that the lights in the OR are bright. Or the OR will be cold, but they can ask for a warm blanket. Unfamiliar sounds and specific smells will be present. Some agencies use photos or videos to familiarize patients before the day of procedure.

Process information includes the general flow of what is going to happen. This information would include the patient's transfer to the holding area, visits by the nurse and the ACP before transfer to the OR, and waking up in the postanesthesia care unit (PACU).

Some patients want specific *procedural information* details. For example, this would include saying an IV line will be started while the patient is in the holding area. Or the surgeon will mark the operative area with an indelible marker to verify the surgical site.[20]

Share the preoperative teaching given to the patient with the nurses providing postoperative care to evaluate patient learning and avoid duplication of teaching. Because there is limited time for teaching, we often use a team approach. Your responsibility is to assess the patient's understanding and fill in the gaps. Record all teaching in the chart. A guide for preoperative patient and caregiver teaching is outlined in Table 18.7. See Chapter 4 for more on patient and caregiver teaching.

General Surgery Information

Unless it is contraindicated (e.g., after craniotomy, tonsillectomy), all patients should receive instruction about deep breathing, coughing, and early ambulation. This is essential because patients may not want to do these activities after surgery unless they know the reasons and practice before surgery. Describe tubes, drains, monitoring devices, or special equipment that will be used after surgery, and explain its purpose. Specific teaching may include how to use incentive spirometers

TABLE 18.7 PATIENT & CAREGIVER TEACHING

Preoperative Preparation

Include the following information in the preoperative teaching plan for the patient and caregiver:

Sensory Information	• Preoperative holding area may be noisy • Medication and cleaning solutions may be odorous • Operating room (OR) can be cold. Forced air warming devices may be used. Warm blankets are available • Talking may be heard but may be distorted because of masks. Ask questions if something is not understood • OR bed will be narrow. Safety straps may be applied • OR lights may be bright • Monitoring machines may be heard (e.g., beeping noises) when awake
Procedural Information	• What to bring and what type of clothing to wear to the surgery center • Any changes in time of surgery • Fluid and food restrictions • Physical preparation needed (e.g., shower, bowel, or skin preparation) • Purpose of frequent vital signs assessment • Pain control and other comfort measures • Why turning, deep breathing, and coughing after surgery are important. Do practice sessions • Insertion of IV lines • Procedure for anesthesia administration • Surgical site may be marked with indelible ink or marker
Process Information	• Admission area • Preoperative holding area, OR, and post-anesthesia care unit (PACU) • Any technology that may be present on awakening, such as monitors, central lines, sequential compression devices
Caregiver Support	• Caregivers can usually stay in preoperative holding area until surgery • Caregivers will be able to see patient after discharge from the PACU or possibly in PACU once the patient is awake or in patient room if the surgery requires a hospital admission • OR staff will update caregivers during surgery and when surgery is over • Surgeon will usually talk with caregivers after surgery

or patient-controlled analgesia pumps. Patients should understand how to rate their pain and how their pain will be managed (see Chapter 9).

The patient should receive surgery-specific information. For example, a patient having a total joint replacement will use a walker after surgery. Tell a patient having open heart surgery about waking up in the intensive care unit.

TABLE 18.8 Preoperative Fasting Recommendations

Liquid and Food Intake	Minimum Fasting Period (h)
Clear liquids (e.g., water, clear tea, black coffee, carbonated beverages, fruit juice without pulp)	2
Breast milk	4
Nonhuman milk, including infant formula	6
Light meal (e.g., toast and clear liquids)	6
Regular meal (may include fried or fatty food, meat)	8 or more

From Practice guidelines for preoperative fasting and the use of pharmacologic agents to reduce the risk of pulmonary aspiration: application to healthy patients undergoing elective procedures, *Anesthesiology* 126:376, 2017.

Many agencies have adopted Enhanced Recovery After Major Surgery (ERAS) protocols to improve patient outcomes.[21] These are based on guidelines for healthy patients of all ages undergoing surgery (except females in labor) from the American Society of Anesthesiologists (Table 18.8).[22] Restricting fluids and food is designed to reduce the risk for pulmonary aspiration, nausea, and vomiting. Guidelines vary for patients having local anesthesia or surgery scheduled late in the day. Most agencies follow the 8-6-2 rule for NPO guidelines. Patients can eat a regular meal up to 8 hours before surgery and a light meal up to 6 hours before surgery. Clear liquids, including carbohydrate energy drinks, are allowed up to 2 hours before surgery. Follow agency protocol. The patient who has not followed the NPO instructions may have surgery delayed or canceled.

Ambulatory Surgery Information

Patients having **ambulatory surgery** or same-day surgery need to receive information before admission. Some ambulatory surgical centers communicate with patients by phone, video, or electronic portal message through their electronic health record (EHR) several days before to obtain health information, give instructions, and answer questions. These patients need information on day-of-surgery events such as arrival time, registration, parking, what to wear, what to bring, and the need to have a responsible adult provide transportation home after surgery. Review safety information related to fall prevention and infection prevention measures. This may include preoperative skin cleansers, oral care, and reviewing current drugs that could affect safety.

LEGAL PREPARATION

Legal preparation for surgery consists of checking that all required forms are correctly signed and are present and that the patient and caregiver clearly understand what is planned. Standard consent forms include the surgical procedure and the need for possible blood transfusions. Some agencies use an anesthesia or sedation consent that is separate from the surgical consent. Follow your agency's policy. Code status, advance directives, and durable power of attorney for health care (see Chapter 10) should be included. For those with advance directives, discuss any new risks associated with the planned surgery. Make sure the approach for treating any potential problems is consistent with the patient's preferences.

Consent for Surgery

The patient must voluntarily sign an informed consent form in the presence of a witness before they can legally have nonemergency surgery. **Informed consent** is an active, shared decision-making process between the HCP and the recipient of care. Three conditions must be met for consent to be valid. First, there must be *adequate disclosure* of the (1) diagnosis; (2) nature and purpose of the procedure; (3) risks and consequences of the procedure; (4) probability of a successful outcome; (5) availability, benefits, and risks of alternative treatments; and (6) prognosis if treatment is not instituted. Second, the patient must show a clear *understanding* of the information before receiving sedating preoperative drugs. If a patient is sedated before signing the consent, surgery may be canceled or delayed. Third, the patient must *give consent voluntarily.* The patient must not be persuaded or coerced by anyone to have the procedure.

The surgeon is ultimately responsible for obtaining the patient's consent for surgical treatment. You may be asked to witness the patient's signature on the consent form. Serve as a patient advocate, verifying that the patient understands the information in the consent and the implications of consent, and gives truly voluntary consent for surgery. If the patient is unclear about the surgical plans, contact the surgeon about the patient's need for more information. The patient should not sign the consent form until all questions have been answered. The patient should be aware that signed consent can be withdrawn at any time (Box 18.1).

If the patient is a minor, unconscious, or mentally incompetent to sign the consent, a legal representative or responsible family member must give written permission. An *emancipated minor* is one who is younger than the legal age of consent but is recognized as having the legal capacity to provide consent. Follow your state's regulations, Nurse Practice Act, and agency policy.

A true medical emergency may override the need to obtain consent. Next of kin may give consent when immediate medical treatment is necessary to preserve life or prevent serious impairment to life or limb, and the patient is incapable of giving consent. If reaching the next of kin is not possible, the HCP may begin emergent treatment without written consent. Follow your agency policy about the process for documenting emergency consent.

BOX 18.1 ETHICAL/LEGAL DILEMMAS

Informed Consent

Situation

J.S., a 72-year-old female, is waiting in the preoperative holding area. You are discussing her impending surgery when you realize that this competent adult does not fully understand her surgery and was not informed of the alternatives to this surgery. Although she has previously signed a consent form, your assessment is that she was not fully informed about her treatment options or does not recall them.

Ethical/Legal Points for Consideration

- Informed consent requires that patients have complete information about the proposed treatment, as well as alternative treatments, risks and benefits of each treatment option, and possible consequences of the surgery. The person (usually the surgeon) performing the procedure usually has this responsibility.
- An opportunity to have questions answered about the various treatment options and their possible outcomes is a crucial element of informed consent.
- A patient can revoke their consent at any time, even at the very last minute. It is essential that you report any circumstance that suggests that the patient does not understand the information or is revoking the informed consent to the person who obtained the consent.
- In most states, the registered nurse's legal role is to witness the signing of the document. As a nurse, you attest to the fact that the patient's signature was valid.

Discussion Questions

1. What do you think you should do next?
2. What is your role as a patient advocate in the informed consent process?
3. What should you do if the patient states that she does not want to know about the surgical procedure or alternatives to surgery?

DAY-OF-SURGERY PREPARATION

Nursing Role

Your responsibilities immediately before surgery include final preoperative teaching, assessment, and communication of pertinent findings. Use your agency's surgical safety checklist to ensure you complete everything (Table 18.9). Make sure all preoperative orders are done and that the chart is complete and goes with the patient to the OR. Verify the presence of a signed informed consent form, laboratory and diagnostic study results, an H&P, a record of any consultations, baseline vital signs, proper skin preparation, and completed nursing notes. The surgical site is identified and marked with an indelible marker by the surgeon and recorded to show that the patient agrees.

Verify the reason the patient is having the procedure with the patient and review their comorbidities. Assess the patient's response to the stress of surgery and clarify any questions or concerns. Last, identify potential risks and complications of the surgical procedure and any special considerations for planning care. The patient is likely to receive care from several different nurses in the preoperative area, OR, PACU, surgical intensive care unit (SICU), and/or surgical unit. Document and directly communicate important findings to health team members, especially during the hand-off process.

Hospitals often require that a patient wear a hospital gown with no underclothes. Surgical centers may allow the patient to wear underwear, depending on the procedure. The patient should remove any cosmetics to allow for observation of skin color. Remove nail polish and artificial nails so you can assess capillary refill and use pulse oximetry. Place an identification

TABLE 18.9 Preoperative Checklist

Preoperative Data	Initials	Day of Surgery	Initials
Height _____ Weight _____		Surgical site marked Y or NA	
Isolation Y or N Type _____		ID band on patient Y or N	
Allergies noted on chart Y or N		Allergy band on patient Y or NA	
Vital signs (baseline) T _____ P _____ R _____ BP _____ Pulse Ox _____		Vital signs Time __________ T _____ P _____ R _____ BP _____ Pulse Ox _____	
Chart Review		**Procedures**	
H&P on chart		NPO since _____	
H&P within 30 days? Y or N		Oral care completed time: __________	
Signed informed consent form on chart Y or N		Capillary glucose Time _______ Result: _____ NA	
Signed consent for blood administration Y or NA		Voided/catheter Time _____	
Blood type and crossmatch Y or NA		Preoperative drugs given Time _____ NA	
Diagnostic Results		Preoperative antibiotics given Time _____ NA	
Hgb/Hct _____ /_____ NA			
PT/INR/PTT _____ /_____ /_____ NA		Preoperative skin prep Y or NA Shower____ Scrub____ Clip____	
CXR _____ NA			
ECG _____ NA hCG _____ Negative _____ Positive _____NA		Makeup, nail polish, false fingernails, and false eyelashes removed Y or NA	
Other labs: (example—test for communicable disease)		Hospital gown applied Y or NA	
Final Chart Review		VTE prophylaxis SCD Y or NA other________	
Additional forms attached:		**Valuables**	
		Dentures Y or N	
		Wig or hairpiece Y or N	
		Eyeglasses Y or N	
Caregiver contact info: __________		Contact lenses Y or N	
Time to OR __________ Date _____		Hearing aid Y or N	
Transported to OR by __________		Prosthesis Y or N	
Final check by __________ RN _____		Jewelry Y or N Piercings with jewelry Y or N	
		Clothing Y or N	
		Disposition of valuables: Hearing aid in place Y or NA	

band on the patient using 2 patient identifiers. Place any allergy and other safety alert bands (Fig. 18.2). Prostheses, dentures, and contact lenses are generally removed to prevent loss or damage. Return patient valuables to a caregiver or secure them according to agency policy. Keep glasses and hearing aids in place to allow the patient to hear instructions and see the staff and environment. Remove them at hand-off with procedure staff and place with patient valuables so they can be easily accessed after sedation.

Encourage the patient to void before you give preoperative drugs and before transfer to the OR. An empty bladder prevents involuntary elimination under anesthesia and reduces the risk for urinary retention during the early postoperative recovery.

Many preoperative drugs interfere with balance and increase the risk for a fall during ambulation. Carefully assess each patient for responses to drugs given and adjust the plan of care as needed.

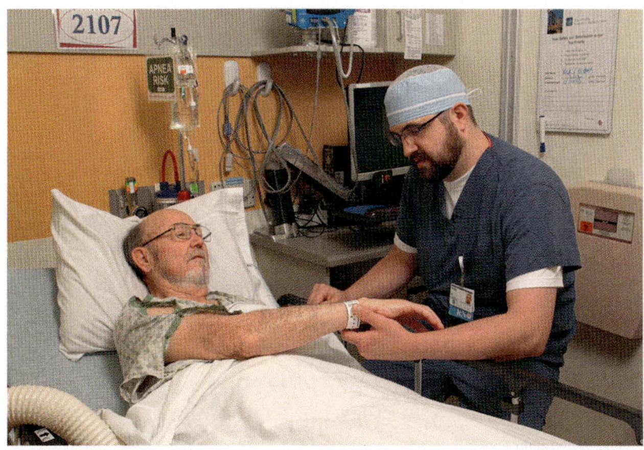

Fig. 18.2 The nurse performs a safety check by verifying that the patient has an identification band (wristband) as part of the preoperative preparations before they go to surgery. (From Stromberg HK: *Medical-surgical nursing*, ed 6, St. Louis, 2026, Elsevier.)

! SAFETY ALERT

Preoperative Checklist

- Use a preoperative checklist to make sure you complete all required preparations.
- This is important to do before the patient receives any sedating drug.

Preoperative Medications

Preoperative medications are used for several reasons (Table 18.10). A patient may receive a single drug or a combination. Benzodiazepines are used for their sedative and amnesic properties. Anticholinergics are sometimes given to reduce secretions. Multimodal pain strategies may be given to decrease pain and anesthetic requirements during surgery. Antiemetics can decrease nausea and vomiting.

Antibiotics are usually given within 30 to 60 minutes of the incision to prevent surgical site infections. They may be repeated during surgery based on length of the case and patient comorbidities. They also may be given when wound contamination is a potential risk (e.g., GI surgery).

Patients may or may not receive medication they routinely take on the day of surgery. To aid patient teaching and remove confusion about which drugs patients are taking, carefully check the preoperative orders. Clarify the orders with the surgeon and/or ACP if needed. People taking β-adrenergic blockers (β-blockers) continue these drugs.[23] Those with diabetes are carefully monitored and may receive insulin in the preoperative period.

Preoperative drugs may be given by mouth (PO), IV, or subcutaneously. Provide PO medication with a small sip of water 60 minutes before the patient goes to the OR unless otherwise ordered. Subcutaneous injections (e.g., insulin) and IV drugs are usually given to the patient after arrival in the preoperative holding area. Teach the patient about the expected effects of the medication (e.g., drowsiness).

Patients having cataract or other eye surgery often receive eyedrops. The patient may need multiple sets of eyedrops given at 5-minute intervals. It is important to give these drugs as prescribed and on time to adequately prepare the eye for surgery.

TABLE 18.10 Drug Therapy

Common Preoperative Agents

Class	Drug	Purpose
Antibiotics	cefazolin	Prevent postoperative infection
Anticholinergics	atropine glycopyrrolate	↓ Oral and respiratory secretions ↓ Vagal activation
	scopolamine (Transderm Scop)	Prevent nausea and vomiting Provide sedation
Antiemetics	ondansetron (Zofran)	Prevent nausea and vomiting
Antihyperglycemics	Insulin	Stabilize glucose
Benzodiazepines	diazepam lorazepam (Ativan) midazolam	↓ Anxiety, induce sedation, amnesic effects
β-Blockers	labetalol	Manage hypertension ↓ Sympathetic response
Histamine (H_2)-receptor antagonists	famotidine	↓ HCl acid secretion, ↑ pH, ↓ gastric volume
Opioids	fentanyl morphine	Relieve pain during preoperative procedures

CHECK YOUR PRACTICE

You are caring for an older patient who received alprazolam for preoperative anxiety. One hour later, they need to use the bathroom. You ask them if they can walk, and they reply, "yes." When helping them to stand, they become dizzy and almost fall. You return them to bed.

- Instead of trying to help the patient ambulate to the bathroom, what could have you done?

Transportation to the Operating Room

Most inpatients go from the nursing unit to the preoperative holding area. Caregivers may go with them to this area. Help the patient move from the bed to the stretcher. This is a good time to quickly assess for any skin issues. Raise the side rails. Make sure the completed chart and any needed equipment go with the patient.

In an ambulatory surgical center, the patient may go from the holding area to the OR by stretcher or wheelchair. If no sedatives have been given, the patient may even walk with someone to the OR. In all cases, ensure patient safety during transport. Record the method of transportation and the person who transports the patient. Provide hand-off communication to the nurse receiving the patient. This allows each of you to ensure you have shared all pertinent patient information. To avoid adverse events related to miscommunication use a hand-off tool or process. AORN recommends the use of an evidence-based tool such as SBAR for the hand-off process in this setting (see Table 1.3).[20]

Show the caregiver where to wait for the patient during surgery. Many hospitals use technology such as a status board that shares patient location. Information about visiting may be communicated electronically through a pager or portable computer. The surgeon may use a consultation room after surgery to discuss the outcome with the caregiver.

Gerontologic Considerations: Preoperative Patient

One of the most important considerations for the older adult is communication. Besides a primary care HCP, older adults often have various specialty providers, including the surgeon. Communication is important among all providers for best outcomes. You may need to coordinate transportation from a long-term care or assisted living facility so that the patient's timely arrival allows for surgery preparation.

An event that has little effect on a younger adult may be overwhelming to the older patient. Older adults may have surgery related to degenerative diseases. Hospitalization may represent a physical decline and loss of health, mobility, and independence. The older adult may view the hospital as a place to die or as a stepping-stone to a nursing home. Help decrease anxieties and fears while maintaining the self-esteem of the older adult undergoing surgery. Involve care coordinators and social workers early to help with discharge planning.

The risks associated with anesthesia and surgery increase in older patients. In general, the older the patient, the greater the risk for complications. In planning care, consider the patient's physiologic status. The surgical risk in the older adult relates to normal aging and changes that compromise organ function, reduce reserve capacity, and limit the body's ability to adapt to stress. This decreased ability to cope with stress, often compounded by the burden of one or more chronic illnesses and the surgery itself, increases the risk for complications.

Older adults may have sensory problems such as reduced vision and hearing. Bright lights may bother those with eye problems. Thought processes and cognitive abilities may be slowed or impaired. Assess and record baseline sensory and cognitive function. Physical reactions are often slowed because of mobility and balance problems. Because of these changes, the older adult may need more time to complete preoperative testing and understand preoperative instructions. These changes require you to pay more attention to promote patient safety and prevent injury.

Finally, determine the presence of or need for caregiver support. Caregiver support is critical for continuity of care after surgery. Planning discharge needs before the procedure improves patient outcomes and promotes timely discharge.

CASE STUDY

Preoperative Patient

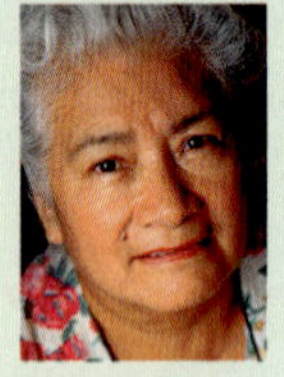

(© Ryan McVay/Photodisc/Thinkstock.)

Patient Profile

N.T., a 66-year-old retired registered nurse, is admitted to the ambulatory surgery center for a hysteroscopy and dilation and curettage (D&C) to obtain uterine biopsies after episodes of postmenopausal bleeding. She has type 2 diabetes, obesity, hypertension, and a history of atrial fibrillation. She has been NPO since midnight and did not take her morning medications. It is now 1200.

Subjective Data

- History of hypertension for 20 years; states, "I can't get my blood pressure under control" despite 2 blood pressure medications (diltiazem, HCTZ)
- History of atrial fibrillation with successful cardioversion 5 years ago, controlled by medications
- Surgical history: cesarean sections at age 30 and 32, gastric banding at age 53. Currently, the band is deflated due to severe acid reflux controlled with omeprazole
- Reports frequent burning in the chest due to reflux. Sleeps with her head elevated
- Lives alone
- Uses herbs to help her sleep
- Former 1 pack/day cigarette smoker × 45 years. Quit 5 years ago
- Drinks 1 glass of wine every night

Objective Data

Physical Assessment

- Alert, cognitively intact, anxious
- Weight 205 lb, height 5 ft 2 in
- BP 180/94, pulse 84 and regular
- Oxygen saturation 95% on room air
- Medications:
  - Diltiazem 240 mg daily
  - Hydrochlorothiazide 25 mg daily
  - ASA 80 mg daily
  - Omeprazole 20 mg daily
- Wears glasses. Has trouble seeing without them

Diagnostic Studies

- CBC, PT, PTT, and urinalysis values within normal limits
- Negative COVID test and MRSA swab
- Chem 12: Glucose 120 mg/dL, HbA1c 5%, potassium 3.4 mEq/L, sodium 145 mEq/L
- Chest x-ray and ECG normal
- Pulmonary function tests within normal limits for age

Interprofessional Care

- D&C scheduled at 1300 today

Discussion Questions

1. ***Recognize:*** What factors may influence N.T.'s response to surgery?
2. ***Analyze:*** What potential perioperative complications may you expect for N.T.?
3. ***Plan:*** What priority topics would you include in N.T.'s preoperative teaching plan?
4. ***Prioritize:*** Based on the assessment data presented, identify the priority clinical problems and related interventions.
5. ***Act:*** Given N.T.'s history, what priority preoperative assessments would you want to complete and why?
6. ***Evaluate:*** What do you need to continually monitor for N.T. before surgery?
7. ***Safety:*** To ensure N.T.'s safety, what preoperative nursing interventions are essential?

Answers available at http://evolve.elsevier.com/Lewis/medsurg.

BRIDGE TO NCLEX EXAMINATION

The number of the question corresponds to the same-numbered outcome at the beginning of the chapter.

1. A patient with obesity (BMI 42.1 kg/m^2) is scheduled for a laparoscopic cholecystectomy in an outpatient surgery setting. Which information would the nurse include in the plan of care?
   - **a.** Surgery will involve removing a part of the liver.
   - **b.** The patient will be in the hospital for several days.
   - **c.** The setting is not appropriate for the planned surgery.
   - **d.** Special equipment may be needed for the patient's care.
2. A patient reports a skin reaction when wearing disposable gloves. Which action would the nurse take *first?*
   - **a.** Notify the surgeon so that the surgery can be canceled.
   - **b.** Ask further questions to assess for a possible latex allergy.
   - **c.** Notify the OR staff at once so they can use latex-free supplies.
   - **d.** No action is needed because the patient's reaction has no bearing on surgery.
3. A patient scheduled for a herniorrhaphy in 2 days reports that they take an anticoagulant agent daily. Which action would the nurse take?
   - **a.** Inform the surgeon since the procedure may have to be rescheduled.
   - **b.** Tell the patient to continue to take the drug up to the day before surgery.
   - **c.** Ask the patient if they have any side effects from taking this drug regularly.
   - **d.** Notify the anesthesia care provider since this drug interferes with anesthetics.
4. A 17-year-old patient with a leg fracture who is scheduled for surgery is an emancipated minor. They have a statement from the court for verification. Which action would the nurse take?
   - **a.** Witness the patient signing the permit after the surgeon obtains consent.
   - **b.** Call a parent or legal guardian to sign the permit since the patient is under 18.
   - **c.** Notify the hospital attorney that an emancipated minor is consenting for surgery.
   - **d.** Obtain verbal consent since written consent is not necessary for emancipated minors.
5. Which intervention would the nurse *prioritize* to aid a preoperative patient in coping with the fear of pain?
   - **a.** Tell the patient that pain medication will be available.
   - **b.** Teach the patient to use guided imagery to reduce pain.
   - **c.** Describe the type of pain expected after the patient's surgery.
   - **d.** Explain the pain management plan and the use of a pain rating scale.
6. A patient is scheduled for surgery requiring general anesthesia at an ambulatory surgical center. The nurse asks them when they ate last. They reply that they had a light breakfast 2 hours before arriving at the surgery center. Which action would the nurse take?
   - **a.** Tell the patient to come back tomorrow since they ate a meal.
   - **b.** Have the patient void before giving any preoperative medication.
   - **c.** Proceed with the preoperative checklist, including site identification.
   - **d.** Notify the anesthesia care provider of when and what the patient last ate.
7. A patient who takes metformin 500 mg every morning for control of type 2 diabetes asks if they should take their medication on the day of surgery. Which recommendation would the nurse make?
   - **a.** Skip their medication on the day of surgery.
   - **b.** Get instructions from the surgeon about adjusting medications.
   - **c.** Take their usual morning dose at bedtime the night before surgery.
   - **d.** Take their medication as usual with a sip of water in the morning.
8. Which preoperative considerations would the nurse plan for the care of an older adult? (**Select all that apply.**)
   - **a.** Using only large-print education materials.
   - **b.** Speaking louder for patients with hearing aids.
   - **c.** Providing warm blankets to prevent hypothermia.
   - **d.** Teaching important information early in the morning.
   - **e.** Assessing for any sensory deficits that may be present.

1. d; 2. b; 3. a; 4. a; 5. d; 6. d; 7. b; 8. c, e.

For rationales to these answers and even more NCLEX review questions, visit http://evolve.elsevier.com/Lewis/medsurg.

REFERENCES

To access the References for this chapter, please scan the QR code with a mobile device.

19

Intraoperative Care

Kim Day

http://evolve.elsevier.com/Lewis/medsurg/

CONCEPTUAL FOCUS

Gas Exchange
Pain
Perfusion
Safety
Tissue Integrity

LEARNING OUTCOMES

1. Describe appropriate attire for areas of the perioperative department.
2. Outline the roles and responsibilities of surgical team members.
3. Prioritize needs of patients undergoing surgery.
4. Analyze the role of a perioperative nurse in managing patients undergoing surgery.
5. Apply basic principles of infection prevention and aseptic technique in the operating room.
6. Recognize operating room safety measures related to patients, equipment, and anesthesia.
7. Describe various anesthesia techniques and common anesthesia drugs.

KEY TERMS

anesthesia care provider (ACP)
anesthesiology
epidural block
general anesthesia
local anesthesia
malignant hyperthermia (MH)
nurse anesthetist
regional anesthesia
spinal anesthesia

Historically, surgery took place in the hospital operating room (OR). Now, many patients have surgery procedures in outpatient settings. More surgeons are using *minimally invasive surgery* (MIS) techniques and advanced technologies such as robotics that decrease blood loss, incision size, pain, recovery time, and hospital length of stay. Hybrid ORs, which allow for MIS and traditional open incision approaches within the same room, are becoming more common. This chapter describes the basics of intraoperative care that apply to all surgical patients, regardless of where or how the surgery is done.

INTRAOPERATIVE CARE

OPERATING ROOM ENVIRONMENT

Department Layout

The surgery department is a controlled environment designed to minimize the spread of pathogens and allow a smooth flow of patients, staff, and equipment for safe surgical patient care. The department is divided into 3 distinct zones: (1) unrestricted, (2) semirestricted, and (3) restricted (Fig. 19.1). The *unrestricted zone* is where people in street clothes interact with those in scrub attire. These areas typically include the points of entry for patients (e.g., holding area), staff (e.g., locker rooms), and information (e.g., nursing station or control desk). The *semirestricted zone* includes the surrounding support areas and corridors. Only authorized staff are allowed access to semirestricted areas. All staff in the semirestricted area should wear clean surgical attire. This includes scrub attire that was laundered in an accredited laundry facility, long-sleeved jacket, shoes dedicated for surgery use or shoe covers, surgical hat that covers all head and facial hair, and personal protective equipment (e.g., face shield). The *restricted zone* is within the semirestricted area. It includes the OR/surgical suite where the procedure takes place and the sterile core (Fig. 19.2). Masks should be worn

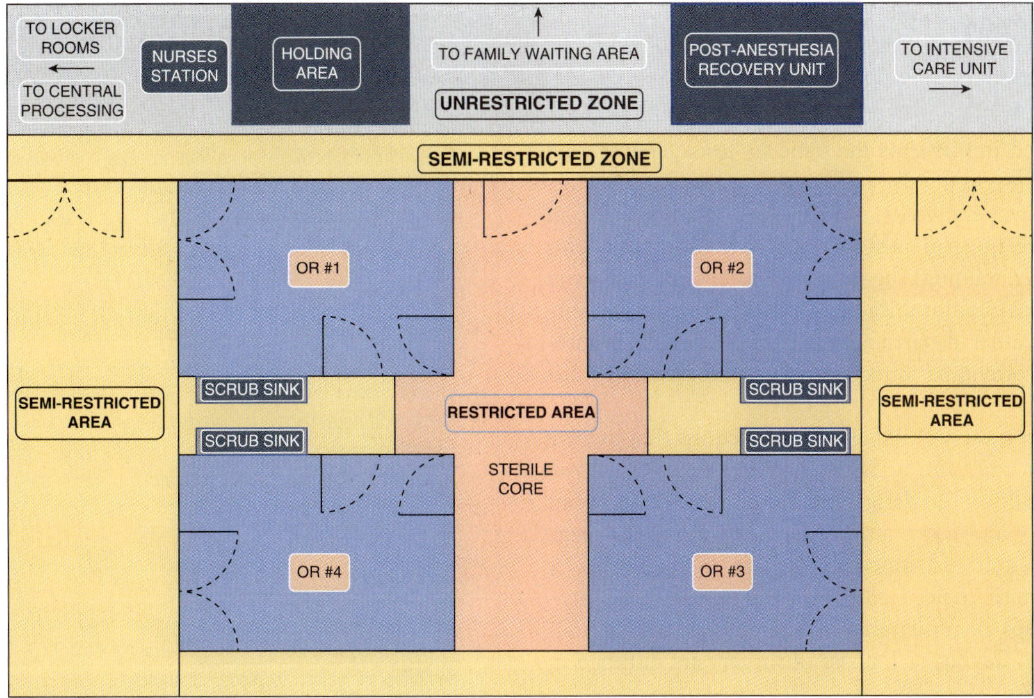

Fig. 19.1 Perioperative department layout.

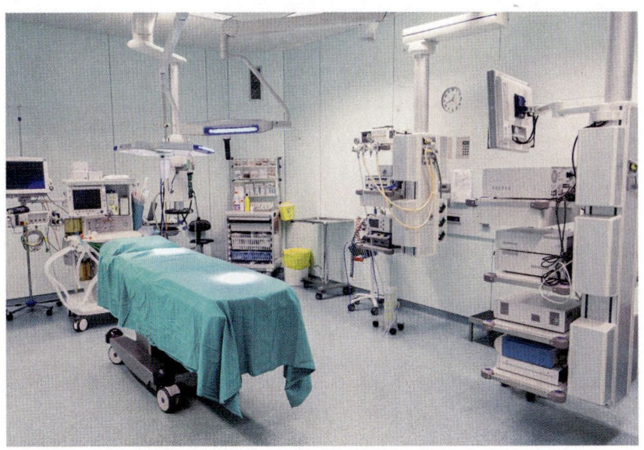

Fig. 19.2 Typical OR. (© iStock.com/windslegend.)

and traffic minimized when sterile supplies are open in the restricted area.[1]

The physical layout is designed to reduce cross-contamination. The flow of clean and sterile supplies and equipment is separate from contaminated supplies, equipment, and waste. Staff move supplies from clean areas, such as the sterile core, through the OR for surgery, and on to the instrument decontamination and sterilization area (e.g., central processing department [CPD]).

Preoperative Holding Area

The preoperative *holding area* is an unrestricted zone where patient identification and assessment take place. In some settings, the holding area is called the *admission, observation, and discharge* (AOD) unit. An AOD unit is designed to allow early morning admission for outpatient surgery, same-day admission, and inpatient holding before surgery. The patient is identified and assessed before and after surgery, before being discharged home or transferred to an inpatient room. The AOD unit is important in outpatient surgery and prevents unnecessary overnight stays in the inpatient setting.

Operating Room

The traditional OR is a unique setting separate from other clinical units. This restricted zone is controlled geographically, environmentally, and aseptically (Fig. 19.1). Having the OR next to the postanesthesia care unit (PACU) and the surgical intensive care unit allows for quick transport of the patient after surgery and close proximity to anesthesia staff if complications occur.

We use several methods to prevent the transmission of infection in the OR. Filters and controlled airflow in the ventilating systems provide dust control. Positive air pressure in the rooms prevents air from entering the OR from the halls and corridors. Temperature and humidity are controlled to prevent bacterial growth. Ultraviolet lighting reduces the number of microorganisms in the air. ORs have strict protocols for cleaning between cases and terminal cleaning at the end of the day.[2]

Furniture that is adjustable, easy to clean, and easy to move promotes safety and comfort. We check equipment frequently to ensure proper functioning and electrical safety. The lighting is designed for a precise view of the surgical site. A communication system offers a way to deliver routine and emergency messages.

SURGICAL TEAM

Registered Nurse

The *perioperative nurse* is an RN who works with the rest of the surgical team and implements the patient's perioperative plan of care. Depending on the size of the OR department, this role may include a preoperative RN, OR RN, and PACU RN. As an OR RN, you are the patient's advocate during surgery. This includes (1) maintaining the patient's safety, dignity, and confidentiality; (2) communicating with the patient, the surgical team, and other departments (e.g., CPD, PACU, laboratory); and (3) providing nursing care as described in this chapter.

During surgery, the OR RN assumes functions that involve either sterile or unsterile activities (Table 19.1). The *scrub nurse* (sterile) follows the designated surgical hand antisepsis with sterile glove and gown attire. They prepare and manage the sterile field and instrumentation. The *circulating nurse* stays in the unsterile field, facilitates the progress of the procedure, and keeps documentation. Examples of nursing activities that occur during each phase of surgery are outlined in Table 19.2.

After meeting specific criteria (e.g., 2 years of experience), perioperative RNs can earn OR certification (CNOR). CNOR certification validates a nurse has essential knowledge and skills in perioperative nursing.[3]

Practical/Vocational Nurse and Surgical Technologist

Depending on a state's nurse practice act, a licensed practical/vocational nurse (LPN/VN) or a surgical technologist may fill the role of the circulating or scrub nurse. Surgical technologists attend an associate degree program or a vocational, hospital, or military training program. The Association of Surgical Technologists sets education standards, provides continuing education, and offers certification for surgical technologists. An RN must supervise the LPN/VN or surgical technologist.

Surgeon and Assistant

The *surgeon* is the physician who does the surgery. The surgeon is primarily responsible for:

- Preoperative medical history and physical assessment, directing preoperative testing, and postoperative management
- Obtaining informed consent
- Leading the surgical team and directing the course of a procedure

The *surgeon's assistant* can be another physician, registered nurse first assistant, physician's assistant, surgical resident or fellow, medical student, or certified surgical first assistant. The assistant usually holds retractors to expose surgical areas and helps with hemostasis and suturing. In some agencies, especially education settings, the assistant may perform some parts of the surgery under the surgeon's direct supervision.

TABLE 19.1 Intraoperative Nursing Activities

Circulating, Nonsterile Activities

Before

- Helps prepare room, ensuring that supplies and equipment are available, in working order, and sterile
- Monitors practices of aseptic technique in self and others
- Checks mechanical and electrical equipment and environment factors
- Conducts a preprocedure verification process
- Confirms informed consent is present and patient has no questions
- Assesses patient's physical and emotional status
- Confirms and implements facility protocols and safety measures
- Checks chart and relates pertinent data to team members
- Helps with applying monitoring devices and insertion of invasive lines and other devices
- Assists with and ensures patient safety in transferring and positioning
- Takes part in surgical time-out

During

- Aids with anesthesia induction
- Records intraoperative care
- Prepares, records, labels, and sends blood, pathology, and any anatomic specimens to proper locations
- Confirms, dispenses, and records drugs used, including local anesthetics
- Coordinates all intraoperative activities with team members and other departments
- Works with scrubbed personnel to keep correct count of sponges, needles, instruments, and medical devices

After

- Facilitates patient transfer to PACU
- Gives hand-off report to PACU nurse with information relevant to care of patient

Scrubbed, Sterile Activities

Before

- Helps prepare the OR
- Completes surgical hand antisepsis; gowns and gloves self and other surgical team members
- Prepares instrument table and arranges sterile equipment for use
- Assists with draping
- Takes part in surgical time-out procedure

During

- Passes instruments to surgeon and assistants by anticipating their needs
- Keeps correct count of sponges, needles, instruments, and medical devices that could be retained in the patient
- Monitors practices of aseptic technique in self and others
- Keeps track of irrigation solutions used for calculation of blood loss
- Accepts, verifies, and reports drugs used by surgeon, including local anesthetics

Registered Nurse First Assistant

The *registered nurse first assistant* (RNFA) works with the surgeon, patient, and surgical team to achieve an optimal patient outcome. The Association of periOperative Registered Nurses (AORN) states that you must have formal education.[4] CNOR nurses or nurse practitioners can complete an RNFA program to assume this expanded role. RNFAs can obtain certification (C-RNFA).

TABLE 19.2 **Common Perioperative Nursing Activities**

Before Surgery	During Surgery	After Surgery
Home, Clinic, Holding Area • Start preoperative assessment • Provide teaching for patient's needs • Involve caregiver **Surgical Unit** • Complete preoperative assessment • Coordinate patient teaching with staff • Develop a plan of care that reflects patient's level of function and ability • Confirm informed consent is present, and patient has no questions • Safely give prescribed drugs **Surgical Suite** • Conduct preprocedure verification • Assess patient's level of consciousness, skin integrity, mobility, emotional status, functional limitations • Review chart • Ensure all supplies and equipment needed are available, functioning, and sterile	**Maintain Safety** • Ensure integrity of sterile field • Ensure correct sponge, needle, instrument, and medical device counts • Position patient to ensure correct alignment, exposure of surgical site, prevention of injury • Prevent chemical injury from prepping solutions, drugs • Ensure safe use of electrical equipment • Safely give ordered drugs **Monitor Physical Status** • Monitor and report changes in vital signs • Monitors blood loss and urine output **Monitor Psychologic Status** • Give emotional support • Ensure patient's right to privacy • Communicate patient's emotional status to surgical team	**Postanesthesia Care Unit, Discharge Area** • Determine patient's response to surgery • Monitor airway, breathing, and circulation (ABCs), vital signs, level of consciousness • Safely give ordered drugs **Clinical Unit** • Evaluate effectiveness of nursing care in OR using patient outcome criteria • Determine patient's level of satisfaction with care • Assess patient's psychologic status • Help with discharge planning **Home, Clinic** • Seek patient's perception of surgery in terms of effects of anesthetic agents, impact on body image, immobilization • Determine caregiver's perceptions of surgery

Anesthesia Care Provider

Anesthesiology is a medical specialty that focuses on clinical management of patients in the perioperative period, pain management, critical care, trauma, airway management, and cardiopulmonary resuscitation. The **anesthesia care provider (ACP)** is responsible for administering anesthetic agents and managing vital life functions (e.g., breathing, BP) during the perioperative period. This can be an anesthesiologist, nurse anesthetist, or anesthesiologist assistant.

A **nurse anesthetist** is a master's or a doctorate prepared RN who graduated from an accredited nurse anesthesia program and completed a national certification examination to become a certified registered nurse anesthetist (CRNA). The CRNA's scope of practice includes[5]:

- Performing and documenting a preanesthetic assessment and evaluation
- Developing and implementing a plan for delivering anesthesia
- Choosing, obtaining, and administering anesthesia, adjuvant drugs, and fluids
- Choosing, applying, and inserting monitoring devices
- Managing patients' airway and pulmonary status
- Managing emergence and recovery from anesthesia
- Releasing or discharging patients from PACU
- Ordering, starting, or modifying pain relief therapy
- Responding to emergency situations by providing airway management

An anesthesiologist assistant (AA) is a master's-prepared health professional who serves under the direction of an anesthesiologist.[2] AAs have completed an accredited program and passed a national certification examination. They take part in all types of anesthesia. This includes giving drugs, obtaining vascular access, applying and interpreting monitors, maintaining airways, and helping with preoperative assessment.

NURSING MANAGEMENT: INTRAOPERATIVE CARE

Before Surgery

Provide physical and emotional comfort for patients and caregivers along with teaching about the procedure. This is particularly important for patients who are anxious and in the same-day surgery settings. There, caregivers must assume greater responsibility for postoperative care. You can usually answer general questions about surgery and anesthesia, such as "Who will be in the room?" "How much of my body will be exposed?" Refer specific questions about the details of the surgery and anesthesia to the surgeon or ACP. For patients who do not speak English, use a qualified interpreter (see Table 2.9).

Separation from caregivers just before surgery can produce patient anxiety. Allowing the caregiver to wait with the patient in the preoperative holding area until the patient is transferred to the OR can reduce anxiety.

Perform a thorough physical assessment during the preoperative preparation of the patient (see Chapter 18).

Chart Review

Required chart data vary with agencies, patient conditions, and procedure. Table 18.5 provides an example of data obtained during the preoperative assessment. This information includes past and present medical history. It allows you to prepare for potential needs during surgery. Discuss abnormal findings or concerns for infection risk and other potential complications with the surgeon or ACP.

CHECK YOUR PRACTICE

Your patient has arrived in the holding area. As you review the chart, you realize the patient has not signed the consent for blood administration. You read that the patient has Alzheimer disease and is not mentally competent to give consent.

- How would you proceed?

Admitting the Patient

Follow your agency's protocol when admitting patients to the preoperative holding area and OR. A general routine includes initial greeting, proper identification, and a supportive welcome to the setting.

The admitting process continues with reassessment of the patient and time for last-minute questions. Complete the chart review and note any problems or changes. Ask the patient about valuables and prostheses. When was their last intake of food and fluid? Confirm that any ordered preoperative drugs were given. Provide a pillow or adjust the patient's position if requested. Most agencies require the patient's hair to be covered just before transfer to the OR suite to contain shed hairs.

You may offer complementary therapies, such as aromatherapy, music therapy, guided imagery, and distraction. These may decrease anxiety, promote relaxation, and reduce pain. Some agencies start these therapies before the patient is admitted to the OR. In others, such as ambulatory settings, they may start after the patient arrives in the holding area.

During Surgery

The circulating nurse is responsible for implementing the intraoperative plan of care and serving as the patient's advocate. The circulating nurse focuses on the whole patient. This involves ongoing assessment, reassessment, and adjusting the care plan to promote the best surgical outcomes.

Room Preparation

Before transferring the patient into the OR, prepare the room to ensure privacy, prevent infection, and promote safety. When a patient has severe obesity, extra staff and special equipment may be needed to safely position and transfer the patient to and from the OR bed. During surgery, special equipment (e.g., extralong instrumentation, bariatric OR bed) may be used.

CHECK YOUR PRACTICE

You are admitting a patient with severe obesity to the holding area before surgery.

- What special considerations are needed to promote a safe surgical experience?

All people entering the OR wear surgical attire (Fig. 19.3). All electrical and mechanical equipment is checked for proper functioning. Each surgical item is opened and placed on the instrument table using sterile technique. Sponges, needles, instruments, and small medical devices (e.g., surgical clip cartridges, universal adapters) are counted according to strict processes to ensure accurate retrieval at the end of the procedure. Any retained surgical supplies, devices, or instruments are sentinel events (never events) or serious reportable events (SREs) that can result in negative patient outcomes.[6] Sentinel events and SREs are discussed in Chapter 1.

During room preparation and the procedure, the scrub person does surgical hand antisepsis, dons sterile gown and gloves, and touches only items in the sterile field. The circulating nurse stays in the unsterile field and does those activities that involve contact with all unsterile items and the patient. This coordinated effort allows for smooth work throughout the procedure.

Transferring the Patient

The patient is moved into the OR after the preoperative assessment is complete and the surgical suite is ready. Always maintain privacy during transfers through public areas. Cover the patient with a gown and/or blanket. Each time a patient is transferred between beds, the wheels of each bed must be locked. Obtain enough staff and ergonomic tools for safe patient handling to lift, guide, and prevent accidental fall or injury to the patient and staff. Once the patient is on the OR bed, prevent falls by ensuring that there is always someone on each side of the patient until a safety strap is secured. The monitor leads (e.g., ECG leads), BP cuff, and pulse oximeter are usually applied after the patient is safely on the OR bed.

Scrubbing, Gowning, and Gloving

All sterile members of the surgical team (scrub nurse, surgeon, assistant) complete surgical hand antisepsis. When wet scrubbing

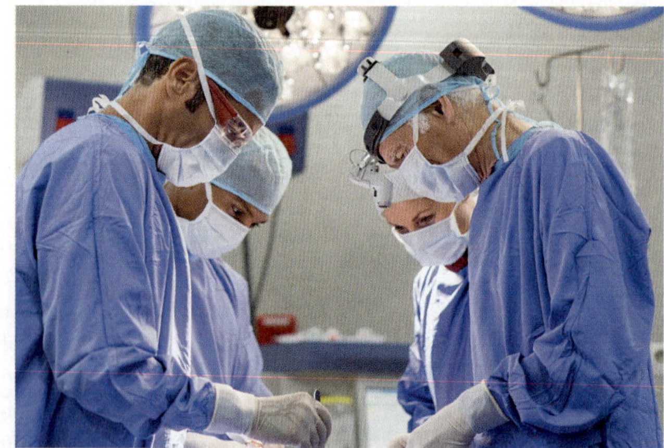

Fig. 19.3 All surgical personnel wear surgical attire. (© iStock.com/Ridofranz.)

is used, clean your fingernails first. Follow with scrubbing each plane of individual fingers, palms, and forearms in the distal to proximal fashion. Always hold your hands away from surgical attire and higher than the elbows. This prevents contamination from clothing or detergent suds and water draining from the unclean area above the elbows to the clean and previously scrubbed areas of the hands and fingers.

Waterless, alcohol-based agents are replacing soap and water in many agencies. When using an alcohol-based surgical hand-scrub product, prewash hands and forearms with soap and dry completely before applying the alcohol-based product. After applying the alcohol-based product, rub hands and forearms thoroughly until dry before donning sterile attire.[1,2]

After completing surgical hand antisepsis, team members enter the OR to put on a sterile gown and 2 pairs of gloves. This protects patients and staff from the transmission of microorganisms. Because the gowns and gloves are sterile, those who have scrubbed can touch and organize sterile items during the procedure.

Basic Aseptic Technique

Aseptic technique is practiced in the OR to prevent infection. This is done by creating and maintaining a sterile field. The center of the sterile field is the site of the surgical incision. Items used in the sterile field, including surgical instruments and equipment, have been sterilized.

Team members must understand specific principles to practice aseptic technique (Table 19.3). If team members do not follow these principles, the patient's safety is compromised and the risk for infection is increased.

The surgical team follows guidelines established by the US Occupational Safety and Health Administration (OSHA) and the AORN to protect the patient and team from exposure to blood-borne pathogens.[7] These guidelines emphasize (1) standard and transmission-based precautions; (2) engineering and work practice controls; and (3) using personal protective equipment, such as gloves, gowns, caps, face shields, masks, and protective eyewear. This is especially important in the OR because of the high risk for exposure to blood-borne pathogens.

Assisting the ACP

While you check the OR to complete the final preparations, the ACP prepares the patient for receiving anesthesia. You need to understand the effects of the anesthetic agents and know the location of all emergency drugs and equipment.

If you are the circulating nurse, you may be involved in placing monitoring devices used during the procedure (e.g., ECG leads). If the patient is having general anesthesia, stay at the patient's side to ensure safety and aid the ACP. These responsibilities may include measuring BP and providing oxygen to the patient before intubation. During the procedure, you are a vital communication link between the ACP and staff in other departments, such as the laboratory or blood bank.

TABLE 19.3 Principles of Aseptic Technique in the Operating Room

- All materials that enter the sterile field must be sterile.
- If a sterile item comes in contact with an unsterile item, it is contaminated.
- Contaminated items are removed at once from the sterile field. If the unsterile item is small (e.g., unopened suture), once it is removed, the area is marked off (i.e., covered with a sterile drape). If the entire field is contaminated, it is set up again with all new materials.
- The surgical team working in the operative field must wear sterile gowns and gloves. Once dressed for the procedure, they must recognize the only parts of the gown considered sterile are the front from chest to table level and sleeves to 2 inches above the elbow.
- A wide margin of safety is maintained between sterile and unsterile fields.
- Tables are sterile only at tabletop level. Items extending beneath this level are contaminated.
- The edges of a sterile package are contaminated once the package has been opened. If a sterile package (e.g., package of sutures) is placed on the sterile field, that entire package stays sterile even when opened.
- Microorganisms travel on airborne particles and will enter the sterile field with excessive air movements and currents.
- Microorganisms travel by capillary action through moist fabrics, resulting in contamination.
- Microorganisms on the patient's and team members' hair, skin, and respiratory tracts must be confined by proper attire.

Positioning the Patient

The surgical team carefully plans the patient's position and monitors the patient throughout the procedure. The ACP says when to begin positioning, usually after induction of anesthesia. The position should allow for accessing the operative site, administering and monitoring of anesthetic agents, and maintaining the airway. There are a variety of surgical positions.[8] Supine is the most common position. It allows access to most body areas, including the abdomen, heart, chest, or head. The prone position is often used in spine surgery (e.g., laminectomy). The lithotomy position is used for some gynecologic, genitourinary, and colon procedures. Other common positions include lateral and sitting.

With any position, take great care to prevent injury to the patient. Improper positioning can result in muscle strain, joint damage, pressure injuries, or nerve damage. Provide correct musculoskeletal alignment. Prevent occlusion of arteries and veins and undue pressure on nerves, skin over bony prominences, earlobes, and eyes.[9] Make sure there is room for adequate thoracic excursion. Take care in positioning older patients. The older adult often has osteoporosis and/or osteoarthritis. Misalignment, pressure, or other insults to arthritic joints desensitized from an anesthetic may create long-term injury and disability.

Provide modesty in exposure. Recognize and respect patient needs, such as previously assessed pain or deformities. It is your responsibility to secure the extremities, provide adequate padding and support, and have physical or mechanical help to avoid unnecessary straining of the staff and patient.

Anesthesia blocks the sensory nerve impulses so the patient will not feel pain, discomfort, or stress placed on nerves, muscles, bones, and skin. General anesthesia causes peripheral vessels to dilate. Position changes affect where the pooling of blood occurs. Pooled prep solutions in dependent areas can quickly create skin burns or abrasions.

If the head of the OR bed is raised, the lower torso will have increased blood volume and the upper torso may become compromised. Hypovolemia and cardiovascular disease can further compromise the patient's status. Because of decreased ability to perceive discomfort or pressure on vulnerable areas and a loss of skin elasticity, the older adult's skin is at risk for injury from tape, electrodes, warming and cooling blankets, and certain types of dressings.

Electrosurgery and Smoke

Care is taken to correctly place the grounding pad and all electrosurgical equipment to prevent injury from burns or fire. When an electrosurgical unit is in use, patients must be properly grounded to prevent unintended injury (Fig. 19.4). Excess hair, adipose tissue, bony prominences, fluid (edema), adhesive failure, and scar tissue can compromise safety. Fire in the OR can have devastating consequences. We can prevent fires with the use of safe practices.[10]

Preparing the Surgical Site

The purpose of skin preparation, or "prepping," is to reduce the number of microorganisms available to migrate to the surgical wound. The circulating nurse, surgeon, or surgical assistant completes the task of prepping before surgery.

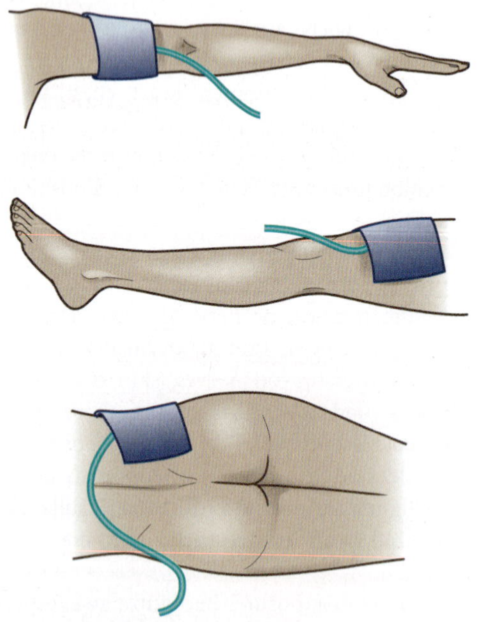

Fig. 19.4 A well-vascularized muscle mass is the best site for grounding. (Courtesy Covidien, Mansfield, MA.)

We prepare the skin by mechanically scrubbing or cleansing the surgical site with an antimicrobial agent specific to the procedure. Follow manufacturer's instructions for proper application of the prepping agent. Follow the principle of scrubbing from the clean area (site of the incision) to the dirty area (distal to the incision).

Antiseptic agents used for skin preparation may contain alcohol and are flammable. Skin injury can occur if these agents pool under the patient. These agents must be properly confined and allowed to fully dry. After the skin is prepped, the fumes are allowed to dispel to reduce the risk for fire. The sterile members of the surgical team then drape the area. Only the site to be incised is left exposed.

Safety Considerations

All surgical procedures put patients at risk for injury. Potential injuries include infection, physical trauma from positioning or equipment, or physiologic effects of surgery itself. Although technical skills, such as operating equipment or proper instrument handling, are a critical part of OR RN competency, nontechnical skills (NTS) have a high impact on outcomes. These include proper and clear communication, teamwork, situational awareness, and stress and fatigue management. Standard approaches and communication tools promote safe patient care and minimize the risk for injury.

Communication. Many team members care for patients in the perioperative process. Chances for error arise whenever team members share information. The Joint Commission requires that all HCPs use a standardized approach to hand-off communication. As an RN, use SBAR (see Table 1.3) to ensure a complete and accurate hand-off every time patient care is transferred to another provider (e.g., change of shift, surgeon to nurse, OR RN to PACU RN).[11]

Surgical Care Improvement Project. The *Surgical Care Improvement Project* (SCIP) is a national quality partnership of organizations focused on improving surgical care by reducing complications. Specific SCIP measures include (1) a prophylactic antibiotic started within 30 to 60 minutes before the surgical incision to decrease risk for infection, (2) applying a warming blanket to prevent unintended hypothermia, and (3) applying intermittent pneumatic compression devices (IPCs) to minimize the risk for venous thromboembolism.

Time-out and surgical checklist. The National Patient Safety Goals (NPSGs) require a preprocedure verification process.[11] This includes verifying relevant documentation (e.g., signed consent forms, nursing and preanesthetic assessment) and the results of any diagnostic studies (e.g., x-rays, biopsy reports). Blood products, implants, devices, and special equipment expected to be used must be available.

The *Universal Protocol,* one of the NPSGs, is followed to prevent wrong patient, wrong site, and wrong surgery.[11] Wrong surgical procedure and surgery on the wrong body part or wrong patient are *sentinel events (never events)* or *SREs* (described in Chapter 1). The surgeon marks the procedure site. If possible, involve the patient in the marking.[1]

A patient safety checklist for ORs is the cornerstone of a major focus to make surgery safer. Using the World Health Organization (WHO) Surgical Safety Checklist has improved compliance with standards and decreased complications from surgery (Fig. 19.5). In addition, OR staff complete a fire risk assessment to identify and reduce the risk of fire.

! SAFETY ALERT

Surgical Time-Out

- Before anesthesia induction, ask the patient to confirm name, birthdate, procedure, site, and consent.
- All surgical team members stop what they are doing just before the procedure starts to verify patient identification, procedure, and surgical site.

After Surgery

Through constant observation of the surgery, the ACP anticipates the end of the procedure. The ACP gives proper types and doses of anesthetic agents so that their effects will be minimal at the end of the surgery. This allows greater physiologic control of patients during the transfer to the PACU.

The ACP and the OR RN or another member of the surgical team go with the patient to the PACU. The hand-off, including the patient's status and the procedure done, is communicated to the nurse receiving the patient in the PACU to promote safe, ongoing care.

ANESTHESIA

The American Society of Anesthesiologists (ASA) defines anesthesia according to the effect that it has on the patient's sensorium and pain perception. These definitions include minimal sedation (e.g., anxiolysis), moderate sedation/analgesia, deep sedation/analgesia, and general anesthesia. The science of providing anesthesia continues to evolve. For example, newer noninvasive technology allows ACPs to track the level of patient awareness (i.e., *awareness monitoring*) during surgery and adjust anesthesia as needed.

The ACP chooses the anesthetic technique and agents in collaboration with the surgeon and patient. The ACP has ultimate responsibility for the choice of anesthesia. Contributing factors include the patient's current physical and mental status, age, allergies, pain history, ACP's expertise, and procedure (e.g., length, site, discharge plans). An absolute contraindication to any anesthetic technique or agent is patient refusal.

The ACP obtains anesthesia consent, writes orders for preoperative and postoperative drugs, and assigns the patient an anesthesia classification. The ASA physical status classification system is based on the patient's physiologic status. It uses a scale of ASA1 to ASA6 (see Table 18.4).[12] An intraoperative complication is more likely to develop when a patient has a higher classification number.

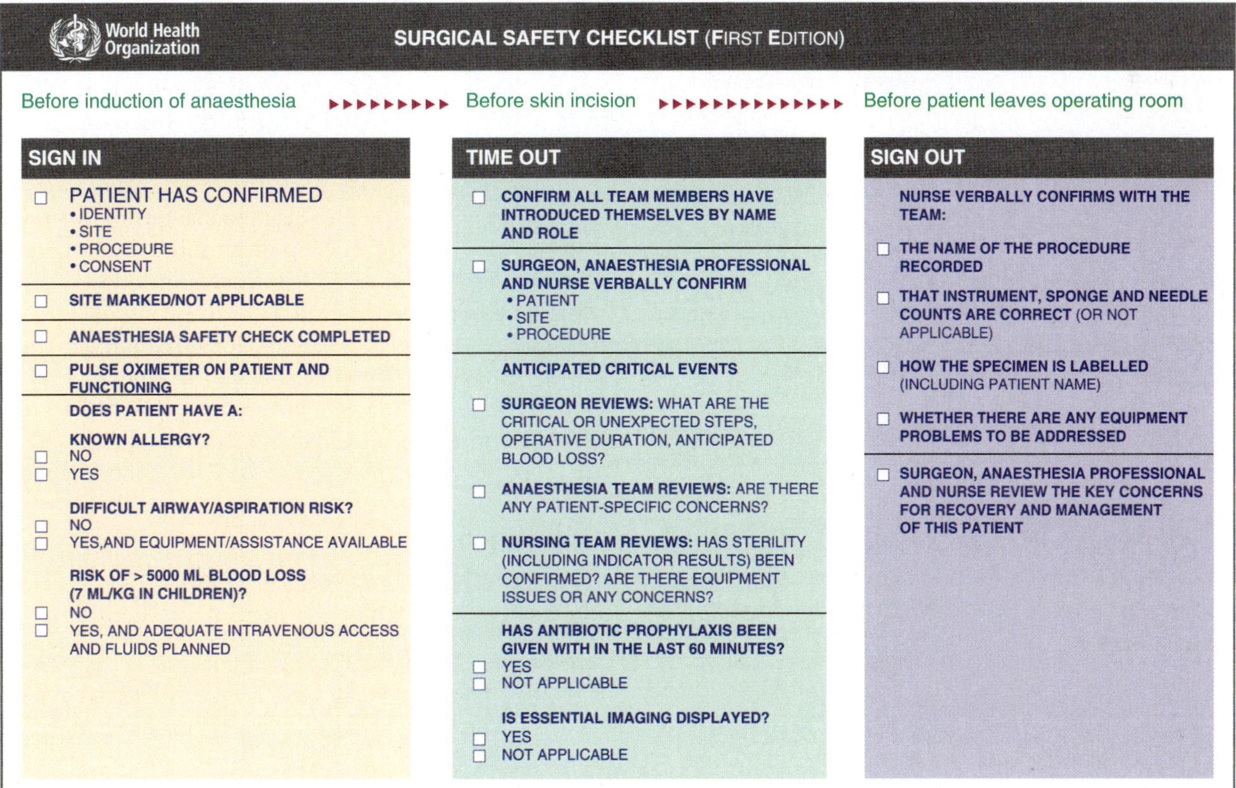
World Health Organization

SURGICAL SAFETY CHECKLIST (FIRST EDITION)

Before induction of anaesthesia ▸▸▸▸▸▸▸▸▸ Before skin incision ▸▸▸▸▸▸▸▸▸▸▸▸▸▸ Before patient leaves operating room

SIGN IN

☐ PATIENT HAS CONFIRMED
- IDENTITY
- SITE
- PROCEDURE
- CONSENT

☐ SITE MARKED/NOT APPLICABLE

☐ ANAESTHESIA SAFETY CHECK COMPLETED

☐ PULSE OXIMETER ON PATIENT AND FUNCTIONING

DOES PATIENT HAVE A:

KNOWN ALLERGY?
☐ NO
☐ YES

DIFFICULT AIRWAY/ASPIRATION RISK?
☐ NO
☐ YES,AND EQUIPMENT/ASSISTANCE AVAILABLE

RISK OF > 5000 ML BLOOD LOSS (7 ML/KG IN CHILDREN)?
☐ NO
☐ YES, AND ADEQUATE INTRAVENOUS ACCESS AND FLUIDS PLANNED

TIME OUT

☐ CONFIRM ALL TEAM MEMBERS HAVE INTRODUCED THEMSELVES BY NAME AND ROLE

☐ SURGEON, ANAESTHESIA PROFESSIONAL AND NURSE VERBALLY CONFIRM
- PATIENT
- SITE
- PROCEDURE

ANTICIPATED CRITICAL EVENTS

☐ SURGEON REVIEWS: WHAT ARE THE CRITICAL OR UNEXPECTED STEPS, OPERATIVE DURATION, ANTICIPATED BLOOD LOSS?

☐ ANAESTHESIA TEAM REVIEWS: ARE THERE ANY PATIENT-SPECIFIC CONCERNS?

☐ NURSING TEAM REVIEWS: HAS STERILITY (INCLUDING INDICATOR RESULTS) BEEN CONFIRMED? ARE THERE EQUIPMENT ISSUES OR ANY CONCERNS?

HAS ANTIBIOTIC PROPHYLAXIS BEEN GIVEN WITH IN THE LAST 60 MINUTES?
☐ YES
☐ NOT APPLICABLE

IS ESSENTIAL IMAGING DISPLAYED?
☐ YES
☐ NOT APPLICABLE

SIGN OUT

NURSE VERBALLY CONFIRMS WITH THE TEAM:

☐ THE NAME OF THE PROCEDURE RECORDED

☐ THAT INSTRUMENT, SPONGE AND NEEDLE COUNTS ARE CORRECT (OR NOT APPLICABLE)

☐ HOW THE SPECIMEN IS LABELLED (INCLUDING PATIENT NAME)

☐ WHETHER THERE ARE ANY EQUIPMENT PROBLEMS TO BE ADDRESSED

☐ SURGEON, ANAESTHESIA PROFESSIONAL AND NURSE REVIEW THE KEY CONCERNS FOR RECOVERY AND MANAGEMENT OF THIS PATIENT

Fig. 19.5 WHO Surgical Safety Checklist.

ANESTHESIA TECHNIQUES

Types of anesthesia techniques include moderate to deep sedation, monitored anesthesia care (MAC), general anesthesia, and local and regional anesthesia (Table 19.4).[12]

Moderate to Deep Sedation

Moderate to deep sedation may be used for procedures outside of the OR (e.g., reducing a dislocated joint in the emergency department). The presence of an ACP is not needed. Trained RNs who are allowed by agency protocols and state nurse practice acts can provide this type of anesthesia under the direct supervision of a physician.

Monitored Anesthesia Care

Monitored anesthesia care (MAC) is used for diagnostic or therapeutic procedures done in or outside of the OR (e.g., endoscopy clinic). MAC includes varying levels of sedation, analgesia, and anxiolysis. A critical part of MAC is the assessment and management of any physiologic problems that may develop. MAC is provided by an ACP because it may be necessary to change to general anesthesia during the procedure.

General Anesthesia

General anesthesia is the technique of choice for patients who are having longer surgeries, need skeletal muscle relaxation, require uncomfortable operative positions because of the location of the incision site, or need control of ventilation. Other reasons include patient refusal of local or regional techniques, contraindications to other techniques, and uncooperative patients. Patients may be uncooperative due to substance use, emotional lability, head injury, impaired cognition, or inability to remain immobile. Phases of general anesthesia are outlined in Table 19.5.

The goals of anesthesia include controlling biologic responses induced by stressors and protecting patients from stress-induced complications. To this end, *total intravenous anesthesia (TIVA)* and newer inhalation agents have a fast onset, fast elimination, and fewer undesirable side effects than earlier agents. These factors promote early discharge from the PACU and ambulatory surgery centers.

General anesthesia may be induced by IV or inhalation and maintained by either or a combination of the two (Table 19.6). A *balanced technique,* using adjunctive drugs to complement the induction, is the most common approach for general anesthesia.

TABLE 19.4 Anesthesia Techniques and Effects

Technique	Effect on Patient
General anesthesia	• Loss of sensation with loss of consciousness • Combination of hypnosis, analgesia, and amnesia • Usually involves use of inhalation agents • Skeletal muscle relaxation • Eliminates coughing, gagging, vomiting, and sympathetic nervous system responsiveness • Requires advanced airway management
Local anesthesia	• Loss of sensation without loss of consciousness • Induced topically or via infiltration, intradermal, or subcutaneously • Topical applications may be aerosolized or nebulized
Moderate sedation/analgesia (formerly called *conscious sedation*)	• Sedative, anxiolytic, and/or analgesic drugs used • Does not typically use inhalation agents • Nitric oxide is used in many protocols (dental procedures) • Patient responsive and breathes without assistance • Not expected to induce level of sedation that would impair patients' ability to protect their airway • Most often used for minor therapeutic procedures (e.g., fracture realignment in the emergency department)
Monitored anesthesia care (MAC)	• Sedative, anxiolytic, and/or analgesic drugs used • Does not usually involve inhalation agents • Patient less responsive and may need airway management • Gives greatest flexibility to match sedation level to patient needs and procedural requirements • Often used in conjunction with regional or local anesthesia • Often used for minor therapeutic and diagnostic procedures (e.g., eye surgery, colonoscopy)
Regional anesthesia	• Loss of sensation to a region of body without loss of consciousness • Involves blocking a specific nerve or group of nerves by administering a local anesthetic • Includes spinal, caudal, and epidural anesthesia and IV and peripheral nerve blocks (e.g., interscalene, axillary, infraclavicular/supraclavicular, popliteal, femoral, sciatic)

From American Society of Anesthesiologists: *Types of anesthesia, 2023.* Retrieved from https://www.asahq.org/madeforthismoment/anesthesia-101/types-of-anesthesia/.

TABLE 19.5 **Phases of General Anesthesia**

Preinduction	Induction	Maintenance	Emergence
Description			
• Period starting with initiation of IV or arterial access, application of monitors (e.g., ECG), administration of preoperative drugs	• Initiation of drugs that make patient unconscious • Airway secured with airway assist devices (ETT, LMA)	• Period during which procedure is done • Patient stays in an unconscious state with measures to ensure airway safety	• Period when procedure is completed • Patient is prepared for return to consciousness and removal of airway assist devices
Role of Anesthesia Care Provider			
• Determine anesthetic care plan • Insert and monitor IV or arterial access • Confirm antibiotic prophylaxis • Give drugs for anxiety, pain, nausea, aspiration prophylaxis	• Give appropriate drugs • Secure airway • Position patient appropriately for procedure	• Monitor patient's physiologic status • Give drugs and titrate fluids as needed	• Reverse residual neuromuscular blocking agents • Assess for return of all protective reflexes • Remove airway assist devices • Assess pain
Role of Perioperative Nurse			
• Complete preoperative assessment • Check and confirm signed informed consent • Complete surgical time-out	• Help with application of monitors (noninvasive and invasive) • Assist with airway management	• Adjust patient position as needed • Monitor patient safety	• Help place dressing • Protect patient during return of reflexes • Prepare to move patient to postanesthesia care unit (PACU)
Classes of Drugs Used			

• Benzodiazepines
• Opioids
• Antibiotics
• Aspiration prophylaxis:
  • H_2 receptor blockers (e.g., famotidine)
  • Anticholinergics (e.g., scopolamine)
  • 5HT3 antagonist (ondansetron)
	• Benzodiazepines
	• Opioids
	• Barbiturates
	• Hypnotics
	• Volatile gases
		• Benzodiazepines
		• Opioids
		• Barbiturates
		• Hypnotics
		• Volatile gases
		• Neuromuscular blocking agents
			• Reversal agents (as needed):
			  • Anticholinesterases (e.g., neostigmine)
			  • Opioid antagonists (e.g., naloxone)
			  • Benzodiazepine antagonists (e.g., flumazenil)
			  • Neuromuscular block reversal of rocuronium and vecuronium (e.g., sugammadex)
			• As-needed opioids
			• Antiemetics

ETT, Endotracheal tube; *LMA,* laryngeal mask airway.

IV Agents

Routine general anesthetics begin with an IV induction agent. This agent may be a hypnotic, anxiolytic, or dissociative agent. When used during the initial period of anesthesia, these agents induce sleep rapidly. A single dose lasts only a few minutes. This is long enough for placement of a laryngeal mask airway (LMA) or an endotracheal (ET) tube. Once this is done, the ACP gives inhalation and/or IV agent(s).[12]

Inhalation Agents

Inhalation agents were the traditional cornerstone of general anesthesia. They may be volatile liquids or gases. Volatile liquids are given through a specially designed vaporizer after being mixed with oxygen. This gas mixture is delivered to the patient through the anesthesia circuit. Waste gases are removed using negative evacuation pressure venting to the outside of the building.

Inhalation agents enter the body through the alveoli in the lungs. These agents are easily administered and rapidly excreted by ventilation. Some inhalation agents (e.g., desflurane) have an irritating effect on the respiratory tract. Complications include coughing, laryngospasm, and increased secretions.[12]

Once the patient has been induced with an IV agent, the inhalation agent is usually delivered through an ET tube or LMA. The ET tube allows control of ventilation and protects the airway from aspiration. LMAs are an important option for patients with difficult airways, but they do not provide access to the trachea or airway protection with the same certainty as ET tubes. Complications of ET tube or LMA use are mainly related to insertion and removal. These include damage to teeth and lips, laryngospasm, laryngeal edema, sore throat, and hoarseness from injury or irritation of the vocal cords or surrounding tissues.

Adjuncts to General Anesthesia

General anesthesia usually requires more than 1 agent. Drugs added to inhalation anesthetic other than an IV induction drug

TABLE 19.6 Drug Therapy

General Anesthesia

Drugs	Advantages	Adverse Effects	Nursing Interventions
IV Agents			
Barbiturates			
methohexital (Brevital)	Rapid induction, duration of action <5 min.	Cardiac effects (e.g., myocardial depression), ↑ HR, ↓ BP, respiratory depression, hiccups, excitation, involuntary movement.	Usually has minimal effect after surgery because of short duration of action. ↑ Nausea in patients with barbiturate sensitivity, histamine-triggered nausea and vomiting.
Nonbarbiturate Hypnotics			
etomidate (Amidate)	Little effect on cardiovascular function. Useful for hemodynamically unstable patients. Minor respiratory depression.	Myoclonia, nausea and vomiting, hiccups, adrenocortical inhibition.	Monitor vital signs. Observe for myoclonia, nausea and vomiting, hiccups, hypoglycemia.
propofol (Diprivan)	Short outpatient procedures because of rapid onset of action, metabolic clearance. May be used for induction and maintenance of anesthesia. ↓ Cerebral blood flow, ↓ intracranial pressure, ↓ intraocular pressure. Has antiemetic and antipruritic properties.	↓ HR, dysrhythmias, ↓ BP, apnea. Transient phlebitis, pain during injection, hiccups. May cause high triglyceride levels.	Monitor vital signs. Monitor brain-injured patients closely for ↓ cerebral perfusion. Monitor serum triglycerides q24h when sedated >24 h.
Inhalation Agents			
Gaseous Agents			
nitrous oxide	Potentiates volatile agents, thus speeding induction and reducing total dosage and side effects. Weak anesthetic, rarely used alone. Good analgesic potency. Anxiolytic properties.	Little or no toxicity at therapeutic concentrations.	Avoid in patients with bone marrow depression. Must give with O_2 to prevent hypoxemia. Avoid in patients with strong history of nausea and vomiting.
Volatile Liquids			
desflurane (Suprane) isoflurane (Forane) sevoflurane (Ultane)	Cause skeletal muscle relaxation. *desflurane:* Fastest onset and emergence, widely used in ambulatory settings. Least postoperative cognitive dysfunction. *isoflurane:* Resistant to metabolic breakdown. Used for surgical cases longer than 2 hours. *sevoflurane:* Predictable effects on cardiovascular and respiratory systems, rapid acting. Preferred for inhalation induction as nonirritating to respiratory tract. Used for procedures less than 2 hours.	Triggers for malignant hyperthermia. Respiratory depression, ↓ BP, myocardial depression. *desflurane and isoflurane:* May be unsuitable for patients with coronary artery disease. *desflurane:* May see longer emergence times. Potential airway irritant. *sevoflurane:* May be associated with emergence delirium, atypical seizure-like activity.	Assess and treat pain during early anesthesia recovery. Assess vital signs. Observe for prolonged respiratory depression. Monitor for nausea and vomiting.
Dissociative Anesthetic			
ketamine (Ketalar)	Given IV or IM. Potent analgesic and amnesic. Used for patients with hypotension from hemorrhage, hypovolemia, sepsis, or severe cardiovascular compromise. Useful in people with asthma to prevent bronchospasm.	May cause hallucinations and nightmares (midazolam decreases these effects), ↑ HR, ↑ BP.	Anticipate use of a benzodiazepine if agitation and hallucinations occur. Calm, quiet environment is essential in postoperative care.

are termed *adjuncts.* Adjuncts are added to achieve unconsciousness, analgesia, amnesia, muscle relaxation, or autonomic nervous system control. They include opioids, benzodiazepines, neuromuscular blocking agents (muscle relaxants), and antiemetics (Table 19.7). These drugs may have synergistic or antagonistic effects. You may see deeper levels of sedation or more drug-related side effects than with inhalation anesthetics alone. If needed, muscle relaxants can be reversed after the surgery is complete. Reversal of other adjuncts (benzodiazepines, opioids) requires prolonged monitoring.

TABLE 19.7 Drug Therapy

Adjuncts to General Anesthesia

Agents	Intended Effect	Adverse Effects	Nursing Interventions
Antiemetics (see Table 46.1)			
aprepitant (Emend) granisetron ondansetron (Zofran) palonosetron	Counteract emetic effects of inhalation agents and opioids. Prevent nausea and vomiting related to histamine release, vagal stimulation, vestibular disturbance, procedure (e.g., abdominal laparoscopy).	Headache, dizziness, IV irritation, dysrhythmias, dysphoria, dystonia, dry mouth, central nervous system sedation.	Monitor heart rhythm, cardiopulmonary status, level of central nervous system excitation or sedation, ability to move limbs, presence of nausea or vomiting.
Benzodiazepines			
diazepam (Valium) lorazepam (Ativan) midazolam (Versed) remimazolam (Byfavo)	Reduce anxiety. Induce and maintain anesthesia. Induce amnesia. Treat emergence delirium. Supplement sedation in local and regional anesthesia, monitored anesthesia care (MAC).	Synergistic effect with opioids, increasing risk for respiratory depression. ↓ BP. Prolonged sedation or confusion.	Monitor level of consciousness. Assess vital signs and note any respiratory depression. Reverse severe benzodiazepine-induced respiratory depression with flumazenil.
Neuromuscular Blocking Agents			
Depolarizing agent: • succinylcholine (Anectine) *Nondepolarizing agents:* • atracurium • cisatracurium (Nimbex) • pancuronium • rocuronium • vecuronium	Promote endotracheal intubation. Promote skeletal muscle relaxation (paralysis) to enhance access to surgical sites. Effects of nondepolarizing agents are usually reversed toward end of surgery by giving anticholinesterase agents (e.g., neostigmine).	Trigger for malignant hyperthermia. Apnea related to respiratory muscle paralysis. Duration of action of nondepolarizing agents may be longer than surgery. Reversal agents may not completely eliminate effects. Confusion and nausea. Recurrence of muscle weakness with correction of hypothermia.	If intubated, monitor return of muscle strength, level of consciousness, and ventilation. Maintain patent airway. Monitor respiratory rate and rhythm until patient can cough and return to previous muscle strength. Ensure availability of nondepolarizing reversal agents (e.g., neostigmine) and emergency respiratory support equipment. Monitor temperature and levels of muscle strength with temperature changes.
Opioids			
alfentanil (Alfenta) fentanyl (Sublimaze) hydromorphone (Dilaudid) morphine sulfate remifentanil (Ultiva) sufentanil (Sufenta)	Induce and maintain anesthesia, reduce stimuli from sensory nerve endings. Provide analgesia during surgery and recovery in postanesthesia care unit (PACU).	Respiratory depression, vomiting, ↓ HR, peripheral vasodilation (when combined with anesthetic). Itching when given regional or IV.	Assess respiratory rate and rhythm, monitor pulse oximetry, protect airway in anticipation of vomiting. Use standing orders for antipruritics, antiemetics. Reverse opioid-induced respiratory depression with naloxone. If used, reversal of analgesic effects also occurs. Monitor closely for recurrent respiratory depression requiring an additional dose of naloxone.
Other Agents			
dexmedetomidine (Precedex)	Induces and maintains sedation before and/or during surgery. Anxiolytic properties.	↓ BP, ↓ HR, sinus arrest, dysrhythmias. Transient ↑ BP during administration of loading dose.	Monitor vital signs.

Dissociative Anesthesia

Dissociative anesthesia interrupts associative brain pathways while blocking sensory pathways. The patient may appear catatonic and amnesic, and has profound analgesia that lasts into the postoperative period. Ketamine (Ketalar) (given IV or IM) is a dissociative anesthetic. It is a potent analgesic and amnesic that does not increase intracranial pressure. Because ketamine is a phenyl cyclohexyl piperidine (PCP) derivative, the drug may cause hallucinations and nightmares, limiting its usefulness. Concurrent use of midazolam (Versed) can reduce or eliminate hallucinations. Providing a quiet, calm environment in the PACU is important for patients receiving dissociative anesthesia.

Local and Regional Anesthesia

Local anesthesia interrupts the generation of nerve impulses by changing the flow of sodium into nerve cells. The result is autonomic nervous system blockade, anesthesia, and skeletal muscle flaccidity or paralysis. Local anesthetics are topical, ophthalmic, nebulized, or injected. They are applied to a specific area of the body by the surgeon or ACP. It does not cause sedation or loss of consciousness.

Some patients report "allergies" to local anesthetics. True allergies to local anesthetics are rare. Allergies are likely to be a result of additives or preservatives in the preparation. Some local anesthetics are combined with epinephrine to provide localized vasoconstriction. This decreases absorption and extends the action of the agent. However, if the local anesthetic is absorbed in the tissues or inadvertently injected IV and enters the general circulation, the patient may have tachycardia, hypertension, and a general feeling of panic.

Regional anesthesia (or block) uses an injected local anesthetic. It involves a central nerve (e.g., spinal) or group of nerves (e.g., plexus) that innervate a site remote to the point of injection. Regional blocks are typically used as preoperative analgesia, during surgery to manage surgical pain, and after surgery to control pain. Indwelling catheters that deliver local anesthetic to the surgical site through an implanted pump can give continuous pain relief up to 7 days after surgery. Continuous catheters are usually removed after 48 to 72 hours to decrease risk of infection.[12]

Advantages of local and regional anesthesia include rapid recovery, continued postoperative analgesia, and no need for sedation. Local and regional routes can safely be used when comorbidities prevent general anesthesia use.

Disadvantages include the risk for technical problems, discomfort at the injection site, and the inability to precisely match the duration of the procedure. Injected local anesthetics may be less successful during prolonged procedures or when infection at the injection site interferes with drug absorption. Another disadvantage is the risk for inadvertent vascular injection leading to local anesthetic systemic toxicity (LAST). LAST may present as confusion, metallic taste, oral numbness, and dizziness.[13] Without treatment, seizures, coma, dysrhythmias, and cardiac arrest may occur. Treatment for LAST involves lipid emulsion infusion along with respiratory and cardiovascular support.[13]

Topical creams, ointments, aerosols, and liquids are standard ways to administer local anesthesia. They are applied directly to the skin, mucous membranes, or open surface. An example is EMLA cream, a combination of prilocaine and lidocaine. It is applied to the site 30 to 60 minutes before a procedure.

In ambulatory or outpatient procedures, you may aid the ACP in administering a peripheral or regional block. You must be familiar with the drugs, including the methods of administration and adverse and toxic effects. Initial patient assessment should include their history with the use of local anesthetics. Have there been any adverse events associated with their use by the patient or blood relatives?

Examples of common regional nerve blocks include brachial plexus block; IV regional anesthesia (IVRA) or Bier block anesthesia; and femoral, axillary, cervical, sciatic, ankle, and retrobulbar blocks. For IVRA or Bier block, the patient has a double-cuff tourniquet applied to prevent absorption of the drug into the systemic circulation.

You can promote the success of regional anesthesia by properly positioning the patient and using supporting devices (e.g., ultrasound imaging, nerve stimulator, tourniquets) as directed by the ACP. Monitor vital signs during block delivery and manage oxygen therapy. Have airway equipment, emergency drugs, and a cardiac monitor/defibrillator available to provide advanced airway and cardiopulmonary support if needed.

Spinal and Epidural Anesthesia

Spinal anesthesia and epidural anesthesia are types of regional anesthesia. **Spinal anesthesia** involves the injection of a local anesthetic into the cerebrospinal fluid in the subarachnoid space, usually below the level of L2 (Fig. 19.6A). The local anesthetic mixes with cerebrospinal fluid. Depending on the extent of its spread, various levels of anesthesia are achieved. Because the local anesthetic is given directly into the cerebrospinal fluid, a spinal anesthetic produces autonomic, sensory, and motor blockade. Patients develop vasodilation and become hypotensive from the autonomic block. They feel no pain because of the sensory block. They cannot move because of the motor block. The duration of action depends on the drug used and the dose given. A spinal anesthetic may be used for procedures involving the lower extremities (e.g., joint replacements) and lower gastrointestinal, prostate, and gynecologic surgeries.

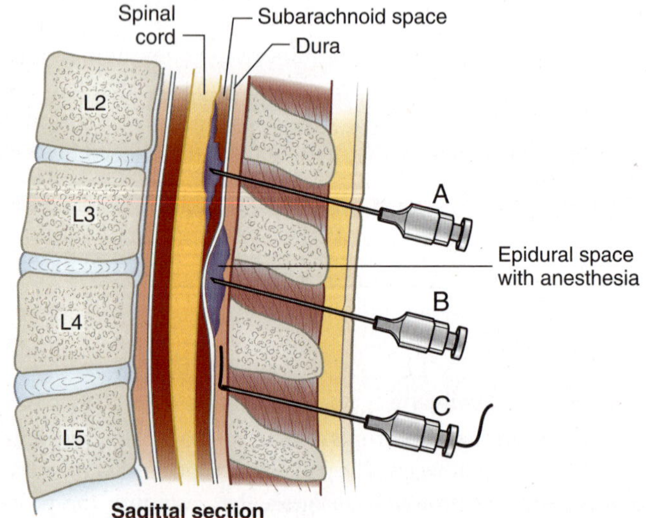

Fig. 19.6 Location of needle point and injected anesthetic relative to dura and spinal cord. (A) Spinal anesthesia. (B) Single-injection epidural. (C) Epidural catheter. (Interspaces most often used are L2–3, L4–5, L3–4.)

An epidural block involves injection of a local anesthetic into the epidural space via a thoracic or lumbar approach (Fig. 19.6B). The anesthetic agent binds to nerve roots as they enter and exit the spinal cord. Anesthetic does not enter the cerebrospinal fluid. Epidural anesthesia may be the sole anesthetic for a procedure. With the use of a low dose or dilute anesthetic, sensory pathways are blocked but motor function remains intact. In higher doses, sensory and motor functions are blocked. An epidural catheter may be placed to allow for continued intraoperative and postoperative analgesia (Fig. 19.6C). Lower doses of epidural local anesthetic are used for postoperative analgesia, usually with an opioid. Epidural anesthesia is often used for analgesia or in combination with sedation or general anesthesia, in obstetrics, vascular procedures involving the lower extremities, lung resections, and renal and midabdominal surgeries. The desirable effects of vasodilation and analgesia contribute to better surgical outcomes.

With spinal or epidural anesthesia, patients can stay fully conscious, receive sedation, or choose general anesthesia. The onset of spinal anesthesia is more rapid than that of epidural anesthesia. With either anesthesia, observe the patient for manifestations of autonomic nervous system blockade. These include nausea and vomiting, hypotension, and bradycardia. There is less autonomic nervous system blockade with epidural anesthesia than with spinal anesthesia. Should "too high" a block be present, the patient may have tingling in the arms and hands, inadequate breathing, or apnea. Other complications include post–dural puncture headache, back pain, urinary retention, isolated nerve injury, and meningitis.

Gerontologic Considerations: Patient Receiving Anesthesia

Aging affects the absorption, distribution, and metabolism of drugs. This results in changes in drug onset, peak, and duration independent of the route of administration. Because of this, anesthetic drugs need to be carefully titrated for older adults. Physiologic changes with aging may change the patient's response to blood and fluid loss and replacement, hypothermia, pain, tolerance of the procedure, and positioning. Monitor the older adult's response to all anesthetic agents. Postoperative delirium is a common complication associated with adverse surgical outcomes.[12] Assess recovery from anesthesia before the patient is transferred out of the PACU.

Some older adults may have a hard time communicating and following directions because of problems with hearing or vision. Give clear and concise communication in the OR, especially when the patient is sedated.

PERIOPERATIVE CRISIS EVENTS

Surgery has inherent risks for an adverse outcome. Some crisis events may be expected (e.g., cardiac arrest in an unstable patient, massive blood loss during trauma surgery). Others occur without warning (e.g., air embolism, hypoxia). Rarer events include anaphylactic reactions and malignant hyperthermia. A crisis demands immediate intervention by all members of the OR team.

Anaphylactic Reactions

Anesthetic agents, antibiotics, blood products, and latex may cause allergic reactions. *Anaphylaxis* is the most severe form of an allergic reaction, with life-threatening pulmonary and circulatory complications. Vigilance and rapid intervention are essential. An anaphylactic reaction causes hypotension, tachycardia, bronchospasm, and pulmonary edema. Anesthesia may mask the initial manifestations of anaphylaxis. Anaphylaxis is discussed in Chapter 13.

Latex allergy is a concern in the surgical setting. Gloves, catheters, and many devices contain natural rubber latex. Latex allergy protocols in each agency help provide a latex-safe environment for susceptible patients. Latex allergies are discussed in Chapter 13.

Malignant Hyperthermia

Malignant hyperthermia (MH) is a rare disorder characterized by hyperthermia with skeletal muscle rigidity. It can result in death. MH occurs in genetically susceptible people exposed to certain anesthetic agents.[14] Succinylcholine (Anectine), especially when given with volatile inhalation agents, is the primary trigger of MH. Other factors include stress, trauma, and heat. When MH does occur, it is usually during general anesthesia. It may occur in the recovery period, too.

MH is an autosomal dominant trait. Predictions based on family history are important but not reliable. Altered control of intracellular calcium causes hypermetabolism of skeletal muscle. This leads to muscle contracture, hyperthermia, hypoxemia, lactic acidosis, and hemodynamic and cardiac problems. Tachycardia, tachypnea, hypercarbia, and ventricular dysrhythmias may occur but are not specific to MH.

MH is diagnosed after ruling out other causes of the hypermetabolism. The rise in body temperature is not an early sign of MH. Unless promptly detected and treated, MH can result in cardiac arrest and death. The definitive treatment of MH is prompt administration of dantrolene (Dantrium, Ryanodex).[14] Dantrolene slows metabolism, reduces muscle contraction, and mediates the catabolic processes associated with MH. Treatment also involves turning off anesthetic agents, providing 100% oxygen, and actively cooling the patient (ice packs in groin and axilla, giving chilled IV fluids). MH can also cause hyperkalemia, disseminated intravascular coagulation, and compartment syndrome.[14] Careful patient monitoring is essential to minimize complications.

To prevent MH, take a careful family history and be alert to the development of MH perioperatively. Patients known or suspected to be at risk for this disorder can receive anesthesia with minimal risk using proper precautions. Teach patients with MH about the condition so that family members may consider being genetically tested.

CASE STUDY

Intraoperative Patient

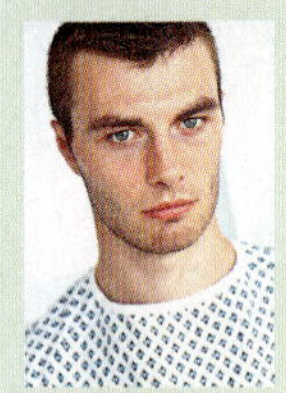

(© wavebreakmedia/ iStock.com.)

Patient Profile

G.S., a 23-year-old college student, came to the emergency department with abdominal pain, nausea, and vomiting. He has no pertinent medical history. A CT scan shows acute appendicitis. He is scheduled for immediate surgery under general anesthesia.

Subjective Data

- Awake and able to identify himself, his birth date, and surgical procedure
- Rates pain as an 8 on a 0 to 10 scale on arrival to the holding area

Objective Data

- Peripheral IV catheter in place with LR at 100 mL/h
- Prescribed cefazolin 1 gm IVPB to be given upon entry into the OR
- Vital signs: HR 88, respiratory rate 20, O_2 saturation 99% on room air, BP 124/86, temp 99.3°F (37.4°C)

Interprofessional Care

- Informed consent obtained for the procedure
- Chlorhexidine bath given for infection prophylaxis

G.S. was taken into the operating room. Induction began with IV medications and inhalation anesthetic followed. G.S. was intubated without difficulty. He is clipped, prepped, and draped for surgery. The surgeon completes the "time-out" and begins the surgery. About 10 minutes into surgery, the ACP notices increasing end-tidal carbon dioxide level and O_2 consumption. Temperature and heart rate are increased. The ACP suspects malignant hyperthermia and tells the surgical team to begin treatment for malignant hyperthermia.

Discussion Questions

1. ***Recognize:*** What are the usual manifestations of malignant hyperthermia? Explain the pathophysiologic process.
2. ***Analyze:*** What complications is G.S. at risk for if they experience malignant hyperthermia?
3. ***Plan:*** What therapy/treatment do you expect?
4. ***Prioritize:*** What is the surgical team's priority for G.S. at this time?
5. ***Act:*** What activities can you delegate to AP?
6. ***Evaluate:*** What do you need to continually monitor?
7. ***Safety:*** Describe specific nursing actions you will take to prevent injury and promote patient safety.

Answers available at http://evolve.elsevier.com/Lewis/medsurg.

BRIDGE TO NCLEX EXAMINATION

The number of the question corresponds to the same-numbered outcome at the beginning of the chapter.

1. Which items would the nurse wear in the semirestricted area of the surgery department?
   - **a.** Street clothing
   - **b.** Surgical attire and head cover
   - **c.** Street clothing and shoe covers
   - **d.** Surgical attire, head cover, shoe covers
2. Which activities might the scrub nurse perform during surgery? **(Select all that apply.)**
   - **a.** Checking electrical equipment
   - **b.** Preparing the instrument table
   - **c.** Assisting with draping the patient
   - **d.** Passing instruments to the surgeon and assistants
   - **e.** Documenting activities occurring in the operating room
3. The nurse is caring for a patient undergoing surgery for a knee replacement. Which factors are critical to the patient's safety during the procedure? **(Select all that apply.)**
   - **a.** Following universal protocol.
   - **b.** The ACP is an anesthesiologist.
   - **c.** The patient has adequate health insurance.
   - **d.** The patient's family is in the surgery waiting area.
   - **e.** The patient's allergies are conveyed to the surgical team.
4. Which action is the nurse's *primary* responsibility for the care of the patient undergoing surgery?
   - **a.** Carrying out tasks related to surgical policies and procedure
   - **b.** Developing and implementing a patient-centered plan of care
   - **c.** Ensuring that the patient has been assessed for safe administration of anesthesia
   - **d.** Performing a preoperative history and physical assessment to identify patient needs
5. Which action would the nurse take when scrubbing at the scrub sink?
   - **a.** Scrub from elbows to hands
   - **b.** Scrub without mechanical friction
   - **c.** Scrub for a minimum of 10 minutes
   - **d.** Hold the hands higher than the elbows
6. Which factors in positioning a patient for surgery increase the risk of patient injury? **(Select all that apply.)**
   - **a.** Loss of pain perception
   - **b.** Incorrect musculoskeletal alignment
   - **c.** Vasoconstriction of the peripheral vessels
   - **d.** Hypovolemia contributing to decreased perfusion
   - **e.** Inability to sense pressure over bony prominences
7. Why is IV induction for general anesthesia the method of choice for *most* surgical patients?
   - **a.** The patient is not intubated.
   - **b.** The agents are nonexplosive.
   - **c.** Induction is rapid and controlled.
   - **d.** Emergence is longer but with fewer complications.

1. d; 2. b, c, d; 3. a, e; 4. b; 5. d; 6. a, b, d, e; 7. c.

For rationales to these answers and even more NCLEX review questions, visit http://evolve.elsevier.com/Lewis/medsurg.

REFERENCES

To access the References for this chapter, please scan the QR code with a mobile device.

20

Postoperative Care

Diane M. Rudolphi

http://evolve.elsevier.com/Lewis/medsurg/

CONCEPTUAL FOCUS

Gas Exchange
Fluid and Electrolytes
Infection
Pain
Perfusion
Safety
Tissue Integrity
Transitions of Care

LEARNING OUTCOMES

1. Prioritize nursing responsibilities related to managing patients in the postanesthesia care unit (PACU).
2. Prioritize nursing responsibilities to maintain patient safety and prevent complications in the PACU and clinical unit.
3. Apply data from the initial nursing assessment to the management of the patient after transfer from the PACU to the clinical unit.
4. Select nursing interventions to manage potential problems during the postoperative period.
5. Distinguish discharge criteria from Phase I and Phase II postanesthesia care.

KEY TERMS

airway obstruction
atelectasis
delayed emergence
emergence delirium
patient-controlled analgesia (PCA)
postoperative ileus (POI)

This chapter focuses on the concepts central to postoperative nursing. The postoperative period begins immediately after surgery and continues until the patient is discharged from care. As the nurse, you play a vital role in supporting ventilation and perfusion, maintaining fluid and electrolyte balance, promoting comfort, reducing infection, and promoting safety.

POSTANESTHESIA CARE

Phases of Care

There are 3 phases of postanesthesia care. During each phase, we provide different levels of care depending on the patient's needs (Table 20.1).[1] Phase I is the immediate postanesthesia period. Close monitoring and attention to basic and vital patient needs are the priority. In Phase II, the priorities focus on preparing the patient for discharge from the hospital or surgical care setting. Phase III or Extended Care is the final phase. It is for patients who need more care after Phase II.[1]

Patients move through the phases of care as determined by their condition and the type of anesthesia received. A patient assigned to Phase I care in the *postanesthesia care unit (PACU)* who is stable and recovering well may rapidly progress to either Phase II care or an inpatient unit. An accelerated system of care called fast-tracking involves admitting ambulatory surgery patients directly to Phase II care. Although fast-tracking can result in time and cost savings, patient safety is the main factor determining where and at what level we provide care.

Postanesthesia Care Unit

The immediate recovery period takes place in the PACU. It is usually next to the operating room (OR). This location reduces patient transportation right after surgery and gives ready access to anesthesia and OR staff. The goals of PACU care are to maintain patient safety during recovery from anesthesia, identify patient problems that may occur because of anesthesia and surgery, and intervene appropriately. This is when patients

TABLE 20.1 Phases of Postanesthesia Care

Phase I—Initial Assessment
- Care during the immediate postanesthesia period
- ECG and more intense monitoring (e.g., arterial BP monitoring, mechanical ventilation)

Goal: Prepare patient for transfer to Phase II level of care, an inpatient unit, or intensive care setting.

Phase II
- Ambulatory surgery patients
- Fast-tracking (i.e., patients who have bypassed Phase I level of care)

Goal: Prepare patient for transfer to extended observation, home, or extended care facility.

Extended Observation
- Extended care or observation after transfer/discharge from Phase I or Phase II levels of care

Goal: Prepare patient for self-care.

Blended Levels of Care
- Various levels of care offered in the same environment

From American Society of PeriAnesthesia Nurses: *2015–2017 Perianesthesia nursing standards, practice recommendations and interpretive statements,* Cherry Hill, NJ, 2015, The Society.

are at greatest risk for respiratory and cardiovascular complications. Patients in the PACU need frequent assessment and intervention.

Phase I Initial Assessment

The patient's admission into the PACU is a joint effort among the health care team. This includes the surgeon, anesthesia care provider (ACP), OR nurse, and PACU nurse. This collaboration fosters a smooth transfer of care to the PACU and helps determine the specific phase of care each patient requires.

The ACP gives a postanesthesia hand-off report (Table 20.2). You may also receive report from an OR nurse. Hand-off reports should be standard and interactive, allowing you to ask questions and clarify information.[2] The ACP should stay in the PACU until you accept responsibility for the care of the patient. Potential problems in the postoperative period are shown in Fig. 20.1.

Begin your initial assessment by evaluating the patient's airway, breathing, and circulation (ABC) status. Table 20.3 describes key parts of a PACU assessment. Be alert for signs of inadequate oxygenation and ventilation (Table 20.4). Any sign of respiratory distress needs prompt intervention.

Plan to obtain vital signs every 15 minutes or more often until stable. Monitor and note any changes in ECG findings from the preoperative baseline. Invasive monitoring (e.g., arterial BP) may be needed. Assess temperature, peripheral pulses, capillary refill, and skin condition (e.g., color, moisture). Any signs of poor tissue perfusion need prompt intervention.

Focus your initial neurologic assessment on level of consciousness; orientation; sensory and motor status; and size, equality, and reactivity of the pupils. Assess for, note, and report any new asymmetric findings. The patient may be awake,

TABLE 20.2 PACU Hand-Off Report

General Information
- Patient name and age
- Surgeon and anesthesia care provider
- Surgical procedure
- Presence of tubes, drains, catheters, and IV lines
- Type of anesthesia (e.g., general, regional, monitored anesthesia care)
- Use of any reversal agents
- Airway status (artificial airway and/or interventions to maintain adequate oxygenation)
- Pain management interventions
- NPO status and postoperative orders that need started

Patient History
- Indication for surgery
- Medical history, medications, allergies
- Preoperative or baseline vital signs, laboratory, and diagnostic findings
- Level of consciousness, orientation
- Specific patient characteristics (e.g., hearing, vision, mobility problems)
- Patient preferences (e.g., cultural, personal beliefs/restrictions)
- Patient emotional status on arrival to OR

Intraoperative Management
- Anesthetic agents
- Other drugs received preoperatively or intraoperatively
- Last dose of opioid administration/pain management plan
- Total fluid replacements, including blood transfusions
- Total fluid losses (e.g., blood, nasogastric drainage)
- Urine output

Intraoperative Course
- Unexpected anesthetic events or reactions
- Unexpected surgical events
- Most recent vital signs and monitoring trends
- Results of laboratory tests and x-rays

drowsy but arousable, or asleep. Because hearing is the first sense to return in the unconscious patient, explain all activities to the patient from the time of admission to the PACU.

If the patient received a regional anesthetic (e.g., spinal, epidural), sensory and motor blockade may still be present. Assess dermatome levels (Fig. 20.2). During recovery from regional anesthesia, sensory and motor function first returns distal to the site where the anesthetic was given. The areas near the site of injections are the last to recover.

! SAFETY ALERT

Regional Anesthesia

- Monitor for complications of regional anesthesia.
- Be alert for respiratory distress, hypotension, dysrhythmias, changes in heart rate, bleeding or hematoma at site, headache, neurologic deficit or prolonged block, urinary retention, nausea, and itching.
- Implement treatment protocols and notify the HCP as needed.

Assess the urinary system and fluid balance by measuring intake and output. Intraoperative fluid totals are part of the

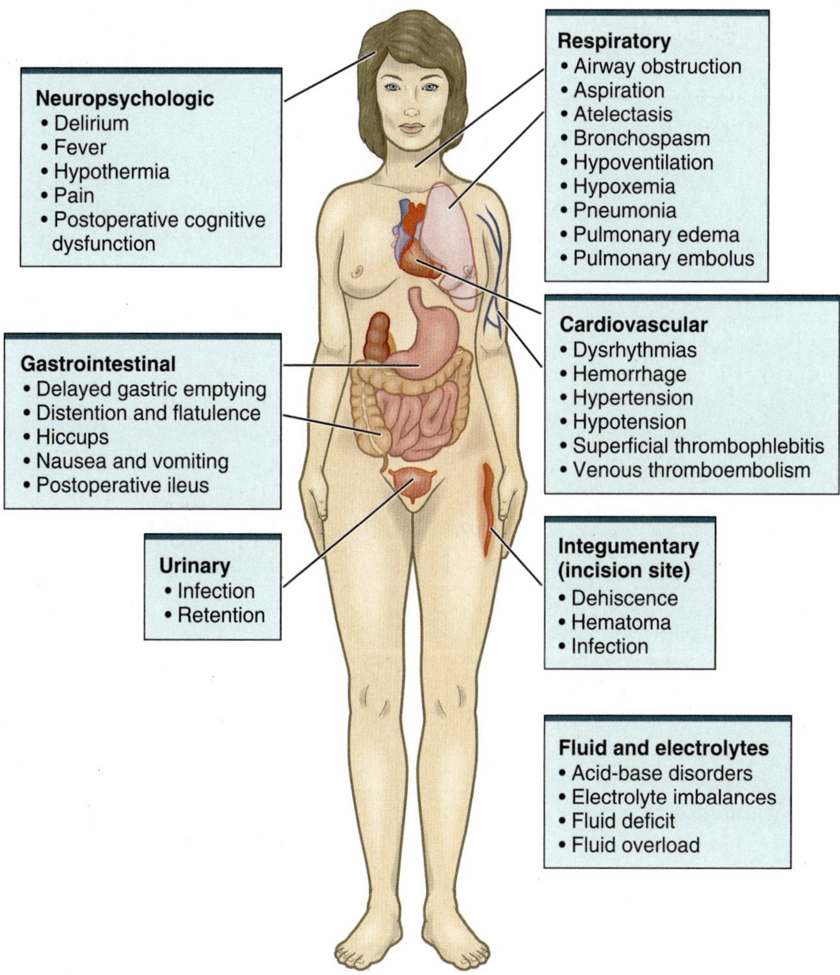

Fig. 20.1 Potential problems in the postoperative period.

ACP report. Note the presence of all IV lines, irrigation solutions and infusions, and output devices, including catheters and wound drains. Assess the surgical site. Note the condition of dressings and the type and amount of drainage. Provide ordered incision care.

POSTOPERATIVE NURSING CARE

The rest of this chapter discusses select patient problems and their nursing management (Table 20.3 and Table 20.5). You can apply this information to postoperative patients in the PACU and clinical unit. A nursing care plan for the postoperative patient (see Nursing Care Plan 20.1) is available on the website for this chapter.

Respiratory Problems

PACU

Respiratory complications pose the greatest risk to patients. High-risk patients should be monitored in the PACU or a critical care unit. Patients at high risk include those who (1) had general anesthesia; (2) are older than 55 years of age; (3) have a history of tobacco use; (4) have preexisting lung problems or sleep breathing impairment; (5) are obese and/or have an unusual body trait (e.g., large or short neck); (6) have comorbidities (e.g., kidney problems, diabetes, hypertension); or (7) had airway, thoracic, or abdominal surgery.

In the initial postanesthesia period, common airway problems include obstruction, hypoxemia, and hypoventilation (Table 20.6). **Airway obstruction** is often caused by the tongue blocking the airway (Fig. 20.3). The base of the tongue falls backward against the soft palate and occludes the pharynx. It is most pronounced in the supine position and in the patient who is very somnolent.

Hypoxemia with respiratory distress is a common complication. It often occurs directly after anesthesia and in the early morning hours during the postoperative period. High acuity patients and those receiving sedating drugs are at highest risk and must be closely monitored. Signs and symptoms of hypoxemia include tachypnea, gasping, anxiety, restlessness, confusion, somnolence, and a rapid or thready pulse.[3]

The most common cause of hypoxemia after surgery is atelectasis. **Atelectasis** (alveolar collapse) may result from bronchial obstruction caused by retained secretions, decreased respiratory excursion, or general anesthesia. Atelectasis occurs when mucus blocks bronchioles or there is not enough alveolar surfactant to hold the alveoli open (Fig. 20.4). Air becomes trapped beyond the mucus blockage. As the air is absorbed, the alveoli collapse. Atelectasis may affect a part of or an entire lobe of the lung.

TABLE 20.3 NURSING MANAGEMENT

Care of the Patient in PACU

Assessment	Interventions
Respiratory	
Airway	
• Patency • Type of O_2 delivery • Presence of an artificial airway • Endotracheal tube with ventilator settings	• Administer and titrate O_2 based on agency protocols. • Position patient appropriately. • Provide respiratory care that supports recovery from anesthesia (e.g., nebulizer treatments, pulmonary drainage procedures, mechanical ventilation, airway support). • Institute extubation protocols. • Encourage deep breathing and coughing.
Breathing	
• Respiratory rate, depth • Auscultate breath sounds • O_2 saturation level • End-tidal carbon dioxide	
Circulation	
• ECG monitoring: rate and rhythm • BP: noninvasive or arterial line • Hemodynamic pressure readings (if applicable) • Temperature • Capillary refill • Color, temperature, moisture of skin • Apical and peripheral pulses • IV assessment: location and condition of sites, solutions infusing	• Give IV fluids, supplemental electrolytes, blood products, and vasoactive drugs as ordered. • Implement rewarming protocols. • Ensure alarms are on and audible. • Encourage to move the legs and arms rhythmically. • Apply pressure dressings as needed.
Neurologic	
• Level of consciousness • Orientation • Sensory and motor status • Pupil size and reaction	• Provide frequent orientation and reassurance. • Apply eyeglasses and hearing aids. • Provide for safety, such as side rails up and beds locked.
Surgical Site	
• Dressings and visible incisions • Drains: type, patency, and drainage	• Provide any incision care needed. • Position the patient to avoid tension on the wound.
Genitourinary	
• Urine output	• Position patient in as normal a position as possible to void.
Pain	
• Incision • Other	• Provide prescribed analgesics. • Implement appropriate nondrug pain management therapies.
Gastrointestinal	
• Nausea, vomiting • Intake (fluids, irrigations) • Bowel sounds	• Administer antiemetics as needed. • Provide oral care. • Maintain NPO status; advance per agency protocol.

Other causes of hypoxemia include pulmonary edema, pulmonary embolism (PE), aspiration, and bronchospasm. An accumulation of fluid in the alveoli can cause *pulmonary edema.*

TABLE 20.4 Signs of Inadequate Oxygenation

Cardiovascular System
- ↑ or ↓ BP
- ↑ or ↓ HR
- Dysrhythmias
- Delayed capillary refill
- ↓ O_2 saturation
- Weak peripheral pulses

Neurologic
- Agitation
- Confusion
- Muscle twitching
- Restlessness
- Seizures
- Somnolence

Renal System
- Urine output <0.5 mL/kg/h

Respiratory System
- Increased to absent respiratory effort
- Use of accessory muscles
- Abnormal breath sounds
- Abnormal ABG values

Skin
- Cool, flushed, or moist skin
- Cyanosis

It may be the result of fluid overload, heart failure, prolonged airway obstruction, sepsis, or aspiration.

Patients are at risk for *aspiration* of gastric contents into the lungs during intubation or after surgery. This can occur with vomiting due to anesthesia depressing the protective airway reflexes. Gastric aspiration may result in laryngospasm, pneumonia, and pulmonary edema. Because of the life-threatening consequences of aspiration, prevention is key. NPO status before surgery has been shown to prevent gastric aspiration.[4]

Bronchospasm is the result of an increase in bronchial smooth muscle tone closing small airways. Airway edema develops, causing secretions to build up in the airway. The patient will have wheezing, dyspnea, hypoxemia, and tachypnea. They may use accessory muscles to try to compensate. Bronchospasm may be due to aspiration, endotracheal intubation, pharyngeal suctioning, or an allergic response. Bronchospasm may occur in any patient. It occurs more often in patients with a history of smoking, asthma, and chronic obstructive pulmonary disease (COPD).

Hypoventilation appears as a decreased respiratory rate or effort, hypoxemia, and increasing hypercapnia (increasing Pa_{CO_2}). It may result from depression of the central respiratory drive (from anesthesia or use of opioids) and/or poor respiratory muscle tone (from neuromuscular blockade or disease).

Clinical Unit

Atelectasis and pneumonia are common respiratory problems, especially in patients with comorbidities (e.g., obstructive sleep

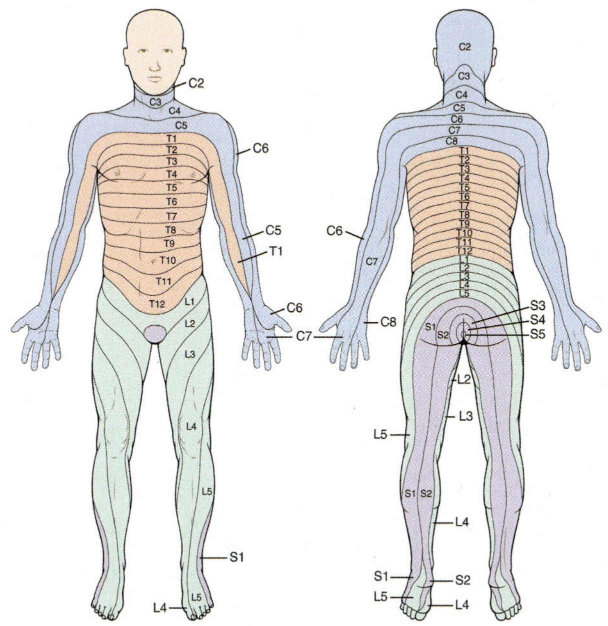

Sensory level anesthesia necessary for surgical procedures

Sensory level	Type of surgery
S2-S5	Hemorrhoidectomy
L2-L3 (knee)	Foot surgery
L1-L3 (inguinal ligament)	Lower extremity surgery
T10 (umbilicus)	Hip surgery Transurethral resection of the prostate Vaginal delivery
T6-T7 (xiphoid process)	Lower abdominal surgery Appendectomy
T4 (nipple)	Upper abdominal surgery Cesarean section

Fig. 20.2 Sensory innervation by spinal nerves and sensory level required for various surgical procedures. (From Pardo M, Miller R: *Basics of anesthesia,* ed 7, St Louis, 2018, Elsevier.)

apnea [OSA], COPD, heart failure) and after abdominal or thoracic surgery.[1,2] Mucous plugs and decreased surfactant production are directly related to hypoventilation, ineffective coughing, history of tobacco use, immobility, and bed rest. Increased bronchial secretions occur when the respiratory passages have been irritated by heavy smoking, COPD, or pulmonary infection, or from dry mucous membranes that occur with intubation, inhalation anesthesia, and dehydration. Without intervention, atelectasis can progress to pneumonia.

Nursing Management: Respiratory Care

Assessment

A thorough respiratory assessment and regular monitoring of vital signs, pulse oximetry, and capnography help you to recognize early signs of respiratory problems. Pay close attention to airway patency, chest symmetry, and the depth, rate, and character of respirations. Impaired ventilation may first be seen as a decreasing pulse oximetry reading, slowed breathing, and/or reduced chest and abdominal movement during breathing. Abdominal or accessory muscle use may occur with respiratory distress. Auscultating breath sounds will alert you to decreased or absent breath sounds. These findings may mean

TABLE 20.5 NURSING MANAGEMENT

Care of the Postoperative Patient on the Clinical Unit

General Care

- Assess patient on initial admission to the unit and an ongoing basis.
- Assess for complications (e.g., atelectasis, hemodynamic instability, cognitive problems, fluid and electrolyte imbalance, fever, nausea and vomiting, urinary retention, infection) and implement appropriate action.
- Develop and implement a patient-specific plan of care based on identified risk factors and potential complications.
- Provide patient and caregiver education, including discharge teaching.

Promoting Patient Recovery

- Have the patient cough and deep breathe and use incentive spirometry as needed.
- Assist the patient to change positions and ambulate as able.
- Provide effective pain management (see Table 9.15).
- Implement measures to reduce nausea and vomiting (see Chapter 46 and Table 46.1).
- Give ordered medications, IV fluids, and blood replacement products.
- Provide wound care, including dressing changes (see Table 12.10).
- Implement measures to reduce delirium (see Table 64.20).
- Advance diet per agency protocol and provide nutrition support.
- Implement VTE prophylaxis.
- Implement measures to address fever (see Table 12.5).

Collaborate With Health Care Team Members

Respiratory Therapist

- Provide respiratory care (e.g., nebulizer treatments, pulmonary drainage procedures).
- Monitor pulse oximetry and capnography and titrate O_2 as needed.
- Perform ABG sampling as needed.
- Assist with O_2 and/or ventilation support during patient transport.

Physical Therapist

- Perform assessment to determine normal functioning level if surgery was emergent.
- Support patient motion and joint mobility.
- Support patient return to baseline functional mobility following surgery.
- Recommend measures for joint positioning, transferring, and/or ambulation.

airflow is diminished or obstructed. Immediately stimulate and wake patients who show poor respiratory effort, noisy respirations, or other signs of respiratory distress. Once patients are awake, coach them to take deep breaths.

! SAFETY ALERT

Hypoventilation

- Always assess for a decreased respiratory rate.
- Use a sedation assessment scale (e.g., Richmond Agitation and Sedation Scale, available at www.icudelirium.org/docs/RASS.pdf) to promote patient safety.
- Begin emergency management protocols if hypoventilation is present.

Pulse oximetry (SpO_2) monitoring is a noninvasive way of assessing arterial O_2 saturation. It provides early warning of

TABLE 20.6 Postoperative Respiratory Complications

Complications	Mechanisms	Manifestations	Interventions
Airway Obstruction			
Laryngeal edema	Allergic drug reaction Mechanical irritation from intubation Fluid overload	Similar to laryngospasm	O_2 therapy Antihistamines Corticosteroids Sedatives Possible intubation
Laryngospasm	Irritation from endotracheal tube, anesthetic gases, or gastric aspiration Most likely to occur after removal of endotracheal tube	Inspiratory stridor (crowing respirations) Sternal retraction Acute respiratory distress	O_2 therapy Positive pressure ventilation IV muscle relaxant Lidocaine Corticosteroids
Retained thick secretions	Secretion stimulation by anesthetic agents Dehydration of secretions	Noisy respirations Coarse crackles	Suctioning Deep breathing and coughing IV hydration Chest PT
Tongue falling back	Muscular flaccidity associated with ↓ consciousness and muscle relaxants	Use of accessory muscles Snoring respirations ↓ Air movement	Patient stimulation Head tilt, jaw thrust (Fig. 20.3) Artificial airway
Hypoxemia			
Aspiration	Inhalation of gastric contents into lungs	Unexplained tachypnea Bronchospasm ↓ O_2 saturation Atelectasis Interstitial edema Alveolar hemorrhage Respiratory failure	O_2 therapy Cardiopulmonary support Antibiotics
Atelectasis	Bronchial obstruction caused by retained secretions or ↓ lung volumes	↓ Breath sounds or Fine crackles ↓ O_2 saturation	Humidified O_2 therapy Deep breathing Incentive spirometry Early mobilization
Pneumonia	Lung infection caused by intubation, aspiration, retained secretions, and/or atelectasis	Dyspnea ↓ Breath sounds or Fine crackles or Coarse crackles or Wheezes ↓ O_2 saturation	Humidified O_2 therapy Deep breathing Incentive spirometry Early mobilization Humidified O_2 therapy Deep breathing Incentive spirometry Mouth care Early mobilization
Bronchospasm	↑ Smooth muscle tone with closure of small airways	Wheezing Dyspnea Tachypnea ↓ O_2 saturation	O_2 therapy Bronchodilators
Pulmonary edema	Fluid overload ↑ Hydrostatic pressure ↓ Interstitial pressure ↑ Capillary permeability	↓ O_2 saturation Crackles Infiltrates on chest x-ray	O_2 therapy Diuretics Fluid restriction
Pulmonary embolism	Thrombus dislodged from peripheral venous system and lodged in pulmonary arterial system	Acute tachypnea Dyspnea Tachycardia Hypotension ↓ O_2 saturation Bronchospasm	O_2 therapy Cardiopulmonary support Anticoagulant therapy

Continued

TABLE 20.6 Postoperative Respiratory Complications—cont'd

Complications	Mechanisms	Manifestations	Interventions
Hypoventilation			
Depressed central respiratory drive	Medullary depression from anesthetics, opioids, sedatives	Shallow respirations ↓ Respiratory rate, apnea ↓ Pa_{O_2} ↑ Pa_{CO_2}	Start capnography or other technology-supported respiratory monitoring Stimulation Reversal of opioids or benzodiazepines Mechanical ventilation
Mechanical restriction	Tight casts, dressings, abdominal binders Positioning and obesity preventing lung expansion	As above	Elevate head of bed Repositioning Loosen dressings
Pain	Shallow breathing to prevent incisional pain	↑ Respiratory rate Hypotension Hypertension ↓ Pa_{CO_2} ↓ Pa_{O_2} Reports of pain Guarding behavior	Opioid analgesic drug therapy NSAID therapy Complementary and alternative therapies (e.g., music, imagery)
Poor respiratory muscle tone	Neuromuscular blockade Neuromuscular disease	As above	Reversal of paralysis Mechanical ventilation

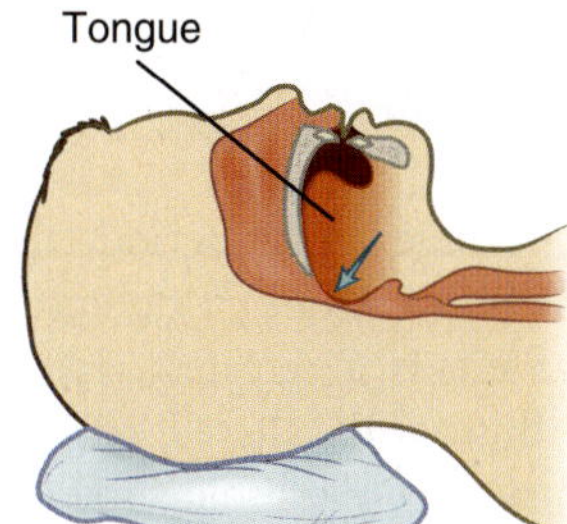

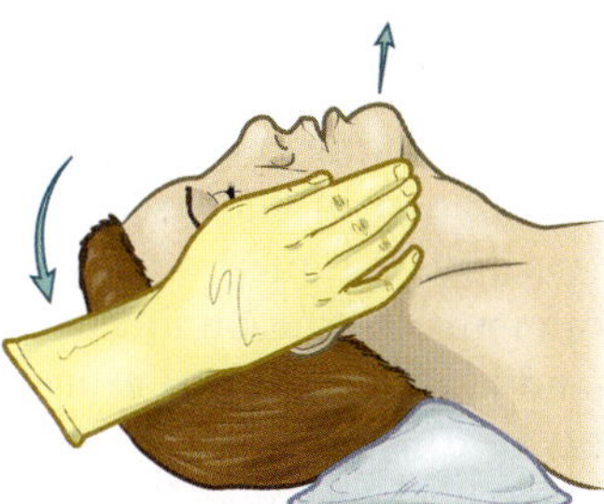

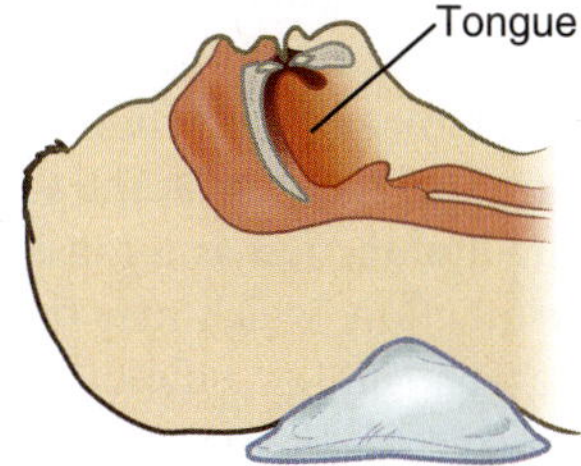

Fig. 20.3 Etiology and relief of airway obstruction.

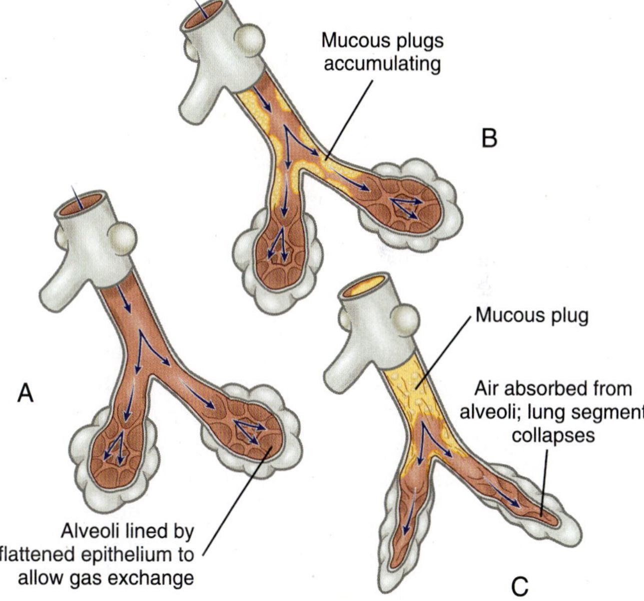

Fig. 20.4 Postoperative atelectasis. (A) Normal bronchiole and alveoli. (B) Mucous plug in bronchiole. (C) Collapse of alveoli resulting from atelectasis after absorption of air.

hypoxemia. High-risk patients should have continuous SpO_2 monitoring.[5] Capnography is used to assess carbon dioxide (CO_2) levels in high acuity patients. This information helps detect respiratory depression and apnea.[1] Pulse oximetry, capnography, $PtcCO_2$, and $PetCO_2$ are discussed in Chapter 27.

Note and record the characteristics of sputum or mucus. Mucus from the trachea and throat is normally colorless and thin. Sputum from the lungs and bronchi is normally thick and

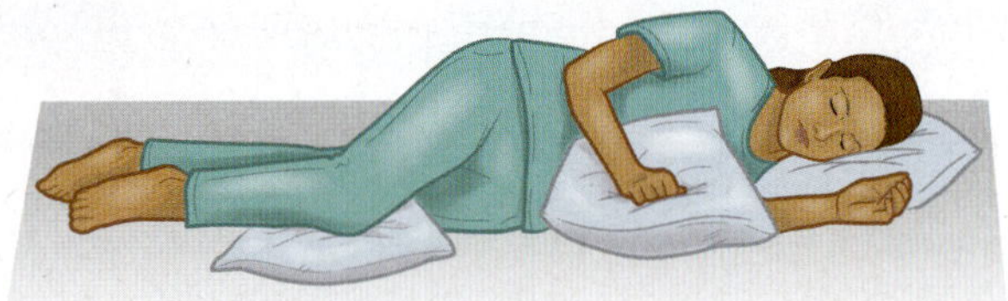

Fig. 20.5 Position of patient during recovery from general anesthesia.

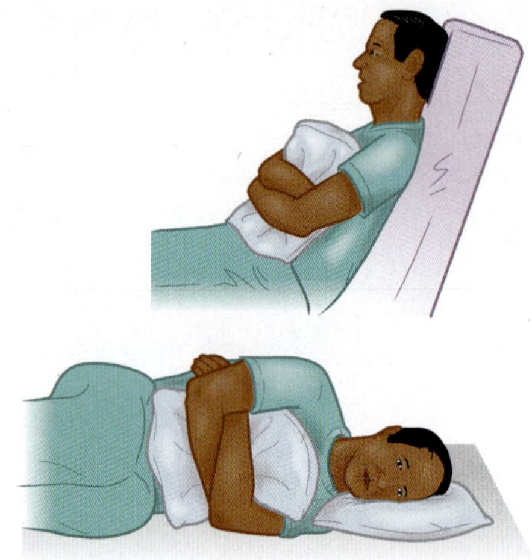

Fig. 20.6 Techniques for splinting incision when coughing.

pale yellow. Changes in sputum color or consistency may indicate a respiratory infection.

◆ Implementation

Nursing interventions for specific respiratory problems are detailed in Table 20.6 and in Chapter 28. In the PACU, nursing interventions are aimed at preventing and treating respiratory problems. Proper patient positioning protects the airway and aids breathing. Place the conscious patient in a supine position with the head of the bed elevated. This position maximizes thoracic expansion by decreasing abdominal pressure on the diaphragm.

! SAFETY ALERT

Postoperative Patient Positioning

- Place the unconscious patient in a lateral "recovery" position (Fig. 20.5).
- This position keeps the airway open and reduces the risk for aspiration if vomiting occurs.

Start O_2 therapy via nasal cannula or face mask if prescribed. O_2 therapy helps to meet the increased demand for O_2 from decreased blood volume or increased metabolism.

Encourage deep breathing to aid gas exchange and promote the return to consciousness. Coughing, deep breathing, and using an incentive spirometer help prevent atelectasis and move respiratory secretions to larger airway passages for expectoration. A technique known as *sustained maximal inspiration* requires the patient to inhale as deeply as possible, hold the breath at the peak of inspiration for a few seconds, and then exhale. This is followed by another deep breath and cough.

Diaphragmatic or abdominal breathing involves inhaling slowly and deeply through the nose, holding the breath for a few seconds, and then exhaling slowly and completely through the mouth. Unless contraindicated, have the patient perform these maneuvers 10 times every hour while awake.

Effective coughing mobilizes secretions. Deep breathing often moves respiratory secretions up and stimulates the cough reflex. Splinting an abdominal or chest incision with a pillow or a rolled blanket supports the incision and aids in coughing up secretions (Fig. 20.6). Reassure the patient that these activities will not cause the incision to open.

Changing the patient's position every 1 to 2 hours improves chest expansion, increases perfusion of both lungs, and prevents pressure injury. Help the patient sit in a chair and ambulate as soon as prescribed. Provide adequate and regular pain medication. Incisional pain often is the greatest barrier to the patient performing effective breathing exercises and ambulation. Adequate oral or IV hydration helps maintain the integrity of mucous membranes and thin secretions for easy expectoration.

Cardiovascular Problems

PACU

In the immediate postanesthesia period, the most common cardiovascular problems include hypotension, hypertension, and dysrhythmias. Patients at greatest risk for cardiovascular problems include those with altered respiratory function, a history of cardiovascular disease, older adults, the debilitated, and critical illness.

The most common cause of hypotension in the PACU is fluid and blood loss. Hemorrhage is always a risk of surgery. The hand-off report and operative report will note the estimated blood loss (EBL) during surgery. Marked blood loss is possible when cauterization or sutures fail. Hemorrhage can occur at the incisional site but most often occurs internally.

Hypotension can impair perfusion to vital organs, especially the brain, heart, and kidneys, and lead to hypovolemic shock. Disorientation, loss of consciousness, chest pain, and oliguria reflect hypoperfusion, hypoxemia, and the loss of physiologic compensation. Intervene promptly to prevent cardiac ischemia or infarction, cerebral ischemia, renal ischemia, and bowel infarction.

Treatment is aimed at addressing any active bleeding and restoring circulating volume with fluid administration or blood products. If there is no response to volume administration, you should consider heart dysfunction as a cause of hypotension.

Primary heart dysfunction, which may occur in myocardial infarction, cardiac tamponade, or pulmonary embolism (PE), results in an acute drop in cardiac output. Secondary heart dysfunction occurs because of the negative *chronotropic* (rate of heart contraction) and negative *inotropic* (force of heart contraction) effects of drugs, such as β-adrenergic blockers or opioids. Other causes of hypotension include decreased systemic vascular resistance and dysrhythmias.

Hypertension most often occurs from sympathetic nervous system stimulation. This may be the result of pain, anxiety, bladder distention, or respiratory distress. Hypertension may be related to hypothermia or preexisting hypertension.

Many problems can cause dysrhythmias. These include hypoxemia, hypercapnia, electrolyte and acid-base imbalances, circulatory instability, preexisting heart disease, hypothermia, pain, surgical stress, and many anesthetic agents.

Clinical Unit

On the clinical unit, fluid and electrolyte imbalances contribute to heart problems. Such imbalances may result from a combination of the body's normal response to the stress of surgery, excess fluid losses, and IV fluid replacement. Fluid status directly affects cardiac output.

Fluid retention during postoperative days 1 to 3 can result from the stress response, which maintains both blood volume and BP. Fluid retention results from the release of antidiuretic hormone (ADH) and adrenocorticotropic hormone (ACTH) and activation of the renin-angiotensin-aldosterone system (RAAS). ADH release leads to increased water reabsorption and decreased urine output, increasing blood volume. ACTH stimulates the adrenal cortex to secrete cortisol and, to a lesser degree, aldosterone (see Figs. 17.9 and 17.10). Fluid losses resulting from surgery decrease kidney perfusion, stimulating the RAAS and causing marked release of aldosterone. Mechanisms that increase aldosterone lead to significant sodium and fluid retention, thus increasing blood volume. Fluid overload may occur during this period of fluid retention if we infuse IV fluids too rapidly, when chronic disease (e.g., heart, kidney) exists, or when the patient is an older adult.

Fluid deficits from untreated preoperative dehydration, blood loss during surgery, or slow or inadequate fluid replacement can decrease cardiac output and tissue perfusion. Losses from vomiting, bleeding, wound drainage, or suctioning can contribute to fluid deficits.

Hypokalemia can result from urinary and gastrointestinal (GI) tract losses. Low serum potassium levels directly affect the heart's contractility and may contribute to decreases in cardiac output and tissue perfusion. Patients with adequate renal function can receive potassium replacement, usually 40 mEq/day. Urine output of at least 0.5 mL/kg/h and a normal serum creatinine and glomerular filtration rate (GFR) indicate adequate renal function.

The state of tissue perfusion or blood flow affects cardiovascular status. The stress response contributes to an increase in clotting tendencies by increasing platelet production. A *venous thromboembolism (VTE)* may form in leg veins because of venous stasis, vein injury, or a hypercoagulable state. VTE is especially common in postoperative patients, older adults, obese persons, immobilized patients, and patients with a history of VTE, PE, or predisposition to clotting. It is a potentially life-threatening complication because it may lead to PE. Suspect PE in any patient with tachypnea, chest pain, hypotension, agitation, tachycardia, and dyspnea, especially when the patient is receiving O_2 therapy.

! SAFETY ALERT

VTE

- Be alert to your patient's risk factors.
- Provide appropriate VTE prophylaxis.
- Monitor for signs/symptoms of VTE.

Syncope (fainting) may result from decreased cardiac output, fluid or blood loss, or defects in cerebral perfusion. Syncope often occurs because of postural hypotension when a patient ambulates. Normally when a patient stands up quickly, the arterial baroreceptors respond to the fall in BP with sympathetic nervous system stimulation. This produces vasoconstriction and maintains BP. These sympathetic and vasomotor functions may be diminished in older adults and immobile, volume depleted, or postanesthesia patients.

❖ Nursing Management: Cardiovascular Care

◆ Assessment

The most important aspect of the cardiovascular assessment is frequent vital sign monitoring. Plan to obtain vital signs every 15 minutes in Phase I, or more often until stabilized, and then less often in Phase II. Compare postoperative vital signs with preoperative and intraoperative findings to determine when the signs are returning to baseline. Notify the ACP or HCP if any of the following occurs:

- Systolic BP <90 mm Hg or >160 mm Hg
- Pulse rate <60 beats/min or >120 beats/min
- Pulse pressure (difference between systolic and diastolic BP) narrows
- BP trends gradually decrease or increase over several consecutive readings
- Change in heart rhythm
- Decreasing trends in hemoglobin, hematocrit, and/or abnormal platelet count

Hypotension accompanied by a normal pulse and warm, dry skin is usually from the residual vasodilating effects of anesthesia. Continue to observe the patient. Hypotension accompanied by a rapid or weak pulse; cold, clammy, pale skin; or trending laboratory findings (decreasing hemoglobin and hematocrit) may indicate hypovolemic shock and needs immediate treatment.

Inspect the surgical area and incisions for bleeding. Look for changes in level of consciousness and vital sign trends of decreasing BP with increasing heart rate. Assess laboratory findings. Decreasing hemoglobin and hematocrit and abnormal platelet count (either decreased or elevated) may indicate bleeding and should be reported to the HCP.

ECG monitoring is recommended for patients who have a history of heart disease and for older patients who have had major surgery. Assess the apical-radial pulse carefully and report any deficits. Valuable information about tissue perfusion is found in assessing peripheral pulses and skin/mucous membrane color, temperature, and moisture.

◆Clinical Problems

Clinical problems related to cardiovascular problems include:

- Altered blood pressure
- Fluid imbalance
- Impaired cardiac function
- Inadequate tissue perfusion

◆Implementation

PACU. Begin treatment of hypotension with O_2 therapy to promote oxygenation of poorly perfused organs. The most common cause of hypotension is fluid loss. Treatment is aimed at addressing any active bleeding and restoring circulating volume with IV fluids or blood products. If there is no response to volume administration, you should consider heart dysfunction as a cause of hypotension. Primary heart dysfunction may require drug intervention. Peripheral vasodilation and hypotension may require vasoconstrictive drugs to increase systemic vascular resistance.

Treatment of hypertension centers on removing the cause of sympathetic nervous system stimulation. This may include giving analgesics, assisting with voiding, and correcting respiratory problems. Rewarming corrects hypothermia-induced hypertension. Patients with preexisting hypertension or who have had heart or vascular surgery usually need drug therapy to reduce BP.

Most dysrhythmias seen in the PACU have identifiable causes. Identifying the cause is a critical first step in correcting the dysrhythmia. With life-threatening dysrhythmias (e.g., ventricular tachycardia), follow your agency's protocol for advanced cardiac life support.

Clinical unit. Continue to monitor vital signs. Keep an accurate intake and output record, monitor laboratory findings (e.g., electrolytes, hematocrit, platelet count), and manage IV therapy after surgery.

VTE prophylaxis often includes early ambulation, pneumatic compression devices, and antiplatelet or anticoagulation drugs.[6] Superficial thrombophlebitis is an uncomfortable but less serious complication that does not lead to PE. It may develop in a superficial leg or arm vein because of venous stasis, vein trauma, and/or irritation from IV catheters or solutions. PE and VTE are discussed in Chapters 30 and 41, respectively.

Early ambulation is the most significant nursing action to prevent complications. Walking (1) increases muscle tone; (2) stimulates circulation, which prevents venous stasis and VTE, and speeds wound healing; (3) increases vital capacity and supports normal respiratory function; and (4) improves feelings of well-being. Begin progression to ambulation by first raising the head of the bed for 1 to 2 minutes. Then help the patient to sit, with legs dangling, while monitoring the pulse rate. If you do not note changes or problems, help the patient ambulate while monitoring the pulse. If you note changes in the pulse or dizziness occurs, sit the patient in a nearby chair until the BP and pulse are stable. Then help the patient back to bed. If dizziness occurs, it may be frightening for the patient. Injury can result from a fall, so take measures to ensure patient and staff safety.

> **CHECK YOUR PRACTICE**
>
> You are caring for an older patient who is 1 day post–colon resection with plans for moving out of the bed to a chair. You help the patient to a sitting position, dangling legs at the bedside. The patient reports feeling dizzy. The patient's BP is 108/64 and apical heart rate is 124.
>
> - What should you do?

Neurologic and Psychologic Problems

PACU

After surgery, some patients develop **emergence delirium**. It is a short-term neurologic change with behaviors such as restlessness, agitation, disorientation, thrashing, and shouting. Causes include anesthetic agents, bladder distention, pain, long duration of preoperative fasting, residual neuromuscular blockade, or the presence of an endotracheal tube. However, if delirium occurs, you should first suspect and assess for hypoxia.

Delayed emergence occurs when a patient takes longer than 90 minutes to awaken from anesthesia. Patients with delayed emergence spend longer periods in the PACU and have prolonged hospital courses. Identifying the cause is critical for determining needed interventions. The most common cause of delayed emergence after anesthesia is drug-related. This includes anesthetic agents and drugs used during the perioperative period. Other causes include hypoxia, hypercapnia, hemorrhage, thrombotic events, metabolic problems, electrolyte imbalances, hypertension, liver problems, uremia, central anticholinergic syndrome, and hypothyroidism.[7]

Clinical Unit

Two types of cognitive impairments in surgical patients are *postoperative cognitive dysfunction* (POCD) and *delirium.* POCD is a decline in the patient's cognitive function (e.g., memory, ability to concentrate) for weeks or months after surgery. POCD occurs most often in the older adult. Preexisting cognitive impairment, duration of anesthesia, complications during surgery, and infection contribute to POCD. Quickly and thoroughly investigate any changes in mental status as the causes may be life threatening.

Postoperative delirium is more common in older patients. Delirium may result from severe pain, fluid and electrolyte imbalances, hypoxemia, organ failure, infection, drug effects, sleep deprivation, and sensory deprivation or overload. Signs include cognitive problems, varying levels of consciousness, altered psychomotor activity, and a disturbed sleep/wake cycle.[8] See Chapter 64 for more about delirium.

Substance use disorder can result in *withdrawal delirium* in patients withdrawing from alcohol, drugs, and/or other substances. Signs and symptoms can include hypertension, tachycardia, irritability, insomnia, nightmares, hallucinations, photophobia, tremors, nausea, vomiting, and/or diaphoresis. Record and report any unusual or disturbed behavior so that a diagnosis can be made and treatment started. Chapter 11 discusses the identification and management of alcohol withdrawal delirium.

Nursing Management: Neurologic and Psychologic Care

Assessment

Assess level of consciousness, orientation, memory, and ability to follow commands. Determine the size, reactivity, and equality of the pupils. Assess the patient's sleep/wake cycle and sensory and motor status. Determine the possible cause if the patient has an altered neurologic status. If the patient who was mentally alert before surgery becomes cognitively impaired after surgery, assess to rule out hypoxia, delirium, or POCD.

Clinical Problems

Clinical problems related to neurologic and psychologic problems include:

- Impaired sleep
- Neurologic problem
- Risk for injury
- Sensory deficit

Implementation

PACU. The most common cause of agitation in the PACU is hypoxemia. Focus attention on evaluating respiratory function. The most common cause of delayed emergence is prolonged drug action. It usually spontaneously resolves with time. If needed, antagonist agents can reverse the effects of benzodiazepines and opioids.

Until the patient is awake and able to communicate effectively, you are responsible for patient safety. This includes monitoring physiologic status, having the side rails up and the call bell available, securing equipment (e.g., IV lines, artificial airways), verifying allergies, and using 2 patient identifiers before giving drugs or completing treatments.

Clinical unit. Interventions to prevent perioperative delirium begin with screening and identification of risk factors. Assistive devices that help promote orientation include clocks, calendars, photos, hearing aids, and eyeglasses. Encourage family to be at the bedside. Choose medications carefully (e.g., avoiding sedatives, antipsychotics, opioids). Manage agitation, pain, or anxiety.[8] Help patients achieve fluid and electrolyte balance, adequate nutrition and sleep, proper bowel and bladder function, and early mobilization.

Provide adequate psychologic support for patients and caregivers. This includes listening to and talking with them, offering explanations and reassurance, and encouraging the presence and aid of caregiver(s). Evaluate the patient's behavior to distinguish a normal reaction to a stressful situation from one that is becoming abnormal or excessive.

Pain and Discomfort

Pain is a common problem and a significant fear for patients. Pain is caused by the interaction of physiologic and psychologic factors. The incision and retraction during surgery traumatize the skin and underlying tissues. There may be reflex muscle spasms around the incision. Anxiety and fear, sometimes related to the anticipation of pain, create tension and further increase muscle tone and spasm.[9] Positioning during surgery and the use of internal devices such as endotracheal tubes or catheters may cause discomfort. The effort and movement associated with coughing, deep breathing, and ambulating may worsen pain by creating tension on the incision area. Other sources of discomfort include nausea and vomiting, environment noise, noxious odors, and shivering.

Patients do not feel pain when the internal viscera are cut. However, pain does result from pressure in the internal viscera. Deep visceral pain may signal a complication such as intestinal distention, bleeding, or abscess formation. Pain may limit respiratory movement, increasing the risk for atelectasis.

Nursing Management: Pain

Assessment

Assess for pain at frequent intervals. A patient's self-report is the single most reliable indicator of pain. Use a pain scale, such as a numeric or FACES pain scale, to assess the severity or intensity of pain. Pain scales are discussed in Chapter 9. Assess pain levels at rest and during activities. If the patient is not able to verbalize pain, assess for other indications of pain (e.g., restlessness, grimacing, changes in vital signs). Where is the pain located? Expect that patients will have incisional pain, especially with movement and with some procedures (e.g., removal of drains). Other causes of pain, such as a full bladder, may be present.

Involve patients in the assessment and management of their pain. Assessing patients from different cultures or those who do not speak English may be challenging. Take extra time and include family in exploring the pain experience with these patients.

Thoroughly assess pain in a patient who does not report any pain. Encourage the use of analgesics as needed. Explain to the patient and caregiver that untreated pain has a negative effect on recovery. Adapt care to meet your patient's unique needs and expectations for pain control.

Implementation

Acute pain from surgery is an individual response that almost always requires the use of analgesics. Safe and effective pain management can be challenging. Patient care should include a multidisciplinary team approach using evidence-based analgesic adjuncts and practices.[10] Begin before surgery to develop a plan for pain control that includes behavioral modalities and control of anxiety. Evaluate adjustments to or continuation of drugs used to treat chronic pain. Teach patients to report pain and how pain will be managed. Share pain management plans during the hand-off report.

Pain control techniques include the use of single modalities (e.g., opioid drugs, patient-controlled analgesia [PCA], regional analgesic [local anesthetic infiltration]), or multimodal analgesia. *Multimodal analgesia,* or the use of 2 or more analgesics with different mechanisms of action (e.g., an opioid and a nonsteroidal antiinflammatory drug [NSAID]), is recommended. Medications such as ibuprofen and acetaminophen are routinely used adjunctively in the pain management plan. This has resulted in a reduced need for opioids. Many medications can be given via various routes based on patient needs. For example, the IV or rectal route would be most effective if a patient has nausea or vomiting.

The HCP often prescribes multimodal pain medications and other comfort measures on an as-needed (PRN) basis. Time analgesic doses to ensure that they are in effect during activities that may be painful, such as ambulation and physical therapy. Manage side effects of opioid analgesic use. The most common include constipation, nausea and vomiting, respiratory and cough depression, and hypotension.

Before giving any analgesic, assess pain, including location, quality, and intensity; vital signs; and level of consciousness. Treat incisional pain as prescribed. If the patient reports chest or leg pain, analgesics may mask a complication (e.g., VTE). If it is gas pain, opioids can worsen it. If the analgesic does not relieve the pain or makes the patient lethargic or somnolent, notify the HCP and request a change.

Patient-controlled analgesia (PCA) allows patients to self-administer preset doses of analgesics by an IV, oral, epidural, or transdermal route. The goals of PCA are to provide immediate analgesia and maintain an acceptable level of pain control. Continuous infusions allow for a steady blood level of analgesia with additional patient doses used before painful events (e.g., walking, deep breathing, and coughing) or for breakthrough pain. Some advantages of PCA are early ambulation, better pain management than with as-needed analgesia, and greater patient satisfaction. PCA is discussed in Chapter 9.

! SAFETY ALERT

PCA

- Assess the patient's pain, sedation status, and the access site.
- Carefully check the HCP's prescription and program the pump for IV or epidural PCA to deliver the prescribed dose of analgesic. Check the right patient, right reason, right medication, right dose (continuous and bolus), right route, and right time.
- Have a second nurse verify the medication programmed into the pump.

Epidural analgesia is the infusion of opioid analgesics through a catheter placed into the epidural space around the spinal cord. The goal of epidural analgesia is delivery of the drug directly to opiate receptors in the spinal cord. Administration methods include intermittent bolus dosing, continuous infusion, and epidural PCA. This results in a constant circulating level and a reduced total dose of medication.

Perineural local anesthesia manages postoperative pain using a small catheter and a mechanical infusion pump to deliver a nonopioid drug directly into the surgical site. A single dose of a long-acting local anesthetic (e.g., bupivacaine, ropivacaine) can provide pain relief that results in the use of less opioids. Patients can be discharged with the catheter in place. It can be maintained for up to 3 days.

Complementary therapies such as music therapy, guided imagery, relaxation exercises, and aromatherapy are effective adjuncts in pain management. Nondrug approaches such as repositioning, massage, and distraction can enhance pain management.

CHECK YOUR PRACTICE

Although PCA analgesia is infusing as prescribed, your postoperative patient reports ongoing pain that is rated 8 on a 0 to 10 scale.

- What steps would you take next to manage this patient's pain more effectively?

Temperature Changes

Knowing your patient's temperature in the postoperative period is important (Table 20.7). Perioperative temperature management can prevent many complications.

Hypothermia

Perioperative *hypothermia* is a core body temperature less than 96.8°F (36°C). Hypothermia may be due to skin exposure, use of cold irrigation solutions, skin preparations, and unwarmed inhaled gases. Although all patients are at risk for postoperative hypothermia, we should closely monitor patients at high risk. This includes patients with hypotension or low preoperative core body temperature, older adults, females, those with pre-existing medical conditions, undergoing open cavity procedures, or having a long procedure.[1]

Complications of hypothermia include vasoconstriction with resulting hypertension, compromised immune function, bleeding, cardiac events, surgical site infection (SSI), altered drug metabolism, increased pain, and shivering. Shivering can increase resting energy expenditure and O_2 consumption up to 500%, causing hypoxemia and myocardial ischemia. Shivering can increase carbon dioxide production; increase heart rate, BP, and intracranial pressure; and significantly affect the patient's comfort level.[1]

Fever

Fever may occur at any time after surgery (Table 20.7). SSI, particularly from aerobic organisms, is often accompanied by a

TABLE 20.7 Postoperative Temperature Changes

Time After Surgery	Temperature	Possible Causes
Up to 12 h	Hypothermia: ≤96.8°F (36°C)	Effects of anesthesia, body heat loss during surgical procedure
First 48 h (postoperative days 1 and 2)	Mild elevation: ≤100.4°F (38°C)	Inflammatory response to surgical stress
	Moderate elevation: >100.4°F (38°C)	Lung congestion, dehydration
After first 48 h (postoperative day 3 and later)	Elevation >100°F (37.8°C)	Infection (e.g., wound, urinary, respiratory)

fever that spikes in the afternoon or evening and returns to near-normal levels in the morning. The respiratory tract may be infected from stasis of secretions with atelectasis. Urinary tract infections (UTIs) may occur from catheterization. Superficial thrombophlebitis may occur at the IV site. A thrombus in the leg veins may raise temperature.

Intermittent high fever accompanied by shaking chills and diaphoresis suggests septicemia. This may occur at any time after surgery. It can result from microorganisms introduced into the bloodstream during surgery, especially in GI or genitourinary (GU) procedures. Septicemia may occur later from a wound or UTI.

Surgical patients who receive broad antibiotic therapy to prevent or treat infection are at risk for *C. difficile* infections (CDIs). Manifestations of CDI may include fever, diarrhea, and abdominal pain.

Malignant hyperthermia (MH) is a rare muscle metabolism disorder triggered by general anesthetic agents. Although often a late sign, it is characterized by a rapid rise in core body temperature and severe muscle rigidity. Other signs include tachycardia, tachypnea, lactic acidosis, hypoxemia, and elevated creatine kinase levels. MH is a life-threatening complication. While most cases of MH occur during general anesthesia, the 1-hour period right after surgery (e.g., in the PACU) is a critical time.[2]

Nursing Management: Temperature

Assessment

Take the patient's temperature on arrival to the PACU and every 15 minutes until normothermic. Use the same route to measure temperature during the patient's stay in the PACU.

Assess the color and temperature of the skin. Communicate risk factors for hypothermia or MH to all members of the perioperative team. Observe the patient for early signs of inflammation and infection that may precede a fever so that we can start treatment promptly.

Implementation

Apply O_2 therapy via nasal cannula or mask to treat the increased demand for O_2 caused by shivering. Shivering can be treated by giving meperidine. *Passive warming measures* include the use of warmed cotton blankets, socks, reflective blankets, and limited skin exposure. *Active warming measures* involve the application of external warming devices, including forced air warmers, heated water mattresses, radiant warmers, heated and humidified O_2, and warmed IV fluids. When using any external warming device, record temperature and the patient's comfort level at 15-minute intervals. Assess skin and prevent skin injuries.

Cooling methods and treatments for MH include the emergent administration of dantrolene (Dantrium), applying ice packs, and providing 100% oxygen.

If fever develops, antipyretic drugs may be prescribed (see Table 12.6). Depending on the suspected cause of the fever, obtain cultures of the wound, sputum, urine, or blood. If a bacterial infection is the source of the fever, start prescribed antibiotics as soon as you obtain cultures. Fever above 103°F (39.4°C) may require body-cooling measures.

Gastrointestinal Problems

Postoperative nausea and vomiting (PONV) are common complications, affecting as many as 80% of high-risk patients. Risk factors include being female, ages 3 to 50 years, history of motion sickness, previous PONV, nonsmoking status, specific anesthetics or opioids, and some durations or types of surgery.[11] Delayed gastric emptying and slowed peristalsis that result from handling the bowel during abdominal surgery contribute to PONV, as does starting oral intake too soon after surgery.

Constipation may occur. It can be due to anesthetics used during surgery that may paralyze the intestine, changes in diet and fluid intake, immobility, and opioids for pain relief. Opioids decrease peristalsis, slow fecal transport, and decrease a patient's urge to defecate.

Postoperative ileus (POI) can be expected as a temporary decrease in gastric and bowel motility after abdominal surgery. It results from the handling or reconstruction of the intestine during surgery. Although there is a decrease in gastric motility, gastric juices continue to be secreted and can result in abdominal distention, nausea, and vomiting. After surgery, motility in the large intestine may be reduced for 2 to 7 days. Motility in the small intestine resumes within several hours after surgery. Risk factors associated with prolonged POI include pharmacologic, neurogenic, mechanical, hormonal, or inflammatory causes.[2] Opioid analgesia may prolong the duration of POI.

Hiccups are intermittent spasms of the diaphragm caused by irritation of the phrenic nerve, which innervates the diaphragm. The phrenic nerve may be irritated by gastric distention, intestinal obstruction, intraabdominal bleeding, or a subphrenic abscess. Indirect irritation of the phrenic nerve may occur with acid-base and electrolyte imbalances. Reflex irritation may be from drinking hot or cold liquids or from the presence of a nasogastric (NG) tube. Hiccups usually last a short time and stop spontaneously.

Nursing Management: Gastrointestinal Care

Assessment

Ask patients about feelings of nausea. Assess the severity using a verbal descriptor or numeric scale. If vomiting occurs, determine the quantity, characteristics, and color of the vomitus. Assess the abdomen for presence of bowel sounds and distention. Because bowel sounds are often absent or diminished right after surgery, auscultate all 4 quadrants to determine the presence, frequency, and characteristics of the sounds. Auscultate for at least 3 to 5 minutes before noting that they are absent. Assess patients regularly to detect the return of normal bowel motility. This is usually accompanied by passing gas or stool and the ability to tolerate oral intake without nausea or vomiting.

Clinical Problems

Clinical problems related to GI problems include:

- Electrolyte imbalance
- Fluid imbalance
- Impaired bowel elimination
- Impaired gastrointestinal function

Implementation

The goal of treatment for POI is the relief of symptoms and return of normal GI function. While the patient is NPO, give IV fluids to maintain fluid and electrolyte balance. Begin oral fluids as prescribed and tolerated. Depending on the surgery, the patient may begin oral intake as soon as bowel sounds and gag reflex return. Offer clear liquids first and advance to solid food while assessing diet tolerance. If the patient tolerates oral intake, IV fluids are decreased or stopped.

Be alert to prevent aspiration if the patient vomits while still lethargic from anesthesia. Position the patient in the lateral recovery position and have suction equipment available. Interventions for PONV include monitoring fluid status and providing antiemetic medications and alternative therapies (see Table 46.1). Prophylactic antiemetic agents may be given to patients at high risk for PONV. Consider alternatives such as essential oils or ice application to the back of the neck to avoid medication side effects.[12] Other interventions include imagery, music, and acupressure.

Constipation may be prevented with bowel protocols that include a stool softener and laxative. Encourage the patient to expel gas. Gas pains tend to become pronounced on the second or third postoperative day. Ambulation and frequent repositioning may provide relief. Positioning the patient on the right side permits gas to rise along the transverse colon and aids its release. Bisacodyl (Dulcolax) suppositories may stimulate colonic peristalsis and expulsion of gas and stool. Resuming a normal diet after bowel sounds have returned also aids the return of normal peristalsis.

An NG tube may be needed to decompress the stomach to provide bowel rest and to prevent nausea, vomiting, and abdominal distention. Provide frequent oral care for comfort and stimulation of salivary glands when the patient is NPO or has an NG tube.

Urinary Problems

Low urine output (800 to 1500 mL) in the first 24 hours after surgery is common regardless of fluid intake. Causes include increased aldosterone and ADH secretion resulting from the stress of surgery; fluid restrictions; and fluid loss through surgery, drainage, and diaphoresis. By the second or third day, expect increased urine output as fluid is mobilized and the immediate stress reaction subsides.

Acute urinary retention can occur for several reasons. Anesthesia depresses the nervous system, including the micturition reflex arc and the higher centers that influence it. The bladder fills more than normal before the patient feels the urge to void. Anesthesia impedes voluntary micturition. Anticholinergic and opioid drugs interfere with the ability to start voiding or to empty the bladder.

Urinary retention is more likely to occur after lower abdominal or pelvic surgery because spasms or guarding of the abdominal and pelvic muscles interferes with micturition. Pain may alter perception and interfere with the awareness of bladder filling. Immobility and bed rest impair voiding ability. The supine position reduces the ability to relax the perineal muscles and external sphincter.

Oliguria, diminished urine output, can be a sign of renal failure. It may result from renal ischemia caused by inadequate renal perfusion.

Nursing Management: Urinary Care

Assessment

Examine the urine for quantity and quality. Urine output should be at least 0.5 mL/kg/h. Note the color, amount, and odor. Most patients void within 6 to 8 hours after surgery. If no voiding occurs, palpate for bladder fullness or percuss the suprapubic area for bladder distention. Scan the bladder with a portable ultrasound to assess volume of urine in the bladder.

Implementation

You can promote voiding by helping the patient into a normal position. Other techniques include providing privacy, running water, offering the patient a drink of water, or pouring warm water over the perineum. Walking, preferably to the bathroom, and the use of a bedside commode are other measures to help with voiding.

The HCP may leave an order to intermittently catheterize the patient in 6 to 8 hours if voiding has not occurred. If catheterization is needed, an intermittent straight catheterization limits the risk for catheter-associated urinary tract infection (CAUTI).

If the patient has an indwelling catheter, maintain patency. To decrease the risk for CAUTI, remove it as soon as possible or within 24 hours unless there is a reason to continue its use.

Surgical Wounds

Surgery generally involves an incision through the skin and underlying tissues, disrupting the protective skin barrier. Wound healing is a major concern after surgery. One of the greatest risks during the perioperative period is SSI. SSIs are associated with prolonged hospitalizations, increased costs, and poor patient outcomes. Most are preventable using evidence-based strategies. These include hand hygiene; selection, timing, and duration of prophylactic antibiotics; surgical site skin preparation; and maintaining perioperative normothermia.[13] Reducing the incidence of SSIs is a major goal of the Surgical Care Improvement Project (SCIP) and prevention of postoperative infections initiative. Prolonged postoperative antibiotic use does not provide any benefit in preventing SSI and may result in antimicrobial resistance.[2]

Surgical wounds may be contaminated from 3 major sources: (1) exogenous flora present in the environment and on the skin, (2) oral flora, and (3) intestinal flora. The incidence of SSI is higher in patients who are malnourished, immunosuppressed, older, or who have had a long hospital stay or a lengthy surgical procedure (more than 3 hours). After bowel surgery, particularly after a traumatic injury, patients are at high risk. SSI may involve the entire incision and extend downward through deeper tissues. A local abscess may spread throughout a body cavity, as in peritonitis.

Evidence of SSI usually does not become clear before the 3rd to 5th postoperative day. Local findings include redness, swelling, and increasing pain and tenderness at the site. Systemic findings are fever and leukocytosis.

Fluid accumulation in a wound creates pressure, impairs circulation and wound healing, and predisposes patients to infection. To allow for drainage, the HCP may place a drain in the incision or make a stab wound next to the incision. Drains may be of soft rubber and drain into a dressing, or firm catheters attached to a Hemovac or other source of gentle suction.

Adequate nutrition is needed for wound healing. Patients who are well nourished before surgery can tolerate the lack of intake for several days. However, patients with nutrition problems due to chronic diseases (e.g., diabetes, ulcerative colitis) are more prone to delayed wound healing. Patients who cannot meet nutrition needs may need enteral or parenteral nutrition to promote healing.

Nursing Management: Surgical Wounds

Assessment

Assess the wound and dressing based on the type of wound, the drains inserted, and expected drainage for the specific type of surgery. Immediately after surgery, check the wound every 15 to 30 minutes or as prescribed. Record the type, amount, color, and odor of drainage. Assess the effect of position changes on drainage. A small amount of serous drainage is common from any type of wound. If a drain is in place, assess the amount of drainage and compare to what is expected. Expected drainage from tubes is shown in Table 20.8. An abdominal incision drain will likely have a moderate amount of serosanguineous drainage in the first 24 hours. In contrast, an inguinal herniorrhaphy should have only minimal serous drainage.

Expect the drainage to change from sanguineous (red) to serosanguineous (pink) to serous (clear yellow) over hours or days, depending on the type of surgery. Purulent drainage may occur with an SSI. *Wound dehiscence* (separation and disruption of previously joined wound edges) may follow a sudden discharge of brown, pink, or clear drainage. Wound dehiscence

TABLE 20.8 Output From Tubes, Drains, and Catheters

Substance	Daily Amount	Color	Odor	Consistency
Indwelling Catheter				
Urine	800–1500 mL for first 24 h Minimum expected output: 0.5 mL/kg/h	Clear, yellow	Ammonia	Watery
Nasogastric Tube or Gastrostomy Tube				
Gastric contents	<1500 mL/day	Pale, yellow-green Bloody after GI surgery	Sour	Watery
Open Drains (e.g., Penrose)				
Wound drainage	Varies with procedure May decrease over hours or days	Varies with procedure Initially may be sanguineous or serosanguineous, changing to serous	Same as wound dressing Foul odor may indicate infection	Thin, watery
Closed Suction Drains (e.g., Hemovac, Jackson-Pratt)				
Wound drainage	Varies with procedure May decrease over hours or days	Varies with procedure Initially may be sanguineous or serosanguineous, changing to serous	Little to no odor Foul odor may indicate infection	Thin, watery
T-Tube				
Bile	500 mL	Bright yellow to dark green	Acid	Thick
Mediastinal Chest Tube				
Wound drainage post cardiothoracic surgery	Varies with procedure Should decrease over several hours after surgery	Sanguineous or serosanguineous	N/A	Thin
Pleural Chest Tube				
Fluid that has collected in the pleural space	Varies with procedure Decreases over hours or days >100 mL/h is considered excessive	Varies with indication for insertion and fluid collected in the pleural spaces	N/A	Varies with reason for insertion

is discussed in Chapter 12. Notify the HCP of excess or abnormal drainage or significant changes in vital signs.

◆ Clinical Problems

Clinical problems related to surgical wounds include:

- Impaired tissue integrity
- Risk for infection

◆ Implementation

The incision may be covered with a dressing after surgery. Many HCPs prefer to change the first postoperative dressing. If the initial operative dressing is saturated, follow agency policy as to changing or simply reinforcing the dressing. Skin graft dressings may stay in place for 3 to 5 days to avoid disturbing the graft site and promote graft acceptance. Specially trained nurses may change these dressings. Skin grafts are discussed in Chapter 25.

To prevent infection, use meticulous care to incisional, wound, and IV sites. When you change a dressing, note the number and type of drains present. Avoid dislodging drains. Inspect the incision site carefully. The area around the sutures may be slightly reddened and swollen, which is an expected inflammatory response. However, the skin around the incision should be of normal color and temperature. If the wound is healing by primary intention, has little or no drainage, or has no drains in place, use a single-layer dressing or no dressing. Use a multilayer dressing when drains are in place, moderate to heavy drainage is occurring, or healing occurs other than by primary intention. Wound care and healing are discussed in Chapter 12.

TRANSITIONS OF CARE

Discharge From the PACU

When the patient has recovered from the effects of anesthesia, vital signs are stable, and no complications have arisen, the patient is ready for discharge from the PACU. The decision is based on written criteria approved by the agency's anesthesiology and medical staff (Table 20.9). We often use a post-anesthesia scoring system (e.g., *Modified Aldrete Scoring System*) to decide if the patient is ready for discharge. The choice of discharge site is based on patient acuity, access to follow-up care, and the potential for complications. A PACU discharge summary note should be done to indicate the patient's condition at the time of transfer.

Discharge to the Clinical Unit

Before discharging the patient from the PACU to the clinical unit, give a hand-off report about the patient to the receiving nurse. Summarize the operative and postanesthesia period. Include information as to where the patient's caregivers are waiting. Nurse-to-nurse communication must be accurate and allow for questions. Using a standard communication tool, such as SBAR, enhances a safe transfer of the patient from the PACU to the clinical unit (Table 20.10).

TABLE 20.9 Surgery Discharge Criteria

PACU Discharge Criteria (Phase I—Initial Assessment)

- Awake, easily arousable (or baseline)
- Vital signs at baseline or stable
- No excess bleeding or drainage
- No respiratory depression
- O_2 saturation 95%–100%
- Pain controlled or acceptable
- Nausea and vomiting controlled
- Report given

Ambulatory Surgery Discharge Criteria (Phase II or Extended Observation)

- All PACU discharge criteria (Phase I) met
- No IV opioid drugs for last 30 min
- Voided if appropriate to surgical procedure or orders
- Able to ambulate if not contraindicated
- Responsible adult present to accompany and drive patient home
- Written discharge instructions given and patient and caregiver understanding confirmed

Admission to the Clinical Unit

When you receive the patient on the clinical unit, assist the PACU transport staff to safely move the patient from the stretcher to the bed. Take care to protect IV lines, drains, and traction devices. Obtain vital signs and compare the patient status with the report from the PACU nurse. After this, perform a more focused assessment and initiate postoperative orders and nursing care (Table 20.11).

Discharge From Ambulatory Surgery

Patients leaving an ambulatory surgery setting must be hemodynamically stable, mobile, alert, and able to provide a degree of self-care when discharged to home (Table 20.9). PONV and pain, common problems after ambulatory surgery, must be under control. These can lead to delirium, prolonged PACU stay, delayed discharge, readmission, delayed return to usual activities, and decreased patient satisfaction.

Overall, patients must be stable and near the level of preoperative functioning for discharge from the unit. They may not drive and must be accompanied by an adult at the time of discharge. Carefully assess the patient's readiness for discharge and home care needs. Determine availability of caregivers (e.g., family, friends) and access to (1) a pharmacy for prescriptions, (2) a phone in the case of an emergency, and (3) follow-up care.

Discharge and Follow-Up Care

As discharge approaches, assess the needs of the patient that may affect teaching (disabilities, reading ability, language). Patients should be given verbal, written, electronic, and/or video instructions with a return appointment and who to call with questions. Standard, preprinted discharge instructions that are surgery specific and easy to read ensure that information is complete. Include the patient and caregiver in discharge planning. Common reasons patients seek help after discharge

TABLE 20.10 Postoperative SBAR Hand-Off Communication

Situation
Patient ________ Date of birth ________
Transferring to Room # ________ Surgeon ________
ACP ________ Type of Anesthesia ________
Procedure ________
Surgical site(s) ________
Estimated Blood Loss (EBL) ________
Medical history ________
Code status ________ Isolation precautions ________

Background
Allergies ________
Medications received in PACU ________
IV site/fluids ________
Dressings and/or drains ________
Significant OR events ________

Assessment
PACU vital signs T ____ P ____ RR ____ BP ____ O_2 Sat ____
O_2 source ________ FiO_2 ________
Pain rating at discharge ________
Method of pain management ________
Last dose of pain medication ________
Mental status ________
Nausea/vomiting at discharge ________
Intake ________ Output ________
Laboratory tests ________
Recovery comments ________

Recommendations
Equipment needed ________
Orders to be completed ________
Family ________
Other notes ________
Transferring RN ________ Phone # for questions ________
Receiving RN ________

include unrelieved pain, questions about drugs, and wound issues (Table 20.12). Patients who are prepared for discharge gradually assume more responsibility for self-care during the postoperative period.

Once the patient and caregiver have reviewed the discharge information, they should provide the nurse with a "teach back" demonstration verifying correct technique and understanding. Document the discharge teaching in the health record. More information about patient teaching is in Chapter 4.

Assessment and evaluation of patients after discharge includes a postoperative return appointment and may also include a follow-up call or visit from a home health nurse who can address any specific questions and concerns. Increasingly, patients are discharged from the hospital with many care needs. They may be transferred to transitional care facilities, to long-term care facilities, or directly home. When discharged directly to home, patients are expected to continue self-care, with help from

TABLE 20.11 NURSING ASSESSMENT

Care of Patient on Admission to Clinical Unit

1. Record time of patient's return to unit and assess airway, breathing, and circulation.
2. Obtain baseline vital signs, including O_2 saturation.
3. Assess neurologic status, including level of consciousness and motor and sensory assessment.
4. Assess level of pain:
   a. Last dose and type of pain control
   b. Current pain rating
5. Assess wound, dressing, and drainage tubes:
   a. Type and amount of drainage
   b. Tubing connected to gravity or suction drainage (per orders)
6. Assess color, temperature, and appearance of skin.
7. Position for airway maintenance, comfort, and safety (bed in low position, side rails up).
8. Check IV infusion:
   a. Type of solution
   b. Amount of fluid remaining
   c. Patency and flow rate
   d. Condition of insertion site and size of catheter
9. Assess urinary status:
   a. Time of voiding
   b. Presence of catheter, patency, and total output
   c. Bladder distention, urge to void, and bladder scan
10. Assess for any nausea or vomiting.
    a. Availability of emesis basin and tissues
11. Position call bell within reach and orient patient to use of call bell.
12. Determine emotional state and provide support as needed.
13. Check for presence of caregiver.
    a. Orient patient and caregiver to immediate environment
14. Check and carry out postoperative orders.

TABLE 20.12 PATIENT & CAREGIVER TEACHING

Surgical Discharge

Provide discharge instructions after surgery verbally, written, or electronically using methods that best meet the patient and caregiver needs. Consider specific disabilities, language, and readability. Include the following information:

- Symptoms to report (e.g., discomfort in other parts of the body, fever, increased incisional pain, swelling, redness, bleeding, drainage)
- When and how to take prescribed drugs and possible side effects (reinforce education about multimodal pain control)
- Care of wound, incision, drain (e.g., dressing change)
- Personal hygiene and showering recommendations
- Activities allowed and prohibited, when various activities can be resumed safely (e.g., driving, return to work, sexual intercourse, leisure activities, lifting restrictions)
- Diet restrictions or modifications
- Where and when to return for follow-up appointment
- Answers to any questions or concerns
- Contact information regarding who to call to report symptoms, ask questions, and address concerns after discharge

caregivers or home health care personnel (e.g., nurses, physical therapists). The care may include dressing changes, wound care, catheter or drain care, antibiotic therapy, or physical therapy. Work with the social worker, discharge planner, or case manager to ensure the patient's safe transition from hospital-based care to community- or home-based care.

CHECK YOUR PRACTICE

You are caring for a young adult patient who had a laparoscopic appendectomy 18 hours ago. The patient meets the discharge criteria, and the HCP has asked you to provide discharge teaching for the patient.

- What information should you prioritize in the discharge teaching plan?

Gerontologic Considerations: Postoperative Patient

Older surgical patients deserve special consideration. Pneumonia is a common complication. The older adult has decreased respiratory function, including decreased ability to cough and decreased thoracic compliance. These changes lead to an increase in the work of breathing and a decreased ability to eliminate drugs. Carefully monitor reactions to anesthetic drugs.

Altered vascular function in the older adult is due to atherosclerosis and decreased elasticity in the blood vessels. Circulating blood volume decreases. Hypertension is common. Cardiac function is often compromised with limited compensatory responses to changes in BP and volume. Monitor cardiovascular status closely throughout the post-operative period.

Drug toxicity is a potential problem in older adults. Renal perfusion normally decreases, along with a reduced ability to remove drugs. Decreased liver function leads to reduced drug metabolism and increased drug activity. Carefully assess renal and liver function to prevent drug overdose and toxicity.

Observe for changes in mental status. Age, alcohol use, poor baseline cognition, hypoxia, metabolic imbalances, hypotension, and polypharmacy can contribute to postoperative delirium. Anesthetics, especially anticholinergic and benzodiazepine drugs, increase the risk for delirium.

Pain control in older patients is challenging because of possible preexisting cognitive deficits, impaired communication, and physiologic changes that affect drug metabolism. Patients may hesitate to ask for pain medication because they believe pain is inevitable after surgery. Some older patients may fear addiction or be nervous about using PCA machines.

CASE STUDY

Postoperative Patient

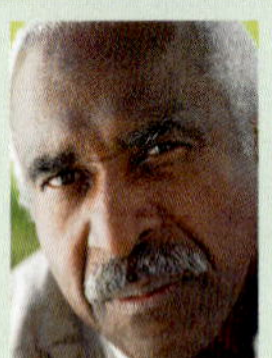

(© BananaStock/ BananaStock/ Thinkstock.)

Patient Profile

E.G., a 74-year-old retired teacher, just had a right total hip replacement to repair a right hip fracture. E.G. fell off a ladder while painting his house. His medical history includes type 2 diabetes and COPD. The surgery was done under general anesthesia and lasted 3 hours.

Subjective Data

- Active walker in his home community
- Smokes 1 pack of cigarettes per day × 58 years
- Always had problems sleeping
- Difficulty hearing, wears hearing aid
- Upset with injury and its impact on life
- Widower; no relatives nearby or friends to assist with care
- Reports pain is 8 on a 0 to 10 scale on arrival to PACU

Objective Data

- Abduction pillow between legs
- Peripheral IV catheter
- Jackson-Pratt drain visible at the site of the hip dressing
- Pneumatic compression boots bilateral lower extremities at 40 mm Hg
- Indwelling urinary catheter in place
- O_2 saturation 95% on 4 L nasal cannula

Interprofessional Care

Postoperative Orders

- Vital signs per PACU routine
- Glucose level on arrival and every 4 hours. Call for glucose level <70 mg/dL or >250 mg/dL. Follow protocol for managing hypoglycemia.
- 0.45% normal saline at 100 mL/h
- Morphine via patient-controlled analgesia 1 mg q10min (20 mg max/4 h) for pain
- Advance diet as tolerated
- O_2 therapy to keep O_2 saturation >90%
- Albuterol 2.5 mg via nebulizer q4h as needed for wheezing
- Encourage coughing, deep breathing, and incentive spirometry q1h × 10 while awake
- Neurovascular checks q1h × 4 h
- Assess, empty, and record output of Jackson-Pratt drain q2h × 8 h
- Maintain strict intake and output
- Pneumatic compression boots at 40 mm Hg
- Ambulate to chair and in halls 3 times daily

Discussion Questions

1. ***Recognize:*** What should be your primary areas of focus when assessing E.G.?
2. ***Recognize:*** What factors predispose E.G. to the following problems: atelectasis, SSI, CAUTI, and VTE?
3. ***Analyze:*** How would you determine E.G. is recovered from general anesthesia and ready to be transferred from the PACU to the clinical unit?
4. ***Analyze:*** What complications is E.G. at risk for developing?
5. ***Plan:*** What referrals may be indicated based on E.G.'s medical history?
6. ***Plan:*** What potential postoperative problems on the clinical unit might you anticipate?
7. ***Prioritize:*** What nursing interventions would be needed in the plan of care to prevent atelectasis, SSI, and VTE?
8. ***Act:*** Identify activities that can be delegated to AP.
9. ***Act:*** What teaching will you provide so that E.G. can successfully self-manage care?
10. ***Evaluate:*** What outcomes would indicate that interprofessional care with respiratory therapy was effective?
11. ***Safety:*** What are risk factors for E.G. developing postoperative delirium? What are the signs and symptoms of delirium?
12. ***Safety:*** Identify 2 areas of risk for injury to E.G. What actions can you take to ensure patient safety?

Answers available at http://evolve.elsevier.com/Lewis/medsurg.

BRIDGE TO NCLEX EXAMINATION

The number of the question corresponds to the same-numbered outcome at the beginning of the chapter.

1. Which assessment is the nurse's *priority* when admitting a patient to the PACU?
   a. The surgical site and character of drainage.
   b. Airway patency and quality of respirations.
   c. The amount of urine output and the presence of bladder distention.
   d. Results of intraoperative laboratory values and medications received.
2. A patient is admitted to the PACU after major abdominal surgery. During the initial assessment the patient tells the nurse, "I think I am going to throw up." Which is the *priority* nursing intervention?
   a. Increase the rate of the IV fluids.
   b. Give antiemetic medication as prescribed.
   c. Obtain vital signs, including O_2 saturation.
   d. Position patient in lateral recovery position.
3. A surgical patient is admitted to the clinical unit. Which assessment data requires attention *first?*
   a. O_2 saturation of 85%
   b. Respiratory rate of 13/min
   c. Temperature of 100.4°F (38°C)
   d. Blood pressure of 90/60 mm Hg
4. A 70-kg postoperative patient has voided 200 mL during the first 8 hours after surgery. Which action would the nurse take *first?*
   a. Encourage additional oral fluids.
   b. Obtain a bladder ultrasound scan.
   c. Perform a straight catheterization.
   d. Continue to monitor this normal finding.
5. Which factor(s) would the nurse include in discharge criteria for a Phase II postanesthetic patient? **(Select all that apply.)**
   a. Ability to drive a vehicle home.
   b. Nausea and vomiting controlled.
   c. No respiratory depression present.
   d. Discharge instructions understood.
   e. Opioid pain medication given 45 minutes ago.

1. b; 2. d; 3. a; 4. b, d; 5. b, c, d, e.

For rationales to these answers and even more NCLEX review questions, visit http://evolve.elsevier.com/Lewis/medsurg.

REFERENCES

To access the References for this chapter, please scan the QR code with a mobile device.

21

Emergency and Disaster Nursing

Samantha J. Bonaduce

http://evolve.elsevier.com/Lewis/medsurg/

CONCEPTUAL FOCUS

Gas Exchange
Interpersonal Violence
Perfusion
Thermoregulation

LEARNING OUTCOMES

1. Apply the steps of emergency triage to a patient who needs emergency care.
2. Relate the pathophysiology to the assessment and interprofessional care of select environment emergencies.
3. Relate the pathophysiology to the assessment and interprofessional care of select toxicologic emergencies.
4. Select appropriate interventions for victims of violence.
5. Distinguish among the responsibilities of health care providers, the community, and select federal agencies in emergency and mass casualty incident preparedness.

KEY TERMS

drowning
emergency
frostbite
heat exhaustion
heatstroke
hypothermia
mass casualty incident (MCI)
primary survey
secondary survey
submersion injury
terrorism
triage
violence

An **emergency** is a serious, unexpected, and often threatening situation needing immediate attention and action.[1] People with emergent needs seek emergency medical services (EMS) or enter emergency departments (EDs). ED nurses care for patients of all ages with a variety of problems. Some EDs specialize in specific patient populations or conditions, such as pediatric ED or trauma ED.

Entire books are dedicated to emergency care. It is a specialty that requires an understanding of specific nursing concepts and approaches to patient problems. The challenge of the ED is that the nurse does not know what patients will come through the doors. The ED nurse must be prepared to meet this challenge. The Emergency Nurses Association (ENA) is the specialty organization aimed at advancing emergency nursing practice. It provides standards of care for nurses working in the ED. The ENA offers a certification process that allows nurses to become certified emergency nurses (CENs).

Postpandemic ED visits are steadily rising to nearly 140 million each year in the United States.[2,3] These increasing numbers have significantly affected ED admission and walkout rates (patients leaving before being seen and treated). Admission rates have increased because of EDs seeing older, sicker patients with more complex needs.[4] Increased walkout rates are attributed to longer wait times. Walking out results in patients not knowing if they have a serious medical concern or not.[5]

This chapter presents an overview of the triage process, use of the primary and secondary survey, and care of select emergency patients. The emergency management of various problems is discussed throughout this book. Emergency management tables

TABLE 21.1 EMERGENCY MANAGEMENT

Emergency Management Tables Throughout the Book

Title	Chapter
Abdominal Trauma	47
Acute Abdominal Pain	47
Acute GI Bleeding	46
Acute Soft Tissue Injury	67
Acute Thyrotoxicosis	54
Anaphylactic Shock	14
Chest Injuries	30
Chest Pain	37
Chest Trauma	30
Depressant Toxicity	11
DKA	53
Dysrhythmias	39
Eye Injury	22
Fractured Extremity	67
Head Injury	61
Hyperthermia	21
Hypoglycemia	53
Hypothermia	21
Inhalation Injury	26
SCI	65
Shock	42
Stimulant Toxicity	11
Stroke	62
Submersion Injuries	21
Tonic-Clonic Seizures	63

outline the acute and emergent care of specific problems. Table 21.1 lists these tables by title and chapter.

EMERGENCY TRIAGE

Recognizing life-threatening illness or injury is one of the most important goals of emergency nursing. Starting treatment to reverse or prevent a crisis is often a priority before making a medical diagnosis. This process begins with your first contact with a patient. Prompt identification of patients who need immediate treatment and determining appropriate interventions are essential nurse competencies.

Triage

Triage refers to the process of rapidly determining patient acuity. It is one of the most important assessment skills needed by ED nurses. ED nurses often confront multiple patients who have a variety of problems. The triage process works on the premise that we treat patients who have a threat to life before other patients.

A *triage system* identifies and categorizes patients so that the most critically ill are treated first. The ENA and American

TABLE 21.2 Examples of Patient Problems at Each ESI Level

ESI Level	Examples of Patient Problems
1	Cardiac arrest, critically injured trauma, intubated head injury, overdose with bradypnea, severe respiratory distress, anaphylactic shock, hypoglycemia with mental status changes
2	Chest pain from ischemia, multiple trauma, suicidal or homicidal, immunocompromised with a fever, acute stroke
3	Abdominal pain or gynecologic disorders unless in severe distress, hip fracture in older adult, vomiting, hypertension
4	Closed extremity trauma, simple laceration, cystitis
5	Cold symptoms, minor burn, poison ivy, recheck (e.g., wound), prescription refill

ESI, Emergency Severity Index.

College of Emergency Physicians support the use of a 5-level triage system.[6] The *Emergency Severity Index* (ESI) is a 5-level triage system that incorporates illness severity and resource use (e.g., ECG, laboratory tests, radiology studies, IV fluids) to determine who we should treat first (Table 21.2). The ESI includes an algorithm that directs how to assign an ESI level to patients coming into the ED. The *ESI Implementation Handbook* details the triage algorithm.[6]

First, assess the patient for any threats to life (ESI-1) (Fig. 21.1). Ask, "Does this patient need lifesaving intervention?" Or, for ESI-2, "Is this a high-risk patient who cannot wait to be seen?" High-risk patients may become unstable or have a high risk for deteriorating. We do not take vital signs for patients assigned ESI-1 or ESI-2 if it will delay immediate lifesaving care. Next, for patients who do not meet the criteria for ESI-1 or ESI-2, take vital signs and determine the number of expected resources they may need. Consider age and current medications (e.g., β-blockers) when evaluating vital signs. Assign patients with normal vital signs to ESI-3 if they require 2 or more resources, ESI-4 for no more than 1 resource, or ESI-5 for no resources. You may reassign patients with abnormal vital signs to ESI-2.[6]

CHECK YOUR PRACTICE

You are working in the ED with your preceptor, who is a triage nurse. A 24-year-old male arrives and states, "I think I have food poisoning. I've been vomiting all night, and now I have diarrhea." The patient reports abdominal cramping that he rates as 6/10. He denies fever or chills. Vital signs: T = 97.8°F (36.6°C), HR = 94, RR = 16, BP = 121/74 mm Hg.

- Assign a triage acuity rating using the ESI.

After you complete the initial focused assessment, proceed with a more detailed assessment. A systematic approach to this assessment decreases the time needed to identify potential threats to life and limits the risk of overlooking a life-threatening problem. A primary and secondary survey is the

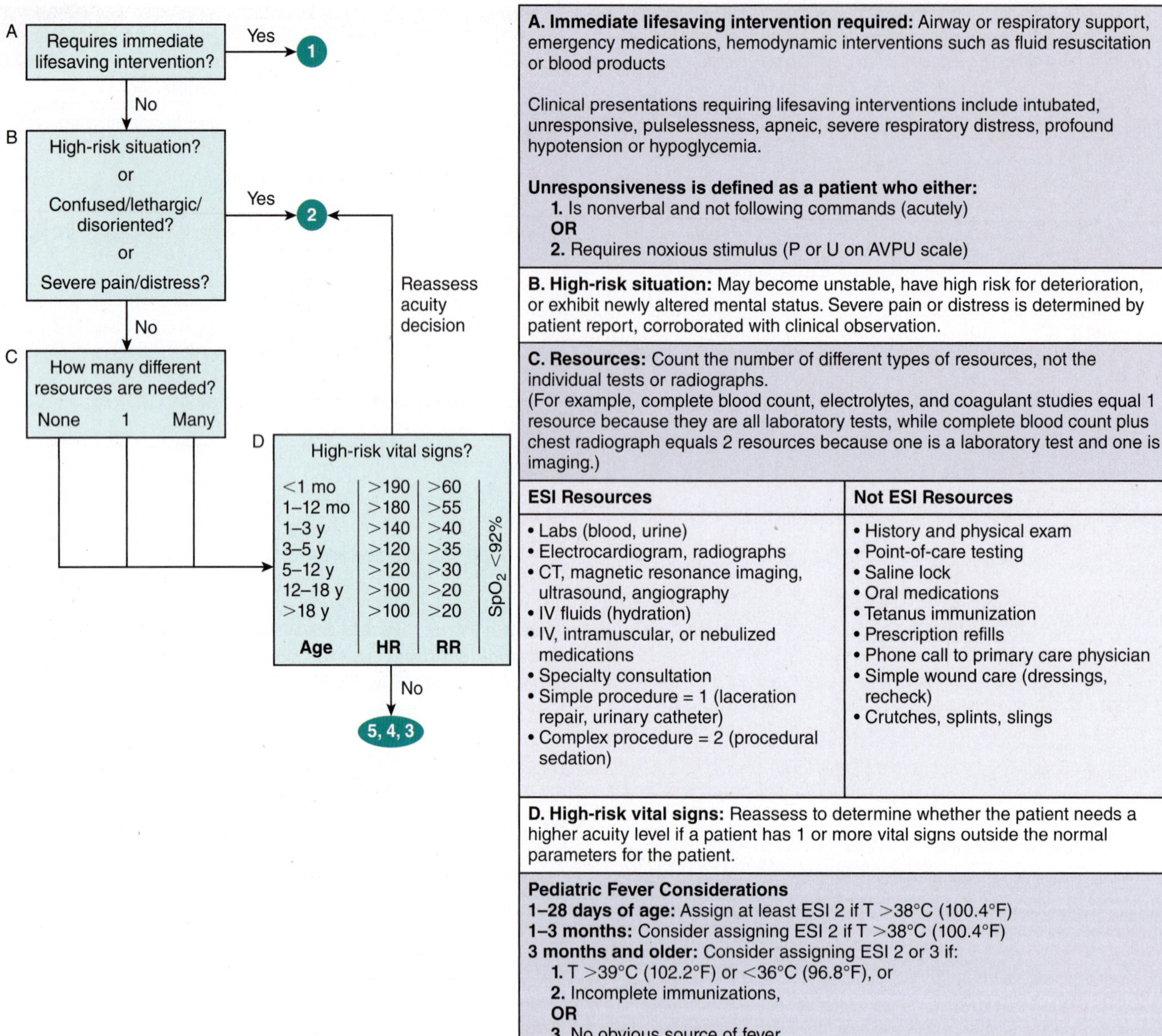

Fig. 21.1 ESI Triage Algorithm, version 5.

approach used for all trauma patients. For nontrauma patients, the primary survey is followed by a focused assessment. Focused assessments are discussed in Chapter 3.

Primary Survey

The **primary survey** (Table 21.3) focuses on airway, breathing, circulation (ABC); disability; exposure; full set of vitals and family presence; and getting other monitoring devices. If there is uncontrolled external hemorrhage, the usual ABC assessment format may be reprioritized to C-A-B-C. The first C stands for *control of hemorrhage.*[7] Apply direct pressure with a sterile dressing followed by a pressure dressing to any obvious bleeding sites.

The primary survey aims to identify life-threatening problems so that we can start treatment (Table 21.4). You may identify life-threatening problems related to ABCs at any point during the primary survey. When this occurs, start interventions at once before moving to the next step of the survey.

A = Alertness and Airway

Many immediate trauma deaths occur because of airway obstruction. Saliva, bloody secretions, vomitus, laryngeal trauma, dentures, facial trauma, fractures, and the tongue can obstruct the airway. Patients at risk for airway compromise include those who drown or have seizures, anaphylaxis, foreign body obstruction, or cardiopulmonary arrest. If an airway is not

TABLE 21.3 EMERGENCY ASSESSMENT

Primary Survey

Assessment	Interventions
Alertness (A_1) and Airway (A_2) With Cervical Spine Stabilization and/or Immobilization	
• Assess alertness (e.g., AVPU). • Assess for respiratory distress. • Determine airway patency. • Check for loose teeth or foreign bodies. • Assess for bleeding, vomitus, or edema.	• Maintain cervical spine stabilization and/or immobilization. • Open airway using jaw-thrust maneuver. • Remove or suction any foreign bodies. • Insert oropharyngeal or nasopharyngeal airway, tracheostomy. • Begin rapid sequence intubation. • Immobilize cervical spine using rigid cervical collar and cervical immobilization device.
Breathing	
• Assess ventilation. • Scan chest for signs of breathing. • Look for paradoxical movement of the chest wall during inspiration and expiration. • Note use of accessory muscles or abdominal muscles. • Observe and count respiratory rate. • Note color of nail beds, mucous membranes. • Auscultate lungs. • Assess jugular venous distention and trachea position.	• Give supplemental O_2 via appropriate delivery system (e.g., nonrebreather mask). • Ventilate with bag-valve-mask with 100% O_2 if respirations are inadequate or absent. • Prepare to intubate if severe respiratory distress (e.g., agonal breaths) or arrest. • Have suction available. • If absent breath sounds, prepare for needle thoracostomy and chest tube insertion.
Circulation and Control of Hemorrhage	
• Assess for uncontrolled bleeding. • Check carotid or femoral pulse. • Palpate pulse for quality and rate. • Assess skin color, temperature, moisture. • Check capillary refill.	• If absent pulse, start CPR and advanced life support measures. • Control bleeding with direct pressure and pressure dressings. • If shock symptoms or hypotensive, start 2 large-bore (14- to 16-gauge) IVs and start infusions of normal saline or lactated Ringer's solution. • Consider intraosseous or central venous access if IV access cannot be rapidly obtained. • Give blood products if ordered.
Disability	
• Assess level of consciousness by determining response to verbal and/or painful stimuli (e.g., Glasgow Coma Scale). • Assess pupils for size, shape, equality, and reactivity.	• Periodically reassess level of consciousness, mental status, and pupil size and reactivity.
Exposure (E_1) and Environment Control (E_2)	
• Assess full body for determination of other or related injuries. • Assess environment.	• Remove clothing for adequate assessment. • Stabilize any impaled objects. • Keep patient warm with blankets, warmed IV fluids, overhead lights to prevent heat loss, if appropriate. • Maintain privacy.
Full Set of Vitals (F_1) and Family Presence (F_2)	
• Assess vital signs and pulse oximetry. • Determine caregiver's desire to be present during invasive procedures and/or CPR.	• Obtain bilateral BP if patient has sustained or is suspected of having sustained chest trauma or if the BP is abnormal. • Assign health team member to support caregiver(s). • Provide emotional support to patient and caregiver.
Get Monitoring Devices (G_1) and Give Comfort (G_2)	
• Determine need for adjunct measures for monitoring the patient's condition: **L**—Laboratory studies **M**—Monitor cardiac status **N**—Naso- or orogastric tube **O**—Oxygen and ventilation assessment **P**—Pain assessment and management	• Obtain laboratory tests, such as type and crossmatch, CBC and metabolic panel, lactate, blood alcohol, toxicology screening, ABGs, coagulation profile, cardiac biomarkers, pregnancy. • Continuously monitor ECG. • Insert NG tube; insert orogastric tube in a patient with significant head or facial trauma. • Monitor oxygenation and ventilation (e.g., continuous pulse oximetry, capnography). • Manage pain with pharmacologic (e.g., NSAIDs, IV opioids) and nonpharmacologic (e.g., distraction, positioning, music) pain management strategies. • Provide comfort measures (e.g., ice, position of comfort, warm blanket).

AVPU, A = alert; V = responsive to voice; P = responsive to pain; U = unresponsive.

TABLE 21.4 Common Life-Threatening Problems Found During Primary Survey

Airway	• Inhalation injury (e.g., fire victim) • Obstruction from foreign bodies, debris (e.g., vomitus), or tongue • Penetrating wounds and/or blunt trauma to upper airway structures
Breathing	• Anaphylaxis • Flail chest with pulmonary contusion • Hemothorax • Pneumothorax
Circulation	• Direct cardiac injury (e.g., myocardial infarction, trauma) • Pericardial tamponade • Shock (e.g., massive burns, hypovolemia) • Uncontrolled external hemorrhage • Hypothermia
Disability	• Head injury • Stroke

maintained, obstruction of airflow, hypoxia, and death will result. Signs of a compromised airway include dyspnea, inability to speak, gasping (agonal) breaths, foreign body in the airway, and trauma to the face or neck. The patient's alertness level is a crucial factor for choosing the right airway interventions. Determine level of consciousness (LOC) by assessing the patient's response to verbal and/or painful stimuli. A simple mnemonic to remember is *AVPU: A* = alert, *V* = responsive to voice, *P* = responsive to pain, and *U* = unresponsive.[8]

Airway maintenance should progress rapidly from the least to the most invasive method. Treatment includes opening the airway using the *jaw-thrust maneuver* (avoiding hyperextension of the neck), suctioning and/or removal of a foreign body, inserting a nasopharyngeal or oropharyngeal airway (in unconscious patients only), and endotracheal intubation. If intubation is impossible because of airway obstruction, an emergency cricothyroidotomy or tracheotomy is done (see Chapter 28). Ventilate patients with 100% O_2 using a bag-valve-mask (BVM) device before intubation or cricothyroidotomy.

Rapid-sequence intubation (RSI) is the way to secure an unprotected airway in the ED by inducing unconsciousness with sedatives (e.g., midazolam, propofol) and paralysis with paralytic drugs (e.g., succinylcholine, rocuronium).[9] These drugs aid in intubation and reduce the risk for aspiration and airway trauma. See Chapter 28 for more about intubation.

If the patient has a suspected spinal cord injury and is not already immobilized, the cervical spine must be stabilized at the same time as the airway assessment. This can be done with manual stabilization or the use of a rigid cervical collar (C collar). Keep the bed flat. Continue to monitor airway patency and breathing effectiveness.

B = Breathing

Adequate airflow through the upper airway does not ensure adequate ventilation. Many problems cause breathing changes. Common ones include fractured ribs, pneumothorax, penetrating injury, allergic reactions, pulmonary emboli, and asthma attacks. Patients with these problems may have a variety of signs and symptoms. There may be dyspnea, paradoxical or asymmetric chest wall movement, decreased or absent breath sounds on the affected side, visible wounds to the chest wall, cyanosis, tachycardia, and hypotension.

Every critically injured or ill patient has increased metabolic and O_2 demand. They should receive supplemental O_2. Give high-flow O_2 (100%) via a nonrebreather mask and monitor the patient's response. Life-threatening problems (e.g., flail chest, tension pneumothorax) can severely and quickly compromise ventilation. Treatment may include BVM ventilation with 100% O_2, needle decompression, intubation, and treatment of the underlying cause.

C = Circulation and Control of Hemorrhage

Uncontrolled internal or external bleeding places a person at risk for hemorrhagic shock (see Chapter 42). Check either a femoral or carotid pulse. Peripheral pulses may be absent because of direct injury or vasoconstriction. Assess the quality and rate of the pulse if found. Assess the skin for color, temperature, and moisture. Altered mental status and delayed capillary refill (longer than 3 seconds) are common signs of shock. When evaluating capillary refill in cold environments, remember that cold temperature delays refill.

Insert IV lines into the upper extremities unless contraindicated, such as an open fracture or an injury that affects limb circulation. Insert 2 large-bore (14- to 16-gauge) IV catheters. Start aggressive fluid resuscitation using normal saline or lactated Ringer's solution. Consider intraosseous or central venous access if unable to rapidly obtain venous access. See Chapter 42 for more about hypovolemic shock and fluid resuscitation.

The HCP may order type-specific packed red blood cells if needed. In an emergency (life-threatening) situation, give blood that is not cross-matched (e.g., O-negative) if immediate transfusion is needed.

D = Disability

Conduct a brief neurologic assessment as part of the primary survey. The patient's LOC is a measure of the degree of disability. Use the Glasgow Coma Scale (GCS) to determine the LOC (see Table 61.5).[8] This allows for consistent communication among the interprofessional care team. Remember: The GCS is not accurate for intubated or aphasic patients. Last, assess pupils for size, shape, equality, and reactivity.

E = Exposure and Environmental Control

Remove the patient's clothing so you can perform a thorough physical assessment. This often requires cutting off the clothing. Be careful not to cut through any area that is forensic evidence (e.g., bullet hole). Do not remove any impaled objects (e.g., knife). Removing these could cause bleeding and further injury. Once the patient is exposed, use warming blankets, overhead warmers, and warmed IV fluids to limit heat loss, prevent hypothermia, and maintain privacy.

F = Full Set of Vitals and Family Presence

Obtain a full set of vital signs, including BP, heart rate, respiratory rate, O_2 saturation, and temperature, after the patient is exposed. If the patient has sustained or is suspected of having sustained chest trauma or if the BP is abnormally high or low, obtain a BP in both arms.

Research supports the benefits for patients, caregivers, and staff of *family presence* during resuscitation and invasive procedures.[10] Patients and caregivers report that caregivers provide comfort. Patients state that caregivers serve as advocates and help remind the care team of their "personhood." Caregivers who are present during invasive procedures and resuscitation view themselves as active participants in the care process. They voice feeling that they receive better information to make decisions. They believe that they comfort the patient and that it is their right to be with the patient. Assign a health care team member to explain the care being delivered and answer questions if a caregiver is present during resuscitation or invasive procedures.

G = Get Monitoring Devices and Give Comfort

Start adjunct measures for monitoring the patient's condition if not already done. Use the memory aid *LMNOP* to remember these resuscitation aids:

L: Laboratory tests, such as type and crossmatch, complete blood count (CBC) and metabolic panel, blood alcohol, toxicology screening, arterial blood gases (ABGs), coagulation profile, cardiac biomarkers, pregnancy test, and urinalysis.

M: Monitor ECG for heart rate and rhythm.

N: Nasogastric (NG) tube to decompress and empty the stomach, reduce the risk for aspiration, and test the contents for blood. Place an orogastric tube in a patient with significant head or facial trauma because an NG tube could enter the brain.

O: Oxygenation and ventilation assessment. Continuously monitor O_2 saturation and end-tidal CO_2 ($EtCO_2$) if the patient is receiving mechanical ventilation (see Chapter 28).

P: Pain assessment and management. Most patients who come to the ED report pain.[8] Providing comfort measures is critical. Many EDs have pain management protocols for nurses to use to treat pain, beginning at triage. Pain management should include a combination of pharmacologic and nonpharmacologic measures. You are the advocate in ensuring comfort measures for the patient.

Secondary Survey

The secondary survey begins after addressing each step of the primary survey and starting any lifesaving care. The **secondary survey** is a brief, systematic process that aims to identify *all* injuries (Table 21.5). It is helpful for discovering unknown problems in patients with a poor or confusing history.[7]

H = History and Head-to-Toe Assessment

Obtain a history and mechanism of the injury or illness. These details provide clues to the cause and guide specific assessments and interventions. The patient may not be able to give a history. Caregivers, friends, bystanders, and prehospital personnel can often provide necessary information.

Use the memory aid *MIST* to help you obtain a prehospital report of the incident or illness:

M: Mechanism of injury

I: Injuries sustained

S: Signs and symptoms before arrival

T: Treatment before arrival

Details of the incident are important because the mechanism of injury and injury patterns can predict specific injuries. For example, a restrained front-seat passenger may have knee or femur fractures from hitting the dashboard and a chest injury from the airbag. Those who fell off a ladder or roof may have fractures, spinal cord injury, or head trauma.

Collect a history. *SAMPLE* is a memory aid that you can use:

S: Symptoms from the injury or illness

A: Allergies (e.g., drugs, food, latex, environment) and tetanus status

M: Medication history

P: Past history (e.g., medical or psychiatric problems, surgeries, smoking history, use of drugs or alcohol, last menstrual period, baseline mental status)

L: Last meal/oral intake

E: Events or environment factors leading to the illness or injury

After you collect the patient's history, a head-to-toe assessment completes the H part of the secondary survey. Note any abnormalities.

Head, neck, and face. Check eyes for extraocular movements. A disconjugate gaze is a sign of neurologic damage. Battle sign, or bruising directly behind the ears, may indicate a fracture of the base or posterior part of the skull. "Raccoon eyes," or periorbital bruising, usually occurs with a fracture of the base of the frontal part of the skull. Check the ears for blood and cerebrospinal fluid. Do not block clear drainage from the ear or nose.

Abdomen and flanks. Frequent evaluation for subtle changes in the abdomen is essential. Motor vehicle crashes and assaults can cause blunt trauma. Penetrating trauma tends to injure specific organs. If the patient has blunt abdominal trauma or you suspect intraabdominal hemorrhage, perform a *focused abdominal sonography for trauma* (FAST).[11] FAST can identify blood in the peritoneal space and assess cardiac function. It is noninvasive and done quickly at the bedside. A FAST cannot rule out a retroperitoneal bleed. If we suspect a bleed, a CT scan is usually done.

Pelvis and perineum. Inspect and gently palpate the pelvis. Do not rock the pelvis. Pain may indicate a pelvic fracture and

TABLE 21.5 EMERGENCY ASSESSMENT

Secondary Survey

Assessment	Interventions
History (H_1) and Head-to-Toe Assessment (H_2)	
History	• Use the mnemonic **MIST** to obtain details of the prehospital report of the incidence or illness: **M**echanism of injury, **I**njuries sustained, **S**igns and symptoms before arrival, and **T**reatment provided before arrival. • Use the mnemonic **SAMPLE** to determine **S**ymptoms from the injury or illness; **A**llergies, including tetanus status; **M**edication history; **P**ast history (e.g., preexisting medical/psychiatric problems, last menstrual period); **L**ast meal/oral intake; and **E**vents/Environment preceding illness or injury.
Head-to-toe assessment	• Note general appearance, including skin color.
Head, neck, and face	• Assess face and scalp for lacerations, bone or soft tissue deformity, tenderness, bleeding, foreign bodies. • Inspect eyes, ears, nose, and mouth for bleeding, foreign bodies, drainage, pain, deformity, bruising, lacerations. • Palpate head for depressions of cranial or facial bones, contusions, hematomas, areas of softness, bony crepitus. • Assess neck for stiffness, pain in cervical vertebrae, tracheal deviation, distended neck veins, bleeding, edema, difficulty swallowing, bruising, subcutaneous emphysema, bony crepitus.
Chest	• Observe rate, depth, and effort of breathing, including chest wall movement and use of accessory muscles. • Palpate for bony crepitus and subcutaneous emphysema. • Auscultate breath sounds. • Obtain 12-lead ECG and chest x-ray. • Inspect for external signs of injury: petechiae, bleeding, cyanosis, bruises, abrasions, lacerations, old scars.
Abdomen and flanks	• Look for symmetry of abdominal wall and bony structures. • Inspect for external signs of injury: bruises, abrasions, lacerations, punctures, old scars. • Auscultate for bowel sounds. • Palpate for masses, guarding, femoral pulses. • Note type and location of pain, rigidity, or distention of abdomen.
Pelvis and perineum	• Gently palpate pelvis. • Assess genitalia for blood at the meatus, priapism, bruising, rectal bleeding, anal sphincter tone. • Determine ability to void.
Extremities	• Inspect for signs of external injury: deformity, bruising, abrasions, lacerations, swelling. • Observe skin color and palpate skin for pain, tenderness, temperature, and crepitus. • Evaluate movement, strength, and sensation in arms and legs. • Assess quality and symmetry of peripheral pulses.
Inspect Posterior Surfaces	• Logroll and inspect and palpate back for deformity, bleeding, lacerations, bruises. Maintain cervical spine immobilization, if appropriate.
Just Keep Reevaluating	• Use the memory aid **VIPP** to reevaluate and assess effectiveness of interventions provided: **V**ital signs, **I**njuries sustained and interventions, **P**rimary survey, and **P**ain level. • Document in the health record. • Keep the process moving along quickly. • More tests may be done, such as bronchoscopy, CT/MRI, angiography.

the need for imaging. Assess for bladder distention, hematuria, dysuria, or inability to void. The HCP may perform a rectal examination to check for blood, prostate gland problems, and loss of sphincter tone (e.g., spinal cord injury).

Extremities. Assess extremities for point tenderness, crepitus, and deformities. If not done prehospital, splint injured extremities above and below the injury to decrease further soft tissue injury and pain. The HCP should realign grossly deformed, pulseless extremities before splinting. Check pulses before and after movement or splinting of an extremity. A pulseless extremity is a time-critical emergency. Immobilize and elevate injured extremities and apply ice packs. Antibiotics are given for open fractures to prevent infection.

Assess for *compartment syndrome.* This occurs over several hours as pressure and swelling increase inside a muscle compartment of an extremity. This compromises the viability of the muscles, nerves, and arteries. Potential causes include crush injuries, fractures, edema, and hemorrhage.

I = Inspect Posterior Surfaces

An often overlooked part of the assessment is the patient's back. Logroll trauma patients while protecting the cervical spine. Up to 4 or more people with 1 person supporting the head may be needed to complete this assessment.

J = Just Keep Reevaluating

After you complete the secondary survey, record all findings. Ongoing monitoring and evaluation are critical. Provide appropriate care and assess the patient's response.

Use the memory aid *VIPP* for the reevaluation process:
V: Vital signs
I: Injuries sustained and interventions
P: Primary survey
P: Pain level

The evaluation of airway patency and the effectiveness of breathing are always the highest priorities. Monitor respiratory rate and rhythm, O_2 saturation, and ABGs (if ordered) to evaluate respiratory status. A portable chest x-ray can confirm the exact placement of tubes. Give tetanus prophylaxis based on vaccination history and the condition of any wounds (Table 21.6).[12]

Closely monitor LOC and vital signs. Note the quality of peripheral pulses and skin temperature, color, and moisture for information about circulation and perfusion. When indicated, insert an indwelling catheter to decompress the bladder, monitor urine output, and check for hematuria. Notify the HCP of any changes that may occur to the patient during this ongoing assessment process.

Depending on their injuries or illness, patients may be (1) transported for diagnostic tests (e.g., CT scan, angiography) or to the operating room for immediate surgery, (2) admitted, or (3) transferred to another facility. You may go with patients on transports. You are responsible for monitoring patients during transport, notifying the HCP if a patient becomes unstable and starting life-support measures as needed.

Cardiac Arrest and Targeted Temperature Management

Many patients arrive at the ED in cardiac arrest. Patients with nontraumatic, out-of-hospital cardiac arrest benefit from a combination of good chest compressions and rapid defibrillation, targeted temperature management (TTM), and supportive care. TTM for at least 24 hours after the return of spontaneous circulation (ROSC) decreases mortality rates and improves neurologic outcomes in many patients.[13] It is recommended for all patients who are comatose or do not follow commands after ROSC.

TTM, or therapeutic hypothermia, involves 3 phases: induction, maintenance, and rewarming. The induction phase begins in the ED. The goal core temperature is 89.6°F to 96.8°F (32°C to 36°C). We use a variety of methods to cool patients. These include icepacks, cooling pads, and blankets. We can perform endovascular cooling with a special central venous catheter.[13] Patients need mechanical ventilation and invasive monitoring and require continuous assessment. Protocols often direct the care of these patients.

Death in the Emergency Department

The loss of life in the ED is a stressful event. Death is often sudden and happens after an accident or unexpected illness. Sudden death is, by its nature, unexpected and thus shocking for family and friends. It is crucial for you to identify and manage your feelings about sudden death so you can help them begin the grieving process (see Chapter 10).

You play a key role in providing comfort. Provide a private area for family and friends to say goodbye. If appropriate, arrange for a visit from a chaplain. Assist the family by collecting personal belongings and making mortuary arrangements. At times, you may need to contact the medical examiner or coroner. An autopsy may be done at the family's request or if death occurred within 24 hours of ED admission, from suspected trauma or violence, or in an unusual way.

Some patients who die in the ED are candidates for organ donation. We can harvest certain tissues and organs (e.g., corneas, liver, pancreas, lungs, kidneys).[14] Organ procurement groups aid in screening potential donors, counseling donor families, obtaining informed consent, and harvesting organs from patients on life support or who die in the ED. Approaching caregivers about donation after an unexpected death can be distressing to both the staff and caregivers. However, for many, donation may be the first positive step in the grieving process.

Gerontologic Considerations: Emergency Care

People over the age of 65 account for a large number of ED visits.[15] Regardless of a patient's age, treatment is provided for all injuries or illnesses unless the patient has a preexisting terminal illness, an extremely low chance for survival, or an advance directive indicating a different course of action.

Understanding the physiologic and psychosocial aspects of aging will improve the care delivered to older adults in the ED (see Chapter 5). Many older adults dismiss their symptoms as

TABLE 21.6 Tetanus Vaccines and TIG for Wound Management

	TYPE OF WOUND	
Vaccination History	**Clean, Minor Wounds**	**All Other Wounds**
Age 11 and Older		
Unknown or <3 doses of tetanus vaccine	Tdap and recommend catch-up vaccination	Tdap and recommend catch-up vaccination TIG
≥3 doses of tetanus vaccine *and* <5 yr since last dose	No indication	No indication
≥3 doses of tetanus vaccine *and* 5–10 yr since last dose	No indication	Tdap preferred (if not yet received) or Td
≥3 doses of tetanus vaccine *and* >10 yr since last dose	Tdap preferred (if not yet received) or Td	Tdap preferred (if not yet received) or Td

Td, Tetanus-diphtheria toxoid absorbed; *Tdap,* tetanus toxoid, reduced diphtheria toxoid, and acellular pertussis vaccine; *TIG,* tetanus immune globulin (human).
From Centers for Disease Control and Prevention: *Tetanus.* Retrieved from www.cdc.gov/tetanus/clinicians.html.

simply "normal for their age." It is important to fully explore any complaint by an older adult.

The older population is at high risk for injury because of changes that occur with aging. Falls are the leading cause of injury.[16] Common causes of falls include weakness, environment hazards, syncope, and orthostatic hypotension. When assessing a patient who has fallen, determine whether the physical findings may have caused the fall or are related to the fall itself. For example, a patient may come to the ED with acute confusion. The confusion may be because of a stroke that caused the patient to fall. Or the patient may have a head injury because of a fall from tripping on a rug.

ENVIRONMENT EMERGENCIES

Emergencies discussed here include heat- and cold-related illnesses, submersion injuries, bites, stings, and envenomation. Increased interest in outdoor activities, such as running, cycling, skiing, and swimming, has increased the number of environment emergencies seen in the ED. Illness or injury may be caused by the activity, exposure to weather, or attack from animals or humans.

HEAT-RELATED ILLNESS

Brief exposure to intense heat or prolonged exposure to less intense heat leads to heat stress. This occurs when thermoregulatory mechanisms, such as sweating, vasodilation, and increased respirations, cannot compensate for exposure to increased ambient temperatures. Ambient temperature is a product of environment temperature and humidity. Strenuous activities in hot or humid environments, clothing that interferes with perspiration, fever, and preexisting illness predispose people to heat stress (Table 21.7). Table 21.8 presents the management of heat-related illnesses.

TABLE 21.7 Risk Factors for Heat-Related Emergencies

Age	• Infants • Older adults
Environment	• High humidity • Lack of access to water, shelter, or shade • Lack of acclimatization • Physical exertion, especially during hot weather • Prolonged exposure to high temperature
Preexisting Illness	• Dehydration • Diabetes • Head injury • Heart disease • Obesity • Sickle cell disease • Skin disorders (e.g., large burn scars) • Spinal cord injury • Stroke or other CNS lesion • Thyrotoxicosis
Prescription Drugs	• Anticholinergics • Antihistamines • Antipsychotics • β-Adrenergic blockers • Benzodiazepines • Calcium channel blockers • Diuretics • Phenothiazines • Thyroid agonists • Tricyclic antidepressants
Substance Use	• Alcohol • Street drugs: Amphetamines, cocaine

Heat Cramps

Heat cramps are severe cramps in large muscle groups fatigued by heavy work.[17] Cramps are brief and intense and tend to occur during rest after exercise or heavy labor. Nausea, tachycardia, pallor, weakness, and profuse sweating are often present. The condition occurs most often in healthy, acclimated athletes with inadequate fluid intake. Cramps resolve rapidly with rest and oral or IV replacement of sodium and water. Elevation, gentle massage, and analgesia minimize pain from heat cramps. Tell the patient to avoid strenuous activity for at least 12 hours. When discharge teaching, emphasize salt replacement during strenuous exercise in hot, humid environments. Recommend the use of commercially prepared electrolyte solutions.

Heat Exhaustion

Prolonged exposure to heat over hours or days leads to **heat exhaustion**. Symptoms include fatigue, nausea and vomiting, and extreme thirst. Hypotension, tachycardia, elevated body temperature, dilated pupils, mild confusion, ashen color, and profuse sweating are present. Heat exhaustion usually occurs in people engaged in strenuous activity in hot, humid weather.

Provide oral and IV fluid replacement as ordered. Implement evaporative cooling measures. Consider hospital admission for older adults, the chronically ill, or those who do not improve within 3 to 4 hours.

Heatstroke

Heatstroke is the most severe form of heat stress. It is a medical emergency. Heatstroke results from failure of hypothalamic thermoregulatory processes. Increased sweating, vasodilation, and increased respiratory rate deplete fluids and electrolytes, specifically sodium. Eventually, sweat glands stop functioning. Core temperature increases rapidly, within 10 to 15 minutes. The brain is highly sensitive to thermal injuries. Cerebral edema and hemorrhage may occur from direct thermal injury to the brain and decreased cerebral blood flow. Death from heatstroke is directly related to the amount of time that the body temperature is high.[17] Prognosis is related to age, health status, and length of exposure. Older adults and those with diabetes, chronic kidney disease, heart disease, or lung disease are more prone.

TABLE 21.8 EMERGENCY MANAGEMENT

Hyperthermia

Assessment Findings	Interventions
Heat Cramps • Severe muscle contractions in exerted muscles • Thirst **Heat Exhaustion** • Altered mental status (e.g., anxiety) • Ashen, pale skin • ↓ BP • Extreme thirst • Fatigue, weakness • ↑ HR • Profuse sweating • Temperature (99.6°F–105.8°F [37.5°C–41°C]) • Weak, thready pulse **Heatstroke** • Altered mental status (ranging from confusion to coma) • ↓ BP • Hot, dry skin • ↑ HR • Tachypnea • Temperature >105.8°F (41°C) • Weakness	**Initial** • Manage and maintain ABCs. • Provide high-flow O_2 via non-rebreather mask or BVM. • Establish IV access. • Begin IV fluid replacement for significant heat injury. • Place patient in a cool environment. • For heatstroke, start rapid cooling measures: remove patient's clothing, place wet sheets over patient, and place in front of fan; immerse in a cool water bath; give cool IV fluids or lavage with cool fluids. • Obtain 12-lead ECG. • Obtain blood for electrolytes and CBC. • Insert urinary catheter. **Ongoing Monitoring** • Monitor ABCs, temperature and vital signs, level of consciousness. • Monitor heart rhythm, O_2 saturation, urine output. • Replace electrolytes as needed. • Monitor urine for myoglobinuria. • Monitor clotting studies for disseminated intravascular coagulation.

Interprofessional Care

Treatment focuses on stabilizing the patient's ABCs, rapidly reducing the core temperature, and monitoring for dysrhythmias. Give 100% O_2 to compensate for the hypermetabolic state. Ventilation with a BVM or intubation and mechanical ventilation may be needed. Place the patient on continuous ECG monitoring and pulse oximetry. Monitor laboratory findings. Correcting electrolyte imbalances and coagulation abnormalities is critical.

The most effective treatment for heatstroke is cold water immersion.[17] You can also place the patient in a cool environment. Other measures to consider include spraying the patient with cool water in front of a large fan, placing a moist sheet over the patient, or applying ice packs to the groin and axillae. In refractory cases, we may perform peritoneal or rectal lavage with iced fluids.

Monitor the patient's temperature and control shivering. Shivering increases core temperature because of the heat generated by muscle activity, which blocks cooling efforts. The HCP may order drugs to control shivering.

Heatstroke places patients at risk for kidney injury because of *rhabdomyolysis*. It is a serious syndrome caused by the breakdown of skeletal muscle. Carefully monitor the urine for color, amount, pH, and myoglobin.

Discharge teaching focuses on how to avoid future problems. Stress the importance of proper hydration and wearing appropriate clothing. Teach patients the early signs of and interventions for heat-related stress. Encourage caregivers to check on those at risk during periods of high temperatures. They should ensure adequate water intake, verify operable air conditioning, and assess for heat-related illness.

COLD-RELATED INJURIES

Cold injuries may be local (e.g., frostbite) or systemic (e.g., hypothermia). Contributing factors include age, duration of exposure, ambient temperature, homelessness, preexisting conditions, drugs that suppress shivering, and alcohol intoxication. Smokers have an increased risk because of the vasoconstrictive effects of nicotine.

Frostbite

Frostbite is true tissue freezing that results in the formation of ice crystals in the tissues and cells. Peripheral vasoconstriction is the first response to cold stress. It results in a decrease in blood flow and vascular stasis. As cell temperature decreases, ice crystals form in intracellular spaces. The organelles are damaged, and the cell membrane is destroyed. This results in edema.

Most (90%) cases involve the hands and feet. The cheeks, nose, ears, and penis are also commonly affected.[18] There are 4 degrees of frostbite (Fig. 21.2). The depth depends on ambient temperature, length of exposure, type and condition (wet or dry) of clothing, wind chill, and contact with metal surfaces. Other factors that affect severity include previous frostbite injury, exhaustion, and poor peripheral vascular status.

Superficial frostbite (grades 1 and 2) involves the skin and subcutaneous tissue, usually the ears, nose, fingers, and toes. The skin appearance ranges from waxy pale yellow, to blue, to mottled. The skin feels crunchy and frozen. Patients may report tingling, numbness, or a burning sensation. Handle the area carefully and never squeeze, massage, or scrub the injured tissue because it is easily damaged. Swelling will occur with thawing. Remove clothing and jewelry, as they may constrict the extremity and decrease circulation.

Immerse the affected area in circulating temperature-controlled water (99.0°F to 102°F) [37.2°C to 38.9°C]).[18] Use warm soaks for the face. Patients often have a warm, stinging sensation as tissue thaws. Blisters form within a few hours. Debride the blisters and apply a sterile dressing. Avoid heavy blankets and clothing because friction and weight can lead to sloughing of damaged tissue. Rewarming is very painful. Residual pain may last weeks or even years. Give prescribed analgesia and tetanus prophylaxis. Assess the patient for systemic hypothermia.

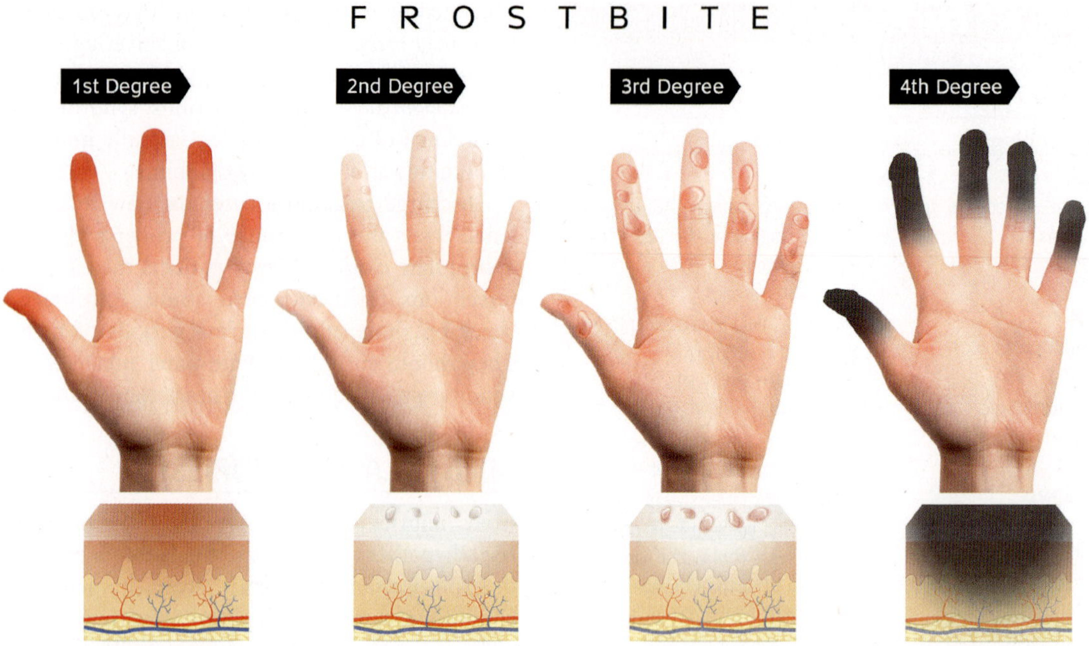

FROSTBITE

1st Degree 2nd Degree 3rd Degree 4th Degree

Fig. 21.2 Grades of frostbite injury. (From Persitz J, Essa A, Ner EB, et al: Frostbite of the extremities: recognition, evaluation, and treatment, *Injury* 53:3088, 2022.)

Deep frostbite (grades 3 and 4) involves muscle, bone, and tendon. The skin is white, hard, and insensitive to touch. The area has the appearance of deep thermal injury with mottling, gradually progressing to gangrene. Immerse the affected extremity in a temperature-controlled, circulating water bath (99.0°F to 102°F) [37.2°C to 38.9°C]) until flushing occurs distal to the injured area.[18]

After rewarming, elevate the extremity to reduce edema. Significant edema may begin within 3 hours, with blistering in 6 hours to days. Give IV analgesia to manage the pain from tissue thawing. All patients should start on nonsteroidal antiinflammatory drugs (NSAIDs) because of their dual role as an analgesic and antiinflammatory. Give tetanus prophylaxis. Assess the patient for systemic hypothermia.

Treatment options to reduce tissue damage with deep frostbite include thrombolytic therapy, anticoagulants, vasodilators, hyperbaric O_2 therapy, and local anesthesia.[18] Amputation may be needed if the injured area is not treated or if treatment is unsuccessful. It may take as long as 90 days to determine the final necrotic area. Prophylactic antibiotics are given if the wound is at risk for infection.

Hypothermia

Hypothermia is a core temperature below 95°F (35°C).[19] It occurs when heat produced by the body cannot compensate for heat lost to the environment. This may occur in a healthy person with environment exposure (primary) or someone with a specific condition that produces hypothermia (secondary). Risk factors include exposure to freezing temperatures, cold winds, and wet terrain; medications (e.g., phenothiazines, neuromuscular blocking agents); alcohol use; traumatic injury; shock; and diabetes.[5] Wet clothing, inadequate clothing, and immersion in cold water (e.g., drowning) increase evaporative heat loss. Older adults are more prone because of decreased body fat, decreased energy reserves, decreased basal metabolic rate, decreased shivering response, and chronic medical problems. Peripheral vasoconstriction is the body's first attempt to conserve heat. As cold temperatures persist, shivering and movement are the body's only way to produce heat.

Assessment findings vary and depend on core temperature (Table 21.9). Patients with *mild hypothermia* (93°F to 95°F [33.9°C to 35°C]) have shivering, lethargy, confusion, behavior changes, and minor heart rate changes. *Moderate hypothermia* (86°F to 93°F [30°C to 33.9°C]) causes rigidity, bradycardia, slowed respiratory rate, BP obtainable only by Doppler, metabolic and respiratory acidosis, and hypovolemia. Shivering decreases or disappears at core temperatures of 86°F (30°C).[19]

As core temperature drops, metabolic rate decreases 2 to 3 times. The cold myocardium is very irritable, making it vulnerable to dysrhythmias (e.g., atrial and ventricular fibrillation). Decreased renal blood flow decreases glomerular filtration rate, which impairs water reabsorption and leads to dehydration. The hematocrit increases as intravascular volume decreases. Cold blood becomes thick and acts as a thrombus, placing patients at risk for stroke, myocardial infarction (MI), pulmonary emboli, and renal failure. Decreased blood flow leads to hypoxia, anaerobic metabolism, lactic acid accumulation, and metabolic acidosis.

Severe hypothermia (below 86°F [30°C]) makes the person appear dead and is a life-threatening situation. Metabolic rate, heart rate, and respirations are so slow that they may be hard to detect. Reflexes are absent. The pupils are fixed and dilated. Profound bradycardia, ventricular fibrillation, or pulseless

TABLE 21.9 EMERGENCY MANAGEMENT

Hypothermia

Cause	Assessment Findings	Interventions

Environment
• Inadequate clothing for environment temperature
• Prolonged exposure to cold
• Prolonged immersion or near-drowning
 	
Health Care Associated
• Blood administration
• Cold IV fluids
• Inadequate warming or rewarming in the ED or operating room
• Receiving neuromuscular blocking agents
 	
Metabolic
• Hypoglycemia
• Hypothyroidism
 	
Other
• Alcohol
• Barbiturates
• Phenothiazines
• Shock
• Trauma
	• Core body temperature:
	  • *Mild hypothermia:* 93°F–95°F (33.9°C–35°C)
	  • *Moderate hypothermia:* 86°F–93°F (30°C–33.9°C)
	  • *Severe hypothermia:* <86°F (30°C)
	• Shivering, ↓ or absent at core body temperatures ≥86°F (30°C)
	• Absence of reflexes
	• Altered mental status
	• Blue, white, or frozen extremities
	• ↓BP
	• Cyanotic, pale skin
	• Dysrhythmias: bradycardia, atrial fibrillation, ventricular fibrillation, asystole
	• Fixed, dilated pupils
	• Hypoventilation
		Initial
		• Remove patient from cold environment.
		• Manage and maintain ABCs.
		• Provide high-flow O_2 via nonrebreather mask or BVM.
		• Anticipate intubation for decreased or absent gag reflex.
		• Establish IV access with 2 large-bore catheters for fluid resuscitation.
		• Rewarm patient:
		  • *Passive:* Remove wet clothing, apply dry clothing and warm blankets, use radiant lights.
		  • *Active external:* Apply heating devices (e.g., air- or fluid-filled warming blankets), use warm water immersion.
		  • *Active internal:* Provide warmed IV fluids; heated, humidified O_2. Peritoneal lavage with warmed fluids. Extracorporeal circulation (e.g., cardiopulmonary bypass, rapid fluid infuser, hemodialysis).
		• Obtain 12-lead ECG.
		• Anticipate need for defibrillation.
		• Warm central trunk first in patients with severe hypothermia to limit rewarming shock.
		• Assess for other injuries.
		• Keep head covered with warm, dry towels or stocking cap to limit loss of heat.
		• Treat patient gently to avoid increased cardiac irritability.
		
		Ongoing Monitoring
		• Monitor ABCs, temperature, level of consciousness, and vital signs.
		• Monitor O_2 saturation, heart rate, and rhythm.
		• Monitor electrolytes, glucose.

electrical activity may be present. Effort is made to warm the patient to at least 86°F (30°C) before pronouncing the person dead. The cause of death is usually ventricular fibrillation.

Interprofessional Care

Treatment focuses on managing and maintaining ABCs, rewarming the patient, correcting dehydration and acidosis, and treating dysrhythmias. Mildly hypothermic patients may be rewarmed with passive and active external measures because their risk for dysrhythmia is low. Those with moderate or severe hypothermia need active internal rewarming measures.

Carefully monitor core temperature during rewarming. Rewarming places patients at risk for *afterdrop*, a further drop in core temperature. This occurs when cold peripheral blood returns to the central circulation. Rewarming shock can produce hypotension and dysrhythmias. Thus patients with moderate to severe hypothermia should have the core warmed before the extremities. Discontinue active rewarming once the core temperature reaches 90°F to 95°F (32.2°C to 35°C).

Patient teaching focuses on how to avoid future cold-related problems. Include dressing in layers for cold weather, covering the head, carrying high-carbohydrate foods for extra calories, and developing a survival plan should an injury occur in an extreme environment.

CHECK YOUR PRACTICE

You are working in the ED when the paramedics arrive with a patient who was found lying on the sidewalk outside the bus station. He is wearing only a lightweight shirt and pants. The outdoor temperature is 12°F (−11.1°C). The patient is unresponsive. Initial vital signs are as follows: rectal temperature = 89.5°F (31.9°C), HR = 38, RR = 8, BP (by Doppler) = 86 mm Hg.

- What are your priority interventions?

SUBMERSION INJURIES

Submersion injury results when a person becomes hypoxic from submersion in a liquid, usually water. Around 4000 deaths from drowning occur each year in the United States.[20] Most victims are children younger than 4 years.[21] The main risk factors include the inability to swim, substance use, poor judgment, trauma, seizures, hypothermia, stroke, and child neglect. Aggressive resuscitation efforts (e.g., airway and ventilation management) improve survival, especially in the prehospital phase.

Drowning is the process of experiencing respiratory impairment after submersion in water or other fluid.[20] Submersion in cold water (below 32°F [0°C]) may slow the progression of hypoxic brain injury. Most drowning victims do not aspirate any liquid because of laryngospasm. If liquid is aspirated, it is in small amounts. Those who do aspirate water develop pulmonary edema, which can cause acute respiratory distress syndrome (see Chapter 32).

The osmotic gradient caused by aspirated fluid leads to fluid imbalances (Fig. 21.3). Hypotonic freshwater is rapidly absorbed into the circulatory system through the alveoli. Freshwater is often contaminated with chlorine, mud, or algae. This causes the breakdown of lung surfactant, fluid seepage, and pulmonary edema.

Hypertonic saltwater draws fluid from the vascular space into the alveoli, impairing alveolar ventilation and causing hypoxia. The body tries to compensate for hypoxia by shunting blood to the lungs. This results in increased pulmonary pressures and deteriorating respiratory status. More and more blood is shunted through the alveoli. Because the blood is not adequately oxygenated, hypoxemia worsens. This causes cerebral injury, edema, and brain death.

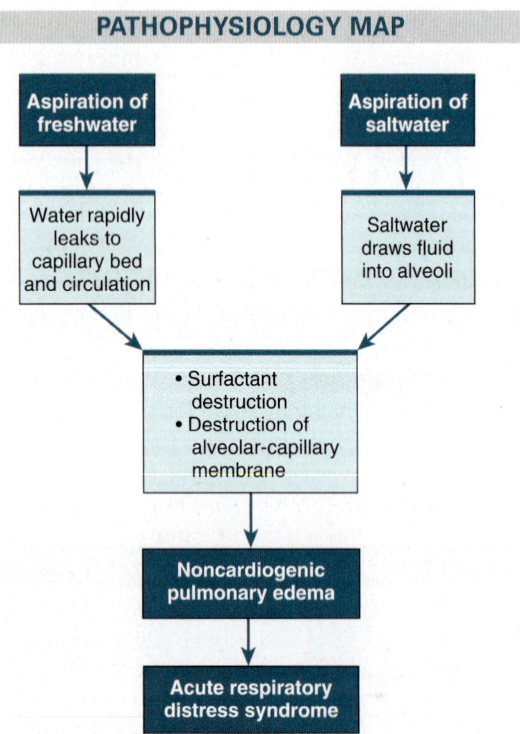

Fig. 21.3 Pathophysiology of submersion injury.

Interprofessional Care

Treatment focuses on correcting hypoxia and fluid imbalances, supporting basic physiologic functions, and rewarming when hypothermia is present. Initial evaluation involves assessing the airway, cervical spine, breathing, and circulation (Table 21.10). Mechanical ventilation with positive end-expiratory pressure or continuous positive airway pressure can improve gas exchange across the alveolar-capillary membrane when pulmonary edema is present (see Chapter 28).

Declining neurologic status suggests cerebral edema, worsening hypoxia, or profound acidosis. Drowning victims may have head and neck injuries that cause changes in the LOC. Complications can develop in patients who are free of symptoms immediately after the drowning episode. Consequently, observe all victims of drowning in a hospital for a minimum of 4 to 8 hours.[20]

Patient teaching focuses on water safety and how to reduce the risks of drowning. Remind patients and caregivers to lock all swimming pool gates; use life jackets on all watercrafts, including inner tubes and rafts; and learn water survival skills. Emphasize the dangers of combining alcohol and drugs with swimming and other water sports.

STINGS AND BITES

Animals, spiders, snakes, and insects cause injury and even death by biting or stinging. Morbidity is a result of either direct tissue damage or lethal toxins. Direct tissue damage is related to the animal's size, teeth characteristics, and jaw strength. Tissue may be lacerated, crushed, or chewed. Teeth, fangs, stingers, spines, or tentacles release toxins that have local or systemic effects. Death from an animal bite is the result of blood loss, allergic reactions, or lethal toxins.

Hymenopteran Stings

The *Hymenoptera* family includes bees, yellow jackets, hornets, wasps, and fire ants. Stings can cause mild discomfort or life-threatening anaphylaxis (see Chapter 42). Venom may be cytotoxic, hemolytic, allergenic, or vasoactive. Symptoms may begin immediately or be delayed up to 48 hours. Reactions are more severe with multiple stings. Most hymenopterans sting repeatedly. However, the domestic honeybee stings only once, usually leaving a barbed stinger with an attached venom sac in the skin so that venom release continues.[22]

African honeybees (killer bees) aggressively swarm if threatened. They can repeatedly sting their victims. These attacks can be fatal.

TABLE 21.10 EMERGENCY MANAGEMENT

Submersion Injuries

Cause	Assessment Findings	Interventions
• Entrapment or entanglement with objects in water • Inability to swim or exhaustion while swimming • Loss of ability to move secondary to trauma, stroke, hypothermia, MI • Poor judgment because of alcohol or drugs • Seizure while in water	**Cardiac** • ↓ BP • Bradycardia • Dysrhythmias • ↑ HR • Cardiac arrest **Respiratory** • Cough with pink-frothy sputum • Crackles, rhonchi • Cyanosis • Dyspnea • Respiratory distress • Respiratory arrest **Other** • Exhaustion • Coma • Coexisting illness (e.g., MI) or injury (e.g., cervical spine injury) • Core temperature slightly elevated or below normal, depending on water temperature and length of submersion • Panic	**Initial** • Manage and maintain ABCs. • Assume cervical spine injury in all drowning victims and stabilize or immobilize cervical spine. • Provide 100% O_2 via nonrebreather mask or BVM. • Anticipate need for mechanical ventilation if airway is compromised (e.g., absent gag reflex). • Establish IV access with 2 large-bore catheters for fluid resuscitation and infuse warmed fluids, if appropriate. • Obtain 12-lead ECG. • Assess for other injuries. • Remove wet clothing and cover with warm blankets. • Obtain temperature and begin rewarming, if needed. • Obtain cervical spine and chest x-rays. • Insert gastric tube and urinary catheter. **Ongoing Monitoring** • Monitor ABCs, vital signs, level of consciousness. • Monitor O_2 saturation, heart rate, and rhythm. • Monitor temperature and maintain normothermia. • Monitor for signs of acute respiratory failure.

! SAFETY ALERT

Hymenopteran Stings

- Remove the stinger using a scraping motion with a thin, flat object, like a fingernail, knife, or credit card.
- Do not use tweezers because they may squeeze the stinger and release more venom.
- Remove rings, watches, or any restrictive clothing around the sting site.

Manifestations of mild reactions include stinging, burning, swelling, and itching. More severe reactions may present with edema, headache, fever, syncope, malaise, nausea, vomiting, wheezing, bronchospasm, laryngeal edema, and hypotension. Treatment depends on the severity of the reaction. Treat mild reactions with elevation, cool compresses, antipruritic lotions, and oral antihistamines. More severe reactions require IM or IV antihistamines, subcutaneous epinephrine, and corticosteroids. Chapter 15 discusses allergic reactions and related patient teaching.

Snake Bites

There are more than 45,000 snakebites each year in the United States. *Envenomation* (poisoning by venom) occurs in about 8000 cases, with only 5 deaths each year.[23] The 2 families of venomous snakes found in the United States are Crotalidae, or pit vipers (rattlesnakes, copperheads, cottonmouths), and Elapidae (coral snakes). Almost all the venomous bites are from pit vipers.

Snake venom may be hemolytic, neurotoxic, vascular toxic, or any combination of these. When bites occur, you will see fang or puncture marks. Patients often have severe pain at the site. There may be swelling, discoloration, and blistering. If moderate envenomation has occurred, the patient will have paresthesias, lymphadenopathy, and nausea and vomiting. Treatment includes wound care and tetanus prophylaxis. Immobilize the affected extremity. Remove potentially constricting clothing. Most bites are minor and resolve without antivenom therapy. We observe the patient for at least 8 hours to ensure no life- or limb-threatening symptoms develop.

Manifestations of severe envenomation include profound edema, tachycardia, blurred vision, headache, chills, paresthesias, hypotension, and muscle twitching. The patient may report a metallic taste in the mouth. As symptoms progress, pulmonary edema, coagulopathy, thrombocytopenia, and hemorrhage may develop.

Snakebites from exotic species are mainly neurotoxic. They cause autonomic dysfunction, paralysis, and dysrhythmias.

Treatment of severe envenomation requires close patient monitoring. The ABCs are most important! Anticipate fluid resuscitation and provide respiratory support. Monitor limb circumference every 30 minutes. Mark any advancing edema. Monitor laboratory results. On rare occasions, the patient will need a fasciotomy.[24] The HCP will discuss the bite with the poison control center. The decision to give antivenom is in consultation with a snake venom expert. There is specific antivenom therapy, often obtained from a zoo, for each species. Antivenom is given only if symptom progression occurs and platelet and coagulation studies are abnormal.

Tick Bites

Ticks live throughout the United States. Specific types are more prevalent in certain regions. Tickborne pathogens can be passed to humans by the bite of an infected tick. Common tickborne illnesses include Lyme disease, Rocky Mountain spotted fever, anaplasmosis, Colorado tick fever, tickborne relapsing fever, and tularemia.[25] Chapter 69 discusses more about Lyme disease.

Ticks transmit pathogens that cause disease through their feeding process. The infected tick attaches to its host and can slowly feed for up to several days. During this time, saliva from the tick can be transferred to the host. Tick saliva may harbor pathogens acquired by the tick from a prior host. The tick should be removed as soon as possible to stop the flow of saliva. Use forceps or tweezers to grasp the tick close to the point of attachment and pull upward in a steady motion (Fig. 21.4). After you remove the tick, clean the skin with soap and water. Do not use a hot match, petroleum jelly, nail polish, or other products to remove the tick. These measures may cause a tick to salivate, thus increasing the risk for infection.

Rocky Mountain spotted fever is the most lethal tick disease.[25] It is caused by *Rickettsia rickettsii,* which is spread to humans by the ixodid tick. The incubation period is 2 to 14 days. A pink macular rash appears on the palms, wrists, soles, feet, and ankles. Other symptoms include fever, chills, malaise, muscle pain, and headache. It is hard to diagnosis in the early stages. Without treatment, the disease can be fatal. Antibiotic therapy with doxycycline is the treatment of choice.

Animal and Human Bites

Every year more than 5 million animal bites are reported in the United States. Animal bites from dogs and cats are the most common. Wild or domestic rodents (e.g., squirrels, hamsters) follow as the third most common offenders. The few bite deaths (15 to 20) are mainly from dogs. The greatest problems from animal bites are infection and destruction of skin, muscle, tendons, blood vessels, and bone. The bite may cause a simple laceration or cause a crush injury, puncture wound, or tearing of multiple layers of tissue (Fig. 21.5). The severity of the injury depends on animal size, victim size, and anatomic location of the bite. Children are at greatest risk.[26]

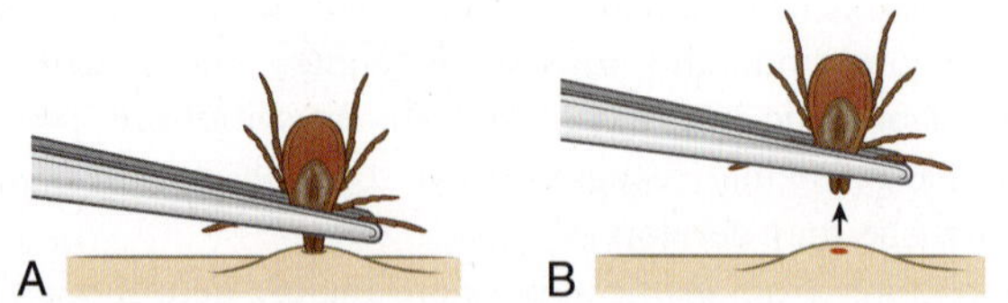

Fig. 21.4 Tick removal. (A) Use tweezers to grasp the tick close to the skin. (B) With a steady motion, pull the tick's body up and away from the skin. Do not be alarmed if the tick's mouthparts stay in the skin. Once the mouthparts are removed from the rest of the tick, it can no longer transmit disease.

Dog bites usually occur on the extremities. Facial bites are common in small children. Cat bites can cause deep puncture wounds. They can involve tendons and joint capsules. There is a greater risk for infection than with dog bites. Septic arthritis, osteomyelitis, and tenosynovitis can occur. The most common infectious organisms from dog and cat bites are the *Pasteurella* species (e.g., *Pasteurella multocida*). Most healthy cats and dogs carry this organism in their mouths.

The human jaw has great crushing ability, causing laceration, puncture, crush injury, soft tissue tearing, and even amputation. Hands, fingers, ears, nose, vagina, and penis are the most common sites of human bites. Often these injuries are the result of violence or sexual activity. There is a high risk of infection from oral bacterial flora, most often *Staphylococcus aureus, Streptococcus* organisms, and hepatitis virus. Infection risk is influenced by the injury's type, location, and extent; patient comorbidities; and time elapsed from the injury to seeking health care.[26] Initial signs of infection include severe pain, edema, and redness at the injury site.

Interprofessional Care

Obtain a history of the bite injury. Note whether an animal was known to the victim or not (and, if not, if it was domestic or wild), the immunization status of the animal and patient, and the patient's comorbidities.[26] Assess the wound. Clean the wound, followed by copious irrigation with sterile saline. Assist

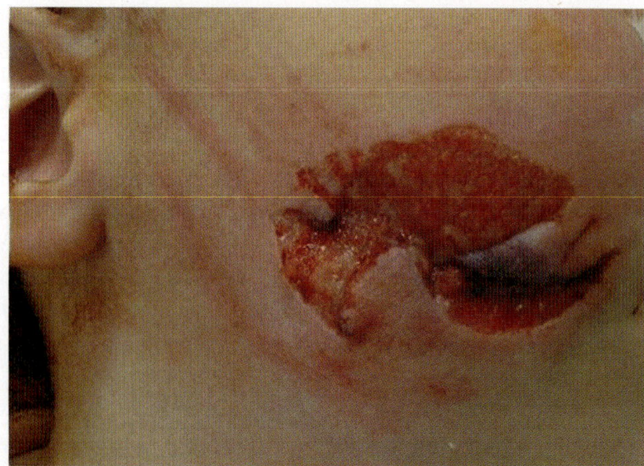
Fig. 21.5 Dog bite wound. (From Khan K, Horswell BB, Samanta D: Dog-bite injuries to the craniofacial region, *J Oral Maxillofac Surg* 78:401, 2020.)

the HCP with any debridement or wound closure. We often leave puncture wounds open. Lacerations may be loosely sutured. Plastic surgery consultation may be needed for disfiguring facial wounds. Splint wounds over joints.

Provide tetanus prophylaxis and analgesics as needed. Prophylactic antibiotics are used for bites at risk for infection. These include wounds over joints, those older than 6 to 12 hours, puncture wounds, and bites of the hand or foot. People at greatest risk for infection are infants, older adults, immunosuppressed patients, patients with substance or alcohol use disorder, people with diabetes, or those taking corticosteroids. Report a bite injury to the police as required.

Consider rabies postexposure prophylaxis in the management of all animal bites. Rabies is caused by a neurotoxic virus in the saliva of an infected animal. Most rabies carriers are wild animals, like raccoons, skunks, bats, foxes, and coyotes. Rabies is usually transmitted through the saliva via a bite by the infected animal. If the saliva from the infected animal has come in contact with its claws, theoretically rabies may be transmitted through a scratch. The virus spreads through the central nervous system (CNS) via peripheral nerves. People who develop rabies may have flulike symptoms, confusion, paresthesias, or numbness, resulting in death.

Consider rabies exposure if an animal attack was not provoked, involves a wild animal, or involves a domestic animal not immunized against rabies. Always provide postexposure vaccinations when the animal is not found or a wild animal caused the bite. The series of 4 rabies vaccine injections (human diploid cell rabies vaccine [HDCV, Imovax Rabies]) are given on days 0, 3, 7, and 14 to provide active immunity.[27] Give an initial, weight-based dose of rabies immune globulin (RIG [HyperRab S/D]) to provide passive immunity at the same time as the first dose of vaccine.

DRUG ALERT

Rabies Postexposure Prophylaxis

- If possible, give the calculated dose of RIG via infiltration around the wound edges.
- Give any remaining volume of RIG IM at a site distant from the vaccine site (e.g., gluteal site for bite wounds on the arm).
- Give the HDCV IM in the deltoid.

POISONING

A poison is any chemical that harms the body. More than 2 million cases of poisoning occur each year in the United States. Poisonings can be accidental, occupational, recreational, or intentional. Poisoning may be caused by toxic plants or contaminated foods (see Chapter 46). Toxins can be ingested, inhaled, injected, splashed in the eye, or absorbed through the skin. Chapter 11 discusses emergencies related to substance use.

The severity of the poisoning depends on the type, concentration, and route of exposure (Table 21.11). Toxins can affect every tissue of the body, so symptoms can be seen in any body system. Specific management of toxins involves decreasing absorption, enhancing elimination, and implementing toxin-specific treatment. Consult the local poison control center (available 24 hours a day) for the current treatment protocols for specific poisons.[28] Binding agents, such as activated charcoal, cathartics, hemodialysis, urine alkalinization, and antidotes, may be given to increase the elimination of poisons.[28] Chelating agents are indicated for poisonings by some metals, such as lead, arsenic, mercury, and iron.

Decontamination takes priority over all care except those needed for life support. Wear personal protective equipment (PPE) for decontamination to prevent secondary exposure. In some cases, decontamination is done by those specially trained in hazardous material decontamination before the patient arrives at the hospital and again at the hospital if needed.

Skin and eye decontamination involves removing toxins from the skin and eyes using copious amounts of water or saline. Most toxins can be safely removed with water or saline. As a rule, brush dry substances from the skin and clothing before using water. Do not remove powdered lime or mustard gas with water. Just brush lime off. Water mixes with mustard gas and releases chlorine gas.

Focus patient teaching on how the poisoning occurred. Arrange for an evaluation and follow-up by a mental health professional for all patients who have poisoning because of a suicide attempt or substance use.

Many health care workers are at risk for exposure to hazardous materials (e.g., antineoplastic drugs, cleaning agents). Consult the Material Safety Data Sheet for specific information about hazardous agents in the workplace. The Occupational Safety and Health Administration (OSHA) should evaluate all poisoning related to a workplace hazard.

VIOLENCE

Violence is physical actions that are intended to hurt or cause harm to someone or something. It may be the result of organic disease (e.g., temporal lobe epilepsy), psychosis (e.g., schizophrenia), or criminal behavior (e.g., assault, murder). A patient cared for in the ED may be the victim or the perpetrator of violence. Violence can take place in a variety of settings, including the home, community, and workplace.

EDs are high-risk areas for *workplace violence*.[29] Measures to protect staff include on-site security personnel, metal detectors, surveillance cameras, staff trained in self-defense, and locked access doors. EDs should have a comprehensive workplace violence prevention program.[29]

An ED nurse must be aware of *family and intimate partner violence* (IPV) or the possibility of a patient being a victim or perpetrator of human trafficking. IPV occurs in all cultures, socioeconomic groups, age groups, and genders. Most victims of family violence and IPV are women, children, and older adults. IPV and human trafficking are coercive behavior

TABLE 21.11 **Common Poisons**

Poison	Manifestations	Treatment
Acetaminophen (Tylenol)	*Phase 1* (within 24 h of ingestion): Malaise, diaphoresis, nausea, vomiting *Phase 2* (24–28 h after ingestion): Right upper quadrant pain, ↓ urine output, ↓ nausea, ↑LFTs *Phase 3* (72–96 h after ingestion): Nausea, vomiting, malaise, jaundice, hypoglycemia, enlarged liver, impaired coagulation including DIC *Phase 4* (7–8 days after ingestion): Recovery, resolution of symptoms or permanent liver damage, LFTs remain high	Activated charcoal, *N*-acetylcysteine (oral form may cause vomiting, IV form can be used).
Acids and Alkalis		
• *Acids:* Toilet bowl cleaners, antirust compounds • *Alkalis:* Drain cleaners, dishwashing detergents, ammonia	Excess salivation, dysphagia, epigastric pain, pneumonitis; burns of mouth, esophagus, and stomach	Immediate dilution (water, milk), corticosteroids (for alkali burns). Do not induce vomiting.
• Aspirin and aspirin-containing drugs	Tachypnea, ↑ HR, fever, seizures, pulmonary edema, occult bleeding or hemorrhage, metabolic acidosis	Activated charcoal, gastric lavage, urine alkalinization, hemodialysis for severe acute ingestion, mechanical ventilation, supportive care.
Bleaches	Irritation of lips, mouth, and eyes, superficial injury to esophagus; chemical pneumonia and pulmonary edema	Washing of exposed skin and eyes, dilution with water and milk, gastric lavage. Do not induce vomiting.
Carbon monoxide	Dyspnea, headache, tachypnea, confusion, impaired judgment, cyanosis, respiratory depression	Remove from source, apply 100% O_2 via nonrebreather mask, BVM, or mechanical ventilation; consider hyperbaric O_2 therapy.
Cyanide	*In small amounts:* Almond odor to breath, headache, dizziness, nausea, confusion, weakness, ↑ BP, ↑ HR, tachypnea *In large amounts:* Seizures, ↓ BP, bradypnea and respiratory arrest, ↓ HR, coma	IV hydroxocobalamin, IV sodium nitrate, IV sodium thiosulfate, supportive care.
Ethylene glycol (antifreeze)	Sweet aromatic odor to breath, nausea, vomiting, slurred speech, ataxia, lethargy, respiratory depression	Activated charcoal, gastric lavage, supportive care.
Iron	Vomiting (often bloody), diarrhea (often bloody), fever, hyperglycemia, lethargy, ↓ BP, seizures, coma	Gastric lavage, chelation therapy (deferoxamine [Desferal]).
NSAIDs	Gastroenteritis, abdominal pain, drowsiness, nystagmus, liver and kidney damage	Activated charcoal, gastric lavage, supportive care.
Tricyclic antidepressants (e.g., amitriptyline)	*In low doses:* Anticholinergic effects, agitation, ↑ BP, ↑ HR *In high doses:* CNS depression, dysrhythmias, ↓ BP, respiratory depression	Multidose activated charcoal, gastric lavage, serum alkalinization with sodium bicarbonate, mechanical ventilation, supportive care. Do not induce vomiting.

patterns in relationships that involve fear, humiliation, intimidation, neglect, or intentional physical, emotional, financial, or sexual injury. See Chapter 58 for information on sexual assault.

Human trafficking involves using force, fraud, or coercion to force the victim to provide labor, services, or a commercial sex act. Risk factors for being a victim include recent migration or relocation, substance use, mental health problems, involvement with the child welfare system, and being a runaway or homeless youth. Traffickers often identify and use their victims' vulnerabilities to create dependency.

It is likely that the ED nurse will come in contact with either a victim or perpetrator of human trafficking. A significant number of human trafficking victims use the ED as their sole source of medical care.[30] Common reasons victims present to the ED include physical injuries, such as fractures and lacerations, infections, reproductive health problems, toxicologic emergencies, and mental health problems such as suicide. ED nurses are uniquely positioned to help identify and report a trafficking victim or perpetrator to the proper authorities.

In the ED, we must screen for family violence and IPV. Ask questions such as, "Do you feel safe at home? Is anyone hurting you?" Barriers to effective screening include lack of privacy, fear of offending the patient, lack of time, and discomfort with the topic. Developing and implementing policies, procedures, and staff education programs improve screening practices.

Be sensitive when gathering information about suspected abuse and trafficking, as it may increase the patient's risk. Start appropriate interventions for patients who you suspect or find are victims of abuse or trafficking. This includes making referrals, notifying appropriate agencies, providing emotional support, and informing victims about their options. The ENA encourages ED nurses to become certified *sexual assault nurse examiners* (SANEs). SANEs provide expert emergency care, collect and document evidence, take part in staff and community education, and advocate for sexual assault and rape victims.

AGENTS OF TERRORISM

Terrorism is the intentional use of violence to cause harm.[31] Terror tactics may include biologic, chemical, nuclear, or explosive events. Prompt recognition and identification of potential health hazards are essential in being prepared.

Biologic agents include bacteria, fungi, viruses, and toxins. Agents most often used include anthrax, smallpox, botulism, plague, tularemia, and hemorrhagic fever. If enough supplies are available, we can treat anthrax, plague, and tularemia with antibiotics, and the organisms are not resistant.[31] Vaccines are available for some agents.

Chemicals can be weapons of mass destruction. We categorize them by their target organ or effect. Nerve agents are the most toxic and rapidly acting chemical agents. For example, sarin is a highly toxic nerve gas that can cause death within minutes of exposure. Radioactive dust and smoke can spread and cause illness if inhaled. *Ionizing radiation*, such as that from a nuclear bomb or damage to a nuclear reactor, is a serious threat to the safety of victims and the environment. Exposure to ionizing radiation may include skin contamination with radioactive material.

Because radiation cannot be seen, smelled, felt, or tasted, you should start measures to limit contamination and provide for decontamination. Begin decontamination procedures immediately if external radioactive contaminants are present.

Explosive devices cause blast, crush, and/or penetrating injuries. Blast injuries result from the supersonic pressurization shock wave caused by the explosion. This shock wave mainly damages the lungs, GI tract, and middle ear. Crush injuries often result from explosions in confined spaces causing structural collapse. Some explosive devices contain materials that are projected during the explosion, leading to penetrating injuries.

PENETRATING TRAUMA

Penetrating trauma is an injury that occurs when an object pierces the skin and enters the body creating an open wound. When the object goes all the way through, creating an entry and exit wound, it is a perforating injury. The most common causes of penetrating and perforating injuries in the United States are gunshot and stab wounds. The severity of the injury largely depends on the body part involved. Patients with penetrating trauma have the best outcome when they are promptly evaluated and treated. All victims must first have a primary assessment to maintain ABC, control bleeding, and evaluate neurologic status.

Penetrating head trauma causes a traumatic brain injury (TBI). It has a high mortality rate. Most deaths from TBI are from gunshot wounds. Other causes include stab wounds, motor vehicle accidents, or occupational accidents. Those who survive penetrating head trauma often have permanent neurologic deficits.

Patients with penetrating neck trauma are at risk for injury to major blood vessels, the airway, and the spinal cord. Anticipate bleeding, respiratory, and neurologic problems. Chest wounds can damage the heart, lungs, esophagus, diaphragm, or trachea. Penetrating wounds to the heart are almost 80% fatal. Lung injury can cause pneumothorax or hemothorax requiring emergent decompression and chest tube insertion (see Chapter 28).

Penetrating wounds to the abdomen often result from gunshot wounds. Severity and prognosis depend on the organs injured. Mortality from abdominal wounds is about 5%. Death usually occurs later because of hemorrhage or infection.

Extremity trauma is usually not life threatening but can cause permanent disability. Blood vessels may be affected, leading to hemorrhage. Angulated fractures can cause penetrating trauma. Nerves, tendons, ligaments, and muscles can be injured. Early interventions include control of bleeding and stabilizing the injured extremity.

EMERGENCY AND MASS CASUALTY INCIDENTS

The term *emergency* usually refers to an extraordinary event that requires a rapid and skilled response and that the community's existing resources can manage. An emergency is different from a **mass casualty incident (MCI)**. With an MCI, the number of people killed or injured in a single incident is large enough to strain or overwhelm a community's ability to respond with existing resources. They always need assistance from resources outside the affected community (Fig. 21.6). MCIs can be human made (e.g., bomb explosion) or natural (e.g., hurricane) events or disasters. MCIs usually involve large numbers of victims, physical and emotional suffering, and permanent changes within a community.

When an emergency or an MCI occurs, first responders go to the scene. Triage of victims of an emergency or an MCI differs from the usual ED triage. Several systems exist. Many use colored tags to designate the seriousness of the injury and the chance for survival (Fig. 21.6). One system uses green for minor injuries and yellow for urgent but not life-threatening injuries. Red means a life-threatening injury requiring immediate intervention. Black indicates those who we expect to die or are deceased.[32]

Triage in an emergency or MCI must be done in less than 15 seconds. Victims need to be treated and stabilized and, if there

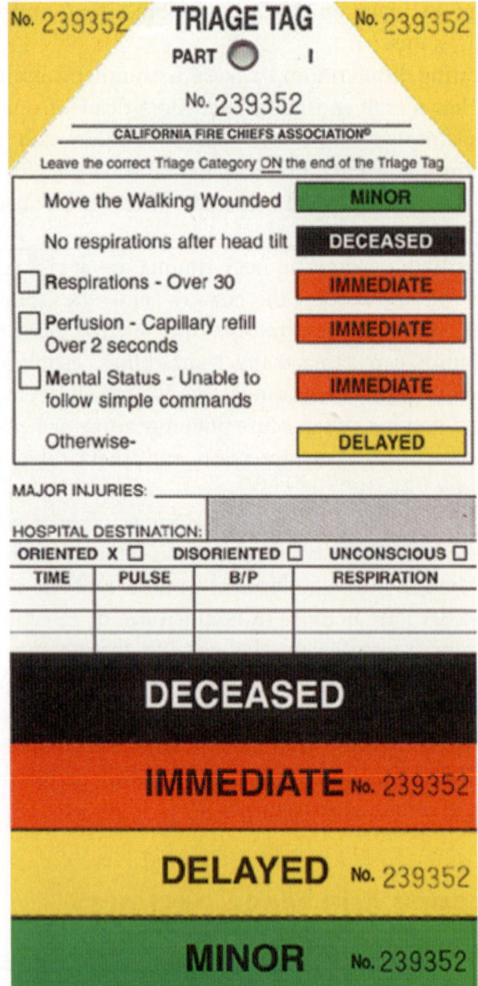

Fig. 21.6 Color-coded triage tag used in mass casualty events. (From Schultz CH, Koenig KL: Disaster preparedness. In *Rosen's emergency medicine: concepts and clinical practice,* ed 9, 2018, Elsevier, pp. 2406–2417.)

is known or suspected contamination, decontaminated at the scene. After this, they are moved to hospitals. Many other victims arrive at hospitals on their own. The total number of victims a hospital can expect is estimated by doubling the number of victims who arrive in the first hour.

Some communities have *community emergency response teams* (CERTs). CERTs are recognized by the Federal Emergency Management Agency (FEMA) as important partners in emergency preparedness. CERT training helps citizens understand their responsibility in preparing for a natural or human-made disaster. They learn what to expect after a disaster and how to safely help themselves, their family, and their neighbors. Training includes lifesaving skills with emphasis on decision making and rescuer safety. CERTs are an extension of the first responder services. They can offer immediate help to victims and organize untrained volunteers to assist until professional services arrive.[33]

BOX 21.1 ETHICAL/LEGAL DILEMMAS

Good Samaritan

Situation

You are employed as a charge nurse at a subacute rehabilitation facility. It is midnight, and you are driving home from work when you see a motor vehicle crash with a person at the side of the road waving and yelling for help. You stop and call 911 to report the incident. What do you do next?

Ethical/Legal Points for Consideration

- As a licensed health care professional, you are under no legal obligation to stop and give aid.
- If you stop, you assume an obligation not to leave the scene until sufficiently trained first responders arrive and assume control.
- Many states encourage health care professionals to stop and give aid by having "Good Samaritan" laws. These laws vary somewhat from state to state. They offer immunity from lawsuits for bystanders who provide aid in emergencies except in the case of gross negligence.
- A Good Samaritan must not be in the place of employment or under employment conditions.
- An example of gross negligence may be refusing to help someone who is seriously bleeding in favor of a person with a minor injury because the bleeding person looked old or disheveled.
- If there is a national disaster, an act of terrorism, or a major emergent need for HCPs, you may need to go to an assigned site to offer aid. The Good Samaritan Act would not cover you under these circumstances.

Discussion Questions

1. What factors do you think contribute to a health care professional's decision whether to stop to provide aid?
2. What basic aid would you feel comfortable providing if you do not have an emergency or trauma background?
3. Would your professional liability insurance cover you if someone claimed that you acted negligently while giving aid?

All health care team members have a role in emergency and MCI preparedness. Know your agency's emergency response plan. This includes knowing your individual and the response team's roles and responsibilities, plus taking part in emergency/MCI preparedness drills. Drills allow us to become familiar with emergency response procedures. These include hospital disaster drills, computer simulations, and tabletop exercises.

Response to MCIs often requires the aid of a federal agency. The National Incident Management System (NIMS), American Red Cross, FEMA, and National Disaster Medical System (NDMS) are examples of federal resources.

All disasters result in stress to those involved. This stress can persist for an extended period. It is influenced by the nature of the event, age, coping mechanisms, role in the event, and medical and mental health history. Many hospitals have a *critical incident stress management unit.* This unit arranges group discussions to allow people to share their feelings about the experience. This is important for emotional recovery.

CASE STUDY

Trauma

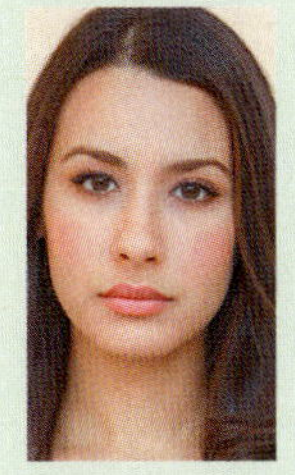
(© Thinkstock.)

Patient Profile

Paramedics bring D.F., a 20-year-old female trauma victim, to the ED by helicopter. She was the driver in a motor vehicle crash and was not wearing a seat belt. Two unrestrained children in the car were pronounced dead at the scene. The paramedics said there was significant damage to the car on the driver's side.

Subjective Data

- Asking "What happened? Where am I?"
- Reports shortness of breath and leg pain

Objective Data

Physical Assessment

- Vital signs: BP = 85/40 mm Hg, HR = 140 beats/min, RR = 36 breaths/min; O_2 saturation = 85% with 100% nonrebreather mask
- Decreased breath sounds on left side of chest
- Asymmetric chest wall movement
- Glasgow Coma Score = 14; pupils slightly unequal
- Badly deformed left lower leg with significant swelling, pedal pulse by Doppler only
- 4-cm head laceration, bleeding controlled

Discussion Questions

1. ***Analyze:*** What are D.F.'s most likely life-threatening injuries?
2. ***Prioritize:*** What is the priority of care for D.F.?
3. ***Prioritize:*** What interventions does she need immediately?
4. ***Plan:*** What other interventions should you consider?
5. ***Plan:*** What are the best practice guidelines for fluid resuscitation in patients with hypovolemic shock?
6. ***Act:*** Several family members have arrived in the ED, including the mother of 1 of the children who died. The second child who died was the patient's child. How would you approach the family?

Answers are available at http://evolve.elsevier.com/Lewis/medsurg.

BRIDGE TO NCLEX EXAMINATION

The number of the question corresponds to the same-numbered outcome at the beginning of the chapter.

1. An older male arrives in triage disoriented and dyspneic. His skin is hot and dry. His wife states that he was fine earlier today. The next *priority* would be to
   a. assess his vital signs.
   b. obtain a brief medical history from his wife.
   c. start supplemental O_2 and have the provider see him.
   d. determine the kind of insurance he has before treating him.
2. A patient has a core temperature of 90°F (32.2°C). The *most* appropriate rewarming technique is
   a. passive rewarming with warm blankets.
   b. active internal rewarming using warmed IV fluids.
   c. passive rewarming using air-filled warming blankets.
   d. active external rewarming by submersing in a warm bath.
3. What interventions does the nurse anticipate for a patient with an aspirin overdose? **(Select 3 responses.)**
   a. Hemodialysis
   b. Corticosteroids
   c. Hyperbaric O_2
   d. Gastric lavage
   e. Activated charcoal
   f. Repeated IV naloxone
4. An older woman arrives in the ED reporting severe pain in her right shoulder. The nurse notes her clothes are soiled with urine and feces. She tells the nurse that she lives with her son and that she "fell." She is tearful and asks you if she can be admitted. What possibility must you consider?
   a. Persons with dementia may be emotional.
   b. Undiagnosed cancer may be causing pain.
   c. The patient may be a victim of family violence.
   d. Orthostatic hypotension likely contributed to her fall.
5. A chemical explosion occurs at a nearby industrial site. First responders report that victims are decontaminated at the scene and about 125 workers will need medical evaluation and care. The first action you would take after receiving this report would be to
   a. issue a code blue alert.
   b. activate the hospital's emergency response plan.
   c. notify the Federal Emergency Management Agency (FEMA).
   d. arrange for the American Red Cross to provide aid to victims.

1. a; 2. b; 3. a, d, e; 4. c; 5. b.

For rationales to these answers and even more NCLEX review questions, visit http://evolve.elsevier.com/Lewis/medsurg.

REFERENCES

To access the References for this chapter, please scan the QR code with a mobile device.

CASE STUDY

Applying Clinical Judgment With Multiple Patients

You have been called into work at 1100 to cover patients for a nurse who had a family emergency. You take over care for the following 3 patients on a surgical unit. You have 1 AP available who is assigned to help you. Two other RNs are on the unit.

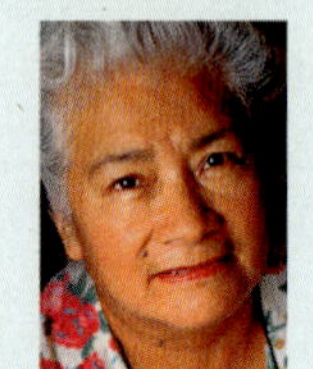 © Ryan Mcvay/Photodisc/Thinkstock	F.D., a 66-year-old female, is scheduled for an abdominal hysterectomy at 1200 for endometrial cancer. She has type 2 diabetes, hypertension, and atrial fibrillation controlled with drug therapy. She has been NPO since midnight. Glucose level at 0730 was 198 mg/dL. She received 4 units of regular insulin at 0800 but no other morning medications. IV of normal saline infusing at 75 mL/h. Weight 205 lb, height 5 ft 2 in. Vital signs: BP 180/94, 84 and regular, 20.
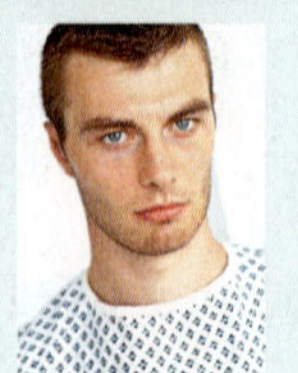 © Wavebreakmedia/iStock.com	G.S., a 23-year-old male, returned to the floor 30 minutes ago after a laparoscopic appendectomy. He experienced malignant hyperthermia during surgery. The AP reports the vital signs as: BP 180/94, 84 and regular, temp 102.2°F (39°C). You have postoperative orders to initiate.
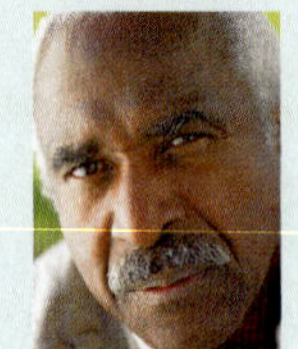 © BananaStock/Thinkstock	E.G., a 74-year-old male, had surgery for a fractured hip yesterday. He is receiving dextrose 5% in 0.45 normal saline at 100 mL/h, morphine via patient-controlled analgesia (PCA) at 1 mg q10min (20 mg max in 4 h) for pain, and heparin 5000 units subcutaneous every 12 h. O_2 to keep O_2 saturation >93%. A self-suction drain is in place at the surgical site. He has good respiratory effort when using his incentive spirometer.

1. Highlight all the findings that require your follow-up.
2. After receiving report, which patient would you see first?
3. You initiate G.S.' postoperative orders and obtain an electrolyte panel and clotting studies. Choose the *best* options for the information missing from the statement that follows by selecting from the list of options provided.

Because G.S. experienced malignant hyperthermia, he is at risk for added postoperative complications, including __________, __________, and __________.

Options:
Delayed wound healing
Delirium
Disseminated intravascular coagulation
Dysrhythmias
Hyperkalemia
Paralytic ileus
Pressure injury
VTE

4. Which tasks should you delegate to the AP? **(Select all that apply.)**
   a. Obtain 1200 vital signs on E.G.
   b. Measure glucose levels on F.D. per protocol.
   c. Review F.D.'s preoperative checklist for completion.
   d. Confirm E.G.'s understanding of how to use the PCA pump.
   e. Remind E.G. and G.S. to use their incentive spirometers every hour.
5. When you enter F.D.'s room, you find her somewhat withdrawn and lethargic. Her face is cool and slightly clammy. What initial action would you perform *first*?
   a. Obtain a stat glucose level.
   b. Give 1 ampule of D50 IV stat.
   c. Increase F.D.'s IV rate to 150 mL/h.
   d. Ask the AP to give F.D. a glass of orange juice.

Case Study Progression

F.D.'s glucose reading was 52 mg/dL. You notify her HCP and give 1 ampule of D_{50} IV dextrose as ordered. You then change her IV infusion to D_5 0.9%. You check her glucose in 15 minutes. It is 104 mg/dL and her symptoms have resolved. You then review the preoperative checklist.

6. A preoperative checklist is used to ensure completion of **(Select all that apply.)**
   a. removal of nail polish and jewelry.
   b. signed and witnessed informed consent.
   c. patient understanding of sensory information.
   d. identification of surgical site with surgical skin marker.
   e. notification of family of where to wait for the surgeon afterward.
7. The laboratory calls to report that E.G.'s activated partial thromboplastin time (aPTT) is 94 seconds. You assess him and find that the hip dressing is saturated with serosanguinous drainage. The next dose of heparin is due at 2100; the last dose was at 0900. Use an X for the nursing actions listed that are indicated (appropriate or necessary) or contraindicated (could be harmful) at this time.

Nursing Action	Indicated	Contraindicated
Initiate bleeding precautions.		
Remove the hip dressing and leave the wound uncovered.		
Obtain a stat ECG.		
Notify the HCP of the aPTT and E.G.'s condition.		
Discontinue the PCA morphine.		
Prepare to administer protamine.		
Obtain a full set of vital signs.		

8. E.G.'s BP is 92/54 with a heart rate of 110 bpm. Respiratory rate is 30 breaths/min, and O_2 saturation is 98% on 2 L of O_2. The *priority* would be to
   a. notify physical therapy that his session today will have to be postponed until evening.
   b. notify the previous RN that a medication error occurred with the heparin dose at 0900.
   c. send an order for stat CBC and type and screen for 4 units of packed red blood cells.
   d. notify the HCP of the laboratory result and anticipate orders for a reversal agent.
9. Which instructions would you give to the AP who will be assisting E.G. with ADLs? **(Select all that apply.)**
   a. Use a soft toothbrush for oral care.
   b. Provide an emery board for nail care.
   c. Avoid overinflating blood pressure cuffs.
   d. Use an electric razor to shave the patient.
   e. Offer mouthwash with alcohol for rinsing.
10. When you encourage G.S. to sit on the edge of the bed for the first time, he tells you that the AP told him that he could do whatever activity he was comfortable doing—to let pain guide his progress. Your *initial* reaction to this statement would be to
   a. ask the AP to clarify what was said to G.S.
   b. report the AP's actions to the nurse manager.
   c. teach G.S. about the reason for postoperative activity.
   d. clarify G.S.'s prescribed activity level with the HCP.

Answers available at http://evolve.elsevier.com/Lewis/medsurg.

22

Assessment and Management: Visual Problems

Aaron M. Sebach

http://evolve.elsevier.com/Lewis/medsurg/

CONCEPTUAL FOCUS

Coping
Functional Ability
Infection
Sensory Perception

LEARNING OUTCOMES

1. Describe the structures and functions of the visual system.
2. Explain the physiologic processes of vision.
3. Obtain subjective and objective assessment data related to the visual system.
4. Perform a physical assessment of the visual system.
5. Distinguish normal from common abnormal findings of the visual system assessment.
6. Link the age-related changes of the visual system to differences in assessment findings.
7. Describe the purpose, significance of results, and nursing responsibilities related to diagnostic studies of the visual system.
8. Compare and contrast the types of refractive errors and appropriate corrections.
9. Describe the common causes and assistive measures for visual impairment.
10. Discuss nursing measures that promote eye health.
11. Explain the pathophysiology, clinical manifestations, and interprofessional and nursing management of the patient with an eye problem.
12. Discuss the general nursing care of patients undergoing eye surgery.

KEY TERMS

age-related macular degeneration (AMD)
astigmatism
cataract
conjunctivitis
enucleation
glaucoma
hordeolum
hyperopia
keratitis
myopia
presbyopia
retinal detachment
retinopathy
strabismus

For people to be independent and engage in fulfilling activities, the visual system must be functional. Decreased visual acuity can significantly affect activities of daily living (ADLs) and independence. Psychosocial consequences can include reduced quality of life, social isolation, depression, and loss of self-esteem. Vision loss also affects caregivers. This makes being involved in vision-loss prevention, detection, and treatment measures important.

STRUCTURES AND FUNCTIONS OF THE VISUAL SYSTEM

The visual system is part of the central nervous system (CNS). It consists of 2 main parts, the eyes, which contain image receptors, and the brain. The brain interprets the information transmitted from receptors into images. Anatomically, the visual system is made up of the periocular structures (orbit, ocular adnexa), eye, and visual pathway.

Periocular Structures

Orbit

The orbits, or eye sockets, are bony structures that contain the eyeballs. Seven bones form the orbit: frontal, zygoma, maxilla, ethmoid, sphenoid, lacrimal, and palatine (Fig. 22.1). In addition to the eye, the orbits contain the associated muscles, nerves, blood vessels, and fat. The average orbit is 35 mm high and 40 mm wide.

Within the orbit are 3 main orbital openings, or *fissures:* optic canal, superior orbital fissure, and inferior orbital fissure. The openings are all channels for arteries, veins, and nerves. The optic canal is at the top of the socket. It provides an entry point for the optic nerve (cranial nerve [CN] II). The superior orbital fissure is a small slit in the posterior orbit. It is the main entry point for several other cranial nerves to enter the orbit from the brain. These include the oculomotor nerve (CN III), trochlear nerve (CN IV), trigeminal nerve (CN V), and abducens nerve (CN VI). The inferior orbital fissure is in the floor of the orbit. It holds the zygomatic branch of the maxillary nerve.

There are 6 extraocular muscles: (1) superior and inferior rectus muscles, (2) medial and lateral rectus muscles, and (3) superior and inferior oblique muscles. They emerge from the apex of the orbit and attach to the eye for stability and movement (Fig. 22.2). Neuromuscular coordination produces simultaneous movement of the eyes in the same direction.

Ocular Adnexa

The ocular adnexa consist of eyebrows, eyelids, eyelashes, and the lacrimal system. These structures protect the eye and serve as a physical barrier to dust and foreign particles. Blinking protects the eye, distributes tears over the anterior surface of the eyeball, and supplies necessary nourishment to surface cells.

Eyelid skin is the thinnest skin in the body. It measures less than 1 mm thick. The upper and lower eyelids join at the medial and lateral canthi. The upper eyelids contain the levator palpebrae superioris muscle. This muscle elevates and retracts the upper eyelid. It is innervated by the superior division of CN III. The eyelids close through the action of the orbicularis muscle. It is innervated by CN VII.

The lacrimal system includes structures for tear production and drainage. The main lacrimal gland and accessory lacrimal glands make tears. Lacrimal glands, in the superotemporal orbit, are exocrine glands. They make and secrete the aqueous layer of tear film and are responsible for reflex tear production. The tear film moistens the eye and supplies oxygen to the cornea.

Accessory lacrimal glands, the *glands of Wolfring* and *glands of Krause,* are found within the conjunctiva of the upper eyelid. They are responsible for baseline tear production. Tears pass over the surface of the eye and then enter the nasolacrimal system. The nasolacrimal drainage system includes the puncta, canaliculi, lacrimal sac, and nasolacrimal duct (Fig. 22.3).

Eye

Eyeball

The eyeball, or globe, is composed of 3 layers (Fig. 22.4). The tough outer layer is composed of the cornea, conjunctiva, and sclera. The middle layer consists of the uveal tract (iris, choroid, and ciliary body) and the innermost layer, the retina. The *anterior cavity* is divided into the anterior and posterior chambers. The anterior chamber lies between the iris and posterior surface of the cornea. The posterior chamber lies between the anterior surface of the lens and posterior surface of the iris. The *posterior cavity* lies in the large space behind the lens and in front of the retina.

External Ocular Structures

The conjunctiva is a transparent mucous membrane covering the inner surface of the eyelids and extends over the sclera. Glands in the conjunctiva secrete mucus and tears. The Tenon capsule, also called the *fascia bulbi,* is a thin layer of fascia that encases the eyeball behind the conjunctiva. The capsule extends posteriorly, ultimately fusing with the optic nerve.

The cornea is transparent and avascular, allowing light to enter the eye. Its curved shape refracts or bends incoming light

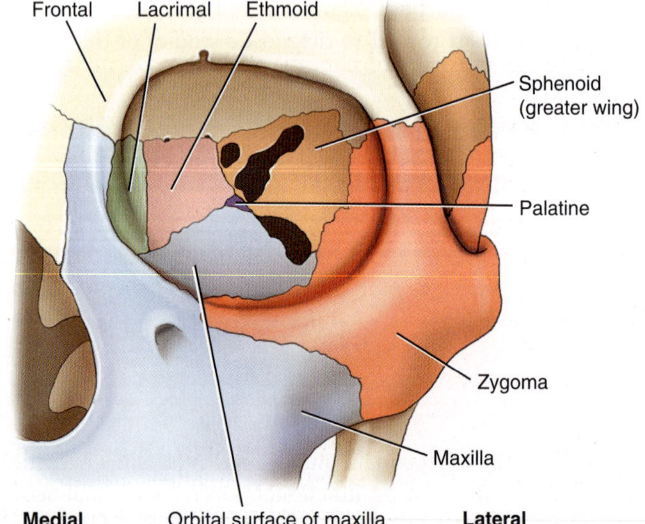

Fig. 22.1 Bones that form the orbit, or eye socket. (From Lampignano J, Kendrick L: *Bontrager's textbook of radiographic positioning and related anatomy,* ed 11, St Louis, 2024, Mosby.)

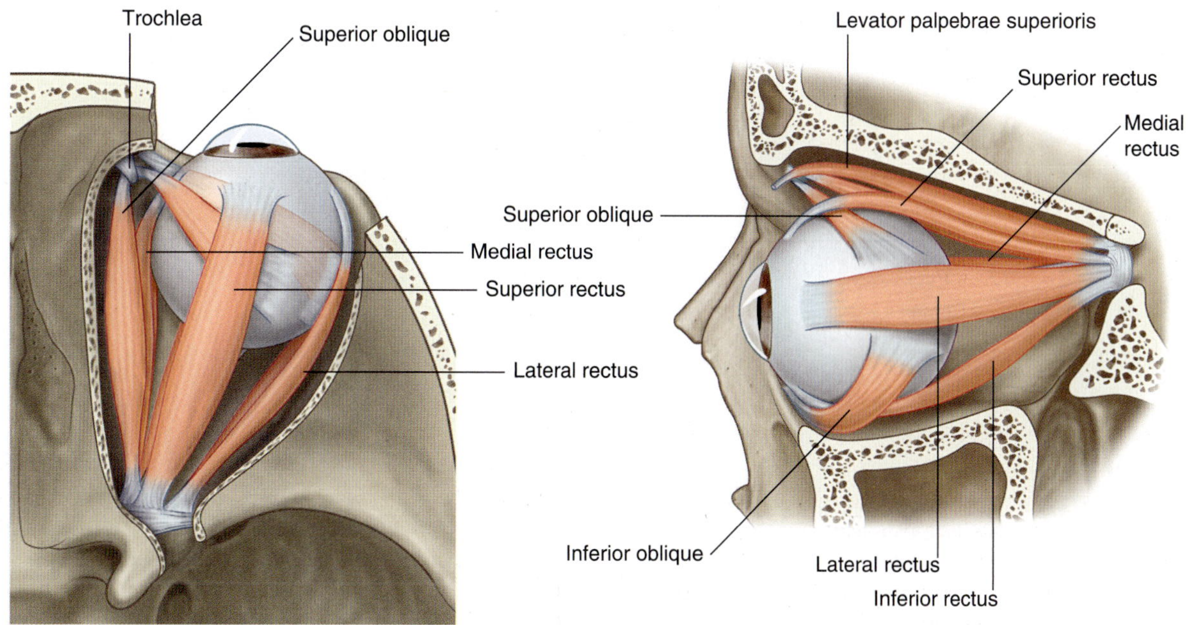

Fig. 22.2 The 6 extraocular muscles. (From Drake R, Vogl AW, Mitchell AWM: *Gray's anatomy for students*, ed 5, Philadelphia, 2023, Elsevier.)

rays to focus them on the retina. The cornea has 6 layers: epithelium, Bowman layer, stroma, Descemet membrane, Dua layer, and endothelium.

The sclera, the white part of the eye, is a fibrous layer of connective tissue. It protects the eye and helps the eye maintain its shape and structure. The sclera extends from the cornea to the optic nerve. The limbus is the junction of the sclera and cornea.

Middle Ocular Structures

The iris gives the eye its color. It has a small round opening in the center called the *pupil.* The pupil allows light to enter the eye. It constricts by action of the iris sphincter muscle (under parasympathetic control) and dilates by action of the iris dilator muscle (under sympathetic control). This controls the amount of light that enters the eye.

The ciliary body is behind the iris. It contains the ciliary muscle and ciliary processes. The ciliary muscle changes the shape of the lens to refract light onto the retina. The ciliary processes make aqueous humor for both the anterior and posterior chamber. The choroid is inside and parallel to the sclera. It is a highly vascular structure that nourishes the ciliary body, iris, and outer part of the retina.

Internal Structures

Aqueous humor. Aqueous humor is a clear watery fluid composed of electrolytes, growth factors, and protein. This fluid fills the anterior chamber of the eye, and it nourishes the nonvascular structures of the anterior chamber, such as the lens. We make aqueous humor from capillary blood in the ciliary body. It is secreted into the posterior chamber and flows through the pupil to enter the anterior chamber. Aqueous humor exits the eye through the *trabecular meshwork* and into the *canal of Schlemm* and venous circulation or through the ciliary muscle. Balanced secretion and excretion of aqueous humor are critical. Excess production or decreased outflow can lead to an increase in intraocular pressure (IOP) greater than 10 to 21 mm Hg.

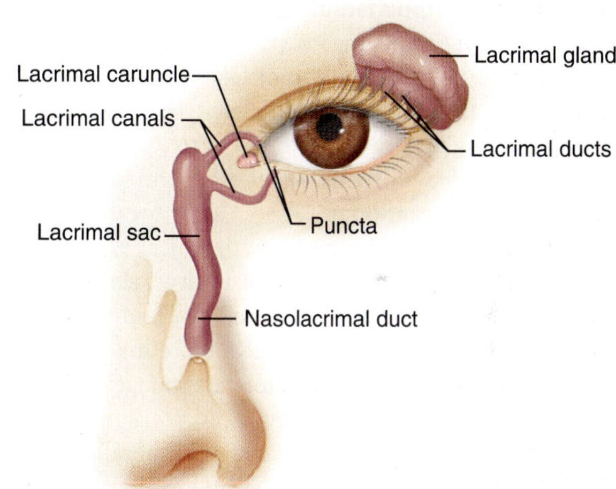

Fig. 22.3 External eye and lacrimal apparatus. Tears made in the lacrimal gland pass over the surface of the eye and enter the lacrimal canal. From there, the tears are carried through the nasolacrimal duct to the nasal cavity. (Modified from Patton KT, Thibodeau GA: *Anatomy and physiology,* ed 8, St Louis, 2013, Mosby.)

Lens. The lens is a biconvex structure behind the iris. Small fibers collectively called the *suspensory ligament,* or the *zonule,* keep the lens in place. The zonule is a series of microscopic wirelike threads that connect the lens to the ciliary body. The main function of the lens is to work with the cornea to refract, or bend, light by changing shape to alter the focal distance of the eye. The action of the ciliary body changes the lens shape as

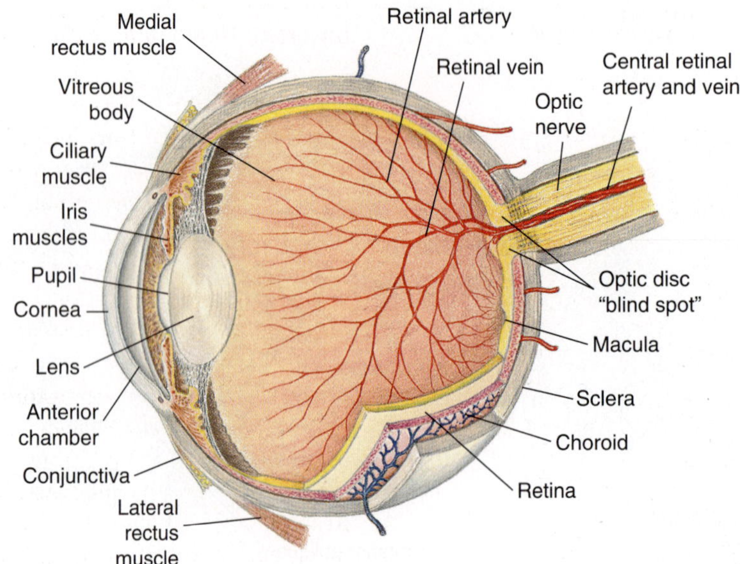

Fig. 22.4 The human eye. (From Seidel H, Ball J, Dains J, et al: *Mosby's guide to physical examination*, ed 9, St. Louis, 2018, Mosby.)

part of accommodation, a process that allows a person to focus. An example of accommodation is the ability to focus on near objects, such as when reading.

Vitreous humor. Vitreous humor is a transparent gel-like substance that fills the posterior cavity (Fig. 22.4). Any nontransparent substance in the vitreous will block light passing through the vitreous. The effect on vision varies, depending on the amount, type, and location of the substance blocking the light.

Retina. The retina lines the back of the eye, extending from the area of the optic nerve to the ciliary body (Fig. 22.4). Neurons make up most of the retina. The retinal cells cannot regenerate if destroyed. The retina converts images into a form that the brain can understand and process.

The retina has 2 main parts: the peripheral retina and central retina. The central retina contains the macula and fovea. The macula is about 6 mm in diameter. It is responsible for the central visual field. The fovea is at the center of the macula. It provides the sharpest visual acuity, which we need for activities in which detail is important, like reading.

The retina contains light-sensitive structures called *photoreceptor cells.* There are 2 types of photoreceptors: rods and cones. Rods and cones convert light to neural signals, which the nervous system translates into vision. Rods are mostly found in the peripheral retina. They are responsible for peripheral vision and night vision. Rods perceive only light and dark. They do not contribute to color vision. Cones are in the central retina, condensed mostly in the fovea. They are responsible for central vision and color vision. There are 3 types of cone cells: red, green, and blue. They all work together to create the full color spectrum.

The retina receives oxygen and nutrients from the choroid and retinal vascular systems. The central retinal artery carries blood and nutrients into the retina. The central retinal vein carries blood away from the retina.

Visual Pathway

The optic nerve, or CN II, transmits vision information from the retina to the brain. The optic nerve begins at the optic disc. That is the region of the retina where the optic nerve and vessels leave the retina. Because there are no photoreceptor cells over the optic disc, it is an anatomic blind spot. In the center of the optic disc is a white, cup-shaped area called the *optic cup*.

For light to reach the retina, it must pass through many structures: the cornea, aqueous humor, lens, and vitreous humor. These structures must be clear for light to reach the retina and stimulate the photoreceptor cells. Once the image travels through the refractive media, it is focused on the retina (Fig. 22.5). From the retina, the impulses travel through the optic nerve to the optic chiasm, where the nasal fibers of each eye cross over to the other side. Fibers from the left field of both eyes form the left optic tract and travel to the left occipital cortex. The fibers from the right field of both eyes form the right optic tract and travel to the right occipital cortex.

Gerontologic Considerations: Effects of Aging on the Visual System

Each structure of the visual system is subject to changes with aging. Many age-related changes are not serious. Table 22.1 shows age-related changes in the visual system and differences in assessment findings.

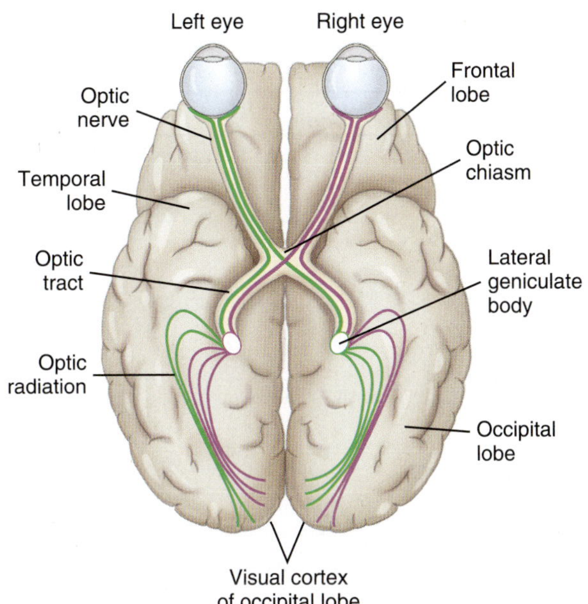

Fig. 22.5 The visual pathway. Fibers from the nasal portion of each retina cross over to the opposite side of the optic chiasma, ending in the lateral geniculate body of the opposite side. The location of a lesion in the visual pathway determines the resulting visual defect.

CASE STUDY

Patient Introduction

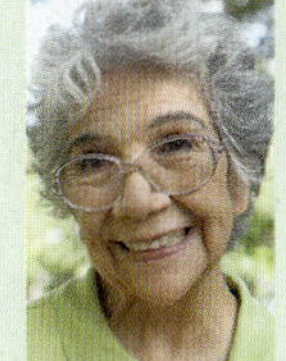

(© Jack Hollingsworth/Photodisc/Thinkstock.)

F.M. is an 81-year-old female who comes to the emergency department with vision changes. F.M. states that her vision "looks like everything is covered with a spider web." She reports seeing periodic light flashes and small white spots "floating" in the air.

Discussion Questions

1. What are some possible causes of F.M.'s vision problems?
2. What assessment questions would you ask her?

You will learn more about F.M. and her condition as you read this assessment chapter.

Answers available at http://evolve.elsevier.com/Lewis/medsurg.

VISUAL SYSTEM ASSESSMENT

Assessing the visual system may be as simple as determining visual acuity or as complex as collecting complete subjective and objective data about the visual system. Patients in a clinic or office setting often seek routine eye care or a change to their eyewear prescription. They may have a concern that they do not mention or even recognize. To perform an assessment, you must determine what is necessary for the specific patient. Although many of these assessments are within your scope of practice, some require special training.

Subjective Data

Important Health Information

Health history. Take a health history, including ocular and nonocular history. A patient's nonocular history can be significant in assessing and treating an eye problem. Ask about systemic diseases that may have eye manifestations. These include diabetes, hypertension, cancer, rheumatoid arthritis, sexually transmitted infections (STIs), AIDS, muscular dystrophy, inflammatory bowel disease, and thyroid disease. Include any history of stroke or neurologic problems (myasthenia gravis, multiple sclerosis), as these have the potential to result in vision problems.

Next, obtain an ocular history. Include the date of the last examination and any change in glasses or contact lenses. Is there a history of strabismus, amblyopia, cataracts, retinal detachment, or glaucoma? Assess for eye pain. Include pain treatment and response. Note any trauma to the eye, its treatment, and sequelae. Obtain a history of all surgeries. Include laser-based eye surgery and invasive treatments, such as retinal injections.

Obtain information about allergies. Allergies often cause eye symptoms, such as itching, burning, watering, drainage, and blurred vision.

Medications. Obtain a complete medication history, including eyedrops. Many drugs affect the eye. These include thyroid agents, antihistamines, oral hypoglycemics, and insulin. Long-term use of corticosteroid preparations can contribute to developing glaucoma or cataracts.[1] Note if the patient is taking β-blockers, because β-blockers used to treat glaucoma can potentiate their effects. Hydroxychloroquine, used to treat rheumatoid arthritis and other autoimmune diseases, can cause retinal toxicity. These patients should have an annual eye examination.

Functional Health Patterns

The functional health pattern assessment depends on the presence or absence of vision loss and whether the loss is permanent or temporary. Table 22.2 lists suggested questions related to functional health patterns.

Health perception–health management. Visual health can affect activities at home or at work. It is important to know how the patient perceives the current health problem. As outlined in Table 22.2, guide the patient in describing the current problem. Assess the patient's ability to perform self-care and eye care.

Patients may not recognize the importance of eye safety practices, such as wearing protective eyewear during potentially hazardous activities or avoiding noxious fumes and other eye irritants. Ask about the use of sunglasses in bright light. Prolonged exposure to ultraviolet (UV) light can affect the retina. Ask about night driving habits and any problems encountered. Millions of people wear contact lenses, but many do not care for them properly. The type of contact lenses and use and care habits may provide an opportunity for teaching.

TABLE 22.1 GERONTOLOGIC ASSESSMENT DIFFERENCES

Visual System

Changes	Differences in Assessment Findings
Eyebrows and Eyelashes	
Loss of pigment in hair	Graying of eyebrows, eyelashes
Eyelids	
Loss of orbital fat, decreased muscle tone	Entropion, ectropion
Tissue atrophy and stretching, prolapse of fat into eyelid tissue, loosening of the levator palpebrae superioris muscle	Dermatochalasis (excess upper lid skin), ptosis
Conjunctiva	
Tissue damage related to chronic exposure to ultraviolet light or to other chronic environmental exposure	Pinguecula (small white or yellowish spot usually on medial aspect of conjunctiva)
Sclera	
Lipid deposition	Scleral color yellowish
Cornea	
Cholesterol deposits in peripheral cornea	Arcus senilis (milky white-gray ring encircling periphery of cornea; Fig. 22.6)
Tissue damage related to chronic exposure	Pterygium (thick, triangular bit of pale tissue that extends from inner canthus of eye to nasal border of cornea)
Decrease in water content, atrophy of nerve fibers	Decreased corneal sensitivity and corneal reflex
Epithelial changes	Loss of corneal luster
Accumulation of lipid deposits	Blurred vision
Lacrimal Apparatus	
Decreased tear secretion	Dryness
Malposition of eyelid and punctal eversion resulting in tears overflowing lid margins instead of draining through puncta	Tearing, irritated eyes
Iris	
Increased rigidity of iris	Decreased pupil size
Dilator muscle atrophy or weakness	Slow recovery of pupil size after light stimulation
Loss of pigment	Change of iris color
Ciliary muscle becoming smaller, stiffer	Decrease in near vision and accommodation
Lens	
Biochemical changes in lens proteins, oxidative damage, chronic exposure to ultraviolet light	Cataracts
Increased rigidity of lens	Presbyopia
Opacities in lens	Reports of glare, night vision impaired
Accumulation of yellow substances	Yellow color of lens
Retina	
Retinal vascular changes from atherosclerosis and hypertension	Narrowed, pale, straighter arterioles. Acute branching
Decrease in number of cones	Changes in color perception, especially blue and violet
Loss of photoreceptor cells, retinal pigment, epithelial cells, and melanin	Decreased visual acuity
AMD caused by vascular changes	Loss of central vision, presence of yellow deposits, atrophy of macular retinal pigment
Vitreous	
Liquefaction and detachment of vitreous	Increased "floaters"

Many refractive errors and other eye problems are hereditary. Hereditary systemic diseases (e.g., sickle cell anemia) can significantly affect eye health. Is there a family history of eye problems? Ask about cataracts, tumors, glaucoma, refractive errors (especially myopia or hyperopia), and retinal degenerative conditions (e.g., age-related macular degeneration [AMD], retinal detachment).

Nutritional-metabolic. High doses of vitamins containing antioxidants, carotenoids, and omega-3 fatty acids (vitamins C and E, beta-carotene, zinc) may be important to eye health. Some patients with AMD may benefit from vitamin supplements.

Elimination. Assess the patient's usual elimination pattern. Straining to defecate (Valsalva maneuver) can raise IOP, which may be a problem after eye surgery.

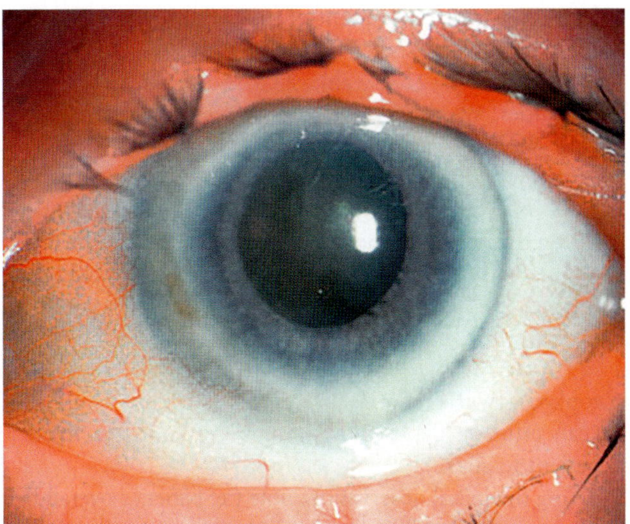

Fig. 22.6 Arcus senilis, or age-related degeneration of the cornea. (From Stein HA, Stein RM, Freeman MI: *Ophthalmic Assistant*, ed 10, 2018, Elsevier.)

Activity-exercise. Reduced vision, symptoms accompanying an eye problem, or activity restrictions after surgery can affect a patient's usual level of activity or exercise. Ask about leisure activities during which an eye injury may occur. For example, gardening, woodworking, or craft activities can result in corneal foreign bodies or penetrating injuries. Sports activities, such as racquetball, baseball, and tennis, carry risks for blunt eye trauma. Protective eyewear should be worn for these sports.

Sleep-rest. Lack of sleep may cause eye irritation, especially in patients who wear contact lenses. Painful eye problems, such as corneal abrasions, may disrupt normal sleep.

Cognitive-perceptual. Assess for other cognitive or perceptual problems. For example, the functional ability of a patient with a vision problem will be further compromised if they also have hearing problems. Patients who cannot see to read may find it harder to follow discharge instructions, especially if they have trouble hearing or remembering verbal instructions.

Self-perception–self-concept. The loss of independence that can follow partial or complete vision loss, even if the condition is temporary, can have devastating effects on a patient's self-concept. Evaluate the potential effect of vision loss on self-image. Disabling glare from a cataract may prevent nighttime driving. Losing the ability to drive can be a significant loss of independence.

Role-relationship. Eye problems can negatively affect the ability to fulfill roles and responsibilities in home, work, and social environments. For example, patients with decreased visual acuity may no longer be able to work. Some occupations predispose workers to eye injuries. For example, factory workers may be at risk from flying debris. Eye safety practices, such as the use of goggles or safety glasses, are now a legal requirement in most workplaces. Ask if the patient's vision has affected their preferred roles and responsibilities.

TABLE 22.2 HEALTH HISTORY

Visual System

Health Perception–Health Management

- Describe the change in your vision and how it affects your daily life.
- Do you wear protective eyewear (sunglasses, safety goggles, hats)?[a]
- Do you wear contact lenses? If so, how do you take care of them?
- Do you use eyedrops? If so, how do you instill them?
- Do you have any allergies that cause eye symptoms?[a]
- Do you have a family history of cataracts, glaucoma, or macular degeneration?[a]

Nutritional-Metabolic

- Do you take any nutrition supplements?[a]
- Describe your diet.
- Does your visual problem affect your ability to obtain and prepare food?[a]

Elimination

- Do you have to strain to urinate or defecate?[a]

Activity-Exercise

- Are your activities limited in any way by your eye problem?[a]
- Do you take part in any leisure activities that have the potential for eye injury?[a]

Sleep-Rest

- Is your vision affected by the amount of sleep you get?[a]
- Does your eye problem affect your sleep?[a]

Cognitive-Perceptual

- Does your eye problem affect your ability to read?[a]
- Do you have any eye pain?[a]
- Do you have any eye itching, burning, or foreign body sensation?[a]

Self-Perception–Self-Concept

- How does your eye problem make you feel about yourself?

Role-Relationship

- Do you have any problems at work or home because of your eyes?[a]
- Have you made any changes in your social activities because of your eyes?[a]

Sexuality-Reproductive

- Has your eye problem caused a change in your sex life?[a]
- For males: Do you use any erectile dysfunction drugs? If so, have you experienced any vision problems with their use?[a]

Coping–Stress Tolerance

- Do you feel able to cope with your eye problem?[a]
- How do you feel that your eye problem has affected your life? How do you cope with these changes?[a]

Value-Belief

- Do you have any conflicts about the treatment of your eye problem?[a]

[a]If yes, describe.

Coping–stress tolerance. Patients with vision problems may have stress. Assess the patient's coping methods and availability of support systems.

CASE STUDY

Subjective Data

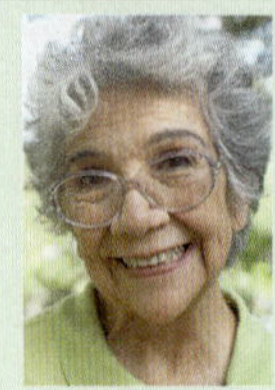

(© Jack Hollingsworth/Photodisc/Thinkstock.)

A focused subjective assessment of F.M. revealed the following information:

- ***History:*** Extraocular extraction of right eye cataract with intraocular lens implant 2 months ago. Type 2 diabetes, hypothyroidism, and hypertension.
- ***Medications:*** Glucophage 500 mg twice daily, levothyroxine 100 mcg daily, metoprolol 50 mg daily.
- ***Health perception–health management:*** Used antibiotic and corticosteroid eyedrops after surgery as directed. Therapy completed 2 weeks ago. She followed up with her eye doctor as directed. Her recovery has been uneventful. No allergies. Reports excellent eyesight until today.
- ***Elimination:*** Reports constipation and increased straining. Has been drinking prune juice daily.
- ***Activity-exercise:*** Walks in the mall at least half a mile 3 times a week. No resistance or isotonic exercises.
- ***Cognitive-perceptual:*** Denies eye pain, itching, or tearing. Reports difficulty reading.
- ***Coping–stress tolerance:*** Afraid she is having a stroke.

Discussion Questions

1. Which subjective assessment findings most concern you?
2. What would you include in your physical assessment? What are you looking for?
3. How will you adjust your assessment based on her age and history?

You will learn more about the physical assessment of the visual system in the next section.

Answers available at http://evolve.elsevier.com/Lewis/medsurg.

Objective Data

Physical Assessment

Physical assessment of the visual system includes inspecting the eye structures and determining the status of how they function. Functional assessment includes (1) assessing the patient's visual acuity, ability to judge closeness and distance, and extraocular muscle function; (2) evaluating visual fields; (3) checking pupil function; and (4) measuring IOP. We examine the ocular adnexa, external eye, and internal structures.

The iris, lens, vitreous, retina, and optic nerve can be seen directly through the clear cornea and pupil opening. This direct inspection requires special observation equipment, such as a slit lamp microscope or ophthalmoscope. The *ophthalmoscope* is a handheld instrument with a light source and magnifying lenses. It allows you to see the posterior part of the eye. It is used to magnify the retina and optic nerves and bring them into crisp focus (Fig. 22.7) and helps obtain vital information about the vascular system and CNS. Skilled use of the ophthalmoscope takes practice.

Normal physical assessment of the visual system is outlined in Table 22.3. Assessment techniques related to vision are described in Table 22.4. Table 22.5 shows select assessment abnormalities. We use a *focused assessment* (Box 22.1) to evaluate the status of previously identified vision problems and to monitor for signs of new problems.

Initial observation. Your initial observation can provide information that will help focus your assessment. Patients dressed in clothing with unusual color combinations may have a color-vision deficit. Note an unusual head position. Patients with diplopia may hold their head in a skewed position to try to see a single image. Patients with a corneal abrasion or photophobia will cover their eyes to block out room light. You can estimate depth perception by extending a hand for the patient to shake.

During the initial observation, note the patient's overall facial and eye appearance. The eyes should be symmetric on the face. The globes should not have a bulging or sunken appearance.

Visual acuity. Always record visual acuity. It is the eye's vital sign. When doing your eye assessment, assess the right eye first and then the left eye. Obtain visual acuity before the patient receives any eye care.

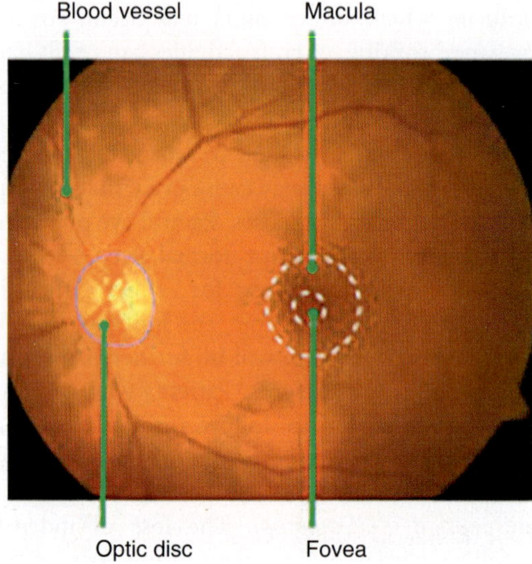

Fig. 22.7 Magnified view of retina. (From Acharya UR, Mookiah MR: Automated screening system for retinal health, *Comput Biol Med,* 75:54, 2016.)

TABLE 22.3 Normal Physical Assessment of Visual System

- Visual acuity 20/20 both eyes. No diplopia.
- External eye structures symmetric and without lesions or deformities.
- Lacrimal apparatus nontender and without drainage.
- Conjunctiva clear. Sclera white.
- PERRLA (pupils equal, round, reactive to light and accommodation).
- Lens clear.
- EOMs intact (extraocular movements intact).

 TABLE 22.4 **NURSING ASSESSMENT**

Assessment Techniques: Visual System

Description	Purpose
Color Vision Testing	
With the Ishihara test, a patient identifies numbers or paths formed by a pattern of dots in a series of color plates.	Determines the ability to distinguish colors
Confrontation Visual Field Test	
Patient faces examiner, covers 1 eye, fixates on examiner's face, and counts the number of fingers that the examiner brings into the field of vision.	Determines whether patient has a full field of vision, without obvious blind spots or vision loss
Intraocular Pressure Testing: Tonometry	
Anesthetized corneal surface is gently touched several times with covered end of probe. Examiner records several readings to obtain a mean IOP.	Measures IOP. Normal pressure is 10–21 mm Hg
Keratometry	
Examiner aligns projection and notes readings of corneal curvature. Often done before fitting contact lenses, before refractive surgery, or after corneal transplantation.	Measures corneal curvature
Ophthalmoscopy	
Examiner holds ophthalmoscope close to the eye, shining light into back of eye and looking through aperture on ophthalmoscope. Examiner adjusts dial to choose the lens that produces needed amount of magnification to inspect retina.	Provides a magnified view of retina and optic nerve (Fig. 22.7)
Pupil Function Testing	
Examiner shines light into the pupil and checks pupillary response. Each pupil is examined independently. Examiner checks for consensual and accommodative response.	Determines pupil response
Visual Acuity Testing	
Patient reads from a Snellen chart at 20 ft (distance vision test), Rosenbaum pocket screener at 14 in (near vision test), or Jaeger chart at 14 in (near vision test). Examiner notes the smallest print patient can read on each chart.	Determines distance and near visual acuity

To assess visual acuity, position the patient on a mark exactly 20 feet (6 m) from the Snellen eye chart. If the patient wears glasses or contacts, leave them on/in. Cover 1 eye at a time. Ask the patient to read down the lines of the chart to the smallest line of letters and numbers possible. Record the result using the numeric fraction at the end of the last successful line read. Indicate whether any letters were missed and if corrective lenses were worn (e.g., "Right eye, 20/30-2, with contacts"). Next ask the patient to cover their other eye and repeat the process. Normal visual acuity is 20/20. The first number indicates the distance the person is standing or sitting from the chart. The second number is the distance at which a normal eye can read that line.

If the patient reports near vision problems or is 40 years of age or older, use a handheld vision screener with varying print sizes (e.g., Jaeger Chart, Rosenbaum Pocket Vision Screener). Hold the card at 14 in (35 cm) from the eye in good light to assess near vision. Examine each eye separately, with glasses on if worn. A normal Rosenbaum Pocket Vision Screener result is 20/20.

A normal Jaeger Chart result is "14/14" in each eye, read without hesitancy, and without the patient moving the card. If you must assess near visual acuity without access to a Jaeger Chart, you can still make an accurate assessment using newsprint or a container label. Record the acuity as "newspaper headline read at X inches." If the patient cannot read any of the lines on both the visual acuity charts, the next step is to assess if they can see hand motion and light perception.

Extraocular muscle function. Assess the corneal light reflex to evaluate for weakness or imbalance of the extraocular muscles. In a darkened room, ask the patient to look straight ahead while shining a penlight directly on the cornea. The light reflection should be in the center of both corneas as the patient faces the light source.

To assess eye movement, hold a finger or an object within 10 to 12 inches of the patient's nose. Ask the patient to follow your finger with their eyes without moving their head through the 6 cardinal positions of gaze. This test can indicate weakness or paralysis in the extraocular muscles and cranial nerves (CN III, CN IV, and CN VI).

Pupil function and intraocular pressure. Assess pupil function by inspecting the pupils and their reactions to light. We often abbreviate the normal finding as PERRL (pupils are equal [in size], round, and reactive to light). The pupils should react to light directly (pupil constricts when a light shines into the eye) and consensually (pupil constricts when a light shines into the opposite eye). In a small number of patients, the pupils are normally unequal in size *(anisocoria)*. Both irises should be of similar color and shape. A color difference between the irises is normal in a small number of people.

To test accommodation, ask the patient to focus on a distant object. This process dilates the eyes. Then have the patient shift the focus to a near object, such as your finger held about 3 inches from their nose. A normal response is constriction of the eyes and convergence (inward movement of both eyes toward each other). When you assess accommodation with the pupil

TABLE 22.5 ASSESSMENT ABNORMALITIES

Visual System

Finding	Description	Possible Etiology and Significance
Subjective Data		
Blurred vision	Gradual or sudden inability to see clearly	Refractive errors, corneal opacities, cataracts, migraine aura, retinal changes (detachment, AMD).
Diplopia	Double vision	Abnormal extraocular muscle action from muscle or cranial nerve problem.
Dryness	Discomfort, sandy, gritty, irritation, burning	Decreased tear formation or changes in tear composition from aging or systemic disease.
Pain	Foreign body sensation	Superficial corneal erosion or abrasion. Can result from contact lens wear or trauma. Conjunctival or corneal foreign body.
	Severe, deep, throbbing	Anterior uveitis, acute glaucoma, infection. Acute glaucoma may cause nausea and/or vomiting.
Photophobia	Persistent abnormal intolerance to light	Inflammation or infection of cornea or anterior uveal tract (iris and ciliary body).
Spots, floaters	Patient describes seeing spots, "spider webs," "curtain," or floaters within the field of vision	Most common cause is vitreous liquefaction. Other causes include hemorrhage into the vitreous humor, retinal holes, and tears.
Objective Data		
Eyelids		
Allergic reactions	Redness, excess tearing, itching of lid margins	Many possible allergens. Associated eye trauma can occur from rubbing itchy eyelids.
Blepharitis	Redness, swelling, and crusting along lid margins	Bacterial invasion of lid margins. Often chronic.
Dermatochalasis	Excess eyelid skin	May eventually obstruct superior and peripheral vision.
Ectropion	Outward turning of lower lid margin	Age-related tissue changes, posttraumatic changes, facial paralysis.
Entropion	Inward turning of upper or lower lid margin, unilateral or bilateral	Age-related tissue changes, posttraumatic changes, facial paralysis.
Hordeolum (stye; Fig. 22.8)	Small, superficial white nodule along lid margin	Infection of the meibomian gland of eyelid. Causative organism is usually bacterial (most often *Staphylococcus aureus*).
Ptosis	Drooping of upper eyelid, unilateral or bilateral	Myasthenia gravis, congenital, or mechanical causes from eyelid tumors or excess skin.
Conjunctiva		
Conjunctivitis	Redness, swelling of conjunctiva May be itchy	Bacterial or viral infection. May be allergic response or inflammatory response to chemical exposure.
Subconjunctival hemorrhage	Appearance of blood spot on sclera May be small or can affect the entire sclera	Conjunctival blood vessels rupture, leaking blood into the subconjunctival space.
Cornea		
Corneal abrasion	Local painful disruption of the epithelial layer of cornea Can be seen with fluorescein dye	Trauma. Overwear or improper fit of contact lenses.
Globe		
Exophthalmos (Fig. 22.9)	Protrusion of globe beyond its normal position within bony orbit Sclera is often visible above iris when eyelids are open	Intraocular or periorbital tumors. Hyperthyroidism.
Pupil		
Abnormal response to light or accommodation	Pupils respond asymmetrically or abnormally to light stimulus or accommodation	CNS problems, general anesthesia.
Anisocoria	Pupils are unequal and constricted	CNS problems. Slight difference in pupil size is normal in some people.
Extraocular Muscles		
Strabismus	Deviation of eye position in 1 or more directions	Overaction or underreaction of 1 or more extraocular muscles.
Lens		
Cataract	Opacification of lens Pupil can appear cloudy or white when opacity is visible behind pupil opening	Aging, trauma, diabetes, long-term systemic corticosteroid therapy.
Visual Field Defect		
Central	Loss of central vision	Macular disease.
Peripheral	Partial or complete loss of peripheral vision	Glaucoma. Interruption of visual pathway (e.g., tumor, stroke). Migraine headache.

AMD, Age-related macular degeneration.

BOX 22.1 FOCUSED ASSESSMENT

Visual System

Use this checklist to make sure the key assessment steps have been done.

Subjective

Ask the patient about the following and note responses:

Changes in vision (e.g., acuity, blurred)
Eye redness, itching, discomfort
Drainage from eyes

Objective: Physical Assessment

Inspect

Eyes for any discoloration or drainage
Conjunctiva and sclera for color and vascularity
Lens for clarity
Eyelid for ptosis

Assess

Vision based on patients looking at the nurse or Snellen chart
Extraocular movements (EOMs)
Peripheral vision
PERRLA

light reflex, a normal response is *PERRLA* (pupils are equal, round, and reactive to light and accommodation).

IOP (Table 22.4) is measured by a variety of methods, including tonometry. Normal IOP ranges from 10 to 21 mm Hg.

Color vision. Test the patient's ability to distinguish colors. There are 2 main types of color blindness. For people with red/green color blindness, reds and greens look similar as a brownish, muted tone. The Ishihara color test assesses the ability to recognize a pattern of color in a series of color plates.

Stereopsis. Stereoscopic vision allows patients to see objects in 3 dimensions. An event that causes a patient to have monocular vision (e.g., enucleation, patching) results in the loss of stereoscopic vision. Without stereopsis, the person's ability to judge distances or the height of a step is impaired. This can have profound consequences if the person trips over a step when walking or follows too closely behind another vehicle when driving.

Eyebrows, eyelashes, and eyelids. All structures should be present and symmetric, without deformity, redness, or swelling. Eyelashes extend outward from the lid margins. With normal closing, the upper and lower eyelid margins barely touch. The lacrimal puncta should be open and positioned properly against the globe.

Conjunctiva and sclera. We can easily assess the conjunctiva and sclera at the same time. Assess the color and smoothness. Look for lesions or foreign bodies. The conjunctiva covering the sclera is normally clear, with fine blood vessels visible mainly in the periphery.

The sclera is normally white. A slight yellow cast may be found in some persons with dark skin or in the older adult from lipid deposition. A pale blue cast caused by scleral thinning can be normal in older adults.

Cornea. The cornea should be clear, transparent, and shiny. The iris should appear flat and not bulge toward the cornea. The area between the cornea and iris should be clear, with no blood or purulent material visible in the anterior chamber.

Retina and optic nerve. Examine the optic nerve or disc for size, color, and abnormalities. The optic disc is creamy yellow with distinct margins. A central depression in the disc, called the *physiologic cup,* may be seen. This area is the exit site for the optic nerve. The cup should be less than half the diameter of the disc. Normally, no hemorrhages or exudates are present in the fundus (retinal background). Inspection of the fundus may show retinal holes, tears, detachments, or lesions. Small hemorrhages can occur with diabetes or hypertension. They appear in various shapes, such as dots or flames. Examine the macula for shape and appearance. This area normally has no blood vessels.

CASE STUDY

Objective Data: Physical Assessment and Diagnostic Studies

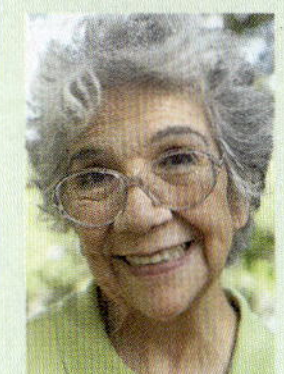

(© Jack Hollingsworth/Photodisc/Thinkstock.)

F.M.'s physical assessment findings were as follows:

- PERRL. No abnormalities of the external eye structures.
- Extraocular movements (EOMs) intact and symmetric.

The HCP performs an ophthalmoscopic examination and finds a partial retinal detachment. Ultrasound confirms the diagnosis.

Discussion Questions

1. What diagnostic studies did you expect to be ordered?
2. Which diagnostic study result most concerns you?

Answers available at http://evolve.elsevier.com/Lewis/medsurg.

DIAGNOSTIC STUDIES OF THE VISUAL SYSTEM

Diagnostic studies provide vital information in monitoring the patient's condition and planning care. Table 22.6 presents common diagnostic studies of the visual system.

VISION PROBLEMS

REFRACTIVE ERRORS

Refraction is the eye's ability to bend light rays so that they fall on the retina. In a normal eye, parallel light rays are focused through the lens into a sharp image on the retina. When the light does not focus properly, it is a refractive error. This defect prevents light rays from converging into a single focus on the retina. Defects are a result of irregularities of the corneal curvature, focusing power of the lens, or length of the eye.

Refractive errors are the most common vision problem. Blurred vision is the major symptom. In some cases, patients may report eye discomfort, eyestrain, or headaches. Most refractive errors can be corrected using eyeglasses or contact

TABLE 22.6 Diagnostic Studies

Visual System

Study	Purpose	Description and Nursing Responsibility
Amsler grid test	Monitors macular problems	Self-administered test using a handheld card printed with a grid of lines (similar to graph paper) (Fig. 22.15). Using 1 eye at a time, the patient fixates on center dot and notes any abnormalities of grid lines, such as wavy, missing, or distorted areas.
Fluorescein angiography	Provides information about flow of blood through retinal vessels	Fluorescein injected IV into peripheral vein followed by serial photographs (over a 10-min period) of retina through dilated pupils. If extravasation occurs, fluorescein is toxic to tissue. The dye can sometimes cause nausea or vomiting. Yellow-orange discoloration of urine and skin may occur.
Perimetry (visual field) testing	Detects changes in central and peripheral vision	Patient sits and looks inside a bowl-shaped instrument called a *perimeter.* While staring at the center of the bowl, a light flashes. The patient presses a button each time a flash is seen, and a computer records the results. A printout shows if there are areas where flashes of light were not seen.
Refractometry	Measures refractive error	Patient sits looking through apertures at a Snellen acuity chart and lenses are changed. Patient chooses lenses that make acuity the sharpest. Eye dilation may help visualize retina and optic nerves. Pupil dilation may last 3–4 h, making it hard to focus on near objects.
Ultrasonography	Assesses size and structure of eye	*A-scan* determines the right power of a lens implant before cataract surgery. *B-scan* can diagnose pathologic problems, including intraocular foreign bodies or tumors, vitreous opacities, and retinal detachments.

lenses, refractive eye laser surgery, or surgical implantation of an artificial lens.

Myopia (nearsightedness) is an inability to accommodate for objects at a distance, causing light rays to be focused in front of the retina. Patients can see near objects, but objects in the distance are blurry. Myopia may occur from excess light refraction by the cornea or lens or an abnormally long eye. It is present in about 30% of Americans.[2] There is strong evidence that many people inherit myopia or the tendency to develop myopia.[2]

Hyperopia (farsightedness) is an inability to accommodate for near objects, causing light rays to focus behind the retina. Patients can see distant objects clearly, but close objects are blurry. This type of error occurs when the cornea or lens does not have adequate focusing power or the eyeball is too short.

Presbyopia is the loss of accommodation associated with age. It usually starts in the early to mid-40s. As the eye ages, the lens becomes larger, firmer, and less elastic. These changes progress with aging and result in an inability to focus on near objects.

Astigmatism is an uneven or irregular curvature of the cornea causing the incoming light rays to be bent unequally. Thus the light rays do not come to a single point of focus on the retina. This results in vision distortion. Astigmatism can occur in conjunction with any of the other refractive errors.

Aphakia is the absence of the lens. It may be removed during cataract surgery. Rarely, the lens may be absent congenitally. A lens that is traumatically injured is removed and replaced with an intraocular lens (IOL) implant. The absence of the lens results in a significant refractive error. Without the focusing ability of the lens, images are projected behind the retina.

Strabismus is a condition in which a person cannot consistently focus both eyes simultaneously on the same object. One eye may deviate in (esotropia), out (exotropia), up (hypertropia), or down (hypotropia). Strabismus in an adult may be caused by thyroid disease, neuromuscular problems of the eye muscles, retinal detachment repair, or cerebral lesions. The main problem is double vision.

Nonsurgical Correction

Corrective Lenses

Corrective lenses can enhance vision in those with myopia, hyperopia, presbyopia, and astigmatism. Many people call glasses for presbyopia "reading glasses" because they are usually worn only for close work. Presbyopic correction may be combined with a correction for another refractive error, such as myopia or astigmatism. In these combined glasses, the presbyopic correction is in the lower part of the glass lens. Traditional bifocals or trifocals have visible lines. Many lenses that correct vision at various distances do not have visible lines. The prescription varies throughout the lens, allowing distance focusing in the top two-thirds and near focus in the bottom one-third of the lens.

Contact Lenses

Contact lenses are another way to correct refractive errors. Contact lenses are made from various plastic and silicone substances. They are highly permeable to oxygen and have a high water content. These features allow for increased wearing time and greater comfort. If the oxygen supply to the cornea is decreased, the cornea can become swollen, resulting in discomfort and decreased visual acuity.

You need to know if a patient wears contact lenses, the pattern of wear (daily or extended), and care practices. Shining a light obliquely on the eyeball can help you see a contact lens. Contact lenses are associated with microbial keratitis, a severe sight-threatening complication. Risk factors for keratitis include poor hand cleaning, poor lens case hygiene, and inadequate lens cleaning. Teach patients to follow recommended cleaning practices and report redness, sensitivity, vision problems, and pain to their eye care provider. Tell patients to remove contact lenses at once if any of these problems occur.

Surgical Therapy

Surgery can eliminate or reduce the need for eyeglasses or contact lenses and correct refractive errors by changing the focus of the eye. Surgical management for refractive errors includes laser surgery and IOL implantation.

Laser-assisted in situ keratomileusis (LASIK) may be considered for patients with low to moderately high myopia or hyperopia. The procedure first involves using a laser or surgical blade to create a flap in the cornea. The flap is folded back, exposing the middle section (stroma) of the cornea. Pulses from a computer-controlled laser vaporize a part of the stroma. The flap is then repositioned, adhering on its own without sutures in a few minutes.[3]

Photorefractive keratectomy (PRK) is indicated for low to moderate myopia or hyperopia. PRK is an option for patients with insufficient corneal thickness for a LASIK flap. With PRK, the epithelium is removed and the laser sculpts the cornea to correct the refractive error. *Laser-assisted subepithelial keratomileusis* (LASEK) is similar to PRK, except that the epithelium is replaced after surgery.

Refractive intraocular lens (refractive IOL) implantation is an option for patients with a high degree of myopia or hyperopia. Like cataract surgery, it involves removing the patient's natural lens and implanting an IOL. The IOL implant used is a special lens designed to correct a refractive error. Refractive IOLs can correct both myopia and presbyopia.

Phakic intraocular lenses (phakic IOLs), or *implantable contact lenses*, are implanted into the eye without removing the eye's natural lens. They are used for patients with high degrees of myopia or hyperopia. Unlike refractive IOLs, phakic IOLs are placed in front of the eye's natural lens. Leaving the natural lens preserves the eye's ability to focus for reading vision.

VISUAL IMPAIRMENT

Visual impairment describes vision that cannot be fully corrected by corrective lenses, medical treatment, or surgery. Visual impairment includes conditions ranging from low vision to the absence of all vision (total blindness) (Table 22.7).

People with severe visual impairment cannot read ordinary print even with correction. They may or may not be legally blind. *Legal blindness* is defined as the best-corrected vision in the better eye of 20/200 or less or 20 degrees or less of remaining visual field. Most blindness in the United States is the result of common eye diseases, including cataracts, glaucoma, AMD, and diabetic retinopathy.

TABLE 22.7 Diagnostic Criteria

Classification of Visual Impairment

Classification is based on the vision in the better eye with the best possible correction.

20/30–20/60	Mild vision loss or near-normal vision
20/70–20/160	Moderate visual impairment
20/200 or worse	Severe visual impairment
20/500–20/1000	Profound visual impairment
Less than 20/1000	Near-total visual impairment
No light perception	Total visual impairment or total blindness

From American Optometry Association: *Low vision and vision rehabilitation.* Retrieved from https://www.aoa.org/healthy-eyes/caring-for-your-eyes/low-vision-and-vision-rehab?sso=y.

NURSING MANAGEMENT: VISUAL IMPAIRMENT

Assessment

It is important to assess how long a patient has had a vision impairment. Recent vision loss has different implications. Determine how the vision impairment affects their functioning. Ask about problems with ADLs. For example, how hard is it for the patient to read, use their phone, move around in their home, or watch television? Other questions can help determine the personal meaning that the patient attaches to their visual impairment. Ask how vision loss has affected specific aspects of their life. What activities does the patient not engage in because of their vision?

Assess the patient's emotional reactions, coping methods, and support systems. The patient may attach many negative meanings to the impairment because of societal views of blindness. For example, the patient may view the impairment as punishment or view themselves as useless and burdensome.

Clinical Problems

Clinical problems for patients with visual impairment include:

- Sensory deficit
- Difficulty coping
- Impaired role performance

Planning

The overall goals are that patients with visual impairment will (1) reach optimal quality of life, (2) discuss feelings related to the loss, (3) identify personal strengths and support systems, and (4) use coping methods. If the patient has been functioning at an acceptable level, the goal is to maintain the current level of function.

Implementation

Health Promotion

Encourage patients with preventable causes of further visual impairment to seek health care (Box 22.2). For example,

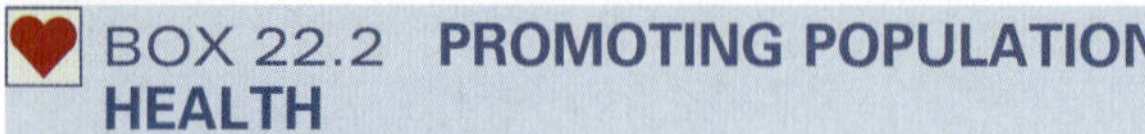

BOX 22.2 PROMOTING POPULATION HEALTH

Responsible Eye Care

- Good hand washing prevents the spread of disease from 1 eye to the other.
- Seeking health care can lead to early detection and prevent further vision loss with certain types of partial vision loss.
- Wearing sunglasses and practicing proper nutrition may help prevent cataracts and age-related macular degeneration.
- Wearing eye protection during potentially hazardous work, hobby, and sport activities reduces the risk for eye injuries.

patients with vision loss from glaucoma may be able to prevent further vision loss with prescribed therapies and regular eye examinations.

Acute Care

Provide emotional support and direct care to patients with acute visual impairment. Allow them to express fear, anger, and grief. Help patients identify positive coping methods. Caregivers are intimately involved in the experiences that occur with vision loss. Include caregivers in discussions and encourage them to express their concerns.

Many people are uncomfortable around someone with visual impairment because they are not sure what behaviors are appropriate. Be sensitive to the patient's feelings without being overly worried or smothering the patient's independence. This will help create a therapeutic nursing presence. Communicate in a normal conversational tone with the patient. Address the patient, not the caregiver. Introduce yourself and everyone who approaches the patient. It is important to say good-bye when leaving the patient's presence.

Make eye contact with the patient. Doing so will ensure you speak facing the patient. It allows you to observe the patient's facial expressions and reactions. Using the *sighted-guide technique* is recommended (Table 22.8).

Chronic Care

Remember that someone classified as legally blind may have some useful vision. Rehabilitation after partial or total vision loss can foster independence, self-esteem, and productivity. Know what services and devices are available and make needed referrals.

For legally blind persons, the primary resource for services is the appropriate state agency for rehabilitation. Legally blind persons are often eligible for federal and state assistance and income tax benefits. A list of agencies that serve partially sighted or blind patients is available from the American Foundation for the Blind (www.afb.org).

Braille, audio books, and a cane or guide dog for ambulation are examples of vision substitution techniques. These are usually best for patients with no functional vision. For most patients who have some remaining vision, vision enhancement techniques can help in learning to ambulate, read printed material, and perform ADLs.

TABLE 22.8 Sighted-Guide Technique

- Ask the patient if they would like help.
- Stand slightly in front and to one side of the patient. Offer your elbow for the patient to hold.
- Walk slightly in front of the patient at a pace that is comfortable for them.
- Serve as the sighted guide. As you walk, describe the environment to help orient the patient. For example, "We're going through an open doorway and approaching 2 steps down."
- Provide advance notice of stairs and if they go up or down.
- Tell the patient when you approach ground level.
- Give advance notice of changes in ground surface (e.g., going from hard flooring to a carpeted area).
- Never guide someone into a seat backward. Help the patient sit by placing 1 of their hands on the back of the chair. Then, allow the patient to orient themselves to the chair independently.

Vision enhancement. A wide range of technologies is available to help people with low vision. These devices include desktop video magnification/closed circuit units, electronic handheld magnifiers, text-to-speech scanners (material read aloud to you), e-readers, and computer tablets (material read aloud, magnification, image zooming, brighter screen, voice recognition). Many of these devices require some training by an assistive technology professional. Encourage patients to practice with the device to ensure they can use it successfully.

Approach magnification is a simple way to enhance residual vision. Recommend that the patient sit closer to the television or hold books closer to the eyes. Contrast enhancement techniques include watching television in black and white, using a black felt-tip marker, and using contrasting colors (e.g., a red stripe at the edge of steps or curbs). Increased lighting can be provided by halogen lamps, direct sunlight, or gooseneck lamps that are aimed directly at the reading material or other near objects. Large-type font is often helpful, especially when used with other vision enhancements.

Non–24-hour sleep/wake disorder. *Non–24-hour sleep/wake disorder (non-24)* is a common problem that occurs in patients with total blindness.[4] This circadian rhythm sleep disorder occurs when a person's biologic clock does not synchronize to a 24-hour day. It is caused by lack of light input to the circadian clock.

People with non-24 have problems falling asleep or staying asleep at night. During the day, they may have an uncontrollable urge to sleep. This may result in severe sleep issues, including insomnia, excess sleepiness, changing patterns of when a person sleeps, and social and work consequences.

Taking melatonin may shift the circadian clock earlier (an advance) or later (a delay). Tasimelteon (Hetlioz), a melatonin receptor agonist, is another treatment. It works by targeting receptors in the brain that control the timing of the sleep/wake cycle.

◆ Evaluation

The overall expected outcomes are that patients with visual impairment will:

- Follow the treatment plan to prevent further vision loss
- Use adaptive coping methods
- Maintain self-esteem and engage in social interactions
- Function safely within their environment

Gerontologic Considerations: Vision Impairment

Older adults are at an increased risk for vision loss caused by eye disease. They may have other deficits, such as limited mobility, that further affect the ability to function in usual ways. Societal devaluation of older adults may compound the self-esteem or isolation issues associated with vision impairment. Financial resources may be inadequate to secure vision services or assistive devices.

Older patients with vision loss are more likely to have cognitive problems.[5] The combination of decreased vision and confusion increases fall risk, which can have serious consequences. Decreased vision may compromise an older patient's ability to function, resulting in concerns about independence and diminished self-image. A major concern is making a potentially dangerous medication error. Taking too much insulin or mistaking one medication for another are examples. Decreased manual dexterity may make instilling prescribed eyedrops hard.

EYE TRAUMA

Many everyday activities can result in eye trauma. The most common eye injuries in the United States are the result of falls and fights. Injuries at home may be caused by cooking, cleaning, gardening, power tool use, and home repair work. Sport- and work-related injuries are other causes of eye trauma.[6]

CHECK YOUR PRACTICE

You are working in your garden when your neighbor comes running into your yard. She is screaming and waving her arms. Her husband was using a chain saw to cut down a tree when a wood chip flew into his eye. You go to your neighbor's yard and find her husband on the ground crying in pain. You assess the wood chip embedded in his left eye.

- What would you do next?

Table 22.9 outlines the emergency management of patients with an eye injury. Chemical burns can be devastating to the eye. They require immediate attention. Alkaline chemicals with a pH greater than 7 are the most harmful, as they can penetrate the eye and damage the inner components. Acidic chemicals with a pH of less than 7 cannot penetrate the eye but can damage the cornea. Both injuries have the potential to result in blindness.

A *Morgan lens* may be used to continuously irrigate an injured eye. This can provide relief for chemical or thermal burns or remove nonembedded foreign materials. A Morgan lens consists of a sterile plastic device resembling a contact lens that floats over the eye (does not physically touch it). It is connected to tubing that delivers the irrigating solution.

Trauma is often a preventable cause of vision loss. Many eye injuries can be prevented by wearing protective eyewear. Your role in providing education is important to reduce the risk of eye trauma.

EXTRAOCULAR PROBLEMS

INFLAMMATION AND INFECTION

One of the most common eye conditions is inflammation or infection of the external eye. Many external irritants or microorganisms can affect the eye, conjunctiva, and cornea.

An external **hordeolum** (or a *stye*) is an infection of the meibomian glands in the lid margin (Fig. 22.8). The most

TABLE 22.9 EMERGENCY MANAGEMENT

Eye Injury

Etiology	Assessment Findings	Interventions
Chemical burn **Foreign bodies** **Thermal burn** • Direct burn from hot surface • Indirect burn from UV light (e.g., welding torch, looking directly at the sun) **Trauma** • Blunt (e.g., fist) • Penetrating (e.g., glass, metal, wood fragments; knife, stick, other objects)	• Abnormal or decreased vision • Abnormal intraocular pressure • Absent eye movements • Blood in the anterior chamber • Fluid drainage from eye (e.g., blood, aqueous humor) • Pain • Photophobia • Prolapsed globe • Redness—diffuse or local • Swelling • Tearing • Visible foreign body • Visual field defect	• Maintain airway, breathing, and circulation. • Determine mechanism of injury. • Assess for other injuries. • Assess for chemical exposure. If present, immediately start eye irrigation with sterile saline or water. • Assess visual acuity. • Stabilize foreign objects. • Cover the eye(s) with dry, sterile patches and a protective shield. Do not put pressure on the eye. • Place patient on NPO status. • Elevate head of bed to 45 degrees. • Monitor pain and give analgesia as prescribed. • Anticipate surgical repair for penetrating injury, globe rupture, or globe avulsion.

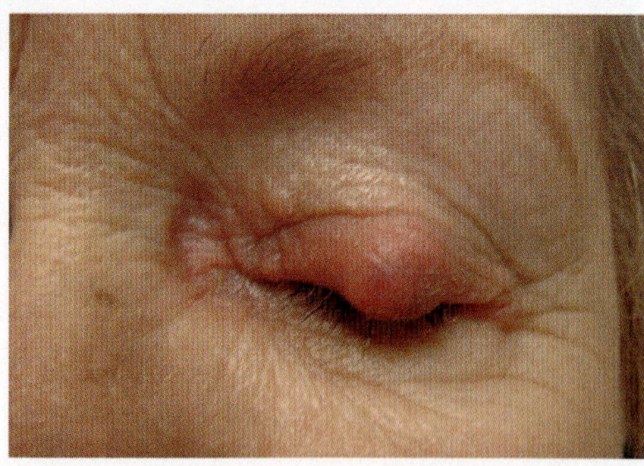

Fig. 22.8 Stye on the upper eyelid caused by staphylococcal infection. (Courtesy Stephen J. Laquis, MD, FACS Ophthalmic Facial Plastic Surgery Specialists, Fort Myers, FL.)

common bacterial infective agent is *Staphylococcus aureus.* A red, swollen, circumscribed, and acutely tender area develops rapidly. Have the patient apply warm, moist compresses at least 4 times a day. This may be the only treatment needed. If the stye recurs, teach the patient to do lid scrubs daily using eye scrub. On occasion, antibiotic ointments or drops may be needed.

A *chalazion* is a chronic inflammatory granuloma of the meibomian glands in the lid. It may evolve from a stye or occur in response to the material released into the lid when a blocked gland ruptures. A chalazion usually appears on the upper lid as a swollen, tender, reddened area that may be painful. Initial treatment is similar to treatment for a stye. If warm, moist compresses are not effective in promoting spontaneous drainage, the HCP may drain the lesion or inject it with corticosteroids.

Blepharitis is a common chronic bilateral inflammation of the lid margins. The lids are red rimmed with many scales or crusts on the lid margins and lashes. Patients mainly have itching. They may also have burning, irritation, and photophobia.

If a staphylococcal infection caused blepharitis, an eye antibiotic ointment must be used. Often blepharitis is caused by both staphylococcal and seborrheal microorganisms. The treatment must be more vigorous to avoid a stye, *keratitis* (inflammation of the cornea), and other eye infections. Emphasize good cleaning practices of the skin and scalp. Gentle cleansing of the lid margins with baby shampoo or lid scrubs can effectively soften and remove crusting.

CONJUNCTIVITIS

Conjunctivitis is an infection or inflammation of the conjunctiva. Infections may be bacterial or viral. Inflammation may result from exposure to allergens or chemical irritants. Careful hand washing and use of individual or disposable towels help prevent spreading.

Bacterial

Acute bacterial conjunctivitis *(pink eye)* is a common infection. Although it occurs in every age group, epidemics are common among children. *S. aureus* is the most common cause. Patients may have discomfort, pruritus, redness, and mucopurulent drainage. Although it typically occurs initially in 1 eye, it generally spreads to the unaffected eye. It is usually self-limiting. Treatment with antibiotic drops may shorten the course. Teach patients the importance of hand washing and avoiding contact with an infected person.

Viral

Many different viruses cause conjunctival infections. Patients may have tearing, foreign body sensation, redness, and mild photophobia. The condition is usually mild and self-limiting. However, it can be severe, with increased discomfort and subconjunctival hemorrhaging. Adenovirus conjunctivitis may be contracted in contaminated swimming pools and through direct contact with an infected patient.

Epidemic keratoconjunctivitis (EKC) is the most serious adenoviral eye disease. EKC is spread by direct contact. Contaminated hands and instruments are the most common sources. Symptoms include tearing, redness, photophobia, and foreign body sensation. In most patients, the disease involves only 1 eye. Treatment is symptomatic and includes ice packs, artificial tears, and dark glasses. Treatment for severe cases may include mild topical corticosteroids to temporarily relieve symptoms and antibiotic ointment. Teach patients the importance of good hygiene practices to avoid spreading the disease.

Chlamydial

Trachoma is a chronic conjunctivitis caused by *Chlamydia trachomatis* (serotypes A through C). It is a major cause of blindness worldwide. Trachoma is most often seen in underdeveloped countries. It is transmitted mainly by the hands and by flies. Adult inclusion conjunctivitis (AIC) is caused by *C. trachomatis* (serotypes D through K).[7] AIC is becoming more prevalent in the United States because of the increase in sexually transmitted chlamydial infection. For unknown reasons, AIC does not carry the long-term consequences of trachoma.

Manifestations of both trachoma and AIC are mucopurulent eye discharge, irritation, redness, and lid swelling. Antibiotic therapy is usually effective for trachoma and AIC. Patients with AIC are at high risk for concurrent chlamydial genital infection and STIs.

Allergic

Conjunctivitis from exposure to an allergen can be mild and transitory or severe enough to cause significant swelling. The main symptom is itching. There may be burning, redness, and tearing. Common allergens include pollen, animal dander, eye solutions, and medications. Teach patients to avoid known allergens if possible. Artificial tears can be effective in diluting the allergen and washing it from the eye. Topical medications include antihistamines and corticosteroids.

KERATITIS

Keratitis is an inflammation or infection of the cornea. It is caused by a variety of microorganisms or by other factors. The condition may involve the conjunctiva and/or the cornea. When it involves both, it is called *keratoconjunctivitis.*

Bacterial

The cornea can become infected by a variety of bacteria. Risk factors include mechanical or chemical corneal epithelial damage, contact lens wear, nutrition deficiencies, immunosuppressed states, and contaminated products (e.g., lens care solutions and cases, topical medications, cosmetics). Treatment includes topical antibiotics. In some cases, patients may need subconjunctival antibiotic injection or, in severe cases, IV antibiotics.

Viral

Herpes simplex virus keratitis (HSK) is the most common cause of corneal blindness in developed countries. It is a growing problem, especially with immunosuppressed patients. The corneal ulcer has a characteristic dendritic (tree-branching) appearance. Pain and photophobia are common.

Current treatment for HSK includes topical ganciclovir or trifluridine or oral or IV acyclovir or valacyclovir.[8] Treatment may involve corneal debridement. Topical corticosteroids are usually contraindicated because they contribute to a longer course and possible deeper corneal ulceration.

The varicella-zoster virus (VZV) that causes chickenpox can affect the eye. Herpes zoster ophthalmicus (HZO) may occur by reactivation of a latent infection that persisted after an earlier attack of varicella or by contact with a patient with chickenpox or herpes zoster. It occurs most often in older adults or immunosuppressed patients. Care of patients with acute HZO includes antiviral agents. Oral antivirals started within 72 hours of symptom onset can reduce disease severity and complications. Other treatments include analgesics for pain, topical corticosteroids to reduce inflammation, and mydriatic agents to dilate the pupil and relieve pain.

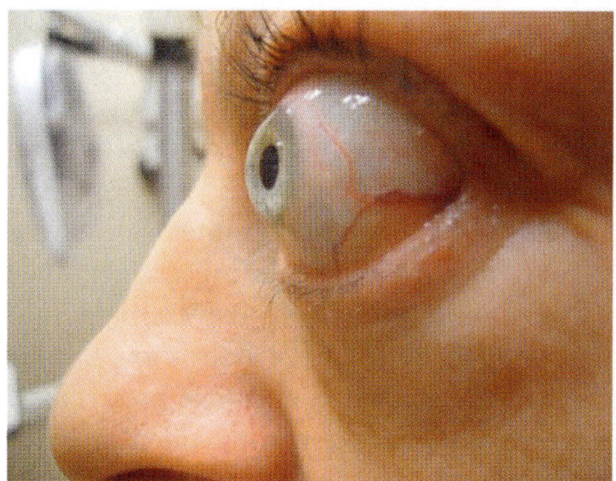

Fig. 22.9 Exophthalmos. (Courtesy Stephen J. Laquis, MD, FACS Ophthalmic Facial Plastic Surgery Specialists, Fort Myers, FL.)

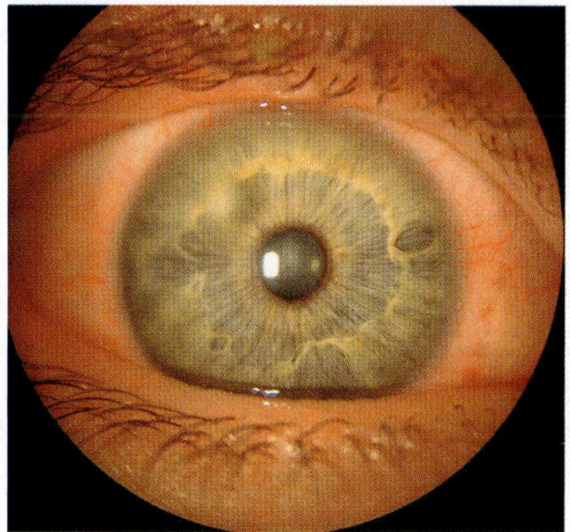

Fig. 22.10 Corneal ulcer. Infection associated with poor contact lens care. (Courtesy Cory J. Bosanko, OD, FAAO, Eye Centers of Tennessee, Crossville, TN.)

Other Causes

Keratitis may be caused by fungi, such as *Aspergillus, Candida,* and *Fusarium* species. This is especially true in the case of eye trauma in an outdoor setting where fungi are prevalent in the soil and moist organic matter.

Acanthamoeba keratitis is caused by a parasite that is associated with contact lens wear, usually from contaminated lens care solutions or cases. Homemade saline solution is particularly susceptible to *Acanthamoeba* contamination. Teach patients who wear contact lenses about good lens care practices. Treatment is difficult because the organism is resistant to most drugs. Antifungal agents (e.g., ketoconazole) may be given. If antimicrobial therapy fails, the patient may need a corneal transplant.

Exposure keratitis occurs when the eyelids cannot adequately close. Patients with *exophthalmos* (protruding eyeball) from thyroid eye disease or masses posterior to the globe are susceptible to exposure keratitis (Fig. 22.9).

Corneal Ulcer

Tissue loss caused by a corneal infection produces a *corneal ulcer* (infectious keratitis) (Fig. 22.10). The infection can be caused by bacteria, viruses, or fungi. Corneal ulcers are often painful. The patient may feel as if there is a foreign body in the eye. Other symptoms may include tearing, purulent or watery discharge, redness, and photophobia. Treatment is aggressive to avoid permanent vision loss. Antibiotic, antiviral, or antifungal eyedrops may be given as often as every hour for the first 24 hours. An untreated corneal ulcer can result in corneal scarring and perforation, or a hole, in the cornea. Depending on the severity of the ulcer and treatment response, a corneal transplant may be needed.

NURSING MANAGEMENT: INFLAMMATION AND INFECTION

Assess for eye problems, including edema, redness, decreased visual acuity, sensation that a foreign body is present, and discomfort. Consider the psychosocial aspects of a patient's condition, especially when vision is impaired.

Patient education about the treatment plan is critical. Careful asepsis and frequent, thorough hand washing are essential to prevent spreading organisms from 1 eye to the other and to other people. Teach patients and caregivers how to avoid sources of eye irritation or infection and how to respond if an eye problem occurs. Patients with an infection related to a sexual mode of transmission need information about that disorder.

Apply warm or cool compresses as needed. Darken the room and give analgesics. If a patient's visual acuity is decreased, modify the environment and activities for safety. Suggest alternative ways to perform daily activities and self-care.

The patient may need eyedrops as often as every hour. If the patient receives 2 or more different drops, stagger the eye drops to promote maximum absorption. For example, if 2 different eyedrops are ordered hourly, give 1 drop on the hour and 1 drop on the half-hour (unless otherwise prescribed). The patient who needs to instill eyedrops often may have sleep deprivation. Review the proper technique for instilling eye drops.

Review the use and care of lenses and lens care products. Teach patients who wear contact lenses and develop infections to discard all opened or used lens care products and cosmetics. This will decrease the risk for reinfection from contaminated products.

DRY EYES

Keratoconjunctivitis sicca (dry eyes) is a common problem, especially in older adults and people with certain systemic autoimmune diseases. These include scleroderma, systemic lupus erythematosus, and Sjögren syndrome. Dry eyes is caused by a decrease in the quality or quantity of the tear film. Patients report irritation or "sand in my eye." The sensation often worsens through the day.

Treatment is aimed at the underlying cause. With decreased tear secretion, the patient may use artificial tears or ointments. Cyclosporine ophthalmic emulsion (Restasis) helps to increase the eyes' natural ability to make tears. In severe cases, closure of the lacrimal puncta may be done.

CORNEAL PROBLEMS

Corneal Scars

Corneal wounds (e.g., trauma, infection) may cause it to become scarred and opacified, thereby decreasing the normal transparency. Treatment is a corneal transplant.

Keratoconus

In *keratoconus,* the anterior cornea thins and bulges forward, forming a cone shape. It usually occurs bilaterally. There is a familial tendency. It appears during adolescence and slowly progresses between ages 20 and 60 years. The main symptom is blurred vision. Early treatment involves glasses or rigid contact lenses.

Intacs inserts are clear plastic lenses surgically inserted on the cornea to help flatten the bulge and improve vision. They are an option when contact lenses or glasses no longer help a patient achieve adequate vision. Collagen cross-linking uses UV light and special eye drops to strengthen collagen fibers in the cornea. Doing so helps to flatten or stiffen the cornea, keeping it from bulging further. Sometimes, the cornea can perforate as central corneal thinning progresses. In these cases, a corneal transplant is done before the cornea can perforate.

Corneal Transplant

More than 50,000 corneal transplants (keratoplasty) are done in the United States each year. These transplants are one of the fastest and safest of all tissue or organ transplant surgeries.[9] Common indications include corneal problems or eye injuries such as ulceration, keratitis, scarring, and keratoconus. Corneal transplants include penetrating (full thickness) and lamellar (partial thickness).

Penetrating (full-thickness) cornea transplant involves transplanting all 3 layers of the cornea. The HCP removes the cornea and replaces it with a donor cornea that is sutured into place (Fig. 22.11). Vision recovery may take up to 1 year.

During a *lamellar cornea transplant,* not all layers of the cornea are replaced. The deepest layer, called the *endothelium* (posterior lamellar cornea transplant), is commonly replaced. Versions of this procedure include Descemet stripping endothelial keratoplasty (DSEK) or Descemet membrane endothelial keratoplasty (DMEK). Lamellar transplants are recommended over full penetrating transplants when the disease process is limited to only part of the cornea.

The time between the donor's death and removal of the tissue should be as short as possible. Eye banks test donors for HIV, syphilis, hepatitis B, and hepatitis C. The tissue is preserved in a special solution. Enhanced tissue procurement and preservation, postoperative topical corticosteroids, and careful follow-up have decreased graft rejection. Matching the blood type of the donor and recipient improves the success rate.

INTRAOCULAR PROBLEMS

CATARACT

A **cataract** is an opacity within the lens. A cataract can occur in 1 or both eyes. If cataracts are present in both eyes, one may affect vision more than the other. Cataract removal is the most common surgery in the United States.

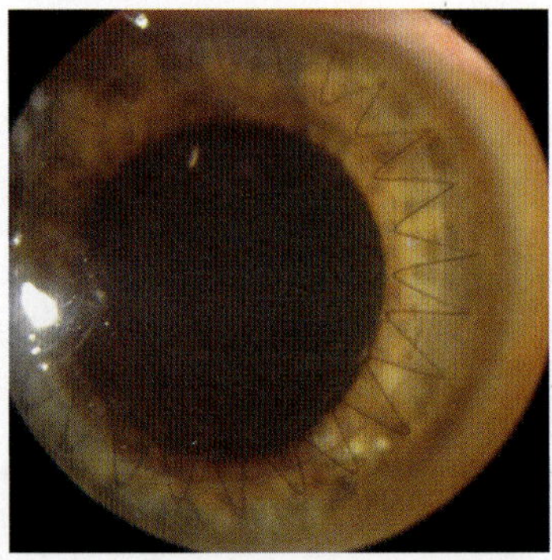

Fig. 22.11 Sutures on a donated cornea after penetrating keratoplasty (corneal transplant). (Courtesy Cory J. Bosanko, OD, FAAO, Eye Centers of Tennessee, Crossville, TN.)

Etiology and Pathophysiology

Most cataracts are age related *(senile cataracts)*. Other risk factors include blunt or penetrating trauma, smoking, alcohol use, radiation or UV light exposure, certain drugs (e.g., steroids), and eye inflammation. The rate of cataract development varies. Patients with diabetes tend to develop cataracts at a younger age.[10]

With senile cataract formation, altered metabolic processes within the lens cause an accumulation of water and changes in the lens fiber structure. These changes affect lens transparency, causing vision changes.

Clinical Manifestations and Diagnostic Studies

Patients with cataracts may have a decrease in vision, abnormal color perception, and glare. Glare is the result of light scatter caused by the lens opacities. It may be significantly worse at night when the pupil dilates. Vision decline is gradual.

Diagnosis is based on decreased visual acuity or another vision problem. The opacity is directly observable by ophthalmoscopic or slit lamp microscopic examination. A totally opaque lens creates the appearance of a white pupil. Table 22.6 lists other diagnostic studies that may be helpful in evaluating a cataract.

Interprofessional Care

Interprofessional care for cataracts is outlined in Table 22.10. Currently, no treatment is available to "cure" cataracts other than surgical removal. Some patients may not have surgery. Changing the eyewear prescription may improve visual acuity, at least temporarily.

Other vision aids, such as reading glasses, may help patients with near vision. Increasing the amount of light to read or do other near-vision tasks is useful. Patients may be willing to adjust their lifestyle to adjust to vision decline. For example, if glare makes it hard to drive at night, a patient may choose to drive only during daylight hours or to have someone else drive at night. Sometimes, informing and reassuring patients about the disease process can make them comfortable about choosing nonsurgical measures, at least temporarily.

Surgical Therapy

When palliative measures no longer provide an acceptable level of vision function, surgery is an option. A patient's occupational needs and lifestyle changes are factors affecting the decision to have surgery. In some instances, factors other than vision influence the need for surgery. Lens-induced problems, such as increased IOP, may require lens removal. Opacities may prevent the HCP from getting a clear view of the retina in patients with diabetic retinopathy or other sight-threatening problems. In these cases, the cataract is removed to allow retinal visualization and adequate management of the problem.

TABLE 22.10 Interprofessional Care

Cataract

Diagnostic Assessment
- History and physical assessment
- Visual acuity measurement
- Ophthalmoscopy
- Slit lamp microscopy
- Glare testing, potential acuity testing in select patients
- Keratometry and A-scan ultrasound (if surgery is planned)
- Other tests (e.g., visual field perimetry) to determine cause of visual loss

Management

Nonsurgical
- Change in eyewear prescription
- Vision aids (reading glasses, magnifiers)
- Increased lighting
- Lifestyle adjustment

Acute Care: Surgical Therapy

Preoperative
- Mydriatic, cycloplegic agents
- Nonsteroidal antiinflammatory drugs
- Topical antibiotics
- Anxiolytic medications

Surgery
- Lens removal
  - Phacoemulsification
  - Extracapsular extraction
- Correction of surgical aphakia
- Intraocular lens implantation (most frequent type of correction)

Postoperative
- Topical antibiotic
- Topical corticosteroid or other antiinflammatory agent
- Mild analgesia, if necessary
- Eye patch or shield and activity as prescribed

DRUG ALERT

Cycloplegics and Mydriatics
- Teach patients to wear dark glasses to decrease photophobia.
- Monitor for signs of systemic toxicity (e.g., tachycardia, CNS effects).

The most common form of cataract surgery is *phacoemulsification*. A small incision is made in the surface of the eye in or near the cornea. Then, a thin ultrasound probe is inserted into the eye and ultrasonic vibrations are used to dissolve the clouded lens into fragments. The lens fragments are then suctioned out through the same ultrasound probe.[10] The small incision is self-sealing and usually does not need sutures.

An *extracapsular cataract extraction procedure* is used for very advanced cataracts where the lens is too dense to dissolve into fragments. The technique requires a larger incision so that the cataract can be removed in 1 piece without being fragmented inside the eye. Sutures are needed to close the larger wound. Vision recovery is often slower. Most patients have an IOL implanted at the time of cataract extraction surgery (Fig. 22.12). A posterior chamber lens is placed in the capsular bag behind the iris.

The patient often receives 3 different eye drops before surgery. A *mydriatic* (α-adrenergic agonist) produces pupil dilation (mydriasis) by contracting the iris dilator muscle. *Cycloplegics*, such as tropicamide (Mydriacyl), block the effects of acetylcholine on the ciliary body and iris sphincter muscles. This produces mydriasis and paralysis of accommodation (cycloplegia).[10] Nonsteroidal antiinflammatory eyedrops reduce inflammation and edema. At the end of the procedure, other drugs, such as antibiotics and corticosteroids, may be given.

NURSING MANAGEMENT: CATARACTS

Assessment

Most patients receive local anesthesia and do not need an extensive physical assessment. However, patients with cataracts are often older adults with medical problems that require preoperative evaluation. Most patients are admitted on an outpatient basis. They present hours before surgery to allow time for preoperative preparation.

Obtain an appropriate history and physical assessment. Assess visual acuity. Note the visual acuity in the unaffected eye. Use this information to determine how visually compromised the patient may be while the operative eye is healing. Assess the psychosocial impact of the problem. What is the patient's level of knowledge about the disease process and treatment options?

Planning

Before surgery, the overall goals are that patients with a cataract will (1) make informed decisions about treatment options and (2) have minimal anxiety. After surgery, the overall goals are that patients with a cataract will (1) have improved vision, (2) understand and follow discharge instructions, and (3) be free of complications.

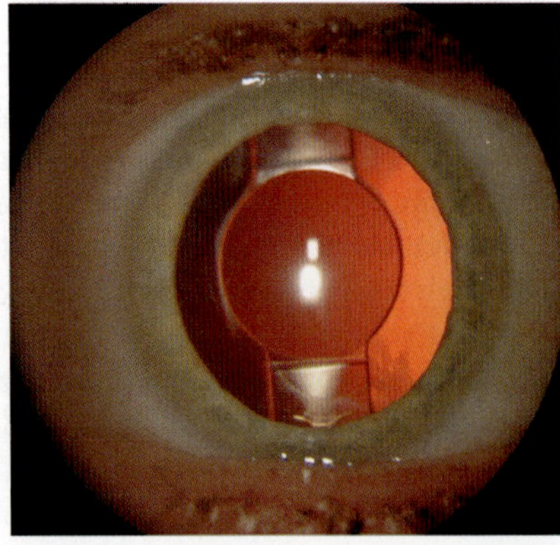

Fig. 22.12 Intraocular lens implant after cataract surgery. (Courtesy Cory J. Bosanko, OD, FAAO, Eye Centers of Tennessee, Crossville, TN.)

Implementation

Health Promotion

There are no proven measures to prevent cataract development. However, suggest that patients wear sunglasses, avoid unnecessary radiation, and maintain appropriate intake of antioxidant vitamins (e.g., vitamins C, E) and good nutrition. Provide information about vision enhancement techniques for those who choose not to have surgery.

Acute Care

Before surgery, patients with cataract need accurate information about the disease process and treatment options because cataract surgery is considered an elective procedure. For patients having surgery, provide information, support, and reassurance about the surgical and postoperative experience to reduce anxiety. Photophobia is common when receiving pupil dilation medications, which can produce transient stinging and burning. Decreasing the room lighting is helpful.

Patients who have cataract surgery remain at the agency for only a few hours unless complications occur. The patient and caregiver are responsible for most postoperative care. Include the caregiver in the instructions because some patients may have difficulty with self-care activities, especially if the vision in the unoperated eye is poor. Table 22.11 outlines patient and caregiver teaching after eye surgery. A nursing care plan for patients after eye surgery (eNursing Care Plan 22.1) is available on the website for this chapter.

Postoperative medications include antibiotic drops to prevent infection and corticosteroid drops to decrease inflammation. The frequency of using eyedrops is gradually reduced and then stopped once the eye has healed. The patient usually has little or no pain. Mild analgesics are usually enough to relieve any pain. If the pain is intense, the patient should notify the HCP because this may indicate hemorrhage, infection, or increased IOP. They may have some scratchiness or blurriness in the operative eye. Remind them not to rub or scratch their eyes.

Activity restrictions and nighttime eye shielding vary based on the HCP's preference. Most prefer that patients avoid activities that increase the IOP. These include bending, straining, coughing, and lifting.

After surgery, HCPs measure visual acuity and IOP, assess anterior chamber depth, and monitor corneal clarity at each visit. Right after surgery, a patient's uncorrected visual acuity in the operative eye may be good. However, it is not unusual for visual acuity to be reduced right after surgery. Some patients may still need glasses or contact lenses to achieve their best visual acuity. Many patients achieve a usable level of visual acuity within a few days after surgery.

Some patients may have significant vision impairment after surgery. They may need several weeks to achieve a usable level of visual acuity. These include patients who do not have an IOL implanted at the time of surgery and those with poor vision in the nonoperative eye. For those patients, the time between surgery and receiving glasses or contacts can be a time of

TABLE 22.11 PATIENT & CAREGIVER TEACHING

After Eye Surgery

Include the following information in the teaching plan for the patient and caregiver after eye surgery:

- Proper hygiene and eye care techniques to ensure that dressings and/or surgical wound is not contaminated during eye care
- Signs and symptoms of infection (e.g., increased or purulent drainage, redness, any decrease in visual acuity) and when and how to report these to allow for early treatment
- Importance of following restrictions on head positioning, bending, coughing, and Valsalva maneuver to optimize visual outcomes and prevent increased intraocular pressure
- How to instill eye medications using aseptic technique and adherence with prescribed eye medication routine to prevent infection
- How to take pain medication and report pain not relieved by medication
- Importance of continued follow-up care
- Measures to cope with visual loss, such as large screens, audiobooks, and additional lighting, and promote safety

significant visual disability. Suggest ways the patient and caregiver can modify activities and the environment to promote safety. Suggestions may include getting help with steps and removing area rugs and other potential obstacles. Audio books and listening to programs are good diversion.

If a patch is used, tell patients that they will not have depth perception until the patch is removed. Measures to avoid falls or other injuries are necessary. Patients with significant vision impairment in the unoperated eye need more help while the operative eye is patched. Some patients may need 1 or 2 weeks for the visual acuity in the operated eye to reach an adequate level for most vision needs. These patients need assistance until the vision improves.

◆ Evaluation

The overall expected outcomes are that patients after cataract surgery will:

- Have improved vision
- Be better able to take care of self
- Have minimal to no pain

RETINOPATHY

Retinopathy is the process of microvascular damage to the retina. It can lead to blurred vision and progressive vision loss. Retinopathy may develop slowly or rapidly. It occurs most often in adults with diabetes or hypertension.

Diabetic retinopathy is a common complication of diabetes, especially in patients with long-standing uncontrolled disease.[11] Nonproliferative retinopathy is the most common form of diabetic retinopathy. It is characterized by capillary microaneurysms, retinal swelling, and hard exudates. Macular edema represents a worsening of retinopathy as plasma leaks from macular blood vessels. As capillary walls weaken, they can rupture, leading to intraretinal "dot or blot"

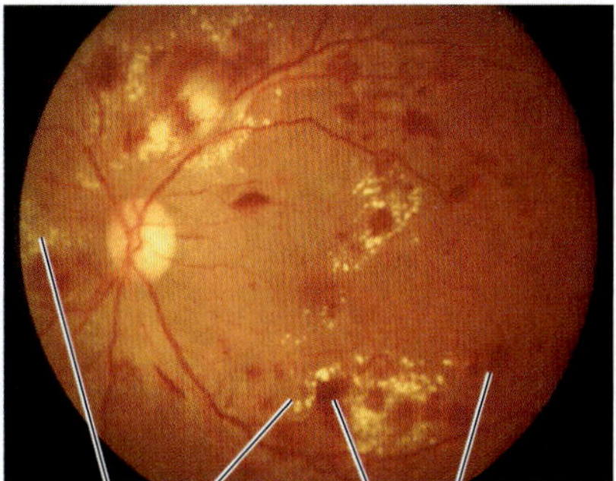

Fig. 22.13 Diabetic retinopathy with extensive hemorrhages, microaneurysms, and exudates. (From Kaiser PK, Freidman NJ: *The Massachusetts Eye and Ear Infirmary illustrated manual of ophthalmology,* ed 5, Elsevier, 2021.)

hemorrhaging (Fig. 22.13) resulting in severe loss in central vision. As the disease advances, *proliferative retinopathy* may occur. New blood vessels grow, but are abnormal, fragile, and predisposed to leaking, thus causing severe vision loss. Diagnosis and treatment of diabetic retinopathy are discussed in Chapter 53.

Hypertensive retinopathy is caused by blockages in retinal blood vessels from hypertension. These changes may not affect vision at first. On routine eye examination, retinal hemorrhages, anoxic cotton-wool spots, and macular swelling can be seen. Sustained, severe hypertension can cause sudden vision loss from swelling of the optic disc and nerve *(papilledema).* Emergent treatment focuses on lowering the patient's BP. Normal vision is usually restored by treating hypertension (see Chapter 36).

RETINAL DETACHMENT

A **retinal detachment** is a separation of the sensory retina and the underlying pigment epithelium, with fluid accumulation between the 2 layers. A retinal detachment is an emergency and requires immediate treatment. There is increased risk of permanent vision loss or blindness if retinal detachment is not treated quickly. Vision prognosis varies depending on the extent, length, and area of detachment.

Etiology and Pathophysiology

We classify retinal detachments based on the cause. The most common cause is a retinal break. *Retinal breaks* are an interruption in the full thickness of the retinal tissue. They can be classified as tears or holes. *Retinal holes* are small breaks that occur spontaneously. *Retinal tears* can occur as the vitreous humor shrinks during aging, pulling on the retina. The retina tears when the traction force exceeds the strength of the retina. Once the retina breaks, liquid vitreous can enter the subretinal space between the sensory layer and the retinal pigment epithelium layer. The fluid lifts the retina away from the underlying tissue, causing a *rhegmatogenous* retinal detachment.

Nonrhegmatogenous detachments include tractional and exudative detachments.[12] Tractional detachments are caused by scar tissue that grows on the surface of the retina, pulling the retina off the back wall of the eye. This may occur from diabetes. Exudative detachments are often caused by AMD, a tumor, blunt injury to the eye, or inflammation.[12] Risk factors for retinal detachment are listed in Table 22.12.

Clinical Manifestations and Diagnostic Studies

Patients with a detaching retina describe symptoms that include flashes of light, floaters (small flecks), and a "cobweb," "hairnet," or ring in the field of vision. Once the retina has detached, patients describe a gradual loss of peripheral or central vision, "like a curtain" coming across the field of vision. There is no pain.

The area of visual loss corresponds inversely to the area of detachment. For example, if the retinal detachment involves the superior retina, the defect is in the inferior visual field. If the detachment is small or develops slowly, the patient may not be aware of a vision problem.

Measuring visual acuity should be the first diagnostic procedure with any report of vision loss (Table 22.13). The HCP can see a retinal detachment using direct and indirect ophthalmoscopy or slit lamp microscopy in conjunction with a special lens to view the periphery of the retina. Ultrasound may be useful in finding a retinal detachment if the eye care provider cannot see the retina (e.g., when the cornea, lens, or vitreous is hazy or opaque).

Interprofessional Care

Some retinal breaks are not likely to progress to detachment. In these situations, the HCP monitors the patient and teaches them to seek immediate evaluation if warning signs and symptoms of impending detachment occur. The goals of treatment are to seal any retinal breaks and reattach the retina. Several techniques are used to meet these goals.

Laser Photocoagulation and Cryopexy

Retinal tears or holes without a detachment may be treated by sealing the retina to the posterior wall using photocoagulation or cryopexy.[12] Photocoagulation uses a laser to make small burns around the retinal tear. Cryopexy uses a special freezing probe to apply intense cold around the tear. With both procedures, the resulting scar tissue seals the retina to prevent a detachment.

Laser photocoagulation and cryopexy therapy are outpatient procedures. Patients typically receive topical anesthesia. There are minimal adverse symptoms during or after the procedure. For retinal breaks accompanied by significant detachment, photocoagulation or cryopexy may be used with scleral buckling.

Scleral Buckling

Scleral buckling is an extraocular surgical procedure that involves placing a band around the globe to move the pigment epithelium, choroid, and sclera toward the detached retina. A silicone implant is sutured against the sclera, causing the sclera to buckle inward. An encircling band may be placed over the implant if there are multiple retinal breaks, if suspected breaks cannot be found, or if there is widespread inward traction on the retina (Fig. 22.14). If present, subretinal fluid may be drained using a small-gauge needle. This promotes contact between the retina and buckled sclera. Scleral buckling is usually an outpatient procedure.

TABLE 22.12 Risk Factors for Retinal Detachment

- Age
- Age-related macular degeneration
- Diabetic retinopathy
- Eye surgery
- Eye trauma
- Family or personal history of retinal detachment
- Severe myopia
- Thinning of the peripheral retina

From National Eye Institute, National Institutes of Health: *Retinal detachment.* Retrieved from https://www.nei.nih.gov/learn-about-eye-health/eye-conditions-and-diseases/retinal-detachment.

TABLE 22.13 Interprofessional Care

Retinal Detachment

Diagnostic Assessment
- History and physical assessment
- Visual acuity measurement
- Ophthalmoscopy
- Slit lamp microscopy
- Ultrasound if cornea, lens, or vitreous is hazy or opaque

Management

Preoperative
- Mydriatic, cycloplegic agents
- Photocoagulation of retinal break that has not progressed to detachment

Surgery
- Laser photocoagulation
- Cryopexy
- Scleral buckling
- Vitrectomy
- Intravitreal bubble

Postoperative
- Topical antibiotics
- Topical corticosteroid
- Analgesia
- Mydriatics
- Positioning and activity as prescribed

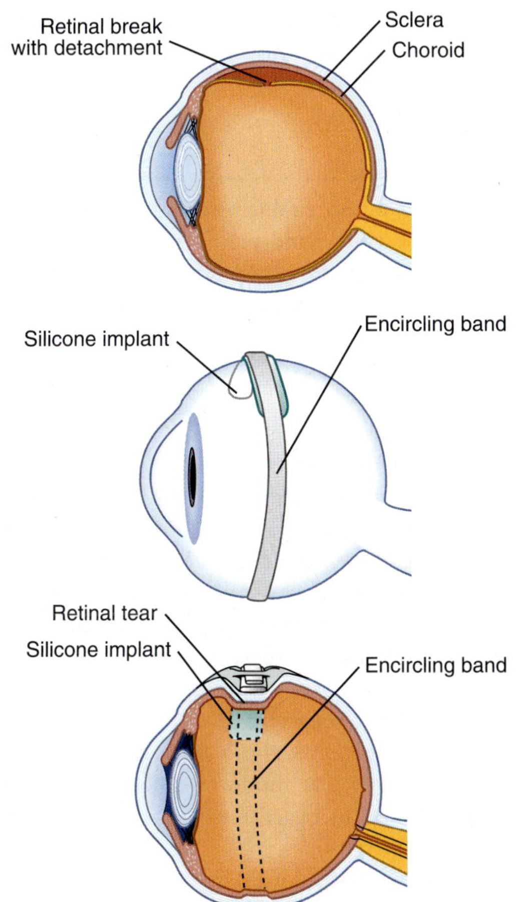

Fig. 22.14 Retinal break with detachment and surgical repair by scleral buckling technique.

Intraocular Procedures

Pneumatic retinopexy is the intravitreal injection of a gas to form a temporary bubble in the vitreous. The intravitreal bubble closes retinal breaks and provides opposition of the separated retinal layers. Because the bubble is temporary, it is combined with laser photocoagulation or cryopexy. Patients with a bubble must position their head so that the bubble is in contact with the retinal break. This position must be maintained for several weeks to allow the retinal break to heal.

Vitrectomy is the surgical removal of the vitreous. It may relieve traction on the retina, especially when the traction results from proliferative diabetic retinopathy. Vitrectomy can be combined with scleral buckling to provide a dual effect in relieving traction.

❖ NURSING MANAGEMENT: RETINAL DETACHMENT

After surgery, patients may be on bed rest and need special positioning to maintain proper position of an intravitreal bubble. The level of activity restriction varies. Verify the prescribed level of activity with the HCP so you can assist patients with activity restrictions.

Patients may need multiple topical medications, including antibiotics, antiinflammatory agents, or dilating agents. Give pain medications as prescribed. Patients may go home within a few hours of surgery or stay in the hospital for several days, depending on the HCP and type of repair. Discharge planning and teaching are important and should begin early. Table 22.11 discusses patient and caregiver teaching after eye surgery. Because patients are at increased risk for retinal detachment in the other eye, teach patients signs and symptoms of retinal detachment. Promote the use of protective eyewear to help avoid eye trauma.

AGE-RELATED MACULAR DEGENERATION

Age-related macular degeneration (AMD) is a leading cause of irreversible central vision loss. AMD is either dry (nonexudative) or wet (exudative). *Dry AMD* is most common, accounting for 90% of all cases. Those with dry AMD often notice that close vision tasks become difficult. In dry AMD, macular cells start to atrophy. This leads to a slowly progressive and painless vision loss.

Wet AMD is the most severe form. It accounts for most cases of AMD-related blindness. Wet AMD has a more rapid onset of vision loss because of the development of abnormal blood vessels in or near the macula. Most patients with wet AMD develop dry AMD first.

Etiology and Pathophysiology

AMD is related to retinal aging. Other risk factors include family history, obesity, hypertension, and being White. Smoking significantly increases the risk of AMD. The risk increases with a higher pack-year exposure.[13] It occurs more often in females.

Dry AMD starts with the abnormal accumulation of yellowish extracellular deposits called *drusen* in the retinal pigment epithelium. Over time, atrophy and degeneration of macular cells occur. In wet AMD, vascular endothelial growth factor (VEGF) promotes the growth of new blood vessels in an abnormal location in the retinal epithelium. As new blood vessels grow, they leak fluid and may bleed, causing scar tissue to develop.

Clinical Manifestations and Diagnostic Studies

Patients may have blurred and darkened vision, *scotomas* (blind spots in the visual field), and *metamorphopsia* (vision distortion). Vision distortion includes the illusion that straight lines, such as the edge of a door or sentences on a page, are wavy or that some objects are smaller than they really are. If only 1 eye is affected, patients may not notice early changes in vision. Acute vision loss may occur from either form.

AMD is diagnosed by visual acuity measurement and ophthalmoscopy. The HCP looks for drusen and other fundus changes associated with AMD. The Amsler grid test may help define the involved area. It provides a baseline for future comparison (Fig. 22.15). Fundus fluorescein angiography and/or indocyanine green dyes may help determine the extent and type of AMD. Optical coherence tomography (OCT), which looks at the macula, or scanning laser ophthalmoscopy can be used.

Interprofessional Care

The goal of care is to reverse or minimize vision loss and improve vision function. Visual prognosis can vary. Treatment options for wet AMD include medications that are injected directly into the vitreous cavity. Ranibizumab (Lucentis), bevacizumab (Avastin), and aflibercept (Eylea) inhibit VEGF. These medications help slow vision loss by halting new vessels from forming.[13] Side effects may include blurred vision, eye irritation, eye pain, and photosensitivity. Injections are given at 4- to 6-week intervals, depending on treatment response. Disease stability is determined by OCT. The findings determine the need for continued intravitreal injections.

Verteporfin (Visudyne) IV is part of photodynamic therapy (PDT) to treat wet AMD. Laser light shone into the eye activates verteporfin and causes it to create blood clots that block abnormal blood vessels. By sealing leaky blood vessels, PDT slows central vision loss. Until the body completely excretes the drug, it can be activated by exposure to sunlight or other high-intensity light, such as halogen. Patients must avoid direct exposure to sunlight and other intense forms of light for 5 days after treatment. Exposing the skin to sunlight could activate the drug in that area, causing a chemical burn.

Antioxidant vitamins (e.g., vitamin C, vitamin E), lutein, zeaxanthin, and zinc may help slow the progression of AMD.[13] Teach patients to eat dark green, leafy vegetables containing lutein (e.g., kale, broccoli, spinach) and foods that are high in zinc (e.g., beef, pork, dairy, whole grains). Smoking cessation may help stop the progression of dry AMD.

The management of patients with visual impairment is appropriate for patients with AMD. Many patients with low-vision assistive devices can continue reading and drive during the daytime and at low speed. The permanent loss of central vision has significant psychosocial implications. Avoid giving the impression that "nothing can be done" when caring for patients with AMD. Although treatment may not recover lost vision, much can be done to augment the remaining vision.

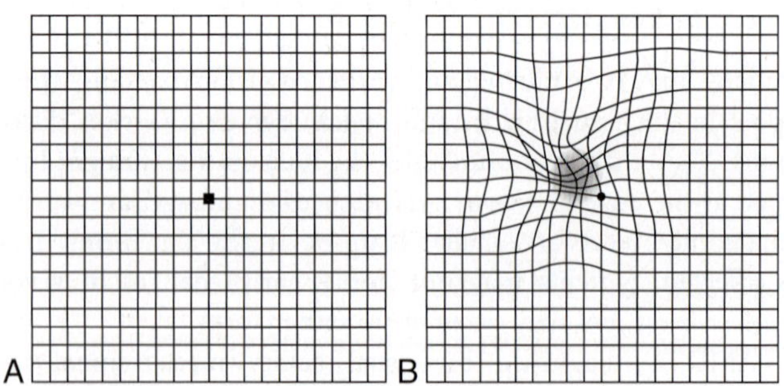

Fig. 22.15 Amsler grid. (A) Normal grid. (B) Abnormal grid as seen by a person with AMD.

GLAUCOMA

Glaucoma is a group of problems characterized by increased IOP, optic nerve atrophy, and peripheral visual field loss. It is the second leading cause of permanent blindness in the United States. Many people with glaucoma are unaware of their condition. The incidence increases with age. Genetic factors play a role in some types of glaucoma.

Etiology and Pathophysiology

A proper balance between the rate of aqueous production *(inflow)* and the rate of aqueous reabsorption *(outflow)* is essential to maintain the IOP within normal limits. The place where outflow occurs is called the *angle* because it is the angle where the iris meets the cornea. When the rate of inflow is greater than the rate of outflow, IOP can increase above normal limits. If IOP stays increased, permanent vision loss may occur.

Primary open-angle glaucoma (POAG) is the most common type of glaucoma. In POAG, the outflow of aqueous humor is decreased in the trabecular meshwork. The drainage channels become clogged, like a clogged kitchen sink.[14] Damage to the optic nerve can then result.

Angle-closure glaucoma (ACG) is caused by a reduction in the outflow of aqueous humor from angle closure. ACG is mainly caused by the lens bulging forward from the aging process. Angle closure may also occur because of pupil dilation in patients with anatomically narrow angles. Acute angle-closure glaucoma (AACG) may be precipitated by situations in which the pupil stays partially dilated long enough to cause an acute and significant rise in the IOP. This may occur with drug-induced mydriasis, emotional excitement, or darkness. Drug-induced mydriasis may occur from topical eye preparations or many systemic medications. Assess medication records before giving medications to patients with ACG. Teach them not to take any mydriatic medications.

Clinical Manifestations

POAG develops slowly and without symptoms of pain or pressure. Patients usually do not notice the gradual visual field loss until peripheral vision is severely reduced.[14] Eventually, patients with untreated glaucoma have "tunnel vision," with only a small center visual field. Peripheral vision is absent.

AACG causes definite symptoms, including sudden, severe pain in or around the eye. Patients often have nausea and vomiting. Vision symptoms include colored halos around lights, blurred vision, and eye redness.

Manifestations of subacute or chronic ACG appear more gradually. Patients who have had a previous unrecognized episode of subacute ACG may report blurred vision, seeing colored halos around lights, eye redness, or eye or brow pain.

Diagnostic Studies

IOP is usually increased in glaucoma above the normal 10 to 21 mm Hg. In POAG, IOP is usually between 22 and 32 mm Hg. In AACG, IOP may exceed 50 mm Hg. Measurements are repeated over time to verify the elevation.

In POAG, slit lamp microscopy reveals a normal angle. In ACG, there may be a markedly narrow or flat anterior chamber angle, an edematous cornea, a fixed and moderately dilated pupil, and ciliary injection (hyperemia of the ciliary blood vessels produces a red color).

Measures of peripheral and central vision provide diagnostic information. Perimetry produces a complete map of the patient's visual field. It may reveal subtle changes in peripheral vision early in the disease process. In ACG, central visual acuity is reduced if there is corneal edema, and the visual fields may be greatly decreased. Central acuity may remain 20/20 even in the presence of severe peripheral visual field loss. As glaucoma progresses, *optic disc cupping* may be one of the first signs of chronic POAG. The optic disc becomes wider, deeper, and paler (light gray or white). This is visible with direct or indirect ophthalmoscopy (Fig. 22.16).

Interprofessional Care

The primary focus of treatment is to maintain the IOP low enough to prevent optic nerve damage. Treatment varies with the type of glaucoma. Diagnostic and interprofessional care of glaucoma is outlined in Table 22.14.

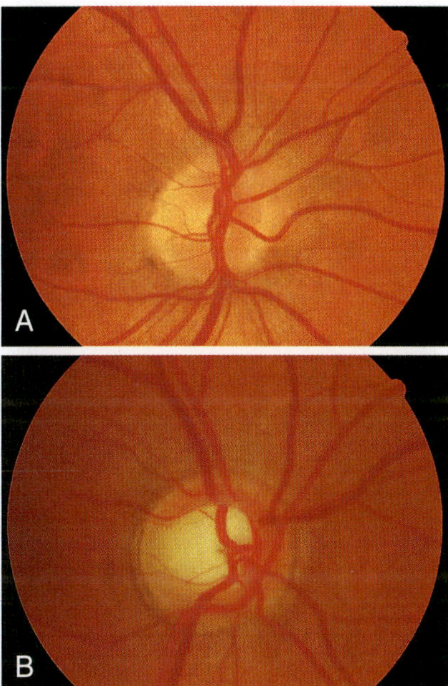

Fig. 22.16 (A) In the normal eye, the optic cup is pink with little cupping. (B) With glaucoma, the optic cup is bleached, and optic cupping is present. Note the retinal vessels, which travel over the edge of the optic cup and appear to dip into it.

Chronic Open-Angle Glaucoma

Drug therapy is the initial treatment in POAG (Table 22.15). Continued treatment and supervision are needed because the drugs control, but do not cure, glaucoma. Because of their superior efficacy and systemic safety, prostaglandin analogs are the preferred initial treatment.

Many patients with glaucoma have other illnesses or take medications that may affect their therapy. Patients taking a β-adrenergic—blocking glaucoma agent may have an additive effect if they also take a systemic β-adrenergic—blocking drug. All β-adrenergic—blocking glaucoma agents are contraindicated in patients with bradycardia, second- or third-degree heart block, cardiogenic shock, and heart failure. Noncardioselective β-adrenergic—blocking glaucoma agents are contraindicated in patients with chronic obstructive pulmonary disease (COPD) or asthma. They may have profound effects in older patients.

Argon laser trabeculoplasty (ALT) is a noninvasive way to lower IOP when medications are not successful or when patients either cannot or will not use drug therapy as prescribed. ALT is an outpatient procedure done with a topical anesthetic. The laser stimulates scarring and contraction of the trabecular meshwork, which opens the outflow channels. Patients need to use topical corticosteroids for 3 to 5 days after the procedure. An acute rise in

TABLE 22.14 Interprofessional Care

Glaucoma

Diagnostic Assessment

- History and physical assessment
- Visual acuity measurement
- Tonometry
- Ophthalmoscopy
- Slit lamp microscopy
- Gonioscopy
- Visual field perimetry

Management

Chronic Open-Angle Glaucoma

Drug Therapy (Table 22.15)

- α-Adrenergic agonists
- β-Adrenergic blockers
- Carbonic anhydrase inhibitors
- Miotics
- Prostaglandin agonists

Surgical Therapy

- Argon laser trabeculoplasty (ALT)
- Trabeculectomy with or without filtering implant

Acute Angle-Closure Glaucoma

- Carbonic anhydrase inhibitors
- Hyperosmotic agent
- Laser peripheral iridotomy
- Surgical iridectomy

TABLE 22.15 Drug Therapy

Acute and Chronic Glaucoma

Drug	Action	Side Effects	Nursing Considerations
α-Adrenergic Agonists			
apraclonidine (Iopidine), brimonidine (Alphagan)	↓ Aqueous humor production	Eye redness, irregular heart rate, dry mouth, fatigue	Topical drops Control or prevent acute postlaser IOP rise (used before and immediately after ALT and iridotomy, Nd:YAG laser capsulotomy) Teach patients at risk for systemic reactions to occlude puncta
β-Adrenergic Blockers			
betaxolol (Betoptic)	β_1 cardioselective ↓ IOP, ↓ aqueous humor production	Eye discomfort Systemic reactions rare but include bradycardia, heart block, pulmonary distress, headache, depression	Topical drugs Contraindicated in patients with bradycardia, cardiogenic shock, heart failure Systemic absorption can have additive effect with systemic β_1-blocking agents
levobunolol (Betagan) timolol maleate (Timoptic, Istalol)	β_1 and β_2 noncardioselective blockers ↓ IOP, ↓ aqueous humor production	Same as betaxolol	Topical drops Same as betaxolol Contraindicated in patients with asthma or COPD
Carbonic Anhydrase Inhibitors			
Systemic			
acetazolamide (Diamox) methazolamide	↓ Aqueous humor production	Paresthesias, hearing problems, tinnitus, anorexia, taste changes, GI problems, headache, drowsiness, depression, kidney stones	Sulfa-type allergic reactions may occur in patients allergic to sulfa Diuretic effect can alter fluid and electrolyte balance Do not give with high-dose aspirin therapy May cause gout attacks
Topical			
brinzolamide dorzolamide (Trusopt)	↓ Aqueous humor production	Transient stinging, blurred vision, redness	Sulfa-type allergic reactions may occur in patients allergic to sulfa
Miotics			
pilocarpine (Isopto Carpine)	Parasympathomimetic Stimulates ciliary muscle contraction, causing miosis and opening of trabecular meshwork, ↑ aqueous outflow Partially inhibits cholinesterase	Eye pain and burning, headache, blurred vision, ↓ adaptation to the dark, syncope, dysrhythmias, hypotension	Topical drops Caution patients about ↓ visual acuity caused by miosis, especially in dim light
Prostaglandin Agonists			
bimatoprost (Lumigan) latanoprost (Xalatan) tafluprost (Zioptan) travoprost (Travatan)	↑ Outflow of aqueous humor between uvea and sclera and usual exit through the trabecular meshwork	↑ Brown iris pigmentation, stinging, redness, dryness, itching, foreign body sensation	Topical drops Teach patients to only use 1 drop per day Remove contact lens 15 min before instilling
Rho Kinase Inhibitors			
netarsudil (Rhopressa)	↓ Aqueous humor production and ↑ outflow	Redness, blurred vision, headache	Topical drops Teach patients to only use 1 drop per day

ALT, Argon laser trabeculoplasty; *COPD,* chronic obstructive pulmonary disease; *IOP,* intraocular pressure; *Nd:YAG,* neodymium-doped yttrium aluminum garnet (laser).

IOP is the most common complication. HCP follow-up occurs at 1 week and again at 4 to 6 weeks after surgery.

Filtration surgery, also called a *trabeculectomy,* may be used if drug and laser therapy are unsuccessful.

Acute Angle-Closure Glaucoma

AACG is an emergency that needs immediate intervention. Carbonic anhydrase inhibitors (Table 22.15) and oral or IV hyperosmotic agents, including isosorbide and mannitol

(Osmitrol), are usually successful in immediately lowering IOP. A laser peripheral iridotomy or surgical iridectomy is necessary for long-term treatment and prevention of recurrence. These procedures allow the aqueous humor to flow through a newly created opening in the iris and into normal outflow channels. A procedure may be done on the other eye as a precaution, as many patients often have an acute attack in the other eye.

NURSING MANAGEMENT: GLAUCOMA

Assessment

Because glaucoma is a chronic condition requiring long-term management, assess the patient's ability to understand and adhere to the treatment plan. Assess the patient's reaction to the diagnosis of a potentially sight-threatening problem. Include any caregivers, because the chronic nature of this problem also affects them. For example, caregivers may need to administer eyedrops if the patient is unable.

Clinical Problems

Clinical problems for patients with glaucoma include:

- Sensory deficit
- Pain
- Impaired role performance

Planning

The overall goals are that patients with glaucoma will (1) have no progression of vision impairment, (2) follow the treatment plan, and (3) be free from complications.

Implementation

Health Promotion

Vision loss from glaucoma is preventable. Provide teaching about the risk for glaucoma and that it increases with age. Stress the importance of early detection and treatment to prevent vision impairment. A comprehensive eye examination is important in identifying patients with glaucoma and those at risk for developing glaucoma. Current recommendations for an eye examination are (1) every 2 to 4 years between ages 40 and 54 years, (2) every 1 to 3 years between ages 55 and 64 years, and (3) every 1 to 2 years for people age 65 years or older.[15] Those at higher risk for glaucoma and other eye issues should have their eyes checked more often.

Acute Care

Acute nursing care is directed mainly toward patients with AACG and surgical patients. Patients with AACG need medication immediately to lower IOP. Most surgeries for glaucoma are done as an outpatient. Administer analgesia to relieve discomfort related to the procedure. Patient and caregiver teaching after eye surgery is discussed in Table 22.11.

Chronic Care

Because of the chronic nature of glaucoma, teach patients to follow the treatment plan and follow-up recommendations prescribed by the HCP. Discuss the disease process and treatment options. Review the purpose, frequency, and technique for administering antiglaucoma drugs. Encourage adherence by helping patients to set up a medication administration schedule. Advocate for a change in therapy if the patient reports unacceptable side effects.

Evaluation

The overall expected outcomes are that patients with glaucoma will:

- Have no further vision loss
- Adhere to the treatment plan
- Safely function within their own environment
- Have relief from pain associated with the disease and surgery

INTRAOCULAR INFLAMMATION AND INFECTION

The term *uveitis* is used to describe inflammation of the uveal tract, retina, vitreous body, or optic nerve. Inflammation may be caused by bacteria, viruses, fungi, or parasites. *Cytomegalovirus retinitis* (CMV retinitis) is an opportunistic infection that occurs in patients with AIDS or immunosuppression. The cause of sterile intraocular inflammation includes autoimmune disorders, AIDS, cancer, or some systemic diseases, such as inflammatory bowel disease. Pain and photophobia are common.

Endophthalmitis is an extensive intraocular inflammation of the vitreous cavity. Bacteria, viruses, fungi, or parasites can induce this serious inflammatory response. The mechanism of infection may be endogenous, in which the infecting agent arrives at the eye through the bloodstream, or exogenous. The infecting agent is often introduced through a surgical wound or a penetrating injury. Although rare, endophthalmitis is a complication of intraocular surgery or penetrating eye injury. It can lead to irreversible blindness within hours or days. Manifestations include eye pain, photophobia, decreased visual acuity, headaches, reddened and swollen conjunctiva, and corneal edema.

Treatment depends on the underlying cause. Intraocular infections require antimicrobial agents. They may be delivered topically, in the subconjunctiva, intravitreally, systemically, or in some combination. Inflammatory responses require antiinflammatory medications (e.g., corticosteroids). Patients are usually uncomfortable and may be anxious or frightened. Provide information and emotional support. In severe cases, patients may need enucleation. When patients have lost visual function, they will grieve the loss. Your role includes supporting patients through the grieving process.

OCULAR TUMORS

Benign and cancerous tumors can occur in many areas of the eye, including the conjunctiva, retina, and orbit. Eyelid cancers include basal cell and squamous cell cancers (see Chapter 25).

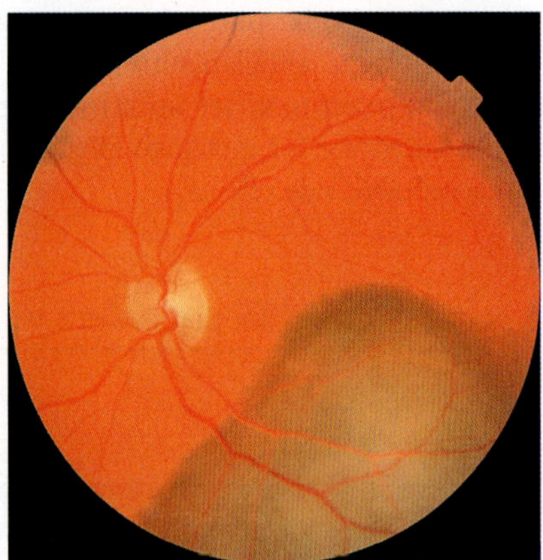

Fig. 22.17 Uveal melanoma. A large tumor in the choroid, the most common location in the eye for melanoma. (Courtesy Cory J. Bosanko, OD, FAAO, Eye Centers of Tennessee, Crossville, TN.)

Uveal melanoma is a cancer of the iris, choroid, or ciliary body (Fig. 22.17). It more often occurs in light-skinned people with light eye color, who are over age 60, and have chronic UV exposure.[16] Uveal melanoma can arise from preexisting nevi in the eye. Tumors may be asymptomatic or there may be vision loss. This depends on the size and location and presence of hemorrhage and retinal detachment. As with other cancers, cancer stage and cell type are important variables in the prognosis. Diagnostic testing may include ultrasound, MRI, angiography, and fine-needle aspiration biopsy. Uveal melanoma often appears as a dome-shaped, well-circumscribed, solid brown to golden pigment in the iris, choroid, or ciliary body.

Depending on the status of the involved eye, treatment options may include radiation therapy, photocoagulation, thermotherapy, resection, and eye removal. Many patients do not lose their eye. Some may have good vision after treatment in the affected eye.

ENUCLEATION

Enucleation is the removal of the eye. The primary reason for enucleation is a blind, painful eye from glaucoma, infection, or trauma. Enucleation may be used to treat ocular cancer. The procedure includes severing the extraocular muscles close to their insertion on the globe, inserting an implant to maintain the intraorbital anatomy, and suturing the ends of the muscles over the implant. The conjunctiva covers the joined muscles. A clear conformer is placed over the conjunctiva until the permanent prosthesis is fitted. A pressure dressing helps prevent bleeding.

After surgery, observe for signs of complications, including excess bleeding or swelling, increased pain, displacement of the implant, and fever. Teaching should include how to instill topical ointments or drops and wound cleansing. Review how to insert the conformer into the socket in case it falls out. The loss of an eye is often devastating, even when enucleation occurs after a lengthy period of painful blindness. Recognize the patient's emotional response and provide support to the patient and caregivers.

About 6 weeks after surgery, the wound will be sufficiently healed for the permanent prosthesis. An ocularist fits the prosthesis and designs it to match the remaining eye. Teach the patient how to remove, cleanse, and insert the prosthesis. Special polishing is needed periodically to remove dried protein secretions.

CASE STUDY

Glaucoma and Diabetic Retinopathy

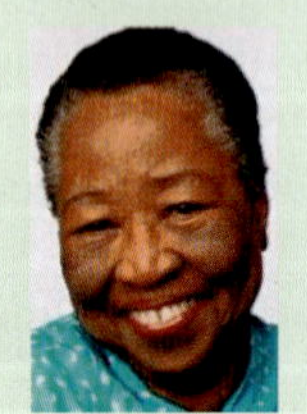

(© Kevin Peterson/ Stockbyte/ Thinkstock.)

Patient Profile

J.K. is a 68-year-old female with a history of osteoarthritis and type 2 diabetes for the past 15 years. J.K. was recently diagnosed with diabetic retinopathy. She returns to the eye clinic with her daughter for continued care of primary open-angle glaucoma (POAG) and reexamination for changes related to diabetic retinopathy. Her current drug therapy for POAG includes topical timolol maleate 0.5% extended release (Timoptic-XE) and latanoprost (Xalatan) 0.005% once daily in both eyes. Her last eye examination showed microaneurysms and hard exudates of the retina.

Subjective Data

- She can no longer read the newspaper and reports that medication labels are difficult to read.
- She is not always able to instill her eyedrops because her hands are gnarled and painful from osteoarthritis.

Objective Data

- Distant and near visual acuity: 20/60 (right eye) and 20/50 (left eye), with a reduction from 20/40 (both eyes) at her last visit
- Intraocular pressure (IOP) 20 mm Hg in each eye
- A new blind spot with visual field testing in the left eye
- Fluorescein angiography shows diabetic macular edema in both eyes

Interprofessional Care

- Brimonidine 0.15% (left eye) 15 min before and immediately after argon laser trabeculoplasty (ALT)
- Argon laser to left eye to seal leaking microaneurysms from macular edema
- Check IOP 1 h after ALT
- Continue previous glaucoma drop regimen
- Follow-up examination in 2 wk for possible ALT of right eye

Discussion Questions

1. ***Recognize:*** Explain the cause of the changes in J.K.'s vision.
2. ***Analyze:*** What main complication is J.K. at risk for?
3. ***Plan:*** Why is ALT an appropriate treatment for J.K.?
4. ***Prioritize:*** Based on the assessment data, what are the priority clinical problems?
5. ***Prioritize:*** What are the priority nursing interventions for J.K.?
6. ***Act:*** Why do we give eyedrops before and immediately after ALT?
7. ***Act:*** What teaching will you provide so J.K. can manage her care?
8. ***Evaluate:*** What outcomes would indicate interprofessional care was effective?

Answers available at http://evolve.elsevier.com/Lewis/medsurg.

BRIDGE TO NCLEX EXAMINATION

The number of the question corresponds to the same-numbered outcome at the beginning of the chapter.

1. In a patient with a hemorrhage in the posterior cavity of the eye, blood is accumulating
   - **a.** in the aqueous humor.
   - **b.** between the lens and retina.
   - **c.** between the cornea and lens.
   - **d.** in the space between the iris and lens.
2. Increased intraocular pressure may occur because of
   - **a.** edema of the corneal stroma.
   - **b.** dilation of the retinal arterioles.
   - **c.** blockage of the lacrimal canals and ducts.
   - **d.** increased aqueous humor production by the ciliary process.
3. Ask patients using eyedrops to treat their glaucoma about
   - **a.** use of corrective lenses.
   - **b.** their usual sleep patterns.
   - **c.** a history of heart or lung disease.
   - **d.** sensitivity to opioids or depressants.
4. The nurse would assess any patient with an eye problem for
   - **a.** visual acuity.
   - **b.** pupil reactions.
   - **c.** intraocular pressure.
   - **d.** confrontation visual fields.
5. When examining a patient's eyes, which finding would be of *most* concern?
   - **a.** Intraocular pressure of 16 mm Hg
   - **b.** Slightly yellowish cast of the sclera
   - **c.** Outward turning of the lower lid margin
   - **d.** Small, white nodule on the upper lid margin
6. Presbyopia occurs in older adults because
   - **a.** the eyeball elongates.
   - **b.** the lens becomes inflexible.
   - **c.** the corneal curvature becomes irregular.
   - **d.** light rays are focusing in front of the retina.
7. Before injecting fluorescein for angiography, it is important for the nurse to (**Select all that apply.**)
   - **a.** administer a topical anesthetic.
   - **b.** ask if the patient is tired or fatigued.
   - **c.** provide the patient with an emesis basin.
   - **d.** inform the patient that skin may turn yellow.
   - **e.** assess for allergies to iodine-based contrast media.
8. Which response would the nurse provide to a patient who asks what astigmatism is?
   - **a.** "It happens because the lens of the eye is absent."
   - **b.** "People with astigmatism have abnormally long eyeballs."
   - **c.** "The cornea of the eye is uneven or irregular with astigmatism."
   - **d.** "Astigmatism occurs because the eye muscles weaken with age."
9. Which intervention would be part of the plan of care for a patient with new vision loss?
   - **a.** Allow the patient to express feelings of grief and anger.
   - **b.** Have the AP perform all self-care activities for the patient.
   - **c.** Address any family present first when discussing care concerns.
   - **d.** Speak loudly and clearly, addressing the patient with each contact.
10. Which patient behaviors would the nurse promote for healthy eyes? (**Select all that apply.**)
    - **a.** Protective sunglasses when bicycling
    - **b.** Taking part in a smoking cessation program
    - **c.** Supplementing diet intake of vitamin C and beta-carotene
    - **d.** Washing hands thoroughly before putting in or taking out contact lenses
    - **e.** A woman avoiding pregnancy for 4 weeks after receiving MMR immunization
11. The *most* important intervention for a patient with epidemic keratoconjunctivitis is
    - **a.** cleansing the affected area with baby shampoo.
    - **b.** monitoring spread of infection to the opposing eye.
    - **c.** regular instillation of artificial tears to the affected eye.
    - **d.** teaching the patient and caregivers good hygiene techniques.
12. What would be included in the discharge teaching for a patient after cataract surgery? (**Select all that apply.**)
    - **a.** Eye discomfort is often relieved with mild analgesics.
    - **b.** A decline in visual acuity is common for the first month.
    - **c.** Stay on bed rest and limit activity for the first few weeks.
    - **d.** Notify the provider if an increase in redness or drainage occurs.
    - **e.** Following activity restrictions is essential to reduce intraocular pressure.

1. b; 2. d; 3. c; 4. a; 5. d; 6. b; 7. c, d; 8. c; 9. a;
10. a, b, c, d; 11. d; 12. a, d, e.

For rationales to these answers and even more NCLEX review questions, visit http://evolve.elsevier.com/Lewis/medsurg.

REFERENCES

To access the References for this chapter, please scan the QR code with a mobile device.

23

Assessment and Management: Auditory Problems

Mariann M. Harding

http://evolve.elsevier.com/Lewis/medsurg/

CONCEPTUAL FOCUS

Functional Ability
Infection
Sensory Perception
Stress and Coping

LEARNING OUTCOMES

1. Describe the structures and functions of the auditory system.
2. Obtain subjective and objective assessment data related to the auditory system.
3. Perform a physical assessment of the auditory system.
4. Distinguish normal from common abnormal findings of the auditory system assessment.
5. Link the age-related changes in the auditory system to differences in assessment findings.
6. Describe the purpose, significance of results, and nursing responsibilities related to diagnostic studies of the auditory system.
7. Explain the pathophysiology, clinical manifestations, and nursing and interprofessional management of common ear problems.
8. Compare the common causes, management, and rehabilitative potential of hearing loss.
9. Explain the use, care, and patient teaching related to assistive hearing devices.
10. Describe measures to assist patients in adapting to hearing loss.

KEY TERMS

acoustic neuroma
benign paroxysmal positional vertigo (BPPV)
external otitis
Ménière disease
nystagmus
otosclerosis
presbycusis
tinnitus
vertigo

Hearing is a complex process that allows us to interact with the environment. It is essential for maintaining relationships with others and experiencing life events. Hearing is the basis for social interaction and communication. It makes it possible to enjoy many of the things that affect quality of life. Hearing loss can have a dramatic impact on the way a person interacts with others and experiences life. This chapter presents an overview of the ear and hearing and discusses care when problems are present.

STRUCTURES AND FUNCTIONS OF THE AUDITORY SYSTEM

The auditory system is composed of the peripheral auditory system and central auditory system. The peripheral auditory system includes the structures of the ear itself: external, middle, and inner ear (Fig. 23.1). This system is involved with the reception and perception of sound. The inner ear functions in hearing and balance.

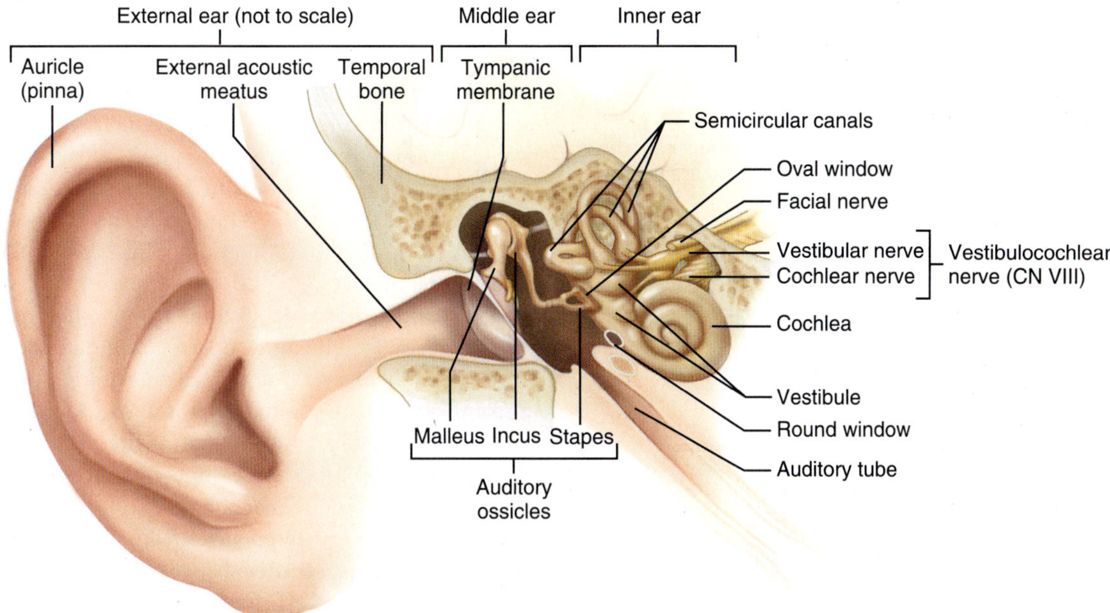

Fig. 23.1 External, middle, and inner ear. (Modified from Patton KT, Thibodeau GA: *Anatomy and physiology,* ed 8, St Louis, 2013, Mosby.)

The central auditory system integrates and assigns meaning to what you hear. This system includes the vestibulocochlear nerve (cranial nerve [CN] VIII) and auditory cortex of the brain. The brain and its pathways transmit and process sound and sensations that maintain equilibrium.

External Ear

The external ear consists of the *pinna* (auricle), external auditory canal (ear canal), and *tympanic membrane (TM),* or eardrum. The pinna is composed of cartilage and connective tissue. It is covered with epithelium, which also lines the ear canal (Fig. 23.1). The *tragus* is the small piece of thick cartilage that is in front of and partly closing the ear canal. The ear canal is a slightly S-shaped tube about 1 inch (2.5 cm) in length in an adult. The lining of the first one-third of the canal contains fine hairs (cilia), sebaceous (oil) glands, and cerumen (wax) glands. The oil and wax lubricate the ear canal, keep it free from debris, and kill bacteria. Thin epithelium lines the distal two-thirds of the canal. It is over bone and very sensitive.

The function of the external ear and canal is to collect and transmit sound waves to the TM. The TM is a shiny, translucent, pearl-gray membrane that separates the outer ear from the middle ear. It is made up of a thin connective tissue membrane covered by skin on the outside and mucosa on the internal surface. The TM transmits sounds between the ear canal and middle ear.

Middle Ear

The middle ear cavity is an air space in the temporal bone. It is lined with mucous membrane. The middle ear contains the *ossicles,* the 3 smallest bones in the body: *malleus, incus,* and *stapes.* The TM is attached to the malleus at the umbo (Fig. 23.2). Vibrations of the TM cause the ossicles to move and transmit sound waves to the oval window. The oval window is a membrane-covered opening between the middle and inner ear.

The eustachian tube connects the middle ear cavity with the nasopharynx. The tube's opening in the nasopharynx is surrounded by the adenoids. The main function of the eustachian tube is maintaining equalized air pressure on both sides of the TM. This allows the TM to move freely. The tube is normally closed, opening only with yawning, swallowing, and chewing. Secretions from the middle ear drain through the tube into the throat. Blockage of the tube can occur with allergies, nasopharyngeal infections, or enlarged adenoids.

The upper part of the middle ear is the epitympanum. It communicates with air cells within the mastoid bone. The mastoid is the posterior part of the temporal bone. The facial nerve (CN VII) passes through the middle ear above the ossicles.

Inner Ear

The inner ear consists of 3 spaces in the temporal bone in a system called the bony labyrinth. The space is filled with watery fluid called perilymph. Within the perilymph is the membranous labyrinth. It follows the shape of the bony labyrinth and holds a thicker fluid called *endolymph.*

The inner ear holds the functional organs for hearing and balance. The receptor organ for hearing is the *organ of Corti.* It lies on the basilar membrane in the *cochlea.* Its tiny hair cells transform fluid vibrations from sounds into electrical impulses. These are transmitted by the acoustic part of CN VIII to the brain.

The *vestibule* and 3 *semicircular canals* make up the organ of balance. The semicircular canals sit at right angles to each other. Structures in each canal and the vestibule generate nerve impulses in response to our movements. The vestibule is beside

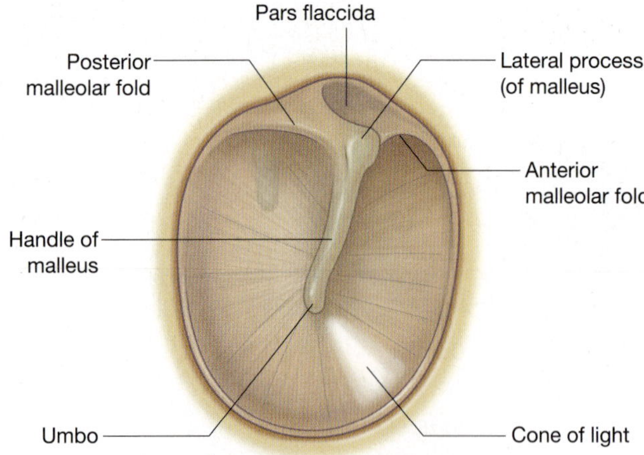

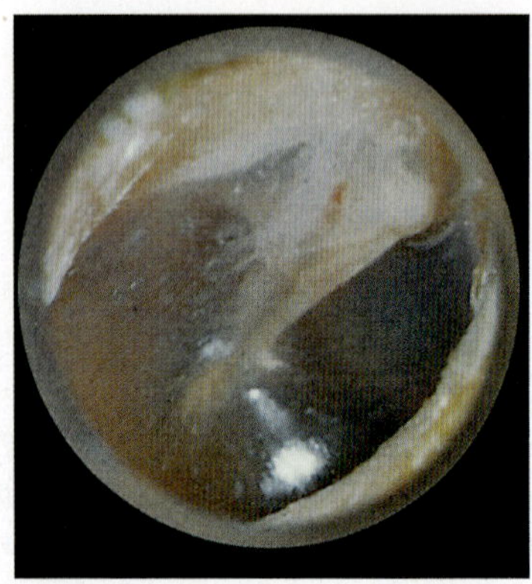

Fig. 23.2 Normal tympanic membrane. (From Vogl AW, Drake RL, Mitchell A: *Gray's basic anatomy,* ed 3, 2023, Elsevier.)

the oval window between the semicircular canals and the cochlea. Nerves from receptors in the vestibule join those from the semicircular canals to form the vestibular nerve. The vestibular nerve joins with the cochlear nerve to form CN VIII.

How Do We Hear?

Hearing depends on a series of complex steps that change sound waves in the air into electrical signals. The role of the external and middle part of the ear is to conduct and amplify sound waves from the environment. Sound waves travel by air and are picked up by the pinna and auditory canal. Sound waves strike the TM, causing it to vibrate. The central part of the TM is connected to the malleus, which then starts to vibrate. The malleus transmits the vibration to the incus and then to the stapes. As the stapes moves back and forth, it pushes the membrane of the oval window in and out.

Movement of the oval window makes waves in the perilymph. These vibrations are picked up by the tiny sensory hair cells of the cochlea, which initiate nerve impulses. These impulses are carried by nerve fibers to the main branch of the acoustic part of CN VIII and then to the auditory cortex in the brain. The bones of the skull can also transmit sound directly to the inner ear (bone conduction).

The auditory cortex translates the impulses into sounds that we know and understand. It processes the volume of sounds and determines the direction they come from. The auditory cortex discriminates relevant sounds from background noise and adjusts the volume of our speech. Last, it filters out unwanted noise so that we can focus on what we are listening to.

We measure sound waves in 2 ways: intensity (or strength) and frequency (or pitch). We measure the intensity in terms of decibels (dB). The lowest hearing decibel level is 0 dB, which is nearly total silence and the softest sound that we can hear. Normal speech is around 40 to 65 dB. A soft whisper is 20 dB. Sounds above 90 dB can lead to hearing damage if people are exposed to them every day or all the time. Hearing becomes uncomfortable if the sound level is above 110 dB.

Frequency is the measurement of the number of sound vibrations in 1 second. We measure it in hertz (Hz). The higher the frequency is, the higher the pitch. Normally, a child and a young adult can hear frequencies from about 16 to 20,000 Hz, but hearing is most sensitive between 500 and 4000 Hz. This is similar to normal speech frequencies.

Gerontologic Considerations: Effects of Aging on the Auditory System

Presbycusis, or age-related hearing loss (ARHL), is the third most common health problem in older adults.[1] Calcification of the ossicles diminishes sound transmission. **Tinnitus**, or ringing in the ears, is common. It may be the first sign of hearing loss. Cerumen glands atrophy, causing cerumen (earwax) to be much drier. The hair in the ear becomes thicker and coarser, trapping the hard, dry earwax in the external canal. This accumulation of dry earwax can interfere with sound transmission. Atrophy of vestibular structures in the inner ear causes a decline in balance and slowing of motor responses.

Age-related changes in the auditory system and differences in assessment findings are outlined in Table 23.1.

CASE STUDY

Patient Introduction

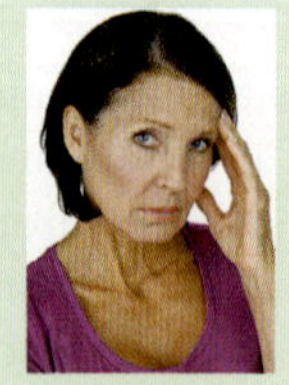

(© Stockphoto4u/iStock.com.)

R.S. is a 57-year-old female who comes to the emergency department with extreme dizziness. She says that she is so dizzy she "can't do anything but lie down." R.S. says her right ear is "plugged," and she has ringing in that ear.

Discussion Questions

1. What are the possible causes of R.M.'s hearing and balance problems?
2. Is her condition stable or an emergency?
3. What assessment questions will you ask?

You will learn more about R.S. and her condition as you read this chapter.

Answers available at http://evolve.elsevier.com/Lewis/medsurg

TABLE 23.1 GERONTOLOGIC ASSESSMENT DIFFERENCES

Auditory System

Changes	Differences in Assessment Findings
External Ear	
Increased hair	Visible hair
Loss of elasticity in cartilage	Collapsed ear canal
Thicker, drier earwax	Impacted earwax, potential hearing loss
Middle Ear	
Rigidity and atrophy of TM	Conductive hearing loss
Inner Ear	
Loss of hair cells in organ of Corti, neuron degeneration in CN VIII and central pathways, reduced blood supply to cochlea, rigidity of ossicles	ARHL, diminished sensitivity to high-pitched sounds, impaired speech reception, tinnitus
Less effective vestibular apparatus in semicircular canals	Changes in balance and body orientation
Brain	
Decline in gray and white matter, auditory orienting reflex slows	Difficulty hearing in a noisy environment, impaired speech perception, decreased ability to locate origin of sound

AUDITORY SYSTEM ASSESSMENT

Assessment of the auditory system should include assessing hearing and balance because the auditory and *vestibular* (balance) systems are closely related. Help the patient describe symptoms to determine the source of the problems. Health history questions to ask the patient are listed in Table 23.2.

Problems with balance may manifest as vertigo or nystagmus. **Vertigo** is a sense that the person or objects around the person are moving or spinning. It is usually stimulated by head movement. *Dizziness* is a sensation of being off-balance that occurs when standing or walking. **Nystagmus** is an abnormal eye movement that may be seen as a twitching of the eyeball or described by patients as a blurring of vision with head or eye movement.

Try to determine symptoms that are related to balance and separate them from those related to hearing loss or tinnitus. The symptoms can be combined later in the assessment to help make a diagnosis and plan patient care.

Subjective Data

Important Health Information

Many ear problems result from childhood illnesses or problems of adjacent organs. This makes a careful assessment of past health problems important. Ask the patient about previous ear problems, especially during childhood. Note (1) the frequency of acute middle ear infections (otitis media); (2) surgeries (e.g., myringotomy, tonsillectomy, tympanoplasty); (3) TM perforations; (4) drainage; and (5) history of mumps, measles, or scarlet fever. Assess for systemic conditions, including diabetes, rheumatoid arthritis, and hypertension, which are associated with hearing loss. Note head injury because it may result in hearing loss. Information about food and environment allergies is important. Allergies can cause edema of the eustachian tube and prevent aeration of the middle ear.

Record symptoms such as vertigo, tinnitus, and hearing loss in the patient's words. Ask for specific details of the sensations and situations that cause them or make them worse. Details about family members with hearing loss and type of hearing loss are important. Hearing loss may be hereditary. The age of onset of ARHL follows a familial pattern. Record the use of and satisfaction with a hearing aid.

Medications

Obtain information about present or past use of ototoxic drugs. More than 200 drugs are ototoxic and have the potential to cause hearing loss, tinnitus, and vertigo. These include aspirin, some antibiotics (aminoglycosides, macrolides, vancomycin), loop diuretics, nonsteroidal antiinflammatory drugs (NSAIDs), salicylates, and certain chemotherapy drugs.[2] Ask about hearing and balance problems in patients receiving these drugs. For many, hearing loss may be reversible if treatment is stopped. Chemical exposure at work (e.g., toluene, carbon disulfide, mercury) may damage the inner ear.

Functional Health Patterns

Hearing and balance problems can affect all aspects of a person's life. To assess the impact of hearing loss, ask health history questions based on functional health patterns (Table 23.2).

Health perception–health management. Note the onset of hearing loss and whether it was sudden or gradual. Who noted the onset (e.g., patient, family, significant others)? Gradual hearing losses are often noted by those who communicate with the patient. The patient often notes sudden losses and those worsened by other problems.

Assess if the patient uses prevention devices. Ask about employment or contact with environments that have high noise levels, such as work with machinery or amplified music. Note if the patient is a swimmer and the frequency and duration of swimming and use of ear protection. Knowing the type of water (pool, lake, ocean) in which the swimming takes place helps identify contact with contaminated water. Assess hygiene practices and ask if the patient places any item in the ear.

Nutritional-metabolic. Ask about ear pain (otalgia) or discomfort when chewing or swallowing. These symptoms may occur with middle ear problems. Note changes in symptoms with food intake. Alcohol and sodium affect the amount of endolymph in the inner ear system. Patients with Ménière disease may notice some symptom improvement with alcohol restriction and a low-sodium diet.

Clenching or grinding of the teeth helps distinguish problems of the ear from referred pain of the temporomandibular joint (TMJ). Ask about dental problems and dentures. Referred pain from the teeth, gums, or throat can cause ear pain.

TABLE 23.2 HEALTH HISTORY

Auditory System

Health Perception–Health Management

Hearing

- Have you had a change in your hearing?[a] If yes, was it sudden or gradual?
- Do you use any devices to improve your hearing, such as a hearing aid?[a]
- Have you had your hearing checked?
- Have you ever had an ear problem such as an infection?
- Describe how you clean your ears.
- How do you protect your hearing?
- Do you have any allergies?[a]
- What medications are you taking?
- Do you have problems following conversations in a noisy environment, such as a restaurant?
- Does a hearing problem cause you difficulty when listening to TV or other device?[a]

Balance

- When did the dizziness or spinning sensation first occur?
- Does this sensation occur when you first stand up, when you are lying down, or both?
- Have you ever fallen because of the dizziness?[a]
- Are there any times of the day when your symptoms are worse?[a]

Tinnitus

- How long have you had ringing in your ears? Has it changed?[a] Describe the ringing (e.g., buzzing, ringing, roaring). Do you also have a feeling of fullness or pressure?[a]
- When does it bother you the most?
- What things have you tried that help or have not helped?

Nutritional-Metabolic

- Do you notice any change in symptoms with changes in diet?[a]
- Does your ear problem cause nausea that interferes with your food intake?[a]
- Does chewing or swallowing cause you ear discomfort?[a]

Activity-Exercise

- Do you need help with certain activities, like lifting or climbing stairs because of symptoms?[a]
- Can you drive or walk alone? If no, elaborate.

Sleep-Rest

- Is your sleep disturbed by noises or ringing in the ears or by a sensation of spinning?[a]

Cognitive-Perceptual

- Do you have ear pain?[a] What relieves the pain? What makes it worse? Does the pain affect your hearing or balance?
- Has anyone around you said that they feel you have hearing loss?[a]

Self-Perception–Self-Concept

- Have changes in your hearing affected how you feel about yourself or your feeling of independence?[a]

Role-Relationship

- What effect has your ear problem had on your work or family life?
- Does a hearing problem cause you to feel embarrassed when you meet new people?
- Does a hearing problem cause you difficulty when visiting friends, relatives, or neighbors?

Coping–Stress Tolerance

- Do you consider your ear problem a source of stress?[a]
- How do you cope when you are having symptoms or with hearing loss?

[a]If yes, describe.

Activity-exercise. Review the patient's activity-exercise pattern when assessing for balance problems. Ask about the onset, duration, and frequency of symptoms. Identify activities that relieve or worsen symptoms and how they relate to the time of the day. For example, patients with Ménière disease are less able to compensate as the day progresses.

Sleep-rest. Ask the patient with chronic tinnitus about sleep problems. Find out if they have tried anything to minimize the tinnitus, such as having a fan on or using white noise devices. Assess for snoring. It can be caused by swelling or hypertrophy of tissue in the nasopharynx. This excess tissue can also impair eustachian tube function and cause ear fullness or pain.

Cognitive-perceptual. Pain occurs with some ear problems, especially those involving the ear canal and middle ear. If pain is present, ask the patient to describe the pain, any drainage present *(otorrhea)*, history of teeth grinding, and treatments used for relief.

Note the patient's ability to pay attention and follow directions. Problems with these tasks may be an early sign of hearing loss. The patient may not recognize a gradual hearing loss. Ask caregivers if they have noted any change in the patient's hearing.

Self-perception–self-concept. Ask how the ear problem has affected their personal life and feelings about themselves. Hearing loss and chronic vertigo are particularly distressing. Hearing loss can result in social situations that affect the patient's self-concept.

Role-relationship. Ask the patient about the effect that an ear problem or vertigo has had on family life, work responsibilities, and social relationships. Hearing loss can interfere with establishing or maintaining a relationship. Loneliness and depression can occur with hearing loss.

Many jobs rely on the ability to hear accurately and respond appropriately. Assess the effect hearing loss has on the patient's job. The unpredictability of vertigo attacks can have devastating effects on all aspects of life. Ordinary activities that require balance, such as driving, cooking, and work, will pose a risk.

Coping–stress tolerance. Ask about coping, stress management, and available support. If the patient seems unable to manage the situation, outside intervention may be needed.

CASE STUDY

Subjective Data

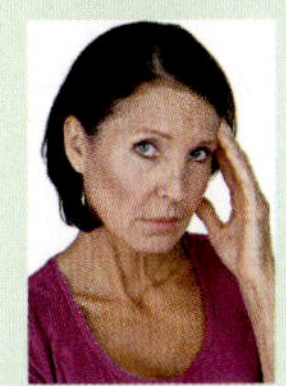

(© Stockphoto4u/ iStock.com.)

A focused subjective assessment of R.S. revealed the following:

- ***History:*** Mild osteoarthritis. Hysterectomy 5 years ago. Last saw her HCP 6 months ago.
- ***Medications:*** Multivitamin 1 oral daily, ibuprofen 200 mg oral every 6 hours as needed.
- ***Health Perception–Health Management:*** She says last night she felt like she had the start of a cold. The symptoms were present this morning when she woke up. She tried to clear her ear by blowing her nose and could not use that ear to talk on the phone. Had excellent hearing until today. Denies any syncope. Does not have allergies.
- ***Nutritional-Metabolic:*** States she is nauseous but has not vomited. Has only had a few sips of water since the symptoms started.
- ***Activity-Exercise:*** Dizziness worse when standing. It is still present when lying down but is less. Her husband drove her to the emergency department because she was unable to drive. Normally walks 1 to 2 miles 5 times a week and attends yoga class 2 times a week.
- ***Cognitive-Perceptual:*** Denies any ear pain, headache.
- ***Coping–Stress Tolerance:*** Concerned she is having a stroke.

Discussion Questions

1. Which subjective assessment findings concern you most?
2. Based on the subjective assessment findings, what would you include in the physical assessment? For what would you be looking?

You will learn more about the physical assessment of the auditory system in the next section.

Answers available at http://evolve.elsevier.com/Lewis/medsurg.

Objective Data

Physical Assessment

During the interview to obtain a health history, obtain objective data about the patient's ability to hear. Look for cues that a patient cannot hear (Table 23.3). Record these observations. This is important if the patient is unaware of hearing loss.

Inspect and palpate the external ear before assessing the external canal and TM. Observe the pinna and surrounding area for symmetry, color, swelling, redness, and lesions. Then palpate the pinna, tragus, and mastoid areas for tenderness and nodules. Gently move the pinna to check for discomfort. Grasping the pinna or pressing on the tragus may cause pain, especially if the external ear or canal is inflamed.

TABLE 23.3 Signs of Possible Hearing Loss

- Does not respond to or understand oral communication
- Has excessively loud or soft speech
- Answers questions inappropriately
- Tilts head, leans forward when listening
- Asking others to speak more slowly, loudly, or clearly
- Misunderstands conversations
- Asking others to repeat what they said
- States other people mumble all the time
- Increases the volume of devices
- Difficulty hearing over the phone

Before inserting an otoscope, inspect the canal opening for patency. Select a speculum slightly smaller than the size of the ear canal. Tip the patient's head to the opposite shoulder. Grasp the top of the pinna and gently pull up and backward to straighten the canal. Hold the otoscope while stabilizing it with your fingers on the patient's cheek, and then insert it slowly. A tight seal of the speculum is essential during this step. Observe the canal for size and shape and the color, amount, and type of earwax.

Inspect the TM for color, fluid behind the membrane, landmarks, contour, and intactness (Fig. 23.2). The TM is normally pearl gray, white, or pink; shiny; and translucent. The handle (manubrium) of the malleus and its short process (umbo) should be visible through the membrane. The position and dome (concave) shape of the TM cause the light from the otoscope to reflect in a cone shape with crisp edges. If the TM is bulging or retracted, the edges of the light reflex will be fuzzy (diffuse) and may spread over the TM. A pneumatic otoscope creates negative pressure to pull at the TM. It is helpful in confirming TM retraction or fluid behind the TM. You cannot examine the middle and inner ear with the otoscope.

A normal assessment of the auditory system is shown in Table 23.4. Table 23.5 summarizes assessment abnormalities of the auditory system. Age-related changes of the auditory system and differences in assessment findings are found in Table 23.1. A *focused assessment* is used to evaluate the status of an existing auditory problem and monitor for new problems. A focused assessment of the auditory system is shown in Box 23.1.

TABLE 23.4 Normal Physical Assessment of Auditory System

- Ears symmetric in location and shape
- Pinna nontender, without lesions
- Canal clear, TM intact, landmarks and light reflex intact
- Able to hear low whisper at 30 cm
- Weber test results, no lateralization. Rinne test results: Air conduction > Bone conduction

CASE STUDY

Objective Data: Physical Assessment

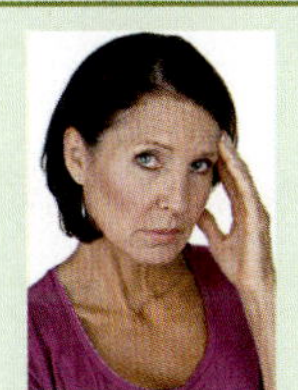

(© Stockphoto4u/ iStock.com.)

Physical assessment findings of R.S. were as follows:

- Neurologic and otoscopic assessments normal
- Unable to hear whisper on the right at 30 cm
- Vision normal. Pupils equal, round, and reactive to light and accommodation (PERRLA) without nystagmus
- Gait unsteady. No motor weakness
- Skin pale, warm, and dry
- Heart rate 84 beats/min, temperature 97.4°F (36.3°C)

Discussion Questions

1. What physical assessment findings concern you most?
2. What diagnostic studies might you expect to be ordered?

As you continue to read this chapter, consider diagnostic studies that you would expect to be performed for R.S.

Answers available at http://evolve.elsevier.com/Lewis/medsurg.

TABLE 23.5 ASSESSMENT ABNORMALITIES
Auditory System

Finding	Description	Possible Cause and Significance
External Ear and Canal		
Discharge	Infection of external ear, usually painful	Swimmer's ear, infection of external ear. Possibly caused by ruptured TM and otitis media
Exostosis	Bony growth extending into canal causing narrowing of canal	May interfere with seeing TM. Usually asymptomatic
Impacted earwax	Wax that was not normally excreted from the ear. Cannot see TM	Decreased hearing possible, pain, sensation of fullness in auditory canal, removal necessary before otoscopic examination
Scaling or lesions	Change in usual appearance of skin	Seborrheic dermatitis, actinic keratosis, basal or squamous cell cancer
Swelling of pinna, pain	Infection of glands of skin, hematoma from trauma	Aspiration (for hematoma)
Tophi	Hard nodules made of uric acid crystals	Occur with gout, metabolic problems. Further treatment needed
Redness, edema in ear canal	Infection of external ear, usually painful	External otitis
Tympanic Membrane (TM)		
Yellow-amber color, air bubbles	Serous fluid in middle	Serous otitis media
Bulging, lack of landmarks (Fig. 23.3)	Fluid-filled middle ear	Acute otitis media, TM perforation
Perforated TM	Previous TM perforation that has failed to heal. Thin, transparent layer of epithelium surrounding TM	Chronic otitis media, mastoiditis, drainage
Retracted TM	Appearance of shorter, more horizontal malleus. Absent or bent cone of light	Vacuum in middle ear, blockage of eustachian tube, negative pressure in middle ear

BOX 23.1 FOCUSED ASSESSMENT
Auditory System

Use this checklist to make sure you have done key assessment steps.

Subjective

Ask the patient about the following and note responses:

Changes in hearing
Ear pain
Ear drainage
Tinnitus

Objective: Physical Assessment

Inspect

Alignment and position of ears on head
Size, shape, symmetry, color, and skin intactness
External ear for discharge or lesions

Assess

Hearing based on ability to respond to conversation, respond to a whisper, or hear a ticking watch

DIAGNOSTIC STUDIES

Table 23.6 describes common diagnostic studies used to assess the auditory system. Several tests are available to determine the cause of certain hearing losses. CT scan and MRI can detect lesions such as a tumor of CN VIII.

Audiometry

Audiometry is used as a screening test for hearing acuity and as a diagnostic test to determine the degree and type of hearing loss. The most common test is pure-tone audiometry. The audiometer produces pure tones at varying intensities to which the person can respond. Hearing loss can affect certain sound frequencies. The specific pattern produced on the audiogram by these losses can help diagnose the type of hearing loss. Threshold refers to the signal level at which pure tones are detected (pure-tone thresholds) or the signal level at which a person correctly hears 50% of the signals (speech detection thresholds).

CASE STUDY
Objective Data: Diagnostic Studies

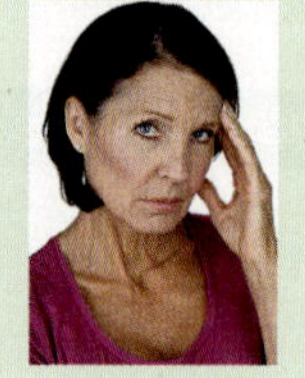

(© Stockphoto4u/iStock.com.)

The Weber test shows lateralization to the left. An audiogram confirms low-frequency, sensorineural hearing loss with normal speech discrimination. An MRI of the head is normal.

Discussion Questions

1. Are these the diagnostic studies that you expected to be ordered?
2. Which diagnostic study results concern you most?

Answers available at http://evolve.elsevier.com/Lewis/medsurg.

TABLE 23.6 Diagnostic Studies

Auditory System

Study	Description, Purpose, and Considerations
Auditory	
Audiometry	*Pure-tone audiometry* quantifies hearing loss. Sounds are presented through earphones in soundproof room. Patient responds when sound is heard. Response is recorded on an audiogram. Determines patient's hearing range in terms of decibels (dB) and hertz (Hz) for diagnosing hearing loss. Tinnitus can cause inconsistent results. *Speech audiometry* includes speech reception threshold (measure of intensity at which speech is recognized) and word recognition score (ability to discriminate among various speech sounds).
Brainstem Auditory Evoked Response (BAER) or Auditory Evoked Potential (AEP)	Measures sound-induced electric signals along auditory pathway of inner ear to brain. Electrodes are placed around the head and signals are rapidly sent from parts of the ear to the brain. *During:* Patient must lie down and be still during entire test.
Electrocochleography	Records electrical activity in cochlea and CN VIII. Electrode placed on or through the TM. Can assess and monitor patients with dizziness.
Tympanometry	Checks middle ear and mobility of TM. Probe is placed snugly into external ear canal, and positive and negative pressures are applied. Measurements made of TM movement.
Tuning Fork Tests	
Rinne test	Compares hearing by bone conduction (BC) and air conduction (AC). Hold stem of vibrating tuning fork against mastoid bone (BC) and note time note. When the sound is no longer heard behind the ear (BC), note time again and move the still-vibrating fork close to the pinna (AC). Have the patient report when they no longer hear sound next to the ear canal (AC) and note time. Normally, sound is heard twice as long in front of the ear as it is on the bone. With conductive hearing loss, the relationship is reversed; BC is longer than AC. With SNHL, AC and BC are reduced, but AC is longer.
Weber test	Place stem of vibrating tuning fork on midline of skull or forehead. Patient then indicates where the sound is heard best. In normal auditory function, the sound is heard equally in both ears. With conductive hearing loss in 1 ear, sound will be louder in that ear. With SNHL, sound is louder in the normal (unaffected) ear.
Vestibular Tests	
Electronystagmography (ENG)	Assesses vestibular problems such as vertigo. Electrodes are placed around each eye. Eye movement is recorded when the inner ear and nearby nerves are stimulated by water or air injected into ear canal. • *Before:* Avoid eating for at least 4 hours before. Avoid caffeine and alcohol for 24 to 48 hours before. • *During:* Observe for vomiting. Ensure patient safety.
Posturography	Group of tests that assess how well person maintains balance control under different conditions when they are upright. Can determine how visual, vestibular, and proprioceptive systems affect balance.
Rotary chair testing	Evaluates peripheral vestibular system. Patient is seated in a chair driven by a motor under computer control. Usually done in the dark. *During:* Observe for vomiting. Ensure patient safety.
Videonystagmography (VNG)	Uses high-speed infrared cameras to record and measure eye movements in response to visual or vestibular stimuli. Detects nystagmus and can identify the site and extent of vestibular lesions and compensation status.

EXTERNAL EAR AND EAR CANAL PROBLEMS

EXTERNAL OTITIS

External otitis involves inflammation, with or without infection, of the ear canal. It may involve the pinna and tragus. Swimming may change the flora of the ear canal because of chemicals and contaminated water. This can result in an infection we often call "swimmer's ear." Other causes include hearing aid use, trauma from foreign objects (e.g., hairpins), and impacted cerumen.[3]

The most common cause is bacterial infection with *Staphylococcus aureus* or *Pseudomonas aeruginosa.*[3] The warm, dark environment of the ear canal provides a good growth medium for microorganisms. Infection may be fungal, such as *Candida albicans* or *Aspergillus.*

Malignant external otitis is a serious infection caused by *P. aeruginosa.* It occurs mainly in older adults with diabetes. The infection, which can spread from the external ear to the parotid gland and temporal bone (osteomyelitis), is usually treated with systemic antibiotics.

Ear pain is an early sign of external otitis. Even in mild cases, patients may have significant pain with chewing, moving the pinna, or pressing on the tragus. Swelling of the ear canal can muffle hearing and cause a sense of fullness. There may be itching and blood-tinged or purulent drainage. Fever and malaise occur if the infection spreads to surrounding tissue.

Interprofessional and Nursing Management

External otitis is diagnosed by otoscopic examination of the ear canal. Take care to avoid pain when pulling on the pinna to straighten out the canal or when inserting the otoscope. The TM may be hard to see due to swelling in the canal. Culture and sensitivity studies of the drainage may be done in rare cases.

The main treatment is topical antibiotic drops for infection and measures for pain control. Moist heat, mild analgesics, and topical anesthetic drops usually control the pain. Some patients receive corticosteroids for inflammation. Improvement should occur in 48 hours. Patients need to adhere to the prescribed therapy for 7 to 10 days for complete resolution (see Table 15.9).

Teach patients how to properly administer ear drops. Wash hands before and after applying eardrops. The drops should be at room temperature. The tip of the dropper should not touch the ear during application to prevent contamination of the entire bottle. The patient should lie down with the affected side up, apply the drops, and then stay in this position for 3 to 5 minutes. This allows the drops to spread. If edema is severe, place the drops on an ear wick. Careful handling and disposal of material saturated with drainage are important. Teach patients ways to reduce the risk for external otitis (Table 23.7).

CERUMEN AND FOREIGN BODIES IN EAR CANAL

The ear canal may be obstructed by cerumen (earwax) or a foreign object. Impacted earwax can cause discomfort and decreased hearing. Other symptoms include tinnitus and vertigo. Remove an impaction by irrigating the canal with body-temperature solutions to soften the earwax. Special syringes may be used. These vary from a simple bulb syringe to special irrigating equipment. Place the patient in a sitting position with an emesis basin under the ear. Pull the pinna up and back, and direct the flow of solution above or below the impaction. Do not completely occlude the ear canal with the syringe tip. If irrigation does not remove the wax, use mild lubricant drops to soften the earwax. The HCP may need to remove severe impactions.

Attempts to remove a foreign object from the ear may result in pushing it farther into the canal. Vegetable matter in the ear tends to swell. This can create a secondary inflammation, making removal more difficult. Mineral oil or lidocaine drops can kill an insect before removal under microscope guidance. The HCP should remove impacted objects.

Avoid using cotton-tipped applicators in the ears. Penetration of the middle ear by a cotton-tipped applicator can cause serious injury to the TM and ossicles. Their use can cause earwax to become impacted against the TM and impair hearing.

TABLE 23.7 PATIENT & CAREGIVER TEACHING

Preventing External Otitis

Include the following instructions when teaching the patient and caregiver.

1. Do not put anything in your ear canal unless requested by your HCP.
2. Report itching if it becomes a problem.
3. Earwax is normal. It lubricates and protects the canal. Report chronic excess earwax if it impairs your hearing.
4. Keep your ears as dry as possible.
   - Use earplugs if you are prone to swimmer's ear.
   - Turn your head to each side for 30 seconds at a time to help water run out of the ears.
   - Do not dry with cotton-tipped applicators.
   - A hair dryer set to low and held at least 6 inches from the ear can speed water evaporation.
   - Try to avoid getting water, soap, or shampoo in your ears when you shower or bathe.

TRAUMA

Trauma to the external ear can cause injury to the subcutaneous tissue and result in a hematoma. If a hematoma is not aspirated, inflammation of the membranes of the ear cartilage (perichondritis) can result. Blows to the ear can cause conductive hearing loss if the ossicles in the middle ear are damaged or the TM is perforated. Head trauma that affects the auditory cortex can impair the ability to understand the meaning of sounds.

CANCER OF EXTERNAL EAR

Skin cancer of the external ear is common. Common types include basal and squamous cell cancers. They often start on the pinna or in the ear canal. If left untreated, they can spread to the TM and invade underlying tissue. Signs include skin ulcers that bleed, pearly white lumps under the skin, and scaly patches of skin. Precancerous actinic keratoses, rough sandpaper-like lesions on the upper border of the pinna, are associated with chronic sun exposure. They are often treated with liquid nitrogen. Teach patients about ways to reduce the dangers of sun exposure. See Chapter 25 for more about skin cancer.

MIDDLE EAR PROBLEMS

ACUTE OTITIS MEDIA

Acute otitis media is an infection of the TM, ossicles, and space of the middle ear. Infection can be due to viruses or bacteria. Swelling of the eustachian tube from colds or allergies can trap bacteria, causing a middle ear infection. Pressure from the inflammation pushes on the TM, causing it to become red, bulging, and painful (Fig. 23.3). Pain, fever, malaise, drainage, and reduced hearing may be present.

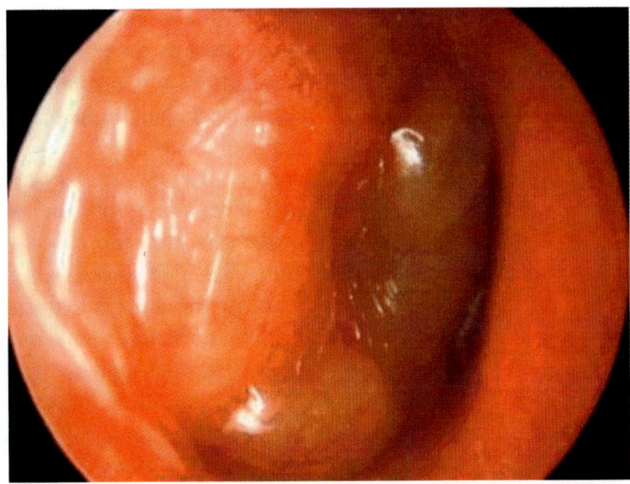

Fig. 23.3 Acute otitis media. (From Pham L-L, Bourayou R, Maghraoui-Slim V, et al: Otitis, sinusitis and related conditions. In Cohen J, Powderly WG, Opal SM [eds]: *Infectious diseases,* ed 4, 2017, Mosby.)

Oral antibiotics and eardrops are used if an infection is present (see Table 15.8). Surgery is reserved for patients who do not respond to medical treatment. A *myringotomy* involves an incision in the TM to release the increased pressure and exudate from the middle ear. A tympanostomy tube may be placed short- or long-term to ventilate the ear. Prompt treatment of acute otitis media can help prevent spontaneous perforation of the TM. If allergies are a causative factor, the patient may receive antihistamines and a nasal corticosteroid spray.

OTITIS MEDIA WITH EFFUSION

Otitis media with effusion is a collection of fluid in the middle ear space without signs of an acute infection. The fluid may be thin, mucoid, or purulent. As fluid builds up in the middle ear and eustachian tube, it places pressure on the TM. The pressure prevents the TM from working properly and therefore results in decreased hearing. Other symptoms include the ear feeling full or "plugged" and popping.

Otitis media with effusion often follows upper respiratory tract or chronic sinus infections, barotrauma (caused by pressure change), or otitis media. It can continue for weeks to months. It usually resolves without treatment but may recur. If the effusion is persistent, myringotomy with tube placement is an effective treatment.

CHRONIC OTITIS MEDIA WITH MASTOIDITIS

Chronic otitis media refers to otitis media that does not improve or keeps returning. There may be a hole, or perforation, in the TM. There is purulent exudate and inflammation that can involve the ossicles, eustachian tube, and mastoid bone. It is often painless. Hearing loss occurs from inflammatory destruction of the ossicles, TM perforation, or accumulation of fluid in the middle ear space. Patients may have nausea and dizziness. A mass of epithelial cells and cholesterol in the middle ear *(cholesteatoma)* may develop. As the cholesteatoma enlarges, it can destroy the adjacent bones. Unless removed surgically, it can cause extensive damage to the ossicles and impair hearing.

Otoscopic examination of the TM may reveal changes in color and mobility or a perforation. Culture and sensitivity tests of the drainage are necessary to identify the organisms involved so patients may receive the right antibiotic therapy. The audiogram may show a hearing loss as great as 50 to 60 dB if the ossicles are damaged or separated. Sinus x-rays, MRI, or a CT scan can assess for mastoiditis and the presence of a mass.

Interprofessional and Nursing Management

The goals of treatment are to clear the middle ear of infection, repair perforations, and preserve hearing (Table 23.8). Topical and systemic antibiotic therapy is started based on the culture and sensitivity results. In many cases of chronic otitis media, antibiotic resistance is present. Patients may need to have frequent evacuation of the drainage and debris.

Often chronic TM perforations do not heal with conservative treatment, and surgery is necessary. *Tympanoplasty (myringoplasty)* involves reconstruction of the TM and/or the ossicles. A *mastoidectomy* is often done with a tympanoplasty to remove infected portions of the mastoid bone. Removal of tissue stops at the middle ear structures that appear capable of conducting sound. Sudden pressure changes in the ear and postoperative infections can disrupt healing or cause facial nerve paralysis.

There may be packing in the ear after surgery. A cotton ball dressing is used if an incision was made through the ear canal. Teach patients to change the packing as needed (Table 23.9). If a postauricular (behind the ear) incision was used and a drain is in place, place a dressing over that area. Then, place a soft outer dressing over the top of that dressing. This will prevent putting pressure on the pinna. Monitor the tightness of the outer dressing to prevent tissue necrosis. Assess the amount and type of drainage. Keep the suture line dry.

TABLE 23.8 Interprofessional Care

Chronic Otitis Media

Diagnostic Assessment
- History and physical assessment
- Otoscopic examination
- Culture and sensitivity of middle ear drainage
- Audiometry
- Imaging: mastoid x-ray, CT scan, MRI

Management
- Ear irrigation
- Otic, oral, or IV antibiotics (see Table 15.8)
- Analgesics
- Antiemetics (see Table 46.1)
- Surgery
  - Tympanoplasty
  - Mastoidectomy

TABLE 23.9 PATIENT & CAREGIVER TEACHING

After Ear Surgery

Include the following information in the teaching plan for the patient and caregiver after ear surgery:

1. Sleep on your back with head slightly elevated for 1 week.
2. Do not bend at the waist.
3. If you need to cough or sneeze, keep your mouth open.
4. Do not strain during bowel movements. You may need a stool softener if constipated.
5. Do not blow your nose or use earplugs for 6 weeks.
6. Keep your ear dry for 6 weeks. No swimming. Place a cotton ball saturated with petroleum jelly in the ear when washing hair.
7. Change your ear dressing daily as prescribed.
8. Do not fly or resume strenuous activity or contact sports until cleared by the HCP.
9. Report excess drainage or severe dizziness to the HCP.

OTOSCLEROSIS

Otosclerosis is a disorder in which abnormal bone growth prevents movement of the footplate of the stapes in the oval window. This reduces the transmission of vibrations to the inner ear fluids and results in conductive hearing loss. Otosclerosis is often hereditary. Hearing loss usually starts in one ear and then in the other. The person may have dizziness or tinnitus.[4]

Otoscopic examination may reveal a reddish blush of the TM (Schwartz sign). It is caused by the vascular and bony changes within the middle ear. Tuning fork tests and an audiogram show good hearing by bone conduction with poor hearing by air conduction (air-bone gap) (Table 23.6). Usually, a difference of at least 20 to 30 dB between air and bone conduction occurs with otosclerosis.

Interprofessional care of otosclerosis is outlined in Table 23.10. Stapedectomy can be a highly effective treatment. It involves part or all the stapes with a laser or microdrill and replacing it with a new, mobile, prosthetic bone. Sodium fluoride and bisphosphonates are given to slow the progression of symptoms.[4] They slow bone resorption and promote the calcification of bony lesions. A hearing aid may be helpful in mild disease.

Nursing management of patients having surgery for otosclerosis is like that of patients having a tympanoplasty (Table 23.9). Place a cotton ball in the ear canal and cover the ear with a small dressing. Patients may have dizziness, nausea, and vomiting because of stimulation of the labyrinth during surgery. Disturbing the perilymph fluid can cause nystagmus. Teach patients to avoid strenuous activities that increase inner ear pressure. Patients with nausea and vomiting may need antiemetic drugs (see Table 46.1).

TABLE 23.10 Interprofessional Care

Otosclerosis

Diagnostic Assessment

- History and physical assessment
- Otoscopic examination
- Rinne and Weber tests
- Audiometry
- Tympanometry

Management

- Hearing aid
- Surgery (stapedectomy, stapes prosthesis)
- Drug therapy (sodium fluoride, bisphosphonates)

INNER EAR PROBLEMS

MÉNIÈRE DISEASE

Ménière disease is a condition defined by spontaneous vertigo attacks (lasting 20 minutes to 12 hours) with low- to mid-frequency sensorineural hearing loss in the affected ear before, during, or after the attack. Patients may have nausea, vomiting, and nystagmus. A sense of fullness in the ear and increasing tinnitus may precede an attack.[5] The person may have the feeling of being pulled to the ground ("drop attacks"). Some report feeling like they are whirling in space. Attacks may occur several times a year. The disease course is variable. Some patients have spontaneous remission while for others, symptoms persist for years.[5]

The cause is unknown. Theories point to viral infections, allergies, trauma, autoimmune reaction, migraine, or genetics as possible causes.[6] The thought is that there is increased pressure from an abnormally large amount of endolymph and/or potassium in the inner ear. Some people have triggers for attacks. Common triggers include stress, fatigue, illness, pressure changes, certain foods, and too much diet salt.

Interprofessional and Nursing Management

Interprofessional care is outlined in Table 23.11. There is no cure. The goal is to reduce the number of attacks, relieve symptoms, and improve quality of life. Medications during an attack can lessen vertigo, nausea, and vomiting. These include antihistamines, anticholinergics, and benzodiazepines.[6,7] Those with severe vomiting may need IV hydration and antiemetics (e.g., ondansetron). Plan nursing interventions to minimize vertigo and maintain safety (Table 23.12).

Frequent and incapacitating attacks are indications for other treatments. Injecting gentamicin through the TM destroys vestibular tissue. Surgical therapies include decompression of the endolymphatic sac by draining fluid from the inner ear and vestibular nerve resection. With single-side involvement, surgical ablation of the labyrinth, resulting in the loss of vestibular and hearing cochlear function, is an option.

TABLE 23.11 Interprofessional Care

Ménière Disease

Diagnostic Assessment
- History and physical assessment
- Audiometry
- Cervical and ocular vestibular evoked myogenic potential

Management

Acute Care

Drug Therapy
- Anticholinergics (scopolamine)
- Antihistamines (e.g., meclizine, diphenhydramine)
- Antiemetics (see Table 46.1)
- Benzodiazepines (e.g., lorazepam)

Surgical Therapy
- Endolymphatic sac decompression
- Endolymphatic shunt
- Labyrinthectomy
- Vestibular nerve section

Chronic Care
- Drug therapy
  - Antihistamines
  - Corticosteroids
  - Diuretics (see Table 36.7)
  - Gentamicin injection
- Diet restriction of sodium, caffeine, alcohol
- Smoking cessation
- Stress reduction strategies
- Vestibular exercises
- Physical therapy

TABLE 23.12 NURSING MANAGEMENT

Care of the Patient With Acute Ménière Disease

- Administer medications and IV hydration as ordered.
- Keep patient in a quiet, darkened room in a comfortable position.
- Have patient avoid sudden head movements and position changes.
- Teach the patient to close the eyes until vertigo stops.
- Avoid fluorescent or flickering lights and television.
- Implement fall precautions.
- Implement measures to address nausea and vomiting.
- Monitor intake and output and daily weights.
- Help the patient with ambulation as needed.

Measures to prevent attacks include diuretics and antihistamines. A low-salt diet with limited caffeine and alcohol often helps. Stress the need to quit smoking. Review ways to avoid allergens and reduce stress.[7] Discuss home safety and ways to decrease fall risk until vertigo is under control. Have the patient sit or lie down at the onset of dizziness.

BENIGN PAROXYSMAL POSITIONAL VERTIGO

Benign paroxysmal positional vertigo (BPPV) is a common cause of vertigo. BPPV is associated with head trauma, infection, and age-related degeneration. However, for many patients, we do not know the cause.

Calcium carbonate particles called otoliths are normally found in a sticky membrane in the part of the inner ear that senses motion. In BPPV, otoliths dislodge and enter the endolymph of the semicircular canals. With motion, the displaced otoliths shift within the fluid, creating unbalance with the opposite ear. This causes the symptoms of dizziness, spinning, and/or swaying.[8] Other symptoms include nystagmus, light-headedness, loss of balance, and nausea. Symptoms tend to be intermittent and may be confused with those of Ménière disease. Diagnosis is based on the results of auditory and vestibular tests.

Although BPPV is bothersome, it is rarely serious unless a person falls. The Epley maneuver, or canalith repositioning procedure, is effective in providing symptom relief for many patients. This maneuver changes the location of the otoliths. It moves them from areas in the inner ear that cause symptoms into less sensitive areas where they do not cause these problems. A trained HCP can teach the patient how to perform the maneuver (Fig. 23.4).

ACOUSTIC NEUROMA

An **acoustic neuroma** is a benign tumor that occurs where CN VIII enters the internal auditory canal. Early diagnosis is important because the tumor can compress the trigeminal and facial nerves and arteries within the internal auditory canal. Symptoms usually begin between 40 and 60 years of age.

Early symptoms are due to CN VIII compression and destruction. They include unilateral, progressive, sensorineural hearing loss, reduced touch sensation in the posterior ear canal, unilateral tinnitus, and mild, intermittent vertigo. Diagnostic tests include neurologic and audiometric tests and MRI.

Radiation therapy for small tumors can preserve hearing and vestibular function. Surgery is an option. Surgery on tumors larger than 3 cm can leave patients with permanent hearing loss and facial paralysis. Stereotactic radiosurgery may slow tumor growth and preserve the facial nerve. Follow-up care after surgery is important to monitor hearing and tumor recurrence. Teach patients to report any clear, colorless discharge from the nose. This may be cerebrospinal fluid (CSF), which increases the risk for infection.

TINNITUS

Tinnitus is the perception of sound when no external noise is present.[9] It is often called "ringing in the ears." It can also present as buzzing, hissing, whistling, swooshing, or clicking. Tinnitus is sometimes the first symptom of hearing loss,

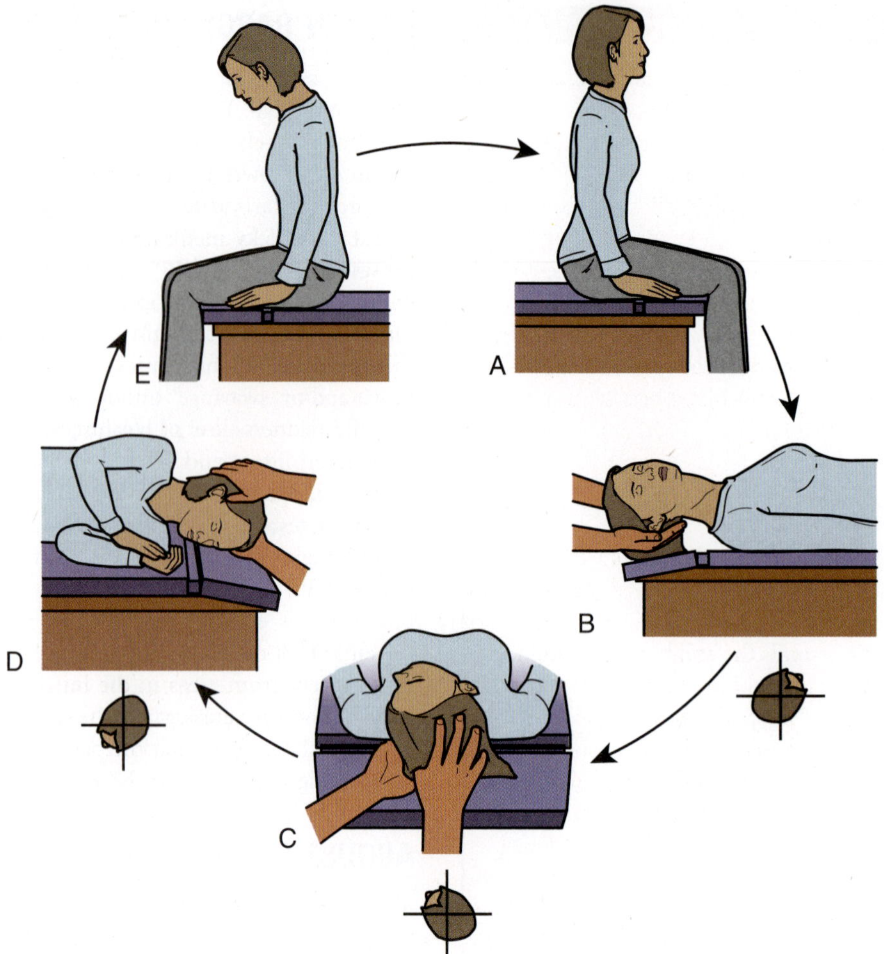

Fig. 23.4 Common steps in the Epley maneuver.

especially in older adults. Often, tinnitus occurs because of noise exposure. There are roughly 200 health problems that are associated with tinnitus. It may be a drug side effect. More than 200 drugs are known to cause tinnitus.

HEARING LOSS AND DEAFNESS

Disabling hearing loss is a common problem. Age is the strongest predictor of hearing loss. In the United States about 25% of those ages 65 to 74 and 50% of those 75 and older have hearing loss.[10] Common causes of hearing loss are shown in Fig. 23.5.

The Deaf community represented by the capital letter D refers to persons with severe to profound hearing loss ("deaf") that impairs communication.[11,12] They use sign language and have their own cultures and practices. For Deaf communities, deafness is considered a way of being, as opposed to a disability that needs correction. The term "Deaf" does not include hard of hearing people, where there may be enough residual hearing that an auditory device, such as a hearing aid, provides adequate assistance to process speech.[11,12]

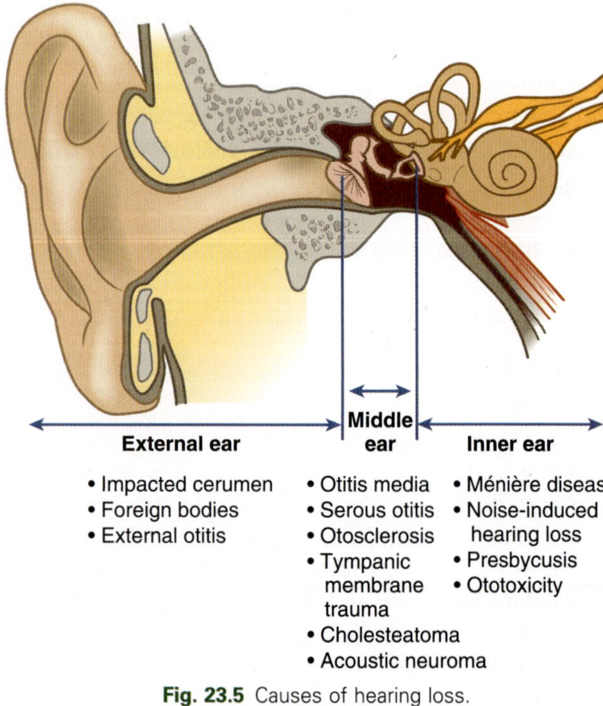

Fig. 23.5 Causes of hearing loss.

Types of Hearing Loss

Conductive Hearing Loss

Conductive hearing loss occurs when outer or middle ear problems impair the transmission of sound waves to the inner ear.[13] There is a decrease in sound intensity and/or a distortion in sound. Common causes in adults include impacted earwax, otitis media, TM perforation, otosclerosis, allergies, and benign tumors.

Symptoms depend on the cause and severity. Speech and other sounds may seem distant or muffled. The audiogram shows better hearing through bone than through air (air-bone gap). The first step is to identify and treat the cause if possible. If correction of the cause is not possible, a hearing aid may be an option.

Sensorineural Hearing Loss

Sensorineural hearing loss (SNHL) is caused by an inner ear or CN VIII problem.[13] Congenital and hereditary factors, noise exposure, aging, Ménière disease, trauma, and ototoxicity can cause SNHL. The main problem is the ability to hear sound but not to understand speech. The ability to hear high-pitched sounds (including consonants) diminishes. Sounds become muffled or faint. They may be distorted and hard to understand. An audiogram shows hearing loss that equally affects air and bone conduction. SNHL can often be treated with a hearing aid or implantable hearing device.

Auditory neuropathy spectrum disorder is a rare type of SNHL where sound is not transmitted properly from the inner ear to CN VIII or from CN VIII to the brain. Hearing loss varies from normal to severe. Speech is generally perceived as distorted and hard to understand.

ARHL is another type of SNHL. Degenerative changes in the inner ear cause ARHL. Noise exposure is a common factor. Hearing loss occurs gradually. People first develop hearing loss at high frequencies. The person hears vowels but cannot distinguish consonants because they are in the high-frequency range. Because consonants help us recognize spoken words, this causes a decreased ability to understand speech. ARHL is associated with poorer cognitive and physical function and higher health care use. It can contribute to feeling isolated as it becomes harder to enjoy talking to family or friends. The prognosis for hearing depends on the cause of the loss. Hearing aids are the main treatment.

Other Types of Hearing Loss

Mixed hearing loss is a combination of conductive damage in the outer or middle ear and sensorineural damage in the inner ear or CN VIII. Anything that causes conductive hearing loss or SNHL can lead to mixed hearing loss. Central hearing loss originates from the CNS or brain. Patients experience poor understanding and slow processing of speech.

An emotional or a psychologic factor can cause functional hearing loss. The patient does not seem to hear or respond to pure-tone subjective hearing tests, but no physical reason for hearing loss exists. Psychologic counseling may help.

Clinical Manifestations

Common early signs of hearing loss are answering questions inappropriately and not responding when not looking at the speaker (Table 23.3). Other behaviors that suggest hearing loss include straining to hear, reading lips, and an increased sensitivity to slight increases in noise level. Often patients are unaware of minimal hearing loss. Family and friends who get tired of repeating or talking loudly are often the first to notice the hearing loss. Pressure by significant others may factor in whether a patient seeks help for impaired hearing.

Sudden hearing loss, or sudden deafness, occurs as an unexplained, rapid loss of hearing (usually in 1 ear) either at once or over several days. It is a medical emergency. The patient should see an HCP at once.

Classification of Hearing Loss

We often classify hearing loss by the decibel level or loss as recorded on the audiogram. Normal hearing is in the 0- to 15-dB range at all frequencies. Most people with a hearing loss of 90 dB or greater have been deaf since birth. Table 23.13 describes the levels of hearing loss.

Interprofessional and Nursing Management

Persons with hearing loss often experience barriers in accessing and receiving health care and achieving optimal health outcomes.[11,12] They have significant problems communicating with the health care team. Hearing loss can affect the ability to understand and follow the advice of HCPs.

You need to establish good communication so the patient has the right health information and feels included in their care. Hearing level, communication style, and language vary greatly. Assess these factors so you are aware of the patient's needs. Confirm the patient's understanding of health teaching. Descriptive visual aids can be helpful. If the patient uses sign language to communicate, use an interpreter when

TABLE 23.13 Diagnostic Criteria

Classification of Hearing Loss

Decibel (dB) Loss	Meaning
0–15	Normal hearing
16–25	Slight hearing loss
26–40	Mild impairment
41–5	Moderate impairment
56–70	Moderately severe impairment
71–90	Severe impairment
>90	Profound deafness

presenting significant information, such as consent or discharge teaching. Use the communication techniques described in Table 23.14.

CHECK YOUR PRACTICE

You offer to help a peer with their caseload by providing teaching to a patient who is being discharged. After you prepare the needed materials, you go to the room, sit down, and start talking with the patient. The patient shakes their head and says, "No, no." You are perplexed until they flash a bracelet that says *I am deaf.*

- How will you proceed?

Health Promotion

Environment noise control. Noise-induced hearing loss is preventable. Three factors affect noise-induced hearing loss: how loud the noise is, how close you are to the noise, and how long you hear the noise. Fig. 23.6 shows the dB levels of common indoor and outdoor sounds. Acoustic trauma, or sudden, severe loud noise, causes hearing loss by destroying the hair cells of the organ of Corti. Noise-induced hearing loss is occurring at an increasing rate. Health teaching about avoiding exposure to noise levels greater than 70 dB is essential (Box 23.2).

In work environments with high noise levels, Occupational Safety and Health Administration (OSHA) standards require employers to implement a hearing conservation program. Programs often include noise exposure analysis, ways to control noise exposure, and employee-employer education. OSHA mandates ear protection for workers in environments where the noise levels consistently exceed 85 dB. Periodic audiometric screening provides baseline data on hearing and a way to measure later hearing loss.

TABLE 23.14 Communicating With Patients With Hearing Impairment

Nonverbal Aids	• Draw attention with hand movements. • Have your face in good light. • Avoid light behind you. • Maintain eye contact. • Use a face shield or clear mask if a face covering is needed. • Avoid chewing, eating, smoking while talking. • Remove background noise. • Move close to better ear.
Verbal Aids	• Speak normally and slowly. Do not shout. • Do not exaggerate facial expressions. • Do not overenunciate. • Use simple sentences. • Rephrase sentence. Use different words. • Write name or difficult words. • Speak in normal voice directly into better ear.

Immunizations. Viral illness during pregnancy can cause deafness from fetal damage and malformations affecting the ear. Promote immunizations, including the measles, mumps, and rubella (MMR) vaccine. Rubella infection during the first 8 weeks of pregnancy is associated with congenital rubella syndrome, which causes SNHL. Females of childbearing age should be tested for antibodies to these viral diseases. Females should avoid pregnancy for at least 3 months after being immunized. Immunization must be delayed if a female is pregnant. Females can be vaccinated safely for rubella during the postpartum period.

Ototoxic substances. Monitor patients who are receiving ototoxic drugs or exposed to ototoxic agents for signs and symptoms of ototoxicity. These include tinnitus, diminished hearing, and balance problems. If symptoms develop, stopping the drug may prevent further damage and allow the symptoms to disappear.

Assistive Technology

Hearing aids. Hearing aids are sound-amplifying devices designed to improve hearing in people with hearing loss. A hearing aid should be fitted by an audiologist or a speech and hearing specialist. Hearing aids differ by design and features, such as wireless connectivity (Table 23.15). They are powered by a regular or rechargeable battery. The type of hearing aid chosen is based on the type and severity of hearing loss, listening needs, and lifestyle.[14]

People who are motivated and optimistic about using a hearing aid are more successful users. Determine the person's readiness for hearing aid therapy. Assess feelings about wearing a hearing aid, the degree to which hearing loss affects life, and any problems manipulating small objects, such as putting a battery in a hearing aid.

Some people are reluctant to use a hearing aid. Reasons cited most often include cost, stigma, difficulty using the technology, amplification of competing noise, and believing they cannot or will not help. Some older adults believe hearing loss is part of getting older. Most hearing aids and batteries are small. Dexterity problems such as stiff fingers may make handling a hearing aid frustrating.

Adjusting to hearing aids takes time (Box 23.3). Most people need a few weeks to a few months to adjust to using hearing aids. Encourage the person to wear them for a few hours the first day, an hour longer the following day, and so on until they are wearing them all day. At first, have them wear the aid at home or in a quiet setting so they can adjust to voices (including their own voice) and background sounds. Then, they should increase the exposure to different sounds and environments. This occurs gradually, depending on the person.

Review the proper care and cleaning of the hearing aid. When the hearing aid is not being worn, it should be stored in a dry, cool area. Cleaning hearing aids before bedtime gives them several hours to dry before they are put in again. Aids should not be worn while bathing or swimming and when using a hair

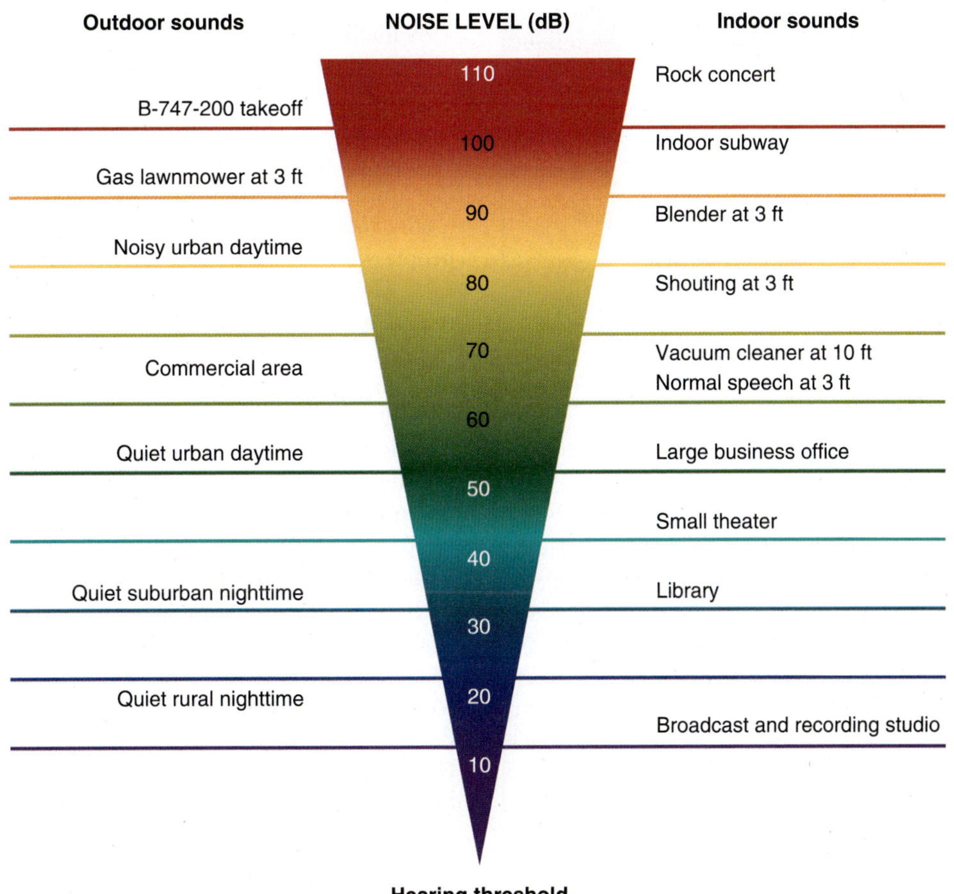

Fig. 23.6 Decibel levels of common sounds.

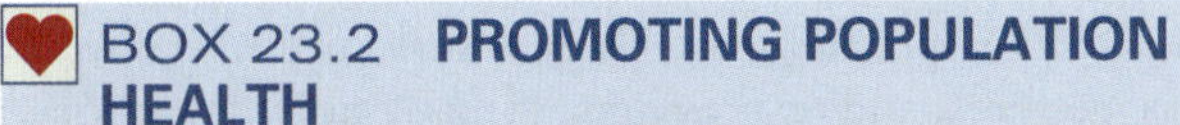

BOX 23.2 PROMOTING POPULATION HEALTH

Promoting Healthy Hearing

- Wear ear protection during recreation and work activities involving high noise levels.
- Monitor your sound level and how long you use personal listening devices.
- Avoid exposure to loud noise whenever possible.
- Listen to music at a reasonable level.
- Undergo screening to detect hearing loss as needed.
- Avoid injury from cotton-tipped applicators and other cleaning materials.

dryer. Encourage use of an umbrella or hat when it is raining. Hair spray, perfume, and shaving cream can clog the microphone opening and build up debris. Have the person take off the aids or cover them before applying these products.

An *implantable hearing device* may be an option for those with mild to severe hearing loss. There are 2 types: bone-anchored and middle ear implant devices. Bone-anchored devices are mainly used for conductive hearing loss or single-sided deafness. They are implanted into the bone of the skull. The sound signal bypasses the middle and outer ear, sending it straight to the cochlea.

TABLE 23.15 Types of Hearing Aids

Type	Considerations
Completely in the canal (CIC)	*Use:* Mild to moderate hearing loss *Advantages:* Smallest and least visible aid. Custom fit. Protected from sounds such as wind noise. *Disadvantages:* No space for add-ons such as volume controls. Small size may be hard to use. Easily clogged by earwax.
In the canal (ITC)	*Use:* Mild to moderate hearing loss *Advantages:* Small, discrete. Custom fit. Has adjustable features such as noise reduction. *Disadvantages:* May be hard to adjust and handle due to size. Not the best in noisy environments. Easily clogged by earwax.
In the ear (ITE)	*Use:* Mild to severe hearing loss *Advantages:* Easy to handle. Several battery options. Have more features. Full or half shell. *Disadvantages:* Visible. May have wind noise. Has several parts.
Behind the ear (BTE) Tube with earmold	*Use:* All types of hearing loss *Advantages:* Strongest. Easy to clean and handle. Longest battery life. Most available features. "Mini" version less visible. *Disadvantages:* Largest, most visible. May have wind noise. Person's voice may sound louder inside their head. Has several parts.

Images with permission by Oticon, Inc., Somerset, NJ.

A middle ear implant can be used as a treatment for SNHL and conductive hearing loss. The implant directly helps move the bones of the middle ear or vibrate the membrane window of the cochlea. This helps increase the transmission of sound vibrations reaching the inner ear. They do not amplify sounds like a hearing aid.

Cochlear implant. A *cochlear implant* may be used for some people with severe to profound hearing loss in one or both ears. The implant bypasses damaged or missing portions of the ear and directly activates CN VIII.[15] The external part of the system consists of a microphone, sound processor, and transmitter. The internal portion includes a receiver and several electrodes (Fig. 23.7). The microphone picks up sounds in the environment. The processor then converts the sounds into electronic signals that are sent to the transmitter. The transmitter sends these signals to the receiver, where they are passed on to the electrodes. The electrodes stimulate CN VIII, which carries the information directly to the brain, where it is interpreted as sound.

An implant does not restore normal hearing but gives a useful representation of sounds. Speech and everyday noises will sound different than what the person remembers. Extensive therapy is needed after receiving an implant to train the brain to understand the sounds heard through the implant. Factors that affect the outcomes include the age when hearing was lost and the length of time between hearing loss and receiving an implant. For adults, the best results occur with a shorter period of hearing loss. Adults with little or no experience with sound tend to benefit less from cochlear implants.

Speech reading. *Speech reading,* or *lip reading,* involves trying to understand speech from watching the speaker's lip movements. It can promote communication by supplementing what the person can hear. It allows for about 40% understanding of the spoken word. Using visual cues with speech, such as gestures and expressions, helps clarify the spoken message.

Sign language. *Sign language* is a visual language for people with profound hearing impairment. It involves specific hand gestures along with facial expressions, head movements, shoulder raises, and other body movements. There are many different sign languages. American Sign Language (ASL) is used in the United States and the English-speaking parts of Canada.

Assistive devices. Assistive listening devices (ALDs) include a variety of technology that amplifies sound. They can be used with a hearing aid or cochlear implant. Amplified telephones are the most common ALD. Special ALDs are used in large areas, like classrooms, theaters, and places of worship. These include hearing loop and FM systems. They send sound directly to a hearing aid or other receiver.

Alerting devices take the place of alarms, such as doorbells and smoke detectors. They use amplified sounds, visual light cues, or vibration to notify the person about their surroundings. Text-telephone alerting systems flash when activated by sound. A specially trained dog can alert their owner to specific sounds within the environment, thus increasing safety.

BOX 23.3 EVIDENCE-BASED PRACTICE

Hearing Aid Education

As a nurse in a community-based vision and hearing health clinic, you work with patients with varying degrees of hearing loss. Patients who need hearing aids can enroll in a 4-week, nurse-led, in-person education program that discusses hearing aid use and equipment care. Over the past 8 months, you have noticed a decrease in program participation with a decrease in the length of daily hearing aid use in patients who do not participate.

Making Clinical Decisions

Synthesis of Best Available Evidence

Providing education about hearing aids significantly increases their use. Patients who understand the benefits and proper use of hearing aids are more likely to wear them regularly. Programs usually include hearing-related information, training in communication skills, and counseling. Research shows that an internet-based program can increase knowledge and self-efficacy about hearing aid use.

Clinician Expertise

You and the other staff contact patients who chose not to enroll and ask them about factors that influenced their decision to not attend the program.

Patient Preferences and Values

A significant number of patients state the long drive to the clinic and the rising cost of gas were major influencing factors for not participating. To address this concern, you develop and implement an interactive education program through a web-based platform. Six months after initiating the web-based program, you note an increase in patients participating in the education program and an increase in their length of daily hearing aid use.

Implications for Nursing Practice

1. What information besides hearing aid use would you include in an education program?
2. What referrals would facilitate patient compliance with hearing aid use and care?

Reference for Evidence

Malmberg M, Anióse K, Skans J, et al: A randomised, controlled trial of clinically implementing online hearing support. *Int J Audiol* 62:472, 2023.

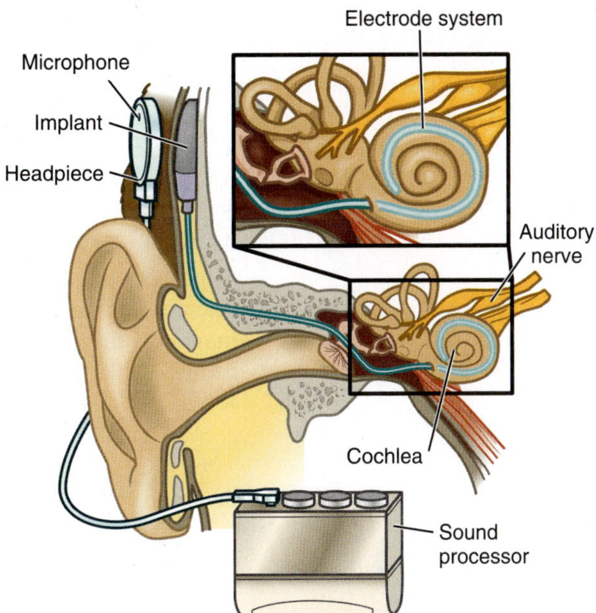

Fig. 23.7 Cochlear implant.

CASE STUDY

Ménière Disease

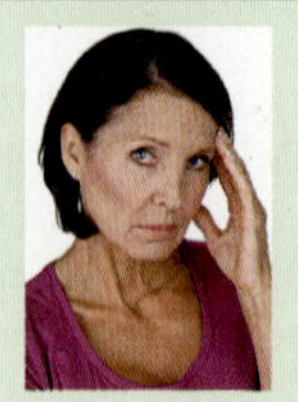

(© Stockphoto4u/ iStock.com.)

Patient Profile

While R.S. is in the emergency department, she starts vomiting violently. She tells you that any movement is making her feel like she is "spinning like crazy." The HCP decides to admit her under observation with plans to administer an intratympanic injection of dexamethasone.

Objective Data

- Skin pale, extremely diaphoretic
- Heart rate 112 beats/min, respirations 22 breaths/min, BP 100/64

Interprofessional Care

- 1000 mg sodium diet as tolerated
- Ondansetron 2 mg IV now
- Lorazepam 1 mg IV every 6 hours
- Meclizine 25 mg orally every 6 hours
- IV dextrose 5% with 0.45% NaCl at 75 mL/h

Discussion Questions

1. ***Analyze:*** Explain the cause of Ménière disease.
2. ***Analyze:*** What manifestations of Ménière disease does R.S. have?
3. ***Plan:*** Give the rationale for each treatment ordered.
4. ***Prioritize:*** Based on the assessment data, what are the priority clinical problems?
5. ***Prioritize:*** What are the priority nursing interventions for R.S.?
6. ***Act:*** Identify interventions that you can delegate to AP.
7. ***Safety:*** Name an area of risk for injury. What actions will you take to ensure patient safety?
8. ***Act:*** What teaching will you provide so R.S. can successfully self-manage her condition after discharge?
9. ***Evaluate:*** What outcomes would indicate care was effective?

Answers available at http://evolve.elsevier.com/Lewis/medsurg.

BRIDGE TO NCLEX EXAMINATION

The number of the question corresponds to the same-numbered outcome at the beginning of the chapter.

1. In a patient with vertigo, the parts of the ear most likely involved are the (**Select all that apply.**)
  a. cochlea.
  b. ossicles.
  c. vestibule.
  d. semicircular canals.
  e. tympanic membrane.

2. A patient reports tinnitus and balance problems. The medication that may be responsible is
  a. propranolol.
  b. warfarin.
  c. furosemide.
  d. acetaminophen.

3. What assessment technique would the nurse use to assess an adult patient's tympanic membrane?
  a. Have the patient tilt the head toward the nurse.
  b. Stabilize the otoscope with your fingers on the patient's cheek.
  c. Pull the pinna down and back to straighten the auditory canal.
  d. Use a speculum slightly larger than the size of the patient's ear canal.

4. A normal finding the nurse would expect when assessing hearing would be
  a. absent cone of light.
  b. bluish purple tympanic membrane.
  c. midline tone heard equally in both ears.
  d. fluid level at hairline in the tympanic membrane.

5. Common age-related changes in the auditory system include (**Select all that apply.**)
  a. drier earwax.
  b. tinnitus in both ears.
  c. auditory nerve degeneration.
  d. atrophy of the tympanic membrane.
  e. greater ability to hear high-pitched sounds.

6. The nurse teaches a patient scheduled for an electronystagmography that the test involves
  a. measuring eardrum movement in response to pressure.
  b. recording eye movements associated with ear irrigation.
  c. wearing headphones and determining which sounds can be heard.
  d. placing an electrode on the tympanic membrane and assessing for dizziness.

7. Care of the patient with an acute attack of Ménière disease includes (**Select all that apply.**)
  a. giving antiemetics as needed.
  b. implementing fall precautions.
  c. keeping the room dark and quiet.
  d. placing the patient on NPO status.
  e. ambulating in the hall independently.

8. Which person is at greatest risk for conductive hearing loss?
  a. 32-year-old with chronic otitis media
  b. 70-year-old receiving furosemide therapy
  c. 52-year-old who experienced head trauma
  d. 48-year-old with new-onset Ménière disease

9. Teach the person who is newly fitted with bilateral hearing aids to (**Select all that apply.**)
   - **a.** replace the batteries monthly.
   - **b.** clean the ear molds weekly or as needed.
   - **c.** clean ears with cotton-tipped applicators daily.
   - **d.** disconnect or remove the batteries when not in use.
   - **e.** initially restrict usage to quiet listening in the home.

10. Which strategies would *best* help the nurse communicate with a patient who has a hearing loss? (**Select all that apply.**)
   - **a.** Overenunciate speech.
   - **b.** Speak normally and slowly.
   - **c.** Exaggerate facial expressions.
   - **d.** Raise the voice to a higher pitch.
   - **e.** Write out names or difficult words.

1. c, d; 2. c; 3. b; 4. c; 5. a, b, c, d; 6. b; 7. a, b, c; 8. a; 9. b, d, e; 10. b, e.

For rationales to these answers and even more NCLEX review questions, visit http://evolve.elsevier.com/Lewis/medsurg.

REFERENCES

To access the References for this chapter, please scan the QR code with a mobile device.

24

Assessment: Integumentary System

Margaret R. Rateau

http://evolve.elsevier.com/Lewis/medsurg/

CONCEPTUAL FOCUS

Health Promotion

Tissue Integrity

LEARNING OUTCOMES

1. Describe the structures and functions of the integumentary system.
2. Link the age-related changes in the integumentary system to differences in assessment findings.
3. Obtain significant subjective and objective data related to the integumentary system.
4. Compare primary and secondary lesions.
5. Perform a physical assessment of the integumentary system.
6. Specify assessment differences in light- and dark-skinned persons.
7. Distinguish normal from common abnormal findings of the integumentary assessment.
8. Describe the purpose, significance of results, and nursing responsibilities related to diagnostic studies of the integumentary system.

KEY TERMS

alopecia
dermis
epidermis
erythema, Table 24.8
hirsutism, Table 24.8
keloid
keratinocytes
melanocytes
mole (nevus), Table 24.8
pruritus
sebaceous glands

The integumentary system is the largest organ of the body. It is composed of the skin, hair, nails, and certain glands. The skin is as complex as any organ but, unlike the others, it is readily visible. Being able to see and touch the skin helps you assess your patients. You can see abnormalities, understand their significance, and intervene early.

STRUCTURES AND FUNCTIONS OF SKIN AND APPENDAGES

Structures

Epidermis

The epidermis is the outer layer of the skin (Fig. 24.1). It is relatively thin. Its thickness ranges from approximately 0.5 mm on the eyelids to 1.5 mm on the palms of the hands and soles of the feet.[1] There are no lymph or vascular structures in the epidermis. It is supported by passive circulation from the dermis.

The epidermis has 5 distinct but interrelated layers. Two of the layers are the stratum corneum (the surface layer) and the stratum germinativum (deepest, basal layer) (Fig. 24.1).

Most epithelial cells are keratinocytes (90%). The remaining cells are melanocytes, Langerhans' cells, and Merkel cells. Keratinocytes form in the basal layer. Initially, they are undifferentiated and shaped like columns. As they mature (keratinize), they move to the surface. There they flatten and die, forming the outer skin layer (stratum corneum). Keratinocytes make a fibrous protein, keratin, which is vital to the skin's protective barrier function. The upward movement of keratinocytes from the basal layer to the outermost levels takes about 14 days. The keratinocytes stay there for another 14 days. This means the epidermis regenerates every 28 days. Thus each month you have a new layer of skin.

Many skin problems result from changes in this cell cycle. If dead cells slough off too rapidly, the skin appears thin and eroded. If new cells form faster than you shed old cells, the skin

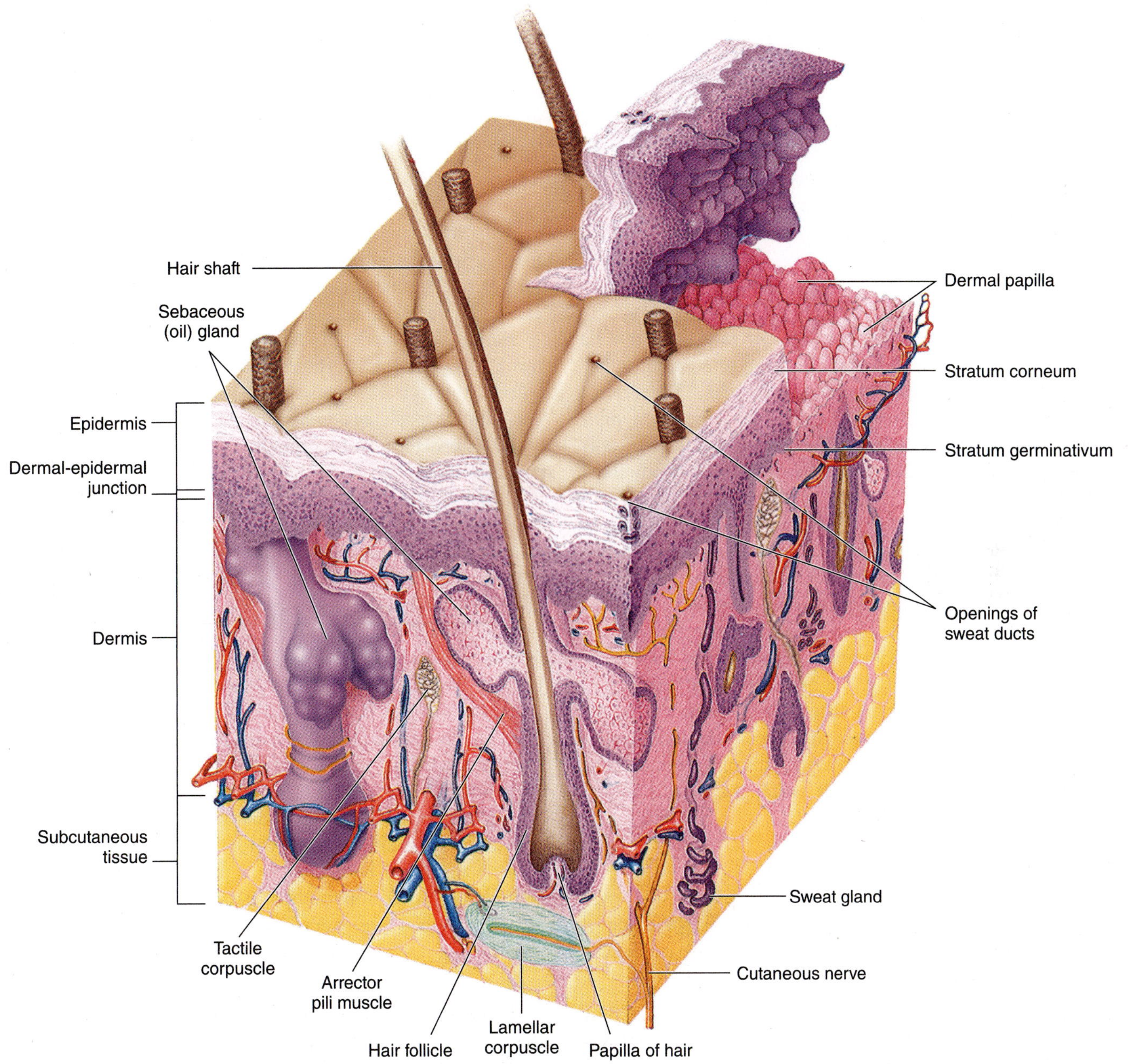

Fig. 24.1 Longitudinal view of the skin. The epidermis is raised at one corner to show the ridges in the dermis. (From Patton K, Bell F, Thompson T, et al: *The human body in health and disease,* ed 8, St Louis, 2024, Elsevier.)

becomes scaly and thickened. The epidermis fails to function normally with skin cancer and psoriasis (see Chapter 25).

Melanocytes are found in the deep, basal layer. They contain melanin, a pigment that gives color to the skin and hair and protects the body from damaging ultraviolet (UV) sunlight. Sunlight and hormones stimulate the melanosome (within the melanocyte) to increase melanin production. All people have similar numbers of melanocytes. In darker skin, the melanosomes are larger and more numerous. They make more eumelanin, a form of melanin that gives us the coloring of our skin. It is primarily responsible for brown and black skin pigmentation.[2] Increased melanin forms a natural sun shield for dark skin and decreases the risk of skin cancer. The distribution of melanocytes varies from one area of the body to another. For example, the face has more melanocytes than the abdomen.

Langerhans' cells are a type of dendritic cell. They are immunocompetent cells that recognize antigens. When they are depleted, the skin cannot initiate an immune response. The Langerhans cells in bioengineered skin grafts are removed to prevent graft rejection. We find decreased numbers of Langerhans cells with skin diseases such as psoriasis and sarcoidosis.

Merkel cells are found in the basal layer. They are involved in the sensation of light touch. We use them when feeling the texture of an object and deciding what it is.

The basement membrane zone is between the epidermis and dermis. It provides for (1) the exchange of fluids between the epidermis and dermis and (2) structural support for the epidermis. The basement membrane helps secure the 2 layers together. Inflammation and separation of the epidermis and dermis result in the blisters seen with problems such as burns, full-thickness wounds, and mechanical trauma.

Dermis

The **dermis** is the connective tissue below the epidermis. Its thickness ranges from 0.6 mm on the eyelid to 3.0 mm on the back, palms of the hands, and soles of the feet.[1] The dermis contains many blood vessels. It also contains nerves, lymph vessels, hair follicles, sebaceous glands, and specialized cells such as mast cells and macrophages that protect the body from external stimuli.

The dermis is made of 3 types of connective tissue: collagen, elastic fibers, and reticular fibers. Collagen forms the greatest part of the dermis. It gives the skin toughness and strength. Collagen is critical in wound healing. The primary cell type in the dermis is the *fibroblast,* which makes collagen and elastin.

The dermis has 2 layers: an upper, thin papillary layer and a deeper, thicker reticular layer. The papillary layer is arranged haphazardly in ridges, or papillae, which extend into the epidermis. These elevated surface ridges form fingerprints and footprints. The reticular layer forms the bulk of the dermis. It is made up of thick collagen bundles arranged parallel to the skin's surface.

Subcutaneous Tissue

The subcutaneous tissue lies below the dermis. It is made of loose connective tissue and fat cells. They provide insulation, cushioning, temperature regulation, and energy storage. The subcutaneous tissue attaches the skin to underlying tissues, such as muscle and bone. The distribution of subcutaneous tissue varies with gender, heredity, age, and nutrition status.

Skin Appendages

Skin appendages include the hair, nails, and glands (sebaceous, apocrine, and eccrine). These appendages are epidermal extensions that have their roots in the dermis. They receive nutrients, electrolytes, and fluids from the dermis. Hair and nails form from special keratin. Systemic diseases can affect the condition and health of hair and nails.

Hair grows on most of the body except for the lips, palms of the hands, interdigital spaces, portions of the genitalia, and soles of the feet. The density and pattern of distribution vary depending on age, sex, and race. Hair color is a result of heredity. It is determined by the type and amount of melanin in the hair shaft. Hair grows about 1 cm per month. People lose about 50 to 100 hairs each day.[3] Baldness, or **alopecia**, results when we do not replace lost hair.

Nails are made of heavily keratinized cells. The part of the nail that you can see is the nail body. The rest is the nail root. A fold of skin hides most of the nail root. The cuticle borders this skinfold. The small part of the nail root you can see is the *lunula.* This white, crescent-shaped area is the site of nail growth (Fig. 24.2). Under the nail is an area of epidermis called the *nail bed.* The nail bed has many blood vessels. Nails grow slowly but continuously. Fingernails grow much faster than toenails, on average of 0.1 mm/day.[4] It takes 4 to 6 months to replace a fingernail. A toenail may take 12 to 18 months to replace. Nail color ranges from pink to yellow or brown depending on skin color. Color and texture variations in nails may be normal or represent an abnormal condition. Pigmented longitudinal bands *(melanonychia striata)* in the nail bed are more likely in people with dark skin (Fig. 24.3).[5]

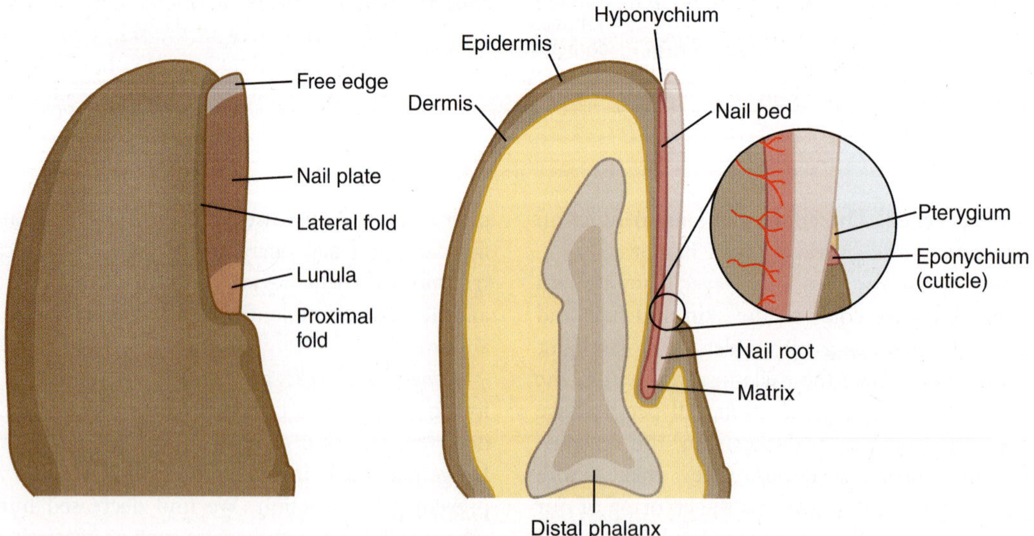

Fig. 24.2 Structure of a nail.

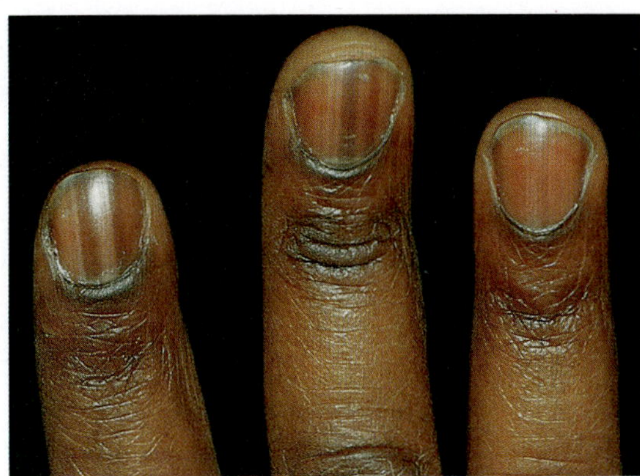

Fig. 24.3 Pigmented nail bands normally seen with dark skin color. (From Ball J, Dains J, Flynn J, et al: *Seidel's guide to physical examination,* ed 10, St Louis, 2023, Mosby.)

There are 2 major types of glands in the skin: sebaceous and sweat (apocrine and eccrine) glands. **Sebaceous glands** secrete *sebum,* which is emptied into the hair follicles. Sebum waterproofs and lubricates the skin and promotes the absorption of fat-soluble substances. Sebum is somewhat bacteriostatic and fungistatic. Sex hormones, particularly testosterone, regulate sebum secretion. Production varies depending on age, sex, and testosterone and estrogen levels. Sebaceous glands are present on all areas of the skin except the palms, soles, and dorsum of the feet. These glands are most abundant on the face, scalp, upper chest, and back.

The *apocrine sweat glands* are mainly found in the axillary, genital, and breast areas. They are always connected to a hair follicle. These glands enlarge and become active at puberty because of reproductive hormones. They secrete a thick, milky substance that is naturally odorless. Odor occurs when skin surface bacteria alter the secretions.

The *eccrine sweat glands* are found on most of the body, except the lips, ear canals, nail beds, labia minora, glans penis, and prepuce. One square inch of skin has about 3000 eccrine sweat glands. Their main function is to cool the body by evaporation, excrete waste products, and moisturize surface cells. Sweat is a transparent, watery solution composed of salts, ammonia, urea, and other wastes. In extreme situations, the body can make 2 to 4 L of sweat per hour or up to 12 L in 24 hours. Heat, certain mental stimuli, and ingesting hot, spicy foods stimulate sweat secretion.

Functions

The skin's main function is to protect the underlying body tissues by serving as a barrier to the external environment. The skin is a barrier against invasion by bacteria and viruses and prevents excess water loss. The fat in the subcutaneous layer insulates the body and provides protection from trauma. Melanin screens and absorbs UV radiation.

The skin with its nerve endings and special receptors collects sensory information from environment stimuli. These special nerve endings give information to the brain about pain, heat and cold, touch, pressure, and vibration.

The skin controls heat regulation by responding to changes in internal and external temperature with vasoconstriction or vasodilation. The skin's excretory function and heat regulation are related. We lose between 600 and 900 mL of water daily through insensible water loss (invisible vaporization from the lungs and skin). This helps regulate body temperature. Sebum and sweat lubricate the skin surface. Endogenous vitamin D synthesis, which is critical to calcium and phosphorus balance, occurs in the epidermis. We make vitamin D in the epidermis when UV light acts on vitamin D precursor cells.

Gerontologic Considerations: Effects of Aging on the Integumentary System

Many skin changes occur with aging. Depending on how you view yourself, the normal, visible effects of aging on the skin and hair may have a profound psychologic effect. Having a youthful look may affect self-image. The appearance of the signs of aging can be a threat to self-concept. Other changes in skin structure related to aging can pose a serious risk. Table 24.1 outlines age-related integumentary changes and differences in assessment findings.

Chronic UV exposure is the major cause of premature aging or photoaging and wrinkling of skin.[6] Sun damage to the skin is cumulative (Fig. 24.4). The wrinkling of sun-exposed areas such as the face and hands is more marked than in a sun-shielded area, such as the buttocks. A photoaged person is more susceptible to skin cancers because UV exposure decreases the ability to repair cellular damage. Other factors that influence skin aging include diabetes, smoking, and alcohol use.

The junction between the dermis and epidermis flattens. This causes the layers to lose their tight bond. Skin tears and other trauma become common as the epidermis slides separately from the dermis. Collagen fibers stiffen, and elastic fibers degenerate. The amount of subcutaneous tissue decreases. These changes, with the added effects of gravity, lead to wrinkling. Fewer free fatty acids in the epidermis result in dry, scaly, itchy skin. Dryness increases the risk for cracks in the skin and secondary infection. Decreased subcutaneous fat increases the risk for traumatic injury, hypothermia, and shearing, which may lead to a pressure injury.

Fewer melanocytes are present. Hair color fades due to decreased melanin. Hormone and vitamin deficiencies can cause dry, thin hair and alopecia. The growth rate of hair and nails decreases. The nail plate thins. Nails become brittle and more prone to splitting and yellowing. Nails, especially toenails, may thicken. The apocrine and eccrine sweat glands atrophy. This causes dry skin and decreased body odor.

Benign growths can occur. These include seborrheic keratoses, vascular lesions such as cherry angiomas, and skin tags. *Actinic keratoses* appear on areas of chronic sun exposure, especially in people with a fair complexion and light eyes. These premalignant skin lesions place a person at increased risk for squamous and basal cell cancers.

TABLE 24.1 GERONTOLOGIC ASSESSMENT DIFFERENCES

Integumentary System

Changes	Differences in Assessment Findings
Skin	
↓ Subcutaneous fat, muscle laxity, degeneration of elastic fibers, collagen stiffening	Wrinkling, sagging breasts and abdomen, redundant flesh around eyes, skin slow to flatten when pinched (tenting)
↓ Extracellular water, surface lipids, sebaceous gland activity	Dry, flaking skin
↓ Apocrine and sebaceous gland activity	Dry skin with minimal to no perspiration, skin color uneven
↑ Capillary fragility and permeability	Bruising
More focal melanocytes in basal layer with pigment accumulation	Solar lentigines on face and back of hands
↓ Blood supply	Less rosy appearance of skin and mucous membranes. Skin cool to touch. ↓ Awareness of pain, touch, temperature, peripheral vibration
↓ Proliferative capacity	Delayed wound healing
↓ Immunocompetence	↑ In skin cancers
Hair	
↓ Melanin and melanocytes	Gray or white hair
↓ Oil	Dry, coarse hair. Scaly scalp
↓ Hair density	Thinning and hair loss
Cumulative androgen effect; ↓ estrogen	Facial hirsutism, baldness
Nails	
↓ Peripheral blood supply	Thick, brittle nails, slow nail growth
↑ Keratin	Longitudinal ridging
↓ Circulation	Prolonged return of blood to nails on blanching

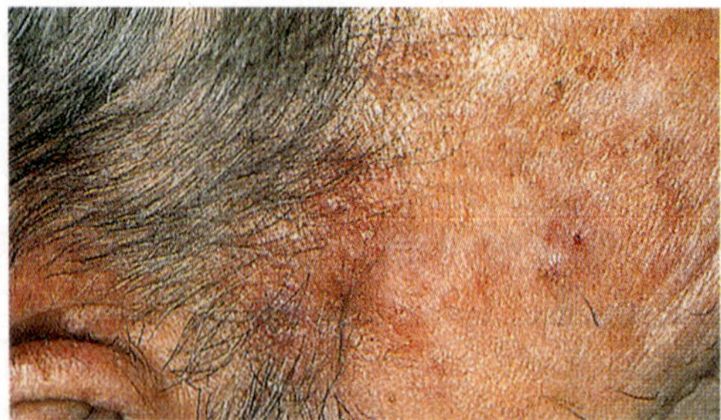

Fig. 24.4 Photoaging. Irregular pigmentation and keratoses occur in sun-damaged skin on forehead. (From Gawkrodger D, Ardern-Jones MR: *Dermatology*, ed 5, Edinburgh, 2012, Churchill Livingstone.)

INTEGUMENTARY SYSTEM ASSESSMENT

The general skin assessment begins with your first contact with the patient and continues throughout the examination. When you meet your patient, take a moment to note the overall condition of their skin and hair. You will assess specific areas of the skin when examining other body systems unless the chief complaint is a skin problem. Record a general statement about the skin's condition (Table 24.2).

TABLE 24.2 Normal Physical Assessment of the Integumentary System

Skin	• Evenly pigmented. No petechiae, purpura, lesions, or excoriations • Warm, good turgor
Nails	• Pink, oval, adhere to nail bed with 160-degree angle
Hair	• Shiny and full; amount and distribution appropriate for age and gender • No flaking of scalp, forehead, or pinna

CASE STUDY

Patient Introduction

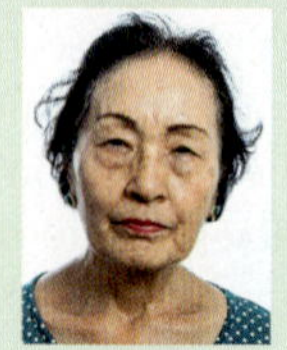

(© andreswd/iStock.com.)

D.A. is a 74-year-old female who comes to the medical clinic with concerns related to "spots" on her face. She says they have been there for a while, and she thought they were just "age spots." She became concerned after her friend was diagnosed with a malignant melanoma.

Discussion Questions

1. What are the possible causes of D.A.'s facial lesions?
2. What questions would you ask D.A. to determine the possible causes?

You will learn more about D.A. and her condition as you read this chapter.

Answers available at http://evolve.elsevier.com/Lewis/medsurg.

Subjective Data

Ask the health history questions outlined in Table 24.3 when you note a skin problem. A thorough health history yields information about possible causes and the effect of the problem on the person's life. Perform the interview with a sensitive and nonjudgmental attitude. The problem may be the result of poor hygiene or unhealthy behaviors. Some problems are highly visible and affect body image and self-concept.

Important Health Information

Health history. Ask about any disease that involves the skin. Many diseases have skin manifestations (Table 24.4). Determine whether the patient has noticed any problems such as jaundice (liver disease), delayed wound healing (diabetes), cyanosis (respiratory, cardiovascular disorder), or pallor (anemia). Obtain specific information related to food sensitivities, pet or drug allergies, and skin reactions to insect bites and stings. Note any history of chronic or unprotected exposure to UV light, including tanning bed use and radiation treatments.

Medications. A thorough medication history is important. Skin-related problems can occur because of taking medication. Many hormones, antibiotics, corticosteroids, and antimetabolites have side effects that manifest in the skin. Medications may contain fragrances and preservatives that can cause skin

TABLE 24.3 **HEALTH HISTORY**

Integumentary System

Health Perception–Health Management
- Describe your daily hygiene practices.
- What skin products are you now using?
- Describe any current skin problems, including onset, course, and treatment (if any).

Nutritional-Metabolic
- Describe any changes in your skin, hair, nails, and mucous membranes.
- Have you noticed any recent changes in the way sores or wounds heal?[a]
- Have you had any weight loss or dietary changes?[a]

Elimination
- Have you noticed recent changes in your skin related to excess sweating, dryness, or swelling?[a]

Activity-Exercise
- Do your leisure or work activities involve using any chemicals that might irritate your skin?[a]
- Do you do anything to protect yourself from the sun?[a]

Sleep-Rest
- Does your skin problem keep you awake or awaken you from sleep?[a]

Cognitive-Perceptual
- Do you have any unusual sensations of heat, cold, or touch?[a]
- Do you have any pain associated with your skin problem?[a]
- Do you have any joint pain?[a]

Self-Perception–Self-Concept
- How does your skin make you feel about yourself?

Role-Relationship
- Has your skin problem changed your relationships with others?[a]
- Have you changed your lifestyle because of your skin problem?[a]

Sexuality-Reproductive
- Has your skin problem changed your intimate relationships with others?[a]
- Has your birth control method (if used) caused a skin problem?[a]

Coping–Stress Tolerance
- Are you aware of any situation or stressor that changes your skin problem?[a]
- Do you think that stress plays a role in your skin problem?[a]
- How do you manage stress?

Value-Belief
- Are there any cultural beliefs that influence your thinking or feelings about your skin problem?[a]
- Are there any treatment options that you would be opposed to using?

[a]If yes, please describe.

reactions. Were medications used to treat a primary skin problem, such as acne or hair loss, or a secondary skin problem, such as itching? Note the drug's name, length of use, method of application, and effectiveness.

Surgery or other treatments. Has the patient had any surgeries, including cosmetic surgery, done on the skin? Record any biopsy results. Note any treatments for a skin problem (e.g., phototherapy) or for a health problem (e.g., radiation therapy). Ask if the patient has had any treatments for cosmetic purposes, such as tanning booth use, laser resurfacing, or cosmetic "peels."

Functional Health Patterns

Health perception–health management. Record a description of any current skin problem, including onset, symptoms, course, and treatment. Ask about health practices, such as self-care habits related to daily hygiene. Assess the frequency of use and sun protection factor (SPF) of sunscreen products. Note the use of personal care products (e.g., shampoos, moisturizing agents, cosmetics), including brand name, quantity, and frequency.

Obtain information about the family history of any skin diseases. Include congenital and familial diseases (e.g., alopecia, psoriasis) and systemic diseases with skin manifestations (e.g., diabetes, thyroid disease, cardiovascular diseases, immune disorders). Note any family and personal history of skin cancer, particularly melanoma. A person has an increased risk for developing melanoma if they have a first-degree relative (e.g., parent, full sibling) who had a melanoma.[7]

Nutritional-metabolic. Ask about the condition of skin, hair, nails, and mucous membranes. Have there been any changes related to diet? A diet history shows the adequacy of nutrients essential to healthy skin and wound healing, such as protein and vitamins A, D, E, and C. Ask if they have areas of chafing or a rash in *intertriginous* areas. This is where skin surfaces overlap and rub on each other (e.g., below the breasts, axillae, groin). Skin in these areas is predisposed to skin tags and yeast, fungal, and bacterial infections. Note any excess or absent sweating. Ask the patient about poor or delayed wound healing.

Elimination. Ask the patient about skin problems, such as dehydration, edema, and pruritus (itching). These can indicate changes in fluid balance. If urinary or fecal incontinence is a problem, ask about the condition of the skin in the anal and perineal areas.

Activity-exercise. Obtain information about environment hazards in relation to hobbies and recreational activities, including exposure to carcinogens, chemical irritants, and allergens. Do any changes occur in the skin during exercise or other activities?

Sleep-rest. Ask the patient about changes in sleep patterns caused by a skin problem. For example, itching can interfere with sleep. Poor sleep and resulting tiredness can be reflected in a patient's face by dark circles under the eyes and a decreased firmness in the facial skin.

Cognitive-perceptual. Assess the perception of the sensations of heat, cold, pain, and touch. Note any discomfort associated with a skin problem, especially when observed in intact skin. Are there any reports of unusual skin sensations? Patients with neuropathy may describe numbness, tingling, or crawling sensations in their arms or legs. Ask about joint pain.

Self-perception–self-concept. Assess any feelings related to having a skin problem, such as sadness, anxiety, despair, or altered body image. These feelings can occur with classic signs

TABLE 24.4 Diseases With Skin Manifestations

Systemic Problem	Skin Manifestations
Cardiovascular	
Peripheral vascular disease	Loss of hair on hands and feet. Delayed capillary filling. Dependent rubor (redness), pain
Rheumatic heart disease	Petechiae, urticaria, nodules, erythema
Thromboangiitis obliterans (Buerger disease)	Pallor or cyanosis, gangrene, ulceration
Venous ulcers	Leathery, brownish skin on lower leg; itching, concave lesion with edema. Scar tissue with healing
Endocrine	
Addison disease	Loss of body hair (especially axillary), general hyperpigmentation (accentuated in folds)
Androgen deficiency	Sparse hair. ↓ Sebum production
Androgen excess	Enlarged facial pores, male sex characteristics, acne, acceleration of coarse hair growth
Diabetes	Reddened plaques of shins, delayed wound healing, neuropathy, acanthosis nigricans (velvety, dark skin on the neck and in skin folds)
Glucocorticoid excess (Cushing syndrome)	Atrophy, striae, epidermal thinning, telangiectasia, acne. ↓ Subcutaneous fat over extremities. Thin, loose dermis. Impaired wound healing. Increased vascular fragility. Mild hirsutism. Excess collection of fat over clavicles, back of neck, abdomen, and face
Hyperpituitarism (acromegaly)	Coarse skin, deepened lines. ↑ Oiliness and sweating, acne. ↑ Number of nevi, hyperpigmentation; hypertrichosis (excess hair growth)
Hyperthyroidism	↑ Sweating, warm skin with persistent flush, thin nails, alopecia. Fine, soft hair
Hypoparathyroidism	Opaque, brittle nails with transverse ridges. Coarse, sparse hair with patchy alopecia
Hypothyroidism	Cold, dry, pale to yellow skin. General nonpitting edema. Dry, coarse, brittle hair. Brittle, slow-growing nails
Gastrointestinal	
Cystic fibrosis	Abnormal sweat gland function
Deficiency of essential fatty acids	Scaly skin
Inflammatory bowel disease	Mouth ulcers, erythema nodosum
Liver disease and biliary tract obstruction	Jaundice, itching, pigmentary abnormalities, changes in nails and hair, spider angiomas, telangiectasia
Malabsorption syndrome	Acquired ichthyosis (dry, scaly skin)
Hematologic	
Anemia	Pallor, hyperpigmentation, pale mucous membranes, hair loss, nail dystrophy
Clotting problems	Purpura, petechiae, bruising
Immune	
HIV infection	Kaposi sarcoma, eosinophilic folliculitis
Hodgkin lymphoma	Itching, sensitive skin
Non-Hodgkin lymphoma	Papules, nodules, plaques, itching
Metabolic	
Nicotinic acid (niacin) deficiency	Redness of exposed areas of skin of hand or foot, face, or neck; infected dermatitis
Vitamin B_1 (thiamine) deficiency	Edema, redness of soles of feet
Vitamin B_2 (riboflavin) deficiency	Red fissures at corner of mouth, glossitis
Vitamin C deficiency	Petechiae, purpura, bleeding gums
Musculoskeletal and Connective Tissue	
Dermatomyositis	Edema; purplish-red upper eyelids; knuckles scaly and red
Scleroderma	Leathery hardening and stiffness of skin
Systemic lupus erythematosus	Discoid lesions, maculopapular semiconfluent rash (butterfly rash), alopecia, mouth ulcers
Neurologic	
Chronic sensory polyneuropathies, spinal cord trauma	Changes in skin from sensory denervation, pressure injuries, anesthesia, paresthesias
Renal	
Chronic kidney disease	Dry skin, itching, uremic frost, pallor, bruises
Reproductive Organs	
Paget disease	Eczematous patch of nipple and areola
Primary syphilis	Chancre
Secondary syphilis	General skin lesions, alopecia
Tertiary syphilis	Gummas
Respiratory	
↓ Oxygenation due to respiratory disease	Cyanosis

of aging or visible skin problems such as acne, rosacea, and psoriasis, which change physical appearance.

Role-relationship. Determine how the skin problem affects relationships with family members, peers, and work associates. Ask about the effect of environment factors on the skin, such as work exposure to irritants, sun, and unusually cold or unhygienic conditions. Contact dermatitis caused by allergens and irritants is a common problem associated with occupation.

Sexuality-reproductive. Assess the effect of the skin problem on sexual activity. Note the reproductive status of the female patient relative to possible therapeutic interventions. For example, isotretinoin used to treat acne, and topical fluorouracil used to treat actinic keratoses, are teratogenic drugs that may cause abnormal fetal development. Pregnant females or females who could become pregnant should not use them.

CASE STUDY

Subjective Data

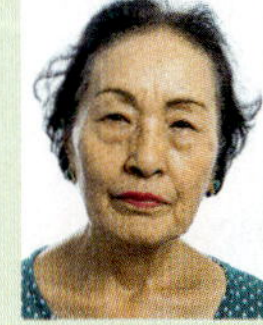

(© andreswd/ iStock.com.)

A focused subjective assessment of D.A. reveals the following:

- ***History:*** Negative except for an appendectomy at age 16.
- ***Medications:*** None at present. No known allergies.
- ***Health Perception–Health Management:*** Washes her face with a skin cleanser in the morning and nighttime. After cleansing, she applies a moisturizer with SPF 15. She has used these facial products for the past 3 years since she first started noticing small age spots appearing. Before that, she just used soap and water.
- ***Nutritional:*** States her skin seems drier as she ages but otherwise no changes besides the "age spots" or "whatever they are." Denies any changes in the way cuts or sores heal. No weight loss. Does not take any vitamins or mineral supplements.
- ***Elimination:*** Although skin is a little dry, D.A. does not perceive it to be excessively dry. Denies excess sweating or any swelling.
- ***Activity-Exercise:*** Loves to garden and go for walks outdoors. Reports a history of frequent, sometimes severe, sunburns as a child. No use of sunscreen growing up but does remember her mother making her wear T-shirts over her bathing suits to help prevent sunburn. Has used sunscreen for the past 20 years when outdoors. Reapplies as needed.
- ***Cognitive-Perceptual:*** Denies any pain or discomfort associated with skin lesions.
- ***Coping–Stress Tolerance:*** Fearful that she might have skin cancer.

Discussion Questions

1. Which subjective assessment findings concern you most?
2. What should you include in the physical assessment? What specific characteristics of the skin lesions would you be looking for?

You will learn more about the physical assessment of the skin in the next section.

Answers available at http://evolve.elsevier.com/Lewis/medsurg.

Objective Data

Physical Assessment

The physical assessment begins with a systematic, general inspection and then a more specific assessment of problem areas. A normal range of differences exists in the skin, hair, and nails. Note normal skin changes related to age, genetic factors, and environment exposures from other changes. Look for changes in the color of the skin, turgor, temperature, dryness, thickness, and vascularity. General principles when assessing the skin are:

- Have a private room of moderate temperature with good lighting. A room with exposure to daylight is best.
- Ensure the patient is comfortable and in attire that allows easy access to all skin areas.
- Perform a general inspection and then a lesion-specific assessment.
- Use the metric system when taking measurements.
- Use the right terminology when documenting.

Clinical photography. Photographs are an adjunct to documentation and promote communication among the interprofessional team. We use them to assess and monitor skin problems and determine whether the problem has improved or declined. They can be used to track moles and precancerous lesions and detect changes early. Follow agency protocol for obtaining the patient's consent to photograph lesions.

Inspection. Inspect the skin for general color and pigmentation, vascularity, bruising, lesions, and discolorations. The critical factor in assessing skin color is change. A skin color that is normal for one patient can be a sign of a pathologic problem in another patient. Skin color depends on the amount of melanin (brown), carotene (yellow), oxyhemoglobin (red), and reduced hemoglobin (bluish-red) present. The best areas to assess erythema, cyanosis, pallor, and jaundice are the areas of least pigmentation. These include the sclera, conjunctivae, nail beds, lips, and buccal mucosa. We see true skin color best in photo-protected areas such as the buttocks. Activity, sun (UV) exposure, emotions, cigarette smoking, and edema, as well as respiratory, renal, cardiovascular, and liver problems, can directly affect skin color.

Note the presence of body art such as piercings and tattoos. The nose, ears, eyebrows, lips, navel, and nipples are common sites of piercing. Examine tattoos and needle-track marks. Note the location and characteristics of the surrounding skin area. Tattoo pigments deposited in the skin may cause itching, pain, and sensitivity for several weeks after the tattoo is placed.

Examine the skin for problems related to vascularity (see Table 33.6). Is there any bruising? Note vascular and purpuric lesions such as *angioma* (benign tumor of blood or lymph vessels), *petechiae* (tiny, flat, purplish-red pinpoint lesions), or *purpura* (purple or reddish areas with bruising that do not blanche). Note the reaction to direct pressure on the lesion. If a lesion blanches on direct pressure and then refills, the redness is due to dilated blood vessels. If the discoloration stays, it is the result of subcutaneous or intradermal bleeding or a nonvascular lesion. Note any pattern of bruising. Is the discoloration in the shape of the hand or fingers? Are bruises at different stages of resolution? These may indicate other health problems or abuse and need further investigation.

Record the color, size, height, distribution, location, and shape of any lesions. Lesions may be primary or secondary lesions. *Primary skin lesions* develop on previously unaltered skin. The common characteristics of primary skin lesions are shown in Table 24.5. *Secondary skin lesions* are lesions that change with time or occur because of scratching or infection (Table 24.6).

TABLE 24.5 Primary Skin Lesions

Lesion	Description
Macule	Circumscribed, flat discoloration that is blue, red, brown, or hypopigmented. <0.5 cm in diameter. If lesion >0.5 cm, it is a patch *Examples:* freckles, petechiae, measles, flat mole (nevus), café-au-lait spots, vitiligo (complete depigmentation)
Papule	Elevated, solid lesion. <0.5 cm in diameter. Color varies. If lesion is >0.5 cm in diameter, it is a nodule *Examples:* wart (verruca), elevated moles, lipoma, basal cell cancer
Plaque	Circumscribed, elevated, superficial, solid lesion. >0.5 cm in diameter *Examples:* psoriasis, seborrheic and actinic keratoses
Pustule	Elevated, superficial lesion filled with purulent fluid *Examples:* acne, impetigo
Vesicle	Circumscribed, superficial collection of serous fluid. <0.5 cm in diameter. If lesion >0.5 cm, it is a bulla *Examples:* varicella (chickenpox), herpes zoster (shingles), second-degree burn
Wheal	Firm, edematous, irregularly shaped area. Size varies. May last only a few hours *Examples:* insect bite, urticaria, angioedema

TABLE 24.6 Secondary Skin Lesions

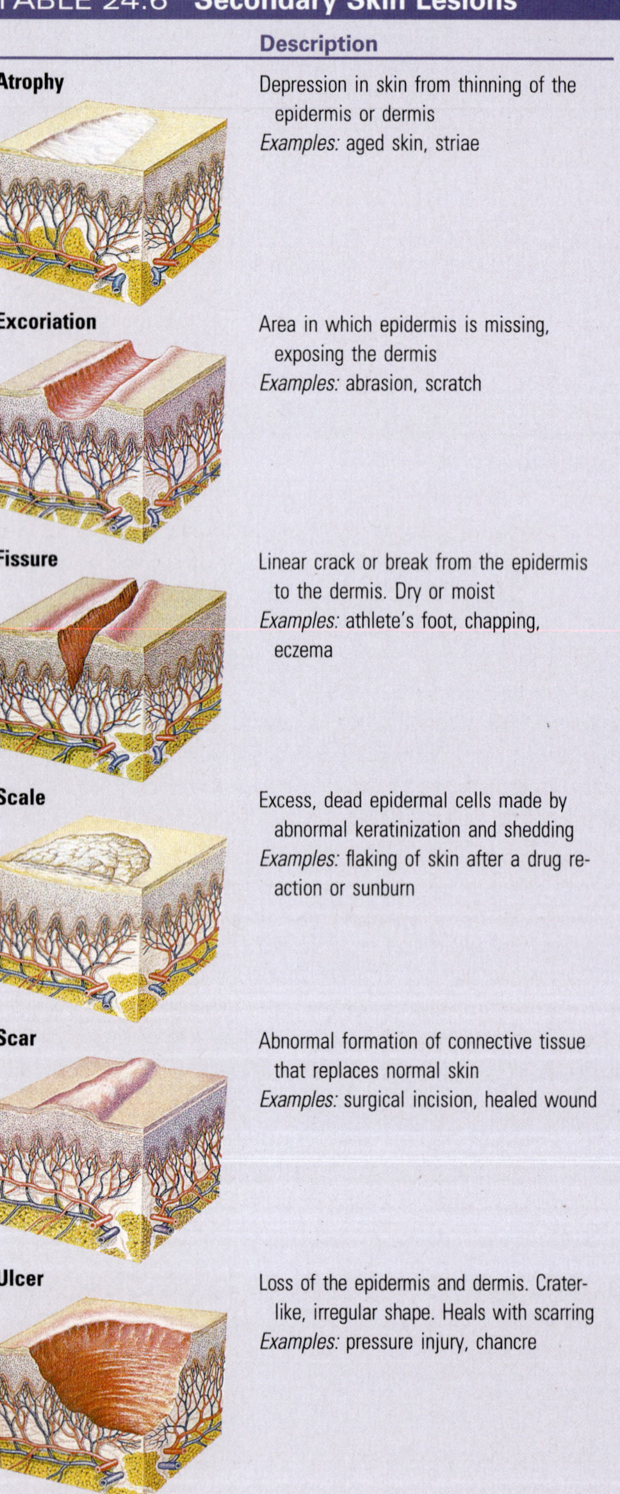

	Description
Atrophy	Depression in skin from thinning of the epidermis or dermis *Examples:* aged skin, striae
Excoriation	Area in which epidermis is missing, exposing the dermis *Examples:* abrasion, scratch
Fissure	Linear crack or break from the epidermis to the dermis. Dry or moist *Examples:* athlete's foot, chapping, eczema
Scale	Excess, dead epidermal cells made by abnormal keratinization and shedding *Examples:* flaking of skin after a drug reaction or sunburn
Scar	Abnormal formation of connective tissue that replaces normal skin *Examples:* surgical incision, healed wound
Ulcer	Loss of the epidermis and dermis. Crater-like, irregular shape. Heals with scarring *Examples:* pressure injury, chancre

TABLE 24.7 Lesion Distribution Terminology

Term	Description
Annular	Circular, begins in center and spreads to periphery (e.g., tinea corporis [ringworm])
Asymmetric	Unilateral distribution
Confluent	Merging together (e.g., urticaria [hives])
Discrete	Distinct individual lesions that are separate (e.g., acne)
Gyrate	Twisted, coiled spiral, snakelike
Grouped	Clusters of lesions (e.g., vesicles of contact dermatitis)
Local	Clearly defined, limited areas of involvement (confined to one area)
Polycyclic	Annular lesions grow together (e.g., psoriasis)
Solitary	Single lesion
Symmetric	Bilateral distribution
Zosteriform	Linear arrangement along a dermatome area (e.g., herpes zoster)

We usually describe skin lesions in terms related to the lesions' configuration (solitary or pattern in relation to other lesions) and distribution (arrangement of lesions over an area of skin) (Table 24.7). Note any unusual odors. Skin sites with lesions, such as rashes, may be colonized with yeast or bacteria, which can cause distinctive odors in areas where skin rubs together (Fig. 24.5).

Inspect all body hair. Note the distribution, texture, and quantity of hair. Changes in the normal distribution of body hair and growth may indicate an endocrine or vascular problem. Inspect the nails, including nail shape, thickness, curvature, and surface. Note any grooves, pitting, ridges, or detachment from the nail bed. Changes in nail smoothness or thickness can occur with anemia, psoriasis, thyroid problems, decreased circulation, and some infections.

Palpation. Palpate the skin to obtain information about temperature, turgor, moisture, and texture. Use the back of your hand to gauge skin temperature. The skin should be warm, not hot; skin temperature increases when blood flow to the dermis increases. A local temperature increase occurs with burns and local inflammation. A general increase occurs when a person has a fever. A decreased body temperature may occur when shock or other circulatory problems, chilling, or infection is present.

Turgor refers to the elasticity of the skin. Assess turgor by gently pinching an area of skin under the clavicle or on the back of the hand. Skin with good turgor should easily move when lifted and immediately return to its original position when released. In older patients or patients with dehydration, a loss of turgor occurs and can cause tenting of the skin.

Skin moisture (dampness or dryness of the skin) increases in areas where skin rubs together. Skin moisture varies with environment temperature, muscular activity, body weight, and body temperature. The skin should be intact with no flaking, scaling, or cracking. Skin generally becomes drier with increasing age.

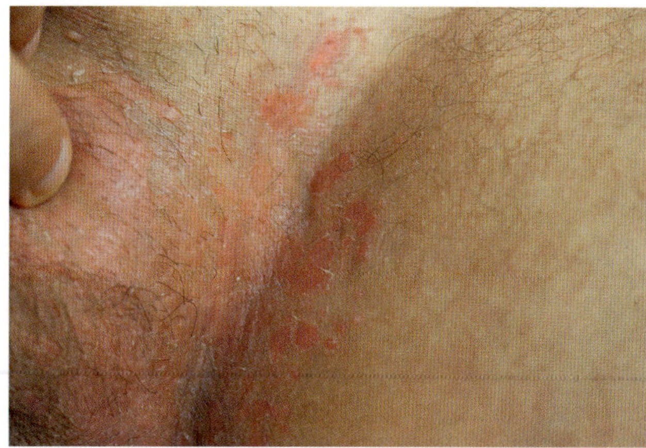

Fig. 24.5 Intertrigo. Rash in body folds with *Candida* infection. (© cunfek/iStock.com.)

BOX 24.1 FOCUSED ASSESSMENT

Integumentary System

Use this checklist to make sure the key assessment steps have been done.

Subjective

Ask the patient about the following and note responses:

Hair loss (unusual or rapid)
Changes in skin (e.g., lesions, bruising)
Nail discoloration

Objective

Inspect

Skin for color, integrity, scars, lesions, signs of breakdown
Facial and body hair for distribution, color, quantity, hygiene
Nails for shape, contour, color, thickness, cleanliness
Dressings, if present

Palpate

Skin for temperature, texture, moisture, thickness, turgor, mobility

Texture refers to the fineness or coarseness of the skin. The skin should feel smooth and firm, with the surface evenly thin in most areas. Thickened callus areas are normal on the soles and palms and relate to weight bearing. Increased skin thickness is often work related and the result of excess pressure. Excess calluses on the soles of patients with neuropathy or diabetes predispose them to developing lesions.

Use a focused assessment (Box 24.1) to evaluate the status of previously identified skin problems and monitor for signs of new problems. Assessment abnormalities of the skin are described in Table 24.8.

Assessment of Dark Skin

The structures of dark skin are often harder to assess (Table 24.9). Color is easiest to assess in areas where the

TABLE 24.8 ASSESSMENT ABNORMALITIES

Integumentary System

Finding	Description	Possible Etiology and Significance
Alopecia	Hair loss	Heredity, friction, rubbing, traction, trauma, stress, infection, inflammation, chemotherapy, pregnancy, emotional shock, tinea capitis, immune factors
Angioma	Tumor consisting of blood or lymph vessels	Normal increase with aging, liver disease, pregnancy, varicose veins
Carotenemia (carotenosis)	Yellow discoloration of skin, no yellowing of sclerae, most noticeable on palms and soles	Vegetables containing carotene (e.g., carrots, squash), hypothyroidism
Comedo (acne lesion)	Enlarged hair follicle plugged with sebum, bacteria, and skin cells; can be open (blackhead) or closed (whitehead)	Heredity, certain drugs, hormone changes with puberty and pregnancy
Cyanosis	Slightly bluish-gray or dark purple discoloration of the skin and mucous membranes caused by excess amounts of reduced hemoglobin in capillaries	Cardiorespiratory problems, vasoconstriction, asphyxiation, anemia, leukemia, some cancers
Cyst	Sac containing fluid or semisolid material	Obstruction of a duct or gland, parasitic infection
Ecchymosis (bruising)	Large, bruise-like lesion caused by collection of extravascular blood in dermis and subcutaneous tissue	Trauma, bleeding disorders
Erythema	Redness in patches of varying size and shape	Heat, certain drugs, alcohol, UV rays, any problem that causes dilation of blood vessels in the skin
Hematoma	Extravasation of blood of enough size to cause visible swelling	Trauma, bleeding disorders
Hirsutism	Male distribution of hair in females	Ovary or adrenal gland problem, decrease in estrogen level, familial trait
Hypopigmentation	Loss of pigmentation resulting in lighter patches than the normal skin	Chemical agents, nutrition, burns, inflammation, infection
Intertrigo	Dermatitis of overlying surfaces of the skin (Fig. 24.5)	Moisture, irritation, obesity; may be complicated by *Candida* infection
Jaundice	Yellow (in light-skinned patients) or yellowish-brown (in dark-skinned patients) discoloration of the skin, best seen in the sclera, due to increased bilirubin in the blood	Liver disease, red blood cell hemolysis, pancreatic cancer, common bile duct obstruction
Keloid	Hypertrophied scar beyond wound margins (Fig. 24.6)	Predisposition more common in dark-skinned persons
Lichenification	Thickening of the skin with accentuated normal skin markings	Repeated scratching, rubbing, and irritation usually because of itching or neurosis
Mole (nevus)	Benign overgrowth of melanocytes	Defects of development; excess numbers and large, irregular moles; often familial
Telangiectasia	Visibly dilated, superficial, small blood vessels, often found on face and thighs	Aging, acne, sun exposure, alcohol, liver failure, corticosteroids, radiation, certain systemic diseases, skin tumors
Tenting	Failure of skin to return immediately to normal position after gentle pinching	Aging, dehydration, cachexia
Varicosity	Increased prominence of superficial veins	Interruption of venous return (e.g., from tumor, incompetent valves, inflammation), often found on lower legs with aging
Vitiligo	Complete absence of melanin (pigment) resulting in chalky-white patch (Fig. 24.7)	Autoimmune, familial, thyroid disease

epidermis is thin, and pigmentation is not influenced by sun exposure, such as the lips, mucous membranes, nail beds, and protected areas (e.g., buttocks). Palmar and plantar surfaces are lighter than other skin areas. Color may not be a reliable indicator of systemic conditions (e.g., flushed skin with fever). Cyanosis may be hard to detect because a normal bluish hue occurs in dark-skinned people. Dark skin rarely shows a blanch response, making it harder to identify pressure injuries. Rashes are often harder to see and may have to be palpated. Wrinkling is less apparent.

Persons with dark skin are predisposed to certain skin and hair problems. **Keloid** is an overgrowth of collagenous tissue at

TABLE 24.9 NURSING ASSESSMENT

Assessment Variations in Light- and Dark-Skinned Persons

Light Skin	Dark Skin
Cyanosis	
Grayish blue tone, especially in nail beds, earlobes, lips, mucous membranes, palms, and soles	Ashen or gray color most easily seen in the conjunctiva of the eye, mucous membranes, and nail beds
Ecchymosis	
Dark red, purple, yellow, or green color, depending on age of bruise	Purple to brownish-black. Hard to see unless in an area of light pigmentation
Erythema	
Reddish tone, increased skin temperature may be present from inflammation	Deeper brown or purple skin tone, increased skin temperature may be present from inflammation
Jaundice	
Yellowish color of skin, sclera, fingernails, palms, and oral mucosa	Yellowish green color most obviously seen in sclera of eye (do not confuse with yellow eye pigmentation, which may be seen in patients with dark skin), palms, and soles
Pallor	
Pale skin color that may appear white or ashen; also seen on lips, nail beds, and mucous membranes	Lack of underlying red tone in brown or black skin. In lighter dark-skinned persons, yellowish-brown skin. In darker dark-skinned persons, ashen or gray skin
Petechiae	
Lesions appearing as small, reddish-purple pinpoints, best seen on abdomen and buttocks	Hard to see. May be seen in the buccal mucosa of the mouth or conjunctiva of the eye
Rash	
May be seen and felt with light palpation	Not easily seen. May be felt with light palpation
Scar	
Generally heals, showing narrow scar line	Higher incidence of keloid development, resulting in a thickened, raised scar (Fig. 24.6)

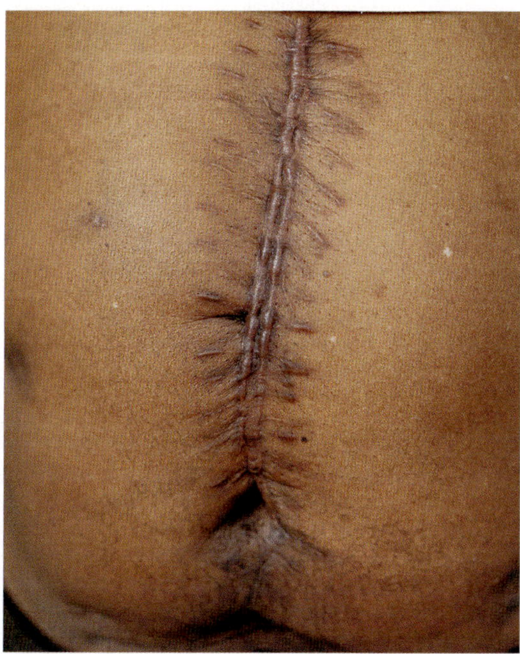

Fig. 24.6 Keloid at a site of former surgery. (© iStock.com/RealPeopleGroup.)

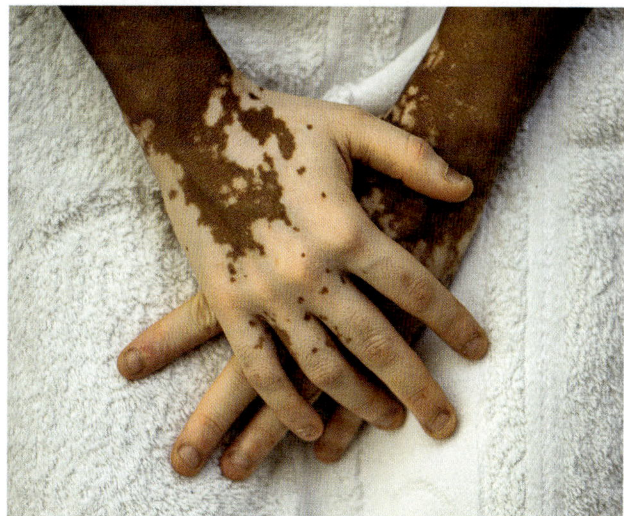

Fig. 24.7 Vitiligo. Total loss of pigment in the affected area. (© Andrea Migliarini/iStock.com.)

the site of a skin injury (e.g., ear piercing) (Fig. 24.6). *Vitiligo* is a total loss of pigment in the affected area (Fig. 24.7). In *dermatosis papulosa nigra,* the person has small, pigmented wart-like papules, often on the face (Fig. 24.8). *Nevus of Ota* is a slate-gray or blue-gray birthmark found on the forehead and face around the eye area. It may involve the sclera. *Traction alopecia* may be the result of trauma from hair rollers or from tight braiding of the hair (Fig. 24.9). The hair loss may be temporary or permanent. *Pseudofolliculitis* occurs when hairs curve back and either reenter or grow under the skin after shaving. This causes an inflammatory response with papules and pustules (Fig. 24.10).

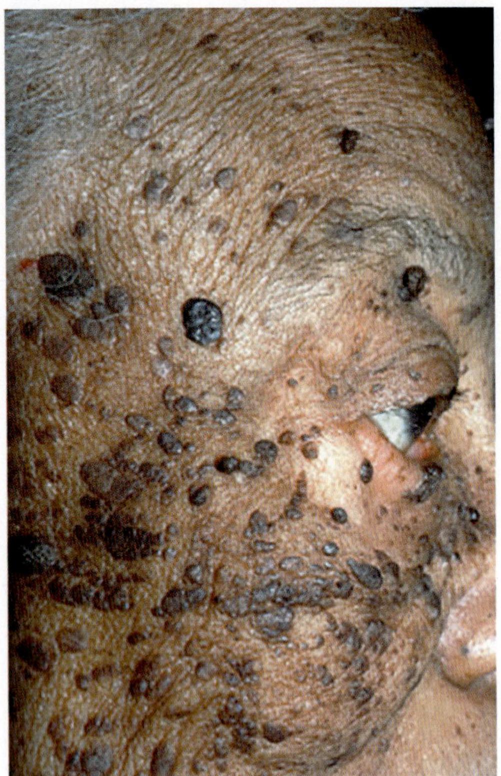

Fig. 24.8 Dermatosis papulosa nigra. Small, pigmented wart-like papules, often on the face. (From James W, Berger T, Elston D: *Andrews' diseases of the skin,* ed 12, Edinburgh, 2016, Elsevier.)

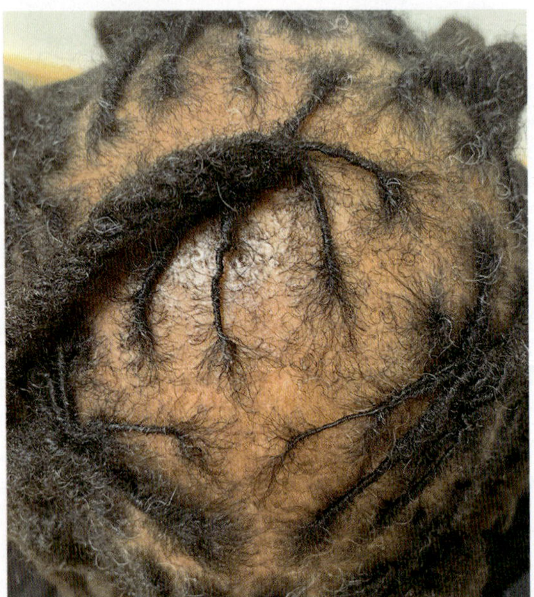

Fig. 24.9 Traction alopecia. (From Micheletti RG, Elson DM, James WD, McMahon PJ: *Andrews' diseases of the skin clinical atlas,* ed 2, St. Louis, 2023, Elsevier.)

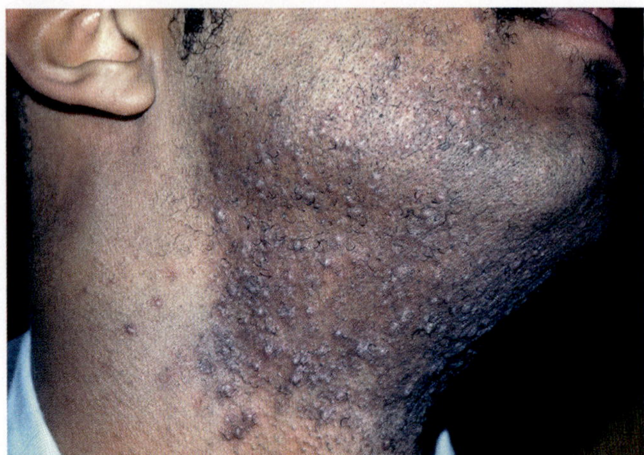

Fig. 24.10 Pseudofolliculitis in the beard area. (From James WD, et al: *Andrews' diseases of the skin,* ed 14, St. Louis, 2026, Elsevier. Courtesy Steven Binnick, MD.)

CASE STUDY

Objective Data: Physical Examination

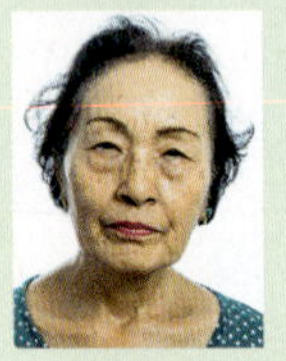

(© andreswd/ iStock.com.)

Physical assessment findings of D.A.'s skin reveal:

- Complexion fair. Wrinkles around eyes, above upper lip, and on sides of cheeks bilaterally. Normal skin temperature and turgor.
- Lesions: on upper right forehead measuring 2 × 3 mm; on left forehead near hairline measuring 1 × 2 mm; and on left lower cheek measuring 2 × 2.5 mm.

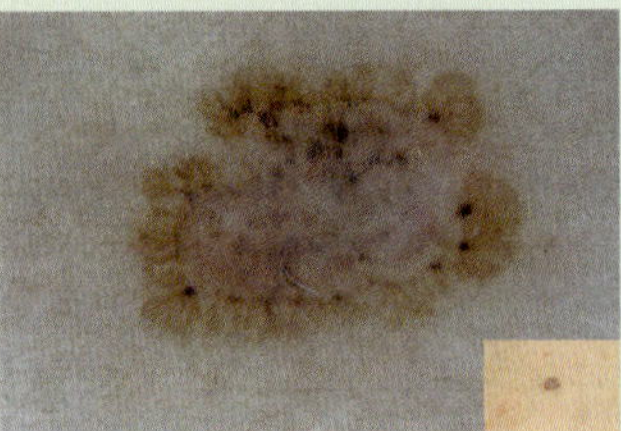

Cheek lesion. (From Peris K, Fargnoli MC, Garbe C, et al: Diagnosis and treatment of basal cell carcinoma, *Eur J Can* 118:10, 2019.)

- The lesions are slightly red and do not blanch with direct pressure. Borders are distinct. The lesions on the forehead have minimal elevation noted on palpation. The lesion on the cheek is slightly elevated.
- No other skin lesions noted.

Discussion Questions

1. Which physical assessment findings concern you most?
2. What diagnostic studies do you think may be ordered for D.A.?

You will learn more about diagnostic studies related to the skin in the next section.

Answers available at http://evolve.elsevier.com/Lewis/medsurg.

DIAGNOSTIC STUDIES OF THE INTEGUMENTARY SYSTEM

Table 24.10 presents common diagnostic studies used for the integumentary system. With *dermatoscopy,* the HCP uses a lighted instrument with optical magnification up to 10 times normal to see skin structures and colors not visible to the naked eye.[8] These devices can help the HCP determine whether a lesion should be biopsied.

Biopsy is a common test used to evaluate a skin lesion. A biopsy is needed when we suspect cancer or the diagnosis is questionable. Techniques include punch, incisional, excisional,

TABLE 24.10 Diagnostic Studies

Integumentary System

Study	Description and Purpose	Nursing Responsibility
Biopsy		
Excisional	Used when good cosmetic results and/or entire lesion removal desired. Skin closed with subcutaneous and skin sutures.	*Before:* Verify consent form is signed (if needed). *During:* Help with site preparation, anesthesia, procedure, and hemostasis. Properly identify specimen. *After:* Apply dressing. Provide discharge teaching
Incisional	Wedge-shaped incision made in lesion too large for excisional biopsy. Done when specimen needed is larger than shave or punch biopsy.	
Punch	Special punch biopsy instrument of appropriate size used. Instrument rotated to appropriate level to include dermis and some fat. Suturing depends on size and site. Provides full-thickness skin for diagnostic purposes.	
Shave	Single-edged razor blade used to shave off superficial lesions or small sample of a large lesion. Provides thin specimen for diagnostic purposes.	
Microscopic Tests		
Culture	Identifies fungi, bacteria, and viruses. For *fungi,* scraping or swab of skin performed. For *bacteria,* material obtained from intact pustules, bullae, or abscesses. For *viruses,* vesicle or bulla and exudate taken from base of lesion.	*Before:* Teach patient the purpose of test. *During:* Properly identify specimen. Follow instructions for storing specimen if not immediately sent to laboratory.
Immunofluorescence studies	Some skin diseases have specific, abnormal antibody proteins that we can identify with fluorescence studies. Can examine both skin tissue and serum.	*Before:* Teach patient the purpose of test. *During:* Help obtain specimen. For punch biopsy, place specimen in special fixative (e.g., Michel's) and not formalin.
Mineral oil slides	Check for infestations by placing scrapings on slide with mineral oil then viewing microscopically.	*Before:* Teach patient the purpose of test. *During:* Prepare slide.
Potassium hydroxide (KOH)	Checks hair, scales, or nails for superficial fungal infection. Put specimen on glass slide and add 10%–20% concentration of KOH.	*Before:* Teach patient the purpose of test. *During:* Prepare slide.
Tzanck test (Wright's and Giemsa's stain)	Fluid and cells from vesicles checked for herpes infections. Specimen put on slide, stained, and examined microscopically.	*Before:* Teach patient the purpose of test. *During:* Use sterile technique for collecting fluid.
Miscellaneous		
Patch test	Assess for allergic dermatitis and photoallergic reactions. Application of allergens to the patient's skin (usually on the back) for 48 h. Test sites examined 48 h later for a reaction, characterized by the presence of erythema, papules, and/or vesicles. May do additional readings beyond 48 h.	*Before:* Teach patient the purpose of test and procedure. *After:* Tell patient to leave patches in place for 48 h. During this time, it is important not to wash the area or play vigorous sports because if the adhesive tape peels off, the process will need to be repeated. Do not expose the patches to sunlight or other sources of UV light.
Wood's lamp (ultraviolet [UV] light)	Examination of skin with long-wave UV light causes specific substances to fluoresce (e.g., *Pseudomonas* organisms, fungal infections, vitiligo).	*Before:* Teach patient the purpose of test and procedure. Tell patient it is not painful. *During:* Darken room.

and shave biopsies. The method used depends on factors such as the site of the biopsy, cosmetic result desired, and type of tissue needed.

Other procedures include stains and cultures for fungal, bacterial, and viral infections. Direct immunofluorescence is a special technique used on biopsy specimens. It may be done in certain conditions such as bullous diseases and systemic lupus erythematosus. Indirect immunofluorescence is done on blood samples.

CASE STUDY

Objective Data: Diagnostic Studies

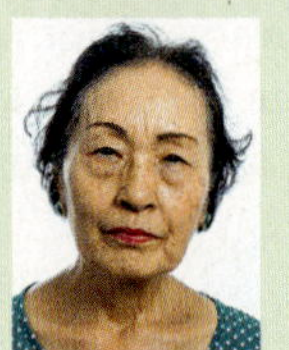

(© andreswd/ iStock.com.)

The HCP examines the lesion via dermatoscopy and uses a Wood's lamp to rule out a fungal infection. The HCP suspects basal cell cancer.

Discussion Questions

1. Are these the diagnostic tests you expected the HCP to perform?
2. What, if any, other diagnostic studies would you expect the HCP to order?
3. What are the interprofessional team's priorities for D.A. at this time?

Answers available at http://evolve.elsevier.com/Lewis/medsurg.

BRIDGE TO NCLEX EXAMINATION

The number of the question corresponds to the same-numbered outcome at the beginning of the chapter.

1. The nurse provides diligent skin care because the primary function of the skin is
   a. insulation.
   b. protection.
   c. sensation.
   d. absorption.
2. Age-related assessment findings of the hair and nails include **(Select all that apply.)**
   a. oily scalp.
   b. scaly scalp.
   c. thinner nails.
   d. thicker, brittle nails.
   e. longitudinal nail ridging.
3. When assessing the nutritional-metabolic pattern in relation to the skin, the nurse asks the patient about
   a. joint pain.
   b. the use of moisturizing shampoo.
   c. recent changes in wound healing.
   d. self-care habits related to daily hygiene.
4. The nurse assessed a patient's skin lesions as firm, edematous, and irregularly shaped with a variable diameter. They would be called
   a. wheals.
   b. papules.
   c. fissures.
   d. plaques.
5. During the physical assessment of a patient's skin, the nurse would
   a. use a flashlight in a poorly lit room.
   b. note cool, moist skin as a normal finding.
   c. pinch up a fold of skin to assess for turgor.
   d. perform a lesion-specific assessment and then a general inspection.
6. Patients with dark skin are more likely to develop
   a. keloids.
   b. wrinkles.
   c. skin rashes.
   d. skin cancer.
7. On inspection of a patient's dark skin, the nurse notes a blue-gray birthmark on the forehead and eye area. This finding is called
   a. vitiligo.
   b. intertrigo.
   c. Nevus of Ota.
   d. telangiectasia.
8. Diagnostic testing is recommended for skin lesions when
   a. a health history cannot be obtained.
   b. a more definitive diagnosis is needed.
   c. percussion reveals an abnormal finding.
   d. treatment with prescribed medication has failed.

1. b; 2. b, d, e; 3. c; 4. a; 5. c; 6. a; 7. c; 8. b.

For rationales to these answers and even more NCLEX review questions, visit http://evolve.elsevier.com/Lewis/medsurg.

REFERENCES

To access the References for this chapter, please scan the QR code with a mobile device.

25

Integumentary Problems

Mary M. Cameron

http://evolve.elsevier.com/Lewis/medsurg/

CONCEPTUAL FOCUS

Cellular Regulation
Coping
Infection
Pain
Self-image
Tissue Integrity

LEARNING OUTCOMES

1. Outline practices to promote skin health.
2. Explain the etiology, clinical manifestations, and interprofessional and nursing management of skin cancers.
3. Relate the etiology, clinical manifestations, and interprofessional and nursing management of skin infections.
4. Describe the prevention and interprofessional and nursing management of infestations and insect bites.
5. Discuss the etiology, clinical manifestations, and interprofessional and nursing management of allergic skin problems.
6. Explain the etiology, clinical manifestations, and interprofessional and nursing management related to benign skin problems.
7. Select nursing interventions to manage patients with a skin problem.
8. Explain the indications and nursing management related to common cosmetic procedures and skin grafts.

KEY TERMS

acne vulgaris, Table 25.10
actinic keratosis (AK)
basal cell carcinoma (BCC)
cellulitis, Table 25.5
cryosurgery
curettage
dysplastic nevi (DN)
herpes zoster, Table 25.6
impetigo, Table 25.5
lichenification
melanoma
psoriasis
rosacea, Table 25.10
squamous cell carcinoma (SCC)
sun protection factor (SPF)

This chapter discusses common skin problems and skin cancer. Impaired skin integrity affects many body functions. The skin reflects physical and psychologic well-being. Many skin problems leave underlying tissues unprotected from infection and chemical dangers. Lesions can be painful because the skin has many sensory nerve endings. Skin problems are often highly visible, potentially affecting body image and causing distress.

PROMOTING SKIN HEALTH

Sun exposure comes with serious risk and results in permanent skin damage. Sunlight is made up of visible light and ultraviolet (UV) light. There are 2 types of UV light: UVA and UVB. Each has different effects on the skin (Table 25.1). UVA light is responsible for tanning, and UVB for sunburn. The damage caused by UV rays is cumulative. It results in degenerative changes in the dermis and premature aging (e.g., loss of elasticity, thinning, wrinkling). Prolonged and repeated sun exposure increases risk for actinic keratosis (AK), basal and squamous cell cancers, and melanoma.

People often do not understand the risks of sun exposure. Following sun safety guidelines beginning early in life can help avoid the damaging effects of the sun and prevent skin cancer. People with fair skin or light-colored eyes should be cautious

TABLE 25.1 Effects of Ultraviolet Light on Skin

Wavelength	Effect
Ultraviolet A (UVA)	Can cause elastic tissue damage and actinic skin damage Contributes to skin cancer
Ultraviolet B (UVB)	Causes sunburn and cumulative effect of sun damage Major factor in developing skin cancer

about sun exposure. They have less melanin and thus less natural protection.

Provide teaching on sun protection. This includes wearing protective clothing, including sunglasses, a large-brimmed hat, and a darker colored, long-sleeved shirt of a tightly woven fabric or carrying an umbrella. The greatest risk is with midday sun, between the hours of 10:00 a.m. and 2:00 p.m., regardless of the latitude. This is when 80% of UV rays occur. Even on overcast days, serious sunburn can occur because up to 80% of the sun's UV rays can penetrate the clouds. Warn people of the dangers of tanning booths and sun lamps, which emit UVA. Tanning booths increase the risk for sunburn, cataracts, and skin cancer.[1]

Sunscreens can filter UVA and UVB light. The 2 types of topical sunscreens are chemical and physical. Chemical sunscreens absorb into the skin. There they absorb or filter UV light, resulting in decreased UV light penetration. Physical sunscreens sit on top of the skin. They reflect UV light away from the skin. Regular sunscreen use decreases the risk for skin cancer.

The U.S. Food and Drug Administration (FDA) rates sunscreen products on their **sun protection factor (SPF)**. The SPF measures the effectiveness of a sunscreen in filtering and absorbing UV light. All sunscreen labels in the United States must say which rays they protect against. Products labeled with "broad spectrum" block UVA and UVB.[2] Sunscreens with broad-spectrum labeling must have an SPF of at least 15. Sunscreens with an SPF of 15 or more filter 92% of the UVB rays. They make sunburn unlikely when applied correctly.

People need to select the right sunscreen for their needs. The general suggestion is that everyone should use daily sunscreen with a minimum SPF of 15. Teach patients to look for the term *broad spectrum* on sunscreen packaging. People with a history of skin cancer or problems with sun sensitivity should use a product with an SPF of at least 30. Sunscreens should be applied 20 to 30 minutes before going outdoors, even in cloudy weather. The SPF value of all sunscreens decreases with time. Sunscreen should be reapplied every 2 hours. You should apply 1 ounce per total body application. The ears, toes, and lips also need sunscreen. Sunscreens are not "waterproof" and must be reapplied after swimming.

Some drugs potentiate the sun's effects, even with brief exposure. The chemicals in these drugs absorb light when exposed to natural sunlight and release energy that harms cells and tissues. Common photosensitizing drugs are shown in Table 25.2. The manifestations of drug-induced photosensitivity (Fig. 25.1) are like those of a sunburn. These include swelling, redness, vesicles, and papular, plaquelike lesions. Assess the photosensitivity of each drug. Teach patients who are taking these drugs about their photosensitizing effect and the need to protect the skin from photosensitivity reactions by using sunscreen products.

TABLE 25.2 Drug Therapy

Drugs That May Cause Photosensitivity

Categories	Examples
Antidepressants	fluoxetine, paroxetine, venlafaxine
Antidysrhythmics	amiodarone, quinidine
Antihistamines	cetirizine, chlorpheniramine, clemastine, diphenhydramine, loratadine
Antimicrobials	tetracycline, azithromycin, ciprofloxacin, sulfonamides
Antifungals	griseofulvin, ketoconazole
Antipsychotics	chlorpromazine, haloperidol
Diuretics	furosemide, thiazides
NSAIDs	diclofenac, ibuprofen, naproxen, piroxicam
Statins	atorvastatin, simvastatin

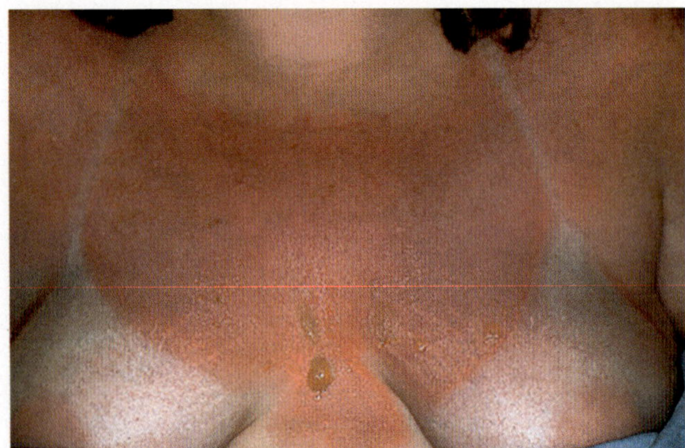

Fig. 25.1 Photosensitivity reaction in a patient taking methotrexate. (From Valeyrie-Allanore L, Obeid O, Revuz J: *Dermatology,* ed 4, St. Louis, 2018, Elsevier.)

Teach patients to assess their skin monthly. They should have a periodic professional assessment of areas that are hard to see. The cornerstone of skin assessment is the ABCDE rule. Assess lesions for ***A****symmetry,* ***B****order* irregularity, ***C****olor* change and variation, ***D****iameter* of 6 mm or more, and ***E****volving* in appearance (Fig. 25.2). Emphasize that a persistent lesion that does not heal and lesions once flat and now raised, once small and recently growing, or changing in appearance are warning signs. Patients should consult their HCP at once if any lesions or moles show any clinical signs (ABCDEs).

SKIN CANCER

Etiology

Skin cancer is the most diagnosed cancer.[3] Skin cancers are either nonmelanoma or melanoma. The fact that skin lesions

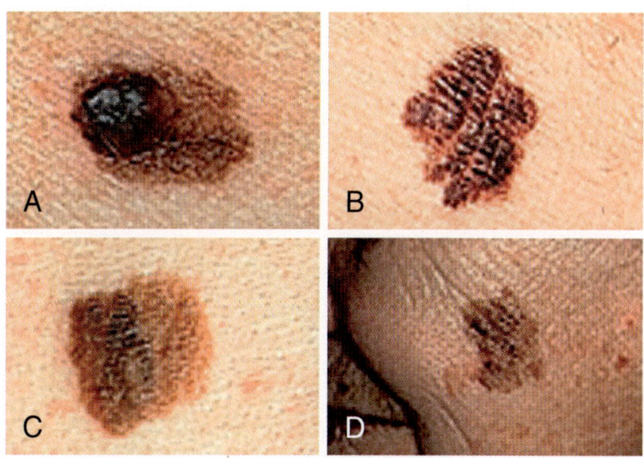

Fig. 25.2 The ABCDEs of melanoma. (A) Asymmetry: one half unlike the other half. (B) Border irregularity: edges are ragged, notched, or blurred. (C) Color: varied pigmentation; shades of tan, brown, and black. (D) Diameter: greater than 6 mm (diameter of a pencil eraser). (E, *not pictured*) Evolving; changing appearance (change in shape, size, color, or other characteristic noted over time). (From The Skin Cancer Foundation, New York, NY.)

are so visible increases the chance of early detection and diagnosis. This often leads to a highly favorable prognosis.

Risk factors for skin cancer include (1) having fair skin and blond or red hair with blue eye color, (2) history of outdoor sunbathing, (3) living near the equator or at high altitudes, (4) family or personal history of skin cancer, (5) having an outdoor occupation, (6) spending a lot of time in outdoor recreation activities, and (7) indoor tanning.[3] The Fitzpatrick Classification of Skin Type can help you determine a person's skin complexion and their risk for skin cancer (Table 25.3). Treatment with oral methoxsalen (psoralen) or psoralen plus UV A radiation (PUVA) increases risk. Persons with dark skin are less susceptible to skin cancer. Their increased melanin is protective. However, there is still a risk, and they need to wear sunscreen.

NONMELANOMA SKIN CANCER

Nonmelanoma skin cancers (basal and squamous cell cancers) are the most common forms of skin cancer. More than 5.4 million new cases are diagnosed each year.[3] Nonmelanoma skin cancers do not develop from melanocytes. They develop in the basement membrane of the skin. Although there are few deaths from nonmelanoma skin cancer, they have the potential for severe local destruction, disfigurement, and disability.

The most common causative factor for nonmelanoma skin cancers is sun exposure. They usually develop in sun-exposed areas, such as the face, head, neck, back of the hands, and arms. There are some differences between basal and squamous cell cancers. Squamous cell cancers usually occur on the head and neck, where there is the highest degree of UV exposure. Basal cell cancers may occur in sun-protected areas.

Actinic Keratosis

Actinic keratosis (AK), or *solar keratosis,* is the most common precancerous skin lesion. They affect most of the older White people. Sun exposure is a key factor. AKs appear most often on skin that has been exposed to the sun or to artificial UV light. They may spontaneously resolve if a person reduces exposure to sunlight.

The clinical appearance of AK can be highly varied. The typical lesion is an irregularly shaped, flat, slightly red papule with indistinct borders and an overlying hard, keratotic scale or horn (Table 25.4). Because AK is impossible to distinguish from squamous cell cancer, treatment should be aggressive. Nonsurgical procedures are the first-line treatment. Any lesion that persists should be evaluated for a biopsy.

Basal Cell Carcinoma

Basal cell carcinoma (BCC) is a locally invasive cancer arising from epidermal basal cells. It is the most common type of skin cancer but the least deadly. BCC usually occurs in middle-aged to older adults. Most occur in the head and neck area (e.g., sun-exposed), followed by the trunk and extremities.[4]

Some BCCs are pigmented, with curled borders and an opaque appearance (Fig. 25.3). They may be hard to distinguish from melanoma. A tissue biopsy is needed to confirm the diagnosis. BCCs rarely metastasize. However, untreated BCC may result in massive tissue destruction. Treatment depends on the location and histologic type, size, history of recurrence, and patient (Table 25.4).

Squamous Cell Carcinoma

Squamous cell carcinoma (SCC) is a cancer arising from keratinizing epidermal cells. SCC can be aggressive and has the potential to metastasize. It may lead to death if not treated early. SCC often occurs at the base of an AK or another lesion. The main risk factors are sun exposure and immunosuppression

TABLE 25.3 Fitzpatrick Classification of Skin Type

Skin Type	Skin Color	Characteristics
I	White, freckles, very fair. Red or blond hair. Blue eyes.	Always burns, never tans
II	White, fair. Red or blond hair. Blue, hazel, or green eyes.	Usually burns, tans with difficulty
III	Cream white, fair. Any eye or hair color.	Sometimes mild burn, gradually tan
IV	Brown, typical Mediterranean skin.	Rarely burns, tans with ease
V	Deep brown, Middle Eastern skin types.	Very rarely burns, tans very easily
VI	Black.	Never burns, tans very easily

TABLE 25.4 Premalignant and Malignant Skin Problems

Etiology and Pathophysiology	Clinical Manifestations	Treatment
Actinic Keratosis		
• Actinic (sun) damage • Premalignant skin lesions • Common in older White individuals • Increase in number with age	• Flat or elevated, dry, hyperkeratotic scaly papule. Often multiple • May be rough or wartlike • Rough adherent scale on red base, which returns when removed • Often on sun-exposed area	• Excision (cryosurgery, laser, chemical peel). Topical fluorouracil, imiquimod, ingenol mebutate. Photodynamic therapy • Recurrence possible even with adequate treatment
Atypical or Dysplastic Nevi (Moles)		
• Morphologically between common acquired nevi and melanoma • May be precursor of melanoma	• Often >5 mm. Irregular border, possibly notched. Frequently multiple • Varying colors of tan, brown, black, red, or pink within single mole • Central part often raised with flat edges • Most common on back, possible in uncommon mole sites such as scalp or buttocks	• Careful monitoring of those with a familial tendency to melanoma or dysplastic nevi • Excisional biopsy for suspicious lesions
Basal Cell Carcinoma		
• Change in epidermal basal cells • No maturation or normal keratinization • Related to sun exposure, skin type, x-ray radiation, scars, some types of nevi • Slow-growing tumor that invades local tissue • Metastasis rare, 90% cure rate with primary lesions	• Small, slowly enlarging papule • Borders semitranslucent or "pearly" with overlying telangiectasia • Erosion, ulceration, and depression of center • Normal skin markings lost (Fig. 25.3)	• Surgical excision, electrodessication and curettage, cryosurgery, radiation therapy, laser therapy, photodynamic therapy • Vismodegib (Erivedge), sonidegib (Odomzo) for metastatic or recurrent locally invasive lesions • Fluorouracil, imiquimod for superficial lesions
Cutaneous T-Cell Lymphoma		
• Origins in skin. Local chronic, slowly progressing disease • Possibly related to environment toxins and chemical exposure • Mycosis fungoides (MF) is most common form • Sézary syndrome is an advanced form of MF • Prevalence twice as high in males	• Classic presentation involves 3 stages: patch (early), plaque, and tumor (advanced) • History of persistent macules followed by gradual appearance of indurated red plaques on trunk • Appears similar to psoriasis • Itching, lymphadenopathy	• Treatment usually controls symptoms but is not curative • Phototherapy, radiation therapy, extracorporeal photopheresis, chemotherapy, biologic therapy (interferon) • Medications include corticosteroids, topical nitrogen mustard, imiquimod, retinoids, romidepsin (Istodax), denileukin diftitox (Ontak), vorinostat (Zolinza)
Melanoma		
• Neoplastic growth of melanocytes anywhere on skin, eyes, or mucous membranes • Classified by major histologic mode of spread • Correlation between survival rate and depth of invasion • Poor prognosis unless diagnosed and treated early • Spreading by local extension, regional lymphatic vessels, and bloodstream	• Irregular color, surface, and border • Variegated color, including red, white, blue, black, gray, brown • Flat or elevated. Eroded or ulcerated • Often <1 cm in size • Most common sites in males are back, then chest. In females are legs, then back (Fig. 25.2)	• Surgical excision and possible sentinel lymph node biopsy • Adjuvant therapy after surgery if lesion >1.5 mm in depth • Key adjuvant therapies include immunotherapy (cytokines, PD-1 inhibitors, CTLA-4 inhibitors), targeted therapy (BRAF and MEK inhibitors)
Squamous Cell Carcinoma (SCC)		
• Cancer of squamous cell of epidermis. Invades dermis, surrounding skin • Often occurs on previously damaged skin (e.g., from sun, radiation, scar) • High cure rate with early detection and treatment	• *Superficial:* Thin, scaly, red plaque without invasion into the dermis (Fig. 25.4) • *Early:* Firm nodules with indistinct borders, scaling, ulceration • *Late:* Covering of lesion with scale or horn from keratinization, ulceration	• Surgery, cryosurgery, radiation therapy, electrosurgery, laser therapy, photodynamic therapy • Untreated lesion may metastasize to regional lymph nodes and distant organs • Fluorouracil, imiquimod for noninvasive SCC • Immunotherapy for metastatic lesions

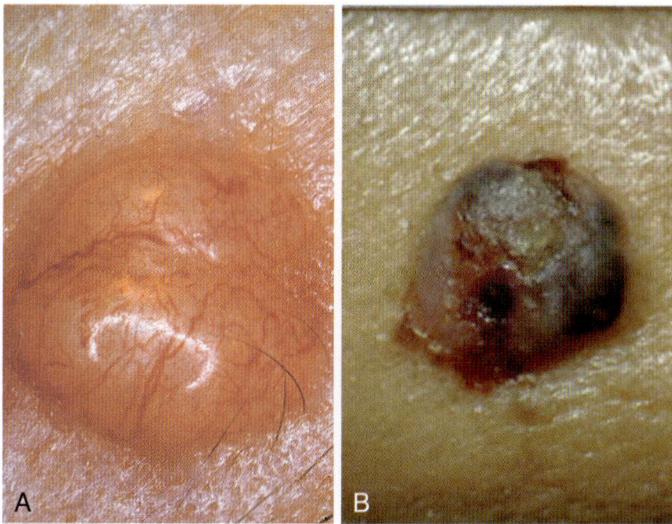

Fig. 25.3 Basal cell carcinoma. (A) On light skin, the lesion typically appears as a smooth-surfaced, pearly papule with telangiectatic vessels. (B) On dark skin, the lesion often appears hyperpigmented. (From Aster JC, Deyrup AT, Das A, et al: *Robbins & Kumar basic pathology,* ed 11, St Louis, 2023, Elsevier.)

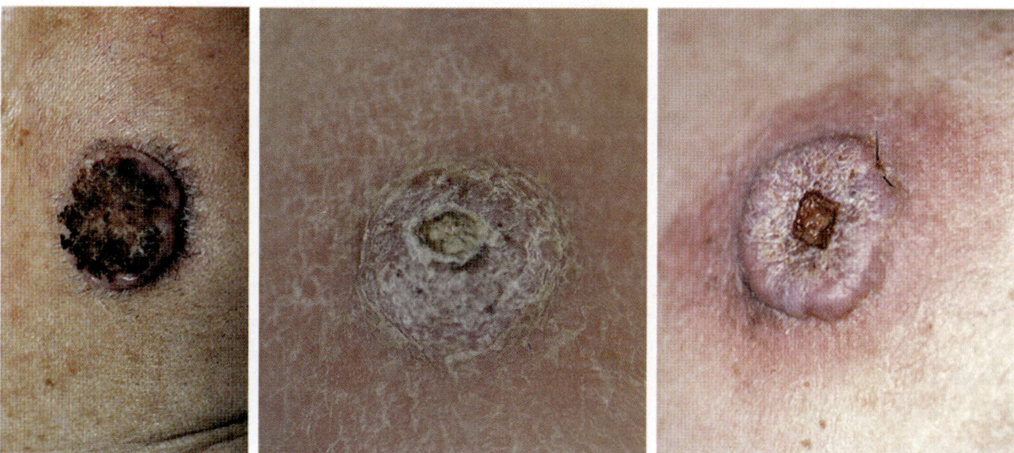

Fig. 25.4 Varying appearances of squamous cell carcinoma. (From Cameron JL, Cameron AM: *Current surgical therapy,* ed 13, St Louis, 2020, Elsevier.)

after an organ transplant.[5] Pipe, cigar, and cigarette smoking contribute to SCC on the mouth and lips. The appearance varies (Fig. 25.4). A biopsy should always be done when a lesion is thought to be SCC. Treatment depends on the location and histologic type, size, history of recurrence, and patient (Table 25.4).

MELANOMA

Melanoma is a tumor arising from melanocytes, the cells that make melanin. It causes most skin cancer deaths. The incidence of melanoma is steadily rising.[1] More than 107,000 new cases are diagnosed each year in the United States, and almost 8000 people die of the disease.[6] Melanoma can metastasize to any organ, including the brain and heart.

A combination of environment and genetic factors is likely involved in developing melanoma. UV light from the sun is the main cause. Artificial sources of UV light, such as sunlamps and tanning booths, also play a role. UV light damages the skin cells, causing "misspellings" (mutations) in their genetic code. This alters the cells. The risk for melanoma is greatest for people who have red or blond hair, blue or light-colored eyes, and light-colored skin that freckles easily. These people have less melanin and thus less protection from UV light. The use of immunosuppressive drugs and a history of dysplastic nevi (DN) increase risk.

A person may have a genetic predisposition toward getting melanoma. Of those with melanoma, 5% to 10% have a first-degree relative (e.g., parent, full sibling) who had melanoma.[1] This risk greatly increases if multiple relatives had melanoma. Mutated genes have been found in some families with a high incidence of melanoma.

Cutaneous melanoma begins in the skin. There are 4 major subtypes: (1) superficial spreading, (2) nodular, (3) lentigo maligna, and (4) acral lentiginous. Ocular melanoma and mucosal melanoma are types of noncutaneous melanoma. They develop in the eye and mucosal linings of the body (such as the mouth or inside the nose), respectively.

Clinical Manifestations

Melanoma often occurs on the lower legs in females and on the trunk and head in males. About 25% occur in existing nevi or moles. About 20% occur in DN. Rarely, it occurs in the mouth, intestines, and eyes. Persons with dark skin often have melanomas on areas with less melanin, such as the palms, soles, mucous membranes, and under the nails.

The cornerstone of skin assessment is the ABCDE rule (Fig. 25.2). Because most melanoma cells continue to make melanin, melanoma tumors are often deep brown or black (Table 25.4). Lesions showing any sudden or progressive change in the ABCDE rule need to be evaluated. Because it is common for people with dark skin to have pigmented, longitudinal bands on their nails, assess for nail discoloration.

Interprofessional Care

One of the first steps in diagnosing a suspicious lesion is dermoscopic examination. Dermoscopy can help the HCP decide if a lesion should be biopsied. Biopsy can determine the type of lesion. A biopsy should be done using an excisional technique. Shave biopsy, shave excision, or electrocauterization are avoided because they do not measure the depth of the lesion.

The most important prognostic factor is tumor thickness at the time of diagnosis. We assess tumor thickness with the *Breslow measurement.* It indicates tumor depth in millimeters. Melanomas less than 1 mm thick have a small chance of spreading. As the melanoma becomes thicker, it has a greater chance of spreading.

Treatment depends on the site of the original tumor and the stage of the cancer. Melanoma staging (stages 0 to IV) is based on tumor size (thickness), node involvement, and metastasis. In stage 0, melanoma is confined to 1 place (in situ) in the epidermis. Melanoma is nearly 100% curable by excision if diagnosed at stage 0. Unfortunately, those with deep tumors or disease that has already spread to lymph nodes often develop metastases. The 5-year survival rate for those with advanced disease is around 27%.[6]

The initial treatment of melanoma is wide surgical excision. Melanoma that has spread to the lymph nodes or nearby sites usually requires additional therapy with combinations of immunotherapy, targeted therapy, chemotherapy, and/or radiation therapy.

Immunotherapy can include cytokines (α-interferon, interleukin-2), PD-1 inhibitors, and CTLA-4 inhibitors. Cytokines enhance the production of many immune system cells, including T cells and B cells. Drugs that block PD-1 or CTLA-4 boost the immune response against melanoma cells.[7] Anti–PD-1 agents include nivolumab (Opdivo) and pembrolizumab (Keytruda). They block PD-1, a protein on T cells that keeps T cells from attacking other cells in the body. Atezolizumab (Tecentriq) targets PD-L1, a protein related to PD-1 that is found on some tumor cells. Ipilimumab (Yervoy) blocks the action of CTLA-4, another protein that normally suppresses the action of T cells.

Targeted therapy for melanoma includes BRAF and MEK inhibitors. About half of melanomas have *BRAF* gene mutations, which make an altered BRAF protein that signals melanoma cells to proliferate. Vemurafenib (Zelboraf), dabrafenib (Tafinlar), and encorafenib (Braftovi) directly target *BRAF* genes. The *MEK* gene works with the *BRAF* gene, so drugs that block MEK proteins also help treat melanomas with *BRAF* gene changes. MEK inhibitors include trametinib (Mekinist), binimetinib (Mektovi), and cobimetinib (Cotellic).[6,7]

Chemotherapy is usually used only with advanced disease. Drugs used include dacarbazine and temozolomide.[6] Radiation therapy has a role in treating lymph node and brain metastases.

Atypical or Dysplastic Nevus

Dysplastic nevi (DN), or atypical moles, are nevi that are larger than usual (greater than 5 mm across) with irregular borders and various shades of color. DN may have the same ABCDE characteristics as melanoma, but they are less pronounced. About 5% to 17% of White persons have DN.[8] Those with DN have an increased risk for developing melanoma in a mole or elsewhere on the body. The more DN a person has, the higher the risk. Those with 10 or more DN have 12 times the risk for developing melanoma.

CHECK YOUR PRACTICE

You are working in an HCP office, and your next patient is a 64-year-old White male. He is worried about the many "brown" spots on his face and arms. He tells you that he worked outside in construction most of his life.

- How would you approach assessing the patient's skin?

SKIN INFECTIONS

Bacterial

Bacterial infection can occur as a primary infection after a break in the skin. A secondary infection can occur in already damaged skin or as a sign of a systemic disease (Table 25.5). Risk factors include the presence of excess moisture, obesity, having atopic dermatitis, systemic corticosteroid or antibiotic use, and having a chronic disease such as diabetes.

Staphylococcus aureus and group A β-hemolytic streptococci are the main types of bacteria that cause primary and secondary skin infections. Streptococci cause impetigo, erysipelas, cellulitis, and lymphangitis. *S. aureus* causes impetigo, folliculitis, cellulitis, and furuncles (Fig. 25.5). When an infection is present, the resulting drainage is infectious. Good skin hygiene and infection control practices help prevent the spread of the infection.

TABLE 25.5 Common Bacterial Skin Infections

Etiology and Pathophysiology	Clinical Manifestations	Treatment and Prognosis
Carbuncle		
• Multiple, interconnecting furuncles	• Many pustules appearing in reddened area • Most common at nape of neck	• Incision and drainage (possibly with packing), antibiotics, meticulous care of involved skin, frequent application of warm, moist compresses • Heal slowly with scar formation
Cellulitis		
• Deep inflammation of subcutaneous tissue from enzymes produced by bacteria • May be a primary infection or secondary complication • Often occurs after break in skin • *Staphylococcus aureus* and streptococci usual causative agents	• Hot, tender, red, edematous area with diffuse borders • Chills, malaise, fever (Fig. 25.5) • Progression to gangrene possible if untreated	*Topical:* • Moist heat, immobilization, and elevation *Systemic:* • Systemic antibiotic therapy • Hospitalization if severe for IV antibiotic therapy based on culture and sensitivity
Erysipelas		
• Superficial cellulitis mainly involving the dermis • Group A β-hemolytic streptococci	• Red, hot, sharply demarcated plaque, indurated, painful • Bacteremia possible • Most common on face and extremities • Toxic signs: fever, ↑ WBC count, headache, malaise	• Systemic antibiotics, usually penicillin • Hospitalization often needed
Folliculitis		
• Usually staphylococci • Present in areas subjected to friction, moisture, rubbing, oil • Increased risk in patients with diabetes	• Small pustule at hair follicle opening with minimal redness • Crusting, tender to touch • Most common on scalp, beard, extremities in males	• Topical antibiotics (e.g., mupirocin) • Cleanse with chlorhexidine • Warm saline compresses • Usually heals without scarring • If lesions extensive and deep, possible scarring, loss of involved hair follicles, and treatment with systemic antibiotics
Furuncle		
• Deep infection with staphylococci around hair follicle • Often occurs with severe acne or seborrheic dermatitis	• Tender, red, painful area around hair follicle • Draining pus and core of necrotic debris on rupture • Most common on face, back of neck, axillae, breasts, buttocks, perineum, thighs	• Same as for carbuncles
Furunculosis		
• Increased risk in patients who are obese, diabetic, chronically ill, regularly exposed to moisture, pressure	• Lesions as noted earlier • Malaise, regional adenopathy, fever	*Topical:* • Incision and drainage • Warm, moist compresses • Measures to reduce surface staphylococci include antimicrobial cream to nares, armpits, groin and antiseptic to entire skin • Meticulous personal hygiene *Systemic:* • Systemic antibiotic effective against MRSA pending culture and sensitivity results • Often recurrent with scarring
Impetigo		
• Streptococci, staphylococci, or a combination • Primary or secondary infection • Contagious	• Vesiculopustular lesions that develop thick, honey-colored crust surrounded by redness • Itches • Most common on face as primary infection	*Topical:* • Wound care with warm saline or aluminum acetate soaks followed by soap-and-water removal of crusts • Topical antibiotic cream or ointment (mupirocin, retapamulin) • Good personal hygiene *Systemic:* • Systemic antibiotics (e.g., cephalexin, doxycycline, dicloxacillin, clindamycin) for widespread infections or systemic manifestations

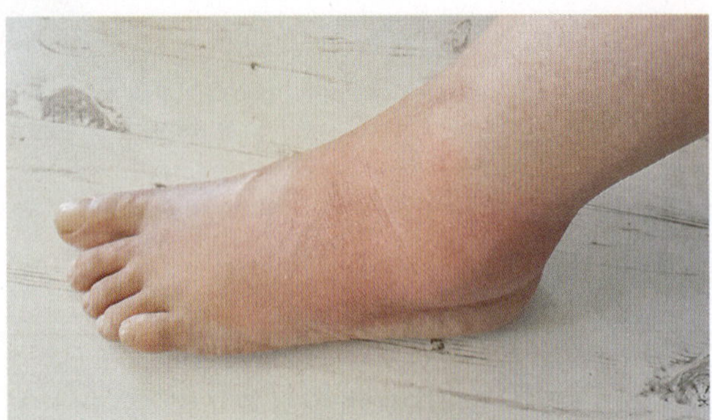

Fig. 25.5 Cellulitis with redness, blistering, and edema. (Suzana Dreno/iStock.com.)

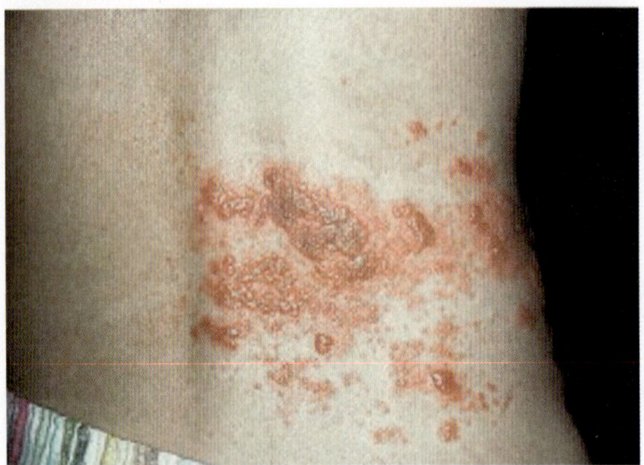

Fig. 25.6 Herpes zoster (shingles) involving the lumbar dermatome. (From Elsevier Point of Care, 2020, Elsevier.)

Viral

A skin lesion may develop when a virus infects a cell or from an inflammatory response to viral infections. Herpes simplex, herpes zoster (Fig. 25.6), and warts are the most common viral skin infections (Table 25.6). Many viral skin infections are hard to treat.

Fungal

Because of the large number of fungi in our environment, exposure to pathologic strains may occur. Skin, hair, and nails can become infected with fungi, including candidiasis and tinea unguium. Common skin fungal infections are described in Table 25.7. Most infections are harmless in healthy adults, but they can cause embarrassment and distress.

Fungal infections are easy to diagnose. A microscopic examination showing the appearance of hyphae (threadlike structures) in a skin scraping mounted in 10% to 20% potassium hydroxide (KOH) indicates a fungal infection. A Wood light examination of hair infected with certain fungi will fluoresce blue to green.

Infestations and Bites

There are many opportunities for exposure to *infestations* (harboring insects or worms) and bites (Table 25.8). In many instances, an allergy to the venom plays a key role in the reaction. In other cases, the manifestations are a reaction to the eggs, feces, or body parts of the invading organism. Some people react with severe hypersensitivity (anaphylaxis), which can be life threatening (see Chapter 14). Blood-feeding insects, such as mosquitos, fleas, and ticks, can transmit infection. Diseases include malaria, Lyme disease, and West Nile virus.

Preventing insect bites by avoiding them or using repellents is somewhat effective. Meticulous hygiene related to care of personal articles, clothing, bedding, and pets can reduce the risk of infestations. Prompt, routine skin inspection is necessary in areas where there is a risk for tick bites.

ALLERGIC SKIN PROBLEMS

Patients often seek treatment for irritant or allergic contact dermatitis, 2 common types of contact dermatitis. *Irritant contact dermatitis* results from direct chemical injury to the skin. *Allergic contact dermatitis* is an antigen-specific, type IV delayed hypersensitivity response. Contact dermatitis is discussed in Chapter 14. Skin problems from allergies and hypersensitivity reactions can be challenging (Table 25.9). A careful history and discussion of exposure to possible offending agents can provide valuable data. Patch testing can help determine possible causative agents. The best treatment of allergic dermatitis is to avoid known irritants. The extreme itching and its potential for chronicity make it a frustrating problem for you and the patient, especially if we cannot find the offending agent.

Skin Drug Reactions

Stevens-Johnson syndrome (SJS) and *toxic epidermal necrolysis* (TEN) are rare, life-threatening diseases. They are violent immune responses that often occur as a severe adverse reaction to either a drug or, more rarely, an infection. The result is the acute destruction of the epithelium of the skin and mucous membranes. SJS, SJS-TEN overlap, and TEN represent a spectrum of disease severity. SJS involves less than 10% of total body surface area, SJS-TEN overlap involves 10% to 29%, and TEN involves more than 30% of total body surface area.[9]

SJS and TEN typically occur 4 to 21 days after starting use of the offending drug. Systemic symptoms, including fever, cough, headache, anorexia, myalgia, and nausea, precede skin and mucous membrane findings by 1 to 3 days. Skin involvement starts as a red, macular rash with purpuric centers. Over a period of hours to days, the rash merges to form blisters with sheetlike epidermal detachment (Fig. 25.7). The lesions usually start on the palms, soles, and trunk, then spread to the face and extremities. They are very painful. Most people have mucosal lesions in the eye, mouth, and genital areas.

Identifying and stopping the offending drug(s) is the most important action in caring for patients with SJS/TEN. Common drugs involved include sulfonamides, fluoroquinolones, NSAIDs, allopurinol, antiseizure drugs, and antiretroviral

TABLE 25.6 Common Viral Skin Infections

Etiology and Pathophysiology	Clinical Manifestations	Treatment and Prognosis
Herpes Simplex Virus (HSV) Types 1 and 2		
• Oral or genital HSV infections serotyped as HSV-1 or HSV-2 • Recurrent, lifelong viral infections • Worsened by sunlight, trauma, menses, stress, systemic infection • Contagious to those not previously infected • Transmitted by respiratory droplets or virus-containing fluid (e.g., saliva, cervical secretions) • Infection in one area readily transmitted to another site by contact	*First episode:* • Symptoms occurring 2 days to 2 weeks after contact • Painful local reaction • Single or grouped vesicles on reddened base • Systemic symptoms (e.g., fever, malaise) possible or no symptoms possible *Recurrent:* • Recurrence in similar spot • Characteristic grouped vesicles on reddened base	• Symptomatic • Soothing, moist compresses; petroleum jelly to lesions • Scarring not usual result • Antiviral agents such as acyclovir (Zovirax), famciclovir, valacyclovir (Valtrex)
Herpes Zoster (Shingles)		
• Activation of varicella-zoster virus • Incidence increases with age • Potentially contagious to anyone who has not had varicella or who is immunosuppressed	• Linear distribution along a dermatome of grouped vesicles and pustules on reddened base (Fig. 25.6) • Usually unilateral on trunk, face, and lumbosacral areas • Burning, pain, and neuralgia preceding outbreak • Mild to severe pain during outbreak	*Topical:* • Wet compresses, silver sulfadiazine (Silvadene) to ruptured vesicles *Systemic:* • Antiviral agents (e.g., acyclovir, famciclovir, valacyclovir) within 72 h of onset to prevent postherpetic neuralgia • Analgesia, mild sedation at bedtime • Gabapentin to treat postherpetic neuralgia • Usually heals without complications, but scarring and postherpetic neuralgia possible • Vaccine (Zostavax) to prevent shingles; one-time dose for adults $\geq$50 yr
Plantar Warts		
• Caused by human papillomavirus (HPV)	• Wart on bottom surface of foot, growing inward because of pressure of walking or standing • Painful when pressure applied • Interrupted skin markings • Cone shaped with black dots (thrombosed vessels) when wart removed	• Topical immunotherapy (imiquimod), cryosurgery • Salicylic acid, cryotherapy, duct tape
Verruca Vulgaris		
• Caused by HPV • May disappear spontaneously in 1 to 2 yr • Mildly contagious by autoinoculation • Specific response depends on area affected • Prevalence greater in youth and immunosuppressed	• Circumscribed, hypertrophic, flesh-colored papule limited to epidermis • Painful on lateral compression	• Surgical dissection • Liquid nitrogen therapy • Blistering agent (cantharidin) • Keratolytic agent (salicylic acid) • CO_2 laser destruction

drugs. Immunotherapy may play a role in slowing disease progression and promoting skin repair.

Patients receive supportive care, often in an intensive care unit. Interventions focus on airway management, preserving kidney function, maintaining fluid and electrolyte balance, and pain control. Fluid replacement is given to maintain urine output. Proper wound care helps prevent infection and promote healing. Dressing with petrolatum gauze or other nonadhesive material provides a barrier and offers moisture to help the skin repair. Because of painful oral lesions, most patients need parenteral or enteral nutrition to meet nutrient needs. Apply eyedrops, lubricating ointment, and antibiotic drops to those with conjunctivitis.

BENIGN SKIN PROBLEMS

The list of benign skin problems is long. Some of the most common and distressing ones include acne (Fig. 25.8), psoriasis, and seborrheic keratoses. Benign skin problems are outlined in Table 25.10.

Psoriasis is a chronic autoimmune disease. It is fairly common, affecting around 7.5 million Americans. The rate is

TABLE 25.7 Common Fungal Infections of the Skin and Nails

Etiology and Pathophysiology	Clinical Manifestations	Treatment and Prognosis
Candidiasis		
• Caused by *Candida albicans* • 50% of adults are symptom-free carriers • Appears in warm, moist areas such as groin, oral mucosa, and submammary folds • Immunosuppression (e.g., from HIV infection, chemotherapy, radiation, organ transplant) allows yeast to become pathogenic	• *Mouth:* White, cheesy plaque; resembles milk curds • *Vagina:* Vaginitis with red, edematous, painful vaginal wall, white patches; vaginal discharge; itching; pain on urination and intercourse • *Skin:* Diffuse, papular, red rash with pinpoint satellite lesions around edges of affected area	• Azole antifungals (e.g., fluconazole, ketoconazole) or other specific medication such as vaginal suppository or oral lozenge • Sexual abstinence or use of condom • Skin hygiene to keep area clean and dry • Powder is effective on nonmucosal surfaces of skin to prevent recurrence
Tinea Corporis		
• Various dermatophytes, often called *ringworm*	• Typical annular (ringlike) scaly appearance, well-defined margins • Redness	• Cool compresses • Topical antifungals for isolated patches; creams or solutions of miconazole, ketoconazole, clotrimazole, butenafine
Tinea Cruris		
• Various dermatophytes • Often called *jock itch*	• Well-defined, scaly plaque in groin area	• Topical antifungal cream or solution
Tinea Pedis		
• Various dermatophytes • Often called *athlete's foot*	• Interdigital scaling and maceration • Scaly plantar surfaces sometimes with redness and blistering • May be itchy and painful	• Topical antifungal cream, gel, solution, spray, powder
Tinea Unguium (Onychomycosis)		
• Various dermatophytes • Incidence increases with age	• May affect only a few nails on 1 hand • Affects toenails most often • Scaliness under distal nail plate • Brittle, thickened, broken, or crumbling nails with yellowish discoloration	• Oral antifungal (terbinafine [Lamisil], itraconazole) • Topical antifungal cream or solution (minimal effectiveness) if unable to tolerate systemic treatment • Thinning of toenails • Nail removal

highest in White persons.[9] It usually develops in those 15 to 35 years old. One-third of people with psoriasis have at least 1 relative with the disease. Psoriasis is associated with metabolic syndrome, heart disease, and type 2 diabetes. Up to 40% of people also have psoriatic arthritis. Psoriatic arthritis is discussed in Chapter 69.

The diagnosis of plaque psoriasis, the most common form, is based on the skin's appearance (Fig. 25.9). Lesions are distinct and appear as red, scaling papules that merge to form plaques. The affected area is normally rounded, with adherent silver scales that bleed easily when removed. Plaques are common on the knees, elbows, scalp, hands, feet, and lower back. They are often itchy and may be painful. The extent of the disease varies. Most people have mild disease. Others have lesions on much of their skin surface.

We tailor treatment to the person's needs. This varies depending on the location of lesions, severity, patient preferences, and comorbidities. Goals range from improved quality of life to complete disease resolution. Psoriasis can erode self-image. The person may be self-conscious and withdraw from social contacts. Quality of life can diminish as people avoid activities. Depression is common.

DRUG ALERT

Isotretinoin

- Used to treat acne (Table 25.10)
- Can cause serious damage to fetus
- Contraindicated in females who are pregnant or want to become pregnant
- Cannot donate blood during treatment and for 1 month after treatment ends
- May cause depression and suicidal ideation

INTERPROFESSIONAL CARE: SKIN PROBLEMS

Many different treatments are used to treat skin problems. A number of these require special equipment. These are usually used by a dermatologist or specially trained nurse. The history, physical assessment, and diagnostic test results guide therapy.

Phototherapy

UV light therapy is a part of treating many skin problems, including psoriasis, cutaneous T-cell lymphoma, atopic

TABLE 25.8 **Common Infestations and Bites**

Etiology and Pathophysiology	Clinical Manifestations	Treatment and Prognosis
Bedbugs		
• *Cimicidae* species • Feeding periodic, usually at night • Present in furniture, walls during day	• Wheal surrounded by vivid flare • Firm hives transforming into persistent lesion • Severe itching • Often grouped in threes on uncovered parts of body	• Lesions usually require no treatment • Antihistamines or topical corticosteroids for severe itching
Bees and Wasps		
• *Hymenoptera* species	• Intense, burning, local pain • Swelling and itching • Severe hypersensitivity may lead to anaphylaxis	• Cool compresses • Antipruritic lotion • Antihistamines • Usually uneventful recovery
Pediculosis (Head Lice, Body Lice, Pubic Lice)		
• *Pediculus humanus* var. *capitis, Pediculus humanus* var. *corporis, Phthirus pubis* • Parasites that suck blood, leave excrement and eggs on skin and hair, live in seams of clothing (if body lice) and in hair as nits; transmission of pubic lice often by sexual contact	• Minute, red, noninflammatory • Points flush with skin; progression to papular wheal-like lesions • Itching • Secondary excoriation, especially parallel linear excoriations in intrascapular region • Nits and eggs firmly attach to hair shaft in head and body	• γ-Benzene hexachloride or pyrethrins to treat various parts of body • Spinosad (Natroba) topical suspension 0.9% to treat scalp and hair • Screen and treat close contacts (e.g., bed partners and playmates) as needed • Do not share head gear
Scabies		
• *Sarcoptes scabiei* • Mite penetrates stratum corneum, deposits eggs • Allergic reaction to eggs, feces, mite parts • Transmission by direct physical contact, sometimes by shared personal items	• Severe itching, especially at night, usually not on face • Presence of burrows, especially in interdigital webs, flexor surface of wrists, genitalia, and anterior axillary folds • Red papules (may be crusted), possible vesiculation, interdigital web crusting	• 5% permethrin topical lotion, 1 overnight application with second application 1 wk later, may yield 95% eradication • Treat all family members, treat environment with plastic covering for 5 days, launder all clothes and linen with bleach • Treat sexual partner • Antibiotics, if secondary infections present • Possible residual itching up to 4 wk after treatment • Recurrence possible if not adequately treated

dermatitis, vitiligo, and itching. Light sources available include broadband UVB, narrowband UVB, and long-wave UV (UVA1). One form of phototherapy combines the use of the photosensitizing drug methoxsalen with UVA light (PUVA). With PUVA, patients receive methoxsalen and then are exposed to UVA.

Treatments are generally given 2 to 3 times a week. Side effects include nausea, itching, and redness. Taking methoxsalen with food and milk may reduce nausea. Caution patients about taking methoxsalen and exposure during therapy to UV rays from sunlight or artificial UV light. Because of the risk for cataracts, patients receiving PUVA need to wear prescription goggles that block 100% of UV light. Teach patients to wear the eyewear for 24 hours after taking the medication when outdoors or near a bright window (UVA penetrates glass). Perform frequent skin assessments on patients receiving phototherapy. The immunosuppressive effects of PUVA increase the risk for skin cancers.

Photodynamic therapy is a special type of phototherapy used to treat AK and some skin cancers. This therapy uses a photosensitizing agent in a different way than other phototherapy treatments. Patients receive the photosensitizing agent IV or topically, depending on the area treated. Time is allowed for the drug to be absorbed by the target cells. Light is then applied to the area, causing the drug to react with oxygen. This starts a reaction that kills the cells.

CHECK YOUR PRACTICE

You are working in a dermatology clinic, preparing a 64-year-old female for phototherapy to treat multiple AK on her nose and both cheeks. She says the first lesion appeared a few years ago. She then started to worry about all the time she spent in her garden without sunscreen. She thought the lesions were just "age spots" and was unconcerned until a few started to grow and periodically bleed.

- What teaching will you provide so she can care for herself after the procedure?

TABLE 25.9 **Common Allergic Skin Problems**

Etiology and Pathophysiology	Clinical Manifestations	Treatment and Prognosis
Allergic Contact Dermatitis		
• Type IV delayed hypersensitivity response (see Chapter 14) • Absorbed agent acts as antigen • Sensitization occurs after 1 or more exposures • Lesions appear 2 to 7 days after contact with allergen	• Red papules and plaques • Sharply circumscribed with occasional vesicles • Itching • Area of dermatitis often takes shape of causative agent (e.g., metal allergy and bandlike dermatitis on ring finger)	• Topical or oral corticosteroids, antihistamines • Skin lubrication • Elimination of contact allergen • Avoid irritating affected area • Systemic corticosteroids if sensitivity severe
Atopic Dermatitis		
• Type 1 hypersensitivity response (see Chapter 14) • Genetically influenced, chronic, relapsing disease • Exaggerated by a skin response to environment allergens • Associated with allergic rhinitis and asthma	• Multiple presentations, including acute, subacute, and chronic stages • *Acute stage:* Redness, oozing vesicles, with extreme itching • *Subacute stage:* Scaly, light red to red-brown plaques; itching • *Chronic stage:* Thickened skin with accentuation of skin markings (lichenification), changes in pigmentation; dry skin; itching; common in antecubital and popliteal space	• Lubricate dry skin • Topical immunomodulators (pimecrolimus [Elidel], tacrolimus [Protopic]) • Stress reduction reduces flares • Corticosteroids, phototherapy for severe inflammation and itching • Antibiotics for secondary infection as needed
Drug Reaction		
• May be caused by any drug that acts as antigen and causes hypersensitivity reaction • Certain drugs (e.g., penicillin) more likely to cause reactions	• Rash; often red, macular and papular, semiconfluent, general rash with abrupt onset • Appearance as late as 14 days after cessation of drug; may be itchy • Some reactions may be life threatening, requiring immediate and intensive care	• Withdrawal of drug if possible • Antihistamines, topical or systemic corticosteroids may be given depending on severity
Urticaria (Hives)		
• Often an allergic event • Redness and edema in upper dermis resulting from a local increase in permeability of capillaries (usually from histamine release)	• Spontaneously occurring, raised or irregularly shaped wheals, varying size, usually multiple • A single lesion usually resolves in 24 h • Can occur anywhere on the body	• Remove triggering agent, if known • Oral antihistamine therapy • Possible systemic corticosteroids

Radiation Therapy

The use of radiation therapy to treat BCC and SCC varies. The best candidates are those with lesions in challenging locations, such as the ear, nose, scalp, neck, and shin; those who may have trouble with wound healing; or those with medical comorbidities who cannot have surgery.[10] Use is limited in those with melanoma to palliative pain control or treating brain metastases.

Radiation therapy requires multiple visits to a radiology department. It can cause permanent hair loss *(alopecia)* of the irradiated areas. Other adverse effects depend on the location and dose of radiation delivered. They include telangiectasia, atrophy, changes in pigmentation, ulceration, hearing loss, eye damage, atrophy, and mucositis. Shielding is needed to prevent lens damage if the irradiated area is around the eyes. See Chapter 16 for more on radiation therapy.

Total-body skin radiation is a treatment for cutaneous T-cell lymphoma. Treatment follows a lengthy course and causes premature skin aging. Patients have varying degrees of permanent alopecia and radiation dermatitis with a transient loss of sweat gland function.

Lasers

Laser treatment is effective for many types of skin problems (Table 25.11). Depending on the type of laser and the wavelength, lasers serve a wide variety of functions. Lasers can make measurable, repeatable, consistent zones of tissue damage. They can cut, coagulate, and vaporize tissue to some degree. Laser light does not accumulate in body cells and cannot cause cumulative cell changes or damage. With less damage to surrounding tissue, there is a decreased risk for scarring.

The surgical use of lasers requires a focusing device to produce a small, high-density spot of energy. Several types of lasers are available. The CO_2 laser, the most common, has many applications as a vaporizing and cutting tool for most tissues. The argon laser emits light that is mainly absorbed by hemoglobin. It helps in the treatment of vascular and other pigmented lesions. Other, less common lasers include copper and gold vapors and neodymium:yttrium-aluminum-garnet (Nd:YAG). Those who work with laser equipment must be familiar with agency procedures on laser safety.

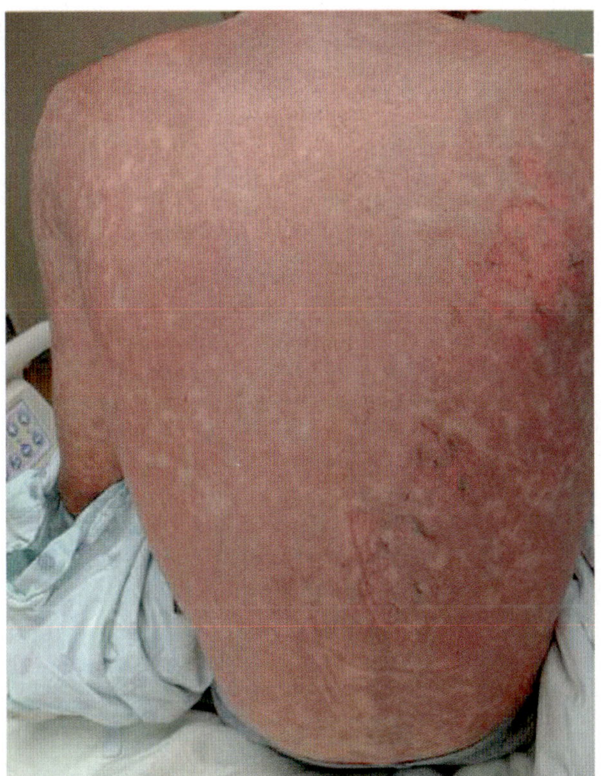

Fig. 25.7 Toxic epidermal necrolysis. (From Dabiri, G, Rüenger T: *Ferri's clinical advisor 2018.* St Louis, 2018, Elsevier, p. 1282.e2.)

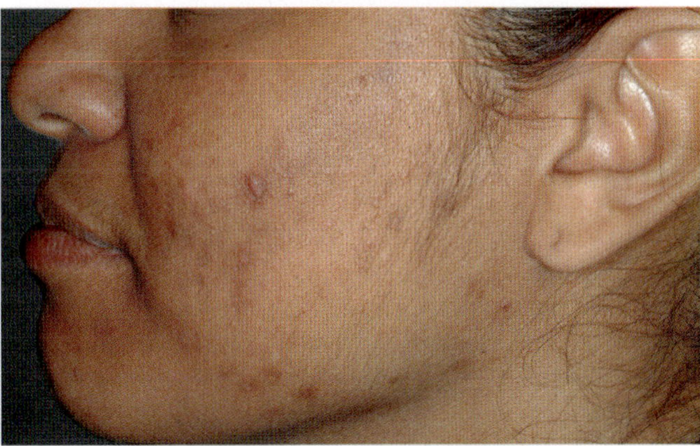

Fig. 25.8 Acne with papules and pustules. (From Miller JJ, Hollins C, Marks JG: *Lookingbill & Marks' principles of dermatology,* ed 7, Philadelphia, 2025, Elsevier.)

Drug Therapy

Antibiotics

We use several topical and systemic antibiotics to treat skin problems. Sometimes they are used concurrently. Common over-the-counter (OTC) topical antibiotics include bacitracin-neomycin-polymyxin (Neosporin), bacitracin, and polymyxin B. Prescription topical antibiotics include (1) mupirocin (for superficial *Staphylococcus* infections such as impetigo), (2) gentamicin (for *Staphylococcus* and many gram-negative organisms), and (3) erythromycin (for gram-positive cocci [staphylococci, streptococci], gram-negative cocci, and bacilli). Metronidazole is a common therapy for rosacea. Topical erythromycin and clindamycin are options for acne.

Systemic infections require systemic antibiotics. They have a role in treating acne and bacterial infections, such as erysipelas, cellulitis, abscesses, and certain wound infections. Frequently used oral drugs include penicillin, erythromycin, doxycycline, clindamycin, and linezolid. Vancomycin is the drug of choice for severe infections.[11]

Corticosteroids

Corticosteroids are effective in treating a wide variety of skin problems. They can be used topically, intralesionally, or systemically. Topical corticosteroids have local antiinflammatory and antipruritic effects. Because corticosteroids may change the manifestations, try to diagnose a skin problem before applying a corticosteroid.

Corticosteroids' potency depends on the drug concentration and delivery system. With prolonged use, high-potency corticosteroids can cause adrenal suppression, especially if a large surface area is covered and occlusive dressings are used. Other side effects include skin atrophy from impaired cell mitosis, capillary fragility, rosacea, acne, and bruising. In general, atrophy does not occur until a corticosteroid has been in use for 2 to 3 weeks. If drug use is stopped at the first sign of atrophy, recovery usually occurs in several weeks. Rebound dermatitis can occur when therapy is stopped. Tapering the use of high-potency topical corticosteroids when improvement is noted reduces the risk.

Low-potency corticosteroids act more slowly. They can be used for a longer time without producing serious side effects. Low-potency corticosteroids are safe to use on the face and areas where skin may touch or rub together, such as the axillae and groin. The most potent delivery system for a topical corticosteroid is an ointment.

Intralesional corticosteroids are injected directly into or just beneath the lesion. This method provides a reservoir of medication with an effect lasting several weeks to months. Intralesional injection is common in the treatment of psoriasis, alopecia areata (patchy hair loss), cystic acne, hypertrophic scars, and keloids. Triamcinolone acetonide (Kenalog) is the most common drug used for intralesional injection.

Systemic corticosteroids can have remarkable results in treating some skin problems. However, they often have undesirable systemic effects. Corticosteroids are helpful in short-term therapy for acute problems such as contact dermatitis caused by poison ivy. Long-term therapy is reserved for those with severe disease, such as bullous (blistering) disorders.

Antihistamines

Oral antihistamines are helpful in treating urticaria (hives), angioedema, and itching that can occur in problems such as atopic dermatitis and other allergic skin reactions. Several antihistamines may be tried before getting an acceptable effect. Antihistamines with sedative effects, such as diphenhydramine, may be better with itching because the tranquilizing and

TABLE 25.10 Common Benign Skin Problems

Etiology and Pathophysiology	Clinical Manifestations	Treatment and Prognosis
Acne Vulgaris		
• Inflammatory disorder of sebaceous glands • More common in teenagers • May begin and persist into adulthood • Flare can occur with corticosteroids and androgen-dominant birth control pills and before menses	• Noninflammatory lesions, including open comedones (blackheads) and closed comedones (whiteheads) • Inflammatory lesions, including papules and pustules • Most common on face, neck, and upper back (Fig. 25.8)	*Topical:* • Mechanical removal of multiple lesions with comedo extractor • Topical benzoyl peroxide, retinoids, antimicrobials (clindamycin, minocycline, erythromycin) *Systemic:* • Systemic antibiotics • Use of isotretinoin for severe nodulocystic acne may provide lasting remission; monitor pregnancy tests, liver function, cholesterol, triglycerides, and for depression • Aim is to suppress new lesions and minimize scarring • Spontaneous remission possible • Often improves with sun exposure
Acrochordons (Skin Tags)		
• Common after midlife • Appearance on neck, axillae, and upper trunk from mechanical friction or redundant skin (associated with obesity)	• Small, skin-colored, soft, pedunculated papules • May become irritated	• No treatment medically necessary • Surgical removal when needed; usually just snipping without anesthesia
Lentigo		
• Increased number of normal melanocytes in basal layer of epidermis from sun exposure and aging • Also called *liver spots* or *age spots*	• Hyperpigmented, brown to black macule or patch (flat lesion) on sun-exposed areas	• Assess for progression • Treatment only for cosmetic purposes: liquid nitrogen, laser resurfacing • May recur • Biopsy when suspicious of melanoma
Lipoma		
• Benign tumor of adipose tissue, often encapsulated • Most common in 40- to 60-yr-old age group	• Rubbery, compressible, round mass of adipose tissue • Single or multiple • Variable in size, may be very large • Most common on trunk, back of neck, forearms	• Usually no treatment • Biopsy to distinguish from liposarcoma • Excision
Nevi (Moles)		
• Grouping of normal cells derived from melanocyte-like precursor cells	• Hyperpigmented areas that vary in form and color • Flat, slightly elevated, verrucoid, polypoid, dome-shaped, sessile, papillomatous • Hair growth possible	• No treatment except for cosmetic reasons • Skin biopsy for suspicious nevi
Psoriasis		
• Autoimmune chronic dermatitis that involves very rapid turnover of epidermal cells • Family predisposition • Usually develops before age 40	• Sharply demarcated, silvery scaling plaques on reddish skin often on the scalp, elbows, knees, palms, soles, and fingernails (Fig. 25.9) • Itching, burning, pain • Local or general, intermittent or continuous • Symptoms vary in intensity from mild to severe	*Goal:* Reduce inflammation and suppress rapid turnover of epidermal cells; no cure, but control is possible *Topical treatments:* • Corticosteroids, tazarotene, calcipotriene, anthralin, tacrolimus, halobetasol propionate and tazarotene (Duobrii) • Intralesional injection of corticosteroids for chronic plaques *Systemic treatments:* • Natural or artificial UVB; PUVA (UVA with topical or systemic photosensitizer) • Traditional and oral therapies: methotrexate, retinoid (acitretin), apremilast (Otezla), cyclosporine • Biologic therapies for moderate to severe plaque disease (see Table 14.18)

TABLE 25.10 Common Benign Skin Problems—cont'd

Etiology and Pathophysiology	Clinical Manifestations	Treatment and Prognosis
Rosacea		
• Common disorder of the central face • Cause is unclear	*Major subtypes:* • Erythematotelangiectatic (ETR): telangiectasia, redness, flushing • Papulopustular (PPR): redness, flushing, papules, pustules • Phymatous (PHY): thickening of the skin, hypertrophy of the nose • Ocular rosacea (OR): tearing, stinging, itching, dryness of the lids	• Avoid triggers: sun, extreme heat/cold, heavy exercise, spicy foods, alcohol use, smoking • Ablative laser surgery • Oral treatments: azithromycin, doxycycline, isotretinoin, minocycline, trimethoprim/sulfamethoxazole • Topical treatments: brimonidine, oxymetazoline hydrochloride cream, azelaic acid, ivermectin, metronidazole, sodium sulfacetamide
Seborrheic Keratoses		
• Benign, familial, exact etiology unknown • Usually occur after age 40, increase in number with age	• Irregularly round or oval, often warty papules or plaques • Well-defined shape, appear being "stuck on" • Increase in pigmentation with time • Usually multiple, may be itchy	• Remove by curettage or cryosurgery for cosmetic reasons or to eliminate source of irritation • Biopsy if unable to distinguish from melanoma

PUVA, Psoralen ultraviolet A; *UVA,* ultraviolet A; *UVB,* ultraviolet B.

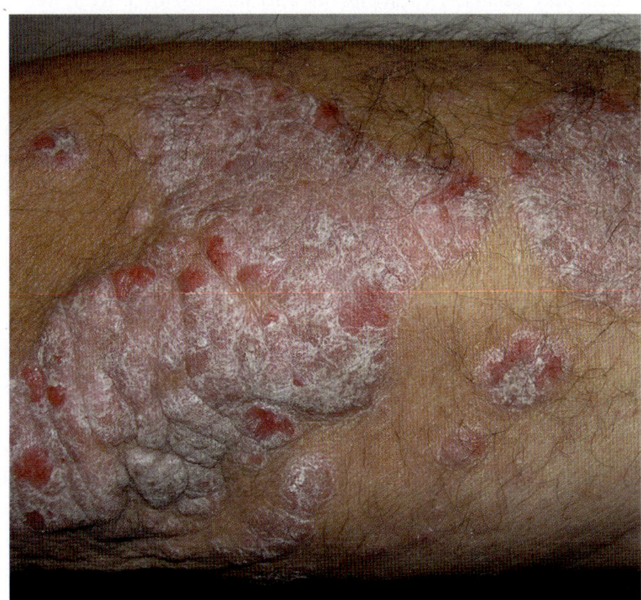

Fig. 25.9 Psoriasis. Characteristic inflammation and scaling. (From Miller JJ, Hollins C, Marks JG: *Lookingbill & Marks' principles of dermatology,* ed 7, Philadelphia, 2025, Elsevier.)

sedative effects enhance symptom relief. Warn patients about sedative effects. They can be a problem when driving or using heavy machinery. Antihistamines, such as loratadine, fexofenadine, and cetirizine, bind to peripheral histamine receptors, giving antihistamine action without sedation. However, they are not effective for controlling itching. Use antihistamines with caution in older adults because of their long half-life and anticholinergic effects.

Fluorouracil

Fluorouracil is a topical cytotoxic agent with selective toxicity for sun-damaged cells. It is used to treat precancerous lesions (especially AK) and some skin cancers. Use causes redness, burning, and itching within 3 to 5 days. Painful, eroded areas over the damaged skin occur within 1 to 3 weeks, depending on skin thickness at the site. Treatment must continue with applications 1 or 2 times a day for 2 to 4 weeks. Healing may take up to 4 weeks after stopping treatment. Afterward, skin should be smooth and free of AK. Multiple courses of therapy may be necessary over the years for those with severely sun-damaged skin. AK may recur in treated areas.

Patient adherence to therapy is important and depends on your teaching. Tell patients they will look worse before they look better. Teach them about the side effects. Reduce redness and itching by applying a low-potency topical corticosteroid 20 minutes after dosing. Because fluorouracil is a photosensitizing drug, patients should avoid sunlight during treatment.

TABLE 25.11 Skin Problems Treated by Laser

- Acne scars
- Hair removal
- Hemangiomas
- Leg veins
- Pigment discoloration in epidermis
- Pigmented nevi
- Port wine stain
- Psoriasis
- Resurfacing of skin
- Rosacea
- Skin lesions
- Tattoo removal
- Vascular lesions
- Warts
- Wrinkles

Immunomodulators

Topical immunomodulators, such as pimecrolimus (Elidel) and tacrolimus (Protopic), are used to treat atopic dermatitis, psoriasis, and rosacea.[12] They work by suppressing the immune system. Side effects are minimal. They include a transient burning or feeling of heat at the application site. Use may increase the risk for skin cancer and precancerous lesions.

The topical immunomodulator imiquimod (Aldara) is used to treat external genital warts, AK, and superficial BCC. It stimulates the production of α-interferon and other cytokines to enhance cell-mediated immunity. Imiquimod boosts the immune response only where applied. Dosing varies depending on the type of lesion treated and the strength prescribed. Most patients have skin reactions, including redness, swelling, blistering, peeling, itching, and burning.

Diagnostic and Surgical Therapy

Skin Scraping

Scraping with a scalpel blade can yield a sample of surface cells for microscopic inspection and diagnosis. The most common tests of skin scrapings are mineral oil examination for scabies and 10% to 20% KOH for fungus.

Electrodessication and Electrocoagulation

Electrical energy can be converted to heat that burns and destroys tissue. The major uses of these therapies are coagulation of bleeding vessels to obtain hemostasis and destruction of small *telangiectasias* (dilation of groups of superficial capillaries and venules). *Electrodessication* usually involves more superficial destruction. It uses a monopolar electrode. *Electrocoagulation* uses a bipolar electrode. It has a deeper effect, with better hemostasis, but an increased chance of scarring. Although minor electrosurgery on patients with a pacemaker poses minimal risk, the electrical energy can affect pacemakers and internal defibrillators.

Curettage

Curettage is the removal and scooping away of tissue using a tool called a *curette.* A curette looks like a small spoon with very sharp edges. It can remove many types of small, soft skin tumors and superficial lesions, such as warts, AK, seborrheic keratosis, and small BCCs and SCCs. The area to be curetted is anesthetized before the procedure. The HCP removes the lesion and then cauterizes the skin. The removed tissue is usually sent for biopsy. A dressing may be applied. Teach patients wound care. A small scar and hypopigmentation can result.

Punch Biopsy

Punch biopsy is a common procedure used to obtain a tissue sample for histologic study or to remove small lesions. The procedure is simple. The HCP marks the biopsy area and then anesthetizes it so that the anesthetic will not obscure the landmarks. The HCP rotates the punch into the skin and removes a small cylinder of skin. Hemostasis is achieved with pressure or absorbable packing. Sites of 4 mm or larger are usually closed with sutures. Punch biopsies are not done below the knee if other sites are available. Circulatory changes can make evaluating the tissue sample difficult.

Cryosurgery

Cryosurgery is the use of subfreezing temperatures to destroy epidermal lesions. It is used to treat common and genital warts, skin tags, thin seborrheic keratoses, AK, BCC, and SCC. Topical liquid nitrogen is the agent most often used for cryosurgery. Damage occurs in treated tissue because of intracellular ice formation. It causes the cell to rupture during thaw, leading to cell death and necrosis. The degree of damage depends on the rate of cooling and the minimum temperature achieved.

Liquid nitrogen is applied directly onto the lesion with a spray or contact probe. Tell patients that they will feel a painful, stinging, cold sensation. The lesion first becomes swollen and red. It may blister. A scab forms and falls off in 1 to 3 weeks. The skin lesion sloughs along with the scab. Growth of new skin follows.

The size of an affected area may limit the use of cryotherapy. Other disadvantages include the potential for harming adjacent healthy tissue and the low temperature of liquid nitrogen destroying melanocytes, leaving an area of hypopigmentation resembling a scar.

Excision

Excision is an option if the lesion involves the dermis. Complete closure of the excised area usually results in a good cosmetic result.

A specific type of excision is *Mohs surgery,* the microscopically controlled removal of skin cancer. In this procedure, the HCP removes tissue sections in thin horizontal layers. All the section's margins are examined to see if cancer cells are present (Fig. 25.10). Any cancer cells not removed by the first excision are removed in serial excisions done on the same day. Benefits of Mohs surgery are that it preserves normal tissue, produces the smallest possible wound, and can completely remove the cancer. Although it can be a lengthy procedure, it is done in an outpatient setting using local anesthesia.

NURSING MANAGEMENT: SKIN PROBLEMS

A careful history is important in diagnosing skin problems. You must be skilled at detecting findings that could help determine the cause of many skin problems. After a careful history and physical assessment, inspect the lesions.

Nursing interventions for skin problems fall into broad categories (Table 25.12). They apply to many problems in inpatient and outpatient settings. A nursing care plan for patients with chronic skin lesions (eNursing Care Plan 25.1) is available on the website for this chapter.

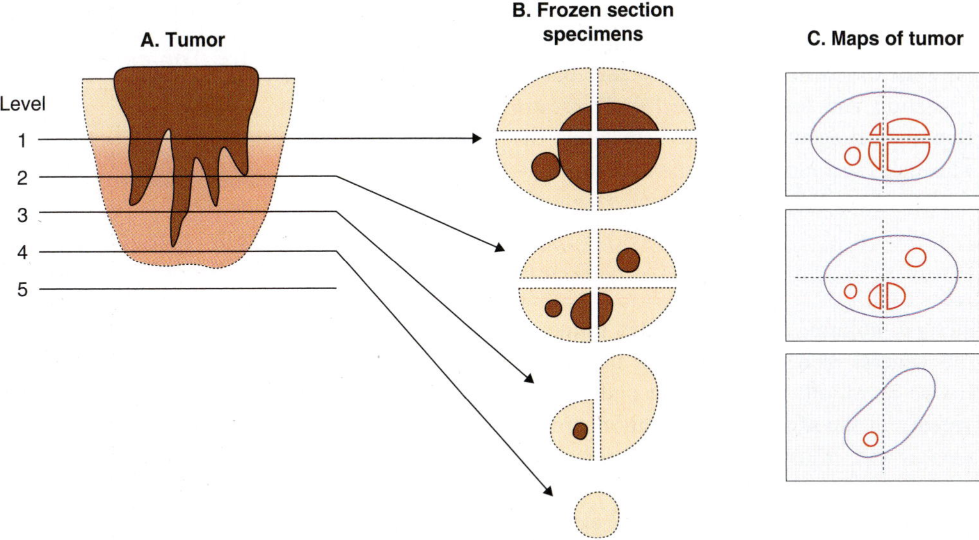

Fig. 25.10 Mohs surgery. (A) BCC with projections in the dermis. (B) Tumor sliced, cut into quadrants before frozen section. Dark areas represent tumor. (C) Map of tumor location drawn from specimens, indicating areas of tumor that need to be removed. (Adapted from Dinulos J: *Habif's clinical dermatology: a color guide to diagnosis and treatment*, ed 7, St Louis, 2021, Elsevier.)

TABLE 25.12 NURSING MANAGEMENT

Skin Problems

- Assess skin for acute and chronic skin problems.
- Assess risk factors for skin problems.
- Document skin problems and risk factor assessment, and develop a plan of care.
- Determine whether patients are taking drugs that increase photosensitivity.
- Teach about risks associated with sun exposure and methods for decreasing exposure to the sun.
- Apply prescribed therapies such as dressings and oral or topical medications.
- Assist patients to discuss feelings about body image.
- Identify ways to reduce the impact of image problems through means such as clothing and cosmetics.
- Clean skin with antibacterial soap, as appropriate.
- Teach about therapies used for skin disorders, including dressings, baths, and oral or topical medications.
- Teach patients treatment measures to control symptoms, such as itching.
- Evaluate treatment for effectiveness and any adverse effects.

TABLE 25.13 NURSING MANAGEMENT

Applying a Wet Compress

- Select compress material that is 4 to 8 layers thick and slightly larger than the area being treated. Use gauze or any clean material. Do not use gauze sponges with fillers, as they retain too much solution.
- Use tap water at room temperature. If drinkable water is not available, use filtered, bottled, or sterile water. Add ordered additives.
- The temperature of the fluid should be tepid. However, when an antiinflammatory effect is desired, the fluid should be cool.
- When using continuous compresses, remove the compress and replace with a new one as needed. Do not add solution to a compress. This can change the fluid's concentration and damage the skin.
- Intermittent compresses are placed for 10 to 30 min, several times a day.
- Assess the skin at regular intervals. If the skin appears macerated, stop the compresses for 2 to 3 days.
- Change and wash daily any material used repeatedly throughout the day.
- Protect the patient from discomfort and chilling.
- Use a water-resistant pad to help protect the mattress, linens, and furniture.

In your patient teaching, stress the duration of the treatment. Review specific instructions about each therapy. Skin problems may be slow to resolve. Tell patients to follow package directions when using OTC drugs. If the package insert says use should not exceed 7 days, patients should heed this warning. Teach patients to stop care and notify the HCP if any systemic signs of inflammation or extensions of the skin problem (e.g., more lesions, increased redness or swelling) develop.

Wet Compresses

It is important to know how to apply a wet compress (Table 25.13). We often apply wet compresses for superficial skin problems that involve inflammation, itching, and infection. They are appropriate for damaged, oozing skin. Wet compresses are a good way to remove crusts and scabs that are adhering to the wound surface. They provide comfort and treatment of problems such as poison ivy, insect bites, and skin infections. Depending on the problem, we may use additives. Common solutions include (1) saline, (2) Burow solution (Domeboro powder [aluminum acetate; calcium acetate]), (3) acetic acid (vinegar), and (4) silver nitrate.

Baths

Baths are an appropriate intervention when large areas of the body need treatment. Baths may be relaxing and will help decrease itching. Agents such as colloidal oatmeal (Aveeno) and sodium bicarbonate can be added directly to bath water. Fill the tub with tepid water to cover the affected areas. Depending on the severity of the problem and the patient's discomfort, have the patient soak for 15 to 20 minutes 3 or 4 times a day. Tell them not to rub the skin dry with a towel but gently pat to prevent increased irritation and inflammation. Apply cream, moisturizers, or other topical agents after the bath while the skin is still damp. This helps seal moisture in the hydrated cells and increases absorption of topical agents.

Hygiene

One's skin type, lifestyle, culture, age, and gender influence hygienic practices. In general, skin and hair must be washed often enough to remove excess oil and excretions and prevent odor. The normal acidity of the skin and perspiration protect against bacterial overgrowth. Most soaps are alkaline and neutralize the skin surface, leading to a loss of protection. Using mild, moisturizing soaps and lipid-free cleansers and avoiding hot water and vigorous scrubbing can noticeably decrease local skin irritation and inflammation. Skin piercings in which jewelry has been inserted can be cared for with antibacterial soaps that do not contain sulfites. Older people should avoid harsh soaps and shampoos and frequent bathing because of the dryness of their skin and scalp.

TABLE 25.14 Drug Therapy

Common Bases for Topical Medications

Agent	Considerations
Cream	Emulsions of oil and water. Most common base for topical medications. Versatile. Lubrication and protection.
Gel	Nongreasy combination of propylene glycol and water. May contain alcohol. Works well on the scalp. Good for acute exudative problems (e.g., poison ivy).
Lotion	Emulsions of water, alcohol, and/or oil. Cooling and drying. Some leave residual powder film after evaporation of water. May cause stinging when used in skinfolds. Useful with subacute itching problems.
Ointment	Oil with differing amounts of water added. Lubrication; prevents dehydration. May be too occlusive for problems with lots of exudate or in body creases. Petrolatum most common.
Paste	Mixture of powder and ointment. Used when drying effect necessary because moisture is absorbed.
Powder	Promotion of dryness. Lubricates skinfold areas to prevent irritation. Base for antifungal preparations. Protect patient from inhaling.

Topical Medications

Topical medications are often used to treat skin problems. The effectiveness of topical therapy depends on which base the medication is prepared in. Table 25.14 describes common bases for topical preparations and their considerations. The base selected depends on the properties needed.

Apply topical agents as directed. As a rule, apply a topical agent in a thin film to clean skin and spread evenly in a downward motion in the direction of hair growth. Thick creams will spread easier if the skin is still damp. If you are using a secondary dressing, you can apply the agent directly onto a dressing. Teach the patient and caregiver proper dosing, application, expected results, and common reactions.

Occlusion with a plastic wrap is an effective way to increase the absorption of topical corticosteroids or simple emollients. The plastic wrap traps perspiration against the outer layer of the epidermis. Applying agents to moist skin increases absorption 10-fold. Use tape or stretch wraps to keep the plastic wrap in place. For lesions on the feet or lower legs, patients can wear socks over the plastic wrap. Wraps applied multiple times daily are kept in place for 2 to 8 hours. Some patients choose to use occlusion at bedtime. Occlusion is not appropriate in areas prone to infection, such as skin creases.

Control of Itching

Many problems cause *pruritus* (itching). This includes dry skin, almost any physical or chemical stimulus to the skin (e.g., drugs or insects), and scaling skin problems. The itch sensation is carried by the same nonmyelinated nerve fibers as pain and temperature. Patients will have pain rather than an itch if the epidermis is damaged or absent. It is important to figure out if itching preceded a skin lesion. Itching can lead to scratching that results in an excoriated and inflamed lesion.

Certain circumstances make itching worse. Teach patients ways to help break the itch/scratch cycle. A cool environment may cause vasoconstriction and decrease itching. Hydration, wet compresses, and moisturizers (including antipruritic lotions) are normally helpful. Apply wet compresses for 30 to 60 minutes, pat the skin dry, and apply a lubricant or medication. Topical and injectable corticosteroids are sometimes used. Topically applied menthol, camphor, or phenol numbs itch receptors. Systemic antihistamines may give relief. The main side effect of most antihistamines is sedation. This may be desirable because itching is often worse at night and can interfere with sleep. Adequate rest increases the ability to tolerate itching, thereby decreasing skin damage from scratching. Have patients avoid anything that causes vasodilation, such as heat or rubbing. Dry skin lowers the itch threshold and increases the itch sensation.

Lichenification is a thickening of epidermis with exaggerated markings resembling a washboard. It is caused by chronic scratching or rubbing of the skin. Lichenification often occurs with atopic dermatitis and other itching problems. The hands, forearms, shins, and nape of the neck are common sites. Scratching may become a habit. Persistent scratching can cause excoriations. Treating the cause of the itching is the key to preventing lichenification.

Preventing Spread

Although most skin problems are not contagious, infection control precautions indicate wearing gloves when working with any open wounds or lesions with drainage. Not all infected drainage is purulent. Careful hand washing and properly disposing of soiled dressings are the best means of preventing the spread of infections or infestations. The most common contagious lesions include impetigo, streptococcal infections, staphylococcal infections (e.g., methicillin-resistant *S. aureus* [MRSA]), fungal infections, primary chancre, scabies, and pediculosis.

Preventing Secondary Infections

Open skin lesions are susceptible to invasion by viral, bacterial, or fungal organisms. Meticulous hygiene, hand washing, and dressing changes are important to minimize the risk for secondary infections. Warn patients about scratching lesions, which can cause excoriations and create a portal of entry for pathogens. Keep the nails short to minimize trauma from scratching.

Cosmetic Camouflage

Cosmetic camouflage is the application of makeup creams, liquids, and/or powders to conceal skin problems. It can do much to mask lesions and scarring and normalize skin appearance. The products are different from normal makeup. They are more opaque, smudge resistant, and water resistant. Persons with skin pigment changes, birthmarks, and healed burns are among the many for whom cosmetic makeup can improve quality of life. A specialist in camouflage cosmetics can help select products and teach patients application techniques.

Postprocedure Care

Provide teaching about skin care after simple procedures, such as skin biopsy, excision, and cryosurgery. In general, review cleansing, dressing changes, topical agent use, and the signs and symptoms of infection. Teach patients how to tell normal inflammation from an infection. A slight red border the first few days after is normal. Signs and symptoms of infection include redness that persists longer than a week or extends beyond a 1-cm border, fever greater than 101°F, increased pain, pronounced swelling, and purulent drainage. If these occur, patients should notify the HCP.

After a skin procedure, cleanse an oozing wound with a saline solution twice daily or as ordered by the HCP. Safe drinking water is an alternative in some situations. Apply antibiotic or ordered ointment with a nonadherent secondary dressing. Wounds that are kept moist and covered heal more rapidly and with less scarring. The initial crust should be left undisturbed. It is a protective coating for the damaged skin beneath it. Healing crusts that have been moisturized and protected will separate naturally from healed epidermis.

We can cover a sutured wound with a variety of dressings. Sutures are removed in 4 to 14 days, depending on the site. Sometimes alternating sutures are removed after the third day. Incision lines may need daily cleansing, usually with plain water. If necessary, a topical antibiotic is applied and the wound is either covered with a dry dressing or left open to air. There may be swelling and discomfort in the first 24 hours. Intermittent application of cold (ice packs) over the dressing may reduce edema. Mild analgesics, such as acetaminophen, should control discomfort.[13]

Psychologic Effects of Skin Problems

The location and visibility of lesions and scars is the key factor with respect to their cosmetic implications. Facial involvement is the most distressing because it is so visible. Patients with chronic skin problems, such as psoriasis, atopic dermatitis, or acne, may have emotional stress. The sequelae could result in social and employment problems with financial implications, a poor self-image, and problems with sexuality. Encourage patients to share their feelings and concerns. Refer patients to dermatology support groups. Many are listed on the American Academy of Dermatology website (www.aad.org). These groups are helpful with patient support and education.

COSMETIC PROCEDURES

Cosmetic procedures are done to enhance, alter, or shape specific parts of the body. The goal is to change one's appearance. A wide range of cosmetic procedures is available. The reasons for having a procedure are as varied as the techniques. The most common is to improve body image. Feeling better about oneself helps boost self-confidence and self-esteem.[14]

Nonsurgical Procedures

Common nonsurgical procedures include chemical peels, toxin injections, fillers, and laser treatment. Topical procedures are described in Table 25.15. Injection of botulinum (e.g., Botox, Dysport) and dermal fillers (e.g., collagen, hyaluronic acid fillers [Restylane, Juvéderm]) can relax or fill in fine lines and wrinkles.[15] Transitory side effects may occur, such as mild redness, pain, swelling, and bruising. Uncommon side effects include allergic reaction, infection, grayish skin discoloration, or lumps at the injection sites. Tell patients that the procedure will need repeating at prescribed intervals to maintain the desired appearance.

Laser treatment is used to treat congenital and acquired vascular lesions (cherry angiomas, spider leg veins, hemangiomas, port-wine stains, tattoo removal) and for skin resurfacing and hair removal. Lasers can reduce scarring and fine wrinkles around the lips or eyes and remove facial lesions (Table 25.11). Swelling, redness, and bruising are common after treatment. The treated areas usually are kept moist with ointment or occlusive dressings for the first few days. Patients must protect treated skin from the sun.

TABLE 25.15 Common Cosmetic Topical Procedures

Tretinoin (Retin-A, Renova)	Chemical Peels (e.g., Jessner, Trichloroacetic Acid [TCA], Salicylic Acid)	Microdermabrasion	α-Hydroxy Acids (e.g., Glycolic Acid, Lactic Acid)
Indications			
Improves appearance of photodamaged skin, especially fine wrinkling. Reduces actinic keratoses.	Improves appearance of photodamaged skin, acne scarring, actinic and seborrheic keratoses.	Smooths appearance of photodamaged and wrinkled skin, acne scarring.	Smooths appearance of photodamaged and wrinkled skin, acne scarring.
Description			
Initially applied every 2 to 3 days. Treatment stopped if severe inflammation occurs. Maximum response in 8 to 12 mo.	Solution applied in varying amounts to the skin, causing a controlled burn with a loss of melanin.	Epidermis and top dermal layer removed by applying aluminum oxide or baking soda crystals. Re-epithelialization of abraded surface then occurs.	Low concentrations (<10%) in many skin care products consumers can apply to the skin. Higher concentrations (50%–70%) applied only by an HCP.
Side Effects			
Redness, swelling, flaking, pigmentation changes. Teratogenic. Increases phototoxicity if taking other photosensitive drugs.	Moderate swelling and crusting for 1 wk. Redness for 6 to 8 wk. Pink tone possible for several months. Photosensitivity.	Light pink tone that resolves within 24 h. Photosensitivity.	Photosensitivity, slight irritation at lower concentrations, severe redness, oozing, and flaking skin possible with higher concentrations.
Patient Teaching			
Apply at night because preparation is inactivated by light. Keep skin moisturized. Use sunscreen and sun avoidance measures. Avoid abrasive or drying facial cleansers.	Use sunscreen. Avoid sun for 6 mo to prevent hyperpigmentation.	Keep skin moisturized. Use sunscreen and sun avoidance measures. Avoid strenuous exercise for 48 h.	Use sunscreen and sun avoidance measures.

Surgical Therapies

Plastic surgery includes cosmetic and reconstructive procedures. Reconstructive surgery is usually medically necessary. It focuses on repairing or reconstructing problems caused by birth disorders, tumor removals, burns, trauma, or other reasons. Common cosmetic surgeries include breast enlargement (see Chapter 56), face lift, eyelid surgery, butt lift, rhinoplasty ("nose job"), abdominoplasty ("tummy tuck"), and liposuction. Eyelid lifts (blepharoplasty) can remove redundant tissue and may improve the field of vision. The surgical approach and incisions vary depending on the procedure and the desired results (Fig. 25.11).

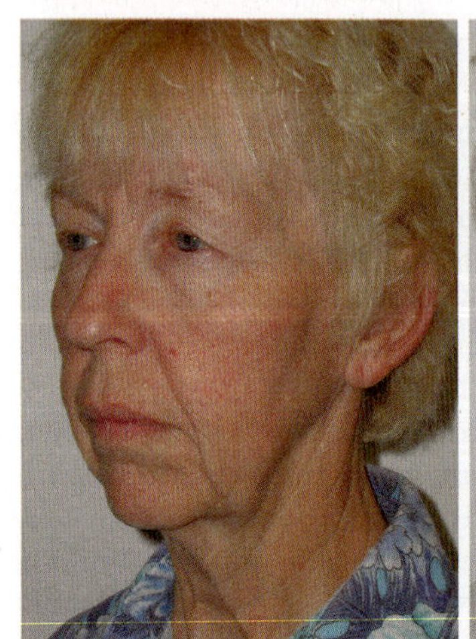
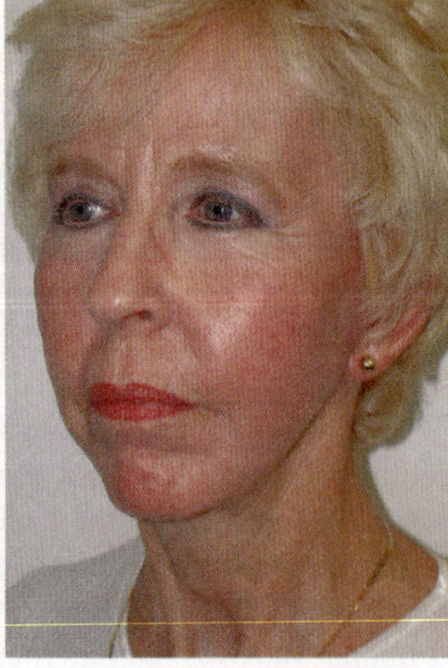

Fig. 25.11 Patient before *(left)* and after *(right)* a face lift, blepharoplasty, and laser resurfacing. (From Niamtu J: *The art and science of facelift surgery*, St Louis, 2025, Elsevier.)

Liposuction

Liposuction is a technique for removing subcutaneous fat to improve facial and body contours. It can remove areas of fat from almost any area that is resistant to other techniques. Liposuction is relatively free of complications. Possible contraindications include anticoagulant use, uncontrolled hypertension, diabetes, and poor cardiovascular status.

The procedure is usually done on an outpatient basis under local anesthesia. One or more sessions may be done, depending on the size of the area. The HCP inserts a blunt-tipped cannula through a small incision and pushes into the fat to break it loose from the fibrous stroma. Multiple repeated thrusts disrupt the fat and create tunnels. The loosened fat is removed with a powerful suction. Afterward, firm pressure is applied to the wounds until drainage stops. It may take several months for the results to be evident.

NURSING MANAGEMENT: COSMETIC SURGERY

Many cosmetic surgeries are done in day-surgery units or in dermatologist or plastic surgeon in-office surgery suites.

Preoperative Management

A major consideration before surgery relates to informed consent and realistic expectations of what cosmetic surgery can accomplish.[15] Although the HCP should provide this information, reinforce as needed and answer questions and concerns. For instance, a face lift has little or no effect on deep wrinkling of the forehead or deep nasolabial grooves. Before-and-after treatment photographs of similar cases are often useful in helping patients set realistic expectations.

Review the time frame for healing. Explain the oozing, crusting stage of an abrasive procedure so patients can plan time off from work if necessary. Because wound healing may not be complete for 1 year, patients should not expect complete results at once. The patient's age, general health, skin type, and the extent (severity) of the problem being treated affect the final result. We try to correct or control any existing health problem before the procedure.

Postoperative Management

Preventing hematoma formation is important after surgery. Ice packs are applied for the first 24 to 48 hours to reduce swelling and bruising. If the surgery involved a change in the skin's circulation, as in a face lift, carefully monitor for adequate circulation. Warm, pink skin that blanches on pressure shows that adequate circulation is present in the surgical area. Supportive, compressive dressings may be applied early in the postoperative period. Complications can occur if the person smokes or does not follow activity restrictions.

Most cosmetic procedures are not very painful. Usually, mild analgesics are enough to keep patients comfortable.[13] Antibiotics are used at the HCP's discretion. Although not common after cosmetic surgery, assess for signs of infection. Teach patients signs and symptoms of infection. Stress that it is important to report them at once so that treatment can be started.

SKIN GRAFTS

Uses

Skin grafts may be done to protect underlying structures or to reconstruct areas for cosmetic or functional purposes. They can facilitate rapid closure and minimize complications. Ideally, wounds heal by primary intention. However, large wounds, surgically created wounds, trauma, and chronic wounds can result in extensive tissue destruction, making healing by primary intention impossible. In these cases, skin grafting can close the defect. Improved surgical techniques make it possible to graft skin, bone, cartilage, fat, fascia, muscles, and nerves. For cosmetically pleasing results, the color, thickness, texture, and hair-growing nature of skin used for grafting should match the recipient site. See Chapter 26 for more about skin grafting for patients with burn injuries.

The 2 types of traditional skin grafts are free grafts and skin flaps. We describe free grafts by how they supply blood to the grafted skin. One method is to transfer the graft (epidermis and part or all of the dermis) to the recipient site from the donor site. The *autograft* (from the patient's own body) or *isograft* (from an identical twin) revascularizes and becomes fixed to the new site. The other method of free skin grafting is *reconstructive microsurgery.* With the use of an operating microscope, the HCP establishes circulation immediately in the graft by connecting blood vessels in the skin flap to vessels in the recipient site.

Skin flaps involve moving a section of skin and subcutaneous tissue from one part of the body to another with the vascular attachment (Fig. 25.12). Skin flaps are used to cover wounds with a poor vascular bed, provide padding when needed, and cover wounds over cartilage and bone. Patients may need intermediate flap placement if the recipient site is far from the donor site. For instance, a skin flap from the thigh to the head would require an intermediate graft. The flap is advanced to the recipient site when circulation is well established at the intermediate site. Patient's needs and the type of defect determine the type of flap and the route of transfer.

Soft tissue expansion is a technique for providing skin for (1) resurfacing a defect, such as a burn scar; (2) removing a disfiguring mark (e.g., a tattoo); or (3) a preliminary step in breast reconstruction. A subcutaneous tissue expander of a proper size and shape is placed under the skin, usually as an outpatient procedure. Weekly expansion with saline solution can be done in a health care setting or by the patient at home. This expansion procedure is repeated until the skin reaches the size needed for the repair. This may take from several weeks to 3 to 4 months. Once enough skin is available, the old incision is opened, the expander is removed, and the soft tissue is ready to be used as an advancement flap. The tissue expander next to a defect has the primary tissue characteristics, such as color and texture.

There are several engineered skin substitutes (e.g., Apligraf, Dermagraft). Each has its own indications and benefits. Some are 2-layered membranes with dermal and epidermal components. Others are only 1 layer. Bioengineered skin is made from neonatal foreskins and cadavers. It does not contain structures such as blood vessels, hair follicles, sweat glands, or cells such as melanocytes and Langerhans cells.[16] Advantages include ready availability, less infection, application in outpatient settings, minimal scarring, and less pain.

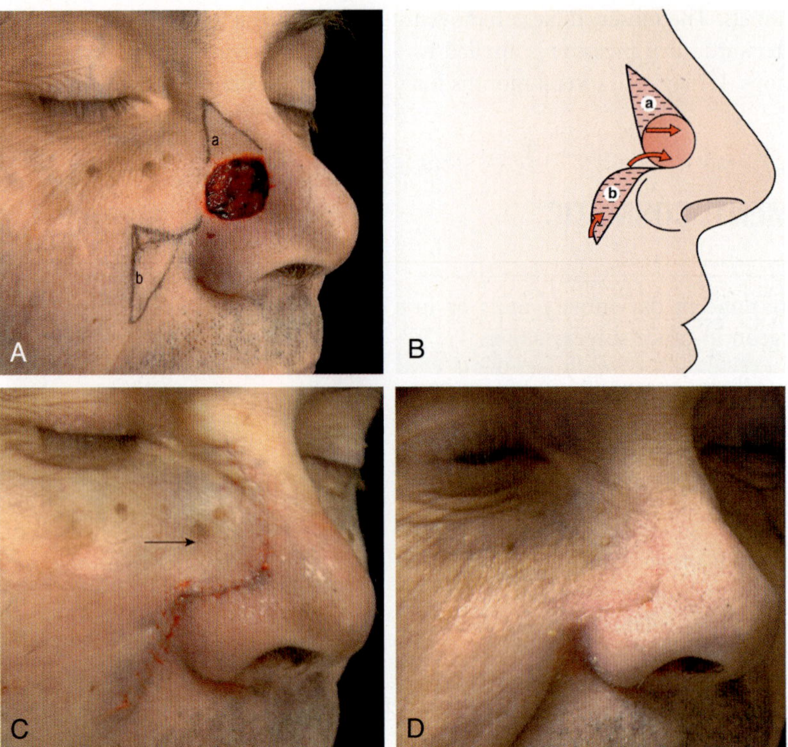

Fig. 25.12 Skin flap. (A) Wound on the nose is covered with a crescent-shaped triangle from the cheek. (B) The crescent fits nicely into the wound. (C) Flap sutured in place. (D) Four-month postoperative appearance. (From Cerroni L, Bolognia JL, Schaffer JV: *Dermatology,* ed 5, St Louis, 2025, Elsevier. Courtesy of the Yale Dermatology Residents' Slide Collection.)

CASE STUDY

Melanoma and Dysplastic Nevi

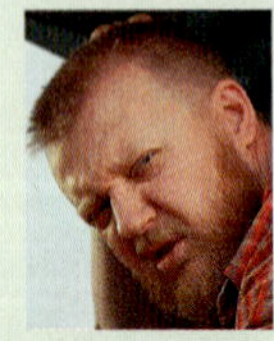

(© Dimedrol68/iStock/Thinkstock.)

Patient Profile

G.L. is a 48-year-old White, fair-skinned male who is a long-distance truck driver. In his leisure time, he enjoys swimming and bicycling. He comes to the clinic because of a changing lesion on his left arm.

Subjective Data

- History of a basal cell cancer (BCC) on his left ear in the last 4 years
- Father treated for metastatic melanoma in the past 2 years
- First noted the lesion 1 month ago when it started changing size
- Anxious that removing the lesion will require extensive, disfiguring surgery

Objective Data

Physical Assessment

- Has a 4-mm lesion, deep brown, scalloped with vaguely defined borders
- 5 dysplastic nevi found on back

Diagnostic Studies

- Excisional biopsy confirmed superficial spreading melanoma
- Sentinel node biopsy results negative
- Determined to be melanoma stage I

Discussion Questions

1. ***Recognize:*** What risk factors for melanoma does G.L. have?
2. ***Recognize:*** What manifestations of melanoma are present?
3. ***Analyze:*** What is the prognosis for a patient with this stage of melanoma?
4. ***Plan:*** What treatment options are available?
5. ***Prioritize:*** What is the priority of care for G.L.?
6. ***Act:*** How would you help G.L. deal with his anxiety over the treatment outcomes?
7. ***Act:*** What would you include in his teaching plan to address future sun exposure?

Answers available at http://evolve.elsevier.com/Lewis/medsurg

BRIDGE TO NCLEX EXAMINATION

The number of the question corresponds to the same-numbered outcome at the beginning of the chapter.

1. Which safe sun practices would the nurse include in a teaching plan for a patient with photosensitivity? (**Select all that apply.**)
   - **a.** Wear protective clothing.
   - **b.** Apply sunscreen liberally and often.
   - **c.** Emphasize the short-term use of a tanning booth.
   - **d.** Avoid exposure to the sun, especially during midday.
   - **e.** Wear any sunscreen that is available from the drugstore.
2. When teaching a patient with melanoma, the nurse recognizes that prognosis is *most* dependent on
   - **a.** the thickness of the lesion.
   - **b.** the degree of asymmetry in the lesion.
   - **c.** the amount of ulceration in the surrounding skin.
   - **d.** how much color variation is present in the lesion.
3. A patient with which disorder is *most* at risk for spreading the disease?
   - **a.** Tinea pedis
   - **b.** Impetigo on the face
   - **c.** Candidiasis of the nails
   - **d.** Psoriasis on the palms and soles
4. A family is diagnosed with pediculosis corporis at a health care center. An appropriate treatment is
   - **a.** applying pyrethrins to the body.
   - **b.** topical application of griseofulvin.
   - **c.** moist compresses applied frequently.
   - **d.** administration of systemic antibiotics.
5. A common site for the lesions caused by atopic dermatitis is the
   - **a.** buttocks.
   - **b.** temporal area.
   - **c.** antecubital space.
   - **d.** plantar surface of the feet.
6. During the assessment of a patient, you note an area of red, sharply defined plaques covered with silvery scales that are mildly itchy on the knees and elbows. You would describe this finding as
   - **a.** lentigo.
   - **b.** psoriasis.
   - **c.** actinic keratosis.
   - **d.** seborrheic keratosis.
7. In teaching a patient who is using topical corticosteroids to treat acute dermatitis, the nurse should tell the patient that (**Select all that apply.**)
   - **a.** the cream form is the most efficient system of delivery.
   - **b.** short-term topical corticosteroid use usually does not cause systemic side effects.
   - **c.** they should use a glove to apply a large amount of topical ointment to prevent further infection.
   - **d.** abruptly stopping the use of topical corticosteroids may cause dermatitis to reappear.
   - **e.** systemic side effects from topical corticosteroids are likely if the patient is malnourished.
8. Important patient teaching after a chemical peel includes
   - **a.** avoiding sun exposure.
   - **b.** applying firm bandages.
   - **c.** limiting vigorous exercise.
   - **d.** using moist heat to relieve discomfort.

1. a, b, d; 2. a; 3. b; 4. a; 5. c; 6. b; 7. b, d; 8. a.

For rationales to these answers and even more NCLEX review questions, visit http://evolve.elsevier.com/Lewis/medsurg.

REFERENCES

To access the References for this chapter, please scan the QR code with a mobile device.

26

Burns

Sylvia Dao

http://evolve.elsevier.com/Lewis/medsurg/

CONCEPTUAL FOCUS

Coping
Fluids and Electrolytes
Gas Exchange
Infection
Nutrition
Pain
Perfusion
Tissue Integrity

LEARNING OUTCOMES

1. Relate the causes of burns to prevention strategies for burn injuries.
2. Distinguish between partial-thickness and full-thickness burns.
3. Apply tools used to determine the severity of burns.
4. Compare the pathophysiology, clinical manifestations, complications, and interprofessional care throughout the burn phases.
5. Outline the nutrition needs of patients with a burn injury.
6. Compare burn wound care techniques and surgical options for partial-thickness and full-thickness burn wounds.
7. Prioritize nursing interventions to manage a burn patient's physiologic and psychosocial needs.
8. Examine the physiologic and psychosocial aspects of burn rehabilitation.
9. Develop a plan of care to prepare the burn patient and caregiver for discharge.

KEY TERMS

chemical burns
debridement
electrical burns
eschar
escharotomy
excision
full-thickness burns
inhalation injuries
partial-thickness burns
thermal burns

The focus of this chapter is the nursing care of patients with burn injuries. In the United States around 398,000 seek treatment each year for burns.[1] Of these, 29,165 people are hospitalized, with 60% receiving care in special burn centers. About 3800 people die each year from their injuries. Burn admissions are most common in summer.

Burns may be caused by thermal injury, chemicals, electric current, or radiation. Injury severity ranges from mild to life threatening. Patients with less serious burns are typically managed in outpatient settings. Those with severe burn injuries are hospitalized in a specialty burn center. The needs of patients with major burns are extensive. They require the expertise of many health care team members. These include nurses, HCPs, occupational therapists (OTs) and physical therapists (PTs), dietitians, social workers, psychologists, and pastoral care. Providing care to patients with burns can be emotionally and physically challenging. It can be rewarding to work as a burn team member and contribute to the recovery of patients with devastating injuries.

As a nurse, you can advocate for and teach about burn prevention (Tables 26.1 and 26.2). Most burn injuries are preventable when safety policies are in place. Coordinated national burn prevention programs in higher-income countries have focused on child-resistant lighters, tap water antiscald devices, stricter building codes, having smoke detectors, and burn safety education.[2]

TABLE 26.1 Common Sources of Burn Injury

Home Hazards
Bathroom and Kitchen
- Water heaters set at 120°F (49°C) or higher
- Microwaved food
- Steam, hot grease, or liquids from cooking

General Household
- Carelessness with cigarettes, matches, candles
- Heat lamps
- Fireplaces (e.g., gas, wood)
- Flammables (e.g., starter fluid, gasoline, kerosene)
- Frayed or defective wiring
- Multiple extension cords per outlet
- Open space heaters
- Outdoor grills (e.g., propane, charcoal)

Occupational Hazards
- Cement
- Chemicals
- Combustible fuels
- Electricity from power lines
- Fertilizers, pesticides
- Hot metals
- Sparks from live electric sources
- Steam pipes
- Tar

TABLE 26.2 PROMOTING POPULATION HEALTH

Strategies to Reduce Burn Injury in Homes

- Install and maintain smoke alarms in your home—on every floor and near all rooms family members sleep in. Test smoke alarms monthly to make sure they are working properly. Use long-life batteries when possible.
- Create and practice a family fire escape plan. Involve kids in the planning. Make sure everyone knows at least 2 ways out of every room. Identify a central meeting place outside.
- Use safe cooking practices, such as never leaving food unattended on the stove. Supervise or restrict children's use of stoves, ovens, and especially microwaves.
- Set your water heater's thermostat to 120°F or lower.
- Store chemicals in approved, labeled containers.
- Replace or repair frayed wiring.
- Avoid outdoor activities during electrical (e.g., lightning) storms.
- Ensure the electrical power source is off before beginning repairs.
- Never use gasoline or other flammable liquids to start a fire.
- Never leave candles unattended or near open windows or curtains.
- Consider a flame-retardant smoking apron for older or "at-risk" people.
- Before placing a child in the bath or getting in the bath yourself, test the water.
- Have a "kid-free zone" of at least 3 feet around the stove and areas where hot food or drink is prepared or carried.
- Never hold a child while you are cooking, drinking a hot liquid, or carrying hot foods or liquids.

BURN INJURY

TYPES OF BURN INJURY

Thermal

Thermal burns are the most common type of burn injury. They are caused by exposure to external heat sources such as flame, scald, or contact with hot material. The severity of the injury depends on the temperature of the burning agent, duration of skin contact, and location and skin thickness. Cold thermal injury, or frostbite, is discussed in Chapter 21.

Chemical

Contact with acids, alkalines, or organic compounds can cause **chemical burns** through absorption, inhalation, or ingestion. Dangerous chemicals are found in homes, businesses, and industries. For example, severe injury can occur with exposure to sulfuric acid, a common chemical used to unclog sinks. Exposure to wet cement, oven cleaners, and heavy industrial cleaners can cause chemical burns. Chemicals such as phenols (chemical disinfectants) and petroleum products (gasoline) cause external burns and systemic toxicity. Acid chemicals cause tissue necrosis. Alkaline chemicals cause liquefaction necrosis, which can be more damaging. Some chemicals will have heat-producing reactions once exposed to the skin, causing superficial blisters or even deep burns. Chemical burns may continue to cause tissue damage long after initial exposure. Severity of chemical burn injury depends on the manner and duration of contact and type, concentration, and quantity of the chemical.

Electrical

Electrical burns result from the intense heat generated from an electric current. Direct damage to nerves and vessels can cause tissue anoxia and cell death. The severity of an electrical injury depends on the voltage, tissue resistance, current pathways, surface area in contact with the current, and length of time that the current flow was sustained (Fig. 26.1). Current that passes through vital organs (e.g., brain, heart, kidneys) causes more life-threatening sequela compared with a current passing through other tissues. The severity can be hard to determine initially because most of the damage is below the skin.

Contact with an electric current can cause muscle contractions strong enough to fracture the long bones and vertebrae. Forceful propulsion of the body from an electrical source can cause injuries such as spinal and limb fractures. For this reason, consider cervical spine injury for all patients with electrical burns.

Electrical injury puts patients at risk for respiratory arrest and metabolic acidosis. An electric shock can cause immediate cardiac standstill or ventricular fibrillation. Massive muscle and blood vessel damage can release myoglobin from injured muscle and hemoglobin from damaged red blood cells (RBCs). Myoglobin can block the renal tubules and cause acute kidney injury (AKI) and rhabdomyolysis (see Chapter 51).

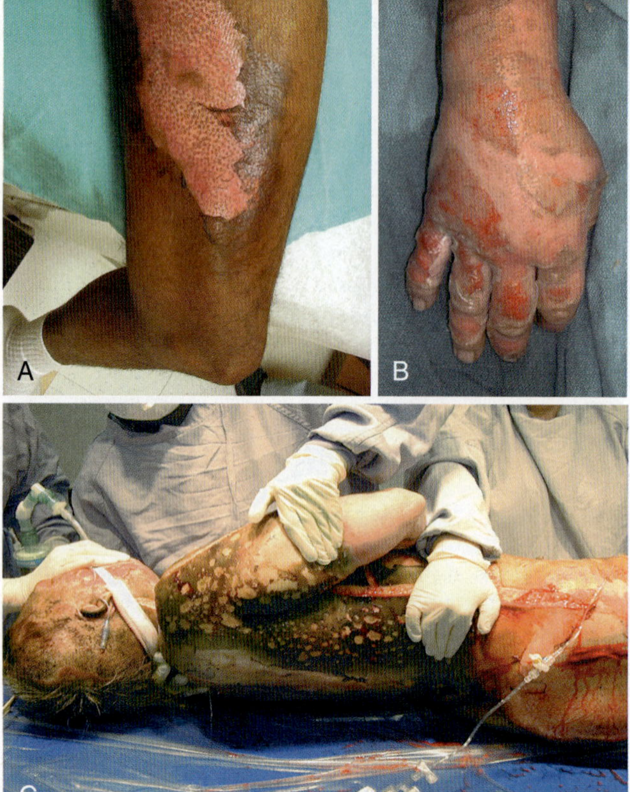

Fig. 26.1 Types of burn injury. (A) Superficial, partial-thickness scald burn to the thigh. (B) Deep, partial-thickness flame burn to the hand. (C) Full-thickness flame burn to posterior chest and arm. (Courtesy Judy Knighton, Toronto, Canada.)

CLASSIFICATION OF BURN INJURY

Severity is determined by (1) depth of burn, (2) extent of burn calculated in percentage of total body surface area (TBSA), (3) location of the burn, (4) preexisting health issues, and (5) associated injuries. The American Burn Association (ABA) provides referral criteria based on injury severity to determine which patients need special treatment in a burn center (Table 26.3).[3]

Burn Depth

Four factors influence burn depth: (1) temperature of the agent, (2) duration of contact, (3) thickness of the epidermis and dermis, and (4) blood supply to the area. Burn injury is determined according to the extent of injury through the epidermis, dermis, and underlying structures. One method describes an injury as first, second, third, or fourth degree. The ABA recommends using the terms *partial-thickness burns* and *full-thickness burns* to classify burns (Figs. 26.2 and 26.3).

TABLE 26.3 Burn Center Referral Criteria

Burn injuries that should be referred to a burn center include the following:

- Partial-thickness burns greater than 10% total body surface area (TBSA).
- Burns that involve the face, hands, feet, genitalia, perineum, or major joints.
- Third-degree burns.
- Electrical burns, including lightning injury.
- Chemical burns.
- Inhalation injury.
- Injury in patients with preexisting health problems that could affect management, prolong recovery, or affect mortality.
- Any patient with burns and concomitant trauma (e.g., fractures) in which the burn injury poses the greatest risk for mortality. In such cases, if the trauma poses a greater immediate risk, the patient may be stabilized in a trauma center before being transferred to a burn unit. HCP judgment is necessary in such situations and would be in concert with triage protocols.
- Burned children in hospitals without qualified personnel or equipment for the care of children.
- Burn injury in patients who will need special social, emotional, or rehabilitative intervention.

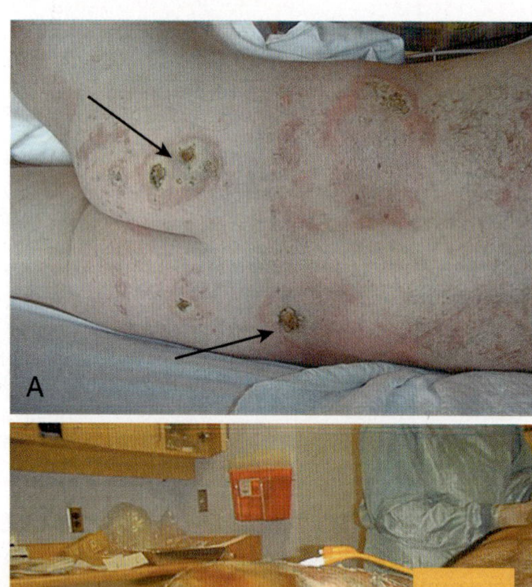

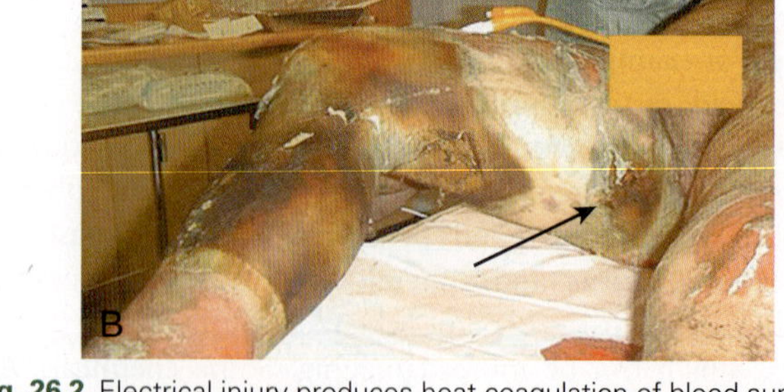

Fig. 26.2 Electrical injury produces heat coagulation of blood supply and contact area as electric current passes through the skin. (A) Back and buttock *(arrows)*. (B) Leg *(arrow)*. (Courtesy Judy Knighton, Toronto, Canada.)

Partial-thickness burns involve the epidermis and sometimes part of the dermis. A **full-thickness injury** occurs if the epidermis and dermis are destroyed. **Eschar** is another name for full-thickness, nonviable burn tissue. Burns can extend beyond the skin and involve tendons, ligaments, muscle, adipose, and bone. Table 26.4 compares the various burn classifications according to the depth of injury.

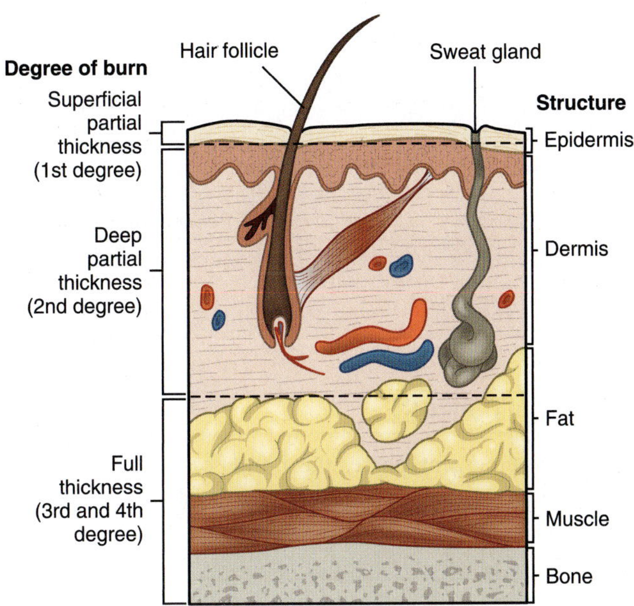

Fig. 26.3 Cross-section of skin showing the depth of burn and structures involved.

Extent of Burn

Calculating the extent of burn injury is critical to ensure appropriate treatment. Incorrect calculation can result in over- or underestimating burn resuscitation. The *Lund-Browder chart* (Fig. 26.4A) and the *Rule of Nines* (Fig. 26.4B) are common methods used to determine burn TBSA. Each has practical limits when taking into consideration sex, age, height, and weight. Emerging technology is available for estimating TBSA.

Location

The location of the burn injury influences the severity. Face, neck, and circumferential torso burns may interfere with gas exchange. Circumferential leathery eschar can restrict chest movement. Edema from inflammation and fluid resuscitation can narrow the airway.

Hand, foot, and joint burns can limit mobility and function. Full-thickness circumferential extremity burns can impair perfusion distal to the injury. Injured hands and feet are challenging to manage because the superficial vascular and nerve supplies require protection. Infection is a risk for patients with ear or nose burns with exposed cartilage because the skin and subcutaneous tissues are thin and there are no blood vessels. Patients with buttocks or perineum burns are at high risk for infection from urine or feces contamination.

Risk Factors

Patients with preexisting chronic diseases have a poorer prognosis for recovery because of the increased demands placed on the body by burn injury. Patients with diabetes or peripheral

TABLE 26.4 Classification of Burn Injury Depth

Classification	Appearance	Possible Cause	Structures Involved
Partial-Thickness Skin Destruction			
Superficial (first-degree) burn	Redness, blanching on pressure, pain and mild swelling, no vesicles or blisters (although after 24 h, skin may blister and peel).	Quick heat flash Superficial sunburn	Superficial epidermal damage with hyperemia. Tactile and pain sensation intact.
Deep (second-degree) burn	Fluid-filled vesicles that are red, shiny, wet (if vesicles have ruptured). Severe pain caused by nerve injury. Mild to moderate edema.	Chemicals Contact burns Electric current Flame Flash Scald Tar, cement	Epidermis and dermis are involved in varying depths. Skin elements, from which epithelial regeneration occurs, remain viable.
Full-Thickness Skin Destruction			
Third- and fourth-degree burns	Dry, waxy white, brown or charred, leathery, or hard skin. Visible thrombosed vessels. Insensitivity to pain because of nerve destruction. Possible muscle, tendon, and bone involvement.	Chemical Electric current Flame Scald Tar, cement	All skin elements and local nerve endings destroyed. Coagulation necrosis present. Surgical intervention required for healing.

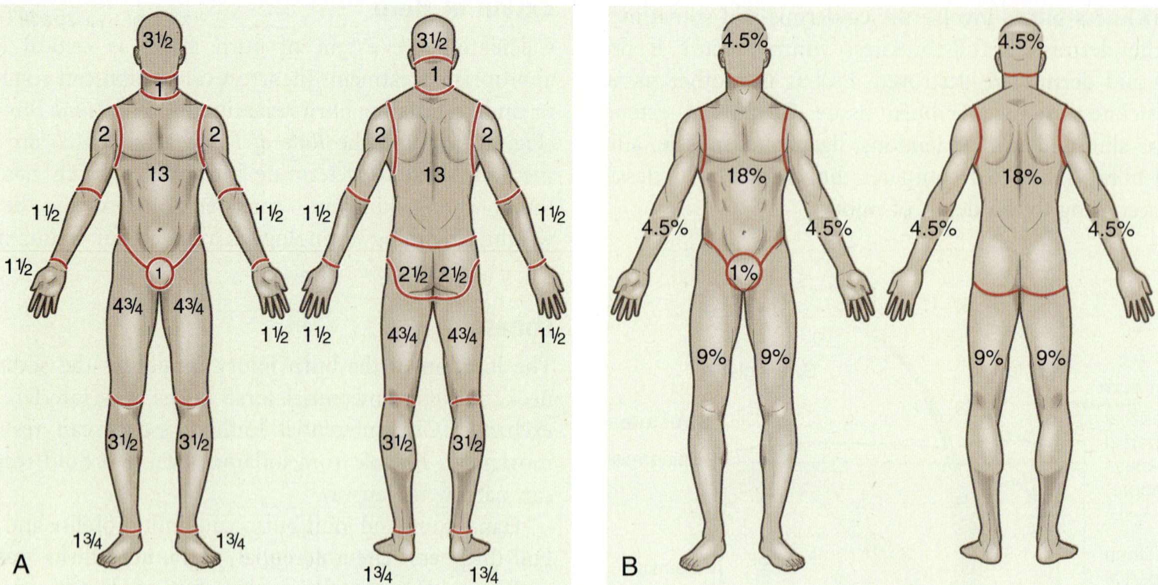

Fig. 26.4 (A) Lund-Browder chart. (B) Rule of Nines chart.

vascular disease are at high risk for delayed healing, especially with foot and leg burns.

PHASES OF BURN MANAGEMENT

Burn management for those with significant injuries can be organized into 4 phases: (1) prehospital and emergency care, (2) emergent (resuscitative), (3) acute (wound healing), and (4) rehabilitative. A nursing care plan for patients with burn injury (eNursing Care Plan 26.1) is available on the website for this chapter.

PREHOSPITAL AND EMERGENCY CARE

Once a burn injury occurs, first responders will arrive at the scene and establish safety. This may involve removing the person from the source of the burn. First responders conduct a primary survey and assess airway, breathing, circulation, disability, and exposure. Airway and breathing are often compromised with severe facial, neck, and torso burns; inhalation injury; and carbon monoxide or cyanide poisoning. Circulation involves stabilizing the heart rate, BP, and temperature. Pulse checks are done in all extremities with an affected burn and to establish large-bore IV access for IV fluid resuscitation. Disability assessment reviews any neurologic problems and/or physical trauma. Exposure assessment requires removing clothing to assess the full extent of injury, in addition to stopping the burning process.

Remember that patients may have other injuries that take priority over the burn injury. First responders must fully explain the circumstances of the injury to the emergency department (ED) team. This is especially important if an injury occurred in an enclosed space or involved hazardous chemicals or a traumatic injury (e.g., fall).

EMERGENT PHASE

During the emergent phase, the health care team prioritizes life-threatening problems. This phase usually lasts up to 72 hours after the initial injury for patients with burns extending over 20% of their bodies. The priority nursing concerns are fluid and electrolyte shifts and gas exchange.

Pathophysiology

Fluid and Electrolyte Shifts

Burn shock is a combination of distributive and hypovolemic shock. It is a significant threat to patients with a major burn (Fig. 26.5). Increased capillary permeability causes a massive shift of fluids that results in a loss of intravascular fluid. Vital signs will begin to change as water, sodium, and plasma proteins move into the interstitial spaces. The progressive loss of protein from the vascular space reduces colloidal osmotic pressure. This causes more fluid to shift out of the vascular space into the interstitial spaces (Fig. 26.6). We call this *third spacing.* Patients may have massive edema and significant wound drainage. Patients can develop AKI and die without adequate resuscitation.

Hemolysis of RBCs from circulating factors released at the time of injury from the burned tissue affects perfusion. Thrombosis in the capillaries of burned tissue causes the loss of additional circulating RBCs. A high hematocrit occurs from hemoconcentration caused by fluid loss. Hematocrit levels will return to normal after burn shock resolves.

Major electrolyte shifts of sodium and potassium occur during this phase. A potassium shift develops first when injured cells and hemolyzed RBCs release potassium into the circulation. Sodium rapidly moves to the interstitial spaces (Fig. 26.7).

PATHOPHYSIOLOGY MAP

BURN

↑ Vascular permeability

Edema → ↓ Blood volume

↓ Intravascular volume → ↑ Hematocrit → ↑ Viscosity

↑ Peripheral resistance

Burn shock

Fig. 26.5 At the time of major burn injury, capillary permeability increases. All fluid components of the blood begin to leak into the interstitium, causing edema and a decreased blood volume. Hematocrit increases. Blood becomes more viscous. The combination of decreased blood volume and increased viscosity increases peripheral resistance. Burn shock, a type of hypovolemic shock, rapidly ensues and, if not corrected, can result in death.

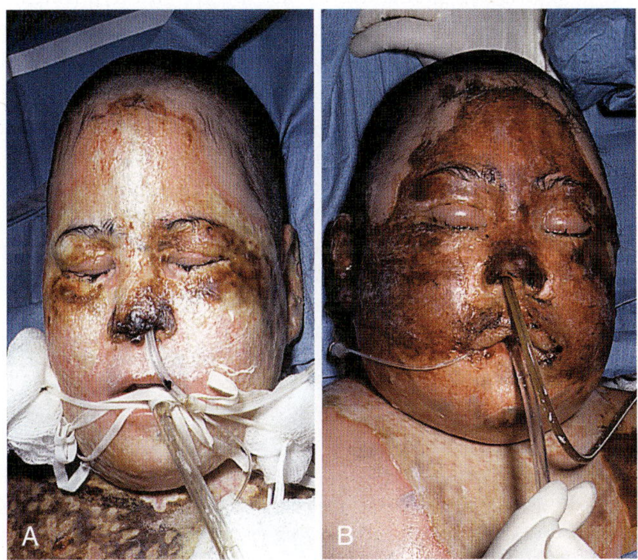

Fig. 26.6 (A) Facial edema before fluid resuscitation. (B) Facial edema after 24 hours. (Courtesy Judy Knighton, Toronto, Canada.)

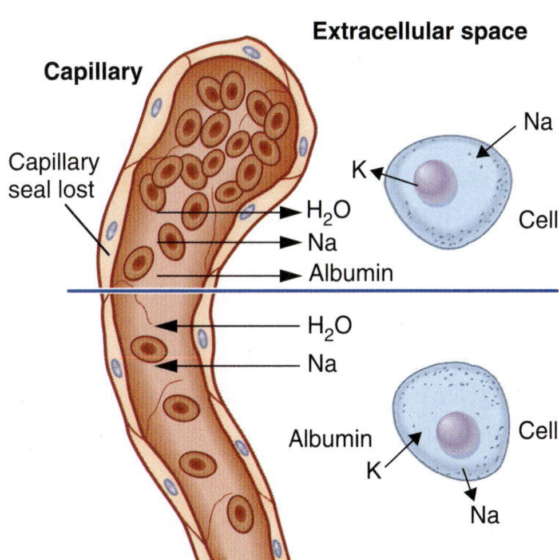

Fig. 26.7 The effects of burn shock are shown above the *blue line*. As the capillary seal is lost, interstitial edema develops. Cellular integrity is altered. Sodium *(Na)* moves into the cell in abnormal amounts, and potassium *(K)* leaves the cell. The shifts after the resolution of burn shock are shown below the *blue line*. Water and sodium move back into the circulating volume through the capillary. Albumin stays in the interstitium. Potassium is transported into the cell, and sodium is transported out as the cellular integrity returns.

The emergent phase ends once capillary membrane permeability is restored after successful fluid resuscitation. Interstitial fluid gradually returns to the vascular space (Fig. 26.7). Potassium levels decline and sodium levels increase.

Inflammation and Healing

Burn injury causes coagulation necrosis. Neutrophils and monocytes accumulate at the site of injury. Fibroblasts and newly formed collagen fibrils appear and begin wound repair within the first 6 to 12 hours after injury.

A burn injury challenges the immune system by changing the skin's barrier to invading organisms. Bone marrow depression occurs and circulating levels of immunoglobulins decrease. Defects occur in white blood cell (WBC) function. The inflammatory cytokine cascade is triggered by tissue damage. This impairs the function of lymphocytes, monocytes, and neutrophils, and the patient is at high risk of infection.

Clinical Manifestations

Seeing patients with major burns can be overwhelming because of the extent of injury and the smell of burned tissue and hair. Patients are normally alert and able to answer questions during admission or until intubated (if there is respiratory compromise). Monitor cognition and report any changes. Unconsciousness or altered mental status usually results from hypoxia caused by inhalation injury. Other possibilities include head trauma, substance use, or the side effects of sedation or pain medication. Patients are often frightened and need your calm reassurance. Give patients simple explanations of what to expect.

Often patients will shiver from heat loss, anxiety, or pain. Provide warm blankets and increase the room temperature or turn on heat lamps. Full-thickness burns are painless because nerves in the dermis are destroyed. Partial-thickness burns are very painful.

Complications

The respiratory, cardiovascular, and renal systems are most susceptible to complications during the emergent phase.

Respiratory

Inhalation injuries from breathing noxious chemicals or hot air will damage the respiratory tract. Three types of inhalation injuries can occur:

- Injury from exposure to toxic gases, including carbon monoxide and/or cyanide
- Above-the-glottis injury from direct heat or chemicals, causing severe mucosal edema
- Below-the-glottis injury leading to airway inflammation and edema, causing atelectasis and pneumonia

The severity of inhalation injury ranges from mild to severe (Table 26.5). Rapid initial and ongoing assessment is critical. Airway compromise and pulmonary edema can quickly develop within hours of injury. Patients may need a fiberoptic bronchoscopy and carboxyhemoglobin blood levels to confirm a suspected inhalation injury. Patients exposed to carbon monoxide from smoke will have elevated carboxyhemoglobin levels. Examine sputum for carbon particles. Watch for signs of respiratory distress, such as increased agitation, anxiety, restlessness, or a change in the rate or character of breathing. Symptoms may not be present at first.

Patients with preexisting lung disease are more likely to develop a respiratory infection. Pneumonia is a common complication of major burns. It is the leading cause of death in patients with an inhalation injury.

Cardiovascular

Cardiac output is often decreased in patients undergoing burn shock resuscitation. Other complications can affect perfusion besides burn shock. Deep circumferential burns and subsequent edema formation can impair blood flow to the extremities. If untreated, ischemia, paresthesia, and necrosis can occur. An **escharotomy** (an incision through the full-thickness eschar) may be done to restore circulation to compromised extremities or improve chest expansion (Fig. 26.8).

Patients are at risk for venous thromboembolism (VTE), especially if other risk factors are present. These include advanced age, obesity, extensive or lower extremity burns, concomitant lower extremity trauma, and prolonged immobility. It is recommended that patients receive low-molecular-weight heparin (enoxaparin) or low-dose unfractionated heparin if there are no contraindications. Apply intermittent pneumatic compression devices if the patient is immobile.

TABLE 26.5 EMERGENCY MANAGEMENT

Inhalation Injury

Etiology	Assessment Findings	Interventions
• Exposure of the respiratory tract to intense heat or flames • Inhalation of noxious chemicals, smoke, or carbon monoxide (CO) • Being trapped in an enclosed space, being in an explosion, or having clothing catch fire	• Altered mental status, including confusion, coma • Carbonaceous sputum • Cherry-red skin color (CO levels >20%) • Coughing • Dark oral or nasal membranes • ↓ O_2 saturation • Difficulty swallowing • Dysrhythmias • Hoarseness • Irritation of upper airways or burning pain in throat or chest • Productive cough with black, gray, or bloody sputum • Rapid, shallow respirations • Restlessness, anxiety • Singed nasal or facial hair • Smoky breath	• If unresponsive, assess circulation, airway, and breathing. • If responsive, monitor the airway, breathing, and circulation. • Assess for a thermal burn. • Provide 100% humidified O_2. • Anticipate endotracheal intubation and mechanical ventilation with inhalation injury. • Monitor vital signs, level of consciousness, O_2 saturation, heart rhythm. • Obtain ABGs, carboxyhemoglobin levels, and chest x-ray. • Remove nonadherent clothing, jewelry, glasses, or contact lenses (if the face was exposed). • Establish IV access with 2 large-bore catheters if burn >20% TBSA. • Begin fluid replacement. • Insert indwelling urinary catheter if burn >20% TBSA and monitor urine output. • Elevate burned limb(s) above the heart to decrease edema. • Give IV analgesia and assess effectiveness frequently. • Identify and treat other injuries (e.g., fractures, pneumothorax, head injury). • Cover concurrent burned areas with dry dressings or clean sheets. • Initiate pain management.

ABGs, Arterial blood gases; *TBSA,* total body surface area.

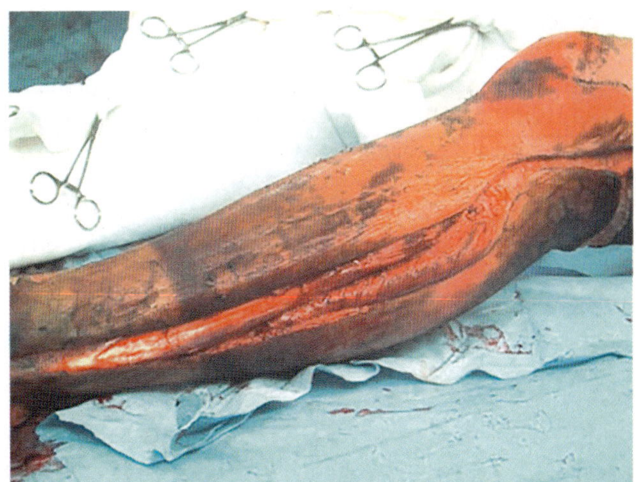

Fig. 26.8 Escharotomies of the lower leg. (From Sheridan R: Medical aspects of trauma and burns. In Goldman L, Schafer A, editors: *Goldman-Cecil medicine,* ed 26, Philadelphia, 2020, Elsevier.)

Renal

The most common renal complication during the emergent phase is AKI.[4] If the patient becomes hypovolemic, blood flow to the kidneys will decrease, causing renal ischemia. If this continues, AKI will develop.

With full-thickness and major electrical burns, released myoglobin (from muscle cell breakdown) and hemoglobin (from RBC breakdown) can block renal tubules. Monitor the adequacy of fluid replacement because this can prevent tubule obstruction.

INTERPROFESSIONAL AND NURSING MANAGEMENT: EMERGENT PHASE

In the emergent phase, survival depends on a rapid and thorough assessment, analyzing findings, planning and prioritizing interventions, and evaluating the results. We initially focus on airway management, fluid and electrolyte balance, wound care, and nutrition (Table 26.6). Patients with significant burns are admitted or transferred to a burn unit after being stabilized.

Airway Management

Work with respiratory therapists to monitor the patient's airway and breathing (Table 26.6). Place patients in a high Fowler's position unless contraindicated (e.g., spinal injury). The treatment for inhalation injury includes administering 100% O_2. Other treatments may include hyperbaric oxygen, aerosolized heparin, N-acetylcysteine, and albuterol. Encourage deep breathing and coughing every hour. Reposition patients every 1 to 2 hours. Suction if needed. Draw arterial blood gases (ABGs) to assess the adequacy of gas exchange. Initiate telemetry. Monitor pulse oximetry and capnography. Evaluate the response to interventions. Report adverse responses or declines to HCPs.

In general, patients with significant face and neck burns need intubation within 1 to 2 hours after injury. Early intubation prevents the need for an emergency cricothyrotomy. Other patients will need intubation if respiratory distress develops. Patients with facial burns need frequent assessment of the endotracheal tube because of swelling. Alternative securement devices, such as twill ties, may be necessary. Measure endotracheal tube placement at the teeth/gums and not the lip because of edema. Extubation may occur at the end of the emergent phase when airway edema resolves. This is usually 3 to 5 days after the initial injury. Patients with extensive lung damage may be intubated for many weeks or months.

! SAFETY ALERT

Pulse CO-Oximetry Monitoring

- Standard pulse oximetry (SpO_2) does not distinguish oxyhemoglobin from carboxyhemoglobin.
- A patient with CO poisoning will have normal SpO_2 readings despite high carboxyhemoglobin levels.
- For patients with suspected or confirmed CO poisoning, use a pulse CO oximetry (SpCO) device.

Fluid Therapy

Nurses have many responsibilities during fluid resuscitation. Insert at least 2 large-bore IVs when burns are greater than 20% TBSA. The HCP may elect to insert a central line. It is critical to select IVs that can handle large volumes of fluid.

You will need to estimate the TBSA of the burn wounds to calculate the initial IV fluid requirements for resuscitation (Fig. 26.4). Use the ABA formula (Table 26.7) or Parkland formula (www.mdcalc.com/parkland-formula-for-burns) to calculate fluid needs for the first 24 hours after injury.[5] Remember formulas are estimates. Fluids are titrated based on the response. Crystalloid solutions and sometimes colloids (albumin) are used for resuscitation. Anticipate an indwelling urinary catheter for patients with burns greater than 20% TBSA. Monitor patients for early signs of fluid overload, especially older patients or those with heart, lung, or kidney problems. Assess for the adequacy of fluid resuscitation hourly using urine output and cardiac parameters and report changes to the HCP:

- *Urine output for adults:* 0.5 to 1 mL/kg/h; *for children:* 1 to 1.5 mg/kg/h.
- *Cardiac parameters:* Mean arterial pressure (MAP) greater than 65 mm Hg, systolic BP greater than 90 mm Hg, heart rate less than 120 beats/min. MAP and BP are best measured by an arterial line. A manual BP is often invalid because of edema and vasoconstriction.

Patients with an electrical injury have greater-than-normal fluid needs to prevent AKI. They often require an osmotic diuretic (mannitol) to increase urine output and overcome hemoglobinuria or myoglobinuria. Continuous renal replacement therapy may be needed.

TABLE 26.6 Interprofessional Care

Burn Injury

	Emergent Phase	Acute Phase	Rehabilitation Phase
Fluid Therapy	• Assess fluid needs. • Begin IV fluid replacement (Table 26.7). • Insert an indwelling urinary catheter. • Monitor urine output.	• Continue to replace fluids, depending on the patient's clinical response. • Monitor for electrolyte imbalance.	
Respiratory Care	• Assess oxygenation needs and respiratory status. • Provide supplemental O_2 as needed. • Intubate if needed. • Encourage deep breathing and coughing. • Reposition every 1 to 2 h. • Initiate telemetry.	• Continue to monitor oxygenation needs and respiratory status. • Monitor for signs of complications (e.g., pneumonia).	
Wound Care	• Start daily shower and wound care. • Debride as needed. • Assess the extent and depth of burns. • Give tetanus toxoid or tetanus antitoxin.	• Continue daily shower and wound care. • Continue debridement (if needed). • Assess wound daily and adjust dressing protocols as needed. • Provide temporary or permanent allografts and care for donor sites. • Administer ordered antibiotics.	• Assess risk for scarring and implement restorative measures. • Continue to teach patients and caregivers about wound care. • Discuss possible reconstructive surgery.
Nutrition	• Assess and provide diet to support wound healing.	• Continue to assess diet to support wound healing. • Administer drugs to prevent stress ulcers.	
Pain	• Assess and manage pain and anxiety.	• Continue to assess for and treat pain and anxiety.	
Physical and Occupational Therapy	• Place the patient in a position that prevents contracture formation and reduces edema. • Assess the need for splints.	• Begin a daily therapy program for maintaining ROM. • Assess the need for splints and anti contracture positioning. • Encourage and aid patients with self-care as needed.	• Continue to prevent or minimize contractures. • Continue to encourage and aid the patient in resuming self-care.
Psychosocial Care	• Provide support to patients and caregivers during the initial crisis phase.	• Provide ongoing support, counseling, and teaching to patients and caregivers about physical and emotional aspects of care and recovery. • Begin discharge planning.	• Prepare for discharge home or transfer to a rehabilitation hospital. • Discuss the possible need for home care nursing.

CHECK YOUR PRACTICE

You are admitting an adult with thermal burns who weighs 72 kg and has 45% TBSA burn. Calculate the fluid requirements for the first 24 h using the ABA formula (2 mL/kg/% total body surface area burn).

Wound Care

Partial-thickness burn wounds appear pink to cherry-red and are wet and shiny with serous exudate. These painful wounds may or may not have intact blisters. Superficial partial-thickness burns will heal within several weeks. Deep partial-thickness burns may take months to heal and require surgical grafting. Full-thickness burns can be white, red, brown, or charred. Patients may not have pain because the nerves in the dermis are destroyed. Large full-thickness burns require skin grafts.

Patients will shower or receive a trolley bath (Fig. 26.9). Patients can lose body heat through their wounds. Prevent hypothermia by keeping the room warm (around 85°F [29.4°C]) and implement other warming measures. Always wear personal protective equipment (PPE) (e.g., disposable hats, masks, gowns, gloves) when burn wounds are exposed.

Use a mild cleanser and washcloths to perform cleansing and gentle wound debridement. **Debridement** is the removal of necrotic tissue from the wound bed. Skilled nurses will use

TABLE 26.7 Fluid Resuscitation Formulas

American Burn Association

2 mL lactated Ringer's solution per kilogram (kg) of body weight per percentage of total body surface area (% TBSA) burned = Total fluid requirements for the first 24 h after burn injury

Application

- ½ of the total in the first 8 h
- ¼ of the total in the second 8 h
- ¼ of the total in third 8 h

Example

For a 70-kg patient with a 50% TBSA burn: 2 mL × 70 × 50 (TBSA burned) = 7000 mL in 24 h

- ½ of the total in first 8 h = 3500 mL (438 mL/h)
- ¼ of the total in second 8 h = 1750 mL (219 mL/h)
- ¼ of the total in third 8 h = 1750 mL (219 mL/h)

American Burn Association Consensus Fluid Resuscitation

2 to 4 mL lactated Ringer's solution per kilogram (kg) of body weight per percentage of total body surface area (% TBSA) burned = Total fluid requirements for the first 24 h after burn

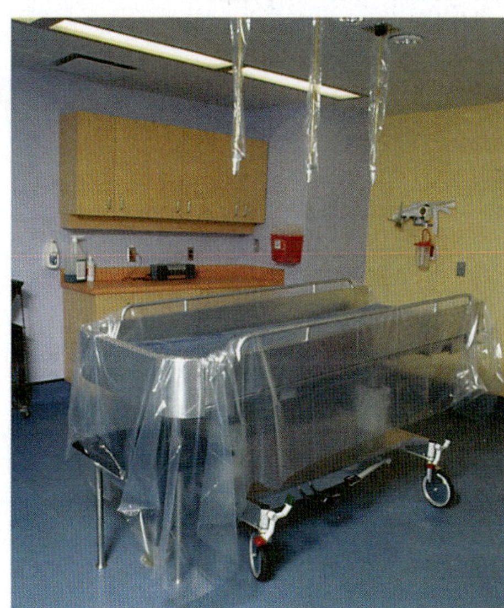

Fig. 26.9 Shower trolley. Showering presents an opportunity for PT and wound care. (Courtesy Judy Knighton, Toronto, Canada.)

scissors and forceps to remove loose burn tissue and blisters. Extensive surgical debridement occurs in the operating room (Fig. 26.10). Nonsurgical debridement relies on collagenase and bromelain-based enzyme ointments for *enzymatic debridement.* The enzymes break down necrotic or nonviable tissue. Once bathing and wound cleansing are finished, assess the skin and burns and reestimate the total burn percentage.

Many types of dressings and topical agents are available. These include antimicrobial creams, hydrocolloids, alginates, hydrogels, collagen, and hyaluronic acid (Fig. 26.11). HCPs will prescribe topical agents based on the burn depth, bacterial

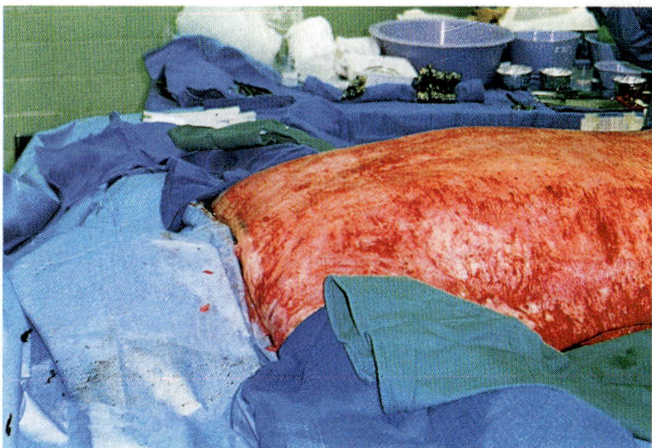

Fig. 26.10 Surgical debridement of full-thickness burns is necessary to prepare the wound for grafting. (Courtesy Judy Knighton, Toronto, Canada.)

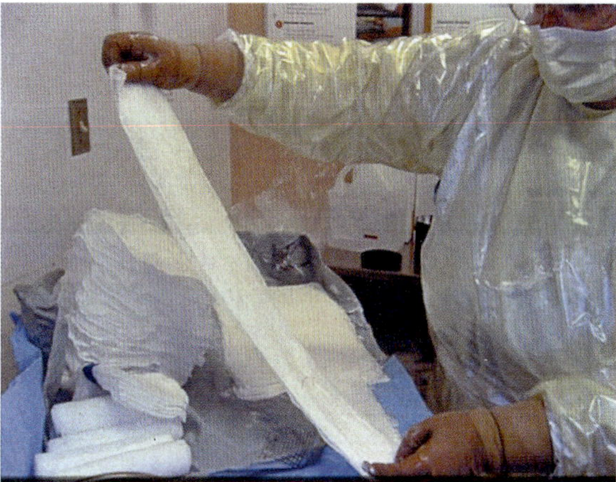

Fig. 26.11 Application of silver sulfadiazine cream to saline-moistened gauze. (Courtesy Judy Knighton, Toronto, Canada.)

count, and cost. Some burns are treated with a topical ointment and left open to the air. Others will be dressed with various products and covered with secondary dressings such as gauze. Dressing change frequency depends on the severity of the burn and the type of dressing. Some dressings are changed twice daily. Others are changed every 5 to 7 days. We may place Ace wraps or tubular elastic dressings to hold burn dressings in place and reduce edema.

Provide adequate analgesia to manage pain during wound cleansing, debridement, and dressing application. This may require anesthesia-assisted dressing changes or moderate sedation. Anticipate patients finding wound care to be physically and emotionally demanding. Provide emotional support during this activity.

! SAFETY ALERT

Drug Allergy Check

- Check for allergies to sulfa, as many burn antimicrobial creams contain sulfa.

Other Care Measures

Certain parts of the body (e.g., face, eyes, hands, arms, ears, perineum) need vigilant nursing care. The face is vascular and can become quite swollen. Facial burns are often covered with ointments and gauze but not wrapped to limit pressure on delicate facial structures. An eye examination should occur soon after admission for all patients with facial burns. Periorbital edema can temporarily prevent eye opening and is often frightening for patients. Assure them the swelling is not permanent. Instill artificial tears into the eyes for moisture and comfort.

Keep the ears free from pressure because of their poor vascularization and the tendency to become infected. Do not use pillows for patients with ear burns. The pressure on the cartilage may cause chondritis. Raise the head using a rolled towel placed under the shoulders to avoid pressure necrosis. Follow the same strategy for patients with neck burns to hyperextend the neck and prevent neck contracture.

Extend burned hands and arms and raise them on pillows or foam wedges to reduce edema. The PT will evaluate and provide splints to keep burned joints in positions of function. Remove the splints often and inspect the skin and bony prominences to avoid pressure areas. Collaborate with the PT/OT to schedule therapy sessions. PTs and OTs can provide range-of-motion (ROM) exercises during dressing changes and throughout the day. ROM helps shift interstitial fluid back into the vascular bed, maintain function, and prevent skin and joint contractures.

Keep the perineum clean and dry after voiding or bowel movements. Remove indwelling catheters used for fluid resuscitation as soon as possible. Consider using a fecal diversion device for patients with frequent, loose stools.

Drug Therapy

Analgesics and Sedatives

Provide analgesics. Early in the postburn period, give IV pain medications. Common drugs used for pain control are shown in Table 26.8. It is standard practice to incorporate multimodal strategies, which include opioids, nonopioids, and nonpharmacologic approaches, in the care of serious burn injuries.[6] When managed appropriately, patients should obtain adequate pain relief.

Remember that the pain level may not directly correlate with the extent and depth of the burn. Analgesic needs vary among patients. Sedatives/hypnotics and antidepressants given with analgesics help with anxiety, insomnia, or depression. Include nondrug methods such as imagery, music, and digital technology distraction.

Tetanus Immunization

Patients routinely receive tetanus toxoid because of the risk of exposure to *Clostridium tetani.* Tetanus immunoglobulin would be considered if the patient has not received an active immunization within 10 years before the burn injury. Tetanus immunization is discussed in Table 21.6.

TABLE 26.8 Drug Therapy

Burns

Drugs	Purpose
Analgesics	
morphine	Relieve pain
hydromorphone (Dilaudid)	
fentanyl (Sublimaze)	
oxycodone and acetaminophen (Percocet)	
nonsteroidal antiinflammatory (e.g., ketorolac)	
adjuvant analgesics (e.g., gabapentin)	
Anticoagulants	
enoxaparin (Lovenox)	Prevent venous thromboembolism
heparin	
Antidepressants	
citalopram (Celexa)	Reduce depression, improve mood
sertraline (Zoloft)	
Gastrointestinal Support	
aluminum hydroxide and magnesium hydroxide (Maalox)	Neutralize stomach acid
calcium carbonate and magnesium carbonate (Mylanta)	
esomeprazole (Nexium)	Decrease stomach acid and risk for stress ulcer
cimetidine (Tagamet)	
nystatin	Prevent overgrowth of *Candida albicans* in oral mucosa
Nutrition Support	
Minerals: zinc, iron (ferrous sulfate)	Promote cell integrity and hemoglobin formation
Vitamins A, C, E, and multivitamin	Promote wound healing
Sedatives/Hypnotics	
lorazepam (Ativan)	Reduce anxiety
midazolam (Versed)	Provide short-acting amnesic effects
zolpidem (Ambien)	Promote sleep

Nutrition Therapy

A hypermetabolic state proportional to the size of the wound occurs after a major burn injury. Resting metabolic rate may increase by 50% to 100% above normal.[7] The core temperature increases. Catecholamine release stimulates catabolism and heat production. Massive catabolism occurs with protein breakdown and increased gluconeogenesis. Failure to supply adequate calories and protein leads to weight loss, malnutrition, and delayed healing.

Early nutrition support within several hours of the burn injury can reduce complications and mortality, optimize burn wound healing, and minimize the negative effects of hypermetabolism and catabolism. Dietitians will calculate nutrition needs and recommend supplements or enteral nutrition (EN). Nonintubated patients with a burn of less than 20% TBSA will usually be able to consume enough calories to meet their nutrition needs. Work with the dietitian to provide a high-protein, high-carbohydrate diet. Patients with major burns may develop an ileus and need a gastrojejunal tube for decompression and EN. Calorie-containing nutrition supplements are given to meet caloric needs. We may give vitamin supplements (Table 26.8).

Intubated patients and those with larger burns need more support. Early EN, usually with smaller-bore tubes, preserves GI function, increases intestinal blood flow, and promotes optimal conditions for wound healing. In general, begin feedings slowly at a rate of 20 to 40 mL/h and increase to the goal rate within 24 to 48 hours. Assess bowel sounds every 8 hours.

ACUTE PHASE

The acute phase of burn care begins with the mobilization of interstitial fluid and subsequent diuresis and continues until wounds are nearly healed. This may take weeks or months depending on the burn severity and the response to treatment.

Pathophysiology

Oxygenation problems may resolve. However, sometimes inhalation injuries will not resolve for many days, weeks, or months. Vital signs are more stable. Wound healing begins as WBCs surround the burn wound and phagocytosis occurs. Necrotic tissue begins to slough. Unfortunately, many patients with major burns will have complications during this phase. They may now become more aware of the enormity of the situation.

Clinical Manifestations

Partial-thickness wounds begin to heal at the wound margins. Epithelial buds, from the hair follicles and glands in the dermal bed, eventually close the wound. Healing is spontaneous and usually occurs within 10 to 21 days. Patients often have more pain during the acute phase because of repeated dressing changes, therapy exercises, opioid tolerance, fatigue, and reduced coping ability.

Fluid and Electrolytes

The body is trying to reestablish fluid and electrolyte balance in the initial acute phase. Monitor serum electrolyte levels and assess for manifestations of electrolyte imbalances (see Chapter 17).

Hyponatremia can develop from excess GI suction and diarrhea. *Dilutional hyponatremia* may occur from excess water intake. Offer fluids other than water, such as juice or nutrition supplements. *Hypernatremia* may occur after successful fluid resuscitation if large amounts of hypertonic solutions were given. EN or inappropriate fluid administration can cause hypernatremia. Restricting sodium in IV fluids and EN can reduce levels.

Hyperkalemia may occur if patients have renal failure, adrenocortical insufficiency, or deep muscle injury (e.g., electrical burn). Damaged cells release large amounts of potassium. Dysrhythmias and arrest can occur. *Hypokalemia* occurs with vomiting, diarrhea, prolonged GI suction, and IV therapy without potassium supplements. Patients lose potassium through their burn wounds.

Complications

Infection

A burn injury destroys the body's first line of defense: the skin. The person's normal flora will quickly colonize the burn wound. The WBCs have functional defects. Patients are immunosuppressed for many months after the burn injury.

Local inflammation, induration, and sometimes purulent drainage can be seen at the burn wound margins. Watch for signs and symptoms of systemic infection, including hypothermia or hyperthermia, increased heart and respiratory rate, decreased BP, and decreased urine output. Patients may have mild confusion, chills, malaise, and loss of appetite. The WBC count can rise over 20,000/μL (20×10^9/L). The causative organisms of sepsis are usually gram-negative bacteria (e.g., *Pseudomonas, Proteus*), increasing the risk for septic shock. Sepsis is a leading cause of death in patients with major burns. It may lead to multiple organ dysfunction syndrome (see Chapter 42).

Fungal infections may develop in the mucous membranes (mouth, genitalia) because of systemic antibiotic therapy and low resistance. In severe cases, fungal infections spread to the blood. The offending organism is usually *Candida albicans.* Administer ordered antifungals such as nystatin and fluconazole.

Cardiovascular and Respiratory

The same cardiovascular and respiratory complications present in the emergent phase may continue into the acute phase of care. New problems, such as pneumonia, might arise, requiring prompt intervention.

Neurologic

Neurologic problems may result because of severe hypoxia from respiratory injuries or as a complication from electrical injuries. Other causes of neurologic problems include electrolyte imbalance, stress, cerebral edema, sepsis, sleep problems, and the use of analgesics and antianxiety drugs.

Some patients may become disoriented, withdraw, or be combative. They may hallucinate or have frequent nightmare-like episodes. Delirium is more acute at night and occurs more often in older patients. Use a screening tool to diagnose delirium (see Table 64.19). Implement measures to prevent delirium. Orient and reassure patients who are confused or agitated. This state is usually transient, lasting from 1 to 2 days to several weeks. However, some complications can last for years and be serious.

Musculoskeletal

The musculoskeletal system is especially prone to complications during the acute phase. As the burns begin to heal and scar tissue forms, the skin is less supple and pliant. ROM may be affected. Skin and joint contractures can occur. Because of pain, patients may prefer a flexed position. Have them stretch and move the burned body parts as much as possible. PT and OT are important. Consult with PTs or OTs about positioning and splinting to prevent or reduce contractures.

Gastrointestinal

Gastrointestinal (GI) complications may develop. Diarrhea may result from the use of EN or antibiotics. Constipation can occur as a side effect of opioids, decreased mobility, and a low-fiber diet. The stress response can decrease blood flow to the GI tract. A stress ulcer may occur.

Aim to prevent stress ulcers by providing feeding as soon as possible after the burn injury. Antacids, H_2-histamine blockers (e.g., cimetidine), and proton pump inhibitors (e.g., omeprazole) are used prophylactically to neutralize stomach acids and inhibit histamine and the secretion of hydrochloric acid (Table 26.8). Patients with major burns may have occult blood in their stools. Monitor them for GI bleeding.

Endocrine

Watch for transient increases in glucose levels because of stress-mediated cortisol and catecholamine release. There is increased mobilization of glycogen stores and gluconeogenesis. Subsequently, glucose is produced with an increase in insulin production. However, insulin's effectiveness decreases because of relative insulin insensitivity. This results in a high glucose level. The increased caloric intake needed to meet metabolic requirements can increase glucose levels. This stress-induced condition reverses as metabolic demands are met and less stress is placed on the entire system. Monitor glucose levels and administer insulin as needed.

INTERPROFESSIONAL AND NURSING MANAGEMENT: ACUTE PHASE

Major interventions in the acute phase are (1) wound care, (2) excision and grafting, (3) pain management, (4) PT and OT, and (5) nutrition therapy.

Wound Care

The goals of wound care are to (1) prevent infection by cleansing and debriding the area of necrotic tissue that would promote bacterial growth and (2) promote wound reepithelialization and/or successful skin grafting. Wound care consists of ongoing observation, assessment, cleansing, debridement, and dressing reapplication. Dressing changes, topical antimicrobial therapy, graft care, and donor site care are done as often as needed, depending on the topical cream or dressing.

Excision and Grafting

Many patients, especially those with major burns, have early excision and grafting. With **excision**, devitalized tissue (eschar) is surgically removed down to the subcutaneous tissue or fascia. Surgical excision can result in massive blood loss.

An autograft uses the patient's skin for grafting. Autografts can be full thickness or split thickness. A *dermatome* is used to remove donor skin for grafting (Fig. 26.12B). The abdomen

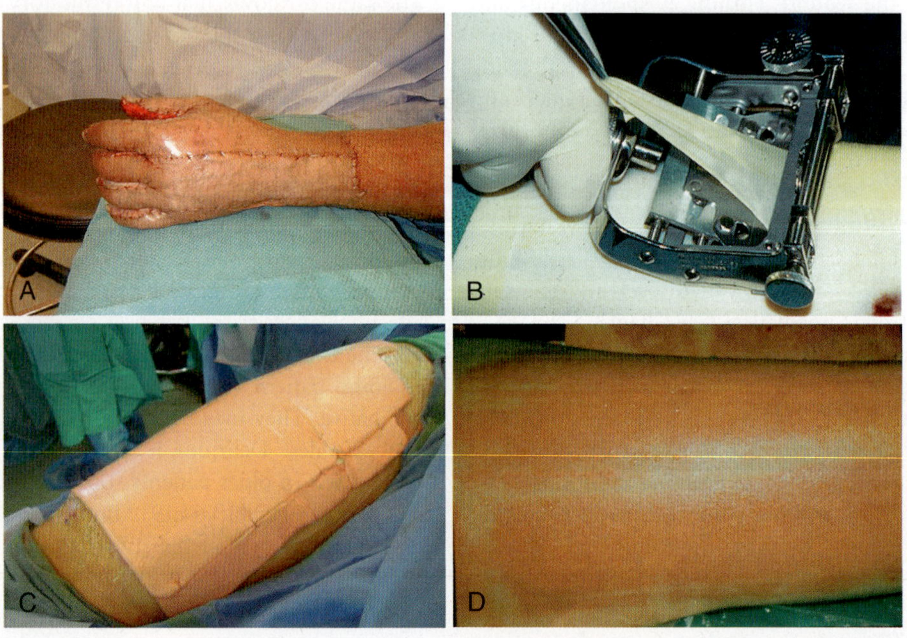

Fig. 26.12 (A) Freshly applied split-thickness sheet skin graft to the hand. (B) Split-thickness skin graft harvested from a patient's thigh using a dermatome. (C) Donor site is covered with a hydrophilic foam dressing after harvesting. (D) Healed donor site. (Courtesy Judy Knighton, Toronto, Canada.)

and thighs are common donor sites. Donor skin can be meshed to allow for greater wound coverage. Sometimes it is applied as an unmeshed sheet for a better cosmetic result when grafting the face, neck, and hands. Sometimes wounds are covered with a biologic dressing or allograft for temporary coverage until permanent grafting can occur (Table 26.9).

The graft is placed on clean, viable tissue to achieve good adherence. Grafts can be stapled or sutured into place (Fig. 26.12A). Negative pressure wound therapy dressings are often placed on top of skin grafts to optimize adherence of the graft to the excised wound bed. Outer occlusive dressings apply just enough pressure to promote adherence of the graft to the wound bed and help control bleeding.

Autologous cell suspension uses a small sample of the patient's skin to produce a sprayed-on suspension of the patient's own cells. The goal is to promote skin growth while reducing the amount of skin needed from donor sites. The suspension is used with meshed split-thickness skin grafts in patients with full-thickness thermal burns.[8]

The goals of donor site care are to promote rapid, moist wound healing, decrease pain at the site, and prevent infection. There are several choices of dressings for donor sites (Fig. 26.12C). Care of the donor site is specific to the dressing. The average healing time for a donor site is 10 to 14 days (Fig. 26.12D). Many newer dressings decrease healing time, which allows earlier harvesting of skin at the same site.

Cultured Epidermal Autografts

In patients with large body burns, only a limited amount of unburned skin may be available as donor sites for grafting. Some of that skin may not be suitable for harvesting. Cultured epidermal autograft (CEA) is a method of getting permanent skin from a person with limited skin available for harvesting.[9] CEA is grown from biopsy samples obtained from the patient's unburned skin. The specimens are sent to a laboratory, where the biopsied keratinocytes are grown in a medium containing epidermal growth factor. After about 18 to 25 days, the keratinocytes have expanded up to 10,000 times. They form sheets that we can use as skin grafts on excised burn wounds (Fig. 26.13A). CEA grafts generally form a seamless, smooth replacement skin tissue (Fig. 26.13B). Problems include poor graft take because of thin epidermal skin, graft loss during healing, infection, and contractures.

Dermal Substitutes

Dermal, or skin, substitutes can be used to close and heal wounds. They can temporarily or permanently fulfill the functions of the skin. There are biologic and synthetic products.[10] Skin substitutes have many advantages, including less need for donor site tissue. They are used in the treatment of life-threatening full-thickness or deep partial-thickness burn wounds when a conventional autograft is not available or advisable, as in older or high-anesthetic-risk patients. They are also used in reconstructive burn surgeries.

Pain Management

Many aspects of burn care cause pain. Eliminating all pain is difficult, but most patients will have acceptable levels of relative comfort if they receive adequate analgesia. To provide effective pain management, you must understand both the physiologic and psychologic aspects of pain. Pain management is discussed in Chapter 9. Evaluate the pain management plan often. The patient's needs may change, and tolerance to drugs may develop.

Patients have 3 types of pain: (1) *continuous, background pain* that might be present throughout the day and night; (2) *treatment-induced pain* caused by dressing changes, ambulation,

TABLE 26.9 Skin Grafts Used for Burn Injury

Graft Type	Source and Description	Coverage
Allograft (or homograft) (same species)	Cadaveric skin	Temporary (3 days to 2 weeks)
Autografts		
Autograft	Patient's skin	Permanent
Cultured epithelial autograft (CEA)—epical	Patient's own skin cell cultures	Permanent
Recell		
Skin Substitutes		
Allover	Acellular dermal matrix derived from donated human skin	Permanent
Apligraf	Donated neonatal foreskin fibroblasts and keratinocytes in bovine collagen gel	Permanent
Biobrane	Semipermeable silicone membrane bonded to nylon fabric	Temporary (10 to 21 days)
Integra	Biodegradable dermal layer made of bovine collagen and glycosaminoglycan bonded to silicone membrane	Permanent
Matriderm	Bovine collagen and elastin matrix	Permanent
OrCel	Donated neonatal foreskin fibroblasts and keratinocytes in bovine collagen sponge	Permanent
Xenograft (or heterograft) (different species)	Porcine skin	Temporary (3 days to 2 weeks)

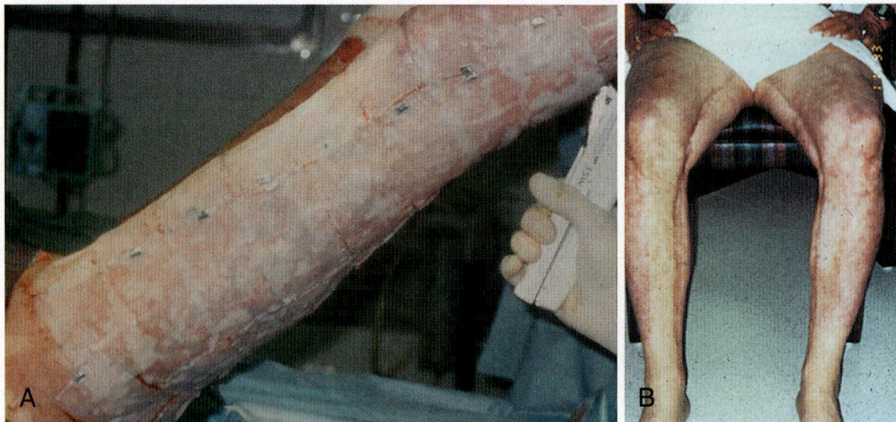

Fig. 26.13 Patient with cultured epithelial autograft (CEA). (A) Intraoperative application of CEA. (B) Healed CEA.

and rehabilitation; and (3) *breakthrough pain.* A multimodal approach is often required. The first line of treatment is medication (Table 26.8). Frequent administration of acetaminophen, NSAID, and/or an opioid (e.g., hydromorphone) provides steady, therapeutic drug levels. Patient-controlled analgesia (PCA) is used in some burn centers. Anxiolytics (e.g., lorazepam, midazolam) and adjuvant analgesics (e.g., gabapentin, pregabalin) can enhance opioid effectiveness. Their use can help reduce opioid dosage and undesirable side effects. Breakthrough doses of analgesia, often opioids, must be available.

CHECK YOUR PRACTICE

A patient with a burn injury is prescribed fentanyl before a dressing change. The patient has multiple IV lines. You are not sure which line to use to give the drug. You know that mixing up IV lines can lead to serious drug errors.

- How would you determine which IV line to use to give the drug?

Provide nonpharmacologic therapy. Relaxation breathing, guided imagery, hypnosis, biofeedback, computer gaming, and music can help patients cope (see Chapter 7).

Remember, the more control patients have in managing pain, the more successful the chosen strategies will be. Active participation in asking for timeouts and scheduling treatments and rest periods can help reduce anticipatory pain.

Physical and Occupational Therapy

Continuous therapy throughout burn recovery is critical to prevent secondary complications and to regain and maintain muscle strength and optimal function. A good time for exercise is during dressing changes when bulky dressings are removed and patients are medicated for pain. Passive and active ROM should be done on all joints. PTs and OTs may provide treatment after dressing changes. Maintain the schedule for wearing custom-fitted splints designed to keep joints in a functional position. Check the skin to make sure the splints are not causing excessive pressure.

Nutrition Therapy

The goal of nutrition therapy during the acute burn phase is to provide adequate calories and protein to promote healing. When the wounds are still open, patients with burns are in a hypermetabolic and catabolic state.

Meeting daily caloric requirements is crucial and should start within the first 1 to 2 days postburn. The dietitian calculates the daily caloric requirements and makes adjustments as the patient's condition changes (e.g., wound healing improves, sepsis develops). Monitor laboratory values (e.g., albumin, prealbumin, total protein, transferrin) as available. Patients may benefit from an antioxidant protocol, which includes selenium, vitamin E, acetylcysteine, ascorbic acid, zinc, and a multivitamin.

Encourage patients to eat high-protein, high-carbohydrate foods to meet caloric goals. Ask caregivers to bring in the patient's favorite foods from home. Appetite is usually reduced. You will need to reinforce the steps being taken to achieve adequate intake. Ideally, weight loss should not be more than 10% of the preburn weight. Record daily caloric intake using calorie count sheets. Review the sheets with the dietitian. Weigh patients often to evaluate progress.

REHABILITATION PHASE

The formal rehabilitation phase begins when wounds have nearly healed and the patient is engaging in some level of self-care. This may happen as early as 2 weeks or as long as 7 to 8 months after a major burn injury. Care goals now are to (1) work toward resuming a functional role in society and (2) rehabilitate from any functional and cosmetic postburn reconstructive surgery.

Clinical Manifestations

Burn wounds heal by either spontaneous reepithelialization or skin grafting. Layers of keratinocytes begin rebuilding the tissue structure destroyed by the burn injury. Collagen fibers, present in the new scar tissue, help with healing and add strength to weakened areas. The new skin appears flat and pink. In about 4 to 6 weeks, the area becomes raised and hyperemic. If adequate ROM is not continued, the new tissue will shorten, causing a contracture. Mature healing is reached in about 12 months when suppleness has returned and the pink or red color has faded to a slightly lighter hue than the surrounding unburned tissue.

Scarring has 2 characteristics: (1) discoloration and (2) contour. Discoloration fades with time. Tell patients with heavily pigmented skin that it will take longer for it to regain tone because of altered melanocytes. Often, the skin does not regain its original tone, though this is impossible to predict. Provide teaching and emotional support to help patients with grieving about body image changes. Cosmetic camouflage or pigment implants can help even out unequal skin tones and improve appearance and self-image.

Scar tissue tends to develop altered contours. That is, it is no longer flat or slightly raised, but becomes elevated and enlarged above the original burned area. Some HCPs believe that pressure and silicone can help keep a scar flat. Burned legs may be wrapped with elastic (e.g., tensor, Ace) bandages to assist with circulation to leg graft and donor sites before ambulation. Burned arms can be wrapped with a layer of tubular elastic gauze (e.g., Tubigrip). This interim pressure prevents blister formation, promotes venous return, and decreases pain and itchiness. Custom-fitted pressure garments replace the elastic bandages and tubular gauze once the skin is healed. Pressure garments and masks should never be worn over unhealed wounds. Pressure garments are worn up to 23 hours a day for as long as 24 months.[11]

Patients typically report discomfort from itching where healing is occurring. Water-based moisturizers and short-term use of oral antihistamines (e.g., hydroxyzine) can help reduce itching. Massage, cooling, emollients, gabapentin, antidepressants, and anesthetic creams may also help.

Skin flaking occurs as the epithelium is replaced by new cells. The newly formed skin is very sensitive to trauma. Blisters and skin tears are likely to develop from slight pressure or friction. These newly healed areas can be more or less sensitive to cold, heat, and touch. Grafted areas are more likely to be less sensitive until peripheral nerve regeneration occurs. Have patients protect healed burn areas from direct sunlight for about 3 months to prevent hyperpigmentation and sunburn injury. Tell patients to wear sunscreen when exposing healed skin to the sun.

Complications

The most common complications during the rehabilitation phase are skin and joint contractures and hypertrophic scarring. Joint contractures may develop because of the shortening of scar tissue in the flexor tissues of a joint. Areas that are most susceptible to contractures include the anterior and lateral neck areas, axillae, antecubital fossae, fingers, groin areas, popliteal fossae, knees, and ankles (Fig. 26.14). Some involve ligaments and tendons.

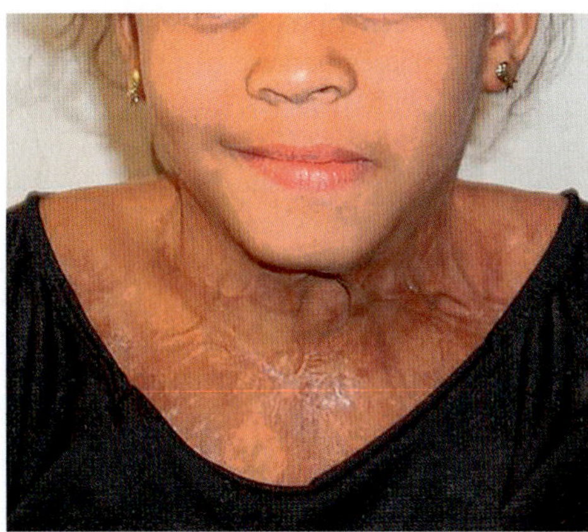

Fig. 26.14 Neck contracture. (Courtesy Linda Bucher, RN, PhD, CEN, CNE, Staff Nurse, Virtua Memorial Hospital, Mt. Holly, NJ.)

Carefully watch for these potential problems. Encourage proper positioning, splinting, and exercise. Teach patients to continue these strategies until the skin matures at around 1-year posthealing. Rehabilitative therapy is aimed at the extension of body parts because the flexors are stronger than the extensors.

NURSING MANAGEMENT: REHABILITATION PHASE

The first step is to ask the patient for their thoughts and feelings about discharge. Encourage both the patient and caregiver to take part in care. They may need wound care instructions. Tell the patient to take a shower, not a bath, to wash the wounds. Have them demonstrate a dressing change. Provide advice on scar management, moisturizing, and sun protection. Suggest using water-based creams that penetrate the dermis (e.g., Vaseline Intensive Rescue) on healed areas to keep the skin supple and moisturized. This will decrease itching and flaking. Antihistamines taken at bedtime may help if itching persists.

Make sure they know when to contact the burn team (e.g., signs of infection, increased pain). Stress the need to keep outpatient visits. The need for further reconstructive surgery is reviewed during follow-up appointments. If needed, work with a social worker or discharge manager to arrange home care services to assist with care.

Assess pain management and nutrition needs during each visit. Encourage the patient to perform the PT and OT exercises. Reassure the patient to maintain morale, especially once they realize that recovery can be slow.

Gerontologic Considerations: Burns

Older patients present many challenges for the burn team. They have thinner dermal layers, a loss of elastic fibers, less subcutaneous adipose tissue, and a decrease in vascularity. As a result, the thinner dermis, with reduced blood flow, sustains deeper burns with poorer rates of healing.

Once injured, the older adult has more complications in the emergent and acute phases because of preexisting comorbidities. Older patients with diabetes, heart failure, or chronic obstructive pulmonary disease (COPD) have higher mortality rates. Burn wounds and donor sites take longer to heal. Recovery from surgical procedures can be more difficult. Weaning from a ventilator can be a challenge, and pneumonia is a frequent complication. It usually takes longer for older patients to rehabilitate to the point at which they can return home. For some, returning home to independent living may not be possible.

EMOTIONAL AND PSYCHOLOGIC CARE

Patients and caregivers have many emotional and psychologic needs during the often lengthy, unpredictable, and complex course of care. They often experience overwhelming emotions, including fear, anger, guilt, or depression. Others fear possible permanent lifestyle changes and disfigurement. You have an important supportive and counseling role as patients struggle to get their lives back on track.

To manage the enormous range of emotional responses that the patient with burns may have, assess the circumstances of the burn (e.g., cause, people involved), family relationships, and ways of coping with stress. At any time, patients may have a variety of emotions. These include fear, anxiety, anger, guilt, and depression (Table 26.10).

Burn survivors often have thoughts and feelings that are frightening and disturbing. There may be guilt about the incident, reliving the burn experience, and fear of dying. They may be frustrated with ongoing discomfort and treatment and feel hopeless about the future. During recovery, new fears may occur: "Can I do this?" "Am I a desirable person?" "How can I go outside looking like this?" These challenges confront patients throughout their recovery and often for years to come.

TABLE 26.10 Common Emotional Responses

Emotion	Possible Verbal Expression
Anger	• Why did this happen to me? • The nurses enjoy hurting me. • I hope the person who did this to me dies.
Anxiety	• I feel out of control. • What is going to happen to me? • When will I look normal again?
Depression	• It is no use going on like this. • I do not care what happens to me. • I wish people would leave me alone.
Fear	• Will I die? • What will happen next? • Will I be disfigured? • Will my family and friends still love me?
Guilt	• If only I had been more careful. • I am being punished because I did something wrong.
Hopefulness	• What do I need to do to survive this injury emotionally and return to my life/family/friends? • What am I meant to learn from this injury?

A burn injury may adversely affect self-esteem. Some fear the loss of relationships because of perceived or actual physical disfigurement. In a society that values physical beauty, changes in body image can result in psychologic distress.

Open and frequent communication among the patient, caregivers, close friends, and burn team members is essential. Because of the tremendous psychologic impact of a burn injury, be sensitive to emotions and concerns. Encourage patients to discuss fears about loss of lifestyle, loss of function, deformity and disfigurement, and return to work and home life. Are there financial burdens from a long and costly hospitalization and rehabilitation?

Encourage independence and an eventual return to preburn activities, such as school or work. Peer counseling and informal interactions with other burn survivors may bring comfort and help restore confidence. Reassure patients that their feelings during this period of adjustment are a normal reaction to an extraordinary event. Frustration and impatience are expected as they establish a new life. Help patients in adapting to a realistic yet positive appraisal of their specific situation. Emphasize what they can do instead of what they cannot do.

Caregivers may share some or all these challenges and feelings. At times, they may feel helpless or too exhausted to help their loved ones. Continued support from trusted and familiar burn team members is essential. Helping caregivers assist with aspects of patient care helps them to reconnect with their loved one and eases the transition home. Many burn survivors and their caregivers remark on the powerful learning experience of the burn and a renewed appreciation of life, despite the ongoing challenges of a prolonged recovery. Acknowledge their feelings are real and common. Most burn survivors speak of satisfaction with their postburn life and are more empowered as time goes on.

Address spiritual and cultural needs because both have a role in treatment decisions and recovery. Pastoral care may be a helpful resource. The need for support, information, and family involvement may vary. Identify what is important to the patient and caregiver and communicate that information in the plan of care.

Discuss sexuality honestly. Acceptance of any changes in physical appearance is hard at first for the patient and their partner. The nature of skin injury can cause modifications in processing sexual stimuli. Touch is an important part of sexuality. Immature scar tissue may make the sensation of touch unpleasant or may dull it. This may be transient. The patient and partner need to know that it is normal and receive anticipatory guidance from the burn team to avoid undue emotional strain.

Burn survivors may have preexisting mental health or substance use issues, which may have contributed to the burn incident. The stress of burn injury can precipitate a crisis. Assessment by a psychiatrist who can prescribe drug therapy and offer counseling may be needed. Early psychiatric intervention is essential if patients have a psychiatric illness or if the injury was a suicide attempt. Many patients have posttraumatic stress disorder. A history of mental health issues can influence the length of hospitalization and the time needed to prepare for discharge. However, distress and trauma symptoms can be a catalyst for positive posttraumatic growth. Coping styles and social support assist in these positive changes postburn.

Support begins in the hospital with links to community resources to ensure continuity of treatment. A referral to a psychiatrist, psychologist, psychiatric advanced practice nurse (APN), mental health counselor, or social worker is discussed if concerns are raised at burn clinic follow-up.

Caregiver and patient support groups may be beneficial in meeting emotional needs at any phase of the recovery process. Speaking with others who have had burn trauma can be beneficial. People with similar experiences can confirm that the patient's feelings are normal and share helpful advice. The Phoenix Society (www.phoenix-society.org) is an international, highly respected burn survivors' support group. For many years, the society has offered valuable support and resources (e.g., the annual World Burn Congress conference) to burn survivors, caregivers, and burn team staff.

SPECIAL NEEDS OF NURSES

Warm, trusting, and mutually satisfying relationships often develop between burn patients and nursing staff during hospitalization and the long-term rehabilitation period. Sometimes the bond can be so strong that patients have difficulty separating from the hospital and staff. The frequency and intensity of family contact can be both rewarding and draining. It may be difficult to cope with the deformities caused by the burn injury, odors, unpleasant sight of wounds, and reality of the pain that accompanies the burn and its treatment. Do not hesitate to seek help from coworkers, a manager, or the employee assistance program should you feel the need.

Ongoing support services or critical incident stress debriefings led by a psychiatrist, psychologist, psychiatric APN, or social worker may be helpful. Peer support groups (e.g., ABA, International Society for Burn Injuries) can serve a similar purpose by helping you cope with difficult feelings from caring for burn patients. Attention to yourself is important to maintain a positive attitude and a healthy work-life balance. Time with family and friends and relaxation at home are essential parts of self-care and a balanced life with purpose and meaning.

CASE STUDY

Burn Injury

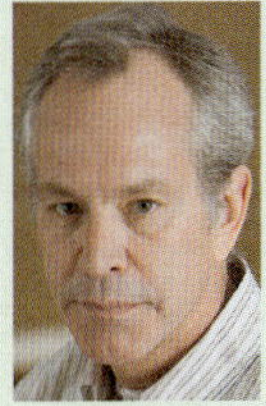

(© Comstock/ Thinkstock.)

Patient Profile

G.M., a 70-year-old male, arrives at the ED with burns to his face, neck, chest, right arm and hand, and right foot. He was burning brush on his farm when the fire went out of control.

Subjective Data

- Reports blurry vision and trouble swallowing.
- States his burns are painful. Pain rated 8/10.
- Says he is a "diabetic" and has "high blood pressure."
- Allergic to sulfa.

Objective Data

Physical Assessment

- Is awake, alert, and oriented but in some distress.
- Eyes are red and irritated.
- Voice is hoarse; nasal hair is singed. Frequent nonproductive cough.
- Face is reddened with blisters noted on the nose and forehead.
- Right arm, right hand, anterior chest, neck, and right foot have shiny, bright red, moist burns.
- Shivering.
- Vital signs: Temp 96.5, pulse 102/min, respiratory rate 26/min, BP 142/84 mm Hg, O_2 saturation 89% with nasal cannula 4 L/min.
- Scattered wheezing throughout all lung fields.

Discussion Questions

1. ***Recognize:*** What subjective and objective findings concern you the most?
2. ***Recognize:*** Which criteria does G.M. meet for admission to the hospital burn unit?
3. ***Analyze:*** What metabolic problems would you expect to develop soon? Explain the physiologic basis for these problems.
4. ***Analyze:*** What complications is G.M. at risk for?
5. ***Prioritize:*** What priority interventions do you need to implement?
6. ***Plan:*** How will you involve other interprofessional team members?
7. ***Act:*** Outline how you would manage G.M.'s pain.
8. ***Act:*** How would you support G.M.'s caregivers?
9. ***Evaluate:*** What outcomes would indicate initial care for the priority problem was effective?

Answers available at http://evolve.elsevier.com/Lewis/medsurg.

BRIDGE TO NCLEX EXAMINATION

The question number corresponds to the same-numbered outcome at the beginning of the chapter.

1. Which instruction would the nurse provide to prevent burn injuries?
   a. Set hot water temperature at 140°F.
   b. Use only hardwired smoke detectors.
   c. Encourage regular home fire exit drills.
   d. Do not allow older adults to cook unattended.
2. Which wound description indicates a need for excision and grafting? **(select all that apply)**
   a. Red, painful blisters
   b. Leathery, brown, exposed tendon
   c. Pearly white color, insensitive to pain, dry
   d. Charred eschar, visible thrombosed blood vessels
   e. Large, fluid-filled vesicles, moderate edema, moist, red

3. Estimate the total body surface area burn injury using the Rule of Nines. Burns involve the entire right arm and upper back.
4. A patient is hospitalized with burns to his head, neck, and anterior and posterior chest. The respiratory therapist applied a nonrebreather mask. On assessment, the nurse auscultates wheezes throughout the lung fields. On reassessment, the wheezes are gone and the breath sounds are greatly decreased. Respiratory rate is 6/min. Oxygen saturation decreases to 88%. The patient is unresponsive. What is the *priority* nursing intervention?
   a. Notify the HCP and prepare for intubation.
   b. Encourage the patient to cough and auscultate the lungs again.
   c. Obtain vital signs, oxygen saturation, and a STAT arterial blood gas.
   d. Document the findings and continue to monitor the patient's breathing.
5. What nutrition intervention promotes wound healing for a patient with a 10% burn injury?
   a. Eat a high-protein, high-carbohydrate diet.
   b. Increase normal caloric intake by about 4 times.
   c. Eat at least 1500 calories/day in small, frequent meals.
   d. Eat a lactose-free diet to reduce the potential for diarrhea.
6. A patient has 25% TBSA burn from a car fire. His wounds have been debrided and covered with a silver-impregnated dressing. What is the *most* important nursing intervention after surgery?
   a. Wash the wound with soap and water 3 times a day.
   b. Medicate for pain relief in between dressing changes.
   c. Reapply a new dressing without disturbing the wound bed.
   d. Assess the wound for signs of infection during dressing changes.
7. What nursing interventions can be used to manage burn pain? (**Select all that apply.**)
   a. Suggest pain management options.
   b. Use a pain-rating tool to monitor the level of pain.
   c. Delay painful dressing changes until the pain is completely relieved.
   d. Use a multimodal approach (e.g., sustained-release and short-acting opioids, NSAIDs, adjuvant analgesics).
   e. Provide nonpharmacologic therapies (e.g., music therapy, distraction) to replace opioids in the acute phase of a burn injury.
8. What intervention prevents hypertrophic scarring during the rehabilitation phase of burn recovery?
   a. Applying pressure garments
   b. Repositioning the patient every 2 hours
   c. Performing active ROM at least every 4 hours
   d. Applying a water-based moisturizer to healed skin
9. A patient is recovering from second- and third-degree burns over 30% of his body, and the burn care team is planning for discharge. The *first* action the nurse would take when meeting with the patient would be to
   a. arrange a return-to-clinic appointment and prescription for pain medications.
   b. give the patient written information and website resources for burn survivors.
   c. teach the patient and the caregiver proper wound care to be performed at home.
   d. review the patient's current health care status and readiness for discharge to home.

1. c; 2. b, c, d; 3. 18% 4. a; 5. a; 6. d 7. a, b, d; 8. a; 9. d.

For rationales to these answers and even more NCLEX review questions, visit http://evolve.elsevier.com/Lewis/medsurg.

REFERENCES

To access the References for this chapter, please scan the QR code with a mobile device.

CASE STUDY

Applying Clinical Judgment With Multiple Patients

You are working the day shift on a medical-surgical unit. The following 3 patients are among the 7 you are assigned to care for today. You have an AP who is assigned to work with you. There are 15 other patients on the unit being cared for by an additional 2 RNs and 2 APs.

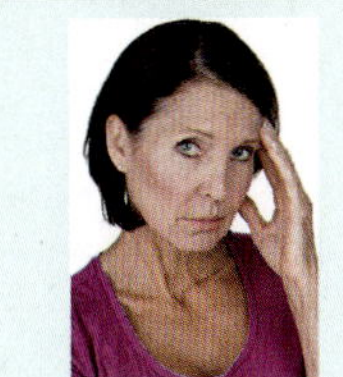 © Stockphoto4u/iStock.com.	R.S., a 57-year-old female, is under observation with Ménière disease. She continues to have extreme dizziness, tinnitus, and nausea. The HCP plans to give an intratympanic injection of dexamethasone today. Vital signs: 100/64, 112, RR 20.
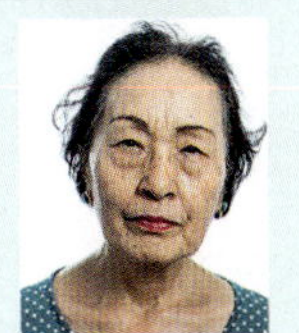 © andreswd/iStock.com.	D.A., a 74-year-old female, is admitted with chest tightness and shortness of breath. Her history is negative except for a recent diagnosis of basal cell carcinoma (BCC) on her face. She is scheduled to have the BCC surgically removed tomorrow. The HCP suspects D.A.'s symptoms are caused by anxiety but wants to rule out coronary artery disease before surgery. The night RN is concerned because her BP is 180/94.
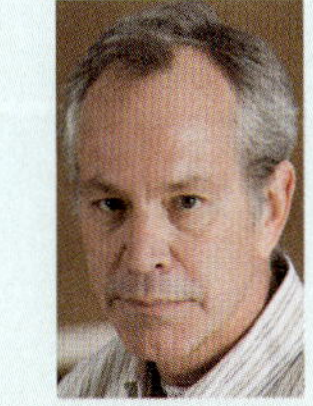 © Comstock/Thinkstock.	G.M., a 70-year-old male, was admitted 12 h ago from the ED with partial-thickness burns to his face, neck, chest, right arm and hand, and right foot (estimated 22% TBSA). Vital signs: 142/84, 102, RR 22, O_2 saturation 94% with O_2 at 6 L/min via nasal cannula. Scattered wheezing throughout all lung fields.

1. Highlight all the findings that require your follow-up.
2. After receiving report, which patient would you see first? Why?
3. Which tasks could you delegate to the AP? **(Select all that apply.)**
   a. Obtain vital signs on R.S.
   b. Take a BP reading on D.A.
   c. Perform a shift assessment on G.M.
   d. Explain planned diagnostic testing to D.A.
   e. Obtain a 12-lead ECG on D.A.
4. When you enter G.M.'s room, he tells you he is not feeling well. He says he has a headache and his legs are "cramping up." He is unaware that he is in the hospital.

   Use an X for the nursing actions listed that are indicated (appropriate or necessary) or contraindicated (could be harmful) at this time.

Nursing Action	Indicated	Contraindicated
Perform a respiratory assessment.		
Direct the AP to stay with G.M. while you contact the HCP.		
Obtain a STAT glucose measurement.		
Administer as-needed acetaminophen for headache relief.		
Place the head of the bed flat.		
Have the AP obtain vital signs with O_2 saturation.		
Review recent laboratory results.		

Case Study Progression

G.M.'s vital signs are BP 114/48 mm Hg, heart rate 112 beats/min, respirations 18 breaths/min, and temperature 98°F (36.8°C). You receive notification that his laboratory results are available. They show the following:

Laboratory Results

Sodium	129 mmol/L
Potassium	5.0 mmol/L
HCO_3	26 mmol/L
BUN	37 mg/dL
Creatinine	2 mg/dL
Glucose	128 mg/dL
Calcium	9.1 mg/dL

5. Choose the *best* option for the information missing from the statement that follows by selecting from the lists of options provided.

   Based on the assessment findings and laboratory results, the nurse determines G.M. is experiencing _____1_____. To manage this problem, you expect that the HCP will order _____2_____.

Options for 1	Options for 2
Hyperglycemia	Furosemide
Hyperkalemia	Insulin
Hyponatremia	IV fluids

6. You notify the HCP, who orders a normal saline IV to infuse at 100 mL/h. Which nursing actions would you include in G.M.'s plan of care at this time? **(Select 4 correct options.)**
   a. Administer IV furosemide.
   b. Administer analgesia as ordered.
   c. Monitor serum electrolyte values.
   d. Initiate daily weights and intake and output.
   e. Maintain IV fluid replacement therapy as ordered.
   f. Obtain a referral to the dietitian for parenteral nutrition.
7. G.M. is thirsty and asks for something to drink. Which fluids would be appropriate to offer him? **(Select 4 correct options.)**
   a. Coffee
   b. Iced tea
   c. Gatorade
   d. Tap water
   e. Apple juice
   f. Orange juice
   g. Oral nutrition supplement
8. D.A. just returned to the unit after a transesophageal echocardiogram. Which action is the highest priority?
   a. Have the AP assist D.A. to lie flat on her back.
   b. Obtain vital signs and pulse oximetry every 4 h.
   c. Maintain D.A. on NPO status until her gag reflex returns.
   d. Assess the lower extremities for signs of circulatory compromise.
9. Which interventions are appropriate for R.S. at this time? **(Select all that apply.)**
   a. Inserting a nasogastric tube
   b. Keeping the room dark and quiet
   c. Placing an emesis basin at the bedside
   d. Elevating the head of the bed to the height desired
   e. Raising the side rails and having the bed in a low position
10. You leave the floor to go to lunch. Which situation would warrant immediate intervention?
    a. The AP is discussing a patient's condition in the cafeteria.
    b. The LPN was off the floor an extra 5 minutes for their lunch break.
    c. A student nurse is administering 1200 medications with the instructor.
    d. Another RN is triaging phone messages and not taking a break at the assigned time.

Answers available at http://evolve.elsevier.com/Lewis/medsurg.

27

Assessment: Respiratory System

Samantha J. Bonaduce

http://evolve.elsevier.com/Lewis/medsurg/

CONCEPTUAL FOCUS

Functional Ability

Gas Exchange

LEARNING OUTCOMES

1. Distinguish the structures and functions of the upper respiratory tract, lower respiratory tract, and chest wall.
2. Describe the processes of inspiration and expiration.
3. Describe the process of oxygenation and ventilation.
4. Identify the respiratory defense mechanisms.
5. Link age-related changes of the respiratory system to differences in assessment findings.
6. Obtain significant subjective and objective assessment data related to the respiratory system.
7. Perform a physical assessment of the respiratory system.
8. Distinguish normal from common abnormal findings of a respiratory physical assessment.
9. Relate the signs and symptoms of inadequate oxygenation to physical assessment findings.
10. Describe the purpose, significance of results, and nursing responsibilities related to diagnostic studies of the respiratory system.
11. Discuss the significance of arterial blood gas values in relation to respiratory function.

KEY TERMS

adventitious breath sounds
chemoreceptor
compliance
crackles, Table 27.5
dyspnea
fremitus
mechanical receptors
oximetry
oxygenation
resistance
surfactant
tidal volume (V_T)
ventilation
wheezes, Table 27.5

The primary purpose of the respiratory system is gas exchange. This involves the transfer of oxygen (O_2) and carbon dioxide (CO_2) between the air and blood. While adequate perfusion is needed to deliver O_2 to the body tissues, adequate ventilation and gas exchange depends on a healthy, functioning respiratory system.

STRUCTURES AND FUNCTIONS OF THE RESPIRATORY SYSTEM

The respiratory system is divided into 2 parts: the upper respiratory tract and lower respiratory tract (Fig. 27.1).

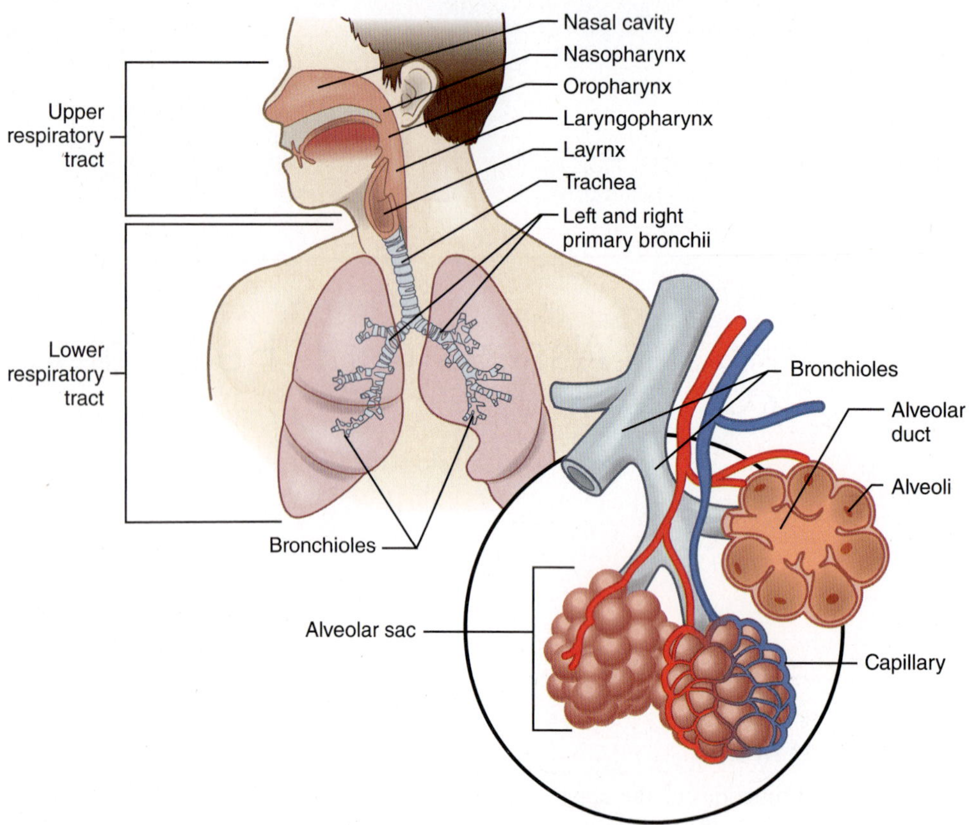

Fig. 27.1 Structures of the respiratory tract.

Upper Respiratory Tract

The *upper respiratory tract* includes the nose, mouth, pharynx, epiglottis, larynx, and trachea. Air enters the respiratory tract through the nose. The nose is made of bone and cartilage. It is divided into 2 nares by the nasal septum. The inside of the nose is shaped into 3 passages by projections called *turbinates.* The turbinates increase the surface area of the nasal mucosa that warms and moistens the air as it enters the nose. The internal nose opens directly into the sinuses. The nasal cavity connects with the pharynx. It is a tubular passageway that is subdivided into 3 parts: *nasopharynx, oropharynx,* and *laryngopharynx.*

The nose protects the lower airway by warming and humidifying air and filtering small particles before air enters the lungs. The olfactory nerve is found within the mucosa of the upper part of the nasal cavity. It is responsible for the sense of smell.[1]

Air moves through the oropharynx to the laryngopharynx. It then travels through the epiglottis to the larynx before moving into the trachea. The *epiglottis* is a small flap behind the tongue that closes over the larynx during swallowing. This prevents solids and liquids from entering the lungs. The vocal cords are in the larynx. Air passes through the glottis (the opening between the vocal cords) and into the trachea.

The trachea is a cylindrical tube about 5 inches (10 to 12 cm) long and 1 inch (1.5 to 2.5 cm) in diameter. U-shaped cartilages keep the trachea open and allow the adjacent esophagus to expand for swallowing. The trachea divides into the right and left mainstem bronchi at a point called the *carina.* The carina is located at the *angle of Louis,* which is at the level of the 5th thoracic vertebrae.[2] The carina is highly sensitive. Stimulation of this area during suctioning causes vigorous coughing.

Lower Respiratory Tract

Once air passes the carina, it is in the lower respiratory tract. The *lower respiratory tract* consists of the bronchi, bronchioles, alveolar ducts, and alveoli. Except for the right and left mainstem bronchi, all lower airway structures are found within the lungs. The right lung is divided into 3 lobes (upper, middle, and lower) and the left lung into 2 lobes (upper and lower) (Fig. 27.2).

The mainstem bronchi, pulmonary vessels, and nerves enter the lungs through a slit called the *hilus.* The right mainstem bronchus is shorter, wider, and straighter than the left mainstem bronchus. That is why aspiration is more likely to occur in the right lung than in the left lung.

The mainstem bronchi subdivide several times to form the lobar, segmental, and subsegmental bronchi. These are called the conducting airways. Further divisions form the bronchioles. The most distant bronchioles are the respiratory bronchioles. The bronchioles are encircled by smooth muscles that constrict and dilate in response to various stimuli. The terms *bronchoconstriction* and *bronchodilation* refer to a decrease or increase in the diameter of the airways caused by contraction or

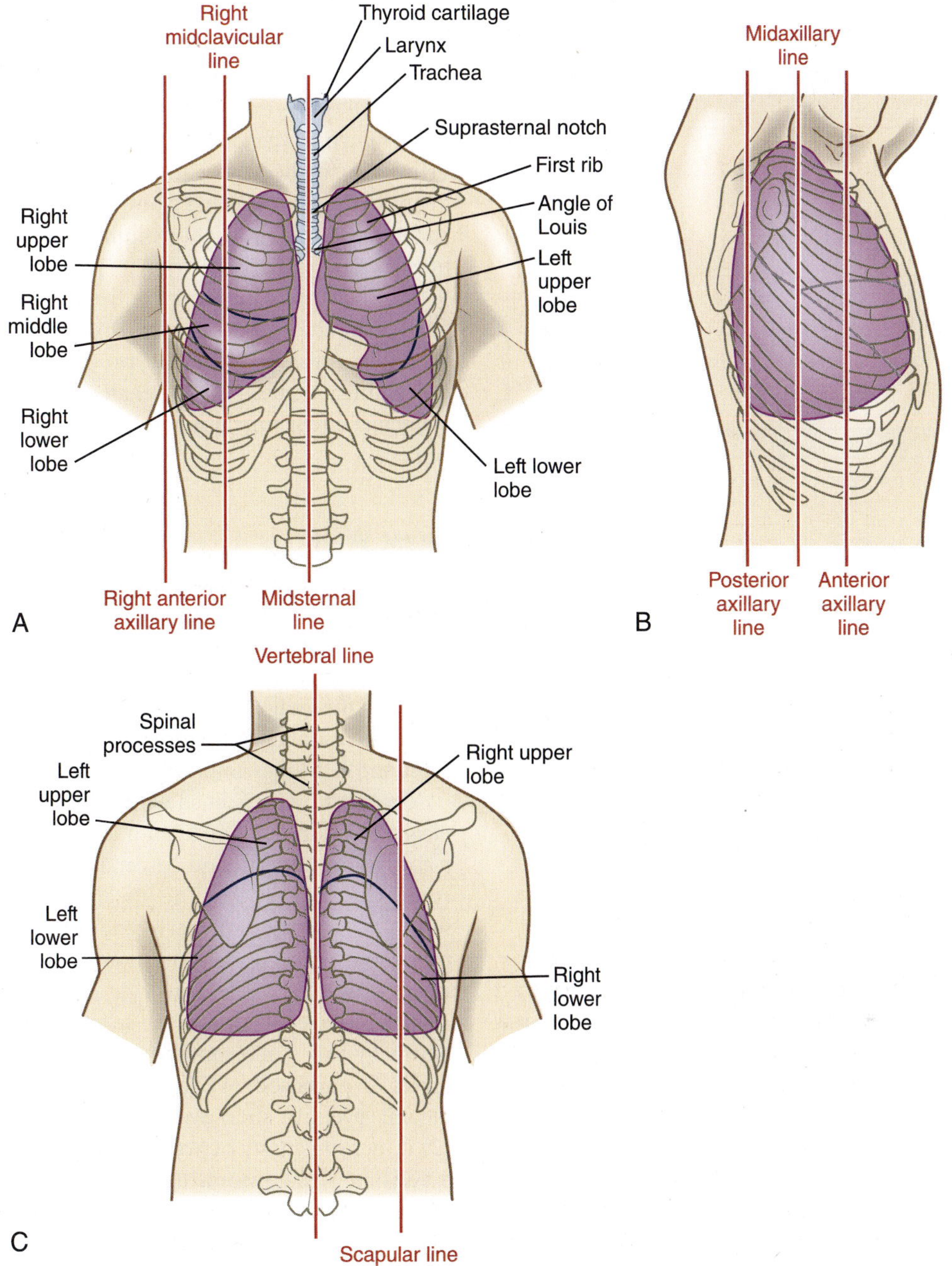

Fig. 27.2 Landmarks and structures of the chest wall. (A) Anterior view. (B) Posterior view. (C) Right lateral view.

relaxation of these muscles. Beyond the bronchioles lie the alveolar ducts and alveoli (Fig. 27.3).

The trachea and bronchi act as a pathway to conduct gases to and from the alveoli. The volume of air in the trachea and bronchi is called the *anatomic dead space* (VD).[3] This air does not take part in gas exchange. In adults, a normal **tidal volume (Vt)**, or volume of air exchanged with each breath, is about 500 mL (in a 150-lb male). Of each 500 mL inhaled, about 150 mL is VD.

The alveoli are the final part of the respiratory tract (Fig. 27.3). *Alveoli* are small sacs in the lungs that are the primary site of gas exchange for O_2 and CO_2. The adult lung has over 300 million alveoli, each 0.3 mm in diameter. The alveoli are interconnected by pores of Kohn.[4] They allow movement of air from alveolus to alveolus (Fig. 27.1). Deep breathing promotes air movement through these pores and helps move mucus out of the respiratory bronchioles. Bacteria can also move through these pores, spreading infection to previously uninfected areas. Alveoli have a total volume of about 2500 mL, with a surface area for gas exchange that is about the size of a tennis court.

Gases are exchanged across the alveolar-capillary membrane, where the alveoli come in contact with pulmonary capillaries (Fig. 27.4). In conditions such as pulmonary edema, excess fluid fills the interstitial space and alveoli. This reduces gas exchange.

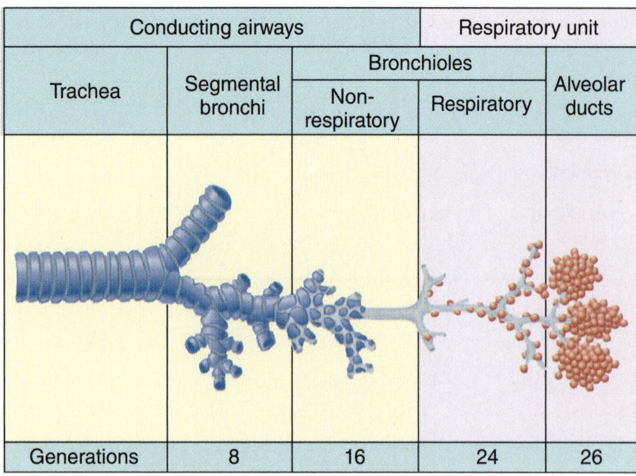

Fig. 27.3 Structures of the lower airways.

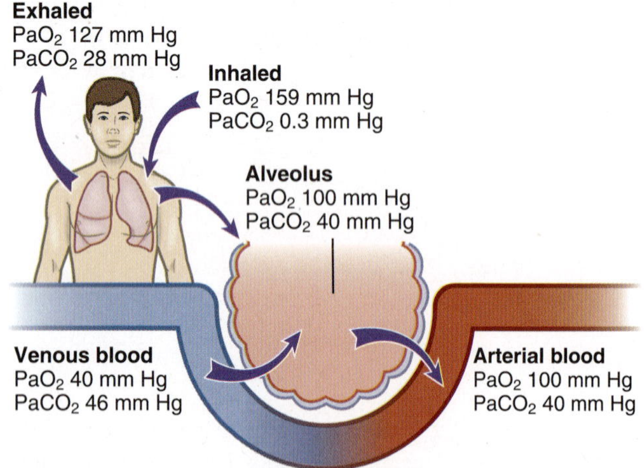

Fig. 27.4 Partial pressure of respiratory gases in normal respiration. The pressures are shown in inhaled and exhaled air from the lungs and at the level of the alveoli and pulmonary venous and arterial blood vessels.

Surfactant

Because alveoli are unstable, they have a natural tendency to collapse. Alveolar cells secrete surfactant. **Surfactant** is a lipoprotein that lowers the surface tension in the alveoli.[5] It reduces the amount of pressure needed to inflate the alveoli and makes them less likely to collapse. Normally, each person takes a slightly larger breath, termed a *sigh,* after every 5 or 6 breaths. This sigh stretches the alveoli and promotes surfactant secretion.

When there is not enough surfactant, the alveoli collapse. The term *atelectasis* refers to collapsed, airless alveoli. Postoperative patients are at risk for atelectasis because of the effects of anesthesia, decreased mobility, and pain, which can alter breathing and lung expansion. In acute respiratory distress syndrome (ARDS), lack of surfactant contributes to widespread atelectasis and collapse of lung tissue (see Chapter 32).

Blood Supply

The lungs have 2 distinct types of circulation: pulmonary and bronchial. Pulmonary circulation provides the lungs with blood that takes part in gas exchange. The pulmonary artery receives deoxygenated blood from the right ventricle of the heart and delivers it to pulmonary capillaries that lie directly alongside the alveoli. O_2—CO_2 exchange occurs at this point. The pulmonary veins return oxygenated blood to the left atrium, which then delivers it to the left ventricle and into systemic circulation. Venous blood is collected from capillary networks of the body and returned to the right atrium by way of the superior and inferior vena cava.

Bronchial circulation starts with the bronchial arteries, which arise from the thoracic aorta. Bronchial circulation does not take part in gas exchange but provides O_2 to the bronchi and other lung tissues. Deoxygenated blood returns from the bronchial circulation through the azygos vein into the superior vena cava.[1]

Chest Wall

The chest wall is shaped, supported, and protected by 24 ribs (12 on each side). The thoracic cage, which consists of the ribs and sternum, protects the lungs and the heart from injury. The *mediastinum* is the space in the middle of the thoracic cavity. It contains the major organs of the chest, including the heart, aorta, and esophagus. The mediastinum physically separates the right and left lungs into 2 separate compartments.

The chest cavity is lined with a membrane called the *parietal pleura.* The lungs are lined with a membrane called the *visceral pleura.* The parietal and visceral pleurae join to form one continuous membrane. The visceral pleura does not have any sensory (pain) fibers or nerve endings. The parietal pleura has pain fibers. This is why irritation or inflammation of the parietal pleura can cause pain with each breath (pleuritic pain).

The *intrapleural space* is the space between the pleural layers. Normally this space contains 10 to 20 mL of fluid. This fluid serves 2 purposes: (1) it provides lubrication, allowing the pleural layers to slide over each other during breathing, and (2) it increases unity between the pleural layers. This promotes expansion of the pleurae and lungs during inspiration.

Fluid drains from the pleural space via lymphatic circulation. Several conditions may cause a pleural effusion, or excess fluid in the pleural space. Pleural fluid may accumulate because of blocked lymphatic drainage (e.g., from cancer) or an imbalance between intravascular and oncotic fluid pressures. This happens with heart failure. Purulent pleural fluid with bacterial infection is called *empyema.*

The *diaphragm* is the major muscle of respiration. During inspiration the diaphragm contracts, moves downward, and increases intrathoracic volume. At the same time, the internal intercostals relax and the external intercostal muscles contract. This increases the lateral and anteroposterior (AP) dimensions of the chest.[6] The scalene muscles also contract on inspiration, raising the first and second ribs. This causes the size of the thoracic cavity to increase and intrathoracic pressure to decrease, pulling air into the lungs.

The diaphragm is made up of 2 hemidiaphragms, each innervated by the right and left phrenic nerves. The phrenic nerves arise from the spinal cord between C3 and C5, the 3rd and 5th cervical vertebrae. Injury to the phrenic nerve results in hemidiaphragm paralysis on the side of the injury. Complete spinal cord injuries above the level of C3 result in total diaphragm paralysis and dependence on a mechanical ventilator (see Chapter 65).

Physiology of Respiration

Oxygenation

Oxygenation refers to the process of obtaining O_2 from the atmospheric air (gas exchange) and making it available to the organs and tissues of the body (perfusion). The lungs' ability to oxygenate arterial blood is evaluated by partial pressure of O_2 in arterial blood (PaO_2), arterial O_2 saturation (SaO_2), and patient assessment.

O_2 is carried in the blood in 2 forms: dissolved O_2 and hemoglobin-bound O_2. The PaO_2 represents the amount of O_2 dissolved in the plasma. It is expressed in millimeters of mercury (mm Hg). The SaO_2 is the amount of O_2 bound to hemoglobin in comparison with the amount of O_2 the hemoglobin can carry. The SaO_2 is expressed as a percent. For example, if the SaO_2 is 90%, this means that 90% of hemoglobin attachments for O_2 have O_2 bound to them.

O_2 and CO_2 move back and forth across the alveolar-capillary membrane by diffusion. The overall direction of movement is from the area of higher concentration to the area of lower concentration. Thus O_2 moves from alveolar gas (atmospheric air) into the arterial blood and CO_2 from the arterial blood into the alveolar gas. Diffusion continues until equilibrium is reached.

Ventilation

Ventilation involves *inspiration,* or inhalation (movement of air into the lungs), and *expiration,* or exhalation (movement of air out of the lungs). Air moves in and out of the lungs because intrathoracic pressure changes in relation to pressure at the airway opening. Contraction of the diaphragm and external intercostal and scalene muscles increases chest dimensions. This decreases intrathoracic pressure. Gas flows from an area of higher pressure (atmospheric) to one of lower pressure (intrathoracic). When **dyspnea** (shortness of breath) occurs, neck, shoulder, and other accessory muscles can aid the effort. Some conditions (e.g., rib fractures, neuromuscular disease) may limit diaphragm or chest wall movement. This causes patients to breathe with smaller tidal volumes. As a result, the lungs do not fully inflate, and gas exchange may be impaired.

Expiration is passive. *Elastic recoil* is the tendency for the lungs to return to their original size after being stretched or expanded. The elasticity of lung tissue is due to the elastin fibers found in the alveolar walls and surrounding the bronchioles and capillaries. The elastic recoil of the chest wall and lungs allows the chest to passively decrease in size (volume). When intrathoracic pressure is greater than atmospheric pressure, air moves out of the lungs.

Exacerbations of asthma or chronic obstructive pulmonary disease (COPD) cause expiration to become an active, labored process (see Chapter 31). Intercostal, scalene, and accessory muscles (e.g., abdominal, trapezius) help expel air during labored breathing.

Compliance and Resistance

Changes in compliance and/or resistance can affect ventilation and oxygenation. **Compliance** refers to the ability of the lungs to expand. This is a result of the elasticity of the lungs and elastic recoil of the chest wall.[7] With decreased compliance, it is harder for the lungs to inflate. This occurs with conditions that increase fluid in the lungs (e.g., pulmonary edema, ARDS, pneumonia), make lung tissue less elastic (e.g., pulmonary fibrosis), or restrict lung movement (e.g., pleural effusion). Compliance increases when there is destruction of alveolar walls and loss of tissue elasticity, as in COPD.

Resistance refers to any obstacle to airflow during inspiration and/or expiration. The main factor affecting airway resistance is changes in the diameter (size) of the airways. For example, patients with an acute asthma attack have narrowed airways, resulting in increased resistance. Bronchodilators decrease resistance by increasing the diameter of the bronchi, promoting air entry. Secretions in the bronchi increase resistance. Secretions can partially block airways, making airways narrower. This makes it harder for patients to get air into their lungs. Removing secretions with mucolytics or expectorants helps decrease resistance.

Control of Respiration

The respiratory center in the medulla responds to chemical and mechanical signals. The medulla sends impulses to the respiratory muscles through the spinal cord and phrenic nerves.

Chemoreceptors

A **chemoreceptor** is a receptor that responds to a change in the chemical content ($PaCO_2$ and pH) of the fluid around it. Central chemoreceptors are found in the medulla. They respond to changes in the hydrogen ion (H^+) concentration.[8] An increase in the H^+ concentration *(acidosis)* causes the medulla to increase the respiratory rate and V_T. A decrease in H^+ concentration *(alkalosis)* has the opposite effect. Changes in $PaCO_2$ regulate ventilation primarily by their effect on the pH of cerebrospinal fluid. When the $PaCO_2$ level is increased, more CO_2 is available to combine with H_2O and form carbonic acid (H_2CO_3). This lowers the cerebrospinal fluid pH and stimulates an increase in respiratory rate. The opposite process occurs with a decrease in $PaCO_2$ level.

Peripheral chemoreceptors are found in the carotid bodies at the bifurcation of the common carotid arteries and in the aortic bodies above and below the aortic arch. The peripheral chemoreceptors respond to decreases in PaO_2 and pH and increases in $PaCO_2$. These changes stimulate the respiratory center.

In a healthy person, an increase in $PaCO_2$ or a decrease in pH causes an immediate increase in the respiratory rate. The $PaCO_2$

does not vary more than about 3 mm Hg if lung function is normal. Some health problems change lung function and result in chronically elevated $Paco_2$ levels. In these instances, patients are not sensitive to further increases in $Paco_2$ as a stimulus to breathe. They may be maintaining ventilation largely because of a hypoxic (decreased O_2) drive from the peripheral chemoreceptors (see Chapter 31).

Mechanical Receptors

Mechanical receptors are found in the conducting upper airways, chest wall, diaphragm, and capillaries of the alveoli. They are stimulated by a variety of physiologic factors, such as irritants, muscle stretching, and alveolar wall distortion. The 3 major types of mechanical receptors are irritant, stretch, and juxtacapillary (J) receptors.[5]

Irritant receptors are found in the conducting airways. These receptors are sensitive to inhaled particles and aerosols. When stimulated, they initiate the cough reflex. Signals from stretch receptors, in the smooth muscle of the airways, aid in the control of respiration. As the lungs inflate, stretch receptors activate the inspiratory center to inhibit further lung expansion. This is the *Hering-Breuer reflex,* which prevents overdistention of the lungs. Stimulation of J receptors, found in the capillaries of the alveoli, occurs with increased pulmonary capillary pressure. This causes rapid, shallow respiration seen in pulmonary edema.

Respiratory Defense Mechanisms

Respiratory defense mechanisms are useful in protecting the lungs from inhaled particles, microorganisms, and toxic gases. The defense mechanisms include air filtration, mucociliary clearance system, cough reflex, reflex bronchoconstriction, and alveolar macrophages.

Air Filtration

Nasal hairs filter inspired air. In addition, the abrupt changes in direction of airflow that occur as air moves through the nasopharynx and larynx increase air turbulence. This causes particles and bacteria to contact the mucosa lining these structures. Most large particles (greater than 5 μm) are less dangerous because they are removed in the nasopharynx or bronchi and do not reach the alveoli.

The velocity of airflow slows greatly after it passes the larynx, aiding the deposit of smaller particles (1 to 5 μm). They settle the way that sand does in a river, a process termed *sedimentation.* Particles less than 1 μm in size are too small to settle in this manner and are deposited in the alveoli. An example of small particles that can build up is coal dust, which can lead to pneumoconiosis (see Chapter 30).

Mucociliary Clearance System

Below the larynx, the mucociliary clearance system, or the *mucociliary escalator,* is responsible for the movement of mucus. Goblet cells and submucosal glands continually secrete mucus at a rate of about 100 mL/day. This mucus forms a blanket that contains the trapped particles and debris from distal lung areas (Fig. 27.1). Secretory immunoglobulin A (IgA) in the mucus helps protect against bacteria and viruses.

Cilia cover the airways from the level of the trachea to the respiratory bronchioles (Fig. 27.1). Each ciliated cell has about 200 cilia. They beat rhythmically about 1000 times per minute in the large airways, moving mucus toward the mouth. We normally swallow the mucus without noticing.

The ciliary beat is slower further down the tracheobronchial tree. As a result, we remove particles that penetrate more deeply into the airways less rapidly. Dehydration, smoking, inhaling high O_2 concentrations, infection, and drugs, such as atropine, anesthetics, alcohol, or cocaine, impair ciliary action. Patients with COPD and cystic fibrosis often have repeated lower respiratory tract infections. These conditions are associated with destroyed cilia, resulting in impaired secretion clearance, a chronic productive cough, and chronic colonization by bacteria. These lead to frequent respiratory tract infections.

Cough Reflex

The cough is a protective reflex that clears the airway by a high-pressure, high-velocity flow of air. It is a backup for mucociliary clearance, especially when this clearance mechanism is overwhelmed or ineffective. Coughing is effective in removing secretions only above the subsegmental level (large or main airways). Secretions below this level must be moved upward by the mucociliary mechanism before we can remove them by coughing.

Reflex Bronchoconstriction

Reflex bronchoconstriction is another defense mechanism. When we inhale large amounts of irritating substances (e.g., dusts, aerosols), the bronchi constrict to prevent entry of the irritants. A person with hyperreactive airways, such as a person with asthma, may have bronchoconstriction after inhalation of triggers, such as cold air, perfume, or other strong odors.

Alveolar Macrophages

The main defense mechanism at the alveolar level is alveolar macrophages. *Alveolar macrophages* rapidly phagocytize inhaled foreign particles, such as bacteria. The debris is moved to the level of the bronchioles for removal by the cilia or removed from the lungs by the lymphatic system. Particles (e.g., coal dust, silica) that cannot be phagocytized tend to remain in the lungs for indefinite periods and can stimulate inflammatory responses. Cigarette smoke impairs alveolar macrophage activity.

Gerontologic Considerations: Effects of Aging on the Respiratory System

Age-related changes in structure, defense mechanisms, and respiratory control occur (Table 27.1). Structure changes

TABLE 27.1 GERONTOLOGIC ASSESSMENT DIFFERENCES

Respiratory System

Changes	Differences in Assessment Findings
Structures	
↑ Anteroposterior diameter ↓ Chest wall compliance Chest wall stiffening Costal cartilage calcification ↓ Elastic recoil ↓ Functioning alveoli ↓ Respiratory muscle strength	Barrel chest appearance, kyphosis, ↓ chest wall movement, ↓ deep breathing, ↓ cough effectiveness ↓ Vital capacity, ↑ residual volume, ↑ functional residual capacity ↓ Breath sounds, particularly at lung bases ↓ Pao_2 and Sao_2, normal pH and $Paco_2$
Defense Mechanisms	
↓ Alveolar macrophage function ↓ Cell-mediated immunity ↓ Cilia function ↓ Cough force ↓ Sensation in pharynx ↓ Specific antibodies	↓ Cough effectiveness, ↓ secretion clearance, thickened mucus ↑ Risk for aspiration, infection, influenza, pneumonia Respiratory infections may be more severe and last longer
Respiratory Control	
↓ Response to hypercapnia ↓ Response to hypoxemia	Slight ↓ Pao_2 and ↑ $Paco_2$ before respiratory rate changes ↓ Ability to maintain acid-base balance Significant hypoxemia or hypercapnia may develop from relatively small incidents Retained secretions, excess sedation, or positioning that impairs chest expansion may change Pao_2 or SpO_2 values

include calcification of the costal cartilages, which can interfere with chest expansion. The outward curvature of the spine is marked, especially with osteoporosis, and the lumbar curve flattens. Therefore the chest may appear barrel shaped, and the person may need to use accessory muscles to breathe. Respiratory muscle strength progressively declines. Overall, the lungs are harder to inflate.

Within the lung, the number of functional alveoli decreases, and they become less elastic. Small airways in the lung bases close earlier in expiration. Therefore more inspired air is distributed to the top of the lung rather than the bottom, and ventilation is less well matched to perfusion, lowering the Pao_2. As a result, older adults have less tolerance for exertion, and dyspnea can occur if their activity exceeds their normal exercise. The older adult who has a significant smoking history, is obese, and has a chronic illness is at greater risk for adverse outcomes.

Respiratory defense mechanisms are less effective because of a decline in immune function and the ability to produce antibodies. The alveolar macrophages are less effective at phagocytosis. Older patients have a less forceful cough and fewer and less functional cilia. Mucous membranes tend to be drier. Poor mucus removal and decreased IgA increase the chance of respiratory tract infections. Swallowing is slower because of transit time in the pharyngeal area. There is reduced sensation in the pharynx. Consequently, the risk for aspiration is greater.

The aging process alters respiratory control, resulting in a more gradual response to changes in blood O_2 or CO_2 level. The Pao_2 may drop to a slightly lower than normal level and the $Paco_2$ may rise to a level slightly higher than normal before the respiratory rate changes.

RESPIRATORY SYSTEM ASSESSMENT

A respiratory assessment can be part of a comprehensive or focused assessment. We use a focused assessment to evaluate the status of previously identified respiratory problems and to monitor for signs of new problems (Box 27.1). Use judgment in determining whether all or part of the history and physical assessment are needed, based on your evaluation of the degree of respiratory distress. If respiratory distress is severe, only obtain pertinent information and defer a thorough assessment until the patient's condition stabilizes.

CASE STUDY

Patient Introduction

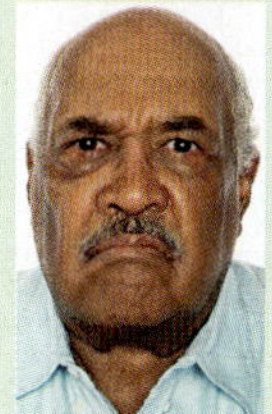

(© Fuse/Thinkstock.)

F.T. is a 70-year-old male who comes to the emergency department (ED) with nausea, fatigue, and increased shortness of breath, which started 3 days ago. He says that he has been using his Advair inhaler 4 times a day instead of 2. He can walk only a few feet in his apartment before he is short of breath. He sleeps in a recliner in the living room. He has noticed some swelling to his hands and feet and has been having trouble urinating.

Discussion Questions

1. What are the possible causes of F.T.'s shortness of breath?
2. What questions would be a priority during the subjective assessment?

You will learn more about F.T. and his condition as you read this assessment chapter.

Answers available at http://evolve.elsevier.com/Lewis/medsurg.

Subjective Data

Important Health Information

Health history. Determine the frequency of upper respiratory problems (e.g., colds, sore throats, sinus problems, allergies). Do seasonal changes influence these problems? Ask about a history of lower respiratory problems, such as asthma, COPD, pneumonia, and tuberculosis (TB).

Ask patients with allergies about possible precipitating factors or triggers, such as medications, pollen, smoke, mold, or pet exposure. Record the characteristics and severity of the allergic reaction, such as runny nose, wheezing, scratchy throat, or chest tightness. Determine the frequency of asthma exacerbations.

Ask about a history of other health problems. Respiratory symptoms are often manifestations of problems that involve

BOX 27.1 FOCUSED ASSESSMENT

Respiratory System

Use this checklist to make sure the key assessment steps have been done.

Subjective

Ask the patient about any of the following and note responses:

Shortness of breath
Pain with breathing
Cough
Sputum production (color, quantity)
Wheezing

Objective: Physical Assessment

Observe

Respirations: Rate, quality, and pattern
Accessory muscle use
Mouth or nose breathing

Inspect

Neck for position of trachea
Shape, symmetry, and movement of chest wall
Skin and nails for integrity and color

Palpate

Chest and back for abnormalities (i.e., masses)

Auscultate

Lung sounds (anterior and posterior)

Objective: Diagnostic

Check the following diagnostic tests for abnormal results:
Arterial blood gases
Chest x-ray
Hemoglobin
Hematocrit

other body systems. For example, patients with heart problems may have dyspnea because of heart failure. Immunocompromised patients may have frequent respiratory tract infections because of decreased immune function.

Medications. Take a medication history. Ask about the dose, frequency, length of time taken, side effects, and the reason for taking the medication. Assess for overuse of short-term bronchodilators as a key indicator of symptom control. Cough is a common side effect of angiotensin-converting enzyme (ACE) inhibitors. Encourage patients to bring all medications and inhalers to each visit.

If the patient is using O_2 for a breathing problem, record the fraction of inspired O_2 concentration (FIO_2), flow rate (liters per minute), method of administration, and number of hours used per day. Assess therapy effectiveness. Review safety practices.

Surgery or other treatments. Find out if the patient has been hospitalized for a respiratory problem. Note the dates, therapy (including surgery), and status of the problem. Has the patient ever been intubated because of a respiratory problem? Ask about the use of and response to respiratory treatments, such as a nebulizer, humidifier, postural drainage, and percussion.

Functional Health Patterns

Health history questions to ask patients with a respiratory problem are outlined in Table 27.2.

Health perception–health management. Ask the patient if there has been a perceived change in health status within the last several days, months, or years. In COPD, lung function declines slowly over many years. The patient may not notice this decline because they have been altering activity to accommodate reduced tolerance. If an upper respiratory tract infection (URI) is superimposed on a chronic problem, dyspnea and decreased exercise tolerance may occur very quickly. In asthma, symptoms may occur or worsen during exercise, in the presence of mold, or with changes in temperature or air pollution.

Explore common manifestations of respiratory problems (e.g., cough, dyspnea). Describe the course of the illness, including when it began, type of symptoms, and factors that worsen or relieve these symptoms. Because of the chronic nature of respiratory problems, patients may relate a change in symptoms (not the onset of new symptoms) when describing the present illness. For example, increased shortness of breath or increased purulence of sputum may suggest an acute COPD exacerbation. Wheezing indicates a degree of airway obstruction, such as asthma, foreign body aspiration, and emphysema.

If a cough is present, assess its quality. For example, a loose-sounding cough occurs with secretions. A dry, hacking cough may mean an airway irritation or obstruction. A harsh, barky cough suggests upper airway obstruction from inhibited vocal cord movement due to subglottic edema. Assess whether the cough is strong enough to clear secretions. Note whether it is productive or nonproductive of secretions. Is the cough acute or chronic (longer than 3 weeks in duration)? Did it begin with a URI? The pattern and cause of the cough are determined by asking questions such as: What has been the pattern of coughing? Has it been regular or paroxysmal (i.e., sudden, periodic onset) or related to a time of day, the weather, certain activities, talking, or deep breathing? Any change over time? Do you clear your throat a lot? What have you tried to relieve the coughing? Did you try any drugs?

If the patient has a productive cough, evaluate the characteristics of sputum: amount, color, consistency, and odor. Quantify the amount of sputum per day. Note any recent increases or decreases in the amount. Sputum is normally clear or slightly whitish. If the patient is a cigarette smoker, the sputum is usually clear to gray with occasional specks of brown. Patients with COPD may have clear, whitish, or slightly yellow sputum, especially in the morning on rising. If the patient reports any change from baseline color, suspect pulmonary complications. Note any changes in consistency of sputum to thick, thin, or frothy and pink tinged. These changes may indicate dehydration, postnasal drip or sinus drainage, or

TABLE 27.2 HEALTH HISTORY

Respiratory System

Health Perception–Health Management
- Describe your daily activities. Have breathing problems prevented you from doing activities that you used to be able to do?[a] Are your breathing problems better, worse, or about the same compared with 6 months ago?
- How do your breathing problems affect your self-care abilities?
- Have you ever smoked? Do you smoke now? If so, what have you smoked? Cigarettes? Cigars? Pipes? Electronic cigarettes?
- If yes, how many cigarettes each day and for how long? Are you interested in stopping smoking? Can we assist your quitting? If you stopped smoking, did you do so because of your health?[a] How did you stop?
- Have you ever used chewing tobacco?
- Have you ever smoked street drugs?[a]
- Do you get the flu shot yearly? When was your last flu shot? Have you had Pneumovax and COVID vaccinations?
- What equipment helps you manage your respiratory problems? How often do you use it? Does it help?

Nutritional-Metabolic
- Have you recently lost weight because of trouble eating related to your respiratory problem? How much weight have you lost? Have you lost this weight voluntarily?
- Do any foods affect your breathing? Sputum production?[a]

Elimination
- Does your breathing problem make it hard for you to get to the toilet?[a]
- Are you inactive because of shortness of breath to the point that you have incontinence? Constipation?[a]

Activity-Exercise
- Are you ever short of breath during exercise? At rest?[a]
- Do you get too short of breath to do the things you want to do?[a]
- Is your home 1 story? 2 stories? How many steps from the street to your door?
- Can you walk up a flight of steps without stopping?
- Are you able to maintain your typical activities of daily living? If not, what are you able to do independently? What do you need help with? What have you had to give up?
- What do you do when you get short of breath? Does this help? How long does it take you to recover after you have been short of breath?

Sleep-Rest
- Do breathing problems cause you to wake up during the night?[a]
- Can you lie flat at night? If not, how many pillows do you use?
- Do you need to sleep upright in a chair?[a]
- Are you or your partner aware of any snoring?
- Do you awaken in the morning feeling rested?
- Do you ever wake up in the morning with a headache?[a]
- Do you fall asleep easily during the day?[a]

Cognitive-Perceptual
- Do you have any pain with breathing?[a] On a scale from 0 to 10, with 0 being "no pain" and 10 being "the worst pain you can imagine," where would you rate your pain? Does it hurt more on inspiration? Expiration? Or both?[a]
- If you are having pain with breathing, describe the pain.
- Has the pain gotten better, worse, or stayed about the same over the past 6 months?
- Do you ever feel restless, irritable, or confused without a reason?[a]
- Do you have difficulty remembering things?[a]

Self-Perception–Self-Concept
- Describe how your respiratory problems have changed your life.
- If you use O_2, do you ever go out without bringing it with you? How often does this occur? Why?

Role-Relationship
- Has your respiratory problem caused any problems in your work, family, or social relationships?[a]

Sexuality-Reproductive
- Has your respiratory problem caused a change in your sexual activity?[a]
- Have you and your partner talked about ways to minimize your breathing problems during sexual activity?

Coping–Stress Tolerance
- On a daily/weekly basis, how often do you leave your home?
- Do you feel under any stress right now?
- Does stress influence your breathing?[a]
- Do you notice if your emotions have any effect on your respiratory problems?
- Are you aware of any respiratory support groups in your area?

Value-Belief
- Do you think the things you have been told to do for your respiratory problems help? If not, why?
- What are you looking for/expecting from the HCP today, in terms of your breathing problem(s)?

[a]If the answer is "yes" to any of these questions, ask the patient to describe.

possible pulmonary edema. Normally sputum should be odorless. A foul odor or exceptionally bad breath or taste in the mouth suggests an infectious process. Ask if sputum production increases or decreases with changes in position (e.g., increased with lying down) or activity.

Determine whether the patient has a history of coughing up blood *(hemoptysis)*. Hemoptysis can range from a slight streaking of blood in the sputum to massive coughing up of blood. The patient may not be able to tell between hemoptysis and *hematemesis* (vomiting blood). Hemoptysis occurs with a variety of conditions such as pneumonia, TB, lung cancer, and severe bronchiectasis.

Smoking is the most important risk factor for COPD and lung cancer. Ask about cigarette use and find out about the use of any tobacco products. This includes cigars, pipes, chewing tobacco, electronic cigarettes (e-cigarettes), and hookah (instrument for vaporizing and smoking flavored tobacco). Find out about exposure to secondhand smoke. Ask if the patient has tried to quit using tobacco products.

Discuss current and past smoking habits. Quantify smoking habits in *pack-years.* Do this by multiplying the number of packs of cigarettes smoked per day by the number of years smoked. For example, a person who smoked 1 pack (20 cigarettes) per day for 15 years has a 15 pack-year history. If they smoked 2 packs for 15 years, then it would be a 30 pack-year history.

Obtain a history of exposure to TB. Ask where the patient has lived and traveled. Risk factors for TB include immigrating from an area with high rates of TB or living in a group setting, such as a prison. Other risk factors include exposure to people with high rates of TB transmission, such as the homeless, IV drug users, and people with HIV infection. Risk factors for fungal lung infections include those exposed to bird and rodent feces or polluted water, those working closely with the soil, and immunocompromised patients.

Review the immunization record for influenza (flu), COVID, and pneumococcal pneumonia. Ask about the use of equipment to manage respiratory symptoms (e.g., home O_2 equipment, inhalers, devices for sleep apnea). Find out the type of equipment used, cleaning of the device, frequency of use, its effect, and any side effects. Have patients show you the use of their inhalers. Many patients do not use these devices correctly (see Chapter 28).

Nutritional-metabolic. Weight loss can be a symptom of respiratory disease. Determine whether weight loss was intentional. If not, was food intake changed by anorexia (from medications), fatigue (from hypoxemia, increased work of breathing), or feeling full quickly (from lung hyperinflation)? Anorexia, weight loss, and chronic malnutrition are common in patients with COPD, lung cancer, TB, and chronic severe infection (bronchiectasis). Assess fluid intake. Dehydration can cause sputum to thicken and obstruct the airway. Rapid weight gain from fluid retention may impair gas exchange.

Elimination. Activity intolerance from dyspnea could result in incontinence if unable to reach a toilet when needed. Dyspnea can be the cause of limited mobility, which can cause constipation. Ask patients with dyspnea about frequency, urgency, and elimination patterns (e.g., day vs. night). People with a chronic cough, especially women, may have urinary incontinence with coughing.

Activity-exercise. Determine whether dyspnea limits activity. Assess whether the patient's home (e.g., number of steps, levels) poses any problems. Ask the patient about the perceived degree of the dyspnea (Table 27.3). For example, can the patient walk up 1 flight of stairs without stopping because of dyspnea? Is dyspnea with activity better, worse, or about the same in the last few days or months? Determine whether the patient has difficulty breathing in a certain position, or if dyspnea is relieved by assuming a different position (e.g., tripod position in COPD).

Discuss whether the patient can carry out activities of daily living without dyspnea or other respiratory symptoms. If unable, record the amount and type of care the patient needs. Immobility and sedentary habits are risk factors for hypoventilation leading to atelectasis or pneumonia.

TABLE 27.3 Dyspnea Rating Scale

Modified Borg Rating Scale for Perceived Dyspnea

Rate	Description
0	Nothing at all
0.5	Very, very slight shortness of breath
1	Very mild shortness of breath
2	Mild shortness of breath
3	Mild shortness of breath or breathing difficulty
4	Somewhat severe
5	Strong or hard breathing
6	
7	Severe shortness of breath or very hard breathing
8	
9	Extremely severe
10	Shortness of breath so severe you need to stop

From Hillegass E: *Essentials of cardiopulmonary physical therapy,* ed 5, Philadelphia, 2022, Saunders.

Sleep-rest. Determine whether the patient wakes up at night because of lung problems. Patients with asthma or COPD may awaken with chest tightness, wheezing, or coughing. This suggests a need for adjunct therapy or other medication changes. Patients may sleep with the head elevated on several pillows to avoid breathing problems from lying flat *(orthopnea).* Excess weight interferes with normal ventilation and may cause hypoventilation or sleep apnea (see Chapter 8). Night sweats may be a sign of TB.

Cognitive-perceptual. Because hypoxia can cause neurologic symptoms, ask about apprehension, restlessness, irritability, and memory changes. These can indicate inadequate cerebral oxygenation. Assess the patient's ability to cooperate with treatment. Hypoxemia interferes with the ability to learn and retain information. Failure or inability to take part in needed therapy may result in worsening of respiratory problems.

Ask about any discomfort or pain with breathing. Explore reports of chest pain to rule out heart involvement. Problems such as pleurisy, fractured ribs, and costochondritis cause chest pain. Assess the patient having pain with breathing, including onset, location of the pain, and factors that make the pain better or worse.

Self-perception–self-concept. Dyspnea limits activity, impairs ability to fulfill normal roles, and often alters self-esteem. Patients may be reluctant to appear in public with a visible nasal cannula and O_2 equipment. A barrel chest, clubbed fingers, pursed-lip breathing, and frequent expectoration of sputum or throat clearing can be embarrassing and lead to social isolation. Explore any body image concerns.

Role-relationship. Respiratory problems can affect performance in work or other activities. Discuss the impact of medications, O_2 therapy, and special routines (e.g., pulmonary hygiene for cystic fibrosis) on the patient's family, job, and social life.

Review the patient's work and frequency and intensity of exposure to fumes, toxins, asbestos, coal, fibers, or silica. Ask whether symptoms are worse in specific situations (e.g., home vs. work). Hobbies, such as woodworking (sawdust) or pottery (silica), and animal exposure (allergies) can cause respiratory problems. Exposure to fumes, smoke, and other chemicals may trigger an attack in patients with asthma.

Coping–stress tolerance. Dyspnea causes anxiety, and anxiety worsens dyspnea. The result is a vicious cycle—patients avoid activities that cause dyspnea, becoming more deconditioned and more dyspneic. The outcome is often physical and leads to social isolation. Assess how often the patient leaves home and interacts with others. The chronic nature of many respiratory problems, such as COPD and asthma, can cause prolonged stress. Ask about coping strategies to manage this stress.

CASE STUDY

Subjective Data

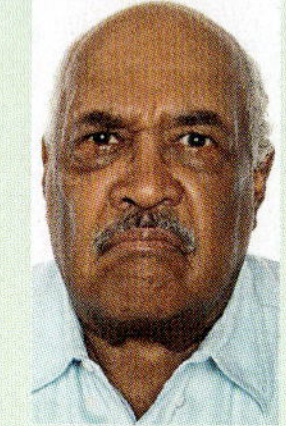

(© Fuse/ Thinkstock.)

A focused subjective assessment of F.T. revealed the following:

- ***History:*** COPD, hypertension, heart failure, benign prostatic hyperplasia. No known allergies.
- ***Medications:*** Metoprolol 50 mg oral daily, furosemide 20 mg oral daily, finasteride 5 mg/day oral, Advair inhaler (fluticasone and salmeterol) 2 puffs twice daily. Uses O_2 at 3 L/min via nasal cannula at home for the past 10 years.
- ***Health Perception–Health Management:*** States he usually manages his COPD well with the Advair inhaler. He thinks he caught a cold from his granddaughter last week. Increasing difficulty breathing. Has a history of 30 pack-years of smoking, quitting 5 years ago.
- ***Nutritional-Metabolic:*** Eating and drinking very little over past 2 to 3 days.
- ***Elimination:*** Voiding small amounts of dark, concentrated urine (mostly at night).
- ***Activity-Exercise:*** At present, cannot walk 100 feet without feeling short of breath. Cannot walk up 1 flight of stairs (21 steps) to get in or out of his apartment without stopping to catch his breath.
- ***Sleep-Rest:*** Difficulty sleeping. Last night he slept upright in his recliner.
- ***Cognitive-Perceptual:*** Denies any pain with the shortness of breath. Feels slightly irritable because of lack of sleep.
- ***Coping–Stress Tolerance:*** Does not know how he will manage to get groceries or clean his apartment. His daughter lives an hour away and has 3 children in school.

Discussion Questions

1. Which subjective assessment findings concern you most?
2. What other information would you ask him about his condition?
3. What will you include in the physical assessment? What would your priorities be in your physical assessment?

You will learn about the physical assessment of the respiratory system in the next section.

Answers available at http://evolve.elsevier.com/Lewis/medsurg.

Objective Data

Physical Assessment

A record of a normal respiratory system physical assessment is shown in Table 27.4. Assessment abnormalities of the thorax and lungs are outlined in Table 27.5. Chest examination findings in common pulmonary problems are described in Table 27.6. Manifestations of inadequate oxygenation are outlined in Table 27.7.

Vital signs. Obtain vital signs before examining the respiratory system. Note the respiratory rate, depth, and rhythm. The normal adult respiratory rate is 12 to 20 breaths/min. Inspiration (I) should take half as long as expiration (E) (I/E ratio = 1:2). Observe for abnormal breathing patterns. Note *Kussmaul* (rapid, deep breathing), *Cheyne-Stokes* (abnormal respirations characterized by alternating periods of apnea and deep, rapid breathing), or *Biot* (irregular breathing with apnea every 4 to 5 cycles) respirations.

Nose. Inspect the nose for patency, inflammation, deformities, symmetry, and discharge. Check each nostril for air patency with respiration while briefly occluding the other nostril. Tilt the head backward and push the tip of the nose upward gently. With a nasal speculum and good light, inspect the interior of the nose. The mucous membrane should be pink and moist, with no edema (bogginess), exudate, or bleeding. Inspect the nasal septum for deviation, perforations, and bleeding. Some septal deviation is normal. Inspect the turbinates for polyps. Polyps are fingerlike projections of swollen nasal mucosa. They may result from long-term irritation of the mucosa (e.g., from allergies). Assess any discharge for color and consistency. Purulent or foul-smelling discharge could occur with a foreign body. Watery discharge could be due to allergies or from cerebrospinal fluid. Bloody discharge could be from trauma or dryness. Thick mucosal discharge could mean an infection.

Mouth and pharynx. Using a good light source, inspect the interior of the mouth for color, lesions, masses, gum retraction, bleeding, and poor dentition. Inspect the tongue for symmetry

TABLE 27.4 Normal Physical Assessment of the Respiratory System

Nose	• Symmetric with no deformities • Nasal mucosa pink, moist with no edema, exudate, blood, or polyps • Nasal septum straight (slight nasal deviation possible) • Nares patent bilaterally
Oral mucosa	• Light pink, moist, no exudate or ulcerations
Pharynx	• Smooth, moist, and pink
Neck	• Trachea midline
Chest	• AP diameter 1:2 • Respirations nonlabored at 12–20 breaths/min • Breath sounds vesicular without crackles or wheezes • Expansion equal bilaterally with no increase in tactile fremitus

TABLE 27.5 ASSESSMENT ABNORMALITIES

Respiratory System

Finding	Description	Common Etiology and Significance
Inspection		
Abdominal paradox	Inward (rather than normal outward) movement of abdomen during inspiration	Inefficient and ineffective breathing pattern; nonspecific sign of severe respiratory distress
Accessory muscle use. Intercostal retractions	Neck and shoulder muscles used to assist breathing; muscles between ribs pull in during inspiration	Chronic obstructive pulmonary disease (COPD), asthma exacerbation, secretion retention Indicates severe respiratory distress/failure, hypoxemia
↑ Anteroposterior (AP) diameter	AP chest diameter equal to lateral Slope of ribs more horizontal (90 degrees) to spine	COPD, asthma, cystic fibrosis, lung hyperinflation, advanced age
Clubbing	↑ Depth, bulk, sponginess of distal part of finger	Chronic hypoxemia, cystic fibrosis, lung cancer, bronchiectasis
Cyanosis	Bluish color of skin best seen in lips and on the palpebral conjunctiva (inside the lower eyelid)	Reflects 5–6 g of hemoglobin not bound with O_2. ↓ O_2 transfer in lungs, ↓ cardiac output
Kussmaul respirations	Regular, rapid, and deep respirations Fruity odor to breath	Metabolic acidosis. Increases CO_2 excretion
Pursed-lip breathing	Exhalation through mouth with lips pursed together to slow exhalation	COPD, asthma. Suggests ↑ breathlessness Strategy taught to slow expiration, ↓ dyspnea
Splinting	Voluntary ↓ in tidal volume to ↓ pain on chest expansion	Thoracic or abdominal incision, chest trauma, pleurisy
Tachypnea	Rate >20 breaths/min	Fever, anxiety, hypoxemia, restrictive lung disease Magnitude of ↑ above normal rate reflects ↑ work of breathing
Tripod position. Inability to lie flat	Leaning forward with arms and elbows supported on overbed table	COPD, asthma exacerbation, pulmonary edema Indicates moderate to severe respiratory distress
Palpation		
Altered chest movement	Unequal or equal but ↓ movement of 2 sides of chest with inspiration	Unequal movement caused by atelectasis, pneumothorax, pleural effusion, splinting Equal but ↓ movement caused by barrel chest, restrictive disease, neuromuscular disease
Altered tactile fremitus	↑ or ↓ in vibrations	↑ in pneumonia, pulmonary edema. ↓ in pleural effusion, lung hyperinflation. Absent in pneumothorax, atelectasis
Tracheal deviation	Leftward or rightward movement of trachea from normal midline position	Nonspecific sign of change in position of mediastinal structures. Medical emergency if caused by tension pneumothorax (trachea deviates to side opposite collapsed lung)
Percussion		
Dullness	Medium-pitched sound over areas that normally make a resonant sound	↑ Density (pneumonia, large atelectasis), ↑ fluid in pleural space (pleural effusion)
Hyperresonance	Loud, lower pitched sound over areas that normally make a resonant sound	Lung hyperinflation (COPD), lung collapse (pneumothorax), air trapping (asthma)
Auscultation		
Absent breath sounds	No sound heard over entire lung or area of lung	Pneumothorax, pleural effusion, mainstem bronchi obstruction, large atelectasis, pneumonectomy, lobectomy
Bronchophony, whispered pectoriloquy	Spoken or whispered syllable more distinct than normal on auscultation	Pneumonia
Coarse **crackles**	Louder, discontinuous, low-pitched sounds caused by air passing through airway intermittently occluded by mucus, unstable bronchial wall. May be heard on inspiration, expiration, or both	Excess fluid within the lungs, heart failure, pulmonary edema, pneumonia with severe congestion, COPD
Egophony	Spoken "E" similar to "A" on auscultation because of altered transmission of voice sounds	Pneumonia, pleural effusion
Fine crackles	Short, discontinuous, high-pitched sounds heard just before the end of inspiration. Result of rapid equalization of gas pressure when collapsed alveoli or terminal bronchioles suddenly snap open	Interstitial edema (early pulmonary edema), alveolar filling (pneumonia), loss of lung volume (atelectasis), early phase of heart failure, idiopathic pulmonary fibrosis
Pleural friction rub	Creaking or grating sound from roughened, inflamed pleural surfaces rubbing together. Evident during inspiration, expiration, or both. No change with coughing. Often uncomfortable, especially on deep inspiration	Pleurisy, pneumonia, pulmonary infarct
Stridor	Continuous musical or crowing sound of constant pitch. Result of partial obstruction of larynx or trachea	Croup, epiglottitis, vocal cord edema after extubation, foreign body
Wheezes	Continuous high-pitched squeaking or musical sound caused by rapid vibration of bronchial walls. First evident on expiration but possibly evident on inspiration as obstruction of airway increases. May be audible without stethoscope	Bronchospasm (caused by asthma), airway obstruction (caused by foreign body, tumor), COPD

TABLE 27.6 Chest Assessment Findings in Respiratory Problems

Problem	Inspection	Palpation	Percussion	Auscultation
Asthma exacerbation	Prolonged expiration, tripod position, pursed lips	↓ Movement	Hyperresonance	Wheezes, ↓ breath sounds ominous sign (severely decreased air movement)
Atelectasis	No change unless involves entire segment, lobe	If small, no change If large, ↓ movement, ↓ fremitus	Dull over affected area	Fine crackles (may disappear with deep breaths) Absent sounds if large
COPD	Barrel chest, cyanosis, tripod position, use of accessory muscles	↓ Movement	Hyperresonant or dull if consolidation	Crackles, wheezes, distant breath sounds
Pleural effusion	Tachypnea, use of accessory muscles	↑ Movement ↑ Fremitus above effusion Absent fremitus over effusion	Dull	↓ or absent over effusion, egophony above effusion
Pneumonia	Tachypnea, use of accessory muscles, duskiness, cyanosis	↑ Fremitus over affected area	Dull over affected areas	*Early:* Bronchial sounds *Later:* Fine and/or coarse crackles, egophony, whispered pectoriloquy
Pulmonary edema	Tachypnea, labored respirations, cyanosis, pink-tinged sputum	↓ Movement or normal movement	Dull or normal depending on amount of fluid	Fine or coarse crackles
Pulmonary fibrosis	Tachypnea	↓ Movement	Normal	Crackles or sounds like Velcro being pulled apart

TABLE 27.7 Manifestations of Inadequate Oxygenation

Manifestations	Onset: Early	Onset: Late
Cardiovascular		
Cool, clammy skin		X
Cyanosis		X
Dysrhythmias	X	X
Hypertension (mild)	X	
Hypotension		X
Tachycardia	X	
Central Nervous System		
Apprehension	X	
Coma		X
Confusion, lethargy	X	X
Restlessness, irritability	X	
Respiratory		
Dyspnea on exertion	X	
Dyspnea at rest		X
Pause for breath between sentences, words		X
Retraction of intercostal spaces on inspiration		X
Tachypnea	X	
Use of accessory muscles		X
Other		
Diaphoresis	X	X
Fatigue	X	X
↓ Urine output	X	X

and lesions. Observe the pharynx by pressing a tongue blade gently against the middle of the back of the tongue. If the oropharynx is tight, have the patient yawn. Yawning usually allows more structures to be visible. The pharynx should be smooth and moist, with exudate, ulcerations, swelling, or postnasal drip. Note the color, symmetry, and any enlargement of the tonsils. Test the gag reflex by placing a tongue blade along the side of the pharynx, at the back of the tongue. A normal response (gagging) means that cranial nerves IX (glossopharyngeal) and X (vagus) are intact, and that the airway is protected.

Neck. Inspect the neck for symmetry and tender or swollen areas. Palpate the lymph nodes while the patient is sitting erect with the neck slightly flexed. Progression of palpation is from the nodes around the ears, to the nodes at the base of the skull, and then to those under the angles of the mandible to the midline. The patient may have small, mobile, nontender nodes *(shotty nodes)*, which are not a sign of a pathologic condition. Tender, hard, or fixed nodes may indicate disease. Describe the location and characteristics of any palpable nodes.

Thorax and lungs. Picture imaginary lines on the chest to help guide your assessment (Fig. 27.2). Describe abnormalities in terms of their location relative to these lines (e.g., 2 cm lateral from the right midclavicular line).

Chest examination is best done in a well-lit, warm room. Take measures to ensure privacy. Expose the patient's chest. Perform all physical assessment maneuvers (inspection, palpation, percussion, auscultation) on either the anterior or posterior chest first rather than moving from anterior to posterior or vice versa with each maneuver. It is best to begin on the posterior chest, particularly with female patients, since you can obtain more information without interference from breast tissue. If the patient tires or you are interrupted, you will obtain baseline data with the most information from examining the posterior chest.

When assessing the *posterior chest,* ask the patient to lean forward with arms folded. This position moves the scapulae away from the spine, exposing more of the area you need to examine. When assessing the *anterior chest,* have the patient sit upright or position the patient supine with the head of the bed elevated to 30 degrees (semi-Fowler's position). The patient may need to lean forward for support on the bedside table to facilitate breathing.

Inspection. First, observe the patient's appearance. Note any sign of respiratory distress, such as tachypnea or use of accessory muscles. Determine the shape and symmetry of the chest. Chest movement should be equal on both sides. The AP diameter should be less than the side-to-side or transverse diameter. Normal AP ratio is 1:2. An increase in AP diameter (e.g., barrel chest) may be due to normal aging or result from lung hyperinflation. Look for abnormalities in the sternum (e.g., *pectus carinatum* [a prominent protrusion of the sternum]) and *pectus excavatum* (an indentation of the lower sternum above the xiphoid process). Note any spinal curvature. Spinal curvatures that affect breathing include kyphosis, scoliosis, and kyphoscoliosis.

Skin color provides clues to respiratory status. Cyanosis, a late sign of hypoxemia, is best seen in light-skinned patients as a bluish tinge to the mucous membranes, lips, and palms of the hands. In dark-skinned persons, cyanosis may be seen as a gray or white discoloration in the conjunctivae or around the mouth. Causes of cyanosis include hypoxemia or decreased cardiac output. Inspect the fingers for *clubbing,* a sign of long-standing hypoxemia. Clubbing is an increase in the angle between the base of the nail and the fingernail to 180 degrees or more. It usually accompanied by an increase in the depth, bulk, and sponginess of the end of the finger.

Palpation. Determine tracheal position by gently placing the index fingers on either side of the trachea just above the suprasternal notch and gently pressing backward. Normal tracheal position is midline; deviation to the left or right is abnormal. Tracheal deviation occurs away from the side of a tension pneumothorax or a neck mass.

Symmetry of chest expansion and extent of movement are determined at the level of the diaphragm. Place your hands over the lower anterior chest wall along the costal margin and move them inward until the thumbs meet at midline. Ask the patient to breathe deeply. Observe the movement of the thumbs away from each other. Normal expansion is 1 inch (2.5 cm). Hand placement on the posterior side of the chest is at the level of the tenth rib. Move the thumbs until they meet over the spine (Fig. 27.5). You can check expansion anteriorly or posteriorly. It is not necessary to check both.

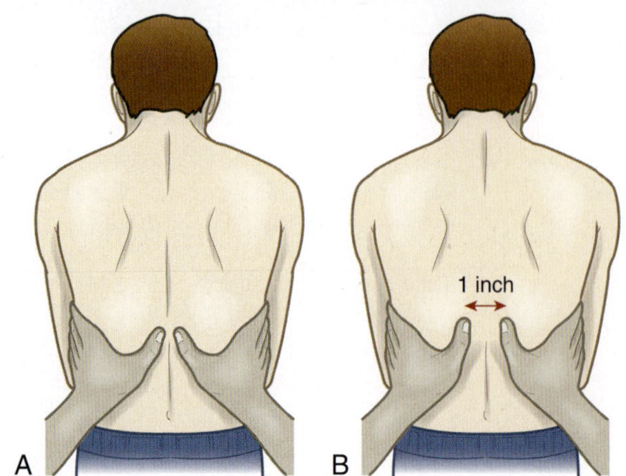

Fig. 27.5 Estimation of thoracic expansion. (A) Exhalation. (B) Maximal inhalation.

Normal chest movement is equal. Unequal expansion occurs when air entry is limited by conditions involving the lung (e.g., atelectasis, pneumothorax) or the chest wall (e.g., incisional pain). Equal but decreased expansion occurs in conditions that produce a hyperinflated or barrel chest or in neuromuscular diseases (e.g., amyotrophic lateral sclerosis, spinal cord lesions). Movement may be absent or unequal over a pleural effusion, an atelectasis, or a pneumothorax.

Fremitus is the vibration of the chest wall made by speech. You can feel tactile fremitus by placing the palmar surface of your hands against the patient's chest with the fingers hyperextended. Ask the patient to repeat a phrase, such as "boy-oh-boy," "toy boat," or "blue balloons," in a deeper, louder-than-normal voice. At the same time, move your hands from top to bottom on the patient's chest (Fig. 27.6). As you palpate, simultaneously compare vibrations (right side vs. left side, from top to bottom). Tactile fremitus is most intense by the sternum and between the scapulae because these areas are closest to the major bronchi. Fremitus is less intense farther away from these areas.

Note any increase, decrease, or absence of fremitus. Increased fremitus occurs when the voice moves through lung filled with fluid or is denser. This happens with pneumonia, lung tumors, thick bronchial secretions, and above a pleural effusion (the lung is compressed upward). Fremitus is decreased if the hand is farther from the lung (e.g., pleural effusion) or the lung is hyperinflated (e.g., barrel chest). Absent fremitus may occur with pneumothorax or atelectasis. The anterior chest is harder to palpate for fremitus because of the large muscles and breast tissue.

Percussion. Percussion is used to assess density or aeration. Percussion sounds are described in Table 27.8. The anterior chest is percussed with the patient in a semisitting or supine position. Starting above the clavicles, percuss downward, intercostal space by intercostal space. The area over lung tissue should be resonant, except for the area of cardiac dullness. To percuss the posterior chest, have the patient sit leaning forward with arms folded. The posterior chest should be resonant over lung tissue to the level of the diaphragm.

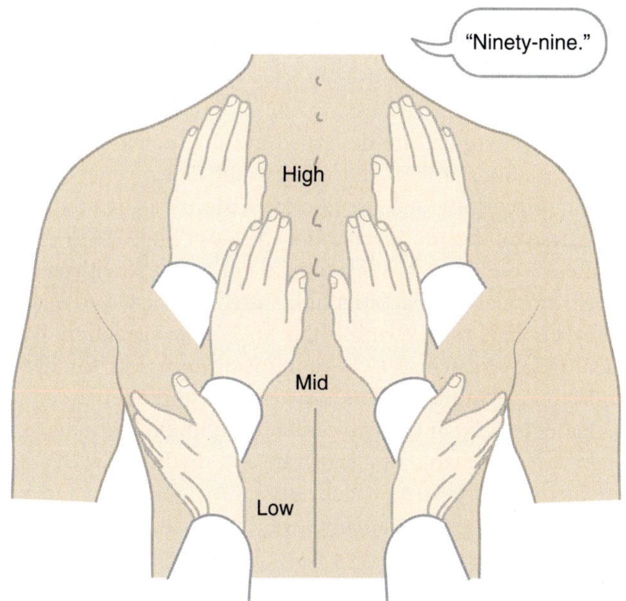

Fig. 27.6 Hand position for tactile fremitus. Place the palms of the hands in the position designated as *"low"* on the right and left sides of the chest. Compare the intensity of vibrations. Continue for all positions in each sequence.

TABLE 27.8 Percussion Sounds

Sound	Description
Dull	Sound with medium-intensity pitch and duration heard over areas of "mixed" solid and lung tissue, such as top area of liver, partially consolidated lung tissue (pneumonia), or fluid-filled pleural space
Flat	Soft, high-pitched sound of short duration heard over very dense tissue where air is not present, such as posterior chest below level of diaphragm
Hyperresonance	Loud, lower pitched sound than normal resonance heard over hyperinflated lungs, such as in chronic obstructive pulmonary disease and acute asthma
Resonance	Low-pitched sound heard over normal lungs
Tympany	Drum-like, loud, empty quality sound heard over pneumothorax

Auscultation. During auscultation, have the patient breathe slowly and a little more deeply than normal through the mouth. Auscultation should proceed from the lung apices to the bases, comparing opposite areas of the chest. If the patient is in mild respiratory distress or you think the patient will tire easily, start at the bases. Place the stethoscope over lung tissue, not over bony prominences. At each placement of the stethoscope, listen to at least 1 cycle of inspiration and expiration. Visualize the location of normal breath sounds (Fig. 27.7).

Lung sounds are heard anteriorly from a line drawn perpendicular from the sternum lateral to the midclavicular line. From the xiphoid process, palpate inferiorly (down) 2 ribs in the midaxillary line and around to the posterior chest. This gives you a fairly accurate and easy way to locate the lung fields. When recording the location of lung sounds, divide the anterior and posterior right lung into thirds (upper, middle, and lower) and the left lung into upper and lower areas. With practice, you will be able to identify which lobes of the lung have particular lung sounds.

The 3 normal breath sounds are bronchial, bronchovesicular, and vesicular (Fig. 27.8). *Bronchial sounds* are loud, high-pitched sounds that resemble air blowing through a hollow pipe. Bronchial sounds have an inspiratory to expiratory (I/E) ratio of 2:3, with a gap between inspiration and expiration. To hear bronchial breath sounds, place the stethoscope next to the trachea in the neck. *Bronchovesicular sounds* have a medium pitch and intensity. They are best heard anteriorly between the first and second intercostal space and posteriorly between the scapulae. Bronchovesicular sounds have a 1:1 ratio, with inspiration equal to expiration. *Vesicular sounds* are relatively soft, low-pitched, gentle, rustling sounds. They are heard over all lung areas except the major bronchi. Vesicular sounds have a 3:1 ratio, with inspiration 3 times longer than expiration.

We classify breath sounds into 2 main categories: normal and abnormal (adventitious). There are a variety of terms that we have used inconsistently to describe abnormal breath sounds. **Adventitious breath sounds** include crackles (fine and coarse), wheezes, stridor, and pleural friction rub (Table 27.5).

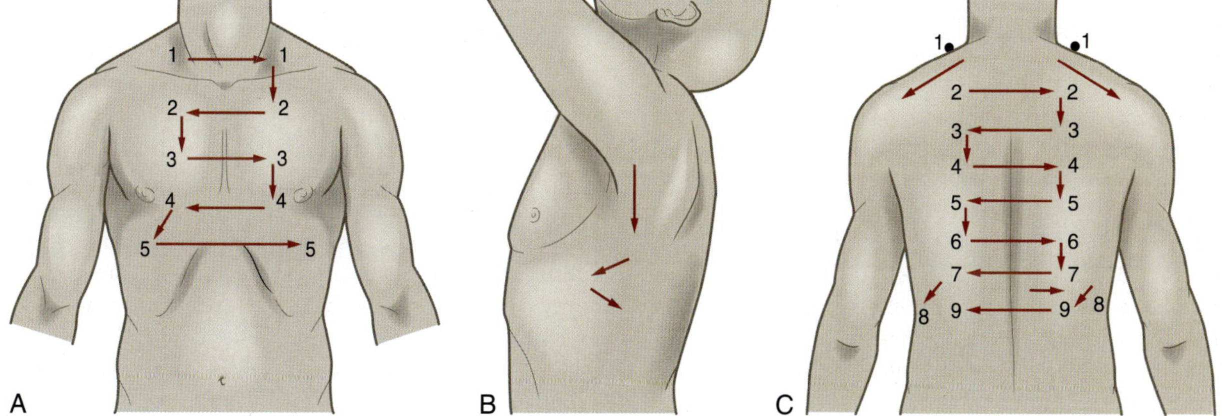

Fig. 27.7 Sequence for auscultation of the chest. (A) Anterior sequence. (B) Lateral sequence. (C) Posterior sequence. Place the stethoscope at each position and listen to at least 1 complete inspiratory and expiratory cycle. Keep in mind that with a female patient the breast tissue will influence the anterior examination.

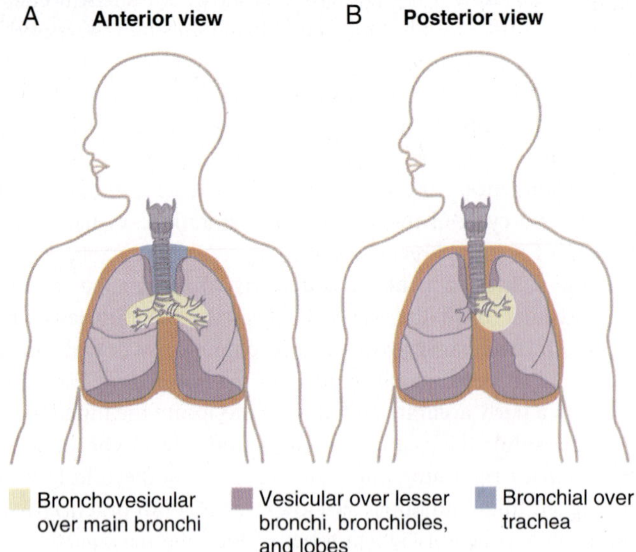

Fig. 27.8 Normal auscultatory sounds. (A) Anterior view. (B) Posterior view.

As you begin assessing lung sounds, first note the air entry, which may be adequate, slightly decreased, or decreased. Absent air entry in any part of the lung is an assessment finding that you should report at once. Next, listen for the breath sounds and the presence of normal and adventitious sounds. Are the normal breath sounds where you would expect to hear them? Focus on the characteristics of any abnormal sound, including the location, pitch (e.g., high, low), duration of sound, and whether the sound is heard on inspiration, expiration, or both.

CASE STUDY

Objective Data: Physical Assessment

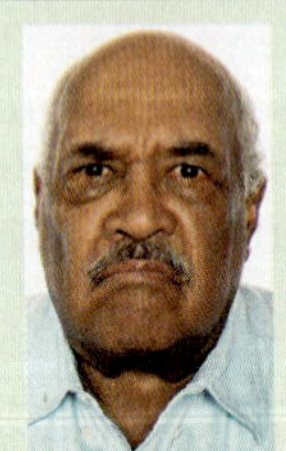

(© Fuse/ Thinkstock.)

Physical assessment findings of F.T. are as follows: Temp: 38°C (100.4°F), apical pulse 110 (irregular), respiratory rate 30 (regular, shallow, slightly labored), BP 170/90 mm Hg. SpO_2 is 87% on room air. Sitting on edge of bed with arms resting on bedside table. Skin color normal for race with no signs of cyanosis. Using accessory muscles in neck and shoulders. Trachea midline. Barrel-shaped chest; chest expansion minimal but equal. Prolonged expiration. Slight clubbing noted. Edema: 3+ pitting edema of both lower legs and feet, bilaterally. Lungs: adequate air entry at apices bilaterally with fine crackles; decreased air entry to right middle lobe and both bases with coarse crackles. Slight expiratory wheeze heard throughout all lung fields. Cough: moist, productive, with yellow-tinged sputum.

Discussion Questions

1. What physical assessment findings concern you most?
2. What diagnostic studies would you expect to be ordered?

You will learn about diagnostic studies of the respiratory system in the next section.

Answers available at http://evolve.elsevier.com/Lewis/medsurg.

DIAGNOSTIC STUDIES OF THE RESPIRATORY SYSTEM

Many diagnostic studies are available to assess the respiratory system. Select studies are described in more detail here.

Two methods are used to assess the effectiveness of gas transfer in the lung and tissue oxygenation: (1) oximetry and (2) analysis of *arterial blood gases* (ABGs) (Table 27.9). These are often used to assess for hypoxia. For patients with normal or near-normal cardiac function, assessing Sao_2 or Pao_2 is usually enough to determine the level of oxygenation. With either one, we can use CO_2 monitoring to assess for hypercapnia to determine patients' oxygenation and ventilatory status. Patients with impaired cardiac output or hemodynamic instability (e.g., changes in heart rate and rhythm, low BP) may have inadequate tissue O_2 delivery and/or abnormal O_2 consumption. For these patients, we can evaluate venous O_2 saturation values.

Oximetry

Oximetry is the measurement of the blood's O_2 saturation.[9] We can measure O_2 saturation in arterial and venous blood. There are noninvasive and invasive oximetry devices.

Arterial

We monitor arterial O_2 saturation (Sao_2) noninvasively and continuously using *pulse oximetry.* We can place the probe on the finger, toe, ear, forehead, or bridge of the nose. The abbreviation SpO_2 is used to indicate the Sao_2. It represents how much O_2 hemoglobin is carrying compared with how much it could carry. SpO_2 and heart rate are displayed on the monitor as digital readings. Normal SpO_2 values are greater than 95% (Table 27.10).[10]

We often assess SpO_2 with each routine vital sign check. SpO_2 values are used during exercise testing and when adjusting flow rates during O_2 therapy. Pulse oximetry is especially valuable in perioperative and critical care situations, in which anesthesia, sedation, or decreased consciousness may mask hypoxia. We can detect changes in SpO_2 and treat patients quickly.

Pulse oximetry values are less accurate when the SpO_2 is less than 70%.[11] At this level, the oximeter may display a value that is ±4% of the actual value. For example, if the SpO_2 reading is 70%, the actual value can range from 66% to 74%. Pulse oximetry is inaccurate if hemoglobin variants (e.g., carboxyhemoglobin, methemoglobin) are present. An accurate SpO_2 may be hard to obtain on patients who are hypothermic, receiving IV vasopressor therapy (e.g., norepinephrine), or have hypoperfusion or vasoconstriction (e.g., shock).[12] If there is doubt about the accuracy of the SpO_2 reading, obtain an ABG analysis to verify the values.

TABLE 27.9 Diagnostic Studies

Oxygenation

Study	Description and Purpose	Nursing Responsibility
Arterial blood gases (ABGs)	Arterial blood obtained through puncture of radial or femoral artery or through arterial catheter. Done to assess acid-base balance, oxygenation/ventilation status, need for and/or change in O_2 therapy, or change in ventilator settings. See Table 27.13 for reference values.	*Before:* Indicate whether patient is using O_2 (flow rate in L/min). Avoid change in O_2 therapy or interventions (e.g., suctioning, position change) for 15 min before obtaining sample. *During:* Assist with positioning (e.g., palm up, wrist slightly hyperextended if radial artery is used). Collect blood in heparinized syringe. To ensure accurate results, expel all air bubbles. *After:* Apply pressure to radial artery for at least 5 min after specimen is obtained to prevent hematoma at the arterial puncture site.
O_2 Monitoring		
Noninvasive oximetry (SpO_2)	Monitors arterial O_2 saturation. Probe attaches to finger, toe, earlobe, bridge of the nose for SpO_2 monitoring. Used for intermittent or continuous monitoring and exercise testing. *Normal SpO_2: >95%.*	*During:* Apply probe. When interpreting SpO_2 values, assess patient status and presence of factors that can alter accuracy of reading. These include motion, low perfusion, cold extremities, bright lights, acrylic nails, dark skin color, carbon monoxide, and anemia.
Invasive oximetry ($ScvO_2$/SvO_2)	Monitors venous O_2 saturation intermittently by obtaining a blood sample from PA catheter or continuously via a fiberoptic sensor as part of a specific central line and monitor. *Normal $ScvO_2$/SvO_2:* 60%–80%.	*During:* Make sure equipment is properly placed and prepped. Changes in values provide an early warning of a change in cardiac output or tissue O_2 delivery. A decrease suggests that less O_2 is being delivered to the tissues or that more O_2 is being consumed.
CO_2 Monitoring		
End-tidal CO_2 ($PetCO_2$) (capnography) (see Fig. 27.9)	Assesses CO_2 level in exhaled air. Graphically displays partial pressure of CO_2. Exhaled gases are sampled from the airway and analyzed by a CO_2 sensor to measure exhaled CO_2. Sensor may be attached to an adaptor on endotracheal or tracheostomy tube. Nasal cannula with a side-stream capnometer can be used in patients without an artificial airway. Can be a diagnostic measure to detect lung disease and for monitoring patients. *Normal difference between $Paco_2$ and $PetCO_2$: 2–5 mm Hg ($Paco_2$: 35–45 mm Hg; $PetCO_2$: 40–50 mm Hg).*	*Before:* Teach patient and caregiver about purpose of capnography monitoring, emphasizing benefit of continuous monitoring. *During:* Make sure sensor is properly attached. Record data per policy.

TABLE 27.10 Normal and Critical Values for Pao_2 and SpO_2

Pao_2 (mm Hg)	SpO_2 (%)	Significance	Manifestations	Management
80–100	≥95	Normal value	Asymptomatic	• Routine patient assessment
60–79	90	Mild hypoxemia	Restlessness, tachycardia, dysrhythmias, dyspnea, hypertension	• Assess patient as needed • Supplemental O_2 may be needed
40–59	88	Moderate hypoxemia	Confusion, lethargy, dysrhythmias, hypotension, respiratory distress, accessory muscle use	• O_2 required • Escalate level of care. Obtain critical care consult • Monitor frequently for sudden deterioration in condition
<40	75	Severe hypoxemia	Cyanosis, coma, respiratory and/or cardiac arrest possible	• High Fio_2, intubation, mechanical ventilation • Continuous patient assessment and evaluation

Venous

Invasive O_2 saturation measurements include venous blood analysis (Table 27.11). Measuring the O_2 saturation of hemoglobin in venous blood helps to determine the adequacy of tissue oxygenation. The O_2 saturation of venous blood from a central venous catheter (CVC) is called *central venous O_2 saturation* ($ScvO_2$). The blood received and measured as $ScvO_2$ from a CVC is primarily from the superior vena cava (SVC), which supplies the upper body (e.g., brain). The O_2 saturation of blood from a pulmonary artery (PA) catheter is the *mixed venous O_2 saturation* (SvO_2). SvO_2 values measured from the PA catheter are a mixture of blood from the SVC, inferior vena cava (IVC), and coronary return.

$ScvO_2$ and SvO_2 reflect the balance among oxygenation of the arterial blood, tissue perfusion, and tissue O_2 consumption (Table 27.12).[13] This gives a global indicator of the balance between O_2 delivery and O_2 consumption. Normal $ScvO_2$ or SvO_2 at rest is 60% to 80%. Even though these values vary slightly, we use both effectively when treating critically ill patients in the intensive care unit (ICU). $ScvO_2$ and SvO_2 are useful in assessing hemodynamic status and response to treatments or activities when considered with SaO_2.

Review sustained decreases and increases in $ScvO_2$ or SvO_2. Decreased $ScvO_2$ or SvO_2 may indicate decreased arterial oxygenation, low cardiac output (CO), low hemoglobin level, or increased O_2 consumption or extraction, which is the ability of tissues to take O_2 from the blood. If the $ScvO_2$ or SvO_2 falls below 60%, determine which factor has changed. Observe for changes in arterial oxygenation (e.g., monitor pulse oximetry, ABGs) and indirectly assess CO and tissue perfusion. This is done by noting any changes in mental status, strength and quality of peripheral pulses, capillary refill, urine output, and skin color and temperature. If arterial oxygenation, CO, and hemoglobin level are unchanged, a fall in $ScvO_2$ or SvO_2 indicates increased O_2 consumption or extraction. This could represent an increased metabolic rate, pain, movement, fever, or shivering. If O_2 consumption increases without a comparable increase in O_2 delivery, more O_2 is extracted from the blood. $ScvO_2$ and SvO_2 will continue to fall.[13]

Increased $ScvO_2$ or SvO_2 may indicate a clinical improvement (e.g., increased arterial O_2 saturation, improved perfusion, decreased metabolic rate) or problem (e.g., sepsis). In sepsis, O_2 is not extracted properly at the tissue level related to the immune response, leaking vessels, and increased fluid build-up, resulting in increased $ScvO_2$ or SvO_2.

TABLE 27.11 Mixed Venous Blood Gas Values

pH	7.31–7.41
PvO_2	38–42 mm Hg
SvO_2	60%–80%
$PvCO_2$	38–55 mm Hg
HCO_3^-	22–26 mEq/L (mmol/L)

$PvCO_2$, Partial pressure of CO_2 in venous blood; *PvO_2*, partial pressure of O_2 in venous blood; *SvO_2*, mixed venous O_2 saturation.

Changes in $ScvO_2$ or SvO_2 guide your interventions. For example, you may note that the heart rate (HR) increased slightly during repositioning but that the $ScvO_2$ remained stable. In this case you would conclude that the patient tolerated the position change. If the $ScvO_2$ dropped, this would be a sign to stop the activity until the $ScvO_2$ returned to baseline.

In many cases, as activity or metabolism increases, HR and CO increase, and $ScvO_2$ or SvO_2 stays constant or varies slightly. However, critically ill patients often have conditions (e.g., heart failure, shock) that prevent substantial increases in CO. In these cases, $ScvO_2$ or SvO_2 can be a useful indicator of the balance between O_2 delivery and consumption.

Arterial Blood Gases

ABGs are obtained to determine oxygenation status and acid-base balance. ABG analysis includes measurement of the PaO_2, $PaCO_2$ (the partial pressure of CO_2 in arterial blood), acidity (pH), bicarbonate (HCO_3^-), and SaO_2. Normal values for ABGs are shown in Table 27.13.

Blood for ABG analysis can be obtained by arterial puncture or from an arterial catheter, which is usually inserted into the radial or femoral artery. Both techniques allow for intermittent analysis. An arterial catheter permits ABG sampling without repeated arterial punctures. The normal PaO_2 decreases with advancing age. It varies in relation to the distance above sea level. At higher altitudes, the barometric pressure is lower, resulting in a lower inspired O_2 pressure and a lower PaO_2.

CO_2 Monitoring

CO_2 can be monitored using transcutaneous CO_2 ($PtCO_2$) and end-tidal CO_2 ($PetCO_2$) capnography. Transcutaneous measurement of CO_2 is a noninvasive method of estimating arterial pressure of CO_2 ($PaCO_2$) using an electrode placed on the skin.[14]

$PetCO_2$ is the noninvasive measurement of alveolar CO_2 during exhalation when CO_2 concentration is at its peak (Fig. 27.9). It is used to monitor and assess trends in patients' ventilatory status. Expired gases are sampled from the patient's airway and are analyzed by a CO_2 sensor that uses infrared light to measure exhaled CO_2. Capnography is usually presented as a graph of expiratory CO_2 plotted against time.[15]

Sputum Studies

Observe sputum for color, volume, viscosity, and presence or absence of blood. We can obtain a sputum sample by expectoration, tracheal suction, or bronchoscopy. When patients are unable to expectorate spontaneously, sputum may be collected by inhaling an irritating aerosol, usually hypertonic saline. This is called *sputum induction.*

A sputum culture and sensitivity can identify an infecting organism (e.g., *Mycobacterium*) or confirm a diagnosis (e.g., cancer). Table 27.14 describes common sputum tests and our responsibilities when obtaining samples.

TABLE 27.12 Interpreting $ScvO_2$ and SvO_2 Measurements

$ScvO_2$ and SvO_2 Measurement[a]	Physiologic Basis for Change in $ScvO_2$ or SvO_2	Clinical Diagnosis and Rationale
High $ScvO_2$ or SvO_2 (80%–95%)	↑ O_2 supply ↓ O_2 demand	• Patient receiving more O_2 than needed by clinical condition • Anesthesia, which causes sedation and ↓ muscle movement • Hypothermia, which ↓ metabolic demand (e.g., with cardiopulmonary bypass) • Sepsis caused by ↓ ability of tissues to use O_2 at the cellular level • False high positive because pulmonary artery catheter is wedged in a pulmonary capillary (SvO_2 only)
Normal $ScvO_2$ or SvO_2 (60%–80%)	Normal O_2 supply and metabolic demand	• Balanced O_2 supply and demand
Low $ScvO_2$ or SvO_2 (<60%)	↓ O_2 supply caused by low hemoglobin ↓ Arterial saturation (Sao_2) ↓ Cardiac output ↑ O_2 demand	• Anemia or bleeding with compromised cardiopulmonary system • Hypoxemia from ↓ O_2 supply or lung disease • Cardiogenic shock caused by left ventricular pump failure • Metabolic demand exceeds O_2 supply in conditions that ↑ muscle movement and metabolic rate (e.g., seizures, fever)

[a]$ScvO_2$ values are generally slightly higher than SvO_2 values.
From Urden LD, Stacy KM, Lough ME: *Critical care nursing: diagnosis and management,* ed 9, St Louis, 2022, Mosby.

TABLE 27.13 Normal Arterial Blood Gas Values

Laboratory Value	Sea Level	1 Mile Above Sea Level
pH	7.35–7.45	7.35–7.45
Pao_2	80–100 mm Hg	65–75 mm Hg
Sao_2	>95%	>95%
$Paco_2$	35–45 mm Hg	35–45 mm Hg
HCO_3^-	22–26 mEq/L (mmol/L)	22–26 mEq/L (mmol/L)

HCO_3^-, Bicarbonate; *$Paco_2$*, partial pressure of arterial CO_2; *Pao_2*, partial pressure of O_2 in arterial blood; *Sao_2*, arterial O_2 saturation.

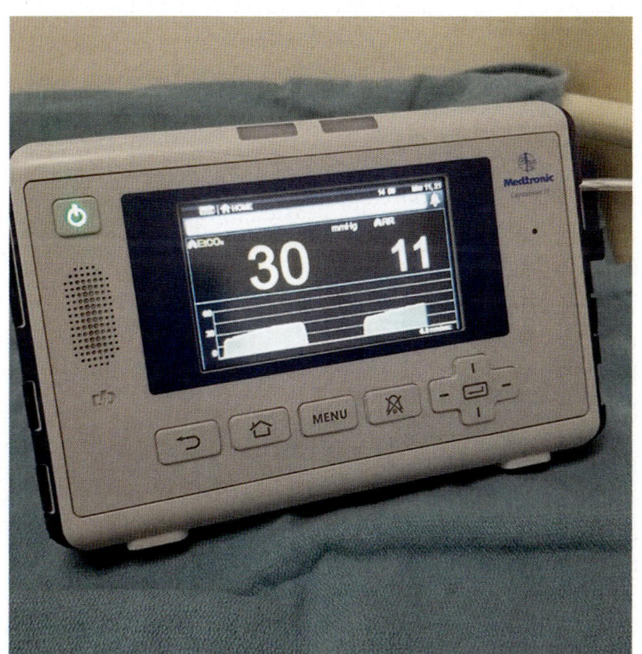

Fig. 27.9 End-tidal CO_2 detector. It is used to measure the exhaled concentration of carbon dioxide.

Skin Tests

Skin tests may be done to assess for allergies (see Chapter 14) or exposure to TB bacilli or fungi. Skin tests involve the intradermal injection of an antigen. Table 27.15 discusses how to interpret tuberculin skin testing. For example, a positive result on a TB skin test means that the patient has been exposed to the antigen. It does not mean that the patient has TB. A negative result means either no exposure or a depression of cell-mediated immunity, which occurs in HIV infection.

Our responsibilities are similar for all skin tests. To prevent a false-negative reaction, be sure that the injection is intradermal and not subcutaneous. After the injection, circle the site(s) and tell the patient not to remove the marks. When charting administration of the antigen, draw a diagram of the forearm and hand, and label the injection site.

When reading test results, use a good light. If an induration is present, use a marking pen to indicate the periphery on all 4 sides of the induration. As the pen touches the raised area, make a mark. Then determine the diameter of the induration in millimeters. Do not measure reddened, flat areas.

Bronchoscopy

Bronchoscopy is a procedure in which the bronchi are seen through a fiberoptic tube (Fig. 27.10). Bronchoscopy may be used for diagnostic purposes (obtain biopsy specimens) and for treatment (e.g., to remove mucous plugs, foreign bodies). Laser therapy, electrocautery, cryotherapy, and stents may be placed through a bronchoscope to achieve patency of an airway that has been partially or nearly fully obstructed by tumors (Table 27.16).

Bronchoscopy can be done in an outpatient procedure room, surgery, or at the bedside in the critical care or medical-surgical unit. Patients may be positioned supine, in low-Fowler's, or even be seated. The HCP inserts the

TABLE 27.14 Sputum Studies

Study	Description and Purpose	Nursing Responsibility
Acid-fast bacteria (AFB) smear and culture	2 different tests used to assess sputum for acid-fast bacilli (e.g., *TB*). In AFB smear (a rapid test), sputum sample spread thinly on glass slide, treated with a fluorochrome stain, and examined under a microscope for AFB. Culture for AFB may take 6 weeks.	*During:* Obtain specimen in early morning after mouth care because secretions collect during night. Have patient expectorate sputum into container after coughing deeply. If unsuccessful, try increasing oral fluid intake unless fluids are restricted. Can collect sputum in sterile container (sputum trap) during suctioning via endotracheal tube or by aspirating secretions from the trachea. If patient cannot produce specimen, they may need bronchoscopy (Fig. 27.10). *After:* Send specimen to laboratory promptly for analysis.
Culture and sensitivity	Diagnose bacterial infection, select antibiotic, and evaluate treatment. Sputum specimen collected in a sterile container. Takes 48–72 h for results.	
Cytology	Determines presence of abnormal cells that may indicate cancer. Single sputum specimen collected in special container with fixative solution.	
Gram stain	Sputum staining allows for classification of bacteria into gram-negative and gram-positive types. Results guide therapy until culture and sensitivity results are complete.	

TABLE 27.15 Interpreting TB Skin Testing

Response	Consider Positive in the Following Groups
Positive Reactions	
≥5-mm induration	• HIV-infected people • People who had recent contact with a person with TB disease • People with fibrotic lesions on chest x-ray consistent with prior TB • Patients with organ transplants • Immunosuppressed persons (e.g., taking the equivalent of ≥15 mg/day of prednisone or those taking tumor necrosis factor—α [TNF-α] antagonists)
≥10-mm induration	• Recent immigrants (<5 years) from high-prevalence countries • Injecting drug users • Residents and employees of high-risk congregate settings • Mycobacteriology laboratory personnel • People with clinical conditions (e.g., diabetes mellitus, end-stage kidney disease) that place them at high risk • People with low body weight (<90% of ideal body weight)
≥15-mm induration	• Any person with no known risk factors for TB
False Reactions	**Possible Causes**
False-negative reactions (do not react even though infected)	• Anergy, immunosuppression • Recent TB infection (within 8–10 weeks of exposure) • Overwhelming TB infection • Recent live virus vaccination (e.g., measles, chickenpox) • Incorrect method of administration or interpretation of tuberculin skin test (TST)
False-positive reactions (react even though not infected)	• Nontuberculous mycobacteria (e.g., *Mycobacterium avium-intracellulare* [MAI] or *Mycobacterium avium* complex [MAC]) • Previous bacille Calmette-Guérin (BCG) vaccine • Incorrect interpretation or antigen of TST

From Centers for Disease Control and Prevention: *Tuberculosis (TB) fact sheet: tuberculin skin testing.* Retrieved from www.cdc.gov/tb/publications/factsheets/testing/skintesting.htm.

bronchoscope through the nose or mouth. Depending on the approach, the nasopharynx or oropharynx is anesthetized with local anesthetic spray. The bronchoscope is coated with water-soluble lubricant and inserted down into the airways. Small amounts (30 mL) of sterile saline may be injected through the scope and withdrawn and examined for cells, a technique termed *bronchoalveolar lavage* (BAL). Bronchoscopy can be done through the endotracheal tube of mechanically ventilated patients.

Lung Biopsy

The purpose of a lung biopsy is to obtain tissue, cells, and/or fluid for evaluation. Specimens can be cultured or examined for cancer cells. Lung biopsy may be done (1) transbronchially, (2) percutaneously or via transthoracic needle aspiration (TTNA), (3) by video-assisted thoracic surgery (VATS), or (4) as an open lung biopsy (Table 27.16).

Transbronchial biopsy involves passing a forceps or needle through the bronchoscope for a specimen. A combination of transbronchial lung biopsy and BAL is used to distinguish infection and rejection in lung transplant recipients. A percutaneous or TTNA biopsy involves inserting a needle through the chest wall, usually under bedside ultrasound or CT guidance. Because of the risk for a pneumothorax, a chest x-ray is done after TTNA.

In VATS, a rigid scope with a lens is passed through a trocar placed into the pleura via 1 or 2 small incisions in the thoracic cavity. The HCP views the lesions in the pleura or peripheral lung on a monitor directly via the scope and can obtain biopsy specimens. A chest tube is kept in place until the lung expands. VATS is much less invasive than open lung biopsy. It is associated with shorter hospital stays and reduced mortality.[16] It is ideal for pleural biopsy and resecting lung nodules.

An open lung biopsy is used when other procedures cannot diagnose pulmonary disease. With patients under anesthesia, the chest is opened with a thoracotomy incision and a biopsy specimen is obtained. Postprocedure care is the same as after thoracotomy (see Chapter 28).

Thoracentesis

Thoracentesis is the insertion of a large-bore needle through the chest wall into the pleural space to obtain specimens for diagnostic evaluation, remove pleural fluid, or instill medication (Fig. 27.11). Patients are positioned sitting upright, leaning on an overbed table with feet supported. The skin is cleansed, and a local anesthetic (lidocaine) is injected subcutaneously. A percutaneous catheter may be left in to allow further drainage of fluid (Table 27.16).

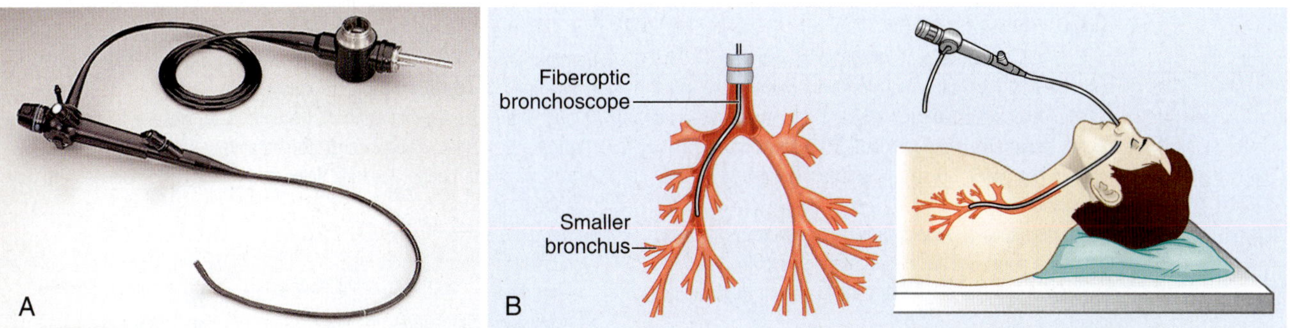

Fig. 27.10 Fiberoptic bronchoscope. (A) The transbronchoscopic balloon-tipped catheter and the flexible fiberoptic bronchoscope. (B) The catheter is introduced into a small airway and the balloon inflated with 1.5 to 2 mL of air to occlude the airway. Bronchoalveolar lavage is done by injecting and withdrawing 30-mL aliquots of sterile saline solution, gently aspirating after each instillation. Specimens are sent to the laboratory for analysis. (A, Courtesy Olympus America Inc., Melville, NY.)

TABLE 27.16 Diagnostic Studies

Respiratory System

Study	Description and Purpose	Nursing Responsibility
Endoscopy		
Bronchoscopy (Fig. 27.10)	Flexible fiberoptic scope used for diagnosis, biopsy, specimen collection, or assessment of changes. May be done to suction mucous plugs, lavage lungs, or remove foreign objects.	*Before:* Obtain signed consent. Have patient be NPO for 6–12 h before the test. Give ordered sedation. *After:* Keep patient NPO until gag reflex returns. Monitor for recovery from sedation. Blood-tinged mucus is not abnormal. If biopsy was done, monitor for hemorrhage and pneumothorax.
Lung biopsy	Specimens may be obtained by transbronchial or percutaneous biopsy or via transthoracic needle aspiration (TTNA), video-assisted thoracoscopic surgery (VATS), or open lung biopsy. Transbronchial biopsy and VATS can be done in the bronchoscopy suite. TTNA done under CT guidance in radiology department. Open lung and VATS done in the operating room (OR). Tests used to obtain specimens for laboratory analysis.	*Before:* Obtain signed consent. Same as bronchoscopy if procedure done with bronchoscope, and same as thoracotomy if open lung biopsy done. *After TTNA:* Check breath sounds q4h for 24 h and report respiratory distress. Check incision site for bleeding. Chest x-ray should be done after TTNA or transbronchial biopsy to check for pneumothorax. *After VATS:* A chest tube may be placed until lung has reexpanded. Monitor breath sounds to follow chest reexpansion. Encourage deep breathing for lung reinflation.
Mediastinoscopy	Scope inserted through a small incision in suprasternal notch and advanced into mediastinum to inspect and biopsy lymph nodes. Used to diagnose lung cancer, non-Hodgkin lymphoma, granulomatous infections, and sarcoidosis.	*Before:* Obtain signed consent. Prepare patient for surgery. Done in OR using a general anesthetic. *After:* Monitor as for bronchoscopy.
Exercise Testing	Diagnose and determine exercise capacity. A *complete test* involves walking on a treadmill while monitoring expired O_2 and CO_2, respiratory rate, heart rate, and heart rhythm. In a *modified test* (desaturation test), only SpO_2 is monitored.	*Before:* Have patient wear comfortable shoes. *During:* Encourage patient to hold handlebars on treadmill and walk as quickly as possible.
Pulmonary Function Tests	Evaluate lung function. Involves use of spirometer to assess air movement as patient performs prescribed respiratory maneuvers (Tables 27.17 and 27.18).	*Before:* Do not schedule immediately after mealtime. Avoid administration of inhaled bronchodilator 6 h before. Assess for respiratory distress. *During:* Assess for respiratory distress. *After:* Assess for respiratory distress. Provide rest after procedure.

Continued

TABLE 27.16 **Diagnostic Studies—cont'd**

Study	Description and Purpose	Nursing Responsibility
Radiology		
Chest x-ray	Screen, diagnose, and evaluate changes in respiratory system. Most common views are anteroposterior (AP) and lateral.	*Before:* Have patient undress to waist, put on gown, and remove any metal between neck and waist.
CT scan	Diagnose suspicious lesions difficult to assess (e.g., mediastinum, hilum, pleura) by conventional x-ray. Common types are helical or spiral CT (contrast medium usually used) and high-resolution CT scan (contrast medium not used). Spiral CT used to diagnose a pulmonary embolism.	*Before:* Before contrast medium used, evaluate renal function. Patient may need to be NPO 4 h before study. *During:* Warn patient that contrast injection may cause a feeling of being warm and flushed. Patient must lie completely still during scan. *After:* Encourage patient to drink fluids to avoid renal problems with any contrast.
MRI	In-depth diagnosis of lesions difficult to assess by CT scan (e.g., lung apex) and for differentiating vascular from nonvascular structures. An IV contrast agent (gadolinium) may be given.	*Before:* Oral and/or IV contrast injection may be used. Check for pregnancy, allergies, and renal function before. Have patient remove all metal objects. Remove metallic foil patches. Contraindicated for persons with implanted metallic devices or other metal fragments unless noted to be MRI safe. Ask about any history of surgical insertion of staples, plates, dental bridges, or other metal appliances. Patient may need to be fasting. Assess for claustrophobia and the need for antianxiety medication. *During:* Patient must lie completely still during scan.
Positron emission tomography (PET) scan	Glucose-containing nuclear tracer substance injected and taken up by metabolically active cells. Follow-up scan shows different-colored tissues based on metabolic rate. Because cancer cells have an increased uptake of glucose, "hot spots" reflecting increased glucose consumption indicate the presence of active cancer. Used to distinguish benign and cancerous lung nodules.	*Before:* Obtain IV access to inject the tracer substance. Patients should be NPO, except for water and medications, for at least 4 h before scan. Hold glucose-containing IV solutions and change to normal saline. Check blood glucose levels. The glucose level must be from 60 —140 mg/dL (3.3—7.8 μmol/L) for accurate glucose metabolic activity. *During:* Patient must lie completely still during scan. *After:* Encourage fluids to excrete radioactive substance.
Pulmonary angiogram	Visualize pulmonary vasculature and locate obstruction or pathologic conditions (e.g., pulmonary embolus). Contrast medium injected through a catheter threaded into pulmonary artery or right side of heart. Series of x-rays taken after contrast medium is injected into pulmonary artery.	*Before:* Assess for allergies, especially to contrast dye. Have patient fast 6—12 h before. Give sedative and other drugs, as ordered. *After:* Check pressure dressing site after procedure. Monitor BP, pulse, and circulation distal to injection site. Place compression device over site. Maintain IV and/or oral fluid intake.
Ventilation-perfusion (V/Q) scan	Assesses ventilation and perfusion of lungs. IV radioisotope given to assess perfusion. To assess ventilation, patient inhales a radioactive gas (xenon or krypton) that outlines alveoli. Normal scans show homogeneous radioactivity. ↓ or absent radioactivity suggests lack of perfusion or airflow. Ventilation without perfusion suggests a pulmonary embolus.	Same as for chest x-ray. *After:* No precautions needed afterward because the gas and isotope transmit radioactivity for only a brief interval.
6-Minute Walk Test	Measure functional capacity and response to treatment in patients with heart or lung disease. Pulse oximetry usually monitored during walk. Distance walked measured and used to monitor progression of disease or improvement after rehabilitation.	*During:* Patient walks as far as possible during 6 min, stopping when short of breath and continuing when able. Continually assess and observe patient tolerance to test.
Thoracentesis (Fig. 27.11)	Obtain specimen of pleural fluid for diagnosis, remove pleural fluid, or instill medication. Do chest x-ray after procedure to check for pneumothorax.	*Before:* Explain procedure and obtain signed consent. *During:* Usually done in patient's room. Position patient upright with elbows on an overbed table and feet supported. Tell patient not to talk or cough during procedure. *After:* Observe for signs of hypoxia and pneumothorax, and verify breath sounds in all fields. Encourage deep breaths to expand lungs. Send labeled specimens to laboratory promptly for analysis.

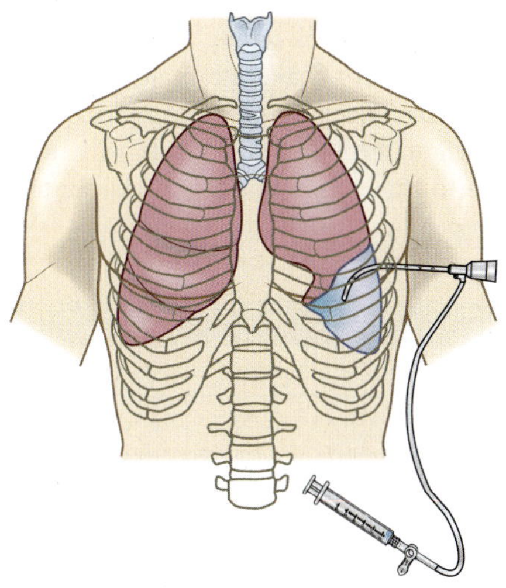

Fig. 27.11 Thoracentesis. A catheter is positioned in the pleural space to remove accumulated fluid.

Pulmonary Function Tests

Pulmonary function tests (PFTs) measure lung volumes and airflow. The results of PFTs can diagnose pulmonary disease, monitor disease progression, assess response to bronchodilators, and evaluate disability. Airflow measurement is obtained by trained personnel using a spirometer. The patient inserts a mouthpiece, takes as deep a breath as possible, and exhales as hard, as fast, and for as long as possible. Verbal coaching is given to ensure that the patient continues blowing out until exhalation is complete.

Computer software calculates the percent of predicted values, that is, how well the performance compares with an average based on age, gender, race, and height.[17] Normal values are 80% to 120% of the predicted value. Normal values for PFTs are shown in Tables 27.17 and 27.18.

Spirometry may be done before and after giving a bronchodilator to determine the response. This helps gauge the reversibility of airway obstruction (e.g., asthma). A positive

TABLE 27.17 Lung Volumes and Capacities

Parameter	Definitions	Normal Value (L)[a]
Volumes		
Expiratory reserve volume (ERV)	Additional air that can be forcefully exhaled after normal exhalation is complete	1.0
Inspiratory reserve volume (IRV)	Maximum volume of air that can be inhaled forcefully after normal inhalation	3.0
Residual volume (RV)	Amount of air remaining in lungs after forced expiration. Air available in lungs for gas exchange between breaths	1.5
Tidal volume (V_T)	Volume of air inhaled and exhaled with each breath. Only a small proportion of total capacity of lungs	0.5
Capacities		
Functional residual capacity (FRC)	Volume of air remaining in lungs at end of normal exhalation (FRC = ERV + RV). Increase or decrease possible with lung disease	2.5
Inspiratory capacity (IC)	Maximum volume of air that can be inhaled after normal expiration (IC = V_T + IRV)	3.5
Total lung capacity (TLC)	Maximum volume of air that lungs can contain (TLC = IRV + V_T + ERV + RV)	6.0
Vital capacity (VC)	Maximum volume of air that can be exhaled after maximum inspiration (VC = IRV + V_T + ERV). Higher VC for males (generally)	4.5

[a]Normal values vary with patient's height, weight, age, race, and gender.

TABLE 27.18 Pulmonary Function Airflow

Measure	Description	Normal Value[a]
Forced vital capacity (FVC)	Amount of air that can be quickly and forcefully exhaled after maximum inspiration	>80% of predicted
Forced expiratory volume in first second of expiration (FEV_1)	Amount of air exhaled in first second of FVC. Grades severity of airway obstruction	>80% of predicted
FEV_1/FVC ratio	Dividing value for FEV_1 by value for FVC. Useful in differentiating obstructive and restrictive pulmonary dysfunction	*Age <50:* ≥75% of predicted *Age ≥50:* ≥70% of predicted
Forced midexpiratory flow rate ($FEF_{25\%-75\%}$)	Measurement of airflow rate in middle half of forced expiration. Early indicator of disease of small airways	*Age <50:* ≥75% of predicted *Age ≥50:* ≥70% of predicted
Peak expiratory flow rate (PEFR)	Maximum airflow rate during forced expiration. Aids in monitoring bronchoconstriction in asthma. Can be measured with peak flow meter	Up to 600 L/min
Maximal voluntary ventilation (MVV)	Deep breathing as rapidly as possible for specified period. Fairly nonspecific test that gives information about exercise capacity. Done with exercise stress test	About 170 L/min

[a]Normal values vary with height, age, race, and gender.

bronchodilator response is an increase of greater than 200 mL or 12% in FEV_1 after administering a bronchodilator.

Home spirometry may be used to monitor lung function in people with asthma, cystic fibrosis, or COPD, as well as before and after lung transplantation or thoracic surgeries. A peak flow meter is the hand-held instrument used at home. The person blows through it forcefully and quickly after taking a deep breath. Spirometry changes can alert to early lung transplant rejection or infection. Data from a peak flow meter provide important feedback to patients with asthma so that they can learn to change activities and medications in response to changes in peak expiratory flow rates.

CASE STUDY

Objective Data: Diagnostic Studies

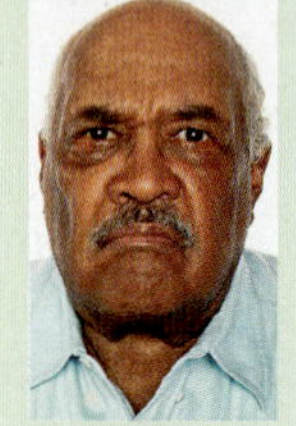

(© Fuse/ Thinkstock.)

The HCP orders the following diagnostic studies for F.T.:

- Chest x-ray
- 12-lead ECG
- Complete blood count (CBC), basic metabolic panel (electrolytes, blood urea nitrogen [BUN], creatinine)
- ABGs
- Sputum for culture and sensitivity

F.T.'s chest x-ray shows a slightly enlarged heart and bilateral consolidation to both lower lobes. The 12-lead ECG reveals sinus tachycardia, rate 110, with no ST segment elevation or depression and no T-wave inversion. The ABGs show compensated respiratory alkalosis with hypoxemia. The white blood cell (WBC) count is 17,350/μL and potassium is 2.9 mEq/L. Sputum results are pending. F.T. is admitted to the medical nursing unit.

Discussion Questions

1. Which diagnostic test results concern you most?
2. What do you think is the cause of F.T.'s problems?
3. What is the interprofessional team's top priority for F.T. at this time?

Answers available at http://evolve.elsevier.com/Lewis/medsurg.

BRIDGE TO NCLEX EXAMINATION

The number of the question corresponds to the same-numbered learning outcome identified at the beginning of this chapter.

1. The key anatomic landmark that separates the upper respiratory tract from the lower respiratory tract is the
   a. carina.
   b. larynx.
   c. trachea.
   d. epiglottis.
2. A patient asks, "How does air get into my lungs?" You base your answer on the knowledge that air moves into the lungs because of
   a. an increase in intrathoracic pressure and decrease atmospheric pressure.
   b. contraction of the accessory abdominal muscles.
   c. stimulation of the respiratory muscles by the chemoreceptors.
   d. a decrease in intrathoracic pressure from an increase in thoracic cavity size.
3. You can *best* determine adequate arterial oxygenation of the blood by assessing
   a. heart rate.
   b. hemoglobin level.
   c. arterial oxygen partial pressure.
   d. arterial carbon dioxide partial pressure.
4. Defense mechanisms that help protect the lung from inhaled particles and microorganisms include the **(select all that apply)**
   a. cough reflex.
   b. mucociliary escalator.
   c. alveolar macrophages.
   d. reflex bronchoconstriction.
   e. alveolar capillary membrane.
5. During the respiratory assessment of an older adult, you would expect to find **(select all that apply)**
   a. a vigorous reflex cough.
   b. increased chest expansion.
   c. increased residual volume.
   d. decreased lung sounds at base of lungs.
   e. increased anteroposterior (AP) chest diameter.
6. When assessing subjective data related to the respiratory health of a patient with emphysema, you would ask about **(select all that apply)**
   a. date of last chest x-ray.
   b. dyspnea during rest or exercise.
   c. pulmonary function test results.
   d. ability to sleep through the entire night.
   e. prescription and over-the-counter medication.
7. When auscultating the chest of a patient in mild respiratory distress, it is *best* to
   a. begin listening at the apices.
   b. begin listening at the lung bases.
   c. begin listening on the anterior chest.
   d. ask the patient to breathe through the nose with the mouth closed.

8. Which respiratory assessment finding would you interpret as abnormal?
   a. Inspiratory chest expansion of 1 inch
   b. Symmetric chest expansion and contraction
   c. Resonance (to percussion) over the lung bases
   d. Bronchial breath sounds in the lower lung fields
9. To detect early signs or symptoms of inadequate oxygenation, you would examine the patient for
   a. dyspnea and hypotension.
   b. apprehension and restlessness.
   c. cyanosis and cool, clammy skin.
   d. increased urine output and diaphoresis.
10. You are preparing the patient for a diagnostic procedure to remove pleural fluid for analysis. You would prepare the patient for which test?
   a. Thoracentesis
   b. Bronchoscopy
   c. Pulmonary angiography
   d. Sputum culture and sensitivity
11. The RN teaches the patient undergoing frequent arterial blood gas analysis that the ABGs can measure **(select all that apply)**
   a. acid-base balance.
   b. bicarbonate (HCO_3^-).
   c. mixed venous O_2 (SvO_2).
   d. compliance and resistance.
   e. partial pressure of O_2 (Pao_2).

1. a; 2. d; 3. c; 4. a, b, c, d; 5. c, d, e; 6. b, d, e; 7. b; 8. d; 9. b; 10. a; 11. a, b, e.

For rationales to these answers and even more NCLEX review questions, visit http://evolve.elsevier.com/Lewis/medsurg.

REFERENCES

To access the References for this chapter, please scan the QR code with a mobile device.

28

Supporting Ventilation

Eugene E. Mondor

http://evolve.elsevier.com/Lewis/medsurg/

CONCEPTUAL FOCUS

Acid-Base Balance
Functional Ability
Gas Exchange
Perfusion

LEARNING OUTCOMES

1. Identify airway clearance techniques that promote gas exchange.
2. Describe the indications for O_2 therapy, including delivery methods and complications.
3. Explain the purpose, function, and nursing responsibilities related to chest tubes and chest drainage systems.
4. Discuss the types of chest surgery and perioperative care.
5. Relate the important aspects of care for patients receiving noninvasive ventilation.
6. Identify the indications for and discern among different modes of mechanical ventilation.
7. Select nursing interventions for patients who are intubated.
8. Identify the steps involved in suctioning patients with an oral endotracheal tube or tracheostomy.
9. Describe complications of mechanical ventilation and corrective actions to ensure optimal ventilation and safe patient care.
10. Describe the process of weaning from mechanical ventilation.
11. Select nursing interventions for patients with a new tracheostomy.
12. Outline the essential teaching for patients with a permanent tracheostomy.

KEY TERMS

assist-control (AC) ventilation
chest physical therapy (CPT)
continuous positive airway pressure (CPAP)
endotracheal (ET) tube
extubation
intubation
mechanical ventilation
negative pressure ventilation
noninvasive ventilation (NIV)
positive end-expiratory pressure (PEEP)
positive pressure ventilation (PPV)
pressure control (PC) ventilation
pressure support (PS) ventilation
pressure ventilation
pursed-lip breathing (PLB)
synchronized intermittent mandatory ventilation (SIMV)
thoracotomy
tracheostomy
volume ventilation
weaning

The exchange of O_2 and carbon dioxide (CO_2) is vital for life. This chapter provides an overview of strategies we use to promote optimal ventilation and oxygenation. Promoting respiratory function is important for best patient outcomes. Without a secure route for ventilation, O_2 therapy will not benefit the patient. Although providing optimal ventilation is no guarantee that oxygenation will improve, without a patent airway, the patient will die.

RESPIRATORY PHYSIOTHERAPY

Respiratory physiotherapy is usually done to enhance ventilation-perfusion matching, improve lung volumes, and promote airway clearance. It consists of breathing and airway clearance techniques. Positioning, mobilization, and using devices like incentive spirometry promote respiratory function.

Breathing Techniques

Deep breathing and using an incentive spirometer help prevent alveolar collapse and move respiratory secretions to larger airway passages for expectoration. An incentive spirometer supports deep breathing by giving patients visual feedback of their respiratory effort.

Two special breathing techniques are diaphragmatic breathing and pursed-lip breathing. *Diaphragmatic (abdominal) breathing* focuses on using the diaphragm instead of the accessory chest muscles to achieve maximum inhalation and slow the respiratory rate. Ideal candidates for diaphragmatic breathing are thoracic and abdominal surgery patients. Patients with chronic obstructive pulmonary disease (COPD) may not tolerate diaphragmatic breathing, as it increases the work of breathing (WOB) and dyspnea.

Pursed-lip breathing (PLB) prolongs exhalation, which prevents bronchiolar collapse and air trapping.[1] PLB is simple, easy to teach, and easy to learn (Table 28.1). It gives patients more control over breathing, especially during exercise and periods of dyspnea. PLB slows the respiratory rate and is easier than diaphragmatic breathing. Teach patients to use "just enough" positive pressure with PLB because excess resistance may increase the WOB. In patients with extreme acute dyspnea, focus on helping them slow the respiratory rate by using PLB.

Airway Clearance Techniques

Many patients with COPD or other respiratory problems who retain secretions, such as cystic fibrosis (CF), need help to clear their airways. Airway clearance techniques (ACTs) loosen mucus and secretions so they can be cleared by coughing. This helps maintain a patent airway. ACTs are often used with other treatments. For example, a patient may receive bronchodilator therapy before ACT. Then the ACT is used, followed by effective coughing (e.g., huff coughing). Respiratory therapists (RTs), physical therapists, and nurses can teach patients and caregivers ACTs.

Huff Coughing

Huff coughing, or *huffing,* is a forced expiratory technique that helps move secretions into the larger airways so they can be expelled. It benefits patients with COPD and emphysema. You can easily teach the patient huff coughing (Table 28.2).[2]

Chest Physical Therapy

Chest physical therapy (CPT) consists of postural drainage, percussion, and vibration. It can be done on spontaneously breathing patients as well as those who are intubated and mechanically ventilated. CPT is used for patients with excessive bronchial secretions who have difficulty clearing them.

CPT should be done by a physiotherapist or other trained person. Complications from improperly performed CPT include fractured ribs, bruising of the chest wall, hypoxemia, and discomfort. The maneuver may be stressful for some patients. Teaching can help ease fear and anxiety and gain trust and cooperation.

Postural Drainage

Postural drainage is the use of positioning techniques that drain secretions from specific segments of the lungs and bronchi into the trachea. The positions used depend on the areas of lung that are involved. This is determined by patient assessment, chest x-rays, chest auscultation, and, when possible, patient preference. For example, patients with left lower lobe involvement need postural drainage of only the affected region. On the other hand, patients with CF may need postural drainage of all lung segments.

TABLE 28.1 PATIENT & CAREGIVER TEACHING

Pursed-Lip Breathing (PLB)

Teach the patient to use PLB before, during, and after any activity that may cause them to be short of breath.

1. Inhale slowly and deeply through the nose.
2. Exhale slowly through pursed lips, as if whistling.
3. Be sure to relax your facial muscles without puffing your cheeks—like whistling—while you are exhaling slowly.
4. Make breathing out (exhalation) 3 times as long as breathing in (inhalation).
5. The following activities can help you get the "feel" of PLB:
   - Blow through a straw in a glass of water, forming small bubbles.
   - Blow a lit candle enough to bend the flame without blowing it out.
   - Steadily blow a table-tennis ball across a table.
   - Blow a tissue held in the hand until it gently flaps.
6. Practice 8 to 10 repetitions of PLB 3 or 4 times a day.

TABLE 28.2 PATIENT & CAREGIVER TEACHING

Effective Huff Coughing

Help the patient assume a sitting position with head slightly flexed, shoulders relaxed, knees flexed, forearms supported by pillow, and, if possible, feet on the floor.

Then teach the patient to:

1. Inhale slowly through the mouth while breathing deeply from the diaphragm.
2. Hold the breath for 2 to 3 seconds.
3. Forcefully exhale quickly as if they are fogging up a mirror with their breath (thus creating a "huff"). This helps move secretions into larger airways.
4. Repeat the "huff" 1 or 2 more times while refraining from a "regular" cough.
5. Cough when mucus is felt in the airways (breathing tubes).
6. Rest for 5 to 10 regular breaths.
7. Repeat the huffs (3 to 5 cycles) until you feel you have cleared mucus or you become tired.

We usually give aerosolized bronchodilators and hydration therapy before postural drainage. The patient stays in the chosen position for about 5 minutes during percussion and vibration. A common order is to perform postural drainage 2 to 4 times a day. In acute situations, we may do postural drainage as often as every 4 hours. Schedule the procedure at least 1 hour before meals or 3 hours after meals.

Postural drainage is best for patients with atelectasis, CF, COPD, and pneumonia. Some commercially available specialty beds can rotate and percuss the patient in various postural drainage positions. Patients with traumatic brain injury, neck injury, chest trauma, hemoptysis, heart disease, or pulmonary embolus should not receive postural drainage. It is contraindicated in hemorrhage and when the patient is not stable.

Percussion

Percussion is done in the appropriate postural drainage position. Place the hands in a cuplike position with the fingers and thumbs closed (Fig. 28.1). The cupped hand should create an air pocket between the patient's chest and the hand. Alternate up and down movement of both hands in a rhythmic fashion. You will hear a hollow sound if done correctly. The air-cushion impact promotes the movement of thick mucus. For patient comfort, place a thin towel over the area you will percuss. The patient may choose to wear a T-shirt or hospital gown.

Vibration

Vibration promotes movement of secretions to the larger airways. Perform vibration by tensing the hand and arm muscles repeatedly, while at the same time pressing mildly with the flat of the hand on the affected area while the patient slowly exhales a deep breath. Commercially available mechanical chest vibrators are available for hospital and home use.

Airway clearance devices. Airway clearance devices are available to help mobilize secretions. They are sometimes easier to tolerate than CPT and often take less time than CPT sessions. Popular devices include the Flutter, Acapella, and TheraPEP Therapy System.

The Flutter mucus clearance device is a handheld device. It is shaped like a small, fat pipe. The Flutter has a mouthpiece, a high-density stainless-steel ball, and a cone that holds the ball. To use the Flutter, the patient takes a slightly bigger-than-normal breath and exhales through the mouth and into the Flutter. As a result, the steel ball moves, which causes vibrations in the airways. The vibration helps loosen mucus in the airways to allow improved expectoration. Use of the Flutter device should be followed by huffing and coughing. Clean the Flutter daily in warm, soapy water.

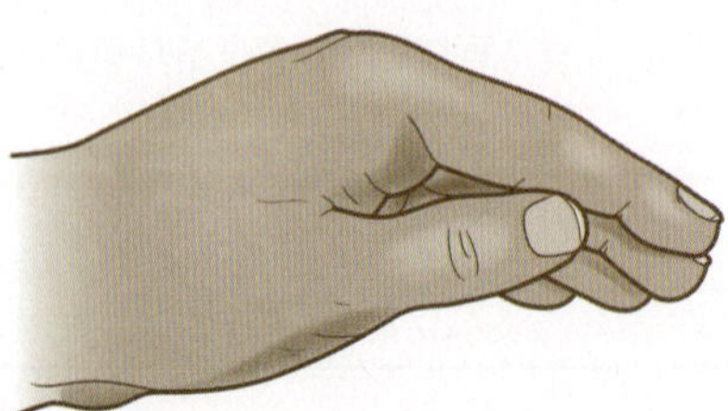

Fig. 28.1 Cupped-hand position for percussion. Cup the hand as though scooping up water.

The Acapella is another small handheld device. It combines positive expired pressure (PEP) and airway vibrations to mobilize secretions. It can be used in any setting. Before use, the resistance dial on the device needs to be set (1 = minimal exhalation resistance, 5 = high exhalation resistance). The patient inhales deeply through the nose or mouth, then seals their lips around the mouthpiece and exhales through the device. You should hear the gentle noise of the rocker inside the device on exhalation. The Acapella can also help deliver aerosolized drugs.

The TheraPEP Therapy System is similar to the Acapella. It uses PEP and can assist with airway clearance and deliver aerosolized drugs. TheraPEP can have either a mouthpiece or mask that is attached to tubing that is connected to a small adjustable resistor and a pressure indicator. The patient inhales through the nose or mouth, holds the breath for a few seconds, then exhales through the resistor. The pressure indicator gives visual feedback about the pressure that the patient needs to hold during exhalation to receive maximal benefit of PEP.

High-frequency chest wall oscillation uses an inflatable vest (e.g., Vest System, Smart Vest) with hoses connected to a high-frequency pulse generator. The pulse generator delivers air to the vest, which vibrates the chest. High-frequency airwaves dislodge mucus from the airways, mobilize the mucus, and move it toward larger airways. The vest is easy to apply and can be used without the aid of another person. The unit weighs 23 to 30 lb (10 to 13 kg), is quiet, comes in a suitcase, and is portable.

O_2 THERAPY

O_2 therapy is a common treatment for hypoxemia and hypoxia. Giving supplemental O_2 increases the partial pressure of O_2 (PO_2) in inspired air. O_2 therapy requires an HCP order. The dose of O_2 administered to patients is the *fraction of inspired oxygen* (FIO_2).

We give O_2 to treat hypoxemia caused by many problems, such as shock, pneumonia, and pulmonary emboli. O_2 therapy is tailored to meet each patient's unique circumstances and physiologic needs. For most patients, the goal of O_2 therapy is to keep either the SaO_2 greater than 92% during rest, sleep, and activity or the PaO_2 greater than 80 mm Hg. We may modify these goals depending on the patient's clinical situation. For example, the HCP may accept a PaO_2 greater than 60 mm Hg and an SpO_2 greater than 88% for patients with long-standing COPD.

DRUG ALERT

O_2

- O_2 is considered a drug.
- Target FIO_2 levels to maintain SpO_2 >92% and PaO_2 between 80 and 100 mm Hg.
- Assess PaO_2 and SpO_2 as needed.
- Administering high levels of O_2 (FIO_2 greater than 60% for more than 24 h) to mechanically ventilated patients can lead to O_2 toxicity.
- Monitor for O_2 toxicity: blurred vision, coughing, chest pain, dyspnea, seizures.

Methods of O_2 Administration

There are various ways to administer O_2 (Table 28.3). Each has advantages and disadvantages. The device used depends on the patient's underlying condition, their FiO_2 requirements, comfort, cost, and financial resources.

We classify O_2 delivery systems as low-flow or high-flow systems. Low-flow O_2 delivery devices are appropriate for patients who are awake, alert, and spontaneously breathing with a stable, intact respiratory drive. These devices provide O_2 in concentrations that do not meet all of a patient's inspiratory demands.[3] Low-flow devices pull in a proportion of room air, which makes the exact FiO_2 unknown. We do know the range of FiO_2 delivered by each device. Examples include nasal prongs, simple masks, and nonrebreather masks.

High-flow O_2 delivery devices deliver fixed O_2 concentrations (e.g., 28%, 35%) independent of a patient's respiratory rate or pattern. High-flow systems provide O_2 in concentrations that meet or exceed a patient's inspiratory demand.[4] These patients are awake, alert, and spontaneously breathing but have higher O_2 requirements that low-flow devices cannot meet. High-flow devices help achieve specific PaO_2 or SpO_2 targets. Examples include the Venturi mask and high-flow nasal cannula.

Humidification

O_2 from O_2 cylinders or wall systems is a dry gas. Dry O_2 has an irritating effect on mucous membranes and dries secretions. Humidification involves adding sterile water attached to the O_2 delivery device to prevent breathing dry air. A common device used for humidification when a patient has a cannula or mask is a small plastic jar filled with sterile water called a *bubble-through humidifier.* It is attached to the O_2 source by a flowmeter.

Many agencies have moved away from providing humidification for low-flow O_2 delivery devices. However, humidification with high-flow O_2 devices (e.g., Vapotherm) is important. Follow agency policy about O_2 therapy and humidification.

Complications

Combustion

O_2 supports combustion and increases the rate of burning. Smoking must be prohibited in any patient care area where O_2 is being used. Display an "Oxygen in Use, No Smoking" sign on the patient's door and in any area where O_2 is in use. Caution patients against smoking with an O_2 cannula in place. It can easily ignite and cause significant burns and life-threatening airway issues.

O_2 Toxicity

O_2 toxicity may result from prolonged exposure to high levels of O_2 (FiO_2). High FiO_2 concentrations can result in a severe inflammatory response because O_2 free radicals damage the alveolar-capillary membrane.[5] This can cause severe pulmonary edema, shunting of blood, and hypoxemia.

Preventing O_2 toxicity is essential. The amount of O_2 administered should be specific for each patient. The most important rule is to provide FiO_2 at the lowest possible level while still maintaining acceptable SpO_2 and PaO_2 values for that specific patient. Monitoring arterial blood gases (ABGs) often helps evaluate the effectiveness of therapy and guides the tapering of O_2.

Absorption Atelectasis

Alveoli contain many different gases, including O_2, CO_2, and nitrogen. Nitrogen helps maintain the size, shape, and structure of the alveolus. If the bronchial tubes become obstructed (e.g., with mucus), the exchange of O_2 and CO_2 cannot occur. Nitrogen will eventually move out of the alveolus and into the bloodstream. This is known as *nitrogen washout.* As a result, the alveolus collapses, and absorption atelectasis occurs. This can worsen hypoxemia.

For patients requiring higher levels of O_2 therapy, monitor ABGs, suction the airway as needed, and give O_2 at the lowest level possible to help avoid this condition.

CO_2 Narcosis

Chemoreceptors control the drive to breathe. They respond to CO_2 and O_2 concentrations in the blood. Normally, an increase in CO_2 in the blood is a major stimulant of the respiratory center. However, some patients (e.g., those with COPD) develop a tolerance for high CO_2 levels. As a result, the respiratory center loses its sensitivity to high CO_2 levels. For these patients, a major "drive" to breathe is hypoxemia. As a result, there is concern about the dangers of giving O_2 to patients with COPD and reducing their drive (stimulus) to breathe.

Not all patients with COPD retain CO_2. Therefore it is good practice to administer O_2 to any patient who will likely benefit from O_2 therapy, whether they need it or not. The danger of not giving O_2 to a patient far outweighs the risk of administering O_2 when it is not needed.

Infection

Infection is a rare complication of O_2 use. It is often related to the device used and how often the device is cleaned or changed. Heated nebulizers present the highest risk. The constant use of humidity supports bacterial growth. When possible, use disposable and single-patient-use equipment. Follow agency policy about cleaning and changing equipment.

NURSING MANAGEMENT: O_2 THERAPY

We use pulse oximetry and/or ABGs to monitor the effectiveness of O_2 therapy and help guide titration of FiO_2. The goal is an O_2 saturation (SpO_2) of at least 92% or a PaO_2 of at least 80 mm Hg (60 mm Hg in the adult ICU). Titrate the O_2 concentration with close monitoring of the PaO_2 and $PaCO_2$. Assess mental status and vital signs before starting O_2 therapy

TABLE 28.3 Methods of O_2 Administration

Description	Nursing Interventions	
Nasal Cannula		
• Most commonly used. • O_2 delivered through plastic tubing (prongs) that fits in the nares. • Used for a patient requiring low O_2 concentrations. • Achieves O_2 concentrations of 24% (at 1 L/min) to 44% (at 6 L/min). • Most patients with COPD can tolerate 2 to 4 L/min through a cannula. • Easy to set up and use. • Allows some freedom of movement.	• Amount of O_2 inhaled depends on room air and patient's breathing pattern. • Assess the nares and ears for skin breakdown. May need to pad tubing where it sits on ears. • Patient can eat, talk, or cough while wearing device. • If flow rates are >5 L/min, nasal membranes may dry and place patient at risk for nosebleeds.	
O_2-Conserving Cannula		
• Looks like a "moustache" (Oxymizer) or "pendant" type. • Cannula has a built-in reservoir that ↑ O_2 concentration and allows patient to use lower FiO_2, which increases comfort and can be increased with activities. • Can deliver O_2 flow rates up to 15 L/min. • Generally indicated for longer-term O_2 therapy at home.	• Cannula is highly visible. • Assess the nares and ears for skin breakdown. May need to pad tubing where it sits behind ears. • Cannot clean cannula. Change cannula every week. • May need ABGs and oximetry to determine correct flow rate. • More expensive than standard nasal cannula.	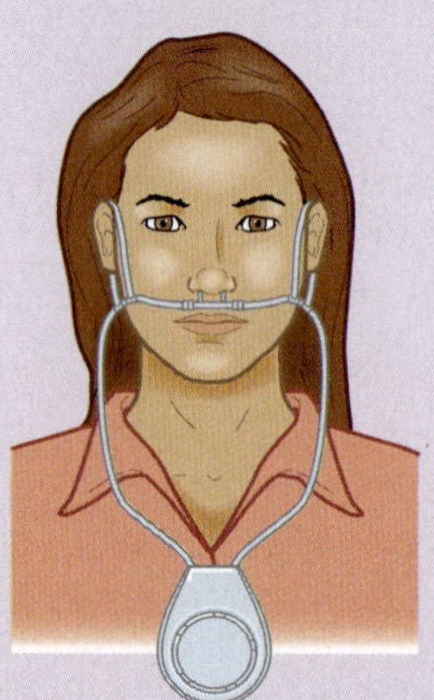
High-Flow Nasal Cannula		
• Blends O_2 with compressed air to generate high FiO_2. • Achieves FiO_2 concentration up to 100% (at flow rate of up to 60 L/min). • Heated humidifier capable of providing 100% humidity. • Soft and flexible nasal prongs. • More comfortable than mask.	• Nasal cannula must be smaller than 50% of nares to allow flow during exhalation and flush out end-expiratory CO_2. • Patients can eat and drink with the device in place. • Patient may describe feeling of always having to blow nose ("rainout") because of humidification.	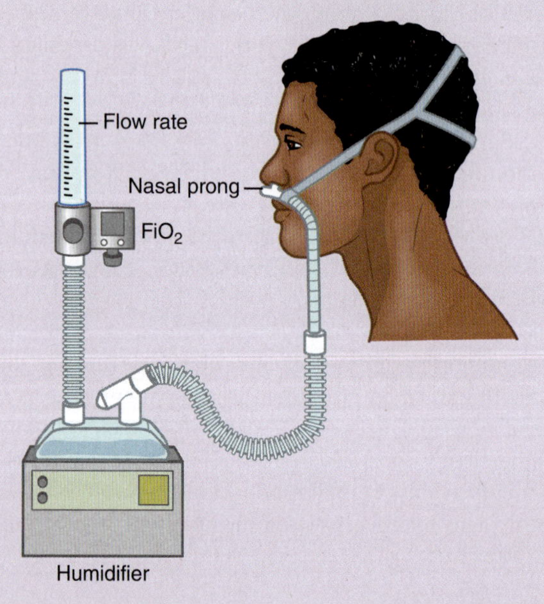

Continued

TABLE 28.3 Methods of O_2 Administration—cont'd

Description	Nursing Interventions
Simple Face Mask	
• Covers the nose and mouth. • Achieves O_2 concentrations of 35% to 50% with flow rates of 6 to 12 L/min. • Provides humidification of inspired air. • Easy to set up and use. • Typically used only for short periods.	• Mask must fit snugly. • Must have flow rates of at least 6 L/min to wash exhaled gases out of mask (if O_2 flow rate not high enough, CO_2 rebreathing is possible). • Watch for pressure injuries behind ears from elastic straps if patient wears for longer periods. Gauze or other padding may alleviate this problem. • Wash and dry under mask q4h and as needed. • May change to nasal cannula while patient is eating.

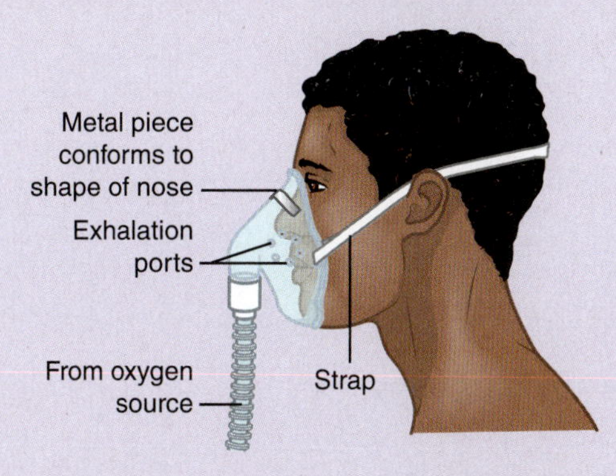

Description	Nursing Interventions
Partial and Nonrebreather Masks	
• Used for short-term therapy for patients with higher O_2 needs than nasal cannula and simple mask. • Achieves O_2 concentrations of 60% to 90% (with flow rates of 10 to 15 L/min). • O_2 flows into reservoir bag and mask during inhalation. • Bag allows patient to rebreathe the first one-third of exhaled air (rich in O_2) in conjunction with delivered O_2. • Vents stay open on partial rebreather. Some agencies prefer this over nonrebreather for patient safety.	• Mask should fit snugly. • O_2 flow rate must be sufficient to keep bag from deflating during inspiration to avoid CO_2 buildup and rebreathing of CO_2. • If deflation occurs, increase flow rate on flowmeter to keep bag inflated. • With nonrebreather masks, make sure valves open during expiration and close during inhalation to prevent decrease in FiO_2 or buildup in CO_2. • Monitor patient closely, because of more advanced interventions such as CPAP, bi-PAP, or intubation and mechanical ventilation may be needed.

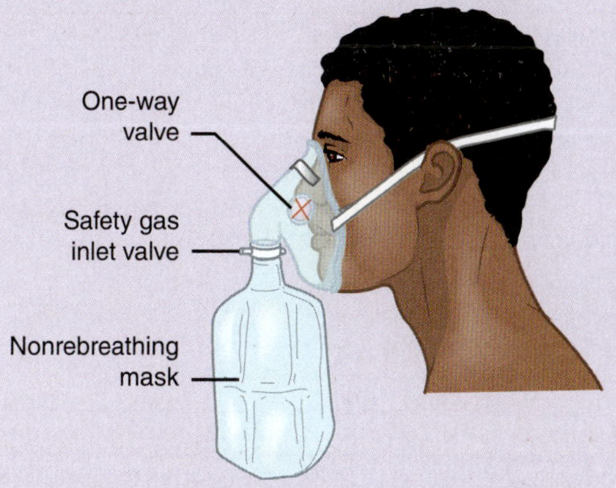

Description	Nursing Interventions
Venturi Mask	
• Lightweight plastic, cone-shaped mask. • Device controls amount of room air that is entrained (drawn in), so precise amounts of O_2 can be delivered. • Adaptors are available for delivery of 24%, 28%, 31%, 35%, 40%, and 50% O_2. • Method is especially helpful for giving constant low O_2 concentrations to patients (e.g., COPD).	• Air ports must not be occluded. • Entrainment device on mask must be changed to deliver different concentrations of O_2. • Must be removed for eating. • Patients can talk, but voice may be muffled.

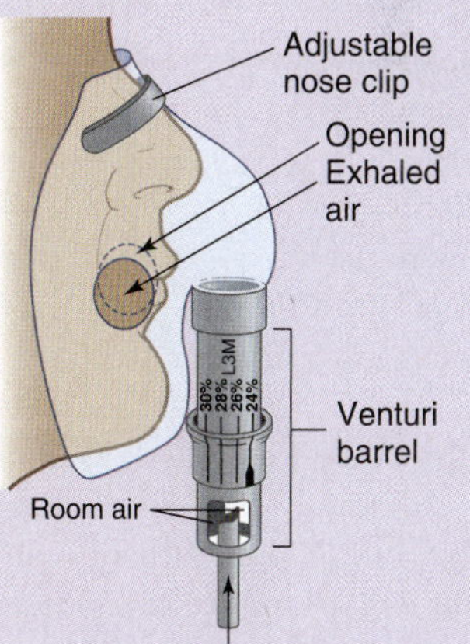

Description	Nursing Interventions
Tracheostomy T-Piece	
• Almost identical to tracheostomy collar but has a T-connector attached to an O_2 blender. • Tight fit allows better O_2 and humidity delivery than tracheostomy collar. • T-piece allows an inline catheter to be connected for suctioning.	• Because T-piece connector can disconnect easily, monitor closely. • T-piece connector may pull on the tracheostomy tube, causing irritation and potential tissue damage. • Monitor for signs of skin breakdown.

TABLE 28.3 Methods of O_2 Administration—cont'd

Description	Nursing Interventions
Tracheostomy Collar	
• Collar attaches to neck with elastic strap and can deliver humidity and O_2 through the tracheostomy. • Because collar does not fit tightly, some O_2 concentration is lost into atmosphere.	• Secretions can collect inside collar and around tracheostomy. • Remove collar and clean q4h and as needed to prevent aspiration and reduce risk of infection.

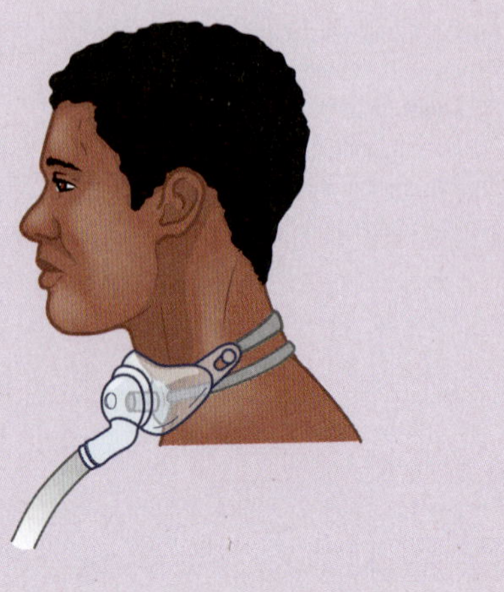

ABG, Arterial blood gas; *Bi-PAP*, bilevel positive airway pressure; *COPD*, chronic obstructive pulmonary disease; *CPAP*, continuous positive airway pressure; *Fio₂*, fraction of inspired oxygen.

and frequently thereafter. Nursing management of patients receiving O_2 therapy is outlined in Table 28.4.

O_2 Therapy at Home

Some patients need O_2 therapy at home to treat hypoxemia associated with chronic conditions. Patients with mild to moderate hypoxemia that persists at discharge from the hospital may need short-term therapy. For example, patients who had COVID pneumonia may need O_2 therapy to treat hypoxemia for a few weeks after discharge. Home health personnel can assess the patient's oxygenation status after an acute episode to see if they still need O_2.

Patients usually rent home O_2 systems. The company then sends an RT to the home. The therapist teaches the patient and caregiver how to use the O_2 system, maintain it, troubleshoot, recognize when the supply is low, and reorder O_2. Table 28.5 shows a patient and caregiver teaching guide for using O_2 at home.

Sources for home O_2 include a liquid O_2 storage system, compressed O_2 in tanks or cylinders, or an O_2 concentrator or extractor. The one chosen depends on the patient's activity level, environment, insurance coverage, and proximity to an O_2 supply company. To increase mobility in the home, patients can use extension tubing with some devices without lowering the O_2 flow delivery. Patients who are active outside the home can use a small, portable system, such as liquid O_2.

Patients may need O_2 only during exercise and/or sleep. Evaluate the need for O_2 during these periods with a 6-minute walk test or overnight oximetry. Patients on long-term therapy need to be assessed at regular intervals (e.g., every 30 to 90 days during the first year, then each year if they are stable).

TABLE 28.4 NURSING MANAGEMENT

O_2 Administration

- Continually assess need for adjustments in O_2 flow rate.
- Evaluate patient response to O_2 therapy, especially when changes are made.
- Provide patient and caregiver teaching about O_2 therapy (see Table 28.5).
- Monitor for adverse effects of O_2 therapy.
- Supervise AP:
  - Use pulse oximetry to measure O_2 saturation and report level to RN.
  - Assist patient with adjustment of O_2 delivery devices (e.g., nasal cannula, simple face mask).
  - Report to RN any change in patient condition.

Collaborate With Respiratory Therapist

- Assist with choosing optimal O_2 delivery device.
- Make sure equipment is clean, working, and replaced as needed.
- Check accuracy of O_2 delivery.
- Frequently assess need for adjustments in O_2 flow rate.

Encourage patients who use home O_2 to remain active and travel normally. If travel is by car, they can plan for O_2 to be available at their destination. O_2 supply companies can help with these arrangements. Patients who are traveling by bus, train, or airplane should inform these agencies when making reservations that they need O_2. O_2 needs for flying can be determined by a pulmonary function test, a 6-minute walk test, hypoxic challenge test, or predictive formula. Portable O_2 concentrators are an immediate source of renewable O_2. They can be available by recharging at home or with a direct current (DC) (e.g., auto) power supply. Several are approved by airlines

TABLE 28.5 PATIENT & CAREGIVER TEACHING

Home O_2 Use

The company that provides the O_2 and equipment will teach the patient about O_2 delivery and equipment care. The following are some general instructions that you may include when teaching the patient and caregiver about the use of home O_2.

Patient Care

- Set the O_2 flow rate at the rate your HCP told you to set it at. Do not change the rate without first talking to your HCP.
- If you have any shortness of breath, are lightheaded or dizzy, or develop wheezing, call the HCP right away.
- Check to make sure you have enough O_2 on hand for weekends and holidays. The company will tell you how to check the O_2 level and when/how you reorder more O_2.

Decreasing Risk for Infection

- Wash hands before and after using your O_2 therapy.
- Wash nasal cannula (prongs) with a liquid soap and thoroughly rinse once or twice a week.
- Brush teeth or use mouthwash several times a day.
- Ask the company providing the equipment how often to change the tubing and filter.
- Replace cannula every 2 to 4 weeks.
- If you have a cold, replace the cannula after your symptoms pass.

Safety

- Keep O_2 tanks at least 5 feet (1.5 m) away from any source of heat (e.g., gas stoves, fireplaces).
- Post "No Smoking—Oxygen in Use" warning signs on the front and back doors of your home.
- Do not allow smoking in the home, and do not smoke yourself while wearing O_2. Nasal cannulas and masks can catch fire and cause serious burns to the face and airways.
- Store O_2 tanks upright.
- Do not use blankets or fabrics that carry a static charge, such as wool or synthetics.
- Do not use flammable liquids such as paint thinners, cleaning fluids, gasoline, kerosene, oil-based paints, or aerosol sprays while using O_2.
- Inform the electric company if you use a concentrator. In case of a power failure, they will know the medical urgency of restoring your power.

for in-flight use. Patients should contact the airline to determine accommodations and policies for in-flight O_2.

ARTIFICIAL AIRWAYS

Patients sometimes need help maintaining a patent airway. Inserting a small, plastic tube into the nose, mouth, or trachea, thereby bypassing upper airway and laryngeal structures, creates a route for ventilation to occur. There are 4 artificial airways we commonly use in practice.

Nasopharyngeal Airway

A nasopharyngeal airway (NPA) is a small, flexible plastic tube inserted into the nostril to help maintain a route for ventilation

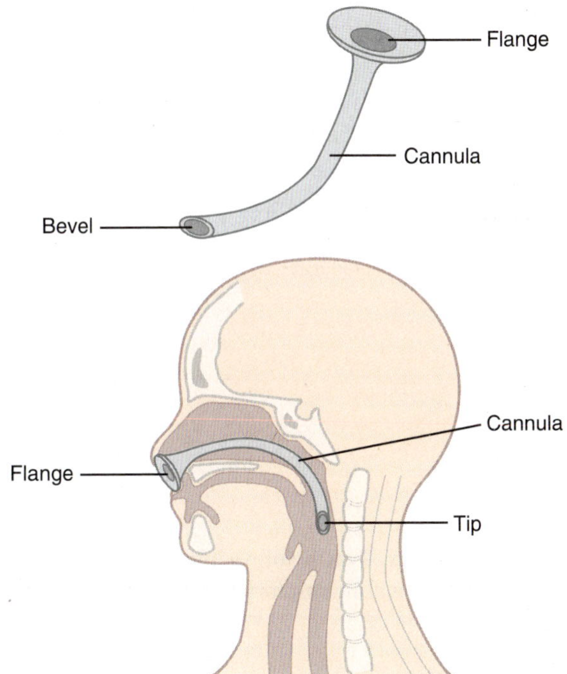

Fig. 28.2 Nasopharyngeal airway.

(Fig. 28.2). The NPA can be placed in conscious or unconscious patients. To measure the length of the tube needed, hold an NPA up to the side of the patient's face. Choose an NPA that correctly measures from the tip of the nose to the tip of the earlobe. To select the right internal diameter, choose a tube with a slightly smaller diameter than the patient's nostril.

Choose the nostril of greatest airflow. Lubricate the tube, and gently insert the tube while rotating it toward the patient's ear. Stop if you encounter any obstruction or difficulty. When correctly positioned, the flange should rest comfortably against the nostril.

Oropharyngeal Airway

The oropharyngeal airway (OPA) is a smaller, shorter tube of firm, hard plastic. The tube is curved, with a flange on one end and blunt opening on the other. Do not insert an OPA in a conscious patient, as this will induce vomiting and risk of aspiration. Only insert the OPA into an unconscious patient.

To measure the length of the OPA needed, hold the OPA up to the side of the patient's face. Measure the tube against the corner of the mouth to the angle of the jaw or earlobe. If the tube is too short, you may push the tongue into the oropharynx and occlude the airway. If the tube is too long, you may damage the posterior oropharynx.

There are a few ways to insert the OPA. The most common way involves inserting the tube with the bevel pointed toward the roof of the mouth. As the flange reaches the lips, rotate the OPA 90 degrees so that the curvature of the OPA fits the natural curvature of the upper airway. Inspect the oral cavity after insertion to ensure you did not push the tongue into the

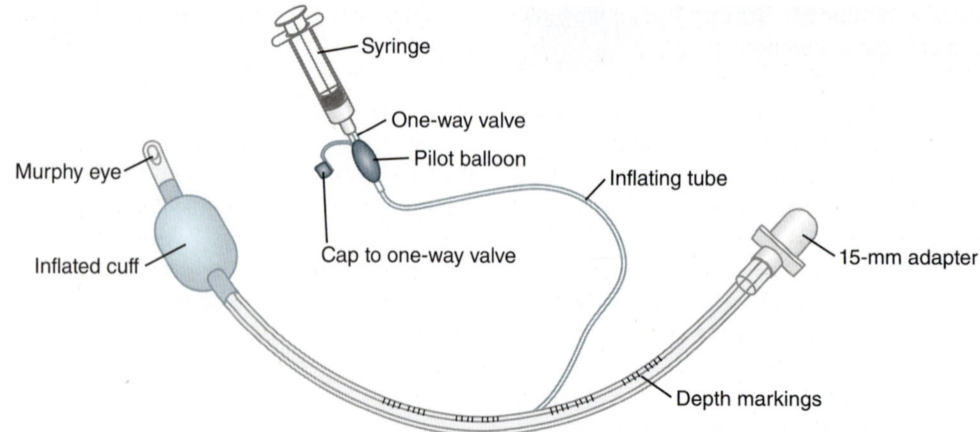

Fig. 28.3 Parts of the endotracheal tube.

posterior oropharynx. Watch for visible chest rise. Correctly inserted, the flange will fit comfortably against the lips.

Tracheostomy

A **tracheostomy** is a surgically created stoma (opening) in the anterior part of the trachea. Tracheostomies and their care are discussed later in this chapter.

Endotracheal Tubes

Intubation is the process of securing the airway with an **endotracheal (ET) tube**, providing an effective route for ventilation. Respiratory indications for intubation include (1) apnea, (2) hypoxemia and/or hypercarbia, (3) upper airway obstruction (e.g., burns, tumor, bleeding), (4) ineffective clearance of secretions, and (5) inability to protect the airway (e.g., altered level of consciousness [LOC]) and/or high risk for aspiration.

The ET tube is a long, flexible, plastic tube that can be placed orally or nasally. An ET consists of a standard adapter (used to attach the bag-valve-mask [BVM] or ventilator), cuff, pilot balloon, and radiopaque markings along the length of the tube. The markings help gauge the distance the tube is inserted. The parts of the oral ET tube are shown in Fig. 28.3. The end of the oral or nasal ET sits 2 to 3 cm above the carina, so that O_2 is delivered to both lungs (Fig. 28.4).

In *oral intubation,* the ET tube is passed into the mouth, enters the posterior oropharynx, through the vocal cords, and into the trachea with the aid of a laryngoscope or a bronchoscope. The most common sizes are 7F and 8F tubes. The size refers to the internal diameter of the tube. Often, females need a 7F tube and males need an 8F tube. Larger-diameter tubes can be used. A larger tube reduces the WOB because of less airway resistance. It is easier to suction and remove secretions and, if needed, perform bronchoscopy.

When oral intubation through the mouth is not possible (e.g., unstable cervical spine injury, dental abscess, epiglottitis), a nasotracheal (NT) tube can help provide a patent airway. The NT tube is slightly longer than the oral ET tube. It is inserted through the nostril and placed blindly (without seeing the larynx).

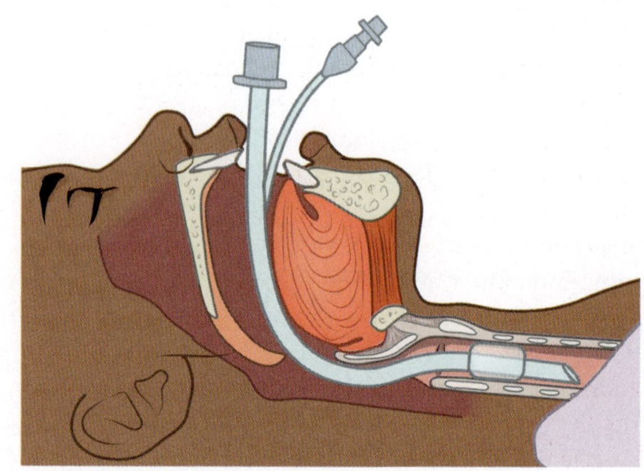

Fig. 28.4 Endotracheal tube placement. The tip of the ET tube is 2 to 3 cm above the carina.

Intubation Procedure

ET intubation is done quickly and safely at the bedside by an HCP or RT. It is common in patients in the ICU. Unless ET intubation is emergent, consent for the procedure is obtained. Tell the patient and caregiver the reason for ET intubation and steps in the procedure. Explain that the patient will not be able to speak while intubated, but that you will provide other means of communication. Tell them that the patient's hands may have removable mitts or the wrists may have soft restraints applied to remind them not to touch the ET tube.

Assemble necessary equipment at the bedside and notify all appropriate personnel. Have the BVM attached to the O_2 outlet and suctioning equipment ready. The BVM has a self-inflating reservoir that, when connected to the O_2 outlet on the wall, delivers FiO_2 concentrations of up to 100%. Remove any dentures or partial plates (for oral intubation) and give premedication drugs as ordered. Premedication varies depending on a patient's LOC (e.g., awake, obtunded), urgency (e.g., emergent, nonemergent), and the HCP's preferences.

For oral intubation, place the patient supine with the head slightly extended and the neck flexed ("sniff position"). This position allows the HCP to see the vocal cords more easily. For nasal intubation, spray the nasal passages with a local anesthetic and vasoconstrictor (e.g., lidocaine with epinephrine) to reduce the risk of trauma and bleeding. Before starting intubation, preoxygenate the patient using the BVM and 100% O_2 for at least 2 minutes. Each intubation attempt is limited to less than 30 seconds. Ventilate the patient between attempts using the BVM and 100% O_2.

Rapid sequence induction (RSI) is the rapid, concurrent administration of both a sedative and a paralytic drug during emergency airway management to induce unconsciousness for intubation. It decreases the risks for aspiration and injury. RSI is not indicated in patients who are in cardiac arrest or have a known difficult airway. The patient receives a sedative-hypnotic-amnesic (e.g., propofol, etomidate) to induce unconsciousness and a rapid-onset opioid (e.g., fentanyl) to blunt the pain of the procedure. This is followed with a neuromuscular blocking agent (NMBA), such as rocuronium, to produce skeletal muscle paralysis. Follow agency policy regarding your role in administering NMBAs.

During intubation, monitor vital signs, including heart rate and rhythm, BP, mean arterial pressure (MAP), and any signs of visible chest movement. Monitor O_2 status with pulse oximetry. Inform the team if the SpO_2 is less than 92%.

Immediately after intubation, inflate the cuff on the ET tube. Help confirm placement of the ET tube while continuing to manually ventilate the patient using the BVM with 100% O_2. Auscultate the lungs for bilateral breath sounds and the epigastrium for the absence of air sounds. Observe for symmetric chest wall movement. SpO_2 should be stable or improved.

A portable end-tidal carbon dioxide ($EtCO_2$) monitor can help confirm the correct placement of the tube. The $EtCO_2$ detector helps confirm placement by noting the presence of exhaled CO_2 from the lungs. A steadily rising CO_2 value and the presence of a waveform confirm correct placement. Or place a colorimetric CO_2 detector between the BVM and ET tube and look for a color change (indicating the presence of CO_2) or a number. At least 5 or 6 exhalations with a consistent CO_2 level must occur to confirm tube placement in the trachea.

If the findings support ET tube placement, help secure the ET per agency policy. Connect the ET tube to the ventilator and closed suctioning system (Fig. 28.5). Assess the need to suction the ET tube and pharynx. Insert a bite block, if needed. Secure it separately from the ET tube to the patient's face. This will help prevent the patient from biting the ET and preventing ventilation.

Obtain a chest x-ray to confirm tube location. Once positioning is confirmed with x-ray, record and mark the position of the oral ET tube at the lip or teeth. For a nasotracheal tube, mark the exit of the tube at the nare.

Obtain ABGs 15 to 30 minutes after intubation. ABG values help determine ventilator settings. Continuous pulse oximetry gives data about arterial oxygenation. $EtCO_2$ monitoring provides data about ventilation.

There are risks with oral ET intubation. It is hard to place the tube with limited head and neck mobility (e.g., spinal cord injury, obesity). Teeth can be accidentally chipped or removed. Patients can obstruct the ET tube by biting down on it. Salivation increases, and swallowing is difficult. Sedation, along with a bite block or oropharyngeal airway, can help prevent obstruction. Mouth care is challenging because of limited space in the oral cavity.

PROCEDURES TO SUPPORT VENTILATION

Many diagnostic, therapeutic, and surgical strategies are available to assist patients with improving oxygenation and promoting more effective ventilation. Bronchoscopy may be used for diagnostic purposes and treatment (e.g., remove mucus plugs, foreign bodies). It can help achieve patency of an airway that has been partially or nearly obstructed by tumors. A thoracentesis can relieve symptoms by draining air or excess fluid from the pleural space. Usually, we remove no more than 1000 to 1200 mL of fluid at one time. Rapid removal of a large volume of pleural fluid can result in hypotension, hypoxemia, or reexpansion pulmonary edema. These procedures are discussed in Chapter 27.

Chest Tubes and Pleural Drainage

If enough fluid or air accumulates in the pleural space, the normally negative subatmospheric pressure becomes positive and 1 or both lungs may collapse. Inserting a chest tube into

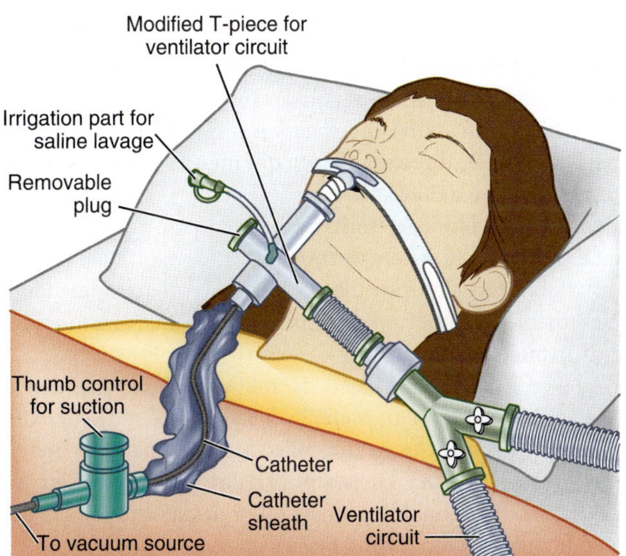

Fig. 28.5 Oral ET tube connected to ventilator circuit and closed tracheal suction system.

the pleural space can reestablish negative pressure, drain the pleural space, and allow for lung expansion.[6]

Chest tubes are about 20 in (51 cm) long and vary in size from 12F to 40F. The size inserted depends on the reason for the chest tube insertion. Large (36F to 40F) tubes are used to drain blood. Medium (24F to 36F) tubes are used to drain fluid. Small (12F to 24F) tubes are used to drain air. Pigtail catheters are very small (10F to 14F) tubes with a curly end designed to keep them in place. Sometimes, they are a safe and effective alternative to larger-bore chest tubes for treatment of pneumothorax.[7]

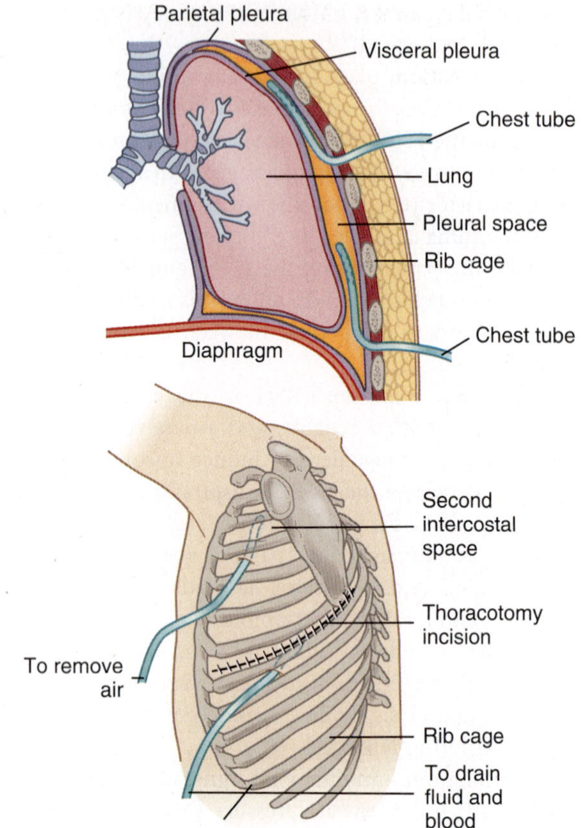

Fig. 28.6 Placement of chest tubes.

Chest Tube Insertion

Chest tube insertion can take place in the ED, during surgery, or at the bedside. Time permitting, a chest x-ray is done to confirm the affected side. The patient is positioned with the arm raised above the head on the affected side to expose the midaxillary area, the standard site for insertion. Elevate the head of bed (up to 45 degrees when possible) to lower the diaphragm and reduce the risk for injury.

The area is cleansed with an antiseptic solution. The HCP injects a local anesthetic and makes a small incision over a rib. The chest tube is advanced up and over the top of the rib to avoid the intercostal nerves and blood vessels that are behind the rib inferiorly (Fig. 28.6). Once inserted, the HCP sutures the tube in place and closes the incision with sutures. The wound is covered with an occlusive dressing. Most HCPs prefer to seal the wound around the chest tube with petroleum (airtight) gauze. The tube is connected to a pleural drainage system. Tube placement is confirmed by chest x-ray.

Chest tube insertion is painful. Assess the need for analgesia and/or sedation and medicate the patient as ordered. Provide emotional reassurance. Monitor vital signs, including heart rate, respiratory rate and rhythm, BP, and SpO_2.

Pleural Drainage System

A chest tube is usually attached to a drainage device or chamber to collect fluid, air, and/or blood from the chest cavity. Many disposable, plastic chest drainage systems are available. Manufacturers include directions for setup and use with each unit. Most units have a 2000-mL capacity.

All chest drainage units have 3 basic compartments (Fig. 28.7). The first compartment, or collection chamber, receives fluid and air from the pleural space. The drained fluid stays in this chamber while expelled air vents to the second compartment.

The second compartment is the water-seal chamber. It contains about 2 cm of water, which acts as a 1-way valve. Incoming air enters from the collection chamber and bubbles up through the water. The water prevents backflow of air into the patient. Brisk bubbling of air often occurs in this chamber when a pneumothorax is first evacuated. Intermittent bubbling during exhalation, coughing, or sneezing (when intrathoracic pressure is increased) may occur as long as there is air in the pleural space. Eventually, as the air leak resolves and the lung becomes more fully expanded, bubbling ceases.

Normal water fluctuation within the water-seal chamber is called *tidaling*. This up and down movement of water with the patient's breathing reflects intrapleural pressure changes during inspiration and expiration. This is normal. If tidaling stops suddenly, assess the chest tube. It may mean the tube is occluded. As the lung reexpands, tidaling gradually slows, then eventually stops.

The third compartment, the suction control chamber, applies suction to the chest drainage unit. There are 2 main types of suction control: wet (water) and dry. For wet suction systems, the suction control chamber uses a column of water to control the amount of suction from the wall regulator. The chamber is filled with a specific amount of water. This amount of water finds the amount of suction applied to the chest drainage unit. You may need to add more water to the suction control chamber as water evaporates. Problems can arise with this chamber if the chest tube unit is tipped or knocked over.

A dry suction chest tube system does not contain water. The amount of suction is determined by turning a dial on the chest tube drainage device to the ordered amount. Suction pressure is usually −20 cm H_2O. A visual alert shows you if the suction is working. Higher pressures (−40 cm H_2O) are sometimes needed to evacuate the pleural space. Lower pressure (−10 cm

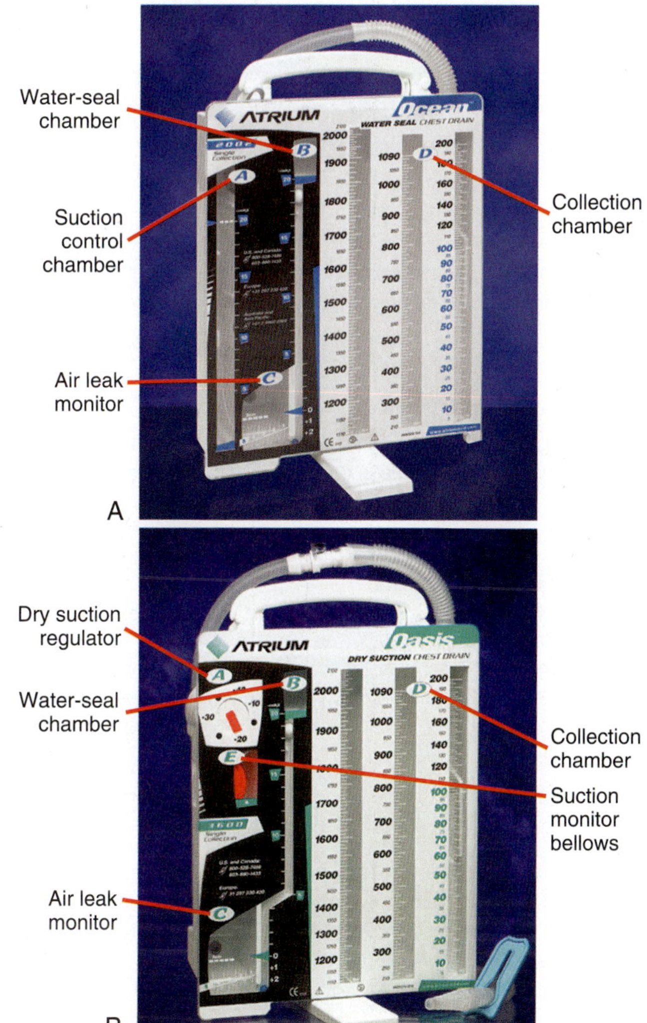

Fig. 28.7 Chest drainage unit. Both units have 3 chambers: (1) collection chamber, (2) water-seal chamber, and (3) suction control chamber. Suction control chamber requires connection to a wall suction source for the suction to work. (A) Water suction. This unit uses water in the suction control chamber to control the suction pressure. (B) Dry suction. We set the desired degree of suction using the control dial. (From Atrium Medical Corporation, Hudson, NH.)

H_2O) may be used for frail and older patients at risk for tissue damage.

A flutter valve (or *Heimlich valve*) is used to remove air from the pleural space (Fig. 28.8). This device consists of a 1-way rubber valve within a rigid plastic tube. It is attached to the external end of the chest tube and has 2 nozzles. The inlet nozzle allows the air to pass into the valve through the chest tube attached to it. The outlet nozzle allows the air to pass to the environment or a collecting device during expiration. During inspiration, when pressure in the chest decreases, the valve closes. This prevents air from going back into the patient's chest. During expiration, when intrathoracic pressure increases, the valve opens.

The flutter valve can be used for a small to moderate-sized pneumothorax. It allows for patient mobility. Patients can

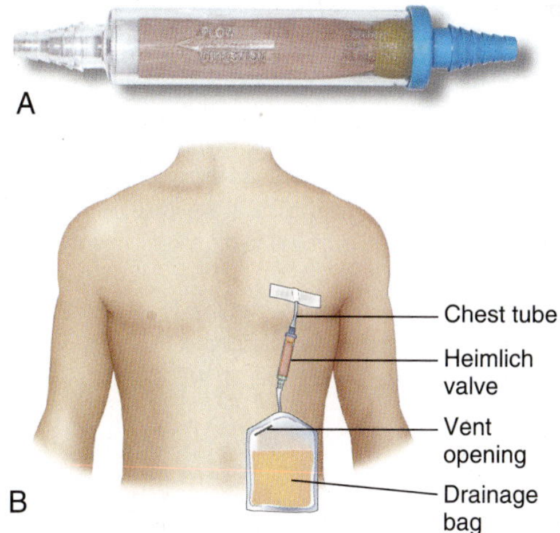

Fig. 28.8 (A) The Heimlich chest drain valve is a specially designed valve that is used in place of a chest drainage unit for small uncomplicated pneumothorax. The valve allows for escape of air but prevents the reentry of air into the pleural space. (B) Placement of valve between chest tube and vented drainage bag, which can be worn under a gown or clothes. (A, Courtesy Becton, Dickinson and Company, Franklin Lakes, NJ.)

hide the smaller drainage bag under clothes when they ambulate. Drainage bags attached to the flutter valve must have a vent to the atmosphere to prevent a tension pneumothorax. This is done by simply cutting a small slit in the top of any drainage bag that does not have a built-in vent. Patients may go home with a flutter valve in place.

NURSING MANAGEMENT: CHEST DRAINAGE

General guidelines for nursing care of patients with chest tubes and chest tube drainage systems are shown in Table 28.6.

Immediately after chest tube insertion, monitor the patient for complications from tube placement and drainage. Monitor vital signs, including respiratory rate and rhythm. Monitor the color and amount of drainage hourly in the first few hours after chest tube insertion. If volumes from 1 to 1.5 L of fluid and/or blood are removed rapidly, reexpansion pulmonary edema or severe, symptomatic hypotension may occur. Ask the HCP how much drainage to expect. Notify them if excess drainage occurs.

Report the development of subcutaneous emphysema or any signs and symptoms of respiratory distress to the HCP at once. Subcutaneous emphysema can occur from air leaking into the tissue surrounding the chest tube insertion site. If present, you will feel a "crackling" sensation when palpating the skin. A small amount of subcutaneous air is harmless and will be reabsorbed. Severe subcutaneous emphysema around the head and neck can potentially cause swelling with airway compromise.

Should clots appear in the tubing and drainage slows or stops, contact the HCP and follow agency policy for reestablishing drainage. Provide adequate pain medication.[8] If a chest tube suddenly becomes disconnected, the immediate priority is to reestablish the water seal. In some agencies, when

TABLE 28.6 NURSING MANAGEMENT

Care of the Patient With a Chest Tube

Clinical Status

- Monitor the patient. Assess vital signs, lung sounds, and need for analgesia.
- Have the patient breathe deeply and use incentive spirometry regularly to promote lung expansion.
- Evaluate for subcutaneous emphysema at the insertion site.
- Encourage range-of-motion exercises to the shoulder on the affected side.
- Provide pain management.
- Assess for complications. Auscultate the lungs (↓ or absent breath sounds may indicate air and/or fluid reaccumulating in chest). Observe color and characteristics of chest tube drainage (significant bleeding >100 mL/h). Observe chest tube insertion site daily (infection may be identified by change in color or amount of drainage, redness at site, patient fever, ↑ WBCs).

Chest Tube Dressings

- Change dressing, maintaining sterile technique according to policy and HCP preference.
- Remove old dressing carefully. Assess the site for inflammation or infection, and culture site as needed. Observe that chest tube sutures are intact.
- Redress with occlusive dressing. Some HCPs prefer a petroleum gauze dressing around the tube to prevent air leak, covered by dry gauze dressing. Date the dressing and document dressing change.

General Chest Tube Management

- Keep all connections between chest tubes, drainage tubing, and the drainage collector tight. Tape all connections.
- Keep all tubing loosely coiled below chest level. Position tubing so that drainage flows freely. Keep the drainage system below the level of the patient's chest because fluid can drain back into the lungs.
- Observe for air fluctuations (tidaling) and bubbling in the water-seal chamber.
- Mark the time of measurement and the fluid level on the drainage unit according to policy. Report any change in the quantity or characteristics of drainage (e.g., clear yellow to bloody) to the HCP. Notify HCP if >100 mL/h drainage.
- Change the unit if the collection chamber is full. Do not try to empty it.
- Never compress, milk, or strip chest tube tubing.

Wet Suction System (see manufacturer's directions for use)

- Keep the suction control chamber at the right water level by adding sterile water as needed to replace water lost to evaporation.
- After filling the suction control chamber to the ordered suction amount (generally 20 cm H_2O suction), connect the suction tubing to the wall suction.
- Dial the wall suction regulator until there is continuous, gentle bubbling in the suction control chamber (no more than 120 mm Hg). Vigorous bubbling is not necessary and will increase the rate of evaporation.
- If there is no bubbling in the suction control chamber, (1) there is no suction, (2) suction is not high enough, or (3) the pleural air leak is so large that suction is not high enough to evacuate it.

Dry Suction System (see manufacturer's directions for use)

- After connecting the patient to the system, turn the dial on the chest drainage system to the amount ordered (generally −20 cm H_2O), and connect the suction tubing to the wall suction source. Increase the suction until the float appears in the window of the drainage unit.
- If ordered to decrease suction, turn the dial down and depress the high-negativity vent. Assess for a rise in the water level of the water-seal chamber.

Managing Complications

1. Loss of tidaling
   - In the spontaneously breathing patient, if fluid does not rise with inspiration or fall with expiration, the drainage system may be blocked, the lungs have reexpanded, or the system is attached to suction.
   - If the chest tube is connected to suction, disconnect momentarily from wall suction to check for tidaling.
2. Air leak
   - If bubbling increases, there may be an air leak in the drainage system or a leak from the patient.
   - Suspect a system leak when bubbling is continuous.
   - Retape tubing connections as needed.
   - Ensure chest tube dressing is air occlusive.
   - If leak persists, briefly clamp the chest tube at the patient's chest. If the leak stops, the air is coming from the patient.
   - If the air leak persists, briefly and methodically move the clamps down the tubing away from the patient until the air leak stops. The leak will then be present between the last 2 clamp points. If the air leak persists all the way to the drainage unit, replace the unit.
3. Drainage system overturned
   - If the drainage system is overturned and the water seal is disrupted, return it to an upright position and encourage the patient to take a few deep breaths.
4. Inadvertent disconnection from patient
   - If the drainage system breaks, place the distal end of the chest tubing (patient-side) in a container of sterile water as an emergency water seal.

disconnection occurs, the exposed end of the chest tube is immersed in sterile water to act as a water seal until a new system can be set up and chest drainage reestablished. Do not clamp the tube. The danger of rapid accumulation of air in the pleural space, causing tension pneumothorax, is far greater than that of a small amount of atmospheric air that enters the pleural space.

You can momentarily clamp a chest tube to change the drainage apparatus or check for air leaks. Appearance of a new air leak warrants assessment of the drainage system to identify whether the air leak is coming from the patient or from the system. Follow your agency policy about specific clinical situations when you may clamp a chest tube.

CHECK YOUR PRACTICE

You are caring for a 37-year-old male patient who has chest injuries from a motorcycle accident. He has 2 chest tubes in place that are each attached to a chest drainage system. While helping him to turn in bed, you accidentally disconnect 1 of the chest tubes from the drainage system.

- What is your most immediate priority?

Chest Tube Removal

Chest tubes are removed when the lungs are reexpanded and fluid drainage has ceased or is minimal. Sometimes, we discontinue the suction and allow the chest tube to drain by gravity for 24 hours before removing the tube.

Give pain medication about 30 minutes before chest tube removal. Gather dressing supplies, including petroleum gauze and dry gauze dressing. Explain the procedure to the patient. The HCP cuts the suture holding the chest tube in place. With the patient holding their breath or bearing down (Valsalva maneuver), the tube is removed. The site is covered with an airtight, occlusive dressing to prevent air from entering the pleural space. A dry gauze dressing is placed over the top. The pleura will seal off, and the wound usually heals in a few days. A chest x-ray is done 30 to 60 minutes after chest tube removal to check for pneumothorax or fluid accumulation.

Observe the wound for drainage and reinforce the dressing if needed. Monitor and record vital signs. Assess the patient for respiratory distress. This may signify a recurrence of the original problem. If respiratory distress occurs, notify the HCP at once.

Chest Surgery

Chest surgery is done for many reasons, including lung, heart, vascular, and esophageal problems. Common chest surgeries are described in Table 28.7.

Thoracotomy

A **thoracotomy** is a surgical incision into the chest to gain access to the heart, lungs, esophagus, thoracic aorta, or anterior spine. Two common approaches to a thoracotomy are the median sternotomy and lateral thoracotomy.

The median sternotomy involves splitting the sternum. It is mainly used for surgery involving the heart. A lateral thoracotomy can be done using a posterolateral or anterolateral incision. A *posterolateral incision* is used for most surgeries involving the lung. The incision is made from front to back at the level of the 4th, 5th, or 6th intercostal space. Strong mechanical retractors are used to separate the ribs and gain access to the lung. An *anterolateral incision* is made in the 4th or 5th intercostal space from the sternal border to the midaxillary line. This procedure is often done for surgery or trauma victims, mediastinal operations, and wedge resections of the upper and middle lobes of the lung.

Video-Assisted Thoracic Surgery

Video-assisted thoracoscopic surgery (VATS) is a widely used, minimally invasive surgical approach for thoracic procedures. It provides a real-time 2-dimensional video image of the inside of the chest cavity. VATS is used for diagnosis and treatment of pleural disease, masses and nodules, and interstitial lung disease. Through incisions just large enough to insert the instruments, the HCP can inspect the chest cavity, biopsy suspicious areas, obtain fluid samples for analysis, and remove tissue.

In patients with chest trauma, the HCP can examine, diagnose, and manage injuries, including injuries to the diaphragm, with VATS. Although most VATS procedures are done on intubated patients, new evidence suggests that VATS in nonintubated, spontaneously breathing patients is of benefit, especially in those with preexisting respiratory problems or who are too debilitated to tolerate an open thoracotomy.[9] The advantages of VATS include less pain, faster return to normal activity, reduced length of hospital stay, lower postoperative morbidity, and fewer complications.[10]

NURSING MANAGEMENT: CHEST SURGERY

Preoperative Care

Assess patients' cardiopulmonary status before surgery to determine their ability to tolerate the procedure and provide a baseline reference for postoperative care. Preoperative evaluation may include chest x-ray, ECG, ABGs, pulmonary function studies, CT, or MRI. Laboratory studies may include CBC, blood glucose, serum electrolytes, blood urea nitrogen (BUN), serum creatinine, prothrombin time/international normalized ratio (PT/INR), and activated partial thromboplastin time (aPTT).

Patients should be in the best possible health and, if applicable, stop smoking before elective surgery. Anxiety associated with anticipated surgery makes smoking cessation difficult. Provide encouragement, support, and teaching about ways to help stop smoking before surgery (see Chapter 11).

TABLE 28.7 Chest Surgeries

Type	Description	Indications
Decortication		
Removal or stripping of thick, fibrous membrane from visceral pleura	Need chest tubes after surgery Allows for improved lung expansion	Empyema or other inflammatory process unresponsive to conservative management
Exploratory Thoracotomy		
Incision into thoracic cavity to look for injured or bleeding tissues and/or vessels	Need chest tubes after surgery	Chest trauma
Lobectomy		
Removal of 1 lobe of lung	Lung tissue expands to fill up space left by resected lobe Need chest tubes after surgery	Lung cancer, bronchiectasis, TB, advanced emphysema, benign lung tumors, fungal infections
Lung Volume Reduction Surgery		
Bronchoscopy procedure	Used to place 1-way valves in airways leading to the diseased parts of the lung Valves let air out, but not in, thus collapsing a certain segment of lung	Advanced emphysema, α_1-antitrypsin emphysema
Open surgical procedure	Involves reducing lung volume by multiple wedge excisions or VATS Removes most diseased lung tissue	Emphysema, lung cancer
Pneumonectomy		
Removal of entire lung	Fluid will gradually fill space where lung was removed May have chest tube after surgery Position patient on operative side to promote expansion of remaining lung	Lung cancer (most common)
Segmental Resection		
Removal of 1 or more lung segments	Indicated for a patient unable to handle more extensive surgery Remaining lung tissue expands to fill space Need chest tubes after surgery	Lung cancer, bronchiectasis
Thoracotomy (Not Involving Lungs)		
Incision into thorax for surgery on other organs	Postoperative care related to thoracotomy and reason for surgical procedure Need chest tubes after surgery	Hiatal hernia repair, open heart surgery, esophageal surgery, tracheal resection, thoracic aorta repair
Video-Assisted Thoracic Surgery (VATS)		
Video-assisted technique with a rigid scope, with a distal lens inserted into pleura and image shown on a monitor screen	Allows HCP to manipulate instruments passed into pleural space through separate small intercostal incisions Done under general anesthesia in operating room May need chest tube after surgery	Lung biopsy, lobectomy, resection of nodules, fistula repair
Wedge Resection		
Removal of small, local lesion that occupies only part of a lung segment	Most conservative approach Done to remove small peripheral nodules or for patients unable to handle more extensive surgery Need chest tubes after surgery	Lung biopsy, excision of small nodules

Teach patients what to expect after surgery. Include the use of O_2, IV fluids, the chance of intubation, possible use of blood products, and the purpose and function of chest tubes. Reassure the patient that they will receive adequate analgesia to reduce pain.

Preoperative teaching should always include exercises for effective deep breathing and incentive spirometry use. If patients practice these techniques before surgery, they will be easier to perform after surgery. Teach patients how to splint the incision with a pillow to promote deep breathing. Have them teach back range-of-motion (ROM) exercises on the affected surgical side.

The thought of losing part of a vital organ is often frightening. Reassure the patient that the lungs have a large degree of functional reserve. Even after the removal of 1 lung, there is enough lung tissue in the remaining lung to maintain adequate oxygenation.

Postoperative Care

The thoracotomy incision is the most painful surgical incision for patients and difficult for nurses to manage. Pain after a thoracotomy is typically intense because respiratory muscles are cut during surgery. For most chest surgeries, chest tubes are placed in the pleural space to allow for lung reexpansion. In a pneumonectomy, chest tubes may be placed in the space where the lung was removed.

Pain management is a priority to prevent respiratory compromise. A multimodal management approach is best after thoracic surgery. This may include the use of oral, subcutaneous, and/or IV opioids; patient-controlled analgesia (PCA); epidural infusions; and/or intercostal nerve blocks. Effective pain management allows patients to breathe deeply, cough, move the arm and shoulder on the operative side, and mobilize.

Nursing care priorities include assessing respiratory function, including observing respiratory rate and effort, breath sounds, and sputum volume and color. Monitor chest tube function. Note amount and type of drainage. Daily chest x-rays are often done. Monitor the patient's temperature. Assess the surgical site as you would for other postoperative patients (see Chapter 20). Care after thoracotomy is described in eNursing Care Plan 28.3 (available on the website for this chapter).

NONINVASIVE VENTILATION

Noninvasive ventilation (NIV) uses a mask instead of an ET tube to help oxygenate and ventilate a patient. The mask can be nasal or full face. NIV is ideal for those who need a higher level of ventilatory support but their condition is not bad enough to need mechanical ventilation. Good candidates for using NIV are patients with COPD exacerbations and heart failure (HF).[11] Patients with cardiac and/or respiratory arrest, acute myocardial infarction, shock, or maxillofacial trauma are not candidates for NIV. Two common modes are continuous positive airway pressure (CPAP) and bilevel positive airway pressure (bi-PAP).

Continuous Positive Airway Pressure

Continuous positive airway pressure (CPAP) helps restore functional residual capacity (FRC). It provides 1 level of pressure that is delivered continuously during both inspiration and expiration. CPAP is a common treatment for obstructive sleep apnea.

CPAP is delivered through a tight-fitting face mask, nasal mask, or nasal pillows. It increases WOB because patients must forcibly exhale against the CPAP. It must be used with caution in patients with heart problems. Monitor the patient closely. Report any decline in their condition to the HCP at once.

Bilevel Positive Airway Pressure

Bi-PAP provides 2 levels of positive pressure support: inspiratory positive airway pressure (IPAP) and expiratory positive airway pressure (EPAP) (Fig. 28.9). IPAP is a higher level of pressure than EPAP. It helps with CO_2 removal. EPAP is a lower level of pressure. It helps keep the alveoli open at end expiration, assisting with oxygenation.

The patient must be awake, alert, able to breathe spontaneously, and tolerate the nose or face piece. Bi-PAP is used for patients with COPD with acute conditions (e.g., pneumonia) or exacerbation of chronic conditions (e.g., HF, acute respiratory failure [ARF]). Its use after extubation from mechanical ventilation can help prevent reintubation.

❖ NURSING MANAGEMENT: NONINVASIVE VENTILATION

Patients with NIV need constant assessment. Assess LOC, hemodynamic stability, and WOB. Patients who have a decreased LOC or increased secretions may not be able to use NIV. The patient must be able to remove the mask independently because of the risk of vomiting and aspiration. In this situation, they may require intubation and mechanical ventilation. Any degree of hemodynamic instability (e.g., tachycardia, hypotension) warrants immediate reevaluation of NIV.

Elevate the head of the bed 30 to 45 degrees. Offer mouth, nare, and eye care frequently. Provide measures to protect the skin from breakdown and ulceration. Any degree of redness constitutes a stage 1 pressure injury. Attempts to alleviate pressure from the tight-fitting mask, including alternating the

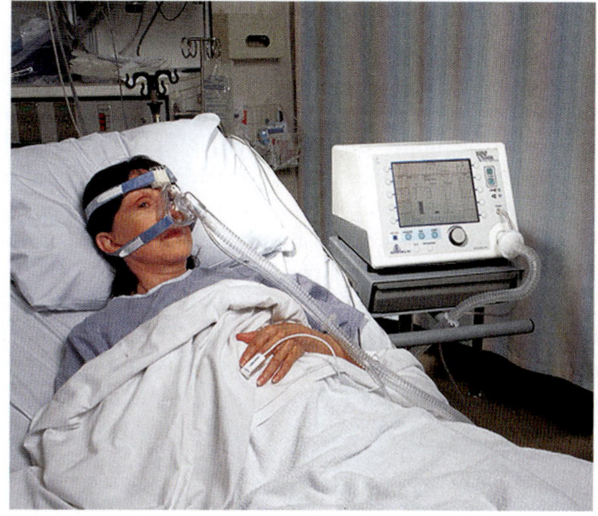

Fig. 28.9 Bi-PAP delivered through a face mask. (Courtesy Respironics, Inc., Murrysville, PA.)

length of time the mask is on, are important. Using masks of different sizes and styles can help. Collaborate with the RT.

MECHANICAL VENTILATION

Mechanical ventilation is the process by which a ventilator is used to deliver O_2 to the lungs. It is a means of supporting oxygenation and ventilation in patients until they recover the ability to breathe independently. It can serve as a bridge to long-term mechanical ventilation or until a decision is made to stop ventilatory support. Mechanical ventilation is not curative.

Indications for mechanical ventilation include (1) ventilatory failure, (2) apnea, (3) inability to protect the airway, (3) obstruction, (4) severe hypoxemia and/or hypercarbia, and (5) respiratory muscle fatigue.[12] Other patients who require mechanical ventilation include those with hemorrhage, trauma, neuromuscular problems, drug overdose, burns, and shock.

Patients with chronic lung disease and their caregivers should discuss mechanical ventilation before a health crisis occurs. Encourage all patients, especially those with chronic illnesses, to discuss the subject of life-sustaining measures, including mechanical ventilation, with their families and HCPs. The patient's wishes about end-of-life treatment should be recorded in an advance directive.

The decision to use, withhold, or stop mechanical ventilation must be made carefully. We must respect the wishes of the patient. When the health care team, patient, and/or caregiver disagree over the treatment that the patient wishes, family conferences are essential to keep the lines of communication open and discuss options. Sometimes, you may need to consult the ethics committee.

Types of Ventilators

Negative Pressure Ventilation

Negative pressure ventilation involves the use of chambers that encase the chest or body and surround it with intermittent subatmospheric (or negative) pressure. It is a form of NIV, as it does not require an artificial invasive airway.

The "iron lung" was the first form of negative pressure ventilation. It was developed in the 1950s during the polio epidemic. Intermittent negative pressure around the chest pulls the chest wall outward, reducing intrathoracic pressure. Air rushes into the upper airway, which is outside the sealed chamber. Expiration is passive. The machine cycles off, allowing chest retraction. This type of ventilation is like normal ventilation in that decreased intrathoracic pressures produce inspiration and expiration is passive.

Though they are rarely used, a few portable negative pressure ventilators are available for home use. They are mainly for patients with chronic neuromuscular diseases and central nervous system problems.

Positive Pressure Ventilation

Positive pressure ventilation (PPV) is the main method of mechanical ventilation used with acutely ill patients (Fig. 28.10). During inspiration, the ventilator pushes air into the lungs under positive pressure. Unlike spontaneous ventilation, intrathoracic pressure is increased during lung inflation, not decreased. Expiration is passive, as occurs in normal expiration. Ventilators can deliver positive pressure breaths to the patient by either volume or pressure.

Volume ventilation. With **volume ventilation**, a predetermined tidal volume (V_T) is delivered with each inspiration.[13] The V_T is consistent from breath to breath. The amount of pressure needed to deliver the breath varies based on the compliance and resistance of the lungs.

Pressure ventilation. With **pressure ventilation**, the peak inspiratory pressure (PIP) is predetermined.[13] The V_T delivered to the patient will vary, based on the pressure selected and the compliance and resistance of the lungs. We monitor the exhaled V_T to prevent hypoventilation, hypoxemia, and alveolar collapse.

Ventilator Settings

Ventilator settings on all modes of mechanical ventilation include FiO_2 and positive end-expiratory pressure (PEEP). Other adjustable ventilator settings include the respiratory rate, V_T, inspiratory:expiratory ratio, inspiratory flow rate and time, and sensitivity (Table 28.8).

Settings are based on the patient's condition, LOC, respiratory muscle strength, chest x-ray, and ABGs. Manipulating ventilator settings (Fig. 28.11) can help correct hypoxemia and hypercarbia. As the patient's condition improves, we can adjust the settings to allow the patient to take more control over their own WOB. Know your responsibility regarding changing ventilator settings. In most settings, this task is the responsibility of the HCP or RT. Always assess the patient's response to any setting changes.

Positive End-Expiratory Pressure

Positive end-expiratory pressure (PEEP) is a ventilator setting in which positive pressure is applied to the airway during

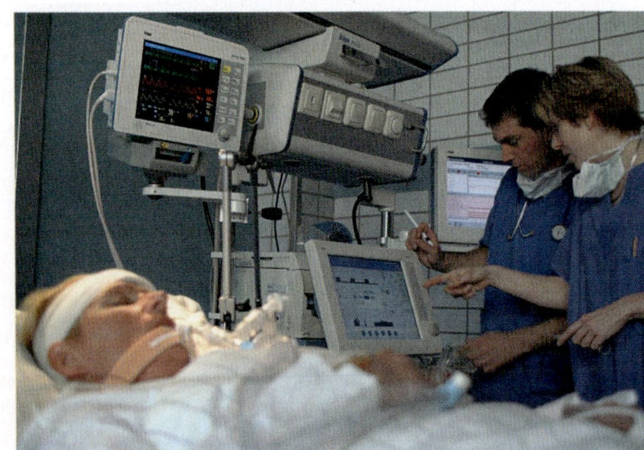

Fig. 28.10 Patient receiving mechanical ventilation. (Courtesy Draeger Medical, Houston, TX.)

exhalation.[14] During exhalation, airway pressure normally drops to near 0. Exhalation occurs passively. With PEEP, exhalation remains passive but pressure falls to the preset PEEP level, often set between 5 and 10 cm H_2O. PEEP increases FRC and can improve oxygenation by enhancing the lung volume that remains at the end of expiration. The mechanisms by which PEEP increases FRC and oxygenation include splinting open of previously collapsed alveoli (increasing the opportunity for O_2 and CO_2 to diffuse across the alveolar-capillary membrane) and preventing alveolar collapse throughout the respiratory cycle.

TABLE 28.8 Adjustable Ventilator Settings

Parameter	Mode	Description
O_2 concentration (Fio_2)	All modes	Fraction of inspired O_2 (Fio_2) delivered to patient Set between 30% and 100% *Usually adjusted* to maintain Pao_2 level >60 mm Hg or SpO_2 level >92%
Positive end-expiratory pressure (PEEP)	All modes	Positive pressure applied at the end of expiration of ventilator breaths *Example:* 5 cm H_2O
Respiratory rate	Full support	Number of breaths ventilator delivers per minute *Example:* 12 to 20 breaths/min
Tidal volume (V_T)	Full support	Volume of gas delivered to patient during each ventilator breath *Example:* 4 to 8 mL/kg
Level of pressure support	Spontaneous breathing mode	Positive pressure used to augment patient's inspiratory pressure during spontaneous breathing *Usual setting:* 5 to 10 cm H_2O
I/E ratio	All modes	Duration of inspiration (I) to duration of expiration (E) *Example:* 1:2 (exhalation twice as long as inspiration)
Inspiratory flow rate and time	Full, partial support	Speed with which V_T is delivered *Example:* 40 to 80 L/min and time is 0.8 to 1.2 seconds
Sensitivity	Full, partial support	Determines amount of effort the patient must generate to initiate a breath from the ventilator; the "trigger" to initiate the breath can be set on the ventilator for either pressure or flow triggering *Example:* Pressure trigger is set 0.5 to 1.5 cm H_2O below baseline pressure; flow trigger is set 1 to 3 L/min below baseline flow
Peak inspiratory pressure (PIP)	Full support	Maximal pressure the ventilator can generate to deliver the V_T; when the PIP limit is reached, the ventilator ends the breath and spills the undelivered volume into the atmosphere *Example:* 30 cm H_2O

PEEP is indicated in all patients who are mechanically ventilated. An intubated patient would never be placed on zero PEEP. PEEP is titrated to the point that oxygenation improves without compromising hemodynamics. We call this *optimal PEEP.* As a rule, 5 cm H_2O PEEP (referred to as *physiologic PEEP*) is used to replace the glottic mechanism, which is bypassed when the patient has an oral ET tube. We can often reduce Fio_2 when PEEP is used.

The classic indication for PEEP therapy is acute respiratory distress syndrome (ARDS). During weaning, PEEP improves gas exchange, vital capacity, and inspiratory force. PEEP is used with caution in patients with traumatic brain injury, increased intracranial pressure (ICP), low CO, and hypovolemia. In these cases, the effects of high PEEP may worsen the patient's condition. Each patient is unique, and mechanical ventilation is specific for each patient.

Modes of Volume Ventilation

The way in which the ventilator delivers effective ventilation is called the *ventilator mode.* It is mainly based on how much WOB the patient can perform. WOB is the inspiratory effort needed to overcome the elasticity and viscosity of the lungs along with airway resistance. Other factors that determine ventilator mode include the patient's condition, LOC, respiratory drive, and ABGs.

Modes of mechanical ventilation can be complex. This is because there are many different manufacturers of ventilators. Similarly, terminology among manufacturers differs, as many

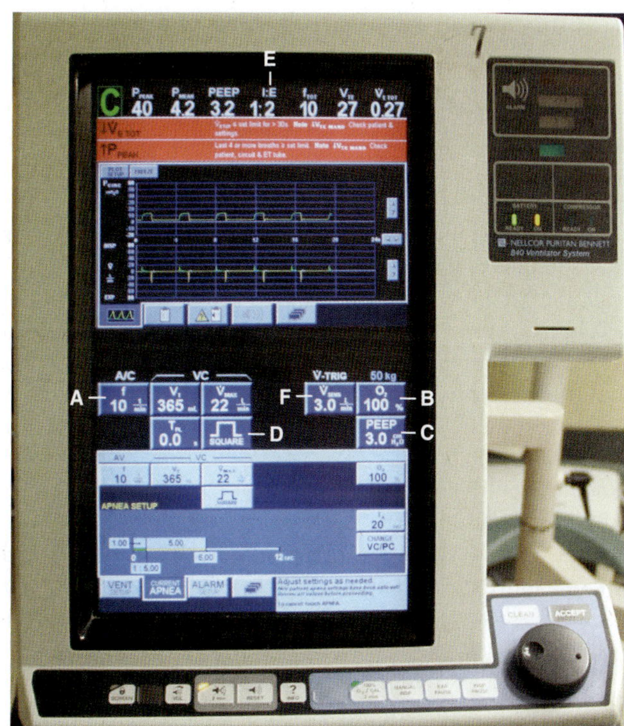

Fig. 28.11 Ventilator control panel. (From Roberts JR: *Roberts and Hedges' clinical procedures in emergency medicine and acute care,* ed 7, St Louis, 2019, Elsevier.)

companies trademark a mode of ventilation with a particular name. To begin to understand mechanical ventilation, focus on 2 key components: (1) how much work the ventilator is doing for the patient (full support, partial support, or spontaneous breathing) and (2) how the breath is being delivered to the patient (volume or pressure).

In *full support* mechanical ventilation, the ventilator does most of the WOB for the patient. The Fio_2, PEEP, respiratory rate V_T, and PIP limit are set. In a *partial support* mode, there is shared responsibility between the patient and ventilator. The Fio_2, PEEP, and respiratory rate are set for some (but not all) breaths, as the patient assumes more responsibility for breathing. In a *spontaneous mode* of mechanical ventilation, the patient assumes responsibility for almost all breathing. Spontaneous modes are often used just before the patient is extubated from the ventilator.

Let us look at the 5 most common modes of mechanical ventilation in North America. These modes include (1) assist control, (2) pressure control, (3) synchronous intermittent mandatory ventilation, (4) pressure support, and (5) CPAP (Table 28.9).

Full support modes

Assist control. In **assist-control (AC)** or **volume-control (VC) ventilation**, the ventilator delivers a preset respiratory rate with a preset V_T.[15] On AC ventilation, breaths can be delivered by the ventilator or triggered by the patient. When the patient initiates a spontaneous breath, the ventilator senses a change in the airflow in the ventilator circuit and then delivers the preset V_T. If the patient breathes over and above the set respiratory rate, the ventilator will deliver the additional breath with the designated V_T. The patient's respiratory rate on AC ventilation will never be below the set respiratory rate.

AC ventilation is the most common mode of full support mechanical ventilation when the patient is first intubated. It is used in patients with a variety of problems. This includes new postoperative patients and those with neuromuscular disorders and ARF.

With AC, the potential for hyperventilation exists. For example, a patient waking up after anesthesia may begin to take more spontaneous breaths above the set respiratory rate. As a result, the patient will receive all additional breaths with the full V_T. This can easily lead to respiratory alkalosis.

Pressure control. **Pressure-control (PC) ventilation** provides patients with a pressure-limited breath.[16] In other words, besides a set respiratory rate, there is a set PIP. When the patient initiates the breath, the ventilator will deliver a volume of gas up to the PIP limit. In PC mode, the PIP limit will never be exceeded. Because there is no preset V_T, the V_T will vary.

Like AC, PC ventilation permits patients to take a breath over and above the set rate anytime they like. When the patient takes a breath above the set rate, the ventilator will deliver the breath based on the current ventilator settings.

PC ventilation is good for patients with decreased compliance and increased resistance ("stiff lungs"). This allows us to have control over the amount of pressure going into the patient, thereby decreasing risk of volutrauma and barotrauma. It is important to monitor the exhaled V_T in PC ventilation. As lungs become stiff and difficult to ventilate, although the PIP limit will not be exceeded, V_T may decrease.

Partial support modes

Synchronized intermittent mandatory ventilation. In **synchronized intermittent mandatory ventilation (SIMV)**, the patient and the ventilator share the WOB. The ventilator delivers a preset V_T at a preset respiratory rate, in synchrony with the patient's spontaneous breathing.[17] In between the ventilator-delivered breaths, the patient can breathe spontaneously and generate their own V_T. In other words, the patient receives the designated V_T for the machine-delivered breaths, but during the spontaneous breaths, the patient can breathe at whatever respiratory rate they wish. Their V_T is variable.

SIMV is used when a patient's condition is too good for a full support mode of mechanical ventilation but they are not yet ready for a spontaneous mode. Benefits of SIMV include improved patient-ventilator synchrony, lower mean airway pressures, and prevention of respiratory muscle atrophy as the patient takes on more responsibility for the WOB.

Spontaneous breathing modes

Pressure support. With **pressure support (PS) ventilation**, positive pressure is applied to the airway only during inspiration. The patient must be able to initiate breathing. The level of positive airway pressure is preset so that the inspiratory flow rate of the gas is greater than the patient's inspiratory flow rate. As the patient starts a breath, the ventilator senses the spontaneous respiratory effort and supplies a rapid flow of gas at the initiation of the breath and then a tapering flow toward the end of inhalation.[14] With PS, the patient determines their own inspiratory length, V_T, and respiratory rate.

PS is the most common mode of spontaneous mechanical ventilation in North America. Its purpose is to help facilitate weaning. PS is not used during ARF because of the risk for hypoventilation and apnea. Advantages include increased patient comfort, decreased WOB (because inspiratory efforts are augmented), decreased O_2 consumption (because inspiratory work is reduced), and improved endurance (because the patient is responsible for initiating their own breaths).

Continuous positive airway pressure. CPAP refers to a mode of spontaneous ventilation where the intubated, mechanically ventilated patient controls almost all aspects of the breath.[18] Do not confuse this with noninvasive CPAP that is used for sleep apnea. With invasive CPAP, all that is set is the Fio_2 and PEEP. There is 1 level of pressure on both inspiration and expiration. There is no set respiratory rate, no set V_T, and no set PIP. The patient determines their respiratory rate and V_T.

CPAP is used to assess the patient's respiratory rate and rhythm, WOB, and hemodynamic status after a period of intubation. In most circumstances, this mode will be used for a short period, around 30 to 120 minutes. If the patient is stable, respiratory assessment parameters stay within normal limits, and there is no increased WOB or desaturation, the patient is often extubated.

TABLE 28.9 **Modes of Mechanical Ventilation**

Mode of Ventilation	Ventilator Settings	Nursing Implications
Full Support		
Assist-control (AC)	• Set FiO_2, PEEP, respiratory rate, V_T, inspiratory time • Ventilator delivers a preset number of breaths with designated V_T • If the patient initiates a spontaneous breath, a full breath with designated V_T is delivered	• V_T is consistent; trend pressure (PIP) • Hyperventilation can occur if patient increases respiratory rate above set rate • To limit spontaneous breaths, sedation may be needed • Example: New surgical patients
Pressure-control (PC)	• Set FiO_2, PEEP, respiratory rate, peak inspiratory pressure (PIP), inspiratory time • Ventilator delivers a preset number of breaths up to a specific PIP (set by HCP) • If the patient initiates a spontaneous breath, a full breath delivered up to the set PIP is delivered	• PIP is never exceeded; trend V_T as will be variable • To limit spontaneous breaths, sedation may be needed • Example: ARDS
Pressure-regulated volume control (PRVC)	• Set FiO_2, PEEP, respiratory rate, V_T, PIP, sensitivity • Ventilator attempts to deliver the desired V_T with the least amount of PIP • Ventilator software analyzes resistance and compliance of each breath and continuously makes adjustments	• Trend V_T and PIP • Monitor for increased WOB
Partial Support Modes		
Synchronized intermittent mandatory ventilation (SIMV)	• Set FiO_2, PEEP, respiratory rate, and V_T for all ventilator-delivered breaths (can be set up with a PIP, but V_T more common) • Inspiratory time and sensitivity also set • Ventilator delivers the preset number of breaths per minute with designated V_T in "synchrony" with patient's own respiratory rate • Between "ventilator-delivered breaths," patient breathes at their own rate and V_T	• A weaning mode • Muscle fatigue may occur because of ↑ WOB
Proportional assist ventilation (PAV)	• Will increase or decrease airway pressure in response to patient's own respiratory effort • Provides a level of support at a percentage of patient effort (e.g., 80%); if patient working hard to initiate a breath, ventilator offers more support • Patient determines own inspiratory volume and inspiratory flow rate	• Monitor WOB • Of no use in the patient who is not spontaneously breathing (will give no support)
Spontaneous Modes		
Pressure support ventilation (PSV)	• Set FiO_2, PEEP, inspiratory pressure level, sensitivity • When the patient initiates a breath, a high flow of gas is delivered to the preselected pressure level, and pressure is maintained throughout inspiration • Patient determines V_T, respiratory rate, inspiratory time • Provides augmented inspiration to a spontaneously breathing patient	• A weaning mode • Patient must be awake and alert and be able to initiate a breath • Observe respiratory rate and V_T • Reduces WOB • Increased ventilator synchrony possible • Monitor for increased WOB • Monitor for apnea
Continuous positive airway pressure (CPAP)	• FiO_2 and PEEP set • One set level of pressure (on inspiration and expiration) • Patient is spontaneously breathing through the ventilator circuit • There is no set respiratory rate, V_T, or inspiratory time	• A weaning mode • Patient must be awake and alert and breathing spontaneously • Observe respiratory rate and V_T • Monitor for increased WOB • Monitor for apnea
Other		
Airway pressure release ventilation (APRV)	• Can be used as a full support or spontaneous mode of ventilation • Set pressure (P-high, P-low) and time (T-high, T-low) • Most of ventilator-delivered breath is spent at P-high and T-high, thus assisting with alveolar recruitment • Quick timed release (P-low, T-low) allows for CO_2 elimination • Permits spontaneous breathing at P-high, T-high	• V_T is not a set variable • Trend ABGs and acid-base balance • APRV increases venous return to the heart • May improve hemodynamics

ABG, Arterial blood gas; *ARDS*, acute respiratory distress syndrome; *WOB*, work of breathing.

Alternative Modes

Advances in technology have led to the development of many other modes of mechanical ventilation. These include (1) pressure-regulated volume control (PRVC), (2) airway pressure release ventilation (APRV), and (3) proportional assist ventilation (PAV) (Table 28.9).

Pressure-regulated volume control. PRVC is a full support mode of mechanical ventilation. It combines features of both volume and pressure delivery of the mechanical breath. There is a set V_T and a set PIP limit. The ventilator tries to deliver the targeted V_T with the least amount of pressure.[19] The ventilator constantly analyzes, breath by breath, resistance and compliance of the lungs, the exhaled V_T, and PIP. Software within the ventilator adjusts the delivery of each breath based on feedback received.

Airway pressure release ventilation. APRV can be used in full support or spontaneous mode, depending on the patient. There are 2 levels of pressure in APRV: pressure-high (P-high) and pressure-low (P-low). There are 2 time values: time-high (T-high) and time-low (T-low). For most of the ventilator breath (inhalation), the patient is at P-high and T-high (e.g., pressure of 30 cm H_2O for around 6 to 8 seconds).[20] This helps with oxygenation and keeping alveoli inflated. During exhalation, pressure drops to near zero (P-low) for a very short period (T-low, about 0.8 second) to promote CO_2 elimination.

APRV allows spontaneous breathing at any point during the inspiratory respiratory cycle (P-high, T-high). We adjust the pressure levels in APRV to meet oxygenation goals. The timed releases are increased or decreased to meet ventilation goals. V_T is not set. It varies depending on the pressure levels, lung compliance and resistance, and degree of spontaneous breathing effort.

APRV is best for patients who need high pressure levels to open collapsed alveoli. It allows for spontaneous respirations. This may reduce the need for deep sedation or paralysis.

Proportional assist ventilation. PAV is a partial support mode of mechanical ventilation. In this mode, the ventilator generates and adjusts inspiratory pressures in proportion to the patient's own respiratory efforts.[21] The patient determines their own inspiratory flow rate and volume. The support that the ventilator provides the patient is a proportion of the patient's effort (e.g., 80%). The ventilator continually monitors compliance and resistance and calculates the degree of support it needs to offer. The patient is an active participant in breathing while receiving PAV. Decreased WOB and less dyssynchrony occur.

NURSING MANAGEMENT: PATIENT RECEIVING MECHANICAL VENTILATION

Care of patients receiving mechanical ventilation requires an interprofessional approach (Table 28.10). Nurses and other team members must constantly synthesize data about a patient's status and collaborate on patient care requirements. This section reviews important aspects to consider when caring for a patient who needs mechanical ventilation.

Artificial Airway Management

Managing an artificial airway is often a shared responsibility between you and the RT. Agency policy dictates which providers perform which task. Nursing responsibilities include (1) maintaining correct tube placement, (2) maintaining proper cuff inflation, (3) maintaining tube patency, and (4) maintaining alarm systems.

Maintaining Correct Tube Placement

Continuously monitor patients with an ET tube for correct placement. Note the exit point from the mouth or nare. Assess the integrity of the tape or securement device. Observe for symmetric chest wall movement. Auscultate to confirm bilateral breath sounds.

If the tube moves or is dislodged, it could easily migrate upward in the pharynx or enter the right or left mainstem bronchus (thus ventilating only 1 lung). This is an airway emergency. Stay with the patient and try to maintain the airway. Support ventilation with a BVM and 100% O_2. Call for help to assess or reposition the tube. If a dislodged tube is not repositioned, little or no O_2 is delivered to the lungs or the entire V_T is delivered to 1 lung. This places the patient at risk for hypoxemia, pneumothorax, and respiratory and/or cardiac arrest.

! SAFETY ALERT

Endotracheal Tube Placement

- Maintain proper ET tube position by recording and marking the position of the tube at the nare (for NT tube) or lip or teeth (for oral ET tube; e.g., oral ET tube 21 cm at the teeth).
- Assess ET tube position at least once per shift and with changes in patient position, early mobility, and before and after patient transport.

Maintaining Proper Cuff Inflation

The cuff is an inflatable, pliable plastic sleeve encircling the lower, outer wall of the ET tube. The cuff stabilizes and "seals" the ET tube within the trachea (Fig. 28.12). This helps prevent the escape of O_2 and helps maintain correct tube position. The cuff "seals off" the lower airways, thus protecting against aspiration.

Excess volume in the cuff can damage the tracheal mucosa. To ensure adequate tracheal perfusion, maintain cuff pressure at 20 to 30 cm H_2O.[22] Measure and record cuff pressure after intubation and on a routine basis (e.g., every 8 hours) using the *minimal occluding volume* (MOV) *technique.*

To perform the MOV technique in mechanically ventilated patients, place a stethoscope over the trachea and inflate the cuff to MOV by adding air until you hear no air at PIP (end of ventilator inspiration). Second, use a manometer to confirm that cuff pressure is between 20 and 30 cm H_2O. Record cuff pressure in the chart. If adequate cuff pressure cannot be maintained or larger volumes of air are needed to keep the cuff inflated, there could be a leak in the cuff or tracheal dilation at the cuff site. In these situations, notify the HCP.

TABLE 28.10 NURSING MANAGEMENT

Care of the Patient Requiring Mechanical Ventilation

- Monitor level of consciousness, hemodynamic stability, patient-ventilator synchrony, patient tolerance to ET or tracheostomy.
- Auscultate breath sounds, assessing for decreased ventilation or adventitious sounds.
- Monitor ventilator settings and alarms.
- Monitor tube placement and cuff pressure.
- Assess respiratory effort and work of breathing (especially on spontaneous modes).
- Determine need for ET tube suctioning, and suction patients as needed.
- Give sedatives, analgesics, and NMBA drugs as ordered.
- Reposition and resecure ET tube (per agency policy).
- Provide ordered VTE and GI prophylaxis.
- Develop plans for communication with the patient.
- Provide oral care per agency policy (Table 28.14).
- Monitor oxygenation level and signs of respiratory fatigue during weaning.
- Teach patients and caregivers about mechanical ventilation and weaning.

Collaborate With Respiratory Therapist

- Maintain ventilator system.
- Change ventilator settings as needed or ordered by HCP.
- Maintain correct tube placement and cuff inflation on ET tube.
- Auscultate breath sounds, assessing for decreased ventilation or adventitious sounds.
- Assess respiratory effort and WOB.
- Determine need for ET tube suctioning, and suction patients as needed.
- Reposition and resecure ET tube (per agency policy).

Collaborate With Dietitian

- Assess and monitor nutrition status.
- Recommend enteral nutrition formulas and optimal diet/caloric intake.

Collaborate With Physical and Occupational Therapist

- Perform range-of-motion exercises.
- Assist with early and progressive ambulation.

Collaborate With Speech Language Therapist

- Assess cognitive function and assist with communication.
- Perform swallowing studies.
- Provide teaching for patients with a long-term tracheostomy.

Collaborate With Social Worker

- Work with the patient and caregiver to identify care needs.
- Help the patient with transitions through the health care system.

ET, Endotracheal tube; *GI,* gastrointestinal; *NMBA,* neuromuscular blocking agent; *VTE;* venous thromboembolism.

Maintaining Tube Patency

Suctioning is needed to clear secretions and to maintain airway patency. Indications for suctioning include (1) visible secretions in the ET tube, (2) increase in respiratory rate or patient coughing, and (3) sudden decrease in SpO_2. Other signs that indicate the patient may need suctioning include an increase in peak airway pressure, auscultating adventitious breath sounds over the trachea or bronchi, or suspected aspiration of secretions.

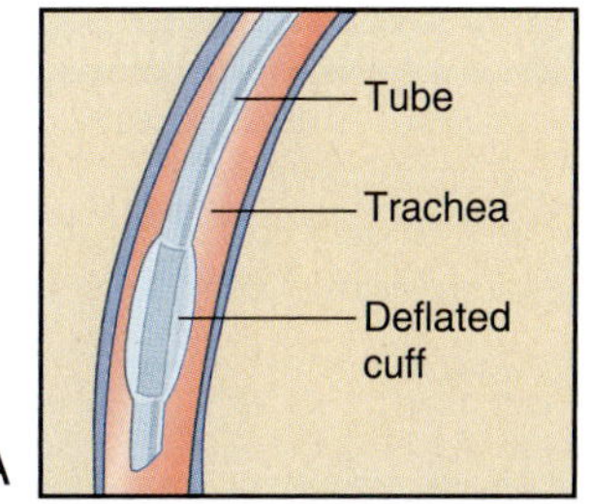

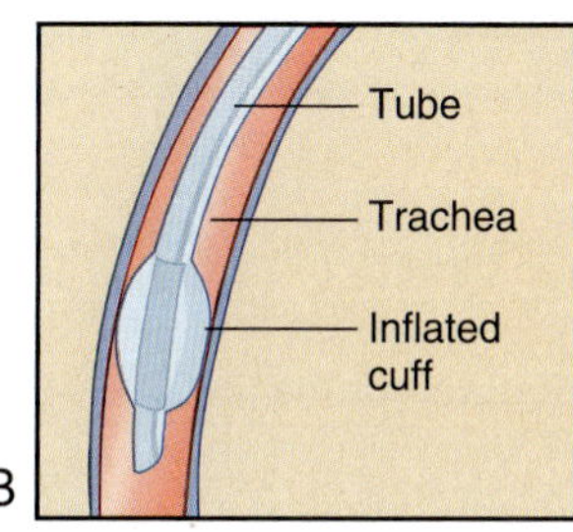

Fig. 28.12 Endotracheal tube cuff. (A) Tube in place with cuff deflated. (B) Tube in place with cuff inflated.

Assess the need for suctioning hourly. Indications may be obvious (as identified earlier), or subtle, such as restlessness or agitation. Do not suction routinely. Suction the patient only when needed. Note the color, character, consistency, and amount of sputum suctioned.

Two common ways we suction are the *closed-suction technique* (CST) and the *open-suction technique* (OST). The CST uses a suction catheter that is enclosed in a plastic sleeve connected directly to the patient-ventilator circuit (Fig. 28.10). With CST, exposure to the patient's secretions and risk of infection are reduced for the HCP and provide patient safety. The CST is the way we suction most intubated patients (Table 28.11).

We perform OST when we need sterile sputum samples or CST is not available. OST is best performed with 2 persons. One person disconnects the patient from the ventilator and uses the BVM while the second person suctions the patient. Table 28.12 describes the OST method.

Potential complications from suctioning include hypoxemia, bronchospasm, increased ICP, dysrhythmias, hypertension, hypotension, airway trauma (mucosal damage), pulmonary bleeding, pain, and infection.[23] Closely assess the patient, including ECG and SpO_2, before, during, and after suctioning. If the patient does not tolerate suctioning (e.g., decreased SpO_2, increased or decreased BP, sustained coughing, dysrhythmias), stop at once. Continue to reassess the patient until they achieve hemodynamic stability, recover, and/or the situation resolves before trying to suction again. Prevent hypoxemia by always hyperoxygenating the patient before and after each suctioning pass and limiting each pass to 10 seconds or less.

Causes of dysrhythmias during suctioning include (1) hypoxemia resulting in myocardial ischemia; (2) vagal stimulation caused by tracheal irritation; and (3) sympathetic nervous system stimulation caused by anxiety, discomfort, or pain. Dysrhythmias include tachydysrhythmias and bradydysrhythmias, premature beats, and asystole. Stop suctioning if any new dysrhythmias develop and monitor the patient.

Tracheal mucosal damage may occur because of suction pressures greater than 120 mm Hg, overly vigorous catheter insertion, and the suction catheter itself. Blood streaks or tissue shreds in aspirated secretions may indicate mucosal damage. This increases the risk for infection and bleeding, especially if the patient is receiving anticoagulants.

TABLE 28.11 Closed Suctioning Technique

The suction technique described here is appropriate for those patients with an oral ET tube or tracheostomy who are receiving invasive mechanical ventilation. Maintaining a closed circuit reduces the risk for infection and limits exposure to bodily fluids during suctioning.

Before You Begin

1. Gather all equipment.
2. Wash hands and don personal protective equipment and gloves.
3. Explain procedure and patient's role in assisting with secretion removal by coughing.
4. Monitor neurologic and cardiopulmonary status (e.g., LOC, vital signs, ECG, SpO_2) before, during, and after suctioning.
5. Check suction source and regulator. Adjust suction pressure to no greater than 120 mm Hg pressure with tubing occluded.

Press [Silence] on the ventilator to pause the alarms while suctioning.

How to Perform the Closed Suction Technique

7. Connect the suction tubing to the end of the in-line suction catheter.
8. Hyperoxygenate the patient by pressing the [100% FiO_2] button on the ventilator. This is the safest way to hyperoxygenate the patient.
   - Another option is to manually increase the FiO_2 to 100%. NOTE: Remember to return FiO_2 to baseline level when suctioning is completed.
   - The least preferred method is to disconnect the ventilator tubing and provide manual ventilation with 100% O_2 using a BVM device. Attach a PEEP valve to the BVM for patients on >5 cm H_2O PEEP. Have a second person give 5 or 6 breaths over 30 seconds.
9. Gently but quickly insert the in-line suction catheter into the oral ET tube/tracheostomy, pausing momentarily to pull back on the plastic sleeve containing the catheter. When the patient begins to cough more forcefully, STOP catheter insertion. NOTE: Do NOT insert the catheter until you meet resistance. This means that the end of the suction catheter is hitting the carina.
10. Apply continuous suction on withdrawal of the catheter (about 10 seconds).
11. Observe patient tolerance to procedure. Stop suctioning the patient and remove the in-line suction catheter from the patient if they become bradycardic or hypotensive. A vagal response may have occurred.
12. Disconnect the suction tubing from the end of the in-line suction catheter and attach the Yankauer. Gently suction the patient's oral cavity.
13. Ask the patient if they need another suction pass. Wait at least 30 seconds (ventilator) or 5 to 6 breaths (BVM) in between each suctioning pass.
14. If the patient does need more suctioning, ensure the ventilator is still providing FiO_2 100%. If not, press the [100% FiO_2] button again.
15. Repeat steps 9 through 13.
16. When the patient does not need more suctioning, ensure the suction tubing is attached to the end of the in-line suction catheter.
17. Rinse the catheter and connecting tubing with the sterile saline solution. Always rinse the tubing away from the patient.
18. Ensure the FiO_2 has returned to its previous setting or manually return the FiO_2 to the desired value.
19. Reassess the patient for hemodynamic stability and that suctioning was effective. Auscultate to assess changes in lung sounds.
20. Record time, amount, character of secretions, number of suction passes, and patient's response to suctioning.

BVM, Bag-valve-mask; *ET,* endotracheal; *LOC,* level of consciousness; *PEEP,* positive end-expiratory pressure.

TABLE 28.12 Open Suctioning Technique

The suction technique described here is appropriate for those patients with an oral ET tube or tracheostomy who are receiving invasive mechanical ventilation. Please note that this is best done with 2 people.

Before You Begin

Follow the same steps (steps 1 to 6) as identified in "Closed Suctioning Technique" (Table 28.11).

How to Perform the Open Suction Technique:

Use sterile technique to open the suction catheter package, using the inside of the package as a sterile field.

1. Fill the sterile solution container with sterile normal saline or water.
2. Don sterile gloves. Designate 1 hand as contaminated for connecting and disconnecting the tubing at the suction catheter and operating the suction control.
3. Pick up the sterile suction catheter with the dominant hand. Attach the catheter to suction tubing. Check the function of equipment by suctioning a small volume of sterile saline solution from the container.
4. Have the second person hyperoxygenate the patient with 100% FiO_2. Disconnect the ventilator tubing from the ET tube/tracheostomy and provide manual ventilation to the patient with 100% O_2 using a BVM device. Attach a PEEP valve to the BVM for patients on >5 cm H_2O PEEP. Have the second person give 5 or 6 breaths over 30 seconds.
5. Once hyperoxygenated, the second person removes the bagger from the end of the oral ET tube or tracheostomy. The first person gently but quickly inserts the in-line suction catheter *without suction* into the airway. When the patient begins to cough more forcefully, STOP catheter insertion. Do not insert the catheter until you meet resistance. This means that the end of the suction catheter is hitting the carina.
6. Apply continuous suction on withdrawal of the catheter (about 10 seconds).
7. Once the catheter is removed, have the second person reattach the BVM to the oral ET tube/tracheostomy and hyperoxygenate the patient.
8. Observe patient tolerance to the procedure. Stop suctioning and remove the in-line suction catheter from the patient if they become bradycardic or hypotensive. A vagal response may have occurred.
9. Ask the patient if they need another suction pass. Wait at least 30 seconds (ventilator) or 5 to 6 breaths (BVM) in between each suctioning pass.
10. Rinse the sterile suction catheter with sterile saline solution between suctioning passes.
11. If the patient needs more suctioning, have the second person remove the BVM from the oral ET tube or tracheostomy and repeat steps 6 through 11.
12. When the patient does not need more suctioning, the second person will reattach the patient to the ventilator. Discard all used suctioning supplies. Dispose of the catheter by wrapping it around the fingers of gloved hand and pulling the glove over the catheter.
13. Reassess the patient for hemodynamic stability and that suctioning was effective. Auscultate to assess changes in lung sounds.
14. Record time, amount, character of secretions, number of suction passes, and patient's response to suctioning.

BVM, Bag-valve-mask; *ET,* endotracheal; *PEEP,* positive end-expiratory pressure.

Secretions may be thick and hard to suction because of inadequate hydration or humidification or infection. Maintain adequate hydration when indicated (e.g., IV fluids). Provide humidification of inspired gases through the ventilator to help thin secretions. Turning (e.g., every 2 hours) and early mobilization help move secretions into larger airways. If infection is the cause of thick secretions, give antibiotics as ordered.

Maintaining Alarm Systems

Ensure that all ventilator alarms are always on. Alarms alert us to potentially dangerous situations, such as patient-ventilator dyssynchrony, ventilator disconnection or malfunction, or unplanned extubation (Table 28.13). Promptly assess any alarm on a mechanical ventilator and correct the cause.

Ventilators sometimes become disconnected from the patient. Most disconnections are discovered by low-pressure alarms. The most frequent site for disconnection is between the tracheal tube and the adapter. This can occur with repositioning or patients touching the ET tube. Push connections together to secure tightly. Teach patients not to touch the ET tube. On many ventilators, we can temporarily suspend or silence alarms for up to 2 minutes for suctioning. After that time, the alarm system automatically turns back on.

! SAFETY ALERT

Alarm Fatigue

- Alarm fatigue can develop in those who hear an excess number of alarms, resulting in sensory overload.
- This can cause a delayed response to alarms or dismissing them altogether and can lead to serious adverse events (e.g., patient death).
- To reduce alarm fatigue, set alarm parameters based on patient-specific needs.

Analgesia and Sedation

Patients receiving PPV may need analgesia (e.g., fentanyl, hydromorphone) and/or sedation (e.g., propofol) to help with ventilation. Before giving analgesia or sedation, try to identify the cause of distress. Common problems that can result in pain, agitation, or anxiety include presence of the ET itself, hypoxemia, hypercapnia, drugs, environment stress (e.g., fear, sleep deprivation), and discomfort from mechanical ventilation.

Assess patient comfort by using a valid pain scale, sedation scale (e.g., Richmond Agitation and Sedation Scale [RASS], Sedation Agitation Scale [SAS]), and/or delirium scale. Consider using relaxation techniques (e.g., music therapy) to complement drug therapy. The goal is to have the patient awake, interacting with their environment, and breathing comfortably and in synchrony with the ventilator.

At times, we may need to paralyze a patient with an NMBA. NMBAs paralyze skeletal muscles, including the diaphragm. The purpose of using NMBA is to remove any WOB and provide more effective synchrony with the ventilator, thereby improving both oxygenation and ventilation. Remember that the paralyzed patient can hear, see, and feel. It is essential to give IV sedation and analgesia concurrently when the patient is paralyzed, as NMBAs possess no analgesic or sedative properties. Given that the patient may or may not be aware of their surroundings, always address them as if they were awake and alert.

The mechanically ventilated patient receiving NMBA is a high-acuity patient in the ICU. Nurses giving these drugs often receive special training. We can assess the depth of paralysis by using the train-of-four (TOF) peripheral nerve stimulator and observing for signs of pain or anxiety (e.g., changes in heart rate [HR] and BP) and ventilator dyssynchrony. The TOF assessment involves delivering 4 successive stimulating currents with the nerve stimulator to elicit muscle twitches (Fig. 28.13). The number of twitches varies with the depth of neuromuscular blockade. The usual goal is 1 or 2 twitches out of 4 currents.

Noninvasive electroencephalogram technology (e.g., bispectral index monitoring [BIS]) can help guide analgesic, sedative, and NMBA therapy.[24] NMBAs should never be given to patients with a cholinesterase deficiency. NMBAs may predispose patients to prolonged paralysis and muscle weakness even after the drugs are stopped.

Hemodynamic Monitoring

Patients receiving invasive mechanical ventilation are hemodynamically monitored. Continuous assessment of the ECG, respiratory rate, BP, MAP, SpO_2, and synchrony with the ventilator provides vital information. Promptly investigate and treat ventilator dyssynchrony, hypertension, hypotension, and decreased O_2 saturations. Patients who cannot maintain heart rate, BP, and CO targets may need IV fluids and drug therapy, such as vasopressors and inotropes.

Oxygenation and Ventilation

Monitoring the respiratory rate and rhythm is important. Is the patient using accessory muscles? Auscultate breath sounds. Assess air entry and breath sound for each lobe, both anteriorly and posteriorly. Is the patient taking any breaths over and above the set rate? Are they initiating spontaneous breaths? Is there an increase in the WOB? Ensure ordered changes to mechanical ventilation (e.g., respiratory rate, FiO_2, PEEP, V_T, minute ventilation) are made. Evaluate the effects of any changes made on patient condition.

Assess for signs of hypoxemia, such as a change in mental status (e.g., confusion), dusky skin, and dysrhythmias. Periodic ABGs and continuous SpO_2 provide data about oxygenation. Central venous or pulmonary artery catheters with $ScvO_2$ or SvO_2 capability provide an indirect measure of tissue oxygenation status.

Indicators of ventilation include $PaCO_2$ and end-tidal carbon dioxide ($EtCO_2$, $PETCO_2$). Changes in $PaCO_2$ reflect alveolar hyperventilation (decreased $PaCO_2$) or hypoventilation (increased $PaCO_2$). $EtCO_2$ monitoring *(capnography)* is done by analyzing exhaled gas directly at the patient-ventilator circuit

TABLE 28.13 NURSING MANAGEMENT

Ventilator Alarms

Alarm	Possible Causes	Interventions
Apnea	• Change in patient condition • Increased work of breathing • Inappropriate mode of ventilation • Loss of airway • Oversedation • Respiratory arrest	• Change mode of ventilation • Disconnect patient from ventilator, attach BVM, call for help • Reassess analgesia and/or sedation if oversedation is primary cause of apnea
High-pressure limit	• ↓ Compliance (e.g., pulmonary edema, ARDS, tension pneumothorax, atelectasis, pneumonia) • Condensation (water) in tubing • Coughing, secretions • Improper alarm setting • Kinked or compressed tubing (e.g., patient biting on ET tube) • Patient fighting ventilator (ventilator dyssynchrony) • ↑ Resistance (e.g., bronchospasm, secretions in airways)	• Suction the patient • Reassure patient • Administer analgesia and/or sedation • Unkink tubing • Insert bite block • Give bronchodilator • Remove water from ventilator tubing • Assess breath sounds, obtain chest x-ray
High V_T, minute ventilation, or respiratory rate	• Anxiety, pain • Change in patient condition (e.g., ↑ metabolic demand, fever, hypoxia, hypercapnia, septic shock, or patient condition improving) • Excess condensation or secretions in tubing	• Reassure patient • Administer analgesia and/or sedation • Assess and reassess patient for change in condition • Change mode of ventilation • Remove water or secretions from tubing
Low-pressure limit	• Disconnection from ventilator or leak in circuit • ET tube or tracheotomy cuff leak (e.g., patient speaking, grunting) • Loss of airway (e.g., partial or total extubation)	• Check all connections • Confirm adequate V_T • Reinflate cuff • Confirm ET tube/tracheostomy position with chest x-ray
Low V_T, minute ventilation, or respiratory rate	• ET tube or tracheotomy cuff leak (e.g., air leak) • Inappropriate mode of ventilation • Insufficient gas flow • Oversedation • Disconnection, loose connection, or leak in circuit	• Reduce sedation • Assess ventilator circuit for leak • Measure cuff pressure to ensure cuff is adequately inflated • Change mode of ventilation • Based on respiratory rate and patient condition, disconnect patient from ventilator, attach BVM, call for help
Ventilator inoperative	• Internal battery not charged • Malfunction • Power failure	• Keep ventilator plugged into correct power source • Disconnect patient from ventilator, attach BVM, call for help

ARDS, Acute respiratory distress syndrome; *BVM,* bag-valve-mask; *ET,* endotracheal.

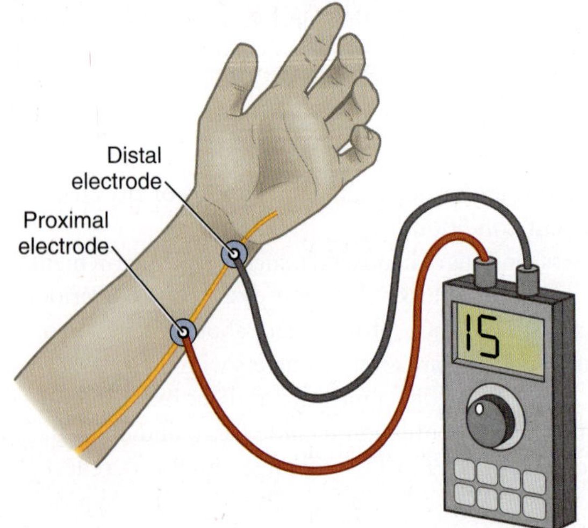

Fig. 28.13 Peripheral nerve stimulator. Placement of electrodes along ulnar nerve.

(mainstream sampling) or by transporting a sample of gas through a small-bore tubing to a bedside monitor *(sidestream sampling).* Continuous $EtCO_2$ monitoring can assess the patency of the airway and presence of breathing. Gradual changes in $EtCO_2$ values may accompany an increase in CO_2 production (e.g., sepsis, hypoventilation) or a decrease in CO_2 production (e.g., hypothermia, decreased CO, metabolic acidosis). $EtCO_2$ is normally 35 to 45 mm Hg.

Oral Care

When an oral ET tube is in place, the patient's mouth is always open. Moisten the lips, tongue, and gums with water swabs to prevent mucosal drying. Oral care provides comfort and prevents injury to the gums and plaque formation (Table 28.14).[25] Follow agency protocol for providing oral care to intubated patients.

TABLE 28.14 Oral Care for a Patient on a Ventilator

General Measures

1. Gather all equipment.
2. Wash hands and don personal protective equipment and gloves.
3. Explain procedure to the patient and caregiver (if present).
4. Perform oral care every 2 to 4 hours using toothettes or a suction toothbrush, a Yankauer suction device, and toothpaste or mouthwash (use 0.12% chlorhexidine oral rinse as per agency protocol).
5. Provide oral care for 1 to 2 minutes, suctioning often.
6. Apply mouth moisturizer to oral mucosa and lips with each cleaning.
7. Suction oral cavity and pharynx only when needed.
8. Dispose of trash and clean equipment. Rinse nondisposable oral suction apparatus with sterile normal saline and place on a dry paper towel.
9. Change all oral suction equipment and suction tubing every 24 hours.

Skin Integrity

Frequent assessment and good care are needed to prevent skin breakdown on the face, lips, tongue, and nares because of pressure from the ET tube or the method used to secure the ET tube. Ongoing assessment is a shared responsibility between the RN and RT. Reposition and retape the ET tube per agency policy as needed to prevent skin breakdown.

Two staff members should always perform repositioning to maintain correct position of the tube and to prevent accidental ET tube dislodgment. Monitor the patient for any signs of respiratory distress throughout the procedure.

For orally intubated patients, remove the bite block (if present) and the old tape. Reposition the ET tube to the opposite side of the mouth. Replace the bite block (if used) and reconfirm proper cuff inflation and tube placement. Secure the ET tube again per agency policy.

We can use a commercial device to secure the ET tube, but some devices increase the risk for skin breakdown. If you use a commercial device, follow the manufacturer's directions for maintaining tube position, providing skin care, and preventing skin breakdown. Always assess the skin under the ET tube, including upper and lower lips and chin, and underneath any securement devices for redness and skin breakdown.

Nutrition Therapy and Gastrointestinal Prophylaxis

Preexisting nutrition problems and being NPO while intubated and mechanically ventilated can produce a unique set of problems. The presence of an ET tube eliminates the normal route for eating. A nasogastric (NG) or an orogastric (OG) tube is inserted and connected to low intermittent suction to decrease risk of aspiration and vomiting. Malnutrition decreases resistance to infection, delays weaning from mechanical ventilation, and slows recovery.

We provide nutrition support to prevent or correct nutrition problems. This goal is achieved through early enteral nutrition (EN) or, if not possible, parenteral nutrition. EN preserves the structure and function of the gut mucosa and stops the movement of gut bacteria across the intestinal wall and into the bloodstream.[26] Patients likely to remain intubated for 3 to 5 days should have a nutrition assessment completed on admission and EN started within 24 hours. Consult the dietitian to determine the patient's caloric and nutrient needs.

Stress from the illness, immobility, or discomfort from the ventilator places patients at risk for developing stress ulcers and GI bleeding. Patients with a preexisting ulcer or those receiving corticosteroids have a higher risk. Any circulatory compromise, including reduced CO caused by PPV, may contribute to ischemia of the gastric and intestinal mucosa and increase the risk for translocation of bacteria from the GI tract. Stress ulcer prophylaxis includes giving histamine (H_2)-receptor blockers (e.g., ranitidine), proton pump inhibitors (PPIs; e.g., esomeprazole), or EN.

Immobility, sedation, impaired circulation, opioid use, and stress contribute to decreased peristalsis. As a result, ventilated patients are at risk for constipation. Start a bowel regimen early to help with gastric motility.

Venous Thromboembolism

Patient mobility is often limited because of presence of the ET and the mechanical ventilator. Altered LOC, analgesia and sedation, and presence of IV infusions further contribute to decreased ability of patients to reposition themselves. As a result, stasis of blood in the lower extremities and the risk of venous thromboembolism (VTE) are of real concern. Start VTE prophylaxis as ordered (see Chapter 41).

Early Mobility

Maintaining muscle strength and preventing complications from immobility are important. With few exceptions (e.g., hemodynamically unstable patients, those receiving NMBA, unstable cervical or thoracic spine fractures, medical contraindications), we encourage most patients receiving invasive mechanical ventilation to exercise and mobilize as soon as possible.

Plan for early and progressive mobility (Box 28.1). Collaborate with physical and occupational therapy. Help the patient perform passive and then active exercises to maintain muscle tone. Simple maneuvers, such as leg lifts or arm circles, are appropriate. Prevent contractures and pressure injuries by proper positioning and using specialized mattresses or beds. Use a portable ventilator or provide manual ventilation with a BVM and 100% O_2 when ambulating patients who are mechanically ventilated.

Communication

Intubated patients have stress from not being able to talk and communicate their needs. Inability to communicate may be because of analgesia, sedation, the ET tube, or neurologic impairment. This lack of communication can be frustrating for patients, caregivers, and health care team. To communicate more effectively, use a variety of methods.

Provide patients with paper and pencil, a whiteboard, or cellphone for texting. A communication board with pictures of common needs is convenient for patients who may speak other languages. A visual alphabet for spelling words is useful for patients who are weak or have difficulty writing.

As part of every procedure, explain what will happen or is happening to the patient. When the patient cannot speak, use picture boards, notepads, magic slates, or computers. When speaking with the patient, look directly at them.

Nonverbal communication is important. Patients have different levels of tolerance for touch, usually related to culture and personal history. If appropriate, use comforting touch with ongoing evaluation of the patient's response. Encourage the caregiver to talk to the patient, even if the patient is intubated, is sedated, or appears comatose.

BOX 28.1 EVIDENCE-BASED PRACTICE

The Mechanically Ventilated Patient and Early Mobilization

W.R. is a 72-year-old female patient who has been in the ICU for 3 days. She failed extubation in the postanesthesia care unit (PACU) after a cholecystectomy, was reintubated, and was admitted to the adult ICU. Weaning trials are planned for today. Yesterday, you started passive exercises and dangling with W.R. Today, you and the physical therapist discuss early mobilization with her and her husband.

Making Clinical Decisions

Best Available Evidence

Implementing an early exercise and mobilization protocol for stable, mechanically ventilated patients is safe and well tolerated. Early mobilization improves patient outcomes. Involving patients and caregivers in decision making around care (e.g., early mobilization) is a priority among this group.

Clinician Expertise

Your unit has successfully implemented an early mobilization protocol for intubated and mechanically ventilated patients in your ICU (part of the ABCDEF Bundle). You are aware that patients and their families often worry about ambulating with complex equipment attached to them.

Patient Preferences and Values

W.R. writes on the computer that she does not want to get out of bed until her "breathing tube is out and she has no more IV lines." Her husband tells you she is "afraid of falling."

Implications for Nursing Practice

1. What will you tell W.R. and her husband about the benefits of early mobilization?
2. How will you help reduce W.R.'s concerns about being "afraid of falling"?
3. How will you involve W.R. and her husband in the decision to take part in the early mobilization program?

Reference for Evidence

Monsees J, Moore Z, Patton D, et al: A systematic review of the effect of early mobilization on length of stay for adults in the intensive care unit, *Nurs Crit Care* 28:499, 2023.

Psychosocial Concerns

Patients receiving mechanical ventilation often have physical and emotional stress. Patients supported by a ventilator cannot speak, move, or breathe normally. Tubes and machines cause pain and fear. Anxiety is common. There is a loss of independence. They may feel helplessness and hopelessness. Usual activities, such as eating and elimination, are complicated. Many patients and caregivers feel uncomfortable in the ICU with its complex equipment, high noise and light levels, and intense pace of activity. Sleeplessness and loss of control enhance anxiety.

Feeling safe is an overpowering need. Work to strengthen the factors that affect feeling safe. Encourage hope as appropriate. Build trusting relationships with both the patient and caregiver. Involve them in decision making as much as possible.

To help reduce anxiety, include patients and caregivers in all conversations. Explain the purpose of equipment and procedures. Encourage them to express concerns, ask questions, and state their needs. Structure the environment in a way that decreases anxiety. For example, encourage caregivers to bring in photographs and personal items. Relaxation techniques (e.g., music therapy) and antianxiety drugs (e.g., lorazepam) may reduce the stress response that anxiety can trigger.

Preventing Delirium

The ABCDEF Bundle is evidence-based practice of providing care that strives to attain an environment in which patients receiving mechanical ventilation are calm, delirium free, and able to express their needs for pain control, positioning, and reassurance. The ABCDEF Bundle ensures **A**ssessment, **B**reathing trials are done daily, correct **C**hoice of analgesia and sedation, **D**elirium prevention and management, **E**arly mobility, and **F**amily engagement.[27]

"Rescue" Therapies

Rescue therapies attempt to alleviate hypoxemia in patients who are not able to maintain reasonable oxygenation despite appropriate mechanical ventilation, high FIO_2, and PEEP. Rescue therapies are tailored to each patient's requirements. Three therapies—inhaled pulmonary vasodilators, proning, and extracorporeal membrane oxygenation (ECMO)—are briefly discussed here.

Inhaled Pulmonary Vasodilators

Inhaled pulmonary vasodilators, such as nitric oxide (NO) and epoprostenol (Flolan), are gas molecules that take part in the regulation of pulmonary vascular tone. For example, inhibiting NO production results in pulmonary vasoconstriction. Continuous delivery of NO results in pulmonary vasodilation. Giving pulmonary vasodilators by inhalation helps increase pulmonary arterial blood flow and decrease pulmonary pressures. As a result, there may be an improvement in gas exchange and arterial oxygenation.

Prone Positioning

Prone positioning is the repositioning of a patient from a supine or lateral position to a prone (on the stomach, face down) position. Proning improves lung recruitment through various mechanisms (see Fig. 32.10). Gravity reverses the effects of fluid in the dependent parts of the lungs. The heart rests on the sternum, away from the lungs, contributing to an overall uniformity of pleural pressures. The prone position requires increased sedation and is labor intensive for the nurse. It can be an effective supportive therapy in critically ill patients with severe ARDS to improve oxygenation. Evidence currently suggests that patients with ARDS should be proned early and remain prone for at least 12 hours per day.[28]

Extracorporeal Membrane Oxygenation

ECMO is an alternative form of pulmonary support for patients with severe respiratory failure (Fig. 28.14). Think of ECMO as a modification of cardiac bypass or kidney dialysis. ECMO involves removing blood from a patient through a large-bore vascular access catheter. When the blood goes through the ECMO unit, it is infused with O_2. CO_2 is removed at the same time. The newly oxygenated blood is then returned to the patient.

ECMO is very labor intensive. It most often occurs in an ICU, with a skilled team of specialists, including a perfusionist and specially trained nurses. Patients must meet specific criteria to receive ECMO. It requires systemic anticoagulation. The risk of bleeding is considered before starting therapy.

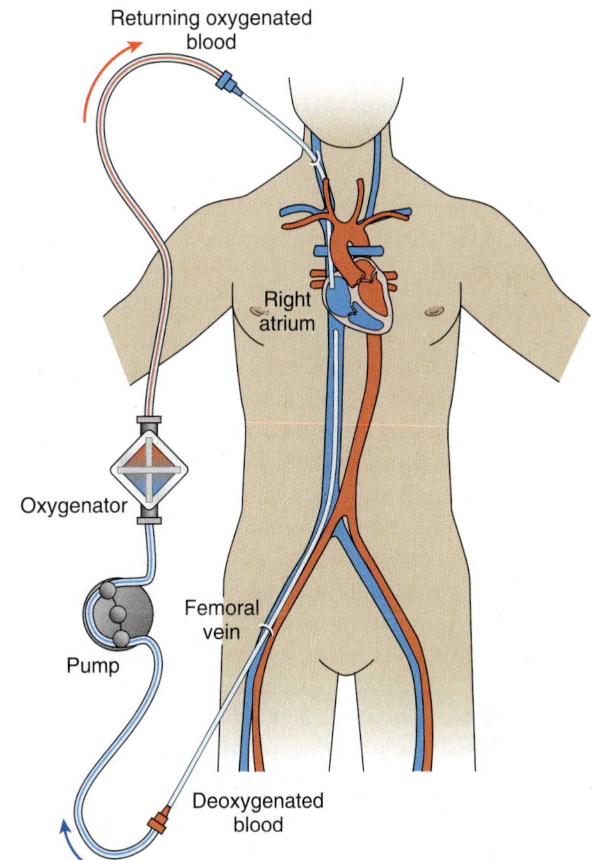

Fig. 28.14 ECMO circuit. The circuit consists of a blood pump and oxygenator. Circulatory access is typically obtained through the femoral vein and artery. Blood is removed from the patient, O_2 is added by the oxygenator and CO_2 is removed, and the blood is reinfused back into the patient. (From Spellman J, Sutherland L: *Cohen's comprehensive thoracic anesthesia,* St Louis, 2022, Elsevier.)

Complications of Mechanical Ventilation

Aspiration

Aspiration is a potential hazard for patients with an ET tube. The ET tube bypasses the epiglottis, keeping it in an open position. As a result, the patient cannot protect the airway from aspiration. The high-volume, low-pressure ET cuff cannot totally prevent the trickle of oral or gastric secretions into the trachea. Secretions can collect above the cuff. When the cuff is deflated, those secretions can move into the lungs.

Oral intubation increases salivation, and swallowing is difficult. Suction the patient's mouth often. Use a Yankauer (tonsil-tip) suction catheter or a sterile single-use catheter. Other factors contributing to aspiration include improper cuff inflation, patient positioning, and decreased gastric mobility and bowel function if receiving EN. Even when the cuff is properly inflated, take precautions to prevent vomiting, which can lead to aspiration. Some newer oral ET tubes provide continuous suctioning of secretions above the cuff. Unless contraindicated, keep the head of the bed elevated at least 30 degrees in all intubated patients who are receiving EN.

Sodium and Water Imbalance

Progressive fluid retention can occur 48 to 72 hours after starting PPV, especially with PEEP. Fluid retention is associated with increased sodium retention and decreased urine output. Fluid balance changes may be the result of decreased CO, which causes decreased renal perfusion. This stimulates the release of renin with the subsequent production of angiotensin and aldosterone. This results in sodium and water retention.

As a part of the stress response, release of antidiuretic hormone (ADH) and cortisol contributes to sodium and water retention. Insensible water loss occurs with an artificial airway because ventilated gases delivered to the patient are humidified. Pressure changes in the thorax decrease release of atrial natriuretic peptide, which contributes to sodium and water retention.

Monitoring intake and output hourly and careful observation of serum electrolytes can help provide early detection of problems to prevent complications.

Adverse Hemodynamic Effects

PPV affects circulation because of the transmission of increased mean airway pressure to various structures in the thorax. Increased intrathoracic pressure compresses the thoracic vessels. This compression decreases venous return to the heart, reducing preload, systolic BP, MAP, and CO. Mean airway pressure increases further when more than 5 cm H_2O of PEEP is being used.

As a result, patients may be hypotensive immediately after intubation, especially because inserting the ET tube is frequently accompanied by analgesia and sedation. However, after a few minutes, most patients adapt to positive pressure ventilation. Continuous monitoring of vital signs and vital sign targets (e.g., keep MAP greater than 65 mm Hg) are essential components of care.

Alveolar Ventilation Changes

Alveolar hypoventilation can be caused by inappropriate ventilator settings, air leaking from the ventilator tubing or around the ET tube or tracheostomy cuff, lung secretions or obstruction, or administering too much analgesia or sedation. A low V_T or respiratory rate decreases minute ventilation. This results in hypoventilation, atelectasis, and respiratory acidosis.

Alveolar hyperventilation can occur if the respiratory rate or V_T is too high (mechanical overventilation) or if a patient receiving assisted ventilation is hyperventilating. Hyperventilation leads to respiratory alkalosis. If hyperventilation is spontaneous, it is important to determine the cause and treat it. Common causes include hypoxemia, pain, anxiety, or compensation for metabolic acidosis. Patients who fight the ventilator or breathe out of synchrony may be anxious or in pain. If the patient is anxious and fearful, sitting with them and coaching them to breathe with the ventilator or weaning the ventilator to a more appropriate setting may help.

Barotrauma

Barotrauma results when increased airway pressure distends the lungs and possibly ruptures fragile alveoli or blebs. The risk for barotrauma increases as lung inflation pressures increase. Patients with noncompliant (stiff) lungs are at greatest risk. This includes those with ARDS.

Increasing inflation pressure places patients at risk for a pneumothorax. With PPV, a simple pneumothorax can become a life-threatening tension pneumothorax. The mediastinum and contralateral lung are compressed, reducing CO. Immediate treatment of a tension pneumothorax includes needle decompression, which is followed by chest tube insertion.

Volutrauma

Volutrauma can occur if too large a volume of air (V_T) is used to ventilate noncompliant lungs. Volutrauma causes alveolar rupture and movement of fluids and proteins into the alveolar spaces. To minimize volutrauma, we use low-tidal volume ventilation in patients with stiff, noncompliant lungs (e.g., ARDS).

Auto-Positive End-Expiratory Pressure

Auto-PEEP is a result of inadequate exhalation time. Auto-PEEP is PEEP over and above what has been set by the HCP.[29] This added PEEP may result in increased WOB, barotrauma, and hemodynamic instability. Interventions to limit auto-PEEP include sedation and analgesia, large-diameter ET tube, decreased respiratory rates, longer exhalation times, and bronchodilators. Reducing water accumulation in the ventilator circuit by frequent emptying or use of heated circuits helps limit auto-PEEP.

Ventilator Malfunction

Ventilator malfunction has been known to occur. Although most agencies have emergency generators in case of a power failure and newer ventilators may have battery backup, power failure is always a possibility. Have a plan for manually ventilating all patients who depend on a ventilator. If at any time you decide the ventilator is malfunctioning (e.g., failure of O_2 supply) or if you cannot determine the cause of an alarm and the patient is in respiratory distress, disconnect the patient from the machine and manually ventilate with a BVM and 100% O_2 until help arrives and the ventilator is fixed or replaced.

CHECK YOUR PRACTICE

You are caring for a 75-year-old female who was orally intubated yesterday for respiratory distress caused by pneumonia. She is on AC (full support) ventilation. Her ventilator settings are RR 14 (set), FiO_2 40%, PEEP 5 cm H_2O, and V_T 400 mL. You respond to the ventilator alarm. You hear audible air escaping from around her mouth as you suction her. The alarm panel shows "low exhaled tidal volume." She appears anxious. Vital signs: HR 112, RR 26, and SpO_2 89%.

- What would be your next steps?

Ventilator-Associated Pneumonia

Ventilator-associated pneumonia (VAP) is pneumonia that occurs 48 hours or more after ET intubation. It occurs in 5% to 40% of all intubated patients.[30] Most patients develop VAP early. COPD, ARDS, and trauma patients are most at risk. Patients who develop VAP have significantly longer days mechanically ventilated and longer hospital stays.[31] Mortality rates are as high as 50%.[30]

The most common organisms that cause VAP are gram-negative bacteria (e.g., *Escherichia coli, Klebsiella, Streptococcus pneumoniae, Haemophilus influenzae*).[32] Others include antibiotic-resistant organisms, such as *Pseudomonas aeruginosa* and oxacillin-resistant *Staphylococcus aureus.*[32] These organisms are abundant in the hospital environment and the patient's GI tract. They can spread in several ways. Examples include contaminated respiratory equipment, inadequate hand washing, adverse environment (e.g., poor room ventilation, high traffic flow), and decreased patient ability to cough and clear secretions. Colonization of the oropharynx by gram-negative organisms predisposes patients to gram-negative pneumonia. Poor nutrition, immobility, and the underlying disease process (e.g., immunosuppression, organ failure) increase risk.

Signs that suggest VAP include a fever, high white blood cell count, change in color and/or amount of sputum, crackles or wheezes on auscultation, and new lung infiltrates on chest x-ray. Obtain sputum cultures. Once VAP is confirmed, start broad-spectrum antibiotics.

Guidelines for VAP prevention include (1) minimizing sedation, including daily spontaneous awakening trials (SATs) or daily spontaneous breathing trials (SBTs); (2) early mobilization; (3) use of ET tubes with subglottic secretion drainage ports; (4) elevating the head of the bed a minimum of 30 to 45 degrees unless contraindicated; and (5) no routine changes of the ventilator circuit tubing.[33]

Other preventive measures include strict hand washing before and after suctioning, whenever ventilator equipment is touched, and after contact with any respiratory secretions (Box 28.2). Always wear gloves when in contact with patients and change gloves between activities (e.g., emptying urinary catheter drainage, hanging an IV drug). As it collects, always drain the water in the ventilator tubing away from the patient.

! SAFETY ALERT

Ventilator-Associated Pneumonia Prevention

- Practice good hand hygiene techniques before and after suctioning and between patient care tasks.
- Keep the head of the bed elevated 30 to 45 degrees.
- Wear gloves when providing oral hygiene.
- Suction patients as needed for comfort.
- Turn patient according to agency policy.
- Begin early mobilization.
- Follow agency policy for limiting sedation with SAT.
- Perform daily SBT unless contraindicated.

Unplanned Extubation

Unplanned extubation can be the result of patient self-removal of the ET tube or accidental removal during movement or a procedure. Sometimes the unplanned extubation is obvious (e.g., the patient is holding the ET tube). Other times, the tip of the ET tube is in the hypopharynx or esophagus, and extubation is not obvious. Signs of unplanned extubation include a low-pressure ventilator alarm, decreased or absent breath sounds, visible respiratory distress, or an audible cuff leak. The patient may be talking to you. Sometimes, an unplanned extubation can be an immediate life-threatening event.

Help prevent unplanned extubation by ensuring that the ET tube is secured and always supported during repositioning, procedures, and patient transfers. Giving adequate sedation and analgesia and following weaning protocols can help decrease the incidence of self-extubation.

Using restraints to immobilize the patient's hands is a deterrent to self-extubation. Explain to the patient and caregiver the purpose of restraints. When you use short-term restraints for patient safety, discuss the use of possible alternatives. Reassess the need for restraints daily, and limit restraint use when possible. Follow agency protocol for the care of patients who are restrained.

BOX 28.2 EVIDENCE-BASED PRACTICE

The Mechanically Ventilated Patient and Early Mobilization

You are working in the ICU in a rural area hospital. Over the past 6 months, you have noted an increase in VAP (ventilator-associated pneumonia) related infections despite having a VAP bundle policy. You question why this trend is happening.

Making Clinical Decisions

Best Available Evidence

Nurses have a major role in preventing VAP in ICU patients. Multiple factors are identified as to why nurses do not follow VAP bundle policies, including insufficient knowledge level regarding VAP prevention protocols, inadequate policy training, and lack of oversight for bundle implementation.

Clinician Expertise

You approach your nurse manager and ask if you can research VAP bundle policies and speak to your colleagues about their implementation of VAP prevention practices.

Patient Preferences and Values

Your colleagues identify a lack of updated or repeated training and unfamiliarity with the current VAP prevention policy. You decide to place VAP bundle policy reminders in each patient room and provide regular training. The nursing team will monitor the incidence of VAP infections for 6 months and compare it with the 6 months prior to implementing the interventions.

Implications for Nursing Practice

1. What outcomes would you expect to see if the new prevention interventions are successfully implemented?
2. In planning care for an ICU patient with VAP, how does VAP influence length of stay and the ability of patients to actively participate in care?

Reference for Evidence

Rehmani A, Au A, Montgomery C, et al: Use of nursing care bundles for the prevention of ventilator-associated pneumonia in low-middle income countries: a scoping review, *Nurs Crit Care* 29(6):1511, 2024.

! SAFETY ALERT

Unplanned Extubation

What to do during an unplanned extubation:

- Stay with the patient.
- Call for help.
- Support oxygenation as needed by applying an adjunct therapy, such as a nasal cannula or manually ventilating the patient with a BVM and 100% O_2.
- Immediately notify the HCP and RT.
- Assess for respiratory distress.
- Assess the need for reintubation.
- If the patient cannot protect their airway or is in respiratory distress, prepare for immediate reintubation.
- Provide emotional support and reassure the patient.

Weaning From Positive Pressure Ventilation

Weaning is the process of gradually reducing ventilator support and allowing the patient to assume greater responsibility for breathing spontaneously. The weaning process typically differs for patients on short-term ventilation (3 to 5 days) versus long-term ventilation (longer than 2 weeks). Those with short-term ventilation (e.g., after heart surgery) usually have a very straightforward weaning process. Patients with prolonged PPV (e.g., patients with COPD who develop respiratory failure, patients with ARDS) often have difficult and lengthy weaning processes that consist of alternating gains and losses. Preparation for weaning begins almost as soon as the patient is intubated and involves a team approach.

Weaning is a complex process. It consists of an assessment of both respiratory and nonrespiratory factors (Table 28.15). First, the primary problem that prompted intubation and mechanical ventilation should be resolving. Second, the lungs should be reasonably clear on auscultation and chest x-ray. Third, the patient needs to be able to breathe spontaneously. The patient who transitions from full support to a spontaneous mode of mechanical ventilation, is hemodynamically stable, and has acceptable ABGs and SpO_2 shows tolerance of the weaning process.

TABLE 28.15 Indicators of Weaning Readiness

Patients receiving mechanical ventilation should have a formal assessment of "readiness for weaning" every 24 hours, if the following are satisfied:

1. Awake, alert, easily rousable
2. Reversal of the underlying cause of respiratory failure
3. Hemodynamically stable:
   - Absence of dysrhythmias, myocardial ischemia
   - Absence of clinical hypotension (low-dose or no vasopressor therapy)
4. Adequate oxygenation
   - $PaO_2/FiO_2 >300$
   - $SpO_2 \geq 92\%$
   - PEEP ≤ 5 to 8 cm H_2O
   - $FiO_2 \leq 40\%$
   - pH ≥ 7.35
5. Stable, intact respiratory drive with ability to initiate spontaneous respirations
6. Other weaning criteria:
   - Hemoglobin ≥ 7 g/dL
   - Temperature $\leq 101.3°F$ (38.5°C)

Nonrespiratory factors include neurologic status, hemodynamic stability, acid-base balance, nutrition status, fluid and electrolyte balance, and hemoglobin. It is important to have an alert, well-rested, and well-informed patient relatively free from pain and anxiety who can cooperate with the weaning plan. This does not mean complete withdrawal from sedatives or analgesics. Instead, drugs should be titrated to achieve comfort without causing excessive drowsiness.

An SAT and SBT help assess the ability of the patient to maintain a stable respiratory drive and adequate O_2 saturation. Unless contraindicated, all patients should have an SAT daily. An SAT should be done by stopping all sedatives and, in patients without active pain, all opioids. Sedation should be restarted at 50% of the previous dose in patients who "fail" the SAT (increased respiratory rate, decreasing O_2 saturations, low V_T) and remain off in patients who "pass." An SBT should occur after a successful SAT and last at least 30 minutes but no more than 120 minutes. It may be completed with low levels of FiO_2, PEEP, or low levels of PS.[34] Tolerating the SBT may lead to extubation. Failure to tolerate an SBT should prompt a search for reversible or complicating factors and a return to the previous mode of mechanical ventilation.

There is no "right" way to wean a patient from mechanical ventilation. Most HCPs will attempt weaning early in the morning after the patient had a good night's rest. The patient should be hemodynamically stable and comfortable. Obtain baseline vital signs and respiratory parameters. Place the patient in bed in a semirecumbent position or sitting in a chair at the bedside.

All health care team members should be familiar with the weaning plan. Weaning approaches include decreasing the number of ventilator-delivered breaths in SIMV. Or we gradually decrease the degree of pressure support daily as ventilatory status permits. PS provides gentle, slow respiratory muscle conditioning. It may be beneficial for patients who are deconditioned or have heart problems.

During the weaning trial, closely monitor the patient for signs and symptoms that may signal a need to end the trial. These include tachypnea, dyspnea, tachycardia, dysrhythmias, sustained desaturation (SpO_2 less than 92%), hypertension or hypotension, agitation, diaphoresis, anxiety, and changes in mental status. Should the patient not tolerate the weaning trial, allow the patient's respiratory muscles to rest between trials. Once the respiratory muscles become fatigued, they may need 12 to 24 hours to recover.

The patient and caregiver need ongoing emotional support. Explain the weaning process to the patient and family to keep them informed of progress and record the patient's tolerance throughout.

Extubation

Extubation is the physical removal of the oral or nasal ET tube. Extubation assessments should include muscle strength (negative inspiratory force) and endurance (spontaneous V_T, vital capacity, minute ventilation, rapid shallow breathing index) (Table 28.16). There should be minimal secretions and the ability to cough and gag.

Before extubation, hyperoxygenate and suction the patient. Have an alternative O_2 delivery device (e.g., nasal prongs) set up. Loosen the ET tapes or commercial holder. Have the patient take a deep breath, and at the peak of inspiration, deflate the ET tube cuff and remove the tube in one smooth motion.

After removal, encourage the patient to take a few slow breaths and cough. Suction the oropharynx as needed. Assess their ability to speak. Give O_2 and provide oral care. Carefully

TABLE 28.16 Diagnostic Criteria

Extubation

Measurement	What It Means	Normal Value	Criteria to Consider Extubation
Spontaneous respiratory rate (RR)	Respiratory rate (number of breaths) over 1 min	12–20 breaths/min	Respiratory rate more than 8–10 breaths/min but less than 30 breaths/min
Spontaneous tidal volume (V_T)	Amount of air moved in and out of the lungs during a single breath (at rest)	>5–7 mL/kg	≥5 mL/kg
Minute ventilation (V_E)	Volume of air moved in and out of the lungs during 1 min (at rest) V_T multiplied by respiratory rate over 1 min *For example:* 0.350 (V_T) × 28 (f) = 9.8 L/min.	3–10 L/min	Between 3 and 15 L/min
Negative inspiratory force or pressure (NIF, NIP)	Amount of negative pressure that a patient can generate Measure of expiratory muscle strength and ability to cough *Measured by clinician:* A pressure manometer (nifometer) is attached to airway or mouth and the patient is asked to take a big deep breath. Clinician observes the values on the nifometer	< −20 to −30 cm H_2O	> −20 cm H_2O The more negative the number, the better indication for extubation
Rapid shallow breathing index, RSBI (f/V_T)	Tobin number Spontaneous respiratory rate (over 1 min) divided by V_T (in liters) *For example:* 30 (f)/0.400 (V_T) = 75	<105	<105
Spontaneous breathing trial (SBT)	If patient passes spontaneous awakening trial (SAT), assess patient during SBT SBT provides little or no ventilator assistance Trial should be at least 30 min to a maximum of 120 min		Successful completion of SBT is based on assessment (e.g., level of consciousness; vital signs; ABG; chest x-ray; intact, stable respiratory drive; stable SpO_2)

monitor vital signs, respiratory status, and oxygenation after extubation and for the first 2 to 3 hours (per agency policy). If the patient does not tolerate extubation (e.g., decreased SpO_2 levels, tachypnea or bradypnea, tachycardia, decreased LOC, decrease in PaO_2, increase in $PaCO_2$), options may include immediate reintubation or a trial of noninvasive ventilation (e.g., bi-PAP).

TRACHEOSTOMY

A tracheostomy is a surgically created stoma (opening) in the anterior part of the trachea (Fig. 28.15A). A tracheostomy may be done to (1) establish a patent airway, (2) bypass an upper airway obstruction, (3) permit long-term mechanical ventilation, and (4) facilitate weaning. When the need for an artificial airway is expected to be prolonged, early tracheotomy (done within 10 to 14 days) appears to have advantages over delayed tracheotomy. These include fewer ventilator-dependent days, reduced length of stay, decreased pain, and improved communication.

The tracheostomy tube is shorter in length and slightly wider in diameter than an ET tube. This makes it easier to keep the tube clean and promotes better oral and bronchial hygiene. A tracheostomy may increase patient comfort because no tube is present in the mouth. There is less risk of long-term damage to vocal cords.

A variety of tracheostomy tubes are available (Table 28.17). They all have a faceplate, or flange, which rests against the neck and an *obturator.* An obturator is used to help insert the tube. Many tracheostomy tubes have an *outer cannula* (which keeps the airway patent) and an *inner cannula.* Inner cannulas can be disposable or nondisposable and removed for cleaning (Fig. 28.15B).

Cuffed and *uncuffed* tracheostomy tubes are available. A tube with an inflated cuff is used the most, especially if the patient needs mechanical ventilation. The cuff is inflated through the balloon inflation port. Cuffs ensure the patient receives the volume of air delivered by the ventilator and decrease the risk of aspiration. Cuffless tubes are often used for patients with long-term tracheostomies or when mechanical ventilation is not needed. With some tracheostomies, talking and eating are possible.

The outer and/or inner cannula may be *fenestrated* or *nonfenestrated.* A *fenestrated tube* has an opening (a hole) on the dorsal surface of the tube. This helps promote spontaneous breathing. With a cuffed, fenestrated tube, when the cuff is deflated and the inner cannula removed, air can pass from the lungs up through the opening in the tracheostomy tube and through the vocal cords (including the larynx) and into the upper airway (including the mouth and nose). This allows the

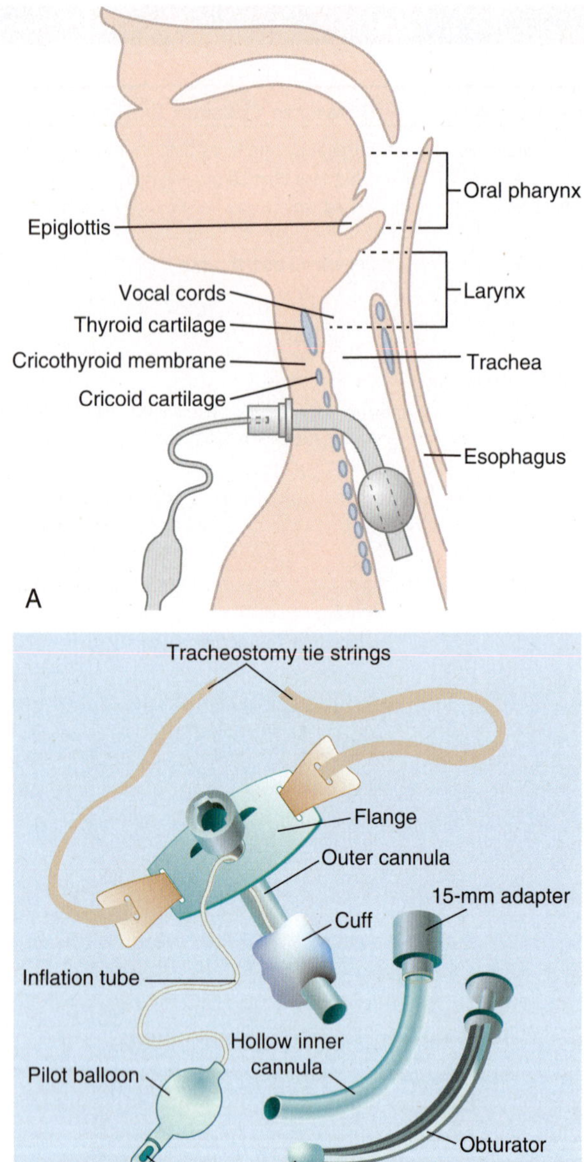

Fig. 28.15 Tracheostomy tube. (A) Placement of a tracheostomy tube. (B) Parts of a tracheostomy tube.

patient to breathe spontaneously and speak with the tube in place. When the inner cannula is reinserted and the cuff reinflated, air cannot pass from the lungs through the vocal cords.

Most patients who need mechanical ventilation have an oral ET tube first. When swelling, trauma, or upper airway obstruction prevents oral ET intubation, an emergent *surgical cricothyroidotomy* (or cricothyrotomy) is needed. This procedure, which can be completed in minutes, involves making an incision through the skin and cricothyroid membrane on the anterior surface of the neck.

Most surgical tracheostomies are done in the operating room using general anesthesia. They may be done electively on intubated patients who need prolonged mechanical ventilation. A horizontal incision is made on the anterior part of the trachea. The tracheostomy tube is inserted, the incision is sutured, and a sterile dressing is applied.

An alternative surgical technique is the *percutaneous tracheostomy*. Using local anesthesia and sedation and under video-assisted guidance, the ET tube is withdrawn up to the level of the glottis. A needle is placed between the second and third tracheal rings, into the middle of the trachea. A dilator is then placed over the top of the needle. The opening is progressively made larger (with increasingly larger dilators) until the hole is big enough for insertion of the tracheostomy tube. Percutaneous tracheostomy approaches have less risk of bleeding and fewer postoperative complications. Surgical and percutaneous tracheostomies may be done in the emergency department or at the bedside in the ICU.

Preparing the Patient for a Tracheostomy

Preprocedure Care

Before the tracheostomy procedure (and time permitting), explain the purpose of the procedure to both the patient and caregiver. If the patient is having the tracheostomy in the operating room, follow all policies for preparing the patient for surgery (see Chapter 18).

If the procedure is being done at the bedside, ensure appropriate personnel, including RTs, are notified and present. Have a BVM, suction, and emergency resuscitation equipment available. Record baseline vital signs. Ensure IV access. Help assemble and set up all the equipment. Position the patient supine. Give analgesia and sedation as ordered by the HCP.

During the Procedure

Monitor hemodynamic status. Observe the patient's response to analgesia and/or sedatives. Note the patient's tolerance to the procedure. Observe the SpO_2. Notify the HCP if the SpO_2 is less than 92%.

Postprocedure Care

The tracheostomy cuff is inflated immediately. We use several methods to confirm correct tracheostomy tube placement: (1) auscultation of the patient's chest for air entry, (2) $EtCO_2$ capnography, (3) video-assisted confirmation for percutaneous tracheostomy, and (4) passage of a suction catheter through the tracheostomy tube. After placement is confirmed, the ET tube is removed. The tracheostomy tube is sutured and secured in place with cotton tracheostomy ties, tracheostomy tapes, or Velcro straps.

Monitor vital signs. SpO_2 readings should remain stable. Obtain a chest x-ray. Note and record the ventilator settings, including mode, FiO_2, and PEEP. Complications of a tracheostomy include airway obstruction, bleeding, infection, and potential tube dislodgment (Table 28.18). Observe the amount of blood on the dressing at the insertion site. Notify the HCP if bleeding persists.

TABLE 28.17 NURSING MANAGEMENT

Specific Types of Tracheostomies

Tube and Characteristics	Nursing Management
Tracheostomy tube with cuff and pilot balloon When properly inflated, low-pressure, high-volume cuff distributes cuff pressure over large area, minimizing pressure on tracheal wall.	**Procedure for cuff inflation:** • *Mechanically ventilated patient:* Minimal occlusion volume (MOV) technique recommended. Place stethoscope over lateral neck (beside trachea). Inflate cuff by slowly injecting air into the cuff until no leak (sound) is heard at peak inspiratory pressure (end of ventilator inspiration). • *Spontaneously breathing patient:* Inflate cuff by slowly injecting air into the cuff until no sound is heard after deep breath or during inhalation with bag-valve-mask. • *Immediately after cuff inflation:* Confirm pressure is within accepted range 20 to 30 cm H_2O (15 to 22 mm Hg) with a manometer. Record cuff pressure and volume of air used for cuff inflation. **Care of patient with an inflated cuff:** • Monitor and record cuff pressure q8h and PRN. Cuff pressure should be 20 to 30 cm H_2O (15 to 22 mm Hg) to allow adequate tracheal capillary perfusion. If needed, remove or add air to the pilot tubing using a syringe. Afterward, confirm cuff pressure is within accepted range with manometer. • Report inability to keep the cuff inflated or need to use progressively larger volumes of air to keep cuff inflated. Potential causes include tracheal dilation at the cuff site or a crack or slow leak in the 1-way inflation valve.
Fenestrated tracheostomy tube (Shiley, Portex) with cuff, inner cannula, and decannulation plug When nonfenestrated inner cannula is removed, cuff is deflated, and decannulation plug inserted, air flows around tube, through fenestration in outer cannula, and up over vocal cords. Patient can then speak. A fenestrated inner cannula can be used to facilitate weaning from mechanical ventilation.	• If possible, assess risk of aspiration before removing inner cannula. A speech pathologist may be able to assist (if available). Deflate cuff. Note coughing. • Never insert decannulation plug in tracheostomy tube until cuff is deflated and nonfenestrated inner cannula removed. Otherwise, patient will not be able to breathe. This will precipitate a respiratory arrest. • Assess for dyspnea and/or respiratory distress when a fenestrated cannula is first used. If this occurs, remove the cap, insert a nonfenestrated inner cannula, reinflate the cuff, and notify the HCP. • A nonfenestrated inner cannula must be used to suction the patient to prevent tracheal damage from the suction catheter passing through fenestrated openings. • Cuff management (as described earlier).
Talking tracheostomy tube (Portex with cuff, 2 external tubings) Has 2 tubes: 1 tube leads to cuff and 1 tube goes to opening above the cuff. When port is connected to air source, air flows out of opening and up over the vocal cords, allowing the patient to speak.	• Patient must be awake, alert, and hemodynamically stable. • Must be able to tolerate cuff deflation. Can exhale around the tracheostomy tube. • When patient wants to speak, deflate cuff and connect port to compressed air (or O_2). Be certain to identify correct tubing. If gas enters the cuff, it will overinflate and rupture, requiring an emergency tube change. • Use lowest flow (typically 4–6 L/min) that results in speech. Patient may not tolerate high flows. • Give O_2 through tracheal collar or adaptor on speaking valve. • Observe for dyspnea and/or respiratory distress. • Cuff management (as described earlier).
Tracheostomy tube (Bivona, Fome-Cuf) with foam-filled cuff Cuff filled with plastic foam. Before insertion, cuff is deflated. After insertion, cuff self-inflates. Pilot tubing not capped. No cuff pressure monitoring needed. Patient cannot speak with this tube.	• Before insertion, withdraw all air from the cuff using a 20-mL syringe. Cap pilot balloon tubing to prevent reentry of air. • After tracheostomy is inserted, remove cap from pilot tubing, allowing cuff to passively reinflate. Cuff is always inflated on this tube. • Do not inject air into tubing or cap pilot balloon tubing while it is in patient. Air will flow in and out in response to pressure changes (head turning). Place tag on tubing to alert staff not to cap or inflate cuff. • Tube tends to collect moisture and secretions while patient is on the ventilator. • Deflate cuff daily to assess integrity of cuff. Assess ease with which cuff deflates. Difficulty deflating cuff indicates a need for tube change. If aspirate returns with air, cuff is no longer intact. • Tube can be used for up to 1 month in patients on home mechanical ventilation. • Good choice for patients who need inflated cuff at home because teaching about cuff pressure is simplified.

TABLE 28.18 Complications of Tracheostomy

Closely monitor patients with a tracheostomy for the following potential complications:

- Air leak
- Airway obstruction
- Altered body image
- Aspiration
- Bleeding
- Fistula formation
- Impaired cough
- Infection
- Subcutaneous emphysema
- Tracheal necrosis
- Tracheal stenosis
- Tube displacement

NURSING MANAGEMENT: PATIENT WITH A TRACHEOSTOMY

Acute Care

This section highlights general guidelines when caring for patients with a tracheostomy (Table 28.19). Suctioning and tracheostomy care are complex activities. Considerable variation exists regarding which health care team member is responsible for patient care tasks. In some places, it is the nurse who is responsible. In others, it is a shared responsibility between nursing and RT. Follow your agency policy. Collaborate with the RT, who will play a key role in the patient's care.

Much of the management of patients receiving mechanical ventilation through a tracheostomy is the same as that of patients with an ET tube. At a minimum, you must assess the tracheostomy site and confirm patency of the tracheostomy tube every shift, or more often based on your assessment. Observe the site for any redness, inflammation, edema, ulceration, or signs of infection. Perform sterile dressing changes every 12 to 24 hours. Have another person to help you with tracheostomy care. Clean around the stoma with normal saline, and apply a sterile precut dressing around the tracheostomy tube site. You can complete dressing changes more often if needed. Care of the stoma and cannula for patients with a tracheostomy is described in Table 28.20.

Because an inflated tracheostomy cuff exerts pressure on the tracheal mucosa, inflate the cuff with the least amount of air needed to obtain an airway seal. Measure cuff inflation pressure with a cuff manometer at least every 8 hours. Cuff inflation pressure should not exceed 20 to 30 cm H_2O (15 to 22 mm Hg). Higher pressures may compress tracheal capillaries, limit blood flow, and predispose patients to tracheal necrosis. The minimal occlusion volume (MOV) is one technique used to inflate the tracheostomy cuff (Table 28.17).

Suction the tracheostomy tube as needed. Try to avoid suctioning through the newly created tracheostomy in the first few hours after the procedure. This may worsen discomfort and promote bleeding. Suctioning may be done using sterile glove and catheter technique or an existing in-line suction catheter (Fig. 28.16). Each time you suction the patient, observe the amount, color, and clarity of secretions. Note patient tolerance.

TABLE 28.19 NURSING MANAGEMENT

Caring for the Patient With a Tracheostomy

Nursing management of the patient with a tracheostomy includes most of the care provided to the patient who is intubated and mechanically ventilated with an oral ET tube.

- Assess tracheostomy site at least once per shift for any signs of inflammation, infection, or skin breakdown.
- Suction the tracheostomy as needed.
- Provide tracheostomy care as per agency guidelines.
- Maintain cuff inflation pressure at 20 to 30 cm H_2O (15–22 mm Hg).
- Teach patient and caregiver about tracheostomy care.

Collaborate With the Respiratory Therapist

- Measure tracheal cuff pressures.
- Maintain cuff inflation pressure at 20 to 30 cm H_2O (15–22 mm Hg).
- Provide tracheostomy care per agency guidelines.
- Ensure equipment is available for suctioning and tracheotomy care.
- Replace the tracheostomy tube or ventilate the patient with a BVM device if accidental dislodgment occurs.
- Assist with decannulation.

Supervise the LPN/VN

- Determine the need for suctioning.
- Suction the tracheostomy.
- Assess patient status after suctioning.
- Provide tracheostomy care using sterile technique.
- Notify the RN of any changes in respiratory status.

Collaborate With the Dietitian

- Assess risk for aspiration.
- Recommend a diet to promote nutrition and decrease aspiration risk.

Collaborate With Physical and Occupational Therapy

- Develop a plan for active range of motion and early mobility.
- Help facilitate any adaptation for patients going home with a tracheostomy.

Collaborate With Speech Language Pathology

- Assess swallowing ability and risk for aspiration.
- Develop plan to avoid aspiration.

BVM, Bag-valve-mask; *ET*, endotracheal.

At first, patients should receive humidified air to compensate for the loss of the upper airway to warm and moisturize secretions. Humidification helps keep secretions thin, decreases formation of mucus plugs, and promotes comfort.

If the inner cannula is disposable, replace per manufacturer and agency guidelines. If nondisposable, clean the inner cannula at least every shift. Cleaning removes mucus from the inside of the tube to prevent airway obstruction.

Change the tracheostomy tapes after the first 24 hours and then as needed (Fig. 28.17). Using a 2-person technique, 1 person stabilizes the tracheostomy while the other person changes the tapes. During the procedure, apply gentle pressure to the flange. Tie the tracheostomy tapes (or Velcro straps) securely

TABLE 28.20 NURSING MANAGEMENT

Stoma and Cannula Care for a Tracheostomy

The following are general guidelines for basic tracheostomy care. Follow the specific policies or procedures in your agency. Clean technique is used for the patient with a tracheostomy at home.

Before You Begin

1. Explain procedure to patient.
2. Use tracheostomy care kit or collect sterile equipment (e.g., suction catheter, 1 pair sterile gloves, 1 pair nonsterile gloves, water basin, tracheostomy ties, tube brush or pipe cleaners, 4 × 4-inch gauze pads, sterile water or normal saline, tracheostomy dressing [optional]).
3. Position patient in semi-Fowler position.
4. Assemble supplies on bedside table.
5. Wash hands. Put on PPE.

Providing Tracheostomy Care

6. Open sterile equipment. Pour sterile H_2O or normal saline into 2 compartments of sterile container or 2 basins, then apply sterile gloves.
7. If present, unlock and remove inner cannula.

NOTE: Some tracheostomy tubes do not have inner cannulas. Care for these tubes includes all steps listed next, except for inner cannula care.

8. Inner cannula care
   - Disposable: If using a disposable inner cannula, replace with new cannula.
   - Nondisposable:
     - Immerse inner cannula in sterile solution and clean inside and outside of cannula using tube brush or pipe cleaners.
     - Rinse cannula in sterile solution. Remove from solution and dry. Insert inner cannula into outer cannula with the curved part downward, and lock in place.
9. Stoma care:
   - Remove dried secretions from stoma using 4 × 4-inch gauze pad soaked in sterile water or saline. Gently pat area around the stoma dry. Be sure to clean under the tracheostomy flange (face plate), using cotton swabs to reach this area.

PPE, Personal protective equipment.

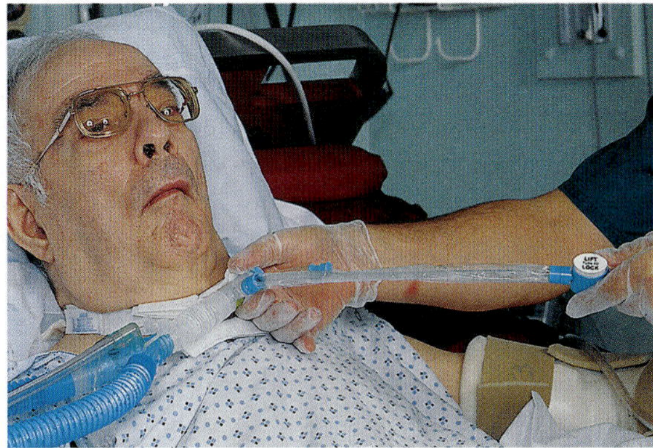

Fig. 28.16 Suctioning a tracheostomy tube with a closed system suction catheter. (From Potter PA, Perry AG: *Basic nursing: essentials for practice,* ed 7, St. Louis, 2011, Mosby.)

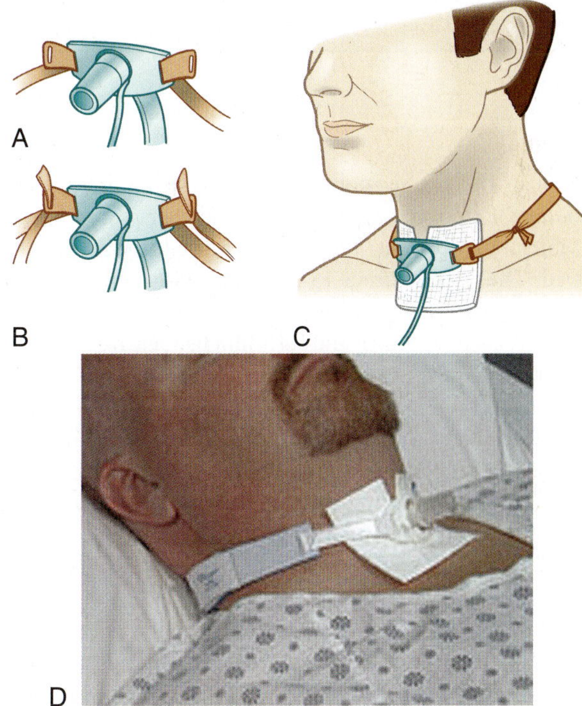

Fig. 28.17 Changing tracheostomy ties. (A) Cut a small slit about 1 inch (2.5 cm) from the end of the tie. Put the slit end into the opening of the flange. (B) Make a loop with the other end of the tape. (C) Tie the tapes together with a double knot on the side of the neck. (D) A Velcro tracheostomy tube holder. (D, Courtesy Dale Medical Products, Franklin, MA.)

with room for 2 fingers between the tapes and the skin. These steps are considered best practice to ensure that the tracheostomy does not become accidentally dislodged during the procedure. In some centers, the HCP or RT may complete this task.

When turning and repositioning the patient, take care not to dislodge the tracheostomy tube. Because the tube may be difficult to reinsert in the immediate postoperative period, several precautions are needed. Keep a replacement tube of equal or smaller size at or near the bedside, readily available for emergency reinsertion. Do not change tracheostomy tapes for at least 24 hours afterward. The HCP often performs the first tube change. This usually happens no sooner than 7 days after the tracheotomy.

Accidental Decannulation

If the tracheostomy tube is accidentally dislodged, call for help. While waiting for the HCP or RT to arrive, you have several options. These depend on agency policy.

Quickly assess the patient's LOC, their ability to breathe, and the presence of any respiratory distress. If respiratory distress is present and it is within your scope of practice, one option is to quickly use a hemostat to spread the opening where the tube was. Insert the obturator in the replacement tube, lubricate with saline, and insert the tube into the stoma. Once the tube is inserted, remove the obturator at once so that air can flow through the tube. Another option is to insert a suction catheter to allow air passage and serve as a guide for insertion. Thread the tracheostomy tube over the catheter and remove the catheter. Trying to reinsert is easier if the stoma tract is mature or more than 1 week old.

If the tube cannot be replaced because of tract immaturity (less than 1 week old) or other circumstances, place the patient in the semi-Fowler position to decrease dyspnea. Cover the stoma with a sterile dressing and ventilate the patient with the BVM over the nose and mouth. If a patient has had a total laryngectomy, there will be complete separation between the upper airway and trachea. Ventilate this patient through the tracheostomy stoma. Loss of the artificial airway can lead to severe dyspnea and hypoxemia, which may quickly progress to respiratory and cardiac arrest.

CHECK YOUR PRACTICE

You are caring for a patient who had a surgically created tracheostomy 6 hours ago. While suctioning the patient, he coughs, dislodging the tracheostomy tube.

- What should you do?

Decannulation

Removal of the tracheostomy from the trachea is called *decannulation*. Removal is possible when the primary condition for which the patient received a tracheostomy has been resolved. The patient needs to (1) be hemodynamically stable, (2) have a stable, intact respiratory drive, (3) be able to adequately exchange air, and (4) independently expectorate secretions.

Explain to the patient what will occur. Monitor vital signs. Suction the patient through the tracheostomy. Clear the mouth of any oral secretions. Loosen and/or cut the tracheostomy ties. Remove any visible sutures holding the tracheostomy in place. Deflate the tracheostomy cuff. Pull the tracheostomy tube outward in one smooth motion. Stop if you meet any resistance and notify the HCP.

After removing the tube, apply a sterile occlusive dressing. Monitor for bleeding. Change the dressing if it gets soiled or wet. If needed, close the stoma with tape strips. Apply an alternative method of O_2 delivery (e.g., nasal prongs) if needed. Monitor respiratory status and O_2 saturation for airway compromise or difficulty breathing. Teach the patient to splint the stoma with the fingers when coughing, swallowing, or speaking. Epithelial tissue begins to form in 24 to 48 hours, and the opening closes within 4 or 5 days. Surgery to close the tracheostomy is usually not needed.

Chronic Care

Some patients have a tracheostomy for life. Care of patients with a long-term tracheostomy includes all the same care as patients with a new tracheostomy. This includes observing the tracheostomy site, cleaning the inner cannula, suctioning, and changing tracheostomy tapes.

The tracheostomy tube should be changed around 1 month after the first tube change and every 1 to 3 months thereafter. When a tracheostomy has been in place for several months, the healed tract should be well formed. Changing the tracheostomy tube is important, as it permits assessment of the stoma and cleaning of the tube. Teach patients the signs and symptoms of infection and how to change the tube at home using a clean technique. Engaging patients to take part in their care helps decrease complications and infection and promotes their feeling of well-being.

Swallowing Problems

An inflated tracheostomy tube cuff may result in swallowing problems by interfering with the normal function of muscles used to swallow. We need to evaluate the patient's swallowing ability and risk for aspiration.

A speech language therapist (SLT) should assess the patient's ability to swallow. To assess for aspiration, the patient receives thickened fluids of different consistencies. If the patient can swallow without aspiration when the cuff is deflated, the cuff may be left deflated, or a cuffless tube may be inserted. At this time, patients may be prescribed varying levels of thickened fluids and soft foods.

Speech With a Tracheostomy Tube

The spontaneously breathing patient may be able to talk with a tracheostomy. Several options are available depending on the type of tracheostomy (Fig. 28.18). For example, if the patient is at low risk of aspiration, (1) remove the inner cannula (if nonfenestrated), (2) deflate the cuff, and (3) place the cap on the tube. When the tracheostomy cuff is deflated, exhaled air can flow upward over the vocal cords and the patient can talk. When a fenestrated cannula is first used, frequently assess the patient for respiratory distress. If the patient cannot tolerate the procedure, remove the cap, insert the nonfenestrated cannula, and reinflate the cuff. Monitor for improvement in patient condition.

The Passy-Muir valve is a simple device that attaches to the hub of the tracheostomy tube (Fig. 28.19). With the cuff deflated, the valve redirects air flow through the vocal cords. On inspiration, the valve on the device opens, allowing the patient to inhale. When the patient exhales, the valve closes and air flows upward around the tracheostomy and through the vocal cords. The patient exhales through the nose and mouth instead of through the tracheostomy, allowing speech. At first, the patient may only tolerate short periods of use until they are used to exhaling through the mouth. Remove the valve if there are any signs of respiratory distress. Speaking devices may help improve self-care and increase self-esteem for the patient with a long-term tracheostomy.

Mechanical Ventilation in the Home

Sometimes, chronically ill ventilated patients who meet specific criteria (e.g., tracheostomy, stabile ventilator settings) are

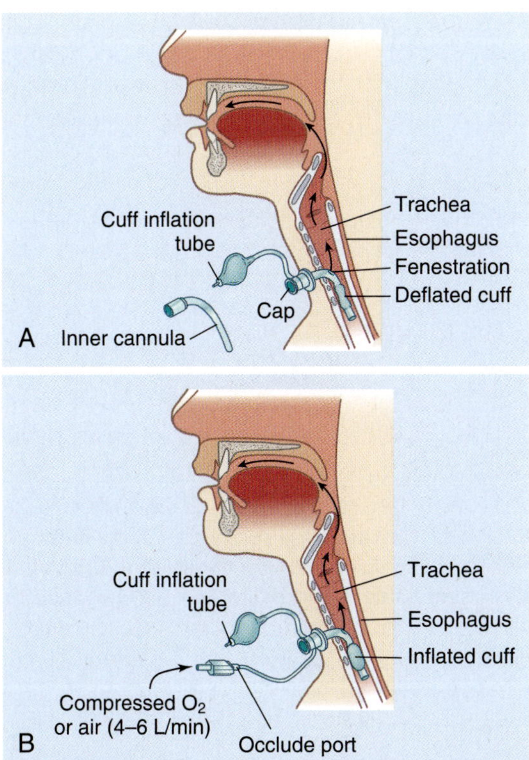

Fig. 28.18 Tracheostomy tubes. (A) Fenestrated tracheostomy tube with cuff deflated, inner cannula removed, and tracheostomy tube capped to allow air to pass over the vocal cords. (B) Speaking tracheostomy tube. One tube is used for cuff inflation. The second tube is connected to a source of compressed air or O_2. When the port on the second tube is occluded, air flows up over the vocal cords, allowing speech with an inflated cuff.

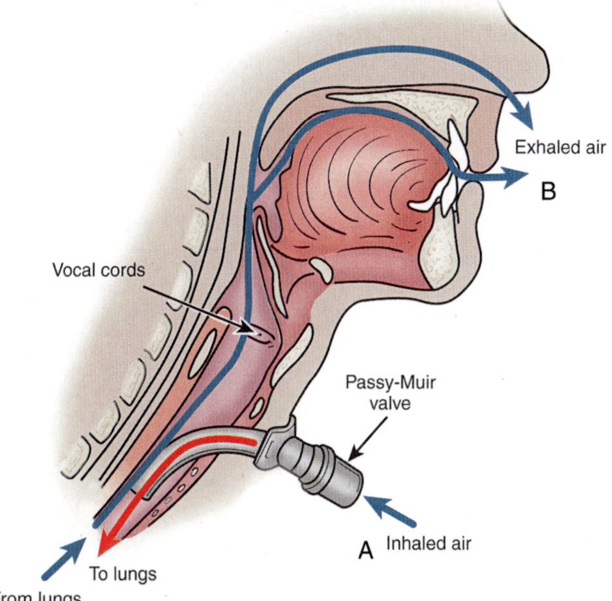

Fig. 28.19 The Passy-Muir valve. The valve attaches to an adaptor. (A) The adaptor allows inspiration through the valve. (B) Expiration must occur through the upper airway to allow speech. (From Hodder RV: A 55-year-old patient with advanced COPD, tracheostomy tube, and sudden respiratory distress, *Chest* 121[1]:279, 2002.)

discharged home. The success of home mechanical ventilation depends, in part, on careful predischarge assessment and planning for the patient and caregivers.

Several types of small, portable, battery-powered positive pressure ventilators are available. They can be attached to a wheelchair or placed on a bedside table. Settings and alarms on these ventilators are simpler to use than standard ventilators.

Home mechanical ventilation has advantages and disadvantages. Having the patient in the home eliminates the strain that the hospital setting imposes on family dynamics. Caregivers may experience many feelings when they first hear about the need for long-term mechanical ventilation. These feelings are often balanced by the chance to care for the patient. At home, the patient may be more mobile and able to take part in more activities of daily living on a personalized schedule.

Disadvantages include problems related to equipment, reimbursement, and caregiver stress and fatigue. Ventilated patients are often dependent and require extensive nursing care, at least at first. Disposable products may not be reimbursable.

Carefully assess financial resources when arranging home ventilation. Social worker involvement may be necessary. Hold a care conference before starting a discharge teaching plan. Caregivers may seem enthusiastic about providing care but may not understand the sacrifices they may have to make financially and in personal time and commitment. Encourage caregivers to consider respite care to periodically relieve their stress and fatigue.

CASE STUDY

Mechanical Ventilation

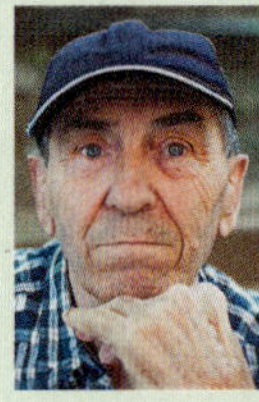

(© Thinkstock.)

Patient Profile

R.K. is a 72-year-old male who collapsed in his home. He was found by the police during a wellness check when his nephew became concerned that he had not heard from him for 3 days. Police activated the emergency response system. On arrival of the paramedics, he was semi-alert, was breathing at 32 breaths/min, had vomited, and was incontinent of a large amount of foul-smelling urine. He was placed on O_2 at 15 L/min with nonbreather mask. A #16G IV was placed in his right lower arm. On admission to the emergency department, R.K. had weak, nonpurposeful movement of all 4 limbs. Vital signs became unstable, with BP 84/49, HR 142, and SpO_2 84%. Assessment revealed no spontaneous respiratory effort, so he was intubated. He received a 500-mL IV fluid bolus. A chest x-ray and ABG were done. An indwelling urinary catheter and OG tube were inserted. R.K. was admitted to the ICU.

Objective Data

Physical Assessment

- Weight: 168 lb (76 kg)
- GCS: 7 (motor: 5; verbal: not scored [patient intubated]; eyes: 2)
- Temperature 102°F (39.3°C); HR 128; BP 85/64 mm Hg (cuff); SpO_2 94%
- ECG: Atrial fibrillation with a rapid ventricular response
- Breath sounds: coarse crackles bilaterally, decreased breath sounds to the right middle and both lower lobes
- Thick, purulent secretions suctioned from ET tube
- Appears dehydrated (dry mucous membranes, cracked lips)

Diagnostic Studies

- Chest x-ray shows right middle and bilateral lower lung lobe consolidation
- ABGs: pH 7.27; Pao_2 75 mm Hg; $Paco_2$ 54 mm Hg; HCO_3 25 mEq/L

Interprofessional Care

- Full support positive pressure ventilation: AC. Settings: Fio_2 100%, V_T 475 mL, respiratory rate 16 breaths/min (no spontaneous respiratory effort), PEEP 5 cm H_2O
- IV 0.9% normal saline at 75mL/h
- EN at 25 mL/h, increase by 20 mL/h every 4 h with a goal of 75 mL/h
- 12 lead ECG in a.m.
- Daily chest x-ray for next 3 days
- Chest physiotherapy and mobilize tomorrow
- Urine for culture and sensitivity
- Drug therapy:
  - Famotidine 10 mg IV q12h
  - Enoxaparin 40 mg subcutaneous daily
  - Ceftriaxone g IV q24h
  - Azithromycin 500 mg IV q24h
  - Fentanyl 50 mcg IV q1h PRN

Discussion Questions

1. ***Recognize:*** Why do you think R.K. collapsed?
2. ***Analyze:*** From a respiratory perspective, what findings from the physical assessment and diagnostic studies concern you most? Which assessment finding needs to be addressed first?
3. ***Plan:*** Identify 2 reasons for intubating and providing mechanical ventilation for R.K.
4. ***Act:*** Based on R.K.'s ABGs, should any ventilator settings be changed? If so, what changes would you suggest?
5. ***Plan:*** R.K.'s condition deteriorates. Pao_2 drops to 58 mm Hg, and SpO_2 is 85%. What can be done to help improve oxygenation?
6. ***Act:*** R.K.'s caregivers want to know why he is receiving tube feedings. What would you tell them? What evidence exists to support the use of EN in intubated patients?
7. ***Safety:*** What safety precautions would be implemented for R.K. while he is a patient in the adult ICU?
8. ***Evaluate:*** What implications would increasing PEEP have for R.K.'s hemodynamic status?

Answers available at http://evolve.elsevier.com/Lewis/medsurg.

BRIDGE TO NCLEX EXAMINATION

The number of the question corresponds to the same-numbered outcome at the beginning of the chapter.

1. Which technique would be most appropriate for a patient with mild COPD to promote airway clearance?
   a. Huff coughing
   b. Postural drainage
   c. Pursed-lip breathing
   d. High-frequency chest wall oscillation

2. The major advantage of a Venturi mask is that it can
   a. deliver up to 80% O_2.
   b. provide continuous 100% humidity.
   c. deliver a precise concentration of O_2.
   d. be used while a patient eats and sleeps.

3. In a spontaneously breathing patient, the nurse notes tidaling of the water level in the water-seal chamber of the chest tube drainage system. The nurse would
   a. continue to monitor the patient.
   b. check all connections for a leak in the system.
   c. raise the collection unit above the level of the heart.
   d. clamp the tubing at a distal point away from the patient.

4. A nursing action to provide a patient after a left lower lobe lobectomy is to
   a. position the patient prone every 2 hours.
   b. monitor the chest tube drainage and functioning.
   c. auscultate lung sounds frequently in the lower left lobe.
   d. administer IV fluid boluses to maintain blood pressure.

5. Which assessment finding concerns you *most* in a patient with pneumonia who is receiving noninvasive ventilation (bi-PAP)?
   a. New onset of confusion to time and place
   b. Fine crackles on auscultation of affected lobe
   c. Patient asks to remove the mask for oral care
   d. HR: 98, RR: 16 bpm, BP: 110/60, SpO_2: 93%
6. A patient with multiple gunshot wounds returns to the ICU from surgery. Vital signs are stable. They are making no spontaneous respiratory effort. Which mode of ventilation would be most appropriate?
   a. Assist control (AC)
   b. Pressure support (PS)
   c. Bilevel positive airway pressure (bi-PAP)
   d. Synchronized intermittent mandatory ventilation (SIMV)
7. Nursing care of a patient with an oral ET tube would include
   a. maintaining ET tube cuff pressure at 35 to 40 cm H_2O.
   b. routine suctioning of the ET tube at least every 2 hours.
   c. observing the patient for spontaneous respiratory effort and work of breathing.
   d. preventing ET tube dislodgment by limiting mouth care to lubrication of the lips.
8. Which nursing action would be the *highest priority* when suctioning a patient with an oral ET tube or tracheostomy?
   a. Hyperoxygenate with 100% Fio_2 before suctioning.
   b. Auscultate lung sounds after suctioning is completed.
   c. Instill 5 mL of normal saline into the tube before suctioning.
   d. Give antianxiety medications 30 minutes before suctioning.
9. The nurse monitors the patient with positive pressure mechanical ventilation for
   a. paralytic ileus because pressure on the abdominal contents affects bowel motility.
   b. diuresis and sodium depletion because of increased release of atrial natriuretic peptide.
   c. signs of cardiovascular insufficiency because pressure in the chest impedes venous return.
   d. respiratory acidosis in a patient with COPD because of alveolar hyperventilation and increased Pao_2 levels.
10. Which findings indicate the patient is ready for weaning from mechanical ventilation? **(Select all that apply.)**
    a. Serum hemoglobin of 15 g/dL
    b. Respirations of 18 breaths/min
    c. Patient is alert and follows commands
    d. Chest x-ray shows large pleural effusion
    e. Mean arterial pressure (MAP) of 55 mm Hg
    f. ABGS: pH 7.38, $Paco_2$ 37 mm Hg, HCO_3^- 24 mEq/L, Pao_2 94.
11. Immediate care priorities in the first few hours for a patient with a new tracheostomy include
    a. encouraging early mobility.
    b. changing the tracheostomy ties.
    c. suctioning the tracheostomy hourly.
    d. observing for bleeding at the insertion site.
12. Discharge teaching for the patient with a permanent tracheostomy after a total laryngectomy would include **(Select all that apply.)**
    a. encouraging regular exercise such as swimming.
    b. washing around the stoma daily with a moist washcloth.
    c. emphasizing the importance of regular follow-up appointments.
    d. providing pictures and "hands-on" instruction for tracheostomy care.
    e. having a list of emergency contact numbers and where to obtain supplies.

1. a; 2. c; 3. a; 4. b; 5. a;
6. a; 7. c; 8. a; 9. c; 10. a, b, c, f; 11. d; 12. b, c, d, e.

For rationales to these answers and even more NCLEX review questions, visit http://evolve.elsevier.com/Lewis/medsurg.

REFERENCES

To access the References for this chapter, please scan the QR code with a mobile device.

29

Upper Respiratory Problems

Janice A. Sarasnick

http://evolve.elsevier.com/Lewis/medsurg/

CONCEPTUAL FOCUS

Cellular Regulation
Functional Ability
Gas Exchange
Infection
Sensory Perception

LEARNING OUTCOMES

1. Describe the clinical manifestations and nursing and interprofessional management of nasal and sinus problems.
2. Describe the clinical manifestations, nursing, and interprofessional management of an upper respiratory infection.
3. Describe the clinical manifestations and nursing and interprofessional management of problems of the pharynx and larynx.
4. Outline the risk factors for and clinical manifestations of head and neck cancer.
5. Discuss the nursing and interprofessional management of patients undergoing surgery for head and neck cancer.
6. Explain essential components of chronic care for patients after head and neck cancer surgery.

KEY TERMS

acute laryngitis
airway obstruction
allergic rhinitis
epistaxis
influenza
laryngectomy, Table 29.7
pharyngitis
rhinoplasty
sinusitis
upper respiratory infection

This chapter discusses problems of the upper respiratory system. The primary concern with upper respiratory problems and cancers of the head and neck is the impact on ventilation and oxygen (O_2) availability. They can affect sleep quality and the ability to have adequate nutrition intake. Sinus and upper respiratory tract infections, allergies, and oral problems can change the senses of smell and taste. Changes in body image and difficulty coping can occur after cancer surgeries.

NASAL AND SINUS PROBLEMS

DEVIATED SEPTUM

Deviated septum is a deflection of the normally straight nasal septum. The cause is usually trauma related or genetic. Up to 80% of adults may have septa that are slightly off-center. The diagnosis of a deviated septum is generally reserved for those whose septa are severely shifted.[1] A deviated septum can interfere with airflow and sinus drainage due to the narrowed passageway.

Symptoms vary depending on the degree of deviation. Minor septal deviations can range from asymptomatic to nasal congestion and frequent sinus infections. Manifestations of severe septal deviation include facial pain, nosebleeds *(epistaxis)*, and obstruction to nasal breathing.

The diagnosis is made during examination with a nasal speculum. Management of minor septal deviation focuses on symptom control. For nasal inflammation and congestion, use saline rinses and decongestants to clear nasal passages and analgesics for pain relief. For severe septal deviation, a nasal septoplasty reconstructs and aligns the deviated septum.

NASAL FRACTURE

Nasal fracture is the most common facial fracture.[2] Nasal fractures often occur from blunt trauma, including fights, automobile accidents, falls, and sports injuries. Using protective sports equipment and safeguarding against falls can prevent many nasal fractures.

We can classify nasal fractures by their fracture pattern (e.g., impacted, comminuted) or the direction of injury (e.g., lateral, frontal). *Simple fractures* may be unilateral or bilateral. They typically have little or no displacement. Powerful frontal blows can cause *complex fractures,* which may involve damage to adjacent facial structures, such as the teeth or eyes. Patients with nasal fractures from blunt force trauma should be evaluated for injury to the cervical spine, orbital sockets, and mandible. Complications include airway obstruction, nosebleeds, meningeal tears causing cerebrospinal fluid (CSF) leakage, septal hematoma, and cosmetic deformity.

Diagnosis of a nasal fracture is based on the history and physical assessment. Although facial deformity is common, a nosebleed may be the only manifestation. Other manifestations include pain, crepitus on palpation, swelling, difficulty breathing out of the nostrils, and bruising.

Assess the patient's ability to breathe through each side of the nose. Note any edema, bleeding, or hematoma. Periorbital bruising involving both eyes is called *raccoon eyes.* It suggests a basilar skull fracture. It increases the chance of CSF leaking into the nasal cavities. Inspect the nose for septal deviation, clear drainage, edema, or bleeding. Clear or pink-tinged persistent drainage after control of bleeding suggests a possible CSF leak. If needed, send a specimen to the laboratory to determine the fluid type.

Goals of nursing care are to maintain a patent airway, reduce edema and pain, prevent complications, and provide support. To maintain the airway, keep the patient sitting upright and slightly forward. Apply ice to the face and nose at 10- to 20-minute intervals to help reduce edema and bleeding. Tell patients not to blow their nose once bleeding has stopped so they do not disrupt the clot or cause further trauma. Give prescribed analgesia to control pain. Acetaminophen is preferred for the first 48 hours to avoid increasing the risk for bleeding. Nasal stuffiness may be relieved with nasal decongestants, saline nasal sprays, and a humidifier. Patients should avoid hot showers and alcohol for the first 48 hours to prevent an increase in swelling.

Not all fractures require further treatment, especially if no deformity is present. If treatment is needed, the bones are realigned using closed reduction or surgery.[3] Closed reduction often uses manipulation to place the bones back into place. Considerable swelling of soft tissues can occur. Antibiotics are considered for a nasal fracture that disrupts the mucosa. The presence of septal hematoma increases the risk for deformity and infection, which may require drainage and antibiotics.

Surgical options include septoplasty and rhinoplasty. Patients have rhinoplasty for several reasons. Both procedures help maintain a patent airway, restore function of the nose, and help reestablish cosmetic appearance. It may be necessary to wait 5 to 7 days to repair the fracture until after edema subsides.

RHINOPLASTY

Rhinoplasty is the surgical reconstruction of the nose. It is done for cosmetic reasons or to improve airway function when trauma or development deformities result in nasal obstruction.

Most rhinoplasty is an outpatient procedure using regional or general anesthesia. Nasal tissue is added or removed, and the nose may be lengthened or shortened. Plastic implants are sometimes used to reshape the nose. Incisions are typically inside the nose and hidden. Sonic rhinoplasty employs an ultrasonic device to gently aspirate bone, enabling a refined cosmetic result.

Before surgery, assess patients' expectations. Actual or perceived changes in body image (e.g., deformed or enlarged nose) can affect self-esteem and interactions with others. The HCP can use digital photographs to show patients their projected appearance after surgery. These images can help patients decide whether to undergo rhinoplasty.

Obtain a medication history. Aspirin-containing drugs and nonsteroidal antiinflammatory drugs (NSAIDs) may need to be stopped for 5 days to 2 weeks before surgery to reduce the risk of bleeding. Encourage smoking cessation to promote postoperative wound healing.

During the immediate postoperative period, the focus of care is (1) ensuring airway patency, (2) continuous assessment of respiratory status, (3) pain management, and (4) observing the surgical site for edema, bleeding, and infection.

After surgery, nasal packing may be inserted to apply pressure and prevent bleeding or septal hematoma formation. An external plastic splint protects and supports the new shape of the nose during the healing process. If present, nasal packing is usually removed 1 or 2 days after surgery. The splint may be left in place for 1 to 2 weeks.

Teaching is important because patients must be able to detect complications at home. Patients typically have temporary nasal and/or facial edema and bruising. Cold compresses and elevating the head can help minimize swelling and discomfort. Teach about activity restrictions aimed at preventing bleeding and injury (no nose blowing, swimming, heavy lifting, strenuous exercise). Sometimes swelling may be slow to resolve, delaying the achievement of a full cosmetic result for up to 1 year.

EPISTAXIS

Epistaxis (nosebleed) can be caused by trauma, low humidity, upper respiratory tract infections, allergies, sinusitis, foreign bodies, chemical irritants (e.g., street drugs), overuse of decongestant nasal sprays, facial or nasal surgery, anatomic malformation, and tumors. Conditions that prolong bleeding time or change platelet counts may predispose patients to nosebleeds. Bleeding time may be prolonged if patients take aspirin, NSAIDs, warfarin, or other anticoagulant drugs.

We describe nosebleeds as anterior or posterior. About 90% of nosebleeds occur in the anterior part of the nasal cavity. They are easy to visualize. Anterior bleeding can be self-treated and usually stops spontaneously. Posterior bleeding occurs more often with older adults with other health problems. Because posterior nosebleeds are closer to the throat, it is often hard to determine how much blood loss has occurred. Posterior bleeding may need medical treatment.

Interprofessional and Nursing Management

Use simple first aid measures to control nosebleeds:

1. Place the patient in a sitting position, leaning slightly forward with head tilted forward.
2. Apply direct pressure by squeezing the entire soft lower part of the nose (nostrils) together for 5 to 15 minutes.
3. If bleeding does not stop within 15 minutes, seek medical assistance.

An anterior bleed may be treated medically by placing a pledget (nasal tampon) impregnated with anesthetic solution (lidocaine) and/or vasoconstrictive agents (epinephrine) into the nasal cavity. Absorbable materials, such as oxidized cellulose (surgical), gelatin foam (Gelfoam), or a gelatin-thrombin combination (Floseal), are another option. Packing for anterior bleeds can stay in place for 48 to 72 hours. Silver nitrate may be used to chemically cauterize a specific bleeding point. Thermal cauterization is reserved for more severe bleeding. Patients may receive local or general anesthesia.[4]

The location of a posterior bleed is harder to find. They often need packing. Packing with compressed nasal sponges or epistaxis balloons is best because of the ease of placement. Packing is inserted into the nares and advanced along the floor of the nasal cavity. The sponge expands with moisture to fill the nasal cavity and tamponade bleeding. An epistaxis balloon inflated with air achieves the same pressure effect (Fig. 29.1). In the absence of a specific nasal device, we may use a size 10F, 12F, or 14F Foley catheter with a 30-mL balloon. A nasal sling (folded 2 × 2–inch gauze pad) may be gently taped under the nares to absorb drainage. If packing does not stop the bleeding, the patient may need arterial embolization.

Nasal sponges, packing, and balloons can impair respiratory status. Monitor level of consciousness, heart rate and rhythm, respiratory rate, and O_2 saturation (SpO_2) using pulse oximetry. Observe for signs of difficulty breathing or swallowing. Because of the increased risk for complications due to the location of the injury, all patients with posterior packing should be on a monitored unit for close observation.

Nasal packing is painful because sufficient pressure must be applied to stop the bleeding. Patients should receive appropriate analgesia. Nasal packing predisposes patients to infection from bacteria (e.g., *Staphylococcus aureus*) present in the nasal cavity. Antibiotics effective against staphylococci may be prescribed. Nasal packing for posterior bleeds may be left in place for 2 to 3 days. Before removal, premedicate for pain as this procedure is uncomfortable. After packing removal, cleanse the nares gently and lubricate them with water-soluble jelly.

Before discharge, provide teaching about follow-up care. Review how to use saline nasal spray and/or a humidifier. Have patients sneeze with the mouth open. They should avoid the use of aspirin-containing products or NSAIDs. Teach them to avoid vigorous nose blowing, engaging in strenuous activity, and lifting and straining for 4 to 6 weeks.

ALLERGIC RHINITIS

Allergic rhinitis is inflammation of the nasal mucosa, often in response to a specific allergen. We usually describe allergic rhinitis by the causative allergen (seasonal or perennial) and the frequency of symptoms (episodic, intermittent, or persistent). *Episodic* refers to symptoms related to sporadic exposure to

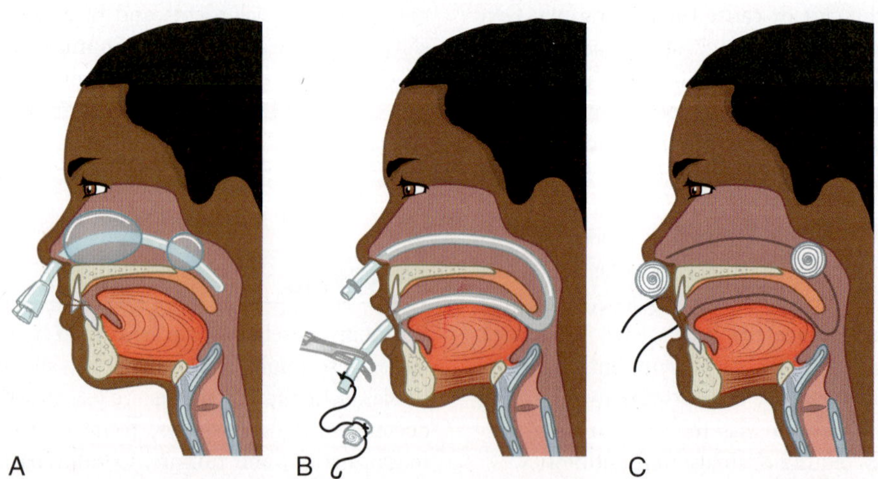

Fig. 29.1 (A) Epistaxis balloon properly inflated and in position. (B) Method for placing posterior nasal pack. A catheter is passed through the bleeding side of the nose and pulled out through the mouth with a hemostat. Strings are tied to the catheter. The pack is pulled up behind the soft palate and into the nasopharynx. (C) Nasal pack in position in the posterior nasopharynx. Dental roll at the nose helps maintain the correct position.

allergens not typically encountered in the person's normal environment. An example is exposure to animal dander when visiting another person's home. *Intermittent* means that the symptoms are present less than 4 days a week or less than 4 weeks per year. *Persistent* means that symptoms are present more than 4 days a week and for more than 4 weeks per year.

Seasonal rhinitis usually occurs in the spring and fall. It is caused by an allergy to pollens from trees, flowers, grasses, or weeds. Attacks may last for several weeks during times when pollen counts are high. Then it disappears and often recurs at the same time the next year. *Perennial rhinitis* occurs year-round from exposure to environment allergens, such as animal dander, dust mites, cockroaches, fungi, and molds. Seasonal and perennial rhinitis can be classified as episodic, intermittent, or persistent, depending on the duration and frequency of symptoms.

Sensitization to an allergen occurs with initial allergen exposure, which results in production of antigen-specific immunoglobulin E (IgE) (see Fig. 14.6). After exposure, mast cells and basophils release histamine, cytokines, prostaglandins, and leukotrienes. These cause the early symptoms of sneezing, itching, rhinorrhea (runny nose), and congestion (stuffy nose).[5] Within 4 to 8 hours after exposure, inflammatory cells infiltrate the nasal tissues, causing and maintaining the inflammatory response. Because symptoms of rhinitis are like those of the common cold, patients may think the condition is a continuous or repeated cold.

Clinical Manifestations

Manifestations of allergic rhinitis are sneezing; watery, itchy eyes and nose; decreased sense of smell; and thin, watery nasal discharge that can lead to more sustained mucus production and congestion. Nasal turbinates appear pale, boggy, and swollen. The turbinates may fill the air space and press against the nasal septum. The posterior ends of the turbinates can become so enlarged that they obstruct sinus aeration or drainage and result in sinusitis. With chronic exposure to allergens, patients may develop a headache, stuffy nose, nasal congestion, and sinus pressure. Nasal polyps, soft, painless growths in the sinus cavity, may form. Postnasal drip occurs when mucus runs down the back of the throat. Nasal polyps and postnasal drip are the most common causes of cough for people with allergies. Patients may report hoarseness and the need to frequently clear the throat to remove the mucus.

Interprofessional and Nursing Management

The key step to managing allergic rhinitis is identifying and avoiding triggers of allergic reactions (Table 29.1). Teach patients to note when allergic reactions occur and keep a diary of activities that precipitate the reaction. Patients are often more aware of intermittent exposure to an allergen, such as pets, than they are of more persistent exposure to allergens, such as dust mites, cockroaches, or mold. Identifying triggers is the first step toward avoiding them.

TABLE 29.1 PATIENT & CAREGIVER TEACHING

Avoiding Allergens in Allergic Rhinitis

Include the following instructions when teaching patients or caregivers about allergic rhinitis:

What to Avoid	Specific Approaches
House dust	• Focus on the bedroom. Remove carpeting. Limit furniture. • Put the pillows and mattress in airtight vinyl bags. • Limit clothing in the bedroom to items worn often. Place clothing in airtight, zipper-sealed vinyl clothes bags. • Install a high-efficiency particulate air (HEPA) filter. • Close the air-conditioning vent into room. • Use blinds rather than draperies.
House dust mites	• Wash bedding in hot water (140°F [60°C]). • Wear a mask when vacuuming. • Install a filter on the outlet port of vacuum cleaner. • Avoid sleeping or lying on upholstered furniture. • Keep house temperature and conditions cool and dry.
Mold spores	• The 3 *D*s that promote growth of mold spores are darkness, dampness, and drafts. • Ventilate closed rooms and open doors. Consider adding windows to dark rooms and keeping a small light on in closets. • Basement light with a timer that provides light several hours a day may decrease mold growth. • Avoid places with high humidity (e.g., basements, clothes hampers, greenhouses, barns).
Pet allergens	• Remove pets from interior of home. • Clean living area thoroughly. • Do not expect instant relief. Symptoms usually do not improve for 1–2 months after pet removal.
Pollens	• Stay inside with doors and windows closed during high-pollen season. • Install an air conditioner with an air filter. Wash filters weekly during high-pollen season. • Use your car's air conditioner "recirculation" feature (circulates air inside the car while shutting off air coming into the vehicle from the outside). • Avoid having plants, especially in the bedroom.
Smoke	• Encourage family and friends to refrain from smoking (if possible) or to go outdoors to smoke. • Presence of a smoker will sabotage any symptom reduction program.

The goal of drug therapy is to reduce inflammation from allergic rhinitis, reduce nasal symptoms, minimize complications, and maximize quality of life. Oral medication options include H_1-antihistamines, decongestants, and leukotriene receptor antagonists (LTRAs). Intranasal medications include antihistamines, anticholinergics, corticosteroids, mast-cell stabilizers, and decongestants (Table 29.2).[6]

TABLE 29.2 Drug Therapy

Rhinitis and Sinusitis

Drug	Mechanism of Action	Side Effects	Nursing Actions
Anticholinergic Nasal Spray			
ipratropium bromide	Blocks nasal cholinergic receptors, reducing nasal secretions in the common cold and nonallergic rhinitis.	Nasal dryness and irritation, nosebleeds.	• May reduce the need for other rhinitis medications.
Antihistamines			
First-Generation Oral Agents			
brompheniramine diphenhydramine	Bind with H_1 receptors on target cells, blocking histamine release. Relieve acute symptoms of allergic response (itching, sneezing, rhinorrhea).	Cross blood-brain barrier, often causing sedation. Can cause paradoxical stimulation (restlessness, nervousness, insomnia). Anticholinergic side effects (palpitations, dry mouth, constipation, urinary hesitancy).	• Warn patient that operating machinery and driving may be dangerous because of sedative effect. • Teach patient to report palpitations, change in heart rate, change in bowel or bladder habits. • Avoid alcohol because of additive depressant effect. • Rapid onset of action, no drug tolerance with prolonged use.
Second-Generation Oral Agents			
cetirizine (Zyrtec) desloratadine (Clarinex) fexofenadine (Allegra) levocetirizine (Xyzal) loratadine (Claritin)	Same as above.	Limited affinity for brain H_1 receptors. Cause minimal sedation, few effects on psychomotor activities or bladder function.	• More expensive than traditional antihistamines. • Rapid onset of action, no drug tolerance with prolonged use.
Second-Generation Nasal Sprays			
azelastine (Astelin, Astepro) olopatadine (Patanase)	Block histamine release. Reduce nasal congestion.	Headache, bitter taste, somnolence, nasal irritation.	• Longer use increases risk for rebound vasodilation, which can increase congestion.
Corticosteroid Nasal Sprays			
beclomethasone budesonide (Rhinocort) ciclesonide (Omnaris) flunisolide fluticasone (Flonase) mometasone (Nasonex) triamcinolone (Nasocort)	Inhibit inflammatory response of allergic rhinitis. Decreases mucosal inflammation and facilitates drainage of sinuses. Systemic effects may occur with higher than recommended doses.	At recommended dose, systemic side effects unlikely. Mild transient nasal irritation, mucosal drying, nosebleeds. In rare instances, local fungal infection with *Candida albicans.*	• Adherence important. Teach patient to use on regular basis. • Have patient clear nasal passages before use. • Reinforce that sprays decrease inflammation and it may take several days or 1–2 wk to achieve maximum effects. • Stop use if nasal infection develops.
Decongestants			
Oral			
pseudoephedrine (Sudafed)	Stimulates adrenergic receptors and promotes vasoconstriction of superficial vessels in the nose and reduces nasal congestion.	Central nervous system (CNS) stimulation, causing insomnia, excitation, headache, irritability, increased blood and ocular pressure, dysuria, palpitations, tachycardia.	• Tolerance variable. • Patient to inform HCP if preexisting cardiovascular disease, hypertension, diabetes, glaucoma, benign prostatic hyperplasia, liver, or kidney disease present before starting therapy. • Rebound nasal congestion may occur with chronic overuse.
Nasal Spray			
oxymetazoline phenylephrine	Same as above.	Same as above.	• Teach not to use for >5 days or >3 or 4 times/day. • Rebound nasal congestion may occur. • Addiction possible.

TABLE 29.2 **Drug Therapy—cont'd**

Rhinitis and Sinusitis

Drug	Mechanism of Action	Side Effects	Nursing Actions
Leukotriene Receptor Antagonists (LTRAs) and Inhibitors			
Antagonists montelukast (Singulair) zafirlukast (Accolate) ***Inhibitors*** zileuton (Zyflo)	Suppress leukotriene activity, thereby inhibiting airway edema, mucus production, bronchoconstriction, and inflammation.	May cause headaches, dizziness, rash, altered liver function, gastrointestinal changes. *Zafirlukast and zileuton:* Monitor prothrombin time (PT) if patient is taking warfarin.	• Monitor liver function tests periodically while on therapy. Stop if elevated. • Give on empty stomach. • Do not stop therapy without consulting HCP. • Do not use for acute attacks.
Mast Cell Stabilizer Nasal Spray			
cromolyn spray	Suppresses release of histamine and other inflammatory mediators from mast cells.	Minimal side effects. Occasional nasal irritation.	• Reinforce that spray prevents symptoms. • Begin 1 week before pollen season starts and use throughout pollen season. • For isolated allergy, use before exposure to allergen. • When used to treat chronic rhinitis, may use with antihistamine and/or nasal decongestant.

Second-generation antihistamines are used before first-generation antihistamines because of their nonsedating effects. Teach patients taking antihistamines to have adequate fluid intake to reduce adverse symptoms and keep secretions thin. Nasal corticosteroid sprays decrease inflammation with little systemic absorption. This makes systemic side effects rare. If monotherapy does not relieve symptoms, a 2-drug combination, such as an oral H_1-antihistamine and an intranasal corticosteroid, may help.

DRUG ALERT

Antihistamines

- First-generation antihistamines (e.g., diphenhydramine) can cause drowsiness and sedation.
- Warn patients that operating machinery and driving may be dangerous because of the sedative effect.
- The sedative effects may lead to hypotension and falls in older adults.

Immunotherapy (allergy shots) may be used when a specific, unavoidable allergen is identified, and drugs are not tolerated or are ineffective in controlling symptoms. Immunotherapy involves controlled exposure to small amounts of the known allergen through frequent (at least weekly) injections with the goal of decreasing sensitivity. Sublingual or intranasal administration of allergen immunotherapy may be an option for some patients. Immunotherapy is discussed in Chapter 14.

NASAL POLYPS

Nasal polyps are soft, painless, benign (noncancerous) growths that form slowly in response to repeated inflammation of the sinus or nasal mucosa. They are most common in adults over age 40 and are twice as likely to occur in men. Polyps, which appear as chronic yellow, gray, or pink semitransparent projections in the naris, can exceed the size of a grape.

Small polyps are typically asymptomatic. Manifestations of larger polyps include nasal obstruction, nasal discharge (usually clear mucus), and speech distortion. Topical and systemic corticosteroids are primary therapies used to shrink nasal polyps. Endoscopic or laser surgery can remove nasal polyps, but recurrence is common.

FOREIGN BODIES

Foreign bodies may potentially lodge in an adult's upper respiratory tract, but it is a rare occurrence. Some foreign bodies, like food, may cause a local inflammatory reaction and nasal discharge. The discharge may become purulent and foul-smelling if the object stays in the nasal cavity for an extended time. Foreign bodies can cause pain, difficulty breathing, and nasal bleeding.

We usually remove foreign bodies from the nose through the route of entry. Sneezing or blowing the nose with the opposite nostril closed may be effective in removing the foreign object. Avoid irrigating the nose or pushing the object backward because these could cause aspiration and airway obstruction. If sneezing or blowing the nose does not remove the object, consult an HCP.

UPPER RESPIRATORY INFECTIONS

ACUTE VIRAL RHINOPHARYNGITIS

An upper respiratory infection (URI) is an infection of the nose, sinuses, and/or throat. Viruses cause most URIs. However, bacterial agents may cause a URI as well. *Acute viral rhinopharyngitis* (nasopharyngitis, common cold) is one type of

URI. Sinusitis and influenza are examples of other types of URI. There are over 200 viruses that may cause a URI.[7] The most typical viruses are the rhinovirus, coronavirus, influenza, parainfluenza, respiratory syncytial virus (RSV), and enterovirus. The most common bacterium is *Streptococcus pyogenes.* It is a group A streptococcus that causes strep throat.[8] Adults may have an average of 2 to 3 colds per year.

Viruses are contagious. They spread by airborne droplets emitted by the infected person while breathing, talking, sneezing, or coughing. Because the pathogens can survive on inanimate objects for up to 3 days, transmission may occur by directly touching the surface and then touching your eyes, nose, or mouth with contaminated hands. Infections increase in winter months when people stay indoors, and overcrowding is more common. Other factors that increase susceptibility include fatigue, physical and emotional stress, allergies affecting the nose and throat, and a compromised immune status.

Clinical Manifestations

Symptoms typically begin 2 or 3 days after infection. They may include runny nose, watery eyes, nasal congestion, sneezing, cough, sore throat, fever, headache, and fatigue. Patients are contagious 1 to 2 days before symptom onset and remain contagious until symptoms have subsided. Symptoms may last 2 to 14 days, with typical recovery in 7 to 10 days.

Interprofessional and Nursing Management

Interventions are directed at relieving symptoms. Care includes rest, oral fluids, antipyretics, and analgesics. Warm saltwater gargles, ice chips, lozenges, or sprays may help ease a sore throat. Saline nasal spray reduces nasal congestion. Antihistamine and decongestant therapy reduces postnasal drip and decreases the severity of cough, nasal obstruction, and nasal discharge. Caution patients to use intranasal decongestant sprays for no more than 5 days to prevent rebound congestion from occurring. Cough suppressants for irritating, bothersome coughs can be used but may not be effective. Patients may ask about vitamin C, echinacea, and zinc products. There is inconclusive evidence to support treatment with these therapies.

DRUG ALERT

Pseudoephedrine

- Large doses may cause tachycardia and palpitations, especially in patients with heart disease.
- Overdose in those over 60 years of age may result in central nervous system depression, seizures, and hallucinations.

Complications include acute bronchitis, sinusitis, otitis media, tonsillitis, and pneumonia. Antibiotics have no effect on viruses. They are an option only if complications are present. Refer to an HCP if there is no improvement in symptoms within 10 to 14 days.

Teach patients the manifestations of a secondary bacterial infection. These include a temperature higher than 103°F (39.4°C); tender, swollen glands; severe sinus or ear pain; or significantly worsening symptoms. Green, purulent nasal drainage during the later stages of a cold is not uncommon and not always indicative of bacterial infection. In patients with lung disease, signs of infection include a change in consistency, color, or volume of the sputum. Because infection can progress rapidly, teach patients with chronic respiratory disease to immediately report sputum changes, increased shortness of breath, and chest tightness.

Exercise, managing stress, adequate sleep, and eating a well-balanced diet may reduce the number and/or severity of URIs.[9] Patients with a chronic illness or a compromised immune system should avoid crowded situations and those with obvious cold symptoms. Frequent handwashing and avoiding hand-to-face contact can help prevent direct spread.

INFLUENZA

Influenza (flu) is a highly contagious respiratory illness that affects millions of people each year. The flu season begins in September and continues through April of each year, peaking from December to February. The flu is responsible for up to 49,000 deaths annually.[10] Vaccination of high-risk groups may help prevent many of these deaths.

Etiology and Pathophysiology

We classify influenza viruses into 4 serotypes (A, B, C, D). Only A and B cause significant illness in humans. Influenza A is subtyped based on the presence of 2 surface proteins: hemagglutinin (H) and neuraminidase (N). The H antigens enable the virus to enter the cell, and the N antigens facilitate cell-to-cell transmission. As a result, we name influenza A viruses by their H and N type (e.g., H3N2).

Influenza A is the most common and most virulent flu virus. It can infect a variety of animals and humans. More than 100 types of influenza A can occur in birds (avian flu), pigs (swine flu), horses, seals, and dogs. When the virus mutates (changes), this allows it to infect different species. When a new viral strain reaches humans, people do not have immunity. The virus can spread quickly around the globe, causing a *pandemic.* For example, type A H1N1 influenza (swine flu) emerged in 2009. It had never been seen in humans before, resulting in a worldwide pandemic. The reemergence of a strain that has not circulated for many years can also trigger a pandemic. *Epidemics* are more local outbreaks, often occurring yearly, caused by variants of already circulating influenza virus strains.

Influenza B and C viruses only infect humans. They do not have subtypes. Outbreaks of influenza B can cause regional epidemics. The disease it produces is milder than that caused by influenza A. Influenza C causes mild illness and does not cause epidemics or pandemics. Influenza D only occurs in animals.

The flu is communicable between humans mainly through infected droplets, inhalation of aerosolized particles, and, to a lesser extent, through direct contact with contaminated surfaces. The virus has an incubation period of 1 to 4 days, with peak transmission risk starting 1 day before the onset of symptoms and continuing for 5 to 7 days after a person first becomes sick.[11]

Clinical Manifestations

For some patients, it may be hard to tell between the common cold and flu (Table 29.3). The onset of flu is abrupt. There may be chills, fever, and generalized myalgia, often accompanied by a headache, cough, sore throat, and fatigue. Assessment findings are usually minimal, with normal breath sounds on chest auscultation. In uncomplicated cases, symptoms often subside within 7 days.

Common complications include pneumonia, which can be primary influenza (viral) pneumonia or secondary bacterial pneumonia, and ear or sinus infections. Dyspnea and diffuse crackles are signs of pulmonary complications. Some patients, especially older adults, have weakness or lethargy that may last for weeks. Patients who develop secondary bacterial pneumonia usually have a gradual improvement of flu symptoms, then worsening cough and purulent sputum. Treatment with antibiotics is usually effective if started early.

Diagnostic Studies

The flu is often diagnosed based on the history, physical assessment, and knowledge of other influenza cases in the community. Testing can help distinguish the flu from other viral and bacterial infections with similar manifestations that may be serious but are treated differently. Nasal or throat cultures may help identify the causative agent. The preferable method of culture collection is from the nasopharyngeal area via a midturbinate nasal swab. This should occur within 4 days of symptom onset. Guidelines for testing include those who are high risk (e.g., immunocompromised) or patients with acute-onset respiratory symptoms. In the hospital, we often test those with cardiopulmonary disease whose condition is worsening.[12]

Rapid influenza diagnostic tests (RIDTs) can help detect the virus in secretions from the respiratory tract. Depending on the method, the test may be completed in the HCP's office, with results available in as little as 15 minutes. RIDTs are best used within the first 48 hours of the onset of symptoms. The main disadvantages of RIDTs are that patients may have a false-negative result, and the test is more sensitive to influenza A than B.[13]

Interprofessional and Nursing Management

The most effective strategy is prevention. Two types of flu vaccines are available: inactivated and live attenuated (Table 29.4). Receiving a flu vaccine results in the production of antibodies against the viruses in the vaccine.

The flu vaccine is changed on a yearly basis. The content depends on the virus strains public health officials determine as being most likely to cause illness in the upcoming flu season. The best time to receive the vaccine is in September or October (before flu exposure) because it takes 2 weeks for antibodies to form and provide full protection from the flu. However, the vaccine can be given at any time during the flu season.

! SAFETY ALERT

Influenza Vaccination

- Advocate for vaccination of all people older than 6 months of age, especially those at high risk (e.g., health care workers, residents of long-term care facilities).
- Give high priority to groups, such as health care workers, who can transmit the flu to high-risk persons.

TABLE 29.3 Comparison of Common Cold and Influenza

Manifestations and Treatment	Common Cold (Viral Rhinitis)	Influenza
Symptom onset	Appear gradually	Abrupt onset. Within 3–6 h
Fever	Rare	Characteristically high 102°–104°F (38.9°–40°C). Lasts 3–4 days
Headache	Uncommon, but may occur	Common (can be severe)
General aches and pains	Slight	Often severe myalgia
Fatigue and weakness	Sometimes. Usually mild	Usual. Starts early and can last up to 2–3 weeks
Exhaustion	Uncommon	Usual at beginning of illness
Stuffy nose	Common	Sometimes
Sneezing	Common	Sometimes
Sore throat	Common	Sometimes
Chest discomfort, cough	Common. Mild to moderate hacking cough	Common
Complications	Sinus congestion. Earache	Bronchitis, pneumonia, acute respiratory failure, and acute respiratory distress syndrome (ARDS). Can be life-threatening
Prevention	Hand washing. Avoid close contact with anyone who has a cold	Handwashing. Annual vaccination. Antiviral drugs. Avoid close contact with anyone who has the flu
Treatment	Temporary relief of symptoms: rest, hydration, decongestants, acetaminophen or ibuprofen for headache, aches, and pains	Antiviral drugs if given within 24–48 h of onset. Rest, hydration, acetaminophen, or ibuprofen for headache, aches, and pains

TABLE 29.4 Types of Influenza Immunization

Trivalent (TIV) or Quadrivalent (QIV) Inactivated Influenza Vaccine	Live Attenuated Influenza Vaccine (LAIV)
Trivalent: Protects against 3 different influenza viruses (2-type A; 1-type B) *Quadrivalent:* Protects against 4 different influenza viruses (2-type A; 2-type B)	Made from weakened influenza virus
Given by injection	Given as an intranasal spray into both nostrils
Approved for use in people ≥6 months of age	Approved for healthy people ages 2–49 years Children 2–8 years and have not had influenza vaccine before need 2 doses (second dose 4 weeks after first dose) Children >9 years need 1 dose
Should NOT be used in: • Infants <6 months in age • Serious allergy/reaction to previous influenza vaccine • Guillain-Barré syndrome diagnosed within previous 6 weeks	Should NOT be used in: • Children <2 years or adults >50 years • Pregnant females or females who plan to become pregnant
Can be used in people at increased risk: • People of any age with chronic medical conditions • Residents of nursing homes and long-term care facilities • People who are immunocompromised • Pregnant females	Before receiving the vaccination, please inform the HCP if you or the person you are caring for have any of the following: • Immunodeficiency • Children or adolescents receiving aspirin or other salicylates • Medical conditions that increase the risk for complications from influenza (chronic heart, lung, liver, kidney, or CNS problems, diabetes; hemoglobinopathies) • HCPs of high-risk patients because of risk for viral transmission from vaccine (should not care for high-risk patients for 7 days after vaccination)
Common side effects are injection site reactions, such as pain, redness, and swelling	Side effects are rare. When effects do occur, may resemble mild flu with runny nose, nasal congestion, cough, and headache

Vaccinating healthy people decreases the incidence and risk for transmitting influenza to those who have less ability to cope with the effects of this illness. Current vaccines are highly purified. Reactions are very rare. Soreness at the injection site is the most reported adverse effect. Contraindications are a history of severe allergic reactions to a previous flu vaccine. Patients with anaphylactic hypersensitivity to eggs should discuss the vaccine with their HCP, as alternatives for vaccinating patients with egg allergies are now available.

The primary nursing goals for those with the flu are symptom relief and preventing secondary infection. Unless patients are at high risk or complications develop, supportive therapy is often all that is needed. Rest, hydration, analgesics, and antipyretics can provide symptom relief. Older adults and those with a chronic illness may need to be hospitalized.

Antiviral medications can shorten the duration of flu symptoms and reduce the risk for complications. Zanamivir (Relenza), oseltamivir (Tamiflu), and peramivir (Rapivab) are neuraminidase inhibitors that prevent the virus from being released and spreading to other cells.[14] Zanamivir is given using an inhaler. Oseltamivir is available as an oral capsule. Peramivir is given IV. The newest drug is baloxavir marboxil (Xofluza). It is a PA endonuclease inhibitor that inhibits viral replication. Patients receive 1 oral dose. Give the tablets with water.

Treatment with antiviral medication should be started as soon as possible in hospitalized patients with influenza, those with severe or complicated illness, or those at high risk for complications. For maximum benefit in treating the flu, therapy should begin within 2 days of the onset of symptoms. It can be started later based on clinical judgment.

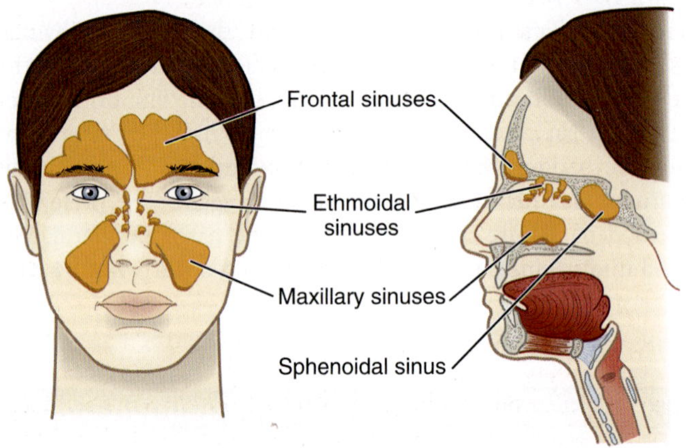

Fig. 29.2 Location of the sinuses.

SINUSITIS

Sinusitis affects 1 in every 7 adults. It develops when inflammation or swelling of the mucosa blocks the openings (ostia) in the sinuses, through which mucus drains into the nose (Fig. 29.2). *Rhinosinusitis,* which may accompany sinusitis, is concurrent inflammation or infection of the nasal mucosa. Nasal polyps, foreign bodies, deviated septa, or tumors can cause obstruction of mucus drainage. Secretions that accumulate behind the blocked ostia provide a rich medium for growth of bacteria, viruses, and fungi, all of which may cause infection.

Viral sinusitis may follow a URI in which the virus penetrates the mucous membrane and decreases ciliary function. Viral infections usually resolve without treatment in less than

14 days. If symptoms worsen after 3 to 5 days or last for longer than 10 days, a secondary bacterial infection may be present. Only 5% to 10% of patients with viral sinusitis develop a bacterial infection and need antibiotic therapy.

Sinusitis can be classified as acute, subacute, recurrent acute, or chronic.[15] *Acute sinusitis* typically begins within 1 week of a URI and lasts less than 4 weeks. *Subacute sinusitis* is present when symptoms progress over 4 to 12 weeks. Recurrent acute rhinosinusitis is defined as having 4 or more sinus infections per year, lasting 7 to 10 days, without having continual symptoms.

Chronic sinusitis (lasting longer than 12 weeks) is a persistent infection usually related to allergies or nasal polyps. It generally results from repeated episodes of acute sinusitis that result in irreversible loss of the normal ciliated epithelium lining the sinus cavity. As many as 50% of patients with moderate to severe asthma have chronic sinusitis. The link between these diseases is unclear. Postnasal drip from sinusitis may trigger asthma by stimulating bronchoconstriction. Gastroesophageal reflux disease (GERD) and smoking may increase the risk for a person with asthma developing sinusitis.

Clinical Manifestations

Acute sinusitis causes significant pain over the affected sinus, purulent nasal drainage, nasal obstruction, congestion, fever, and malaise. Patients may appear acutely ill. Inspect the nasal mucosa and palpate the paranasal sinuses for pain. Findings that indicate acute sinusitis include edematous mucosa, discolored purulent nasal drainage, enlarged turbinates, tenderness over the involved frontal and/or maxillary sinuses, and *halitosis* (bad breath). Recurrent headaches are common. They may change in intensity with position changes or when secretions drain.

The symptoms of chronic sinusitis are often nonspecific. They may have facial or dental pain, nasal congestion, and increased drainage. Fever, severe pain, and purulent drainage are rare. Some symptoms mimic those seen with allergies. X-rays or CT scans of the sinuses may help confirm the diagnosis. CT scans may show sinuses filled with fluid or a thickened mucous membrane. Nasal endoscopy with a flexible scope may be used to examine the sinuses, obtain a specimen for culture, and restore normal drainage.

Interprofessional and Nursing Management

Patient and caregiver teaching for acute and chronic sinusitis is shown in Table 29.5.

If allergies are the precipitating cause of sinusitis, review ways to reduce sinus inflammation and infection. Discuss environment control of allergens and drug therapy.

Initial treatment for acute sinusitis focuses on symptom relief. Medications include oral or topical decongestants to promote drainage, intranasal corticosteroids to decrease inflammation, analgesics to relieve pain, and saline nasal spray to relieve congestion. Teach patients using topical decongestants to use the medication for no longer than 5 days to prevent rebound congestion caused by vasodilation. Saline irrigation of the nasal cavity can rinse nasal passages, promote drainage, and decrease inflammation. Saline nasal spray is available over the counter. If symptoms worsen or last longer than 1 week, antibiotic therapy may be prescribed.

With chronic sinusitis, mixed bacterial flora is often present, and infections are hard to eliminate. Broad-spectrum antibiotics may be used for 4 to 6 weeks.

Medical therapy may not relieve the symptoms of some patients with persistent, recurrent, or chronic sinus illnesses. Patients may need nasal endoscopic surgery to relieve blockage caused by hypertrophy or septal deviation. This is usually an outpatient procedure under local anesthesia. Propel, a self-expanding implant, can be placed directly in the sinus during surgery. Propel helps maintain patency to the sinus cavity after surgery and provides local corticosteroid delivery directly to the sinus lining before dissolving after 30 days.

TABLE 29.5 PATIENT & CAREGIVER TEACHING

Acute or Chronic Sinusitis

Include the following instructions when teaching patients and caregivers about managing sinusitis:

1. Get plenty of rest to help the body fight infection and promote recovery.
2. Keep well hydrated by drinking 6–8 glasses of water per day to thin secretions.
3. Take hot showers. Use a steam inhaler (15-min vaporization of boiled water), bedside humidifier, or nasal saline spray to promote secretion drainage.
4. Apply warm, damp towels around nose, cheeks, and eyes to ease facial pain.
5. Sleep with head elevated to help sinuses drain and reduce congestion.
6. Report a temperature of 100.4°F (38°C) or higher, which indicates infection.
7. Follow prescribed medication plan:
   - Take analgesics to relieve pain.
   - Take decongestants/expectorants to relieve swelling.
   - Take antibiotics (as prescribed) for infection. Take the entire prescription and report continued symptoms or a change in symptoms.
   - Use nasal sprays to relieve congestion.
8. Perform nasal saline washes once or twice a day to wash sinuses.
9. Do not smoke and avoid exposure to smoke. It will irritate and worsen symptoms.
10. If allergies predispose to sinusitis, follow instructions about environment control, drug therapy, and immunotherapy to reduce the inflammation and prevent sinus infection.

PHARYNGEAL AND LARYNGEAL PROBLEMS

ACUTE PHARYNGITIS

Acute **pharyngitis** is an acute inflammation of the pharyngeal walls. It may include the tonsils, palate, and uvula. It can be caused by a viral, bacterial, or fungal infection. Viral pharyngitis accounts for about 90% of cases. Bacterial pharyngitis ("strep throat") usually results from group A β-hemolytic streptococci and accounts for 5% to 10% of cases.

Fungal pharyngitis, such as candidiasis, can develop with the prolonged use of antibiotics or inhaled corticosteroids. It can also occur in immunosuppressed patients, especially those with HIV infection. Other causes of pharyngitis include dry air, smoking, GERD, allergy, postnasal drip, endotracheal tube (ET) intubation, chemical fumes, and cancer.

Clinical Manifestations

Symptoms of acute pharyngitis range in severity from a "scratchy" throat to pain so severe that swallowing is difficult. Because viral and streptococcal infections appear as a red and edematous pharynx (with or without patchy exudates), it may be hard to tell between them.

Four classic manifestations present in bacterial pharyngitis include (1) fever greater than 100.4°F (38°C); (2) anterior cervical lymph node enlargement; (3) tonsillar or pharyngeal exudate; and (4) absence of cough. However, appearance is not always diagnostic. When 2 or 3 of these criteria are present, a rapid antigen detection test and/or a throat culture can help with the diagnosis. White, irregular patches on the oropharynx suggest fungal infection with *Candida albicans.*

Interprofessional and Nursing Management

The goals of treatment are infection control, symptom relief, and preventing secondary complications. Patients with viral pharyngitis receive symptomatic care. For bacterial pharyngitis caused by group A β-hemolytic streptococci, penicillin is the drug of choice. This antibiotic must be taken several times a day for a full 10 days to prevent complications, such as rheumatic fever. For patients allergic to penicillin, erythromycin and clindamycin are substitutes. Other antibiotics, such as azithromycin or a 1st-generation cephalosporin, are options. Most people with streptococcal infections are contagious until they have been on antibiotics for 24 to 48 hours. Repeat throat cultures after antibiotic therapy are not needed.

Candida infections are treated with nystatin, an antifungal antibiotic. Teach patients to swish the preparation in their mouths for as long as possible before swallowing it. Treatment should continue until symptoms are gone. Patients taking inhaled corticosteroids are at risk for infection with *Candida* organisms. Rinsing the mouth with water after using corticosteroids can prevent this infection.

Teach patients to use ibuprofen or acetaminophen for pain relief. Encourage patients to increase fluid intake. For symptom relief, have patients gargle with warm salt water (½ tsp of salt in 8 oz of water). Have them drink warm or cold, bland liquids; and suck on popsicles, hard candies, or throat lozenges. Encourage the use of a cool-mist vaporizer or humidifier.

PERITONSILLAR ABSCESS

Peritonsillar abscess is a complication of tonsillitis. It is most often caused by group A β-hemolytic streptococci. The abscess causes pain, swelling, and blockage of the throat (when severe), threatening airway patency. Patients may have a high fever, chills, leukocytosis, difficulty swallowing, and a muffled voice. Treatment consists of IV antibiotic therapy and needle aspiration or incision and drainage of the abscess. In some cases, an emergency tonsillectomy is done. An elective tonsillectomy is scheduled after the infection has subsided.

LARYNGEAL POLYPS

Laryngeal polyps develop on the vocal cords from vocal abuse (e.g., excess talking, singing) or irritation (e.g., intubation, cigarette smoking). The most common sign is hoarseness. Conservative treatment involves voice rest and adequate hydration. Large polyps may cause dysphagia, dyspnea, and stridor. They may need to be surgically removed. Polyps are usually benign but may be removed because they can become cancerous.

ACUTE LARYNGITIS

Acute laryngitis is swelling and inflammation of the voice box (larynx). A virus (e.g., flu, common cold) is the most common cause. Other causes include inflammatory or infectious conditions of the upper respiratory tract (e.g., tonsillitis, acute bronchitis), vocal overuse (e.g., yelling loudly at a concert or a sporting event), exposure to smoke, or chemical inhalation.

The classic hallmark signs include a tingling or burning sensation at the back of the throat, a persistent need to clear the throat, and hoarseness, which may be accompanied by complete loss of voice. There may be a low-grade fever, persistent cough, or feeling of fullness in the throat. Symptoms will appear suddenly, increase in severity over 2 to 3 days, then gradually subside over the next 7 to 10 days as the condition improves. It usually resolves within 21 days.

Diagnosis is made based on the history, physical assessment, and changes in voice. Treatment is supportive. Encourage patients to limit using their voice. This includes talking and whispering. Whispering places increased strain on the vocal cords that may worsen the pain. Acetaminophen, cough suppressants, throat lozenges, and using a humidifier are helpful for discomfort.

Have patients increase fluid intake. They should avoid caffeine and alcohol, which may worsen a sore throat. Encourage smoking cessation. If a bacterial cause is known, such as acute bronchitis or tonsillitis, antibiotics are prescribed. If symptoms last longer than 3 weeks, patients should return to their HCP for further assessment and treatment.

AIRWAY OBSTRUCTION

Acute **airway obstruction** is a medical emergency. Airway obstruction can be caused by aspiration of food or a foreign body, allergic reactions, edema, and inflammation caused by infections or burns, peritonsillar or retropharyngeal abscesses, cancer, laryngeal or tracheal stenosis, and trauma.

Airway obstruction may be partial or complete. The presentation often depends on the cause of the obstruction and/or location of the blockage. For example, objects lodged within the larynx may cause voice hoarseness or complete airway obstruction. Tracheal obstruction may cause wheezing. Objects lodged within the lower respiratory system (e.g., bronchus) may cause a cough or decreased air entry on the affected side.

Manifestations include choking, stridor, flaring nostrils, wheezing, restlessness, tachycardia, cyanosis, and changes in level of consciousness. Prompt assessment and treatment are essential. A partial obstruction may quickly progress to complete obstruction. Complete airway obstruction can result in permanent brain damage or death if not corrected within 3 to 5 minutes.

Your immediate priority is to ensure the patient has a patent airway. Interventions to reestablish a patent airway include the obstructed airway (Heimlich) maneuver, cricothyroidotomy, ET intubation, or tracheostomy. Unexplained partial airway obstruction or recurrent symptoms indicate the need for more tests, including a chest x-ray, laryngoscopy, and rigid bronchoscopy.

HEAD AND NECK CANCER

Head and neck cancer is classified according to the area where it occurs. These cancers may involve the nasal cavity and paranasal sinuses, nasopharynx, oropharynx, larynx, oral cavity, and/or salivary gland. Cancer of the oral cavity is discussed in Chapter 46. Most head and neck cancers arise from squamous cells that line the mucosal surfaces of the head and neck.

More than 53,000 new cases of head and neck cancer are diagnosed each year in the United States.[16] Tobacco use causes 85% of head and neck cancers. Excess alcohol use is another major risk factor. Head and neck cancer most often occurs in people over age 50 and twice as often in men. Head and neck cancers in those younger than 50 years are often related to human papillomavirus (HPV) infection. Other risk factors include exposure to the sun, asbestos, industrial chemicals, marijuana use, radiation therapy to the head and neck, and poor oral hygiene.[17]

Unfortunately, most patients have locally advanced disease at the time of diagnosis. Disability from the disease and its treatment is significant because of the potential loss of voice, adverse effects from chemotherapy and/or radiation, disfigurement, and social concerns.

Clinical Manifestations

The early manifestations vary with the location of the tumor. For example, patients with pharyngeal cancer may have what feels like a lump in the throat or a sore throat that does not get better with treatment. Some have white or red patches in the mouth or a change in their voice. Hoarseness that lasts more than 2 weeks may be a symptom of early laryngeal cancer.

Other manifestations may include ear pain or ringing in the ears, swelling or lumps in the neck, constant coughing, and coughing up blood. Swelling of the jaw can cause dentures to fit poorly or become uncomfortable. Unintentional weight loss and difficulty with chewing, swallowing, moving the tongue or jaw, and breathing are typically late symptoms. A partially or fully obstructed airway is often a late manifestation of head and neck cancer.

Diagnostic Studies

Early detection is key to patient survival. Physical assessment involves a focused assessment of the ears, nose, throat, mouth, and neck. Examine the mouth, including the area under the tongue and dentures, with a flashlight. There may be thickening of the normally soft and pliable oral mucosa. Inspect the floor of the mouth and tongue. *Leukoplakia* (white patch) or *erythroplakia* (fiery red patch) may be present. Leukoplakia and carcinoma in situ (local to a defined area) may precede invasive carcinoma by many years. Palpate the lymph nodes in the neck.

If lesions are suspected, the HCP may examine upper airways using indirect pharyngoscopy and laryngoscopy (which involves using a laryngeal mirror). The larynx and vocal cords are visually inspected for lesions and tissue mobility. Typically, multiple biopsy specimens are obtained to help determine the extent of the disease. A CT scan or MRI may be done to detect local and regional spread. Positron emission tomography (PET) scanning is also used in diagnosis. The interprofessional care of head and neck cancer is outlined in Table 29.6.

Staging of Head and Neck Cancer

Head and neck cancer is staged based on the size of the tumor (T), number and location of involved lymph nodes (N), and extent of metastasis (M). This is referred to as *TNM staging.*

TABLE 29.6 Interprofessional Care

Head and Neck Cancer

Diagnostic Assessment

- History and physical assessment
- Indirect pharyngoscopy and laryngoscopy
- Endoscopy
- Biopsy
- Chest x-ray
- Barium swallow

Management

- Surgery (Table 29.7)
- Radiation therapy
- Chemotherapy
- Targeted therapy
- Respiratory therapy
- Physical therapy
- Occupational therapy
- Speech therapy

Staging is slightly different for each type of cancer. Generally, stage 0 is in situ, or confined to where it began, through stage 4, with more advanced disease. TNM staging is discussed in Chapter 16.

Interprofessional Care

Treatment for head and neck cancer is based on many factors. These include the tumor location, TNM stage, age and overall general health, cosmetic and functional considerations (e.g., ability to talk, swallow, chew), and patient choice. Treatment options include surgery, radiation therapy, chemotherapy, targeted therapy, or any combination of these therapies.

Surgical Therapy

Surgery is often the first-line treatment option for head and neck cancers. Some patients may be treated with surgery alone. For other patients, combining surgery with radiation therapy and/or chemotherapy may be appropriate. Surgical options depend on the location and stage of cancer (Table 29.7). After extensive surgery to remove head and neck cancer, reconstructive operations can help restore the structure and function of the affected areas.

TABLE 29.7 Surgical Procedures for Head and Neck Cancer

Cordectomy	Removal of part or all the vocal cords May be changes in tone of voice Removing part of a vocal cord may lead to a hoarse voice If both vocal cords are removed, speech will no longer be possible
Laser surgery	An endoscope with a laser is inserted down the throat, and the tumor can be vaporized or removed
Laryngectomy	Removal of part (partial) or all (total) the larynx Total laryngectomy changes airflow in and out of the lungs, and normal voice production will not be possible (Fig. 29.3)
Lymph node removal	Amount of tissue and number of lymph nodes removed depend on how far cancer has spread
Pharyngectomy	Removal of part or all the throat
Tracheostomy	Creates an alternate pathway for breathing by creating a stoma in the trachea
Vocal cord stripping	Removal of outer layers of tissue on the vocal cords May be used for a biopsy or to treat some cancers confined to the vocal cords Rarely affects speech
Neck Dissection Surgery	
Modified radical neck dissection	Most common type of neck dissection Removal of all lymph nodes Less neck tissue removed than with radical dissection May spare the nerves in the neck and, sometimes, the blood vessels or muscle
Radical neck dissection	Removal of all the tissue on the side of the neck from the mandible to the clavicle Removes the muscle, nerve, salivary gland, major blood vessels
Selective neck dissection	If cancer has not spread far, fewer lymph nodes are removed May save muscle, nerve, blood vessels in the neck

Radiation Therapy

Radiation therapy is often preferred for patients with early head and neck cancer because it offers patients good results with voice preservation. Some patients refuse surgery for advanced lesions because of the extent of the procedure and potential risks involved. In this situation, radiation therapy is used as the sole treatment or in combination with chemotherapy. Other patients may opt for surgery and a combination of radiation and/or chemotherapy treatments.

Radiation therapy can be delivered by external-beam therapy or internal implants (brachytherapy). Brachytherapy delivers high doses of radiation to the target area while limiting the exposure of surrounding tissues. Thin, hollow, plastic needles are inserted into the tumor area, and radioactive seeds are placed in the needles. The seeds emit continuous radiation. Radiation therapy and brachytherapy are discussed in Chapter 16.

Chemotherapy and Targeted Therapy

Chemotherapy is used in combination with radiation therapy for patients with stage 3 or 4 head and neck cancers. Chemotherapy agents currently recommended are nivolumab, pembrolizumab (Keytruda), carboplatin, docetaxel (Taxotere), methotrexate sodium, and bleomycin.[18]

Cetuximab (Erbitux), a targeted therapy, is used with chemotherapy to treat patients with late-stage head and neck cancer. The drug targets epidermal growth factor receptor (EGFR), a specific protein within cancer cells, and stops the cells from growing. Targeted therapy is discussed in Chapter 16 and Table 16.12.

Nutrition Therapy

Many patients with head and neck cancer are malnourished even before treatment begins. Treatment modalities increase the risk for malnutrition. For example, after radical neck surgery, patients may be unable to consume nutrients orally because of swelling, the incisions, or difficulty with swallowing. Side effects from chemotherapy and radiation therapy can impair a patient's ability to maintain adequate nutrition. Painful oral mucositis often leads to breaks in treatment if a patient is relying on oral intake for nutrition. Antiemetics or analgesics given before meals can reduce nausea and mouth pain.

A thorough nutrition assessment and prophylactic placement of a gastrostomy tube in high-risk patients are vital to maintaining adequate nutrition. Enteral nutrition (EN) may be started before treatment to obtain and maintain optimal nutrition needed for tissue repair (see Chapter 44). Teach

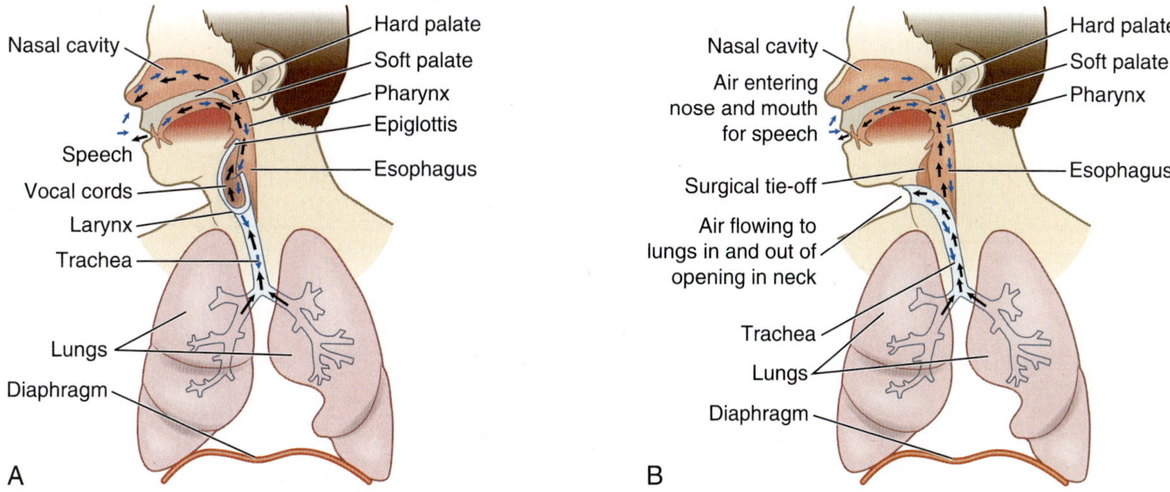

Fig. 29.3 Airflow in and out of the lungs (A) before and (B) after total laryngectomy. There is no anatomic connection between the nose, mouth, and throat. Inhaled and exhaled air enters the lungs through a surgically created stoma (hole) in the neck.

patients and caregivers about EN. Patients who are not candidates for or who refuse EN need to be monitored closely for weight loss.

Bland foods are easier for patients to tolerate. Patients can increase caloric intake by adding dry milk to foods during preparation, eating foods high in calories, and using oral supplements. It is helpful to add mild sauces and gravy to food. This adds calories and moistens food so that it is easier to swallow.

Expect swallowing problems when patients resume eating after surgery. The type and degree of difficulty vary depending on the surgery. A video-fluoroscopic swallowing study may evaluate the safety of swallowing after surgery. When patients can successfully swallow with low or no risk for aspiration, they may have small amounts of thickened liquids or pureed foods while in high-Fowler's position. Avoid thin, watery fluids because they are hard to swallow and increase the risk for aspiration. Closely monitor and observe for any signs or symptoms of respiratory distress and/or choking when eating resumes. Oral suctioning can help prevent aspiration.

Physical Therapy

After surgery for head and neck cancer, the physical therapist will help teach patients how to use the upper extremities to assist with support and movement of the head. In the immediate postoperative period, patients should begin an exercise program to maintain strength and movement in the shoulders and neck. Without exercise, patients may develop a "frozen" shoulder and limited range of neck motion. Patients should continue the exercise program after discharge to prevent future functional disabilities.

Speech Therapy

Before surgery, a speech therapist should meet with the patient and caregiver to discuss any effect that surgery will have on the voice and potential adaptations or voice restoration options. The International Association of Laryngectomees, a group for laryngectomy patients, focuses on helping patients reestablish speech. Local groups, such as "Lost Chord" or "New Voice," often have volunteers to visit patients before surgery.

We use 3 major approaches to restore oral communication: (1) electrolarynx, (2) tracheoesophageal puncture (TEP) voice restoration, and (3) esophageal speech. An *electrolarynx* is a hand-held, battery-powered device that creates speech with the use of sound waves (Fig. 29.4A). This option allows for speech immediately after surgery. It needs little maintenance and is easy to learn. The primary disadvantage is the mechanical sound quality, which many patients do not like.

In TEP, a fistula is created in the tracheoesophageal wall. It diverts pulmonary air across the pharyngoesophageal mucosa for phonation when the tracheostoma is occluded. A one-way prosthetic valve is placed in the tract. The valve prevents aspiration of food or saliva from the esophagus into the tracheostomy. To speak, the patient manually blocks the stoma with the finger. Air moves from the lungs, through the prosthesis, into the esophagus, and out the mouth. Speech is made by the air vibrating against the esophagus and is formed into words by moving the tongue and lips. A common voice prosthesis is the Blom-Singer prosthesis (Fig. 29.4B). TEP offers the best speech quality with the highest degree of patient satisfaction.

Esophageal speech depends on air entering the esophagus and then being expelled past the pharyngoesophageal segment, the vibratory source for sound production. Disadvantages of developing esophageal speech are the length of time needed to learn the technique and the reduction in voice quality.

❖ NURSING MANAGEMENT: HEAD AND NECK CANCER

◆ Assessment

Table 29.8 presents subjective and objective data to obtain from patients with head and neck cancer.

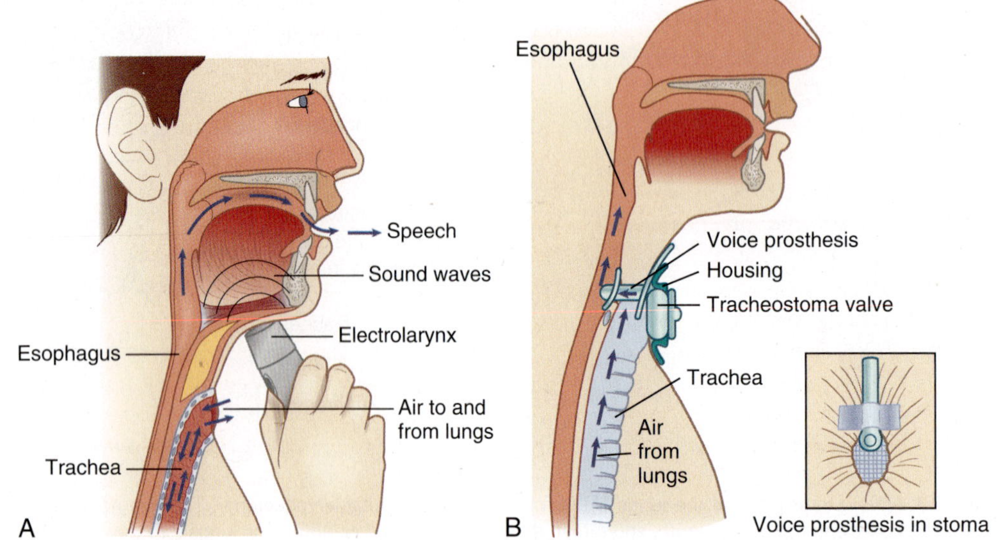

Fig. 29.4 (A) The sound waves created by the electrolarynx allow the person to speak. (B) The Blom-Singer voice prosthesis and valve.

◆ Clinical Problems

Clinical problems for patients with head and neck cancer include:

- Impaired respiratory function
- Risk for aspiration
- Difficulty coping
- Impaired communication

More information on clinical problems and the care of patients with head and neck cancer is presented in eNursing Care Plan 29.1 on the website for this chapter.

◆ Planning

The overall goals are that patients will have (1) a patent airway, (2) an acceptable body image, (3) no complications related to therapy, (4) adequate nutrition intake, (5) minimal pain, and (6) the ability to communicate.

◆ Implementation

Health Promotion

Many head and neck cancers can be prevented. Their development is closely related to personal habits, mainly tobacco use and excess alcohol use. Poor oral hygiene and HPV infection are also risk factors for head and neck cancer.

Include information about risk factors in health teaching. Encourage good oral hygiene. Teach patients about safe sex practices to prevent HPV infection (e.g., use condoms, encourage vaccination). When cancer has been diagnosed, tobacco and alcohol cessation are still important. The chance of a cure, by any treatment modality, for patients who continue to smoke and use alcohol is decreased. Also, the risk for a second

TABLE 29.8 NURSING ASSESSMENT

Head and Neck Cancer

Subjective Data

Important Health Information

- *Health history:* Positive family history; prolonged tobacco use (cigarettes, pipes, cigars, chewing tobacco, smokeless tobacco); prolonged, heavy alcohol use; poor intake of fruits and vegetables
- *Medications:* Prolonged use of over-the-counter medication for sore throat, decongestants

Functional Health Patterns

- *Health perception–health management:* Does not take part in preventive health measures, long history of alcohol and tobacco use
- *Nutritional-metabolic:* Mouth ulcer that does not heal, change in fit of dentures, change in appetite, sudden or unexplained weight loss, swallowing difficulty (e.g., sensation of a lump in throat, pain with swallowing, aspiration when swallowing)
- *Activity-exercise:* Fatigue with minimal exertion
- *Cognitive-perceptual:* Sore throat, pain on swallowing, referred ear pain

Objective Data

Respiratory

Hoarseness, change in voice quality, chronic laryngitis, nasal voice, palpable neck mass and lymph nodes (tender, hard, fixed), tracheal deviation; dyspnea, stridor (late sign)

Gastrointestinal

White (leukoplakia) or red (erythroplakia) patches inside mouth, ulceration of mucosa, asymmetric tongue, exudate in mouth or pharynx, mass or thickening of mucosa

Possible Diagnostic Findings

Mass on direct or indirect laryngoscopy; tumor on soft tissue x-ray, CT scan, or MRI; positive biopsy

primary cancer is significantly increased. Give patients information about smoking cessation and techniques for success. If needed, refer to an alcohol treatment program. Smoking and alcohol cessation are discussed in Chapter 11.

Acute Care

Preoperative care. Preparation is the same as for any major surgery. Assess understanding of the planned surgery and clarify information as needed. Teach patients and caregivers about the type of treatment, care needed, and reason for treatment and care. Tailor teaching to the planned surgery. For example, include information about expected changes in speech after a laryngectomy. Help prepare them to deal with the psychologic impact of the diagnosis of cancer, change in physical appearance, possible need for EN, and use of other communication methods because of loss of voice. Assess their support system. The patient may not have someone to help after discharge or may have a job that cannot be continued, leaving the patient unemployed.

Postoperative care. Immediately after surgery, nursing care priorities include airway management, wound care, nutrition, communication, and psychosocial issues related to body image changes. Maintaining a patent airway is essential. Inflammation in the surgical area may compress the trachea. Keep the patients in a semi-Fowler's position to decrease edema and limit tension on suture lines.

Give analgesic drugs as needed for pain control. Because patients may not be able to speak, have them nonverbally rate their pain (e.g., visual pain scale) to help assess the effectiveness of the medication. Pain management is discussed in Chapter 9. Monitor vital signs frequently. Be alert for hemorrhage, as many of the structures in the head and neck area are very vascular. Pay attention to heart rate, BP, SpO_2, and hemoglobin values.

Patients with a laryngectomy need frequent suctioning via the tracheostomy tube. Secretions typically change in amount and consistency over time. Patients may initially have a large amount of blood-tinged secretions that gradually diminish and thicken. Maintain adequate fluid intake (IV, enteral) and humidification of inspired gases to keep secretions liquid and mucous membranes moist. Encourage deep breathing and coughing.

Establish communication so that patients can share information about their basic needs. Alphabet boards, writing materials, pictorial guides, laptops, and hand signals are useful methods for communicating. Programmable speech-generating devices allow the use of recorded messages that are matched with a graphic representing each message.

Pressure dressings, packing, or drainage tubes may be present, depending on the surgery. Do not change any dressing unless you have a specific order from the HCP. Dressings are typically not present with skin flaps. This allows better visualization of the flap and avoids excess pressure on tissue. Initially, check skin flaps hourly for color and any change in size or edema. We may use Doppler ultrasound to determine the presence of a pulse, depending on the location of the skin flap.

Care for any wound drains that are in use. Drainage may be bloody at first. It should gradually decrease in volume and become more clear over 24 to 48 hours. Monitor patency of drainage tubes every hour in the first few hours after surgery, then every 4 hours to ensure proper functioning. If tubing becomes obstructed, fluid will accumulate under the skin flap. This predisposes patients to hematomas or seromas, impaired wound healing, and increased risk for infection. After removal of the drainage tubes, monitor for any swelling. Assess incision sites for signs of infection.

Patients may have a nasogastric (NG) tube inserted during surgery to remove gastric contents via intermittent suction for the first 24 to 48 hours until peristalsis returns. Because the NG tube lies close to internal incision lines, do not manipulate or move the tube. When bowel sounds return, start EN slowly and advance to meet nutrition needs.

Radiation therapy. Dry mouth *(xerostomia)*, a frequent and annoying problem, typically occurs within a few weeks of treatment. The saliva decreases in volume and becomes thick. This change may be temporary or permanent. Pilocarpine hydrochloride (Salagen) is often effective in increasing saliva production.

CHECK YOUR PRACTICE

Your 64-year-old male patient with oral cancer has been receiving radiation therapy for 3 weeks. He has developed xerostomia and oral mucositis. He asks if you have any suggestions to help relieve his symptoms.

- How would you respond?

Once patients can have foods or fluids by mouth, they can get symptom relief by increasing fluid intake, chewing sugarless gum or sugarless candy, using nonalcoholic mouth rinses (baking soda, glycerin solutions), and using artificial saliva. Teach them to carry a water bottle with them. Fluoride gels or treatments can help prevent dental deterioration caused by xerostomia.

Oral mucositis can cause irritation, ulceration, and pain. Teach patients oral care basics, including the use of a soft toothbrush and regular flossing. Patients can wear empty fluoride gel trays, bite blocks, athletic mouth guards, or gauze pads during radiation treatments. This prevents radiation scatter to the tongue and cheek from metal work in the mouth. Warm bland rinses, like those with salt and baking soda, 4 to 6 times daily may be helpful. Sucking on ice chips can help with the pain. Patients should avoid commercial mouthwashes and hot, spicy, or acidic foods because they are irritating.

Skin over the irradiated area often becomes reddened and sensitive to touch. Teach patients to use only prescribed lotions and skin products while undergoing radiation therapy and to not use any lotions within 2 hours before treatment. Skin care for patients having radiation therapy is discussed in Chapter 16.

Fatigue is a common side effect of radiation therapy and chemotherapy. Encourage patients to walk 15 to 30 minutes each day because regular exercise can give them more energy. Teach patients to do activities that are most important to them and to rest during periods of low energy. Identify support systems. Encourage patients to ask for help.

Chronic Care

Patients may be discharged with a tracheostomy and an NG or gastrostomy feeding tube. Some may need a home health care referral and assessment to evaluate the patient's ability to perform self-care activities. Teach them how to manage tubes and whom to call if there are problems. Provide pictorial instructions for tracheostomy care, suctioning, stoma, and skin care, and EN as appropriate. Encouraging patients to take part in self-care is an important part of rehabilitation.

Teach patients the importance of wearing a Medic Alert bracelet or other identification that alerts emergency personnel of the possible changes in breathing status because of surgery. Because patients no longer breathe through the nose, they often lose the ability to smell smoke. Have them install smoke and carbon monoxide detectors in the home. The loss of smell and radiation therapy may lead to decreased taste. Encourage eating food that is colorful, attractive, and nutritious. Refer to a dietitian as needed. Patients can resume exercise, recreation, and sexual activity when able. Most can return to work 1 to 2 months after surgery.

Stoma care. If patients have a stoma after surgery, teach them stoma care (see Chapter 28). Patients should wash the area around the stoma daily with a moist cloth. A nasal wash spray is used every 1 to 2 hours to keep the stoma moist and prevent crusting. Dried secretions can be removed with tweezers. If a laryngectomy tube is in place, remove the entire tube at least daily and clean it in the same manner as a tracheostomy tube. The inner cannula may have to be removed and cleaned more often. A scarf or loose shirt can hide the stoma.

Patients should cover the stoma when coughing (because mucus may be expectorated) and during any activity (e.g., shaving, applying makeup) that may lead to inhalation of foreign materials. Because water can easily enter the stoma, have them wear a plastic collar when taking a shower. Swimming is contraindicated. Humidification is given with mechanical ventilation or after extubation with a tracheostomy mask. After discharge, patients can use a bedside humidifier.

Psychosocial needs. Psychosocial care is of utmost importance. Issues concerning depression, change in body image, and sexuality are common. Although we discuss changes before surgery, patients may not be psychologically prepared for the extent of these changes. If the patient has a significant other, this person's reaction to the altered appearance is important. Acceptance by another person can promote an improved self-image.

Depression may occur for many reasons: inability to speak because of the surgery and/or presence of a tracheostomy tube, altered physical appearance, edema, loss of independence and reliance on others, and feelings of helplessness and hopelessness. Depression also may be related to concern about the prognosis.

Allow patients and caregivers to express their feelings and emotions. Convey acceptance to help patients regain positive feelings about their body image and self-concept. Encourage participation in support groups. Provide information about groups available through the local branch of the American Cancer Society. Provide a psychiatric referral for patients who have prolonged or severe depression.

Xerostomia and fatigue can physically affect sexuality. It may be hard for patients to talk about sexual problems because of changes in communication. Help the patient and partner by allowing them to talk about their sexuality and how surgery and treatment may affect their relationship. Helping them see that sexuality involves much more than appearance may relieve some anxiety.

However, many never return to a full-time job. The changes that follow a total laryngectomy can be upsetting. Loss of speech, loss of the ability to taste and smell, inability to make audible sounds (including laughing and weeping), and the presence of a permanent tracheal stoma that produces undesirable mucus are often overwhelming to patients.

◆ Evaluation

Expected outcomes for patients with head and neck cancer who are treated surgically are that patients will:

- Have effective coughing and secretion clearance
- Swallow oral foods without aspiration
- Use effective coping strategies
- Use effective communication techniques

CASE STUDY

Laryngeal Cancer

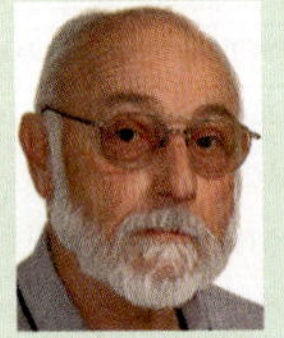

(© iStockphoto/ Thinkstoc.)

Patient Profile

M.R., a 69-year-old retired baker, is on your medical floor with influenza. He told his HCP that he has "a cough that just won't go away," difficulty swallowing, and "a sore throat that really hasn't gotten better" over the past year. His wife passed away 6 years ago. He has 3 adult children. One daughter lives in the same city. He has a history of hypertension, smoking, alcohol use, gastroesophageal reflux disease (GERD), and type 2 diabetes.

Subjective Data

- States that his symptoms worsened in the past 3 months
- Has used various cough and cold remedies over the past 6 months to relieve symptoms without relief
- Has lost weight because of decreased appetite and difficulty swallowing
- Has smoked 3 packs of cigarettes a day for the past 50 years
- Consumes 4 to 6 cans of beer a day

Objective Data

Physical Assessment

- Temp 102.4°F (39.1°C), heart rate 99 beats/min, BP 176/84 mm Hg
- Respiratory rate 24 breaths/min; respirations short, shallow, slightly labored; SpO_2 87% on room air
- Awake and alert
- Appears gray, malnourished, dehydrated
- Small, irregular white patches on the sides of oral cavity
- Enlarged cervical nodes bilaterally, nontender
- Lung sounds diminished at bases with occasional fine crackles on expiration

Diagnostic Studies

- Chest x-ray: lung fields clear
- Laryngoscopy: mass in subglottic area (requires further evaluation)
- CT scan: subglottic lesion with lymph node involvement
- Diagnosis: laryngeal cancer

Continued

CASE STUDY—cont'd

Interprofessional Care

- Scheduled for a total laryngectomy with radiation and chemotherapy after surgery
- Percutaneous gastrostomy tube preoperatively for EN

Discussion Questions

1. ***Recognize:*** What assessment information suggests M.R. was at risk for laryngeal cancer?
2. ***Analyze:*** What factors may affect wound healing after surgery?
3. ***Prioritize:*** What are your priority teaching strategies before his total laryngectomy?
4. ***Act:*** How would you explain the gastrostomy tube to M.R.?

Case Progression

M.R. is transferred to the clinical unit after 24 hours in the ICU. He is awake, alert, but slightly confused. His BP is 168/94 mm Hg. A tracheostomy tube is in place with O_2 via tracheal mask. Enteral feeding transfusing at 30 mL/h via gastrostomy tube. The indwelling catheter is patent and draining a moderate amount of amber urine. M.R. is picking at his surgical drains. When you try to reassure him, he just starts waving his hands at you.

5. ***Analyze:*** What information would you want to know from the ICU nurse who transported M.R. to the clinical unit?
6. ***Prioritize:*** Based on the assessment data, what are your priority clinical problems?
7. ***Plan:*** How would you plan to meet M.R.'s communication needs during the first few postoperative days?
8. ***Act:*** Four hours after transfer to the clinical unit, M.R. is tearful and is staring at the wall. What would you do?
9. ***Act:*** What teaching does M.R. need to help him assume self-care after his surgery?
10. ***Safety:*** What precautions should he take because of his stoma?

Answers available at http://evolve.elsevier.com/Lewis/medsurg.

BRIDGE TO NCLEX EXAMINATION

The number of the question corresponds to the same-numbered outcome at the beginning of the chapter.

1. A patient with allergic rhinitis reports severe nasal congestion; sneezing; and watery, itchy eyes and nose at various times of the year. When teaching patients how to control these symptoms, the nurse teaches patients to
  a. avoid all intranasal sprays and oral antihistamines.
  b. limit the usage of nasal decongestant spray to 10 days.
  c. use oral decongestants at bedtime to prevent symptoms during the night.
  d. keep a diary of when the allergic reaction occurs and what precipitates it.

2. A patient is seen at the clinic with fever, muscle aches, sore throat with yellowish exudate, and headache. The nurse anticipates that their care will include (**Select all that apply.**)
  a. providing antipyretic for fever
  b. immediate treatment with antibiotics.
  c. a throat culture or rapid strep antigen test.
  d. supportive care, including cool, bland liquids.
  e. comprehensive history to determine possible cause.

3. A 19-year-old patient arrives at the clinic with a sore throat and fever of 102.4°F (39.1°C). Assessment findings include enlarged anterior cervical lymph nodes and exudate at the back of the throat. What is the priority nursing action?
  a. Administer morphine 1 mg IV for pain.
  b. Administer acetaminophen for pain and fever.
  c. Increase hydration by providing oral and IV fluids.
  d. Document the assessment findings in the nursing notes.

4. When planning health care teaching to prevent or detect early head and neck cancer, which people would be the *priority* to target? (**Select all that apply.**)
  a. 65-year-old male who has used chewing tobacco most of his life
  b. 45-year-old rancher who uses chewing tobacco while driving his herds of cattle
  c. 21-year-old college student who drinks beer on weekends with his fraternity brothers
  d. 78-year-old female who has been drinking liquor since her husband died 15 years ago
  e. 22-year-old female who has been diagnosed with human papillomavirus of the cervix

5. While in the recovery room, a patient with a total laryngectomy is suctioned and has bloody mucus with some clots. Which nursing interventions would apply? (**Select all that apply.**)
  a. Notify the health care provider at once.
  b. Place the patient in semi-Fowler's position.
  c. Use a bag-valve-mask (BVM) and begin rescue breathing.
  d. Instill 10 mL of normal saline into the tracheostomy tube to loosen secretions.
  e. Continue assessment, including O_2 saturation, respiratory rate, and breath sounds.

6. Discharge teaching for patients after surgery for head and neck cancer would include (**Select all that apply.**)
  a. encouraging regular exercise such as swimming.
  b. washing around the stoma daily with a moist washcloth.
  c. encouraging participation in a postlaryngectomy support group.
  d. providing pictures and "hands-on" instruction for tracheostomy care.
  e. teaching how to hold breath and trying to gag to promote swallowing reflex.

1. d; 2. a, c, d, e; 3. b; 4. a, b, d, e; 5. b, e; 6. b, c, d.

For rationales to these answers and even more NCLEX review questions, visit http://evolve.elsevier.com/Lewis/medsurg.

REFERENCES

To access the References for this chapter, please scan the QR code with a mobile device.

30

Lower Respiratory Problems

Eugene E. Mondor

http://evolve.elsevier.com/Lewis/medsurg/

CONCEPTUAL FOCUS

Cellular Regulation
Clotting
Functional Ability
Gas Exchange
Infection

LEARNING OUTCOMES

1. Compare the clinical manifestations and nursing and interprofessional management of patients with acute bronchitis and pertussis.
2. Distinguish among the types of pneumonia and their etiology and pathophysiology.
3. Describe the clinical manifestations, diagnostic studies, and interprofessional and nursing management of patients with pneumonia.
4. Explain the pathophysiology, clinical manifestations, complications, diagnostic studies, and interprofessional and nursing management of patients with tuberculosis.
5. Describe the pathophysiology, clinical manifestations, and nursing and interprofessional management of patients with a lung abscess.
6. Identify the etiology, clinical manifestations, and nursing and interprofessional management of patients with a pleural effusion.
7. Compare the pathophysiology, clinical manifestations, and nursing and interprofessional management of fractured ribs, flail chest, and pneumothorax.
8. Describe the pathophysiology, clinical manifestations, and nursing and interprofessional management of pulmonary embolism, pulmonary hypertension, and cor pulmonale.
9. Identify the causative factors, clinical manifestations, and nursing and interprofessional management of patients with environment lung diseases.
10. Describe disorders in which a lung transplant is a treatment option, explaining the nursing and interprofessional management of the transplant recipient.
11. Explain the etiology, risk factors, pathophysiology, clinical manifestations, and interprofessional and nursing management of patients with lung cancer.

KEY TERMS

acute bronchitis
community-acquired pneumonia (CAP)
cor pulmonale
empyema
flail chest
hemothorax
hospital-acquired pneumonia (HAP)
lung abscess
pertussis
pleural effusion
pleurisy (pleuritis)
pneumoconiosis
pneumonia
pneumothorax
pulmonary arterial hypertension
pulmonary edema
pulmonary embolism (PE)
tension pneumothorax
tuberculosis (TB)

A variety of problems can affect the lower respiratory system. This chapter discusses lower respiratory tract diseases that influence gas exchange. We focus on infectious, restrictive, traumatic, vascular, environment, and oncologic problems. Left untreated, many of these problems will have profound and possibly life-threatening consequences, as oxygenation and ventilation are both essential for life.

LOWER RESPIRATORY TRACT INFECTIONS

Lower respiratory tract infection is a common and serious problem. It is the reason for thousands of clinic and emergency department visits and hospital admissions each year. In the United States in 2023, pneumonia and influenza caused around 42,000 deaths.[1]

ACUTE BRONCHITIS

Acute bronchitis is a self-limiting inflammation of the bronchi in the lower respiratory tract. Viruses cause most acute bronchial infections. Air pollution, dust, chemical inhalation, smoking, chronic sinusitis, and asthma are other triggers.

Cough is the most common symptom. It may last for up to 3 weeks and be more frequent at night. When present, sputum is often clear, although some patients have purulent sputum. Other symptoms may include headache, fever, malaise, hoarseness, myalgias, dyspnea, and chest pain.

Diagnosis is based on the assessment. Assessment may reveal normal breath sounds or crackles or wheezes, usually on expiration and with exertion. Chest x-rays are normal and not needed unless we suspect pneumonia or some other lung problem.

The goal of care is to relieve symptoms and prevent pneumonia. Treatment is supportive. It includes cough suppressants (e.g., dextromethorphan), encouraging oral fluid intake, and using a humidifier. Throat lozenges, hot tea, and honey may help relieve cough. β_2-Agonist (bronchodilator) inhalers are useful for patients with wheezes or underlying lung problems. Antibiotics may be given to patients with underlying chronic conditions who are at risk for or have a prolonged infection with systemic symptoms. If acute bronchitis is due to influenza, we may start treatment with antiviral drugs.

Encourage patients to not smoke, avoid secondhand smoke, and wash their hands often (Box 30.1). If patients with acute bronchitis develop a fever, have trouble breathing, or have symptoms that last longer than 4 weeks, they should see their HCP.

PERTUSSIS

Pertussis is a highly contagious respiratory infection. It is caused by the gram-negative bacillus *Bordetella pertussis.* The bacteria attach to the cilia of the respiratory tract and release toxins that damage the cilia, causing inflammation and swelling. Cases of pertussis have been steadily increasing in the United States since the 1980s.[2] The largest increase is in teens and adults. We think that immunity from childhood tetanus, diphtheria, and pertussis vaccine (Tdap) vaccination may decrease over time, allowing a milder (but still contagious) infection to occur. The Centers for Disease Control and Prevention (CDC) currently recommends that all adolescents (11 years and older) and adults who have not received a dose of Tdap receive a 1-time vaccination as soon as possible.[3]

Manifestations of pertussis occur in stages. The 1st stage, lasting 1 to 2 weeks, manifests as a mild upper respiratory tract infection (URI) with a low-grade or no fever, runny nose, watery eyes, malaise, and mild, nonproductive cough. The 2nd stage, from the 2nd to 10th weeks of infection, is characterized by paroxysms of cough. The last stage lasts 2 to 3 weeks. The cough is less severe. The patient may still be weak.

The hallmark characteristic of pertussis is uncontrollable, violent coughing. Inspiration after each cough produces the typical "whooping" sound as patients try to breathe in air against an obstructed glottis. The "whoop" is often not present in teens and adults, especially those who are vaccinated. Coughing is more frequent at night. Vomiting may occur with coughing. The cough may last from 6 to 10 weeks.

In the community, diagnosis is mainly by history and assessment. In the acute care setting, the CDC recommends nasopharyngeal cultures, polymerase chain reaction (PCR) of nasopharyngeal secretions, or serology testing.[4] The treatment is macrolide (erythromycin, azithromycin) antibiotics to minimize symptoms and prevent disease spread (see Table 15.8). Patients who cannot take macrolides are given trimethoprim/sulfamethoxazole.

Patients are infectious from the beginning of the 1st stage through the 3rd week after onset of symptoms or until 5 days after starting antibiotic therapy. Place hospitalized patients on droplet precautions. Patients should not use cough suppressants, bronchodilators, or antihistamines as they are ineffective and may worsen coughing. The CDC recommends antibiotic therapy for those who had close contact with the patient.

BOX 30.1 PROMOTING POPULATION HEALTH

Preventing Respiratory Diseases

- Wash hands often to prevent and avoid spreading infections.
- Get Tdap, pneumococcal, COVID, and flu vaccines as directed by the HCP.
- Avoid smoking and exposure to second-hand and environment smoke.
- Wear proper personal protective equipment (PPE) when working in an occupation with prolonged exposure to dust, fumes, or gases.
- Avoid exposure to allergens, indoor pollutants, and air pollutants.

PNEUMONIA

Pneumonia is an acute infection of the lung parenchyma. Despite progress in antibiotic therapy to treat pneumonia, pneumonia still has significant morbidity and mortality. Pneumonia and lower respiratory tract infections were the 4th leading cause of death worldwide in 2019.[5]

Etiology

Normally, various defense mechanisms protect the airway distal to the larynx from infection. Mechanisms that create a mechanical barrier to prevent microorganisms from entering the tracheobronchial tree include air filtration, epiglottis closure over the trachea, cough reflex, mucociliary clearance, and reflex

TABLE 30.1 Risk Factors for Pneumonia

- Abdominal or chest surgery
- Age >65 years
- Air pollution
- Altered level of consciousness (e.g., head injury, seizures, anesthesia, drug overdose, stroke)
- Bed rest, prolonged immobility
- Chronic diseases: chronic lung and liver disease, asthma, diabetes, heart disease, cancer, chronic kidney disease
- Debilitating illness
- Enteral feedings via nasogastric or orogastric tubes
- Exposure to bats, birds, rabbits, and farm animal feces
- Immunosuppressive conditions and/or therapy (e.g., corticosteroids, chemotherapy, HIV infection, immunosuppressive therapy)
- Inhalation or aspiration of noxious substances
- IV drug use
- Malnutrition
- Resident of a long-term care facility
- Smoking
- Tracheal intubation (endotracheal intubation, tracheostomy)
- URI

bronchoconstriction. Immune defense mechanisms include secretion of immunoglobulins A and G and alveolar macrophages.

Pneumonia is more likely to occur when defense mechanisms become incompetent or are overwhelmed by the virulence or quantity of infectious agents. A weakened cough or epiglottal reflex may allow aspiration of oropharyngeal contents into the lungs. Tracheal intubation bypasses normal filtration processes and interferes with the cough reflex and mucociliary clearance. Air pollution, smoking, viral URIs, and normal changes that occur with aging can impair mucociliary clearance. Chronic diseases can suppress the immune system's ability to inhibit bacterial growth. Risk factors for pneumonia are listed in Table 30.1.

Pathogens that cause pneumonia reach the lung in 3 ways:

1. *Aspiration* of normal flora from the nasopharynx or oropharynx. Many organisms that cause pneumonia are normal inhabitants of the mouth and pharynx in healthy adults.
2. *Inhalation* of microbes present in the air. Examples include *Mycoplasma pneumoniae* and fungal pneumonias.
3. *Hematogenous spread* from a primary infection elsewhere in the body. One example is *Staphylococcus aureus* from infective endocarditis.

Classifications of Pneumonia

There is no universally accepted classification system for pneumonia. Some classify pneumonia by the causative pathogens (e.g., bacterial, viral, fungal), disease characteristics, or appearance on chest x-ray. The most widely used way to classify pneumonia is as either *community-acquired* or *hospital-acquired* pneumonia. This classification helps the HCP identify the most likely cause (Table 30.2) and choice of antimicrobial therapy.

TABLE 30.2 Organisms Causing Pneumonia

Community-Acquired Pneumonia (CAP)

Typical

- *Escherichia coli*
- *Haemophilus influenzae*[a]
- *Klebsiella pneumoniae*[a]
- Methicillin-resistant *Staphylococcus aureus* (MRSA)
- *Moraxella catarrhalis*
- *Staphylococcus aureus*[a]
- *Streptococcus pneumoniae*[a]

Atypical

- *Chlamydophila pneumoniae*
- *Coxiella burnettii*
- *Legionella pneumophilia*
- *Mycoplasma pneumoniae*
- *Mycobacterium tuberculosis*

Respiratory Viruses

- Adenoviruses
- Influenza A and B
- Parainfluenza virus
- Respiratory syncytial virus
- Rhinovirus
- Severe acute respiratory syndrome coronavirus—2 (SARS-CoV-2)

Other Causes of CAP

- Fungi
- Oral anaerobes

Hospital-Acquired Pneumonia (HAP)

- Acinetobacter[b]
- Enterobacter
- *Escherichia coli*[b]
- *Haemophilus influenzae*
- *Klebsiella pneumoniae*[b]
- Microaspiration of bacteria that colonize the mouth, oropharynx
- *Pseudomonas aeruginosa*[b]
- *Proteus* species
- *Serratia marcescens*
- *Staphylococcus aureus* (both methicillin-resistant and methicillin-sensitive)

[a]Most common causes of CAP.
[b]Most common causes of HAP.

Community-Acquired Pneumonia

Community-acquired pneumonia (CAP) is an acute lung infection that occurs in patients who have not been hospitalized or lived in a long-term care facility within 14 days of symptom onset. The decision to treat the patient at home or admit to a hospital is based on several factors. These include the patient's age, vital signs, mental status, comorbid conditions, and overall condition. We can use various tools (Table 30.3) to support clinical judgment.

TABLE 30.3 Pneumonia Severity Index (PSI)

The PSI can supplement clinical judgment to determine the severity of pneumonia and whether patients need to be hospitalized.

DEMOGRAPHICS/INFORMATION

Factor	Points	
Age (in years)	For each year, score 1 point (e.g., 65 years = 65 points)	
	Yes	**No**
Women	10	0
Extended care resident	10	0
Associated Conditions and/or Illnesses		
Heart failure	10	0
Cardiovascular disease	10	0
Kidney disease	10	0
Active cancer	30	0
Liver disease	20	0
Assessment Findings		
Altered mental status	20	0
Respiratory rate ≥30/min	20	0
BP <90 mm Hg	20	0
Pulse >125/min	10	0
Temperature <95°F (35°C) or ≥103.8°F (40°C)	15	0
Diagnostics and Lab Results		
Pleural effusion	10	0
pH <7.35	30	0
BUN ≥30 mg/dL (11 mmol/L)	20	0
Sodium <130 mEq/L	20	0
Glucose >250 mg/dL (14 mmol/L)	10	0
Hematocrit <30%	10	0
PaO_2 <60 mm Hg or SpO_2 <90%	10	0

SCORING

Points	Class	Risk	Associated Mortality
50 or less	I	Low	0.1%
51–70	II	Low	0.6%
71–91	III	Low	0.9%
91–130	IV	Moderate	9.3%
131–395	V	High	27%

Hospital-Acquired Pneumonia

Hospital-acquired pneumonia (HAP) is pneumonia in non-intubated patients that begins 48 hours or longer after admission to hospital and was not present when they were admitted. *Ventilator-associated pneumonia (VAP),* a type of HAP, refers to pneumonia that occurs more than 48 hours after endotracheal intubation.[6] VAP is discussed in Chapter 28. Both HAP and VAP are associated with longer hospital stays, increased costs, and increased mortality.

Types of Pneumonia

There are several types of pneumonia. *Viral pneumonia* is the most common type. It occurs in one-third of all pneumonia cases. It may be mild and self-limiting or cause potentially life-threatening problems, such as acute respiratory failure (ARF) in influenza. Patients with *bacterial pneumonia* may be extremely ill and need hospital admission. *Mycoplasma pneumonia,* which has traits of both bacteria and viruses, is often called "atypical" pneumonia. It is mild and often occurs in people younger than 40 years of age.

Aspiration Pneumonia

Aspiration pneumonia results from the abnormal entry of material from the mouth or stomach into the trachea and lungs. Conditions that increase aspiration risk include decreased level of consciousness (e.g., seizure, anesthesia, head injury, stroke, opioid overdose), swallowing problems, and having a nasogastric (NG) tube with or without enteral feeding. With loss of consciousness, the gag and cough reflexes are depressed, making aspiration more likely.

The aspirated material (food, water, vomitus, oropharyngeal secretions) triggers an inflammatory response. The most common form of aspiration pneumonia is a bacterial infection. The sputum culture often shows more than 1 organism, including aerobes and anaerobes, since they both make up the flora of the oropharynx.

Until cultures are done and results obtained, antibiotic therapy is based on an assessment of probable cause, severity of illness, and patient factors (e.g., malnutrition, current antibiotic therapy). For patients who aspirate in hospitals, antibiotic coverage should include both gram-negative organisms and methicillin-resistant *Staphylococcus aureus* (MRSA). Aspiration of acidic gastric contents can cause *chemical (noninfectious) pneumonitis,* which may not need antibiotic therapy. However, secondary bacterial infection can occur in these patients 48 to 72 hours later.

Necrotizing Pneumonia

Necrotizing pneumonia is a rare complication of bacterial lung infection. It causes the lung tissue to turn into a thick, liquid mass. Cavitation and lung abscesses can occur. This sometimes happens with CAP. We do not know the exact mechanisms involved. Common causative organisms include *Staphylococcus, Klebsiella,* and *Streptococcus.* Signs and symptoms include respiratory insufficiency and/or failure, leukocytosis, and abnormalities on chest imaging. Treatment includes long-term antibiotic therapy and possible surgery.

Opportunistic Pneumonia

Opportunistic pneumonia is infection of the lower respiratory tract in immunocompromised patients. Persons most at risk are those with altered immune responses. This includes people with severe malnutrition, immunodeficiency (e.g., HIV infection), and those receiving radiation therapy, chemotherapy, and immunosuppressive therapy. The immunocompromised person may develop infection from organisms that do not normally cause disease, such as *Pneumocystis jiroveci* pneumonia (PJP) or cytomegalovirus (CMV).

PJP is occurring with greater frequency in HIV-negative, immunocompromised persons. The onset is slow and subtle. Symptoms include fever, tachypnea, tachycardia, dyspnea, nonproductive cough, and hypoxemia. The chest x-ray usually shows diffuse bilateral infiltrates. In widespread disease, the lungs have massive *consolidation* (fluid accumulation).

PJP can be life-threatening, causing ARF and death. Infection can spread to other organs, including the liver, bone marrow, lymph nodes, spleen, and thyroid. Although the causative agent is fungal, PJP does not respond to antifungal agents. Treatment consists of IV or oral trimethoprim/sulfamethoxazole, depending on the severity of disease, overall clinical condition, and the patient's response.

CMV, a herpes virus, can cause viral pneumonia. Most CMV infections are asymptomatic or mild. Severe disease can occur in people with an impaired immune response. CMV is one of the most important life-threatening complications after hematopoietic stem cell transplant.[7] Antiviral medications (e.g., ganciclovir) and high-dose immunoglobulin are part of treatment.

Pathophysiology

Pathophysiologic changes related to pneumonia vary depending on the offending pathogen. Almost all pathogens trigger an inflammatory response in the lungs (Fig. 30.1). Inflammation, characterized by an increase in blood flow and vascular permeability, activates neutrophils to engulf and kill the offending pathogens. As a result, the inflammation attracts more neutrophils. Airway edema occurs, and fluid leaks from the capillaries and tissues into alveoli. Normal O_2 transport is affected, leading to manifestations of hypoxia (e.g., tachypnea, dyspnea, tachycardia).

Atelectasis, the absence of gas or air in 1 or more areas of the lung, may occur with pneumonia. *Consolidation* occurs when the normally air-filled alveoli become filled with water, fluid, and/or debris (Fig. 30.2). This can partially obstruct airflow, impair gas exchange, and cause significant increased work of breathing. Over time and with appropriate antibiotic therapy, macrophages lyse and remove the debris. This allows lung tissue to recover and gas exchange to return to normal.

Clinical Manifestations

The most common presenting symptoms are cough, fever, chills, dyspnea, tachypnea, and pleuritic chest pain. The cough may or may not be productive. Sputum may be green, yellow, or even rust colored (bloody). Viral pneumonia initially appears with cough, sore throat, and headache, with worsening respiratory symptoms 12 to 36 hours after onset.

Older or debilitated patients may not have classic symptoms of pneumonia. Confusion or stupor (possibly related to hypoxia) may be the only finding. The older adult may have hypothermia, rather than fever. Nonspecific manifestations include diaphoresis, anorexia, fatigue, myalgias, and headache.

There may be fine or coarse crackles over the affected region. If consolidation is present, bronchial breath sounds, egophony (an increase in the sound of the patient's voice), and increased fremitus (chest wall vibrations made by vocalization) may be present. Patients with pleural effusion may have dullness to percussion over the affected area.

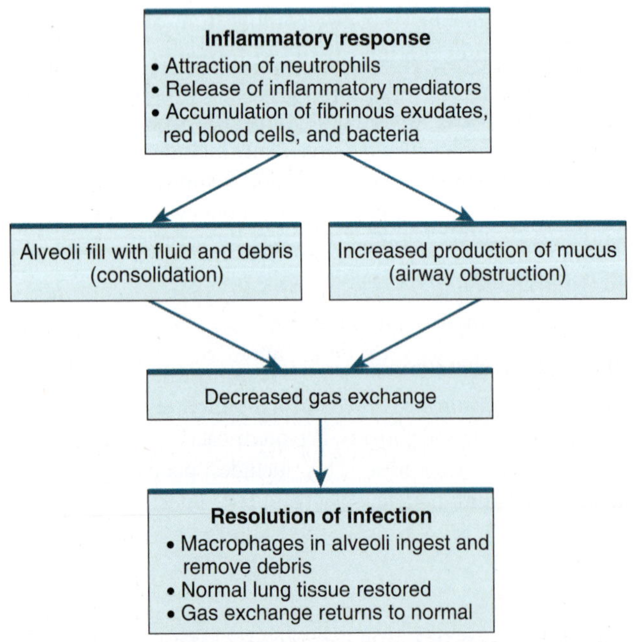

Fig. 30.1 Pathophysiology of pneumonia.

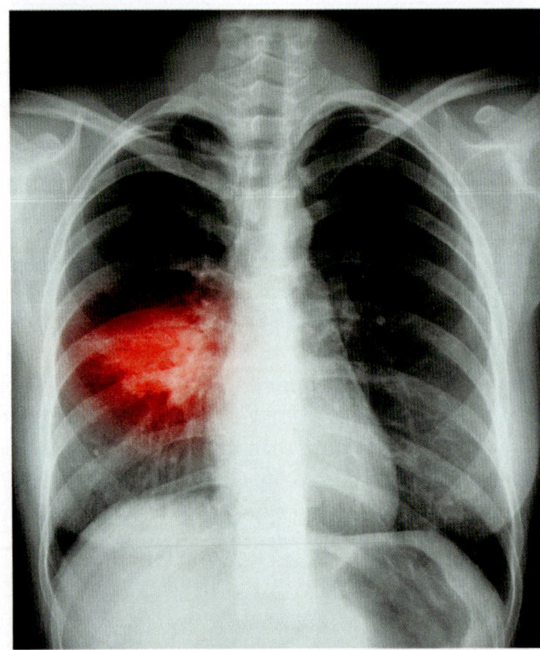

Fig. 30.2 Chest x-ray of a patient with acute bacterial pneumonia. (© iStock.com/stockdevil.)

Complications

A major problem today is pneumonia caused by multidrug-resistant (MDR) pathogens. Common culprits include MRSA and gram-negative bacilli. Risk factors for MDR pneumonia include advanced age, immunosuppression, history of antibiotic use, and prolonged mechanical ventilation.[8] Antibiotic susceptibility tests can help identify MDR pathogens. The virulence of MDR pathogens can severely limit options for antimicrobial therapy. MDR pathogens increase mortality from pneumonia.

Other complications from pneumonia develop more often in older adults and those with underlying chronic diseases. These can include:

- *Pleurisy,* inflammation of the pleura.
- *Pleural effusion,* or fluid in the pleural space. In most cases, the effusion is sterile and reabsorbed in 1 to 2 weeks. Sometimes, effusions require aspiration by thoracentesis.
- *Bacteremia,* bacterial infection in the blood. It is more likely to occur in infections with *Streptococcus pneumoniae* and *Haemophilus influenzae.*
- *Pneumothorax* occurs when air collects in the pleural space, causing the lungs to collapse.
- *ARF* is a leading cause of death in patients with severe pneumonia. ARF occurs when pneumonia damages the lungs' ability to exchange O_2 and CO_2 across the alveolar-capillary membrane.
- *Sepsis* can occur when bacteria within alveoli enter the bloodstream. Severe sepsis can lead to shock and multisystem organ dysfunction syndrome (MODS) (see Chapter 42).

Lung abscess is not a common complication of pneumonia. It may occur with pneumonia caused by *S. aureus* and gram-negative organisms. *Empyema,* the accumulation of purulent exudate in the pleural cavity, occurs in up to 20% of cases. It requires antibiotic therapy and drainage of the exudate by a chest tube or surgery. Pleurisy, pleural effusion, and lung abscess are discussed later in this chapter.

Diagnostic Studies

The common diagnostic studies are outlined in Table 30.4. History, physical assessment, and chest x-ray often give enough information to make decisions about early treatment. Chest x-ray often shows patterns characteristic of the infecting pathogen and is important in diagnosing pneumonia. X-ray may show pleural effusions. Bronchoscopy with bronchial washings or thoracentesis may be done to obtain cell and fluid samples from patients not responding to initial therapy.

Arterial blood gases (ABGs) may show hypoxemia, hypercapnia, and/or acid-base imbalance. Leukocytosis occurs in most patients with bacterial pneumonia. The white blood cell (WBC) count is usually greater than 15,000/μL (15×10^9/L) with the presence of bands (immature neutrophils). Ideally, we should obtain a sputum specimen for culture and Gram stain to identify the organism before starting antibiotic therapy. However, we should not delay starting antibiotic therapy if we cannot obtain a specimen. Delays in antibiotic therapy can increase mortality. Blood cultures are done for patients who are seriously ill.

TABLE 30.4 Interprofessional Care

Pneumonia

Diagnostic Assessment

- History and physical assessment
- Chest x-ray
- Sputum: Gram stain, culture and sensitivity test
- Pulse oximetry and/or ABGs
- CBC, white blood cell differential, and routine blood chemistries
- Blood cultures (if indicated)

Management

- O_2 therapy with mechanical ventilation (as needed)
- IV fluids, increased fluid intake (at least 2–3 L/day)
- VTE prophylaxis
- Physiotherapy, early mobility
- Balance between activity and rest

Drug Therapy

- Antibiotic therapy (see Table 15.8)
- Antipyretics (see Table 12.5)
- Analgesics

Interprofessional Care

Once the diagnosis of pneumonia is made, we start treatment based on risk factors, underlying medical conditions, assessment findings, most likely causative pathogen, and risk for MDR infection. *Empiric antibiotic therapy,* the initiation of treatment before a definitive diagnosis or causative agent is made, should be started as soon as pneumonia is suspected. It is based on the drugs known to be effective for the most likely cause. Antibiotic therapy is adjusted after sputum cultures identify the exact pathogen causing the infection.

Antibiotics are highly effective for both bacterial and mycoplasma pneumonia. In uncomplicated cases, patients should respond to drug therapy within 48 to 72 hours. Signs of improvement include decreased temperature, improved breathing, and less chest discomfort. Patients who do not respond to therapy or deteriorate need evaluation for noninfectious causes, complications, coexisting infectious processes, or pneumonia caused by an MDR pathogen.

Although cough suppressants, mucolytics, bronchodilators, and corticosteroids are often prescribed as adjunctive therapy, the use of these drugs is debatable. However, they may be prescribed for patients with underlying chronic conditions.

Currently, there is no definitive treatment for most viral pneumonias. Care is generally supportive. In most cases, viral pneumonia is self-limiting and will often resolve in 3 to 4 days. Antiviral therapy may be used to treat pneumonia caused by influenza (e.g., oseltamivir, zanamivir) or a few other viruses (e.g., acyclovir for herpes simplex virus).

Drug Therapy

The HCP selects empiric therapy based on the likely pathogen. Table 30.5 presents the drug therapy for bacterial CAP. Multiple regimens exist. All treatment should initially include antibiotics that are effective against both resistant gram-negative and resistant gram-positive organisms.

We switch patients from IV to oral antibiotic therapy as soon as they are improving clinically and able to take oral medication. Stable patients can be discharged on oral antibiotics. Total treatment time for patients with CAP should be a minimum of 5 days. Patients should be afebrile for 48 to 72 hours before stopping treatment. Longer treatment time may be needed if initial therapy was not active against the identified pathogen or complications occurred.

Clinical Problems

Clinical problems for patients with pneumonia may include:

- Impaired respiratory function
- Infection
- Fluid imbalance
- Activity intolerance
- Altered body temperature

Additional information on clinical problems and interventions for patients with pneumonia is shown in eNursing Care Plan 30.1 on the website for this chapter.

NURSING MANAGEMENT: PNEUMONIA

Assessment

Table 30.6 presents subjective and objective data to obtain from patients with pneumonia.

TABLE 30.5 Drug Therapy

Bacterial Community-Acquired Pneumonia

Patient Variable	Treatment Options
Outpatient	
Healthy	Oral β-lactam *OR* oral doxycycline
No comorbidities, healthy, <65 years, no risk factors for antibiotic-resistant infection	*ADD* oral macrolide if infection with atypical organism is suspected
Comorbidities	Oral β-lactam *PLUS* oral macrolide or oral doxycycline
Diabetes; chronic liver, lung, heart, or renal disease; cancer; alcohol use; no spleen	OR Oral fluoroquinolone
Inpatient (Depends on Whether MRSA or Pseudomonas Present)	
Nonsevere; MRSA or Pseudomonas not present	IV β-lactam *PLUS* IV/oral macrolide or IV/oral doxycycline OR IV or oral fluoroquinolone
Severe; MRSA or Pseudomonas not present	IV β-lactam *PLUS* IV macrolide or IV fluoroquinolone
Known MRSA or Pseudomonas, recent (within 90 days) hospitalization with IV antibiotics	MRSA: IV vancomycin *OR* IV linezolid Pseudomonas: IV piperacillin-tazobactam *OR* IV cefepime *OR* IV carbapenem
Special Considerations	
Pseudomonas infection in patient with penicillin allergy	Substitute aztreonam for β-lactam
Pregnancy	Outpatient: amoxicillin *OR* amoxicillin/clavulanate *PLUS* azithromycin Inpatient: IV β-lactam *PLUS* azithromycin

MRSA, Methicillin-resistant *Staphylococcus aureus*.
From *Antibacterial drugs for community acquired pneumonia.* Retrieved from https://secure.medicalletter.org/TML-article-1616b.

TABLE 30.6 NURSING ASSESSMENT

Pneumonia

Subjective Data

Important Health Information

Health history: Lung cancer, COPD, diabetes, chronic debilitating disease, malnutrition, immunosuppression, exposure to chemical toxins, dust, or allergens

Medications: Antibiotics, corticosteroids, chemotherapy, immunosuppressants

Surgery or other treatments: Recent abdominal or chest surgery, splenectomy, endotracheal intubation, enteral feedings, or any surgery with general anesthesia

Functional Health Patterns

Health perception–health management: Smoking, alcohol use, drug use, recent tract URI, malaise

Nutritional-metabolic: Anorexia, nausea, vomiting

Activity-exercise: Prolonged bed rest or immobility. Fatigue, weakness. Dyspnea, cough

Cognitive-perceptual: Pain with breathing, nasal congestion, chest pain, sore throat, headache, abdominal pain, muscle aches

Objective Data

Cardiovascular

- Tachycardia

General

- Fever, restlessness, lethargy. Splinting of thoracic cavity

Neurologic

- Changes in mental status, ranging from confusion to delirium

Respiratory

- Tachypnea, pharyngitis
- Asymmetric chest movements or retraction, decreased excursion
- Nasal flaring, use of accessory muscles (neck, abdomen)
- Crackles, friction rub, dullness on percussion over consolidated areas, ↑ tactile fremitus on palpation
- Pink, rusty, purulent, green, yellow, or white sputum (amount may be scant to copious)

Possible Diagnostic Findings

- Leukocytosis, positive sputum on Gram stain and culture. Patchy or diffuse infiltrates, abscesses, pleural effusion, or pneumothorax on chest x-ray
- Abnormal ABGs (changes in Pa_{O_2}, Pa_{CO_2}, and/or pH depending on severity)

Planning

The overall goals for patients with pneumonia include (1) no signs of hypoxemia, (2) normal breathing patterns, (3) clear breath sounds, (4) normal chest x-ray, (5) normal WBC count, and (6) no complications.

Implementation

Health Promotion

To reduce the risk for pneumonia, teach patients to practice good health habits, such as frequent handwashing, good nutrition, adequate rest, regular exercise, and coughing or sneezing into the elbow rather than hands. Smoking cessation is one of the most important health-promoting behaviors. Identifying patients at risk and taking measures to prevent pneumonia are important. Encourage those at risk for pneumonia (e.g., chronically ill, older adult, immunosuppressed) to obtain needed vaccines. Pneumococcal vaccine is used to prevent *S. pneumoniae* infection (Table 30.7).

Acute Care

Nursing care for patients with pneumonia is outlined in Table 30.8. Essential nursing care for hospitalized patients includes monitoring trends in assessment findings and the response to therapy. Prompt collection of specimens and timely administration of antibiotics are critical. Supportive care is provided according to patient needs. This might include O_2 therapy to treat hypoxemia and measures to reduce fever (see Table 12.5). Practice strict medical asepsis and adherence to infection control guidelines to reduce transmission among staff, visitors, and patients. Work with the respiratory therapist to monitor the patient and provide chest physiotherapy. Proper positioning can help improve oxygenation, ease breathing, and promote lung drainage.

TABLE 30.7 Pneumococcal Vaccines

Vaccine[a]	Recommendations for Use
Pneumococcal conjugate vaccine (PCV15, PCV20) Protects against 15 and 20 types of pneumococcal bacteria	• Children <5 years • Persons 5–64 years old with certain medical conditions (e.g., sickle cell disease, asplenia, immunodeficiencies, HIV infection, chronic kidney disease, leukemia, cancer, long-term immunosuppressive therapy) and never received PCV • Adults ≥65 years who never received PCV
Pneumococcal polysaccharide vaccine (PPSV23, Pneumovax 23) Protects against 23 types of pneumococcal bacteria	• Adults 19–64 years old who get PCV15 • Persons 2–18 years old at high risk of pneumococcal disease (e.g., heart disease, lung disease, diabetes, alcohol use, cirrhosis, sickle cell disease, immunocompromised, cancer) • If PCV15 was given, it should be followed by a dose of PPSV23.

From CDC: *Pneumococcal vaccination.* Retrieved from https://www.cdc.gov/vaccines/vpd/pneumo/index.html.

Hydration is important to prevent dehydration and thin and loosen secretions. Monitor fluid intake. If the patient is an older adult, has heart failure (HF), or has a known preexisting respiratory condition, administer IV fluids carefully to avoid fluid overload. Evaluate intake and output. Monitor and replace electrolytes as needed.

Weight loss may occur because of increased metabolic needs, difficulty eating due to dyspnea, nonspecific abdominal symptoms, and activity intolerance. Small, frequent meals are easier for patients with dyspnea to tolerate. Offer foods high in calories and nutrients. A nutrition assessment by a dietitian may be done on admission to acute care.

Balance rest and activity to each patient's tolerance. Benefits of early mobility include improved lung and chest expansion, mobilization of secretions, and preventing venous stasis. Treat pain to a comfort level that permits the patient to deep breathe and cough yet be awake and alert and able to achieve optimum mobility.

TABLE 30.8 NURSING MANAGEMENT

Care of the Patient With Pneumonia

- Monitor respiratory status:
  - Breath sounds: Assess for decreased or absent air entry and presence of adventitious sounds.
  - Rate, rhythm, depth, and effort of respirations (work of breathing).
  - Characteristics of any secretions.
  - Ability to cough effectively and clear secretions.
  - Fatigue.
- Keep the head of the bed elevated at least 30 degrees.
- Assess for signs of hypoxemia, administer O_2 as ordered.
- Administer antibiotic and IV fluid therapy as ordered.
- Administer medications (e.g., bronchodilators and inhalers) to promote airway patency and gas exchange.
- Encourage the patient to cough, deep breathe, and use the incentive spirometer.
- Turn and reposition the patient every 2 h to promote lung expansion and mobilize secretions.
- Administer analgesics as ordered to relieve pain.
- Implement measures to manage fever (see Table 12.5).
- Monitor intake and output.
- Provide ordered VTE and GI prophylaxis.
- Supervise AP:
  - Obtain vital signs and report to RN.
  - Provide personal hygiene, skin care, and oral care.
  - Assist with frequent position changes, including early mobility.

Collaborate With Respiratory Therapist

- Apply O_2 therapy as ordered.
- Perform chest physiotherapy (e.g., percussion, postural drainage).

Collaborate With Dietitian

- Assess and monitor nutrition status.
- Recommend optimal diet.

Collaborate With Physical and Occupational Therapist

- Perform range-of-motion (ROM) exercises.
- Assist with early and progressive ambulation.

Implement measures to reduce the incidence of pneumonia in patients at high risk. Elevate the head-of-bed to at least 30 degrees in patients at risk of aspiration. Assess for presence of a gag reflex before giving food or fluids. In the ICU, strictly adhere to the ventilator bundle (see Table 28.10), a group of interventions aimed at reducing the risk for VAP.

Teaching includes the importance of taking all the prescribed antibiotic (see Table 15.9). Tell patients to drink plenty of liquids (at least 6 to 10 glasses/day, unless contraindicated) and avoid alcohol and smoking. A cool mist humidifier or warm bath may help them breathe easier. Share that it may be several weeks before their usual sense of well-being returns. Explain that a follow-up chest x-ray may be done in 6 to 8 weeks to evaluate resolution of pneumonia. Older adult or chronically ill patients may have a prolonged period of convalescence. Provide teaching about available influenza and pneumococcal vaccines.

◆ Evaluation

The expected outcomes are that patients with pneumonia will have:

- Effective respiratory rate, rhythm, and depth of respirations
- Lungs clear to auscultation
- No complications

TUBERCULOSIS

Tuberculosis (TB) is an infectious disease caused by *Mycobacterium tuberculosis.* It usually involves the lungs, but can infect any organ, including the brain, kidneys, and bones. About 25% of the world's population is infected with TB.[9] The incidence of TB worldwide declined until the mid-1980s. We are now seeing increasing rates of TB. This is attributed to HIV and the emergence of drug-resistant strains of *M. tuberculosis.*

TB occurs disproportionately in the poor, underserved, and minorities. People most at risk include the homeless, residents of inner-city neighborhoods, foreign-born people, those living or working in institutions (long-term care facilities, prisons, shelters, hospitals), IV drug users, overcrowded living conditions, less than optimal sanitation, and those with poor access to health care. Immunosuppression from any cause (e.g., HIV, cancer, long-term corticosteroid use) increases the risk for active TB infection.

Etiology and Pathophysiology

M. tuberculosis is a gram-positive, aerobic, acid-fast bacillus (AFB). It is usually spread from person to person by airborne droplets expectorated when breathing, talking, singing, sneezing, and coughing. TB is not highly infectious. Transmission requires close contact and frequent or prolonged exposure. TB does not spread by touching, sharing food utensils, kissing, or any other physical contact.

Factors that influence transmission include the (1) number of organisms expelled into the air, (2) concentration of organisms (small spaces with limited ventilation would mean higher concentration), (3) length of time of exposure, and (4) immune system of the exposed person. Once inhaled, these small droplets lodge in bronchioles and alveoli. A local inflammatory reaction occurs, and the infection is established. This is called the *Ghon lesion* or *focus.* It represents a calcified TB granuloma, the hallmark of a primary TB infection. The formation of a granuloma is a defense mechanism aimed at walling off the infection and preventing further spread. Bacillus replication is inhibited, stopping the infection.

Most immunocompetent adults infected with TB can completely kill the mycobacteria. Some people have mycobacteria in a nonreplicating dormant state. Of these people, 5% to 10% develop active TB infection when the bacteria begin to multiply months or years later. While *M. tuberculosis* is aerophilic (O_2 loving) and has an affinity for the lungs, the infection can spread through the lymphatic system and find good environments for growth in other organs. These include the cerebral cortex, spine, bone epiphyses, liver, kidneys, lymph nodes, and adrenal glands.

Once a strain of *M. tuberculosis* develops resistance to the first-line drug therapy (isoniazid and rifampin), it is called *multidrug-resistant tuberculosis (MDR-TB).*[10] Extensively drug-resistant TB (XDR-TB) is an even rarer type of MDR-TB. XDR-TB is resistant to fluoroquinolones and at least 1 second-line drug.[11] Resistance results from several problems, including incorrect prescribing, poor follow-up, and nonadherence to the prescribed regimen.

Classification

We use several systems to classify TB. The American Thoracic Society classifies TB based on disease development (Table 30.9).

TABLE 30.9 Classification of Tuberculosis

Class	Exposure or Infection	Description
0	No TB exposure, not infected	No history of exposure, negative tuberculin skin test (TST) or interferon-γ release assay (IGRA)
1	TB exposure, no infection	Negative TST or IGRA (if given 8 wk after exposure)
2	TB infection, no disease	Positive TST or IGRA, negative bacterial studies, no clinical or bacterial evidence of TB, no TB on chest x-ray
3	TB, clinically active	Positive bacterial studies or positive reaction to TST or IGRA and TB on chest x-ray
4	TB, not clinically active	History of TB or abnormal but stable chest x-ray in patient with a positive TST or IGRA. Negative bacterial studies. No clinical signs and symptoms of active TB or abnormal chest x-ray
5	Suspected TB	Diagnosis pending. Person should not be in this classification for >3 months

We also classify TB by (1) its presentation (primary, latent, reactivated) and (2) whether it is pulmonary or extrapulmonary.

Primary TB infection starts when the bacteria are inhaled and trigger an inflammatory reaction. Most people have effective immune responses that encapsulate the organisms for the rest of their lives, preventing the initial infection from progressing to disease. If the initial immune response is not adequate, the body cannot contain the organism. As a result, the bacteria replicate and *active TB disease* results. When active disease develops within the first 2 years of infection, it is called *primary TB*. People coinfected with HIV are at greatest risk for developing active TB.

Postprimary TB, or *reactivation TB*, is defined as TB disease occurring 2 or more years after the initial infection. If the site of TB is pulmonary or laryngeal, the person is infectious and can transmit the disease to others.

Latent TB infection (LTBI) occurs in a person who does not have active TB disease (Table 30.10). People with LTBI have a positive skin test but are asymptomatic. They cannot transmit the TB bacteria to others but can develop active TB disease later. Immunosuppression, diabetes, poor nutrition, HIV, glucocorticoid therapy, pregnancy, stress, and chronic disease can reactivate the disease. Treatment of LTBI is as important as primary TB.

Clinical Manifestations

Symptoms of pulmonary TB usually do not develop until 2 to 3 weeks after infection or reactivation. The primary manifestation is an initial dry cough. The cough becomes productive with mucoid or mucopurulent sputum. Active TB may present with constitutional symptoms (e.g., fatigue, malaise, anorexia, unexplained weight loss, low-grade fevers, night sweats). Dyspnea and hemoptysis are late symptoms that may signify substantial disease or a pleural effusion.

Sometimes, TB has a more acute, sudden presentation. Patients may have a high fever, chills, flu-like symptoms, pleuritic pain, productive cough, and ARF. Auscultation may be normal or reveal adventitious sounds, such as crackles. Hypotension and hypoxemia may be present.

Immunosuppressed people and older adults are less likely to have fever and other signs of an infection. In patients with HIV, classic TB manifestations, such as fever, cough, and weight loss, may be wrongly attributed to PJP or other opportunistic diseases. Respiratory problems in patients with HIV are assessed to determine the cause. A change in cognitive function may be the only initial presenting sign of TB in an older person.

The manifestations of extrapulmonary TB depend on the organs infected. For example, renal TB can cause dysuria and hematuria. Bone and joint TB may cause severe pain. Headaches, vomiting, and lymphadenopathy may be present with TB meningitis.

TABLE 30.10 Comparison of Latent Tuberculosis Infection (LTBI) and Active Tuberculosis

LTBI	TB Disease
Has no symptoms	Symptomatic
Does not feel sick	Usually feels sick
Cannot spread TB bacteria to others	May spread TB bacteria to others
Usually has a positive TST or blood test result showing TB infection	Usually has a positive TST or blood test result showing TB infection
Normal chest x-ray and negative sputum smear	May have an abnormal chest x-ray or positive sputum smear or culture
Needs treatment for latent TB infection to prevent active TB disease	Needs treatment for active TB disease

From CDC: *Tuberculosis (TB) fact sheets: the difference between latent TB infection and TB disease.* Retrieved from https://www.cdc.gov/tb/publications/factsheets/general/ltbiandactivetb.htm.

Complications

Properly treated, pulmonary TB typically heals without complications, except for scarring and residual cavitation within the lung. Significant lung damage, though rare, can occur in patients who are poorly treated or who do not respond to TB treatment.

Miliary TB is widespread dissemination of the mycobacterium through the bloodstream to several distant organs. The infection may be fatal if untreated. It can occur with primary disease or reactivation of LTBI. Manifestations slowly progress over a period of days, weeks, or even months. Symptoms vary depending on the organs that are affected. Fever, cough, and lymphadenopathy are present. Hepatomegaly and splenomegaly may occur.

Pleural TB, a specific type of extrapulmonary TB, can result from either primary disease or reactivation of LTBI. Chest pain, fever, cough, and a unilateral pleural effusion are common. The pleural effusion is caused by bacteria in the pleural space, which triggers an inflammatory reaction and produces protein-rich fluid. Empyema is less common but may occur from large numbers of TB organisms in the pleural space. Diagnosis is confirmed by AFB cultures and a pleural biopsy.

Because TB can infect organs throughout the body, other acute and long-term complications can result. Spinal TB (Pott disease) can cause destruction of the intervertebral disc and adjacent vertebrae. Central nervous system (CNS) TB can cause bacterial meningitis. Abdominal TB can lead to peritonitis, especially in HIV-positive patients. The kidneys, adrenal glands, lymph nodes, and urogenital tract can be affected.

Diagnostic Studies

Tuberculin Skin Test

The tuberculin skin test (TST) (Mantoux test) using purified protein derivative (PPD) is the standard method to screen people for *M. tuberculosis.* The test is given by injecting 0.1 mL of PPD intradermally on the ventral surface of the forearm. We read the test by inspection and palpation 48 to 72 hours later for the presence or absence of induration. Induration, a palpable, raised, hardened area or swelling (not redness) at the injection site, means the person has been exposed to TB and has developed antibodies. Antibody formation occurs 2 to 12 weeks after initial exposure to the bacteria. Any indurated area is measured and recorded in millimeters. Based on the size of the induration and risk factors, we make an interpretation based on CDC standards for determining a positive test (see Table 27.15).

Two-step testing with the Mantoux test is recommended for baseline or initial screening for health care workers and those who have a decreased response to allergens. If the 1st test is positive, the person does not need the 2nd test. They do, however, need further evaluation for active disease. If the 1st test is negative, a 2nd test is done 1 to 3 weeks later. Some people with LTBI or who were previously infected with TB may have a false-negative result with the 1st test. Repeating the test may boost the body's ability to react in future tests. A positive reaction to a subsequent test could be a new infection or the result of the boosted reaction to an old infection. A previously negative 2-step test ensures that any future positive results are interpreted as being caused by a new infection.

Interferon-γ Release Assays

Interferon-γ (INF-γ) release assays (IGRAs) are another screening tool for TB. IGRAs are blood tests that detect INF-γ release from T cells in response to *M. tuberculosis.*[12] Examples of IGRAs include QuantiFERON-TB Gold In-Tube test (QFT-GIT) and the T-SPOT.TB test. Test results are available in a few hours.

IGRAs have several advantages over TST. IGRAs require a single patient visit, are not subject to reader bias, have no "booster" phenomenon, and are not affected by bacillus Calmette-Guérin (BCG) vaccination. IGRA costs much more than TST. The choice of test should be based on context and reasons for testing. Neither IGRAs nor TST can tell between LTBI and active TB infection. LTBI can only be diagnosed by excluding active TB.

Chest X-Ray

Although chest x-ray findings are important, it is not possible to make a diagnosis of TB based solely on chest x-ray. A chest x-ray may appear normal in patients with TB. Findings that suggest TB include upper lobe infiltrates, cavitary infiltrates, lymph node involvement, and pleural and/or pericardial effusion.

Bacterial Studies

Sputum culture is the gold standard for diagnosing TB. We need 3 consecutive sputum specimens, each collected at 8- to 24-hour intervals, with at least 1 early morning specimen. The initial test involves microscopic examination of stained sputum smears for AFB. A definitive diagnosis of TB requires mycobacterial growth, which can take up to 6 weeks. For patients in whom suspicion of TB is high, we start treatment while waiting for culture results. We can obtain samples of other suspected TB sites from gastric washings, cerebrospinal fluid (CSF), or fluid from an effusion or abscess.

Interprofessional Care

Most patients with TB are treated on an outpatient basis (Table 30.11). Many people can continue to work and maintain their lifestyles with few changes. Patients with sputum smear–positive TB are considered infectious for the first 2 weeks after starting treatment. These patients should restrict visitors, and avoid travel, public transportation, and trips to public places. Teach them the importance of good handwashing and oral hygiene. Hospitalization may be needed for severely ill or debilitated patients.

Drug Therapy

Active disease. The mainstay of TB treatment is drug therapy (Table 30.12). Because of the growing prevalence of MDR-TB, it is important to manage patients with active TB aggressively. Many different drug schedules are possible. Choice of treatment depends on the clinical situation, presence of underlying health conditions, and perceived adherence with drug therapy.

Drug therapy is divided into 2 phases: intensive and continuation (Table 30.13). In most circumstances the treatment regimen for patients with previously untreated TB consists of a plan with 4 drugs (isoniazid, rifampin, pyrazinamide, ethambutol). If the patient develops a toxic reaction to the primary drugs, other drugs can be used, including rifabutin and rifapentine (Priftin).

TABLE 30.11 Interprofessional Care

Pulmonary Tuberculosis

Diagnostic Assessment
- History and physical assessment
- Tuberculin skin test (TST)
- IGRA: QuantiFERON-TB Gold In-Tube test (QFT-GIT) or T-SPOT.TB test
- Chest x-ray
- Bacterial studies
  - Sputum smear for acid-fast bacilli (AFB)
  - Sputum culture

Management
- Long-term treatment with antimicrobial drugs (Tables 30.13 and 30.14)
- Follow-up AFB smears, cultures, and chest x-rays
- Follow-up care, addressing needs of patient and close contacts

IGRA, Interferon-γ release assay.

TABLE 30.12 Drug Therapy

Tuberculosis

Drug	Common Side Effects
For Active TB	
ethambutol	Loss of visual acuity (e.g., color blindness), blurred vision, confusion, liver toxicity, peripheral neuropathy
isoniazid	Rash, nausea, vomiting, confusion, liver toxicity
pyrazinamide	Liver toxicity, joint pain, hyperuricemia
rifampin	Behavior changes, liver toxicity, thrombocytopenia, orange discoloration of bodily fluids (sputum, urine, sweat, tears), anorexia, nausea, abdominal discomfort
For Drug-Resistant TB	
aminoglycosides (e.g., amikacin)	Hepatitis, GI effects, ototoxicity, kidney toxicity
bedaquiline (Sirturo)	Nausea, vomiting, liver problems, joint and muscle pain, dysrhythmias
fluoroquinolones (e.g., levofloxacin)	GI problems, neurologic effects (dizziness, headache, peripheral neuropathy), rash, dysrhythmias, prolonged QT interval, liver toxicity
pretomanid	Peripheral neuropathy, headache, vision changes, GI effects
streptomycin	Ototoxicity, neurotoxicity, kidney toxicity
Other Drugs Used	
rifabutin (Mycobutin)	Liver toxicity, thrombocytopenia, neutropenia, orange discoloration of bodily fluids (sputum, urine, sweat, tears); GI effects
rifapentine (Priftin)	Like those of rifampin

DRUG ALERT

Isoniazid

- Alcohol may increase risk for liver toxicity.
- Teach patients to avoid drinking alcohol during treatment.
- Monitor for signs of hepatitis before and while taking drug.

Sensitivity testing guides the treatment for MDR-TB. MDR-TB therapy in the initial phase typically includes 5 drugs: 1 or 2 first-line agents, a fluoroquinolone, an injectable antibiotic, and 1 or more second-line agents for 4 to 6 months. This is followed by at least 4 drugs, minus the injectable antibiotic, for 18 to 24 months. Two newer drugs, bedaquiline (Sirturo) and delamanid (Deltyba), are used in combination with other drugs to treat MDR-TB and XDR-TB.

Nonadherence is a major factor in the emergence of MDR-TB and treatment failures (Box 30.2). *Directly observed therapy* (DOT) involves providing the prescribed drugs directly to patients and watching as they swallow the drugs. DOT ensures adherence, especially for those at risk for nonadherence. VDOT, a form of DOT using digital technology, has emerged as an alternative to in-person observation. DOT is an expensive but essential public health measure. In many areas, the public health nurse administers DOT at a clinic site.

Fixed-dose combination drugs may enhance adherence. Combinations of isoniazid and rifampin and of isoniazid, rifampin, and pyrazinamide are available to simplify therapy. The therapy for people with HIV uses the same medications as outlined in Table 30.13, but in a slightly different schedule. In the intensive phase, HIV patients take isoniazid, ethambutol, pyrazinamide, and rifamycin for the 1st 2 months, then isoniazid and rifamycin for the last 4 months.

Teach patients about the adverse effects of drug therapy and when to seek medical care. The major side effect of isoniazid, rifampin, and pyrazinamide is nonviral hepatitis. Baseline liver function tests are done at the start of treatment and checked every 2 to 4 weeks, especially if results are abnormal.

Latent tuberculosis infection. In people with LTBI, drug therapy helps prevent a TB infection from developing into active TB disease. Because a person with LTBI has fewer bacteria, treatment is much easier. Drug regimens for LTBI are outlined in Table 30.14. The standard treatment regimen for LTBI is 9 months of daily isoniazid. This plan is recommended for patients with HIV and those with fibrotic lesions on chest x-ray. Because of risk of severe liver injury and death, the CDC does not recommend the combination of rifampin and pyrazinamide for treatment of LTBI.

Bacille Calmette-Guérin vaccine. Bacille Calmette-Guérin (BCG) vaccine is a live, attenuated strain of *Mycobacterium bovis.* The vaccine is given to infants in parts of the world with a high prevalence of TB. In the United States it is rarely used because of the low risk for TB and the vaccine's variable effectiveness against adult pulmonary TB. BCG vaccination can result in a false-positive TST. IGRA results are not affected. The BCG vaccine should be considered only for select persons who meet specific criteria (e.g., health care workers who are continually exposed to patients with MDR-TB and when infection control precautions are not successful).

NURSING MANAGEMENT: TUBERCULOSIS

Assessment

Ask patients about a history of TB, chronic illness, or any immunosuppressive disease or medications. Obtain a social and occupational history to assess for risk factors. Assess for productive cough, night sweats, fever, weight loss, pleuritic chest pain, and abnormal lung sounds. If the patient has a productive cough, early morning is the best time to collect sputum specimens for an AFB smear.

Clinical Problems

Clinical problems for patients with TB may include:

- Impaired respiratory function
- Infection

TABLE 30.13 Drug Therapy

Tuberculosis Treatment Regimens

4-MONTH TREATMENT PLAN

INTENSIVE MEDICATION PHASE			CONTINUATION MEDICATION PHASE			
Drug	**Time**	**Frequency**	**Drug**	**Time**	**Frequency**	**TOTAL DOSES**
INH	8 wk	7 days/wk for 56 doses*	INH	9 wk	7 days/wk for 63 doses*	119
MOX			MOX			
PZA			RPT			
RPT						

6- TO 9-MONTH TREATMENT PLAN

INTENSIVE MEDICATION PHASE				CONTINUATION MEDICATION PHASE				
		FREQUENCY				FREQUENCY		
Drug	**Time**	**No DOT**	**DOT**	**Drug**	**Time**	**No DOT**	**DOT**	**TOTAL DOSES**
EMB	8 wk	7 days/wk	5 days/wk	INH	18 wk	7 days/wk 126 doses	5 days/wk 90 doses	130–182[a]
INH		56 doses	40 doses	RIF				
PZA								
RIF								
EMB	8 wk	7 days/wk	5 days/wk	INH	18 wk	3 times/wk for 54 doses		94–110[b]
INH		56 doses	40 doses	RIF				
PZA								
RIF								
EMB	8 wk	3 times/wk for 24 doses		INH	18 wk	3 times/wk for 54 doses		78
INH				RIF				
PZA								
RIF								

*At least 5 of the 7 weekly doses should be given under DOT.

[a]Preferred regimen for newly diagnosed TB.

[b]Preferred regimen when adherence may be difficult.

EMB, Ethambutol; *INH,* isoniazid; *MOX,* moxifloxacin; *PZA,* pyrazinamide; RIF, rifampin; *RPT,* rifapentine.

From Centers for Disease Control and Prevention: *Tuberculosis (TB): treatment for TB disease.* Retrieved from https://www.cdc.gov/tb/topic/treatment/tbdisease.htm.

◆ Planning

The overall goals are that patients with TB will (1) have normal lung function, (2) adhere to the treatment plan, (3) take measures to prevent the spread of TB, and (4) have no recurrence.

◆ Implementation

Health Promotion

The goal is to eradicate TB worldwide. Screening programs in known risk groups are valuable in detecting people with TB. For example, the person with a positive TST should have a chest x-ray to assess for active TB disease. Report people diagnosed with TB to public health authorities for identification and assessment of contacts and risk to the community. Treatment of LTBI reduces the number of TB carriers in the community.

Programs that address social factors influencing TB are essential for reducing transmission. Lowering rates of HIV infection, poverty, overcrowded housing, malnutrition, smoking, and drug and alcohol use can help decrease TB infection rates. Improving access to health care and providing education on preventing TB are important.

Acute Care

Patients admitted with respiratory symptoms should be assessed for the possibility of TB. Those strongly suspected of having TB should (1) be placed on airborne isolation; (2) receive a medical workup, including chest x-ray, sputum smear, and culture; and (3) start drug therapy. Airborne infection isolation is needed for patients with pulmonary or laryngeal TB until they are not infectious. Place patients in a single-occupancy room with negative pressure and airflow of 6 to 12 exchanges per hour. Everyone entering the room should wear a high-efficiency particulate air (HEPA) or N95 mask.

Teach patients to cover their nose and mouth with paper tissues every time they cough, sneeze, or produce sputum. Have them throw tissues into a paper bag and dispose of them with the trash or flush them down the toilet. Emphasize good handwashing after handling sputum and soiled tissues. If

BOX 30.2 ETHICAL/LEGAL DILEMMAS

Patient Adherence

Situation

While working at a health clinic at a homeless shelter, you discover that L.B., a 60-year-old male with TB, has not been taking his drug therapy. He tells you that it is hard for him to get to the clinic to obtain his medications. He tells you he has a hard time remembering his appointments. L.B. confides in you that he cannot read or write very well at all and cannot understand all the information that has been given to him about his condition. You are concerned about L.B. and the risk he poses for the other people at the shelter and at the meal sites where he often visits.

Ethical/Legal Points for Consideration

- Adherence is a complex issue involving culture, values, and beliefs, perceived risk for disease, access to treatment, availability of resources, and perceived consequences of failure to adhere to treatment.
- State emergency detention laws provide public health officials with the legal authority to take action to apprehend and hold a person with TB who we believe to be a threat to public health.
- The federal government and many states have provisions for quarantine, detention, and treatment of patients with TB who do not adhere to treatment.
- Advocacy for both the patient and the community obliges you to involve other health care team members, such as social services, to aid in obtaining resources or support for the patient to complete a course of treatment.
- With the threats of bioterrorism and the globalization of infectious disease, it seems unlikely that the government's power to detain will change anytime soon.

Discussion Questions

1. How would you begin your initial conversation with L.B. about your concerns?
2. How might being unable to effectively read and/or write affect L.B. and the treatment plan that has been developed? What alternatives of care can we offer that may help?
3. Under what circumstances, if any, are HCPs justified in overriding a patient's autonomy or decision making?

TABLE 30.14 Drug Therapy

LTBI Regimens

Drug	Time	Frequency	Indications
isoniazid and rifapentine	12 wk	Once weekly[a]	Only for healthy patients not at risk for MDR-TB
rifampin	16 wk	Daily	For patients who are resistant to isoniazid
isoniazid	24 wk	Daily or twice weekly	Alternate plan if adherence is a concern
	36 wk	Daily or twice weekly	36 wk, daily dosing is preferred treatment plan

[a]Use directly observed therapy (DOT).

From Centers for Disease Control and Prevention: *Tuberculosis (TB): treatment regimens for latent tuberculosis infections (LTBI).* Retrieved from https://www.cdc.gov/tb/topic/treatment/ltbi.htm.

patients need to be out of the negative-pressure room, they must wear a standard surgical mask to prevent exposure to others. Minimize prolonged visitation to other parts of the hospital.

Other care for hospitalized patients with TB includes monitoring vital signs, providing adequate nutrition, maintaining a balance between activity and rest, and monitoring for complications. Identify and screen close contacts of the person with TB. Anyone testing positive for TB infection needs further evaluation and treatment for either LTBI or active TB disease.

Chronic Care

Patients who respond clinically are discharged home if their household contacts have already been exposed and they are not posing a risk to others. A sputum specimen for AFB smear and culture are done monthly until 2 consecutive specimen cultures are negative. More frequent AFB smears may be done to assess the early response to treatment and determine infectiousness. Negative cultures are needed to declare the patient not infectious.

Teach patients how to minimize exposure to close contacts and household members. Homes should be well ventilated, especially the areas where the infected person spends a lot of time. While still infectious, patients should sleep alone and spend as much time as possible outdoors. Teach them to minimize time in congregate settings and public transportation.

Teach patients and caregivers about adherence with the treatment plan. Most treatment failures occur because the patient does not take the drug, stops taking it too soon, or takes it irregularly. Strategies to improve adherence include teaching and counseling, reminder systems, incentives or rewards, contracts, and DOT.

Notify the public health department. They are responsible for follow-up on household contacts and assessing patients for adherence. If adherence is an issue, the public health department may be responsible for DOT (Box 30.3). Most patients are considered adequately treated when drug therapy has been completed, cultures are negative, there is improvement in their condition, and improvement on chest x-ray.

Because about 5% of patients have relapses, teach patients to recognize the symptoms that occur with recurrent TB. If these symptoms occur, patients should seek immediate medical attention. Teach patients about factors that could reactivate TB, such as immunosuppressive therapy, cancer, and prolonged debilitating illness. If patients have any of these, we must notify the HCP so that they can be monitored for TB reactivation. In some situations, it is necessary to put a patient on anti-TB therapy. Because smoking is associated with poor outcomes, encourage patients who smoke to quit. Provide patients with teaching and resources to help them stop smoking.

◆ Evaluation

The expected outcomes are that patients with TB will have:

- Resolution of the disease
- Normal lung function

BOX 30.3 EVIDENCE-BASED PRACTICE

Adherence to TB Treatment Program

You are a nurse working in an outpatient health clinic with C.J., a 42-year-old female diagnosed 2 months ago with active TB. She is on directly observed therapy (DOT). In the past 2 weeks, you notice C.J. has started to miss and has been late for her appointments. She tells you it is hard to make her appointments as a new job requires long work hours. She asks if she needs to continue with her visits to get her drugs. She says she is *"feeling better"* and does not understand *"what all the fuss over the drugs is about."* She adds that she is *"perfectly capable of taking my own pills."*

Making Clinical Decisions

Best Available Evidence

Guidelines for effective case management of patients with TB include education, home visits, patient reminders, and incentives. TB clinic attendance and treatment completion rates are higher when patients take part in DOT compared with self-administered therapy. When appointments are missed, phone calls, Web-based videos, or home visits can engage patients resulting in improved attendance and treatment completion.

Clinician Expertise

You are aware that patient-centered care includes being responsive to patients' needs. You know that TB therapy is required for at least 4 months to help control TB. Nurses are aware that patients may stop attending appointments and taking their drugs when feeling well again. This can lead to treatment failure, the need to restart therapy, and multidrug resistance.

Patient Preferences and Values

C.J. tells you she has a busy job and cannot always remember her appointments. She stated that she would like to be responsible for taking her drugs.

Implications for Nursing Practice

1. What factors may be contributing to C.J.'s lack of adherence to her treatment program?
2. What teaching would you provide to C.J. about taking her own medications?
3. How might you incorporate digital technology to help increase medication compliance?
4. How will you determine whether C.J. is adhering to the drug treatment plan?

Reference for Evidence

Sazali MF, Rahim SA, Mohammad AH, et al: Improving tuberculosis medication adherence, *Tuberc Resp Disease* 86:82, 2023.

- Increased knowledge about TB
- No further transmission of TB

ATYPICAL MYCOBACTERIA

There are more than 30 acid-fast mycobacteria that cause diseases other than TB. These include lung disease, lymphadenitis, skin or soft tissue disease, and disseminated disease. Atypical mycobacteria are not airborne or transmitted by droplets. They can be found in tap water, soil, bird feces, and house dust.

People who are immunosuppressed or have chronic lung disease are most susceptible to infection. Pulmonary symptoms include cough, shortness of breath, weight loss, fatigue, and blood-tinged sputum.

TABLE 30.15 Fungal Lung Infections

Infection	Organism
Endemic Fungal Infections	
Blastomycosis	*Blastomyces dermatitidis*
Coccidioidomycosis	*Coccidioides immitis*
Histoplasmosis	*Histoplasma capsulatum*
Opportunistic Fungal Infections	
Aspergillosis	*Aspergillus fumigatus*
Candidiasis	*Candida albicans*
Cryptococcosis	*Cryptococcus neoformans, Cryptococcus gattii*

Diagnosis is challenging and differs based on the site of the infection. We cannot tell this type of lung disease from TB either clinically or radiologically. Diagnostic studies done include a chest x-ray and 3 sputum specimens tested for AFB. Treatment may include a prolonged course of antibiotics, depending on the organism cultured and the patient's condition.

PULMONARY FUNGAL INFECTIONS

Pulmonary fungal pneumonia is an infectious process in the lungs caused by endemic (native and common) or opportunistic fungi (Table 30.15). Endemic fungal pathogens cause infection in healthy people and immunocompromised people in certain areas. For example, *Coccidioides,* which causes coccidioidomycosis, is a fungus found in the soil of dry, low-rainfall areas.[13] It is endemic in many areas of the southwestern United States. Opportunistic fungal infections occur in immunocompromised patients and in patients with cystic fibrosis. These infections can be life-threatening.

Pulmonary fungal infections are acquired by inhaling spores. They are not transmitted from person to person. Patients do not need to be placed in isolation. The manifestations are like those of bacterial pneumonia. Skin testing, serology, and biopsy methods help identify the infecting organism.

The choice of antifungal agent is based on the pathogen identified on culture or most likely suspected. Amphotericin B IV is the standard therapy for treating serious systemic fungal infections. Less serious infections can be treated with oral antifungals, such as ketoconazole, fluconazole (Diflucan), voriconazole (Vfend), and itraconazole (Sporanox).

LUNG ABSCESS

Etiology and Pathophysiology

A **lung abscess** is necrosis of lung tissue. It typically results from bacteria aspirated from the oral cavity in patients with periodontal disease. Lung abscess can also result from IV drug use, cancer, pulmonary emboli, TB, and various parasitic and fungal diseases. The abscess usually develops slowly, beginning with an enlarging area of infection that becomes necrotic and eventually forms a cavity filled with purulent material.

Abscesses usually contain more than 1 type of microbe, most often anaerobic flora of the mouth and pharynx.

The lung area most often affected due to aspiration is the posterior segment of the upper lobes. The abscess may erode into the bronchial system, causing foul-smelling or sour-tasting sputum. It may grow toward the pleura and cause pleuritic pain. Multiple small abscesses, sometimes referred to as *necrotizing pneumonia,* can occur within the lung.

Clinical Manifestations and Complications

Manifestations usually occur slowly over a period of weeks to months, especially if anaerobic organisms are the cause. Symptoms of abscess caused by aerobic bacteria develop more acutely and resemble bacterial pneumonia. Most common is cough-induced, purulent sputum (often dark brown), that is foul smelling and foul tasting. Hemoptysis is common, especially when an abscess ruptures into a bronchus. Other manifestations include fever, chills, weakness, night sweats, pleuritic pain, dyspnea, anorexia, and weight loss.

Assessment reveals decreased breath sounds over the involved segment of lung. Bronchial breath sounds may be transmitted to the periphery if the communicating bronchus becomes patent and the segment begins to drain. Crackles may be present in the later stages as the abscess drains.

The infection can spread through the bloodstream and cause several possible complications. Pulmonary abscess, bronchopleural fistula, bronchiectasis, and empyema from perforation of the abscess into the pleural cavity can occur.[14]

Diagnostic Studies

A chest x-ray is often the only test needed to diagnose a lung abscess. The presence of a single cavitary lesion with an air-fluid level and local infiltrates confirms the diagnosis. CT scanning may be helpful if the abscess is not clear on chest x-ray. If there is drainage via the bronchus, sputum will contain the microorganisms that are present in the abscess.

Bronchoscopy may be used to collect a specimen or assess for underlying cancer. Pleural fluid and blood cultures may help identify the offending organisms. An elevated neutrophil count may indicate an infection. Necrotic pulmonary lesions also can be caused by lung infarction, pulmonary embolism, and sarcoidosis.

Interprofessional and Nursing Management

Monitor vital signs, level of consciousness (LOC), and respiratory rate and rhythm. Note any signs and symptoms of respiratory distress. Observe for any signs of hypoxemia. Apply O_2 as needed.

IV antibiotic therapy should be started immediately. Clindamycin is a first-line therapy for its effectiveness against *Staphylococcus* and anaerobic organisms. IV antibiotics are switched to oral antibiotics once a patient shows clinical and chest x-ray signs of improvement.

Because of the need for prolonged antibiotic therapy, teach patients to take antibiotics as directed for the entire prescribed period (see Table 15.9). Sometimes patients must return periodically during the course of antibiotic therapy for repeat cultures and sensitivity tests to ensure that the infecting organism is not becoming resistant to the antibiotic. When antibiotic therapy is complete, the patient is reevaluated.

Patients who do not respond to antibiotic treatment may need percutaneous drainage of the abscess. Surgery is sometimes done when reinfection of a large cavitary lesion occurs, when an empyema develops, or to establish a diagnosis when there is evidence of an underlying problem, such as cancer. The usual procedure in such cases is a lobectomy. A pneumonectomy may be needed when multiple abscesses exist.

Teach patients how to cough effectively. Chest physiotherapy and postural drainage are not recommended because they may promote movement of microorganisms into adjacent bronchi and other lobes of the lungs, extending infection. Rest, optimal nutrition, and adequate fluid intake promote recovery. If dentition is poor or dental hygiene is not adequate, encourage patients to obtain dental care. Collaborate with the social worker to evaluate options for dental care if a patient has limited resources.

RESTRICTIVE RESPIRATORY DISORDERS

Disorders that impair the ability of the chest wall and diaphragm to move with respiration are called *restrictive respiratory disorders.* There are 2 categories: *extrapulmonary conditions,* in which the lung tissue is normal, and *intrapulmonary conditions,* in which the primary cause is the lung or pleura. Examples of extrapulmonary and intrapulmonary conditions are listed in Table 30.16.

The hallmark characteristic of a restrictive lung disorder is a reduced total lung capacity (TLC). Mixed obstructive and

TABLE 30.16 Common Causes of Restrictive Lung Disease

Intrapulmonary Causes

Parenchymal Disorders

- Acute respiratory distress syndrome (ARDS)
- Atelectasis
- Chronic empyema
- Idiopathic pulmonary fibrosis (IPF)
- Interstitial lung diseases
- Pneumonia

Pleural Disorders

- Pleural effusion
- Pleurisy (pleuritis)
- Pneumothorax

Extrapulmonary Causes

- Head injury, central nervous system lesion (e.g., tumor, stroke)
- Kyphoscoliosis
- Neuromuscular disorders: amyotrophic lateral sclerosis, muscular dystrophy, myasthenia gravis
- Obesity
- Opioid and barbiturate overdose

restrictive disorders sometimes occur together. For example, a patient may have both asthma (an obstructive problem) and pulmonary fibrosis (a restrictive problem).

ATELECTASIS

Atelectasis is a lung condition characterized by collapsed, airless alveoli. It may be asymptomatic. Other patients have extreme shortness of breath and chest pain. There may be decreased or absent breath sounds and dullness to percussion over the affected area. The most common cause is obstruction of the small airways with secretions. This is common in patients on bed rest and in almost all postoperative patients. Deep-breathing exercises, coughing, incentive spirometry, and early mobility are important to prevent atelectasis and treat patients at risk (see Chapter 20).

PLEURISY

Pleurisy (pleuritis) is an inflammation of the pleura. It can be caused by infection, cancer, autoimmune disorders, chest trauma, GI disease, and some drugs. The inflammation usually subsides once we treat the cause. The pain of pleurisy is typically abrupt, sharp in onset, and worse with inspiration. Breathing is short, shallow, and rapid to avoid unnecessary pleura and chest wall movement. A pleural friction rub may occur. It is usually loudest at peak inspiration.

Treatment is directed at the underlying cause and providing pain relief. Teach patients to splint the rib cage when coughing. If the pain is severe, intercostal nerve blocks may be considered.

PLEURAL EFFUSION

A **pleural effusion** is an abnormal collection of fluid in the pleural space. It is a sign of another condition. A balance among hydrostatic pressure, oncotic pressure, and capillary membrane permeability governs movement of fluid in and out of the pleural space. Fluid accumulation can be due to increased pulmonary capillary pressure, decreased oncotic pressure, increased pleural membrane permeability, or obstruction of lymphatic flow.

Types of Pleural Effusions

We classify pleural effusions as transudative or exudative depending on the protein content. A *transudate effusion* occurs mainly in noninflammatory conditions. It is an accumulation of protein-poor, cell-poor fluid. The fluid is usually clear, pale yellow. Causes include (1) increased hydrostatic pressure found in HF or (2) decreased oncotic pressure from hypoalbuminemia (e.g., with chronic liver or renal disease). An *exudative effusion* results from increased capillary permeability due to an inflammatory reaction. This fluid is rich in protein. Exudative effusions most often occur with an infection or cancer.

An **empyema** is a collection of purulent fluid in the pleural space. Common causes include pneumonia, TB, lung abscess, and infected surgical chest wounds.

Clinical Manifestations

Common manifestations are dyspnea, cough, and occasional sharp, nonradiating chest pain that may be worse on inhalation. Breath sounds may be decreased over the affected area. A chest x-ray may show decreased chest movement on the affected side. A chest x-ray and CT reveal the volume and location of the effusion. Additional manifestations seen with empyema include fever, night sweats, cough, and weight loss.

Interprofessional and Nursing Management

Management focuses on treating the underlying cause. For example, adequate treatment of HF with diuretics and sodium restriction may result in a decreased incidence of pleural effusion. The treatment of malignant effusions is more difficult. These effusions often reoccur and reaccumulate quickly after thoracentesis.

Treatment options for an empyema include antibiotic therapy, percutaneous drainage, chest tube insertion, and intrapleural fibrinolytic therapy. Some patients may need surgery. Surgical options include drainage, decortication, or an open window thoracostomy.

Chemical pleurodesis is sometimes done to obliterate the pleural space and prevent reaccumulation of effusion fluid. This procedure first requires chest tube drainage of the effusion. Once the fluid is drained, a chemical agent is instilled into the pleural space. The chest tube is clamped for 8 hours while the patient is turned in different positions. This allows the chemical to contact the entire pleural space. After 8 hours, the chest tube is unclamped and attached to a drainage unit. Chest tubes are left in place until fluid drainage is less than 150 mL/day and no air leaks are noted. Fever and chest pain are common side effects after pleurodesis.

We provide supportive nursing care as needed. This may include O_2 therapy to treat hypoxemia and analgesics to relieve chest pain. Implement measures to manage fever (see Table 12.5). Hydration, nutrition support, and positioning are part of the care plan. Work with the respiratory therapist to monitor the patient's condition and provide chest physiotherapy. Care of patients with a chest tube is described in Chapter 28.

INTERSTITIAL LUNG DISEASES

Interstitial lung disease (ILD), or *diffuse parenchymal lung disease,* refers to more than 200 lung disorders in which the tissue between the air sacs of the lungs (the interstitium) is affected by inflammation or scarring (fibrosis). Most ILDs are rare.

Many times, the cause of ILD is unknown. Known causes include inhalation of occupational and environment toxins, certain drugs, radiation therapy, connective tissue disorders, infection, and cancer. Treatment is aimed at reducing exposure to the causative agent or treating the underlying disease process. While scarring is not reversible, treatment with corticosteroids and immunosuppressant drugs can minimize progression. A lung transplant may be an option for some patients.

IDIOPATHIC PULMONARY FIBROSIS

Idiopathic pulmonary fibrosis (IPF) is a progressive disorder characterized by chronic inflammation and formation of scar tissue in the connective tissue.[15] Risk factors include smoking and exposure to wood and metal dust. IPF affects more men. It typically first appears between the ages of 50 and 70 years. We do not know the cause of IPF.

Manifestations include exertional dyspnea, a dry, nonproductive cough, clubbing, and inspiratory crackles. Fatigue, weakness, anorexia, and weight loss may occur as the disease progresses. Chest x-ray findings are often nonspecific. Pulmonary function tests may be abnormal, with reduced vital capacity and impaired gas exchange. Open lung biopsy using video-assisted thoracic surgery (VATS) often helps to confirm the pathology. It is the gold standard for diagnosis.

The course is variable, and the prognosis is poor. The median survival rate is 2.5 to 3.5 years after diagnosis. There is no known cure. Many people are first treated with a corticosteroid, sometimes in combination with other drugs that suppress the immune system (e.g., methotrexate, cyclosporine). Kinase inhibitor drugs, which block multiple pathways that are involved with scarring, include nintedanib (Ofev) and pirfenidone (Esbriet). O_2 therapy and pulmonary rehabilitation should be prescribed. A lung transplant may be an option.

SARCOIDOSIS

Sarcoidosis is a chronic, multisystem granulomatous disease of unknown cause. It mainly affects the lungs. The disease may also involve the skin, eyes, liver, kidney, heart, and lymph nodes. Signs and symptoms vary depending on what organs are affected. Pulmonary symptoms include dyspnea, cough, and chest pain. Many patients do not have symptoms.

Staging and treatment decisions are based on chest x-ray, pulmonary function tests, and severity of symptoms. Some patients have a spontaneous remission. Treatment is aimed at suppressing the inflammatory response. Patients are followed every 3 to 6 months with pulmonary function tests, chest x-ray, and CT scan to monitor disease progression.

CHEST TRAUMA AND THORACIC INJURY

Traumatic injuries to the chest contribute to many deaths. Chest injuries range from simple rib fractures to cardiorespiratory arrest. We classify the primary mechanisms of injury as either blunt trauma or penetrating trauma.

Blunt trauma occurs when the chest strikes or is struck by an object. The impact can cause shearing and compression of chest structures. The external injury may appear minor, but internally, organs may be severely damaged. Rib and sternal fractures can easily tear lung tissue. In a high-velocity impact, shearing forces can result in tearing of the aorta. Compression of the chest may result in heart or lung contusion, crush injury, and organ rupture.

In *penetrating trauma*, a foreign object impales or passes through the body tissues, creating an open wound. Examples include knife wounds, gunshot wounds, and injuries with other sharp objects. Emergency care of patients with a chest injury is outlined in Table 30.17. The most common chest emergencies and their management are described in Table 30.18.

FRACTURED RIBS

Rib fractures are the most common type of chest injury from blunt trauma. Ribs 5 through 9 are most often fractured because they are the least protected by chest muscles. A splintered or displaced fractured rib can damage the pleura, lungs, heart, and other internal organs.

Manifestations include pain at the site of injury, especially during inspiration and with coughing. The patient splints the affected area. They take shallow breaths to try to decrease the discomfort. Atelectasis and pneumonia may develop because of pain, decreased chest wall movement, and retained secretions.

The goal of treatment is to decrease pain so that patients can breathe adequately and clear secretions. Strapping the chest with tape or using a thoracic binder is not recommended. These limit chest expansion and predispose the person to atelectasis and hypoxemia. NSAIDs, opioids, and thoracic nerve blocks can reduce pain and assist with deep breathing and coughing. Surgical plating of fractured ribs may be done for patients with extreme chest wall deformity. Teaching should emphasize deep breathing, coughing, incentive spirometry, and pain management.

FLAIL CHEST

Flail chest results from the fracture of 3 or more consecutive ribs, in 2 or more separate places, causing an unstable segment (Fig. 30.3). It also can be caused by fracture of the sternum and several consecutive ribs. The resulting chest wall instability causes paradoxic movement during breathing. During inspiration, the affected part is sucked in, and during expiration, it bulges out. In other words, the affected (flail) area moves in the opposite direction with respect to the intact part of the chest. This paradoxic chest movement may prevent adequate ventilation and increase the work of breathing.

A flail chest is usually apparent on assessment. Patients have rapid, shallow respirations and tachycardia. Thorax movement is asymmetric and uncoordinated. Patients may try to splint the chest to assist with breathing. The history, mechanism of injury, abnormal chest movement, crepitus near the rib fractures, and chest x-ray assist in the diagnosis.

The goal is to promote lung expansion and ensure adequate ventilation and oxygenation. The underlying injured lung may be contused, worsening hypoxemia. Administer supplement O_2, monitor vital signs, and record SpO_2. Assess respiratory rate, rhythm, and depth. Some patients may need mechanical ventilation. Analgesia can help promote adequate respiration. Patients with extreme deformity may need surgical fixation of

TABLE 30.17 EMERGENCY MANAGEMENT

Chest Trauma

Etiology	Assessment Findings	Interventions
Blunt • Assault with blunt object • Crush injury • Explosion • Fall • Motor vehicle collision • Pedestrian accident • Sports injury **Penetrating** • Arrow • Gunshot • Knife • Stick	**Respiratory** • Audible air escaping from chest wound • ↓ Breath sounds on side of injury • Cough with or without hemoptysis • Cyanosis of mouth, face, nail beds, mucous membranes • Dyspnea, respiratory distress • Frothy secretions • ↓ O_2 saturation • Tracheal deviation **Cardiovascular** • Asymmetric BP values in arms • ↓ BP • Chest pain • Distended neck veins • Dysrhythmias • Muffled heart sounds • Narrowed pulse pressure • Rapid, thready pulse **Surface Findings** • Abrasions • Asymmetric chest movement • Bruising • Contusions • Lacerations • Open chest wound • Subcutaneous emphysema	**Initial** • If unresponsive, immediately assess circulation, airway, and breathing. • If responsive, monitor airway, breathing, and circulation. • Apply high-flow O_2 to keep SpO_2 >90%. • Establish IV access with 2 large-bore catheters. Begin IV fluid resuscitation. • Remove clothing to assess injury. • Cover sucking chest wound with nonporous dressing taped on 3 sides (vent dressing). • Stabilize impaled objects with bulky dressings. *Do not remove object.* • Assess for life-threatening injuries and treat appropriately. • Place patient in a semi-Fowler's position if breathing is easier *after* cervical spine injury has been ruled out. • Give analgesia as needed for pain and to help with breathing. • Prepare for emergency needle decompression if tension pneumothorax or cardiac tamponade present. **Ongoing Monitoring** • Monitor LOC, vital signs, O_2 saturation, cardiac rhythm, respiratory rate and rhythm, urine output. • Assess for increased work of breathing and respiratory distress; anticipate possible intubation. • Release vent dressing if tension pneumothorax develops after sucking chest wound is covered.

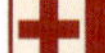

TABLE 30.18 EMERGENCY MANAGEMENT

Chest Injuries

Injury and Description	Manifestations	Interventions
Cardiac Tamponade Blood rapidly collects in pericardial sac, compresses myocardium because pericardium does not stretch, and prevents ventricles from filling.	Muffled, distant heart sounds, hypotension, neck vein distention, ↑ central venous pressure	Medical emergency. Immediate pericardiocentesis. Follow-up with surgical repair as required.
Flail Chest Fracture of 3 or more adjacent ribs in 2 or more places with loss of chest wall stability (see Fig. 30.3).	Paradoxic movement of chest wall, respiratory distress. May be associated hemothorax, pneumothorax, pulmonary contusion	O_2 as needed to maintain O_2 saturation, analgesia. Positive pressure mechanical ventilation for acute respiratory distress; will also help stabilize flail segment. Treat associated injuries. Possible surgical fixation for severe damage to chest wall.
Hemothorax Blood in the pleural space, may or may not occur in conjunction with pneumothorax.	Dyspnea, decreased or absent breath sounds, dullness to percussion, ↓ Hgb, shock (depending on blood volume lost)	Chest tube insertion with chest drainage system. Autotransfusion of collected blood. Treatment of hypovolemia with IV fluid, packed red blood cells.
Pneumothorax Air in pleural space (see Fig. 30.4).	Dyspnea, ↓ movement of involved chest wall, decreased or absent breath sounds on the affected side, hyperresonance to percussion	Chest tube insertion with chest drainage system.
Tension Pneumothorax Air in pleural space that does not escape. Increased air in the pleural space shifts organs and increases intrathoracic pressure (see Fig. 30.5).	Cyanosis, air hunger, extreme agitation, subcutaneous emphysema, neck vein distention, hyperresonance to percussion, tracheal deviation away from affected side (late sign)	Medical emergency: needle decompression followed by chest tube insertion with chest drainage system.

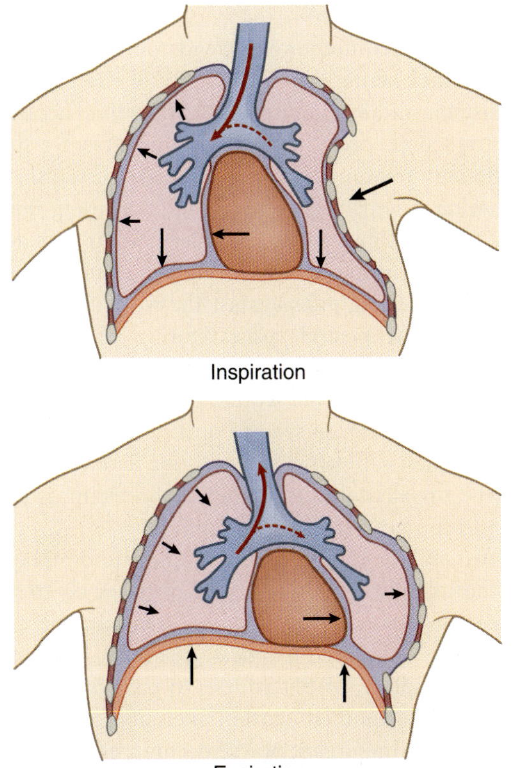

Fig. 30.3 Flail chest causes paradoxic respiration. On inspiration, the flail section moves inward with mediastinal shift to the uninjured side. On expiration, the flail section bulges outward with mediastinal shift to the injured side.

the flail segment. The lung parenchyma and fractured ribs heal with time. Some patients continue to have intercostal pain several weeks after the flail chest has resolved.

PNEUMOTHORAX

A **pneumothorax** is caused by air entering the pleural cavity. Normally, negative (subatmospheric) pressure exists between the visceral pleura (surrounding the lung) and parietal pleura (lining the chest cavity), known as the *pleural space.* The pleural space has a few milliliters of lubricating fluid to reduce friction when the tissues move. When the volume of air that enters this normally subatmospheric space increases, lung volume decreases. As a result, the change to positive pressure causes a partial or complete lung collapse.

We can describe a pneumothorax as *open* (air entering through an opening in the chest wall) or *closed* (no external wound). Penetrating trauma allows air to enter the pleural space through an opening in the chest wall (Fig. 30.4). A penetrating chest wound is also called a *sucking chest wound,* since air enters the pleural space through the chest wall during inspiration. A pneumothorax should be suspected after any trauma to the chest wall.

If a pneumothorax is small, mild tachycardia and dyspnea may be the only manifestations. With a larger pneumothorax, respiratory distress may be present, including short, shallow,

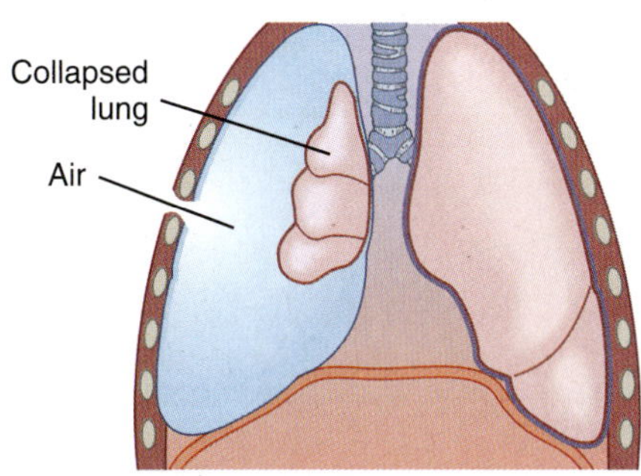

Fig. 30.4 Open pneumothorax. Collapse of lung results from disruption of chest wall and outside air entering the thoracic cavity.

rapid respirations, dyspnea, and low O_2 saturation. Breath sounds are absent over the affected area. A chest x-ray will show air or fluid in the pleural space and reduced lung volume.

Types of Pneumothoraxes

Spontaneous Pneumothorax

A spontaneous pneumothorax typically occurs due to the rupture of small blebs (air-filled sacs) on the surface of the lung. These blebs can occur in healthy young people or from lung disease, such as chronic obstructive pulmonary disease (COPD), asthma, cystic fibrosis, and pneumonia. Smoking increases the risk for bleb formation. Other risk factors include being tall and thin, male gender, family history, and previous spontaneous pneumothorax.

Iatrogenic Pneumothorax

Iatrogenic pneumothorax can occur due to laceration or puncture of the lung during a procedure. For example, transthoracic needle aspiration, subclavian catheter insertion, pleural biopsy, and transbronchial lung biopsy all have the potential to injure the lung. Tearing of the esophageal wall during insertion of a gastric tube can allow air from the esophagus to enter the mediastinum and pleural space. Barotrauma from excessive ventilatory pressure during manual or mechanical ventilation can rupture alveoli, creating a pneumothorax.

Tension Pneumothorax

Tension pneumothorax occurs when air enters the pleural space but cannot escape. The continued accumulation of air in the pleural space causes increasingly elevated intrapleural pressures. This results in compression of the lung on the affected side and pressure on the heart and great vessels, pushing them away from the affected side (Fig. 30.5). The mediastinum shifts toward the unaffected side, compressing the "good" lung, which further compromises oxygenation and ventilation. As the pressure increases, venous return decreases and cardiac output falls.

Tension pneumothorax may result from either an open or a closed pneumothorax. In an open chest wound, a flap may act as a 1-way valve. Thus air can enter on inspiration but cannot escape. Tension pneumothorax can occur with mechanical

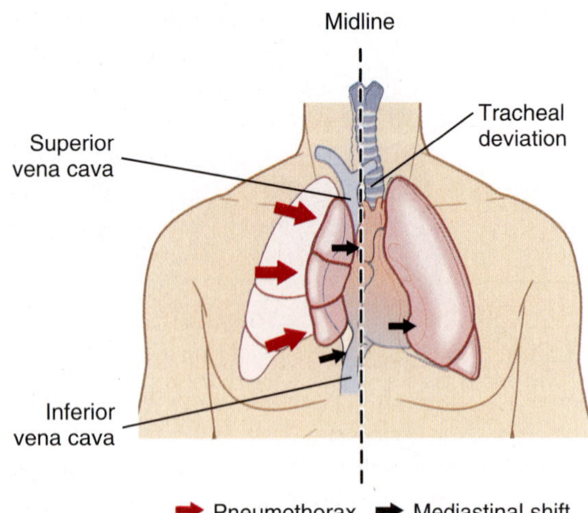

Fig. 30.5 Tension pneumothorax. As pleural pressure on the affected side increases, mediastinal displacement occurs, causing respiratory and cardiovascular compromise. Tracheal deviation is an external but late sign of mediastinal shift.

ventilation and resuscitative efforts. It can also occur if chest tubes are clamped or become blocked in patients with a pneumothorax. Unclamping the tube or relieving the obstruction may correct this situation.

Tension pneumothorax is a medical emergency. It affects both the respiratory and cardiovascular systems. Manifestations include severe dyspnea, marked tachycardia, neck vein distention, and profuse diaphoresis. Decreased or absent breath sounds will be present on the affected side. Tracheal deviation is a very late sign. If we do not quickly identify the problem and relieve the pressure in the pleural space, patients are likely to die of inadequate cardiac output and severe hypoxemia.

Hemothorax

Hemothorax is an accumulation of blood in the pleural space from injury to the chest wall, diaphragm, lung, blood vessels, or mediastinum. When it occurs with pneumothorax, it is called a *hemopneumothorax*. Patients with a traumatic hemothorax need immediate insertion of a chest tube for evacuation of the blood. Sometimes, blood drained from a chest tube can be reinfused back into the patient (autotransfusion) after the injury. However, this requires special equipment and set-up before chest tube insertion.

Chylothorax

Chylothorax is the presence of lymphatic fluid in the pleural space. The thoracic duct is disrupted either traumatically or from cancer, allowing lymphatic fluid to fill the pleural space. Some cases heal with conservative treatment (chest drainage, bowel rest, diet). Octreotide may reduce the flow of lymphatic fluid. Surgery (thoracic duct ligation) and pleurodesis (the artificial production of adhesions between the parietal and visceral pleura) are options for some patients.

Interprofessional Care

Treatment of a pneumothorax depends on its severity, underlying cause, and hemodynamic stability of the patient. If the patient is stable and has minimal air and/or fluid accumulation in the intrapleural space, the condition may resolve spontaneously. The only treatment would then be observation.

Prehospital emergency care consists of covering the wound with an occlusive dressing that is secured on 3 sides (vent dressing). During inspiration, as negative pressure is created in the chest, the dressing pulls against the wound, preventing air from entering the pleural space. During expiration, as the pressure rises in the pleural space, the dressing is pushed out and air escapes through the wound and from under the dressing. If the object that caused the open chest wound is still in place, prehospital care providers will not remove it. They will stabilize the impaled object with a bulky dressing and arrange transport to the nearest medical facility.

In acute care, the most definitive and common treatment of pneumothorax and hemothorax is to insert a chest tube and connect it to water-seal drainage. Repeated spontaneous pneumothorax may need surgical treatment with a partial pleurectomy, stapling, or pleurodesis to promote adherence of the pleurae to one another. Tension pneumothorax is a medical emergency, requiring urgent needle decompression followed by chest tube insertion to water-seal drainage. Care of patients with chest tubes is described in Chapter 28.

VASCULAR LUNG DISORDERS

PULMONARY EDEMA

Pulmonary edema is an abnormal accumulation of fluid in the alveoli and interstitial spaces of the lungs. It is a complication of various heart and lung problems (Table 30.19). In severe cases,

TABLE 30.19 Causes of Pulmonary Edema

Cardiac
- Acute myocardial infarction
- Aortic and/or mitral regurgitation
- Cardiomyopathy
- Dysrhythmias
- Left ventricular (heart) failure

Noncardiac
- Acute respiratory distress syndrome (ARDS)
- Altered capillary permeability of lungs: aspiration, inhaled toxins, inflammation (e.g., pneumonia), severe hypoxia, near-drowning
- Anaphylactic (allergic) reaction
- Hypoalbuminemia: nephrotic syndrome, liver disease, nutrition problems
- Lymph system cancer (e.g., non-Hodgkin lymphoma)
- Multiple blood transfusions
- Opioid overdose
- Overhydration with IV fluids
- O_2 toxicity
- Sepsis
- Traumatic injury, shock
- Unknown causes: neurogenic condition, high altitude

pulmonary edema can be a life-threatening medical emergency. The most common cause of pulmonary edema is left-sided HF.

Patients often present with varying degrees of dyspnea, diaphoresis, and wheezing, depending on the severity of pulmonary edema and underlying medical condition. A 3rd heart sound may be present. Sputum may be blood-tinged and frothy. A chest x-ray is the best option for confirming the diagnosis.

Treatment is directed toward finding the underlying cause of the edema and reducing the amount of fluid in the lungs. Goals include simultaneously improving oxygenation, ventilation, and cardiac output, which enhances tissue perfusion.

Place the patient in a semi- or high Fowler's position. Administer O_2 to keep SpO_2 greater than 90%. This may require low- or high-flow O_2 delivery devices, noninvasive ventilation (e.g., Bi-PAP), or mechanical ventilation. Preload reduction may be accomplished by giving IV diuretics (e.g., furosemide) or nitroglycerine. Cardiac output can be supported with IV dobutamine. Monitor vital signs, work of breathing, breath sounds, urinary output, electrolyte balance, and response to treatment.

PULMONARY EMBOLISM

Etiology and Pathophysiology

Pulmonary embolism (PE) is the blockage of 1 or more pulmonary arteries by a thrombus, fat or air embolus, or tumor tissue. PE consists of material that gains access to the venous system and then to the pulmonary circulation. PE travels with blood flow through ever-smaller blood vessels until it lodges and obstructs perfusion of the alveoli. The lower lobes are most often affected.

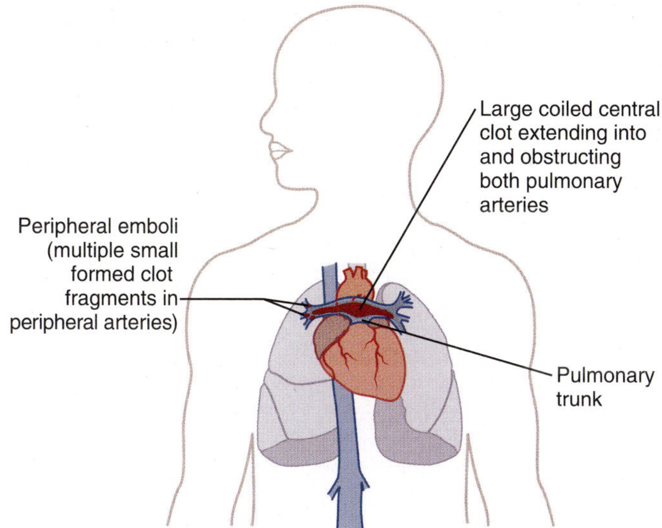

Fig. 30.6 Saddle pulmonary embolus. This embolus straddles the bifurcation of a major artery, with the clot extending down into both right and left branches of the major vessel.

Most PEs arise from deep vein thrombosis (DVT) in the deep veins of the legs. *Venous thromboembolism (VTE)* is the preferred term to describe the spectrum from DVT to PE. Other sites of origin of PE include femoral or iliac veins, right side of the heart (atrial fibrillation), and pelvic veins (especially after surgery or childbirth). Upper extremity DVT sometimes occurs in the presence of central venous catheters or arterial lines. These cases may resolve with catheter removal. A *saddle embolus* refers to a large thrombus lodged at an arterial bifurcation (Fig. 30.6).

Less common causes include fat emboli (from fractured long bones), air emboli (from improperly administered IV therapy), bacterial vegetation on heart valves, amniotic fluid, and cancer.[16] Risk factors for PE include immobility or reduced mobility, surgery within the last 3 months (especially pelvic and lower extremity surgery), history of VTE, oral contraceptive or hormone therapy, smoking, prolonged air travel, HF, pregnancy, and clotting disorders.

Clinical Manifestations

The signs and symptoms are varied and nonspecific, making diagnosis difficult. Manifestations depend on the type, size, and extent of emboli. Small emboli may go undetected or cause vague, transient symptoms. Symptoms may begin slowly or appear suddenly. Dyspnea is the most common presenting symptom in patients with PE. Mild to moderate hypoxemia may occur. Other manifestations include tachypnea, cough, chest pain, hemoptysis, crackles, wheezing, fever, accentuation of pulmonic heart sound, tachycardia, and syncope. Massive PE may cause a sudden change in mental status, hypotension, feelings of impending doom, and cardiorespiratory arrest.

Complications

About 10% of patients with massive PE die within the 1st hour. Treatment with anticoagulants significantly reduces mortality.

Complications include pulmonary infarction and pulmonary hypertension. *Pulmonary infarction* (death of lung tissue) is most likely when there is (1) occlusion of a large or medium-sized pulmonary vessel (more than 2 mm in diameter), (2) insufficient collateral blood flow from the bronchial circulation, or (3) preexisting lung disease. Infarction results in alveolar necrosis and hemorrhage. Sometimes the necrotic tissue becomes infected, and an abscess may develop. Pleural effusions are common.

Pulmonary hypertension results from hypoxemia or from involvement of a large surface area of the pulmonary bed. As a single event, PE rarely causes pulmonary hypertension. Recurrent PEs or PEs that do not completely resolve gradually reduce capillary bed blood flow over time. This may eventually cause *chronic thromboembolic pulmonary hypertension.* Dilation and hypertrophy of the right ventricle occur. Depending on the severity of pulmonary hypertension and how quickly it develops, outcomes can vary. Some patients die within months while others live for decades.

Diagnostic Studies

A *spiral (helical) CT scan* (CT angiography or CTA) is the most common test to diagnose PE. An IV injection of contrast media is needed to view the pulmonary blood vessels. The scanner continuously rotates around the patient while obtaining views of the lung vasculature. This allows us to see all anatomic regions of the lungs. Computer reconstruction gives a 3-D picture and assists in seeing PE.

If a patient cannot have contrast media, a ventilation-perfusion (V/Q) scan is done. The V/Q scan has 2 parts. It is most accurate when both are done:

1. *Perfusion scanning* involves IV injection of a radioisotope. A scanning device images the pulmonary circulation.
2. *Ventilation scanning* involves inhalation of a radioactive gas, such as xenon. Scanning reflects the distribution of gas through the lung. This requires the patient's cooperation. It may not be possible to perform in critically ill patients, especially if the patient is intubated.

ABG analysis is important but does not diagnose PE. Pao_2 may be low because of inadequate oxygenation from occluded pulmonary vessels preventing matching of perfusion to ventilation. The pH is often normal unless respiratory alkalosis develops because of prolonged hyperventilation or to compensate for lactic acidosis caused by shock.

Abnormal findings may be seen on a chest x-ray (atelectasis, pleural effusion) and ECG (nonspecific ST segment, T wave changes), but they are not diagnostic for PE. Serum troponin levels and b-type natriuretic peptide (BNP) levels are often high.

D-dimer is a laboratory test that measures the amount of cross-linked fibrin fragments. These fragments are the result of clot degradation. The disadvantage of D-dimer testing is that it is neither specific (many other conditions cause increases) nor sensitive, because up to 50% of patients with a small PE have normal results. Patients with suspected PE and an elevated D-dimer level but normal venous ultrasound may need a spiral CT or lung scan.

Interprofessional Care

To reduce mortality, we start treatment as soon as we suspect PE (Table 30.20). The goals are to (1) promote optimal cardiorespiratory function, (2) ensure adequate blood flow, (3) prevent further growth or extension of thrombi, and (4) prevent and avoid complications and recurrence.

Immediate assessment should focus on cardiorespiratory status, which varies by the size and location of the PE. Initiate O_2 by mask or cannula when hypoxemia is present. Titrate the Fio_2 based on ABG analysis. In some situations, mechanical ventilation is needed to maintain adequate oxygenation. Respiratory measures—including turning, coughing, deep breathing, and incentive spirometry—are important to help prevent atelectasis. Pain from pleural irritation or reduced coronary blood flow is treated with opioids. If HF is present, diuretics are used. If manifestations of shock are present, IV fluids and vasopressor agents are given as needed to support circulation.

Drug Therapy

Patients with PE need immediate anticoagulation. Drug therapy for patients with acute PE occurs in 3 phases: initial (for the first 7 days), longer (up to 6 weeks), and extended (6 months and beyond). Subcutaneous low-molecular-weight heparin (LMWH) (e.g., enoxaparin, fondaparinux) is the recommended treatment for patients with acute PE. LMWH is safer and more effective than unfractionated heparin. Unfractionated IV heparin is effective but hard to titrate to therapeutic levels.

Warfarin should be started at the time of diagnosis. Therapy continues for at least 3 to 6 months and then reevaluated. Alternatives to warfarin include apixaban (Eliquis), dabigatran (Pradaxa), and edoxaban (Savaysa). Anticoagulant therapy may be contraindicated if the patient has complicating factors, such as liver problems (causing changes in the clotting), bleeding, a history of hemorrhagic stroke, heparin-induced thrombocytopenia (HIT), or other blood dyscrasias.

TABLE 30.20 Interprofessional Care

Acute Pulmonary Embolism

Diagnostic Assessment

- History and physical assessment
- Chest x-ray
- Continuous ECG monitoring
- Pulse oximetry, ABGs
- Spiral (helical) CT scan; if unavailable, CTA or pulmonary angiography
- Ventilation-perfusion (V/Q) lung scan (for nonventilated patient)
- Useful lab tests (but not diagnostic); D-dimer, troponin, b-natriuretic peptide levels
- Ultrasound of upper or lower extremities (based on likely source)

Management

- Monitor hemodynamic status (HR, BP)
- Supplemental O_2, intubation if needed
- Monitor hemoglobin, assess patient for bleeding
- Monitor activated partial thromboplastin time and international normalized ratio levels
- Balance activity and rest
- Inferior vena cava filter
- Life-threatening situation: pulmonary embolectomy

Drug Therapy

- Unfractionated heparin IV
- Low-molecular-weight heparin (e.g., enoxaparin [Lovenox]) SC
- Factor Xa inhibitors (e.g., apixaban [Eliquis], edoxaban)
- Thrombin inhibitors (e.g., dabigatran [Pradaxa])
- Warfarin (Coumadin) for long-term therapy
- Thrombolytics (e.g., alteplase rt-PA) for life-threatening situation
- Analgesia

Some HCPs use direct thrombin inhibitors (see Table 41.10) to treat PE. Similarly, fibrinolytic agents, such as tissue plasminogen activator (tPA) or alteplase (Activase), may help dissolve the PE and the source of the thrombus in the pelvis or deep leg veins, thus decreasing the risk for recurrent emboli. Fibrinolytic therapy is discussed in Chapter 37.

Surgical Therapy

Hemodynamically unstable patients with massive PE in whom thrombolytic therapy is contraindicated may be candidates for pulmonary embolectomy. Embolectomy, the removal of emboli, can help decrease right ventricular afterload. It can be done through a diagnostic imaging (vascular catheter) or surgical approach. Embolectomy can help decrease right ventricular afterload.

Percutaneous intervention techniques, ultrasound-guided catheter thrombolysis, and aspiration thrombectomy are newer, moderately invasive procedures for PE. In patients who are high risk and for whom anticoagulation is contraindicated, an inferior vena cava (IVC) filter may be the treatment of choice (Fig. 30.7). This device, inserted through the femoral vein, is placed at the level of the renal veins in the inferior vena cava. Once inserted, the filter expands and prevents the movement of large clots upward and into the pulmonary system. Complications are rare but include misplacement, migration, and perforation.

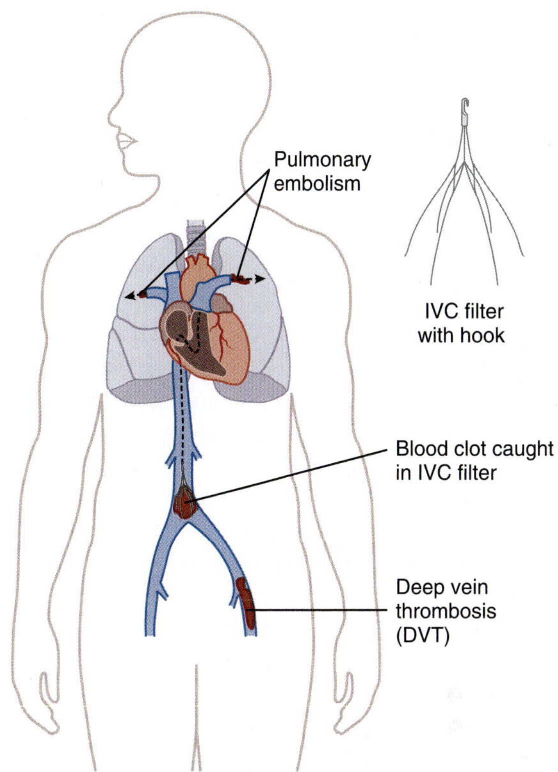

Fig. 30.7 Inferior vena cava *(IVC)* filter. This small device is placed in the inferior vena cava. It helps trap blood clots that may travel from the lower extremities up toward the brain and heart.

NURSING MANAGEMENT: PULMONARY EMBOLISM

Prevention of PE begins with preventing DVT. Identifying patients at risk is essential. Nursing measures aimed at prevention of PE are similar to those for prophylaxis of VTE. These include the use of intermittent pneumatic compression devices, early ambulation, and anticoagulant therapy.

Initially, keep the patient on bed rest in a semi-Fowler's position. Assess cardiopulmonary status with monitoring of vital signs, cardiac rhythm, pulse oximetry, ABGs, and lung sounds. Apply O_2 therapy as directed. Maintain a patent IV line for medications and fluid therapy. Monitor laboratory results to ensure therapeutic ranges of INR (for warfarin) and aPTT (for IV heparin). Monitor platelet counts for thrombocytopenia and the development of HIT. Observe the patient for complications of anticoagulant and fibrinolytic therapy (e.g., bleeding, bruising).

The patient may be anxious because of pain, inability to breathe, and fear of death. Provide emotional support and reassurance to help relieve anxiety.

Teaching about long-term anticoagulant therapy is essential. Anticoagulant therapy often continues for at least 3 months. Patients with large or recurrent emboli may be treated indefinitely with anticoagulants. INR levels are drawn at intervals and warfarin dosage is adjusted. Some patients are monitored by nurses in an anticoagulation clinic.

Long-term management of PE is similar to that for patients with VTE (see Chapter 41). Discharge planning is aimed at preventing worsening of the current condition and avoiding complications and recurrence. Reinforce the need for patients to return to the HCP for regular follow-up care.

PULMONARY ARTERIAL HYPERTENSION

In **pulmonary arterial hypertension** (PAH) there is an elevated pulmonary artery pressure (greater than 20 mm Hg) from an increase in resistance to blood flow through the pulmonary circulation.[17] Pulmonary hypertension can occur as a primary disease *(idiopathic pulmonary arterial hypertension)* or as a secondary complication of a respiratory, heart, autoimmune, liver, or connective tissue problem *(secondary pulmonary arterial hypertension).*

There are 5 classes of pulmonary hypertension.[18] Each is based on cause:

Group 1: Attributed to medication, specific diseases, genetic (inherited) link, or idiopathic

Group 2: Related to left-sided heart disease

Group 3: Related to the lung disease or hypoxia

Group 4: Related to the cardiovascular system and thromboembolism

Group 5: Multifactorial (and often unclear) origins (e.g., hematologic, metabolic, renal involvement)

Idiopathic Pulmonary Arterial Hypertension

Etiology and Pathophysiology

Idiopathic pulmonary arterial hypertension (IPAH) is related to connective tissue diseases, cirrhosis, and HIV. The exact relationship between these disorders and IPAH is unclear, as is the pathophysiology of IPAH. We believe that some type of insult (e.g., hormonal, mechanical) to the pulmonary endothelium may occur, causing a cascade of events leading to vascular scarring, endothelial dysfunction, and smooth muscle proliferation (Fig. 30.8). IPAH affects more females.

Clinical Manifestations and Diagnostic Studies

The classic symptoms are dyspnea on exertion and fatigue. Exertional chest pain, dizziness, and syncope may occur. These are related to the inability of cardiac output to increase in response to increased O_2 demand. Abnormal heart sounds may be heard, including an S_3. Eventually, as the disease progresses, dyspnea occurs at rest. Pulmonary hypertension increases the workload of the right ventricle, and over time causes right ventricular hypertrophy (cor pulmonale) and, eventually, HF.

Right-sided cardiac catheterization is the definitive test to diagnose any type of pulmonary hypertension. It gives an accurate measurement of pulmonary artery pressures, cardiac output, and pulmonary vascular resistance. Diagnostic evaluation often includes ECG, chest x-ray, pulmonary function tests, echocardiogram, and CT scan. Confirmation of IPAH requires a workup to exclude conditions that may cause secondary pulmonary hypertension.

The mean time between onset of symptoms and the diagnosis is about 2 years. By the time patients become symptomatic, the disease is already in the advanced stages and the pulmonary artery pressure is often 2 to 3 times normal values.

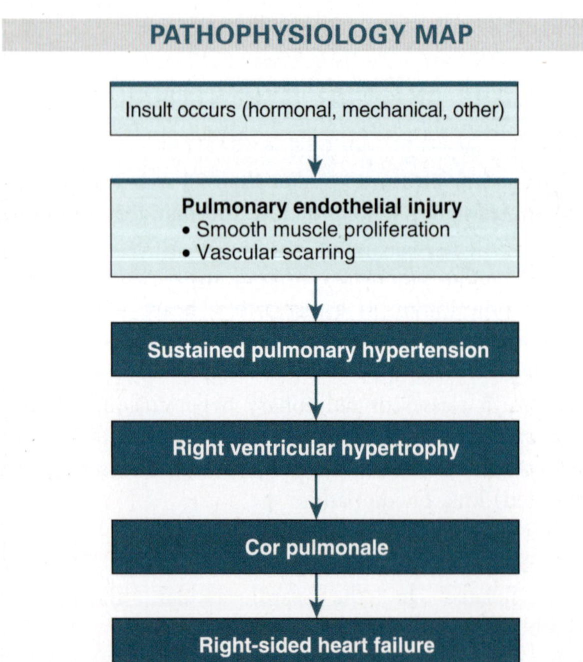

Fig. 30.8 Pathogenesis of pulmonary hypertension and cor pulmonale.

Interprofessional and Nursing Management

Although IPAH has no cure, treatment can relieve symptoms, improve quality of life, and prolong life. Left untreated, IPAH can rapidly progress, causing right-sided HF and death within a few years. New drug therapy has greatly improved survival. Drug therapy consists of agents that dilate the pulmonary blood vessels, reduce right ventricular overload, and reverse remodeling (Table 30.21). Diuretics are used to manage peripheral edema. Anticoagulants reduce the risk of thrombus formation. Because hypoxia is a potent pulmonary vasoconstrictor, low-flow O_2 gives symptomatic relief. The goal is to keep O_2 saturation 90% or greater.

Surgical therapy includes pulmonary thromboendarterectomy (PTE), in which clots are removed from the pulmonary arteries. It is a technically demanding, high-risk procedure, done only at certain centers. Atrial septostomy is a palliative procedure. It involves the creation of an intraatrial right-to-left shunt to decompress the right ventricle. It is used for some patients awaiting a lung transplant. A lung transplant is an option for some patients who do not respond to drug therapy and progress to severe right-sided HF. Recurrence has not been reported in persons who had a lung transplant.

Secondary Pulmonary Arterial Hypertension

Secondary pulmonary arterial hypertension (SPAH) occurs when another disease causes a chronic increase in pulmonary artery pressures. The primary disease can cause anatomic or vascular changes that result in pulmonary hypertension. SPAH can develop due to parenchymal lung disease, left ventricular dysfunction, intracardiac shunts, chronic PE, or systemic connective tissue disease.[19]

The symptoms can reflect the underlying disease, but some are directly related to SPAH. These include dyspnea, fatigue, lethargy, and chest pain. Findings can include right ventricular hypertrophy and signs of right-sided HF (increased pulmonic heart sound, S_4 heart sound, peripheral edema, hepatomegaly).

Diagnosis of SPAH is like that of IPAH. With SPAH, we treat the underlying primary disorder. When irreversible pulmonary vascular damage has occurred, therapies for IPAH are started. A PTE may offer a cure for patients with chronic pulmonary hypertension caused by PE.

COR PULMONALE

Cor pulmonale is enlargement of the right ventricle caused by a primary respiratory disorder. Almost any disorder that affects the respiratory system can cause cor pulmonale. The most common cause is COPD. Pulmonary hypertension is usually a preexisting condition in the person with cor pulmonale. Overt

TABLE 30.21 **Drug Therapy**

Pulmonary Hypertension

Drug	Mechanism of Action	Considerations
Endothelin Receptor Antagonists		
ambrisentan (Letairis) bosentan (Tracleer) macitentan (Opsumit)	• Inhibits binding of endothelin to receptor on smooth muscle in pulmonary system • Promotes relaxation of pulmonary arteries • ↓ Pulmonary artery pressure	• Given orally • Bosentan: Hepatotoxicity • Macitentan: low hemoglobin • Contraindicated in females who are or want to become pregnant
Phosphodiesterase (Type 5) Enzyme Inhibitors		
sildenafil (Revatio) tadalafil (Adcirca) riociguat (Adempas)	• Promote smooth muscle relaxation in lung vasculature • ↑ Blood flow to lungs	• Given orally • Contraindicated in patients taking nitroglycerin (may cause refractory hypotension) • Side effects: headache, back pain, flushing • Drug interactions with antibiotics, alpha blockers, verapamil
Vasodilators		
iloprost (Ventavis) treprostinil (Tyvaso)	• Synthetic analogs of prostacyclin (PGI_2) • Dilate systemic and pulmonary arterial vasculature • Help relieve dyspnea	• Depending on drug, may be given by inhalation (nebulizer), oral, subcutaneously, or IV • Inhalation: given 6–9 times a day using a disk inserted into a nebulizer • Can cause orthostatic hypotension. Do not give to patients with systolic BP <85 mm Hg • Use cautiously in asthma and emphysema (can make cough and breathing worse)
Prostacyclin Analogs		
epoprostenol (Flolan, Veletri) treprostinil (Remodulin)	• Promote pulmonary vasodilation and reduce pulmonary vascular resistance • ↓ Dyspnea and chest congestion • Inhibits platelets	• Flolan: most effective for advanced pulmonary arterial hypertension • Most often given by continuous IV (central line) • Half-life of epoprostenol is short • Potential clinical deterioration from abrupt withdrawal if infusion disrupted • Side effects: headache, rash, GI upset

HF may be present. Fig. 30.8 outlines the cause and pathogenesis of pulmonary hypertension and cor pulmonale.

Clinical Manifestations and Diagnostic Studies

Common symptoms include exertional dyspnea, tachypnea, cough, and fatigue. ECG may show right ventricular hypertrophy and an increase in intensity of S_2. Chronic hypoxemia leads to polycythemia and increased total blood volume and viscosity. Polycythemia is often present in cor pulmonale from COPD.

If HF accompanies cor pulmonale, peripheral edema, weight gain, distended neck veins, full, bounding pulse, and enlarged liver may occur. Various laboratory tests and imaging studies are used to confirm the diagnosis (Table 30.22).

Interprofessional and Nursing Management

Early identification is essential before changes to the heart occur that may be irreversible. Management is directed at determining the cause and treating the underlying problem.

Long-term O_2 therapy, the mainstay of treatment to correct hypoxemia, reduces vasoconstriction and pulmonary hypertension. Any fluid, electrolyte, and/or acid-base imbalances are corrected. Diuretics may help decrease plasma volume and reduce the workload on the heart but are used with caution. In some cases, decreases in fluid volume from diuresis can worsen heart function. Bronchodilator therapy is needed if the underlying respiratory problem is due to an obstructive disorder.

Other treatments may include vasodilator therapy, calcium channel blockers, anticoagulants, digitalis, and phlebotomy. All have varying degrees of success. Chronic management of cor pulmonale from COPD is like that described for COPD (see Chapter 31).

ENVIRONMENT LUNG DISEASE

Environment or occupation-induced lung diseases result from inhaled dust or chemicals. The extent of lung damage is influenced by the toxicity of the inhaled substance, amount and duration of exposure, and individual susceptibility.

TABLE 30.22 Interprofessional Care

Cor Pulmonale

Diagnostic Assessment
- History and physical assessment
- ABGs, SpO_2
- Serum electrolytes (including BUN and creatinine)
- b-Type natriuretic peptide (BNP)
- ECG
- Chest x-ray
- Echocardiography
- CT scan, MRI, ventilation-perfusion (VQ) scan
- Cardiac catheterization

Management
- Treat the cause (may be difficult, often involves improving O_2 delivery and right ventricular function)
- O_2 therapy
- Low-sodium diet

Drug Therapy (Depending on Cause and Patient Condition)
- Bronchodilators
- Diuretics (use with caution)
- Pulmonary vasodilators
- Calcium channel blockers
- Inotropic agents
- Digitalis
- Anticoagulation therapy

Environment lung diseases include pneumoconiosis, chemical pneumonitis, and hypersensitivity pneumonitis.

Pneumoconiosis is a general term for a group of lung diseases caused by inhalation and retention of mineral or metal dust particles. The literal meaning of *pneumoconiosis* is "dust in the lungs." We classify these diseases by the origin of the dust (e.g., silicosis, asbestosis, berylliosis). For example, silicosis occurs from inhaling silica from sand and rock. Coal worker's pneumoconiosis (CWP), or *black lung,* is caused by inhaling large amounts of coal dust. The inhaled substance is ingested by macrophages, which release substances that cause cell injury and death. Fibrosis occurs from tissue repair after inflammation. Breathing problems become evident after many years of repeated exposure, resulting in diffuse *pulmonary fibrosis* (excess connective tissue).

Asbestos is a group of minerals composed of microscopic fibers. For many years, asbestos was used for insulation and to help fireproof buildings. When disturbed, asbestos releases tiny filament particles into the air. Once inhaled, the tiny fibers become deposited within the lung. Asbestosis causes chronic lung inflammation. People with repeated exposure to asbestos are at a greater risk for disease. Lung cancer and mesothelioma, both pleural and peritoneal, are associated with asbestos exposure.[20]

Chemical pneumonitis results from exposure to toxic chemical fumes. There are 2 types of chemical pneumonitis: acute and chronic. In the acute form, there is diffuse lung injury with pulmonary edema. Chronically, the clinical picture is that of *bronchiolitis obliterans* (obstruction of the bronchioles due to inflammation and fibrosis). The chest x-ray is normal or shows hyperinflation.

Hypersensitivity pneumonitis, or extrinsic allergic alveolitis, is a form of parenchymal lung disease seen when a person inhales an antigen to which they are allergic. There are acute, subacute, and chronic forms. Examples include bird fancier's lung (exposure to particles in feathers and droppings of birds) and farmer's lung (inhalation of hay dust particles).

Clinical Manifestations

Symptoms of many environment lung diseases may not occur until at least 10 to 15 years after the initial exposure to the inhaled irritant. Manifestations common to all pneumoconiosis include dyspnea, cough, wheezing, and weight loss. Pulmonary function studies often show reduced vital capacity. A chest x-ray often shows lung involvement specific to the primary problem. CT scans have been useful in detecting early lung involvement.

COPD is the most common complication. Other associated problems include acute pulmonary edema, lung cancer, mesothelioma, and TB. The appearance of symptoms and complications is often the reason patients seek medical care. Cor pulmonale is a late complication. It is more common when there is diffuse pulmonary fibrosis.

Interprofessional and Nursing Management

The best approach is to prevent or decrease exposure. Teach those at risk about the use of PPE. Wearing masks and ensuring well-designed, effective ventilation systems are in place are appropriate for some occupations. Smoke inhalation by nonsmokers has led to laws requiring a smoke-free workplace. Periodic inspections and monitoring of workplaces by agencies such as the Occupational Safety and Health Administration (OSHA) and the National Institute for Occupational Safety and Health (NIOSH) reinforce employers' obligations to provide a safe work environment.

Encourage regular medical check-ups for those in high-risk occupations. Early diagnosis is essential to halting the disease process. Care is directed toward preventing disease progression and monitoring, improving, or controlling respiratory symptoms. Treatment depends on the cause and severity of the condition. Acute care may include O_2 therapy, IV fluid, inhaled bronchodilators, corticosteroids, and NSAIDs. Some patients need mechanical ventilation. Longer-term care includes pulmonary rehabilitation. Patients should be immunized against pneumococcal pneumonia and influenza. Discontinuing exposure to the offending agent and smoking cessation may or may not be effective in stopping disease progression.

LUNG TRANSPLANTS

Lung transplants have become an important option for patients with end-stage lung disease. Unfortunately, the limiting factor is the lack of donors. A variety of pulmonary problems are potentially treatable with a lung transplant (Table 30.23). Better selection criteria, improved surgical techniques, enhanced immunosuppression, and better postoperative care have resulted in improved survival rates.

Four types of lung transplant procedures are available: single-lung, bilateral lung, heart-lung, and transplantation of lobes from a living-related donor. *Lobar transplantation* from living donors is reserved for those who urgently need a transplant and are unlikely to survive until a donor becomes available. Most of these recipients are patients with cystic fibrosis. The donors are their parents or relatives.

Preoperative Care

Patients being considered for a lung transplant have an extensive evaluation. Absolute contraindications include cancer within the past 2 years (excluding some types of skin cancer), untreatable advanced dysfunction of another major organ system (e.g., heart, liver, renal failure), uncorrectable bleeding condition, TB, severe obesity (BMI >35 kg/m^2), and significant psychosocial problems.[21] The patient and family must be able to cope with complex postoperative care. Many transplant centers require outpatient pulmonary rehabilitation before surgery to maximize physical conditioning.

In the United States the United Network for Organ Sharing (UNOS) designates recipients of donor lungs based on a lung allocation score (LAS). The LAS helps prioritize waiting list recipients based on the urgency of need and expected post-transplant survival expectations.

Postoperative Care

Immediate postoperative care often includes mechanical ventilation and hemodynamic monitoring in the ICU. IV therapy, immunosuppression, nutrition support, detection of early rejection, and preventing or treating complications, including infection, are priorities. Once hemodynamic stability has been achieved and mechanical ventilation discontinued, patients are transferred to a high-acuity or surgical unit.

Lung transplant recipients are at risk for multiple complications. Infections are the leading cause of death, especially within the 1st year after transplant.[22] Bacterial bronchitis and pneumonia are the most common infections. CMV, fungi, viruses, and mycobacteria are also causative agents. Noninfectious issues may include VTE, diaphragmatic dysfunction, and cancer.

Immunosuppressive therapy usually includes a 3-drug regimen of tacrolimus, mycophenolate mofetil (CellCept), and prednisone (see Table 14.17). Lung transplant recipients usually receive higher levels of immunosuppressive therapy than other organ recipients.

Acute rejection is common. The risk of infection is highest in the first 30 days post–lung transplant and between the 6th and 12th months. Signs include low-grade fever, fatigue, dyspnea, dry cough, and O_2 desaturation. A diagnosis of rejection is made by transbronchial biopsy, via bronchoscopy. Treatment consists of high doses of IV corticosteroids for 3 days, followed by high doses of oral prednisone. In patients with persistent or recurrent acute rejection, antilymphocyte therapy may be useful.

Bronchiolitis obliterans syndrome (BOS) is a manifestation of chronic rejection. BOS is characterized by airflow obstruction that progresses over time. The onset is often subacute, with gradual development of exertional dyspnea, nonproductive cough, wheezing, and/or low-grade fever. Airway obstruction is not responsive to bronchodilators and corticosteroid therapy. Additional immunosuppressive agents can treat chronic rejection. Because acute rejection is a major risk factor for BOS, preventing acute rejection is key to decreasing chronic rejection.[23]

Before discharge, patients need to be able to perform self-care activities, including managing their medication plan and knowing when to call the transplant team. Teach patients pulmonary clearance measures, including chest physiotherapy and deep-breathing and coughing techniques, to help minimize complications. Home spirometry is used to monitor trends in lung function. Teach patients to keep medication logs, laboratory results, and spirometry records. An outpatient rehabilitation program can improve physical endurance.

After discharge, the transplant team follows patients for transplant-related issues. Patients return to their HCP for health maintenance and routine illnesses. Care coordination among the transplant team, inpatient team, and primary care team is essential for ongoing successful management. Information about organ transplants, histocompatibility, rejection, and immunosuppressive therapy is in Chapter 14.

TABLE 30.23 Common Indications for a Lung Transplant

- Progressive lung disease and greater than 50% chance of death in the next 2 years without a lung transplant
- Chronic obstructive pulmonary disease (COPD)
- Cystic fibrosis (CF)
- Emphysema with α_1-antitrypsin deficiency
- Idiopathic pulmonary fibrosis (IPF)
- Interstitial lung disease (ILD)
- Pulmonary arterial hypertension (PAH)

LUNG CANCER

Lung cancer is the leading cause of cancer-related deaths in the United States.[24] In 2022, over 350 deaths per day occurred from lung cancer.[25] Although lung cancer has a high mortality and low cure rate, advances in medical treatment are improving the response to treatment.

Etiology

Smoking causes 80% to 90% of all lung cancers.[26] There is no safe form of tobacco or tobacco product. Using smokeless tobacco, pipes and cigars, hookah and waterpipe, bidis, and kreteks all pose significant risk for lung cancer. Tobacco smoke contains over 7000 chemicals, of which 250 are harmful. Of the harmful substances in tobacco smoke, 70 interfere with normal cell development and are linked to lung cancer.[27]

The risk for developing lung cancer is directly related to total exposure to tobacco smoke. Measures of exposure include the total number of cigarettes smoked in a lifetime, age of smoking onset, depth of inhalation, tar and nicotine content, and the use of unfiltered cigarettes. The risk for lung cancer gradually decreases with smoking cessation, reaching that of nonsmokers within 10 to 15 years of quitting.

Nonsmokers can develop lung cancer. Sidestream smoke (smoke from burning cigarettes, cigars) has the same carcinogens found in mainstream smoke (smoke inhaled and exhaled by the smoker). This exposure to secondhand smoke creates a health risk for nonsmoking adults and children.

Other risk factors include exposure to high levels of pollution, radiation (especially radon exposure), and asbestos. Heavy or prolonged exposure to industrial agents, such as radon, coal dust, asbestos, chromium, silica, arsenic, and diesel exhaust, increases risk, especially in smokers.[28]

Differences in incidence, risk factors, and survival exist between males and females. Not only are more males diagnosed with lung cancer, but they also tend to have a higher-grade tumor at the time of diagnosis. Females are more likely to be diagnosed at a younger age, have a family history of cancer, and lack a smoking history. Genetic, hormonal, and molecular factors may explain these differences.

The incidence and survivability vary between racial and ethnic populations. Black persons have the highest incidence of lung cancer and are more likely to die of lung cancer.

Pathophysiology

We think most primary lung tumors arise from mutated epithelial cells. The growth of mutations, which are caused by carcinogens, is influenced by various genetic factors. Once underway, epidermal growth factor promotes tumor development. Tumor cells grow slowly, taking 8 to 10 years for a tumor to reach 1 cm in size, the smallest lesion detectable on x-ray. Lung cancers often occur in the segmental bronchi or beyond and in the upper lobes. Lung cancers metastasize mainly by direct extension and through the blood and lymph system. Common sites for metastasis are the lymph nodes, liver, brain, bones, and adrenal glands.

Types of Lung Tumors

There are 2 broad subtypes of primary lung cancer: non–small cell lung cancer (NSCLC) and small cell lung cancer (SCLC) (Table 30.24).[29] They account for most lung tumors. Other tumor types include:

- *Hamartomas* are the most common benign tumor. They are a slow-growing congenital tumor made up of fibrous tissue, fat, and blood vessels.
- *Mucous gland adenoma* is a benign tumor arising in the bronchi. It consists of columnar cystic spaces.
- *Mesotheliomas* can be malignant or benign. They start in the visceral pleura. Malignant mesotheliomas are related to asbestos exposure.

Secondary metastases from other cancers can occur. Cancer cells from another part of the body reach the lungs through the pulmonary capillaries or lymphatic network. The main cancers that spread to the lungs often start in the breast, GI tract, or genitourinary tract.

Paraneoplastic Syndrome

Lung cancer can cause *paraneoplastic syndrome.* This rare condition may be initiated by hormones, cytokines, enzymes (secreted by tumor cells), or antibodies (made by the body in response to the tumor) that destroy healthy cells. Sometimes, paraneoplastic syndrome manifests before the cancer is diagnosed. SCLC is most often associated with paraneoplastic syndrome.

Examples of paraneoplastic syndrome include hypercalcemia, hypercoagulability, syndrome of inappropriate antidiuresis (SIAD), subacute cerebellar degeneration, adrenal hypersecretion, Cushing syndrome, and Eaton-Lambert syndrome. The conditions may stabilize with treatment of the underlying cancer.

Clinical Manifestations

The manifestations of lung cancer are usually nonspecific. They may appear late in the disease process. Symptoms may be masked by a chronic cough attributed to smoking or smoking-related lung disease. Manifestations depend on the type of lung cancer, its location, and extent of metastasis. Lung cancer often presents as lobar pneumonia that does not respond to treatment.

A persistent cough is the most common symptom and often the one that is reported first. Patients may have dyspnea or wheezing. Blood-tinged sputum may be present because of bleeding caused by the cancer. Chest pain, if present, is often worse with deep breathing, coughing, or laughing.

Later manifestations include nonspecific systemic symptoms, such as anorexia, nausea and vomiting, fatigue, and weight loss. Hoarseness may be present due to laryngeal nerve involvement. Dysphagia, unilateral paralysis of the diaphragm, and superior vena cava obstruction may occur because of intrathoracic spread of the cancer. Lymph nodes are often palpable in the neck or axillae. Mediastinal involvement may lead to pericardial effusion, cardiac tamponade, and dysrhythmias.

Diagnostic Studies

A chest x-ray is the first diagnostic test done for patients with suspected lung cancer. The x-ray may be normal or identify a lung mass or infiltrate (Fig. 30.9). Evidence of metastasis to the

TABLE 30.24 Types of Primary Lung Cancer

Type	Growth Rate	Characteristics	Response to Therapy
Non–Small Cell Lung Cancer (NSCLC)			
Adenocarcinoma	Moderate	• 40% of lung cancers • Most common lung cancer in the United States • More common in women • Most common cancer in people who have not smoked • Found in peripheral areas of lung • Often has no manifestations until widespread metastasis is present	• Surgical resection may be tried depending on staging • Does not respond well to chemotherapy
Large cell (undifferentiated) cancer	Rapid	• 10%–15% of lung cancers • Composed of large cells that are anaplastic • Can appear in any part of lung, but often arise in bronchi • Highly metastatic via lymphatics and blood	• Surgery is not usually done because of high rate of metastases • Tumor may be radiosensitive but often recur
Squamous cell cancer	Slow	• 25%–30% of lung cancers • Centrally located (bronchi) • Early symptoms of nonproductive cough and hemoptysis • Does not have a strong tendency to metastasize	• Surgical resection may be tried • Adjuvant chemotherapy and radiation • Depending on the staging, life expectancy is better than for SCLC
Small Cell Lung Cancer (SCLC)			
Small cell cancer (oat cell cancer)	Very rapid	• 10%–15% of lung cancers • Very aggressive • Spreads early via lymphatics and bloodstream • Frequent brain metastasis • Associated with endocrine problems	• Chemotherapy mainstay of treatment; more responsive to chemotherapy than NSCLC • Radiation used as adjuvant therapy and palliative measure • Often associated with paraneoplastic syndromes • Overall poor prognosis

ribs or vertebrae and a pleural effusion may be seen on chest x-ray. CT scans can identify the location and extent of masses in the chest, any mediastinal involvement, and lymph node enlargement.

Sputum cytology can identify cancer cells, but sputum samples are rarely used in diagnosing lung cancer because cancer cells are not always present in the sputum. A definitive diagnosis requires a biopsy. Cells for biopsy can be obtained by CT-guided needle aspiration, bronchoscopy, mediastinoscopy, or VATS. If a thoracentesis is done to relieve a pleural effusion, the fluid is analyzed for cancer cells.

Accurate assessment is critical for staging and determining treatment. Bone scans, CT scans of the brain, pelvis, and abdomen, MRI, and/or PET scans assess for metastases. A CBC with differential, electrolyte panel, and liver and renal function tests is done. Sometimes pulmonary function tests may be done. Table 30.25 outlines the diagnostic assessment and management of lung cancer.

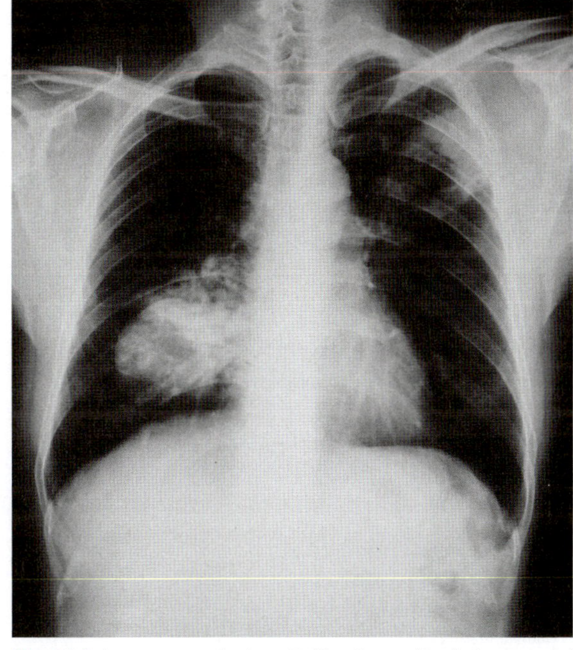

Fig. 30.9 Lung cancer lesion. (© iStock.com/Sutthaburawonk.)

Staging

Staging of NSCLC is done using the TNM staging system.[30] Under the TNM system, cancer is grouped into 4 stages with A or B subtypes. A simplified version of staging of NSCLC is shown in Table 30.26. Patients with stages I, II, and IIIA disease may be surgical candidates. Stage IIIB or IV disease is usually inoperable and has a poor prognosis. Many NSCLCs are not resectable at the time of diagnosis.

Staging of SCLC by TNM has not been useful because this cancer is aggressive and always considered systemic. The stages of SCLC are *limited* and *extensive. Limited* means that the tumor is only on 1 side of the chest and regional lymph nodes. *Extensive* SCLC means that the cancer extends beyond the limited stage. Unfortunately, most patients with SCLC have extensive disease at the time of diagnosis.

Interprofessional Care

Surgical Therapy

Surgical resection is the treatment of choice in NSCLC stages I to IIIA without mediastinal involvement. Resection gives the best chance for a cure. Factors that affect survival include the size of the primary tumor and preexisting comorbidities. For other NSCLC stages, patients may have surgery in conjunction with radiation therapy, chemotherapy, and targeted therapy.

Surgical procedures include segmental or wedge resection, lobectomy (removal of 1 or more lobes of the lung), or pneumonectomy (removal of a lung). VATS may be used to treat lung cancers near the outside of the lung. Surgery is generally not done for SCLC because of its rapid growth and dissemination at the time of diagnosis.

When the tumor is operable, we must evaluate the patient's cardiopulmonary status to determine their ability to have surgery. Pulmonary function studies, ABGs, anesthesia, and critical care consults are often done to assess cardiopulmonary status and overall surgical risk.

TABLE 30.25 Interprofessional Care

Lung Cancer

Diagnostic Assessment

- History and physical assessment
- Chest x-ray
- Bronchoscopy
- Cytology studies: Bronchial washings or pleural space fluid
- Transbronchial or percutaneous fine-needle aspiration
- CT scan, MRI, PET
- Mediastinoscopy
- Video-assisted thoracoscopic surgery (VATS)
- Laboratory tests: CBC, electrolytes, BUN, creatinine, WBC and differential, liver function tests, calcium chemistries

Management

- Surgery (segmental or wedge resection, lobectomy, pneumonectomy)
- Radiation therapy
- Chemotherapy
- Targeted therapy and immunotherapy
- Prophylactic cranial radiation
- Bronchoscopic laser therapy
- Photodynamic therapy
- Airway stenting
- Radiofrequency ablation

Radiation Therapy

Radiation therapy is a treatment for both NSCLC and SCLC. Radiation therapy may be given as curative, palliative, or adjuvant therapy in combination with surgery, chemotherapy, or targeted therapy.

TABLE 30.26 Staging of Non–Small Cell Lung Cancer

Stages		Characteristics
Occult		Cancer cells may be found in sputum or lung fluid samples, but not in any other test; cannot determine location
0		Cancer cells found in first layer of cells in the respiratory airway or alveoli
I		Tumor is small, local to lung. No lymph node involvement; no spread to other organs
	A	A1: Tumor <1 cm. Minimally invasive (<0.5 cm into lung tissue). No lymph node involvement; no spread to other organs A2: Tumor 1–2 cm. Minimally invasive. No lymph node involvement; no spread to other organs A3: Tumor 2– 3 cm. Minimally invasive. No lymph node involvement; no spread to other organs
	B	Tumor 3–4 cm and invades main airway and visceral pleura (but not into right or left bronchi)
II		Increased tumor size. One or more tumors but only in one lung and on same side. May/may not involve lymph nodes; no spread to other organs
	A	Tumor 4–5 cm with invasion of main airway and visceral pleura (but not right or left bronchi)
	B	Tumor 5–7 cm involving bronchus, visceral and parietal pleura, diaphragm, phrenic nerve involvement. May be 2 or more tumors in same lobe of lung. May/may not involve lymph nodes near bronchi on same side of chest
III		Increased spread of tumor(s)
	A	2 or more tumors ≤5 cm in one lung spread to nearby (same side) structures (chest wall, pleura, pericardium). Metastases into diaphragm, visceral pleura, mediastinum, heart, bone. Regional lymph nodes (below carina) involved
	B	2 or more tumors 5–7 cm in the same lung. Metastases into diaphragm, visceral pleura, mediastinum, heart, bone, chest wall, phrenic nerve. Regional lymph nodes (same side or opposite side, above clavicle) involved
	C	Tumor >7 cm and more than 2 tumors in a different lobe of the same lung. Metastases into diaphragm, visceral pleura, mediastinum, heart, bone, chest wall, phrenic nerve, spine. Regional lymph nodes (above clavicle) on opposite side involved
IV		Distant metastasis (to the other lung) and tumors often vary in size
	A	Metastases to the other lung, pleura, pericardium; 1 new tumor outside of chest
	B	Metastases widespread and 2 or more tumors outside of the chest

From American Cancer Society: *Non-small cell lung cancer stages.* Retrieved from https://www.cancer.org/cancer/types/lung-cancer/detection-diagnosis-staging/staging-nsclc.html.

Radiation therapy may be the primary therapy in the person who cannot undergo surgical resection because of comorbidities. Radiation therapy relieves dyspnea and hemoptysis from bronchial obstructive tumors and treats superior vena cava syndrome. It can treat pain from metastatic bone lesions or brain metastasis. Radiation before surgery can reduce the tumor mass before surgical resection. Complications of radiation therapy include esophagitis, skin irritation, nausea and vomiting, anorexia, and radiation pneumonitis (see Chapter 16).

Stereotactic body radiotherapy (SBRT), or *stereotactic radiosurgery (SRS),* is a type of radiation therapy. It uses high doses of radiation and special positioning to deliver radiation to the tumor while exposing only a small part of healthy lung. It does not destroy the tumor, but damages tumor DNA. Therapy is given over 1 to 3 days. SBRT is an option for patients with early-stage lung cancers who cannot have surgery.

Chemotherapy

Chemotherapy is the main treatment for SCLC. In NSCLC, chemotherapy may be used to treat nonresectable tumors or as adjuvant therapy to surgery. A variety of chemotherapy drugs and multidrug protocols are used. Chemotherapy for lung cancer typically consists of combinations of 2 of these drugs: etoposide, carboplatin, cisplatin, paclitaxel, vinorelbine, docetaxel, gemcitabine, and pemetrexed.[31]

Targeted Therapy

Targeted therapies block the growth of molecules involved in specific aspects of tumor growth (see Chapter 16). Because they inhibit growth rather than directly killing cancer cells, targeted therapy may be less toxic than chemotherapy. They are used alone or in combination with chemotherapy agents. There are 10 classes of targeted therapies used in treating lung cancer. The agents given are specific to the patient.

Angiogenesis inhibitors inhibit the growth of new blood vessels by targeting vascular endothelial growth factor, which helps blood vessels develop.[32] KRAS inhibitors, such as sotorasib and adagrasib, attach to mutated KRAS proteins on cancer cells to prevent them from reproducing. Epidermal growth factor (EGFR) inhibitors block signals from this protein, which stops cells from growing.

Immunotherapy

Nivolumab (Opdivo), atezolizumab (Tecentriq), and pembrolizumab (Keytruda) are drugs that target PD-L1, a protein on T cells that normally helps keep these cells from attacking other cells in the body. By blocking PD-L1, these drugs boost the body's immune system to fight the cancer cells. This can shrink some tumors or slow their growth. Nivolumab and pembrolizumab can be used in people with metastatic NSCLC whose cancer has stopped responding to or has returned after chemotherapy. Atezolizumab can be given alone, in combination with other chemotherapy agents, and after surgery.

Other Therapies

Prophylactic cranial irradiation. Patients with SCLC have early metastases, especially to the CNS. Most chemotherapy does not penetrate the blood-brain barrier. As a result, after successful systemic treatment, the patient is at risk for brain metastases. Prophylactic radiation can decrease the incidence of brain metastases and may improve survival rates in patients with limited SCLC.

Bronchoscopic laser therapy. Bronchoscopic laser therapy makes it possible to remove obstructing bronchial tumors. It is a safe and effective treatment. Symptoms of airway obstruction are relieved due to thermal necrosis and tumor shrinkage. The procedure may be repeated as needed.

Photodynamic therapy. Photodynamic therapy (PDT) is a form of treatment for early-stage lung cancers that uses a combination of a drug and specific type of light. It is a 2-step process. First, we give the patient a drug called a photosynthesizer. The drug is absorbed into the cancer cells. Then, after 24 to 48 hours, the cells are exposed to a specific wavelength of laser light via bronchoscopy. The light activates the drug, causing cell death. Necrotic tissue is removed with bronchoscopy a few days later. This process can be repeated as needed. PDT can affect nutrient delivery to cancer cells and stimulate the immune system to attack the cancer cells.

Airway stenting. Stents are used alone or in combination with other techniques for relief of dyspnea, cough, or respiratory insufficiency. The stent is inserted during a bronchoscopy. The advantage of a stent is that it supports the airway wall against collapse or external compression and can delay extension of tumor into the airway lumen.

Radiofrequency ablation. Radiofrequency ablation therapy is used to treat small NSCLC lung tumors that are near the outer edge of the lungs. This therapy is an alternative to surgery in patients who cannot or choose not to have surgery. A thin, needle-like probe is inserted through the skin into the tumor. CT scans are used to guide placement. An electric current is then passed through the probe, which heats and destroys cancer cells. Local anesthesia is used.

NURSING MANAGEMENT: LUNG CANCER

Assessment

Determine the patient and caregiver's understanding of the condition, diagnostic tests, treatment options, and prognosis. Assess their anxiety level and support available from family and significant others. Subjective and objective data that you should obtain are described in Table 30.27.

Clinical Problems

Clinical problems for patients with lung cancer may include:

- Impaired respiratory function
- Difficulty coping
- Pain

TABLE 30.27 NURSING ASSESSMENT

Lung Cancer

Subjective Data

Important Health Information

Health history: Exposure to secondhand smoke, airborne carcinogens (e.g., asbestos, radon, hydrocarbons), other pollutants. Urban living environment. Chronic lung disease (e.g., TB, COPD, bronchiectasis). History of cancer

Medications: Cough medicines, bronchodilators, expectorants, other respiratory medications

Functional Health Patterns

Health perception—health management: Smoking history, including what was smoked, amount per day, and number of years. Family history of lung cancer. Frequent respiratory tract infections

Activity-exercise: Fatigue. Persistent cough (productive or nonproductive). Dyspnea at rest or with exertion, hemoptysis (late symptom)

Cognitive-perceptual: Chest pain or tightness, shoulder and arm pain, headache, bone pain (late symptom)

Objective Data

Cardiovascular

- Pericardial effusion, cardiac tamponade, dysrhythmias (late signs)

General

- Fever, nose and/or throat infection, neck and axillary lymphadenopathy, paraneoplastic syndrome (e.g., syndrome of inappropriate antidiuresis)

GI

- Anorexia, nausea, vomiting, weight loss, dysphagia (late)

Musculoskeletal

- Pathologic fractures, muscle wasting (late)

Neurologic

- Confusion, disorientation, unsteady gait (brain metastasis)

Respiratory

- Wheezing, hoarseness, stridor, dyspnea on exertion (unilateral diaphragm paralysis), pleural effusions (late signs)

Skin

- Edema of neck and face (superior vena cava syndrome), clubbing. Jaundice (liver metastasis)

Possible Diagnostic Findings

- Lesions and any metastases on chest x-ray, CT scan, MRI, PET scan
- Positive sputum or bronchial washings for cytologic studies
- Positive fiberoptic bronchoscopy and biopsy findings

◆ Planning

The overall goals are that patients with lung cancer will have (1) a patent airway, (2) adequate tissue oxygenation, (3) minimal discomfort, (4) an understanding about the type of lung cancer, and (5) a realistic outlook about treatment and prognosis.

◆ Implementation

Health Promotion

The best way to halt the epidemic of lung cancer is to prevent people from smoking, help smokers stop smoking, and decrease exposure to pollutants. Because most smokers start in the teenage years, preventing teen smoking has the most significant role in reducing the incidence of lung cancer. A wealth of material is available to the smoker who is interested in smoking cessation (see Chapter 10).

Many medical groups recommend cancer screening for high-risk patients. Adults ages 50 to 80 with a history of smoking (20 pack-year smoking history or currently smoke) or who quit smoking but less than 15 years ago should have annual screening for lung cancer.[33] Screening is done using low-dose CT.

Acute Care

Nursing care initially involves support and reassurance during diagnostic evaluation. It is important to assess for the multiple stressors that can occur when someone receives a lung cancer diagnosis. Patients have the stress of their symptoms, including dyspnea and cough. Diagnostic and therapeutic interventions provide more stress by placing patients in unfamiliar environments with unusual and perhaps painful procedures. Emotional stress includes waiting for test results and awareness of the high mortality rate. Further worries involve role performance and ability to care for their family while undergoing cancer treatment.

Patient-centered care depends on the diagnosis and plan for treatment. Teach signs and symptoms to report (e.g., hemoptysis, dysphagia, chest pain, hoarseness). Provide comfort. Teach ways to reduce pain and monitor for drug side effects. Be available to listen to patients and their family. Encourage them to share their thoughts, fears, and concerns. Help the patients and caregivers cope with the stress of both illness and treatment. Foster coping strategies for both patient and caregivers and help them access resources to deal with the illness.

CHECK YOUR PRACTICE

You are completing discharge teaching with E.S., a 72-year-old patient who had a lobectomy for NSCLC. She tells you, "I'm not going to give up my cigarettes because I am just going to die anyhow. I might as well enjoy smoking while I can."

- How would you respond?

Chronic Care

Assess patients who smoke for smoking cessation readiness. Some patients may not perceive value in quitting smoking once they have a diagnosis of lung cancer. We can encourage patients to perhaps quit or decrease the number of cigarettes smoked per day. We might be able to gain support from family members who may wish to quit smoking with the patient. Explain the importance of maintaining a smoke-free environment in the home, particularly if O_2 will be in use. If the treatment plan includes home O_2, the teaching plan must include the safe use of O_2.

For many patients with lung cancer, little can be done to significantly prolong their lives. Radiation therapy and chemotherapy can provide palliative relief from distressing symptoms. Constant pain may become a major problem. Measures used to relieve pain are discussed in Chapter 9. Care of patients with cancer is discussed in Chapter 16. The palliative care team should be involved as the patient and family move toward the end of life (see Chapter 10). Social workers and spiritual care advisors are invaluable in end-of-life situations. The team can provide information about disability, financial planning, and community resources for end-of-life care, such as hospice and home care.

◆ Evaluation

The expected outcomes are that patients with lung cancer will:

- Have adequate breathing patterns
- Maintain adequate oxygenation
- Have minimal to no pain
- Convey feelings, with a realistic attitude about prognosis

CASE STUDY

Pneumonia and Lung Cancer

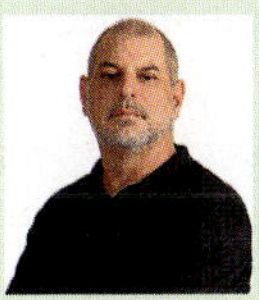

(© Giovanni-Seabra/ iStock.com.)

Patient Profile

J.H. is a 59-year-old male plumber who comes to the ED with shortness of breath. J.H. says his shortness of breath "has really increased over the past few months." J.H. has not been to a doctor for many years, as he is often "too busy with work." His son, a 4th-year nursing student, thinks that it may be something serious. His wife told him to get his "cough checked out."

Subjective Data

- 43 pack-year history of cigarette smoking
- Has had 25-lb weight loss despite a normal appetite in the past 2 months
- Admits to an occasional "smoker's cough" for the past 2 to 3 years
- Increased shortness of breath recently, and coughing up a small amount of blood-tinged sputum on occasion
- Married and the father of 3 adult children

Objective Data

Physical Assessment

- Thin, pale male who looks older than stated age
- Height 6 ft (182.9 cm); weight 135 lb (61.2 kg)
- Intermittently confused, looks anxious
- Vital signs: temperature 102.6°F (39.2°C), heart rate 110, respiratory rate 32 (shallow, slightly labored), BP 98/54
- Lungs have coarse crackles (left upper and left lower lobes) that clear with cough; decreased breath sounds (right middle lobe and right lower lobe)
- Chest wall has limited excursion on right side

Diagnostic Studies

- ABGs: pH 7.51, Pa_{O_2} 62 mm Hg, Pa_{CO_2} 30 mm Hg, HCO_3^- 22 mEq/L
- SpO_2 saturation 86% (room air)
- Chest x-ray: right lung (RML, RLL) consolidation, with small, visible mass around right bronchus; small pleural effusion (<150 mL) on the right side
- Bronchoscopy: Biopsy of mass reveals small cell lung cancer (SCLC)

Interprofessional Care

- Diagnosis: pneumonia with SCLC
- Follow up and discuss with patient and family treatment options

Discussion Questions

1. ***Recognize:*** How would you classify J.H.'s pneumonia? Why is this important?
2. ***Analyze:*** Which findings concern you?
3. ***Analyze:*** What is your analysis of J.H.'s ABG results?
4. ***Plan:*** How would other members of the health care team be involved in J.H.'s care?
5. ***Prioritize:*** Based on the assessment data presented, what are the priority clinical problems?
6. ***Prioritize:*** What are the priority nursing interventions for J.H.?
7. ***Act:*** Identify activities that you can delegate to AP.
8. ***Act:*** You are planning a meeting with J.H. and his family to discuss their needs. The morning of the meeting, the HCP informs you that bronchoscopy results reveal J.H. is terminally ill. How will the test results be disclosed to the patient and his family? Who would you include in this meeting?
9. ***Act:*** J.H.'s children tell you that they are worried they will get lung cancer, since their father has it and they grew up around his secondhand smoke. They want to know what kind of screening is available for them. How will you respond?
10. ***Evaluate:*** How would radiation therapy help J.H.?

Answers available at http://evolve.elsevier.com/Lewis/medsurg.

BRIDGE TO NCLEX EXAMINATION

The number of the question corresponds to the same-numbered outcome at the beginning of the chapter.

1. Priority nursing interventions for a patient with acute bronchitis include
   a. auscultating lung sounds.
   b. encouraging fluid restriction.
   c. administering antibiotic therapy.
   d. teaching the patient to avoid cough suppressants.
2. Which patient(s) have the greatest risk for aspiration pneumonia? **(Select all that apply.)**
   a. Patient who had thoracic surgery
   b. Patient with acute opioid overdose
   c. Patient who had a myocardial infarction
   d. Patient who is receiving enteral feeding
   e. Patient who had a stroke with dysphagia
3. Nursing interventions for the newly admitted patient with pneumonia would include
   a. perform postural drainage every hour.
   b. provide analgesics every 2 hours to promote comfort.
   c. administer O_2 as prescribed to maintain optimal O_2 levels.
   d. teach them how to cough effectively and expectorate secretions.
4. A patient with TB is admitted to the hospital and placed in a single-patient room on airborne precautions. What would the nurse teach the patient? **(Select all that apply.)**
   a. No visitors will be allowed while in airborne isolation.
   b. Expect regular TB skin testing to evaluate for infection.
   c. Adherence to precautions includes coughing into a paper tissue.
   d. Take all medications for full length of time to prevent drug-resistant TB.
   e. Wear a standard isolation mask if leaving the airborne isolation room.
5. What is the priority intervention for a patient with a lung abscess?
   a. Postural drainage
   b. Antibiotic administration
   c. Obtaining a sputum specimen
   d. Asking the patient about a family history of lung cancer
6. The patient with a right-side pleural effusion has a chest tube attached to straight drainage and O_2 at 6 L/min via nasal cannula. Vital signs are stable. Which actions would the nurse include in the plan of care? **(select all that apply)**
   a. Placing the patient on NPO status
   b. Administering analgesia as ordered
   c. Maintaining high-Fowler's position
   d. Encouraging deep breathing and coughing
   e. Monitoring color and amount of chest tube drainage
7. Which assessment finding would lead you to suspect a flail chest in a trauma patient with multiple injuries?
   a. Chest tube is draining bright red blood.
   b. Tracheal deviation to the unaffected side.
   c. Paradoxic chest movement during respiration.
   d. Little to no movement of the involved chest wall.
8. When planning care for a patient at high risk for pulmonary embolism, the nurse prioritizes
   a. maintaining the patient on strict bed rest.
   b. using intermittent pneumatic compression devices.
   c. encouraging the patient to cough and deep breathe.
   d. encouraging a fluid intake of 2000 mL per 8-hour shift.
9. You are assessing a 76-year-old retired building inspector with a long-standing dry cough, increasing periods of shortness of breath, and infrequent chest discomfort. On examination, his vital signs are stable. You note fine crackles over all lung lobes. Which condition would you suspect?
   a. Environment lung disease
   b. Acute myocardial infarction
   c. Shock and respiratory acidosis
   d. Acute respiratory distress syndrome (ARDS)
10. Management of a patient after a lung transplant includes which measures? **(Select all that apply.)**
   a. IV fluid therapy accompanied by intake and output.
   b. Mechanical ventilation in the early postoperative period.
   c. Preparing for chest tube insertion if acute rejection is suspected.
   d. Immunosuppressant therapy, which usually involves a 3-drug regimen.
   e. Pulmonary clearance measures, including deep-breathing and coughing.
11. Nursing care of a patient with Stage 4 lung cancer would include
   a. coordinating a referral to palliative care.
   b. limiting visitors to decrease infection risk.
   c. NPO status and starting parenteral nutrition.
   d. avoiding talking about the cancer diagnosis.

1. a; 2. b, d, e; 3. d; 4. c, d, e; 5. b; 6. b, d, e; 7. c;
8. b; 9. a; 10. a, b, d, e; 11. a.

For rationales to these answers and even more NCLEX review questions, visit http://evolve.elsevier.com/Lewis/medsurg.

REFERENCES

To access the References for this chapter, please scan the QR code with a mobile device.

31

Obstructive Pulmonary Diseases

Eugene E. Mondor

http://evolve.elsevier.com/Lewis/medsurg/

CONCEPTUAL FOCUS

Fatigue
Functional Ability
Gas Exchange
Infection
Self-Management

LEARNING OUTCOMES

1. Describe the pathophysiology, clinical manifestations, and interprofessional and nursing management of patients with bronchiectasis.
2. Describe the pathophysiology, clinical manifestations, and interprofessional and nursing management of patients with cystic fibrosis.
3. Describe the etiology, pathophysiology, and clinical manifestations of asthma.
4. Explain the difference between acute asthma exacerbation and status asthmaticus.
5. Describe the interprofessional care and nursing management of patients with asthma.
6. Identify the drug classes used in the treatment of asthma and chronic obstructive pulmonary disease (COPD).
7. Describe the etiology, pathophysiology, clinical manifestations, and interprofessional care of patients with COPD.
8. Explain the nursing management of patients with COPD.

KEY TERMS

α_1-antitrypsin deficiency (AATD)
asthma
bronchiectasis
chronic bronchitis
chronic obstructive pulmonary disease (COPD)
cystic fibrosis (CF)
emphysema
peak expiratory flow (PEF)
status asthmaticus

Imagine needing to think about every breath that you take every day of your life. People with obstructive lung diseases live with this unsettling experience. Obstructive pulmonary diseases are the most common chronic lung conditions. The 4 obstructive lung diseases discussed in this chapter are bronchiectasis, cystic fibrosis (CF), asthma, and chronic obstructive pulmonary disease (COPD). Knowing common terms used in discussing respiratory care will help you better understand this content (Table 31.1).

BRONCHIECTASIS

Bronchiectasis is a chronic respiratory condition. It can exist on its own or with many other conditions, including CF, asthma, and COPD. Bronchiectasis affects more than 500,000 people in the United States.[1]

Etiology and Pathophysiology

The hallmark characteristic of bronchiectasis is permanent, abnormal dilation of medium-sized bronchi. It results from inflammatory changes that destroy elastic and muscle structures supporting the bronchial wall. There is an ongoing, continuous cycle of inflammation, airway wall damage, impaired secretion clearance, and infection.[2] The bronchial walls weaken, and the mucociliary mechanism is impaired. This allows bacteria and thick mucus to accumulate within the bronchial walls. Bacteria attract neutrophils, which increases inflammation and causes edema. The excess mucus and edema decrease expiratory airflow.

As a result, airways become colonized with microorganisms, and pockets of infection form (Fig. 31.1). Patients often have *Pseudomonas aeruginosa* (most common), *Hemophilus influenzae,*

TABLE 31.1 Common Terms Used in Respiratory Care

Respiratory Terms	
FeNO	Fractional exhaled nitric oxide; measures levels of nitric oxide (NO) in your breath
FEV_1	Forced expiratory volume in 1 second
FEV_1/FVC	Volume of air exhaled during the 1st second of a forced exhalation; is a ratio, expressed as a percentage (%), of FVC
FVC	Forced vital capacity; after inhaling as much as possible, the total amount of air that can be exhaled
PEF	Peak expiratory flow; the maximal rate a person can exhale after a full inspiration; provides measurement of airflow limitation in asthma
Pharmacologic Terms	
ICS	Inhaled corticosteroid
LABA	Long-acting β_2-agonist
LAMA	Long-acting muscarinic antagonist
LTRA	Leukotriene receptor antagonist
SABA	Short-acting β_2-agonist
SAMA	Short-acting muscarinic antagonist

or *Staphylococcus aureus.*[3] *P. aeruginosa* is associated with frequent exacerbations, more hospital admissions, rapid decline in lung function, poor quality of life, and higher mortality.[3]

While 40% of cases have no known cause, bacterial infection of the lungs is the main cause in adults.[4] It can follow a single episode of severe pneumonia or infection that was either not treated or received inadequate or delayed treatment. Other risk factors include airway obstruction with mucus plugs, impaired pulmonary defenses, and repeated aspiration. Several systemic problems, such as diabetes, inflammatory bowel disease, rheumatoid arthritis, immune deficiency, and α-1 antitrypsin deficiency (AATD) may be present.[5]

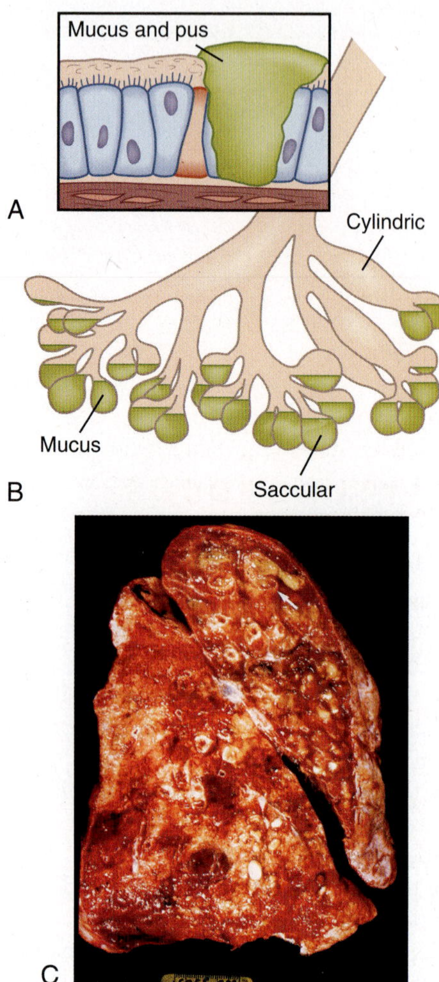

Fig. 31.1 Pathologic changes in bronchiectasis. (A) Longitudinal section of bronchial wall where chronic infection has caused damage. (B) Collection of purulent material in dilated bronchioles, leading to persistent infection. (C) Bronchiectasis in a patient with CF who underwent lung transplantation. Cut surfaces of the lung show markedly distended peripheral bronchi filled with mucopurulent secretions. (C, From Kumar V, Abbas AK, Aster JC: *Robbins and Cotran pathologic basis of disease,* ed 10, Philadelphia, 2021, Saunders.)

Clinical Manifestations

The key sign is a persistent, chronic cough with thick, tenacious, purulent sputum. In rare situations, some patients with severe disease and upper lobe involvement may have no sputum production and little cough. Recurrent infections can injure blood vessels. Large connections (anastomoses) may develop between blood vessels in the lungs, and hemoptysis may occur. In severe cases, bleeding can be life-threatening. Other manifestations include pleuritic chest pain, dyspnea, wheezing, clubbing, weight loss, and anemia. Adventitious sounds are heard (e.g., crackles, wheezes) over the lung fields.

Complications

Pulmonary hypertension can occur. Repeated exacerbations are often accompanied by chronic inflammation and hypoxemia. Colonization with multidrug-resistant organisms can occur, especially if the patient has received antibiotic therapy over long periods. Neovascularization of the bronchial arteries can lead to hemoptysis and, in some situations, hemorrhage. Massive hemoptysis can be life-threatening.

Diagnostic Studies

A CT scan is the gold standard for diagnosing bronchiectasis. Chest x-rays may show nonspecific abnormalities. Pulmonary function tests (PFTs) usually show an obstructive pattern, with decreases in FEV_1 and FEV_1/FVC. Sputum cultures may confirm an infection.

Interprofessional Care

There is no cure for bronchiectasis. Most patients are managed on an outpatient basis. Contact with the health care system is often related to exacerbations. When the patient is not responding to care, hospitalization may be needed for monitoring and treatment.

Therapy is aimed at controlling symptoms, treating acute flare-ups, and preventing a decline in lung function. Antibiotics are the mainstay of treatment. They are often given for a minimum of 14 days. Antibiotics may be given orally, IV, or inhaled (nebulizer). Choice and route of antibiotic therapy depend on culture results and patient condition. Long-term antibiotic therapy is given to patients who have symptoms that recur a few days after stopping antibiotics. Bronchodilator therapy with short-acting β_2-agonists (SABAs), long-acting β_2-agonists (LABAs), or anticholinergics can prevent bronchospasm and promote mucus clearance.

For a small number of patients who have poor control despite maximal therapy, a surgical resection or a lung transplant may be an option.

NURSING MANAGEMENT: BRONCHIECTASIS

Assessment

For patients not in immediate distress, obtain a patient and family history. If possible, identify onset, risk factors, and any complications. Review current drug therapy and treatments the patient is receiving.

Implementation

Acute Care

Priorities for patients in immediate distress include maintaining a patent airway, ensuring an adequate route for ventilation, and stabilizing vital signs. Notify the HCP immediately if the patient is expectorating large amounts of blood.

Monitor vital signs and respiratory status, including rate, rhythm, and SpO_2. Apply ordered O_2 therapy if O_2 saturation is less than 90% on room air. Elevate the head of the bed to at least 30 degrees. Place patients who may be bleeding from the airways in a side-lying position with the suspected bleeding side down. Have oral suction available. Ensure there is a valid type and crossmatch available.

One important goal is to promote drainage and removal of mucus. Various airway clearance techniques (ACTs) can help with secretion removal. Provide chest physiotherapy (CPT) with postural drainage unless the patient is actively bleeding. Hydration may help with expectorating secretions. Hyperosmolar agents (e.g., hypertonic saline) given by nebulizer can liquefy secretions.

Good nutrition is important. It may be hard to maintain because patients are often anorexic. Oral hygiene to cleanse the mouth and remove dried sputum may improve appetite. Foods that are appealing, provided in smaller quantities, and offered more often may increase the desire to eat.

Chronic Care

Patient teaching is important. Encourage patients to follow as healthy a lifestyle as possible. Stress the need to follow a healthy diet. Encourage them to engage in regular exercise. Rest is important to prevent overexertion. Discuss how to prevent exacerbations and review ACTs. Stress the need to quit smoking or, at minimum, reduce the amount smoked. Help them develop a routine that permits as much functional independence as possible with activities of daily living (ADLs).

Maintaining hydration is important to liquefy secretions. Unless contraindicated, patients should drink at least 2 to 3 L of fluid daily. Have the patient drink low-sodium fluids to avoid fluid retention. A steamy shower can be effective in helping loosen thick secretions.

Teach the patient and caregiver signs and symptoms to report to the HCP. These include increased work of breathing (WOB), change in sputum production, or dyspnea. Fever, chills, and chest pain may or may not occur with exacerbations. Teach patients when to contact the HCP if hemoptysis occurs. Some patients expectorate a "spot" of blood at times. This is usual for them and does not require urgent attention. However, if the patient coughs a moderate to large amount of blood, they should contact the HCP at once.

CYSTIC FIBROSIS

Cystic fibrosis (CF) is an inherited genetic disorder characterized by altered transport of sodium and chloride ions in and out of epithelial cells. This changes exocrine gland secretions, causing increased mucus production and airway obstruction. This defect also affects the gastrointestinal (GI) system (pancreas, biliary tract) and reproductive organs.

CF affects all ages and races. The severity and progression of CF vary. Many cases are diagnosed during newborn screening. Other patients are not diagnosed until they are adults. With early diagnosis and improvements in therapy, the prognosis has significantly improved. There are about 30,000 people in the United States living with CF.[6] More than 60% of the CF population are adults.[7]

Genetic Link

CF is an autosomal recessive disorder (Box 31.1). The CF gene is found on chromosome 7, which makes a protein called *CF transmembrane conductance regulator (CFTR).*[8] The CFTR protein is found on the epithelial surface of the airways, GI tract, and ducts of the liver, pancreas, and sweat glands. CFTR controls the channel that moves sodium, chloride, and fluid in and out of epithelial cells. Mutations in the *CFTR* gene change this protein so that the channels are blocked. As a result, cells that line the passageways of the lungs, pancreas, intestines, and other organs have secretions that are low in water content. This makes the secretions abnormally thick and sticky (Fig. 31.2). The thick secretions plug the ducts in these organs. This can cause scarring in organs and organ failure.

Pathophysiology

CF has a significant effect on the airways. It can affect both the upper and lower respiratory tracts. CF progresses from being a

BOX 31.1 GENETICS IN CLINICAL PRACTICE

Cystic Fibrosis

Genetic Basis

- Autosomal recessive disorder
- Caused by mutations in CF transmembrane regulator *(CFTR)* gene
- There are more than 2500 different mutations of the *CFTR* gene
- The most common mutation is the *F508del* mutation in the *CFTR* gene, where a single amino acid is removed

Incidence

- Most common in White persons
- In the United States, 1 in 2500 to 3500 White births
- One in every 25 to 30 White persons are carriers of the gene
- 1000 new cases diagnosed each year, most before 1 year of age

Clinical Implications

- Most people who have a child with CF are not aware of the family history of the condition
- All people of reproductive age, regardless of family history, should be offered CF screening

Genetic Testing

- Can identify if a person is a carrier of the mutation for the *CFTR* gene
- Can screen relatives of family members who have CF
- Prenatal fetal testing (e.g., amniocentesis) can be done if parents are known carriers
- All 50 states require newborn CF screening
- Testing is usually done in children if CF is suspected or if parents are possible carriers

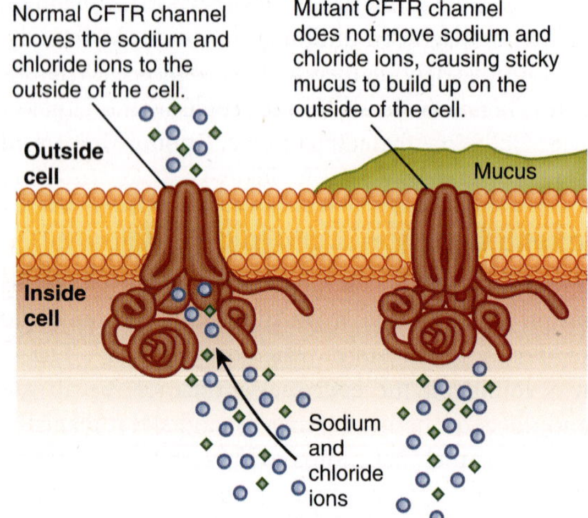

Fig. 31.2 Cystic fibrosis transmembrane conductance regulator *(CFTR)* is a protein of the cell membrane that normally helps sodium and chloride move in and out of cells. People with CF inherit a defective gene. As a result, movement of sodium and chloride is blocked. Abnormally thick sticky mucus is produced on the outside of the cell.

disease of the small airways to involving the larger airways with destruction of lung tissue. The mucus lining the airways becomes dehydrated and tenacious. Cilia become overwhelmed with thick secretions. As a result, cilia motility is decreased, allowing mucus to adhere to the airways. At the same time, the bronchioles become obstructed with thick mucus, leading to air trapping, hyperinflation of the lungs, and eventually, airway scarring.

With CF, there are acute and, over time, chronic pulmonary infections. *Pseudomonas* is the most common organism in adults.[9] Antibiotic resistance can develop after multiple exposures to antibiotics. Lung inflammation occurs. It can narrow airways and cause a decrease in lung function. An increase in inflammatory mediators (e.g., interleukins, oxidants, proteases released by neutrophils) contributes to disease progression.

Over a long period, local hypoxia and arteriolar vasoconstriction cause pulmonary vascular remodeling. Blebs and large cysts are severe manifestations of lung destruction. Pneumothorax may occur. There is a proliferation of capillaries in response to chronic infection. During exacerbations, there may be erosion of these capillaries with hemoptysis. Hemoptysis may range from scant streaking to major bleeding, which can be fatal. Patients may develop heart problems, including hypertension and heart failure (HF).[10] This is related to changes in lung function and respiratory failure as CF evolves

Plugging of the pancreatic exocrine ducts with mucus causes pancreatic insufficiency. The pancreas does not make enough pancreatic enzymes, such as lipase, amylase, and proteases (trypsin, chymotrypsin), to allow for nutrient absorption. Malabsorption of fat, protein, and fat-soluble vitamins occurs. Fat malabsorption causes steatorrhea (large, oily, frequent bowel movements). Protein malabsorption results in the failure to grow and gain weight. Over time, atrophy and progressive fibrosis of the pancreas occur. The exocrine function of the pancreas may be completely lost. Pancreatitis may be present.

CF-related diabetes (CFRD) occurs in up to 50% of patients with CF. It is caused by the underdevelopment of pancreatic islet cells in utero and destruction of beta cells over the person's lifetime.[11] CFRD has characteristics of type 1 and type 2 diabetes. The pancreas makes insulin, but there is reduced and delayed insulin secretion. Insulin deficiency contributes to a decline in lung function and nutrition. All the complications associated with diabetes affect patients with CFRD.

GI problems include gastroesophageal reflux disease (GERD), gallstones, and constipation. Mucus deposits in the ducts can damage the liver and gallbladder. Liver enzymes may be chronically increased. Cirrhosis and portal hypertension can develop over time. Colorectal cancer may occur.

Distal intestinal obstruction syndrome (DIOS) results from an intermittent obstruction, often in the terminal ileum at the point of the ileocecal junction. It is caused by defective water and chloride secretion, absence of bile salts, and increased GI acidity. Risk factors include under- or overdosing of pancreatic replacement enzyme supplements, change in diet, dehydration, previous abdominal surgery, and opioid use.[12]

Clinical Manifestations

The manifestations vary depending on the severity of the disease. Severity may vary greatly, both within families and among different families. Carriers do not have symptoms.

Adult patients often present with atypical symptoms, such as new-onset diabetes or infertility problems. A common symptom in adults is a frequent cough. With time, the cough becomes persistent and produces thick, purulent sputum. Upper respiratory infection (URI) manifestations may include chronic sinusitis and nasal polyposis. Other lung problems include recurring lung infections, such as bronchiolitis, bronchitis, and pneumonia. With advanced lung disease, clubbing occurs. As the disease progresses, periods of clinical stability are interspersed by exacerbations. The patient may have increased cough, increased sputum production, decreased lung function, and weight loss. Over time, exacerbations become more frequent, bronchiectasis worsens, and the recovery of lost lung function is less complete. These changes may lead to respiratory failure.

Patients with DIOS may have right lower quadrant pain, nausea, vomiting, and a palpable mass. Insufficient pancreatic enzyme release causes the typical pattern of protein and fat malabsorption. Many people are thin with a low body mass index (BMI). They may have frequent bulky, foul-smelling stools.

Both males and females have delayed puberty. Some females have difficulty conceiving. The cervical mucus may be thick. During exacerbations, menstrual irregularities and secondary amenorrhea are common. Most females with CF can become pregnant. Most pregnancies result in viable infants.

Nearly all males with CF have reproductive issues. Because the vas deferens fails to develop in utero, there is no transport of sperm from storage in the testes to the penile urethra. However, they make sperm normally and can father a child with assisted reproductive technology.

Complications

Most adult patients with CF die of complications from lung infection. Early intervention with antibiotics is key when infection is present. Antibiotic choice is based on sputum culture results. *P. aeruginosa* and *S. aureus* are most frequently reported.[13]

Other complications include CFRD and bone, sinus, and liver disease. Respiratory and left ventricular HF caused by pulmonary hypertension are late complications. Pneumothorax, a rare but serious complication, is caused by the formation of bullae and blebs on the surface of the lung. Liver failure and bowel obstruction may occur. Massive hemoptysis, though rare, can be life-threatening.

Diagnostic Studies

The diagnostic criteria for CF include a combination of clinical presentation, family history, and laboratory and genetic testing. The sweat glands of patients with CF do not absorb sodium chloride from the sweat as it moves through the sweat duct. As a result, there is excess chloride in the sweat. The sweat chloride test is the gold standard for diagnosing CF. It is done with the pilocarpine iontophoresis method. Pilocarpine is placed on the skin (usually the arm) and carried by a small electric current to stimulate sweat production. This part of the test takes about 5 minutes. Next, gauze, filter paper, or a coil is placed on the skin for up to 30 minutes. The sweat is collected and analyzed for sweat chloride concentrations. A sweat chloride value above 60 mmol/L is considered positive for the diagnosis of CF.[8] However, a second sweat chloride test on another day is recommended to confirm the diagnosis.

Laboratory testing is often done if the results from a sweat chloride test are uncertain. We can send a blood or cell sample to a place that specializes in genetic testing. Most laboratories test for the most common mutations of the CF gene. Because more than 2000 mutations cause CF, screening for all mutations is difficult and done only at special laboratories.

Interprofessional Care

An interprofessional team should be involved in the care of patients with CF. The Cystic Fibrosis Foundation funds more than 130 CF care centers nationwide. The high-quality, special care from CF care centers has led to an improved length and quality of life for people with CF. These centers offer the best care, treatments, and support for those with this condition. The teams include a nurse, physician, respiratory therapist, physical therapist, dietitian, social worker, and often a nurse practitioner.

Management of lung problems aims at relieving airway obstruction and controlling infection. Aerosol and nebulizer treatments promote drainage of thick bronchial mucus. The drugs we use dilate the airways, liquefy mucus, and promote clearance of secretions.

The abnormal viscosity of secretions is increased by concentrated DNA from neutrophils involved in chronic infection. Drugs that degrade the DNA in CF sputum (e.g., inhaled dornase alfa [Pulmozyme]) increase airflow and reduce the number of exacerbations.[14] Inhaled hypertonic saline (7%) increases osmolality, allowing water to collect on inner airway surfaces. It is effective in clearing mucus and decreases exacerbations. It is given as maintenance therapy 2 to 4 times per day. Some patients need bronchodilators (e.g., β_2-adrenergic agonists) to control bronchospasm, but the long-term benefit is not known. Bronchodilators may be given with hypertonic saline to decrease bronchospasms.

Respiratory care includes ACTs because the normal ciliary motion in CF airways is impaired. CPT (postural drainage with percussion and vibration) and high-frequency chest wall oscillation loosen mucus. Special expiratory techniques that use airflow to remove the loosened secretions help clear secretions. Examples include pursed-lip breathing, forced expiration, huff coughing, and regular exercise. No ACT is better than the others. Patients may prefer a certain technique or device that works well for them in their daily routine.

With infections, antibiotics are generally prescribed for 10 to 14 days. Longer therapy may be needed with severe infections. No antibiotic is superior to another in CF treatment. In many situations, a combination of antibiotics is necessary. Oral agents used for mild exacerbations include fluoroquinolones such as ciprofloxacin. In more severe cases, an antipseudomonal beta-lactam (e.g., piperacillin/tazobactam, ceftazidime, aztreonam) with an aminoglycoside or fluoroquinolone is recommended. Patients with CF metabolize drugs differently, especially aminoglycosides and beta-lactam antibiotics. Renal clearance of these drugs is higher with a decreased half-life. As a result, higher doses are often needed.

All patients with CF should have CFTR genotyping. This will help see if they carry a mutation that is a target of CFTR modulator therapy. The specific CFTR variant a person has determines whether 1 drug or a combination of drugs will be needed to treat the disease.

Evidence suggests a triple (3-drug) combination improves lung function and decreases exacerbations in 90% of CF patients. Trikafta is an oral therapy that consists of tezacaftor, ivacaftor, and elexacaftor.[15] This drug targets the defective CFTR protein and normalizes the transport of ions through the membrane. Triple Ivacaftor, a CFTR modulator, may be effective in CF exacerbations. However, less than 5% of patients respond to this drug.[13]

Most CF patients have *Pseudomonas* infection. It can be hard to treat because this organism develops resistance to antibiotics. Thus a common class of antibiotic used to treat chronic *Pseudomonas* infection is aminoglycosides, such as tobramycin. Other commonly used drugs include colistin and aztreonam. Aerosolized antibiotics improve lung function and decrease exacerbations. Alternating a combination of 2 different antibiotics given over many weeks or months is common.

Patients with hypoxemia, pulmonary hypertension, or HF may need home O_2 therapy. Those with a large pneumothorax need chest tube drainage, sometimes repeatedly. Sclerosing of the pleural space or partial pleural stripping and pleural abrasion may be done for recurrent episodes of pneumothorax. With massive hemoptysis, bronchial artery embolization is necessary. Lung transplant may be an option for patients with severe CF unresponsive to usual therapy.

Nutrition management includes increasing calories, fats, and salts. Calorie supplements improve nutrition status. Extra salt is needed when sweating is increased, such as during hot weather, with a fever, or from intense physical activity. Pancreatic insufficiency necessitates pancreatic enzyme replacement of lipase, protease, and amylase (e.g., pancrelipase [Pancreaze]) taken before each meal and snack. An adequate intake of protein and vitamins is important. Fat-soluble vitamins (A, D, E, and K) must be supplemented since they are malabsorbed. Hyperglycemia may need insulin treatment.

If the patient develops DIOS with a bowel obstruction, we make every attempt to manage the obstruction medically. Patients may be NPO, receive IV fluids, and have a nasogastric (NG) tube for decompression. Drug therapy may include prokinetic agents (e.g., macrolide antibiotics, metoclopramide), mucolytics (oral N-acetylcysteine [NAC]), stimulant laxatives, lactulose, and polyethylene glycol (PEG) electrolyte solution. Careful monitoring of bowel habits and patterns is essential. If DIOS does not resolve with medical treatment, surgery may be necessary to prevent ischemic bowel.

NURSING MANAGEMENT: CYSTIC FIBROSIS

Assessment

Subjective and objective data you should obtain from patients with CF are shown in Table 31.2.

Clinical Problems

Clinical problems for patients with CF may include:

- Impaired respiratory function
- Infection
- Nutritionally compromised

TABLE 31.2 NURSING ASSESSMENT

Cystic Fibrosis

Subjective Data

Important Health Information

- *Health history:* Recurrent respiratory and/or sinus infections, persistent cough with excess sputum production
- *Medications:* Use of and compliance with bronchodilators, antibiotics

Functional Health Patterns

- *Health perception–health maintenance:* Family history of cystic fibrosis, when diagnosed, genetic testing
- *Nutritional-metabolic:* Diet intolerances, voracious appetite, weight loss, heartburn
- *Elimination:* Intestinal gas; large, frequent bowel movements; constipation
- *Activity-exercise:* Fatigue, ↓ exercise tolerance, amount and type of exercise; dyspnea, cough, excess mucus or sputum production, coughing up blood, ACTs
- *Cognitive-perceptual:* Abdominal pain
- *Sexuality-reproductive:* Delayed menarche, menstrual problem, infertility
- *Coping–stress tolerance:* Anxiety, depression, difficulty coping

Objective Data

Cardiovascular

- ↑ Heart rate

Eyes

- Scleral icterus

General

- Restlessness, failure to thrive

GI

- Protuberant abdomen; abdominal distention; foul, fatty stools

Respiratory

- Sinus congestion, postnasal drip, persistent runny nose
- Decreased breath sounds, adventitious breath sounds (crackles, wheezes)
- Sputum (thick, tenacious)
- ↑ Work of breathing, accessory muscle use, barrel chest

Skin

- Salty skin; clubbing; cyanosis (circumoral, nail bed)

Possible Diagnostic Findings

- Abnormal sweat chloride test, abnormal ABGs, and pulmonary function tests
- Abnormal chest x-ray, fecal fat analysis

ABG, Arterial blood gas; *ACT,* airway clearance technique.

Planning

The overall goals are that patients with CF will have (1) adequate airway clearance, (2) absence of respiratory infection, (3) adequate nutrition to maintain appropriate weight, (4) ability to perform optimal ADLs, (5) recognize and treat complications related to CF, and (6) actively take part in their treatment plan.

Implementation

Acute Care

Acute care for patients with CF focuses on relief of bronchoconstriction and improving airflow. Interventions include aggressive CPT, antibiotics, and O_2 therapy in severe disease. Measures to optimize nutrition are essential.

In severe cases, patients may be cared for in the intensive care unit (ICU). Reasons for ICU admission include acute respiratory insufficiency, acute respiratory failure (ARF), and hemoptysis. Patients may need mechanical ventilation and hemodynamic monitoring.

Chronic Care

Chronic care focuses on ACTs, treating infection with antibiotic therapy, nutrition support (including pancreatic enzymes), and psychosocial support.

Encourage patients to take part in aerobic exercise. It is effective in clearing the airways. Considerations when planning an exercise program include (1) meeting increased nutrition demands of exercise, (2) drinking large amounts of fluid, (3) replacing salt losses, and (4) observing for dehydration.

Help patients maintain independence by allowing them to assume more responsibility for their care and life goals. Discuss sexuality. Delayed development of secondary sex characteristics and irregular menses are common. The issue of marrying and having children is complicated. Genetic counseling is appropriate when the patient is considering having children. Another concern is uncertainty surrounding the shortened life span of the parent with CF.

Other crises and life transitions that must be dealt with in adult patients include identifying employment goals, developing motivation, coping with treatment, and adjusting to the need for dependence if health fails. Disclosing the CF diagnosis to friends, potential spouses, and/or employers may pose significant social, emotional, and financial challenges.

CF imposes a significant emotional and financial burden on both the patient and family. In many situations, the cost of drugs, special equipment, and health care poses financial hardship. Issues related to costs of health care, burden of self-care, career choices, fertility, and decreased life expectancy may lead to anxiety and depression. Referral to counseling may help depending on the patient's ability to cope with the condition and availability of support networks. Community resources are available to help patients and caregivers. The Cystic Fibrosis Foundation is a source of information and support.

ASTHMA

Asthma is a diverse disease characterized by bronchial hyperreactivity with reversible expiratory airflow limitation, either spontaneously or with treatment. The clinical course of asthma is unpredictable. It ranges from periods of adequate control to frequent attacks with poor control of symptoms. Signs and symptoms can be variable. For example, there may be mild shortness of breath and chest tightness with a minor asthma attack. In a major asthma attack, severe shortness of breath, accessory muscle use, stridor, and severe hypoxemia appear. Respiratory and/or cardiac arrest can occur.

Asthma affects around 25 million adult Americans.[16] It is a major public health concern. In 2021 there were over 1 million emergency department (ED) visits and 104,805 hospitalizations.[17] In 2020 the mortality rate for asthma increased for the first time in over 20 years.[17] A total of 3941 deaths occurred.

Risk Factors and Triggers

Risk factors for asthma and triggers of asthma attacks are related to the patient (e.g., genetic factors) or the environment

TABLE 31.3 Triggers of Asthma Attacks

Air Pollutants	• Aerosol sprays • Cigarette smoke • Exhaust fumes • Oxidants • Perfumes • Sulfur dioxide
Allergen Inhalation	• Animal dander (e.g., dogs, cats, mice, guinea pigs) • Cockroaches • House dust mite • Molds • Pollens
Drugs	• Aspirin • β-Adrenergic blockers • NSAIDs
Food Additives	• Beer, wine, dried fruit, shrimp, processed potatoes • Monosodium glutamate • Sulfites (bisulfites and metabisulfites) • Tartrazine
Occupation Exposure	• Agriculture, farming • Industrial chemicals and plastics • Laundry detergents • Metal salts • Paints, solvents • Wood and vegetable dusts
Pulmonary	• Sinusitis, allergic rhinitis • Viral upper respiratory infection
Other Factors	• Exercise and cold, dry air • Gastroesophageal reflux disease • Hormones, menses • Stress

(e.g., pollen) (Table 31.3). Let us look at some of the key risk factors and triggers of asthma attacks.

Nose and Sinus Problems

Most patients have a history of allergic rhinitis. Treatment of allergic rhinitis usually improves asthma symptoms. Acute and chronic sinusitis, especially bacterial rhinosinusitis, may worsen asthma. Chronic sinus problems that cause inflammation of the mucous membranes can trigger an asthma attack. Sinusitis must be treated and large nasal polyps removed for the patient to have good control of their asthma.

Allergens

Allergens cause varying degrees of allergic reactions in susceptible persons. Indoor and outdoor allergens, such as cockroaches, furry animals, fungi, pollen, and molds, can trigger asthma attacks. We are not clear, though, about their role in causing asthma.

Cigarette Smoke

The American Lung Association (ALA) estimates that 18% of persons with asthma smoke.[18] In a person with asthma, smoking is associated with a faster decline of lung function, increased severity, more frequent HCP visits, and a decreased response to treatment. *Passive smoking*, or secondhand smoke, is a risk factor for asthma.

Air Pollutants

Various air pollutants, such as wood smoke or vehicle exhaust, can trigger asthma attacks. In heavily industrial or densely populated areas, climate conditions can lead to concentrated pollution in the atmosphere, especially with thermal inversions and stagnant air masses. News sources often report ozone alert days. Patients with breathing problems should minimize outdoor activity during these times.

Respiratory Tract Infections

Respiratory tract infections are a major trigger for an acute asthma attack. Acute URIs can decrease the diameter of the airways and induce airway hyperresponsiveness. Viral-induced changes in epithelial cells, the accumulation of cells that enhance inflammation, and edema of airway walls contribute to altered respiratory function. These changes may worsen asthma.

Immune Response

People who have a lower incidence of asthma were exposed to certain infections early in life. They received fewer antibiotics, were around other children (e.g., siblings, day care), or lived in rural settings or with pets. The *hygiene hypothesis* suggests that in extremely clean environments, the immune system of newborns and children will not fully mature and develop. In other words, exposure to different germs and various infections during infancy and childhood helps strengthen your immune system.

Genetics

The genetics of asthma are complex. Many genes may be involved. They are likely responsible for different responses to triggers and asthma drugs. Atopy, the genetic predisposition to develop an allergic (immunoglobulin E [IgE]—mediated) response to common allergens, is a major risk factor.

Gastroesophageal Reflux Disease

GERD is more common in people with asthma. It can worsen asthma symptoms because reflux may trigger bronchoconstriction and cause aspiration. Asthma drugs can worsen GERD symptoms. β_2-Agonists, especially when given orally, relax the lower esophageal sphincter. This allows stomach contents to reflux into the esophagus and potentially be aspirated. Treatment can improve nocturnal asthma control, improve quality of life, and prevent asthma symptoms in some patients. GERD is discussed in Chapter 46.

Drugs and Food Additives

Some people with asthma have what we call *asthma-exacerbated respiratory disease (AERD).* This chronic condition is characterized by nasal polyps, asthma, and sensitivity to aspirin and nonsteroidal antiinflammatory drugs (NSAIDs).[19] People with AERD who use salicylic acid (e.g., aspirin) or NSAIDs can develop coughing, wheezing, and rhinorrhea within a few hours. Angioedema can occur. Management of AERD consists of nasal polyp removal and aspirin desensitization. If this is not possible, teach patients to avoid salicylic acid and NSAIDs. Other options include corticosteroids, leukotriene modifiers, and biologic therapy.[20]

β-Adrenergic blockers in oral form (e.g., metoprolol) or eye drops (e.g., timolol) may trigger an asthma attack because they can cause bronchospasm. Asthma attacks can occur after the use of sulfite-containing preservatives found in eye solutions, IV corticosteroids, and some inhaled bronchodilators. ACE inhibitors (e.g., lisinopril) may cause a dry, hacking cough, making asthma symptoms worse.

Food and drug additives that may trigger asthma include tartrazine (yellow dye no. 5) and sulfiting agents. They are common preservatives and sanitizing agents. Sulfiting agents are in fruits, beer, and wine. They are used in salad bars to protect vegetables from oxidation. Food allergies triggering asthma reactions in adults are rare.

Exercise

We call asthma that is induced by or becomes worse during physical exertion *exercise-induced bronchoconstriction (EIB).*[21] Typically, symptoms of EIB are worse during activities in which there is exposure to cold, dry air. For example, skiing is more likely to cause EIB than swimming in an indoor heated pool.

Varying degrees of bronchoconstriction and inflammation may occur because of changes in airway mucosa caused by hyperventilation during exercise. The type of sport, training environment, and genetics contribute to EIB. EIB frequently occurs after less than 10 minutes of vigorous exercise. It often resolves within 90 minutes.

Occupation Factors

Occupational asthma is the most common job-related respiratory problem. Irritants cause a change in airway responsiveness. Symptoms may not occur until the patient has had months to years of exposure. These agents are diverse. They include wood dusts, laundry detergents, metal salts, chemicals, paints, solvents, and plastics. People with occupational asthma often give a history of arriving at work feeling well but gradually develop symptoms, which may become progressively worse, by the end of the day.

Psychologic Factors

Many people report that symptoms worsen with stress. An asthma attack caused by any trigger can cause panic, stress, and anxiety. These emotions, and other psychologic factors, can lead to bronchoconstriction through stimulation of the cholinergic reflex pathways. Extreme behavior expressions (e.g., crying, laughing, anger, fear) can lead to hyperventilation and hypocapnia, which can cause airway narrowing and trigger an asthma attack.

Pathophysiology

The main pathophysiologic process in asthma is persistent but variable inflammation of the airways. Airflow is limited because inflammation results in bronchoconstriction, airway hyperresponsiveness (hyperreactivity), and edema of the airways. Exposure to allergens or irritants starts the inflammatory cascade (Fig. 31.3). A variety of inflammatory cells are involved, including mast cells, macrophages, eosinophils, neutrophils, T and B lymphocytes, and epithelial cells of the airways.

As the inflammatory process begins, mast cells (beneath the basement membrane of the bronchial wall) degranulate and release multiple inflammatory mediators. These include leukotrienes, histamine, cytokines, prostaglandins, and nitric oxide (Fig. 31.4). Inflammatory mediators have effects on the (1) blood vessels, causing vasodilation and increasing capillary permeability (runny nose); (2) nerve cells, causing itching; (3)

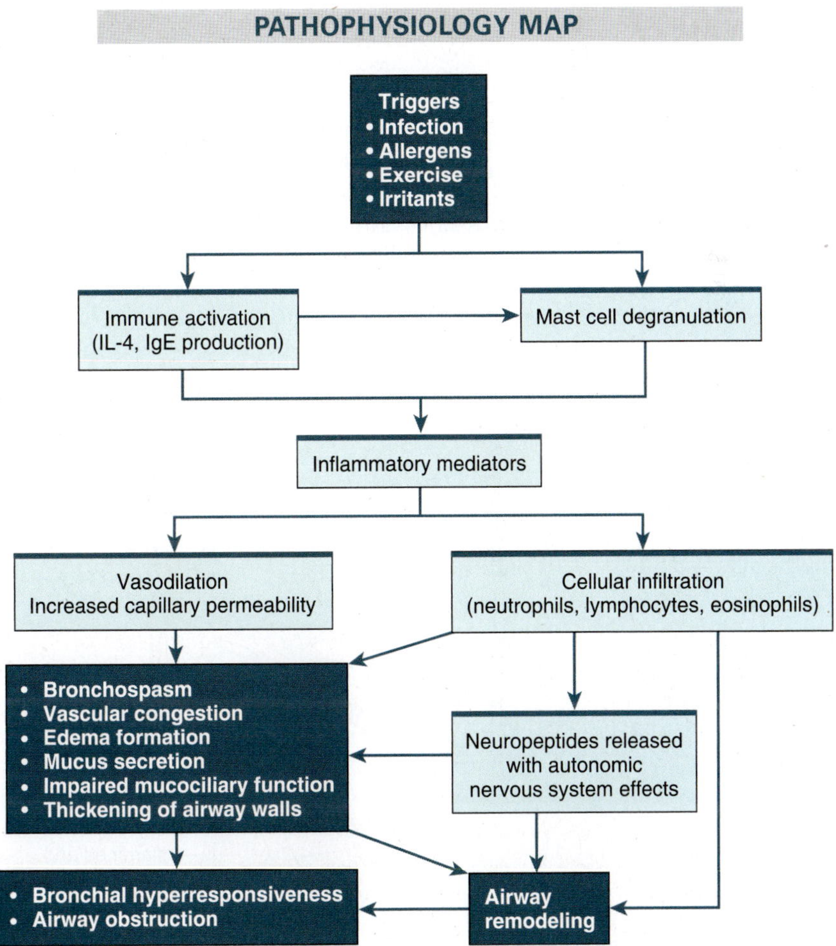

Fig. 31.3 Pathophysiology of asthma. *IL,* Interleukin; *IgE,* immunoglobulin E. (Adapted from McCance KL, Huether SE: *Pathophysiology: the biologic basis for disease in adults and children,* ed 8, St. Louis, 2022, Elsevier.)

smooth muscle cells, causing bronchial spasm and airway narrowing; and (4) goblet cells, causing mucus production. As a result, edema of airway mucosa, muscle spasm, and accumulation of secretions produce varying degrees of expiratory airflow obstruction (Fig. 31.5). This causes the characteristic wheezing, air trapping, and hyperinflation of the lungs. Expiration may be difficult and prolonged.

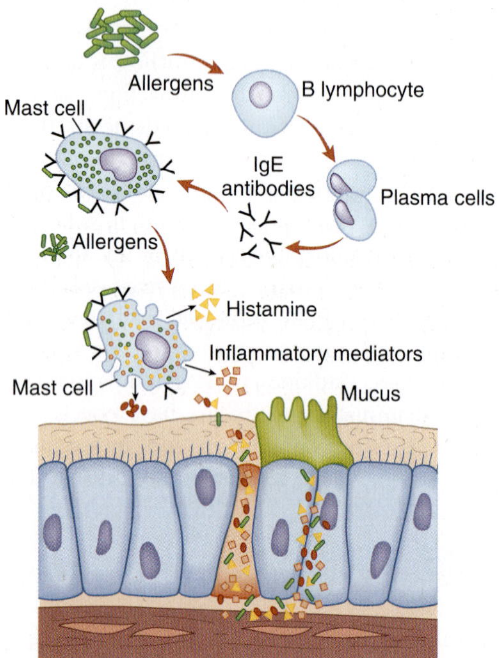

Fig. 31.4 Allergic asthma is triggered when an allergen cross-links immunoglobulin E *(IgE)* receptors on mast cells, which are then activated to release histamine and other inflammatory mediators (early-phase response). A late-phase response may occur as a result of further inflammation and edema.

This process is the *early-phase response* of asthma. Clinically, it occurs within minutes after exposure to an allergen or irritant. It generally resolves within 1 to 2 hours.

The *late-phase response* occurs in about 50% of people with asthma. With the late response, symptoms recur 4 to 6 hours after the early response and last 24 hours or more. There is an ongoing influx of inflammatory cells, which were set in motion by the initial response with continuing airway inflammation. Corticosteroids are often effective in treating inflammation in this late phase. Chronic inflammation may cause structural changes in the bronchial wall, known as *remodeling*. Over time, a progressive loss of lung function occurs that therapy cannot fully reverse. Structural changes include fibrosis of the subepithelium, hypertrophy of the smooth muscle of the airways, thickening of the basement membrane, mucus hypersecretion, continued inflammation, cartilage changes, and angiogenesis.[22] Remodeling and genetic factors may explain why some persons have persistent asthma and limited response to therapy.

Clinical Manifestations

Asthma attacks range from minor interferences in breathing to life-threatening episodes. Depending on a person's physiologic response, asthma can rapidly progress from normal breathing to an acute, severe attack or a life-threatening medical emergency within a few minutes.

The characteristic manifestations of an asthma attack are wheezing, cough, dyspnea, and chest tightness after exposure to a risk factor or trigger. The most common finding during an acute asthma event is wheezing. For wheezing to occur, the patient must be able to move enough air to make the sound. Wheezing

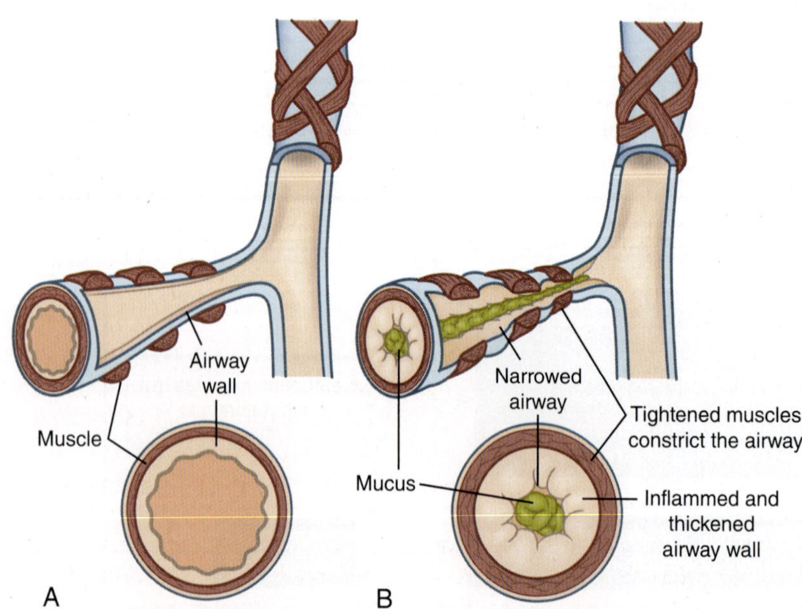

Fig. 31.5 Factors causing expiratory obstruction in asthma. (A) Cross section of a bronchiole occluded by muscle spasm, edema of mucosa, and mucus in the lumen. (B) Longitudinal section of a bronchiole.

usually occurs first on exhalation. As asthma progresses, the patient may wheeze during inspiration and expiration.

However, wheezing is an unreliable sign to gauge the severity of an attack. Many patients with minor attacks wheeze loudly. Others with severe attacks do not wheeze. Patients with a severe asthma attack may wheeze only during forced expiration or have no audible wheezing because of the marked reduction in airflow.

Decreased or absent breath sounds may signal a significant decrease in air movement resulting from exhaustion and an inability to generate enough muscle force to breathe. Severely decreased breath sounds, or a "silent chest," are an ominous sign. This often means severe airway obstruction and impending ARF.

! SAFETY ALERT

Silent Chest

- If the patient with asthma who has been wheezing suddenly stops (e.g., silent chest) and struggles to breathe, this is a life-threatening emergency.
- Call for help.
- The patient may need intubation and mechanical ventilation.

Hyperventilation occurs during an asthma attack as lung receptors respond to the increase in lung volume from trapped air and airflow limitation. Decreased alveolar perfusion and ventilation and increased alveolar gas pressure lead to V/Q mismatch. The patient may be hypoxemic early, with decreased $Paco_2$ and increased pH (respiratory alkalosis) because they are hyperventilating. As airflow limitation worsens with subsequent air trapping, the patient works much harder to breathe. The $Paco_2$ normalizes as the patient tires but eventually rises to produce respiratory acidosis. Increasing $Paco_2$ and decreasing pH are ominous signs of ARF.

In some patients, cough is the only symptom. This is termed *cough variant asthma (CVA)*. Bronchospasm is not present or may not be severe enough to cause airflow obstruction or wheezing, but it can increase bronchial tone and cause irritation with stimulation of the cough receptors. The cough may be nonproductive or with secretions. PEF or FEV_1 values may be normal to near normal. Seasonal flare-ups, increased eosinophils in sputum, and airway remodeling can occur.[23]

CHECK YOUR PRACTICE

A patient with an acute asthma attack is in the ED with moderate respiratory distress. He has been receiving therapy and seems to be responding. You suddenly notice he is no longer wheezing.

- Should you consider this a sign that the patient is doing better?

Asthma Classifications

Several sets of national and international guidelines exist for classifying asthma. Each guideline has a slightly different perspective about asthma and how to classify the severity of an attack. The severity of an asthma attack guides treatment. All the major guidelines emphasize the importance of assessing the severity of the disease at the time of diagnosis, with initial treatment, and with periodic monitoring to determine control of symptoms. Patient history before the asthma attack is important.

Many HCPs use the 2012 National Heart, Lung, and Blood Institute (NHLBI) guidelines for classifying asthma severity (Table 31.4). They describe asthma as intermittent, mild persistent, moderate persistent, or severe persistent.[23]

Complications

In some people, airway remodeling causes respiratory-related issues. As bronchi become thicker and less elastic and airways become narrower, this may increase WOB. Compromised lung function may lead to a state of continuous symptoms and chronic debilitation, including fatigue, headaches, and lack of activity. Asthma predisposes patients to pneumonia, worse episodes of the flu, and, in rare situations, tension pneumothorax. ARF and status asthmaticus are the most severe complications of an asthma attack.

Status Asthmaticus

A life-threatening medical emergency, **status asthmaticus** is the most extreme form of an acute asthma attack. It is characterized by hypoxia, hypercapnia, and ARF. The patient is unresponsive to treatment with bronchodilators and corticosteroids. They may have chest tightness, a severely marked increase in shortness of breath, or suddenly be unable to speak. Hypotension, bradycardia, and respiratory and/or cardiac arrest may occur if we do not recognize that the patient is getting worse.

Diagnostic Studies

Tests used to diagnose asthma are shown in Table 31.5. In general, the HCP should consider a diagnosis of asthma if various indicators (e.g., manifestations, health history, peak flow variability, spirometry) are positive. The history is important to determine whether a person has had similar attacks, which are often precipitated by a known trigger. Because wheezing and cough occur with a variety of disorders (e.g., COPD, GERD, vocal cord problems, HF), it is important to determine whether asthma or another disease is the cause. Table 31.6 shows a comparison of asthma and COPD.

Peak expiratory flow (PEF), measured by peak flow meter, is a test of lung function. PEF measures the maximum rate of airflow after a forceful exhalation. When monitored routinely, PEF measurements can provide a baseline of the patient's health status. PEF can help predict an asthma attack or monitor the severity of disease. Test results depend on age, gender, and height. Because peak flow meters vary, we should compare PEF with the patient's previous best measurements using their meter.

TABLE 31.4 Diagnostic Criteria

Asthma Severity Classification

	ASTHMA SEVERITY			
		PERSISTENT		
Components	**Intermittent**	**Mild**	**Moderate**	**Severe**
Symptoms	≤2 days/wk	>2 days/wk, not daily	Daily	Continuous
Flare-ups	Brief, vary in intensity	Noticeable	More frequent	Daily
Interference with ADLs	None	May affect ADLs	Some limitations, may affect ADLs	Often restricts ADLs
Nighttime awakenings	≤2/mo	3–4/mo	>1/wk, but not nightly	Every night (7/wk)
Lung function	FEV_1 >80% Normal FEV_1 between attacks; FEV_1/FVC normal	FEV_1 >80% predicted; FEV_1/FVC normal	FEV_1 60%–80% predicted; FEV_1/FVC reduced by 5%	FEV_1 <60% predicted; FEV_1/FVC reduced by >5%
Risk				
	Consider severity and interval since last attack. →			
	More frequently occurring attacks with increasing intensity often indicate higher severity of condition. →			
	Relative annual risk for exacerbation may be related to FEV_1. →			
Recommended Step for Initiating Treatment	**Step 1**	**Step 2**	**Step 3**	**Step 4 or 5**
	Reevaluate asthma control in 2–6 wk and adjust therapy as needed			

Guidelines for Using Table

- This stepwise approach is meant to help guide the HCP. It is not a substitute for patient assessment and clinical decision making.
- Assign patients to the most severe step in which any feature occurs.
- Clinical features may overlap across steps.
- Determine level of severity by assessing impairment and risk. Assess impairment by recall of previous 2–4 wk spirometry results.
- Classification should change over time with treatment. After treatment, the focus switches to the level of control, not the classification of severity.

ADL, Activities of daily living.
Data from Cloutier MM, Baptist AP, Blake KV, et al., 2020 focused updates to the asthma management guidelines: a report from the National Asthma Education and Prevention Program Coordinating Committee Expert Panel Working Group. *J Allergy Clin Immunol* 146:1217, 2020.

Spirometry is usually normal between asthma attacks if the patient has no other underlying lung disease. The patient may show an obstructive pattern, including a decrease in forced vital capacity (FVC), PEF, FEV_1, and FEV_1/FVC ratio.

When a spirometry test is scheduled, patients must stop taking any bronchodilator drugs for 6 to 12 hours before the test. Spirometry can be done before and after the administration of a bronchodilator to assess the response. This helps determine the reversibility of airway obstruction, which is important in diagnosing asthma. A positive (favorable) response to the bronchodilator is an increase of more than 200 mL and an increase of more than 12% between preadministration and postadministration values.[24]

We can use a handheld, point-of-care device to measure fractional exhaled nitric oxide (FeNO). FeNO levels are increased in asthma from eosinophilic-induced airway inflammation. FeNO is not used to diagnose asthma. It is used to help evaluate and guide therapy and gauge loss of asthma control and risk of attacks.[25]

Increased serum eosinophil counts and IgE levels suggest an allergen or genetic link. Allergy skin testing can assess sensitivity to specific allergens. A positive skin test does not necessarily mean that the allergen is causing asthma. On the other hand, a negative allergy test does not mean that asthma is not allergy related.

A chest x-ray in asymptomatic patients with asthma is usually normal. Chest x-rays are usually not done unless systemic symptoms, such as fever or chills, are present. It can show if something else is causing symptoms (e.g., pneumonia, foreign body in the airway). A sputum specimen for culture may be done to rule out bacterial infection, especially if the patient has purulent sputum, a history of URI, a fever, or an increased white blood cell (WBC) count.

Interprofessional Care

The goal of care is to achieve and maintain asthma control. The Global Initiative for Asthma (GINA) guidelines are the most widely recognized evidence-based strategies for addressing asthma worldwide.[26] All current guidelines, including GINA, suggest a stepwise approach to drug therapy. They provide directions about drug therapy based on steps (Fig. 31.6). The HCP will "step up" drug therapy as asthma symptoms worsen and "step down" therapy as the patient achieves control. The level of control is determined by medication use, symptoms, and PEF or FEV_1 (Table 31.7).

TABLE 31.5 Interprofessional Care

Asthma

Diagnostic Assessment
- History and physical assessment
- Spirometry, including response to bronchodilator therapy
- Peak expiratory flow (PEF)
- Chest x-ray
- Pulse oximetry
- Allergy skin testing (if indicated)
- Eosinophil and IgE levels (if indicated)

Management
- Identify and avoid or eliminate triggers
- Patient and caregiver teaching
- Drug therapy (Tables 31.8 and 31.9 and Figs. 31.6 and 31.7)
- Written asthma action plan (Fig. 31.10)
- Desensitization (immunotherapy) if indicated
- Assess for control (e.g., Asthma Control Test [ACT])

Acute Attacks
- Inhaled corticosteroids (alternatives: IV or oral corticosteroids)
- Inhaled β_2-adrenergic agonists
- Inhaled anticholinergics
- Position upright (semi- to high-Fowler's)
- Supplemental O_2
- SpO_2 monitoring
- ABGs
- IV fluids
- IV magnesium
- As required: Mechanical ventilation

ABG, Arterial blood gas.

GINA's recommended drug therapy for asthma in adults and adolescents is shown in 2 "tracks." There is strong research favoring track 1, in which low-dose inhaled corticosteroid (ICS)-formoterol is the preferred reliever across all treatment steps, compared with track 2, in which SABA is the alternative reliever. The reason for this change was the reported risks of 'SABA-only' treatment. Regular use of SABA (even for as short as 1 to 2 weeks) is associated with airway hyperresponsiveness, downregulation of beta receptors with decreased bronchodilator effect, increased allergic response, and eosinophilia. Reliance on SABA alone frequently leads to overuse. Overuse of SABA is associated with increased number of exacerbations and ED and hospital visits and increased mortality.

All groups endorse having a written "action plan" to help prevent future attacks. They promote patient teaching and emphasize adherence to the treatment plan. As no two patients with asthma are alike, it is important to remember that drug therapy must be specific for the patient.

TABLE 31.6 Comparison of Asthma and COPD[a]

	Asthma	COPD
Feature		
Age	Usually <40 yr (onset)	Usually 30–45 yr (onset)
Smoking history	No causal relationship	Causal relationship: Often long history (>10–20 pack-yr)
Health and family history	Presence of allergy, rhinitis, eczema. Family history of asthma	Infrequent allergies. May have exposure to environment pollutants. With AATD, family history of lung or liver disease without smoking
Clinical symptoms	Intermittent, vary day to day. Often worse at night (nocturnal asthma)	Slowly progressive, persistent. Worsening of condition over time
Dyspnea	Absent except in attacks or poor control	Dyspnea during exercise and/or daily activities
Sputum	Infrequent	Often
Disease course	Often stable (with varying number and severity of attacks each year)	Progressive worsening (with increasingly more frequent exacerbations)
Diagnostic Study Results		
ABGs	Normal between or during attacks	Between exacerbations in advanced COPD • Often low-normal pH and Pa_{O_2} • High-normal Pa_{CO_2} with normal to high HCO_3^- (may be fully or partially compensated respiratory acidosis)
pH	↑ Early in attack, then ↓ if prolonged or severe attack	Normal → ↓
Pa_{O_2}	↓	N→ ↓
Pa_{CO_2}	↓ Early in attack, then ↑ if prolonged or severe attack	N→ ↑
Chest x-ray	May be normal or show some degree of hyperinflation	Hyperinflation, flattened diaphragm. May have cardiac enlargement
Lung volumes	Often normal	Usually not normal as disease progresses
• Total lung capacity	↑	↑
• Functional residual capacity	↑	↑
• FEV_1	↓ → N	↓
• FEV_1/FVC	N→ ↓	↓ (<70%)

[a]Patients may have features of both asthma and COPD.
AATD, α-1 Antitrypsin deficiency.

Drug Therapy

Drug therapy for asthma can be complex. Asthma drugs are divided into 2 general types: (1) *short-term controller* ("rescue") agents to treat attacks and (2) *preferred reliever* agents

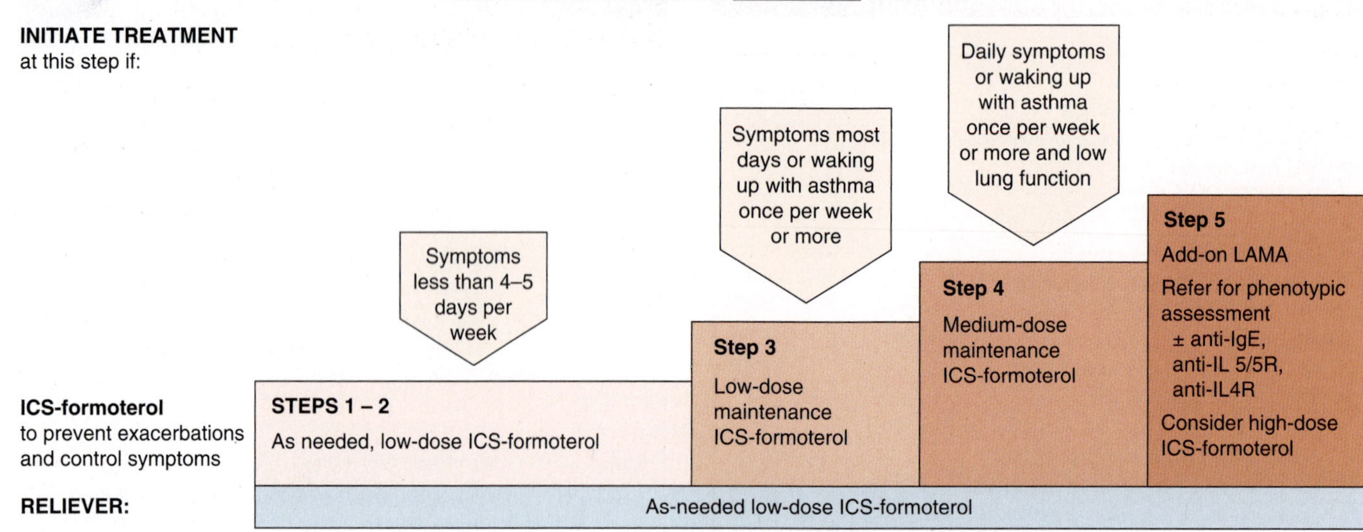

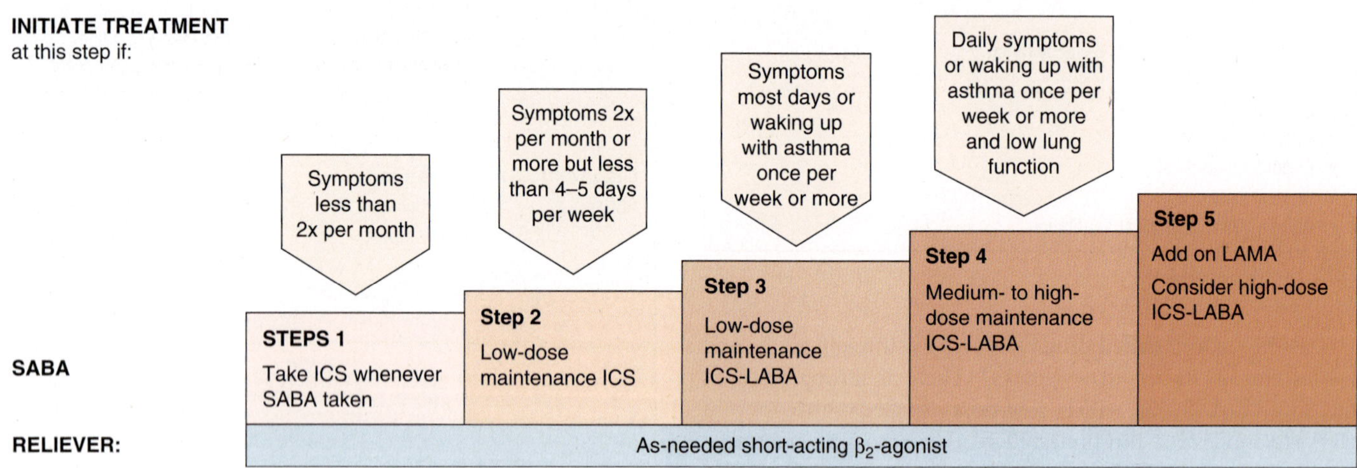

Fig. 31.6 Stepwise approach to asthma treatment. *ICS,* Inhaled corticosteroid; *IL,* interleukin; *LABA,* long-acting β_2-agonist; *LTRA,* leukrotriene receptor agonist; *SABA,* short-acting β_2-agonist.

(Table 31.8). You need to understand the different classes of drugs used to treat asthma and asthma attacks, their desired effects, side effects, and when to use different drugs. Patient history, drug therapy, and frequency and severity of attacks help the HCP decide which drugs are best suited to control asthma symptoms. Common drugs used in asthma therapy are shown in Table 31.9.

Corticosteroids. GINA guidelines recommend using ICS as first-line agents in an acute asthma attack and as the first step in acute asthma management (Fig. 31.7).[26] While this recommendation has been accepted globally for some time, it has only recently become part of the standard of asthma care in the United States.

Corticosteroids are antiinflammatory drugs. They reduce bronchial hyperresponsiveness, block the late-phase response, and inhibit the migration of inflammatory cells. They are the most effective short-term controller drugs for asthma and improve asthma control better than any other drug.

Side effects of ICSs include easy bruising and decreased bone mineral density. Oropharyngeal candidiasis, hoarseness, and dry cough are local side effects. These problems can be reduced or prevented by using a spacer with the metered-dose inhaler (MDI) and by gargling with water or mouthwash after each use. Using a spacer or holding device can help get more drug into the lungs.

TABLE 31.7 Components of Asthma Control

	CLASSIFICATION OF ASTHMA CONTROL		
Components	**Well Controlled**	**Not Well Controlled**	**Poorly Controlled**
Impairment			
Symptoms	≤2 days/wk	>2 days/wk	Throughout the day
Nighttime awakenings	≤2/mo	1–3/wk	≥4/wk
Interference with normal activity	None	Some limitation	Extremely limited
FEV_1	>80% predicted/personal best	60%–80% predicted/personal best	<60% predicted/ personal best
Risk			
Attacks requiring additional drug therapy	0–1/yr	≥2/yr	≥2/yr
Progressive loss of lung function	Evaluation requires long-term follow-up. →		
Treatment-related adverse effects	Can vary in intensity from none to very troublesome and worrisome. Level of intensity does not correlate to specific levels of control but is considered in the overall assessment of risk. →		
Recommended action for treatment (based on assessment of control)	• Maintain current step. • Regular follow-up every 1–6 mo to maintain control. • Consider step down if well controlled for at least 3 mo.	• Step up 1 step. • Reevaluate in 2–6 wk. • Review medication adherence, inhaler technique. • For side effects, consider alternative treatment options.	• Step up 1 or 2 steps. • Reevaluate in 2 wk. • Review medication adherence, inhaler technique. • For side effects, consider alternative treatment options.

From U.S. Department of Health and Human Services, National Heart, Lung, and Blood Institute: Asthma care quick reference: diagnosing and managing asthma. Adapted from *Guidelines from the National Asthma Education and Prevention Program – expert panel report 3*. September 2012. NIH Publication No. 12-5075.

Bronchodilators. The 3 classes of bronchodilator drugs used in asthma therapy are β_2-adrenergic agonists (β_2-agonists), methylxanthines, and anticholinergics.

β_2-Adrenergic agonist drugs. β_2-adrenergic agonists may be SABAs or LABAs. While inhaled SABAs remain effective drugs for relieving acute bronchospasm (as seen in an acute asthma attack), they are no longer recommended as first-line therapy. This is perhaps the biggest change in asthma management in the past several years. However, they do play a key role in asthma management. These drugs have an onset of action within minutes and are effective for 4 to 8 hours. They stimulate β-adrenergic receptors in the bronchioles, producing bronchodilation. They also increase mucociliary clearance.

β_2-adrenergic agonists can prevent bronchospasm caused by different triggers because they prevent the release of inflammatory mediators from mast cells. They do not inhibit the late-phase response of asthma or have antiinflammatory effects. If used often, inhaled β_2-adrenergic agonists may cause tremors, anxiety, nausea, tachycardia, and palpitations.

Too frequent use of β_2-adrenergic agonists indicates poor asthma control and may mask the severity of the condition. Drug effectiveness can be reduced. SABAs should not be used alone for recurrent, repeated asthma attacks or for long-term control. The GINA guidelines suggest that they be used as an alternative reliever medication when a patient does not respond to low-dose ICSs.

TABLE 31.8 Drug Therapy

Asthma

Types of Drugs	Drug Class
Controller Drugs	**Inhaled Corticosteroids** Short-acting β_2-adrenergic agonists (SABA)
Single Maintenance, Reliever and Alternate Reliever Drugs (SMART)	Anticholinergics • Short-acting muscarinic antagonist (SAMA) • Long-acting muscarinic antagonist (LAMA) β_2-Adrenergic agonists • SABA • Long-acting β-adrenergic agonist (LABA)
	Oral Corticosteroids Leukotriene modifiers • Leukotriene receptor antagonist • Leukotriene inhibitor
	Methylxanthines Monoclonal antibody immune modulators • Anti-IgE • Anti–interleukin 5
	Phosphodiesterase Inhibitors Combination preparations • ICS/SABA • ICS/LABA • ICS/LAMA/LAB

TABLE 31.9 Drug Therapy
Asthma and COPD

Drug	Use	Route	Considerations
Anticholinergics			
Short-Acting Muscarinic Antagonists (SAMAs)			
ipratropium (Atrovent HFA)	Asthma, COPD	Nebulizer, MDI	Can be monotherapy. Produces bronchodilation within minutes. Side effects: Headache, dry mouth, cough, dizziness, palpitations.
Long-Acting Muscarinic Antagonists (LAMAs)			
aclidinium bromide (Tudorza, Tudorza Pressair)	COPD	DPI	Side effects: Headache, cough, cold symptoms. Do not take with other anticholinergics.
revefenacin (Yupelri)	COPD	Nebulizer	Dosed once daily as maintenance treatment. Does not cause usual side effects of other anticholinergics. Do not take with other anticholinergics.
tiotropium bromide (Spiriva, Spiriva HandiHaler, Spiriva Respimat)	Asthma, COPD	DPI	Typically used with ICS. Dosed once daily as maintenance treatment. Do not take with other anticholinergics. Effects of drug last >24 h. Side effects: Headache, dry mouth, dizziness, palpitations. Blurred vision if powder comes in contact with eyes. Maximum effect 1 wk after starting drug.
umeclidinium (Incruse Ellipta)	COPD	DPI	Typically used with ICS. Dosed once daily as maintenance treatment. Do not take with other anticholinergics. Side effects: Cough, cold symptoms, sore throat, arthralgia, diarrhea.
β_2-Adrenergic Agonists			
Inhaled: Short-Acting β-Adrenergic Agonists (SABAs)			
albuterol (Accuneb, Ventolin HFA, ProAir HFA, ProAir DigiHaler)	Asthma COPD	Nebulizer, MDI Oral	Produces bronchodilation within 5 min; effects last 3–6 h. Oral tablets (long-acting, extended-release) not for acute situation. Side effects: Tremors, headache, tachycardia, nausea. MDI may be more effective than nebulizer, as drug delivered more quickly to the lungs. Use with caution in patients with cardiac problems because of ↑ BP and heart rate, CNS stimulation, and ↑ risk for dysrhythmias. Can cause hypokalemia.
levalbuterol (Xopenex, Xopenex HFA)	Asthma COPD	Nebulizer, MDI	MDI: Response in 15 min, peak effect in 75 min; Neb: Response in 10–17 min; peak effect in 1.5 h. Do not use if solution discolored. Side effects: Tremors, headache, lightheadedness, tachycardia.
Inhaled: Long-Acting β-Adrenergic Agonists (LABAs) In asthma: Never use as monotherapy. Use only in combination with ICSs. In COPD: Some drugs used as monotherapy. Not used for rapid relief of dyspnea.			
arformoterol (Brovana)	COPD	Nebulizer	Not used in acute situations. Monitor for paradoxical bronchospasm at high doses. Side effects: Back pain, GI distress, edema, leg cramps, hypokalemia.
formoterol (Foradil Perforomist)	COPD	DPI, nebulizer	Side effects: Tremors, headache, wheezing, tachycardia, GI distress, hypokalemia. Use with caution in diabetes, can increase glucose levels.
indacaterol (Arcapta Neohaler)	COPD	DPI	Once-daily use. Use with caution in diabetes, can increase glucose levels. Side effects: Tremors, cough, upset stomach, wheezing, rash, hypokalemia.
olodaterol (Stiolto, Striverdi Respimat)	COPD	MDI	Once-daily use. Side effects: Dizziness, cold symptoms.
salmeterol (Serevent)	COPD	DPI	Do not use more than twice daily. Side effects: Tremors, tachycardia, muscle pain, wheezing. Helps prevent exercise-induced asthma in those with persistent asthma.

TABLE 31.9 Drug Therapy—cont'd

Asthma and COPD

Drug	Use	Route	Considerations
Corticosteroids			
Oral, Inhaled			
hydrocortisone (Solu-Cortef)	Asthma	IV	Oral preferred over IV. IV therapy preferred for patients undergoing surgery.
methylprednisolone (Medrol, Solu-Medrol)	Asthma	Oral, IV	Side effects: hyperglycemia, ↑ BP, fluid retention, ↑ risk of infection. May take a few days for results to be seen in severe COPD exacerbation.
prednisone	Asthma COPD	Oral	Take oral dose in morning with food or milk. High dose may cause GI distress. Long-term therapy requires vitamin D and calcium supplements to prevent osteoporosis. Long-term steroid therapy: discontinue gradually to prevent adrenal insufficiency.
Inhaled			
beclomethasone (Beclovent, Qvar RediHaler)	Asthma	MDI	Used with SABA in acute attack; may need to increase dosage. Side effects: Headache, cough, hoarseness, oral candidiasis (thrush). Rinse mouth with water or mouthwash after use to prevent oral fungal infections.
budesonide (Pulmicort Flexhaler, Pulmicort Respules, Rhinocort)	Asthma	DPI, nebulizer	Spacer device with MDI may decrease incidence of oral candidiasis. May not see effects until after at least 2–4 wk of regular treatment.
ciclesonide (Alvesco)	Asthma	MDI	
fluticasone (Flovent HFA, Flovent Diskus, Arnuity Ellipta)	Asthma	MDI, DPI	
mometasone (Asmanex HFA, Asmanex Twisthaler)	Asthma	DPI	
Leukotriene Modifiers			
Leukotriene Receptor Antagonists (LRAs)			
montelukast (Singulair)	Asthma	Oral	Do not use in acute attack. May prevent wheezing and dyspnea caused by asthma during exercise. Side effects: Headache, stuffy/runny nose, sore throat, fever, GI distress. Linked to agitation, mood changes, hallucination, depression, thoughts of suicide.
zafirlukast (Accolate)	Asthma	Oral	Do not use in acute attack. No specific side effects. Take at least 1 h before or 2 h after meals. Contraindicated in cirrhosis. Reduces clearance of warfarin (drug ↑ prothrombin time).
Leukotriene Inhibitor			
zileuton (Zyflo, Zyflo CR)	Asthma	Oral	Do not use in acute attack. Extended-release tablets: Do not crush, chew, or cut. Side effects: Headache, fever, cough, stuffy/runny nose, nausea. Use with caution in liver disease; monitor liver enzymes. May interfere with metabolism of warfarin and theophylline. Monitor for changes in sleep and behavior.
Methylxanthines			
Oral: theophylline (Theo-24, Elixophyllin Theochron) *IV agent:* aminophylline (no longer recommended)	Asthma, COPD	Oral, IV	Very limited use. Used as adjunct to ICS and β_2-adrenergic agonists for exacerbations. Theophylline may be helpful for nighttime asthma attacks. Side effects: CNS stimulation, headache, tachycardia, dysrhythmias, nausea, vomiting, altered glucose levels. Nicotine ↑ liver clearance of methylxanthines; dosage increase needed for those who smoke. Many drug interactions. Taking drug with food or antacids may help GI effects.
Phosphodiesterase Inhibitors			
roflumilast (Daliresp)	COPD	Oral	Do not use in acute attack. Used in severe COPD to reduce exacerbation frequency. Side effects: Headache, insomnia, GI distress, unexplained weight loss, suicidal thoughts. Numerous drug interactions; do not take with amiodarone, theophylline, phenytoin.

Continued

TABLE 31.9 Drug Therapy—cont'd

Asthma and COPD

Drug	Use	Route	Considerations
Biologics			
• Target cells and proteins that cause inflammation. • Usually an "add-on" to existing drug regimen in severe asthma. • Treats source of the inflammation (not symptoms), helping patients achieve better control in long-term asthma.			
Anti-IgE			
omalizumab (Xolair)	Asthma	Subcutaneous	Add-on therapy in patients receiving other asthma drugs. Dose and frequency based on total IgE levels and body weight. Total IgE levels elevated up to 1 yr after therapy stopped; do not use as a guide for dosing drug. Side effects: Dizziness, joint pain, fatigue, stuffy/runny nose. Pain, burning at injection site, anaphylactic reaction possible. Give only under direct medical supervision every 2–4 wk.
Anti–Interleukin 5			
mepolizumab (Nucala)	Asthma	Subcutaneous	Add-on therapy in patients receiving other asthma drugs. Side effects: Headache, back pain. Hypersensitivity reactions may occur. Give only under direct medical supervision every 4 wk.
reslizumab (Cinqair)	Asthma	IV	Add-on therapy in patients receiving other asthma drugs. Given every 4 wk as an IV infusion over 1 h. Risk for anaphylactic reactions. Monitor for infection.
Combination Agents			
• Combine 2 or 3 different medications into one inhaler. • Combinations may include corticosteroids, SABA, LABA, or LAMA. • Most often used once daily. • No one combination drug is superior to another.			
Inhaled Corticosteroid and SABA			
budesonide and albuterol (Airsupra)	Asthma	MDI	Not a maintenance treatment for asthma. No more than 6 doses (12 puffs) in 24 h.
Inhaled Corticosteroid and LABA			
budesonide and formoterol (Symbicort)	Asthma, COPD	MDI	Do not use in acute attack. Daily or q12h. Side effects: Dry mouth, hoarseness, possible oral yeast infections. Rinse oral cavity after use. Reduce risk of thrush by using spacer.
fluticasone and salmeterol (Advair HFA, Advair Diskus, Airduo DigiHaler)	Asthma, COPD	MDI	Do not use in acute attack. Daily or q12h. Space doses at least 12 h apart.
fluticasone and vilanterol (Breo-Ellipta)	Asthma, COPD	MDI	Do not use in acute attack. Use daily or q12h. Do not take another LABA. May affect glucose and potassium levels. Do not take extra doses if symptoms worsen; consult HCP immediately.
mometasone and formoterol (Dulera)	Asthma	MDI	Do not use in acute attack. Daily or q12h. Fewest side effects of all the combination inhalers. May notice increase in wheezing after receiving drug.
Inhaled Corticosteroid, LABA, and LAMA			
fluticasone, umeclidinium, and vilanterol (Trelegy-Ellipta)	Asthma, COPD		Do not use in acute attack. Once-daily treatment. Side effects: Headache, joint pain, stuffy/runny nose, nausea, diarrhea. Do not use if severe allergy to milk protein. May need to decrease or eliminate caffeine intake.

COPD, Chronic obstructive pulmonary disease; *DPI,* dry powder inhaler; *ICS,* inhaled corticosteroid; *MDI,* metered-dose inhaler.

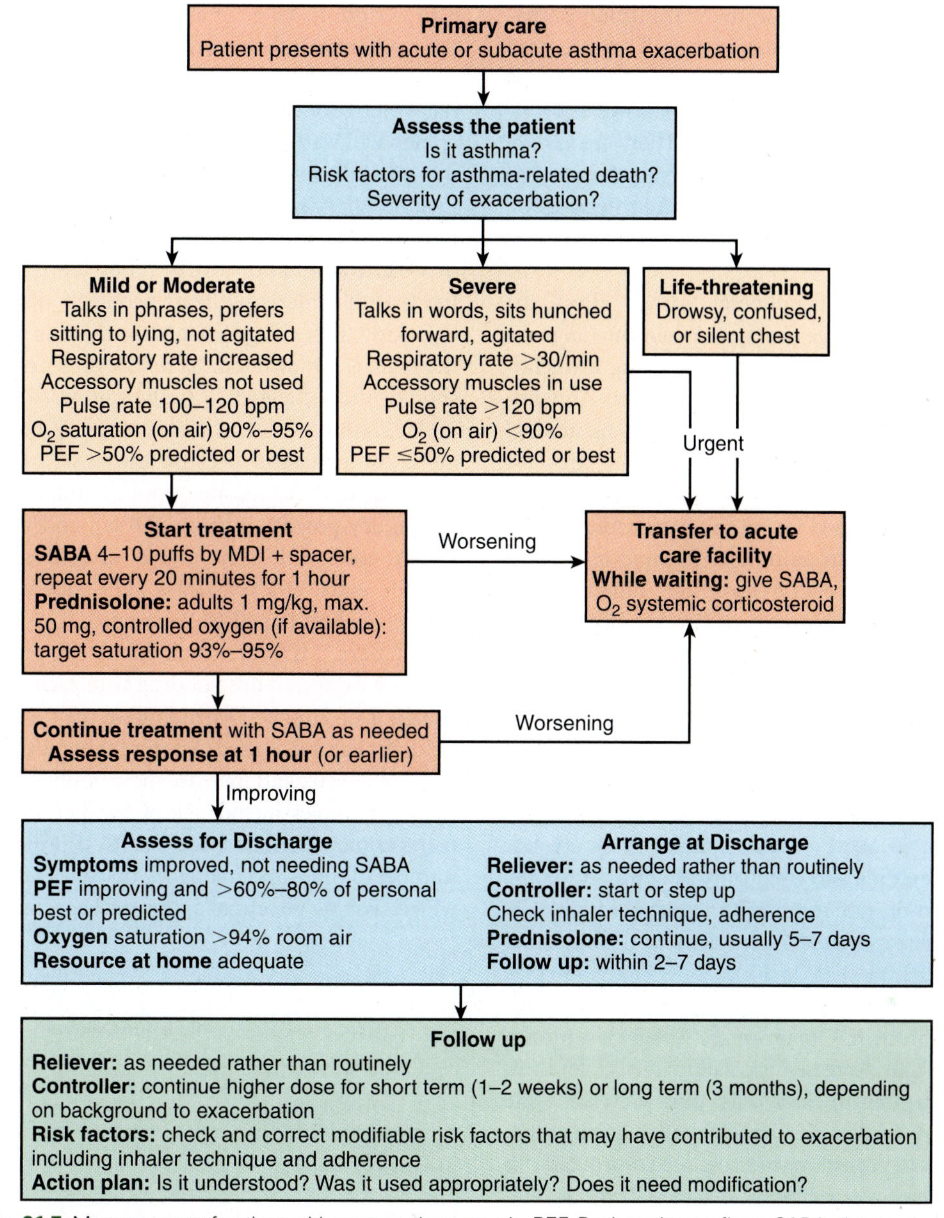

Fig. 31.7 Management of patient with acute asthma attack. *PEF,* Peak expiratory flow; *SABA,* short-acting β_2-agonist (doses are for salbutamol). (Modified from *GINA evidence-based strategy document, 2021.* https://ginasthma.org.)

Like SABAs, LABAs should not be used alone as primary treatment. They should be used only if the patient does not respond to medium-dose ICSs. In other words, LABAs can be used as an adjunct to treatment. Examples of LABAs used to treat asthma attacks include salmeterol and formoterol.

LABAs are effective for 12 hours. Tell patients that LABAs should not be used to treat acute symptoms or to obtain quick relief from bronchospasm. LABAs are used only once every 12 hours. Combination therapy using an ICS and a LABA is available in several inhalers (e.g., fluticasone/salmeterol [Advair], budesonide/formoterol [Symbicort]). Combinations are more convenient, improve adherence, and ensure that patients receive the LABA with an ICS.

DRUG ALERT

β_2-Adrenergic Agonists

- Use with caution in patients with heart problems.
- Both SABAs and LABAs may cause increased BP and heart rate, central nervous system stimulation, and dysrhythmias.

DRUG ALERT

Long-Acting β_2-Adrenergic Agonists (LABAs)

- Should not be the first or only drug used to treat asthma.
- Should be added to the treatment plan only if other drugs do not control asthma.
- Do not use to treat wheezing that is getting worse.

Methylxanthines. Sustained-release methylxanthine preparations are not a first-line controller medication. They are used only as an alternative therapy. GINA no longer recommends theophylline as a part of asthma treatment. It is a weak bronchodilator with mild antiinflammatory effects. There are several problems with theophylline. There are many side effects and drug interactions. It has a very narrow margin of safety, so we must check serum blood levels regularly to see if drug levels are within therapeutic range.

Anticholinergic drugs. Anticholinergic drugs affect the muscles around the bronchi (large airways). When the lungs are irritated, these bands of muscle can tighten, causing bronchoconstriction via the parasympathetic nervous system. Anticholinergics work by preventing these muscles from tightening. Thus these drugs promote bronchodilation. They are less effective than equivalent doses of SABAs. Therefore short-acting anticholinergic drugs are not used except in severe acute asthma attacks. Examples include ipratropium and tiotropium.

Leukotriene modifiers. Leukotrienes are inflammatory mediators produced from arachidonic acid metabolism. They are potent bronchoconstrictors. Some leukotrienes cause airway edema and inflammation, worsening symptoms of an acute asthma attack.

Leukotriene receptor agonists (LTRAs) block the release of some substances from mast cells and eosinophils, producing bronchodilator and antiinflammatory effects. LTRAs do not reverse bronchospasm in acute asthma attacks. They are less effective than corticosteroids and used only as adjunct therapy for those patients who do not respond to treatment with ICS. LTRAs include zafirlukast (Accolate), montelukast (Singulair), and zileuton (Zyflo CR).

Biologics.

Anti–immunoglobulin E. Omalizumab (Xolair) is a monoclonal antibody to IgE that decreases circulating free IgE levels. It prevents IgE from attaching to mast cells, thus preventing the release of inflammatory mediators. Omalizumab is given to patients with moderate to severe asthma or those not controlled with ICSs alone. There is a risk for anaphylaxis, so patients must receive the injection in a setting where this emergency can be treated.

Anti–interleukin 5. Interleukin (IL)-5 is a cytokine involved in the inflammatory response in asthma by promoting eosinophil activity.[27] Monoclonal antibodies that inhibit IL-5 decrease the production and survival of eosinophils. As a result, inflammation and edema of the airway subside. They are mainly used for patients with a history of severe asthma attacks and as an adjunct with other asthma medication. These drugs include mepolizumab (Nucala), reslizumab (Cinqair), and benralizumab (Fasenra).

Nonprescription combination drugs. Several combination drugs are available over the counter (OTC). They are usually combinations of a bronchodilator (ephedrine) and an expectorant (guaifenesin). Often, patients seek OTC drugs because they are less expensive than prescription drugs. Many people consider these drugs safe because they can be obtained without a prescription. In general, they should be avoided because of their potential side effects.

OTC inhalers containing epinephrine are advertised as relieving bronchospasm. Those containing ephedrine and epinephrine are potentially dangerous because they stimulate the central nervous and cardiovascular systems. Side effects include nervousness, palpitations, dysrhythmias, tremors, insomnia, and increased BP. Teach patients about the dangers of OTC combination drugs. They are possibly unsafe for patients with underlying heart problems. For patients who insist on taking these drugs, encourage them to discuss their use with the HCP. Caution them to follow directions on the label. They should notify their HCP if any untoward reaction occurs.

Inhalation devices for drug delivery. Many asthma drugs are given by inhalation because the onset of action is faster and systemic side effects are reduced. Inhalation devices include MDIs, dry powder inhalers (DPIs), and nebulizers (Fig. 31.8). When used with comparable drug doses, MDIs and DPIs provide equal efficacy. Costs vary widely. Patients should use the device best suited to their needs.

Inhalers. MDIs are small, handheld, pressurized devices that deliver a measured dose of drug with each activation. The dose is usually 1 or 2 puffs. Depending on the specific MDI, a spacer or holding chamber is used to reduce the amount of drug delivered to the oropharynx and increase the amount of drug delivered to the lungs. Examples include AeroChamber and InspirEase. Spacers help people who have hand-breath coordination problems. The number of times and frequency that an MDI must be primed vary widely. Follow directions in the package insert.

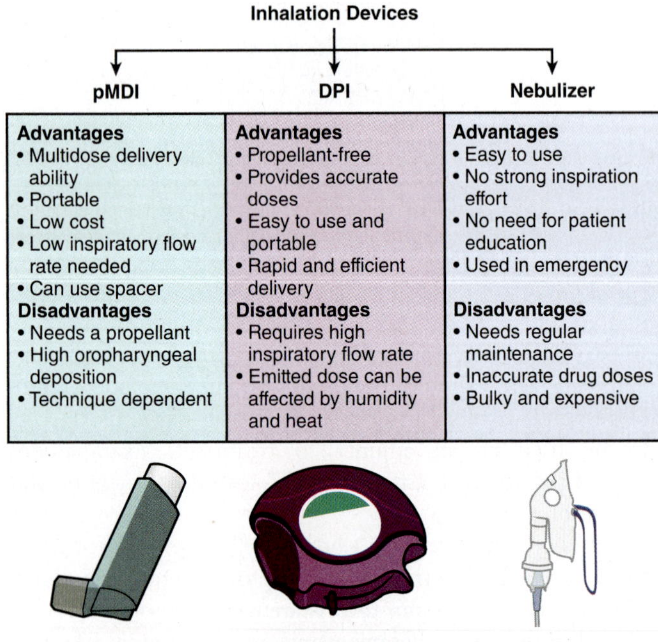

Fig. 31.8 Inhalation devices.

Patients using several MDIs are often unclear about the order in which to use them. In most circumstances, the controller drug (e.g., ICS) is used first, followed by reliever medications (as needed) for clinical conditions that do not improve. Teach patients about the different drugs used to treat asthma, how they work, and the indications for use. Review the order in which patients should take their medications.

An MDI drug is effective only if taken properly. Review MDI technique during each visit. Patients need to know how to use the MDI correctly (Fig. 31.9), how to determine whether the MDI is empty, and how to effectively clean and care for the device. Problems using an MDI are listed in Table 31.10.

Dry powder inhalers. DPIs contain dry, powdered medication. They are breath activated. DPIs have several advantages over MDIs. They require less manual dexterity. There is no need to coordinate device puffs with inhalation. Some disadvantages are that some common drugs are not available in DPIs. The medication may clump if exposed to humidity. Because the medicine is delivered only by the patient's inspiratory effort, patients with a low FEV_1 (less than 1 L) may not be able to inspire the medication. Table 31.11 describes how to use a DPI.

Nebulizers. Nebulizers are small machines used to convert drug solutions into mist. The mist can be inhaled through a face mask or mouthpiece held between the teeth with the lips closed around the device. Nebulizers are usually used for those who have severe asthma or difficulty with the MDI inhalation. They do not provide better delivery of medication than a spacer with an inhaler.

Using an inhaler seems simple, but most patients do not use it the right way. When you use your inhaler the wrong way, less medicine gets to your lungs. (Your physician may give you other types of inhalers.)

For the next 2 weeks, read these steps aloud as you do them or ask someone to read them to you. Ask your physician or nurse to check how well you are using your inhaler.

Use your inhaler in one of the three ways pictured here (**A** or **B** is best, but **C** can be used if you have trouble with **A** or **B**).

Steps for Using Your Inhaler

Getting ready
1. Take off the cap and shake the inhaler.
2. Breathe out all the way.
3. Hold your inhaler the way your doctor said (**A, B,** or **C**).

Breathe in slowly
4. As you start breathing in **slowly** through your mouth, press down on the inhaler **one** time. (If you use a holding chamber, first press down on the inhaler. Within 5 seconds, begin to breathe in slowly.)
5. Keep breathing in **slowly,** as deeply as you can.

Hold your breath
6. Hold your breath as you count to 10 slowly, if you can.
7. For inhaled quick-relief medicine (β_2-agonists), wait about 1 minute between puffs. There is no need to wait between puffs for other medicines.

A. Hold inhaler 1 to 2 inches in front of your mouth (about the width of two fingers).

B. Use a spacer/holding chamber. These come in many shapes and can be useful to any patient.

C. Put the inhaler in your mouth.

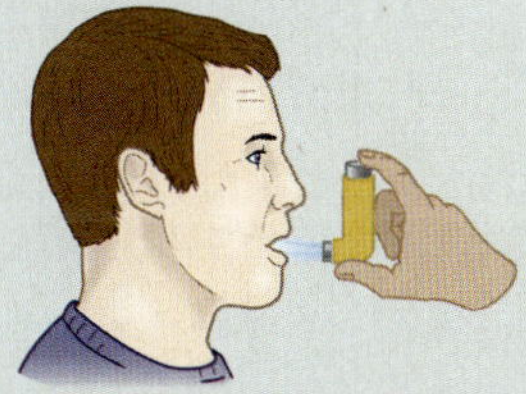

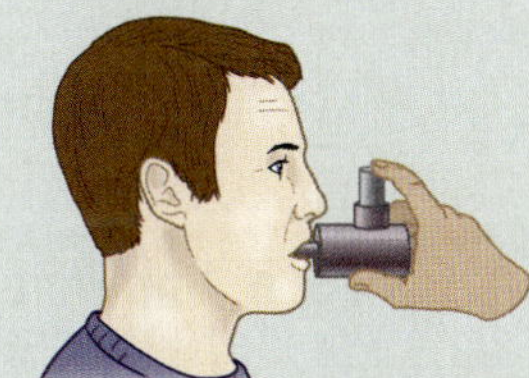

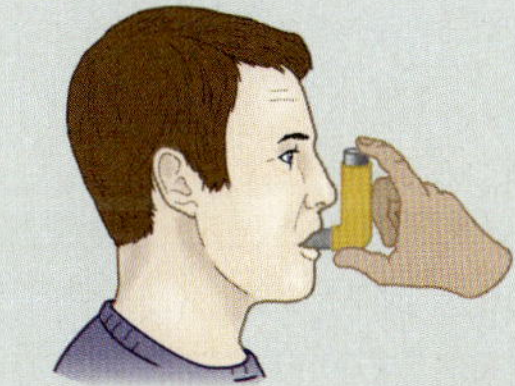

Clean Your Inhaler as Needed

Look at the hole where the medicine sprays out from your inhaler. If you see "powder" in or around the hole, clean the inhaler. Remove the metal canister from the L-shaped plastic mouthpiece. Rinse only the mouthpiece and cap in warm water. Let them dry overnight. In the morning, put the canister back inside. Put the cap on.

Know When to Replace Your Inhaler

For medicines you take each day (an example): Say your new canister has 200 puffs (number of puffs is listed on canister) and you are told to take 8 puffs per day.

$$\frac{200 \text{ puffs in canister}}{8 \text{ puffs per day}} = 25 \text{ days}$$

So this canister will last 25 days. If you started using this inhaler on May 1, replace it on or before May 25.

You can write the date on your canister.

For **quick-relief medicine take as needed** and count each puff.

Do not put your canister in water to see if it is empty as water may enter the MDI and impair the inhaler.

Fig. 31.9 How to use your metered-dose inhaler.

TABLE 31.10 Problems Using a Metered-Dose Inhaler (MDI)

- Need to coordinate activation with inspiration
- Activating MDI in the mouth while breathing through nose
- Inhaling too rapidly
- Breathing in too early or too late
- Not holding the breath for 10 sec (or as close to 10 sec as possible)
- Holding MDI upside down or sideways
- Inhaling more than 1 puff with each inspiration
- Not shaking MDI before use (if indicated)
- Not waiting enough time between each puff
- Not opening mouth wide enough (if using open mouth technique), causing medication to bounce off teeth, tongue, or palate
- Not having adequate strength to activate MDI
- Not being able to understand and/or follow directions
- Inadvertently using an empty container

TABLE 31.11 PATIENT & CAREGIVER TEACHING

How to Use a Dry Powder Inhaler (DPI)

Include the following instructions when teaching a patient to use a DPI:

1. Remove mouthpiece cap or open the device according to manufacturer's instructions. If there is an external counter, note the number of doses remaining.
2. Load the medicine into the inhaler or engage the lever to allow the medicine to become available. Some DPIs are held upright while loading. Others are held sideways or in a horizontal position.
3. Do not shake your medicine.
4. Stand up or sit up straight. Breathe out, getting as much air out of your lungs as you can. Do not breathe into your inhaler because this could affect the dose.
5. Place the inhaler's mouthpiece into your mouth. Close your lips tightly around the mouthpiece.
6. Inhale deeply and quickly. This will ensure that the medicine moves down deeply into your lungs. You may not taste or sense the medicine going into your lungs.
7. Remove the inhaler from your mouth.
8. Hold your breath for 5 to 10 sec to disperse the medicine into your lungs. Then, slowly exhale.
9. If there is an external counter, note the number of doses left. It should be 1 less than the number in step 1.
10. Repeat these steps if you need to take a second dose.

Nebulizers are usually powered by compressed air or O_2 generator. At home, the patient may have an air-powered compressor. In the hospital, wall O_2 or compressed air powers the nebulizer.

Aerosolized medication orders must include the drug, dose, diluent, and whether it is to be nebulized with O_2 or compressed air. The advantage of nebulized therapy is that it is easy to use. Common nebulized agents include albuterol and ipratropium. Place the patient upright. This position allows for efficient breathing and helps ensure adequate penetration and deposition of the aerosolized drug into the lungs. The patient must breathe slowly and deeply through the mouth and hold each inspiration for 2 to 3 seconds. Deep diaphragmatic breathing helps ensure delivery of the drug. Tell the patient to breathe normally in between large, inhaled breaths. After treatment, have the patient cough effectively.

To reduce the potential for bacterial growth, review cleaning procedures for respiratory equipment. An effective home-cleaning method is to wash the nebulizer daily in soap and water, rinse it with water, and soak it for 20 to 30 minutes in a 1:1 white vinegar–water solution, followed by a water rinse and air drying.

NURSING MANAGEMENT: ASTHMA

Assessment

Subjective and objective data you should obtain from patients with asthma are outlined in Table 31.12. If a patient is not in acute distress, obtain a detailed health history. Include information about when asthma was first diagnosed, triggers, and what helped relieve past asthma attacks. Assessment of patients with asthma may be normal, especially between attacks.

Clinical Problems

Clinical problems for patients with asthma may include:

- Impaired respiratory function
- Activity intolerance
- Anxiety

Additional information on clinical problems and interventions is presented in eNursing Care Plan 31.1 on the website for this chapter.

Planning

The overall goals are that patients with asthma will achieve asthma control, as evidenced by (1) minimal symptoms during the day and night, (2) acceptable activity levels (including exercise), (3) maintaining greater than 80% of personal best PEF, (4) few or no adverse effects of drug therapy, (5) no acute asthma attacks, and (6) adequate knowledge to carry out the treatment plan.

Implementation

Health Promotion

Your role in preventing asthma attacks or decreasing their severity focuses mainly on teaching the patient and caregiver. Teach patients to identify and avoid known personal triggers for asthma (e.g., cigarette smoke, pet dander) and irritants (e.g., cold air, aspirin, foods, cats, indoor air pollution) (Table 31.3).

When cold air cannot be avoided, dressing properly with scarves or using a mask helps reduce the risk for an asthma attack. Aspirin and NSAIDs should be avoided if they are known to trigger an attack. Many OTC drugs contain aspirin. Teach patients to read all labels carefully. Nonselective β-blockers (e.g., propranolol) are contraindicated because they inhibit bronchodilation. Selective β-blockers (e.g., atenolol)

TABLE 31.12 NURSING ASSESSMENT

Asthma

Subjective Data

Important Health Information

Health history: Allergic rhinitis, sinusitis, or skin allergies. Previous asthma attacks (frequency, severity) and any required hospitalization. Symptoms worsened by triggers in the environment. GERD. Occupational exposure to chemical irritants (e.g., paints, dust).

Medications: Use of medications. Adherence, inhaler technique. Use of antibiotics. Pattern and amount of "controller" and "preferred" or "alternative" reliever used per week. Drugs that may trigger an attack in susceptible persons, such as aspirin, NSAIDs, β-adrenergic blockers.

Functional Health Patterns

Health perception–health management: Family history of allergies and/or asthma. Recent upper respiratory or sinus infection.

Activity-exercise: Fatigue, decreased or absent exercise tolerance. Dyspnea, cough (especially at night), productive cough with white, yellow, or other colored sputum. Chest tightness, feelings of suffocation, air hunger, talking in short sentences or words or phrases, sitting upright to breathe.

Sleep-rest: Awakened from sleep because of cough or breathing difficulties, insomnia.

Coping–stress tolerance: Stress in work environment or home.

Objective Data

Cardiovascular

↑ Heart rate, pulsus paradoxus, jugular venous distention, hypertension or hypotension, premature ventricular contractions

General

Restlessness, exhaustion, confusion, upright or forward-leaning body position

Respiratory

Nasal discharge, nasal polyps, mucosal swelling

Crackles, decreased or absent breath sounds, and wheezes (inspiratory, expiratory, or both)

Hyperresonance on percussion

Sputum (thick, white, tenacious)

↑ work of breathing with use of accessory muscles

Intercostal and supraclavicular retractions

Tachypnea with hyperventilation

Prolonged expiration

Skin

Diaphoresis, cyanosis (circumoral, nail bed), eczema

GERD, Gastroesophageal reflux disease.

should be used with caution. Desensitization (immunotherapy) may be partially effective in decreasing sensitivity to known allergens.

Prompt diagnosis and treatment of sinusitis and URIs may help prevent an asthma attack. If occupation irritants are involved, the patient may need to consider changing jobs. Those who are obese often find that weight loss improves asthma control. If exercise is planned or if the patient had an asthma attack previously with exercise, they may need a pretreatment or long-term control plan to prevent bronchospasm.

Acute Care

During an acute attack, signs and symptoms, medication use, and PEF or FEV_1 measurements can be used to help identify the severity of an asthma attack and guide us in providing treatment. The goal is to achieve rapid control of the symptoms and return patients to their previous level of functioning as quickly as possible. Therapy is specific to the patient, considering their history, severity of symptoms, frequency of exacerbations, asthma action plan (including medications), and patient response. Management of patients with an acute asthma attack is shown in Fig. 31.7.

Patients with mild or moderate asthma attacks may be seen in an outpatient clinic or ED. These attacks occur no more than twice per week, with minimal interference in day-to-day activity. The patient is alert, oriented, and speaks in sentences. The patient may describe chest tightness, varying degrees of difficulty breathing, and a slight increase in the use of asthma drugs. O_2 saturation is usually greater than 90% on room air and PEF greater than 50% of predicted or personal best.

ICS are the mainstays of treatment for mild to moderate asthma attacks. Monitor vital signs and monitor for a change in patient condition. Most patients improve shortly after receiving medication. When the patient improves, review the asthma action plan with them. Teach them the importance of a follow-up appointment with the HCP. If the patient's condition is slow to respond, does not respond, or the HCP suspects another condition may be occurring or contributing to the acute attack, we should transfer the outpatient to an acute care facility.

A severe attack is usually frightening enough for most patients to go to the ED. In many cases, a severe asthma attack will call for hospital admission. Managing patients with a severe attack focuses on maintaining ventilation, correcting hypoxemia, and monitoring patient condition.

In a severe attack, continuously monitor vital signs and WOB. Patients may be tachycardic and focused on breathing. Respiratory rates greater than 30 breaths/min may be present. They may use accessory muscles. They may be agitated, restless, or confused from hypoxemia. Patients often sit forward to maximize diaphragm movement.

IV magnesium sulfate has a bronchodilator effect. It may be given to patients with a very low FEV_1 or peak flow (less than 40% of predicted or personal best) or those who do not respond to initial treatment. IV magnesium should not delay intubation if needed.

Patients with status asthmaticus may need mechanical ventilation. Hemodynamic monitoring is critical. Continuous analgesic infusions (e.g., ketamine, morphine) and sedation with drugs such as propofol help decrease WOB and promote synchrony with the ventilator. In some circumstances, neuromuscular blocking agents (e.g., rocuronium) may be used. Inhaled anesthetics, such as isoflurane, are an option for those not responding to conventional treatment. These patients are cared for in the ICU.

Bedside PEF may be used to monitor airflow obstruction in mild to moderate asthma attacks. Obtaining a PEF during a severe asthma attack is usually not possible. However, if it can be obtained, PEF less than 200 L/min or 50% or less of predicted or of personal best indicates severe obstruction. Serial PEF results, oximetry, and measurement of arterial blood gases (ABGs) give information about the severity of the attack and the response to therapy.

O_2 therapy is given to achieve a PaO_2 of at least 80 mm Hg or O_2 saturation greater than 90%. O_2 monitoring should be continuous with pulse oximetry. Give prescribed drugs. If the patient can swallow, oral corticosteroids will be part of the treatment plan. Otherwise, IV steroids will be given. SABAs may be part of the treatment plan. Ongoing monitoring is important. Symptoms may gradually diminish after medication therapy but often recur.

Auscultate lung sounds and assess for wheezing. Loud wheezing may occur in airways that are responding to therapy as airflow increases. As improvement continues and airflow increases, breath sounds increase and wheezing decreases. The "silent chest" is an ominous clinical finding. It often signals impending ARF. Immediately notify the HCP.

The resolution of edema, cell infiltration of airway mucosa, elimination of mucous plugs, and disappearance of bronchospasm may take several days to improve after a severe attack. As a result, therapy must be continued even after clinical improvement. Continue to evaluate the patient's response to therapy.

Implement measures during an acute attack to decrease the patient's anxiety and sense of panic. Assess anxiety level. Position the patient comfortably (usually sitting in semi- to high-Fowler's position) to maximize chest expansion. A calm, quiet, reassuring attitude may help the patient relax. A technique called "talking down" can help the patient remain calm. In talking down, you gain eye contact with the patient. In a firm, calm voice, coach the patient to use pursed-lip breathing. Pursed-lip breathing keeps the airways open by maintaining positive pressure (see Table 28.1). Stay with the patient until the respiratory rate has slowed.

When the acute attack subsides, encourage rest. Provide a quiet, calm environment. When the patient is less exhausted, can breathe easier, and is beginning to recover, try to obtain a history and do a physical assessment. If caregivers are present, they may be able to provide information about the health history. This information is important in planning and implementing a patient-centered plan of care.

Chronic Care

A major goal in asthma care is to maximize the patient's ability to safely manage an acute asthma episode using an asthma action plan (Fig. 31.10). Action plans are important for all people with asthma, especially those who have frequent, acute attacks. They are based on the patient's asthma symptoms and PEF. The action plan dictates what symptoms or PEF necessitate a change in asthma drug therapy to gain control.

Patients must measure PEF at least daily. PEF monitoring, when done correctly, is a reliable, objective measure of asthma control (Table 31.13). Some patients may not perceive minimal but important changes in their breathing. They may have a significant decrease in lung function without any symptoms other than a change in PEF.

If PEF is in the green zone (usually 80% to 100% of the patient's personal best), the patient should take their usual medications. A PEF within the yellow zone (usually 50% to 80% of personal best) indicates caution. A PEF in the red zone (50% or less of personal best) indicates a serious problem. In other words, something is triggering asthma symptoms (e.g., viral infection). The patient should seek health care as soon as possible.

The written asthma action plan needs to clearly identify the "step-up" increase in medications during the acute phase of an infection. For example, the patient can use different strategies, such as using the low-dose ICS more often. Although it may happen, it is unusual for a patient's PEF to drop from the green zone to the red zone quickly. Usually, the patient has time to make changes in medications, avoid triggers, and notify the HCP. The dose is "stepped down" once the symptoms subside. Some patients may benefit from keeping a diary to record medication use, wheezing or coughing, PEF, side effects of drugs, and activity level. This information will help the HCP adjust therapy and the action plan as needed.

Involve caregivers in asthma action plans. They should know where to find the patient's medications. Teach them how to decrease the patient's anxiety if an asthma attack occurs. When the patient is stabilized or controlled, the caregiver can gently remind the patient about monitoring daily PEF by asking questions, such as "What zone are you in?" or "How's your peak flow today?" A patient and caregiver teaching guide for patients with asthma is shown in Table 31.14.

Exercise (e.g., swimming, walking, cycling) within the patient's limit of tolerance is beneficial. It may require pretreatment with medication. Good nutrition and uninterrupted sleep are important. If a patient with asthma reports poor sleep because of symptoms, their asthma is not under good control and their plan should be reevaluated. Encourage patients to maintain a fluid intake of 2 to 3 L/day.

Validated questionnaires (e.g., Asthma Control Test [ACT] available at www.asthmacontroltest.com) can be used to assess quality of life. Patients may have frequent absences from school or work. They may have psychologic issues, such as stress, anxiety, and depression. Asthma support groups are available online and around the country. Relaxation therapies (e.g., yoga, meditation, breathing techniques) may help lessen respiratory muscle workload and decrease respiratory rate.

Disparities in socioeconomic status and access to health care may be part of the reason some people have poorly controlled asthma. Explore and try to eliminate any potential barriers to health care. Use culturally appropriate resources and education material in the patient's language to improve knowledge about asthma. A social service referral can help lower-income patients obtain access to care.

Drug Therapy Teaching

Two factors that promote successful asthma management include knowing about asthma drugs and taking them correctly. The drug regimen for asthma can be confusing and

ASTHMA ACTION PLAN

For: Doctor: Date:

Doctor's Phone Number: Hospital/Emergency Department Phone Number:

GREEN ZONE

DOING WELL

- No cough, wheeze, chest tightness, or shortness of breath during the day or night
- Can do usual activities

And, if a peak flow meter is used,

Peak flow: more than
(80 percent or more of my best peak flow)

My best peak flow is:

Daily Medications

Medicine	How much to take	When to take it

Before exercise ☐ ☐2 or ☐4 puffs 5 minutes before exercise

YELLOW ZONE

ASTHMA IS GETTING WORSE

- Cough, wheeze, chest tightness, or shortness of breath, or
- Waking at night due to asthma, or
- Can do some, but not all, usual activities

-Or-

Peak flow: to
(50 to 79 percent of my best peak flow)

1st **Add: quick-relief medicine—and keep taking your GREEN ZONE medicine.**

(quick-relief medicine) Number of puffs or ☐Nebulizer, once Can repeat every minutes up to maximum of doses

2nd **If your symptoms (and peak flow, if used) return to GREEN ZONE after 1 hour of above treatment:**

☐Continue monitoring to be sure you stay in the green zone.

-Or-

If your symptoms (and peak flow, if used) do not return to GREEN ZONE after 1 hour of above treatment:

☐Take: (quick-relief medicine) Number of puffs **or** ☐Nebulizer

☐Add: (oral steroid) mg per day For (3-10) days

☐Call the doctor ☐before/ ☐within hours after taking the oral steroid.

RED ZONE

MEDICAL ALERT!

- Very short of breath, or
- Quick-relief medicines have not helped, or
- Cannot do usual activities, or
- Symptoms are same or get worse after 24 hours in Yellow Zone

-Or-

Peak flow: less than
(50 percent of my best peak flow)

Take this medicine:

☐ (quick-relief medicine) Number of puffs **or** ☐Nebulizer

☐ (oral steroid) mg

Then call your doctor NOW. Go to the hospital or call an ambulance if:

- You are still in the red zone after 15 minutes AND
- You have not reached your doctor.

DANGER SIGNS

- **Trouble walking and talking due to shortness of breath**
- **Lips or fingernails are blue**

- **Take puffs of (quick relief medicine) AND**
- **Go to the hospital or call for an ambulance (phone) NOW!**

Fig. 31.10 Asthma action plan. (From National Heart, Lung, and Blood Institute: *Asthma action plan.* https://www.nhlbi.nih.gov/health-topics/all-publications-and-resources/asthma-action-plan-2020.)

complex. Reinforcement and frequent repetition of key learning points are often needed.

Teach patients about their medications. Include the name, purpose, dose, method of administration, and when to use. Help them understand the differences between "controller," "preferred reliever," and "alternative reliever" drugs. They need to be able to monitor their response to therapy, know when symptoms are not improving, and know when they need help. Review side effects and what to do if they occur. Teach patients about how to prime, use, and clean devices. Review package inserts. At each visit, assess device technique and the asthma action plan.

Several factors can affect the correct use of inhalation devices. These include advanced age, changes in dexterity (e.g., arthritis in hands, coordination), cognition, convenience, administration time and preference, and affordability.

Adherence with drug therapy is a major challenge in chronic asthma management. Lack of adherence often occurs when patients are symptom free and do not use drug therapy regularly because they do not feel an immediate benefit. They do not realize that the medications treat the ongoing inflammation that accompanies asthma. Explain the importance and purpose of taking long-term agents. Stress that maximum improvement may take some time. Stress that without regular use, swelling in the airways may increase and asthma will likely worsen over time.

◆ Evaluation

The expected outcomes are that patients with asthma will:

- Maintain a patent airway and effectively remove secretions
- Have normal respiratory rate, unlabored breathing, and adequate breath sounds
- Correctly use medications
- Manage asthma and acute asthma attacks with a written asthma action plan
- Report decreased anxiety with increased control of breathing

CHRONIC OBSTRUCTIVE PULMONARY DISEASE

Chronic obstructive pulmonary disease (COPD) is a progressive lung disease characterized by persistent airflow

TABLE 31.13 PATIENT & CAREGIVER TEACHING

How to Use Your Peak Flow Meter

Include the following instructions when teaching patients to use a peak flow meter:

Why Use a Peak Flow Meter?

- A peak flow meter is a handheld device that measures how well air moves out of your lungs.
- During an asthma attack, the airways of the lungs usually begin to narrow slowly. The peak flow meter may tell you if there is narrowing in the airways, sometimes even before asthma symptoms occur.
- By taking your medicines early (before symptoms), you may be able to stop an acute episode quickly and avoid a severe asthma attack.
- The peak flow meter is used to help you and your HCP:
  - Learn what makes your asthma worse.
  - Decide if your treatment plan is working well.
  - Decide when to add or stop medicine.
  - Decide when to seek emergency care.

How to Use Your Peak Flow Meter

1. Move the indicator to the bottom of the numbered scale.
2. Stand up.
3. Take a deep breath, filling your lungs completely.
4. Place the mouthpiece in your mouth and close your lips around it. Do not put your tongue inside the hole.
5. Blow out as hard and fast as you can in a single blow.
   - Write down the number you get. But if you cough or make a mistake, do not write down the number. Perform the action again.
   - Repeat steps 1 through 5 two more times. Write down the best (highest number) of the 3 blows in your asthma diary.

What Is Your Personal Best Peak Flow Number?

- Your personal best peak flow number is the highest (peak flow) number you can achieve over a 2- to 3-week period when your asthma is under good control. Good control is when you feel good and have no asthma symptoms.
- Asthma is different for every patient. Your best peak expiratory flow (PEF) may be higher or lower than the peak flow of someone of your height, weight, and gender. This means that it is important for you to test yourself. Everyone has their own personal best peak flow number, which is the basis for your treatment plan.
- To find your personal best peak flow number, take peak flow readings:
  - At least twice a day for 2–3 weeks, between 12 noon and 2 PM when your peak flow is the highest
  - Before (if possible) and about 15–20 minutes after taking your prescribed medication
  - And as instructed by your HCP

The Peak Flow Zone System

Once you know your personal best peak flow number, your HCP will help you place the peak flow numbers into zones. Zones are set up like a traffic light (red, yellow, green). As you trend your peak flow numbers over time, this will help you know what zone you are in and what to do when the number changes. For example:

- *Green Zone* (more than __L/min [80% or higher of your personal best number]). This means good control. No asthma symptoms are present. Take your medicine as usual.
- *Yellow Zone* (between __ and __L/min [50% to <80% of your personal best number]). This means caution. Follow your plan, including taking any reliever medications. Are you still in the yellow zone after treatment? If so, your asthma may not be under good control. Contact your HCP and ask if you need to change or increase your daily medicines.
- *Red Zone* (<__L/min [<50% of your personal best number]). This signals a medical alert. Take your preferred or alternative reliever medication right away. Call your HCP and ask what to do, or go directly to the ED.

Use a Logbook to Keep Track of Your Peak Flow

- Record your personal best peak flow number and peak flow zones in your asthma logbook daily.
- Measure your peak flow when you wake up, *before* taking medicine. Write down your peak flow number in the diary every day, or as instructed by your HCP.

limitation. It is associated with an enhanced chronic inflammatory response in the airways and lungs. In 2021 COPD was the 6th leading cause of death in the United States. It was responsible for 138,825 deaths.[28]

Previous definitions of COPD have included such terms as *chronic bronchitis* and *emphysema*. Each condition has features of COPD, but neither by itself is COPD. **Chronic bronchitis** is the presence of cough and sputum production for at least 3 months in each of 2 consecutive years. It is an independent disease that may precede or follow the development of airflow limitation. **Emphysema**, the destruction of alveoli without fibrosis, describes one of several structural changes in COPD.

Risk Factors

Many factors affect the development and progression of COPD. Next, let us discuss the most common risk factors.

TABLE 31.14 PATIENT & CAREGIVER TEACHING

Asthma

Include the following information in a teaching plan for patients with asthma and the caregiver to help improve the quality of life and promote lifestyle changes that support successful living with asthma:

What Is Asthma?
- Basic anatomy and physiology of lung
- Pathophysiology of asthma
- Relationship of pathophysiology to signs and symptoms
- Measurement and correlation of spirometry and peak expiratory flow (PEF)

What Is Good Asthma Control?
- Personal ideas of good control
- Use the Asthma Control Test available at www.asthmacontroltest.com

Obstacles to Asthma Treatment and Control
- Discuss with patient and caregiver possible obstacles (e.g., denial, poor perception of asthma severity by patient, cost of medications)

Environment and Trigger Control
- Identify triggers and preventive measures (use trigger diary)
- Avoiding allergens and other triggers
- Need to maintain good hydration

Medications
- Classes and how drugs work
- Terms: Controller and preferred and alternative reliever
- Correct use of inhalers, spacer, and nebulizer
- Write out the medication list, and create a drug schedule

Pursed-Lip Breathing (see Table 28.1)

Correct Use of Peak Flow Meter (Table 31.13)

Asthma Action Plan (Fig. 31.10)
- Purpose of action plan and how to use
- Patient-centered plan developed between HCP and patient
- HCP and emergency contact information
- Peak flow zones
- Early recognition of infection
- Building a partnership with the HCP

For more information, visit the American Lung Association website at www.lung.org/lung-disease/asthma.

Cigarette Smoking

The major risk factor for developing COPD is cigarette smoking. Of the 16 million people in the United States who have COPD, around 38% report that they currently smoke.[29] COPD should be considered in any person who is over the age of 40 with a smoking history of 10 or more pack-years. It is the leading cause of death in females who smoke.

Cigarette smoke has several direct effects on the respiratory tract (Table 31.15). The irritating effect of smoke causes hyperplasia of cells, including goblet cells, increasing mucus production. Hyperplasia reduces airway diameter and makes it harder to clear secretions. Smoking reduces ciliary activity and may cause actual loss of cilia. Smoking causes abnormal dilation of the distal air space and destruction of alveolar walls. Many cells develop large, atypical nuclei, which we consider precancerous. Smoking is the source of chronic, enhanced inflammation of various parts of the lung with structural changes and remodeling over time.

TABLE 31.15 Effects of Tobacco Smoke on the Respiratory System

Area of Defect	Acute Effects	Long-Term Effects
Respiratory mucosa		
• Nasopharyngeal	↓ Sense of smell	Cancer
• Tongue	↓ Sense of taste	Cancer
• Vocal cords	Hoarseness	Chronic cough, cancer
• Bronchus and bronchioles	Bronchospasm, cough	Chronic bronchitis, asthma, cancer
Cilia	Paralysis, sputum accumulation, cough	Chronic bronchitis, cancer
Mucous glands	↑ Secretions, ↑ cough	Hyperplasia and hypertrophy of glands, chronic bronchitis
Alveolar macrophages	↓ Function	↑ Infections
Elastin and collagen fibers	↑ Destruction by proteases ↓ Antiproteases (α_1-antitrypsin) function ↓ Synthesis and repair of elastin	Emphysema

Cigarette smoking causes oxidative stress and an imbalance between proteases that break down connective tissue in the lung and antiproteases that protect the lungs. These changes increase with more severe disease and persist even after a patient has stopped smoking. In adults, environmental tobacco smoke (ETS) can cause decreased lung function, increased respiratory symptoms, and severe lower respiratory tract infections (e.g., pneumonia). ETS increases the risk for nasal sinus and lung cancer.

Infection

Severe recurring respiratory tract infections in childhood are associated with reduced lung function and increased respiratory symptoms in adulthood. We are not sure if COPD is related to recurrent respiratory or other infections in adults. People with HIV infection who smoke develop COPD faster.[30] Tuberculosis is also a risk factor.

Asthma

Patients with COPD may have asthma, and asthma may be a risk factor for COPD. There is a considerable pathologic and functional overlap between asthma and COPD, especially among older adults, who may have components of both. We call this *asthma-COPD overlap syndrome.*

Air Pollution

High levels of urban air pollution are harmful to people with existing lung disease. Exposure to coal and other biomass fuels people use for indoor heating and cooking is another risk factor. Many people who have never smoked are at increased risk because of cooking with these fuels in poorly ventilated areas.

Occupation Chemicals and Dusts

If a person has intense or prolonged exposure to various dusts, vapors, irritants, or fumes in the workplace, symptoms of lung impairment consistent with COPD can develop. If a person has occupation exposure and smokes, the risk for COPD increases significantly.

Aging

Many believe aging is a risk factor for COPD, but the research is not conclusive. Does the aging process lead to COPD? Or is COPD a result of cumulative exposures that occur over a lifetime? Some normal changes associated with aging (see Table 27.1) are like those seen in patients with COPD.

BOX 31.2 GENETICS IN CLINICAL PRACTICE

α_1-Antitrypsin Deficiency (AATD)

Genetic Basis

- Autosomal recessive disorder
- Gene provides instructions for the liver to make the protein *α_1-antitrypsin* (AAT), which protects the lungs and liver from proteolytic enzymes
- Over 100 reported mutations of *SERPINA1,* the gene that causes AATD, but not all mutations cause the disease
- Without enough functional AAT, proteolytic enzymes destroy alveoli and cause lung disease

Incidence

- Occurs in 1 in 3000 to 5000 live births in the United States
- Persons of Northern or Central European descent most affected

Clinical Implications

- Disease onset and first diagnosis usually occur between ages 30 and 45 years of age
- Disease predisposes to early-onset emphysema
- Can cause lung and liver disease
- Smoking and alcohol use appear to accelerate severity of disease
- Augmentation therapy includes once-per-week infusion of purified AAT replacement therapy to help prevent worsening of the condition

Genetic Testing

- All patients with COPD, asthma, and unexplained liver disease should be considered for DNA testing
- Serum assay is available to measure the AAT level in blood

Genetics

An intriguing question is why some smokers develop COPD and others do not. This suggests genetic factors may play a role in who develops it. Genetics may also play a role in why people who never smoked but were exposed to ETS over long periods develop COPD. We have identified 1 genetic factor: the "Z" allele of the AAT protein.[31]

Alpha-1 Antitrypsin Deficiency

Alpha-1 (α1) antitrypsin deficiency (AATD) is an autosomal recessive disorder that may affect the lungs and liver (Box 31.2). AAT is a protein made by the liver and normally found in the lungs. The main function is to protect lung tissue from attack by proteases during inflammation caused by smoking and infections. Unfortunately, few people are tested for AATD until symptoms are present and they are seeking medical care. About 2% of all people diagnosed with COPD in the United States have AATD. Smoking speeds the disease process in these patients. Genetic counseling may be appropriate for patients with AATD who plan to have children.

Pathophysiology

COPD is characterized by chronic inflammation of the airways, lung parenchyma (respiratory bronchioles and alveoli), and pulmonary blood vessels (Fig. 31.11). The defining feature of COPD is airflow limitation that is not fully reversible during forced exhalation. The main cause is the loss of elastic recoil and airflow obstruction from mucus hypersecretion, mucosal edema, and bronchospasm. COPD has an uneven distribution of pathologic changes. Severely impaired and/or destroyed areas of lung tissue exist alongside areas of relatively normal lung.

The inflammatory process most often starts with inhaling oxidants in noxious particles and gases (e.g., cigarette smoke). Oxidants adversely affect the lungs as they inactivate antiproteases (which prevent destruction of the lungs), stimulate mucus secretion, and increase fluid in the lungs. The activity of proteases (which break down connective tissue of the lungs) increases, and antiproteases are inhibited. So, the natural balance of protease/antiprotease is tipped in favor of alveolar destruction and loss of the lungs' elastic recoil.

The predominant inflammatory cells in COPD are neutrophils, macrophages, and lymphocytes. Inflammatory cells attract other inflammatory mediators (e.g., leukotrienes) and proinflammatory cytokines (e.g., tumor necrosis factor). Repeated exposure and chronic inflammation cause tissue destruction and disrupt the normal defense mechanisms and repair process of the lung. Permanent structural changes occur. Chronic inflammation can contribute to other health problems, including osteoporosis and diabetes.

Inability to expire air is a main characteristic of COPD. The main site of the airflow limitation is in the smaller airways. As

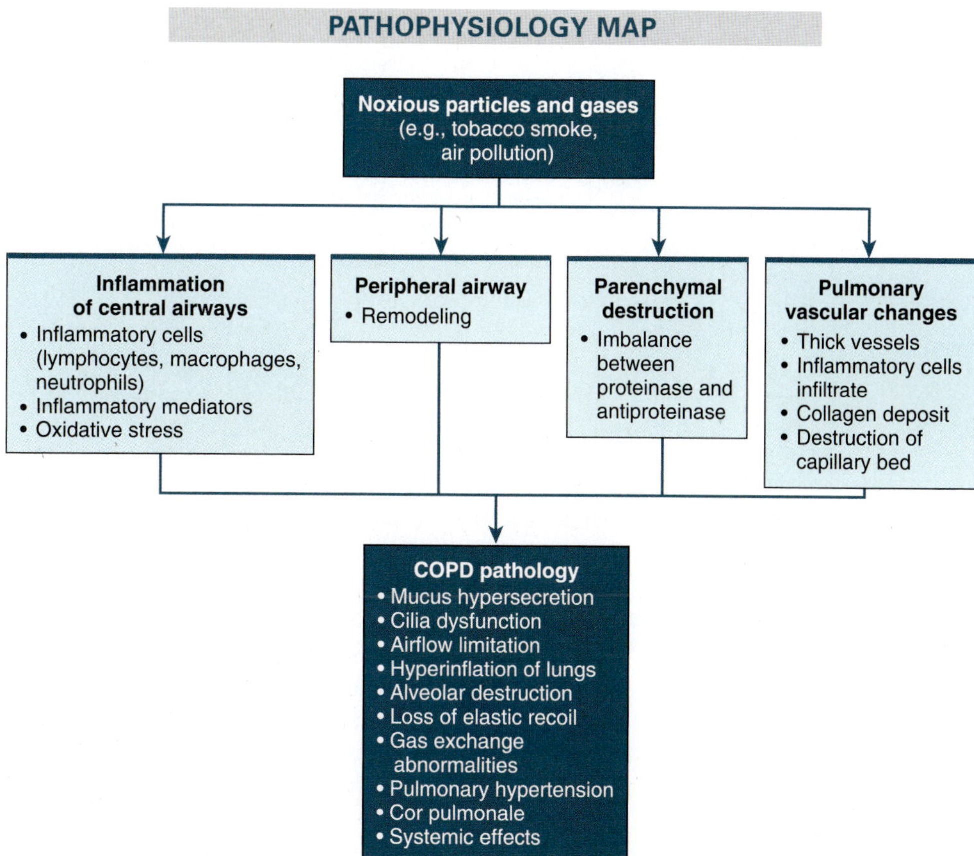

Fig. 31.11 Pathophysiology of COPD.

the smaller airways become obstructed, air is progressively trapped during expiration. The volume of residual air in the lungs at end expiration becomes greatly increased in severe COPD. As the air remains trapped, the chest hyperexpands and becomes barrel shaped because the respiratory muscles lose their elasticity. Functional residual capacity (FRC) increases. The residual air, combined with the loss of elastic recoil, makes passive expiration of air difficult. The patient must now inhale when the lungs are in an "overinflated" state. As a result, the patient becomes dyspneic with limited exercise capacity.

Typically, patients do not have problems with hypoxemia at rest until late in the disease. At first, hypoxemia may develop during exercise and patients may benefit from supplemental O_2. Gas exchange problems result in hypoxemia and hypercapnia (increased CO_2) as the disease worsens. As the air trapping increases, walls of alveoli are destroyed (Fig. 31.12). Bullae (large air spaces in the parenchyma) and blebs (air spaces next to pleurae) can form in and on the lungs. Bullae and blebs are not effective in gas exchange because they do not contain a capillary that normally surrounds each alveolus. Therefore a significant V/Q mismatch and hypoxemia result. Peripheral airway obstruction also results in V/Q imbalance and, combined with respiratory muscle impairment, leads to CO_2 retention, particularly in severe forms of the disease.

Excess mucus production, resulting in a chronic productive cough, is a feature of persons with predominant chronic bronchitis. However, not all patients with COPD have sputum production. When present, excess mucus production results from an increased number of mucus-secreting goblet cells, enlarged submucosal glands, cilia dysfunction, and stimulation from inflammatory mediators.

Classification of COPD

We classify COPD as mild, moderate, severe, and very severe (Table 31.16). An FEV_1/FVC ratio of less than 70% establishes the diagnosis. The severity of obstruction (as shown by FEV_1) determines the stage of COPD. Management is based on the patient's symptoms, classification, and exacerbation history.

Clinical Manifestations

The manifestations of COPD typically develop slowly. A clinical diagnosis should be considered in any patient who has chronic cough or sputum production, dyspnea, and a history of exposure to risk factors for the disease (e.g., tobacco smoke, dusts). It is sometimes hard to tell COPD from asthma, especially if the person has a history of smoking.

A chronic intermittent cough is often the first symptom. Patients may dismiss the cough, as they associate it with smoking or environment exposure. The cough may be productive. Significant airflow limitation can exist without cough or sputum. Typically, dyspnea is progressive, usually occurs with exertion, and is present every day.

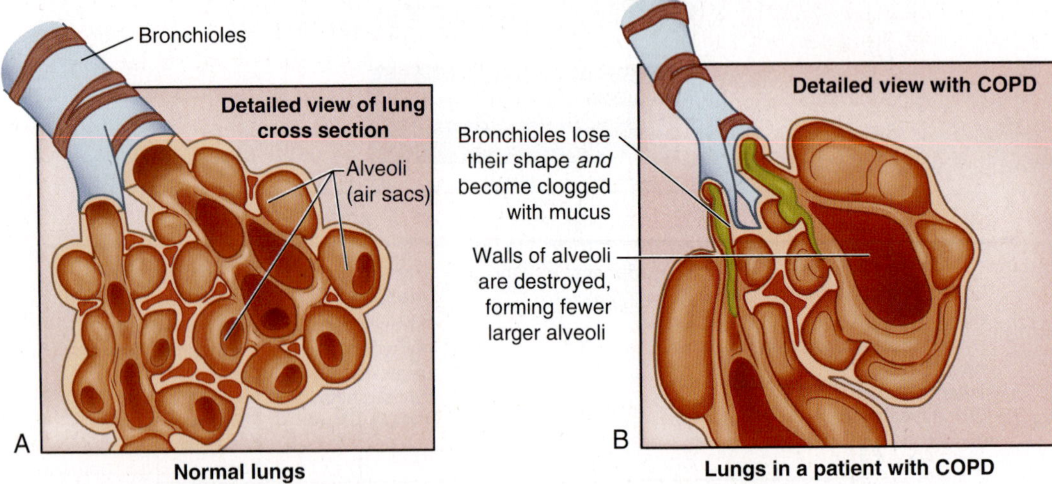

Fig. 31.12 (A) Normal lungs showing bronchioles and alveoli. (B) Changes in the bronchioles and alveoli in the lungs of a patient with COPD.

TABLE 31.16 Diagnostic Criteria

Severity of Airflow Obstruction in COPD

In patients who have been diagnosed with COPD and have a postbronchodilator $FEV_1/FVC < 0.7$:

Classification	Level of Severity	FEV_1 Results
GOLD 1	Mild	$FEV_1 \geq 80\%$ predicted
GOLD 2	Moderate	FEV_1 50%–80% predicted
GOLD 3	Severe	FEV_1 30%–50% predicted
GOLD 4	Very severe	$FEV_1 < 30\%$ predicted

From the Global Strategy for Diagnosis, Management and Prevention of COPD 2024. © Adapted from Global Initiative for Chronic Obstructive Lung Disease: 2024 Report. Retrieved from https://goldcopd.org/2024-gold-report/.

Patients may report chest heaviness, not being able to take a deep breath, gasping, increased effort to breathe, and air hunger. They tend to ignore symptoms and rationalize that "I'm getting older" or "I'm out of shape." Some change behaviors to avoid dyspnea, such as taking the elevator instead of the stairs. Patients will seek medical care when dyspnea becomes severe or impairs their ability to complete ADLs.

In the late stages of COPD, dyspnea is almost always present, even at rest. Patients must work harder to breathe. As more alveoli become overdistended, increasing amounts of air are trapped. This causes the diaphragm to flatten. Effective abdominal breathing is decreased because of the flattened diaphragm. As a result, the patient becomes more of a chest breather, relying on the intercostal and accessory muscles. Chest breathing is not particularly efficient, especially over long periods. Patients may sit upright with their arms supported on a fixed surface, such as an overbed table *(tripod position)*.

Wheezing and chest tightness may be present. These symptoms can vary by time of the day or from day to day, especially in those with severe disease. Chest tightness, which often follows activity, may feel like muscle contractions. We may hear decreased breath sounds and/or wheezes in all lung fields. Because the anteroposterior diameter of the chest increases ("barrel chest") from the chronic air trapping, patients may need to breathe louder than normal for us to hear breath sounds with a stethoscope. The expiratory phase is prolonged. They may naturally purse lips on expiration (pursed-lip breathing).

Persons with advanced COPD often have fatigue, weight loss, and anorexia. Even with adequate caloric intake, they may still lose weight. Fatigue is a highly prevalent symptom that affects ADLs.

Over time, hypoxemia (Pao_2 less than 80 mm Hg or O_2 saturation less than 88% on room air) may develop with hypercapnia ($Paco_2$ over 45 mm Hg). Bluish-red skin color results from polycythemia and cyanosis. Polycythemia develops from increased red blood cell (RBC) production as the body tries to compensate for chronic hypoxemia. Hemoglobin concentrations may reach 20 g/dL (200 g/L) or more. Some persons, though, have low hemoglobin and hematocrit because of chronic anemia.

Complications

Primary complications of COPD include acute exacerbations, pulmonary hypertension, cor pulmonale, and ARF.

Acute Exacerbations

An exacerbation of COPD is an acute event characterized by a worsening of respiratory symptoms. Exacerbations are signaled by a sudden change in the patient's usual dyspnea, cough, and/or sputum (e.g., something different from the usual daily pattern). Respiratory infections are a common cause. Exacerbations are common and increase in frequency (on average 1 or 2 per year) as the disease progresses. As the severity of COPD increases, repeated exacerbations are associated with poorer outcomes.

Pulmonary Hypertension and Cor Pulmonale

In COPD, the main cause of pulmonary hypertension is constriction of the pulmonary vessels because of alveolar hypoxia. As the disease advances, the structure of the pulmonary arteries changes, resulting in thickening of the vascular smooth muscle. Because of the loss of alveolar walls and the capillaries surrounding them, pressure in the pulmonary circulation increases. Chronic hypoxia stimulates RBC production, which causes polycythemia. This results in increased blood viscosity. These patients have increased pulmonary vascular resistance and, as a result, develop pulmonary hypertension.

The pressure within the lungs increases. Thus the right side of the heart must work harder to push blood into the lungs, causing right ventricular hypertrophy. The right ventricle dilates, and right HF develops. Cor pulmonale is a late manifestation of COPD (Fig. 31.13). Once a patient develops cor pulmonale, the prognosis worsens. However, not all patients with COPD develop cor pulmonale.

Dyspnea is the most common symptom of cor pulmonale. Lung sounds are normal, or crackles may be present in the bases. Heart sounds may include S_3, S_4, and systolic murmurs. Manifestations of right HF may develop. These include distended neck veins, hepatomegaly with right upper quadrant tenderness, peripheral edema, and weight gain. Typically, chest x-rays show large pulmonary vessels.

The treatment of cor pulmonale includes continuous, long-term, low-flow O_2 therapy. Diuretics may be given if left HF or pulmonary edema is present but must be used with caution. In some cases, decreases in fluid volume from diuresis can worsen heart function. Long-term anticoagulation therapy is started to help decrease the risk for venous thromboembolism (VTE). HF is the focus of Chapter 38.

Acute Respiratory Failure

Patients with severe COPD who have serious exacerbations are at risk for ARF. All too often, patients wait too long to contact their HCP when they first develop symptoms suggestive of exacerbation. By the time they seek out medical attention, their condition has worsened to the point that they need ICU admission and mechanical ventilation. ARF is discussed in Chapter 32.

Diagnostic Studies

History and physical assessment are important in the diagnostic workup. Validated questionnaires such as the COPD Assessment Test (www.catestonline.org) help assess symptoms.

Spirometry confirms the diagnosis in those suspected of having COPD. It also confirms the presence of airflow obstruction and determines the severity. A diagnosis of COPD is made

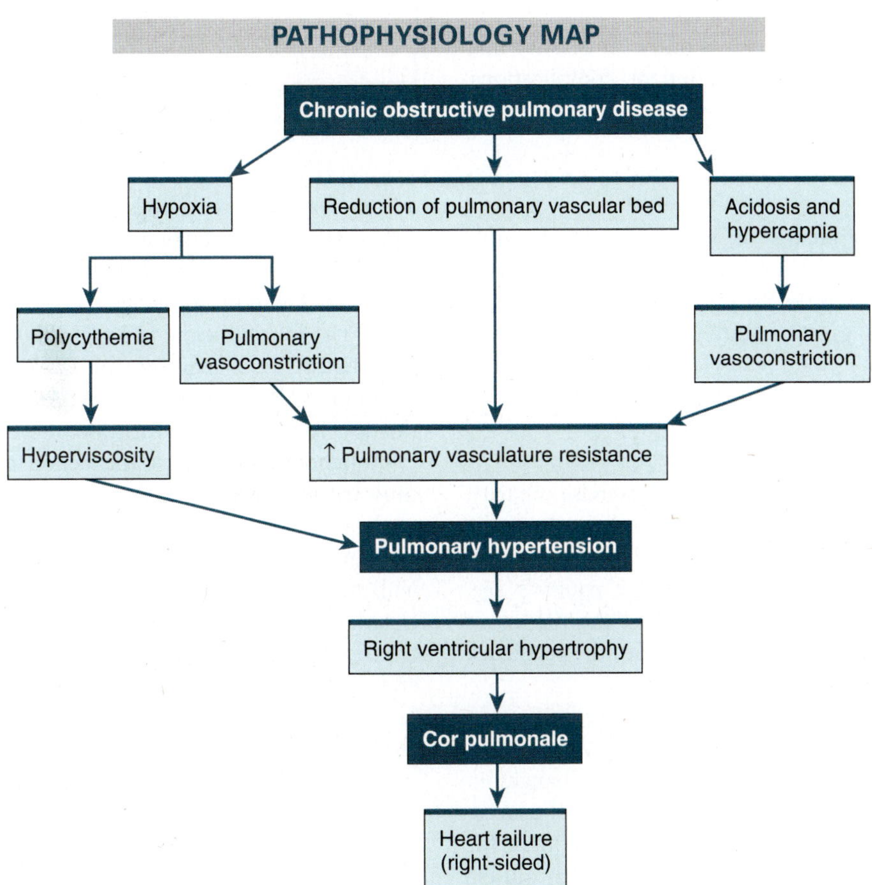

Fig. 31.13 Mechanisms involved in the pathophysiology of pulmonary hypertension and cor pulmonale from COPD.

when the postbronchodilator FEV_1/FVC ratio is less than 70%.[32] The FEV_1 value is a guideline for the degree of severity of COPD. The lower the FEV_1, the more the airways are obstructed.

Other diagnostic studies that may be done are outlined in Table 31.17. Chest x-rays often show a flat diaphragm because of hyperinflated lungs. Patients often have exercise-induced hypoxemia. A physical or respiratory therapist may do a 6-minute walk test to assess the severity of COPD (see Table 27.16). Walking less than 350 meters and an O_2 saturation of 88% or lower is associated with increased mortality.[33]

We usually monitor ABGs in patients hospitalized with acute COPD exacerbations. ABGs do not diagnose the condition but help identify the severity of the exacerbation by assessing oxygenation. In early stages, there may be a normal or only slightly decreased Pao_2 and usually a normal or slightly increased $Paco_2$ level. In the later stages of COPD, typical findings are a low-normal pH, high-normal or above-normal $Paco_2$, and high-normal bicarbonate (HCO_3^-). This may indicate either partially or fully compensated respiratory acidosis. In a fully compensated state, the kidneys conserve HCO_3^- to increase the pH to within normal range.

An ECG may be normal or show signs of right HF. An echocardiogram or multigated acquisition (MUGA) scan can evaluate heart function. Sputum for culture and sensitivity may be done if an infection such as pneumonia is suspected.

TABLE 31.17 Interprofessional Care

COPD

Diagnostic Assessment

- History and physical assessment, including COPD Assessment Test
- Chest x-ray
- Spirometry
- Arterial blood gases (ABGs)
- 6-Minute walk test
- Serum α_1-antitrypsin levels

Management

- Smoking cessation
- Drug therapies (Tables 31.9 and 31.19)
- Airway clearance techniques (ACTs)
- Breathing exercises and retraining
- Hydration of 2–3 L/day (if not contraindicated)
- Immunizations: Influenza, pneumococcal, COVID-19
- Long-term O_2 (if indicated)
- Progressive exercise plan, especially walking and upper body strengthening
- Pulmonary rehabilitation program
- Nutrition assessment, supplementation
- Treat complications
  - Pulmonary hypertension
  - Cor pulmonale
  - Acute exacerbations
  - Acute respiratory failure
- Surgery (if suitable candidate, based on age, medical history, severity and stage of COPD)
  - Lung volume reduction surgery
  - Bullectomy
  - Lung transplant

Interprofessional Care

Many patients with COPD are treated as outpatients. They may be hospitalized for an acute exacerbation or complications, such as pneumonia, HF, or ARF.

Oxygen Therapy

O_2 therapy is often part of the treatment of COPD. It is the only treatment linked to improved survival. For most patients, the goal of O_2 therapy is to keep the Sao_2 greater than 88% to 92% during rest, sleep, and exertion and the Pao_2 greater than 60 mm Hg.[34]

Drug Therapy

Drug therapy can reduce symptoms, increase exercise capacity, and improve overall health. This will hopefully reduce the number and severity of exacerbations. Choice of drug therapy is based on several factors. These include the patient's age, symptoms and how quickly they occur, FEV_1, the risk of or number of exacerbations, and coexisting health problems. Table 31.18 shows suggestions for drug therapy.

Like asthma, medications are given in a stepwise fashion. In COPD, they are usually "stepped up." Because continual symptoms are present, "stepping down" is rare. Changes in therapy are usually based on symptoms and repeated exacerbations. Bronchodilator therapy is the first-line treatment for most patients. Bronchodilators relax bronchial smooth muscle in the airway and improve ventilation, thus reducing dyspnea and increasing FEV_1. Drugs commonly used are β_2-adrenergic agonists, anticholinergics, and, to a rare extent, methylxanthines. The choice of bronchodilator depends on the patient's response. These drugs are given on a scheduled or as-needed basis. The inhaled route is preferred.

A SABA is a mainstay of COPD treatment. The most common SABA is albuterol. LABAs are often used as monotherapy. Salmeterol and formoterol are widely used LABAs.

Anticholinergics block the action of acetylcholine on the muscarinic receptors in the smooth muscle of the bronchotracheal tree. The most common short-acting muscarinic agent (SAMA) is ipratropium bromide. For patients who need a drug with a more prolonged effect, long-acting muscarinic agents (LAMAs) such as tiotropium are an option.

Combining short-acting bronchodilators with anticholinergic agents into 1 combination drug may help improve bronchodilation and decrease side effects. For example, albuterol and ipratropium can be nebulized together or delivered by inhalation spray (Combivent Respimat).

Depending on the severity of symptoms and stage of COPD, regular treatment with an ICS may be prescribed. An ICS is not used as monotherapy because of the side effects. An ICS is often combined with a LABA for enhanced effect. Examples of

TABLE 31.18 Drug Therapy

Options for COPD Treatment

Medication	Possible Options
Bronchodilators	SABA
	LABA
	LAMA
	LABA + LAMA
Corticosteroids	ICS + LABA
	ICS + LABA + LAMA
Antibiotics	Macrolides (some evidence to suggest macrolides may reduce incidence of exacerbation in COPD)
Antiinflammatory	Roflumilast
Antimucolytics	N-Acetylcysteine
Vaccinations	COVID-19
	Influenza
	Pneumococcal
	Respiratory syncytial virus (RSV)

ICS, Inhaled corticosteroid; *LABA,* long-acting β_2-agonist; *LAMA,* long-acting muscarinic agent; *SABA,* short-acting β_2-agonist.

combination ICSs with LABAs are fluticasone/salmeterol (Advair) and budesonide/formoterol (Symbicort). Inhaled LAMAs, LABAs, and ICSs all help reduce COPD exacerbations. Some patients with COPD are on "triple therapy," which includes a LABA, LAMA, and ICS. Fluticasone/umeclidinium/vilanterol is one example of a "triple therapy" agent.

We rarely use methylxanthines such as theophylline. They have serious side effects. Theophylline interacts with many drugs and has a very narrow therapeutic window. A low dose of theophylline with an ICS may help a few patients who do not respond to other inhaled medications.

Roflumilast (Daliresp) is an oral agent used to decrease exacerbations in patients with severe COPD and chronic bronchitis. It is an antiinflammatory drug used for long-term therapy. It does not treat acute problems.

Oral corticosteroids are effective for short-term use to treat acute exacerbations. They should not be used for long-term therapy in COPD. Mucolytic agents, such as NAC, may be used for patients with COPD who have an acute exacerbation. They have antiinflammatory and mucolytic properties. NAC may help improve overall health and quality of life in some patients.

Respiratory Care

Teaching patients with COPD breathing retraining exercises is important. The 2 main types of breathing retraining exercises are (1) pursed-lip breathing (see Table 28.1) and (2) diaphragmatic breathing. Diaphragmatic breathing in some patients with COPD may increase the WOB and dyspnea.

Many patients have ineffective coughing patterns that do not clear their airways of sputum. Teach patients ways to cough effectively to bring the secretions to the central airways to expectorate them (see Table 28.2). ACTs are helpful in patients with a COPD exacerbation. They are often used in conjunction with other treatments. Typically, patients receive bronchodilator therapy through an inhaler device (e.g., nebulizer) before ACT. Then, the ACT is used, followed by effective coughing (e.g., huff coughing). Airway clearance devices can also help mobilize secretions (see Chapter 28).

Nutrition Therapy

Many patients with advanced COPD are underweight with loss of muscle mass and cachexia. Weight loss, malnutrition, and muscle dysfunction can affect quality of life and contribute to increased mortality. Factors that contribute to malnutrition include increased inflammatory mediators, increased metabolic rate from ventilatory effort, and lack of appetite. Other factors include taste changes caused by chronic mouth breathing, excess sputum, fatigue, anxiety, depression, and drug side effects.

There is no specific diet for patients with COPD. A well-balanced diet that includes fresh fruits, whole grains, and vegetables is best.[35] A diet high in protein, moderate in carbohydrates, and moderate to high in fat is recommended for most patients. Meals can be divided into 5 or 6 small portions a day. Offer high-protein and moderate-calorie nutrition supplements between meals. The dietitian is an excellent resource for what combinations of nutrients and supplements are best.

Underweight patients need extra protein and calories. They may need 25 to 45 kcal/kg body weight and more than 1.5 g of protein/kg body weight to maintain their weight. Patients with malnutrition may need up to 2.5 g of protein/kg of body weight to maintain muscle mass.

To decrease dyspnea and conserve energy, patients should rest for at least 30 minutes before eating and use a bronchodilator before meals. Teach patients to avoid exercise and treatments for at least 1 hour before and after eating. If a patient desaturates while eating, O_2 therapy by nasal cannula may help. Encourage activity, such as walking, to stimulate appetite.

Getting patients to eat adequate amounts of nutritionally sound foods may be difficult. Teach patients or those responsible for meal preparation ways to make mealtime easier and more nutritious by increasing calories and protein without increasing the amount of food eaten (Table 31.19).

TABLE 31.19 NUTRITION THERAPY

Maximizing Food Intake in COPD

- Rest before meals.
- Make meals that are easy to prepare.
- Eat while sitting up.
- Eat high-calorie foods first.
- Drink liquids at the end of your meal.
- Try more frequent meals and snacks during the day.
- Cold foods can make you feel less full than hot foods.
- If you use O_2, wear oxygen during mealtimes (e.g., nasal cannula).
- Keep ready-prepared meals available for times when you have increased shortness of breath.

Surgical Therapy

Various surgical procedures can help manage severe COPD. However, it is important to remember that many patients with severe COPD are not candidates for surgery.

One type of surgery is *lung volume reduction surgery* (LVRS). The goal of LVRS is to reduce the size of the lungs by removing some of the diseased lung tissue so that the remaining healthy lung tissue can perform better. Reducing the diseased lung tissue by about 20% to 35% results in decreased airway obstruction and increased room for the remaining normal alveoli to expand and function.[36] Besides improving lung and chest wall mechanics, LVRS allows the diaphragm to return to its normal shape. This allows the patient to breathe more efficiently.

Another surgical procedure is *bronchoscopic lung volume reduction (BLVR)*. It involves placing multiple 1-way valves by bronchoscopy in the airways leading to the diseased parts of the lung. The valves allow air to leave the lung during exhalation and prevent air from entering during inspiration. By completely occluding a specific area of the lung, this collapses that area. BLVR produces a result similar to LVRS. Pneumothorax is a common complication.

In a *bullectomy*, 1 or more very large bullae are removed. Their removal helps decrease WOB. A lung transplant helps a very small number of patients with advanced COPD. Although single-lung transplants are most common because of a shortage of donors, a bilateral transplant can be done. Lung transplants are discussed in Chapter 30.

NURSING MANAGEMENT: COPD

Assessment

Subjective and objective data that you should obtain from patients with COPD are outlined in Table 31.20.

Clinical Problems

Clinical problems for patients with COPD may include:

- Impaired respiratory function
- Activity intolerance
- Nutritionally compromised
- Ineffective coping

Additional information on clinical problems and interventions is presented in eNursing Care Plan 31.2 available on the website for this chapter.

Planning

The overall goals are that patients with COPD will have (1) relief from symptoms, (2) ability to perform ADLs and improved exercise tolerance, (3) no complications related to COPD, (4) knowledge to implement a long-term treatment plan, (5) no disease progression, and (6) improved quality of life.

TABLE 31.20 NURSING ASSESSMENT

COPD

Subjective Data

Important Health Information

Health history: Long-term exposure to chemical pollutants, respiratory irritants, occupational fumes, dust; recurrent respiratory tract infections; previous hospitalizations

Medications: Use of O_2 (include frequency and duration of O_2 use), bronchodilators, corticosteroids, antibiotics, anticholinergics, OTC drugs, illicit substances

Functional Health Patterns

Health perception—health management: Smoking (pack-years, including passive smoking, willingness to stop smoking, and previous attempts); what is/was smoked (e.g., cigarettes, pipes, cigars, e-cigarettes); family history of respiratory disease AATD)

Nutritional-metabolic: Anorexia, weight loss or gain

Activity-exercise: Increasing dyspnea and/or presence of sputum; fatigue, ability to perform ADLs; swelling of hands or feet; progressive dyspnea, especially on exertion; ability to walk up 1 flight of stairs without stopping; wheezing; recurrent cough; sputum volume, purulence (especially in the morning); orthopnea

Elimination: Constipation, gas, bloating; urine leakage, incontinence

Sleep-rest: Insomnia; sitting up position for sleeping, paroxysmal nocturnal dyspnea

Cognitive-perceptual: Headache, chest or abdominal soreness

Coping—stress tolerance: Anxiety, depression

Objective Data

Cardiovascular

↑ Heart rate, dysrhythmias, jugular venous distention, distant heart tones, right heart failure, S_3 (cor pulmonale), pedal edema

General

Debilitation, restlessness, upright position

GI

Ascites, hepatomegaly (cor pulmonale)

Musculoskeletal

Muscle atrophy, ↑ anteroposterior diameter (barrel chest)

Respiratory

Rapid, shallow breathing

Prolonged expiratory phase; pursed-lip breathing

Use of accessory muscles

↓ Chest excursion and diaphragm movement

Wheezing, crackles, decreased or bronchial breath sounds, inability to speak

Skin

Cyanosis (bronchitis), pallor or ruddy color, digital clubbing, poor skin turgor, thin skin, easy bruising; peripheral edema (cor pulmonale)

Possible Diagnostic Findings

Abnormal ABGs (compensated respiratory acidosis, ↓ Pa_{O_2} or Sa_{O_2}, ↑ Pa_{CO_2}), pulmonary function tests showing expiratory airflow obstruction (e.g., low FEV_1, low FEV_1/FVC. Chest x-ray: flattened diaphragm and hyperinflation with/without infiltrates. Echocardiogram: large right ventricle, polycythemia

AATD, α_1-Antitrypsin deficiency; *ABG,* arterial blood gas; *ADL,* activity of daily living; *OTC,* over the counter.

◆ Implementation

Health Promotion

The incidence of COPD would decrease dramatically if people did not smoke, did not begin to smoke, or would stop smoking. Smoking cessation is vital but challenging. Many patients with COPD will have smoked for most of their lives. It is the only way to slow disease progression. After a person stops smoking, the decline in lung function that occurred with smoking slows. The sooner the smoker stops, the less chance lung function is lost and the sooner the symptoms decrease, especially cough and sputum production. Smoking cessation is discussed in Chapter 11.

Avoiding or controlling exposure to occupation and environment pollutants and irritants is another preventive measure to maintain healthy lungs. Assess exposure to irritants. Determine ways to control or avoid them. For example, teach patients to avoid smoke-filled rooms and air pollutants.

Acute Care

Patients with COPD may need hospitalization for other complications, such as cor pulmonale, ARF, or acute exacerbation. Exacerbations may be treated at home or in the hospital, depending on severity. The severity is determined by the history leading up to the exacerbation, symptoms, hemodynamic stability, O_2 requirements, WOB, ABGs, and the presence of coexisting diseases. The presence of other problems often complicates exacerbations.

The nursing management of patients with an acute COPD exacerbation is outlined in Table 31.21. Assess patients for manifestations of exacerbation, including increased dyspnea, increased sputum volume, or increased sputum purulence. They may have malaise, insomnia, fatigue, depression, confusion, decreased exercise tolerance, increased wheezing, or fever. Are these new symptoms or worsening of usual symptoms?

Be alert for signs of severity, such as using accessory muscles, central cyanosis, edema in the lower extremities, unstable BP, right HF, and altered alertness. Assess ABGs for respiratory acidosis and worsening hypoxemia, indicating an "acute-on-chronic" respiratory failure. Ask about the number of exacerbations per year and if treatment occurred in the home or hospital.

SABAs and oral corticosteroids are the usual treatments for exacerbations. SABAs with SAMAs are another option. Drug administration by MDI or nebulizer works equally well. Sicker patients may need a nebulizer. Antibiotics are given if the exacerbation is caused by a bacterial infection (e.g., pneumonia). Patients with HF may receive small doses of diuretics.

In the hospital, most patients receive O_2 therapy. We try to use noninvasive mechanical methods (e.g., bilevel positive airway pressure [BiPAP]) to support ventilation rather than invasive ventilatory support. If needed, the patient will be intubated and mechanically ventilated.

Once the immediate crisis has resolved, reassess the degree and severity of any underlying problems. The information obtained will help in planning care going forward and assist with changes in the treatment plan that may be needed after discharge.

TABLE 31.21 NURSING MANAGEMENT

Acute COPD Exacerbation

- Regularly monitor indicators of respiratory function:
  - Vital signs with SpO_2
  - Auscultate lung sounds; note respiratory rhythm and WOB
  - ABGs (as needed)
  - Manifestations of hypoxia
- Give ordered drug therapy, including bronchodilators, steroids, diuretics, antibiotics
- Place the patient in high-Fowler's to optimize respiratory function
- Give ordered IV fluids
- Encourage oral fluids as tolerated
- Promote adequate rest periods, such as 90 minutes of undisturbed sleep, and limit visitors (as needed)
- Ensure adequate nutrition with small frequent meals and between-meal supplements
- Provide measures to promote comfort and reduce anxiety
- Evaluate the patient's response to treatment
- Know the patient's resuscitation status, and be prepared to initiate immediate resuscitation protocols and respiratory support if condition worsens
- Notify the HCP of significant changes in condition
- Provide patient and caregiver teaching about COPD (Table 31.22)

Supervise AP

- Obtain daily weights, vital signs, and intake and output
- Provide frequent oral hygiene and encourage oral fluids
- Assist with hygiene, ADLs, and pulmonary rehabilitation exercises as needed

Collaborate With Interprofessional Team Members

Respiratory Therapist

- Administer O_2 therapy
- Provide chest physiotherapy
- Monitor respiratory status

Dietitian

- Assess nutrition status
- Recommend interventions to meet patient's nutrition needs
- Provide instructions for diet changes as needed

Physical Therapist

- Assess current level of fitness
- Assist with ambulation and pulmonary rehabilitation exercises

Social Worker

- Assist with obtaining medical equipment after discharge
- Assist with financial resources

ABG, Arterial blood gas; *ADL*, activity of daily living; *WOB*, work of breathing.

Chronic Care

The health care team works together to formulate a patient-centered treatment plan. The most important aspect in the long-term care of patients with COPD is teaching. A large part of your role is to help patients self-manage their disease. A patient and caregiver teaching guide is shown in Table 31.22.

Stress the importance of regular follow-up appointments. Regular follow-ups help us monitor response to treatment and see if any changes must be made. Each visit is an opportunity for you to discuss nonpharmacologic approaches to manage COPD to further enhance the treatment plan. Early treatment of respiratory tract infections and COPD exacerbations helps prevent progression and complications. Teach the patient and caregiver early recognition of the 3 main manifestations of exacerbations: increased dyspnea, increased sputum volume, and increased sputum purulence. Early identification of respiratory problems may prevent hospitalization and ARF.

People with COPD should avoid others who are sick, practice good hand-washing techniques, take drugs as prescribed, exercise regularly, and maintain a healthy weight. Patients are very susceptible to lung infections. They should receive influenza, pneumococcal, and COVID-19 vaccinations.

Patients often ask whether moving to a warmer or drier climate will help. In general, such moves are generally not beneficial. Discourage moves to places with an elevation of 4000 ft or more because of the lower partial pressure of O_2 found in the air at higher elevations. Other disadvantages of moving may be that a person leaves a job, friends, and familiar environment, which could be stressful. This may outweigh any advantage gained from being in a different climate.

Pulmonary rehabilitation. Pulmonary rehabilitation usually includes smoking cessation, nutrition counseling, exercise training, and teaching. Physical therapists or nurses with experience in respiratory care are often responsible for managing the program. Pulmonary rehabilitation works best if patients start when COPD is in a moderate stage, but even patients who have advanced COPD can benefit. Outcomes include relief of dyspnea and fatigue, improved emotional function, and enhanced sense of control that people have over their COPD.

Activity. Patients with severe COPD typically use upper thoracic and neck muscles to breathe rather than the diaphragm. Thus they may have difficulty with upper extremity activities, especially those that require raising the arm above the head. Exercise training may improve muscle function and help reduce dyspnea. It also leads to energy conservation, which is an important part of COPD rehabilitation.

Review alternative energy-saving practices for ADLs. Explore how alternative methods of hair care, shaving, showering, and reaching are working. In severe COPD, patients should try to sit as much as possible when performing activities. If the patient uses home O_2 therapy, O_2 should be used during hygiene because these tasks are energy consuming. The occupational therapist is an excellent resource for activity suggestions.

Regular exercise is important (Box 31.3). Encourage patients to make a schedule and plan daily and weekly activities, leaving time for rest periods. To ensure long-term adherence, the exercise plan must be appropriate, safe for the patient, and easy to perform. Walking or other endurance exercises (e.g., stationary cycling, treadmills at a slow rate) combined with strength training are the best ways to strengthen muscles and improve endurance. Developing exercise endurance is important. If it takes longer than 5 minutes to return to baseline, the patient has most likely "overdone it." They should go at a slower pace during the next exercise period. Keeping a diary or log of the exercise program may help.

TABLE 31.22 PATIENT & CAREGIVER TEACHING

COPD

Include the following information in the teaching plan to assist patients with COPD and their caregivers to improve quality of life through promoting lifestyle practices that support successful living with COPD:

What Is COPD?
- How the lung works (basic anatomy and physiology)
- How the lungs change with COPD (basic pathophysiology)
- Signs and symptoms of COPD, acute exacerbations
- How to tell COPD from the common cold, flu, pneumonia
- Tests to assess breathing

Breathing and Airway Clearance Exercises
- Pursed-lip breathing (see Table 28.1)
- Airway clearance technique: huff cough (see Chapter 28)

Energy Conservation Techniques
- Daily activities (e.g., waking up, bathing, grooming, shopping, traveling)
- Use of oxygen equipment (if required)
- Consult with physical therapist, occupational therapist

Medications
- Types (include class, mechanism of action, types of devices)
- Medication schedule
- Correct use of inhalers, spacer, nebulizer (Fig. 31.8)
- Guide for home O_2 use and equipment

Psychosocial Support
- Worries about dependency
- Psychosocial issues (e.g., depression, anxiety, panic)
- Concerns about interpersonal relationships (e.g., intimacy)
- Worry about chronic condition and fear of dying
- Treatment decisions and end-of-life issues
- Support and rehabilitation groups

COPD Self-Management
- Reduce risk factors, especially smoking cessation
- Exercise program of walking and arm strengthening
- Recognition of signs and symptoms of respiratory infection, HF, acute exacerbation
- Need to report changes in condition in a timely manner
- Importance of annual flu vaccinations
- Importance of yearly follow-up

Nutrition Support (Table 31.20)
- Dietitian consult
- Ways to lose or gain weight if needed

For more information, see American Lung Association at www.lung.org/lung-disease/copd.

BOX 31.3 EVIDENCE-BASED PRACTICE

Physical Activity and COPD

You are working as a nurse in a pulmonary clinic with N.T., a 71-year-old male who was just discharged from the hospital with an exacerbation of COPD. He tells you he has been inactive for most of the past 8 months because "my breathing seems to worsen with any type of activity."

Making Clinical Decisions

Best Available Evidence

Patients with COPD who take part in regular moderate activity (e.g., brisk walking) have fewer severe flare-ups and are less likely to be admitted or readmitted to the hospital. Activity improves lung function and lessens depressive symptoms. The season of the year and temperature can be barriers to outdoor exercise.

Clinician Expertise

Physical inactivity is common in patients with COPD. You are aware that inactivity may place N.T. at a greater risk for functional decline and readmission.

Patient Preference and Values

N.T. tells you that he misses taking walks every day with his wife and dog. He is wondering if he would be able to resume this activity at a slower pace.

Implications for Practice

1. What factors will you discuss with N.T. about activity and COPD?
2. How would you assess N.T.'s willingness and motivation to engage in activity?
3. How would you involve interprofessional team members to assist N.T. in regular activity?

Reference

Ribeiro Moço VJ, Gulart AA, Lopes AJ, et al: Minimal-resource home exercise program improves activities of daily living, perceived health status, and shortness of breath in individuals with COPD Stages GOLD II to IV. *COPD* 20:298, 2023.

Many patients with moderate or severe COPD are anxious and fearful of walking or performing exercise. Teach patients coordinated walking with slow, pursed-lip breathing. Both patients and caregivers need support while they build the confidence they need to walk, perform daily exercises, or help with these activities.

Psychosocial care. Coping is a challenge for both patient and family. As COPD progresses, patients are often confronted with many lifestyle changes that may involve decreased ability to care for themselves, decreased energy for social activities, and loss or change in a job.

When a patient is first diagnosed or has complications that require hospitalization, expect a variety of responses. Emotions often expressed include denial, anger, frustration from real or perceived increased dependence, and loneliness from social isolation. Guilt may result if the disease is related to smoking.

Patients experience many losses as the disease progresses. Because many patients have depression and anxiety, assess for both. Ask patients if they "feel down" or "feel blue." Do they appear anxious about being able to control their breathlessness? Do they know what to do if they have an exacerbation? Are they showing concern over more difficulty in self-care activities, such as preparing meals and bathing? How is the family coping?

It is important to convey a sense of thoughtfulness and care. Teach patients about COPD and their treatment, which can help provide a sense of control. They may benefit from stress management techniques (e.g., massage, muscle relaxation). Include caregivers so they can be a source of support. Support groups at local ALA chapters (e.g., the Better Breathers Club), hospitals, and clinics can be helpful.

A mental health referral may be needed for proper screening and diagnosis of depression or other problems. Cognitive and behavior therapy may improve quality of life. Drugs may be used to treat both depression and anxiety. When patients are anxious because of dyspnea, pursed-lip breathing and SABAs may be appropriate.

Sexuality and sexual activity. Modifying sexual activity can contribute to well-being. Assess if the patient has any concerns related to sexuality and functioning. Ask open-ended questions to assess whether they want or are willing to discuss their concerns with you. For example, you could ask, "How does your shortness of breath affect your desire for intimacy with your partner?" This type of general, open-ended question gives the patient an opportunity to discuss concerns with you.

Dyspnea should not be a major problem in sexual activity except for patients in severe late stages. Generally, if the patient can walk up 2 flights of stairs or walk briskly, they should have enough energy for sexual activity. Using an inhaled bronchodilator before sexual activity can help ventilation. Other suggestions that may be helpful: (1) plan sexual activity during the part of the day when breathing is best, which is usually late morning or early afternoon; (2) use slow pursed-lip breathing; (3) refrain from sexual activity after eating or drinking alcohol; (4) choose less stressful positions (e.g., side-lying); and (5) use O_2 if prescribed.

Most patients with COPD are older. Their sexual performance issues may be related to aging. This is a good opportunity to teach patients about normal age-related changes. Encourage open communication between partners about their needs, expectations, and any problems they encounter.

Sleep. Adequate sleep is important to maintain quality of life and productivity. Most patients with COPD have sleep problems. Current tobacco use, depression, and anxiety are all common in COPD and lead to more trouble sleeping. β_2-Agonists may cause restlessness and insomnia. Postnasal drip or nasal congestion may cause coughing and wheezing at night.

Hyperinflation of the lungs and reduction in ventilation can result in severe drops in O_2 saturation (down to 60% or less) during sleep. This leads to an increased workload on the heart. Hypercapnia may contribute to more frequent awakening. The net result is sleeping poorly and waking up unrefreshed and fatigued.

Nasal saline sprays or rinses before sleep and in the morning may help. If the patient is prescribed O_2 therapy, using it at night may decrease insomnia. If the patient is a restless sleeper, snores, stops breathing while asleep, and tends to fall asleep during the day, they may need testing for sleep apnea (see Chapter 8).

End-of-Life Care

The trajectory of COPD is a gradual decline in health with increasing exacerbations. In the later, severe stages, palliative, end-of-life, and hospice care are important components of patient care.

End-of-life issues and advance directives are important topics for discussion. This may be hard for the patient and family to consider because of the uncertainty of the disease.

◆ Evaluation

The expected outcomes are that patients with COPD will

- Maintain a patent airway by effectively coughing
- Maintain an effective rate, rhythm, and depth of respirations
- Have clear breath sounds
- Return to preexacerbation baseline respiratory function
- Have $Paco_2$ and Pao_2 values within normal for the patient
- Have an optimal level of functioning with ADLs

Gerontologic Considerations: COPD

Older adults have physiologic changes, including reduced lean body mass, decreased respiratory muscle strength, increased dyspnea, and lower exercise tolerance that may increase the burden of disease from COPD. They may have difficulty handling increased secretions during an exacerbation. Smoking cessation is a key intervention but may be hard to achieve. This may lead to a higher incidence of acute exacerbations and hospitalization.

COPD is often complicated by the presence of other problems, such as diabetes, heart disease, hypertension, osteoporosis, impaired cognition, and lung cancer. These problems can make it harder for patients to cope with the stress of an exacerbation. Some drugs used to treat common problems, such as hypertension, can worsen COPD symptoms. If possible, we avoid using nonspecific β-blockers Because they can block the β_2 receptors in the airway and cause bronchoconstriction. Angiotensin-converting enzyme (ACE) inhibitors may cause a dry cough or worsen a present cough.

Drugs used to manage an exacerbation can complicate disease management and increase the chance of adverse events. Assess for potential drug-drug interactions, especially in patients being treated for other problems.

Impaired cognition and complex medication plans can contribute to nonadherence. Writing action plans in large font and setting reminders can help patients with poor memory and vision problems. Arthritis can hinder a person from using proper techniques for MDIs. Review MDI technique during visits. Have a DPI or spacers prescribed (if possible) because they are easier to use.

Older patients with COPD often have impaired quality of life. An important measure is to focus on ways to improve quality of life. Psychologic support becomes imperative to help patients achieve successful outcomes. In the later stages of COPD, palliative and hospice care can help manage symptoms and improve the quality of the rest of their lives (Box 31.4).

BOX 31.4 ETHICAL/LEGAL DILEMMAS

Advance Directives

Situation

L.H., an 84-year-old male with end-stage COPD, is admitted to the hospital in acute respiratory failure (ARF). He is intubated, placed on full-support mechanical ventilation, and transferred to the ICU. L.H. is taking no spontaneous breaths. He infrequently responds by opening his eyes, sometimes to the sound of voice and other times only to painful stimuli. A chest x-ray shows pneumonia in both lungs. Antibiotics are ordered. A Foley drains a small amount of cloudy, dark amber urine.

L.H. had his advance directive (AD) drawn up 5 years ago. Copies were given to his wife and HCP at that time. His wife brings the documents to the ICU and tells you that the hospital must stop treating her husband. She insists that per his AD, the health care team should allow him to die. However, their oldest son, who lives out of state and is currently on his way to see his dad, tells you over the telephone that he will file a lawsuit against the hospital if they do not provide full care to his father.

Ethical/Legal Points for Consideration

- A living will permits people to share their preferences and refusals should they become terminally ill or be in a situation in which there is no hope of recovery and they cannot speak for themselves.
- The durable power of attorney for health care permits persons to name a proxy to make health care decisions in the event the person is incapacitated.
- AD laws vary from state to state concerning the need for witnesses and naming the proxy.
- Families may be divided about decisions for their loved ones. Conflicts often arise when feelings of remorse or guilt and money and/or property are involved. This situation requires you to notify the HCP, engage social work and spiritual care, and ask for a family conference. In some circumstances, consultation from the ethics committee may be needed.
- HCPs are obligated to follow the patient's AD when a patient is no longer able to speak for themselves.
- In your scope of nursing practice, you may need to (1) teach patients and families about ADs; (2) make AD documents available to patients; (3) determine whether all involved HCPs are aware of the patient's AD; (4) assist the patient and family in communicating with the HCP when a "no code" or "DNR" (do not resuscitate) order is requested; and (5) assist the conflicted family in obtaining counseling when needed.
- You need to be aware and informed about the decision-making laws and regulations in your state about ADs and your role with respect to ADs.

Discussion Questions

1. What should you do with the information provided by L.H.'s wife?
2. The HCP asks that you organize a family conference. How would you address the family's needs at the conference? What would you identify as a priority at this meeting?
3. What other health care team members could you invite to the conference to help facilitate discussion and decision making?
4. The family conference does not go well. While L.H.'s wife accepts her husband's end-stage COPD diagnosis, the son does not. The wife and son have different views on how L.H. is to be managed. What would be your approach to L.H.'s plan of care? How might you involve the family members in L.H.'s plan of care?

CASE STUDY

COPD

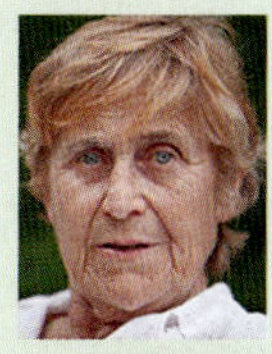

(© iStockphoto/ Thinkstock.0)

Patient Profile

H.M., a 68-year-old female, has been in the hospital for 6 days with an acute COPD exacerbation (GOLD 3 [severe]). She was admitted after 4 days of increasing shortness of breath. She noted an increased volume of sputum. It was initially white but turned "greenish." H.M. is scheduled for discharge tomorrow. Her 73-year-old husband will care for her at home.

Subjective Data

Preadmission

- Husband said her skin tone looked "bluish"
- Increased Ventolin HFA use at home to 5 or 6 times a day for dyspnea
- Described having "jitters" and "racing heart"

Medical History

- Had 3 or 4 COPD exacerbations in the past year that were managed at home
- A 30 pack-year history of smoking; smokes half a pack per day now to "clear out lungs" in the morning
- Eats a regular diet but "gets full fast"
- Cannot climb 1 flight of stairs without stopping; is able to walk down the flat driveway about 20 ft (6 m) without difficulty
- Awakens 2 to 3 times per night coughing and short of breath
- Sleeps in the recliner sitting upright
- Last spirometry: decreased FEV_1 (48%) and FEV_1/FVC (62%)

Objective Data

Emergency Department

Physical Assessment

- Weight 129 lb (58.5 kg), height 5 ft 8 in (172 cm), BMI 20 kg/m^2
- Temp 100°F (37.8°C), pulse 86 (regular), respiratory rate 28 (shallow, slightly labored), BP 136/76 mm Hg
- Increased anteroposterior diameter of chest
- Slight use of accessory neck muscles with breathing
- Distant breath sounds with occasional expiratory wheezes
- 2+ nonpitting pedal edema

Diagnostic Studies

- ABG: pH 7.34, $Paco_2$ 59 mm Hg, HCO_3^- 27 mEq/L, Pao_2 68 mm Hg
- WBC: 16,500/μL
- Chest x-ray: hyperinflation, flat diaphragm, no sign of pneumonia
- Sputum: negative (no organisms present)

24 Hours Postadmission to Hospital

- ABG: pH 7.30, $Paco_2$ 63 mm Hg, HCO_3^- 29 mEq/L, Pao_2 64 mm Hg

Interprofessional Care

- O_2 4 L/min via nasal cannula
- Prednisone 40 mg/day orally daily for 5 days
- Doxycycline 100 mg/day orally daily for 10 days
- Ipratropium HFA MDI 2 puffs 4 times a day
- Lasix 10 mg orally twice daily

Discussion Questions

1. ***Recognize:*** What manifestations show H.M. had an exacerbation of COPD?
2. ***Analyze:*** What is the most likely cause of her exacerbation?
3. ***Analyze:*** Why would H.M. "feel full fast" when eating? What could you do to address this issue?
4. ***Analyze:*** What symptoms indicate overuse of inhalers? Which drug would cause the symptoms described?
5. ***Analyze:*** Interpret the ABG on admission and 24 hours postadmission. In comparing both ABGs, do you see a pattern?
6. ***Prioritize:*** Based on the assessment data presented, what are the priority clinical problems?
7. ***Act:*** What is one suggestion you could make to H.M. that could slow the progression of her COPD?
8. ***Act:*** What would you include in her discharge planning and teaching?
9. Develop a conceptual care map for H.M.

Answers available at http://evolve.elsevier.com/Lewis/medsurg.

BRIDGE TO NCLEX EXAMINATION

The number of the question corresponds to the same-numbered outcome at the beginning of the chapter.

1. The nurse teaches a patient with bronchiectasis that which problem would warrant a call to the clinic?
- **a.** Blood clots in the sputum
- **b.** Sticky sputum on a hot day
- **c.** Producing large amounts of sputum daily
- **d.** Increased shortness of breath after eating a large meal

2. Which treatments would the nurse expect to implement in the management plan of an adult patient with cystic fibrosis? **(Select all that apply.)**
- **a.** Airway clearance techniques
- **b.** Bronchodilators and mucolytics
- **c.** Pancreatic enzyme replacement
- **d.** IV corticosteroids on a chronic basis
- **e.** Inhaled tobramycin for *Pseudomonas* infection

3. Which symptoms in a patient's history suggest asthma or risk factors for asthma? **(Select all that apply.)**
- **a.** Prolonged inhalation
- **b.** Gastric reflux or heartburn
- **c.** Cough worse at night or early in the morning
- **d.** History of allergic rhinitis or chronic sinusitis
- **e.** Chest pain and syncope after exercising with a stationary bicycle for 5 minutes

4. Which finding indicates that a patient with asthma is developing status asthmaticus? **(Select all that apply.)**
- **a.** Anxiety and panic
- **b.** Positive sputum culture
- **c.** Unable to speak in complete sentences
- **d.** Chest x-ray shows hyperinflated lungs
- **e.** Lack of response to conventional treatment

5. Which statement indicates the patient with asthma requires further teaching before discharge?
   a. "I use my corticosteroid inhaler every time I feel short of breath."
   b. "I get a flu shot every year and see my HCP if I have an upper respiratory tract infection."
   c. "I use my inhaler before I visit my aunt who has a cat, but I only visit for a few minutes because of my allergies."
   d. "I walk 30 minutes every day, but sometimes I have to use my bronchodilator inhaler before walking to prevent me from getting short of breath."
6. Which two medications would be administered to a patient experiencing an acute asthma attack?
   a. Cough suppressant, antibiotic
   b. Long-acting muscarinic agent, methylxanthine
   c. Phosphodiesterase inhibitor, biologic
   d. Inhaled corticosteroid, short-acting beta-agonist
7. The plan of care for the patient with chronic obstructive pulmonary disease (COPD) would include **(Select all that apply.)**
   a. exercise such as walking.
   b. high flow rate of O_2 administration.
   c. low-dose oral corticosteroid therapy.
   d. use of monthly chest x-rays to monitor the progression of COPD.
   e. breathing exercises, such as pursed-lip breathing, that focus on exhalation.
8. What would the nurse include when teaching a patient how to use a metered-dose inhaler (MDI)?
   a. After activating the MDI, breathe in as quickly as you can.
   b. Estimate the amount of remaining medicine in the MDI by floating the canister in water.
   c. Disassemble the plastic canister from the inhaler and rinse both pieces under running water every week.
   d. To determine how long the canister will last, divide the total number of puffs in the canister by the puffs needed per day.

1. a; 2. a, b, c, e; 3. b, c, d; 4. a, c, e; 5. a; 6. d; 7. a, c, e; 8. d.

For rationales to these answers and even more NCLEX review questions, visit http://evolve.elsevier.com/Lewis/medsurg.

REFERENCES

To access the References for this chapter, please scan the QR code with a mobile device.

32

Acute Respiratory Failure and Acute Respiratory Distress Syndrome

Eugene E. Mondor

http://evolve.elsevier.com/Lewis/medsurg/

CONCEPTUAL FOCUS

Acid-Base Balance
Anxiety
Gas Exchange

LEARNING OUTCOMES

1. Discuss the etiology, pathophysiology, and clinical manifestations of hypoxemic and hypercapnic acute respiratory failure (ARF).
2. Describe the nursing and interprofessional management of respiratory failure.
3. Discuss the pathophysiology and clinical manifestations of acute respiratory distress syndrome (ARDS).
4. Describe the nursing and interprofessional management of ARDS.
5. Identify interventions to prevent and manage complications of ARF and ARDS.

KEY TERMS

acute respiratory distress syndrome (ARDS)
acute respiratory failure (ARF)
chronic respiratory failure (CRF)
hypercapnia
hypercapnic respiratory failure
hypoxemia
hypoxemic respiratory failure
hypoxia
PaO_2/FiO_2 (P/F) ratio
permissive hypercapnia
refractory hypoxemia
shunt
V/Q mismatch

This chapter discusses acute respiratory failure (ARF) and acute respiratory distress syndrome (ARDS). The management of patients with ARF and ARDS focuses on interventions to promote adequate oxygenation, ensure effective ventilation, identify and treat the underlying cause(s), and prevent complications. When the respiratory system fails, it affects all body systems.

ACUTE RESPIRATORY FAILURE

Acute respiratory failure (ARF) occurs when oxygenation, ventilation, or both are inadequate. ARF is not a disease. It is a symptom that reflects insufficient and/or failure of lung function (Fig. 32.1). In ARF, not enough O_2 is transferred to the blood, or inadequate CO_2 is removed from the lungs. ARF occurs with problems involving the lungs or other body systems (Table 32.1).

Conditions that interfere with diffusion of O_2 result in **hypoxemia**. This is a decrease in arterial O_2 (PaO_2) and saturation (SaO_2) to less than normal values. Insufficient CO_2 removal results in **hypercapnia**. This is an increase in arterial CO_2 ($PaCO_2$). We use arterial blood gases (ABGs) to assess changes in pH, PaO_2, $PaCO_2$, bicarbonate, and SaO_2. We use pulse oximetry to assess arterial O_2 saturation (SpO_2).

We can classify ARF as hypoxemic or hypercapnic (Fig. 32.2). **Hypoxemic respiratory failure** is a PaO_2 less than 60 mm Hg in arterial blood (on room air and at sea level) with normal or slightly subnormal $PaCO_2$ levels.[1] The main problem is inadequate exchange of O_2 between the alveoli and pulmonary capillaries. This low PaO_2 level may exist despite O_2 therapy.

Hypercapnic respiratory failure (or *ventilatory failure*) is a $PaCO_2$ greater than 50 mm Hg, which may be accompanied by hypoxemia and/or acidosis (arterial pH less than 7.35).[1] The main problem is generally not the lungs (which are often normal), but the body's inability to remove CO_2. This causes the $PaCO_2$ to be higher than normal. As the $PaCO_2$ level climbs,

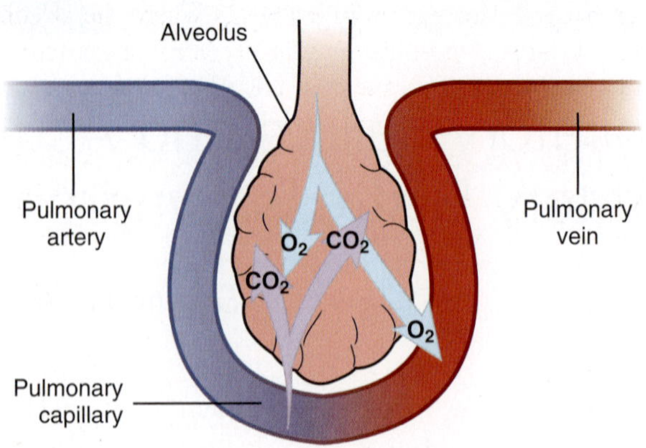

Fig. 32.1 The alveolus and pulmonary capillary: normal gas exchange unit in the lung.

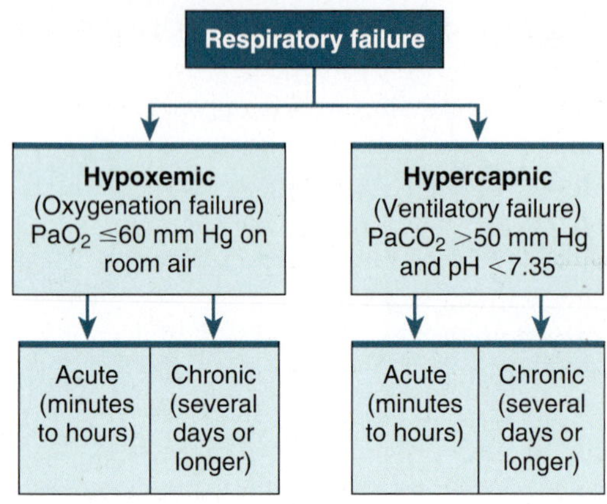

Fig. 32.2 Classification of acute respiratory failure.

TABLE 32.1 Common Causes of ARF

Hypoxemic Respiratory Failure	Hypercapnic Respiratory Failure
Respiratory Problems	**Respiratory Problems**
ARDS	ARDS
Asthma	Asthma
Bronchiectasis	Chronic bronchitis
Chronic bronchitis	COPD
Emphysema	Cystic fibrosis
Pneumonia	Emphysema
Pneumothorax	Pulmonary edema
Pulmonary edema	Upper airway obstruction
Pulmonary embolism	
Toxic inhalation (e.g., smoke)	
Cardiac	**Chest Wall**
Anatomic shunt (e.g., ventricular septal defect)	Kyphoscoliosis
	Pain
Cardiogenic pulmonary edema	Severe obesity
Cardiogenic shock	Thoracic trauma (e.g., flail chest)
Heart failure (HF)	
High-CO states with diffusion limitation	**CNS**
	Brainstem injury or infarction
	Sedative and opioid overdose
	Severe head injury (TBI)
	Spinal cord injury
	Neuromuscular
	Amyotrophic lateral sclerosis
	Critical illness polyneuropathy
	Guillain-Barré syndrome
	Muscular dystrophy
	Multiple sclerosis
	Myasthenia gravis
	Phrenic nerve injury
	Poliomyelitis
	Toxin exposure

the body is eventually unable to compensate for the increase. This causes acidosis to worsen. It puts patients at risk of hemodynamic instability and respiratory and/or cardiac arrest.

When respiratory failure is acute in onset, significant changes in Pa_{O_2} and Pa_{CO_2} can occur quickly. Changes develop over several minutes to a few hours to 1 or 2 days. Patients may have hemodynamic instability (e.g., tachycardia, hypotension), increased respiratory effort, and decreased level of consciousness. Urgent intervention is needed. **Chronic respiratory failure (CRF)** develops more slowly, over days to weeks. Patients are usually more stable as the body has time to compensate for the small but subtle changes. CRF does not typically present as an immediate, life-threatening condition.

Patients may have both types of respiratory failure at the same time. For example, a patient with chronic obstructive pulmonary disease (COPD) who has pneumonia can have "acute-on-chronic" respiratory failure. Here, the patient has an underlying chronic respiratory problem. The new infection, when added to the chronic problem, results in the "acute-on-chronic" clinical picture.

Etiology and Pathophysiology

Hypoxemic Respiratory Failure

Four mechanisms may cause hypoxemia and contribute to the development of acute hypoxemic respiratory failure: (1) mismatch between ventilation (V) and perfusion (Q), referred to as **V/Q mismatch**; (2) shunt; (3) diffusion impairment or limitation; and (4) alveolar hypoventilation. The most common causes are V/Q mismatch and shunt.

Ventilation-perfusion mismatch. In normal lungs, the volume of blood perfusing the lungs and the amount of gas reaching the alveoli are fairly constant. When you compare normal alveolar ventilation (around 4 L/min) to pulmonary blood flow (around 5 L/min), you have a V/Q ratio of 0.8.[2] In a perfect match, ventilation and perfusion yield a V/Q ratio of 1:1, expressed as V/Q = 1. When the match is not 1:1, a V/Q mismatch occurs.

Ventilation and perfusion are not perfectly matched in all areas of the lung. Some regional variation, or mismatch, occurs. For example, at the apex of the lung, V/Q ratios are greater than 1 (more ventilation than perfusion). At the base of the lung, V/Q ratios are less than 1 (less ventilation than perfusion).

Because changes at the lung apex balance changes at the base, the net effect is a close overall match (Fig. 32.3).

Many problems can cause a V/Q mismatch (Fig. 32.4). The most common are those in which increased secretions are present in the airways (e.g., COPD) or alveoli (e.g., pneumonia) or bronchospasm is present (e.g., asthma). V/Q mismatch may result from pain, alveolar collapse (atelectasis), or pulmonary emboli.

Pain can interfere with chest and abdominal wall movement and compromise ventilation. Patients may be unwilling to take big, deep breaths. As a result, short, shallow respirations contribute to the development of atelectasis. This is the beginning of a V/Q mismatch. At the same time, pain activates the stress response, increasing baseline metabolic state. O_2 consumption and CO_2 production (as a by-product of cell and tissue metabolism) increase. Increased O_2 demand, increased CO_2 levels, and decreased O_2 supply increase ventilation demands. Since there is no effect on blood flow to the lungs, the V/Q mismatch worsens.

When a pulmonary embolus occurs, it limits blood flow distal to the occlusion. While some areas of normal lung ventilation remain, a decrease in perfusion to other parts of the lung occurs from the vessel occlusion. This results in a V/Q mismatch. If the embolus is large enough to block a major pulmonary artery, it can cause severe hemodynamic instability.

The best way to treat hypoxemia caused by a V/Q mismatch is to treat the cause. O_2 therapy is often the first step. Most patients with a hypoxemic V/Q mismatch will respond to O_2 therapy. Frequent ABG analysis, pulse oximetry, and continuous assessment of level of consciousness, respiratory rate and rhythm, and response to O_2 therapy are essential.

Shunt. A **shunt** occurs when blood exits the heart without having taken part in gas exchange. A shunt is an extreme form of a V/Q mismatch. There are 2 types: *anatomic* and *physiologic*. An *anatomic shunt* occurs when blood passes through an anatomic channel in the heart (e.g., a ventricular septal defect) and bypasses the lungs. A *physiologic shunt* occurs when blood flows through the pulmonary capillaries without taking part in gas exchange.[3] This occurs in problems where the alveoli fill with fluid (e.g., pneumonia) and the exchange of gas across the alveolar-capillary membrane is severely impaired.

Patients with a shunt are usually more hypoxemic than patients with V/Q mismatch. O_2 therapy alone is often not effective at increasing the $Pa{O_2}$. They often need mechanical ventilation with a high fraction of inspired O_2 ($Fi{O_2}$) to improve gas exchange.

Diffusion impairment. *Diffusion impairment* occurs when gas exchange across the alveolar-capillary membrane is compromised by a process that damages or destroys the alveolar membrane or affects blood flow through the pulmonary capillaries (Fig. 32.5).[4] Conditions that cause the alveolar-capillary membrane to become thicker (fibrotic) slow gas transport. These include pulmonary fibrosis, interstitial lung disease, and ARDS. The accumulation of fluid, white blood cells, or protein in the alveoli contributes to a decrease in gas exchange between the alveolus and capillary bed. This occurs with pulmonary edema.

The classic sign of diffusion impairment is hypoxemia that worsens mostly with exercise. During exercise, blood moves quickly through the lungs. This decreases the time for O_2 diffusion across the alveolar-capillary membrane. With less time for gas exchange, hypoxemia occurs. Diffusion impairment can occur in conditions where CO is markedly increased (e.g., high-output heart failure [HF]).

Alveolar hypoventilation. *Alveolar hypoventilation* is a decrease in ventilation that increases $Pa{CO_2}$. Common causes include central nervous system (CNS) problems, chest wall dysfunction, acute asthma, or restrictive lung disease. Although

V/Q	PaO_2	$PaCO_2$
3.3	132	28
1.0	108	39
0.63	89	42

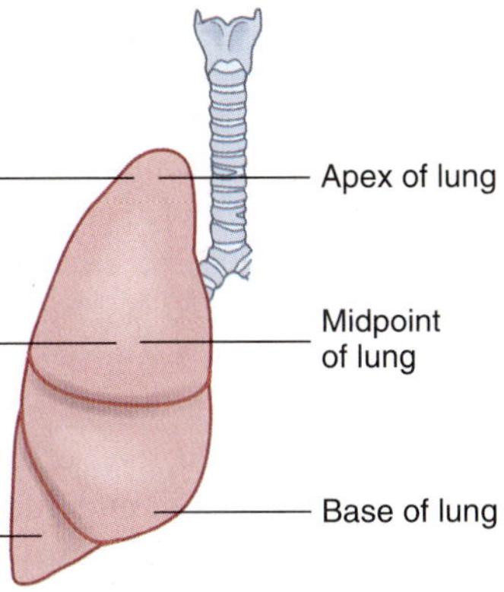

Apex of lung
Midpoint of lung
Base of lung

Fig. 32.3 Regional V/Q differences in the normal lung. The $Pa{O_2}$ is higher at the apex of the lung and lower at the base. Values for $Pa{CO_2}$ are the opposite (i.e., lower at the apex and higher at the base). Blood that exits the lung is a mixture of these values.

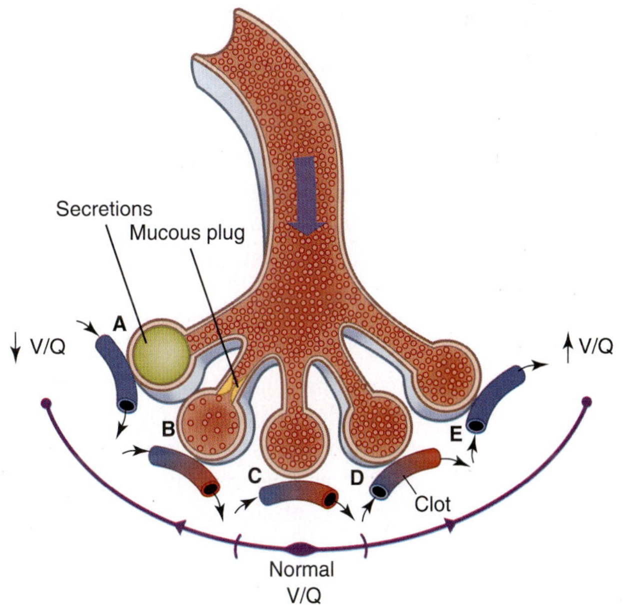

Fig. 32.4 Causes of V/Q mismatch. (A) Absolute shunt: no ventilation occurs because of fluid filling the alveoli. (B) Ventilation partially compromised by secretions in the airway. (C) Normal lung unit. (D) Perfusion partially compromised by emboli obstructing blood flow. (E) Dead space, no perfusion because of obstruction of the pulmonary capillary.

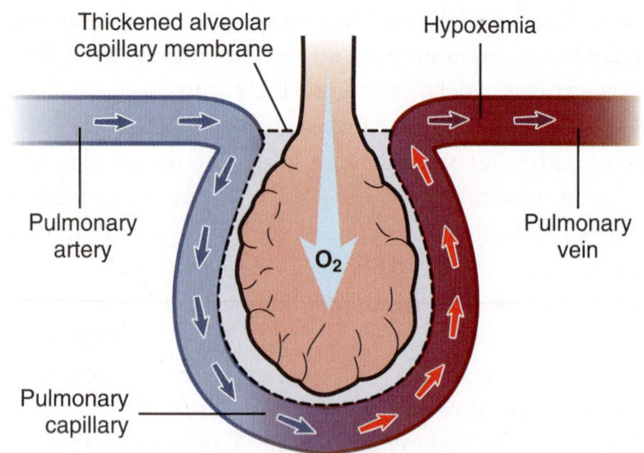

Fig. 32.5 Diffusion impairment. Reduced exchange of CO_2 and O_2 because of the thickened alveolar-capillary membrane.

alveolar hypoventilation is mainly a mechanism of hypercapnic respiratory failure, it can also contribute to hypoxemia.

Interrelationship of mechanisms. Rarely is acute hypoxemic respiratory failure caused by a single factor. More often, it is a combination of 2 or more factors. For example, patients with ARF from pneumonia may have a V/Q mismatch and shunt. Inflammation, edema, and exudate obstruct the airways (V/Q mismatch) and fill the alveoli with exudate (shunt). Contributing factors include increases in O_2 demand from anxiety, dyspnea, and pain.

Consequences of Hypoxemia

Hypoxemia can lead to hypoxia if not corrected. **Hypoxia**, a decrease in O_2 supply at the cell level, occurs when the PaO_2 falls enough to cause signs and symptoms of inadequate oxygenation. If hypoxia is severe, the cells shift from aerobic to anaerobic metabolism. Anaerobic metabolism uses more fuel, produces less energy, and is less efficient than aerobic metabolism. The waste product of anaerobic metabolism is lactic acid. Lactic acid is harder to remove from the body than CO_2 because it must be buffered with sodium bicarbonate. When the body does not have enough sodium bicarbonate to buffer the lactic acid, metabolic acidosis occurs. Left uncorrected, tissue and cell dysfunction, and ultimately cell death, occurs.

Hypercapnic Respiratory Failure

In acute hypercapnic respiratory failure, or *ventilatory failure*, the respiratory system cannot maintain CO_2 levels within normal limits. This condition occurs from an increase in CO_2 production or a decrease in alveolar ventilation. Hypercapnic respiratory failure can be acute or chronic.

Many problems can cause hypercapnic respiratory failure. We group these into 4 categories: (1) CNS, (2) neuromuscular, (3) chest wall, and (4) respiratory. Hypercapnic ARF due to CNS, neuromuscular, and/or chest wall problems can occur in the presence of normal lungs.

CNS problems. Several CNS problems can suppress the drive to breathe. An example is opioid overdose. It decreases CO_2 reactivity in the brainstem. This allows arterial CO_2 levels to rise. Brainstem infarction or traumatic brain injury (TBI) may interfere with the function of the respiratory center in the medulla. The medulla does not sense a change in $PaCO_2$, and as a result, an increase in respiratory rate does not occur. High-level spinal cord injuries (SCIs) can affect nerve supply to the respiratory muscles of the chest wall and diaphragm.

Neuromuscular problems. Various neuromuscular problems place patients at risk for respiratory failure. For example, patients with Guillain-Barré syndrome and multiple sclerosis may present with varying respiratory muscle weakness and/or paralysis. As a result, they cannot eliminate CO_2 and are unable to maintain normal $PaCO_2$ levels. Exposure to toxins can interfere with the nerve supply to muscles. Respiratory muscle weakness can occur from muscle wasting during critical illness.

Chest wall problems. Several conditions contribute to ARF by preventing normal chest wall or diaphragm movement or limiting lung expansion. With flail chest, fractures prevent the rib cage from expanding normally. In severe obesity, the weight of the chest and abdominal contents limit lung expansion. With kyphosis, spine changes compress the lungs and prevent adequate chest wall expansion.

Respiratory problems. Obstructive lung disease, lower respiratory tract infection, and HF increase risk for hypercapnic respiratory failure.[5] This is because the underlying pathophysiology results in airflow limitations and airflow obstruction. Respiratory muscle fatigue and ventilatory failure occur from the added work of breathing (WOB) needed to inspire air against increased airway resistance and air trapped within the alveoli.

Clinical Manifestations

Respiratory failure may develop suddenly (acute, minutes or hours) or gradually (chronic, several days or weeks). A sudden decrease in PaO_2 and/or a rapid rise in $PaCO_2$ implies a serious respiratory problem, which can quickly become a life-threatening emergency. An example is a patient with asthma who develops severe bronchospasm and a marked decrease in airflow. This can result in respiratory muscle fatigue, acidosis, and ARF.

Signs of respiratory failure are related to the extent of change in PaO_2 or $PaCO_2$, the speed of change (acute or chronic), underlying medical problem, and the patient's ability to compensate for this change. When compensatory mechanisms fail, respiratory failure occurs. Because clinical signs vary, frequent and repeated assessment of the patient's overall condition is a priority.

A lack of O_2 affects all body systems (Table 32.2). For example, a decreased level of consciousness may occur when not enough blood, O_2, and glucose are supplied to the brain. Permanent brain damage can result if hypoxia is severe and prolonged. Gastrointestinal (GI) system changes include tissue ischemia and increased intestinal wall permeability. Bacteria can migrate from the GI tract into systemic circulation. Renal

TABLE 32.2 Common Manifestations of Hypoxemia and Hypercapnia

Specific	Nonspecific
Hypoxemia	
Respiratory	**Cardiovascular**
Accessory muscle use	↑ BP (early), ↓ BP (late)
Cyanosis (late)	Dysrhythmias
Dyspnea	↑ HR
Intercostal muscle retraction	Skin cool, clammy, diaphoretic
Nasal flaring	**CNS**
Pallor	Anxiety
Paradoxical chest or abdominal wall movement with respiratory cycle (late finding)	Agitation
	Confusion
	↓ Level of consciousness
Prolonged expiration	Restlessness, combative behavior
SpO_2 (<90%)	**Other**
Tachypnea	Fatigue
	Inability to speak in complete sentences without pausing to breathe
Hypercapnia	
Respiratory	**Cardiovascular**
Dyspnea	↑ BP or ↓ BP
Limited chest wall movement	Dysrhythmias
Pursed-lip breathing	↑ HR
Tripod position	**CNS**
Respiratory rate (↑ initially, as condition worsens ↓ rate with shallow respirations)	Agitation
	Confusion
	Morning headache
	Progressive somnolence
	Neuromuscular
	↓ Deep tendon reflexes
	Muscle weakness
	Tremors, seizures (late)

function may be impaired. Sodium retention, peripheral edema, and acute kidney injury (AKI) may occur.

One of the first signs of hypoxemic ARF is a change in mental status. Mental status changes occur early because the brain is sensitive to changes in O_2 (and to a lesser degree CO_2) levels and acid-base balance. Restlessness, confusion, and agitation suggest inadequate O_2 delivery to the brain. A morning headache and low respiratory rate with a decreased level of consciousness may indicate problems with CO_2 removal.

Tachycardia, tachypnea, pallor, and a mild increase in WOB are early signs of ARF. These changes indicate attempts by the heart and lungs to compensate for decreased O_2 delivery and rising CO_2 levels. It is important to understand that cyanosis is an unreliable indicator of hypoxemia. It is a late sign in ARF. It often does not occur until deoxygenated hemoglobin concentration in the capillaries is around 5 g/dL.[6]

Observing the patient's position helps assess the effort associated with WOB. Patients with mild respiratory distress may be able to lie down. In moderate distress, patients may prefer to sit. With severe distress, they may be unable to breathe unless sitting upright. The tripod position helps decrease WOB in patients with moderate to severe COPD and ARF. The patient sits with the arms propped on the overbed table or the knees. Propping the arms increases the anteroposterior (AP) diameter of the chest and changes pressure in the thorax.

Patients in ARF may initially have a rapid, shallow breathing pattern. Increased respiratory rates require a substantial amount of work and increased energy. This can lead to respiratory muscle fatigue. A change from a rapid rate to a slower rate in a patient in respiratory distress suggests worsening of patient condition. It often means CO_2 levels are rising. There is an increased chance of respiratory arrest.

Assess their ability to speak. Patients with dyspnea may be able to speak only a few words at a time between breaths. For example, they may have "2-word" or "3-word" dyspnea. This means they can say only 2 or 3 words before pausing to breathe.

Patients with dyspnea may use pursed-lip breathing (see Table 28.1). This technique increases Sa_{O_2} by slowing respirations, increasing time for expiration, and preventing small bronchioles from collapsing. You may see *retraction* (inward movement) of the intercostal spaces or supraclavicular area and accessory muscle use during inspiration or expiration. Using accessory muscles often signifies a moderate to high degree of respiratory distress.

Paradoxical breathing occurs with severe respiratory distress. Normally, the thorax and abdomen move outward on inspiration and inward on exhalation. With paradoxical breathing, the abdomen and chest each move in the opposite direction. Paradoxical breathing results from maximal use of the accessory muscles of respiration.

Auscultate breath sounds. Note the presence and location of any abnormal breath sounds. Fine crackles may occur with pulmonary edema. Coarse crackles heard on expiration indicate fluid in the airways. This may be a sign of pneumonia or HF. Absent or decreased breath sounds occur with atelectasis, pleural effusion, or hypoventilation. Bronchial breath sounds over the lung periphery occur with lung consolidation from pneumonia. You may hear a pleural friction rub if pneumonia involves the pleura.

Diagnostic Studies

The most common diagnostic studies used to evaluate ARF are chest x-ray and ABG analysis. A chest x-ray helps identify the cause (e.g., atelectasis, pneumonia). ABGs assess oxygenation (Pa_{O_2}) and ventilation (Pa_{CO_2}) status and acid-base (pH, bicarbonate) balance. Pulse oximetry (SpO_2) monitors oxygenation status indirectly.

Other diagnostic studies that may be done include a complete blood cell count (CBC), electrolytes, urinalysis, and 12-lead ECG. Other tests can help identify other problems contributing to ARF. Examples include a d-dimer (pulmonary emboli), troponin I and/or T (myocardial infarction), or brain natriuretic peptide (HF). Blood and sputum cultures may reveal infection. A CT scan or V/Q scan may be done if a pulmonary embolus is suspected. For patients in moderate to severe ARF, end-tidal CO_2 ($EtCO_2$) monitoring can assess trends in ventilation.

NURSING AND INTERPROFESSIONAL MANAGEMENT: ARF

Because many different problems cause ARF, management and care are specific to the patient. Factors considered include patient age, underlying comorbidities, severity of onset, and suspected or most likely cause of ARF. In acute care settings, collaboration among the health care team (e.g., nurses, physicians, respiratory therapists, pharmacists) is essential.

For mild to moderate ARF, patients may be hospitalized. O_2 administration via a high-flow O_2 delivery device may be started. Noninvasive ventilation, such as bilevel positive airway pressure (Bi-PAP), may be an option for patients who are awake, alert, able to maintain a patent airway and clear their own secretions.

In severe ARF, patients receive care in an intensive care unit (ICU). ICU care will include mechanical ventilation. Continuous pulse oximetry and arterial BP monitoring will occur. ABGs will be drawn often. Central venous pressure (CVP) monitoring may be ordered. Patients may need advanced hemodynamic monitoring to evaluate parameters such as ejection fraction, CO, and pulmonary capillary wedge pressure (PCWP). Central or mixed venous O_2 saturation ($ScvO_2$ or SvO_2) data help determine the adequacy of tissue perfusion and response to treatment.

Assessment

Table 32.3 presents subjective and objective data that you should obtain from patients with ARF. A thorough assessment may result in the early detection of respiratory insufficiency or failure. This allows us to intervene sooner and may prevent worsening in respiratory condition. Monitor patients with preexisting cardiac and/or respiratory disease. Any change in their overall status may cause significant respiratory and hemodynamic decompensation.

The priority is assessing the ability to maintain a patent airway and breathe (ventilate). Observe trends in ABGs, pulse oximetry, and assessment findings. Remain alert to subtle changes that can occur in your patient's condition from hypoxemia or hypercarbia. Your ability to detect problems, notify the HCP, implement treatment, and evaluate response to therapy is essential.

Clinical Problems

Clinical problems for patients with ARF may include:

- Impaired respiratory system function
- Inadequate tissue perfusion
- Acid-base imbalance

Additional information on clinical problems and interventions for patients with ARF is presented in eNursing Care Plan 32.1 (available on the website for this chapter).

TABLE 32.3 NURSING ASSESSMENT

ARF

Subjective Data

Important Health Information

Health history: Age, tobacco, alcohol, or drug use. Hospitalizations related to lung disease, thoracic or spinal cord trauma, occupational exposures to lung toxins

Medications: Use of home O_2, respiratory medications, immunosuppressant (e.g., corticosteroid) therapy, CNS depressants, illicit substances

Surgery or other treatments: Past mechanical ventilation, recent surgery

Functional Health Patterns

Health perception–health management: Exercise, self-care activities, immunizations (flu, pneumonia, RSV, COVID)

Nutritional-metabolic: Eating habits; history of bloating, indigestion; recent weight gain or loss, change in appetite. Use of vitamins or herb supplements

Activity-exercise: Fatigue, dizziness, dyspnea at rest or with activity, wheezing, cough (productive or nonproductive), sputum (volume, color, viscosity), palpitations, swollen feet, change in exercise tolerance

Sleep-rest: Changes in sleep pattern, use of CPAP

Cognitive-perceptual: Headache, chest pain or tightness, chronic pain. Cognition, level of consciousness

Coping–stress tolerance: Anxiety, depression, feelings of hopelessness

Objective Data

Cardiovascular

↑ HR, dysrhythmias, extra heart sounds (S_3, S_4). Bounding pulse. ↑ BP progressing to ↓ BP. Pulsus paradoxus, jugular venous distention, edema

GI

Abdominal distention, ascites, epigastric tenderness, hepatojugular reflex

Neurologic

Somnolence, confusion, slurred speech, restlessness, delirium, agitation, tremors, seizures, ↓ deep tendon reflexes, papilledema

Respiratory

↑ Respiratory rate (shallow, labored), ↑ WOB. Accessory muscle use with retractions, ↑ diaphragmatic excursion or asymmetric chest expansion, paradoxical chest and abdominal wall movement. Tactile fremitus, crepitus, or deviated trachea (late sign). Absent, decreased, or adventitious breath sounds. Pleural friction rub. Bronchial or bronchovesicular sounds heard in other than normal location, inspiratory stridor

Skin

Pale, cool, clammy skin or warm, flushed skin. Peripheral and/or central cyanosis. Peripheral dependent edema

Possible Diagnostic Findings

↓/↑ pH, ↑/↓ $PaCO_2$, ↑/↓ bicarbonate, ↓ PaO_2, ↓ SaO_2, ↓ SpO_2, abnormal hemoglobin, ↑ WBC count, abnormal electrolytes. Abnormal chest x-ray. Abnormal CVP, bedside echocardiogram, and/or pulmonary artery pressures. Initially, CO may be ↑ due to the stress response. As hypoxemia, hypercapnia, and acidosis become more severe, CO will ↓.

Planning

The overall goals for patients with ARF include (1) independently maintain a patent airway, (2) absence of dyspnea or return to baseline breathing patterns, (3) effectively cough and able to clear secretions, and (4) normal ABG values or values within the patient's baseline.

◆ Implementation

Health Promotion

For patients at risk for ARF, prevention and early recognition of respiratory problems is important. This is especially crucial for patients with neuromuscular, cardiac, or respiratory problems (e.g., COPD). Assess patients at high risk often and implement preventive measures. Preventing atelectasis, pneumonia, and complications of immobility and optimizing hydration and nutrition can decrease the risk for ARF. Early strategies may include deep breathing and coughing, incentive spirometry, and early ambulation.

Acute Care

Interventions to improve oxygenation and ventilation status are essential to improving O_2 delivery and patient outcomes (Table 32.4). The primary aim is to identify and treat the underlying cause of ARF. Patients with V/Q mismatch, shunting, or diffusion impairment may be managed slightly differently, depending on the underlying cause. The nursing management of patients with ARF is outlined in Table 32.5.

Respiratory Care

The goals of respiratory care include maintaining a patent airway, adequate oxygenation and ventilation, and correcting acid-base imbalance. Interventions include O_2 therapy, mobilizing secretions, and noninvasive or invasive positive pressure ventilation (PPV).

O_2 therapy. The main goal of O_2 therapy is to correct hypoxemia with O_2 administration. We apply O_2 at the lowest possible O_2 concentration needed to keep the PaO_2, SpO_2, and SaO_2 within patient-specific goals. Observe the response to O_2 therapy. Monitor for changes in mental status, respiratory rate, and ABGs. A trend toward a normal PaO_2 level lets you know that the patient is responsive to O_2.

There are several ways to provide O_2. Chapter 28 and Table 28.3 discuss O_2 delivery devices. The device selected depends on the patient's condition, degree of ARF, ability to maintain a patent airway, the amount of FiO_2 the device delivers, and their ability to breathe spontaneously. The selected O_2 delivery device must help maintain PaO_2 at 60 mm Hg or higher and SaO_2 at 90% or higher.

High-flow nasal cannula O_2 therapy is gaining more attention in treating hypoxemic and hypercapnic ARF. One advantage of this method is the ability to deliver very precise amounts of O_2 (e.g., up to 80 L/min with FiO_2 of 100%) with little effect from room air.[7] Humidification helps both loosen and facilitate removal of secretions, while enhancing patient comfort.

Breathing high O_2 concentrations for prolonged periods is not without potential adverse effects. Exposure to higher FiO_2 (greater than 60%) for longer than 48 hours poses a risk for *O_2 toxicity.* In this situation, the high O_2 levels cause inflammation and cell death by disrupting the alveolar-capillary membrane. *Absorption atelectasis* is another risk. O_2 can replace nitrogen and other gases normally present in the alveoli. Without nitrogen to help maintain the size and shape of the alveolus, structural support is lost, and the alveolus collapses. Other effects of prolonged exposure to high O_2 levels include activation of neutrophils, increased pulmonary capillary permeability, alveolar edema, atelectasis, and impaired tissue perfusion.[8]

Another risk of O_2 therapy is specific to patients with chronic hypercapnia (e.g., patients with COPD). Chronic hypercapnia blunts the response of chemoreceptors to high CO_2 levels as a respiratory stimulant. Initial O_2 therapy may be provided through a low-flow device, such as a nasal cannula at 1 to 2 L/min or a Venturi mask at 24% to 28%. Those who do not respond to O_2 therapy or other interventions may need mechanical ventilation with higher FiO_2.

Mobilizing secretions. Retained pulmonary secretions may cause or worsen ARF. This occurs because the movement of O_2

TABLE 32.4 Interprofessional Care

ARF

Diagnostic Assessment

- Vital signs with pulse oximetry (SpO_2)
- History and physical assessment
- Arterial blood gases (ABGs)
- Chest x-ray
- CBC with differential, electrolytes
- 12-Lead ECG
- Blood, sputum, and/or urine cultures (if indicated)
- Hemodynamic monitoring (if indicated)

Management

Respiratory Therapy

- O_2 therapy
- Mobilization of secretions
  - Positioning
  - Effective coughing
  - Chest physiotherapy
  - Suctioning of the airway
  - Humidification
  - Oral and/or IV hydration
  - Ambulation
- Positive pressure ventilation (PPV)
  - Noninvasive positive pressure ventilation (e.g., BiPAP)
  - Intubation with positive pressure ventilation

Drug Therapy

- Reduce pain, anxiety, restlessness (e.g., fentanyl, morphine, lorazepam)
- Relieve bronchospasm (e.g., albuterol)
- Reduce pulmonary congestion (e.g., furosemide, morphine)
- Treat pulmonary infections (e.g., antibiotics)
- Reduce airway inflammation (e.g., corticosteroids)

TABLE 32.5 NURSING MANAGEMENT

Care of Patients With ARF

- Monitor patients continuously for their response to therapy:
  - Respiratory and oxygenation status
  - Clinical signs of improved or worsening condition
  - Symptoms of respiratory failure
- Monitor hemodynamic status, including CVP, MAP, PAP, PAWP
- Implement measures to enhance oxygenation
  - Position patient to maximize ventilation
  - Encourage slow, deep breathing; turning; and coughing
  - Perform chest physiotherapy
  - Provide oral and IV hydration
  - Optimize balance between rest and activity
- Administer prescribed medications, including bronchodilators, diuretics, corticosteroids
- Monitor for and correct acid-base and electrolyte imbalances
- Maintain continuous ECG monitoring
- Obtain daily weight and maintain intake and output
- Prevent complications by providing prophylaxis for:
  - VAP (Table 32.9)
  - Stress ulcer (see Chapter 28)
  - VTE (see Chapter 41)
- Provide measures to reduce pain and anxiety
- Maintain open communication with patients and caregivers

Collaboration

Respiratory Therapy

- Apply supplemental O_2 as prescribed and titrate to maintain SpO_2
- Implement measures to provide optimal mechanical ventilation (see Chapter 28)
- Monitor the effects of position change on vital signs, ABGs, SpO_2, $ScvO_2$/SvO_2, end-tidal CO_2
- Perform suctioning
- Administer humidified air or O_2
- Administer prescribed aerosol treatments

Dietitian

- Determine, with dietitian, number of calories and type of nutrients needed
- Provide needed nutrition within limits of prescribed diet
- Select nutrition supplements
- Administer EN, PN

into the alveoli and the removal of CO_2 is severely limited or blocked. Secretions can be mobilized by proper positioning, effective coughing, chest physiotherapy, suctioning, humidification, hydration, and, when possible, early ambulation.

Positioning. Patients with ARF should always be positioned upright. Elevate the head of the bed at least 30 degrees or use chair-bed position. This helps maximize respiratory expansion, decrease dyspnea, and mobilize secretions. In a sitting position, ventilation and perfusion are best in the lung bases. If there is a chance for aspiration, position the patient side-lying.

We may place patients with a 1-sided lung problem in a lateral or side-lying position. This position, called *good lung down,* allows for improved V/Q matching in the affected lung. Pulmonary blood flow and ventilation are better in dependent lung areas. Secretions can drain out of the affected lung so they can be removed with suctioning. For example, place a patient with right-sided pneumonia on the left side. This will maximize ventilation and perfusion in the "good" lung and aid in secretion removal from the affected lung (postural drainage). Patients with ARF often have problems with both lungs. They may need to be repositioned to both sides at regular intervals to optimize air movement and secretion drainage.

As a result of the pandemic, placing patients in a prone position is more widely used. The purpose is to help improve oxygenation. Proning was often only undertaken with mechanically ventilated and heavily sedated patients in the ICU. Awake proning can achieve many benefits for patients who are not mechanically ventilated.[9] While beneficial in some situations, awake patients may have difficulty staying in the prone position and have significant discomfort.[10] Teaching about proning, positioning, and ensuring patient comfort may help.

Effective coughing. When secretions are present, encourage patients to cough. Unfortunately, not all patients will have enough strength or force to produce a cough that will clear the airway of secretions. *Augmented coughing (quad coughing)* may benefit some patients. To aid with augmented coughing, place 1 or both hands at the anterolateral base of the lungs. As you encourage the patient to breathe as deeply as possible, when expiration begins, move your hands forcefully upward. This increases abdominal pressure and helps the patient cough. It also increases expiratory flow and promotes removal of secretions.

Huff coughing and the *staged cough* can mobilize secretions. *Huff coughing* is a series of coughs performed while saying the word "huff." This technique prevents the glottis from closing, forcing air and mucus from the airways.[11] Huff coughing is described in Chapter 28. To perform a staged cough, the patient assumes a sitting position. They breathe in and out 3 or 4 times through the mouth, then cough while bending forward and pressing a pillow inward against the diaphragm.

Chest physiotherapy. Chest physiotherapy is indicated for all patients producing sputum or with severe atelectasis or pulmonary infiltrates on chest x-ray.[12] Postural drainage, percussion, and vibration to the affected lung segments help move secretions to the larger airways. Then they can be removed by coughing or suctioning. See more about chest physiotherapy in Chapter 28.

Suctioning. Suctioning may be needed if the patient is unable to expectorate secretions. Inserting a soft-tip suction catheter through a nasopharyngeal tube in the awake, nonintubated patient may help remove secretions at the back of the throat. Perform suctioning on a nonintubated patient with caution, as stimulating the gag reflex may induce vomiting. Suction through an artificial airway (e.g., endotracheal tube, tracheostomy) as needed (see Chapter 28).

Humidification. Humidification is an adjunct in secretion management. We can thin secretions with aerosols of sterile normal saline or mucolytic drugs (e.g., acetylcysteine mixed with a bronchodilator) given by nebulizer. O_2 given by aerosol mask can thin secretions and promote their removal. Aerosol therapy may cause bronchospasm and severe coughing, decreasing PaO_2. Frequent assessment of the patient's tolerance to therapy is needed.

Hydration. Thick, viscous secretions are hard to expel. Unless contraindicated, adequate fluid intake (2 to 3 L/day) keeps secretions thin and easier to remove. Patients who are unable to take enough fluids orally need IV hydration. Assess cardiac and renal status to determine whether the patient can tolerate the IV fluid volume and avoid HF and pulmonary edema. Regularly assess for signs of fluid overload (e.g., crackles, dyspnea, weight gain, increased CVP).

CHECK YOUR PRACTICE

You are caring for a 72-year-old male patient with hypoxemic ARF. He has a history of atrial flutter and COPD. A chest x-ray shows left-sided pneumonia. Your patient is awake but mildly confused. He has a productive cough with thick, yellow-green purulent sputum.

- What interventions would you expect to be ordered?

Positive pressure ventilation. If initial measures do not improve oxygenation and ventilation, the patient may need enhanced ventilatory assistance. Noninvasive positive pressure ventilation (NIPPV) is one option for the patient who is awake, alert, and able to maintain spontaneous ventilation, but requires a higher level of respiratory support. With NIPPV, it is possible to provide O_2 and decrease WOB, avoiding the need for intubation (Fig. 32.6).[12]

NIPPV is most useful in managing patients with CRF who have a secondary medical problem. For example, it may help patients with CRF that is worse due to cardiac problems or infection. It is an option for patients who refuse intubation but still want some degree of ventilatory support (e.g., patients with end-stage COPD). NIPPV is not appropriate for patients with a decreased level of consciousness, high O_2 requirements, hemodynamic instability, excess secretions, or GI bleeding.[13] NIPPV after extubation can help avoid reintubation. If respiratory status worsens with NIPPV, mechanical ventilation with higher O_2 concentrations is needed. Nursing management for patients with NIPPV is discussed in Chapter 28.

There are 2 forms of NIPPV used for patients with ARF: CPAP and BiPAP. Continuous positive airway pressure (CPAP) delivers 1 constant level of pressure during inspiration and expiration. The most frequently used NIPPV for ARF is BiPAP. BiPAP uses 2 different levels of positive pressure (one on inspiration, another on expiration). BiPAP provides O_2 therapy and humidification, decreases WOB, and reduces respiratory muscle fatigue. It helps open collapsed airways and decrease shunt.

Drug Therapy

Goals of drug therapy include (1) reduce airway inflammation and bronchospasm, (2) relieve pulmonary congestion, (3) treat infection (if present), and (4) reduce anxiety, pain, and restlessness. Drug therapy depends on several factors. These include the cause and severity of ARF, any comorbidities, and whether an infection is present.

Reduce airway inflammation and bronchospasm. Relief of bronchospasm increases alveolar ventilation. In acute bronchospasm, short-acting bronchodilators may be given at 15- to 30-minute intervals until a response occurs. Side effects include tachycardia and hypertension. Prolonged use increases the risk for dysrhythmias and cardiac ischemia. Monitor vital signs and ECG for any changes.

Corticosteroids (e.g., IV methylprednisolone) may be used with other drugs, such as bronchodilators, to relieve inflammation and bronchospasm. It may take several hours to see their effects. Inhaled corticosteroids may take 4 to 5 days for optimum therapeutic effects, so they will not relieve dyspnea or increased WOB quickly.

DRUG ALERT

IV Corticosteroids

- Monitor potassium levels. Corticosteroids worsen hypokalemia caused by diuretics.
- Prolonged use causes adrenal insufficiency.
- Hyperglycemia, especially in those with diabetes, is common.

Relieve pulmonary congestion. Interstitial fluid can accumulate in the lungs because of injury to the alveolar-capillary membrane. IV diuretics (e.g., furosemide), morphine, or nitroglycerin can decrease pulmonary congestion by helping remove excess fluid from the body, reducing afterload, and decreasing WOB. Use caution when giving these drugs, especially in older adults. Changes in heart rate and rhythm and significant decreases in BP are common.

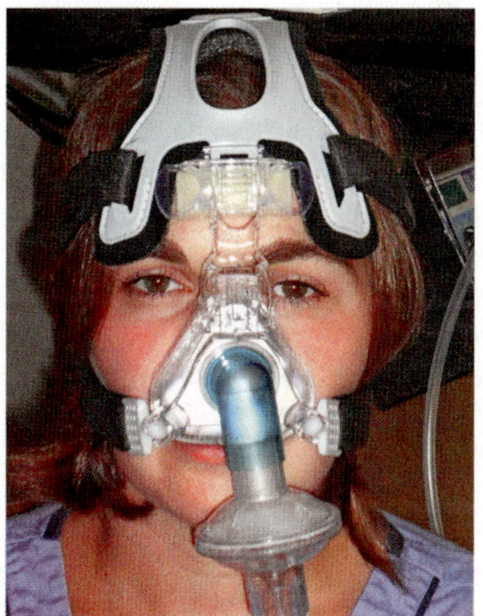

Fig. 32.6 Noninvasive BiPAP ventilation. A mask is placed over the nose or nose and mouth. Positive pressure from a mechanical ventilator aids the patient's breathing efforts, decreasing the work of breathing. (Courtesy Richard Arbour, RN, MSN, CCRN, CNRN, CCNS, FAAN, and Anna Kirk, RN, MSN.)

Treat infection. Lung infections (e.g., pneumonia, acute bronchitis) can cause or worsen ARF. They can result in excess mucus production, fever, increased O_2 consumption, and inflamed, fluid-filled, and/or collapsed alveoli. Alveoli that are fluid filled or collapsed cannot take part in gas exchange. IV antibiotics are given to treat infection. Chest x-rays can show the location and extent of infection. Sputum cultures identify the organisms causing the infection and their sensitivity to antimicrobial drugs.

Reduce anxiety, pain, and restlessness. Anxiety, pain, and restlessness may result from hypoxemia and dyspnea. They increase O_2 consumption and CO_2 production (from an increased metabolic rate) and increase WOB. For nonintubated patients, this may cause tachypnea and ineffective ventilation. For intubated patients, this may cause ventilator dyssynchrony and increase the risk for unplanned extubation (see Chapter 28).

We promote patient comfort in several ways. Frequently turn and reposition the patient. Provide reassurance and emotional support to patients and caregivers. IV benzodiazepines (e.g., lorazepam) and opioids (e.g., morphine) in small doses may decrease anxiety, restlessness, and pain. Assess for treatable causes of restlessness (e.g., hypoxemia, pain, delirium) and manage as needed. Do not depend solely on the use of analgesics and sedatives.

! SAFETY ALERT

Managing Restlessness and Sedation

- Monitor patients closely for CNS, cardiac, and respiratory depression when giving sedative and analgesic drugs, especially in nonintubated patients.
- Sedative and analgesic drugs may have a prolonged effect in critically ill and older adult patients. This can delay weaning from mechanical ventilation and increase ICU and hospital length of stay.

Nutrition Therapy

Maintaining protein and energy stores is important. The hypermetabolic state increases the calories needed to maintain a stable body weight and muscle mass. Nutrition depletion causes a loss of muscle mass, including the respiratory muscles, which may delay recovery. The dietitian often determines the best method of feeding and optimal calorie and fluid requirements. Ideally, enteral nutrition (EN) should be started within 24 to 48 hours (see Chapter 44).

◆ Evaluation

The expected outcomes are that patients with ARF will

- Independently maintain a patent airway
- Maintain adequate oxygenation and ventilation
- Demonstrate hemodynamic stability
- Achieve a return to baseline respiratory system function

Gerontologic Considerations: ARF

Many factors contribute to an increased risk for ARF in older adults. The reduced ventilatory capacity that accompanies aging increases the risk for ARF. Physiologic changes in the lungs include fewer functioning alveoli, decreased elasticity within the airways, and connective tissue changes.[14] Decreased chest wall compliance, decreased respiratory muscle strength, decreased cough, and increased risk of aspiration occur.[15]

In older adults, the $Pa{O_2}$ falls further, and the $Pa{CO_2}$ rises to a higher level before the respiratory system is stimulated to change the rate and depth of breathing. This delayed response contributes to respiratory insufficiency. A history of tobacco use can accelerate age-related respiratory changes. Poor nutrition status and less physiologic reserve in the cardiopulmonary system increase the risk for further compromising respiratory function.

ACUTE RESPIRATORY DISTRESS SYNDROME

Acute respiratory distress syndrome (ARDS) is a sudden and progressive form of ARF in which the alveolar-capillary membrane becomes damaged and more permeable to intravascular fluid (Fig. 32.7). ARDS accounts for about 10% of adult ICU admissions and almost 25% of patients who need mechanical ventilation. ARDS causes over 74,500 deaths each year in the United States.[16] The mortality rate is closely aligned to the severity of ARDS. Up to 45% of patients with severe cases die.[17]

Etiology

Table 32.6 lists conditions that predispose patients to ARDS. The most common cause is sepsis. ARDS may develop because of multisystem organ dysfunction syndrome (MODS). Patients with multiple risk factors are 3 or 4 times more likely to develop ARDS.

Initially, a direct or indirect lung injury sets the stage for ARDS. In direct lung injury, the pathogen comes into contact with the lung tissue. For example, aspiration of GI contents into the lung initiates the inflammatory response. In an indirect injury, ARDS develops due to a problem somewhere else in the body. For example, bowel obstruction with perforation causes widespread inflammation and infection. As a result, septic mediators enter the bloodstream and move toward the lungs. The lungs provide a favorable environment for their proliferation. This is the beginning of ARF, which, left untreated, can progress to ARDS.

Pathophysiology

The pathophysiologic changes in ARDS are divided into 3 phases: (1) injury or exudative phase, (2) reparative or proliferative phase, and (3) fibrotic or fibroproliferative phase. The pathophysiology of ARDS is shown in Fig. 32.8.

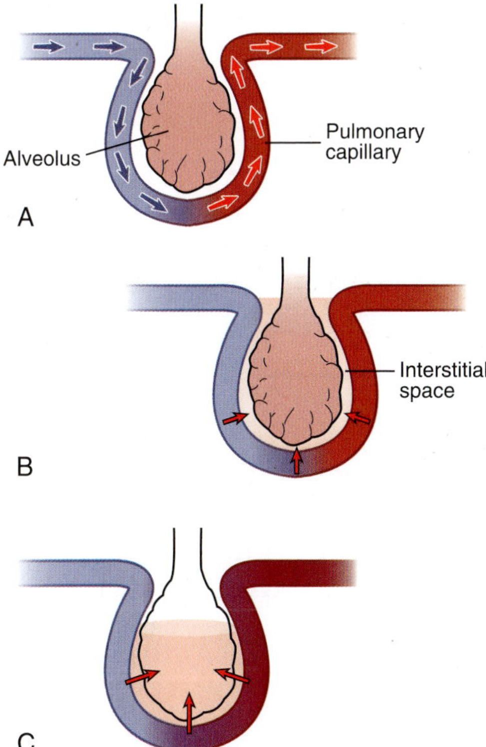

Fig. 32.7 Stages of edema formation in ARDS. (A) Normal alveolus and pulmonary capillary. (B) Interstitial edema occurs with accumulation of and increased flow of fluid into the interstitial space. (C) Alveolar edema occurs when the fluid crosses the alveolar-capillary membrane, causing severe impairment in gas exchange.

TABLE 32.6 Predisposing Conditions to ARDS

Direct Lung Injury	Indirect Lung Injury
Common Causes	
• Aspiration (gastric contents or other substances) • Bacterial or viral pneumonia	• Massive trauma • Other shock states (hypovolemic, cardiogenic) • Sepsis and septic shock (especially gram-negative infection) • Severe TBI
Less Common Causes	
• Chest trauma (blunt or penetrating) • Embolism: fat, air, amniotic fluid, thrombus • Inhalation of toxic substances • Near-drowning • O_2 toxicity • Radiation pneumonitis	• Acute pancreatitis • Cardiopulmonary bypass • Disseminated intravascular coagulation • Opioid drug overdose • Transfusion-related acute lung injury (e.g., multiple blood transfusions) • Urosepsis

Injury or Exudative Phase

The *injury or exudative phase* usually occurs 24 to 72 hours after the initial insult (direct or indirect). It generally lasts 7 to 10 days.[18] Engorgement of the peribronchial and perivascular interstitial space causes interstitial edema. Fluid in the lung tissue surrounding the alveoli crosses the alveolar membrane and enters the alveolar space. V/Q mismatch and shunt develop because alveoli begin to fill with fluid. Blood in the capillary network cannot be oxygenated.

We do not know the exact cause of alveolar-capillary membrane damage. Some think it is caused by the inflammatory response and stimulation of immune system. These events attract neutrophils to the lung tissues. Neutrophils release biochemical, humoral, and cellular mediators that damage the lung. Changes that occur from mediator activity include increased pulmonary capillary membrane permeability, collagen destruction, formation of pulmonary microemboli, and pulmonary artery vasoconstriction.

Hypoxemia and the stimulation of juxtacapillary receptors in the stiff lung tissue *(J reflex)* initially cause an increase in respiratory rate and a decrease in tidal volume (V_T). This breathing pattern increases CO_2 removal, causing respiratory alkalosis. CO increases in response to hypoxemia, a compensatory effort to increase pulmonary blood flow. As atelectasis increases, and pulmonary edema and pulmonary shunt worsen, the body's ability to compensate fails. Hypoventilation, decreased CO, and decreased tissue O_2 perfusion occur.

The changes caused by ARDS damage alveolar type I and II cells. This damage, in addition to fluid and protein accumulation, results in surfactant dysfunction. When surfactant synthesis is decreased or surfactant becomes inactivated, alveoli collapse, and atelectasis occurs. Widespread atelectasis further decreases lung compliance, compromises gas exchange, and contributes to hypoxemia. The hyaline membrane that lines the inside of each alveolus thickens, impairing diffusion. This worsens hypoxemia and causes even more atelectasis, which further impairs gas exchange.

Severe V/Q mismatch and shunting of pulmonary capillary blood result in hypoxemia unresponsive to increasing O_2 concentrations. This classic sign of ARDS is called **refractory hypoxemia**. In other words, despite receiving higher O_2 concentrations, the patient does not respond. There is no increase in PaO_2, SaO_2, or SpO_2. The patient's condition continues to get worse. As the lungs become less compliant because of decreased surfactant, pulmonary edema, and atelectasis, the patient must generate higher airway pressures to inflate "stiff" lungs. Reduced lung compliance increases WOB. When the patient can no longer maintain spontaneous ventilation, they need mechanical ventilation.

Reparative or Proliferative Phase

The *reparative* or *proliferative phase* of ARDS begins 1 to 2 weeks after the initial lung injury.[19] During this phase, there continues to be an influx of neutrophils, monocytes, lymphocytes, and fibroblasts as part of the inflammatory response. Increased pulmonary vascular resistance and pulmonary hypertension may occur because fibroblasts and inflammatory cells damage the pulmonary vasculature. Lung compliance continues to decrease due to interstitial fibrosis. Hypoxemia continues because of the thickened alveolar membrane. This

PATHOPHYSIOLOGY MAP

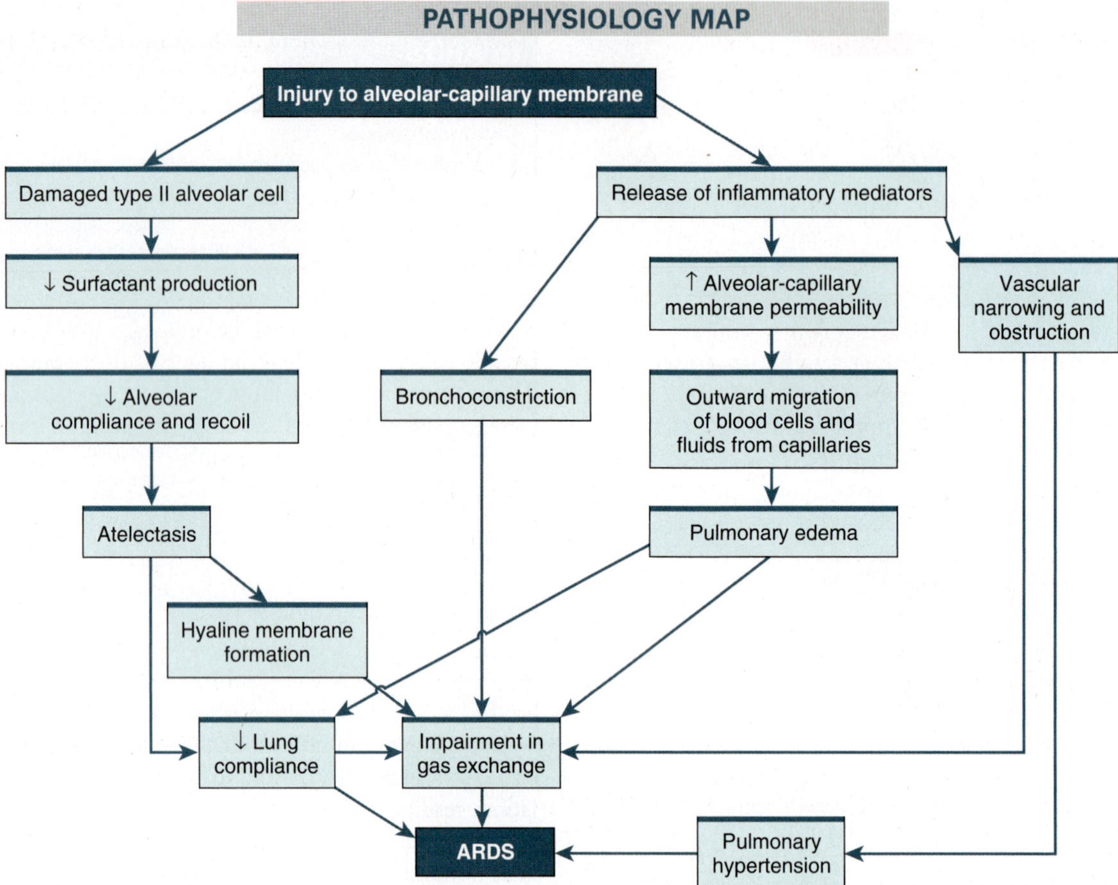

Fig. 32.8 Pathophysiology of ARDS.

causes V/Q mismatch, diffusion limitation, and shunting. Fluid in the lungs and secretions in the airways increase airway resistance. The proliferative phase is complete when dense, fibrous tissue replaces the diseased lung. If the reparative phase persists, widespread fibrosis results. If the reparative phase stops, the lesions may resolve.

Fibrotic or Fibroproliferative Phase

The *fibrotic phase* (*chronic* or *late phase*) of ARDS may start as early as 24 hours after the initial lung injury and may last several weeks.[2] Not all patients who develop ARDS enter the fibrotic stage. For those who do, it is associated with a poorer prognosis. Collagenous and fibrous tissues remodel the lung. Diffuse scarring of the lungs, interstitial fibrosis, and enlarged alveoli result in decreased lung compliance. Fibrosis reduces the surface area for gas exchange. Hypoxemia is common, even as the patient improves. Pulmonary hypertension may result from pulmonary vascular changes and fibrosis.

Clinical Progression

The progression of ARDS varies. Some survive the acute phase of lung injury. Pulmonary edema resolves, and recovery occurs within 1 or 2 weeks. The chance for survival is poorer in those who enter the fibrotic stage. Some patients may need several weeks of long-term mechanical ventilation. It is not known why injured lungs repair and recover in some patients and worsen in others. Several factors affect the course and outcome of ARDS. These include the nature of the initial injury, extent, and severity of comorbidities, how quickly the patient received medical care, and additional pulmonary complications (e.g., pneumothorax).

Most patients completely recover from ARDS within a year. Not all patients regain normal lung function. Abnormal lung function can persist for years. Patients may have fatigue, chest pain, and persistent dyspnea. The severity of scarring and changes within the lungs are key factors. Mechanical ventilation, duration of time ventilated, and use of extracorporeal membrane oxygenation (ECMO) may be contributing factors.[20]

Clinical Manifestations and Diagnostic Studies

The initial presentation of ARDS is often subtle. At the time of the initial injury, and for the first 24 to 72 hours, the patient may not have respiratory symptoms or have only mild dyspnea, tachypnea, cough, and restlessness. Lung auscultation may be normal or reveal fine, scattered crackles. ABGs may show mild hypoxemia and respiratory alkalosis caused by hyperventilation. The chest x-ray may be normal or reveal diffusely scattered, but minimal interstitial infiltrates.

As ARDS evolves, symptoms worsen because of hypoxemia (Table 32.2). Respiratory distress becomes evident as WOB increases. Tachypnea and intercostal and suprasternal retractions may be present. Tachycardia, diaphoresis, mental status changes, and pallor may occur. Lung auscultation usually reveals scattered to diffuse crackles and coarse crackles on expiration. After 72 hours, the chest x-ray often shows diffuse and extensive bilateral interstitial and alveolar infiltrates (Fig. 32.9). We often refer to this as a "whiteout" because consolidation and infiltrates are widespread, leaving few recognizable air spaces. Pleural effusions may be present.

As ARDS progresses, ABGs reflect changes in oxygenation and ventilation. Refractory hypoxemia is the hallmark characteristic of ARDS. Hypercapnia often signifies that respiratory muscle fatigue and hypoventilation have severely affected gas exchange. Respiratory failure is imminent.

The Berlin definition of ARDS helps us identify patients with ARDS and determine its severity (Table 32.7).[21] To help evaluate the severity of hypoxemia, we can calculate the **Pao_2/Fio_2 (P/F) ratio**. This measure reflects the ratio of the Pao_2 to the Fio_2 that the patient is receiving. Under normal circumstances (e.g., Pao_2 80 to 100 mm Hg; Fio_2 0.21 [room air]), the P/F ratio is greater than 400 (e.g., 95/0.21 = 452). With lung injury and impaired O_2 delivery, the Pao_2 often is lower than expected despite increased Fio_2. The P/F ratio distinguishes among mild (<300), moderate (<200), and severe (<100) ARDS.

CHECK YOUR PRACTICE

You are caring for a 26-year-old female with ARDS who experienced near-drowning 4 days ago. She is mechanically ventilated and receiving IV sedation. Ventilator settings: full support (control mode), Fio_2 0.90 (90%), PEEP +15 cm H_2O, V_T 350 mL, respiratory rate 18 breaths/min (patient taking no breaths above the ventilator rate), peak pressure 35 cm H_2O. Pao_2 is 83 mm Hg.

- Calculate and interpret the Pao_2/Fio_2 (P/F) ratio.

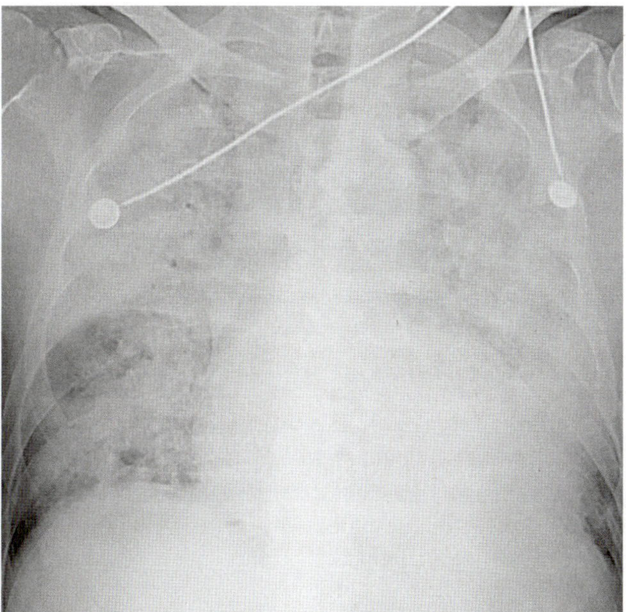

Fig. 32.9 Chest x-ray of a patient with ARDS. The x-ray shows extensive areas of consolidation. (From Walker CM, Chung JH: *Muller's imaging of the chest,* ed 2, St Louis, 2019, Elsevier.)

Complications

Complications may develop because of ARDS itself or its treatment (Table 32.8). Besides the lungs, the organs most often involved are the kidneys, liver, and heart. The main cause of death in ARDS is MODS, often accompanied by sepsis.

Complications of Mechanical Ventilation

Patients with ARDS are at risk for all the complications associated with mechanical ventilation as any other patient. These include volutrauma (when too large of tidal volume is used to deliver air to stiff, noncompliant lungs), barotrauma, stress ulcers, and ventilator-associated pneumonia (VAP). Implement a ventilator bundle to reduce the incidence of VAP (Table 32.9).[22] Complications of mechanical ventilation are discussed in Chapter 28.

Venous Thromboembolism (VTE)

Patients receiving mechanical ventilation are at risk for venous thromboembolism (VTE), which includes deep vein thrombosis (DVT) and pulmonary emboli. Care includes intermittent pneumatic compression devices, anticoagulation, active and passive range of motion, and, when possible, early ambulation (see Chapter 41).

Acute Kidney Injury

AKI occurs from decreased renal perfusion, with subsequent decreased O_2 delivery. This most often occurs because of hypotension from shock. It may also result from hypoxemia or nephrotoxic drugs (e.g., vancomycin) used to treat ARDS-related infections.

TABLE 32.7 Diagnostic Criteria

Berlin Definition of ARDS

Timing
Acute onset; within 1 week (7 days) of a known clinical insult or new or worsening respiratory symptoms

Pulmonary Edema
Respiratory failure cannot be explained by cardiac failure or intravascular volume overload

Chest X-Ray
Bilateral opacities: not fully explained by effusions, lobar/lung collapse, or nodules

Oxygenation
- *Mild ARDS:* Pao_2/Fio_2 ratio $\leq$300 with PEEP or CPAP $\geq$5 cm H_2O
- *Moderate ARDS:* Pao_2/Fio_2 ratio $\leq$200 with PEEP or CPAP $\geq$5 cm H_2O
- *Severe ARDS:* Pao_2/Fio_2 ratio <100 with PEEP or CPAP $\geq$5 cm H_2O

From Fujishima S: Guideline-based management of acute respiratory failure and acute respiratory distress syndrome, *J Intens Care* 11:10, 2023.

TABLE 32.8 Complications of ARDS

Cardiovascular
- Dysrhythmias
- Hypotension

CNS and Psychologic
- Delirium
- PTSD

GI
- Hypermetabolic state, ↑ nutrient requirements
- Paralytic ileus
- Pneumoperitoneum
- Stress ulcers and GI bleeding

Hematologic
- Disseminated intravascular coagulation
- Thrombocytopenia
- Venous thromboembolism (VTE)

Infection
- Antibiotic resistance
- Catheter-related infection (e.g., central and peripheral IV catheters, urinary)

Musculoskeletal
- Muscle weakness
- Critical illness polyneuropathy

Renal
- Acute kidney injury (AKI)

Respiratory
- Mechanical ventilation: barotrauma, volutrauma
- Pneumothorax
- Prolonged mechanical ventilation, tracheostomy
- Pulmonary fibrosis
- Ventilator-associated pneumonia (VAP)

Monitoring intake and output hourly, tracking daily weights, and observing trends in daily creatinine and BUN levels are important. When AKI occurs, many patients receive continuous renal replacement therapy (CRRT) (see Chapter 51). They cannot tolerate losing the large volumes of fluid with traditional hemodialysis. The overall mortality rate for patients with ARDS is higher in those who need CRRT.

Psychologic Issues

Patients who survive ARDS may have anxiety, memory problems, inability to focus, nightmares, depression, and in some instances, posttraumatic stress disorder (PTSD). PTSD can occur in ARDS survivors up to 5 years later. It is important to identify and address these issues in ARDS survivors.

TABLE 32.9 Essential Components of a Ventilator Bundle

- Avoid intubation (if possible), prevent reintubation
  - High-flow nasal cannula or NIPPV (e.g., Bi-PAP)
- Minimize use of sedation
  - Decrease use of benzodiazepines
  - Implement protocols to minimize analgesia and sedation and facilitate extubation
  - Daily assessment of readiness for extubation (see Table 28.16)
- Elevate head of the bed 30–45 degrees
- Oral care without chlorhexidine
- Early enteral nutrition
- Establish regular physical therapy plan
- Change the mechanical ventilator circuit only if visibly soiled

From Klompas M, Branson R, Cawcutt K, et al: Strategies to prevent ventilator-associated pneumonia, ventilator-associated events, and non-ventilator hospital-acquired pneumonia in acute care hospitals: 2022 update, *Infect Control Hosp Epidemiol* 43:687, 2022.

NURSING AND INTERPROFESSIONAL MANAGEMENT: ARDS

Patients with ARDS will receive care in an ICU. Management of patients with ARF (Tables 32.4 and 32.5) and the nursing care plan for ARF (eNursing Care Plan 32.1 available on the website for this chapter) apply to patients with ARDS. The next section discusses additional care for patients with ARDS (Table 32.10). Even with appropriate therapy, the clinical course of ARDS is complex and unpredictable.

Assessment

Because ARDS is the most severe form of ARF, the subjective and objective data you would obtain from patients with ARDS are the same as those for ARF (Table 32.3).

Planning

Overall goals for patients with ARDS include maintaining a Pa_{O_2} of 60 mm Hg or higher, maintaining hemodynamic stability, correcting acid-base and/or electrolyte imbalances, reducing WOB, and identifying and treating the cause. Longer-term goals include (1) Pa_{O_2} within normal limits for age or at baseline on room air, (2) Sa_{O_2} greater than 90%, (3) resolution of the cause(s), and (4) avoiding complications.

Implementation

Respiratory Management

Best practices in respiratory care for patients with ARDS include (1) O_2 administration, (2) mechanical ventilation with low V_T ventilation, permissive hypercapnia, and PEEP, (3) prone positioning, and (4) ECMO.[23]

O_2 administration. The primary goal of O_2 therapy is to correct hypoxemia. Initially, high-flow O_2 delivery, including

TABLE 32.10 Interprofessional Care

ARDS

General Care

- Hemodynamic monitoring
- Identify and treat underlying cause

Respiratory Therapy (see Chapter 28)

- O_2 administration
- Mechanical ventilation
  - Low V_T ventilation
  - Permissive hypercapnia
  - PEEP
- Positioning (e.g., prone)
- Extracorporeal membrane oxygenation (ECMO)

Supportive Care

- Analgesia and sedation
- Neuromuscular blocking agents
- IV fluids
- Inotropic and vasopressor drugs
  - norepinephrine
  - vasopressin
  - dopamine
  - dobutamine
- VAP prophylaxis (Table 32.9)
- Nutrition therapy
- Stress ulcer prophylaxis
- VTE prophylaxis

BiPAP, that delivers higher O_2 concentrations to maximize O_2 delivery may be all that is needed. Continuously monitor SpO_2 to assess the effectiveness of O_2 therapy. If respiratory function worsens, high-flow O_2 will not be able to keep the Pao_2 within acceptable ranges. Patients with moderate to severe ARDS and refractory hypoxemia need mechanical ventilation to maintain an acceptable Pao_2. Even with mechanical ventilation, patients with severe ARDS may need an Fio_2 of 100% to keep the Pao_2 at least 60 mm Hg. Most HCPs agree that in the injury and reparative phases, they may have to accept a lower-than-normal Pao_2 (e.g., Pao_2 55 to 80 mm Hg) and SpO_2 (88% to 95%).

Mechanical ventilation. Patients often need several days of mechanical ventilation to allow time for the overwhelming inflammation and fluid accumulation in the lungs to begin resolving. All mechanically ventilated patients with ARDS in the ICU will have continuous heart rate, respiratory rate, BP, and SpO_2 monitoring. $EtCO_2$ monitoring is standard.

Patients usually receive full support, pressure-control (PC) mechanical ventilation. PC helps keep the inspiratory and plateau pressures from becoming too high. This prevents alveolar overdistention and rupture. By reducing the amount of pressure going into the stiff, noncompliant lungs, hopefully we can help prevent further lung injury.

Patients are ventilated with a low V_T of 4 to 8 mL/kg.[2] Delivering a large V_T into stiff lungs can cause volutrauma and barotrauma. Volutrauma causes *alveolar fractures* (damage or tears in the alveolar-capillary membrane) and the movement of fluids and protein into the alveolar spaces. Low V_T ventilation reduces mortality and the risk for volutrauma.[24]

As a result of delivering a lower-than-normal V_T to a patient with ARDS, the $Paco_2$ level will slowly rise above normal limits. This is known as **permissive hypercapnia**. A $Paco_2$ of up to 70 mm Hg has been accepted in ARDS management.[23] Patients may not tolerate this rise in $Paco_2$, even if it is gradual. We do not use permissive hypercapnia with patients who are pregnant, have TBI, or have increased ICP.

Frequent ABG samples are needed with monitoring of pH, Pao_2, and $Paco_2$ values. The pH is kept greater than 7.30.[23] Acidosis and rising CO_2 levels are powerful stimulants to breathe. As a result, when permissive hypercapnia is used, patients usually receive continuous IV analgesia and sedation. If the patient continues to breathe over and above the set respiratory rate on the ventilator, neuromuscular blocking agents (NMBAs) are often given.

During PPV, it is common to apply PEEP in increments of 3 to 5 cm H_2O until oxygenation is adequate. PEEP increases the volume of air left in the lungs at the end of a normal expiration and helps open collapsed alveoli. PEEP may improve ventilation, thus allowing the Fio_2 to be lowered. Patients with ARDS may need higher levels of PEEP (e.g., 10 to 20 cm H_2O).

The added intrathoracic and intrapulmonic pressures generated by positive pressure in the lungs and transmitted to surrounding structures (e.g., inferior vena cava, heart) at end expiration can decrease venous return. Dramatic reductions in preload, cardiac output (CO), and BP can occur. High levels of PEEP or excess inspiratory pressures can cause barotrauma and volutrauma.

Prone positioning. Proning is an option for patients with refractory hypoxemia and ARDS who do not respond to other strategies to increase Pao_2. By turning the patient prone, perfusion may be better matched to ventilation (Fig. 32.10). Air-filled alveoli in the anterior part of the lung become dependent. Alveoli in the posterior part of the lungs are "recruited" (given the opportunity to reexpand), hopefully improving oxygenation. Early prone positioning (within the first 48 hours if possible) has been associated with reduced mortality in patients with moderate and severe ARDS.[25] They can stay in the prone position for up to 16 hours per day. We do not know the optimal length of time that a patient should be prone.

Placing a patient prone requires an ICU intensivist, respiratory therapist, and at least 3 nurses. It is labor intensive. Attention must be given to securing and maintaining the airway before, during, and after proning. Once prone, the patient needs to be reattached to hemodynamic monitoring equipment. Complications, including loss of airway, brachial plexus and pressure injuries, and cardiac arrest, can occur at any stage of proning or supination (returning the patient to a face-up position).

Some patients have a big improvement in Pao_2 soon after being proned. The improvement in oxygenation may be enough to allow a reduction in Fio_2 or PEEP. You may see hemodynamic instability (dysrhythmias, a decrease in BP) from

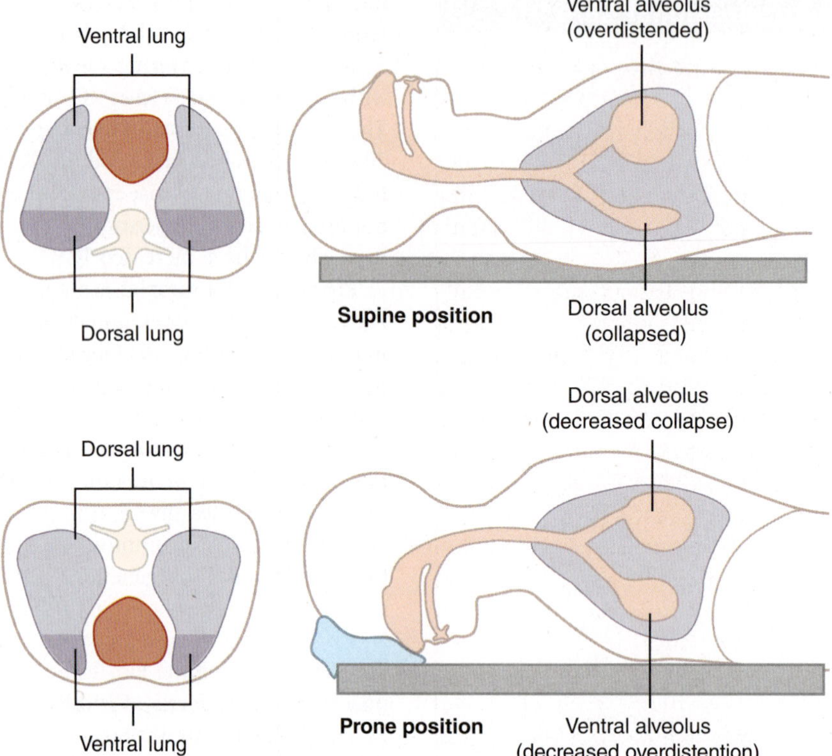

Fig. 32.10 Changes in the lung that occur because of prone positioning.

fluid shifts while patients are prone. There may be more need for airway suctioning as secretions are mobilized.

Alternatives to proning include continuous lateral rotation therapy (CLRT) and kinetic therapy. CLRT provides continuous, slow, side-to-side turning by rotating the actual bed frame less than 40 degrees. The bed moves laterally for 18 of every 24 hours to simulate postural drainage and help mobilize pulmonary secretions. Some beds have a vibration feature that provides chest physiotherapy. This assists with secretion mobilization and removal. Kinetic therapy is like CLRT, in that patients rotate side-to-side 40 degrees or more.

Whether your patient is proned or another option is chosen, obtain baseline assessments of their pulmonary status (e.g., respiratory rate and rhythm, breath sounds, ABGs, SpO_2). Continue to monitor the patient throughout the duration of therapy.

Extracorporeal membrane oxygenation (ECMO). ECMO is used most often in special ICUs in major cities. Like hemodialysis, a catheter is inserted into a large blood vessel (most often the internal jugular, femoral artery, or femoral vein). Blood exits the body through the catheter and enters the ECMO unit. There, O_2 is delivered into the blood, and CO_2 is removed. Oxygenated blood is returned to the patient. $ECCO_2R$ (extracorporeal CO_2 removal) is like ECMO. It does not require as high blood flow rates. It is only used to remove CO_2. ECMO and $ECCO_2R$ are expensive and require specially trained nurses and other personnel.

Supportive Care

Analgesia and sedation. Analgesia and sedation, by direct or continuous IV infusion, are essential. Analgesia and sedation decrease the discomfort from having an ET tube, help reduce WOB, and prevent patient-ventilator dyssynchrony.

Patients who breathe asynchronously with mechanical ventilation may benefit from adjusting ventilator inspiratory flow rates or other settings. Patients who stay asynchronous with mechanical ventilation despite aggressive analgesia and sedation may need an NMBA. NMBAs relax skeletal muscles and promote synchrony with mechanical ventilation. Remember that patients receiving an NMBA can appear to be asleep but still be awake and in pain. For this reason, simultaneous administration of analgesia and sedation with NMBAs is essential.

! SAFETY ALERT

Neuromuscular Blockade

- Always give concurrent analgesia and sedation to patients receiving an NMBA.
- This eliminates patient awareness, ensures patient comfort, and avoids the terrifying experience of being awake and in pain while pharmacologically paralyzed.
- Use an NMBA for the shortest duration and at the lowest dose possible to avoid complications.

Monitoring sedation levels in patients receiving NMBAs is challenging. Observe the patient's respiratory rate and whether they are taking breaths above the ventilator rate. If so, the patient may require an increase in analgesia, sedation, and/or NMBA. $EtCO_2$ monitoring can help detect spontaneous breathing by changes in $EtCO_2$ waveforms. A peripheral nerve stimulator is an additional adjunct used in some settings to help assess the depth of paralysis in patients receiving an NMBA.

Maintaining hemodynamic stability. Patients are frequently hemodynamically unstable and need vasopressors and/or inotropes to maintain heart rate and BP. Hemodynamic monitoring (e.g., arterial BP monitoring, CVP, SpO_2) is essential. BP and mean arterial pressure (MAP) are important indicators of CO. Bedside echocardiogram can evaluate cardiac function and fluid volume status. We may monitor stroke volume variation, CO, and mixed venous O_2 saturation ($ScvO_2$ or SvO_2) noninvasively. Dysrhythmias are common. Maintain continuous ECG monitoring. A decrease in CO is treated with IV fluids, drugs, or both. Chapter 42 discusses drugs used to treat decreased CO and shock. Monitoring trends in hemodynamic status over time allows us to adjust therapy as needed.

Maintaining fluid balance. Maintaining fluid balance is challenging. Increasing pulmonary capillary permeability results in fluid in the lungs and causes pulmonary edema. At the same time, patients may be intravascularly volume depleted and have hypotension and decreased CO (from mechanical ventilation and PEEP).

Monitor hemodynamic parameters and daily weights to assess fluid volume status. Monitor intake and output hourly. Keep patients with ARDS on the "dry" side. In other words, avoid aggressive resuscitation with IV fluids. Since ARDS is an inflammatory process, diuretics play a minimal role. Dialysis therapy, such as CRRT, can help by removing small amounts of fluid hourly.

Optimizing nutrition. Meeting nutrition needs of patients with ARDS is difficult. Maintaining protein and energy stores is important. Nutrition depletion causes a loss of muscle mass, including the respiratory muscles. This may prolong mechanical ventilation and delay recovery. Consult the dietitian. We should start EN as soon as possible, ideally within 24 to 48 hours. Sometimes we measure patients' resting energy expenditure using a metabolic cart to determine their ideal nutrition requirements. This noninvasive procedure involves measuring the patient's resting O_2 consumption and CO_2 production.

◆ Evaluation

The expected outcomes for patients with ARDS are like those for patients with ARF. Patients with ARDS should be able to maintain and sustain adequate oxygenation and ventilation with decreasing amounts of O_2, be hemodynamically stable, and be free of complications.

CASE STUDY

Acute Respiratory Distress Syndrome

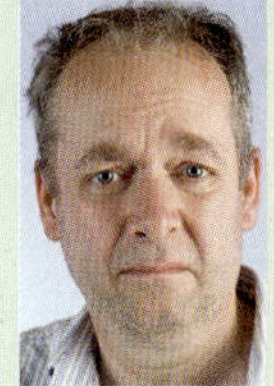

(© Thinkstock.)

Patient Profile

J.N., a 67-year-old male, was admitted 36 hours ago to the surgical ICU after emergent surgery for a small bowel obstruction, acute ischemic bowel, and perforated colon. During surgery, the HCP resected 2 feet of intestine, repaired perforated colon, and irrigated the abdominal cavity. J.N.'s BP decreased to 70 mm Hg for 6 minutes during surgery. He received 4 units of packed red blood cells and 5 L of 0.9% normal saline.

Postoperative Status

After surgery, J.N. was hemodynamically unstable (tachycardic, hypotensive) and unable to be extubated (weaned) from mechanical ventilation. His condition worsened over the first 24 hours in the ICU. He became more tachycardic and hypotensive. J.N. continued to have declining Sao_2 levels, increased WOB, and worsening hemodynamic status. Despite direct IV analgesia and sedation, his respiratory rate increased. He was often "out-of-sync" with the ventilator and required progressively higher Fio_2. A chest x-ray revealed bilateral pleural effusions and a right-sided pneumothorax, requiring chest tube placement. J.N. stayed dyssynchronous with the ventilator, so continuous IV analgesia and sedation infusions were ordered. NMBA was started to decrease his WOB and achieve ventilator synchrony.

Current Status

J.N. is hemodynamically unstable and requires IV norepinephrine to support BP. He is receiving 100% Fio_2 with PEEP 15 cm H_2O. Oxygenation continues to worsen. J.N. was diagnosed with AKI, and CRRT is being considered. His wife has brought in a copy of his advance directive. It states he does not want to be kept alive by artificial means. J.N.'s wife and adult children are at the bedside and voicing concerns to you about his condition and treatment.

Objective Data

Physical Assessment

- *CNS:* Sedated, paralyzed. Head of bed elevated 30 degrees. Temp 101°F (38.3°C) rectally
- *Cardiovascular:* BP 96/54 mm Hg. MAP 68 mm Hg. 2+ carotid, radial, and femoral pulses; 1+ dorsalis pedis pulses. Skin cool, slow capillary refill (greater than 5 seconds). ECG shows:

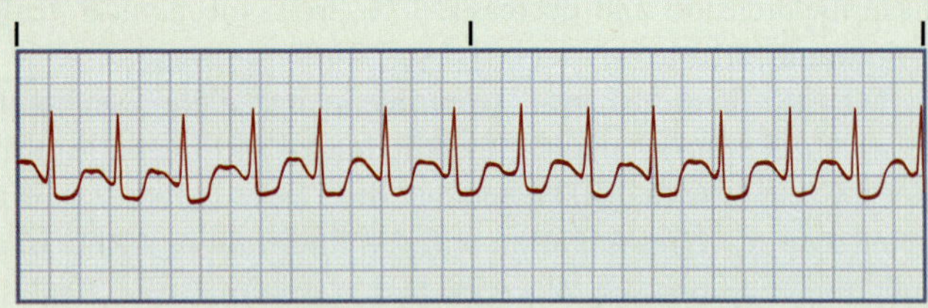

- *Ventilator settings:* V_T 350 mL, Fio_2 100%, rate 24/min, PEEP 15 cm H_2O, peak inspiratory pressure 35 cm H_2O
- *Respiratory:* Respiratory rate 24 breaths/min and in sync with ventilator. SpO_2 88%, coarse crackles bilaterally throughout all lung fields
- *GI:* Surgical dressing intact but shows small amount of "shadow" oozing; colostomy draining a moderate amount of serosanguineous drainage. NG tube draining a small amount of dark brown fluid. Currently NPO. Orders received to initiate EN at 10 mL/h
- *Renal:* Indwelling Foley catheter draining concentrated, dark amber urine less than 30 mL/h

Diagnostic Findings

- *Chest x-ray:* Bilateral, scattered interstitial infiltrates compatible with ARDS
- *Current ABGs:* pH 7.23, Pao_2 59 mm Hg, $Paco_2$ 57 mm Hg, HCO_3^- 16 mEq/L, O_2 saturation 88%
- Hemoglobin 6.9 g/dL (69 g/L), WBC 20.6/μL (20.6 × 10^9/L)
- Increased BUN and creatinine

Discussion Questions

1. ***Recognize:*** What is the cause of ARDS for J.N.? Is this a direct or indirect cause?
2. ***Recognize:*** How does the pathophysiology of ARDS predispose J.N. to refractory hypoxemia?
3. ***Analyze:*** What signs and symptoms does J.N. have that support a diagnosis of ARDS?
4. ***Analyze:*** Calculate the Pao_2/Fio_2 ratio. What does this value tell you about the seriousness of his condition?
5. ***Analyze:*** What other complications is J.N. at risk for from ARDS?
6. ***Plan:*** You are orienting a new nurse who asks you why you allowed J.N.'s family to stay at the bedside during the assessment and morning rounds with the ICU team. How would you respond?
7. ***Prioritize:*** What priority interventions should be implemented to improve J.N.'s respiratory status and hypoxemia?
8. ***Act:*** What information would you give to J.N.'s family about his status?
9. ***Act:*** Given J.N.'s advance directive, what ethical/legal issues could you encounter?

Answers available at http://evolve.elsevier.com/Lewis/medsurg.

BRIDGE TO NCLEX EXAMINATION

The number of the question corresponds to the same-numbered outcome at the beginning of the chapter.

1. Which signs and symptoms lead the nurse to suspect hypoxemic respiratory failure? **(Select all that apply.)**
   - **a.** Cyanosis
   - **b.** Tachypnea
   - **c.** Morning headache
   - **d.** Paradoxical breathing
   - **e.** Use of pursed-lip breathing
2. An important consideration in selecting an O_2 delivery device for the patient with acute hypoxemic respiratory failure is to
   - **a.** always start with noninvasive positive pressure ventilation.
   - **b.** apply a low-flow device, such as a nasal cannula or face mask.
   - **c.** be able to correct the Pao_2 to a normal level as quickly as possible.
   - **d.** base the selection on the patient's condition and amount of Fio_2 needed and delivered by the device.
3. The *most* common early manifestations of ARDS are:
   - **a.** dyspnea and tachypnea.
   - **b.** cyanosis and apprehension.
   - **c.** respiratory distress and frothy sputum.
   - **d.** bradycardia and increased work of breathing.
4. Interventions used in managing patients with ARDS include **(Select all that apply.)**
   - **a.** prone positioning.
   - **b.** IV injection of surfactant.
   - **c.** low tidal volume ventilation.
   - **d.** aggressive IV fluid resuscitation.
   - **e.** positive end expiratory pressure (PEEP).
5. Which intervention is *most* likely to limit volutrauma in patients with ARDS who are intubated and mechanically ventilated?
   - **a.** Increasing PEEP
   - **b.** Increasing the inspiratory flow rate
   - **c.** Use of low tidal volume ventilation
   - **d.** Suctioning the patient via endotracheal tube hourly

1. a, b, d; 2. d; 3. a; 4. a, c, e; 5. c.

For rationales to these answers and even more NCLEX review questions, visit http://evolve.elsevier.com/Lewis/medsurg.

REFERENCES

To access the References for this chapter, please scan the QR code with a mobile device.

CASE STUDY

Applying Clinical Judgment With Multiple Patients

You are assigned to care for the following 4 patients on a medical-surgical unit. You are sharing 1 AP with another RN.

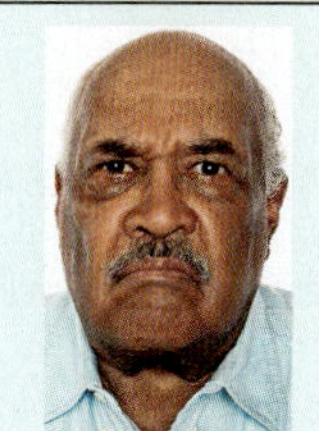 © Fuse/Thinkstock.	F.T., a 70-year-old male with COPD, was admitted 2 days ago with bilateral lower lobe pneumonia. He is receiving IV antibiotics. Vital signs: 150/70, 94, RR 24, 99.4°F (37.4°C), O_2 saturation 96% on O_2 at 3 L/min via nasal cannula.
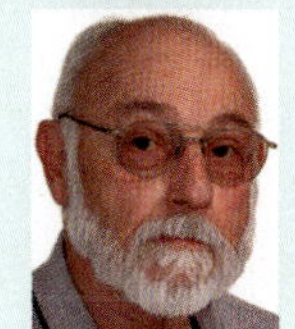 © iStockphoto/Thinkstock.	M.R., a 69-year-old male, is 3 days postoperative after a total laryngectomy with tracheostomy for laryngeal cancer. He developed pneumonia after surgery. He transferred from ICU at 0200 to accommodate a new patient. His last pain medication was 4 hours ago. He is awake, alert, but slightly confused. A tracheostomy tube is in place with O_2 via tracheal mask. Enteral nutrition running at 30 mL/h via gastrostomy tube. Vital signs: 168/94, 84, RR 22, O_2 saturation 96%.
© GiovanniSeabra/iStock.com	J.H. is a 59-year-old male with right lower lobe pneumonia and Stage 4 small cell lung cancer. He is intermittently confused and anxious. Vital signs: 118/62, 106, RR 28 and shallow, 102.6°F (39.2°C), O_2 saturation 92% on O_2 at 4 L/min via nasal cannula.
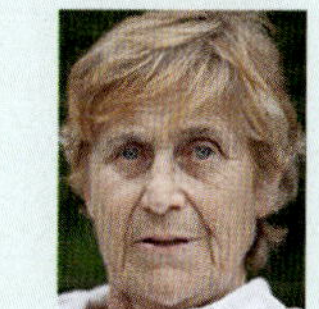 © iStockphoto/Thinkstock.	H.M. is a 68-year-old female admitted 6 days ago with a COPD exacerbation. She has not been able to ambulate much because of her shortness of breath. She is on oral prednisone and ipratropium. She is being discharged later today. She is starting Advair Diskus and O_2 therapy at home.

1. Highlight all the findings above that require your follow-up.
2. After receiving report, which patient would you see first?
3. Which morning tasks can you delegate to the AP? **(Select all that apply.)**
   a. Take vital signs and a pulse oximetry reading on F.T.
   b. Assess M.R.'s pain level and show him how to administer his feeding.
   c. Assist H.M. with AM care and gather belongings in anticipation of discharge.
   d. Provide coffee for J.H.'s family as they await a family meeting with the HCP.
   e. Teach F.T. how to do pursed-lip breathing and titrate O_2 to maintain saturation >95%.
4. While you are assessing J.H., the AP tells you that H.M. is reporting chest pain and worsening shortness of breath. M.R. is requesting pain medication. What is your best option?
   a. Ask the AP to get H.M.'s vital signs while you give M.R. pain medication.
   b. Ask the AP to increase H.M.'s O_2 to L/min while you assess M.R.'s pain.
   c. Ask the AP to obtain a stat 12-lead ECG on H.M. while you perform a focused cardiac and respiratory assessment.
   d. Ask the AP to have another RN give M.R. his pain medication while you go directly to H.M.'s room.

Case Study Progression

After assessing H.M., you notify the HCP. A stat 12-lead ECG is done, and a blood sample is drawn to check cardiac enzymes. H.M.'s chest pain is not relieved by sublingual nitroglycerin. You then give 1 mg IV morphine. H.M. states that the pain is "a little better" but continues to report dyspnea. The 12-lead ECG and cardiac enzyme results are all within normal limits.

5. Based on these findings, you recognize that H.M. may be experiencing _____1_____ and anticipate the HCP will order _____2_____ to determine the cause of her symptoms.

Options for 1	Options for 2
Acute heart failure	BNP and echocardiogram
Pneumothorax	D-dimer and spiral CT scan
Pulmonary embolism	ABGs and chest x-ray

6. While the transport nurse goes with H.M. to the radiology department, you turn your attention back to your remaining 3 patients. You see that you need to complete M.R.'s medication reconciliation after his transfer and prepare his morning medications. Complete the information missing from the table below by selecting from the lists of options provided.

Medication	Dose, Route, Frequency	Drug Class	Indication
acetaminophen	**1**	Analgesic; antipyretic	Reduce pain and fever
2	40 mg subcut daily	Anticoagulant	VTE prophylaxis
ceftriaxone	1 gram IV q12hr	Cephalosporin	**3**
omeprazole	40 mg IV daily	**4**	Stress ulcer prophylaxis
Options for 1	***Options for 2***	***Options for 3***	***Options for 4***
325 mg rectal q4h as needed 650 mg PEG q6h as needed 1000 mg PEG q6h as needed	Enoxaparin Heparin Warfarin	Chemotherapy for laryngeal cancer Relieve dry mouth Treat postoperative pneumonia	Antacid Histamine receptor blocker Proton pump inhibitor

7. Before giving M.R.'s 0900 enteral feeding, you find his PEG tube clogged. Which action would you take *next*?
   a. Flush the tube with warm water, using a back-and-forth motion.
   b. Obtain an x-ray to confirm the tube is still placed in the stomach.
   c. Notify the HCP so that surgery to insert new tube can be scheduled.
   d. Instill 30 mL of cranberry juice into the tube and recheck in 1 hour.

CASE STUDY—cont'd

Applying Clinical Judgment With Multiple Patients

8. You perform F.T.'s assessment and update his plan of care.
For each assessment finding, use an X to indicate whether the interventions were *Effective* (helped meet expected outcomes) or *Ineffective* (did not help meet expected outcomes).

Assessment Finding	Effective	Ineffective
Lungs have bibasilar coarse crackles		
Peripheral edema is 3+ bilaterally		
Performs active range of motion without dyspnea		
Heart rate 80/min, regular		
Restlessness, slightly confused		
Afebrile		
Anorexia with weight loss		
Clear sputum		

9. J.H.'s son calls you on the telephone to ask about his father's condition and long-term prognosis. Which initial response would be *most* appropriate?
   a. Ask the person what the code word is to identify himself as family.
   b. Empathize with the son's need to know his father's long-term prognosis.
   c. Tell him you are not allowed to discuss any information over the telephone.
   d. Ask J.H.'s son what the HCP has told him to clarify his understanding of the situation.
10. Which 2 interprofessional team members would be most appropriate to involve in caring for J.H. right now and why?
   a. Lawyer
   b. Dietitian
   c. Social worker
   d. Physical therapist
   e. Respiratory therapist
   f. Occupational therapist

Answers available at http://evolve.elsevier.com/Lewis/medsurg.

33

Assessment: Hematologic System

Sandra Irene Rome

http: //evolve.elsevier.com/Lewis/medsurg/

CONCEPTUAL FOCUS

Clotting
Functional Ability
Gas Exchange
Infection
Perfusion

LEARNING OUTCOMES

1. Describe the structures and functions of the hematologic system.
2. Distinguish between the different types of blood cells and their functions.
3. Explain the process of hemostasis.
4. Link the age-related changes in the hematologic system to differences in findings of hematologic studies.
5. Obtain subjective and objective assessment data related to the hematologic system.
6. Perform a physical assessment of the hematologic system.
7. Distinguish normal from common abnormal findings of a hematologic physical assessment.
8. Describe the purpose, significance of results, and nursing responsibilities related to diagnostic studies of the hematologic system.

KEY TERMS

ecchymoses
erythropoiesis
fibrinolysis
hematopoiesis
hemolysis
leukopenia
neutropenia
pancytopenia
petechiae
reticulocyte
thrombocytopenia
thrombocytosis

Hematology is the study of blood and blood-forming tissues. This includes the bone marrow, blood, spleen, and lymph system. You need basic knowledge of hematology to be able to assess several important concepts in the clinical setting. A functioning hematologic system supports our ability to transport oxygen (O_2), carbon dioxide (CO_2), nutrients, wastes, and electrolytes. It maintains intravascular volume, coagulates blood, and combats infections.[1]

STRUCTURES AND FUNCTIONS OF THE HEMATOLOGIC SYSTEM

Bone Marrow

Blood cell production (**hematopoiesis**) occurs within the bone marrow. *Bone marrow* is the soft material that fills the central core of bones. There are 2 types of bone marrow, yellow (adipose) and red (hematopoietic). Red marrow actively makes blood cells. In adults, we find red marrow mainly in the flat and irregular bones. These include the ends of long bones, pelvic bones, vertebrae, sacrum, sternum, ribs, flat cranial bones, and scapulae.

All 3 types of blood cells (red blood cells [RBCs], white blood cells [WBCs], platelets) develop from a common hematopoietic stem cell in the bone marrow. The hematopoietic *stem cell* is best described as an immature blood cell that can self-renew and differentiate into hematopoietic precursor cells. Several types of blood cells form as the cells mature and differentiate (Fig. 33.1).

The bone marrow responds by a negative feedback system to the need for specific blood cells by increasing that cell's production. Various factors or cytokines (e.g., erythropoietin, granulocyte colony-stimulating factor [G-CSF], stem cell factor, thrombopoietin) stimulate the bone marrow. This results in stem cells differentiating into one of the committed hematopoietic cells (e.g., RBC). For example, when tissue hypoxia occurs, the kidney secretes erythropoietin. It circulates to the bone marrow and causes proerythroblasts to differentiate in the bone marrow.

Blood

Blood is a type of connective tissue. It has 3 major functions: transportation, regulation, and protection (Table 33.1). Blood

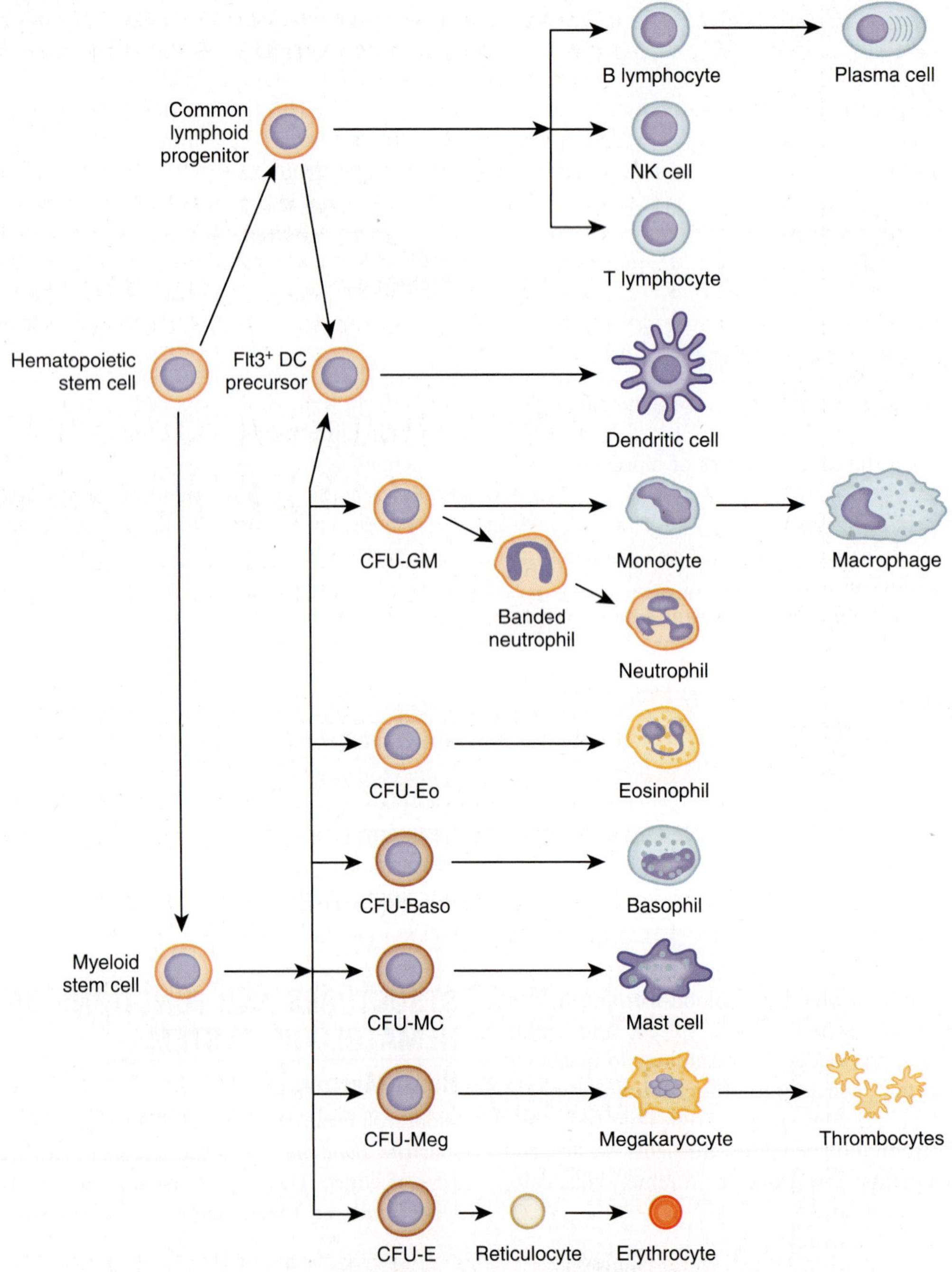

Fig. 33.1 Development of blood cells.

has 2 major components: plasma and blood cells. In an adult weighing between 150 and 180 lb, the volume of blood is between 4.7 and 5.5 L (5 to 6 quarts).

Plasma

About 55% of blood is plasma (Fig. 33.2).[1] Plasma is composed mainly of water. It also contains proteins, electrolytes, gases, nutrients (e.g., glucose, amino acids, lipids), and waste. The term *serum* refers to plasma minus its clotting factors. Plasma proteins include albumin, globulin, and clotting factors (mostly fibrinogen). Albumin is a protein that helps maintain oncotic pressure in the blood.[1] The liver makes most plasma proteins. The exception is antibodies (immunoglobulins). They are made by plasma cells.

TABLE 33.1 Functions of Blood

Function	Examples
Protection	• Maintain appropriate blood coagulation • Combating invasion of pathogens and other foreign substances
Regulation	• Fluid and electrolyte balance • Acid-base balance • Body temperature • Intravascular oncotic pressure
Transportation	• O_2 from lungs to cells • Nutrients from GI tract to cells • Hormones from endocrine glands to tissues and cells • Metabolic waste products (e.g., CO_2, NH_3, urea) from cells to lungs, liver, kidneys

Blood Cells

About 45% of the blood (Fig. 33.2) is composed of blood cells. The 3 types of blood cells are *erythrocytes* (RBCs), *leukocytes* (WBCs), and *thrombocytes* (platelets). The main function of RBCs is O_2 transportation. WBCs help protect the body from infection. Platelets promote blood coagulation.

Erythrocytes. The main functions of RBCs include transport of gases (both O_2 and CO_2) and assistance in maintaining acid-base balance. RBCs are flexible with a biconcave shape. This flexibility allows them to change shape so they can easily pass through tiny capillaries. The cell membrane is thin to promote diffusion of gases.

RBCs are mainly composed of a large molecule called *hemoglobin.* Hemoglobin is a complex protein-iron compound composed of heme (an iron compound) and globin (a simple

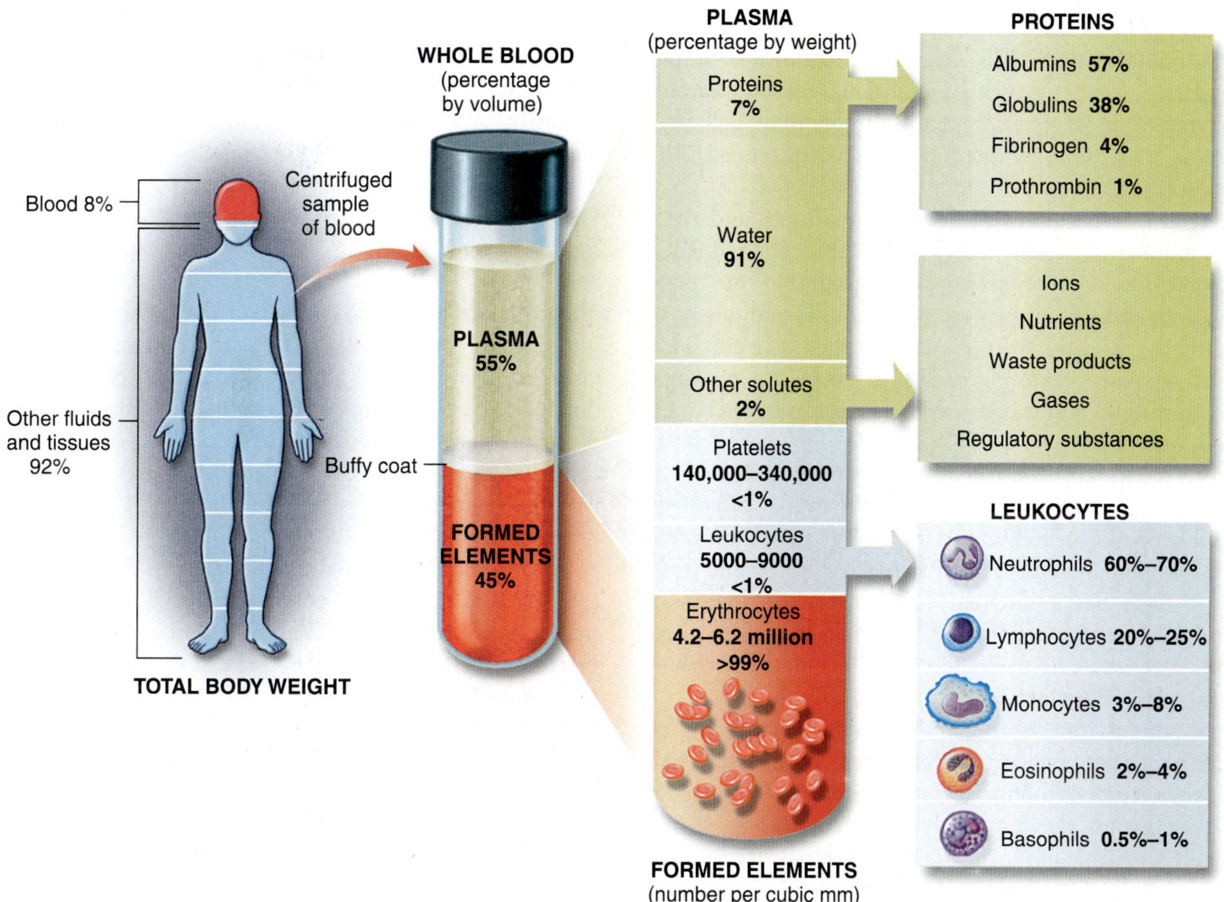

Fig. 33.2 Blood components in a healthy adult. Normally, 45% of the blood is composed of blood cells and 55% is composed of plasma. (From Patton KT, Thibodeau GA: *The human body in health and disease,* ed 8, St Louis, 2024, Mosby.)

protein). It binds with O_2 and CO_2. As RBCs circulate through the capillaries surrounding alveoli within the lung, O_2 attaches to iron on the hemoglobin. We refer to this O_2-bound hemoglobin as *oxyhemoglobin.* It gives arterial blood its bright red appearance. As RBCs flow to body tissues, O_2 detaches from the hemoglobin and diffuses from the capillary into tissue cells. CO_2 diffuses from tissue cells into the capillary, attaches to the globin part of hemoglobin, and is transported to the lungs for removal. Hemoglobin acts as a buffer and plays a role in maintaining acid-base balance. This buffering function is described in Chapter 17.

Erythropoiesis is the process of RBC production. It is regulated by cell O_2 requirements and general metabolic activity. Erythropoiesis is stimulated by hypoxia and controlled by *erythropoietin,* a glycoprotein growth factor made and released mainly by the kidney. Erythropoietin stimulates the bone marrow to increase RBC production. We make about 2.5 million RBCs per second. The normal life span of RBCs is about 120 days. We need many essential nutrients to make RBCs. These include protein, iron, folate (folic acid), cobalamin (vitamin B_{12}), riboflavin (vitamin B_2), pyridoxine (vitamin B_6), pantothenic acid, niacin, ascorbic acid (vitamin C), copper, and vitamin E. Endocrine hormones, such as thyroxine, corticosteroids, and testosterone, affect RBC production. For example, hypothyroidism may cause anemia.[2]

Several distinct cell types evolve during RBC maturation (Fig. 33.1). The **reticulocyte** is an immature RBC. Reticulocytes can develop into mature RBCs within 48 hours of release into the circulation. A mature RBC lacks a nucleus and cannot undergo mitotic division. Assessing the number of reticulocytes is a useful way to assess the rate and adequacy of RBC production.[1]

Hemolysis (destruction of RBCs) by monocytes and macrophages removes abnormal, defective, damaged, and old RBCs from circulation. Hemolysis normally occurs in the bone marrow, liver, and spleen. Because bilirubin is a component of RBCs, hemolysis results in increased bilirubin that our body must process. When hemolysis occurs by normal mechanisms, the liver conjugates and excretes all the bilirubin in bile.

Leukocytes. *Leukocytes* (WBCs) appear white when separated from blood. Like the RBCs, WBCs originate from stem cells within the bone marrow (Fig. 33.1). They may eventually reside in the thymus or secondary lymphoid tissues, such as the spleen, lymph nodes, and Peyer patches. There are several types of WBCs. Each has a different function. WBCs that have granules in the cytoplasm are *granulocytes* (or *polymorphonuclear leukocytes*). Granulocytes include neutrophils, basophils, and eosinophils.

WBCs that do not have granules in the cytoplasm are *agranulocytes.* They include lymphocytes, monocytes, and natural killer cells. Lymphocytes and monocytes are *mononuclear cells* because they have only 1 discrete nucleus. WBCs have a widely variable life span. Granulocytes may live for only hours. Some T lymphocytes may live for years.

Granulocytes. The main function of granulocytes is *phagocytosis.* This is the process by which WBCs engulf any unwanted organism and then digest and kill it. They can migrate through vessel walls and to the sites where they are needed. The *neutrophil* is the most common type of granulocyte. They make up 65% to 75% of WBCs. Neutrophils are the main phagocytic cells involved in acute inflammatory responses. Once they engulf a pathogen, the neutrophil dies in 1 to 2 days.[1] Hematopoietic growth factors (e.g., G-CSF, granulocyte-macrophage colony-stimulating factor [GM-CSF]) stimulate neutrophil production and maturation.

We call a mature neutrophil a *segmented neutrophil* ("seg," polysegmented neutrophil) because the nucleus is segmented into 2 to 5 lobes connected by strands. An immature neutrophil is a *band* (for the band appearance of the nucleus). Although band cells are sometimes found in the peripheral circulation of normal people and are capable of phagocytosis, the mature neutrophil is much more effective. An increase in neutrophils is a common sign of infection and tissue injury.

Eosinophils make up only 2% to 5% of WBCs. One of their main functions is to engulf antigen-antibody complexes formed during an allergic response. We think they are involved in inflammation. High eosinophil levels occur with some cancers, such as Hodgkin lymphoma, in parasitic infections, and in various skin diseases and connective tissue disorders.[1]

Basophils make up less than 1% of WBCs. They have cytoplasmic granules that contain chemical mediators, such as histamine. A basophil responds to stimulation by an antigen or by tissue injury by releasing substances from the granules. This is part of the response seen in allergic and inflammatory reactions. *Mast cells* are like basophils, but they reside in connective tissues. They play a key role in inflammation, blood vessel permeability, and smooth muscle contraction.

Lymphocytes. Lymphocytes make up 20% to 25% of the WBCs in the blood.[1] They form the basis of cellular and humoral immune responses. Two lymphocyte subtypes are B cells and T cells. T-cell precursors originate in the bone marrow. They migrate to the thymus gland for further differentiation into T cells. *Natural killer (NK) cells* are lymphocytes that kill virus-infected cells and activate T cells and phagocytes. They do not need prior exposure to antigens. Dendritic cells are the main phagocytic cells in the peripheral organs and skin. Most lymphocytes briefly circulate in the blood and reside in lymphoid and other tissues. See Chapter 14 for more about lymphocyte function.

Monocytes. Monocytes make up about 3% to 8% of the total WBCs.[1] They are potent phagocytic cells that ingest matter, such as bacteria, dead cells, tissue debris, and old or defective RBCs. These cells are present in the blood for only a brief time before they migrate into the tissues and become macrophages. In addition to macrophages that have differentiated from monocytes, tissues have resident macrophages. These resident macrophages have special names (e.g., Kupffer cells in the liver, osteoclasts in the bone, alveolar macrophages in the lung). They protect the body from pathogens at these entry points and are more phagocytic than monocytes. Macrophages interact with lymphocytes to promote humoral and cellular immune responses.

Thrombocytes. The main function of thrombocytes, or *platelets*, is to start the clotting process by producing an initial platelet plug at the site of injury. Platelets circulate suspended in plasma in an unactivated state. They must be available in enough numbers and structurally and metabolically sound for blood clotting to occur. Platelet activation starts at the site of any capillary damage. Increasing numbers of platelets accumulate to form an initial platelet plug that is stabilized with clotting factors. We store about one-third of our platelets in the spleen.

Platelets originate from stem cells within the bone marrow (Fig. 33.1). The stem cell undergoes differentiation by transforming into a *megakaryocyte*, which fragments into platelets. Platelet production is partly regulated by *thrombopoietin* (TPO). TPO is a growth factor that acts on bone marrow to stimulate platelet production. It is mainly made in the liver. During inflammation, interleukin 6 (IL-6) causes the liver to make more TPO, which increases platelet production and potential thrombosis. Typically, platelets have a life span of only 8 to 11 days.

Iron Metabolism

Our iron requirement is 25 mg daily. We get iron from food and supplements. Our body absorbs only 1 to 2 mg of iron from our diet. The rest comes from the continued recycling of iron from RBCs. As part of normal iron metabolism, iron is recycled after macrophages in the liver and spleen phagocytize, or ingest and destroy, old and damaged RBCs.

After diet iron is absorbed in the duodenum and proximal jejunum, transferrin transports it through the plasma (Fig. 33.3). Transferrin is made in the liver. How much iron is bound to transferrin is a reliable indicator of the iron supply for developing RBCs.

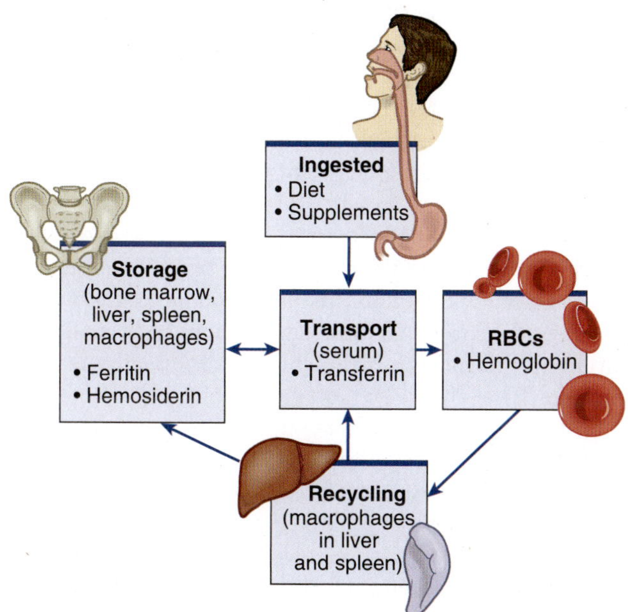

Fig. 33.3 Normal iron metabolism. Iron is ingested in the diet or from supplements. Macrophages break down ingested RBCs. Iron is returned to blood bound to transferrin or stored as ferritin or hemosiderin.

About two-thirds of total body iron is bound to heme in RBCs (hemoglobin) and muscle cells (myoglobin). We store the other one-third as ferritin and hemosiderin (degraded form of ferritin) in the bone marrow, spleen, liver, and macrophages (Fig. 33.3). When we do not replace stored iron, hemoglobin production is reduced. Normally, there is very little iron loss except from blood loss. We lose about 3% daily in urine, sweat, bile, and epithelial cells from the skin and gastrointestinal (GI) tract.[1]

Clotting Mechanisms

Hemostasis describes the arrest of bleeding (Fig. 33.4). This process is important in minimizing blood loss when body structures are injured. The sequence of events includes (1) vascular injury, endothelial sloughing, subendothelial exposure, vasoconstriction; (2) adhesion; (3) platelet activation with conformational change, allowing them to bind adhesive proteins; (4) aggregation and coagulation factor activation leading to stabilization of the clot; (5) platelet plug formation; and (6) clot retraction and dissolution.

Vascular Injury, Endothelial Sloughing, Subendothelial Exposure, and Vasoconstriction

When a blood vessel is injured, it begins to slough and exposes the endothelium. This causes the release of substances such as thromboxane A_2 (TXA_2), von Willebrand factor (vWF), and clotting factor VIII. Platelets then begin to fill endothelial gaps. An immediate local vasoconstrictive response occurs. Vasoconstriction reduces blood leakage from the vessel by restricting the vessel size and pressing the endothelial surfaces together. The latter reaction enhances vessel wall stickiness and keeps the vessel closed after vasoconstriction subsides.

Adhesion

The loss of endothelial cells exposes adhesive glycoproteins, such as collagen and vWF, to which more platelets adhere. The stickiness is termed *adhesiveness*. The formation of clumps is termed *aggregation* or *agglutination*.

Activation and Conformational Change

The interactions thus far cause the platelets to undergo an activation process. This leads to changes in platelet shape. The platelets then can bind adhesive proteins, including fibrinogen and vWF. Release of various platelet granules (including adenosine diphosphate [ADP]) recruits and activates other platelets, clotting factors, and growth factors.

Aggregation

Platelet aggregation is stimulated by TXA_2 and ADP, which induce fibrinogen receptors on the platelet. The formation of a visible fibrin clot on the platelet plug is the conclusion of a

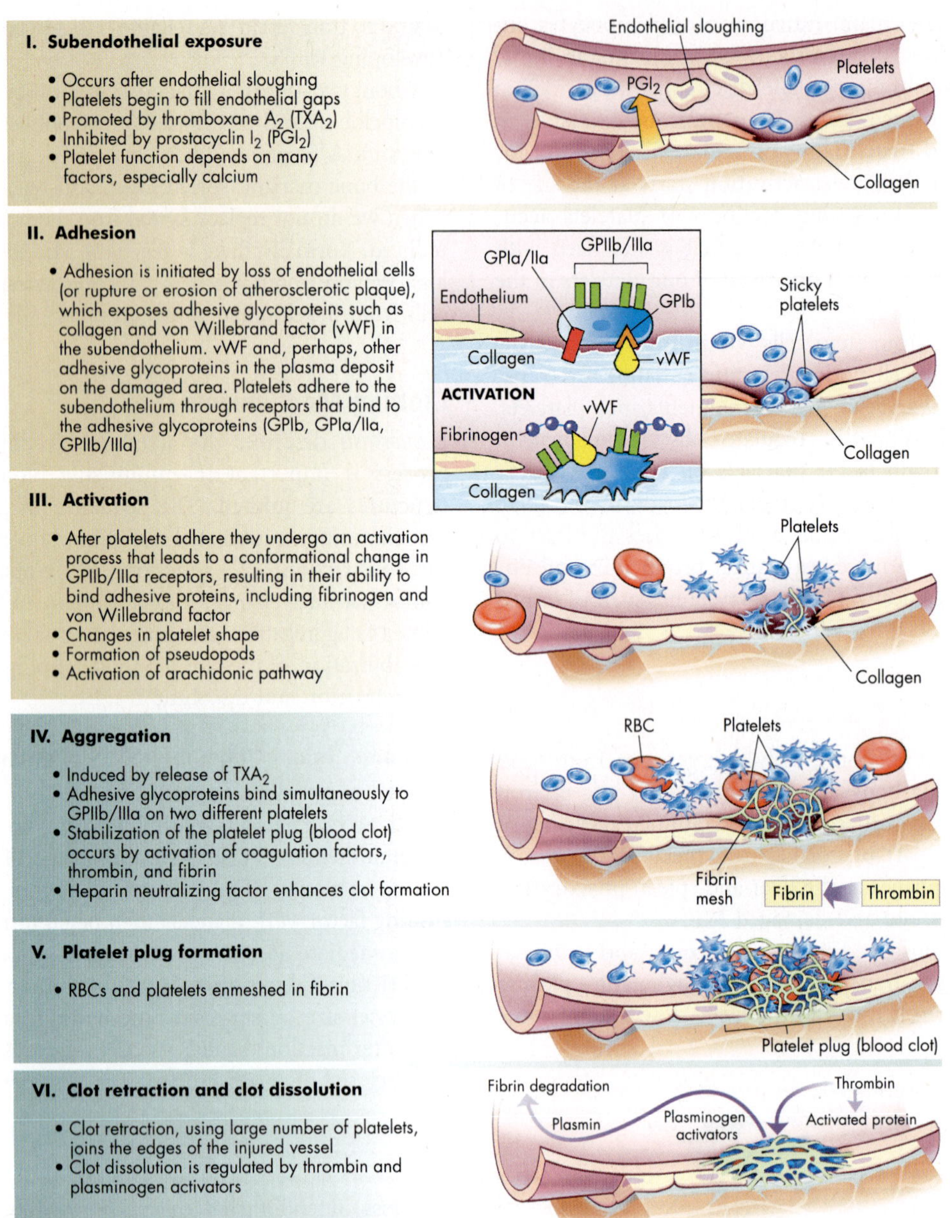

Fig. 33.4 Blood vessel damage, platelet activation, blood clot formation and dissolution. (From McCance KL et al: *Pathophysiology: the biological basis for disease in adults and children,* ed 8, St. Louis, 2019, Elsevier.)

complex series of reactions involving different clotting (coagulation) factors. Plasma clotting factors are labeled with both names and Roman numerals (Table 33.2).[3] Most are glycoproteins made in the liver. Monocytes, endothelial cells, and megakaryocytes make a few clotting factors. Some are enzymes that circulate in an inactive form (zymogens).

Plasma proteins circulate in inactive forms until stimulated to start clotting through the intrinsic or extrinsic pathway (Fig. 33.5). The *intrinsic pathway* is activated by collagen exposure from endothelial injury when the blood vessel is damaged. The *extrinsic pathway* is activated when tissue factor or tissue thromboplastin is released from injured tissues.

Coagulation follows the same final common pathway of the clotting cascade. Thrombin, in the common pathway, is the most powerful enzyme in the coagulation process (Fig. 33.5). It converts fibrinogen to fibrin, which is an essential part of a blood clot.[4]

Platelet Plug Formation

The final blood clot is a meshwork of protein strands that stabilizes the platelet plug and traps other cells, such as RBCs, phagocytes, and microorganisms.

TABLE 33.2 Coagulation Factors

Coagulation Factor	Action
I Fibrinogen	Source of fibrin to form a clot
II Prothrombin	Converted to thrombin, which then activates fibrinogen into fibrin as well as factors V, VII, VIII, XI, XIII, protein C, for clot stabilization
III Tissue factor, thromboplastin	Released from damaged endothelial cells and activates the extrinsic pathway by reacting with factor VII
IV Calcium	Required cofactor at several points in the coagulation cascade
V Labile factor	Binds with factor X to activate prothrombin
VII Stable factor, proconvertin	Forms a complex with factor III (tissue factor) and activates factors IX and X
VIII Antihemophilic factor	Works with factor IX and calcium to activate factor X. Von Willebrand factor is the carrier for factor VIII
IX Christmas factor (antihemophilic factor B)	Together with factor VIII, activates factor X
X Stuart-Prower factor	Activates conversion of factor II (prothrombin) to thrombin
XI Plasma thromboplastin antecedent (antihemophilic factor C)	Activates factor IX when calcium is present
XII Hageman factor	Activates factor XI, which starts the intrinsic pathway
XIII Fibrin-stabilizing factor	Cross-links fibrin strands and stabilizes fibrin clot

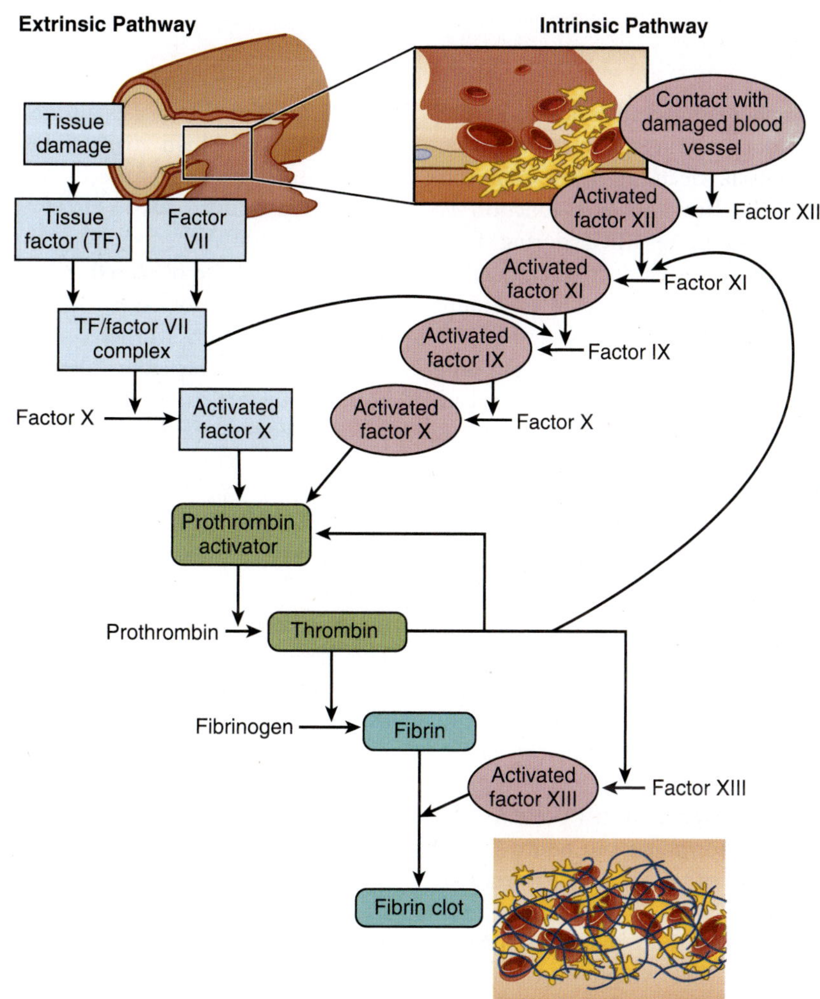

Fig. 33.5 Coagulation mechanism showing steps in the intrinsic pathway and extrinsic pathway as they would occur in the test tube.

Clot Retraction and Dissolution

Just as some blood elements foster coagulation *(procoagulants)*, others interfere with clotting *(anticoagulants)*. This counter mechanism to blood clotting keeps blood in its fluid state.

Antithrombin activity, vessel and platelet activity, and fibrinolysis contribute to anticoagulation. As the name implies, antithrombins keep blood in a fluid state by antagonizing thrombin, a powerful coagulant. Endogenous heparin, antithrombin III, protein C, and protein S are examples of anticoagulants.

The second way we keep blood in its fluid form is fibrinolysis, a process resulting in the dissolution of the fibrin clot. The fibrinolytic system starts when plasminogen is activated by substances such as tissue plasminogen activator (t-PA) and urokinase-like plasminogen activator (u-PA) to plasmin. Thrombin can activate the conversion of plasminogen to plasmin, promoting fibrinolysis. Plasmin attacks either fibrin or fibrinogen by splitting the molecules into smaller elements called *fibrin split products* (FSPs) or *fibrin degradation products* (FDPs). You can find more about FSPs in Table 33.8 and in the section on disseminated intravascular coagulation (DIC) in Chapter 34.

Excess fibrinolysis predisposes patients to bleeding. In this situation, bleeding results from the destruction of fibrin in platelet plugs or from the anticoagulation effects of increased FSPs. Increased FSPs lead to impaired platelet aggregation, reduced prothrombin, and an inability to stabilize fibrin.

Spleen

The spleen is the largest lymphoid organ. It is found in the upper left quadrant of the abdomen. The spleen has 6 major functions: hematopoietic, filtration, cleansing, waste removal, immunologic, and storage.[1] The hematopoietic function is shown by the spleen's ability to make RBCs during fetal development. It filters blood-born antigens, such as circulating bacteria, especially encapsulated organisms such as gram-positive cocci. It cleanses the blood through the action of the mononuclear phagocyte system. The spleen removes old and defective RBCs from the circulation. In doing so, the spleen can catabolize hemoglobin released by hemolysis and return the iron part of the hemoglobin to the bone marrow for reuse. The spleen's rich supply of lymphocytes, monocytes, and stored immunoglobulins plays a role in immunologic function. The spleen is a storage site for RBCs and platelets. It can store more than 300 mL of blood. We store about one-third of platelets in the spleen.[1]

Lymph System

The lymph system, consisting of lymph, lymphatic capillaries, ducts, and lymph nodes, carries fluid from the interstitial spaces to the blood. It is through the lymph that proteins and fat from the GI tract and certain hormones can return to the circulatory system. The lymph system returns excess interstitial fluid to the blood.

Lymph is pale yellow interstitial fluid that has diffused through lymphatic capillary walls. The lymph vessels collect interstitial fluid from the tissues and transport it as lymph through vessels. Eventually, lymph enters the thoracic duct, which drains into the superior vena cava. Lymph formation increases when interstitial fluid increases. This forces more fluid into the lymph system. When too much interstitial fluid develops or when something interferes with lymph reabsorption, *lymphedema* develops. Lymphedema may occur as a complication of mastectomy or lumpectomy with dissection of axillary nodes. In this case lymphedema is caused by the obstruction of lymph flow from the removal of lymph nodes.

The lymphatic capillaries are thin-walled vessels that have an irregular diameter. They are larger than blood capillaries and do not have valves.

The *lymph nodes* are part of the lymph system. Their main function is to filter pathogens and foreign particles that are carried by lymph to the nodes. They are the main site for the first encounter between antigen and lymphocytes.[1] Structurally, the nodes are small clumps of lymph tissue. They are found in groups along lymph vessels at various sites. There are more than 200 lymph nodes throughout the body. The greatest number is in the abdomen surrounding the GI tract. They vary in size according to their location. We have both superficial and deep lymph nodes. We can palpate superficial nodes. Evaluating deep nodes requires radiologic examination.[5]

Liver

The liver has metabolic, secretory, vascular, immune, and storage functions. It makes all the procoagulants we need for hemostasis and blood coagulation and secretes bilirubin and bile. It stores iron that exceeds tissue needs, which can occur with blood transfusions or diseases that cause iron overload. *Hepcidin,* made by the liver, is a key regulator of iron balance. It inhibits the release of stored iron from enterocytes in the intestines and macrophages. Iron overload or inflammation stimulates hepcidin synthesis.[6] When iron is deficient, hepatocytes make less hepcidin. This results in the release of stored iron and an increase in diet absorption. Other liver functions are described in Chapters 43 and 48.

Gerontologic Considerations: Effects of Aging on the Hematologic System

Hematopoietic stem cell function and the number of bone marrow cells declines with age. Bone marrow fat increases.[7] This leads to an inability to respond to increased demands of hematopoiesis, an increased incidence of myeloid cancer, and compromised immunity.[8] Although the older adult can still maintain adequate blood cell levels, the reduced reserve capacity leaves them more vulnerable to possible problems with clotting, transporting O_2, and fighting infection, especially during periods of increased demand. This contributes to their having a decreased ability to compensate for an acute or chronic illness.

Total serum iron, total iron-binding capacity, and iron absorption are all decreased. The RBC plasma membranes are more fragile. This may account for a slight increase in mean corpuscular volume (MCV) and a slight decrease in mean corpuscular hemoglobin concentration (MCHC) of RBCs in some older adults.[3] Healthy older patients are not able to make reticulocytes in response to hemorrhage or hypoxemia as well as younger adults. This is likely due to a blunted response to erythropoietin.[3] Table 33.3 outlines the effects of aging on hematologic studies.

TABLE 33.3 GERONTOLOGIC ASSESSMENT DIFFERENCES

Effects of Aging on Hematologic Studies

Study	Changes
CBC Studies	
Mean corpuscular hemoglobin concentration (MCHC)	May be slightly ↓
Mean corpuscular volume (MCV)	May be slightly ↑
Platelets	May be slightly ↓; possible ↑ in adhesiveness
White blood cell (WBC) count	↓ Response to infection
Clotting Studies	
D-dimers	↑
Erythrocyte sedimentation rate (ESR)	↑ Significantly
Factors V, VII, IX	May be ↑
Fibrinogen	May be ↑
Partial thromboplastin time	May be ↓
Iron Studies	
Erythropoietin	May be ↑
Ferritin	↑
Serum iron	↓
Total iron-binding capacity	↓

The function of lymphocytes decreases, blunting the response to infection.[8] Immune changes related to aging are detailed in Chapter 14.

Platelets may have increased adhesiveness and clotting factors increase. Thus aging is associated with an increased chance of clotting problems, such as venous thromboembolism.[1] Changes in vascular integrity related to aging can manifest as easy bruising.

CASE STUDY

Patient Introduction

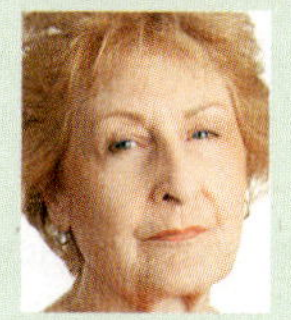
(© Lisa F. Young/ iStock.)

A.J. is a 63-year-old female who presents to the emergency department with her husband. He came home from work and found her at home, weak and in bed after she worked. She says she has been slowly getting more "cold and tired," but "that is what happens when you work at my age." Her husband states that she has become more tired over the last couple of weeks and "she looks pale." She has been having trouble working all day and even gets short of breath when doing simple errands. She recently had a "bad cold and sinus infection" that only improved after 2 courses of antibiotics. A.J. says, "I've noticed I've had a lot of bruising lately."

Discussion Questions

1. What are the possible causes of A.J.'s weakness, pallor, and shortness of breath?
2. Is her condition stable or an emergency?
3. What key assessment questions would you ask A.J.?

You will learn more about A.J. and her condition as you read this chapter.

Answers available at http://evolve.elsevier.com/Lewis/medsurg.

HEMATOLOGIC SYSTEM ASSESSMENT

Subjective Data

Important Health Information

Health history. Determine whether patients had prior hematologic problems. Ask about anemia, bleeding problems, and blood disorders. Are there related medical conditions, such as malabsorption or liver (e.g., hepatitis, cirrhosis), kidney, or spleen problems? A history of recent or recurrent infections or blood clotting problems is important.

Medications. Obtain a complete medication history. Ask about the use of vitamins, herbal products, or diet supplements. Many medications may interfere with normal hematologic function.[6] Those on long-term anticoagulant therapy, such as warfarin, are at risk for bleeding problems. Chemotherapy drugs and antiretroviral agents may cause bone marrow depression. Patients previously treated with chemotherapy agents, particularly alkylating agents, have a higher risk for developing a secondary cancer of leukemia or lymphoma. Many drugs used to treat cardiovascular disease can cause problems with hematopoietic cell production or coagulation.

Surgery. Obtain a surgical history. This includes splenectomy, tumor removal, prosthetic heart valve placement, and GI surgeries. A partial or total gastrectomy removes parietal cells, thus reducing intrinsic factor needed for the absorption of cobalamin (vitamin B_{12}). Duodenal excision (where iron absorption occurs), gastric bypass (the duodenum may be bypassed and parietal cell surface area decreased), and ileal resection (reduces area where cobalamin absorption takes place) can result in problems. Assess wound healing and if there were any bleeding problems. Determine the number of previous blood transfusions and any complications. The risk for transfusion reactions and iron overload increases with the number of blood transfusions.

Functional Health Patterns

Key questions to ask patients with a hematologic problem are outlined in Table 33.4.

Health perception–health management. Ask patients to describe their state of health. Obtain a family history of hematologic problems. Ask about anemia, cancer, RBC disorders, such as sickle cell disease, and bleeding disorders, such as hemophilia and clotting problems.

Assess risk factors, such as alcohol and cigarette use. Persons with alcohol use disorder often have vitamin deficiencies. Alcohol exerts a damaging effect on platelet function and the liver, where we make clotting factors. Bleeding problems can develop and should be expected. Illicit drug use is important because many of these drugs may affect hematopoiesis.

Cigarette smoking increases low-density lipoprotein (LDL) cholesterol and levels of CO_2. This leads to hypoxia and changing the anticoagulant properties of the endothelium. Smoking increases platelet reactivity, plasma fibrinogen, hematocrit, and blood viscosity.

Nutritional-metabolic. Determine whether patients have anorexia, nausea, vomiting, or oral discomfort. A diet history

TABLE 33.4 HEALTH HISTORY

Hematologic System

Health Perception–Health Management

- Do you have any problem performing daily activities because of a lack of energy?[a]
- Do you take any prescribed or over-the-counter medications?[a]
- Are you taking any herbs?[a] Home remedies?[a]
- Do you smoke cigarettes or drink alcohol?[a]
- Have you in the past or are you currently consuming illegal drugs? What agents? What route? How often? When did you last use?
- Have you ever received a blood transfusion?[a]
- Is there any family history of anemia, cancer, bleeding, or clotting problems?[a]
- Have you had any surgeries or gastric procedures?[a]

Nutritional-Metabolic

- Do you have any problems with eating, chewing, or swallowing?[a]
- Have you had any mouth sores, sore tongue, swollen or sore gums, oral bleeding?[a]
- Describe your typical diet. If vegetarian, do you eat eggs, milk products, fish?
- How has your appetite been?
- Have you had any changes in your weight in the past year?[a]
- Do you take any vitamins, nutrition supplements, or iron?[a]
- Is nausea and vomiting a problem for you?[a]
- Have you ever had any unusual bleeding or bruising?[a]
- Have there been recent changes in the condition or color of your skin?[a]
- Have you had night sweats or fevers?[a]
- Have you noticed any swelling in your armpits, neck, or groin?[a]

Elimination

- Have you had black or tarry stools?[a] Have you had light, clay-colored stools?[a]
- Have you noticed any blood or dark "tea color" in your urine?[a]
- Has your urine had a foul odor or cloudiness?
- Have you had any decrease in urine output?[a]

Activity-Exercise

- Do you have any shortness of breath at rest? With activity?[a]
- Do you have any limitations in joint motion?[a] Have any of your joints been swollen?[a]
- Do you have a problem with unsteady gait? Have you fallen recently?[a]
- Do you exercise regularly? What type and how often?[a]
- After activity, do you ever notice bleeding or bruising?[a]

Sleep-Rest

- Have you been overly fatigued recently?[a]
- Are you more tired than usual?[a]
- Do you feel rested on awakening? If no, explain.

Cognitive-Perceptual

- Have you had any numbness or tingling?[a]
- Have you had any problems with your vision, hearing, or taste?[a]
- Have you noticed any changes in your mental function?[a]
- Do you have any pain, such as bone, joint, or abdominal pain, or abdominal fullness?[a]
- Do you have pain when moving your joints?[a]
- Have your muscles been sore or achy recently?[a]

Role-Relationship

- Does your occupation bring you into contact with hazardous substances?[a]
- Has your present illness caused a change in your roles and relationships?[a]

Sexuality-Reproductive

- Has your problem caused any sexual or intimacy problems that concern you?[a]
- *Females:* When was your last menses? Do you consider your cycle normal? How long does your bleeding usually last? Have you had any increase in cramping or clotting?[a] Have there been any changes in the amount of flow?[a]
- *Males:* Do you ever have impotence?[a]
- Have you had unprotected sex in the past 6 months?[a] Was your partner someone new or a person with whom you have had a long-term sexual relationship?

Coping–Stress Tolerance

- Do you have a support system to help you when needed?
- What coping strategies do you use when your symptoms are worse?
- Do you have any specific symptoms when you feel stressed?[a]

Value-Belief

- Do you have any personal or religious objection to receiving blood or blood products?[a]
- Do you have any conflicts between your planned therapy and your value-belief system?[a]

[a]If yes, describe.

may give clues about the cause of anemia. We need an adequate intake of iron, cobalamin, and folic acid for RBC development.[9]

Explore any change in skin texture, color, or temperature. Ask about bleeding gum tissue or bleeding from anywhere on the body. Ask about any lumps or swelling in the neck, armpits, or groin. Specifically, ask what the lumps feel like (i.e., hard or soft, tender or nontender). Are they mobile or fixed? Primary lymph tumors are usually not painful. A nontender, consistently swollen lymph node may be a sign of cancer, such as Hodgkin or non-Hodgkin lymphoma. An acute infection may cause enlarged, tender lymph nodes.[5] Explore any reports of fever. Ask if patients have chills or night sweats.

Ask about a history of heart or lung diseases. Cardiovascular problems, such as valvular disease or hypertension, may predispose patients to hemolysis. Lung problems that lead to hypoxemia may cause chronic stimulation of erythropoietin and result in *polycythemia* (excess RBCs).

Activity-exercise. Because fatigue is a prominent symptom in many hematologic problems, ask about feelings of tiredness. Is there any weakness or feelings of heavy extremities? Assess for apathy, malaise, dyspnea, or palpitations. Note any change in the ability to perform regular exercise and/or activities of daily living (ADLs).

Sleep-rest. Determine whether patients feel rested after a night's sleep. Fatigue from a hematologic problem often does not resolve after sleep.

Cognitive-perceptual. Assess for any joint pain. Joint pain in the joint may occur with an autoimmune disorder, such as rheumatoid arthritis. It may occur with gout from increased uric acid production due to hematologic cancer or hemolytic anemia. Aching bones may result from pressure of expanding bone marrow with diseases such as leukemia. *Hemarthrosis* (blood in a joint) occurs in patients with bleeding disorders and can be painful. Note any paresthesias, numbness, and tingling.

Role-relationship. Ask about any past or present occupation or household exposures to radiation or chemicals. If such exposure has occurred, determine the type, amount, and duration of the exposure. A person who was exposed to radiation, as a treatment modality or by accident, has a higher incidence of certain hematologic problems. The same is true of a person who was exposed to certain chemicals (e.g., benzene, vinyl chloride, pesticides). These chemicals are often used by those in the military, mechanics, and workers in the petroleum, construction, farming, and transportation industries. Assess the effect of the present illness on the patient's usual roles and responsibilities.

Sexuality-reproductive. Take a careful menstrual history. Include the age at which menarche and menopause began, duration and amount of bleeding, incidence of clotting and cramping, and any associated problems. Ask males if they have any erectile problems. Has sexual behavior increased the risk for HIV infection?

Coping–stress tolerance. Patients with a hematologic problem often need help with ADLs. Ask patients if adequate support is available to meet daily needs. Explore their usual methods of handling stress. With platelet disorders or hemophilia, the potential for hemorrhage can be so frightening that usual life patterns may be drastically curtailed, affecting quality of life.

Value-belief. Treatment for some hematologic problems involves blood transfusions or a bone marrow transplant. Assess whether these treatments conflict with the patient's value-belief system, including cultural and religious beliefs related to blood and blood transfusions. Notify the HCP if you identify any conflicts.

Objective Data

Physical Assessment

A complete physical assessment is needed to examine all systems that affect or are affected by the hematologic system. Presenting symptoms may not immediately point to a hematologic problem (Table 33.5). For example, paresthesias of the lower extremities may not appear to be a hematologic problem. But when combined with other findings and risk factors, it may indicate cobalamin deficiency and resulting pernicious anemia. Certain aspects of the assessment are specifically relevant. These include skin, lymph nodes, spleen, and liver.

A *focused assessment* is used to assess the status of previously identified hematologic problems and to monitor for signs of new problems. A focused assessment of the hematologic system is shown in Box 33.1.

Lymph node assessment. Assess lymph nodes symmetrically. Note location, size (in centimeters), degree of fixation (e.g., movable, fixed), tenderness, and texture. Lightly palpate the superficial lymph nodes using the pads of the fingers (Fig. 33.6). Gently roll the skin over the area and feel for lymph node enlargement. Lymph nodes are usually not palpable in adults. If a node is palpable, it should be small (0.5 to 1 cm), mobile, firm, and nontender to be considered a normal finding. A node that is tender, hard, fixed, or enlarged (whether it is tender or not) is an abnormal finding and needs further investigation. Tender nodes are usually a result of inflammation. Firm or fixed nodes suggest cancer.[5] We cannot palpate deep lymph nodes. They are evaluated by radiologic examination.

Develop a sequence to examine lymph nodes. A convenient sequence is to start at the head and neck. First, palpate the preauricular, posterior auricular, occipital, tonsillar, submandibular, submental, superficial cervical, posterior cervical chain, deep cervical chain, and supraclavicular nodes. Next,

CASE STUDY

Subjective Data

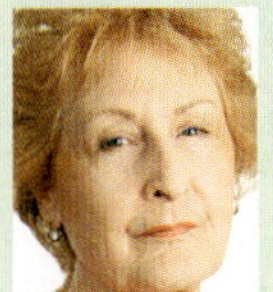
(© Lisa F. Young/ iStock.)

A focused subjective assessment of A.J. revealed the following information:

Medical History: History of mild osteoarthritis. No surgical history. Prefers to take care of self with "natural therapy" and has not seen an HCP for 5 years, except for the recent sinus infection.

Medications: Metamucil 1 Tbsp/day; vitamins C, E, and D with calcium.

Health Perception–Health Management: Denies family or personal history of anemia, cancer, or bleeding disorders. Believes she comes from family longevity because they "eat organic foods." Drinks 1 glass of red wine with her evening meal "because it's good for your heart." Reporting a gradual increase in shortness of breath with exertion. Says she really cannot do anything anymore without having to stop and catch her breath. Says, "It's tough getting old."

Nutritional-Metabolic: Eat a lot of pasta "because it is cheap." Uses a lot of garlic for flavoring and the "health benefit of it." Although not a vegetarian, eats little meat.

Elimination: Denies black or tarry stool. Occasional constipation. No problems with urination.

Activity-Exercise: Having a hard time performing ADLs without having to stop and catch her breath. Denies dyspnea at rest. States joints are stiff on arising in morning and after sitting but able to get around OK and work at her secretarial job. States her walking is steady but weak. No history of falling.

Sleep-Rest: Typically sleeps 8 to 9 hours per night with no trouble falling asleep. Still feels tired and needs to nap during her lunch break and during her days off.

Cognitive-Perceptual: Denies any numbness or tingling. Admits to being a little hard of hearing but can still see "pretty good."

Value-Belief: Prefers natural therapies over traditional medication.

Discussion Questions

1. What subjective assessment findings concern you most?
2. What would you include in the physical assessment? For what would you be looking?

You will learn more about the physical assessment of the hematologic system in the next section.

Answers available at http://evolve.elsevier.com/Lewis/medsurg.

TABLE 33.5 ASSESSMENT ABNORMALITIES

Hematologic System

Finding	Description	Possible Cause and Significance
Abdomen		
Distended abdomen	Larger than normal abdominal profile. May be soft or firm, tender or nontender, and accompanied by other symptoms, such as nausea, vomiting, rebound tenderness	Lymphoma or some leukemias may present as abdominal adenopathy, mass(es), or bowel obstruction
Hepatomegaly	Palpable liver	Leukemia, cirrhosis, fibrosis due to iron overload from long-term RBC transfusions
Splenomegaly	Palpable spleen	Anemia, thrombocytopenia, leukemia, lymphoma, leukopenia, mononucleosis, malaria, cirrhosis, trauma, portal hypertension
Eyes		
Blurred vision, diplopia, visual field cuts	Decreased visual acuity or areas of blindness (field cuts)	Anemia, extreme leukocytosis, polycythemia, hyperviscosity may cause vision problems. Thrombocytopenia may cause intraocular hemorrhage with vision changes. Excess clotting may cause thromboses in circulation to the brain that cause visual field cuts
Conjunctival pallor	Paleness. Decreased or absence of coloration in the conjunctiva	Anemia
Jaundiced sclera	Yellow appearance of sclera	Accumulation of bile pigment resulting from rapid or excess hemolysis or liver disease or infiltration
Heart and Chest		
Altered blood pressure	*Hypertension:* >140/90 mm Hg	May occur initially as a compensatory mechanism for anemia
	Hypotension: <90 mm Hg systolic or >40 mm Hg drop from baseline	Infection, blood loss, compromised cardiovascular compensatory mechanisms
	Orthostasis: HR >20 beats/min increase or BP >20 mm Hg decrease from baseline when moving from a lying position to either sitting or standing	Common with anemia, especially if accompanied by low blood volume
Low O_2 saturation	O_2-carrying capacity as reflected by O_2 saturation by pulse oximetry	O_2 saturation may be decreased in cases of severe anemia
Palpitations	Feeling the heartbeat, flutter, or pound in chest	Anemia, fluid volume overload, hypotension with impending syncope, hypertension, dysrhythmias
Sternal tenderness	Abnormal sensitivity to touch or pressure on sternum	Leukemia resulting from increased bone marrow cellularity, causing increase in pressure and bone erosion Multiple myeloma because of lytic bone lesions
Tachycardia	Heart rate >100 beats/min	Compensatory mechanism in anemia to increase cardiac output. May be present with fever, infection
Lymph Nodes		
Lymphadenopathy	Lymph nodes enlarged (>1 cm). May be tender to touch	Infection, foreign infiltrations, leukemia, lymphoma, Hodgkin lymphoma, metastatic cancer
Mouth		
Gingival and mucous membrane changes	Pallor, gingival and mucosal ulceration or infection, swelling, bleeding	Anemia, neutropenia thrombocytopenia. Inability of impaired leukocytes to combat oral infections. Gingival hyperplasia may be present with some types of leukemia
Smooth tongue	Tongue surface smooth and shiny. Mucosa thin and red from decreased papillae	Pernicious anemia, iron-deficiency anemia
Musculoskeletal System		
Arthralgia	Joint pain	Bleeding into joints from sickle cell disease, hemophilia
Bone pain	Pain in pelvis, ribs, spine, sternum	Multiple myeloma related to lytic bone lesions. Bone invasion by leukemia cells, bone demineralization resulting from various cancers, sickle cell disease
Joint swelling	Fluid-filled spaces surrounding joints	Hemophilia and sickle cell anemia as hemarthrosis causes inflammation
Nervous System		
Headache, nuchal rigidity	Pain in the cranium, potentially involving one area or extending from frontal area to back of neck	Headache common in mild to moderate anemia. Severe headache with or without vision changes may signal intracranial hemorrhage due to thrombocytopenia. CNS disease with acute lymphoblastic leukemia, CNS lymphoma

TABLE 33.5 ASSESSMENT ABNORMALITIES—cont'd

Hematologic System

Finding	Description	Possible Cause and Significance
Paresthesias of feet and hands, ataxia	Numbness sensation and extreme sensitivity in central and peripheral nerves. Impaired muscle movement	Cobalamin (vitamin B_{12}) deficiency or folate deficiency
Weakness	Lacking physical strength or energy	Anemia
Nose		
Nosebleeds	Spontaneous bleeding from nares	Low platelet counts, clotting problem, leukemia
Skin		
Chloroma	Tumor arising from myeloid tissue. Contains a pale green pigment	Acute myelogenous leukemia that has infiltrated the skin, rare forms of lymphoma
Cyanosis	Bluish discoloration of skin and mucous membranes	Anemia, excess concentration of deoxyhemoglobin in blood
Flushing	Transient, episodic redness of skin (usually around face and neck)	Increase Hgb (polycythemia), congestion of capillaries Flushing of palms of hands or soles of feet sign of anemia
Jaundice	Yellow appearance of skin and mucous membranes	Accumulation of bile pigment caused by rapid or excessive hemolysis or liver damage
Leg ulcers	Prominent on the malleoli on the ankles	Sickle cell disease
Pallor of skin or nail beds	Paleness. Decreased or absence of skin coloration	Anemia
Plasmacytoma	Tumor arising from abnormal plasma cells	Multiple myeloma that has infiltrated tissue
Pruritus	Unpleasant cutaneous sensation that provokes the desire to rub or scratch skin	Hodgkin lymphoma, cutaneous lymphomas, infiltrative leukemias, increased bilirubin

palpate the axillary lymph nodes and pectoral, subscapular, and lateral groups of nodes. Then examine the epitrochlear nodes found in the antecubital fossa between the biceps and triceps muscles. Last, palpate the inguinal lymph nodes found in the groin.

Liver and spleen palpation. The liver and spleen are normally not detectable by palpating the abdomen. An enlarged liver or spleen may be detectable by percussion or palpation. How to palpate and percuss the liver and spleen are described in Chapter 43.

Skin assessment. Examine the skin over the entire body. In patients with RBC disorders, the skin may be pale or pasty. It may have a cyanotic tinge in severe anemia. Erythrocytosis often causes small vessel occlusions, causing a purple, mottled appearance of the face, nose, fingers, or toes. You can best assess color changes in persons with dark skin in the sclera, conjunctiva, buccal mucosa, tongue, lips, nail beds, and palms.[5] *Clubbing of the fingers* can be seen with chronic anemia. Skin assessment is discussed in Chapter 24.

WBC disorders may cause infectious or cancerous skin lesions. These may occur anywhere and have a variable distribution pattern.

Look for findings that can indicate bleeding problems. Assess for petechiae (small purplish red pinpoint lesions), ecchymoses (bruising), and *spider nevus* (a form of *telangiectasia*) (Table 33.6). The location of petechiae can indicate an accumulation of blood in the skin or mucous membranes. Small vessels leak under pressure, and the platelet numbers are not enough to stop the bleeding. Petechiae are more likely to occur where clothing constricts the circulation. In general, skin and mucosal bleeding means a platelet disorder. Spontaneous bleeding into joints or muscles means a coagulation factor problem.

CASE STUDY

Objective Data: Physical Assessment

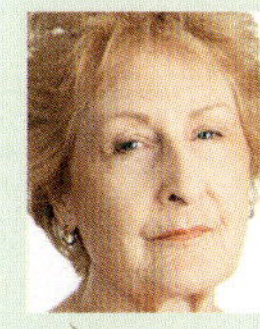

(© Lisa F. Young/iStock.)

Physical assessment findings of A.J. are as follows:

BP 100/70 (lying), 88/60 (standing); apical pulse 110 (lying), 124 (standing), regular. Respiratory rate 26, temp 96.8°F (36°C), O_2 saturation 90% on room air. Weight 106 lb (48 kg). Height 5 ft 1 in. Skin pale. 2 bruises on her right arm; 1 on the left lower leg. A few scattered petechiae on both ankles. No jaundice noted. Conjunctivae pale. Tongue smooth and shiny. Lungs clear with diminished breath sounds in the bases bilaterally. No visible bleeding. No enlarged lymph nodes, spleen, or liver noted. General weakness with dyspnea on exertion. No numbness or tingling or peripheral edema.

Discussion Questions

1. Which physical assessment findings are of most concern to you?
2. Based on the assessment findings, what diagnostic studies do you think may be ordered for A.J.?

You will learn more about diagnostic studies in relation to the hematologic system in the next section.

Answers available at http://evolve.elsevier.com/Lewis/medsurg.

BOX 33.1 FOCUSED ASSESSMENT

Hematologic System

Use this checklist to make sure the key assessment steps have been done.

Subjective

Ask the patient about the following and note responses:

Unusual bleeding or bruising
Black, tarry stool
Blood in vomitus
Swelling in neck, armpits, or groin
Dark-colored or blood in urine
Fatigue
Heart palpitations

Objective: Diagnostic

Check the following laboratory results for critical values:

CBC
WBC count with differential
Clotting: PT, INR, aPTT, platelets
Hgb, Hct

Objective: Physical Assessment

Inspect

Skin for lesions or color changes

Auscultate

BP for change or orthostasis

Palpate

Pulse for tachycardia
Liver and spleen for enlargement
Lymph nodes for lymphadenopathy

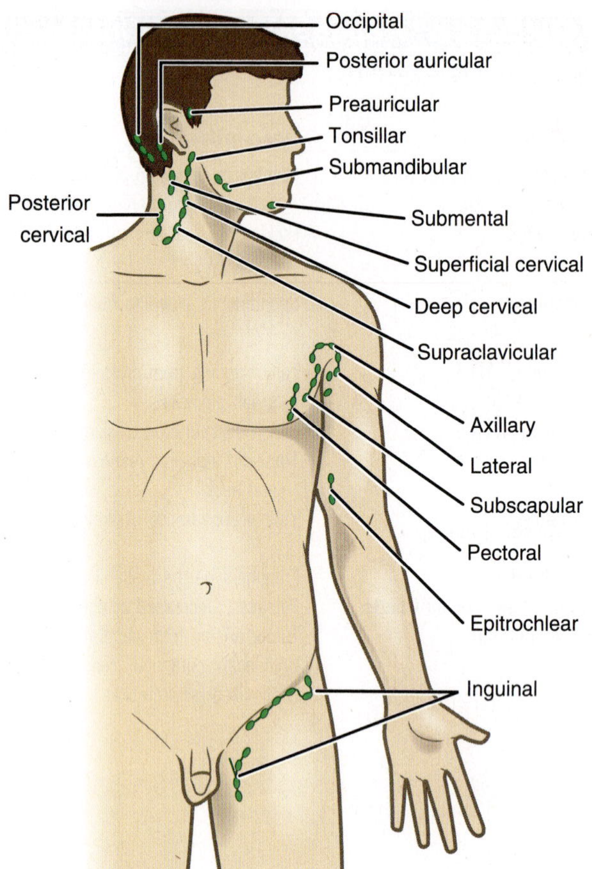

Fig. 33.6 Palpable superficial lymph nodes.

DIAGNOSTIC STUDIES

Laboratory Studies

Complete Blood Count

The complete blood count (CBC) involves several laboratory tests (Table 33.7). In addition to the CBC, a *peripheral smear* may be done. The smear is used to look at the *morphology* (shape and appearance) of the blood cells and may help with the diagnosis. For example, many immature blast WBCs may indicate acute leukemia. Diseases or treatments can disrupt the entire system. When the entire CBC is suppressed, a condition termed **pancytopenia** (marked decrease in the number of RBCs, WBCs, and platelets) exists.

Red blood cells. The total RBC count is reported as RBC $\times$ 10^6/μL. However, the total RBC count is not fully reliable in determining the adequacy of RBC function. We must assess other data, such as hemoglobin, hematocrit, and RBC indices. Normal values of some RBC tests are different for males and females because normal values are based on body mass. Males usually have a larger body mass than women.

The *hemoglobin (Hgb) value* is reduced with anemia, hemorrhage, and hemodilution, such as that occurring with excess fluid volume. Increased hemoglobin occurs in polycythemia or hemoconcentration, which can develop from volume depletion (dehydration). Increases and decreases of the hematocrit value and RBC count occur with the same conditions that raise and lower the hemoglobin value.

The *hematocrit (Hct) value* is determined by spinning blood in a centrifuge. This causes RBCs and plasma to separate. The RBCs, being the heavier elements, settle to the bottom (Fig. 33.2). The hematocrit value is the percent of RBCs compared with the total blood volume. The hematocrit value generally is 3 times the hemoglobin value. *RBC indices* are special indicators that reflect RBC volume, color, and hemoglobin saturation (Table 33.7).[10] These parameters give insight into the cause of anemia.

White blood cells. The WBC count gives 2 sets of information. The first is a total count of WBCs in 1 μL of peripheral blood. A WBC count over 10,000/μL occurs with infection, inflammation, tissue injury or death, and cancer (e.g., leukemia, lymphoma). Although the degree of WBC elevation does not necessarily predict the severity of illness, it can give clues to the cause. Extremely high WBC counts (e.g., greater than 25,000/μL) occur with certain types of leukemia. A WBC count less than 5000/μL (**leukopenia**) occurs with bone marrow depression, severe or chronic illness, and other types of leukemia.

The second aspect of the WBC count, the *differential count,* measures the percent of each type of WBC. The WBC differential gives valuable clues about the cause of illness. When infections are

TABLE 33.6 ASSESSMENT ABNORMALITIES

Vascular Skin Lesions

Finding	Description	Possible Cause and Significance
Angioma 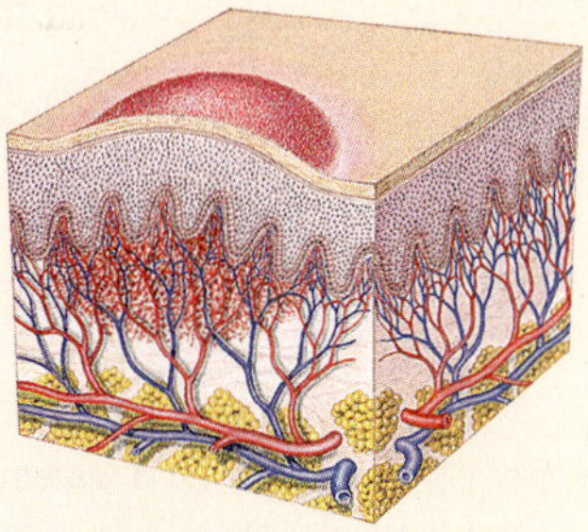	Benign tumor. Consists of blood or lymph vessels	Most are congenital. May disappear spontaneously
Ecchymosis (bruise) 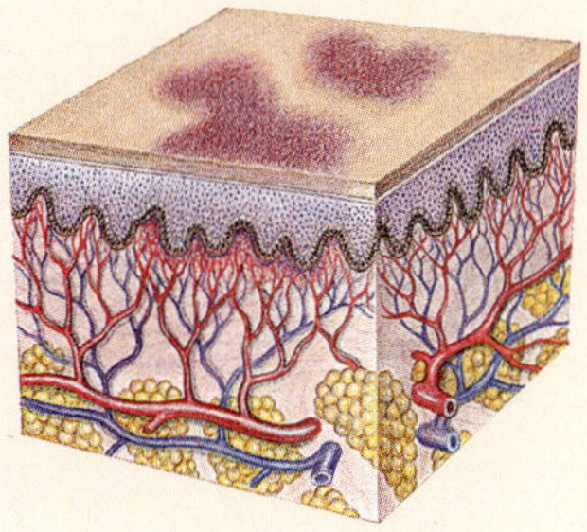	Hemorrhagic spots of varied size. Flat. Round or irregular	Decreased platelets or clotting factors resulting in hemorrhage into skin. Vascular abnormalities. Break in blood vessel walls from trauma
Petechiae 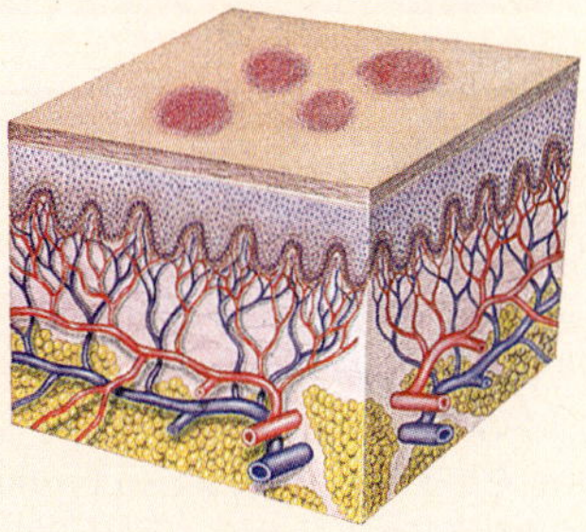	Pinpoint, flat, round area >2 mm. Purple, dark red, or brown	Same as above
Purpura 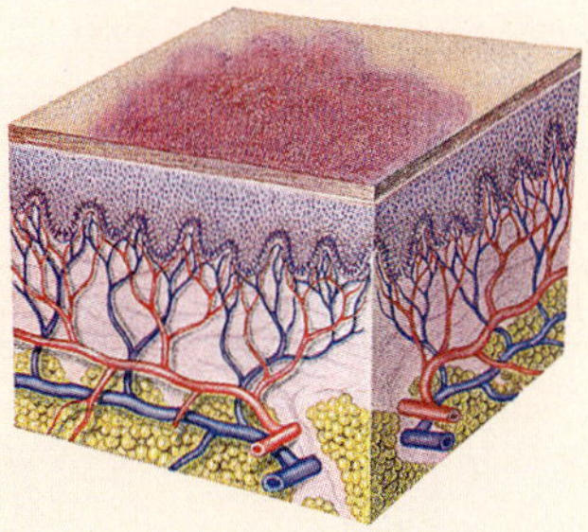	Flat purple or reddish discoloration. <5 mm. Do not blanche.	Same as above

Continued

TABLE 33.6 ASSESSMENT ABNORMALITIES—cont'd

Vascular Skin Lesions

Finding	Description	Possible Cause and Significance
Spider nevus (spider angioma)	Has a round, red, central part and branching radiations resembling a spider's web. Usually found on face, neck, or chest	High estrogen levels as in pregnancy or liver disease
Telangiectasia	Fine, irregular red lines	Permanently dilated small blood vessels. Usually caused by sun damage or aging. May be seen with varicose veins, scleroderma, rosacea

Figures from Ball JW et al: *Seidel's guide to physical examination,* ed 10, St Louis, 2023, Mosby.

TABLE 33.7 Diagnostic Studies

CBC Studies

Study	Description and Purpose	Reference Intervals
Hemoglobin (Hgb)	Amount of total Hgb in peripheral blood	*Female:* 12–16 g/dL (120–160 g/L) *Male:* 14–18 g/dL (140–180 g/L)
Hematocrit (Hct)	Measures packed cell volume of RBCs. Expressed as a percentage of the total blood volume	*Female:* 37%–47% (0.37–0.47) *Male:* 42%–52% (0.42–0.52)
Platelet count	Number of circulating platelets	150,000–400,000 $\times$ 10^3/L (150–400 $\times$ 10^9/L)
Total RBC count (erythrocyte count)	Number of circulating RBCs per volume of blood	*Female:* 4.2–5.4 $\times$ $10^6/\mu L$ (4.2–5.4 $\times$ 10^{12}/L) *Male:* 4.7–6.1 $\times$ $10^6/\mu L$ (4.7–6.1 $\times$ 10^{12}/L)
Red cell indices		
Mean corpuscular volume (MCV): $MCV = \frac{Hct \times 10}{RBC \times 10^6}$	Determines relative size of RBCs. Low MCV reflection of microcytosis. High MCV reflection of macrocytosis	80–95 fL
Mean corpuscular hemoglobin (MCH): $MCH = \frac{Hgb \times 10}{RBC \times 10^6}$	Measures average amount of Hgb in an RBC. Low MCH indicates microcytosis or hypochromia. High MCH indicates macrocytosis	27–31 pg
Mean corpuscular hemoglobin concentration (MCHC): $MCHC = \frac{Hgb \times 100}{Hct}$	Evaluates RBC saturation with Hgb. Low MCHC indicates hypochromia. High MCHC occurs with spherocytosis	32%–36% (0.32–0.36)
RBC morphology	Examines shape and size of RBCs	No variation in RBC morphology
Reticulocyte count	Number of immature RBCs released from the bone marrow into the blood	0.5%–2.0% of RBC
WBC count	Total number of WBCs	5000–10,000/mm^3 (5–10 $\times$ 10^9/L)
WBC differential	Determines whether each kind of WBC is present in proper proportion. Determines absolute value of each type of WBC by multiplying the percentage of cell type by total WBC count and dividing by 10	*Segmented neutrophils:* 55%–70% (0.55–0.70) *Banded neutrophils:* 0%–5% (0–0.08) *Eosinophils:* 1%–5% (0.01–0.04) *Basophils:* 0.5%–1% (0.005–0.01) *Lymphocytes:* 20%–40% (0.20–0.40) *Monocytes:* 2%–8% (0.02–0.08)

TABLE 33.8 Diagnostic Studies

Clotting Studies

Study	Description and Purpose	Reference Intervals
Activated clotting time (ACT)	Evaluates intrinsic coagulation status. More accurate than aPTT. Used during dialysis, coronary artery bypass procedure, arteriograms	70–120 sec
Activated partial thromboplastin time (aPTT)	Assesses intrinsic coagulation by measuring factors I, II, V, VIII, IX, X, XI, XII. Higher in patients receiving heparin	30–40 sec
Antithrombin (antithrombin III)	Naturally occurring protein made by liver that inhibits coagulation by inactivating thrombin and other factors. Lower in DIC and hypercoagulable disorders	17–30 mg/dL (170–300 mg/L) or 80%–130%
D-dimer	Assay to measure a fragment of fibrin that forms because of fibrin degradation and clot lysis. Used as an adjunctive measure in diagnosis of hypercoagulable conditions (e.g., DIC, pulmonary embolism)	<250 ng/mL (<250 μg/L)
Fibrin split products (FSPs) or fibrin degradation products (FDPs)	Reflects degree of fibrinolysis and predisposition to bleed (if present). Screening test for DIC. High levels occur with DIC, advanced cancer, severe inflammation	<10 μg/mL (<10 mg/L)
Fibrinogen (factor I)	Reflects fibrinogen level. Increase is a possible sign of enhancement of fibrin formation, making patient hypercoagulable. Decrease means patient may be predisposed to bleeding	200–400 mg/dL (2–4 g/L)
International normalized ratio (INR)	Standard system of reporting prothrombin time (PT) based on a reference calibration model. Calculated by comparing PT with a control value	0.8–1.1
Plasminogen	Assesses for plasminogen deficiency in patients who have multiple thromboembolic episodes	2.4–4.4 units/mL
Platelet count	Number of circulating platelets	150,000–400,000 × 10^3/L (150–400 × 10^9/L)
Prothrombin time (PT)	Assesses extrinsic coagulation by measuring factors I, II, V, VII, X	11–12.5 sec
Thrombin time	Reflects adequacy of thrombin and time to clot. Prolonged thrombin time means that coagulation is inadequate due to decreased thrombin activity	<21 sec

severe, we release more granulocytes from the bone marrow as a compensatory mechanism. To meet the increased demand, many young, immature polymorphonuclear neutrophils *(bands)* are released into circulation. More mature neutrophils are called *polymorphonuclear segmented neutrophils (segs)*. Together, bands and segs make up the *absolute neutrophil count* (ANC).

The WBC differential is very important because it is possible for the total WBC count to be essentially normal despite a marked change in one type of WBC. For example, a patient may have a normal WBC count of 8800/μL, but the differential count may show that the proportion of lymphocytes is only 10%. This is an abnormal finding that needs investigation.

When the bone marrow does not make enough neutrophils, neutropenia occurs. **Neutropenia** is a condition in which the ANC is less than 1000 cells/μL. Calculate the ANC by multiplying the total WBC count by the percentage of neutrophils. Neutropenia results from many disease processes, such as leukemia, or from bone marrow suppression. Severe neutropenia is associated with an ANC of less than 500 cells/μL. It is associated with a high risk for infection and death from sepsis.

Platelet count. The platelet count is the number of platelets per microliter of blood. Normal platelet counts are between 150,000 and 400,000/μL. Counts below 100,000/μL signify a condition termed **thrombocytopenia**. Bleeding may occur with thrombocytopenia. Spontaneous hemorrhage is possible once platelet counts fall below 10,000/μL, depending on the clinical situation.[6] A description of clotting studies is given in Table 33.8.[10]

Thrombocytosis is too many platelets. It occurs with inflammation and some cancers (Chapter 34). The most likely complication of thrombocytosis is excess clotting.

Blood Typing and Rh Factor

Blood group antigens (A and B) are found only on RBC membranes. They form the basis for the ABO blood typing system (Table 33.9). The presence or absence of 1 or both inherited antigens is the basis for the 4 blood groups: A, B, AB, and O. Blood group A has A antigens, group B has B antigens, group AB has both antigens, and group O has neither A nor B antigens. Each person has antibodies in the serum termed *anti-A* and *anti-B* that react with A or B antigens. These antibodies are found when the corresponding antigen is absent from the RBC surface. For example, there are B antibodies in the serum of people with blood group A.[1]

Blood reactions based on ABO incompatibilities result from RBC hemolysis. RBCs *agglutinate* (or clump) when an antibody is present to react with the antigens on the RBC membrane. For example, agglutination will occur in the blood of a person with type A blood if they receive blood transfused from a person with

TABLE 33.9 ABO and Rh Blood Groups

	ANTIGENS PRESENT ON RBC		ANTIBODIES POSSIBLY PRESENT IN PLASMA		
Blood Type	**A or B**	**Rh (D)**	**A or B**	**Rh (D)**	**Percent of General Population**
0	—	—	A, B	Rh	7
0+	—	Rh	A, B	—	38
A	A	—	B	Rh	6
A+	A	Rh	B	—	34
B	B	—	A	Rh	2
B+	B	Rh	A	—	9
AB	A, B	—	—	Rh	1
AB+	A, B	Rh	—	—	3

B antigens (i.e., type B or AB). The anti-B antibodies in the type A blood would react with the B antigens, starting the process that results in RBC hemolysis. Blood component compatibilities for transfusions are outlined in Table 34.33.

The *Rh system* is based on a third antigen, D. It is also on the RBC membrane. Rh-positive people have the D antigen, while Rh-negative people do not. Rh-positive blood is indicated with a "+" after the ABO group (e.g., AB+). Rh status is determined by a Coombs test (Table 33.10).

Because of transfusion therapy or during childbirth, a Rh-negative person may be exposed to Rh-positive blood. After exposure during childbirth, a Rh-negative mother forms an antibody, anti-D, which acts against Rh antigens (Rh-positive people normally have no anti-D). In future pregnancies, the mother's anti-D antibodies can cross the placenta and attack the RBCs of an Rh-positive fetus, causing hemolysis of the RBCs. A pregnant Rh-negative female should receive Rho(D) immune globulin (RhoGAM) injections to prevent anti-D antibodies from forming.[4]

Iron Metabolism

Laboratory tests used to assess iron metabolism include serum iron, transferrin saturation, ferritin, and total iron-binding capacity. We may do tests for nutrition problems that can lead to defective RBC production (Table 33.10).[10]

Serum iron is a measurement of the amount of protein-bound iron circulating in the serum. *Transferrin saturation* is a good indicator of iron available for erythropoiesis. Unlike serum iron, the iron bound to transferrin is readily available for the body to use. You calculate transferrin saturation by dividing serum iron by total iron binding capacity (TIBC) and multiplying by 100. For example, a patient with a serum iron level of 100 µg/dL and a TIBC of 300 µg/dL would have a transferrin saturation of about 33%.

Under normal conditions, ferritin concentration correlates closely with body iron stores. In normal patients, 1 ng/mL of ferritin corresponds to 8 to 10 mg of stored iron.

TIBC gives an indirect measure of all proteins that bind or transport iron between the tissues and bone marrow. However, it overestimates transferrin levels by 16% to 20% because it measures other proteins that can bind iron. These other proteins only bind iron when transferrin is more than half saturated. TIBC varies inversely with tissue iron stores. It is higher when iron stores are low and lower when iron stores are high.

Biopsies

Biopsy procedures specific to hematologic assessment are bone marrow examination and lymph node biopsy. A biopsy provides information needed for diagnosis and treatment planning. In general, these procedures are done when a peripheral blood smear is nonspecific.

Bone Marrow Examination

Bone marrow examination is important in evaluating many hematologic problems. It may involve aspiration only or aspiration with biopsy (Table 33.11).[10] The benefits gained from bone marrow examination are (1) a full evaluation of hematopoiesis and (2) the ability to get specimens for cytopathologic and chromosomal analysis. The preferred site for both aspiration and biopsy of bone marrow is the posterior iliac crest. A physician, nurse practitioner, or physician's assistant can perform the procedure. Patients may receive local anesthesia and sedation to minimize anxiety and pain.

For bone marrow aspiration, the skin over the puncture site is cleansed with a bactericidal agent. The skin, subcutaneous tissue, and periosteum are injected with a local anesthetic agent. Once the area is anesthetized, a bone marrow needle is inserted through the cortex of the bone (Fig. 33.7). The stylet of the needle is removed. The hub is attached to a 10-mL syringe, and 0.2 to 0.5 mL of the fluid marrow is aspirated. Patients will have pain when the periosteum is penetrated and with aspiration. Although the pain will last only a few seconds, it can be quite uncomfortable. After the marrow aspiration, the needle is removed. Pressure is applied over the aspiration site to ensure hemostasis. We then cover the site with a sterile pressure dressing.

Complications of bone marrow aspiration are minimal. There is a chance of damaging underlying structures. Other complications include infection if the patient is neutropenic. Hemorrhage may occur in patients with severe thrombocytopenia.

Monitor the patient's vital signs until stable. Assess the site for excess drainage or bleeding. If bleeding is present, have the patient lie supine for 30 to 60 minutes to keep pressure on the site. If the bed is too soft, have the patient lie on a rolled towel

TABLE 33.10 **Diagnostic Studies**

Miscellaneous Blood Studies

Study	Description and Purpose	Normal Values
Bilirubin	Measures degree of RBC hemolysis or liver's inability to excrete normal quantities of bilirubin. Increase in indirect (unconjugated) bilirubin with hemolysis. Increase in direct (conjugated) bilirubin with obstructive problems (e.g., gallstones, liver tumor)	*Total:* 0.3–1.0 mg/dL (5.1–17.0 μmol/L) *Direct:* 0.1–0.3 mg/dL (1.7–5.1 μmol/L) *Indirect:* 0.2–0.8 mg/dL (3.4–12.0 μmol/L)
Blood smear (peripheral blood smear)	Reviews color, size, shape, quantity of cells in peripheral blood. Provides information about problems affecting RBCs, WBCs, or platelets	Normal quantity of each cell type, normal size, shape, and color of RBCs, normal WBC differential count and platelets
Coombs test	Differentiates among types of hemolytic anemias and investigates hemolytic transfusion reactions. Detects immune antibodies and Rh factor	Negative
• Direct	Detects antibodies that are attached to RBCs	Negative
• Indirect	Detects circulating antibodies against red cells in serum	Negative
Cobalamin (vitamin B_{12})	Level of cobalamin available for production of new RBCs	160–950 pg/mL (118–701 pmol/L)
Erythrocyte sedimentation rate (ESR)	Measures sedimentation or settling of RBCs in 1 h. Inflammatory process causes a change in plasma proteins, resulting in aggregation of RBCs and making them heavier. The faster the sedimentation rate, the higher the ESR	<20 mm/h (some gender variation)
Erythropoietin	Measures degree of hormonal stimulation to bone marrow to stimulate the release of RBCs	5–35 IU/mL (5–30 U/L)
Ferritin	Major iron storage protein. Is normally present in blood in concentrations directly related to iron storage	10–300 ng/mL (10–300 μg/L)
Folic acid (folate)	Amount of folic acid (folate) available for RBC production	5–25 ng/mL (11–57 nmol/L)
Haptoglobin	Glycoprotein that binds to Hgb released into the bloodstream by hemolysis. Decreased with red cell hemolysis. Increased with infection, inflammation, cancer	50–220 mg/dL
Hemoglobin (Hgb) electrophoresis	Proteins involved in development of Hgb molecule have a definitive pattern of separation on electrophoresis. This pattern is changed with abnormal Hgb synthesis (e.g., thalassemia) or sickle cell anemia (where Hgb S is increased)	Normal Hb A1: >95% Hb A2: 2%–3% Hb F: 0.8%–2% Hb S: 0 Hb C: 0
Homocysteine	Intermediate amino acid formed during the metabolism of the essential amino acid methionine. Rapidly metabolized through pathways that require cobalamin (vitamin B_{12}) and folic acid. Increased in cobalamin and folic acid deficiency	*Normal:* 4–14 μmol/L
Iron		
• Iron total	Reflects amount of iron combined with proteins in serum. Indicates status of iron storage and use	*Male:* 80–180 μg/dL (14–32 μmol/L) *Female:* 60–160 μg/dL (11–29 μmol/L)
• (Total) iron-binding capacity (TIBC)	Measures all proteins available for binding iron. Transferrin represents the largest quantity of iron-binding proteins. Thus TIBC is an indirect measure of transferrin, an evaluation of the amount of extra iron that can be carried	250–460 μg/dL (45–82 μmol/L)
Lactic dehydrogenase (LDH)	Intracellular enzyme present in almost all body tissues. Levels rise in response to cell damage. Increased levels confirm diagnosis of injury or disease. Used as a nonspecific marker of hematologic cancer growth and response to treatment	100–190 U/L
Methylmalonic acid (MMA)	Indirect test for cobalamin (vitamin B_{12}). MMA metabolism requires cobalamin. Increased levels with cobalamin deficiency. Helps distinguish cobalamin deficiency from folic acid deficiency	<3.6 μmol/mmol creatinine
Microglobulin (beta$_2$ microglobulin)	Protein found on the surface of all cells. Increased in chronic infection, inflammatory diseases, or cancers such as lymphoma, leukemia, multiple myeloma. May be used as a tumor marker	*Blood:* 0.7–1.8 μg/mL *Urine:* ≤300 μg/L Spinal fluid: ≤2.4 mg/L
Serum protein electrophoresis (SPEP)	Separates proteins in blood on basis of electric charge. Helps detect hyperglobulinemic states, such as in multiple myeloma or some lymphomas	Normal banding pattern of albumin and globulins. Increase in any protein *(protein spike)* is abnormal
Transferrin	Largest of proteins that bind to iron. Increased in most people with iron-deficiency anemia	*Male:* 215–365 mg/dL (2.15–3.65 g/L) *Female:* 250–380 mg/dL (2.5–3.8 g/L)
Transferrin saturation (%)	Decreased in iron-deficiency anemia. Increased in hemolytic and megaloblastic anemia	*Male:* 20%–50% *Female:* 15%–50%

TABLE 33.11 Diagnostic Studies

Hematologic System

Study	Description and Purpose	Nursing Responsibility
Molecular, Cytogenetic, and Gene Analysis Studies		
Cancer genomics (genotyping) **Cell surface immunophenotyping (flow cytometry)** **Chromosomal karyotyping (PCR)** **Fluorescence in situ hybridization (FISH)** **Next-generation sequencing**	Assesses for genetic or chromosome abnormalities of cancer cells. Uses peripheral blood (e.g., leukemia), biopsy specimen (bone marrow, lymph node, tissue), or CSF. Used to confirm diagnosis and determine treatment, prognosis, and response to therapy	*Before:* Explain purpose of testing. HCP will provide specific significance.
Procedures		
Bone marrow biopsy (Fig. 33.7)	Removal of bone marrow through a locally anesthetized site to assess blood-forming tissue. Used to diagnose and monitor aplastic anemia, multiple myeloma, myelodysplastic syndromes, leukemia, and some lymphomas	*Before:* Explain procedure. Obtain signed consent. Perform a surgical time-out before procedure. Analgesics may be given to enhance patient comfort and cooperation. *After:* Apply pressure dressing. Assess biopsy site for bleeding and apply pressure as needed. Tenderness at the puncture site for a few days may be normal. Assess for infection.
Lumbar puncture (LP)	Done to obtain CSF for testing for cancer, infection, and degenerative brain diseases. May be used to give chemotherapy to the central nervous system	*Before:* Have patient empty bladder. *During:* Help position patient and provide support. *After:* Watch site for bleeding and infection. Spinal headaches may occur. Follow HCP orders for how long the patient should lie flat. Encourage the patient to drink fluids.
Lymph node biopsy	Used to obtain lymph tissue for histologic examination to determine diagnosis and therapy	*Before:* Explain procedure. Obtain signed consent. *After:* Watch site for bleeding. Monitor vital signs, especially if platelet count is low. Change sterile dressing as ordered. Inspect wound for healing and infection.
• Closed (needle) or fine needle	Done at the bedside or in an outpatient area. A very small needle is used to reduce risk for tracking cancer cells through normal subcutaneous tissue	
• Open	Done in operating room or procedure area using either local or general anesthesia. After making an incision, the lymph node and surrounding tissue are excised whenever possible	
Radioisotope Studies		
Bone scan	Radioactive isotope is injected IV and taken up by the bones. Uniform uptake is normal. Increased uptake seen in osteomyelitis, certain fractures, and bone cancer	*Before:* Patient may be asked to drink 4–6 glasses of water and then void before imaging (to see pelvic bones). Obtain IV access for injection of isotope.
Radiologic Studies		
CT scan	Noninvasive radiologic examination using computer-assisted x-ray can evaluate many structural abnormalities: tumors, fluid collections, inflammation, obstruction. May be used as a guide for biopsies. Contrast medium may be used. Spiral (helical) CT scans can obtain many images in a short amount of time	*Before:* Assess for iodine sensitivity if contrast medium used. IV and/or oral contrast may be given prior depending on the area being studied. Patient may need to be NPO for 4 h. *After:* Have patient drink fluids to avoid renal problems with contrast.
MRI	Noninvasive procedure produces sensitive images of soft tissue (central nervous system, neck and back, bones and joints, heart, breasts). An IV contrast agent (gadolinium) may be given. May provide a better contrast between normal tissue and pathologic tissue than CT	*Before:* Oral and/or IV contrast injection may be used. Check for pregnancy, allergies, and renal function before test. Have patient remove all metal objects. Ask about any history of surgical insertion of staples, plates, dental bridges, or other metal appliances. Remove metallic foil patches. Patient may need to fast. Assess for claustrophobia and the need for antianxiety medication. Have patient urinate. *During:* Patient must lie completely still during scan.

Continued

TABLE 33.11 Diagnostic Studies
Hematologic System— cont'd

Study	Description and Purpose	Nursing Responsibility
Positron emission tomography (PET)	Glucose-containing nuclear tracer substance is injected and taken up by metabolically active cells. Follow-up scan shows different-colored tissues based on metabolic rate. Because cancer cells have an increased uptake of glucose, "hot spots" reflecting increased glucose consumption indicate the presence of active cancer. CT scanning may be done in conjunction or images fused	*Before:* Obtain IV access to inject the tracer substance. Patients should be NPO, except for water and medications, for at least 4 h prior. Hold glucose-containing IV solutions and change to normal saline. Check glucose levels as high levels may interfere with test. May need bowel preparation depending on area being studied. Have patient urinate. *After:* Encourage fluids to excrete radioactive substance.
Ultrasound (abdominal, liver, spleen)	Noninvasive probe is lubricated and slid across the abdomen to detect density and borders of the abdominal organs. Can detect irregular borders, masses, vascular structure, fluid collections, and biliary tree	*During:* Patient must be comfortable lying flat and having probe compress abdomen.
Urine Studies		
Bence Jones protein (free kappa and lambda light chains)	An electrophoretic measurement used to detect Bence Jones protein, which is found in most cases of multiple myeloma. May be present in some other hematologic disorders and metastatic cancers. Negative finding is normal	*During:* Obtain random urine specimen early in the morning. If a 24-h urine collection is done, discard first specimen, and collect all urine voided during the 24 h, keeping on ice or refrigerated. Remind patient not to put toilet paper in urine collection container.

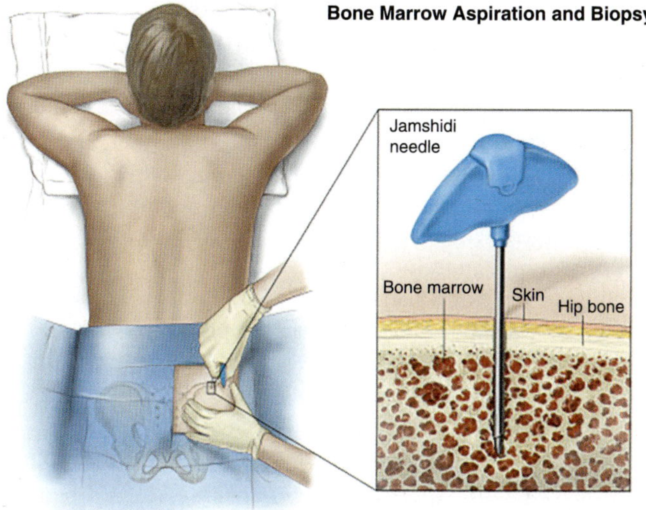

Fig. 33.7 Bone marrow aspiration from the posterior iliac crest.

to provide more pressure. Notify the HCP if bleeding continues. You may give analgesics for postprocedure pain. Soreness over the puncture site for 3 to 4 days after the procedure is normal.

Lymph Node Biopsy

Lymph node biopsy involves obtaining lymph tissue for histologic examination to determine the diagnosis and help plan therapy. This may be done by either an open or a closed (needle) biopsy.

If the results from a needle biopsy are negative, it may only mean that the cancer cells were not part of the tissue in the biopsy specimen. However, a positive finding may be enough evidence to confirm a diagnosis. This technique is rarely used to confirm an initial diagnosis because larger specimens, such as excisional biopsies, are usually needed to perform cytopathologic tests.

Molecular Cytogenetics and Gene Analysis

Testing for specific chromosomal variations with hematologic problems is essential to diagnosis (Table 33.11). Results determine treatment options, prognosis, and response to therapy. If a large number of abnormal cells are circulating in the blood, such as in acute leukemia, these tests may be done on peripheral blood. However, testing is usually done on samples from bone marrow, lymph node biopsies, and sometimes cerebrospinal fluid (CSF).[3]

There are many molecular tests. Flow cytometry can detect specific cell populations and their cell surface antigens.[3] Fluorescence in situ hybridization (FISH) identifies genetic defects using nucleic probes that are complementary to a targeted region of deoxyribonucleic acid (DNA). FISH can identify an abnormal extra chromosome 8, which is common in certain leukemias.[3] Reverse transcription polymerase chain reaction (PCR) is another way to detect specific mutations and amount. PCR can detect the Philadelphia chromosome translocation t(9;22) seen in chronic myeloid leukemia and some cases of acute lymphoblastic leukemia.[3]

CASE STUDY

Objective Data: Diagnostic Studies

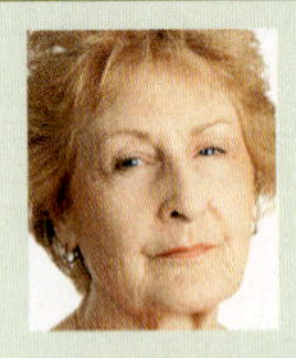
(© Lisa F. Young/iStock.)

The HCP orders the following diagnostic studies for A.J.:

- CBC, basic metabolic panel (electrolytes, BUN, creatinine), PT/PTT
- Arterial blood gases
- Chest x-ray

A.J.'s CBC reveals an Hgb of 5.9 g/dL, Hct of 18.2%, WBC of 2600/μL (2.6×10^9/L), platelet count of 72,000/μL, PT = 18 seconds, aPTT = 37. Arterial blood gases and chest x-ray are normal. The HCP orders more blood work, including a WBC differential and RBC indices, and admits her to the hospital for further evaluation and potential treatment.

Discussion Questions

1. Are these the diagnostic studies that you expected to be ordered?
2. Which diagnostic study results concern you most? What other studies may be ordered on admission?

This case study is continued in Chapter 34.

Answers available at http://evolve.elsevier.com/Lewis/medsurg.

BRIDGE TO NCLEX EXAMINATION

The number of the question corresponds to the same-numbered outcome at the beginning of the chapter.

1. A person who lives at a high altitude may normally have an increased Hgb and RBC count because
 a. high altitudes cause vascular fluid loss, leading to hemoconcentration.
 b. hypoxia caused by decreased atmospheric O_2 stimulates erythropoiesis.
 c. the function of the spleen in removing old RBCs is impaired at high altitudes.
 d. impaired production of platelets leads to proportionally higher red cell counts.

2. A patient with cancer arising from granulocytic cells in the bone marrow will have
 a. a risk for bleeding.
 b. altered oxygenation.
 c. decreased production of antibodies.
 d. decreased phagocytosis of bacteria.

3. An anticoagulant such as warfarin that interferes with prothrombin production will alter the clotting mechanism during
 a. platelet aggregation.
 b. activation of thrombin.
 c. the release of tissue thromboplastin.
 d. stimulation of factor activation complex.

4. When reviewing laboratory results of an older patient with an infection, the nurse would expect to find
 a. mild leukocytosis.
 b. decreased platelet count.
 c. increased hemoglobin and hematocrit levels.
 d. decreased erythrocyte sedimentation rate (ESR).

5. Key information from the health history that relates to the hematologic system includes
 a. jaundice.
 b. bladder surgery.
 c. early menopause.
 d. multiple pregnancies.

6. While assessing the lymph nodes, the nurse would
 a. apply gentle, firm pressure to deep lymph nodes.
 b. palpate the deep cervical and supraclavicular nodes last.
 c. lightly palpate superficial lymph nodes with the pads of the fingers.
 d. use the tips of the second, third, and fourth fingers to apply deep palpation.

7. A normal finding when palpating lymph nodes in an adult patient is
 a. hard, fixed nodes.
 b. firm, mobile nodes.
 c. enlarged, tender nodes.
 d. hard, nontender nodes.

8. Nursing care for a patient after a bone marrow biopsy and aspiration includes (**Select all that apply.**)
 a. giving analgesics as needed.
 b. preparing to start a blood transfusion.
 c. keeping the sterile pressure dressing intact.
 d. giving preprocedure and postprocedure antibiotic medications.
 e. monitoring vital signs and assessing the site for excess drainage or bleeding.

1. b; 2. d; 3. b; 4. a; 5. a; 6. c; 7. b; 8. a, c, e.

For rationales to these answers and even more NCLEX review questions, visit http://evolve.elsevier.com/Lewis/medsurg.

REFERENCES

To access the References for this chapter, please scan the QR code with a mobile device.

34

Hematologic Problems

Sandra Irene Rome

http://evolve.elsevier.com/Lewis/medsurg/

CONCEPTUAL FOCUS

Cellular Regulation
Clotting
Fatigue
Functional Ability
Gas Exchange
Immunity
Infection
Perfusion

LEARNING OUTCOMES

1. Describe the general clinical manifestations and complications of anemia.
2. Distinguish the etiologies, clinical manifestations, diagnostic findings, and interprofessional and nursing management of iron deficiency, megaloblastic, and aplastic anemias.
3. Explain the nursing management of anemia from blood loss.
4. Describe the pathophysiology, clinical manifestations, and interprofessional and nursing management of anemia from increased erythrocyte destruction.
5. Describe the pathophysiology and nursing and interprofessional management of polycythemia.
6. Explain the pathophysiology, clinical manifestations, and interprofessional and nursing management of various types of thrombocytopenia.
7. Describe the types, clinical manifestations, diagnostic findings, and interprofessional and nursing management of hemophilia and von Willebrand disease.
8. Explain the pathophysiology, diagnostic findings, and interprofessional and nursing management of disseminated intravascular coagulation.
9. Describe the etiology, clinical manifestations, and interprofessional and nursing management of neutropenia.
10. Describe the pathophysiology, clinical manifestations, and interprofessional and nursing management of myelodysplastic syndromes.
11. Explain the nursing and interprofessional management of acute and chronic leukemias.
12. Compare Hodgkin lymphoma and non-Hodgkin lymphoma in terms of clinical manifestations, staging, and interprofessional and nursing management.
13. Describe the pathophysiology, clinical manifestations, and interprofessional and nursing management of multiple myeloma.
14. Discuss spleen disorders and their interprofessional care.
15. Describe the nursing management of patients receiving blood products.

KEY TERMS

anemia
aplastic anemia
disseminated intravascular coagulation (DIC)
hemochromatosis
hemolytic anemia
hemophilia
Hodgkin lymphoma
iron deficiency anemia
leukemia
lymphomas
megaloblastic anemias
multiple myeloma
myelodysplastic syndromes (MDS)
neutropenia
non-Hodgkin lymphomas (NHLs)
pernicious anemia
polycythemia
sickle cell disease (SCD)
thalassemia
thrombocytopenia

This chapter discusses common hematologic problems and their associated concepts. There is a wide range of blood conditions and cancers. Because blood has so many essential functions, hematologic problems affect patients in many ways. Patients with anemia and hematologic cancer often cope with fatigue. Impaired immunity and the risk for infection are concerns among patients with hematologic cancer and common side effects of therapy. Clotting is a protective mechanism that supports homeostasis when injury occurs. Excess clotting can impair perfusion. Inadequate clotting can lead to blood loss and fluid volume deficit.

ANEMIAS

ANEMIA

Definition and Classification

Anemia is a deficiency in the number of erythrocytes (red blood cells [RBCs]), the quantity or quality of hemoglobin (Hgb), and/or volume of packed RBCs (hematocrit). It is not a specific disease but rather a manifestation of a pathologic process. It is a common problem with many diverse causes. These include blood loss, impaired RBC production, or increased RBC destruction (Fig. 34.1). The diagnosis of anemia is based on a complete blood count (CBC), reticulocyte count, and peripheral blood smear. Once identified, further research is done to find the specific cause.[1]

Anemia can result from primary hematologic problems or develop because of diseases or disorders of other body systems. We classify the types of anemia by either *morphology* (cell characteristic) or *etiology* (cause). Morphologic classification is based on RBC size and color (Table 34.1). Etiologic classification is based on the clinical condition causing the anemia (Table 34.2). Although the morphologic system is the most accurate way to classify anemia, it is easier to discuss patient care by focusing on the cause of the anemia.

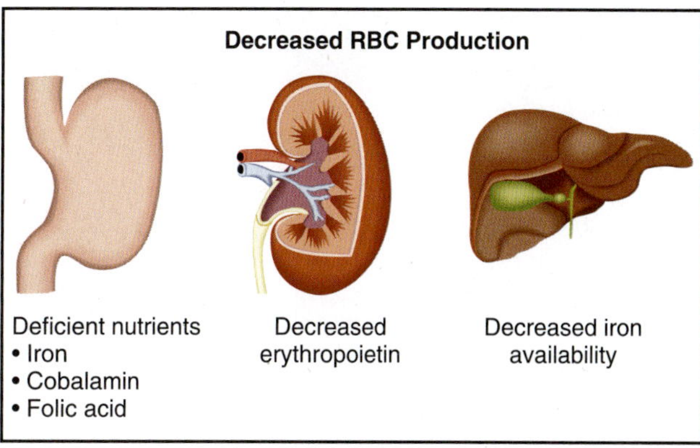

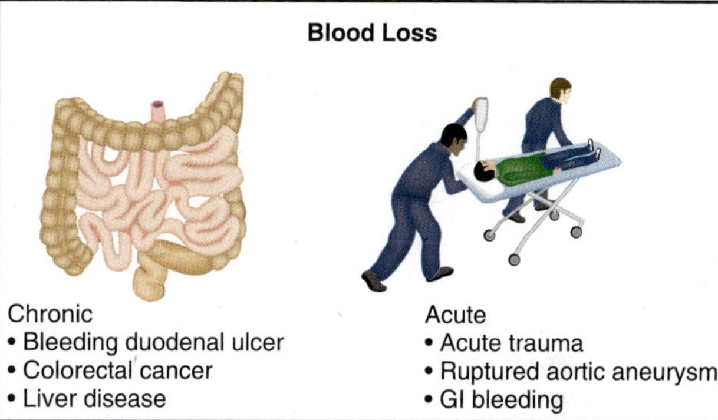

Increased RBC Destruction

Hemolysis
- Sickle cell disease
- Medication (e.g., methyldopa [Aldomet])
- Incompatible blood
- Trauma (e.g., cardiopulmonary bypass)

Fig. 34.1 Causes of anemia.

TABLE 34.1 Morphologic Classification of Anemia

Morphology	Etiology
Normocytic, normochromic (normal size and color) MCV 80–95 fL, MCH 27–31 pg	Acute blood loss, hemolysis, chronic kidney disease, chronic disease, cancer, endocrine problems, starvation, aplastic anemia, sickle cell anemia, pregnancy
Microcytic, hypochromic (small size, pale color) MCV <80 fL, MCH <27 pg	Iron deficiency anemia, vitamin B_6 deficiency, copper deficiency, thalassemia, lead poisoning
Macrocytic (megaloblastic), normochromic (large size, normal color) MCV >95 fL, MCH >31 pg	Cobalamin (vitamin B_{12}) deficiency, folic acid deficiency, liver disease (including effects of alcohol use)

MCH, Mean corpuscular hemoglobin; *MCV,* mean corpuscular volume.

Clinical Manifestations

Because RBCs transport O_2, RBC disorders can lead to tissue hypoxia. The manifestations of anemia result from the body's response to hypoxia. Specific manifestations vary depending on how fast the anemia has evolved, its severity, and any coexisting disease. We often use Hgb levels to determine the severity of anemia.

Mild anemia (Hgb 10 to 12 g/dL [100 to 120 g/L]) may exist without causing symptoms (Table 34.3). If symptoms develop, it is because the patient has an underlying disease or has a compensatory response to heavy exercise. In moderate anemia (Hgb 6 to 10 g/dL [60 to 100 g/L]), there is an increase in cardiopulmonary symptoms. The patient may have them while resting and with activity. In severe anemia (Hgb less than 6 g/dL [60 g/L]), the patient has many manifestations involving multiple body systems.

Skin manifestations include pallor, jaundice, and itching. Pallor results from low Hgb levels and reduced blood flow to the skin. Jaundice occurs when RBC hemolysis increases the serum bilirubin concentration. Hemolysis also causes itching from the increased serum and skin bile concentrations.

Cardiopulmonary manifestations result from the heart and lungs trying to provide adequate amounts of O_2 to the tissues.

TABLE 34.2 Etiologic Classification of Anemia

Decreased RBC Production

Decreased Hemoglobin Synthesis
- Iron deficiency
- Sideroblastic anemia (↓ porphyrin)
- Thalassemia (↓ globin synthesis)

Decreased Number of RBC Precursors
- Aplastic anemia and inherited disorders (e.g., Fanconi syndrome)
- Anemia of myeloproliferative diseases (e.g., leukemia) and myelodysplasia
- Chronic diseases or disorders
- Medications and chemicals (e.g., chemotherapy, lead)
- Radiation

Defective DNA Synthesis
- Cobalamin (vitamin B_{12}) deficiency
- Folic acid deficiency

Blood Loss

Acute
- Blood vessel rupture
- Splenic sequestration crisis
- Trauma

Chronic
- Gastritis
- Hemorrhoids
- Menstrual flow

Increased RBC Destruction (Hemolytic Anemias)

Acquired (Extrinsic)
- Antibodies against RBCs
- Cancer
- DIC
- Extracorporeal circulation
- HELLP syndrome (hemolysis, ↑ liver enzymes, ↓ platelets associated with pregnancy)
- Infectious agents (e.g., malaria) and toxins
- Physical destruction
- Prosthetic heart valves
- Thrombotic thrombocytopenic purpura (TTP)

Hereditary (Intrinsic)
- Abnormal hemoglobin (sickle cell disease)
- Enzyme deficiency (glucose-6-phosphate dehydrogenase [G6PD])
- Membrane abnormalities (paroxysmal nocturnal hemoglobinuria, hereditary spherocytosis)

Cardiac output is maintained by increasing the heart rate (HR) and stroke volume. Low blood viscosity contributes to systolic murmurs and bruits. In extreme cases or when heart disease is present, angina and myocardial infarction (MI) may occur if myocardial O_2 needs are not met. Heart failure (HF), cardiomegaly, pulmonary and systemic congestion, ascites, and peripheral edema may develop if the heart is overworked.

NURSING MANAGEMENT: ANEMIA

This section discusses general management of anemia. Specific care for various types of anemia is discussed later in this chapter. More information on the nursing care of patients with anemia is discussed in eNursing Care Plan 34.1.

Assessment

Table 34.4 outlines the subjective and objective data you should obtain from patients with anemia. Assess the patient's knowledge about proper nutrition and adherence to precautions to prevent cardiopulmonary stress, falls, and injury.

Clinical Problems

Clinical problems for patients with anemia include:
- Fatigue
- Nutritionally compromised
- Impaired tissue perfusion

Planning

The overall goals are that patients with anemia will (1) assume normal activities of daily living, (2) maintain adequate nutrition, and (3) develop no complications from anemia.

Implementation

The goal is to correct the cause of the anemia. Implement nursing interventions specific to the patient's needs and type of anemia. Acute interventions may include blood transfusions, drug therapy (e.g., iron supplements), and O_2 therapy to stabilize the patient. Diet and lifestyle changes (described in sections on specific types of anemia) can reverse some anemias.

For patients with fatigue, encourage alternate rest and activity periods. Help patients to prioritize activities according to energy levels. Arrange activities (e.g., avoid activity right after meals) to reduce competition for O_2 supply to vital functions. Aid with regular activities (e.g., ambulation, transfers, personal care) to minimize fatigue and risk for injury from falls. Monitor cardiorespiratory response to activity (e.g., tachycardia, dysrhythmias, dyspnea, diaphoresis, pallor, tachypnea).

Collaborate with the dietitian to determine the number of calories and type of nutrients needed to meet nutrition requirements. Encourage increased intake of foods listed in Table 34.5 that are high in the nutrients needed for RBC production.[2,3]

Gerontologic Considerations: Anemia

Modest changes in RBC mass occur in older adults. Healthy older adults have a modest decline in Hgb of about 1 g/dL after age 70. This is partly because of the decreased production of testosterone in males and estrogen in females.[1]

TABLE 34.3 Manifestations of Anemia

	SEVERITY OF ANEMIA		
Body System	**Mild (Hgb 10–12 g/dL [100–120 g/L])**	**Moderate (Hgb 6–10 g/dL [60–100 g/L])**	**Severe (Hgb <6 g/dL [<60 g/L])**
Cardiovascular	Palpitations	Palpitations, bounding pulse	↑ HR, ↑ pulse pressure, systolic murmurs, intermittent claudication, angina, heart failure, myocardial infarction
Eyes	None	None	Icteric conjunctiva and sclera, retinal hemorrhage, blurred vision
GI	None	None	Anorexia, hepatomegaly, splenomegaly, problems swallowing, sore mouth
General	None or mild fatigue	Fatigue	Sensitivity to cold, weight loss, lethargy
Mouth	None	None	Glossitis, smooth tongue
Musculoskeletal	None	None	Bone pain
Pulmonary	Exertional dyspnea	Dyspnea	Tachypnea, orthopnea, dyspnea at rest
Neurologic	None	"Roaring in the ears"	Headache, vertigo, irritability, depression, impaired thought processes
Skin	None	None	Pallor, jaundice, itching

TABLE 34.4 NURSING ASSESSMENT

Anemia

Subjective Data

Important Health Information

Health history: Recent blood loss or trauma; chronic liver, endocrine, or renal disease (including dialysis); GI disease (malabsorption syndrome, ulcers, gastritis); inflammatory disorders (especially Crohn disease); smoking, exposure to radiation or chemical toxins (arsenic, lead, benzenes, copper); infectious diseases; recent travel with possible exposure to infection; angina, myocardial infarction; history of falling

Medications: Use of vitamin and iron supplements; aspirin, anticoagulants, oral contraceptives, phenobarbital, penicillins, NSAIDs, omeprazole, phenytoin, sulfonamides, herbal products

Surgery or other treatments: Recent surgery, small bowel resection, gastrectomy, prosthetic heart valves, chemotherapy, radiation therapy

Diet history: General diet patterns, alcohol use

Functional Health Patterns

Health perception–health management: Family history of anemia; malaise

Nutritional-metabolic: Nausea, vomiting, anorexia, weight loss; dysphagia, dyspepsia, heartburn; night sweats, cold intolerance

Elimination: Hematuria, ↓ urine output; diarrhea, constipation, flatulence, tarry stools, bloody stools

Activity-exercise: Fatigue, muscle weakness, ↓ strength; dyspnea, orthopnea, cough, hemoptysis; palpitations; shortness of breath with activity

Cognitive-perceptual: Headache; abdominal, chest, and bone pain; painful tongue; paresthesias of feet and hands; itching; changes in vision, taste, or hearing; vertigo; hypersensitivity to cold; dizziness

Sexuality-reproductive: Menorrhagia, metrorrhagia; recent or current pregnancy; male impotence

Objective Data

General

Lethargy, apathy, general lymphadenopathy, fever

Cardiovascular

↑ HR, systolic murmur, dysrhythmias; postural hypotension, widened pulse pressure, carotid bruits, intermittent claudication, ankle edema

GI

Hepatosplenomegaly; glossitis; beefy, red tongue; stomatitis; abdominal distention; anorexia

Neurologic

Headache, roaring in the ears, confusion, impaired judgment, irritability, ataxia, unsteady gait, paralysis, loss of vibration sense

Respiratory

Tachypnea

Skin

Pale skin and mucous membranes; blue, pale white, or icteric sclera; cheilitis (inflammation of the lips); poor skin turgor; brittle, spoon-shaped fingernails; jaundice; petechiae; bruising; nose or gingival bleeding; poor healing; dry, brittle, thinning hair

Possible Diagnostic Findings

↓ RBCs, ↓ Hgb; ↓ Hct; ↑ or ↓ reticulocytes, ↑ or ↓ MCV; possible ↓ iron, ferritin, folate, or cobalamin (vitamin B_{12}); heme-positive stools; ↓ EPO level; ↑ or ↓ LDH, bilirubin, transferrin (Table 34.6)

EPO, Erythropoietin; *LDH,* lactate hydrogenase; *MCV,* mean corpuscular volume; *RBC,* red blood cell.

Anemia is not a normal finding in older adults. For many, anemia is due to an underlying cause, such as iron deficiency, bleeding, chronic disease, renal problems, or a hematologic problem. For those with no identifiable cause, it may be the result of cytokine dysregulation with aging.[1]

Manifestations of anemia in older adults may include pallor, confusion, ataxia, fatigue, and worsening cardiovascular and respiratory problems. Unfortunately, anemia may go unrecognized in older adults because we mistake the manifestations for normal aging changes or overlook them because of another

TABLE 34.5 NUTRITION THERAPY

Nutrients for Red Blood Cell (RBC) Production

Role in RBC Production	Food Sources
Amino Acids (Protein)	
Heme and plasma membrane synthesis and structure	Eggs, meat, milk and milk products (cheese, ice cream), poultry, fish, legumes, nuts, soy
Cobalamin (Vitamin B_{12})	
Synthesis of DNA, RBC maturation, facilitates folate metabolism	Meat, eggs, enriched grain products, milk and dairy foods, fish
Copper	
Mobilizes iron from tissues to plasma	Shellfish, whole grains, nuts, potatoes, organ meats, dark leafy greens, dried fruits
Folic Acid	
Synthesis of DNA and RNA, RBC maturation	Green leafy vegetables, enriched grain products and breakfast cereals, orange juice, peanuts, beans
Iron	
Hemoglobin synthesis	Lean beef, turkey, pork and chicken, fish, legumes, dark green leafy vegetables, whole-grain and enriched bread and cereals, beans
Niacin	
RBC maturation	Peanut butter, beef, poultry, fish; enriched and fortified grains; nuts and legumes
Pantothenic Acid (Vitamin B_5)	
Heme synthesis	Beef, poultry, seafood and organ meats; potatoes, avocado, cereal grains, legumes, eggs, milk
Pyridoxine (Vitamin B_6)	
Heme synthesis	Poultry, fish, organ meats, fortified cereals, potatoes, bananas
Riboflavin (Vitamin B_2)	
Oxidative reactions	Milk and dairy foods, enriched bread and other grain products, lean meats, eggs, green leafy vegetables
Vitamin C (Ascorbic Acid)	
Maintains iron in its ferrous form, aids in iron absorption	Citrus fruits, green leafy vegetables, strawberries, potatoes, kiwi fruit, tomatoes, green and red bell peppers
Vitamin E	
Heme synthesis. Protection against oxidative damage to RBCs	Vegetable oils, salad dressings, margarine, wheat germ, whole-grain products, seeds, nuts, peanut butter

health problem. By recognizing signs of anemia, you can play a key role in the care of older adults with this condition.

ANEMIA CAUSED BY DECREASED RBC PRODUCTION

Normally RBC production (*erythropoiesis*) is in equilibrium with RBC destruction and loss. This balance ensures that an adequate number of RBCs is always available. The normal life span of an RBC is 120 days. Three problems lead to decreased RBC production: (1) decreased Hgb synthesis from iron deficiency anemia, thalassemia, and sideroblastic anemia; (2) defective deoxyribonucleic acid (DNA) synthesis in RBCs (e.g., cobalamin deficiency, folic acid deficiency) may lead to megaloblastic anemias; and (3) diminished availability of RBC precursors may result in aplastic anemia and anemia of chronic disease (Table 34.2).

IRON DEFICIENCY ANEMIA

Iron deficiency anemia is the most common nutrition disorder in the world. Those most susceptible to iron deficiency anemia are the very young, those on poor diets, and females in their reproductive years.[4]

Etiology

Iron deficiency anemia may develop from inadequate diet intake, malabsorption, blood loss, or red cell hemolysis. Normal iron intake is usually enough to meet the needs of males and older females. It may be inadequate for people with higher iron needs (e.g., menstruating or pregnant females).

Iron malabsorption may occur after certain types of gastrointestinal (GI) surgery and in malabsorption syndromes. Iron absorption occurs in the duodenum. Thus malabsorption may occur after surgery that involves removal or bypass of the duodenum. It may occur if duodenal disease alters or destroys the absorption surface.

Blood loss is a major cause of iron deficiency in adults. The major sources of chronic blood loss are from the GI and genitourinary (GU) systems. GI bleeding is often not obvious. It may exist for a long time before the problem is found. Loss of 50 to 75 mL of blood from the upper GI tract is enough for stools to appear black *(melena)*. The black color results from the iron in the RBCs.

Common causes of GI blood loss are peptic ulcer, gastritis, esophagitis, diverticula, hemorrhoids, and cancer. GU blood loss occurs mainly from menstrual bleeding. Postmenopausal bleeding can contribute to anemia in susceptible older females. Dialysis treatment may cause iron deficiency anemia because of the blood lost in the dialysis equipment and frequent blood sampling.

Clinical Manifestations

In the early course of iron deficiency anemia, patients may not have any symptoms. As the disease becomes chronic, any of the general manifestations of anemia may develop (Table 34.3). Specific manifestations may occur with iron deficiency anemia. Pallor is the most common finding. *Glossitis* (inflammation of the tongue) is the second most common. Another finding is *cheilitis* (inflammation of the lips). Patients may report headache, paresthesias, and a burning sensation of the tongue.

Diagnostic Studies

Laboratory values seen with iron deficiency anemia are shown in Table 34.6.[4] Other diagnostic studies (e.g., stool occult blood

TABLE 34.6 Laboratory Results in Anemia

Etiology	Hgb/ Hct	Mean Corpuscular Volume (MCV)	Reticulocytes	Iron	Total Iron Binding Capacity (TIBC)	Transferrin	Ferritin	Bilirubin	B_{12}	Folate
Acute blood loss	↓	N or ↓	N or ↑	N	N	N	N	N	N	N
Aplastic anemia	↓	N or slight ↑	↓	N or ↓	N or ↑	N	N	N	N	N
Chronic blood loss	↓	↓	N or ↑	↓	↓	N	N	N or ↓	N	N
Chronic disease	↓	N or ↓	N or ↓	↓	↓	N or ↓	N or ↑	N	N	N
Cobalamin deficiency	↓	↑	N or ↓	N or ↑	N	Slight ↑	↑	N or slight ↑	↓	N
Folic acid deficiency	↓	↑	N or ↓	N or ↑	N	Slight ↑	↑	N or slight ↑	N	↓
Hemolytic anemia	↓	N or ↑	↑	N or ↑	N or ↓	N	N or ↑	↑	N	N
Iron deficiency	↓	↓	N or slight ↓ or ↑	↓	↑	N or ↓	↓	N or ↓	N	N
Sickle cell anemia	↓	N	↑	N or ↑	N or ↓	N	N	↑	N	↓
Thalassemia major	↓	N or ↓	↑	↑	↓	↓	N or ↑	↑	N	↓

N, normal.

test) are done to find the cause of the iron deficiency. Endoscopy and colonoscopy may detect GI bleeding. A bone marrow biopsy may be done if other tests are inconclusive.

Interprofessional and Nursing Management

The main goal is to treat the underlying problem that is causing iron loss, reduced intake (e.g., malnutrition, alcohol use), or poor iron absorption. We also direct efforts toward replacing iron (Table 34.7). Teach patients which foods are good sources of iron (Table 34.5). If nutrition is already adequate, increasing iron intake through diet may not be enough. Patients may need oral, or occasionally, IV iron supplements. If the iron deficiency is from acute blood loss, patients may need a packed RBC transfusion.

Drug Therapy

Many oral iron preparations are available. When giving iron, consider the following:

1. Iron is absorbed best from the duodenum and proximal jejunum. Enteric-coated or sustained-release capsules, which release iron farther down in the GI tract, are counterproductive and expensive.
2. The daily dose should provide 100 to 200 mg of elemental iron. This can be taken in divided daily doses or on alternate days, depending on tolerability and response.
3. Iron is best absorbed in an acidic environment. For this reason and to avoid binding the iron with food, iron should be taken an hour before meals, when the duodenal mucosa is most acidic. Taking iron with vitamin C (ascorbic acid) or orange juice enhances iron absorption. Iron may be taken with meals if absolutely needed to decrease GI side effects.
4. Undiluted liquid iron may stain the teeth. Dilute liquid iron, and have the patient drink it through a straw.
5. GI side effects may occur, including heartburn, constipation, and diarrhea. Have the patient stay upright for 30 minutes after taking oral forms. If side effects develop, the dose and type of supplement may need to be adjusted. For example, someone may not be able to tolerate ferrous sulfate because of the effects of the sulfate base. Ferrous gluconate may be better for them. Tell patients that iron will cause their stools to become black because the GI tract excretes excess iron. Constipation is common. The patient should start on stool softeners and laxatives, if needed, when started on iron.

TABLE 34.7 Interprofessional Care

Iron Deficiency Anemia

Diagnostic Assessment

- History and physical assessment
- Hgb and Hct (hematocrit) levels
- RBC count, including morphology
- Reticulocyte count
- Serum iron, ferritin, transferrin
- Total iron-binding capacity (TIBC)
- Stool examination for occult blood

Management

- Identify and treat underlying cause
- Drug therapy
- Oral: ferrous sulfate or ferrous gluconate
- IM or IV: iron dextran, sodium ferrous gluconate, iron sucrose
- Nutrition therapy (Table 34.5)
- Packed RBC transfusion

DRUG ALERT

Iron

- Some IV and IM iron preparations have a risk for an allergic reaction, so monitor the patient accordingly.
- The patient should be upright for 30 minutes after taking iron orally.

In some situations, we may need to give parenteral iron. Parenteral iron is indicated for malabsorption, intolerance of oral iron, a need for iron beyond oral limits, or poor adherence in taking oral iron. Parenteral iron can be given IM or IV. Administer IV iron dextran slowly, per orders (over at least 15 minutes). Take baseline vital signs, then observe the patient for at least 30 minutes so we can monitor for anaphylaxis.

Because IM iron solutions may stain the skin, use separate needles for withdrawing the solution and injecting the medication. Use a Z-track injection technique.

Assess the Hgb and RBC count to evaluate the response to therapy. Stress adherence with diet and drug therapy. To replenish the body's iron stores, patients need to take iron therapy for 2 to 3 months after the Hgb level returns to normal. Monitor patients who need lifelong iron therapy for potential liver problems from iron storage.

THALASSEMIA

Etiology

Thalassemia is a group of diseases involving inadequate production of normal Hgb, which decreases RBC production. Thalassemia is caused by an absent or reduced globulin protein. α-Globin chains are absent or reduced in α-thalassemia. β-Globin chains are absent or reduced in β-thalassemia. Thalassemia is commonly found in persons whose ethnic origins are near the Mediterranean Sea and equatorial or near-equatorial regions of Southeastern Asia, the Middle East, India, Pakistan, China, Southern Russia, and Africa.[4]

Genetic Link

Thalassemia has an autosomal recessive genetic basis. A person with thalassemia may have a heterozygous or homozygous form of the disease. A person who is heterozygous has 1 thalassemic gene and 1 normal gene. They have *thalassemia minor* (or thalassemic trait), which is a mild form of the disease. A homozygous person has 2 thalassemic genes. This causes the more severe form known as *thalassemia major.*

Pathophysiology

Hemolysis occurs as mononuclear phagocytes in the marrow destroy most erythroblasts. Those released into the blood are rapidly destroyed by macrophages in the spleen. The bone marrow responds to the reduced O_2-carrying capacity of the blood by increasing RBC production. The marrow becomes packed with immature erythroid precursors that die. This stimulates further RBC production, leading to chronic bone marrow hyperplasia and expansion of the marrow space. This may cause thickening of the cranium and maxillary cavity. Thrombocytosis after spleen dysfunction and/or removal may occur.

Clinical Manifestations and Diagnostic Studies

Patients with thalassemia minor are often asymptomatic. They have mild to moderate anemia with *microcytosis* (small cells) and *hypochromia* (pale cells), mild splenomegaly, bronzed skin color, and bone marrow hyperplasia.

Thalassemia major is a life-threatening disease. Symptoms develop in childhood by age 2. They can cause growth and development deficits. The person is pale and has other general symptoms of anemia (Table 34.3). Jaundice from RBC hemolysis is prominent. There is pronounced splenomegaly because the spleen continuously tries to remove the damaged RBCs. Hepatomegaly and cardiomyopathy occur from iron deposition.

Cardiac complications from iron overload, lung disease, and hypertension contribute to early death. Endocrine problems (diabetes, growth retardation, hypogonadism), osteoporosis, pulmonary hypertension, and thrombosis may occur.

Laboratory values seen with thalassemia major are shown in Table 34.6.

Interprofessional Care

Thalassemia minor does not need treatment because the body adapts to the reduction of normal Hgb. Treatment of thalassemia major includes blood transfusions or exchange transfusions in conjunction with chelating agents that bind to iron. Transfusions are generally given when the Hgb drops to less than 7 g/dL (100 g/L), depending on the manifestations.[1] Chelating agents reduce the iron overloading that occurs with chronic transfusion therapy. Drugs used include oral deferasirox or deferiprone or IV or subcutaneous deferoxamine.[1] A new therapy, luspatercept-aamt, is given subcutaneously every 21 days. It improves Hgb levels and reduces transfusion needs. It blocks inhibitors of late-stage RBC production.[2]

Because an enlarged spleen sequesters RBCs, patients may need a splenectomy. Monitor liver, heart, and lung function and provide treatment as needed.

Up until recently hematopoietic stem cell transplantation (HSCT) was the only cure for thalassemia. However, the risks of this procedure may outweigh its benefits. It requires a healthy donor. In new gene therapy, stem cells are collected from the patient and edited with a modified β-globin gene. The patient receives chemotherapy to suppress the bone marrow before the stem cell infusion. The stem cells then grow new healthy blood cells over time. This therapy has risks related to temporary low blood counts, leading to potential infection and bleeding.[5]

MEGALOBLASTIC ANEMIAS

Megaloblastic anemias are characterized by the presence of abnormally large *(macrocytic)* RBCs. We call them *megaloblasts.* Macrocytic RBCs are easily destroyed because they have fragile cell membranes. Megaloblastic anemias are caused by impaired DNA synthesis, which results in defective RBC maturation. Most result from cobalamin (vitamin B_{12}) and folic acid deficiencies. They can occur with congenital disorders, suppression of DNA synthesis by drugs, inborn errors of cobalamin and folic acid metabolism, and *erythroleukemia* (malignant blood disorder characterized by a proliferation of erythropoietic cells in bone marrow) (Table 34.8).

COBALAMIN DEFICIENCY

The most common cause of cobalamin deficiency is **pernicious anemia**. It is caused by an absence of *intrinsic factor* (IF). Pernicious anemia is a disease of insidious onset. Although the average age of onset is 60 years of age, it can occur at any age. About 30% of patients have a family history. There is a strong relationship with other autoimmune diseases, such as Graves disease.

Etiology

Normally, the parietal cells of the gastric mucosa secrete IF. IF is required for cobalamin (extrinsic factor) absorption. We absorb cobalamin in the distal ileum. In pernicious anemia, the gastric mucosa does not secrete IF because of either gastric mucosal atrophy or autoimmune destruction of parietal cells. In the autoimmune process, antibodies are directed against the gastric parietal cells and/or IF itself. Because parietal cells also secrete hydrochloric acid (HCl), in pernicious anemia, there is a decrease in HCl in the stomach. An acid environment in the stomach is needed for IF secretion.

Cobalamin deficiency can occur in patients who had GI surgery (e.g., gastrectomy, gastric bypass) or a small bowel resection involving the ileum. Others at risk include those with Crohn disease, ileitis, celiac disease, diverticula of the small intestine, or chronic atrophic gastritis (Table 34.8). In these cases, cobalamin deficiency results from the loss of IF-secreting gastric mucosal cells or impaired absorption of cobalamin in the distal ileum. Cobalamin deficiency also occurs with excess alcohol or hot tea ingestion, smoking, long-term users of H_2-histamine receptor blockers and proton pump inhibitors, and those who are strict vegetarians.[4]

Because there is a familial predisposition for pernicious anemia, assess patients who have a positive family history for symptoms. Although the disease cannot be prevented, early detection and treatment can lead to reversal of symptoms.

TABLE 34.8 Causes of Megaloblastic Anemia

Cobalamin (Vitamin B_{12}) Deficiency
- Chronic alcohol use
- Diet deficiency
- Gastric intrinsic factor deficiency
  - Celiac disease
  - Chronic gastritis
  - GI surgery: Gastrectomy, gastric bypass
  - *Helicobacter pylori*
- Increased requirement (pregnancy)
- Malabsorption: Celiac disease, inflammatory bowel

Folic Acid Deficiency
- Chronic alcohol use
- Chronic hemodialysis (folic acid lost during dialysis)
- Diet deficiency (e.g., leafy green vegetables, citrus fruits)
- Drugs interfering with absorption or use of folic acid (e.g., metformin phenytoin)
- Increased requirement (pregnancy)
- Malabsorption: Celiac disease, Crohn disease, small bowel resection

Drug-Induced Suppression of DNA Synthesis
- Alkylating agents
- Folate antagonists
- Metabolic inhibitors

Inherited Defects
- Defective folate metabolism (deficiency of folate transporter protein)
- Defective transport of cobalamin (intrinsic factor deficiency)

Myelodysplastic Syndromes

Clinical Manifestations

General manifestations of anemia caused by cobalamin deficiency are a result of tissue hypoxia (Table 34.3). GI manifestations include a sore, red, beefy, and shiny tongue; anorexia, nausea, and vomiting; and abdominal pain. Typical neuromuscular manifestations include weakness, paresthesias of the feet and hands, reduced vibratory and position senses, ataxia, muscle weakness, and impaired cognition. Because cobalamin deficiency–related anemia has an insidious onset, it may take several months or years for manifestations to develop.

Diagnostic Studies

Laboratory data reflective of cobalamin deficiency anemia are shown in Table 34.6. The RBCs appear large (macrocytic) and have abnormal shapes. This structure contributes to RBC destruction because the cell membrane is fragile. Normal serum folate levels and low cobalamin levels suggest anemia from cobalamin deficiency. A serum anti-IF antibody test is specific for pernicious anemia. Patients have an increased risk for gastric cancer. They may have an upper GI endoscopy and biopsy of the gastric mucosa at the time of diagnosis and at appropriate intervals afterward.

Serum methylmalonic acid (MMA) (high in cobalamin deficiency) and serum homocysteine (high in cobalamin and folic acid deficiencies) help determine the cause of the anemia.

Interprofessional and Nursing Management

Without cobalamin administration, the patient will die in 1 to 3 years. Oral treatments may be effective for those with a poor diet intake. However, most patients need parenteral vitamin B_{12} (cyanocobalamin, hydroxocobalamin) or intranasal cyanocobalamin because of the absorption problem. A typical treatment schedule consists of 1 mg of cobalamin SQ or IM daily (week 1), then 1 mg/week for 4 weeks, then 1 mg/month for life.[2]

The nursing measures discussed in eNursing Care Plan 34.1 for patients with anemia are appropriate for patients with cobalamin deficiency anemia. Assess for neurologic problems that are not corrected by replacement therapy. Implement measures to reduce the risk for injury from the decreased sensitivity to heat and pain. Protect patients from falling, burns, and trauma. In some people, neuromuscular problems may not be reversible. They may need physical therapy.

FOLIC ACID DEFICIENCY

Folic acid (folate) deficiency can cause megaloblastic anemia. Folic acid is needed for DNA synthesis leading to RBC formation and maturation. Common causes of folic acid deficiency are shown in Table 34.8.

The manifestations of folic acid deficiency are similar to cobalamin deficiency. It develops insidiously. Symptoms may be attributed to other coexisting problems (e.g., cirrhosis, esophageal varices). GI problems may include stomatitis, cheilosis, dysphagia, flatulence, and diarrhea. Thiamine deficiency, which is often present with folate deficiency, can cause neurologic symptoms.

The diagnostic findings for folic acid deficiency are shown in Table 34.6. The serum folate level is low (normal 5 to 25 ng/mL [11 to 57 nmol/L]), with a normal serum cobalamin level.

We treat folic acid deficiency with replacement therapy. The usual dosage is 1 to 5 mg/day by mouth.[2] The duration of treatment depends on the reason for the deficiency. Teach patients to eat foods high in folic acid (Table 34.5). The nursing measures discussed in eNursing Care Plan 34.1 for patients with anemia are appropriate for patients with folic acid deficiency anemia.

ANEMIA OF CHRONIC DISEASE

Anemia of chronic disease usually develops after 1 to 2 months of disease activity. Causes include cancer, autoimmune and infectious disorders (HIV, hepatitis, malaria), HF, or chronic inflammation. Bleeding episodes can contribute to anemia of chronic disease.

Anemia of chronic disease is associated with an underproduction of RBCs and mild shortening of RBC survival. The RBCs are usually normocytic, normochromic, and hypoproliferative. The anemia is usually mild. It can become more severe if the underlying disorder is not treated.

This type of anemia has an immune basis. The cytokines released in these problems, especially interleukin-6 (IL-6), cause an increased uptake and retention of iron within macrophages (see Fig. 33.3). This leads to a diversion of iron from circulation into storage sites, limiting the iron available for RBC production. There is reduced RBC life span, decreased erythropoietin (EPO) production, and an ineffective bone marrow response to EPO.

Anemia of chronic disease must be recognized and distinguished from anemia of other causes. High serum ferritin and increased iron stores distinguish it from iron deficiency anemia. There are normal folate and cobalamin blood levels.

The best treatment is to correct the underlying problem. If the anemia is severe, blood transfusions may be needed. They are not recommended for long-term treatment. EPO therapy is used for anemia from renal disease (see Chapter 51) and cancer and its therapies (see Chapter 16). Use is limited because of the increased risk for thromboembolism and death.

APLASTIC ANEMIA

Aplastic anemia is a disease in which patients have peripheral blood *pancytopenia* (decrease of all blood cell types—RBCs, white blood cells [WBCs], platelets) and hypocellular bone marrow. The spectrum can range from a moderate condition managed with hematopoietic growth factors or blood transfusions to very severe with potentially fatal bleeding and sepsis. The incidence of aplastic anemia is rare, with an annual rate of 2 new cases per million people in the United States per year.[6]

Etiology

We think most aplastic anemias are the result of autoimmune activity by autoreactive T lymphocytes. The cytotoxic T cells target and destroy the patient's own hematopoietic stem cells. Other causes include toxic injury to bone marrow stem cells or an inherited stem cell defect (Table 34.9).

Clinical Manifestations

Aplastic anemia can manifest abruptly (over days) or insidiously over weeks to months. It can vary from mild to very

TABLE 34.9 Causes of Aplastic Anemia

- Idiopathic
- Chemical agents and toxins (e.g., benzene, insecticides)
- Drugs (e.g., alkylating agents, antiseizure drugs, antimetabolites, antimicrobials, gold, NSAIDs, antithyroid medications)
- Inherited stem cell defect (e.g., Fanconi anemia)
- Radiation
- Toxic injury to bone marrow stem cells
- Viral and bacterial infection

severe. Patients may have symptoms caused by suppression of any or all bone marrow elements. General manifestations of anemia, such as fatigue and dyspnea, in addition to cardiovascular and cerebral responses, may occur (Table 34.3). Patients with neutropenia (low neutrophil count) are susceptible to infection. They are at risk for septic shock and death. Thrombocytopenia can lead to bleeding (e.g., petechiae, bruising, nosebleeds).

Diagnostic Studies

Laboratory studies confirm the diagnosis. Because aplastic anemia affects all marrow elements, Hgb, WBC, and platelet values are decreased. Other RBC indices are generally normal (Table 34.6). Thus we classify the condition as a normocytic, normochromic anemia. The reticulocyte count is low. Serum iron and total iron-binding capacity (TIBC) may be high as initial signs of decreased RBC production. Bone marrow biopsy, aspiration, and pathologic examination will be done to confirm the laboratory findings. The marrow in aplastic anemia is hypocellular (<30%) with increased yellow marrow (fat content).

Interprofessional and Nursing Management

Management is based on identifying and removing the causative agent (when possible) and providing supportive care until the pancytopenia resolves. Nursing actions are aimed at preventing complications from infection and bleeding. Nursing interventions appropriate for patients with pancytopenia from aplastic anemia are discussed in eNursing Care Plan 34.1 for anemia, eNursing Care Plan 34.2 for thrombocytopenia, and Table 34.23 (later in this chapter).

The prognosis of severe untreated aplastic anemia is poor. Early consideration of HSCT is critical. The best treatment outcomes for those who receive HSCT occur in younger patients who have had limited blood transfusions. Prior transfusions increase the risk for HSCT graft rejection. HSCT is discussed in Chapter 16.

Those in the interim or ineligible for HSCT may receive immunosuppressive therapy with antithymocyte globulin (ATG) and cyclosporine.[2] Eltrombopag, an oral thrombopoietin receptor agonist, can increase platelet counts. High-dose cyclophosphamide, alemtuzumab, or androgens may be helpful in some patients who do not respond to other treatments.[2] Patients not undergoing HSCT who need ongoing supportive blood transfusion should receive an iron-binding agent to prevent iron overload.

ANEMIA CAUSED BY BLOOD LOSS

An acute or chronic problem can cause anemia from blood loss.

ACUTE BLOOD LOSS

Acute blood loss occurs with sudden bleeding. Causes of acute blood loss include trauma, surgery complications, and problems that disrupt vascular integrity. There are 2 clinical concerns in such situations. First, a sudden reduction in the total blood volume can lead to hypovolemic shock. Second, if the acute loss is more gradual, the body maintains its blood volume by slowly increasing the plasma volume. Although this preserves circulating fluid volume, the number of RBCs available to carry O_2 is decreased.

Clinical Manifestations

The manifestations of anemia from acute blood loss are caused by the body's attempts to maintain an adequate blood volume and meet O_2 requirements. Table 34.10 outlines the manifestations of patients with varying degrees of blood volume loss. The patient's signs and symptoms are more important than the laboratory values. For example, an adult with a bleeding peptic ulcer who had a 750-mL hematemesis (15% of normal total blood volume) within the past 30 minutes may have postural hypotension and normal Hgb and hematocrit values. Over the next 36 to 48 hours, fluid moving from the extravascular into the intravascular space will replace most of the blood volume deficit. Only then will the Hgb and hematocrit reflect the blood loss.

Assess patients for pain. Internal bleeding may cause pain because of tissue distention, organ displacement, and nerve compression. Pain may be local or referred. In the case of retroperitoneal bleeding, patients may not have abdominal pain. Instead, there may be numbness and pain in a lower extremity from compression of the lateral cutaneous nerve (in the region of the 1st to 3rd lumbar vertebrae). The major complication is shock (see Chapter 42).

Diagnostic Studies

When blood volume loss is sudden, plasma volume has not yet had a chance to increase. Laboratory data do not reflect the RBC loss. Values may seem normal or high for 2 to 3 days. However, once the plasma volume is replaced, the RBC mass is less concentrated. Then, RBC, Hgb, and hematocrit levels are low and reflect the actual blood loss.

TABLE 34.10 Manifestations of Acute Blood Loss

VOLUME LOST[a]		
%	**mL**	**Manifestations**
10	500	None or rare vasovagal syncope
20	1000	No detectable signs or symptoms at rest. ↑ HR with exercise and slight postural hypotension
30	1500	Normal supine BP and HR at rest. Postural hypotension and ↑ HR with exercise
40	2000	BP, central venous pressure, and cardiac output below normal at rest; air hunger; rapid, thready pulse; cold, clammy skin
50	2500	Shock, lactic acidosis, potential death

[a]Based on an adult with a total blood volume of 5 L.

Interprofessional and Nursing Management

Interprofessional care is initially concerned with (1) replacing blood and intravascular volume to prevent shock; (2) promoting coagulation to prevent further bleeding; and (3) finding the source of the bleeding and stopping the blood loss. Blood transfusions (packed RBCs) can be used depending on the volume lost. If a large volume of blood is lost, such as in trauma, a "massive transfusion protocol" is employed with a rapid transfuser/warmer. If a warmer is not used, life-threatening hypothermia, acidosis, and coagulopathy can occur. Plasma, RBCs, and platelets are infused in a 1:1:1 ratio. Cryoprecipitate may be given because large volumes of RBCs dilute the coagulation system. IV fluids are used in emergencies to provide volume replacement fluids (e.g., 0.9% NaCl).[7,8] The amount of infusion varies with the solution used.

The body needs 2 to 5 days to make more RBCs in response to increased EPO. Patients may need iron supplements because iron availability affects the marrow production of RBCs. When anemia exists after acute blood loss, diet iron may not be enough to maintain iron stores. We may need to give oral or parenteral iron preparations.

The anemia should begin to correct itself once we find the source of bleeding, control the blood loss, and replace fluid and blood volumes. There should be no need for long-term treatment.

CHRONIC BLOOD LOSS

The sources of chronic blood loss are similar to those of iron deficiency anemia (e.g., bleeding ulcer, hemorrhoids, menstrual and postmenopausal blood loss). The effects of chronic blood loss are usually caused by depleted iron stores. We consider it an iron deficiency anemia. Management of chronic blood loss anemia involves identifying the source and stopping the bleeding. Patients may need iron supplements.

ANEMIA CAUSED BY INCREASED RBC DESTRUCTION

Hemolytic anemia is a condition caused by the destruction or hemolysis of RBCs at a rate that exceeds production. Hemolysis can occur with problems intrinsic or extrinsic to the RBCs. *Intrinsic hemolytic anemias,* which are usually hereditary, result from defects in the RBCs themselves (Table 34.2).

More common is *acquired hemolytic anemia.* In this type of anemia, the RBCs are normal but external factors are causing damage (Table 34.2). Macrophages, particularly those in the spleen, liver, and bone marrow, destroy RBCs that are old, defective, or moderately damaged. Fig. 34.2 shows the sequence of events involved in extravascular hemolysis.

Patients with hemolytic anemia have the general manifestations of anemia with some specific manifestations (Table 34.3). Jaundice occurs because the increased RBC destruction causes increased bilirubin levels. The spleen and liver may enlarge from hyperactivity. This is the result of macrophage phagocytosis of the defective RBCs.

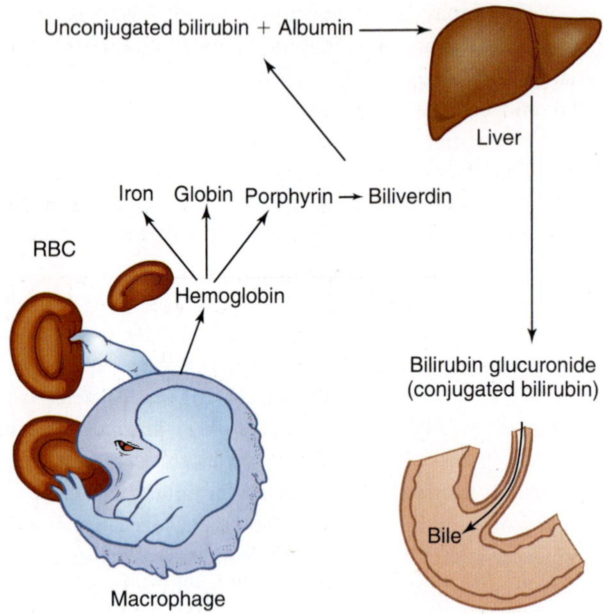

Fig. 34.2 Sequence of events in extravascular hemolysis.

A focus of treatment is to maintain renal function. When RBCs are hemolyzed, the Hgb molecule is released and filtered by the kidneys. The accumulation of Hgb molecules can obstruct the renal tubules and lead to acute tubular necrosis (see Chapter 51).

SICKLE CELL DISEASE

Sickle cell disease (SCD) is a group of inherited, autosomal recessive disorders characterized by an abnormal form of Hgb in the RBC (Box 34.1). Because this is a genetic disorder, SCD is usually found during routine neonatal screening. Although median survival can now exceed 50 years old, SCD often results in irreversible damage of the lungs, kidneys, brain, retina, or bones that affect patients' quality of life.

Etiology and Pathophysiology

In SCD, the abnormal Hgb, *hemoglobin S* (Hgb S), results from the substitution of valine for glutamic acid on the β-globin chain of Hgb (see Fig. 13.3). Hgb S causes the RBC to stiffen and elongate, taking on a sickle shape in response to low O_2 levels (Fig. 34.3).

Types of sickle cell disorders include sickle cell anemia, sickle cell–thalassemia, sickle cell Hgb C disease, and sickle cell trait.[9] *Sickle cell anemia* is the most severe of the SCD syndromes. It occurs when a person is homozygous for hemoglobin S (Hgb SS), meaning the person has inherited Hgb S from both parents. *Sickle cell–thalassemia* and *sickle cell Hgb C* occur when a person inherits Hgb S from 1 parent and another type of abnormal Hgb (e.g., thalassemia or Hgb C) from the other parent. Both these forms of SCD are less common and

BOX 34.1 GENETICS IN CLINICAL PRACTICE

Sickle Cell Disease

Genetic Basis

- Autosomal recessive disorder
- Mutation in β-globin *(HBB)* gene found on chromosome 11
- Various versions of β-globin result from different mutations in the *HBB* gene
- Hgb S variant involves substitution of valine for glutamic acid in the β-globin gene

Incidence

- Most common inherited blood disorder in the United States
- Affects around 100,000 Americans
- Occurs in about 1 of every 365 African American births
- Occurs in about 1 of every 16,300 Hispanic American births
- Affects people of Mediterranean, Caribbean, Arabian, East Indian, South and Central American, and South African descent
- 1 in 13 African American babies is born with sickle cell trait

Clinical Implications

- DNA testing is available; electrophoresis of hemoglobin and sickling screening test are common
- Sickle cell trait is the carrier state for sickle cell disease (SCD) and is a mild type of SCD
- If both parents have the trait, there is a 1 in 4 chance that their baby will have SCD
- Genetic counseling is recommended for people with a family history of SCD so they can understand the risks for transmitting the genetic mutation

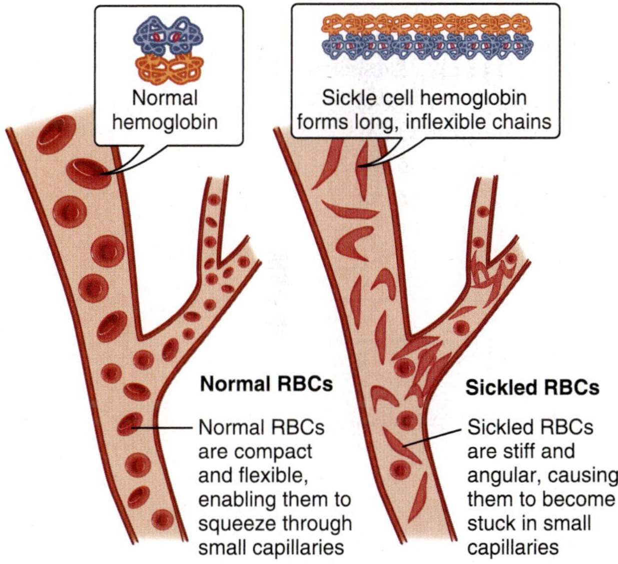

Fig. 34.3 In sickle cell disease, the hemoglobin forms long, inflexible chains and alters the shape of the red blood cells *(RBCs)*. The sickled RBCs can become stuck in the capillaries and occlude the blood flow.

less severe than sickle cell anemia. *Sickle cell trait* occurs when a person is heterozygous for hemoglobin S (Hgb AS). This means the person has inherited Hgb S from 1 parent and normal hemoglobin (Hgb A) from the other parent. Sickle cell trait is typically a mild to asymptomatic condition.

Sickling Episodes

The major pathophysiologic event of SCD is the sickling of RBCs (Fig. 34.3). The main trigger of sickling episodes is low O_2 tension in the blood. Infection is the most common cause of hypoxia or deoxygenation of RBCs. Other causes include high altitude, emotional or physical stress, surgery, and blood loss. Events that can trigger or sustain a sickling episode include dehydration, increased hydrogen ion concentration (acidosis), increased plasma osmolality, decreased plasma volume, and low body temperature. A sickling episode can occur without an obvious cause.

Sickled RBCs become rigid and take on an elongated, crescent shape (Fig. 34.3). Sickled cells cannot easily pass through capillaries or other small vessels and can cause vascular occlusion, leading to acute or chronic tissue injury. The resulting hemostasis promotes a self-perpetuating cycle of local hypoxia, deoxygenation of more RBCs, and more sickling. Circulating sickled cells are hemolyzed by the spleen, leading to anemia. At first, sickling is reversible with reoxygenation. It eventually becomes irreversible because of cell membrane damage from recurrent sickling. Vasoocclusive phenomena and hemolysis are the clinical hallmarks of SCD.

Sickle cell crisis is a severe, painful, acute exacerbation of RBC sickling, causing a vasoocclusive crisis. As sickled cells impair blood flow, vasospasm occurs, further restricting blood flow. Severe capillary hypoxia causes changes in membrane permeability, leading to plasma loss, hemoconcentration, thrombi, and further circulatory stagnation. Tissue ischemia, infarction, and necrosis eventually occur from lack of O_2. Shock is a possible life-threatening consequence because of severe O_2 depletion of the tissues and decreased circulating fluid volume. Sickle cell crisis can begin suddenly and persist for days to weeks.

The frequency, extent, and severity of sickling episodes are highly variable and unpredictable. They depend on the percentage of Hgb S present. People with sickle cell anemia have the most severe form because the RBCs have a high percentage of Hgb S.

Clinical Manifestations

The effects of SCD vary from person to person. The severity may be caused by genetic variants. Many people with sickle cell anemia are in fairly good health most of the time. However, they may have chronic health problems and pain from organ tissue hypoxia and damage (e.g., involving the kidneys or liver).

The typical patient is anemic but asymptomatic except during sickling episodes. Because most people with sickle cell anemia have dark skin, pallor is easier to detect by examining the mucous membranes. The skin may have a grayish cast. Because of hemolysis, jaundice is common.

The main symptom associated with sickling is pain. The pain severity can range from minor to excruciating. During sickle cell crisis, the pain is severe because of tissue ischemia. The episodes can affect any area of the body or several sites simultaneously. The back, chest, extremities, and abdomen are affected most often. Pain episodes are often accompanied by other manifestations, such as fever, tachypnea, hypertension, nausea, and vomiting.

Complications

With repeated episodes of sickling, there is gradual involvement of all body systems, especially the spleen, lungs, kidneys, and brain.[9] Organs that need large amounts of O_2 are most often affected and form the basis for many of the complications of SCD (Fig. 34.4). Infection is a major cause of mortality. One reason for this is the spleen does not phagocytize foreign substances as it becomes infarcted and dysfunctional (usually by 2 to 4 years of age) from the sickled RBCs. The spleen becomes small from the repeated scarring, termed *autosplenectomy.*

Pneumonia is the most common infection. It often is of pneumococcal origin. Infections can be so severe that they cause aplastic and hemolytic crisis and gallstones. *Aplastic crisis* can be so severe that it causes a temporary shutdown of RBC production in the bone marrow.

Acute chest syndrome is a term used to describe acute pulmonary complications that include pneumonia, tissue infarction, and fat embolism. There may be fever, chest pain, cough, lung infiltrates, and dyspnea. Pulmonary infarctions may cause pulmonary hypertension, MI, and cor pulmonale. The heart may become ischemic and enlarged, leading to HF. Retinal vessel obstruction may result in bleeding, scarring, retinal detachment, and blindness. The increased blood viscosity and the lack of O_2 can injure the kidneys. Renal failure may occur. Pulmonary embolism or stroke can result from thrombosis and infarction of cerebral blood vessels. Bone changes may include osteoporosis and osteosclerosis after infarction. Chronic leg ulcers can result from hypoxia and are especially prevalent around the ankles. *Priapism* (persistent penile erection) may occur if penile veins become occluded.

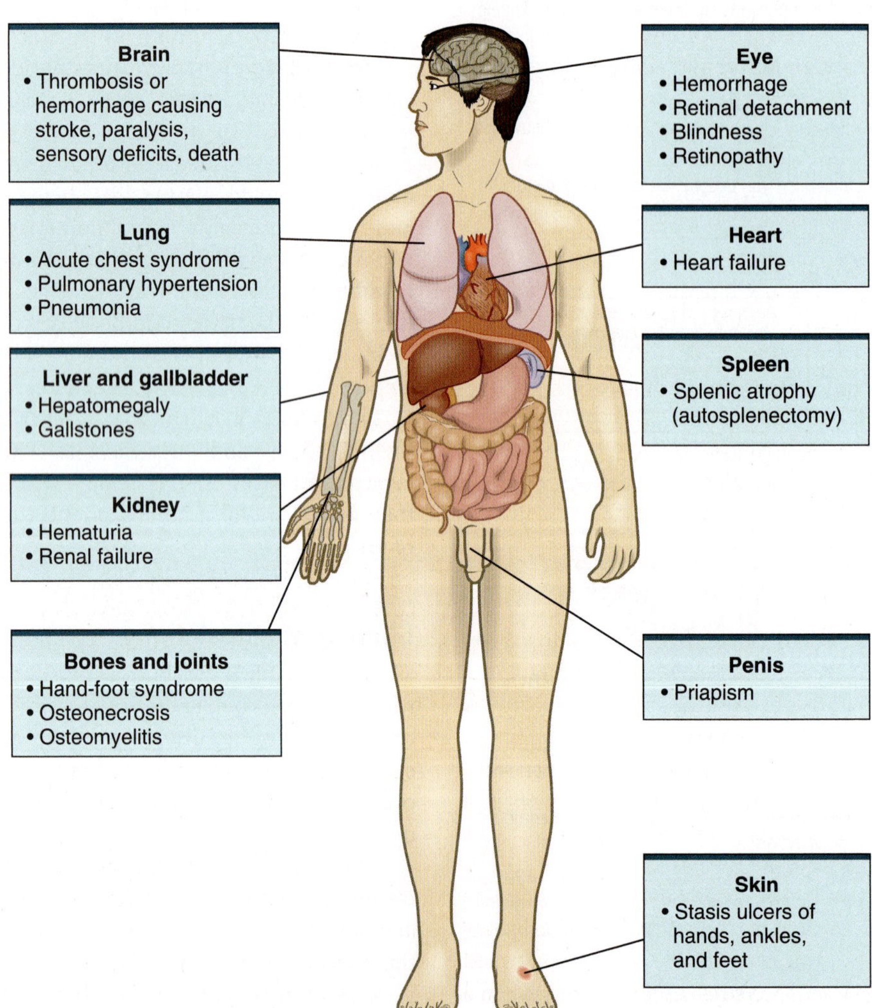

Fig. 34.4 Clinical manifestations and complications of sickle cell disease. (Modified from Rogers JL, Brashers VL: *Understanding pathophysiology*, ed 9, St Louis, 2023, Elsevier.)

Diagnostic Studies

A peripheral blood smear may reveal sickled cells and increased, abnormal reticulocytes. Hgb electrophoresis can determine the amount of Hgb S and SCD from other variants.

The accelerated RBC breakdown gives the patient the characteristic findings of hemolysis (high serum bilirubin levels) and abnormal laboratory test results (Table 34.6). Skeletal x-rays show bone and joint deformities and flattening. MRI can diagnose a stroke caused by blocked cerebral vessels from sickled cells. Doppler studies can assess for deep vein thromboses (DVTs). A chest x-ray can diagnose infection.

Interprofessional and Nursing Management

Goals of care include (1) alleviating the manifestations from complications of SCD, (2) minimizing end organ damage, (3) optimizing treatment strategies, and (4) preventing and treating serious sequelae, such as infection.

Patients in sickle cell crisis may need to be hospitalized. O_2 therapy treats hypoxia and controls sickling. Assess respiratory status. Encourage incentive spirometry. Rest can reduce metabolic requirements. Provide DVT prophylaxis. Fluids will reduce blood viscosity and maintain renal function. Priapism is managed with pain medication and fluids. If it does not resolve within a few hours, a urologist may be called.[2]

Transfusion therapy is needed with an aplastic crisis. Patients who have frequent crises or serious complications, such as acute chest syndrome, may need aggressive RBC exchange transfusion programs. They may need iron chelation therapy to reduce transfusion-produced iron overload.

CHECK YOUR PRACTICE

A 21-year-old Black female presents to the emergency department (ED) after a ski trip to Colorado. She is in excruciating pain in her chest and abdomen. She is short of breath, and her O_2 saturation is 86%. Vital signs show her heart rate is 110 beats/min and respiratory rate 28/min. She has crackles in the lungs. You note 6 previous ED admissions for sickle cell crises.

- What are your priorities for her nursing care?

Use a holistic approach to address the pain and its impact on quality of life (see Chapter 9). Patients may have different types and sites of pain. Undertreatment of sickle cell pain is a major problem (Box 34.2). Patients with SCD may develop tolerance. They may need larger doses of pain medication to reduce pain to an acceptable level. Pain can cause patients to have central sensitization, hyperalgesia, and altered opioid metabolism. This can cause mood and emotional problems.

During an acute crisis, optimal pain control usually includes large doses of continuous opioid analgesics, along with breakthrough analgesia, often in the form of patient-controlled analgesia (PCA). Adjunctive measures include nonsteroidal antiinflammatory drugs (NSAIDs), antineuropathic pain drugs (e.g., antidepressants, antiseizure drugs), local anesthetics, or nerve blocks. Occupational and physical therapy can optimize functioning. Social and chaplain services can help address social, emotional, and spiritual needs.

BOX 34.2 ETHICAL/LEGAL DILEMMAS

Pain Management

Situation

N.C., a 21-year-old African American male in the emergency department (ED) in sickle cell crisis, reports excruciating pain. He is known to several of the ED staff members. A nurse remarks to you that it must be time for his "fix" of pain drugs.

Ethical/Legal Points for Consideration

- The standard of care for pain management requires that (1) a pain assessment is done based on the patient's self-report, (2) the patient receives the best possible pain relief under the circumstances, and (3) we provide competent and compassionate care to all patients.
- The pain assessment includes reviewing the medical record to see if there are health care issues or conditions that may affect the response to pain and pain management.
- Document behaviors related to pain management. Be objective rather than subjective, such as labeling ("the patient is in withdrawal").
- When pain relief is inadequate, you must notify the HCP. Make sure the HCP has assessed the patient and based the plan of care on that assessment.

Discussion Questions

1. How can you teach your peers about pain assessment and management?
2. What factors do you need to include in your assessment and management of N.C.?

Infection is a frequent complication. Any febrile illness is an emergency. Wound infections, such as chronic leg ulcers, may be treated with rest, antibiotics, and proper wound care (see Chapter 12). Patients with acute chest syndrome receive broad-spectrum antibiotics, O_2 therapy, fluid therapy, and exchange transfusion. Blood transfusions are done sparingly between crises because patients develop antibodies to RBCs and iron overload. Because chronic hemolysis results in decreased folic acid stores, patients should take an oral folic acid supplement.

Various drugs can reduce sickling episodes. Hydroxyurea (Hydrea) increases the production of fetal hemoglobin (Hgb F) and alters the adhesion of sickled RBCs to the endothelium. The increase in Hgb F is accompanied by a reduction in hemolysis, an increase in Hgb concentration, and a decrease in sickled cells and painful crises. Crizanlizumab (Adakveo) reduces sickle cell and blood vessel adhesion. Oxbryta (Voxelotor) stabilizes an oxygenated Hgb cell, reducing sickling. Oral glutamine, an amino acid, decreases endothelial adhesion and can reduce the number and frequency of pain crises and hospitalizations.[10]

Allogeneic HSCT was the only available treatment that could cure some patients with SCD. The selection of recipients, donor scarcity, risk, and cost-effectiveness limit its use. Newer gene therapies are now available. The treatment process is similar to HSCT except that the patient's own apheresed stem cells are modified using a viral vector. The patient receives myeloablative chemotherapy, the cells are infused, and the stem cells produce healthy blood cells. Temporary low blood counts warrant supportive care for infection, bleeding, and anemia.[11]

Patient teaching and support are important in the long-term care of patients with SCD. The patient and caregiver must understand the basis of SCD and the reasons for supportive care and ongoing screening tailored to SCD manifestations. Teach patients ways to avoid crises and to seek medical attention quickly to counteract problems, such as upper respiratory tract infections. Teach patients to maintain adequate fluid intake. Encourage routine immunizations, such as pneumococcal, influenza, and hepatitis. Screening for retinopathy should begin at age 10. Each person with SCD should have a reproductive life plan.[2] Provide teaching about pain control because the pain during a crisis may be severe and often requires considerable analgesia. Minor pain episodes that are not associated with infection or other symptoms that need medical attention can sometimes be managed at home.

ACQUIRED HEMOLYTIC ANEMIA

Acquired hemolytic anemia results from hemolysis of RBCs from extrinsic factors. These factors include (1) physical destruction, (2) antibody reactions, and (3) infectious agents and toxins (Table 34.2).[4]

Physical destruction of RBCs results from the exertion of extreme force on the cells. Traumatic events that disrupt the RBC membrane include hemodialysis, extracorporeal circulation used in cardiopulmonary bypass, and prosthetic heart valves. The force needed to push blood through abnormal vessels, such as those that have been burned, irradiated, or affected by vascular disease (e.g., diabetes), may physically damage RBCs.

RBCs can be fragmented and destroyed as they try to pass through abnormal arterial or venous microcirculation. The RBCs are sheared as they try to pass by excess platelet aggregation and/or fibrin polymer formation, such as is seen in thrombotic thrombocytopenic purpura (TTP) and disseminated intravascular coagulation (DIC).

Antibodies may destroy RBCs by the mechanisms involved in antigen-antibody reactions. In blood transfusion reactions, the recipient's antibodies attack and hemolyze donor cells. Autoimmune antibody reactions occur when people develop antibodies against their own RBCs. This can be idiopathic (no prior hemolytic history) or from other autoimmune diseases (e.g., systemic lupus erythematosus [SLE]) or medications (clopidogrel, tacrolimus).[2]

Infectious agents cause hemolysis in 3 ways: (1) invading the RBC and destroying its contents (e.g., parasites, such as in malaria), (2) releasing hemolytic substances (e.g., *Clostridium perfringens*), and (3) generating an antigen-antibody reaction (e.g., *Mycoplasma pneumoniae*). Various agents may be toxic to RBCs and cause hemolysis. Hemolytic toxins include chemicals, such as oxidative drugs, arsenic, lead, copper, and bee stings or spider bites.

Laboratory findings in hemolytic anemia are shown in Table 34.6. Treatment and management involve general supportive care until the causative agent can be eliminated or at least made less injurious to the RBCs. Because a hemolytic crisis is a potential consequence, be ready to institute emergency therapy. This includes aggressive hydration and electrolyte replacement to reduce the risk for kidney injury caused by Hgb (from RBC lysis) clogging the kidney tubules and subsequent shock. Supportive care may include giving corticosteroids and blood products or removing the spleen.

Patients with chronic hemolytic anemia may need folate replacement. To suppress the RBC destruction, immunosuppressive agents may be used, such as glucocorticoids or rituximab, a monoclonal antibody to B-cell CD20. For severe cases associated with hemolysis, thrombocytopenia, and acute kidney injury, additional immunosuppressants (e.g., cyclosporine) may be used. Plasma exchange and complement inhibitors such as eculizumab and sutimlimab are options.[4]

RED BLOOD CELL DISORDERS

HEMOCHROMATOSIS

Hemochromatosis is an iron overload disorder characterized by increased intestinal iron absorption. A genetic defect is the most common cause (Box 34.3).[12] It may occur with diseases such as sideroblastic anemia and liver disease or chronic blood transfusions used to treat thalassemia and SCD. Symptoms usually do not develop until after age 40 years in males and 50 years in females.

The amount of iron in plasma in adults is about 2 to 4 mg. People with hemochromatosis accumulate iron at an increased rate. Clinical symptoms usually present when iron exceeds 4 to 5 g total body content.[2]

Early symptoms are nonspecific. They include fatigue, arthralgia, impotence, abdominal pain, and weight loss. Later, the excess iron accumulates in the liver and causes liver enlargement and cirrhosis. Excess iron deposits in the liver, pancreas, heart, joints, and endocrine glands cause diabetes, skin pigment changes (bronzing), heart problems (e.g., cardiomyopathy), arthritis, and testicular atrophy. There may be an enlarged liver and spleen and skin pigmentation changes. Laboratory values show a high serum iron, TIBC, and ferritin. Testing for known genetic mutations confirms the diagnosis. MRI can measure liver and cardiac iron.

The goal of treatment is to remove excess iron from the body and minimize any symptoms the patient may have. Iron removal is achieved by removing 350 to 450 mL of blood each week until the iron stores are depleted.[2] Then blood is removed less often to maintain iron levels within normal limits.

Iron-chelating drugs may be used. They form a complex with iron and promote its excretion from the body. Deferoxamine chelates and removes iron via the kidneys. It is given IV or subcutaneously. Deferasirox and deferiprone are oral drugs.

Diet changes include avoiding vitamin C and iron supplements, alcohol, uncooked seafood, and iron-rich foods.

We manage problems from organ involvement (e.g., diabetes, HF) with the usual treatment for these problems. The most common causes of death are cirrhosis, liver failure, liver cancer, and HF. With early diagnosis and treatment, life expectancy is normal. However, many cases go undetected and untreated.

BOX 34.3 GENETICS IN CLINICAL PRACTICE

Hemochromatosis

Genetic Basis

- Autosomal recessive disorder
- Caused by mutations in the *HFE, HAMP, SLC40A1,* and *TFR2* genes and others
- These genes play a key role in regulating iron absorption, transport, and storage
- Gene mutations impair the control of iron absorption during digestion and change iron distribution in the body, causing iron accumulation in tissues and organs

Incidence

- Most common genetic disease in people of European ancestry
- The C282Y mutation of the *HFE* gene is the most common
- About 1 in 15 people of Northern European ancestry have at least 1 copy of the *C282Y* mutation in the *HFE* gene
- Affects 1 in 300 non-Hispanic White persons in the United States

Clinical Implications

- DNA testing is recommended for all first-degree relatives of people with the disease
- Many people who have the gene mutation do not know it until the disease becomes apparent
- Clinical expression is variable and depends on iron intake, blood loss, and other modifying factors
- Early treatment can prevent serious complications

POLYCYTHEMIA

Polycythemia is the production and presence of increased numbers of RBCs. The increase in RBCs can be so great that blood circulation is impaired because of the increased blood viscosity *(hyperviscosity)* and volume *(hypervolemia).*

Etiology and Pathophysiology

There are 2 types of polycythemia: primary and secondary (Fig. 34.5). Their causes and pathogenesis differ, although their complications and manifestations are similar.

Primary Polycythemia

There are 2 main types of primary polycythemia. *Congenital polycythemia* is a rare autosomal dominant disorder caused by hemoglobin mutation or hypersensitivity to EPO. *Polycythemia vera* is a chronic myeloproliferative disorder. It involves increased production of RBCs, WBCs, and platelets. This leads to enhanced blood viscosity and blood volume and congestion of organs and tissues with blood. Splenomegaly and hepatomegaly are common. Patients have hypercoagulopathy that predisposes them to clotting and abnormal platelet function that can lead to bleeding. The disease develops insidiously and follows a chronic, vacillating course. The median age at diagnosis is between 60 and 80 years old.[4]

Secondary Polycythemia

Secondary polycythemia can be either hypoxia driven or hypoxia independent. In hypoxia-independent secondary polycythemia,

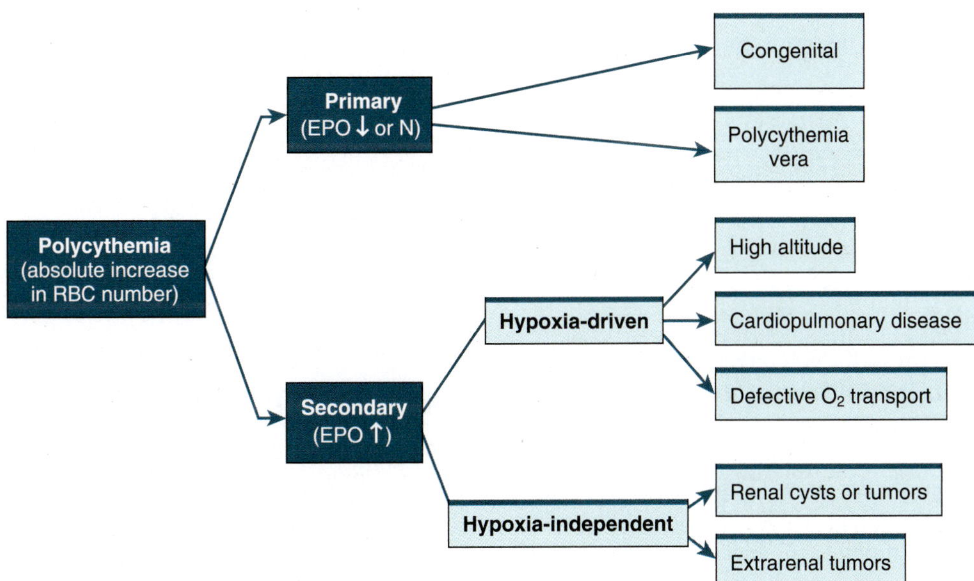

Fig. 34.5 Differentiating between primary and secondary polycythemia. *EPO,* Erythropoietin; *N,* normal.

cancer or benign tumor tissue makes EPO. Serum EPO levels often stay increased in these situations.

In hypoxia-driven secondary polycythemia, hypoxia stimulates the kidneys to make EPO, which stimulates RBC production. The need for O_2 may result from high altitude, lung disease, cardiovascular disease, alveolar hypoventilation, defective O_2 transport, or tissue hypoxia. EPO levels may return to normal once the Hgb stabilizes at a higher level. Thus secondary polycythemia is a physiologic response in which the body tries to compensate for a problem. Chapter 31 discusses hypoxia-driven secondary polycythemia in chronic obstructive pulmonary disease (COPD).

Clinical Manifestations and Complications

Circulatory manifestations are often the first signs. Hypertension caused by hypervolemia and hyperviscosity can cause headache, vertigo, dizziness, tinnitus, and visual changes. General itching (often exacerbated by a hot bath) may be present. It is related to histamine release from an increased number of basophils. Paresthesias and *erythromelalgia* (painful burning and redness of the hands and feet) can occur. Patients may have angina, HF, intermittent claudication, and thrombophlebitis, which may be complicated by embolization. These manifestations are caused by blood vessel distention, impaired blood flow, circulatory stasis, thrombosis, and tissue hypoxia from hypervolemia and hyperviscosity. The most common acute complication and major cause of mortality is stroke from a thrombosis.

Hemorrhagic phenomena caused by either vessel rupture from overdistention or inadequate platelet function may result in petechiae, bruising, nosebleeds, or GI bleeding. Bleeding can be acute and catastrophic. Hepatomegaly and splenomegaly from organ engorgement may contribute to satiety and fullness. Patients may have pain from peptic ulcers caused either by increased gastric secretions or liver and spleen engorgement. *Plethora* (ruddy complexion) may be present. Uric acid is a product of RBC destruction. As RBC destruction increases, uric acid production increases. This leads to hyperuricemia and gout.

Although the incidence is low, myelofibrosis and leukemia develop in some patients with polycythemia vera. These disorders may be caused by the chemotherapy drugs used to treat the disease or by a disorder in the stem cells that progresses to erythroleukemia.

Diagnostic Studies

The major diagnostic criteria for polycythemia vera include (1) high Hgb, hematocrit, and RBC mass; (2) bone marrow examination showing hypercellularity of RBCs, WBCs, and platelets; and (3) presence of gene mutations (*JAK2* V617F, *JAK2* exon 12).[2] Other studies show (1) low EPO level (secondary polycythemia has a high level); (2) high WBC count with basophilia and neutrophilia; (3) high platelet count and platelet dysfunction; and (4) normal or high leukocyte alkaline phosphatase, uric acid, and cobalamin levels.

Interprofessional and Nursing Management

Treatment aims to reduce blood volume and viscosity and bone marrow activity. Phlebotomy is the mainstay of treatment. The aim of phlebotomy is to reduce the hematocrit and keep it less than 45%.[2] At the time of diagnosis, 300 to 500 mL of blood may be removed every few days until the hematocrit is reduced to acceptable levels. Phlebotomy then may be needed every 2 to 3 months, reducing the blood volume by about 500 mL each time. A person managed with repeated phlebotomies eventually becomes iron deficient, although they are rarely symptomatic. Hydration therapy can reduce blood viscosity. Low-dose aspirin can prevent clotting.[2]

Myelosuppressive agents, such as hydroxyurea or busulfan, may be given. Ruxolitinib, which inhibits expression of the *JAK2* mutation, is given to those who do not respond to hydroxyurea. α-Interferon (α-IFN)-2b and pegylated IFN alfa-2a are options for females of childbearing age or those with intractable itching.

When acute exacerbations develop, you have several nursing responsibilities. Depending on your agency, you may either assist with or perform the phlebotomy. Assess intake and output during hydration therapy to avoid fluid overload (which worsens circulatory congestion) or fluid deficit (which makes the blood more viscous). Give prescribed myelosuppressive agents. Observe the patient and teach them about drug side effects.

Assess nutrition status. Inadequate food intake can result from GI symptoms of fullness, pain, and dyspepsia. Begin activities and any drug therapy to decrease thrombus formation.

Because of its chronic nature, polycythemia vera requires ongoing evaluation. Assess the patient for complications with each encounter.

PROBLEMS OF HEMOSTASIS

Hemostasis involves the vascular endothelium, platelets, and coagulation factors. They normally work together to stop bleeding and repair vascular injury. These mechanisms are described in Chapter 33. Disruption in any component may result in bleeding or thrombotic disorders.

Three major problems discussed in this section are (1) thrombocytopenia (low platelet count), (2) hemophilia and von Willebrand disease (inherited disorders of specific clotting factors), and (3) DIC.

THROMBOCYTOPENIA

Etiology and Pathophysiology

Thrombocytopenia is a reduction of platelets to less than 150,000/μL (150 × 10^9/L). Acute, severe, or prolonged decreases from normal can result in abnormal hemostasis that presents as prolonged bleeding from minor trauma or spontaneous bleeding without injury.

Platelet disorders occur from impaired production, increased destruction, or abnormal distribution (Table 34.11).[5] Although they can be inherited (e.g., Wiskott-Aldrich syndrome), most are acquired. Acquired thrombocytopenia is often caused by an underlying condition (e.g., aplastic anemia, leukemia), infection, nutrition deficiencies, or therapy used to treat another problem.[2] Drugs are a common cause of acquired disorders. Some drugs are directly myelosuppressive (e.g., chemotherapy). Another mechanism of drug-related thrombocytopenia is accelerated platelet destruction caused by antibodies. Antibodies attack the platelets when the drug binds to the platelet surface.

Immune Thrombocytopenia

The most common acquired thrombocytopenia is *immune thrombocytopenia* (ITP). ITP is an acquired immune disorder where there is abnormal platelet destruction. In general, ITP presents as an acute condition in children and a chronic condition in adults.

ITP results from antiplatelet antibodies, impaired platelet production, and T cell–mediated destruction of platelets. In ITP, antibodies coat the platelets. These platelets function normally. When they reach the spleen, the antibody-coated platelets are mistaken as foreign and destroyed by macrophages. Decreased platelet production contributes to ITP. Sometimes autoimmune disease (e.g., SLE) or infection, such as *Helicobacter pylori* or viral infection (HIV), contributes to ITP. Platelets normally survive 8 to 10 days. In ITP, platelet survival is shortened.

TABLE 34.11 Causes of Acquired Thrombocytopenia

Impaired Platelet Production
- Cancers and other disorders
  - Aplastic anemia
  - Leukemia, lymphoma, myeloma, myelodysplastic disorders
  - Marrow metastases by solid tumors
- Drugs (chemotherapy, ganciclovir)
- Immune thrombocytopenia (ITP)
- Infections, bacterial, fungal, viral (hepatitis C virus, HIV, cytomegalovirus)
- Nutrition deficiencies, alcohol use
- Radiation

Increased Platelet Destruction
- Artificial surfaces (e.g., cardiopulmonary bypass, hemodialysis)
- Disseminated intravascular coagulation (DIC)
- Heparin-induced thrombocytopenia (HIT)
- Pregnancy-related
- Thrombotic microangiopathy
  - Atypical hemolytic uremic syndromes (aHUSs)
  - Thrombotic thrombocytopenic purpura (TTP)

Abnormal Platelet Distribution
- Dilution (massive blood transfusion, fluids)
- Spleen sequestration

Thrombotic Thrombocytopenic Purpura

TTP is an uncommon syndrome characterized by microangiopathic hemolytic anemia (MAHA), thrombocytopenia, neurologic changes, fever, and renal problems. Not all features are present in all patients. Because it is almost always associated with hemolytic-uremic syndrome (HUS), TTP is often referred to as *TTP-HUS*.

In most cases, TTP is caused by the deficiency of a plasma enzyme (ADAMTS13) that breaks down the von Willebrand clotting factor (von Willebrand factor [vWF]) into normal size. vWF is the most important factor that mediates platelet adhesion to damaged endothelial cells. Without the enzyme, unusually large amounts of vWF attach to activated platelets, promoting platelet aggregation. Microthrombi form that deposit in arterioles and capillaries. There are fewer platelets circulating to prevent bleeding. TTP is a medical emergency because bleeding and clotting occur at the same time.

TTP may be idiopathic. It is thought to be caused by an autoimmune disorder against ADAMTS13. It may occur because of certain drug toxicities (e.g., chemotherapy, cyclosporine, oral contraceptives, valacyclovir, clopidogrel), pregnancy or preeclampsia, infection, or a known autoimmune disorder, such as SLE or scleroderma.[2]

Heparin-Induced Thrombocytopenia

One of the risks associated with heparin is the life-threatening condition called *heparin-induced thrombocytopenia* (HIT), or *heparin-induced thrombocytopenia and thrombosis syndrome* (HITTS). Typically, patients develop thrombocytopenia 7 to 14 days after the onset of heparin therapy. We suspect HIT if the platelet count decreases by more than 50% or is less than 150,000/µL. About up to 3% of postoperative patients and 0.5% of medical patients who receive unfractionated heparin may develop HIT.[2]

In HIT, platelet destruction and vascular endothelial injury are the 2 major responses to an immune-mediated response to heparin. Platelet factor 4 (PF4; a protein made and released by platelets) binds to heparin. This PF4-heparin complex then binds to the platelet surface, leading to further platelet activation and release of more PF4, thus creating a positive feedback loop. The body makes antibodies against the PF4-heparin-platelet complex. They are removed prematurely from circulation, leading to thrombocytopenia and platelet-fibrin thrombi.

Although the major problem of HIT is venous thrombosis, arterial thrombosis can occur. DVT and pulmonary emboli most often result as a complication of the thromboses. Other complications include arterial vascular infarcts, causing skin necrosis, stroke, and end organ damage (e.g., kidneys). Bleeding symptoms are unusual because the platelet count is rarely less than 20,000/µL.

Clinical Manifestations

Many patients with thrombocytopenia are asymptomatic. The most common symptom is bleeding. Bleeding may be insidious or acute and internal or external. It may occur in any area of the body, including the mucosa, skin, joints, retina, and brain. Mucosal bleeding may manifest as nosebleeds and gingival bleeding. Large bullous hemorrhages may appear on the buccal mucosa because of the lack of vessel protection by the submucosal tissue. Bleeding into the skin is seen as petechiae, purpura, or bruising (Fig. 34.6). Pain and tenderness are sometimes present.

Prolonged bleeding from trauma or injury does not usually occur until platelet counts are under 50,000/μL (50×10^9/L).[2] When the count is under 20,000/μL (20×10^9/L), spontaneous, life-threatening bleeding (e.g., intracranial bleeding) can occur.

Insidious bleeding may be first detected by discovering anemia from blood loss. Be aware of manifestations of internal blood loss, including weakness, fainting, dizziness, tachycardia, abdominal pain, and hypotension. Prolonged bleeding after routine procedures such as venipuncture or IM injection may indicate thrombocytopenia.

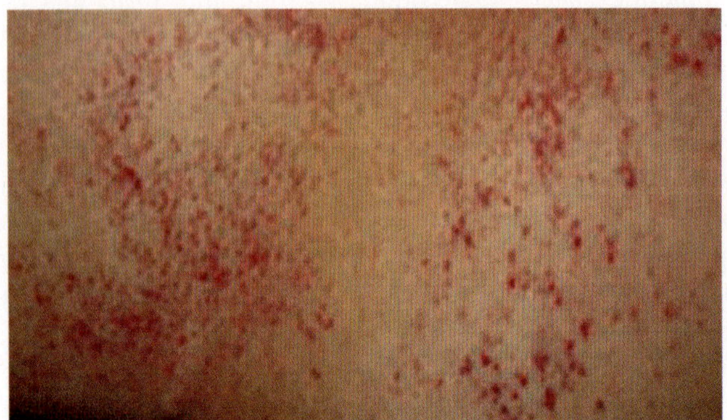

Fig. 34.6 Acute immune thrombocytopenic purpura often presents with purpuric lesions. (From Mousdi M, Pegka S, Skouteli M, et al: COVID-19 vaccination associated severe immune thrombocytopenia, *Atherosclerosis* 355:193, 2022.)

Because vascular thromboses may occur with thrombocytopenia (e.g., TTP, HIT), assess for signs and symptoms of vascular ischemic problems (see Chapter 41).

Diagnostic Studies

Thrombocytopenia exists when the platelet count is under 150,000/μL (150×10^9/L). The history and assessment, along with laboratory studies, help determine the cause. Table 34.12 compares results for types of thrombocytopenia.

Laboratory tests that assess secondary hemostasis or coagulation, such as the prothrombin time (PT) and activated partial thromboplastin time (aPTT), can be normal even in severe thrombocytopenia. If they are increased, this may point toward DIC.

Specific assays, such as ITP antigen–specific assay, platelet activation/function assay, or PF4-heparin complex for HIT, can help with the diagnosis. In TTP, testing for ADAMTS13 deficiency is not always diagnostic. Thrombocytopenia may be severe in TTP, but coagulation studies are normal. Lactate dehydrogenase (LDH) may be increased. With TTP, altered RBC morphology, including *spherocytes* (small, globular, completely hemoglobinated RBCs), fragmented cells (schistocytes), and pronounced reticulocytosis, may be present. These findings are partially a result of intravascular fibrin deposition causing a "slicing" of RBCs.

Bone marrow examination may be done to see if production problems (e.g., leukemia, aplastic anemia, other myeloproliferative disorders) are the cause of thrombocytopenia or when other tests are inconclusive. When destruction of circulating

TABLE 34.12 Laboratory Results in Thrombocytopenia and DIC

Laboratory Test	ITP	TTP	HIT	DIC
Platelets	↓↓↓↓	↓↓↓	↓↓	↓↓↓
Hemolysis				
Haptoglobin	N	↓	N	↓
Hgb	N	↓↓	N	N or ↓
Indirect bilirubin	N	↑	N	N or ↑
Lactate dehydrogenase	N	↑↑↑	N	↑
Reticulocytes	N	↑	N	N or ↑
Schistocytes	N	↑↑↑	N or ↑	N or ↑
Coagulopathy				
PT (prothrombin time)	N	N	N	Prolonged
aPTT	N	N	N	Prolonged
D dimer	N	N or ↑	↑	↑↑
Other tests	ITP IgG assay, platelet activation/function assay, *Helicobacter pylori*, hepatitis C, HIV, bone marrow biopsy	ADAMTS13 Urinalysis (for proteinuria, hematuria), creatinine	Platelet activation/function assay, PF4-heparin complex (antigen assay)	Fibrin split products (FSPs)

aPTT, Activated partial thromboplastin time; *DIC,* disseminated intravascular coagulation; *HIT,* heparin-induced thrombocytopenia; *ITP,* immune thrombocytopenia; *N,* normal; *TTP,* thrombotic thrombocytopenic purpura.

platelets is the cause, bone marrow analysis shows *megakaryocytes* (precursors of platelets) to be normal or increased, even though circulating platelets are reduced. The absence or decreased number of megakaryocytes on bone marrow biopsy is consistent with thrombocytopenia caused by decreased bone marrow production (e.g., aplastic anemia).

Interprofessional Care

Interprofessional care differs based on the cause. Removal or treatment of the underlying cause is sometimes sufficient. Patients with thrombocytopenia should avoid aspirin and other drugs that affect platelet function or production. The following sections discuss management strategies for the different causes of thrombocytopenia (Table 34.13).

Immune Thrombocytopenic Purpura

Multiple therapies are part of managing ITP. If the patient is asymptomatic, they may not be treated unless the platelet count is under 30,000/μL.[2] Corticosteroids are used initially to treat ITP because they suppress the phagocytic response of splenic macrophages. This alters the spleen's recognition of platelets and increases platelets' life span. Corticosteroids depress antibody formation and reduce capillary leakage. High doses of IV immunoglobulin (IVIG) and a component of IVIG, anti-Rh_0(D) (anti-D, WinRho), may be used.[2]

Thrombopoietin receptor agonists that increase platelet production are used for patients with chronic ITP who have an insufficient response to steroids. Rituximab lyses activated B cells, thus reducing the immune recognition of platelets.

Immunosuppressive therapy (e.g., azathioprine) or a splenic tyrosine kinase inhibitor, fostamatinib, may be used in refractory cases (Table 34.13).[2] Platelet transfusions can increase platelet counts in cases of life-threatening bleeding, a platelet count less than 10,000/μL, or with bleeding before a procedure. Platelets should not be given prophylactically because of the risk for antibody formation.

Patients may need a splenectomy if they do not respond to treatment. The spleen normally sequesters about one-third of the platelets, so its removal increases the number of platelets in circulation. Because some antibody synthesis occurs in the spleen, antiplatelet antibodies decrease after splenectomy. The spleen has an abundance of macrophages that destroy platelets. Thus removing the spleen can increase platelets.

Thrombotic Thrombocytopenic Purpura

We treat TTP in a variety of ways. The first step is to treat the underlying disorder or remove the causative agent, if known. If untreated, TTP usually results in irreversible renal failure and death. Plasma exchange (plasmapheresis) can reverse platelet consumption by supplying the right vWF and enzyme (ADAMTS13) and removing the large vWF molecules that bind with platelets. Treatment should continue daily until platelet counts normalize and hemolysis has ceased. Corticosteroids are used with this treatment.[2]

Caplacizumab is an anti-VWF antibody that blocks VWF binding to platelets. It can reduce platelet aggregation and thrombosis and normalize the platelet count.[2] Rituximab is another option. It decreases the level of inhibitory ADAMTS13 immunoglobulin G (IgG) antibodies. Splenectomy may be done in patients who are refractory to plasma exchange or immunosuppression. Platelet administration is contraindicated unless life-threatening bleeding is occurring because it may lead to new vWF-platelet complexes and increased clotting.[2]

TABLE 34.13 Interprofessional Care

Thrombocytopenia

Diagnostic Assessment
- History and physical assessment
- Bone marrow aspiration and biopsy
- Complete blood count (CBC), including platelet count
- Specific laboratory studies (Table 34.12)

Management

Immune Thrombocytopenic Purpura
- Corticosteroids
- IV immunoglobulin (IVIG)
- Anti-Rh_0(D)
- Thrombopoietin receptor antagonists
  - Avatrombopag (Doptelet)
  - Eltrombopag (Promacta)
  - Romiplostim (Nplate)
- Fostamatinib
- Rituximab (Rituxan)
- Splenectomy
- Immunosuppressives (e.g., azathioprine, cyclophosphamide)

Thrombotic Thrombocytopenic Purpura
- Identify and treat or remove cause
- Plasmapheresis (plasma exchange)
- Corticosteroids
- Caplacizumab
- Rituximab (Rituxan)
- Splenectomy

Heparin-Induced Thrombocytopenia
- Direct thrombin inhibitors (see Table 41.10)
- Factor Xa inhibitors (see Table 41.10)
  - Direct: rivaroxaban (Xarelto), apixaban (Eliquis)
  - Indirect: fondaparinux, danaparoid
- Plasmapheresis
- High-dose IVIG

Decreased Platelet Production
- Identify and treat or remove cause
- Thrombopoietin receptor agonists (avatrombopag, eltrombopag, romiplostim)
- Platelet transfusions
- Immune therapies (corticosteroids, cyclosporine)

Heparin-Induced Thrombocytopenia

We stop all forms of heparin when HIT is present. To maintain anticoagulation, patients should receive a direct thrombin inhibitor (e.g., argatroban) or factor Xa inhibitor (e.g., rivaroxaban) (see Table 41.10). If clotting is severe, the most common treatments are plasmapheresis to clear the platelet-aggregating IgG from the blood, thrombolytic agents to treat the thromboembolic events, and surgery to remove clots. Platelet transfusions are not given because they may enhance thromboembolic events. Patients who have had HIT should never receive heparin or low-molecular-weight heparin (LMWH) again. This should be noted in the medical record.

Thrombocytopenia From Decreased Platelet Production

The management of acquired thrombocytopenia is based on finding the cause and treating the disease or removing the causative agent. Platelet transfusions are given if life-threatening bleeding develops. Platelet transfusions are generally not done unless the count is under 10,000/μL (10×10^9/L) or the patient is actively bleeding, has an active infection, or is having an invasive procedure.

NURSING MANAGEMENT: THROMBOCYTOPENIA

Assessment

Subjective and objective data that you should obtain from patients with thrombocytopenia are outlined in Table 34.14.

TABLE 34.14 NURSING ASSESSMENT

Thrombocytopenia

Subjetctive Data

Important Health Information

Health history: Recent or excess bleeding; viral illness; cancer (especially leukemia or lymphoma); aplastic anemia; SLE; cirrhosis; exposure to radiation or toxic chemicals; DIC

Medications: Many medications, including chemotherapy agents, valproic acid, furosemide, NSAIDs, penicillin

Functional Health Patterns

Health perception–health management: Family history of bleeding problems; malaise

Nutritional-metabolic: Coffee-ground or bloody vomitus; easy bruising

Elimination: Hematuria, dark or bloody stools

Activity-exercise: Fatigue, weakness, fainting; nosebleeds, hemoptysis; dyspnea

Cognitive-perceptual: Pain and tenderness in bleeding areas (e.g., abdomen, head, extremities); headache

Sexuality-reproductive: Menorrhagia, metrorrhagia

Objective Data

General

Fever, lethargy

GI

Splenomegaly, abdominal distention; heme-positive stools; bleeding gingiva

Skin

Petechiae, bruising, purpura

Possible Diagnostic Findings

Platelet count <150,000/μL (150×10^9/L), prolonged bleeding time, ↓ Hgb and Hct; normal or ↑ megakaryocytes in bone marrow examination

DIC, Disseminated intravascular coagulation; *SLE,* systemic lupus erythematosus.

Clinical Problems

The main clinical problem for patients with thrombocytopenia is impaired tissue perfusion.

Planning

The overall goals are that patients with thrombocytopenia will (1) have no bleeding, (2) maintain vascular integrity, and (3) manage self-care related to an increased risk for bleeding.

Implementation

Acute Care

The goal during acute episodes of thrombocytopenia is to prevent or control bleeding (see eNursing Care Plan 34.2 on the website for this chapter). Bleeding is usually from superficial sites. Deep bleeding (into muscles, joints, and the abdomen) usually occurs only when clotting factors are decreased. Bleeding from the posterior nasopharynx may be hard to detect because the person swallows the blood. If you cannot avoid a subcutaneous injection, use a small-gauge needle. Apply direct pressure for at least 5 to 10 minutes after the injection. An ice pack may be helpful. Avoid IM injections.

Note that many of these disorders may be accompanied by vascular clotting. As bleeding occurs, RBCs and coagulation factors are consumed along with platelets. Monitor all blood cell and coagulation studies. Administering platelet transfusions is a key nursing role.

Chronic Care

Help patients understand the importance of adhering to self-care measures that reduce the risk for bleeding (Table 34.15). Encourage people to seek care if manifestations of bleeding (e.g., prolonged nosebleeds, petechiae) develop. Stress that a minor nosebleed or new petechiae may indicate potential bleeding and to notify the HCP. Discourage using drugs known to be causes of acquired thrombocytopenia and reduced platelet function. Aspirin reduces platelet adhesiveness, thus contributing to bleeding.

Monitor patients with ITP who are receiving treatment for their response to therapy. Teach the person with acquired thrombocytopenia to avoid causative agents when possible

(Table 34.11). If patients cannot avoid causative agents (e.g., chemotherapy), teach them to avoid injury or trauma during these periods and the signs and symptoms of bleeding (Table 34.15).

In a female with thrombocytopenia, menstrual blood loss may exceed the usual amount and duration. Suppressing menses with hormonal agents may be needed during predictable periods of thrombocytopenia (e.g., during chemotherapy and HSCT) to reduce menstrual blood loss.

Patients with either ITP or acquired thrombocytopenia should have planned periodic medical evaluations to assess and treat situations in which exacerbations and bleeding are likely to occur. Address the impact of the condition on quality of life.

TABLE 34.15 PATIENT & CAREGIVER TEACHING

Thrombocytopenia

Include the following instructions when teaching a patient or caregiver the precautions to take when the platelet count is low:

1. Notify your HCP of any symptoms of bleeding. These include:
   - Black, tarry, or bloody bowel movements
   - Black or bloody vomit, sputum, or urine
   - Bleeding from the mouth or anywhere in the body
   - Bruising or small red or purple spots on the skin
   - Difficulty talking, sudden weakness of an arm or leg, confusion
   - Headache or changes in how well you can see
2. Ask your HCP about restrictions in your normal activities, such as vigorous exercise or lifting weights. In general, walking is safe. Wear sturdy shoes or slippers. If you are weak and at risk for falling, get help or supervision when getting out of bed or a chair.
3. Do not blow your nose forcefully; gently pat it with a tissue if needed. For a nosebleed, keep your head up and apply firm pressure to the nostrils and bridge of your nose. If bleeding continues, place an ice bag over the bridge of your nose and the nape of your neck. If you are unable to stop a nosebleed after 10 min, call your HCP.
4. Do not bend down with your head lower than your waist.
5. Prevent constipation by drinking plenty of fluids. Do not strain when having a bowel movement. Your HCP may prescribe a stool softener. Do not use a suppository, an enema, or a rectal thermometer without the permission of your HCP.
6. Shave only with an electric razor. Do not use blades.
7. Do not tweeze your eyebrows or other body hair.
8. Do not puncture your skin, such as getting tattoos or body piercing.
9. Do not use any medication that can prolong bleeding, such as aspirin. If you are unsure about a medication, ask your HCP or pharmacist about it.
10. Use a soft-bristle toothbrush or disposable mouth sponge to prevent injuring the gums. Flossing is usually safe if done gently using thin tape floss. Do not use oral hygiene products containing glycerin, alcohol, or other drying agents.
11. Women who are menstruating should keep track of the number of pads used per day. When you use more pads per day than usual or bleed more days, notify your HCP. Do not use tampons.
12. Ask your HCP before you have any invasive procedures done, such as a dental cleaning, manicure, or pedicure.
13. Decrease irritation of the oral mucosa by avoiding spicy, salty, acidic, dry, rough, or hard foods.

◆ Evaluation

The expected outcomes are that patients with thrombocytopenia will:

- Have no evidence of bleeding or bruising
- State needed knowledge and skills to manage the disease process

HEMOPHILIA AND VON WILLEBRAND DISEASE

Hemophilia is an X-linked recessive genetic disorder caused by a defective or deficient coagulation factor. There are 2 major types: *hemophilia A* (classic hemophilia, factor VIII deficiency) and *hemophilia B* (Christmas disease, factor IX deficiency). *Von Willebrand disease* is a related disorder involving a deficiency of the von Willebrand coagulation protein. Factor VIII is made in the liver and circulates as a complex with vWF.

Hemophilia A is 4 times as common as hemophilia B.[13] Although rare, there are cases of *acquired hemophilia A* that are caused by the body developing antibodies against its own factor VIII. Von Willebrand disease is the most common congenital bleeding disorder. The inheritance patterns of hemophilia and von Willebrand disease are discussed in Table 34.16 and Box 34.4.

Clinical Manifestations and Complications

The manifestations of hemophilia A and B are similar. All manifestations relate to bleeding. Any bleeding episode in people with hemophilia may be life threatening. Manifestations include (1) slow, persistent, prolonged bleeding from minor trauma and small cuts; (2) delayed bleeding after minor injuries (the delay may be several hours or days); (3) uncontrollable bleeding after dental extractions or gingival irritation with a hard-bristle toothbrush; (4) nosebleeds, especially after a blow to the face; (5) GI bleeding from ulcers and gastritis; (6) hematuria and potential renal failure from GU trauma; (7) spleen rupture from falls or abdominal trauma; (8) bruising and subcutaneous hematomas (Fig. 34.7) and possible compartment syndrome; (9) neurologic signs, such as pain, anesthesia, and paralysis, which may develop from nerve compression caused by hematoma formation; and (10) hemarthrosis

TABLE 34.16 Types of Hemophilia

Type	Inheritance Pattern
Hemophilia A	
Factor VIII	Recessive sex-linked. Transmitted by female carriers, occurs almost exclusively in males.
Hemophilia B	
Factor IX	Recessive sex-linked. Transmitted by female carriers, occurs almost exclusively in males.
von Willebrand Disease	
vWF, variable factor VIII deficiencies and platelet dysfunction	Autosomal dominant, seen in both genders. Recessive, in severe forms of the disease.

(bleeding into the joints) (Fig. 34.8). This can lead to joint injury and deformity severe enough to cause crippling.[4]

In children, these manifestations may lead to the diagnosis. In adults, these may be the first sign of a mild form of the disease that escaped detection through a childhood free of major injuries, dental procedures, or surgeries.

Diagnostic Studies

Laboratory studies determine the type of hemophilia present. Any factor deficiency within the intrinsic system (factor VIII, IX, XI, or XII or vWF) will yield the laboratory results outlined in Table 34.17.

BOX 34.4 GENETICS IN CLINICAL PRACTICE

Hemophilia A and B

Genetic Basis

- X-linked recessive disorder
- *Hemophilia A:* Caused by mutations in the *F8* gene that provides instructions for making coagulation factor VIII
- *Hemophilia B:* Caused by mutations in the *F9* gene that provides instructions for making coagulation factor IX
- Mutations in the *F8* or *F9* gene lead to the production of an abnormal version or reduced amounts of coagulation factors

Incidence

- *Hemophilia A:* 1 in 5600 male births
- *Hemophilia B:* 1 in 1400 male births

Clinical Implications

- Female carriers transmit the genetic defect to 50% of their sons; 50% of their daughters are carriers
- Males with hemophilia do not transmit the genetic defect to their son; all their daughters are carriers
- Although rare, female hemophilia can occur if a male with hemophilia mates with a female carrier

Interprofessional Care

The goals of interprofessional care are to prevent and treat bleeding. Care for persons with hemophilia or von Willebrand disease requires (1) preventive care, (2) replacement therapy during acute bleeding episodes and as prophylaxis, and (3) treating complications of the disease and its therapy. Most patients can expect almost normal life spans free of bloodborne illnesses because of improvements in the blood donation process and the use of recombinant replacement factors.[14] Designated treatment centers provide interprofessional care of hemophilia and related disorders.

Replacement of deficient clotting factors is the primary means to support patients with hemophilia. Regular prophylaxis is preferred over on-demand treatment. The most common problem with acute management is starting factor replacement therapy too late and stopping it too soon. Minor bleeding episodes should be treated for at least 72 hours.

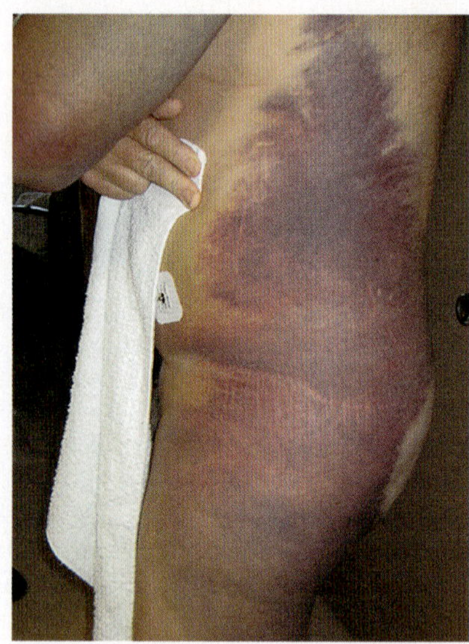

Fig. 34.7 Severe bruising in a person with hemophilia after a fall. (Courtesy Peter Bonner.)

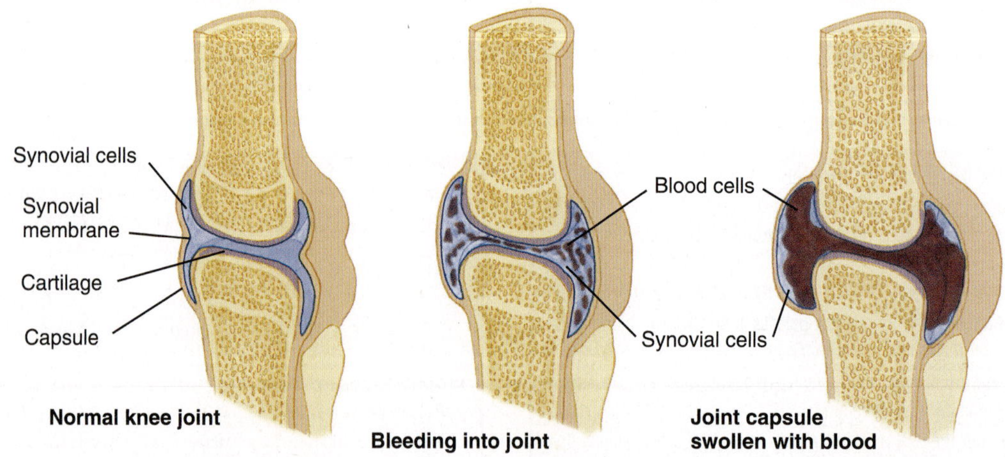

Fig. 34.8 Hemarthrosis of the knee is a common complication of hemophilia. (From McKinney ES, James SR, Murray SS, et al: *Maternal-child nursing,* ed 6, St. Louis, 2022, Elsevier.)

TABLE 34.17 Laboratory Results in Hemophilia

Test	Results
Bleeding time	Prolonged in von Willebrand disease because of structurally defective platelets. Normal in hemophilia A and B because platelets not affected.
Factor assays	Reductions of factor VIII in hemophilia A, factor IX in hemophilia B, vWF in von Willebrand disease.
Partial thromboplastin time	Prolonged because of deficiency in intrinsic clotting system factor.
Platelet count	Normal. Adequate platelet production.
Prothrombin time	Normal. No involvement of extrinsic system.
Thrombin time	Normal. No impairment of thrombin-fibrinogen reaction.

TABLE 34.18 Drug Therapy

Examples of Replacement Factors for Hemophilia

Factor VIII	Factor IX	Von Willebrand	Patients Who Have Inhibitors
Advate	Alphanine SD	Alphanate	Bebulin
Adynovate	Alprolix	HumateP	Emicizumab
Afstyla	Bebulin	Vonvendi	FEIBA (Factor Eight Inhibitor Bypassing Activity)
Alphanate	BeneFix	Wilate	
Eloctate	Idelvion		
Esperoct	Ixinity		Eptacog alfa
Emicizumab	Mononine		Eptacog beta
Hemofil M	Profilnine		Hemlibra
Humate-P	Rixubis		Profilnine
Jivi			
Kogenate FS			
NovoEight			
Wilate			
Xyntha			

Surgery and traumatic injuries may need longer therapy. Patients may need prophylactic replacement therapy before surgery and dental care. Table 34.18 lists examples of replacement therapy.

For mild hemophilia A and certain subtypes of von Willebrand disease, desmopressin acetate (DDAVP), a synthetic analog of vasopressin, can stimulate an increase in factor VIII and vWF.[2] This drug acts on platelets and endothelial cells to cause the release of vWF. vWF then binds with factor VIII, thus increasing its concentration. DDAVP can be given IV, subcutaneously, or by intranasal spray. Beneficial effects (e.g., decreased bleeding time) are seen within 30 minutes when given IV and can last for more than 12 hours. Because the drug's effect is short lived, monitor the patient closely. They may need repeated doses. It is an appropriate therapy for minor bleeding episodes and dental procedures. The intranasal form may be used as home therapy for some patients with mild to moderate forms of the disease.

Antifibrinolytic therapy (tranexamic acid) reduces fibrinolysis by inhibiting plasminogen activation in the fibrin clot, thus enhancing clot stability.[2] These agents stabilize clots in areas of increased fibrinolysis, such as the oral cavity, and in patients with difficult episodes of nosebleeds and menorrhagia. Topical thrombin and fibrin sealants can treat mucosal bleeding.

Complications of hemophilia treatment include development of inhibitors to factors VIII or IX, allergic reactions, and thrombotic complications with using factor IX because it contains activated coagulation factors. Patients with vWF may develop antibodies against vWF concentrates, the infusion of which could cause life-threatening anaphylaxis. Replacement factors for these patients should not contain vWF. Chronically, the development of inhibitors to the factor products can occur and needs expert management. Emicizumab is an option to address the problem of inhibitors for hemophilia A. It is a monoclonal antibody that binds factors IX and X, causing activation of factor X. This leads to thrombin generation, bypassing the need for factor VIII.[15] Gene transfer therapy is available for patients with hemophilia A (valoctogene roxaparvovec) and hemophilia B (etranacogene dezaparvovec) without inhibitors. Each is a one-time infusion that promotes the production of normal clotting factors in the liver. Patients receiving gene therapies have fewer bleeding episodes and less need for factor replacement.[15]

❖ NURSING MANAGEMENT: HEMOPHILIA

◆ Implementation

Health Promotion

Because of the hereditary nature of hemophilia, refer affected persons for genetic counseling before reproduction. This is important because many people with hemophilia live into adulthood. Include reproductive concerns and long-term effects in the care plan.

Acute Care

We implement measures to control bleeding. They include the following:

1. Stop the topical bleeding as quickly as possible. Apply direct pressure or ice, pack the area with Gelfoam or fibrin foam, and apply topical hemostatic agents, such as thrombin.
2. Give the specific coagulation factor to raise the level of the deficient coagulation factor. Monitor the patient for signs and symptoms, such as hypersensitivity.
3. When joint bleeding occurs, add the "RICE" protocol: Rest the involved joint to prevent crippling deformities from hemarthrosis, ice the joint for 20 minutes every 3 to 4 hours, compress/wrap the joint, and elevate. Give analgesics to reduce severe pain. Do not use aspirin and aspirin-

containing compounds. As soon as bleeding stops, encourage mobilization of the affected area through range-of-motion exercises and physical therapy. Avoid weight bearing until all swelling has resolved and muscle strength has returned. Orthotics may be prescribed.

4. Manage life-threatening complications that may develop from bleeding or side effects from coagulation factors. Examples include measures to prevent or treat airway obstruction from bleeding into the neck and pharynx, recognizing compartment syndrome in an extremity, and early assessment and treatment of intracranial bleeding.

Chronic Care

Home management is a primary consideration because the disease follows a progressive, chronic course. The patient's knowledge of the illness and how to live with it influences their quality and length of life (Box 34.5). Refer the patient and caregiver to a local chapter of the National Hemophilia Foundation to encourage networking with others who are dealing with hemophilia.[13] Perform ongoing assessment of the patient's adaptation to the illness. Provide psychosocial support and assistance as needed.

Most of the long-term care measures are related to patient teaching. Teach patients to recognize disease-related problems and which problems can be treated at home and which require hospitalization. Immediate medical attention is needed for severe pain or swelling of a muscle or joint that restricts movement or inhibits sleep and for a head injury, swelling in the neck or mouth, abdominal pain, hematuria, melena, and wounds in need of suturing.

Teach patients to perform daily oral hygiene without causing trauma. Discuss how to prevent injuries. Teach patients to take part only in noncontact sports (e.g., golf). Patients should wear a Medic Alert tag to ensure that HCPs know about the hemophilia in case of an accident. Teach patients or caregivers to self-administer factor replacement therapies.

BOX 34.5 EVIDENCE-BASED PRACTICE

Depression in Patients With Hemophilia

K.S. is a 47-year-old female admitted with hematuria and hypertension. She was diagnosed with hemophilia A as an infant. She has a history of chronic joint disease and pain from bleeding into joints. You note that she is identified as an "inhibitor" although she has been doing better with self-injections of emicizumab. In discussion with the clinical nurse specialist, you learn that inhibitors are people with hemophilia A who develop antibodies to attack clotting factors provided in disease treatment. Their management is complex because their immune system resists standard treatments. When you perform your admission interview, you identify behaviors suggesting anxiety and depression. K.S. seems apathetic, responding briefly to questions about her history and symptoms. Then she unexpectedly asks, "Do we have to do this again? After all these trips to the hospital, I've had it with all these questions."

Making Clinical Decisions

Synthesis of Best Available Evidence

Persons with hemophilia often experience pain and impaired function, leading to a decreased quality of life and depression. Anxiety can be related to the risk of bleeding.

Clinician Expertise

You realize an appropriate approach to the admission interview is to slow the interaction with the patient, speak in a low tone, and demonstrate empathy about the repeated hospitalizations. If she continues to show irritability or expresses anger, you will remain calm and supportive. Assure K.S. you are interested in understanding her health concerns so you can provide the best possible care and support her in her disease management. Encourage K.S. to share her feelings about the chronic nature of hemophilia and the years of living with its uncertainty. Ask questions about pain management, disability, and social support with empathy. Allow K.S. to steer the conversation as much as possible.

Patient Preferences and Values

K.S. expresses concern about failed treatments. She tells you she is hopeful that she will be eligible for a treatment with a new gene therapy even though she has inhibitors now.

Implications for Nursing Practice

1. How should you discuss gene therapy treatment with K.S.?
2. What else do you want to know about her depression and anxiety?
3. What strategies can you suggest to improve her quality of life?

Reference for Evidence

Fletcher S, Jenner K, Holland M, et al: Barriers to gene therapy, understanding the concerns people with haemophilia have: an exigency sub-study, *Orphanet J Rare Dis* 19:59, 2024.

DISSEMINATED INTRAVASCULAR COAGULATION

Disseminated intravascular coagulation (DIC) is a serious bleeding and thrombotic disorder that results from abnormally initiated and accelerated clotting. Subsequent decreases in clotting factors and platelets ensue, which may lead to uncontrollable, profuse bleeding. DIC is not a disease. It is always caused by an underlying disease or condition. That underlying problem must be treated for DIC to resolve.

Etiology and Pathophysiology

DIC is an abnormal response of the normal clotting cascade stimulated by a disease process or disorder.[4] Table 34.19 lists diseases and disorders known to predispose a patient to DIC. DIC can occur as an acute, catastrophic condition, or it may exist at a subacute or chronic level. Chronic and subacute DIC is most often seen in patients with long-standing illnesses, such as cancer or autoimmune disease. Occasionally these patients have subclinical disease manifested only by laboratory abnormalities. Each condition may have 1 or multiple triggering mechanisms to start the clotting cascade. For example, tumors and traumatized or necrotic tissue release tissue factors into circulation. Endotoxin from gram-negative bacteria activates several steps in the coagulation cascade.

The manifestations of DIC result from (1) consumption and depletion of platelets and coagulation factors, and (2) clot lysis and formation of fibrin split products (FSPs) that have anticoagulant properties (Fig. 34.9). Tissue factor is released at the site of tissue injury and by some cancers, such as leukemia. It enhances normal coagulation mechanisms. Abundant intravascular thrombin, the most powerful coagulant, is made. It speeds the conversion of fibrinogen to fibrin and enhances platelet aggregation. There is widespread fibrin and platelet deposition in capillaries and arterioles, causing thrombosis. This process can lead to multiorgan failure.

TABLE 34.19 Risk Factors for DIC

Acute DIC

- **Cancers**
  - Acute leukemia
  - Metastatic solid tumors
- **Hemolytic Processes**
  - Acute hemolysis from infection or immunologic disorders
  - Transfusion of mismatched blood
- **Obstetric Conditions**
  - Abruptio placentae
  - Amniotic fluid embolism
  - HELLP syndrome
  - Retained dead fetus
  - Septic abortion or pregnancy
- **Septicemia**
- **Shock**
  - Anaphylactic
  - Cardiogenic
  - Hemorrhagic
- **Tissue Damage**
  - Acute anoxia (e.g., after cardiac arrest)
  - Extensive burns and trauma
  - Heatstroke
  - Hepatitis
  - Postoperative damage, especially after extracorporeal membrane oxygenation
  - Prosthetic devices
  - Severe head injury
  - Snakebites
  - Transplant rejections
  - Vascular disorders (e.g., aortic aneurysm)

Subacute DIC

- Metastatic cancer
- Myeloproliferative/lymphoproliferative cancers

Chronic DIC

- Cancer
- Liver disease
- Systemic lupus erythematosus (SLE)

Clotting inhibitory mechanisms, such as antithrombin III (AT III) and protein C, are depressed. Excess clotting activates the fibrinolytic system, which in turn breaks down the newly formed clot, creating FSPs. FSPs have anticoagulant properties. They inhibit normal blood clotting by (1) coating the platelets and interfering with platelet function; (2) interfering with thrombin and thus disrupting coagulation; and (3) attaching to fibrinogen, which interferes with the process needed to form a stable clot. As FSPs accumulate and clotting factors are depleted, the blood loses its ability to clot. A stable clot cannot form at injury sites, which predisposes the patient to bleeding.

Clinical Manifestations

DIC has bleeding and thrombotic manifestations. Question bleeding in a person with no history or obvious cause because it may be the first manifestation of acute DIC. Bleeding manifestations include manifestations in the (1) skin, such as pallor, petechiae, purpura, oozing blood, venipuncture site bleeding, hematomas, and occult bleeding; (2) respiratory system (e.g., tachypnea, hemoptysis); (3) cardiovascular system, such as tachycardia and hypotension; (4) GI tract, such as upper and lower GI bleeding, abdominal distention, and bloody stools; (5) GU tract (e.g., hematuria); (6) neurologic system, such as vision changes, dizziness, headache, and mental status changes; and (7) musculoskeletal system (e.g., bone and joint pain).

Thrombotic manifestations are a result of fibrin or platelet deposition in the microvasculature (Fig. 34.9). These manifestations affect the (1) skin (e.g., cyanosis, ischemic tissue necrosis, hemorrhagic necrosis); (2) respiratory system (e.g., tachypnea, dyspnea, pulmonary emboli); (3) cardiovascular system

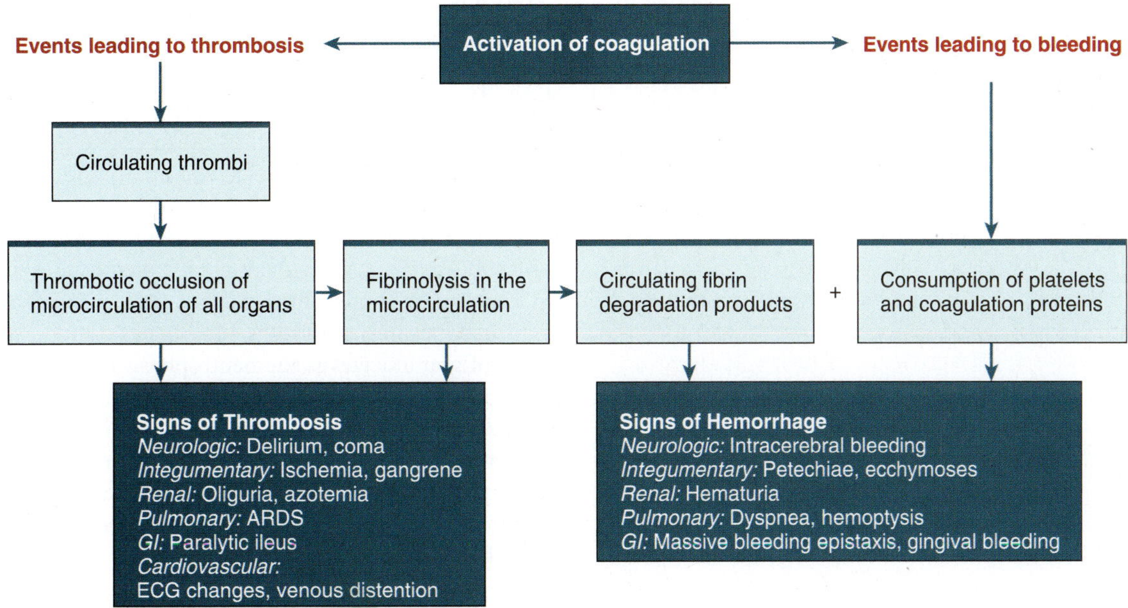

Fig. 34.9 Sequence of events that occur during DIC.

(e.g., ECG changes, venous distention); (4) GI tract (e.g., abdominal pain, paralytic ileus); (5) kidneys (damage and oliguria, leading to failure); and (6) neurologic system (e.g., delirium, coma).

Diagnostic Studies

Table 34.20 lists tests used to diagnose acute DIC. D-dimer, a polymer resulting from the breakdown of fibrin, is a specific marker for the degree of fibrinolysis. In general, tests that measure raw materials needed for coagulation (e.g., platelets, fibrinogen) are reduced and values that measure clotting times are prolonged. Fragmented RBCs (schistocytes), indicative of partial occlusion of small vessels by fibrin thrombi, may be found on blood smears.

Interprofessional Care

It is important to diagnose DIC quickly, stabilize the patient (e.g., oxygenation, volume replacement), treat the underlying cause, and control the ongoing thrombosis and bleeding. Depending on its severity, we use a variety of measures to manage DIC (Fig. 34.10). First, if chronic DIC is diagnosed in a patient who is not bleeding, no treatment is needed. Treating the underlying cause may be enough to reverse the DIC (e.g., chemotherapy with DIC caused by cancer). When the patient with DIC is bleeding, therapy is directed toward providing support with needed blood products while treating the cause.

Blood products are given cautiously based on specific component deficiencies to patients who have serious bleeding, are at high risk for bleeding (e.g., surgery), or require invasive procedures. Blood product support with platelets, cryoprecipitate, and fresh frozen plasma (FFP) is usually reserved for a patient with life-threatening bleeding.[2] Therapy stabilizes a patient, prevents severe blood loss or massive thrombosis, and gives time to treat the underlying cause. Cryoprecipitate replaces factor VIII and fibrinogen. It may be given if the fibrinogen level is low and there is potentially dangerous or active bleeding.[2] FFP is given only to patients with significant bleeding and a prolonged PT and aPTT. It replaces all clotting factors except platelets and is a source of antithrombin.

Patients with thrombosis are often treated by anticoagulation with heparin or LMWH. Heparin is used to treat DIC only when the benefit (reduce clotting) outweighs the risk (further bleeding). AT III (Atnativ) may be useful in severe DIC, although it increases the risk for bleeding.[2] Chronic DIC does not respond to oral anticoagulants. It is controlled with long-term use of heparin.

TABLE 34.20 Laboratory Results in Acute DIC

Test	Finding in Acute DIC
Screening Tests	
Prothrombin time (PT)	Prolonged
Partial thromboplastin time (PTT)	Prolonged
Activated partial thromboplastin time (aPTT)	Prolonged
Fibrinogen	↓
Platelets	↓
Thrombin time	Prolonged
Special Tests	
Antithrombin III (AT III)	↓
D-dimers (cross-linked fibrin fragments)	↑
Factor assays (prothrombin and factors V, VIII, X, XIII)	↓ but may be misleading because V and VIII ↑ with inflammation
Fibrin split products (FSPs)	↑
Peripheral blood smear	Schistocytes present
Plasminogen, tissue plasminogen activator	↓
Proteins C and S	↓

NURSING MANAGEMENT: DISSEMINATED INTRAVASCULAR COAGULATION

Be alert to the development of DIC, especially with the risk factors listed in Table 34.19. Early detection of bleeding and clotting, both occult and overt, is important. Assess for signs of external bleeding (e.g., petechiae, oozing at IV sites), signs of internal bleeding (e.g., increased heart rate, change in mental status, increasing abdominal girth), and any signs that microthrombi may be causing clinically significant organ damage (e.g., decreased urine output, increased creatinine).

Remember that because DIC is caused by an underlying disease, that problem must be managed while providing supportive care for the manifestations of DIC. Minimize tissue damage and protect patients from sources of bleeding. Prompt administration of prescribed therapies is crucial. Give blood products and medications. Table 34.14 and eNursing Care Plan 34.2 provide assessments and interventions for patients with DIC.

NEUTROPENIA

Pathophysiology

Leukopenia refers to a decrease in the total WBC count (granulocytes, monocytes, and lymphocytes). *Granulocytopenia* is a deficiency of granulocytes, which include neutrophils, eosinophils, and basophils. Neutrophilic granulocytes (neutrophils) play a key role in phagocytizing pathogenic microbes. They are closely monitored in clinical practice as an indicator of infection risk. A reduction in neutrophils is termed **neutropenia**. Some clinicians use the terms *granulocytopenia* and *neutropenia* interchangeably because the largest constituency of granulocytes is the neutrophils.

Normally, neutrophils range from 3000 to 7000 cells/μL. Calculate the *absolute neutrophil count* (ANC) by multiplying the total WBC count by the percentage of neutrophils (segmented and banded). *Neutropenia* is defined as ANC less than 1000 cells/μL (1×10^9/L). *Severe neutropenia* is an ANC less than 500 cells/μL.[2]

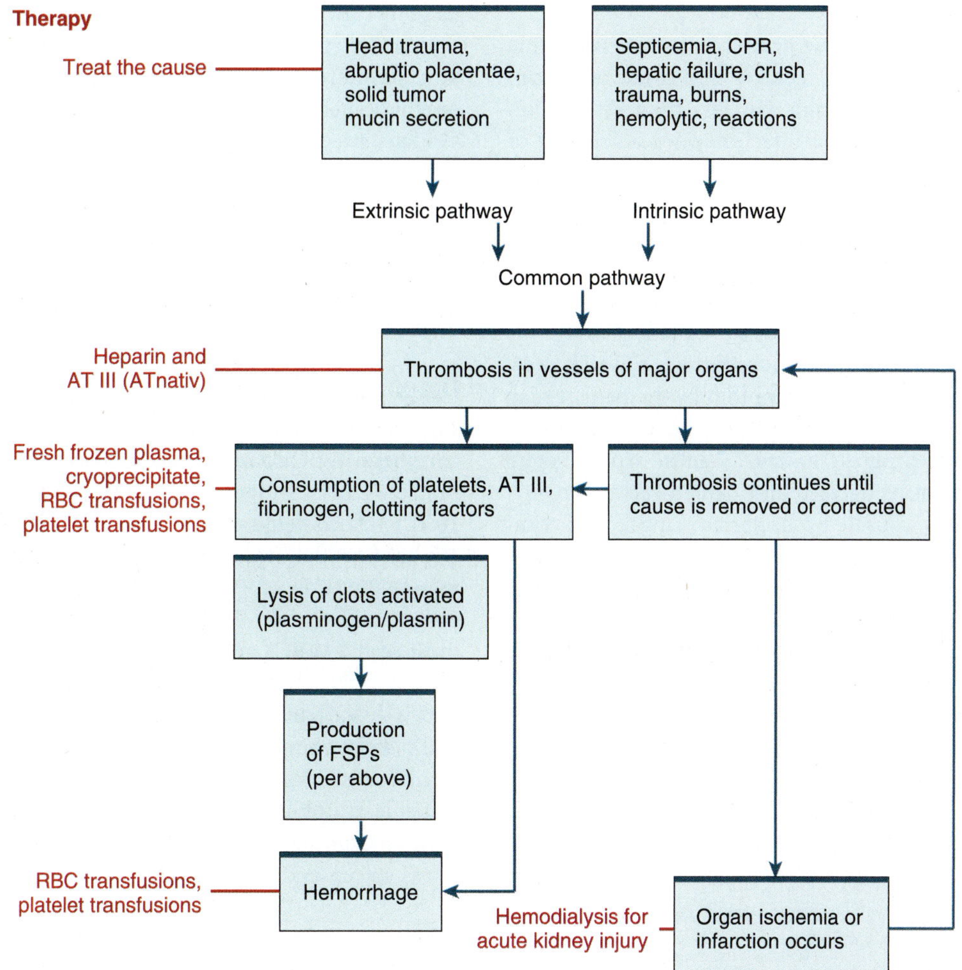

Fig. 34.10 Sites of action for therapies in DIC. *AT III,* Antithrombin III; *FSP,* fibrin split product.

It is important to know whether the decrease in the neutrophil count was gradual or rapid, the degree of neutropenia, and the duration. The faster the drop and the longer the duration, the greater the chance of life-threatening infection, sepsis, and death. Patients with an ANC between 500 and 1000/μL are at moderate risk for a bacterial infection. Severe neutropenia (under 500/μL) places patients at severe risk. Other factors and comorbid conditions can increase the risk of life-threatening consequences. These include immune disorders or treatments (e.g., SLE, steroids), being older than age 60, and having an existing infection or previous fungal infection.[16]

Neutropenia is a clinical consequence of several conditions or diseases (Table 34.21). It can be an expected effect, a side effect, or an unintentional effect of certain drugs. The most common cause of neutropenia is chemotherapy and immunosuppressive therapy for the treatment of cancer and autoimmune disease. A term we use to describe the lowest point of neutropenia (and other blood cells) in patients treated with chemotherapy is *nadir.*

Clinical Manifestations

Patients with neutropenia are predisposed to infection with opportunistic pathogens and nonpathogenic organisms from the normal body flora. The classic manifestations of inflammation—redness, heat, and swelling—may not occur. WBCs are the major component of pus. Therefore in patients with neutropenia, pus formation (e.g., visible skin lesion) is absent.

! SAFETY ALERT

Neutropenia

- A low-grade fever in neutropenic patients is of great significance. It may indicate infection and lead to septic shock and death unless treated promptly.
- Neutropenic fever (≥100.4°F [38°C] and/or new signs or symptoms (tachycardia, chills) suggesting infection and a neutrophil count <500/μL) is a medical emergency.
- Blood cultures should be drawn STAT (within 1 h) and antibiotics started within 1 h.

Assume that fever or any new symptom in a neutropenic patient is caused by infection. It requires immediate attention. Immunocompromised, neutropenic patients have little or no ability to fight infection. A minor infection can lead rapidly to sepsis and death. The mucous membranes of the throat and mouth, skin, perineal area, and pulmonary system are common entry points for pathogenic organisms in susceptible hosts.

Manifestations related to infection may include sore throat and dysphagia, ulcerative lesions of the pharyngeal and buccal mucosa, diarrhea, rectal tenderness, vaginal itching or discharge, shortness of breath, and nonproductive cough. Any report of minor pain or any other symptom by the patient may be significant and should be reported to the HCP at once. Minor problems can progress to fever, chills, sepsis, septic shock, and death if not recognized and treated early.

Systemic infections caused by bacterial, fungal, and viral organisms are common in patients with neutropenia. The patient's own flora (normally nonpathogenic) contributes significantly to life-threatening infections. Organisms known to be common sources of infection include gram-positive coagulase-negative *Staphylococcus* and *Staphylococcus aureus,* viridans streptococci and gram-negative *Escherichia coli, Klebsiella, Enterobacter,* and *Pseudomonas aeruginosa.*[16] Fungi involved include *Candida* (usually *C. albicans*) and *Aspergillus* organisms. Viral infections caused by reactivation of herpes simplex and zoster are common after prolonged periods of neutropenia, such as in patients undergoing HSCT.[16]

TABLE 34.21 Common Causes of Neutropenia

Autoimmune Disorders
- Felty syndrome
- Systemic lupus erythematosus

Drugs
- Anticancer agents (busulfan, methotrexate, mercaptopurine, cytarabine, rituximab, combination therapies)
- Anticonvulsants (phenytoin, carbamazepine, valproic acid)
- Antiinflammatory drugs (indomethacin)
- Antimicrobial agents (linezolid, levamisole, penicillin G, trimethoprim/sulfamethoxazole)
- Antipsychotics (clozapine, olanzapine, chlorpromazine)
- Antithyroid drugs (methimazole, propylthiouracil)
- Cardiovascular drugs (ticlopidine, procainamide)
- $Histamine_2$ blockers (cimetidine, ranitidine)

Hematologic Disorders
- Aplastic anemia
- Congenital (cyclic neutropenia)
- Idiopathic neutropenia
- Leukemia
- Myelodysplastic syndrome

Infections
- Fulminant bacterial infection (e.g., typhoid fever, miliary tuberculosis)
- Parasitic
- Rickettsial
- Viral (e.g., hepatitis, influenza, HIV, measles)

Other
- Bone marrow infiltration (e.g., cancer, tuberculosis, lymphoma)
- Hemodialysis
- Hypersplenism (e.g., portal hypertension, storage diseases [e.g., Gaucher disease])
- Nutrition deficiencies (cobalamin, folic acid)
- Severe sepsis

Diagnostic Studies

The primary diagnostic tests for assessing neutropenia are the peripheral WBC count and bone marrow aspiration and biopsy (Table 34.22). A total WBC count of less than 4000/μL (4×10^9/L) reflects leukopenia. However, only a differential count can confirm the presence of neutropenia (neutrophil count less than 1000/μL [1×10^9/L]). Patients with acute leukemia who present with a high WBC may in fact have neutropenia, because most of the WBCs are ineffective leukemia blast cells.

A peripheral blood smear assesses for immature forms of WBCs (e.g., bands). The hematocrit level, reticulocyte count, and platelet count are done to evaluate bone marrow function. Review past and current drug history. If the cause of neutropenia is unknown, bone marrow aspiration and biopsy are done to examine cell numbers and morphology. Other studies assess spleen and liver function.

TABLE 34.22 Interprofessional Care

Neutropenia

Diagnostic Assessment
- History and physical assessment
- Medication review
- Risk assessment for severity and duration of neutropenia
- WBC count with differential count, morphology
- Hgb and Hct
- Reticulocyte and platelet count
- Bone marrow aspiration and biopsy
- Cultures of nose, throat, sputum, urine, stool, obvious lesions, blood
- Chest x-ray, liver function tests, and other diagnostic tests

Management
- Identify and remove cause of neutropenia (if possible)
- Identification of site of infection (if present) and causative organism
- Blood cultures drawn STAT, before antibiotics
- Antimicrobial therapy STAT (within 1 h)
- Prophylactic hematopoietic myeloid growth factors after myelosuppressive chemotherapy
- Strict hand hygiene
- Single-patient room, positive-pressure or high-efficiency particulate air (HEPA) filtration, depending on risk
- Community isolation and home precautions (if outpatient)
- Safe activity and ambulation to maintain physical and pulmonary function

Interprofessional and Nursing Management

The nursing and interprofessional care of neutropenia includes (1) determining the cause of neutropenia, (2) instituting antibiotic therapy, (3) identifying the offending organisms if an infection has developed, and (4) implementing protective practices (e.g., strict hand washing, skin and oral hygiene) Table 34.22 and Table 34.23 describe the care of patients with neutropenia. We can often treat patients on an outpatient basis if the patient and caregiver can monitor for fever and signs of infection and seek care promptly if needed (Table 34.24).

Sometimes, the cause of neutropenia can be easily treated (e.g., nutrition deficiencies). However, neutropenia can be a side effect that must be tolerated as a necessary step in therapy (e.g., chemotherapy, radiation therapy). In some situations, neutropenia resolves when the primary problem is treated (Table 34.21). Myeloid growth factors (see Table 16.14) can be used to prevent neutropenia or to reduce its severity and duration.[17] Once neutropenia has occurred, these agents are generally not as effective.

Ongoing monitoring is essential. Early identification and management can prevent death from sepsis. Monitor neutropenic patients for signs and symptoms of infection (e.g., any fever 100.4°F [38°C] or greater, unexplained tachycardia, chills) and early septic shock. Obtain frequent vital signs (e.g., every 15 minutes to 1 hour) and assess mental status. See Chapter 42 for more information on signs of septic shock. Identifying the infective organism depends on obtaining cultures from various sites. Serial blood cultures (at least 2 or 1 from a peripheral site and 1 from a venous access device) should be done promptly and antibiotics started within 1 hour.

Prophylactic antibiotic, antiviral, and antifungal medications may be started, then switched to treatment doses depending on the risk of specific infections and diagnostic results. We usually give broad-spectrum antibiotics by the IV route because of the rapidly lethal effects of infection. However, some oral antibiotics are highly effective. We may give them to patients who do not have severe or prolonged neutropenia. Using a third- or fourth-generation cephalosporin with broad microorganism coverage (e.g., cefepime, ceftazidime) or a carbapenem (e.g., imipenem/cilastatin) depends on the response and diagnostic tests.

Begin therapy promptly and observe for side effects of antimicrobial agents. Ongoing febrile episodes or a change in assessment requires a call to the HCP for assessment or more cultures, diagnostic tests, or antimicrobial therapies. The longer the neutropenia, the greater the risk for a fungal infection. Antifungal therapy is started whenever a culture is positive or in

TABLE 34.23 NURSING MANAGEMENT

Caring for the Patient With Neutropenia

- Make sure that hand hygiene is done before, during, and after patient care by everyone caring for the patient.
- Maintain appropriate isolation precautions.
- Assess for signs and symptoms of infection and report suspected infections promptly.
- Screen visitors for infectious diseases.
- Place the patient on a diet that observes food safety guidelines (well-washed fruits and vegetables; keep hot foods hot and cold foods cold; no undercooked eggs, meats, soft/mold cheeses, yogurt) to protect them from bacteria found in some foods.
- Obtain ordered cultures; monitor results of cultures and laboratory tests for absolute granulocyte count, WBC count, and differential.
- Give prescribed antimicrobials and hematopoietic growth factors.
- Implement measures to manage fever (see Table 12.5).
- Provide daily skin care and frequent oral hygiene.
- Remove fresh flowers and plants from patient areas.
- Teach patient and caregivers about
  - Hand hygiene.
  - How to avoid infection, including the need for skin care and oral hygiene (Table 34.24).
  - Signs and symptoms of infection and what to do if they occur.

TABLE 34.24 PATIENT & CAREGIVER TEACHING

Neutropenia

Include the following instructions when teaching a patient or caregiver the precautions to take when the neutrophil count is low:

1. Clean your hands often with soap and water. Make sure those around you wash their hands often, especially if they help with your care. You may also use an antibacterial hand gel.
2. Notify your nurse or HCP if you have any of the following:
   - Fever ≥100.4°F (38°C)[a]
   - Chills or feeling hot
   - Redness, swelling, discharge, or new pain on or in your body
   - Changes in urination or bowel movements
   - Cough, sore throat, mouth sores, or blisters
3. If you are at home, take your temperature as directed and follow instructions on what to do if you have a fever or any other symptoms of infection.
4. Avoid crowds and people with colds, flu, or infections. If you are in a public area, wear a mask and use hand sanitizing gel frequently.
5. Avoid uncooked meats, seafood, or eggs and unwashed fruits and vegetables. Ask your HCP about your specific diet guidelines.
6. Avoid prolonged contact with soil, such as gardening, and household renovation.
7. Bathe or shower daily. Use moisturizer to prevent skin from drying and cracking.
8. Maintain some daily activity as instructed by your health care team. This may include walking and moderate exercise while avoiding crowds.
9. Brush your teeth with a soft toothbrush 4 times daily. You may floss once daily if it does not cause excess pain or bleeding. Avoid alcohol-based mouthwashes.
10. Do not clean up after pets. Litter boxes, reptile cages, fish tanks, and bird cages have specific risks for infection. You may feed and pet your dog or cat if you wash your hands well after handling.

[a]Confirm the cut-off temperature with the HCP.

patients who do not become afebrile with broad-spectrum antibiotic coverage.

Sputum, throat, lesions, wounds, urine, and fecal cultures may be part of surveillance. Depending on the clinical situation, the patient may need CT scans, bronchoscopy with bronchial brushings, or lung biopsy to diagnose the cause of pneumonic infiltrates. Invasive diagnostic studies are often contraindicated because of the concern of introducing infection and the fact that patients are often thrombocytopenic. Despite these many tests, we find the causative organism only 50% of the time.[2] Thus the priority is to obtain the blood cultures and begin the antibiotic at once.

Hand hygiene is the single most important preventive measure to minimize the risk for infection in neutropenic patients. Strict hand hygiene by staff and visitors using an antiseptic hand wash or sanitizing gel before and after contact is the major method to prevent transmission of harmful pathogens.

Keep immunocompromised patients separate from those with infections. Place hospitalized patients in a private room. High-efficiency particulate air (HEPA) filtration is an air-handling method with a high-flow filtering system that can reduce the number of aerosolized pathogens (especially molds) in the environment. Teach the patient and caregiver to avoid potentially hazardous foods, such as raw and undercooked meats and eggs, and to make sure fruits and vegetables are washed well before eating.

Do not overlook quality-of-life issues for patients with neutropenia. Fatigue, malaise, a decrease in functioning, and social isolation require coaching on safe activity.

MYELODYSPLASTIC SYNDROME

Myelodysplastic syndrome (MDS) is a group of hematopoietic stem cell disorders that results in peripheral blood cytopenia, abnormal cell morphology in 1 or more cell lines, and increased risk of acute myeloid leukemia (AML). Although it can occur in all age groups, the highest prevalence is in people older than 80 years of age.[18]

Etiology and Pathophysiology

The cause of MDS is unknown. Persons at risk are those who had radiation therapy, had chemotherapy with alkylating agents, or were exposed to industrial solvents (e.g., benzene, vinyl chloride). Around 50% of patients with MDS have an acquired chromosome abnormality.[2] Rarely, genetic disorders cause the disease.

We refer to MDS as a *clonal disorder* because some bone marrow stem cells continue to function normally, while others do not. The abnormal clone of the stem cells is usually found in the bone marrow. Eventually, it may be found in the circulation.

Sometimes, one type of MDS transforms into another. Depending on the subtype, MDS may progress to AML. In contrast to AML, in which the leukemic cells show little normal maturation, the clonal cells in MDS always have some degree of maturity. Disease progression is slower than in AML. Sometimes treatment is not needed.

Clinical Manifestations

Manifestations result from neoplastic transformation of the immature hematopoietic stem cells in the bone marrow. MDS often presents as infection and bleeding caused by inadequate numbers of ineffectively functioning circulating granulocytes or platelets. It may be found in the older adult during testing for the symptoms of anemia, thrombocytopenia, or neutropenia. It may be diagnosed incidentally from a routine CBC. During the advanced stage of MDS, life-threatening anemia, thrombocytopenia, and neutropenia occur.

Diagnostic Studies

Bone marrow biopsy with aspirate analysis is essential for the diagnosis and classification of the type of MDS. The patient has peripheral cytopenia and changes in the bone marrow (hypocellular or hypercellular). Laboratory data and bone marrow studies rule out other causes of dysplasia, such as nonmalignant disorders, cobalamin and folate deficiencies, and infection.

Interprofessional and Nursing Management

Treatment is based on the premise that treatment aggressiveness should match disease aggressiveness. This is based on the amount and type of dysplasia in the bone marrow, specific genetic mutations, anticipated patient tolerance, and patient preference. Supportive treatment consists of hematologic monitoring (serial bone marrow and peripheral blood examinations), antibiotic therapy, or transfusions with blood products along with chelators to prevent iron overload. Aminocaproic acid or other antifibrinolytic drugs may be used for patients who are refractory to platelet transfusions.

Low-risk patients may be treated with EPO, myeloid growth factors, or lenalidomide.[2] Azacitidine (Vidaza) and decitabine (Dacogen) are drugs that help restore normal growth control and differentiation of hematopoietic cells. They reduce the frequency of transformation of MDS to acute leukemia. Side effects include myelosuppression, GI distress, and renal problems.

Other treatments include cytarabine with or without antitumor antibiotics (anthracyclines), ATG, and cyclosporine.[18] Chemotherapy and allogeneic HSCT are used in appropriate patients to treat bone marrow dysfunction of MDS and restore it with normal hematopoiesis.

Nursing care of patients with MDS is like that of patients with manifestations of anemia, thrombocytopenia, and neutropenia. See eNursing Care Plan 34.1 for patients with anemia, eNursing Care Plan 34.2 for the patient with thrombocytopenia, and Table 34.23 for managing patients with neutropenia.

LEUKEMIA

Etiology and Pathophysiology

Leukemia is the general term used to describe a group of cancers affecting the blood and blood-forming tissues of the bone marrow, lymph system, and spleen. Leukemia occurs in all age groups. It results in an accumulation of dysfunctional cells because of a loss of regulation in cell division. An estimated 62,770 new cases are diagnosed each year. Leukemias account for 28% of all childhood cancers.[19] The disease follows a progressive course that is fatal if untreated. Progress in successful cancer treatments has been rapid in the last 50 years.

Leukemia has no single cause. It begins as a mutation in the DNA of certain cells. Most leukemias result from a combination of factors, including genetic and environment influences. Chemical agents (e.g., benzene), chemotherapy drugs (e.g., alkylating agents, topoisomerase II inhibitors), viruses, radiation, and immunologic deficiencies increase the risk. Depending on the type of leukemia, other potential causes are exposure to pesticides (farmworkers) and smoking. Leukemia occurs more often in those with certain congenital or inherited abnormalities (e.g., Down syndrome).[2]

Classification

We classify leukemia based on acute versus chronic disease and the type of WBC involved. The terms *acute* and *chronic* refer to cell maturity and nature of disease onset. With acute leukemia, there is clonal proliferation of immature hematopoietic cells. The leukemia develops after malignant transformation of one type of immature hematopoietic cell, followed by cellular replication and expansion of that malignant clone (Fig. 34.11).[4] Chronic leukemias involve more mature forms of the WBC. The disease onset is more gradual.

Leukemia classified by the type of leukocyte involved is either myelogenous or lymphocytic in origin. By combining the acute and chronic categories with the cell type involved, we identify 4 major types of leukemia: acute lymphocytic leukemia

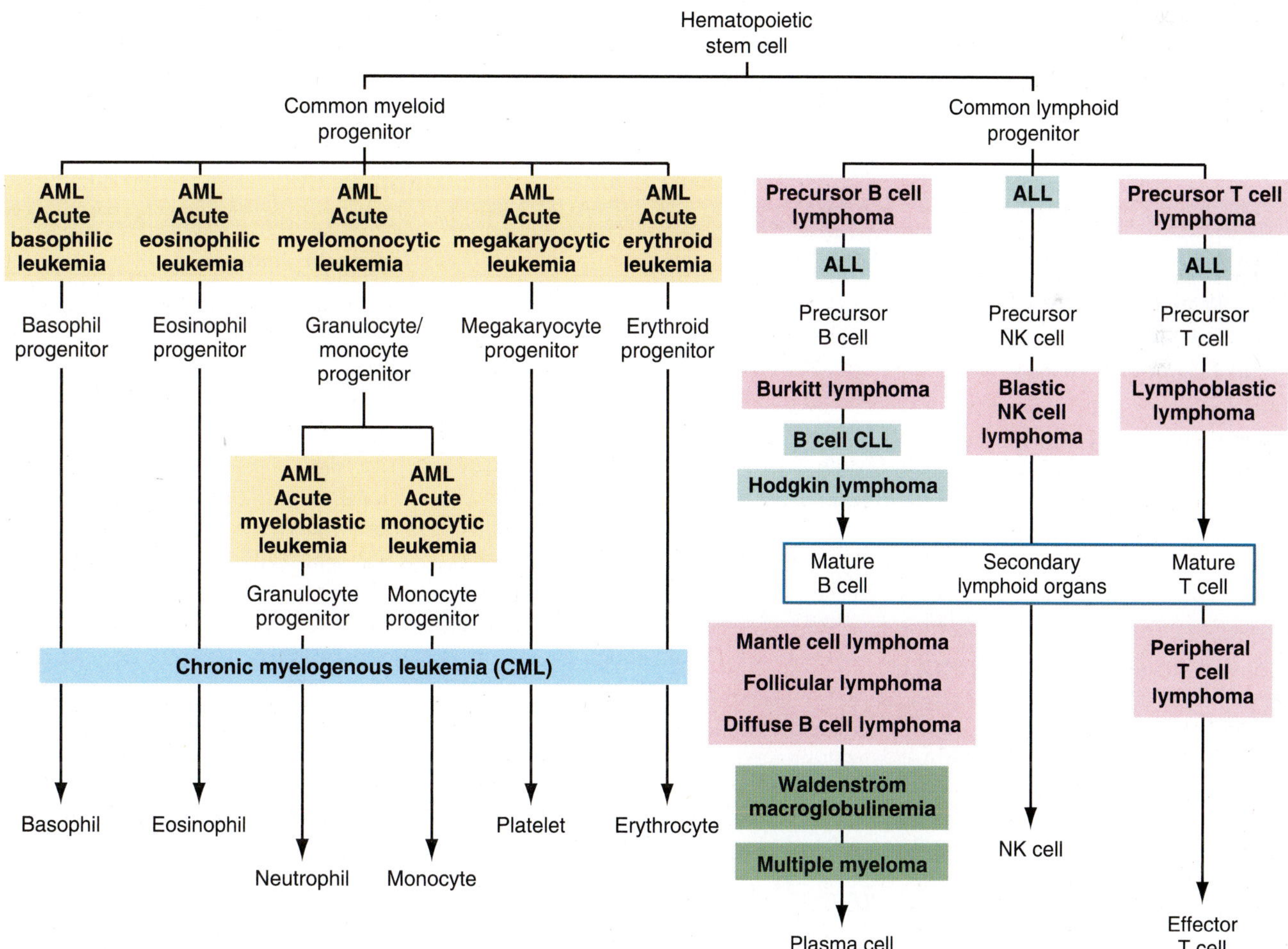

Fig. 34.11 Origins of leukemias, lymphomas, and myeloma. Differentiation pathways of blood-forming cells and the point at which the malignant clone originates. *AML,* Acute myeloid leukemia; *CLL,* chronic lymphocytic leukemia; *NK,* natural killer. (Modified from Rogers JL, Brashers VL: *McCance & Huether's pathophysiology,* ed 9, St Louis, 2023, Elsevier.)

(ALL), AML, chronic myelogenous (granulocytic) leukemia (CML), and chronic lymphocytic leukemia (CLL). Table 34.25 shows other defining features of these subtypes.

Acute Myeloid Leukemia

AML represents about one-third of all leukemias. It makes up about 76% of the acute leukemias in adults.[19] With AML there is uncontrolled proliferation of myeloblasts, the precursors of granulocytes. There is hyperplasia of the bone marrow. The manifestations are usually related to replacement of normal hematopoietic cells in the marrow by leukemic myeloblasts and, to a lesser extent, infiltration of other organs and tissue (Table 34.25). Its onset is often abrupt and dramatic. Patients may have serious infections and abnormal bleeding from the onset of the disease.

Acute Lymphocytic Leukemia

ALL is the most common type of leukemia in children. It accounts for around 23% of acute leukemia cases in adults.[19] In ALL, immature small lymphocytes proliferate in the bone marrow. Most are of B-cell origin. Most patients have fever at the time of diagnosis. Signs and symptoms may appear abruptly with bleeding or fever, or they may be insidious with progressive weakness, fatigue, bone and/or joint pain, and bleeding. Central nervous system (CNS) infiltration is especially common. Infiltration into other tissues and lymph nodes can occur.

Chronic Myelogenous Leukemia

CML is caused by excess development of neoplastic granulocytes in the bone marrow. These granulocytes are in all stages of development. They move into the peripheral blood in massive numbers and infiltrate the liver and spleen.

The natural history of CML is a chronic stable phase followed by a more acute, aggressive phase called the *blastic phase.* The chronic phase of CML can last for several years with current therapies. Once CML transforms to an acute or blastic phase, it must be treated more aggressively, similar to acute leukemia. For younger patients and those who stop responding to maintenance therapy, HSCT is done.

Genetic Link. The *Philadelphia chromosome* originates from the translocation between the *BCR* gene on chromosome 22 and the *ABL* gene on chromosome 9. The protein that is encoded by the newly created *BCR-ABL* gene on the Philadelphia chromosome interferes with normal cell cycle events, such as the regulation of cell proliferation.

CML is defined by the presence of the Philadelphia chromosome in the setting of a chronic myeloproliferative neoplasm.[20] It is a diagnostic hallmark of CML and an important indicator of residual disease or relapse after

TABLE 34.25 Types of Leukemia

Age of Onset	Clinical Manifestations	Diagnostic Findings
Acute Myeloid Leukemia (AML)		
Median age at diagnosis 68 yr.	Fatigue, weakness, headache, mouth sores, anemia, bleeding, fever, infection; gingival hyperplasia, mild splenomegaly.	↓ RBC count, Hgb, Hct, platelet count. ↓ to ↑ WBC count with myeloblasts. ↑ LDH. Hypercellular bone marrow with myeloblasts.
Acute Lymphocytic Leukemia (ALL)		
Most patients are older than 50 yr.	Fever, pallor, bleeding, anorexia, fatigue, and weakness. Bone, joint, and abdominal pain. General lymphadenopathy, infections, weight loss, hepatosplenomegaly, mouth sores. Neurologic manifestations: Headache, ↑ intracranial pressure (nausea, vomiting, lethargy, cranial nerve dysfunction) from meningeal infiltration. Painless enlargement of the scrotum.	↓ RBC, Hgb, Hct, platelet count. ↓, normal, or ↑ WBC count. ↑ LDH. Hypercellular bone marrow with lymphoblasts. Lymphoblasts may be in cerebrospinal fluid. Presence of Philadelphia chromosome (up to 19% of patients).
Chronic Myelogenous Leukemia (CML)		
Increase in incidence with advancing age. Median age at diagnosis is above 60. Rare in children.	No symptoms early in disease. Fatigue and weakness, fever, night sweats, sternal tenderness, weight loss, joint pain, bone pain, massive splenomegaly.	↓ RBC count, Hgb, Hct. ↑ platelet count early, ↓ count later. ↑ WBCs, including a wide variety of myeloid cells and basophils. Nucleated RBCs common. Philadelphia chromosome present.
Chronic Lymphocytic Leukemia (CLL)		
Median age at diagnosis is 70. Predominance in males.	Frequently no symptoms. Detection of disease often during examination for unrelated condition. Fatigue, anorexia, splenomegaly, lymphadenopathy, hepatomegaly. May progress to fever, night sweats, weight loss, fatigue, and frequent infections.	Mild anemia and thrombocytopenia with disease progression. Total WBC count >100,000/μL. ↑ in peripheral lymphocytes and lymphocytes in bone marrow. May have autoimmune hemolytic anemia, idiopathic thrombocytopenic purpura, hypogammaglobulinemia.

treatment. However, the presence of the Philadelphia chromosome is not specific to diagnose CML. It is also found in ALL and occasionally in AML.

Chronic Lymphocytic Leukemia

CLL presents in older persons. With CLL there are production and accumulation of functionally inactive but long-lived small, mature-appearing lymphocytes. B cells are usually involved. The lymphocytes infiltrate the bone marrow, spleen, and liver. Lymph node enlargement (lymphadenopathy) is present throughout the body.

Complications are rare in early CLL but may develop as the disease advances. Pressure on nerves from enlarged lymph nodes causes pain and even paralysis. Mediastinal node enlargement leads to pulmonary symptoms. Because CLL is usually a disease of older adults, treatment decisions must consider disease progression and treatment side effects. Many patients in the early stages of CLL do not need treatment. Others are followed closely and receive treatment only when the disease progresses.

Other Leukemias

Occasionally we cannot determine the subtype of leukemia. The leukemic cells may have lymphoid, myeloid, or mixed characteristics. Often these patients do not respond to treatment and have a poor prognosis. Other rare types include hairy cell and biphenotypic (both abnormal myeloid and lymphoid clones) leukemias.

Clinical Manifestations

The manifestations of leukemia vary (Table 34.25). They relate to problems caused by bone marrow failure and, sometimes, leukemic infiltrates in tissues (Fig. 34.12). Bone marrow failure results from (1) bone marrow overcrowding by abnormal cells and (2) inadequate production of normal marrow elements. Patients are predisposed to anemia, thrombocytopenia, and decreased number and function of WBCs.

As leukemia progresses, the body makes fewer normal blood cells. The abnormal WBCs continue to accumulate because they do not go through the normal cell life cycle to death *(apoptosis)*. The leukemic cells may infiltrate the organs, leading to splenomegaly, hepatomegaly, lymphadenopathy, bone pain, meningeal irritation, and oral lesions. Solid masses from collections of leukemic cells, called *chloromas*, can occur. A high leukemic white count in the peripheral blood (more than 100,000 cells/μL) can cause the blood to thicken and potentially block circulatory pathways. This is called *leukostasis*. It can be life threatening.

Diagnostic Studies

Peripheral blood evaluation and bone marrow examination are the primary methods used to diagnose and classify the type of

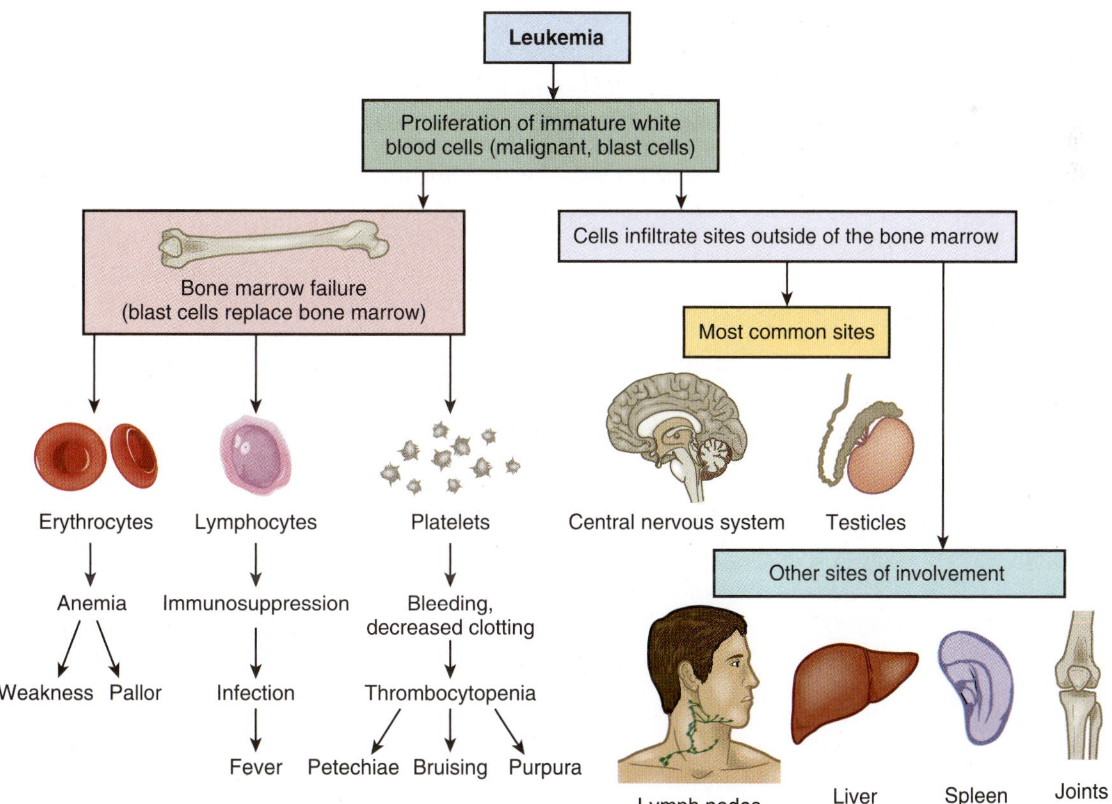

Fig. 34.12 Pathophysiology of leukemia. (Modified from McKinney ES, James SR, Murray SS, et al: *Maternal-child nursing*, Philadelphia, 2000, Saunders.)

leukemia. We use various morphologic, histochemical, immunologic, and cytogenetic methods to identify leukemic cell types, stage of development, and genetic mutations. Knowing the type of leukemia is important because each type has a different prognosis and treatment options. For example, in CML, the finding of the Philadelphia chromosome is an important diagnostic indicator. It is sometimes present in ALL and affects treatment.[21] Other studies, such as lumbar puncture and PET/CT scans, can detect leukemic cells outside of the blood and bone marrow.

Interprofessional Care

For many patients, cure is a realistic goal. For others, the goal is to attain remission or disease control. In *complete remission,* there is no evidence of disease on physical assessment, the bone marrow and peripheral blood appear normal, and molecular analysis shows no residual problems. *Minimal residual disease* is when tumor cells cannot be detected by morphologic examination but can be identified by molecular testing. With *partial remission,* there is a lack of symptoms and a normal peripheral blood smear, but there is still evidence of disease in the bone marrow. *Molecular remission* means that all molecular studies are negative for residual leukemia.

The prognosis is related to the ability to maintain remission. The prognosis becomes more unfavorable with each relapse. After each relapse, the succeeding remission may be harder to achieve and shorter in duration.

Treatment decisions are tailored to the patient's age and fitness, presence of other conditions, and genetic analysis. Because chemotherapy is the mainstay of the treatment, you need to understand the principles of cancer chemotherapy (see Chapter 16). Radiation and biologic therapies may be used. Sometimes patients have such a high WBC count (e.g., 100,000 cells/μL or more) that initial emergent treatment may include leukapheresis and hydroxyurea. The purpose of these treatments is to reduce the WBC count and risk for leukemia cell–induced thrombosis. In some cases, such as asymptomatic patients with CLL, watchful waiting with active supportive care may be appropriate.

Chemotherapy Stages

We often think about chemotherapy as 3 stages: induction, postinduction or postremission (consolidation), and maintenance.

Induction therapy. The first stage, *induction therapy,* is the attempt to bring about a remission. Induction is aggressive treatment that seeks to destroy leukemic cells in the tissues, peripheral blood, and bone marrow to eventually restore normal hematopoiesis on bone marrow recovery. During induction therapy, patients may become critically ill because the bone marrow is severely depressed by chemotherapy. Nursing interventions focus on neutropenia, thrombocytopenia, and anemia. Common chemotherapy drugs for AML induction therapy include cytarabine and an antitumor antibiotic (anthracycline), such as daunorubicin or idarubicin.[22] Oral therapies that can target specific genetic mutations may be prescribed. After 1 course of induction therapy, 50% to 70% of newly diagnosed patients achieve complete remission.[2] We assume that leukemic cells persist undetected after induction therapy. This could lead to relapse within a few months without more therapy.

Postinduction or postremission therapy. Terms used to describe postinduction or postremission chemotherapy include *intensification* and *consolidation. Intensification therapy,* or high-dose therapy, may start immediately after induction therapy and last for several months. Other drugs that target the cell differently from those given during induction may be added.

Consolidation therapy is started after a remission is achieved. It may consist of 1 or 2 more courses of the same drugs given during induction or involve high-dose therapy (intensive consolidation). The purpose of consolidation therapy is to eliminate remaining leukemic cells that may not be evident.

Maintenance therapy. The goal of maintenance therapy is to keep the body free of leukemic cells. It may be used for acute leukemia, depending on the presence of specific cytogenetic markers and therapies that can target them.

Drug Therapy Regimens

Combination drug therapy is the mainstay of treatment for leukemia. The purposes for using multiple drugs are to (1) decrease drug resistance, (2) minimize the drug toxicity by using multiple drugs with varying toxicities, and (3) interrupt cell growth at multiple points in the cell cycle. The drugs used vary. Table 34.26 gives examples of treatment regimens used in various types of leukemia.

Some drugs target small molecules that promote the growth and differentiation of leukemic cells. For example, midostaurin, a multikinase inhibitor, inhibits a growth pathway in patients with AML with the *FLT3* mutation.[2] Imatinib (Gleevec) and other tyrosine kinase inhibitors target the BCR-ABL protein that is present in nearly all patients with CML and some patients with ALL.[20] This drug kills only cancer cells, leaving healthy cells alone.

Monoclonal antibodies are an important treatment for hematopoietic cancers. However, cures with these therapies alone are rare. Rituximab binds to the B-cell antigen (CD20) and is a treatment for ALL and CLL. Alemtuzumab (Campath), a treatment for CLL, binds to CD52, an antigen present on T and B cells.[22]

Other Treatments

Radiation therapy and corticosteroids may have a role in treating leukemia. Total body radiation can prepare patients for bone marrow transplantation. Radiation may be restricted to certain areas, such as the liver and spleen, or other organs affected by infiltrates. In ALL, prophylactic intrathecal methotrexate or cytarabine is given to decrease the CNS involvement, which is common. When CNS leukemia does occur, cranial radiation is an option. Immunotherapy and targeted therapy,

TABLE 34.26 **Drug Therapy**

Leukemia

Drug Therapy	Other Therapy
Acute Myeloid Leukemia (AML)	
arsenic trioxide, azacitidine, cytarabine, daunorubicin, decitabine, enasidenib, etoposide, fludarabine, gemtuzumab ozogamicin, gilteritinib, glasdegib, idarubicin, ivosidenib, midostaurin, mitoxantrone, quizartinib, sorafenib, tretinoin, venetoclax	Allogeneic hematopoietic stem cell transplant (HSCT) (see Chapter 16)
Combination chemotherapy of cytarabine and antitumor antibiotic (most common initial therapy for younger fit patients)	
Acute Lymphocytic Leukemia (ALL)	
asparaginase, blinatumomab, bosutinib, clofarabine, cyclophosphamide, cytarabine, dasatinib, daunorubicin, dexamethasone, doxorubicin, etoposide, fludarabine, imatinib, inotuzumab ozogamicin, 6-mercaptopurine, methotrexate, nelarabine, nilotinib, pegaspargase, ponatinib, prednisone, rituximab, vincristine	Cranial radiation therapy, intrathecal methotrexate or cytarabine, allogeneic HSCT, tisagenlecleucel (CAR-T cell therapy) (see Chapter 16)
Combination chemotherapy of several agents is common over a prolonged time	
Chronic Myelogenous Leukemia	
bosutinib, dasatinib, imatinib, nilotinib, omacetaxine, ponatinib	HSCT, α-interferon, leukapheresis
Combination chemotherapy for progression to acute phase as per either AML or ALL therapy	
Chronic Lymphocytic Leukemia	
Acalabrutinib, alemtuzumab, chlorambucil, bendamustine, cyclophosphamide, duvelisib, fludarabine, ibrutinib, idelalisib, lenalidomide, obinutuzumab, ofatumumab, pirtobrutinib, prednisone, rituximab, venetoclax, zanubrutinib	Radiation, splenectomy, colony-stimulating factors, allogeneic HSCT

such as monoclonal antibodies and chimeric antigen receptor (CAR) T cells, may be indicated for specific leukemias. These therapies are discussed in Chapter 16.

Hematopoietic Stem Cell Transplantation

HSCT is another option for treating leukemia. The goal of HSCT is to eliminate all leukemic cells from the body using combinations of chemotherapy with or without total body irradiation. This treatment eradicates the patient's hematopoietic stem cells, which are then replaced with those of a human leukocyte antigen (HLA)–matched sibling, HLA-half-matched relative, volunteer donor *(allogeneic)*, or identical twin *(syngeneic)*. HSCT is discussed in Chapter 16. Serious complications after allogeneic HSCT are graft-versus-host disease (GVHD), relapse of leukemia, and infection. Because HSCT has serious risks, patients must weigh the risks for treatment-related death or treatment failure (relapse) with the hope of cure.

NURSING MANAGEMENT: LEUKEMIA

Assessment

Subjective and objective data that you should obtain from patients with leukemia are outlined in Table 34.27.

Planning

The overall goals are that patients with leukemia will (1) understand and adhere to the treatment plan; (2) have minimal side effects and complications associated with the disease and its treatment; and (3) establish realistic hope and goals, feeling supported during periods of treatment, relapse, or remission.

Implementation

Acute Care

The nursing role during acute phases of leukemia is challenging. Patients with leukemia have many physical and psychosocial needs. The diagnosis of leukemia can evoke great fear and be equated with death. It may be viewed as a hopeless, horrible disease with many painful and undesirable consequences. The treatment and prognosis are driven by many factors, such as age, type of leukemia, coexisting conditions, and the presence of certain genetic mutations. You must understand the type of leukemia, prognosis, treatment plan, and goals. By doing this, you can help patients to realize that although the future may be uncertain, they can have a meaningful quality of life while in remission or with disease control and that, in some cases, there is reasonable hope for cure.

You are an advocate in helping the patient and family understand the complexities of treatment decisions and manage the side effects and toxicities. The diagnosis often brings with it the need to make difficult decisions at a time of profound stress. The patient and family may need help adjusting to the stress of the onset of serious illness and losses imposed by the sick role (e.g., dependence, changes in role responsibilities).

Encourage patients to discuss quality-of-life issues. Patients may need a long hospitalization or to temporarily relocate to an appropriate treatment center. This can lead a patient to feeling deserted and isolated at a time when support is most needed. You can help reverse feelings of abandonment and loneliness by

TABLE 34.27 NURSING ASSESSMENT

Leukemia

Subjective Data

Important Health Information

Health history: Exposure to chemical toxins (e.g., benzene, arsenic), radiation, or viruses (HTLV-1); chromosome abnormalities (Down syndrome, Klinefelter syndrome, Fanconi syndrome), immunologic deficiencies; organ transplantation; frequent infections; bleeding tendencies

Medications: Chemotherapy

Surgery or other treatments: Radiation exposure; prior radiation and chemotherapy for cancer

Functional Health Patterns

Health perception–health management: Family history of leukemia; malaise

Nutritional-metabolic: Mouth sores, weight loss; chills, night sweats; nausea, vomiting, anorexia, dysphagia, early satiety; easy bruising

Elimination: Hematuria, ↓ urine output; diarrhea, dark or bloody stools

Activity-exercise: Fatigue with progressive weakness; dyspnea, nosebleeds, cough

Cognitive-perceptual: Headache; muscle cramps; sore throat; sternal tenderness, bone, joint, abdominal pain; paresthesias, numbness, tingling, visual changes

Sexuality-reproductive: Prolonged menses, menorrhagia, metrorrhagia, impotence

Objective Data

General

Fever, lymphadenopathy, lethargy

Cardiovascular

↑ HR, systolic murmurs

GI

Gingival bleeding and hyperplasia; oral ulcerations, herpes and *Candida* infections; perirectal irritation and infection; hepatomegaly, splenomegaly

Musculoskeletal

Muscle wasting, bone pain, joint pain

Neurologic

Seizures, disorientation, confusion, impaired coordination, cranial nerve palsies, papilledema

Skin

Pallor or jaundice; petechiae, bruising, purpura, reddish brown to purple cutaneous infiltrates, macules, and papules

Possible Diagnostic Findings

↓, normal, or ↑ WBC count with shift to the left (↑ blast cells) and neutropenia; anemia, ↓ hematocrit and hemoglobin, thrombocytopenia, specific chromosome abnormalities; hypercellular bone marrow aspirate or biopsy with myeloblasts, lymphoblasts, and markedly ↓ normal cells

balancing the demanding technical needs with a humanistic, caring approach. The patient's needs are best met by care from an interprofessional team (e.g., psychiatric and oncology clinical nurse specialists, case managers, dietitians, chaplains, social workers).

Quality nursing care significantly affects survival and comfort during aggressive chemotherapy. You need to make astute assessments and plan care to help patients manage the severe side effects. Life-threatening results of bone marrow suppression (neutropenia, thrombocytopenia, and anemia) require prompt nursing interventions. Other critical aspects of care include anticipating, monitoring for, and helping to treat emergencies, such as DIC, tumor lysis syndrome, and leukostasis. Complications of chemotherapy may affect the GI tract, nutrition status, skin and mucosa, cardiopulmonary status, liver, kidneys, and neurologic system. Nursing interventions related to chemotherapy are discussed in Chapter 16.

Implement measures to maximize safety and physical function. Review all drugs being given. Assess laboratory data reflecting drug effects and sequelae of the disease. Unlike treatments for solid tumors, patients with leukemia often receive chemotherapy even if they have severe myelosuppression because the underlying disorder is causing the problem and will not resolve unless treated.

Ongoing care is needed to monitor for signs and symptoms of disease control or relapse. For patients receiving long-term or maintenance chemotherapy, the fatigue of long-term chronic disease management can become discouraging. Teach the patient and caregiver the importance of continued diligence in disease management and the need for follow-up care. Review drug information, self-care measures, and when to seek medical care.

Chronic Care

The goals of rehabilitation for long-term survivors of leukemia are to manage the physical, psychologic, social, and spiritual consequences and delayed effects from the disease and its treatment. Involving patients in survivor networks and support groups or services may help them adapt to living after a life-threatening illness. Exploring national and community resources (e.g., American Cancer Society, Leukemia & Lymphoma Society) may reduce the financial burden and the feelings of dependence. Provide resources for spiritual support.

Vigilant follow-up care helps to ensure that we recognize and treat the survivor's unique needs. Patients often need a referral or consultation. For example, physical therapy personnel may develop an exercise program to address post-treatment deficits from drug-induced peripheral neuropathy. Patients should follow the advice of their HCP about receiving vaccines.

◆ Evaluation

The expected outcomes are that patients with leukemia will:

- Cope effectively with the diagnosis, treatment regimen, and prognosis
- Have no life-threatening complications related to the disease or treatment
- Feel supported throughout treatment

LYMPHOMAS

Lymphomas are cancers originating in the bone marrow and lymphatic structures resulting in the proliferation of lymphocytes. Lymphomas make up 4% to 5% of all cancers in the United States.[19] Two major types of lymphoma are Hodgkin lymphoma and non-Hodgkin lymphoma (NHL). A comparison of these 2 types of lymphoma is shown in Table 34.28.

HODGKIN LYMPHOMA

Hodgkin lymphoma, or *Hodgkin disease,* makes up about 10% of all lymphomas. There is a proliferation of abnormal giant, multinucleated cells, called *Reed-Sternberg cells,* or its variant, *Hodgkin cells* (mononucleated), which proliferate in the lymph nodes. The disease has a bimodal age-specific incidence, occurring most often in persons from 15 to 30 years of age and older than 55 years of age.[23] Each year, about 8570 new cases of Hodgkin lymphoma are diagnosed.[19] Up to 96% of patients may be cured depending on stage and risk factors.

Etiology and Pathophysiology

Although the cause of Hodgkin lymphoma is unknown, several key factors play a role in its development. The main interacting factors include infection with Epstein-Barr virus (EBV), genetic predisposition, and exposure to occupational toxins. The incidence is increased in those with HIV infection.

The disease likely starts in a single location and then spreads along adjacent lymphatics. However, in recurrent disease, it may spread more diffusely. It eventually infiltrates other organs, especially lungs, spleen, and liver. When the disease begins above the diaphragm, it stays confined to lymph nodes for a variable time. Disease originating below the diaphragm often spreads to extra lymphoid sites, such as the liver. There are 5 histologic subtypes. Nodular sclerosis classic Hodgkin lymphoma is the most common.

TABLE 34.28 Comparison of Hodgkin and Non-Hodgkin Lymphoma

	Hodgkin Lymphoma	Non-Hodgkin Lymphoma
Cell origin	B lymphocytes	B lymphocytes (85%) T or natural killer lymphocytes (15%)
Extent of disease	Local to regional but may be more widespread. Spreads to adjacent tissues	Disseminated, can spread to other areas of the body
B symptoms (fever, drenching night sweats, weight loss)	Common	Uncommon
Extranodal involvement	Rare	Common

Clinical Manifestations

The onset of symptoms is usually gradual. The initial sign is often enlargement of cervical, axillary, or inguinal lymph nodes (Fig. 34.13). Subsequent lymph node involvement is generally by spread to adjacent lymph nodes. The nodes are movable and nontender. Enlarged nodes are not painful unless they exert pressure on adjacent nerves.

Patients may have weight loss, fatigue, weakness, fever, chills, tachycardia, or night sweats. A group of initial findings, including fever (>100.4°F [38°C]), drenching night sweats, and weight loss (exceeding 10% in 6 months), are termed *B symptoms.* They correlate with a worse prognosis. After having even small amounts of alcohol, patients with Hodgkin lymphoma may have a rapid onset of pain at the site of disease. The cause for the alcohol-induced pain is unknown. General itching without skin lesions may develop. Cough, dyspnea, stridor, and dysphagia may occur with mediastinal node involvement.

In more advanced disease, there may be hepatomegaly and splenomegaly. Anemia results from increased destruction and decreased production of RBCs. Other signs vary depending on the site of disease. For example, intrathoracic involvement may lead to superior vena cava syndrome. Enlarged retroperitoneal nodes may cause palpable abdominal masses or interfere with renal function. Jaundice may occur from liver involvement. Bone pain occurs from bone involvement.

Diagnostic and Staging Studies

Peripheral blood analysis, lymph node biopsy, bone marrow examination, and radiologic studies are important in evaluating Hodgkin lymphoma. Abnormalities in the CBC, such as microcytic hypochromic anemia, are variable and not diagnostic. Leukopenia and thrombocytopenia may develop, but they are usually a consequence of treatment, advanced disease, or hypersplenism. Other blood studies may show increased erythrocyte sedimentation rate and LDH, high leukocyte

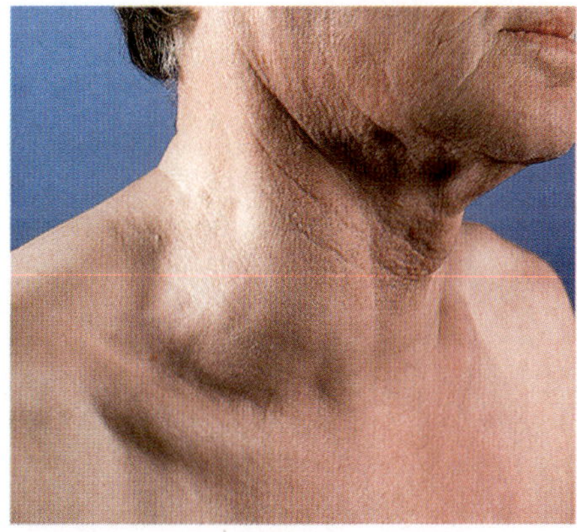

Fig. 34.13 Enlarged cervical lymph node in the neck of a male with Hodgkin lymphoma. (From Howard MR, Hamilton PJ: *Haematology: an illustrated colour atlas,* ed 4, London, 2013, Churchill Livingston.)

alkaline phosphatase from liver and bone involvement, hypercalcemia from bone involvement, and hypoalbuminemia from liver involvement.

Radiologic evaluation can define the sites and determine the clinical stage of the disease. Staging is based on the extent of the disease, presence of B symptoms, and prognostic features (Fig. 34.14). PET and CT scans are used to stage and then assess the response to therapy and to distinguish residual tumor from fibrotic masses after treatment. Scans can show masses, such as renal displacement caused by retroperitoneal node enlargement, abdominal or mediastinal lymph node enlargement, and liver, spleen, bone, and brain infiltration.

Interprofessional and Nursing Management

Treatment depends on the nature and extent of the disease. Combination chemotherapy works well because the drugs used have an additive antitumor effect without increasing side effects. As with leukemia, therapy must be aggressive. The standard for chemotherapy is the ABVD regimen: doxorubicin (**A**driamycin), **b**leomycin, **v**inblastine, and **d**acarbazine. Bleomycin may be substituted with brentuximab vedotin to reduce pulmonary toxicity. Patients with favorable early-stage disease receive 2 to 4 cycles of chemotherapy.[23] Patients with early-stage disease but unfavorable prognostic features (e.g., B symptoms) or intermediate-stage disease receive 4 to 6 cycles of chemotherapy. Advanced-stage Hodgkin lymphoma is treated more aggressively using 6 to 8 cycles of chemotherapy. A common regimen is BEACOPP (**b**leomycin, **e**toposide, doxorubicin [**A**driamycin], **c**yclophosphamide, vincristine [**O**ncovin], **p**rocarbazine, and **p**rednisone).[23] The role of involved-site radiation as a supplement to chemotherapy varies depending on the extent of disease and the presence of resistant disease after chemotherapy.

A variety of chemotherapy and immunotherapy regimens are options for patients who have relapsed or refractory disease. A common regimen is "ICE" (ifosfamide, carboplatin, etoposide).[2] Sometimes we give a single drug palliatively to someone who cannot tolerate intensive combination therapy. Ideally, once in remission, a curative option may be intensive chemotherapy with HSCT. HSCT has allowed patients to receive higher, potentially curative chemotherapy while reducing life-threatening leukopenia. Maintenance chemotherapy does not contribute to increased survival after achieving remission.

A serious consequence of treatment is the later development of secondary cancers and potential long-term treatment toxicities, such as endocrine, heart, and lung problems. Secondary solid tumor cancers may occur 10 years after ending treatment. The most common secondary cancers are lung and breast cancer, especially with radiation therapy. Patients should have close follow-up and screening for early detection of these problems.

Nursing care focuses on managing problems related to the disease (e.g., pain caused by a tumor, superior vena cava syndrome), pancytopenia, and other side effects of therapy. Because patient survival depends on their response to treatment, supporting the patient through the consequences of treatment is important.

Psychosocial considerations are important. Address the physical and spiritual consequences. Fertility issues may be of concern because this disease occurs in adolescents and young adults. Help ensure that these issues are addressed soon after diagnosis and before treatment is initiated.

NON-HODGKIN LYMPHOMA

Non-Hodgkin lymphomas (NHLs) are a broad group of cancers of primarily B, T, and natural killer (NK) cells. NHL is

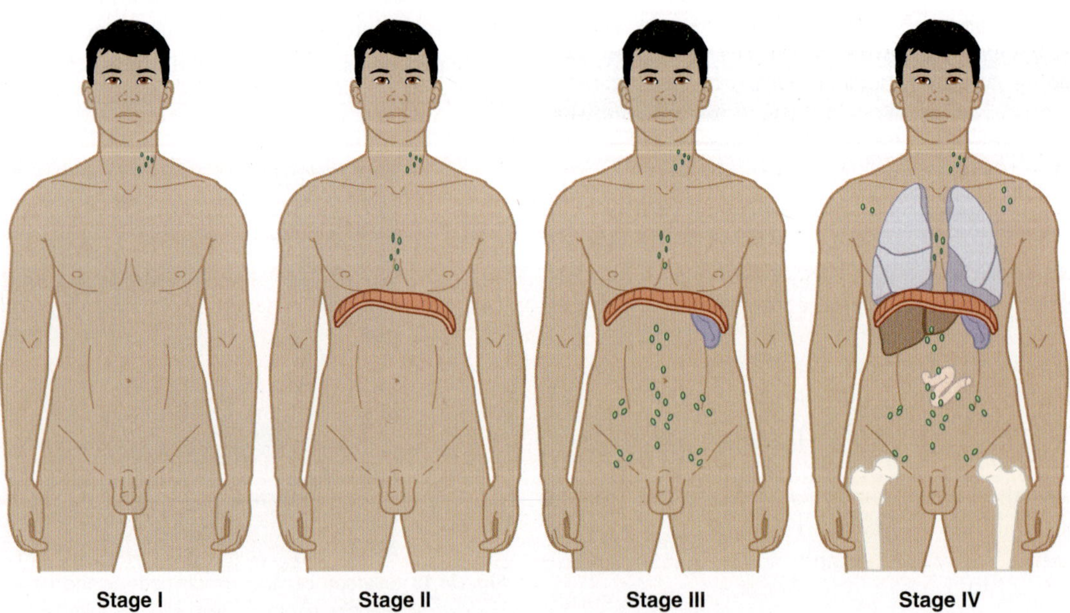

Fig. 34.14 Staging system for Hodgkin lymphoma and non-Hodgkin lymphoma.

TABLE 34.29 Common Classifications of Non-Hodgkin Lymphoma

B-Cell Lymphomas
- Burkitt lymphoma
- Diffuse large B-cell lymphoma (DLBCL)
- Follicular lymphoma
- Mantle cell lymphoma
- Marginal zone B-cell lymphoma (MALT)
- Plasmablastic lymphoma
- Small lymphocytic lymphoma/chronic lymphocytic leukemia

T-Cell and Natural Killer (NK)–Cell Lymphomas
- Anaplastic large T-cell lymphoma
- Extranodal NK/T cell lymphoma
- Mycosis fungoides and Sézary syndrome
- Peripheral T-cell lymphoma, not otherwise specified (NOS)

Posttransplant Lymphoproliferative Disorders (PTLD)
- Infectious mononucleosis–like PTLD

Histiocytic and Dendritic Cell Tumors
- Langerhans cell histiocytosis

the most common hematologic cancer. Each year about 80,620 new cases are diagnosed and 20,140 deaths occur.[19] There are more than 75 types. We classify NHL by the level of differentiation (maturity), cell of origin, immunophenotype (cell surface antigens, CD20, CD52), and genetic and clinical features. The most common subtypes are diffuse large B-cell lymphoma and follicular lymphoma. Burkitt lymphoma is the most aggressive form. A simplified example of the classification system is shown in Table 34.29.

Etiology and Pathophysiology

The cause of NHL is usually unknown. NHLs may result from chromosomal translocations, infections, environment factors, and immunodeficiency. Chromosomal translocations have a key role in the pathogenesis of many NHLs. Viruses and bacteria implicated in the pathogenesis of NHL include human T-cell leukemia virus, type 1 (HTLV-1), EBV, human herpesvirus 8, hepatitis C, and *H. pylori*.[2] Chemicals linked to NHL include pesticides, herbicides, solvents, and organic chemicals. NHL is more common in people who have inherited immunodeficiency syndromes, have used immunosuppressive agents (e.g., to prevent rejection after an organ transplant or to treat autoimmune problems), or received chemotherapy or radiation therapy.

All NHLs involve lymphocytes arrested in various stages of development and may mimic leukemia. For example, small lymphocytic lymphoma (SLL) and CLL result from malignant proliferation of small B lymphocytes, with most CLL disease occurring within the bone marrow versus the lymph nodes. Some NHLs begin outside the lymph nodes. Diffuse large B-cell lymphoma is usually found in lymph nodes in the neck or abdomen.

Clinical Manifestations

A variety of presentations and courses occur, from indolent (slowly developing) to rapidly progressive disease. The method of spread can be unpredictable. Most patients have widespread disease at the time of diagnosis. The primary manifestation is painless lymph node enlargement.[2] The lymphadenopathy can wax and wane in indolent disease. Some patients with NHL present with skin manifestations. Patients with high-grade lymphomas may have lymphadenopathy and B symptoms, such as fever, night sweats, and weight loss. Because the disease has usually spread, other symptoms depend on where the disease is present (e.g., hepatomegaly with liver involvement, neurologic symptoms with CNS disease). There may be airway obstruction, hyperuricemia and renal failure from tumor lysis syndrome, pericardial tamponade, or GI symptoms.

Diagnostic and Staging Studies

Diagnostic studies used for NHL resemble those used for Hodgkin lymphoma. However, because NHL is more often in extranodal sites, more diagnostic studies may be done. These include an MRI or lumbar puncture to rule out CNS disease, a bone marrow biopsy to determine bone marrow infiltration, or a barium enema or upper endoscopy to look for GI involvement. In early NHL, the CBC may be normal, but some lymphomas manifest in a "leukemic" phase.

Clinical staging, as described for Hodgkin lymphoma, helps to guide therapy (Fig. 34.14). Establishing the precise histologic subtype through biopsy is important. The prognosis is based on histopathology. Treatment is guided by the cell type, cytogenetic studies, and clinical behavior: *indolent* (low grade), *aggressive* (high grade), or *highly aggressive* (very high grade). Other factors, known as the *International Prognostic Index (IPI)*, may be considered for each subtype. These include the clinical stage, number of extranodal sites, serum LDH, and patient's age and performance status. Immunologic, cytogenetic, and molecular studies are used for making treatment decisions and assessing prognosis. Other studies might include blood tests for tumor lysis; screening for hepatitis, HIV, and other infections; skin biopsies; bone marrow biopsies; and lumbar punctures.

Interprofessional and Nursing Management

Treatment involves chemotherapy, biotherapy, radiation, and sometimes phototherapy and topical therapy (Table 34.30). More aggressive lymphomas (diffuse large B cell) are generally more responsive to treatment. In contrast, indolent lymphomas have a naturally long course but are hard to effectively treat.

Patients with low-grade (indolent) lymphoma may live 10 years or more without treatment. However, some early therapies can be well tolerated and may reduce the time to progression of the disease. Those that have an infectious basis, such as *H. pylori* gastric lymphomas, may be treated with antibiotic or antiviral therapy. HSCT may help in certain subtypes of aggressive or refractory lymphomas. CAR T-cell immunotherapy may be used.

TABLE 34.30 Treatment of Non-Hodgkin Lymphoma[a]

Recommended Therapies	Common Chemotherapy Combinations
Indolent (Low-Grade) Follicular Lymphoma, Marginal Zone B-Cell Lymphoma, Mucosa-Associated Lymphoid Tissue (MALT)	
• External beam irradiation for local, limited disease • Single-agent rituximab, obinutuzumab • Rituximab or obinutuzumab with another agent (bendamustine, chlorambucil, cyclophosphamide, lenalidomide) • Combination chemotherapy (R-CHOP or other) • Targeted therapies (ibrutinib, tazemetostat, zanubrutinib) • Radioimmunotherapy • Hematopoietic stem cell transplant (HSCT) • Anti-CD19 CAR T-cell therapy • Bispecific monoclonal antibody therapy (mosunetuzumab)	**R-CHOP:** **r**ituximab, **c**yclophosphamide, **d**oxorubicin hydrochloride, **v**incristine (**O**ncovin), **p**rednisone **R-CVP:** **r**ituximab, **c**yclophosphamide, **v**incristine, **p**rednisone
Aggressive (Intermediate- or High-Grade) Mantle Cell, Diffuse Large B-Cell, T-Cell, Natural Killer–Cell Lymphomas	
• Combination chemotherapy with local radiation if needed • Aggressive combination chemotherapy for 3–8 cycles with local radiation if needed • Intrathecal chemotherapy if needed • Single agent or other combination treatment, depending on subtype and response (e.g., acalabrutinib, alemtuzumab, belinostat, bendamustine, bortezomib, brentuximab vedotin, etoposide, gemcitabine, ibrutinib, ifosfamide, lenalidomide, methotrexate, nivolumab, oxaliplatin, pegaspargase, pembrolizumab, polatuzumab vedotin, romidepsin, venetoclax, vinorelbine, zanubrutinib) • HSCT (autologous or allogeneic) • Anti-CD19 CAR T-cell therapy	**CHOP** ± rituximab (see earlier) **ICE** ± rituximab: **i**fosfamide, **c**yclophosphamide, **e**toposide **R-EPOCH:** **r**ituximab, **e**toposide, **p**rednisone, vincristine (**O**ncovin), **c**yclophosphamide, doxorubicin **h**ydrochloride **ESHAP ± R:** **e**toposide, methylprednisolone (**S**olu-Medrol), **h**igh-dose cytarabine (**A**ra-C), cisplatin (**P**latinol), with or without **r**ituximab **Hyper-CVAD ± R:** hyperfractionated **c**yclophosphamide, **v**incristine, doxorubicin (**A**driamycin), **d**examethasone alternating with high-dose methotrexate and cytarabine with or without rituximab **DHAP ± R:** **d**examethasone, **h**igh-dose cytarabine (**A**ra-C), cisplatin (**P**latinol), with or without **r**ituximab
Highly Aggressive (e.g., Burkitt Lymphoma)	
• Aggressive combination chemotherapy for 3–8 cycles • HSCT	**R-EPOCH:** **r**ituximab, **e**toposide, **p**rednisone, vincristine (**O**ncovin), **c**yclophosphamide, doxorubicin **h**ydrochloride **Hyper-CVAD ± R** (see earlier) **CODOX-M:** **c**yclophosphamide, vincristine (**O**ncovin), **doxo**rubicin, high-dose **m**ethotrexate, with or without rituximab (includes intrathecal methotrexate) **ICE** ± rituximab (see earlier)

[a]The acronym for some drug regimens uses the trade name of chemotherapy drugs. In some cases, the trade name drug has been discontinued, and the drug currently used is the generic version.

Rituximab, a monoclonal antibody against the CD20 antigen on the surface of normal and cancer B cells, treats NHL in combination with other agents. Once bound to the cells, rituximab causes lysis and cell death. Numerous chemotherapy combinations are used to try to overcome the resistant nature of this disease. Targeted therapies are becoming more prevalent (Table 34.30).

DRUG ALERT

Rituximab (Rituxan)

- Monitor for signs of severe hypersensitivity infusion reactions, especially with the first infusion.
- Manifestations may include hypotension, bronchospasm, dysrhythmias, angioedema, and cardiogenic shock.
- Screen for history of hepatitis because the drug may reactivate hepatitis.

In general, T-cell lymphomas are harder to cure. We treat them aggressively up-front, often followed by HSCT. Treatment of cutaneous T-cell lymphomas includes topical corticosteroids or topical chemotherapy for limited-stage disease. For more diffuse disease, treatment may include more aggressive combination therapies.

The nursing care for NHL is similar to that for Hodgkin lymphoma. It is based on managing problems related to the disease (e.g., pain caused by the tumor, obstruction, spinal cord compression, tumor lysis syndrome), pancytopenia, and other side effects of therapy. However, because NHL can be more extensive and involve specific organs (e.g., CNS, spleen, liver, GI tract, bone marrow), it is important to understand the subtype and extent of the disease. For example, a patient with colon involvement may have acute abdominal pain, guarding, and an enlarged abdomen. A patient with a Burkitt NHL beginning chemotherapy is at high risk for tumor lysis syndrome and needs frequent laboratory monitoring. See Chapter 16 for more on cancer therapies and their effects.

Patients undergoing external beam radiation therapy have special nursing needs. The skin in the radiation field needs special care. Include concepts related to safety issues with radiation therapy in the plan of care (see Chapter 16).

Psychosocial considerations are important. Help the patient and family to understand the disease, treatment, and expected and potential side effects. Some aggressive treatments need close follow-up and even inpatient admission. Fertility issues may be of concern in young patients. Evaluate patients with NHL for long-term effects of therapy because the delayed consequences of disease and treatment may not be apparent for many years.

MULTIPLE MYELOMA

Multiple myeloma, or *plasma cell myeloma,* is a condition in which cancerous plasma cells proliferate in the bone marrow and destroy bone. Multiple myeloma accounts for about 1.8% of all cancers and 19% of hematologic cancers.[19] The disease is more common in males and in African Americans. The median age at diagnosis is 69 years. Outcomes vary. Twenty percent of patients survive less than 2 years, and 40% survive more than 10 years.[2]

Etiology and Pathophysiology

The cause is unknown. It is possible that exposure to organic chemicals (e.g., benzene), herbicides, and insecticides plays a role. Viral infections, such as HIV, may increase the risk.

The disease process involves excess production of plasma cells. Normal plasma cells are activated B cells, which make immunoglobulins (antibodies) that protect the body. In multiple myeloma, instead of a variety of plasma cells making antibodies to fight different infections, myeloma tumors make monoclonal antibodies. *Monoclonal* means they are all of 1 type, making them ineffective and even harmful. Not only do they not fight infections, but they infiltrate the bone marrow. These monoclonal proteins (called *M proteins*) are made up of 2 light chains and 2 heavy chains. *Bence Jones proteins* are the light chain part of these monoclonal antibodies. They may show up in the urine of patients with multiple myeloma.

Cancerous plasma cells build up in the bone marrow. They produce nuclear factor-κβ (NF-κβ) ligand (RANKL), which binds to RANK receptors on the osteoclast surface, causing activation and osteolytic lesions. As myeloma protein increases, normal plasma cells are reduced. This further compromises normal immune responses. Proliferation of cancerous plasma cells and the overproduction of immunoglobulin and proteins may result in the end organ effects of myeloma on the bone marrow, bone, and kidneys and possibly the spleen, lymph nodes, liver, and heart.

Clinical Manifestations

Multiple myeloma develops slowly and insidiously. Patients often do not have symptoms until the disease is advanced. Skeletal pain is the major symptom. Pain in the pelvis, spine, and ribs is common and triggered by movement. Diffuse osteoporosis develops as the myeloma protein destroys bone. Osteolytic lesions occur in the skull, vertebrae, long bones, and ribs. Vertebral destruction can lead to vertebral collapse with spinal cord compression. Loss of bone integrity can lead to pathologic fractures.

Bony degeneration causes calcium loss from bones, eventually causing hypercalcemia. Hypercalcemia may cause renal, GI, or neurologic problems, such as polyuria, anorexia, confusion, and heart problems. *Hyperviscosity syndrome* leading to cerebral, lung, renal, and other organ dysfunction can occur. High protein levels caused by the myeloma protein can result in renal tubular obstruction, interstitial nephritis, and renal failure. Patients may have anemia, thrombocytopenia, neutropenia, and immune dysfunction from the replacement of normal bone marrow with plasma cells. Neurologic problems may be caused by regional myeloma cell growth compressing the spinal cord or cranial nerves or by perineuronal or perivascular deposition of the abnormal protein.

Diagnostic Studies

Evaluation involves laboratory, radiologic, and bone marrow examination. M protein is often found in the blood and urine. Possible findings include pancytopenia, hypercalcemia, Bence Jones protein in the urine, and a high serum creatinine. Bone marrow analysis shows significantly increased numbers of plasma cells in the bone marrow. Skeletal bone surveys, MRI, and/or PET and CT scans show distinct areas of destroyed bone; general thinning of the bones; or fractures, especially in the vertebrae, ribs, pelvis, and bones of the thigh and upper arms.

The simplest measure of staging and prognosis in multiple myeloma is based on blood levels of 2 markers: β_2-microglobulin and albumin. Higher levels of β_2-microglobulin and lower levels of albumin are associated with a poorer prognosis.[24] Cytogenetic studies of the bone marrow also play a role in prognosis. For example, deletion of chromosome 17p is a high-risk (poor prognostic) feature.

Interprofessional and Nursing Management

Interprofessional care involves managing the disease and its symptoms. Current treatment options include corticosteroids, chemotherapy, immunotherapy, targeted therapy, and HSCT.[24] Multiple myeloma is seldom cured. Treatment can relieve symptoms, produce remission, and prolong life. Controlling pain and preventing pathologic fractures are goals of management. Most patients need therapy off and on during the course of the disease.

Zoledronic acid and denosumab inhibit bone breakdown. They are given for skeletal pain and hypercalcemia. They inhibit bone resorption without inhibiting bone formation and mineralization. A major focus of nursing care relates to patient safety because of the bone involvement and sequelae from bone breakdown. Because of the potential for pathologic fractures, use caution when moving and ambulating the patient. A slight twist or strain in the wrong area (e.g., a weak area in the bones) may cause a fracture.

DRUG ALERT

Zoledronic Acid (Zometa)

- Make sure the patient is hydrated before giving the drug.
- Renal toxicity may occur if the IV infusion is given in less than 15 minutes.
- Patients should have a dental examination before the first dose and ongoing monitoring for osteonecrosis of the jaw.

Kyphoplasty may be used to control spine vertebral disease. It is a minimally invasive procedure in which cement is injected to stabilize vertebral compression.

Initial treatment includes a corticosteroid plus 2 chemotherapy agents, such as lenalidomide and bortezomib or carfilzomib.[24] The goal is to reduce the number of plasma cells. Initial treatment depends on whether the patient is a stem cell transplant candidate and predicted tolerance of therapy. High-dose chemotherapy followed by HSCT has evolved as the standard of care in eligible patients.

Immunotherapy and targeted therapy are options. Immunomodulator drugs (described in Chapter 16) include lenalidomide and pomalidomide. Proteosome inhibitors include bortezomib, carfilzomib, and ixazomib. Aggressive myeloma may be treated with chemotherapy, such as cyclophosphamide, etoposide, and others. Daratumumab and isatuximab are monoclonal antibodies against CD38, a protein found on the surface of myeloma cells. CAR T-cell therapy targeting the B-cell maturation antigen (BCMA) on the myeloma cell is an option for some patients after prior therapies. Monoclonal antibodies targeting cell surface antigens on myeloma cells link a patient's T cell to kill the myeloma. These therapies can cause cytokine release syndrome (mimicking sepsis) and neurologic toxicities. Thus we closely monitor patients.

Other drugs can treat some complications of multiple myeloma. For example, IV furosemide promotes renal excretion of calcium. Although tumor lysis is rare, once chemotherapy is started, allopurinol may be given to prevent any renal damage from uric acid accumulation from cell breakdown. The myeloma proteins increase the risk for renal problems and electrolyte and fluid imbalances.

Ambulation and adequate hydration are used to treat hypercalcemia, dehydration, and potential renal damage. Weight bearing helps the bones resorb some calcium. Maintaining adequate hydration helps minimize problems from hypercalcemia and prevent protein precipitates from causing renal tubular obstruction. IV fluids help maintain a urine output of 1.5 to 2 L/day if the patient does not already have renal problems.

In some patients, the levels of plasma proteins are so high that it causes a hyperviscosity of the blood leading to neurologic changes, renal insufficiency, and other problems related to lack of blood flow. In this instance plasmapheresis is used.

As in any pain management situation, assess the patient and implement measures to control pain (see Chapter 9). Nonopioids or an acetaminophen/opioid combination may be more effective than opioids alone in diminishing bone pain. Braces, especially for the spine, may help control pain. Peripheral neuropathy is common with several therapies for multiple myeloma. It contributes to discomfort, the inability to do basic activities of daily living, and the risk for injury from falling.

Patients are at risk for DVT related to chemotherapy and immobility. They should receive preventive measures unless their platelet count is low.

Assessment and prompt treatment of infection are important. Recurrent infections may be caused by decreased normal immunoglobulin production, the ineffectiveness of the overproduced and abnormal immunoglobulins, corticosteroids, and/or neutropenia from bone marrow infiltration or side effects of treatment.

Psychosocial needs require sensitive, skilled management. Help the patient and significant others adapt to changes fostered by chronic illness and adjust to the losses related to the disease process, while helping to maximize functioning and quality of life. The patient may have remissions and exacerbations. Patients may be on dialysis because of myeloma-induced renal failure. Acute care is needed at various times during the illness.

The final, acute phase is unresponsive to treatment and usually short in duration. Help the patient and family navigate needed resources, such as palliative or hospice care, social services, and spiritual care, as appropriate.

SPLEEN PROBLEMS

Many illnesses can affect the spleen. Most can cause some degree of *splenomegaly* (enlarged spleen) (Table 34.31). However,

TABLE 34.31 Common Causes of Splenomegaly

Congestion and Hematologic Disorders

- Acquired hemolytic anemia
- Cirrhosis of the liver
- Heart failure (portal hypertension)
- Portal or splenic vein thrombosis
- Sickle cell disease
- Thalassemia

Infections and Inflammation

- Autoimmune disorders: Rheumatoid arthritis, systemic lupus erythematosus
- Bacterial infections: brucellosis, endocarditis, salmonella, tuberculosis, spleen abscess
- Fungal infections: histoplasmosis, systemic candidiasis
- Parasitic infections: malaria
- Viral infections: cytomegalovirus, hepatitis, cytomegalovirus

Infiltrative Diseases and Tumors or Cysts

- Acute and chronic leukemia
- Amyloidosis
- Gaucher disease
- Lymphomas
- Polycythemia vera
- Other primary or secondary tumors and cysts
- Sarcoidosis

an enlarged spleen may be present in some people without any evidence of disease. The term *hypersplenism* refers to the presence of splenomegaly and peripheral cytopenias (anemia, leukopenia, thrombocytopenia) with normal bone marrow. The degree of spleen enlargement varies. For example, massive spleen enlargement may occur with viral infections, CML, and thalassemia major. Mild spleen enlargement occurs with HF and SLE.

The normal spleen holds 350 mL of blood. It stores about one-third of our platelet mass. When the spleen enlarges, its normal filtering and storage capacity increases. Consequently, there is often a reduction in the number of circulating blood cells as they engorge the spleen. In addition, there are unusual findings in the peripheral smear. These include abnormally shaped RBCs, Howell-Jolly bodies (a dark purple granule in the RBC), and siderotic granules (Pappenheimer bodies) clustering near the edge of the RBC.[25] These findings aid in diagnosing a malfunctioning spleen. A slight to moderate enlargement of the spleen is usually asymptomatic and found during routine abdominal assessment. Although massive splenomegaly can be well tolerated, patients may have abdominal discomfort and early satiety. Other ways we assess the size of the spleen include ultrasound, CT or PET scan, MRI, and liver/spleen nuclear scan.

Treating the underlying condition may be warranted. Sometimes a splenectomy is part of the evaluation or treatment of splenomegaly. A major reason for splenectomy is spleen rupture. The spleen may rupture from trauma; inadvertent tearing during another surgery; and diseases such as mononucleosis, malaria, and lymphoid tumors. After a splenectomy, there can be a dramatic increase in peripheral RBC, WBC, and platelet counts.

Nursing care for patients with spleen disorders depends on the problem. Splenomegaly may be painful. Patients may need analgesics and care in moving, turning, and positioning. Promote lung expansion because spleen enlargement may impair diaphragmatic expansion. If anemia, thrombocytopenia, or leukopenia develops from spleen enlargement, institute measures to support the patient and prevent life-threatening complications.

After a splenectomy, observe the patient for bleeding and shock. Immune deficiencies may develop, such as low IgG levels. Patients have a lifelong risk for infection, especially from encapsulated organisms, such as *Pneumococcus* species. Pneumococcal vaccination reduces this risk.

BLOOD COMPONENT THERAPY

Blood component therapy is often used to manage hematologic diseases. Many therapeutic and surgical procedures depend on blood product support. Blood component therapy only temporarily supports the patient until the underlying problem is resolved. Because transfusions are not free from hazards, they should be used only if needed. The HCP should discuss the risks, benefits, and alternatives with the patient. This should be recorded in the medical record (Box 34.6).

BOX 34.6 ETHICAL/LEGAL DILEMMAS

Religious Beliefs

Situation

W.D., an 81-year-old female with dementia, comes to the hospital with lower gastrointestinal (GI) bleeding. During colonoscopy, the HCP cauterized the source of the bleed; however, her Hgb is 5.4 g/dL. Her family tells you that she is a Jehovah's Witness and must not receive blood products. If she does not have transfusions, her HCP is concerned she will have cardiopulmonary failure.

Ethical/Legal Points for Consideration

- Competent adults have the right to make health care decisions, including the right to refuse treatment, based on their religious beliefs.
- If the patient is determined to be incompetent and a guardian is appointed, the guardian has the legal right to make the consent or refusal.
- If the HCP believes that the treatment is essential to preserve life and health and there is no legal decision maker, a request is made for a legal determination of whether the patient is incapable of consent or refusal. If the judge agrees, the patient is made a ward of the court for this issue. Usually, the HCP is directed to make a decision based on the patient's best interests.

Discussion Questions

1. What resources do you have available to consult about religious practices?
2. How could you determine whether the family was acting in W.D.'s best interest or their own?
3. What nonblood alternatives are available for Jehovah's Witnesses?

Traditionally, the term *blood transfusion* meant the administration of whole blood. Blood transfusion now has a broader meaning because of the ability to give specific components of blood, such as platelets, packed RBCs, or plasma. Usually, a specific component is ordered. Whole blood may be used in cases of massive bleeding, severe coagulopathy, or shock or in trauma and military settings (Table 34.32). In severe hemorrhage situations, a "mass transfusion protocol" may be employed. This is the infusion of FFP, platelets, and RBCs done quickly in a 1:1:1 ratio with a warming infusion device.[7]

Administration Procedure

In general, we use 18- to 20-gauge IV catheters to give blood products to adults. Smaller gauges, such as 25 gauge, may be used in neonates. Larger sizes (e.g., 14 or 16 gauge) in adults may be preferred when giving rapid transfusions or if the infusion is sluggish. Smaller needles can be used for platelets, albumin, and clotting factor replacement. In emergencies when we cannot establish IV access, we may use the intraosseous route. Verify the patency of the access before requesting the blood product from the blood bank. Most blood product administration tubing is of a "Y type" with a macroaggregate filter (150 to 260 μm; filters out particulate). One arm of the Y is for the isotonic saline solution and the other arm of the Y for the blood product. You may use infusion pumps or syringes approved by your agency for blood administration.

TABLE 34.32 Common Blood Products

Description	Special Considerations	Indications for Use
Albumin		
Prepared from plasma. Available in 5% or 25% solution. Hyperosmolar solution acts by moving water from extravascular to intravascular space.	Albumin 25% expands the blood volume by ≈3.5 times. Can be stored several years, according to manufacturer. Dispensed in a bottle for infusion by pharmacy.	Hypovolemic shock, hypoalbuminemia, after large-volume paracentesis, replacement in plasmapheresis.
Cryoprecipitates and Commercial Concentrates		
Prepared from fresh frozen plasma. Has other clotting factors, especially factor VIII, factor XIII, fibronectin, von Willebrand factor.	Table 34.18. 10–15 mL/bag. Can be stored for 1 yr. Once thawed, must be used within 4–6 h.	Replacement for fibrinogen deficiency, usually because of DIC, severe liver disease, or massive transfusion.
Fresh Frozen Plasma		
Liquid part of whole blood is separated from cells and frozen. Rich in clotting factors but has no platelets.	1 unit is ≈300 mL. Can be stored for up to 1 yr, depending on storage. Must be used within 24 h after thawing.	Use in treating hemorrhagic shock. Bleeding caused by deficiency in clotting factors (e.g., DIC, bleeding, massive transfusion) and sometimes when PT or PTT are greater than 1.5 –1.7 times normal and the presence of bleeding.
Frozen RBCs		
Prepared from RBCs using glycerol for protection and frozen. Successive washings with saline solution remove most WBCs and plasma proteins.	Can be stored for up to 10 yr.	Autotransfusion. Stockpiling or rare donors for patients with alloantibodies.
Packed RBCs		
Prepared from whole blood by sedimentation or centrifugation. Leukocyte depletion (leukoreduction) by filtration, washing is frequently used. Decreases nonhemolytic febrile or mild allergic reactions in patients who receive frequent transfusions. Reduces transmission of viruses.	1 unit is 250–350 mL. Can be stored up to 42 days depending on processing (anticoagulants, preservatives). Use of RBCs for treatment allows remaining components of blood (e.g., platelets, albumin, plasma) to be used for other purposes. Irradiation prevents graft-versus-host disease in immunocompromised patients.	Severe or symptomatic anemia, acute blood loss. 1 unit of RBCs can be expected to ↑ Hgb by 1 g/dL or Hct by 3% in a typical adult. Preferred RBC source because they are more component specific. Less risk of fluid overload.
Platelets		
Prepared from fresh whole blood. For patients who receive frequent transfusions and become refractory, may give leukocyte reduced, HLA, or type specific to prevent alloimmunization to HLA antigens.	Can obtain multiple units from 1 donor by plateletpheresis. An apheresed single donation is usually 200–400 mL in volume. May be pooled from multiple donors. Can be kept at room temperature in the blood bank under gentle agitation for 1–5 days depending on type of collection and storage.	Bleeding caused by thrombocytopenia. May be contraindicated in TTP and HIT except in life-threatening hemorrhage. Average expected corrected count increment (1 h post infusion) is 30,000–60,000/μL. Failure to have an increase may be due to fever, sepsis, splenomegaly, or DIC or development of antibodies *(refractory).*

DIC, Disseminated intravascular coagulation; *HIT, heparin-induced thrombocytopenia; HLA,* human leukocyte antigen; *PT,* prothrombin time; *PTT,* partial thromboplastin time.

! SAFETY ALERT

Blood Transfusions

- Do not use any solution other than 0.9% sodium chloride for giving blood because they will cause RBC hemolysis.
- Exceptions to these restrictions may be appropriate, such as in trauma situations. These solutions include ABO-compatible plasma and 5% albumin. Follow agency policy.
- Do not give any additives, including medications, in the same tubing as the blood unless you first clear the tubing with saline solution.

After obtaining the blood product from the blood bank, make a positive identification of the blood product and recipient. Improper product-to-patient identification is the most common cause of hemolytic transfusion reactions. This places a great responsibility on nurses to conduct the identification procedure correctly. Follow agency procedure. Most have a dual-checking system with 2 licensed persons checking the patient identification with the labeled blood product and/or a bar-code scanning system. The blood bank does the typing and crossmatching of the donor's blood with the recipient's blood.

TABLE 34.33 **Blood Component Compatibilities for Transfusions**

	DONOR PRODUCT			
Recipient's Type	**Packed Red Blood Cells**	**Plasma**	**Platelets**	**Cryoprecipitate**
O+	O+, O−	All groups	O, B, A, AB	Any group is safe to transfuse
O−	O−			
A+	A+, A−, O+, O−	A, AB	A, AB, B, O	
A−	A−, O−			
B+	B+, B−, O+, O−	B, AB	B, AB, A, O	
B−	B−, O−			
AB+	All groups	Only AB	Any group	
AB−	AB− B−, A−, O−			

TABLE 34.34 **NURSING MANAGEMENT**

Blood Transfusions

- Complete a baseline physical assessment as a basis to assess changes during and after the transfusion.
- Ensure that the IV line is appropriate and patent.
- Double-check patient identification and blood product identification data with another licensed nurse (consider state Nurse Practice Act and agency policy).
- Adjust the transfusion rate according to the HCP orders and agency policy.
- Assess for signs of transfusion reactions.
- Delegate AP to take vital signs as directed.
- Evaluate for therapeutic effect of blood product (improvement in CBC, ↑ BP, ↓ bleeding).
- Monitor for circulatory overload (e.g., shortness of breath) if the transfusion is given rapidly.

Collaborate With Other Team Members

Blood Bank Personnel

- Perform type and crossmatch of the donor's blood with the recipient's blood.
- Note the result of the compatibility testing on the product bag or tag.
- When handing off blood products to nursing personnel, ensure that a positive identification is made with product and patient's information.
- Assist the HCP in evaluating transfusion reactions.

The result of any compatibility testing and the expiration date should be on the product bag or tag.

Table 34.33 outlines blood component compatibilities for transfusions. ABO compatibility is not a prerequisite for platelet transfusions. However, after multiple platelet transfusions, a patient may develop anti-HLA antibodies to the transfused platelets. With the use of lymphocyte typing to match HLA types of the donor and recipient, multiple platelet transfusions can be given with fewer complications to those who develop antibodies to platelets. The patient may be premedicated with an antihistamine and hydrocortisone to decrease the chance of reacting to platelet transfusions if there is a history of reactions.

Take vital signs before beginning the transfusion so that you have a baseline in case an acute reaction occurs (Table 34.34). If the patient has abnormal vital signs (e.g., high fever), call the HCP to clarify if you should give the blood product. Start the blood as soon as you have it. Do not refrigerate it on the nursing unit. You must start to transfuse the unit before the expiration date and time have passed.[7] During the first 15 minutes or 50 mL of blood infusion, stay with the patient. Reactions are most likely to occur during this time. The infusion rate during this period should be no more than 2 mL/min. Do not infuse packed RBCs quickly except in an emergency. Rapid infusion of cold blood may cause the patient to become chilled. If rapid replacement of large amounts of blood is needed, you might use a blood-warming device. Other blood components, such as FFP and platelets, may be given over 15 to 30 minutes. Refer to your agency's policy and the HCP's orders.

After the first 15 minutes, retake vital signs to assess patient tolerance. The rate of the rest of the infusion is determined by the HCP's orders, the patient's clinical condition, and the product being infused. Observe the patient periodically throughout the transfusion (e.g., every 30 minutes) and up to 1 hour after the transfusion. Most patients not at risk of fluid overload can tolerate the infusion of 1 unit of packed RBCs over 2 hours. The transfusion should not take more than 4 hours to give because of the increased risk for bacterial growth in the product once it is out of refrigeration.

Blood Transfusion Reactions

A *blood transfusion reaction* is an adverse reaction to blood transfusion therapy. It can range in severity from mild symptoms to a life-threatening condition. Because reactions can be significant, perform a careful assessment. Common signs and symptoms are associated with more than 1 type of adverse reaction. We describe blood transfusion reactions as acute or delayed (Tables 34.35 and 34.36). The attending HCP and blood bank HCPs are responsible for identifying the type of reaction. A transfusion reaction is a *serious reportable event* (SRE) and a *sentinel event* (see Chapter 1).

Acute Transfusion Reactions

The most common cause of hemolytic reactions is transfusion of ABO-incompatible blood (Table 34.35). This is an example of a type II cytotoxic hypersensitivity reaction (see Chapter 14). Severe hemolytic reactions are rare. Mislabeling specimens and giving blood to the wrong person cause most acute hemolytic reactions. This points to the importance of using proper patient identifiers when drawing blood samples and when giving medications and blood products.

TABLE 34.35 Acute Transfusion Reactions

Cause	Manifestations	Management	Prevention
Acute Hemolytic Reaction			
Infusion of ABO-incompatible whole blood, RBCs, or components containing as little as 10 mL of RBCs. Antibodies in the recipient's plasma attach to antigens on transfused RBCs, causing RBC destruction.	Reactions usually develop in first 15 min. May occur up to 24 h after. Fever with or without chills; back, abdominal, chest, or flank pain; infusion site pain, ↑ HR, dyspnea, tachypnea, ↓ BP, hemoglobinuria, acute jaundice, dark urine, bleeding, acute kidney injury, shock, cardiac arrest, DIC, death.	Monitor and maintain BP with IV fluids. Treat shock and DIC if present. Draw blood samples for serologic testing slowly to avoid hemolysis from the procedure. Send other specimens. Give prescribed diuretics to maintain urine flow. Insert indwelling urinary catheter or measure voided amounts to monitor hourly urine output. Dialysis may be needed if renal failure occurs. Do not transfuse more RBC-containing components until blood bank has provided newly crossmatched units.	Verify and document patient identification from sample collection to product infusion (e.g., visually compare label on sample collection and blood product with patient identification). Before transfusion, perform a 2-person verification of recipient and product identification and compatibility.
Allergic Reaction (Mild)			
Sensitivity to foreign plasma proteins. More common in people with history of allergies.	Flushing, itching, hives.	Give ordered antihistamine, corticosteroid, epinephrine. If symptoms are mild and transient, transfusion may be restarted slowly with HCP's order. Do not restart transfusion if fever or pulmonary symptoms develop.	Treat prophylactically with antihistamines or steroids. Consider washed RBCs and platelets.
Anaphylactic and Severe Allergic Reaction			
Sensitivity to donor plasma proteins. Infusion of IgA proteins to IgA-deficient recipient who has developed IgA antibody.	Anxiety, abdominal pain, hives, dyspnea, wheezing, progressing to angioedema, bronchospasm, ↓ BP, shock, and possible cardiac arrest.	Monitor VS frequently. Start CPR, if indicated. Administer O_2. Have epinephrine ready for injection. Give ordered antihistamines, corticosteroids, β_2-agonists. Do not restart transfusion.	Transfuse extensively washed RBC products from which all plasma has been removed. Use blood from IgA-deficient donor. Use autologous components.
Circulatory Overload			
Fluid given faster than the circulation can accommodate. People with heart or renal disease at risk.	Cough, dyspnea, pulmonary congestion, adventitious breath sounds, headache, hypertension, ↑ HR, distended neck veins.	Monitor VS. Place patient upright with feet in dependent position. Obtain chest x-ray. Give prescribed diuretics, O_2.	Adjust transfusion volume and flow rate based on patient size and clinical status. Have blood bank divide future units into smaller aliquots for better spacing of fluid infused.
Febrile, Nonhemolytic Reaction			
Patient antibodies react to donor antigens present on WBCs (most common), platelets, or plasma proteins; or donor plasma antibodies react against cellular antigens in recipient's blood.	Sudden chills, rigors, and fever (rise in temperature of >1°C), headache, vomiting.	Give antipyretics as prescribed (acetaminophen). Do not restart transfusion unless HCP orders.	Consider leukocyte-reduced blood products.

Continued

TABLE 34.35 Acute Transfusion Reactions—cont'd

Cause	Manifestations	Management	Prevention
Massive Blood Transfusion Reaction			
Can occur with replacement of 10 or more RBC units within 24 h. RBC transfusions do not contain clotting factors, albumin, and platelets.	Hypothermia and dysrhythmias (from rapid infusion of large quantities of cold blood). Citrate toxicity and hypocalcemia (from the citrate, a storage solution). Hypocalcemia (citrate binds calcium). Hyperkalemia or hypokalemia.	Monitor frequent vital signs. Draw labs to monitor clotting status and electrolyte levels. Monitor ECG for changes from electrolyte problems.	Use blood-warming equipment. Infuse ordered 10% calcium gluconate. Because of dilution effect on coagulation because of massive RBC transfusion, platelets and plasma will be given.
Sepsis			
Transfusion of bacterially infected blood components.	Rapid onset of chills, rigors, fever, vomiting, diarrhea, marked ↓ BP, shock.	Monitor VS. Obtain blood cultures. Other tests may be ordered to discern from a hemolytic reaction. Treat septicemia as directed with antibiotics, IV fluids, vasopressors.	Collect, process, store, and transfuse blood products according to blood banking standards and complete transfusion within 4 h of starting time.
Transfusion-Related Acute Lung Injury (TRALI) Reaction			
Reaction between transfused antileukocyte antibodies and recipient's leukocytes, causing pulmonary inflammation and capillary leak.	Fever, chills, hypotension, tachypnea, frothy sputum, dyspnea, hypoxemia, respiratory failure. Noncardiogenic pulmonary edema. A leading cause of transfusion-related deaths. Arises within 1—6 h of transfusion.	Monitor VS frequently. Provide O_2. Start CPR if needed, and provide ventilatory and BP support if needed. Draw blood for arterial blood gases and HLA or antileukocyte antibodies and other tests to discern from hemolysis or circulatory overload. Obtain chest x-ray.	Provide leukocyte-reduced products. Blood bank personnel will identify donors who are implicated in TRALI reactions and will not allow them to donate.

DIC, Disseminated intravascular coagulation; *HLA,* human leukocyte antigen; *VS,* vital signs.

TABLE 34.36 Delayed Transfusion Reactions

Manifestations	Prevention and Management
Delayed Hemolytic	
Fever, mild jaundice, ↓ hemoglobin. Occurs as early as 3 days or as late as several months posttransfusion as the result of destruction of transfused RBCs by alloantibodies not detected during crossmatch.	Monitor patients with supportive care. Hemolysis may be severe enough to warrant further transfusions with antigen-negative RBCs. Eculizumab may be beneficial.
Graft-Versus-Host Disease	
Rash, diarrhea, hepatitis, fever.	Irradiation of blood products to reduce the risk of donor lymphocytes attacking an immunocompromised patient.
Infection	
Specific product testing has greatly reduced the risk of infection. Potential risk of infection includes: *Babesia* species (babesiosis), Creutzfeldt-Jakob disease, cytomegalovirus (CMV), dengue fever virus, hepatitis B and C, herpesvirus type 6, HIV, herpesvirus 8, Epstein-Barr virus (EBV), HTLV-I/II, malaria, *Trypanosoma cruzi* (Chagas disease), West Nile virus, Zika virus.	Treatment based on cause. Ways of detecting some infectious agents before product release are now used, such as surface antigen testing and nucleic acid tests for *Babesia,* hepatitis, HIV, HTLV, *Treponema pallidum* and *T. cruzi,* West Nile virus, and Zika virus. Donor screening is only available method to reduce the risk for donor-contaminated blood for dengue fever virus, malaria, and Creutzfeldt-Jakob disease. Leukocyte-reduced components or processing may reduce virus transmission. Patients may be monitored serologically (e.g., CMV titers after allogeneic stem cell transplant).
Iron Overload	
Excess iron is deposited in heart, liver, pancreas, and endocrine organs, causing dysfunction. HF, dysrhythmias, impaired thyroid and gonadal function, diabetes, arthritis, cirrhosis. Occurs in patients receiving ≥20 units for chronic anemia (e.g., sickle cell anemia, β-thalassemia) over time. Ferritin level values should be no greater than 1000—1500 ng/mL.	May be prevented by iron chelators, which chelate and remove accumulated iron via the kidneys. Given IV, subcutaneously, or orally. Phlebotomy may be used.

! SAFETY ALERT

Transfusion Reaction

If a transfusion reaction occurs, take the following steps:

1. Stop the transfusion and stay with the patient.
2. Maintain a patent IV line with saline solution.
3. Notify the blood bank and the HCP.
4. Recheck identifying tags and numbers.
5. Monitor vital signs and urine output.
6. Treat symptoms per HCP order.
7. Save the blood bag and tubing and send them to the blood bank.
8. Collect ordered blood and other specimens to evaluate for the reaction.
9. Document according to agency policy.

Delayed Transfusion Reactions

Delayed transfusion reactions include delayed hemolytic reactions, infections, GVHD, and iron overload (Table 34.36).

CHECK YOUR PRACTICE

Your 82-year-old male patient with severe iron deficiency anemia is receiving his second unit of packed RBCs. He received the first transfusion without any problems. He is now reporting chills and feels like his heart is racing.

- What should you do?

Autotransfusion

Autotransfusion, or autologous transfusion, involves removing whole blood from a person and transfusing that blood back into the same person. This avoids problems of incompatibility, allergic reactions, and disease transmission. Methods of autotransfusion include:

- *Autologous donation* or *elective phlebotomy* (predeposit transfusion). A person donates blood before a planned surgery. The blood can be frozen and stored for up to 10 years. Usually, the blood is stored without being frozen and given to the person within a few weeks of donation. This technique is beneficial to patients with a rare blood type or for any patient who may need limited blood product support during a major surgery (e.g., elective orthopedic surgery).
- *Autotransfusion.* A method for replacing blood volume that involves safely and aseptically collecting, filtering, and returning the patient's own blood lost during a major surgery or from a traumatic injury. Autotransfusion collection devices are most often used in surgery. Some allow blood to be automatically and continuously reinfused. Others require collecting the blood for a time (usually no longer than 4 hours) and then reinfusing it. Drainage after the first 24 hours or drainage that may contain pathogens is generally not reinfused. Anticoagulants may be added before reinfusion.

CASE STUDY

Leukemia

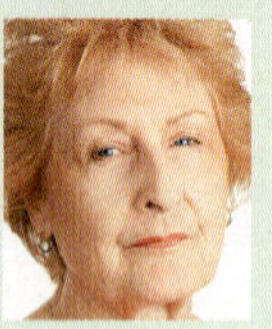

(© Lisa F. Young/iStock.)

Patient Profile

A.J. is a 63-year-old female who is brought to the ED by her husband (see the Chapter 33 Case Study). She has become progressively weaker and was admitted for further evaluation.

Subjective Data

- Progressive weakness over the last couple of weeks
- Had a recent sinus infection that resolved after 2 courses of antibiotics
- Reports periodic shortness of breath
- Has noticed a lot of bruising lately

Objective Data

Physical Assessment

- Scattered petechiae on both ankles and 2 bruises on arms and 3 on left lower leg
- Skin is very pale
- BP 100/70 (lying), 88/60 (standing); temperature 96.8°F (36°C); respiratory rate 26/min; apical pulse 110/min (lying), 124/min (standing); O_2 saturation 90% on room air

Laboratory Results

- Hct 18.2%
- Hgb 5.9 g/dL, WBC count 2600/μL (2.6×10^9/L)
- Platelet count 72,000/μL (72×10^9/L)
- Peripheral blood smear shows that 80% of the WBCs are blasts
- PT 18 sec, aPTT 37 sec
- LDH 560 units/L

Bone Marrow Biopsy

- Multiple myeloblasts (>50%)

Interprofessional Care

- Consultation with a hematologist-oncologist
- 2 units of packed RBCs
- Diagnosis: acute myeloid leukemia (AML)

Discussion Questions

1. ***Recognize:*** What laboratory and bone marrow biopsy results suggest AML?
2. ***Recognize:*** How is AML treated?
3. ***Analyze:*** What is A.J.'s prognosis?
4. ***Plan:*** What life-threatening problems can happen with AML and its treatment? How can you anticipate and assess for these problems?
5. ***Prioritize:*** Based on the assessment data presented, what are the priority clinical problems?
6. ***Prioritize:*** What are the priority nursing interventions for A.J.?
7. ***Prioritize:*** What are the patient teaching priorities for an adult newly diagnosed with AML?
8. ***Act:*** What interprofessional team members are likely to be involved in A.J.'s care?
9. ***Act:*** A.J. becomes fatigued after starting chemotherapy. She wants to know if she can still work and do household chores even if she is so fatigued. What is your best advice for her?
10. Develop a conceptual care map for A.J.

Answers available at http://evolve.elsevier.com/Lewis/medsurg.

BRIDGE TO NCLEX EXAMINATION

The number of the question corresponds to the same-numbered outcome at the beginning of the chapter.

1. In a severely anemic patient, the nurse would expect to find
   a. cyanosis and hypertension.
   b. pulmonary edema and fibrosis.
   c. dyspnea and increased heart rate.
   d. dysrhythmias and expiratory wheezing.
2. When obtaining assessment data from a patient with a microcytic, hypochromic anemia, the nurse would ask the patient about
   a. folic acid intake.
   b. diet intake of iron.
   c. a history of gastric surgery.
   d. a history of sickle cell anemia.
3. Nursing care for a patient with severe anemia from peptic ulcer disease includes **(Select all that apply.)**
   a. instructions for high-iron diet.
   b. taking vital signs every 8 hours.
   c. monitoring stools for occult blood.
   d. teaching self-injection of erythropoietin.
   e. administering cobalamin (vitamin B_{12}) injections.
4. The nursing management of a patient in sickle cell crisis includes **(Select all that apply.)**
   a. monitoring CBC and electrolytes.
   b. optimal pain management and O_2 therapy.
   c. blood transfusions if needed and iron chelation.
   d. rest as needed and deep vein thrombosis prophylaxis.
   e. administration of IV iron and diet high in iron content.
5. A complication of the hyperviscosity of polycythemia is
   a. thrombosis.
   b. cardiomyopathy.
   c. pulmonary edema.
   d. disseminated intravascular coagulation (DIC).
6. The nurse instructs the patient with thrombocytopenia to
   a. dab their nose instead of blowing.
   b. be careful when shaving with a safety razor.
   c. continue with physical activities to stimulate thrombopoiesis.
   d. avoid aspirin because it may mask the fever that occurs with thrombocytopenia.
7. The nurse would expect that a patient with von Willebrand disease undergoing surgery would be treated with administration of vWF and
   a. thrombin.
   b. factor VI.
   c. factor VII.
   d. factor VIII.
8. A patient with a head injury develops petechiae across the chest and abdomen and oozing from venipuncture sites. Which measures would the nurse include in the plan of care? **(Select all that apply.)**
   a. Avoid other venipunctures.
   b. Apply dressings to the sites.
   c. Use an electric razor for shaving.
   d. Provide oral care with glycerin swabs.
   e. Administer ordered warfarin sodium.
9. Priority nursing actions when caring for a hospitalized patient with a new-onset temperature of 102.2°F (39°C) and severe neutropenia include **(Select all that apply.)**
   a. start the prescribed antibiotic STAT.
   b. draw ordered blood cultures STAT.
   c. ongoing monitoring of vital signs for septic shock.
   d. take a full set of vital signs and notify the HCP immediately.
   e. administer transfusions of WBCs treated to decrease immunogenicity.
10. Because myelodysplastic syndrome arises from immature hematopoietic stem cells in the bone marrow, laboratory results the nurse would expect to find include a(n)
    a. excess of T cells.
    b. excess of platelets.
    c. deficiency of granulocytes.
    d. deficiency of all cell blood components.
11. Combination drug therapy is often used to treat leukemia and lymphoma because
    a. there are fewer toxic and side effects.
    b. the chance that 1 drug will be effective is increased.
    c. the drugs are more effective without causing side effects.
    d. the drugs work by different mechanisms to maximize killing of cancer cells.
12. The nurse is aware that a major difference between Hodgkin lymphoma and non-Hodgkin lymphoma is that
    a. Hodgkin lymphoma occurs only in young adults.
    b. Hodgkin lymphoma is considered potentially curable.
    c. non-Hodgkin lymphoma can manifest in multiple areas.
    d. non-Hodgkin lymphoma is treated only with radiation therapy.
13. A patient with multiple myeloma becomes confused with an increased urine output. The laboratory finding that may explain these findings is:
    a. hyperkalemia.
    b. hyperuricemia.
    c. hypercalcemia.
    d. hypocalcemia.
14. When reviewing a patient's hematologic laboratory values after a splenectomy, the nurse would expect to find
    a. RBC abnormalities.
    b. increased WBC count.
    c. decreased hemoglobin.
    d. decreased platelet count.

15. Transfusion complications that can be decreased with leukocyte depletion or reduction of RBC transfusion are
  a. chills and hemolysis.
  b. leukostasis and neutrophilia.
  c. fluid overload and pulmonary edema.
  d. transmission of cytomegalovirus and fever.

1. c; 2. b; 3. a, c; 4. a, b, c, d; 5. a; 6. a; 7. d; 8. a, b, c; 9. a, b, c, d; 10. d; 11. d; 12. c; 13. c; 14. b; 15. d.

For rationales to these answers and even more NCLEX review questions, visit http://evolve.elsevier.com/Lewis/medsurg.

REFERENCES

To access the References for this chapter, please scan the QR code with a mobile device.

Case Study

Applying Clinical Judgment With Multiple Patients

You are working on the oncology unit and have been assigned to care for the following 4 patients. You have 1 AP who is assigned to help you, and there are 2 other RNs on your clinical unit.

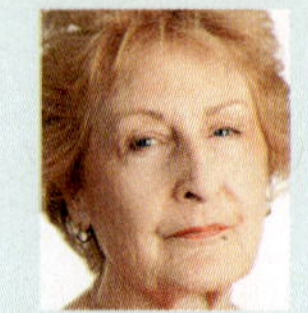 © Lisa F. Young/iStock.	A.J. is a 63-year-old female admitted with severe anemia (Hgb 5.9 g/dL, Hct 18.2%) and acute myelocytic leukemia (AML). Her WBC count is 2600/μL, and platelet count is 72,000/μL. A.J. has dyspnea on exertion. She has received the first of 2 units of RBCs. Vital signs: 102/60, 100, RR 22, temp 96.8°F (36°C), O_2 saturation 94% with O_2 at 2 L/min via nasal cannula. She starts chemotherapy tomorrow.
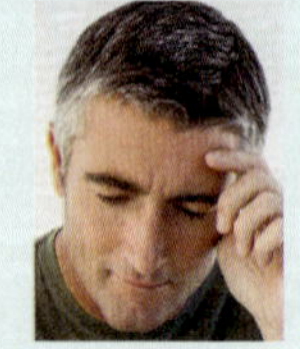 © g-stockstudio/iStock/ Thinkstock.	J.J. is a 52-year-old male newly diagnosed with acute lymphocytic leukemia (ALL). Laboratory results reveal Hgb 6.9 g/dL, Hct 20%, WBC count 120,000/μL (120 × 109/L), and platelet count 9000/μL (25 × 109/L). Vital signs: 100/70, 110, RR 26, temperature 102.2°F (39°C). He is having a port placed today after he receives platelet transfusions.
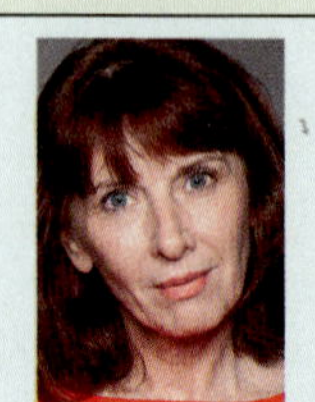 © Studio Grand Ouest/ iStock/Thinkstock.	P.H. is a 45-year-old female who is receiving chemotherapy for ovarian cancer. She was admitted with fever and chills. Her WBC count is 2200/μL (2.2 × 109/L), with an absolute neutrophil count (ANC) of 400/μL (0.4 × 109/L). She needs to receive her 1st dose of IV antibiotic therapy. Vital signs: 118/60, 98, RR 20, temperature 99.2°F (37.3°C).

1. Highlight all the findings that require your follow-up.
2. After receiving report, which patient would you see first?
3. Which tasks could you delegate to the AP? **(Select 4 correct options.)**
   a. Assist A.J. to a chair after completing her AM care.
   b. Obtain the 1st unit of platelets for J.J. from the blood bank.
   c. Explain the importance of isolation to P.H. and her family.
   d. Obtain vital signs for A.J. in between blood transfusions.
   e. Provide teaching to J.J. about the port placement procedure.
   f. Obtain reverse isolation carts from supply for J.J. and P.H.
   g. Ensure that J.J. and A.J. have patent IV infusion lines.

Case Study—cont'd

4. When you enter J.J.'s room, you find him confused and lethargic. His family states he had just had a severe coughing episode.

Use an X for the nursing actions that are indicated (appropriate or necessary), contraindicated (could be harmful), or nonessential (makes no difference or not necessary) for J.J. at this time.

Nursing Action	Indicated	Contraindicated
Perform a focused neurologic assessment.		
Direct the AP to stay with J.J. while you contact the HCP.		
Ask family members for a copy of his living will.		
Call respiratory therapy to give him a breathing treatment.		
Place him flat, in a side-lying position.		
Obtain vital signs with O_2 saturation.		
Initiate NPO status.		
Insert an indwelling urinary catheter.		

Case Study Progression

J.J.'s HCP orders a repeat CBC and an emergency CT scan of the head. Your supervisor arranges for another RN to accompany J.J. to the CT scan so you can administer the 2nd unit of blood to A.J. and the IV antibiotic to P.H.

5. Based on P.H.'s condition, the priority need will be prevention of ________1______. To reduce this risk, the most important intervention is to ______2_____.

Options for 1	Options for 2
Bleeding	encourage ambulation as tolerated
Infection	initiate bleeding precautions
VTE	perform hand hygiene

6. While waiting for A.J.'s blood, you complete her assessment and begin to develop her plan of care. Indicate which nursing action(s) listed in the far-left column is appropriate for each potential complication. Actions may be used more than once. Note that not all actions will be used.

Nursing Action	Complication	Appropriate Nursing Action(s) for Each Complication
a. Implement neutropenic precautions	Anemia	
b. Administer ferrous sulfate 325 mg TID.	Dehydration	
c. Provide a nutrition supplement with each meal.	Infection	
d. Titrate O_2 therapy.		
e. Obtain daily weights.		
f. Reposition every 2 hours while in bed.		
g. Alternate rest and activity periods.		
h. Monitor laboratory results as available.		

7. The RN from the float pool arrives to accompany J.J. to the CT scan at the same time the AP arrives with the platelet infusion. Which intervention would be *most* appropriate?
   a. Put the unit platelets in the refrigerator to start when J.J. returns to the floor.
   b. Ask the RN to verify the correct unit of platelets with you and start the infusion.
   c. Give the RN an SBAR report and ask her to start the platelets on the way to CT scan.
   d. Ask the RN if she would prefer to give the platelets or hold it for J.J.'s return to the unit.
8. The HCP orders ferrous sulfate 325 mg TID for A.J. You teach A.J. to take her iron **(Select all that apply.)**
   a. at breakfast time in the morning.
   b. with orange juice to increase absorption.
   c. 1 hour before meals to facilitate absorption.
   d. 2 hours after eating to minimize side effects.
   e. whenever she feels tired or is short of breath with activity.

Answers available at http://evolve.elsevier.com/Lewis/medsurg.

35

Assessment: Cardiovascular System

Debra Hagler and Diana Rabbani Hagler

http://evolve.elsevier.com/Lewis/medsurg/

CONCEPTUAL FOCUS

Health Promotion
Nutrition
Perfusion

LEARNING OUTCOMES

1. Describe the anatomic location and function of the heart.
2. Relate the coronary circulation to the areas of heart muscle supplied by the major coronary arteries.
3. Distinguish the structure and function of arteries, veins, capillaries, and endothelium.
4. Describe the mechanisms involved in blood pressure regulation.
5. Relate the various waveforms on a normal electrocardiogram to the associated cardiac events.
6. Obtain significant subjective and objective assessment data related to the cardiovascular system.
7. Perform a physical assessment of the cardiovascular system.
8. Distinguish normal from common abnormal findings of a cardiovascular physical assessment.
9. Link the age-related changes of the cardiovascular system to the differences in assessment findings.
10. Apply the principles of hemodynamic monitoring to the nursing and interprofessional management of patients.
11. Describe the purpose, significance of results, and nursing responsibilities related to diagnostic studies of the cardiovascular system.

KEY TERMS

afterload
arterial blood pressure
arterial pressure–based cardiac output (APCO)
cardiac index (CI)
cardiac output (CO)
cardiac reserve
coronary angiography
diastole
diastolic blood pressure (DBP)
ejection fraction (EF)
hemodynamic monitoring
Korotkoff sounds
mean arterial pressure (MAP)
murmur
point of maximal impulse (PMI)
preload
pulse pressure
systole
systolic blood pressure (SBP)

STRUCTURES AND FUNCTION OF THE CARDIOVASCULAR SYSTEM

Heart

Structure

The heart is a 4-chambered hollow muscular organ normally about the size of a fist. It lies within the thorax, in the mediastinal space that separates the right and left pleural cavities. The heart is composed of 3 layers: a thin inner lining, the *endocardium;* a layer of muscle, the *myocardium;* and an outer layer, the *epicardium.* A fibroserous sac called the *pericardium* covers the heart. The pericardium consists of 2 layers: the inner *(visceral)* layer (part of the epicardium) and the outer *(parietal)* layer. A small amount of pericardial fluid (around 10 to 15 mL) lubricates the space between the pericardial layers *(pericardial space)* and prevents friction between the surfaces as the heart contracts.

The septum vertically divides the heart. The interatrial septum creates a right and left atrium. The interventricular septum creates a right and left ventricle. The wall thickness of each heart chamber is different. The atrial myocardium is thinner than that of the ventricles. The left ventricular wall is 2 to 3 times thicker than the right ventricular wall. The thickness of the left ventricle is needed for the strength to pump the blood into the systemic circulation.[1]

Blood Flow Through the Heart

Fig. 35.1 shows the blood flow through the heart. The 4 valves of the heart keep blood flowing forward. The cusps of the mitral and tricuspid valves are attached to thin strands of fibrous tissue called *chordae tendineae* (Fig. 35.2). Chordae are anchored in the papillary muscles of the ventricles. This support prevents the eversion of the valve leaflets into the atria during ventricular contraction. The pulmonic and aortic valves *(semilunar valves)* prevent blood from flowing backward into the ventricles at the end of each ventricular contraction.

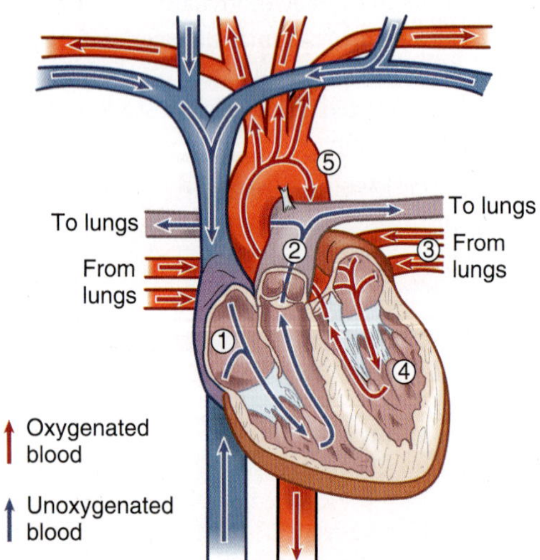

Fig. 35.1 Diagram of blood flow through the heart. *Arrows* show direction of flow. *1,* The right atrium receives venous blood from the inferior and superior venae cava and the coronary sinus. The blood then passes through the tricuspid valve into the right ventricle. *2,* With each contraction, the right ventricle pumps blood through the pulmonic valve into the pulmonary artery and to the lungs. *3,* Oxygenated blood flows from the lungs to the left atrium by way of the pulmonary veins. *4,* It then passes through the mitral valve and into the left ventricle. *5,* As the heart contracts, blood is ejected through the aortic valve into the aorta and enters the systemic circulation.

Blood Supply to the Myocardium

The myocardium has its own blood supply, the *coronary circulation* (Fig. 35.3). Blood flow into the 2 major coronary arteries occurs primarily during **diastole** (relaxation of the myocardium). The left coronary artery arises from the aorta and divides into 2 main branches: the left anterior descending artery and left circumflex artery. These arteries supply the left atrium, left ventricle, interventricular septum, and part of the right ventricle. The right coronary artery arises from the aorta, and its branches supply the right atrium, right ventricle, and part of the posterior wall of the left ventricle. In 90% of people, the atrioventricular (AV) node and the bundle of His receive blood supply from the right coronary artery. For this reason, blockage of this artery often causes serious defects in cardiac conduction.

The divisions of coronary veins parallel the coronary arteries. Most of the blood from the coronary system drains into the coronary sinus (a large channel). It empties into the right atrium, near the entrance of the inferior vena cava.

Conduction System

The conduction system consists of specialized tissue that creates and transports the electrical impulse, or action potential. This impulse starts depolarization of the heart cells, leading to heart muscle contraction (Fig. 35.4A). The electrical impulse normally begins in the sinoatrial (SA) node

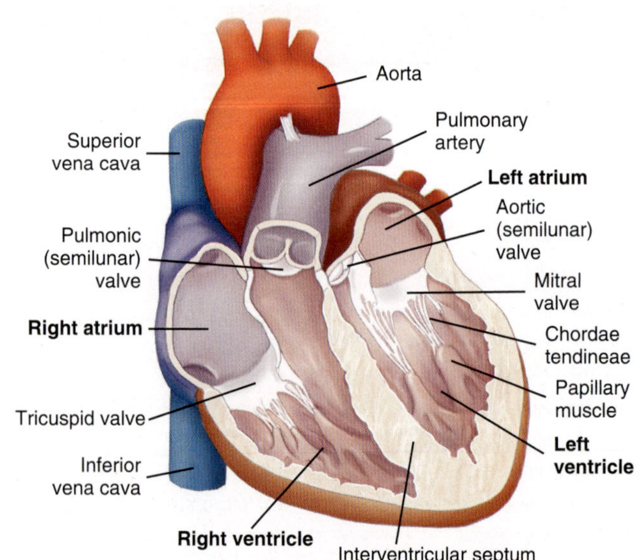

Fig. 35.2 Anatomic structures of the heart and heart valves.

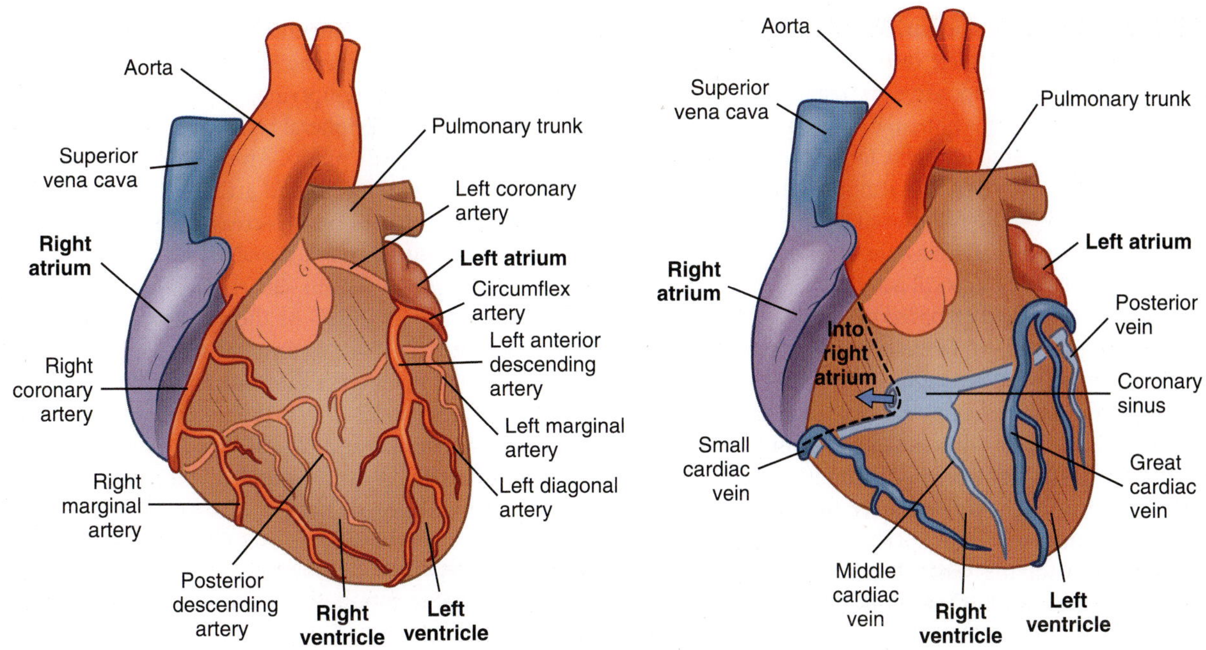

Fig. 35.3 Coronary arteries and veins.

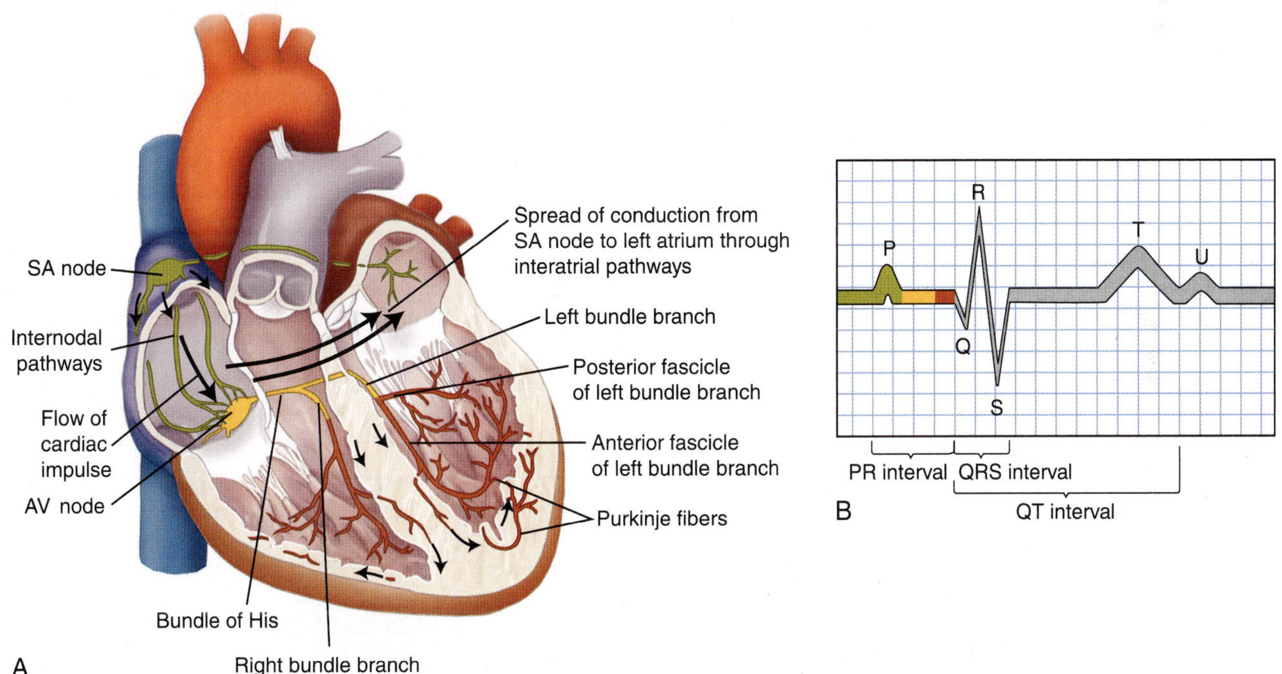

Fig. 35.4 (A) Conduction system of the heart. *AV*, Atrioventricular; *SA*, sinoatrial. (B) The normal ECG pattern. The *P* wave represents depolarization of the atria. The *QRS* complex indicates depolarization of the ventricles. The *T* wave represents repolarization of the ventricles. The *U* wave, if present, may represent repolarization of the Purkinje fibers or be associated with hypokalemia. The PR, QRS, and QT intervals reflect the time it takes for the impulse to travel from one area of the heart to another.

(pacemaker of the heart). Impulses from the SA node travel through interatrial pathways to depolarize the atria, resulting in a contraction.

The electrical impulse travels from the atria to the AV node through internodal pathways. The signal then moves through the bundle of His and the left and right bundle branches. The left bundle branch has 2 divisions: anterior and posterior. The action potential moves through the walls of both ventricles via *Purkinje fibers.* The ventricular conduction system delivers the impulse within 0.12 second. This triggers a synchronized right and left ventricular contraction and ejection of blood into the pulmonary and systemic circulations.

Last, repolarization occurs when the contractile and conduction pathway cells regain their resting polarized condition. Heart muscle cells are unresponsive or *refractory* to restimulation during the action potential. During ventricular contraction, there is an *absolute refractory period* when heart muscle does not respond to any new stimuli. After this period, heart muscle gradually recovers its excitability, and a *relative refractory period* occurs by early diastole.[2]

Electrocardiogram. The electrical activity of the heart can be detected using electrodes and recorded on an ECG. We use the letters *P, QRS, T,* and *U* to name the separate waveforms (Fig. 35.4B). The first waveform, the P wave, begins with the firing of the SA node. It represents depolarization of the atria. The QRS complex represents depolarization from the AV node through the ventricles. A delay of impulse transmission through the AV node accounts for the time between the beginning of the P wave and the beginning of the QRS wave. The T wave represents repolarization of the ventricles. The U wave, if seen, may represent repolarization of the Purkinje fibers. A large U wave may occur with hypokalemia.

Intervals between these waves (PR, QRS, and QT intervals) reflect the time it takes for the signal to travel from 1 area of the heart to another. Changes in the timing often indicate a pathologic condition.[3] See Chapter 39 for a complete discussion of ECG monitoring.

Mechanical System

Depolarization triggers mechanical activity. **Systole**, contraction of the heart muscle, results in ejection of blood from the ventricles. Relaxation of the heart muscle, *diastole,* allows for filling of the ventricles. **Cardiac output (CO)** is the amount of blood pumped by each ventricle in 1 minute. For the normal adult at rest, CO ranges from 4 to 8 L/min. Calculate CO by multiplying the amount of blood ejected from the ventricle with each heartbeat—*stroke volume* (SV) times heart rate (HR) per minute:

$$CO = SV \times HR$$

Factors affecting cardiac output. Many factors can affect either HR or SV and thus the CO. HR is controlled mainly by the autonomic nervous system. It can reach as high as 180 beats/min for short periods without harmful effects. With rapid HRs, there is less time for diastolic filling and perfusion of the coronary arteries. The factors affecting the SV are preload, contractility, and afterload. Increasing preload, contractility, and afterload increases the workload of the heart muscle, resulting in increased O_2 demand.

The Frank-Starling law states that, to a point, the more the myocardial fibers are stretched, the greater their force of contraction. The volume of blood stretching the ventricles at the end of diastole, before the next contraction, is called **preload**. Preload can be increased by conditions such as hypertension, aortic valve disease, and hypervolemia. Preload is decreased when a rapid HR or hypovolemia reduces ventricular filling during diastole. Contractility can be increased by epinephrine and norepinephrine released by the sympathetic nervous system. Increasing contractility raises the SV by increasing ventricular emptying.[1]

Afterload is the peripheral resistance, or force, against which the left ventricle must pump. Afterload depends on the size of the ventricle, wall tension, and arterial BP. If the arterial BP is elevated, the ventricles meet increased resistance to ejection of blood, increasing the work demand. Eventually this results in *ventricular hypertrophy,* an enlargement of the heart muscle without an increase in CO or the size of chambers. Both right and left ventricles work against resistance. The right ventricle pumps against the afterload of pulmonary arterial resistance.[2]

The cardiovascular (CV) system must respond to many situations in health and illness (e.g., exercise, stress, hypovolemia). The ability to respond to these demands by maintaining or increasing CO is the **cardiac reserve**.

Vascular System

Blood Vessels

The 3 major types of blood vessels are the arteries, veins, and capillaries. Arteries, except for the pulmonary artery (PA), carry oxygenated blood away from the heart. Veins, except for the pulmonary veins, carry deoxygenated blood toward the heart. Small branches of arteries and veins are arterioles and venules, respectively. Blood circulates from the left side of the heart into arteries, arterioles, capillaries, venules, and veins and then back to the right side of the heart.

Arteries and arterioles. The arterial system differs from the venous system by the amount and type of tissue that make up arterial walls (Fig. 35.5). The large arteries have thick walls composed mainly of elastic tissue. This elastic property cushions the impact of the pressure from ventricular contraction and provides recoil that propels blood forward into the circulation. Large arteries contain some smooth muscle. Examples of large arteries are the aorta and PA.

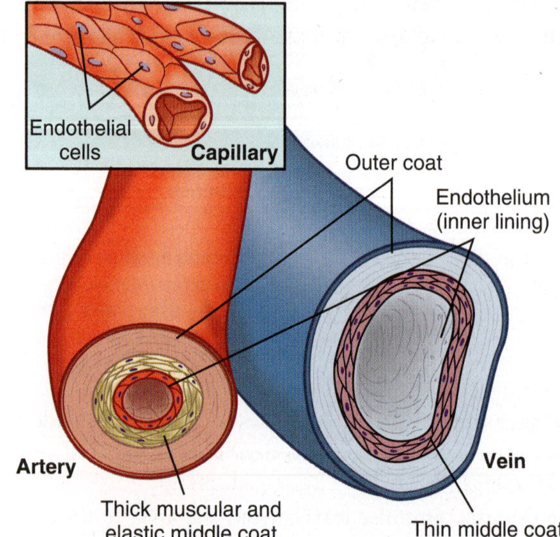

Fig. 35.5 Comparative thickness of layers of the artery, vein, and capillary.

Arterioles have more smooth muscle and little elastic tissue. Arterioles control arterial BP and distribution of blood flow. They respond readily to local conditions such as low O_2 and increasing levels of carbon dioxide (CO_2) by dilating or constricting.

The innermost lining of the arteries is the endothelium. The endothelium maintains hemostasis, promotes blood flow, and, under normal conditions, inhibits blood coagulation. When the endothelial surface is disrupted (e.g., rupture of an atherosclerotic plaque), the coagulation cascade results in the formation of a fibrin clot.

Capillaries. The thin capillary wall made up of endothelial cells has no elastic or muscle tissue (Fig. 35.5). Exchange of cell nutrients and metabolic end products takes place through these thin-walled vessels. Capillaries connect the arterioles and venules.

Veins and venules. Venules are small vessels with a minor amount of muscle and connective tissue. Venules collect blood from the capillary beds and channel it to the larger veins.

Veins are large-diameter, thin-walled vessels that return blood to the right atrium (Fig. 35.5). The venous system is a low-pressure, high-volume system. The larger veins have semilunar valves at intervals to maintain the blood flow toward the heart and to prevent backward flow. Several factors affect the amount of blood in the venous system. These include arterial flow, compression of veins by skeletal muscles, changes in thoracic and abdominal pressures, and right atrial pressure.

The largest veins are the *superior vena cava,* which returns blood to the heart from the head, neck, and arms, and the *inferior vena cava,* which returns blood to the heart from the lower part of the body. Pressure in the right side of the heart affects these large vessels. Elevated right atrial pressure can cause distended neck veins or liver engorgement because of resistance to blood flow.[1]

Regulation of the Cardiovascular System

Autonomic Nervous System

The autonomic nervous system consists of the sympathetic nervous system and parasympathetic nervous system (see Chapter 60).

Effect on the heart. Stimulation of the sympathetic nervous system increases HR, speed of impulse conduction through the AV node, and force of atrial and ventricular contractions. This effect is mediated by specific sites in the heart called *beta (β)-adrenergic receptors.* They are receptors for norepinephrine and epinephrine. Parasympathetic system stimulation (mediated by the vagus nerve) slows the HR by decreasing the impulses from the SA node and conduction through the AV node.

Effect on blood vessels. The source of neural control of blood vessels is the sympathetic nervous system. Alpha$_1$ (α_1)-adrenergic receptors are found in vascular smooth muscles. Stimulation of α_1-adrenergic receptors results in vasoconstriction. Decreased stimulation to α_1-adrenergic receptors causes vasodilation. Sympathetic nervous system receptors that influence BP are described in Table 36.1.

Baroreceptors

Baroreceptors in the aortic arch and carotid sinus (at the origin of the internal carotid artery) are sensitive to stretch or pressure within the arterial system. Stimulation of these receptors (e.g., volume overload) sends information to the vasomotor center in the brainstem. This results in temporary inhibition of the sympathetic nervous system and enhancement of the parasympathetic influence. The result is a decreased HR and peripheral vasodilation. Decreased arterial pressure has the opposite effect.

Chemoreceptors

Chemoreceptors are found in the aortic and carotid bodies and the medulla. They can cause changes in respiratory rate and BP in response to increased arterial CO_2 pressure (hypercapnia) and, to less degree, decreased plasma pH (acidosis) and arterial O_2 pressure (hypoxia). Chemoreceptors in the medulla stimulate the vasomotor center to increase BP.[2]

Blood Pressure

The **arterial blood pressure** is a measure of the force exerted by blood against the walls of the arterial system. The **systolic blood pressure (SBP)** is the peak pressure exerted against the arteries when the heart contracts. The **diastolic blood pressure (DBP)** is the residual pressure in the arterial system during ventricular relaxation (or filling).

The main factors influencing BP are CO and *systemic vascular resistance* (SVR):

$$BP = CO \times SVR$$

SVR is the force opposing the movement of blood. This force is created mainly in small arteries and arterioles. BP is recorded as the ratio of SBP to DBP (e.g., 120/80 mm Hg). Normal BP is SBP less than 120 mm Hg and DBP less than 80 mm Hg (see Chapter 36).[4] Sometimes, an *auscultatory gap* occurs, which is a loss of sound between the SBP and DBP.

Pulse Pressure and Mean Arterial Pressure

Pulse pressure is the difference between the SBP and DBP. It is normally about one-third of the SBP. If the BP is 120/80 mm Hg, the pulse pressure is 40 mm Hg. An increased pulse pressure and SBP may occur when a person exercises or has atherosclerosis of the larger arteries. A decreased pulse pressure may occur with heart failure (HF) or hypovolemia.

Another measurement related to BP is **mean arterial pressure (MAP)**. The MAP refers to the average pressure within the arterial system. It is not the average of the DBP and SBP, because the length of diastole is about twice that of systole at normal HRs. MAP is calculated as follows:

$$MAP = (SBP + 2DBP) \div 3$$

A person with a BP of 120/60 mm Hg has an estimated MAP of 80 mm Hg. The MAP must be greater than 60 mm Hg to perfuse the vital organs under most conditions. When the MAP is low for a period of time, vital organs become ischemic.

Gerontologic Considerations: Effects of Aging on the Cardiovascular System

Age-related changes in the CV system and differences in assessment findings are found in Table 35.1. Many of the changes are a result of the combined effects of the aging process, disease, environment, and health behaviors. With increased age, collagen in the heart increases and elastin decreases. These changes affect the heart muscle's ability to stretch and contract. The older adult has a decreased CV response to stress and is less sensitive to β-adrenergic agonist drugs. Exercise results in a much smaller increase in CO for older adults.[5]

Heart valves thicken and stiffen from lipid accumulation, collagen degeneration, and fibrosis. The aortic and mitral valves are most often affected. These changes result in either regurgitation of blood when the valve should be closed or narrowing of the orifice of the valve *(stenosis)* when the valve should be open.

The number of pacemaker cells in the SA node and conduction cells in the internodal tracts, bundle of His, and bundle branches decrease. The decrease contributes to the development of sinus and atrial dysrhythmias and heart blocks. Many older adults have an abnormal resting ECG that shows increases in the PR and/or QT intervals.[6] The number and function of β-adrenergic receptors in the heart decrease with age.[7]

With age, arteries and veins thicken and become less elastic. Arteries become more sensitive to vasopressin (antidiuretic hormone). Both changes increase SBP and pulse pressure with a decreased or unchanged DBP. Valves in the large leg veins return the blood to the heart less effectively, often resulting in dependent edema.

When an older adult changes position (e.g., sits upright), the sympathetic nerve pathway produces a blunted (reduced) HR response, which may lead to a drop in BP and sense of lightheadedness on arising (orthostatic hypotension). *Postprandial hypotension* (decrease in BP of at least 20 mm Hg that occurs within 75 minutes after eating) may occur in otherwise healthy older adults. Both orthostatic and postprandial hypotension increase fall risk in older adults.

TABLE 35.1 GERONTOLOGIC ASSESSMENT DIFFERENCES

Cardiovascular System

Changes	Differences in Assessment Findings
Chest Wall	
Kyphosis	Altered chest landmarks for palpation, percussion, and auscultation. Distant heart sounds
Heart	
Myocardial hypertrophy, ↑ collagen and scarring, ↓ elastin	↓ Cardiac reserve, HF. S_4 may be present
Downward displacement	Difficulty in isolating apical pulse.
↓ CO, HR, SV in response to exercise or stress	↓ Response to exercise and stress. Slowed recovery from activity
↓ Number of cells in conduction system	↓ Amplitude of QRS complex and slight lengthening of PR, QRS, and QT intervals. Irregular rhythms, ↓ maximal HR, ↓ HR variability
↓ Number and function of beta (β)-adrenergic receptors	
Valve rigidity from calcification, sclerosis, or fibrosis, impeding complete closure of valves	Systolic murmur (aortic or mitral) possible without a sign of CVD
Blood Vessels	
Arterial stiffening caused by loss of elastin in arterial walls, thickening of intima of arteries, and progressive fibrosis of media	↑ In SBP and possible ↑ or ↓ in DBP. Possible widened pulse pressure. ↓ Pedal pulses. Intermittent claudication
↑ Venous tortuosity	Inflamed, painful, or cord-like varicosities. Dependent edema

CASE STUDY

Patient Information

(© Jupiterimages/Banana-Stock/Thinkstock.)

L.P., a 63-year-old male, is brought to the hospital by ambulance at 0600 after reporting chest tightness, shortness of breath, and "heart pounding" (palpitations). The paramedics started an IV and O_2 at 2 L/min via nasal cannula. They obtained a 12-lead ECG and gave him 4 low-dose ASA to chew and a sublingual nitroglycerin tablet. L.P. is pain free on arrival to the emergency department but still has palpitations.

Discussion Questions

1. What are the possible causes of L.P.'s symptoms?
2. Is L.P.'s condition stable or unstable?

You will learn more about L.P. and his condition as you read this assessment chapter.

Answers available at http://evolve.elsevier.com/Lewis/medsurg.

CARDIOVASCULAR SYSTEM ASSESSMENT

Subjective Data

The health history and physical assessment will help you distinguish symptoms of a CV problem. Ask patients what problem has led to seeking health care. Evaluate all symptoms patients report. Explore all cues that alert you to the possibility of underlying cardiovascular disease (CVD).

Important Health Information

Health history. Many illnesses affect the CV system directly or indirectly. Obtain a history of angina, diabetes, anemia, rheumatic fever, streptococcal throat infections, congenital heart disease, stroke, hypertension, thrombophlebitis, dysrhythmias, and varicosities. Fully explore any symptoms patients report. Ask about dyspnea, fatigue, dizziness with position changes, syncope, edema, intermittent claudication, and palpitations.

Assess for allergies to drugs, food, or the environment. Has the patient ever had a drug reaction or an allergic or anaphylactic reaction? Ask about any allergic reaction to contrast media. Note alcohol and tobacco use.

Medications. Obtain a complete medication history. Record the dose and time last taken for each. Include over-the-counter (OTC) and prescription drugs and herbal supplements. For example, aspirin prolongs the blood clotting time. Assess for use of noncardiac drugs that can adversely affect the CV system (Table 35.2).

Surgery and other treatments. Ask about treatments, surgeries, or hospital admissions related to CV problems. Have any procedures been done for CV symptoms? Note whether patients have had an ECG or a chest x-ray.

Functional Health Patterns

Review each functional health pattern for connections between lifestyle and CV health. Key questions to ask a person with a CV problem are listed in Table 35.3.

Health perception–health management. Ask patients about major CV risk factors. These include abnormal serum lipids, hypertension, sedentary lifestyle, diabetes, obesity, and tobacco use. Estimate the number of pack-years of tobacco use (number of packs smoked per day multiplied by the number of years the patient has smoked). Note their attitude about tobacco use and attempts and methods used to stop. Record the type of alcohol used, amount, and frequency. Note any use of habit-forming or recreational substances.

Confirmed illnesses of blood relatives can highlight any genetic tendencies toward coronary artery disease (CAD), hypertension, varicosities, bleeding, diabetes, cardiomyopathy, and stroke. Note any family members who had heart disease at an early age (<50 years of age for men; <55 years of age for women). Is there a family health history of noncardiac problems that affect the CV system such as lung, kidney, or liver disease?

Nutritional-metabolic. Being underweight or overweight may indicate a CV problem. Assess the patient's weight over the past year in relation to height. Review their food habits. What is the amount of salt and saturated fats in their typical diet? Explore patients' attitudes and plans about diet and weight management.

Elimination. Patients taking diuretics may report increased voiding and/or nocturia. Ask about incontinence or constipation, including use of prescribed and OTC drugs for constipation. Teach patients with heart problems to avoid straining *(Valsalva maneuver)* during a bowel movement. Ask if they have swelling of the lower extremities and if it resolves when they elevate their feet.

TABLE 35.2 Potential Cardiovascular Effects of Select Noncardiac Drugs

Drug Classification	Examples	Cardiovascular Effects
Anticancer agents	daunorubicin doxorubicin	Dysrhythmias, cardiomyopathy
Antipsychotics	chlorpromazine haloperidol	Dysrhythmias, orthostatic hypotension
Antirheumatics	hydroxychloroquine	Dysrhythmias, cardiomyopathy, heart block, prolonged QT interval,
Corticosteroids	cortisone prednisone	Hypotension, edema, potassium depletion
Hormone therapy, oral contraceptives	estrogen + progestin	MI, thromboembolism, stroke, hypertension
Nonsteroidal antiinflammatory drugs (NSAIDs)	celecoxib diclofenac ibuprofen	MI, stroke, hypertension, HF
Psychostimulants	amphetamines cocaine	Tachycardia, angina, MI, hypertension, dysrhythmias
Tricyclic antidepressants	amitriptyline doxepin	Dysrhythmias, orthostatic hypotension

Activity-exercise. The benefit of exercise for CV health is clear, with aerobic exercise being most beneficial. Record the types, duration, intensity, and frequency of exercise. Ask about symptoms during exercise (e.g., chest pain, dyspnea, claudication) that may indicate a CV problem.

Sleep-rest. CV problems often disrupt sleep. *Paroxysmal nocturnal dyspnea* (attacks of shortness of breath, especially at night that awaken the patient) and *Cheyne-Stokes respiration* (periods of very shallow breaths to alternating periods of apnea and deep, rapid breathing) are associated with HF. Note the number of pillows needed to sleep or the need to sleep upright in a chair *(orthopnea)*.

Sleep apnea is associated with an increased risk for life-threatening dysrhythmias, especially in patients with HF. Nocturia, a common finding in CVD, interrupts normal sleep patterns.

Cognitive-perceptual. Ask patients and caregivers about cognitive-perceptual problems. CV problems such as dysrhythmias, hypertension, and stroke may cause difficulties with syncope, language, and memory. Report pain associated with the CV system (e.g., chest pain, claudication).

Role-relationship. The patient's marital status, role in the household, employment status, number of children and their ages, living environment, and caregivers help you to identify strengths and support systems in the patient's life.

Sexuality-reproductive. Ask patients about the effect of the CV problem on sexual activity. Because some patients fear sudden death during sexual intercourse, they may change their sexual behavior. Fatigue, chest pain, or dyspnea may limit

TABLE 35.3 HEALTH HISTORY

Cardiovascular System

Health Perception–Health Management

- What measures do you practice to decrease risk factors for heart disease?
- Have you noticed an increase in heart symptoms such as chest pain or dyspnea?[a]
- Does your heart problem cause you to be less able to care for yourself?[a]
- Do you foresee any potential self-care problems because of your heart problem?[a]
- Have you ever used tobacco? If yes, in what form, how much, and for how long? Have you tried to quit? If yes, what methods have you tried? Are you interested in learning about quitting?
- How often and how much alcohol do you drink?

Nutritional-Metabolic

- Describe your usual daily diet, including salt, fat, and liquid intake.
- What is your present weight? What was your weight 1 year ago? If different, explain.
- Does eating cause fatigue or shortness of breath?[a]

Elimination

- Do your feet or ankles ever swell?[a] If yes, how far up your legs? Does it go away after sleeping all night?
- Have you ever taken drugs to help you get rid of excess fluid or to relieve constipation?[a]
- Are you having any problems related to urination?[a]
- Do you ever strain to have a bowel movement?

Activity-Exercise

- Are your daily activities or exercise limited because of your heart problem?[a]
- When were you last able to comfortably perform your usual activities or exercise?
- Do you have any discomfort or symptoms during exercise or activity?[a]
- Can you comfortably walk and talk at the same time?
- How often do you attend activities outside your home?
- What was your most strenuous activity in the past few weeks compared with 6 months ago?

Sleep-Rest

- How many pillows do you sleep on at night? Has this changed recently?[a]
- Do you ever wake up suddenly and feel as if you cannot catch your breath?[a]
- Do you have a history of sleep apnea?[a]
- Do you ever sleep in a chair at night? If yes, how often?
- How many times a night do you awaken to urinate?

Cognitive-Perceptual

- Do you ever have dizziness or fainting?[a]
- Do you ever find it hard to express yourself or to remember things?[a]
- Do you have any pain (e.g., chest pain, leg pain with activity) because of your heart problem?[a]

Self-Perception–Self-Concept

- Have your perceptions of yourself changed since you were diagnosed with heart disease?[a]
- How has your heart disease affected the quality of your life?

Role-Relationship

- Has this illness affected any of the roles that you play in your daily life?[a]
- How has your heart disease affected your significant others?

Sexuality-Reproductive

- Has your heart disease caused a change in your sexual activity?[a]
- Do you have any heart-related symptoms during sexual activity?[a]
- Do any of your drugs affect your ability to take part in sexual activities?[a]
- *Females:* Are you currently taking oral contraceptives, hormonal therapy, or drug therapy for breast cancer?
- *Males:* Are you taking any drugs to treat erectile dysfunction?

Coping–Stress Tolerance

- Describe your normal coping mechanisms during times of stress or anxiety.
- To whom or where would you turn during a time of stress? Are these people or services helping you now?[a]
- Do you practice any stress reduction techniques?[a]
- Do you have a history of depression?[a]
- Do you feel capable of handling your present health situation?
- Do you have any heart symptoms (e.g., chest pain, palpitations) during times of stress or anger?[a]

Values-Beliefs

- What influence have your values or beliefs had during your illness?
- Do you feel any conflicts between your values or beliefs and the plan of care?[a]
- Describe any cultural or spiritual beliefs that may influence managing your heart problem.

[a]If yes, describe.

activity. Erectile dysfunction (ED) may be a symptom of peripheral vascular disease (PVD) and/or a side effect of some drugs used to treat CVD (e.g., β-blockers, diuretics). Ask male patients about the use of drugs such as phosphodiesterase inhibitors for ED. These drugs are contraindicated if the patient is taking a nitrate because the combination can cause significant hypotension.[6]

Ask female patients if they use oral contraceptives, hormone therapy (HT) for symptoms of menopause, or drug therapy for breast cancer. Females who smoke tobacco and use oral contraceptives are at increased risk for blood clots (e.g., venous thromboembolism). There is an increased risk for CVD with the use of HT and selective estrogen-receptor modulators (e.g., tamoxifen).[6]

Coping–stress tolerance. Work-related stress, depression, and inadequate social support are risk factors for CVD and heart events. Ask the patient about these factors. Information about support systems such as family, extended family and friends, counselors, or religious groups is useful in planning care.

CASE STUDY

Subjective Data

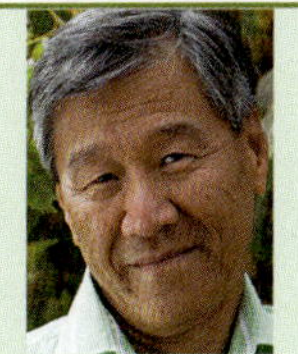

(© Jupiterimages/ Banana-Stock/ Thinkstock.)

A focused subjective assessment of L.P. revealed the following:

- ***Medical History:*** History of hypertension, mitral valve prolapse with mild regurgitation, HF, and type 2 diabetes.
- ***Oral Medications:*** Lisinopril 10 mg/day, metoprolol 50 mg twice daily, aspirin 81 mg/day, furosemide 40 mg/day, and glipizide 5 mg/day.
- ***Health Perception–Health Management:*** L.P. denies any history of chest pain or coronary artery disease. He reports feeling fine until this morning when he awoke and developed shortness of breath (SOB), chest tightness, and palpitations while walking to the bathroom. He thought he was having a heart attack, so his wife called 911. Denies smoking or alcohol intake. SOB and chest tightness are now gone, but he continues to feel palpitations.
- ***Elimination:*** Denies edema or nocturia. States he takes furosemide in the morning and typically "passes urine until lunchtime."

Discussion Questions

1. Which subjective assessment findings most concern you?
2. How will you conduct a patient-centered assessment?
3. Is this a good time to teach him about how to use nitroglycerin tablets?
4. What should you include in the physical assessment? What cues would you be looking for?

You will learn more about the physical assessment of the CV system in the next section.

Answers available at http://evolve.elsevier.com/Lewis/medsurg

BOX 35.1 FOCUSED ASSESSMENT

Cardiovascular System

Use this checklist to remind you of the key assessment steps.

Subjective

Ask the patient about the following and note responses:

Chest pain, discomfort
Palpitations
Shortness of breath (especially when lying down or at rest)
Edema in legs or any part of body
Leg pain during exercise
Excess urination at night

Objective: Diagnostic

Check the following for critical values or changes:

Cardiac biomarkers
Hematocrit, hemoglobin, platelets
Glucose, electrolytes, BUN, creatinine
ECG
Chest x-ray

Objective: Physical Assessment

Inspect and Palpate

Anterior chest wall for pulsations and heaves
Pulses for symmetry, quality, and rhythm

Auscultate

Bilateral BP
Heart for rate, rhythm, and sounds

Objective Data

Physical Assessment

Abnormal assessment findings are described in Table 35.4. A method of recording data from the CV assessment is shown in Table 35.5. A focused assessment is used to evaluate the status of previously identified CV problems and to monitor for new problems. A focused assessment of the CV system is outlined in Box 35.1.

Vital signs. Observe the patient's general appearance and obtain vital signs. Measure BP bilaterally. Readings can vary from 5 to 15 mm Hg between arms. Use the arm with the highest BP for later measurements. Obtain an orthostatic (postural) BP and HR while the patient is supine, sitting with legs dangling, and standing. SBP should not decrease more than 20 mm Hg from the supine to the standing position. HR should not increase more than 20 beats/min from the supine to the standing position.

Blood pressure measurement. We can measure BP with invasive or noninvasive techniques. The invasive technique requires catheter insertion into an artery. The catheter is attached to a transducer, and the pressure is measured directly. Invasive arterial BP monitoring is discussed later in this chapter.

Noninvasive, indirect measurement of BP is done with a sphygmomanometer and stethoscope. The sphygmomanometer has an inflatable cuff and a pressure gauge. We measure BP by auscultating for sounds of turbulent blood flow through a compressed artery (termed **Korotkoff sounds**). The brachial artery is the recommended site for taking a BP.

Proper BP technique, such as using the correct cuff and positioning arm at heart level, is essential for correct readings (Table 35.6). Another noninvasive way to measure BP indirectly is with an automated oscillometric device.

We can assess SBP and pulse using a Doppler ultrasonic flowmeter. The hand-held transducer is positioned over the artery (identified by audible, pulsatile sounds). The cuff is applied above the artery, inflated until the sounds disappear, and then inflated another 20 to 30 mm Hg beyond that point. The cuff is then slowly deflated. The point where sounds return is the SBP.[4]

Peripheral vascular system

Inspection. Inspect the skin for color, hair distribution, and venous pattern. Check the extremities for edema, dependent rubor, clubbing of the nail beds, varicosities, and lesions such as stasis ulcers. Edema in the legs can be caused by gravity, varicosities, or right-sided HF.

Inspect the large neck veins (internal and external jugular) while gradually moving the patient from a supine position to an upright (30 to 45 degrees) position. Right-sided HF can cause distention and prominent pulsations of the neck veins referred to as *jugular venous distention* (JVD).

Palpation. Palpate the upper and lower extremities for temperature, moisture, pulses, and edema bilaterally to assess for symmetry. Look for edema by depressing the skin over the tibia or medial malleolus for 5 seconds. Normally, there is no depression after you release pressure. If pitting edema is present, grade it from 1+ (mild pitting, slight brief indentation) to 4+ (very deep pitting, indentation that lasts a long time).

Palpate the pulses in the neck and extremities for rhythm and force of arterial blood flow. Palpate each carotid pulse

TABLE 35.4 ASSESSMENT ABNORMALITIES

Cardiovascular System

Finding[a]	Description	Possible Etiology[a] and Significance
Inspection		
Central cyanosis	Bluish or purplish tinge in tongue, conjunctivae, inner surface of lips	Inadequate O_2 saturation of arterial blood because of pulmonary or cardiac disorders
Clubbing of nail beds	Loss of normal angle between base of nail and skin	Endocarditis, congenital defects, prolonged O_2 deficiency
Color changes in extremities with postural change	Pallor, cyanosis, mottling of skin after limb elevation. Dependent rubor (reddish blue discoloration). Glossy skin	Chronic decreased arterial perfusion
Jugular venous distention (JVD)	Distended neck (jugular) veins with patient sitting at 30- to 45-degree angle	↑ Right atrial pressure, right-sided HF
Peripheral cyanosis	Bluish or purplish tinge in extremities or in nose and ears	↓ Blood flow from HF, vasoconstriction, cold environment
Splinter hemorrhages	Small red to black streaks under fingernails	Infective endocarditis
Ulcers	*Venous:* Necrotic crater-like lesion, usually at medial malleolus. Slowly healing wound	Poor venous return, varicose veins, incompetent venous valves
	Arterial: Pale ischemic base, well-defined edges usually found on toes, heels, lateral malleoli	Arteriosclerosis, diabetes
Varicose veins	Visible dilated, discolored, tortuous vessels in legs	Incompetent valves in vein
Palpation		
Pulse		
<60 beats/min	Bradycardia	Rest, sleep, athletic conditioning, SA or AV node damage, side effect of drugs (e.g., β-blockers), hypothyroidism
>100 beats/min	Tachycardia	Exercise, anxiety, hypovolemia, shock, need for increased CO, hyperthyroidism
Absent	Lack of pulse	Local atherosclerosis, trauma, embolus
Bounding	Sharp, brisk, pounding pulse	Hyperkinetic states (e.g., anxiety, fever), anemia, hyperthyroidism
Displaced point of maximal impulse (apical pulse)	Palpate (or auscultate) the point of maximal impulse below the 5th ICS and to the left of the MCL	Cardiac enlargement because of coronary artery disease, HF, cardiomyopathy
Irregular	Regularly irregular or irregularly irregular. Skipped beats	Dysrhythmias
Pulsus alternans	Regular rhythm, but strength of pulse varies with each beat	HF, cardiac tamponade
Rigidity	Stiff or inflexible vessel wall	Atherosclerosis
Thready	Weak, slowly rising pulse easily obliterated by pressure	Blood loss, ↓ CO, aortic valve disease, peripheral arterial disease
Thrill	Vibration of vessel or chest wall	Aneurysm, aortic regurgitation, arteriovenous fistula
Extremities		
Asymmetry in limb circumference	Measurable swelling of involved limb	Venous thromboembolism, varicose veins, lymphedema
Cold extremities	Hands and/or feet cold to touch. External covering needed for comfort	Peripheral arterial disease, ↓ CO, severe anemia
Delayed capillary refill	Blanching of nail bed for ≥ 2 sec after release of pressure	↓ Perfusion, anemia
Pitting edema of lower extremities or sacral area	Visible finger indentation after firm pressure, weight gain, tightening of clothing (including shoes), marks or indentations from constricting garments	Interruption of venous return to heart, right-sided HF
Unusually warm extremities	Hands and feet warmer than normal	Thyrotoxicosis
Auscultation		
3rd heart sound (S_3)	Extra heart sound, low pitched, heard in early diastole. Similar to sound of a gallop	Left ventricular failure. Volume overload. Mitral, aortic, or tricuspid regurgitation. Hypertension
4th heart sound (S_4)	Extra heart sound, low pitched, heard in late diastole. Similar to sound of a gallop	Forceful atrial contraction from resistance to ventricular filling (e.g., in left ventricular hypertrophy, aortic stenosis, hypertension, coronary artery disease)

TABLE 35.4 ASSESSMENT ABNORMALITIES—cont'd

Cardiovascular System

Arterial bruit	Turbulent flow sound in peripheral artery	Arterial obstruction or aneurysm
Heart murmurs	Turbulent sounds between normal heart sounds. Note loudness, pitch, shape, quality, duration, timing	Heart valve disorder, abnormal blood flow patterns
Pericardial friction rub	High-pitched, scratchy sound during S_1 and/or S_2 at the apex. Heard best with patient sitting and leaning forward while holding breath at end expiration	Pericarditis
Pulse deficit	Apical HR exceeding peripheral pulse rate	Dysrhythmias, most often atrial fibrillation/flutter or premature ventricular contractions

[a]Limited to common abnormal assessment findings and etiologic factors. (Further discussion of conditions listed is found in Chapters 36 to 42.)

TABLE 35.5 Normal Physical Assessment of Cardiovascular System

Inspection	No pallor or cyanosis. PMI not visible. No JVD with patient at 45-degree angle
Palpation	Skin warm. Capillary refill <2 sec. PMI palpable in 4th ICS at left MCL. No thrills or heaves. Slight palpable pulsations of abdominal aorta in epigastric area. Carotid and extremity pulses 2+ and equal bilaterally. No pedal or sacral edema
Auscultation	S_1 and S_2 heard. Apical-radial pulse rate equal, 72, and regular. No murmurs or extra heart sounds

MCL, Midclavicular line; *PMI,* point of maximal impulse.

separately to avoid vagal stimulation and dysrhythmias. Compare the characteristics of the arteries in the right and left extremities simultaneously to determine symmetry.

When palpating the arteries identified in Fig. 35.6, rate the force of the pulse using the following scale:

0 = Absent
1+ = Weak
2+ = Normal
3+ = Increased, full, bounding

Note the rigidity (hardness) of the artery. The normal pulse feels like a tap, but a narrowed or bulging vessel wall vibrates. The term for a palpable vibration is *thrill.*

We use *capillary refill* to assess arterial flow to the extremities. Position the patient's hands near the level of the heart and squeeze a nail bed briefly to produce blanching. Color should return to the nail bed in less than 2 seconds after release.

Auscultation. Auscultate the carotid arteries, abdominal aorta, and femoral arteries as part of the initial CV assessment. An artery that is narrowed or has a bulging wall may create turbulent blood flow. This abnormal flow can cause a buzzing or humming termed a *bruit.* We can hear it with the bell of the stethoscope over the vessel.

TABLE 35.6 Blood Pressure Measurement

The patient should not have smoked, exercised, or ingested caffeine within 30 min before measurement.

1. Seat patient with legs uncrossed, feet on the floor, and back supported. Bare patient's arm and support it at heart level. There are conditions when an extremity should not be used to measure BP. These include deep venous thrombosis, arteriovenous fistula or graft, peripherally inserted central line (PICC), lymphedema, and limb ischemia.
2. Begin measurement after the patient has rested quietly for 5 min. Ask patient to relax as much as possible and not to talk during the measurement.
3. Use the right cuff size. Follow instructions for fit and placement according to manufacturer's recommendations.
4. Measure and record BP in both arms initially and note any differences. Use the arm with the highest BP and verify the reference point is at the heart.
5. BP should preferably be taken with an oscillometric device. The accuracy of oscillometric devices may be limited if patients are hypertensive, hypotensive, or have dysrhythmias (e.g., atrial fibrillation).
6. Patients with atrial fibrillation may HR variations causing variations in BP, so it is recommended to take 3 different measurements over several minutes to confirm the BP.
7. For manual measurement, inflate the cuff to a pressure 20–30 mm Hg above the patient's usual SBP. If the SBP is not known, estimate the pressure by palpating the brachial pulse and inflating the cuff until the pulse ceases. The pressure noted at this time is the estimated SBP. Inflate the BP cuff 20–30 mm Hg above this number. Deflate the cuff at a rate of 2–3 mm Hg/sec and listen for Korotkoff sounds. There are 5 phases of Korotkoff sounds. The 1st phase is a tapping sound caused by the spurt of blood into the constricted artery as the pressure in the cuff is gradually deflated. This sound is the SBP. The 5th phase occurs when the sound disappears, which is the DBP.
8. Record the SBP and DBP.
9. Provide the patient verbally and in writing with the BP reading, BP goal, and recommendations for follow-up.

Thorax

Inspection and palpation. Begin with a general inspection and palpation. Next, inspect and palpate the areas where the heart valves project their sounds by finding the intercostal spaces (ICSs). The raised notch, the *angle of Louis,* is where the manubrium and body of the sternum join at the level of the 2nd rib. It is palpable in the midline of the sternum. Palpate for the 2nd ICS, then count each ICS to find specific auscultatory areas (Fig. 35.7).

Locate the following auscultatory areas: aortic area in the 2nd ICS to the right of the sternum, pulmonic area in the 2nd ICS to the left of the sternum, tricuspid area in the 5th left ICS close to the sternum, and mitral area in the left midclavicular line at the 5th ICS. A 5th auscultatory area is the *Erb point,* located at the 3rd left ICS near the sternum. Normally, we cannot feel pulsations in these areas unless the patient has a thin chest wall. A heart valve disorder may be present if you feel abnormal pulsations or thrills.

Inspect and palpate the epigastric area on either side of the midline just below the xiphoid process. In a thin person, you may see abdominal aortic pulsations. Normally, you can palpate the aorta here. Next, inspect the precordium, which is over the heart, for heaves. *Heaves* are sustained lifts of the chest wall in the precordial area that you can see or palpate. They may be caused by left ventricular hypertrophy.

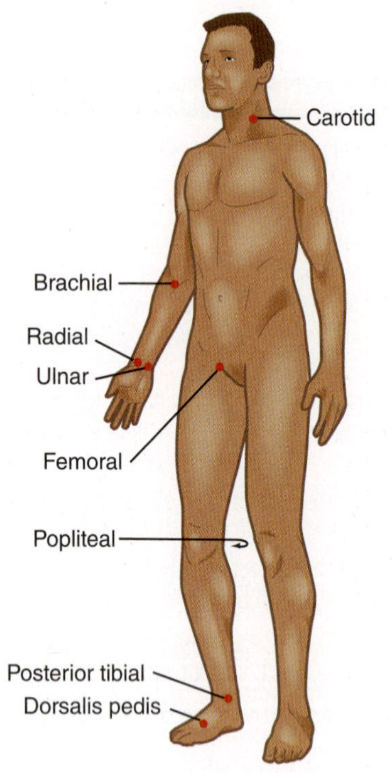

Fig. 35.6 Common sites for palpating arteries.

When the patient is supine, palpate the mitral valve area for the **point of maximal impulse (PMI)** (called the *apical pulse*). This reflects the pulsation of the apex of the heart. The PMI lies medial to the midclavicular line in the 4th or 5th ICS. If you can palpate the PMI, record its position in relation to the midclavicular line and ICSs. If the PMI is below the 5th ICS and left of the midclavicular line, the heart may be enlarged.

Auscultation. Normal heart sounds are made by the movement of blood through the heart valves. We can hear these sounds through a stethoscope placed on the chest wall. The first heart sound (S_1) represents closure of the tricuspid and mitral valves. It has a soft lubb sound. The second heart sound (S_2) represents closure of the aortic and pulmonic valves. It has a sharp dupp sound. S_1 signals the beginning of systole. S_2 signals the beginning of diastole (Fig. 35.8). Listen to the auscultatory areas in sequence (Fig. 35.7).

S_1 and S_2 are heard best with the diaphragm of the stethoscope because they are high pitched. Extra heart sounds (S_3 or S_4), if present, are heard best with the bell of the stethoscope because they are low pitched. Have the patient lean forward while sitting to enhance the sounds from the 2nd ICSs (aortic and pulmonic areas). Place the patient in a left side-lying position to enhance the sounds at the mitral area.

When auscultating the apical area, simultaneously palpate the radial pulse. Determine whether the rhythm is regular or

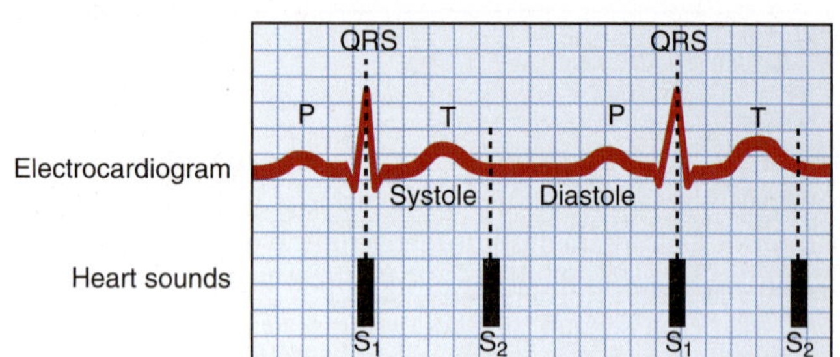

Fig. 35.8 Relationship of ECG, cardiac cycle, and heart sounds.

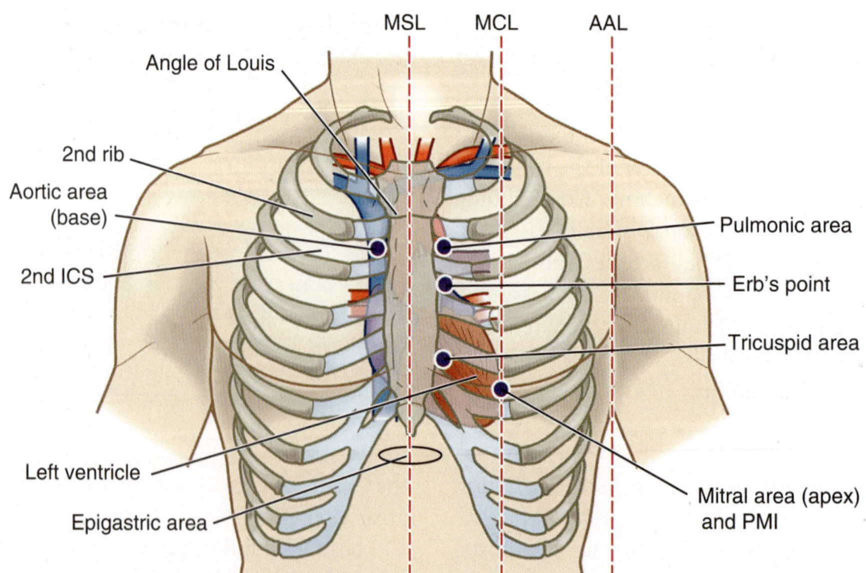

Fig. 35.7 Orientation of the heart within the thorax and cardiac auscultatory areas. *Red lines* indicate the midsternal line *(MSL),* midclavicular line *(MCL),* and anterior axillary line *(AAL). ICS,* Intercostal space; *PMI,* point of maximal impulse.

irregular while listening and feeling. If the apical and radial pulses are not equivalent, count the apical pulse while a 2nd person simultaneously counts the radial pulse for 1 full minute. A difference between the 2 numbers, called a *pulse deficit*, can indicate dysrhythmias.

Normally no sound is heard between S_1 and S_2. An exception to this is a normal splitting of S_2, which is best heard at the pulmonic area during inspiration. Splitting of S_2 can be abnormal if it is heard during expiration or if it is constant (fixed) during the respiratory cycle. Describe any sounds heard in addition to S_1 and S_2.

The S_3 heart sound is a low-intensity vibration of the ventricular walls usually from decreased compliance of the ventricles during filling. An S_3 heart sound may be normal (physiologic) in young adults. It is pathologic in patients with left-sided HF or mitral valve regurgitation. S_3 is heard closely after S_2. It is known as a ventricular gallop.

The S_4 heart sound is a low-frequency vibration caused by atrial contraction. It precedes S_1 of the next cycle and is known as an atrial gallop. An S_4 heart sound may be normal in older adults with no evidence of heart disease. It is pathologic in patients with CAD, cardiomyopathy, left ventricular hypertrophy, or aortic stenosis.

Turbulent blood flow across valve is heard as a whooshing sound or **murmur** between heartbeats. We grade murmurs on a 6-point Roman numeral scale based on loudness and recorded as a ratio. I/VI means a murmur that is barely audible with the stethoscope, heard only in a quiet room and then not easily. VI/VI means a murmur that you can hear with the stethoscope lifted just off the chest wall.

Pericardial friction rubs are sounds that occur when inflamed surfaces of the pericardium (pericarditis) move against each other. They are high-pitched, scratchy sounds that may be intermittent and may last several hours to days. Friction rubs are heard best at the apex with patients upright, leaning forward, and holding their breath after expiration.[5]

Record the characteristics of any abnormal sounds. This includes the timing (during systole or diastole), location (the anatomic site on the chest where it is heard the loudest), and position (heard best when the patient is supine, sitting and leaning forward, or in the left side-lying position).[5] Note any other findings (irregular apical pulse, palpable chest wall heaves) associated with the sound.

HEMODYNAMIC MONITORING

Hemodynamic monitoring is the measurement of pressure, flow, and oxygenation within the CV system. The purpose of hemodynamic monitoring is to assess heart function, fluid balance, and the effects of fluids and drugs on CO. Both invasive (internally placed) and noninvasive (externally placed) devices measure hemodynamic parameters (values). These include systemic and pulmonary arterial pressures, central venous pressure (CVP), pulmonary artery wedge pressure (PAWP) (pulmonary artery occlusive pressure [PAOP]), CO/cardiac index (CI), SV/SV index (SVI), O_2 saturation of the hemoglobin of arterial blood (SaO_2), and mixed venous O_2 saturation (SvO_2).

From these measurements, you can calculate other values. These include the resistance of the systemic and pulmonary arterial vasculature and O_2 content, delivery, and consumption. The combined data provide a picture of the patient's hemodynamic status and the effects of therapy over time (trends). Pay attention to accuracy of measurement to help guide effective treatment.

CASE STUDY

Objective Data: Physical Assessment

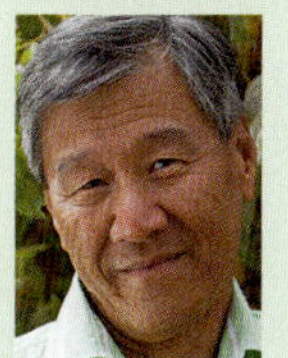

(© Jupiterimages/ Banana-Stock/ Thinkstock.)

Physical assessment findings of L.P. are as follows:

- BP 100/54, HR 154 and irregular, respiratory rate 20, temperature 98.2°F (36.8°C), O_2 saturation 94% on room air
- Awake, alert, and oriented ×3
- Lungs clear on auscultation; systolic murmur present
- Heart monitor shows atrial fibrillation with a rapid ventricular response
- +1 pedal pulses bilaterally
- No peripheral edema, JVD, or heaves noted

Discussion Questions

1. Which physical assessment findings most concern you?
2. Based on the results of the subjective and physical assessment findings, what diagnostic studies do you think will be ordered for L.P.?

You will learn more about diagnostic studies related to the CV system in the next section.

Answers available at http://evolve.elsevier.com/Lewis/medsurg.

Hemodynamic Measurements

Cardiac Output and Cardiac Index

CO is the volume of blood in liters pumped by the heart in 1 minute. **Cardiac index (CI)** is the measurement of CO adjusted for body surface area (BSA). CI reflects the relative CO for the body size. The normal CI is 2.8 to 4.2 L per minute per meter squared ($L/min/m^2$). The volume ejected with each heartbeat is the SV. Like CI, *stroke volume index* (SVI) is the measurement of SV adjusted for BSA.

CO and the forces opposing blood flow determine BP. SVR (opposition encountered by the left ventricle) or *pulmonary vascular resistance* (PVR) (opposition encountered by the right ventricle) is the resistance to blood flow by the vessels. Preload, afterload, and contractility determine SV and thus CO. Table 35.7 presents the formulas and values for common hemodynamic parameters.

TABLE 35.7 Resting Hemodynamic Parameters

Indicators	Normal Range
Preload	
Pulmonary artery diastolic pressure (PADP)	4–12 mm Hg
Pulmonary artery wedge pressure (PAWP) or left atrial pressure (LAP)	6–12 mm Hg
Right atrial pressure (RAP) or central venous pressure (CVP)	2–8 mm Hg
Right ventricular end-diastolic volume (RVEDV) $= \frac{\text{Stroke volume (SV)}}{\text{Right ventricular ejection fraction (RVEF)}}$	100–160 mL
Afterload	
$\text{MAP}^a = \frac{\text{Systolic blood pressure} + 2(\text{Diastolic blood pressure})}{3}$	70–105 mm Hg
$\text{PAMP}^a = \frac{\text{Pulmonary artery systolic pressure (PASP)} + 2(\text{PADP})}{3}$	10–20 mm Hg
Pulmonary vascular resistance (PVR) $= \frac{(\text{PAMP} - \text{PAWP}) \times 80}{\text{Cardiac output (CO)}}$	<250 dynes/sec/cm^{-5}
Pulmonary vascular resistance index (PVRI) $= \frac{(\text{PAMP} - \text{PAWP}) \times 80}{\text{Cardiac index (CI)}}$	160–380 dynes/sec/cm^{-5}/m^2
Systemic vascular resistance (SVR) $= \frac{(\text{Mean arterial pressure [MAP]} - \text{CVP}) \times 80}{\text{CO}}$	800–1200 dynes/sec/cm^{-5}
Systemic vascular resistance index (SVRI) $= \frac{(\text{MAP} - \text{CVP}) \times 80}{\text{CI}}$	1970–2390 dynes/sec/cm^{-5}/m^2
Other	
Heart rate	60–100 beats/min
$\text{CI} = \frac{\text{CO}}{\text{Body surface area (BSA)}}$	2.2–4 L/min/m^2
$\text{CO} = \text{SV} \times \text{HR}$	4–8 L/min
$\text{RVEF} = \frac{\text{SV}}{\text{RVEDV} \times 100}$	40%–60%
Stoke volume $= \frac{\text{CO}}{\text{Heart rate}}$	60–150 mL/beat
Stoke volume index (SVI) $= \frac{\text{CI}}{\text{Heart rate}}$	30–65 mL/beat/m^2
Stoke volume variation (SVV) $= \frac{SV_{max} - SV_{min}}{SV_{mean}}$	<13%
Oxygenation	
Arterial hemoglobin O_2 saturation	95%–100%
Mixed venous hemoglobin O_2 saturation	60%–80%
Venous hemoglobin O_2 saturation	70%

[a]This formula is an approximation because it does not take the heart rate into consideration. The monitor measures the area under the pressure curve and HR to calculate MAP and PAMP.

Preload

Preload is the volume in the ventricle at the end of diastole. Chamber volume measurements are hard to obtain so we use pressure measurements to estimate the volume. Left ventricular preload is the *left ventricular end-diastolic pressure.* PAWP reflects left ventricular end-diastolic pressure under normal conditions (i.e., when there is no mitral valve dysfunction, intracardiac defect, or dysrhythmia). CVP is measured in the right atrium or in the vena cava close to the heart. It is the right ventricular preload or right ventricular end-diastolic pressure when there is no tricuspid valve dysfunction, intracardiac defect, or dysrhythmia.

The clinical measurement of preload is not a direct measure of muscle stretch. The measurement is of the pressure at the time of the peak stretch (end diastole). This pressure indirectly indicates the amount of stretch and the volume. Diuresis and vasodilation decrease preload. Fluid administration increases preload.

Afterload

Afterload refers to the forces opposing ventricular ejection of blood. These forces include systemic arterial pressure, aortic valve resistance, and blood volume and density. SVR and arterial pressure are indices of left ventricular afterload, but they do not include all the components of afterload. SVR is the resistance of the systemic vascular bed. Similarly, PVR and pulmonary arterial pressure are indices of right ventricular afterload. PVR is the resistance of the pulmonary vascular bed (Table 35.7).

Increased afterload often results in a decreased CO and increased O_2 demand. CO can be improved and myocardial O_2 needs reduced by decreasing afterload (i.e., decreasing forces opposing contraction). For example, vasodilator drug therapy (e.g., milrinone) can reduce afterload.

Contractility

Contractility describes the strength of contraction. Increased contractility results in increased SV and increased myocardial O_2 needs. Epinephrine, norepinephrine, isoproterenol, dopamine, dobutamine, digitalis-like drugs, calcium, and milrinone increase or improve contractility. We call these drugs *positive inotropes. Negative inotropes* reduce contractility. These include certain drugs (e.g., calcium channel blockers, β-adrenergic blockers) and clinical conditions (e.g., acidosis).

There are no direct clinical measures of cardiac contractility. Measuring preload (PAWP) and CO and graphing the results indirectly indicate contractility. If preload, HR, and afterload remain constant and CO changes, then contractility changed. Contractility is reduced in the failing heart and with cardiac ischemia.[7]

Noninvasive Hemodynamic Monitoring

Major uses of noninvasive hemodynamic monitoring include (1) detecting early signs and symptoms of pulmonary or cardiac problems, (2) determining cardiac or pulmonary cause of dyspnea, (3) evaluating the cause and managing hypotension, (4) monitoring after removing a PA catheter or justifying insertion of a PA catheter, (5) evaluating drug therapy, and (6) diagnosing rejection after heart transplantation.

Methods to estimate CO noninvasively include pulse wave analysis, thoracic electrical bioimpedance or bioreactance, and pulse wave transit time. Noninvasive finger cuff devices or a sensor over the radial artery provide continuous monitoring through pulse wave analysis. CO and BP are calculated from pulsation and pressure waveform analysis in the distal arteries. Bioimpedance methods use electrodes to sense changes in electrical conductivity of the blood and estimate SV. Pulse wave transit time is the time the pulse wave takes to travel from the heart to the peripheral arteries. It can be measured with a device that includes electrodes and pulse oximetry.[8]

CO can be measured using ultrasound (US) technology. Both transesophageal echocardiography (TEE) and ultrasonic CO monitoring provide consistent values similar to the standard method of thermodilution CO.

Some methods of measuring hemodynamic parameters are less accurate than invasive methods. Noninvasive CO measurement is less reliable when patients have structural changes in the heart anatomy.[9] However, these methods decrease the risks (i.e., sepsis) from invasive methods.[10]

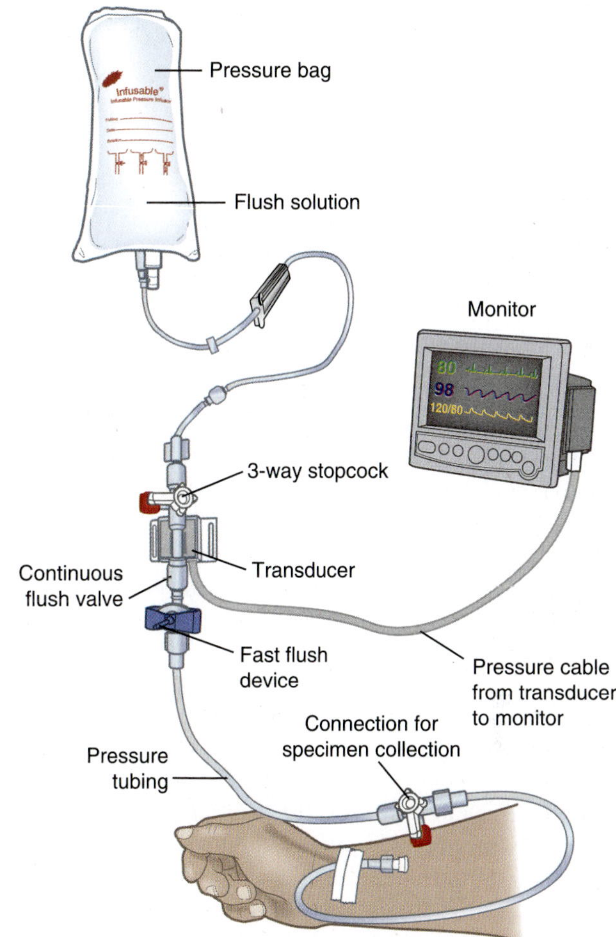

Fig. 35.9 Parts of a pressure monitoring system. The cannula, shown entering the radial artery, is connected via pressure (nondistensible) tubing to the transducer. The transducer converts the pressure wave into an electronic signal. The transducer is wired to the electronic monitoring system, which amplifies, conditions, displays, and records the signal. Stopcocks allow for specimen withdrawal and referencing and zero-balancing procedures. A flush system, consisting of a pressurized bag of IV fluid, tubing, and a flush device, is connected to the system. The flush system provides continuous slow (~3 mL/h) flushing and a mechanism for fast flushing of lines.

Invasive Pressure Monitoring

Invasive lines are used in the ICU to measure systemic and pulmonary BPs. Fig. 35.9 shows the parts of a typical invasive arterial BP monitoring system. The catheter, pressure tubing, flush system, and transducer are disposable.

Pressure monitoring equipment is referenced and zero-balanced to the environment, and dynamic response characteristics are optimized for accuracy. *Referencing* means placing the transducer so that the zero-reference point is at the level of the atria of the heart. The stopcock nearest the transducer is used for the zero reference. To place this level with the atria, use an external landmark, the phlebostatic axis. To find the *phlebostatic axis,* draw 2 imaginary lines with the patient supine

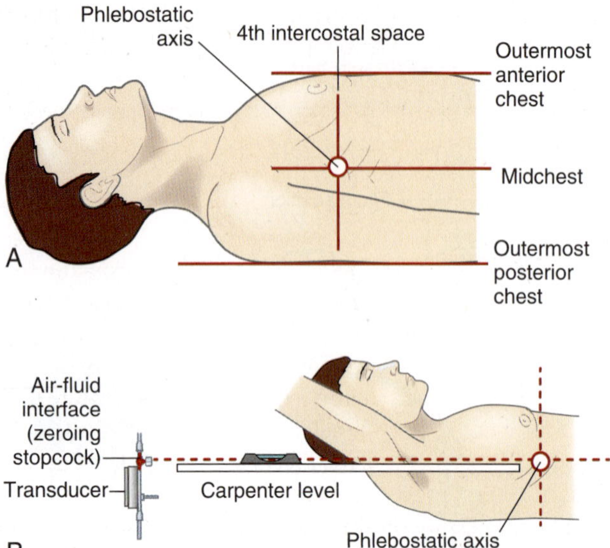

Fig. 35.10 Identification of the phlebostatic axis. (A) Phlebostatic axis is an external landmark used to identify the level of the atria in the supine patient. It is defined as the intersection of 2 imaginary lines: 1 drawn horizontally from the axilla, midway between the anterior and posterior chest walls, and the other drawn vertically through the 4th ICS along the lateral chest wall. (B) Air-fluid interface (zeroing the stopcock) is level with the phlebostatic axis using a carpenter's or laser level.

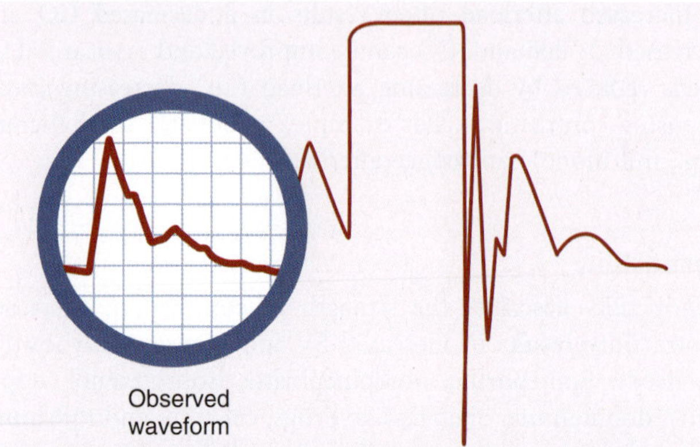

When the fast flush of the continuous flush system is activated and quickly released, a sharp upstroke terminates in a flat line at the maximal indicator on the monitor and hard copy. This is then followed by an immediate rapid downstroke extending below baseline with just 1 or 2 oscillations within 0.12 second (minimal ringing) and a quick return to a baseline. The patient's pressure waveform is also clearly defined with all components of the waveform, such as the dicrotic notch on an arterial waveform, clearly visible.

Fig. 35.11 Optimally damped system. Dynamic response test using the fast flush system: normal response. No adjustment in the monitoring system is needed. (From Darovic GO, Vanriper S, Vanriper J: Fluid-filled monitoring systems. In Darovic GO, editor: *Hemodynamic monitoring,* ed 2, Philadelphia, 1995, Saunders.)

(Fig. 35.10A). Draw a horizontal line from the axilla, midway between the anterior and posterior chest walls. Draw a vertical line laterally through the 4th ICS along the chest wall. The phlebostatic axis is the intersection of the 2 imaginary lines. Mark this location on the patient's chest with a permanent marker. Position the port of the stopcock nearest the transducer level at the phlebostatic axis. Tape the transducer to the patient's chest at the phlebostatic axis, or ideally mount it on a bedside pole (Fig. 35.10B).

Zeroing confirms that when pressure within the system is zero, the monitor reads 0. To do this, open the reference stopcock to room air (off to the patient) and observe the monitor for a reading of 0. This allows the monitor to use the atmospheric pressure as a reference for 0. Zero the transducer during the initial setup, immediately after insertion of the arterial line, when the transducer has been disconnected from the pressure cable or the pressure cable has been disconnected from the monitor and when the accuracy of the measurements is questioned. Always follow the manufacturer's guidelines.

Optimizing dynamic response characteristics involves checking that the equipment reproduces, without distortion, a signal that changes rapidly. Perform a *dynamic response test (square wave test)* every 8 to 12 hours, when the system is opened to air, or when you question the accuracy of the measurements. It involves activating the fast flush and checking that the equipment reproduces a distortion-free signal (Fig. 35.11).[7]

! SAFETY ALERT

Positioning the Zero Reference Stopcock

- Mark the location of the phlebostatic axis on the patient's chest with a permanent marker.
- Recheck the leveling of the zero-reference stopcock to the phlebostatic axis with any change in the patient's position.
- Transducers higher than the phlebostatic axis will produce falsely low BP readings.
- Transducers lower than the phlebostatic axis will produce falsely high BP readings.

Types of Invasive Pressure Monitoring

Arterial BP. Continuous arterial BP monitoring is indicated for patients in many situations. These include acute hypotension and hypertension, respiratory failure, shock, neurologic injury, coronary interventional procedures, continuous infusion of vasoactive drugs (e.g., norepinephrine), and frequent arterial blood gas (ABG) sampling. A nontapered catheter is typically used to cannulate an artery (e.g., radial, femoral) using a percutaneous approach. After insertion, the HCP usually sutures the catheter in place. Immobilize the insertion site to prevent dislodging or kinking the catheter line.

Measurements. Use the arterial line to obtain systolic, diastolic, and mean arterial pressure (MAP) (Fig. 35.12). Table 35.8 outlines the steps in obtaining BP measurements with an invasive line. Values with the head of the bed elevated up to 45 degrees are generally equal to measurements with the patient supine unless the patient's BP is extremely sensitive to orthostatic changes. Keep the zero-reference stopcock level with the phlebostatic axis to ensure accurate continuous measurements.

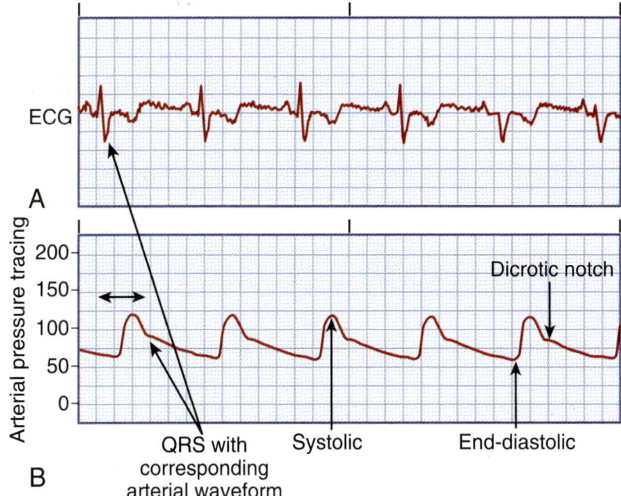

Fig. 35.12 (A) Simultaneously recorded ECG tracing. (B) Systemic arterial pressure tracing. Systolic pressure is the peak pressure. The *dicrotic notch* indicates aortic valve closure. Diastolic pressure is the lowest value before contraction. Mean pressure is the average pressure over time calculated by the monitoring equipment. (Modified from Urden LD, Stacy KM, Lough ME: *Critical care nursing: diagnosis and management,* ed 6, St Louis, 2010, Mosby.)

TABLE 35.8 Invasive Arterial Blood Pressure Measurement

1. Explain the procedure to the patient.
2. Position the patient supine and flat or, if appropriate, with the head of the bed less than 45 degrees or prone.
3. Confirm that the zero reference (port of the stopcock nearest the transducer) is at the level of the phlebostatic axis (Fig. 35.10). If the reference stopcock is not taped to the patient's chest, use a leveling device to position the stopcock on a bedside pole at the point level with the phlebostatic axis.
4. Observe the monitor tracing and assess the quality of the tracing. Perform a dynamic response test (Fig. 35.11).
5. Obtain an analog printout (if available) and measure the systolic and diastolic pressures at end expiration (Fig. 35.12). If no printout is available, freeze the tracing on the oscilloscope screen. Use the cursor to measure the pressures at end expiration.
6. Record the pressure measurements promptly. Include (if available) the printout marked to identify the points read.

Set the high- and low-pressure alarms based on the patient's status. Various patient conditions will change the pressure tracings. In HF, the systolic upstroke may be slower. In volume depletion, systolic pressure varies with mechanical ventilation, decreasing during inspiration. Tracings of the arterial wave may be recorded in the health record. Observe simultaneous ECG and pressure tracings with dysrhythmias. Urgently address dysrhythmias that significantly decrease arterial BP.

Complications. Arterial lines carry the risk for hemorrhage, infection, thrombus formation, neurovascular impairment, and loss of limb. Hemorrhage is most likely to occur if the catheter dislodges or the line disconnects. To avoid this complication, use Luer-Lok connections, monitor the arterial waveform, and activate alarms. If the pressure in the line falls (e.g., when the line is disconnected), the low-pressure alarm sounds immediately, notifying you to promptly correct the problem.

To limit the risk for catheter-related infection, inspect the insertion site for local signs of inflammation. Monitor for signs of systemic infection. Change the pressure tubing, flush bag, and transducer according to agency policy. If you suspect infection, contact the HCP to discuss removing the catheter.

Circulatory impairment can result from formation of a thrombus around the catheter, release of an embolus, spasm, or occlusion of the circulation by the catheter. Before inserting a line into the radial artery, perform an *Allen test* to confirm that ulnar circulation to the hand is adequate. Apply pressure to the radial and ulnar arteries simultaneously. If the patient is able, ask them to open and close the hand repeatedly. The hand should blanch. Release the pressure on the ulnar artery while maintaining pressure on the radial artery. If pinkness does not return within 6 seconds, the ulnar artery is not adequate. You should not use the radial artery on that limb for line insertion.

Once the catheter is inserted, assess the neurovascular status distal to the arterial insertion site hourly. The limb with compromised arterial flow looks cool and pale, with capillary refill time longer than 3 seconds. The patient may have symptoms of neurovascular impairment (e.g., paresthesia, pain, paralysis). This is an emergency and must be reported to the HCP at once to avoid the loss of a limb.

To maintain line patency and limit thrombus formation, assess the flush system every 1 to 4 hours to determine that the (1) pressure bag is inflated to 300 mm Hg, (2) flush bag contains fluid, and (3) system is delivering a continuous slow (1 to 3 mL/h) flush. Follow agency policy for adding heparin to the flush solution.[7]

Arterial pressure–based cardiac output. Arterial pressure–based cardiac output (APCO) measurement is a minimally invasive technique to determine *continuous CO* (CCO)/*continuous CI* (CCI). This technology uses a sensor attached to a standard invasive arterial pressure line and a monitor.

APCO can assess a patient's ability to increase SV in response to fluids *(preload responsiveness)* (Table 35.7). This is determined by using stroke volume variation (SVV) or measuring the percent increase in SV after a fluid bolus. SVV is the variation of the arterial pulsation caused by the heart-lung interaction. It is a sensitive indicator of preload responsiveness in some patients. SVV helps predict whether a patient would benefit from additional IV fluid boluses.[11]

Measurements. *Arterial pressure* is the force generated by the ejection of blood from the left ventricle into the arterial circulation. The heart's contractions (systole) produce pulsatile pressure waves. The sensor measures the arterial pulse pressure, which is proportional to SV. APCO monitoring uses the arterial waveform characteristics, along with demographic data (e.g., gender, age, height, weight), to calculate SV, and HR to calculate CCO/CCI and SV/SVI every 20 seconds. CO is calculated by multiplying the HR and calculated SV. It is displayed on a continuous basis. APCO monitoring is often used with a central venous oximetry catheter. Together, these allow for continuous monitoring of central venous O_2 saturation ($ScvO_2$) and SVR that is derived from the CVP.

Pulmonary artery flow-directed catheter. PA pressure monitoring guides the management of patients with complicated heart and lung problems (Table 35.9). Pulmonary artery diastolic pressure (PADP) and PAWP are sensitive indicators of heart function and fluid volume status. PADP and PAWP increase in HF and fluid volume overload. They decrease with volume depletion. PA pressures can guide fluid therapy volume.

TABLE 35.9 Common Indications and Contraindications for Pulmonary Artery Catheterization

Indications
- Assessment of response to therapy in mixed types of shock
- Cardiogenic shock
- Differential diagnosis and response to therapy in pulmonary hypertension
- MI with complications (e.g., HF, cardiogenic shock)
- Potentially reversible systolic HF
- Severe chronic HF requiring vasoactive drug therapy
- Transplantation workup

Contraindications
- Coagulopathy
- Endocardial pacemaker
- Endocarditis
- Mechanical tricuspid or pulmonic valve
- Right heart mass (e.g., thrombus, tumor)

A PA flow-directed catheter (e.g., Swan-Ganz) is used to measure PA pressures, including PAWP. The standard PA catheter has multiple lumens (Fig. 35.13). When properly positioned, the distal lumen port (catheter tip) is within the PA. We use this port to monitor PA pressures and sample mixed venous blood (e.g., to monitor O_2 saturation).

A balloon connected to an external valve surrounds the distal lumen port. Balloon inflation has 2 purposes: (1) to allow blood to "float" the catheter forward and (2) to allow PAWP measurement. There are 1 or 2 proximal lumens, with exit ports in the right atrium or right atrium and right ventricle (if 2). The right atrium port is used for CVP measurement, injecting fluid for CO measurement, and withdrawing blood specimens. The 2nd proximal port (if available) is for infusing fluids and drugs or for blood sampling. A sensor near the distal tip monitors core temperature and is used for the thermodilution method of measuring CO.

An advanced technology PA catheter can continuously monitor SvO_2. CCO and right ventricular ejection fraction (RVEF) can be measured using advanced thermodilution technology. RVEF gives information about right ventricular function and helps to assess right heart contractility. Right ventricular end-diastolic volume, a key indicator of preload, is assessed by dividing SV by RVEF (Table 35.7).

The HCP often inserts a PA catheter at the bedside. Preparation includes arranging the monitor, cables, and infusion and pressurized flush solutions. The system is leveled and zero-referenced to the phlebostatic axis. Note the patient's electrolyte, acid-base, oxygenation, and coagulation status. Imbalances such as hypokalemia, hypomagnesemia, hypoxemia, or acidosis can make the heart more irritable. This can increase the risk for ventricular dysrhythmia during

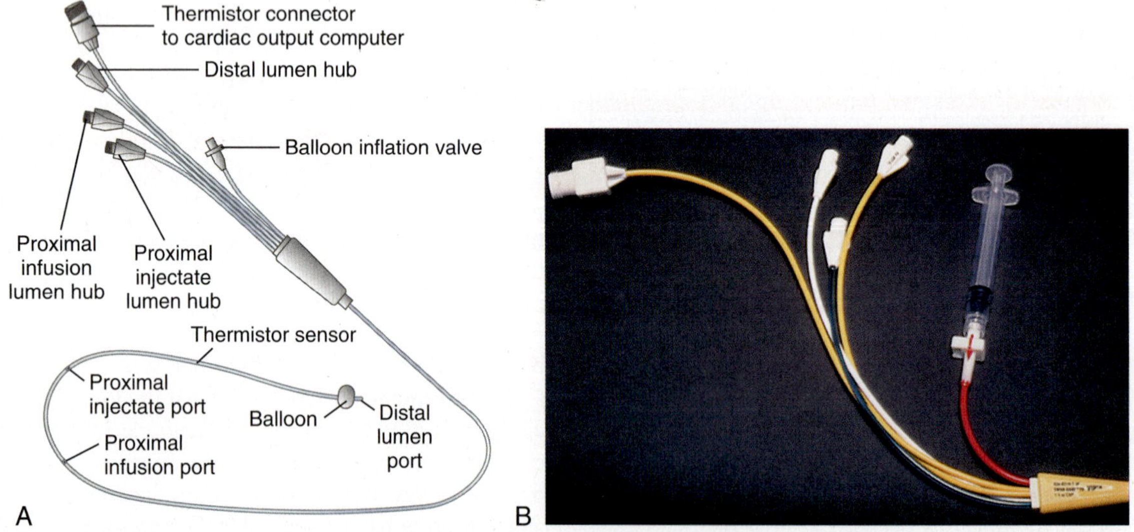

Fig. 35.13 Pulmonary artery (PA) catheter. (A) Catheter with 5 lumens. When properly positioned, the distal lumen exit port is in the PA and the proximal lumen ports are in the right atrium and right ventricle. The distal and 1 of the proximal ports are used to measure PA and CVP, respectively. A balloon surrounds the catheter near the distal end. The balloon inflation valve is used to inflate the balloon with air to allow reading of the PAWP. A thermistor near the distal tip senses PA temperature and measures thermodilution cardiac output when solution cooler than body temperature is injected into a proximal port. (B) Photo of an actual catheter. (B, Courtesy Edwards Critical Care Division, Baxter Healthcare Corporation, Santa Ana, CA.)

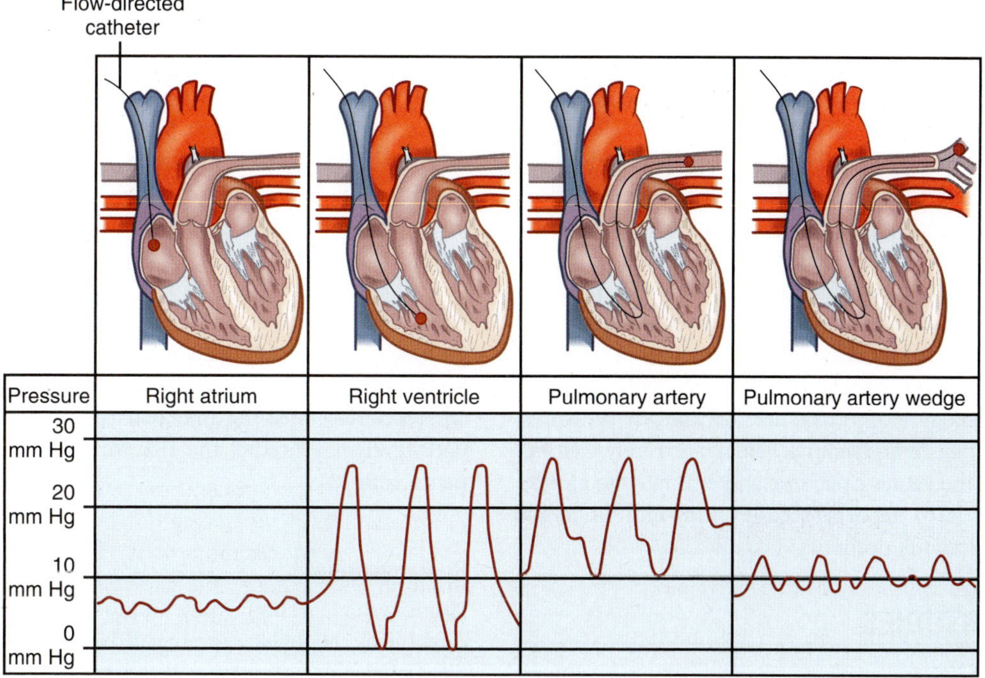

Fig. 35.14 Position of the pulmonary artery flow-directed catheter during progressive stages of insertion with corresponding pressure waveforms. (Modified from Urden LD, Stacy KM, Lough ME: *Critical care nursing: diagnosis and management,* ed 6, St Louis, 2010, Mosby.)

catheter insertion. Coagulopathy increases the risk for hemorrhage.

During insertion, a key nursing role is to observe the characteristic waveforms on the monitor as the HCP moves the catheter through the heart to the PA (Fig. 35.14). Monitor the ECG continuously because of the risk for dysrhythmias, especially when the catheter reaches the right ventricle. After insertion and before using the PA catheter, obtain a chest x-ray to confirm catheter placement. Note and record the measurement at the exit point. Apply an occlusive sterile dressing and change it according to agency policy.[7]

Central venous or right atrial pressure measurement. CVP measures right ventricular preload and reflects fluid volume status. We most often measure it with a central venous catheter placed in the internal jugular or subclavian vein. It can be measured with a PA catheter using the proximal lumen in the right atrium. CVP waveforms (Fig. 35.15) are similar to PAWP waveforms. CVP is measured as a mean pressure at the end of expiration. A high CVP indicates right ventricular failure or volume overload. A low CVP indicates hypovolemia.[11]

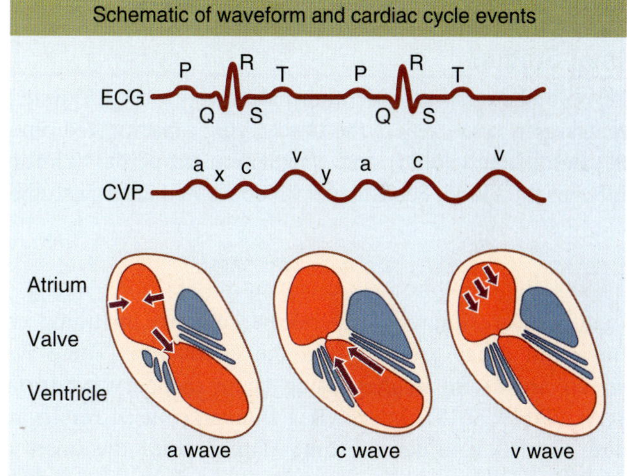

Fig. 35.15 Cardiac events that produce the CVP waveform with *a, c,* and *v* waves. The *a* wave represents atrial contraction. The *x* descent represents atrial relaxation. The *c* wave represents the bulging of the closed tricuspid valve into the right atrium during ventricular systole. The *v* wave represents atrial filling. The *y* descent represents opening of the tricuspid valve and filling of the ventricle. (Modified from Urden LD, Stacy KM, Lough ME: *Critical care nursing: diagnosis and management,* ed 6, St Louis, 2010, Mosby.)

NURSING MANAGEMENT: HEMODYNAMIC MONITORING

Assessment of hemodynamic status requires integrating data from many sources and trending data over time. Comprehensive nursing observations give important clues about the patient's hemodynamic status.

Obtain baseline data about the patient's general appearance, level of consciousness, skin color and temperature, vital signs, peripheral pulses, capillary refill, and urine output. Does the patient appear tired, weak, or exhausted? There may be too little cardiac reserve to sustain even minimum activity. Pallor, cool skin, and decreased pulses may indicate decreased CO.

Changes in mental status may reflect problems with cerebral perfusion or oxygenation. Monitor urine output to determine the adequacy of perfusion to the kidneys. Patients with decreased perfusion to the GI tract may develop hypoactive or absent bowel sounds. If the patient is bleeding and developing shock, the BP may be stable at first. The patient may become increasingly pale and cool from peripheral vasoconstriction. Conversely, patients with septic shock may be warm and pink yet have tachycardia and BP instability. Increased HRs are common in stressed, compromised, critically ill patients. However, sustained tachycardia increases myocardial O_2 demand and can result in decreased CO.

Always correlate your patient observations with data obtained from technology (e.g., ECG, arterial and PA pressures, $ScvO_2$, SvO_2). Single hemodynamic values are rarely helpful. Monitor trends in the values over time and evaluate the clinical picture. The goal is to recognize early clues and intervene before the patient's status declines.[7]

DIAGNOSTIC STUDIES

Many diagnostic tests are available to assess the CV system. Select studies are discussed in detail in this section. Table 35.10 describes common serology studies. Tests that provide information about the structure and function of the heart and CV system are outlined in Table 35.11.

Blood Studies

Many blood studies provide information about the CV system. For example, some reflect the O_2-carrying capacity (red blood cell count, hemoglobin) and coagulation properties (clotting times) of the blood. See Chapter 33 about hematology studies.

Cardiac Biomarkers

When cells are injured, they release contents including enzymes and other proteins into the circulation. These *biomarkers* are useful in diagnosing acute coronary syndrome (ACS) (Table 35.10). Interpreting biomarker level results requires you to consider the time elapsed from the onset of symptoms. Other data (patient symptoms, history, and ECG changes) complete the diagnostic picture for patients with suspected ACS.

Cardiac-specific troponin is a heart muscle protein released into circulation after injury or infarction. Two subtypes, cardiac-specific troponin T (cTnT) and cardiac-specific troponin I (cTnI), are specific to heart muscle. Normally the troponin level in the blood is very low. A rise in level is diagnostic of myocardial infarction (MI) or injury. cTnT and cTnI are detectable within hours (on average 4 to 6 hours) of MI or injury, peak at 10 to 24 hours, and can be detected for up to 10 to 14 days. Troponin is the biomarker of choice in diagnosing ACS. High-sensitivity troponin (hs-cTnT, hs-cTnI) assays provide even earlier detection of a heart event, within 1 to 3 hours.[12]

Copeptin, a substitute marker for arginine vasopressin (AVP), can be detected in patients with an acute MI, ischemic stroke, or HF. Considering both troponin and copeptin levels together may provide increased sensitivity for rapidly diagnosing acute MI. High copeptin levels are associated with increased mortality in patients with acute MI.[13]

C-Reactive Protein

C-reactive protein (CRP) is made by the liver during periods of acute inflammation. Increased CRP levels are linked with atherosclerosis and the first occurrence of a heart event. The CRP level may predict the risk for future heart events in patients with MI.

Homocysteine

Homocysteine (Hcy) is an amino acid made during protein catabolism. High Hcy levels can be either hereditary or from diet deficiencies of vitamin B_6, vitamin B_{12}, or folate. They are linked to a higher risk for CVD, PVD, and stroke. Hcy testing is recommended for patients with a family history of early CVD or a history of CVD in the absence of common risk factors.

Cardiac Natriuretic Peptide Markers

There are 3 natriuretic peptides: (1) atrial natriuretic peptide (ANP) from the atrium, (2) b-type natriuretic peptide (BNP) from the ventricles, and (3) c-type natriuretic peptide from endothelial and renal epithelial cells. BNP is the marker of choice for distinguishing between a cardiac or respiratory cause of dyspnea. N-terminal pro–brain natriuretic peptide (NT-pro-BNP) is secreted in the ventricles and is more sensitive but less specific than BNP as a diagnostic marker of HF. When DBP increases (e.g., HF), BNP and NT-pro-BNP are released and increase natriuresis (excretion of sodium in the urine). ANP and BNP are discussed in Chapter 36 and Chapter 38.

Serum Lipids

Serum lipids consist of triglycerides, cholesterol, and phospholipids (Table 35.10). These *lipoproteins* circulate in the blood bound to protein. A lipid panel usually measures cholesterol, triglyceride, low-density lipoprotein (LDL), and high-density lipoprotein (HDL).

Triglycerides, the main storage form of lipids, make up about 95% of fatty tissue. Cholesterol, a structural part of cell membranes and plasma lipoproteins, is a precursor of corticosteroids, sex hormones, and bile salts. It is absorbed from food in the gastrointestinal tract and synthesized in the liver. Phospholipids contain glycerol, fatty acids, phosphates, and a

TABLE 35.10 Serology Studies

Cardiovascular System

Study	Reference Interval[a]	Description and Purpose
Biomarkers		
b-Type natriuretic peptide (BNP)	<100 pg/mL (100 pmol/L)	Peptide that causes natriuresis. ↑ in HF. Levels ↑ after nesiritide (Natrecor) infusion and for 1 month after cardiac surgery.
CK-MB	Concentrations <4%–6% of total creatine kinase (CK)	Tests for myocardial cell injury. No longer used for diagnosis of acute injury. Serum levels ↑ within 3–6 h after MI, peak after 12–24 hours, normalize within 48 hours.
Copeptin	<10 pmol/L	Reflects arginine vasopressin (AVP) concentration. ↑ Levels highly indicative of MI. Higher in men, after exercise, and with stress. Influenced by fasting and water load.
C-reactive protein (CRP)	High-sensitivity CRP assay. *Lowest risk:* <1 mg/dL *Moderate risk:* 1–3 mg/dL *High risk:* >3 mg/dL	Marker of inflammation. May help predict risk for cardiac disease and cardiac events such as an acute MI. ↑ in bacterial infections and inflammatory disorders.
Homocysteine	4–14 μmol/L Levels may ↑ with age	Amino acid made during protein catabolism. Risk factor for CVD. Associated with vitamin B_{12} and folate deficiencies.
N-terminal (NT)-pro-BNP	*≤74 years:* 124 pg/mL *>75 years:* 449 pg/mL	Helps assess severity of HF. Levels are higher in females and patients with renal insufficiency.
Troponin (cardiac)	*Troponin T (cTnT)* <0.1 ng/mL (<0.1 mcg/L) *High sensitivity Troponin T (hsTnT):* <14 ng/L for women <22 ng/L for men *Troponin I (cTnI)* *Negative:* <0.03 ng/mL (<0.03 mcg/L)	Preferred test for cardiac injury/ischemia: hsTnT assays detect troponins at lower concentrations as early as 90 min, speeding triage in possible MI. After the initial blood sample, blood is collected at 12 h, then daily for 3–5 days.
Lipids		
Cholesterol	<200 mg/dL (<5.2 mmol/L) (varies with age and gender)	Blood lipid associated with arteriosclerosis. ↑ Level is a risk factor for CVD. Nonfasting or fasting.
Lipoprotein (a) (Lp[a])	<30 mg/dL (<0.3 g/L)	↑ Level indicates an increased risk for atherosclerosis, MI, and stroke. Nonfasting or fasting.
Lipoprotein-associated phospholipase A_2 (Lp-PLA_2)	*Low risk:* ≤151 ng/mL *Moderate risk:* 152–194 ng/mL *High risk:* ≥195 ng/mL	Indicates inflammation and increased risk for CAD. Nonfasting or fasting.
Lipoproteins (HDL, LDL)	HDL Recommended *Male:* >45 mg/dL *Female:* >55 mg/dL *Low risk for CAD:* ≥60 mg/dL *High risk for CAD:* <40 mg/dL LDL <130 mg/dL *Moderate risk for CAD:* 130–159 mg/dL *High risk for CAD:* >160 mg/dL	Marked day-to-day fluctuations, so more than 1 level is needed for accurate diagnosis. Nonfasting or fasting. Assess risk for heart disease by dividing the total cholesterol level by the HDL level and obtaining a ratio. *Low risk:* Ratio <3 *Average risk:* Ratio 3–5 *Increased risk:* Ratio >5
Triglycerides	*Male:* 40–160 mg/dL *Female:* 35–135 mg/dL	Mixtures of fatty acids. Elevation associated with CVD and diabetes. Avoid alcohol for 24 h before testing. Nonfasting or fasting.

[a]Reference ranges for the laboratory tests vary by agency because of differences in equipment and reagents used.

nitrogenous compound. Although formed in most cells, phospholipids usually enter the circulation as lipoproteins synthesized by the liver. Apoproteins are water-soluble proteins that combine with most lipids to form lipoproteins.

Different classes of lipoproteins contain varying amounts of naturally occurring lipids. These include:

- Chylomicrons: mainly exogenous triglycerides from fat intake

TABLE 35.11 Diagnostic Studies

Cardiovascular System

Study	Description and Purpose	Nursing Responsibility
Electrocardiography		
12-lead ECG	Electrodes on the chest and extremities record cardiac electrical activity from 12 different views. A resting 12-lead ECG can identify conduction problems, dysrhythmias, position of heart, cardiac hypertrophy, pericarditis, myocardial ischemia or infarction, pacemaker activity, and effectiveness of drug therapy at 1 point in time.	*Before:* Prepare skin. Apply electrodes and leads. Place patient supine (or with head of bed elevated, if short of breath). Tell patient that no discomfort is involved and to lie still to decrease motion artifact. *During:* Ensure the patient lies still to decrease motion artifact.
ECG event monitor or loop recorder	Records rhythm changes that are not frequent enough to be recorded in a 24-h period. Can aid in diagnosing the cause of chest pain, palpitations, dyspnea, and syncope. It allows more freedom than a regular Holter monitor. Some units have electrodes that attach to the chest and have a loop of memory that captures the onset and end of an event. Other types are placed directly on the wrist, chest, or fingers and record the ECG in real time. Recordings may be transmitted over the phone to a receiving unit.	*Before:* Teach how to use equipment for recording and transmitting events. Teach patient about skin preparation for lead placement or steady skin contact to ensure quality tracings. Tell patient to start recording when symptoms begin or as soon after as possible.
ECG Holter monitoring	Recording of ECG rhythm for 24–48 h to correlate with symptoms and activities recorded in diary. Encourage normal patient activity to simulate conditions that produce symptoms. Electrodes are placed on chest. A recorder stores information until it is recalled, printed, and analyzed for any rhythm changes.	*Before:* Prepare skin. Apply electrodes and leads. Explain need to keep an accurate diary of activities and symptoms. Tell patient there is no bathing and showering during monitoring. Skin irritation may develop from electrodes. If device has an event marker, teach patient to push that button when having symptoms.
Signal-averaged ECG (SAECG)	High-resolution ECG that can identify electrical activity called late potentials. Their presence indicates a patient is at risk for developing ventricular dysrhythmias (e.g., ventricular tachycardia).	Same as for 12-lead ECG.
Functional		
6-Minute walk test	Distance patient can walk on a flat surface in 6 min. Measures response to treatments and determines functional capacity for activities of daily living. Useful in those who are debilitated or unable to perform treadmill or exercise bike testing. May be a better measure of fitness for older adults than exercise testing.	*Before:* Tell patient to wear comfortable shoes. Inform patient to carry or pull O_2 if used routinely. *During:* Encourage patient to walk as quickly as possible.
Exercise or stress testing	Provides information on cardiac function and exercise tolerance. A common protocol uses 3-min stages at set speeds and elevation of treadmill belt. The patient can exercise to either predicted peak HR (calculated by subtracting the person's age from 220) or peak exercise tolerance, at which time the test is ended. The test is ended for chest discomfort, significant changes in vital signs from baseline, or significant ECG changes (e.g., ischemia, dysrhythmias). The ECG is monitored after exercise for ischemia and rhythm changes or, if ECG changes occurred with exercise, for return to baseline. Important diagnosing CAD. An exercise bike may be used if the patient is unable to walk on the treadmill.	*Before:* Patient must wear comfortable clothes and shoes for walking or running. Tell patient to report any symptoms. β-Blockers may be held 24 h before the test because they blunt the HR and limit the patient's ability to achieve maximal HR. Caffeine is held for 24 h. Patients must refrain from smoking and strenuous exercise for 3 h before test. Obtain baseline vital signs and 12-lead-ECG. *During:* Monitor vital signs and ECG during each stage of exercise and after until all vital signs and ECG changes have returned to normal or baseline. Monitor patient for any signs of distress (e.g., angina, dyspnea).
Noninvasive hemodynamic monitoring	Obtained using a continuous finger cuff or by thoracic bioreactance/bioimpedance methods. Possible to obtain repeated measurements of SV, CO, and systemic BP.	Minimal to no risk. Patients who need hemodynamic monitoring are likely to be in perioperative settings, critical care units, and emergency departments.

Continued

TABLE 35.11 Diagnostic Studies—cont'd

Cardiovascular System

Study	Description and Purpose	Nursing Responsibility
Imaging		
Chest x-ray	Patient is placed in lateral and posteroanterior (PA) positions to examine lung fields and heart size (Fig. 35.16). Helps diagnosis HF and pulmonary edema and visualize heart size and contour.	*Before:* Ask about frequency of recent x-rays and chance of pregnancy. Provide lead shielding to areas not being viewed. Remove jewelry or metal objects that may obstruct the view of heart and lungs.
Cardiac CT; electron beam CT (EBCT)	Heart-specific imaging technology with or without IV contrast medium. Used to evaluate heart anatomy, coronary circulation, and blood vessels. EBCT, or ultrafast CT, uses a scanning electron beam to quantify calcification in coronary arteries and heart valves (Fig. 35.18). IV contrast may be used if calcium scoring is below threshold level. Used for risk assessment in asymptomatic patients and to assess for heart disease in patients with atypical symptoms potentially related to cardiac causes.	*Before:* Assess for contrast allergy. Explain that patient may feel a warm sensation, salty taste after IV contrast injection, nausea. *During:* Patient must lie still during test.
Cardiovascular magnetic resonance imaging (CMRI)	Noninvasive imaging technique obtains information about heart tissue, EF, aneurysms, CO, and patency of proximal coronary arteries. Measures regurgitant fraction that may determine valve repair or replacement. It does not involve ionizing radiation. Provides images in multiple planes with uniformly good resolution.	*Before:* Check for pregnancy, allergies, and renal function before test. Have patient remove all metal objects. Remove metallic foil patches. Patient may need to fast. Assess for claustrophobia and need for antianxiety medication. Contraindicated for persons with implanted metallic devices or other metal fragments unless noted to be MRI safe. Ask about the presence of staples, plates, dental bridges, or other metal appliances. *During:* Patient must lie completely still during test.
Coronary CT angiography (CTA)	Use of CT with injected IV contrast medium to obtain images of coronary vessels and diagnose CAD. Used to evaluate chest pain and monitor progression of coronary vascular disease.	*Before:* Assess for contrast allergy. Obtain IV access. Remove metal objects before test. The patient may need to fast for several hours prior. A β-blocker may be given before the test to control HR. *During:* Patients must have a regular heart rhythm for accurate testing.
Echocardiogram • Contrast • M-mode • 2-dimensional • Color-flow imaging (duplex) • Real-time 3-dimensional • Pharmacologic echocardiogram	Ultrasound transducer is placed in 4 positions on the chest to record sound waves bounced off the heart. Records direction and flow of blood through the heart and transforms it to audio and graphic data. Measures valve abnormalities, congenital heart defects, wall motion, EF, and heart function. IV contrast agent may be used to enhance images (Fig. 35.17). Pharmacologic echocardiogram is a substitute for the exercise stress test in persons unable to exercise. IV adenosine, dobutamine, or dipyridamole is given over several minutes or regadenoson (Lexiscan) is given as a single bolus over 10 sec while echocardiogram is performed to detect wall motion abnormalities.	*Before:* Place patient in a left side-lying position. Tell patient about procedure and sensations (pressure and mechanical movement from head of transducer). May be difficult to obtain in patients with COPD due to large amount of air between heart and chest cavity. Pharmacologic echocardiogram: *Before:* Obtain baseline vital signs and IV access for injection of drugs. *During:* Monitor vital signs until baseline achieved. Assess for signs and symptoms of distress or side effects (e.g., dyspnea, dizziness, nausea). Aminophylline may be given to prevent or reverse side effects of dipyridamole.
Exercise (stress) nuclear imaging	Identifies cardiac symptoms and rhythm changes and simulates in a safe environment. Nuclear imaging images are taken at rest. Injection is given at maximum HR (usually 85% of age-predicted maximum) on bicycle or treadmill. Patient then continues exercise for 1 min to circulate the radioactive isotope. Scanning is done 15–60 min after exercise. A resting scan is done 60–90 min after initial infusion or 24 h later.	*Before:* Tell patient to eat only a light meal between scans. Some drugs may need to be held for 1–2 days before the scan. Patients should not have caffeine 12 h prior. Obtain IV access. *During:* If targeted maximum HR is not achieved with exercise, test may be changed to pharmacologic imaging.
Magnetic resonance angiography (MRA)	Used for imaging vascular occlusive disease and abdominal aortic aneurysms. Same as MRI but with use of gadolinium as IV contrast medium.	*Before:* Contraindications include allergies to contrast medium and implanted metallic devices or other metal fragments unless noted to be MRA safe. Discuss any implants before scan. Obtain IV access.

Continued

TABLE 35.11 Diagnostic Studies—cont'd

Cardiovascular System

Study	Description and Purpose	Nursing Responsibility
Multigated acquisition (MUGA) (cardiac blood pool) scan	Small amount of blood is removed, mixed with a radioactive isotope (e.g., Technetium-99m [^{99m}Tc sestamibi]), and reinjected IV. With the ECG used for timing, images are obtained during the cardiac cycle. Indicated for patients with MI, HF, or valve disease. Can evaluate the effect of various cardiac or cardiotoxic drugs on the heart and the cardiac EF.	*Before:* Explain procedure to patient. Obtain IV access for removal of blood sample and reinjection of isotope. Start ECG monitoring.
Nuclear imaging	Involves IV injection of radioactive isotopes (^{99m}Tc sestamibi [Cardiolite]). Radioactive uptake is counted over the heart by scintillation camera. Gives information about heart contractility, myocardial perfusion, and acute injury.	*Before:* Remove bra to decrease artifact. Obtain IV access for injection of isotopes. Explain that radioactive isotope used is a small, diagnostic amount and will lose most of its radioactivity in a few hours. Tell patient that they will be lying still on back with arms extended overhead for 20 min. *During:* Repeat scans are done within a few minutes to hours after the injection.
Pharmacologic nuclear imaging	Regadenoson, dipyridamole, or adenosine are given to produce vasodilation for patients unable to tolerate exercise. Vasodilation increases blood flow to well-perfused coronary arteries. Scanning procedure is same. Aminophylline may be given to prevent or reverse side effects of dipyridamole (e.g., dyspnea, dizziness, nausea). Dobutamine is used if vasodilators are contraindicated.	*Before:* Tell patient to avoid caffeine products and theophylline (for regadenoson or dipyridamole testing) for 12 h before. Hold calcium channel blockers and β-blockers for 24 h before the test. *During:* Assess for side effects (dyspnea, dizziness, nausea).
Positron emission tomography (PET)	Highly sensitive in distinguishing viable and nonviable heart tissue. Uses 2 radionuclides. Nitrogen-13-ammonia is injected IV first and scanned to evaluate myocardial perfusion. A second radioactive isotope, fluoro-18-deoxyglucose, is then injected and scanned to show myocardial metabolic function. In the normal heart, both scans match, but in an ischemic or damaged heart, they differ. The patient may or may not be stressed. A baseline resting scan is usually done for comparison.	*Before:* Obtain IV access to inject the tracer substance. Patients should be NPO, except for water and medications, for at least 4 h prior. If exercise is part of testing, patient must fast and refrain from tobacco and caffeine for 24 h before test. Hold glucose-containing IV solutions and change to normal saline. Check blood glucose levels. The glucose level must be between 60 and 140 mg/dL (3.3–7.8 μmol/L) for accurate glucose metabolic activity. *During:* Patient must lie completely still during scan. *After:* Encourage fluids to excrete radioactive substance.
Single-photon emission computed tomography (SPECT)	Determine risk for infarction and any infarction size. Small amounts of a radioactive isotope (e.g., ^{99m}Tc tetrofosmin [Myoview], thallium-201) are injected IV, and recordings are made of the radioactivity emitted over a specific area of the body. Circulation of the isotope can detect coronary artery blood flow, intracardiac shunts, motion of ventricles, EF, and size of the heart chambers.	*Before:* Short fasting period may be needed. Obtain IV access for injection of isotope. Remove all jewelry from chest wall. Start ECG monitoring. *During:* Patient must lie completely still during scan. *After:* Encourage fluids to excrete radioactive substance.
Stress echocardiogram	Combination of exercise test and echocardiogram. Evaluates differences in left ventricular wall motion and thickening before and after exercise with ultrasound. Postexercise images taken within 1 min of stopping exercise.	*Before:* Prepare patient for treadmill or exercise bicycle. Tell patient of importance of timely return to examination table for imaging after exercise.
Transesophageal echocardiogram (TEE)	A probe with an ultrasound transducer at the tip is swallowed while the HCP controls angle and depth. As it passes down the esophagus, it sends back clear images of heart size, wall motion, valve abnormalities, endocarditis vegetation, and possible source of thrombi without interference from lungs or chest ribs. A contrast medium may be injected IV for evaluating direction of blood flow if an atrial or ventricular septal defect is suspected. Doppler ultrasound and color flow imaging can be used concurrently.	*Before:* Tell patient to fast for at least 6 h before test. Remove dentures. *During:* IV sedation is given and throat locally anesthetized. A bite block is placed in the mouth. Monitor vital signs, specifically O_2 saturation and BP. Perform suctioning as needed. *After:* Patient may not eat or drink until gag reflex returns. Monitor patient until sedation resolves. Sore throat is temporary. A designated driver is needed if test is done in the outpatient department.

- Low-density lipoproteins (LDLs): mostly cholesterol with moderate amounts of phospholipids
- High-density lipoproteins (HDLs): about 50% protein and 50% phospholipids and cholesterol
- Very-low-density lipoproteins (VLDLs): mainly endogenous triglycerides with moderate amounts of phospholipids and cholesterol

Increases in triglycerides and LDL are strongly associated with CAD. An increased HDL level is associated with a decreased risk of CAD. HDLs serve a protective role by mobilizing cholesterol from tissues. Although a relationship exists between high serum cholesterol levels and CAD, total cholesterol alone is not enough for an assessment of CAD. A risk assessment is calculated by comparing the total cholesterol to HDL ratio over time. An increase in the ratio means increased risk.

Plasma levels of apolipoprotein A-I (apo A-I) (the major HDL protein) and the ratio of apo A-I to apolipoprotein B (apo B) (the major LDL protein) are stronger predictors of CAD than the HDL cholesterol level alone. Measuring these lipoproteins can be useful in identifying patients at risk for CAD.

Lipoprotein (a), or Lp(a), has been studied for its role as a risk factor for CAD. Increased levels of Lp(a), especially with increased levels of lactate dehydrogenase (LDH), have been linked with atherosclerosis, especially in women.

Lipoprotein-associated phospholipase A_2 (Lp-PLA_2) is an inflammatory enzyme expressed in atherosclerotic plaques. High levels of Lp-PLA_2 are related to an increased risk for CAD.[14]

Electrocardiography

Electrocardiogram

The basic P, QRS, and T waveforms (Fig. 35.4B) are used to assess heart activity. Deviations from the normal sinus rhythm can indicate problems in heart function. There are many types of ECG monitoring, including a resting 12-lead ECG, ambulatory ECG monitoring, and exercise or stress testing (Table 35.11). Continuous ambulatory ECG monitoring provides diagnostic information over a period of time. See Chapter 39 for a complete discussion of ECG monitoring.

Event Monitor

An event monitor is used to record less-frequent ECG events. An event monitor is a portable unit that uses electrodes to store and/or send ECG data. There are 2 types, external and implantable. External event recorders are worn for 1 to 4 weeks. They require electrodes continuously attached to the skin. The patient pushes a button or uses a telephone software application to make a note when symptoms occur. The electrocardiographic activity can be sent in real time to an HCP or analyzed at the end of the wearing period. These devices also can perform a routine pacemaker check over the phone.

An implantable loop recorder is used for patients who may have serious yet infrequent dysrhythmias. This small recorder is implanted through a small incision into the chest wall and can continuously monitor heart activity for several years.

ECG applications are available from a smartphone. By touching special sensors or wearing a smartphone watch, patients can see and record their cardiac rhythms for routine monitoring or for later discussion with the HCP.

Functional Studies

Exercise or Stress Testing

Heart symptoms may occur only with activity because of the demand on the coronary arteries to supply more O_2 to the heart muscle. Exercise testing can evaluate the heart's response to physical stress. This helps to assess CVD and set limits for exercise programs. Exercise testing is used for people who can walk unassisted or use a bicycle. It is also helpful for those with ECGs that limit diagnostic interpretation (e.g., pacemakers) (Table 35.11). ECG and BP are monitored throughout the exercise period for signs of cardiac stress.

Imaging

Chest X-Ray

A radiographic picture of the chest shows heart shape and size and anatomic changes in individual chambers (Fig. 35.16). A chest x-ray records any displacement or enlargement of the heart, extra fluid around the heart (pericardial effusion), and pulmonary congestion (Table 35.11).

Echocardiography

The echocardiogram uses US waves to record the movement of the structures of the heart. US waves directed at the heart are reflected back patterns. *Contrast echocardiography* involves

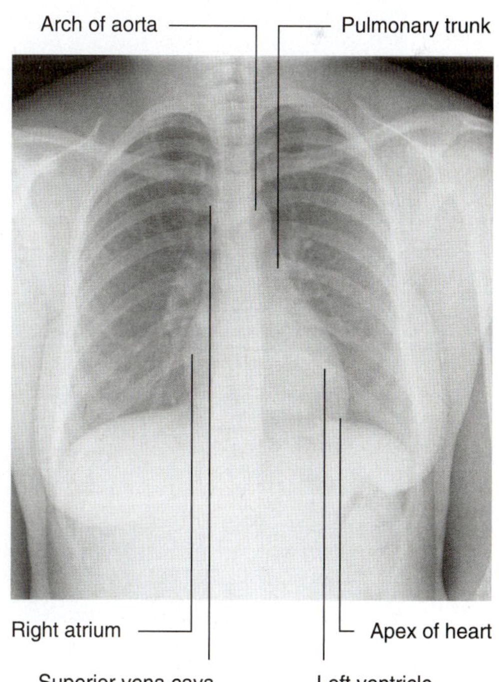

Fig. 35.16 Chest x-ray: standard posterior-anterior view. (From Drake RL, Vogl AW, Mitchell AWM: *Gray's anatomy for students,* ed 2, Philadelphia, 2010, Churchill Livingstone.)

adding an IV contrast agent (e.g., agitated saline) to help define the images, especially in patients with increased body mass.

The echocardiogram provides information about abnormalities of (1) valvular structures and motion, (2) heart chamber size and contents, (3) ventricular and septal motion and thickness, (4) pericardial sac, and (5) ascending aorta. The **ejection fraction (EF)**, or the percentage of end-diastolic blood volume that is ejected during systole, can be measured. The EF provides information about the function of the left ventricle during systole.

The 2D echocardiogram sweeps the US beam through an arc showing correct spatial relationships among the structures. *Color-flow imaging (duplex)* is the combination of 2D echocardiography and Doppler technology (Fig. 35.17). It uses color changes to show the speed and direction of blood flow. This helps to diagnose pathologic conditions, such as valvular leaks and congenital defects. *Real-time 3D ultrasound* uses multiple images with computer technology to provide information about how the structures of the heart change during the cardiac cycle.

Stress echocardiography combines a stress test with an echocardiogram. A digital computer compares images before and after exercise, showing heart wall motion and function. For those persons unable to exercise, IV drugs are used. These include dobutamine, which produces pharmacologic stress on the heart, and dipyridamole, which vasodilates healthy arteries. Unhealthy arteries do not respond as well, which can be seen on the echocardiogram.

A *bubble study* is a type of contrast echocardiography used to check for a defect in the wall between the 2 upper chambers of the heart, such as a patent foramen ovale (PFO). Tiny bubbles in sterile solution are injected into a vein while an echocardiogram scans to detect any passage of the bubbles from the right to left heart. The bubbles are very small, and the bubble solution is absorbed into the bloodstream without endangering the patient.

TEE provides more precise echocardiography of the heart than surface echocardiography. It removes interference from the chest wall and lungs (Table 35.11). The TEE uses a flexible endoscope with a US transducer in the tip to image the heart and great vessels. The scope is passed into the esophagus to the level of the heart. M-mode, 2D, Doppler, and color flow imaging can be obtained.

TEE is used often in an outpatient setting for evaluation of mitral valve disease and for identification of endocarditis vegetation, thrombus before cardioversion, or the source of heart emboli. In addition, TEE is used in the operating room to assess intraoperative heart function and in the emergency department to detect suspected aortic dissection.

The risks of TEE are low. However, complications include perforation or tearing of the esophagus, hemorrhage, dysrhythmias, vasovagal reactions, and transient hypoxemia. TEE is contraindicated if patients have a history of esophageal disorders, dysphagia, or radiation therapy to the chest wall. Patients are sedated during a TEE.

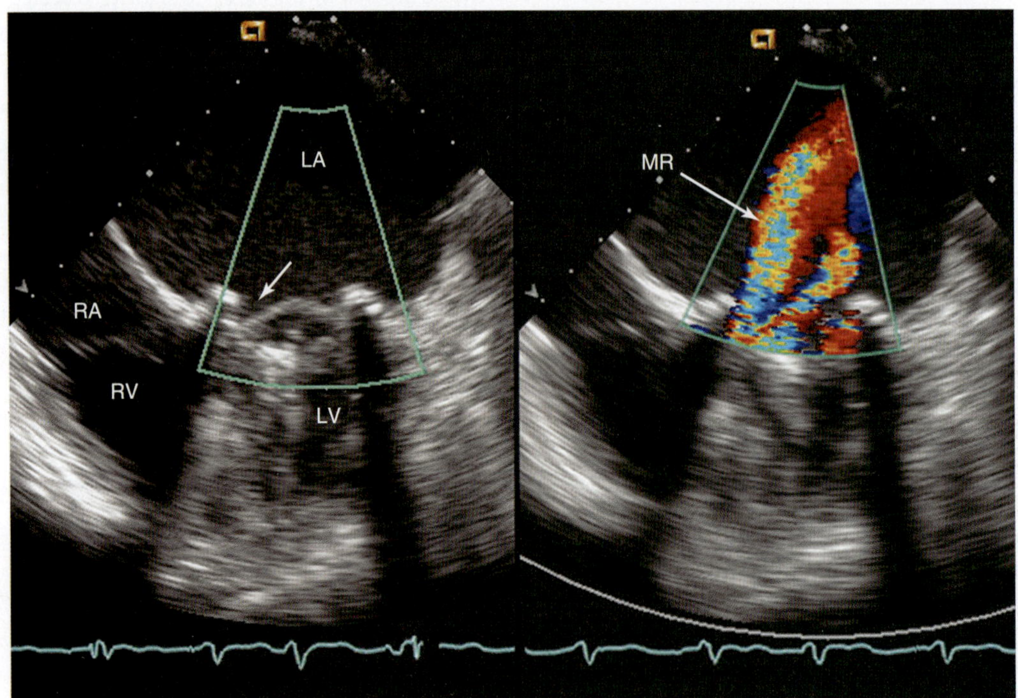

Fig. 35.17 Echocardiogram. Left side, Two-dimensional echocardiography (*black and white*). Right side, Color Doppler echocardiography. The heart is oriented with the ventricles on the lower portion of the picture and the atria on the upper portion. The 4 chambers of the heart are easily identified. The right side of the heart is seen on the left side of the figure. *LV,* Left ventricle; *RV,* right ventricle; *RA,* right atrium; *LA,* left atrium; *MV,* mitral valve leaflets *(white line)* closed during systole. On the color Doppler echocardiogram, the *blue* indicates abnormal reversal of blood flowing from the left ventricle and into the left atrium during systole because of mitral valve regurgitation. *MR,* Mitral regurgitation. (From Pagana KD, Pagana TJ: *Mosby's manual of diagnostic and laboratory tests,* ed 7, St. Louis, 2022, Mosby.)

Cardiac Computed Tomography

Cardiac CT is a heart-imaging test that uses CT technology with or without IV contrast (dye) to see the heart anatomy, coronary circulation, and great blood vessels (e.g., aorta, pulmonary veins, artery). *Multidetector CT (MDCT)* scanning is very fast and provides detailed images. Types of CT scans used to diagnose heart disease include coronary CT angiography (CTA) and calcium-scoring CT scan (Table 35.11).

Coronary CTA is a noninvasive test. It is faster, is less risky, and requires less radiation exposure than cardiac catheterization. Patients must have a normal sinus rhythm for this test. Although the use of coronary CTA is increasing, cardiac catheterization is the gold standard to diagnose CAD. If coronary blockages are found during cardiac catheterization, treatment (e.g., angioplasty, stent placement) can be done during the same procedure.

The calcium-scoring CT scan is used to find calcium deposits in plaque in the coronary arteries. The most common method used is the electron beam CT (EBCT) (Fig. 35.18). It can detect early coronary calcification before symptoms develop and confirm suspected CAD. The amount of coronary calcium predicts the risk of future cardiac events.

Cardiovascular Magnetic Resonance Imaging

Cardiovascular magnetic resonance imaging (CMRI) can detect areas of MI in a 3D view. It is sensitive enough to find even small MIs that are not apparent with single-photon emission computed tomography (SPECT). CMRI aids in the final diagnosis of MI and the assessment of EF. It plays a role in predicting recovery from MI and diagnosing congenital heart and aortic disorders and CAD. One major advantage of CMRI is that it does not expose patients to radiation.

Patients with coronary stents can undergo CMRI 6 weeks after stent placement. CMRI is discouraged in those with older model pacemakers and implantable cardioverter defibrillators (ICDs) because the magnets can change the function of the devices. However, when there is a strong clinical need and the benefits outweigh the risks, CMRI can be done at centers experienced in this procedure. Most newer pacemakers and ICDs are approved for use with MRI.

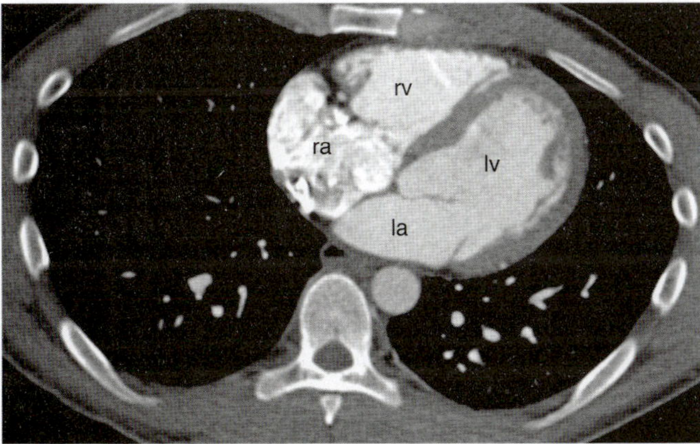

Fig. 35.18 CT scan. At the level of the heart, contrast material is seen filling the right atrium *(ra)* and crossing the atrioventricular (tricuspid) valve into the right ventricle *(rv)*. The thick, muscular left ventricular *(lv)* wall is visualized as it contracts. The left atrium *(la)* is seen anterior to the esophagus. (Kacmarek RM et al: *Egan's fundamentals of respiratory care,* ed 12, St. Louis, 2020, Elsevier.)

Nuclear Cardiology

A common nuclear imaging test is the multigated acquisition (MUGA) or cardiac blood pool scan. This test provides information on wall motion during systole and diastole, heart valves, and EF (Table 35.11).

Perfusion imaging is used with exercise testing to determine whether the coronary blood flow changes with increased activity. This procedure is used to diagnose CAD, make a prognosis in existing CAD, distinguish viable heart muscle from scar tissue, and determine the potential for success of interventions (e.g., coronary artery bypass surgery, percutaneous coronary intervention) (see Chapter 37).

Exercise stress perfusion imaging is an option if a patient cannot exercise. IV regadenoson, dipyridamole, or adenosine can be given to dilate the coronary arteries and simulate the effect of exercise. After the drug takes effect, the isotope (technetium, thallium, sestamibi) is injected for imaging. Patients who are obese or have large breasts may have false-positive results. Patients with severe multivessel coronary disease or blockages in their left main coronary artery may have false-negative results.

Positron emission tomography (PET) stress testing is used due to its high sensitivity for revealing myocardial ischemia. This type of myocardial perfusion imaging is often done using rubidium-82.

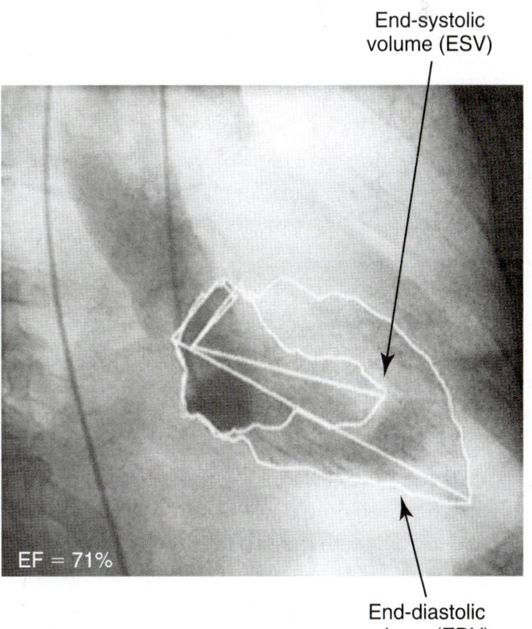

Fig. 35.19 Cardiac catheterization. End-diastolic volume and end-systolic volume used to determine ejection fraction *(EF)*. (From Lough M: *Hemodynamic monitoring: evolving technologies and clinical practice,* St Louis, 2016, Elsevier.)

TABLE 35.12 Interventional Studies

Cardiovascular System

Study	Description and Purpose	Nursing Responsibility
Cardiac catheterization; coronary angiography	Involves insertion of catheter into heart via a vein (for right side of heart) and/or an artery (for left side of heart). Done to evaluate chest pain and obtain information about the heart and major vessels. Measures pressures within the heart chambers. Contrast medium is injected to help see structures and motion of heart. With coronary angiography, contrast medium is injected directly into coronary arteries to evaluate patency and collateral circulation.	Table 35.13.
Electrophysiology study (EPS)	Invasive study to record intracardiac electrical activity using catheters (with multiple electrodes) inserted via the femoral or jugular veins into right side of heart. Catheter electrodes record the electrical activity in different heart structures. Can induce and stop dysrhythmias. Insertion of a pacemaker or implantable cardioverter defibrillator (ICD) or ablation of a dysrhythmia pathway may be done during or right after the EPS. See Chapter 36 for more details.	*Before:* Antidysrhythmic drugs may be stopped several days before. Keep patient NPO 6–8 h before test. Give premedication to promote relaxation if ordered. Obtain IV access. IV sedation often given. *After:* Assess vital signs often. Monitor ECG continuously per agency protocol. Patient will be on bed rest for 6–8 h after procedure.
Fractional flow reserve (FFR)	During cardiac catheterization, a specialized wire is inserted into coronary arteries to measure pressure and flow. Information is used to determine need for angioplasty or stenting on nonsignificant blockages.	Same as for cardiac catheterization.
Intravascular ultrasound (IVUS)	During cardiac catheterization a small ultrasound probe is introduced into coronary arteries. Used to assess blood vessel patency, size and consistency of plaque, arterial walls, and effectiveness of intracoronary artery treatment.	Same as for cardiac catheterization.
Peripheral arteriography and venography	Peripheral vessel blood flow is assessed by injecting contrast media into appropriate arteries or veins (arteriography and venography). Serial x-ray studies done to detect atherosclerotic plaques, occlusion, aneurysms, venous abnormalities, or traumatic injury. Table 41.9 for more peripheral vascular diagnostic studies.	*Before:* Assess for contrast allergy. Explain that patient may feel a warm sensation, salty taste after contrast injection. Patient may have nausea. Give mild sedative, if ordered. *During:* Observe for allergic reaction to contrast media. *After:* Inspect insertion site for bleeding or swelling. Check extremity with puncture site for pulsation, warmth, color, and motion. Encourage fluids to excrete radioactive substance.

Interventional Studies

Cardiac Catheterization

Cardiac catheterization provides information about CAD, coronary spasm, congenital and valvular heart disease, and ventricular function. Cardiac catheterization is used to measure intracardiac pressures and O_2 levels, as well as CO and EF (Fig. 35.19). With injection of contrast media and fluoroscopy, the coronary arteries can be seen, chambers of the heart can be outlined, and wall motion assessed (Table 35.12).

Cardiac catheterization is done by inserting a radiopaque catheter into the right and/or left side of the heart. For the right side of the heart, the HCP inserts a catheter into the femoral, internal jugular, subclavian, or antecubital vein. Pressures are recorded as the catheter is moved into the vena cava, right atrium, right ventricle, and PA. The catheter is then moved until it is wedged or lodged in position. This blocks the blood flow and pressure from the right side of the heart and detects pressure through the pulmonary capillary bed to the left side of the heart (PAWP).

Left-sided heart catheterization is done by inserting a catheter into a radial, femoral, or brachial artery. The catheter is passed in a retrograde manner up to the aorta, across the aortic valve, and into the left ventricle.

Coronary angiography is done with a left-sided heart catheterization. The catheter is positioned at the origin of the coronary arteries (Fig. 35.3), and contrast medium is injected into the arteries. Patients often feel a temporary flushed sensation with dye injection. The images show the location and severity of any coronary blockages (Fig. 35.20 and Fig. 37.15).

Complications of cardiac catheterization include bleeding or hematoma at the puncture site; allergic reactions to the contrast media; looping or kinking of the catheter; infection; thrombus formation; aortic dissection; dysrhythmias; MI; stroke; and puncture of the ventricles, septum, or lung tissue.[15]

Intravascular Ultrasound

Intravascular ultrasound (IVUS), or intracoronary ultrasound (ICUS), is an invasive procedure done in the catheterization laboratory with coronary angiography. The US images provide a

TABLE 35.13 NURSING MANAGEMENT

Care of the Patient Undergoing Cardiac Catheterization

Preprocedure

- Assess for allergies, especially to contrast dye.
- Perform baseline assessment, including vital signs, pulse oximetry, heart and breath sounds, neurovascular assessment of extremities (e.g., distal pulses, skin temperature, skin color, sensation).
- Withhold food and fluids for 6 hours before.
- Assess baseline laboratory values (e.g., cardiac biomarkers, creatinine).
- Teach patient and caregiver about procedure and postprocedure care. Explain the use of local anesthesia at insertion site. Describe the flushed feeling when dye is injected and possible fluttering sensation of heart as catheter is passed.
- Give sedative and other drugs, as ordered.

Postprocedure

- Perform assessment and compare to baseline: vital signs, pulse oximetry, and heart and breath sounds. Note hypotension or hypertension and signs of pulmonary emboli (e.g., respiratory difficulty).
- Assess neurovascular status, including peripheral pulses, color, and sensation, of extremity per agency protocol.
- Place compression device over arterial site to achieve hemostasis, if indicated.
- Observe insertion site for hematoma and bleeding every 15 min for the first hour, then according to agency policy.
- Monitor ECG for dysrhythmias or other changes (e.g., ST segment elevation).
- Monitor patient for chest pain and other sources of pain or discomfort.
- Maintain bed rest as prescribed after femoral access, depending on hemostasis method.
- Maintain IV and/or oral fluid intake and monitor urine output.
- Teach patient and caregiver about discharge care, including signs and symptoms to report to HCP (e.g., site complications, return of chest pain), and any activity restrictions.

cross-sectional view of the arterial walls of the coronary arteries. In IVUS, a miniature transducer attached to a small catheter is moved into the artery to be studied for US imaging. The health of the arterial layers is assessed, including the composition, location, and thickness of any plaque. IVUS can evaluate vessel response to treatments such as stent placement and atherectomy.[15] Patients often have IVUS in addition to angiography or a coronary intervention. Nursing care after IVUS is similar to that for patients after a cardiac catheterization.

Electrophysiology Study

The electrophysiology study (EPS) records and manipulates the heart's electrical activity using electrodes placed inside the heart chambers. It provides information on SA node, AV node, and ventricular conduction. It is helpful in determining the source and treatment of dysrhythmias (Table 35.12). In EPS, catheters are inserted like a right-sided heart catheterization. Nursing care after EPS is similar to that for patients after a cardiac catheterization.[15]

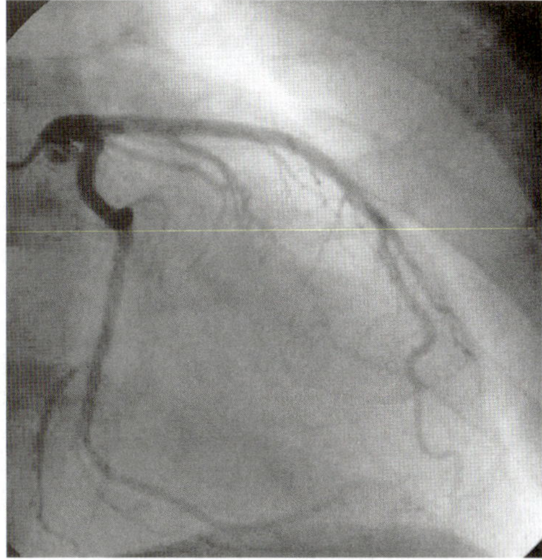

Fig. 35.20 Angiogram showing a normal left coronary and circumflex artery. (From Drake RL, Vogl AW, Mitchell AWM: *Gray's anatomy for students,* ed 2, Philadelphia, 2010, Churchill Livingstone.)

CASE STUDY

Objective Data: Diagnostic Studies

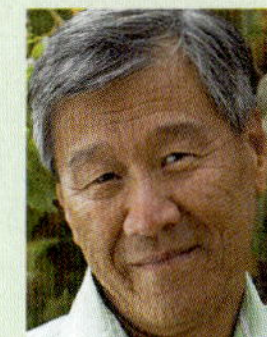

(© Jupiterimages/ Banana-Stock/ Thinkstock.)

The HCP orders the following diagnostic studies for L.P.: f0130

- 12-lead ECG
- CBC, basic metabolic panel (glucose, electrolytes, BUN, creatinine)
- PTT, PT, INR
- Pro-BNP and troponin
- Chest x-ray

The ECG shows atrial fibrillation with a rapid ventricular response. L.P.'s initial troponin levels are within normal limits. Chest x-ray, CBC, and coagulation studies are all within normal limits. The potassium level is 3.1 mEq/L and pro-BNP is high (1204 pg/mL). The HCP orders 250 mL NSS IV bolus; an oral dose of potassium, a loading dose of IV diltiazem followed by a continuous infusion, and weight-based heparin to be started in the emergency department. L.P. will be admitted to the progressive care unit and have a cardiology consult.

Discussion Questions

1. Are these the diagnostic studies that you expected to be ordered?
2. Which diagnostic study results are abnormal?
3. Which diagnostic study results most concern you?

Answers available at http://evolve.elsevier.com/Lewis/medsurg.

BRIDGE TO NCLEX EXAMINATION

The number of the question corresponds to the same-numbered outcome at the beginning of the chapter.

1. Where is the blood flow altered when a patient has a tricuspid valve problem?
   a. Vena cava and right atrium
   b. Left atrium and left ventricle
   c. Right atrium and right ventricle
   d. Right ventricle and pulmonary artery
2. A patient has a severe blockage in the right coronary artery. Which heart structures would the nurse expect to be affected by this blockage? **(Select all that apply.)**
   a. AV node
   b. Left ventricle
   c. Coronary sinus
   d. Right ventricle
   e. Pulmonic valve
3. Which part of the vascular system provides hemostasis?
   a. Thin vessels of the capillaries
   b. Endothelial layer of the arteries
   c. Elastic middle layer of the veins
   d. Smooth muscle of the arterial walls
4. Which homeostatic mechanism is stimulated to compensate for a rise in blood pressure?
   a. Baroreceptors that inhibit the sympathetic nervous system, causing vasodilation
   b. Chemoreceptors that inhibit the sympathetic nervous system, causing vasodilation
   c. Baroreceptors that inhibit the parasympathetic nervous system, causing vasodilation
   d. Chemoreceptors that stimulate the sympathetic nervous system, causing an increased heart rate
5. Which action does the P wave on an ECG represent?
   a. Firing of the SA node and repolarizing the atria
   b. Firing of the SA node and depolarizing the atria
   c. Conduction through the AV node and depolarizing the atria
   d. Conduction through the AV node and spreading to the bundle of His
6. Which subjective data related to the cardiovascular system would the nurse plan to obtain? **(Select all that apply.)**
   a. Annual income
   b. Smoking history
   c. Spiritual preferences
   d. Number of pillows used to sleep
   e. Blood for basic laboratory studies
7. Which heart valve sound is heard best at the left midclavicular line at the level of the 5th ICS?
   a. Aortic
   b. Mitral
   c. Tricuspid
   d. Pulmonic
8. Which condition is likely to cause a pulse deficit of 23 beats?
   a. Dysrhythmia
   b. Heart murmur
   c. Gallop rhythm
   d. Pericardial friction rub
9. Which finding is expected in the assessment of an 81-year-old patient?
   a. Narrowed pulse pressure
   b. Diminished carotid artery pulses
   c. Difficulty isolating the apical pulse
   d. Increased heart rate in response to stress
10. Which patient structure would the nurse align with the transducer to establish accurate hemodynamic monitoring?
   a. Left ventricle
   b. Phlebostatic axis
   c. Inferior vena cava
   d. Midclavicular line
11. Which nursing responsibilities are priorities when caring for a patient returning from a cardiac catheterization? **(Select all that apply.)**
   a. Monitoring vital signs and ECG
   b. Checking the catheter insertion site and distal pulses
   c. Helping the patient to ambulate to the bathroom to void
   d. Teaching the patient about the risks of the isotope injection
   e. Telling the patient that they will be sleepy from the general anesthesia

1. c; 2. a, b, d; 3. b; 4. a; 5. b; 6. b, c, d; 7. b; 8. a;
9. c; 10. b; 11. a, b.

For rationales to these answers and even more NCLEX review questions, visit http://evolve.elsevier.com/Lewis/medsurg.

REFERENCES

To access the References for this chapter, please scan the QR code with a mobile device.

36 Hypertension

Rita Wermers

http://evolve.elsevier.com/Lewis/medsurg/

CONCEPTUAL FOCUS

Adherence
Fluids and Electrolytes
Perfusion
Self-Management

LEARNING OUTCOMES

1. Relate the pathophysiology of primary hypertension to the clinical manifestations and complications.
2. Choose strategies for the prevention of primary hypertension.
3. Describe the interprofessional care for primary hypertension.
4. Explain the interprofessional care of the older adult with primary hypertension.
5. Prioritize the nursing management of patients with primary hypertension.
6. Describe the nursing and interprofessional care of patients with a hypertensive crisis.

KEY TERMS

blood pressure (BP)
elevated blood pressure, Table 36.2
hypertension
hypertensive crisis
orthostatic hypotension
primary hypertension
secondary hypertension
systemic vascular resistance (SVR)

Hypertension, or high blood pressure (BP), is one of the most important modifiable risk factors for the development of cardiovascular disease (CVD). As BP increases, so does the risk for myocardial infarction (MI), heart failure (HF), stroke, renal disease, and vision loss. This chapter discusses the nursing and interprofessional care of patients with or at risk for hypertension. Providing comprehensive care requires you to collaborate with many members of the health care team. Patient education is key to hypertension management. Proper nutrition and exercise are important health promotion behaviors.

Current guidelines reveal that around half of adults in the United States meet the criteria for the diagnosis of hypertension. Heart disease, often directly related to hypertension, accounts for 23.7% of all deaths each year in the United States.[1,2]

Most people with high BP need a combination of medication and lifestyle modifications.[3] Of the 108 million U.S. adults with hypertension, at least 25% do not have their BP in control. Of those with uncontrolled BP, 49% are untreated.

The American College of Cardiology Foundation and the American Heart Association (AHA) provide performance measures for hypertension management. Target goals are based on evidence-based guidelines. These goals consider age and comorbidities when recommending treatment options.[4,5]

National guidelines are designed to apply to all racial and ethnic groups. However, specific groups have higher incidences of risk factors. BP control is strongly affected by social determinants of health. These include lack of access to health care, poverty, and chronic stress.[6] Emerging research highlights the need to include underrepresented populations in clinical and genetic studies.[7]

BLOOD PRESSURE REGULATION

Blood pressure (BP) is the force exerted by the blood against the walls of the blood vessel. It must be adequate to maintain tissue perfusion during activity and rest. Maintaining normal BP and tissue perfusion requires the integration of systemic factors and local peripheral vascular effects. BP is mainly a function of cardiac output (CO) and systemic vascular resistance (Fig. 36.1).

CO is the total blood flow through the systemic or pulmonary circulation per minute. It is determined by the

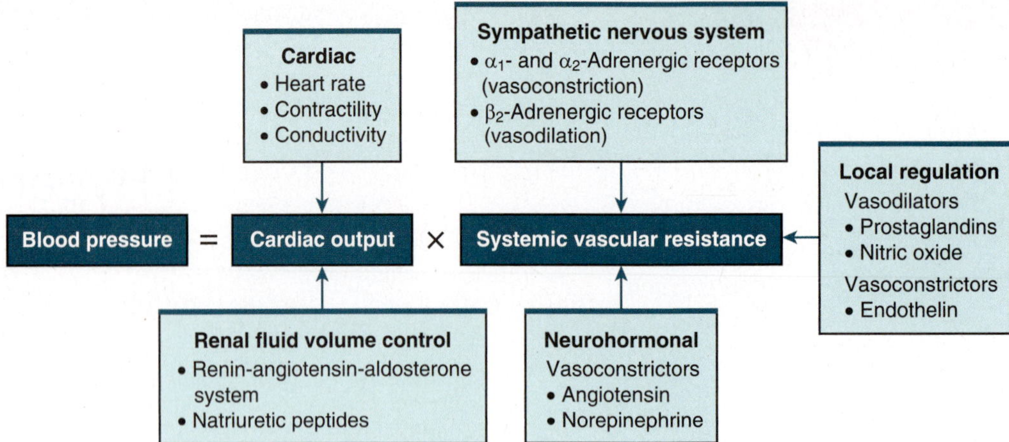

Fig. 36.1 Factors influencing BP. Hypertension develops when one or more of the BP-regulating mechanisms are defective.

stroke volume (SV) or the amount of blood pumped out of the left ventricle per beat (about 70 mL) multiplied by the heart rate (HR).

Systemic vascular resistance (SVR) is the force opposing the movement of blood within the blood vessels. The radius of the small arteries and arterioles is the principal factor determining SVR. As arteries narrow, resistance to blood flow increases. As arteries dilate, resistance to blood flow decreases. A small change in the radius of the arterioles creates a significant change in the SVR. If SVR is increased and CO stays constant or increases, arterial BP will increase.

The mechanisms that regulate BP can affect CO or SVR or both. Regulation of BP is a complex process involving both short-term (seconds to hours) and long-term (days to weeks) mechanisms. Short-term mechanisms, including the sympathetic nervous system (SNS) and vascular endothelium, are active within a few seconds. Long-term mechanisms include renal and hormonal processes that regulate arteriolar resistance and blood volume. In a healthy person, these regulatory mechanisms work in response to the body's demands.

Sympathetic Nervous System

The nervous system, which reacts within seconds after a drop in BP, increases BP by activating the SNS. Increased SNS activity increases HR and cardiac contractility. It causes widespread vasoconstriction in the peripheral arterioles and promotes the release of renin from the kidneys. The net effect of SNS activation is to increase BP by increasing both CO and SVR.

Specialized nerve cells called *baroreceptors* are found in the carotid arteries and arch of the aorta. These cells sense changes in BP and send this information to the vasomotor centers in the brainstem. The brainstem sends this information through complex networks of neurons that excite or inhibit efferent nerves. SNS efferent nerves innervate cardiac and vascular smooth muscle cells. Under normal conditions, a low level of continuous SNS activity maintains vascular tone. BP may be reduced by the withdrawal of SNS activity or by stimulation of the parasympathetic nervous system (PNS). The PNS decreases the HR (via the vagus nerve) and thereby decreases CO.

The neurotransmitter norepinephrine (NE) is released from SNS nerve endings. NE activates receptors in the sinoatrial node, myocardium, and vascular smooth muscle. The response to NE depends on the type of receptors present. SNS receptors are classified as α_1, α_2, β_1, and β_2 (Table 36.1). The smooth muscle of the blood vessels has α-adrenergic and β_2-adrenergic receptors. α-Adrenergic receptors found in the peripheral vasculature cause vasoconstriction when stimulated by NE. β_1-Adrenergic receptors in the heart respond to NE and epinephrine with increased HR (chronotropic), increased force of contraction (inotropic), and increased speed of conduction (dromotropic). β_2-Adrenergic receptors are activated mainly by epinephrine released from the adrenal medulla. They cause vasodilation (Fig. 36.1).

The sympathetic vasomotor center interacts with many areas of the brain to maintain normal BP under various conditions. It is activated during times of pain, stress, and exercise. The SNS response causes an increase in CO and BP to adjust to the body's increased O_2 demands. During the postural change from lying to standing, there is a transient decrease in BP. The vasomotor center is stimulated. The SNS response causes peripheral vasoconstriction and increased venous return to the heart. If this reaction did not occur, blood flow to the brain would be inadequate, resulting in dizziness or syncope.

Baroreceptors

Baroreceptors have a vital role in maintaining BP stability during normal activities. They are sensitive to stretching. When stimulated by an increase in BP, they send inhibitory impulses to the sympathetic vasomotor center. SNS inhibition results in decreased HR, decreased force of contraction, and vasodilation in peripheral arterioles.

When baroreceptors sense a fall in BP, the SNS is activated. The result is constriction of the peripheral arterioles, increased HR, and increased contractility of the heart. In long-standing

TABLE 36.1 Sympathetic Nervous System Receptors Affecting BP

Receptor	Location	Response When Activated
α_1	Vascular smooth muscle	Vasoconstriction
	Heart	↑ Contractility (positive inotropic effect)
α_2	Presynaptic nerve terminals	Inhibit norepinephrine release
	Vascular smooth muscle	Vasoconstriction
β_1	Heart	↑ Contractility (positive inotropic effect) ↑ HR (positive chronotropic effect) ↑ Conduction (positive dromotropic effect)
	Juxtaglomerular cells of the kidney	↑ Renin secretion
β_2	Smooth muscle of blood vessels in heart (e.g., coronary arteries), lungs (e.g., bronchi), and skeletal muscle	Vasodilation
Dopamine receptors	Primarily renal blood vessels	Vasodilation

hypertension, the baroreceptors become adjusted to increased BP levels and recognize this level as their new "normal."

Vascular Endothelium

The vascular endothelium is a single-cell layer that lines the blood vessels. The endothelium is responsible for several critical functions. These include platelet adhesion, coagulation regulation, immune function, and regulating fluid control within the vessel and extravascular space. The endothelium can cause adhesion and aggregation of neutrophils and stimulate smooth muscle growth.

The endothelium is essential to the regulation and maintenance of vasodilating and vasoconstricting substances. Endothelium-derived vasoactive substances include *nitric oxide* (NO) and *prostacyclin*. Both are vasodilators. Another product of the endothelium is *endothelin* (ET). It is a potent vasoconstrictor (Fig. 36.1). CVD risk factors, such as smoking and diabetes, can reduce functional endothelial cells. This can cause arterial tone changes (excess constriction or dilation), which are early warning signals of CVD.

Renal System

The kidneys contribute to BP regulation by controlling sodium excretion and extracellular fluid (ECF) volume (see Chapter 49). Sodium retention results in water retention, which increases ECF volume. This action increases venous return to the heart and SV. Together, these increase CO and BP.

The renin-angiotensin-aldosterone system (RAAS) plays an essential role in BP regulation (Fig. 36.1). The juxtaglomerular apparatus in the kidney secretes renin in response to SNS stimulation, decreased blood flow through the kidneys, or decreased sodium concentration. Renin is an enzyme that converts angiotensinogen to angiotensin I. Angiotensin I is then converted to angiotensin II (A-II) by angiotensin-converting enzyme (ACE). A-II increases BP by 2 different mechanisms (see Fig. 49.4). First, A-II is a potent vasoconstrictor and increases SVR. This results in an immediate increase in BP. Second, over a period of hours or days, A-II increases BP indirectly by stimulating the adrenal cortex to secrete aldosterone.

A-II acts at a local level within the heart and blood vessels. These effects include vasoconstriction and tissue growth that result in remodeling of the vessel walls. These changes are linked to the development of primary hypertension and the long-term effects of hypertension (e.g., atherosclerosis, renal disease, cardiac hypertrophy).

Prostaglandins (PGE_2 and PGI_2) secreted by the renal medulla have a vasodilator effect on the systemic circulation. This results in decreased SVR and lower BP. Heart cells secrete the natriuretic peptides (atrial natriuretic peptide [ANP] and b-type natriuretic peptide [BNP]). They oppose the effects of antidiuretic hormone (ADH) and aldosterone. This results in *natriuresis* (excretion of sodium in urine) and diuresis, resulting in reduced blood volume and BP.

Endocrine System

SNS stimulation results in the release of epinephrine along with a small fraction of NE by the adrenal medulla. Epinephrine increases CO by increasing HR and myocardial contractility. Epinephrine activates β_2-adrenergic receptors in peripheral arterioles of skeletal muscle, causing vasodilation. In peripheral arterioles with only α_1-adrenergic receptors (skin and kidneys), epinephrine causes vasoconstriction.

A-II stimulates the adrenal cortex to release aldosterone. Aldosterone stimulates the kidneys to retain sodium and water, which increases blood volume and CO (see Fig. 49.4).

Increased blood sodium and osmolarity levels stimulate the release of ADH from the posterior pituitary gland. ADH increases the ECF volume by promoting water reabsorption in the distal and collecting tubules of the kidneys. The resulting increase in blood volume causes an increase in CO and BP.

HYPERTENSION

Classification

Table 36.2 shows the BP classifications for people 18 years of age and older.[5] If either the systolic BP (SBP) or diastolic BP (DBP) is outside of a range, the higher measurement determines the classification. For example, 115/86 would be classified as hypertension stage 1 even though the SBP is within normal limits.

TABLE 36.2 Diagnostic Criteria

Classification of Hypertension

Category	Systolic BP (mm Hg)		Diastolic BP (mm Hg)
Normal BP	<120	and	<80
Elevated BP	120–129	and	<80
Hypertension, stage 1	130–139	or	80–89
Hypertension, stage 2	≥140	or	≥90

From Whelton PK, Carey RM, Aronow WS, et al: 2017 ACC/AHA/AAPA/ABC/ACPM/AGS/APhA/ASH/ASPC/NMA/PCNA guideline for the prevention, detection, evaluation, and management of high blood pressure in adults: a report of the American College of Cardiology/AHA Task Force on Clinical Practice Guidelines, *J Am Coll Cardiol* 71:e127, 2018.

TABLE 36.3 Common Causes of Secondary Hypertension

- Cirrhosis
- Coarctation or congenital narrowing of the aorta
- Drug-related: estrogen replacement therapy, oral contraceptives, corticosteroids, nonsteroidal antiinflammatory drugs (e.g., COX-2 inhibitors), sympathetic nervous system stimulants (e.g., cocaine, monoamine oxidase)
- Endocrine problems (e.g., pheochromocytoma, Cushing syndrome, thyroid disease)
- Neurologic problems (e.g., brain tumors, stroke, traumatic brain injury)
- Obstructive sleep apnea
- Pregnancy-induced hypertension
- Renal disease (e.g., renal artery stenosis, glomerulonephritis)

SBP increases with age. DBP rises until around 55 years old and then declines. BP classification is based on 2 or more readings, accurately performed on both arms, on 2 separate occasions.

Etiology

Hypertension can result from primary or secondary causes.

Primary Hypertension

Primary hypertension (*essential* or *idiopathic)* is elevated BP without an identified cause. It accounts for 90% to 95% of all cases of hypertension. There are many contributing factors. These include changes in endothelial function related to vasoconstricting or vasodilating agents, increased SNS activity, overproduction of sodium-retaining hormones, increased sodium intake, greater than ideal body weight, age, family history, ethnicity, diabetes, tobacco use, and excess alcohol use.

Secondary Hypertension

Secondary hypertension is elevated BP with a specific cause that often can be identified and corrected (Table 36.3). It accounts for 5% to 10% of hypertension in adults. Secondary hypertension should be suspected in people who suddenly develop high BP. It is often present in patients with obstructive sleep apnea. Findings in secondary hypertension relate to the underlying cause. For example, an abdominal bruit heard over the renal arteries may indicate renal disease. Treatment is aimed at removing or treating the underlying cause. Secondary hypertension is a contributing factor to hypertensive crisis.

Pathophysiology of Primary Hypertension

BP rises with increased CO or SVR. As hypertension progresses from elevated to stage 1, increases in both blood volume and CO are often present, leading to an increase in SVR. As hypertension progresses, SVR rises, and CO returns to normal. The hemodynamic hallmark of hypertension is a persistently increased SVR. This persistent increase in SVR may occur in several ways. Table 36.4 shows factors that relate to the development or consequences of primary hypertension. Abnormalities of any of the mechanisms involved in maintaining normal BP can result in hypertension (Fig. 36.1).

Water and Sodium Retention

Excess sodium intake is linked to the development of hypertension. Although most people consume a high-sodium diet, only 1 in 3 will develop hypertension. When sodium is restricted in people with hypertension, their BP usually falls. This suggests that some degree of sodium sensitivity may exist for high sodium intake to trigger the development of hypertension. A high sodium intake may activate a number of systemic mechanisms. Fig. 36.2 shows the relationships among salt intake, BP, and changes in heart structure.

In clinical practice, there is not an easy or straightforward test to identify people whose BP will rise with even a small increase in salt intake *(salt sensitive)* versus those who can ingest large amounts of sodium without much change in BP *(salt resistant).* The effect of sodium on BP has a strong genetic component. The effect of sodium is more significant in Black persons and middle-aged and older adults. Salt sensitivity increases the risk of renal problems, endothelial dysfunction, and HF.[8]

Altered Renin-Angiotensin-Aldosterone Mechanism

High plasma renin activity (PRA) increases the conversion of angiotensinogen to angiotensin I (see Fig. 49.4). This change in the RAAS may contribute to the development of hypertension. Any rise in BP inhibits the release of renin from the renal juxtaglomerular cells. Based on this feedback loop, we would expect low levels of PRA in patients with primary hypertension. However, only about 30% have low PRA, 50% have normal levels, and 20% have high PRA. These normal or high PRA levels may be related to excess renin secretion from ischemic nephrons.

Stress and Increased Sympathetic Nervous System Activity

Factors such as anger, fear, and pain influence BP. Physiologic responses to stress are typically protective but may persist,

TABLE 36.4 Risk Factors for Primary Hypertension

Risk Factor	Description
Age	• Systolic BP rises progressively with age • After age 50, SBP >140 mm Hg is a more important risk factor than diastolic BP
Alcohol	• Excess alcohol use is a risk factor • Moderate alcohol use has cardioprotective properties; males should limit their daily intake of alcohol to 2 drinks per day, and 1 drink per day for females
Diabetes	• Hypertension is more common in patients with diabetes • When hypertension and diabetes coexist, complications (e.g., target organ disease) are more severe
Ethnicity	• Incidence of hypertension and resistant hypertension is higher in Black persons • Black persons are more likely to develop hypertension at a younger age and have more severe end organ damage • Black persons have the highest death rate from hypertension
Excess sodium intake	• High sodium intake can • Contribute to hypertension in salt-sensitive patients • ↓ Effectiveness of certain antihypertensive drugs
Family history	• History of a close blood relative (e.g., parents, sibling) with hypertension ↑ risk
Gender	• Before early middle age, hypertension is more common in males. • After age 64, hypertension is more common in females. This is due in part to menopause-related factors, such as estrogen withdrawal, overproduction of pituitary hormones, and weight gain
Increased lipids	• ↑ Cholesterol and triglyceride levels are primary risk factors for atherosclerosis • Hyperlipidemia is more common in people with hypertension
Obesity	• Weight gain ↑ frequency of hypertension • Risk increases with central abdominal obesity
Sedentary lifestyle	• Regular physical activity can help control weight and reduce risk • Physical activity may ↓ BP
Socioeconomic status	• More prevalent in lower socioeconomic groups and among the less educated
Stress	• People exposed to repeated stress may develop hypertension more often • People with hypertension may respond differently to stress than those who do not develop hypertension
Tobacco use	• Smoking tobacco greatly ↑ risk • People with hypertension who smoke tobacco are at even greater risk for CVD

resulting in a prolonged increase in SNS activity. Increased SNS stimulation causes increased vasoconstriction, increased HR, and increased renin release. Increased renin activates the RAAS, leading to elevated BP. People with high levels of repeated stress develop hypertension more often.

Insulin Resistance and Hyperinsulinemia

Defects in glucose, insulin, and lipoprotein metabolism are common in primary hypertension. These defects are not present in secondary hypertension and do not improve when primary hypertension is treated. Insulin resistance is a risk factor in the development of hypertension and CVD. High insulin levels stimulate SNS activity, impair nitrous oxide–mediated vasodilation, promote vascular hypertrophy, and increase renal sodium reabsorption.

Endothelial Dysfunction

Hypertension can manifest as a prolonged vasoconstriction response or as a reduced vasodilator response. High levels of ET may cause prolonged vasoconstriction. Vasodilation effects can be altered by oxygen free radicals, which impair the bioavailability of NO. This leads to cellular dysfunction and an imbalance of the vasodilation and vasoconstriction mechanisms in the endothelium.

Genetic Link

Genetic variations are associated with the development of hypertension. For example, genetic abnormalities can cause a rare form of hypertension characterized by excess potassium levels. Several genetic variants of substances on the endothelium affect BP and the development of hypertension by influencing the body's sensitivity to salt. When endothelial surface proteins are activated, proinflammatory properties are stimulated. This impairs the endothelial cells' ability to activate vasodilatory effects, leading to hypertension.

Research is currently ongoing to understand the complicated role of endothelial dysfunction and genetics in the formation and progression of hypertension. We recommend screening children and siblings of people with hypertension and advising them to adopt healthy lifestyles to minimize their risk for developing hypertension.

Clinical Manifestations

Hypertension is called the "silent killer" because it is often asymptomatic until it becomes severe and target organ disease occurs. Patients with severe hypertension may have a variety of symptoms from the effects on blood vessels in the various organs and tissues or due to the increased workload of the heart. These secondary symptoms include fatigue, dizziness, palpitations, angina, and dyspnea.[9]

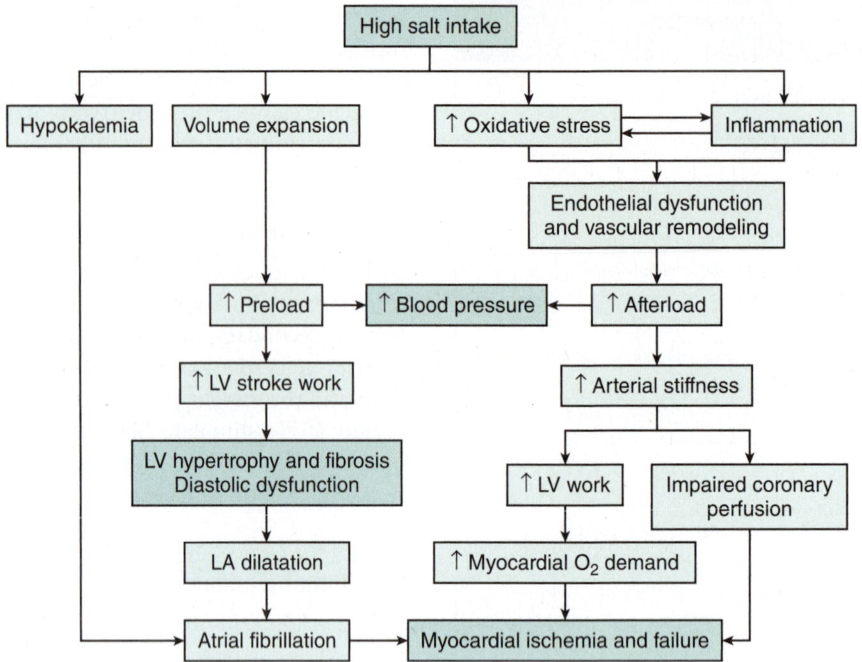

Fig. 36.2 Link among salt intake, BP, and changes in the heart.

Complications

The most common complications of hypertension are *target organ diseases* occurring in the heart (hypertensive heart disease), brain (cerebrovascular disease), peripheral vessels (peripheral vascular disease [PVD]), kidneys (nephrosclerosis), and eyes (retinal damage) (Fig. 36.3).

Hypertensive Heart Disease

Coronary artery disease. Hypertension is a significant risk factor for coronary artery disease (CAD). The "response-to-injury" theory of atherogenesis suggests that hypertension disrupts the coronary artery endothelium (see Fig. 37.1). This results in a rigid arterial wall with a narrowed lumen and may account for the high rate of CAD, angina, and MI.

Left ventricular hypertrophy. Sustained high BP increases the cardiac workload and causes left ventricular hypertrophy (LVH). Initially, LVH is a compensatory mechanism that strengthens cardiac contraction and increases CO. However, increased contractility increases myocardial work and O_2 demand. Progressive LVH, especially in the presence of CAD, can cause HF.

Heart failure. HF occurs when the heart's compensatory mechanisms are overwhelmed, and the heart can no longer pump enough blood to meet the body's demands (see Chapter 38). Contractility is depressed. SV and CO are decreased. Patients may have shortness of breath on exertion, paroxysmal nocturnal dyspnea, and fatigue.

Cerebrovascular Disease

Atherosclerosis is the most common cause of cerebrovascular disease. Hypertension is a significant risk factor for cerebral atherosclerosis and stroke. Even in mildly hypertensive people, the risk for stroke is 4 times higher than in normotensive people. Adequate BP control decreases the risk for stroke.

Atherosclerotic plaques are often found at the bifurcation of the common carotid artery and in the internal and external carotid arteries. Portions of the atherosclerotic plaque or the blood clot that forms with disruption of the plaque may break off and travel to cerebral vessels, producing thromboembolism. Patients may have transient ischemic attacks or a stroke. These conditions are discussed in Chapter 62.

Hypertensive encephalopathy may occur after a marked rise in BP if autoregulation does not decrease the cerebral blood flow. *Autoregulation* is a physiologic process that keeps cerebral blood flow constant despite fluctuations in BP. Typically, as pressure in the cerebral blood vessels rises, the vessels constrict to maintain constant flow. When BP exceeds the body's ability to autoregulate, the cerebral vessels suddenly dilate, capillary permeability increases, and cerebral edema develops. This causes a rise in intracranial pressure. If left untreated, patients can die quickly from brain damage. Chapter 60 reviews cerebral blood flow and autoregulation.

Peripheral Vascular Disease

Hypertension speeds up the process of atherosclerosis in the peripheral blood vessels. This leads to PVD, aortic aneurysm, and aortic dissection (see Chapter 41). *Intermittent claudication* (ischemic leg pain precipitated by activity and relieved by rest) is a classic symptom of PVD.

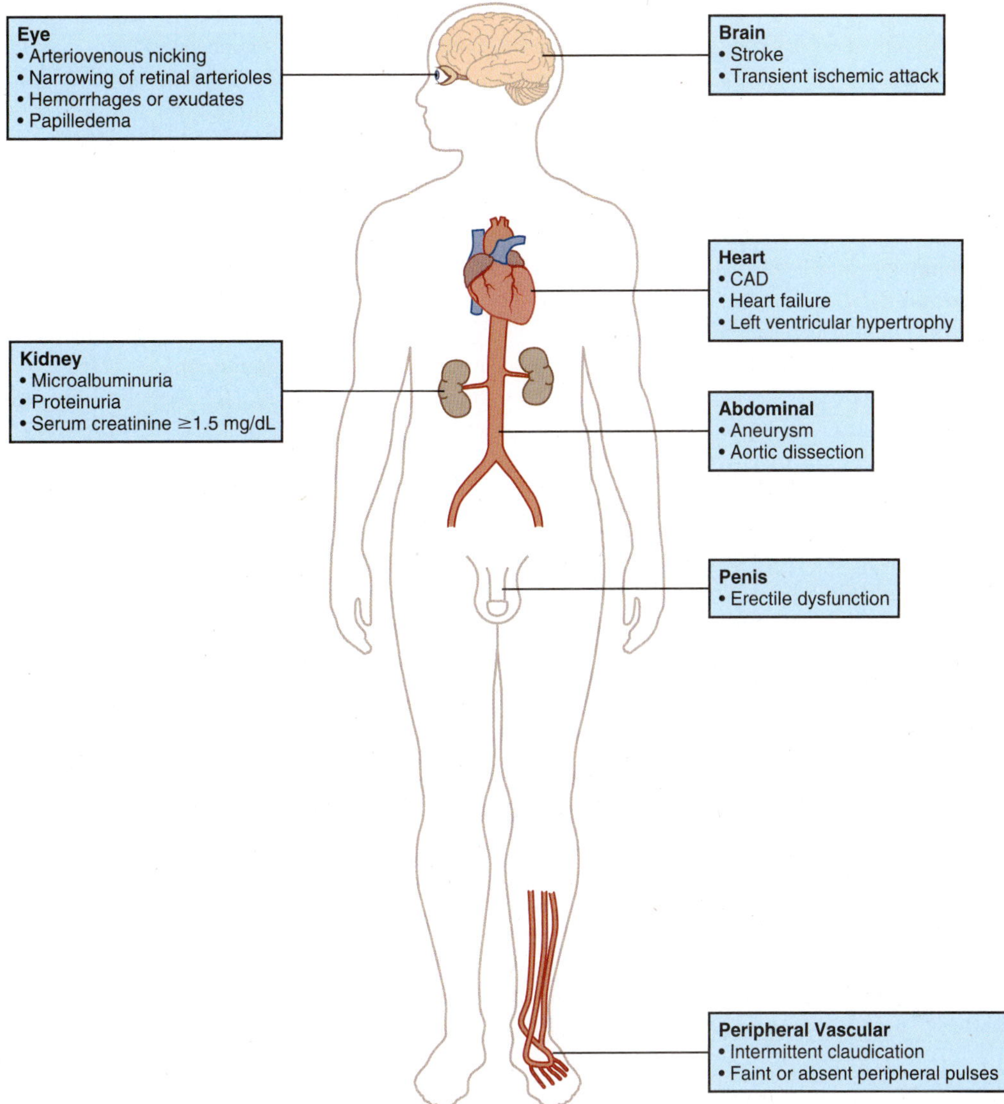

Fig. 36.3 Common complications of hypertension.

Nephrosclerosis

Hypertension is one of the leading causes of chronic kidney disease (CKD). Some degree of renal disease is usually present even with mild hypertension. Renal disease results from ischemia caused by the narrowing of the renal blood vessels. This leads to atrophy of the tubules, destruction of the glomeruli, and eventual death of nephrons. The remaining intact nephrons can compensate, but changes may eventually lead to renal failure. Laboratory signs of renal disease are albuminuria, proteinuria, microscopic hematuria, and high creatinine and blood urea nitrogen (BUN) levels. Nocturia is an early symptom of renal disease (see Chapter 50).

Retinal Damage

Damage to the retinal vessels can be seen with an ophthalmoscope. Manifestations of retinal damage include blurred vision, retinal hemorrhage, and vision loss (Fig. 36.4).

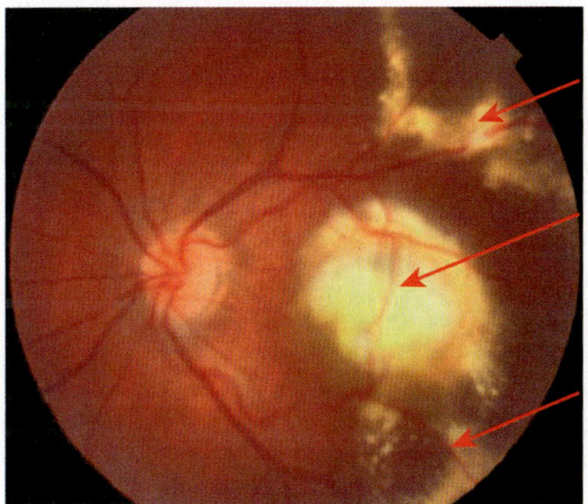

Fig. 36.4 Massive retinal exudates (indicated by *arrows*) from hypertensive retinopathy. To see what a normal retina looks like on ophthalmoscopic examination, see Fig. 22.7. (From Kliegman RM, Behrman RE, Jenson HB, et al: *Nelson textbook of pediatrics,* ed 18, Philadelphia, 2011, Saunders.)

Diagnostic Studies

Measurement of BP is essential in assessing and monitoring hypertension. Chapter 35 and the Nursing Management section later in this chapter discuss BP measurement.

Table 36.5 lists diagnostic studies performed in a person with hypertension. Basic laboratory studies may be done to (1) identify or rule out causes of secondary hypertension, (2) evaluate target organ disease, (3) determine overall cardiovascular risk, or (4) establish baseline levels before starting therapy. Routine urinalysis and BUN and creatinine levels are used to screen for renal involvement. Decreases in creatinine clearance indicate renal insufficiency. Chapter 49 discusses serum creatinine and creatinine clearance.

Measurement of serum electrolytes, especially potassium, is essential to detect hyperaldosteronism, a cause of secondary hypertension. Glucose levels aid in the diagnosis of diabetes. A lipid profile gives information about risk factors related to atherosclerosis and CVD. An ECG can identify the presence of LVH, cardiac ischemia, or previous MI. If LVH is suspected, echocardiography is often done. If the history, physical assessment, or severity of hypertension points to a secondary cause, further testing is needed.

TABLE 36.5 Interprofessional Care

Hypertension

Diagnostic Assessment

- History and physical assessment, including an ophthalmic examination
- Fasting glucose
- Routine urinalysis
- Basic metabolic panel with estimated glomerular filtration rate (eGFR)
- Complete blood count
- Lipid profile (total lipids, triglycerides, HDL and LDL cholesterol, total-to-HDL cholesterol ratio)
- Serum uric acid, calcium, and magnesium
- 12-Lead ECG

Optional

- 24-hour urinary creatinine clearance
- Echocardiography
- Liver function studies
- Thyroid-stimulating hormone (TSH)

Management

- Periodic BP monitoring
  - Home BP monitoring
  - Ambulatory BP monitoring every 3–6 months by an HCP once goal BP is achieved and stabilized
- Nutrition therapy
  - Restrict salt and sodium
  - Restrict cholesterol and saturated fats
  - Maintain adequate potassium and calcium intake
  - Weight management
- Regular, moderate physical activity
- Tobacco cessation (see Tables 11.3 through 11.5)
- Moderate alcohol use
- Stress management techniques (see Chapter 7)
- Antihypertensive drugs (Tables 36.6–36.8)
- Patient and caregiver teaching

Ambulatory Blood Pressure Monitoring

Some patients have high BP readings in a clinical setting and normal readings when BP is measured elsewhere. This phenomenon is referred to as "white coat" hypertension. Ambulatory BP monitoring (ABPM) is one method for diagnosing white coat hypertension. It is a noninvasive, fully automated system that measures BP at preset intervals over a 12- to 24-hour period. The equipment is worn continuously for 24 hours, and results are reviewed by the provider. The monitoring equipment includes a BP cuff and a microprocessing unit that fits into a pouch worn on a shoulder strap or belt. Tell patients to hold their arm still by their side when the device is taking a reading. Have them keep a diary of activities that may affect BP. Other applications for ABPM include suspected antihypertensive drug resistance, hypotensive symptoms with antihypertensive therapy, episodic hypertension, or SNS dysfunction.

BP has diurnal variability. For day-active people, BP is highest in the early morning, decreases during the day, and is lowest at night. BP at night (during sleep) usually drops by 10% or more from daytime (awake) BP.[5] ABPM verifies the presence of diurnal variability.

Some patients with hypertension do not show a typical nocturnal dip in BP. They are referred to as "nondippers." Patients at highest risk for CVD are "reverse dippers." They have an increase in nighttime SBP. Current research is focused on using drugs to optimize cardioprotective effects and convert nondippers and reverse dippers to dippers.

Interprofessional Care

The 2021 scientific statement from the AHA recommends team-based care to control risk factors for atherosclerotic cardiovascular disease (ASCVD).[7] Table 36.5 outlines the interprofessional care for patients with hypertension. Goals include achieving and maintaining goal BP and reducing CVD risk and target organ disease. Lifestyle modifications are a part of therapy for all patients with elevated BP and hypertension.

Lifestyle Modifications

Lifestyle modifications are directed toward reducing patients' BP and overall CVD risk. The AHA's "Life's Simple 7" steps support ways to modify and improve health. These are (1) manage BP, (2) control cholesterol, (3) reduce glucose, (4) get active, (5) eat better, (6) lose weight, and (7) stop smoking. Other modifications address sodium restrictions and alcohol use. Assess social determinants of health as part of lifestyle modifications (see Chapter 2).[7]

Weight loss. Persons who are overweight have an increased incidence of hypertension and increased risk for CVD. Weight loss can have a significant effect on lowering BP. The effect is seen with even moderate weight loss. A rule of thumb is for every 1 kg of weight lost, BP will decrease by 1 mm Hg. When a person decreases caloric intake, sodium and fat intake are usually reduced. Although reducing diet fat content has not shown sustained benefits in BP control, it may slow the progress of atherosclerosis and reduce overall CVD risk. Weight loss through a combination of calorie restriction and moderate physical activity is recommended for patients with hypertension who are overweight.

Nutrition and diet. Plant-based and Mediterranean diets with increased fruit, nut, vegetable, legumes, and lean proteins from fish and vegetables decrease BP and mortality rates from CVD.[10] The Dietary Approaches to Stop Hypertension (DASH) eating plan has been shown to decrease BP.[11]

Sodium reduction. The average adult sodium intake in the United States is around 4200 mg/day in males and 3300 mg/day in females. Healthy adults should restrict sodium intake to 2300 mg/day or less.[8] Adults who consume less than 1500 mg of sodium lower their BP even further.[7]

The patient and caregiver, especially the person who prepares the meals, need to learn about low-sodium diets. Review the patient's typical diet to identify foods high in sodium. The AHA calls 6 food groups that are the highest sodium sources in the United States the "Salty Six." They recommend not adding salt and reducing intake of foods in these groups: bread products, lunch meat and cured meats, pizza, soup, sandwiches, and poultry. Teaching should include reading labels of over-the-counter (OTC) drugs, prepared and packaged foods, and health products (e.g., toothpaste containing baking soda) to identify hidden sources of sodium.

Sodium restriction may be enough to control BP or allow for lower drug dosages in some patients. Moderate sodium restriction lessens the risk for hypokalemia from diuretic therapy. However, the response differs between patients who are salt sensitive or salt resistant.

Increased diet potassium and calcium are associated with lower BP. People with hypertension should receive adequate intake of these from food sources. Calcium supplements are not recommended to lower BP.

Moderate alcohol use. Excess alcohol use is strongly associated with hypertension. Drinking 3 or more alcoholic drinks a day is a risk factor for CVD and stroke. Males should limit their intake of alcohol to no more than 2 drinks per day and females and lighter-weight males to no more than 1 drink per day. One drink is defined as 12 oz of regular beer, 5 oz of wine (12% alcohol), or 1.5 oz of 80-proof distilled spirits. Excess alcohol use that results in cirrhosis is a frequent cause of secondary hypertension.

Physical activity. A physically active lifestyle is essential to promote good health. Adults should perform a minimum of 150 minutes of moderate exercise or 75 minutes of vigorous exercise per week. For those unable to do the minimum recommendation, even some exercise improves BP.[12,13]

Physical activity guidelines are different for adults age 18 to 65 years, adults over 65 years, and adults age 50 to 64 years with functional limitations. The differences relate to the definition of moderate and vigorous aerobic activity. For adults ages 18 to 65, walking briskly at a pace that noticeably increases the pulse defines moderate-intensity aerobic activity. Jogging at a pace that substantially increases the pulse and causes rapid breathing is an example of vigorous activity for this age group. For all other adults, individual fitness levels guide aerobic intensity.[12]

All adults should perform muscle-strengthening activities using the major muscles of the body at least twice a week. This helps to maintain or increase muscle strength and endurance. Flexibility and balance exercises are recommended at least twice a week for older adults, especially for those at risk for falls.[13] Moderate-intensity activities can lower BP, promote relaxation, and decrease or control body weight. Regular activity of this type can reduce SBP by 4 to 9 mm Hg.[5]

Physical activity is more likely to become a habit if it is safe and enjoyable, fits easily into one's daily schedule, and is inexpensive. Many shopping malls open early in the morning, offering a warm, safe, flat area for walking. Some health clubs offer special "off-peak" rates to encourage physical activity among older adults. Some health insurance carriers offer health club discounts as a benefit to encourage member fitness. Cardiac rehabilitation programs offer supervised exercise and education about reducing CVD risk factors.

Help people with hypertension to increase their physical activity by explaining the need for physical activity, describing the types of physical activities, and aiding them in starting an exercise plan. Tell sedentary people to increase activity levels gradually. Those with CVD or other serious health problems need a thorough examination and possibly a stress test before beginning an exercise program.

Avoiding tobacco products. Nicotine contained in tobacco causes vasoconstriction and increases BP, especially in people with hypertension. Smoking tobacco is a major risk factor for CVD. Strongly encourage everyone, especially patients with hypertension, to avoid tobacco use. We see the cardiovascular benefits of stopping tobacco use within a year. Teach those who continue to use tobacco products to monitor their BP regularly. Chapter 11 discusses tobacco use and smoking cessation.

Other risk factors. Risk for hypertension can be related to social determinants of health and psychosocial factors. These factors can contribute to the risk for developing CVD and to a poorer prognosis and clinical course in those with CVD. Social determinants of health include socioeconomic status, resources to meet daily needs, support systems, stress at work and in family life, education, health care access, safe housing, and exposure to violence.[14] These factors have direct effects on the cardiovascular system by activating the SNS and stress hormones. They can contribute to CVD indirectly by their impact on lifestyle behaviors and choices.

Screening is essential so appropriate referrals can be given to help the patient and family. Referrals might include counseling, behavior interventions such as community or religious support systems, social work assistance for finding resources such as fresh fruits and vegetables, or information on housing assistance. Once basic needs are met, beneficial options might include relaxation training, stress management, support groups, and exercise training.[15]

Drug Therapy

These are the current recommendations for antihypertensive drug therapy[5]:

- In patients 65 years or older with an average SBP of more than 130 mm Hg who are ambulatory and living in a community setting rather than living in a skilled agency, treatment goals should be to obtain an SBP less than 130 mm Hg.
- In patients 65 years or older with an average SBP of more than 130 mm Hg who live in a skilled agency, and/or have multiple comorbidities or limited life expectancy, treatment should be based on patient preference, clinical experiences, and team input.
- In patients over 18 years old with hypertension, known CVD, or other risk factors, a BP of 130/80 mm Hg is the goal of treatment.
- In all other patients without CVD or other risk factors, a BP of less than 130/80 mm Hg may be reasonable.

Drugs currently available for treating hypertension have 2 primary actions: (1) decrease the volume of circulating blood and (2) reduce SVR (Tables 36.6, 36.7, and 36.8).[5]

TABLE 36.6 Drug Therapy

Antihypertensive Agents

Drug	Mechanism of Action	Nursing Considerations
Adrenergic Inhibitors		
Central-Acting α-Adrenergic Agonists		
clonidine (Catapres) clonidine patch (Catapres-TTS)	↓ Sympathetic outflow from central nervous system ↓ Peripheral sympathetic tone, produces vasodilation, ↓ SVR and BP	Sudden discontinuation may cause withdrawal syndrome, including rebound hypertension, ↑ HR, headache, tremors, apprehension, sweating Chewing gum or hard candy may relieve dry mouth Alcohol and sedatives ↑ sedation Transdermal patch may be related to fewer side effects and better adherence
guanfacine	Same as clonidine	Same as clonidine, but not available in the transdermal formulation
methyldopa	Same as clonidine	Teach patient about daytime sedation and avoiding hazardous activities Taking a single daily dose at bedtime minimizes the sedative effect Avoid use in older adults
α_1-Adrenergic Blockers		
doxazosin (Cardura) prazosin (Minipress) terazosin	Block α_1-adrenergic effects, producing peripheral vasodilation (↓ SVR and BP) Beneficial effects on lipid profile	↓ Resistance to the outflow of urine in benign prostatic hyperplasia Take at bedtime to reduce risk associated with orthostatic hypotension
phentolamine	Blocks α_1-adrenergic receptors, resulting in peripheral vasodilation (↓ SVR and BP)	Used short-term to manage pheochromocytoma Used locally to prevent necrosis of skin and subcutaneous tissue after extravasation of adrenergic drug No oral formulation
β-Adrenergic Blockers		
Cardioselective Blockers		
acebutolol atenolol (Tenormin) betaxolol bisoprolol esmolol (Brevibloc) metoprolol (Lopressor)	Block β_1-adrenergic receptors (Table 36.1) ↓ BP by blocking β-adrenergic effects ↓ CO and sympathetic vasoconstrictor tone ↓ Renin secretion by kidneys	Monitor pulse and BP regularly Use with caution in patients with diabetes because may depress the tachycardia associated with hypoglycemia and adversely affect glucose metabolism Use with caution in patients with bronchospastic disease Drug of choice for patients with a history of an MI or HF Esmolol is for IV use only Lose cardioselectivity at higher doses
Noncardioselective Blockers		
nadolol (Corgard) pindolol propranolol (Inderal)	Block β_1- and β_2-adrenergic receptors (Table 36.1) ↓ BP by blocking β_1- and β_2-adrenergic effects	Same as cardioselective, except may cause bronchospasm, especially in patients with a history of asthma Sudden discontinuation may cause withdrawal syndrome
Mixed α-Blockers and β-Blockers		
carvedilol (Coreg) labetalol	α_1-, β_1-, and β_2-adrenergic blocking properties producing peripheral vasodilation and ↓ HR (Table 36.1) ↓ CO, SVR, and BP	Same as β-blockers IV form is available for hypertensive crisis in hospitalized patients Keep patient supine during IV administration Assess for severe orthostatic hypotension before allowing upright activities (e.g., commode)

TABLE 36.6 Drug Therapy—cont'd

Antihypertensive Agents

Drug	Mechanism of Action	Nursing Considerations
Angiotensin Inhibitors		
Angiotensin-Converting Enzyme (ACE) Inhibitors		
benazepril (Lotensin) captopril enalapril (Vasotec) fosinopril lisinopril (Zestril) moexipril perindopril quinapril (Accupril) ramipril (Altace) trandolapril	Inhibit ACE, ↓ conversion of angiotensin I to angiotensin II (A-II) Inhibit A-II—mediated vasoconstriction	Aspirin and NSAIDs may ↓ effectiveness Adding a diuretic enhances effect, but should not be used with potassium-sparing diuretics Risk for adverse renal effects and/or hyperkalemia when taken with NSAIDs aldosterone antagonists Can ↑ creatinine Inhibit breakdown of bradykinin, which may cause a dry, hacking cough that can occur at any point during treatment, even years later With pregnancy, discontinue as soon as possible Captopril may be given orally for hypertensive crisis
Angiotensin II Receptor Blockers (ARBs)		
azilsartan (Edarbi) candesartan (Atacand) irbesartan (Avapro) losartan (Cozaar) olmesartan (Benicar) telmisartan (Micardis) valsartan (Diovan)	Prevent action of A-II Produce vasodilation ↑ Na^+ and water excretion	Full effect on BP may not be seen for 3–6 weeks Do not affect bradykinin levels, therefore an acceptable alternative to ACE inhibitors in people who develop a dry cough In patients with kidney disease, ACE inhibitors and ARBs should not be used together due to adverse renal effects With pregnancy, discontinue as soon as possible Risk for adverse renal effects and/or hyperkalemia when taken with NSAIDs
Calcium Channel Blockers (CCBs)		
Non-Dihydropyridines		
diltiazem extended release (Cardizem LA) verapamil intermediate release (Calan SR) verapamil timed-release (Verelan PM)	Inhibit movement of Ca^{2+} across cell membrane, resulting in vasodilation Cardioselective resulting in a ↓ in HR and slowing of AV conduction	Use with caution in patients with HF Grapefruit juice may ↑ concentrations and toxicity of certain CCBs; avoid concurrent use Used for supraventricular tachydysrhythmias Avoid in patients with second- or third-degree AV block or left ventricular systolic dysfunction
Dihydropyridines		
amlodipine (Norvasc) clevidipine (Cleviprex) felodipine isradipine nicardipine sustained release nifedipine long acting (Procardia XL) nisoldipine (Sular)	Cause vascular smooth muscle relaxation resulting in ↓ SVR and arterial BP	More potent peripheral vasodilators Clevidipine is for IV use only; change solution every 12 h Serious adverse events (e.g., stroke, acute MI) have occurred IV nicardipine is available for hypertensive crisis in hospitalized patients Change peripheral IV infusion site every 12 h
Direct Vasodilators		
fenoldopam (Corlopam)	Activates dopamine receptors, resulting in systemic and renal vasodilation	IV use only for hypertensive crisis in hospitalized patients Use cautiously in patients with glaucoma Patient should remain flat for 1 h after administration
hydralazine	↓ SVR and BP by direct arterial vasodilation	IV use for hypertensive crisis in hospitalized patients Twice-daily oral dosage Not used as monotherapy because of side effects Contraindicated in patients with CAD
minoxidil	↓ SVR and BP by direct arterial vasodilation	Reserved for treatment of severe hypertension associated with renal failure and resistant to other therapy Once- or twice-daily dosage
nitroglycerin	Relaxes arterial and venous smooth muscle, reducing preload and SVR At a low dose, venous dilation predominates; at a higher dose, arterial dilation is present	IV use for hypertensive crisis in hospitalized patients with myocardial ischemia Given by continuous IV infusion
sodium nitroprusside	Direct arterial vasodilation ↓ SVR and BP	IV use for hypertensive crisis in hospitalized patients Given by continuous IV infusion Arterial BP monitoring recommended Wrap IV solutions with an opaque material to protect from light Stable for 24 h then metabolized to cyanide, then thiocyanate Monitor thiocyanate levels with prolonged use (>3 days) or doses ≥4 mcg/kg/min

TABLE 36.7 Drug Therapy

Diuretic Agents

Drug	Mechanism of Action	Nursing Considerations
Aldosterone Receptor Blockers		
eplerenone (Inspra) spironolactone (Aldactone)	Inhibit the Na^+-retaining and K^+-excreting effects of aldosterone in the distal and collecting tubules	Monitor for orthostatic hypotension and hyperkalemia Do not combine with potassium-sparing diuretics or potassium supplements Use with caution in patients on ACE inhibitors or angiotensin II blockers Classified as potassium-sparing diuretics Risk for adverse renal effects and/or hyperkalemia when taken with NSAIDs
Loop Diuretics		
bumetanide (Bumex) furosemide (Lasix) torsemide	Inhibit NaCl reabsorption in the ascending limb of the loop of Henle ↑ Excretion of Na^+ and Cl^- More potent diuretic effect than thiazides, but shorter duration of action	Monitor for orthostatic hypotension and electrolyte abnormalities Remain effective despite renal insufficiency ↑ Diuretic effect at higher doses Less effective for hypertension
Potassium-Sparing Diuretics		
amiloride (Midamor) triamterene (Dyrenium)	↓ K^+ and Na^+ exchange in the distal and collecting tubules ↓ Excretion of K^+, H^+, Ca^{2+}, and Mg^{2+}	Monitor for orthostatic hypotension and hyperkalemia Contraindicated in patients with renal failure Use with caution in patients on ACE inhibitors or angiotensin II blockers Avoid potassium supplements
Renin Inhibitors		
Aliskiren hemifumarate (Tekturna)	Directly inhibits renin, thus reducing the conversion of angiotensinogen to angiotensin I	May cause angioedema of the face, extremities, lips, tongue, glottis, and/or larynx Not used during pregnancy
Thiazide and Related Diuretics		
chlorothiazide chlorthalidone hydrochlorothiazide indapamide metolazone (Zaroxolyn)	Inhibit NaCl reabsorption in the distal convoluted tubule ↑ Excretion of Na^+ and Cl^- Initial ↓ in ECF Sustained ↓ in SVR Lower BP moderately in 2–4 weeks	Monitor for orthostatic hypotension, hypokalemia, and alkalosis May potentiate cardiotoxicity of digoxin by producing hypokalemia Sodium restriction ↓ the risk for hypokalemia NSAIDs can ↓ diuretic and antihypertensive effects and potentially cause renal problems Teach patient to supplement with potassium-rich foods

Fig. 36.5 shows the various sites and methods of action of antihypertensive agents. Drugs used in the treatment of hypertension include:

- *Adrenergic-inhibiting agents* act by decreasing SNS effects—centrally on the vasomotor center and peripherally to inhibit NE release or to block the adrenergic receptors on blood vessels.
- *ACE inhibitors* prevent the conversion of angiotensin I to angiotensin II and reduce angiotensin II (A-II)—mediated vasoconstriction and sodium and water retention.
- *A-II receptor blockers (ARBs)* prevent angiotensin II from binding to its receptors in the walls of the blood vessels.
- *Calcium channel blockers (CCBs)* increase sodium excretion and cause arteriolar vasodilation by preventing the movement of calcium into cells.
- *Direct vasodilators* decrease the BP by relaxing the vascular smooth muscle and reducing SVR.
- *Diuretics* promote sodium and water excretion, reduce plasma volume, and reduce the vascular response to catecholamines.

The preferred first-line therapy for patients with stage 1 hypertension includes nonpharmacologic treatment and one first-line drug. The preferred first-line drug classes are a thiazide diuretic, a CCB, an ACE inhibitor, or an ARB. For most patients, a diuretic should be the first drug ordered.[5,7] Patients with stage 2 hypertension receive nonpharmacologic treatment and 2 antihypertensive agents from different classifications. If a drug is not tolerated or is contraindicated, then a drug from another class is used.

Once antihypertensive therapy begins, patients should return for follow-up and dosage adjustments monthly until the goal BP is reached. More frequent visits are needed for patients with stage 2 hypertension or with comorbidities. After BP is at

TABLE 36.8 Drug Therapy

Combination Therapy for Hypertension

Combinations	Trade Names
ACE Inhibitors and Diuretics	
benazepril/hydrochlorothiazide	Lotensin HCT
enalapril/hydrochlorothiazide	Vaseretic
lisinopril/hydrochlorothiazide	Zestoretic
Angiotensin II Receptor Blockers and CCBs	
olmesartan/amlodipine	Azor
telmisartan/amlodipine	Twynsta
valsartan/amlodipine	Exforge
Angiotensin II Receptor Blockers and Diuretics	
candesartan/hydrochlorothiazide	Atacand HCT
losartan/hydrochlorothiazide	Hyzaar
olmesartan medoxomil/hydrochlorothiazide	Benicar HCT
valsartan/hydrochlorothiazide	Diovan HCT
Angiotensin II Receptor Blocker, Diuretic, and CCB	
amlodipine/hydrochlorothiazide/valsartan	Exforge HCT
β-Blockers and Diuretics	
metoprolol/hydrochlorothiazide	Lopressor HCT
nadolol/bendroflumethiazide	Corzide
olmesartan medoxomil/amlodipine/hydrochlorothiazide	Tribenzor
CCB and ACE Inhibitor	
amlodipine/benazepril	Lotrel
Diuretics and Diuretics	
spironolactone/hydrochlorothiazide	Aldactazide
triamterene/hydrochlorothiazide	Dyazide, Maxzide

goal and stable, follow-up visits are usually at 3- to 6-month intervals. Comorbidities (e.g., HF), associated diseases (e.g., diabetes), and the need for ongoing monitoring (e.g., laboratory testing) influence the frequency of visits.

DRUG ALERT

Doxazosin

- Use caution when giving the first dose. It is best to give the first dose at bedtime to reduce the first dose BP drop.
- Syncope occasionally occurs 30 to 90 minutes after the first dose, a too-rapid increase in dose, or addition of another antihypertensive agent to therapy.
- Severe hypotension can occur with patients taking phosphodiesterase inhibitors, such as sildenafil or tadalafil.

Resistant hypertension. Carefully explore all reasons why a patient may not be at goal BP (Table 36.9). *Resistant hypertension* is the failure to reach goal BP in patients who are taking full doses of an appropriate 3-drug therapy regimen that includes a diuretic. Resistant hypertension carries a 2- to 6-fold increase in complications including MI and stroke. Treatments focus on identifying risk factors that could contribute to hypertension, assessing adherence, and evaluating alternative drug therapies. Overactive renal nerves can be a cause of resistant hypertension. *Renal denervation* may be used to help lower BP and SNS activity in patients with resistant hypertension.

NURSING MANAGEMENT: PRIMARY HYPERTENSION

Assessment

Table 36.10 presents subjective and objective data to obtain from patients with hypertension.

Clinical Problems

Clinical problems for patients with hypertension include:

- Altered blood pressure
- Body weight problem
- Difficulty coping
- Health maintenance alteration
- Impaired cardiac function
- Impaired sexual function
- Inadequate tissue perfusion
- Nutritionally compromised

Planning

Nursing care focuses on the priority problems of maintaining BP at a level that decreases complications and supporting patients to manage what may be a complicated drug regimen with many side effects. The overall goals for patients with hypertension are that patients will (1) achieve and maintain the goal BP; (2) have minimal side effects of therapy; and (3) manage and cope with this condition.

Implementation

Health Promotion

Primary prevention of hypertension is a cost-effective approach. Current recommendations for primary prevention include the lifestyle modifications that avoid or delay the rise in BP in at-risk people described earlier. Teaching about risk factors is appropriate for all patients. Modifiable risk factors include obesity, diabetes, tobacco use, and physical inactivity. Discuss lifestyle modifications based on identified risk factors.

The National Heart, Lung, and Blood Institute provides Web-based educational materials in several languages for HCPs, patients, and the public to raise awareness about the dangers of high BP. Search available publications at https://catalog.nhlbi.nih.gov/.

Patient evaluation. You are in an ideal position to assess for the presence of hypertension, identify the risk factors for hypertension and CAD, and teach patients about these conditions. Hypertension is usually discovered through community programs or routine screening for insurance, employment, and military physical examinations.

In addition to BP measurement, a health assessment should include such factors as age; gender; diet history (including salt and alcohol intake); weight patterns; tobacco use; and family history of CVD, stroke, renal disease, and diabetes. Note all drugs taken: prescribed, OTC, and recreational. Ask the patient about a history of high BP and the results of any treatment.

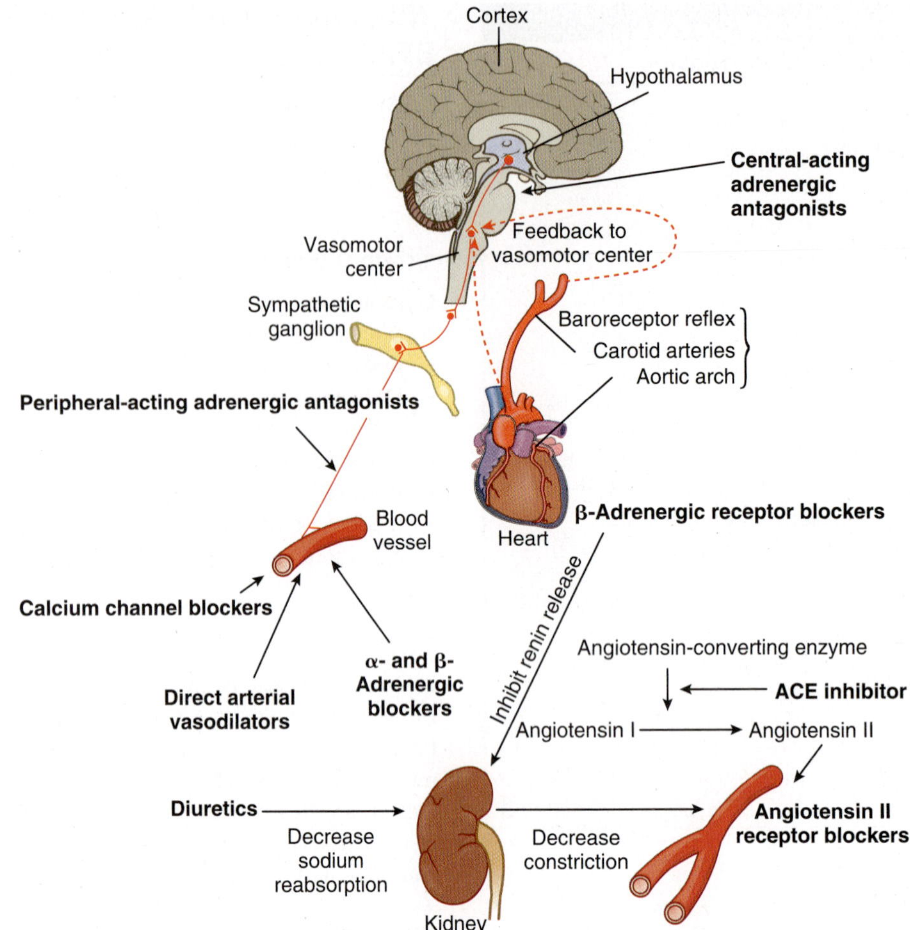

Fig. 36.5 Site and method of action of various antihypertensive drugs (**bold** type). (From U.S. Department of Health and Human Services: *Seventh report of the Joint National Committee on Prevention, Detection, Evaluation, and Treatment of High Blood Pressure [JNC 7]*, Washington, DC, 2003, National Institutes of Health.)

Blood pressure measurement. Proper size and correct placement of the BP cuff are critical for accurate measurement (see Table 35.6).[16] Place the patient's arm at the level of the heart during BP measurement. For BP measurements taken in the sitting position, raise and support the arm at the level of the heart. For measurements taken in a supine position, raise and support (e.g., with a small pillow) the arm at heart level. If the arm is resting on the bed, it will be below heart level. Note any differences in measurements between each arm. At the time of the BP measurement, give each person a written, numeric value of the reading. If further evaluation is needed, explain why.

If neither upper arm can be used to measure the BP (e.g., the presence of IV lines, fistula), or if a maximum size BP cuff does not fit the upper arm, use the forearm. In this case position the proper size cuff midway between the elbow and the wrist. Auscultate Korotkoff sounds over the radial artery or use a Doppler device to note SBP. Use of an oscillometric device on the forearm is acceptable. Forearm and upper arm BPs are not interchangeable.

! SAFETY ALERT

BP Measurement

- If using the forearm rather than the upper arm for BP measurement, document the site.
- BP cuffs that are too small or too large will result in readings that are falsely high or low, respectively.
- If bilateral BP measurements are not equal, record this finding and use the arm with the highest BP for all future measurements.

Assess for orthostatic (or postural) changes in BP and HR in older adults, people taking antihypertensive drugs, and patients who report symptoms consistent with reduced BP on standing (e.g., lightheadedness, dizziness, syncope). Measure BP and HR in the supine, sitting, and standing positions at every visit. Start by having the person rest in the supine position for 3 minutes. Take baseline readings for BP and pulse. Have the patient sit and repeat the BP and pulse. Then have the patient stand and

TABLE 36.9 Causes of Resistant Hypertension

Causes of Pseudoresistant Hypertension
- Improper BP measurements (i.e., inappropriate BP cuff size)
- Inadequate drug doses
- Inappropriate drug therapy
- Poor adherence to drug regimen (e.g., due to side effects, finances)
- White coat syndrome

Volume Overload
- Drug-induced
  - Corticosteroids
  - Cyclosporine and tacrolimus (Prograf)
  - Erythropoietin
  - Nonsteroidal antiinflammatory drugs
  - Oral contraceptives
  - Sympathomimetics (e.g., decongestants, diet pills)
  - Illegal drugs (e.g., cocaine, amphetamines)
  - Herbal supplements (e.g., ma huang, bitter orange)
- Excess salt intake
- Inadequate diuretic therapy
- Licorice
- Volume retention from kidney disease

Associated Conditions
- Excess alcohol use
- Increasing obesity
- Obstructive sleep apnea

From Brandani L: Resistant hypertension: a therapeutic challenge, *J Clin Hypertens* 20:76, 2018.

assess BP and pulse. After the patient has been standing for 3 minutes, measure BP and pulse again. Usually, the SBP decreases slightly (less than 10 mm Hg) on standing, while the DBP and pulse increase slightly.[17]

Orthostatic hypotension occurs when patients move from a supine to standing position, and there is a decrease of 20 mm Hg or more in SBP, a decrease of 10 mm Hg or more in DBP, and/or an increase in the HR of 20 beats/min. Patients may feel lightheaded, dizzy, and faint. It results from a change in the autonomic nervous system's mechanisms for regulating BP during position changes. Other causes include dehydration and inadequate vasoconstrictor mechanisms related to disease or drug therapy.

Some people have a wide gap between the first Korotkoff sound and subsequent beats. We call this an *auscultatory gap*. Failure to inflate the cuff high enough may result in an inaccurate SBP, a reading lower than the patient's actual BP.

Trends in BP are more important than a single value. In acute care settings, BP measurement is usually done to assess volume status and effects of drugs rather than diagnose hypertension. Inform the HCP of any patient with a persistent elevated BP. They should be evaluated for hypertension.[5]

Chronic Care

Your primary role in the long-term management of hypertension is to assist patients to reach the goal BP and adhere to the treatment plan (Table 36.11). Your actions include evaluating therapeutic effectiveness, detecting and reporting any adverse treatment effects, assessing and enhancing adherence, and teaching patients and caregivers. Discuss lifestyle modifications based on identified risk factors. Table 36.12 contains general information and health-promoting behaviors for patients with hypertension.

Teaching related to drug therapy. Side effects of antihypertensive therapy are common. They may be so severe or undesirable that a patient does not adhere to the therapy.[5,7] Telling patients about side effects that may reduce with time may help the person to continue with therapy. The number or severity of side effects may relate to the dose. It may be necessary to change the drug or decrease the dose. Teach

TABLE 36.10 NURSING ASSESSMENT

Hypertension

Subjective Data

Important Health Information

Health history: Known duration and past workup of high BP; cardiovascular, cerebrovascular, renal, or thyroid disease; diabetes; pituitary disorders; obesity; dyslipidemia; menopause or hormone replacement status

Medications: Use of any prescription, OTC, recreational, or herbal products; use of antihypertensive drug therapy

Functional Health Patterns

Health perception–health management: Family history of hypertension or CVD; tobacco use, alcohol use; sedentary lifestyle; health literacy; readiness for change

Nutritional-metabolic: Usual salt and fat intake; weight gain or loss

Elimination: Nocturia

Activity-exercise: Fatigue; dyspnea on exertion, palpitations, exertional chest pain; intermittent claudication, muscle cramps; usual pattern and type of exercise

Cognitive-perceptual: Dizziness; blurred vision; paresthesias

Sexual-reproductive: Erectile dysfunction, decreased libido

Coping–stress tolerance: Stressful life events

Objective Data

Cardiovascular

SBP consistently >130 mm Hg or DBP >80 mm Hg; orthostatic changes in BP and HR; bilateral BPs significantly different; abnormal heart sounds; laterally displaced apical pulse; decreased or absent peripheral pulses; carotid, renal, or femoral bruits; peripheral edema

Gastrointestinal

Obesity (BMI $\geq$30 kg/m^2); abnormal waist-hip ratio

Neurologic

Mental status changes

Possible Diagnostic Findings

Abnormal electrolytes (especially potassium); ↑ BUN, creatinine, glucose, cholesterol, and triglyceride levels; proteinuria, albuminuria, microscopic hematuria

Evidence of ischemic heart disease and left ventricular hypertrophy on ECG; structural heart disease and left ventricular hypertrophy on echocardiogram; arteriovenous nicking, retinal hemorrhages, and papilledema on funduscopic examination

TABLE 36.11 NURSING MANAGEMENT

Caring for the Patient With Hypertension

You will need to collaborate with many health care team members to deliver, delegate, and coordinate care based on the patient's status.

- Develop and conduct hypertension screening programs.
- Assess patients for hypertension risk factors and develop risk modification plans.
- Teach patients about lifestyle management and drug therapy.
- Monitor for adverse effects of antihypertensive drugs.
- Evaluate the effectiveness of lifestyle management and drug therapy in decreasing BP to acceptable levels.
- Teach about home BP monitoring, including the correct use of automatic BP monitors.
- Make referrals to other HCPs and programs, such as dietitians or stress management programs.
- Monitor for complications of hypertension, such as CAD, HF, cerebrovascular disease, PVD, and renal disease.
- Assess the patient with a hypertensive crisis for evidence of target organ disease (e.g., encephalopathy, renal insufficiency, cardiac decompensation).
- Manage the patient with hypertensive urgency or emergency, including giving drugs and evaluating for resolution of the crisis.
- Supervise AP in measuring BP.
  - Obtain accurate BP readings in outpatient and inpatient settings.
  - Report high or low BP readings at once to RN.
  - Check postural BPs as directed.

Collaborate With Other Team Members

Dietitian

- Obtain a diet history from the patient.
- Teach the components of the DASH diet.
- Provide instructions for any diet changes needed.

Physical Therapist

- Assess current fitness level.
- Develop an exercise plan with the patient.

patients to report all side effects to the HCP. There are many options for treating hypertension. A plan that is acceptable to the patient should be the goal.

A common side effect of several antihypertensive drugs is orthostatic hypotension. Table 36.12 presents specific measures to teach patients to control or decrease orthostatic hypotension.

Sexual problems may occur with many antihypertensive drugs. This can be a significant reason that patients do not adhere to the treatment plan. Problems can range from reduced libido to erectile dysfunction. Rather than discussing a sexual problem with an HCP, the patient may decide to stop therapy. The sexual problems may be easier for a patient to discuss once you explain that the drug may be the source of the problem. Changing to another antihypertensive drug can decrease or relieve these side effects. Encourage patients to discuss sexual issues with the HCP. If the patient is reluctant to do so, offer to alert the HCP to the patient's side effects.

Some unpleasant side effects result from a drug's therapeutic effect, but these can be decreased. For example, diuretics cause dry mouth and frequent voiding. Sugarless gum or hard candy may help ease the dry mouth. Taking diuretics earlier in the day may limit frequent voiding during the night and preserve sleep.

TABLE 36.12 PATIENT & CAREGIVER TEACHING

Hypertension

When teaching the patient and/or caregiver about hypertension, include the following:

General Instructions

- Give the patient the BP reading and explain what it means (e.g., high, low, goal, borderline).
- Encourage the patient to monitor BP at home and teach the patient to call the HCP if BP exceeds high or low limits set by HCP.
- Hypertension is usually asymptomatic, and symptoms (e.g., nosebleeds) do not reliably indicate BP levels.
- Long-term therapy and follow-up care are necessary to treat hypertension. Therapy involves lifestyle changes (e.g., weight management, sodium reduction, smoking cessation, regular physical activity) and, in most cases, drugs to regulate the BP.
- Therapy will not cure but should control hypertension.
- Controlled hypertension usually results in an excellent prognosis.
- Explain the potential dangers of uncontrolled hypertension (e.g., stroke, heart attack).

Instructions Related to Medication Therapy

- Be specific about the names, actions, dosages, and side effects of prescribed drugs.
- Help the patient plan regular and convenient times for taking medications and measuring BP.
- Do not stop drugs abruptly because withdrawal may cause a severe hypertensive reaction.
- Do not double up on a dose when a dose is missed.
- If BP increases or decreases, do not change the dose of the drug without consulting the HCP.
- Do not take any drugs belonging to someone else.
- Supplement diet with foods high in potassium (e.g., citrus fruits, green leafy vegetables) if taking potassium-wasting diuretics.
- Avoid hot baths, excess amounts of alcohol, and strenuous exercise within 3 h of taking drugs that promote vasodilation.
- Many drugs cause orthostatic hypotension. Reduce the effects of orthostatic hypotension by rising slowly from the bed, sitting on the side of the bed for a few minutes, standing slowly, and beginning to move if no symptoms develop (e.g., dizziness, lightheadedness).
- Do not stand still for prolonged periods. Lie or sit down when dizziness occurs.
- Do leg exercises to increase venous return.
- Some drugs cause sexual problems (e.g., erectile dysfunction, decreased libido). Consult with the HCP about changing drugs or dosages if sexual problems develop.
- Some side effects, like fatigue and diarrhea, may decrease with time.
- Be careful about taking potentially high-risk OTC drugs, such as high-sodium antacids, appetite suppressants, and cold and sinus medications. Read warning labels and consult with a pharmacist. Nonselective NSAIDs (e.g., ibuprofen) and selective NSAIDs (e.g., celecoxib) can cause loss of BP control and HF.

Home BP monitoring. Most patients with known or suspected hypertension should monitor their BP at home. The readings are often lower than those taken in the office setting and are a better predictor of CVD risk. Home BP readings may help achieve patient adherence by reinforcing the need for therapy. Provide information that will help patients understand what their goal or target BP is and why.

CHECK YOUR PRACTICE

You are making a home visit for a 78-year-old female who is recovering from a hip replacement after she fractured her femur. She currently takes a combination of lisinopril/hydrochlorothiazide. The patient's daughter (her caregiver) tells you that her mother's BP that morning was 150/88. She took it 2 more times, and it was the same. They are both worried and anxious that something is wrong because they heard that a BP over 130/80 is very bad.

- What should you do? What teaching would you provide?

Patient teaching is critical to ensure accuracy. Tell patients to buy an oscillometric BP monitor that uses a cuff for the upper arm or wrist. The patient should bring the BP monitor to the office to verify proper cuff size, the accuracy of the device, and the patient's technique.

Teach patients to obtain a BP according to the steps in Table 35.6. Tell patients to measure BP in the nondominant arm, or arm with the higher BP if there is a known difference between arms. Tell patients to measure BP first thing in the morning (if possible, before taking any drugs) and at night before going to bed. Have patients record all BP measurements and bring the record to office visits.

For clinical decision making (e.g., changes in dosage, starting a new drug), tell patients to take BP readings as described for 1 week. Stable, normotensive patients should measure morning and evening BP for at least 1 week every 3 months. Devices that have memory or printouts of the readings are convenient for reporting.[5]

Patient adherence. A significant problem in the long-term management of patients with hypertension is poor adherence to the treatment plan. The reasons for nonadherence are complicated. They can include inadequate patient teaching, low health literacy, drug side effects, the BP returning to normal range with the therapy, the high cost of drugs, and lack of insurance.

Determine the reasons when a patient is not adhering to treatment. Assess the patient's diet, activity level, and lifestyle as other indicators of adherence. Develop a plan with the patient and caregiver to improve adherence (Box 36.1). The plan should consider the patient's habits, cultural beliefs, and lifestyle. Active patient participation increases adherence to the plan. Measures include involving patients in choosing drugs that are affordable and involving caregivers. Substituting combination drugs for multiple drugs once the BP is stable may promote adherence. Combination drugs are shown in Table 36.8. They reduce the number of pills that the patient must take each day and may reduce costs.

Help the patient and caregiver understand that primary hypertension is a chronic illness that cannot be cured. Stress that it can be controlled with drug therapy, diet changes, physical activity, periodic follow-up, and other relevant lifestyle modifications.

BOX 36.1 EVIDENCE-BASED PRACTICE

Medication Adherence in Hypertension

You are caring for a 67-year-old male admitted to your unit after surgery. The health record states the patient has stage 2 hypertension and is prescribed hydrochlorothiazide and lisinopril. The patient's current BP is 160/88 mm Hg.

Making Clinical Decisions

Synthesis of Best Available Evidence

Medication adherence is important for hypertension control. Patients with stage 2 hypertension receive nonpharmacologic treatment and 2 antihypertensive agents from different classifications. Research shows that adherence is influenced by patient knowledge and beliefs, support systems, access to health care resources, and previous negative experiences with treatment.

Clinician Expertise

You know that a primary nursing role in hypertension management is to provide education to help patients reach their goal BP and adhere to the treatment plan. You ask the patient about his use of prescribed medications. He states he often "forgets" to take his medication and occasionally "runs out" of medication. The patient says he does not understand your concern as he always "feels fine." You question if this patient has a solid understanding of his hypertension and whether he can obtain his medications.

Patient Preferences and Values

The patient agrees to a referral to the cardiac clinic for hypertension management. The 6-week program includes education about hypertension and medications, which has shown to be successful in increasing adherence. The patient's BP will be monitored throughout and after the program. He will also be enrolled in a free medication program.

Implications for Nursing Practice

1. Besides family support, what other elements of social support could you explore?
2. How would you measure medication adherence and determine if adherence has improved?

Reference for Evidence

Zhou X, Zhang X, Gu N, et al: Barriers and facilitators of medication adherence in hypertension patients: a meta-integration of qualitative research, *J Patient Exp* 11, 2024.

Evaluation

The overall expected outcomes are that patients with hypertension will

- Achieve and maintain goal BP as defined for the person
- Understand, accept, and implement the treatment plan
- Report minimal side effects of drug therapy

Gerontologic Considerations: Hypertension

The prevalence of hypertension increases with age. The lifetime risk for developing hypertension is around 90% for normotensive persons over age 55. Older adults are more likely to have white coat hypertension.[5]

The pathophysiology of hypertension in the older adult involves several age-related physical changes: (1) loss of elasticity in large arteries from atherosclerosis, (2) increased collagen content and stiffness of the myocardium, (3) increased peripheral vascular resistance, (4) decreased adrenergic receptor sensitivity, (5) blunting of baroreceptor reflexes, (6) decreased renal function, and (7) decreased renin response to sodium and water depletion.

In the older adult who is taking antihypertensive drugs, absorption of some agents may be altered because of decreased blood flow to the gut. Metabolism and excretion may be prolonged. Care should be taken to assess for orthostatic hypotension and acute kidney injury in patients over 65 years old. Older adults who have multiple comorbidities and do not live independently (i.e., skilled agency) should have gradual dosage changes to minimize complications.[5]

Orthostatic hypotension often occurs in older adults because of impaired baroreceptor reflexes. It may also be related to volume depletion or chronic disease states, such as decreased renal and liver function or electrolyte imbalance. Drugs should be started at low doses and increased slowly to reduce the chance of orthostatic hypotension.

Older adults may have drops in BP after meals. The most significant decrease occurs about 1 hour after eating. BP returns to preprandial levels 3 to 4 hours after eating.

HYPERTENSIVE CRISIS

Hypertensive crisis is a term that indicates either a hypertensive urgency or emergency. A hypertensive crisis occurs at systolic BP greater than 180 mm Hg and/or DBP greater than 120 mm Hg. BPs can be greater than 220/140 mm Hg. The differences between hypertensive urgency and emergency are the presence of target organ damage and the type of treatment the patient will receive.

Hypertensive emergencies have evidence of target organ disease. They most often require hospitalization for immediate, controlled BP reduction. Without prompt treatment, complications include encephalopathy, intracranial or subarachnoid hemorrhage, HF, MI, renal failure, dissecting aortic aneurysm, and retinopathy.[9,18] Untreated hypertensive emergencies have a 1-year mortality rate of more than 79%. Prompt recognition and treatment are essential.

Hypertensive urgency is more common. There is no clinical evidence of target organ disease. Hospitalization may not be needed. It may be associated with chronic, stable complications such as stable angina, chronic HF, or prior MI or cerebrovascular accident with no threat of an acute event.

A hypertensive crisis occurs more often in patients with a history of hypertension who have not adhered to their medication regimens or who have been undermedicated. Rapidly increasing BP with turbulent blood flow can cause shearing of the endothelial surfaces, leading to further vascular damage and the release of more vasoconstricting substances. A vicious cycle of increased BP follows, leading to life-threatening damage to target organs.

Hypertensive crisis can be related to illicit drug use. Drugs such as cocaine, amphetamines, phencyclidine (PCP), and lysergic acid diethylamide (LSD) can cause a hypertensive crisis. Complications include drug-induced seizures, stroke, MI, or encephalopathy. Table 36.13 lists common causes of hypertensive crisis.

TABLE 36.13 EMERGENCY MANAGEMENT

Hypertensive Crisis

Etiology	Assessment Findings	Interventions
• Acute aortic dissection • Acute kidney problems • Drug use (cocaine, amphetamines) • Exacerbation of chronic hypertension • Head injury • Monoamine oxidase inhibitors are taken with tyramine-containing foods • Myocardial infarction • Pheochromocytoma • Preeclampsia, eclampsia • Rebound hypertension (from abrupt withdrawal of some antihypertensive drugs)	• Systolic BP greater than 180 mm Hg and/or diastolic BP greater than 120 mm Hg • Chest pain • Confusion • Dyspnea • Headache • Nausea and vomiting • Renal symptoms (nocturia, hematuria, polyuria) • Seizures • Vision changes (blurry or double vision)	• Obtain baseline vital signs, including O_2 saturation. • Start continuous BP and ECG monitoring. • Auscultate heart and breath sounds. • Insert IV. • Administer IV antihypertensive medications as ordered (e.g., sodium nitroprusside). • Obtain baseline blood work. • Give O_2 per agency protocol. **Ongoing Monitoring** • Monitor vital signs, level of consciousness, heart and breath sounds, neurologic function, heart rhythm, and O_2 saturation. • Titrate the drug according to MAP or SBP as ordered. • Assess and record response to drugs (e.g., decrease in chest pain). • Measure urine output hourly. • Maintain bed rest. • Provide reassurance and emotional support to patient and caregiver. • Explain all interventions to patient and caregiver.

Clinical Manifestations

A hypertensive emergency often presents as *hypertensive encephalopathy.* This is a syndrome in which a sudden rise in BP is associated with a severe headache, nausea, vomiting, seizures, confusion, and coma (Table 36.13). The manifestations of encephalopathy are the result of increased cerebral capillary permeability, which can lead to cerebral edema and disruption in cerebral function. Retinal examination shows exudates, hemorrhages, and/or papilledema.

Renal insufficiency ranging from minor injury to complete renal failure can occur. Rapid cardiac decompensation ranges from unstable angina to MI and pulmonary edema. Patients can have chest pain and dyspnea. Aortic dissection can cause sudden, severe chest and back pain with reduced or absent pulses in the extremities.

Interprofessional and Nursing Management

Hypertensive emergencies require hospitalization, IV administration of antihypertensive drugs, and intensive monitoring. BP level alone is not the major factor in deciding treatment. The link between elevated BP and signs of new or progressive target organ disease determines the seriousness of the situation.

When treating hypertensive emergencies, we often use the mean arterial pressure (MAP) instead of BP readings to guide and evaluate therapy. The initial goal is to decrease MAP by no more than 20% to 25% or to decrease MAP to 110 to 115 mm Hg. If the patient is clinically stable, drugs can be titrated to gradually lower BP over the next 24 hours. Lowering the BP too quickly or too much may decrease cerebral, coronary, or renal perfusion. A rapid decrease could cause a stroke, MI, or renal failure.

CHECK YOUR PRACTICE

A 68-year-old male presents to the emergency department with a BP of 210/118. He reports a severe headache and vomiting. You know that his BP is dangerously high and must be lowered.

- Calculate his MAP.
- What treatments would you expect to be ordered?

There are a few exceptions. Patients with aortic dissection should have their SBP lowered to less than 100 to 120 mm Hg as soon as possible (if tolerated). BP is lowered in patients with acute ischemic stroke to allow the use of thrombolytic agents. With acute intracranial hemorrhage and an SBP between 150 and 220 mm Hg, antihypertensive therapy may be given if there are no contraindications.[18]

IV agents used for hypertensive emergencies include vasodilators (e.g., sodium nitroprusside, fenoldopam, nicardipine), adrenergic inhibitors (e.g., phentolamine, labetalol, esmolol), and the CCB clevidipine (Cleviprex).[18] Sodium nitroprusside is the most effective IV drug to treat hypertensive emergencies. Oral agents may be given along with IV drugs to help make an earlier transition to long-term therapy.

DRUG ALERT

Labetalol

- Teach the patient not to stop the drug abruptly.
- Abrupt cessation may precipitate angina or HF.

Antihypertensive drugs given IV have a rapid (within seconds to minutes) onset of action. Assess the patient's BP and HR every 2 to 3 minutes during their initial administration. Use an arterial line (see Chapter 35) or an automated, noninvasive BP machine to monitor the BP. Titrate the drug according to MAP or SBP as ordered. Monitor the ECG for dysrhythmias and signs of ischemia or MI. Use extreme caution in treating patients with CAD or cerebrovascular disease. Measure urine output hourly to assess renal perfusion. Patients receiving IV agents may be kept on bed rest. Getting up (e.g., to use the commode) may cause severe cerebral ischemia and fainting.

Ongoing assessment is essential to evaluate the effectiveness of and the patient's response to therapy. Monitor cardiac, lung, and renal systems for decompensation caused by the severe increase in BP (e.g., angina, pulmonary edema, renal failure).

Frequent neurologic checks, including the level of consciousness, pupillary size and reaction, and movement of extremities, help detect any changes in the patient's condition. The neurologic changes of a hypertensive crisis are often like those of a stroke but without the focal or lateralizing signs often seen with a stroke. In a stroke, impairments affect a specific region or side of the body.

Hypertensive urgencies usually can be managed with oral agents and outpatient follow-up care within 24 hours. The initial decision for oral antihypertensive agents should be made based on the underlying cause of the hypertensive urgency, the patient characteristics, and comorbidities. A disadvantage of oral drugs is the inability to regulate the dosage moment to moment, as can be done with IV therapy. Some of the most commonly used oral drugs are captopril, labetalol, clonidine, and amlodipine (Table 36.6).

Once the hypertensive crisis is resolved, it is essential to determine the cause. Patients will need appropriate management and teaching to avoid future crises.

DRUG ALERT

Clonidine

- Teach the patient to change positions slowly to limit orthostatic hypotension.
- Avoid hazardous activities because the drug may cause drowsiness.
- Do not stop abruptly as this may cause a rebound increase in BP.

Not every patient with an elevated BP needs emergent drug therapy or hospitalization. Allowing the patient to sit for 20 or 30 minutes in a quiet environment may significantly reduce BP. Oral drugs may be started or adjusted. Other interventions include encouraging patients to share any concerns or fears, answering questions about hypertension, and reducing any adverse stimuli (e.g., excess noise) in the environment.

CASE STUDY

Primary Hypertension

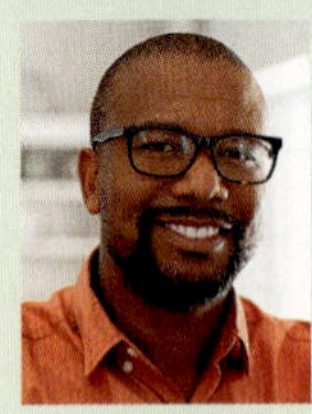
(© Ridofranz/ iStock.com.)

Patient Profile

R.L. is a 45-year-old male with no history of hypertension. At a screening clinic 2 months ago, his BP was 150/95 mm Hg. His HCP has followed him for the past month. During this time, he has been taking hydrochlorothiazide 12.5 mg/day. He is here today for a follow-up visit.

Subjective Data

- Father died of a stroke at age 60
- Mother is alive but has hypertension and a history of MI
- States that he feels fine
- Smokes 1 pack of cigarettes daily for the past 28 years
- Drinks 5–6 beers on most Friday and Saturday nights with work colleagues
- Has heard that BP drugs "make you impotent"

Objective Data

Physical Assessment

- Mild retinopathy (retinal arteriolar narrowing on ophthalmoscopic examination)
- BP: 166/108 mm Hg (highest of 2 readings, 2 min apart)
- Sustained apical impulse palpable in the 4th intercostal space just lateral to the midclavicular line
- Heart rate is regular with a pulse of 84

Diagnostic Studies

- ECG: mild left ventricular hypertrophy
- Urinalysis: protein 30 mg/dL (0.3 g/L)
- Serum creatinine level: 1.6 mg/dL (141 mmol/L)

Interprofessional Care

- Low-sodium, DASH diet
- Hydrochlorothiazide 25 mg/day oral (dose increase)
- Lisinopril 5 mg once daily (second drug added)

Discussion Questions

1. ***Recognize:*** What risk factors does R.L. have for hypertension?
2. ***Recognize:*** What stage of hypertension does R.L. have?
3. ***Analyze:*** What are the abnormal findings in the objective data?
4. ***Analyze:*** Based on the assessment, what target organ disease may be present?
5. ***Analyze:*** What additional assessment would be done?
6. ***Plan:*** What medications would you expect to see ordered?
7. ***Plan:*** What referrals may be indicated for R.L.?
8. ***Prioritize:*** Based on your assessment, which teaching points about hypertension are the most important?
9. ***Prioritize:*** What is the most important problem to manage for R.L. right now?
10. ***Act:*** What would you teach R.L. about the medications he is prescribed?
11. ***Act:*** What other teaching is needed?
12. ***Evaluate:*** What follow-up is needed to assess his response to your plan?

Answers available at http://evolve.elsevier.com/Lewis/medsurg.

BRIDGE TO NCLEX EXAMINATION

The number of the question corresponds to the same-numbered outcome at the beginning of the chapter.

1. A defect in which BP-regulating mechanisms can result in the development of hypertension? **(Select all that apply.)**
   - **a.** Release of norepinephrine
   - **b.** Secretion of prostaglandins
   - **c.** Stimulation of the sympathetic nervous system
   - **d.** Stimulation of the parasympathetic nervous system
   - **e.** Activation of the renin-angiotensin-aldosterone system

2. Which item in a patient history would the nurse recognize as a modifiable risk factor for the development of hypertension?
   - **a.** Low-calcium diet
   - **b.** Excess alcohol use
   - **c.** Family history of hypertension
   - **d.** Consumption of a high-protein diet

3. Which information would the nurse apply to a teaching plan for a patient with hypertension?
   - **a.** All patients with elevated BP need drug therapy.
   - **b.** Obese persons must achieve a normal weight to lower BP.
   - **c.** It is not necessary to limit salt in the diet if taking a diuretic.
   - **d.** Lifestyle modifications are needed for persons with elevated BP.

4. Which consideration would the nurse include in the management of the older adult with hypertension?
   - **a.** Preventing primary hypertension from converting to secondary hypertension
   - **b.** Recognizing that the older adult is less likely to adhere to the drug therapy regimen than a younger adult
   - **c.** Ensuring that the patient receives larger initial doses of antihypertensive drugs because of impaired absorption
   - **d.** Using a precise technique in assessing the BP of the patient because of the possible presence of orthostatic hypertension

5. A patient with newly discovered high BP has an average reading of 158/98 mm Hg after 3 months of exercise and diet modifications. Which management strategy would the nurse expect?
   - **a.** Drug therapy will be needed because the BP has not reached the goal.
   - **b.** BP monitoring should continue for 3 months to confirm a diagnosis of hypertension.
   - **c.** Lifestyle changes are less important because they were not effective, and drugs will be started.
   - **d.** More changes in the patient's lifestyle are needed for a longer time before starting drug therapy.

6. A patient is admitted in a hypertensive emergency (BP 244/142 mm Hg). Sodium nitroprusside is started to treat the elevated BP. Which management strategies would the nurse anticipate? **(Select all that apply.)**
   a. Measuring hourly urine output
   b. Continuous BP monitoring with an arterial line
   c. Decreasing the MAP by 50% within the first hour
   d. Maintaining bed rest and giving tranquilizers to lower the BP
   e. Assessing the patient for signs of heart failure and changes in mental status

1. a, c, e; 2. b; 3. d; 4. d; 5. a; 6. a, b, e.

For rationales to these answers and even more NCLEX review questions, visit http://evolve.elsevier.com/Lewis/medsurg.

REFERENCES

To access the References for this chapter, please scan the QR code with a mobile device.

37

Coronary Artery Disease and Acute Coronary Syndrome

Rose B. Shaffer and Julia B. Corbo

http://evolve.elsevier.com/Lewis/medsurg/

CONCEPTUAL FOCUS

Activity Intolerance
Fatigue
Glucose Regulation
Pain
Perfusion
Sexuality

LEARNING OUTCOMES

1. Relate the etiology and pathophysiology of coronary artery disease (CAD), chronic stable angina, and acute coronary syndrome (ACS) to the clinical manifestations of each disorder.
2. Describe the nursing role in promoting lifestyle changes in patients at risk for CAD.
3. Distinguish the precipitating factors, clinical manifestations, and interprofessional and nursing care of patients with CAD and chronic stable angina.
4. Explain the clinical manifestations, diagnostic studies, complications, and interprofessional and nursing care of patients with ACS.
5. Outline drug therapy used to treat patients with CAD, chronic stable angina, and ACS.
6. Prioritize key components to include in the rehabilitation of patients recovering from ACS and coronary revascularization procedures.
7. Distinguish the precipitating factors, clinical manifestations, and interprofessional and nursing care of patients who are at risk for or have had sudden cardiac death.

KEY TERMS

acute coronary syndrome (ACS)
angina
angina with nonobstructive coronary arteries (ANOCA)
atherosclerosis
chronic stable angina
collateral circulation
coronary artery disease (CAD)
coronary revascularization
ischemia with nonobstructive coronary arteries (INOCA)
metabolic equivalent (MET)
microvascular angina
myocardial infarction (MI)
myocardial infarction with nonobstructive coronary arteries (MINOCA)
percutaneous coronary intervention (PCI)
stent
sudden cardiac death (SCD)
unstable angina (UA)
vasospastic angina

Cardiovascular disease (CVD) is the leading cause of death worldwide. CVD encompasses several disorders of the heart and blood vessels, including coronary artery disease (CAD), cerebrovascular disease, and heart failure (HF), among others. Globally in 2019, an estimated 17.9 million people died from CVD. Heart attacks and strokes accounted for 85% of those deaths.[1]

CAD, the most common type of CVD, was the leading cause of death in the United States in 2020.[2] CAD is a condition of plaque buildup in the arteries that supply blood to the heart. It can have both acute and chronic manifestations. Patients with CAD may be asymptomatic or develop chest pain, which we refer to as *angina*. CAD can progress to unstable angina (UA) and myocardial infarction (MI), which we refer to as *acute coronary syndrome (ACS)*. The process of perfusion depends on the heart's ability to generate enough cardiac output (CO) to distribute blood to all body tissues. Significant CAD negatively affects heart function, resulting in impaired CO and decreased perfusion. This chapter discusses the care of patients with CAD, chronic stable angina, and ACS along with measures to promote optimal perfusion.

CORONARY ARTERY DISEASE

Coronary artery disease (CAD) is a type of blood vessel disorder in the general category of atherosclerosis. The term **atherosclerosis** comes from 2 Greek words: *athere,* meaning "gruel or fatty mush," and *skleros,* meaning "hard." Atherosclerosis begins as soft deposits of fat that harden with age, often referred to as *hardening of the arteries.* Atherosclerosis can occur in any artery in the body. When *atheromas* (fatty deposits) form in the coronary arteries, we call the disease CAD. Other terms used to describe CAD include *arteriosclerotic heart disease (ASHD), cardiovascular heart disease (CVHD), ischemic heart disease (IHD), coronary heart disease (CHD),* and *chronic coronary disease (CCD).*

Etiology and Pathophysiology

With atherosclerosis, there are lipid deposits within the intima, the innermost layer of the arterial wall. A layer of endothelial cells lines the intima to provide a barrier between blood and the arterial wall. Endothelium is normally nonreactive to platelets and leukocytes, in addition to coagulation, fibrinolytic, and complement factors. Endothelial injury and inflammation play a key role in developing atherosclerosis. Damage to the endothelial lining can result from tobacco use, hyperlipidemia, hypertension, toxins, diabetes, inflammation, and infection (Fig. 37.1A).[3]

Increased levels of C-reactive protein (CRP), lipoprotein(a), and homocysteine may increase the risk of CAD. CRP is a nonspecific marker of inflammation made by the liver. Levels rise when there is systemic inflammation, such as rheumatoid arthritis or inflammatory bowel disease. High-sensitivity CRP (hs-CRP) levels may be increased in people at risk for CAD. Lipoprotein(a) is a type of low-density lipoprotein (LDL) attached to a protein called apo(a). It is "stickier" than other types of LDL particles, increasing the risk for developing CAD.

Homocysteine is made by the breakdown of the essential amino acid methionine, found in diet protein. High homocysteine levels can lead to endothelial dysfunction. High lipoprotein(a) and homocysteine levels may contribute to atherosclerosis by (1) damaging the inner lining of blood vessels, (2) promoting plaque buildup, and (3) changing the clotting mechanism to make clots more likely to occur. Folic acid supplements can lower homocysteine levels, but lowering homocysteine levels with folic acid does not lower the risk of CAD.

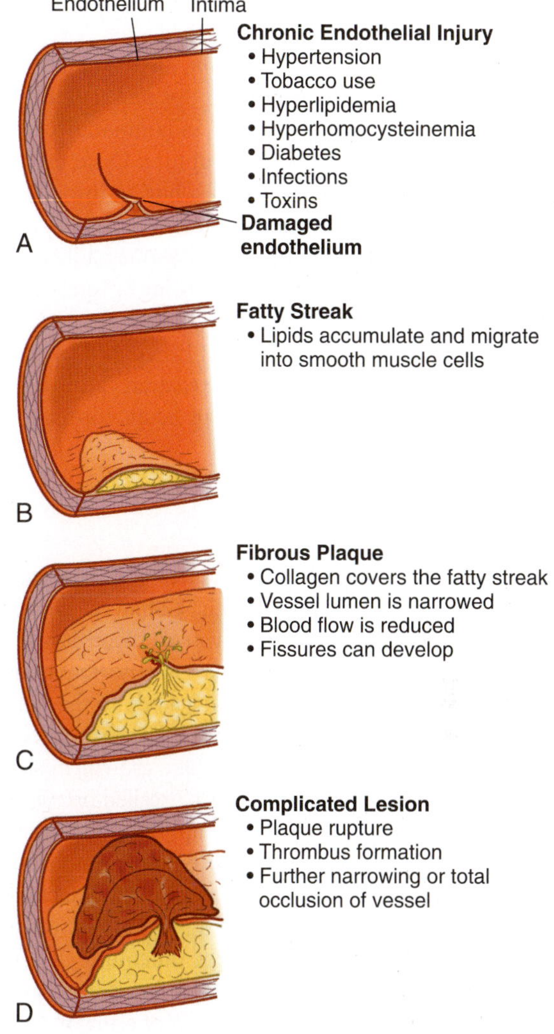

Fig. 37.1 Pathogenesis of atherosclerosis. (A) Chronic endothelial injury damages endothelium. (B) Fatty streak and lipid core formation. (C) Plaque progression with collagen fibrous cap covering lipid core. (D) Plaque disruption: Plaque rupture with thrombus formation.

Stages of Development

CAD is a progressive disease that develops in stages over many years. By the time the patient becomes symptomatic, the disease usually is well advanced. The stages of development in atherosclerosis are (1) fatty streak, (2) plaque progression, and (3) plaque disruption.[3]

Fatty streak. *Fatty streaks,* the earliest form of atherosclerosis, are lipid-filled smooth muscle cells. As streaks of fat develop within the smooth muscle cells, a yellow tinge appears. Fatty streaks appear in the coronary arteries by age 20. They involve more surface area as one ages. Medications that lower LDL cholesterol may slow this process (Fig. 37.1B).

Plaque progression. The *plaque progression* stage is the beginning of progressive changes in the endothelium of the arterial wall. These changes can appear in the coronary arteries by age 30 and increase with age.

Normally, the endothelium repairs itself immediately. This does not occur in a person with CAD. Once endothelial injury takes place, lipoproteins (carrier proteins within the bloodstream) transport cholesterol and other lipids into the arterial intima. Collagen covers the fatty buildup and forms a fibrous cap with a grayish or whitish appearance (the fibrous cap covers a lipid core). These plaques can form on one side of the artery or in a circular fashion involving the entire lumen. The borders can be smooth or irregular with rough, jagged edges. The end result is narrowing of the vessel lumen and reduced blood flow to the distal tissue (Fig. 37.1C).

Plaque disruption. *Plaque disruption,* the last stage in the development of the atherosclerotic lesion, is the most dangerous. As the fibrous plaque grows, inflammation can result in plaque instability, ulceration, and rupture. Once the plaque ruptures, many platelets accumulate, leading to thrombus formation. Platelet aggregation and adhesion is the body's attempt to "heal" the ruptured area. The thrombus may adhere to the wall of the artery, leading to further narrowing or total occlusion of the artery. Activation of the exposed platelets causes expression of glycoprotein IIb/IIIa (GP IIb/IIIa) receptors that bind fibrinogen. More platelet aggregation and adhesion enlarge the thrombus. This leads to an acute coronary event (Fig. 37.1D).

Collateral Circulation

Coronary collaterals are preformed connections, or *anastomoses,* between the main epicardial vessels. **Collateral circulation** allows for an alternative supply of coronary blood flow during an episode of acute or chronic ischemia.[4] In a normal heart, the anastomoses are numerous but small in caliber. In the setting of significant coronary artery blockage, collateral circulation consists of fewer larger-caliber vessels. The growth in size of a few smaller arterioles into larger arteries is called *arteriogenesis.* Collateral circulation can also develop via the process of *angiogenesis,* where new vessel growth occurs around areas of ischemia in response to locally released growth factors and inflammatory mediators.[5] Collateral circulation after acute MI is associated with improved long-term outcomes (Fig. 37.2). Collateral circulation can be seen during a coronary angiogram when there is a total or subtotal occlusion of a major coronary artery (Fig. 37.3).[5]

Risk Factors

Table 37.1 shows risk factors associated with CAD. Several assessment tools calculate risk for CAD based on a person's health information and risk factors. Common data used to generate a risk score include (1) age, (2) gender, (3) race, (4) tobacco use, (5) diabetes, (6) weight, (7) BP, (8) use of BP drugs, (9) cholesterol levels, and (10) family history. A 10-year risk calculator for people between the ages of 40 and 79 who have not been diagnosed with CAD, MI, or stroke is available at https://tools.acc.org/ascvd-risk-estimator-plus/#!/calculate/estimate/.

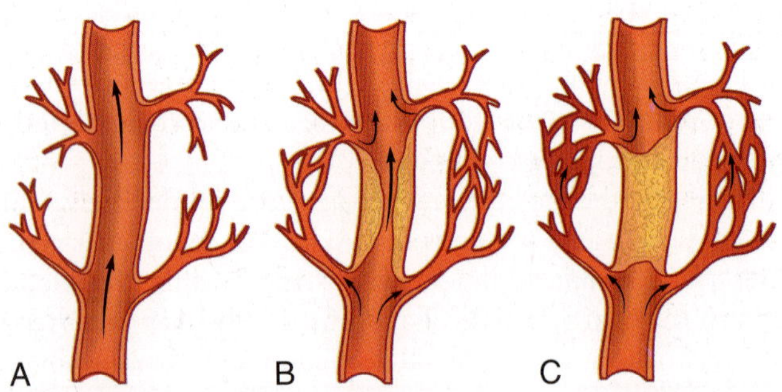

Fig. 37.2 Vessel occlusion with collateral circulation. (A) Open, functioning coronary artery. (B) Partial coronary artery closure with collateral circulation being established. (C) Total coronary artery occlusion with collateral circulation bypassing the occlusion to supply blood to the myocardium.

Nonmodifiable Risk Factors

The incidence of CAD is highest among middle-aged males. However, the risk for CAD increases for males over age 45 and females over age 55.[6] One possible reason females are diagnosed later may be the cardioprotective effects of estrogen.[7]

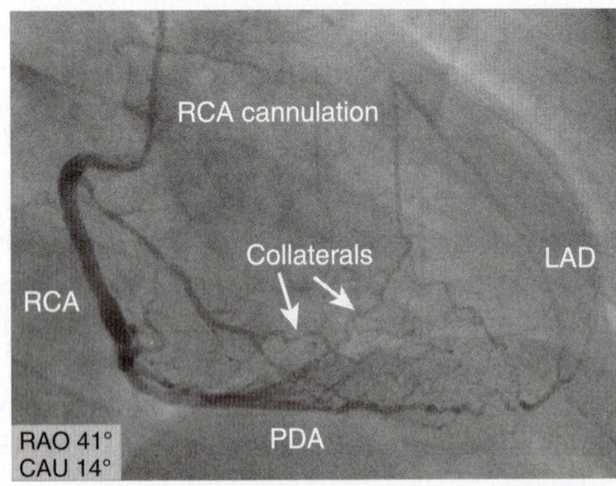

Fig. 37.3 Coronary angiogram showing collateral circulation from the right coronary artery (RCA) to the left anterior descending artery, which is 100% occluded proximally. The left anterior descending artery fills retrograde up to the100% occlusion. (From Libby P: *Braunwald's heart disease: a textbook of cardiovascular medicine,* ed 12, St Louis, 2022, Elsevier.)

TABLE 37.1 Risk Factors for Coronary Artery Disease

Nonmodifiable Risk Factors	Modifiable Risk Factors

• Increasing age
• Ethnicity
• Biologic sex
• Genetic predisposition and family history of heart disease
	Major
	• BP >120/80 mm Hg
	• Diabetes
	• Lipid levels:
	  • Total cholesterol >200 mg/dL
	  • Triglycerides ≥150 mg/dL
	  • LDL cholesterol >130 mg/dL
	  • HDL cholesterol <40 mg/dL in males or <50 mg/dL in females
	• Metabolic syndrome
	• Obesity (see Chapter 45)
	• Physical inactivity
	• Tobacco use
	Contributing Risk Factors
	• ↑ Homocysteine, CRP, lipoprotein(a) levels
	• Psychosocial risk factors (e.g., depression, hostility)
	• Substance use

CK-MM, Creatinine kinase-MM; *HDL,* high-density lipoprotein; *FH,* familial hypercholesterolemia; *LDL,* low-density lipoprotein; *VLDL,* very low-density lipoprotein.

Because females are older at the time of CAD diagnosis, they are more likely to have other risk factors (e.g., hypertension, diabetes, high lipids). Females carry added risk factors including early menarche, early menopause, gestational diabetes, hypertension during pregnancy, eclampsia, preeclampsia, preterm delivery, oral contraceptive use, and an increased tendency for systemic inflammatory disorders (e.g., scleroderma, rheumatoid arthritis).[8]

Heart disease is the leading cause of death in females in the United States. It accounts for 7 times more deaths in females compared with breast cancer. When females present to an HCP, their symptoms may be unrecognized as heart related because the symptoms are often atypical.[9] These atypical symptoms include fatigue, weakness, shortness of breath, upper back pain, nausea, indigestion, lightheadedness, palpitations, and anxiety. This lack of recognition of symptoms as a heart problem leads to delays in seeking treatment and HCPs recognizing the symptoms.

Although chest pain or an MI in males is most often caused by a significant blockage in a major coronary artery, chest pain or an MI in females can occur without a significant blockage in a major coronary artery.[9] Microvascular dysfunction or vasospasm occurs more frequently in females, which can cause ischemia with resultant angina.

CAD data show racial and ethnic disparities. The prevalence of most CAD and acute MI is higher in Black adults. Overall, Asian males and females have a lower prevalence of CAD.[10]

Family history is a risk factor for CAD and MI. Often patients with angina or MI can name a parent or sibling who has CAD or died from CAD. A family history of a first-degree relative with premature CAD (under age 55 for a male or under age 65 for a female) puts the patient at even greater risk for developing CAD.[3] Advances in genotyping and genetic sequencing have increased understanding of the inherited risk of developing CAD. It is very complex because multiple genetic mutations are related to CAD.

Familial hypercholesterolemia (FH), a genetic disorder where the body is unable to adequately remove LDL from the blood, results in extremely high LDL levels. These patients are at a higher risk for premature CAD and events, such as an MI, if not identified and treated early. FH involves a single gene mutation, allowing for genetic testing for the disease. So, we can refer patients for genetic testing if we suspect FH.

Major Modifiable Risk Factors

High lipids. High lipid levels, except for high-density lipoprotein (HDL), are a major risk factor for CAD (see Table 35.10). Increased risk for CAD is associated with a total cholesterol level greater than 200 mg/dL (5.2 mmol/L), an LDL level greater than 130 mg/dL (3.4 mmol/L), a fasting triglyceride level greater than 150 mg/dL (1.7 mmol/L), and/or an HDL level less than 40 mg/dL (1.0 mmol/L) in males and less than 50 mg/dL (1.3 mmol/L) in females. Adults in the United States with a total cholesterol in the range of 150 mg/dL, which corresponds to an LDL level of about 100 mg/dL, have low rates of CAD.[11]

For the body to be able to use and transport lipids, they must become soluble in blood by combining with proteins to form lipoproteins. Lipoproteins are vehicles for fat mobilization and transport. They vary in composition. The 2 main lipoproteins are HDLs and LDLs. Most refer to HDL as the "good cholesterol" and LDL as the "bad cholesterol."

HDLs contain more protein by weight and fewer lipids than any other lipoprotein. They carry lipids away from arteries to the liver for metabolism through a process called *reverse cholesterol transport*.[3] This helps prevent lipid accumulation within the arterial walls, making high HDL levels desirable. Premenopausal females usually have higher HDL levels than males. This may be related to the protective effects of natural estrogen. After menopause, females' HDL levels decrease to levels near those of males. In general, HDL levels are higher in females, decrease with age, and are low in those with CAD. Physical activity, eating more healthy fats, losing excess weight, moderate alcohol use (up to 1 drink/day for females and 2 drinks/day for males), and quitting smoking increase HDL levels.

LDLs contain more cholesterol than any other lipoproteins and have an affinity for arterial walls. High LDL levels correlate closely with an increased incidence of atherosclerosis and CAD. This is why low LDL levels are desirable. We cannot calculate LDL levels if the triglyceride levels are greater than 400 mg/dL (>4.35 mmol/L).

Triglycerides are the most common type of fat in the blood. High triglyceride levels (hypertriglyceridemia) increase the risk for CAD. Triglyceride levels of 150 to 199 mg/dL are considered borderline. Levels ≥200 are considered high. Certain diseases (e.g., type 2 diabetes, chronic kidney disease [CKD]), drugs [e.g., corticosteroids, hormone therapy]), and genetic disorders (e.g., familial hypertriglyceridemia) are associated with high triglyceride levels. Lifestyle factors that contribute to high levels include high alcohol use, high intake of refined carbohydrates and simple sugars, and physical inactivity.

Hypertension. Hypertension increases the risk for CAD, stroke, HF, and death.[12] It is more common in postmenopausal females than in males. This may be related to the decrease in estrogen associated with menopause.

The shearing stress of an elevated BP causes endothelial injury, increasing the risk of atherosclerosis. Atherosclerosis, in turn, causes narrowed, thickened arterial walls and decreases the distensibility and elasticity of vessels. The left ventricle (LV) must generate more force to pump blood through diseased arteries. This increased force is reflected in a higher BP. This added workload on the heart muscle can result in LV hypertrophy.

Elevated BP and hypertension are controlled with lifestyle changes and medications. Those with stage 1 or 2 hypertension often need more than 1 drug to reach therapeutic goals (see Tables 36.6, 36.7, and 36.8). Teach patients the importance of achieving and maintaining target BP goals. See Chapter 36 for a complete discussion of hypertension.

Tobacco use. Tobacco use is a major CAD risk factor. Although the rate of cigarette smoking has decreased in the

United States, the use of new tobacco products such as electronic cigarettes (e-cigarettes) has increased. Using any tobacco product (e.g., cigarettes, e-cigarettes, cigars, pipes, smokeless tobacco) carries an increased risk for cardiovascular disease.[13] Tobacco smoking decreases estrogen levels, placing premenopausal females who use tobacco at greater risk for CAD.

Tobacco smoke affects endothelial function and promotes atherosclerosis and blood clots.[7] There is an increase in LDL levels and a decrease in HDL levels, which add to vessel inflammation and thrombosis. Nicotine in tobacco smoke causes catecholamine (e.g., epinephrine, norepinephrine) release, which leads to increases in heart rate (HR), contractility, BP, and peripheral vasoconstriction. These changes increase the heart's workload.[13] Carbon monoxide in tobacco smoke can injure the endothelium and reduce the number of hemoglobin sites available for O_2 transport. Thus the effects of an increased cardiac workload and the O_2-depleting effect of carbon monoxide decrease the O_2 available to the heart muscle.

At any age, the benefits of smoking cessation are dramatic. CAD risk and mortality rates drop within weeks to months after quitting. The risk goes down even further the longer one abstains from tobacco use.[2] People usually need intensive intervention to quit. Individual and group counseling, nicotine replacement therapy, and smoking cessation drugs (e.g., bupropion, varenicline) are examples of smoking cessation strategies. See Chapter 11 and Tables 11.3, 11.4, and 11.5 for information on smoking cessation.

Nonsmokers exposed to secondhand tobacco smoke increase their risk for CAD by 25% to 30%.[2] People who live in the same house as the person who smokes should encourage that person to quit or smoke outside to decrease others' exposure to environment smoke.

Some states in the United States have legalized marijuana (cannabis) for recreation and/or medical use. Cannabis contains tetrahydrocannabinol (THC) and cannabidiol (CBD). THC can increase BP, heart rate, and myocardial O_2 demand. It can cause platelet activation and endothelial dysfunction. Smoking or inhaling cannabis can increase levels of carbon monoxide in the blood, which can lead to endothelial dysfunction and impaired O_2 binding. Heavier cannabis use (more days per month) is associated with CAD.[14]

Diabetes. Diabetes is a major modifiable risk factor for CAD. Undiagnosed diabetes is often discovered when a person has an MI. The incidence of CAD is greater among people who have diabetes, even with well-controlled glucose levels.[7] Patients with diabetes manifest CAD at an earlier age, likely related to endothelial dysfunction and changes in lipid metabolism. Patients with diabetes often have high cholesterol and triglyceride levels. Diabetes management should aim to achieve a glycosylated hemoglobin (HbA1c) level of less than 7%.[7]

In patients with CAD and diabetes, diabetic medications, including sodium-glucose cotransporter-2 (SGLT2) inhibitors and glucagon-like peptide-1 (GLP-1) receptor agonists, can decrease major adverse cardiac events (MACEs) such as MI and stroke.[7] Examples of SGLT2 inhibitors include dapagliflozin (Farxiga) and empagliflozin (Jardiance), among others. Dulaglutide (Trulicity) and semaglutide (Ozempic) are examples of GLP-1 receptor agonists.

Physical inactivity. Physical inactivity increases the risk for CAD. Physical inactivity means a lack of adequate physical exercise on a regular basis. Exercise training for those who are physically inactive reduces the risk for CAD through more efficient lipid metabolism, increased HDL production, a decreased risk of thrombus formation, and more efficient O_2 extraction by the muscles. This decreases the heart's workload. For people with CAD, regular physical activity may improve functional capacity and quality of life and improve other risk factors, such as insulin resistance, glucose intolerance, and obesity.[7]

Obesity and metabolic syndrome. The death rate from CAD is higher in persons who are obese. *Obesity* is defined as a body mass index (BMI) of greater than 30 kg/m^2. Severe obesity is defined as a BMI of greater than 40 kg/m^2.[7] We calculate BMI by dividing a person's weight in kilograms by the height in meters squared (see Fig. 45.6). A way to determine central obesity is to measure waist circumference. Males with a waist circumference more than 40 inches or females with a waist circumference more than 35 inches have central obesity. People who tend to store fat in the abdomen (an "apple" figure) rather than in the hips and buttocks (a "pear" figure) have a higher incidence of CAD (see Table 45.5). Obese people may have increased levels of LDL and triglycerides, which are strongly related to the development of atherosclerosis. Obesity is linked with hypertension, insulin resistance, and diabetes.

Metabolic syndrome refers to a cluster of risk factors for CAD that may be related to insulin resistance. It is defined as the presence of any 3 of the following 5 risk factors: (1) central obesity, (2) hypertension, (3) hypertriglyceridemia, (4) low HDL levels, and (5) high fasting glucose levels (see Table 45.12). Chapter 45 discusses metabolic syndrome.

Contributing Modifiable Risk Factors

Psychologic states. Certain behaviors and lifestyles may contribute to the development of CAD. Psychologic risk factors for CAD include depression, acute and chronic stress, anxiety, hostility and anger, and lack of social support. Stressful states contribute to the progression of CAD through sympathetic nervous system (SNS) stimulation. An increased release of catecholamines from SNS stimulation increases BP and may contribute to endothelial injury, inflammation, and platelet activation. SNS stimulation increases HR and the force of myocardial contraction, which increases myocardial O_2 demand. Stress-induced mechanisms may increase lipid and glucose levels and cause changes in blood coagulation, which contribute to atherosclerosis.

Substance use. The use of illegal drugs such as cocaine and methamphetamine can cause coronary artery spasm with angina. This can result in increased myocardial O_2 demand, myocardial ischemia, or infarction. In addition to chest pain, patients often present with sinus tachycardia and high BP. An MI may occur in the setting of prolonged, severe vasoconstriction. Cardiac biomarkers (e.g., troponin levels) and an ECG help determine whether the patient is experiencing an MI. A drug screen may identify if illegal drugs precipitated the cardiac event.

INTERPROFESSIONAL AND NURSING MANAGEMENT: CORONARY ARTERY DISEASE

Health Promotion

Management of CAD risk factors may prevent, modify, or slow disease progression. In the United States CAD-related deaths have gradually declined. This is related to our efforts to become healthier and advance CAD treatment. Prevention and early treatment of heart disease involves a multifaceted approach throughout the life span. In fact, healthy lifestyle behaviors should begin in childhood.

Identifying High-Risk Persons

Clinical signs of CAD are not apparent in the early stages of the disease. Therefore it is critical to identify people at risk for the condition. Risk screening involves obtaining a thorough health history. Ask patients about a family history of heart disease in parents and siblings, especially a premature history of CAD. Ask females about any problems during pregnancy and age of menarche and menopause. Note the presence of any cardiovascular symptoms. Assess environment factors, such as eating habits, type of diet, and level of exercise, to elicit lifestyle patterns. Include a psychosocial history to determine tobacco use, alcohol intake, recent stressful events (e.g., loss of a spouse), and psychologic states (e.g., anxiety, depression, anger). The place and type of employment provide vital information on the kind of activity performed, exposure to pollutants or toxins, and degree of stress associated with work. For patients between ages 40 and 79 who have never been diagnosed with CAD, we can use the 10-year risk calculator to help identify high-risk persons: https://tools.acc.org/ascvd-risk-estimator-plus/#!/calculate/estimate/.

Assess patients' attitudes and beliefs about health and illness. Their attitude gives insight to how disease and lifestyle changes may affect them. It can reveal misconceptions about heart disease. Knowing a patient's education background and health literacy helps determine teaching needs. If the patient has prescribed drugs, assess their knowledge of the medications and adherence to drug therapy.

Managing High-Risk Persons

Recommend preventive measures for all persons at risk for CAD. The person with nonmodifiable risk factors (e.g., age, gender, ethnicity) can still reduce their risk by controlling modifiable risk factors. For example, a young person with a family history of premature heart disease can decrease the risk for CAD by maintaining an ideal body weight, getting adequate physical exercise, reducing saturated fat intake, and avoiding tobacco and substance use.

Encourage people who have modifiable risk factors to make lifestyle changes to reduce their risk for CAD. You play a key role in teaching health-promoting behaviors (Table 37.2). For highly motivated people, just knowing how to reduce their risk may be all the information they need to start.

Other people may be unable to perceive a threat of CAD. Few people want to make lifestyle changes, especially in the absence of symptoms. First, help them to clarify their personal values. Then, discuss risk factors and have them identify their individual risks. Help them set realistic goals and choose which risk factor(s) to change first. Recommend working on one risk factor at a time. Some people are reluctant to change until they have symptoms or have an MI. Others, having had an MI, still may find the idea of changing lifelong habits unacceptable. Help them review options and respect their decisions.

Physical Activity

For patients with CAD, encourage regular physical activity because it can help with weight reduction and reducing systolic BP and may help increase HDL cholesterol. The AHA recommends 30 to 60 minutes per day of moderate aerobic activity (e.g., brisk walking, biking, recreational swimming) or 15 to 30 minutes per day of higher-intensity aerobic activity (e.g., jogging, singles tennis, swimming laps) for patients with no contraindications.[7] Basic physical activity guidelines for patients with CAD follow the FITT formula (Table 37.3). In addition, strength training (e.g., resistance or weight training) is recommended at least 2 days a week to improve muscle strength and functional capacity. For sedentary patients with CAD, even lower-intensity exercise (e.g., gardening, walking at a slow pace) can improve overall metabolic and cardiovascular health. Step counters or walking prompts may help reduce sedentary time.[7]

Nutrition Therapy

Diet recommendations focus on lowering LDL cholesterol by decreasing saturated fat and cholesterol intake and increasing complex carbohydrates (e.g., whole grains, fruit, vegetables) and fiber (Tables 37.4 and 37.5). Fat intake should be about 20% to 35% of total calories, with most coming from monounsaturated and polyunsaturated fats. Foods high in unsaturated fat include unsalted nuts (e.g., walnuts, peanuts, almonds) and avocado. Examples of oils low in saturated fat include canola, olive, and avocado.

Following a Mediterranean diet including lean protein (e.g., salmon) and plant-based foods with decreased intake of saturated fat (e.g., red meat) reduces multiple cardiac risk factors. For patients who have already had a cardiac event, switching to a Mediterranean-style diet can lower rates of secondary events and reduce mortality rate.[7]

TABLE 37.2 PATIENT & CAREGIVER TEACHING

Reducing Risk Factors for Coronary Artery Disease

Include the following instructions when teaching risk reduction for coronary artery disease:

Risk Factor	Health-Promoting Behaviors
Hypertension	• Monitor home-based BP and obtain regular checkups. • Take prescribed drugs for BP control. • Reduce salt intake. • Stop tobacco use. Avoid exposure to environmental tobacco (secondhand) smoke. • Control or reduce weight. • Perform physical activity daily.
High lipids	• Reduce total fat intake. • Reduce saturated fat intake. • Take prescribed drugs to reduce lipids. • Adjust total caloric intake to achieve and maintain ideal body weight. • Engage in daily physical activity. • Increase amount of complex carbohydrates, fiber, and vegetable proteins in diet. • Follow up with HCP for regular lipid panel assessments.
Tobacco use (see Chapter 11)	• Begin a tobacco cessation program. • Change daily routines associated with tobacco use to reduce desire to smoke. • Substitute other activities for smoking. • Ask caregivers to support efforts to stop smoking. • Avoid exposure to environmental tobacco smoke.
Physical inactivity	• Develop and maintain at least 30 min of moderate physical activity daily (minimum 5 days a week). • Increase activities to a fitness level.
Psychologic state	• Increase awareness of behaviors that are harmful to health. • Change patterns that add to stress (e.g., get up 30 min earlier so that breakfast is not eaten on way to work). • Set realistic goals. • Reassess priorities considering identified risk factors. • Learn effective stress management strategies (see Chapter 7). • Seek professional help if feeling depressed, angry, or anxious. • Plan time for adequate rest and sleep (see Chapter 8).
Obesity (see Chapter 45)	• Change eating patterns and habits. • Reduce caloric intake to achieve body mass index of 18.5–24.9 kg/m^2. • Increase physical activity to increase caloric expenditure. • Avoid fad and crash diets, which are not effective over time. • Avoid large, heavy meals. Consider smaller, more frequent meals.
Diabetes (see Chapter 53)	• Follow the recommended diet. • Control or reduce weight. • Take prescribed drugs for diabetes. • Monitor glucose and HbA1C levels regularly and follow up with HCP.

Omega-3 fatty acids reduce triglyceride levels and can slow the progression of CAD. They do not affect LDL levels. The AHA recommends eating fatty fish twice a week (e.g., salmon, albacore tuna, and mackerel) because they are high in omega-3 fatty acids. Omega-3 fatty acids can be hard to get by diet alone. Over-the-counter fish oils have not been shown to reduce cardiovascular events. The HCP may recommend a prescription fish oil called icosapent ethyl (Vascepa), which can lower triglyceride levels. Patients with a high triglyceride level should reduce or eliminate alcohol and simple sugars.

Simple carbohydrates (e.g., sugar, high fructose corn syrup), sugar-sweetened beverages, and refined grains (those <25% whole grain by weight) should be avoided. Sugar-sweetened beverages (e.g., 100% fruit juices, sports and energy drinks, soda, sweetened coffees/teas) increase the risk of cardiac events in those with CAD.[7]

Restricting diet sodium to a daily intake of <1500 mg per day helps maintain a healthy BP and reduce the risk of CVD events. Teach patients about hidden sources of sodium such as processed, smoked, cured, and/or salted meats. Following the popular Dietary Approaches to Stop Hypertension (DASH) diet can reduce cardiac inflammation and injury.[7]

Drug Therapy

Patients diagnosed with CAD usually take a cholesterol medication (Table 37.6) and an antiplatelet medication (e.g., low-dose aspirin). Patients already on cholesterol medication because they were at high risk for developing CAD may need an increased dose or second drug. See "Drug Therapy" in the "Chronic Stable Angina" section for more details about cholesterol and antiplatelet medications.

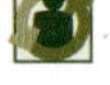

Gerontologic Considerations: Coronary Artery Disease

Heart disease is common in people over age 75. In the older adult, CAD is often a result of nonmodifiable risk factors (e.g., age) and lifelong modifiable behaviors that have not been modified (e.g., inactivity, tobacco use). ACS should be considered when a person over age 75 presents with symptoms such as shortness of breath, syncope, acute delirium, or an unexplained fall.[15]

Most research on patients with CAD has not included older adults or enrolled only relatively healthy older adults. Therefore

TABLE 37.3 PATIENT & CAREGIVER TEACHING

FITT Activity Guidelines for CAD, Chronic Stable Angina, and ACS

Include the following information in the teaching plan for the patient with chronic stable angina and acute coronary syndrome (ACS) and the caregiver:

Warm-Up/Cool-Down

Perform mild stretching for 3–5 min before the physical activity and 5 min after the activity. Do not abruptly start or stop the planned activity.

Frequency

Perform physical activity on most days of the week.

Intensity

Heart rate (HR) determines the activity intensity. If an exercise stress test has not been done, the HR of the patient recovering from a myocardial infarction (MI) should not exceed 20 beats/min over the resting HR. Patients taking β-blockers may not be able to achieve the same HR with exercise as those not taking β-blockers. They should discuss specific HR targets with their HCP.

Type of Physical Activity

Select physical activity that is regular, rhythmic, and repetitive, using large muscles to build up endurance (e.g., walking, cycling, swimming, rowing).

Time

Physical activity sessions should be at least 30 min long. Begin slowly at personal tolerance (perhaps only 5–10 min) and build up to 30 min.

it is difficult to generalize results to the older adult with multiple comorbidities and functional/cognitive decline. Because of changes in the heart, liver, kidneys, and brain of older adults (see Table 35.1), they are at risk for treatment complications.[16] However, strategies to reduce CAD risk and treat CAD can be effective in this age group. Treatment of hypertension and hyperlipidemia helps stabilize plaque in the coronary arteries. Tobacco cessation helps to decrease the risk for CAD at any age. Physical activity improves functional ability, endurance, and ability to tolerate stress. Heat intolerance results from a decreased ability to sweat efficiently. Teach older patients to maintain a moderate pace and to avoid physical activity in extreme temperatures. Recommend (1) longer warm-up periods, (2) longer periods of low-level activity, and/or (3) longer rest periods between sessions. For the older adult who is obese, making modest diet changes and slowly increasing physical activity (e.g., walking) results in more positive benefits than aiming for a significant weight loss.

Encouraging older patients to adopt a healthy lifestyle may increase quality of life and reduce the risk for CAD and fatal cardiac events. Older adults face many of the same challenges in making lifestyle changes as younger people. First, assess for health literacy and the readiness to change. Then, help the patient select the lifestyle changes most likely to reduce risk for CAD.

TABLE 37.4 NUTRITION THERAPY

Therapeutic Lifestyle Changes to Diet

Diet Recommendations	Recommended Daily Intake

Combined total fat calories from:
• *Saturated fats:* Limit fats that are usually solid at room and refrigerator temperature (e.g., lard, butter, whole-milk products, fatty cuts of meat, bacon)
• *Trans fats:* Mainly in foods made with hydrogenated vegetable oils, such as many hard margarines and shortenings
• *Unsaturated fats:* In oils that are usually liquid at room and refrigerator temperature (e.g., olive, corn, sunflower, soybean). There are 2 types of unsaturated fats:
  • *Monounsaturated fats:* In greatest amounts in foods from plants, including olives; avocadoes; and canola, sunflower, and peanut oils.
  • *Polyunsaturated fats:* Found mostly in nuts, seeds, fish, seed oils, and oysters. Omega-3 fatty acid is a type of polyunsaturated fat that may help reduce the risk of coronary artery disease (CAD).
	25%–35% of total daily calories (including <7% from saturated fat)

Cholesterol	<200 mg
Plant stanols or sterols (e.g., margarines, nuts, seeds, legumes, vegetable oils)[a]	2 g
Diet soluble fiber[a]	10–25 g of soluble fiber
Total calories	Only enough calories to reach or maintain a healthy weight

[a]Diet options for lowering low-density lipoprotein (LDL).

CHRONIC STABLE ANGINA

CAD is a chronic and progressive disease. Patients who are asymptomatic for many years may eventually develop angina. **Angina**, or chest pain, is the clinical symptom of myocardial ischemia. It is caused by either an increased demand for O_2 or a decreased supply of O_2 to the heart muscle (Table 37.7). When the demand for myocardial O_2 exceeds the ability of the coronary arteries to supply the heart with O_2, *myocardial ischemia* occurs. The most common reason for angina to develop is significant narrowing of 1 or more coronary arteries by atherosclerosis. This leads to insufficient blood flow to the heart muscle. When ischemia occurs from an atherosclerotic plaque, the artery is usually narrowed 70% or more (50% or more for the left main coronary artery).[17]

Chronic stable angina refers to chest pain that occurs intermittently over a long period with a similar predictable pattern of onset, duration, and intensity of symptoms. It is often provoked by physical exertion, stress, or emotional upset. Obtain an accurate assessment of angina (Table 37.8). Some

TABLE 37.5 NUTRITION THERAPY

Tips to Make Diet and Lifestyle Changes

General Tips

1. Know your calorie needs to achieve and maintain a healthy weight.
2. Know the calorie content of the foods and beverages you eat.
3. Track your weight, physical activity, and calorie intake.
4. Prepare and eat smaller, more frequent meals.
5. Track your activities and, whenever possible, decrease sedentary activities (e.g., watching television, computer time).
6. Incorporate physical movement into daily activities (e.g., take stairs and extra steps whenever possible).
7. Do not smoke or use any type of tobacco product.
8. If you drink alcohol, do so in moderation (e.g., no more than 1 drink for females or 2 drinks for males a day).
9. Aim for 7 to 9 hours of sleep per night.

Tips Related to Food Choices and Preparation

1. Use the Nutrition Facts panel on food labels and ingredients lists when choosing foods to buy.
2. Use fresh or frozen vegetables and fruits in place of canned vegetables and fruits.
3. Replace high-calorie foods with fresh fruits and vegetables.
4. Increase fiber intake by eating beans (legumes), whole-grain products, fruits, and vegetables.
5. Use liquid vegetable oils in place of solid fats.
6. Limit beverages and foods high in added sugars (e.g., sucrose, glucose, fructose, maltose, dextrose, corn syrups, concentrated fruit juice, honey). Water should be your primary drink.
7. Choose foods made with whole grains (e.g., whole wheat, oats, rye, barley, brown rice, wild rice, buckwheat).
8. Avoid pastries and high-calorie bakery products (e.g., muffins, doughnuts).
9. Select milk and dairy products that are either fat free or low fat.
10. Reduce salt intake by:
    - Comparing the sodium content of products (e.g., different brands of tomato sauce) and choosing products with less sodium.
    - Choosing versions of processed foods with reduced salt, including cereals, canned products, and baked goods.
    - Limiting condiments (e.g., soy sauce, ketchup).
11. Use lean cuts of meat and remove skin from poultry before cooking or eating.
12. Avoid processed meats that are high in saturated fat and sodium (e.g., deli meats).
13. Grill, bake, or broil fish, meat, and poultry.
14. Incorporate plant-based meat substitutes into recipes (e.g., soy, tofu, quinoa).
15. Consume whole vegetables and fruits in place of juices.

From NIH Publication No. 24-HL-8218: *Take action for your heart: get started!* January 2024.
Retrieved from https://www.nhlbi.nih.gov/resources/take-action-your-heart-get-started-fact-sheet.

patients deny feeling pain. Instead, they may describe pressure, heaviness, or discomfort in the chest or a squeezing, tight, or suffocating sensation. Other symptoms, such as dyspnea or fatigue, may occur. Chronic angina pain usually does not change with position or breathing.

Most angina pain is substernal. It may radiate to the jaw, neck, shoulders, and/or arms. Many people with angina describe a feeling of indigestion or a burning sensation in the epigastric region. The sensation may be felt between the shoulder blades (Fig. 37.4). Often, people who describe pain between the shoulder blades or indigestion-type pain dismiss it as not being heart related. Some patients, especially females and older adults, report atypical symptoms of angina, including dyspnea, nausea, abdominal/epigastric discomfort, and/or fatigue.[15] We refer to this as an *anginal equivalent.*

The pain of chronic stable angina usually lasts only a few minutes. It often subsides when the precipitating factor is resolved (e.g., by resting, calming down, using sublingual nitroglycerin [SL NTG]) (Table 37.9). Pain at rest is unusual and may indicate UA. With ischemia, the 12-lead ECG often shows ST segment depression and/or T wave inversion. These changes represent an inadequate supply of blood and O_2 to the heart muscle. In the normal ECG, the ST segments should be isoelectric or flat on the isoelectric line (Fig. 37.5A). ST depression is significant if it is at least 1 mm (1 small box) below the isoelectric line in at least 2 contiguous leads (2 leads that look at the same wall of the heart). The ECG changes return to baseline when adequate blood flow is restored and pain is relieved.

We treat patients with chronic stable angina with drug therapy. Because chronic stable angina is often predictable, drugs are timed to provide peak effects during the time of day when angina is likely to occur. For example, if angina occurs when rising, patients can take medication as soon as awakening and wait 30 minutes to 1 hour before engaging in activity. A comparison of the major types of angina is shown in Table 37.10.

Angina With Nonobstructive Coronary Arteries

Angina can occur from ischemia related to vasomotor dysfunction in the coronary vasculature. The O_2 supply to the heart muscle is limited not by plaque, but by coronary vasospasm and/or microvascular dysfunction. This is referred to as **angina with nonobstructive coronary arteries (ANOCA)**. There are 2 categories of ANOCA: (1) vasospastic angina and (2) microvascular angina. **Ischemia with nonobstructive coronary arteries (INOCA)** is the term used when there is documented ischemia in a person without obstructive CAD. **Myocardial infarction with nonobstructive coronary arteries (MINOCA)** is the term used when an MI occurs without obstructive CAD. These 3 conditions are more common in females.[9]

Vasospastic Angina

Vasospastic angina *(Prinzmetal angina)* is a rare form of angina that often occurs at rest. Risk factors include a history of migraine headaches, Raynaud phenomenon, and heavy smoking. It usually is caused by hyperreactivity of the smooth muscle of a major coronary artery resulting in strong contraction (spasm) of the vessel.[18] The spasm may occur with or without CAD.

Contributing factors include increased levels of certain substances (e.g., cocaine, methamphetamine), exposure to medications that narrow blood vessels (e.g., sumatriptan), and cold weather exposure. When spasms occur, the patient has

TABLE 37.6 Drug Therapy

Antihyperlipidemics

Drug	Mechanism of Action	Side Effects	Nursing Considerations
ATP-Citrate Lyase Inhibitor			
bempedoic acid (Nexletol)	↓ Liver synthesis of cholesterol ↓ LDL	Tendon rupture Gout Muscle spasms Upper respiratory tract infection	Monitor uric acid levels because of risk of gout. Use in caution with patients who have had a previous tendon rupture.
Fibric Acid Derivatives			
fenofibrate (Tricor) gemfibrozil (Lopid)	↓ Liver synthesis and secretion of VLDL ↓ VLDL ↓ Triglycerides ↓ LDL ↑ HDL	Rashes GI problems (e.g., nausea, diarrhea) ↑ Liver enzymes Myopathy, rhabdomyolysis	May ↑ effects of warfarin and some antihyperglycemic drugs. When used in combination with statins, may increase adverse effects of statins, especially myopathy.
HMG-CoA Reductase Inhibitors (Statins)			
atorvastatin (Lipitor) fluvastatin (Lescol XL) lovastatin (Mevacor) pitavastatin (Livalo) pravastatin (Pravachol) rosuvastatin (Crestor) simvastatin (Zocor)	Block synthesis of cholesterol and ↑ LDL receptors in liver ↓ LDL ↓ Triglycerides ↑ HDL (small)	Rash GI problems ↑ Liver enzymes Myopathy, rhabdomyolysis	Well tolerated with few side effects. Monitor liver enzymes and recheck them after any increase in dosage. Assess CK-MM if symptoms of myopathy (e.g., muscle aches, weakness) occur.
Niacin			
niacin (Niaspan)	↓ Synthesis and secretion of VLDL and LDL ↓ LDL ↓ Triglycerides ↑ HDL	Flushing and itching in upper torso and face GI problems (e.g., nausea, vomiting, dyspepsia, diarrhea) Orthostatic hypotension	Most side effects subside with time. Taking aspirin or ibuprofen 30 min before drug may reduce flushing. Take drug with food. Decreased liver function may occur with high doses.
Omega-3 Fatty Acid			
icosapent ethyl (Vascepa) eicosapentaenoic acid (EPA)	↓ Synthesis and/or secretion of triglycerides	Arthralgia Bleeding	For patients with severe hypertriglyceridemia (levels ≥500 mg/dL). Used with statin therapy for patients with CAD who have high triglyceride levels. High risk of bleeding when taken with drugs that increase the risk of bleeding, such as aspirin or warfarin.
omega-3 acid ethyl esters (Lovaza)	↓ Triglycerides ↑ HDL	Anaphylaxis Rash Taste changes GI problems (e.g., constipation, vomiting)	Give with meals and do not open or dissolve capsules.
Bile Acid Sequestrants			
colesevelam (Welchol) colestipol (Colestid) cholestyramine (Questran)	Binds with bile acids in intestine, forming insoluble complex and excreted in feces Binding results in removal of LDL and cholesterol ↓ LDL	Unpleasant quality to taste GI problems (e.g., indigestion, constipation, bloating)	Side effects lessen with time. Interferes with absorption of many drugs, including digoxin, thiazides, warfarin, thyroid hormones, β-adrenergic blockers, some antibiotics (e.g., penicillin). Take other drugs 1 h before or 3–4 h after bile acid sequestrants.

Continued

TABLE 37.6 Drug Therapy—cont'd

Antihyperlipidemics

Drug	Mechanism of Action	Side Effects	Nursing Considerations
Proprotein Convertase Subtilisin/Kexin 9 (PCSK9) Inhibitors			
alirocumab (Praluent) evolocumab (Repatha)	Inactivate PCSK9 protein ↓ LDL	Injection site reactions Muscle pain, limb pain, and fatigue	Monoclonal antibodies. Used with diet and maximum statin therapy to treat FH, those who need further LDL lowering, or are statin intolerant. Given by subcutaneous injection every 2 wk or every 4 wk at a higher dose.
Small Interfering Ribonucleic Acid (siRNA)			
inclisiran (Leqvio)	Inactivate PCSK9 protein ↓ LDL	Injection site reactions	Used with diet and statin therapy to treat FH. Given by subcutaneous injection.
Cholesterol Absorption Inhibitor			
ezetimibe (Zetia)	↓ Intestinal absorption of cholesterol ↓ LDL ↑ HDL	Infrequent, headache and mild GI distress	When used with a statin, further reduces LDL. Avoid use by patients with liver problems.

CK-MM, Creatinine kinase-MM; *HDL,* high-density lipoprotein; *FH,* familial hypercholesterolemia; *LDL,* low-density lipoprotein; *VLDL,* very low-density lipoprotein.

TABLE 37.7 Select Conditions Influencing Myocardial O_2 Needs

Decreased O_2 Supply	Increased O_2 Demand or Consumption
Cardiac	
• Coronary artery atherosclerosis	• Aortic stenosis
• Coronary artery spasm	• Cardiomyopathy
• Coronary artery thrombosis	• Dysrhythmias
• Dysrhythmias	• Left ventricular hypertrophy
• Heart failure	• Tachycardia
• Valve disorders	
Noncardiac	
• Anemia	• Anxiety
• Asthma	• Hypertension
• Chronic obstructive pulmonary disease	• Hyperthermia
	• Hyperthyroidism
• Hypovolemia	• Physical exertion
• Hypoxemia	• Substance (stimulant) use (e.g., cocaine, amphetamines)
• Pneumonia	

TABLE 37.8 PQRST Assessment of Angina

Use the following memory aid to obtain information from the patient who has chest pain:

	Factor	Questions to Ask Patient
P	Precipitating events	What events or activities precipitated the pain or discomfort (e.g., argument, exercise, resting)?
Q	Quality of pain	What does the pain or discomfort feel like (e.g., pressure, dull, aching, tight, squeezing, heaviness)?
R	Region (location) and radiation of pain	Can you point to where the pain or discomfort is located? Does the pain or discomfort radiate to other areas (e.g., back, neck, arms, jaw, shoulder, elbow)?
S	Severity of pain	On a scale of 0–10, with 0 indicating no pain and 10 being the most severe pain you could imagine, what number would you give the pain or discomfort?
T	Timing	When did the pain or discomfort begin? Has it changed since this time? Have you had pain/discomfort like this before?

angina and transient ST segment elevation (Fig. 37.5B). The spasm can cause severe ischemia leading to infarction (MINOCA). The pain may occur at rest or during rapid eye movement (REM) sleep when myocardial O_2 consumption increases between midnight and early morning. Some patients have short bursts of pain at the same time each day. The pain may be relieved with SL NTG or it may disappear spontaneously. Treatment includes calcium channel blockers (CCBs) and/or nitrates.[18] Encourage patients to stop the use of any offending substances. Regular, moderate exercise may reduce the number of episodes.

Microvascular Angina

With **microvascular angina**, chest pain occurs in the absence of significant CAD or major coronary artery spasm. The small distal branches of the coronary microcirculation develop atherosclerosis or spasm leading to ischemia. This is known as *coronary microvascular disease or dysfunction* (MVD). Often the angina is prolonged and brought on by physical exertion. Patients usually have a positive stress test, yet no obstructive coronary disease is found

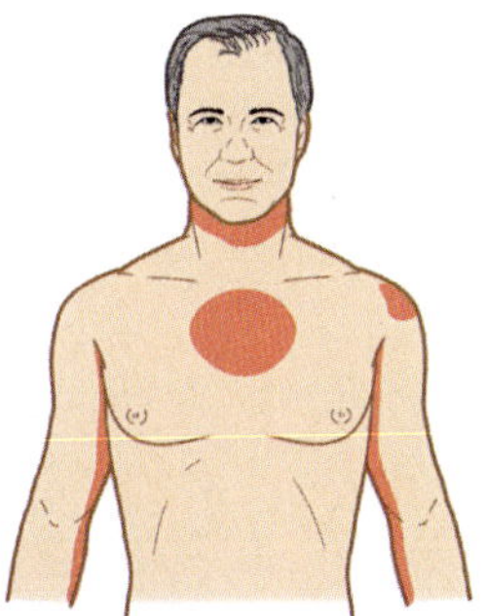

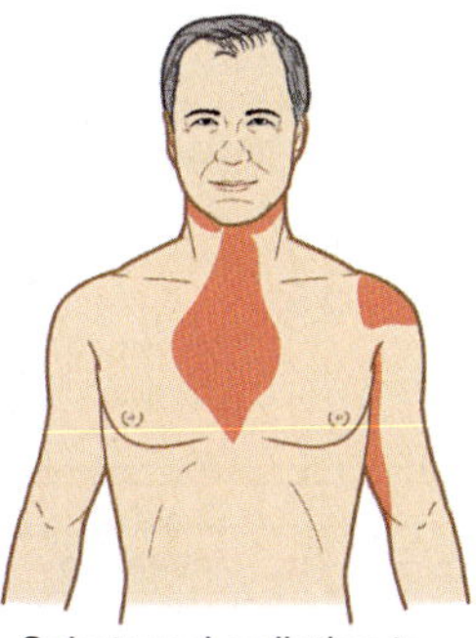

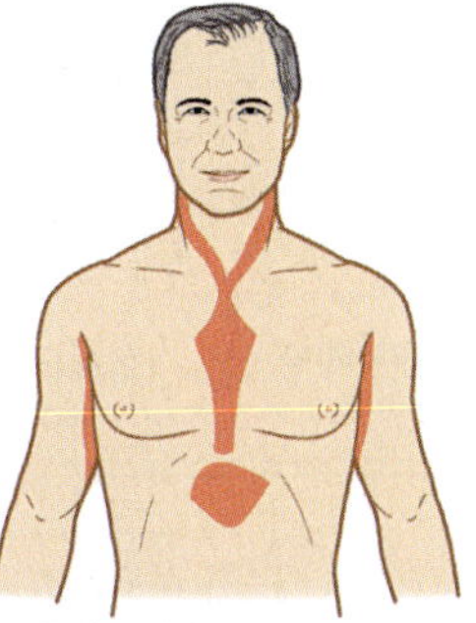

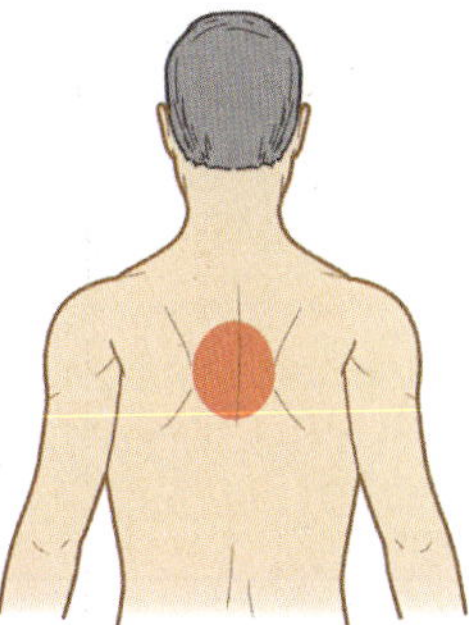

Fig. 37.4 Common locations and patterns of pain during angina or myocardial infarction (MI).

TABLE 37.9 Precipitating Factors of Angina

Circadian Rhythm Patterns
- Manifestations of CAD tend to occur in the early morning and within the first few hours after awakening

Consuming a Heavy Meal (e.g., holiday meals)
- Can increase the workload of the heart
- During the digestive process, blood is diverted to the GI system, reducing blood flow in the coronary arteries

Physical Exertion
- Increases HR, reducing the time the heart spends in diastole (the time of greatest coronary blood flow), resulting in an increase in myocardial O_2 demand
- Isometric arm exercise (e.g., raking, lifting heavy objects, snow shoveling) can cause exertional angina

Sexual Activity
- Increases cardiac workload and sympathetic stimulation
- In a person with CAD, extra cardiac workload may precipitate angina

Stimulants (e.g., cocaine, amphetamines)
- Increase HR and BP and increase myocardial O_2 demand
- Stimulate vasoconstriction and decrease myocardial O_2 supply
- May precipitate dysrhythmias

Strong Emotions
- Stimulate the sympathetic nervous system, activating the stress response
- Increase workload of the heart

Temperature Extremes
- Increase workload of the heart
- Blood vessels constrict in response to a cold stimulus
- Blood vessels dilate and blood pools in the skin in response to a hot stimulus

Tobacco Use and Environment Tobacco Smoke
- Decrease available O_2 by increasing the level of carbon monoxide
- Nicotine stimulates catecholamine release, causing vasoconstriction and an increased HR

CAD, Coronary artery disease; *HR,* heart rate.

in the major coronary arteries during coronary angiography. β-Blockers and CCBs are first-line treatment options.

Silent Ischemia

Silent ischemia refers to myocardial ischemia without subjective symptoms. There is no way to diagnose silent ischemia without ECG monitoring. When silent ischemia occurs in a monitored patient (e.g., 12-lead ECG or when using ST segment monitoring), we can see ST-T wave changes in leads facing the ischemic wall (Fig. 37.5A). Patients with diabetes have an increased prevalence of silent ischemia. This is likely the result of diabetic neuropathy affecting the nerves of the cardiovascular system. We treat ischemia with pain or without pain the same. They have the same prognosis.

INTERPROFESSIONAL AND NURSING MANAGEMENT: CHRONIC STABLE ANGINA

Chronic stable angina can progress or develop into ACS (UA or MI). Therefore any change in the usual pattern of angina should be evaluated. Patients with chronic stable angina may be admitted with a change in the angina pattern. Until an assessment and diagnostic studies are completed, it may be unclear if a patient is having typical chronic stable angina, UA, or an MI.

The goal of treatment for patients admitted with angina is to decrease O_2 demand and/or increase O_2 supply. Nursing care focuses on the priority problems of managing acute pain and anxiety while increasing O_2 delivery to the myocardium. The overall goals for patients who present with angina include (1) pain relief, (2) immediate treatment, (3) preservation of heart muscle if an MI is suspected, (4) effective coping with illness-associated anxiety, (5) participation in a rehabilitation plan, and (6) reduction of risk factors.

Acute Care

If your patient has chest pain and you are unsure if the pain is from chronic stable angina, UA, or an MI, plan to perform the following measures: (1) position the patient upright unless contraindicated and apply supplemental O_2 if the O_2 saturation is under 90% or the patient is dyspneic; (2) assess vital signs; (3) obtain a 12-lead ECG; (4) apply a continuous ECG

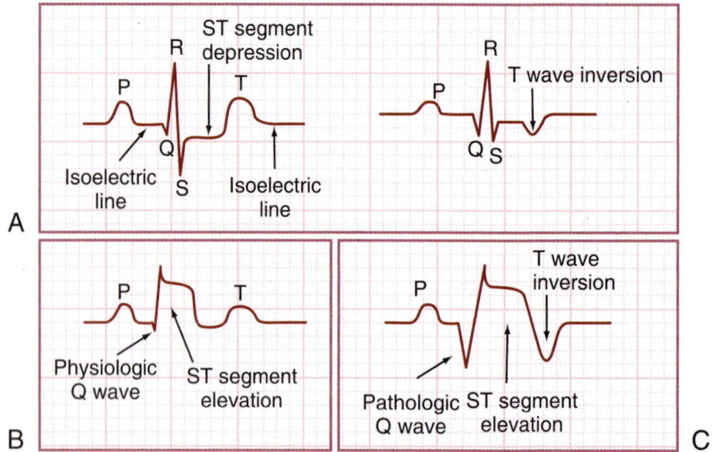

Fig. 37.5 ST segment, T wave, and Q wave changes associated with myocardial ischemia (A), injury or coronary spasm (B), and infarction (C).

TABLE 37.10 Comparison of Major Types of Angina

Type	Etiology	Characteristics
Chronic stable angina	Myocardial ischemia (usually from CAD) caused by an O_2 supply/demand mismatch	• Episodic pain lasting a few minutes • Provoked by exertion or stress • Relieved by rest or nitroglycerin
Microvascular angina (ANOCA)	Myocardial ischemia from microvascular disease affecting the small, distal branches of coronary arteries	• More common in females • Triggered by activities of daily living (e.g., shopping, work) vs. physical exercise (exertion) • Treatment may include β-blockers or calcium channel blockers
Vasospastic angina (ANOCA)	Coronary vasospasm	• Occurs mainly at rest • Triggered by smoking and increased levels of some substances (e.g., epinephrine, cocaine), drugs that narrow blood vessels (e.g., sumatriptan), cold weather • May occur in presence or absence of CAD • Treatment may include long-acting nitrates and/or calcium channel blockers
Unstable angina	Rupture of unstable plaque, exposing thrombogenic surface	• New-onset angina • Chronic stable angina that increases in frequency, duration, or severity • Occurs at rest or with minimal exertion • Lasts more than 10 min

ANOCA, Angina with nonobstructive coronary arteries; *CAD,* coronary artery disease.

monitor; (5) start an IV; (6) provide prompt pain relief, first with SL or IV NTG, followed by an IV opioid analgesic (e.g., fentanyl), if needed; (7) obtain cardiac biomarkers (e.g., troponin); (8) assess heart and breath sounds; and (9) obtain a chest x-ray. The patient may be anxious and may have pale, cool, clammy skin. BP and HR may be high. There may be an atrial (S_4) or a ventricular (S_3) gallop. A new systolic murmur heard during angina may indicate ischemia of a papillary muscle of the mitral valve, causing mitral regurgitation (the mitral valve does not close properly, causing blood to leak back into the left atrium). The murmur may be transient and disappear when symptoms resolve.

Ask patients to describe the pain and rate it on a scale of 0 to 10 before and after treatment to evaluate the effectiveness of the interventions. Use the same words the patient used to describe the symptoms (e.g., tightness, pressure). Assess for other signs of pain, such as restlessness; ECG changes; high HR, respiratory rate, or BP; clutching the chest or bed linens; or other nonverbal cues. Support and reassure the patient. Use a calm approach to help reduce the patient's anxiety. If the chest pain is not related to ACS, the patient may be discharged within 1 or 2 days. Further testing may be done during hospitalization or as an outpatient.

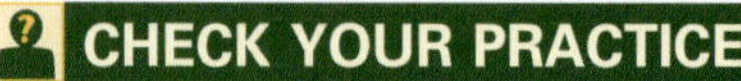

CHECK YOUR PRACTICE

A visitor finds you in the hallway and tells you that her father is having chest pain. You are not assigned to the patient.

- How would you proceed?

Patient Teaching

Reassure patients with a history of angina that a long, active life is possible. Preventing or at least reducing the frequency of

TABLE 37.11 Treatment of Chronic Stable Angina and Acute Coronary Syndrome

Strategies for the patient with chronic stable angina should address all the treatment elements and related patient teaching in the following mnemonic:

Element	Treatment
A	Antiplatelet/anticoagulant therapy Antiangina therapy ACE inhibitor/angiotensin receptor blocker
B	β-Blocker BP control
C	Cigarette smoking cessation Cholesterol (lipid) management Calcium channel blockers Cardiac rehabilitation
D	Diet (weight management) Diabetes management Depression screening
E	Education Exercise
F	Flu vaccination

ACE, Angiotensin-converting enzyme.
Modified from Smith SC, Benjamin EJ, Bonow RO, et al: AHA/ACCF secondary prevention and risk reduction therapy for patients with coronary and other atherosclerotic vascular disease: 2011 update, *J Am Coll Cardiol* 58:2432, 2011.

angina is key, so teaching is essential. Emphasize risk factor modification to slow the progression of CAD. Help patients to identify their risk factors for CAD and ways to reduce modifiable risk factors (Tables 37.1 and 37.2). Give patients information about CAD, angina, precipitating factors for angina (Table 37.9), and medications to treat angina (Tables 37.11 and 37.12 and Fig. 37.6).

Teach the patient and caregiver about diets low in salt and saturated fats (Tables 37.4 and 37.5). Maintaining ideal body weight is important in controlling angina because excess weight increases the heart's workload. Give the patient a regular, individualized program of physical activity that conditions rather than stresses the heart.

Help the patient to identify and avoid factors that precipitate angina (Table 37.9). For example, teach the patient to avoid exposure to extremes of weather and eating large, heavy meals. Tell the patient to rest for 1 to 2 hours after a heavy meal because blood shifts to the GI tract.

If needed, arrange for counseling to assess the psychologic adjustment of the patient and caregiver to the diagnosis of CAD and the resulting angina. Many patients feel a threat to identity, self-esteem, and their usual roles in society.

Drug Therapy

Drug therapy for chronic stable angina aims to reduce angina and the risk for MI and death. The most common medications to optimize myocardial perfusion in chronic stable angina include nitrates, angiotensin-converting enzyme (ACE) inhibitors, β-blockers, and CCBs (Tables 37.11 and 37.12 and Fig. 37.6). Lipid-lowering drugs are given to slow progression of plaque buildup. Low-dose aspirin is given for secondary prevention (patients with diagnosed CAD) in the absence of contraindications (Table 37.12).

Nitrates

Short-acting nitrates are first-line therapy for an acute episode of angina. Nitrates produce their principal effects by the following mechanisms:

Dilating peripheral blood vessels: This results in decreased systemic vascular resistance (SVR), venous pooling, and decreased venous blood return to the heart (preload). Myocardial O_2 demand then decreases because of the reduced cardiac workload.

Dilating coronary arteries and collateral vessels: This may increase blood flow to the ischemic areas of the heart.

Relief of chest pain after use of NTG is not diagnostic of myocardial ischemia. The broad vasodilatory effects of NTG will relieve chest pain caused by conditions such as esophageal spasm.

Orthostatic hypotension is common. Monitor the BP because vasodilation may cause a drop in BP, especially in volume-depleted patients.

Short-acting nitroglycerin preparations. Sublingual NTG tablets or translingual sprays (Nitrolingual) usually relieve pain in about 5 minutes. The recommended dose of short-acting NTG is 1 tablet under the tongue or 1 to 2 metered sprays of translingual NTG on or under the tongue. If symptoms are unchanged or worse after 5 minutes, the patient can take a second dose. If there is no relief within the next 5 minutes, tell the patient to contact the emergency response system (e.g., 911).

Teach the patient and caregiver the proper storage and use of NTG. It should always be easily accessible to the patient. Store the tablets away from light and heat sources, including body heat, to protect them from degradation. Keep tablets in their original bottles. Once opened, the tablets lose potency. They should be replaced every 6 months.

Tell the patient to sit down and place the NTG tablet under the tongue and allow it to dissolve. If using the spray, the patient should direct it on or under the tongue, not inhale it. SL NTG tablets should cause a tingling sensation when taken; if not, they may be outdated. Warn the patient that a headache, dizziness, or flushing may occur. Caution the patient to change positions slowly after NTG use because orthostatic hypotension may occur.

Patients can use NTG prophylactically before starting an activity that is known to cause angina (e.g., emotionally stressful situation, sexual intercourse). In these cases, the patient can take a tablet or spray 5 to 10 minutes before beginning the activity. Tell patients to report any changes in the usual pattern of pain, such as increasing frequency, nighttime angina, or angina at rest.

Long-acting nitrates. Oral nitrates, such as isosorbide dinitrate (e.g., Isordil) and isosorbide mononitrate (e.g., Imdur),

TABLE 37.12 Drug Therapy

Chronic Stable Angina and Acute Coronary Syndrome

Drug	Mechanism of Action and Considerations
Angiotensin-Converting Enzyme (ACE) Inhibitors (see Table 36.6)	
benazepril (Lotensin) captopril (Capoten) enalapril (Vasotec) fosinopril (Monopril) lisinopril (Zestril) quinapril (Accupril) ramipril (Altace)	• Prevent conversion of angiotensin I to angiotensin II, resulting in vasodilation • May prevent or limit ventricular remodeling • Decrease endothelial dysfunction • Treat HF, decreased LV function, tachycardia, MI, hypertension, diabetes, and chronic kidney disease
Angiotensin II Receptor Blockers (see Table 36.6)	
candesartan (Atacand) irbesartan (Avapro) losartan (Cozaar) olmesartan (Benicar) telmisartan (Micardis) valsartan (Diovan)	• Inhibit binding of angiotensin II to angiotensin I receptors, resulting in vasodilation • For patients intolerant of ACE inhibitors
Anticoagulant Agents (see Table 41.10)	
Direct Thrombin Inhibitors	
IV agents argatroban bivalirudin (Angiomax) **Oral agent** dabigatran (Pradaxa)	• Direct inhibition of the clotting factor thrombin • IV agents can be used during PCI • Argatroban is used mainly for patients with or at risk for heparin-induced thrombocytopenia • Dabigatran is approved to prevent strokes in patients with nonvalvular atrial fibrillation
Low-Molecular-Weight Heparin	
dalteparin (Fragmin) enoxaparin (Lovenox)	• Binds to antithrombin III, enhancing its effect • Heparin–antithrombin III complex inactivates activated factor X and thrombin • Prevents conversion of fibrinogen to fibrin
Unfractionated Heparin	
heparin	• Prevents conversion of fibrinogen to fibrin and prothrombin to thrombin
Vitamin K Antagonist	
warfarin (Coumadin)	• Interferes with liver synthesis of vitamin K–dependent clotting factors • Treats patients with atrial fibrillation, those at risk for thromboembolism (large anterior wall infarctions or ventricular aneurysms), and those with mechanical heart valves • Patients need regular blood work (prothrombin time [PT] with international normalized ratio [INR]) to assess therapeutic range
Factor Xa Inhibitors	
Oral agents apixaban (Eliquis) rivorixaban (Xarelto) **Subcut/IV agent** fondaparinux (Arixtra)	• Block the clotting activity of Factor Xa to prevent clot formation • Oral agents used to prevent stroke in patients with nonvalvular atrial fibrillation; not FDA approved to prevent thromboembolism (large anterior wall infarctions or ventricular aneurysms) or in patients with mechanical heart valves • Fondaparinux may be used for patients with UA or NSTEMI
Antiplatelet Agents	
aspirin	• Inhibits cyclooxygenase, which in turn produces thromboxane A_2, a potent platelet activator • Given as soon as ACS is suspected, unless truly allergic
cangrelor (Kengreal)	• Inhibits platelet aggregation • Given IV • Approved for use in patients during a PCI procedure
clopidogrel (Plavix)	• Inhibits platelet aggregation • Used in combination with low-dose aspirin to treat ACS with or without PCI and after elective PCI for CAD • An alternative for patients who cannot take aspirin
prasugrel (Effient)	• Inhibits platelet aggregation • Used with aspirin for patients with ACS who had PCI • Not approved to treat patients with ACS who do not undergo PCI • Caution in patients ≥75 years old or weight <60 kg • Contraindicated in patients with prior stroke or TIA
ticagrelor (Brilinta)	• Inhibits platelet aggregation • Used with low-dose aspirin to treat ACS with or without PCI • Effectiveness decreased by aspirin dosages >100 mg/day
vorapaxar (Zontivity)	• Inhibits platelet aggregation • Increases risk for bleeding, including life-threatening and fatal bleeding (boxed warning) • Must not be used in people who have had a stroke, TIA, or bleeding in the head, because the risk for bleeding in the head is too great
Glycoprotein IIb/IIIa Inhibitors	
eptifibatide (Integrilin) tirofiban (Aggrastat)	• Prevents the binding of fibrinogen to platelets, thereby blocking platelet aggregation • Used with aspirin for patients with ACS or during PCI
β-Adrenergic Blockers (see Table 36.6)	
Cardioselective β-Blockers	
atenolol (Tenormin) bisoprolol (Zebeta) metoprolol (Lopressor) nebivolol (Bystolic)	• Inhibits sympathetic nervous stimulation of the heart • Reduces heart rate, contractility, and BP • Reduces ischemia • Decreases afterload
Nonselective β-Blockers	
carvedilol (Coreg) nadolol (Corgard) propranolol (Inderal) labetalol (Trandate)	

TABLE 37.12 Drug Therapy—cont'd

Chronic Stable Angina and Acute Coronary Syndrome

Drug	Mechanism of Action and Considerations
Calcium Channel Blockers (see Table 36.6)	
Dihydropyridines amlodipine (Norvasc) felodipine (Plendil) nifedipine (Procardia) nicardipine (Cardene) **Nondihydropyridines** diltiazem (Cardizem) verapamil (Calan)	• Prevents calcium entry into vascular smooth muscle cells and myocytes (cardiac cells) • May prevent or control coronary vasospasm • Promotes coronary and peripheral vasodilation • Reduces HR, contractility, and BP • Dihydropyridines are more potent vasodilators • Nondihydropyridines have greater effect on reducing heart rate and contractility
Nitrates (see Table 36.6)	
isosorbide dinitrate (Isordil) isosorbide mononitrate (Imdur) Sublingual nitroglycerin (Nitrostat) Translingual spray nitroglycerin (Nitrolingual) Nitroglycerin ointment Transdermal nitroglycerin IV nitroglycerin	• Promotes peripheral vasodilation, decreasing preload and afterload • Promotes coronary artery vasodilation • May prevent or control coronary vasospasm • Monitor for hypotension • Headache is a common side effect • Avoid use of erectile dysfunction drugs while taking nitrates
Opioids	
fentanyl	• Functions as an analgesic and sedative
morphine	• Functions as an analgesic and sedative • Acts as a vasodilator to reduce preload and myocardial O_2 consumption
Sodium Current Inhibitor	
ranolazine (Ranexa)	• Treats chronic angina in patients who have not had an adequate response with other antianginal medications • No effect on BP or HR
Thrombolytic Agents	
reteplase (Retavase) alteplase (Activase) tenecteplase (TNKase)	• Breaks up fibrin meshwork in clots • Used only in STEMI when access to a hospital with PCI capability is not available or is too far away

ACS, Acute coronary syndrome; *HF,* heart failure; *LV,* left ventricular; *MI,* myocardial infarction; *NSTEMI,* non-ST segment elevation myocardial infarction; *PCI,* percutaneous coronary intervention; *STEMI,* ST segment elevation myocardial infarction; *TIA,* transient ischemic attack; *UA,* unstable angina.

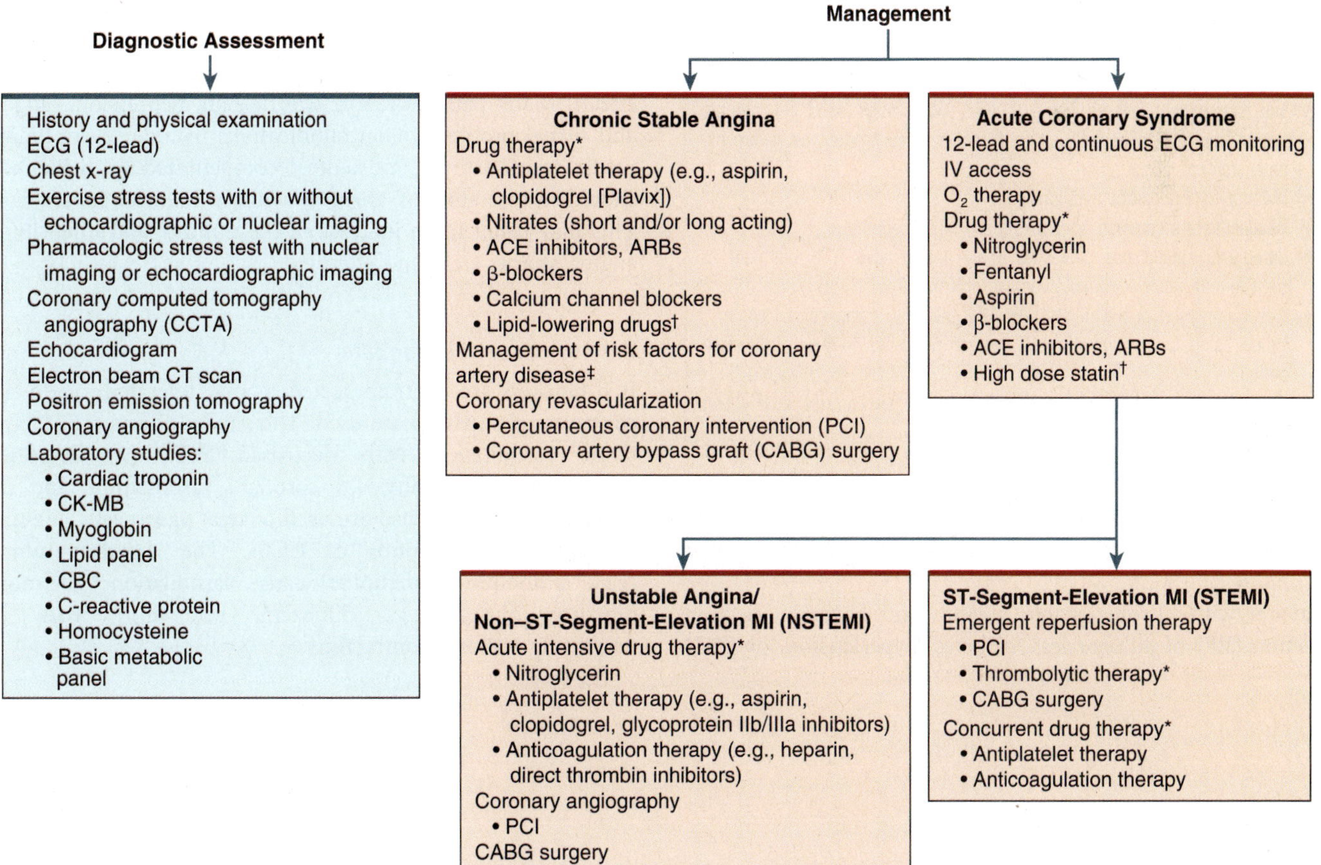

Fig. 37.6 Interprofessional care: Chronic stable angina and acute coronary syndrome. *Table 37.12. †Table 37.6. ‡Tables 37.2, 37.4, and 37.5.

are longer acting than SL or translingual NTG. They can reduce the frequency of angina attacks and may be used to treat vasospastic angina. The main side effect is headache from the dilation of cerebral blood vessels. Tell patients to take acetaminophen to relieve the headache. Over time, headaches may decrease. Remind patients that taking a long-acting NTG preparation should not keep them from using translingual or SL NTG if chest pain develops.

Nitroglycerin paste is a 2% NTG topical ointment dosed by the inch. It is placed on the upper body or arm over a flat muscular area that is free of hair and scars. Once absorbed, it prevents or reduces angina frequency for 3 to 6 hours. The ointment should be wiped off each evening to allow for a 10- to 14-hour nitrate-free interval to prevent nitrate tolerance.

Transdermal NTG is a single patch applied once a day to the upper body or upper arms for timed release of NTG over a 24-hour period. Patches should be worn for 12 to 14 hours and removed in the evening to allow for a 10- to 14-hour nitrate-free interval to prevent nitrate tolerance.

Teach male patients using drugs for erectile dysfunction (e.g., sildenafil, tadalafil) not to use these drugs within 48 hours of using nitrates because severe hypotension has been reported.[7] Tell patients to discuss the use of these drugs with their HCP.

DRUG ALERT

Nitrates

- Keep SL NTG tablets in a dark, airtight container to maintain potency.
- Tell the patient to sit down before using short-acting nitrates.
- Place SL NTG under the tongue.
- Spray translingual NTG onto or under the tongue.
- Tell the patient not to combine NTG with drugs used for erectile dysfunction (e.g., sildenafil) within 48 hours of each other, as severe hypotension can occur.
- Monitor for orthostatic hypotension.
- Headaches are common after taking any NTG preparation.
- Caregivers should use gloves to apply and remove NTG ointment or transdermal patches to avoid contact with the drug.
- Never cardiovert or defibrillate over NTG paste or a transdermal patch.
- When using long-acting nitrates, provide a 10- to 14-hour nitrate-free period.
- Remind patients using long-acting nitrates that they can use short-acting nitrates when needed.

Angiotensin-Converting Enzyme Inhibitors and Angiotensin Receptor Blockers

Patients with chronic stable angina who have an ejection fraction (EF) of 40% or less, diabetes, hypertension, or CKD should take an ACE inhibitor (e.g., ramipril) indefinitely unless contraindicated. Patients with chronic stable angina with a normal EF, diabetes, and 1 other CAD risk factor also should take an ACE inhibitor to decrease the risk of MI, stroke, and death.[7]

These drugs result in vasodilation, which is why we use them to treat hypertension. More importantly, they can prevent or reverse ventricular remodeling in patients who have had an MI. For patients who are intolerant of ACE inhibitors (e.g., cough, angioedema), angiotensin receptor blockers (ARBs) are used (e.g., losartan). ACE inhibitors and ARBs are discussed in Chapter 36 and Table 36.6.

β-Adrenergic Blockers

β-Blockers are used to relieve angina in patients with chronic stable angina. These drugs decrease myocardial contractility, HR, SVR, and BP to reduce the myocardial O_2 demand and prevent angina. β-Blockers work by blocking β-1 receptors (mostly found in cardiac tissue) and β-2 receptors (mostly found in bronchial and smooth muscle tissue). β-Blockers are categorized as nonselective (block β-1 and β-2 receptors) or selective (block β-1 receptors). Selective β-blockers include metoprolol and bisoprolol. Patients who have LV dysfunction (LVEF $\leq$40%) may take β-blockers indefinitely unless contraindicated because of asthma or severe bradycardia. β-Blockers that are proven to reduce the risk for death in patients with LV dysfunction, HF, or MI include carvedilol, metoprolol succinate, and bisoprolol.

β-Blockers have many side effects. These include bradycardia, hypotension, wheezing from bronchospasm, and GI effects. Many patients report weight gain, depression, fatigue, and sexual problems. Contraindications include severe bradycardia, severe asthma, and acute decompensated HF. β-Blockers should not be stopped abruptly without medical supervision. This may result in an increase in the number and intensity of angina attacks (rebound effect).

Calcium Channel Blockers

If β-blockers are contraindicated, poorly tolerated, or do not control angina, CCBs are used. Their main effects are (1) systemic vasodilation with decreased SVR, (2) decreased myocardial contractility, (3) coronary vasodilation, and (4) decreased HR. They also are used to treat vasospastic angina.

There are 2 groups of CCBs. The dihydropyridines (e.g., amlodipine, nifedipine) cause vasodilation. The nondihydropyridines (e.g., diltiazem, verapamil) work by decreasing HR and contractility.

Side effects include fatigue, headache, dizziness, flushing, hypotension, and peripheral edema. The nondihydropyridines increase digoxin levels. We closely monitor digoxin levels after starting these agents. Teach patients the signs and symptoms of digoxin toxicity (e.g., GI symptoms, confusion, visual disturbances). Verapamil can cause severe constipation by relaxing GI smooth muscle and slowing peristalsis, especially in older adults.

Sodium Current Inhibitor

Ranolazine, a sodium current inhibitor, is used to treat chronic angina in patients who have not had an adequate response with other medications. Ranolazine does not affect BP or HR. It can prolong the QT interval. Use it very cautiously in patients with a long QT interval or who are taking other QT-prolonging drugs (e.g., fluoxetine). Common side effects include dizziness, nausea, constipation, and headache.

Select Antiinflammatory Agent

Colchicine is an antiinflammatory drug that was added to the guideline recommendations.[7] In patients with chronic stable angina, colchicine may be added for secondary prevention to reduce future cardiac events. GI side effects are common.

Lipid-Lowering Drugs

High LDL and triglyceride levels are one of the biggest risk factors for developing CAD. The treatment of high cholesterol focuses mostly on lowering LDL cholesterol and triglyceride levels (Table 37.6). Guidelines for treating high LDL levels are based on known risk factors and a person's 10-year risk for having heart disease or stroke. In people who do not have CAD, an LDL level of <100 mg/dL is desirable.[2] If there is any evidence of CAD, an LDL of <70 mg/dL is the goal.[7]

HMG-CoA reductase inhibitors (statins). The statin drugs are the most widely used lipid-lowering drugs (Table 37.6). They inhibit cholesterol synthesis in the liver and increase the number of hepatic LDL receptors, removing more LDL from the blood. Statins reduce the lipid content in atherosclerotic lesions and promote plaque stability, reducing the chance of plaque rupture. They can cause a small decrease in triglyceride levels and a very small increase in HDL.[3] Statins are prescribed for secondary prevention with ACS to reduce future cardiac events and strokes and can decrease mortality, even if LDL levels are in the "normal" range.

Patients who should receive statin therapy include:

- Those with known CAD
- Those at very high risk for CAD with an LDL greater than 70 mg/dL
- Those with primary elevations of LDL cholesterol levels of ≥190 mg/dL
- Those 40 to 75 years of age with diabetes and LDL cholesterol levels greater than 70 mg/dL
- Those 40 to 75 years of age without diabetes with LDL cholesterol levels ≥70 mg/dL plus a 10-year risk for CAD of 7.5% or greater

Treatment goals include (1) treating patients with known CAD but no clinical events with a high-dose statin (e.g., atorvastatin 80 mg) to reduce the LDL by 50% and (2) treating very high-risk patients (patients with a history of 1 or more major events and multiple high-risk conditions) with a high-dose statin to lower the LDL to less than 70 mg/dL. People without known CAD who are 40 to 75 years of age should discuss with the HCP their 10-year risk before starting a statin.[11]

Drug therapy continues for a lifetime. Lipid levels should be reassessed after 4 to 8 weeks of therapy. If they are still high, drug therapy may be changed. If the patient becomes intolerant, we may change the drug. Intolerance to one statin does not mean intolerance to all statins. Adverse effects include liver damage and myalgia (muscle ache or weakness without breakdown of skeletal muscle) that can progress to rhabdomyolysis (breakdown of skeletal muscle).[3]

Review the rationale and goals of treatment, along with the safety and side effects of lipid-lowering drugs. Treatment includes weight loss, if overweight, and increased physical activity.

DRUG ALERT

Simvastatin

- Prothrombin time may increase in patients taking warfarin.
- Use with caution in patients on amiodarone because it can increase the risk of myopathy.

Niacin. Niacin, a water-soluble B vitamin, is effective in lowering triglyceride levels and mildly lowering LDL levels (Table 37.6). At high doses, niacin may increase HDL levels. Research shows that adding niacin does not reduce the risk of CAD and MI in patients who are on a statin.[7]

Fibric acid derivatives (fibrates). Fibric acid derivatives (e.g., fenofibrate, gemfibrozil) are used to lower triglyceride levels (Table 37.6). They can increase HDL levels and indirectly lower LDL through their effect on HDL and triglycerides. Most patients tolerate the drugs well.

DRUG ALERT

Gemfibrozil

- May increase the risk of bleeding in patients taking warfarin.
- Use cautiously in patients taking statins because of an increased risk of myopathy.

Bile acid sequestrants. Bile acid sequestrants (e.g., colesevelam) bind bile acids in the intestine and prevent their reabsorption in the liver (Table 37.6). This stimulates the production of more LDL receptors to reduce LDL levels. Bile acid sequestrants decrease absorption of many other drugs (e.g., warfarin, thiazides). Tell patients to take those drugs 1 hour before or 3 to 4 hours after bile acid sequestrants to decrease this adverse effect.[3]

Proprotein convertase subtilisin/kexin 9 inhibitors. Proprotein convertase subtilisin/kexin 9 (PCSK9) is a protein secreted into the blood by the liver. Receptors in the liver are responsible for removing LDL cholesterol from the blood. The

LDL receptors do this over and over. When the PCSK9 protein binds to an LDL receptor, it destroys the receptor, thus reducing the number of available receptors (Table 37.6). Inhibiting the PCSK9 enzyme allows more LDL receptors to be available, thus decreasing LDL levels. They can cut LDL levels by 50% to 60%.[3] Evolocumab (Repatha) and alirocumab (Praluent) are the approved PCSK9 inhibitors. They are not first-line therapy. They are used with diet and maximum statin therapy for adults with FH and those with CAD who have an inadequate response to statins.[7,11] For those who are intolerant of statins, it may be used as the sole therapy.

Adenosine triphosphate—citrate lyase inhibitor. Bempedoic acid decreases the liver's ability to make cholesterol by inhibiting a liver enzyme called adenosine triphosphate—citrate lyase (ACL). This drug should be avoided in patients receiving more than 20 mg of simvastatin or 40 mg of pravastatin because it can increase levels of both drugs.

Small interfering ribonucleic acid. Inclisiran is for patients on the maximum statin dose who need additional LDL lowering. It is approved for adults with FH and works by breaking down the PCSK9 protein, allowing more LDL receptors to be available. It is given as a one-time subcutaneous injection that is repeated in 3 months. It is then dosed subcutaneously every 6 months.

Cholesterol absorption inhibitor. Ezetimibe selectively inhibits diet and biliary cholesterol absorption across the intestinal wall (Table 37.6). It is usually added with a statin to achieve an even greater reduction in LDL.

Omega-3 fatty acids (fish oil). Research on over-the-counter fish oil supplements has not shown any cardiovascular benefit. The prescription drug icosapent ethyl has been shown to reduce the risk of cardiovascular events.[7] Side effects are rare but include bleeding. This is why fish oil is often held before surgery.

Antiplatelet Therapy

Antiplatelet therapy with daily low-dose aspirin (81 mg) is used for secondary prevention (e.g., people with known CAD). Aspirin for primary prevention (e.g., people without known CAD) is controversial because of the potential risk for bleeding. Low-dose aspirin may be used for primary prevention in adults ages 40 to 70 years who are at high risk of developing CAD but do not have an increased risk for bleeding. It should not be started as primary prevention in adults over age 70.[19] Enteric-coated aspirin is recommended to help with GI protection. If a patient has a true allergy to aspirin, another antiplatelet medication can be used such as clopidogrel.

Diagnostic and Interventional Studies

When a patient describes new-onset chest pain and we suspect CAD, or when a patient with chronic stable angina has a change in the angina pattern, a variety of studies are done (Fig. 37.6). After a detailed health history and physical assessment, we compare a 12-lead ECG with a previous ECG for changes that may indicate an ACS. Laboratory tests (e.g., cardiac biomarkers [troponin]) can determine whether the patient is having an ACS event. Other laboratory tests (e.g., lipid profile, lipo(a), HbA1c) can identify risk factors for CAD. A chest x-ray may show cardiac enlargement, aortic calcifications, or pulmonary congestion. An echocardiogram can detect resting LV wall motion abnormalities suggestive of CAD.

If the ECG and troponin levels are negative, the patient may have an exercise stress test (walking on a treadmill) with or without imaging. Imaging techniques include echocardiography to look for wall motion abnormalities or nuclear imaging to look for perfusion abnormalities. Nuclear perfusion images can be obtained using either single photon emission CT (SPECT) or positron emission tomography (PET). For those with physical limitations in walking, a pharmacologic (e.g., adenosine, dipyridamole) stress test with nuclear imaging or a pharmacologic (dobutamine) stress echocardiogram are options. Stress testing with imaging may be abnormal if coronary blockages are greater than 50% in the left main coronary artery or 70% in other vessels. Coronary artery calcium (CAC) scoring or coronary computed tomography angiography (CCTA, CTA) testing may be done if there is no evidence of ACS and the patient remains free of chest pain. See Table 35.10 for more about these studies. Cardiovascular magnetic resonance (CMR) can evaluate ventricular function, identify myocardial ischemia and infarct, and assess myocardial viability. CMR can detect microvascular obstruction.[15]

Coronary Angiography and Percutaneous Coronary Intervention

For patients with increasing angina, cardiac catheterization with coronary angiography is the gold-standard test to directly visualize the coronary arteries. It can be done via radial or femoral artery access using contrast and fluoroscopy. It may be done for a patient with chest discomfort who has a normal ECG and biomarkers but has an abnormal stress test. Coronary angiography should be done only if the patient is a candidate for percutaneous or surgical coronary revascularization. Depending on the findings and patient factors, some patients are treated with medical therapy. Others are referred for percutaneous or surgical intervention.

Coronary revascularization with **percutaneous coronary intervention (PCI)** may be done at the same time as the coronary angiography or at a later time. During PCI, a catheter with a deflated balloon tip is inserted into the blocked coronary artery. The deflated balloon is positioned inside the blockage and inflated. This compresses the plaque against the artery wall, resulting in vessel dilation and a larger vessel diameter. This procedure is a *balloon angioplasty.*

Intracoronary stents are usually placed after a balloon angioplasty. A **stent** is an expandable meshlike structure designed to keep a coronary artery open (Figs. 37.7 and 37.8). There are 2 types of stents: bare metal stents (BMSs) and drug-eluting stents (DESs). A DES is coated with a drug (e.g., everolimus, zotarolimus) to reduce the risk for overgrowth of the intimal lining *(neointimal hyperplasia)* within the stent.

Because stents are thrombogenic, drugs are used to prevent platelet aggregation and thrombosis within the stent. Drugs commonly used during PCI are unfractionated heparin (UH) or low-molecular-weight heparin (LMWH), a direct thrombin inhibitor (e.g., bivalirudin), and/or a GP IIb/IIIa inhibitor (e.g., tirofiban) (Table 37.12). After PCI, the patient receives dual antiplatelet therapy (DAPT) (e.g., aspirin plus clopidogrel) until the intimal lining grows over the metal stent and provides a smooth vascular surface. Clopidogrel is given as a 600-mg loading dose followed by 75 mg daily.

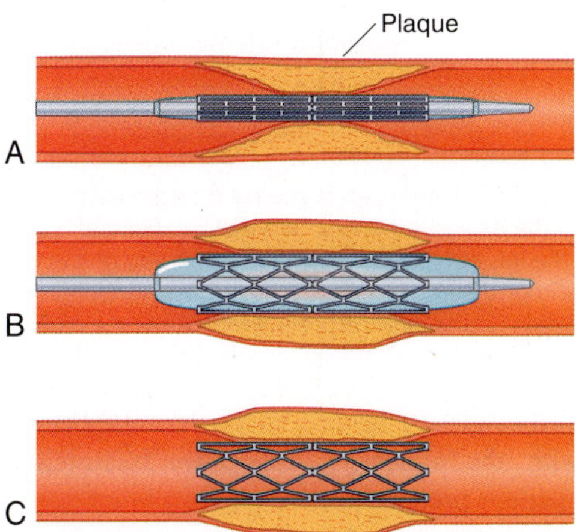

Fig. 37.7 Placement of a coronary artery stent. (A) The stent is placed at the site of the lesion. (B) The balloon is inflated, expanding the stent. The balloon is then deflated and removed. (C) The implanted stent is left in place.

After DES placement, DAPT is typically continued for a minimum of 12 months to prevent thrombosis inside the stent. With the newer-generation DESs, 6 months of DAPT is enough to prevent stent thrombosis; however, patients remain on 1 antiplatelet medication after DAPT is stopped (either low-dose coated aspirin or clopidogrel).[17] The duration of DAPT for patients with a BMS is a minimum of 1 month after PCI, then 1 antiplatelet medication is continued.

Potential complications from coronary angiography with PCI include (1) abrupt closure from coronary artery dissection or rupture, (2) vascular injury at the artery access site (e.g., femoral, radial), (3) acute MI from acute stent thrombosis or from plaque dislodging and blocking the vessel distal to the original blockage, (4) stent embolization, (5) failure to cross the blockage with a balloon or stent, (6) coronary spasm, (7) dye allergy, (8) renal injury, (9) bleeding (e.g., hematoma or retroperitoneal bleeding), (10) infection, (11) stroke, and (12) the need for emergent coronary artery bypass graft (CABG) surgery. The risk for dysrhythmias during and after PCI is high, so monitor the ECG afterward. Before and after coronary angiography and PCI, patients need frequent monitoring and interventions (Table 37.13).

More PCIs than CABGs are done in the United States.[2] The advantages of PCI include (1) it is done with IV sedation and local anesthesia; (2) the patient is ambulatory shortly after the procedure; (3) the length of stay for patients with stable coronary disease who undergo elective PCI is less than 24 hours compared with 4 to 6 days after CABG surgery, thus reducing hospital costs; and (4) the patient can return to work several

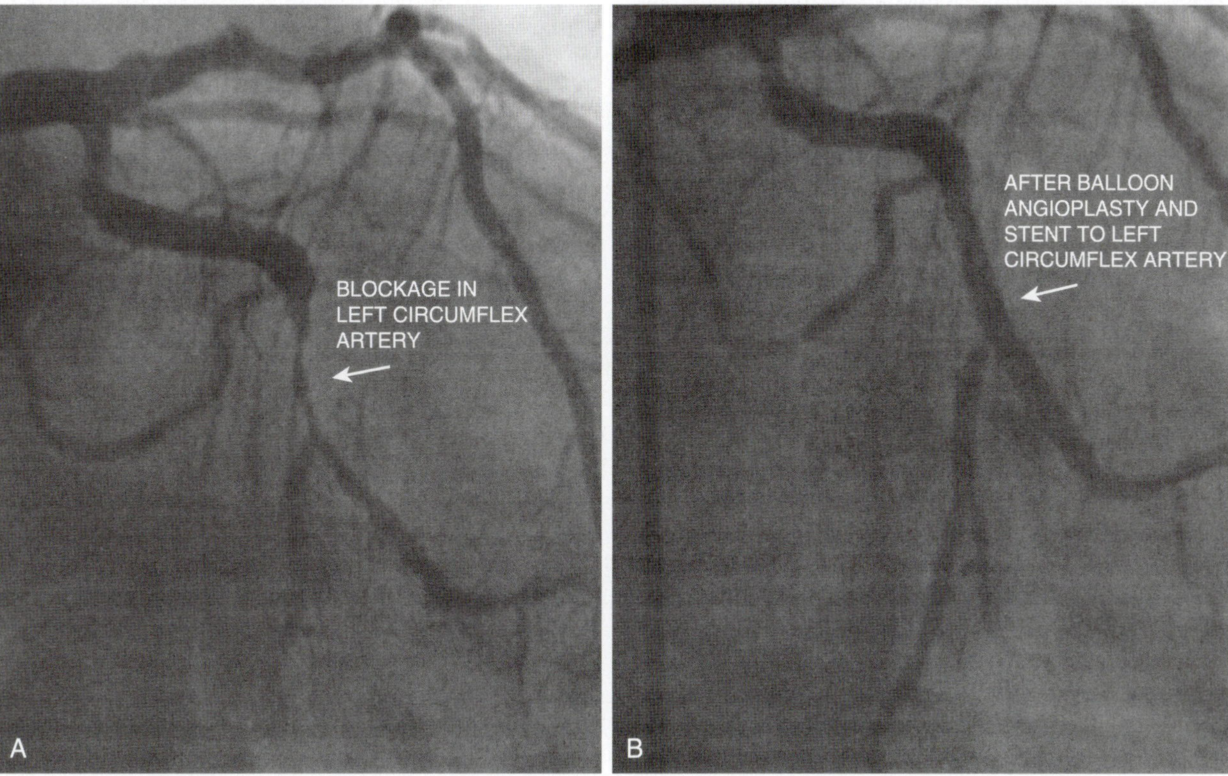

Fig. 37.8 (A) Ninety percent occlusion of the left circumflex artery *(arrow)*. (B) Left circumflex artery is opened after balloon angioplasty and drug-eluting stent (DES) placement.

TABLE 37.13 NURSING MANAGEMENT

Percutaneous Coronary Intervention

Preprocedure

- Assess for allergies, especially to contrast dye.
- Perform baseline assessment, including vital signs, pulse oximetry, heart and breath sounds, neurovascular assessment of extremities (e.g., distal pulses, skin temperature, skin color, sensation).
- Withhold food and fluids for 6–12 h before planned procedures.
- Assess baseline laboratory values (e.g., CBC, BMP).
- Give ordered drugs before the procedure and stop drugs not needed for the procedure.
- Teach patient and caregiver about procedure and postprocedure care.

Postprocedure

- Perform assessment and compare to baseline: vital signs, pulse oximetry, heart and breath sounds, neurovascular assessment of extremity used for procedure, assessment of catheter insertion site for hematoma, bleeding, and bruit.
- Assess compression device over arterial site to assure hemostasis per agency policy.
- Assess neurovascular status of accessed extremity every 15 min for the first hour, then according to agency policy.
- Check for bleeding or hematoma at catheter insertion site every 15 min for the first hour, then according to agency policy.
- Report changes in neurovascular status of involved extremity or any bleeding.
- Monitor ECG for dysrhythmias or other changes (e.g., ST segment elevation or depression).
- Monitor for chest pain and other sources of pain or discomfort (e.g., back, vascular access site).
- Monitor IV infusions of antianginals (e.g., nitroglycerin) and antiplatelet medications (e.g., tirofiban).
- Maintain bed rest as prescribed after femoral artery access.
- Teach patient and caregiver about discharge drugs and DAPT therapy.
- Teach patient and caregiver about discharge care, including signs and symptoms to report to HCP (e.g., access site complications, return of chest pain).

Assistive Personnel

- Supervise AP:
  - Take vital signs and report increases or decreases in HR or BP to RN.
  - Report patient descriptions of chest pain, shortness of breath, and/or any other discomfort or distress to RN.
  - Report changes in neurovascular status of the involved extremity or any bleeding to the RN.
  - Help with oral hygiene and hydration, meals, and toileting.
  - Record oral intake and urine output as ordered.

BMP, Basic metabolic panel; *CBC,* complete blood count.

weeks sooner after PCI, compared with 6- to 8-weeks after CABG.

PCI may not be feasible for all patients. CABG surgery provides a survival benefit in some groups of patients (e.g., 3-vessel CAD, 3-vessel CAD with diabetes and/or LV dysfunction).[17] If the optimal treatment (PCI or CABG) for CAD is not clear (e.g., patients with complex disease or serious comorbid conditions), a heart team approach is recommended. The heart team should include cardiac surgeons and interventional and general cardiologists. They review the risks and benefits of each option with the patient. Collaborative treatment decisions consider patient preferences.[17]

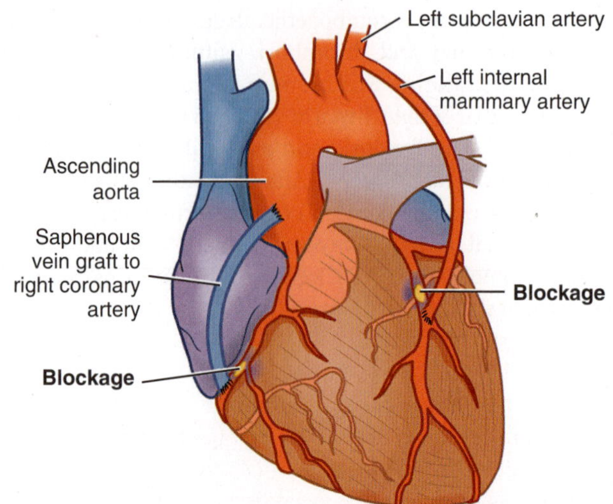

Fig. 37.9 Proximal end of the left internal mammary artery (LIMA) is left attached to the subclavian artery, and the distal end of the LIMA is sutured into the left anterior descending (LAD) artery below the blockage. Proximal end of the saphenous vein is sutured to the aorta. The distal end is sutured into the right coronary artery below the area of blockage.

Surgical Coronary Revascularization

Coronary revascularization with CABG surgery is generally recommended for patients with chronic stable angina who (1) do not respond well to medical management, (2) have 3-vessel CAD with or without diabetes, (3) have ischemic cardiomyopathy and/or significant left main CAD, (4) are not candidates for PCI (e.g., blockages are long or difficult to access), or (5) continue to have chest pain after PCI. CABG surgery and PCI do not cure CAD. Both procedures are done to alleviate angina. Even after CABG, the bypass grafts are subject to the same progressive disease process as native coronary arteries. Lifestyle changes and medications may help slow the progression of plaque buildup in the bypass grafts and reduce the risk for recurrent events.

CABG surgery consists of placing 1 or more arterial or venous grafts distal to the blocked coronary artery to provide blood to the heart muscle. Vessels used as bypass grafts include the (1) saphenous vein from the leg, (2) radial artery from the forearm, and (3) internal mammary artery (IMA), also known as the internal thoracic artery (ITA). It is a branch of the subclavian artery (Fig. 37.9).

Traditional Coronary Artery Bypass Graft Surgery

Traditional CABG surgery requires a sternotomy (opening of the chest cavity) and *cardiopulmonary bypass* (CPB). During CPB, blood is diverted from the heart to a machine. There it is oxygenated and returned (via a pump) to the patient. This allows the HCP to operate on a quiet, nonbeating, bloodless heart while vital organs are perfused. CPB can cause postoperative neurologic problems (e.g., cognitive issues, stroke), renal problems, dysrhythmias, and bleeding.[20]

The left IMA (LIMA) is the most common artery used as a bypass graft. The proximal part remains attached to its origin (the left subclavian artery). The distal end of the LIMA is dissected from the chest wall and sutured to the coronary artery distal to the blockage. It usually is used to bypass the left anterior descending (LAD) artery because the LAD supplies blood to the largest part of the heart muscle (anterior wall). IMAs also tend to have longer patency rates than saphenous veins (Fig. 37.9). Using the right IMA and LIMA carries an increased risk of sternal wound infection, especially in patients with diabetes or obesity.[17]

Saphenous veins can be used for bypass grafts. The HCP endoscopically removes the saphenous vein from 1 or both legs. A section is sutured into the ascending aorta near the opening of the native coronary artery and then anastomosed to the coronary artery distal to the blockage (Fig. 37.9). Saphenous vein grafts are more prone to developing diffuse intimal hyperplasia, future stenosis, and graft occlusion.

The radial artery, another potential graft, is a thick muscular artery prone to spasm. Perioperative CCBs or long-acting nitrates are used to control the spasms.[20] Patency rates are not as good as the IMA but are better than saphenous veins. Serious extremity complications (e.g., hand ischemia, wound infection) are rare after removal of the radial artery. The nondominant hand is usually used because patients may develop paresthesia and impaired sensation in the hand after radial artery harvest.

Minimally Invasive Direct Coronary Artery Bypass

Minimally invasive direct coronary artery bypass (MIDCAB) offers patients an approach to surgical treatment that does not involve a sternotomy and CPB. The technique requires several small incisions between the ribs or a minithoracotomy. Because this procedure is done on a beating heart, a mechanical stabilizer immobilizes the heart so bypass grafts can be sewn into the native artery.

Off-Pump Coronary Artery Bypass

The off-pump coronary artery bypass (OPCAB) procedure uses a median sternotomy to access all coronary vessels. CPB is not used, thus the name "off-pump coronary bypass." OPCAB is performed on a beating heart using mechanical stabilizers.

Totally Endoscopic Coronary Artery Bypass (Robotic-Assisted Coronary Artery Bypass)

Totally endoscopic coronary artery bypass (TECAB) uses robotic technology to perform CABG surgery. It requires several instrument ports in the chest cavity so there is no surgical incision. CPB may or may not be used. This procedure is done mostly for patients with LAD disease where a LIMA graft can be used. TECAB is not widely accepted because of increased time and personnel needed.[20]

Benefits of MIDCAB, OPCAB, and TECAB include potential reductions in blood loss, postoperative pain, risk of sternal wound infection, bed rest time, renal and neurologic issues, inflammatory response (if CPB is not used), hospital stays, and recovery times.[20]

Postoperative Care After CABG Surgery

Care after CABG surgery is provided in the intensive care unit (ICU) for 24 to 48 hours. Ongoing intensive monitoring of hemodynamic status is critical. The patient will have continuous ECG monitoring and invasive lines for monitoring vital functions (see Chapter 35). These may include (1) hemodynamic monitoring (e.g., CO), (2) an arterial line for continuous BP monitoring, (3) pleural and mediastinal chest tubes for chest drainage, (4) an endotracheal tube connected to mechanical ventilation, (5) epicardial pacing wires for emergency pacing of the heart, (6) a urinary catheter to monitor urine output, and (7) a nasogastric tube for gastric decompression. Most patients are extubated within 6 hours and transferred to a step-down unit within 24 to 48 hours for continued monitoring.

Many of the complications that develop after CABG surgery relate to the use of CPB. Major complications of CPB are bleeding and anemia from damage to red blood cells and platelets, fluid and electrolyte imbalances, infection, and hypothermia. Focus your care on assessing the patient for bleeding (e.g., chest tube drainage, incision sites), monitoring hemodynamics, checking fluid status, replacing blood and electrolytes as needed, and restoring temperature (e.g., warming blankets).

Postoperative dysrhythmias, especially atrial fibrillation (AF), are common. New-onset AF occurs in about 18% of patients after CABG surgery.[17] β-Blockers and amiodarone should be started before CABG surgery and restarted as soon as possible after surgery (unless contraindicated) to reduce the incidence of AF.[17] See Chapter 39 for information on treating AF.

Sternal wound infections are a serious and deadly complication that occur in <1% of patients undergoing CABG surgery. Patients with diabetes or stress-induced hyperglycemia should have an insulin infusion to maintain a glucose of <180 mg/dL to help reduce the risk of sternal wound infection.[17]

Provide wound care for the surgical sites (e.g., leg, chest, arm). Chest and radial site incisions often do not need dressings after 24 hours. Management of the chest wound is like that of other chest surgeries (see Chapter 28). Care of the leg incision is minimal because endoscopy is used to harvest the vein.

Care of a radial artery harvest site includes monitoring sensory and motor function of the hand. Patients with a radial artery harvest may take a CCB and/or a long-acting nitrate after surgery to reduce the incidence of arterial spasm.[20]

Other nursing interventions include strategies to manage pain and prevent venous thromboembolism (e.g., early ambulation, sequential compression device) and respiratory complications (e.g., incentive spirometry, splinting during coughing and deep-breathing exercises). Chapter 20 details care of postoperative patients.

Postoperative cognitive dysfunction (POCD) can manifest days to weeks after surgery. It usually improves within a few months after surgery. For some, POCD can become a chronic problem. This includes impairment of memory, concentration, language comprehension, and social integration. Depression and anxiety are common.

Older patients (>75 years) can often undergo elective CABG with good results. Many have multiple preoperative comorbidities, so the incidence of postoperative complications (e.g., dysrhythmias, stroke, POCD, infection) is higher. Although older patients may benefit from PCI or CABG surgery, any decisions should incorporate the informed patient's wishes.[17]

Postoperative nursing care of patients with a MIDCAB, OPCAB, or TECAB procedure is similar to caring for patients who undergo traditional CABG surgery, although the recovery time usually is shorter. Patients often resume routine activities sooner than patients who have traditional CABG surgery. Patients often report higher levels of pain with a thoracotomy incision than with a sternotomy incision. Bleeding; AF; infection; and renal, pulmonary, and neurologic complications can occur with MIDCAB, OPCAB, and TECAB surgery, although less commonly than with traditional CABG surgery.[20]

Enhanced External Counterpulsation

Patients with refractory angina sometimes use *enhanced external counterpulsation* (EECP).[7] Inflatable BP cuffs are placed around the calves and thighs. The cuffs sequentially inflate during diastole and deflate during systole from the calves to the thighs. This action increases venous return (increases preload) and decreases aortic pressure (decreases afterload), so the LV does not need to work as hard to push the blood out into the aorta. This increases coronary perfusion, improves LV diastolic filling, and helps with collateral circulation.[21] Patients go for treatment 5 days a week for a total of 35 sessions. EECP is contraindicated in patients with decompensated HF, severe peripheral artery disease, and severe aortic regurgitation.

ACUTE CORONARY SYNDROME

Acute coronary syndrome (ACS) is caused by the rupture or erosion of an atherosclerotic plaque with partial or complete coronary artery thrombosis. The thrombus may decrease blood flow to the myocardium, leading to myocardial ischemia and infarction.[22] A **myocardial infarction (MI)** is necrosis of myocardial tissue due to ischemia.[22] ACS includes the spectrum of non-ST elevation ACS (*UA and non–ST segment elevation myocardial infarction* [NSTEMI]) and *ST segment elevation myocardial infarction* (STEMI) (Fig. 37.10). The severity of ACS depends on the degree of narrowing caused by the thrombus. Patients with NSTEMI may have a partially occluded coronary artery, which leads to subendocardial ischemia. Those with STEMI often have a completely occluded artery.[22]

It is unclear what causes the plaque to become unstable in a MI, but systemic inflammation may play a role. When the plaque ruptures, the lipid core spills into the artery. Platelets accumulate in large numbers at the site, causing a thrombus, which in turn, creates an abrupt partial or complete stoppage of blood flow. This can cause irreversible myocardial cell death (necrosis) in the heart muscle beyond the blockage (Fig. 37.11). Most MIs occur in the person with preexisting CAD. MINOCA occurs in about 5% to 6% of patients presenting with an acute MI.

Heart muscle cells become hypoxic within seconds to minutes of a coronary occlusion as they are deprived of O_2 and glucose. The O_2-depleted myocardium uses anaerobic metabolism, causing glucose levels to increase and lactic acid to accumulate. In ischemic conditions, heart cells are viable for about 20 minutes. Irreversible heart damage starts after 20 minutes if there is no collateral circulation (Figs. 37.2 and 37.3).[3] Cardiac biomarkers are released into the blood when there is myocardial necrosis. If blood flow can be reestablished (reperfusion), aerobic metabolism resumes, contractility is restored, and cell repair begins.

The acute MI process evolves over hours to days. The earliest heart muscle tissue to become ischemic is the subendocardium,

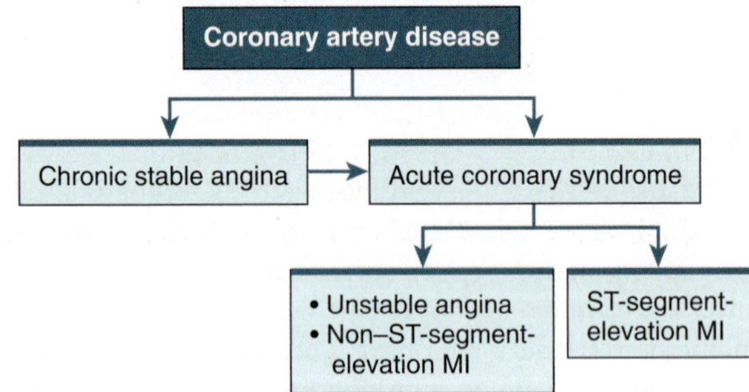

Fig. 37.10 Relationships among coronary artery disease, chronic stable angina, and acute coronary syndrome.

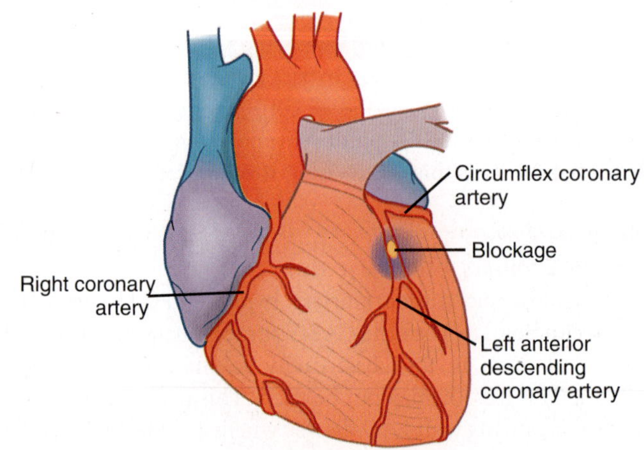

Fig. 37.11 Occlusion of the left anterior descending (LAD) coronary artery, resulting in acute myocardial infarction (MI).

the innermost layer. If ischemia persists, it takes about 4 to 6 hours for the entire thickness of the heart muscle to necrose. In the case of NSTEMI, where a thrombus is partially blocking the artery, the time to complete necrosis may be as long as 12 hours.[22]

Most MIs affect the LV. They are described based on the location of infarction (e.g., anterior, inferior, lateral, septal, or posterior wall). The location of the MI and ECG changes correlate with the involved coronary artery (Table 37.14). For example, in most people, the right coronary artery (RCA) supplies blood to the inferior and posterior LV walls. Blockage of the RCA results in an inferior wall and/or posterior wall MI. Anterior wall infarctions result from blockages in the LAD artery. Blockages in the left circumflex artery usually cause lateral wall MIs. Damage can occur in more than 1 location if more than 1 coronary artery is involved (e.g., anterolateral MI). We often see reciprocal changes (e.g., ST segment depression and/or T wave inversion) in ECG leads near the infarcted wall, which represent ischemia in that area. Right ventricular (RV) MIs are much less common and treated differently from LV MIs. Suspect an RV MI in patients who have an inferior wall STEMI because the RCA supplies both the RV and the inferior wall of the LV.

With either STEMI or NSTEMI, an echocardiogram may show *hypokinesis* (worsening myocardial contractility) or *akinesis* (absent myocardial contractility) in the infarcted area(s). The degree of LV dysfunction depends on the area of the heart involved and size of the infarction.

ST Elevation Myocardial Infarction

A STEMI, caused by a complete occlusive thrombus, results in ST elevation in the ECG leads facing the area of infarction (Figs. 37.5B, 37.12, and 37.13). ST segment elevation is significant if it is 1 mm (1 small block) or more above the isoelectric line in at least 2 contiguous leads (2 leads that look at the same wall of the heart) except in V_2 and V_3. In those leads, the ST elevation must be 2 mm (2 small blocks) or more to be significant.[23] ST elevation represents myocardial injury that is potentially reversible but, if not treated emergently, likely will evolve to permanent necrosis (tissue death) of the myocardium.

A STEMI is an emergency. The artery must be opened within 90 minutes of presentation to restore blood and O_2 to the heart muscle and limit the infarct size. This can be done either by PCI or with thrombolytic (fibrinolytic) therapy. PCI is the first-line treatment, if available (Fig. 37.7). Thrombolytic therapy is done in hospitals that do not have a catheterization laboratory for PCI. If the patient does not seek treatment quickly, the STEMI will evolve to cause potentially significant and irreversible heart muscle damage. A pathologic Q wave will be seen on the ECG if the patient does not seek immediate treatment. A pathologic Q wave is a new Q wave not seen on a previous ECG or a deep Q wave that is greater than or equal to one-third the height of the R wave in the same lead (Fig. 37.5C).

TABLE 37.14 ECG Evidence in Acute Coronary Syndrome

Involvement Left Ventricle	Leads Facing Area	Associated Coronary Artery
Septal wall	V_1, V_2	Left anterior descending (LAD)
Anterior wall	V_3, V_4	LAD
Lateral wall, low	V_5, V_6	LAD, circumflex
Lateral wall, high	I, aVL	Circumflex
Inferior wall	II, III, aVF	Right coronary artery, posterior descending coronary artery (in rare circumstances, it can be the left circumflex artery)

Non–ST Elevation Acute Coronary Syndromes

Non–ST Elevation Myocardial Infarction

NSTEMI, caused by a nonocclusive thrombus, does not cause ST segment elevation on the 12-lead ECG. The ECG may show ST depression and/or T wave inversion in the leads facing the area of infarction (Figs. 37.5A and 37.14). They do not develop a pathologic Q wave. Cardiac biomarkers are increased. Patients with an NSTEMI do not undergo emergent angiography but usually have the procedure within 24 hours of presentation to diagnose and evaluate the extent of the disease.[17] Thrombolytic therapy is not a treatment option for patients with an NSTEMI.

Unstable Angina

Unstable angina (UA) is chest pain that is new in onset, occurs at rest, or occurs with increasing frequency, duration, or less effort than the patient's chronic stable angina pattern. UA may be the first clinical sign of CAD. The pain usually lasts 10 minutes or more. Unlike chronic stable angina, UA is unpredictable. It may occur during sleep or even at rest. Patients may describe chest pain that has progressed rapidly in the last few hours, days, or weeks, often ending in pain at rest. UA must be assessed and treated immediately (e.g., aspirin, nitrates) to prevent further ischemia. ECG changes that may occur with UA include ST depression and/or T wave inversion in the leads facing the ischemic wall(s) (Figs. 37.5A and 37.14). These patients will have *negative* cardiac biomarkers because of the lack of myocardial necrosis. A coronary angiogram may be done during the hospitalization or as an outpatient.

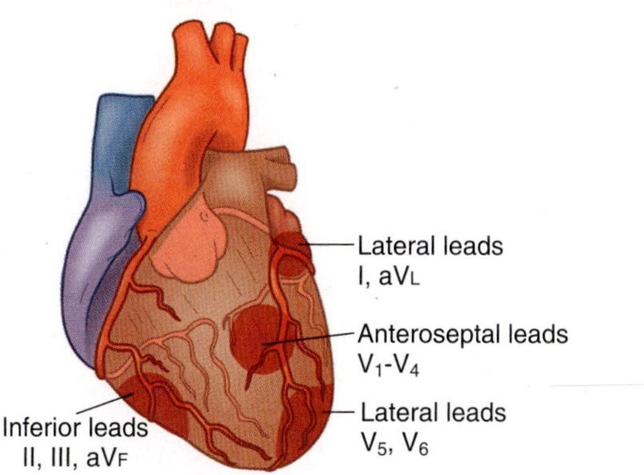

Fig. 37.12 Definitive ECG changes occur in leads that face the area of ischemia, injury, or infarction. Reciprocal changes may occur in leads facing walls near the area of injury or infarction.

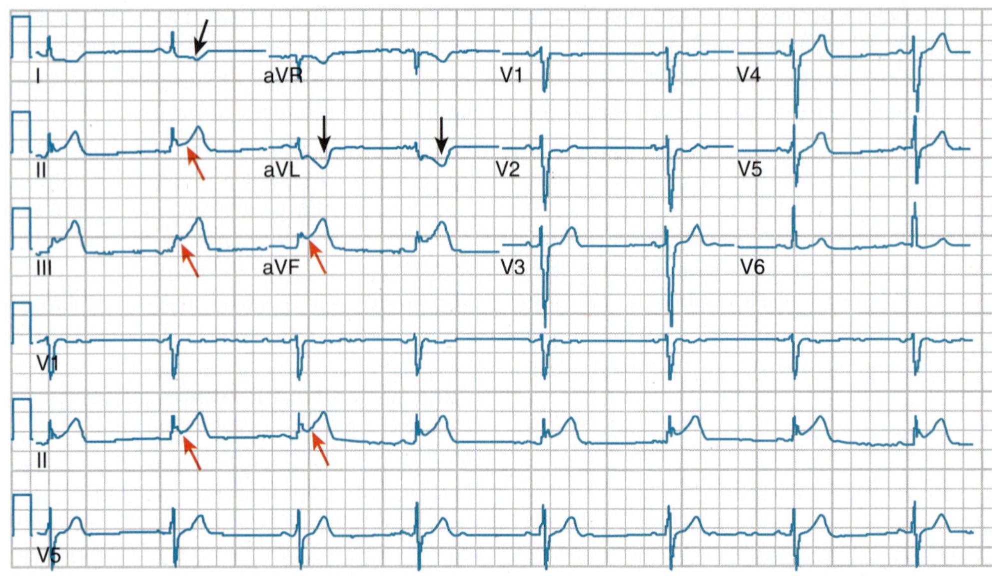

Fig. 37.13 ECG findings with an inferior ST segment elevation myocardial infarction (STEMI). Note the ST segment elevation in the inferior leads: leads II, III, and aVF *(red arrows)*. Also note the ST depression with T wave inversion in leads I and aVL *(black arrows)*, which are the reciprocal changes in the lateral leads (lateral wall ischemia). (From Ruedy J, Marshal SA: *On call principles and protocols,* ed. 7, Philadelphia, 2025, Elsevier.)

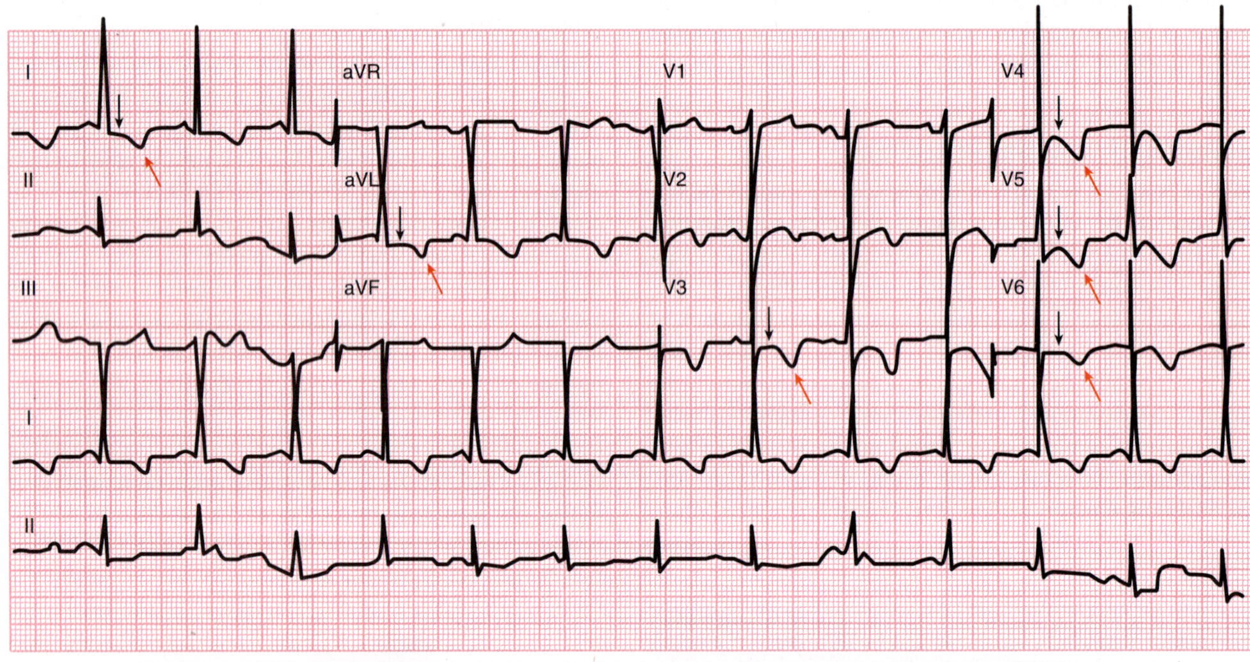

Fig. 37.14 ECG findings with anterior and lateral ischemia or non–ST segment elevation myocardial infarction (NSTEMI). Note the ST depression in the lateral leads (lead I, aVL, V_5, and V_6 *[black arrows]*) and the T wave inversion in I, aVL, V_5, and V_6 (*red arrows*). These leads face the lateral wall. Note the ST depression in 2 anterior leads (V_3 and V_4 *[black arrows]*) and the T wave inversion in V_3 and V_4 (*red arrows*). These leads face the anterior wall. Cardiac biomarkers will determine whether this patient had unstable angina (UA) or an NSTEMI.

Clinical Manifestations

Pain

Chest pain with an MI may or may not be different from previous episodes of angina. It is often described as a persistent heavy pressure or a tight, burning, constricted, or crushing feeling. Common locations are the substernal or epigastric area. The pain may radiate to the neck, lower jaw, arms, or back (Fig. 37.4). When epigastric pain is present, patients may relate it to indigestion, take antacids without relief, and therefore delay seeking treatment. It may occur while the patient is active or resting, asleep, or awake. Pain often occurs in the early morning hours related to circadian rhythms and hormone fluctuations.

Not everyone who has an MI has classic symptoms. Some patients may not describe chest "pain" but may use the word "discomfort." They may report nausea, indigestion, or shortness of breath. Some females may present with symptoms such as fatigue, weakness, shortness of breath, nausea, or indigestion. Patients with diabetes may have silent (asymptomatic) MIs because of cardiac neuropathy or have atypical symptoms (e.g., shortness of breath). Older patients may have a change in mental status (e.g., confusion, delirium), shortness of breath, dizziness, or an unexplained fall.[15]

Sympathetic Nervous System Stimulation

During the initial phase of MI, the ischemic heart cells release catecholamines. This results in diaphoresis, increased HR and BP, and vasoconstriction of peripheral blood vessels. The skin may be ashen, clammy, and cool to the touch.

Cardiovascular Manifestations

In response to the release of catecholamines, BP and HR may be high initially. Later, the BP may drop because of decreased CO. If severe enough, this may result in decreased renal perfusion and urine output. Crackles, if present, suggest LV dysfunction. Jugular venous distention (JVD), hepatic engorgement, and peripheral edema are related to RV dysfunction.

Your patient may have abnormally distant heart sounds. Other abnormal sounds suggesting LV dysfunction include an S_3 and/or S_4. A loud holosystolic murmur may occur with a ventricular septal defect or papillary muscle rupture resulting in mitral regurgitation.

Nausea and Vomiting

Your patient may have nausea and vomiting. These symptoms can result from reflex stimulation of the vomiting center by severe pain. They can also result from vasovagal reflexes initiated in the area of the infarcted heart muscle, especially with inferior wall MIs.

Fever

A low-grade fever may occur within 24 to 48 hours and last 4 to 5 days. This is the result of a systemic inflammatory process caused by the death of myocardial cells.

Healing Process

The body's response to cell death is the inflammatory process (see Chapter 12). The dead heart cells release enzymes (e.g., troponins) that are important diagnostic indicators of MI. Within hours, lymphocytes, neutrophils, and macrophages infiltrate the infarcted area to clean up the necrotic cells (myocytes). Within days to weeks, a collagen scar replaces the dead myocytes.

The necrotic zone of a STEMI is identified by ECG changes (e.g., lowering of the initially elevated ST segments, T wave inversion, and/or a pathologic Q wave) within 1 or 2 days. At this point, the lymphocytes, neutrophils, and macrophages have cleared the necrotic debris from the injured area. The collagen matrix that will eventually form scar tissue is laid down.

At 10 to 14 days after MI, the new scar tissue is still weak. The heart muscle is vulnerable to increased stress during this time. The patient's activity level may be increasing, so special caution and assessment are necessary. By 6 weeks after MI, scar tissue has completely replaced necrotic tissue and the injured area is considered healed. Often the scarred area is less compliant than the surrounding area. This may be manifested by abnormal wall motion on an echocardiogram or nuclear imaging (e.g., hypokinesis, akinesis), decreased LV function, altered conduction patterns, dysrhythmias, or HF. Years later, the scarred area may become an irritable focus for life-threatening dysrhythmias causing sudden cardiac death (SCD).

These changes in the infarcted heart muscle also cause changes in the unaffected areas. To try to compensate for the damaged muscle, the normal myocardium hypertrophies and dilates. This process is called *ventricular remodeling.* Remodeling can lead to the development of late HF, especially after an anterior wall MI. ACE inhibitors or ARBs are given to limit ventricular remodeling.

Diagnostic Studies

The 12-lead ECG and cardiac biomarkers are the primary diagnostic studies used to determine whether a person has had an ACS event.

Electrocardiogram Findings

The ECG is one of the primary tools to diagnose UA, NSTEMI, and STEMI. Whenever possible, compare a new ECG to a previous ECG. Changes in the QRS complex, ST segment, and T wave caused by injury, ischemia, and infarction can develop slowly or quickly in ACS. The pattern of ECG changes among the 12 leads provides information on the coronary artery involved in ACS (Table 37.14).

ECG changes can be absent or subtle at first. Because an MI is a dynamic process that evolves over time, serial ECGs are done to show the progression of ischemia, injury, infarction, and resolution of the infarction. For diagnostic and treatment purposes, it is important to distinguish between STEMI and UA/NSTEMI. Patients with STEMI usually have a complete coronary occlusion and go to the catheterization laboratory emergently. You will see ST elevation in the leads facing the infarcted wall on the 12-lead ECG (Figs. 37.5B, 37.12, and 37.13 and Table 37.14). ST segment elevation is significant if it is 1 mm or more above the isoelectric line (2 mm or more in V_2 and V_3) in at least 2 contiguous leads.[23] Within a few hours to days, the ST segments begin to lower and the T wave inverts. Pathologic Q waves develop in the same leads if reperfusion is delayed or not done (Fig. 37.5C). The pathologic Q waves will remain on the ECG forever. With early reperfusion, pathologic Q waves do not develop. T wave inversion may persist for months after a STEMI.

Patients with UA or NSTEMI usually have transient thrombosis or incomplete coronary occlusion. They both may present with angina and have the same ECG changes, which include ST depression and/or T wave flattening/inversion in the leads facing the area of ischemia or infarction (Figs. 37.5A, 37.12, and 37.14 and Table 37.14). Patients with NSTEMI do not develop pathologic Q waves on the ECG. The only way to distinguish UA from NSTEMI is by drawing cardiac biomarkers. Biomarkers will be high in patients with NSTEMI but normal in patients with UA.

Cardiac Biomarkers

Cardiac biomarkers are proteins released into the blood from necrotic heart muscle after an MI (see Table 35.10). These biomarkers are important in the diagnosis of MI. The presence of biomarkers helps distinguish between UA (negative biomarkers) and NSTEMI (positive biomarkers).

Cardiac-specific troponin biomarkers are explicit indicators of MI. There are 2 conventional subtypes: cardiac-specific troponin T (cTnT) and cardiac-specific troponin I (cTnI). cTnI and cTnT levels increase 4 to 6 hours after the onset of MI, peak at 10 to 24 hours, and return to baseline over 10 to 14 days. Serial sets of conventional cardiac-specific troponins are drawn 3 to 6 hours after the first draw.[15] Once the levels drop off, we can stop drawing them.

A high-sensitivity cardiac troponin test (hs-cTn) provides more rapid detection of MI compared with the conventional cardiac-specific troponin assays. This allows for a quicker diagnosis. hs-cTn levels rise within 1 hour of cardiac injury and stay high for 7 to 14 days. A second hs-cTn is drawn 2 to 3 hours after the first one if STEMI is ruled out.[15] These tests are the standard cardiac biomarkers used to identify MI.

Coronary Angiography

Patients with a STEMI must undergo coronary angiography within 90 minutes of presentation to the emergency department (ED) to identify the involved artery. PCI is performed to facilitate reperfusion (Fig. 37.15).

Interprofessional Care

It is important to quickly diagnose and treat a patient with ACS. Fig. 37.6 shows the interprofessional care of ACS. Initial management of the patient with chest pain most often occurs in the ED (Table 37.15). Obtain vital signs and a 12-lead ECG. Compare the ECG with a previous ECG whenever possible. Draw cardiac biomarkers and start continuous ECG monitoring. Position the patient in an upright position unless contraindicated and start O_2 by nasal cannula to keep O_2 saturation above 90%.[22] Obtain IV access for drug administration. Give SL NTG and a 165- to 325-mg loading dose of aspirin if not given before arrival at the ED. Give an IV opioid (e.g., fentanyl) for pain unrelieved by NTG. Give a high-dose statin (e.g., atorvastatin 80 mg). Obtain baseline laboratory studies.

If the ECG shows ST elevation, the patient is taken directly for coronary angiography in PCI-capable hospitals. Thrombolytic therapy is started if the patient is unable to be quickly transported to a PCI-capable hospital. If the ECG shows ST depression and/or T wave inversion, we admit the patient to an ICU or telemetry unit. Dysrhythmias are treated according to agency protocols. Serial cardiac biomarkers are drawn until the peak level drops off. Patients with UA or NSTEMI are started

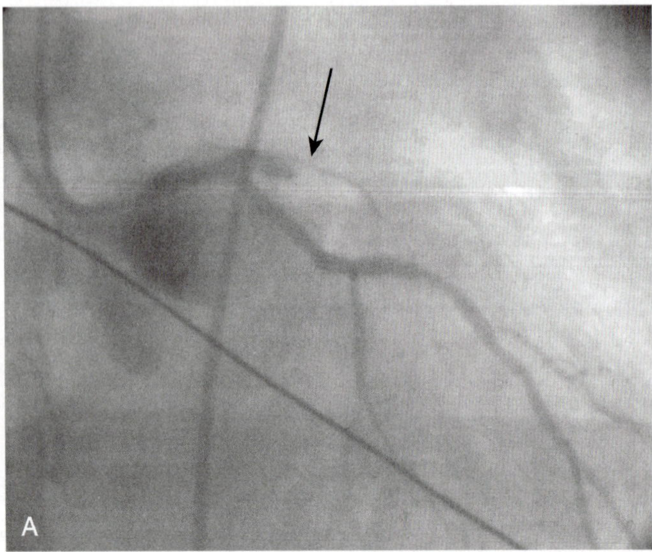

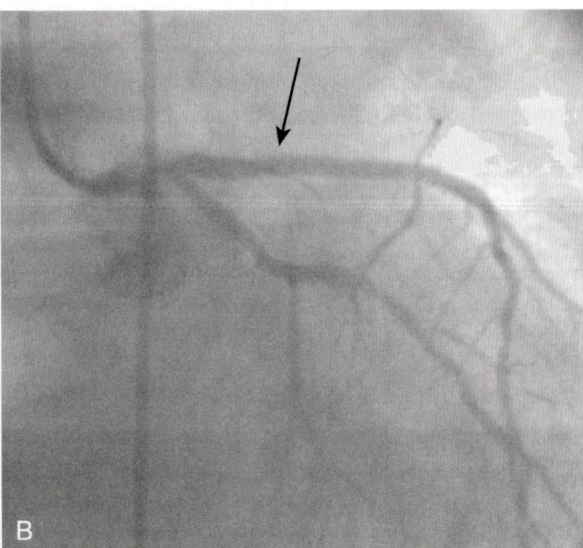

Fig. 37.15 (A) One hundred percent thrombotic occlusion of the left anterior descending (LAD) artery *(arrow)* causing an ST segment elevation myocardial infarction (STEMI). (B) After percutaneous coronary intervention (PCI) with a drug-coated stent to the LAD artery *(arrow)*. Blood flow is restored to the entire LAD artery.

TABLE 37.15 EMERGENCY MANAGEMENT

Chest Pain

Etiology	Assessment Findings	Interventions
Cardiovascular • Aortic aneurysm • Aortic valve disease • Dysrhythmia • MI • Myocardial ischemia • Pericarditis **Respiratory** • Costochondritis • Pleurisy • Pneumonia • Pneumothorax, hemothorax • Pulmonary edema • Pulmonary embolus **Chest Trauma** • Cardiac tamponade • Flail chest • Great vessel injury • Hemothorax • Pulmonary contusion • Rib/sternal fracture **Gastrointestinal** • Cholecystitis • Esophagitis • GERD • Hiatal hernia • Peptic ulcer **Other** • Acute anxiety • Drugs (e.g., cocaine) • Strenuous exercise • Stress	• Angina; pain in chest, neck, jaw, arm, shoulder • Anxiety • Decreased or ↑ BP • Cold, clammy skin • Decreased O_2 saturation • Diaphoresis • Dyspnea, tachypnea • Dysrhythmias • Epigastric pain • Feeling of impending doom • Indigestion, heartburn • Murmurs • Narrow pulse pressure • Nausea and vomiting • Palpitations • Pericardial friction rub • Syncope, loss of consciousness • Tachycardia, bradycardia • Unequal BP readings in upper extremities • Weakness	**Initial** • Monitor airway, breathing, and circulation (ABC). • Position patient upright unless contraindicated. • Give O_2 by nasal cannula or nonrebreather mask to maintain O_2 saturation over 90%. • Obtain baseline vital signs. • Obtain 12-lead ECG. • Auscultate heart and breath sounds. • Insert 2 IV catheters. • Assess pain using PQRST mnemonic (Table 37.8). • Medicate for pain as ordered (e.g., nitroglycerin, fentanyl). • Start continuous ECG monitoring and identify underlying rhythm. • Obtain baseline blood work (e.g., cardiac biomarkers, CBC, basic metabolic panel, coagulation studies). • Obtain portable chest x-ray. • Assess for contraindications for antiplatelet, anticoagulant, or thrombolytic therapy or percutaneous coronary intervention. • Give aspirin unless contraindicated. • Give a high-dose statin. • Give antidysrhythmic drugs for life-threatening dysrhythmias. **Ongoing Monitoring** • Monitor ABCs, vital signs, level of consciousness, heart and breath sounds, heart rhythm, and O_2 saturation. • Assess and record response to drugs (e.g., decrease in chest pain) and remedicate or titrate drugs (e.g., nitroglycerin) as needed. • Provide reassurance and emotional support to patient and caregiver. • Explain all interventions and procedures to patient and caregiver in simple terms. • Anticipate need for intubation if respiratory distress is evident. • Prepare for CPR and defibrillation if cardiac arrest is evident. • Anticipate need for transcutaneous pacing for symptomatic bradycardia or heart block.

CBC, Complete blood count; *GERD,* gastroesophageal reflux disease; *MI,* myocardial infarction.

on systemic anticoagulation with either subcutaneous LMWH or IV UH to reduce the risk of further clot formation. Antiplatelet medications (e.g., ticagrelor) are typically started in the cardiac catheterization laboratory when a large thrombus or no reflow/slow flow is seen on the coronary angiogram.[17] A common side effect of these drugs is bleeding.

Emergent Percutaneous Coronary Intervention

Emergent coronary angiography with PCI is the first line of treatment for patients with confirmed STEMI. The goal is to open the blocked artery within 90 minutes of arrival to an agency that has an interventional cardiac catheterization laboratory to limit the infarction size. The patient undergoes coronary angiography to (1) locate the infarct-related vessel, (2) assess the other coronary arteries for significant blockage(s), and (3) determine the presence or absence of collateral circulation. During the procedure, a DES is inserted into the infarct-related coronary artery (Figs. 37.7 and 37.15). If the patient is hemodynamically stable and other coronary arteries are found to have significant blockage during the emergent catheterization, a second PCI on the noninfarct artery is usually done at another time to reduce the risk of MI or death.[17] Patients with severe LV dysfunction may require an intraaortic balloon pump (IABP), percutaneous LV assist device, and/or inotropes (e.g., dobutamine).

After PCI for any ACS, DAPT (low-dose aspirin plus either ticagrelor, prasugrel, or clopidogrel) is continued for 1 year. Clopidogrel, prasugrel, and ticagrelor are oral P2Y12 inhibitors. Ticagrelor and prasugrel are the preferred agents in patients with ACS to reduce ischemic events and prevent stent thrombosis.[22] After 1 year, the patient continues to take a single antiplatelet agent. Some patients remain on DAPT longer if there are no bleeding complications.

Complications of PCI that may lead to emergent CABG include dissection or rupture of the coronary artery, abrupt artery closure, acute stent thrombosis, and failure to cross the blockage with a balloon or stent. There is a risk that the infarction could be extended if a part of the plaque dislodges and blocks the vessel distal to the catheter.

Thrombolytic Therapy

Thrombolytic therapy is indicated only for patients with STEMI in agencies that do not have an interventional cardiac catheterization laboratory or when one is too far away to transfer the patient quickly. Patients admitted to non–PCI-capable hospitals should be moved to a PCI-capable hospital if the time from hospital presentation to balloon inflation (PCI) time can be under 120 minutes.[17] Treatment of STEMI with thrombolytic therapy aims to limit the infarction size by dissolving the thrombus in the coronary artery to restore blood flow to the heart muscle. The goal is to give the thrombolytic within 30 minutes of the patient's arrival to the ED.

CHECK YOUR PRACTICE

Your patient had an emergent PCI 2 days ago for a STEMI. You are about to give him his morning medications, which include ticagrelor and aspirin. The patient asks you if he will need to take these medications forever.

- What would you tell the patient?

Indications and contraindications. All thrombolytics are given IV (Table 37.12). Although they have different pharmacokinetics, they all open the blocked artery by lysing the thrombus. Because thrombolytics lyse the pathologic clot, they may lyse other clots (e.g., a postoperative site). Patient selection is important because minor or major bleeding can be a complication of therapy. Inclusion criteria for thrombolytic therapy are (1) chest pain less than 12 hours with 12-lead ECG findings consistent with a STEMI and (2) no absolute contraindications (Table 37.16).

Procedure. Each hospital has a protocol for giving thrombolytic therapy. We complete 2 common steps before starting thrombolytic therapy: (1) draw blood to obtain baseline laboratory values and (2) start 2 or 3 lines for IV therapy. Perform all other invasive procedures before giving the thrombolytic agent to reduce the risk of bleeding.

We give thrombolytics either by an IV bolus or via an infusion over up to 3 hours. Note the time when therapy begins. Monitor the patient during and after the thrombolytic. Assess heart rhythm, vital signs, and pulse oximetry. Assess the heart and lungs often to evaluate the response to therapy. Regularly assess for changes in neurologic status that may indicate cerebral bleeding.

When reperfusion occurs (e.g., a blocked coronary artery is opened and blood flow is restored to the heart muscle), several clinical signs can be seen. The most reliable sign is the return of the ST segment to baseline on the ECG. Other signs include resolution of chest pain and an early, rapid rise of cardiac biomarkers. These levels increase as the necrotic heart cells release proteins into the circulation after perfusion is restored to the area. The presence of *reperfusion dysrhythmias* (e.g., accelerated idioventricular rhythm) is a less reliable sign of reperfusion. These dysrhythmias are generally self-limiting and do not require aggressive treatment.

TABLE 37.16 Contraindications for Thrombolytic Therapy

Absolute Contraindications

- Active internal bleeding (excluding menses)
- History of intracranial hemorrhage
- Intracranial cancer
- Known structural or vascular abnormality (e.g., arteriovenous malformation)
- Recent (within last 3 months) ischemic stroke
- Significant closed-head or facial trauma within last 3 months
- Suspected aortic dissection

Relative Contraindications

- Active peptic ulcer
- Anticoagulant therapy with INR >1.7 or PT >15 sec
- Dementia
- History of chronic, severe, poorly controlled hypertension
- Noncompressible vascular punctures
- Pregnancy
- Prior ischemic stroke (>3 months ago)
- Recent (within 2–4 weeks) internal bleeding
- Severe hypertension on presentation (SBP >180 mm Hg or DBP >110 mm Hg)
- Traumatic or prolonged (>10 min) CPR
- For streptokinase: Prior exposure (>5 days ago), prior allergic reaction

DBP, Diastolic blood pressure; *INR,* international normalized ratio; *PT,* prothrombin time; *SBP,* systolic blood pressure.

From Rao SV, O'Donoghue ML, Ruel M, et al: 2025 ACC/AHA/ACEP/NAEMSP/SCAI guideline for the management of patients with acute coronary syndromes, *Circulation* 151:e00, 2025.

A major concern with thrombolytic therapy is reocclusion of the artery. The site of the thrombus is unstable, and another clot may form. Therefore IV heparin therapy is started. If another clot forms, the patient may have similar chest pain symptoms, and ECG changes will return. Patients receiving thrombolytic therapy should be transferred to an agency with PCI capabilities in case thrombolytic therapy fails.

Bleeding is the main complication of thrombolytic therapy. Ongoing nursing assessment is essential. Minor bleeding (e.g., surface bleeding from IV sites or gingival bleeding) is expected. Control bleeding by applying manual pressure followed by a pressure dressing or ice packs. Intracranial bleeding is a rare and extreme emergency. Monitor neurologic status closely.

SAFETY ALERT

Thrombolytic Therapy

- Minor or major bleeding can occur with thrombolytic drugs.
- Place 2 or 3 IV lines before starting thrombolytic therapy.
- If signs and symptoms of major bleeding occur (e.g., drop in BP, increase in HR, sudden change in mental status, blood in the urine or stool), stop the drug and notify the HCP.

Complications of Myocardial Infarction

Dysrhythmias. Dysrhythmias are the most common complication after an MI, seen in 80% to 90% of patients. Ventricular tachycardia (VT) and ventricular fibrillation (VF) are the most common cause of death in patients in the prehospital period. VT or VF most often occurs within the first 4 hours after the onset of chest pain. Premature ventricular contractions (PVCs) may precede VT and VF.

Bradycardias (e.g., complete heart block) can develop when key areas of the conduction system such as the sinus or atrioventricular node are destroyed. A patient who is symptomatic with bradycardia may need an external pacemaker or a temporary transvenous pacemaker.

With reperfusion (thrombolytic therapy or PCI), it is common to see PVCs, asymptomatic nonsustained VT, and idioventricular rhythms. These rhythms are not associated with an increased risk for SCD. Patients are not treated unless they are symptomatic.[22] See Chapter 39 for information about dysrhythmias and their management.

Heart failure. HF is a complication that occurs when the right or left ventricle's pumping action is reduced. Depending on the severity and extent of the injury, left-sided HF occurs initially with subtle signs, such as mild dyspnea, restlessness, agitation, or slight tachycardia. Other signs indicating the onset of left-sided HF include pulmonary congestion on chest x-ray, an S_3 heart sound, crackles on auscultation of the lungs, paroxysmal nocturnal dyspnea (PND), and orthopnea. Signs of right-sided HF include JVD, abdominal distention, or lower extremity edema. See Chapter 38 for information about the treatment of acute decompensated HF.

Cardiogenic shock. *Cardiogenic shock* occurs when O_2 and nutrients supplied to the tissues are inadequate because of severe LV failure, papillary muscle rupture, ventricular septal rupture, LV free wall rupture, or RV infarction.[22] This occurs less often when STEMI is treated early and rapidly with PCI or thrombolytic therapy. Cardiogenic shock, which has a high death rate, requires aggressive management. This includes control of dysrhythmias, mechanical circulatory devices (e.g., IABP, extracorporeal membrane oxygenation [ECMO]), and support of contractility with vasoactive drugs (e.g., dobutamine). Goals of therapy are to maximize O_2 delivery, reduce O_2 demand, and prevent complications (e.g., acute kidney injury). See more about cardiogenic shock in Chapter 42.

Papillary muscle dysfunction or rupture. *Papillary muscle dysfunction* may occur if the infarcted area includes or is near the papillary muscle that attaches to the mitral valve (see Fig. 35.2). Suspect papillary muscle dysfunction if you hear a new systolic murmur suggestive of mitral regurgitation at the heart apex. An echocardiogram confirms the diagnosis.

Papillary muscle rupture is a rare and life-threatening complication. It causes acute and massive mitral valve regurgitation. Dyspnea, pulmonary edema, and decreased CO result from the backup of blood in the left atrium. This condition aggravates an already damaged LV by reducing CO even further. Patients undergo rapid clinical decline. Treatment includes afterload reduction (e.g., nitroprusside) and/or mechanical support (e.g., IABP) therapy with immediate surgery to repair or replace the mitral valve.[22] See Chapter 40 for information on valve problems.

Left ventricular aneurysm. *Left ventricular aneurysm* results when the infarcted heart wall thins and bulges out during contraction. This is a late complication that can develop within days, weeks, or months after the infarction. It is more common with anterior MIs.[22] Patients with a left ventricular aneurysm may develop HF because of loss of forward output as the aneurysm fills during systole, dysrhythmias related to stretched myofibers, and angina. Stagnant blood flow within the aneurysm can promote thrombus formation and distal embolization. An LV aneurysm can lead to ventricular rupture, which is usually fatal. Anticoagulation therapy is recommended unless contraindicated. Suspect LV aneurysm if ST elevations persist on ECG weeks after MI or a bulge is noted along the LV border on chest x-ray. Echocardiogram can confirm the diagnosis.

Ventricular septal wall rupture and left ventricular free wall rupture. A new loud systolic murmur heard in patients with acute MI may signal ventricular septal wall rupture. Depending on the size of the defect and degree of RV and LV dysfunction, HF and cardiogenic shock may occur. The patient must undergo emergency repair, either surgically or percutaneously. The defect can quickly expand and lead to hemodynamic compromise.[22]

LV free wall rupture is an emergency. Rapid hemodynamic compromise and death ensue if not treated immediately. Although this is a rare complication, death rates are high. Free wall rupture occurs more often in patients after their first MI, patients with anterior MIs, older adults, and females.[22]

Pericarditis. *Acute pericarditis,* an inflammation of the visceral and/or parietal pericardium, may occur 2 or 3 days after an acute MI. The key sign is mild to severe chest pain that increases with inspiration, coughing, and movement of the upper body. Sitting in a forward position often relieves the pain. The pain is usually different from pain caused by an MI.

If you suspect pericarditis, assess for the presence of a friction rub over the pericardium. You can hear the sound best with the diaphragm of the stethoscope at the mid to lower left sternal border. It may be persistent or intermittent. Fever may be present. Patients may have hypotension and/or a narrow pulse pressure if there is a significant pericardial effusion or cardiac tamponade. Asymptomatic pericardial effusions are common after STEMI.[22]

Besides physical findings, a 12-lead ECG is helpful in making a diagnosis. Typical ECG changes include diffuse ST segment elevations in many unrelated leads (with STEMI, ST elevation occurs in the leads facing the infarcted wall). This reflects the inflammation of the pericardium. Treatment includes pain relief with high doses of aspirin (e.g., 650 mg every 4 to 6 hours). Nonsteroidal antiinflammatory drugs (NSAIDs) and cyclooxygenase II (COX-2) inhibitors are avoided after MI because they can increase the risk of reinfarction, cardiac rupture, and death.[22] Pericarditis is discussed in Chapter 40.

Dressler syndrome. *Dressler syndrome* is a rare form of pericarditis that can develop 1 to 8 weeks after MI. We do not know the cause. It may be an autoimmune reaction to the necrotic heart muscle. Patients have pleuritic chest pain, fever, and malaise. A pericardial friction rub may be heard. A pericardial effusion may be present on echocardiogram. Laboratory findings include a high white blood cell count (leukocytosis) and erythrocyte sedimentation rate (ESR). Aspirin is the treatment of choice.[3]

Drug Therapy

See Table 37.12 and Fig. 37.6 for drug therapy prescribed for patients with chronic stable angina and ACS. When a patient presents with suspected ACS, they receive a loading dose of 165 to 325 mg of aspirin, SL or IV NTG, and high-dose atorvastatin (80 mg). Patients with UA and NSTEMI receive systemic anticoagulation. Because patients with STEMI go directly to a cardiac catheterization laboratory for coronary angiography, they do not get systemic anticoagulation. If a coronary stent is placed, then DAPT is initiated. Oral β-blockers and ACE inhibitors/ARBs are started within the first 24 hours if there are no contraindications. CCBs are used if the patient cannot tolerate β-blockers. They are used cautiously after MI because they can decrease myocardial contractility. Nitrates and fentanyl may be given for pain relief.[22]

Antiplatelet medications. DAPT with ticagrelor or prasugrel plus low-dose aspirin is prescribed after a STEMI or NSTEMI whether the patient does or does not get a stent.[22] DAPT is recommended for a year if there is no bleeding. After that, monotherapy with either aspirin or a P2Y12 drug is recommended. Monotherapy with 75 to 100 mg of aspirin daily is prescribed for patients with UA.

Intravenous nitroglycerin. IV NTG is used in the initial treatment for patients with ACS. SL NTG can be used until the IV NTG is prepared. The goal of therapy is to reduce angina pain and improve coronary blood flow. IV NTG decreases preload and afterload while increasing the myocardial O_2 supply. The onset of action is immediate. Titrate NTG to eliminate chest pain. Because hypotension is a common side effect, closely monitor BP. Patients who become hypotensive may be volume depleted and may benefit from an IV fluid bolus. Closely assess for volume overload after the bolus (e.g., crackles on lung auscultation).

Opioid analgesics. Rapid and effective pain relief is important to prevent sympathetic activation. Fentanyl is the drug of choice for chest pain that is unrelieved by NTG.[22] Morphine is an alternative therapy. As a vasodilator, it decreases cardiac workload by lowering myocardial O_2 consumption, reducing contractility, and decreasing BP and HR. Both can help reduce anxiety and fear. In rare situations, opioids can depress respirations. Monitor for signs of bradypnea or hypotension, which could worsen myocardial ischemia and infarction.

β-Adrenergic blockers. β-Blockers decrease myocardial O_2 demand by reducing HR, BP, and contractility. They help reduce the risk of reinfarction, HF, and death. β-Blockers are given to patients who do not have complications from their MI (e.g., decompensated HF, cardiogenic shock, bradycardia, hypotension). If the EF remains <50%, the drugs are continued indefinitely.[7]

Angiotensin-converting enzyme inhibitors and angiotensin receptor blockers. ACE inhibitors should be started within the first 24 hours if the BP is stable and there are no contraindications (e.g., hypotension, worsening renal impairment). They are taken indefinitely in patients after STEMI or NSTEMI, with HF, or with an EF less than 40% if there are no contraindications. ACE inhibitors can help prevent ventricular remodeling, thereby preventing or slowing the development of HF. ARBs are an option if patients cannot tolerate ACE inhibitors.

Antidysrhythmic drugs. Dysrhythmias are the most common complication after an MI. In general, they are self-limiting and not treated aggressively unless they are life threatening (e.g., sustained VT). Chapter 39 discusses the drugs used to treat dysrhythmias.

Lipid-lowering drugs. All patients with ACS need a baseline lipid panel. Patients with ACS who are not on a lipid-lowering agent should receive a high-dose lipid-lowering drug and remain on it indefinitely unless contraindicated (Table 37.6). Patients on a lipid-lowering drug at the time of the MI should have the dose maximized and/or start a second lipid-lowering drug.[22]

Aldosterone antagonists. Aldosterone antagonists (e.g., spironolactone, eplerenone) can decrease mortality after a STEMI in patients with decreased LV function (<40%) and either symptomatic HF or diabetes. There also are data to support a mortality benefit in patients with STEMI and an LVEF greater than 40% without HF.[24] One of these drugs should be added if there are no contraindications (e.g., hyperkalemia, increased creatinine).

Stool softeners. After an MI, the patient may be predisposed to constipation because of bed rest and opioid drugs. Stool softeners (e.g., docusate sodium) prevent straining and the resultant vagal stimulation from the Valsalva maneuver. Vagal stimulation produces bradycardia and can provoke dysrhythmias. A laxative may be used, if needed.

Nutrition Therapy

Initially, patients may be NPO except for water until stable (e.g., pain free, nausea resolved). Advance oral intake as tolerated to a low-salt, low-saturated-fat, and low-cholesterol diet (Tables 37.4 and 37.5).

NURSING MANAGEMENT: ACUTE CORONARY SYNDROME

Assessment

Table 37.17 presents the subjective and objective data to obtain from patients with ACS.

Clinical Problems

Clinical problems for patients with ACS may include:

- Impaired cardiac function
- Pain
- Anxiety
- Activity intolerance

More information on clinical problems of patients with ACS is in eNursing Care Plan 37.1 available on the website for this chapter.

Planning

Nursing care focuses on the priority problems of pain and impaired cardiac function. The immediate goals for patients with ACS include (1) pain relief, (2) immediate treatment, and (3) preservation of heart muscle. During the hospitalization, the overall goals include (1) effective coping with anxiety, (2) participation in rehabilitation planning, and (3) discussion about risk factor reduction.

Implementation

Monitor vital signs and pulse oximetry frequently according to agency protocol during the first few hours after admission to the ICU or telemetry unit. Maintain continuous ECG monitoring. Obtain serial 12-lead ECGs and draw serial cardiac biomarkers. Maintain bed rest according to agency policy and gradually increase activity unless contraindicated.

For patients with UA and NSTEMI, we use heparin (UH or LMWH) to prevent microemboli from forming and causing further chest pain. DAPT (e.g., aspirin and ticagrelor) is recommended for patients with STEMI and NSTEMI (with or without a stent) (Table 37.12). Patients with UA only receive aspirin. If a patient with UA has a stent placed, we use DAPT.

TABLE 37.17 NURSING ASSESSMENT

Acute Coronary Syndrome

Subjective Data

Important Health Information

Health history: Previous history of coronary artery disease (CAD), chest pain/angina, myocardial infarction (MI), valve disease (e.g., aortic stenosis), heart failure, or cardiomyopathy. History of hypertension, diabetes, anemia, lung disease, hyperlipidemia. History of premature CAD in a family member

Medications: Use of antiplatelets, anticoagulants, nitrates, angiotensin-converting enzyme (ACE) inhibitors, β-blockers, calcium channel blockers, antihypertensive drugs, lipid-lowering drugs, over-the-counter drugs (e.g., vitamin and herb supplements)

History of present illness: Description of precipitating events related to current illness (Table 37.9), including any self-treatments and response. Description of current symptoms (Table 37.8).

Functional Health Patterns

Health perception–health management: Sedentary lifestyle, tobacco use, exposure to environment smoke, drug use

Nutritional-metabolic: Indigestion, heartburn, nausea, belching, vomiting

Elimination: Urinary urgency or frequency, straining at stool

Activity-exercise: Palpitations, dyspnea, dizziness, weakness

Cognitive-perceptual: Substernal chest pain or pressure (squeezing, constricting, aching, sharp, tingling), radiation to jaw, neck, shoulders, back, or arms

Coping–stress tolerance: Stressful lifestyle, depression, anger, anxiety, feeling of impending doom

Objective Data

General

Anxious, fearful, restless, distressed

Cardiovascular

Tachycardia or bradycardia, pulsus alternans (alternating weak and strong heartbeats), pulse deficit, dysrhythmias (especially ventricular), murmur, S_3, S_4, ↑ or ↓ BP

Skin

Cool, clammy, pale skin

Possible Diagnostic Findings

Positive cardiac biomarkers, ↑ lipids; ↑ white blood cell (WBC) count. Pathologic Q wave, ST segment elevation, and/or ST-T wave abnormalities on ECG. Heart enlargement, calcifications, or pulmonary congestion on chest x-ray. Abnormal wall motion on resting echocardiogram. Positive findings on cardiac catheterization.

Coronary angiography is an option for patients with UA and NSTEMI after being stabilized or if angina returns. Depending on the results, options include risk factor reduction with medical management, PCI, or CABG surgery.

For patients with STEMI, reperfusion therapy begins as soon as possible. *Reperfusion therapy* includes emergent PCI (preferred in PCI-capable hospitals) or thrombolytic therapy (in hospitals not capable of performing PCI). The goal in the treatment of STEMI is to save as much heart muscle as possible. Technical advances in PCI technology have almost eliminated CABG surgery as the primary treatment for patients with STEMI unless there is another reason to perform surgery (e.g., ventricular septal rupture, papillary muscle rupture).[17]

Pain

Provide NTG and opioid analgesia as needed to eliminate or reduce chest pain. Ongoing evaluation and documentation of the effectiveness of the interventions are important. Once pain is relieved, some patients interpret the absence of pain as an absence of heart disease. Teach about the importance of continued therapy to limit myocardial damage.

Monitoring

Maintain continuous ECG monitoring. Treat life-threatening dysrhythmias quickly. During the initial period after MI, sustained VT and VF are the most common lethal dysrhythmias.[22] In many patients, PVCs precede these dysrhythmias. We usually do not treat isolated PVCs. VT is treated if it is sustained VT. Treatment of nonsustained VT depends on the hemodynamic status.

Assess the ST segments for shifts above or below the baseline of the ECG (signals reinfarction or ischemia). Silent ischemia, noted only by ST segment depression and/or T wave inversion, occurs without subjective symptoms (e.g., chest pain). Notify the HCP if you see ST segment changes with or without clinical symptoms.

Perform a physical assessment to detect changes from baseline findings. Assess for signs and symptoms of early HF (e.g., dyspnea, tachycardia, crackles, distended neck veins, an S_3 heart sound). Monitor intake and output. Obtain a daily weight.

Rest and Comfort

Promoting rest and comfort for patients with any degree of heart damage is important. There is no evidence for prolonged bed rest for patients with an uncomplicated MI (e.g., angina resolved, no signs of complications). Their activity should slowly increase. Patients with UA and NSTEMI may sit in a chair when angina is resolved if there are no complications. Patients with an uncomplicated STEMI may sit in a chair within a few hours after the event, especially if the radial artery was used for the PCI. The use of the bathroom, a commode, or a bedpan is based on patient preference and hemodynamic status. Bed rest may be ordered for the first few days after a complicated MI, depending on the patient's condition.

Teach patients why activity is limited. Gradually increase the patient's heart workload and activity level (e.g., walking in the hall or walking steps). Before discharge, it is important that the patient achieves an activity level adequate for life at home. Discuss and encourage outpatient cardiac rehabilitation. Table 37.18 outlines the phases of cardiac rehabilitation.

When sleeping or resting, the body requires less work from the heart than it does when active. Plan nursing and other interventions to ensure adequate rest periods free from interruption. Comfort measures that can promote rest include a quiet environment, use of relaxation techniques (e.g., music therapy, guided imagery), and assurance that staff is nearby and responsive to the patient's needs.

Anxiety

A degree of anxiety is present in all patients with ACS. Identify the source of anxiety and assist the patient in reducing it. If the patient is afraid of being alone, allow a caregiver to sit by quietly and check the patient frequently. If a source of anxiety is the unknown, explore these concerns with the patient. For anxiety caused by lack of information, provide teaching based on the patient's stated need and level of understanding. Answer questions with clear, simple explanations.

TABLE 37.18 Phases of Rehabilitation After Acute Coronary Syndrome

Phase I: Hospital
- Occurs while the patient is still hospitalized
- Activity level depends on severity of angina or MI
- Patient may first sit up in bed or chair, perform range-of-motion exercises and self-care (e.g., washing, shaving), and progress to walking in hallway and limited stair climbing
- Attention focuses on management of chest pain, anxiety, dysrhythmias, and complications

Phase II: Early Recovery
- Begins after discharge
- Usually lasts from 2 to 12 weeks and is held in an outpatient facility but may be done in the home
- Activity level is gradually increased under the supervision of the cardiac rehabilitation team and with ECG monitoring
- Team may suggest that physical activity (e.g., walking program) be started at home
- Teaching about risk factor reduction is provided

Phase III: Late Recovery
- Long-term maintenance program
- Individual physical activity programs are designed and implemented at home, a local gym, or the rehabilitation center
- Patient and caregiver restructure lifestyles and roles
- Therapeutic lifestyle changes should become lifelong habits
- Medical supervision recommended

CHECK YOUR PRACTICE

You are walking in the hallway with a 64-year-old female who had an MI 3 days ago. She is being discharged tomorrow. She is visibly anxious and irritable, wringing her hands and talking very fast. She tells you, "My heart is pounding." You do not know if she is anxious or about to have another MI.
- What should you do?

Begin teaching at the patient's level. For example, many patients are not ready to learn about the pathology of CAD. The earliest questions usually relate to how the disease affects perceived control and independence. Examples include:

- When will I leave the ICU?
- When can I get out of bed?
- When will I be discharged?
- When can I return to work?
- How many changes will I have to make in my life?
- Will this happen again?

Tell patients that more complete teaching will begin once they are feeling stronger. Often the patient with ACS may not be able to ask the most serious concern: Am I going to die? Even if a patient denies this concern, it is helpful for you to start a conversation by remarking that fear of dying is a common concern among most patients who have had this condition. This gives the patient "permission" to talk about an uncomfortable and fearful topic.

Emotional and Behavior Reactions

Patients' emotional and behavior reactions vary, but often follow a predictable pattern (Table 37.19). Your role is to understand what the patient is experiencing and to support the use of constructive coping styles.

Assess the support structure of the patient and caregiver. Determine how you can help maximize the support system. Often the patient is separated from their support system during hospitalization. With patient permission, you can talk with the caregivers about the patient's progress and support the caregivers who will be helping the patient. Open visitation is helpful in decreasing anxiety and increasing support for patients with ACS. If a visitor is unable to get to the hospital, a video chat with a tablet or phone could be arranged. Help patients identify additional support systems (e.g., spiritual care, Mended Hearts) to assist during the hospital stay and/or after discharge.

Patient Teaching

Patient teaching is needed at every stage of hospitalization and recovery. Give patients and caregivers the tools they need to make informed decisions about their health (Box 37.1). Careful assessment of the patient's health literacy and learning needs helps you set realistic goals (see Chapter 4). Table 37.20 presents a teaching guide for the patient and caregiver.

The timing of the teaching is important. When patients and caregivers are in crisis, they may not be ready to learn new information. Answer questions in simple, brief terms. The answers often need repetition. When the shock accompanying a crisis subsides, the patient and caregiver are better able to focus on detailed information.

TABLE 37.19 Psychosocial Responses to Acute Coronary Syndrome

Anger and Hostility • Often expressed as "Why did this happen to me?" • May be directed at family, staff, or medical regimen
Anxiety and Fear • Fears long-term disability and death • Overtly displays apprehension, restlessness, insomnia, tachycardia • Less overtly displays increased verbalization, projection of feelings to others, hypochondriasis • Fears activity • Fears recurrent chest pain, heart attacks, and sudden death
Denial • May have history of ignoring signs and symptoms related to heart disease • Minimizes severity of problem • Ignores restrictions • Avoids discussing illness or its significance
Dependency • Totally reliant on staff • Unwilling to perform tasks or activities unless approved by HCP • Wants ECG monitoring to continue • Hesitant to leave the ICU, telemetry unit, or hospital
Depression • Mourns loss of health, altered body function, and changes in lifestyle • Realizes seriousness of situation • Begins to worry about future implications of health problem • Shows manifestations of withdrawal, crying, apathy • May be more evident after discharge
Realistic Acceptance • Focuses on optimum rehabilitation • Plans changes compatible with altered cardiac function • Actively engages in lifestyle changes to address risk factors

Limit your use of medical terms. For example, you are caring for a patient with UA who asks you why he has chest tightness when he climbs stairs. Begin by explaining that the heart is a muscle that works as a pump. Like all muscles, it needs O_2 to work (or pump) properly. When fat and cholesterol block the blood vessels supplying the heart muscle with O_2, less O_2 is available to the muscle. As a result, the pump cannot work well. Tell the patient that the chest tightness (angina) is the heart's message that it is having trouble doing its work. If possible, use visual aids to support what you are explaining.

Patients must recognize that CAD is a chronic disease. It is not curable. Therefore they may need basic lifestyle changes to promote recovery and future health. Tell patients that recovery takes time, and resuming physical activity after ACS or heart surgery is slow and gradual. However, with adequate supportive care, recovery is likely.

Anticipatory guidance involves preparing the patient and caregiver for what to expect during recovery and rehabilitation. By learning what to expect, the patient gains a sense of control.

BOX 37.1 EVIDENCE-BASED PRACTICE

Nurse-Led Programs for CAD

You are a nurse working on a telemetry unit. At the most recent meeting, administration reported that patients newly diagnosed with CAD are often readmitted within 3 to 4 weeks after their initial hospitalization due to recurring symptoms. Unit practice standards outline the discharge teaching that nurses provide about CAD management and health promotion. Teaching sessions include watching a brief video and reviewing a packet of written materials with the patient.

Making Clinical Decisions

Synthesis of Best Available Evidence

Evidence supports a strong link between nurse-led clinics and positive patient outcomes, including reduced hospital readmission rates. In addition, nurse-led clinics have been shown to enhance care delivery, support effective management of CAD, and expand access to health care.

Clinician Expertise

Since you know that you play a key role in teaching health-promoting behaviors, you decide to research effective strategies to reduce hospital readmissions following a diagnosis of CAD. Based on your findings, you present a proposal to the facility practice council for a nurse-led interactive education program to be delivered during the first 3 weeks after patient discharge. The program goal is to decrease the rate of repeat admissions within the first 6 months following a diagnosis of CAD.

Patient Preferences and Values

Patients who participated in the nurse-led group activities had a 38% decrease in hospital readmissions compared with those who did not participate. Patient participants reported greater satisfaction with their ability to manage their CAD.

Implications for Nursing Practice

1. What strategies may be useful when developing a nurse-led program?
2. Other than the readmission rate, how can the nurse evaluate the effectiveness of the nurse-led education program?

Reference for Evidence

Qui X: Nurse-led intervention in management of patients with cardiovascular diseases: A brief literature review, *BMC Nurs* 23:6, 2024.

For example, a middle-aged male who smokes 2 packs of cigarettes a day, is 20 pounds overweight, and gets no physical exercise may feel overwhelmed with the idea of changes. He may decide that he can live with a weight reduction plan and will get some exercise but that it is not possible for him to quit smoking. He believes that because he is changing 2 of his 3 risk factors, he will be healthier. Ideally, the tobacco risk factor should be a priority for this patient. However, if the patient is not ready to accept information about risks and effects of tobacco use, you must respect their choices.

Physical Activity

Physical activity supports optimal physiologic functioning and psychologic well-being. It has a direct, positive effect on maximal O_2 uptake, increasing CO, decreasing blood lipids, decreasing BP, increasing blood flow through the coronary arteries, increasing muscle mass and flexibility, improving the psychologic state, and assisting in weight loss and control. A regular schedule of physical activity, even after many years of sedentary living, is beneficial.

TABLE 37.20 PATIENT & CAREGIVER TEACHING

Acute Coronary Syndrome

Include the following information in the teaching plan for the patient with acute coronary syndrome and the caregiver:

- Signs and symptoms of angina and MI and what to do should they occur (e.g., how to take nitroglycerin)[a]
- When and how to seek help (e.g., contact 911)[a]
- Anatomy and physiology of the heart and coronary arteries
- Cause and effect of CAD
- Definition of terms (e.g., CAD, angina, heart failure)
- Identification of and plan to decrease risk factors[a] (Tables 37.1, 37.2, 37.3, 37.4, and 37.5)
- Reasons for tests and treatments (e.g., ECG monitoring, blood work, coronary angiography), activity limitations and rest, diet, and drugs[a]
- Expectations about recovery (anticipatory guidance)
- Resumption of work, physical activity, sexual activity
- Measures to promote recovery and health (e.g., cardiac rehabilitation)
- Importance of the gradual, progressive resumption of activity[a]

[a]Identified by patients as important to learn before discharge.
CAD, Coronary artery disease; *MI,* myocardial infarction.

One method of identifying levels of physical activity is by using **metabolic equivalent (MET)** units: 1 MET is the amount of O_2 needed by the body at rest—3.5 mL of O_2 per kilogram per minute, or 1.4 cal/kg of body weight per minute. The MET determines the energy costs of various exercises (Table 37.21).

In the hospital, we gradually increase the activity level so that by the time of discharge the patient can tolerate moderate-energy activities of 3 to 6 METs. Many patients with an uncomplicated MI are in the hospital for 3 or 4 days. By day 2, the patient can walk in the hallway and begin climbing a few steps. Give the patient specific guidelines for physical activity to avoid overexertion. Tell the patient to always "listen to what your body is saying"—the most important aspect of recovery.

Teach patients that the AHA recommends 30 minutes of moderate-intensity aerobic activity (e.g., brisk walking) at least 5 days a week (150 minutes/week).[7] Patients who have been hospitalized for a coronary event (e.g., PCI, UA, NSTEMI, STEMI) should "work up" to 30 minutes of exercise per day. An exercise stress test may be done after hospitalization to determine whether chest pain occurs with activity and guide physical activity. Patients who have been physically inactive and just starting an exercise program should do so under supervision. Cardiac rehabilitation, either in a group or home setting, is recommended.[22,25]

Teach patients to check their HR. Some patients may use technology (e.g., cell phone applications, fitness trackers) to check their HR. Patients should know the limits within which to exercise. Tell patients that the HR should return to the resting HR within a few minutes of stopping the exercise. Tell patients to stop exercising and rest if chest pain or shortness of breath occurs. Recommend that they carry SL NTG with them. Teach them to respond to physical activity in terms of symptoms rather than absolute HR, because many patients are taking β-blockers, which blunt the HR response to exercise. You cannot overstress

TABLE 37.21 Energy Expenditure in Metabolic Equivalents (METs)

Low-Energy Activities (<3 METs or <3 cal/min)

Activities in Hospital

- Eating
- Resting supine
- Washing hands, face

Activities Outside Hospital

- Driving a car
- Painting, seated
- Sewing by machine
- Sweeping floor

Moderate-Energy Activities (3–6 METs or 3–5 cal/min)

Activities in Hospital

- Showering
- Sitting on bedside commode
- Using bedpan
- Walking at 3–4 mph

Activities Outside Hospital

- Cycling at 5.5 mph on level ground
- Going up a flight of stairs
- Golfing
- General gardening
- Ironing, standing
- Painting, standing

High-Energy Activities (6–8 METs or 6–8 cal/min)

- Mowing lawn using walking mower
- Performing carpentry
- Walking 5 mph

Very-High-Energy Activities (>9 METs or >9 cal/min)

- Cross-country skiing
- Cycling at >13 mph
- Running at >6 mph
- Shoveling heavy snow (not recommended for any patient with CAD)

this point. Basic physical activity guidelines for patients after ACS follow the FITT formula (Table 37.3).

The basic categories of physical activity are aerobic and anaerobic activities. Most daily activities are a mixture of the two. *Aerobic activities* involve increasing your heart rate and breathing for a long period. Walking, swimming, and bicycling are examples of *aerobic* activities. *Aerobic* exercise can put a safe, steady load on the heart and lungs and improve the circulation to other organs.

Anaerobic activities involve quick bursts of energy for short periods with maximum effort (e.g., weightlifting, pushing heavy objects). These activities may be associated with the Valsalva maneuver and may cause a vasovagal response. Because the HR and BP change rapidly during anaerobic exercise, patients should limit these exercises.

Females who have an MI often have poor adherence to a regular physical activity program.[8] They are less likely to be referred for cardiac rehabilitation.[6] In many cases, females are caregivers for everyone but themselves. They may prioritize a physical activity program as less important than caring for others.[6]

Another factor linked to poor adherence to a physical activity program is depression. Depression is common among patients who suffer an ACS, especially in females.[6] Routinely screen for depression and recommend referral for treatment as appropriate. Many patients recover physically from ACS or CABG surgery but do not attain psychologic well-being.

Cardiac Rehabilitation

Cardiac rehabilitation is the restoration of a person to an optimal state of function in 6 areas: (1) physiologic, (2) psychologic, (3) mental, (4) spiritual, (5) economic, and (6) vocational. It is an evidence-based intervention encompassing patient education, behavior modification, and exercise training to reduce death, reduce readmissions, and improve quality of life. All patients who have had UA, an MI, a PCI, or CABG surgery should receive a referral for outpatient or home-based cardiac rehabilitation (Table 37.18). Cardiac rehabilitation is a Class I recommendation from the AHA for any patient with HF or a cardiac event.

Unfortunately, cardiac rehabilitation is not often recommended, and participation is less than optimal. Females, those from minority populations, people with low income, and those who are uninsured or underinsured often do not get referrals to cardiac rehabilitation.[25] Outpatient in-person programs are helpful, but not all patients are able to take part in them because of cost, location, and travel limitations. Home-based cardiac rehabilitation programs can provide an alternative. Wearable devices to track heart rate during exercise and maintaining contact with the patient (e.g., telehealth, exercise logs, Internet) may help with the success of these programs.

Resuming Sexual Activity

It is important to include sexual counseling for heart patients and their partners. This area of discussion may be difficult for both the patient and HCP to approach. Concern about resumption of sexual activity after hospitalization for ACS often produces more stress than the physiologic act. Most patients change their sexual behavior because they are concerned about sexual inadequacy, death during intercourse, and impotence. A concerned and knowledgeable HCP can clarify any misconceptions with specific counseling.

Before providing guidelines on resumption of sexual activity, review the patient's physiologic status, the physiologic effects of sexual activity, and the psychologic effects of having an MI. Sexual activity with the usual partner is a moderate-energy activity equivalent to 3 to 5 METS.[7] You may be uncertain of how and when to begin counseling about resuming sex. It is helpful to consider sex a physical activity and to discuss or explore feelings in this area when discussing other physical activities. One helpful approach is, "Many people who have had a heart attack wonder when they will be able to resume sexual activity. Has this been of concern to you?" You may also state, "Sexual activity, like other forms of activity, should be gradually resumed after MI." Facilitate discussion by providing patients with reading material on resuming sexual activity. Say something such as, "If resuming sexual activity has been of concern to you, this information should be helpful." This type of nonthreatening statement brings up the topic, allows the patient to explore personal feelings, and gives the patient an opportunity to raise questions with you or another HCP. Table 37.22 outlines common guidelines.

Tell patients that the inability to perform sexually after an MI or bypass surgery is common and that sexual problems usually disappear after several attempts. Reinforce the idea that patience and understanding usually solve the problem. Male patients may be interested in using drugs to correct erectile dysfunction. Warn the patient not to use these drugs within 48 hours of using nitrates because severe hypotension has been reported. Tell patients to discuss the use of these drugs with their HCP.

It is common for a patient who has chest pain on physical exertion to have some angina during sexual stimulation or intercourse. Patients may take SL NTG before sexual activity to help prevent angina. Tell the patient to delay sex after a heavy meal or excess alcohol intake, when extremely tired or stressed, or with unfamiliar partners. Patients should avoid anal intercourse because of the chance of eliciting a vasovagal response.

Tell the patient that resumption of sex depends on the patient's and partner's emotional readiness and on the HCP's assessment of the extent of recovery. It is generally safe to resume sexual activity when a patient can exercise between 3 and 5 METS (e.g., showering, walking 3 to 4 miles per hour) without chest pain or excessive shortness of breath.[7]

◆ Evaluation

The expected outcomes are that patients with ACS will:

- Maintain stable signs of adequate CO
- Have relief of pain and/or shortness of breath
- Report decreased anxiety and increased sense of self-control
- Achieve a realistic program of activity that balances physical activity with energy-conserving activities
- Describe the disease process, measures to reduce risk factors, and rehabilitation activities necessary to manage the therapeutic regimen

TABLE 37.22 PATIENT & CAREGIVER TEACHING

Sexual Activity After Acute Coronary Syndrome

Include the following information in the teaching plan for the patient and their partner after acute coronary syndrome (ACS):

- Resume sexual activity at a level that relates to sexual activity before experiencing ACS.
- Physical training may improve the physiologic response to intercourse. Encourage daily physical activity during recovery.
- Reduce food and alcohol intake before intercourse is anticipated (e.g., waiting 3–4 h after eating a large meal before engaging in sexual activity).
- Familiar surroundings and a familiar partner reduce anxiety.
- Masturbation may be useful and may reassure the patient that sexual activity is still possible.
- Avoid hot or cold showers just before and after intercourse.
- Foreplay is desirable because it allows a gradual increase in HR before orgasm.
- Positions during intercourse are a matter of personal choice.
- Orogenital sex places no undue strain on the heart.
- A relaxed atmosphere free of fatigue and stress is optimal.
- Prophylactic use of nitrates to decrease chest pain during sexual activity may be needed.
- Use of erectile agents within 48 h is contraindicated if taking nitrates in any form.
- Avoid anal intercourse because of the chance of inducing a vasovagal response.

SUDDEN CARDIAC DEATH

Sudden cardiac death (SCD) is a cardiac arrest, most often caused by a lethal cardiac dysrhythmia. Death occurs because of an abrupt loss of CO and cerebral blood flow. The dysrhythmia can be caused by a variety of cardiac causes. About 350,000 adults in the United States suffer cardiac arrest every year. Most of these occur outside of the hospital. This is why all public facilities should have automatic external defibrillators (AEDs).

Etiology and Pathophysiology

SCD is defined as the sudden unexpected death occurring within 1 hour of symptom onset in an apparently healthy person. If the death was not witnessed, SCD is defined as occurring in a person who was in good health 24 hours before the event. Some people have symptoms within 1 hour of the event (e.g., angina, palpitations, dizziness, or lightheadedness).

Common causes of SCD are acute or prior MI, CAD, and HF with a reduced ejection fraction (HFrEF). Less common causes can be grouped into 2 categories: (1) structural or infiltrative diseases (e.g., hypertrophic cardiomyopathy, amyloidosis) and (2) primary electrical diseases with a structurally normal heart (e.g., long QT syndrome, Brugada syndrome). Acute ventricular dysrhythmias (e.g., VT or VF) account for most cases of SCD. VT and VF are often reversible with early defibrillation (an electrical shock to the heart). A VT or VF arrest may or may not be associated with an acute MI. Many SCD survivors have a history of a prior (old) MI that caused LV dysfunction, electrical instability from scarred heart muscle, and a reduced LVEF. Some patients who have a sudden cardiac arrest have nonshockable rhythms such as asystole or pulseless electrical activity. Survival rates for these patients are low.

Interprofessional and Nursing Care

Survivors of SCD should have targeted temperature management to help improve survivability and neurologic outcomes. People who survive an SCD event need a diagnostic workup to determine whether an acute MI was the cause. We obtain serial cardiac biomarkers and ECGs. Anyone who survives an SCD event should undergo coronary angiography to identify if significant CAD was the cause. PCI or CABG surgery is usually recommended because significant CAD may be a reversible cause of SCD.

If no reversible cause of the SCD event is identified and the EF is low-normal, it is useful to know if these patients are likely to have a recurrence. Assessment of life-threatening dysrhythmias in these patients may include obtaining an electrophysiology (EP) study.[26] An EP study is done under fluoroscopy. Pacing electrodes are placed in various cardiac areas and stimuli are selectively used to reproduce life-threatening dysrhythmias. See Chapters 35 and 39 for a discussion of EP studies.

For patients who had a syncopal episode thought to be caused by ventricular dysrhythmias, an outpatient wearable cardiac monitor (e.g., Holter monitor) can be used for up to 48 hours or a Mobile Cardiac Outpatient Telemetry monitor may be worn up to 30 days. An implantable cardiac loop recorder (e.g., LINQ) can be left in place up to 3 years and monitored remotely.

The most common approach to preventing a recurrence of SCD and improving survival is the use of an implantable cardioverter-defibrillator (ICD).[26] ICDs are implanted devices, similar to pacemaker implants, that recognize VT or VF within seconds and deliver an internal shock to terminate the dysrhythmia. They are used for primary prevention (those at high risk for a cardiac arrest, like those with decreased LV function) and for secondary prevention (those who survived cardiac arrest). An EF of less than 35% is the most common criterion to help guide decisions about placing an ICD.[26] Patients who had SCD from an acute MI should receive at least 40 days of maximal medical therapy to see if there is recovery in the EF before an ICD is implanted. See Chapter 39 for a discussion of ICDs. Drug therapy with an antiarrhythmic (e.g., amiodarone) may be used with an ICD to decrease or eliminate episodes of ventricular dysrhythmias.

Some patients at risk for SCD (e.g., during the time when a patient with an MI and low EF must wait at least 40 days on maximum medical therapy to see if there is improvement in LV function) may use a wearable cardioverter-defibrillator (e.g., LifeVest) as a bridge to ICD implantation. The wearable cardioverter-defibrillator is an external defibrillator that is worn under clothing. It has electrodes that continuously record the patient's ECG and deliver a shock if VT or VF is detected by the device. The patient wears the device 24 hours a day. It is removed only for bathing or showering.

Be alert to the patient's psychosocial adaptation to this sudden "brush with death." Many patients develop a "time bomb" mentality. They and their caregivers fear the recurrence of cardiac arrest. They may become anxious, angry, and depressed. The grief response varies. Patients and caregivers may need to deal with other issues, such as driving restrictions, role reversal, and change in occupation. Be attuned to the specific needs of the patient and caregiver. Provide information and emotional support.

Teach caregivers and community members about the actions needed to save lives. Rapid, high-quality CPR and defibrillation with an AED, combined with early advanced cardiac life support (ACLS), has improved long-term survival rates for a witnessed arrest caused by ventricular dysrhythmias.

CASE STUDY

Myocardial Infarction

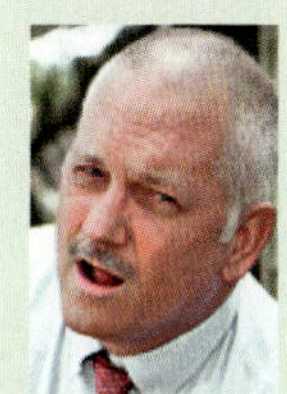

(© iStockphoto/ Thinkstock.)

Patient Profile

D.M., a 51-year-old White male, is rushed to the ED by ambulance with crushing, substernal chest pain that radiates down his left arm. He reports dizziness and nausea.

Subjective Data

- Short of breath, nauseous
- History of chronic stable angina and hypertension
- States he is "borderline diabetic"
- Overweight, but recently lost 10 lb.
- Does not exercise
- Has 3 teenage children who are causing "problems"
- Small business owner; recently lost his best friend and business partner, who died from cancer

Objective Data

Physical Assessment

- Diaphoretic
- BP 165/100 mm Hg, pulse rate 120/min, respiratory rate 26/min

Diagnostic Studies

- 12-lead ECG shows sinus tachycardia with occasional PVCs and ST elevation in leads II, III, aVF, V_5, and V_6 consistent with an inferolateral wall MI
- High troponin level
- Total cholesterol 350 mg/dL (9.1 mmol/L)
- HbA1c 9.0%

Interprofessional Care

- ED: Notify the cardiac catheterization laboratory of a patient with STEMI
- O_2 2 L/min via nasal cannula, titrate to keep O_2 saturation above 90%
- Continuous ECG monitoring
- 2 IV access sites
- Aspirin 325 mg (chewable) orally now
- Atorvastatin 80 mg orally
- SL NTG until an IV line is placed, then titrate nitroglycerin IV to relieve chest pain; hold for symptomatic hypotension
- Fentanyl 100 mcg IV; may repeat in 15 min as needed for chest pain unrelieved by NTG
- Vital signs (including pulse oximetry) every 10 min
- Prepare patient for coronary angiography with possible PCI

Discussion Questions

1. ***Recognize:*** Explain the pathogenesis of CAD. What risk factors contribute to its development? What risk factors were present in D.M.'s life?
2. ***Analyze:*** Which coronary artery(ies) is (are) most likely occluded in D.M.'s coronary circulation?
3. ***Analyze:*** Explain the significance of the results of the laboratory tests and the 12-lead ECG finding.
4. ***Plan:*** Give a rationale for each treatment measure ordered for D.M.
5. ***Prioritize:*** What are the priority nursing interventions for D.M. before PCI? Immediately after PCI?
6. ***Act:*** Identify activities you can delegate to AP.
7. ***Evaluate:*** What outcomes would show that interprofessional care was successful?
8. Develop a conceptual care map for D.M.

Answers and a corresponding conceptual care map available at http://evolve.elsevier.com/Lewis/medsurg.

BRIDGE TO NCLEX EXAMINATION

The number of the question corresponds to the same-numbered outcome at the beginning of the chapter.

1. Which information would the nurse include in teaching a patient about CAD? **(Select all that apply.)**
   - **a.** Diffuse involvement of plaque formation in coronary veins
   - **b.** Abnormal levels of cholesterol, especially low-density lipoproteins
   - **c.** Accumulation of lipid and fibrous tissue within the coronary arteries
   - **d.** Development of angina because of a decreased blood supply to the heart muscle
   - **e.** Chronic vasoconstriction of coronary arteries leading to permanent vasospasm
2. After teaching a patient about ways to decrease risk factors for CAD, which patient statement indicates that further instruction is needed?
   - **a.** "I can keep my blood pressure normal with medication."
   - **b.** "I would like to add weightlifting to my exercise program."
   - **c.** "I can change my diet to decrease my intake of saturated fats."
   - **d.** "I will change my lifestyle to reduce activities that increase my stress."
3. A hospitalized patient with a history of chronic stable angina tells the nurse they are having chest pain. Which information about ischemia would the nurse use as a basis for planning care?
   - **a.** It will always progress to myocardial infarction.
   - **b.** It can be relieved by rest, nitroglycerin, or both.
   - **c.** It is often associated with vomiting and extreme fatigue.
   - **d.** It indicates that irreversible myocardial damage is occurring.
4. The nurse is caring for a patient who is 2 days post MI. The patient reports chest pain when taking a deep breath. Which action would be a *priority*?
   - **a.** Notify the provider STAT and obtain a 12-lead ECG.
   - **b.** Obtain vital signs and auscultate for a pericardial friction rub.
   - **c.** Apply high-flow O_2 by face mask and auscultate breath sounds.
   - **d.** Medicate the patient with an opiate analgesic and reevaluate in 30 minutes.
5. A patient is in the ICU with a diagnosis of NSTEMI. Which drugs would the nurse expect the patient to receive? **(Select all that apply.)**
   - **a.** Oral statin therapy
   - **b.** Antiplatelet therapy
   - **c.** Thrombolytic therapy
   - **d.** Prophylactic antibiotics
   - **e.** Intravenous nitroglycerin
6. A patient is recovering from an uncomplicated MI. Which rehabilitation guideline is a *priority* to include in the teaching plan?
   - **a.** Refrain from sexual activity for a minimum of 3 weeks.
   - **b.** Plan a diet program that aims for a 1- to 2-lb. weight loss per week.
   - **c.** Begin an exercise program that aims for at least five 30-minute sessions per week.
   - **d.** Consider the use of erectile agents and prophylactic NTG before sexual activity.
7. Which finding is the strongest predictor of risk for sudden cardiac death?
   - **a.** Atrial fibrillation
   - **b.** Aortic valve disease
   - **c.** Mitral valve disease
   - **d.** Left ventricular dysfunction

1. b, c, d; 2. b; 3. b; 4. b; 5. a, b, e; 6. c; 7. d.

For rationales to these answers and even more NCLEX review questions, visit http://evolve.elsevier.com/Lewis/medsurg.

REFERENCES

To access the References for this chapter, please scan the QR code with a mobile device.

38

Heart Failure

Vera Barton-Maxwell

http://evolve.elsevier.com/Lewis/medsurg/

CONCEPTUAL FOCUS

Fatigue
Fluids and Electrolytes
Functional Ability
Gas Exchange
Perfusion
Self-Management

LEARNING OUTCOMES

1. Compare the pathophysiology of heart failure with reduced ejection fraction (HFrEF) and heart failure with preserved ejection fraction (HFpEF).
2. Relate the compensatory mechanisms involved in heart failure (HF) to the development of acute decompensated heart failure (ADHF) and chronic HF.
3. Describe nursing and interprofessional care to manage patients with ADHF.
4. Describe nursing and interprofessional care to manage patients with chronic HF.
5. Discuss the nursing and interprofessional care of patients with a circulatory assist device.
6. Describe the indications for a heart transplant and the nursing care of heart transplant recipients.

KEY TERMS

acute decompensated heart failure (ADHF)
cardiac resynchronization therapy (CRT)
heart failure (HF)
heart failure with preserved ejection fraction (HFpEF)
heart failure with reduced ejection fraction (HFrEF)
heart transplant
intraaortic balloon pump (IABP)
ventricular assist device (VAD)

HEART FAILURE

Heart failure (HF) is a complex clinical syndrome that develops in response to myocardial insult. The heart is not able to provide sufficient blood to meet the oxygen (O_2) needs of tissues and organs. The decreased cardiac output (CO) leads to decreased tissue perfusion, impaired gas exchange, fluid imbalance, and decreased functional ability. HF is a major health problem in the United States. Patients with HF need a multidisciplinary team of providers. Nurses have a key role in caring for people with HF. This chapter describes the nursing and interprofessional care of patients with HF.

The number of people with HF in the United States has increased from 5.7 million (2009–2012) to 6.5 million. That number is projected to rise to over 8 million adults by 2030.[1] The complex, progressive nature of HF often results in poor outcomes. Twenty percent of HF patients die within the first year of diagnosis. The 5-year mortality is 52.6%.[1] Non-Hispanic Black patients with HF have the highest rates of hospitalizations and death.[2]

HF places a significant economic burden on the health care system. HF is a leading cause for hospital admission in the United States, accounting for almost 6.5 million hospital days each year.[3] HF is the most common cause of hospitalization for patients 65 years or older. Patients with HF are at high risk of readmission.[4]

Classifications of Heart Failure

New York Heart Association Classes

The New York Heart Association (NYHA) Functional Classification places patients in 1 of 4 categories (I–IV) based on physical activity limitation and symptoms.[5] NYHA class designation changes when symptoms worsen or improve.

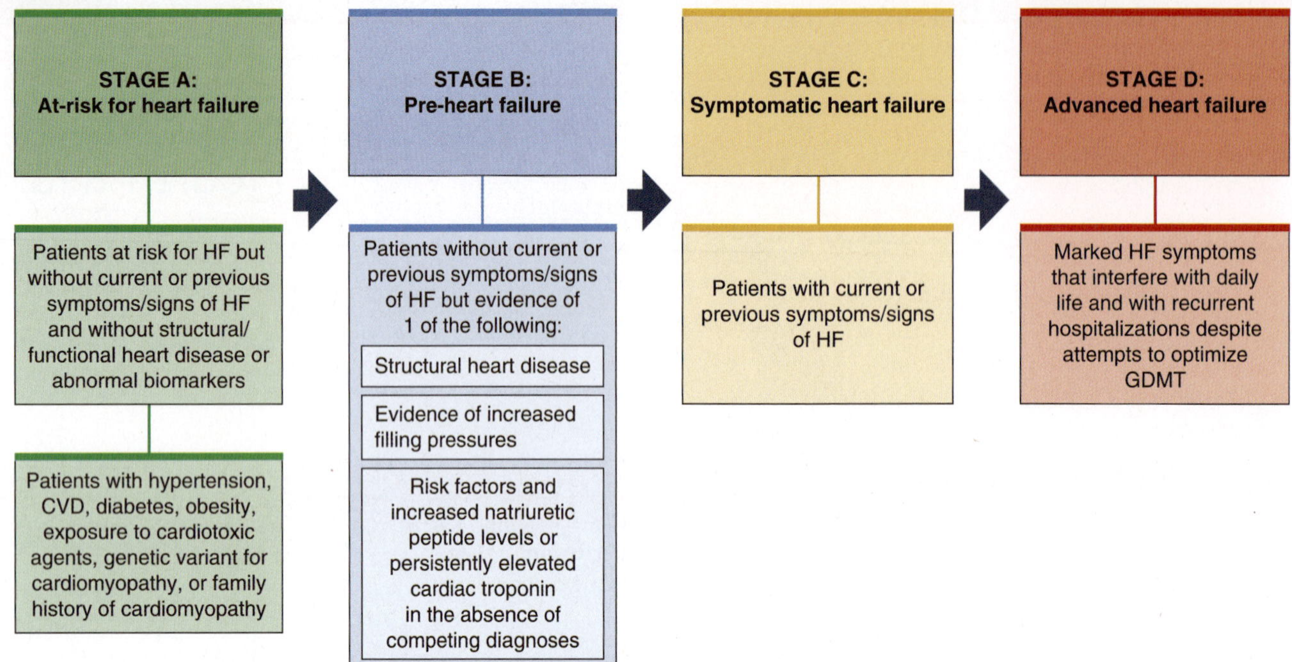

Fig. 38.1 The ACC/AHA stages of HF. *ACC,* American College of Cardiology; *AHA,* American Heart Association; *CVD,* cardiovascular disease; *GDMT,* guideline-directed medical therapy; *HF,* heart failure.

Stages of Heart Failure

The American College of Cardiology Foundation and the American Heart Association (ACCF/AHA) staging system (A–D) emphasizes the evolution, progression, and treatment of HF (Fig. 38.1).[6] This system identifies people at risk for developing HF in the future (stage A). This encourages addressing risk factors and treating existing conditions. The ACCF/AHA staging is progressive and unidirectional. Patients advance to a higher (worse) stage as the disease progresses. Table 38.1 compares the NYHA classification and ACC/AHA staging system.

Classification by Left Ventricular Ejection Fraction

Left ventricular ejection fraction (LVEF) is the percentage of the total blood volume in the left ventricle (LV) at the end of diastole that is pumped out of the LV with the next systole. LVEF is important to how we classify HF. Prognoses and treatment guidelines are based on LVEF.

HF involves a defect in either ventricular systolic function/ LV contraction (**heart failure with reduced ejection fraction [HFrEF]**) and/or a defect in ventricular diastolic function/ filling (**heart failure with preserved ejection fraction [HFpEF]**). There are 4 HF categories based on LVEF (Table 38.2). HFrEF is defined as LVEF ≤40%. HFpEF, present in about 50% of the HF population, is defined as LVEF ≥50%. The other 2 categories represent those with an LVEF in the midrange (41%–49%) and those with previously low LVEFs that have improved.[7]

Etiology

Table 38.3 describes the main causes of HF. Risk factors for developing HF include the largely modifiable conditions of diabetes and obesity. Thus many people in the United States can be categorized as having stage A HF.[7] Other causes include hypertension (HTN), myocardial infarction (MI), atherosclerotic heart disease, valvular heart disease, and familial or genetic cardiomyopathies; amyloidosis; cardiotoxicity with cancer or other treatments; or substance abuse such as alcohol, cocaine, or methamphetamine.[1]

Genetic Link

Cardiomyopathies that weaken the heart muscle and cause HF can be acquired or inherited. The inherited forms involve autosomal dominant traits. Such mutations are typically found in genes encoding sarcomeric proteins.[8] The body's largest known protein, *titin,* responds to such a mutated gene. Titin mutations impair sarcomere function and disrupt chemical signaling, which weakens ventricular structure and stability.[9] Other genes and gene mutations are linked to the development of HTN and CAD, known risk factors for HF (see Chapters 36 and 37).

Pathophysiology

HF develops in response to myocardial injury from various sources and results in decreased heart function. Signs of HF are the result of neurohormonal compensatory mechanisms in response to myocardial dysfunction, leading to remodeling of myocardial structure and changes in function (Fig. 38.2).

Left-Sided Heart Failure

The most common form of HF, left-sided HF, results from either HFrEF or HFpEF or a combination of the two.

TABLE 38.1 Diagnostic Criteria

ACCF/AHA Stage of Heart Failure and NYHA Functional Classification

ACCF/AHA Stages		NYHA Functional Classification	
A	At high risk for HF, but no heart disease or symptoms	None	
B	Heart disease is present but there are no signs or symptoms	I	No limitation of physical activity. Ordinary physical activity does not cause symptoms of HF.
C	Heart disease is present with prior or current symptoms	I	No limitation of physical activity. Ordinary physical activity does not cause symptoms of HF.
		II	Slight limitation of physical activity. Comfortable at rest, but ordinary physical activity results in symptoms of HF.
		III	Marked limitation of physical activity. Comfortable at rest, but less than ordinary activity causes symptoms of HF.
		IV	Inability to carry out any physical activity without discomfort. Symptoms may be present at rest.
D	Advanced heart disease with continued HF requiring specialized therapy	IV	Inability to carry out any physical activity without discomfort. Symptoms may be present at rest.

ACCF, American College of Cardiology Foundation; *AHA,* American Heart Association; *NYHA,* New York Heart Association.

Heart failure with reduced ejection fraction (HFrEF). HFrEF results from an inability of the heart to pump blood effectively (e.g., MI), increased afterload (e.g., HTN), cardiomyopathy, and mechanical problems (e.g., heart valve disease). The hallmark of HFrEF is a decrease in LVEF. Normal LVEF is 55% to 65%. Patients with HFrEF have an LVEF of 40% or less. The LVEF can be as low as 5% to 10%. The LV in HFrEF does not generate enough pressure to eject blood forward through the aorta. Over time, the LV dilates and hypertrophies. The weakened heart muscle cannot generate adequate SV, which impairs CO. Because the LV cannot effectively push blood forward, end diastolic volumes and pressures in the LV increase. When the LV fails, blood backs up into the left atrium (LA). This causes fluid accumulation in the lungs. The increased pulmonary hydrostatic pressure causes fluid leakage from the pulmonary capillary bed into the interstitium and then the alveoli. This results in pulmonary congestion and edema (Fig. 38.3).

Heart failure with preserved EF. HFpEF results from the inability of the ventricles to relax and fill during diastole. HTN, diabetes, obesity, CAD, and chronic kidney disease contribute to

TABLE 38.2 Heart Failure Classifications Based on LVEF

HF Classification	LVEF Criteria
HFrEF (HF with reduced EF)	≤40%
HFimpEF (HF with improved EF)	Previous LVEF ≤40% and a follow-up measurement of LVEF >40%
HFmrEF (HF with mildly reduced EF)	LVEF 41%–49%
HFpEF (HF with preserved EF)	≥50%

Data from Yancy CW, Jessup M, Bozkurt B, et al, 2013 ACCF/AHA guideline for the management of heart failure: a report of the American College of Cardiology Foundation/American Heart Association Task Force on Practice guidelines, *Circulation* 128:e240, 2013.

TABLE 38.3 Primary Causes of Heart Failure

- Amyloidosis
- Atherosclerotic heart disease
- Cardiomyopathies (peripartum, genetic, acquired)
- Cardiotoxic substances
- Hemochromatosis
- Hypertension
- Myocardial infarction
- Myocarditis
- Sarcoidosis
- Substance use (alcohol, cocaine, amphetamine)
- Thyroid disease
- Valvular heart disease

HFpEF.[10] The LV is stiff and noncompliant, causing high filling pressures in HFpEF. Decreased filling volume in the ventricles results in decreased SV. The eventual result of HFpEF is the same as that of HFrEF, a reduced CO leading to fluid congestion. The diagnosis of HFpEF is based on (1) signs and symptoms of HF, (2) normal LVEF, and (3) evidence of LV diastolic dysfunction by echocardiography or cardiac catheterization.

Patients with borderline HFpEF (LVEF 41% to 49%) have similar characteristics and receive similar therapies to those for patients with HFpEF. Patients with ventricular failure of any type may have low BP, low CO, and poor renal perfusion. Poor exercise tolerance and dysrhythmias are common. Patients may present acutely from an MI or chronically from worsening cardiomyopathy or HTN.

Right-Sided Heart Failure

Right-sided HF occurs when the right ventricle (RV) does not pump effectively. When the RV fails, fluid backs up into the venous system. This causes movement of fluid into the tissues and organs (e.g., peripheral edema, ascites, hepatomegaly, jugular venous distention [JVD]).

The most common cause of right-sided HF is left-sided HF. As the LV fails, fluid backs up into the pulmonary system, increasing pressures in the lungs. The RV works harder to push blood to the pulmonary system. Over time, this increased workload weakens the RV, and gradually it fails. Causes of

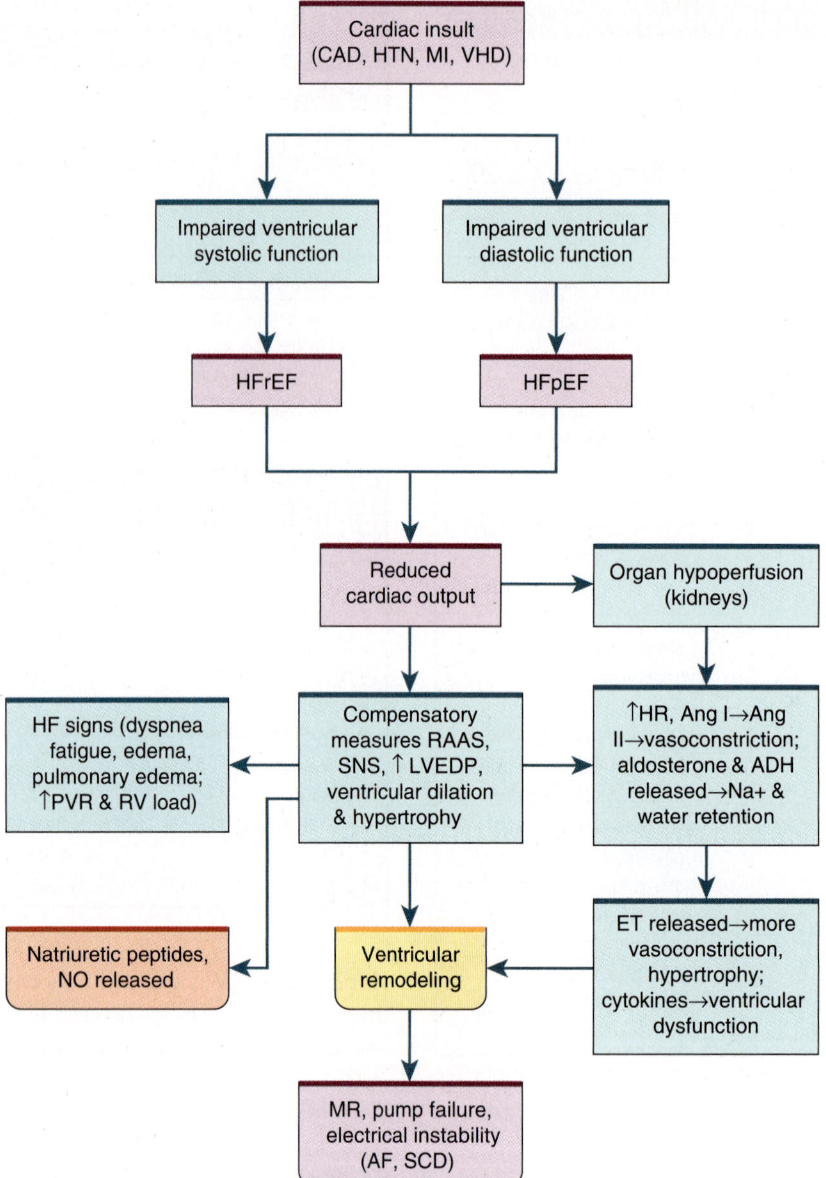

Fig. 38.2 Pathophysiology of HF. *Ang I,* Angiotensin I; *Ang II,* angiotensin II; *ADH,* antidiuretic hormone; *ET,* endothelin; *HFpEF,* HF with preserved ejection fraction; *HFrEF,* HF with reduced ejection fraction; *LVEDP,* left ventricular end-diastolic pressure; *MR,* mitral regurgitation; *NO,* nitric oxide; *PVR,* pulmonary vascular resistance; *RAAS,* renin-angiotensin-aldosterone system; *SCD,* sudden cardiac death; *SNS,* sympathetic nervous system; *VHD,* valvular heart disease.

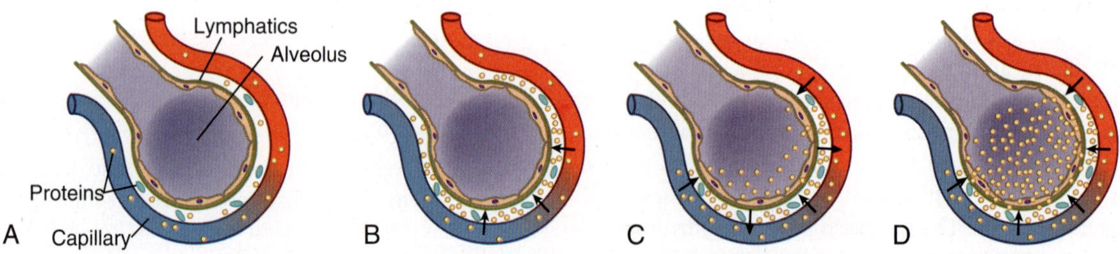

Fig. 38.3 Pulmonary edema. As pulmonary edema progresses, it inhibits O_2 and CO_2 exchange at the alveolar-capillary interface. (A) Normal relationship. (B) Increased pulmonary capillary hydrostatic pressure causes fluid to move from the vascular space into the pulmonary interstitial space. (C) Lymphatic flow increases to try to pull fluid back into the vascular or lymphatic space. (D) Failure of lymphatic flow and worsening of left-sided HF result in further movement of fluid into the interstitial space and into the alveoli. (Modified from Urden LD, Stacy KM, Lough ME: *Critical care nursing: diagnosis and management,* ed 6, St Louis, 2010, Mosby.)

right-sided HF independent of LV function include RV infarction, pulmonary embolism, and *cor pulmonale* (RV dilation and hypertrophy from lung disease) (see Chapter 31).

Biventricular Failure

Biventricular failure includes both LV and RV dysfunction. Neither ventricle pumps effectively. Fluid builds up and systemic veins are engorged. Inadequate CO results in decreased perfusion to vital organs.[3]

Compensatory Mechanisms

HF can have an abrupt onset as with acute MI, or it can be a subtle process of slow, progressive changes. The overloaded heart uses compensatory mechanisms to try to maintain adequate CO. The main compensatory mechanisms include neurohormonal responses and ventricular adaptations.

Neurohormonal response

Renin-angiotensin-aldosterone system. Activation of the renin-angiotensin-aldosterone system (RAAS) increases preload and ventricular contractility to maintain CO. RAAS activation promotes retention of fluid and sodium. The juxtaglomerular apparatus in the kidneys senses decreased renal perfusion from a falling CO. In response, the kidneys release renin, which converts angiotensinogen to angiotensin I (see Chapter 49 and Fig. 49.1). Angiotensin I is next converted to angiotensin II by a converting enzyme made in the lungs. Angiotensin II, a potent vasoconstrictor, stimulates renal water and sodium retention and the release of aldosterone from the adrenal gland. Aldosterone acts in the nephron to stimulate sodium retention and potassium excretion and promotes myocardial fibrosis in the failing heart.

Continuous activation of the RAAS and SNS in HF leads to increased levels of antidiuretic hormone (ADH). ADH regulates water retention by stimulating renal tubular reabsorption. It is released via baroreceptor signals in response to arterial low pressure/underfilling. ADH causes vasoconstriction and increases BP and central venous pressure (CVP). The consequences are fluid congestion and hyponatremia.[11] Chronic activation of the RAAS can have harmful effects. These include cardiac myocyte apoptosis (programmed cell death), hypertrophy, and fibrosis. They cause the signs and symptoms of HF.

Sympathetic nervous system. Baroreceptors sense low arterial pressure, stimulating the sympathetic nervous system (SNS) to try to maintain CO. Catecholamines (epinephrine and norepinephrine) are released. Stimulation of β-adrenergic receptors increases HR *(chronotropy)* and ventricular contractility *(inotropy)*. Chronic SNS stimulation increases myocardial O_2 demand on the already weakened heart.

Peptides and cytokines. Continuous activation of the neurohormonal responses (RAAS and SNS) leads to high levels of endothelin and proinflammatory cytokines. These high levels increase the heart's workload, causing progressive LV dysfunction, myocyte hypertrophy, and ventricular remodeling.[11]

Endothelin is a vasoconstrictor peptide made by the vascular endothelial cells. Endothelin release is stimulated by hypoxia, ischemia, neurohormones, and inflammatory cytokines. Although endothelin stimulates contraction in most smooth muscles, it has the opposite effect on the heart. It acts as a negative inotrope, decreasing ventricular contractility in the failing heart.

Myocytes release proinflammatory cytokines in response to heart injury (e.g., MI, HF). Two cytokines, tumor necrosis factor (TNF) and interleukin-1 (IL-1), further depress heart function through a negative inotropic effect, causing myocyte hypertrophy and apoptosis. Over time, a systemic inflammatory response occurs.

Ventricular adaptations

Dilation. *Dilation* is an enlargement of the heart chambers (Fig. 38.4A). It occurs when pressure in the heart chambers (usually the LV) is elevated over time. The heart muscle fibers stretch in response to the volume of blood in the heart at the end of diastole. According to the *Frank-Starling Law,* the strength of the heart's contraction is directly proportional to its diastolic stretch. The implication is that increased preload (a greater influx of blood into the ventricle during diastole) will cause a more forceful contraction. This increased contraction initially leads to increased CO and maintains BP and perfusion. Dilation starts as an adaptive mechanism to cope with increasing blood volume. However, excess preload exhausts the Frank-Starling mechanism, and overstretched heart muscle fibers no longer increase CO.

Hypertrophy. *Hypertrophy* is an adaptive increase in the heart muscle thickness as a slow response to overwork and strain (Fig. 38.4B). It takes time for this increased muscle tissue to develop. Initially, the increased contractile power of the muscle fibers leads to increased CO and maintains tissue perfusion. Over time, hypertrophic heart muscle has poor contractility, needs more O_2 to perform work, has poor coronary artery circulation, becomes ischemic more easily, and is prone to dysrhythmias.

Remodeling. Pathologic *ventricular remodeling* is a change in the structure (dimensions, mass, shape) of the heart. Ventricular remodeling in HF occurs over time in response to pressure or volume overload and/or cardiac injury and compensatory mechanisms. These include neurohormonal, ET, cytokine activation, and ventricular adaptations, including dilation and hypertrophy. This altered shape of the ventricles eventually leads to increased ventricular mass, increased wall tension, increased O_2 consumption, and impaired contractility. The heart becomes less elliptical and more spherical. The ventricles become larger but less effective pumps. LVEF further declines. Increases in angiotensin II, aldosterone, and cytokines stimulate collagen synthesis leading to fibrosis and further impaired pumping ability. Ventricular remodeling is associated with sudden cardiac death and a worse prognosis in HF.

Beneficial Counterregulatory Mechanisms

The body tries to maintain balance through counterregulatory processes. Natriuretic peptides (atrial natriuretic peptide [ANP] and brain [b-type] natriuretic peptide [BNP]) are hormones made by the heart muscle. ANP is released from the atria and

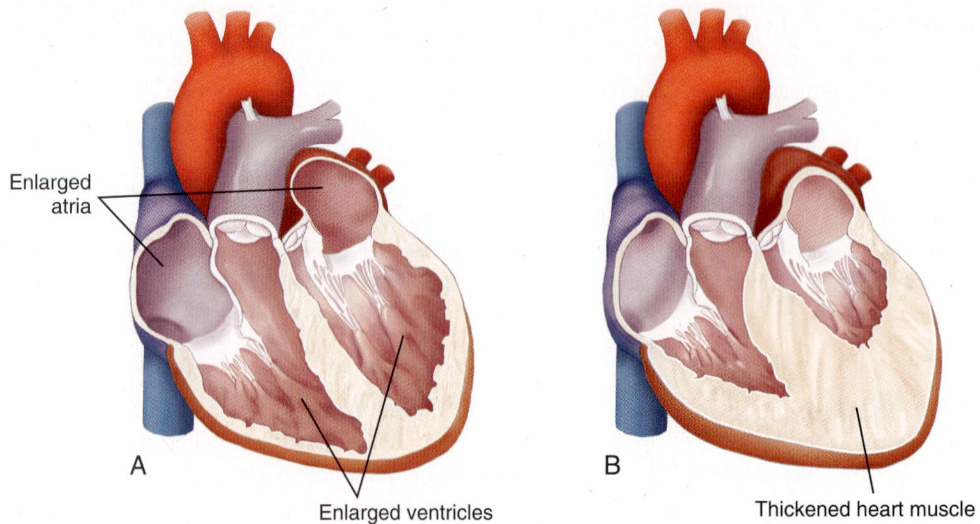

Fig. 38.4 (A) Dilated heart chambers. (B) Hypertrophied heart chambers.

BNP is released from the ventricles in response to increased blood volume and cardiac wall stretching.[12]

Natriuretic peptides have beneficial renal, cardiovascular, and hormonal effects. Renal effects include (1) increased glomerular filtration rate and diuresis and (2) sodium excretion (natriuresis). Cardiovascular effects include (1) vasodilation and (2) decreased BP. Hormonal effects include (1) inhibition of aldosterone and renin secretion and (2) interference with ADH release. The combined effects of ANP and BNP help counter the adverse effects of the SNS and RAAS.[12] We can measure BNP levels. High BNP occurs with fluid retention and is a predictor of death in HF.

Nitric oxide (NO) and prostaglandin are counterregulatory substances released from the vascular endothelium in response to the compensatory mechanisms activated in HF. NO and prostaglandin work to relax the arterial smooth muscle. This results in vasodilation and decreased afterload.[13]

Compensated HF occurs when compensatory mechanisms succeed in maintaining an adequate CO for tissue perfusion. *Decompensated HF* occurs when these mechanisms can no longer maintain adequate CO and inadequate tissue perfusion results.

Clinical Manifestations: Acute Decompensated Heart Failure

Acute decompensated heart failure (ADHF) is an increase (usually sudden) in symptoms of HF with a decrease in functional status. ADHF often requires rapid escalation of therapy and hospital admission. A diagnosis of ADHF is corroborated by increased natriuretic peptide levels and/or objective signs of pulmonary or systemic congestion.[14]

ADHF typically presents with findings related to pulmonary congestion and volume overload. Neurohormonal activation leads to impaired sodium excretion through the kidneys that results in sodium and fluid accumulation. To help compensate, the lymphatic system increases its flow to help maintain a constant volume of the pulmonary extravascular fluid (Fig. 38.3A and B). The lungs become less compliant. There is increased resistance in the small airways. We often see a mild increase in respiratory rate (RR) and a decrease in partial pressure of O_2 in arterial blood (PaO_2).

If pulmonary venous pressure continues to increase, more fluid moves into the interstitial space than the lymphatics can remove, causing *interstitial edema* (Fig. 38.3C). Tachypnea and coughing develop, and the patient becomes symptomatic (e.g., short of breath). If the pulmonary venous pressure increases further, the alveolar lining is disrupted. Fluid moves into the alveoli *(alveolar edema)*. Arterial blood gas values worsen (lower PaO_2, increased $PaCO_2$, respiratory acidosis). Auscultation may reveal crackles and wheezes.

ADHF can manifest as pulmonary edema. Lung alveoli fill with serosanguineous fluid (Fig. 38.3D). Findings include acute manifestations of left HF, such as dyspnea, *orthopnea,* and *paroxysmal nocturnal dyspnea.* The RR is often over 30 breaths per minute. You may see accessory respiratory muscle use and pink, frothy sputum.

JVD is often present due to elevated LV filling pressures. Patients are usually anxious and pale and may be cyanotic. The HR is often rapid with an abnormal S_3 or S_4 heart sound (see Table 35.4). BP may be high or decreased depending on the severity of the HF. Hypotension indicates severe LV systolic dysfunction and possible cardiogenic shock. Cool extremities occur with low CO and poor perfusion. Skin pallor, ashy color, or mottling may be present from peripheral vasoconstriction.

We categorize patients with ADHF into 1 of 4 groups based on hemodynamic and clinical status: dry-warm, dry-cold, wet-warm, and wet-cold (Table 38.4). The most common presentation is a wet and warm patient. A patient is "wet" due to volume overload (e.g., congestion, dyspnea) but "warm" due to maintaining adequate perfusion (warm skin, positive pulses).

TABLE 38.4 Clinical Profile in Acute Decompensated Heart Failure

		CONGESTION (WET)	
		No	**Yes**
LOW PERFUSION (COLD)	**No**	**Dry-Warm** • PAWP normal • CO normal • Signs and symptoms: none	**Wet-Warm** • PAWP ↑ • CO normal • Signs and symptoms: dyspnea, edema, orthopnea
	Yes	**Dry-Cold** • PAWP ↓ or normal • CO ↓ • Signs and symptoms: edema, hypotension, cool extremities	**Wet-Cold** • PAWP ↑ • CO ↓ • Signs and symptoms: altered mental status, ↓ O_2 saturation, ↓ urine output, shock

PAWP, Pulmonary artery wedge pressure.

CHECK YOUR PRACTICE

You are assigned to a patient with ADHF who is in the HF unit. The patient has bilateral crackles in the midlower lung fields and dyspnea when moving from the bed to the commode. The skin is warm. Pulses are present in all extremities. Your preceptor asks you to categorize your patient based on the classification systems in Fig. 38.1 and Tables 38.1 and 38.2.

- In what NYHA class would you place your patient?
- In what ACCF/AHA stage would you place your patient?
- What ADHF clinical profile does your patient best fit?

Clinical Manifestations: Chronic Heart Failure

Chronic HF is a progressive syndrome of reduced CO and increased venous pressure associated with the death of cardiac muscle cells. Neurohormonal and hemodynamic mechanisms to compensate for reduced CO include vasoconstriction and SNS stimulation, an inflammatory response involving cytokines, and ventricular remodeling. These responses are responsible for the manifestations of chronic HF. Table 38.5 lists the manifestations of right-sided and left-sided chronic HF.

Fatigue

Fatigue from usual daily activities is an early symptom of chronic HF. As CO decreases, fatigue eventually limits activities. Anemia can cause fatigue in HF.

Pulmonary Manifestations

Dyspnea is the most common manifestation of chronic HF. It is caused by increased pulmonary pressures from interstitial and alveolar edema. Dyspnea can occur early in the HF disease process with mild exertion. As HF progresses, dyspnea develops with less exertion or at rest.

TABLE 38.5 Manifestations of Heart Failure

Right-Sided Heart Failure	Left-Sided Heart Failure
Signs	
• Right ventricular heaves • ↑ HR • Anasarca (massive general edema) • Ascites • Edema (e.g., pedal, scrotum) • Hepatomegaly • JVD • Murmurs • Weight gain	• Left ventricular heaves • ↑ HR • S_3 and S_4 heart sounds • ABGs: ↓ Pao_2, slight ↑ $Paco_2$ • Confusion, restlessness • Dry, hacking cough • Crackles (pulmonary edema) • Pleural effusion • PMI displaced inferiorly and left of the midclavicular line (LV hypertrophy) • Pulsus alternans • Shallow respirations up to 32–40/min • Frothy, pink-tinged sputum (advanced pulmonary edema)
Symptoms	
• Anorexia and GI bloating • Anxiety, depression • Fatigue • Nausea • RUQ pain	• Anxiety, depression • Dyspnea • Fatigue, weakness • Nocturia • Orthopnea • Paroxysmal nocturnal dyspnea

Orthopnea occurs due to redistribution of fluid from the legs into the lungs while lying down. Dyspnea is usually relieved by sitting up. Ask about the number of pillows used under the head while sleeping or about sleeping in a recliner to aid breathing.

A chronic, nonproductive cough that is worse when lying down is often from pulmonary congestion. Paroxysmal nocturnal dyspnea (PND) is caused by fluid accumulation entering the alveoli while the patient is supine. The patient awakens in a panic with feelings of suffocation and a strong desire to sit or stand to aid breathing.

Tachycardia

Tachycardia is an early sign of HF. To compensate for a reduced CO, the body increases the HR via SNS activation. Over time, persistent tachycardia is harmful and may worsen HF symptoms. Adequate HR control in patients with chronic HF is associated with better outcomes, including decreased hospitalizations and death.[3] Patients may report a fast or irregular heartbeat, a fluttering sensation, or "skipped beats."

Edema

Edema can indicate volume overload. Common sites include dependent body areas (peripheral edema), liver (hepatomegaly), abdominal cavity (ascites), and lungs (pulmonary edema, pleural effusion). If the patient is in bed, dependent sacral and scrotal edema may develop. Pressing the edematous skin with the finger may leave a depression *(pitting edema).*

Changes in Urine Output

Urine output may be low because of decreased renal perfusion. HF patients often develop resistance to diuretics, which can result in a drop in urinary output. *Nocturia* is excess urination at night. It is due to increased renal perfusion in the supine position.

Skin Changes

Low CO can decrease perfusion to the extremities with *mottling,* a blue or gray skin coloring. The skin may appear dusky because tissue capillary O_2 extraction is increased with chronic HF. Chronic edema can result in pigment changes. A cool or clammy feeling to touch can occur with poor perfusion. The skin may be dry from diuretic therapy.

Mental Status and Behavior Changes

Cerebral hypoperfusion may occur because of hypoxia to the brain from decreased CO. Hypotension from HF medications and hypovolemia are also causes of neurologic changes in chronic HF.

The patient or caregiver may report confusion, forgetfulness, inattentiveness, and restlessness. Assess for neurologic problems, such as stroke or transient ischemic attack (TIA) and mental health problems. The prevalences of depression and anxiety are high. Having depression increases the risk of death and readmission.[15] Patients with mental health problems have poor adherence to treatment and decreased quality of life.

Sleep Problems

Snoring and daytime sleepiness can indicate sleep apnea, a common condition with chronic HF. Screening for sleep apnea is an important part of HF care (see Chapter 8). Insomnia could be related to mental health, including anxiety or depression, or daytime napping. Nocturia may disturb sleep.

Chest Pain

Chest pain or angina can be the result of the reduced CO associated with HF in patients with CAD. Chest pain in HF can also occur due to myocardial stretch from volume overload.

Weight Changes

Many factors contribute to weight changes. Progressive weight gain in chronic HF may indicate fluid retention. Renal failure may contribute to fluid retention. Abdominal fullness from ascites and hepatomegaly often causes anorexia and nausea. As HF advances, cardiac *cachexia* with muscle wasting and fat loss can be masked by edema.

Complications of Heart Failure

Pleural Effusion

A pleural effusion is a common complication. Increased capillary hydrostatic pressure in the circulation causes fluid leakage into the pleural space. Pleural effusions may cause dyspnea, cough, and chest pain. Pleural effusion is discussed in Chapter 30.

Dysrhythmias and Dyssynchronous Contraction

Atrial and ventricular dysrhythmias can occur. Structural changes, including myocardial stretch, fibrosis, and chamber dilation, alter the electrical paths of the heart. Early or delayed depolarizations can trigger dysrhythmias. AF is common. The prevalence of AF increases as the severity of HF increases. Loss of "atrial kick" during systole contributes to decreased CO and worsening HF symptoms. Dizziness, lightheadedness, or syncope from hypoperfusion to the brain can occur if dysrhythmias further decrease CO.

AF promotes thrombus formation within the atria. Thrombi can break loose and form emboli, placing patients at significant risk for stroke. An enlarged LV and very low LVEF increase the risk for thrombus formation in the LV. Treatment with anticoagulation is a priority if there are no significant contraindications. Treatment with drugs to achieve HR control is important. Other options include cardioversion and ablation. Atrial fibrillation is discussed in Chapter 39.

Patients with HF are at risk for dangerous ventricular dysrhythmias (e.g., ventricular tachycardia [VT], ventricular fibrillation [VF]). SCD (sudden loss of cardiac function due to a fatal ventricular tachyarrhythmia) is a major cause of death. Patients with HFrEF are at greatest risk for SCD. Guidelines recommend consideration of an implantable cardioverter-defibrillator (ICD) for patients with an LVEF less than 35% who are NYHA Class II or III.[7] SCD is discussed in Chapter 37. Dysrhythmias are discussed in Chapter 39.

Ventricular remodeling can lead to dyssynchrony in ventricular contractions. One ventricle may contract before the other ventricle, leading to poor ventricular filling (preload), reduced force of ventricular contraction (systole), and severe mitral regurgitation (MR). This worsens HF symptoms. **Cardiac resynchronization therapy (CRT)** with implantable cardiac devices can significantly improve morbidity and mortality. Many patients with HF receive a combination ICD and CRT device, discussed later in the chapter.

Hepatomegaly

HF can lead to hepatomegaly as the liver becomes congested with venous blood. This congestion can lead to impaired liver function. Eventually liver cells die, fibrosis occurs, and cirrhosis can develop (see Chapter 48).

Cardiorenal Syndrome

Reduced CO results in decreased renal perfusion, decreased glomerular filtration rate, and increased creatinine. Neurohormonal activation causes sodium and water retention, worsening HF symptoms, and renal function.

Anemia

The main cause of anemia in chronic HF is chronic kidney insufficiency. Renal vasoconstriction results in the kidney making less erythropoietin. Excess cytokine production can reduce erythropoietin secretion. The anemia itself can worsen heart function due to increased cardiac workload through tachycardia, fluid retention, and increased SV. This worsens fatigue and other HF manifestations.

Diagnostic Studies

Diagnostic tests for ADHF and chronic HF are outlined in Table 38.6. A key goal is to find the underlying cause of HF.

An echocardiogram is a valuable, noninvasive diagnostic tool used in patients with HF. The echocardiogram gives information about chamber size and function, LVEF, heart valve function, wall thickness and motion, presence of effusion or thrombus, and intracardiac and pulmonary pressures. This test helps to distinguish between HFrEF and HFpEF. Other useful tests include 12-lead ECG, ambulatory heart monitors, chest x-ray, nuclear imaging studies, and heart catheterization. An endomyocardial biopsy may be done during heart catheterization to evaluate for infective or infiltrative disease in patients who develop unexplained, new-onset HF.

Laboratory studies aid in the diagnosis of HF. In general, BNP and N-terminal prohormone of BNP (NT-proBNP) levels correlate positively with the degree of LV failure.[7] Increases in BNP or NT-proBNP levels can be caused by conditions other than HF, including pulmonary embolism, renal failure, and acute coronary syndrome.

Interprofessional Care: Acute Decompensated Heart Failure

Many persons with HF have episodes of ADHF. Common precipitating factors include respiratory infections, dysrhythmias, acute coronary syndrome, uncontrolled HTN, and nonadherence to drug and diet therapy. Stable patients with ADHF may be treated in the emergency department (ED) or admitted to a telemetry unit. Unstable patients are managed in an intensive care unit (ICU).

Goals of therapy for patients hospitalized with ADHF include (1) relieving symptoms; (2) optimizing volume status; (3) supporting oxygenation, ventilation, CO, and end organ perfusion; (4) identifying and addressing the cause of the ADHF; and (5) avoiding complications.

Drug Therapy

Drug therapy is essential in treating ADHF (Table 38.7).

TABLE 38.6 Interprofessional Care

Heart Failure

Both ADHF and Chronic HF	ADHF	Chronic HF
Diagnostic Assessment		
• History and physical assessment • Determine underlying cause • Electrolytes, cardiac biomarkers, BNP or NT-proBNP (see Table 35.10), liver function tests, thyroid function tests, CBC, lipid profile, kidney function tests, urinalysis • Chest x-ray • 12-lead ECG • Echocardiogram (see Table 35.11) • Nuclear imaging studies (see Table 35.11) • Cardiac catheterization (see Tables 35.12 and 35.13)	• Measure LV function • Hemodynamic monitoring • Endomyocardial biopsy in select patients	• Cardiopulmonary exercise stress test • 6-min walk test • Sleep studies in select patients
Management		
• Treat underlying cause • Drug therapy (Table 38.7) • Circulatory assist devices (e.g., ventricular assist device) • Daily weights • Sodium- and possibly fluid-restricted diet • O_2 by mask or nasal cannula if indicated	• High-Fowler's position • Noninvasive positive pressure ventilation • Circulatory assist device: IABP, ECMO, LVAD • Mechanical ventilation • Vital signs, urine output at least q1h until stable • Continuous ECG and pulse oximetry monitoring • Hemodynamic monitoring (e.g., intraarterial BP, PAWP, CO) • Cardioversion (e.g., atrial fibrillation) • Ultrafiltration	• Cardiac resynchronization therapy with biventricular pacing and internal cardioverter-defibrillator • Heart transplant • Rest-activity periods • Dietitian consult • Physical/occupational therapy consult • Cardiac rehabilitation • Home health nursing care (e.g., telehealth monitoring) • Palliative and end-of-life care

TABLE 38.7 Drug Therapy

Heart Failure

Drug	Mechanism of Action
Anticoagulants (see Table 41.10)	
	• Prevent thromboembolism • Recommended for patients with an ejection fraction <20% and/or atrial fibrillation
Antidysrhythmic Drugs (see Table 39.9)	
	• Prevent or treat dysrhythmias
β-Adrenergic Blockers (see Table 36.6)	
bisoprolol carvedilol (Coreg) metoprolol succinate (Toprol-XL)	• ↓ Afterload • Inhibit SNS • Reverse cardiac remodeling • ↓ Death in patients with chronic HF
Diuretics (see Table 36.7)	
Loop Diuretics	
bumetanide (Bumex) furosemide (Lasix)	• Block sodium absorption in the kidneys at the loop of Henle • ↑ Urine output • ↓ Fluid volume • ↓ Preload • ↓ Pulmonary venous pressure • Relieve symptoms of fluid congestion
Thiazide Diuretics	
hydrochlorothiazide metolazone (Zaroxolyn)	• Block sodium reabsorption at the distal renal tubule • ↑ Urine output (milder diuretic effect than loop diuretics) • ↓ BP
Aldosterone Antagonists	
eplerenone (Inspra) spironolactone (Aldactone)	• Inhibit aldosterone that causes sodium and water retention and antiinflammatory responses in HF • Prevent potassium loss by inhibiting sodium and potassium exchange in the distal tubule • Mild diuretic effect • ↓ Death and hospitalizations in patients with chronic HF
Morphine	
morphine (MS Contin, Duramorph)	• Bind to opioid receptors • May decrease the chemoreceptor response to hypoxia and/or cause vasodilation, reducing pulmonary congestion • ↓ Reduce anxiety
Neprilysin-Angiotensin Receptor Inhibitors	
sacubitril/valsartan (Entresto)	• Sacubitril inhibits neprilysin, decreasing natriuretic degradation which promotes diuresis, natriuresis • Valsartan selectively blocks angiotensin II receptors • ↓ BP • Dilate venules and arterioles • ↑ Renal blood flow • ↓ Death and hospitalizations in patients with chronic HF
Positive Inotropes	
β-Adrenergic Agonists	
dobutamine dopamine	• ↑ Contractility (positive inotropic effect) • ↑ CO • May reduce PAWP • May cause dysrhythmias • ↑ Myocardial O_2 demand
Digitalis Glycoside	
digoxin	• Weak positive inotrope mostly at higher doses • ↓ Effects of RAAS and SNS • May reduce HF symptoms and hospitalization if added to standard therapy for chronic HF
Phosphodiesterase Inhibitor	
milrinone[a]	• Produce mild vasodilation • ↑ SV and CO • Promote vasodilation
Renin-Angiotensin-Aldosterone System Inhibitors (see Table 36.6)	
ACE Inhibitors benazepril (Lotensin) captopril enalapril (Vasotec) ***Angiotensin II Receptor Blockers*** losartan (Cozaar) valsartan (Diovan)	• Dilate venules and arterioles • ↓ Afterload and SVR • ↑ Renal blood flow • May relieve HF symptoms • Promote reverse remodeling • May ↓ death and hospitalizations in patients with chronic HF
Selective SA Node Inhibitor	
ivabradine (Corlanor)	• Selectively inhibits the I *f*-current in the SA node • ↓ HR • May ↓ death and hospitalizations in patients with HFrEF in sinus rhythm with a HR ≥ 70 bpm • Only for patients with chronic HF
Sodium-Glucose Cotransporter Inhibitors	
dapagliflozin (Farxiga) empagliflozin (Jardiance)	• Inhibit SGLT2 activity and modulate reabsorption of glucose in the kidneys, causing glucose excretion in the urine • Osmotic diuretic in HF • ↓ Blood volume and preload, which relieves congestion and HF symptoms • ↓ Oxidative stress and inflammation • ↑ Endothelial function, ↑ nitric oxide (NO) availability, vasodilation • ↓ Death and hospitalization in HFrEF
Soluble Guanylate Cyclase Stimulators	
vericiguat (Verquvo)	• Stimulates relaxation of smooth muscle cells • ↑ Sensitivity to nitric oxide • ↓ Hypertrophy, inflammation, fibrosis • ↓ Death and HF hospitalization after an HF hospitalization or need for IV diuretics in HFrEF
Vasodilators	
isosorbide dinitrate/hydralazine (BiDil) nitrates (e.g., nitroglycerin, isosorbide dinitrate [Isordil]) nitroprusside (Nitropress)[a]	• ↓ Afterload • Dilate the arterioles of the kidneys, leading to ↑ renal perfusion and fluid loss • ↓ BP • ↓ Preload • Nesiritide may reduce PAWP • May relieve HF symptoms (e.g., dyspnea) • Isosorbide dinitrate/hydralazine, fixed dose, may ↓ death in Black people with HFrEF and NYHA Class III–IV symptoms

[a]Used for ADHF only.

Diuretics. Diuretics are the first line for treating patients with volume overload (see Table 36.7). Diuretics decrease sodium reabsorption at various sites within the kidneys, enhancing sodium and water loss. Decreasing intravascular volume reduces fluid returning to the LV (preload). This allows for more efficient LV pumping, decreased pulmonary vascular pressures, and improved alveolar gas exchange. Loop diuretics (e.g., furosemide) are given by IV bolus or infusion. Thiazide diuretics or mineralocorticoids (e.g., spironolactone) may be added. Increased urine output, decreased symptoms, and fluid weight loss indicate effective diuretic therapy.

Vasodilators. Patients with ADHF who are not hypotensive may receive vasodilators. They are used to relieve dyspnea.[7] Patients on IV vasodilators may have an indwelling arterial line or continuous noninvasive blood pressure monitoring.

IV nitroglycerin (NTG) is a primary vasodilator. It reduces blood return to the right side of the heart, thus reducing preload. It improves coronary artery blood flow by dilating the coronary arteries. This increases myocardial O_2 supply. In high doses, NTG slightly reduces afterload. Tolerance often develops with continued IV use, requiring higher doses. When titrating IV NTG, monitor BP every 5 to 10 minutes to avoid hypotension.

Sodium nitroprusside (Nitropress) is a potent IV arterial vasodilator that reduces preload and afterload, thus improving myocardial contraction, increasing CO, and reducing pulmonary congestion. Complications of therapy include hypotension and, at high doses, thiocyanate (cyanide) toxicity.

DRUG ALERT

Sodium Nitroprusside

- Record baseline BP and continuously monitor during administration.
- Arterial BP monitoring is recommended during infusion.
- Rapid IV infusion can reduce BP too quickly and cause hypotension.
- Headache, dizziness, nausea, agitation, and restlessness can occur.
- Monitor for thiocyanate toxicity if infusion is greater than 3 mcg/kg/min.

Morphine. Morphine dilates pulmonary and systemic blood vessels, reducing preload and afterload. It can be given in small IV boluses to relieve dyspnea with ADHF. Monitor the patient closely. Morphine has serious adverse effects, including respiratory depression.

Positive inotropes. Patients with signs of hypoperfusion may receive inotropic agents. Inotropic drugs increase myocardial contractility. They are used for patients with low CO despite adequate fluid volume. Current evidence recommends inotropic therapy only for the short-term treatment of patients with ADHF who have not responded to conventional drug therapy (e.g., diuretics, vasodilators, morphine).[1]

Drugs include β-agonists (e.g., dopamine, dobutamine, norepinephrine [Levophed]) and phosphodiesterase inhibitors (milrinone). In addition to increasing myocardial contractility and SVR, dopamine dilates the renal blood vessels and enhances urine output. Unlike dopamine, dobutamine is a selective β-agonist that works mainly on the β_1-receptors in the heart. It does not increase SVR. We evaluate therapy effectiveness by assessing for improved CO, BP, urine output, and reduced filling pressures.

DRUG ALERT

IV Inotropic Therapy

- Use continuous ECG monitoring as they can cause life-threatening dysrhythmias.
- Monitor IV site. Tissue necrosis and sloughing can occur with drug extravasation.

Milrinone is an inotrope and vasodilator. Milrinone improves myocardial contractility, increases CO, decreases afterload, and reduces BP. It is only given IV. Adverse effects include dysrhythmias, thrombocytopenia, and liver toxicity.

Digitalis is a weaker positive inotrope that can be added if symptoms persist after other drugs have been started. Digoxin can mildly increase contractility but also increases myocardial O_2 consumption. It can reduce heart rate, especially in those with atrial fibrillation. Monitor digoxin levels if toxicity is suspected and make dose adjustments based on renal function. Potassium and magnesium levels must be maintained.

SAFETY ALERT

Infusion Pumps

- To control the rate and assist with titration, use an infusion pump whenever you are giving IV vasodilators and inotropes.
- Pumps with drug libraries can help avoid rates and doses that are out of the safe range.

Nonpharmacologic Therapies

Ultrafiltration, or *aquapheresis,* can treat volume overload when diuretics have not been effective.[16] Ultrafiltration removes fluid volume and excess sodium from the blood while maintaining hemodynamic stability. Hemodialysis can reduce volume overload with renal failure. These treatments are discussed in Chapter 51.

Implantation of CRT, a biventricular pacemaker, may be done for patients with ADHF who meet specific criteria and do not respond to more traditional therapies. Mechanical circulatory support devices can be used temporarily in patients with NYHA class IV symptoms who are dependent on inotropes. These devices are discussed later in this chapter.

Interprofessional Care: Chronic Heart Failure

Evidence-based medication and device therapies have dramatically improved outcomes for patients with chronic HFrEF (Table 38.6). The Heart Failure Society of America (HFSA) and the AHA regularly update guidelines on HF therapies.

The goals of chronic HF therapies include (1) symptom management, (2) decreased mortality and morbidity, and (3) minimizing side effects. These therapies treat the underlying cause and contributing factors, maximize CO, improve ventricular function, improve quality of life (QOL), and preserve target organ function. Symptom management depends heavily on adherence to self-management protocols (e.g., daily weights, diet, exercise) and drug and device therapies.

Drug Therapy

Guideline-directed drug therapy for HFrEF, targeting neurohormonal blockade of the SNS and RAAS, has improved survival and reduced hospitalizations.[6] Neurohormonal blockade decreases plasma aldosterone levels and SNS activity, while promoting vasodilation and sodium and water excretion. Drug therapy for chronic HF is outlined in Table 38.7. Four priority drug classes are referred to as the 4 pillars of heart failure: angiotensin receptor/neprilysin inhibitors (ARNIs), beta-blockers (BBs), mineralocorticoid receptor antagonists (MRAs), and sodium-glucose cotransporter-2 inhibitors (SGLT2i) (Fig. 38.5).[17]

Angiotensin receptor/neprilysin inhibitors. Sacubitril/valsartan (Entresto) is a combination of a neprilysin inhibitor (sacubitril) and an ARB (valsartan). It is now considered the first-line therapy and the first pillar of HF treatment.[7] This drug provides dual blockade of the RAAS and the natriuretic peptide system. Sacubitril, a recombinant form of BNP, inhibits neprilysin, an enzyme that degrades natriuretic peptides. Sacubitril inhibition allows for more available circulating BNP. This results in decreased SVR, afterload, and CVP and increased natriuresis and diuresis. Monitor patients for hypotension, renal insufficiency, and angioedema.

β-Adrenergic blockers. β-Blockers are one of the 4 pillars of HF drugs.[17] They directly block the negative effects of the SNS (e.g., increased HR) on the failing heart. Three β-blockers have been found to decrease death in patients with HFrEF: carvedilol (Coreg), metoprolol succinate (Toprol-XL), and bisoprolol. They can increase LVEF. The improvement in LVEF is dose related, so the highest tolerated dose is prescribed.[6] However, because β-blockers can reduce myocardial contractility, care must be taken in patients with volume overload. After a low starting dose, the dose is increased every 2 weeks as tolerated. Side effects include worsening of HF symptoms, hypotension, fatigue, and bradycardia.

DRUG ALERT
Carvedilol

- Obtain standing BP 1 hour after dosing to assess tolerance.
- Overdose can cause bradycardia, hypotension, bronchospasm, and cardiogenic shock.
- Abrupt withdrawal may result in sweating, palpitations, and headaches.

Mineralocorticoids (aldosterone antagonists). Mineralocorticoids are the third pillar of HF drugs. Spironolactone (Aldactone) and eplerenone (Inspra) are potassium-sparing diuretics that inhibit aldosterone activation. They bind to receptors at the aldosterone-dependent sodium-potassium exchange site in the distal renal tubule, where they have a mild diuretic effect. Monitor potassium levels and renal function.

DRUG ALERT
Spironolactone

- Monitor potassium levels during treatment.
- Use with caution in patients taking digoxin, since hyperkalemia may reduce the effects of digoxin.
- Teach patients to avoid foods high in potassium (e.g., bananas, oranges).
- Assess male patients for gynecomastia, a common side effect of long-term use.

Sodium–glucose cotransporter-2 inhibitors (SGLT2i). SGLT2i make up the fourth pillar of drug therapy for HFrEF. They were developed for diabetes treatment. With use, they were found to have profound CV benefits for patients with HFrEF. SGLT2i promote diuresis by inhibiting glucose and sodium reabsorption in the renal tubules. This reduces blood volume and preload. SGLT2i reduce oxidative stress and inflammation in HF. They improve endothelial function, enhancing nitric oxide (NO) bioavailability and vasodilation. SGLT2i reduce intraglomerular pressure and mitigate the risk of acute kidney injury.[18]

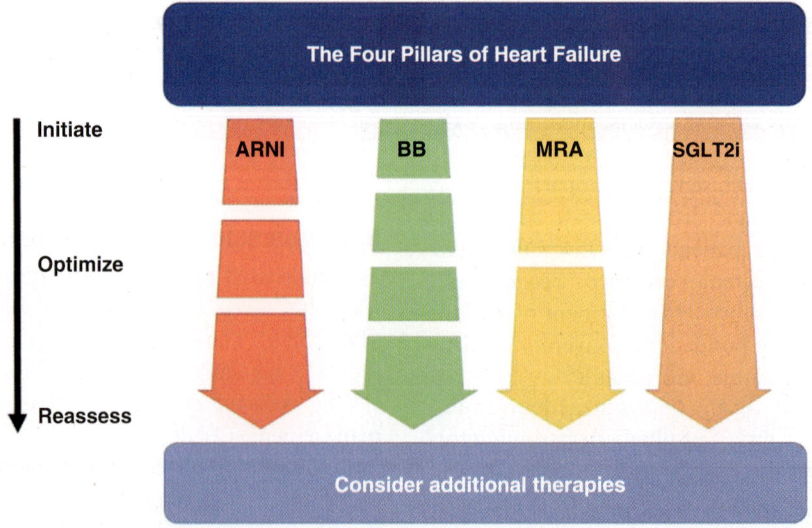

Fig. 38.5 The 4 pillars of heart failure drug therapy. All agents are started in parallel. This is followed by up-titration in 1, 2, or 3 steps, as needed. Additional therapies are considered as a final step. *ARNI,* Angiotensin receptor-neprilysin inhibitor; *BB,* beta-blocker; *MRA,* mineralocorticoid receptor antagonists; *SGLT2i,* sodium-glucose cotransporter 2 inhibitors. (From National Heart, Lung, and Blood Institute; National Institutes of Health; U.S. Department of Health and Human Services.)

Other agents

ACE inhibitors. ACE inhibitors block the RAAS by reducing the conversion of angiotensin I to angiotensin II. They decrease afterload and SVR and slow ventricular remodeling by inhibiting ventricular hypertrophy. Examples of ACE inhibitors are shown in Table 38.7. More information about ACE inhibitors can be found in Chapter 36 and Table 36.6.

DRUG ALERT

Captopril

- May cause severe hypotension and hyperkalemia.
- Monitor patients for first-dose hypotension (first-dose syncope).
- Skipping doses or stopping the drug can result in rebound HTN.
- Angioedema, a rare adverse effect, can be sudden and life-threatening.

Angiotensin II receptor blockers (ARBs). For patients who are unable to tolerate neprilysin inhibitors or ACE inhibitors, ARBs are recommended.[6] ARBs prevent the vasoconstrictor and aldosterone-secreting effects of angiotensin II by binding to the angiotensin II receptor sites. ARBs promote afterload reduction and vasodilation. Monitoring is similar to that for ACE inhibitors.

Ivabradine (Corlanor). Ivabradine selectively inhibits a particular sodium/potassium current in the SA node, decreasing HR. Patients with HFrEF who are in sinus rhythm with HR greater than 70 bpm and have symptoms despite optimal doses of other drugs may have fewer hospitalizations when taking ivabradine. Monitor patients for bradycardia and lightheadedness.[19]

Hydralazine/isosorbide dinitrate combination (BiDil). This drug is a combination of 2 vasodilators: hydralazine and isosorbide dinitrate. It can significantly reduce death and improve LVEF and exercise tolerance by reducing afterload through vasodilation. The drug is specifically effective in Black people with HFrEF already receiving optimal doses of other evidence-based medications.[2] Side effects include hypotension and headache. It should not be used with phosphodiesterase inhibitors, such as sildenafil.

Digitalis. Digitalis (digoxin), a weak positive inotrope, acts mainly as a neurohormonal modulator that reduces the effects of the SNS and suppresses renin secretion from the kidneys. Low-dose digitalis decreases HF hospitalizations and symptoms in patients who are still symptomatic despite standard HF therapies.[7] Better outcomes occur with digoxin levels under 0.9 ng/mL. Higher levels are associated with death and digoxin toxicity. Dose is based on body mass, renal function, and concurrent medications. The usual daily dose in HF is 0.125 mg. Monitor renal function and potassium levels.

Diuretics. Diuretics reduce symptoms of fluid overload in HFrEF and HFpEF. They reduce edema, pulmonary venous pressure, and preload by promoting renal excretion of sodium and water (see Table 36.7). In chronic HF, patients receive the lowest effective dose of diuretic. Diuretic resistance in patients with HF may require increasing doses and adding different types of diuretics.

Novel agents. In patients with progressive HFrEF despite guideline-directed therapy, novel drug agents are considered. The effects of oral soluble guanylyl cyclase stimulator (vericiguat) include vasodilation, improved endothelial function, and decreased fibrosis of the heart.[7] Studies of omega-3 polyunsaturated fatty acids (PUFAs) supplements provided impressive data on risk reduction in CV events when used with evidence-based therapies.[7]

Device Therapy

Patients with HFrEF may benefit from implantable cardiac devices after other therapies are used. In patients with an LVEF less than 35%, neurohormonal effects and cardiac remodeling can result in dyssynchronous contraction of the LV and RV, contributing to poor ventricular filling and reduced CO. CRT (biventricular pacing) is recommended for these patients.[6,7] With CRT, an extra pacing lead placed through the coronary sinus to a coronary vein of the LV coordinates right and left ventricular contractions (Fig. 38.6). Patients with low LVEF are at significant risk for SCD. An ICD is recommended for primary prevention of SCD.[6,7] Patients with symptomatic HFrEF often need both CRT and an ICD. Combination implantable devices are available. Pacemakers and defibrillators are discussed in Chapter 39. Mechanical assist devices available to sustain HF patients with deteriorating function and those awaiting heart transplant are discussed later in the chapter.

CHECK YOUR PRACTICE

Your patient is scheduled for a biventricular pacemaker for worsening HF. The patient has a demand pacemaker and asks you why they need a new one.

- How would you respond to the question?

Invasive Remote Patient Monitoring (RPM)

Implanted ICD and CRT devices can be used to remotely monitor patients. This information can predict HF decompensation and help with clinical decision making. RPM includes BP, weight, activity level, dysrhythmias, and HR. HR trends can evaluate therapy. An increasing HR can indicate worsening HF. A reduced HR variability is associated with higher risk for exacerbation and hospitalization. Intrathoracic impedance is an indicator of intrathoracic fluid level providing

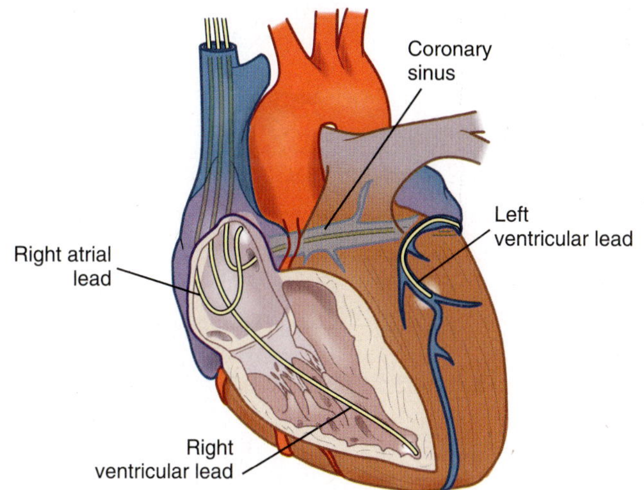

Fig. 38.6 Placement of pacing leads in cardiac resynchronization therapy.

early detection of impending ADHF.[20] Implantable remote hemodynamic monitoring is also possible. A PA sensor can be implanted during a right heart catheterization. It can provide information about HR, systolic, diastolic, and mean pulmonary artery pressure (PAP). Early detection of increases in intracardiac pressures, PAP, and fluid status allows for proactive management and fewer hospitalizations.[20]

Therapies for HFpEF

Comorbidities including HTN, diabetes, obesity, CAD, and CKD contribute significantly to HFpEF. Optimal management of these comorbidities is vital. Recommended management to reduce symptoms is similar to that with HFrEF including the use of diuretics to reduce congestion.[7] SGLT2i have shown significant benefit with decreased HF hospitalizations and death in symptomatic people with HFpEF.[21] ARNIs, MRAs, and ARBs are other options.

End-Stage Heart Failure Therapy

Therapeutic options for stage D HF patients include (1) inotropic therapy, (2) mechanical circulatory support (MCS) devices, (3) palliative care and hospice (with or without ICD deactivation), and (4) heart transplant. Patients who are not eligible for heart transplant may be candidates for lifelong MCS. These devices have significantly improved outcomes and QOL for patients with end-stage HF.

Nutrition Therapy

Excess sodium may worsen HF symptoms and lead to an exacerbation. The AHA recommends a sodium intake of <2300 mg/d for general CV health promotion. There is no evidence to support a more restrictive level in patients with HF. Excess sodium restriction can result in poor diet quality. The DASH diet is rich in antioxidants and potassium. It can achieve sodium restriction without compromising nutrition. It may reduce hospitalizations for HF (Fig. 38.7).[22]

Take a detailed diet history. Review what foods the patient eats, and when, where, and how often the patient dines out. Assess the cultural value of food. Use this information to help the patient and caregiver in making diet choices in an individualized and culturally sensitive diet plan. The AHA website has helpful diet guidelines for patients with HF.

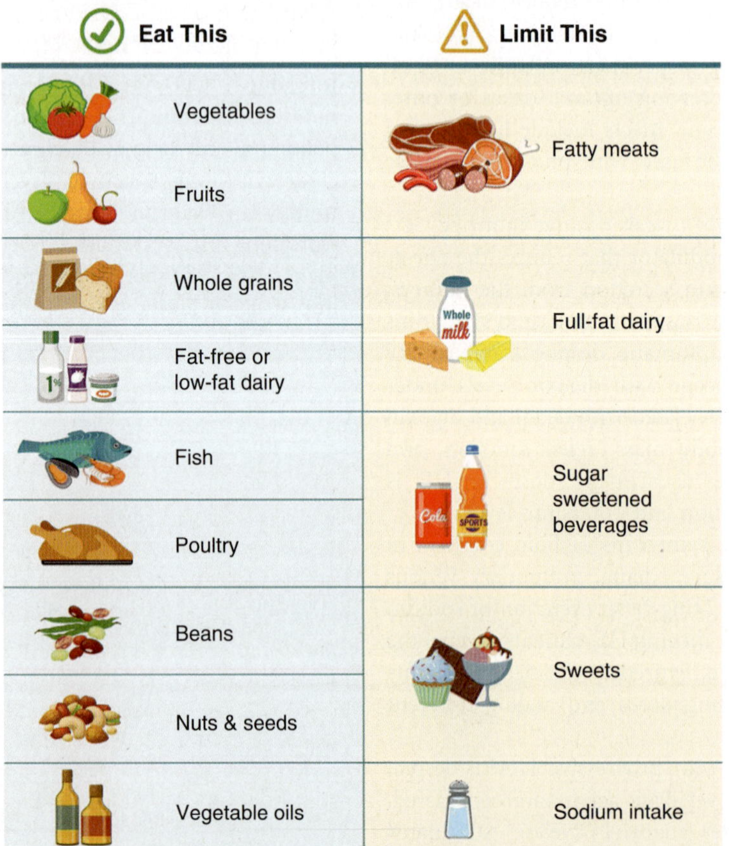

Fig. 38.7 DASH diet. (From National Heart, Lung, and Blood Institute; National Institutes of Health; U.S. Department of Health and Human Services.)

Review how to find sodium content per serving and the number of servings per package. Teach ways to enhance food flavors (e.g., lemon juice, spices) without the use of added salt. Discuss the high sodium content of most restaurant foods.

NURSING MANAGEMENT: HEART FAILURE

Assessment

Subjective and objective data that you should obtain from patients with HF are shown in Table 38.8. Obtain a complete medication list. Patients with chronic HF often take multiple drugs for coexisting conditions. OTC drugs that pose a risk to people with HF include nonsteroidal antiinflammatory drugs (NSAIDs), high-dose aspirin, ephedrine, pseudoephedrine, and diet pills. NSAIDs can increase sodium retention and worsen HF.

Explore chronic health problems as they may exacerbate HF, affecting the plan of care and the timing and choice of therapies. For example, a patient with sleep apnea might be able to minimize some HF symptoms by using a continuous positive airway pressure device at night.

Clinical Problems

Clinical problems for patients with HF include:

- Activity intolerance
- Fatigue
- Fluid imbalance
- Health maintenance alteration
- Impaired cardiac function
- Impaired respiratory function
- Inadequate tissue perfusion

More information on clinical problems and interventions for patients with HF is presented in eNursing Care Plan 38.1 on the website for this chapter.

Planning

Nursing care focuses on the priority problems of decreased CO, impaired oxygenation, fluid overload, activity intolerance, and managing a complex drug regimen. The overall goals of care include (1) decrease in symptoms (e.g., shortness of breath, fatigue), (2) decrease in peripheral edema, (3) increase in exercise tolerance, (4) adherence with the treatment plan, and (5) no complications related to HF.

Implementation

Health Promotion

Healthy lifestyle habits such as maintaining regular physical activity, normal weight, and optimal BP and glucose levels; healthy eating; and not smoking reduce the lifetime risk of developing HF.[23] Managing risk factors is vital for those with stage A HF to prevent progression to symptomatic HF. A treatment goal of <130/80 mm Hg is recommended for those with HTN.[7] Patients with diabetes who take an SGLT2i for glucose control gain cardiovascular benefits.

TABLE 38.8 NURSING ASSESSMENT

Heart Failure

Subjective Data

Important Health Information

Health history: CAD (including recent MI), HTN, cardiomyopathy, valve or congenital heart disease, diabetes, hyperlipidemia, renal disease, thyroid or lung disease, rapid or irregular heart rate

Medications: Use of and adherence with any heart drugs. Use of diuretics, estrogens, corticosteroids, NSAIDs, OTC drugs, herbal supplements

Functional Health Patterns

Health perception–health management: Fatigue, depression, anxiety

Nutritional-metabolic: Usual sodium intake. Nausea, vomiting, anorexia, stomach bloating. Weight gain, ankle swelling

Elimination: Nocturia, decreased daytime urine output, constipation

Activity-exercise: Dyspnea, orthopnea, cough. Palpitations, dizziness, fainting

Sleep-rest: Number of pillows used for sleeping. Paroxysmal nocturnal dyspnea, insomnia, sleep apnea

Cognitive-perceptual: Chest pain or heaviness. RUQ pain, abdominal discomfort. Behavior changes, visual changes

Objective Data

Cardiovascular

Tachycardia, S_3, S_4, murmurs. Pulsus alternans. PMI displaced inferiorly and posteriorly, lifts and heaves, jugular venous distention

Gastrointestinal

Abdominal distention, hepatomegaly, ascites

Neurologic

Restlessness, confusion, decreased attention or memory

Respiratory

Tachypnea, crackles, wheezes. Frothy, blood-tinged sputum

Skin

Cool, diaphoretic skin. Cyanosis or pallor. Peripheral edema (right-sided HF)

Possible Diagnostic Findings

Altered electrolytes (especially Na^+ and K^+), ↑ BUN, creatinine, or liver function tests. ↑ NT-proBNP or BNP. Chest x-ray shows cardiomegaly, pulmonary congestion, and interstitial pulmonary edema. Echocardiogram shows ↑ chamber size, decreased wall motion, decreased LVEF or normal LVEF with evidence of diastolic dysfunction (abnormal relaxation/filling). Atrial and ventricular enlargement on ECG. ↓ O_2 saturation

Acute Care

Nursing care for patients in ACDH is shown in Table 38.9. Patients with ADHF need ongoing assessment and evaluation of vital signs, O_2 saturation, mentation, ECGs, and indicators of volume overload and decreased perfusion. Signs of decreased perfusion include hypotension, decreased urine output, cool extremities, altered mentation, dysrhythmias, and worsening renal and liver function tests. Record intake, output, and daily weights to evaluate fluid status. Be alert for signs of fluid volume overload. These include edema, ascites, JVD, an S_3 heart sound, crackles, hypoxia, and worsening renal function.

TABLE 38.9 NURSING MANAGEMENT

Patients With ADHF

- Monitor vital signs, neurologic status, peripheral circulation, and laboratory results.
- Auscultate breath sounds, respiratory effort, and work of breathing.
- Use pulse oximetry to monitor oxygenation status.
- Monitor ECG and hemodynamic status, including MAP, PAP, PAWP, CO, and CI, if available.
- Evaluate fluid balance. Obtain daily weight.
- Give prescribed medications to reduce preload and evaluate effectiveness.
- Identify and mitigate factors precipitating ADHF.
- Provide ordered VTE prophylaxis.
- Position patient to ease dyspnea. Maintain Fowler's position.
- Provide small, frequent meals to decrease oxygen needed for digestion.
- Alternate any rest and activity periods. Maintain ordered activity and exercise restrictions and monitor response to activity.
- Provide emotional rest to decrease O_2 consumption.
- Teach patients and caregivers about therapy regimen and self-care (Table 38.10).

Collaborate With Respiratory Therapist

- Administer supplemental O_2 or other noninvasive ventilator support as needed.
- Assist with choosing optimal O_2 delivery device.
- Frequently assess need to adjust O_2 flow rate.

Collaborate With Dietitian

- Assess and monitor nutrition status.
- Recommend restricted diet and review diet plans.

Collaborate With Physical Therapist

- Perform ROM exercises.
- Assist with early and progressive ambulation.

Collaborate With Social Worker

- Work with the patient and caregiver to identify care needs.
- Help the patient with transitions through the health care system.

In addition to continual ECG and O_2 saturation monitoring, patients may have hemodynamic monitoring, including arterial BP. If a pulmonary artery (PA) catheter is placed, we monitor CO and pulmonary artery wedge pressure (PAWP). A normal PAWP, an indirect measure of LA filling pressure, is 6 to 15 mm Hg. Patients with ADHF may have a PAWP as high as 30 mm Hg. Drug therapies are adjusted to maximize CO and reduce PAWP. Hemodynamic monitoring is discussed in Chapter 35.

In a person with HF, the blood may not be adequately oxygenated. Supplemental O_2 helps increase the $Pa{O_2}$ and helps meet tissue O_2 needs. This helps to relieve patient dyspnea and fatigue. In severe pulmonary edema, patients may need noninvasive positive pressure ventilation (e.g., bilevel positive airway pressure [BiPAP]) or intubation and mechanical ventilation. BiPAP decreases preload. O_2 therapy and ventilatory support are discussed in Chapter 28.

Place the patient who has dyspnea in a high-Fowler's position with feet horizontal in the bed or dangling at the bedside with arms supported. The sitting position helps decrease venous return by pooling the blood in the extremities and increases the capacity for breathing.

Physical and emotional rest allow patients to conserve energy and decrease the need for more O_2. The degree of rest needed depends on the severity of HF. Patients with severe HF may be on bed rest. Patients with mild to moderate HF can be ambulatory with monitored activity.

Patients with mild to moderate HF usually do not need fluid restrictions. Fluid restrictions may be needed for stage D HF patients with persistent fluid retention despite moderate sodium intake.

Chronic Care

HF is a chronic and progressive condition that requires lifelong therapy. Transitional care programs and protocols help ensure coordination and continuity of health care as patients transfer between settings. HF management programs that include patient education on self-management and exercise and close home surveillance follow-up by nurses can reduce short-term readmission rates in high-risk patients (Box 38.1).[24]

Home health (HH) professionals can be a vital part of the chronic and transitional care HF team. HH nurses often use care protocols coordinated with the patient and HCP to identify worsening HF (e.g., weight gain, increased dyspnea). Many HH agencies offer special HF programs.

Telehealth and device RPM (e.g., electronic scale, BP cuff, pulse oximeter) can collect physiologic and symptom data (Fig. 38.8).[20] Results can be sent to the HCP via telephone or secure website. In response to collected data, therapeutic interventions, such as a temporary increase in diuretic therapy, can be implemented to improve function and prevent hospitalization.

HF care should include symptom management and monitoring responses to therapies. Include the patient and caregivers in the overall care plan. Help them develop a clear action plan for response to signs and symptoms of impending exacerbation. A patient and caregiver guide for patients with HF is shown in Table 38.10.

Teach patients the basic mechanism of action of medications and signs of toxicity. Effective self-care includes proper technique in taking a pulse (for a full minute) and use of RPM. Patients should understand when to hold heart rate–lowering drugs, such as β-blockers and digoxin. Teach patients taking diuretic and/or potassium supplements signs and symptoms of hypokalemia and hyperkalemia.

Exercise training can improve symptoms of chronic HF. Exercise is safe and improves overall sense of well-being. It is associated with reduced death.[25] Tailor exercise programs based on what the patient most enjoys doing. Teach them about the importance of rest periods, especially after exertion, and energy-conserving behaviors. Changes may be needed if the environment involves an increased cardiac workload (e.g., frequent climbing of stairs). Consult with a physical therapist or occupational therapist as needed.

Palliative and End-of-Life Care

Palliative care should be part of the care of all patients with HF.[6,7] Palliative care has a role across the stages of HF, starting early after diagnosis and intensifying in end-stage HF.[7]

BOX 38.1 EVIDENCE-BASED PRACTICE

Heart Failure and Quality of Life

You are part of the rehabilitation team working with HF patients. Many patients who had frequent hospital admissions over the past year admit "difficulty with" or "having little control" over their management of their HF. Patients share that they do feel they are "enjoying" their life as much as hoped due to their health. A variety of reasons were identified as to why these outcomes are occurring. You question whether more could be done to decrease the frequency of hospitalizations with these patients and improve their quality of life.

Making Clinical Decisions

Synthesis of Best Available Evidence

Patients experiencing HF often have negative perceptions of the overall effects of life quality. Poorer quality of life is associated with higher mortality rates, lower self-care adherence, and an increase in hospitalizations for symptom management. Patients who practice self-care regarding HF management and health promoting activities have decreased hospital readmissions and better health outcomes. HF management programs that include patient education on self-management (e.g., daily weights, diet, exercise) and close home surveillance by nurses can reduce readmission rates and improve health outcomes.

Clinician Expertise

Nursing staff started to provide follow-up phone calls for the first 6 months following discharge from rehabilitation to patients who were admitted to the hospital for HF 3 or more times in the past year. The calls reinforced routine self-care education for condition management and health promoting activities and provided support for the patient and family members.

Patient Preferences and Values

Patients shared in survey data that they appreciated the follow-up phone calls and support from nursing staff. They felt less overwhelmed with managing their HF and thought they were doing "better" with adherence. Some patients asked about including in-person visits or text messages as another means of support.

Implications for Nursing Practice

1. What are important topics related to HF management that should be discussed in the follow-up phone calls with the patient?
2. Other than a decreased number of hospital readmissions, what might indicate an improvement in the patient's quality of life?

Reference for Evidence

Seid S, Amendoeira J, Ferreira M: Self-care and quality of life among adult patients with heart failure: scoping review, *Sage Open Nurs*, 9, 2023.

The ACCF and AHA provide guidelines for patients with end-stage HF (stage D). End-of-life discussions include advance directives and information about advanced HF therapies (e.g., VADs, heart transplants), palliative care, and hospice. Repeated hospitalizations and ED visits for ADHF predict end-stage HF.[6,7]

Patients are eligible for hospice when (1) an HCP certifies that a life expectancy of 6 months or less is expected assuming the disease takes its normal course, (2) the patient has received optimal medical treatment and is not a candidate for further invasive procedures, and (3) the patient is assessed at NYHA Class IV.

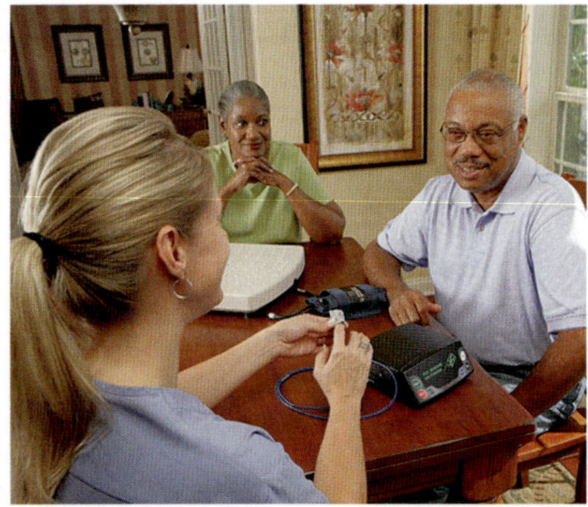

Fig. 38.8 Home-based telehealth monitoring unit. (Used with permission from Honeywell HomMed.)

End-of-life nursing care of patients with HF includes ongoing assessment and evaluation of interventions for effectiveness. Strategies include patient and caregiver support, drug therapies, and nondrug therapies. Palliative and end-of-life care are discussed in Chapter 10.

◆ Evaluation

The expected outcomes are that patients with HF will:

- Maintain adequate O_2/CO_2 exchange at the alveolar-capillary membrane to meet O_2 needs
- Maintain adequate blood pumped by the heart to meet metabolic demands
- Have a reduction or absence of edema and stable baseline weight
- Achieve a realistic program of activity that balances physical activity with energy-conserving activities

MECHANICAL CIRCULATORY SUPPORT

MCS is an option for patients with advanced HFrEF to prolong life and improve functional capacity.[7] Temporary MCS can be used to stabilize patients with decompensated HF in cardiogenic shock.[26] MCS devices decrease cardiac work and improve organ perfusion when conventional drug therapy is no longer adequate. The type of device used depends on the extent and nature of the problem. These devices are used in 3 situations: (1) supporting the left, right, or both ventricles while recovering from acute injury; (2) stabilizing the patient before heart surgery; and (3) awaiting a heart transplant.

Short-term MCS devices include the intraaortic balloon pump (IABP) and extracorporeal membrane oxygenation (ECMO), Impella, and TandemHeart. The limitations of bed rest and the risk for infection and vascular complications prevent their long-term use. Long-term MCS ventricular assist devices (VADs) include percutaneous devices (PVADs) and transplanted devices (LVADs, BiVADs). VADs provide highly

TABLE 38.10 PATIENT & CAREGIVER TEACHING

Heart Failure

Include the following instructions when teaching the patient and caregiver about managing heart failure:

Diet Therapy

- Consult the diet plan and list of permitted and restricted foods.
- Adhere to any sodium restriction guidelines outlined by your HCP.
- Read labels to assess sodium content. Check the labels of over-the-counter drugs, such as laxatives, cough medicines, and antacids for sodium content.
- Avoid using salt when preparing foods or adding salt to foods.
- Weigh yourself at the same time each day, preferably in the morning, using the same scale and wearing similar clothes.
- Eat small, frequent meals.

Exercise and Activity

- Plan your regular daily rest and activity program. After exertion, such as exercise and ADLs, plan a rest period.
- Increase walking and other activities gradually, provided they do not cause fatigue or dyspnea.
- Consider a cardiac rehabilitation program.
- Avoid extremes of heat and cold.
- Consider shorter working hours or schedule rest period during working hours.

Ongoing Monitoring

- Know the signs and symptoms of worsening HF. These include increasing dyspnea, cough, orthopnea, PND, weight gain, edema, fluid retention, fatigue, and tiredness with physical activity.
- Report at once any of the following to the HCP:
  - Weight gain of 3 lb (1.4 kg) in 2 days, or 3–5 lb (2.3 kg) in a week
  - Difficulty breathing, especially with activity or when lying flat
  - Waking up breathless at night
  - Frequent dry, hacking cough, especially when lying down
  - Fatigue, weakness
  - Swelling of ankles, feet, or abdomen. Swelling of face or difficulty breathing (if taking ACE inhibitors)
  - Nausea with abdominal swelling, pain, and tenderness
  - Dizziness or fainting
- Follow up with HCP on regular basis.
- Consider joining a local support group with your family members and/or caregiver(s).

Health Promotion

- Obtain annual influenza vaccination.
- Obtain pneumococcal and COVID-19 vaccines.
- Develop plan to reduce risk factors (e.g., BP control, tobacco cessation, blood glucose/HbA_{1c} control, weight reduction).
- Avoid emotional upsets. Share any concerns, fears, feelings of depression, with HCP.

Drug Therapy

- Take each drug as prescribed.
- Develop a system (e.g., daily chart, weekly pillbox) to ensure drugs are taken.
- Count pulse rate each day before taking drugs (if appropriate). Know the limits that your HCP wants for your pulse rate.
- Take BP at determined intervals (if appropriate). Know your target BP limits.
- Know signs and symptoms of orthostatic hypotension and how to prevent them.
- If taking anticoagulants, know signs and symptoms of bleeding (bleeding gums, increased bruises, blood in stool or urine) and what to do.
- Know your INR and target range if taking warfarin (Coumadin) and how often to have blood checked.

effective long-term support as standard care in many heart transplant centers.

Any form of MCS device will eventually be turned off. This may be at the time of transplant or recovery, or when a patient no longer wishes to continue support.

Intraaortic Balloon Pump

The **intraaortic balloon pump (IABP)** has been used for patients in cardiogenic shock since the 1970s, but its use is decreasing in favor of newer therapies. The IABP provides temporary circulatory assistance in hemodynamically unstable patients by decreasing PA pressures and systemic vascular resistance (SVR), leading to improved CO. The IABP can increase coronary blood flow to the heart muscle and decrease the heart's workload through counterpulsation.

The IABP consists of a sausage-shaped balloon, a pump that inflates and deflates the balloon, and a control panel for synchronizing the balloon inflation to the cardiac cycle. The balloon is inserted percutaneously or surgically into the femoral artery. It is placed in the descending thoracic aorta just below the left subclavian artery and above the renal arteries (Fig. 38.9). After placement, an x-ray confirms the position.

The pump fills the balloon with helium at the start of diastole (immediately after aortic valve closure) and deflates it just before the next systole. The ECG triggers deflation on the upstroke of the R wave (of the QRS) and inflation on the T wave. The dicrotic notch of the arterial pressure tracing is used to refine timing (Fig. 38.10).

Table 38.11 describes the hemodynamic effects of IABP therapy. We refer to IABP therapy as *counterpulsation* because the timing of balloon inflation is opposite the ventricular contraction. The IABP assist ratio is 1:1 in the acute phase of treatment. This means that 1 IABP cycle of inflation and deflation occurs for every heartbeat. In late diastole when the balloon is totally inflated, blood is forcibly displaced distal to the extremities and proximal to the coronary arteries and main branches of the aortic arch. Diastolic arterial pressure rises (diastolic augmentation). This increases coronary artery perfusion pressure and perfusion of vital organs. The rise in coronary artery perfusion pressure increases blood flow to the myocardium. The balloon is rapidly deflated just before systole. This creates a vacuum that causes aortic pressure to drop. When aortic resistance to left ventricular ejection is reduced (reduced afterload), the left ventricle empties more easily and completely. SV increases while myocardial O_2 consumption decreases.

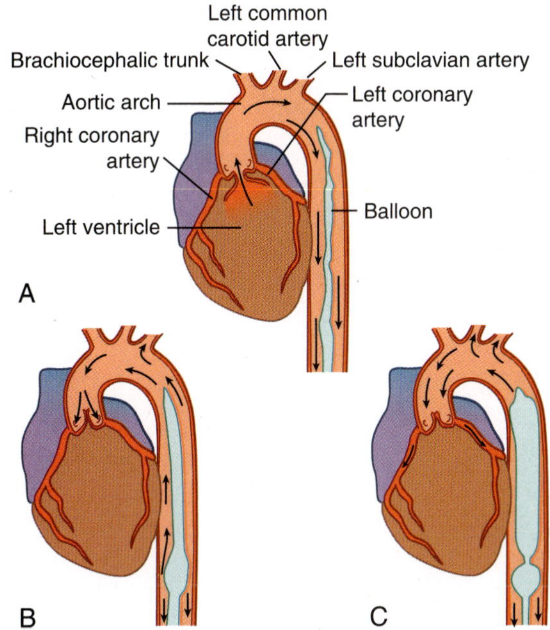

Fig. 38.9 IABP. (A) During systole the balloon is deflated, which helps with ejection of blood into the periphery. (B) In early diastole, the balloon begins to inflate. (C) In late diastole, the balloon is totally inflated, which augments aortic pressure and increases the coronary perfusion pressure. This increases coronary and cerebral blood flow.

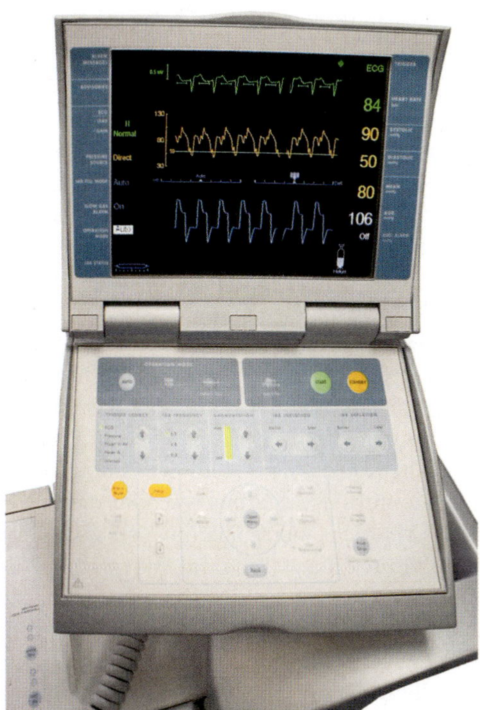

Fig. 38.10 Monitoring on an IABP machine. A photo of the IABP machine with a monitor. The monitor shows the ECG wave pattern in different colors and the numerical value with heart rate. (© beerkoff/iStock.com.)

TABLE 38.11 Hemodynamic Effects of Counterpulsation

Effects of Inflation During Diastole

- ↓ Angina
- ↑ Coronary artery perfusion pressure
- ↑ Diastolic pressure (may exceed systolic pressure)
- ↓ ECG evidence of ischemia
- ↑ O_2 delivery to the myocardium
- ↑ Pressure in the aortic root during diastole
- ↓ Ventricular ectopy

Effects of Deflation During Systole

- ↓ Afterload
- Improved mentation
- ↓ Peak systolic pressure
- ↓ Myocardial O_2 consumption
- ↑ Stroke volume, possibly associated with:
  - Warm skin
  - ↑ Urine output
  - ↓ HR
  - ↓ Pulmonary artery pressures
  - ↓ Crackles

As the patient improves, circulatory support provided by the IABP is gradually reduced. Weaning involves reducing the IABP assist ratio from 1:1 to 1:2 and assessing the response.

An iVAC uses the IABP counterpulsation console for driving. It unloads the left ventricle by aspirating blood from the left ventricle during systole and ejecting the same blood into the aorta during diastole.[27] The iVAC offers circulatory support of 2.5 to 3.0 L/min. This is more support than an IABP but less than a conventional VAD. Side effects include hemolysis and platelet consumption from shear and fragmentation.

Complications of IABP Therapy

Vascular injuries, such as aortic dissection and compromised distal circulation, can occur with IABP therapy. Thrombus and embolus formation add to the risk for circulatory compromise to the extremity. The action of the IABP can destroy platelets and cause thrombocytopenia. Balloon movement can block the left subclavian, renal, or mesenteric arteries. This can result in a weak or absent radial pulse, decreased urine output, and reduced or absent bowel sounds. To reduce complications, perform cardiovascular, neurovascular, and hemodynamic assessments every 15 to 60 minutes, depending on the patient's status (Table 38.12). Mechanical complications from IABP can occur. Improper timing of balloon inflation may cause increased afterload, decreased CO, myocardial ischemia, and increased myocardial O_2 demand.

Extracorporeal Membrane Oxygenation (ECMO)

ECMO has become the first-line therapy in cardiogenic shock unresponsive to standard therapy. It provides respiratory and

TABLE 38.12 NURSING MANAGEMENT

IABP Complications

Potential Complication	Nursing Interventions
Arterial trauma caused by insertion or balloon displacement	• Assess and mark peripheral pulses before inserting balloon to use as baseline for assessing pulses after insertion. • Assess perfusion to upper and lower extremities at least every hour. • Measure urine output at least every hour (occlusion of renal arteries causes severe ↓ in urine output). • Observe arterial waveforms for sudden changes. • Keep head of bed no higher than 45 degrees. • Do not flex cannulated leg at the hip. • Immobilize cannulated leg to prevent flexion using a draw sheet tucked under the mattress, soft ankle restraint, or knee immobilizer.
Balloon leak or rupture	• Prepare for emergent removal and possible reinsertion.
Hematologic problems due to platelet aggregation along the balloon (e.g., thrombocytopenia)	• Monitor coagulation profiles, hematocrit, and platelet count.
Hemorrhage from insertion site	• Check site for bleeding at least every hour. • Monitor vital signs and assess for hypovolemia.
Infection at site	• Use strict aseptic technique for insertion and dressing changes for all lines. • Cover all insertion sites with occlusive dressings. • Give prescribed prophylactic antibiotic for entire course of therapy.
Issues related to immobilization (e.g., pressure injuries)	• Reposition patient at least q2h, being careful to maintain proper positioning. • Use appropriate pressure-relieving devices.
VTE caused by trauma, balloon obstruction of blood flow distal to catheter	• Give prophylactic heparin therapy (if ordered). • Assess pulses, urine output, and level of consciousness at least every hour. • Check circulation, sensation, and movement in both legs at least every hour.

cardiac support. ECMO does not "treat" HF. It is a temporary form of life support that can stay in place for several days as a bridge. ECMO involves removing blood from a patient through a large-bore vascular access catheter. When the blood goes through the ECMO unit, it is infused with O_2. CO_2 is removed at the same time. The newly oxygenated blood is then returned to the patient.

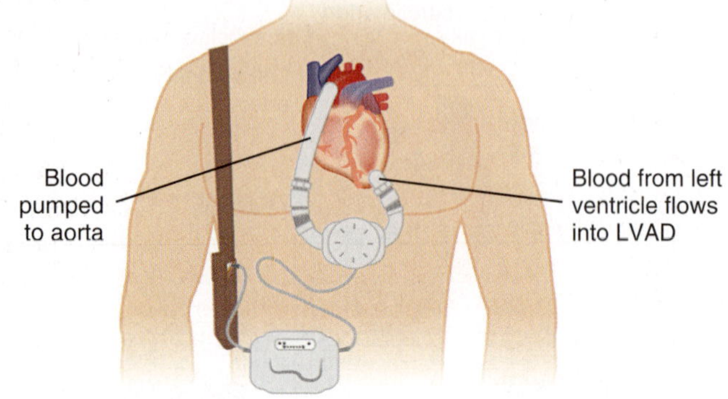

Fig. 38.11 Schematic diagram of a biventricular assist device (BVAD). (From Urden LD, Stacy KM, Lough ME: *Critical care nursing: diagnosis and management,* ed 8, St Louis, 2018, Mosby.)

Ventricular Assist Devices

A **ventricular assist device (VAD)** provides short- and long-term support for the failing heart. VADs are inserted into the path of flowing blood to augment or replace the action of the ventricle. Some VADs are implanted internally (e.g., peritoneum). Others are placed externally. A typical VAD shunts blood from the left atrium or ventricle to the device and then to the aorta. Some VADs provide right or biventricular support (Fig. 38.11). VADs operate on AC current or batteries.

Failure to wean from cardiopulmonary bypass (CPB) after surgery is a key indicator for VAD support. Other indications include (1) postcardiotomy cardiogenic shock, (2) a bridge to recovery or a heart transplant, and (3) patients with NYHA Class IV heart disease who do not respond to medical therapy. Relative contraindications for VAD therapy include (1) body surface area (BSA) less than manufacturer's limit (e.g., 1.2 m^2), (2) irreversible end-stage organ damage, and (3) comorbidities limiting life expectancy to under 3 years.

Impella systems are a commonly used percutaneous VAD (pVAD). They offer various levels of support depending on the model used. The Impella LV system draws blood from the left ventricle and pumps it into the ascending aorta, effectively unloading the ventricle and maintaining systemic perfusion. It can pump between 2.5 and 5 L/min. Patients can receive support for up to 14 days.[28]

The TandemHeart and ProtekDuo are pVADs that, in some configurations, support ECMO. The TandemHeart withdraws oxygenated blood from the left atrium and returns it to the systemic circulation through a cannula in the femoral artery, thereby bypassing the left ventricle. The ProtekDuo provides right ventricular support. It is inserted via the internal jugular vein and uses a dual-lumen cannula to draw blood from the right atrium and return it to the pulmonary artery, thereby bypassing the right ventricle.

Implantable Artificial Heart

A fully implantable artificial heart can provide a bridge to a transplant or replace the hearts of patients who are not eligible for a transplant and have no other treatment options. A major advantage of the artificial heart is that patients do not need immunosuppression therapy. Risks include infection, thrombus, and stroke. Patients need lifelong anticoagulation and ongoing care.

Interprofessional and Nursing Management

Patients with an MCS device need highly skilled care. Perform frequent and thorough cardiovascular assessments. These include measuring hemodynamic parameters (e.g., arterial BP, CO, SVR), auscultating the heart and lungs, and evaluating the ECG (e.g., rate, rhythm). Assess for adequate tissue perfusion (e.g., skin color and temperature, mental status, capillary refill, peripheral pulses, urine output, bowel sounds) at regular intervals. MCS should improve these findings.

Observe for signs of bleeding, cardiac tamponade, ventricular failure, infection, dysrhythmias, renal failure, hemolysis, and VTE. Patients with VAD may be mobile and need an activity plan. In some cases, patients with VADs may go home. Preparation for discharge is complex with in-depth teaching about the device and support equipment (e.g., battery chargers). A competent caregiver must always be present.

Patients with an IABP are relatively immobile. They are limited to side-lying or supine positions with the head of bed elevated less than 45 degrees. They may be receiving mechanical ventilation and often have multiple invasive lines. All of this increases the risk for pressure injury and makes it hard to find a comfortable position. Patients may have sleep problems and anxiety. Adequate sedation, pain relief, skin care, and comfort measures are essential.

HEART TRANSPLANTS

A **heart transplant** is the transfer of a healthy donor heart to a patient with a diseased heart. In the United States, more than 3500 patients are awaiting heart transplants. Although the number of patients in need of a transplant has increased, the number of donors has remained about the same. The 1-year heart transplant survival rate is close to 90%.

Criteria for Selection

A careful selection process ensures that hearts are distributed fairly and to those who will benefit most. Donor and recipient matching is based on body and heart size and immunologic assessment. That assessment includes ABO blood type, antibody screen, panel of reactive antibody (PRA) level, and human leukocyte antigen typing. The United Network for Organ Sharing (UNOS) manages a system to assign donor organs. This process is discussed in Chapter 14.

Indications and contraindications for a heart transplant are outlined in Table 38.13. Once a person meets the criteria for a transplant, a thorough physical examination and diagnostic workup are done. We assess heart function and vascular and immune systems. The patient and caregiver undergo a psychologic evaluation of coping skills, support systems, and commitment to follow a rigorous lifelong regimen. The complexity of the transplant process may be overwhelming to a patient without an adequate support system and understanding of the needed lifestyle changes.

A person accepted as a transplant candidate is placed on a transplant list. This may happen quickly during an acute illness or after a longer period. Stable patients may wait at home and receive ongoing medical care. If unstable, a patient may be hospitalized for more intensive therapy. Unfortunately, the overall waiting period for a new heart is long. Many patients die while waiting for a transplant.

TABLE 38.13 Common Indications and Contraindications for a Heart Transplant

Indications
- End-stage HF refractory to medical care
- Severe, decompensated, inoperable, heart valve disease
- Recurrent life-threatening dysrhythmias not responsive to maximal interventions, including defibrillators
- Any other heart problems that severely limit normal function and/or have a mortality risk of more than 50% within 2 years

Contraindications

Absolute
- Active infection, including HIV infection
- Age over 70 years
- Advanced cerebral or peripheral vascular disease not amenable to correction
- Life-threatening illness (e.g., cancer) that will limit survival to <5 years despite therapy
- Severe lung disease that will likely result in the patient being ventilator-dependent after transplant

Relative
- Severe obesity
- Psychologic impairment
- Evidence of noncompliance with therapy
- Active substance use (e.g., alcohol, drugs, tobacco)
- Liver or kidney failure not explained by HF
- Diabetes with vascular and neurologic complications
- Unrealistic expectations about transplant, its risks, and its benefits
- Lack of social support network that can make long-term commitment for patient's welfare

Surgical Procedure

A retrieved heart is placed on ice until it can be implanted. For the heart, this is optimally less than 4 hours. Donor hearts are implanted using 1 of 2 approaches. In the biatrial approach, the recipient's damaged heart is removed at the midatrial level. The donor heart is connected at the LA, PA, aorta, and RA. In the bicaval approach, the RA of the recipient's heart (with the SA node and atrial conduction intact) is preserved and then the donor heart is connected. CPB during surgery maintains oxygenation and perfusion to vital organs.

Posttransplant Care

A number of complications can occur after a transplant. In the first year after a transplant, the major causes of death are infection and acute rejection. There is a risk for SCD.

Immunosuppressive therapy is the key in posttransplant care. Most immunosuppressive regimens include corticosteroids, calcineurin inhibitors (tacrolimus), and antiproliferative drugs (mycophenolate mofetil). The mechanisms of action and side effects of these and other immunosuppressants are discussed in Chapter 14. Infection is a concern with immunosuppressive therapy. Long-term immunosuppressive therapy increases the risk for cancers, especially lymphomas, and cardiac vasculopathy (accelerated CAD).

To detect rejection, an endomyocardial biopsy is done weekly for the first month, monthly for the next 6 months, and yearly thereafter. In this procedure, the HCP inserts a catheter into the jugular vein and moves it into the RV. The catheter uses a bioptome, a device with 2 small cups that can be closed, to remove small samples of heart muscle for analysis.

Nursing care focuses on promoting patient adaptation to the transplant process, monitoring heart function, managing lifestyle changes, and ongoing teaching and support of the patient and caregiver.

CASE STUDY

Heart Failure

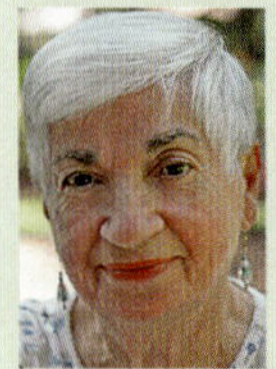
(© iStockphoto/ Thinkstock.)

Patient Profile

J.E. is a 70-year-old female who was admitted to the HF care unit with increasing shortness of breath, fatigue, and weight gain.

Subjective Data

- HTN for 20 years
- MI at 58 years of age
- Has increasing shortness of breath, fatigue, and an unexplained 11-lb weight gain during the past 2 weeks
- Had a respiratory tract infection 2 weeks ago; has persistent cough and edema in legs
- Cannot climb a flight of stairs without getting short of breath
- Sleeps with head elevated on 3 pillows
- Lives alone, does not always remember to take medication

Objective Data

Physical Assessment

- Moderate respiratory distress, use of accessory muscles, respiratory rate 36 breaths/min
- Systolic heart murmur
- Heart rate 110/min
- Bilateral crackles in all lung fields
- Cyanotic lips and extremities
- Skin cool and diaphoretic

Diagnostic Studies

- Chest x-ray results: cardiomegaly with right and left ventricular hypertrophy; fluid in lower lung fields
- Echocardiogram results: ejection fraction 20%
- ECG: Sinus tachycardia

Interprofessional Care

- Furosemide 40 mg IV twice daily
- Potassium 40 mEq orally twice daily
- Sacubitril/valsartan (Entresto) 97 mg/103 mg orally twice daily
- Nitroglycerin IV drip starting at 5 mcg/min
- Continuous ECG monitoring
- Nutrition: DASH diet
- Titrate O_2 to keep O_2 saturation >93%
- Monitor intake and output, and daily weights
- Electrolytes; NT-proBNP level; cardiac biomarkers q8h × 3

Discussion Questions

1. ***Recognize:*** What clinical manifestations of ADHF did J.E. exhibit?
2. ***Analyze:*** How would an NT-proBNP level be beneficial in the diagnosis of ADHF?
3. ***Plan:*** Give the rationale for each of the HCP's orders prescribed for J.E.
4. ***Prioritize:*** What are your priority nursing interventions for J.E.?
5. ***Act:*** Which interventions can you delegate to AP or other members of the interprofessional team?
6. ***Evaluate:*** What outcomes would indicate that goals were not met?
7. Develop a conceptual care map for J.E.

Answers and a corresponding concept map available at http://evolve.elsevier.com/Lewis/medsurg.

BRIDGE TO NCLEX EXAMINATION

The number of the question corresponds to the same-numbered outcome at the beginning of the chapter.

1. Which statements accurately describe heart failure with preserved ejection fraction (HFpEF)? **(Select all that apply.)**
   - a. Uncontrolled hypertension is a primary cause.
   - b. Left ventricular ejection fraction may be within normal limits.
   - c. The pathophysiology involves ventricular relaxation and filling.
   - d. Multiple evidence-based therapies have been shown to decrease mortality.
   - e. Therapies focus on symptom control and treatment of underlying conditions.
2. Which compensatory mechanism involved in both chronic heart failure and acute decompensated heart failure leads to fluid retention and edema?
   - a. Ventricular dilation
   - b. Ventricular hypertrophy
   - c. Increased systemic blood pressure
   - d. Renin-angiotensin-aldosterone activation
3. What are the expected actions of IV dobutamine in a patient with acute decompensated heart failure? **(Select all that apply.)**
   - a. Raises the heart rate
   - b. Dilates renal blood vessels
   - c. Increases heart contractility
   - d. Acts as a selective β-agonist
   - e. Increases systemic vascular resistance
4. Which actions would the nurse take to prevent complications in a patient with chronic heart failure and atrial fibrillation receiving low-dose digitalis and a loop diuretic? **(Select all that apply.)**
   - a. Monitor potassium levels.
   - b. Teach the patient how to take a pulse rate.
   - c. Keep an accurate measure of intake and output.
   - d. Withhold digitalis if the pulse rhythm is irregular.
   - e. Teach the patient about diet potassium restrictions.
5. Which hemodynamic changes would the nurse expect after successful initiation of intraaortic balloon pump therapy? **(Select all that apply.)**
   - a. Decreased SV
   - b. Decreased SVR
   - c. Decreased PAWP
   - d. Increased diastolic BP
   - e. Decreased myocardial O_2 consumption
6. Which are the greatest risks for patients in the first year after a heart transplant? **(Select all that apply.)**
   - a. Cancer
   - b. Infection
   - c. Rejection
   - d. Vasculopathy
   - e. Sudden cardiac death

1. a, b, c, e; 2. d; 3. c, d; 4. a, b; 5. b, c, d, e; 6. b, c, e.

For rationales to these answers and even more NCLEX review questions, visit http://evolve.elsevier.com/Lewis/medsurg.

REFERENCES

To access the References for this chapter, please scan the QR code with a mobile device.

39

Dysrhythmias

Kimberly Day

http://evolve.elsevier.com/Lewis/medsurg/

CONCEPTUAL FOCUS

Fluids and Electrolytes

Perfusion

LEARNING OUTCOMES

1. Examine the nursing care of patients needing continuous electrocardiographic monitoring.
2. Distinguish the clinical characteristics and ECG patterns of normal sinus rhythm, common dysrhythmias, and pacemaker rhythms.
3. Describe the nursing and interprofessional management of patients with common dysrhythmias.
4. Compare and contrast defibrillation and cardioversion.
5. Describe the nursing and interprofessional management of patients with pacemakers and implantable cardioverter-defibrillators.
6. Select interventions for patients undergoing electrophysiologic testing and radiofrequency catheter ablation therapy.

KEY TERMS

asystole
atrial fibrillation
atrial flutter
automatic external defibrillator (AED)
cardiac pacemaker
complete heart block
dysrhythmias
premature atrial contraction (PAC)
premature ventricular contraction (PVC)
telemetry monitoring
ventricular fibrillation (VF)
ventricular tachycardia (VT)

This chapter describes basic principles of electrocardiographic monitoring and the recognition and treatment of common dysrhythmias. Adequate perfusion to the body tissues requires the heart to generate sufficient cardiac output (CO). Abnormal heart rhythms, called **dysrhythmias**, can directly decrease CO by changing stroke volume and heart rate (HR). For example, tachycardia from a fever may decrease CO and cause hypotension. Your ability to recognize normal heart rhythms and dysrhythmias is an essential nursing skill.[1] Prompt recognition of a dysrhythmia and assessment of a patient's response to the rhythm is critical to maintaining adequate perfusion.

ELECTROPHYSIOLOGY

Conduction System

Four properties of heart cells allow the conduction system to start an electrical impulse, send it through the heart tissue, and stimulate muscle contraction (Table 39.1). The heart's conduction system consists of specialized neuromuscular tissue found throughout the heart (see Fig. 35.4A). A normal impulse starts in the sinoatrial (SA) node in the upper right atrium near the entrance of the vena cava. It spreads over the atrial myocardium via interatrial and internodal pathways, causing atrial contraction. The impulse then travels to the atrioventricular (AV) node, through the bundle of His, and down the left and right bundle branches to the Purkinje fibers in the ventricles, causing ventricular contraction.[2]

Nervous Control of the Heart

The autonomic nervous system plays a vital role in the rate of impulse formation, speed of conduction, and strength of cardiac contraction. The parts of the autonomic nervous system that affect the heart are the vagus nerve fibers of the parasympathetic nervous system and the nerve fibers of the sympathetic nervous system.

Stimulation of the vagus nerve slows firing of the SA node and slows impulse conduction through the AV node. This decreases HR. Stimulation of the sympathetic nerves increases SA node firing, AV node impulse conduction, and cardiac contractility. This increases HR.[3]

Electrocardiographic Monitoring

The ECG is a graphic tracing of the electrical impulses in the heart. The waveforms on the ECG represent the electrical activity of depolarization and repolarization produced by the movement of ions across the membranes of heart cells (see Fig. 35.4B).

The membrane of a heart cell is semipermeable. This allows it to maintain a high concentration of potassium and a low concentration of sodium inside the cell. Outside the cell, a high concentration of sodium and a low concentration of potassium exist. The inside of the cell, when at rest or in the polarized state, is negatively charged compared with the outside. When a cell or groups of cells are stimulated, the cell membrane changes its permeability. This change allows sodium to move rapidly into the cell. The inside of the cell is then positively charged compared with the outside *(depolarization)*. A slower movement of ions across the membrane restores the cell to the polarized state, called *repolarization*. Fig. 39.1 describes the phases of the cardiac action potential.

A 12-lead ECG view of the heart is helpful in assessing dysrhythmias. Six of the leads measure electrical forces in the frontal plane. These are bipolar (positive and negative) leads I, II, and III and unipolar (positive) leads aVR, aVL, and aVF (Fig. 39.2A and B). The 6 unipolar leads (V_1 through V_6) measure the electrical forces in the horizontal plane (precordial leads) (Fig. 39.2C). The 12-lead ECG may show signs of structural changes, conduction changes, damage (e.g., ischemia, infarction), electrolyte imbalance, or drug toxicity. Fig. 39.3 is an example of a normal 12-lead ECG.

We can use 1 or more ECG leads to continuously monitor a patient. The most common leads used are leads II and V_1 (Fig. 39.4). We use a modified chest lead (MCL_1) when only 3

TABLE 39.1 Properties of Heart Cells

Property	Definition
Automaticity	Ability to initiate an impulse spontaneously and continuously
Excitability	Ability to be electrically stimulated
Conductivity	Ability to transmit an impulse along a membrane in an orderly manner
Contractility	Ability to respond mechanically to an impulse

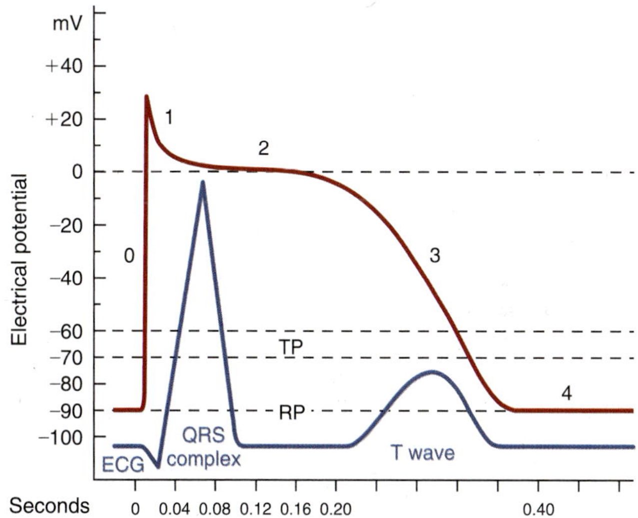

Fig. 39.1 Phases of the cardiac action potential. The electrical potential, measured in millivolts *(mV)*, is indicated along the vertical axis of the graph. Time, measured in seconds (sec), is indicated along the horizontal axis. The action potential has 5 phases, labeled *0* through *4*. Each phase represents a specific electrical event or combination of electrical events. Phase 0 is the upstroke of rapid depolarization and corresponds with ventricular contraction. Phases 1, 2, and 3 represent repolarization. Phase 4 is known as complete repolarization (or the polarized state) and corresponds to diastole. *RP*, Resting membrane potential; *TP*, threshold membrane potential.

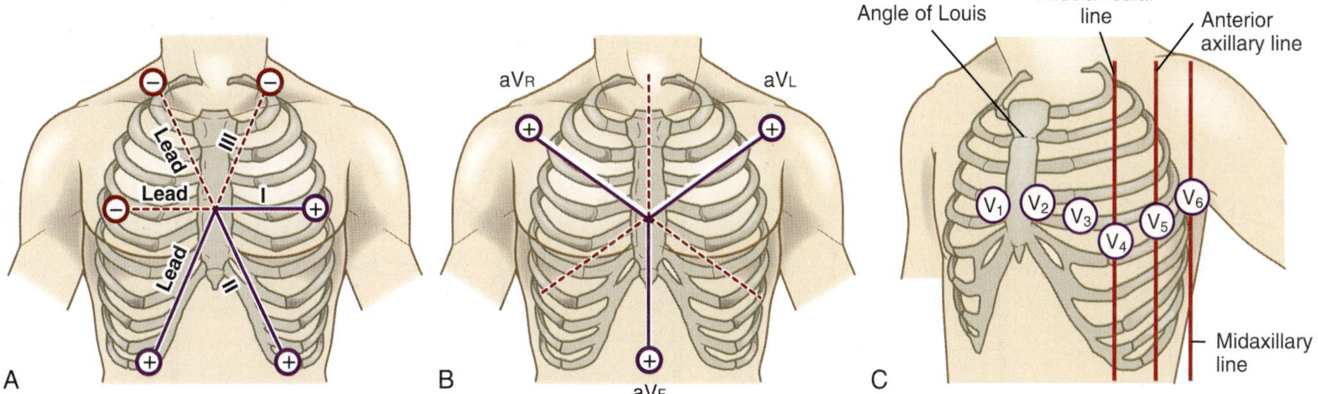

Fig. 39.2 (A) Limb leads I, II, and III. These bipolar leads are placed on the extremities. Shown are the angles from which these leads view the heart. (B) Limb leads aVR, aVL, and aVF. These unipolar leads use the center of the heart as their negative electrode. (C) Placement for the unipolar chest leads: V_1, 4th intercostal space at the right sternal border; V_2, 4th intercostal space at the left sternal border; V_3, halfway between V_2 and V_4; V_4, 5th intercostal space at the left midclavicular line; V_5, 5th intercostal space at the left anterior axillary line; V_6, 5th intercostal space at the left midaxillary line.

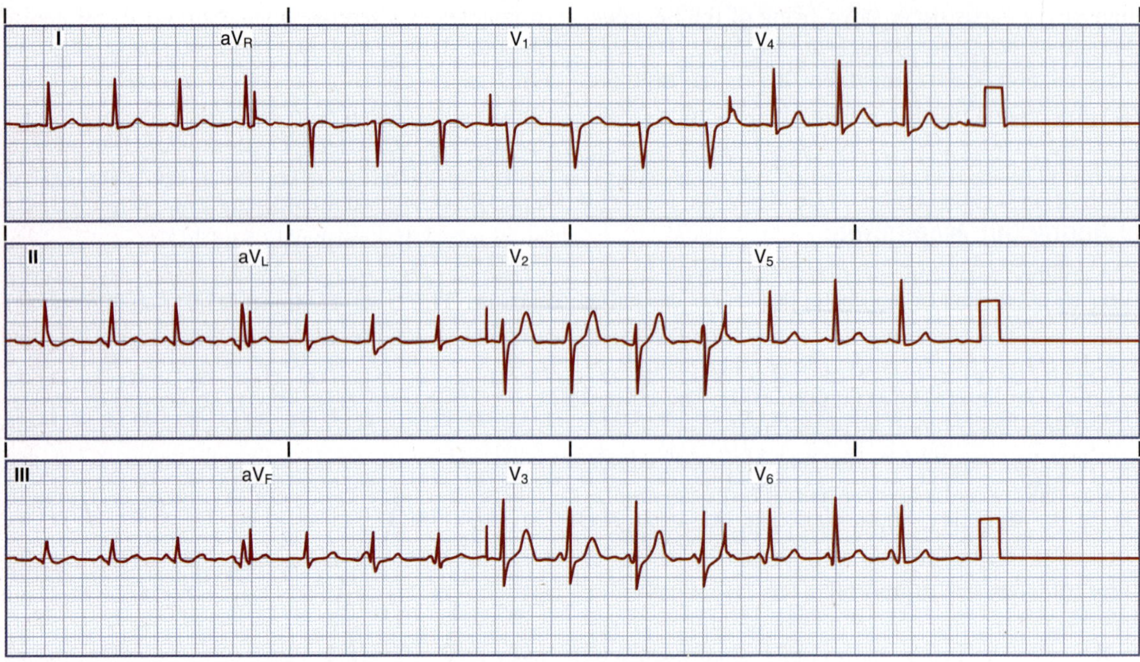

Fig. 39.3 12-lead ECG showing a normal sinus rhythm.

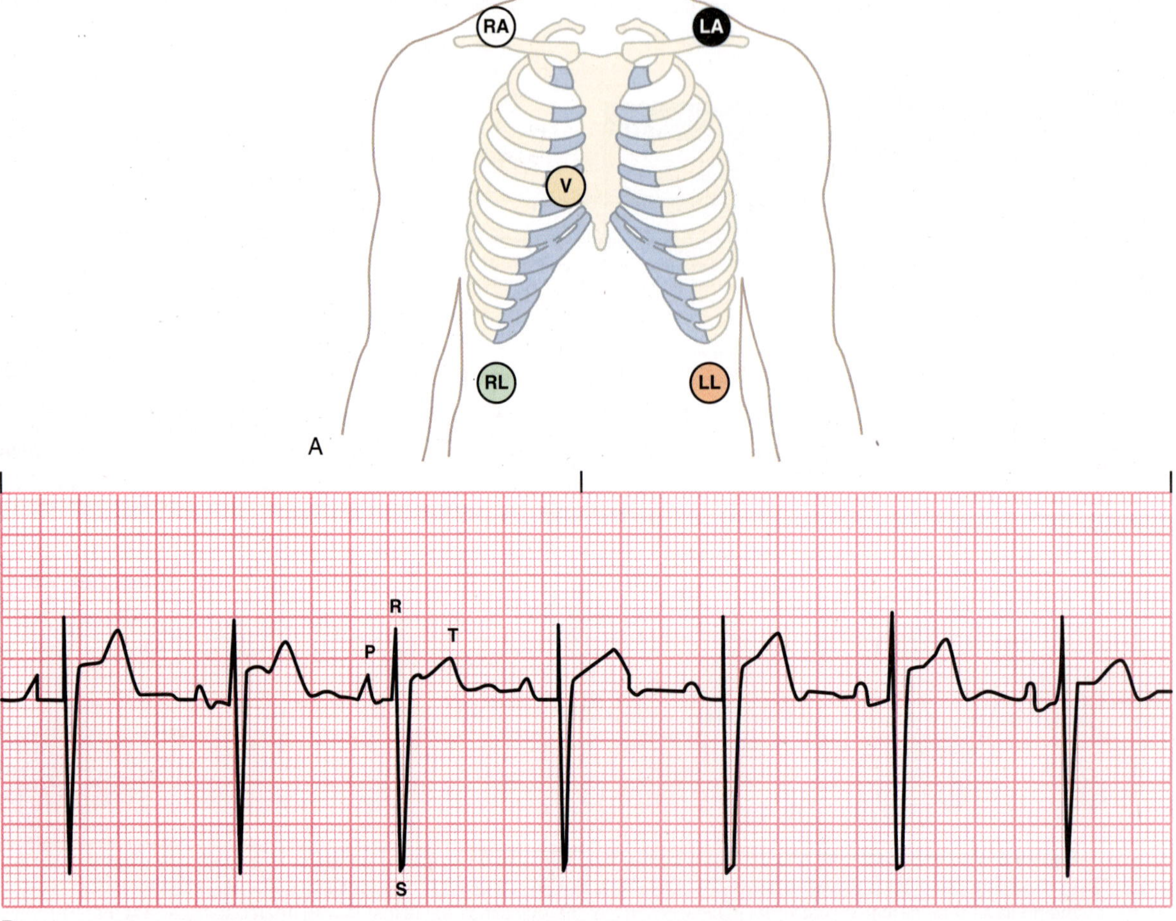

Fig. 39.4 (A) Lead placement for V_1 using a 5-lead system. (B) Typical ECG tracing in lead V_1. *LA,* Left arm; *LL,* left leg; *RA,* right arm; *RL,* right leg; *V,* chest lead.

leads are available for monitoring. MCL_1 is similar to V_1. Accurate ECG interpretation depends on the correct placement of the leads on the patient. The patient's clinical status determines which monitoring leads we use.[4]

The ECG monitor continuously displays the heart rhythm. Paper attached to the monitor records the ECG (rhythm strip) to provide a record of the patient's rhythm. It allows us to measure complexes and intervals and assess dysrhythmias.

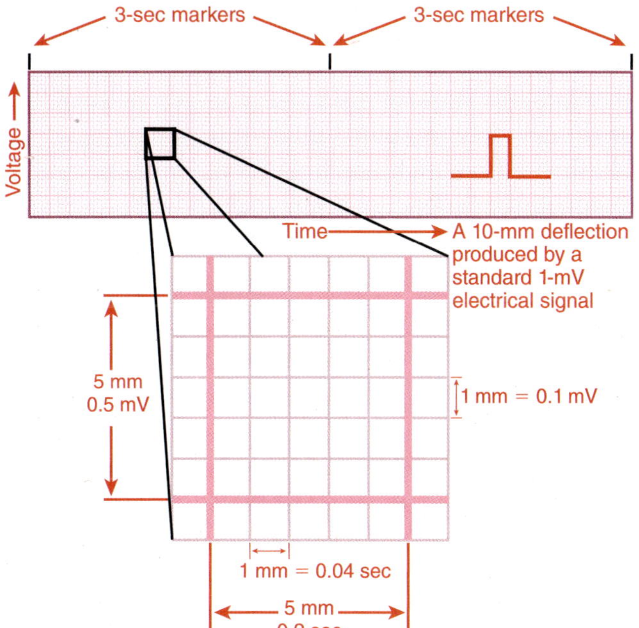

Fig. 39.5 Time and voltage on the ECG; 6-sec strip.

To correctly interpret an ECG, measure time and voltage on the ECG paper. ECG paper consists of large (heavy lines) and small (light lines) squares (Fig. 39.5). Each large square consists of 25 smaller squares (5 horizontal and 5 vertical). Horizontally, each small square (1 mm) represents 0.04 second. This means that 1 large square equals 0.20 second and that 300 large squares equal 1 minute. Vertically, each small square (1 mm) represents 0.1 millivolt (mV). This means that 1 large square equals 0.5 mV. Use these squares to calculate the HR and measure time intervals for the different ECG complexes.

You can use a variety of methods to calculate the HR from an ECG. The most accurate way is to count the number of QRS complexes in 1 minute. A simpler way is to note that every 3 seconds, a marker appears on the ECG paper (Fig. 39.5). Count the number of QRS complexes in 6 seconds and multiply that number by 10. This is the estimated number of beats per minute (Fig. 39.6).

Another method to calculate the HR is to count the number of small squares between 1 R-R interval. Divide this number into 1500 to get the HR. Last, you can count the number of large squares between 1 R-R interval and divide this number into 300 to get the HR (Fig. 39.6). All these methods are more accurate when the rhythm is regular.

Another way to measure distances on the ECG strip is to use calipers. Often a P or R wave will not fall directly on a light or heavy line. Place the fine points of the calipers exactly on the parts you need to measure and then move to another part of the strip for a more precise time measurement.

Fig. 39.7 shows the components of a normal ECG tracing. Table 39.2 describes ECG waveforms and intervals, normal

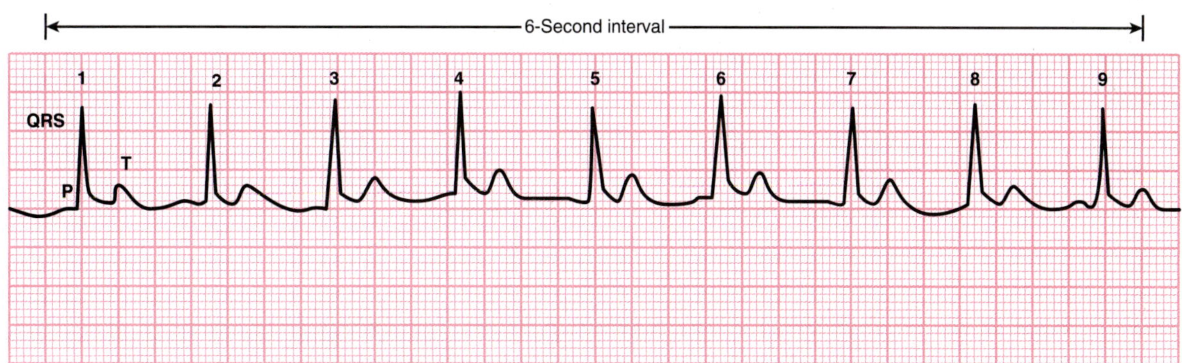

Fig. 39.6 When the rhythm is regular, heart rate can be determined by counting the number of "R" waves. The estimated heart rate is 90 beats/min. Note: Recorded from lead II.

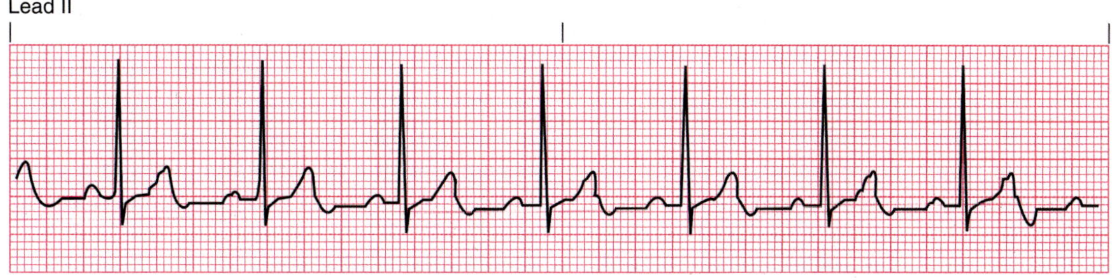

Fig. 39.7 Normal sinus rhythm. Note: Recorded from lead II.

TABLE 39.2 **ECG Waveforms and Intervals**[a]

Description	Normal Duration (sec)	Source of Possible Variation
P Wave		
Represents time for the passage of the electrical impulse through the atrium causing atrial depolarization (contraction). Should be upright	0.06–0.12	Problem in conduction within atria
PR Interval		
Measured from beginning of P wave to beginning of QRS complex. Represents time taken for impulse to spread through the atria, AV node and bundle of His, bundle branches, and Purkinje fibers to a point immediately before ventricular contraction	0.12–0.20	Problem in conduction usually in AV node, bundle of His, or bundle branches but can be in atria as well
QRS Complex		
Q wave: First negative (downward) deflection after the P wave, short and narrow, not present in several leads	<0.03	MI may result in development of a pathologic Q wave that is wide (≥0.03 sec) and deep (≥25% of the height of the R wave)
R wave: First positive (upward) deflection in the QRS complex	Not usually measured	
S wave: First negative (downward) deflection after the R wave	Not usually measured	
QRS Interval		
Measured from beginning to end of QRS complex. Represents time taken for depolarization (contraction) of both ventricles (systole)	<0.12	Problem in conduction in bundle branches or in ventricles
ST Segment		
Measured from the S wave of the QRS complex to the beginning of the T wave. Represents the time between ventricular depolarization and repolarization (diastole). Should be isoelectric (flat)	0.12	Changes (e.g., elevation, depression) usually caused by ischemia, injury, MI
T Wave		
Represents time for ventricular repolarization. Should be upright	0.16	Changes (e.g., tall, peaked; inverted) usually caused by electrolyte imbalances, ischemia, MI
QT Interval[b]		
Measured from beginning of QRS complex to end of T wave. Represents time taken for entire electrical depolarization and repolarization of the ventricles. Normal adult females have slightly longer QT intervals	0.34–0.43	Problems usually affecting repolarization more than depolarization and caused by drugs, electrolyte imbalances, and changes in heart rate

[a]HR influences the duration of these intervals, especially the PR and QT intervals (e.g., QT interval shortens in duration as heart rate increases).
[b]A corrected QT interval (QTc) is calculated to account for the influence of heart rate.

durations, and possible sources of changes. Table 39.3 presents a systematic approach to assessing a heart rhythm.

ECG leads consist of an electrode pad fixed with conductive gel. Before placing these on the patient, properly prepare the skin. Clip excess hair on the chest wall with scissors. Gently rub the skin with dry gauze until slightly pink. If the skin is oily, wipe with alcohol first. If the patient is diaphoretic, apply a skin protectant before placing the electrode.

Artifact is a distortion of the baseline and waveforms seen on the ECG (Fig. 39.8). It is hard to accurately interpret an ECG when artifact is present. You may see artifact on the monitor when leads and electrodes are not secure, the conductive gel is becoming dry, there is muscle activity (e.g., shivering, ambulating), or electrical interference. If artifact occurs, check the connections in the equipment. Replace the electrodes if the conductive gel has dried out.

Telemetry Monitoring

Telemetry monitoring is the observation of a patient's HR and rhythm at a site distant from the patient. This technology can help rapidly identify dysrhythmias, ischemia, or myocardial infarction (MI). There are 2 types of systems for telemetry monitoring. The first type is a centralized monitoring system. It requires you or a telemetry technician to continuously observe a group of patients' ECGs at a central location. The second system of telemetry monitoring does not require constant surveillance. These systems have the capability of detecting and storing data. Advanced alarm systems provide different levels of detection of dysrhythmias, ischemia, or MI.

Electrophysiology of Dysrhythmias

Dysrhythmias result from disorders of impulse formation, impulse conduction, or both. The heart has specialized cells in the SA node, atria, AV node, bundle of His, and Purkinje fibers (His-Purkinje system), which can fire (discharge) spontaneously. This is termed *automaticity.* Normally, the SA node is the natural pacemaker of the heart. It spontaneously fires 60 to 100 times per minute (Table 39.4). A secondary pacemaker from another site may fire in 2 ways. If the SA node fires more slowly than a secondary pacemaker, the electrical signals from the secondary pacemaker may "escape." The secondary pacemaker will then fire automatically at its intrinsic rate. These secondary pacemakers may start from the AV node at a rate of 40 to 60 times per minute or the His-Purkinje system at a rate of 20 to 40 times per minute.

Another way that secondary pacemakers can start is when they fire more rapidly than the normal pacemaker of the SA node. *Triggered beats* (early or late) may come from an *ectopic focus* or *accessory pathway* (area outside the normal conduction pathway) in the atria, AV node, or ventricles. This results in a dysrhythmia, which replaces the normal sinus rhythm.

The impulse started by the SA node, or an ectopic focus, is conducted to the heart cells. The property of myocardial tissue that allows it to be depolarized by a stimulus is called *excitability.* The level of excitability is determined by the length of time after depolarization before the tissues can be restimulated. The recovery period after stimulation is the *refractory phase* or period. The *absolute refractory phase* or period occurs when excitability is zero, and the heart cannot be stimulated. The *relative refractory period* occurs slightly later in the cycle, and excitability is more likely. In states of *full excitability,* the heart is completely recovered. Fig. 39.9 shows the relationship between the refractory period and ECG.

If conduction is depressed and some areas of the heart are blocked (e.g., by infarction), the unblocked areas are activated earlier than the blocked areas. When the block is unidirectional, this uneven conduction may allow the initial impulse to reenter areas that were previously not excitable but have recovered. The reentering impulse may be able to depolarize the atria and ventricles, causing a premature beat or rapid rhythm.

TABLE 39.3 Approach to Assessing Heart Rhythm

When assessing a heart rhythm, use a consistent and systematic approach. One such approach includes the following:

1. Look for the P wave. Is it upright or inverted? Is there 1 for every QRS complex or more than 1? Are atrial fibrillatory or flutter waves present?
2. Evaluate the atrial rhythm. Is it regular or irregular?
3. Calculate the atrial rate.
4. Measure the duration of the PR interval. Is it normal duration or prolonged? Is the duration consistent before each QRS?
5. Evaluate the ventricular rhythm. Is it regular or irregular?
6. Calculate the ventricular rate.
7. Measure the duration of the QRS complex. Is it normal duration or prolonged?
8. Assess the ST segment. Is it isoelectric (flat), elevated, or depressed?
9. Measure the duration of the QT interval. Correct for heart rate (QTc) to determine whether it is normal or prolonged.
10. Note the T wave. Is it upright or inverted?
11. *Other questions to consider include:*
    What is the dominant or underlying rhythm and/or dysrhythmia?
    What is the clinical significance of your findings?
    What is the treatment for the particular rhythm?

TABLE 39.4 Intrinsic Rates of the Conduction System

Part of Conduction System	Rate
SA node and atria	60–100 times/min
AV node and bundle of His	40–60 times/min
Bundle branches and Purkinje fibers	20–40 times/min

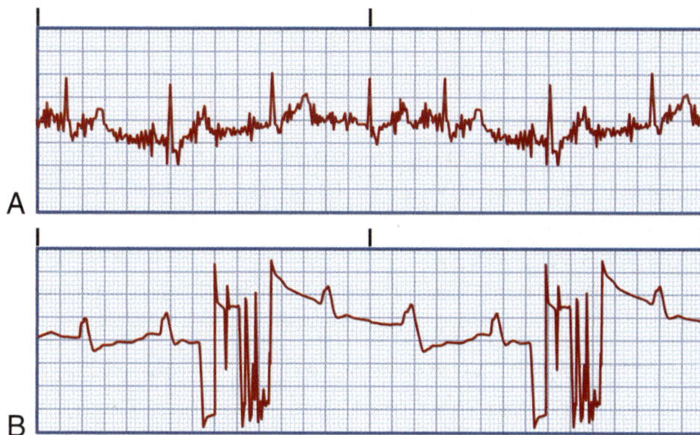

Fig. 39.8 Artifact. (A) Muscle tremor. (B) Loose electrodes.

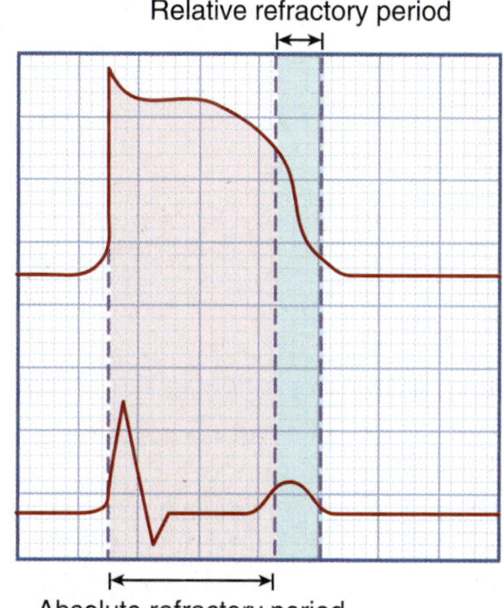

Fig. 39.9 Absolute and relative refractory periods correlated with the heart muscle's action potential and with an ECG tracing. (Modified from Urden LD, Stacy KM, Lough ME: *Critical care nursing: diagnosis and management,* ed 6, St Louis, 2010, Mosby.)

Evaluating Dysrhythmias

Dysrhythmias occur as the result of various abnormalities and disease states. Assess the patient's clinical status, the heart rhythm, and any changes in rhythm. Determining the cause of dysrhythmias is a priority. The cause influences the treatment. Table 39.5 presents common causes of dysrhythmias.

Dysrhythmias occurring in nonmonitored settings present management challenges. If the patient becomes symptomatic (e.g., chest pain, syncope), determining the rhythm by heart monitoring is a high priority. Activate the emergency response system (ERS). Table 39.6 outlines the emergency care of patients with a dysrhythmia.

In addition to continuous ECG monitoring during hospitalization, several other tests can assess dysrhythmias and the effectiveness of antidysrhythmic drug therapy. These include an electrophysiologic study (EPS), Holter monitoring, event monitoring (or loop recorder), exercise treadmill testing, and signal-averaged ECG. They can be done on an inpatient or outpatient basis. See Tables 35.11 and 35.12 for nursing care related to these tests.

An *electrophysiologic study* can identify the causes of heart blocks, tachydysrhythmias (dysrhythmias with rates greater than 100 beats/min), bradydysrhythmias (dysrhythmias with rates less than 60 beats/min), and syncope. An EPS study can locate accessory pathways and determine the effectiveness of antidysrhythmic drugs.

The Holter monitor continuously records the ECG while a patient is ambulatory and performing daily activities. The patient keeps a diary and records activities and any symptoms. Events in the diary are correlated with any dysrhythmias seen on the ECG.

Use of event monitors has improved the evaluation of dysrhythmias in outpatients. Event monitors are recorders that the patient activates only when they have symptoms. New technology using smartphone apps can obtain and save ECG recordings and even detect some dysrhythmias.

Exercise treadmill testing evaluates the patient's heart rhythm during exercise. Any exercise-induced dysrhythmias or ECG changes that occur can be evaluated for treatment. The signal-averaged ECG identifies *late potentials.* Their presence suggests the patient may be at risk for developing serious ventricular dysrhythmias.

CARDIAC RHYTHMS

This section reviews common normal rhythms and dysrhythmias and gives an example of an ECG tracing. Table 39.7 presents the characteristics of each.

Normal Cardiac Rhythms

Normal Sinus Rhythm

Normal sinus rhythm refers to a rhythm that starts in the SA node at a rate of 60 to 100 beats/min and follows the normal conduction pathway (Fig. 39.10). The P wave is normal,

TABLE 39.5 Common Causes of Dysrhythmias

Heart Conditions
- Accessory pathways
- Cardiomyopathy
- Conduction defects
- Heart failure
- Myocardial ischemia, infarction
- Valve disease

Other Conditions
- Acid-base imbalances
- Alcohol
- Caffeine, tobacco
- Connective tissue disorders
- Drowning
- Drug effects (e.g., antidysrhythmic drugs, stimulants, β-blockers) or toxicity
- Electric shock
- Electrolyte imbalances (e.g., hyperkalemia, hypocalcemia)
- Emotional crisis
- Herbal or diet supplements (e.g., bitter orange, fish oil)
- Hypoxia
- Metabolic conditions (e.g., thyroid problems)
- Sepsis, shock
- Toxins

TABLE 39.6 EMERGENCY MANAGEMENT
Dysrhythmias

Assessment Findings	Interventions
• Irregular rate and rhythm; ↑ HR, bradycardia • Chest, neck, shoulder, back, jaw, or arm pain • Cold, clammy skin • ↓ Level of consciousness, confusion • ↓ or ↑ BP • ↓ O_2 saturation • ↓ Peripheral pulses • Diaphoresis • Dizziness, syncope • Dyspnea • Extreme restlessness, anxiety • Feeling of impending doom • Nausea and vomiting • Numbness, tingling of arms • Pallor • Palpitations • Weakness and fatigue	**Initial** • If unresponsive, assess circulation, airway, and breathing (CAB). • If responsive, monitor airway, breathing, and circulation (ABC). • Apply O_2 via nasal cannula or nonrebreather mask. • Take baseline vital signs with O_2 saturation. • Obtain 12-lead ECG. • Begin continuous ECG monitoring. • Identify underlying rate and rhythm. • Identify dysrhythmia. • Establish IV access. • Obtain baseline laboratory studies (e.g., CBC, electrolytes). **Ongoing Monitoring** • Monitor ABCs, vital signs, level of consciousness, O_2 saturation, and heart rhythm. • Anticipate need for antidysrhythmic drugs and analgesics. • Anticipate need for intubation if respiratory distress occurs. • Anticipate need to begin advanced cardiovascular life support (e.g., CPR, defibrillation, transcutaneous pacing).

TABLE 39.7 Characteristics of Common Dysrhythmias

Pattern	Rate and Rhythm	P Wave	PR Interval	QRS Complex
Normal sinus rhythm (NSR)	60–100 beats/min and regular	Normal	Normal	Normal
Sinus bradycardia	<60 beats/min and regular	Normal	Normal	Normal
Sinus tachycardia	101–180 beats/min and regular	Normal	Normal	Normal
Premature atrial contraction (PAC)		Abnormal shape	Normal	Normal (usually)
Paroxysmal supraventricular tachycardia (PSVT)	150–220 beats/min and regular	Abnormal shape, may be hidden in the preceding T wave	Normal or shortened	Normal (usually)
Atrial flutter	*Atrial:* 200–350 beats/min and regular *Ventricular:* > or <100 beats/min and may be regular or irregular	Flutter (F) waves (saw-toothed pattern); more flutter waves than QRS complexes. May occur in a 2:1, 3:1, 4:1, etc., pattern	Not measurable	Normal (usually)
Atrial fibrillation	*Atrial:* 350–600 beats/min and irregular *Ventricular:* > or <100 beats/min and irregular	Fibrillatory (f) waves	Not measurable	Normal (usually)
Junctional dysrhythmias	40–180 beats/min and regular	Inverted, may be hidden in QRS complex or behind the S wave	Shortened, if present	Normal (usually)
First-degree AV block	Normal and regular	Normal	>0.20 sec	Normal
Second-degree AV block				
• **Type I** (Mobitz I, Wenckebach heart block)	*Atrial:* Normal and regular *Ventricular:* Slower and irregular	Normal	Progressive lengthening (longer, longer, longer, drop, now you have a Wenckebach)	Normal QRS width, with pattern of 1 nonconducted (blocked) QRS complex
• **Type II** (Mobitz II heart block)	*Atrial:* Usually normal and regular *Ventricular:* Slower and regular or irregular	More P waves than QRS complexes (e.g., 2:1, 3:1)	Normal or prolonged but consistent for every QRS	Widened QRS, preceded by 2 or more P waves, with nonconducted (blocked) QRS complex
Third-degree AV block (complete heart block)	*Atrial:* Regular but may appear irregular due to P waves hidden in QRS complexes *Ventricular:* 20–60 beats/min and regular	Normal, but no connection with QRS complex	Inconsistent	Normal or widened, no relationship with P waves
Premature ventricular contraction (PVC)	Underlying rhythm can be any rate, regular or irregular rhythm, PVCs occur at variable rates	Not usually visible, hidden in the PVC	Not measurable	Wide and distorted
Ventricular tachycardia (VT)	150–250 beats/min and regular or irregular	Not usually visible	Not measurable	Wide and distorted
Accelerated idioventricular rhythm	40–100 beats/min and regular	Not usually visible	Not measurable	Wide and distorted
Ventricular fibrillation (VF)	Not measurable and irregular	Absent	Not measurable	Not measurable

precedes each QRS complex, and has a normal shape and duration. The PR interval is normal. The QRS complex has a normal shape and duration. Normal sinus rhythm implies that cardiac electrical activity is normal.

Sinus Arrhythmia

In *sinus arrhythmia,* the conduction pathway is the same as that in sinus rhythm, but the SA node fires irregularly. This often results from changes in intrathoracic pressure during breathing.

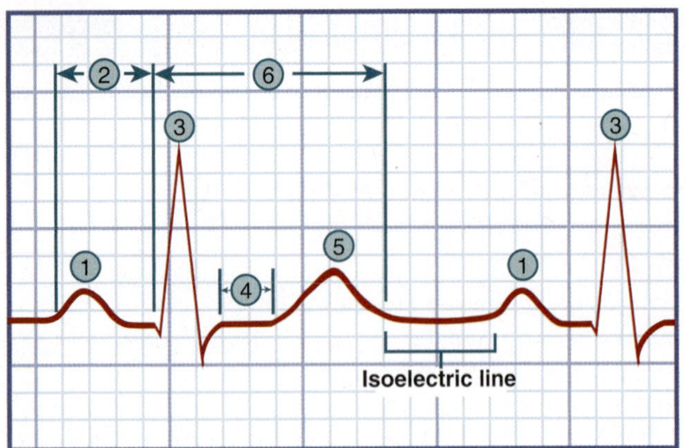

Fig. 39.10 The ECG tracing as seen in normal sinus rhythm. *1,* P wave; *2,* PR interval; *3,* QRS complex: Q wave, R wave, S wave; *4,* ST segment; *5,* T wave; *6,* QT interval. Isoelectric (flat) line or baseline represents the absence of electrical activity in the heart cells.

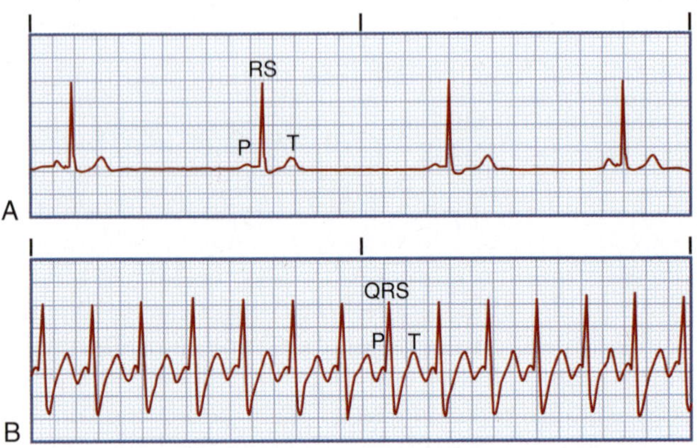

Fig. 39.11 (A) Sinus bradycardia. (B) Sinus tachycardia.

The HR increases slightly during inspiration and decreases slightly during exhalation. It remains 60 to 100 beats/min. It is common in healthy adults.

Types of Dysrhythmias

Sinus Bradycardia

In *sinus bradycardia,* the conduction pathway is the same as in sinus rhythm, but the SA node fires at a rate less than 60 beats/min (Fig. 39.11A). *Symptomatic bradycardia* refers to an HR that is less than 60 beats/min and causes a patient to have symptoms of inadequate perfusion (e.g., fatigue, dizziness, chest pain, syncope).[5]

Clinical associations. Sinus bradycardia may be a normal rhythm in aerobically trained athletes and in some people during sleep. It occurs in response to a Valsalva maneuver, hypothermia, increased intraocular pressure, vagal stimulation, and certain drugs (e.g., β-blockers, calcium channel blockers). Common diseases associated with sinus bradycardia are hypothyroidism, increased intracranial pressure, and inferior MI.

ECG characteristics. In sinus bradycardia, the HR is less than 60 beats/min, and rhythm is regular. The P wave precedes each QRS complex and has a normal shape and duration. The PR interval is normal. The QRS complex has a normal shape and duration.

Clinical significance. The significance depends on how the patient tolerates it. Manifestations of symptomatic bradycardia include pale, cool skin, hypotension, weakness, angina, dizziness, confusion, and shortness of breath.

Treatment. If bradycardia is due to drugs, these may have to be held, stopped, or reduced. For patients with symptoms, treatment consists of giving IV atropine (anticholinergic drug).[6] If atropine is ineffective, transcutaneous pacing or a dopamine or epinephrine infusion are options. The patient may need a permanent pacemaker.

Sinus Tachycardia

The conduction pathway is the same in *sinus tachycardia* as in normal sinus rhythm. The discharge rate from the sinus node increases because of vagal inhibition or sympathetic stimulation. The sinus rate is 101 to 180 beats/min (Fig. 39.11B).

Clinical associations. Sinus tachycardia can occur with many physiologic and psychologic stressors. These include exercise, fever, pain, hypotension, hypovolemia, anemia, hypoxia, hypoglycemia, myocardial ischemia, heart failure (HF), hyperthyroidism, anxiety, and fear. It can be an effect of drugs, such as epinephrine, norepinephrine (Levophed), atropine, caffeine, theophylline, or hydralazine. Many over-the-counter cold remedies have active ingredients (e.g., pseudoephedrine) that can cause tachycardia.

ECG characteristics. In sinus tachycardia, the HR is 101 to 180 beats/min, and rhythm is regular. The P wave is normal and precedes each QRS complex. The PR interval is normal. The QRS complex has a normal shape and duration.

Clinical significance. The significance depends on a patient's tolerance of the increased HR. The patient may have dizziness, dyspnea, and hypotension because of decreased CO. An increased HR increases myocardial oxygen (O_2) consumption. Angina or an increase in infarction size may occur with sinus tachycardia in those with coronary artery disease (CAD) or acute MI.

Treatment. The underlying cause guides the treatment. For example, if the patient has tachycardia from pain, effective pain management is important to treat the tachycardia. In clinically stable patients, we may try vagal maneuvers. IV β-blockers (e.g., metoprolol) or calcium channel blockers (e.g., diltiazem) can reduce HR and decrease myocardial O_2 consumption.[6] Clinically unstable patients may need synchronized cardioversion.

Premature Atrial Contraction

A **premature atrial contraction (PAC)** is a contraction starting from an ectopic focus in the atrium (a location other than the SA node) sooner than the next expected sinus beat. The ectopic signal starts in the left or right atrium and travels across the atria by an abnormal pathway. This creates a distorted P wave (Fig. 39.12). At the AV node, the ectopic signal may be stopped (nonconducted PAC), delayed (lengthened PR interval), or conducted normally. If the signal moves through the AV node, in most cases, it is conducted normally through the ventricles.

Clinical associations. In a normal heart, a PAC can result from emotional stress, fatigue, or from caffeine, tobacco, or alcohol use. A PAC can also result from hypoxia, electrolyte imbalances, hyperthyroidism, chronic obstructive pulmonary disease (COPD), and heart disease, including CAD and valvular disease.

ECG characteristics. HR varies with the underlying rate and frequency of the PAC. The rhythm is irregular. The P wave has a different shape from that of a P wave originating in the SA node. It may be hidden in the preceding T wave. The PR interval may be shorter or longer than the PR interval coming from the SA node but is within normal limits. The QRS complex is usually normal. If the QRS interval is 0.12 second or more, abnormal conduction through the ventricles is occurring.

Clinical significance. In a person with a healthy heart, isolated PACs are not significant. Patients may report palpitations or a sense that the heart "skipped a beat." In a person with heart disease, frequent PACs may indicate enhanced automaticity of the atria or a reentry mechanism. Such PACs may warn of or start more serious dysrhythmias (e.g., supraventricular tachycardia [SVT]).

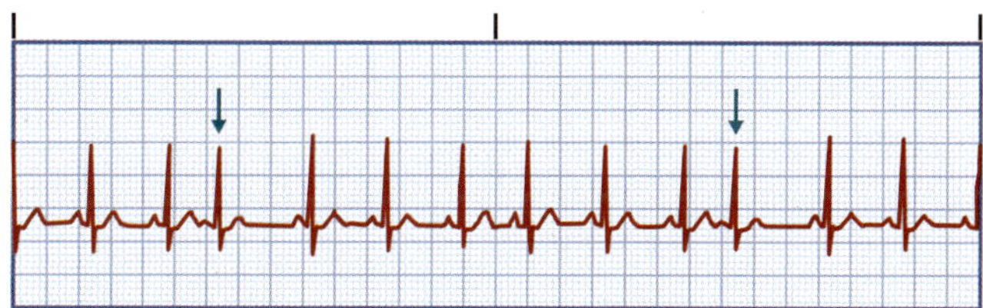

Fig. 39.12 Premature atrial contractions *(arrows)*.

Treatment. Treatment depends on the patient's symptoms. Sources of stimulation, such as caffeine or sympathomimetic drugs (e.g., epinephrine, dopamine), may be withdrawn. β-Blockers may be used to decrease PACs.

Paroxysmal Supraventricular Tachycardia

Paroxysmal supraventricular tachycardia (PSVT), also called supraventricular tachycardia or atrial tachycardia, is a dysrhythmia starting in an ectopic focus anywhere above the bifurcation of the bundle of His (Fig. 39.13).[7] Identifying the ectopic focus is often hard even with a 12-lead ECG since it requires recording the dysrhythmia as it starts.

PSVT occurs because of a reentrant phenomenon (reexcitation of the atria when there is a 1-way block). Usually, a PAC triggers a run of repeated premature beats. *Paroxysmal* refers to an abrupt onset and ending. A brief period of *asystole* (absence of all cardiac electrical activity) may follow the termination. AV block may prevent some of the impulses from being conducted to the ventricles. PSVT can occur with Wolff-Parkinson-White (WPW) syndrome or "preexcitation" with extra conduction or accessory pathways.

Clinical associations. In the normal heart, PSVT may occur with overexertion, emotional stress, deep inspiration, and stimulants, such as caffeine and tobacco. PSVT is associated with rheumatic heart disease, digitalis toxicity, CAD, and cor pulmonale.

ECG characteristics. In PSVT, the HR is 150 to 220 beats/min. The rhythm is regular or slightly irregular. The P wave may have an abnormal shape or be hidden in the preceding T wave. The PR interval may be shortened or normal. The QRS complex is usually normal.

Clinical significance. The significance depends on the symptoms. A prolonged episode and HR greater than 180 beats/min will reduce stroke volume and decrease CO.

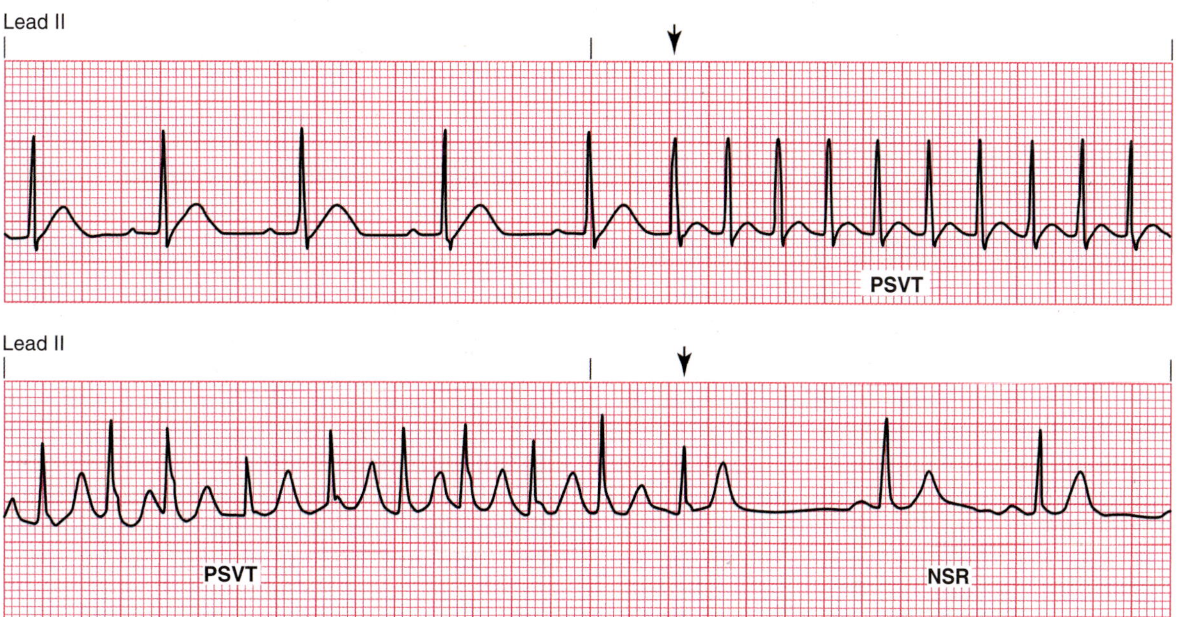

Fig. 39.13 Paroxysmal supraventricular tachycardia (PSVT). *Arrows* indicate beginning and ending of PSVT.

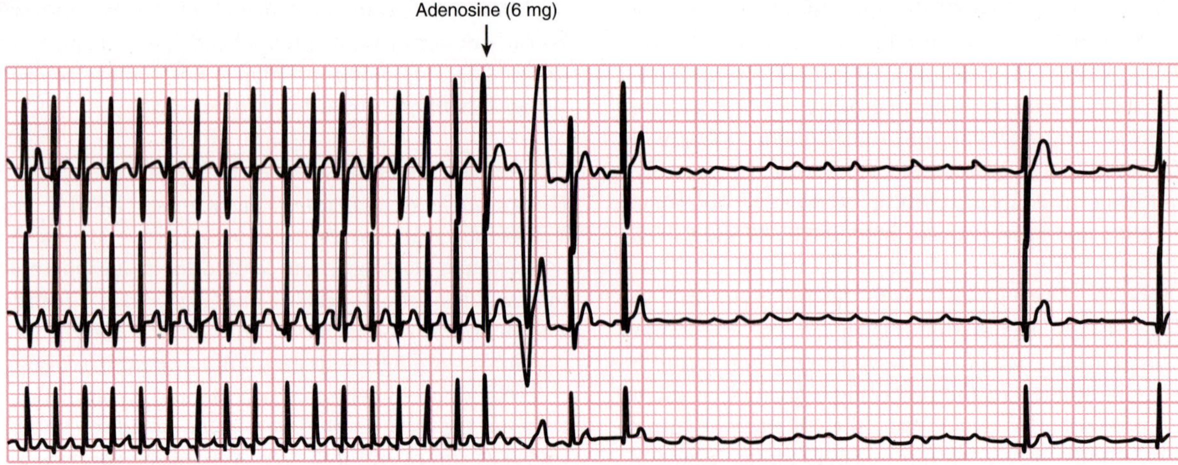

Fig. 39.14 Administration of adenosine rapid IV push. Note that SVT is followed by a brief period of asystole before the return to normal sinus rhythm. This is a common occurrence after adenosine.

Manifestations include hypotension, palpitations, dyspnea, and angina.

Treatment. Treatment includes vagal stimulation and drug therapy. Common vagal maneuvers include Valsalva and coughing. IV adenosine is the drug of choice to convert PSVT to a normal sinus rhythm (Fig. 39.14).[6,7] This drug has a short half-life (10 seconds) and is well tolerated. IV β-blockers and calcium channel blockers (e.g., diltiazem, verapamil) are options. Patients who become hemodynamically unstable undergo synchronized cardioversion. Treatment of recurring PSVT and PSVT in patients with WPW syndrome includes radiofrequency catheter ablation of the accessory pathway.

DRUG ALERT

Adenosine

- Explain that the patient may feel chest pressure after receiving the medication.
- Injection site should be as close to the heart as possible (e.g., antecubital area).
- Give IV dose rapidly (over 1 to 2 sec) and follow with a rapid 20-mL normal saline flush. Use a stopcock setup to make sure adenosine gets to the heart quickly.
- Monitor patient's ECG continuously. Brief period of asystole is common (Fig. 39.14).
- Assess the patient for flushing, dizziness, chest pain, or palpitations.

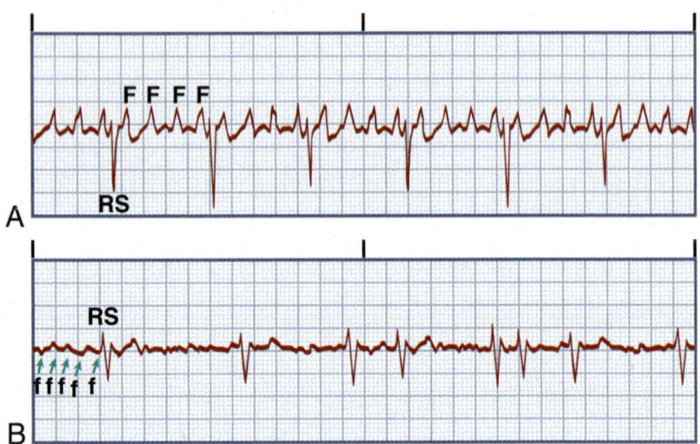

Fig. 39.15 (A) Atrial flutter with a 4:1 conduction (4 flutter *[F]* waves to each QRS complex). (B) Atrial fibrillation with a controlled ventricular response. Note the chaotic fibrillatory *(f)* waves *(arrows)* between the RS complexes. NOTE: Recorded from lead V_1.

Atrial Flutter

Atrial flutter is an atrial tachydysrhythmia identified by recurring, regular, sawtooth-shaped flutter waves originating from a single ectopic focus in the right atrium or, less often, the left atrium (Fig. 39.15A).

Clinical associations. Atrial flutter rarely occurs in a healthy heart. It can occur with CAD, hypertension, mitral valve disorders, pulmonary embolus, COPD, cor pulmonale, cardiomyopathy, hyperthyroidism, and the use of drugs, such as digoxin, quinidine, and epinephrine.

ECG characteristics. Atrial rate is 200 to 350 beats/min. The ventricular rate varies based on the conduction ratio. In 2:1 conduction, the ventricular rate is typically around 150 beats/min. Atrial and ventricular rhythms are usually regular. The atrial flutter waves represent atrial depolarization followed by repolarization. The PR interval is variable and not measurable. The QRS complex is usually normal. There is usually some AV block in a fixed ratio of flutter waves to QRS complexes because the AV node can delay signals from the atria.

Clinical significance. The high ventricular rates (greater than 100 beats/min) and loss of the atrial "kick" (atrial contraction coordinated with ventricular contraction) in atrial flutter decrease CO. This can cause serious problems, such as HF, especially in patients with underlying heart disease. Patients with atrial flutter have an increased risk for stroke because thrombi (clots) can form in the atria from the stasis of blood.

Patients receive an anticoagulant to prevent stroke.[8] See Chapter 41 for discussion of anticoagulation therapy.

Treatment. The primary goal in treatment is to slow the ventricular response by increasing AV block. Drugs used to control ventricular rate include calcium channel blockers and β-blockers.[6,8] Electrical cardioversion may convert the atrial flutter to sinus rhythm in an emergency (e.g., when the patient is clinically unstable) or electively. Antidysrhythmic drugs can convert atrial flutter to sinus rhythm (e.g., ibutilide [Corvert]) or maintain sinus rhythm (e.g., amiodarone, flecainide).[8]

Radiofrequency catheter ablation in an EPS laboratory is the treatment of choice for atrial flutter. Low-voltage, high-frequency electrical energy is used to ablate (or destroy) the ectopic foci through a catheter in the right atrium. This should restore normal sinus rhythm.

Atrial Fibrillation

Atrial fibrillation is characterized by total disorganization of atrial electrical activity because of multiple ectopic foci. It results in loss of effective atrial contraction (Fig. 39.15B). The dysrhythmia may be paroxysmal (beginning and ending spontaneously) or persistent (lasting more than 7 days). Atrial fibrillation is the most common, clinically significant dysrhythmia with respect to morbidity and mortality rates and economic impact. Its prevalence increases with age.

Clinical associations. Atrial fibrillation usually occurs in patients with underlying heart disease, such as CAD, valvular heart disease, cardiomyopathy, hypertensive heart disease, HF, and pericarditis. It often develops acutely with thyrotoxicosis, alcohol intoxication, caffeine use, electrolyte problems, stress, and after heart surgery.

ECG characteristics. During atrial fibrillation, the atrial rate may be as high as 350 to 600 beats/min. Chaotic, fibrillatory waves replace the P waves. Ventricular rate varies, and the rhythm is usually irregular. When the ventricular rate is between 60 and 100 beats/min, atrial fibrillation has a *controlled ventricular response.* Atrial fibrillation with a ventricular rate greater than 100 beats/min is atrial fibrillation with a *rapid (or uncontrolled) ventricular response.* The PR interval is not measurable. The QRS complex usually has a normal shape and duration. At times, atrial flutter and atrial fibrillation coexist.

Clinical significance. Atrial fibrillation results in a decrease in CO because of ineffective atrial contractions (loss of atrial kick) and/or a rapid ventricular response (RVR). Thrombi may form in the atria because of blood stasis. An embolized clot may move through arteries to the brain, causing a stroke. Atrial fibrillation accounts for 1 in 7 strokes.[9]

Treatment. The goals of treatment are to decrease the ventricular response (to less than 100 beats/min), prevent stroke, and convert to sinus rhythm, if possible. Ventricular rate control is a priority. Drugs used for rate control include calcium channel blockers (e.g., diltiazem), β-blockers (e.g., metoprolol), amiodarone, and digoxin (Lanoxin).[8]

Some patients need drug or electrical conversion of atrial fibrillation to a normal sinus rhythm (e.g., reduced exercise tolerance with rate control drugs, contraindications to warfarin). The most common antidysrhythmic drug used for conversion to and maintenance of sinus rhythm is amiodarone.[8]

Electrical cardioversion may convert atrial fibrillation to a normal sinus rhythm. If a patient is in atrial fibrillation for longer than 48 hours, anticoagulation therapy is needed for 3 weeks before the cardioversion.[8] Anticoagulation therapy continues for several weeks because the procedure can cause the clots to dislodge, placing the patient at risk for stroke. A transesophageal echocardiogram may be done to rule out clots in the atria. If no clots are present, anticoagulation therapy may not be needed before cardioversion.

If drugs or cardioversion does not convert atrial fibrillation to normal sinus rhythm, the patient needs long-term anticoagulation therapy (Table 39.8). Warfarin requires monitoring for therapeutic levels (e.g., international normalized ratio [INR]). Alternatives to warfarin are available that do not require routine laboratory testing. Examples include dabigatran (Pradaxa), apixaban (Eliquis), and rivaroxaban (Xarelto).[8] See Chapter 41 for more on anticoagulation therapy.

For symptomatic patients with atrial fibrillation refractory to drugs or electrical conversion, radiofrequency catheter ablation, AV nodal ablation, and the Maze procedure are further options. AV nodal ablation involves destruction of the AV node and insertion of a permanent ventricular pacemaker. The Maze procedure stops atrial fibrillation by interrupting the ectopic foci that are causing the dysrhythmia. Incisions are made in both atria, and *cryoablation* (cold therapy) is used to stop the formation and conduction of ectopic signals and restore normal sinus rhythm.[8]

TABLE 39.8 Drug Therapy

Antithrombotic Therapy for Atrial Fibrillation and Atrial Flutter

Risk Category	Recommended Therapy
Mechanical heart valve	Warfarin (target INR 2.5–3.5)
CHA_2DS_2-VASc[a] score of 0	No therapy recommended
CHA_2DS_2-VASc score of 1	No therapy recommended. An oral anticoagulant or aspirin (e.g., 81–325 mg/day) may be considered
CHA_2DS_2-VASc score of ≥2 or a history of prior stroke or transient ischemia attack (TIA)	Warfarin (target INR 2.0–3.0) Apixaban (Eliquis) Dabigatran (Pradaxa) Edoxaban (Savaysa) Rivaroxaban (Xarelto)
CHA_2DS_2-VASc score of ≥2 and end-stage kidney disease or on hemodialysis	Warfarin (INR 2.0–3.0) Apixaban (Eliquis)

[a]CHA_2DS_2-VASc refers to congestive heart failure, hypertension, age, diabetes, prior stroke or TIA or thromboembolism, vascular disease, age, sex category.

Modified from January CT, Wann LS, Calkins H, et al: 2019 AHA/ACC/HRS focused update on the 2014 AHA/ACC/HRS guideline for the management of patients with atrial fibrillation, *Circulation* 140:e125, 2019.

Left atrial appendage occlusion. The left atrial appendage (LAA) is a pouch that extends off the left atrium. The LAA is a common source of blood clots in patients with atrial fibrillation. LAA occlusion is a treatment strategy to prevent blood clot formation in patients who have atrial fibrillation. Removing or occluding the LAA can decrease the incidence of strokes.

A special stapler can be used to remove the LAA, or the LAA can be occluded manually with sutures or an LAA occlusion device.[8] These devices are positioned around the LAA and then closed like a clamp to prevent blood from flowing into and out of the LAA. LAA occlusion is an alternative for patients who cannot use oral anticoagulants.

CHECK YOUR PRACTICE

You are caring for a 72-year-old female patient who was admitted with chest pain. She has continuous EGG monitoring. You are concerned because you think the ECG tracing is hard to interpret, and she may be in atrial fibrillation. Your preceptor tells you a lot of artifact is present.

- What can you do to improve the ECG tracing?
- How would you determine the patient's rhythm?

Junctional Dysrhythmias

Junctional dysrhythmias start in the area of the AV node to the bundle of His known as the AV junction. When the SA node does not fire, or the signal is blocked, the AV node becomes the pacemaker of the heart. The impulse from the AV node usually moves in a retrograde (backward) fashion through the atria. This produces an abnormal P wave that occurs just before or after the QRS complex or is hidden in the QRS complex. The impulse usually moves normally through the ventricles.

Junctional premature beats may occur. They are treated like PACs. Other junctional dysrhythmias include junctional escape rhythm (Fig. 39.16), accelerated junctional rhythm, and junctional tachycardia. Their treatment depends on the patient's tolerance of the rhythm and their clinical condition.

Clinical associations. Junctional dysrhythmias are often associated with CAD, HF, cardiomyopathy, electrolyte imbalances, inferior MI, and rheumatic heart disease. Certain drugs (e.g., digoxin, nicotine, amphetamines, caffeine) can also cause junctional dysrhythmias.

ECG characteristics. In junctional escape rhythm, the HR is 40 to 60 beats/min. HR is 61 to 100 beats/min in accelerated junctional rhythm and 101 to 180 beats/min in junctional tachycardia. The rhythm is regular. The P wave is abnormal in shape and inverted. It can be hidden in the QRS complex (Fig. 39.16). The PR interval is less than 0.12 second when the P wave precedes the QRS complex. The QRS complex is usually normal.

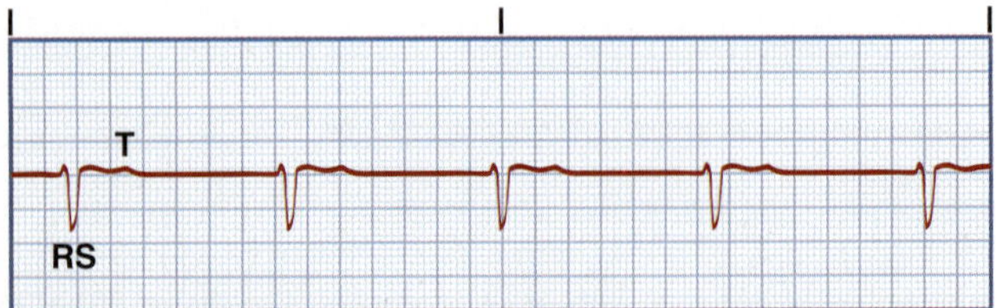

Fig. 39.16 Junctional escape rhythm. P wave is hidden in the RS complex. NOTE: Recorded from lead V_1.

Clinical significance. Junctional escape rhythms serve as a safety mechanism when the SA node has not been effective. Escape rhythms should not be suppressed. Accelerated junctional rhythm is due to sympathetic stimulation to improve CO. Junctional tachycardia indicates a more serious problem. This rhythm may reduce CO, causing the patient to become hemodynamically unstable (e.g., hypotensive).

Treatment. Treatment varies by the type of junctional dysrhythmia. If a patient has symptoms with a junctional escape rhythm, atropine can be used. If accelerated junctional rhythm or junctional tachycardia are caused by drug toxicity, the drug is stopped. In the absence of digitalis toxicity, β-blockers, calcium channel blockers, and amiodarone are used for rate control.

First-Degree AV Block

First-degree AV block is a type of AV block in which every impulse is conducted to the ventricles, but the time of AV conduction is prolonged (Fig. 39.17A). After the impulse moves through the AV node, the ventricles usually respond normally.

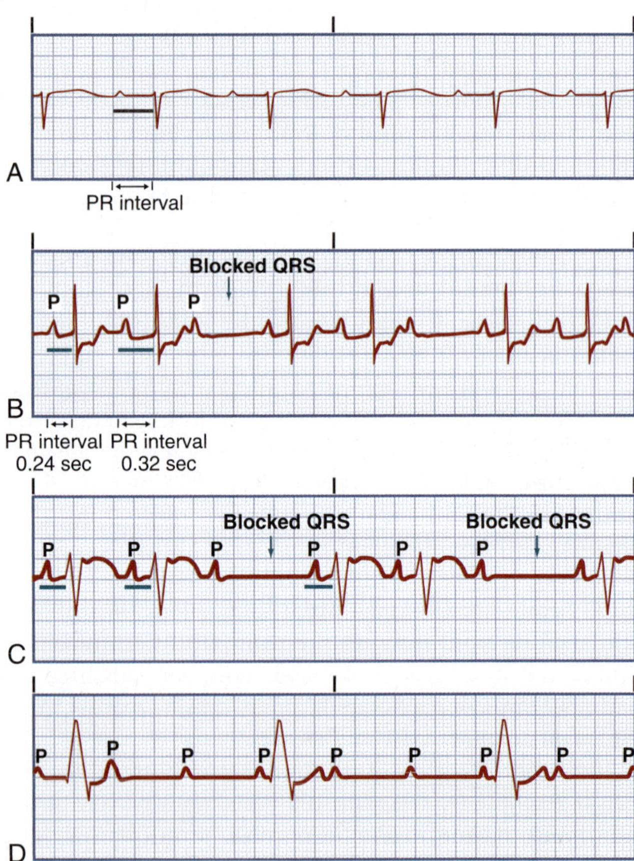

Fig. 39.17 Heart block. (A) First-degree AV block with a PR interval of 0.40 sec. (B) Second-degree AV block, type I, with progressive lengthening of the PR interval until a QRS complex is blocked. (C) Second-degree AV block, type II, with constant PR intervals and variable blocked QRS complexes. (D) Third-degree AV block. Note that there is no relationship between P waves and QRS complexes.

Clinical associations. First-degree AV block is associated with increasing age, MI, CAD, rheumatic fever, hyperthyroidism, electrolyte imbalances (e.g., hypokalemia), vagal stimulation, and drugs, such as digoxin, β-blockers, calcium channel blockers, and flecainide.

ECG characteristics. In first-degree AV block, the HR is normal. The rhythm is regular. The P wave is normal. The PR interval is prolonged (greater than 0.20 second). The QRS complex usually has a normal shape and duration.

Clinical significance. First-degree AV block is usually not serious. Patients are asymptomatic.

Treatment. There is no treatment for first-degree AV block. Treatment of associated conditions may be considered. Monitor patients for changes in heart rhythm (e.g., more serious AV block).

Second-Degree AV Block, Type I

Type I second-degree AV block (Mobitz I or *Wenckebach heart block)* includes a gradual lengthening of the PR interval. AV conduction time is increasingly prolonged until an atrial impulse is not conducted and a QRS complex is blocked (missing) (Fig. 39.17B). Type I AV block most often occurs in the AV node, but it can occur in the His-Purkinje system.

Clinical associations. Type I AV block may result from drugs, such as digoxin or β-blockers. It can occur with CAD and other diseases that can slow AV conduction.

ECG characteristics. Atrial rate is regular, but ventricular rate may be slower because of nonconducted or blocked QRS complexes resulting in bradycardia. Once a ventricular beat is blocked, the cycle repeats itself with progressive lengthening of the PR intervals until another QRS complex is blocked. Think of the phrase, "longer, longer, longer, drop, now you have a Wenckebach." The rhythm appears on the ECG in a pattern of grouped beats. Ventricular rhythm is irregular. The P wave has a normal shape. The QRS complex has a normal shape and duration.

Clinical significance. Type I AV block is usually a result of myocardial ischemia or inferior MI. It is generally transient and well tolerated. However, in some patients (e.g., acute MI), it may be a warning sign of a more serious AV conduction problem (e.g., complete heart block).

Treatment. Symptomatic patients may need atropine or a temporary pacemaker to increase HR, especially if they have had an MI. If the patient is asymptomatic, observe the rhythm closely. Have a transcutaneous pacemaker (TCP) on standby. Bradycardia is more likely to become symptomatic when hypotension, HF, or shock is already present.

Second-Degree AV Block, Type II

In *type II second-degree AV block (Mobitz II heart block)*, a P wave is nonconducted without progressive PR lengthening. This usually occurs when a block in 1 of the bundle branches is present (Fig. 39.17C). On conducted beats, the PR interval is constant. Type II second-degree AV block is a more serious type of block because a certain number of impulses from the SA node are not conducted to the ventricles. This occurs in ratios of 2:1, 3:1, and so on (e.g., 2 P waves to 1 QRS complex, 3 P waves to 1 QRS complex). It may occur with varying ratios.[2]

Clinical associations. Type II AV block is associated with rheumatic heart disease, CAD, anterior MI, and drug toxicity.

ECG characteristics. Atrial rate is usually normal. Ventricular rate depends on the degree of AV block. Atrial rhythm is regular, but ventricular rhythm may be irregular. The P wave has a normal shape. The PR interval may be normal or prolonged in duration and remains constant on conducted beats. The QRS complex is usually greater than 0.12 second because of bundle branch block.

Clinical significance. Type II AV block often progresses to third-degree AV block. It has a poor prognosis. The reduced HR often results in decreased CO with subsequent hypotension and myocardial ischemia. Type II AV block is an indication for a permanent pacemaker.

Treatment. Transcutaneous pacing or the insertion of a temporary pacemaker may be needed before inserting a permanent pacemaker if the patient is symptomatic (e.g., hypotension, angina).[2,6]

Third-Degree AV Block

Third-degree AV block, or **complete heart block**, is a form of AV dissociation in which no impulses from the atria are conducted to the ventricles (Fig. 39.17D). The atria are stimulated and contract independently of the ventricles. The ventricular rhythm is an escape rhythm. The ectopic pacemaker may be above or below the bifurcation of the bundle of His.

Clinical associations. Third-degree AV block can occur with severe heart disease, including CAD, MI, myocarditis, cardiomyopathy, and some systemic diseases, such as scleroderma. Some drugs can cause third-degree AV block, such as digoxin, β-blockers, and calcium channel blockers.

ECG characteristics. The atrial rate is usually a sinus rate of 60 to 100 beats/min. The ventricular rate depends on the site of the block. If it is in the AV node, the rate is 40 to 60 beats/min. If it is in the His-Purkinje system, it is 20 to 40 beats/min. Atrial and ventricular rhythms are regular but unrelated to each other. The P wave has a normal shape. The PR interval is variable. There is no relationship between the P wave and the QRS complex. The QRS complex is normal if the escape rhythm starts at the bundle of His or above. It is widened if the escape rhythm starts below the bundle of His.

Clinical significance. Third-degree AV block usually results in reduced CO with ischemia, HF, and shock. Syncope from third-degree AV block may result from severe bradycardia or even periods of asystole.

Treatment. Symptomatic patients need a TCP until a temporary transvenous pacemaker can be inserted.[6] Drugs such as dopamine and epinephrine are interim measures to increase HR and support BP until temporary pacing is started. Patients need a permanent pacemaker as soon as possible. Atropine is not an effective treatment.

Premature Ventricular Contractions

A **premature ventricular contraction (PVC)** is a contraction coming from an ectopic focus in the ventricles. It is the premature (early) occurrence of a QRS complex. A PVC is wide and distorted in shape compared with a QRS complex coming down the normal conduction pathway (Fig. 39.18). PVCs that have the same shape are *unifocal* PVCs. PVCs that arise from different foci appear different in shape from each other. These are *multifocal* PVCs. When every other beat is a PVC, the rhythm is *ventricular bigeminy*. When every third beat is a PVC, it is *ventricular trigeminy*. We call 2 consecutive PVCs a *couplet*.

Ventricular tachycardia (VT) occurs when there are 3 or more consecutive PVCs. *R-on-T phenomenon* occurs when a PVC falls on the T wave of a preceding beat (Fig. 39.19). This is especially dangerous because the PVC is firing during the relative refractory phase of ventricular repolarization. Excitability of the heart cells increases during this time. The risk for the PVC to start VT or ventricular fibrillation (VF) is great.

Clinical associations. PVCs are associated with stimulants, such as caffeine, alcohol, nicotine, aminophylline, epinephrine, and isoproterenol. They can occur with electrolyte imbalances, hypoxia, fever, exercise, and emotional stress. Disease states associated with PVCs include MI, mitral valve prolapse, HF, cardiomyopathy, and CAD.

ECG characteristics. HR varies according to intrinsic rate and number of PVCs. Rhythm is irregular because of premature beats. The P wave is rarely visible. It is usually lost in the QRS complex of the PVC. Retrograde conduction may occur with the P wave seen after the ectopic beat. The PR interval is not measurable. The QRS complex is wide and distorted in shape, lasting more than 0.12 second. The T wave is generally large and opposite in direction to the major direction of the QRS complex.

Clinical significance. PVCs are usually not harmful in patients with a normal heart. PVCs in CAD or acute MI indicate ventricular irritability. PVCs may reduce CO and lead to angina and HF for those with heart disease, so assess the patient's physiologic response. Take the apical-radial pulse rate and determine the pulse deficit since PVCs often do not generate a sufficient ventricular contraction to result in a peripheral pulse.

Treatment. Treatment relates to the cause of the PVCs (e.g., O_2 therapy for hypoxia, electrolyte replacement). Assessing the patient's hemodynamic status is important to determine whether treatment with drug therapy is needed. Drug therapy includes β-blockers, lidocaine, or amiodarone.

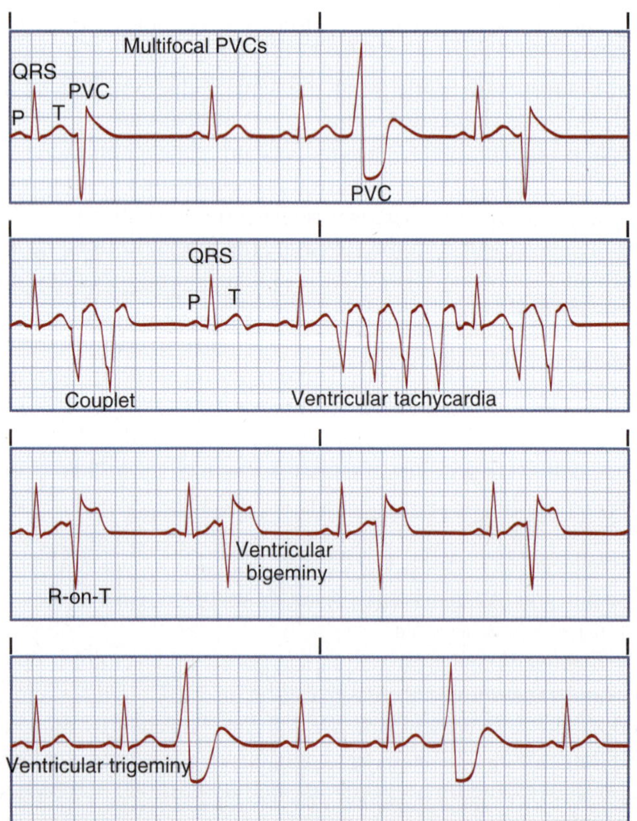

Fig. 39.18 Various types of premature ventricular contractions *(PVCs)*.

Accelerated Idioventricular Rhythm

An *accelerated idioventricular rhythm* (AIVR) can develop when the intrinsic pacemaker (SA node or AV node) rate is slower than that of a ventricular ectopic pacemaker. The rate is between 40 and 100 beats/min.

Clinical associations. AIVR is often associated with acute MI and reperfusion of the myocardium after thrombolytic therapy or percutaneous coronary interventions (e.g., angioplasty). It can occur with digitalis toxicity.

Treatment. In the setting of acute MI, AIVR is usually self-limiting and well tolerated, and it needs no treatment. If the patient becomes symptomatic (e.g., hypotensive, chest pain), atropine is an option. Temporary pacing may be needed. Drugs that suppress ventricular rhythms (e.g., amiodarone) should not be used because they can further reduce the HR.

Ventricular Tachycardia

A run of 3 or more PVCs defines **ventricular tachycardia (VT)**. It occurs when an ectopic focus or foci fire repeatedly and the ventricle takes control as the pacemaker. Different forms of VT

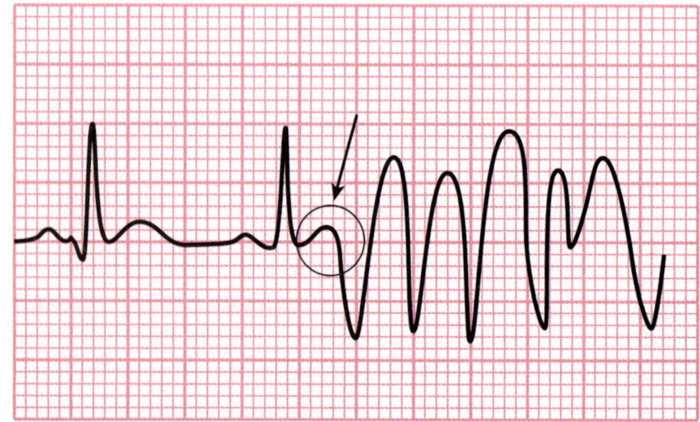

Fig. 39.19 R-on-T phenomenon. The "shock" occurred on the T wave leading to ventricular tachycardia.

exist, depending on QRS configuration. *Monomorphic* VT (Fig. 39.20A) has QRS complexes that are the same in shape, size, and direction. *Polymorphic* VT occurs when the QRS complexes gradually change back and forth from one shape, size, and direction to another over a series of beats. *Torsades de pointes* (French for "twisting of the points") is polymorphic VT with a prolonged QT interval of the underlying rhythm (Fig. 39.20B).

We describe VT as sustained (longer than 30 seconds) or nonsustained (less than 30 seconds). The development of VT is an ominous sign. It is a life-threatening dysrhythmia because of decreased CO and the possible development of VF, which is lethal.

Clinical associations. VT is associated with MI, CAD, significant electrolyte imbalances, cardiomyopathy, long QT syndrome, drug toxicity, and central nervous system disorders. It can occur in patients who have no evidence of heart disease.

ECG characteristics. Ventricular rate is 150 to 250 beats/min. Rhythm may be regular or irregular. AV dissociation may be present, with P waves occurring independently of the QRS complex. The ventricles may depolarize the atria in a retrograde fashion. The P wave is usually buried in the QRS complex. The PR interval is not measurable. The QRS complex appears distorted and wide (greater than 0.12 second in duration). The T wave is in the opposite direction of the QRS complex (Fig. 39.20).

Clinical significance. VT can be stable (patient has a pulse) or unstable (patient is pulseless). Sustained VT causes a severe decrease in CO because of decreased ventricular diastolic filling times and loss of atrial contraction. This results in hypotension, pulmonary edema, decreased cerebral blood flow, and cardiopulmonary arrest. VT must be treated quickly, even if it occurs only briefly and stops abruptly. Episodes may recur if prophylactic treatment is not started. VF may develop.

Treatment. Precipitating causes (e.g., electrolyte imbalances, ischemia) must be identified and treated. If the VT is monomorphic and the patient is clinically stable (e.g., pulse is present) with preserved left ventricular function, options include IV procainamide, lidocaine, or amiodarone.[6] These drugs can be given if VT is polymorphic with a normal baseline QT interval.

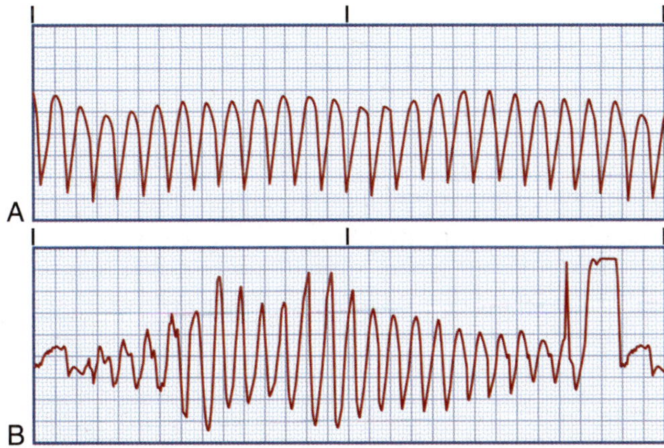

Fig. 39.20 Ventricular tachycardia. (A) Monomorphic. (B) Torsades de pointes (polymorphic).

Treatment for polymorphic VT with a prolonged baseline QT interval includes IV magnesium, phenytoin, or antitachycardia pacing (discussed later in this chapter). Drugs that prolong the QT interval (e.g., dofetilide [Tikosyn]) should be stopped. Cardioversion is used if drug therapy is ineffective.

VT without a pulse is a lethal dysrhythmia. It is treated the same as VF. Cardiopulmonary resuscitation (CPR) and rapid defibrillation are the first lines of treatment (Box 39.1). This is followed by administering epinephrine and antidysrhythmics (e.g., amiodarone or lidocaine) if defibrillation is unsuccessful.[6]

CHECK YOUR PRACTICE

You are assigned to a 69-year-old male patient on a telemetry unit who is recovering from colon surgery. He has a history of 2 MIs, and he has 3 coronary stents in place. You hear his ECG monitor alarm and see what looks like ventricular tachycardia.

- What should you do?

Ventricular Fibrillation

Ventricular fibrillation (VF) is a severe derangement of the heart rhythm characterized on ECG by irregular waveforms of varying shapes and amplitude (Fig. 39.21). This represents the firing of multiple ectopic foci in the ventricle. Mechanically, the

BOX 39.1 ETHICAL/LEGAL DILEMMAS

Scope and Standards of Practice

Situation

A young female with a history of viral cardiomyopathy is admitted to the intensive care unit (ICU) after having several episodes of nonsustained ventricular tachycardia (VT). While she is being stabilized, she codes (pulseless VT) and needs intubation. A nurse anesthetist tries to intubate her 3 times unsuccessfully. There is an unforeseen delay in the arrival of the anesthesiologist. P.F., an ICU nurse who is a paramedic certified in advanced trauma life support (ATLS) and advanced cardiovascular life support (ACLS), intubates the patient. The next day the nursing supervisor questions P.F. about intubating the patient since this is not within the scope of practice for an ICU nurse in that agency.

Ethical/Legal Points for Consideration

- Each state board of nursing defines their own RN *Scope of Practice,* including rules and regulations that guide practice. They can vary from state to state.
- Individual agencies have policies and procedures that describe the scope of practice for nurses. These can be more restrictive than those of the state.
- P.F. has training, education, and certification beyond the usual nursing role.
- The life-threatening situation is an extenuating circumstance.
- Negligence may have been a factor if P.F., who is a nurse with training and experience, had not acted.

Discussion Questions

1. What would you have done in this situation?
2. How would you respond to the nursing supervisor?
3. What are the legal ramifications for P.F. in this situation?
4. What are the ethical issues in this situation?

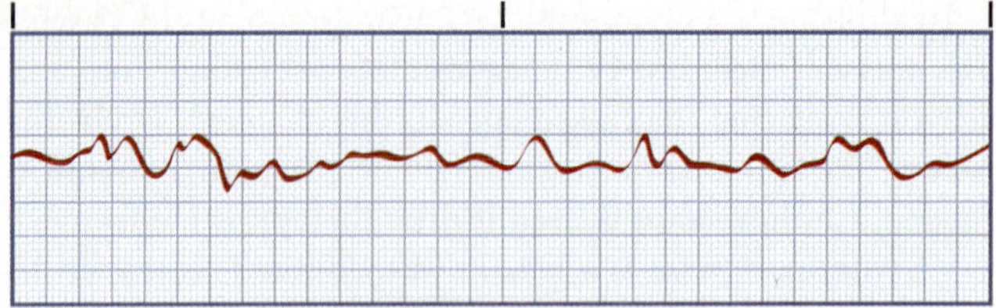

Fig. 39.21 Ventricular fibrillation.

ventricle is simply "quivering," with no effective contraction, so no CO occurs. VF is a lethal dysrhythmia.

Clinical associations. VF occurs in acute MI, myocardial ischemia, and chronic diseases such as HF and cardiomyopathy. It may occur during cardiac pacing or cardiac catheterization procedures because of catheter stimulation of the ventricle. It may happen with coronary reperfusion after thrombolytic therapy. Other causes are electric shock, hyperkalemia, hypoxemia, acidosis, and drug toxicity.

ECG characteristics. HR is not measurable. Rhythm is irregular and chaotic. The P wave is not visible. The PR interval and the QRS interval are not measurable.

Clinical significance. VF results in an unresponsive, pulseless, and apneic state. If VF is not treated quickly, the patient will not recover.

Treatment. Treatment consists of immediate initiation of CPR and ACLS with the use of defibrillation and definitive drug therapy (e.g., epinephrine, amiodarone). There should be no delay in starting chest compressions and using a defibrillator once available.

Asystole

Asystole is the total absence of ventricular electrical activity. Occasionally, P waves are seen. No ventricular contraction occurs because depolarization does not occur. Patients are unresponsive, pulseless, and apneic. Asystole is a lethal dysrhythmia that needs immediate treatment. VF may masquerade as asystole. Always assess the rhythm in more than 1 lead. The prognosis of a patient with asystole is very poor.

Clinical associations. Asystole is usually a result of advanced heart disease, a severe cardiac conduction system problem, or end-stage HF.

Clinical significance. Generally, patients with asystole have end-stage heart disease or have had prolonged arrest and cannot be resuscitated.

Treatment. Treatment consists of CPR with ACLS measures. These include definitive drug therapy with epinephrine, intubation, and efforts to determine the underlying cause.

Pulseless Electrical Activity

Pulseless electrical activity (PEA) is a situation in which organized electrical activity is seen on the ECG, but there is no mechanical heart activity, and the patient has no pulse. It is the most common dysrhythmia seen after defibrillation. Prognosis is poor unless we quickly identify and treat the underlying cause. Common causes of PEA include hypovolemia, hypoxia, metabolic acidosis, hyperkalemia, hypokalemia, hypoglycemia, hypothermia, toxins (e.g., drug overdose), cardiac tamponade, thrombosis (e.g., MI, pulmonary embolus), tension pneumothorax, and trauma. Treatment begins with CPR, followed by drug therapy (e.g., epinephrine) and intubation. Correcting the underlying cause is critical to prognosis.

Sudden Cardiac Death

The term *sudden cardiac death* (SCD) refers to death from a cardiac cause. Most SCDs result from ventricular dysrhythmias, specifically VT or VF. SCD is discussed in Chapter 37.

INTERPROFESSIONAL AND NURSING MANAGEMENT: DYSRHYTHMIAS

Antidysrhythmic Drug Therapy

Table 39.9 shows antidysrhythmic drugs by their primary effects on the heart cells and the ECG.

Before giving any *antidysrhythmic drug,* perform a thorough assessment with a complete physical assessment, health history, medication allergies, and medication history. Assess for contraindications, cautions, and drug interactions. Obtain a baseline ECG. Assess vital signs, heart and lung sounds, and pulse rate, rhythm, and quality. Assess for signs and symptoms from the decreased CO because of the dysrhythmia, such as restlessness, syncope, chest pain, dyspnea, and crackles. Review laboratory studies, including electrolytes and liver and kidney function tests.

When giving antidysrhythmics, monitor the ECG and vital signs, especially BP and pulse rate. Assess for changes in the physical assessment. Monitor laboratory studies as needed. Give specific instructions for each drug. Teach patients that oral forms are often better tolerated if taken with food to help decrease GI upset. Tell patients to avoid alcohol, caffeine, and tobacco.

Defibrillation

Defibrillation is the treatment of choice to end VF and pulseless VT. It is most effective when the myocardial cells are not yet anoxic or acidotic. Rapid defibrillation (within 2 minutes) is critical to a successful patient outcome. Defibrillation involves passing an electric shock through the heart to depolarize the myocardial cells. The goal is that, after repolarization, the SA node will be able to resume the role of pacemaker.

Defibrillators deliver energy using a monophasic or biphasic waveform. Monophasic defibrillators deliver energy in 1 direction. Biphasic defibrillators deliver energy in 2 directions (Fig. 39.22). The shocks delivered are at lower energies and with fewer postshock dysrhythmias than monophasic defibrillators.

We measure the output of a defibrillator in *joules,* or watts per second. The recommended energy for initial shocks in defibrillation depends on the type of defibrillator. Biphasic defibrillators deliver the first and any successive shocks using

TABLE 39.9 Drug Therapy

Antidysrhythmic Drugs

Drug	Effects on the Action Potential	Effects on ECG
Class I: Sodium Channel Blockers	Decrease impulse conduction in the atria, ventricles, and His-Purkinje system	
Class IA		
disopyramide (Norpace) procainamide quinidine	Delay repolarization	Widened QRS and prolonged QT interval
Class IB		
lidocaine mexiletine phenytoin (Dilantin)	Accelerate repolarization	Little or no effect on ECG
Class IC		
flecainide propafenone (Rythmol SR)	Decrease impulse conduction	Pronounced prodysrhythmic actions, widened QRS, prolonged QT interval
Class II: β-Adrenergic Blockers		
esmolol (Brevibloc) metoprolol (Lopressor) propranolol (Inderal)	Decrease automaticity of the SA node, slow impulse conduction in AV node, reduce atrial and ventricular contractility	Bradycardia, prolonged PR interval, AV block
Class III: Potassium Channel Blockers		
amiodarone dofetilide (Tikosyn) ibutilide (Corvert) sotalol[a] (Betapace)	Delay repolarization, resulting in prolonged duration of action potential and refractory period	Prolonged PR and QT intervals, widened QRS, bradycardia
Class IV: Calcium Channel Blockers		
diltiazem (Cardizem) verapamil	Decrease automaticity of SA node, delay AV node conduction. Reduce myocardial contractility	Bradycardia, prolonged PR interval, AV block
Other Agents		
adenosine (Adenocard) digoxin (Lanoxin)	Decrease conduction through AV node, reduce automaticity of SA node	Prolonged PR interval, AV block
dronedarone (Multaq)[b]	Suppress atrial dysrhythmias though mechanism is unknown	Prolonged QT interval
magnesium	Decrease impulse conduction through AV node	AV block

[a]Sotalol has both class II and class III properties.
[b]Dronedarone has class I through IV properties.

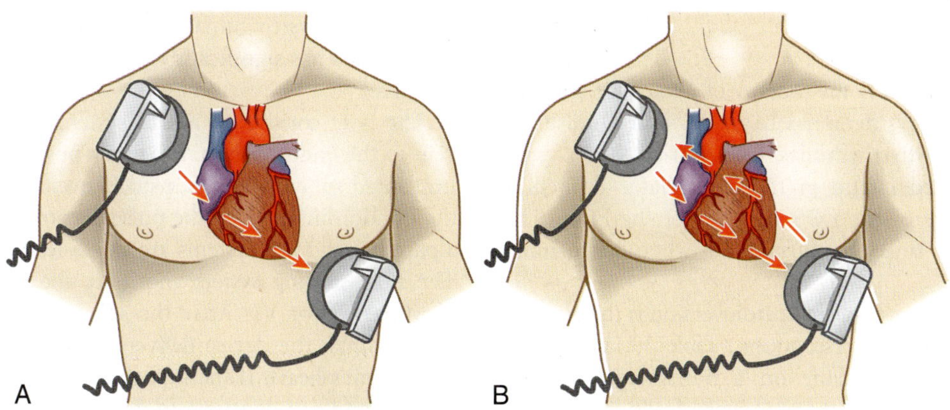

Fig. 39.22 Paddle placement and current flow in monophasic defibrillation (A) and biphasic defibrillation (B).

TABLE 39.10 Defibrillation

The following general steps are taken for defibrillation:

1. Continue CPR until the defibrillator is charged.
2. Apply hands-free defibrillator pads to the chest, one on the upper right chest above the nipple and the other on the left side below the breast tissue. If hands-free pads are not available, apply conductive material (e.g., gel pads) to the chest.
3. Turn the defibrillator on and select the proper energy level.
4. Make sure the synchronizer switch is turned off.
5. Charge the defibrillator using the button on the defibrillator.
6. Call and look to see that everyone is "all clear." Ensure staff are not touching the patient or the bed at the time of discharge, and the O_2 source is away from the patient.
7. Deliver the charge by depressing the shock button on the defibrillator or the buttons on the paddles simultaneously while pushing down with at least 15 pounds of pressure (7.5 kg).

120 to 200 joules. Recommendations for monophasic defibrillators include an initial shock at 360 joules. After the first shock, start CPR immediately, beginning with chest compressions.

We can perform rapid defibrillation using a manual or automatic device. Manual defibrillators require you to interpret heart rhythms, determine the need for a shock, and deliver a shock. An **automatic external defibrillator (AED)** can detect heart rhythms and tell the user to deliver a shock using hands-free defibrillator pads. Proficiency in AED use is part of the basic life support course for health care professionals. Be familiar with the operation of the type of defibrillator used in your clinical setting.

The general steps taken for defibrillation are listed in Table 39.10.

! SAFETY ALERT

Defibrillation and Cardioversion

- Check that the synchronizer switch is OFF for defibrillation.
- Turn the synchronizer switch ON for cardioversion.
- Never apply defibrillator pads over a pacemaker or implantable cardioverter-defibrillator.
- Be certain that personnel and O_2 equipment are "all clear" before discharging the device.

Synchronized Cardioversion

Synchronized cardioversion is the therapy of choice for patients with ventricular tachydysrhythmias (e.g., VT with a pulse) or supraventricular tachydysrhythmias (e.g., atrial flutter with RVR). A synchronized circuit in the defibrillator delivers a shock on the R wave of the QRS complex of the ECG. The synchronizer switch must be turned on when performing cardioversion.

The procedure for synchronized cardioversion is the same as for defibrillation with a few exceptions (Table 39.11). If synchronized cardioversion is done on a nonemergency basis (e.g., the patient is awake and hemodynamically stable), we sedate the patient with IV agents (e.g., midazolam, fentanyl) beforehand. Pay strict attention to maintaining the patient's airway. If a patient with SVT or VT with a pulse becomes hemodynamically unstable, synchronized cardioversion should be done as quickly as possible. Start the initial energy for synchronized cardioversion at 50 to 100 joules (biphasic defibrillator) and 100 joules (monophasic defibrillator) and increase if needed. Atrial fibrillation requires a higher starting energy level in joules than SVT or VT with a pulse. If the patient becomes pulseless or the rhythm changes to VF, turn the synchronizer switch off and perform defibrillation.

TABLE 39.11 NURSING MANAGEMENT

Assisting With Cardioversion

Preprocedure

- Obtain 12-lead ECG and initiate ECG monitoring.
- Perform baseline assessment, including vital signs, pulse oximetry. Note any manifestations of the dysrhythmia.
- Withhold food and fluids per institution policy.
- Assess baseline laboratory values (e.g., cardiac biomarkers, electrolytes).
- Teach patient and caregiver about procedure and postprocedure care.
- Remove all metallic objects, dentures, and transdermal patches. You may need to clip or remove chest hair.
- Establish IV access.
- Give sedative and other drugs, as ordered.

Postprocedure

- Maintain patent airway and administer O_2 as needed.
- Monitor ECG for dysrhythmias or other changes (e.g., ST segment elevation).
- Perform assessment and compare to baseline: vital signs, pulse oximetry, and heart and breath sounds.
- Assess level of consciousness and reorient as needed.
- Administer IV dysrhythmic and analgesic medications as ordered.
- Assess for burns and provide skin care.

Implantable Cardioverter-Defibrillator

The *implantable cardioverter-defibrillator* (ICD) is an important technology for patients who (1) have survived SCD, (2) have spontaneous sustained VT, (3) have syncope with inducible VT or VF during EPS, or (4) are at high risk for future life-threatening dysrhythmias (e.g., have cardiomyopathy). The use of ICDs has significantly decreased mortality rates in these patients.[10]

The ICD consists of a lead system placed via a subclavian vein to the endocardium. A battery-powered pulse generator is implanted subcutaneously, usually over the pectoral muscle on the nondominant side. The pulse generator is similar in size to a pacemaker. Most systems are single-lead systems (Fig. 39.23). The ICD sensing system monitors the HR and rhythm and identifies VT or VF. After the sensing system detects a lethal dysrhythmia, the device delivers a 25-joule or lower shock to the patient's heart. If the first shock is unsuccessful, the device recycles and can continue to deliver shocks.

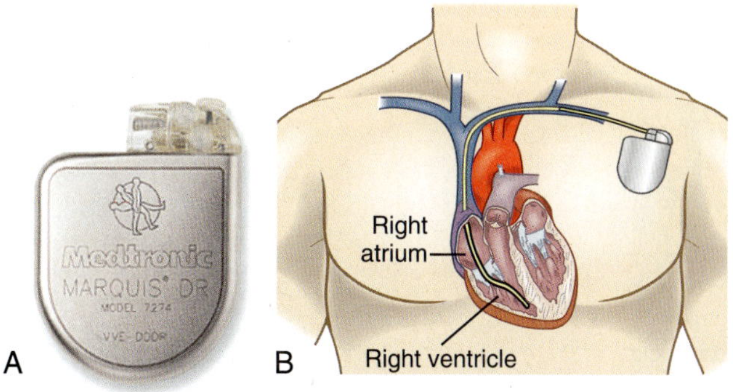

Fig. 39.23 (A) The implantable cardioverter-defibrillator (ICD) pulse generator from Medtronic, Inc. (B) The ICD is placed in a subcutaneous pocket over the pectoral muscle. A single-lead system is placed transvenously from the pulse generator to the endocardium. The single lead detects dysrhythmias and delivers an electric shock to the heart muscle. (Courtesy Medtronic, Inc., Minneapolis, MN.)

In addition to defibrillation capabilities, ICDs have *antitachycardia* and *antibradycardia pacing* capabilities. These devices use algorithms that detect dysrhythmias and determine the appropriate response. They can start *overdrive pacing* of SVT and VT, sparing the patient painful defibrillator shocks. They can provide backup pacing for bradydysrhythmias that may occur after defibrillation. Nursing care of patients undergoing ICD placement is similar to the care of patients undergoing permanent pacemaker implantation.

Patients with structural or congenital cardiac anomalies may receive a subcutaneous ICD (S-ICD).[10] The S-ICD pulse generator is placed under the skin on the left side of the chest with the electrode under the skin above the sternum. The system delivers a shock if it detects VT or VF. Since the S-ICD does not have any electrodes implanted in the heart, it has no pacing capability.

Teaching patients receiving an ICD and the caregiver is important. Patients may have a variety of emotions. These include fear of body image change, fear of recurrent dysrhythmias, expectation of pain with ICD discharge (described as a feeling of a blow to the chest), and anxiety about going home. Encourage patients and caregivers to take part in local or online ICD support groups. Table 39.12 presents a teaching guide for patients with an ICD and their caregivers.

Pacemakers

The artificial **cardiac pacemaker** is an electronic device used to pace the heart when the normal conduction pathway is damaged. The basic pacing circuit consists of a power source (battery-powered pulse generator) with programmable circuitry, 1 or more pacing leads, and the myocardium. The electrical signal (stimulus) travels from the pulse generator, through the leads, to the wall of the myocardium. The heart muscle is "captured" and stimulated to contract (Fig. 39.24).

Current pacemakers are small, sophisticated, and precise. They pace the atrium and/or 1 or both ventricles. Most pacemakers are *demand pacemakers*. This means that they sense the heart's electrical activity and fire only when the HR drops below a preset rate. Demand pacemakers have 2 distinct features: (1) a sensing device that inhibits the pacemaker when the HR is adequate and (2) a pacing device that triggers the pacemaker when no QRS complexes occur within a preset time.

In addition to antibradycardia pacing, devices now include antitachycardia and overdrive pacing. *Antitachycardia pacing*

TABLE 39.12 PATIENT & CAREGIVER TEACHING

Implantable Cardioverter-Defibrillator (ICD)

Include the following information in the teaching plan for a patient receiving an ICD and the patient's caregiver:

1. Follow up with your HCP for routine checks of the function of the ICD. This is often done by interrogating the device using a telephone.
2. Report any signs of infection at incision site (e.g., redness, swelling, drainage) or fever to your HCP at once.
3. Keep incision dry for 4 days after insertion or as instructed.
4. Avoid lifting arm on ICD side above shoulder until approved.
5. Discuss resuming sexual activity with your HCP. It is usually safe to resume sexual activity once your incision is healed.
6. Do not drive until cleared by your HCP. This decision is usually based on the ongoing presence of dysrhythmias, the frequency of ICD firings, your overall health, and state laws about drivers with ICDs.
7. Avoid direct blows to ICD site.
8. Avoid large magnets and strong electromagnetic fields because these may interfere with the device.
9. You should not have an MRI unless the ICD is approved as MRI safe or there is a protocol in place for patient safety during the procedure.
10. Travel is not restricted. Tell security (e.g., airport, train station, public buildings) of presence of ICD because it may set off the metal detector. Hand-held screening wands should not be placed directly over the ICD. Manufacturer information may vary about the effect of metal detectors on the function of the ICD.
11. Do not stand near antitheft devices in doorways of stores and public buildings. Walk through them at a normal pace.
12. If your ICD fires once, call your HCP right away. If you feel sick or if it fires more than once, contact the emergency response system.
13. Always wear a Medic Alert ID device.
14. Always carry the ICD identification card and a current list of your drugs.
15. Consider joining an ICD support group.
16. Caregivers should learn cardiopulmonary resuscitation (CPR).

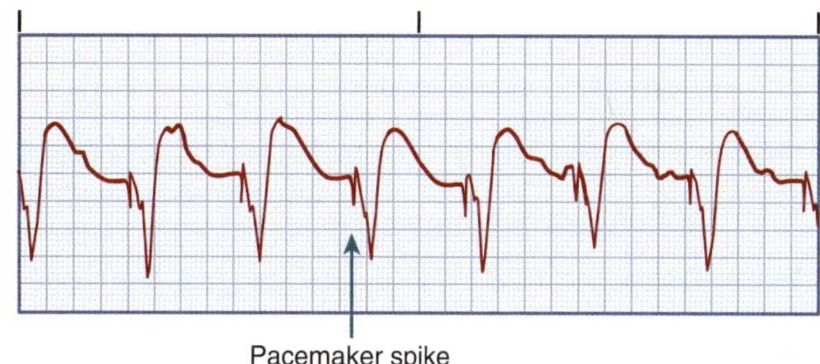

Fig. 39.24 Ventricular capture (depolarization) from signal *(pacemaker spike)* from pacemaker lead in the right ventricle.

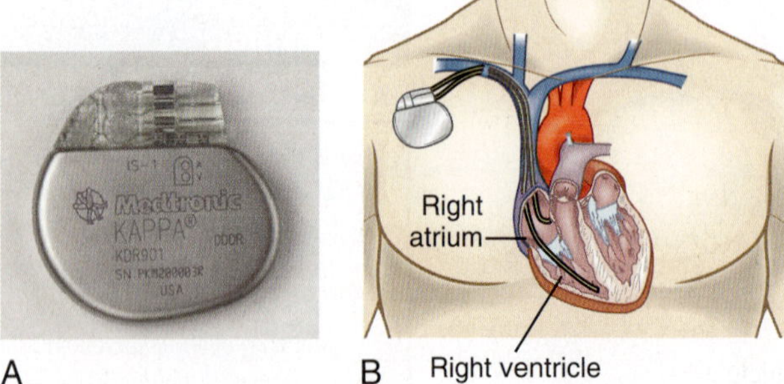

Fig. 39.25 (A) A dual-chamber rate-responsive pacemaker from Medtronic, Inc., is designed to treat patients with chronic heart problems in which the heart beats too slowly to support the body's circulation needs. (B) Pacing leads in both the atrium and the ventricle enable a dual-chamber pacemaker to sense and pace in both heart chambers. (Courtesy Medtronic, Inc., Minneapolis, MN.)

TABLE 39.13 Indications for Permanent Pacemakers

- Acquired AV block
- Second-degree AV block
- Third-degree AV block
- Atrial fibrillation with a slow ventricular response
- Bundle branch block
- Cardiomyopathy
  - Dilated
  - Hypertrophic
- HF
- SA node dysfunction
- Symptomatic bradycardia with unknown cause
- Tachydysrhythmias (e.g., ventricular tachycardia)

involves the delivery of a stimulus to the ventricle to end tachydysrhythmias (e.g., VT). Overdrive pacing involves pacing the atrium at rates of 200 to 500 impulses per minute to try to stop atrial tachycardias (e.g., atrial flutter with an RVR).

Permanent Pacemaker

A *permanent pacemaker* is totally implanted within the body (Fig. 39.25). The power source is placed subcutaneously, usually over the pectoral muscle on the nondominant side. The pacing leads are placed transvenously to the right atrium and/or 1 or both ventricles and attached to the power source. Common reasons for insertion of a permanent pacemaker are found in Table 39.13.

New technology and research are focused on miniaturized, leadless permanent pacemakers. Single-component devices have the battery, sensors, electronics, and stimulating electrodes in a small capsule that is placed in the ventricle using a deflatable sheath. A multicomponent device has a small "seed" that is placed in a cardiac chamber. It acts as an energy transducer while an outside piece beams ultrasound (or radio waves) to the seed. The seed converts the energy to a pacing pulse. The lack of a transvenous lead and subcutaneous pulse generator is a major shift in cardiac pacing.[11] Other research is focusing on making permanent pacemakers without batteries.

TABLE 39.14 Common Indications for Temporary Pacemakers

- Maintain adequate HR and rhythm during special circumstances
  - During surgery and postoperative recovery
  - During cardiac catheterization or coronary angioplasty
  - With drug therapy that may cause bradycardia
  - Before implantation of a permanent pacemaker
- Prophylaxis after open heart surgery
- Acute anterior MI with second- or third-degree AV block or bundle branch block
- Acute inferior MI with symptomatic bradycardia and AV block
- EPS to evaluate patient with bradydysrhythmias and tachydysrhythmias

Cardiac Resynchronization Therapy

Cardiac resynchronization therapy (CRT) is a pacing technique that resynchronizes the heart cycle by pacing both ventricles *(biventricular pacing)*. This promotes improvement in ventricular function. Most patients with HF have intraventricular conduction delays causing abnormal ventricular contraction. This causes dyssynchrony between the right and left ventricles and results in reduced systolic function, pump inefficiency, and worsened HF. Patients with severe left ventricular dysfunction may have devices that combine CRT with an ICD.

Temporary Pacemaker

A *temporary pacemaker* is one that has the power source outside the body. There are 3 types of temporary pacemakers: transvenous, epicardial, and transcutaneous. Table 39.14 lists common reasons for temporary pacing.

A *transvenous pacemaker* consists of a lead or leads that are threaded transvenously to the right atrium and/or right ventricle and attached to the external power source (Fig. 39.26). Most of these pacemakers are inserted in the ED or ICU in emergency situations. They provide a bridge to inserting a permanent pacemaker or resolving the underlying cause of the dysrhythmia.

Epicardial pacing involves attaching an atrial and a ventricular pacing lead to the epicardium during heart surgery. The leads are passed through the chest wall and attached to the external power source. Epicardial pacing leads are placed in case a bradydysrhythmia or tachydysrhythmia occurs in the early postoperative period.

A *transcutaneous pacemaker* can provide adequate HR and rhythm to the patient in an emergency. Placement of a TCP is a noninvasive, temporary procedure used until a transvenous pacemaker is inserted or more definitive therapy is available.[6]

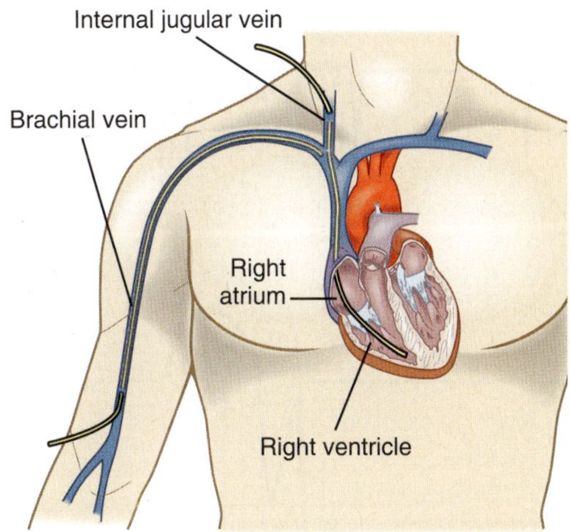

Fig. 39.26 Temporary transvenous pacemaker catheter insertion. A single lead is positioned in the right ventricle through the brachial, subclavian, jugular, or femoral vein.

The TCP consists of a power source and a rate- and voltage-control device that attaches to 2 large, multifunction electrode pads. Position 1 pad on the anterior part of the chest, usually on the V_4 lead position. Place the other pad on the back between the spine and left scapula at the level of the heart (Fig. 39.27). When programming the TCP, use the lowest current that results in a ventricular contraction (capture) to minimize patient discomfort.

Before starting TCP therapy, it is important to tell the patient what to expect. Explain that the muscle contractions created by the pacemaker when the current passes through the chest wall are uncomfortable. Reassure the patient that the TCP is temporary and that it will be replaced by a transvenous or permanent pacemaker as soon as possible. If possible, provide analgesia and/or sedation while the TCP is in use.

Monitoring Patients With Pacemakers

Patients with temporary or permanent pacemakers are ECG monitored to evaluate the status of the pacemaker. Pacemaker malfunction involves a failure to sense, a failure to capture, or a failure to pace. *Failure to sense* occurs when the pacemaker does not recognize spontaneous atrial or ventricular activity, and it fires inappropriately (Fig. 39.28A). This can result in the pacemaker firing during the excitable period of the cardiac cycle and the potential for VT. Causes of failure to sense include fibrosis around the tip of the pacing lead, battery failure, sensing set too high, or dislodgment of the electrode.

Failure to capture occurs when the electrical charge to the myocardium is insufficient to produce atrial or ventricular contraction (Fig. 39.28B). This can result in serious bradycardia or asystole. Common causes include pacer lead damage, battery

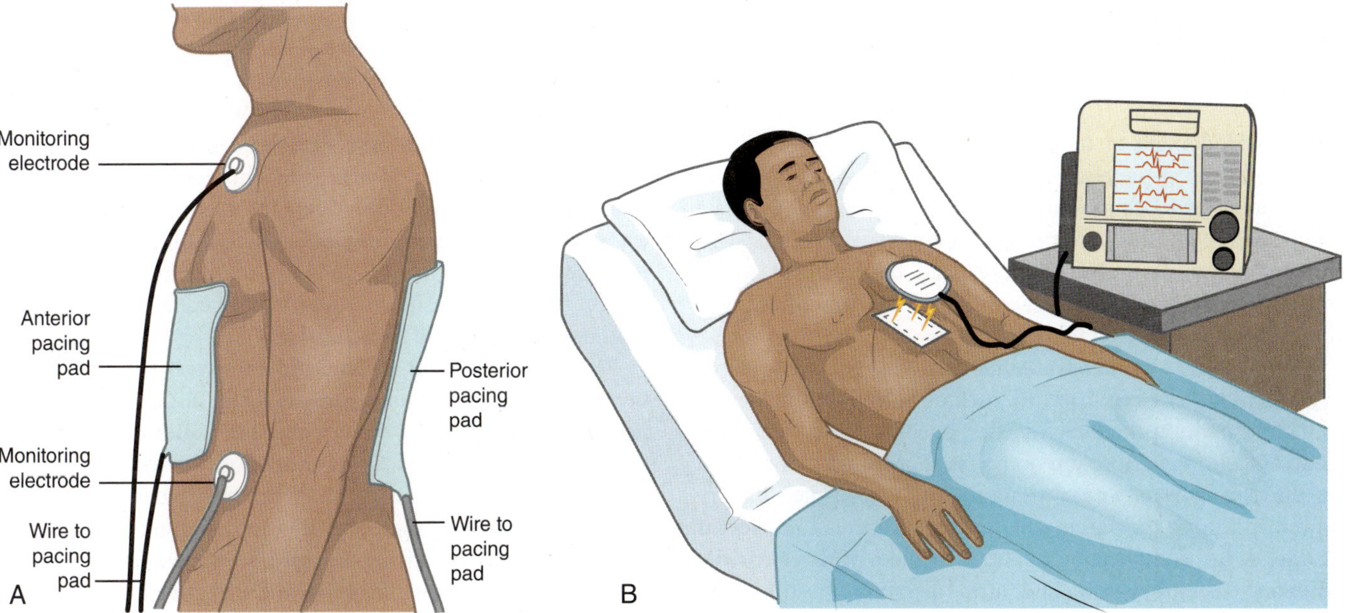

Fig. 39.27 Transcutaneous pacemaker. Pacing electrodes are placed on the anterior and posterior chest walls (A) and attached to an external pacing unit (B).

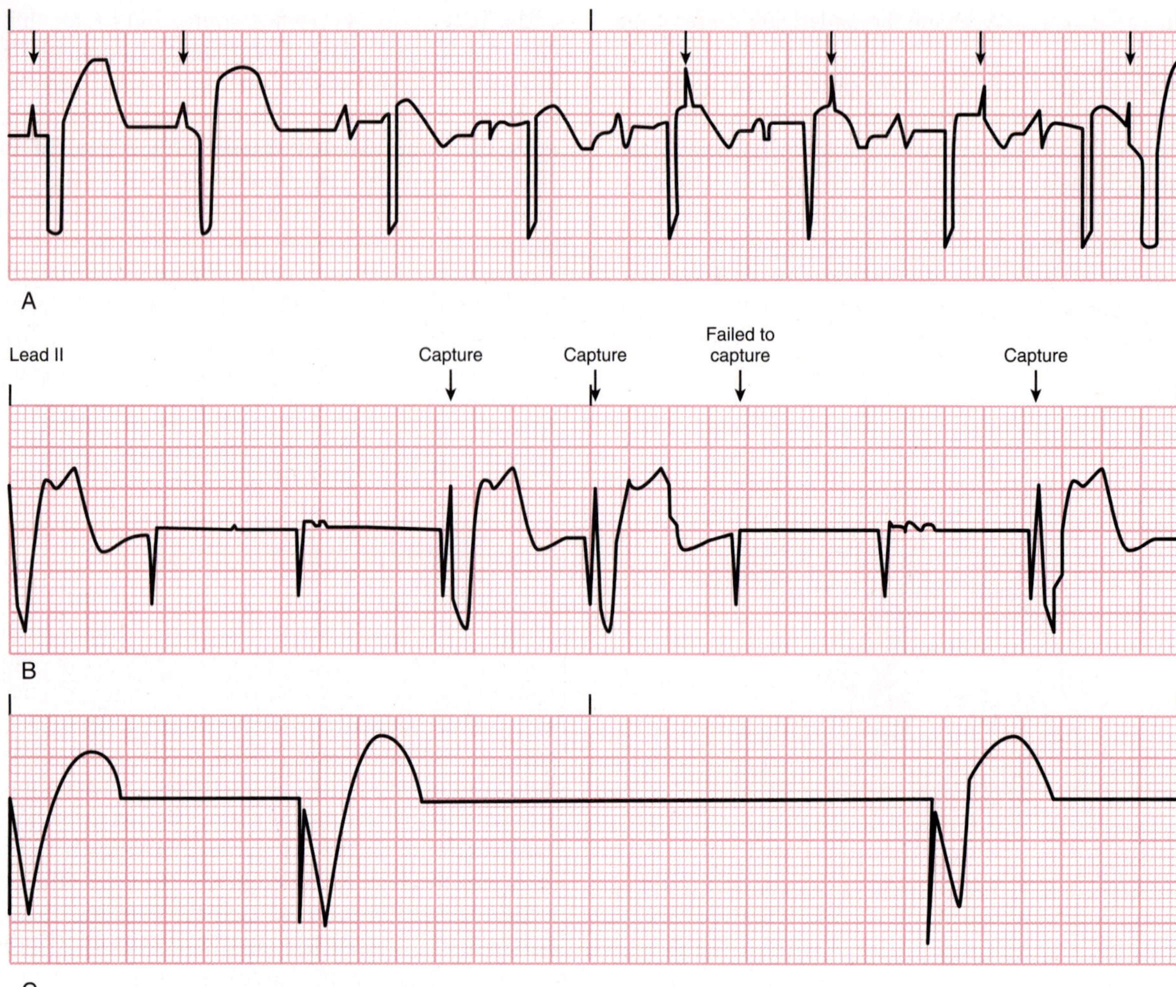

Fig. 39.28 Causes of pacemaker malfunction. (A) Failure to sense: the pacemaker does not sense the patient's own cardiac rhythm and initiates an electrical impulse. Failure to sense manifests as pacer spikes that fall too closely to the patient's own rhythm, earlier than the programmed rate (see *arrows*). (B) Failure to capture: a pacer spike is noted but is not followed by a P wave (atrial pacemaker) or a QRS complex (ventricular pacemaker). (C) Failure to pace: the pacemaker fails to initiate an electrical stimulus when it should fire.

failure, dislodgment of the electrode, electrical charge set too low, or fibrosis at the electrode tip.

Failure to pace occurs when the pacemaker does not initiate an electrical stimulus when it should fire (Fig. 39.28C). This can happen from a wire fracture, lead displacement, oversensing, or electrical interference. Table 39.15 describes pacemaker troubleshooting.

Complications of invasive temporary (e.g., transvenous) or permanent pacemaker insertion include infection and hematoma formation at the insertion site, pneumothorax, failure to sense or capture, perforation of the atrial or ventricular septum by the pacing lead, and appearance of "end-of-life" battery power on testing the pacemaker. Several measures can prevent or assess for complications. These include prophylactic IV antibiotic therapy before and after insertion, postinsertion chest x-ray to check lead placement and to rule out a pneumothorax, careful observation of insertion site, and continuous ECG monitoring of the patient's rhythm.

After pacemaker insertion, patients can be out of bed once stable. Have them limit arm and shoulder activity on the operative side to prevent dislodging the newly implanted pacing leads. Observe the insertion site for signs of bleeding and check that the incision is intact. Note any temperature elevation or pain at the insertion site and treat as ordered. Most patients are discharged by the next day if stable.

Table 39.16 outlines patient and caregiver teaching for patients with a pacemaker. Patients with a newly implanted pacemaker and their caregivers may have questions about activity restrictions and concerns about body image. The goals of pacemaker therapy include enhancing physiologic functioning and quality of life. Emphasize this to patients and caregivers and provide specific advice on activity restrictions.

After discharge, patients need to check pacemaker function on a regular basis. This can include outpatient visits to a pacemaker clinic or home monitoring using telephone transmitter devices. Another method to evaluate pacemaker

TABLE 39.15 NURSING MANAGEMENT

Troubleshooting Pacemakers

Problem	Potential Solution
General concern about pacemaker function	• Monitor continuous ECG and patient's vital signs while troubleshooting pacemaker problems • Call emergency response services if needed • Contact HCP if basic troubleshooting does not work, as patient could have a lead wire displaced or a defective lead wire
Temporary pacemaker not firing	• Check to make sure all connections are hooked up correctly and tight • Ensure that hands-free pads have contact with the skin (shave excess hair, dry off perspiration) • Check that the generator has power (plug in the equipment or use a new battery each time)
Temporary pacemaker not capturing	• Check connections • Check for generator power • Turn up the milliamps on the generator, look for capture, and set 10 milliamps above capture • Place patient on left side to promote contact of the transvenous pacing wire with the epicardium
Temporary pacemaker not sensing patient's underlying rhythm	• Check connections • Check for generator power • Turn up sensitivity • Place patient on left side
Permanent pacemaker not working	• Contact HCP • Contact pacemaker company for service if requested by HCP

performance is noninvasive program stimulation. This procedure is done on an outpatient basis in the EPS laboratory.

TABLE 39.16 PATIENT & CAREGIVER TEACHING

Pacemaker

Include the following information in the teaching plan for a patient with a pacemaker and the patient's caregiver:

1. Maintain follow-up care with your HCP to begin regular pacemaker function checks. This is often done by checking the device using a telephone.
2. Report any signs of infection at incision site (e.g., redness, swelling, drainage) or fever to your HCP at once.
3. Keep incision dry for 4 days after implantation, or as ordered.
4. Avoid lifting arm on pacemaker side above shoulder until approved by your cardiologist.
5. Avoid direct blows to pacemaker site.
6. Avoid proximity to high-output electric generators because these can interfere with the function of the pacemaker.
7. You should not have an MRI unless the pacemaker is approved as MRI safe or there is a protocol in place for patient safety during the procedure.
8. Microwave ovens are safe to use and do not interfere with pacemaker function.
9. Avoid standing near antitheft devices in doorways of department stores and public libraries. Walk through them at a normal pace.
10. Travel is not restricted. Tell security (e.g., airport, train station, public buildings) of presence of pacemaker because it may set off the metal detector. Hand-held screening wands should not be placed directly over the pacemaker. Manufacturer information may vary about the effect of metal detectors on the function of the pacemaker.
11. Monitor pulse and tell your HCP if heart rate drops below predetermined rate.
12. Always carry your pacemaker information card and a current list of drugs.
13. Always wear a Medic Alert ID device.
14. Consider joining a pacemaker support group (e.g., www.pacemakerclub.com/).

Radiofrequency Catheter Ablation Therapy

Radiofrequency catheter ablation therapy uses electrical energy to "burn" or ablate areas of the conduction system. Ablation therapy is done after EPS has identified the source of the dysrhythmia. An electrode-tipped ablation catheter ablates accessory pathways or ectopic sites in the atria, AV node, and ventricles. Catheter ablation is a definitive treatment for tachydysrhythmias. It is the nonpharmacologic treatment of choice for atrial dysrhythmias resulting in rapid ventricular rates and AV nodal reentrant tachycardia refractory to drug therapy.

The ablation procedure is an effective treatment with a low complication rate. Nursing care of patients after ablation therapy is similar to that of patients undergoing cardiac catheterization (see Chapter 35 and Table 35.12).

SYNCOPE

Syncope is a brief lapse in consciousness accompanied by a loss in postural tone (fainting). The causes of syncope can be cardiovascular or noncardiovascular. The most common cause of syncope is cardioneurogenic syncope, or "vasovagal" syncope (e.g., carotid sinus sensitivity). Other cardiovascular causes relate to dysrhythmias (e.g., tachycardias, bradycardias), prosthetic valve malfunction, pulmonary emboli, and HF. Noncardiovascular causes vary and include stress, hypoglycemia, dehydration, stroke, and seizure.[12]

A diagnostic workup for patients with syncope from a suspected heart cause begins with ruling out structural and ischemic heart disease. This is done with echocardiography and stress testing. EPS is used to diagnose atrial and ventricular tachydysrhythmias and conduction problems causing bradydysrhythmias, all of which can cause syncope. These problems can be treated with antidysrhythmic drug therapy, pacemakers, ICDs, and/or catheter ablation therapy.

Patients without structural heart disease or in whom EPS testing is not diagnostic may have a *head-up tilt-test.* Normally, an upright position results in gravity displacing 300 to

800 mL of blood to the lower extremities. Specialized nerve fibers called mechanoreceptors are found throughout the vascular system. These respond to the increased blood volume with a reflex increase in sympathetic stimulation and decrease in parasympathetic output. The end results are a slight increase in HR and diastolic BP and a slight decrease in systolic BP.

In cardioneurogenic syncope, the increased venous pooling in the upright position reduces venous return to the heart. This results in a sudden, compensatory increase in ventricular contraction. The brain mistakenly thinks this is a hypertensive state and stops sympathetic stimulation. This produces a paradoxical vasodilation and bradycardia (vasovagal response). The end results are bradycardia, hypotension, cerebral hypoperfusion, and syncope.

In the head-up tilt-test, the patient is placed on a table supported by a belt across the torso and feet. We obtain baseline ECG, BP, and HR with the patient in the horizontal position. Next, the table is tilted 60 to 80 degrees. The patient stays in this upright position for 20 to 60 minutes. We record ECG and HR continuously. BP is measured every 3 minutes throughout the test.

If the patient's BP and HR responses are abnormal and clinical symptoms occur (e.g., faintness), the test is positive. If after 30 minutes there is no response, the table is returned to the horizontal position, and an IV infusion of low-dose isoproterenol may be given to test for a response.

Other diagnostic tests for syncope use recording devices (e.g., Holter monitor or event monitor/loop recorder; see Table 35.11), blood volume determination, hemodynamic testing, and autonomic reflex testing. About 30% of those who have 1 episode of syncope have a recurrence. The underlying cause of syncope and the patient's age and comorbidities affect the treatment and prognosis.[12]

CASE STUDY

Ventricular Dysrhythmias

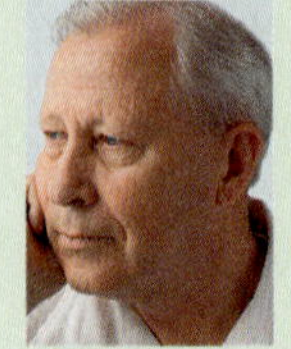

(© iStockphoto/ Thinkstock.)

Patient Profile

J.M., a 54-year-old teacher, came to the emergency department with shortness of breath, chest discomfort, and a "racing heart." J.M. is alert and oriented and able to answer all your questions with short responses.

Subjective Data

- History of hypertension, diabetes type 2
- No known drug allergies
- Takes 500 mg metformin twice daily
- States this has never happened before, and he is scared
- Reports 7/10 midsternal chest pain

Objective Data

Physical Assessment

- Appears anxious, scared, diaphoretic
- BP 86/54 mm Hg, HR 230 beats/min, respirations 24/min
- Lungs clear bilaterally
- Heart: no murmurs or gallops, regular

Diagnostic Studies

- 12-Lead ECG shows wide complex ventricular tachycardia
- Serum cardiac biomarkers negative
- Serum potassium 2.8 mEq/L (2.8 mmol/L)
- Glucose 162 mg/dL

One hour after arrival, J.M. suddenly becomes unresponsive with no heart rate or respirations.

The ECG shows that the rhythm has changed to the irregular waves of ventricular fibrillation.

Discussion Questions

1. ***Recognize:*** Interpret the rhythm J.M. is currently in.
2. ***Analyze:*** What are the important findings now and from J.M.'s history?
3. ***Plan:*** What treatment would you expect based on J.M.'s condition?
4. ***Prioritize:*** What is the most important intervention that needs to be done immediately for J.M.?
5. ***Act:*** What other interventions would you need to implement for J.M.?
6. ***Evaluate:*** What outcome would indicate the immediate interventions were successful?
7. ***Safety:*** What safety precautions should be considered when performing interventions?

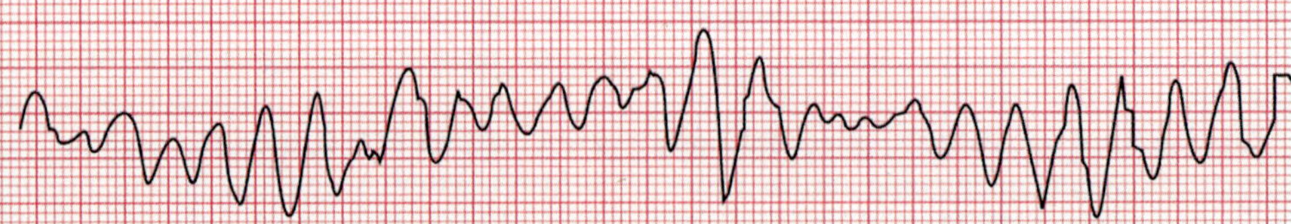

Answers available at http://evolve.elsevier.com/Lewis/medsurg.

BRIDGE TO NCLEX EXAMINATION

The number of the question corresponds to the same-numbered outcome at the beginning of the chapter.

1. A patient with syncope has continuous ECG monitoring. The rhythm strip shows: atrial rate 74 beats/min and regular; ventricular rate 62 beats/min and irregular; P wave normal shape; PR interval lengthens progressively until a P wave is not conducted; QRS normal shape. Which action would the nurse *prioritize?*
   a. Administer epinephrine 1 mg IV push.
   b. Prepare the patient for synchronized cardioversion.
   c. Observe for symptoms of hypotension and angina.
   d. Apply transcutaneous pacemaker pads on the patient.
2. The ECG monitor of a patient in the cardiac care unit after an MI shows ventricular bigeminy with a rate of 50 beats/min. Which action would the nurse take?
   a. Perform defibrillation.
   b. Administer IV amiodarone.
   c. Prepare for pacemaker insertion.
   d. Assess the patient for symptoms.
3. Which findings indicate decreased cardiac output in a patient with supraventricular tachycardia?
   a. Hypertension and dyspnea
   b. Chest pain and palpitations
   c. Abdominal distention and tachypnea
   d. Bounding pulses and a systolic murmur
4. Which information would the nurse consider when preparing a patient for elective synchronized cardioversion?
   a. Defibrillation delivers a lower dose of electrical energy.
   b. Cardioversion is a treatment for atrial bradydysrhythmias.
   c. Defibrillation delivers a shock during the QRS complex.
   d. Cardioversion is painful for an awake patient.
5. Which patient teaching points would the nurse include when providing discharge instructions to a patient with a new permanent pacemaker? **(Select all that apply.)**
   a. Avoid or limit air travel.
   b. Take and record a daily pulse rate.
   c. Obtain and wear a Medic Alert ID device at all times.
   d. Avoid lifting arm on the side of the pacemaker above the shoulder.
   e. Do not use a microwave oven because it interferes with pacemaker function.
6. Which information would the nurse teach the patient scheduled for a radiofrequency catheter ablation procedure?
   a. Ventricular bradycardia may be induced and treated during the procedure.
   b. A catheter will be placed in both femoral arteries to allow double-catheter intervention.
   c. The procedure will destroy areas of the conduction system that are causing rapid heart rhythms.
   d. General anesthetic will be given to prevent the awareness of any "sudden cardiac death" experiences.

1. c; 2. d; 3. b; 4. d; 5. b, c, d; 6. c.

For rationales to these answers and even more NCLEX review questions, visit http://evolve.elsevier.com/Lewis/medsurg.

REFERENCES

To access the References for this chapter, please scan the QR code with a mobile device.

40

Inflammatory and Structural Heart Disorders

Patricia Keegan and Leslie Ogburn

http://evolve.elsevier.com/Lewis/medsurg/

CONCEPTUAL FOCUS

Functional Ability
Infection
Inflammation
Perfusion

LEARNING OUTCOMES

1. Describe the pathophysiology, clinical manifestations, and interprofessional and nursing management of patients with infective endocarditis and pericarditis.
2. Describe the pathophysiology, clinical manifestations, and interprofessional and nursing management of patients with myocarditis.
3. Distinguish the etiology, pathophysiology, and clinical manifestations of rheumatic fever and rheumatic heart disease.
4. Describe the interprofessional and nursing management of patients with rheumatic heart disease.
5. Describe the pathophysiology, clinical manifestations, and interprofessional and nursing management of patients with heart valve disease.
6. Relate the pathophysiology, clinical manifestations, and interprofessional and nursing management of patients with different types of cardiomyopathy.

KEY TERMS

aortic regurgitation (AR)
aortic stenosis (AS)
cardiac tamponade
cardiomyopathy (CMP)
dilated cardiomyopathy
hypertrophic cardiomyopathy
infective endocarditis (IE)
mitral valve prolapse (MVP)
myocarditis
pericardiocentesis
pericarditis
regurgitation
rheumatic fever (RF)
rheumatic heart disease (RHD)
stenosis

This chapter focuses on patients with select inflammatory and structural heart problems. Inflammatory, infectious, and structural problems impair cardiac output (CO), which leads to decreased tissue perfusion. Patients may have pain, fever, and decreased functional and cognitive ability. The nurse plays a key role in providing patients with the education needed to manage problems and their effects.

INFLAMMATORY HEART PROBLEMS

INFECTIVE ENDOCARDITIS

Infective endocarditis (IE) is a disease of the *endocardium* (the innermost layer of the heart) and the heart valves (Fig. 40.1). The number of IE cases and deaths has increased sharply during the last 30 years.[1] Despite advances in antimicrobial and surgical therapy, IE remains a major clinical problem with mortality rates of 20% to 25%.[2] IE is a therapeutic challenge, as treatment approaches are often ineffective.

Classification

We often classify IE based on the cause (e.g., IV drug use IE [IVDA IE], fungal IE) or site of involvement (e.g., prosthetic valve endocarditis [PVE]). We also describe IE as subacute or acute. *Subacute IE* affects those with preexisting valve disease over a period of months. *Acute IE* affects those with healthy valves and appears as a rapidly progressive illness.

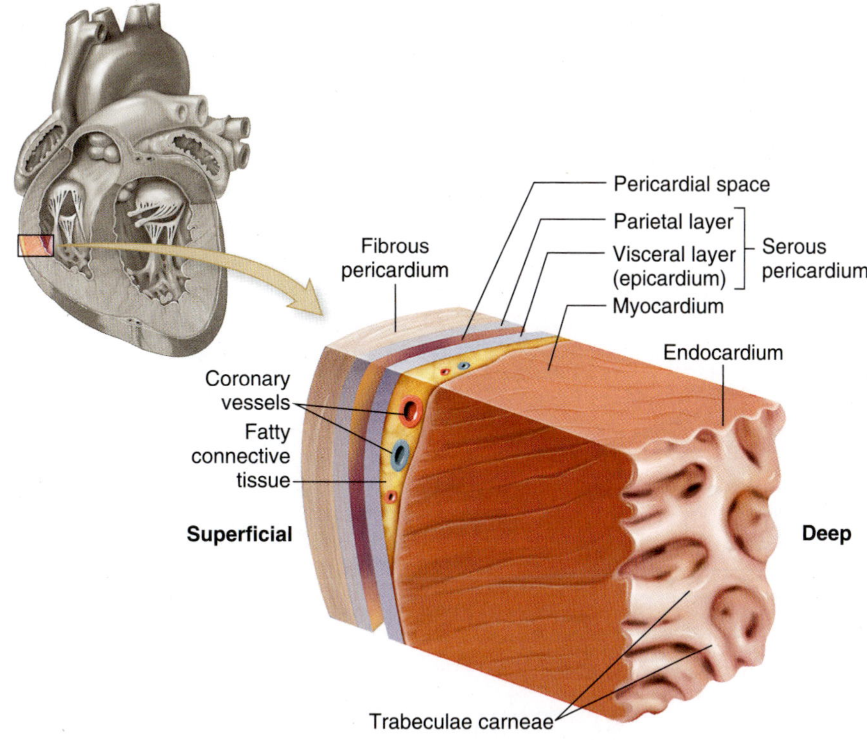

Fig. 40.1 Layers of the heart muscle and pericardium. The section of the heart wall shows the fibrous pericardium, the parietal and visceral layers of the serous pericardium (with the pericardial sac between them), the myocardium, and the endocardium. (Modified from Patton KT, Bell FB, Thompson T, et al: *Anatomy & physiology,* ed 11, St Louis, 2022, Elsevier.)

TABLE 40.1 Common Risk Factors for Endocarditis

Cardiac Conditions
- Cardiomyopathy
- Congenital heart disease
- Heart lesions (e.g., ventricular septal defect, asymmetric septal hypertrophy)
- Marfan syndrome
- Pacemaker
- Prior infective endocarditis
- Prosthetic heart valve(s)
- Rheumatic heart disease
- Valve disease

Noncardiac Conditions
- Hospital-acquired bacteremia
- IV drug use

Procedure-Associated
- Intravascular devices (e.g., central venous catheter)
- Procedures listed in Table 40.2

Etiology and Pathophysiology

Persons with a number of cardiac and noncardiac conditions can develop IE (Table 40.1). The main risk factors include (1) history of IE, (2) IV drug use, (3) having a prosthetic valve, (4) health care–associated infection from an intravascular device (e.g., methicillin-resistant *Staphylococcus aureus* [MRSA]), and (5) dialysis.[3]

IE occurs when blood flow allows organisms to contact and infect previously damaged heart valves or other endothelial surfaces (Fig. 40.2). About 50% of cases are caused by *S. aureus.*[3] Other bacterial causes include *Streptococcus viridans* and coagulase-negative staphylococci. Besides streptococci, other colonizers of the oropharynx, such as the HACEK organisms (*Haemophilus, Actinobacillus, Cardiobacterium, Eikenella, Kingella*) can cause IE.[1] Bacterial biofilm forms on the endocardium, most often on the aortic and mitral valves. The biofilm protects bacteria from systemic antibiotics and host phagocytic defenses while the bacteria continue to damage the valve tissue.

IE typically develops in 3 stages: (1) bacteremia, (2) adhesion, and (3) vegetation. *Vegetations,* the primary lesions of IE, consist of fibrin, leukocytes, platelets, and microbes that stick to the valve surface or endocardium. The loss of parts of these fragile vegetations into the circulation results in *emboli.* Up to 10.5% of persons with IE develop embolization.[4] Left-sided heart vegetations move to various organs (e.g., brain, kidneys, spleen) and the extremities, causing local infarction. Right-sided heart lesions move to the lungs, causing pulmonary emboli.

The infection may spread locally and damage the valves and their supporting structures. This can cause dysrhythmias and valve dysfunction. Invasion of the myocardium can lead to heart failure (HF), sepsis, and heart block.

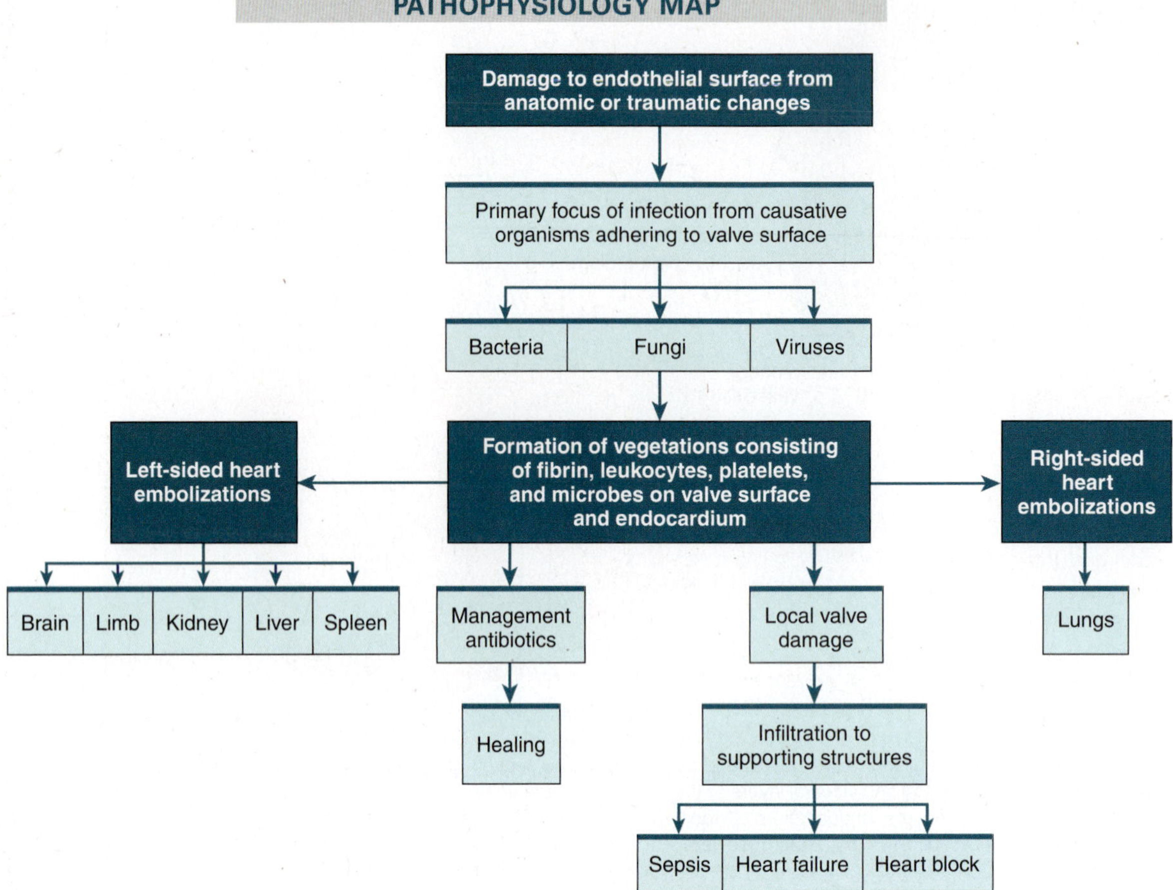

Fig. 40.2 Pathogenesis of IE.

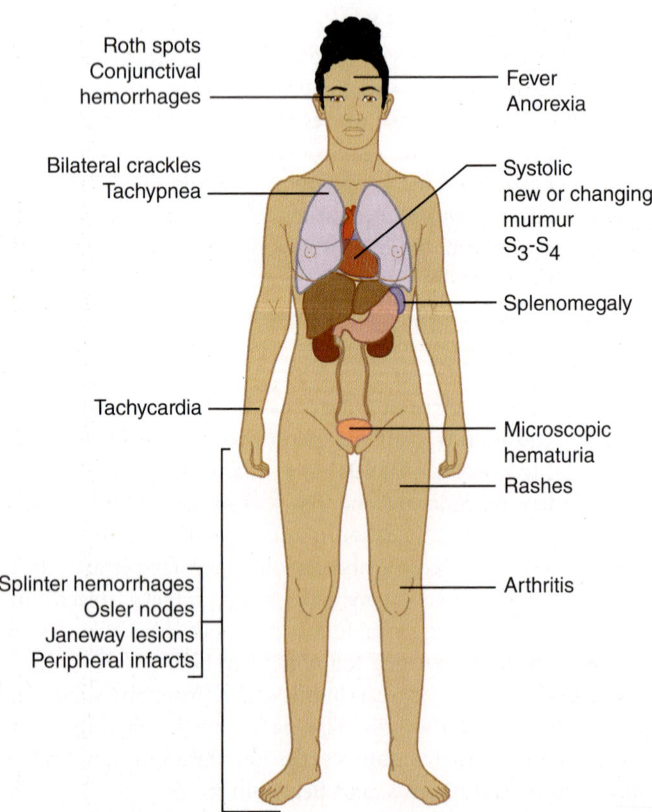

Fig. 40.3 Manifestations of infective endocarditis.

Clinical Manifestations

The manifestations of IE are nonspecific and involve multiple organ systems (Fig. 40.3). Most patients have a fever. Fever may be low grade or absent in older adults or those who are immunocompromised. Other symptoms include chills, weakness, malaise, fatigue, and anorexia.

Vascular signs include *splinter hemorrhages* (black longitudinal streaks) in the nail beds. Petechiae from microembolization of vegetative lesions can occur on the conjunctivae, lips, buccal mucosa, palate, ankles, feet, and antecubital and popliteal areas. *Osler nodes* (painful, tender, red or purple, pea-size lesions) are found on the fingertips or toes. *Janeway lesions* (flat, painless, small, red spots) may be seen on the fingertips, palms, soles of feet, and toes. Eye examination may show hemorrhagic retinal lesions called *Roth spots.*

HF is common. It occurs in up to 80% of patients with aortic valve IE and 50% of those with mitral valve IE. Most patients have a new or worsening systolic murmur. Murmurs are usually absent in tricuspid IE because right-sided heart sounds are too low to be heard. Three in ten patients present with an embolic event such as stroke.[4]

Diagnostic Studies

The diagnosis of IE relies on the assessment, laboratory results, imaging, and cultures.[1] The history is important. Ask patients if they have had any recent (within the last 3 to 6 months) dental, urologic, surgical, or gynecologic procedures, including childbirth. Note a history of IVDA, heart disease, or infections (e.g., skin, respiratory, urinary tract). Have they had a heart catheterization, heart surgery, intravascular device placement, or dialysis?

Three blood cultures drawn over a period of 1 hour from 3 different venipuncture sites will be positive in most patients with IE.[5] Culture-negative IE is associated with antibiotic use within the previous 2 weeks or results from a pathogen not easily detected by standard cultures. Mild leukocytosis occurs in acute IE. The erythrocyte sedimentation rate (ESR) and C-reactive protein (CRP) levels may be increased. Echocardiography can show vegetations.

Guidelines for the diagnosis of IE are based on the Duke criteria. Patients must have 2 major criteria and 1 minor criterion, or 1 major and 3 minor, or 5 minor criteria. Major criteria include positive blood cultures, typical microorganism for IE from 2 separate blood cultures, and evidence of endocardial involvement, such as new valve vegetation. Minor criteria include predisposing heart problem or IV drug use, fever, vascular phenomena, immunologic phenomena, microbiologic evidence, or echocardiogram findings consistent with IE but not meeting major criteria.

Interprofessional Care

Prophylactic Treatment

Situations and conditions that require antibiotic prophylaxis are detailed in Table 40.2.

TABLE 40.2 Antibiotic Prophylaxis to Prevent Endocarditis

Target Groups for Prophylactic Antibiotics

People with the following heart conditions should receive prophylactic antibiotics when they have the conditions or procedures listed here:

- Congenital heart disease (CHD)
  - Unrepaired cyanotic CHD (including palliative shunts and conduits)
  - Repaired congenital heart defect with prosthetic material or device for 6 months after the procedure
  - Repaired CHD with residual defects at the site or next to the site of prosthetic patch or prosthetic device
- Heart transplant recipients who develop heart valve disease
- History of infective endocarditis (IE)
- Prosthetic heart valve or prosthetic material used to repair heart valve

Conditions or Procedures Requiring Antibiotic Prophylaxis

When the target groups have the following conditions or procedures, they need prophylactic antibiotics:

- Dental manipulation involving the gums, roots of the teeth, or puncture of the oral mucosa
- Respiratory
  - Respiratory tract incisions (e.g., biopsy)
  - Tonsillectomy and adenoidectomy
- Surgery involving infected skin, skin structures, or musculoskeletal tissue

Modified from Nishimura RA, Otto CM, Bonow RO, et al: 2017 focused update of the 2014 AHA/ACC guidelines for the management of patients with valvular heart disease, *Circulation* 135:e1159, 2017.

Drug Therapy

Identifying the causative organism is the key to successfully treating IE. Long-term treatment is needed to kill dormant bacteria within the bacterial biofilm and valve vegetations. Complete removal of the organism generally takes weeks. Relapses are common.

Antibiotic therapy is based on blood culture results. The effectiveness of therapy is assessed with subsequent blood cultures. Cultures that stay positive indicate inadequate or inappropriate antibiotics, an aortic root or myocardial abscess, or the wrong diagnosis (e.g., an infection elsewhere). It is reasonable to obtain 2 sets of blood cultures every 24 to 48 hours until the infection is cleared.[5] After completing antibiotics, follow-up echocardiogram and inflammatory markers are done at 1, 3, 6, and 12 months.

Fungal IE and PVE respond poorly to antibiotic therapy alone. Early valve replacement followed by prolonged (6 weeks or more) antibiotics is needed in these situations. Valve replacement surgery is done in 50% to 60% of cases of IE. Three reasons for surgery are valve dysfunction causing HF, to prevent embolization, or for uncontrolled infection.[1]

! SAFETY ALERT

Communicating Test Results

- If blood culture results for a patient diagnosed with IE show that the organism is not susceptible to the ordered antibiotic, immediately notify the HCP.
- A National Patient Safety Goal stresses the importance of communicating critical test results to the right HCP in a timely manner.

NURSING MANAGEMENT: INFECTIVE ENDOCARDITIS

Assessment

Subjective and objective data to obtain from patients with IE are found in Table 40.3. Assess vital signs together with heart sounds to detect a new murmur, a change in a preexisting murmur, and extra sounds (e.g., S_3).

Arthralgia (joint pain) and myalgias *(muscle pain)* are common. Assess patients for joint or muscle tenderness and decreased range of motion (ROM). Examine patients for petechiae, splinter hemorrhages, and Osler nodes. Complete an assessment for hemodynamic or embolic complications.

Clinical Problems

Clinical problems for patients with IE include:

- Impaired cardiac function
- Infection
- Fatigue
- Substance use

More information on clinical problems and interventions for patients with IE is in eNursing Care Plan 40.1 on the website for this chapter.

TABLE 40.3 NURSING ASSESSMENT

Infective Endocarditis (IE)

Subjective Data

Important Health Information

Health history: Valve, congenital, or syphilitic heart disease, including valve repair or replacement. Previous IE, childbirth, staphylococcal or streptococcal infections, hospital-acquired bacteremia

Medications: Immunosuppressive therapy

Surgery or other treatments: Recent obstetric or gynecologic procedures. Invasive procedures, including catheterization, cystoscopy. Recent dental or surgical procedures, GI procedures (e.g., endoscopy)

Functional Health Patterns

Health perception—health management: IV drug use, alcohol use; malaise

Nutritional-metabolic: Weight gain or loss, anorexia; chills, diaphoresis

Elimination: Bloody urine

Activity-exercise: Exercise intolerance, weakness, fatigue; cough, dyspnea on exertion, orthopnea, palpitations

Sleep-rest: Night sweats

Cognitive-perceptual: Chest, back, or abdominal pain; headache, joint tenderness, muscle tenderness

Objective Data

Cardiovascular

Dysrhythmia, tachycardia, new murmurs, S_3, S_4; retinal hemorrhages

General

Fever

Respiratory

Tachypnea, crackles

Skin

Osler nodes on extremities, splinter hemorrhages under nail beds, Janeway lesions on fingertips, palms, soles of feet, and toes. Petechiae of skin, mucous membranes, or conjunctivae. Purpura, peripheral edema, finger clubbing.

Possible Diagnostic Findings

Leukocytosis, anemia, ↑ ESR, ↑ CRP, and cardiac biomarkers. Positive blood cultures, hematuria. Echocardiogram showing chamber enlargement, valve dysfunction, and vegetations. Chest x-ray showing cardiomegaly and pulmonary infiltrates. ECG showing ischemia and conduction defects. Signs of systemic embolization or pulmonary embolism

◆ Planning

The overall goals for patients with IE include (1) normal or baseline cardiac function, (2) ability to perform activities of daily living (ADLs) without fatigue, and (3) an understanding of the treatment plan to prevent recurrence.

◆ Implementation

Health Promotion

Teach patients at high risk for IE (Tables 40.1 and 40.2) to help reduce the incidence and recurrence of IE. Tell patients to avoid people with infections, especially upper respiratory tract infections, and to report cold, flu, and cough symptoms. Stress the importance of avoiding fatigue, planning rest periods, using good oral hygiene, and scheduling regular dental visits.

Tell patients to inform HCPs scheduling invasive procedures about the history of IE (Table 40.2). Prophylactic antibiotic therapy may be needed. Refer patients with IVDA IE for drug rehabilitation.

Acute Care

Patients with IE have many problems that need nursing management. IE generally requires treatment with antibiotics for 4 to 6 weeks. After initial treatment in the hospital, patients may continue treatment at home if hemodynamically stable and adherent. Assess the home setting for adequate support. Patients who receive outpatient IV antibiotics need vigilant home nursing care.

Monitor laboratory data, including blood cultures, to determine antibiotic effectiveness. Fever is managed with aspirin, acetaminophen, fluids, and rest (see Table 12.5). Teach the patient and caregiver about the importance of monitoring temperature. Persistent fever may mean that the antibiotic is ineffective. Administer analgesia and implement measures to manage pain.

Patients need adequate physical and emotional rest. Bed rest may be needed for patients with fever or complications (e.g., HF). Otherwise, patients may perform moderate activity. To prevent problems related to decreased mobility, have patients wear elastic compression stockings, perform ROM exercises, and deep-breathe and cough every 2 hours. Patients may have anxiety and fear. Offer strategies to help them cope with the illness.

Teach the patient and caregiver the nature of the disease and how to reduce the risk for reinfection. Explain the relationship between follow-up care, good nutrition and dental care, and prompt treatment of common infections (e.g., colds) to stay healthy. Teach patients symptoms to report that may indicate another infection (e.g., fever, fatigue, chills) or a complication (e.g., dyspnea, chest pain, weight gain).

◆ Evaluation

The expected outcomes are that patients with IE will:

- Maintain adequate tissue and organ perfusion
- Maintain normal body temperature
- Report an increase in physical and emotional comfort

ACUTE PERICARDITIS

Pericarditis refers to inflammation of the pericardial layers (Fig. 40.1). It is the most common form of pericardial disease. The cause may be infectious or noninfectious. Common causes of acute pericarditis are listed in Table 40.4. Most often, the cause of acute pericarditis is *idiopathic* (unknown) or viral.[6] About 20% of cases are caused by postcardiac injury.

TABLE 40.4 Common Causes of Pericarditis

Infectious

- Bacterial: Pneumococci, staphylococci, streptococci, *Neisseria gonorrhoeae, Legionella pneumophila, Mycobacterium tuberculosis,* septicemia from gram-negative organisms
- Fungal: Histoplasma, *Candida* species
- Viral: Coxsackie A and B virus, echovirus, adenovirus, mumps, hepatitis, Epstein-Barr, varicella-zoster, HIV
- Others: Toxoplasmosis, Lyme disease

Noninfectious

- Acute MI
- Cancers: Lung, breast, leukemia. Hodgkin lymphoma, non-Hodgkin lymphoma
- Dissecting aortic aneurysm
- Myxedema
- Radiation
- Renal failure
- Trauma: Thoracic surgery, pacemaker insertion, cardiac diagnostic procedures

Hypersensitive or Autoimmune

- Dressler syndrome
- Drug reactions (e.g., procainamide, hydralazine)
- Postpericardiotomy syndrome
- Rheumatic fever
- Rheumatologic diseases: Rheumatoid arthritis, systemic lupus erythematosus, scleroderma, ankylosing spondylitis

Pathophysiology

There are 3 types of pericarditis: acute, subacute, and chronic. Acute pericarditis develops rapidly, causing the pericardial sac to become inflamed and leak fluid (pericardial effusion). The characteristic pathologic finding in acute pericarditis is inflammation. There is an influx of neutrophils, increased pericardial vascularity, and, eventually, fibrin deposition on the epicardium. Subacute pericarditis occurs weeks to months after an event. Pericarditis lasting more than 6 months is considered chronic. Recurrent pericarditis may occur in up to 30% of patients after an initial episode of acute pericarditis.[6]

Post–myocardial infarction (MI) syndrome (Dressler syndrome) pericarditis can occur 4 to 6 weeks after transmural MI (see Chapter 37). This syndrome is more common after a large anterior infarct. Viral pericarditis is often seen after respiratory or GI illness.[6]

Clinical Manifestations

Symptoms include progressive, severe, sharp chest pain.[7] The pain is often worse with deep inspiration and when lying flat. Sitting up and leaning forward relieves the pain. The pain may radiate to the neck, arms, or left shoulder, making it hard to distinguish from angina. One distinction is that the pain from pericarditis can be referred to the trapezius muscle (shoulder, upper back). Dyspnea is related to the patient's breathing in rapid, shallow breaths to avoid chest pain. Fever and anxiety may worsen dyspnea.

TABLE 40.5 Measuring Pulsus Paradoxus

1. Position the patient in a semirecumbent position.
2. Have patient breathe normally.
3. Using a manually operated BP cuff, measure systolic BP.
4. Inflate BP cuff at least 20 mm Hg above systolic BP.
5. Deflate cuff slowly until you hear sounds throughout the respiratory cycle (inspiration and expiration) and note the pressure.
6. Determine the difference between the measurements taken in steps 3 and 5. This will equal the amount of paradox. The difference is normally <10 mm Hg. If the difference is >10 mm Hg, cardiac tamponade may be present.

For example:

Sounds heard on expiration at	110 mm Hg
Sounds heard throughout cycle at	−82 mm Hg
Amount of paradox	28 mm Hg

The hallmark finding in acute pericarditis is a *pericardial friction rub.* The rub is a scratching, grating, high-pitched sound believed to result from friction between the roughened pericardial and epicardial surfaces. It is best heard with the stethoscope at the lower left sternal border of the chest with the patient leaning forward. Because it is hard to tell a pericardial friction rub from a pleural friction rub, ask the patient to hold their breath for a few seconds. If you still hear the rub, it is cardiac. Pericardial friction rubs may be intermittent.

Complications

The major complications are pericardial effusion and cardiac tamponade. *Pericardial effusion* is excess fluid in the pericardium. It can occur rapidly (e.g., chest trauma) or slowly (e.g., tuberculosis pericarditis). Large effusions compress nearby structures. Pulmonary tissue compression can cause cough, dyspnea, and tachypnea. Phrenic nerve compression can cause hiccups. Compression of the laryngeal nerve may cause hoarseness. Heart sounds are distant and muffled. BP is usually maintained.

Cardiac tamponade develops as the pericardial effusion volume increases and compresses the heart. The speed of fluid accumulation affects the severity of clinical signs. Tamponade can be acute (e.g., rupture of heart, trauma) or subacute (e.g., from renal failure, cancer).

Patients may report chest pain. They are often confused, anxious, and restless. As the compression of the heart increases, there is decreased CO, muffled heart sounds, narrowed pulse pressure, tachypnea, and tachycardia. Increased jugular venous pressure causes jugular venous distention (JVD). *Pulsus paradoxus,* if present, is a large decrease in systolic BP during inspiration (Table 40.5). In patients with a slow-onset tamponade, dyspnea may be the only sign.

Diagnostic Studies

Diagnosis of acute pericarditis is based on the presence of at least 2 of these 4 criteria: (1) characteristic chest pain, (2)

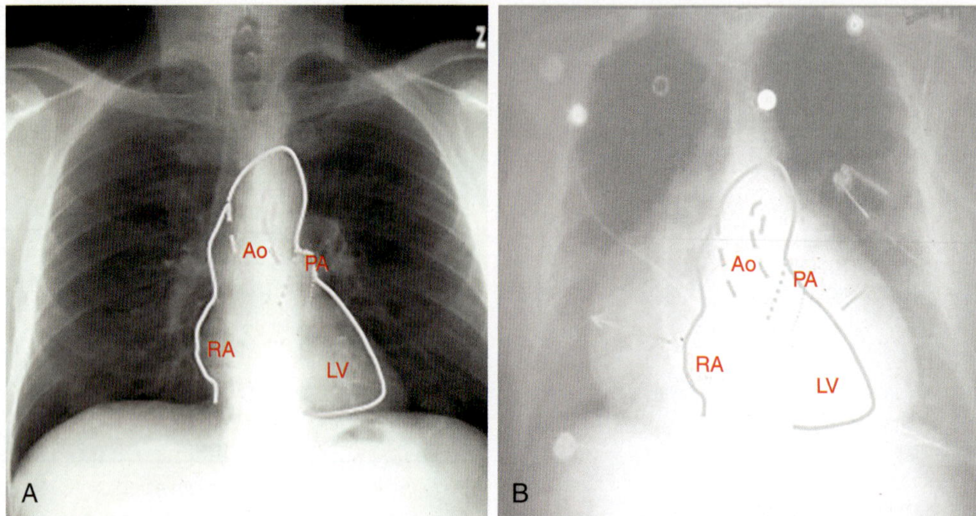

Fig. 40.4 (A) X-ray of a normal chest. (B) Pericardial effusion is present. Note the classic "water bottle shape" heart *(arrows)*. Select structures and great vessels are labeled: *Ao*, ascending aorta; *LV*, left ventricle; *PA*, pulmonary artery; *RA*, right atrium. (From Appleton C, Gilliam L: Cardiac tamponade, *Cardiol Clin* 35:525, 2017.)

pericardial friction rub, (3) new or worsening pericardial effusion, and (4) characteristic ECG changes. The ECG is useful in diagnosing acute pericarditis. ECG changes related to inflammation are noted in 90% of cases. Diffuse (widespread) ST segment elevation reflects abnormal ventricular repolarization. PR segment depression may be present, reflecting atrial injury.

An echocardiogram can determine the presence of a pericardial effusion or cardiac tamponade. Doppler imaging and color M-mode can assess diastolic function and diagnose constrictive pericarditis. A CT scan or cardiac MRI can visualize the pericardium and pericardial space. Chest x-ray findings are often normal. A large pericardial effusion may appear as cardiomegaly (Fig. 40.4).

Laboratory findings include leukocytosis and increased CRP and ESR. Troponin levels may be increased in patients with ST segment elevation and acute pericarditis, which could indicate concurrent heart damage. Fluid obtained during pericardiocentesis or tissue from a pericardial biopsy may be studied to determine the cause of pericarditis.

Interprofessional Care

Most cases are managed in the outpatient setting. Patients with high-risk features should be admitted for treatment. These include a high fever (>38°C), subacute onset, large pericardial effusion or tamponade, lack of response to therapy after 1 week of treatment, or evidence of myocardial involvement. Other predictors of high risk include immunosuppression, oral anticoagulation, and trauma.

Management is aimed at identifying and treating the underlying problem and symptoms (Table 40.6). Antibiotics treat bacterial pericarditis. Nonsteroidal antiinflammatory drugs (NSAIDs) control pain and inflammation. Corticosteroids are used for patients with pericarditis from systemic lupus erythematosus, patients already taking corticosteroids for autoimmune conditions, or patients who do not respond to NSAIDs. Aspirin is recommended for treatment of pericarditis after an ST elevation MI. Colchicine, an antiinflammatory drug used for gout, may help patients with pericarditis for more than 10 days or who have recurrent pericarditis.[8]

Pericardiocentesis is usually done for pericardial effusion with acute cardiac tamponade, purulent pericarditis, or suspected cancer (Fig. 40.5). Hemodynamic support for a patient before the procedure may include giving volume expanders and

TABLE 40.6 Interprofessional Care

Acute Pericarditis

Diagnostic Assessment

- History and physical assessment (note pericardial friction rub, pulsus paradoxus)
- Laboratory: CRP, ESR, white blood cell count
- ECG
- Chest x-ray
- Echocardiogram
- CT scan
- MRI
- Pericardiocentesis, pericardial biopsy

Management

- Treatment of underlying disease
- Bed rest
- Drug therapy
  - NSAIDs
  - Corticosteroids
  - Antibiotics (for bacterial infection)
- Pericardiocentesis (for tamponade)
- Pericardial window (for tamponade or ongoing pericardial effusion)

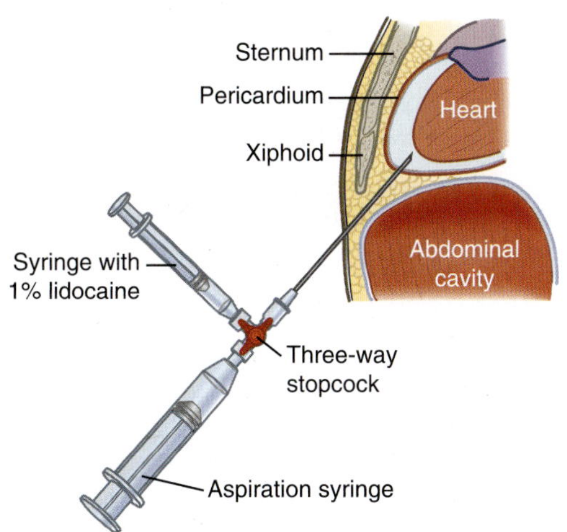

Fig. 40.5 Pericardiocentesis performed under sterile conditions in conjunction with ECG and hemodynamic measurements.

inotropic agents (e.g., norepinephrine) and stopping anticoagulants. A needle is inserted into the pericardial space to remove fluid for analysis and relieve heart pressure. Complications include dysrhythmias, further cardiac tamponade, pneumomediastinum, pneumothorax, myocardial laceration, and coronary artery laceration.

A *pericardial window* is a surgical procedure for diagnosis or drainage of excess fluid. Cutting a "window" into part of the pericardium allows the fluid to drain into the peritoneum or chest.

NURSING MANAGEMENT: ACUTE PERICARDITIS

Managing pain and anxiety during acute pericarditis is a key nursing consideration. Assess the pain to distinguish angina (myocardial ischemia) from pericarditis (see Table 37.8). Pericarditis pain is usually found in the precordium or left trapezius region. It has a sharp quality that increases with inspiration. Pain is often relieved when the patient sits up or leans forward and is worse when lying flat. Patients with acute pericarditis are at risk for cardiac tamponade and decreased CO. Monitor for signs of tamponade and prepare for possible pericardiocentesis.

Pain relief measures include keeping patients on bed rest with the head of the bed raised to 45 degrees and providing an overbed table for support. Antiinflammatory drugs can help control the pain. Give these drugs with food or milk. Tell patients to avoid alcohol because of the risk of GI bleeding. Other drugs, such as a proton pump inhibitor (e.g., pantoprazole, omeprazole), can reduce stomach acid.

Provide simple, complete explanations of procedures and possible causes of the pain to help reduce anxiety. These explanations are particularly important for patients undergoing testing and for patients who have previously had angina or an MI.

CHECK YOUR PRACTICE

You are assigned to a 58-year-old male patient who had an MI 3 days ago. He has now developed pericarditis. When you are making rounds, you assess that the patient is slightly confused and has prominent neck veins. His heart rate is 118 beats/min.

- What should you do next?

CHRONIC CONSTRICTIVE PERICARDITIS

Chronic constrictive pericarditis is a condition in which fibrosis and rigidity of the pericardium result in decreased pericardial elasticity and restricted ventricular filling. The cause may be infection, heart surgery, mediastinal radiation therapy, or idiopathic.[9] The condition is characterized by pericardial effusion that is slowly reabsorbed with progression to fibrous scarring, thickening of the pericardium from calcium deposits, and destruction of the pericardial space. The fibrotic, thickened, and adherent pericardium encases the heart. This prevents adequate atrial and ventricular stretch.

Manifestations of chronic constrictive pericarditis mimic HF and cor pulmonale. Decreased CO accounts for many of the manifestations. These include dyspnea on exertion, peripheral edema, ascites, fatigue, anorexia, and weight loss. The most prominent finding is JVD.

Echocardiography is recommended to diagnose constrictive pericarditis.[9] CT and MRI can be used to measure pericardial thickness and assess diastolic filling patterns. ECG changes are often nonspecific. The heart on the chest x-ray may be normal or enlarged. Cardiac catheterization can evaluate diastolic filling pressures and confirm diagnosis.

The treatment of choice for symptomatic chronic constrictive pericarditis is a *pericardiectomy.* This involves complete resection of the pericardium through a median sternotomy with cardiopulmonary bypass (see Chapter 37). Some patients show immediate improvement. Others may take weeks. The prognosis improves when the patient has surgery before becoming clinically unstable. Diuretics are used in patients who are not surgical candidates.[9]

MYOCARDITIS

Etiology and Pathophysiology

Myocarditis is an inflammatory process of the heart muscle (myocardium). It can present in acute, subacute, or chronic phases with focal or diffuse myocardial involvement. Myocarditis has various causes. Viral infections are the most frequent cause of myocarditis in the United States and developed countries. The most frequently implicated viruses are parvovirus B-19 and human herpesvirus 6 (HHV 6), followed by Epstein-Barr virus, enterovirus, human cytomegalovirus, and adenovirus. Other pathogens include various bacteria, fungi, protozoa, and helminths. Many reports of COVID-19 and influenza-associated myocarditis have occurred.[10]

In developing countries, rheumatic carditis, Chagas disease, and complications related to advanced HIV/AIDS are important causes. Common noninfectious causes include autoimmune disorders such as systemic lupus erythematosus, Wegener granulomatosis, and giant cell arteritis. In 50% to 80% of cases, no cause is found.

Myocardial infection causes cell damage and necrosis, activating the immune response. Cytokines and O_2 free radicals are released. As the infection progresses, an autoimmune response causes further destruction of myocytes and heart dysfunction.

Clinical Manifestations and Diagnostic Studies

Diagnosis is based on clinical presentation and confirmed by endomyocardial biopsy.[10] The features vary from a benign course without overt symptoms to HF, dysrhythmias, or sudden cardiac death (SCD). Fever, fatigue, malaise, myalgias, pharyngitis, dyspnea, lymphadenopathy, and nausea and vomiting are early manifestations of the viral form.

Cardiac signs appear 7 to 10 days after viral infection. Pericarditis may be present. Signs include pleuritic chest pain with a pericardial friction rub and effusion. Late signs relate to the development of HF. They include crackles, S_3 heart sound, JVD, syncope, peripheral edema, and angina. The ECG changes are often nonspecific but reflect pericardial involvement (e.g., diffuse ST segment changes). Dysrhythmias and conduction problems may be present.

Patients with mild myocarditis usually have a good prognosis. Poor prognostic factors include low ejection fraction (EF), left bundle branch block, and syncope. Patients may develop varying degrees of heart block and require permanent pacing. Dilated cardiomyopathy may occur. Cardiogenic shock is the most common cause of death, with the highest mortality rates in postpartum cardiomyopathy.[10]

Laboratory findings are often inconclusive. They may include mild to moderate leukocytosis and atypical lymphocytes, high viral titers, and increased ESR, CRP, and cardiac biomarkers, such as troponin. The virus is often present in tissue and pericardial fluid samples only during the first 8 to 10 days of illness.

Endomyocardial biopsy provides histologic confirmation of myocarditis.[10] A biopsy is most diagnostic during the first 6 weeks of acute illness, when lymphocytic infiltration and myocyte damage are present. Nuclear scans, echocardiography, and MRI assess heart function.

Interprofessional and Nursing Management

Treatment consists of managing symptoms. Angiotensin-converting enzyme (ACE) inhibitors and β-adrenergic receptor blockers (β-blockers) are used if the heart is enlarged or to treat HF (see Chapter 38). Diuretics reduce fluid volume and preload. If the patient is not hypotensive, IV drugs such as nitroprusside and milrinone reduce afterload and improve CO by decreasing systemic vascular resistance. Digoxin improves heart contractility and reduces heart rate (HR). It is used with caution because of increased sensitivity to adverse effects (e.g., dysrhythmias) and potential toxicity. Anticoagulation reduces the risk for clot formation from blood stasis in patients with a low EF.

DRUG ALERT

Digoxin

- Use cautiously in patients with myocarditis.
- Myocarditis predisposes to drug-related dysrhythmias and toxicity.

Myocarditis with an autoimmune basis is treated with immunosuppressive agents to reduce heart inflammation and damage. Antivirals may be used as adjunct therapy.

Supportive care includes O_2 therapy, bed rest, and restricted activity. In cases of severe HF, intraaortic balloon pump therapy and ventricular assist devices (VADs) may be needed (see Chapter 38). In some cases, the patient may need a heart transplant.

Focus your interventions on improving CO and managing the signs and symptoms of HF. Select nursing measures to decrease cardiac workload. These include placing the patient in a semi-Fowler's position, spacing activity and rest periods, and providing a quiet environment. Monitor drugs that increase the heart's contractility and decrease preload, afterload, or both. Evaluate the effectiveness of interventions on an ongoing basis.

The patient may be anxious about the diagnosis. Assess the level of anxiety and take measures to decrease it. Keep the patient and caregiver informed about the therapeutic plan.

Patients who receive immunosuppressive therapy are at increased risk for infection. Monitor for complications and provide patients with proper infection control procedures.

RHEUMATIC FEVER AND RHEUMATIC HEART DISEASE

Rheumatic fever (RF) is an acute inflammatory disease that can involve all the heart layers. **Rheumatic heart disease (RHD)** is chronic scarring and deformity of the heart valves resulting from RF. Over 40.5 million people worldwide have evidence of RHD.

Etiology and Pathophysiology

RF occurs as a complication 2 to 3 weeks after a bout of group A streptococcal (GAS) pharyngitis.[11] It affects the heart, skin, joints, and central nervous system (CNS). Painless subcutaneous nodules, arthralgias or arthritis, and chorea may develop. About 50% of RF episodes are *rheumatic pancarditis,* involving all layers of the heart (endocardium, myocardium, and pericardium; Fig. 40.1). RHD is the result of valve damage from an abnormal immune response to *Streptococcus.*

RHD is found mainly in the valves, with swelling and erosion of the valve leaflets. Vegetation forms from deposits of fibrin and blood cells in areas of erosion. The lesions initially create a thickening of the valve leaflets, fusion of commissures and chordae tendineae, and fibrosis of the papillary muscle. Valve leaflets may become calcified, resulting in stenosis. The less mobile valve leaflets may not close properly, causing regurgitation.

RHD often affects left-sided valves, particularly the mitral valve. Isolated aortic disease occurs in 2% of cases.[11] Right-sided valve disease often involves the tricuspid valve as primary valvulitis or a consequence of left-sided valve disease. It rarely affects the pulmonic valve.

Nodules, called *Aschoff bodies,* are formed by a reaction to inflammation with swelling and destruction of collagen fibers. As Aschoff bodies age, they become more fibrous, and scar tissue forms in the myocardium. Rheumatic pericarditis develops and affects both layers of the pericardium. The layers become thick and covered with fibrinous exudate. A serosanguineous pericardial effusion may develop. When healing occurs, fibrosis and adhesions develop that partially or completely destroy the pericardial sac. Damage to the heart begins during the first attack of RF. Recurrent infections cause further structural damage. *Chronic rheumatic carditis* results from changes in valve structure months to years after an episode of RF.

Clinical Manifestations and Diagnostic Studies

Jones criteria are used to diagnose acute RF.[11] The presence of 2 major criteria or 1 major and 2 minor criteria plus evidence of a preceding GAS infection indicates a high probability of acute RF (Table 40.7). The minor criteria confirm the presence of RF when only 1 major criterion is present.

TABLE 40.7 Diagnostic Criteria

Revised Jones Criteria for Rheumatic Fever

These criteria apply to the initial episode of rheumatic fever in moderate- or high-risk populations.

Major Criteria
- Carditis: Clinical and/or subclinical
- Arthritis
  - Monoarthritis or polyarthritis
  - Polyarthralgia
- Erythema marginatum
- Subcutaneous nodules
- Sydenham chorea

Minor Criteria
- Monoarthralgia
- Fever
- Laboratory findings: ↑ ESR and/or ↑ CRP
- ECG findings: Prolonged PR interval after accounting for age variability (unless carditis is a major criterion)

Evidence of Group A Streptococcal Infection
- ↑ Antistreptolysin-O titer, positive throat culture, positive rapid antigen test for group A streptococci

Modified from Gewitz MH, Baltimore RS, Tani LY, et al: Revision of the Jones criteria for the diagnosis of acute rheumatic fever in the era of Doppler echocardiography: a scientific statement from the AHA, *Circulation* 131:1806, 2015.

Major Criteria

Carditis (inflammation of the heart) is the most important manifestation of RF. It results in 3 signs: (1) heart murmur or murmurs of mitral or aortic regurgitation, or mitral stenosis; (2) heart enlargement and HF from myocarditis; and (3) pericarditis resulting in muffled heart sounds, chest pain, pericardial friction rub, or signs of effusion.

Monoarthritis or polyarthritis is the most common finding in RF. It occurs in up to 75% of patients. The inflammatory process affects the synovial membranes of the joints. This causes swelling, heat, redness, tenderness, and limitation of motion. The larger joints, particularly the knees, ankles, elbows, and wrists, are most often affected.

Sydenham chorea is the major CNS manifestation. Patients have involuntary movements, especially of the face and limbs; muscle weakness; and speech and gait problems.

Erythema marginatum lesions occur in less than 10% of patients with RF. The bright pink, nonpruritic, maplike macular lesions occur mainly on the trunk and proximal extremities. They intensify with heat (e.g., warm bath). *Subcutaneous nodules* associated with severe carditis are small, hard, painless swellings found over extensor surfaces of joints, particularly the knees, wrists, and elbows.

No single diagnostic test exists for RF. An ECG and chest x-ray can help in the initial assessment of RHD. The most consistent ECG change is a prolonged PR interval from delayed atrioventricular (AV) conduction. In older patients, atrial fibrillation may be present.[11] A chest x-ray may show an enlarged heart.

Echocardiogram can show thickening of the valve apparatus (presence of either or both valvular and chordal thickening) and changes in valve mobility. There may be either or both restricted and excess leaflet motion.

Interprofessional Care

Treatment consists of drug therapy and supportive care (Table 40.8). Antibiotic therapy does not change the course of acute RHD or the development of carditis. It eliminates

TABLE 40.8 Interprofessional Care

Rheumatic Fever

Diagnostic Assessment
- History and physical assessment
- Laboratory studies (Table 40.7)
- Chest x-ray
- Echocardiogram
- ECG

Management
- Bed rest or limited activity
- Drug therapy
  - Antibiotics
  - NSAIDs
  - Salicylates
  - Corticosteroids

residual GAS in the tonsils and pharynx and prevents the spread of infection. Salicylates, NSAIDs, and corticosteroids are used to control fever and joint manifestations.

NURSING MANAGEMENT: RHEUMATIC FEVER AND RHEUMATIC HEART DISEASE

Assessment

Table 40.9 presents the subjective and objective data to obtain from patients with RF and RHD.

Inspect the skin. Palpate for subcutaneous nodules over all bony surfaces and along extensor tendons of the hands and feet. The nodules range in size from 1 to 4 cm and are hard, painless, and freely movable. Inspect the trunk and inner aspect of the upper arm and thigh for erythema marginatum. Assess for these bright pink maculae in good light because the rash is hard to see, especially in patients with dark skin.

TABLE 40.9 NURSING ASSESSMENT

Rheumatic Fever and Rheumatic Heart Disease

Subjective Data

Important Health Information

Health history: Recent streptococcal infection, history of RF or rheumatic heart disease

Functional Health Patterns

Health perception–health management: Family history of RF. Malaise.

Nutritional-metabolic: Anorexia, weight loss

Activity-exercise: Palpitations, weakness, fatigue, impaired coordination

Cognitive-perceptual: Chest pain, widespread joint pain, and tenderness (especially large joints)

Objective Data

Cardiovascular

Tachycardia, pericardial friction rub, muffled heart sounds, murmurs, peripheral edema

General

Fever

Musculoskeletal

Signs of monoarthritis or polyarthritis, including swelling, heat, redness, limitation of motion (especially of knees, ankles, elbows, shoulders, wrists)

Neurologic

Chorea (involuntary, purposeless, rapid motions; facial grimaces)

Skin

Subcutaneous nodules and erythema marginatum

Possible Diagnostic Findings

Cardiomegaly on chest x-ray. Prolonged PR interval on ECG. Valve abnormalities, chamber dilation, and pericardial effusion on echocardiogram. ↑ Antistreptolysin-O titer, positive throat culture, positive rapid antigen test for group A streptococci, ↑ ESR, ↑ CRP, leukocytosis

Clinical Problems

Clinical problems for patients with RF and RHD include:

- Fatigue
- Impaired cardiac function
- Infection

Planning

The goals for patients with RF and RHD include (1) normal or baseline heart function, (2) resumption of daily activities without joint pain, and (3) ability to manage the long-term antibiotic therapy.

Implementation

Health Promotion

Early detection and immediate treatment of GAS pharyngitis can prevent RF. Treatment with penicillin is the most widely used antibiotic. If a patient is allergic to penicillin, a narrow-spectrum cephalosporin (e.g., cephalexin), clindamycin, or azithromycin is used.[12] Therapy requires strict adherence to the full course of treatment. Teach people in the community to seek prompt medical care for symptoms of streptococcal pharyngitis.

Acute Care

Give antibiotics as prescribed to treat the streptococcal infection. Teach patients that completing the full course of antibiotics is vital to successful treatment (see Table 15.9).

Promote optimal rest. This reduces cardiac workload and metabolic needs. Position painful joints for proper alignment and apply heat for comfort. Give salicylates, NSAIDs, and corticosteroids as prescribed for joint pain. Implement measures to manage fever (see Table 12.5). Stress the importance of gentle activities during recovery.

CHECK YOUR PRACTICE

Your 28-year-old male patient is recovering from carditis after RF. As you are preparing him for discharge from the hospital, he is pacing the floor and seems quite upset. You ask him to sit down so you can talk. He tells you, "I'm a heart cripple. I will never be able to play ball with my sons or go skiing again. I might as well just go to bed and stay there."

- What are the key elements to include in your teaching plan?

Chronic Care

The goal of care is to prevent a recurrence of RF. A prior history of RF makes a patient more susceptible to a second attack after a streptococcal infection. The best prevention is treatment with prophylactic antibiotics. The drug of choice is penicillin. Patients with RF without carditis need prophylaxis until age 20 and for a minimum of 5 years. Those with acute RF with carditis and residual valve damage may need prophylaxis until age 40 or for 10 years after the last RF episode, whichever is longer. Some need lifelong prophylaxis. Patients with rheumatic carditis and residual heart disease (e.g., persistent valve disease) need lifelong dental prophylaxis.[12]

Teach patients with a history of RF about the disease process and the need for ongoing antibiotic prophylaxis. Review good nutrition, hygiene practices, and adequate rest. Caution the patient about the possible development of valve disease. Tell patients to seek medical care for symptoms such as fatigue, dizziness, palpitations, unexplained weight gain, or exertional dyspnea.[12]

◆ Evaluation

The expected outcomes are that patients with RF and RHD will:

- Be able to perform ADLs with minimal fatigue and pain
- Adhere to the treatment plan
- Express confidence in managing the disease
- Use measures to prevent complications

HEART VALVE DISEASE

Two AV valves (mitral and tricuspid) and 2 semilunar valves (aortic and pulmonic) control blood flow through the heart (see Fig. 35.2). The pressure on either side of an open valve is normally equal. However, in a stenotic valve, the valve opening is smaller because of limited leaflet opening. The forward flow of blood is impaired. This creates a difference in pressure on the 2 sides of the open valve. The amount of **stenosis** (constriction or narrowing) is seen in the pressure differences (the higher the difference, the greater the stenosis). When **regurgitation** occurs (referred to as *incompetence* or *insufficiency*), there is incomplete closure of the valve and backward flow of blood (Fig. 40.6).

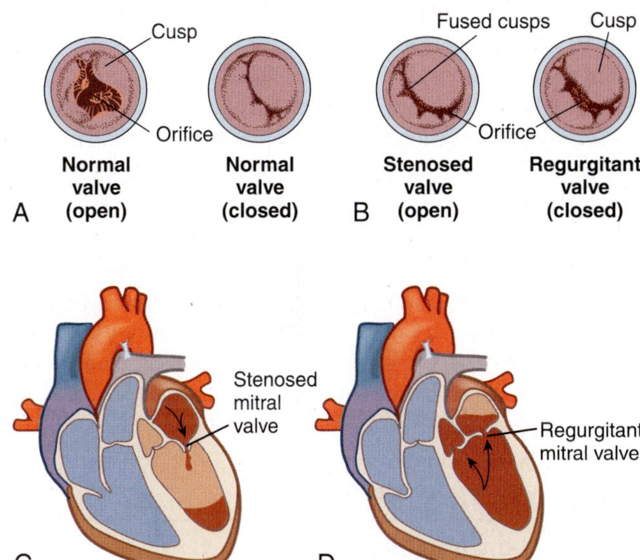

Fig. 40.6 Valve stenosis and regurgitation. (A) Normal position of the valve leaflets when the valve is open and closed. (B) Open position of a stenosed valve *(left)* and closed position of regurgitant valve *(right)*. (C) Hemodynamic effect of mitral stenosis. The stenosed valve is unable to open sufficiently during left atrial systole, inhibiting left ventricular filling. (D) Hemodynamic effect of MR. The mitral valve does not close completely during left ventricular systole, letting blood reenter the left atrium. At the same time, blood is moving forward through the aortic valve. (From McCance KL, Huether SE: *Pathophysiology: the biologic basis for disease in adults and children*, ed 6, St Louis, 2010, Mosby.)

Congenital heart disease (CHD) is the most common cause of valve disorders in children and teens. Aortic stenosis and mitral regurgitation (MR) often occur in older adults who have some form of heart disease. Other causes of valve disease in adults are related to aging, endocarditis, RHD, hypertension, and autoimmune disorders.

MITRAL VALVE STENOSIS

Etiology and Pathophysiology

The most common cause of mitral stenosis is RHD.[13] Less common causes are congenital mitral stenosis, rheumatoid arthritis, radiation exposure, and systemic lupus erythematosus. RHD causes scarring of the valve leaflets and the chordae tendineae. Contractures and adhesions develop between the commissures (the junctional areas). The stenotic mitral valve takes on a "fish mouth" shape from the thickening and shortening of the mitral valve structures. Severe mitral annular calcification can cause stenosis in older adults.

These deformities block the blood flow and create a pressure difference between the left atrium and left ventricle during diastole. As a result, left atrial pressure and volume increase. This causes higher pulmonary vasculature pressure. The overloaded left atrium places patients at risk for atrial fibrillation. In chronic mitral stenosis, pressure overload occurs in the left atrium, pulmonary bed, and right ventricle.

Clinical Manifestations

The main symptom is exertional dyspnea from reduced lung compliance (Table 40.10). Heart sounds include a loud 1st heart sound and a low-pitched, diastolic murmur (best heard at the apex with the stethoscope). Less often, patients may have hoarseness (from atrial enlargement pressing on the laryngeal nerve), hemoptysis (from pulmonary hypertension), and chest pain (from decreased CO and coronary perfusion). Emboli can form in the left atrium from atrial fibrillation and cause a stroke. Fatigue and palpitations from atrial fibrillation may occur.

MITRAL VALVE REGURGITATION

Etiology and Pathophysiology

Mitral valve function depends on intact mitral leaflets, mitral annulus, chordae tendineae, papillary muscles, left atrium, and left ventricle. A defect in any of these structures can cause regurgitation. MR may result from problems with the leaflets or from the surrounding structures. In primary (degenerative) MR, there is a problem with the leaflets. In secondary (functional) MR, the cause is myocardial disease.[13] Most cases are caused by MI, chronic RHD, mitral valve prolapse, ischemic papillary muscle dysfunction, and IE. MI with left ventricular failure increases the risk for rupture of the chordae tendineae and acute MR.

MR allows blood to flow backward from the left ventricle to the left atrium because of incomplete valve closure during

TABLE 40.10 Manifestations of Valve Heart Disease

Type	Manifestations
Mitral valve prolapse	Palpitations, dyspnea, chest pain, activity intolerance, syncope, holosystolic murmur.
Mitral valve regurgitation	*Acute:* New systolic murmur with pulmonary edema. Cardiogenic shock. *Chronic:* Weakness, fatigue, exertional dyspnea, edema. Palpitations, S_3, holosystolic murmur.
Mitral valve stenosis	Dyspnea on exertion. Hoarseness, hemoptysis, fatigue, chest pain. Atrial fibrillation. Palpitations. Loud, accentuated S_1. Low-pitched, diastolic murmur.
Aortic valve regurgitation	*Acute:* Abrupt onset of profound dyspnea, chest pain, left ventricular failure, and cardiogenic shock. *Chronic:* Fatigue, exertional dyspnea, orthopnea. Water-hammer pulse, heaving precordial impulse, ↓ or absent S_1, S_3, or S_4. Soft, high-pitched diastolic murmur, Austin Flint murmur.
Aortic valve stenosis	Angina, syncope, dyspnea on exertion, HF, normal or soft S_1, ↑ or absent S_2, systolic murmur, prominent S_4.
Tricuspid and pulmonic stenosis	*Tricuspid:* Peripheral edema, ascites, fatigue, JVD. Diastolic low-pitched murmur with increased intensity during inspiration. *Pulmonic:* Fatigue, dyspnea, syncope. Loud midsystolic murmur.

systole. Both the left ventricle and left atrium must work harder to preserve CO. In acute MR, the sudden increase in pressure and volume transmits back to the pulmonary bed. This results in pulmonary edema and, if not treated, cardiogenic shock. In chronic MR, the added volume results in left atrial enlargement, left ventricular dilation and hypertrophy, and, finally, a decrease in CO.

Clinical Manifestations

The nature of its onset determines the clinical course of MR (Table 40.10). Patients with acute MR have thready peripheral pulses and cool, clammy extremities. A low CO may mask a new systolic murmur. Rapid assessment (e.g., heart catheterization) and intervention (e.g., valve repair or replacement) are critical.

Patients with chronic MR may remain asymptomatic for years. Early symptoms of left ventricular failure may include weakness, fatigue, palpitations, and dyspnea. These gradually progress to orthopnea, paroxysmal nocturnal dyspnea, and peripheral edema. Increased left ventricular volume leads to an audible 3rd heart sound (S_3), even with normal left ventricular function. The murmur is a loud holosystolic murmur at the apex radiating to the left axilla. Patients with asymptomatic MR must be monitored carefully.

Treatment for MR depends on the cause of the regurgitation. Primary MR typically requires valve repair or replacement before significant left ventricular failure or pulmonary hypertension develops.[13] Medical management includes guideline-directed medical therapy (GDMT).

MITRAL VALVE PROLAPSE

Etiology and Pathophysiology

Mitral valve prolapse (MVP) is an abnormality of the mitral valve leaflets and the papillary muscles or chordae that allows the leaflets to prolapse, or buckle, back into the left atrium during systole (Fig. 40.6). MVP affects 2% to 3% of the population. It is usually benign, but serious complications can occur, including MR, IE, SCD, HF, and cerebral ischemia.

The cause of MVP is unknown. There is an increased familial incidence. The genetic inheritance is often autosomal dominant (see Chapter 13). MVP in this group results from a connective tissue defect affecting only the valve, as part of Marfan syndrome, or another hereditary condition that affects collagen structure.

Clinical Manifestations

MVP has a broad range of severity. Most patients are asymptomatic for their entire lives. About 10% of those with MVP become symptomatic. A characteristic of MVP is a regurgitation murmur that is louder during systole. Severe MR is an uncommon but serious complication.

Echocardiography can confirm MVP. Dysrhythmias, such as premature ventricular contractions, paroxysmal supraventricular tachycardia, and ventricular tachycardia, may cause palpitations, lightheadedness, and syncope. IE may occur in patients with MR associated with MVP.

Patients may have chest discomfort caused by abnormal tension on the papillary muscles.[14] Chest pain episodes tend to occur in clusters, especially during periods of stress. Dyspnea, palpitations, and syncope sometimes accompany chest pain. β-Blockers are given to control palpitations and chest pain. Encourage patients to stay hydrated, exercise regularly, and avoid caffeine.

Most patients with MVP have a benign, manageable course. For those who do develop symptomatic MR, no current therapy delays the need for valve surgery. A teaching plan for patients with MVP is outlined in Table 40.11.

AORTIC VALVE STENOSIS

Etiology and Pathophysiology

Congenital **aortic stenosis (AS)** is generally found in childhood, adolescence, or young adulthood. In older adults, it is a result of RF or degeneration, similar to coronary artery disease. AS is the most frequent degenerative valve disorder, affecting 3% of people over 65 years of age.[15] In RHD, fusion and calcification cause the valve leaflets to stiffen and retract, resulting in stenosis. AS caused by RHD accompanies mitral valve disease. Isolated AS is usually nonrheumatic.

TABLE 40.11 PATIENT & CAREGIVER TEACHING

Mitral Valve Prolapse (MVP)

Include the following information in the teaching plan for a patient with MVP and the patient's caregiver:

- Take drugs as prescribed (e.g., β-blockers to control palpitations, chest pain).
- Adopt healthy eating habits.
- Avoid caffeine. It is a stimulant and may worsen symptoms.
- If you use diet pills or other over-the-counter drugs, check for common ingredients that are stimulants (e.g., caffeine, ephedrine) because these can worsen symptoms.
- Begin, or maintain, an exercise program to achieve optimal health.
- Contact the HCP or emergency response system (ERS) if symptoms develop or worsen (e.g., palpitations, fatigue, shortness of breath, anxiety).

AS causes obstruction of blood flow from the left ventricle to the aorta during systole. The result is left ventricular hypertrophy. Myocardial O_2 consumption increases because of the increased myocardial mass. As the disease progresses and compensation fails, reduced CO leads to decreased tissue perfusion, pulmonary hypertension, and HF. Left untreated, severe AS has a poor prognosis.

Clinical Manifestations

Manifestations (Table 40.10) develop when the valve orifice becomes about one-third of its normal size. They include the classic triad of angina, syncope, and exertional dyspnea, reflecting left ventricular failure.[15] Auscultation often reveals a crescendo-decrescendo, holosystolic murmur that may radiate to the carotids.

Some patients may be asymptomatic. The prognosis is poorer for patients with symptoms and those whose valve obstruction is not fixed. Nitroglycerin is used cautiously to treat angina in patients with AS. It can significantly reduce BP and worsen chest pain.

DRUG ALERT

Nitroglycerin

- Use cautiously in patients with AS because significant hypotension may occur.
- The drug can worsen chest pain as a result of the decrease in preload and drop in BP.

AORTIC VALVE REGURGITATION

Etiology and Pathophysiology

Aortic regurgitation (AR) may be the result of primary disease of the aortic valve leaflets, the aortic root, or both.[16] Trauma, IE, or aortic dissection can cause acute AR, which is a life-threatening emergency. Chronic AR generally results from RHD, a congenital bicuspid aortic valve, syphilis, a connective tissue problem, or a postsurgical cause.[16]

AR causes retrograde (backward) blood flow from the ascending aorta into the left ventricle during diastole. This results in volume overload. The left ventricle initially compensates for chronic AR by dilation and hypertrophy. Myocardial contractility eventually declines, and blood volume in the left atrium and pulmonary bed increases. This leads to pulmonary hypertension and right ventricular (RV) failure.

Clinical Manifestations

Patients with acute AR have sudden signs of cardiovascular collapse (Table 40.10). They develop severe dyspnea, chest pain, and hypotension, indicating left ventricular failure and cardiogenic shock, a life-threatening emergency.

Patients with chronic, severe AR develop a *water-hammer pulse* (strong, quick beat that collapses immediately). Heart sounds may include a soft or absent S_1, S_3, or S_4 and a soft, high-pitched diastolic murmur.

Patients with chronic AR often are asymptomatic for years.[16] Exertional dyspnea, orthopnea, and paroxysmal nocturnal dyspnea develop only after considerable heart dysfunction has occurred (Table 40.10). Angina occurs less often than in AS.

TRICUSPID AND PULMONIC VALVE DISEASE

Etiology and Pathophysiology

Tricuspid regurgitation (TR) can be primary or secondary. Primary TR is less common. It is typically caused by IE or congenital malformation. Secondary TR is caused by RV dilatation from pulmonary hypertension, cor pulmonale, or pulmonary outflow tract obstruction. Patients do not show JVD, enlarged liver, and peripheral edema until regurgitation is severe. Diagnosis is made by history, physical, and echocardiogram. The prognosis is poor for severe TR.

Tricuspid stenosis is usually caused by RF. Signs and symptoms include a fluttering discomfort in the neck, fatigue, and possible right upper quadrant pain.

Pulmonic regurgitation is often asymptomatic. A crescendo-decrescendo murmur is present. Potential causes include pulmonary hypertension, surgical repair of tetralogy of Fallot (TOF), or congenital valve disease. It can cause RV dilation.

Pulmonic stenosis is often caused by CHD. It results in RV hypertension and hypertrophy (Table 40.10). It is largely asymptomatic. When symptoms develop, they are similar to those of AS (syncope, dyspnea, angina). Symptoms typically do not present until adulthood.

DIAGNOSTIC STUDIES: HEART VALVE DISEASE

Diagnosis of heart valve disease includes information from the history and physical assessment and a variety of tests (Table 40.12). An echocardiogram shows valve structure, function, and heart chamber size. Transesophageal echocardiography and Doppler color flow imaging help diagnose and monitor disease progression. 3D echocardiography can help assess mitral valve problems and CHD.

Chest x-ray shows the heart size, altered pulmonary circulation, and valve calcification. An ECG identifies HR, rhythm, and any ischemia or ventricular hypertrophy. Heart catheterization detects pressure changes in the heart chambers, records pressure differences across the valves, and measures the size of valve openings.

TABLE 40.12 Interprofessional Care

Heart Valve Disease

Diagnostic Assessment
- History and physical assessment
- Chest x-ray
- Complete blood count
- ECG
- Echocardiography (Doppler, transesophageal)
- Heart catheterization

Management

Conservative Therapy
- Prophylactic antibiotic therapy (Table 40.2)
- Sodium restriction
- Drug therapy to treat or control HF
  - Vasodilators (e.g., sacubitril/valsartan, ACE inhibitors, ARBs, nitrates)[a]
  - Positive inotropes (e.g., digoxin)
  - Diuretics
  - β-Blockers
- Anticoagulation (see Table 41.10)
- Antidysrhythmic drugs (see Table 39.9)
- Percutaneous transluminal balloon valvuloplasty
- Percutaneous valve replacement

Surgical Therapy
- Valve repair
  - Annuloplasty
  - Commissurotomy (valvulotomy)
  - Valvuloplasty
- Valve replacement

[a]Use cautiously in patients with aortic stenosis.

INTERPROFESSIONAL CARE: HEART VALVE DISEASE

Conservative Therapy

Overall treatment focuses on preventing HF exacerbations, acute pulmonary edema, thromboembolism, and recurrent RF and IE (Table 40.12). HF is treated with vasodilators, positive inotropes, β-blockers, diuretics, and a low-sodium diet (see Chapter 38). Atrial dysrhythmias are common. They are treated with calcium channel blockers, β-blockers, antiarrhythmic drugs, or electrical cardioversion (see Chapter 39). Anticoagulant therapy is used in patients with atrial fibrillation to prevent systemic or pulmonary emboli.

Percutaneous Transluminal Balloon Valvuloplasty

An alternative treatment for some patients is *percutaneous transluminal balloon valvuloplasty* (PTBV). During PTBV, the fused commissures are split open. Balloon valvuloplasty can treat disease in any valve.[13] It is not a permanent fix for stenosis. This procedure is typically done in patients who cannot undergo aortic valve replacement.

The PTBV procedure is typically done in the cardiac catheterization laboratory (Fig. 40.7). It involves threading a balloon-tipped catheter from the femoral artery or vein to the stenotic valve. The balloon is inflated to separate the valve leaflets. A single- or double-balloon technique may be used. Using a single Inoue balloon with an hourglass shape allows sequential inflation.

Surgical Therapy

The decision for valve repair or replacement depends on a patient's symptoms using the New York Heart Association classification system for functional disability (see Table 38.2).[13] The procedure used depends on the (1) valves involved,

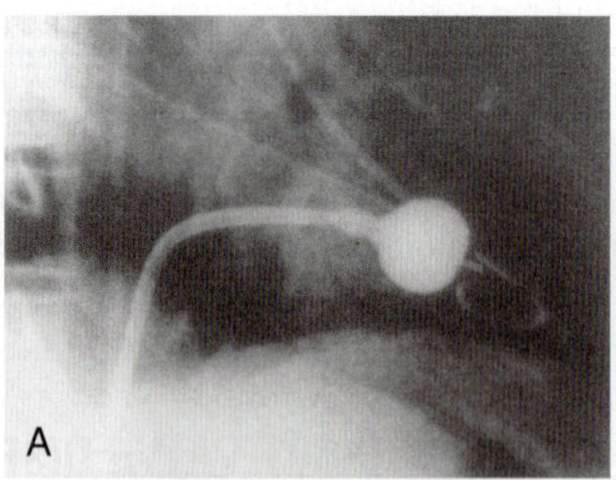

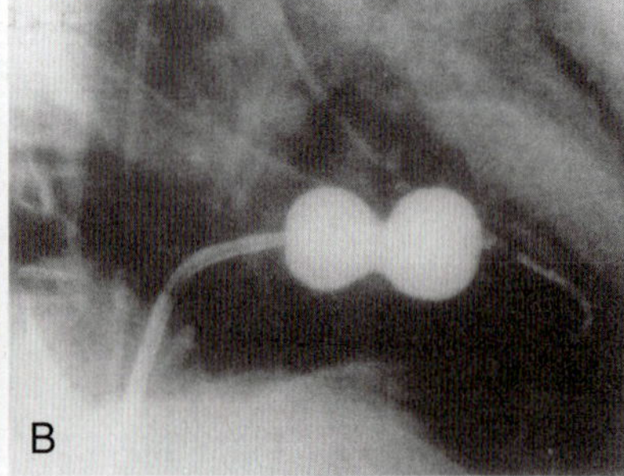

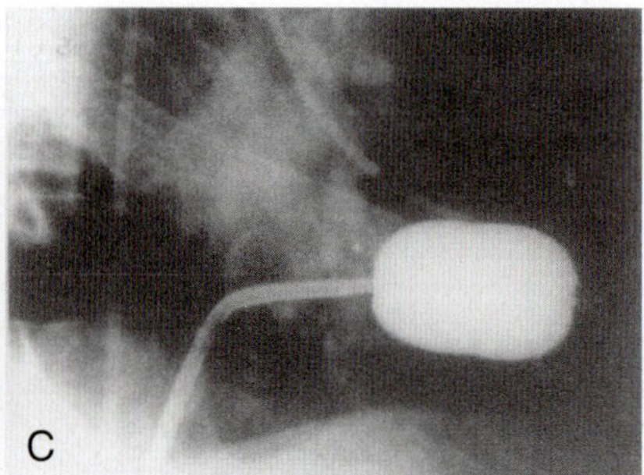

Fig. 40.7 Mitral valvuloplasty performed by the Inoue technique. The catheter is placed in the mitral valve and the distal part of the Inoue balloon inflated (A). The balloon is then pulled back in the mitral valve and inflated for 10 to 15 seconds under fluoroscopic control (B) until the waist of the balloon is no longer visible (C) and the balloon falls back into the left atrium. (From Crawford MH, DiMarco JP, Paulus WJ: *Cardiology,* ed 3, Edinburgh, 2010, Mosby.)

(2) pathology and severity of the disease, and (3) the patient's clinical condition (Box 40.1).

Valve Repair

Valve repair is preferred over replacement when possible. Repair has a lower operative mortality rate than valve replacement. It is often used in mitral or tricuspid valve disease. Although repair avoids the risks of replacement, it may not restore total valve function.

Open surgical *valvuloplasty* involves repair of the valve by suturing the torn leaflets, chordae tendineae, or papillary muscles. It is mainly used to treat MR or TR.

Minimally invasive valve surgery involves a ministernotomy or parasternal approach. It may include robotic and thoracoscopic surgical systems. Advantages include shorter lengths of stay, fewer blood transfusions, less pain, and lower risk for sternal infection and postoperative atrial fibrillation. For patients with MR or TR, further valve repair or reconstruction using annuloplasty is an option. *Annuloplasty* involves reconstruction of the annulus, with or without the aid of prosthetic rings.

BOX 40.1 ETHICAL/LEGAL DILEMMAS

Do Not Resuscitate

Situation

J.L., a 68-year-old male, is admitted for a second mitral valve repair and coronary artery bypass graft surgery. He did not adhere to the treatment plan after his original surgery 7 years ago. You are worried about his future adherence to the drug, diet, and exercise plan. He is on dialysis, making him a high-risk open surgical patient. J.L. and his caregiver request all treatment and decline to discuss advance directives (ADs) or do-not-resuscitate (DNR) orders.

Ethical/Legal Points for Consideration

- Adherence to past treatment plans is not a factor when considering DNR decisions. Many circumstances are outside the patient's control, such as finances, transportation, availability of help, and declining physical status.
- Based on their expertise, HCPs have the right to refuse to provide treatment that offers no benefit to the patient.
- ADs do not include a DNR order. If the patient is unable to speak for themselves, the HCP can start a DNR order only after a conversation with the health care proxy and/or nearest kin. The decision usually depends on evidence of the patient's preferences (substituted judgment standard) or what is thought to be in the patient's best interest.
- The HCP is not compelled to enact a DNR without clear direction from the patient or proxy.
- If the involved parties disagree about the patient's treatment plan, a referral can be made to an ethics committee, they can seek treatment from another HCP, or they may seek legal intervention by way of a court order.

Discussion Questions

- How can a lack of understanding or limited financial resources contribute to nonadherence with the plan of care?
- What type of information should be given to a patient and caregiver in discussions about ADs and DNR orders? Who should provide this information?
- Who can initiate a referral to an ethics committee?

Valve Replacement

Valve replacement may be needed. Desirable valves are nonthrombogenic, durable, and create minimal stenosis. A wide variety of prosthetic mechanical or biologic (tissue) valves are available.

Mechanical valves are made from artificial materials. They consist of combinations of metal alloys, pyrolytic carbon, and Dacron. Mechanical valves are more durable and last longer. However, they have an increased risk for thromboembolism. Patients need long-term anticoagulation therapy, which increases the risk of bleeding.

Biologic valves are made from bovine, porcine, or human (cadaver) heart tissue. They usually contain some human-made materials. A "decellularizing" process allows for decreased calcification of the bioprosthetic valve. They produce a more natural pattern of blood flow compared with mechanical valves. However, they are less durable and tend to cause early calcification, tissue degeneration, and stiffening of the leaflets. Both valve types are subject to leaking and risk of IE.

Anticoagulation therapy is not needed with biologic valves because of their low thrombogenicity. However, patients with atrial fibrillation need long-term anticoagulation. Some patients with biologic valves or annuloplasty with prosthetic rings may need anticoagulation the first few months after surgery until endothelial cells cover the suture lines (endothelialized).

Transcatheter therapies are another option. They are used as an alternative to surgery or for patients who have aortic or mitral prosthetic valve failure. Transcatheter edge-to-edge repair is available for patients with severe MR who are at very high risk for open surgery. Transcatheter pulmonary valve replacement is approved for use in patients with pulmonary valve disease caused by CHD. The newest therapy is the Edwards Evoque tricuspid valve. This self-expanding valve is delivered via femoral vein to replace the tricuspid valve without open heart surgery.[17]

Transcatheter aortic valve replacement (TAVR) is an option for patients with severe, symptomatic AS. It can also be done to repair failing surgical valves (valve-in-valve TAVR). In most patients, the procedure is done using a transfemoral approach. The evaluation for TAVR may include an echocardiogram, cardiac CT angiogram, and heart catheterization.[13] Imaging can determine valve size and help in planning the procedure. There are 3 available TAVR valves in the United States. The Edwards Sapien 3 valve is made of bovine pericardial tissue. It is a balloon-expandable valve (Fig. 40.8).[18] The CoreValve transcatheter aortic valve is a self-expanding valve made of porcine pericardial tissue.[19] The last valve, the Abbott Navitor, is a self-expanding valve for patients at high risk for open surgery.[20]

The choice of valves depends on many factors. A mechanical valve may be best for younger patients because it is more durable. If a patient cannot take an anticoagulant (e.g., females of childbearing age), a biologic valve is an option. Frail patients

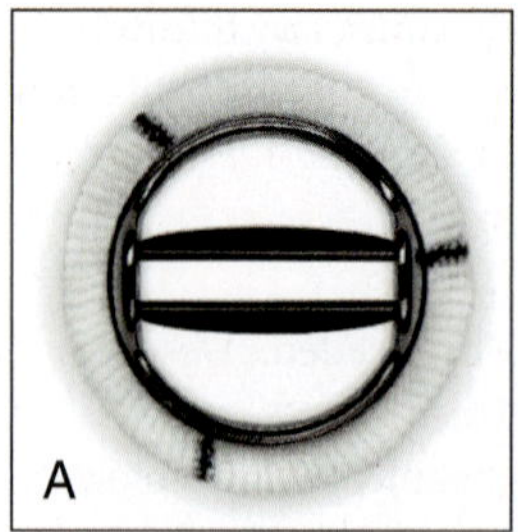

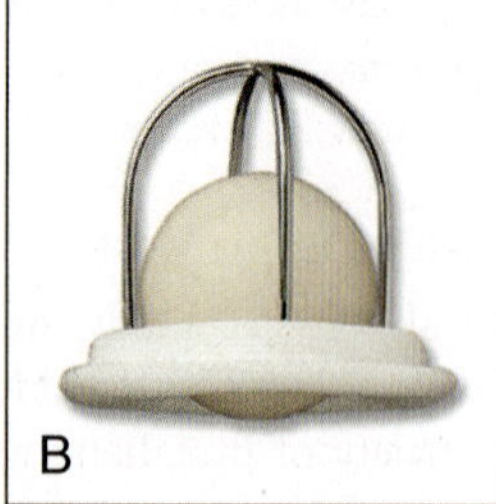

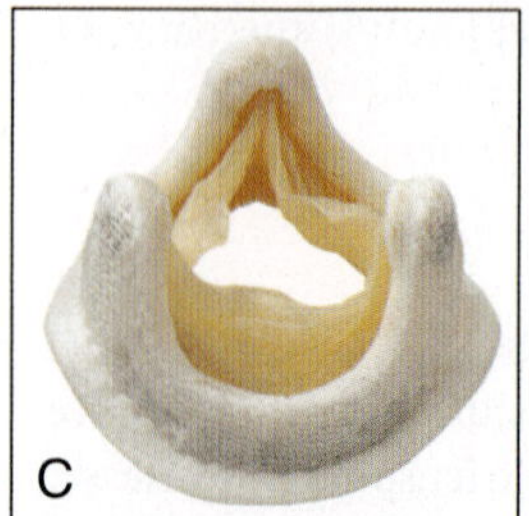

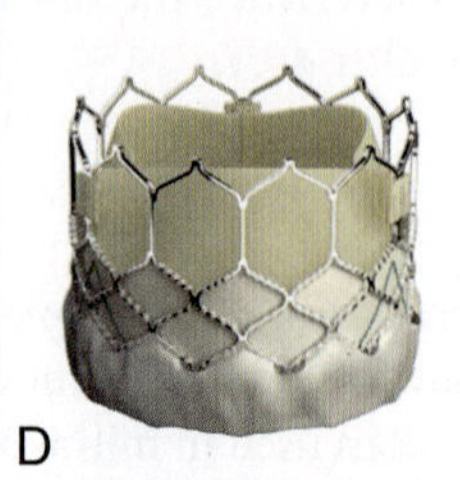

Fig. 40.8 Types of prosthetic heart valves. (A) St. Jude bileaflet mechanical valve. (B) Starr-Edwards caged ball valve. (C) Stented porcine Medtronic Mosaic bioprosthetic valve. (D) Transcatheter balloon-expandable Edwards SAPIEN 3 bioprosthetic valve. (From Bonow RO, Mann DL, Zipes DP, et al: *Braunwald's heart disease: a textbook of cardiovascular medicine*, ed 12, Philadelphia, 2012, Saunders.)

with comorbidities need to be evaluated by a qualified heart team for a full evaluation before considering surgery.[20] Encourage patients to discuss short- and long-term consequences of valve choices with their HCPs.

NURSING MANAGEMENT: HEART VALVE DISEASE

Assessment

Table 40.13 presents the subjective and objective data to obtain from patients with valve disease.

Clinical Problems

Clinical problems for patients with heart valve disease include:

- Impaired cardiac function
- Fatigue
- Fluid imbalance

More information on clinical problems and interventions is in eNursing Care Plan 40.2, available on the website for this chapter.

Planning

The overall goals for patients with valve disease include (1) normal heart function, (2) improved activity tolerance, and (3) an understanding of the disease process and health maintenance.

Implementation

Health Promotion

Encourage early treatment of streptococcal infections to prevent acquired RHD. Patients at risk for IE and any patient with certain heart conditions must receive prophylactic antibiotics (Table 40.2). Teach the person with a history of RF, IE, or CHD to report symptoms of heart valve disease.

Chronic Care

Patients with progressive heart valve disease may need outpatient care or hospitalization for management of HF, IE, embolic disease, or dysrhythmias. HF is the most common reason for ongoing medical care.

Develop the care plan to emphasize conserving energy, setting priorities, and taking planned rest periods. An

TABLE 40.13 NURSING ASSESSMENT

Heart Valve Disease

Subjective Data

Important Health Information

Health history: IE, congenital defects, chest trauma, cardiomyopathy, syphilis, Marfan syndrome, myocardial infarction, rheumatic fever, streptococcal infections

Functional Health Patterns

Health perception–health management: IV drug use, fatigue

Activity-exercise: Palpitations, weakness, activity intolerance, dizziness, fainting, dyspnea on exertion, cough, hemoptysis, orthopnea

Sleep-rest: Paroxysmal nocturnal dyspnea

Cognitive-perceptual: Angina, atypical chest pain

Objective Data

Cardiovascular

Abnormal heart sounds, including murmurs, S_3, and S_4. Dysrhythmias, including atrial fibrillation, premature ventricular contractions. Tachycardia. ↑ or ↓ in pulse pressure, ↓ BP, water-hammer or thready peripheral pulses.

Gastrointestinal

Ascites, hepatomegaly, weight gain

General

Fever

Respiratory

Crackles, wheezes, hoarseness

Skin

Diaphoresis, flushing, cyanosis, clubbing, peripheral edema

Possible Diagnostic Findings

Cardiomegaly on chest x-ray. ECG abnormalities specific to involved valve. Echocardiogram (valve disorders, chamber dilation), heart catheterization (abnormal valves, chamber pressures, cardiac output, blood flow, depending on involved valve).

IE, Infective endocarditis; *MI,* myocardial infarction; *RF,* rheumatic fever.

appropriate exercise plan can increase cardiac tolerance. Discourage tobacco use. Consider a referral to a vocational counselor if the patient has a physically or emotionally demanding job.

Perform ongoing assessments to monitor the effectiveness of drugs. Teach the actions and side effects of drugs to increase adherence. Emphasize the importance of prophylactic antibiotic therapy to prevent IE (Table 40.2).

When heart valve disease cannot be managed medically, surgery is needed. See Chapter 37 for the care of patients having heart surgery. Patients on warfarin after surgery for valve replacement must have the international normalized ratio (INR) checked regularly to determine proper dosage and adequacy of therapy. INR values of 2.5 to 3.5 are therapeutic for patients with most mechanical valves.[21]

Table 41.15 outlines teaching related to anticoagulant therapy. Teach patients to follow up with an HCP regularly and when to seek urgent medical care. Tell patients to notify the HCP of any signs of infection, HF, or bleeding and any planned invasive or dental work. Encourage patients to wear a Medic Alert device or bracelet and carry the valve information card.

◆ Evaluation

The expected outcomes are that patients with heart valve disease will:

- Maintain adequate tissue and organ perfusion
- Achieve fluid balance
- Achieve an optimal level of activity
- Describe the disease process and measures to prevent complications

CARDIOMYOPATHY

Cardiomyopathy (CMP) is a group of diseases that directly affect myocardial structure or function. We classify CMP as primary or secondary. *Primary CMP* refers to idiopathic conditions involving only the heart muscle. In *secondary CMP*, another disease process causes myocardial disease. Common causes of secondary CMP are shown in Table 40.14.

TABLE 40.14 Causes of Cardiomyopathy

Dilated CMP	Hypertrophic CMP
• Cardiotoxic agents: alcohol, cocaine, doxorubicin • Coronary artery disease • Genetic (autosomal dominant) • Hypertension • Metabolic problems • Muscular dystrophy • Myocarditis • Pregnancy • Valve disease	• Aortic stenosis (AS) • Genetic (autosomal dominant) • Hypertension **Restrictive CMP** • Amyloidosis • Cancer • Endomyocardial fibrosis • Postradiation therapy • Sarcoidosis • Ventricular thrombus

Three major types of CMP are dilated, hypertrophic, and restrictive. Each type has its own pathogenesis, clinical presentation, and treatment (Tables 40.15 and 40.16). CMP that leads to cardiomegaly and HF is the main reason for heart transplants.

Takotsubo cardiomyopathy is a transient heart condition that causes apical akinesis and mimics acute coronary syndrome. This acute, stress-related syndrome is more common in postmenopausal females. Patients often have chest pain, ST segment elevation, and increased cardiac biomarkers consistent with an MI. However, when a patient undergoes heart catheterization, there is no significant coronary artery disease. Treatment is largely supportive. Around 5% of patients need anticoagulation.[22]

DILATED CARDIOMYOPATHY

Etiology and Pathophysiology

Dilated cardiomyopathy is the most common type of CMP. It causes HF in 20% to 45% of cases. Dilated CMP is a primary myocardial disorder with genetic or acquired origins. Alcohol-related dilated CMP has its own unique presentation and treatment. Other common causes of dilated CMP are shown in Table 40.14.

Dilated CMP appears with diffuse inflammation and rapid degeneration of heart fibers. This results in ventricular

TABLE 40.15 Types of Cardiomyopathy

Dilated	Hypertrophic	Restrictive
Cardiac Output		
↓	Normal or ↓	Normal or ↓
Cardiomegaly		
Moderate to severe	Mild to moderate	Mild
Contractility		
↓	↑ or ↓	Normal or ↓
Dysrhythmias		
Sinus tachycardia, atrial and ventricular dysrhythmias	Atrial and ventricular dysrhythmias	Atrial and ventricular dysrhythmias
Major Manifestations		
Fatigue, weakness, palpitations, dyspnea	Exertional dyspnea, fatigue, angina, syncope, palpitations	Dyspnea, fatigue
Outflow Tract Obstruction		
None	↑	None
Valve Incompetence		
Atrioventricular (AV) valves, especially mitral	Mitral valve	AV valves

dilation, impaired systolic function, atrial enlargement, and blood stasis in the left ventricle. SCD from dysrhythmias is a leading cause of death in idiopathic dilated CMP. Ventricular dilation causes *cardiomegaly* (Fig. 40.9) and contractile dysfunction. In contrast to HF, the walls of the ventricles do not hypertrophy.

TABLE 40.16 Interprofessional Care

Cardiomyopathy

Diagnostic Assessment

- History and physical assessment
- ECG
- b-Type natriuretic peptide (BNP)
- Chest x-ray
- Echocardiogram
- Nuclear imaging studies
- Heart catheterization
- Endomyocardial biopsy

Management

- Drug therapy
  - Nitrates (except in hypertrophic cardiomyopathy)
  - β-Blockers
  - Antidysrhythmics
  - ACE inhibitors
  - Calcium channel blockers
  - Diuretics
  - Digitalis (except in hypertrophic cardiomyopathy unless used to treat atrial fibrillation)
  - Anticoagulants (if indicated)
- Ventricular assist device
- Cardiac resynchronization therapy
- Implantable cardioverter-defibrillator
- Surgical repair
- Heart transplant
- Cardiac rehabilitation
- Palliative and hospice care

Clinical Manifestations

The signs and symptoms of dilated CMP may develop acutely after an infection or slowly over time. Symptoms can include decreased exercise capacity, fatigue, dyspnea at rest, paroxysmal nocturnal dyspnea, and orthopnea. As the disease progresses, patients may have a dry cough, palpitations, abdominal bloating, nausea, vomiting, and anorexia. Signs can include an abnormal S_3 and/or S_4, dysrhythmias, heart murmurs, pulmonary crackles, edema, weak peripheral pulses, pallor, hepatomegaly, and JVD. Decreased blood flow through an enlarged heart promotes stasis and blood clot formation and may lead to systemic embolization.

Diagnostic Studies

Echocardiography is usually the basis for diagnosing dilated CMP. Chest x-ray may show cardiomegaly with signs of pulmonary venous hypertension and pleural effusion. The ECG may show tachycardia, bradycardia, and dysrhythmias with conduction problems. Laboratory studies may show increased B-type natriuretic peptide (BNP) levels if HF is present.

Heart catheterization evaluates the patient for coronary artery disease. An endomyocardial biopsy done during right-sided heart catheterization can identify infectious organisms or other causes of disease.

Interprofessional and Nursing Management

Interventions focus on controlling HF by enhancing heart contractility and decreasing preload and afterload. This is similar to how we manage chronic HF. Treatment guidelines are based on the stage of disease progression (see Table 38.6). Nutrition and drug therapy and cardiac rehabilitation may help lessen symptoms of HF and improve CO and quality of life.

Several types of drugs are given to manage HF (see Table 38.7). Sacubitril/valsartan, ACE inhibitors, and/or vasodilators reduce afterload. Nitrates (e.g., nitroglycerin) and

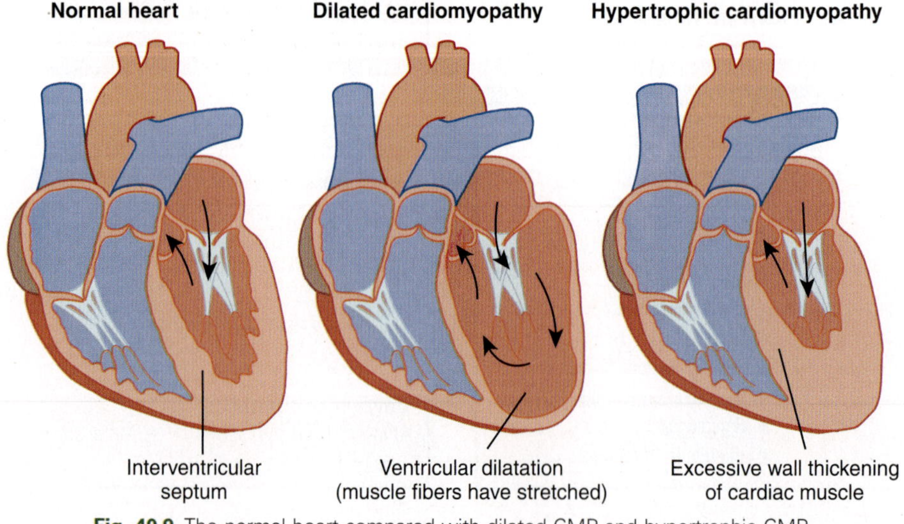

Fig. 40.9 The normal heart compared with dilated CMP and hypertrophic CMP.

diuretics (e.g., furosemide) decrease preload. β-Blockers (e.g., metoprolol) and aldosterone antagonists (e.g., spironolactone) control the neurohormonal stimulation that occurs in HF. Dysrhythmias are treated with an antidysrhythmic (see Chapter 39). Anticoagulation therapy reduces the risk for systemic embolization from clots that form in the heart chambers. For patients with a reduced EF, guidelines recommend adding an SGLT2 inhibitor.[23]

Statins may be helpful (see Table 37.6). Patients with secondary dilated CMP are treated for the underlying disease process. For example, teach patients with alcohol-related dilated CMP to abstain from alcohol.

Unfortunately, dilated CMP does not respond well to therapy, and patients have multiple episodes of HF. Patients may receive infusions of dobutamine or milrinone along with aggressive diuresis in a hospital, an outpatient setting, or in the home under nursing supervision. After treatment, many patients see an improvement in symptoms for several weeks.

Patients may benefit from nondrug therapies. A VAD allows the heart to rest and recover from acute HF or serves as a bridge to a heart transplant. Other options include cardiac resynchronization therapy and an implantable cardioverter-defibrillator (ICD) (see Chapter 38). A heart transplant may be an option in end-stage CMP. A permanent, implantable VAD, known as *destination therapy,* is an option for patients with advanced disease who are not candidates for a heart transplant (see Chapter 38). Currently, about 50% of heart transplants are done to treat CMP. Heart transplant recipients have a good prognosis. However, donor hearts are scarce. Many patients with dilated CMP die before receiving a heart.

Patients with dilated CMP are very ill and have a grave prognosis. Your expert nursing care is critical. Observe for worsening HF, dysrhythmias, and embolus formation. Monitor drug effectiveness. The goals of therapy are to keep the patient at an optimal level of functioning and out of the hospital. Include caregivers when planning care. Encourage caregivers to learn CPR. Teach them when and how to access emergency care. Home health and hospice nursing can provide patients and caregivers with palliative care. This includes strategies to maximize functional status or end-of-life care to prepare for a peaceful death.

HYPERTROPHIC CARDIOMYOPATHY

Etiology and Pathophysiology

Hypertrophic cardiomyopathy is a genetic disorder that causes asymmetric left ventricular hypertrophy without ventricular dilation.[24] In one form of the disease, the septum between the 2 ventricles becomes enlarged and blocks the blood flow from the left ventricle. We call this *hypertrophic obstructive cardiomyopathy* (HOCM) or *asymmetric septal hypertrophy* (ASH).

Hypertrophic CMP occurs less often than dilated CMP. It is more common in males. It is usually diagnosed in young adults and, most often, in active, athletic people. Hypertrophic CMP is the most common cause of SCD in otherwise healthy young people. It accounts for 3% of deaths in young competitive athletes. First-degree relatives of patients with HOCM need to be screened for the disease.

Early identification is important (Table 40.14). The 4 main characteristics of hypertrophic CMP are (1) massive ventricular hypertrophy; (2) rapid, forceful contraction of the left ventricle; (3) impaired relaxation (diastole); and (4) obstruction to aortic outflow (not present in all patients). Ventricular hypertrophy is associated with a thickened intraventricular septum and ventricular wall (Fig. 40.9). The result is poor filling of the stiff ventricle. Decreased ventricular filling and obstruction to outflow decrease CO, especially during exertion.

Clinical Manifestations

Some patients with hypertrophic CMP may be asymptomatic. Others have dyspnea, fatigue, angina, and syncope. The most common symptom is dyspnea caused by increased left ventricular diastolic pressure.[24] Fatigue occurs because of the decrease in CO and exercise-induced flow obstruction. Increased left ventricular mass or compression of the small coronary arteries by the hypertrophic myocardium causes angina. Patients may have syncope during increased activity from obstruction to aortic outflow. Syncope can be caused by dysrhythmias, such as supraventricular tachycardia, atrial fibrillation, ventricular tachycardia, and ventricular fibrillation (see Chapter 39).

Diagnostic Studies

Clinical findings may be unremarkable. On chest palpation, the apical impulse can be exaggerated and displaced to the left. Auscultation may reveal an S_4 and a systolic murmur between the apex and sternal border at the 4th intercostal space. ECG findings usually show ventricular hypertrophy, ST-T wave abnormalities, prominent Q waves in the inferior or precordial leads, and dysrhythmias (see Chapter 39).

The echocardiogram is the main diagnostic tool used to confirm hypertrophic CMP. It may show wall motion abnormalities and diastolic dysfunction. Heart catheterization and nuclear stress testing may help diagnose and guide the treatment of hypertrophic CMP.

Interprofessional and Nursing Management

The goals of care are to improve ventricular filling by reducing ventricular contractility and relieving left ventricular outflow obstruction. These can be achieved with β-blocker (e.g., metoprolol) or calcium channel blocker (e.g., verapamil) therapy.[21] Mavacamten inhibits myosin action to reduce contractibility.[25] Amiodarone or sotalol are effective antidysrhythmic drugs. Patients at risk for SCD need a cardioverter-defibrillator (see Chapter 39).

AV pacing is helpful for patients with hypertrophic CMP and outflow obstruction. When the ventricles are paced from the apex of the right ventricle, septal depolarization occurs first. This allows the septum to move away from the left ventricular wall and reduces the degree of obstruction of the outflow tract.

Some patients with severe symptoms unresponsive to therapy may be candidates for surgical treatment of their hypertrophied septum. A *ventriculomyotomy and myectomy* involve cutting into the thickened septal muscle and removing some of the ventricular muscle. Most patients have an improvement in symptoms and exercise tolerance after surgery.

An alternative nonsurgical procedure to reduce symptoms and the left ventricular outflow obstruction is *percutaneous transluminal septal myocardial ablation* (PTSMA). This procedure consists of injecting alcohol into the first septal artery branching off the left anterior descending artery to cause ischemia and septal wall infarction. Ablation of the septal wall decreases the obstruction to flow, and the patient's symptoms decrease. The procedure can improve HF symptoms and exercise capacity. Potential complications include conduction problems (e.g., heart block) and MI.

Interventions for hypertrophic CMP focus on relieving symptoms, observing for and preventing complications, and providing emotional support. Teach patients to avoid strenuous activity and dehydration. Any activity that causes an increase in systemic vascular resistance (thus increasing the obstruction to forward flow) is dangerous. Rest and elevation of the feet to improve venous return to the heart can help manage chest pain. Vasodilators, such as nitroglycerin, may worsen chest pain by decreasing venous return and further increasing obstruction of blood flow from the heart.

RESTRICTIVE CARDIOMYOPATHY

Etiology and Pathophysiology

Restrictive cardiomyopathy is the least common type of CMP. It is a disease of the myocardium that impairs diastolic filling and stretch. Systolic function stays unchanged. The specific cause of restrictive CMP is unknown, but several processes may be involved. Myocardial fibrosis, hypertrophy, and infiltration stiffen the ventricular wall with loss of ventricular compliance. Secondary causes of restrictive CMP include amyloidosis, endocardial fibrosis, sarcoidosis, and thoracic radiation. With restrictive CMP, the ventricles are resistant to filling and require high diastolic filling pressures to maintain CO.

Clinical Manifestations and Diagnostic Studies

Classic manifestations are fatigue, exercise intolerance, and dyspnea. The heart cannot increase CO by increasing the HR without further compromising ventricular filling. Other symptoms may include angina, orthopnea, syncope, and palpitations. Patients may have signs of HF, including dyspnea, peripheral edema, weight gain, ascites, hepatomegaly, and JVD.

The chest x-ray may be normal, or it may show cardiomegaly from atrial enlargement. Pleural effusions and pulmonary congestion may occur as a patient progresses to HF. The most common dysrhythmias are supraventricular (atrial fibrillation) or AV block. Echocardiography may show a left ventricle that is normal size with a thickened wall, slightly dilated right ventricle, and dilated atria. Endomyocardial biopsy, CT scan, and nuclear imaging may help in the diagnosis.

Interprofessional and Nursing Management

There is no specific treatment for restrictive CMP. Treatments aim to improve diastolic filling and the underlying disease process using conventional therapy and nursing care for HF and dysrhythmias. A heart transplant may be an option. Teach patients to avoid situations, such as strenuous activity and dehydration, which impair ventricular filling and increase systemic vascular resistance. Nursing care of patients with CMP includes patient-specific teaching based on their manifestations. A guide for patient and caregiver teaching is outlined in Table 40.17.

TABLE 40.17 PATIENT & CAREGIVER TEACHING

Cardiomyopathy

Include the following information in the teaching plan for a patient with cardiomyopathy and the patient's caregiver:

- Take all drugs as prescribed and regularly follow up with HCP.
- Follow a low-sodium diet (if prescribed) and read all product labels (food and over-the-counter drugs) for sodium content.
- Drink 6 to 8 glasses of water a day unless fluids are restricted.
- Achieve and maintain a reasonable weight and avoid large meals.
- Avoid alcohol, caffeine, diet pills, and over-the-counter cold medicines that may contain stimulants.
- Balance activity and rest periods.
- Avoid heavy lifting or vigorous isometric exercises and check with HCP for exercise guidelines.
- Use stress management techniques: relaxation breathing, guided imagery.
- Report any signs of heart failure to HCP, including weight gain, edema, shortness of breath, and increased fatigue.
- Encourage caregivers to learn CPR because of the potential for cardiac arrest.
- Access emergency response system (ERS) according to the HCP's instructions.

CASE STUDY

Heart Valve Disease

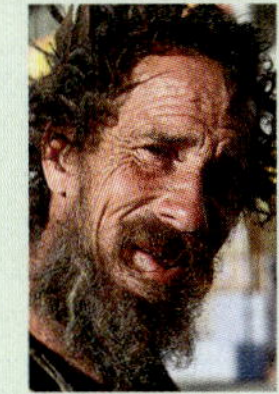

(© JennaDub/ iStock/Thinkstock.)

Patient Profile

R.B. is a 50-year-old male admitted to the hospital for acute decompensated HF caused by heart valve disease.

Subjective Data

- History of IV drug use.
- Reports regular alcohol use of 1 pint of whiskey per day.
- States, "I'm short of breath all the time. I can't sleep when I lay down."
- Describes chest pain with minimal exertion.
- Recently unemployed.
- States, "I'm always tired."
- States, "The prescribed drugs are too expensive. I can't afford them."
- A 35-pack-year history.

Objective Data

Physical Assessment

- A 3rd heart sound (S_3)
- Loud holosystolic murmur of mitral regurgitation
- Missing all teeth from periodontal disease
- Vital signs: Temp 99.0°F (37.2°C); apical-radial pulse equal at 110 beats/min, irregular; respirations 24; BP 104/58 mm Hg

Diagnostic Studies

- ECG shows atrial fibrillation with a rapid ventricular response
- Chest x-ray shows pulmonary congestion and cardiomegaly
- Transesophageal echocardiography shows left atrial and ventricular hypertrophy and mitral and aortic regurgitation; EF 30%

Discussion Questions

1. ***Recognize:*** Distinguish the consequences of mitral and aortic regurgitation.
2. ***Analyze:*** Which information in R.B.'s history indicates a risk factor for valve disease?
3. ***Plan:*** What therapy do you expect will be planned for R.B.?
4. ***Prioritize:*** Identify the priority interventions for R.B.
5. ***Act:*** Identify the tasks that you would delegate to AP.
6. ***Evaluate:*** What information would indicate that R.B. understands why he will need to continue taking anticoagulants after the valve replacement surgery?
7. ***Safety:*** What safety precautions should we consider for R.B.?

Answers available at http://evolve.elsevier.com/Lewis/medsurg.

BRIDGE TO NCLEX EXAMINATION

The number of the question corresponds to the same-numbered outcome at the beginning of the chapter.

1. Which findings would the nurse expect when assessing a patient with infective endocarditis? **(Select all that apply.)**
   - **a.** Retinal hemorrhages
   - **b.** Splinter hemorrhages
   - **c.** Presence of Osler nodes
   - **d.** Painless nodules over bony prominences
   - **e.** Erythematous macules on the palms and soles
2. Which intervention is *the highest priority* in nursing management of a patient with myocarditis?
   - **a.** Providing meticulous skin care
   - **b.** Assuring tight glycemic control
   - **c.** Administering antibiotic prophylaxis
   - **d.** Monitoring oxygenation and ventilation
3. Which condition would the nurse teach the patient is a possible long-term consequence of rheumatic fever?
   - **a.** Heart valve disease
   - **b.** Pulmonary hypertension
   - **c.** Superior vena cava syndrome
   - **d.** Hypertrophy of the right ventricle
4. Which is a *priority* intervention for a patient during the acute phase of rheumatic fever?
   - **a.** Giving IV antibiotics as prescribed
   - **b.** Managing pain with opioid analgesics
   - **c.** Encouraging fluid intake for hydration
   - **d.** Performing frequent active range-of-motion exercises
5. Which interventions could the nurse delegate to AP when caring for a patient with mitral stenosis and new-onset atrial fibrillation? **(Select all that apply.)**
   - **a.** Obtain and record daily weight.
   - **b.** Determine apical-radial pulse rate.
   - **c.** Observe for overt signs of bleeding.
   - **d.** Teach the patient how to avoid bruising and bleeding.
   - **e.** Obtain and record vital signs, including pulse oximetry.
6. Which intervention would be a *priority* when caring for a patient newly admitted with heart failure secondary to dilated cardiomyopathy?
   - **a.** Encourage caregivers to learn CPR.
   - **b.** Consider a consult with hospice for palliative care.
   - **c.** Monitor the patient's response to prescribed medications.
   - **d.** Arrange for the patient to enter a cardiac rehabilitation program.

1. a, b, c, e; 2. d; 3. a; 4. a; 5. a, c, e; 6. c.

For rationales to these answers and even more NCLEX review questions, visit http://evolve.elsevier.com/Lewis/medsurg.

REFERENCES

To access the References for this chapter, please scan the QR code with a mobile device.

41

Vascular Disorders

Kimberly Day

http://evolve.elsevier.com/Lewis/medsurg/

CONCEPTUAL FOCUS

Perfusion

Tissue Integrity

LEARNING OUTCOMES

1. Relate the etiology and pathophysiology of peripheral artery disease (PAD) to the major risk factors.
2. Describe the clinical manifestations and interprofessional and nursing management of patients with lower extremity PAD.
3. Plan nursing and interprofessional management for patients with acute arterial ischemia.
4. Distinguish the pathophysiology, clinical manifestations, and nursing and interprofessional management of patients with thromboangiitis obliterans and Raynaud phenomenon.
5. Distinguish the pathophysiology, clinical manifestations, and interprofessional and nursing management of patients with different types of aortic aneurysms.
6. Select nursing interventions for patients undergoing an aortic aneurysm repair.
7. Describe the pathophysiology, clinical manifestations, and interprofessional and nursing management of patients with aortic dissection.
8. Evaluate risk factors for superficial vein thrombosis or venous thromboembolism (VTE).
9. Distinguish between the clinical characteristics of superficial vein thrombosis and VTE.
10. Outline the interprofessional and nursing management of patients with superficial vein thrombosis and VTE.
11. Prioritize the nursing management for patients receiving anticoagulant therapy.
12. Relate the pathophysiology and clinical manifestations to the interprofessional care of patients with varicose veins, chronic venous insufficiency, and venous leg ulcers.

KEY TERMS

acute arterial ischemia
aneurysm
aortic dissection
chronic venous insufficiency (CVI)
critical limb ischemia
deep vein thrombosis (DVT)
intermittent claudication
peripheral artery disease (PAD)
postthrombotic syndrome (PTS)
superficial vein thrombosis
thromboangiitis obliterans (Buerger disease)
varicose veins
venous thromboembolism (VTE)
venous thrombosis
Virchow triad

Vascular system problems include disorders of the arteries, veins, and lymphatic vessels. This chapter discusses peripheral artery disease, aortic aneurysm and dissection, and venous diseases.

These problems can result in decreased perfusion and ischemia of the peripheral tissues. Patients often have pain and difficulties with mobility and activities of daily living. Education is a key part of management. Proper nutrition, smoking cessation, and exercise are important health promotion behaviors. Following measures to promote safety, especially for those on anticoagulant therapy, is critical.

ARTERIAL DISEASE

LOWER EXTREMITY PERIPHERAL ARTERY DISEASE

Peripheral artery disease (PAD) involves thickening of artery walls. This results in a progressive narrowing of the arteries of the upper and lower extremities. PAD prevalence increases with age. It typically becomes symptomatic between ages 50 and 70 years. In people with diabetes, PAD occurs earlier. In the United

States about 6.5 million people over age 40 have PAD. The prevalence is highest in Black people.[1]

PAD is strongly related to other types of cardiovascular disease (CVD) and their risk factors. Patients with PAD have a higher risk for general mortality, CVD mortality, major coronary events, and stroke.[2] It is a marker of systemic atherosclerosis. Patients with PAD are more likely to have coronary artery disease (CAD) and/or cerebral artery disease.

Etiology and Pathophysiology

The leading cause of PAD is *atherosclerosis.* Atherosclerosis often affects certain segments of the arterial tree. These include the coronary, carotid, and lower extremity arteries. Symptoms occur when vessels are 60% to 75% blocked.

Other risk factors for PAD are similar, but not identical, to those for CAD. Key risk factors for PAD are tobacco use (most important), diabetes, hypertension, high lipid levels, and age over 60.[1] Having multiple risk factors dramatically increases the risk. Diabetes is associated with more severe below-the-knee PAD. Those with advanced PAD often have multiple arterial occlusions.

Clinical Manifestations

Lower extremity PAD may affect the iliac, femoral, popliteal, tibial, or peroneal arteries or any combination of these arteries (Fig. 41.1). The severity of symptoms depends on the site and extent of the blockage and the amount of collateral circulation.

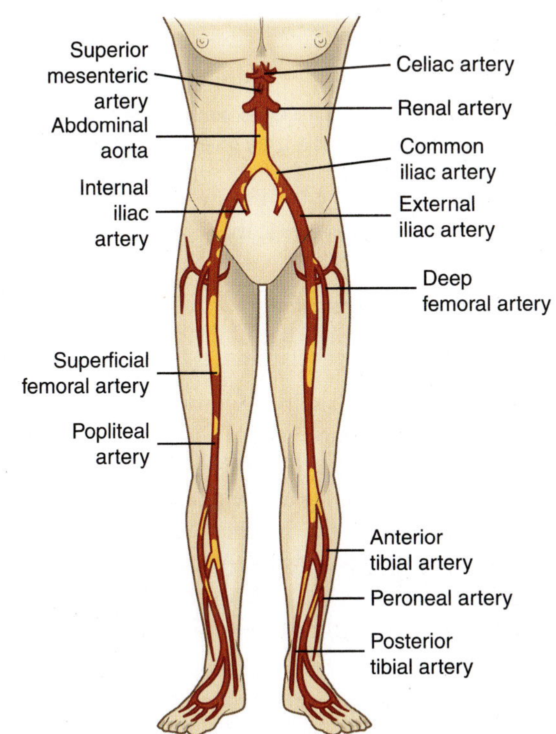

Fig. 41.1 Common anatomic locations of atherosclerotic lesions (shown in *yellow*) of the abdominal aorta and lower extremities.

The classic symptom of lower extremity PAD **is intermittent claudication.** This ischemic muscle pain is caused by exercise, resolves within 10 minutes with rest, and is reproducible. The pain results from the buildup of lactic acid from anaerobic metabolism. Once the patient stops exercising, the lactic acid clears, and the pain subsides. PAD of the iliac arteries causes pain in the buttocks and thighs. Calf pain occurs with femoral or popliteal artery involvement.

As many as one-third of patients with PAD have classic symptoms. Others have no symptoms or atypical leg symptoms (e.g., burning, heaviness, pressure, soreness, tightness, weakness) in atypical locations (e.g., ankle, foot, hamstring, hip, knee, shin). PAD involving the internal iliac arteries may cause erectile dysfunction.

Paresthesia (numbness or tingling) in the toes or feet may result from nerve tissue ischemia. True peripheral neuropathy occurs more often in patients with diabetes and in those with long-standing ischemia. Neuropathy causes severe shooting or burning pain in the extremity. It does not follow particular nerve roots and may be present near ulcerated areas. Gradual, reduced blood flow to neurons causes loss of sensation to pressure and deep pain. So, patients may not notice lower extremity injuries.

The limb's appearance gives vital information about reduced blood flow. The skin becomes thin, shiny, and taut. The lower legs lose their hair. Pedal, popliteal, or femoral pulses are decreased or absent. Pallor develops when the leg is elevated *(elevation pallor).* Conversely, *reactive hyperemia* (redness of the foot) develops when the limb is in a dependent position *(dependent rubor)* (Table 41.1).

As PAD progresses and involves multiple arterial segments, continuous pain develops at rest. Rest pain most often occurs in the foot or toes. It is worse with limb elevation. Rest pain occurs when blood flow does not meet basic metabolic needs of the distal tissues. It occurs more often at night because cardiac output tends to drop during sleep and the limbs are at heart level. Patients often try to relieve pain by gravity. They dangle their legs over the side of the bed or sleep in a chair.

Critical limb ischemia (CLI) is a condition characterized by chronic ischemic rest pain lasting more than 2 weeks, nonhealing arterial leg ulcers, or gangrene of the leg from PAD. Patients with PAD who have diabetes, heart failure (HF), and a history of a stroke have a higher risk for CLI.[2]

Complications

Lower extremity PAD progresses slowly. Prolonged ischemia leads to atrophy of the skin and underlying muscles. Minor trauma to the feet (e.g., stubbing one's toe, blister from shoes) can result in delayed healing, wound infection, and tissue necrosis, especially in patients with diabetes. Arterial (ischemic) ulcers most often occur over bony prominences on the toes, feet, and lower legs (Table 41.1). Nonhealing ulcers and gangrene are the most serious complications. If PAD develops over an extended period, collateral circulation may prevent gangrene.

Amputation may be needed if adequate blood flow is not restored or if severe infection occurs. Uncontrolled pain and

TABLE 41.1 Comparison of Peripheral Artery and Venous Disease

Characteristic	Peripheral Artery Disease	Venous Disease
Ankle-brachial index	≤0.90	>0.90
Capillary refill	>3 sec	<3 sec
Dermatitis	Rare	Often
Edema	Absent unless leg constantly in dependent position	Lower leg edema
Hair	Loss of hair on legs, feet, toes	Hair may be present or absent
Nails	Thickened, brittle	Normal or thickened
Pain	Intermittent claudication or rest pain in foot Ulcer may be painful	Dull ache or heaviness in calf or thigh Ulcer often painful
Peripheral pulses	Decreased or absent	Present, may be hard to palpate with edema
Pruritus	Rarely occurs	Often occurs
Skin color	Dependent rubor, elevation pallor	Bronze-brown pigmentation Varicose veins may be visible
Skin temperature	Cool, temperature gradient down the leg	Warm, no temperature gradient
Skin texture	Thin, shiny, taut	Skin thick, hardened, and indurated
Ulcer		
• Location	Tips of toes, foot, or lateral malleolus	Near medial malleolus
• Margin	Rounded, smooth, looks "punched out"	Irregularly shaped
• Drainage	Minimal	Moderate to large amount
• Tissue	Black eschar or pale pink granulation	Yellow slough or dark red, "ruddy" granulation

TABLE 41.2 Interprofessional Care

Peripheral Artery Disease

Diagnostic Assessment

- Health history and physical assessment, including palpation of peripheral pulses
- Doppler ultrasound studies
- Segmental BPs
- Ankle-brachial index (ABI) (Table 41.3)
- Duplex imaging
- Angiography
- Magnetic resonance angiography

Management

Conservative Therapy

- Cardiovascular disease risk factor modification
  - Tobacco cessation
  - Regular physical exercise
  - Achieve or maintain ideal body weight
  - Follow dietary approaches to stop hypertension (DASH) diet or Mediterranean diet
  - Tight glucose control with diabetes, including HbA1c monitoring
  - Tight control of BP and lipid and triglyceride levels
  - Antiplatelet agent (aspirin, clopidogrel)
  - ACE inhibitors (see Table 36.6)
- Treat claudication symptoms
  - Structured walking or exercise program
  - Cilostazol or pentoxifylline
- Nutrition therapy (DASH or Mediterranean diet)
- Physical/occupational therapy
- Proper foot care (see Table 53.16)

Surgical Therapy

- Percutaneous transluminal balloon angioplasty with or without stent
- Percutaneous transluminal atherectomy
- Percutaneous transluminal cryoplasty
- Peripheral artery bypass surgery
- Patch graft angioplasty, often in conjunction with bypass surgery
- Endarterectomy (for local stenosis; rarely done as a stand-alone procedure)
- Thrombolytic therapy or mechanical clot extraction therapy (for acute ischemia only)
- Sympathectomy (for pain management only)
- Amputation

ACE, Angiotensin-converting enzyme.

severe, spreading infection are indicators for amputation in people who are not candidates for revascularization. Diabetes increases the risk of amputation.

Diagnostic Studies

Various tests assess blood flow and the vascular system (Table 41.2). Doppler ultrasound with duplex imaging maps blood flow throughout an entire arterial region. It can determine the degree of blood flow. Angiography and magnetic resonance angiography show the location and extent of PAD (see Table 35.11).

Segmental BPs are obtained using Doppler ultrasound and a sphygmomanometer at the thigh, below the knee, and at ankle level while the patient is supine. A drop in segmental BP of greater than 30 mm Hg suggests PAD.

The *ankle-brachial index* (ABI) is a PAD screening tool. Calculate the ABI for each leg by dividing the ankle systolic BP (SBP) by the higher of the brachial SBPs. PAD guidelines recommend uniform reporting of ABI results (Table 41.3).[2] Calcified and stiff arteries in patients who are older or have diabetes often show a falsely elevated ABI.

Interprofessional Care

Table 41.2 outlines the interprofessional care for patients with PAD.

TABLE 41.3 Interpreting Ankle-Brachial Index Results

ABI	Clinical Significance
>1.30	Noncompressible arteries
1.00–1.30	Normal ABI
0.91–0.99	Borderline ABI
≤0.90	Abnormal ABI
Classification of PAD Severity	
0.90–0.71	Mild PAD
0.70–0.41	Moderate PAD
≤0.40	Severe PAD

Risk Factor Modification

The first treatment goal for patients with PAD is to reduce CVD risk factors. This may require lifestyle changes and drug therapy (see Tables 37.2 to 37.5). Hypertension is a well-known risk factor for PAD progression. Encourage reduced sodium intake and following the dietary approaches to stop hypertension (DASH) or Mediterranean diet. Chapter 36 discusses hypertension. Support aggressive lipid management with diet interventions and drug therapy (see Table 37.6).

Tobacco cessation is essential to reduce the risk for CVD events, PAD progression, and death. This is a difficult process with a high incidence of relapse. Suggest tobacco cessation strategies (see Tables 11.3 to 11.6). Patients with diabetes should maintain a glycosylated hemoglobin (A1c) below 7.0%.[3] Chapter 53 discusses diabetes.

Drug Therapy

Angiotensin-converting enzyme (ACE) inhibitors (e.g., ramipril) can reduce PAD symptoms. Antiplatelet agents reduce the risks for CVD events and death. Oral antiplatelet therapy should include low-dose aspirin therapy. Aspirin-intolerant patients may take clopidogrel bisulfate (Plavix) daily. Combination antiplatelet therapy with aspirin and clopidogrel bisulfate may be used by select high-risk patients. Anticoagulants (e.g., warfarin) are not recommended for preventing CVD events in patients with PAD.

DRUG ALERT

Clopidogrel Bisulfate and Omeprazole

- Taking omeprazole with clopidogrel bisulfate reduces the antiplatelet effect by half.
- This reduced effect increases the risk for myocardial infarction (MI) and stroke.

Two drugs are available to treat intermittent claudication: cilostazol and pentoxifylline. Cilostazol—a phosphodiesterase inhibitor—inhibits platelet aggregation and increases vasodilation. Pentoxifylline—a synthetic dimethylxanthine derivative—improves the flexibility of red blood cells (RBCs) and decreases fibrinogen concentration, platelet adhesiveness, and blood viscosity. It is not as effective as cilostazol and should only be used if a patient has a contraindication to cilostazol.[4]

Exercise Therapy

A supervised exercise program is recommended as part of the initial treatment for patients with intermittent claudication. Patients should exercise for 30 to 45 min/day, at least 3 times/week, for a minimum of 3 months. Although we most often prescribe walking, other modes of exercise (e.g., cycling) improve walking ability and quality of life.[2]

Encouraging exercise is especially important for females because they have faster functional decline and greater mobility loss than males with PAD. Overall, patients with PAD who have higher levels of daily physical activity have better survival rates.[4]

Nutrition Therapy

Teach patients to maintain a body mass index (BMI) less than 25 kg/m^2 and a waist circumference less than 40 inches for males and less than 35 inches for females. Even modest, sustained weight loss of 3% to 5% yields important reductions in triglycerides, glucose, A1c, and the risk for developing type 2 diabetes. Greater weight loss has greater benefits. Recommend a diet reduced in calories and salt for persons who are obese or overweight.

Management of Critical Limb Ischemia

Optimal therapy for patients with CLI is revascularization via bypass surgery using an *autogenous* (native) vein. An alternative is percutaneous transluminal angioplasty (PTA).[2] Patients with CLI should continue optimal drug therapy (e.g., statin, antiplatelet, ACE inhibitor, β-blocker) to reduce the risk for a CVD event.

Conservative management includes protecting the extremity from trauma, decreasing ischemic pain, preventing and controlling infection, and improving perfusion. Inspect, cleanse, and lubricate feet to prevent skin cracking and infection. Avoid lubrication between the toes and soaking the patient's feet to prevent skin breakdown. Keep the affected foot clean and dry. Cover any ulcers with a dry, sterile dressing. We use a variety of wound care products to treat deep ulcers. Healing is unlikely without increasing the blood flow.

Encourage patients to wear soft, roomy, and protective footwear and avoid extremes of heat and cold. Keep the heels free of pressure. Place a pillow under the calves so that the heels are off the mattress or use a heel protection device. Giving analgesics and placing the bed in the reverse Trendelenburg position may control pain and increase perfusion to the lower extremities.

Spinal cord stimulation may help patients with CLI to manage pain. Other promising strategies include growth factors and gene and stem cell therapy to stimulate blood vessel growth *(angiogenesis)*. Unfortunately, almost half of the patients with CLI will die within 5 years.[5]

Interventional Radiology Procedures

Interventional radiology catheter-based procedures are alternatives to surgery for treating lower extremity PAD. These procedures take place in a catheterization laboratory. They are similar to angiography in that they involve inserting a special catheter into the femoral artery. The PTA procedure uses a catheter with a balloon at the tip. The tip of the catheter is moved to the narrowed (stenotic) area of the artery. The balloon is then inflated, compressing the atherosclerotic intimal lining.[4] We give antiplatelet agents afterward to reduce the risk for restenosis. Long-term, low-dose aspirin therapy or clopidogrel is recommended.

Stents—expandable metallic devices—are placed within the artery after balloon angioplasty. The stent holds the artery open. Angioplasty balloons and peripheral stents coated with a drug (e.g., paclitaxel) can limit new tissue growth in the treated area and improve long-term patency rates.[4]

Atherectomy is the removal of the obstructing plaque. A directional atherectomy device uses a high-speed cutting disk that cuts long strips of the atheroma. Laser atherectomy uses ultraviolet energy to break up the atheroma. Another type of atherectomy catheter has a diamond-coated tip that rotates at a high speed like a drill.

Cryoplasty combines PTA and cold therapy. A special balloon is filled with liquid nitrous oxide, which changes to gas as it enters the balloon. Expansion of the gas results in cooling to 14°F (−10°C). The cold temperature limits restenosis by reducing smooth muscle cell activity.

Surgical Therapy

Various surgical approaches are used to improve blood flow beyond a blocked artery. When possible, peripheral artery bypass surgery is done with an autogenous vein to bypass (carry blood around) the lesion (Fig. 41.2). Synthetic grafts are used for long routes, such as an axillary-femoral bypass. When a person's own vein is not available, a human umbilical vein or a composite sequential bypass graft (native vein plus synthetic graft) can be used.[2] PTA with stenting may be done in combination with bypass surgery.

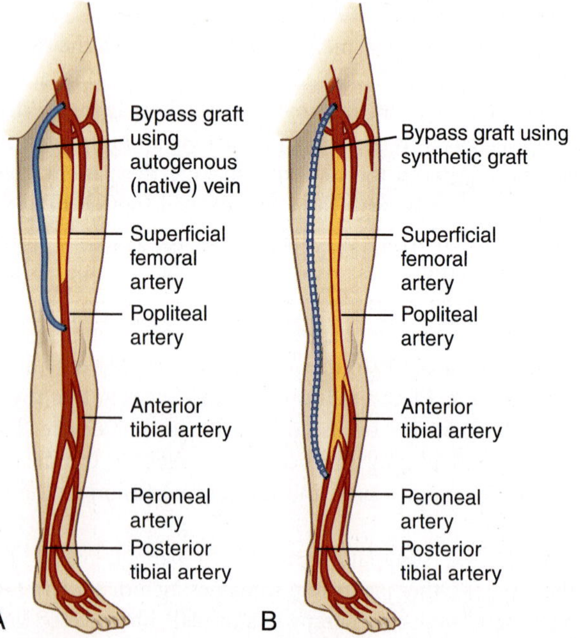

Fig. 41.2 (A) Femoral-popliteal bypass graft around an occluded superficial femoral artery. (B) Femoral-posterior tibial bypass graft around occluded superficial femoral, popliteal, and proximal tibial arteries.

Other options include *endarterectomy* (opening the artery and removing the obstructing plaque) and *patch graft angioplasty* (opening the artery, removing plaque, and sewing a patch to the opening to widen the lumen).

Amputation may be needed if tissue necrosis is extensive, gangrene or osteomyelitis develops, or all major arteries in the limb are blocked. Preserving as much of the limb as possible improves rehabilitation potential. Amputation is discussed in Chapter 67.

NURSING MANAGEMENT: LOWER EXTREMITY PAD

Assessment

Table 41.4 presents subjective and objective data to obtain from patients with PAD.

TABLE 41.4 NURSING ASSESSMENT

Peripheral Artery Disease

Subjective Data

Important Health Information

Health history: Diabetes, hypertension, hyperlipidemia, hypertriglyceridemia, hyperuricemia, impaired renal function, obesity.

Functional Health Patterns

Health perception–health management: Family history of cardiovascular disease. Tobacco use, including exposure to environment smoke.

Nutritional-metabolic: High sodium, saturated fat, and cholesterol intake. Elevated HbA1c.

Activity-exercise: Exercise intolerance, sedentary lifestyle.

Cognitive-perceptual: Buttock, thigh, or calf pain that is precipitated by exercise and subsides with rest (intermittent claudication) or progresses to pain at rest. Burning pain in feet and toes at rest. Numbness, tingling, sensation of cold in legs or feet. Progressive loss of sensation and deep pain in extremities.

Sexuality-reproductive: Erectile dysfunction.

Objective Data

Cardiovascular

Decreased or absent peripheral pulses. Feet cool to touch. Capillary refill >3 sex. Bruits may be present at pulse sites.

Neurologic

Impaired mobility or sensation.

Skin

Loss of hair on legs and feet. Thick toenails. Pallor with elevation. Dependent rubor. Thin, cool, shiny skin with muscle atrophy. Skin breakdown and arterial ulcers, especially over bony areas. Gangrene.

Possible Diagnostic Findings

Arterial stenosis evident with duplex imaging, ↓ Doppler pressures, ↓ ABI, angiography shows peripheral atherosclerosis. ↑ High-sensitivity C-reactive protein, homocysteine, or lipoprotein (a) [Lp(a)] levels.

◆ Clinical Problems

Clinical problems for patients with PAD may include:

- Activity intolerance
- Impaired tissue integrity
- Inadequate tissue perfusion
- Pain

Additional information on clinical problems and interventions for patients with PAD of the lower extremities is presented in eNursing Care Plan 41.1 on the website for this chapter.

◆ Planning

Nursing care focuses on the priority problems of poor tissue perfusion and pain. The overall goals include (1) adequate tissue perfusion; (2) pain relief; (3) increased exercise tolerance; (4) intact, healthy skin on the extremities; and (5) knowledge of disease and treatment plan.

◆ Implementation

Health Promotion

Assess patients for and provide instructions on how to control CVD risk factors (see Table 37.2). Teach diet modification to reduce cholesterol, saturated fat, and salt (see Tables 37.4 and 37.5). Teach proper foot care and injury prevention. Encourage patients with family histories of cardiac, diabetes, or vascular disease to obtain regular follow-up care.

Acute Care

After surgical or radiologic intervention, observe the patient in a recovery area. Check the operative extremity every 15 minutes initially and then hourly. Assess color, temperature, capillary refill, peripheral pulses, and sensation and movement. Immediately notify the HCP of any loss of palpable pulses or change in the Doppler sound over a pulse. Do not obtain ABI measurements, as they place the patient at risk for graft thrombosis. Compare assessment findings with the patient's baseline and with findings in the opposite limb.

Patients with a history of chronic ischemic rest pain may have tolerance to opioids. Thus aggressive pain management may be needed after surgery.

After the patient leaves the recovery area, continue to monitor extremity perfusion. Assess for complications, such as bleeding, hematoma, thrombosis, embolization, and compartment syndrome. A dramatic increase in pain, loss of previously palpable pulses, extremity pallor or cyanosis, numbness or tingling, or a cold extremity suggests graft or stent blockage. Report these findings to the HCP at once.

CHECK YOUR PRACTICE

You are caring for a 74-year-old male patient who is recovering from left femoral-popliteal bypass graft surgery. When you respond to the patient's call light, the patient reports severe pain in the operative leg. On assessment, you cannot palpate the dorsalis pedis and posterior tibial pulses. The foot is cold to touch.

- What are your next actions?

Do not place the patient in a knee-flexed position except for exercise. Turn the patient and position frequently with pillows to support the incision. On postoperative day 1, help the patient out of bed several times. Walking even short distances is desirable. A walker may be helpful, especially for frail, older patients. Discourage prolonged sitting with legs lowered, because it may cause pain and edema, increase the risk for venous thrombosis, and place stress on the suture lines. Graduated compression stockings may help control leg edema. If edema develops, position the patient supine, and elevate the leg above heart level.

Surgical site infection (SSI) is a serious complication. Careful postoperative assessment and wound care are important. SSIs are associated with early graft loss, longer hospitalization, reoperation, and sepsis.

Chronic Care

Assess for CVD risk factors and teach health promotion strategies (Table 41.5). Continued tobacco use dramatically decreases graft and stent patency and increases the risk for MI and stroke.

TABLE 41.5 PATIENT & CAREGIVER TEACHING

Peripheral Artery Bypass Surgery

Include the following information in the teaching plan for a patient undergoing peripheral artery bypass surgery and the patient's caregiver:

1. Reduce risk factors. Stop tobacco use, control glucose levels with diabetes, control BP, lower lipid and triglyceride levels, achieve or maintain ideal body weight, and exercise regularly.
2. Basic mechanism of action (why prescribed for patient), side effects, and safety precautions for drugs such as antiplatelets, antihypertensives, lipid-lowering therapy, and pain medication.
3. Eat healthy—it is essential to recovery. Drink plenty of fluids. Eat a well-balanced diet (e.g., foods high in protein, vitamins C and A, and zinc; high-fiber foods; fresh fruits and vegetables). Eat fewer high-fat foods and reduce salt intake.
4. Take part in a supervised exercise program or take a daily walk. In the beginning, take several short walks a day and rest between activities. Gradually increase your walking to 30–40 min/day, 3 to 5 days/week.
5. Care for feet and legs. Inspect feet and wash them daily. Wear clean cotton or wool socks and well-fitting shoes. File toenails straight across. Avoid sitting with legs crossed, extreme hot and cold temperatures, and prolonged standing.
6. Follow routine postoperative wound care that includes keeping incision clean and dry; do not disturb adhesive bandages (if present).
7. Monitor for signs and symptoms of impaired healing or infection of the leg incision, and notify HCP if any of the following occur:
   - Prolonged drainage or pus from the incision
   - Increased redness, warmth, pain, or hardness along incision
   - Separation of wound edges
   - Fever >100°F (37.8°C)
8. Keep all follow-up appointments with HCP.
9. Notify HCP at once of increased leg or foot pain or a change in the color or temperature of leg or foot.

Long-term antiplatelet therapy with aspirin or clopidogrel is used after surgery. Patients having distal peripheral bypass surgery (i.e., below the knee) using synthetic graft materials receive dual antiplatelet therapy (clopidogrel plus aspirin) for 1 to 3 months, followed by lifelong single antiplatelet therapy. Clopidogrel is preferred over aspirin.[4]

Encourage supervised exercise training after revascularization. Explain that exercise decreases CVD risk factors, including hypertension, hyperlipidemia, obesity, and glucose levels. Foot care is especially important in patients with diabetes and PAD (see Table 53.16). Diabetic neuropathy increases the risk for injury. Tell patients to inspect their legs and feet daily for changes in skin color or texture. Show patients how to palpate pulses and check skin temperature and capillary refill. Stress reporting any changes or the presence of ulceration or inflammation to the HCP.

Thick or overgrown toenails and calluses are potentially serious and need regular attention by an HCP (e.g., podiatrist). Patients with poor eyesight, back problems, obesity, or arthritis may need help with foot care. Encourage patients to wear clean, all-cotton or all-wool socks and comfortable shoes with round toes and soft insoles. Tell patients to lace shoes loosely and break in new shoes gradually.

◆ Evaluation

The expected outcomes are that patients with PAD of the lower extremities will have:

- Adequate peripheral tissue perfusion
- Increased activity tolerance
- Effective pain management

ACUTE ARTERIAL ISCHEMIA

Etiology and Pathophysiology

Acute arterial ischemia is a sudden interruption in the arterial blood supply to a tissue, an organ, or an extremity. If left untreated, it can result in tissue death. Causes include embolism, thrombosis of an atherosclerotic artery, or trauma. *Embolization* of a thrombus from the heart is the most frequent cause of acute arterial occlusion. Heart conditions in which thrombi can develop include infective endocarditis, mitral valve disease, atrial fibrillation, cardiomyopathies, and prosthetic heart valves. Noncardiac sources of emboli include aneurysms, ulcerated atherosclerotic plaque, recent endovascular procedures, and venous thrombi.

Thrombi that originate in the left side of the heart may dislodge and travel anywhere in the systemic circulation. Most emboli block an artery of the leg where vessels branch (e.g., iliofemoral, popliteal, tibial) or narrow. Sudden local thrombosis may occur at the site of an atherosclerotic plaque. Hypovolemia (e.g., shock), hyperviscosity (e.g., polycythemia), and hypercoagulability (e.g., chemotherapy) predispose a person to thrombotic arterial occlusion.

Traumatic injury to an extremity may cause partial or total arterial blockage. Acute arterial occlusion may develop from arterial dissection in the carotid artery or aorta or from a procedure-related arterial injury (e.g., after angiography).

Clinical Manifestations

Manifestations of acute arterial ischemia include the *6 Ps: pain, pallor, pulselessness, paresthesia, paralysis,* and *poikilothermia* (adaptation of the limb to the environment temperature, most often cool). If you detect these signs, immediately notify the HCP. Without immediate intervention, ischemia may progress to tissue necrosis and gangrene within a few hours.

Paralysis is a late sign of acute arterial ischemia and signals the death of nerves supplying the extremity. Foot drop occurs from nerve damage. Because nerve tissue is very sensitive to hypoxia, limb paralysis or ischemic neuropathy may persist even after revascularization.

Interprofessional Care

Early diagnosis and treatment are essential to keep the affected limb viable during acute arterial ischemia. Anticoagulant therapy with IV unfractionated heparin (UH) prevents thrombus growth and inhibits further embolization. In patients undergoing embolectomy, UH is followed by long-term anticoagulation.

To restore blood flow, the thrombus is removed as soon as possible. Options consist of surgical thrombectomy (recommended procedure), percutaneous catheter-directed thrombolytic therapy, percutaneous mechanical thrombectomy with or without thrombolytic therapy, or surgical bypass.[4]

Percutaneous catheter-directed thrombolytic therapy using alteplase (Activase) is an option for acute arterial ischemia of less than 14 days. The HCP inserts a catheter into the femoral artery and moves it to the site of the clot. The thrombolytic drug is continuously infused to directly dissolve the clot over 24 to 48 hours. (Chapter 37 discusses thrombolytic therapy.) Close monitoring is required to make sure the catheter does not move and the patient does not bleed from the catheter insertion site.

Surgical revascularization may be used in patients with trauma (e.g., lacerated artery) or with significant arterial blockage. Amputation is done for patients with ischemic rest pain and tissue loss if limb salvage is not possible. If a patient is at risk for further embolization from a persistent source (e.g., chronic atrial fibrillation), long-term anticoagulation is prescribed.

THROMBOANGIITIS OBLITERANS

Thromboangiitis obliterans (Buerger disease) is a nonatherosclerotic, segmental, recurrent inflammatory disorder of the small and medium arteries and veins of the arms and legs. Cerebral, coronary, mesenteric, pulmonary, and/or renal arteries are rarely involved. The disease occurs mostly in males between 20 and 50 years of age with a long history of tobacco and/or marijuana use without other CVD risk factors (e.g., hypertension, hyperlipidemia, diabetes).[6]

In the acute phase of Buerger disease, an inflammatory thrombus blocks the vessel. Over time, the thrombus becomes more organized and the inflammation in the vessel wall subsides. During the chronic phase, thrombosis and fibrosis in the vessel cause tissue ischemia.

The symptoms of Buerger disease often are confused with PAD and other autoimmune diseases (e.g., scleroderma). Patients may have intermittent claudication of the feet, hands, or arms. As the disease progresses, rest pain and ischemic ulcerations develop. Other signs and symptoms may include color and temperature changes of the limbs, paresthesia, superficial vein thrombosis, and cold sensitivity.

There are no laboratory or diagnostic tests specific to Buerger disease. The diagnosis is based on age of onset; history; symptoms; involvement of distal vessels; presence of ischemic ulcerations; and exclusion of autoimmune disease, diabetes, thrombophilia (inherited tendency to clot), and other sources of emboli, such as atherosclerosis and aneurysm.[6]

The main treatment is the complete cessation of tobacco and marijuana use in any form. Use of nicotine replacement products is contraindicated. Conservative management includes avoiding limb exposure to cold temperatures, a supervised walking program, antibiotics to treat any infected ulcers, and analgesics to manage the ischemic pain. Teach patients to avoid trauma to the extremities.

Surgical options include lumbar sympathectomy (transection of a nerve, ganglion, and/or plexus of the sympathetic nervous system), implanting a spinal cord stimulator, and bypass surgery.[6] Sympathectomy and a spinal cord stimulator can improve distal blood flow, reduce pain, and decrease the rate of amputation. Neither alters the inflammatory process. Bypass surgery may be used in select patients with severe ischemia. Stem cell therapy promotes ulcer healing, new blood vessel formation, and nerve cell regeneration.[6]

Painful ulcerations may require finger or toe amputations. Amputation below the knee may be needed in severe cases. The rate of amputation in those who continue tobacco or marijuana use after diagnosis is much higher than in those who stop.

RAYNAUD PHENOMENON

Raynaud phenomenon is an episodic vasospastic disorder of small cutaneous arteries, most often involving the fingers and toes. Abnormalities in the vascular, intravascular, and neuronal mechanisms cause vasoconstriction.[7] It occurs more often in females between 15 and 30 years of age.

Raynaud phenomenon may occur in isolation (primary Raynaud phenomenon) or with an underlying disease (e.g., scleroderma, systemic lupus erythematosus; secondary Raynaud phenomenon). Other risk factors include using vibrating machinery or work in cold environments, exposure to heavy metals (e.g., lead), and certain infections (e.g., hepatitis B).

Raynaud phenomenon is characterized by vasospasm-induced color changes (white, blue, and red) of fingers, toes, ears, face, knees, and nipples.[8] Decreased perfusion results in pallor (white/gray). The areas then appear cyanotic (bluish purple) (Fig. 41.3). These changes are followed by rubor (red), a hyperemic response when blood flow is restored. Patients usually describe coldness and numbness in the vasoconstrictive phase. This is followed by throbbing, aching pain, tingling, and swelling in the hyperemic phase. An episode usually lasts 20 minutes but may last for several hours. Triggers include cold exposure, emotional upsets, tobacco use, and caffeine.

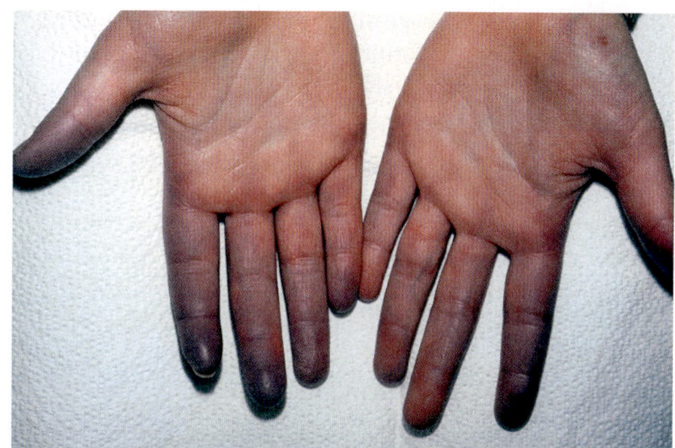

Fig. 41.3 Raynaud phenomenon. (From James WD, Elston DM, Dirk M: *Andrews' diseases of the skin clinical atlas,* St Louis, 2018, Elsevier.)

After frequent, prolonged attacks, the skin may become thickened and the nails brittle. Complications include *punctate* (small hole) lesions of the fingertips and superficial gangrenous ulcers.[8] Patients should have follow-up to monitor for development of connective tissue or autoimmune diseases.

Preventing episodes is the focus of care. Tell patients to avoid temperature extremes and wear loose, warm clothing as protection from the cold, including gloves when handling cold objects. Immersing hands in warm water often decreases the vasospasm. Patients should stop using all tobacco products and avoid caffeine and other drugs that have vasoconstrictive effects (e.g., amphetamines, ergotamine, pseudoephedrine). Suggest stress management strategies.

Sustained-release calcium channel blockers (e.g., nifedipine) are the first-line drug therapy. They relax smooth muscles of the arterioles by blocking the influx of calcium into the cells. This reduces the frequency and severity of vasospastic attacks. If symptoms persist, other vasodilators (e.g., phosphodiesterase-5 inhibitors [sildenafil]) or topical nitroglycerin 2% ointment may be used.[7] Calcium channel blockers can be taken with nitroglycerin topical ointment. Phosphodiesterase-5 inhibitors are not used with topical nitroglycerin because of the risk for hypotension.

Prompt intervention is needed for patients with digital ulceration or CLI. Treatment options include antibiotics, analgesics, and surgical debridement of necrotic tissue. Botulinum toxin A and statins may lessen the severity of Raynaud phenomenon.[8] Sympathectomy is done only in severe cases refractory to medical treatment when digit survival is threatened.

AORTIC ANEURYSMS

Etiology and Pathophysiology

One of the most common problems affecting the aorta is an **aneurysm,** which is a permanent, local outpouching or dilation of the vessel wall. Aortic aneurysms may involve the aortic arch and thoracic and/or abdominal aorta. Three-fourths of aortic aneurysms occur in the abdominal aorta. Most abdominal aortic aneurysms (AAAs) occur below the renal arteries. Aneurysms may occur in more than 1 location.

We classify the main causes as degenerative, congenital, infectious, mechanical (e.g., penetrating or blunt trauma), or inflammatory (e.g., aortitis). Aneurysms occur more often in males and in White people. The incidence increases with age.[9] Tobacco use is the most important modifiable risk factor.[9] Other risk factors include hypertension, CAD, family history, high cholesterol, lower extremity PAD, carotid artery disease, prior stroke, and obesity.

Genetic Link

Both aortic aneurysm and aortic dissection have a strong genetic component. The familial tendency is related to several congenital anomalies. Examples include bicuspid aortic valve, coarctation of the aorta, Turner syndrome, autosomal dominant polycystic kidney disease, specific collagen defects (e.g., Ehlers-Danlos syndrome), and premature breakdown of vascular elastic tissue (e.g., Marfan syndrome).[9]

Classification

There are several types of aneurysms (Fig. 41.4A to C). A *true aneurysm* is one in which the wall of the artery forms the aneurysm, with at least 1 vessel layer still intact. True aneurysms are described as fusiform or saccular. A *fusiform aneurysm* is circumferential and relatively uniform in shape. A *saccular aneurysm* is pouchlike with a narrow neck connecting the bulge to 1 side of the arterial wall.

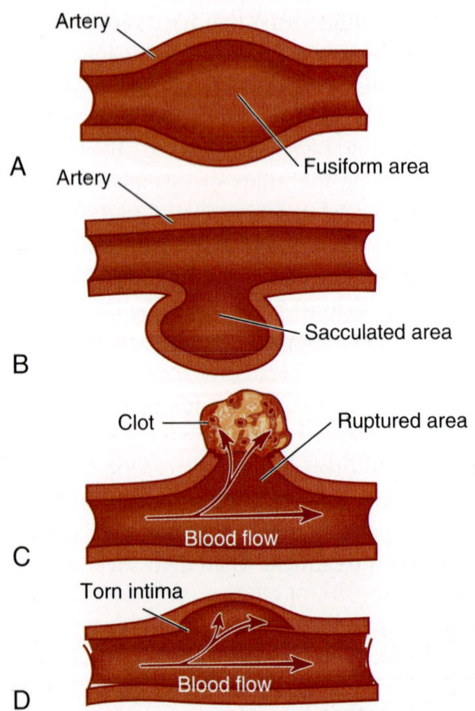

Fig. 41.4 (A) True fusiform abdominal aortic aneurysm. (B) True saccular aortic aneurysm. (C) False aneurysm, or pseudoaneurysm. (D) Aortic dissection.

A *false aneurysm,* or *pseudoaneurysm,* is not an aneurysm. It is a disruption of all arterial wall layers with bleeding that is contained by surrounding anatomic structures. False aneurysms may result from trauma, infection, peripheral artery bypass graft surgery (at the site of the graft-to-artery anastomosis), or arterial leakage after removing a cannula (e.g., femoral artery catheter, intraaortic balloon pump).

Clinical Manifestations

Thoracic aortic aneurysms (TAAs) are often asymptomatic. When present, symptoms include deep, diffuse chest pain that may extend to the interscapular area. Ascending aorta and aortic arch aneurysms can cause (1) angina from decreased blood flow to the coronary arteries; (2) transient ischemic attacks from decreased blood flow to the carotid arteries; and (3) coughing, shortness of breath, hoarseness, and/or difficulty swallowing from pressure on the laryngeal nerve. If the aneurysm presses on the superior vena cava, decreased venous return can result in jugular venous distention and edema of the face and arms.

AAAs are often asymptomatic. They are often found during routine physical assessment or evaluation for another problem (e.g., abdominal x-ray, CT scan). A pulsatile mass in the periumbilical area slightly to the left of the midline may be present. Bruits may be auscultated over the aneurysm. Physical findings may be hard to detect in obese persons.

AAA symptoms may mimic pain associated with abdominal or back disorders. Compression of nearby anatomic structures and nerves may cause symptoms, such as back pain, epigastric discomfort, altered bowel elimination, and intermittent claudication. Sometimes, aneurysms spontaneously embolize plaque, causing "blue toe syndrome" (patchy mottling of the feet and toes in the presence of palpable pedal pulses).

Complications

The most serious complication is the risk for aneurysm rupture. The larger the aneurysm, the greater the risk for rupture. Risk is also higher in persons who smoke.[9] If rupture occurs into the thoracic or abdominal cavity, patients can die of massive hemorrhage. Patients who reach the hospital will be in hypovolemic shock. In this situation, simultaneous resuscitation and immediate surgical repair are needed. For patients admitted to the hospital with a ruptured AAA, in-hospital mortality is high at 53%.[9]

If rupture occurs into the retroperitoneal space, bleeding may be controlled by surrounding structures, preventing exsanguination and death. In this case patients often have severe back pain. Back or flank bruising *(Grey Turner sign)* may be present.

Diagnostic Studies

Chest x-rays may show abnormal widening of the thoracic aorta. An abdominal x-ray may show calcification within the aortic wall. An ECG may rule out myocardial infarction (MI), because thoracic aneurysm or dissection symptoms can mimic angina. Echocardiography assesses the function of the aortic valve. Ultrasound is useful for aneurysm screening and to monitor aneurysm size. A CT scan or MRI can diagnose and assess the location and severity of aneurysms. Angiography gives helpful information by using contrast imaging to map the entire aortic system (see Table 35.11).

Interprofessional Care

The main goal of care is to prevent aneurysm rupture. Early detection and prompt treatment are essential. Conservative medical therapy of small, asymptomatic AAAs (less than 5.4 cm) is the best practice.[9] This consists of managing hypertension, hyperlipidemia, diabetes, and other CVD risk factors.[9] A statin and an ACE inhibitor may be prescribed. Those with small aneurysms—4.0 to 5.4 cm—should have monitoring of aneurysm size using ultrasound or CT every 6 to 12 months. Ultrasound every 3 years is done for patients with AAAs smaller than 4.0 cm in diameter.

Surgical repair is recommended in patients with asymptomatic aneurysms 5.5 cm in diameter or larger. Surgical intervention may occur sooner if the patient has a genetic disorder (e.g., Marfan, Ehlers-Danlos syndrome), the aneurysm expands rapidly, the patient becomes symptomatic, or the risk for rupture is high.

Surgical Therapy

If the aneurysm ruptures, the patient needs emergent surgery. For elective aneurysm repair surgery, we identify any comorbidities that affect surgical risk. The patient should be well hydrated with normal electrolytes, coagulation, and hematocrit. Carotid or coronary artery blockages may be corrected before aneurysm repair.

Open aneurysm repair (OAR) involves a large abdominal incision through which the surgeon (1) cuts into the diseased aortic segment, (2) removes any thrombus or plaque, (3) sutures a synthetic graft to the aorta proximal and distal to the aneurysm, and (4) sutures the native aortic wall around the graft to act as a protective cover (Fig. 41.5). For iliac artery aneurysms, a bifurcated graft replaces the entire diseased segment. With saccular aneurysms, it may be possible to excise only the bulbous lesion and repair the artery by primary closure (suturing the artery together) or with an autogenous or synthetic patch graft.

All OARs require aortic cross-clamping proximal and distal to the aneurysm. Most resections are done in 30 to 45 minutes. After removing the clamps, blood flow is restored. The risk for postoperative complications, such as acute kidney injury, increases in patients who have OAR of AAAs above the level of the renal arteries.

Minimally invasive endovascular aneurysm repair (EVAR) is an alternative to OAR for select patients. EVAR involves placing a sutureless aortic graft into the abdominal aorta inside the

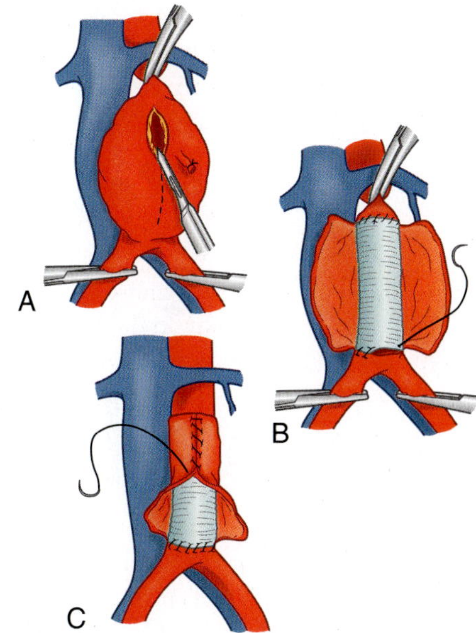

Fig. 41.5 Surgical repair of an abdominal aortic aneurysm. (A) Incising the aneurysmal sac. (B) Inserting synthetic graft. (C) Suturing native aortic wall over synthetic graft.

aneurysm via the femoral artery. Grafts are made of various materials, such as a Dacron cylinder consisting of several sections, and supported with multiple rings of flexible wire. Eligibility criteria include iliofemoral vessels that allow for safe graft insertion and vessels of sufficient length and width to support the graft.[9]

The main section of the graft is bifurcated. It is delivered through a femoral artery catheter. The second part of the graft is inserted through the opposite femoral artery. When all graft components are in place, they are deployed against the vessel wall by balloon inflation. The blood then flows through the endovascular graft, preventing further expansion of the aneurysm (Fig. 41.6).

Angiography is done afterward to check for leaks and to confirm patency of all stent-graft components. The aneurysmal wall shrinks over time because the blood is diverted through the endograft. EVAR is less invasive than OAR and requires a shorter hospital stay. EVAR also has fewer complications, such as paraplegia and death.

Surgical complications. The most common complication of AAA repair is *endoleak,* the seepage of blood back into the old aneurysm. This may result from an inadequate seal at either graft end, a tear through the graft fabric, or leakage between overlapping graft segments. Repair may require coil embolization (insertion of beads) for hemostasis.

Other complications include aneurysm growth above or below the graft, aneurysm rupture, aortic dissection, bleeding, renal artery occlusion caused by stent migration, graft thrombosis, incisional site hematoma, and incisional infection. Patients undergoing EVAR need periodic imaging for the rest of their lives to monitor for an endoleak, assess stability of the aneurysm, and determine the need for surgery.

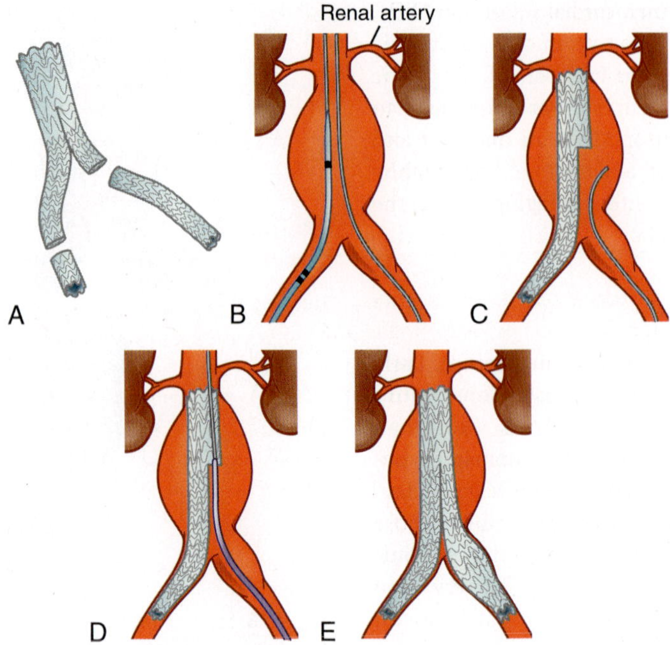

Fig. 41.6 Bifurcated (2-branched) endovascular stent grafting of an aneurysm. (A) Insertion of a woven polyester graft covered by a tubular metal web (stent). (B) The stent graft is inserted through a large blood vessel (e.g., femoral artery) using a delivery catheter. The catheter is positioned below the renal arteries in the area of the aneurysm. (C) The stent graft is slowly released into the blood vessel. When the stent comes in contact with the blood vessel, it expands to a preset size. (D) A second stent graft can be inserted in the opposite vessel if needed. (E) Fully deployed bifurcated stent graft.

A potentially lethal complication in an emergency repair of a ruptured AAA is the development of *intraabdominal hypertension* (IAH) with associated *abdominal compartment syndrome.* Persistent IAH reduces blood flow to the viscera. Abdominal compartment syndrome refers to the impaired organ perfusion caused by IAH and resulting multisystem organ failure. IAH is confirmed by measuring intraabdominal pressure indirectly through a catheter and transducer system.

Treatment goals include controlling situations that lead to IAH. Interventions include open (surgical) decompression, percutaneous drainage, and percutaneous drainage combined with a thrombolytic infusion. Conservative measures, such as mechanical ventilation, positioning, gastric decompression, cautious fluid resuscitation, pain management, and temporary hemofiltration, are used.

NURSING MANAGEMENT: AORTIC ANEURYSMS

Assessment

Begin with a history and physical assessment. Because atherosclerosis is a systemic disease, look for signs of cardiac, pulmonary, cerebral, and lower extremity vascular problems. Monitor patients for signs of aneurysm rupture. Patients often report severe, increased abdominal, back, groin, or periumbilical pain. Signs of shock include diaphoresis, pallor, weakness, tachycardia, hypotension, and changes in level of consciousness.

Obtain baseline data to compare with later assessments. Pay attention to the character and quality of the peripheral pulses and renal and neurologic status. Before surgery, mark pedal pulse sites (dorsalis pedis, posterior tibial) with a marker. Note any skin lesions on the lower extremities.

Planning

The overall goals for patients undergoing aortic surgery include (1) normal tissue perfusion; (2) intact motor and sensory function; and (3) no complications related to surgical repair, such as thrombosis, infection, or rupture.

Implementation

Health Promotion

To promote overall health, encourage patients to reduce CVD risk factors (see Table 37.2). These include controlling BP, ceasing tobacco use (see Chapter 11), increasing physical activity, and maintaining normal body weight and lipid levels. These measures help ensure continued graft patency after surgical repair. Counsel patients about taking part in moderate physical activity.

Acute Care

Before surgery, provide emotional support and teaching to the patient and caregiver (see Chapter 18). In general, aortic surgery patients have a bowel preparation and skin cleansing with an antimicrobial agent the day before surgery. They are NPO after midnight on the day of surgery and receive IV antibiotics before the first incision. Patients with a history of CVD receive a β-blocker (e.g., metoprolol).

After surgery, patients are often in the ICU for 24 to 48 hours. Various devices are in place, such as an endotracheal tube for mechanical ventilation, an arterial line, and a central venous pressure (CVP) catheter. Patients need continuous ECG and pulse oximetry monitoring. If the thorax is opened during surgery, chest tubes will be in place. Patients may have a lumbar catheter draining cerebrospinal fluid to prevent neurologic problems. Pain medication is given via subcutaneous infusion into the incision site, epidural catheters, or IV patient-controlled analgesia (PCA).

In addition to the usual goals of care for postoperative patients (e.g., maintaining adequate respiratory function, fluid and electrolyte balance, and pain control [see Chapter 20]), check for graft patency and renal perfusion. Watch for and intervene to limit or treat cardiac ischemia, dysrhythmias, infections, venous thromboembolism (VTE), and neurologic complications. eNursing Care Plan 41.2 for patients with an aneurysm repair or other aortic surgery is available on the website for this chapter.

Graft patency. An adequate BP is important to maintain graft patency. Prolonged low BP may result in graft thrombosis. Give IV fluids and blood components as ordered to maintain adequate blood flow. Monitor CVP or pulmonary artery (PA) pressures and urine output hourly in the immediate postoperative period to assess hydration and perfusion status.

Avoid severe hypertension, which may stress the arterial anastomoses. This can result in leakage of blood or rupture at the suture lines. Drug therapy with IV diuretics (e.g., furosemide) or IV antihypertensive agents (e.g., labetalol, hydralazine, sodium nitroprusside) may be indicated.

Cardiovascular status. Myocardial ischemia or infarction may occur in the perioperative period from decreased myocardial O_2 supply or increased myocardial O_2 demands. Dysrhythmias may occur because of electrolyte imbalances, hypoxemia, hypothermia, or myocardial ischemia. Maintain continuous ECG monitoring. Administer O_2 per protocol. Other care includes frequent electrolyte and arterial blood gas determinations and giving IV antidysrhythmics, antihypertensives, and electrolytes as needed. Provide adequate pain control.

Infection. A prosthetic vascular graft infection is a rare but life-threatening complication. Nursing interventions to prevent infection include giving a broad-spectrum antibiotic as prescribed (see Table 15.8). Assess temperature regularly, and promptly report fever. Monitor laboratory results for a high white blood cell (WBC) count, which may be the first sign of an infection. Ensure adequate nutrition. Assess the surgical incision for signs of infection (e.g., redness, swelling, drainage). Keep surgical incisions clean and dry and perform wound care as prescribed (Box 41.1).

Use good hand-washing and strict aseptic technique in the care of all peripheral, arterial, and CVP catheter insertion sites. These are ports of entry for bacteria. Meticulous perineal care for patients with an indwelling urinary catheter and early catheter removal are essential to minimize the risk for urinary tract infection.

Gastrointestinal care. After OAR, postoperative ileus may develop because of anesthesia and the handling of the bowel during surgery. The intestines may become swollen and bruised. Peristalsis ceases for variable intervals. A retroperitoneal surgical approach decreases the risk for bowel complications.

A nasogastric (NG) tube may be present and connected to low, intermittent suction to decompress the stomach, prevent aspiration of stomach contents, and decrease pressure on suture lines. Record the amount and character of the NG output. While the patient is NPO, provide frequent oral care. Ice chips or lozenges can help soothe a dry or irritated throat. Assess bowel sounds every 4 hours. Note the passing of flatus as it signals returning bowel function. Encourage early ambulation to help the return of bowel function. A postoperative ileus rarely lasts beyond the fourth postoperative day.

BOX 41.1 EVIDENCE-BASED PRACTICE

Use of Negative Pressure Wound Therapy

Your surgical step-down unit cares for many patients recovering from abdominal aortic aneurysm repair surgeries. Your colleagues and you have noticed an increase in wound infections over the last 6 months despite adherence to a strict protocol of traditional sterile dressing changes. You are asked to participate in an evidence-based practice project investigating wound care practices.

Making Clinical Decisions

Synthesis of Best Available Evidence

Negative pressure wound therapy (NPWT) has been used to treat acute and chronic open wounds. It has now been adapted for the treatment of closed wounds, such as closed surgical incisions. NPWT promotes tissue granulation, pulls excess fluid from the wound, reduces bacterial load, and increases blood flow into the wound.

Clinician Expertise

Chart review showed that many patients experienced complications, particularly infections, that you believe contributed to impaired wound healing. Since research showed a reduction in wound infections and other complications with the use of NPWT, you determine this approach is the best solution.

Patient Preferences and Values

Your unit implemented NPWT for all patients having abdominal aortic aneurysm repair surgeries for 6 months. After the 6-month period, the nurse manager reported a 35% decrease in wound infections from the previous 6 months.

Implications for Nursing Practice

1. How could you use evidence to change a practice on your unit?
2. What unit/hospital personnel should be made aware of this information?

Reference for Evidence

Yu X, Xie P, Li J-Z, Cao L, Ye J: Effects of negative-pressure wound therapy in the prevention of surgical-site wound infection after vascular surgery: a meta-analysis, *Int Wound J* 21:2, 2024.

If the blood supply to the bowel is disrupted during surgery, ischemia or death of intestinal tissue may result. Manifestations of this rare, but serious, complication include absent bowel sounds, fever, abdominal distention and pain, diarrhea, and bloody stools. If bowel infarction occurs, immediate reoperation is needed to restore blood flow and resect the infarcted area.

Neurologic status. Neurologic complications can occur. When the ascending aorta and aortic arch are involved, assess level of consciousness, pupil size and response to light, facial symmetry, tongue position, speech, upper extremity movement, and quality of hand grasps. When the descending aorta is involved, perform a neurovascular assessment of the lower extremities. Report changes from baseline to the HCP immediately.

Peripheral perfusion. The location of the aneurysm determines the type of peripheral perfusion assessment. Check and record all peripheral pulses hourly for several hours and then routinely (based on agency policy). When the ascending aorta and aortic arch are involved, assess the carotid, radial, and temporal artery pulses. For surgery of the descending aorta, assess the femoral, popliteal, posterior tibial, and dorsalis pedis pulses. You may need a Doppler to assess peripheral pulses. Check skin temperature and color, capillary refill time, and sensation and movement of the extremities.

Sometimes, lower extremity pulses may be absent for a short time after surgery because of vasospasm and hypothermia. A decreased or absent pulse together with a cool, pale, mottled, or painful extremity may indicate embolization or graft occlusion. Report these findings to the HCP at once. Early graft occlusion requires reoperation. It is essential to compare your findings with the preoperative status to determine the cause of a decreased or absent pulse and the proper treatment. In some patients, pulses may have been absent before surgery because of coexistent PAD.

Renal perfusion. Patients will have an indwelling urinary catheter after surgery. In the immediate postoperative period, record hourly urine output. Further evaluate renal function by monitoring daily blood urea nitrogen (BUN) and serum creatinine levels. CVPs give vital information about hydration status. Maintain accurate fluid intake and output and record daily weights until the patient resumes a regular diet.

Decreased renal perfusion can occur from embolization of an aortic thrombus or plaque to either or both renal arteries. Hypotension, dehydration, prolonged aortic clamping during surgery, or blood loss can lead to kidney ischemia. Irreversible renal failure may occur after surgery, particularly in high-risk people (e.g., patients with diabetes).

Discharge teaching. Teach patients to gradually increase activities and avoid heavy lifting for 6 weeks. Fatigue, poor appetite, and irregular bowel patterns are common. Teach the patient and caregiver to look for changes in color or warmth of the extremities. They can learn to palpate peripheral pulses to assess changes in pulse quality. Report any redness, swelling, increased pain, drainage from incisions, or fever greater than 100°F (37.8°C) to the HCP.

Sexual problems in male patients are common after aortic surgery. A referral to a urologist and counseling may be useful if erectile dysfunction occurs.

◆ Evaluation

Expected outcomes are that patients who undergo aortic surgery will have:

- Patent arterial graft with adequate distal perfusion
- Adequate urine output
- No signs of infection

AORTIC DISSECTION

Aortic dissection, often called *dissecting aneurysm,* is not a type of aneurysm. Rather, dissection results from the creation of a false lumen between the intima (inner lining) and the media (middle layer) of the arterial wall (Fig. 41.4D and Fig. 41.7). We classify aortic dissection based on its location and duration of onset. *Type A dissection* affects the ascending aorta and arch, requiring emergency surgery. *Type B dissection* begins in the descending aorta, allowing for potential conservative management.[10] Dissections are acute (first 14 days), subacute (14 to 90 days), or chronic (greater than 90 days) based on symptom onset.[11]

Etiology and Pathophysiology

Nontraumatic aortic dissection is caused by weakened elastic fibers in the arterial wall. Chronic hypertension hastens this

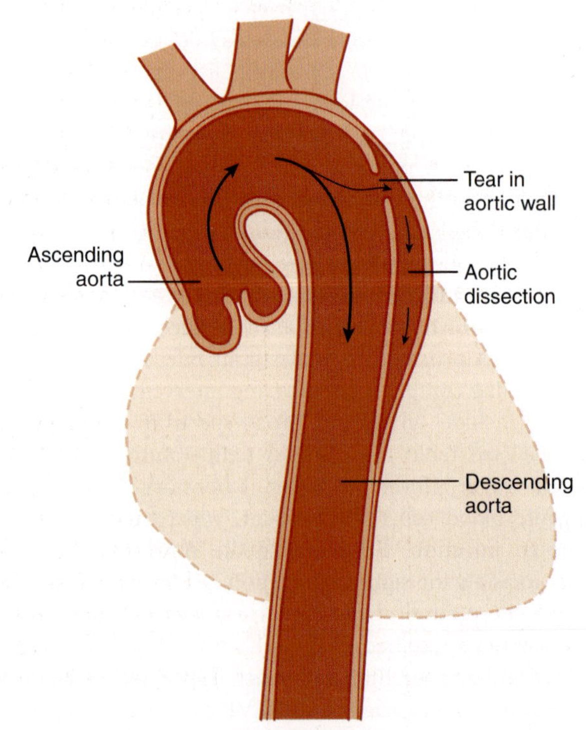

Fig. 41.7 Aortic dissection.

process. In aortic dissection, a tear develops in the inner layer of the aorta. Blood surges through this tear into the middle layer of the aorta, causing the inner and middle layers to separate (dissect). If the blood-filled channel ruptures through the outside aortic wall, aortic dissection is often fatal.

As the heart contracts, each pulsation increases the pressure on the damaged area and worsens the dissection. Extension of the dissection may cut off blood supply to the brain, kidneys, spinal cord, and extremities. The false lumen may remain patent, become thrombosed (clotted), rejoin the true lumen by way of a distal tear, or rupture.

Males have an overall higher risk.[12] Females who develop aortic dissection are older and have reduced weight, height, and hemoglobin levels.[12] Hypertension is the most important risk factor for aortic dissection.[10] Other risk factors include age, aortic diseases (e.g., aortitis, coarctation, arch hypoplasia), atherosclerosis, blunt trauma, tobacco use, cocaine or methamphetamine use, congenital heart disease (e.g., bicuspid aortic valve), connective tissue disorders (e.g., Marfan syndrome), family history, history of heart surgery, and pregnancy.

Clinical Manifestations

About 80% of patients with an acute type A aortic dissection report an abrupt onset of severe anterior chest or back pain. Patients with acute type B aortic dissection are more likely to report pain in their back, abdomen, or legs. Pain location may overlap between type A and B dissections. The pain may be described as "sharp" and "worst ever" or as "tearing," "ripping," or "stabbing." As the dissection progresses, pain may follow the path of the dissection. Older patients are less likely to have an abrupt onset of pain and more likely to have hypotension and vague symptoms. Some patients have no pain, emphasizing the importance of the physical assessment.

If the aortic arch is involved, the patient may have neurologic problems. These include altered level of consciousness, weakened or absent carotid and temporal pulses, dizziness, and syncope. Type A aortic dissection usually disrupts blood flow in the coronary arteries and causes aortic valve insufficiency. When either subclavian artery is involved, the radial, ulnar, and brachial pulse quality and BP readings may be different between the left and right arms. As the dissection progresses down the aorta, the abdominal organs and lower extremities show signs of decreased tissue perfusion.

Complications

A severe and life-threatening complication of an acute ascending aortic dissection is *cardiac tamponade.* This occurs when blood from the dissection leaks into the pericardial sac. Manifestations of tamponade include hypotension, narrowed pulse pressure, jugular venous distention, muffled heart sounds, and pulsus paradoxus (see Chapter 40).

An aorta weakened by dissection may rupture. Hemorrhage may occur into the mediastinal, pleural, or abdominal cavities. Aortic rupture typically results in exsanguination and death.

Aortic dissection can lead to occlusion of the blood supply to vital organs. Spinal cord ischemia leads to weakness and decreased sensation. Rarely, lower extremity paralysis may occur. Renal ischemia can lead to renal failure. Abdominal (mesenteric) ischemia can occur and cause abdominal pain, decreased bowel sounds, altered bowel function, and bowel necrosis.

Diagnostic Studies

Diagnostic studies to detect aortic dissection are similar to those for suspected aneurysms (Table 41.6). An ECG can help rule out cardiac ischemia. A chest x-ray may show a widening of the mediastinum and pleural effusion. MRI, 3D CT scanning, and transesophageal echocardiography (TEE) are equally reliable for diagnosing acute aortic dissection. A CT scan or MRI can give detailed information on the severity of the dissection and related complications (e.g., pericardial effusions, carotid dissection). TEE is preferred in very unstable patients or those with contraindications to CT or MRI (e.g., those with metal implants).

Interprofessional Care

Patients with acute aortic dissection are managed in the ICU. The initial goals of therapy for acute aortic dissection without complications are heart rate (HR) and BP control and pain management. Lowering HR and BP reduces aortic wall stress by decreasing SBP and myocardial contractility (Table 41.6). This limits extension of the dissection. An IV β-blocker (e.g., esmolol) is titrated to a target HR under 60 beats/min or SBP between 100 and 110 mm Hg. A calcium channel blocker

TABLE 41.6 Interprofessional Care

Aortic Dissection

Diagnostic Assessment
- Health history and physical assessment
- ECG
- Chest x-ray
- CT scan
- Transesophageal echocardiogram
- MRI

Management
- Bed rest
- Pain relief with opioids
- Blood transfusion (if needed)

Drug Therapy (see Table 36.6)
- IV β-blockers
- IV calcium channel blockers
- ACE inhibitors

Surgical Therapy
- Endovascular aortic dissection repair
- Open surgical repair

(e.g., diltiazem) can be used to lower HR if a β-blocker is contraindicated. Morphine decreases sympathetic nervous system stimulation and relieves pain. Supportive treatment for an acute aortic dissection is a bridge to surgery.

Conservative Therapy

Patients with an acute or chronic type B aortic dissection without complications can be treated conservatively. Treatment includes pain relief, HR and BP control, and CVD risk factor modification with close surveillance imaging with CT or MRI.

Endovascular Dissection Repair

Endovascular repair is a treatment option for acute type B aortic dissections with complications (e.g., hemodynamic instability) and chronic type B aortic dissection with complications (e.g., peripheral ischemia). Thoracic endovascular aortic repair (TEVAR) is similar to EVAR. Fewer postsurgical complications occur with TEVAR. However, TEVAR does not prevent the risk for renal failure, paraplegia, or stroke.[11] If a lumbar spinal drain is inserted to help decrease or prevent neurologic complications, strict aseptic technique is used to prevent infection.

Surgical Therapy

An acute type A aortic dissection is a surgical emergency. Mortality rate is 50% within 48 hours of symptom onset. Otherwise, surgery is indicated when conservative therapy is ineffective or when complications (e.g., HF) occur. Open surgical repair is recommended for patients with a chronic dissection who have a connective tissue disorder or an aneurysm greater than 5.5 cm.[9]

The aorta is fragile after dissection. Surgery is delayed, when possible, to allow time for edema to decrease and to permit blood clotting in the false lumen. Surgery involves resecting the aortic segment with the intimal tear and replacing it with a synthetic graft. Even with prompt surgical intervention, the in-hospital mortality is high.[10] Causes of death include aortic rupture, mesenteric ischemia, MI, sepsis, stroke, and multiorgan failure.

❖ NURSING MANAGEMENT: AORTIC DISSECTION

Preoperatively, keep the patient in bed in a semi-Fowler position and maintain a quiet environment. Manage pain and anxiety, giving opioids and sedatives as prescribed. These measures help keep the HR and SBP at the lowest possible level that maintains vital organ perfusion (typically HR less than 60 beats/min; SBP between 100 and 120 mm Hg).

Titrating IV antihypertensive agents requires careful supervision. Maintain continuous ECG and arterial BP monitoring. Monitor vital signs frequently, sometimes as often as every 2 to 3 minutes, until target HR and BP are reached. Look for changes in peripheral pulses and signs of increasing pain, restlessness, and anxiety.

Postoperative care is similar to that after OAR. In preparation for discharge, focus on patient and caregiver teaching. Help patients understand the need to take antihypertensive drugs daily for the rest of their lives. β-Blockers are used to control HR and BP and decrease myocardial contractility. ACE inhibitors (e.g., lisinopril) are given if the patient cannot tolerate β-blockers. It is important that patients understand the drug regimen and side effects (e.g., dizziness, depression, fatigue, erectile dysfunction). Tell patients to discuss any side effects with the HCP before stopping medication.

Follow-up with regularly scheduled MRIs or CTs is essential. The most common cause of death in long-term survivors is aortic rupture from redissection or aneurysm formation. Tell patients to activate the emergency response system (ERS) for immediate care if the pain or other symptoms return.

VENOUS DISORDERS

PHLEBITIS

Phlebitis is an acute inflammation of the walls of small, cannulated veins. Manifestations include pain, tenderness, warmth, redness, swelling, and a palpable cord. Risk factors are mechanical irritation from an IV catheter, infusion of irritating drugs, and IV catheter location in an area of flexion (e.g., wrist and antecubital area). Avoid IV catheter insertion in these areas whenever possible.

Phlebitis usually resolves quickly after catheter removal. If edema is present, elevate the extremity to promote fluid reabsorption. Apply warm, moist heat and give oral NSAIDs (e.g., ibuprofen) or topical NSAIDs (e.g., diclofenac gel) to relieve pain and inflammation.

VENOUS THROMBOSIS

Venous thrombosis involves the formation of a *thrombus* (blood clot) with vein inflammation. It is the most common disorder of the veins. We classify it as either superficial vein thrombosis or deep vein thrombosis. **Superficial vein thrombosis** is the formation of a thrombus in a superficial vein, usually the greater or lesser saphenous vein. **Deep vein thrombosis (DVT)** involves a thrombus in a deep vein, most often the iliac and/or femoral veins. **Venous thromboembolism (VTE)** is the preferred terminology. It represents the spectrum from DVT to pulmonary embolism (PE) (Table 41.7). Chapter 30 discusses PE. Nearly 25% of patients with superficial vein thrombosis also have a DVT or PE at the time of diagnosis.[13] These patients are at risk for developing recurrent VTE.

Etiology

The 3 key factors (called **Virchow triad**) that cause venous thrombosis are (1) venous stasis, (2) damage of the endothelium (inner lining of the vein), and (3) hypercoagulability

TABLE 41.7 Comparison of Superficial Vein Thrombosis and Venous Thromboembolism

	Superficial Vein Thrombosis	Venous Thromboembolism (VTE)
Usual location	Typically, superficial leg veins (e.g., varicosities). Sometimes superficial arm veins.	Deep veins of arms (e.g., axillary, subclavian), legs (e.g., femoral), pelvis (e.g., iliac), vena cava, and pulmonary system.
Clinical findings	Tenderness, itchiness, redness, warmth, pain, inflammation, and induration along the course of superficial vein. Vein appears as a palpable cord. Edema rarely occurs.	Tenderness to pressure over involved vein, induration of overlying muscle, venous distention. Edema. May have mild to moderate pain, deep reddish color to area caused by venous congestion. Some have no obvious physical changes in the affected extremity.
Sequelae	If untreated, clot may extend to deeper veins and VTE may occur.	Embolization to lungs (PE) may occur and may result in death. Pulmonary hypertension and postthrombotic syndrome with or without venous leg ulceration may develop.

PE, Pulmonary embolism.

(Fig. 41.8). Patients at risk for developing VTE usually have predisposing conditions to these 3 factors (Table 41.8).

Venous Stasis

Normal venous blood flow depends on the action of muscles in the extremities and the function of venous valves, which allow flow in one direction. *Venous stasis* occurs when the valves are dysfunctional or the muscles of the extremities are inactive. Venous stasis occurs most often in people who are obese or pregnant, have chronic HF or atrial fibrillation, have been traveling on long trips without regular exercise, have a prolonged surgical procedure, or are immobile for long periods (e.g., spinal cord injury, fractured hip, limb paralysis).

Endothelial Damage

Damage to the endothelium may be caused by direct (e.g., surgery, intravascular catheterization, trauma, burns, prior VTE) or indirect (chemotherapy, diabetes, sepsis) injury. Damaged endothelium stimulates platelet activation and starts the coagulation cascade. This predisposes patients to thrombus development.

Blood Hypercoagulability

Blood hypercoagulability occurs with many problems. These include severe anemias, polycythemia, cancers (e.g., breast, brain, pancreas, GI tract); nephrotic syndrome; high homocysteine levels; and protein C, protein S, and antithrombin deficiency. Patients with sepsis are predisposed to hypercoagulability because of endotoxins released from bacteria. Some drugs

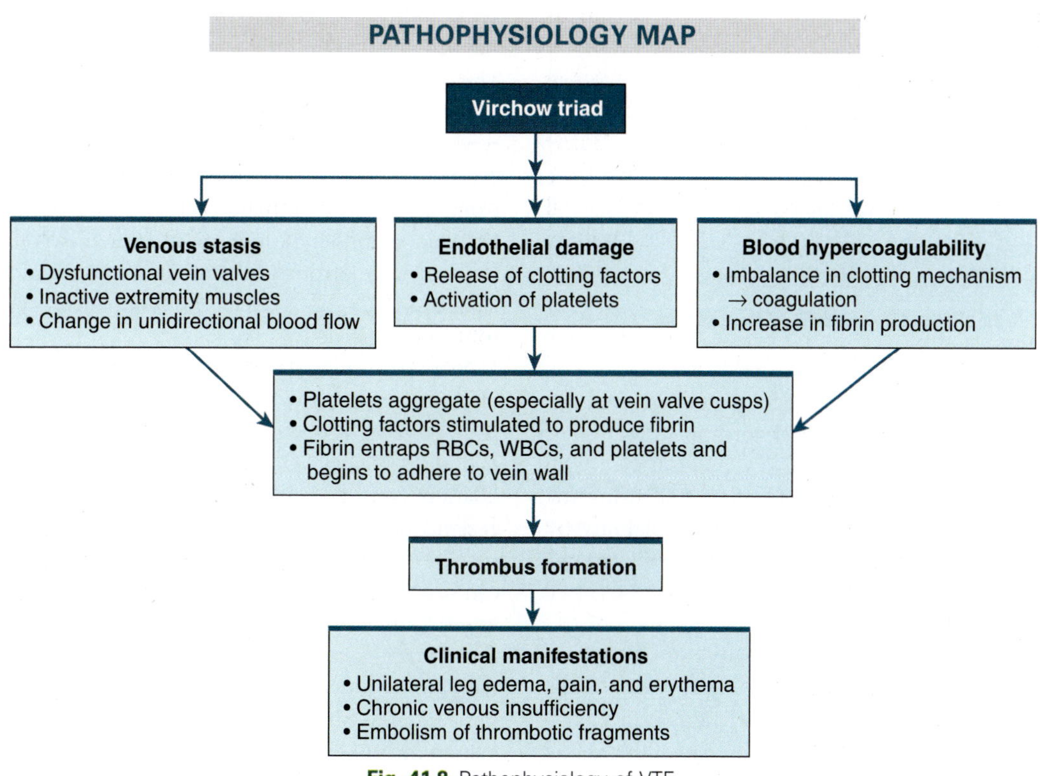

Fig. 41.8 Pathophysiology of VTE.

TABLE 41.8 Risk Factors for VTE

Endothelial Damage
- Abdominal and pelvic surgery (e.g., gynecologic, urologic surgery)
- Caustic or hypertonic IV drugs
- History of VTE, chronic venous insufficiency
- Indwelling, peripherally inserted central vein catheter
- IV drug use
- Trauma

Venous Stasis
- Advanced age
- Atrial fibrillation
- Bed rest
- Fractured leg, pelvis, hip
- Heart failure
- Long trips without adequate exercise
- Obesity
- Orthopedic surgery (especially hip or lower extremity)
- Pregnancy and postpartum period
- Prolonged immobility
- Spinal cord injury or limb paralysis
- Stroke
- Varicose veins, sclerotherapy treatment

Hypercoagulability of Blood
- Antiphospholipid antibody syndrome
- Antithrombin III deficiency
- Cancer (especially breast, brain, hepatic, pancreatic, GI)
- Dehydration, malnutrition
- Elevated (clotting) factor VIII or lipoprotein(a)
- Erythropoiesis-stimulating drugs (e.g., epoetin alfa)
- High altitude
- Hormone therapy
- High homocysteine level
- Nephrotic syndrome
- Oral contraceptives, especially in females older than 35 years who use tobacco
- Polycythemia vera
- Pregnancy and postpartum period
- Protein C deficiency
- Protein S deficiency
- Sepsis
- Severe anemia
- Tobacco use

(e.g., corticosteroids, estrogens) predispose patients to thrombus formation.

Females who use tobacco, take estrogen-based oral contraceptives, are postmenopausal and on oral hormone therapy, are over 35 years old, or have a family history of VTE have a very high risk for VTE.[13] Taking oral contraceptives and using tobacco doubles the risk. Smoking causes hypercoagulability by increasing plasma fibrinogen and homocysteine levels and activating the intrinsic coagulation pathway.

Pathophysiology

Local platelet aggregation and fibrin entrap RBCs, WBCs, and more platelets to form a thrombus. A frequent site of thrombus formation is the valve cusp of a vein, where venous stasis occurs. As a thrombus enlarges, more blood cells and fibrin collect behind it. This makes a larger clot with a "tail" that eventually blocks the lumen of the vein.

If a thrombus only partially blocks the vein, endothelial cells cover the thrombus and stop the thrombotic process. If the thrombus does detach, it undergoes lysis or becomes firmly organized within 5 to 7 days. The organized thrombus may detach and result in an embolus. Turbulent blood flow is a major factor in embolization. The thrombus can become an embolus that flows through the venous circulation to the heart and lodges in the pulmonary circulation, becoming a PE.

Clinical Manifestations

Patients with superficial vein thrombosis may have a palpable, firm, subcutaneous cordlike vein (Table 41.7). The surrounding area may be itchy, painful to the touch, reddened, and warm. A mild fever and leukocytosis may be present. Extremity edema may occur. Lower extremity superficial vein thrombosis often involves varicose veins.

Patients with lower extremity VTE may have unilateral leg edema, pain, tenderness with palpation, dilated superficial veins, a sense of fullness in the thigh or the calf, paresthesias, warm skin, redness, or a fever greater than 100.4°F (38°C) (Table 41.7). If the inferior vena cava is involved, both legs may be edematous and cyanotic. About 10% of VTEs involve the upper extremity veins. They may extend into the internal jugular vein or superior vena cava. If the superior vena cava is involved, similar symptoms may occur in the arms, neck, back, and face.

Complications

The most serious complications of VTE are PE, chronic thromboembolic pulmonary hypertension, postthrombotic syndrome, and phlegmasia cerulea dolens. **Postthrombotic syndrome (PTS)** occurs in 8% to 70% of patients. It results from chronic inflammation and chronic venous hypertension. Chronic venous hypertension is caused by vein wall and vein valve damage (from acute inflammation and thrombus reorganization), venous valve reflux, and persistent venous (outflow) obstruction.

Symptoms include pain, aching, fatigue, heaviness, sensation of swelling, cramps, pruritus, tingling, paresthesia, bursting pain with exercise, and venous claudication. Manifestations include persistent edema, spider veins (telangiectasia), venous dilation (ectasia), redness, cyanosis, increased pigmentation, eczema, pain during compression, atrophie blanche (white scar tissue), and *lipodermatosclerosis* (Fig. 41.9). Venous ulceration can occur with severe PTS. Signs of PTS typically begin months to years after a VTE. Risk factors include persistent leg symptoms 1 month after VTE, proximal VTE location (e.g., near the iliofemoral junction), extensive VTE, recurrent VTE on the same side, asymptomatic VTE, and residual thrombus. Other factors include obesity, older age, poor anticoagulation control,

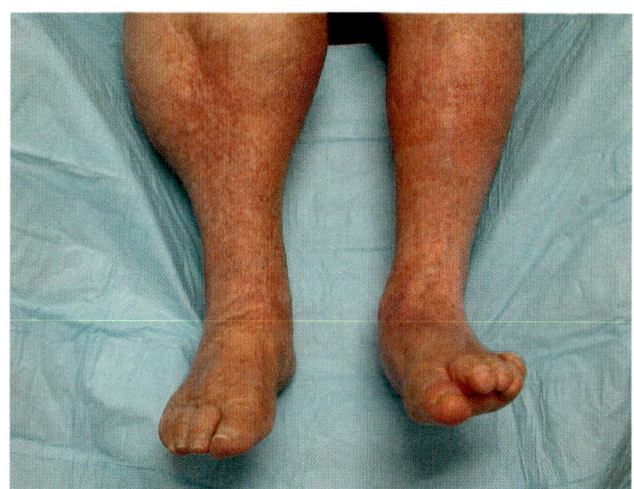

Fig. 41.9 Lipodermatosclerosis. The leg becomes tapered like an "inverted bottle." Skin becomes scarred and leathery with brown discoloration and changes in pigmentation. (From Etufugh CN, Phillips TJ: Venous ulcers, *Clin Dermatol* 25:125, 2007.)

daily tobacco use before pregnancy, increased D-dimer levels, elevated inflammatory markers, and varicose veins.

Phlegmasia cerulea dolens (swollen, blue, painful leg) is a rare complication of severe lower extremity VTE. It involves the major leg veins, causing near-total occlusion of venous outflow. Patients typically have sudden, massive swelling; deep pain; and intense cyanosis of the extremity. If untreated, the venous obstruction causes arterial occlusion and gangrene, requiring amputation.

Diagnostic Studies

Diagnosis of an initial VTE is based on the assessment combined with D-dimer testing and/or ultrasound. Table 41.9 presents the diagnostic studies used to determine the site or location and extent of a VTE.

Interprofessional Care

VTE Prevention

All health care team members have important roles in VTE prevention. Prevention is a core measure of high-quality health care by The Joint Commission (TJC) and the National Quality Forum. TJC recommends that hospitals have a policy addressing VTE prevention on admission of all adult patients. Interventions are based on bleeding and thrombosis risk, medical history, current drugs, medical diagnoses, scheduled procedures, and patient preferences.

Early and aggressive mobilization is the easiest and most cost-effective method to decrease VTE risk. Patients on bed rest should change position at least every 2 hours. Unless contraindicated, teach patients to flex and extend their feet, knees, and hips at least every 2 to 4 hours while awake. Patients who are able should be out of bed in a chair for meals and walk at least 4 to 6 times per day. Teach the patient and caregiver about the importance of these measures. Early and frequent ambulation is sufficient prophylaxis for patients at very low risk for VTE who had minor surgical procedures.

Graduated compression stockings (e.g., thromboembolic deterrent [TED] hose) are a part of VTE prevention in hospitalized patients. VTE prevention is enhanced if the stockings are used along with anticoagulation. Proper stocking use means any toe hole is under the toes, the heel patch is over the heel, a thigh gusset is on the inner thigh (thigh length only), and there

TABLE 41.9 Diagnostic Studies
VTE

Study	Description and Abnormal Findings
Blood Laboratory Studies	
ACT, aPTT, INR, bleeding time, Hgb, Hct, platelet count	Altered with underlying blood dyscrasia (e.g., increased Hgb and Hct in patient with polycythemia).
D-dimer	Fragment of fibrin formed from fibrin degradation and clot lysis. High results suggest VTE. *Normal results:* <250 ng/mL (<250 mcg/L)
Fibrin monomer complex	Forms when concentration of thrombin exceeds that of antithrombin. Presence is sign of thrombus formation and suggests VTE. *Normal results:* <6.1 mg/L.
Noninvasive Venous Studies	
Duplex ultrasound	Combination of compression ultrasound with spectral and color flow Doppler. Veins examined for compressibility and intraluminal filling defects to help determine location and extent of thrombus (most widely used test to diagnose VTE).
Venous compression ultrasound	Evaluation of deep femoral, popliteal, and posterior tibial veins. *Normal finding:* Veins collapse with application of external pressure. *Abnormal finding:* Veins do not collapse with application of external pressure. Failure to collapse suggests a thrombus.
Invasive Venous Studies	
Computed tomography venography (CTV)	Uses spiral CT to evaluate veins in pelvis, thighs, and calves after injection of contrast material. May be done simultaneously with CT angiography of pulmonary vessels for patients being evaluated for VTE.
Contrast venography (phlebogram)	X-ray determination of location and extent of clot using contrast media to outline filling defects. Identifies presence of collateral circulation. Once the gold standard, but now rarely done.
Magnetic resonance venography	Uses MRI with special software to evaluate blood flow through veins. Can be done with or without contrast. Highly accurate for pelvic and proximal veins. Less accurate for calf veins. Can distinguish acute and chronic thrombus.

ACT, Activated clotting time; *aPTT,* activated partial thromboplastin time; *INR,* international normalized ratio.

are no wrinkles. The stockings should not be rolled down, cut, or otherwise altered. Stockings that are not fitted and worn correctly can impede venous return or can cause arterial ischemia, edema, skin breakdown, and VTE. Stockings are not recommended if a patient already has a VTE.[13]

Intermittent pneumatic compression devices (IPCs) use inflatable sleeves or boots to compress the calf and thigh and/or foot and ankle to improve venous return. The sleeves apply external pressure through an electric pump. IPCs may be used with graduated compression stockings. Ensure correct fit of IPCs by accurately measuring the extremities. IPCs are not effective if they are not fitted and applied correctly or if the patient does not wear the device continuously while at rest. The IPCs can be removed for bathing, skin assessment, and ambulation. IPCs are not worn when a patient has an active VTE because of the risk for PE.

Drug Therapy

Anticoagulants are used routinely for VTE prevention and treatment. The regimen depends on the patient's VTE risk. The goal of anticoagulant therapy for VTE prevention is to prevent clot formation. The goals for treatment of a confirmed VTE are to prevent new clot development, spread of the clot, and embolization.

The 3 major classes of anticoagulants available are (1) vitamin K antagonists (VKAs), (2) thrombin inhibitors (both indirect and direct), and (3) factor Xa inhibitors (Table 41.10).[13,14] Anticoagulant therapy does not dissolve the clot. Clot lysis begins naturally through the body's intrinsic fibrinolytic system (see Chapter 33).

Vitamin K antagonists. The oral anticoagulant for long-term or extended anticoagulation is warfarin, a VKA. Warfarin inhibits activation of the vitamin K–dependent coagulation factors II, VII, IX, and X and the anticoagulant proteins C and S. Fig. 33.4 shows the clotting pathways. Warfarin begins to take effect in 48 to 72 hours and achieves maximum effect several days later. Thus an overlap of a parenteral anticoagulant (e.g., UH or low-molecular-weight heparin [LMWH]) and warfarin is needed for 5 days. We monitor the level of anticoagulation daily using the INR. The INR is a standard system of reporting prothrombin time (PT) (Table 41.11).

Take a careful history before starting warfarin. Do not give antiplatelet drugs or NSAIDs with warfarin, as these increase bleeding risk.[14] Many other drugs, vitamins, minerals, and herbal supplements interact with warfarin. A diet that varies in vitamin K intake (e.g., green leafy vegetables) can make it hard to achieve and maintain a target INR level. Genetic variants in the genes *VKORC1* and cytochrome P450 2C9 *(CYP2C9)* may influence how some people respond to warfarin. See Table 13.5 and Fig. 13.7.

Thrombin inhibitors. There are 2 major classes of *indirect thrombin inhibitors:* UH and LMWHs. UH (e.g., heparin) affects antithrombin. Antithrombin inhibits thrombin-mediated conversion of fibrinogen to fibrin by affecting factors II (prothrombin), IX, X, XI, and XII (see Fig. 33.4). Heparin can be given subcutaneously for VTE prevention or by continuous IV infusion for VTE treatment. IV heparin use requires frequent monitoring of clotting status by measuring activated partial thromboplastin time (aPTT) (Table 41.11).

One serious adverse effect of heparin is *heparin-induced thrombocytopenia* (HIT). An immune reaction to heparin causes a severe, sudden decrease in the platelet count along with a paradoxical increase in venous or arterial thrombosis. We diagnose HIT by measuring the presence of heparin antibodies in the blood. Treatment includes immediately stopping heparin therapy. If further anticoagulation is needed, we give a non-heparin anticoagulant (e.g., fondaparinux).[14] Another side effect of long-term heparin therapy is osteoporosis.

LMWHs (e.g., enoxaparin) are derived from UH. They have more predictable dose responses, longer half-lives, and fewer bleeding complications than UH. LMWHs are less likely to cause HIT and osteoporosis. LMWHs typically do not require ongoing anticoagulant monitoring and dose adjustment. Their antiinflammatory properties may help prevent PTS and venous ulcer development.

Direct thrombin inhibitors are either hirudin derivatives or synthetic thrombin inhibitors (Table 41.11). Hirudin is made using recombinant deoxyribonucleic acid (DNA) technology. It binds specifically with thrombin and directly inhibits its function without causing plasma protein and platelet interactions. Hirudin derivatives (e.g., bivalirudin) are given by continuous IV infusion. Bivalirudin is given to patients with or at risk for HIT having a percutaneous coronary intervention.

Argatroban—a synthetic direct thrombin inhibitor—hinders thrombin. It is an alternative to heparin for the prevention and treatment of HIT and for patients with or at risk for HIT needing percutaneous coronary interventions.

Dabigatran (Pradaxa) is an oral direct thrombin inhibitor. It is used for VTE prevention after elective joint replacement, for stroke prevention in nonvalvular atrial fibrillation, and as a treatment for VTE. Dabigatran has 5 major advantages compared with warfarin: rapid onset, no need to monitor anticoagulation, few drug-food interactions, lower risk for major bleeding, and predictable dose response.

Factor Xa inhibitors. *Factor Xa inhibitors* inhibit factor Xa directly or indirectly, producing rapid anticoagulation. These include fondaparinux (Arixtra), rivaroxaban (Xarelto), apixaban (Eliquis), and edoxaban (Savaysa). All are used for both VTE prevention and treatment. Fondaparinux is contraindicated in patients with severe renal disease. Although coagulation monitoring or dose adjustment is not needed, anticoagulant activity can be measured using anti-Xa assays (Table 41.11).

Anticoagulant therapy for VTE prevention. For VTE prevention in hospitalized medical patients at risk for thrombosis who are not bleeding, low-dose UH, LMWH, or fondaparinux is used. If a patient is at low VTE risk, drug prophylaxis is not needed. Patients with moderate VTE risk (e.g., general, gynecologic, urologic surgery) should receive either UH or LMWH. Patients with high VTE risk (e.g., trauma) should receive UH or LMWH until discharge. Patients having abdominal or pelvic surgery for cancer or major orthopedic surgery (e.g., total knee or hip replacement) should receive VTE prophylaxis.[13]

TABLE 41.10 Drug Therapy

Anticoagulants

Drug	Route of Administration	Considerations
Thrombin Inhibitors: Indirect		
Low-Molecular-Weight Heparin (LMWH)		
dalteparin (Fragmin) enoxaparin (Lovenox)	Subcut	Routine coagulation tests typically not needed. Monitor CBC count at regular intervals. Do not expel air bubble from prefilled syringe. Inject deep into subcutaneous tissue (preferably abdominal fatty tissue or above iliac crest), inserting entire length of needle. Hold skinfold during injection but release before removing needle. Do not aspirate. Do not rub site after injection. Rotate sites. Reduced dosage needed in patients with renal problems. Monitor platelet count for HIT. *Antidote:* Protamine
Unfractionated Heparin (UH)		
heparin sodium	Continuous IV Intermittent IV Subcut	Therapeutic effects measured at regular intervals by the aPTT or ACT. Monitor platelet count for HIT. Follow administration guidelines for LMWH if giving subcut. IV given as an adjunct for existing blood clots. SQ given to prevent clot development. *Antidote:* Protamine
Factor Xa Inhibitors		
apixaban (Eliquis) edoxaban (Savaysa) fondaparinux (Arixtra) rivaroxaban (Xarelto)	Oral Oral Subcut Oral	VTE prevention and treatment. Routine coagulation tests not needed. Monitor CBC and creatinine at regular intervals. May cause thrombocytopenia. Do not expel air bubble before giving fondaparinux. Follow administration guidelines as described for subcutaneous LMWHs. *Antidote:* Andexanet alfa (Andexxa) reverses the effects of all factor Xa inhibitors
Thrombin Inhibitors: Direct		
Hirudin Derivatives		
bivalirudin (Angiomax)	IV	Therapeutic effect measured by ACT or aPTT. Used in patients with HIT who need anticoagulation. Antidote: None
Synthetic Thrombin Inhibitors		
argatroban	IV	Therapeutic effect measured by aPTT. Antidote: None
dabigatran (Pradaxa)	Oral	No routine coagulation tests needed. *Antidote:* Idarucizumab (Praxbind)
Vitamin K Antagonists (VKAs)		
warfarin (Coumadin)	Oral	INR used to monitor therapeutic levels. Give at the same time each day. Variations of certain genes (e.g., *CYP2CP, VKORC1*) may influence response to drug. *Antidote:* Vitamin K. IV vitamin K and/or fresh frozen plasma is recommended

ACT, Activated clotting time; *aPTT,* activated partial thromboplastin time; *CBC,* complete blood count; *HIT,* heparin-induced thrombocytopenia.

Anticoagulant therapy for VTE treatment. Patients with confirmed VTE should receive initial treatment with either LMWH, UH, or an oral factor Xa drug. Oral VKA therapy may be an option. A therapeutic INR is maintained between 2.0 and 3.0 if VKA therapy is used. Active treatment of VTE should continue for at least 3 months.

Patients with multiple comorbidities, complex medical issues, or a large VTE usually are hospitalized for parenteral UH administration. Depending on the presentation and home situation, patients may be safely managed as outpatients.

Thrombolytic therapy for VTE treatment. Another treatment option is catheter-directed administration of a thrombolytic drug (e.g., alteplase). It dissolves the clot(s), reduces the acute symptoms, improves deep venous flow, reduces valvular reflux, and may help decrease the incidence of PTS. Catheter-directed thrombolysis is an option for patients who have a

TABLE 41.11 **Blood Coagulation Tests**

Test	Normal Value	Therapeutic Value	Drugs Monitored
Activated clotting time (ACT)	70–120 sec[a]	>300 sec	• Hirudin derivatives (e.g., bivalirudin) • Synthetic thrombin inhibitors (e.g., argatroban) • Unfractionated heparin (e.g., heparin)
Activated partial thromboplastin time (aPTT)	30–40 sec	46–70 sec	• Hirudin derivatives • Synthetic thrombin inhibitors • Unfractionated heparin
Anti-factor Xa	0 units/mL	0.6–1.0 units/mL	• Factor Xa inhibitors (e.g., fondaparinux, rivaroxaban)
	0 units/mL	0.2–1.5 units/mL	• Low-molecular-weight heparin (e.g., enoxaparin)
International normalized ratio (INR)	0.75–1.25	2–3	• Vitamin K antagonists (e.g., warfarin)

[a]Varies based on type of system and test reagent or activator used.

low risk of bleeding and present with an acute, extensive, symptomatic, proximal VTE. Systemic anticoagulation is needed before, during, and after catheter-directed thrombolysis. Chapter 37 discusses thrombolytic therapy.

CHECK YOUR PRACTICE

Your 55-year-old female patient is admitted with an extensive VTE in her right leg. She is receiving weight-based IV heparin per agency protocol: 18 units/kg/h. You receive the following critical laboratory result: aPTT 122 seconds.

- Describe your next actions.

Surgical and Interventional Radiology Procedures

A few patients with extensive, acute, proximal VTE who are not candidates for catheter-directed thrombolysis and/or interventional radiology therapies (because of bleeding risk) may have surgery.[13] Surgical options include open venous thrombectomy and inferior vena cava interruption. *Venous thrombectomy* involves removing the clot through a vein incision. Anticoagulant therapy is used after venous thrombectomy.

Vena cava interruption devices (e.g., Greenfield, Vena Tech, TrapEase filters) can be placed percutaneously through the right femoral or right internal jugular veins. The filter device is opened, and the spokes penetrate the vessel walls (Fig. 41.10). The filters act as a "sieve-type" device. They filter clots without interrupting blood flow. Complications after the insertion are rare but include air embolism, improper placement, migration of the filter, and perforation of the vena cava with retroperitoneal bleeding. Over time, clots can clog the filter and

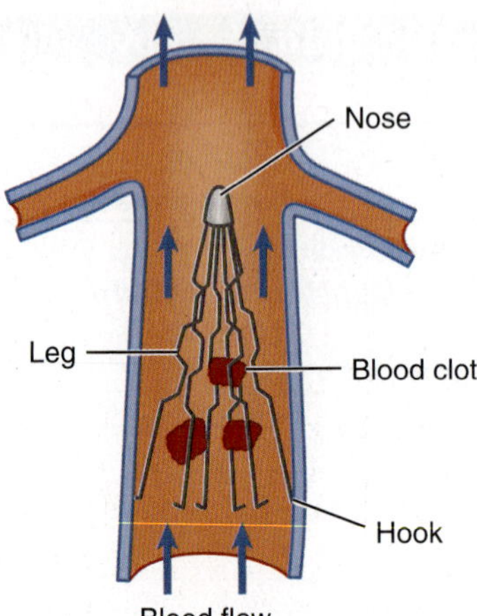

Fig. 41.10 Inferior vena cava interruption technique using Greenfield stainless-steel filter to prevent pulmonary embolism. As blood travels up the vena cava, clots are trapped in the filter.

completely block the vena cava, requiring filter removal and replacement. A filter device is recommended with acute PE or proximal VTE of the leg in patients with active bleeding or if anticoagulant therapy is contraindicated or ineffective.

Percutaneous endovascular interventional radiology procedures can be used along with catheter-directed thrombolytic therapy, especially for severely symptomatic patients with iliocaval (systemic veins of the abdomen) or iliofemoral obstruction. The procedures are like those used in the treatment of lower extremity PAD. The difference is accessing an occluded vein instead of an artery. Options include mechanical thrombectomy, pharmacomechanical devices, postthrombus extraction, angioplasty, and/or stenting.[13] Anticoagulation therapy is recommended after an iliofemoral interventional procedure. Postprocedure nursing care focuses on (1) maintaining catheter systems (if continuous infusions); (2) monitoring for bleeding, embolization, and impaired perfusion; and (3) VTE prevention teaching.

NURSING MANAGEMENT: VTE

Assessment

Table 41.12 presents the subjective and objective data to obtain from patients with VTE.

Clinical Problems

Clinical problems for patients with VTE include:

- Inadequate tissue perfusion
- Pain
- Impaired tissue integrity

Planning

The overall goals for patients with VTE include (1) pain relief, (2) decreased edema, (3) knowledge of disorder and treatment plan, (4) intact skin, (5) no bleeding, and (6) no PE.

TABLE 41.12 NURSING ASSESSMENT

VTE

Subjective Data

Important Health Information (Table 41.8)

Assess for risk factors listed in Table 41.8.

Functional Health Patterns

Health perception–health management: IV drug abuse, tobacco use, obesity

Activity-exercise: Inactivity

Cognitive-perceptual: Pain in area on palpation or ambulation

Objective Data

Cardiovascular

Distention and warmth of superficial veins in affected area. Edema and cyanosis of extremities, neck, back, and face (if superior vena cava involvement).

General

Fever, anxiety, pain

Skin

Increased size of extremity compared with other side. Taut, shiny, warm skin; redness; tender to palpation. No physical changes in the affected extremity in some patients.

Possible Diagnostic Findings

Leukocytosis, abnormal coagulation, anemia or ↑ hematocrit and RBC count, ↑ D-dimer level, positive venous compression on duplex ultrasound study; positive CT venogram, magnetic resonance venogram, or contrast venogram study

TABLE 41.13 NURSING MANAGEMENT

Care for the Patient With VTE

- Assess patients for VTE risk and monitor for VTE in at-risk patients (Table 41.8).
- Assess for use of medications and substances that may affect the coagulation status.
- Give prescribed oral, subcutaneous, and IV anticoagulants.
- Evaluate effect of anticoagulant drugs by monitoring laboratory results and side effects of therapy (Table 41.11).
- Titrate doses of unfractionated heparin (UH), warfarin, and direct thrombin inhibitors based on results of blood studies and agency protocols.
- Assess for complications of VTE, including pulmonary embolism (PE) and chronic venous insufficiency.
- Apply graduated compression stockings or intermittent pneumatic compression devices (IPCs) with attention to proper size, application, and use.
- Provide patient and caregiver teaching:
- Teach the patient and caregiver:
    - Manifestations of PE and the need to contact the emergency response system if these occur
    - Need for laboratory testing
    - Preventive measures, including diet, leg exercises, ambulation, graduated compression stockings and IPCs, avoiding nicotine, and taking anticoagulant drugs (Table 41.15).
- Supervise AP:
    - Reposition patients who are on bed rest at least every 2 h.
    - Remind patients to flex and extend the legs and feet at least every 2 h while in bed.
    - Help ambulatory patients to walk at least 4–6 times daily.
    - Apply graduated compression stockings and/or IPCs.
- Collaborate with the physical therapist:
    - Assess mobility status.
    - Develop exercise/muscle strengthening program as needed.
- Collaborate with the dietitian:
    - Assess diet and nutrition status.
    - Provide diet teaching as needed.

◆ Implementation

Acute Care

Focus your nursing care for patients with VTE on preventing thrombi and reducing inflammation (Table 41.13). Review with patients any drugs, vitamins, minerals, and herbal supplements that may interfere with anticoagulant therapy. Depending on the anticoagulant ordered, monitor INR, aPTT, ACT, anti–factor Xa levels, complete blood count (CBC), creatinine, factor X levels, hemoglobin, hematocrit, platelet levels, and/or liver enzymes. Monitor platelet counts for patients getting UH or LMWH to assess for HIT. Direct thrombin inhibitors may need adjustment for patients with renal or liver disease. Check the results of pertinent tests before starting, giving, or changing anticoagulant therapy.

Monitor for and reduce the risk for bleeding with anticoagulant therapy (Table 41.14). Bleeding risk is greater in people receiving LMWH or UH with an active gastroduodenal ulcer, prior bleeding history, low platelet count, hepatic or renal failure, rheumatic disease, cancer, or age greater than 85 years. Patients receiving warfarin with an INR of 5.0 or more have a higher risk for bleeding. In case of anticoagulation above target goals, give reversal agents (e.g., protamine, vitamin K) or make dosage adjustments as prescribed.

Early ambulation after acute VTE results in a more rapid decrease in edema and limb pain, fewer PTS symptoms, and better quality of life. It does not increase the short-term risk of a PE. Teach the patient and caregiver the importance of physical activity. Help patients ambulate several times a day. For patients with acute VTE with severe edema and limb pain, bed rest with limb elevation may initially be prescribed.

If a superficial vein thrombosis affects a short vein segment (less than 5 cm) and is not near the saphenofemoral junction, anticoagulants may not be needed. Oral NSAIDs can ease symptoms. Other interventions include having patients wear graduated compression stockings or bandages, apply warm compresses, elevate the affected limb above the level of the heart, apply topical NSAIDs, and perform mild exercise, such as walking.

Chronic Care

Focus teaching on modifying VTE risk factors, monitoring laboratory values, diet, and drug instructions. Recommend that

TABLE 41.14 NURSING MANAGEMENT

Patients Receiving Anticoagulants

Assessment
- Perform frequent assessments for signs and symptoms of bleeding (e.g., hypotension, tachycardia) or clotting.
- Examine urine and stool for overt and occult signs of blood.
- Inspect skin often, especially under any splinting devices.
- Evaluate platelet count for signs of thrombocytopenia.
- Evaluate coagulation tests for target therapeutic levels.
- Evaluate lower extremity for bruising or hematoma development if IPC device used.
- Notify the HCP of any abnormalities in assessments, vital signs, or laboratory values.

Injections
- Avoid IM injections.
- Minimize venipunctures.
- Use small-gauge needles for venipunctures unless therapy requires a larger gauge.
- Apply manual pressure for at least 10 min (or longer if needed) on venipuncture sites.

Patient Care
- Avoid restrictive clothing.
- Humidify any supplemental O_2.
- Apply moisturizing lotion to skin.
- Use electric razors, not straight razors.
- Perform physical care in a gentle manner.
- Tell patient not to forcefully blow nose.
- Avoid removing or disrupting established clots.
- Use soft toothbrushes or foam swabs for oral care.
- Reposition the patient carefully at regular intervals.
- Limit tape application. Use paper tape as appropriate.
- Give stool softeners to avoid hard stools and straining.
- Use support pads, mattresses, bed cradles, and therapeutic beds as indicated.
- Perform risk for fall and skin breakdown assessments per agency policy and implement safety and preventive measures as needed.

IPC, Intermittent pneumatic compression.

DRUG ALERT

Anticoagulant Therapy

- Observe closely for any signs of bleeding: hypotension; tachycardia; hematuria; melena; hematemesis; petechiae; and bruising, oozing, or visible bleeding from trauma site or surgical incision.
- Tell patients to report bleeding: black or bloody stools, bleeding gums, bloody urine or sputum, coffee-ground or bloody vomit, excessive bruising, nosebleeds, excessive menstrual bleeding.
- Assess for mental status changes, especially in older patients, since this may indicate cerebral bleeding.
- Tell patients to avoid taking aspirin, NSAIDs, fish oil supplements, garlic supplements, ginkgo biloba, and certain antibiotics (e.g., sulfamethoxazole and trimethoprim).

TABLE 41.15 PATIENT & CAREGIVER TEACHING

Anticoagulant Therapy

Include the following information in the teaching plan for a patient receiving anticoagulant therapy and the patient's caregiver:

1. Drug dosage, actions, side effects, and how long therapy will last.
2. Take drug at the same time each day (preferably in afternoon or evening).
3. Depending on drug, obtain blood tests to assess therapeutic effect and whether change in dosage is needed.
4. How to perform subcutaneous injection (if needed).
5. Contact emergency response system immediately for any of the following adverse side effects of drug therapy:
   - Blood in urine or stool; black, tarry stools
   - Vomiting blood, coffee-ground emesis
   - Unusual bleeding from gums, skin, or nose or heavy menstrual bleeding
   - Severe headaches or stomach pain
   - Chest pain, shortness of breath, palpitations (heart racing)
   - Weakness, dizziness, mental status changes
   - Cold, blue, or painful feet
6. Avoid activities with a high risk for injury that may cause bleeding (e.g., contact sports, rollerblading, use of straight razor).
7. Avoid all aspirin-containing drugs and NSAIDs.
8. Limit alcohol use to small to moderate amounts (12 oz beer, 4 oz wine, 1 oz hard liquor/day).
9. Wear a medical alert device saying the anticoagulant drug being taken.
10. If taking warfarin, avoid frequent or dramatic changes in eating foods high in vitamin K.
11. Consult with HCP before beginning or stopping any drug, vitamin, mineral, or diet or herbal supplement. Do not take vitamin K.
12. Inform all HCPs, including dentist, of anticoagulant therapy.
13. Implement safety precautions to prevent falls (e.g., avoid use of throw rugs).
14. Apply pressure for 10 to 15 min if bleeding occurs (e.g., nosebleed).

patients stop smoking and avoid all nicotine products. Teach patients to avoid constrictive clothing. Tell females with a history of VTE to stop oral contraceptives or hormone therapy.

Patients need to limit standing or sitting in a motionless, leg-dependent position. When traveling long distances, they should frequently exercise the calf muscles, take short walks, and maintain hydration with nonalcoholic, noncaffeinated beverages. For those at high risk for VTE who are planning a long trip, recommend properly fitted, knee-high graduated compression stockings during travel to decrease edema and VTE risk. Aspirin or anticoagulant use is not suggested for long-distance travelers. Teach the patient and caregiver to contact ERS for signs and symptoms of PE, such as sudden onset of dyspnea, tachypnea, and pleuritic chest pain.

Review drug dosage, actions, and side effects; the need for routine blood tests; and what symptoms need immediate medical attention (Table 41.15). Devices are available for home monitoring of INR. Teach patients taking LMWH or fondaparinux and their caregivers how to give the drug subcutaneously.

Teach patients taking warfarin to follow a consistent diet of foods containing vitamin K. They should avoid any supplements containing vitamin K (e.g., vitamins, green tea). Tell patients to limit alcohol intake. Proper hydration reduces hypercoagulability, which may occur with dehydration.

Patients who are overweight need to implement a diet plan and increase physical activity to achieve and maintain desired weight. Exercise may help patients with VTE and PTS and improve quality of life. Help patients develop an exercise program with an emphasis on leg strength training and aerobic activity.

Graduated compression stockings reduce swelling in patients with a proximal VTE.[13] Alternatively, IPCs may be used for patients with significant edema and moderate to severe PTS. The long-term use of graduated compression stockings may not prevent PTS development.

◆ Evaluation

The expected outcomes are that patients with VTE will have:

- Minimal to no pain
- Intact skin
- Increased knowledge of disorder and treatment plan
- No signs of hemorrhage or occult bleeding

VARICOSE VEINS

Varicose veins, or *varicosities,* are dilated (3 mm or larger in diameter), tortuous superficial veins. They are often found in the saphenous vein system. Varicosities may be small and harmless or large and bulging. *Primary varicose veins* are caused by a weakness of the vein walls. *Secondary varicose veins* result from direct injury, a previous VTE, or excess vein distention. Secondary varicose veins may occur in the esophagus (esophageal varices), vulva, spermatic cords (varicoceles), and anorectal area (hemorrhoids) and as abnormal arteriovenous (AV) connections.

Congenital varicose veins result from chromosomal defects that cause abnormal development of the venous system. *Reticular veins* are smaller varicose veins that appear flat, less tortuous, and blue-green in color. *Telangiectasias* (often called *spider veins*) are small visible vessels (generally less than 1 mm in diameter) that appear bluish black, purple, or red.

Etiology and Pathophysiology

Superficial veins in the lower extremities become dilated and tortuous in response to backward (retrograde) blood flow and increased venous pressure. They are more common in females. Risk factors include family history of chronic venous disease, weak vein structure, tobacco use, age, obesity, multiparity, history of VTE, venous obstruction from extrinsic pressure by tumors, thrombophilia, phlebitis, leg injury, and occupations that require prolonged standing or sitting.

In primary varicose veins, weak vein walls allow the vein valve ring to enlarge, so the leaflets no longer fit together properly (incompetent). Incompetent vein valves allow backward blood flow, particularly when the patient is standing. This results in increased venous pressure and further venous distention. High pressure in the superficial veins can be caused by vein valve dysfunction in the deep veins or perforator veins (veins that perforate the deep fascia of muscles to connect the superficial veins to the deep veins).

Clinical Manifestations

Discomfort from varicose veins varies among people. It tends to be worse after episodes of superficial vein thrombosis. Symptoms affect females more often. The most common symptoms include a heavy, achy feeling or pain after prolonged standing or sitting. Walking or limb elevation relieves pain. Some patients feel pressure or an itchy, burning, tingling, throbbing, or cramplike leg sensation. Swelling, restless or tired legs, fatigue, and nocturnal leg cramps may occur.

Superficial venous thrombosis is the most frequent complication of varicose veins. It may occur spontaneously or after trauma, surgery, or pregnancy. Rare complications include rupture of the varicose veins resulting in external bleeding and skin ulcers.

Diagnostic Studies and Interprofessional Care

Superficial varicose veins often can be diagnosed by physical assessment. Duplex ultrasound imaging is the gold standard to evaluate venous anatomy, valvular competence, and venous obstruction.[15] Conservative treatment involves rest with limb elevation; graduated compression stockings; leg strengthening exercise, such as walking; and weight loss.

Drug Therapy

Venoactive drugs work by stimulating release of chemicals within the vein walls to strengthen the circulation and reduce inflammation and edema. Several natural and synthetic venoactive agents have been used to treat varicose veins and advanced chronic venous disease. These include micronized purified flavonoid fraction, rutosides (e.g., horse chestnut seed extract), proanthocyanidins (from grapes and apples), and *Ruscus* (butcher's broom).[14] Benefits of venoactive drugs include pain relief, edema reduction, and decreased leg cramping and restless legs. These drugs are widely used in Europe. They are not approved by the FDA. However, many are available over the counter as diet or herbal supplements.

Interventional and Surgical Therapies

Sclerotherapy involves the direct IV injection of a liquid or foam sclerosing substance (e.g., hypertonic saline, polidocanol, glycerin) that chemically ablates (destroys) the treated veins. Sclerotherapy can be used on telangiectasias, perforator veins, reticular veins, smaller varicose veins, and venous malformations (Fig. 41.11). This procedure is done in an office setting and causes minimal discomfort.

The most common complications of sclerotherapy are residual pigmentation, thrombophlebitis, and ulcers.[15] After

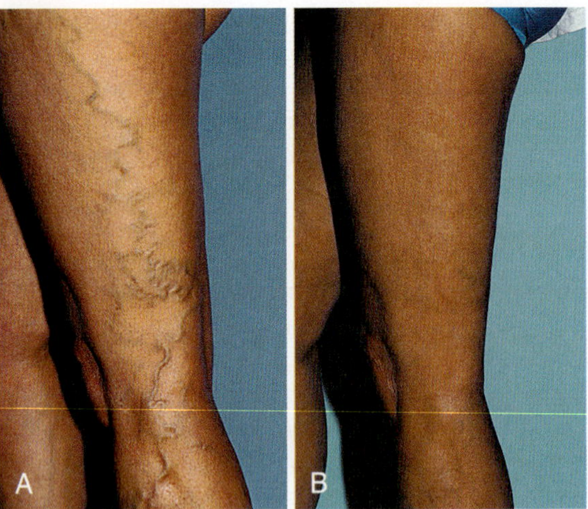

Fig. 41.11 (A) Varicose veins before treatment. (B) Appearance after treatment with sclerotherapy. (From Goldman MP, Guex JJ, Weiss RA: *Sclerotherapy: treatment of varicose and telangiectatic leg veins,* ed 5, Philadelphia, 2011, Mosby.)

injection, a graduated compression stocking or bandage is worn. Patients should not travel long distances during the first week after sclerotherapy to minimize the risk for a VTE.

Transcutaneous laser or light therapy is used for patients with telangiectasias in whom sclerotherapy is contraindicated or has been ineffective. High-intensity pulsed-light therapy can target reticular veins. These lasers work by heating the hemoglobin in the vessels, causing vessel sclerosis. Complications of these therapies include pain, blistering, hyperpigmentation, and superficial erosions.

A minimally invasive treatment for saphenous vein reflux is endovenous ablation using thermal energy from radiofrequency or laser therapy. The HCP inserts a catheter into the vein to heat the vein wall, which then causes the vein to collapse. Complications include bruising, skin burns, hyperpigmentation, infection, paresthesia, superficial or deep vein thrombosis, and PE. Graduated compression stockings or bandages are worn afterward. Endovenous thermal ablation may be done in combination with surgical ligation or phlebectomy.

Surgical intervention is needed for recurrent superficial venous thrombosis or when symptoms cannot be controlled with other therapy. The traditional surgery involves ligation of the entire vein (usually the greater saphenous vein) and removing its incompetent branches. An alternative but time-consuming technique is *ambulatory phlebectomy.* This involves pulling the varicosity through a "stab" incision followed by excision of the vein. *Transilluminated powered phlebectomy* involves using a tissue resector to destroy clusters of varicosities and then removing the pieces via aspiration. Complications include bleeding, bruising, and infection.

❖ NURSING MANAGEMENT: VARICOSE VEINS

Prevention is a key factor related to varicose veins. Tell patients to avoid sitting or standing for long periods, maintain ideal body weight, take precautions against injury to the extremities, avoid wearing constrictive clothing, and walk daily.

After vein ligation surgery, encourage patients to deep-breathe, which promotes venous return. Check the extremities regularly for color, movement, sensation, temperature, edema, and quality of pedal pulses. Some bruising and discoloration are normal. Elevate the legs 15 degrees to limit edema. Remove graduated compression stockings or bandages every 8 hours for short periods and then reapply them.

Long-term management is directed toward improving circulation and appearance, relieving discomfort, and avoiding complications. Varicosities can recur in other veins after surgery. Teach patients the proper use and care of custom-fitted graduated compression stockings. Patients should apply stockings in bed before rising in the morning.

Emphasize the importance of periodic positioning of the legs above the heart. Overweight patients may need help with weight loss. Patients with a job that requires long periods of standing or sitting need to frequently flex and extend the hips, legs, and ankles and change positions.

CHRONIC VENOUS INSUFFICIENCY AND VENOUS LEG ULCERS

Chronic venous insufficiency (CVI) describes abnormalities of the venous system that result in advanced signs and symptoms, such as edema, skin changes, and/or venous leg ulcers.[16] CVI can lead to *venous leg ulcers* (also called *venous stasis ulcers* or *varicose ulcers*). Although CVI and venous leg ulcers are not life-threatening diseases, they are painful, slow to heal, debilitating, and costly conditions that adversely affect patients' quality of life. They are a common problem in older adults.

Etiology and Pathophysiology

Both long-standing primary varicose veins and PTS can progress to CVI. *Ambulatory venous hypertension* causes serous fluid and RBCs to leak from the capillaries and venules into the tissue. This causes edema and chronic inflammatory changes. Enzymes in the tissue eventually break down RBCs. This releases *hemosiderin,* which causes brownish skin discoloration. Over time, fibrous tissue replaces the skin and subcutaneous tissue around the ankle. This results in thick, hardened, contracted skin. Although the causes of CVI are known, the exact pathophysiology of venous leg ulcers is unknown.

Clinical Manifestations

In patients with CVI, the skin of the lower leg is leathery, with a characteristic brownish or "brawny" appearance from the hemosiderin deposition. Edema usually has been persistent for a prolonged period. Eczema with itching and scratching is often present (Table 41.1).

Venous ulcers classically occur above the medial malleolus (Fig. 41.12). The ulcer is often quite painful, particularly when edema or infection is present. Pain may be worse when the leg is in a dependent position. If the venous ulcer is untreated, the wound becomes wider and deeper, increasing the risk for infection.

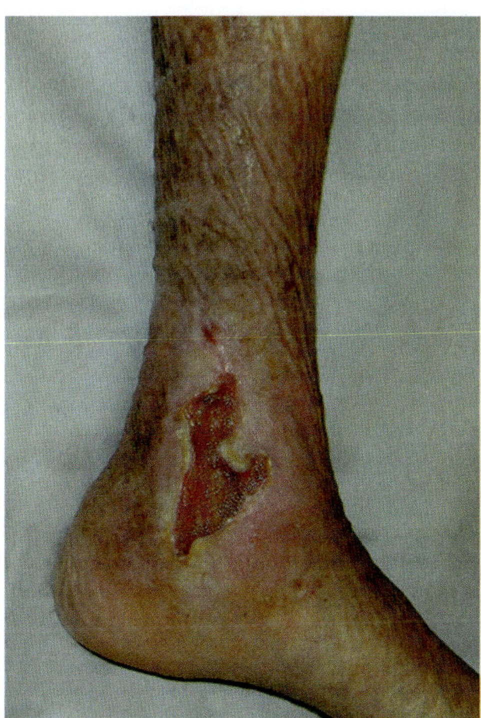

Fig. 41.12 Venous leg ulcer. (From Quick C, Biers SM: *Essential surgery: problems, diagnosis, and management*, St Louis, 2020, Elsevier.)

Interprofessional and Nursing Management

Compression is essential for venous ulcer healing and preventing recurrence. A variety of options are available for compression therapy. These include custom-fitted graduated compression stockings, elastic tubular support bandages, a Velcro wrap (CircAid), IPCs, and multilayer (3 or 4) bandage systems (e.g., Profore). Evaluate patients when choosing a compression method. Before starting compression therapy, assess the arterial status to make sure PAD is not present. An ABI of 0.4 or less suggests severe PAD, and patients should not have any type of compression therapy.[2] Show how to correctly apply the compression therapy and have the patient "show back" the skill. Stockings should be worn daily to prevent recurrent leg ulcers. Tell patients to replace stockings every 4 to 6 months.

Discuss activity guidelines and proper limb positioning. Tell patients with CVI to avoid standing or sitting for long periods, which decreases blood return from the lower extremities. Teach patients to frequently elevate their legs above the level of the heart to reduce edema. Encourage patients to begin a daily walking program once an ulcer heals. Tell the patient and caregiver to avoid trauma to the limbs. Teach proper foot and leg care to avoid more skin trauma.

Moist environment dressings are the basis of wound care. A variety of dressings are available. These include transparent film dressings, hydrocolloids, hydrogels, foams, alginates, gauze, and combination dressings. Dressing decisions should be based on wound characteristics, cost, best evidence, and clinician judgment. Chapter 12 and Table 12.14 discuss dressings.

Assess nutrition status. A balanced diet with adequate protein, calories, and nutrients is essential. Foods high in protein (e.g., meat, beans, tofu), vitamin A (green leafy vegetables), vitamin C (citrus fruits, tomatoes), and zinc (meat, seafood) are most important for healing. For patients with diabetes, maintaining normal glucose levels aids the healing process.

Though venous leg ulcers are colonized by bacteria, routine use of antibiotics is not indicated. Signs of infection include change in quantity, color, or odor of the drainage; pus; redness of the wound edges; change in sensation around the wound; and warmth around the wound. There may be increased local pain, edema, or both; dark-colored granulation tissue; induration around the wound; delayed healing; and cellulitis. If signs of infection occur, obtain a wound culture. Culture results guide antibiotic therapy. The usual treatment for infection is wound debridement, wound excision, and systemic antibiotics.

If the ulcer does not heal with conservative therapy, drug therapy is an option. Pentoxifylline combined with compression therapy can improve healing. Pentoxifylline minimizes WBC activation and adhesion to capillary endothelium and decreases oxidative stress.

Other treatments are considered for large venous leg ulcers that do not respond to standard therapy after 4 to 6 weeks. These include coverage with a skin replacement or substitute, such as split-thickness skin grafts or artificial bioengineered skin. Chapter 26 discusses skin grafting. Although grafts help with healing, they do not replace the need for lifelong compression therapy.

Patients with CVI have dry, flaky, itchy skin. Daily moisturizing decreases itching and prevents skin cracking. Contact dermatitis may result from contact with sensitizing products. These include topical antimicrobial agents (e.g., gentamicin); additives in bandages or dressings (e.g., adhesives); ointments containing lanolin, alcohols, or benzocaine; and creams or lotions with fragrance or preservatives. Assess wounds for signs of infection with each dressing change (Table 41.16).

TABLE 41.16 NURSING MANAGEMENT

Care for the Patient With Chronic Venous Insufficiency

- Assess the patient for increases in edema, eczema, and venous leg ulcers.
- Assess diet and nutrition status and make referrals as needed.
- Assess for the use of venoactive diet supplements or herbs that may adversely affect comorbid conditions and/or prescription drugs.
- Choose best options for compression therapy and wound care.
- Give prescribed analgesics, antibiotics, or other drugs.
- Apply compression therapy.
- Provide wound care for venous leg ulcers.
- Evaluate the effectiveness of therapies and need for alternative approaches.
- Teach patient and caregivers about the manifestations, complications, and treatment of venous insufficiency.
- Supervise the AP:
  - Aid patients in elevating legs to reduce edema and pain.
  - Apply graduated compression stockings.
- Collaborate with the dietitian:
  - Assess diet and nutrition status.
  - Provide diet education as needed.

CASE STUDY

Peripheral Artery Disease

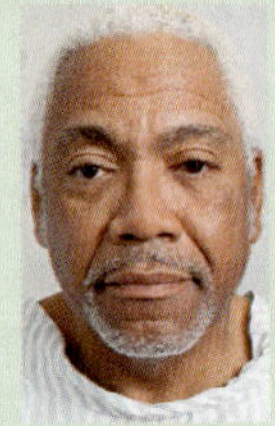
(© IPGGutenbergUKLtd/iStock/Thinkstock.)

Patient Profile

S.J., a 73-year-old male, is admitted to the hospital with rest pain in both legs and a nonhealing ulcer of the big toe on the right foot.

Subjective Data

- History of an MI, stroke, hypertension, HF, type 1 diabetes
- Had a left femoral-popliteal bypass 5 years ago
- Has a 45-pack-year history of tobacco use
- Has been using insulin for 30 years
- Reports sudden, intense increase in right foot pain for past 2 h
- Has slept in recliner with right leg in dependent position for several months to decrease leg pain

Current Medications

- Oral medications: Furosemide 40 mg/day, isosorbide dinitrate/hydralazine hydrochloride 1 tablet every 8 h, aspirin 325 mg/day, diltiazem sustained release 240 mg/day
- Aspart (NovoLog) insulin with meals (sliding scale)
- Glargine insulin 50 units/day subcutaneously

Objective Data

Physical Assessment

- BP 148/92 mm Hg, irregular apical HR 90/min, respiratory rate 22/min, temp 97.9°F (36.6°C)
- Alert and oriented, anxious, with no apparent physical or mental deficits from stroke
- Has 1+ right femoral pulse, popliteal pulse by Doppler only, posterior tibial pulse by Doppler only, and dorsalis pedis pulse absent (not palpable or present by Doppler). Left leg pulses are 1+.
- Right leg ABI: 0.20. Left leg ABI: 0.68.
- Has a 2-cm necrotic ulcer on tip of right big toe.
- Has thickened toenails. Shiny, thin skin on legs. No hair on both lower legs.
- Right foot is very cool, pale, and mottled in color with decreased sensation.
- No peripheral edema.
- Bedside glucose measurement 298 mg/dL (last meal 4 h before admission).

Discussion Questions

1. ***Recognize:*** What risk factors do you identify that led to S.J. having PAD?
2. ***Analyze:*** What are the important findings from S.J.'s assessment?
3. ***Plan:*** What treatment options are possible?
4. ***Prioritize:*** What is the most important thing the team can do for S.J.?
5. ***Act:*** What role do APs have in providing care?
6. ***Evaluate:*** What do you need to continually monitor?
7. ***Safety:*** What safety precautions should we consider for S.J.?

Answers available at http://evolve.elsevier.com/Lewis/medsurg.

BRIDGE TO NCLEX EXAMINATION

The number of the questions corresponds to the same-numbered outcome at the beginning of the chapter.

1. A 50-year-old female who weighs 95 kg has a history of high blood pressure, high sodium intake, tobacco use, and sedentary lifestyle. Which is the *most important* risk factor for peripheral artery disease (PAD) to address in the nursing plan of care?
   - **a.** Salt intake
   - **b.** Tobacco use
   - **c.** Excess weight
   - **d.** Sedentary lifestyle
2. Which information would the nurse include when explaining the cause of rest pain with PAD?
   - **a.** Vasospasm of cutaneous arteries in the feet
   - **b.** Decrease in blood flow to the nerves of the feet
   - **c.** Increase in retrograde venous perfusion to the lower legs
   - **d.** Constriction in blood flow to leg muscles during exercise
3. A patient with infective endocarditis develops sudden left leg pain with pallor, paresthesia, and a loss of peripheral pulses. Which action would the nurse take *first*?
   - **a.** Notify the HCP of the change in perfusion.
   - **b.** Start anticoagulant therapy with IV heparin.
   - **c.** Elevate the leg to improve the venous return.
   - **d.** Position the patient in reverse Trendelenburg.
4. Which clinical manifestations can the nurse expect to see in both patients with Buerger disease and patients with Raynaud phenomenon? (**Select all that apply.**)
   - **a.** Intermittent low-grade fevers
   - **b.** Sensitivity to cold temperatures
   - **c.** Gangrenous ulcers on fingertips
   - **d.** Color changes of fingers and toes
   - **e.** Episodes of superficial vein thrombosis
5. Which signs and symptoms would suggest aneurysm rupture in a patient with an abdominal aortic aneurysm?
   - **a.** Rapid onset of shortness of breath and hemoptysis
   - **b.** Sudden low back pain and bruising along the flank
   - **c.** Patchy blue mottling on feet and toes and rest pain
   - **d.** Gradually increasing substernal chest pain and diaphoresis
6. Which nursing interventions are the *priority* immediately after an abdominal aortic aneurysm repair?
   - **a.** Assessing nutrition status and diet preferences
   - **b.** Starting IV heparin and monitoring anticoagulation
   - **c.** Administering IV fluids and watching kidney function
   - **d.** Elevating the legs and applying compression stockings
7. Which goal is the *priority* of interprofessional care for a patient with a suspected acute aortic dissection?
   - **a.** Reduce anxiety
   - **b.** Monitor chest pain
   - **c.** Control blood pressure
   - **d.** Increase myocardial contractility

8. Which patient is at *highest* risk for venous thromboembolism?
   a. A 62-year-old male with spider veins who is having arthroscopic knee surgery
   b. A 32-year-old female who smokes, takes oral contraceptives, and is planning a long flight
   A 26-year-old female who is 3 days postpartum and received maintenance IV fluids for 12 hours during her labor
   d. An active 72-year-old male at home recovering from transurethral resection of the prostate for benign prostatic hyperplasia
9. Which clinical findings would the nurse expect in a person with an acute lower extremity VTE? **(Select all that apply.)**
   a. Pallor and coolness of foot and calf
   b. Mild to moderate calf pain and tenderness
   c. Grossly decreased or absent pedal pulses
   d. Unilateral edema and induration of the thigh
   e. Palpable cord along a superficial varicose vein
10. Which treatment would the nurse anticipate for an otherwise healthy person with an initial VTE?
    a. IV argatroban as an inpatient
    b. IV unfractionated heparin as an inpatient
    c. Subcutaneous unfractionated heparin as an outpatient
    d. Subcutaneous low-molecular-weight heparin as an outpatient
11. Which instruction is a *key* aspect of teaching for a patient on anticoagulant therapy?
    a. Monitor for and report any signs of bleeding.
    b. Do not take acetaminophen (Tylenol) for a headache.
    c. Decrease your diet intake of foods containing vitamin K.
    d. Arrange to have blood drawn twice a week to check drug effects.
12. The nurse is planning care and teaching for a patient with venous leg ulcers. Which patient action is the *most* important in promoting healing and control?
    a. Following activity guidelines
    b. Using moist environment dressings
    c. Taking horse chestnut seed extract daily
    d. Applying graduated compression stockings

1. b; 2. b; 3. a; 4. b, c, d; 5. b; 6. c; 7. c; 8. b;
9. b, d; 10. d; 11. a; 12. d.

For rationales to these answers and even more NCLEX review questions, visit http://evolve.elsevier.com/Lewis/medsurg.

REFERENCES

To access the References for this chapter, please scan the QR code with a mobile device.

42

Shock, Sepsis, and Multiple Organ Dysfunction Syndrome

Helen Miley

http://evolve.elsevier.com/Lewis/medsurg/

CONCEPTUAL FOCUS

Fluid and Electrolytes
Gas Exchange
Inflammation
Perfusion

LEARNING OUTCOMES

1. Relate the pathophysiology to the clinical manifestations of the different types of shock.
2. Compare the effects of shock, sepsis, systemic inflammatory response syndrome, and multiple organ dysfunction syndrome (MODS) on the major body systems.
3. Compare the interprofessional care, drug therapy, and nursing management of patients with different types of shock.
4. Describe the interprofessional care and nursing management of patients with MODS.

KEY TERMS

cardiogenic shock
distributive shock
hypovolemic shock
multiple organ dysfunction syndrome (MODS)neurogenic shock
obstructive shock
sepsis
septic shock
shock
systemic inflammatory response syndrome (SIRS)

Shock, systemic inflammatory response syndrome (SIRS), sepsis, and multiple organ dysfunction syndrome (MODS) are serious and interrelated problems (Fig. 42.1). **Shock** is a syndrome characterized by decreased tissue perfusion and impaired cell metabolism. This results in an imbalance between the supply of and demand for O_2 and nutrients. The exchange of O_2 and nutrients at the cell level is essential to life. When cells are hypoperfused, the demand for O_2 and nutrients exceeds the supply at the microcirculatory level. Ischemia can occur, leading to cell injury and death. Thus shock is life-threatening. This chapter provides an overview of the different types of shock, SIRS, sepsis, and MODS and their related management.

SHOCK

Classification of Shock

There are 4 main categories of shock: cardiogenic, hypovolemic, distributive, and obstructive (Table 42.1).[1] Although the cause, initial presentation, and management vary for each type, physiologic responses to hypoperfusion are similar.

Cardiogenic Shock

Cardiogenic shock occurs when either systolic or diastolic dysfunction of the heart's pumping action results in reduced cardiac output (CO), stroke volume (SV), and BP. These changes compromise myocardial perfusion, further depress myocardial function, and decrease CO and perfusion. Causes of cardiogenic shock are shown in Table 42.1. It is the leading cause of death from acute myocardial infarction (MI). Although the in-hospital mortality has improved due to aggressive intervention (early revascularization, mechanical circulatory support), the 6- to 12-month mortality remains high.[2]

Fig. 42.2 shows the pathophysiology of cardiogenic shock. The heart's inability to pump the blood forward is called *systolic dysfunction.* This inability results in a low CO (less than 4 L/min) and *cardiac index* (less than 2.5 L/min/m^2). Systolic dysfunction

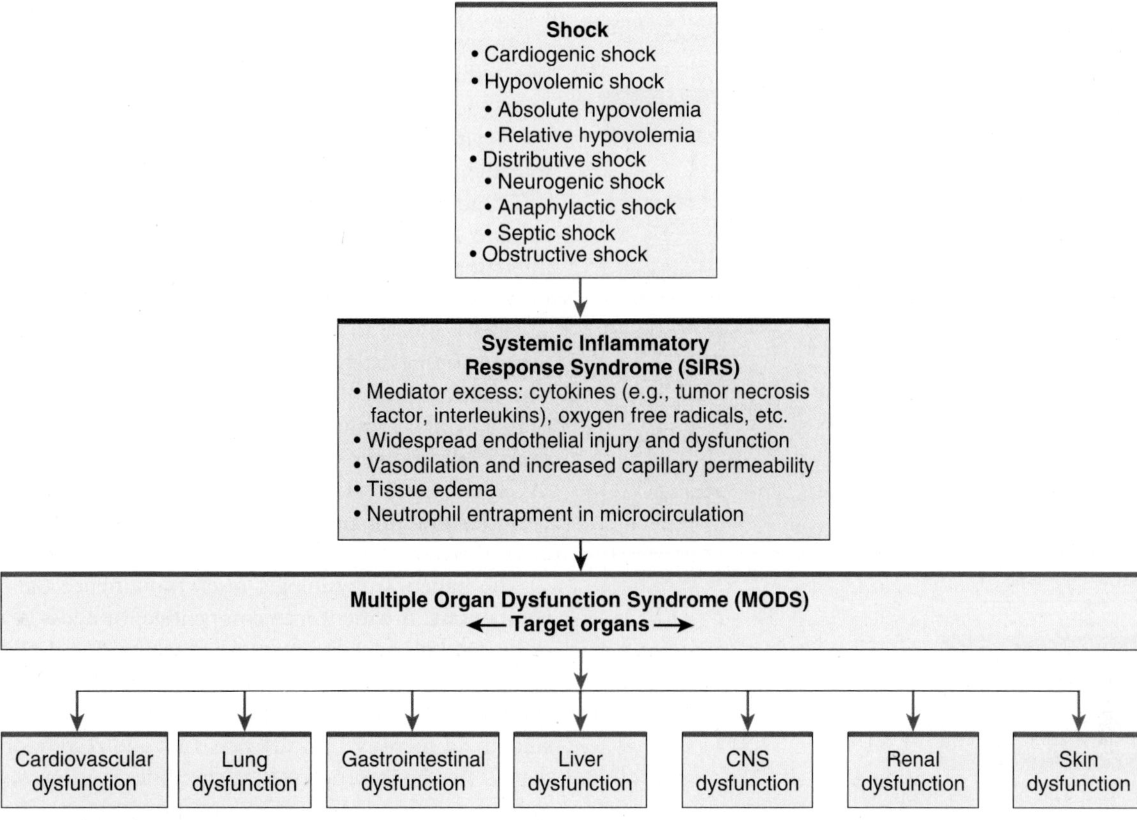

Fig. 42.1 Relationship of shock, systemic inflammatory response syndrome, and multiple organ dysfunction syndrome.

TABLE 42.1 Classification of Shock States

Types and Causes	Associated Conditions
Cardiogenic Shock	
• Diastolic dysfunction: inability of the heart to fill	Cardiac tamponade, ventricular hypertrophy, cardiomyopathy
• Dysrhythmias	Bradydysrhythmias, tachydysrhythmias
• Structural problems	Valvular stenosis or regurgitation, ventricular septal rupture, tension pneumothorax
• Systolic dysfunction: inability of the heart to pump blood forward	MI, cardiomyopathy, blunt cardiac injury, severe systemic or pulmonary hypertension, myocardial depression from metabolic problems
Hypovolemic Shock	
Absolute Hypovolemia	
• External loss of whole blood	Hemorrhage from trauma, surgery, GI bleeding
• Loss of other body fluids	Vomiting, diarrhea, excess diuresis, diabetes, arginine vasopressin disorder (AVP disorder)
Relative Hypovolemia	
• Fluid shifts	Burn injuries, ascites
• Internal bleeding	Fracture of long bones, ruptured spleen, hemothorax, severe pancreatitis
• Massive vasodilation	Sepsis
• Pooling of blood or fluids	Bowel obstruction
Distributive Shock	
Anaphylactic Shock	
• Hypersensitivity (allergic) reaction to a sensitizing substance	Contrast media, blood, blood products, drugs, insect bites, anesthetic agents, food, food additives, vaccines, environmental agents, latex
Neurogenic Shock	
• Hemodynamic consequence of spinal cord injury and/or disease at or above T5	Severe pain, drugs, hypoglycemia, injury
• Spinal anesthesia	
• Vasomotor center depression	
Septic Shock	
• At-risk patients	Older adults, diabetes, chronic kidney disease, HF, immunosuppression, malnutrition, debilitation, burns, major surgery, trauma
• Infection	Pneumonia, peritonitis, urinary tract, invasive procedures, indwelling lines and catheters
Obstructive Shock	
• Physical obstruction impeding the filling or outflow of blood resulting in reduced CO	Cardiac tamponade, tension pneumothorax, superior vena cava syndrome, abdominal compartment syndrome, pulmonary embolism

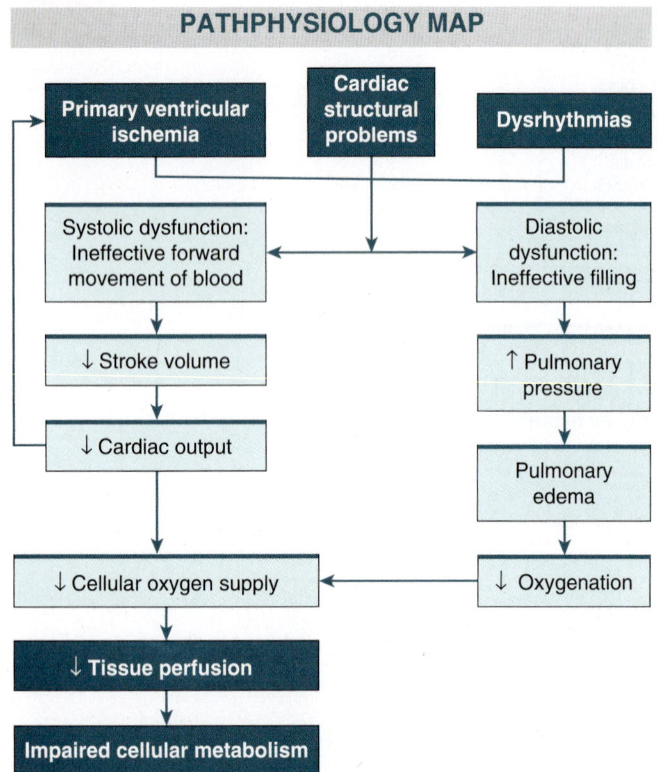

Fig. 42.2 The pathophysiology of cardiogenic shock.

primarily affects the left ventricle because systolic pressure is greater on the left side of the heart. The most common cause of systolic dysfunction is acute MI. When systolic dysfunction affects the right side of the heart, blood flow through the pulmonary circulation is reduced. Decreased filling of the heart results in decreased SV. Table 42.1 lists causes of diastolic dysfunction.

The early presentation of patients with cardiogenic shock is similar to that of patients with acute decompensated heart failure (HF) (see Chapter 38). Patients may have tachycardia and hypotension. Pulse pressure may be narrowed due to the heart's inability to pump blood forward during systole and increased volume during diastole. An increase in systemic vascular resistance (SVR) increases the workload of the heart. This increases myocardial O_2 consumption.

Patients are tachypneic. Crackles are present from pulmonary congestion. The hemodynamic profile shows an increase in the pulmonary artery (PA) wedge pressure (PAWP), stroke volume variation (SVV), and pulmonary vascular resistance.

Signs of peripheral hypoperfusion (e.g., cyanosis, pallor, weak peripheral pulses, cool and clammy skin, delayed capillary refill) occur. Decreased renal blood flow results in sodium and water retention and decreased urine output. Anxiety, confusion, and agitation may develop with impaired cerebral perfusion. Tables 42.2 and 42.3 describe the laboratory findings and clinical presentation of patients with cardiogenic shock.

Hypovolemic Shock

Hypovolemic shock occurs from inadequate fluid volume in the intravascular space to support adequate perfusion (Table 42.1).[3] The volume loss may be either an absolute or a relative volume loss. *Absolute hypovolemia* results when fluid is lost through hemorrhage, gastrointestinal (GI) loss (e.g., vomiting, diarrhea), fistula drainage, or diuresis. In *relative hypovolemia,* fluid volume moves out of the vascular space into the extravascular space (e.g., intracavitary space). We call this type of fluid shift *third spacing.* One example of relative volume loss is fluid leaking from the vascular space to the interstitial space from increased capillary permeability, as seen in burns (see Chapter 26).

The response to acute volume loss depends on several factors, including extent of injury, age, and general state of health. The clinical presentation of hypovolemic shock is consistent (Table 42.3). Reduced intravascular volume results in a decreased venous return to the heart, with decreased preload, SV, and CO. A cascade of events results in decreased tissue perfusion and impaired cell metabolism, the hallmarks of shock (Fig. 42.3).

The patient's physiologic reserves influence their ability to compensate. A patient may compensate for a loss of up to 15% of the total blood volume (approximately 750 mL). Further loss of volume (15% to 30%) results in a sympathetic nervous system (SNS)–mediated response.[3] At first, this response results in an increase in heart rate, CO, and respiratory rate and depth. As shock progresses, tachycardia continues, but mean arterial pressure (MAP), CO, and urine output decrease. The patient may appear anxious.

If the shock is due to hypovolemia, crystalloid fluid replacement is the key. With blood loss, prompt control of the bleeding and administering blood products is essential. In both instances, if the patient is resuscitated early, tissue dysfunction is generally reversible. If volume loss is greater than 30%, compensatory mechanisms may fail. Loss of autoregulation in the microcirculation and irreversible tissue destruction occur with loss of more than 40% of the total blood volume. Common laboratory studies and assessments include serial measurements of hemoglobin and hematocrit, electrolytes, lactate, arterial blood gases (ABGs), mixed central venous O_2 saturation (SvO_2), and hourly urine outputs (Table 42.2).

Distributive Shock

Distributive shock has many causes. It is a condition of relative hypovolemia due to intravascular volume redistribution from loss of vascular tone or disordered permeability. The 3 subsets of distributive shock are neurogenic, anaphylactic, and septic.[4]

Neurogenic shock. **Neurogenic shock** is a hemodynamic phenomenon that can occur within 30 minutes of a spinal cord injury. It can last up to 6 weeks or be irreversible. Neurogenic shock related to spinal cord injuries is generally associated with a cervical or high thoracic injury. The injury results in massive vasodilation without compensation from the loss of SNS vasoconstrictor tone.[5] This massive vasodilation leads to pooling of blood in the blood vessels, tissue hypoperfusion, and impaired cell metabolism (Fig. 42.4).

TABLE 42.2 Diagnostic Studies

Shock

Study	Finding	Significance
Arterial blood gases	Respiratory alkalosis	Found in early shock due to hyperventilation
	Metabolic acidosis	Occurs later in shock when lactate accumulates in blood from anaerobic metabolism
Base deficit	>−6	Acid production due to hypoxia
Blood cultures	Growth of organisms	May show cause of infection
BUN	↑	Impaired kidney function caused by hypoperfusion from severe vasoconstriction, cell catabolism (e.g., trauma, infection)
Creatine kinase	↑	Trauma, MI. Response to cell damage and/or hypoxia
Creatinine	↑	Impaired kidney function caused by hypoperfusion from severe vasoconstriction
DIC screen		Disseminated intravascular coagulation (DIC) can develop within hours to days after initial assault on the body (e.g., shock)
• D-dimer	↑	
• Fibrin split products (FSPs)	↑	
• Fibrinogen	↓	
• INR	↑	
• Platelet count	↓	
• PTT and PT	↑	
• Thrombin time	↑	
Glucose	↑	Found in early shock due to release of liver glycogen stores in response to sympathetic nervous system stimulation and cortisol. Insulin insensitivity develops
	↓	Depleted glycogen stores with liver dysfunction possible as shock progresses
Electrolytes		
• Sodium	↑	Found in early shock because of ↑ secretion of aldosterone, causing renal retention of sodium
	↓	May be iatrogenic if excess hypotonic fluid is given after fluid loss
• Potassium	↑	Results when dead cells release potassium. Occurs in acute kidney injury and acidosis
	↓	Found in early shock because of ↑ secretion of aldosterone, causing renal potassium excretion
Lactate	↑	Usually ↑ once significant hypoperfusion and impaired O_2 use at the cell level have occurred. By-product of anaerobic metabolism
Liver enzymes (ALT, AST, GGT)	↑	Liver cell destruction in progressive stage of shock
Procalcitonin (PCT)	↑	Biomarker released in response to bacterial infections
RBC count, hematocrit, hemoglobin	Normal	Remains within normal limits in shock because of relative hypovolemia and pump failure and in hemorrhagic shock before fluid resuscitation
	↓	Hemorrhagic shock after fluid resuscitation when fluids other than blood are used
	↑	Nonhemorrhagic shock caused by actual hypovolemia and hemoconcentration
Troponin	↑	MI
White blood cell count	↑, ↓	Infection, septic shock

ALT, Alanine aminotransferase; *AST,* aspartate aminotransferase; *GGT,* γ-glutamyl transferase; *INR,* international normalized ratio; *PT,* prothrombin time; *PTT,* partial thromboplastin time.

In addition to spinal cord injury, spinal anesthesia can block transmission of impulses from the SNS. Depression of the vasomotor center of the medulla from drugs (e.g., opioids, benzodiazepines) can decrease vasoconstrictor tone of the peripheral blood vessels, resulting in neurogenic shock (Table 42.1).

The classic manifestations are hypotension (from the massive vasodilation) and bradycardia (from unopposed parasympathetic stimulation).[5] Vasodilation along with the inability to regulate temperature promotes heat loss. At first, the skin is warm due to the massive vasodilation. As the heat disperses, the patient is at risk for hypothermia. Later, the skin may be cool or warm depending on the ambient temperature (*poikilothermia,* taking on the temperature of the environment). The skin is usually dry. Tables 42.2 and 42.3 further describe the laboratory findings and clinical presentation of patients with neurogenic shock.

Although spinal shock and neurogenic shock often occur in the same patient, they are not the same disorder. *Spinal shock* is a transient condition that is present after an acute spinal cord injury (see Chapter 65). Patients with spinal shock have an absence of all voluntary and reflex neurologic activity below the level of the injury.

Anaphylactic shock. *Anaphylactic shock* is an acute, life-threatening hypersensitivity (allergic) reaction to a sensitizing substance (e.g., drug, chemical, vaccine, food, insect venom).[6] The reaction quickly causes massive vasodilation, release of vasoactive mediators, and an increase in capillary permeability. As capillary permeability increases, fluid leaks from the vascular space into the interstitial space.

Anaphylactic shock can lead to respiratory distress due to laryngeal edema or severe bronchospasm and circulatory failure

TABLE 42.3 Clinical Presentation of Types of Shock

Cardiogenic Shock	Hypovolemic Shock	Neurogenic Shock	Anaphylactic Shock	Septic Shock	Obstructive Shock
Cardiovascular					
↑ HR ↓ BP ↓ SV, CO ↑ SVR, PAWP, CVP ↓ Capillary refill	↑ HR ↓ Preload ↓ CO, CVP, PAWP ↑ SVR ↓ Capillary refill	↓ HR ↓ BP ↓ CO, CVP, SVR ↓/↑ Temperature	↑ HR ↓ CO, CVP, PAWP Chest pain Third spacing of fluid	↑ HR ↓/↑ Temperature Myocardial dysfunction Biventricular dilation ↓ Ejection fraction	↑ HR ↓↓ BP ↓ Preload ↓ CO ↑ SVR, CVP
Gastrointestinal					
↓ Bowel sounds Nausea, vomiting	Absent bowel sounds	Bowel dysfunction	Abdominal pain Cramping Diarrhea Nausea Vomiting	GI bleeding Paralytic ileus	↓ To absent bowel sounds
Neurologic					
Anxiety Confusion Agitation	Anxiety Confusion Agitation	Flaccid paralysis below the level of the lesion Loss of reflex activity	Anxiety Confusion Feeling of impending doom ↓ LOC Metallic taste	Anxiety Confusion Agitation Coma (late)	Anxiety Confusion Agitation
Renal					
↑ Na^+ and H_2O retention ↓ Renal blood flow ↓ Urine output	↓ Urine output	Bladder dysfunction	Incontinence	↓ Urine output	↓ Urine output
Respiratory					
Tachypnea Crackles Cyanosis	Tachypnea → bradypnea (late)	Dysfunction related to level of injury	Shortness of breath Edema of larynx and epiglottis Stridor Wheezing	Hyperventilation Crackles Respiratory alkalosis → respiratory acidosis Hypoxemia Respiratory failure ARDS Pulmonary hypertension	Tachypnea → bradypnea (late) Shortness of breath
Skin					
Pallor Cool, clammy	Pallor Cool, clammy	↓ Skin perfusion Cool or warm Dry	Flushing Pruritus Urticaria Angioedema	Warm and flushed → cool and mottled (late)	Pallor Cool, clammy
Diagnostic Findings (see Table 42.2)					
↑ b-Type natriuretic peptide (BNP) ↑ Glucose ↑ BUN ↑ Cardiac biomarkers Chest x-ray (e.g., pulmonary infiltrates) ECG (e.g., dysrhythmias) Echocardiogram (e.g., left ventricular dysfunction	Electrolyte changes ↓ Hematocrit ↓ Hemoglobin ↑ Lactate ↑ Urine specific gravity		History of allergies Exposure to contrast media	↑ Glucose ↑ Lactate ↓ Platelets Positive blood cultures ↑ Procalcitonin ↑ Urine specific gravity ↓ Urine Na^+ ↑/↓ WBC	Specific to cause of obstruction

PATHOPHYSIOLOGY MAP

Hypovolemia relative
Hypovolemia absolute
↓ Circulating volume
↓ Venous return
↓ Stroke volume
↓ Cardiac output
↓ Cellular oxygen supply
Decreased blood pressure
↓ Tissue perfusion
Impaired cellular metabolism

Fig. 42.3 The pathophysiology of hypovolemic shock.

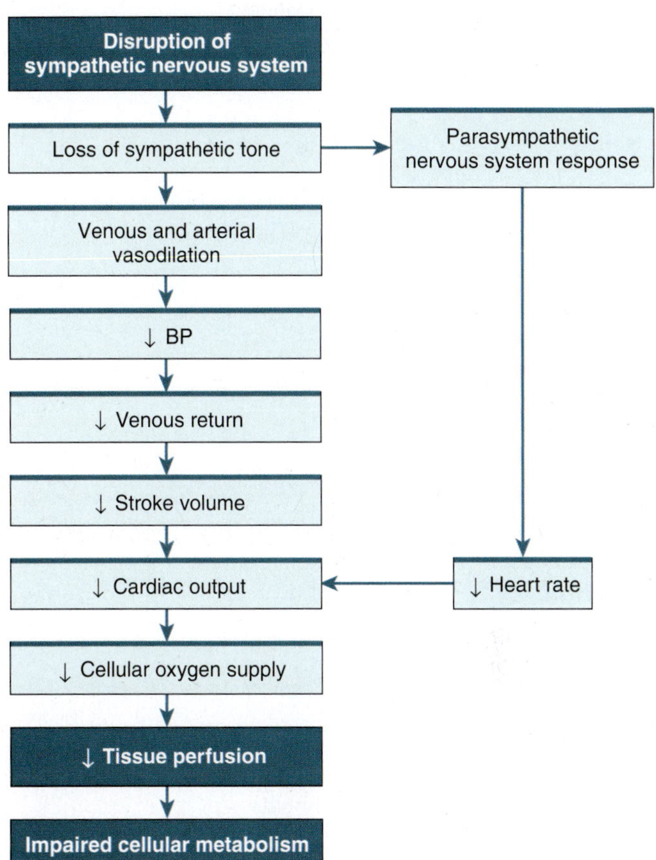

Fig. 42.4 The pathophysiology of neurogenic shock.

from the massive vasodilation. Patients have a sudden onset of symptoms, including dizziness, chest pain, incontinence, swelling of the lips and tongue, wheezing, and stridor. Skin changes include flushing, pruritus, urticaria, and angioedema. Patients may be anxious and confused and have a sense of impending doom.

A patient can have a severe allergic reaction, leading to anaphylactic shock, after contact, inhalation, ingestion, or injection with an antigen (allergen) to which the person has previously been sensitized (Table 42.1). IV administration of the antigen (allergen) is the route most likely to cause anaphylaxis. However, oral, topical, and inhalation routes can cause anaphylactic reactions. Tables 42.2 and 42.3 describe the laboratory findings and clinical presentation of patients in anaphylactic shock. Quick action with epinephrine administration is critical to prevent an allergic reaction from progressing to anaphylactic shock.[6] Anaphylaxis is discussed in Chapter 14.

Septic shock. Sepsis is a life-threatening syndrome in response to infection. It is characterized by a dysregulated response along with new organ dysfunction related to the infection (Table 42.4).[7] In as many as 30% of patients with sepsis, a causative agent is not identified. Sepsis and septic shock have a high incidence, with a mortality rate of 15% or higher.[8]

Septic shock is a subset of sepsis. It has an increased mortality risk due to profound circulatory, cell, and metabolic changes. With septic shock, there is persistent hypotension despite adequate fluid resuscitation and inadequate tissue perfusion that results in tissue hypoxia.[7] Bacteria are the most common cause of sepsis. Parasites, fungi, and viruses can also cause sepsis and septic shock.[9] Fig. 42.5 presents the pathophysiology of septic shock.

A microorganism entering the body triggers normal immune and inflammatory responses. In sepsis and septic shock, the body's response to the microorganism is exaggerated. Both proinflammatory and antiinflammatory responses are activated. Coagulation increases, and fibrinolysis decreases.[10] Endotoxins from the microorganism cell wall stimulate the release of cytokines. These include tumor necrosis factor (TNF), interleukin-1 (IL-1), and other proinflammatory mediators that act through secondary mediators, such as platelet-activating factor, IL-6, and IL-8.[10] The release of platelet-activating factor results in the formation of microthrombi and microvasculature obstruction. The combined effects of the mediators result in endothelial damage, vasodilation, increased capillary permeability, and neutrophil and platelet aggregation and adhesion to the endothelium.

Septic shock has 3 major pathophysiologic effects: vasodilation, maldistribution of blood flow, and myocardial depression. Acute vasodilation and fluids shifting out of the intravascular space lead to relative hypovolemia and hypotension. Blood flow in the microcirculation is decreased, causing poor O_2 delivery and tissue hypoxia. The combination of TNF

TABLE 42.4 Diagnostic Criteria

Sepsis

Infection, documented or suspected, and some of the following:

General Variables

- Altered mental status
- Fever (temperature >100.9°F [38.3°C])
- Heart rate >90 beats/min
- Hyperglycemia (glucose >140 mg/dL) in the absence of diabetes
- Hypothermia (core temperature <97.0°F [36°C])
- SBP ≤100 mm Hg
- Significant edema or positive fluid balance (>20 mL/kg over 24 h)
- Tachypnea (respiratory rate ≥22/min)

Inflammatory Variables

- ↑ C-reactive protein
- Leukocytosis (WBC count >12,000/μL)
- Leukopenia (WBC count <4000/μL)
- Normal WBC count with >10% immature forms (bands)
- ↑ Procalcitonin

Hemodynamic Variables

- Arterial hypotension (SBP <90 mm Hg, MAP <70 mm Hg, or a decrease in SBP >40 mm Hg)

Organ Dysfunction Variables

- Acute oliguria (urine output <0.5 mL/kg/h for at least 2 h despite adequate fluid resuscitation)
- Arterial hypoxemia (Pao_2/Fio_2 <300)
- Coagulation abnormalities (INR >1.5 or PTT >60 s)
- Hyperbilirubinemia (total bilirubin >4 mg/dL)
- Ileus (absent bowel sounds)
- Creatinine increase >0.5 mg/dL
- Thrombocytopenia (platelet count <100,000/μL)

Tissue Perfusion Variables

- Hyperlactatemia (>1 mmol/L)
- Mottling, ↓ capillary refill

INR, International normalized ratio; *PTT,* partial thromboplastin time.

and IL-1 has a role in sepsis-induced myocardial dysfunction. The ejection fraction (EF) is decreased for the first few days after the initial insult. Because of a decreased EF, the ventricles dilate to maintain the SV. The EF typically improves, and ventricular dilation resolves over 7 to 10 days. Persistent high CO and a low SVR beyond 24 hours is an ominous finding. Coronary artery perfusion and myocardial O_2 metabolism are not primarily altered in septic shock.

Respiratory failure is common. The patient initially hyperventilates as a compensatory mechanism, causing respiratory alkalosis. Once the patient tires and can no longer compensate, respiratory acidosis develops. Respiratory failure develops in 85% of patients with sepsis; 40% develop acute respiratory distress syndrome (ARDS) (see Chapter 32). These patients may need mechanical ventilation.

Other signs of septic shock include changes in neurologic status, decreased urine output, and GI problems, such as GI bleeding and paralytic ileus. Table 42.3 gives the clinical presentation of patients with septic shock.

Obstructive Shock

Obstructive shock develops when a physical obstruction to blood flow occurs with a decreased CO (Fig. 42.6). This can be caused by restricted diastolic filling of the right ventricle from compression (e.g., cardiac tamponade, tension pneumothorax, superior vena cava syndrome).[1] In *abdominal compartment syndrome,* increased abdominal pressures compress the inferior vena cava and decrease venous return to the heart. Pulmonary embolism and right ventricular thrombi cause an outflow obstruction as blood leaves the right ventricle through the PA. This leads to decreased blood flow to the lungs and decreased blood return to the left atrium.

Patients have a decreased CO, increased afterload, and variable left ventricular filling pressures. Other signs include jugular venous distention and pulsus paradoxus. Rapid assessment and treatment are important to prevent further hemodynamic compromise and possible cardiac arrest (Fig. 42.6).

Stages of Shock

Management of shock depends on understanding the pathogenesis of the type of shock the patient has and where the patient is on the shock "continuum." We categorize shock into 4 overlapping stages: (1) initial stage, (2) compensatory stage, (3) progressive stage, and (4) refractory stage.[7]

Initial Stage

The *initial stage* of shock occurs at the cell level and is not clinically apparent. Metabolism changes at the cell level from aerobic to anaerobic, causing lactic acid buildup. Lactic acid is a waste product that is removed by the liver.[7] However, this process requires O_2, which is unavailable because of the decrease in tissue perfusion.

Compensatory Stage

In the *compensatory stage* the body activates neural, hormone, and biochemical compensatory mechanisms to try to maintain homeostasis. The patient's clinical presentation begins to reflect the body's responses to the imbalance in O_2 supply and demand (Table 42.5).

A classic sign of shock is a drop in BP and a narrowing of the pulse pressure. The baroreceptors in the carotid and aortic bodies immediately respond by activating the SNS. The SNS stimulates vasoconstriction and the release of the potent vasoconstrictors epinephrine and norepinephrine. Blood flow to the heart and brain is maintained. Blood flow to nonvital organs, such as kidneys, GI tract, skin, and lungs, is diverted or shunted.

The myocardium responds to the SNS stimulation and the increased O_2 demand by increasing the heart rate and contractility. Increased contractility increases myocardial O_2 consumption. The coronary arteries dilate to try to meet the increased O_2 demands of the myocardium.

Shunting blood away from the lungs has an important clinical effect. Decreased blood flow to the lungs increases the

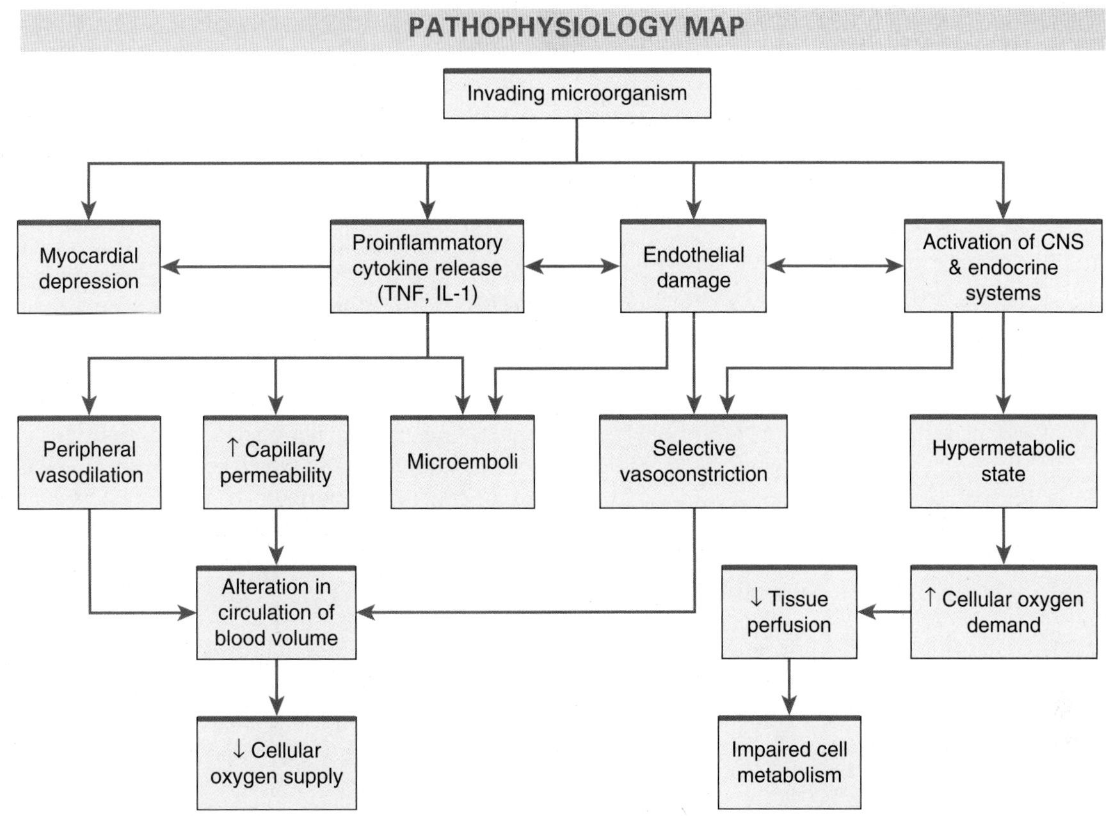

Fig. 42.5 The pathophysiology of septic shock. *IL,* Interleukin; *TNF,* tumor necrosis factor.

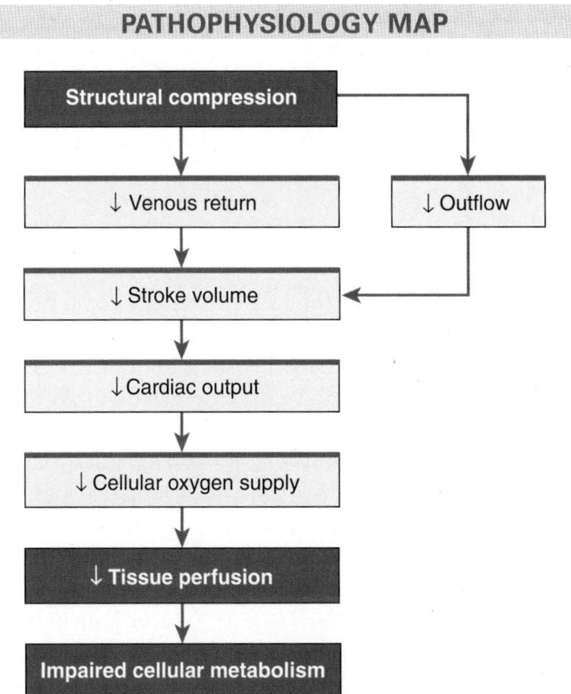

Fig. 42.6 The pathophysiology of obstructive shock.

physiologic dead space. *Physiologic dead space* is the anatomic dead space (the amount of air that will not reach gas-exchanging units) and any inspired air that cannot take part in gas exchange. The clinical result of an increase in dead space ventilation is a *ventilation-perfusion mismatch.* Some areas of the lungs that are being ventilated will not be perfused because of the decreased blood flow to the lungs. Arterial O_2 levels decrease, and the patient increases the rate and depth of respirations in compensation.

The shunting of blood from other organ systems results in clinically important changes. The decrease in blood flow to the GI tract results in impaired motility and slowed peristalsis. This increases the risk for paralytic ileus.

Decreased blood flow to the skin results in a patient feeling cool and clammy. The exception is a patient in early septic shock who may feel warm and flushed because of a hyperdynamic state.

Decreased renal blood flow activates the renin-angiotensin system. Renin stimulates angiotensinogen to make angiotensin I, which is then converted to a potent vasoconstrictor, angiotensin II. The net result is an increase in venous return to the heart and an increase in BP. Angiotensin II stimulates the adrenal cortex to release aldosterone. This results in sodium and water reabsorption and potassium excretion by the kidneys. The increase in sodium reabsorption raises the serum osmolality and stimulates the release of antidiuretic hormone (ADH). ADH increases water reabsorption by the kidneys, further increasing blood volume. The increase in total circulating volume results in an increase in CO and BP.

A multisystem response to decreased tissue perfusion starts during the compensatory stage of shock. If the cause of the shock is corrected, the patient will recover with little or no

TABLE 42.5 Manifestations of Stages of Shock

Compensatory Stage	Progressive Stage	Refractory Stage
Cardiovascular		
Sympathetic nervous system response: • Epinephrine/norepinephrine (vasoconstriction) release • ↑ Myocardial O_2 consumption • ↑ Contractility • ↑ HR • Coronary artery dilation • Narrowed pulse pressure • ↓ BP	↑ Capillary permeability → systemic interstitial edema ↓ CO → ↓ BP and ↑ HR MAP <60 mm Hg (or 40 mm Hg drop in BP from baseline) ↓ Coronary perfusion → dysrhythmias, myocardial ischemia, MI ↓ Peripheral perfusion → ischemia of distal extremities, ↓ pulses, ↓ capillary refill	Profound hypotension ↓ CO Bradycardia, irregular rhythm ↓ BP inadequate to perfuse vital organs
Gastrointestinal		
↓ Blood supply ↓ GI motility Hypoactive bowel sounds ↑ Risk for paralytic ileus	Vasoconstriction and ↓ perfusion → ischemic gut (e.g., stomach, intestines, gallbladder, pancreas): • Erosive ulcers • GI bleeding • Translocation of GI bacteria • Impaired nutrient absorption	Ischemic gut
Hematologic		
	DIC: • Thrombin clots in microcirculation • Consumption of platelets and clotting factors	DIC progresses
Liver		
	Failure to metabolize drugs and waste products Cell death (↑ liver enzymes) Jaundice (↓ clearance of bilirubin) ↑ Ammonia and lactate	Metabolic changes from accumulation of waste products (e.g., NH_3, lactate, CO_2)
Neurologic		
Oriented Restless, apprehensive, confused Change in level of consciousness	↓ Cerebral perfusion pressure ↓ Cerebral blood flow ↓ Responsiveness to stimuli Delirium	Unresponsive Areflexia (loss of reflexes) Pupils nonreactive and dilated
Renal		
↓ Renal blood flow ↑ Renin resulting in release of angiotensin (vasoconstrictor) ↑ Aldosterone causing Na^+ and H_2O reabsorption ↑ Antidiuretic hormone causing H_2O reabsorption	Renal tubules become ischemic → acute tubular necrosis ↓ Urine output ↑ BUN-to-creatinine ratio ↑ Urine sodium ↓ Urine osmolality and specific gravity ↓ Urine potassium Metabolic acidosis	Anuria
Respiratory		
• ↓ Blood flow to the lungs: • ↑ Physiologic dead space • ↑ Ventilation-perfusion mismatch • Hyperventilation • ↑ Minute ventilation (V_E) • Tachypnea	ARDS: • ↑ Capillary permeability • Pulmonary vasoconstriction • Pulmonary interstitial edema • Alveolar edema • Diffuse infiltrates • Tachypnea • ↓ Compliance • Crackles	Severe refractory hypoxemia Respiratory failure
Skin		
Pale and cool Warm and flushed	Cold and clammy	Mottled, cyanotic
Temperature		
Normal or abnormal	Hypothermia or hyperthermia	Hypothermia

residual effects. If the cause of the shock is not corrected and the body is unable to compensate, the patient enters the progressive stage of shock.

Progressive Stage

The *progressive stage* of shock begins as compensatory mechanisms fail. Changes in mental status are important findings in this stage. Patients may be moved to the intensive care unit (ICU) for advanced monitoring and treatment.

The cardiovascular system is now profoundly affected. CO falls, causing a decrease in BP and coronary artery, cerebral, and peripheral perfusion. Decreased cell perfusion continues. Altered capillary permeability allows fluid and protein to leak out of the vascular space into the surrounding interstitial space. Circulating volume decreases with an increase in edema. Patients may have *anasarca* (diffuse profound edema). Fluid leakage from the vascular space further decreases perfusion to the solid organs (e.g., liver, GI tract, lungs) and peripheral tissues.

Myocardial dysfunction from decreased perfusion results in dysrhythmias, myocardial ischemia, and possibly MI. The result is complete deterioration of the cardiovascular system. Sustained hypoperfusion results in weak peripheral pulses. Ischemia of the distal extremities eventually occurs.

The pulmonary system is often the first system to show signs of critical dysfunction. Blood flow to the lungs is reduced. In response to the decreased blood flow and SNS stimulation, the pulmonary arterioles constrict. This increases PA pressure. As the pressure within the pulmonary vasculature increases, blood flow to the pulmonary capillaries decreases and ventilation-perfusion mismatch worsens.

Another key response in the lungs is fluid movement from the pulmonary vasculature into the interstitial space. As capillary permeability increases, fluid moving into the interstitial spaces results in interstitial edema, bronchoconstriction, and decreased functional residual capacity. With further increases in capillary permeability, fluid moves into the alveoli, causing alveolar edema and a decrease in surfactant production. The combined effects of pulmonary vasoconstriction and bronchoconstriction are impaired gas exchange, decreased lung compliance, and worsening ventilation-perfusion mismatch. Clinically, patients have tachypnea, crackles, and an increased work of breathing.

The GI system is affected by prolonged decreased tissue perfusion. As the blood supply to the GI tract is decreased, the normally protective mucosal barrier becomes ischemic. This ischemia predisposes patients to ulcers and GI bleeding (see Chapter 46). It increases the risk for bacterial migration from the GI tract to the blood and lungs. There is a decreased ability to absorb nutrients.

The loss of liver function leads to a failure of the liver to metabolize drugs and waste products (e.g., lactate, ammonia). Jaundice results from the buildup of bilirubin. As the liver cells die, liver enzymes increase. The liver loses its ability to function as an immune organ. Kupffer cells no longer destroy bacteria from the GI tract. Instead, they are released into the bloodstream, increasing the risk of bacteremia.

Prolonged hypoperfusion of the kidneys causes renal tubular ischemia. The resulting acute tubular necrosis may lead to acute kidney injury (AKI). This can be worsened by nephrotoxic drugs (e.g., certain antibiotics, anesthetics, diuretics) (see Table 49.3). Patients have decreased urine output and increased blood urea nitrogen (BUN) and creatinine. Metabolic acidosis occurs from the kidneys' inability to excrete acids (especially lactic acid) and reabsorb bicarbonate.

Hematologic dysfunction adds to the complexity of the clinical picture. Patients are at risk for disseminated intravascular coagulation (DIC). The consumption of platelets and clotting factors with secondary fibrinolysis results in significant bleeding from the GI tract, lungs, and puncture sites (see Chapter 34). Table 42.3 shows laboratory values in DIC. Aggressive interventions are needed to prevent the development of MODS.

Refractory Stage

In this last stage of shock, decreased perfusion from peripheral vasoconstriction and decreased CO worsen anaerobic metabolism. Lactic acid accumulation contributes to increased capillary permeability and dilation. Increased capillary permeability allows fluid and plasma proteins to leave the vascular space and move to the interstitial space. Blood pools in the capillary beds due to the constricted venules and dilated arterioles. The loss of intravascular volume worsens hypotension and tachycardia and decreases coronary blood flow. Decreased coronary blood flow leads to worsening myocardial depression and a further decline in CO. Cerebral blood flow cannot be maintained and cerebral ischemia results.

The patient now has profound hypotension and hypoxemia. The failure of the liver, lungs, and kidneys results in an accumulation of waste products, such as lactate, urea, ammonia, and CO_2. The failure of an organ system affects several other organ systems. Recovery is unlikely in this stage. The organs are in failure, and the body's compensatory mechanisms are overwhelmed (Table 42.5).

Diagnostic Studies

The diagnosis of a specific type and cause of shock starts with a history and physical assessment. A medical and surgical history and history of recent events (e.g., surgery, chest pain, trauma) provide valuable data. Basic laboratory investigations include a CBC, CMP, ABG, PT/PTT, lactate, and procalcitonin.[11,12] Other diagnostic studies include a 12-lead ECG, continuous ECG monitoring, chest x-ray, continuous pulse oximetry, and hemodynamic monitoring. Chapter 35 discusses hemodynamic monitoring. Bedside ultrasound can provide valuable information regarding fluid status, cardiac function, and bleeding.[13] Decreased tissue perfusion in shock leads to an increased lactate with a base deficit (the amount needed to bring the pH back to normal). These laboratory changes reflect an increase in anaerobic metabolism.[11] Table 42.2 outlines laboratory findings seen in shock.

Interprofessional Care

Successful management of patients in shock depends on early recognition and treatment. Many times, the nurse at the bedside looking at trends in the patient's condition identifies an early stage of shock. Prompt intervention in the early stages of shock may prevent the decline to the progressive or irreversible stage. Successful management includes (1) identifying patients at risk for developing shock; (2) integrating the history and clinical findings to establish a diagnosis; (3) implementing interventions to control or eliminate the cause; (4) protecting target and distal organs from dysfunction; and (5) providing multisystem supportive care. Table 42.6 provides an overview of the initial assessment findings and interventions for the emergency care of patients in shock.

General management strategies begin with ensuring that the patient is responsive and has a patent airway. Once the airway is established O_2 delivery must be optimized. Supplemental O_2 and noninvasive or invasive mechanical ventilation may be needed to maintain an arterial O_2 saturation of 90% or more (PaO_2 greater than 60 mm Hg) (see Chapter 28). The MAP and circulating blood volume are optimized with fluid replacement and drug therapy.

Oxygen and Ventilation

There are 3 components to assure efficient O_2 delivery: CO, available hemoglobin, and arterial O_2 saturation (SaO_2). Methods to optimize O_2 delivery are directed at increasing supply and decreasing demand. Supply is increased by (1) optimizing the CO with fluid replacement and/or drug therapy, (2) increasing the hemoglobin through blood transfusions, and/or (3) increasing the arterial O_2 saturation with supplemental O_2 and mechanical ventilation.

Plan care to avoid disrupting the balance of O_2 supply and demand. Space activities that increase O_2 consumption (e.g., suctioning, position changes) to allow for O_2 conservation. Intermittent or continuous $ScvO_2$ monitoring by a central venous catheter or mixed venous O_2 saturation (SvO_2) may be helpful. Both reflect the dynamic balance between O_2 supply and demand. Assess these values along with related hemodynamic measures (e.g., arterial pressure–based cardiac output [APCO], O_2 consumption, hemoglobin) to evaluate the patient's response to treatments and activities (see Chapters 28 and 35).

Fluid Resuscitation

The cornerstone of therapy for septic, hypovolemic, and anaphylactic shock is volume expansion with fluid

TABLE 42.6 EMERGENCY MANAGEMENT

Shock

Common Causes	Assessment Findings	Interventions
Medical • Addisonian crisis • AVP disorder • Dehydration • Diabetes • MI • Pulmonary embolus • Sepsis **Surgical** • Aortic dissection • GI bleeding • Postoperative bleeding • Ruptured ectopic pregnancy or ovarian cyst • Ruptured organ or vessel • Vaginal bleeding **Trauma** • Fractures, spinal injury • Multiorgan injury • Ruptured or lacerated vessel or organ (e.g., spleen)	• Anxiety • Chills • Confusion • Cool, clammy skin (warm skin in early onset of septic and neurogenic shock) • Cyanosis • Dysrhythmias • Extreme thirst • Feeling of impending doom • Hypotension • ↓ Level of consciousness • Narrowed pulse pressure • Nausea and vomiting • Obvious hemorrhage or injury • ↓ O_2 saturation • Pallor • Rapid, weak, thready pulses • Restlessness • Tachypnea, dyspnea, or shallow, irregular respirations • Temperature dysregulation • Weakness	**Initial** • If unresponsive, assess circulation, airway, and breathing (CAB). • If responsive, monitor airway, breathing, and circulation (ABC). • Stabilize cervical spine as appropriate. • Control any external bleeding with direct pressure or pressure dressing. • Give high-flow O_2 (100%) by nonrebreather mask or bag-valve-mask. • Anticipate need for intubation and mechanical ventilation. • Establish IV access with 2 large-bore catheters (14- to 16-gauge) or an intraosseous access device; aid with central line insertion. • Begin fluid resuscitation with crystalloids (e.g., 30 mL/kg repeated until hemodynamic improvement is seen). • Draw blood for laboratory studies (e.g., blood cultures, lactate, WBC). • Assess for life-threatening injuries (e.g., cardiac tamponade, liver laceration, tension pneumothorax). • Consider vasopressor therapy if hypotension persists after fluid resuscitation. • Insert an indwelling urinary catheter and nasogastric tube. • Start antibiotic therapy after blood cultures if sepsis is suspected. • Obtain 12-lead ECG and treat dysrhythmias. **Ongoing Monitoring** • ABCs • Level of consciousness • Vital signs, including pulse oximetry; peripheral pulses, capillary refill, skin color, and temperature • Respiratory status • Heart rate and rhythm • Urine output

administration (Table 42.7).[14] The goal for fluid resuscitation is to restore tissue perfusion. Fluid resuscitation should start using 1 or 2 large-bore (e.g., 14- to 16-gauge) IV catheters, an intraosseous (IO) access device, or a central venous catheter. The initial amount of fluid recommended is 30 mL/kg of crystalloid over the first 3 hours, with frequent reassessment.[7]

! SAFETY ALERT

Intraosseous (IO) Access

- Use an IO access device for emergency resuscitation when IV access cannot be obtained.
- Insertion sites include the sternum, proximal and distal tibia, and proximal and distal humerus.
- Remove IO devices within 24 h of insertion or as soon as possible after peripheral or central IV access is obtained.
- Monitor for complications: extravasation of drugs and fluids into the soft tissue, fractures caused during insertion, and osteomyelitis.

The choice of fluid is based on the type and volume of fluid lost and the patient's clinical status. The ideal fluid is controversial.[14] Currently, we use normal saline most often in the initial resuscitation of shock. Large-volume resuscitation with normal saline can lead to hyperchloremic metabolic acidosis. Lactated Ringer solution can cause lactate levels to increase because the failing liver cannot convert lactate to bicarbonate.[14] Transfusions of red blood cells (RBCs) may be given to treat hypovolemic shock due to bleeding.

Fluid responsiveness is determined by clinical assessment. Although BP helps to determine whether the CO is adequate, an assessment of end organ perfusion (e.g., urine output, neurologic function, peripheral pulses) provides more relevant data. Monitor vital signs, cerebral and abdominal perfusion pressures, capillary refill, neurologic status, and skin temperature. Evaluate trends in BP with an automatic BP cuff or an arterial catheter. Use an indwelling urinary catheter to monitor urine output during resuscitation. Hemodynamic parameters, such as SVV or CO, are also used.

Other interventions we use to monitor fluid response include a passive leg raise (PLR) challenge and inferior vena cava evaluation.[15] A PLR challenge provides a transient increase in fluid volume of 300 to 500 mL by placing the patient supine and raising the legs to 45 degrees (Fig. 42.7). Response is monitored within 1 to 2 minutes by measuring CO, CI, SV,

TABLE 42.7 Fluid Therapy in Shock

Fluid Type	Mechanism of Action	Type of Shock	Nursing Implications
Crystalloids			
Isotonic			
• 0.9% NaCl, normal saline solution (NSS) • Lactated Ringer (LR) solution	Primarily stays in the intravascular space, ↑ intravascular volume.	Initial volume replacement in most types of shock.	Monitor patient closely for circulatory overload. Do not use LR in patients with liver failure. LR may be used if hyperchloremic acidosis develops from use of NSS in fluid resuscitation.
Hypertonic			
• 1.8%, 3%, 5% NaCl	Stays in the intravascular space, increases serum osmolarity, shifts fluid volume from intracellular space to extracellular space to intravascular space.	Initial volume expansion in hypovolemic shock.	Monitor patient closely for signs of hypernatremia (e.g., disorientation, seizures). Central line preferred for infusing saline solutions ≥3%, since these may damage veins.
Blood or Blood Products			
Packed red blood cells Fresh frozen plasma Platelets	Replaces blood loss, increases O_2-carrying capability. Replaces coagulation factors. Helps control bleeding caused by thrombocytopenia.	All types.	Same precautions as any blood administration (see Table 34.34).
Colloids			
Human serum albumin (5% or 25%)	Can increase plasma colloid osmotic pressure. Rapid volume expansion.	All types except cardiogenic and neurogenic shock.	Use 5% solution in hypovolemic patients. Use 25% solution in patients with fluid and sodium restrictions. Monitor for circulatory overload. Mild side effects of chills, fever, and urticaria may develop. More expensive than crystalloids.
Dextran (dextran 40)	Hyperosmotic glucose polymer.	Limited use due to side effects, including reducing platelet adhesion, diluting clotting factors.	Increases risk for bleeding. Monitor patient for allergic reactions and acute kidney injury. Has maximum volume recommendations per manufacturer.

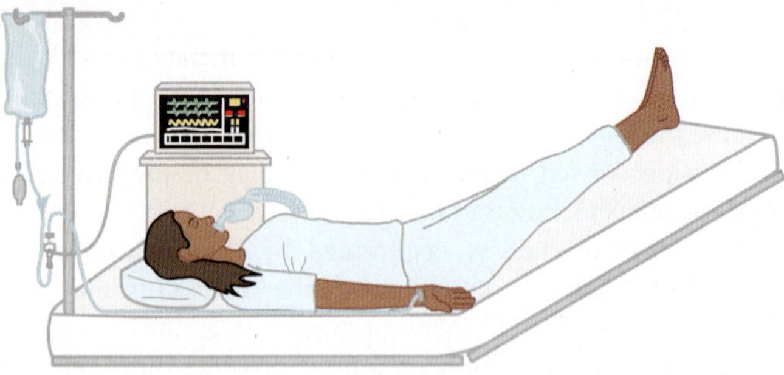

Fig. 42.7 Passive leg raise challenge in a patient with septic shock.

SVV, or other parameters for improvement. If the response is positive, the patient is fluid responsive and should receive more fluids.

! SAFETY ALERT

Complications of Fluid Resuscitation

- Warm crystalloid and colloid solutions during massive fluid resuscitation to prevent hypothermia.
- When giving large volumes of packed RBCs, remember that they do not contain clotting factors.
- Assess for hypocalcemia and disseminated intravascular coagulation (DIC).
- Replace clotting factors based on the clinical status and laboratory studies.
- Observe for fluid overload and respiratory compromise.

Drug Therapy

The goal of drug therapy is to correct decreased tissue perfusion. We give IV drugs used to improve perfusion via an infusion pump and central venous line. Many of these drugs have vasoconstrictor properties that are harmful if the drug leaks into the tissues while being infused peripherally (Table 42.8).

Sympathomimetic drugs. Drugs that mimic the action of the SNS are called *sympathomimetic.* Their effects are mediated through their binding to α- or β-adrenergic receptors. They differ in their relative α- and β-adrenergic effects.[7]

Drugs that cause peripheral vasoconstriction are called *vasopressor drugs* (e.g., norepinephrine, dopamine, phenylephrine). Severe peripheral vasoconstriction decreases peripheral tissue perfusion. Vasoconstriction increases SVR, the workload of the heart, and myocardial O_2 demand. It can harm patients in cardiogenic shock by causing further myocardial damage and increasing the risk for dysrhythmias.[7] Use of vasopressor drugs is limited to patients who do not respond to fluid resuscitation. Adequate fluid resuscitation must be achieved before starting vasopressors because the vasoconstrictor effects in patients with low blood volume will further reduce tissue perfusion. Typically, if hypotension persists after adequate fluid resuscitation, we then give a vasopressor (e.g., norepinephrine, dopamine) and/or an inotrope (e.g., dobutamine).

The goal of vasopressor therapy is to achieve and maintain an MAP of greater than 65 mm Hg.[7] Continuously monitor end organ perfusion (e.g., urine output, level of consciousness) and lactate levels (e.g., every 3 hours for the first 6 hours) to ensure tissue perfusion is adequate.

Vasodilator drugs. Patients in cardiogenic shock have decreased myocardial contractility. Vasodilators may be needed to decrease afterload, myocardial workload, and O_2 needs. Although vasoconstriction is a useful compensatory mechanism for maintaining BP, excess constriction reduces tissue blood flow and increases the cardiac workload. Vasodilator therapy can break the harmful cycle of vasoconstriction causing a decrease in CO and BP, resulting in further sympathetic-induced vasoconstriction.

The goal of vasodilator therapy, as in vasopressor therapy, is to maintain the MAP greater than 65 mm Hg. Monitor hemodynamic parameters (e.g., CVP, CO, $ScvO_2/SvO_2$, SV, PA pressures) and assessment findings so that fluids can be increased, or vasodilator therapy decreased if a serious fall in CO or BP occurs. The vasodilator agent most often used for patients in cardiogenic shock is nitroglycerin. Vasodilation may be enhanced with nitroprusside or nitroglycerin in noncardiogenic shock.

Nutrition Therapy

Protein-calorie malnutrition is common because of hypermetabolism. Nutrition is vital to reducing mortality.[16] Enteral nutrition (EN) should be started within the first 24 hours. However, full calorie replacement is not recommended for previously well-nourished adults early in a critical illness. Start the patient on a *trophic feeding.* This is a small amount of EN (e.g., 10 mL/h). Early EN enhances perfusion of the GI tract and helps maintain the integrity of the gut mucosa. Advance feedings as tolerated and as prescribed. We use parenteral nutrition (PN) only if EN is contraindicated. Chapter 44 discusses EN and PN.

Weigh the patient daily on the same scale at the same time of day. If the patient has a significant weight loss, rule out dehydration before adding more calories. Weight gain is common because of third spacing of fluids. Monitor protein, total albumin, prealbumin, BUN, glucose, and electrolytes to assess nutrition status.

Measures Specific to Type of Shock

Cardiogenic Shock

For patients in cardiogenic shock, the overall goal is to restore heart function and the balance between O_2 supply and demand in the myocardium. Cardiac catheterization is done as soon as possible after the initial insult.[2] Specific measures to restore blood flow include angioplasty with stenting, emergency revascularization, and valve replacement. Until these interventions are done, we optimize SV and CO to achieve adequate perfusion (Tables 42.8 and 42.9).

Hemodynamic management aims to reduce the workload of the heart through drug therapy and/or mechanical interventions. Drugs can decrease the workload of the heart by dilating coronary arteries (e.g., nitrates) and reducing preload (e.g., diuretics), afterload (e.g., vasodilators), and heart rate and contractility (e.g., β-adrenergic blockers).

TABLE 42.8 Drug Therapy

Shock

Drug[a]	Mechanism of Action	Type of Shock	Nursing Implications
angiotensin II (Giapreza)	↑ BP, ↑ MAP ↑ SVR	Septic and other distributive shock	Give through central line. Monitor for thromboembolic events. Provide VTE prophylaxis.
dobutamine	↑ Myocardial contractility ↓ Ventricular filling pressures ↓ SVR, PAWP ↑ CO, SV, CVP ↑/↓ HR	Cardiogenic shock with severe systolic dysfunction Septic shock to increase O_2 delivery and raise $ScvO_2$ or SvO_2 to 70% if Hgb >7 g/dL or Hct ≥30%	Give through central line (infiltration leads to tissue sloughing). Do not give in same line with $NaHCO_3$. Monitor HR, BP (hypotension may worsen, requiring addition of a vasopressor). Stop infusion if tachydysrhythmias develop.
dopamine	Positive inotropic effects: ↑ Myocardial contractility ↑ Automaticity ↑ Atrioventricular conduction ↑ HR, CO ↑ BP, ↑ MAP ↑ MVO_2 Can cause progressive vasoconstriction at high doses	Cardiogenic shock	Give through central line (infiltration leads to tissue sloughing). Do not give in same line with $NaHCO_3$. Monitor for tachydysrhythmias. Monitor for peripheral vasoconstriction (e.g., paresthesias, coldness in extremities) at moderate to high doses.
epinephrine (Adrenalin)	*Low doses:* β-adrenergic agonist (cardiac stimulation, bronchodilation, peripheral vasodilation) ↑ HR, contractility, CO ↓ SVR *High doses:* α-adrenergic agonist (peripheral vasoconstriction) ↑ SV, SVR ↑ Systolic/↓ diastolic BP, widened pulse pressure ↑ CVP, PAWP	Cardiogenic shock Anaphylactic shock Septic shock if 2nd agent needed after norepinephrine Cardiac arrest, pulseless ventricular tachycardia, ventricular fibrillation, asystole	Monitor for HR >110 beats/min. Monitor for dyspnea, pulmonary edema. Monitor for chest pain, dysrhythmias from ↑ MVO_2. Monitor for renal failure due to ischemia.
hydrocortisone (Solu-Cortef)	↓ Inflammation, reverses ↑ capillary permeability ↑ BP, HR	Septic shock requiring vasopressor therapy (despite fluid resuscitation) to maintain adequate BP Anaphylactic shock if hypotension persists after initial therapy	Monitor for hypokalemia, hyperglycemia. Consider use as continuous infusion.
nitroglycerin	Venous dilation Dilates coronary arteries ↓ Preload, MVO_2, SVR, BP	Cardiogenic shock	Continuously monitor BP and HR, since reflex tachycardia may occur. Glass bottle recommended for infusion.
norepinephrine (Levophed)	β_1-Adrenergic agonist (cardiac stimulation) α-Adrenergic agonist (peripheral vasoconstriction) Renal and splanchnic vasoconstriction ↑ BP, MAP, CVP, PAWP, SVR ↑/↓ CO	Cardiogenic shock after MI Septic shock—first drug of choice for BP unresponsive to adequate fluid resuscitation	Give through central line (infiltration leads to tissue sloughing). Monitor for dysrhythmias due to ↑ MVO_2 requirements.
phenylephrine	α-Adrenergic agonist (peripheral vasoconstriction) Renal, mesenteric, splanchnic, cutaneous, and pulmonary blood vessel constriction ↑ HR, BP, SVR ↑/↓ CO	Neurogenic shock	Monitor for reflex bradycardia, headache, restlessness. Monitor for renal failure from ↓ renal blood flow. Give through central line (infiltration leads to tissue sloughing).
sodium nitroprusside	Arterial and venous vasodilation ↓ Preload, afterload ↓ CVP, PAWP ↑/↓ CO ↓ BP	Cardiogenic shock with ↑ SVR	Continuously monitor BP. Protect solution from light. Wrap infusion bottle with opaque covering. Give with D_5W only. Monitor cyanide levels and signs of cyanide toxicity (e.g., metabolic acidosis, tachycardia, altered level of consciousness, seizures, coma, almond smell on breath).
vasopressin	Antidiuretic hormone Nonadrenergic vasoconstrictor ↑ MAP ↑ Urine output	Shock states (most often septic shock) refractory to other vasopressors	Given with norepinephrine and in low doses. Infusions are not titrated. Monitor hemodynamic pressures and urine output.

CVP, Central venous pressure; *MVO_2,* myocardial O_2 consumption; *PAWP,* pulmonary artery wedge pressure; *SVR,* systemic vascular resistance.

TABLE 42.9 Interprofessional Care

Shock

Oxygenation	Circulation	Drug Therapies	Supportive Therapies
Cardiogenic Shock			
• Supplemental O_2 (e.g., nasal cannula, nonrebreather mask) • Intubation and mechanical ventilation, if needed • Monitor $ScvO_2$ or SvO_2	• Restore blood flow with angioplasty with stenting, emergent coronary revascularization • Reduce workload of heart with circulatory assist devices: IABP, VAD	• Nitrates (e.g., nitroglycerin) • Inotropes (e.g., dobutamine) • Diuretics (e.g., furosemide) • β-Adrenergic blockers (contraindicated with ↓ ejection fraction)	• Treat dysrhythmias
Hypovolemic Shock			
• Supplemental O_2 • Monitor $ScvO_2$ or SvO_2	• Rapid fluid replacement using 2 large-bore (14–16 gauge) peripheral IV lines, an intraosseous access device, or central venous catheter • Restore fluid volume (e.g., blood, blood products, crystalloids) • End points of fluid resuscitation: • CVP 15 mm Hg • PAWP 10–12 mm Hg	• No specific drug therapy	• Correct the cause (e.g., stop bleeding, GI losses) • Use warmed IV fluids, including blood products (if appropriate)
Septic Shock			
• Supplemental O_2 • Intubation and mechanical ventilation, if needed • Monitor $ScvO_2$ or SvO_2	• Aggressive fluid resuscitation (e.g., 30 mL/kg of crystalloids repeated if hemodynamic improvement is noted) • End points of fluid resuscitation are based on: • Focused assessment including vital signs, cardiopulmonary assessment, capillary refill, peripheral pulses, and skin or any 2 of the following: • $ScvO_2$ >70 or SvO_2 >65 • CVP 8–12 mm Hg • Cardiovascular ultrasound • Fluid responsiveness with passive leg raise or fluid challenge	• Prescribed antibiotics • Vasopressors (e.g., norepinephrine) • Inotropes (e.g., dobutamine) • Anticoagulants (e.g., low-molecular-weight heparin)	• Obtain cultures (e.g., blood, wound) before beginning antibiotics • Monitor temperature • Control glucose • Stress ulcer prophylaxis
Neurogenic Shock			
• Maintain patent airway • Supplemental O_2 • Intubation and mechanical ventilation (if needed)	• Cautious fluid administration	• Vasopressors (e.g., phenylephrine) • Atropine (for bradycardia)	• Minimize spinal cord trauma with stabilization • Monitor temperature
Anaphylactic Shock			
• Maintain patent airway • Supplemental O_2 • Intubation and mechanical ventilation, if needed	• Aggressive fluid resuscitation with colloids	• Epinephrine (IM or IV) • Antihistamines (e.g., diphenhydramine) • Histamine (H_2)-receptor blockers • Bronchodilators: nebulized (e.g., albuterol) • Corticosteroids (if hypotension persists)	• Identify and remove offending cause • Prevent by avoiding known allergens • Premedicate with history of prior sensitivity (e.g., contrast media)
Obstructive Shock			
• Maintain patent airway • Supplemental O_2 • Intubation and mechanical ventilation, if needed	• Restore circulation by treating cause of obstruction • Fluid resuscitation may provide temporary improvement in CO and BP	• No specific drug therapy	• Treat cause of obstruction (e.g., pericardiocentesis for cardiac tamponade, needle decompression or chest tube insertion for tension pneumothorax, embolectomy for pulmonary embolism)

Patients may benefit from a circulatory assist device (e.g., intraaortic balloon pump, ventricular assist device [VAD]) (see Chapter 39). The goals are to decrease SVR and left ventricular workload so that the heart can heal. A VAD may be used as a temporary measure for patients in cardiogenic shock who are awaiting a heart transplant. A heart transplant is an option for a small group of patients with cardiogenic shock.

Hypovolemic Shock

Managing hypovolemic shock focuses on stopping the fluid loss and restoring circulating volume. We often plan the initial fluid resuscitation using a 3:1 rule (3 mL of isotonic crystalloid for every 1 mL of estimated blood loss). Table 42.7 describes fluids used for volume resuscitation, their mechanism of action, and specific nursing implications.

Septic Shock

Patients in septic shock receive fluid replacement and broad-spectrum antibiotics within the first hour (Fig. 42.8). The goal of fluid resuscitation is to restore the intravascular volume and organ perfusion. We achieve initial volume resuscitation by giving 30 mL/kg of an isotonic crystalloid solution over the first 3 hours and then reevaluating fluid status.[17] A fluid challenge may be repeated until hemodynamic improvement (e.g., increase in MAP and/or CVP) is seen. To evaluate large-volume fluid resuscitation, hemodynamic monitoring is needed. Table 42.9 shows predetermined end points of fluid resuscitation along with methods to reassess volume status.

If the patient is hypotensive after initial volume resuscitation and no longer fluid responsive, a vasopressor is added. The first drug of choice is norepinephrine.[7] Vasodilation and low CO, or vasodilation alone, can cause low BP despite adequate fluid resuscitation. Vasopressin may be added for those who are refractory to initial vasopressor therapy.[7] Exogenous vasopressin can replace the stores of physiologic vasopressin that are often depleted in septic shock.

DRUG ALERT

Vasopressin

- Given along with norepinephrine.
- Infuse at low doses (e.g., 0.03 units/min) using an IV pump.
- Do not titrate infusion.
- Use cautiously in patients with coronary artery disease.

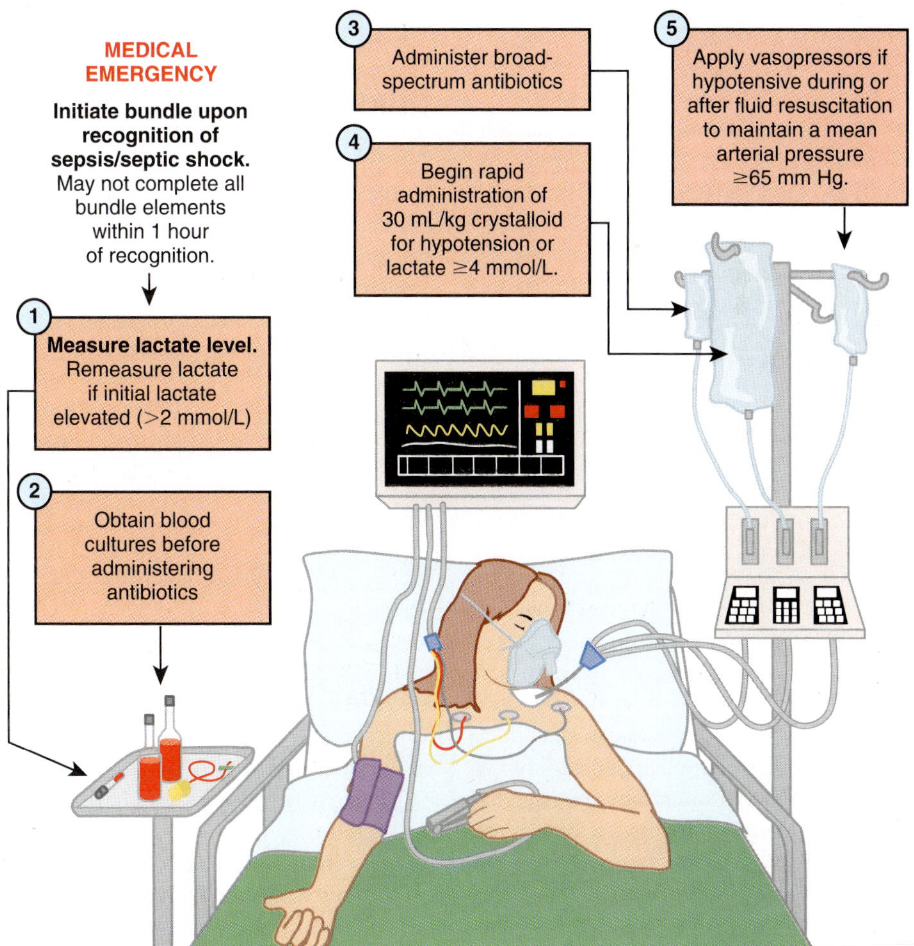

Fig. 42.8 Hour-1 bundle for sepsis and septic shock. (From Institute for Healthcare Improvement: Surviving Sepsis campaign.)

Vasopressor drugs may increase BP but can decrease SV. Giving an inotropic agent (e.g., dobutamine) can offset the decrease in SV and increase tissue perfusion (Table 42.8). IV corticosteroids may be considered for patients in septic shock who cannot maintain an adequate BP despite vasopressor therapy and fluid resuscitation.

Patients with septic shock initially have a normal or high CO. If a patient is unable to achieve and maintain an adequate CO and has unmet tissue O_2 demands, CO may be increased using drug therapy (e.g., dopamine). $ScvO_2$ or SvO_2 monitoring is used to assess the balance between O_2 delivery and consumption, and adequacy of the CO (see Chapter 35). If balance is maintained, tissue demands will be met.

Broad-spectrum antibiotics should be started within the first hour of sepsis or septic shock.[7] Obtain cultures (e.g., blood, wound, urine, stool, sputum) before starting antibiotics. However, this should not delay the start of antibiotics within the first hour. Specific antibiotics may be ordered after we identify the organism.

Other aspects of care are initiated to prevent complications. Glucose should be maintained below 180 mg/dL (10.0 mmol/L) for patients in shock.[7] Monitor glucose according to agency policy. Stress ulcer prophylaxis with proton pump inhibitors (e.g., pantoprazole) and venous thromboembolism (VTE) prophylaxis (e.g., heparin, enoxaparin) are recommended.[7]

Neurogenic Shock

The specific treatment of neurogenic shock is based on the cause. If the cause is spinal cord injury, we use measures to promote spinal stability (e.g., spinal precautions, cervical stabilization with a collar). Once the spine is stabilized, treating hypotension and bradycardia is essential to prevent further ischemic spinal cord damage. Treatment involves vasopressors (e.g., phenylephrine) to maintain BP and organ perfusion (Table 42.8). Bradycardia may be treated with atropine. Infuse fluids cautiously because hypotension is not related to fluid loss. Monitor patients with a spinal cord injury for hypothermia caused by hypothalamic dysfunction (Table 42.9).

Anaphylactic Shock

The first strategy in managing patients at risk for anaphylactic shock is prevention. The history is key to avoiding risk factors for anaphylaxis (Table 42.1). The clinical presentation of anaphylactic shock is dramatic. Immediate intervention is required. Epinephrine is the drug of choice to treat anaphylactic shock.[6] It causes peripheral vasoconstriction and bronchodilation and opposes the effect of histamine. Diphenhydramine and histamine receptor blockers (e.g., famotidine) are given as adjunctive therapies to block the ongoing release of histamine from the allergic reaction.

Maintaining a patent airway is important. Patients can quickly develop airway compromise from laryngeal edema or bronchoconstriction. Nebulized bronchodilators are highly effective. Aerosolized epinephrine can reduce laryngeal edema. Endotracheal intubation may be needed to secure and maintain a patent airway.

Hypotension results from fluid leaking out of the intravascular space into the interstitial space due to increased vascular permeability and vasodilation. Aggressive fluid resuscitation, usually with crystalloids, is needed. IV corticosteroids may be helpful in anaphylactic shock if significant hypotension persists after 1 to 2 hours of aggressive therapy (Tables 42.8 and 42.9).

Obstructive Shock

The main strategy in treating obstructive shock is early recognition and treatment to relieve or manage the obstruction (Table 42.1). Mechanical decompression for pericardial tamponade, tension pneumothorax, and hemopneumothorax may be done by needle or tube insertion. A pulmonary embolism requires immediate anticoagulation therapy, thrombolytic therapy, or pulmonary embolectomy. Superior vena cava syndrome, a compression or obstruction of the outflow tract of the mediastinum, may be treated by radiation, debulking, or removal of the mass or cause. A decompressive laparotomy may be done for abdominal compartment syndrome for patients with high intraabdominal pressures and hemodynamic instability.

NURSING MANAGEMENT: SHOCK

Assessment

Focus your assessment on the ABCs: airway, breathing, and circulation.[8] Next, assess for tissue perfusion. This includes evaluating vital signs, level of consciousness, peripheral pulses, capillary refill, skin (e.g., temperature, color, moisture), and urine output. As shock progresses, neurologic status declines, urine output decreases, skin becomes cooler and mottled, and peripheral pulses decrease.

To understand the complexity of the patient's clinical status, integrate all the assessment data. Obtain a brief history from the patient or caregiver. Include a description of the events leading to the shock state, time of onset and duration of symptoms, and health history (e.g., medications, allergies). Obtain details about any care the patient received before hospitalization.

Clinical Problems

Clinical problems for patients in shock may include:

- Impaired cardiac function
- Impaired respiratory function
- Altered BP

More information on nursing diagnoses and interventions for patients with shock is presented in eNursing Care Plan 42.1 (available on the website for this chapter).

◆ Planning

The overall goals for patients in shock include (1) adequate tissue perfusion, (2) restoration of normal or baseline BP, (3) recovery of organ function, (4) avoiding complications from prolonged states of hypoperfusion, and (5) preventing health care–associated complications.

◆ Implementation

Health Promotion

You play a key role in the prevention of shock by identifying patients at risk. In general, patients who are older, are immunocompromised, or have chronic illnesses are at an increased risk. Surgery or trauma increases the risk for shock from hemorrhage, spinal cord injury, sepsis, and other problems (Table 42.1).

Planning is essential to help prevent shock in at-risk patients. For example, patients with an acute anterior wall MI are at high risk for cardiogenic shock.[2] The main goal for these patients is to limit the infarct size by restoring coronary blood flow. Rest, analgesics, and sedation can reduce the myocardial demand for O_2. Modify the ICU environment to provide care at intervals that will not increase the patient's O_2 demand. For example, if the patient becomes tired with bathing, perform this care at a time that does not interfere with other activities that increase O_2 demand.

A person with certain severe allergies, such as to drugs, shellfish, insect bites, and latex, is at increased risk for anaphylactic shock. This risk can be decreased by carefully assessing the patient for allergies.

! SAFETY ALERT

Preventing Allergic Reactions

- Confirm allergies before giving drugs or starting diagnostic procedures (e.g., CT scan with contrast media).
- Premedicate (e.g., diphenhydramine, methylprednisolone) patients who need a drug to which they are at high risk for an allergic reaction (e.g., contrast media).
- Encourage patients with allergies to obtain and wear a medical alert device and report all allergies to their HCPs.
- Teach patients about kits that contain equipment and drugs (e.g., epinephrine) for the treatment of acute allergic reactions.

Careful monitoring of fluid balance can help prevent hypovolemic shock. Ongoing monitoring of intake and output and daily weights is important. Identifying trends in the patient's condition is more meaningful than any single piece of clinical information.

Monitor all patients for infection. Progression from an infection to sepsis and septic shock depends on the patient's defense mechanisms. Patients who are immunocompromised are at high risk for opportunistic infections. Strategies to decrease the risk for health care–associated infections (HAIs) include decreasing the number of invasive catheters (e.g., central lines, bladder catheters), using aseptic technique during invasive procedures, and paying strict attention to hand washing. Change equipment per agency policy. Thoroughly sanitize or discard (if disposable) equipment between patient use.

Evidence-based guidelines are available to reduce the risk for HAIs (e.g., ventilator-associated pneumonia, central line infections, catheter-associated urinary tract infections). These guidelines, called *care bundles,* outline key interventions aimed at reducing infections.[17]

Acute Care

Your role in shock involves (1) monitoring the patient's ongoing status, (2) identifying trends to detect changes in the patient's condition, (3) planning and implementing nursing interventions and therapy, (4) evaluating the response to therapy, (5) providing emotional support to the patient and caregiver, and (6) collaborating with other health care team members to coordinate care.

Neurologic status. Assess orientation and level of consciousness, using a valid tool, at least every 1 to 2 hours. Neurologic status is the best indicator of cerebral blood flow. Be aware of findings of neurologic involvement (e.g., changes in behavior, restlessness, blurred vision, confusion, paresthesias). Note subtle changes in mental status (e.g., mild agitation) and report them to the HCP.

Orientation in the ICU environment is especially important. Reorient the patient to person, place, time, and events on a regular basis. Reduce noise and light levels to control sensory input. Keep a day-night cycle of activity. Promote rest as much as possible. Sensory overload and disruption of the patient's diurnal cycle may contribute to delirium (see Chapter 64).

Cardiovascular status. We base most of the therapy for shock on information about cardiovascular status. If the patient is unstable, continuously assess heart rate and rhythm, BP, CVP, and PA pressures, including CO, SVR, SV, and SVV (if available). Monitoring trends in hemodynamic parameters provides more important information than single values. Integrating hemodynamic with assessment data is essential in planning strategies to manage patients with shock. Chapter 35 discusses cardiovascular monitoring.

Continuously monitor the ECG. Dysrhythmias may result from cardiovascular and metabolic problems. Assess heart sounds for an S_3 or S_4 sound or new murmurs. An S_3 sound usually indicates HF. Monitor the skin for signs of adequate perfusion. Changes in temperature, pallor, flushing, cyanosis, diaphoresis, and piloerection indicate hypoperfusion.

Assess the response to fluid and drug administration as often as every 5 to 10 minutes. Make adjustments (e.g., drug titration) as needed. Once tissue perfusion is restored and the patient is stable, you can decrease the frequency of monitoring and slowly wean the patient off drugs that support BP and tissue perfusion.

CHECK YOUR PRACTICE

You are admitting a 69-year-old male patient to the ICU with a diagnosis of sepsis. Your findings show that he is confused, with weak peripheral pulses and a BP of 84/50.

- What fluids would you expect to be ordered?
- How much fluid would you expect to infuse to improve his BP?
- Despite aggressive fluid resuscitation, the patient is still hypotensive. What drug would you expect to give to improve tissue perfusion?

Respiratory care. Frequently assess respiratory status to ensure adequate oxygenation, detect complications, and provide data about acid-base status. At first, monitor the rate, depth, and rhythm of respirations as often as every 15 to 30 minutes. Increased rate and depth of respirations reflect the patient's attempts to compensate for metabolic acidosis. Assess breath sounds every 1 to 2 hours and as needed for any changes that may indicate fluid overload or accumulated secretions.

Use pulse oximetry to continuously monitor O_2 saturation. Pulse oximetry using a finger probe may not be accurate because of poor peripheral circulation. Instead, attach the probe to the ear, nose, or forehead (according to the manufacturer's guidelines). ABGs give definitive information on ventilation and oxygenation status and acid-base balance. Initial interpretation of ABGs is often your responsibility. A $Pa{O_2}$ less than 60 mm Hg (in the absence of chronic lung disease) indicates hypoxemia and the need for higher O_2 concentrations or a different mode of O_2 administration. Low $Pa{CO_2}$ with a low pH and low bicarbonate level may mean that the patient is trying to compensate for metabolic acidosis from high lactate levels.

A rising $Pa{CO_2}$ with a persistently low pH and $Pa{O_2}$ indicates the need for advanced pulmonary management. Many patients in shock are intubated and on mechanical ventilation. Maintaining a patent airway and monitoring for ventilator-related complications are critical. Chapter 28 discusses mechanical ventilation.

Renal status. At first, measure urine output every 1 to 2 hours to assess renal perfusion. An indwelling urinary catheter helps to measure output during resuscitation. Urine output less than 0.5 mL/kg/h indicates inadequate renal perfusion. Use trends in creatinine to assess renal function. Creatinine is a better indicator of renal function than BUN because the catabolic state affects BUN.

Temperature. Monitor temperature every 4 hours if normal. In the presence of a high or subnormal temperature, obtain hourly core temperatures (e.g., urinary, esophageal, PA catheter). Use light covers and control the room temperature to keep the patient comfortably warm. If the patient's temperature increases to greater than 101.5°F (38.6°C) and the patient becomes uncomfortable or shows cardiovascular compromise, treat the fever with antipyretic drugs (e.g., ibuprofen) and remove some of the bed covers. Consider a cooling device to decrease metabolism and myocardial oxygen needs if fever persists despite treatment (see Table 12.5).

Gastrointestinal status. Auscultate bowel sounds at least every 4 hours. Monitor for abdominal distention. If a nasogastric tube is present, measure drainage and check for occult blood. Check all stools for occult blood.

Skin integrity. Hygiene is especially important because impaired tissue perfusion predisposes patients to skin breakdown and infection. Perform bathing and other nursing measures carefully because patients in shock have problems with O_2 delivery to tissues. Use clinical judgment in determining priorities of care to limit the demands for increased O_2. Monitor trends in O_2 consumption (e.g., SpO_2, $ScvO_2/SvO_2$) during all interventions to assess the patient's tolerance of activity.

The increased O_2 demand that occurs during repositioning makes preventing pressure injuries challenging for those with limited O_2 reserves. Turn the patient at least every 1 to 2 hours. Maintain good body alignment. Use a pressure-relieving or pressure-reducing mattress or a specialty bed as needed. Perform passive range of motion 3 or 4 times a day to maintain joint mobility and help prevent tissue breakdown.

Oral care is essential because mucous membranes may become dry and fragile in volume-depleted patients. Intubated patients usually have difficulty swallowing, causing pooled secretions in the mouth. Apply a water-soluble lubricant to the lips to prevent drying and cracking. Brush the teeth or gums with a soft toothbrush every 8 to 12 hours. Swab the lips and oral mucosa with a moisturizing solution every 2 to 4 hours.

Emotional support. Fear, anxiety, and pain may worsen respiratory distress and increase catecholamine release. Monitor mental state and pain level. Give drugs to decrease anxiety and pain as needed. Continuous infusions of a benzodiazepine (e.g., lorazepam) and an opioid or sedative (e.g., morphine, propofol) are helpful in decreasing anxiety and pain.

Patients may want a visit from a spiritual or religious leader. One way to provide support is to offer to call the leader rather than wait for patients or caregivers to express a wish for counseling.

CHECK YOUR PRACTICE

Your patient is a 74-year-old male recovering from septic shock after a perforated diverticulum. He has been in the ICU for 7 days. His condition is finally stable. His wife has been at his bedside for his entire ICU stay. While caring for him, you suggest that she take a brief walk and get a snack. She bursts out with tears, "I can't leave him. You know that he almost died."

- How can you support this caregiver?

Caregivers need to be informed of the patient's condition. Give the patient and caregiver simple explanations of all procedures before you carry them out and information about the plan of care. If they ask questions about progress and prognosis, give simple and honest answers.

Continuity of care is important to decrease anxiety, limit conflicting information, and increase trust. If the prognosis becomes grave, support the caregiver when making tough decisions, such as withdrawing life support. The health care team must promote realistic expectations and outcomes. Remember, compassion is as essential as scientific and technical expertise in providing care.

Ensure that the caregiver can spend time with the patient if the patient perceives this time as comforting. Explain in simple terms the purpose of any tubes and equipment attached to or surrounding the patient. Tell them what they may and may not touch. If possible, place the patient's hands and arms outside the sheets to encourage therapeutic touch. Encourage caregivers to perform simple comfort measures if desired. Provide privacy as much as possible while assuring them that help is readily available should it be needed. Always position the call light in reach of the patient or caregiver.

Chronic Care

Rehabilitation of patients who have a critical illness requires prevention or early treatment of complications and teaching focused on disease management and preventing recurrence of shock. Continue to monitor patients for complications throughout the recovery period. These may include decreased range of motion, muscle weakness, decreased physical endurance, AKI (see Chapter 51), and fibrotic lung disease from ARDS (see Chapter 32). Patients recovering from shock often need care coordination of diverse services after discharge. These can include admission to transitional care units (e.g., for mechanical ventilation weaning), rehabilitation centers (inpatient or outpatient), or home health care agencies. Start planning for a safe transition from hospital to home as soon as a patient is admitted to the hospital.

◆ Evaluation

The expected outcomes are that patients with shock will have:

- Adequate tissue perfusion with restoration of normal or baseline BP
- Normal organ function with no complications from hypoperfusion
- Decreased fear and anxiety

SYSTEMIC INFLAMMATORY RESPONSE SYNDROME AND MULTIPLE ORGAN DYSFUNCTION SYNDROME

Etiology

Systemic inflammatory response syndrome (SIRS) is a systemic inflammatory response to an insult, including infection (sepsis), ischemia, infarction, and injury.[10] General inflammation in organs remote from the initial insult characterizes SIRS. Many different mechanisms can trigger SIRS. These include:

- Mechanical tissue trauma: burns, crush injuries, surgery
- Abscess formation: intraabdominal, extremities
- Ischemic or necrotic tissue: pancreatitis, vascular disease, MI
- Microbial invasion: bacteria, viruses, fungi, parasites
- Endotoxin release: gram-negative and gram-positive bacteria
- Global perfusion deficits: postcardiac resuscitation, shock states
- Regional perfusion deficits: local distal perfusion deficits

Multiple organ dysfunction syndrome (MODS) is the failure of 2 or more organ systems in acutely ill patients such that homeostasis cannot be maintained without intervention.[10] MODS results from SIRS. These 2 syndromes represent the ends of a continuum. Transition from SIRS to MODS does not occur in a clear-cut manner (Fig. 42.1).

Pathophysiology

When the inflammatory response is activated, consequences include the release of mediators, direct damage to the endothelium, and hypermetabolism. Increased vascular permeability allows mediators and protein to leak out of the endothelium and into the interstitial space. White blood cells begin to digest the foreign debris, and the coagulation cascade is activated. Hypotension, decreased perfusion, microemboli, and redistributed or shunted blood flow compromise organ perfusion.

The respiratory system is often the first system to show signs of dysfunction in SIRS and MODS.[10] Inflammatory mediators damage the pulmonary vasculature endothelium and cause increased capillary permeability. Fluid moves from the pulmonary vasculature into the pulmonary interstitial spaces, then moves to the alveoli, causing alveolar edema. Type I pneumocytes (alveolar cells) are destroyed. Type II pneumocytes are damaged. Surfactant production is decreased. The alveoli collapse, creating an increase in *shunt* (blood flow to the lungs that does not take part in gas exchange) and worsening ventilation-perfusion mismatch. The result is ARDS. Patients with ARDS need aggressive pulmonary management with mechanical ventilation. See Chapter 32 for a discussion of ARDS.

Cardiovascular changes include myocardial depression and massive vasodilation in response to increasing tissue demands. Vasodilation results in decreased SVR and BP. The baroreceptor reflex causes release of *inotropic* (increasing force of contraction) and *chronotropic* (increasing heart rate) factors that enhance CO. To compensate for hypotension, CO increases by an increase in heart rate and SV. Increases in capillary permeability cause a shift of albumin and fluid out of the vascular space. This further reduces venous return and preload. Patients become warm and tachycardic with a high CO and a low SVR. Other signs include decreased capillary refill, skin mottling, decreased CVP and PAWP, and dysrhythmias. $ScvO_2$ or SvO_2 may be abnormally high because the patient is perfusing areas not consuming much O_2 (e.g., skin, nonworking muscle). Other areas may have blood shunted away from them. Eventually, either perfusion of vital organs becomes insufficient or the cells are unable to use O_2 and their function is further compromised.

Neurologic dysfunction in SIRS and MODS often presents as mental status changes. These acute changes can be an early sign of SIRS or MODS. Patients may be confused and agitated, combative, disoriented, lethargic, or comatose. These changes are due to hypoxemia, the effects of inflammatory mediators, and impaired perfusion.

AKI from hypoperfusion and the effects of the mediators are common. Decreased renal perfusion activates the SNS and the renin-angiotensin system. Stimulating the renin-angiotensin system causes systemic vasoconstriction and aldosterone-mediated sodium and water reabsorption. Another risk factor for AKI is the use of nephrotoxic drugs. Many antibiotics used to treat gram-negative bacteria (e.g., aminoglycosides) can be nephrotoxic. Careful monitoring of drug levels is essential to avoid nephrotoxic effects.

The GI tract plays a key role in the development of MODS. GI motility is often decreased in critical illness, causing abdominal distention and paralytic ileus. In the early stages of SIRS and MODS, blood is shunted away from the GI mucosa. This makes it highly vulnerable to ischemic injury. Decreased perfusion leads to a breakdown of the normally protective mucosal barrier. This increases the risk for ulceration, GI bleeding, and bacterial movement from the GI tract into circulation.

Metabolic changes are pronounced. Both SIRS and MODS trigger a hypermetabolic response. Glycogen stores are rapidly converted to glucose (glycogenolysis). Once glycogen is depleted, amino acids are converted to glucose (gluconeogenesis), reducing protein stores. Fatty acids are used for fuel. Catecholamines and glucocorticoids are released and cause hyperglycemia and insulin resistance. The net result is a catabolic state with a loss of lean body mass (muscle).

Hypermetabolism may last for several days and cause liver dysfunction. Protein synthesis is impaired. The liver cannot make albumin, a key protein in maintaining plasma oncotic pressure. This changes plasma oncotic pressure, causing fluid and protein to leak from the vascular spaces to the interstitial space. At this point, giving IV albumin does not normalize oncotic pressure.

As hypermetabolism persists, patients cannot convert lactate to glucose and lactate accumulates (lactic acidosis). Despite increases in glycogenolysis and gluconeogenesis, eventually the liver cannot maintain an adequate glucose level and patients become hypoglycemic. Hypoglycemia can also develop due to acute adrenal insufficiency.

DIC may result from dysfunction of the coagulation system. DIC causes microvascular clotting and bleeding at the same time because of the depletion of clotting factors and excess fibrinolysis. Chapter 34 discusses DIC.

Electrolyte imbalances are common. They result from hormone and metabolic changes and fluid shifts. These changes worsen mental status changes, neuromuscular problems, and dysrhythmias. ADH and aldosterone release results in sodium and water retention. Aldosterone increases urinary potassium loss. Catecholamines cause potassium to move into the cell, causing hypokalemia. Hypokalemia can cause dysrhythmias and muscle weakness. Metabolic acidosis results from impaired tissue perfusion, hypoxia, and the shift to anaerobic metabolism. This increases lactate levels. Progressive renal dysfunction contributes to metabolic acidosis. Hypocalcemia, hypomagnesemia, and hypophosphatemia are common.

Clinical Manifestations

The clinical manifestations of SIRS and MODS are described in Table 42.10.

Interprofessional and Nursing Management

The prognosis for patients with MODS is poor, with mortality rates of 40% to 60%. Mortality increases as more organ systems fail. The most common cause of death is sepsis. Maintain communication between the health care team and the patient's caregiver about realistic goals and outcomes for patients with MODS.

Survival improves with early, goal-directed therapy to prevent SIRS from progressing to MODS. Your key role is vigilant assessment and ongoing monitoring to detect early signs of deterioration or organ dysfunction. Interprofessional care focuses on (1) preventing and treating infection, (2) maintaining tissue oxygenation, (3) nutrition and metabolic support, and (4) support of failing organs. Table 42.10 outlines the management for patients with SIRS and MODS.

Preventing and Treating Infection

Aggressive infection control strategies are essential to decrease the risk for HAIs. Early, aggressive surgery is recommended to remove necrotic tissue (e.g., early debridement of burn tissue) that can provide a culture medium for microorganisms. Aggressive pulmonary management, including early mobilization, can reduce the risk for infection. Strict asepsis can decrease infections related to intraarterial lines, endotracheal tubes, indwelling urinary catheters, IV lines, and other invasive devices or procedures. Daily assessment of the ongoing need for invasive lines and other devices is an important strategy to prevent or limit HAIs.

Despite aggressive strategies, infection may develop. Once an infection is suspected, begin interventions to treat the cause. Send cultures and start prescribed broad-spectrum antibiotic therapy. Adjust therapy based on the culture results, if needed.

Tissue Oxygenation

Hypoxemia often occurs because patients have greater O_2 needs and decreased O_2 supply to the tissues. Interventions that decrease O_2 demand and increase O_2 delivery are essential. Sedation, mechanical ventilation, analgesia, and rest may decrease O_2 demand and should be considered. Treating fever, chills, and pain decreases O_2 demand. O_2 delivery may be optimized by individualizing tidal volumes with positive end-expiratory pressure, increasing preload (e.g., fluids) or myocardial contractility to enhance CO, or reducing afterload to increase CO.

Nutrition

Hypermetabolism can result in profound weight loss, cachexia, and further organ failure. Protein-calorie malnutrition is a key sign of hypermetabolism. Total energy expenditure is often increased 1.5 to 2.0 times the normal metabolic rate. Because of

TABLE 42.10 Manifestations and Management of SIRS and MODS

Manifestations	Management	Manifestations	Management
Cardiovascular		**Neurologic**	
Biventricular failure	Volume management to ↑ preload	Acute change in neurologic status	Evaluate for hepatic or metabolic encephalopathy
↓ BP, MAP, SVR	Hemodynamic monitoring	Confusion, disorientation, delirium	Optimize cerebral blood flow
↑ HR, CO, SV	Arterial pressure monitoring to maintain MAP >65 mm Hg	Fever	↓ Cerebral O_2 requirements
Massive vasodilation	Vasopressors	Hepatic encephalopathy	Prevent secondary tissue ischemia
Myocardial depression	Intermittent or continuous $ScvO_2$ or SvO_2 monitoring	Seizures	Calcium channel blockers (reduce cerebral vasospasm)
Systolic, diastolic dysfunction	Balance O_2 supply and demand		
	Continuous ECG monitoring		
	Circulatory assist devices	**Renal**	
	VTE prophylaxis	*Prerenal:* renal hypoperfusion	Diuretics
Endocrine		• BUN/creatinine ratio >20:1	• Loop diuretics (e.g., furosemide)
Hyperglycemia → hypoglycemia	Provide continuous insulin infusion and glucose to maintain blood glucose 140–180 mg/dL (7.77–10.0 mmol/L)	• ↓ Urine Na^+ <20 mEq/L	• May need to ↑ dosage due to ↓ glomerular filtration rate
		• ↑ Urine osmolality	
		• Urine specific gravity >1.020	
		Intrarenal: acute tubular necrosis	Continuous renal replacement therapy (see Chapter 51)
Gastrointestinal		• BUN/creatinine ratio <10:1–15:1	
GI bleeding	Stress ulcer prophylaxis	• ↑ Urine Na^+ >20 mEq/L	
Hypoperfusion → ↓ peristalsis, paralytic ileus	• Antacids (e.g., Maalox)	• ↓ Urine osmolality	
Mucosal ischemia	• Proton pump inhibitors (e.g., omeprazole)	• Urine specific gravity ~1.010	
• ↓ Intramucosal pH	• sucralfate (Carafate)	**Respiratory**	
• Potential translocation of gut bacteria	Monitor abdominal distention, intraabdominal pressures	ARDS (see Chapter 32):	Optimize O_2 delivery and minimize O_2 consumption
• Potential abdominal compartment syndrome	Dietitian consult	• Bilateral fluffy infiltrates on chest x-ray	Mechanical ventilation (see Chapter 28)
Mucosal ulceration on endoscopy	Enteral nutrition	• ↓ Compliance	• Positive end-expiratory pressure
	Stimulate mucosal activity	• Dyspnea (severe)	• Lung protective modes (e.g., pressure-control inverse ratio ventilation, low tidal volumes)
	Provide essential nutrients and optimal calories	↑ C-reactive protein	• Permissive hypercapnia
		• Minute ventilation	• Positioning (e.g., continuous lateral rotation therapy, prone positioning)
		• PaO_2/FIO_2 ratio <200	
Hematologic System		• PAWP <18 mm Hg	
↑ Bleeding times, ↑ PT, ↑ PTT	Observe for bleeding from obvious and/or occult sites	• Pulmonary hypertension	
↑ D-dimer	Replace factors being lost (e.g., platelets)	• Refractory hypoxemia	
↑ Fibrin split products	Minimize traumatic interventions (e.g., IM injections, multiple venipunctures)	• Tachypnea	
↓ Platelet count (thrombocytopenia)		• Ventilation-perfusion (V/Q) mismatch	
Liver			
Bilirubin >2 mg/dL (34 μmol/L)	Maintain adequate tissue perfusion		
Hepatic encephalopathy	Provide nutrition support (e.g., enteral nutrition)		
Jaundice	Careful use of drugs metabolized by liver		
↑ Liver enzymes (ALT, AST, GGT)			
↓ Albumin, prealbumin, transferrin			
↑ Ammonia			

ALT, Alanine aminotransferase; *AST,* aspartate aminotransferase; *GGT,* γ-glutamyl transferase; *PA,* pulmonary artery; *PAWP,* pulmonary artery wedge pressure; *PT,* prothrombin time; *PTT,* partial thromboplastin time.

their short half-life, monitor transferrin and prealbumin levels to assess liver protein synthesis.

The goal of nutrition support is to preserve organ function. Providing early and optimal nutrition decreases morbidity and mortality rates. EN is preferred. If we cannot use EN, then consider PN (see Chapter 44). Provide glycemic control using insulin with a goal of glucose levels of 180 mg/dL or less.[1]

Support of Failing Organs

Support of any failing organ is a goal of therapy. For example, patients with ARDS require aggressive O_2 therapy and mechanical ventilation. DIC should be treated appropriately (e.g., blood products). Renal failure may require dialysis. Continuous renal replacement therapy is better tolerated than hemodialysis, especially in patients with hemodynamic instability.

CASE STUDY

Shock

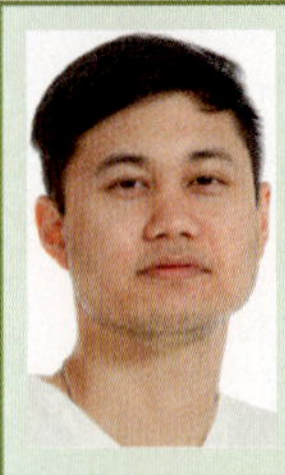

((© Thinkstock.))

Patient Profile

K.L., a 25-year-old Korean American male, was driving a motor vehicle involved in a crash. K.L. was ejected through the windshield and found 10 feet from his car. He was face down, conscious, and moaning. His wife and daughter were in the car with their seat belts on. They sustained minor injuries and are very frightened and upset. All passengers were taken to the ED. This information pertains to K.L.

Subjective Data

- States, "I can't breathe"
- Cries out when abdomen is palpated

Objective Data

Physical Assessment

- *Cardiovascular:* BP 80/56 mm Hg; apical pulse 138 but no palpable radial or pedal pulses; carotid pulse 1+. ECG shows:

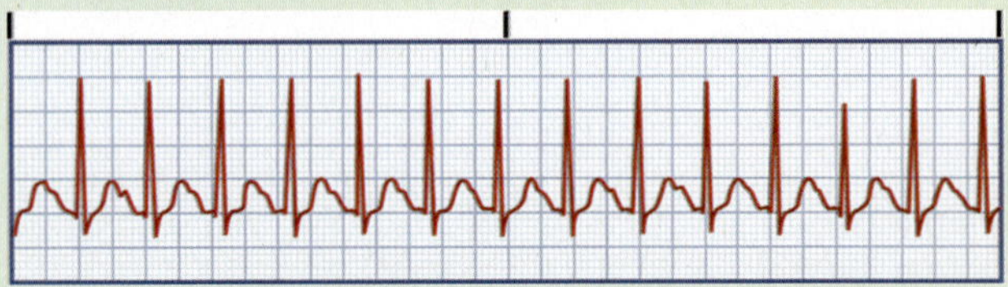

- *Respiratory:* respiratory rate 35 breaths/min; labored breathing with shallow respirations; asymmetric chest wall movement; absence of breath sounds on left side. Trachea deviated slightly to the right
- *Abdomen:* slightly distended and left upper quadrant painful on palpation
- *Musculoskeletal:* open compound fracture of the lower left leg

Diagnostic Studies

- Chest x-ray: hemothorax with 6 rib fractures
- Hematocrit: 28%

Interprofessional Care (in the ED)

- Intraosseous access in right proximal tibia placed prehospital
- Left chest tube placed, draining bright red blood
- Fluid resuscitation started with crystalloids
- High-flow O_2 by nonrebreather mask

Emergency Surgical Procedures

- Splenectomy
- Repair of torn intercostal artery
- Repair of compound fracture

Discussion Questions

1. ***Recognize:*** What types of shock is K.L. at high risk for experiencing?
2. ***Analyze:*** Based on the assessment data, what types of shock is K.L. experiencing?
3. ***Analyze:*** What potential complications is K.L. at risk for?
4. ***Prioritize:*** Based on the assessment data presented, what are the priority clinical problems?
5. ***Prioritize:*** What are the priority nursing responsibilities for K.L. before he goes to surgery?
6. ***Act:*** K.L.'s parents arrive. English is their second language. They are very anxious and asking about their son. What can you do to provide culturally respectful, competent, family-centered care?
7. ***Act:*** Identify the tasks that could be delegated to AP.

Answers available at http://evolve.elsevier.com/Lewis/medsurg.

BRIDGE TO NCLEX EXAMINATION

The number of the question corresponds to the same-numbered outcome at the beginning of the chapter.

1. A patient with a spinal cord injury at T4 has a decreasing blood pressure with bradycardia. Which condition is the patient likely experiencing?
- **a.** Relative hypervolemia.
- **b.** Absolute hypovolemia.
- **c.** Neurogenic shock from vasodilation.
- **d.** Obstructive shock from traumatic injury.

2. A 78-year-old male with a history of diabetes has confusion and temperature of 104°F (40°C). There is a wound on his right heel with purulent drainage. After an infusion of 3 L of normal saline solution, his assessment findings are BP 84/40 mm Hg; heart rate 110; respiratory rate 42 and shallow; CO 8 L/min; and PAWP 4 mm Hg. Which condition is the patient likely experiencing?
- **a.** Septic shock.
- **b.** Neurogenic shock.
- **c.** Multiple organ dysfunction syndrome.
- **d.** Systemic inflammatory response syndrome.

3. Which interventions are treatments for cardiogenic shock? **(Select all that apply.)**
- **a.** Dobutamine to increase myocardial contractility.
- **b.** Vasopressors to increase systemic vascular resistance.
- **c.** Circulatory assist devices such as an intraaortic balloon pump.
- **d.** Corticosteroids to stabilize the cell wall in the infarcted myocardium.
- **e.** Trendelenburg positioning to facilitate venous return and increase preload.

4. Which assessment parameters are the *most* accurate for assessing tissue perfusion in the patient with MODS?
   a. Blood pressure, pulse, and respirations
   b. Breath sounds, blood pressure, and body temperature
   c. Pulse pressure, level of consciousness, and pupil response
   d. Level of consciousness, urinary output, and skin temperature

1. c; 2. a; 3. a, c; 4. d.

For rationales to these answers and even more NCLEX review questions, visit http://evolve.elsevier.com/Lewis/medsurg.

REFERENCES

To access the References for this chapter, please scan the QR code with a mobile device.

CASE STUDY

Applying Clinical Judgment With Multiple Patients

You are working on the cardiovascular stepdown unit and have been assigned to care for the following 4 patients. You have 1 AP assigned to help you.

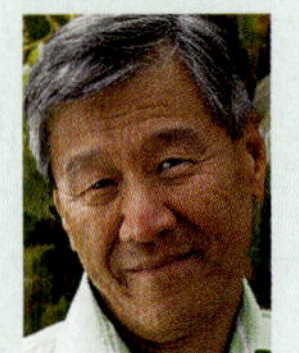 (© Jupiterimages/Banana-Stock/Thinkstock.)	L.P. is a 63-year-old male who came to the ED with chest pain, dyspnea, and palpitations. Cardiac enzymes were normal. ECG showed atrial fibrillation with a rapid ventricular response. He has been on IV diltiazem and IV heparin for 24 h. Although his heart rate has decreased, the atrial fibrillation persists. Vital signs: 124/72, 102, RR 18, O_2 saturation 98% on 2 L/min via nasal cannula.
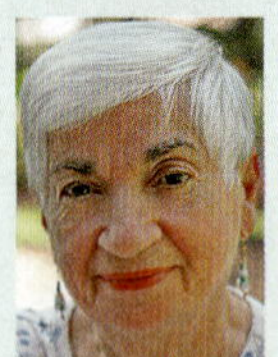 (© iStockphoto/Thinkstock.)	J.E. is a 70-year-old female admitted with dyspnea, fatigue, and weight gain. She has a systolic murmur and bilateral crackles. Her ejection fraction is 20%. She is receiving IV furosemide, oral potassium and enalapril, and IV nesiritide infusion. Cardiac enzymes are normal. Vital signs: 108/62, 92, RR 22, O_2 saturation 94% on 6 L/min via nasal cannula.
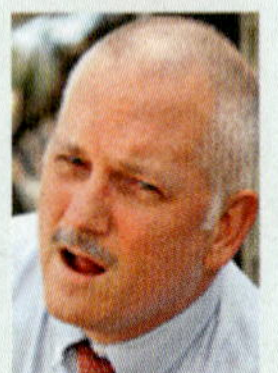 (© iStockphoto/Thinkstock.)	D.M. is a 51-year-old male who was admitted 2 days ago with a suspected inferolateral wall MI. Cardiac catheterization showed a 90% blockage of his left anterior descending (LAD) artery. Angioplasty was done, and 2 stents inserted. While admitted, he has been diagnosed with diabetes and hypertension. He is now 2 days post-PTCA, has had no recurrence of his chest pain, and is to be discharged this evening.
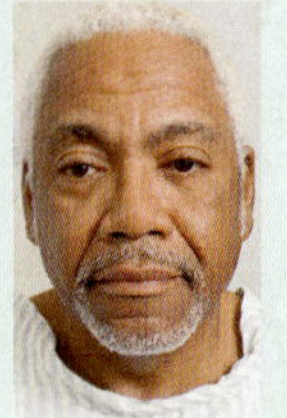 (© iStockphoto/Thinkstock.)	S.J. is a 73-year-old male admitted with rest pain in both legs and a nonhealing ulcer of the big toe on the right foot. He has a history of MI, stroke, hypertension, and type 1 diabetes. He had a left femoral-popliteal bypass 5 years ago. Right foot is cool, pale, and mottled with decreased sensation. He has a 1+ right femoral pulse, right posterior tibial pulse only obtained by Doppler. Right dorsalis pedis pulse absent by Doppler. Left leg pulses are 1+. Vital signs: 148/92, 90 and irregular, RR 22.

1. Highlight all the findings above that require your follow-up.
2. After receiving report, which patient would you see first? Second?
3. Which tasks could you delegate to the AP? **(Select all that apply.)**
   a. Calculate intake for L.P.'s heparin infusion.
   b. Report changes in pain or sensation of S.J.'s legs.
   c. Teach D.M. about activity restrictions after PTCA.
   d. Obtain vital signs and O_2 saturation for L.P. and S.J.
   e. Obtain a telemetry monitor for S.J. and apply the electrodes.
4. As you are assessing L.P., the AP tells you that S.J. is diaphoretic and reports chest pain. Use an X for the nursing actions listed below that are *Indicated* (appropriate or necessary) or *Contraindicated* (could be harmful) for S.J. at this time.

Nursing Action	Indicated	Contraindicated
Administer prescribed as-needed nitroglycerin.		
Obtain a wound culture and place a dressing on the right foot.		
Obtain a 12-lead ECG and start continuous ECG monitoring per protocol.		
Call respiratory therapy to give him a breathing treatment.		
Perform focused heart and lung assessments.		
Apply O_2 per nasal cannula per protocol.		
Obtain vital signs with O_2 saturation.		

Case Study Progression

S.J. rates his chest pain as a 9/10. His BP is 110/70, heart rate 110, respiratory rate 26, and SpO_2 93% on room air. You administer 0.4 mg SL nitroglycerin with minimal pain relief after 5 minutes. The 12-lead ECG shows new ST elevation in leads II, III, and aVF.

5. Which interventions would you expect the HCP to order for S.J.? **(Select all that apply.)**
   a. Cardiac biomarkers
   b. IV fentanyl now, repeat × 1 dose
   c. Emergent cardiac catheterization
   d. Furosemide 40 mg IV push STAT
   e. Increase the O_2 flow rate to 12 L/min
6. Choose the *best* option for the information missing from the statement below by selecting from the lists of options provided.

Because J.E is receiving nesiritide, she is at risk of experiencing _______1______. To detect this complication, you will need to monitor _____2_____.

Options for 1	Options for 2
Hypokalemia	Blood pressure
Hypotension	Respiratory rate
Respiratory depression	Serum potassium levels

7. You are preparing to give morning medications. Which patient should receive medications first?
   a. Oral potassium and enalapril to J.E.
   b. Oral metoprolol, aspirin, and clopidogrel to D.M.
   c. IV furosemide, oral omeprazole, and metoprolol to L.P.
   d. Subcut Novolog, oral diltiazem, and furosemide to S.J.
8. You are reviewing J.E.'s assessment findings to evaluate her progress. For each assessment finding, use an X to indicate whether the interventions were *Effective* (helped to meet expected outcomes) or *Ineffective* (did not help meet expected outcomes).

Assessment Finding	Effective	Ineffective
Peripheral edema is 3+ bilaterally		
Lung sounds with fewer crackles		
Heart rate 101/min, regular		
Restlessness, inattentive		
Weight has decreased by 6 lb in 2 days		
Increased BNP this am		
Reports no chest pain past 24 h		

10. You ask the AP to take D.M.'s vital signs before and after having him walk 300 feet. When reviewing the chart, you note record of the walk but not his vital signs. What is your initial action?
    a. Report the incident to the charge nurse for follow-up.
    b. Talk to the AP about why the vital signs were not recorded.
    c. Walk D.M. yourself and take his vital signs before and after.
    d. Ask the AP to walk with D.M. again and obtain vital signs before and after.

Answers available at http://evolve.elsevier.com/Lewis/medsurg.

43

Assessment: Gastrointestinal System

Kara Ann Ventura

http://evolve.elsevier.com/Lewis/medsurg/

CONCEPTUAL FOCUS

Elimination
Fluids and Electrolytes
Nutrition

LEARNING OUTCOMES

1. Describe the structures and functions of the gastrointestinal (GI) tract.
2. Describe the structures and functions of the liver, gallbladder, biliary tract, and pancreas.
3. Distinguish the processes of ingestion, digestion, absorption, and elimination.
4. Explain the processes of biliary metabolism, bile production, and bile excretion.
5. Link the age-related changes of the GI system to the differences in assessment findings.
6. Obtain significant subjective and objective assessment data related to the GI system.
7. Perform a physical assessment of the GI system.
8. Distinguish normal from abnormal findings of a GI physical assessment.
9. Describe the purpose, significance of results, and nursing responsibilities related to diagnostic studies of the GI system.

KEY TERMS

absorption
bilirubin
borborygmi, Table 43.9
cheilosis, Table 43.9
digestion
endoscopy
hematemesis, Table 43.9
ingestion
Kupffer cells
melena, Table 43.9
steatorrhea, Table 43.9
tenesmus, Table 43.9
Valsalva maneuver

The gastrointestinal (GI) system, or the *digestive system,* consists of the GI tract and its associated organs and glands. Included in the GI tract are the mouth, esophagus, stomach, small intestine, large intestine, rectum, and anus. The associated organs are the liver, pancreas, and gallbladder (Fig. 43.1). GI problems that change physiologic processes affect a person's ability to maintain nutrition status and eliminate waste.

STRUCTURE AND FUNCTION OF THE GI SYSTEM

The GI tract extends around 30 ft (9 m) from the mouth to the anus. The GI tract is essentially a tube composed of 4 layers. From the inside to the outside, these layers are (1) mucosa lining; (2) submucosa connective tissue, which contains glands, blood vessels, and lymph nodes; (3) muscle; and (4) serosa. There are 3 smooth muscle layers: the oblique (inner) layer, circular (middle) layer, and longitudinal (outer) layer.

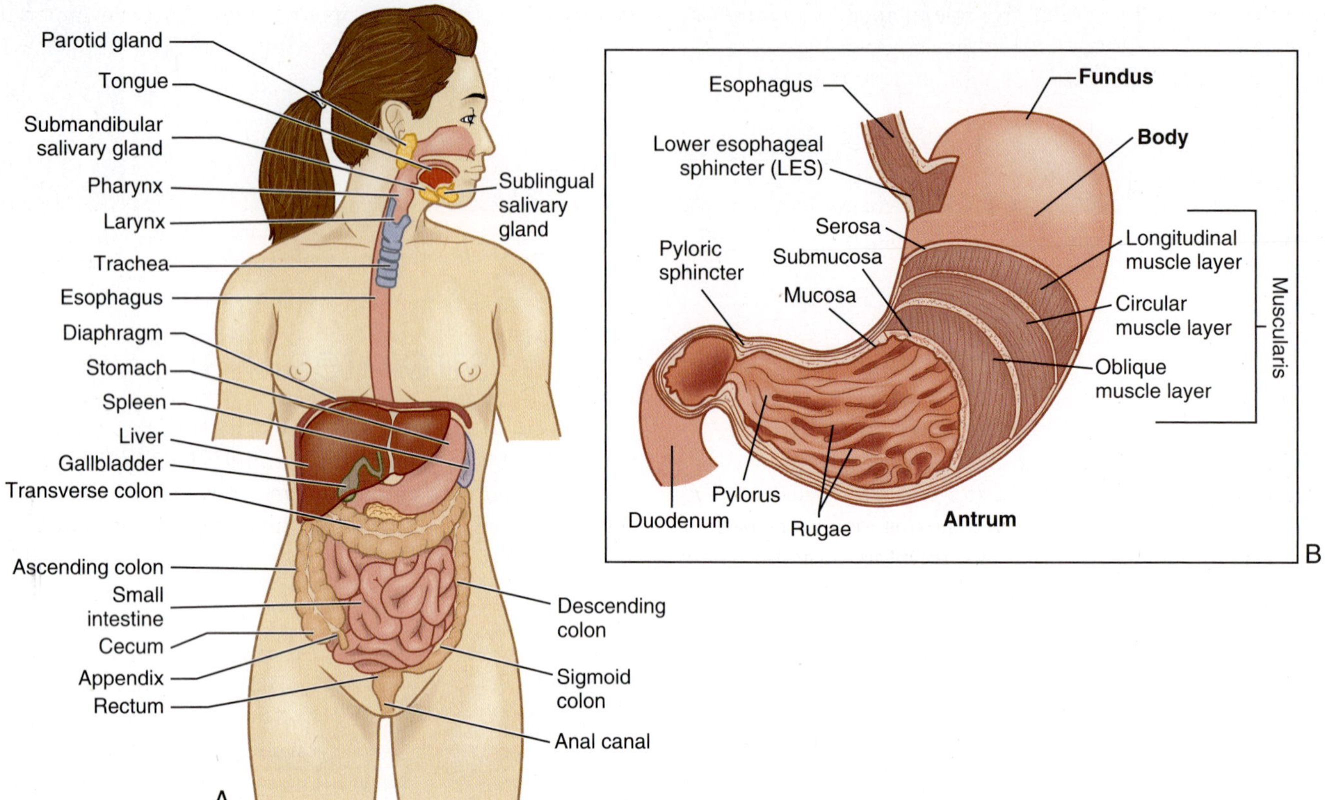

Fig. 43.1 (A) Location of organs of the GI system. (B) Parts of the stomach.

Parasympathetic and sympathetic branches of the autonomic nervous system (ANS) innervate the GI tract. The parasympathetic (cholinergic) system is mainly excitatory. The sympathetic (adrenergic) system is mainly inhibitory. For example, parasympathetic stimulation increases peristalsis, and sympathetic stimulation decreases it. Both sympathetic and parasympathetic afferent fibers relay sensory information.

The GI tract has its own nervous system: the enteric nervous system (ENS) or intrinsic nervous system. The ENS system regulates motility and secretion along the entire GI tract. The ENS is composed of 2 networks: (1) Meissner plexus in the submucosa and (2) Auerbach (myenteric) plexus between the muscle layers. The submucosal plexus controls secretion and is involved in many sensory functions. The myenteric plexus is the major nerve supply to the GI tract and controls GI movements. Although the ENS receives innervation from the ANS, it functions independently of the brain and spinal cord.

Circulation in the GI system is unique in that venous blood draining the GI tract organs empties into the portal vein, which then perfuses the liver. This allows the liver to clean the blood of bacteria and toxins from the GI tract. The celiac artery, superior mesenteric artery (SMA), and inferior mesenteric artery (IMA) supply arterial blood to the GI tract. The stomach and duodenum receive their blood supply from the celiac axis. The distal small intestine to mid large intestine receives its blood supply from branches of the hepatic and SMA. The distal large intestine through the anus receives its blood supply from the IMA. The GI tract and accessory organs receive 25% to 30% of the cardiac output at rest and 35% or more after eating. Because such a large percentage of the cardiac output perfuses these organs, the GI tract is a major source from which to divert blood flow during exercise, stress, or injury.

The peritoneum almost completely covers the abdominal organs. The 2 layers of the peritoneum are the *parietal layer,* which lines the abdominal cavity wall, and the *visceral layer.* It covers the abdominal organs. The peritoneal cavity is the potential space between the parietal and visceral layers. The 2 folds of the peritoneum are the mesentery and omentum. The mesentery attaches the small intestine and part of the large intestine to the posterior abdominal wall. It contains blood and lymph vessels. The omentum hangs like an apron from the stomach to the intestines. It contains fat and lymph nodes.

The main function of the GI system is to supply nutrients to body cells. This is accomplished through the processes of (1) *ingestion* (taking in food), (2) *digestion* (breaking down food), and (3) *absorption* (transferring food products into circulation). *Elimination* is the process of excreting the waste products of digestion.

Ingestion

Ingestion is the intake of food. *Appetite,* the desire to ingest food, influences how much food a person eats. We have an appetite center in the hypothalamus. Several factors, including hypoglycemia, an empty stomach, and a decrease in body temperature, stimulate appetite. The hormone *ghrelin* released from the stomach mucosa plays a role in appetite stimulation. Another hormone, *leptin,* is involved in appetite suppression. The sight, smell, and taste of food can stimulate appetite. Stomach distention, illness (especially accompanied by fever), hyperglycemia, nausea, vomiting, and certain drugs (e.g., amphetamines) inhibit appetite.

Deglutition, or swallowing, is the mechanical portion of ingestion. The mouth, pharynx, and esophagus are involved in swallowing.

Mouth

The mouth consists of the lips and oral (buccal) cavity. The lips surround the opening of the mouth and function in speech. The hard and soft palates form the roof of the oral cavity. The oral cavity contains the teeth and tongue. The tongue is a solid muscle mass. It aids in chewing and moving food to the back of the throat for swallowing. The taste receptors (taste buds) are on the sides and tip of the tongue. The tongue is also important in speech.

Within the oral cavity are 3 pairs of salivary glands: parotid, submaxillary, and sublingual glands. These glands produce saliva. Saliva consists of water, protein, mucin, inorganic salts, and salivary amylase.

Pharynx

The pharynx is a muscular tube lined with mucous membrane. It has 3 sections: nasopharynx, oropharynx, and laryngeal pharynx. The mucous membrane is continuous with the nasal cavity, mouth, auditory tubes, and larynx. During ingestion, the oropharynx is the route for food from the mouth to the esophagus. Food or liquid stimulates receptors in the oropharynx, initiating the swallowing reflex. During swallowing, the epiglottis closes over the opening to the larynx and prevents food from entering the respiratory tract. The tonsils and adenoids, composed of lymphoid tissue, help the body prevent infection.

Esophagus

The esophagus is a hollow, muscular tube that receives food from the pharynx and moves it to the stomach. It is 7 to 10 in (18 to 25 cm) long and 0.8 in (2 cm) in diameter. The esophagus is in the thoracic cavity. It is structurally composed of 4 layers: inner mucosa, submucosa, muscularis propria, and outermost adventitia. The upper third of the esophagus is composed of striated skeletal muscle. The distal two-thirds are composed of smooth muscle.

Between swallows, the esophagus is collapsed and the *upper esophageal sphincter* (UES) closed. With swallowing, the UES relaxes, and a peristaltic wave moves the bolus into the esophagus. The muscular layers contract *(peristalsis)* and propel the food to the stomach. The *lower esophageal sphincter* (LES) at the distal end of the esophagus controls the opening of the esophagus into the stomach. It stays contracted except during swallowing, belching, or vomiting. The LES is an important barrier that normally prevents reflux of acidic gastric contents into the esophagus.

Digestion and Absorption

Stomach

The stomach's functions are to store food, mix food with gastric secretions, and empty contents in small boluses into the small intestine. The stomach absorbs only small amounts of water, alcohol, electrolytes, and certain drugs.

The stomach is usually J shaped and lies obliquely in the epigastric, umbilical, and left hypochondriac regions of the abdomen (Fig. 43.5, later in the chapter). It always contains gastric fluid and mucus. The 3 main parts of the stomach are the fundus (cardia), body, and antrum (Fig. 43.1). The pylorus is a small portion of the antrum proximal to the pyloric sphincter. The LES and pyloric sphincter guard the entrance to and exit from the stomach.

The stomach wall has 4 layers. The serous (outer) layer of the stomach is continuous with the peritoneum. The muscular layer consists of the longitudinal (outer) layer, circular (middle) layer, and oblique (inner) layer. The mucosal layer forms folds called rugae that have many small glands. In the fundus, the glands contain (1) chief cells, which secrete pepsinogen, and (2) parietal cells, which secrete hydrochloric (HCl) acid, water, and intrinsic factor. HCl acid makes gastric juice acidic. This acidic pH helps protect us against ingested organisms. Intrinsic factor promotes cobalamin (vitamin B_{12}) absorption in the small intestine.

Small Intestine

The main functions of the small intestine are digestion and **absorption**, the uptake of nutrients from the gut lumen to the bloodstream. The small intestine is a coiled tube about 23 ft (7 m) in length and 1 to 1.1 in (2.5 to 2.8 cm) in diameter. It extends from the pylorus to the ileocecal valve. The small intestine is composed of the duodenum, jejunum, and ileum. The ileocecal valve prevents reflux of large intestine contents into the small intestine.

The mucosa of the small intestine is thick, vascular, and glandular. The functional units of the small intestine are *villi.* They are minute, fingerlike projections in the mucous membrane. Villi contain epithelial cells that produce the intestinal digestive enzymes. The epithelial cells on the villi also have *microvilli.* The circular folds in the mucous and submucous layers, along with the villi and microvilli, increase the surface area for digestion and absorption.

The digestive enzymes on the brush border of the microvilli chemically break down nutrients for absorption. Between the bases of the villi lie the crypts of Lieberkühn. They contain stem cells that are the precursors for the other epithelial cells. Brunner's glands in the submucosa of the duodenum secrete an alkaline fluid containing bicarbonate that neutralizes acidic fluids and protects the mucosa. Intestinal goblet cells secrete mucus that protects the mucosa.

Physiology of Digestion

Digestion is the physical and chemical breakdown of food into absorbable substances. The timely movement of food through the GI tract and the secretion of specific enzymes promote digestion. These enzymes break down food to particles of appropriate size for absorption (Table 43.1).

The process of digestion begins in the mouth, where food is chewed, mechanically broken down, and mixed with saliva. Saliva helps us swallow by lubricating food. Saliva contains amylase, which breaks down starches to maltose. Chewing and the sight, smell, thought, and taste of food stimulate the release of saliva. A person makes about 1 L of saliva each day. After swallowing, food moves through the esophagus to the stomach. No digestion or absorption occurs in the esophagus.

GI secretion and motility are under neural and hormonal control. Food entering the stomach and small intestine triggers the release of hormones into the bloodstream (Tables 43.2 and 43.3). These hormones play important roles in the control of HCl acid secretion, production and release of digestive enzymes, and motility.

In the stomach, muscle action mixes the food with gastric secretions to form *chyme,* which is now ready for absorption. Protein digestion begins with the release of pepsinogen from chief cells. The stomach's acidic environment results in the conversion of pepsinogen to its active form, pepsin. Pepsin begins the breakdown of proteins. There is minimal digestion of starches and fats. The stomach also serves as a reservoir for food, releasing it slowly into the small intestine. The length of time that food stays in the stomach depends on the composition of the food. The average meal stays in the stomach for 3 to 4 hours.

In the small intestine, the physical presence and chemical nature of chyme stimulates motility and secretion. Secretions involved in digestion include enzymes from the pancreas, bile from the liver, and enzymes from the small intestine (Table 43.1). Carbohydrates are broken down to monosaccharides, fats to glycerol and fatty acids, and proteins to amino acids. Enzymes on the brush border of the microvilli complete the digestion process. These enzymes break down disaccharides to monosaccharides and peptides to amino acids for absorption.

The absorption of most of the end products of digestion occurs in the small intestine. The movement of the villi enables these end products to come in contact with the absorbing membrane. Monosaccharides, fatty acids, amino acids, water, electrolytes, vitamins, and minerals are absorbed.

TABLE 43.1 GI Secretions

Daily Amount (mL)	Secretions/ Enzymes	Action
Salivary Glands		
1000–1500	Salivary amylase	Initiates starch digestion
Stomach		
2500	HCl acid	Activation of pepsinogen to pepsin
	Intrinsic factor	Essential for cobalamin absorption in ileum
	Lipase	Fat digestion
	Pepsinogen	Protein digestion
Small Intestine		
3000	Aminopeptidases	Protein digestion
	Amylase	Carbohydrate digestion
	Enterokinase	Activation of trypsinogen to trypsin
	Lactase	Lactose to glucose and galactose
	Lipase	Fat digestion
	Maltase	Maltose to 2 glucose molecules
	Peptidases	Protein digestion
	Sucrase	Sucrose to glucose and fructose
Pancreas		
700	Amylase	Starch to disaccharides
	Chymotrypsin	Protein digestion
	Lipase	Fat digestion
	Trypsinogen	Protein digestion
Liver and Gallbladder		
1000	Bile	Emulsifies fats and aids in absorption of fatty acids and fat-soluble vitamins (A, D, E, K)

TABLE 43.2 Phases of Gastric Secretion

Stimulus to Secretion	Secretion
Cephalic (Nervous)	
Sight, smell, taste of food (before food enters stomach). Initiated in the CNS and mediated by the vagus nerve.	HCl acid, pepsinogen, mucus
Gastric (Hormonal and Nervous)	
Food in antrum of stomach, vagal stimulation.	Release of gastrin from antrum into circulation to stimulate gastric secretions and motility
Intestine (Hormonal)	
Presence of chyme in small intestine.	*Acidic chyme* (pH <2): Release of secretin, gastric inhibitory polypeptide, cholecystokinin into circulation to decrease HCl acid secretion *Chyme* (pH >3): Release of gastrin from duodenum to increase acid secretion

Elimination

Large Intestine

The large intestine is a hollow, muscular tube around 5 to 6 ft (1.5 to 1.8 m) long and 2 in (5 cm) in diameter. The 4 parts of the large intestine are shown in Fig. 43.2.

The essential functions of the large intestine are water and electrolyte absorption. The large intestine also forms feces and serves as a reservoir for the fecal mass until defecation occurs. Feces are composed of water (75%), bacteria, unabsorbed minerals, undigested foodstuffs, bile pigments, and epithelial cells. The large intestine secretes mucus, which acts as a lubricant and protects the mucosa.

Microorganisms in the colon contribute to digestion by (1) producing vitamin K and some B vitamins and (2) breaking down proteins that are not digested or absorbed in the small intestine into amino acids. Bacteria deaminate the amino acids, resulting in ammonia. Ammonia is carried to the liver, where it is converted to urea. Urea is excreted by the kidneys. Bacteria produce gas that escapes the colon through the anus as *flatulence* or *flatus.* If an infection or antibiotics alter the normal microbiome, an overgrowth of pathogenic bacteria can occur and cause disease.

The large intestine movements are usually slow. However, propulsive (mass movements) peristalsis does occur. Food entering the stomach and duodenum triggers gastrocolic and duodenocolic reflexes, resulting in peristalsis in the colon. These reflexes are more active after the first daily meal and often result in bowel evacuation.

Defecation is a reflex action involving voluntary and involuntary control. Feces in the rectum stimulate sensory nerve endings that produce the desire to defecate. The reflex center for defecation is in the parasympathetic nerve fibers in the sacral part of the spinal cord. These fibers produce contraction of the rectum and relaxation of the internal anal sphincter.

TABLE 43.3 Hormones Controlling GI Secretion and Motility

Hormone	Source	Activating Stimuli	Function
Gastrin	Gastric and duodenal mucosa	Stomach distention, partially digested proteins in pylorus	Stimulates gastric acid secretion and motility. Maintains LES tone.
Cholecystokinin	Duodenal mucosa	Fatty acids and amino acids in small intestine	Contracts gallbladder and relaxes sphincter of Oddi. Allows increased flow of bile into duodenum. Release of pancreatic digestive enzymes.
Gastric inhibitory peptide	Duodenal mucosa	Fatty acids and lipids in small intestine	Inhibits gastric acid secretion and motility.
Secretin	Duodenal mucosa	Acid entering small intestine	Inhibits gastric motility and acid secretion. Stimulates pancreatic bicarbonate secretion.

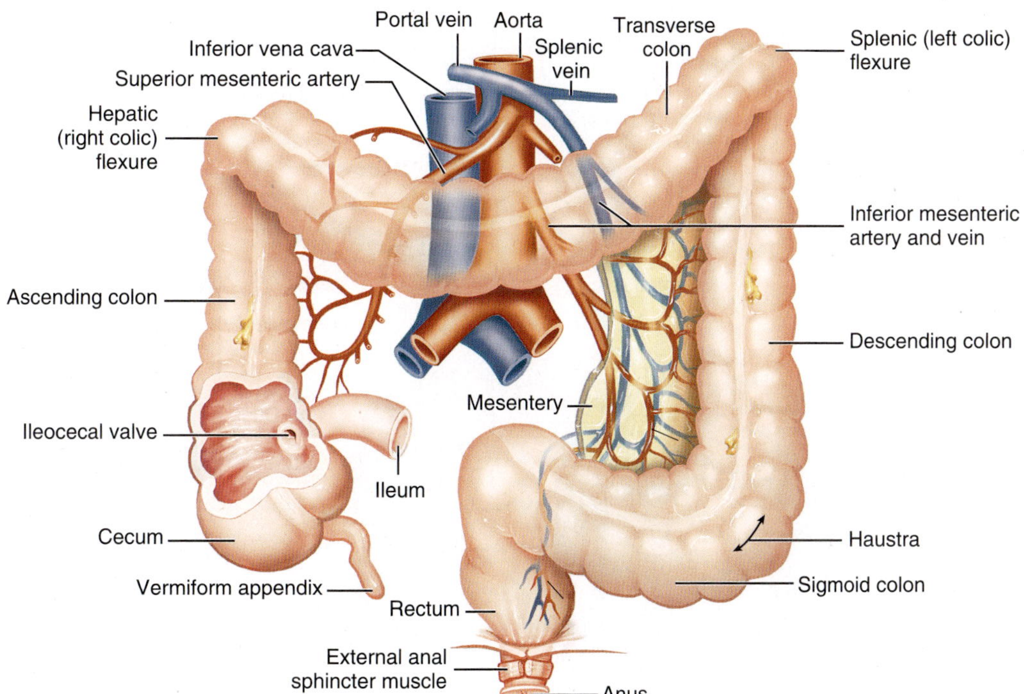

Fig. 43.2 Anatomic locations of the large intestine. (From Patton KT, Thibodeau GA: *Anatomy and physiology,* ed 7, St Louis, 2018, Mosby.)

When a person feels the desire to defecate, they can voluntarily relax the external anal sphincter. An acceptable environment for defecation is usually needed or the urge to defecate will be ignored. If a person suppresses defecation for long periods, problems can occur, such as constipation or fecal impaction.

The **Valsalva maneuver**, often referred to as "bearing down," can promote defecation. During this maneuver, the person inspires deeply and holds the breath, closing the airway, while contracting abdominal muscles and bearing down. This increases intraabdominal and intrathoracic pressures and reduces venous return to the heart. The heart rate temporarily decreases along with a decrease in cardiac output. This results in a transient drop in BP. When the patient relaxes, thoracic pressure falls, resulting in a sudden flow of blood into the heart, increased heart rate, and an immediate rise in BP. The Valsalva maneuver may be contraindicated in patients with a head injury, eye surgery, heart problems, hemorrhoids, abdominal surgery, or liver cirrhosis with portal hypertension.

Liver, Biliary Tract, and Pancreas

Liver

The liver is the largest internal organ in the body, weighing around 3 lb (1.36 kg). It lies in the right epigastric region (Fig. 43.5, later in the chapter). Most of the liver is enclosed in peritoneum. It has a fibrous capsule that divides it into right and left lobes (Fig. 43.3).

The functional units of the liver are lobules. A lobule consists of rows of hepatic cells *(hepatocytes)* arranged in cords that radiate out from a central vein. Capillaries called *sinusoids* lie between the rows of hepatocytes. Sinusoids are lined with **Kupffer cells**. They carry out phagocytic activity, removing bacteria and toxins from the blood. The hepatic cells secrete

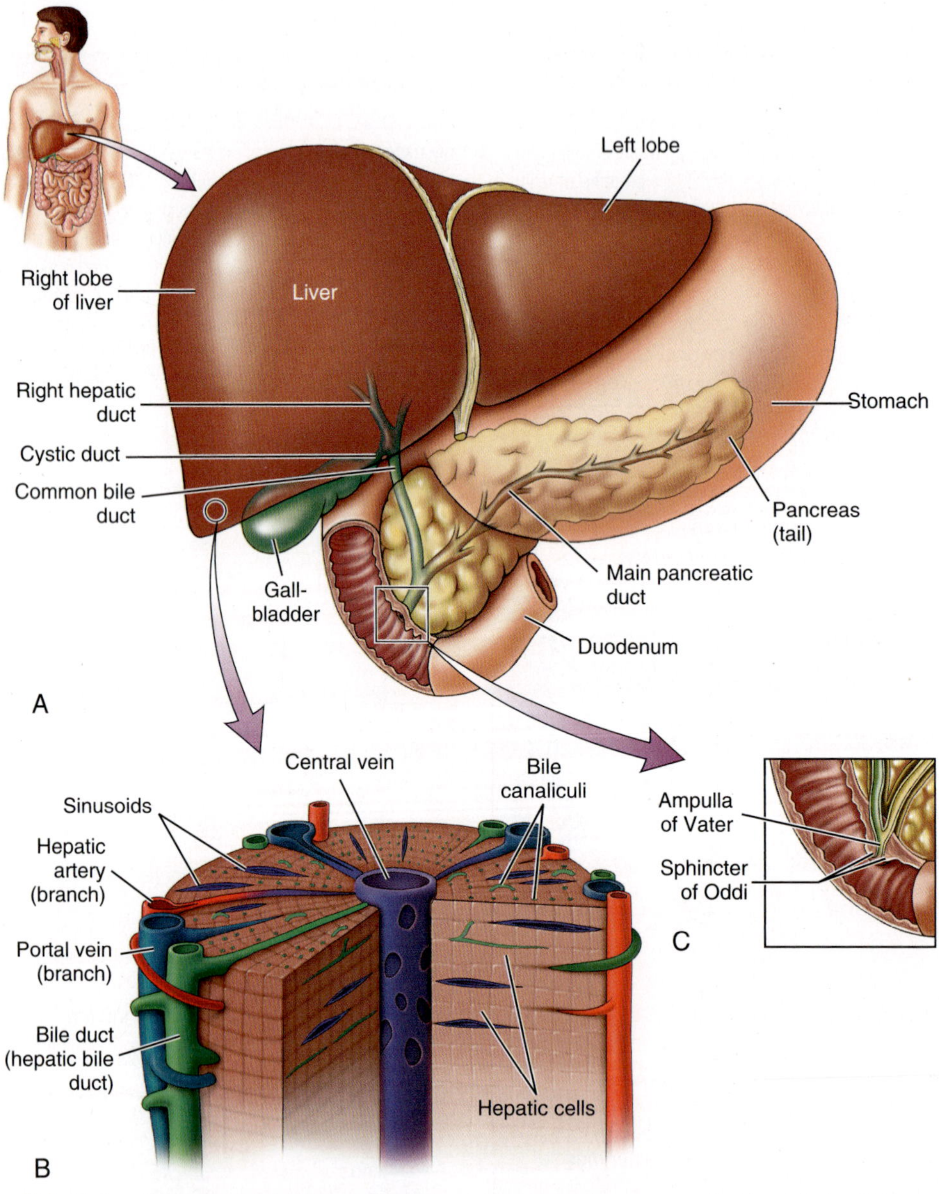

Fig. 43.3 (A) Gross structure of the liver, gallbladder, pancreas, and duct system. (B) Liver lobule. (C) Entrance of the common bile duct into the duodenum.

bile into tiny canals called *canaliculi.* These merge with other canals to form larger, interlobular bile ducts, which unite into the 2 main left and right hepatic ducts.

The liver has a rich blood supply. The portal circulatory system brings blood to the liver from the stomach, intestines, spleen, and pancreas. About 25% of the blood supply comes from the hepatic artery, a branch of the celiac artery. The other 75% comes from the portal vein. The portal vein carries absorbed products of digestion directly to the liver. Once in the liver, the portal vein branches and comes in contact with each lobule.

The liver has many functions. It has metabolic, secretory, vascular, and storage functions (Table 43.4). The hepatic cells constantly make bile. Bile consists of water, cholesterol, bile salts, electrolytes, fatty acids, and bilirubin. It provides the alkaline medium needed for the action of pancreatic lipase. Bile salts are needed for fat emulsification and digestion.

Bilirubin metabolism. The liver constantly makes **bilirubin**, a pigment derived from the breakdown of hemoglobin (Fig. 43.4). When released into the bloodstream, it binds to albumin. This form of bilirubin is called *unconjugated.* It is insoluble in water and transported to the liver. In the liver, unconjugated bilirubin is conjugated with glucuronic acid and excreted in bile into the intestine. *Conjugated* bilirubin is soluble in water. In the intestines, bacterial action reduces bilirubin to stercobilinogen and urobilinogen. Stercobilinogen accounts for the brown color of stool. A small amount of urobilinogen is reabsorbed into the blood. It then is returned to the liver through the portal circulation. There, it is excreted again in the bile or entered into circulation and excreted by the kidneys.

TABLE 43.4 Liver Functions

Function	Description
Metabolic Functions	
Blood clotting	Synthesis of prothrombin (factor I), fibrinogen (factor II), and factors V, VII, IX, and X.
Carbohydrate metabolism	Glycogenesis (conversion of glucose to glycogen), glycogenolysis (process of breaking down glycogen to glucose), gluconeogenesis (formation of glucose from amino acids and fatty acids).
Detoxification	Inactivate drugs and harmful substances and excrete their breakdown products.
Fat metabolism	Synthesis of lipoproteins, breakdown of triglycerides into fatty acids and glycerol, formation of ketone bodies, synthesis of fatty acids from amino acids and glucose, synthesis and breakdown of cholesterol.
Protein metabolism	Synthesis of nonessential amino acids, synthesis of plasma proteins (except gamma globulin), synthesis of clotting factors. Bacteria in colon deaminate amino acids to form ammonia (NH_3), which is then changed to urea (NH_4).
Secretory Functions	
Bile production	Formation of bile, which contains bile salts, bile pigments (mainly bilirubin), and cholesterol.
Bilirubin	Conjugation and secretion of bilirubin.
Vascular Functions	
Blood filtration	Breakdown of old RBCs, WBCs, bacteria, and other particles. Breakdown of hemoglobin from old RBCs to bilirubin and biliverdin.
Blood reservoir	Temporary storage for blood within general circulation.
Storage Functions	
Storage	Store glucose in form of glycogen; vitamins, including fat-soluble (A, D, E, K) and water-soluble (B_1, B_2, cobalamin, folic acid); fatty acids; minerals (iron, copper); and amino acids in form of albumin and β-globulins.

Biliary Tract

The biliary tract consists of the gallbladder and ducts that connect the liver, gallbladder, and duodenum. The gallbladder is a pear-shaped sac found below the liver. Its function is to concentrate and store bile. It holds around 45 mL of bile. The presence of fat in the upper duodenum triggers the release of cholecystokinin, which causes the gallbladder to contract and release bile.

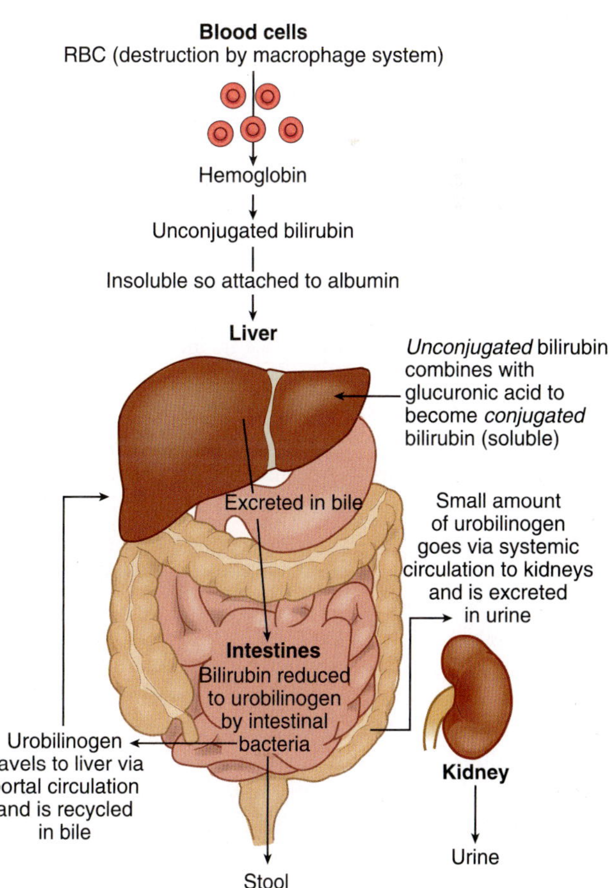

Fig. 43.4 Bilirubin metabolism and conjugation.

The hepatic ducts receive bile from the canaliculi in the liver lobules. The left and right hepatic ducts merge with the cystic duct from the gallbladder to form the common bile duct. Bile moves down the common bile duct to enter the duodenum at the ampulla of Vater (Fig. 43.3). The pancreatic duct also enters the duodenum at this point.

Pancreas

The pancreas is a long, slender gland lying behind the stomach and in front of the first and second lumbar vertebrae. It consists of a head, body, and tail. The peritoneum covers the anterior surface of the pancreas. The pancreas has lobes and lobules. The pancreatic duct extends along the gland and enters the duodenum through the common bile duct at the ampulla of Vater (Fig. 43.3).

The pancreas has exocrine and endocrine functions. The exocrine function contributes to digestion through the production and release of enzymes (Table 43.1). The endocrine function occurs in the islets of Langerhans, whose β cells secrete insulin and amylin; α cells secrete glucagon; δ cells secrete somatostatin; and F cells secrete pancreatic polypeptide.

Gerontologic Considerations: Effects of Aging on the GI System

The process of aging changes the functional ability of the GI system. Age-related changes in the GI system and differences in assessment findings are outlined in Table 43.5.

Many factors can lead to a decrease in appetite and make eating less pleasurable. Caries and periodontal disease can lead to loss of teeth. Taste buds decline in number and the sense of smell lessens, leading to decreased ability to taste. With less saliva, a very dry mouth *(xerostomia)* is common.[1]

Age-related changes in the esophagus include delayed emptying, resulting from smooth muscle weakness; reduced UES opening; and an incompetent LES. Although GI motility decreases with age, secretion and absorption are less affected. The older adult often has a decrease in intrinsic acid and HCl acid secretion *(hypochlorhydria)*.[2]

Chronic constipation affects 30% to 40% of adults over age 60.[3] Factors that increase the risk for constipation include slower peristalsis, anorectal dysfunction, inactivity, decreased fiber intake, inadequate fluid intake, and constipating medications. Neurologic, cognitive, and metabolic problems may play a role. See Chapter 47 for more about constipation.

The liver size decreases after 50 years of age. Age-related enzyme changes in the liver decrease the liver's ability to metabolize drugs and hormones. The pancreas undergoes structural changes, such as fibrosis, fatty acid deposits, and atrophy. Gallbladder diseases increase with age.[4]

Older adults, especially those over 85, are at risk for decreased food intake. The inability to obtain food affects nutrition intake. Economic constraints may reduce the number of fresh fruits and vegetables consumed and thus the amount of fiber. Immobility limits the ability to prepare meals.

CASE STUDY

Patient Introduction

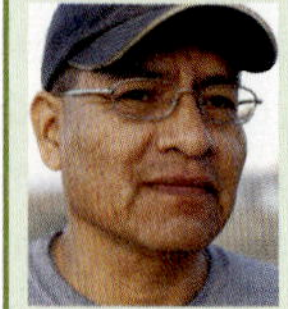
(© iStockphoto/ Thinkstock.)

Patient Profile

L.C. is a 58-year-old Native American male from a Pueblo tribe in northern New Mexico. L.C.'s wife and family drove 50 miles to take him to the Indian Health Service hospital. He comes into the emergency department (ED) doubled over with abdominal pain. He is grimacing and holding his abdomen with both arms. You are working as the triage nurse that morning.

Discussion Questions

1. What are the possible causes for L.C.'s acute abdominal pain?
2. What assessment questions will you ask him?
3. How will you individualize the assessment based on his ethnic/cultural background?

You will learn more about L.C. and his condition as you read this assessment chapter.

Answers available at http://evolve.elsevier.com/Lewis/medsurg.

GI SYSTEM ASSESSMENT

Subjective Data

Important Health Information

Health history. Obtain information about the history or presence of the problems related to GI functioning and fully explore any symptoms. Ask about any abdominal pain, nausea, vomiting, abdominal distention, jaundice, heartburn, dyspepsia, changes in appetite, hematemesis, indigestion, bloating, and trouble swallowing. Review the patient's bowel habits. Ask about diarrhea, constipation, melena, rectal bleeding, hemorrhoids, and excess gas. Has the patient had any GI problems such as reflux, gastritis, hepatitis, colitis, gallstones, peptic ulcer, cancer, diverticuli, or hernias?

Obtain a weight history. Explore in detail any unexplained or unplanned weight loss or gain within the past 6 to 12 months. Discuss any history of chronic dieting and repeated weight loss and gain.

Medications. Obtain a medication history. Note the reason for taking the medication, the dose and frequency, length of time taken, route, its effect, and any side effects. Include information about probiotics and nutrition supplements. Many drugs cause side effects in the GI system. GI problems can affect drug absorption and effectiveness. Antacids and laxatives may affect medication absorption. Ask the patient about laxative or antacid use, including the type and frequency.

Many chemicals, supplements, and drugs may be hepatotoxic (see livertox.nih.gov). They can result in significant harm unless monitored closely. Examples include chronic high doses of acetaminophen and nonsteroidal antiinflammatory drugs (NSAIDs). NSAIDs may also cause upper GI bleeding, with an increasing risk as the person ages. Other medications, such as antibiotics, may change the normal bacterial composition in the GI tract, resulting in diarrhea.

Surgery or other treatments. Obtain information about hospitalizations for any problems related to the GI system.

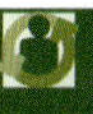

TABLE 43.5 GERONTOLOGIC ASSESSMENT DIFFERENCES

GI System

Expected Aging Changes	Differences in Assessment Findings
Mouth	
Atrophy of gingival tissue	Poor-fitting dentures
↓ Number of taste buds, ↓ sense of smell	↓ Sense of taste (especially salty and sweet)
↓ Volume of saliva	Dry oral mucosa
Gingival retraction	Loss of teeth, dental implants, dentures, difficulty chewing
Esophagus	
↓ LES pressure, ↓ motility	Epigastric distress, dysphagia, potential for hiatal hernia and aspiration
Abdominal Wall	
↓ Number and sensitivity of sensory receptors	Less sensitivity to surface pain
Thinner and less taut	More visible peristalsis, easier palpation of organs
Stomach	
Atrophy of gastric mucosa, ↓ blood flow	Food intolerances, signs of anemia from cobalamin malabsorption, slower gastric emptying
Small Intestines	
Slightly ↓ motility and secretion of most digestive enzymes	Indigestion, slowed intestinal transit, delayed absorption of fat-soluble vitamins
Liver	
↓ Protein synthesis, ↓ ability to regenerate	↓ Drug and hormone metabolism
↓ Size and lowered position	Easier palpation because of lower border extending past costal margin
Large Intestine, Anus, Rectum	
↓ Anal sphincter tone and nerve supply to rectal area	Fecal incontinence
↓ Muscular tone, ↓ motility	Flatulence, abdominal distention, relaxed perineal musculature
↓ Transit time, ↓ sensation to defecation	Constipation, fecal impaction
Pancreas	
Pancreatic ducts distended, ↓ lipase production, ↓ pancreatic reserve	Impaired fat absorption, ↓ glucose tolerance

Record any abdominal or rectal surgery, including the year, reason for surgery, postoperative course, and blood transfusions. Terms related to common GI surgeries are listed in Table 43.6.

TABLE 43.6 GI Surgeries

Procedure	Description
Appendectomy	Removal of appendix
Cholecystectomy	Removal of gallbladder
Choledochojejunostomy	Opening between common bile duct and jejunum
Choledocholithotomy	Opening into common bile duct for removal of stones
Colectomy	Removal of colon
Colostomy	Opening into colon
Esophagoenterostomy	Removal of part of esophagus with segment of colon attached to remaining part
Esophagogastrostomy	Removal of esophagus and anastomosis of remaining part to stomach
Gastrectomy	Removal of stomach
Gastrostomy	Opening into stomach
Glossectomy	Removal of tongue
Hemiglossectomy	Removal of half of tongue
Herniorrhaphy	Repair of a hernia
Ileostomy	Opening into ileum
Mandibulectomy	Removal of mandible
Pyloroplasty	Enlargement and repair of pyloric sphincter area
Vagotomy	Resection of branch of vagus nerve

Functional Health Patterns

Key questions to ask patients with a GI problem are outlined in Table 43.7.

Health perception–health management. Ask about any health practices related to the GI system. This includes maintaining normal body weight, proper dental care, adequate nutrition, and effective elimination habits.

Ask about recent foreign travel with possible exposure to hepatitis or parasitic infestation. Explore any sexual and drug use behaviors that may increase risk for hepatitis exposure. Determine whether the patient has received hepatitis A and B vaccination.

Assess the patient for habits that affect GI functioning. Drinking alcohol in large quantities or for long periods has harmful effects on the stomach mucosa.[5] Chronic alcohol exposure causes fatty infiltration of the liver and liver damage, leading to cirrhosis and liver cancer. Obtain a history of cigarette smoking. Nicotine is irritating to the GI tract mucosa. Cigarette smoking is related to GI cancers (especially mouth and esophageal cancer), esophagitis, and ulcers. Smoking delays the healing of ulcers.

Family history is important. About one-third of cases of colorectal cancer (CRC) occur in patients with a family history. Because of the relationship between CRC and breast cancer, ask about a history of either type of cancer in the family.

Nutritional-metabolic. A thorough nutrition assessment is essential. Take a diet history and ask about content and amount or portion size. Food preferences and preparation may vary by culture and religion. Open-ended questions allow patients to express beliefs and feelings about the diet. For example, you can say, "Please tell me about your food and beverage intake over the past 24 hours." You can use a 24-hour diet recall to analyze the adequacy of the diet. Help the patient recall the

TABLE 43.7 HEALTH HISTORY

GI System

Health Perception–Health Management

- Describe any measures used to treat GI symptoms such as diarrhea or constipation.
- Do you smoke?[a] Do you drink alcohol?[a]
- Are you exposed to any chemicals on a regular basis?[a] Have you been exposed in the past?[a]
- Have you recently traveled outside the United States?[a]

Nutritional-Metabolic

- Describe your usual daily food and fluid intake.
- Do you take any vitamin or mineral supplements?[a]
- Have you had any changes in appetite or food tolerance?[a]
- Has there been any weight change in the past 6–12 months?[a]
- Are you allergic to any foods?[a]

Elimination

- Describe the frequency and time of day you have bowel movements. What is the consistency of the bowel movement?
- Do you use laxatives or enemas?[a] If so, how often?
- Have there been any recent changes in your bowel pattern?[a]
- Do you have any pain with bowel movements or pain relieved by bowel movements?
- Describe any skin problems caused by GI problems.
- Do you need any assistive equipment, such as ostomy equipment, raised toilet seat, or commode?

Activity-Exercise

- Do you have limitations in mobility that make it hard for you to obtain and prepare food?[a]

Sleep-Rest

- Do you have any problem sleeping because of a GI problem?[a]
- Are you awakened by symptoms such as gas, abdominal pain, diarrhea, or heartburn?[a]

Cognitive-Perceptual

- Have you had any change in taste or smell that have affected your appetite?[a]
- Do you have any heat or cold sensitivity that affects eating?[a]
- Does pain interfere with food preparation, appetite, or chewing?[a]
- Do pain medications cause constipation, diarrhea, or appetite suppression?[a]

Self-Perception–Self-Concept

- Describe any changes in your weight that have affected how you feel about yourself.
- Have you had any changes in normal elimination that have affected how you feel about yourself?[a]
- Do you have any symptoms of GI disease caused physical changes that are a problem for you?[a]

Role-Relationship

- Describe the impact of any GI problem on your usual roles and relationships.
- Have any changes in elimination affected your relationships?[a]
- Do you live alone? Describe how your family or others assist you with your GI problems.

Sexuality-Reproductive

- Describe the effect of your GI problem on your sexual activity.

Coping–Stress Tolerance

- Do you have GI symptoms in response to stressful or emotional situations?[a]
- Describe how you deal with any GI symptoms that result.

Value-Belief

- Describe any cultural or religious beliefs about food and food preparation that may influence the treatment of your GI problem.

[a]If yes, describe.

preceding day's food intake, including early morning and nighttime intake, snacks, and liquids. Then evaluate the diet in relation to recommended servings for diet intake using a guide such as MyPlate (www.choosemyplate.gov). A 1-week recall may provide more information on usual diet patterns. Compare weekday and weekend diet intake patterns in relation to the quality and quantity of food.

Ask the patient about the use of sugar and salt substitutes, caffeine intake, and amount of fluid and fiber intake. Note any changes in appetite, food tolerance, and weight. Anorexia and weight loss may indicate cancer or inflammation. Decreased food intake can be the consequence of economic problems or depression.

Ask about food allergies and intolerances, including lactose and gluten. Have the patient describe the allergic response and any GI symptoms.

Elimination. Elicit a detailed account of the patient's bowel elimination pattern. Note the frequency, time of day, and usual stool consistency. Ask about the presence of pain with bowel movements, if bowel movements relieve pain, and any recent changes in bowel patterns. Explore the use of laxatives and enemas, including type, frequency, and results. Assess for access to a toilet. Identify the use of and access to items such as a commode or ostomy supplies.

Record the amount and type of fluid and fiber intake. These influence the frequency and consistency of stools. Inadequate fiber intake can be associated with constipation. Look for any association between a skin and GI problem. Food allergies can cause skin lesions, pruritus, and edema. Diarrhea can result in redness, irritation, and pain in the perianal area. External drainage systems, such as an ileostomy or ileal conduit, may cause local skin irritation.

Activity-exercise. Activity and exercise affect GI motility. Immobility is a risk factor for constipation. Assess ambulatory status to determine whether the patient can secure and prepare food. If the patient is unable to do these tasks, see if a family member or an outside agency is meeting this need. Note any limitation in the ability to feed oneself.

Sleep-rest. Ask the patient if GI symptoms affect sleep or rest. Nausea, vomiting, diarrhea, indigestion, and bloating can cause sleep problems. For example, a patient with gastroesophageal reflux disease (GERD) may wake with burning epigastric pain.

The patient may have a bedtime ritual that involves a specific food or beverage. Herbal teas may be sleep inducing. Note the patient's routines and comply with these whenever possible to avoid sleeplessness. Hunger can prevent sleep. A light, easily digested snack may help.

Cognitive-perceptual. Sensory changes can result in problems related to acquiring, preparing, and ingesting food. Changes in taste or smell can affect appetite and eating pleasure. Vertigo can make shopping or standing at a stove difficult and dangerous. Heat or cold sensitivity can make some foods painful to eat. Problems in expressive communication limit the patient's ability to state personal food preferences.

Acute and chronic pain influence intake. Behaviors associated with pain include avoiding activity, fatigue, and disrupted eating patterns. For patients receiving opioid medications, assess for decreased appetite, constipation, nausea, and sedation.

Self-perception–self-concept. Many GI and nutrition problems affect self-perception. Overweight and underweight people may have problems related to self-esteem and body image. Repeated attempts to achieve a personally acceptable weight can be discouraging and depressing for some people. The way a person recounts a weight history can alert you to potential problems in this area.

The need for external devices to manage elimination, such as a colostomy or an ileostomy, may be challenging for some patients. The patient's willingness to engage in self-care and to discuss this situation provides you with valuable information related to body image and self-esteem.

Physical changes from advanced liver disease can be disturbing for patients. Jaundice, muscle wasting, and ascites cause significant changes in external appearance. Assess the patient's attitude about these changes.

Sexuality-reproductive. Changes related to sexuality and reproductive status can result from problems of the GI system. For example, obesity, jaundice, and ascites could decrease the acceptance of a potential sexual partner. An ostomy can affect a patient's confidence related to sexual activity.

Anorexia can affect the reproductive status of female patients. Obesity leads to reduced fertility and increased miscarriage rates in women.

Coping–stress tolerance. Determine what is stressful for the patient and what coping mechanisms the patient uses. Factors outside the GI tract can influence its functioning. Psychologic and emotional factors, such as stress and anxiety, influence GI functioning in many people. Stress can manifest as anorexia, nausea, epigastric and abdominal pain, or diarrhea. It can worsen some GI problems, such as peptic ulcer disease, irritable bowel syndrome, and IBD.

Value-belief. Assess spiritual, religious, and cultural beliefs about food and food preparation. When possible, respect these preferences. Determine whether any value or belief could interfere with planned interventions. For example, if the patient with anemia is a vegetarian, you will need to consider how to increase their intake of iron-rich foods other than meat.

CASE STUDY

Subjective Data

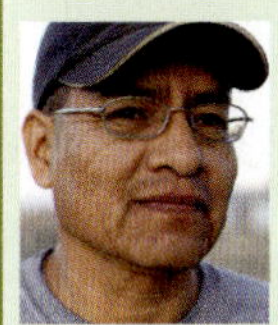

(© iStockphoto/Thinkstock.)

A focused subjective assessment of L.C. revealed the following information:

- ***Health History:*** Negative history for medical or surgical problems.
- ***Medications:*** None.
- ***Health Perception–Health Management:*** L.C. states he has not been feeling well for the past several weeks. He feels weak and fatigues easily. Denies exposure to chemicals. No recent travel outside of the United States. Smokes 1 pack of cigarettes per day for 20 years. Drinks 3 to 4 bottles of beer per day.
- ***Nutritional-Metabolic:*** L.C. is 5 ft, 9 in tall and weighs 140 lb (BMI: 20.7 kg/m^2). States has been losing weight over the past several months and does not have an appetite. No food allergies.
- ***Elimination:*** Reports alternating episodes of constipation and diarrhea. He noticed some bright red blood in stools. Has not had a bowel movement for 4 days.
- ***Cognitive-Perceptual:*** Rates pain as a 9 on a scale of 0 to 10. States pain comes and goes in waves. Prefers to lie still with knees flexed and drawn into his abdomen.

Discussion Questions

1. Which subjective assessment findings concern you most?
2. Based on these subjective assessment findings, what should you include in the physical assessment? What would you be looking for?
3. What would be your priority assessment?

You will learn more about physical assessment of the GI system in the next section.

Answers available at http://evolve.elsevier.com/Lewis/medsurg.

Objective Data

Physical Assessment

Findings of a normal physical assessment of the GI system are shown in Table 43.8. Table 43.9 outlines assessment abnormalities. A *focused assessment* (Box 43.1) evaluates the status of previously identified GI problems and monitors for signs of new problems.

Mouth. Inspect the mouth for symmetry, color, and size. Observe for abnormalities, cracking, ulcers, or fissures. The dorsum (top) of the tongue should have a thin white coating. The undersurface should be smooth. Observe for any lesions. Using a tongue blade, inspect the buccal mucosa. Note the color, any areas of pigmentation, and any lesions. Dark-skinned persons normally have patchy areas of pigmentation. Palpate any suspicious areas. Note ulcers, nodules, indurations, and areas of tenderness.

In assessing the teeth and gums, look for caries, loose teeth, abnormal shape and position of teeth, and swelling, bleeding, discoloration, or gingival inflammation. Note any distinctive breath odor. Pay attention to dentures (e.g., fit, condition). Ask patients with dentures to remove them during an oral exam to allow for good visualization and palpation of the area.

TABLE 43.8 Normal Physical Assessment of GI System

Mouth
- Moist and pink lips
- Pink and moist buccal mucosa and gingivae without plaques or lesions
- Teeth in good repair
- Protrusion of tongue in midline without deviation or twitches
- Pink uvula (in midline), soft palate, tonsils, and posterior pharynx
- Swallows smoothly without coughing or gagging

Abdomen
- Flat without masses or scars. No bruises
- Bowel sounds present in all quadrants
- No abdominal tenderness; nonpalpable liver and spleen
- Liver 10 cm in right midclavicular line
- General tympany

Anus
- Absence of lesions, fissures, and hemorrhoids
- Good sphincter tone
- Rectal walls smooth and soft
- No masses
- Stool soft, brown, and heme negative

BOX 43.1 FOCUSED ASSESSMENT

GI System

Use this checklist to make sure the key assessment steps have been done.

Subjective

Ask the patient about any of the following and note responses:

Loss of appetite
Abdominal pain
Changes in stools (color, blood, consistency, frequency, pain)
Nausea, vomiting
Painful swallowing

Objective: Diagnostic

Check the following results for critical values:

Endoscopy
CT scan
Radiologic series: upper GI, lower GI
Stool for occult blood or ova and parasites
Liver function tests

Objective: Physical Assessment

Inspect

Skin for color, scars, petechiae, and other lesions
Abdominal contour for symmetry and distention
Perianal area for intact skin, hemorrhoids

Auscultate

Bowel sounds

Palpate

Abdominal quadrants using light touch
Abdominal quadrants using a deep technique

Inspect the pharynx by tilting the patient's head back and depressing the tongue with a tongue blade. Observe the tonsils, uvula, soft palate, and anterior and posterior pillars. Tell the patient to say "ah." The uvula and soft palate should rise and remain midline. Assess the ability to swallow.

Abdomen. We use 2 systems to anatomically describe the surface of the abdomen. One system divides the abdomen into 4 quadrants by a perpendicular line from the sternum to the pubic bone and a horizontal line across the abdomen at the umbilicus (Fig. 43.5A and Table 43.10). The other system divides the abdomen into 9 regions (Fig. 43.5B). We often assess only the epigastric, umbilical, and suprapubic or hypogastric regions.

For the abdominal assessment, good lighting should shine across the abdomen. The patient should be supine and as relaxed as possible. To help relax the abdominal muscles, have the patient slightly flex the knees and raise the head of the bed slightly. The patient should have an empty bladder. Use warm hands when doing the abdominal assessment to avoid eliciting muscle guarding. Ask the patient to breathe slowly through the mouth.

Inspection. Assess the abdomen for skin changes (color, texture, scars, striae, dilated veins, rashes, lesions), umbilicus (location and contour), symmetry, and contour (flat, rounded [convex], concave, protuberant, distended). Note observable hernias or masses. Is there any movement (pulsations, peristalsis)? A normal aortic pulsation may be seen in the epigastric area. Look across the abdomen tangentially (across the abdomen in a line) for peristalsis. Peristalsis is not normally visible in an adult. It may be visible in a very thin person.

Auscultation. When you examine the abdomen, auscultate before percussion and palpation because these latter procedures may alter the bowel sounds. Use the diaphragm of the stethoscope to auscultate bowel sounds because they are high pitched. Use the bell of the stethoscope to detect lower pitched sounds. Warm the stethoscope in your hands before auscultating to help prevent abdominal muscle contraction. Listen in the epigastrium and in all 4 quadrants. Start in the right lower quadrant because bowel sounds are normally present there. Listen for bowel sounds for at least 2 minutes. Do not count bowel sounds. Determine whether they are normal, hypoactive, or hyperactive.

The frequency and intensity of bowel sounds vary depending on the phase of digestion. Normal sounds are high pitched and gurgling. Stomach growling or loud gurgles *(borborygmi)* indicate hyperperistalsis. The bowel sounds are high pitched (rushes and tinkling) when the intestines are under tension, as in intestinal obstruction. Listen for decreased or absent bowel sounds. If you are patient and listen for several minutes, you will often find the bowel sounds are not absent but are hypoactive. If you do not hear bowel sounds, note the amount of time you listened in each quadrant without hearing bowel sounds.

Listen for vascular sounds. A *bruit,* best heard with the bell of the stethoscope, is a swishing or buzzing sound and indicates turbulent blood flow. Normally, you should not hear aortic bruits.

TABLE 43.9 ASSESSMENT ABNORMALITIES

GI System

Finding	Description	Possible Etiology and Significance
Mouth		
Acute marginal gingivitis	Friable, edematous, painful, bleeding gingivae	Irritation from ill-fitting dentures or orthodontic appliances, calcium deposits on teeth, food impaction
Candidiasis	White, curdlike lesions surrounded by erythematous mucosa	Candida albicans
Cheilitis	Inflammation of lips (usually lower) with fissuring, scaling, crusting	Often unknown
Cheilosis	Softening, fissuring, and cracking of lips at angles of mouth	Riboflavin deficiency
Geographic tongue	Scattered red, smooth (loss of papillae) areas on dorsum of tongue	Unknown
Glossitis	Reddened, ulcerated, swollen tongue	Exposure to streptococci, irritation, injury, vitamin B deficiencies, anemia
Herpes simplex	Vesicular lesion	Herpesvirus
Leukoplakia	Thickened white patches	Premalignant lesion
Pyorrhea	Recessed gingivae, purulent pockets	Periodontitis
Smooth tongue	Red, slick appearance	Cobalamin deficiency
Ulcer, plaque on lips or in mouth	Sore or lesion	Cancer, viral infections
Esophagus and Stomach		
Dyspepsia	Burning or indigestion	Peptic ulcer disease, gallbladder disease
Dysphagia	Difficulty swallowing, sensation of food sticking in esophagus	Esophageal problems, cancer of esophagus
Eructation	Belching	Various GI problems, GERD, dyspepsia, rumination
Hematemesis	Vomiting of blood	Esophageal varices, bleeding peptic ulcer
Nausea and vomiting	Feeling of impending vomiting, expulsion of gastric contents through mouth	GI infections, common manifestation of many GI problems, stress, fear, and pathologic conditions
Odynophagia	Painful swallowing	Cancer of esophagus, esophagitis
Pyrosis	Heartburn, burning in epigastric or substernal area	Hiatal hernia, esophagitis, incompetent LES
Abdomen		
Absence of liver dullness	Tympany on percussion	Air from viscus (e.g., perforated ulcer)
Absent bowel sounds	No bowel sounds on auscultation	Peritonitis, paralytic ileus, obstruction
Ascites	Accumulated fluid within abdominal cavity, eversion of umbilicus (usually)	Peritoneal inflammation, heart failure, metastatic cancer, cirrhosis
Borborygmi	Waves of loud, gurgling sounds	Hyperactive bowel from eating
Bruit	Humming or swishing sound heard through stethoscope over vessel	Partial arterial obstruction (narrowing of vessel), turbulent flow (aneurysm)
Distention	Excessive gas accumulation, enlarged abdomen, generalized tympany	Obstruction, paralytic ileus
Hepatomegaly	Enlargement of liver, liver edge >1–2 cm below costal margin	Metastatic cancer, hepatitis, venous congestion, cardiac congestion
Hernia	Bulge or nodule in abdomen, usually appearing on straining	Inguinal (in inguinal canal), femoral (in femoral canal), umbilical (herniation of umbilicus), diastasis rectus (deformity) or incisional (defect in muscles after surgery)
Hyperresonance	Loud, tinkling rushes	Intestinal obstruction
Masses	Lump on palpation	Tumors, cysts
Nodular liver	Enlarged, hard liver with irregular edge or surface	Cirrhosis, focal nodular hyperplasia, cancer
Rebound tenderness	Sudden pain when fingers withdrawn quickly	Peritoneal inflammation, appendicitis
Splenomegaly	Enlarged spleen	Chronic leukemia, hemolytic states, portal hypertension, some infections
Rectum and Anus		
Fissure	Ulceration in anal canal	Straining, irritation
Hemorrhoids	Thrombosed veins in rectum and anus (internal or external)	Portal hypertension, chronic constipation, prolonged sitting or standing, pregnancy
Mass	Firm, nodular edge	Tumor, cancer
Melena	Abnormal, black, tarry stool containing digested blood	Cancer, bleeding in upper GI tract from ulcers, varices
Pilonidal cyst	Opening of sinus tract, cyst in midline just above coccyx	Probably congenital
Steatorrhea	Fatty, frothy, foul-smelling stool	Chronic pancreatitis, biliary obstruction, malabsorption problems
Tenesmus	Painful and ineffective straining, sense of incomplete evacuation	Inflammatory bowel disease, irritable bowel syndrome, diarrhea from GI infection (e.g., food poisoning)

TABLE 43.10 **Structures Located in Abdominal Regions**

Right Upper Quadrant	Left Upper Quadrant	Right Lower Quadrant	Left Lower Quadrant
• Liver • Gallbladder • Pylorus • Duodenum • Head of pancreas • Right adrenal gland • Portion of right kidney • Hepatic flexure of colon • Portion of ascending and transverse colon	• Left lobe of liver • Spleen • Stomach • Body of pancreas • Left adrenal gland • Portion of left kidney • Splenic flexure of colon • Portion of transverse and descending colon	• Lower pole of right kidney • Cecum and appendix • Portion of ascending colon • Bladder (if distended) • Right ovary and fallopian tube • Uterus (if enlarged) • Right spermatic cord • Right ureter	• Lower pole of left kidney • Sigmoid flexure • Part of descending colon • Bladder (if distended) • Left ovary and fallopian tube • Uterus (if enlarged) • Left spermatic cord • Left ureter

Percussion. The purpose of percussing the abdomen is to estimate the size of the liver and spleen and determine the presence of fluid, distention, and masses. Sound waves vary according to the density of underlying tissues. Air produces a higher pitched, hollow sound termed *tympany.* Fluid or masses produce a short, high-pitched sound with little resonance termed *dullness.* Lightly percuss all 4 quadrants of the abdomen and assess the distribution of tympany and dullness (Fig. 43.6). Tympany is the predominant percussion sound of the abdomen.

To percuss the liver, start below the umbilicus in the right midclavicular line and percuss lightly upward until you hear dullness. This is the lower border of the liver. Next, start at the nipple line in the right midclavicular line and percuss downward between ribs to the area of dullness indicating the upper border of the liver. Measure the height or vertical space between the 2 borders to determine the size of the liver. The normal range of liver height in the right midclavicular line is 2.4 to 5 in (6 to 12.7 cm).

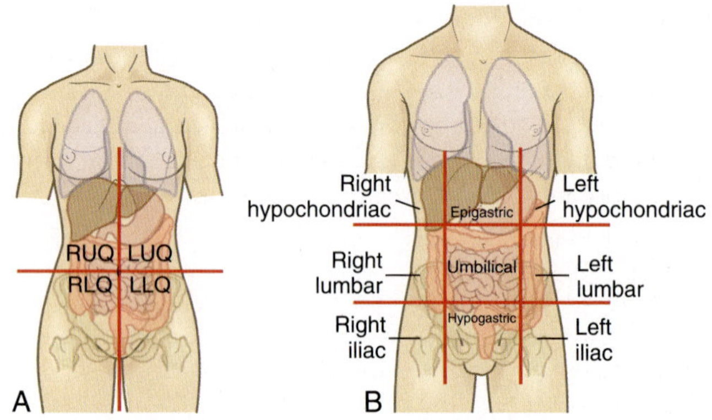

Fig. 43.5 (A) Abdominal quadrants. (B) Abdominal regions. *LLQ,* Left lower quadrant; *LUQ,* left upper quadrant; *RLQ,* right lower quadrant; *RUQ,* right upper quadrant.

Palpation. Use palpation to assess the abdominal organs and detect any tenderness, distention, masses, or fluid. Palpate any areas in which the patient reports tenderness last. As you palpate, observe the patient's facial expression because it will provide nonverbal cues of discomfort or pain.

Begin with light palpation. Note any tenderness, muscular resistance, masses, and swelling. Keep your fingers together and press gently with the pads of the fingertips, depressing the abdominal wall about 0.4 in (1 cm). Use smooth movements and palpate all quadrants.

Use *deep palpation* to delineate abdominal organs and masses. Use the palmar surfaces of your fingers to press more deeply. Again, palpate all quadrants. Note the location, size, and shape of masses, as well as the presence of tenderness. Another method for deep abdominal palpation is the 2-hand method. Place one hand on top of the other and apply pressure to the bottom hand with the fingers of the top hand. With the fingers of the bottom hand, feel for organs and masses. Practice both methods of palpation to determine which is most effective.

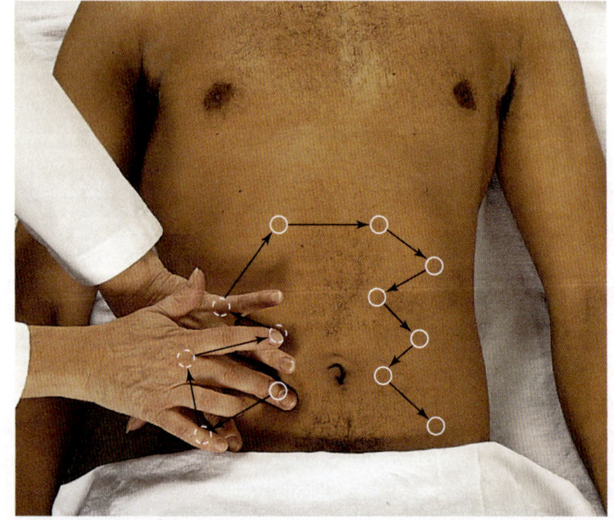

Fig. 43.6 Technique for percussion of the abdomen. Moving clockwise, percuss lightly in all 4 quadrants. (From Jarvis C: *Physical examination and health assessment,* ed 8, St Louis, 2020, Saunders.)

Check a problem area on the abdomen for rebound tenderness by pressing in slowly and firmly over the painful site. Withdraw the palpating fingers quickly. Pain on withdrawal of the fingers indicates peritoneal inflammation. Because assessing for rebound tenderness may produce pain and severe muscle spasm, it should be done at the end of the assessment and only by an experienced practitioner.

To palpate the liver, place your left hand behind the patient to support the right eleventh and twelfth ribs (Fig. 43.7). The patient may relax on your hand. Press the left hand forward and place the right hand on the right abdomen lateral to the rectus muscle. The fingertips should be below the lower border of liver dullness and pointed toward the right costal margin. Gently press in and up. The patient should take a deep breath with the abdomen so the liver drops and is in a better position for palpation. Try to feel the liver edge as it comes down to the fingertips. During inspiration, the liver edge should feel firm, sharp, and smooth. Describe the surface and contour and any tenderness. If the patient has chronic obstructive pulmonary disease, large lungs, or a low diaphragm, the liver may be palpated 0.4 to 0.8 in (1 to 2 cm) below the right costal margin.

To palpate the spleen, move to the patient's left side. Place your right hand under the patient, and support and press the left lower rib cage forward. Place your left hand below the left costal margin and press it in toward the spleen. Ask the patient to breathe deeply. The fingertips can feel the tip or edge of an enlarged spleen. The normal spleen size range is about 5 in long (12.7 cm), 3 in wide (7.6 cm), and 1.5 in (3.8 cm) thick. It is normally not palpable. If it is palpable, do not continue, because manual compression of an enlarged spleen may cause it to rupture.

Rectum and anus. Inspect perianal and anal areas for color, texture, masses, rashes, scars, erythema, fissures, and external hemorrhoids. Palpate any masses or unusual areas with a gloved hand.

For the digital examination of the rectum, place a gloved, lubricated index finger against the anus while having the patient gently bear down (Valsalva maneuver). Then, as the sphincter relaxes, insert the finger. Point the finger toward the umbilicus. Try to get the patient to relax. Insert the finger into the rectum as far as possible and palpate all surfaces. Assess any nodules, tenderness, or irregularities. Use the gloved finger to remove a stool sample and check it for occult blood. However, a single guaiac-based fecal occult blood test has limited sensitivity in detecting CRC.

CASE STUDY

Objective Data: Physical Assessment

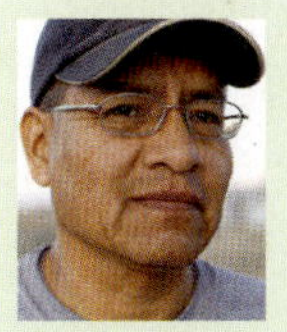

(© iStockphoto/ Thinkstock.)

A focused assessment of L.C. reveals the following: BP 120/74, HR 110, respiratory rate 24, temperature 100.4°F (43°C). Abdomen firm and slightly distended. High-pitched bowel sounds in upper quadrants. No bowel sounds auscultated in left lower quadrant. Mild abdominal palpation elicits pain.

Discussion Questions

1. Which physical assessment findings concern you most?
2. What diagnostic studies do you think may be ordered for L.C.?

You will learn more about diagnostic studies related to the GI system in the next section.

Answers available at http://evolve.elsevier.com/Lewis/medsurg.

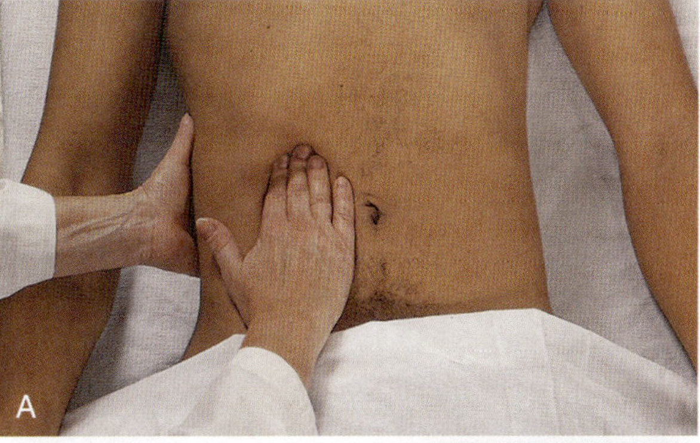

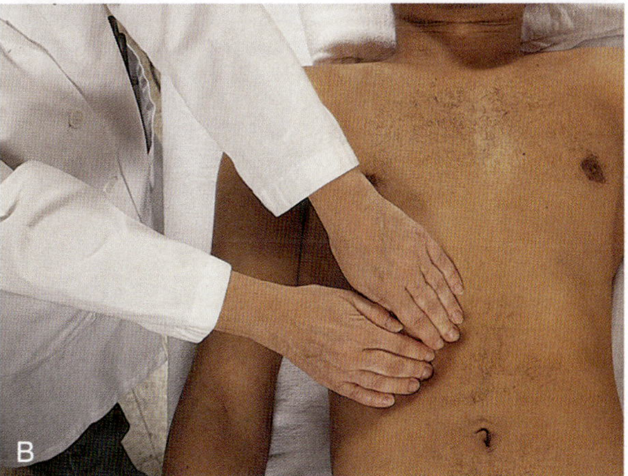

Fig. 43.7 (A) Technique for liver palpation. (B) Alternative technique to palpate liver with fingers hooked over the costal region. (From Jarvis C: *Physical examination and health assessment,* ed 8, St Louis, 2020, Saunders.)

DIAGNOSTIC STUDIES

Table 43.11 describes select laboratory studies related to GI problems. LFTs are blood studies that reflect hepatic disease. Table 43.12 describes common LFTs. Table 43.13 presents common diagnostic studies of the GI system. Select studies are described in more detail here.

Many GI diagnostic studies require (1) measures to cleanse the GI tract and (2) ingestion or injection of a contrast medium or a radiopaque tracer. When preparing the patient, it is important to ask about any known allergies to drugs, iodine, shellfish, or contrast media. Often, the patient has a series of GI diagnostic tests done. Monitor the patient closely to avoid problems, such as dehydration from prolonged fluid restriction and diarrhea from bowel-cleansing procedures. Ensure adequate hydration and nutrition during the testing period. Adjustments may be needed during the preparation, especially for those with certain health problems (e.g., diabetes). Consider any physical limitations and pressure points when positioning a patient during testing.

Radiologic Studies

Upper GI Series

An upper GI series with small bowel follow-through provides visualization of the oropharyngeal area, esophagus, stomach,

TABLE 43.11 Laboratory Studies

GI System

Test	Reference Interval	Description and Purpose
Blood Studies		
Amylase	60–120 U/L (30–220 U/L)	Enzyme secreted by pancreas. Important in diagnosing acute pancreatitis. Level peaks in 24 h and then returns to normal in 48–72 h
Gastrin	25–100 pg/mL when fasting	Hormone secreted by cells of the antrum of the stomach, the duodenum, and the pancreatic islets of Langerhans
Lipase	0–160 U/L	Enzyme secreted by pancreas. Important in diagnosing pancreatitis. Level stays higher longer than serum amylase in acute pancreatitis
Fecal Tests		
Fecal analysis	Note form, consistency, and color. Specimen examined for mucus, blood, pus, parasites, and fat content	Keep diet free of red meat for 24–48 h before occult blood test
Fecal DNA testing	Negative	Detects shredded cell debris from polyps, adenomas, and cancers
Fecal occult blood	Negative	Detects blood in stool related to the presence of inflammatory bowel disease, diverticulosis, ulcers, cancer, and other GI problems
Stool culture	Normal intestinal flora	Tests for the presence of bacteria, including *C. difficile*

TABLE 43.12 Liver Function Tests

Test	Reference Interval	Description and Purpose
Bile Formation and Excretion		
Serum bilirubin		Measures liver's ability to conjugate and excrete bilirubin, distinguishing between unconjugated (indirect) and conjugated (direct) bilirubin in plasma
• Total	0.3–1.0 mg/dL (5.1–17 μmol/L)	Measures direct and indirect total bilirubin
• Direct	0.1–0.3 mg/dL (1.7–5.1 μmol/L)	Measures conjugated bilirubin. High in obstructive jaundice
• Indirect	0.2–0.8 mg/dL (3.4–12 μmol/L)	Measures unconjugated bilirubin. High in liver and hemolytic problems
Urine bilirubin	0 or negative	Measures urine excretion of conjugated bilirubin
Hemostatic Function		
Prothrombin time (PT)	11–12.5 s	Determination of prothrombin activity
Vitamin K	0.1–2.2 ng/mL (0.22–4.88 nmol/L)	Essential cofactor for many clotting factors
Lipid Metabolism		
Cholesterol (serum)	200 mg/dL (<5.2 mmol/L), varying with age	Synthesized and excreted by liver. High in biliary obstruction. Low in cirrhosis and malnutrition
Protein Metabolism		
α-Fetoprotein	<10 ng/mL (<10 mcg/L)	Sign of liver cancer
Ammonia	10–80 mcg/dL (6–47 μmol N/L)	Conversion of ammonia to urea normally occurs in liver. Increase can result in hepatic encephalopathy due to cirrhosis
Protein (serum)	*Albumin:* 3.5–5.0 g/dL (35–50 g/L) *Globulin:* 2.3–3.4 g/dL (23–34 g/L) *Total protein:* 6.4–8.3 g/dL (64–83 g/L)	Measures serum proteins made by liver
Serum Enzymes		
Alanine aminotransferase (ALT)	4–36 U/L	High in liver damage and inflammation
Alkaline phosphatase (ALP)	30–120 U/L (0.5–2.0 μkat/L)	Originates from bone and liver. Levels rise when excretion is impaired because of biliary tract obstruction
γ-Glutamyl transpeptidase (GGT)	Male and female: >45: 8–38 U/L Female: <45: 5–27 U/L	High in hepatitis, cholestatic liver diseases and alcoholic liver diseases. More sensitive for liver dysfunction than ALP
Aspartate aminotransferase (AST)	0–35 U/L (0.0–0.58 μkat/L)	High in liver damage and inflammation

TABLE 43.13 Diagnostic Studies

GI System

Study	Description and Purpose	Nursing Responsibility
Endoscopy		
Colonoscopy	Visualize entire colon up to ileocecal valve with flexible fiberoptic scope. Patient's position is changed frequently during procedure to assist with advancement of scope to cecum. Diagnose or detect inflammatory bowel disease, polyps, tumors, and diverticulosis and dilate strictures. Allows for biopsy and removal of polyps without laparotomy	*Before:* Bowel preparation prior varies depending on HCP. Should avoid fiber for up to 72 h prior, then either a clear or full liquid diet 24 h before. Bowel cleansing should follow a split-dose regimen. The evening before the procedure, the patient should use a cleansing solution. The second dose should begin 4–6 h before the procedure. A split-dose regimen started early morning the day of a procedure provides better cleansing for patients scheduled in the afternoon. Encourage the patient to drink all the solution. Stools will be clear or clear yellow liquid when the colon is clean. Bisacodyl tablets or suppositories may be given before the cleansing solution to remove the bulk of the stool. Explain to patient that a flexible scope will be inserted while patient in side-lying position and sedation will be given. *After:* May have abdominal cramps caused by stimulation of peristalsis because the bowel is constantly inflated with air during procedure. Teach patients about pain afterward. Tell patients if pain lasts longer than 24 h to notify HCP. Check vital signs. Assess for rectal bleeding and perforation (e.g., malaise, abdominal distention, tenesmus).
Endoscopic retrograde cholangiopancreatography (ERCP)	Fiberoptic endoscope (using fluoroscopy) is orally inserted into descending duodenum. Then common bile and pancreatic ducts are cannulated. Contrast medium is injected into ducts to allow for direct visualization of structures. Can retrieve a gallstone from distal common bile duct, dilate strictures, biopsy, and diagnose pseudocysts	*Before:* Explain procedure. Keep NPO 8 h before. Ensure consent form is signed. Give sedation immediately before and during procedure. Give ordered antibiotics. *After:* Check vital signs. Assess for perforation, pancreatitis, or infection. Keep NPO until gag reflex returns.
Esophagogastroduodenoscopy (EGD)	Visualize mucosal lining of esophagus, stomach, and duodenum with flexible endoscope. May use video imaging to visualize stomach motility. Detects inflammation, ulcerations, tumors, varices, or Mallory-Weiss tears. Biopsies may be taken. Varices can be treated with band ligation or sclerotherapy	*Before:* Keep NPO for 8 h. Ensure consent form is signed. Give ordered preoperative medication. Explain to patient that local anesthesia may be sprayed on throat before insertion of scope and that patient will be sedated during procedure. *After:* Keep NPO until gag reflex returns. Use warm saline gargles for relief of sore throat. Assess for signs of perforation.
Laparoscopy (peritoneoscopy)	Visualize peritoneal cavity and contents with laparoscope. Double-puncture peritoneoscopy permits better visualization of abdominal cavity, especially liver. Done in operating room. Can obtain biopsy specimen	*Before:* Ensure consent form is signed. Keep NPO 8 h. Give preoperative sedative medication. Ensure bladder and bowels are emptied. *After:* Observe for complications of bleeding and bowel perforation.
Sigmoidoscopy	Visualize rectum and sigmoid colon with lighted flexible endoscope. Sometimes a special table is used to tilt patient into knee-chest position. Detect tumors, polyps, inflammatory and infectious diseases, fissures, hemorrhoids	*Before:* Bowel preparation similar to colonoscopy. Explain to patient knee-chest position, need to take deep breaths during insertion of scope, and possible urge to defecate as scope is passed. Encourage patient to relax and let abdomen go limp. *After:* Observe for rectal bleeding after polypectomy or biopsy.
Video capsule endoscopy	Patient swallows a vitamin-sized capsule with camera, which provides endoscopic visualization of GI tract (Fig. 43.10). Camera takes >50,000 images during test, relaying them to monitoring device that patient wears on a belt. Images then downloaded to computer. Used to look at areas of GI tract not accessible by upper and lower endoscopy	*Before:* Keep NPO for 8 h. May have bowel preparation similar to colonoscopy. After swallowing capsule, clear liquids resumed in 2 h and food in 4 h. *After:* 8 h after swallowing device, patient returns to have monitoring device removed. Tell patient that capsule is disposable and will be present in a bowel movement.

Continued

TABLE 43.13 **Diagnostic Studies—cont'd**

Study	Description and Purpose	Nursing Responsibility
Radiology		
Cholangiography		
• Magnetic resonance cholangiopancreatography (MRCP)	Use of MRI technology to obtain images of biliary and pancreatic ducts	Same as MRI.
• Percutaneous transhepatic catheter (PTC)	Under local anesthesia and monitored anesthesia care, a long needle is passed into liver (under fluoroscopy) and into bile duct. Bile is removed. Radiopaque contrast medium directly injected into biliary system. Used to determine filling of hepatic and biliary ducts	*Before:* Assess for contraindications, precautions, or complications with use of contrast medium. Keep NPO for 8–12 h before test. Start prophylactic IV antibiotics 1 h prior. *After:* Observe patient for signs of hemorrhage, bile leakage, and infection. Observe safety precautions until sedation wears off. Maintain bed rest for 6 h.
• Surgical cholangiogram	Contrast medium is injected into common bile duct during surgery on biliary structures	*Before:* Explain that anesthetic will be used. Assess for contraindications or precautions with use of contrast medium.
CT scan	Noninvasive radiologic examination allows for exposures at different depths. Using oral and IV contrast medium accentuates density differences. Detects biliary tract, liver, and pancreatic disorders	*Before:* Before contrast medium used, evaluate renal function. Assess if patient is allergic to shellfish since the contrast is iodine based. Patient may need to be NPO prior. *During:* Warn patient that contrast injection may cause a feeling of being warm and flushed. Patient must lie completely still during scan. *After:* Encourage fluid intake to avoid renal problems with any contrast.
Defecography	Uses fluoroscopy or MRI to assess the shape and position of the rectum during defecation. Using a lubricated small plastic tip, fill rectum and anus with barium. Oral barium allows small bowel to be visualized. The person then sits on a toilet-like seat attached to the x-ray table. They are asked to push and empty the rectum. Images are taken while person is sitting at rest, straining, squeezing, and during defecation. Detects pelvic floor abnormalities	*Before:* Keep patient NPO for 2 h. 2 enemas are given 2 h before, 15 min apart. Oral barium is given 1 h before.
Gastric emptying breath test (GEBT)	Noninvasive test that measures CO_2 in a patient's breath. Used to diagnose delayed gastric emptying. Baseline breath test done. Then patient eats a special test meal that includes *Spirulina platensis,* a protein enriched with carbon-13. It is measured in breath samples collected after the meal	*Before:* Need to be NPO 8 h prior. *During:* Test takes 4–5 h. Breath samples taken at multiple time points.
Lower GI or barium enema	Fluoroscopic x-ray exam of colon using contrast medium given rectally (enema) (Fig. 43.8). Double-contrast or air-contrast barium enema is test of choice. Air is infused after the barium flows through transverse colon. Used to detect the presence of tumors, diverticula, and polyps	*Before:* Give laxatives and enemas until colon is clear of stool evening before. Follow clear liquid diet evening before. Keep patient NPO for 8 h before test. Teach patient that cramping and urge to defecate may occur during procedure and patient may be placed in various positions on tilt table. *After:* Give fluids, laxatives, or suppositories to help in expelling barium. Observe stool for passage of contrast medium. Tell patient that stool may be white for up to 72 h.
MRI	Noninvasive procedure using radiofrequency waves and a magnetic field. IV contrast medium (gadolinium) may be used. Used to detect hepatobiliary disease, liver lesions, and sources of GI bleeding and stage GI cancers	*Before:* Check for pregnancy, allergies, and renal function. Have patient remove all metal objects. Ask about any staples, plates, dental bridges, or other metal appliances. Remove metallic foil patches. Patient may need to be fasting. Assess for claustrophobia and the need for antianxiety medication. *During:* Must lie completely still during scan.

TABLE 43.13 **Diagnostic Studies—cont'd**

Study	Description and Purpose	Nursing Responsibility
Nuclear imaging scans (scintigraphy)	Tracer doses of a radioactive isotope are injected IV, and a scanning device picks up radioactive emission, which is recorded on paper. Shows size, shape, and position of organ. Identifies functional disorders and structural defects	*Before:* Tell patient that the substance used contains only traces of radioactivity and poses little to no danger. Schedule no more than 1 radionuclide test a day. Explain to patient need to lie flat during scanning.
• Gastric emptying studies	Assesses ability of stomach to empty solids. Patient eats special food containing ^{99m}Tc and with water. Images are obtained at 0, 1, 2, and 4 h later. Used to study gastric emptying disorders caused by ulcers, ulcer surgery, diabetes, cancer, or functional disorders	*Before*: Need to be NPO 4 h prior.
• Hepatobiliary scintigraphy (HIDA)	Patient is given IV injection of ^{99m}Tc. Imaging then records distribution of tracer in liver, biliary tree, gallbladder, and proximal small intestine. Used to identify obstructions of bile ducts (gallstones, tumors), gallbladder disease, and bile leaks	*Before*: Need to be NPO 4 h prior.
• Scintigraphy of GI bleeding	^{99m}Tc-labeled sulfur colloid or ^{99m}Tc labeling of patient's own RBCs to determine site of active GI blood loss. Sulfur colloid or patient's RBCs are injected, then images of abdomen taken at intermittent intervals	Same as above.
Small bowel series	Contrast medium is ingested, and films taken every 30 min until medium reaches terminal ileum	*Before:* Explain procedure, including the need to drink contrast medium and assume various positions on x-ray table. NPO for at least 8 h. Avoid smoking after midnight. *After:* Take measures to prevent contrast medium impaction (fluids, laxatives). Stool may be white for up to 72 h.
Upper GI or barium swallow	Fluoroscopic x-ray study using contrast medium. Used to diagnose structural abnormalities of esophagus, stomach, and duodenum	Same as for small bowel series.
Ultrasound	Noninvasive procedure. High-frequency ultrasound waves are passed into body structures and recorded as they are reflected. Used to show size and shape of an organ	
• Abdominal ultrasound	Conductive gel is applied to skin, and a transducer is placed on the area. Detects abdominal masses (tumors, cysts), gallstones, biliary and liver disease, ascites	*Before:* NPO for 8–12 h. Air or gas can reduce quality of images. Food intake can cause gallbladder contraction, resulting in suboptimal study.
• Endoscopic ultrasound (EUS)	Small ultrasound transducer is installed on tip of endoscope. Because EUS transducer gets close to the organ(s) being examined, images obtained are more accurate and detailed than those provided by traditional ultrasound Detects and stages esophageal, gastric, rectal, biliary, and pancreatic tumors and abnormalities	Same as EGD.
• Ultrasound elastography (Fibroscan)	Transient elastography uses an ultrasound transducer to assess level of liver fibrosis. Used to monitor patients with chronic liver disease	*Before:* Explain the need to lie in dorsal decubitus position with right arm in extreme abduction.
Virtual colonoscopy	Combines CT scanning or MRI with computer virtual reality software. Air is introduced via a tube placed in rectum to enlarge colon to enhance visualization. Images obtained while patient is on back and abdomen. Computer combines images to form 2D and 3D pictures that are viewed on monitor. Detects intestine and colon diseases, including polyps, cancer, diverticulosis, and lower GI bleeding	*Before:* Bowel preparation similar to colonoscopy.

and small intestine. The procedure consists of the patient swallowing contrast medium (a thick barium solution or gastrografin) and then assuming different positions on the x-ray table. The movement of the contrast medium is observed with fluoroscopy, and a series of x-rays are taken. An upper GI series can identify esophageal strictures, polyps, tumors, hiatal hernias, foreign bodies, and ulcers.

Lower GI Series

The purpose of a lower GI series, or barium enema, is to observe (using fluoroscopy) the colon filling with contrast medium and to observe (by x-ray) the filled colon. The patient receives an enema of contrast medium. This procedure identifies polyps, tumors, and other lesions in the colon. Adding air contrast after the barium provides better visualization (Fig. 43.8). Because the patient must retain the barium, an older or immobile patient may not tolerate it very well.

Virtual Colonoscopy

Virtual colonoscopy combines CT scanning or MRI to produce images of the colon and rectum less invasively. It requires radiation and prior cleansing of the colon but no sedation.

Compared with conventional colonoscopy, virtual colonoscopy provides a better view inside the colon that is narrow from inflammation or a growth.[6] If a polyp is found, it will have to be removed by conventional colonoscopy. Virtual colonoscopy may be less sensitive in obtaining information on the details and color of the mucosa and in detecting small (less than 10 mm) or flat polyps.

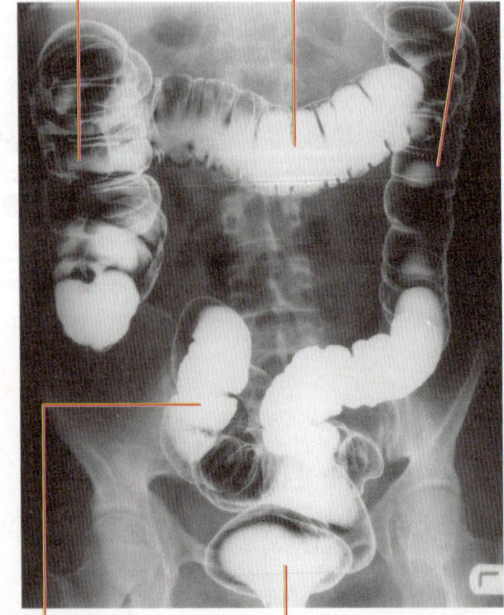

Fig. 43.8 Barium enema x-ray showing the large intestine. (From Drake RL, Vogl W, Mitchell AWM: *Gray's anatomy for students,* ed 4, St Louis, 2020, Elsevier.)

Endoscopy

Endoscopy refers to the direct visualization of a body structure through an endoscope. An endoscope is a fiberoptic instrument with a light and camera attached, allowing the ability to take video and still pictures (Fig. 43.9). Some endoscopes have a channel through which to pass instruments, such as biopsy forceps and cytology brushes.

Endoscopy can examine the esophagus, stomach, duodenum, and colon. *Endoscopic retrograde cholangiopancreatography* (ERCP) visualizes the pancreatic, hepatic, and common bile ducts. Endoscopy is often combined with diagnostic procedures, including biopsy, cytologic studies, invasive, and therapeutic procedures. Examples include polypectomy, sclerosis or banding of varices, cauterization of bleeding sites, common bile duct stone removal, and balloon dilation.

The major complication of GI endoscopy is perforation through the structure being studied. Many endoscopic procedures require short-acting IV sedation. All endoscopic procedures require informed, written consent. Specific endoscopy procedures are discussed in Table 43.13.

Capsule endoscopy is a noninvasive approach to visualize the GI tract (Fig. 43.10). Colon capsule endoscopy is useful in diagnosing small bowel disease and monitoring inflammation in patients with IBD. Its sensitivity in detecting colon polyps and CRC is being researched.[6]

Liver Biopsy

The purpose of a liver biopsy is to obtain hepatic tissue. The tissue is used to establish a diagnosis of cancer or liver disease or assess and stage fibrosis and cirrhosis. It may be done to follow the progression of liver disease.

A liver biopsy can be open or closed. The *open method* involves making an incision and removing a wedge of tissue. It is done in the operating room with the patient under general anesthesia, often with another surgical procedure. The *closed,* or *needle, biopsy* can be done in 2 ways. A percutaneous procedure is often done with ultrasound or CT guidance. The HCP administers a local anesthetic, then inserts a needle between 6th and 7th or 8th and 9th intercostal spaces on the right side to

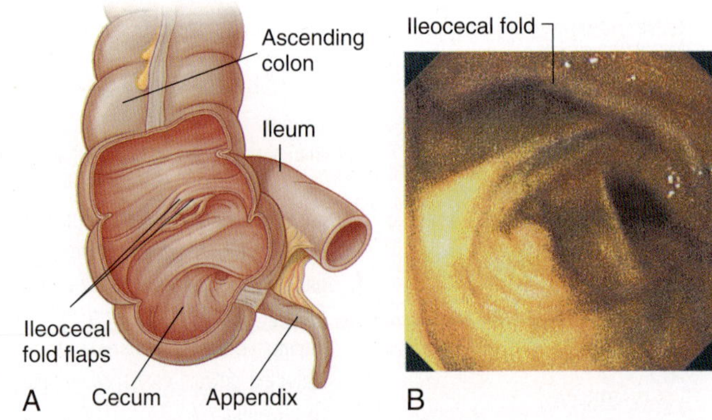

Fig. 43.9 (A) Illustration showing the ileocecal junction and the ileocecal fold. (B) Endoscopic image of the ileocecal fold. (From Drake RL, Vogl W, Mitchell AWM: *Gray's anatomy for students,* ed 4, 2020, Elsevier.)

obtain specimen of hepatic tissue. Table 43.14 outlines the nursing management of patients undergoing a liver biopsy. A liver biopsy done in interventional radiology can be obtained through a transjugular approach. The HCP enters the jugular vein and advances a small sheath into the hepatic vein. A biopsy needle is passed through the sheath, into the vein wall, then into the liver tissue.

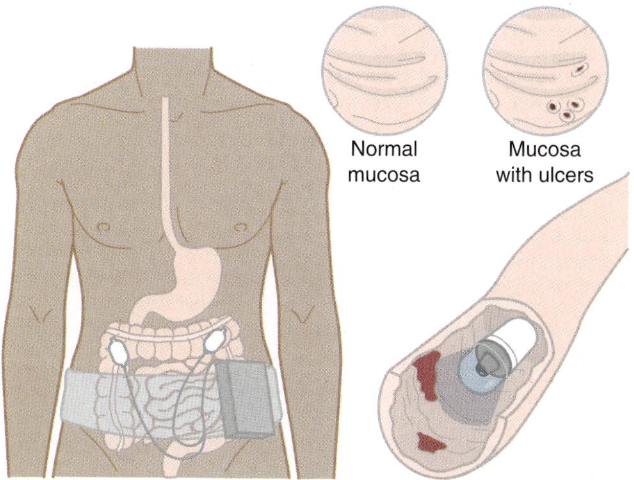

Fig. 43.10 Capsule endoscopy. The pill-sized video capsule has its own camera and light source. As it travels through the GI tract, it sends messages through sensing electrodes placed on the chest and abdomen to a data recorder worn on a waist belt. After the test, the images are viewed on a computer.

TABLE 43.14 NURSING MANAGEMENT

Care of the Patient Undergoing Closed Liver Biopsy

Preprocedure

- Perform baseline assessment, including vital signs, pulse oximetry.
- Withhold food and fluids for 8–12 h before.
- Check coagulation status (prothrombin time, clotting or bleeding time).
- Give sedative and other drugs, as ordered.
- Obtain type and crossmatch (in event patient bleeds and requires blood).
- Teach patient and caregiver about procedure and postprocedure care. Explain need to hold breath after expiration when needle is inserted.
- Ensure informed consent has been signed.

Postprocedure

- Check vital signs to detect internal bleeding q15min × 2, q30min × 4, q1h × 4.
- Notify HCP of dyspnea, cyanosis, and restlessness, which may occur with pneumothorax.
- Keep patient lying on right side for minimum of 2 h to splint puncture site. Then maintain bed rest for 12–14 h, as ordered.
- Apply a small dressing over the needle insertion site.
- Teach patient and caregiver about discharge care, including signs and symptoms to report to HCP (e.g., site complications) and any activity restrictions. Tell patient to avoid straining or coughing, which increase intraabdominal pressure.

CASE STUDY

Objective Data: Diagnostic Studies

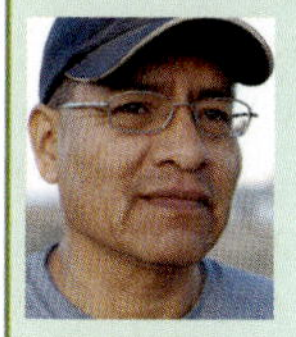

(© iStockphoto/ Thinkstock.)

The ED physician performs a rectal examination and finds a palpable mass. The following diagnostic tests are ordered:

- CBC
- Electrolytes
- Liver function tests
- Urinalysis
- CT scan of the abdomen
- Colonoscopy

The CBC reveals an Hgb of 6.8 g/dL and an Hct of 20%. The WBC count is normal. The electrolytes, liver function tests, and urinalysis are within normal limits. The CT scan reveals pockets of gas and fluid in the ascending colon and 2 medium-sized tumors in the transverse colon.

Discussion Questions

1. Which diagnostic study results concern you most?
2. With this information, what other diagnostic studies would you expect to be ordered for L.C.?
3. What are the interprofessional team's priorities for L.C. at this time?

Case study continued in Chapter 47.

Answers available at http://evolve.elsevier.com/Lewis/medsurg.

BRIDGE TO NCLEX EXAMINATION

The number of the question corresponds to the same-numbered outcome at the beginning of the chapter.

1. A patient is admitted with diarrhea and dehydration. The increased peristalsis resulting in diarrhea can be related to
   a. sympathetic inhibition.
   b. mixing and propulsion.
   c. sympathetic stimulation.
   d. parasympathetic stimulation.
2. A patient has a high level of indirect (unconjugated) bilirubin. One cause of this finding is
   a. the gallbladder is unable to contract to release stored bile.
   b. bilirubin is not being conjugated and excreted into the bile by the liver.
   c. the Kupffer cells in the liver are unable to remove bilirubin from the blood.
   d. there is an obstruction in the biliary tract preventing flow of bile into the small intestine.

3. As gastric contents move into the small intestine, the bowel is normally protected from the acidity of gastric contents by the
   a. inhibition of secretin release.
   b. secretion of mucus by goblet cells.
   c. release of pancreatic digestive enzymes.
   d. release of gastrin by the duodenal mucosa.
4. A patient has jaundice with pale colored stools. This is *most* likely related to
   a. decreased bile flow into the intestine.
   b. increased production of urobilinogen.
   c. increased bile and bilirubin in the blood.
   d. increased production of cholecystokinin.
5. An 80-year-old male states that, although he adds a lot of salt to his food, it still does not have much taste. The nurse's response is based on the knowledge that the older adult
   a. should not have any changes in taste.
   b. has a loss of taste buds, especially for sweet and salt.
   c. has some loss of taste but no problems chewing food.
   d. loses some sense of taste related to the increased ability to smell.
6. An appropriate question for the nurse to ask when assessing the health perception–health maintenance pattern related to gastrointestinal function is
   a. "What is your usual bowel elimination pattern?"
   b. "What percentage of your income is spent on food?"
   c. "Have you traveled to a foreign country in the last year?"
   d. "Do you have diarrhea when you are under a lot of stress?"
7. When assessing the abdomen, the nurse would
   a. listen for bowel sounds in all 4 quadrants for 2 minutes.
   b. place the patient supine with the bed flat and knees straight.
   c. describe bowel sounds as absent if no sound is heard in a quadrant after 2 minutes.
   d. use the following order of techniques: inspection, palpation, percussion, auscultation.
8. Normal physical assessment findings of the gastrointestinal system are **(Select all that apply.)**
   a. nonpalpable spleen.
   b. borborygmi in upper right quadrant.
   c. tympany on percussion of the abdomen.
   d. liver edge 2 to 4 cm below the costal margin.
   e. finding of a firm, nodular edge on the rectal examination.
9. In preparing a patient for a colonoscopy, the nurse explains that
   a. a signed permit is not needed.
   b. sedation will be used during the procedure.
   c. one cleansing enema part of the required preparation.
   d. light meals should be eaten for 3 days before the procedure.

1. d; 2. b; 3. b; 4. a; 5. b; 6. c; 7. b; 8. a, c; 9. b.

For rationales to these answers and even more NCLEX review questions, visit http://evolve.elsevier.com/Lewis/medsurg.

REFERENCES

To access the References for this chapter, please scan the QR code with a mobile device.

44

Nutrition Problems

Mariann M. Harding

http://evolve.elsevier.com/Lewis/medsurg/

CONCEPTUAL FOCUS

Functional Ability
Health Promotion
Nutrition

LEARNING OUTCOMES

1. Relate the components of a well-balanced diet to their impact on health outcomes.
2. Describe the etiology and clinical manifestations of malnutrition.
3. Describe the components of a nutrition assessment.
4. Discuss nutrition care interventions for patients with malnutrition.
5. Explain the indications, complications, and nursing management related to the use of enteral nutrition.
6. Explain the indications, complications, and nursing management related to the use of parenteral nutrition.

KEY TERMS

enteral nutrition (EN)
food insecurity
malabsorption syndrome
malnutrition
parenteral nutrition (PN)
refeeding syndrome
tube feeding

This chapter focuses on nutrition problems. Many factors affect nutrition by changing the way we ingest, absorb, digest, and metabolize nutrients. These changes can lead to malnutrition and health problems that affect functional status and quality of life. This makes assessment and interventions aimed at promoting optimal nutrition important nursing roles.

NUTRITION

Nutrition is the sum of processes by which one takes in and uses nutrients. Optimal nutrition, in the absence of any underlying disease process, results from eating a balanced diet. Any change in nutrient intake or use can cause nutrition problems. Nutrition problems occur in all ages, cultures, and socioeconomic classes.

Many factors influence nutrition. We establish our attitudes toward food and eating habits early. Diet intake often reflects culture or religious practices. Financial status and community resources affect the food someone can buy. Body type, age, gender, medications, physical activity, and health problems influence daily caloric requirements. Adjustments in caloric intake are necessary depending on changes in health status and daily activity level.

There are several ways to estimate daily caloric needs based on resting metabolic rate. One way is to use the Mifflin–St. Jeor equation (Table 44.1).[1] Another way to estimate daily calories needed is by multiplying kilocalories per kilogram (kcal/kg). An average adult should consume 20 to 25 cal/kg body weight to lose weight and 25 to 30 cal/kg to maintain weight. Those with injury or illness may need at least 30 to 35 cal/kg.

Carbohydrates, the body's main source of energy, yield about 4 cal/g. We classify them as either simple or complex depending on the number of sugars they have. Simple carbohydrates come in 2 forms: monosaccharides, such as glucose and fructose, which are found in fruits and honey, and disaccharides, such as sucrose, maltose, and lactose. Sucrose is found in foods made with table sugar and some fruit. Most dairy products contain lactose. Complex carbohydrates are called *polysaccharides.* They include whole grains, rice, potatoes, pasta, and beans.

Carbohydrates are the chief protein-sparing ingredient in a nutritionally sound diet. The Dietary Reference Intake (DRI) recommendations are that 45% to 65% of total calories should

TABLE 44.1 Estimating Daily Calorie Requirements

Mifflin–St. Jeor Equation

For each gender, use this formula to calculate energy expenditure:

Males: 10 × weight (kg) + 6.25 × height (cm) − 5 × age (year) + 5

Females: 10 × weight (kg) + 6.25 × height (cm) − 5 × age (year) − 161

To determine total daily calorie needs, multiply the energy expenditure by the appropriate activity factor:

1.200 = sedentary (little or no exercise)
1.375 = lightly active (light exercise/sports 1–3 days/week)
1.550 = moderately active (moderate exercise/sports 3–5 days/week)
1.725 = very active (hard exercise/sports 6–7 days a week)
1.900 = extra active (very hard exercise/sports and physical job)

Example

Male: Weight 180 lb (82 kg); height 5 ft, 10 in (178 cm); age 50, very active

Energy expenditure = 10 (82) + 6.25 (178) − 5 (50) + 5 × 1.725 = 2911

Female: Weight 150 lb (68 kg); height 5 ft, 6 in (168 cm); age 60; lightly active

Energy expenditure = 10 (68) + 6.25 (168) − 5 (60) −161 × 1.375 = 1745

TABLE 44.2 NUTRITION THERAPY

Foods High in Protein

Complete Proteins
- Eggs
- Fish
- Meats
- Milk and milk products
- Poultry

Incomplete Proteins
- Grains
- Legumes
- Nuts
- Seeds

come from carbohydrates.[2] A person should consume around 14 g of fiber per 1000 calories per day from fruits, vegetables, and whole grains. This is roughly 28 to 30 g for a 2000-calorie diet.

Fats are a major source of energy. One gram of fat yields 9 calories. Fats are stored in adipose tissue and the abdominal cavity. They act as carriers of essential fatty acids and fat-soluble vitamins. Fats help us feel full after eating. Diets high in excess calories, usually in the form of fats and sugars, contribute to obesity.

Fats can be divided into (1) potentially harmful (saturated fat and trans fat) and (2) healthier diet fat (monounsaturated and polyunsaturated fat). Fat intake should be no more than 20% to 35% of total calories.[2] Less than 10% of calories should be from saturated fatty acids. This is about 20 g of saturated fat per day in a 2000-calorie diet. We should avoid foods with trans fat.[2]

Proteins are needed for tissue growth, repair, and maintenance; body regulatory functions; and energy production. Ideally, 10% to 35% of daily caloric needs should come from protein.[2] The DRI of protein is 0.8 to 1 g/kg of body weight. For the normal healthy person of average body size, this is about 45 to 65 g of protein daily. One gram of protein yields 4 calories. Amino acids are the basic units of protein structure. We classify the 22 amino acids as essential or nonessential. The body can make nonessential amino acids if an adequate supply of protein is available. The body cannot make the 9 essential amino acids. Their availability depends totally on one's diet. We obtain amino acids from animal and plant sources. *Complete proteins* contain all the essential amino acids. Proteins that lack one or more of the essential amino acids are *incomplete proteins.* Table 44.2 lists foods high in protein.

Vitamins are organic compounds needed in small amounts for normal metabolism. Vitamins function in enzyme reactions that facilitate amino acid, fat, and carbohydrate metabolism. A diet consisting of foods from the 5 basic food groups is essential for obtaining the recommended intake of essential vitamins (Table 44.3). There are 2 categories of vitamins: *water-soluble* vitamins (vitamin C and the B-complex vitamins) and *fat-soluble* vitamins (vitamins A, D, E, and K). Because the body stores excess fat-soluble vitamins, consuming too much can result in toxicity. There are upper limits for vitamins A, D, and E. Vitamin deficiencies are rare in most developed countries. When they do occur, they often involve several vitamins. This may happen with a person who is chronically ill or had surgery on the GI tract.

Mineral salts make up about 4% of body weight. The body needs minerals to build and repair tissues, regulate body fluids, and assist in various functions. Minerals needed in amounts greater than 100 mg/day are *major minerals.* They include calcium, phosphorus, and sodium. Minerals that we need in small amounts are *trace minerals.* Table 44.4 lists the major and trace minerals. A well-balanced diet usually meets the DRI of minerals. However, deficiency and excess states can occur. Some minerals are stored and can be toxic if taken in excess amounts. Many patients are prone to anemia from low iron intake. Table 44.5 lists examples of foods high in iron.

MALNUTRITION

Malnutrition is an imbalance in a person's intake of energy and/or nutrients that has adverse outcomes.[3] It affects body composition and functional status. The term malnutrition describes 3 broad problems. *Undernutrition* occurs when nutrition reserves are depleted and nutrient and energy intake are not sufficient to meet daily needs or added metabolic stress. Most use the term malnutrition to refer to undernutrition. We use the terms interchangeably here.

The other 2 problems are obesity and micronutrient malnutrition. Micronutrient malnutrition is present when there is a lack of key vitamins and minerals. Iodine, vitamin A, and iron deficiencies are the most common.[3] Chapter 45 discusses obesity.

Malnutrition is a growing concern. Disease-related malnutrition (DRM) is common in patients with acute and chronic

TABLE 44.3 Adult Vitamin Intake and Manifestations of Deficiencies

Vitamin	Dietary Reference Intake	Manifestations of Deficiency
Fat Soluble		
A (retinol)	*Males:* 900 mcg *Females:* 700 mcg	Night blindness, dry eyes, cornea ulcers or scarring. Impaired immunity, respiratory infections. Dry, scaly skin
D	*Adults age 19–70:* 600 IU *Adults age >70:* 800 IU	Muscle weakness, muscle aches, bone pain. GI problems, tetany, osteomalacia
E	*Adults:* 15 mg	Neurologic deficits, anemia
K	*Males:* 120 mcg *Females:* 90 mcg	Bleeding, easy bruising
Water Soluble		
B_1 (thiamine)	*Males:* 1.2 mg *Females:* 1.1 mg	Anorexia, fatigue, irritability, constipation, paresthesia, insomnia
B_6 (pyridoxine)	*Males age 19–50:* 1.3 mg *Males age >51:* 1.7 mg *Females age 19–50:* 1.3 mg *Females age >51:* 1.5 mg	Seizures, dermatitis, anemia, neuropathy with motor weakness, mouth ulcers
B_{12} (cobalamin)	*Adults:* 2.4 mcg	Megaloblastic anemia, anorexia, glossitis, sore mouth, pallor, neurologic problems, weight loss, nausea, constipation
C	*Males:* 90 mg *Females:* 75 mg	Bleeding gums, loose teeth, easy bruising, poor wound healing. Weakness, muscle and joint pain
Folate (folic acid)	*Adults:* 400 mcg	Megaloblastic anemia, anorexia, fatigue, sore tongue, diarrhea, confusion

TABLE 44.4 Mineral Salts

Major Minerals
- Calcium
- Chloride
- Magnesium
- Phosphorus
- Potassium
- Sodium
- Sulfur

Trace Minerals
- Chromium
- Copper
- Fluoride
- Iodine
- Iron
- Manganese
- Molybdenum
- Selenium
- Zinc

TABLE 44.5 NUTRITION THERAPY

Foods High in Iron

Food	Selected Serving Size	% of Daily Value
Breakfast cereal, fortified	1 serving	100
Clams: steamed, boiled, or canned (drained)	3 oz	13
Oatmeal, instant, fortified, prepared (enriched)	⅔ cup	19–58
Organ meats (liver, giblets)	3 oz	28
Oysters: baked, broiled, steamed	3 oz	44
Soybeans, cooked	½ cup	24
Spinach, boiled and drained	½ cup	17
Tofu, firm	½ cup	17
White beans, canned	½ cup	22

illness. Rates for DRM for hospitalized patients vary from 10% to 70%. Rates are higher in older adults and those who are critically ill.[4] DRM is associated with poor health outcomes. Malnutrition in older adults increases with dependency. It affects around 30% of those in long-term care facilities.[5]

Etiology

Malnutrition is not one specific and well-defined illness but a syndrome with several potential mechanisms.[6] There are 3 cause-based terms we use in clinical practice to describe malnutrition in adults (Fig. 44.1).[7]

- *Starvation-related malnutrition* occurs when nutrition needs are not met through diet. There is no inflammation (e.g., anorexia).
- *Chronic DRM* occurs when diet intake or nutrient uptake does not meet tissue needs but would under normal conditions. It is related to mild to moderate chronic inflammation. Associated health problems include liver disease, chronic kidney disease, arthritis, and cancer.[8]
- *Acute DRM* is related to acute disease or injury states with severe inflammation. Examples include major infection, burns, trauma, and surgery.

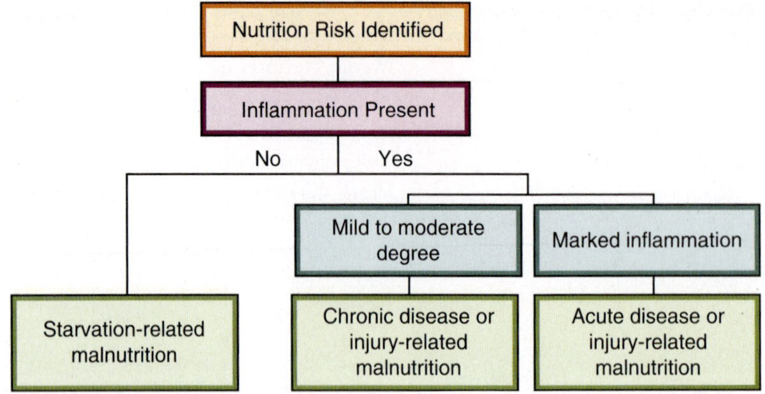

Fig. 44.1 Cause-based malnutrition definitions. (Adapted from Jensen GL, Bistrian B, Roubenoff R, et al: Malnutrition syndromes: a conundrum vs continuum, *JPEN J Parenter Enteral Nutr*, 33:710, 2009.)

TABLE 44.6 Risk Factors for Malnutrition

- Alcohol use
- Anorexia, impaired oral intake
- Cancer and its treatment
- Decreased mobility
- Dementia
- Depression
- Eating disorder (e.g., anorexia nervosa, bulimia)
- Endocrine problems
- Excess dieting to lose weight
- Food insecurity
- Impaired dentition
- Impaired GI function, GI surgery
- Increased metabolic requirements (e.g., infection, trauma, fever, burns)
- Kidney disease
- Liver disease
- Medications: Corticosteroids, chemotherapy, diet aids, supplements
- Neurologic impairment
- No oral intake and/or receiving standard IV solutions for 10 days (adults) or for 5 days (older adults)
- Nutrient losses from malabsorption, dialysis, diarrhea, wounds
- Sensory deficits with taste, smell
- Swallowing problems (e.g., head and neck cancer, stroke)

Contributing Factors

Many factors contribute to malnutrition. These include health problems and food insecurity. Table 44.6 lists risk factors for malnutrition.

Health Problems

Malnutrition is a common consequence of illness, surgery, injury, or hospitalization. Hospitalized patients, especially the older adult, are at risk for DRM. Prolonged illness, sepsis, draining wounds, burns, hemorrhage, fractures, and immobilization can contribute to malnutrition. Existing malnutrition is likely to become more severe with illness. Likewise, patients who are nutritionally fit on entering the hospital can develop DRM because of their health problems.

Symptoms that occur with gastrointestinal (GI) problems, like anorexia, nausea, vomiting, and diarrhea, interfere with normal food intake and metabolism. **Malabsorption syndrome** is the impaired absorption of nutrients from the GI tract. Decreases in digestive enzymes or bowel surface area can quickly lead to malnutrition. For example, after a gastrectomy, patients need cobalamin supplements because intrinsic factor (normally made in the stomach) is not available to promote cobalamin absorption. Poor oral health from gum disease, missing teeth, or dry mouth can impair the ability to chew and swallow food.

Many drugs have GI side effects and alter normal GI processes. For example, antibiotics can change the normal flora of the intestines. This decreases the body's ability to make biotin, a B-complex vitamin whose production depends on gut flora.

Fever, which occurs with illnesses, injuries, and infections, increases basal metabolic rate (BMR) and nitrogen loss. Each degree of temperature increase on the Fahrenheit scale raises the BMR by about 7%. Without an increase in caloric intake, the body uses protein stores to supply calories, and protein depletion develops. After the body temperature returns to normal, the rate of protein breakdown and resynthesis may stay increased for several weeks.

A *drug-nutrient interaction* occurs when a drug affects how the body uses nutrients. Many drug and food or beverage interactions may occur. Potential adverse interactions include incompatibilities and altered drug effectiveness. Drug side effects include nausea, dry mouth, a change in the taste of food, or a decrease in appetite. You need to monitor for these effects.

Eating disorders include *anorexia nervosa (AN)* and *bulimia nervosa (BN)*. AN is characterized by restricting intake, difficulty maintaining an appropriate weight, intense fear of gaining weight or being fat, and distorted body image. Persons with AN restrict the number of calories and the types of food they eat. Some exercise compulsively, purge via vomiting and laxatives, and/or binge eat. There may be an unwillingness to maintain a healthy weight, refusal to eat, continuous dieting, detailed food rituals, and avoiding social situations. They often go to great lengths to conceal their eating habits. BN is characterized by recurrent episodes of binge eating. To prevent weight gain, the person then engages in compensatory behaviors (vomiting, laxative or diuretic misuse, overexercise). Like those with AN, the person with BN is concerned with body image.

Food Insecurity

Food insecurity is a limitation in the accessibility and/or lack of resources (e.g., income, transportation, ability) to secure safe and nutritious food.[9] Household food insecurity often stems from limited resources. Poverty, underemployment, and high housing costs are related to food insecurity.[9] Persons living in food-insecure homes often follow diets that are inadequate in nutrients. There may be an unequal distribution of food within the home or limited intake. Available food may be unsafe, not culturally appropriate, or of poor quality.

Pathophysiology

The speed at which malnutrition develops depends on the quantity and quality of the protein and calorie intake, illness, and person's age. During the early phase of starvation, the body selectively uses carbohydrates (glycogen) rather than fat and protein to meet metabolic needs. These carbohydrate stores, found in the liver and muscles, are minimal. They may be depleted within 18 hours. The body uses protein only in its normal role in cellular metabolism.

Once carbohydrate stores are depleted, the body converts skeletal protein to glucose for energy. Alanine and glutamine are the first amino acids used in *gluconeogenesis,* the process by which the liver forms glucose. The resulting plasma glucose allows metabolic processes to continue. When these amino acids are used as energy sources, the person may be in negative nitrogen balance (nitrogen excretion exceeds nitrogen intake).

Within 5 to 9 days, the body uses fat to supply much of the needed energy. In prolonged starvation, fat provides up to 97% of calories, conserving protein. Depletion of fat stores depends on the amount available. Fat stores are generally used up in 4 to 6 weeks. Once fat stores are gone, the body uses proteins, including those in internal organs and plasma. They rapidly decrease because they are the only remaining body source of energy available.

As protein depletion continues, muscles (the largest store of protein in the body) become wasted and flabby. Liver function becomes impaired, and protein synthesis decreases. The decreased protein synthesis lowers plasma oncotic pressure. As oncotic pressure decreases, body fluids shift from the vascular space into the interstitial compartment. Eventually, albumin leaks into the interstitial space along with the fluid. Edema becomes observable. Edema in the face and legs can mask underlying muscle wasting.

As the total blood volume decreases, the skin appears dry and wrinkled. As fluids shift to the interstitial space, ions also move. Sodium concentration increases in the cell. Potassium and magnesium shift to the extracellular space. The sodium-potassium exchange pump has high-energy needs, using 20% to 50% of all calories ingested. When the diet is extremely deficient in calories and essential proteins, the pump will fail. This leaves sodium inside the cell, along with water, and the cell expands.

The liver is the body organ that loses the most mass during protein deprivation. Fat gradually infiltrates the liver because of decreased synthesis of lipoproteins. Death will rapidly ensue if the person does not receive protein and necessary nutrients.

Inflammation

Inflammation is a key driver in DRM, leading to anorexia and decreased food intake, which results in catabolism.[6,10] In DRM with acute and chronic inflammation, the sympathetic nervous, immune, and endocrine systems interact. The result is the release of stress hormones, including cortisol and catecholamines, and proinflammatory cytokines (e.g., interleukin-6 [IL-6]). BMR increases. Cytokine effects include insulin resistance, increased muscle breakdown, and decreased protein synthesis.[10]

Clinical Manifestations

Malnutrition affects the function of every organ system and can alter body composition (Table 44.7). This results in muscle wasting, weakness, fatigue, loss of fat, and reduced strength. The skin can be dry and scaly with brittle nails and hair loss. Crusting and ulcerations with changes in the tongue may be seen in the mouth.

Decreased protein is available for tissue repair, causing delayed wound healing. The person is more susceptible to infections. Both humoral and cell-mediated immunity are deficient. Leukocytes decrease in the peripheral blood. Impaired phagocytosis occurs because of the lack of energy needed to drive the process. The lack of iron and folic acid, the building blocks for red blood cells (RBCs), causes anemia.

There are no specific laboratory tests for malnutrition. Electrolyte levels reflect changes taking place between the intracellular and extracellular spaces. The potassium level often increases. The RBC count and hemoglobin level may show anemia. The total lymphocyte count decreases. Liver enzyme levels may increase. Levels of both fat-soluble and water-soluble vitamins usually decrease. Low levels of fat-soluble vitamins correlate with *steatorrhea* (fatty stools).

Albumin and prealbumin are *negative acute-phase proteins.* This means that during an inflammatory response, the liver decreases synthesis of these proteins. Low or below-normal levels occur with inflammation. Because of the strong relationship between inflammation and malnutrition, they are useful in identifying patients at risk for poor outcomes.[11]

NURSING MANAGEMENT: MALNUTRITION

Assessment

Malnutrition is diagnosed in a 2-step approach. The first step consists of nutrition screening to identify patients who are malnourished or at risk of malnutrition. As a nurse, you are responsible for nutrition assessment and screening across care settings. The Joint Commission requires nutrition screening for

TABLE 44.7 NURSING ASSESSMENT

Malnutrition

Subjective Data

Important Health Information: Table 44.6

Assess for risk factors listed in Table 44.6.

Functional Health Patterns

Health perception–health management: Alcohol or drug use. Malaise, apathy.

Nutritional-metabolic: Weight change over past 6–12 months. Change in appetite, typical diet intake, food preferences, food allergies or intolerance. Ill-fitting or absent dentures. Dry mouth, problems chewing or swallowing, bloating, or gas. ↑ Sensitivity to cold, poor wound healing. Nausea, anorexia.

Elimination: Constipation, diarrhea, nocturia, ↓ urine output.

Activity-exercise: Change in activity. ↓ Functional ability. Weakness, fatigue, poor endurance.

Cognitive-perceptual: Pain in mouth. Paresthesias, loss of position and vibratory sense.

Role-relationship: Change in family (e.g., loss of a spouse), food insecurity.

Sexual-reproductive: Amenorrhea, impotence, ↓ libido, infertility.

Objective Data

General

Underweight for height. Listless, cachectic.

Cardiovascular

↑ or ↓ heart rate, ↓ BP, dysrhythmias, peripheral edema

Eyes

Pale or red conjunctiva. Dryness and dull appearance of conjunctivae and cornea, soft cornea. Blood vessel growth in cornea. Redness and fissuring of eyelid corners.

GI

Swollen, smooth, raw, beefy red tongue (glossitis); hypertrophic or atrophic papillae. Dental cavities, absent or loose teeth, discolored tooth enamel. Spongy, pale, receded gums with a tendency to bleed easily; periodontal disease. Ulcerations, white patches, or plaques. Redness, swelling of oral mucosa. Distended, tympanic abdomen. Ascites, hepatomegaly, ↓ bowel sounds, steatorrhea.

Musculoskeletal

↓ Muscle mass with poor tone, "wasted" appearance, ↓ hand grip strength, bowlegs, chest deformity, prominent bony structures, loss of subcutaneous tissue.

Neurologic

↓ Reflexes, tremor; irritability, confusion, syncope, peripheral neuropathy

Respiratory

↓ Respiratory rate, ↓ vital capacity, crackles, weak cough

Skin

Dry, brittle, sparse, dull hair; alopecia. Dry, scaly lips. Fever blisters, crusts and lesions at corners of mouth (cheilosis). Brittle, ridged nails. ↓ Skin tone and elasticity. Cool, rough, dry, scaly skin with pigment changes; jaundice. Dermatitis. Pressure injuries, poor wound healing.

Diagnostic Findings

↓ Hemoglobin and hematocrit, ↓ mean corpuscular volume (MCV), mean corpuscular hemoglobin (MCH), and mean corpuscular hemoglobin concentration (MCHC). Abnormal electrolyte levels. ↓ Blood urea nitrogen (BUN) and creatinine, ↓ albumin, transferrin, and prealbumin. ↑ C-reactive protein, ↓ lymphocytes, liver enzymes, ↓ vitamin levels.

all patients within 24 hours of admission with a detailed nutrition assessment if a patient is at risk. Use a valid and reliable nutrition screening tool. Many screening tools are available. Hospital-specific screening tools review common admission assessment data, including a history of weight loss, intake before admission, use of nutrition support, chewing or swallowing issues, and skin breakdown.

The Malnutrition Screening Tool (Fig. 44.2) and Nutrition Risk Score are common tools used with adults in acute care.[12] The Mini Nutrition Assessment assesses nutrition status in older adults. In long-term care, we use the Minimum Data Set (MDS) form to obtain nutrition information. In home care settings, the OASIS E is used to collect information on diet, intake, dental health, swallowing problems, and need for meal assistance.

Assess nutrition when performing the physical assessment. Often, a patient's nutrition state is not the reason for seeking medical care. It may be a contributing factor to health problems and have an impact on management and recovery. With increased stress, such as surgery or trauma, patients will need more calories and protein. Wound healing requires increased protein. Patients having major surgery who have DRM or are at risk for DRM need increased protein and calorie intake to promote healing after surgery.

Identify risk factors for malnutrition and why they exist. Take medical, nutrition, and medication histories. Obtain a complete diet history from the patient or caregiver. Assessing the foods eaten over the past week shows the patient's diet habits. Is the person living in a home with food insecurity?

If screening identifies a person at risk, they need a complete assessment. Table 44.7 outlines the assessment of patients with malnutrition. To diagnose malnutrition using the Global Leadership Initiative on Malnutrition (GLIM) tool, at least 1 phenotype criteria (unintentional weight loss, low body mass index (BMI), and reduced muscle mass) and at least 1 etiologic criteria (reduced food intake and inflammation or disease) must be present.[6]

Measure weight and height on admission. Make sure the measurements are accurate. When possible, measure the actual height rather than use a self-report. Other options include arm demi-span and knee-height measurements. The *arm demi-span* is the distance from a point on the midline at the suprasternal notch to the web between the middle and ring fingers with the arm horizontally outstretched. For people confined to bed, using a Luft ruler is another option.

Obtain a detailed weight history, noting weight loss. Ask whether weight loss was intentional and the period over which it took place. A loss of more than 5% of usual body weight over

Malnutrition Screening Tool (MST)

STEP 1: Screen with the MST

1 Have you recently lost weight without trying?

No	0
Unsure	2

If yes, how much weight have you lost?

2-13 lb	1
14-23 lb	2
24-33 lb	3
34 lb or more	4
Unsure	2

Weight loss score: ______

2 Have you been eating poorly because of a decreased appetite?

No	0
Yes	1

Appetite score: ______

Add weight loss and appetite scores

MST SCORE: ______

STEP 2: Score to determine risk

MST = 0 OR 1
NOT AT RISK
Eating well with little or no weight loss

If length of stay exceeds 7 days, then rescreen, repeating weekly as needed.

MST = 2 OR MORE
AT RISK
Eating poorly and/or recent weight loss

Rapidly implement nutrition interventions. Perform nutrition consult within 24-72 hrs, depending on risk.

STEP 3: Intervene with nutritional support for your patients at risk of malnutrition.

Notes: ______

Ferguson, M et al. *Nutrition* 1999 15:458-464

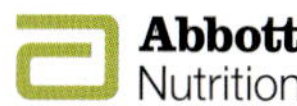

Fig. 44.2 Malnutrition Screening Tool. (From Ferguson M, Capra S, Bauer J, et al: Development of a valid and reliable malnutrition screening tool for adult acute hospital patients, *Nutrition* 15:458–464, 1999.)

6 months (whether intentional or unintentional) is a key indicator for further assessment. If an involuntary weight loss exceeds 10% of the usual weight, explore the reason. Unintentional weight loss is important to consider in the obese person. Malnutrition can be present despite excess body weight. Assess the current weight in relation to ideal body weight. We often use waist circumference and hip-to-waist ratio to assess nutrition status (see Chapter 45).

Calculate the BMI. *Body mass index* is a measure of weight for height (see Fig. 45.6). A BMI of less than 18.5 kg/m^2 is considered underweight. Normal weight is a BMI between 18.5 and 24.9 kg/m^2. Overweight is a BMI between 25 and 29.9 kg/m^2. A BMI of 30 kg/m^2 or greater is obese. BMIs outside the normal range are associated with increased mortality.

Measure skinfold thickness at various sites and calf and midarm circumference.[13] The sites most reflective of body fat are those over the biceps and triceps, below the scapula, above the iliac crest, and over the upper thigh. Compare the measures obtained with standards for healthy persons of the same age and gender. Both skinfold thickness and circumferences may decrease in malnutrition. Shifts in hydration status influence these measurements. The measurements are most beneficial when done serially and by someone trained in anthropometry.

Functional assessment focuses on activities of daily living (ADLs) tools. The tools used most often are the Katz Index and Lawton Scale. Muscle strength reflects physical functional status.[13] Muscle strength measures include handgrip strength and knee extension. Timed gait and chair stands are markers of lower extremity strength.

◆ Clinical Problems

Clinical problems for patients with malnutrition include:

- Nutritionally compromised
- Body weight problem
- Risk for impaired tissue integrity
- Inadequate community resources

◆ Planning

The overall goals are that patients with malnutrition will (1) achieve balanced nutrition and optimal weight, (2) consume a nutritionally balanced diet, (3) have no adverse effects from malnutrition, and (4) recognize factors that lead to malnutrition and take preventive action.

◆ Implementation

Health Promotion

It is part of your role to teach and reinforce healthy eating habits. Use MyPlate, the Dietary Guidelines for Americans, and Nutrition Facts food labels to promote healthy nutrition. The MyPlate approach is a visual guide for sensible meal planning. It helps someone eat healthfully and make good food choices. MyPlate focuses on the proportions of 5 food groups (grains, protein, fruits, vegetables, and dairy) that you should eat at each meal (Fig. 44.3 and Table 44.8). At the health professionals' link at www.myplate.gov, you can download daily food plans, sample menus, and tips for how to be physically active. These materials are valuable to use in patient teaching. MyPlate materials for older adults are available at https://www.myplate.gov/life-stages/older-adults.

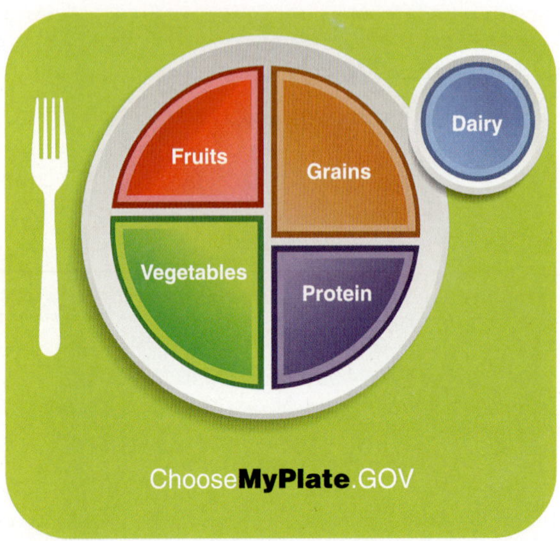

Fig. 44.3 MyPlate is the primary food group symbol that serves as a reminder to make healthy food choices and to build a healthy plate at mealtimes. For more information, see www.myplate.gov. (From U.S. Department of Agriculture, Center for Nutrition Policy and Promotion: Guidance on use of USDA's MyPlate and statements about amounts of food groups contributed by foods on food product labels, Washington, DC, U.S. Department of Agriculture.)

People with food insecurity use many strategies to obtain sufficient food. These include taking part in federal food assistance programs, obtaining food from community feeding systems (food pantries, soup kitchens, shelters), and gardening. Consult with social workers and dietitians about available resources. Help patients make food choices that meet nutrition requirements while considering their resources. Advocate in your community for access to healthy food (Box 44.1).

There are many education resources. Electronic and print sources are available for determining nutrition information in commonly consumed foods. Many food products have Nutrition Facts labels (Fig. 44.4). Consumer and health professional education materials on Nutrition Facts labels are available on the U.S. Food and Drug Administration (FDA) website (www.fda.gov/Food/LabelingNutrition/ucm20026097.htm).

Interactive web-based programs and mobile device applications are available to track physical activity, calories, nutrients, and foods eaten. Some applications use built-in barcode scanners to scan foods quickly and give their nutrition facts. Users can compare items for their nutrition benefit and cost. Other applications give information on portion sizes and adjustments needed to reduce calories, sodium, or fat in the diet based on the user's height, weight, and activity level.

Acute Care

Collaborate with the HCP and dietitian to implement nutrition therapy specific to patients' needs, preferences, and goals

TABLE 44.8 NUTRITION THERAPY

Tips for Balanced Nutrition

1. Balance calories	• Find out how many calories you need for a day as a first step in managing your weight. Go to www.myplate.gov to find your calorie level. • Being physically active helps you balance calories.
2. Enjoy your food, but eat less	• Take the time to enjoy your food as you eat it. • Eating too fast or when your attention is elsewhere may lead to eating too many calories. • Pay attention to hunger and fullness cues before, during, and after meals. Use them to recognize when to eat and when you have had enough.
3. Avoid oversized portions	• Use a smaller plate, bowl, and glass. • Portion out foods before you eat. • When eating out, choose a smaller size portion, share a dish, or take home part of your meal.
4. Foods to eat more often	• Eat more vegetables, fruits, whole grains, and fat-free or 1% milk and dairy products. • These foods have the nutrients you need for health, including potassium, calcium, vitamin D, and fiber. Make them the basis for meals and snacks. • Choose beverages with little added sugar or caloric sweeteners.
5. Make half your plate fruits and vegetables	• Choose red, orange, and dark-green vegetables such as tomatoes, sweet potatoes, and broccoli, along with other vegetables, for your meals. • Add fruit to meals as part of main or side dishes or as dessert.
6. Use fat-free or low-fat (1%) milk	• They have the same amount of calcium and other essential nutrients as whole milk. • They have fewer calories and less saturated fat.
7. Make half your grains whole grains	• To eat more whole grains, substitute a whole-grain product for a refined product. For example, eat whole-wheat bread instead of white bread or brown rice instead of white rice.
8. Foods to eat less often	• Cut back on foods high in solid fats, added sugars, and salt. • Limit cakes, cookies, ice cream, candies, sweetened drinks, pizza, and fatty meats such as ribs, sausages, bacon, and hot dogs. • Use these foods as occasional treats, not everyday foods.
9. Compare sodium in foods	• Use the Nutrition Facts label (Fig. 44.4) to choose lower-sodium versions of foods, such as soup, bread, and frozen meals. • Select foods labeled "low sodium," "reduced sodium," or "no salt added."
10. Drink water instead of sugary drinks	• Cut calories by drinking water or unsweetened beverages. • Limit your intake of soda, energy drinks, and sports drinks.

MyPlate Tips for a Healthy Lifestyle from U.S. Department of Agriculture Center for Nutrition Policy and Promotion: *Nutrition education series, DG tips sheet no 1, June 2011*. Retrieved from www.myplate.gov and www.health.gov/dietaryguidelines.

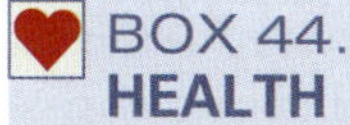

BOX 44.1 PROMOTING POPULATION HEALTH

Access to Nutritional Food

- Identify community risk factors for food insecurity
- Teach community members about solutions to food insecurity
- Provide nutrition education to prevent chronic health problems
- Recommend resources and education programs
- Be involved in advocating for food-insecure persons in your community

(Table 44.9). Nutrition care is therapy and not just supportive care.[14] Some agencies have nutrition support teams. Their function is to manage patients' nutrition support. The nutrition support nurse on that team is a key resource for issues about patients' nutrition and nutrition access. Managing DRM includes a combination of nutrition care interventions. These include diet teaching, special diets, oral nutrition supplements (ONSs), enteral nutrition (EN), parenteral nutrition (PN), special nutrient supplements such as vitamin D, and other interventions, such as exercise. Fig. 44.5 shows a decision-making tree for nutrition support.

Obtain weight daily. In conjunction with food and fluid intake, weight gives the best picture of fluid and nutrition state. Evaluate changes in weight. Rapid changes are usually the result of shifts in fluid balance. If the patient can take food by mouth, obtain a daily calorie count and diet diary. These give a record of food intake. Help patients select appropriate foods for their diet plan. Offering foods preferred by the patient enhances intake. You may have caregivers bring in favorite foods. Some patients benefit from appetite stimulants, such as megestrol acetate or dronabinol (Marinol), to improve intake.

Patients may need ONS. These may be items prepared in the facility or commercially prepared. ONSs provide extra calories, proteins, fluids, and nutrients. They are widely used as an adjunct to meals and fluid intake when intake is deficient. They provide advanced nutrition and calories. These include a wide variety of puddings and shakes, such as Ensure or Boost. In long-term care, using an ONS for oral medication administration increases caloric intake. EN may be an option in patients who are still unable to take in enough calories. If EN is not possible, consider starting PN.

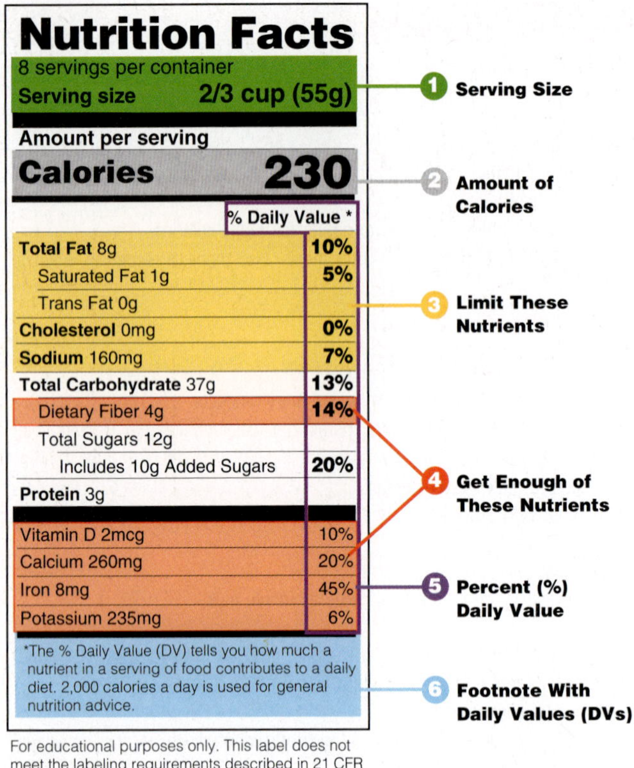

Fig. 44.4 Sample of a Nutrition Facts label. (From U.S. Department of Health and Human Services, Nutrition facts label, Silver Spring, U.S. Department of Health and Human Services.)

TABLE 44.9 NURSING MANAGEMENT

Nutrition Care Interventions

1. Provide prescribed diet for nutrition goals.
   - Offer a variety of appropriate drinks and foods.
   - Encourage the family to bring the patient's favorite foods from home.
   - Offer and help with diet selection.
2. Administer medications as prescribed. These may include nutrition supplements; electrolyte, vitamin, and mineral supplements; appetite stimulants; and antiemetics.
3. Obtain a daily weight and calorie count. Evaluate intake and output.
4. Promote a positive meal experience:
   - Offer oral hygiene and provide hand hygiene.
   - Help the patient to the proper position. Place the bedside table at the right height.
   - Clear the bedside table of clutter. Remove urinals and bedpans from sight.
   - If needed, open cartons and packages.
   - Protect mealtime from unnecessary interruptions by performing nonurgent care before or after meals.
5. Offer patients with impaired mental status fluids and food at regular intervals.
6. Help patients with eating as needed. Encourage caregiver involvement.
7. Coordinate referrals as needed:
   - Speech therapy: Swallowing evaluations
   - Occupational therapy: Functional ability and adaptive devices
   - Social workers: Resources for obtaining healthy food and obtaining dental care
8. Teach the patient and caregiver the role of diet and nutrition in health. Discuss the reason for interventions, including daily weights, intake and output, and diet. Review foods and fluids for their diet plan.

Refeeding syndrome. Refeeding syndrome is a range of metabolic and electrolyte changes that occur when calories are reintroduced after a period of decreased or absent caloric intake.[15] Conditions that predispose patients to refeeding syndrome include chronic alcohol use, cancer, trauma, inflammatory bowel disease, and major surgery. Hypophosphatemia is the hallmark of refeeding syndrome. Other manifestations include hyperglycemia, fluid retention, hypokalemia, and hypomagnesemia. Serious outcomes include dysrhythmias and respiratory arrest.

In at-risk patients, we should restart feeding slowly. Many recommend taking 7 to 10 days to achieve target intake.[15] Monitor electrolyte values and fluid balance. Maintain ECG monitoring. Many receive phosphate, potassium, magnesium, and B vitamin supplements.

Chronic Care

Many patients are discharged on a diet plan. Discharge preparation for both patients and caregivers is essential. If access to a dietitian is limited, you may be the main source of nutrition information. Consider eating habits, religious beliefs, cultural values, age, resources, and state of health. Is there a need for accessing resources, such as federal food assistance programs or community feeding systems (food pantries, soup kitchens, shelters)?

Teach them about the cause of malnutrition. They need to be aware that malnourishment, whatever the cause, can recur and that adhering to the diet for a few weeks cannot fully restore balanced nutrition. It may take many months to reach this goal. Emphasize the need for follow-up care to achieve and maintain balanced nutrition. Ensure proper follow-up, such as visits by the home health nurse and outpatient dietitian referrals. Some patients, such as those with an eating disorder, will need a referral for psychiatric counseling. Encourage self-assessment of progress by having patients weigh themselves once or twice a week and keep a weight record. A diet diary is one way to analyze and reinforce eating patterns. These records are helpful in follow-up care.

◆ Evaluation

The expected outcomes are that patients who are malnourished will:

- Achieve balanced nutrition and optimal weight
- Consume a nutritionally balanced diet
- Have no adverse effects from malnutrition
- Take action to maintain balanced nutrition

Gerontologic Considerations: Malnutrition

Nutrition affects quality of life, functional status, and health in older adults. They are particularly vulnerable to malnutrition across care settings. Older hospitalized adults with malnutrition are more likely to have poor wound healing, pressure injuries,

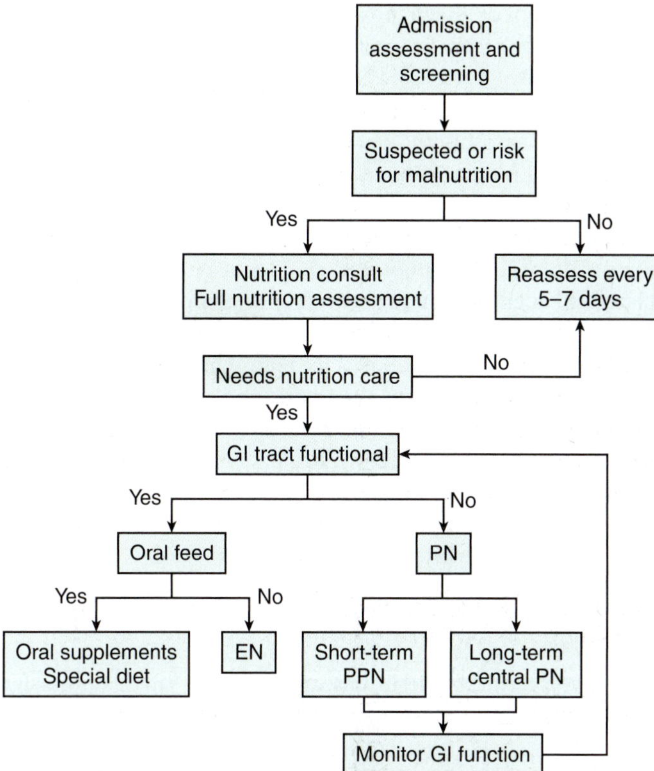

Fig. 44.5 Nutrition support algorithm.

infections, postoperative complications, and increased mortality. They are less able to regain body weight lost after illness or surgery.

You play a key role in assessing older adults' nutrition risk. Assess for appetite, problems with eating or swallowing, and inadequate servings of nutrients. Someone with limited income may restrict the number of meals or the nutrient quality of meals. Social isolation may be a problem. Those who live alone may lose their desire to cook and report decreased appetite. Functional limitations may affect the ability to feed oneself, buy food, or cook and prepare meals. Some may lack transportation to buy food. Chronic illnesses can affect nutrition status. Older adults with dementia (see Chapter 64) or a stroke (see Chapter 62) have unique challenges with eating.

Physiologic changes associated with aging include a decrease in lean body mass, which can decrease caloric requirement and affect muscle strength and function. Older adults on bed rest or prolonged inactivity lose more lean body mass than younger adults. Changes in smell and taste affect appetite.

General nutrition guidelines apply to older adults. Requirements vary depending on the degree of malnutrition and health status. To prevent loss of muscle mass and maintain function, older adults may need to increase protein intake and ingest a moderate amount of high-quality protein at each meal. Daily vitamin D requirements are higher for older adults (Table 44.3). Focus your initial care on improving oral intake and providing a pleasant, social environment for meals (Table 44.9).

Many older adults are vulnerable when discharged from the hospital to the home. They may not be able to shop for or prepare food during their recovery. Consult with the social worker and dietitian to ensure there is access to food on discharge. Many community-based organizations address food and nutrition needs. These include home-delivered meals or groceries and senior congregate meals. Improving the social setting of a meal often improves intake.

TABLE 44.10 Common Indications for Enteral Nutrition

- Anorexia
- Burns
- Chemotherapy
- Critical illness
- Facial fractures, surgery
- Neurologic problems
- Prolonged NPO
- Radiation therapy

ADVANCED NUTRITION SUPPORT

Enteral Nutrition

Enteral nutrition (EN), or **tube feeding,** is nutrition delivered through a tube, catheter, or stoma directly into the GI tract. EN is used with patients who have a functioning GI tract but cannot take any or enough oral nourishment or when it is unsafe to do so. EN helps maintain gut integrity by maintaining normal digestion and absorption.

The decision to start EN is based on several factors (Table 44.10). Can the patient obtain adequate nourishment by mouth? Do they have dysphagia, chewing problems, GI problems, or preexisting malnutrition? Review the duration of expected poor intake. Is the patient critically ill, under sedation, or have advanced untreatable cancer? If a patient is not able to give consent, review their advance directives about artificial nutrition and hydration.

There is a wide variety of EN formulas. Their concentration, osmolality, and amounts of nutrients vary.[16] There are formulas with and without fiber. Disease-specific formulas target patients with diabetes or liver, kidney, or lung disease. Blenderized foods are options. Standard formulas provide between 1 and 2 cal/mL. They are nutritionally complete when the patient receives 1000 to 1500 mL.[16] The number and size of particles in the formula determine its osmolality. The more hydrolyzed or broken down the nutrients, the greater the osmolality.

Delivery options are continuous infusion, intermittent, and bolus feedings. Feedings may be given by infusion pump, gravity, and syringe. Critically ill patients often receive EN by continuous infusion.[17] Intermittent and bolus feeding may be an option if the patient improves or is receiving EN at home.

EN Access

Access can be obtained through the nose or mouth, with the end destination being the stomach or below the pyloric sphincter (into the small intestine).[17] The type of access depends on the patient's (1) expected length of time EN will be needed, (2) risk for aspiration, (3) clinical status, (4) GI tract function, and (5) anatomy (e.g., extreme obesity). Fig. 44.6 shows the locations of commonly used EN tubes.

The default location for feeding is the stomach. It has a large reservoir, allows for gastric digestion, and is closest to physiologic eating. Placement into the small intestine decreases the chance of regurgitating gastric contents into the esophagus and aspiration.[17] These feedings are given continuously or intermittently by pump.[18]

Orogastric, nasogastric, nasoduodenal, and nasojejunal tubes. Nasal and oral placed tubes are used for short-term feeding (less than 4 weeks). Nasoduodenal and nasojejunal tubes are used when feeding patients into the small intestine.

Polyurethane or silicone feeding tubes of various lengths, diameters, and features are used depending on patients' needs. The tubes are soft and flexible. This decreases the risk for mucosal damage. The tubes are also radiopaque, making their position readily identified by x-ray.

Although smaller feeding tubes have many advantages over larger tubes, such as the standard nasogastric (NG) tube, there are disadvantages. Because of the small diameter and length, these tubes clog easily. They are prone to occlusion if you do not thoroughly crush and dissolve drugs before administration. Not flushing the tube before and after giving drugs can cause tube occlusion. Checking gastric residual volume (GRV) is harder. Vomiting or coughing can dislodge the tube. The tube can become knotted or kinked. Problems may require removal and insertion of a new tube, adding to cost and patient discomfort.

Gastrostomy and jejunostomy tubes. If feedings are needed for an extended time, tubes can be placed in the stomach (gastrostomy) or small bowel (jejunostomy). A gastrostomy tube (G-tube) can be placed surgically, radiologically, or endoscopically (Fig. 44.7). Percutaneous endoscopic gastrostomy (PEG) tube and radiologically placed G-tube procedures have fewer risks than surgical placement. The procedure requires IV sedation and local anesthesia. IV antibiotics are given before the procedure.

For patients with chronic reflux, feeding through a jejunostomy (J-tube) can reduce the risk for aspiration. J-tubes are placed either endoscopically or with open or laparoscopic surgery. Combination gastrojejunostomy (G-J) tubes allow for gastric decompression and small bowel feeding. When a patient has a G-J tube, know which port is the gastric and which is the jejunal.

The tube is either premarked or marked at the skin insertion site. Feedings can start within 24 hours after a surgically placed G- or J-tube without waiting for flatus or a bowel movement. Most other PEG tube feedings can start within 4 hours of insertion, although agency policies vary.

EN Safety

You have a critical role in ensuring that we safely administer EN. Aspiration and dislodged tubes are important safety

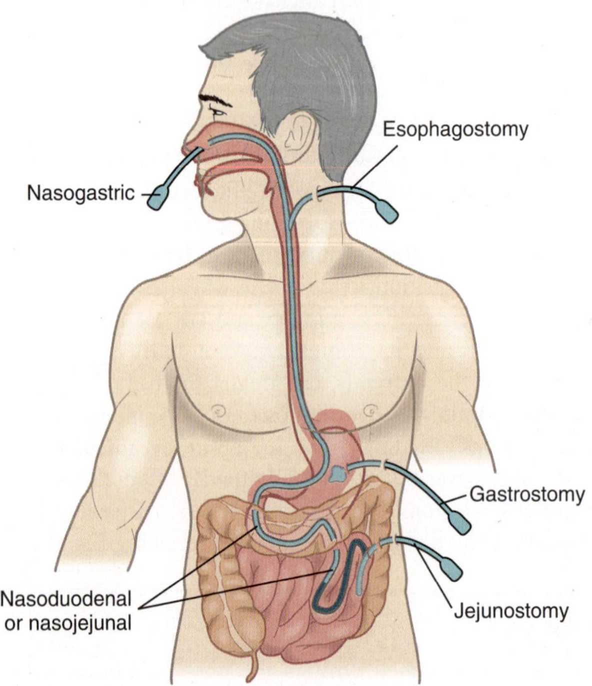

Fig. 44.6 Common enteral feeding tube placement locations.

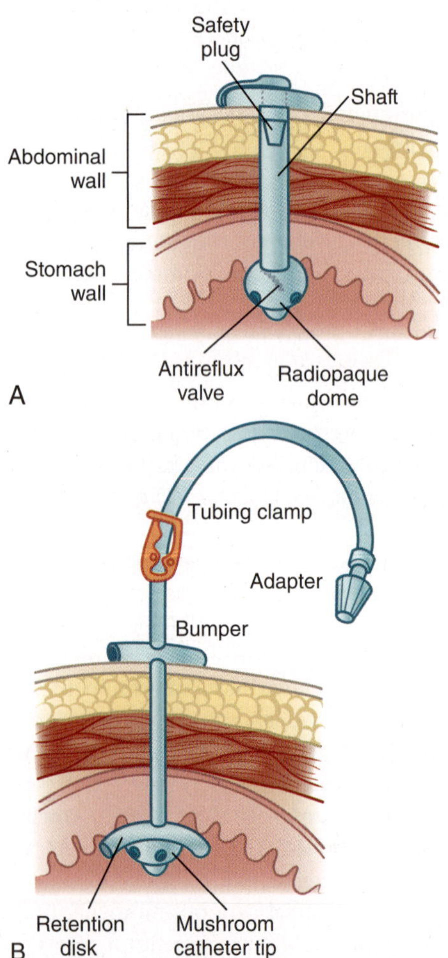

Fig. 44.7 (A) Gastrostomy feeding button in place. (B) Gastrostomy tube with retention disk and bumper.

concerns. Nursing management of EN is shown in Table 44.11. Managing common problems in patients receiving EN is outlined in Table 44.12. A nursing care plan for patients receiving EN (eNursing Care Plan 44.1) is available on the website for this chapter.

Tube position. Obtain x-ray confirmation of newly inserted nasal or orogastric tubes to confirm proper position before starting feedings or medications. Tubes can pass directly into the bronchus without any obvious respiratory manifestations. Placing a tube under electromagnetic guidance reduces the risk for misplacement with blind insertion. Capnography can help determine tube placement in the respiratory tract.[19]

Maintain proper placement of the tube after starting feedings. Mark the exit site of the tube at the time of the initial x-ray. To check if a tube is still in the proper position, assess the tube's external length at regular intervals.

A small bowel tube can migrate upward into the stomach or esophagus. If you see a significant increase in the external length, use other bedside tests to help determine whether the

TABLE 44.11 NURSING MANAGEMENT

Enteral Nutrition

Safe Administration

- Give medications in the safest form possible.
  - Use liquid medications only if they are labeled safe for enteral use.
  - Dilute thick liquid medications.
  - Do not combine medications with the enteral formula.
  - Crush drugs to a fine powder and dissolve in purified water.
  - Use an ENFit syringe to administer medications.
- Employ measures to decrease aspiration risk.
  - Check tube placement before feeding and each medication administration.
  - Keep head of bed elevated to 30- to 45-degree angle.
- Assess patient's tolerance of feeding.
  - Perform a regular abdominal assessment.
- Avoid contamination of formula and equipment.
- Assess for complications related to EN (Table 44.12).
- Assess tube insertion site for signs of pressure injury and skin breakdown. Cleanse and protect area as needed.
- Use measures to prevent tubing misconnections (Table 44.13).
- Maintain patency by flushing tubes before and after medication administration or at least once per shift. Flush continuous feeding at regular intervals.

Delegate to Licensed Practical/Vocational Nurse (LPN/VN)

- Insert nasogastric (NG) tube for stable patient.
- Flush NG and gastrostomy tubes.
- Give medications and bolus or continuous feeding for stable patient.
- Remove NG tube.
- Provide skin care around tube sites.

Supervise AP

- Provide routine oral care.
- Weigh patient and obtain intake and output.
- Keep the head of bed elevated 30–45 degrees.
- Report symptoms that may indicate problems with EN to RN or LPN.
- Alert RN or LPN about pump alarms.

Collaborate With Dietitian

- Evaluate nutrition status.
- Select EN formula.
- Monitor for and manage complications related to EN.
- Teach patient and caregiver about home EN and tube care.

Collaborate With Pharmacist

- Select appropriate form of each drug that patient is receiving.
- Decide best practice for giving each enteral drug.

TABLE 44.12 NURSING MANAGEMENT

Enteral Nutrition Problems

Problems and Causes	Management
Constipation	
Decreased fluid intake	• Increase fluid intake if not contraindicated. • Maintain fluid intake of 30 mL/kg body weight.
Fiber	• Change formula to one with more fiber content. • Give laxative as ordered.
Dehydration	
Diarrhea, vomiting	• Decrease rate or change formula. • Review other drugs that patient is receiving.
Fluid intake	• Increase EN intake. • Administer supplemental tube, oral, or IV fluid intake if appropriate.
Hyperglycemia	• Check glucose levels often. • Maintain glucose level with as-needed insulin.
Diarrhea	

Contamination	• Refrigerate unused formula and record date opened.
	• Discard outdated formula.
	• Discard formula left standing for longer than manufacturer's guidelines.
	  • 8 h for ready-to-feed formulas (cans)
	  • 4 h for reconstituted formula
	  • 24 h for closed-system formulas
	• Use a closed system.

Feeding too fast	• Dilute or decrease rate of feeding. • Change to continuous feedings. • Decrease water boluses.
Formula	• Change to a formula that has more fiber or is less hypertonic. • Change to continuous feedings.
Infection	• Obtain stool culture for fecal leukocyte determination, *C. difficile,* and/or toxin assay.
Medications	• Check for drugs that may cause diarrhea (e.g., drugs in sorbitol suspension, antibiotics).
Tube moving distally	• Properly secure tube before beginning feeding. • Check placement before each bolus feeding or at least every 4 h if continuous feedings.
Vomiting	
Delayed gastric emptying	• Consult with HCP about a prokinetic drug. • Discontinue drugs that interfere with GI motility. • Consider formula with less fiber and/or fat.
Improper tube placement	• Replace tube in proper position. • Check tube position before each bolus feeding and every 4 h with continuous feedings.

tube has moved. These measures include assessing aspirate color and pH. Because each measure has limitations, confirm placement with more than one test.

! SAFETY ALERT

Do not use auscultation to confirm feeding tube placement.

Aspiration risk. Evaluate all patients for risk for aspiration. Proper patient positioning decreases the risk for aspiration. Always keep the head of the bed elevated 30 to 45 degrees. If the patient does not tolerate a backrest elevation, use reverse Trendelenburg position to elevate the head of the bed unless contraindicated. If you need to lower the head of the bed for a procedure, quickly return the patient to at least 30 degrees. Follow agency policy for stopping feeding while the patient is supine. Keep the head elevated for 30 to 60 minutes after intermittent and bolus feedings.

! SAFETY ALERT

Keep the head of the bed elevated 30 to 45 degrees in a patient receiving EN to prevent aspiration.

There is no agreement about whether to check GRV. Some think an increased GRV increases the risk for aspiration. Other research does not support the practice. Follow your agency policy for checking GRV. Common protocols call for checking it every 6 to 8 hours and before each bolus or intermittent feeding.

Before starting feeding, ensure the tube is in the right position. Other measures to decrease aspiration risk include giving feedings continuously, minimizing sedation, and performing frequent oral suctioning. Promotility drugs, such as erythromycin or metoclopramide, improve gastric emptying and may reduce aspiration risk.

Site care. Skin care around gastrostomy and jejunostomy tube sites is important because digestive juices irritate the skin. Assess the skin around the site daily for redness and maceration. Monitor bumper tension and routinely check for pressure injury.

Keep the skin clean and dry. At first, rinse it with sterile water and dry it. Apply a dressing until the site is healed. After that, wash with mild soap and water. You may apply a protective ointment (zinc oxide, petroleum gauze) or skin barrier (Karaya, Stomahesive) around the tube. If the skin is irritated, consider using other types of drain or tube pouches. Consult a wound, ostomy, and continence nurse (WOCN) if problems occur.

Tube patency. All tubes require routine flushing. Generally, flush tubes in adults with at least 30 mL of purified water every 4 hours during continuous feedings or before and after each bolus feeding. Use sterile water in immunocompromised and critically ill patients. Flush tubes between each medication and after giving any medications. Flush clogged tubes with warm water, using a back-and-forth motion. If that does not work, an enzyme declogging solution or mechanical devices for clearing feeding tubes are options.[17]

CHECK YOUR PRACTICE

You are caring for a patient who has a PEG tube placed for EN after a stroke. As you prepare to flush the tube with water before giving their scheduled medications, you find that you cannot flush the tube.

- What should your next actions be?

Misconnection. An *enteral feeding misconnection* is an inadvertent connection between an enteral feeding system and a nonenteral system, such as an IV line, peritoneal dialysis catheter, or tracheostomy tube cuff. With an enteral feeding misconnection, EN formula intended for the GI tract is given IV or into the respiratory tract. Severe injury and death can result from a misconnection. Table 44.13 gives tips to decrease the risk for enteral feeding misconnections.

Gerontologic Considerations: Enteral Nutrition

EN can improve nutrition status in older patients. Because of physiologic changes, older adults are more vulnerable to complications from EN, especially fluid and electrolyte imbalances. Complications such as diarrhea can leave patients dehydrated. Decreased thirst perception or impaired cognitive function decreases patients' ability to seek needed fluids.

With aging, there is an increased risk for glucose intolerance. As a result, older patients are more susceptible to hyperglycemia from the high carbohydrate load of some EN formulas. Older adults with compromised cardiovascular function (e.g., heart failure) will have a decreased ability to handle large volumes of formula. If this happens, patients may need a more

TABLE 44.13 NURSING MANAGEMENT

Decreasing Enteral Feeding Misconnections

These tips will help you decrease your risk for making an enteral feeding misconnection:

1. Use products that have an ENFit feeding connector system.
2. Use an ENFit syringe to administer all enteral drugs.
3. Teach visitors, LPN/VNs, and AP to notify the nurse if an enteral feeding line becomes disconnected and not to reconnect any line.
4. Do not change or adapt IV or feeding devices because it may compromise the safety features.
5. Do not use an IV pump or IV tubing to deliver EN.
6. When making a reconnection or connecting a new infusion, trace lines back to their origins and make sure connections are secure.
7. As part of the handoff process, recheck connections and trace all tubes to their origin.
8. Route tubes and catheters that have different purposes in unique and standard directions (e.g., route IV lines toward the patient's head and enteral lines toward the feet).
9. Label or color-code feeding tubes and connectors.
10. When there are multiple access points and/or several bags hanging, place proximal and distal labels on all tubing.
11. Check vital signs after making any connection.
12. Label the bags with large, bold statements such as "WARNING! For Enteral Use Only—NOT for IV Use."
13. Make tubing connections under proper lighting.

concentrated formula (2.0 cal/mL). Older adults have an increased risk for aspiration caused by gastroesophageal reflux disease (GERD) and delayed gastric emptying.

Parenteral Nutrition

Parenteral nutrition (PN) is the administration of nutrients directly into the bloodstream. It is used when oral intake or EN is not possible or is insufficient. Table 44.14 lists common reasons for PN.

Composition

PN contains many different ingredients. It is customized to meet the needs of each patient. The composition is reformulated as a patient's condition changes. This requires you to collaborate with the health care team.

PN components include fluids, macronutrients (amino acids, dextrose, lipids), and micronutrients (electrolytes, vitamins, trace elements). PN base solutions include a 2-in-1 with dextrose and amino acids or a 3-in-1 with a lipid emulsion (ILE), dextrose, and amino acids.[20] Electrolytes (sodium, potassium, chloride, calcium, magnesium, phosphate) are available in some premixed solutions or added by the pharmacy. The pharmacy also can add vitamins and trace elements (zinc, copper, chromium, selenium, manganese).

Calories. Calories in PN mainly come from carbohydrates in the form of dextrose and fats in the form of ILE. Dextrose 100 to 150 g/day (1 g provides 3.4 calories) has a protein-sparing effect.[21] Providing adequate calories via glucose and fat allows the use of amino acids for wound healing and not for energy. However, dextrose and ILE overfeeding can lead to metabolic complications. To minimize these problems, the recommended energy intake is 12 to 25 cal/kg/day.[20]

ILE solutions of 10%, 20%, and 30% are available. ILE supplies about 1 cal/mL (10% solution) or 2 cal/mL (20% solution). They primarily contain soybean, safflower, coconut, or olive oil with egg phospholipids added as an emulsifier.[20,21] ILE supplies a large number of calories in a small amount of fluid. This is helpful when patients are at risk for fluid overload.

ILE provides 20% to 30% of the total calories of PN.[20] Most patients receive 1 g/kg/day to avoid lipid overload. Triglyceride levels are done at the beginning of PN and then closely monitored. Give ILE administered separately over a minimum of 12 hours. The initial infusion rate should not exceed 0.5 mL/kg/h. If no reactions occur, the rate can increase to 1 mL/h.

ILE is contraindicated in patients with a problem with fat metabolism, such as hyperlipidemia. They are used cautiously in patients at risk for fat embolism (e.g., fractured femur) and patients with an allergy to eggs or soybeans.

Protein. Protein is provided at the rate of 0.8 to 1.5 g/kg/day depending on a patient's needs. Protein requirements can exceed 150 g/day (2 g/kg/day) to ensure a positive nitrogen balance in septic, critically ill, burn, or multiple trauma patients. Protein needs may be lower than 0.8 g/kg in those with liver problems or end-stage renal disease who are not on dialysis.[22]

Micronutrients. Micronutrients include electrolytes, vitamins, and trace elements. The exact amounts depend on a patient's health problem and laboratory levels. Assess requirements daily at the beginning of therapy and then several times a week as PN progresses. Adding a daily multivitamin preparation to PN often meets the vitamin requirements.

TABLE 44.14 Common Indications for Parenteral Nutrition

- Chronic severe diarrhea and vomiting
- Complicated surgery or trauma
- Enteritis from chemotherapy or radiation
- GI obstruction, cancer
- GI tract anomalies and fistulae
- Inaccessible GI tract
- Inflammatory bowel disease
- Pancreatitis
- Severe malabsorption
- Short bowel syndrome

Methods of Administration

PN is given as central PN or peripheral parenteral nutrition (PPN). Central PN and PPN differ in nutrient content and tonicity. Tonicity is measured in milliosmoles (mOsm) or the concentration of particles in a fluid.

Central parenteral nutrition. *Central PN* is delivered through a central vein via a central venous access device (CVAD) (see Chapter 17). It is indicated when long-term support is needed or when a patient has high protein and caloric requirements. Central PN solutions are hypertonic, measuring at least 1600 mOsm/L. The high glucose content ranges from 20% to 50%. Central PN must be infused in a large central vein so that rapid dilution can occur. Using a peripheral vein for hypertonic, central PN solutions would cause irritation and thrombophlebitis.

Peripheral parenteral nutrition. PPN is given through a peripherally inserted catheter or vascular access device into a large vein. It is used when (1) nutrition support is needed for only a short time, (2) protein and caloric requirements are not high, (3) the risk for a central catheter is too great, or (4) oral intake is inadequate.

Compared with central PN, PPN has fewer nutrients. Although this makes PPN less hypertonic, it still has an osmolality between 750 and 900 mOsm/L.[20] This increases the risk for phlebitis. Another potential complication is fluid overload. PPN requires large volumes of fluid, which many patients cannot tolerate.

NURSING MANAGEMENT: PARENTERAL NUTRITION

Nursing management of patients receiving PN is outlined in Table 44.15 and eNursing Care Plan 44.2, available on the

TABLE 44.15 NURSING MANAGEMENT

Parenteral Nutrition

PN Solutions

- Add nothing to PN solutions after they are prepared in the pharmacy.
- Limit number of people involved in preparing and administering PN to reduce risk for infection.
- PN solutions are ordered daily to adjust to the patient's current needs.
- PN solution label must show the nutrient content, all additives, time mixed, and expiration date and time.
- Refrigerate solutions until 30 min before use. They are good for 24 h at room temperature.

Maintain Infusions

- Follow proper aseptic techniques to reduce infection risk.
- Use a 0.22-micron filter with solutions not containing ILE and a 1.2-micron filter with solutions containing ILE.
- Change filters and IV tubing with each new PN container or every 24 h.
- Label tubing and filter with date and time they are put into use.
- If a multilumen catheter is present, use a dedicated line for PN.
- Do not draw blood from a line dedicated for PN unless necessary.
- Give PN using an infusion pump.
- Set an alarm to alert for tubing obstruction.
- Protect the PN solution from light.

Ensure Safety

- Before starting PN, check label and ingredients in solution to make sure they match the order.
- Verify infusion pump settings with a second RN before starting PN.
- Trace the administration tubing to the point of origin at the start of the infusion and at all handoffs.
- Check the solution for leaks, color changes, particles, clarity, and fat emulsions separating. If present, promptly return it to the pharmacy.
- Discontinue a PN solution and replace it with a new solution if bag is not empty at the end of 24 h.
- Infuse separate fat emulsions over 12 h.
- If a bag is empty or contaminated before more solution is available, give 10% or 20% dextrose (based on the amount of dextrose in central PN) or 5% dextrose solution (based on the amount of dextrose in PPN) to prevent hypoglycemia.

Hyperglycemia

- Check glucose levels at bedside q4–6h.
- Maintain a glucose range of 140–180 mg/dL. Give sliding-scale insulin to keep the glucose level in the normal range.

Catheter-Related Problems

- Assess the catheter site for inflammation and infection.
- Immunosuppressed patients have a high risk for infection. Note subtle signs in patients receiving chemotherapy, corticosteroids, or antibiotics, which can mask signs of infection.
- Follow agency policy for changing catheter dressings and other central line infection prevention measures (see Chapter 17).
- If you suspect an infection, notify the HCP.

Transitioning to Oral Nutrition

- Encourage oral nourishment and keep a careful record of intake. A general rule is that 60% of caloric needs should be met orally or through EN before discontinuing PN.
- Begin with clear liquids and advance as tolerated to a soft diet.

Assess Effectiveness

- Monitor initial vital signs q4–8h.
- Obtain daily weight as a measure of hydration and nutrition.
- Maintain intake and output record.
- Determine the cause of any weight changes (e.g., fluid gained from edema, actual change in weight).
- Assess glucose, electrolytes, and urea nitrogen.
- CBC and liver function studies are done a minimum of 3 times per week until stable and then weekly as needed.

TABLE 44.16 Complications of Parenteral Nutrition

Catheter-Related Problems

- Bleeding
- Catheter-related infection
- Dislodgment
- Embolism, thrombosis
- Occlusion
- Pneumothorax

Metabolic Problems

- Abnormal electrolyte levels
- Hyperglycemia, hypoglycemia
- Hyperlipidemia
- Kidney problems
- Liver problems
- Refeeding syndrome
- Vitamin and mineral deficiencies

website for this chapter. Complications from PN are related to either the catheter or the PN infusion itself (Table 44.16).

Home Nutrition Support

Home PN or EN is an accepted mode of nutrition therapy for patients who are at risk for malnutrition or are malnourished and need continued nutrition support. Some patients receive home therapy for many months, even years. Home nutrition care is expensive. Specific criteria must be met for expenses to be reimbursed. The discharge planning team must be involved early to help plan for such issues.

Teach patients and caregivers about catheter or tube care, proper technique in mixing and handling of the solutions and tubing, and side effects and complications. Home nutrition support may be a burden for patients and caregivers and affect the quality of life. Tell the family about support groups, such as the Oley Foundation (www.oley.org).

CASE STUDY

Malnutrition

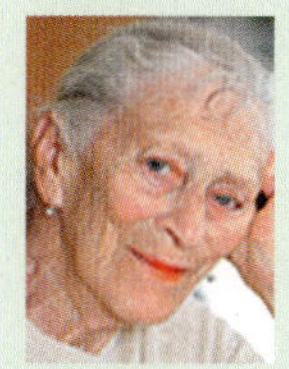
(© iStockphoto/ Thinkstock.)

Patient Profile

M.S. is a 70-year-old female who was recently admitted with malnutrition.

Subjective Data

- Reports 30-lb weight loss in past 2 months
- Recently had a thrombotic stroke with hemiparesis and dysphagia
- History of rheumatoid arthritis
- Has had nothing by mouth for the past 24 h and just started EN via PEG tube
- Lives with her daughter, who is at her bedside

Objective Data

Physical Assessment

- Has left-sided weakness
- BP is 150/90 mm Hg
- 5 ft, 4 in tall, weight 100 lb
- PEG tube recently placed

Laboratory Results

- Albumin 2.9 g/dL
- Prealbumin 11.0 mg/dL
- C-reactive protein 0.9 mg/L

Discussion Questions

1. ***Recognize:*** What are M.S.'s risk factors for malnutrition?
2. ***Analyze:*** Which complications of EN is M.S. at risk for?
3. ***Plan:*** What would we include in a nutrition program for M.S.?
4. ***Prioritize:*** Based on the assessment data presented, what are the priority clinical problems?
5. ***Act:*** Outline the priority nutrition care interventions for M.S.
6. ***Act:*** Which interventions can you delegate to AP?
7. ***Evaluate:*** What assessment data would you collect to decide if care was effective?

Answers available at http://evolve.elsevier.com/Lewis/medsurg.

BRIDGE TO NCLEX EXAMINATION

The number of the question corresponds to the same-numbered outcome at the beginning of the chapter.

1. The nurse would counsel a healthy person that their daily diet intake should consist of
- **a.** 30% to 40 % fat, which should all be from foods high in saturated fats.
- **b.** 10 grams of fiber, mainly from fruits, vegetables, and diet supplements.
- **c.** 80 grams of protein, including foods that are complete and incomplete proteins.
- **d.** 45% to 65% carbohydrates, making sure to include a variety of fruits and vegetables.

2. Place in order the substrates the body uses for energy during starvation, beginning with 1 for the first component and ending with 4 for the last component.
- **a.** Skeletal protein
- **b.** Glycogen
- **c.** Visceral protein
- **d.** Fat stores

3. A complete nutrition assessment is *most* important for the patient who
- **a.** has a BMI of 25.5 kg/m^2.
- **b.** reports episodes of nightly nocturia.
- **c.** reports a 5-year history of chronic constipation.
- **d.** reports unintentional weight loss of 10 lb in 2 months.

4. Which data *best* supports that nutrition care is effective for a patient with malnutrition?
- **a.** The patient's family is bringing in their favorite foods.
- **b.** The patient selects menu items according to their diet plan.
- **c.** The patient's weight is steadily increasing toward the set goal.
- **d.** The social worker provided the patient with meal options post discharge.

5. Which method is *best* to use when confirming initial placement of a blindly inserted small-bore NG feeding tube?
- **a.** X-ray
- **b.** Air insertion
- **c.** Observing patient for coughing
- **d.** pH measurement of gastric aspirate

6. A patient is receiving peripheral parenteral nutrition. The solution is complete before the new solution arrives on the unit. The nurse gives
- **a.** 20% intralipids.
- **b.** 5% dextrose solution.
- **c.** 0.45% normal saline solution.
- **d.** 5% lactated Ringer's solution.

1. d; 2. b, a, d, c; 3. d, 4. c; 5. a; 6. b.

For rationales to these answers and more NCLEX review questions, visit http://evolve.elsevier.com/Lewis/medsurg.

REFERENCES

To access the References for this chapter, please scan the QR code with a mobile device.

45

Obesity

Lori Ann Wenz

http://evolve.elsevier.com/Lewis/medsurg/

CONCEPTUAL FOCUS

Health Promotion
Nutrition
Self-Management

LEARNING OUTCOMES

1. Discuss the epidemiology and etiology of obesity.
2. Explain the health risks associated with obesity.
3. Discern among classification systems for obesity.
4. Discuss interprofessional care for patients with obesity.
5. Describe the nursing and interprofessional management related to patients with obesity undergoing surgery.
6. Describe the etiology, clinical manifestations, and nursing and interprofessional management of metabolic syndrome.

KEY TERMS

body mass index (BMI)
lipectomy
metabolic syndrome
obesity
overweight
waist-to-hip ratio (WHR)

EPIDEMIOLOGY

Obesity is a major public health issue in the United States. Currently, about 42% of adults in the United States have obesity. Geographic, racial and ethnic, and income disparities exist. Obesity rates are highest in the South and Midwest (Fig. 45.1), among Black and Hispanic persons (Fig. 45.2), and among those with lower income and less education.[1]

Obesity in adulthood is often a problem that begins in childhood or adolescence. More than 1 in 10 children develop obesity.[1] Reversing childhood obesity is a key part of addressing the obesity epidemic.

ETIOLOGY

Obesity is a complex, multifactorial, progressive neuroendocrine disease resulting in excess adipose tissue.[2] It is caused by an imbalance among energy intake, energy storage, and energy expenditure. Many factors, including genetic and environment influences, contribute to obesity. Personal factors involve decisions about nutrition and physical activity. Other factors include stress, sleep problems, medications, and socioeconomic status.[3]

In obesity, there is an increase in the number of adipocytes, or fat cells, and an increase in their size *(hypertrophy)*. Fat cells can increase their volume several thousand times to accommodate large increases in lipid storage. The increase in size and number of adipocytes results in adiposopathy, or "sick fat" disease. Excess energy is stored in fat deposits in the viscera, abdomen, and pericardium. Fat deposited within other organs, including the liver, kidney, heart, muscle, and pancreas, causes damage. The result is metabolic problems such as hypertension (HTN), type 2 diabetes (T2DM), dyslipidemia, inflammatory diseases, and sex hormone problems.

Genetic Link

A family history of obesity is the greatest predictor of developing the condition. We have found over 500 genes linked to obesity. Genes influence factors such as appetite, satiety (the sense of fullness), food cravings, body fat distribution, and how we store calories. The most common form of obesity, polygenic, results from multiple genes interacting with nutrition and lifestyle factors.[4] Having 1 or more of these genes means the person is at increased risk to develop obesity, but it does not mean that they will develop obesity.

Monogenic obesity and syndromic obesity are rare forms of severe obesity that begin in early childhood. Monogenic obesity is associated with a single gene variant that affects the ability to regulate weight. Syndromic obesity is associated with one or more genetic variants. Other features include development delays and endocrine problems. Examples of genetic obesity syndromes include Bardet-Biedl syndrome (BBS), Alstrom syndrome, and Prader-Willi syndrome.

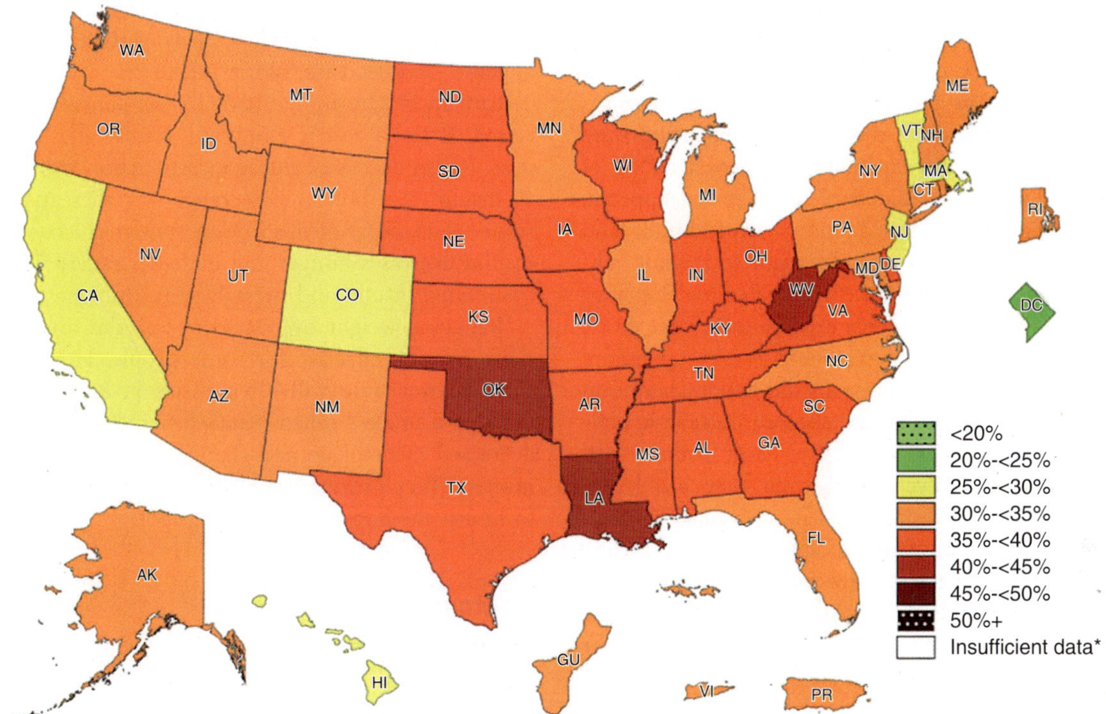

Fig. 45.1 Prevalence of obesity among U.S. adults by state and territory. (From *Behavioral Risk Factor Surveillance System.* Retrieved from https://www.cdc.gov/obesity/php/data-research/adult-obesity-prevalence-maps.html.)

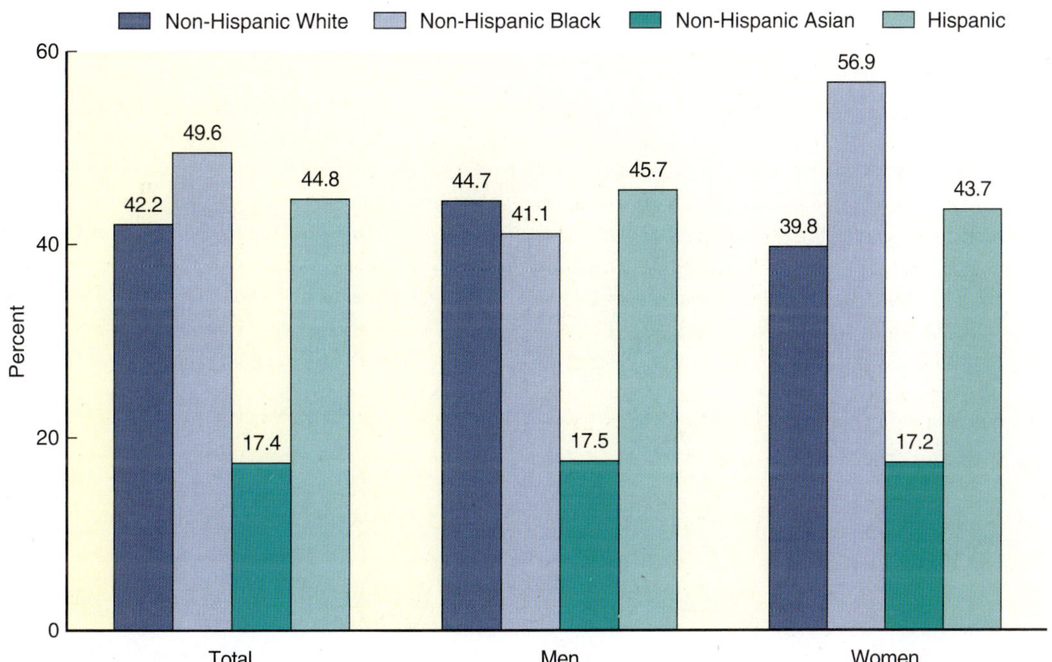

Fig. 45.2 Obesity affects some groups disproportionately. Among U.S. adults, Black and Hispanic populations have the highest rates of obesity. (From Centers for Disease Control and Prevention: *Prevalence of obesity and severe obesity among adults: US, 2017–2018.* Retrieved from https://www.cdc.gov/nchs/products/databriefs/db360.htm.)

Physiologic Regulatory Mechanisms in Obesity

Weight is regulated by complex processes involving the hypothalamus and multiple body organs. These include adipose tissue, the pancreas, stomach, intestines, and skeletal muscles.[5] The hypothalamus, gut, and adipose tissue make hormones and peptides that stimulate or inhibit appetite (Fig. 45.3). The hypothalamus makes neuropeptide Y, agouti-related peptide, and γ-aminobutyric acid. They are powerful appetite stimulants that reduce energy expenditure and weight increase. Proopiomelanocortin (POMC), also made in the hypothalamus, suppresses appetite and increases energy expenditure. When signaling of neurohormones is ineffective, the result is increased appetite, increased caloric intake, decreased energy expenditure, and weight increase. Hormones and peptides made in the gut, adipocytes, and skeletal muscles affect the hypothalamus. Thus they have a key role in appetite and energy expenditure (Table 45.1).

There are several peripheral mediators of weight regulation. Leptin is made in adipocytes. It acts in the hypothalamus to suppress appetite and increase fat metabolism. A genetic deficiency of leptin causes extreme obesity. Most people with obesity have high leptin levels, suggesting they are leptin resistant.[6] This may be the result of a failure to make enough leptin receptors or producing faulty receptors.

Ghrelin, a gut hormone, regulates appetite by inhibiting leptin. It acts in the hypothalamus and the brain's pleasure centers to stimulate hunger. Normally, ghrelin levels are higher when a person is hungry and decrease after eating. Some gastric bypass patients do not have the premeal increase in ghrelin.[3] The low ghrelin levels help suppress appetite and contribute to the surgery's effectiveness.

Adipocytes make substances we call *adipokines*. Adipokines play roles in glucose and lipid metabolism, insulin sensitivity, energy homeostasis, inflammation, immunity, and vascular function. Excess visceral fat is associated with adipokine dysfunction, which leads to insulin resistance, dyslipidemia, and high blood pressure.

Glucagon-like peptide-1 (GLP-1) and glucose-dependent insulinotropic polypeptide (GIP) are made in the small and large intestines in response to carbohydrates. These hormones stimulate insulin production in the pancreas, thus contributing to glucose regulation. They delay gastric emptying, reduce appetite, and decrease caloric intake.

Amylin is a hormone made by the pancreas in response to eating. It slows gastric emptying, resulting in feelings of fullness. It also decreases glucagon production from the pancreas.

Insulin is a hormone secreted by pancreatic beta cells in response to nutrient absorption. When glucose is controlled, insulin decreases hunger and increases satiety. In the presence of elevated insulin and hypoglycemia, hunger increases.

Reducing weight by restricting calories and increasing activity may be effective for some people. However, restricting calories over time will often result in an increased appetite through a process called *metabolic adaptation*.[5] This results in decreased metabolism and changes in appetite-regulating hormones. The person then increases caloric intake in an attempt to return the body to a higher weight.

Environment Factors

In today's culture, people have greater access to high-calorie, ultra-processed, energy-dense foods and sugar-sweetened drinks. Eating these items is associated with obesity. Portion size has increased dramatically (Fig. 45.4). Lack of physical exercise contributes to weight gain and obesity. We expend less energy in our everyday lives because of economic growth, technology use, and social changes. Increased time spent gaming, surfing the Internet, and watching TV contributes to the increase in sedentary habits.

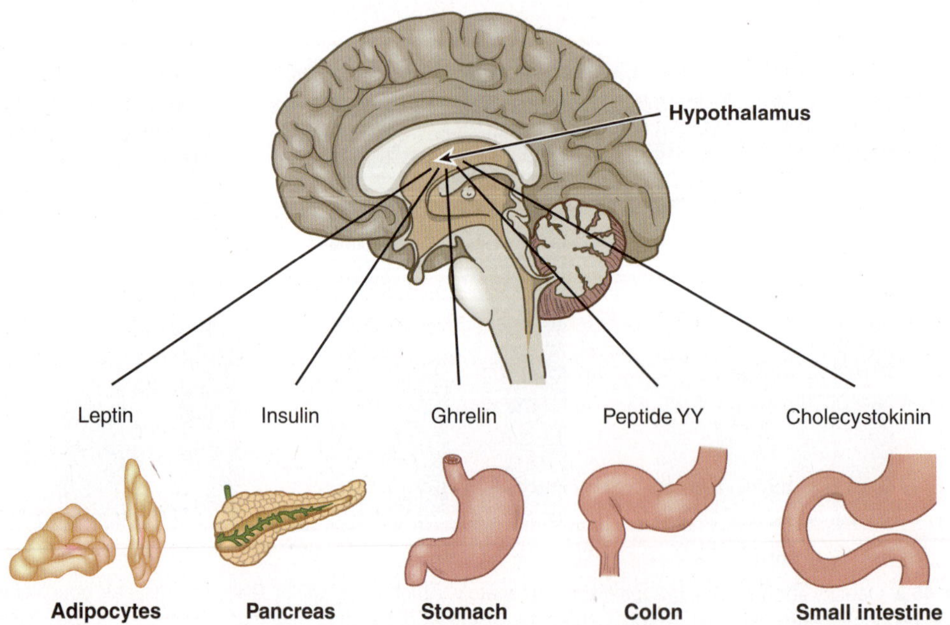

Fig. 45.3 Common hormones and peptides that interact with the hypothalamus to control and influence eating patterns, metabolic activities, and digestion. Disruption in these interactions results in obesity.

TABLE 45.1 Hormones and Peptides in Obesity

Where Produced	Normal Function	Alteration in Obesity
Anorexins (Suppress Appetite)		
Cholecystokinin		
Small intestine	Inhibits gastric emptying Sends satiety signals to hypothalamus	Unknown
Glucagon-Like Peptide-1 (GLP-1)		
Large intestine Small intestine	↑ Insulin secretion Increases satiety (mediated by GLP-1 receptors in brain)	Unknown
Insulin		
Pancreas	Decreases appetite	↑ Insulin secretion, which stimulates ↑ liver synthesis of triglycerides and ↓ HDL production
Leptin		
Adipocytes	Suppresses appetite and hunger Regulates eating behavior	Obesity is associated with high levels Leptin resistance develops with potential loss of appetite suppression
Peptide YY		
Colon	Inhibits appetite by slowing GI motility and gastric emptying	↓ Circulating levels ↓ Release after eating
Orexins (Stimulate Appetite)		
Ghrelin		
Stomach (primarily)	Stimulates appetite ↑ After food deprivation ↓ In response to food in the stomach	Normal postprandial decline does not occur, which can lead to increased appetite and overeating
Neuropeptide Y		
Hypothalamus	Stimulates appetite	Imbalance causes increased appetite

HDL, High-density lipoprotein.

Socioeconomic status is a risk factor for obesity in several ways.[2] There may be a lack of access to affordable and nutritious food at full-service grocers and farmers' markets. People with low incomes stretch their limited food dollars by buying less expensive foods that often have poor nutrition quality with greater caloric content. Low-income neighborhoods may lack safe locations for exercise, such as parks, playgrounds, walking trails, and swimming pools.

Psychologic Factors

People use food for many reasons besides nutrition. Associations with food begin in childhood, such as the use of food for comfort or rewards. The social component of eating begins early in life when food is associated with pleasure and fun at such events as birthday parties and holidays. Stress, sadness, anxiety, and other emotions can lead people to eat too much. Eating while watching television, working, studying, or browsing the Internet can lead to consuming unnecessary calories and an increase in weight.

Weight-Promoting Drugs

Several drugs contribute to weight increase (Table 45.2). The way they do so varies. Some increase insulin resistance, lipogenesis, and liver glucose production. Others decrease glucose uptake in the muscle, change the gut microbiome, or change appetite hormone production.

COMPLICATIONS

Over 200 complications are associated with obesity (Fig. 45.5). Mortality rates rise as weight increases, especially when there is excess visceral adiposity. Fortunately, most conditions improve or resolve when obesity is treated effectively (Box 45.1).

Cardiovascular Disease

Obesity is a significant risk factor for cardiovascular disease (CVD) and stroke. Android obesity is the strongest predictor. It is linked with increased low-density lipoproteins (LDLs), high triglycerides, and decreased high-density lipoproteins (HDLs).[7] HTN can occur because of increased circulating blood volume, abnormal vasoconstriction, and increased risk for sleep apnea (raises BP). Excess body fat can lead to chronic inflammation throughout the body, especially in blood vessels, thus increasing the risk for CVD.[2]

Diabetes

Obesity is the greatest risk factor for developing T2DM. Excess weight decreases the effectiveness of insulin.[7] When insulin does not work effectively, too much glucose stays in the blood. The body then makes more insulin to compensate. Pancreatic cells that make insulin may get overworked and become worn out. Over time, the pancreas is no longer able to keep glucose in the normal range.

Obesity complicates T2DM management by increasing insulin resistance and glucose intolerance.[8] Adiponectin, an adipokine that increases insulin sensitivity, is decreased with obesity.[5] These factors make obesity in patients with T2DM harder to treat.

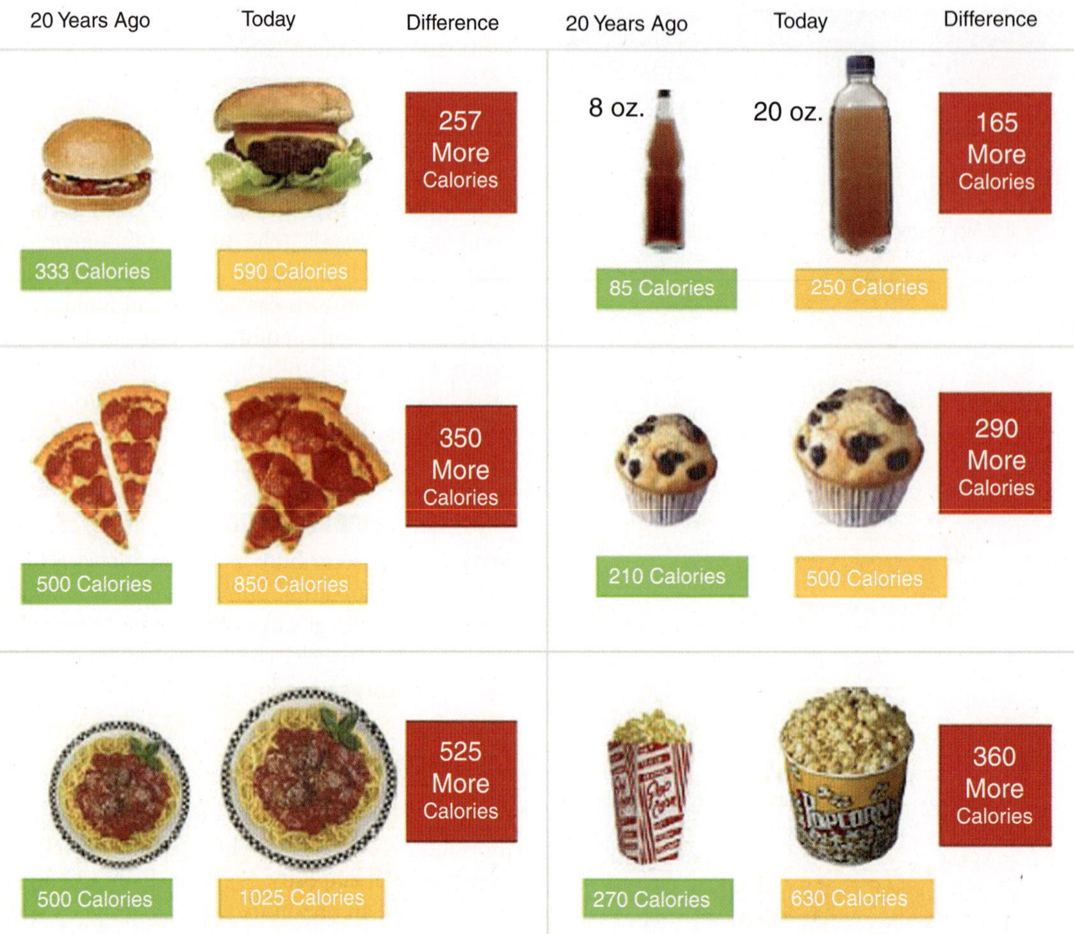

Fig. 45.4 Changes in portion size over the years. (Modified from https://www.nhlbi.nih.gov/health/educational/wecan/portion/documents/PD1.pdf.)

TABLE 45.2 Weight-Promoting Medications
Antihyperglycemics: Insulins, sulfonylureas
Antidepressants
Antipsychotics
Anticonvulsants: Gabapentin, valproic acid
Clonidine
Corticosteroids
Diphenhydramine
Hormone replacement therapy: Estrogen, progesterone

Gastrointestinal and Liver Problems

Gastroesophageal reflux disease (GERD) and gallstones are more prevalent in people with obesity. Metabolic dysfunction–associated steatotic disease (MASLD) is a condition in which lipids are deposited in the liver, resulting in a fatty liver. MASLD may increase liver glucose production. It can eventually progress to cirrhosis. Weight loss can improve MASLD.

Respiratory and Sleep Problems

The increased fat mass may lead to sleep apnea and obesity hypoventilation syndrome. Sleep apnea results from increased fat around the neck and in the tongue, leading to a narrowed airway, snoring, and hypoventilation while sleeping. The increased distribution of fat around the diaphragm and lungs causes reduced chest wall compliance, increased work of breathing, and decreased total lung capacity.

Poor sleep may increase appetite. Building up a sleep debt over a matter of days can impair metabolism, increase insulin resistance, and disrupt appetite hormone levels. Leptin levels fall in people who are sleep deprived, thus increasing appetite.

Musculoskeletal Problems

Obesity is associated with an increased risk of osteoarthritis. It puts stress on weight-bearing joints, especially the knees and hips. Increased body fat triggers inflammatory mediators and contributes to cartilage deterioration. Hyperuricemia and gout often occur in people with obesity and metabolic syndrome.

Cancer

Cancers most strongly linked to excess body fat are breast, colorectal, endometrial, esophagus, gallbladder, kidney, liver, ovarian, stomach, and thyroid cancer.[9] The links between

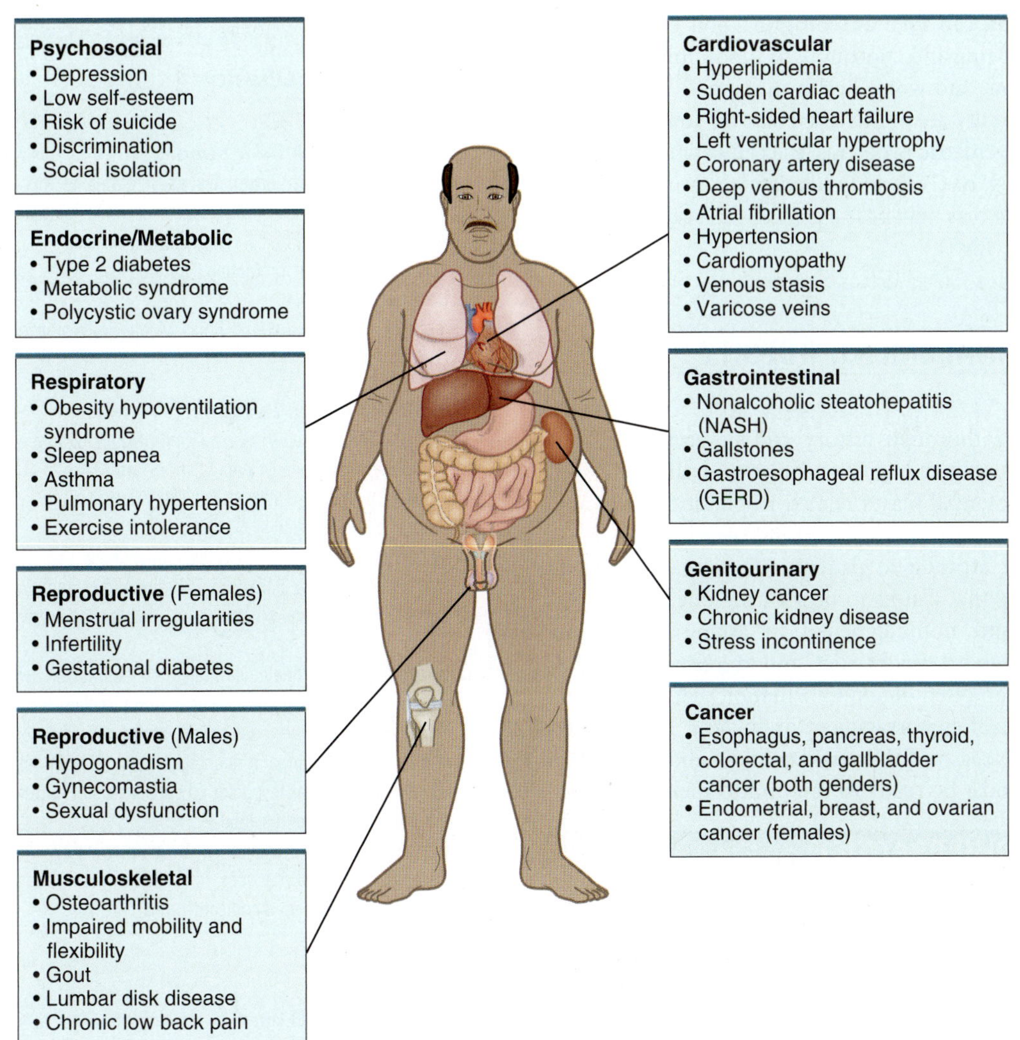

Fig. 45.5 Health risks associated with obesity.

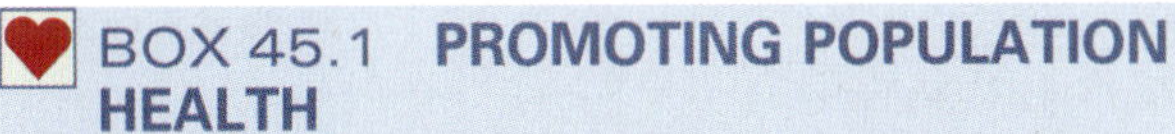

BOX 45.1 PROMOTING POPULATION HEALTH

Health Impact of Maintaining a Healthy Weight

- Lowers the risk for hypertension and high cholesterol
- Increases chance for longevity and better quality of life
- Reduces the risk for developing type 2 diabetes
- Reduces the risk for heart disease, stroke, and gallbladder disease
- Reduces the risk for breathing problems, including sleep apnea and asthma
- Decreases the risk for developing osteoarthritis, low back pain, and some types of cancers

obesity and cancer are complex. Several hormones and factors often present in obesity increase the risk for cancer. Adipokines from fat cells may stimulate cell and blood vessel growth. For example, leptin promotes cell proliferation. Fat tissue plays a role in changing androgens into estrogens. The resulting increased estrogen levels, especially after menopause, may lead to breast and endometrial cancer. Esophageal cancer may be related to acid reflux caused by abdominal obesity.

Stress and Psychosocial Problems

The consequences of obesity extend beyond the physical aspects. Many have a reduced quality of life. They often experience stigma, and in some cases discrimination, in 3 important areas: employment, education, and health care. *Weight bias* refers to negative attitudes, beliefs, and stereotypes associated with a person's weight. There may be explicit bias, such as blaming a person for obesity, or implicit bias, which involves making assumptions about the person based on their weight. Many people struggle with internal weight bias, believing they are responsible for developing and treating their disease. Patients often relate negative experiences, for example, having been judged and told to simply "eat less and move more." Such statements are often rooted in a lack of understanding of obesity as a chronic disease.

Bias and stigma can take an emotional toll on a person's psychologic well-being and contribute to suboptimal treatment, disease progression, and worse health outcomes.[10]

People with obesity are at increased risk for low self-esteem, loneliness, and psychiatric problems. Bias and stigma are linked to an increased risk of CVD and maladaptive eating behaviors. Alarmingly, weight bias may pose a greater threat to health than body mass index (BMI).

NURSING MANAGEMENT: OBESITY

Assessment

The first step is a thorough history and physical assessment (Table 45.3). Before you begin, examine your own personal beliefs and any potential biases related to obesity. If you associate obesity with a lack of willpower and overindulgence, you may convey your attitude to patients. They may experience shame in a setting that claims to be a caring one.

Be sensitive and nonjudgmental in asking specific and leading questions about weight, diet, and exercise (Table 45.4). In doing so, you can often obtain information that patients may have withheld out of embarrassment or shyness. Patients need to understand the reason for questions asked about weight or diet habits. You must be ready to respond to their concerns.

CHECK YOUR PRACTICE

You are working in the clinic, and the provider has asked you to do an assessment on a 54-year-old male for referral to a weight loss program. He is 5 ft, 9 in and weighs 282 lb. His BP has been hard to control with drugs and diet. While you are trying to do an assessment, he interrupts you and asks if he can leave. He angrily tells you, "I am not going to give up my favorite foods, quit drinking, or exercise. Do you understand that?"

- How would you respond?

Assess patients' willingness to change and potential for change. If people are not ready for change, offer them the opportunity to return for further discussion when they are ready to discuss their weight again and make lifestyle changes.

We need to determine whether any physical problems may be causing or contributing to obesity. When obtaining the history, explore genetic and endocrine factors, such as hypothyroidism, hypothalamic tumors, Cushing syndrome, hypogonadism in males, and polycystic ovary syndrome in females. A fasting glucose level, lipid panel (triglyceride level, LDL and HDL cholesterol levels), and liver and thyroid function tests aid in evaluating the cause and effects of obesity. Assess for any comorbid problems related to obesity, such as HTN, sleep apnea, and T2DM. These problems will require special treatment.

Obtain a medication history. Identify drug therapy that may be contributing to weight increase and/or preventing weight loss (Table 45.2). Changing a drug to one that is weight neutral or weight-loss promoting can improve obesity.

TABLE 45.3 NURSING ASSESSMENT

Patients With Obesity

Subjective Data

Important Health Information

Health history: Obesity onset; diseases related to metabolism and obesity, including HTN, CVD, stroke, cancer, chronic joint pain, respiratory problems, T2DM, cholelithiasis, metabolic syndrome

Medications: Weight promoting, antiobesity, herb products, weight loss treatments

Surgery or other treatments: Prior weight loss procedures (metabolic and bariatric surgery)

Functional Health Patterns

Health perception—health management: Family history of obesity; perception of problem; methods of weight loss tried

Nutritional-metabolic: Table 45.4

Elimination: Constipation

Activity-exercise: Typical exercise; drowsiness, somnolence; dyspnea on exertion, orthopnea, paroxysmal nocturnal dyspnea; type and hours of work

Sleep-rest: Snoring, hours of sleep, waking feeling rested, sleep apnea, CPAP use

Cognitive-perceptual: Feelings of rejection, depression, isolation, guilt, internal bias or shame; meaning or value of food; feeling full, difficulty staying full between meals, emotional eating, eating out of boredom

Role-relationship: Change in financial status or family relationships; personal, social, and financial resources to support a diet pattern; food environment, including who prepares food

Sexuality-reproductive: Menstrual irregularity, heavy menstrual flow in females, birth control practices, infertility; effect of obesity on sexual activity and attractiveness to significant other

Objective Data

General

Body mass index $\geq$30 kg/m^2; waist circumference: female >35 in (89 cm), male >40 in (102 cm); neck circumference female <16 in, male <17 in

Respiratory

↑ Work of breathing; rapid, shallow breathing

Cardiovascular

↑ BP, tachycardia, dysrhythmias

Musculoskeletal

Decreased joint mobility and flexibility; knee, hip, and low back pain

Reproductive

Gynecomastia and hypogonadism in males

Skin

Acanthosis nigricans of neck, axillae, under breasts, abdominal skin folds, and groin; dark coarse hair on chest, chin, cheeks, abdomen of females. Pink-purple striae on breasts, abdomen, hips, thighs, arms

Possible Diagnostic Findings

↑ Glucose, LDL cholesterol, triglycerides, A1C, fasting insulin; TSH, CRP; ↓ HDL, vitamin D. Chest x-ray showing enlarged heart; ECG showing dysrhythmia; abnormal liver function tests

CPAP, Continuous positive airway pressure; *CRP,* C-reactive protein; *CVD,* cardiovascular disease; *LDL,* low-density lipoprotein; *TSH,* thyroid-stimulating hormone; *T2DM,* type 2 diabetes.

TABLE 45.4 Nutrition Assessment

Patients With Obesity

When assessing patients with obesity and before selecting a weight loss strategy, ask the following questions:

- What is your history with weight gain and weight loss?
- Are other family members overweight?
- How has your body weight affected your health?
- What do you think contributes to your weight?
- What does food mean to you? How do you use food, such as stress relief, provide comfort, boredom?
- Describe your normal diet. What types of foods do you usually eat? What types of beverages and how much are you drinking?
- Describe your motivation for losing weight.
- What have you already tried to lose weight? Was it successful? If not, why not?
- Would you like to manage your weight differently? If so, how?
- What barriers do you think impede your weight loss efforts?
- Are there any major stresses that will make it hard to focus on weight control?
- How much time do you have for exercise on a daily or weekly basis?
- Describe the support you have from family and/or friends for losing weight.

TABLE 45.5 Relationship Between Body Shape and Health Risks

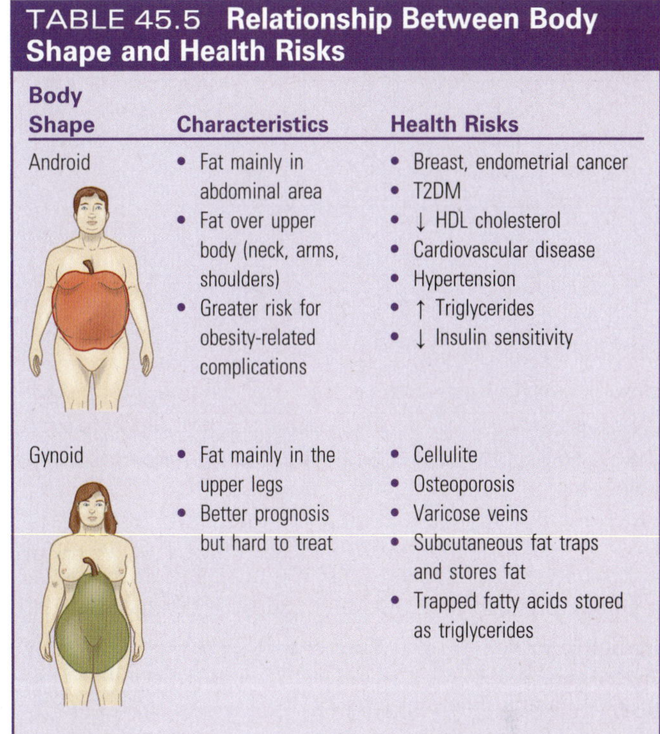

Body Shape	Characteristics	Health Risks
Android	• Fat mainly in abdominal area • Fat over upper body (neck, arms, shoulders) • Greater risk for obesity-related complications	• Breast, endometrial cancer • T2DM • ↓ HDL cholesterol • Cardiovascular disease • Hypertension • ↑ Triglycerides • ↓ Insulin sensitivity
Gynoid	• Fat mainly in the upper legs • Better prognosis but hard to treat	• Cellulite • Osteoporosis • Varicose veins • Subcutaneous fat traps and stores fat • Trapped fatty acids stored as triglycerides

HDL, High-density lipoprotein; *T2DM,* type 2 diabetes.

Classifications of Body Weight and Obesity

An important part of the assessment is to determine and classify body weight. Common assessment methods include BMI, waist circumference, waist-to-hip ratio (WHR), and percent body fat. The most widely used and endorsed measures are BMI and waist circumference. They are cost-effective, reliable, and easily used in all practice settings. Other methods for measuring body fat include skinfold calipers and bioelectrical impedance. Their accuracy can vary based on a variety of patient and technician factors.

Obesity can be described by the location of adipose depots (Table 45.5). Android obesity occurs when fat is mainly deposited in the abdominal area. Those with fat distribution in the upper legs and hips are considered to have gynoid obesity. Genetics play a key role in determining a person's body shape and weight.

Body mass index. The most common way we classify weight is **body mass index (BMI)**. We calculate BMI by dividing a person's weight (in kilograms) by the square of the height in meters (Fig. 45.6). Table 45.6 shows the classification of overweight and obesity by BMI. Persons with a BMI less than 18.5 kg/m^2 are considered underweight. A BMI between 18.5 and 24.9 kg/m^2 reflects a normal body weight. A BMI of 25 to 29.9 kg/m^2 is classified as **overweight**. Those with a BMI of 30 kg/m^2 or above are considered to have obesity. Obesity is grouped into 3 classes. Class 1 obesity is a BMI of 30 to 34.9 kg/m^2, class II obesity is a BMI of 35 to 39.9 kg/m^2, and class III obesity is a BMI of 40 or greater.

There are some limitations to using BMI. You need to consider it in relation to age, race, gender, and body build. For example, in a person with high muscle mass, such as an athlete, BMI will be higher and will not provide an accurate assessment of weight. This is why we combine other measures with BMI for an accurate evaluation of weight.

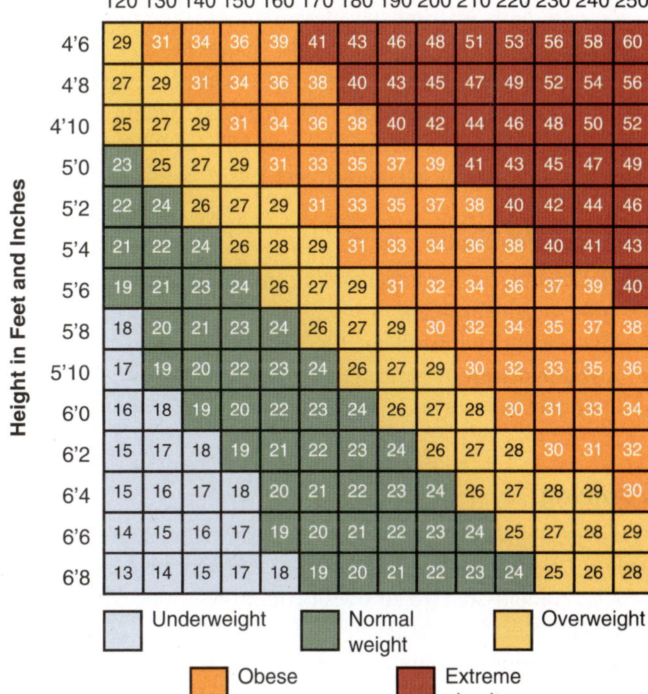

$$\text{BMI (kg/m}^2\text{)} = \frac{\text{Weight (pounds)} \quad 703}{\text{Height (inches)}^2}$$

Weight in Pounds (columns); Height in Feet and Inches (rows)

Height	120	130	140	150	160	170	180	190	200	210	220	230	240	250
4'6	29	31	34	36	39	41	43	46	48	51	53	56	58	60
4'8	27	29	31	34	36	38	40	43	45	47	49	52	54	56
4'10	25	27	29	31	34	36	38	40	42	44	46	48	50	52
5'0	23	25	27	29	31	33	35	37	39	41	43	45	47	49
5'2	22	24	26	27	29	31	33	35	37	38	40	42	44	46
5'4	21	22	24	26	28	29	31	33	34	36	38	40	41	43
5'6	19	21	23	24	26	27	29	31	32	34	36	37	39	40
5'8	18	20	21	23	24	26	27	29	30	32	34	35	37	38
5'10	17	19	20	22	23	24	26	27	29	30	32	33	35	36
6'0	16	18	19	20	22	23	24	26	27	28	30	31	33	34
6'2	15	17	18	19	21	22	23	24	26	27	28	30	31	32
6'4	15	16	17	18	20	21	22	23	24	26	27	28	29	30
6'6	14	15	16	17	19	20	21	22	23	24	25	27	28	29
6'8	13	14	15	17	18	19	20	21	22	23	24	25	26	28

Fig. 45.6 Body mass index *(BMI)* chart. Healthy weight: BMI 18 to 24.9 kg/m^2; overweight: BMI 25 to 29.9 kg/m^2; obesity: BMI 30 kg/m^2. BMI = weight (kg)/height (m^2).

TABLE 45.6 Diagnostic Criteria

Classification of Overweight and Obesity

	BMI (kg/m²)	Obesity Class	DISEASE RISK RELATIVE TO NORMAL WEIGHT AND WAIST CIRCUMFERENCE: Males ≤40 in (102 cm) Females ≤35 in (89 cm)	Males >40 in (102 cm) Females >35 in (89 cm)
Underweight	<18.5	—	—	—
Normal	18.5–24.9	—	—	—
Overweight	25.0–29.9	—	Increased	High
Obesity	30.0–34.9	Class I	High	Very high
	35.0–39.9	Class II	Very high	Very high
Extreme obesity	≥40.0	Class III	Extremely high	Extremely high

From National Heart, Lung, and Blood Institute: *Classification of overweight and obesity by BMI, waist circumference, and associated disease risks.* Retrieved from www.nhlbi.nih.gov/health/public/heart/obesity/lose_wt/bmi_dis.htm.

Waist circumference. *Waist circumference* is a measure of visceral adiposity. Measure waist circumference at the highest point of the iliac crest after the patient has exhaled. Health risks, including CVD and metabolic syndrome, increase if the waist circumference is greater than 40 inches in males and greater than 35 inches in females.[11]

Waist-to-hip ratio. The waist-to-hip ratio (WHR) is another way to assess obesity. Calculate the WHR by dividing the waist measurement by the hip measurement. In females, the ratio should be 0.8 or less, and in males, it should be 1.0 or less. This means that in females, the waist should be narrower than the hips, and in males, the waist should be narrower than or the same as the hips. A higher WHR indicates abdominal adiposity, which puts a person at a greater risk for health problems.

Percent body fat. Body fat measurement is the most specific assessment of body fat. The gold standard for measuring percent body fat is dual energy x-ray absorptiometry (DEXA). Females naturally have higher fat mass. A healthy body fat range is 25% to 31% for females and 18% to 24% for males. This is influenced by age and fitness level.

◆ Clinical Problems

Clinical problems for patients with obesity may include:

- Body weight problem
- Musculoskeletal problem
- Risk for disease
- Negative self-image

◆ Planning

The overall goals for patients with obesity include (1) improved health, (2) improved quality of life, (3) minimize or prevent health problems related to obesity, and (4) achieve and maintain weight loss to a specified level.

◆ Implementation

Treatment begins with recognizing obesity as a chronic, progressive disease that requires long-term treatment and monitoring. It is rare to find a person with obesity who has not tried to lose weight. Some people have met with limited and temporary success, and others have met only with failure. Understanding a person's weight history, identifying factors contributing to their obesity, and knowing treatments that have or have not been effective are essential in developing the treatment plan.

TABLE 45.7 Interprofessional Care

Obesity

Diagnostic Assessment

- History and physical assessment
- Family history
- BMI, waist circumference, waist-to-hip ratio
- Assessment of health risks and comorbidities

Management

- Manage comorbidities
- Lifestyle interventions
  - Behavior therapy
  - Nutrition therapy (Table 45.8)
  - Drug therapy (Table 45.9)
  - Physical activity
  - Social support
  - Surgical therapy (Table 45.10)

A holistic approach to weight loss is most effective. A comprehensive plan should address nutrition, physical activity, behavior therapy, and medical management (Table 45.7). Achieving an "ideal" BMI is not necessary and may not be a realistic goal. Even modest weight loss of 5% or more can have health benefits.[12] Greater weight losses produce greater benefits. With the introduction of effective antiobesity drugs, comprehensive obesity treatment can result in the loss of 15% to 20% of body weight.

You have a key role in planning for and managing the care of patients with obesity. You can help patients by being a source of information. Motivational interviewing (see Chapter 4) helps patients understand why they want to improve their health and helps them gain confidence in their ability to do so. Focusing on the reasons for wanting to change may help patients develop strategies for improving their health and reducing their weight. Encourage healthy eating habits and adequate exercise as lifestyle patterns to develop and maintain (Box 45.2).

A weekly check of body weight is a good method of monitoring progress. Daily weighing is not recommended because of fluctuations that result from retained water (including urine) and feces. Teach patients to obtain the weight at the same time of the day, wearing the same type of clothing. Encourage them to keep an electronic or paper journal. Have them record their daily food and drink consumption and exercise. They should note where they eat and with whom. This can give insight into factors that influence eating habits that patients can control or change. Reviewing the journal can help find relationships among food intake, exercise, and weight loss. Apps can give immediate access to nutrition information and track nutrient intake.

Weight loss will slow over time in response to treatment interventions. A person may have periods of days to weeks without any change in weight. Make patients aware that this is normal and expected. Weight loss will decrease over time as the body adapts to the treatment intervention. Eventually body weight will plateau as the body establishes a new weight setpoint.[13] The patient and HCP should discuss intensifying treatment when a weight plateau is reached or obesity or related complications are not controlled.

BOX 45.2 PROMOTING POPULATION HEALTH

Maintaining a Healthy Weight

- Keep a food journal.
- Weigh yourself regularly.
- Eat 5 or more servings of fruits and vegetables daily.
- Choose whole-grain foods, such as brown rice and whole-wheat bread.
- Avoid highly processed foods made with refined white sugar, flour, and saturated fat.
- Avoid foods that are high in "energy density" or have a lot of calories in a small amount of food.
- Take part in exercise:
  - 150 min of moderate-intensity aerobic activity (i.e., brisk walking) every week
  - Muscle-strengthening activities on 2 or more days a week

Nutrition Therapy

Nutrition therapy with calorie restriction is the cornerstone of obesity treatment. There is no standard diet plan. A variety of plans are effective in treating obesity and can be sustained long term. Diet plans involve restricting fats, carbohydrates, or both.[13] Carbohydrate restriction is recommended for patients with obesity and T2DM to reduce weight and improve glucose control. Reducing caloric intake by 500 to 1000 kcal per day will result in a body weight loss of 1 to 2 lb per week for most people. A summary of diet plans and their effects on health are described in Table 45.8.

TABLE 45.8 NUTRITION THERAPY

Diet Plans for Obesity

Diet Plan	Components	Metabolic Effects
Carbohydrate restricted	Foods high in protein and fat Low: Less than 130 g of carbohydrate/day Very low: Less than 50 g of carbohydrate/day	↓ Glucose, triglycerides ↑ LDL, HDL
Fat restricted	Less than 30% daily caloric intake (33 g fat for every 1000 cal) Healthy carbohydrates (fruits, vegetables, whole grains)	↓ LDL, BP
High protein (Atkins)	1.6 g/kg/day or more than 25% of daily caloric intake	↓ LDL, triglycerides
Intermittent fasting	Calories consumed during limited time each day Multiple options: • Alternate-day fasting • 16/8 (16 h fasting, 8 h restricted eating) • 12/12 (12 h fasting, 12 h restricted eating) • 18/6 (18 h fasting, 6 h restricted eating)	↓ Inflammatory markers, visceral fat, BP ↓ Insulin resistance Improved gut microbiome
Ketogenic (high fat)	Less than 20 g/day carbohydrates for 12 wk (induction) then increase to up to 100 g/day (maintenance) More than 50% of total daily calories from fat	↑ HDL, LDL
Mediterranean	Daily intake of vegetables, fruit, whole grains, healthy fats Weekly intake of fish, poultry, beans, eggs Moderate dairy intake Limited red meat	↓ Cardiovascular disease, inflammatory markers Protects against Parkinson, dementia, Alzheimer disease
Reduced calorie	Low-calorie: 500 cal decrease in total caloric intake, total 1000–1600 cal/day Very low-calorie: Under 800 cal/day	↑ HDL ↓ BP, LDL, glucose, triglycerides
Vegetarian, vegan	Plant based, whole foods; no animal, processed, or ultra-processed food products	↓ BP, visceral fat

HDL, High-density lipoprotein; *LDL*, low-density lipoprotein.

An assessment of eating habits will provide the basis for making nutrition changes. When developing a diet plan, consider food allergies and sensitivities, cultural and social traditions, food access and availability, and time and resources necessary for preparing and cooking meals.[13] Calorie and specific nutrient needs will vary based on lifestyle, health, and disease status. Diet changes can also target improvements in complications of obesity, such as T2DM.[8] A diet plan that accommodates patient preferences and daily routines will increase adherence and sustainability.

In general, the food choices should emphasize vegetables, fruits, and whole grains, which are sources of diet fiber.[13] Recommended daily fiber intake is 25 to 30 g per day. Lean meat, fish, poultry, beans, eggs, and dairy products provide sufficient protein, healthful fats, and the B-complex vitamins. Protein recommendations are 0.8 to 2.0 g/kg of ideal body weight per day.

Encourage patients to limit the intake of calorie-dense, highly processed foods and foods high in saturated trans fats, salt, and added sugars. Encourage the appropriate fluid intake in the form of water. Have them limit or avoid alcohol, sugar-sweetened beverages, and fruit juices. These increase caloric intake and are low in nutrition value.

A very low-calorie meal plan—less than 800 kcal/day—should be medically supervised and is intended for short-term use.[13] Such a meal plan often consists of meal replacement soups, shakes, and bars. People on very low-calorie diets need frequent monitoring. The severe energy restriction places them at risk for vitamin and nutrition deficiencies and other health complications. This type of meal plan is commonly used before surgery to promote weight loss and reduce the size of the liver.

Many people try to lose weight by following a fad diet. A *fad diet* promises fast weight loss with minimal effort and quick results. They are often promoted widely on social media and on television. Often, fad diets advocate eliminating a category of foods, such as carbohydrates. People who follow a fad diet may lose a large amount of weight in a short time, but it is not sustainable. Most regain the weight they lost, if not more. Therefore discourage using a fad diet.

The amount of weight loss achieved by nutrition changes is highly variable and depends in part on the starting weight. Because males have a higher percentage of lean body mass, they are often able to lose weight more quickly than females. Females have a higher percentage of body fat, which is metabolically less active than muscle tissue. Postmenopausal females are particularly prone to an increase in adiposity and a decrease in muscle mass. These changes are associated with a decline in estrogen and changes in appetite hormones.

When a person first starts a weight loss program, measuring food portion sizes can help ensure they are eating appropriate portions. Food portions can be weighed using a scale. Everyday objects can be used as a visual cue to determine portion sizes. The size of a female's fist or a baseball is equivalent to a serving of vegetables or fruit. The recommended portion size of meat is 3 oz. This is about the size of a person's palm or a deck of cards. A serving of cheese is about the size of a thumb or 6 dice. The standard size for chopped vegetables is a ½ cup. A portion size quiz is available at www.nhlbi.nih.gov/health/educational/wecan/eat-right/portion-distortion.htm.

Physical Activity

Exercise plays a key role in treating obesity, improving health, and maintaining a healthy weight. Consider the patient's current level of activity, capacity for activity, and physical limitations when developing a plan for physical activity.[13] Patients should aim for at least 150 minutes of moderate exercise or 75 minutes a week of vigorous exercise per week and incorporate resistance exercises or strength training. That works out to 30 minutes of brisk walking or 15 minutes of running for 5 days a week. The type of exercise (high vs. low intensity) does not seem to affect overall weight loss. More intensive exercise may result in weight loss with a reduced time commitment, making it preferable for some people. A total of 200 to 300 minutes per week of moderate exercise is recommended to maintain weight loss or prevent weight regain after weight loss.[5]

Increasing activity gradually to accommodate the patient's current fitness level and addressing physical or structural barriers to access will increase success. Explore ways to incorporate exercise in daily routines. It may be as simple as parking farther from entry doors or taking the stairs. Digital health technologies that track and monitor activity and incorporate goal setting are effective tools to increase physical activity and weight loss. Joining a health club can help with getting exercise. Stress that engaging in weekend exercise only or in spurts of strenuous exercise is not helpful and can be dangerous.

Behavior Therapy

Behavior therapy promotes a collaborative and patient-centered approach to supporting nutrition and lifestyle changes. One effective strategy for managing obesity is cognitive-behavior therapy (CBT). By addressing the underlying emotional and psychologic factors contributing to obesity, CBT helps patients develop healthy coping mechanisms and make lasting lifestyle changes.

The 5 A's framework is a widely used method in behavior therapy for obesity. Steps of the 5 A's framework include Ask, Assess, Advise, Agree, and Assist. Treatment begins by asking permission to discuss a person's weight. Assessing readiness for change, giving the person control over their health, and fostering trust can improve outcomes. Once permission is granted, the assessment is completed and the patient advised on treatment options. Together the patient and HCP agree on a treatment plan. The HCP can assist patients with identifying and overcoming any challenges with treatment and arranging for follow-up.

Motivational interviewing is an effective behavior therapy that allows patients to explore their reasons for change and empowers them to take an active role in their health journey. It encourages patients to recognize their potential and build skills necessary for successful behavior change.

Drug Therapy

Drugs to treat obesity are approved for use as an adjunctive treatment to nutrition and lifestyle changes. The role of drug therapy is to overcome any contributing pathophysiology.[14] Using drugs to treat obesity promotes and sustains weight loss, increasing adherence to nutrition and lifestyle changes. Drug therapy is indicated for adults with a BMI of 30 kg/m^2 or greater (obesity) or adults with a BMI of 27 kg/m^2 or greater (overweight) with at least 1 weight-related condition, such as HTN, T2DM, or dyslipidemia.[5] FDA-approved drugs for treating obesity are shown in Table 45.9.

Your role related to drug therapy is to provide teaching about proper administration, side effects, and how the drugs fit into the overall treatment plan. Patients must understand that stopping treatment will result in a return of most, if not all, of the weight lost. Review with patients their insurance coverage for obesity treatments. Many insurance companies do not pay for medications to treat obesity. Tell patients not to change drug dosages without consulting with the HCP. Finally, discourage patients from buying over-the-counter diet aids and drug treatments available online unless recommended by an HCP.

◆ Evaluation

The expected outcomes are that patients with obesity will:
- Achieve and maintain optimal weight
- Have improvement in obesity-related comorbidities
- Integrate healthy practices into daily routines
- Have an improved self-image

METABOLIC AND BARIATRIC SURGERY AND DEVICES

A number of metabolic and bariatric surgery (MBS) procedures and bariatric devices are used to treat obesity (Table 45.10). They are indicated for weight loss along with nutrition and lifestyle changes.[15] Most bariatric devices are short-term

TABLE 45.9 Drug Therapy

Obesity

Drug	Mechanism of Action	Nursing Considerations
bupropion/naltrexone (Contrave)	*bupropion:* antidepressant *naltrexone:* opioid antagonist	• Side effects: nausea, constipation, headache, dizziness, insomnia, dry mouth • Monitor for suicidal thoughts and neuropsychiatric reactions • ↑ BP and heart rate. Should not use in patients with uncontrolled hypertension • Can cause seizures
liraglutide (Saxenda, Victoza)	Glucagon-like peptide 1 (GLP-1) agonist Induces satiety	• Used to treat T2DM • Daily injection • Side effects: nausea, diarrhea, headache, fatigue, dizziness • Monitor for suicidal ideation, pancreatitis
orlistat (Xenical, Alli [low-dose form available over the counter])	Inhibits gastrointestinal (GI) lipase Blocks fat breakdown and absorption in intestine	• Side effects: stool leakage, flatulence, diarrhea, abdominal bloating, especially if a high-fat diet is consumed • Liver injury, kidney stones may occur • May need daily multivitamin supplement • Taken with each main meal containing fat
phentermine/topiramate ER (Qsymia)	*phentermine:* Sympathomimetic; decreases appetite *topiramate:* Decreases appetite and food cravings	• Side effects: dizziness, insomnia, dry mouth, headache, high blood pressure • Do not use in patients with glaucoma or hyperthyroidism • Avoid pregnancy • ↑ Heart rate. Do not use in patients with hypertension, heart disease
semaglutide (Wegovy)	Mimics GLP-1 Induces satiety Slows gastric emptying ↑ Insulin production in response to carbohydrate intake ↓ Liver gluconeogenesis	• Side effects: GI distress • Used to treat T2DM • Weekly injection
tirzepatide (Zepbound)	Mimics GLP1 and GIP Reduces appetite Reduces caloric intake	• Side effects: GI distress • Used to treat T2DM • Weekly injection • Increase risk of thyroid cancer • Decrease effect of oral contraceptive agents

T2DM, Type 2 diabetes.
Data from Gudzune KA, Kushner RF: Medications for obesity: a review, *JAMA* 332(7): 571–984, 2024.

treatments for patients with less severe obesity. MBS is the most effective long-term treatment for obesity. It often results in significant improvement in metabolic diseases such as hyperlipidemia, HTN, and T2DM. MBS is associated with improved quality of life and increased longevity. Other outcomes include decreased total cholesterol and triglycerides, decreased GERD, and decreased sleep apnea.

The procedure or device selected depends on several factors. These include the severity of obesity, medical history, medication taken, age, and nutrition and lifestyle preferences. Criteria

TABLE 45.10 Surgical Therapy for Obesity

Description	Advantages	Disadvantages
Restrictive Surgery		
Adjustable Gastric Banding (AGB) (Lap-Band, Realize Band) (Fig. 45.7A)		
• Inflatable band encircles stomach • Creation of gastric pouch with about 30 mL (1 oz) capacity • Later stretches to 60–90 mL (2–3 oz) • Upper gastric pouch connected by very narrow channel to lower section of stomach	• Food digestion occurs normally • Band can be adjusted to ↑ or ↓ restriction • Can be reversed • No dumping syndrome • No malabsorption • Low complication rate	• Some nausea and vomiting initially (eating too much too quickly) • May have food intolerance, gastric dysmotility, regurgitation • Problems with adjusting device • Band may slip or erode into stomach wall • Gastric perforation or obstruction may occur, requiring surgery • Weight loss may be more limited than with other types of surgery
Sleeve Gastrectomy (Gastric Sleeve) (Fig. 45.7B)		
• About 75% of stomach removed • Creation of sleeve-shaped stomach with 60–150 mL (2–5 oz) capacity	• Preserves stomach function • Does not bypass intestines • Weight loss can occur rapidly	• Leakage related to stapling • Not reversible • Nutrition problems common
Gastric Plication		
• Adapted version of sleeve gastrectomy (gastric sleeve) • Sleeve created by suturing rather than removing stomach	• Minimal surgery compared with sleeve gastrectomy • Does not bypass intestines	• Requires hospital stay of 24–48 h • Nausea common after procedure • Risks include stomach leakage from sutured areas, blockage of stomach from swelling or fold too tight
Intragastric Balloon		
• Involves placing a deflated balloon into stomach • Balloon then filled with saline and occupies space in stomach	• Most are placed endoscopically as an outpatient procedure	• Left in place up to 6 months • Once device is in stomach, nausea, vomiting, abdominal pain, indigestion, gastric ulcers can occur
Malabsorptive Surgery		
Biliopancreatic Diversion (BPD) With or Without Duodenal Switch (Fig. 45.7C)		
• 70% of stomach removed • Anastomosis between stomach and intestine • Decreases amount of small intestine available for nutrient absorption • Duodenal switch cuts stomach vertically and is shaped like a tube	• Able to eat larger meals than with gastric bypass or banding procedures • Less food intolerance • Rapid weight loss • Greater long-term weight loss	• Abdominal bloating, foul-smelling gas (steatorrhea) common • Often have 3 or 4 loose bowel movements a day • Nutrition problems include malabsorption of fat-soluble vitamins, iron deficiency anemia, protein-calorie malnutrition • Dumping syndrome common • Most complicated of weight loss surgeries
Combination of Restrictive and Malabsorptive Surgery		
Roux-en-Y Gastric Bypass (RYGB) (Fig. 45.7D)		
• Surgery on stomach to create a pouch (restrictive) • Small gastric pouch connected to jejunum • Remaining stomach and first segment of small intestine are bypassed (malabsorptive)	• Better weight loss results than with restrictive procedures • Lower incidence of malnutrition and diarrhea • Rapid improvement of weight-related comorbidities • Good long-term results	• Leak at site of anastomosis can occur • Nutrition problems include anemia (iron deficiency, cobalamin deficiency, folic acid deficiency); calcium deficiency • Dumping syndrome common • Not reversible

for bariatric surgery include having a BMI of 35 kg/m^2 or more or a BMI of 30 kg/m^2 or more with at least 1 weight-related comorbidity, such as T2DM, HTN, sleep apnea, or CVD.[15] Insurance coverage for MBS varies. Those who cover surgery often require extensive documentation. This often includes taking part in a supervised nutrition and lifestyle program, which can vary from 1 to 6 months or more.

There are changes in neuroendocrine hormones affecting appetite, the gut microbiome, and bile salts affecting absorption. The changes in anatomy result in decreased nutrient absorption.

Although it offers an effective treatment, MBS does not cure obesity. Monitoring and a lifetime of diet and lifestyle changes are essential to improve long-term outcomes for patients after MBS. These include monitoring of weight, diet patterns, and laboratory tests for metabolic health and vitamin and nutrition deficiencies. Changes in anatomy result in decreased nutrient absorption. Daily multivitamin and calcium supplements are necessary for life. Dosing varies based on the surgery.

Despite the efficacy of MBS, not every response is the same. A small number of patients will have a less-than-expected amount of weight loss. Up to 30% of patients will have a relapse of obesity and an increase in weight after surgery. Factors contributing to long-term disease control after MBS include regular follow-up, adherence to the diet plan, and regular physical activity.

The risks of MBS are low, caused in part by the extensive presurgical workup.[16] The preoperative workup includes a comprehensive physical and psychologic assessment to identify those at higher surgical risk. Surgical candidates are screened for psychologic, physical, and psychiatric problems that are associated with poor surgical outcomes or interfere with ability to sustain lifelong behavior changes. These include unstable mood disorders, suicidal ideation, and active substance use. Other contraindications include illnesses that are known to reduce life expectancy and are not likely to improve after surgery. These include advanced cancer; end-stage kidney, liver, heart, and lung disease; or inability to comply with medical care.

Bariatric Devices

Adjustable Gastric Banding

Adjustable gastric banding (AGB) involves limiting the stomach size with an inflatable band placed around the fundus of the stomach (Fig. 45.7A). The band is connected to a subcutaneous port that can be inflated or deflated (by fluid injection in the HCP's office) to meet patients' needs. The band divides the stomach into 2 unequal parts. The upper part acts as the new stomach. Because it holds much less, patients feel full more quickly. The band causes a delay in stomach emptying, providing patients with further satiety.

AGB can be reversed or converted to an MBS. Although no longer commonly performed, many patients still have AGB in place. Postoperative risks include adhesions, band slipping, and dysphagia. Dysphagia can be a surgical emergency if patients are unable to swallow their saliva. Revision surgery involves removing the AGB and converting to a laparoscopic sleeve gastrectomy (LSG) or Roux-en-Y gastric bypass (RYGB). Because it is a restrictive device, there is less risk for nutrition problems. The impact on weight and metabolic health is less than that of MBS. Expected weight loss is 15% to 20% of body weight.

Intragastric Balloons

Intragastric balloon systems use an inflated balloon to occupy space in the stomach. The balloon does not change the stomach's anatomy. It is meant to help patients feel full and reduce the amount of food and fluid they can consume. Balloons are indicated for patients with a BMI of 30 to 40 kg/m^2.

Balloons are less invasive than MBS, and there is less risk for nutrition deficiencies. Several different balloons are available. They differ in volume, means of insertion and removal, duration used, and adjustability. Some balloons are placed endoscopically with the patient under mild sedation. Once in place, the balloon is filled with 400 to 900 cc of saline or gas.

With air balloons, the patient swallows the balloon in a capsule that is attached to a thin catheter. The balloon is inflated with nitrogen gas through the catheter. After inflation, the catheter is detached and removed, leaving the balloon in the stomach.

Balloons can remain in place for up to 6 months. When it is time to remove a balloon, it is first deflated and then removed under endoscopy. Expected weight loss is 10% at the end of 6 months. Most patients have an average of 7% weight loss at the end of 1 year. The intragastric balloon may be used as an adjunctive treatment for obesity in combination with drug therapy.

Balloons are contraindicated in patients who had GI surgery or have inflammatory bowel disease, large hiatal hernia, delayed gastric emptying, or active *H. pylori* infection. Patients may have vomiting, nausea, abdominal pain, and indigestion. Other risks are gastric ulcers and changes in balloon size.

Endoscopic Sleeve Gastroplasty

The *endoscopic sleeve gastroplasty* (ESG) is a minimally invasive procedure performed with an endoscopic suturing device. It is indicated for those with a BMI of 30 to 50 kg/m^2. Similar to a gastric sleeve, the ESG is performed by folding the stomach wall inward and then placing sutures to secure the folded stomach wall. The expected weight loss of 13% to 20% is similar to the LSG. There are no incisions. The procedure requires less time and anesthesia. For these reasons it may be considered as an initial treatment in those with higher surgical risk or as adjunctive treatment for those experiencing relapse of obesity after LSG.

Surgical Procedures

Laparoscopic Sleeve Gastrectomy (Gastric Sleeve)

The LSG (gastric sleeve) is the most common MBS. The procedure involves removing about 75% of the stomach, leaving a

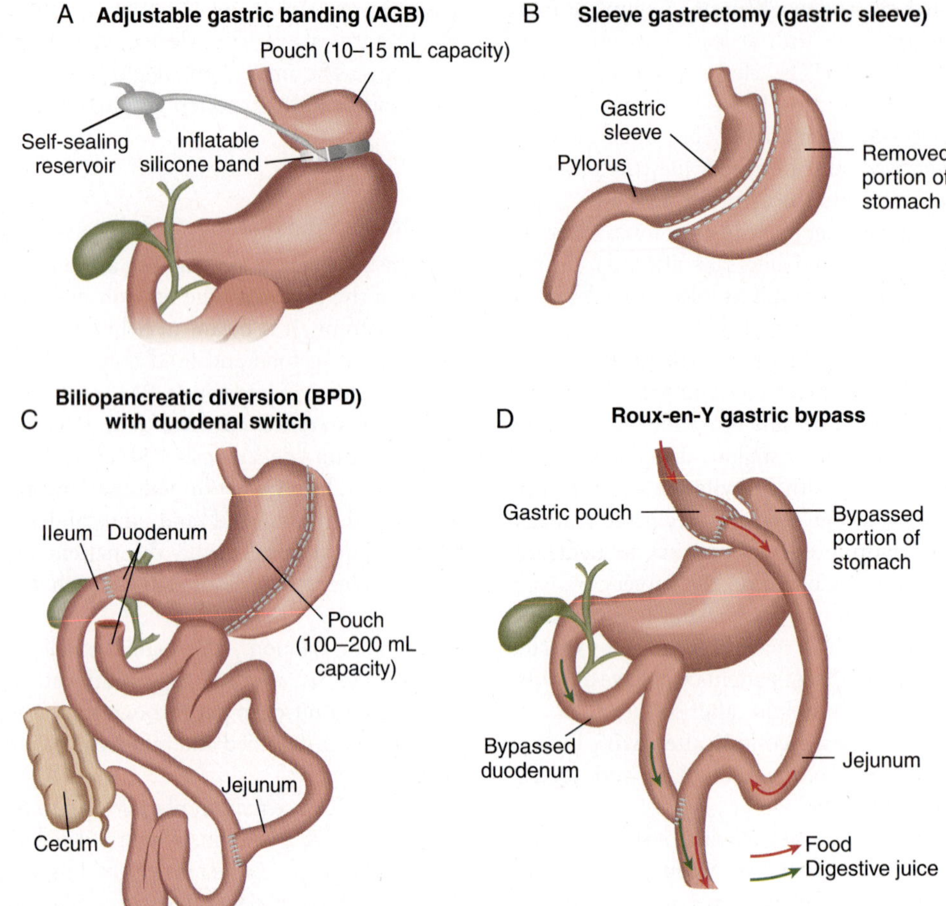

Fig. 45.7 Bariatric surgical procedures. (A) Adjustable gastric banding *(AGB)* uses a band to create a gastric pouch. (B) Sleeve gastrectomy involves creating a sleeve-shaped stomach by removing about 75% of the stomach. (C) Biliopancreatic diversion *(BPD)* with duodenal switch procedure creates an anastomosis between the stomach and intestine. (D) Roux-en-Y gastric bypass procedure involves constructing a gastric pouch whose outlet is a Y-shaped limb of small intestine.

sleeve-shaped stomach (Fig. 45.7B). The stomach is drastically reduced in size, limiting food portions that a person can eat. Metabolic and hormone changes include a decrease in nutrient absorption caused by a reduction in the stomach's surface area. There are also changes in the production of appetite hormones. Weight loss is between 20% and 25% of body weight. Because it is a shorter surgery, it may be more tolerable for medically complex patients. LSG is associated with a 20% to 30% risk of new-onset or worsening GERD. Thus it may not be best for patients with GERD or a known hiatal hernia.

Roux-en-Y Gastric Bypass

The RYGB involves separating the esophagus from the stomach, creating a 15- to 30-mL gastric pouch, and separating the small intestine at the jejunum. The distal jejunum is then attached to the gastric pouch. The proximal jejunum is attached to the common channel of the small intestine at the jejunum, creating a Y-shaped limb of the small bowel (Fig. 45.7D). After the procedure, food bypasses 90% of the stomach, the duodenum, and a small segment of the jejunum. There are significant changes in the absorption of calories and nutrients, appetite-regulating hormones, and the gut microbiome. These changes contribute to weight loss and improvement in metabolic diseases such as HTN, T2DM, and liver disease. Patients can expect a loss of 30% to 35% of body weight. This procedure is an effective treatment for GERD or hiatal hernia. The risk for complications within the first 30 days after surgery is low. They include leaks at the anastomosis, vitamin and nutrition deficiencies, nausea, vomiting, and dehydration. Long-term complications include vitamin and nutrition deficiencies; ulcers, fistula, stenosis, or stricture at the anastomosis; and internal hernia.

Another complication is *dumping syndrome.* It often results from a rapid emptying of high-carbohydrate foods into the intestines followed by a rapid influx of fluid. Symptoms can include vomiting, nausea, weakness, shakiness, sweating, faintness, irritability, abdominal cramping, and urgent diarrhea. Patients are encouraged to limit or avoid sugar-sweetened foods and drinks and to avoid drinking fluids within

30 minutes before or after a meal to reduce the risk of dumping syndrome.

Other Surgical Procedures

The most malabsorptive surgical procedures include the biliopancreatic diversion with duodenal switch (BPD-DS, Fig. 47.7C) and the single anastomosis with duodenal-ileal bypass with sleeve gastrectomy (SADI). Both surgeries involve an LSG and bypassing the duodenum to reduce the length of the small intestine where absorption occurs. The common channel in BPD-DS is shorter than that of the SADI and results in greater risk for malabsorption. These procedures result in the greatest amount of weight reduction at 35% to 45% total body weight loss. They offer the greatest improvement in glucose control and potential for T2DM remission. These procedures may be considered as an initial surgery for those with more severe obesity or as a second surgery for those seeking additional treatment of their obesity after LSG.

NURSING MANAGEMENT: PERIOPERATIVE CARE FOR PATIENTS WITH OBESITY

This section discusses general nursing considerations for the care of patients with obesity who are having surgery. Special nursing considerations are described for patients who are having bariatric surgery (Table 45.11). See Chapters 18 through 20 for more on the care of surgical patients.

Perioperative Care

Special considerations are needed for patients with obesity who are having surgery. Before surgery, interview patients to obtain health information. Do they currently use any assistive devices? Focus on identifying comorbidities that increase the risk for complications in the perioperative period. You may need to coordinate care with the specialty providers.

Have a plan in place before the patients arrive so that they receive optimal care and feel welcomed and expected. Have available appropriately sized hospital gowns, beds, and commodes. Use a large or thigh BP cuff size to avoid measurement errors. Ensure that the cuff is available and placed in the room.

Consider how the patient will be weighed and transported throughout the hospital. A wheelchair with removable arms that is large enough to safely accommodate the patient and pass easily through doorways should be available.

You may need to use different assessment techniques to assess heart, lung, and bowel sounds. For example, because of the large chest wall, breath and heart sounds are often distant. You can use an electronic stethoscope to amplify lung, heart, and bowel sounds. Excess adipose tissue may make obtaining venous access difficult. A longer IV catheter is helpful (longer than 1 in) to go through the overlying tissue to the vein. It is important that the cannula is far enough into the vein, so it does not dislodge or infiltrate.

Teach coughing and deep breathing techniques and methods of turning and positioning to prevent pulmonary complications after surgery. If possible, show how to use a spirometer before surgery. Spirometer use helps prevent and treat postoperative lung congestion. Practicing these strategies beforehand can help patients perform them after surgery. If a patient uses CPAP at home for sleep apnea, arrange for CPAP use while the patient is hospitalized.

Use necessary transfer equipment. The transfer from surgery may require many staff members. During the transfer, keep the airway stabilized.

TABLE 45.11 NURSING MANAGEMENT
Care of Patients Undergoing Bariatric Surgery

Preoperative
- Assess for use of assistive devices. Note any physical limitations or mobility issues.
- Perform baseline assessment, including vital signs, pulse oximetry, height, weight, BMI, skin condition, nutrition status, and heart, lung, and bowel sounds.
- Assess baseline laboratory values and diagnostic test results (e.g., pulmonary function tests).
- Teach patient and caregiver about the procedure and postoperative care. Review coughing and deep breathing techniques, incentive spirometer use, and methods of turning and positioning to prevent pulmonary complications.
- Explain the need for frequent assessment and interventions to prevent VTE.
- Have available proper-sized hospital gowns, beds, BP cuffs, and transfer equipment.

Immediate Postoperative
- Perform assessment and compare with baseline: vital signs, pulse oximetry, and heart and lung sounds.
- Assess abdominal wound for the amount and type of drainage, condition of the incision, and signs of infection.
- Observe for anastomosis leak (tachycardia, fever, tachypnea, chest and abdominal pain).
- Help patient turn, cough, and deep-breathe, and use incentive spirometer at least every 2 h.
- Protect the incision against any straining that accompanies turning and coughing.
- Give pain medications as needed.
- Position the patient upright at a minimum of a 45-degree angle.
- Maintain IV and/or oral fluid intake and monitor urine output.
- Institute measures to prevent VTE.
- Nutrition
  - Start with room-temperature water and low-sugar clear liquids.
  - Begin with 15 mL every 10–15 min, gradually increase to 90 mL every 30 min.
  - Move to a low-fat, full liquid diet after 48 h if tolerating clear liquids.
  - Observe for dehydration (thirst, decreased urine output, headache, dizziness).

VTE, Venous thromboembolism.

The initial postoperative care focuses on careful assessment and immediate intervention for cardiopulmonary complications. The body stores anesthetics in adipose tissue. As adipose cells release anesthetics back into the bloodstream, patients may become resedated after surgery. If this happens, be prepared to perform a head-tilt or jaw-thrust maneuver. Keep the oral and nasal airways open.

Obesity can cause breathing to become shallow and rapid. The extra adipose tissue in the chest and abdomen compresses the diaphragm, thoracic, and abdominal structures. This compression restricts the chest's ability to expand, preventing the lungs from working as efficiently as they would otherwise. Patients retain more CO_2 with less O_2 delivered to the lungs. This results in hypoxemia. Keep the head of the bed elevated to reduce abdominal pressure and increase lung expansion. Administer O_2 therapy as needed.

Implement venous thromboembolism (VTE) precautions. Diligence in turning and ambulation postoperatively will help prevent complications. Help patients as needed. They may not have the stamina to walk even a short distance. Have proper help and equipment available.

Wound infection, dehiscence, and delayed healing are potential problems. Assess the skin often. Keep skin folds clean and dry to prevent dermatitis and bacterial or fungal infections. Implement measures to reduce the risk of pressure injury.

Care of Patients Undergoing Bariatric Surgery

Acute Care

Ensure that patients scheduled for bariatric surgery understand the procedure. Your teaching depends on the type of procedure and surgical approach. Stress that we will frequently assess vital signs and general assessment to monitor for complications. Tell patients that we will help them with ambulation soon after surgery. They will be encouraged to cough and deep breathe to prevent pulmonary complications.

Patients may have abdominal pain after bariatric surgery. Give pain medications as needed. Be aware that pain could be from an anastomosis leak rather than typical surgical pain. Abdominal wounds require frequent observation for the amount and type of drainage, condition of the incision, and signs of infection. Monitor vital signs to help identify problems, such as infection or anastomosis leak.

Patients usually start a low-sugar, clear liquid diet within 24 hours after surgery. Begin with 15-mL increments every 10 to 15 minutes. If the patient does not have any nausea or other problems, gradually increase intake to a goal of 90 mL every 30 minutes. Teach patients to avoid gulping fluids or drinking with a straw to reduce air swallowing. Avoid drinks with caffeine or carbonation. Patients who tolerate clear liquids are advanced to a low-calorie, full liquid diet.

Chronic Care

Patients having bariatric surgery must drastically change their drinking and diet patterns because of the anatomic changes from surgery. They must clearly understand their diet. A dietitian is a key member of the bariatric team. They help patients with the transition to the new diet.

Patients usually are discharged on a full liquid diet. Over the next several weeks patients transition to pureed foods, then soft foods, and begin vitamin supplements.[17] Most patients transition to the usual diet 4 to 6 weeks after surgery.

The usual diet is high in protein with some carbohydrates and fiber. Meals will be smaller portions. Encourage patients to eat slowly to prevent symptoms of nausea, vomiting, and stomach pain that can occur with overfilling the smaller stomach. Techniques to slow consumption include chewing food thoroughly, not swallowing until food is liquid enough to pass through a straw, placing the fork or spoon down on the table between bites of food, and making a meal last at least 15 to 20 minutes. Many need a protein supplement once or twice a day for the first few months after surgery to meet protein needs. Patients should not consume fluids with meals. Fluids and foods high in sugar or total carbohydrates tend to promote diarrhea and dumping syndrome. Calorie-dense foods should be avoided to permit more nutritious food to be consumed.

Stress the importance of long-term follow-up care to monitor obesity response to treatment and potential complications. Teach patients to inform the HCP of any changes in their physical or emotional condition. Nutrition deficiencies are common after MBS, including anemia, vitamin deficiencies, and diarrhea. Patients should take multivitamins with folate, calcium, vitamin D, iron, and vitamin B_{12} for life.[17] Peptic ulcer formation, dumping syndrome, and small bowel obstruction may be seen late in the rehabilitation stage.

Several potential psychologic problems may arise after surgery. Assess social functioning, self-esteem, sexual life, and activities of daily living in follow-up care. Some patients feel guilty that they had to achieve weight loss by having surgery rather than the "willpower" of reduced diet intake and exercise. Be ready to provide support and assist patients in moving away from such negative feelings.

By 6 to 8 months after surgery, most patients have lost considerable weight and are able to see how much their appearance has changed. The greatest amount of weight loss is achieved between 1 and 2 years after surgery. Help patients adjust to a new body image. Massive weight loss may leave patients with large quantities of excess skin that can result in problems with irritation and breakdown and contribute to altered body image (Fig. 45.8). Discuss this possible outcome before surgery and again during the rehabilitation phase. Cosmetic surgery may help with this situation. Do not hesitate to encourage counseling for unresolved psychologic issues.

Often one result of MBS is the return of fertility in females. Females must carefully consider the risk for pregnancy after bariatric surgery. Pregnancy complications can result from anemia and nutrition deficiencies. Depending on the type of surgery, intestinal obstructions and hernias may occur with pregnancy. In general, encourage females to postpone pregnancy for 12 to 18 months after bariatric surgery.

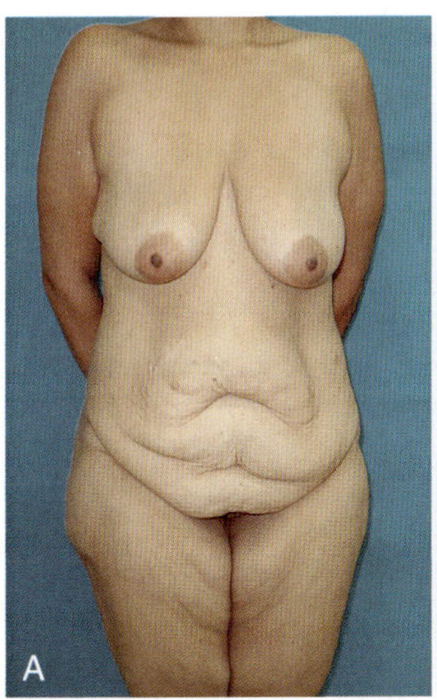

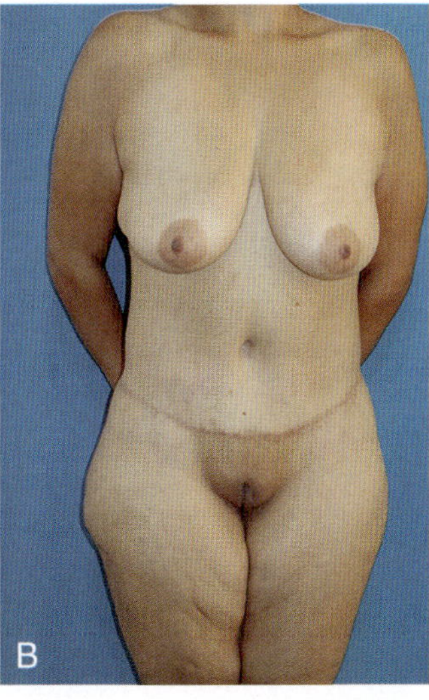

Fig. 45.8 (A) Preoperative view of a female with massive weight loss who had gastric bypass surgery. (B) View after abdominoplasty. (From Villegas-Alza FJ: *TULUA Abdominoplasty,* Philadelphia, 2025, Elsevier.)

Some patients will have less-than-expected weight loss after MBS. Others may not sustain weight loss. Up to 30% of patients will increase their weight from their lowest weight after surgery.

CHECK YOUR PRACTICE

You are working in the bariatric surgery outpatient clinic. When you walk into the clinic room where a 36-year-old female is waiting for her follow-up visit, you find her distraught and crying. You ask her what is wrong. She responds, "I am a total failure. I have been fat all my life, and I had to have this horrible surgery to help me. Why couldn't I do it on my own?"

- How can you handle this situation?

Gerontologic Considerations: Obesity in Older Adults

The prevalence of obesity is increasing in older people. Contributing factors include chronic health conditions, medications, and changes in nutrition and metabolism. A decrease in energy expenditure is an important contributor to a gradual increase in body fat with age. Obesity is more common in older females than in older males. Sarcopenic obesity, a condition of decreased muscle mass and increased fat mass with normal BMI, is more common in older adults.

Obesity in older adults can worsen age-related declines in physical function and lead to frailty and disability. Obesity is associated with increased mortality. Those who have obesity live 6 to 7 years less than people of normal weight.

Obesity worsens many changes associated with aging. Excess body weight places more demands on arthritic joints. The mechanical strain on weight-bearing joints can lead to premature immobility. Excess intraabdominal weight can cause problems with urinary incontinence. Excess weight may contribute to hypoventilation and sleep apnea.

Obesity affects the quality of life for older adults. Weight loss can improve physical functioning and obesity-related health complications. The same therapeutic approaches for obesity discussed earlier also apply to older adults.

COSMETIC SURGERY

Lipectomy

Effective obesity treatment with significant weight loss can lead to the presence of excess skin. This skin can limit mobility, create challenges with the fit of clothing, and contribute to skin irritation and skin breakdown. A **lipectomy** (adipectomy) is the surgical removal of excess skin and adipose tissue. Targeted areas often include the abdomen, hips, back, buttocks, breasts, and arms. It is recommended that patients achieve their lowest weight and sustain that weight for at least 3 months before having a lipectomy. Body image and self-esteem may improve after surgery as mobility, skin issues, and the fit of clothing improve. A lipectomy is not without complications. There is a risk for poor wound healing and infection. Tissue removal does not prevent obesity from recurring.

Liposuction

Another cosmetic procedure is liposuction, a suction-assisted lipectomy. This surgery helps improve facial appearance or body contour. A good candidate is a person who has excess fat under the chin, along the jawline, in the nasolabial folds, over the abdomen, or around the waist and upper thighs. A long, hollow, stainless steel cannula is inserted through a small incision over the fatty tissue to be suctioned. This procedure is not usually recommended for an older person because the skin is less elastic and will not accommodate the new underlying shape.

METABOLIC SYNDROME

Metabolic syndrome is not a disease, but a group of conditions that increase a person's chance of developing CVD, stroke, and T2DM. Just over 1 in 3 adults have metabolic syndrome. The prevalence is 50% for those 60 years of age and older. The number of persons aged 20 to 39 years with metabolic syndrome is steadily increasing. Metabolic syndrome is diagnosed if a person has 3 or more of the conditions listed in Table 45.12. These include obesity, HTN, abnormal lipid levels, and high glucose.

Etiology and Pathophysiology

The main underlying risk factor for metabolic syndrome is insulin resistance related to excess visceral fat (Fig. 45.9). Insulin resistance is the decreased ability of the body's cells to respond to the action of insulin. The pancreas compensates by secreting more insulin, resulting in hyperinsulinemia. Other characteristics include HTN, increased risk for clotting, and

TABLE 45.12 Diagnostic Criteria

Metabolic Syndrome

Any 3 of the 5 measures are needed to diagnose metabolic syndrome:

Measure	Criteria
Waist circumference	≥40 in (102 cm) in males ≥35 in (89 cm) in females
Triglycerides	>150 mg/dL (1.7 mmol/L) *OR* Drug treatment for high triglycerides
HDL cholesterol	<40 mg/dL (0.9 mmol/L) in males <50 mg/dL (1.1 mmol/L) in females *OR* Drug treatment for high cholesterol
BP	≥130 mm Hg systolic BP *OR* ≥85 mm Hg diastolic BP *OR* Drug treatment for hypertension
Fasting glucose	≥100 mg/dL *OR* Drug treatment for elevated glucose

HDL, High-density lipoprotein.
From National Heart, Lung, and Blood Institute: *How is metabolic syndrome diagnosed?* Retrieved from www.nhlbi.nih.gov/health/health-topics/topics/ms/diagnosis.

abnormal cholesterol levels. The net effect of these states is an increased prevalence of CVD.

Clinical Manifestations

The signs of metabolic syndrome are impaired fasting glucose, HTN, abnormal cholesterol levels, and obesity. Medical problems develop over time if the condition is not addressed. Patients are at a higher risk for CVD, stroke, T2DM, renal disease, and polycystic ovary syndrome. Patients with metabolic syndrome who smoke have an even higher risk.

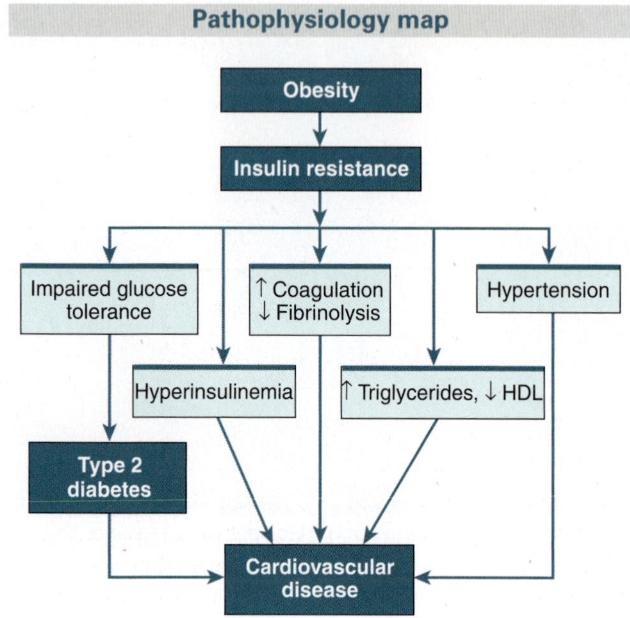

Fig. 45.9 Relationship among insulin resistance, obesity, diabetes, and cardiovascular disease.

Nursing and Interprofessional Management

Treatment of metabolic syndrome includes changes in nutrition and activity with behavior therapy. Weight loss will often result in improvement or remission of metabolic syndrome and reduce the risk for CVD and T2DM.

You can help patients by giving information on healthy diet patterns, exercise, and smoking cessation. Because sedentary lifestyles contribute to metabolic syndrome, increasing regular exercise will lower patients' risk. In addition to helping with weight loss, regular exercise decreases triglyceride levels and increases HDL cholesterol levels in those with metabolic syndrome. There are no specific medications for metabolic syndrome. Patients may receive drugs to lower cholesterol and BP as needed. Metformin can lower glucose levels and enhance the cells' sensitivity to insulin.

CASE STUDY

Obesity

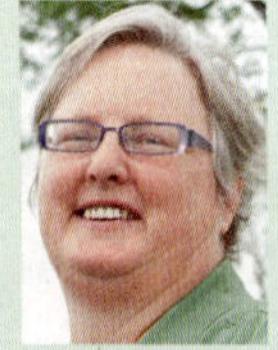

(© Thinkstock.)

Patient Profile

S.R. is a 48-year-old female who comes to the clinic reporting hip pain.

Subjective Data

- States that it is "getting hard to get around"
- Reports gradual weight gain of 40 lb over past 20 years
- Lives in a rural community with no sidewalks
- Spends her free time streaming movies
- Reports a history of T2DM, shortness of breath, HTN, osteoarthritis
- Had knee replacement surgery at age 46 for osteoarthritis
- Tried orlistat but hated the side effects

Objective Data

Physical Assessment

- 5 ft, 6 in tall; weighs 230 lb; BMI 37 kg/m^2, waist circumference of 40 in
- Excess adiposity; nontender, soft abdomen
- BP 160/100 mm Hg
- Moderate pain with range of motion of both hips

Laboratory Results

- Fasting glucose 250 mg/dL (13.9 mmol/L)
- Total cholesterol 205 mg/dL (5.3 mmol/L)
- Triglyceride 298 mg/dL (3.36 mmol/L)
- HDL cholesterol 31 mg/dL (0.8 mmol/L)
- LDL cholesterol 114 mg/dL

Continued

CASE STUDY—cont'd

Obesity

Interprofessional Care

- Referral to a community weight loss program
- Consult with bariatric surgeon
- Diagnosed with bilateral osteoarthritis of the hips

Discussion Questions

1. ***Recognize:*** What risk factors may have led to S.R.'s obesity?
2. ***Analyze:*** Based on the assessment, what complications of obesity does S.R. have? Why did she develop them?
3. ***Analyze:*** Describe the significance of her laboratory results.
4. ***Plan:*** Is S.R. a candidate for bariatric surgery? Why or why not?
5. ***Plan:*** How could a comprehensive community weight loss program be beneficial to S.R.?
6. ***Prioritize:*** What are her priority clinical problems?
7. ***Act:*** What teaching would you provide as part of an effective weight loss program?
8. ***Evaluate:*** What parameters do you need to continue to monitor?

Answers available at http://evolve.elsevier.com/Lewis/medsurg.

BRIDGE TO NCLEX EXAMINATION

The number of the question corresponds to the same-numbered outcome at the beginning of the chapter.

1. Which statement *best* describes the cause of obesity?
   a. Obesity primarily results from a genetic predisposition.
   b. Psychosocial factors can override the effects of genetics in causing obesity.
   c. Genetic factors are more important than environment factors in causing obesity.
   d. Obesity is the result of complex interactions between genetic and environment factors.
2. Health risks associated with obesity include **(select all that apply)**
   a. colorectal cancer.
   b. rheumatoid arthritis.
   c. polycystic ovary syndrome.
   d. nonalcoholic steatohepatitis.
   e. systemic lupus erythematosus.
3. The nurse is screening a new male patient for obesity. Which assessment findings support the diagnosis of obesity? **(Select all that apply.)**
   a. BMI 32.71
   b. Percent body fat 28%
   c. Waist-to-hip ratio 0.79
   d. Weight 248 lb, height 6′1″
   e. Waist circumference 48 inches
4. A patient who is interested in starting antiobesity medication asks if they are a candidate for treatment. You would respond based on the knowledge that drug therapy is for adults
   a. with a BMI $\geq$35 kg/m^2
   b. with a BMI $\geq$40 kg/m^2
   c. with a BMI $\geq$27 kg/m^2 with at least 1 comorbidity
   d. who cannot lose weight with nutrition and lifestyle changes
5. A patient with obesity has undergone Roux-en-Y gastric bypass surgery. In planning postoperative care, the nurse expects that the patient
   a. may have severe diarrhea early in the postoperative period.
   b. will not be allowed to ambulate for 1 to 2 days postoperatively.
   c. will have small amounts of oral liquids within the first 24 hours.
   d. will require nasogastric suction until the drainage is pale yellow.
6. Which criteria must be met for a diagnosis of metabolic syndrome? **(Select all that apply.)**
   a. Hypertension
   b. High triglycerides
   c. Elevated plasma glucose
   d. Increased waist circumference
   e. Decreased low-density lipoproteins

1. d; 2. a, c, d; 3. a, b, d, e; 4. c; 5. c; 6. a, b, c, d.

For rationales to these answers and even more NCLEX review questions, visit http://evolve.elsever.com/Lewis/medsurg.

REFERENCES

To access the References for this chapter, please scan the QR code with a mobile device.

46

Upper Gastrointestinal Problems

Kara Ann Ventura

http://evolve.elsevier.com/Lewis/medsurg/

CONCEPTUAL FOCUS

Cellular Regulation
Fluid and Electrolytes
Nutrition
Pain
Sleep
Tissue Integrity

LEARNING OUTCOMES

1. Describe the etiology, complications, and interprofessional and nursing management of nausea and vomiting.
2. Discuss the etiology, clinical manifestations, and interprofessional and nursing management of common oral inflammations and infections.
3. Describe the etiology, clinical manifestations, complications, and interprofessional and nursing management of oral cancer.
4. Explain the types, pathophysiology, clinical manifestations, complications, and interprofessional and nursing management of gastroesophageal reflux disease and hiatal hernia.
5. Relate the pathophysiology, clinical manifestations, complications, and interprofessional management of esophageal cancer, diverticula, achalasia, and strictures.
6. Compare acute and chronic gastritis, including the etiology, pathophysiology, and interprofessional and nursing management.
7. Distinguish gastric and duodenal ulcers, including the etiology, pathophysiology, clinical manifestations, complications, and interprofessional and nursing management.
8. Outline the clinical manifestations and interprofessional and nursing management of stomach cancer.
9. Explain the common etiologies, clinical manifestations, and interprofessional and nursing management of upper gastrointestinal bleeding.
10. Identify nursing responsibilities related to food poisoning.

KEY TERMS

achalasia
Barrett esophagus
dysphagia
esophageal cancer
esophagitis
gastritis
gastroesophageal reflux disease (GERD)
hiatal hernia
nausea
peptic ulcer disease (PUD)
stomach (gastric) cancer
stress-related mucosal disease (SRMD)
vomiting

This chapter reviews several upper gastrointestinal (GI) problems and the care of patients undergoing upper GI surgery. Conceptually, patients with impaired upper GI function may have malnutrition from decreased intake. Many are at risk for altered fluid, electrolyte, and acid-base balance. Problems with eating, drinking, or talking may cause pain and impair the ability to communicate. Pain can disrupt sleep and cause fatigue. Problems swallowing increase the risk for aspiration.

NAUSEA AND VOMITING

Etiology and Pathophysiology

Nausea and vomiting are the most common manifestations of GI disease. Although nausea and vomiting can occur independently, they are closely related and usually treated as one problem. **Nausea** is a feeling of discomfort in the epigastrium with a conscious desire to vomit. **Vomiting** is the forceful ejection of partially digested food and secretions *(emesis)* from the upper GI tract.

Nausea and vomiting occur in a wide variety of GI problems and in many conditions unrelated to GI disease. These include pregnancy, infection, central nervous system (CNS) problems (e.g., meningitis, tumor), and cardiovascular disease (CVD) (e.g., myocardial infarction, heart failure). They can occur with psychologic states (e.g., stress, fear) or when the GI tract becomes overly irritated, excited, or distended. Patients may have nausea and vomiting after surgery with general anesthesia or as a drug side effect (e.g., chemotherapy, opioids). Females are more likely to have nausea and vomiting associated with anesthesia and motion sickness.[1]

The vomiting center in the medulla coordinates the multiple components involved in vomiting (Fig. 46.1). This center receives input from various stimuli. Neural impulses reach the vomiting center via afferent pathways through branches of the autonomic nervous system. Receptors for these afferent fibers are found in the GI tract, kidneys, heart, and uterus. When stimulated, these relay information to the vomiting center, which initiates the vomiting reflex.

Vomiting is a complex act. It requires the coordinated activity of several structures: closure of the glottis, deep inspiration with contraction of the diaphragm in the inspiratory position, closure of the pylorus, relaxation of the stomach and lower esophageal sphincter (LES), and contraction of the abdominal muscles with increasing intraabdominal pressure. These simultaneous activities force the stomach contents up through the esophagus, into the pharynx, and out the mouth.

The chemoreceptor trigger zone (CTZ), found in the brainstem, responds to chemical stimuli from drugs, toxins, and labyrinthine stimulation (e.g., motion sickness). Once stimulated, the CTZ transmits impulses directly to the vomiting center. This activates the autonomic nervous system, resulting in parasympathetic and sympathetic stimulation. Sympathetic activation causes tachycardia, tachypnea, and diaphoresis. Parasympathetic stimulation causes relaxation of the LES, an increase in gastric motility, and increased saliva.

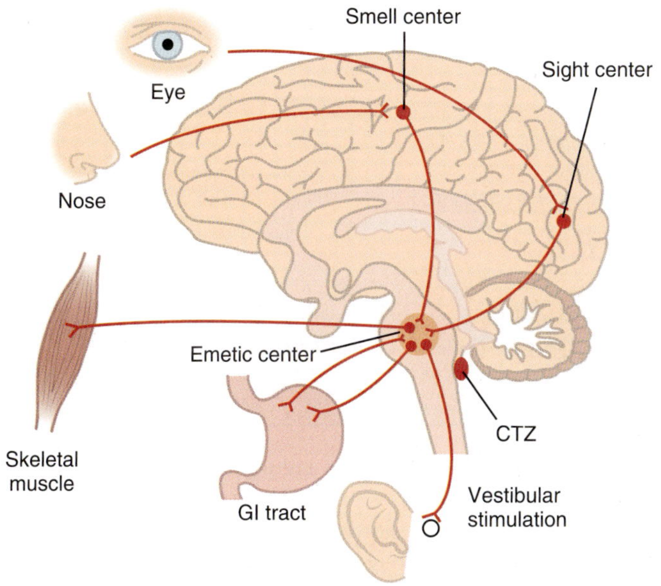

Fig. 46.1 Stimuli involved in the act of vomiting. *CTZ*, Chemoreceptor trigger zone.

Clinical Manifestations

Nausea is subjective. *Anorexia* (lack of appetite) usually accompanies nausea. When nausea and vomiting occur over a long period, dehydration can develop rapidly. Water and essential electrolytes (e.g., potassium, sodium, chloride) are lost. As vomiting persists, the patient may have severe electrolyte imbalances, fluid volume loss, and circulatory failure. Weight loss resulting from fluid loss can occur in a short time with severe vomiting. Metabolic alkalosis can result from loss of gastric hydrochloric (HCl) acid.

Interprofessional Care

The goals of care in treating nausea and vomiting are to determine and treat the underlying cause, recognize and correct any complications, and provide symptomatic relief.

Drug Therapy

The use of drug therapy depends on the cause (Table 46.1). Many antiemetic drugs act in the CNS via the CTZ to block the neurochemicals that trigger nausea and vomiting. When the cause has not been determined, use drugs with caution. Using antiemetics before knowing the cause can mask the underlying problem and delay diagnosis and treatment. Older adults are especially susceptible to the CNS side effects of antiemetic drugs. These drugs may cause confusion and increase fall risk. Doses should be reduced, and efficacy closely evaluated. Use safety precautions. 5-HT_3 (serotonin) receptor antagonists are effective in reducing chemotherapy-induced nausea and vomiting (CINV), postoperative nausea and vomiting (PONV), and nausea and vomiting related to migraine headache and anxiety.[2]

NURSING MANAGEMENT: NAUSEA AND VOMITING

Assessment

Patients with prolonged or persistent nausea or vomiting need a thorough assessment. You need to be able to identify patients who are at high risk. Assess for risk factors and describe the contents of the emesis. Table 46.2 presents subjective and objective data to obtain from patients with nausea and vomiting.

When food is the precipitating cause of nausea and vomiting, help patients identify the specific food. Determine when it was eaten, prior history with the food, and whether anyone else who ate the food is sick. Emesis containing partially digested food several hours after a meal indicates gastric outlet obstruction or delayed gastric emptying. The presence of fecal odor and bile after prolonged vomiting suggests intestinal obstruction below the level of the pylorus. Bile in the emesis suggests obstruction below the ampulla of Vater.

The color of the emesis helps determine the presence and source of any bleeding. Bright red blood occurs with active

TABLE 46.1 Drug Therapy

Nausea and Vomiting

Drug	Mechanism of Action	Side Effects	Considerations
Anticholinergics			
scopolamine transdermal	Block cholinergic pathways to vomiting center	Dry mouth, somnolence	Postoperative nausea and vomiting (PONV), motion sickness Wash hands after applying Wear only 1 patch at a time
Antihistamines			
dimenhydrinate (Dramamine) diphenhydramine hydroxyzine meclizine (Antivert)	Block histamine receptors that trigger nausea and vomiting	Dry mouth, hypotension, sedation, rashes, constipation	Motion sickness, PONV Avoid with glaucoma Take 1 h before travel begins
Cannabinoids			
dronabinol (Marinol) nabilone (Cesamet)	Inhibit vomiting control mechanism in the medulla	Dry mouth, amnesia, ataxia, confusion, coordination problems, dizziness, somnolence	May be part of the plan to manage chemotherapy-induced nausea and vomiting (CINV) Option only when other therapies are not effective because of potential for abuse and sedation
Corticosteroids			
dexamethasone	Not well understood how it works	Hyperglycemia, insomnia, euphoria	Given with other antiemetics to manage acute and delayed CINV
Dopamine D2/D3 Receptor Antagonist			
amisulpride (Barhemsys)	Block dopaminergic receptors in the CTZ	Chills, hypokalemia, hypotension, abdominal distention	PONV IV route Monitor ECG
5-HT$_3$ (Serotonin) Antagonists			
granisetron ondansetron (Zofran) palonosetron (Aloxi)	Block action of serotonin	Constipation, diarrhea, headache, fatigue, malaise, ↑ liver function tests	PONV, CINV, hyperemesis Oral, IV routes
Phenothiazines			
chlorpromazine prochlorperazine promethazine	Act in the CNS level of the CTZ. Block dopamine receptors that trigger nausea and vomiting	Dry mouth, hypotension, sedation, rashes, constipation, photosensitivity	PONV Oral, IV, rectal routes preferred Parenteral route can cause severe tissue injury May discolor urine reddish-brown
Prokinetic			
metoclopramide (Reglan)	Inhibit action of dopamine. ↑ Gastric motility and emptying	CNS side effects ranging from anxiety to hallucinations, extrapyramidal side effects, including tremor and dyskinesias	PONV, CINV Monitor for suicidal ideation Do not use if GI stimulation would be dangerous (e.g., UGI)
Substance P/Neurokinin-1 Receptor Antagonists			
aprepitant (Emend) netupitant and palonosetron (Akynzeo) rolapitant (Varubi)	Block interaction of substance P at NK-1 receptor	Headache, hiccups, fatigue, constipation, diarrhea, anorexia	CINV, PONV Reduces effectiveness of oral contraceptives Oral, IV routes

bleeding. This could be due to a *Mallory-Weiss tear* (disruption of the mucosal lining near the esophagogastric junction), esophageal varices, gastric or duodenal ulcer, or cancer. Emesis with a "coffee-grounds" appearance is related to gastric bleeding. The blood changes to dark brown because of its interaction with HCl acid.

Discern among vomiting, regurgitation, and projectile vomiting. *Regurgitation* is an effortless process in which partially digested food slowly comes up from the stomach. Retching or vomiting rarely occurs before it. *Projectile vomiting* is a forceful expulsion of stomach contents without nausea. It often occurs with brain and spinal cord tumors.

TABLE 46.2 NURSING ASSESSMENT

Nausea and Vomiting

Subjective Data

Important Health Information

Health history: GI problems, chronic indigestion, food allergies, pregnancy, infection, CNS problems, recent travel, eating disorders, metabolic problems, cancer, CVD, renal disease

Medications: Antiemetics, digitalis, opioids, ferrous sulfate, aspirin, aminophylline, alcohol, antibiotics, chemotherapy. General anesthesia

Surgery or other treatments: Recent surgery

Functional Health Patterns

Nutritional-metabolic: Amount, frequency, timing, character, and color of emesis. Dry heaves. Anorexia, weight loss. Food intake

Activity-exercise: Weakness, fatigue

Cognitive-perceptual: Abdominal tenderness or pain

Coping–stress tolerance: Stress, fear

Objective Data

General

Lethargy, sunken eyeballs

GI

Amount, frequency, character (e.g., projectile), content (undigested food, blood, bile, feces), and color of emesis (red, coffee-grounds, green-yellow)

Skin

Pallor, dry mucous membranes, poor skin turgor

Urinary

↓ Output, concentrated urine

Possible Diagnostic Findings

Altered electrolytes (especially hypokalemia), metabolic alkalosis, abnormal upper GI findings on endoscopy or abdominal x-rays

The timing of nausea and vomiting can help determine its cause. Early morning vomiting is common in pregnancy. Emotional stressors may elicit vomiting during or right after eating. Those with *cyclic vomiting syndrome* have recurring episodes of nausea, vomiting, and fatigue that last from a few hours up to many days without any evidence of functional or infectious illness.

◆ Clinical Problems

Clinical problems for patients with nausea and vomiting may include:

- Fluid imbalance
- Electrolyte imbalance
- Nutritionally compromised
- Impaired GI function

More information on clinical problems and interventions is in eNursing Care Plan 41.1 (available on the website for this chapter).

◆ Planning

The overall goals are that patients with nausea and vomiting will (1) have minimal or no nausea and vomiting, (2) have normal electrolyte levels and hydration status, and (3) return to their normal fluid and nutrient intake.

◆ Implementation

Most people with nausea and vomiting are at home. When symptoms persist, patients may need to be hospitalized to diagnose the underlying problem. Until we confirm a diagnosis, patients are NPO and given IV fluids. Patients with persistent vomiting, a possible bowel obstruction, or paralytic ileus may need a nasogastric (NG) tube connected to suction to decompress the stomach. Secure the NG tube to prevent its movement in the nose and back of the throat. This can stimulate nausea and vomiting.

With prolonged or severe vomiting, there is a chance of dehydration, and acid-base and electrolyte imbalances. Patients need IV fluid therapy with electrolyte and glucose until they can tolerate oral intake. Monitor patients with heart or renal problems. They are at greater risk for life-threatening fluid and electrolyte imbalances. They are also at greater risk for adverse consequences from excess fluid and electrolyte replacement.

Record intake and output. Monitor vital signs and assess for signs of dehydration. Maintain a quiet, odor-free environment. Provide oral care. Observe for changes in mentation. Pulmonary aspiration is a concern when vomiting occurs in older or unconscious patients or in those with an impaired gag reflex. To prevent aspiration, put patients who cannot manage self-care in a semi-Fowler or side-lying position.

Nutrition Therapy

When symptoms occur, stop all foods and drugs. Start oral nutrition with clear liquids once symptoms have subsided. Water is the initial fluid of choice for oral rehydration. Have patients sip small amounts of room temperature fluids (5 to 15 mL) every 15 to 20 minutes. Other options include carbonated beverages with the carbonation removed at room temperature and warm tea. Very hot or cold liquids are often hard to tolerate. Broth and sports drinks (e.g., Gatorade) are high in sodium, so give them with caution. Dry toast, crackers, and plain gelatin may be helpful.

As the patient's condition improves, provide a diet high in carbohydrates and low in fat. Bland foods, such as a baked potato, rice, cooked chicken, and cereal, are ideal. Many patients do not tolerate coffee, spicy foods, highly acidic foods, and those with strong odors. Tell patients to eat food slowly and in small amounts to prevent stomach distention. Liquids taken between meals rather than with meals reduce distention. Consult a dietitian about nutritious foods that the patient can tolerate.

CHECK YOUR PRACTICE

You are caring for a newly admitted 76-year-old male who reports vomiting for the past 3 days. He says, "I cannot keep anything down, not even water."

- What assessment do you need to perform?
- What findings would show he is dehydrated?
- What are your priority nursing interventions?

Teach patients and caregivers (1) how to manage nausea, (2) ways to prevent nausea and vomiting, and (3) how to maintain fluid and nutrition intake. Tell them to keep the immediate environment quiet, free of noxious odors, and well ventilated. Avoiding sudden changes of position and unnecessary activity is helpful. Encourage the use of relaxation techniques, frequent rest periods, and diversion. Changes in body position or exercise may help some patients. Provide pain management measures. Cleansing the face and hands with a cool washcloth and providing mouth care between episodes increases the person's comfort level.

If you suspect a medication is the cause, notify the HCP at once. The HCP may change the dose or prescribe a new drug. Tell patients that stopping the drug without consulting the HCP may have adverse effects on their health. Patients should take an antiemetic drug only if prescribed by the HCP. Taking over-the-counter (OTC) drugs to relieve symptoms may make the problem worse.

◆ Evaluation

Expected outcomes for patients with nausea and vomiting include:

- Be comfortable, with minimal or no nausea and vomiting
- Have normal electrolyte levels
- Maintain adequate intake of fluids and nutrients

ORAL PROBLEMS

INFLAMMATIONS AND INFECTIONS

Oral inflammations and infections are shown in Table 46.3. They may be due to specific mouth diseases or related to systemic problems, such as leukemia or vitamin deficiency. Patients who are immunosuppressed (e.g., receiving chemotherapy) or using corticosteroid inhalant treatment for asthma are at risk for oral infections (e.g., candidiasis). Oral infections may predispose patients to infections in other body organs. For

TABLE 46.3 Oral Infections and Inflammation

Infection or Inflammation	Cause	Manifestations	Treatment
Aphthous stomatitis (canker sore)	• Recurrent and chronic form of infection • Related to systemic disease, trauma, stress, or unknown causes	• Painful ulcers of mouth and lips • White or gray shallow ulcer surrounded by redness	• Corticosteroids (topical or systemic) • Tetracycline oral suspension
Gingivitis	• Poor oral hygiene • Malocclusion, missing or irregular teeth, faulty dentistry • Eating soft rather than fibrous foods	• Inflamed gingivae and interdental papillae • Bleeding during tooth brushing • Pus, abscess formation with loosening of teeth (periodontitis)	• Prevention through health teaching, dental care, gingival massage, professional teeth cleaning • Eat fibrous foods • Good brushing habits with flossing
Herpes simplex (cold sore, fever blister) (see Table 25.6)	• Herpes simplex virus (type 1 or 2) • Risk factors: upper respiratory tract infections, excess exposure to sunlight, food allergies, stress, onset of menstruation	• Lip lesions, mouth lesions, vesicle formation (single or clustered) • Shallow, painful ulcers	• Spirits of camphor, corticosteroid cream, mild antiseptic mouthwash, viscous lidocaine • Remove or control risk factors • Antiviral agents (e.g., acyclovir, valacyclovir)
Oral candidiasis (moniliasis or thrush)	• *Candida albicans* (yeastlike fungus) • Debilitation • Prolonged high-dose antibiotic or corticosteroid therapy	• Pearly, bluish white "milk-curd" membranous lesions on mucosa of mouth and larynx • Sore mouth, yeasty halitosis	• Miconazole buccal tablets (Oravig) • Nystatin or amphotericin B as oral suspension or buccal tablets • Good oral hygiene
Parotitis (inflammation of parotid gland, surgical mumps)	• *Staphylococcus* species usually • *Streptococcus* species occasionally • Debilitation and dehydration with poor oral hygiene • Extended NPO status	• Pain in area of gland and ear • Absent salivation • Purulent exudate from gland, redness, ulcers	• Antibiotics, mouthwashes, warm compresses • Preventive measures, such as chewing gum, sucking on hard candy • Adequate fluid intake
Stomatitis (inflammation of mouth)	• Trauma, pathogens, irritants (tobacco, alcohol) • Renal, liver, hematologic diseases • Side effect of chemotherapy and radiation	• ↑ Saliva • Halitosis • Sore mouth	• Remove or treat cause • Oral hygiene with soothing solutions, topical medications • Soft, bland diet
Vincent's infection (acute necrotizing ulcerative gingivitis, trench mouth)	• Fusiform bacteria, Vincent spirochetes • Risk factors: Stress, excess fatigue, poor oral hygiene • B and C vitamin deficiencies	• Painful, bleeding gingivae • Eroding necrotic lesions of interdental papillae • Ulcers that bleed • ↑ Saliva with metallic taste, fetid mouth odor • Anorexia, fever, malaise	• Physical and mental rest • Avoid smoking and alcohol • Soft, nutritious diet • Good oral hygiene • Topical antibiotics • Mouth irrigations with chlorhexidine and saline solutions

example, the oral cavity is a potential reservoir for respiratory pathogens. Oral pathogens are associated with diabetes and heart disease.[3]

Managing oral problems focuses on identifying the cause, eliminating infection, providing comfort measures, and maintaining intake. They can severely impair oral intake. Regular and good oral and dental hygiene reduces oral infections and inflammation.

ORAL CANCER

There are 2 types of oral cancer: *oral cavity cancer,* which starts in the mouth, and *oropharyngeal cancer.* It develops in the part of the throat just behind the mouth (the oropharynx). *Head and neck squamous cell carcinoma* (HNSCC) is a broad term used for cancers of the oral cavity, pharynx, and larynx. Most oral cancer lesions occur on the lower lip. Other common sites are the lateral border and undersurface of the tongue, labial commissure, and buccal mucosa. Each year 51,540 Americans are diagnosed with oral cancer. An estimated 10,030 people die.[4]

Oral cancer is more common after age 35. The average age at diagnosis is 65 years. It is 2 times more common in men. The 5-year survival rate is 84% for local cancer and 65% for all stages of oral cavity and pharynx cancer combined.[4] Lip cancer has the most favorable prognosis. The visibility of lip lesions usually leads to an earlier diagnosis.

Etiology and Pathophysiology

We do not know the exact cause of oral cancer. There are several risk factors (Table 46.4). About 75% to 90% report a history of tobacco or frequent alcohol use. More than 30% of patients with lip cancer have outdoor occupations, showing that prolonged exposure to sunlight is a risk factor. Irritation from the pipe stem resting on the lip is a factor in pipe smokers. Human papillomavirus (HPV) contributes to 25% of oral cancer cases. HPV-associated oropharyngeal cancer is associated with multiple sexual partners, especially multiple oral sex partners.[5]

Clinical Manifestations

Common manifestations are shown in Table 46.4. Patients may report nonspecific symptoms such as chronic sore throat, sore mouth, and voice changes. *Leukoplakia,* called "smoker's patch," is a white patch on the mouth mucosa or tongue. It is a precancerous lesion, with 15% transforming into cancer. The patch becomes *keratinized* (hard and leathery), which is called hyperkeratosis. Leukoplakia results from chronic irritation, especially from smoking. *Erythroplasia* (erythroplakia), a red velvety patch on the mouth or tongue, is another precancerous lesion. More than 50% of cases of Erythroplasia progress to squamous cell cancer. About 30% of patients have an asymptomatic neck mass.

Lip cancer usually appears as an indurated, painless ulcer on the lip. The first sign of tongue cancer is an ulcer or area of thickening. The tongue may be sore or painful, especially when eating hot or highly seasoned foods. Lesions are most likely to develop in the proximal half of the tongue. Some patients have limited tongue movement. Later symptoms include increased saliva, slurred speech, dysphagia (difficulty swallowing), toothache, and earache.

Diagnostic Studies

Diagnostic tests can identify cancer and oral dysplasia, a precursor to oral cancer (Table 46.5). Once cancer is diagnosed, imaging tests such as CT scan, MRI, and PET are used for staging. HPV testing is done as HPV status affects staging. If the cancer is HPV-positive, the same tumor size and node involvement leads to a lower staging compared with HPV-negative cases. This is due to a difference in prognosis and cancer behavior.

Interprofessional Care

Management usually consists of surgery, radiation, chemotherapy, or a combination of these. The curative treatments are usually surgery and radiation.

Surgical Therapy

Surgery is the most effective treatment, especially for early-stage disease.[6] The procedure done depends on the location and

TABLE 46.4 Types and Characteristics of Oral Cancer

Location	Risk Factors	Manifestations	Treatment
Lip	Constant overexposure to sun, ruddy and fair complexion, recurrent herpetic lesions, pipe stem irritation, syphilis, immunosuppression	Indurated, painless ulcer	Surgery, radiation
Oral cavity	Poor oral hygiene, tobacco use (pipe and cigar smoking, snuff, chewing tobacco), chronic alcohol use, chronic irritation (jagged tooth, ill-fitting prosthesis, chemical or mechanical irritants), HPV	Leukoplakia, erythroplakia, ulcers, sore spot, rough area, pain, dysphagia, a lump or thickening in the cheek A sore throat or a feeling that something is stuck Difficulty chewing and speaking (later signs)	Surgery (mandibulectomy, radical neck dissection, resection of buccal mucosa), internal and external radiation
Tongue	Tobacco and alcohol use, chronic irritation, syphilis	Ulcer or area of thickening, soreness, or pain Limited tongue movement ↑ Saliva, slurred speech, dysphagia, toothache, earache (later signs)	Surgery (hemiglossectomy or glossectomy), radiation

TABLE 46.5 Interprofessional Care

Oral Cancer

Diagnostic Assessment

- History and physical assessment
- Biopsy
- Oral exfoliative cytology
- Toluidine blue test
- CT, MRI, PET scans
- HPV test

Management

- Surgical excision
- Radiation therapy
- Chemotherapy
- Nutrition therapy

extent of the tumor. Some patients with small tumors in the mouth and throat are candidates for minimally invasive robotic-assisted surgery. Many surgeries are radical procedures involving extensive resections. Some examples are partial *mandibulectomy* (removal of the mandible), *hemiglossectomy* (removal of half of the tongue), *glossectomy* (removal of the tongue), resections of the buccal mucosa and floor of the mouth, and radical neck dissection.

Radical neck dissection includes wide excision of the primary tumor with removal of the regional lymph nodes, the deep cervical lymph nodes, and their lymphatic channels. Other structures that are removed depend on the extent of the primary tumor. They include the sternocleidomastoid muscle and other close muscles, internal jugular vein, mandible, submaxillary gland, part of the thyroid and parathyroid glands, and spinal accessory nerve. Patients usually have a tracheostomy. Head and neck surgery is described in more detail in Chapter 29.

Nonsurgical Therapy

Radiation therapy may be used alone to treat small cancers or when tumors cannot be removed. Patients usually do not have radiation before surgery because it is hard to remove radiated tissue. The tissue becomes fibrotic and heals slower. Most patients begin radiation about 6 weeks after surgery.

Chemotherapy can shrink tumors before surgery, decrease metastasis, sensitize cancer cells to radiation, or treat distant metastases. Common chemotherapy drugs include fluorouracil, cisplatin, carboplatin, paclitaxel, docetaxel, and hydroxyurea. A common combination is cisplatin and fluorouracil.[7] This combination is more effective than either drug alone. Chemotherapy is discussed in Chapter 16.

Palliative treatment is considered when the prognosis is poor, the cancer is inoperable, or a patient decides against surgery. Palliation aims to treat the symptoms and make patients more comfortable. If it becomes hard for a patient to swallow, placing a gastrostomy tube will allow for adequate nutrition intake. Frequent suctioning of the oral cavity is needed when swallowing becomes difficult. Other palliative and end-of-life nursing measures are discussed in Chapter 10.

TABLE 46.6 NURSING ASSESSMENT

Oral Cancer

Subjective Data

Important Health Information

Health history: Recurrent oral herpetic lesions, HPV infection or vaccination, syphilis, exposure to sunlight

Medications: Immunosuppressants

Surgery or other treatments: Removal of prior tumors or lesions

Functional Health Patterns

Health perception—health management: Alcohol and tobacco use, pipe smoking. Poor oral hygiene

Nutritional-metabolic: Reduced oral intake, weight loss, difficulty chewing food, ↑ saliva, intolerance to some foods or temperatures of food

Cognitive-perceptual: Mouth or tongue soreness or pain, toothache, earache, neck stiffness, dysphagia, difficulty speaking

Objective Data

GI

Areas of thickening or roughness, ulcers, leukoplakia, or erythroplakia on the tongue or oral mucosa. Limited tongue movement. ↑ Saliva, drooling. Slurred speech. Foul breath odor

Skin

Indurated, painless ulcer on lip. Painless neck mass

Possible Diagnostic Findings

Positive exfoliative smear cytology, positive biopsy, positive HPV test

Nutrition Therapy

Many patients are malnourished before surgery. They may need a percutaneous endoscopic gastrostomy (PEG) and enteral nutrition (EN) before radiation treatment or surgery. After surgery, patients may be unable to ingest nutrients orally because of mucositis, swelling, location of sutures, or problems swallowing. Parenteral nutrition (PN) is given for the first 24 to 48 hours. After that time, EN is given via NG, gastrostomy, or jejunostomy tube. Cervical esophagostomy and pharyngostomy are options for some patients. See Chapter 44 for information on EN and PN.

Assess for feeding tolerance. Adjust the amount, time, and formula if nausea, vomiting, diarrhea, or distention occurs. Give small amounts of water when the patient can swallow. Observe for choking. Suction as needed to prevent aspiration.

NURSING MANAGEMENT: ORAL CANCER

Assessment

Subjective and objective data to obtain from patients with oral cancer are outlined in Table 46.6.

◆ Planning

The overall goals are that patients with cancer of the oral cavity will (1) have a patent airway, (2) be able to communicate, (3) have adequate intake to maintain nutrition, and (4) have relief of pain and discomfort.

◆ Implementation

You play a key role in the early detection and treatment of oral cancer. Identify patients at risk (Table 46.4). Review information about smoking cessation with patients who smoke or use snuff or chewing tobacco. Provide information about promoting oral health (Box 46.1).

Early detection is important. Teach patients to report unexplained pain or soreness of the mouth, unusual bleeding, dysphagia, sore throat, voice changes, or swelling or lump in the neck. Refer any person with an ulcerative lesion that does not heal within 2 to 3 weeks to the HCP.

Preoperative care must consider patients' physical and psychosocial needs. Physical preparation is the same as that for any major surgery, with special emphasis on oral hygiene (see Chapter 18). Include information on postoperative communication and feeding. See Chapter 29 for more information about the nursing care of patients undergoing a radical neck dissection.

BOX 46.1 PROMOTING POPULATION HEALTH

Health Impact of Good Oral Hygiene

- Improves quality of life
- Lowers risk for loss of teeth
- Reduces pain and disability
- Aids in early detection of oral and craniofacial cancers
- Decreases cost of care needed from dental professionals
- Decreases risk for periodontal disease, gingivitis, and dental caries

◆ Evaluation

Expected outcomes for patients with oral cancer include:

- No respiratory complications
- Be able to communicate
- Maintain adequate intake and nutrition status
- Have minimal pain and discomfort with eating, drinking, and talking

ESOPHAGEAL PROBLEMS

GASTROESOPHAGEAL REFLUX DISEASE

Gastroesophageal reflux disease (GERD) is a symptom of mucosal damage caused by reflux of stomach acid into the lower esophagus. GERD is not a disease but a syndrome. It is the most common upper GI problem. About 15 million Americans have GERD symptoms each day.[8]

Etiology and Pathophysiology

GERD has no one single cause (Fig. 46.2). GERD results when the reflux of acidic gastric contents into the esophagus overwhelms the esophageal defenses. Gastric HCl acid and pepsin secretions in reflux cause esophageal irritation and inflammation *(esophagitis)*. If it contains intestinal proteolytic enzymes (e.g., trypsin) and bile, this further irritates the esophageal mucosa. The degree of inflammation depends on the amount and composition of the gastric reflux and on the esophagus's mucosal defense mechanisms.

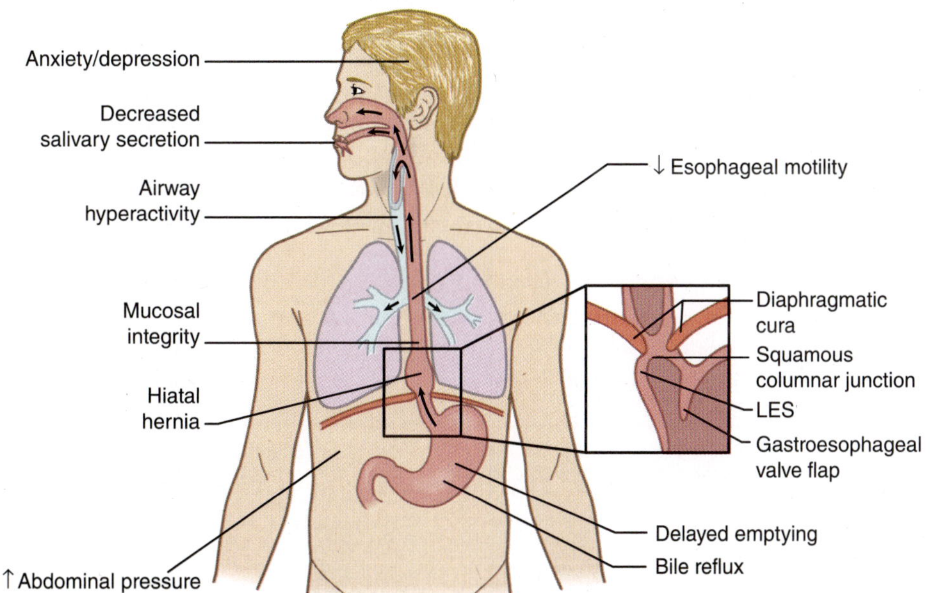

Fig. 46.2 Factors involved in the pathogenesis of GERD.

Several factors contribute to GERD (Table 46.7). A key factor causing GERD is an incompetent LES. Normally, the LES acts as an antireflux barrier. An incompetent LES lets gastric contents move from the stomach to the esophagus when the patient is supine or has an increase in intraabdominal pressure. In an obese person the intraabdominal pressure increases, which can worsen GERD. Certain foods and drugs decrease LES pressure. Some drugs, such as nonsteroidal antiinflammatory drugs (NSAIDs) and potassium, can irritate the esophageal mucosa, causing *medication-induced esophagitis.*

Clinical Manifestations

The symptoms of GERD vary from person to person. We consider persistent mild symptoms (more than twice a week) or moderate to severe symptoms once a week as GERD.

Heartburn *(pyrosis)* is the most common symptom. Heartburn is a burning, tight sensation felt intermittently beneath the lower sternum and spreading upward to the throat or jaw. It may occur after ingesting food or drugs that decrease the LES pressure or directly irritate the esophageal mucosa. An HCP should evaluate heartburn that occurs more than twice a week, is severe, is associated with dysphagia, or occurs at night and wakes a person from sleep. Older adults who report the recent onset of heartburn should receive medical evaluation.

GERD-related chest pain can mimic angina. It is described as burning, squeezing, or radiating to the back, neck, jaw, or arms. Chest pain is more common in older adults with GERD. Unlike angina, antacids relieve GERD-related chest pain.

Patients may have dyspepsia or regurgitation. *Dyspepsia* is pain or discomfort centered in the upper abdomen (mainly in or around the midline). Regurgitation is described as hot, bitter, or sour liquid coming into the throat or mouth.

A person with GERD may report respiratory symptoms, including wheezing, coughing, and dyspnea. Nighttime discomfort and coughing can awaken the person, resulting in disturbed sleep. Otolaryngologic symptoms include hoarseness, sore throat, a *globus sensation* (sense of a lump in the throat), hypersalivation, and choking.

TABLE 46.7 Factors Contributing to GERD

- **Decreased LES pressure**
  - Alcohol
  - Chocolate (theobromine)
  - Drugs
    - Antidepressants
    - Anticholinergics
    - β-Adrenergic blockers
    - Calcium channel blockers
    - Diazepam
    - Morphine sulfate
    - Nitrates
    - Progesterone
  - Fatty foods
  - Nicotine
  - Peppermint, spearmint
  - Tea, coffee (caffeine)
- **Hiatal hernia**
- **Incompetent LES**
- **Medication-induced esophagitis**
  - NSAIDs
  - Potassium
- **Obesity**

Complications

Complications are due to the direct local effects of gastric acid on the esophageal mucosa. **Esophagitis** (inflammation of the esophagus) is a common complication of GERD. Ulcers with esophagitis may be present (Fig. 46.3). Repeated esophagitis may lead to scar tissue formation, stricture, and dysphagia.

About 5% to 30% of people with chronic GERD have **Barrett esophagus** (BE). BE is a precancerous lesion that increases the risk for esophageal cancer. Because of this risk, those with BE undergo surveillance endoscopy or radiofrequency ablation as needed. Other risk factors for BE include being over age 60, being male, being White, and having central obesity.

Respiratory complications include cough, bronchospasm, laryngospasm, and cricopharyngeal spasm. These are due to gastric secretions irritating the upper airway. Asthma, chronic bronchitis, and pneumonia may develop from aspiration. Dental erosion, especially in the posterior teeth, may result from acid reflux into the mouth.

Diagnostic Studies

GERD is often diagnosed based on symptoms and the response to behavior and drug therapies. Diagnostic tests are done when usual therapy is ineffective or when we suspect complications (Table 46.8).

Endoscopy is used to assess LES competence and the degree of any inflammation, scarring, and strictures. Biopsy and cytologic specimens can distinguish stomach or esophageal cancer from BE. In addition, the degree of dysplasia (low grade versus high grade) is determined. Manometric studies measure

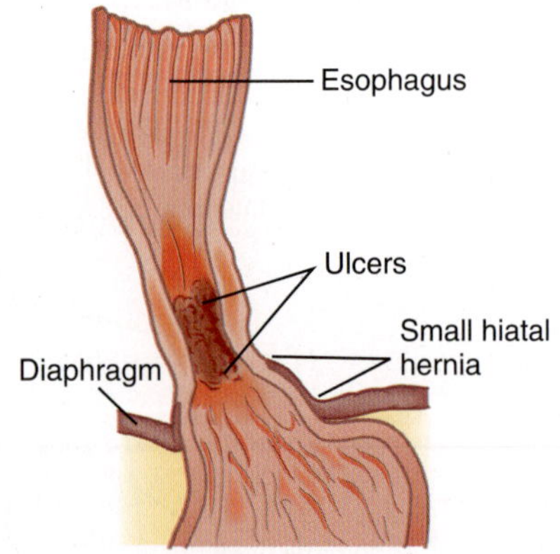

Fig. 46.3 Esophagitis with esophageal ulcers.

TABLE 46.8 Interprofessional Care

GERD and Hiatal Hernia

Diagnostic Assessment
- History and physical assessment
- Upper GI endoscopy with biopsy and cytologic analysis
- Esophagram
- Motility (manometry) studies
- pH monitoring (laboratory or 24 h ambulatory)
- Radionuclide studies

Management

Conservative
- Elevate head of bed 30 degrees
- Avoid reflux-inducing foods (fatty foods, chocolate, peppermint)
- Avoid alcohol
- Reduce or avoid acidic pH beverages (colas, red wine, orange juice)

Drug Therapy (Table 46.10)
- PPIs
- H_2 receptor blockers
- Antacids
- Prokinetics

Surgical Therapy
- Nissen fundoplication
- Toupet fundoplication

Endoscopic Therapy
- Intraluminal valvuloplasty
- Radiofrequency ablation

pressure in the esophagus and LES and esophageal motility function. Ambulatory esophageal pH monitoring is an option for those with refractory symptoms and no mucosal inflammation. Radionuclide tests can detect reflux of gastric contents and the rate of esophageal clearance.

Nursing and Interprofessional Management

Most patients with GERD can successfully manage the condition through lifestyle modifications, drug therapy, and nutrition therapy. These approaches require patient teaching and adherence to therapies. When these therapies are ineffective, surgery is an option (Table 46.8).

Lifestyle Modifications

A patient and caregiver teaching guide is shown in Table 46.9. Teach patients with GERD to avoid factors that trigger symptoms. They should elevate the head of the bed 30 degrees. This can be done using pillows, blocks, or automatic bed frames. Patients should not be supine for 2 to 3 hours after a meal.

Encourage patients who smoke to stop. If needed, refer the patient to community resources for help in stopping smoking. If stress causes symptoms, teach ways to cope with stress (see Chapter 7). Discuss ways to maintain healthy weight, decrease

TABLE 46.9 PATIENT & CAREGIVER TEACHING

GERD

Include the following topics when teaching patients and caregivers about managing GERD:
- Follow a low-fat diet
- Eat small, frequent meals to prevent gastric distention
- Avoid alcohol and beverages that contain caffeine
- Smoking cessation causes an almost immediate, marked decrease in lower esophageal sphincter pressure
- Do not lie down for 2–3 h after eating, wear tight clothing around the waist, or bend over, especially after eating
- Avoid eating within 3 h of bedtime
- Sleep with head of bed elevated 30 degrees
- Implement measures to reduce weight, if needed
- Concerns about lifestyle changes and living with a chronic illness

alcohol use, and increase physical activity. Increased saliva production by chewing gum and oral lozenges may help with mild symptoms.

Drug Therapy

Drug therapy focuses on decreasing the volume and acidity of reflux, improving LES function, increasing esophageal clearance, and protecting the esophageal mucosa (Table 46.10). Proton pump inhibitors (PPIs) and histamine (H_2) receptor blockers are the most common treatments for symptomatic GERD.[9] The goal of HCl acid suppression treatment is to reduce the acidity of the gastric refluxate. Patients with symptomatic GERD but not esophagitis *(nonerosive GERD)* achieve symptom relief with PPIs and H_2 receptor blockers. Have patients contact the HCP if symptoms persist.

PPIs are more effective in healing esophagitis than H_2 receptor blockers. PPIs should start with once-daily dosing, taken before the first meal of the day. PPIs decrease the incidence of esophageal strictures, a complication of chronic GERD. Long-term PPI use may decrease bone density and increase risk of GI cancer, kidney disease, and vitamin B_{12} and magnesium deficiency.[10]

DRUG ALERT

PPIs
- Long-term use or high doses may increase the risk for hip, wrist, and spine fractures.
- Patients should take the lowest dose for the shortest duration needed to treat their condition.

Adjunctive treatments include antacids and prokinetic drugs. Antacids produce quick, short-lived relief of heartburn. Common antacids consist of magnesium hydroxide or aluminum hydroxide as single preparations or in various combinations (Table 46.10). Some preparations combine an H_2

TABLE 46.10 Drug Therapy

GERD and Peptic Ulcer Disease

Drug	Mechanism of Action	Side Effects	Considerations
Potassium Channel Acid Blockers (PCABs)			
vonoprazan (Voquezna)	↓ HCl acid by blocking potassium-binding sites on the H^+-K^+-ATPase enzyme responsible for acid production ↓ Irritation of esophageal mucosa	Abdominal pain, bloating, diarrhea, nausea, URI, rash	Do not crush tablets Take capsules whole Take at the same time each day Do not stop without checking with the HCP
Proton Pump Inhibitors (PPIs)			
dexlansoprazole (Dexilant) esomeprazole (Nexium) lansoprazole (Prevacid) omeprazole (Prilosec) omeprazole and sodium bicarbonate (Zegerid) pantoprazole (Protonix) rabeprazole (AcipHex)	↓ HCl acid by inhibiting the proton pump (H^+-K^+-ATPase) responsible for H^+ secretion ↓ Irritation of esophageal and gastric mucosa	Headache, abdominal pain, nausea, diarrhea, vomiting, flatulence	Prescription and OTC Do not stop without checking with the HCP Esomeprazole, lansoprazole, pantoprazole have IV form
Histamine (H_2) Receptor Blockers			
cimetidine famotidine (Pepcid) nizatidine	Block the action of histamine on the H_2 receptors to ↓ HCl acid secretion ↓ Conversion of pepsinogen to pepsin ↓ Irritation of esophageal and gastric mucosa	Headache, abdominal pain, constipation, diarrhea	Prescription and OTC Do not to stop without checking with the HCP Onset of action is 1 h Effects last up to 12 h depending on drug Famotidine and cimetidine given oral, IV Nizatidine IV only
Antacids, Acid Neutralizers			
Single Substance aluminum hydroxide (Amphojel) calcium carbonate (Tums) sodium bicarbonate (Alka-Seltzer) ***Aluminum and Magnesium*** Maalox, Mylanta aluminum/magnesium trisilicate (Gaviscon)	Neutralize HCl acid	*Aluminum hydroxide:* Constipation, phosphorus depletion with chronic use *Calcium carbonate:* Constipation or diarrhea, hypercalcemia, milk-alkali syndrome, renal calculi *Magnesium preparations:* Diarrhea, hypermagnesemia. Use with caution in patients with renal problems *Sodium preparations:* Milk-alkali syndrome if used with large amounts of calcium. Use with caution in patients on sodium restrictions	Neutralizing effects of antacids taken on an empty stomach last 20–30 min Most effective taken 1–3 h after meals and at bedtime Avoid magnesium in patients with kidney disease Many adverse drug interactions Take with 8 ounces of water
Cholinergic			
bethanechol	↑ LES pressure, ↑ esophageal emptying, ↑ gastric emptying	Lightheadedness, syncope, flushing, diarrhea, stomach cramps, dizziness	Give on empty stomach 1 h before or 2 h after meals
Cytoprotective			
sucralfate (Carafate)	Act to form a protective layer and serve as a barrier against acid, bile salts, and enzymes in the stomach	Constipation	Give on empty stomach 1 h before or 2 h after meals Give 1 h before or after antacids
Prokinetic			
metoclopramide (Reglan)	Block effect of dopamine ↑ Gastric motility and emptying ↓ Reflux	CNS side effects ranging from anxiety to hallucinations Extrapyramidal side effects (tremor and dyskinesias similar to Parkinson disease)	Monitor for suicidal ideation Do not use if GI stimulation would be dangerous (e.g., UGI)
Prostaglandin (Synthetic)			
misoprostol (Cytotec)	Protect lining of stomach *Cytoprotective:* ↑ Production of gastric mucus and mucosal secretion of bicarbonate *Antisecretory:* ↓ HCl acid secretion	Abdominal pain, diarrhea, GI bleeding, uterine rupture if pregnant	Teratogenic; use with caution in females of childbearing age

receptor blocker with an antacid. For example, Pepcid Complete includes famotidine, calcium carbonate, and magnesium hydroxide.

Antacids may be useful in patients with mild, intermittent heartburn. In patients with moderate to severe or frequent symptoms or patients with esophagitis, antacids are not effective in relieving symptoms or healing lesions. After an acute phase of bleeding, antacids may be given hourly, either orally or through the NG tube. If an NG tube is in place, periodically aspirate the stomach contents and test the pH level. If pH is less than 5, intermittent suction may be used, or the frequency or dosage of the antacid or antisecretory agent increased.

The type and dosage of antacid given depend on side effects and potential drug interactions. Antacids high in sodium are used cautiously in older adults and patients with CVD, liver, and renal disease. Antacids can interact adversely with many drugs. They enhance the effects of some drugs, like benzodiazepines and pseudoephedrine. Antacids can decrease the absorption rates of other drugs, such as thyroid hormones, phenytoin, and tetracycline. Adjust the timing of other medications as needed.

Prokinetics increase LES pressure and improve gastric emptying, which may result in a small improvement in regurgitation and vomiting. Common agents include cisapride, metoclopramide (Reglan), bethanechol, and baclofen. Many have significant side effects, so their use is limited only to those with delayed gastric emptying.

DRUG ALERT

Metoclopramide

- Chronic use or high doses carry the risk for tardive dyskinesia.
- Tardive dyskinesia (TD) is a neurologic condition characterized by involuntary and repetitive movements of the body (e.g., extremity movements, lip smacking).
- TD may persist after stopping the drug.

Nutrition Therapy

No specific diet is used to treat GERD. Some patients may need to avoid foods that decrease LES pressure. These include chocolate, peppermint, fatty foods, coffee, and tea (Table 46.7). Some foods (e.g., tomato-based products, orange juice, cola, red wine) and soda may irritate the esophagus. Tell patients to avoid late evening meals, nighttime snacking, and milk, especially at bedtime, since these increase gastric acid secretion. Small, frequent meals and drinking fluids between meals help prevent stomach distention. Weight loss is recommended in patients with excess adiposity.

Surgical Therapy

Antireflux surgery is reserved for patients with complications, such as esophagitis, medication intolerance, stricture, BE, and persistent severe symptoms. The goal of surgery is to reduce reflux by enhancing LES integrity. Most procedures are done laparoscopically. The fundus of the stomach is wrapped around the lower part of the esophagus to reinforce and repair the defective barrier. Nissen and Toupet fundoplication are common laparoscopic antireflux surgeries (Fig. 46.4).

Laparoscopic fundoplication is often an outpatient procedure. Patients at risk for complications, including those with prior upper abdominal surgeries or comorbidities (e.g., cardiac disease, obesity), may be hospitalized afterward. Complications include gastric or esophageal injury, splenic injury, pneumothorax, perforation, bleeding, infection, and pneumonia.

After surgery, reflux symptoms should decrease. However, recurrence is possible. In the first month after surgery, patients may report mild dysphagia. This is caused by edema and should resolve. Teach patients to report persistent symptoms, such as heartburn and regurgitation.

A LINX Reflux Management System is an option for patients who have symptoms despite maximum medical management. A LINX system is a ring of small, flexible magnets enclosed in

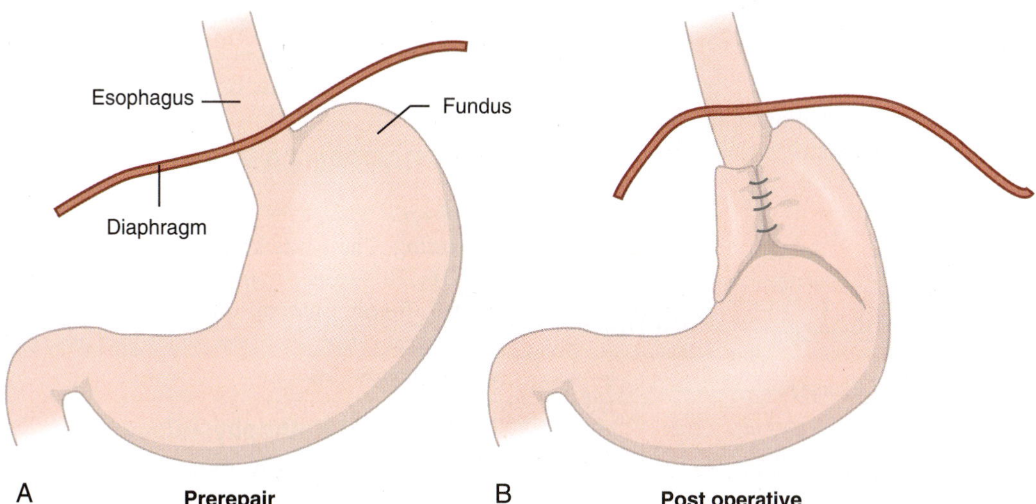

Fig. 46.4 Nissen fundoplication. (A) Fundus of stomach is wrapped around distal esophagus. (B) The fundus is then sutured to itself.

titanium beads and connected by titanium wires. Once implanted laparoscopically into the LES, the ring strengthens the weak LES. Under resting (nonswallowing) conditions, the magnetic attraction between the beads helps keep a weak LES closed to prevent reflux. When the person swallows, the force of pressure from the movement of fluids or foods overwhelms the magnetic forces and the fluid or food passes to the stomach. Problems with the system include nausea, swallowing problems, and pain when swallowing food. Patients who have a LINX system cannot have an MRI as it could cause serious harm.

Endoscopic Therapy

Alternatives to surgery include endoscopic mucosal resection (EMR) and radiofrequency ablation. The heat energy delivered through radiofrequencies creates lesions that we think thicken the LES. For patients with high-grade dysplasia, EMR can be used as a diagnostic test to obtain biopsy samples. Biopsy results determine whether cancer is present.

HIATAL HERNIA

Hiatal hernia is herniation of part of the stomach into the esophagus through an opening, or hiatus, in the diaphragm. We also call it a *diaphragmatic hernia* or *esophageal hernia.* Hiatal hernias are the most common abnormality found on x-ray examination of the upper GI tract. They are common in older adults and occur more often in women.

Hiatal hernias are divided into 4 types:

1. Type I, or sliding type, occurs when the gastroesophageal junction (GEJ) is displaced upwards toward the hiatus. Accounts for 95% of hernias (Fig. 46.5A).
2. Type II is a paraesophageal hiatal hernia. It occurs when part of the stomach migrates into the mediastinum parallel to the esophagus Fig. 46.5B).
3. Type III is both a paraesophageal hernia and a sliding hernia. The GEJ and a portion of the stomach have migrated into the mediastinum.
4. Type IV is when the stomach, as well as an additional organ such as the colon, small intestine, or spleen, herniates into the chest.[11]

Etiology and Pathophysiology

Hiatal hernia is associated with weakening of the muscles in the diaphragm around the esophagogastric opening. Factors that increase intraabdominal pressure may predispose patients to developing a hiatal hernia. These include excess adiposity, pregnancy, ascites, tumors, intense physical exertion, and heavy lifting on a continual basis.

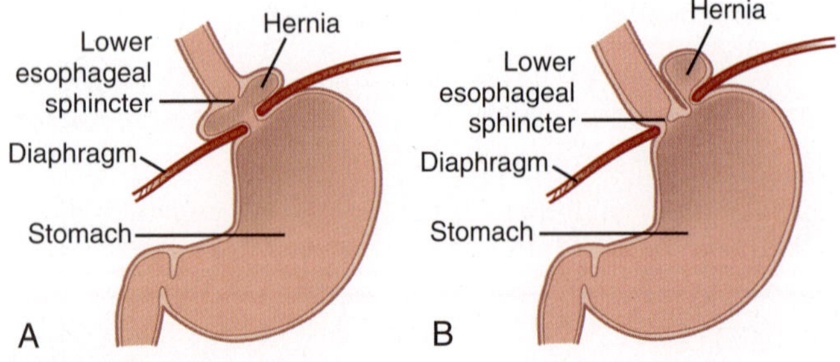

Fig. 46.5 (A) Type I sliding hiatal hernia. (B) Type II rolling or paraesophageal hernia.

Clinical Manifestations and Complications

Some people with hiatal hernia are asymptomatic. When present, manifestations of hiatal hernia are similar to those of GERD. For a few patients, the first sign may be a serious problem, such as esophageal bleeding from esophagitis or respiratory complications (e.g., aspiration pneumonia) due to aspiration of gastric contents.

Complications that may occur include GERD, esophagitis, bleeding from erosion, stenosis (narrowing of the esophagus), ulcerations of the herniated part of the stomach, strangulation of the hernia, and regurgitation with tracheal aspiration.

Diagnostic Studies

An esophagram (barium swallow) may show the protrusion of gastric mucosa through the esophageal hiatus. Endoscopy of the lower esophagus gives information on the degree of mucosal inflammation or other abnormalities. Other tests done are the same as those for GERD (Table 46.8).

Nursing and Interprofessional Management

Conservative therapy of hiatal hernia is similar to that described for GERD. Teach patients to reduce intraabdominal pressure by eliminating constricting garments and avoiding lifting and straining.

Acute paraesophageal hernia is a medical emergency. Surgical treatment includes reducing the herniated stomach into the abdomen, *herniotomy* (excision of the hernia sac), *herniorrhaphy* (closure of the hiatal defect), fundoplication, and *gastropexy* (attachment of the stomach below the diaphragm to prevent reherniation). The goals are to reduce the hernia, provide an acceptable LES pressure, and prevent movement of the gastroesophageal junction. Surgery to repair hiatal hernia is often done laparoscopically by Nissen or Toupet techniques (Fig. 46.4). The approach used (thoracic or abdominal) depends on the patient.

ESOPHAGEAL CANCER

Esophageal cancer is not common. However, the rates are increasing. The United States had 23,370 new cases diagnosed and 16,170 deaths occur from esophageal cancer in 2024. The overall 5-year survival rate is 21.7%.[12] The incidence of esophageal cancer increases with age. Those between 65 and 75 are at greatest risk.

Etiology and Pathophysiology

The cause of esophageal cancer is unknown. Key risk factors include BE, age, smoking, excess alcohol use, and obesity. Current smoking or a history of smoking has a twice greater risk for esophageal cancer. Those with injury to the esophageal mucosa (e.g., from occupational exposure to asbestos and cement dust) are at greater risk.[13] *Achalasia,* a condition marked by delayed emptying of the lower esophagus, is associated with squamous cell cancer.

Most esophageal cancers are adenocarcinomas. The others are squamous cell tumors. Adenocarcinomas arise from the glands lining the esophagus and resemble cancers of the stomach and small intestine. Most esophageal tumors occur in the middle and lower portions of the esophagus. The tumor usually appears as an ulcerated lesion. It may penetrate the muscular layer and extend outside the wall of the esophagus. Many patients have advanced disease at the time of diagnosis. The cancer spreads via the lymph system. The liver and lung are common sites of metastasis.

Clinical Manifestations and Complications

By the time a patient has symptoms, the tumor is often advanced. Progressive dysphagia is the most common symptom. Patients may describe a substernal feeling that food is not passing. At first dysphagia occurs only with meat, then with soft foods, and eventually with liquids.

Pain develops late. It occurs in the substernal, epigastric, or back areas. Pain usually increases with swallowing. It may radiate to the neck, jaw, ears, and shoulders. If the tumor is in the upper third of the esophagus, symptoms, such as sore throat, choking, and hoarseness, may occur. Most patients lose weight. When esophageal stenosis (narrowing) is severe, regurgitation of blood-flecked esophageal contents is common.

Bleeding occurs if the cancer erodes through the esophagus and into the aorta. Esophageal perforation with fistula formation into the lung or trachea sometimes develops. The tumor may enlarge enough to cause esophageal obstruction, especially in the later stages.

Diagnostic Studies

Endoscopic biopsy is needed to diagnose esophageal cancer. Endoscopic ultrasonography (EUS) is important in staging esophageal cancer. Esophagram may show narrowing of the esophagus at the tumor site (Table 46.11).

Interprofessional Care

Treatment depends on the tumor's location and whether invasion or metastasis is present. Esophageal cancer usually has a poor prognosis because it is often diagnosed at an advanced stage. The best results occur with a multimodal approach, including surgery, endoscopic ablation, chemotherapy, and radiation therapy. Depending on the location and cancer spread, only chemotherapy and radiation may be used. Palliative therapy consists of restoring swallowing function and maintaining nutrition and hydration.

TABLE 46.11 Interprofessional Care

Esophageal Cancer

Diagnostic Assessment
- History and physical assessment
- Endoscopy of esophagus with biopsy
- Endoscopic ultrasonography
- Esophagram
- Bronchoscopy
- CT, MRI, PET scans

Management

Conservative
- Radiation therapy
- Chemotherapy

Surgical Therapy
- Esophagectomy
- Esophagoenterostomy
- Esophagogastrostomy

Endoscopic Therapy
- Dilation, stents
- Endoscopic mucosal resection
- Laser therapy
- Photodynamic therapy
- Radiofrequency ablation

Surgical Therapy

Surgical treatments include (1) removal of part or all the esophagus *(esophagectomy)* with use of a Dacron graft to replace the resected part, (2) resection of a portion of the esophagus and anastomosis of the remaining portion to the stomach *(esophagogastrostomy),* and (3) resection of a portion of the esophagus and of a segment of colon to the remaining portion *(esophagoenterostomy).* The surgical approaches may be open (thoracic, abdominal incision) or laparoscopic.

Minimally invasive esophagectomy (e.g., laparoscopic vagal nerve—sparing surgery) is being done more often. The smaller incisions result in decreased intensive care unit (ICU) and hospital stays with fewer complications.

Endoscopic Therapy

Endoscopic therapy includes photodynamic therapy, EMR, and radiofrequency ablation. In photodynamic therapy, the patient receives an IV injection of porfimer sodium (Photofrin), a photosensitizer. Although most tissues absorb porfimer, cancer tissue absorbs it to a greater degree. The HCP directs light toward the cancer using a fiber passed through an endoscope. The light reacts with porfimer, starting a reaction that destroys the cancer cells. Patients must avoid direct sunlight for up to 6 weeks afterward.

EMR is an option for some small, very early-stage cancers. It involves removing cancer tissue using an endoscope.

Radiofrequency ablation uses electric currents to kill cancer cells by heating them.

Dilation, stent placement, or both can relieve obstruction. Dilation increases the lumen of the esophagus. There are various types of dilators. Placement of stents or expandable stents may help when dilation is no longer effective. Self-expandable metal stents are available with features to prevent stent migration and tumor ingrowth. Stents and dilators often relieve dysphagia by allowing food and liquid to pass through the stenotic area. They may be placed before surgery may help improve nutrition status.

Endoscopic laser therapy may be used in combination with dilation. Laser therapy can be repeated if obstruction recurs as the tumor grows. Sometimes these procedures are combined with radiation therapy.

Chemotherapy

Many different chemotherapy drugs can be used to treat esophageal cancer. Regimens include carboplatin and paclitaxel, cisplatin and irinotecan, and oxaliplatin, paclitaxel, or cisplatin with fluorouracil or capecitabine. DCF (docetaxel, cisplatin, fluorouracil) is an option for metastatic disease. New therapy focuses on combining chemotherapy with gene therapy. Chemotherapy is discussed in Chapter 16.

Radiation Therapy

Depending on the type and stage of esophageal cancer, radiation therapy may be given with chemotherapy. Concurrent therapy is given for palliation of symptoms, especially dysphagia, and to increase survival. Some patients receive radiation therapy before surgery.

Targeted Therapy

Some esophageal cancers have too much HER-2 protein on their cell surfaces, which helps cancer cells to grow. Trastuzumab (Herceptin) is a drug that targets the HER-2 protein and kills cancer cells.

Ramucirumab (Cyramza), an angiogenesis inhibitor, binds to the receptor for *vascular endothelial growth factor* (VEGF). It prevents VEGF from binding to the receptor and signaling the body to make more blood vessels. This can help slow or stop the growth and spread of cancer. Ramucirumab treats advanced cancers that start at the gastroesophageal junction. Targeted therapies are discussed in Chapter 16.

NURSING MANAGEMENT: ESOPHAGEAL CANCER

Assessment

Ask patients about a history of GERD, hiatal hernia, achalasia, BE, and tobacco and alcohol use. Assess patients for progressive dysphagia and *odynophagia* (burning, squeezing pain while swallowing). Are there foods or liquids that cause dysphagia? Assess for pain (substernal, epigastric, or back areas), choking, heartburn, hoarseness, cough, anorexia, weight loss, and regurgitation.

Clinical Problems

Clinical problems for patients with esophageal cancer include:

- Pain
- Nutritionally compromised
- Impaired GI function
- Difficulty coping

Planning

The overall goals are that patients with esophageal cancer will (1) have relief of symptoms, including pain and dysphagia, (2) achieve optimal nutrition intake, and (3) have a quality of life appropriate to stage of disease and prognosis.

Implementation

Health Promotion

Counsel patients with GERD, BE, or hiatal hernia about the importance of regular follow-up evaluation. Health counseling should focus on smoking cessation and reducing risk factors for GERD (Table 46.7). Encourage patients to seek medical attention for any esophageal problems, especially dysphagia.

Acute Care

Preoperative care. Patients and caregivers usually react with shock, disbelief, and depression when given the diagnosis of esophageal cancer. Provide emotional and physical support. Clarify test results and provide information. Maintain a positive attitude with respect to the patient's immediate recovery and long-term survival.

Pay attention to the patient's nutrition needs. Many are poorly nourished because of the inability to ingest adequate amounts of food and fluids. A high-calorie, high-protein diet is recommended. Some patients need a liquid form of this diet. Others may need IV fluid replacement or PN. Teach the patient and caregiver how to keep an intake and output record. Assess for signs of fluid and electrolyte imbalance. Some treatment protocols include preoperative radiation and chemotherapy.

Meticulous oral care is essential. Cleanse the mouth thoroughly, including the tongue, gingivae, and teeth or dentures. It may be necessary to use swabs or a gauze pad and to scrub the mouth, including the tongue.

Include information about chest tubes (with a planned open thoracic approach), IV lines, NG tubes, pain management, EN, turning, coughing, and deep breathing in preoperative teaching. General preoperative care is discussed in Chapter 18.

Postoperative care. During the immediate postoperative period, patients usually receive care in the ICU for 1 to 2 days. In addition to usual postoperative complications, dysrhythmias may result from the proximity of the pericardium to the surgical site. Other complications include anastomotic leaks, fistula formation, interstitial pulmonary edema, and acute respiratory distress related to the disruption of the mediastinal lymph nodes.

Patients usually have an NG tube in place for 5 to 7 days. The drainage may be bloody for 8 to 12 hours. The drainage gradually changes to greenish yellow. Key nursing actions include assessing the drainage, maintaining the tube, and providing oral and nasal care. Do not irrigate the NG tube, reposition it, or reinsert it without consulting the HCP.

If the chest cavity is entered, postoperative drainage is achieved with chest tube insertion. Assess the amount and type of drainage. Notify the HCP of excess drainage (e.g., over 400 to 600 mL in 8 hours). Chest surgery and drainage tubes are discussed in Chapter 28.

Implement measures to prevent respiratory complications. Have the patient turn, cough and deep breathe, and use an incentive spirometer every 2 hours. Follow VTE prophylaxis measures. Provide effective pain management.

A feeding tube may be placed depending on the type of surgery (e.g., esophagogastrectomy). Patients often have a swallowing study before starting oral fluids. When starting fluids, give water (30 to 60 mL) hourly and gradually progress to small, frequent, bland meals. Keep the patient in an upright position for 2 hours after to prevent reflux and aspiration. With EN, observe the patient for signs of intolerance to the feeding or leakage of the feeding into the mediastinum. Symptoms of leakage include pain, fever, and dyspnea (see Chapter 44).

Chronic Care

Most patients need long-term follow-up care after surgery for esophageal cancer. Patients may need chemotherapy and radiation. Encourage and assist patients in maintaining adequate nutrition. A permanent feeding gastrostomy may be in place. Patients usually are afraid and anxious about the cancer diagnosis. Know what the HCP has told the patient about the prognosis and provide support.

Referral to a palliative care or home health nurse may be needed. See Chapter 16 for the care of cancer patients and Chapter 10 for a discussion of palliative and end-of-life care.

◆ Evaluation

Expected outcomes for patients with esophageal cancer include:

- Maintain a patent airway
- Have relief of pain
- Be able to swallow comfortably and consume adequate intake
- Have a quality of life appropriate to stage of disease and prognosis

OTHER ESOPHAGEAL PROBLEMS

Eosinophilic Esophagitis

Eosinophilic esophagitis (EoE) is characterized by swelling of the esophagus from an infiltration of *eosinophils.* People with EoE often have a personal or family history of other allergic diseases. The most common food triggers are milk, egg, wheat, rye, and beef. Environment allergens, such as pollens, molds, cats, dogs, and dust mite allergens, may be involved.

Patients may have severe heartburn, difficulty swallowing, food impaction in the esophagus, nausea, vomiting, and weight loss. The diagnosis is based on symptoms and biopsy findings of eosinophils infiltrating esophageal tissue obtained from endoscopy. Allergy skin testing helps to determine the person's allergens.

Avoiding the foods to which the person has positive allergy tests is the first treatment. Other common treatments include PPIs (Table 46.10) and corticosteroids. Corticosteroids are used to treat EoE when avoiding allergic triggers does not relieve symptoms.

Corticosteroids may be used orally (prednisone) or as a topical therapy with inhaled corticosteroids (e.g., fluticasone). The patient takes a puff of fluticasone, and rather than inhaling it, swallows the medication. This directly delivers the drug to the esophagus. The most common side effect is a yeast infection of the throat (esophageal candidiasis).

Esophageal Diverticula

Esophageal diverticula are saclike outpouchings of 1 or more layers of the esophagus. They occur in 3 main areas: (1) above the upper esophageal sphincter *(Zenker diverticulum),* (2) near the esophageal midpoint (traction diverticulum), and (3) above the LES (epiphrenic diverticulum) (Fig. 46.6). Zenker diverticula are the most common. They occur most often in people older than 60 years.

Symptoms include dysphagia, regurgitation, chronic cough, aspiration, and weight loss. Food becomes trapped in

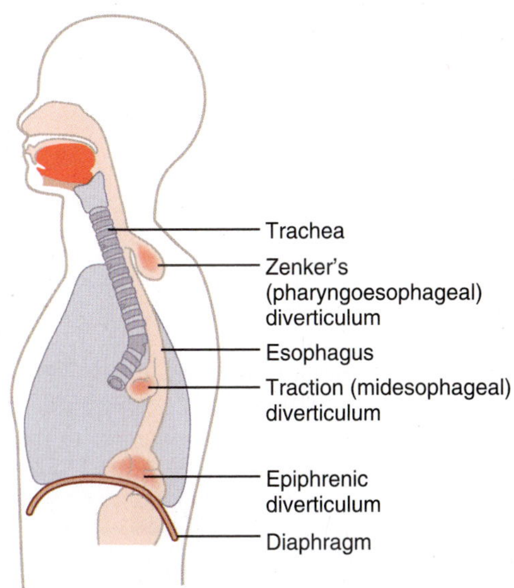

Fig. 46.6 Sites for esophageal diverticula. These hollow outpouchings may occur just above the upper esophageal sphincter (Zenker's), near the midpoint of the esophagus (traction), and just above the LES (epiphrenic).

outpouches. This causes food to taste sour and gives breathe a foul odor. Complications include malnutrition, aspiration, and perforation. Endoscopy or barium studies can easily establish a diagnosis.

Some patients find that they can empty the pocket of food by applying pressure at a certain point on the neck. The diet may have to be limited to foods that pass more readily, such as pureed foods. Surgery may be needed if nutrition is disrupted. The type of surgery depends on the diverticulum's size and location and the patient's condition. Diverticula can either be cut out (diverticulectomy) or repaired through an open approach or endoscopy. The most serious surgical complication is esophageal perforation.

Esophageal Strictures

The most common cause of *esophageal strictures* (or narrowing) is chronic GERD. Ingesting strong acids or alkalis, external beam radiation, and surgical anastomosis can also cause strictures. Trauma, such as throat lacerations and gunshot wounds, can lead to strictures from scar formation. Strictures can cause dysphagia and regurgitation, leading to weight loss.

Strictures can be dilated using dilating instruments or balloons. Dilation may be done with or without endoscopy or with fluoroscopy. Surgical excision with anastomosis is sometimes needed. Patients may have a temporary or permanent gastrostomy.

Achalasia

In **achalasia**, peristalsis of the smooth muscle of the lower two-thirds of the esophagus is absent. Achalasia is a rare, chronic disorder. The exact cause is unknown. With achalasia, the pressure in the LES increases along with incomplete relaxation. Esophageal obstruction at or near the diaphragm occurs. Food and fluid accumulate in the lower esophagus. The result is dilation of the esophagus above the tapered affected segment of the lower esophagus (Fig. 46.7). There is a selective loss of inhibitory neurons, resulting in unopposed contraction of the LES.

The onset of achalasia is usually slow. Dysphagia is the most common symptom. It occurs with liquids and solids. Patients may report a globus sensation and/or substernal chest pain (similar to angina pain) during or right after a meal. About a third have nighttime regurgitation. *Halitosis* (foul-smelling breath) and the inability to eructate (belch) can occur. Patients may report symptoms of GERD and regurgitation of sour-tasting food and liquids, especially when they are lying down. Weight loss is common.

Diagnosis is made with esophagram, high-resolution manometry, and/or endoscopy. Treatment focuses on symptom management. The goals of treatment are to relieve dysphagia and regurgitation, improve esophageal emptying by disrupting the LES, and prevent the development of mega-esophagus (enlargement of the lower esophagus).

Endoscopic pneumatic dilation involves dilating the LES muscle using balloons of progressively larger diameter (3.0, 3.5, and 4.0 cm) (Fig. 46.8). It is an outpatient procedure. If this is ineffective, the next option is a Heller myotomy, done laparoscopically. In this procedure, the HCP cuts through the muscles of the LES, allowing food to pass. Because GERD with esophagitis and stricture is a common complication, patients often have antireflux surgery at the same time. They typically return to usual activities 1 to 2 weeks afterward.

Medical therapy is less effective than invasive procedures. The injection of botulinum toxin endoscopically into the LES gives short-term relief of symptoms and improves esophageal emptying. It works by promoting relaxation of the smooth muscle. This treatment is used for older patients for whom surgery and pneumatic dilation is not an option due to other chronic illnesses.

Nitrates (e.g., isosorbide dinitrate) and calcium channel blockers (e.g., nifedipine) relax the LES and may improve dysphagia. They are taken sublingually 10 to 30 minutes before

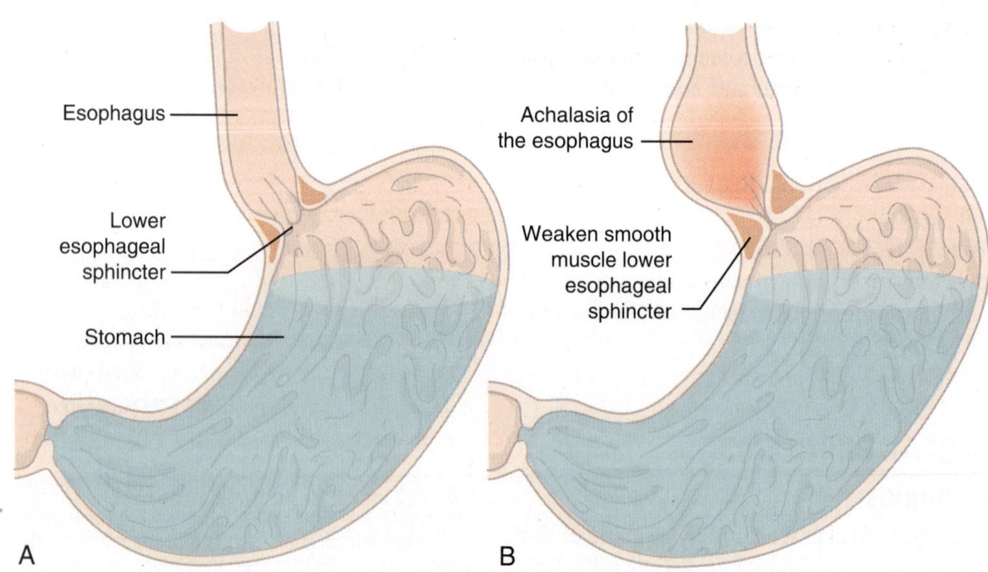

Fig. 46.7 Esophageal achalasia. (A) Healthy esophagus. (B) Achalasia.

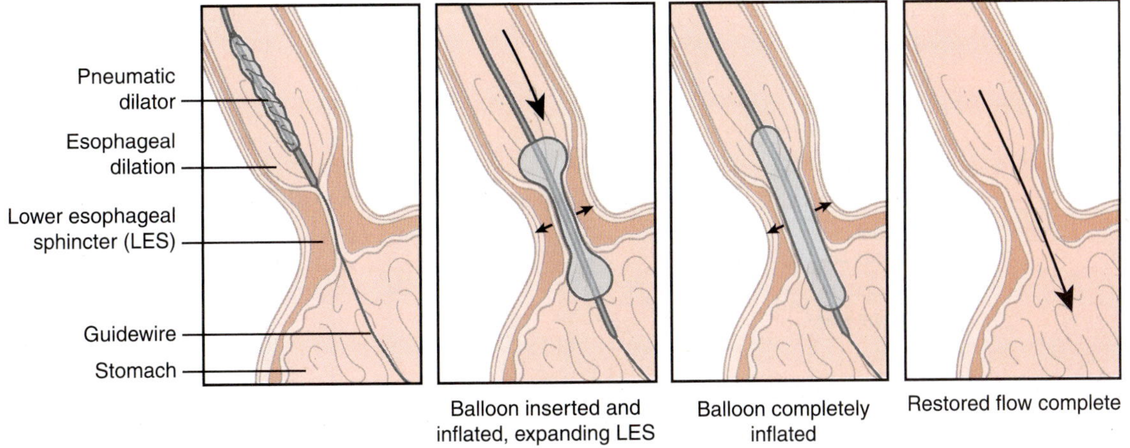

Fig. 46.8 Pneumatic dilation can treat achalasia by maintaining an adequate lumen.

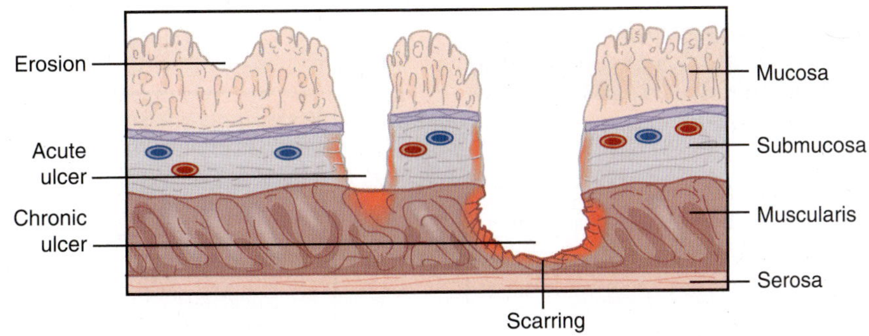

Fig. 46.9 Peptic ulcers, including an erosion, an acute ulcer, and a chronic ulcer. The acute ulcer and the chronic ulcer may penetrate the entire wall of the stomach.

meals. Side effects, drug tolerance, and short duration of action limit their use. Lifestyle measures include a semisoft diet, eating slowly, drinking fluid with meals, and sleeping with the head elevated.

Esophageal Varices

Esophageal varices are dilated, tortuous veins occurring in the lower part of the esophagus. They are due to portal hypertension. Esophageal varices are a common complication of liver cirrhosis. They are discussed in Chapter 48.

STOMACH AND UPPER SMALL INTESTINE PROBLEMS

PEPTIC ULCER DISEASE

Peptic ulcer disease (PUD) is a condition characterized by erosion of the GI mucosa from the digestive action of HCl acid and pepsin. Any part of the GI tract that is in contact with gastric secretions is susceptible to ulcer development. This includes the lower esophagus, stomach, duodenum, and margin of a gastrojejunal anastomosis after surgical procedures. PUD affects about 4.6 million people in the United States each year and 8.9 million globally.[14]

Types

We classify peptic ulcers as acute or chronic (depending on the degree and duration of mucosal involvement) and by location (gastric or duodenal). *Acute ulcers* (Fig. 46.9) cause superficial erosion and minimal inflammation. They are of short duration and resolve quickly when the cause is identified and removed. Chronic ulcers (Fig. 46.10) are of long duration, present continuously for many months or intermittently throughout the person's lifetime. They can erode through the muscular wall with the formation of fibrous tissue. Chronic ulcers are more common.

Gastric and duodenal ulcers differ in their incidence and presentation (Table 46.12). Gastric ulcers can occur in any part of the stomach. They most often occur in the antrum. Gastric ulcers are less common than duodenal ulcers. Because of the peak incidence of gastric ulcers in older adults, the mortality rate from gastric ulcers is greater than that from duodenal ulcers. They are also more likely to cause an obstruction. *H. pylori*, NSAIDs, and bile reflux are the main risk factors.

Duodenal ulcers account for about 80% of all PUD. *H. pylori* is the most common risk factor. Duodenal ulcers are often related to high HCl acid secretion. Those at high risk include people with chronic obstructive pulmonary disease (COPD), cirrhosis, pancreatitis, hyperparathyroidism, chronic kidney disease, and *Zollinger-Ellison syndrome* (ZES). ZES is a rare condition characterized by severe peptic ulceration and HCl acid hypersecretion. Duodenal ulcers tend to occur

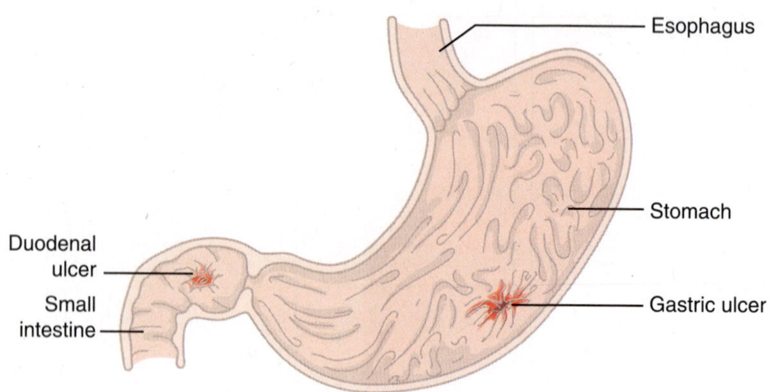

Fig. 46.10 Common sites for gastric and duodenal ulcers.

TABLE 46.12 Comparison of Gastric and Duodenal Ulcers

Gastric Ulcers	Duodenal Ulcers
Lesion	
Superficial, smooth margins. Round, oval, or cone shaped	Penetrating (deformity of duodenal bulb from healing of recurrent ulcers)
Location of Lesion	
Any part of stomach; most often in antrum	First 1–2 cm of duodenum
Gastric Secretion	
Normal to ↓	↑
Incidence	
↑ In females	↑ In males, but increasing in females (especially postmenopausal)
Peak age 50–60 years	Peak age 35–45 years
↑ Cancer risk	No ↑ in cancer risk
H. pylori infection in 80%	*H. pylori* infection in 90%
↑ With incompetent pyloric sphincter and bile reflux	Associated with other diseases (e.g., COPD, pancreatic disease, hyperparathyroidism, ZES, chronic renal failure)
Clinical Manifestations	
Burning or gaseous pressure in epigastrium	Burning, cramping, pressure-like pain across midepigastrium and upper abdomen. Back pain with posterior ulcers
Pain 1–2 h after meals. If penetrating ulcer, aggravation of discomfort with food	Pain 2–5 h after meals and midmorning, midafternoon, middle of night. Periodic and episodic. Pain relief with antacids and food
Recurrence Rate	
High	High

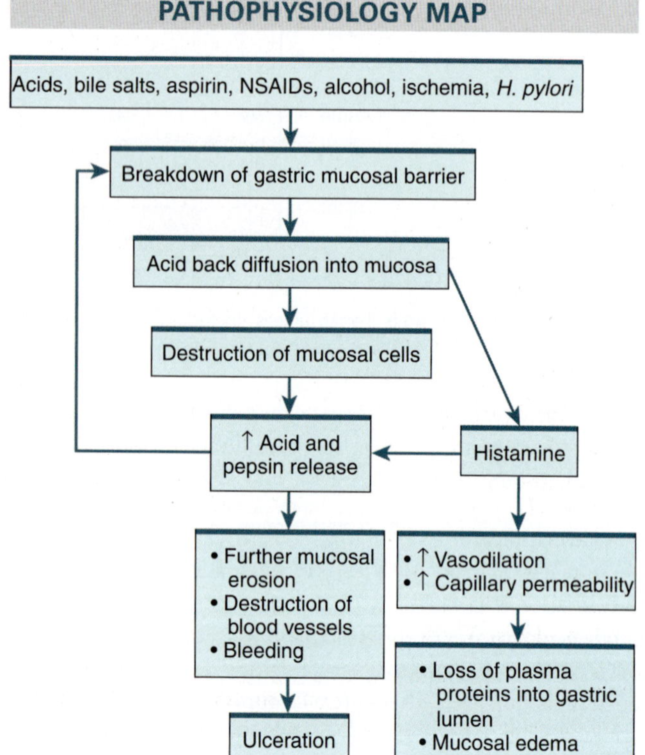

Fig. 46.11 Disruption of gastric mucosa and pathophysiologic consequences of back diffusion of acids.

continuously for a few weeks or months and then disappear for a time, only to recur some months later.

Etiology and Pathophysiology

The pathophysiology of ulcer development is outlined in Fig. 46.11. The back diffusion of HCl acid into the gastric mucosa results in cell destruction and inflammation. Histamine is released from the damaged mucosa. This results in vasodilation, increased capillary permeability, and further secretion of

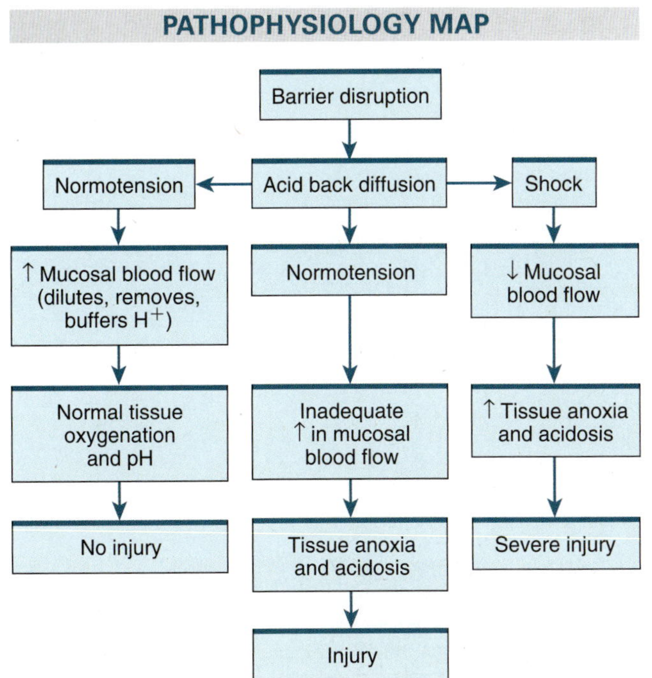

Fig. 46.12 Relationship between mucosal blood flow and disruption of the gastric mucosal barrier.

acid and pepsin. Fig. 46.12 shows the interrelationship between the mucosal blood flow and disruption of the gastric mucosal barrier. Several factors damage the mucosal barrier.

Helicobacter pylori

The major risk factor is infection with *Helicobacter pylori.*[15] 80% of gastric and 90% of duodenal ulcers are related to *H. pylori. H. pylori* affects 30% to 40% of persons in North America. Infection likely occurs during childhood with transmission from family members to the child, possibly through a fecal-oral or oral-oral route. Most people with *H. pylori* do not develop ulcers. Those infected with *CagA*-positive strains are more likely to have PUD.

In the stomach, the bacteria can survive a long time by colonizing the gastric epithelial cells within the mucosal layer. The bacteria make urease, which metabolizes urea-producing ammonium chloride and other damaging chemicals. Urease activates the immune response with antibody production and the release of inflammatory cytokines. This leads to increased gastric acid secretion and causes tissue damage, leading to PUD.

Medication-Induced Injury

NSAID use is responsible for most non—*H. pylori* peptic ulcers. NSAIDs inhibit prostaglandin synthesis, increase gastric acid secretion, and reduce the integrity of the mucosal barrier. NSAID use in the presence of *H. pylori* further increases the risk for PUD. Patients taking corticosteroids or anticoagulants with NSAIDs have a higher risk for PUD. Corticosteroids affect mucosal cell renewal and decrease its protective effects.

Lifestyle

High alcohol use can cause acute mucosal lesions. Alcohol, coffee, and smoking stimulate acid secretion. Smoking, stress, and depression can delay ulcer healing after they have developed.

Clinical Manifestations

In gastric ulcers, the discomfort is generally high in the epigastrium. It occurs about 1 to 2 hours after meals. The pain is described as "burning" or "gaseous." If the ulcer has eroded through the gastric mucosa, food tends to worsen the pain. For some patients, the earliest symptoms are due to a serious complication, such as perforation.

In duodenal ulcers, symptoms occur when gastric acid comes in contact with the ulcers. With meals, food is present to help buffer the acid. Symptoms occur generally 2 to 5 hours after a meal. The pain is described as "burning" or "cramplike." It is most often in the midepigastric region beneath the xiphoid process. Duodenal ulcers can cause back pain.

Some patients have bloating, nausea, vomiting, and early feelings of fullness. Not all patients with ulcers will have pain or discomfort. *Silent* peptic ulcers are more likely to occur in older adults and those taking NSAIDs. The presence or absence of symptoms is not related to the size of the ulcer or the degree of healing.

Diagnostic Studies

Endoscopy is the most accurate procedure to determine the presence and location of an ulcer. It allows for direct viewing of the gastric and duodenal mucosa (Fig. 46.13). During endoscopy, tissue specimens are taken to determine whether *H. pylori* is present and rule out stomach cancer.

Several tests are available to confirm *H. pylori* infection. The gold standard for diagnosing *H. pylori* infection is a biopsy of the antral mucosa with testing for urease (rapid urease testing). Urea is a byproduct of the metabolism of *H. pylori* bacteria. Noninvasive tests include serology, stool, and breath testing. Urea breath and stool antigen tests can identify active infection. Breath tests are more accurate than stool tests. Antibody tests for *H. pylori* can remain positive for years. They are not good for evaluating treatment results.

A barium contrast study may be used to diagnose gastric outlet obstruction or for ulcer detection in those who cannot undergo endoscopy. High fasting gastrin levels may show the presence of a possible gastrinoma (ZES). A secretin stimulation test can discern a gastrinoma from other causes of hypergastrinemia.

Laboratory tests, including a CBC, liver enzyme studies, amylase, and stool examination, may be done. A CBC may show anemia from ulcer bleeding. Liver enzyme studies help detect any liver problems (e.g., cirrhosis) that may complicate ulcer treatment. Stools are tested for blood. Amylase evaluates pancreatic function if we suspect posterior duodenal ulcer penetration of the pancreas.

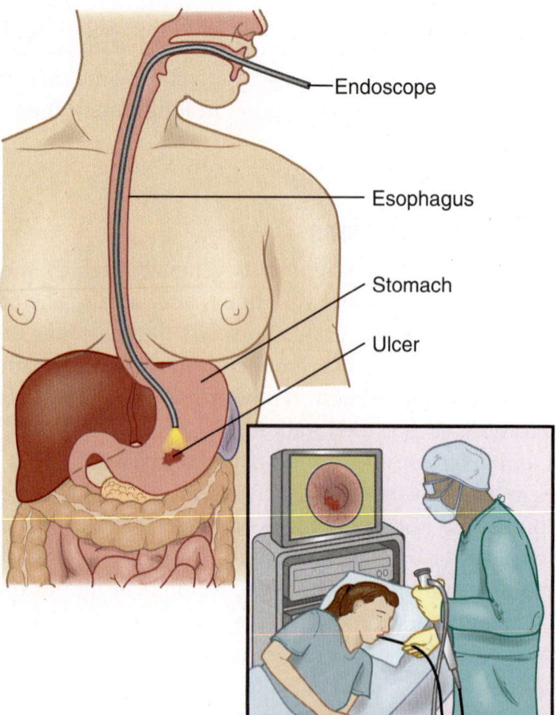

Fig. 46.13 Esophagogastroduodenoscopy (EGD) directly visualizes the mucosal lining of the stomach with a flexible endoscope. Ulcers or tumors can be directly seen, and biopsies obtained.

Interprofessional Care

Conservative Care

Treatment consists of adequate rest, drug therapy, smoking cessation, and diet changes (if needed) (Table 46.13). The goals are to decrease gastric acidity and enhance mucosal defense mechanisms.

Patients are generally treated in ambulatory care. Pain disappears after 3 to 6 days. Ulcer healing is much slower. Complete healing may take 3 to 9 weeks, depending on ulcer size, treatment, and patient adherence. Endoscopy is the most accurate way to monitor ulcer healing. Follow-up endoscopy is usually done 3 to 6 months after diagnosis and treatment.

Aspirin and nonselective NSAIDs are stopped for 4 to 6 weeks. When aspirin must be continued, coadministration with a PPI, H_2 receptor blocker, or misoprostol may be prescribed. Patients receiving low-dose aspirin for CVD and stroke risk who have a history of ulcer disease may need long-term treatment with a PPI. Enteric-coated aspirin decreases local irritation but does not reduce the overall risk for GI bleeding.

Smoking has an irritating effect on the mucosa and delays mucosal healing. Patients should stop or severely reduce smoking. Adequate rest is important for healing and may require some changes in a patient's daily routine. Avoiding or restricting alcohol use will enhance healing.

TABLE 46.13 Interprofessional Care

Peptic Ulcer Disease

Diagnostic Assessment

- History and physical assessment
- Upper GI endoscopy with biopsy
- Endoscopic ultrasound
- *H. pylori* testing of breath, urine, blood, tissue
- Complete blood cell count
- Liver enzymes
- Amylase
- Stool testing for blood

Management

Conservative Therapy

- Adequate rest
- Smoking and alcohol cessation
- Stress management (see Chapter 7)

Drug Therapy (Tables 46.10 and 46.14)

- Antibiotics for *H. pylori*
- Proton pump inhibitors (PPIs)
- Adjunctive therapy
  - H2-receptor blockers
  - Cytoprotective drugs
  - Antacids

Surgical Therapy

- Gastric outlet obstruction: pyloroplasty and vagotomy
- Perforation: simple closure with omentum graft
- Ulcer removal or reduction
  - Billroth I and II
  - Vagotomy and pyloroplasty

Acute Exacerbation Without Complications

- NPO
- NG suction
- Adequate rest
- IV fluid replacement

Drug Therapy (Tables 46.10 and 46.14)

- Antibiotics for *H. pylori*
- PPIs
- Adjunctive therapy
  - PCABs
  - Cytoprotective drugs
  - Antacids
  - Sedatives

Acute Exacerbation With Complications (Bleeding, Perforation, Obstruction)

- NPO
- NG suction
- IV PPI
- Bed rest
- IV fluid replacement
- Blood transfusions
- Stomach lavage (possible)

Drug Therapy

Medications are a key part of therapy (Table 46.10). Drug therapy involves a combination of drugs to reduce gastric acid secretion, protect the GI mucosa and, if needed, eliminate *H. pylori* infection. After the ulcer has healed, many patients can stop acid-blocking therapy. Some may need to continue low-dose maintenance therapy.

Antibiotic therapy. Patients with *H. pylori* infection need antibiotic therapy. Bismuth-based quadruple therapy (BQT) for 14 days is the recommended treatment (Table 46.14).[15] Because of antibiotic-resistant organisms, a growing number of patients do not have *H. pylori* eradicated with a single round of therapy. Talicia is a rifabutin-based treatment for those with resistant *H. pylori* infection. Each capsule contains omeprazole, amoxicillin, and rifabutin. Vonoprazan with amoxicillin and clarithromycin are other alternatives.

Acid-blocking therapy. Acid-blocking therapy, particularly with PPIs, is an effective treatment. They reduce gastric acid secretion and promote ulcer healing. PPIs can be given alone to treat ulcers not caused by *H. pylori.* They are given with antibiotics to treat ulcers caused by *H. pylori.* Potassium-competitive acid blockers (PCABs) such as vonoprazan are given for patients who do not respond to PPI therapy.[15]

Cytoprotective drug therapy. Sucralfate is used for short-term ulcer treatment. It provides mucosal protection for the esophagus, stomach, and duodenum. Sucralfate does not have acid-neutralizing capabilities. Adverse side effects are minimal. It binds with cimetidine, digoxin, warfarin, phenytoin, and tetracycline, reducing their bioavailability.

Adjunct drugs. H_2 receptor blockers and antacids may be used as adjunct therapy to promote ulcer healing. Antacids increase gastric pH by neutralizing HCl acid. As a result, they reduce the acid content of chyme reaching the duodenum. Some antacids (e.g., aluminum hydroxide) can bind to bile salts, thus decreasing the damaging effects of bile on the gastric mucosa.

TABLE 46.14 Drug Therapy

H. pylori *Infection*

Regimen	Drugs	Dosing Per Day
Optimized bismuth quadruple therapy	PPI	20–40 mg, 2 times
	Metronidazole	500 mg, 3 or 4 times
	Tetracycline	500 mg, 4 times
	Bismuth compound	4 times
Rifabutin triple therapy (Talicia)	Amoxicillin	1 g, 3 times
	Omeprazole	40 mg, 3 times
	Rifabutin	50 mg, 3 times
PCAB dual therapy (Voquezna Dual Pak)	Vonoprazan	20 mg, 3 times
	Amoxicillin	1 g, 3 times
PCAB triple therapy (Voquezna Triple Pak)	Vonoprazan	20 mg, 2 times
	Amoxicillin	1 g, 2 times
	Clarithromycin	500 mg, 2 times

Misoprostol is a synthetic prostaglandin analog prescribed to prevent gastric ulcers caused by NSAIDs and LDA. It has protective, and some antisecretory, effects on gastric mucosa. People who need chronic NSAID therapy, such as those with osteoarthritis, may benefit from its use.

Some patients may receive tricyclic antidepressants (e.g., imipramine, doxepin). They may contribute to overall pain relief through their effects on afferent pain fiber transmission. Their anticholinergic properties result in reduced acid secretion. Anticholinergic drugs are sometimes used for PUD treatment.

Nutrition Therapy

There is no specific diet used to treat PUD. Patients should eat and drink foods and fluids that do not cause any distressing symptoms. Foods that may cause gastric irritation include pepper, carbonated beverages, broth (meat extract), and hot, spicy foods. Caffeine-containing beverages and foods can increase symptoms in some patients. Teach patients to avoid alcohol use because it can delay healing.

Surgical Therapy

With the use of drug therapy and endoscopic therapy to treat PUD, surgery is less common. Surgery is an option for those with complications that are unresponsive to medical management or concerns about stomach cancer. Gastric surgeries are described later in this chapter.

Complications

The 3 major complications of chronic PUD are GI bleeding, perforation, and gastric outlet obstruction.[17] These complications are emergency situations. Patients may need surgical intervention.

GI Bleeding

GI bleeding is the most common complication of PUD. Duodenal ulcers cause more bleeding episodes than gastric ulcers.

Perforation

Perforation is the most lethal complication of PUD. Perforation risk is highest with large penetrating duodenal ulcers (Fig. 46.14). However, the mortality rate from a perforated gastric ulcer is higher. Patients with gastric ulcers are often older and have concurrent medical problems, which accounts for the higher mortality rate.

With perforation, the ulcer penetrates the serosal surface with spillage of gastric or duodenal contents into the peritoneal cavity. The contents entering the peritoneal cavity may contain air, saliva, food particles, HCl acid, pepsin, bacteria, bile, and pancreatic fluid and enzymes.

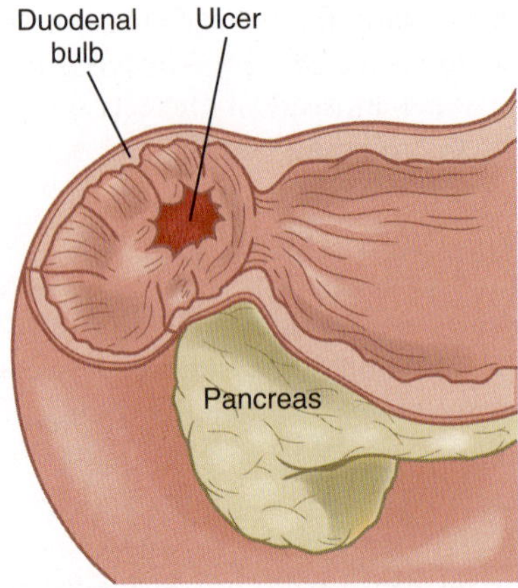

Fig. 46.14 Duodenal ulcer of the posterior wall penetrating the head of the pancreas, resulting in walled-off perforation.

The manifestations of perforation are sudden and dramatic. During the initial phase (up to 2 hours after perforation), patients have sudden, severe upper abdominal pain that quickly spreads throughout the abdomen. The pain radiates to the back and shoulders. Food or antacids do not relieve pain. The abdomen appears rigid and board-like. Bowel sounds are usually absent. Nausea and vomiting may occur. Pulse is increased and weak. Without treatment, bacterial peritonitis may occur within 6 to 12 hours. The intensity of peritonitis is proportional to the amount and duration of the spillage through the perforation. Broad-spectrum antibiotic therapy is prescribed.

The immediate focus of managing patients with a perforation is to stop the spillage of GI contents into the peritoneal cavity and restore blood volume. Small perforations may spontaneously seal themselves and symptoms cease. Spontaneous sealing occurs because of fibrin production in response to the perforation. This can lead to fibrinous fusion of the duodenum or gastric curvature to adjacent tissue (mainly the liver) and strictures that can obstruct the flow of intestinal contents and the passage of stool.

Larger perforations need immediate surgical closure. Whether the patient has an open or laparoscopic repair depends on the ulcer's location and HCP preference. The procedure with the least risk is simple oversewing of the perforation and reinforcement of the area with a graft of omentum. Excess gastric contents are suctioned from the peritoneal cavity during the surgical procedure.

Gastric Outlet Obstruction

Acute and chronic PUD can cause gastric outlet obstruction. Obstruction in the distal stomach and duodenum is the result of edema, inflammation, pylorospasm, or fibrous scar tissue formation. With obstruction the discomfort or pain is worse toward the end of the day as the stomach fills and dilates. Belching or self-induced vomiting may provide some relief. Vomiting is common and often projectile. Emesis may contain food particles that were ingested hours or days before. Constipation occurs from dehydration and decreased diet intake from anorexia. Over time, dilation of the stomach and visible swelling in the upper abdomen may occur.

The aim of therapy for obstruction is to decompress the stomach and correct any existing fluid and electrolyte imbalances. Constant NG aspiration of stomach contents can help relieve symptoms. This allows edema and inflammation to subside and permits normal flow of gastric contents through the pylorus.

IV fluids and electrolytes are replaced according to the degree of dehydration, vomiting, and electrolyte imbalance shown by laboratory studies. A PPI or H_2 receptor blocker is used if the obstruction is due to an active ulcer. Balloon dilation can open a pyloric obstruction. Surgery may be needed to remove scar tissue.

NURSING MANAGEMENT: PEPTIC ULCER DISEASE

Assessment

Subjective and objective data to obtain from patients with PUD are outlined in Table 46.15.

TABLE 46.15 NURSING ASSESSMENT

Peptic Ulcer Disease

Subjective Data

Important Health Information

Health history: Chronic kidney disease, pancreatic disease, COPD, serious illness or trauma, hyperparathyroidism, cirrhosis, Zollinger-Ellison syndrome

Medications: Aspirin, corticosteroids, NSAIDs

Surgery or other treatments: Complicated or prolonged surgery

Functional Health Patterns

Health perception—health management: Alcohol use, smoking, caffeine use. Family history of PUD

Nutritional-metabolic: Weight loss, anorexia, nausea and vomiting, hematemesis, dyspepsia, heartburn, belching

Elimination: Black, tarry stools

Cognitive-perceptual:

- *Duodenal ulcers:* Burning, midepigastric or back pain occurring 2–5 h after meals and relieved by food; nighttime pain common
- *Gastric ulcers:* High epigastric pain occurring 1–2 h after meals. Food may precipitate or worsen pain

Coping—stress tolerance: Acute or chronic stress

Objective Data

General

Anxiety, irritability

Gastrointestinal

Epigastric tenderness

Possible Diagnostic Findings

Anemia. Guaiac-positive stools. Positive blood, urine, breath, or stool tests for *H. pylori.* Abnormal upper GI endoscopic and barium studies

Clinical Problems

Clinical problems for patients with PUD may include:

- Impaired GI function
- Pain

Additional information on clinical problems and interventions for patients with PUD is in eNursing Care Plan 46.2 available on the website for this chapter.

Planning

The overall goals are that patients with PUD will (1) adhere to the treatment plan, (2) achieve pain relief, (3) be free from complications, (4) have complete healing of the peptic ulcer, and (5) make lifestyle changes to prevent recurrence.

Implementation

Health Promotion

You play a key role in identifying those at risk for PUD. Early detection and treatment of ulcers are important in reducing morbidity. Patients who are taking ulcerogenic drugs (e.g., NSAIDs, LDA) are at risk for PUD. Encourage patients to take these drugs with food. Teach patients to report symptoms related to gastric irritation, including epigastric pain, to their HCP.

Acute Care

During an acute exacerbation, patients often report increased pain, nausea, and vomiting. Some may have bleeding. Many patients try to cope with the symptoms at home before seeking medical care.

Patients may be NPO for a few days, have an NG tube connected to intermittent suction, and receive IV fluid replacement. The volume of fluid lost, signs and symptoms, and laboratory test results (hemoglobin, hematocrit, electrolytes) determine the type and amount of IV fluids given. Take vital signs initially and then at least hourly to detect and treat shock. Give IV fluids as ordered. Maintain intake and output, especially of the gastric aspirate.

Maintain patency of the NG tube. When the stomach is empty of gastric secretions, pain decreases, and ulcer healing begins. Regularly irrigate the NG tube with a normal saline solution per agency policy. It may be helpful to reposition the patient from side to side so that the tube tip is not constantly lying against the mucosal surface. Cleaning and lubricating the nares decreases soreness. Analysis of gastric contents may include pH testing and analysis for blood, bile, or other substances.

Physical and emotional rest is helpful to ulcer healing. The environment should be quiet and restful. Pain medications provide comfort. A mild sedative may help if patients are anxious and apprehensive. Use good judgment before sedating a patient who is becoming increasingly restless because the drug could mask the signs of shock from GI bleeding. Regular mouth care relieves the dry mouth.

GI bleeding. Changes in vital signs and an increase in the amount and redness of aspirate often signal massive upper GI bleeding. With bleeding, the pain often decreases because the blood helps neutralize the acidic gastric contents. Maintain the patency of the NG tube so that blood clots do not obstruct the tube. If the tube becomes blocked, the patient can develop abdominal distention. Use interventions similar to those described for upper GI bleeding.

Perforation. If manifestations of a perforation develop, notify the HCP immediately. Take vital signs promptly and record them every 15 to 30 minutes. Temporarily stop all oral or NG drugs and feedings. If perforation exists, anything taken orally can add to the spillage into the peritoneal cavity and increase discomfort.

An NG tube can provide continuous aspiration and gastric decompression to stop spillage through the perforation. For duodenal aspiration, the tube is placed as near to the perforation site as possible to promote decompression.

Give IV fluid as ordered. Circulating blood volume is replaced with lactated Ringer's and albumin solutions. These solutions substitute for the fluids lost from the vascular and interstitial space as peritonitis develops. Packed RBCs may be needed. A central venous pressure line and an indwelling urinary catheter may be inserted and monitored hourly. Patients with heart disease need ECG monitoring or a pulmonary artery catheter for assessment of left ventricular function. Give prescribed antibiotic therapy for bacterial peritonitis.

Gastric outlet obstruction. To check for obstruction, clamp the NG tube intermittently and measure the gastric residual volume. The frequency and amount of time the tube is clamped are related to the amount of aspirate obtained and the patient's comfort level. A common method is to clamp the tube overnight (usually 8 to 12 hours) and measure the gastric residual volume in the morning. When the aspirate falls below 200 mL, it is within a normal range and the patient can begin oral intake of clear liquids. Oral fluids begin at 30 mL/h and then gradually increase in amount. As the amount of gastric residual decreases, solid foods are added, and the tube is removed.

If the patient resumed oral feedings and you note symptoms of obstruction, promptly inform the HCP. Generally, all that is needed to treat the problem is to resume gastric aspiration until the edema and inflammation resulting from the acute episode resolve. IV fluids with electrolyte replacement keep the patient hydrated during this period. If conservative treatment is not successful, surgery is done after the acute phase has passed.

Chronic Care

PUD is a chronic, recurring disorder. Patients with PUD have specific teaching needs to prevent recurrence and complications. Table 46.16 provides a patient and caregiver teaching guide for PUD. Teaching should cover aspects of the disease process, drugs, lifestyle changes (alcohol use, smoking), and need for regular follow-up care. Discuss potential complications. Some patients have repeated exacerbations. Review what to do if pain or other symptoms recur or there is blood in emesis or stools. Work with the dietitian to plan ways to incorporate diet modifications.

TABLE 46.16 PATIENT & CAREGIVER TEACHING

Peptic Ulcer Disease

Include the following instructions when teaching patients and caregivers about management of PUD:

1. Avoid foods that cause epigastric distress, such as acidic foods.
2. Avoid cigarettes. Smoking promotes ulcer development and delays ulcer healing.
3. Reduce or stop alcohol use.
4. Avoid OTC drugs unless approved by the HCP. Many preparations contain ingredients, such as aspirin, which should not be taken unless approved by the HCP. Check with the HCP about the use of NSAIDs.
5. Do not interchange brands of PPIs, antacids, or H_2 receptor blockers that you can buy OTC without checking with the HCP. This can lead to harmful side effects.
6. Follow prescribed drug therapy to prevent a relapse. This includes antisecretory and antibiotic drugs.
7. Report any of the following:
   - Increased nausea or vomiting
   - Increased epigastric pain
   - Bloody emesis or tarry stools
8. Stress can be related to PUD. Learn and use stress management strategies (see Chapter 7).
9. Share concerns about lifestyle changes and living with a chronic illness.

Because ulcers often recur, interrupting or stopping therapy can have harmful results. Strict adherence to drug therapy is important. Teach patients about prescribed drugs, including their actions, side effects, and dangers if omitted for any reason. Make sure they know not to take OTC drugs (e.g., NSAIDs, LDA) unless approved by the HCP. Some H_2 receptor blockers and PPIs are available without a prescription. Tell patients to check with the HCP before switching from a prescription to an OTC preparation to avoid side effects and incorrect dosing.

Patients may be reluctant to talk about personal stress, their usual ways of coping, smoking habits, or alcohol use. Provide information about the negative effects of alcohol and cigarettes on PUD and ulcer healing. Changes such as smoking cessation and alcohol abstinence are hard for many people. Patients may do better in reducing, rather than eliminating, use of these substances. However, the goal is total cessation.

◆ Evaluation

Expected outcomes for patients with PUD include:

- Have pain controlled without the use of analgesics
- Commit to self-care and management of the disease
- Be free from complications

STOMACH CANCER

Stomach (gastric) cancer is an adenocarcinoma of the stomach wall (Fig. 46.15). It accounts for more than 26,890 new cancer cases and 10,880 deaths annually.[16] In the United States the number of new cases of stomach cancer has been dropping by about 1.5% each year over the last 10 years. In the United States the incidence is higher in males by a 2:1 ratio. The average age at the time of diagnosis is 68.[16]

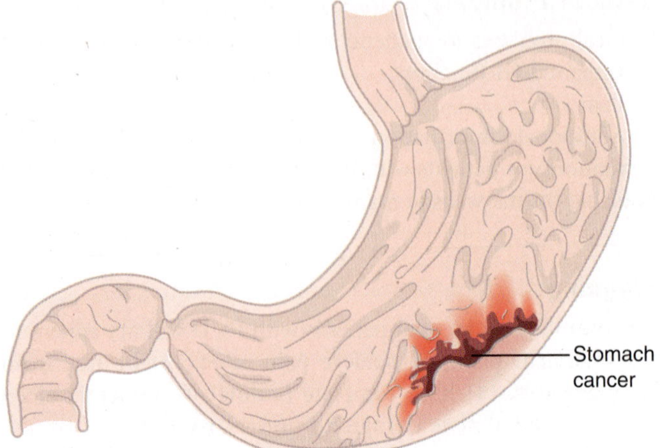

Fig. 46.15 Stomach cancer often begins in cells that line the stomach.

At the time of diagnosis, only 10% to 20% of patients have disease confined to the stomach. The 5-year survival rate in this group is 75%. However, more than 50% have advanced metastatic disease. The overall 5-year survival rate of all people with stomach cancer is about 36%.[16]

Etiology and Pathophysiology

We do not know the exact cause of stomach cancer. It likely begins with a nonspecific mucosal injury because of infection (*H. pylori*), autoimmune-related inflammation, or repeated exposure to irritants such as bile or NSAIDs. It is possible that *H. pylori* and resulting cell changes induces a sequence of transitions from dysplasia to cancer. Lifestyle factors include smoking, obesity, and diets high in smoked foods, salted fish and meat, and pickled vegetables. Whole grains and fresh fruits and vegetables reduce stomach cancer risk.

Other risk factors include atrophic gastritis, pernicious anemia, stomach polyps, *achlorhydria* (absent or low production of gastric HCl), and stomach lymphoma (mucosa-associated lymphoid tissue). Although first-degree relatives of patients with stomach cancer are at increased risk, only about 10% of stomach cancers have an inherited component. About 1% of stomach cancers are hereditary diffuse gastric cancer (HDGC).[17]

Stomach cancer spreads by direct extension. It typically infiltrates rapidly to the surrounding tissue and liver. Seeding of tumor cells into the peritoneal cavity occurs late in the course of the disease.

Clinical Manifestations

Manifestations include unexplained weight loss, indigestion, and abdominal discomfort or pain. Anemia is common. It is caused by chronic blood loss as the lesion erodes through the mucosa or from pernicious anemia (caused by loss of intrinsic factor). The person appears pale and weak. They may report fatigue, weakness, dizziness, and, in extreme cases, shortness of breath. The stool may be positive for occult blood. Patients may report *early satiety,* or a sense of being full sooner than usual. Hard and enlarged supraclavicular lymph nodes suggest metastasis via the thoracic duct. The presence of ascites is a poor prognostic sign.

Diagnostic Studies

Table 46.17 outlines the diagnostic studies for stomach cancer. Upper GI endoscopy is the best diagnostic tool. The stomach can be distended with air during the procedure, stretching the mucosal folds. Tissue biopsy and histologic examination are important in diagnosing stomach cancer.

Endoscopic ultrasound, CT, MRI, and PET scanning can be used to stage the disease. Laparoscopy is done to determine peritoneal spread.

Blood studies detect anemia and determine its severity. Increased liver enzymes and amylase levels may mean liver and pancreas involvement. Stool examination provides evidence of occult or gross bleeding. The presence of tumor markers can help diagnose cancer.

Interprofessional Care

Surgical Therapy

The treatment of choice for stomach cancer is surgical removal of the tumor. The aim is to remove as much of the stomach as needed to remove the tumor and a margin of normal tissue. The location and extent of the lesion, the patient's physical condition, and the HCP's preference determine the surgery done (e.g., open versus laparoscopic).

TABLE 46.17 Interprofessional Care

Stomach Cancer

Diagnostic Assessment	Management

• History and physical assessment
• Endoscopy and biopsy
• CT, MRI, PET scans
• Upper GI barium study
• Exfoliative cytologic study
• Endoscopic ultrasonography
• CBC
• Liver enzymes
• Urinalysis
• Stool examination
• Amylase
• Tumor markers
  • α-Fetoprotein
  • Carbohydrate antigen (CA)-19-9, CA-125, CA 72-4
  • Carcinoembryonic antigen (CEA)
	• Surgical therapy
	  • Subtotal gastrectomy (Billroth I or II procedure)
	  • Total gastrectomy with esophagojejunostomy
	• Chemotherapy
	• Radiation therapy
	• Targeted therapy

Patients with lesions in the antrum or pyloric region generally have a Billroth I or II procedure (Fig. 46.16). When the lesion is in the fundus, a total gastrectomy with esophagojejunostomy is done (Fig. 46.17). When metastasis has occurred to adjacent organs, such as the spleen, ovaries, or bowel, the surgical procedure is extended as needed. If the tumor extends into the transverse colon, partial colon resection is done.

Preoperative management focuses on correcting nutrition deficits and treating anemia. Packed RBC transfusions correct the anemia. If gastric outlet obstruction occurs, gastric decompression may be needed before surgery.

Chemotherapy and Radiation Therapy

Many chemotherapy drugs can be used to treat stomach cancer. These include fluorouracil, capecitabine, carboplatin, cisplatin, docetaxel, epirubicin, irinotecan, oxaliplatin, and paclitaxel. Combination therapies offer better outcomes. Examples include ECF (epirubicin, cisplatin, fluorouracil) and

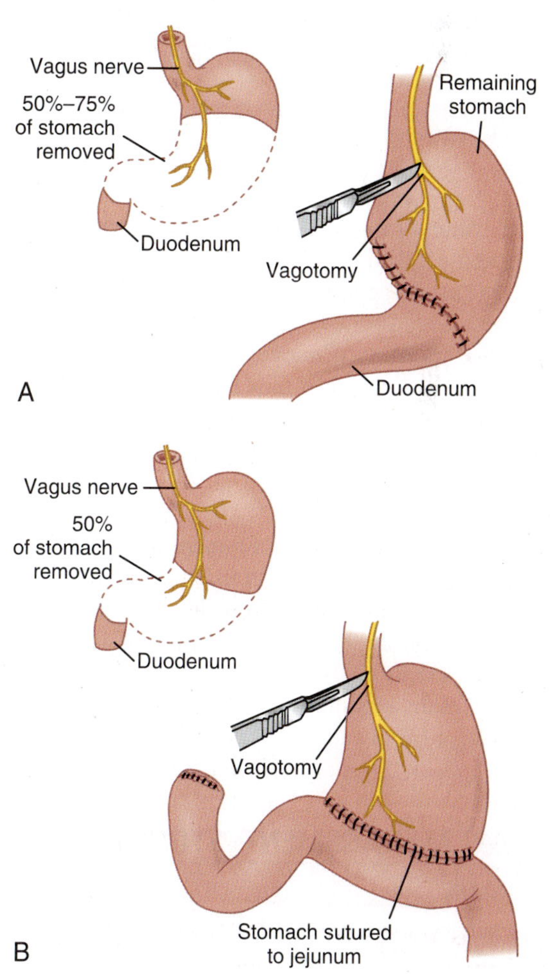

Fig. 46.16 (A) Billroth I procedure (subtotal gastric resection with gastroduodenostomy anastomosis). (B) Billroth II procedure (subtotal gastric resection with gastrojejunostomy anastomosis).

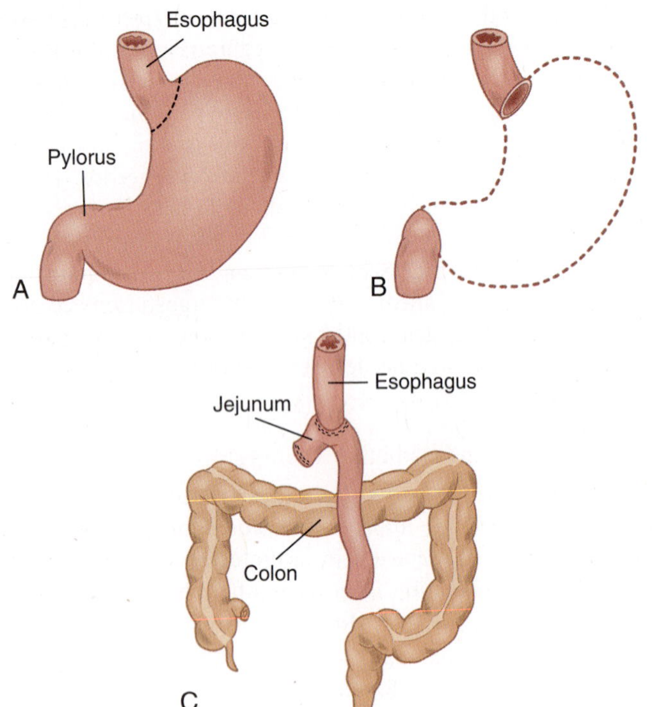

Fig. 46.17 Total gastrectomy for stomach cancer. (A) Normal anatomic structure of the stomach. (B) Removal of the stomach (total gastrectomy). (C) Anastomosis of the esophagus with the jejunum (esophagojejunostomy).

docetaxel, irinotecan, oxaliplatin, or cisplatin with fluorouracil or capecitabine.[18] Intraperitoneal chemotherapy may be used to treat metastatic disease. Chemotherapy is discussed in Chapter 16.

Combined radiation therapy and chemotherapy can reduce recurrence or be a palliative measure to decrease tumor mass and provide temporary relief of obstruction.

Targeted Therapy

Trastuzumab (Herceptin) and ramucirumab (Cyramza) are targeted therapies used to treat stomach cancer. About 20% of patients have too much HER-2 on the surface of the cancer cells. Trastuzumab targets the HER-2 protein and kills cancer cells. Ramucirumab binds to the receptor for VEGF and prevents VEGF from binding to the receptor. This prevents the growth and spread of cancer.[19]

NURSING MANAGEMENT: STOMACH CANCER

Assessment

The assessment of patients with stomach cancer is similar to that for PUD (Table 46.15). Obtain a nutrition assessment, psychosocial history, and physical assessment. Assess how the patient and caregiver are coping with the cancer diagnosis.

The nutrition assessment includes information about appetite and changes in eating patterns over the previous 6 months. Determine the patient's normal weight and any recent weight changes. Unexplained weight loss and anorexia are common. Evaluate nutrition status. Cachexia may be present if oral intake was reduced for an extended period. Malnourished patients do not respond well to chemotherapy or radiation therapy and are a poor surgical risk. There may be vague abdominal symptoms, including dyspepsia and intestinal gas, discomfort, or pain. Explore where any pain is, when it occurs, and how it is relieved.

Determine the patient's usual method of coping. A cancer diagnosis and a treatment plan that may include surgery, chemotherapy, or radiation treatment is stressful. If surgery is planned, assess expectations about surgery (cure or palliation) and how they responded to previous surgical procedures.

Planning

The overall goals are that patients with stomach cancer will (1) have minimal discomfort, (2) achieve optimal nutrition status, and (3) maintain a degree of spiritual and psychologic well-being appropriate to the disease stage.

Implementation

When diagnostic tests confirm cancer, the patient and family generally react with shock, disbelief, and depression. Provide emotional and physical support, provide information, and clarify test results. Maintain a positive attitude with respect to their immediate recovery and long-term survival.

Because of changes in appetite and early satiety, the patient may be malnourished. Surgery may be delayed until the patient is more physically able to withstand it. A positive nutrition state enhances wound healing and the ability to deal with infection and other possible postoperative complications. Some patients better tolerate several small meals a day than 3 regular meals. It may be challenging to persuade patients to eat when they have no appetite and are depressed. Getting the caregiver to help with meals and encourage intake may be helpful. Commercial liquid supplements and vitamins may supplement the diet. If a patient is unable to ingest oral feedings, the HCP may prescribe EN or PN (see Chapter 44).

If needed, packed RBCs and fluid volume restoration may be given during the preoperative period. Preoperative teaching and the postoperative care of patients having stomach cancer surgery are described in the gastric surgery section.

Radiation therapy or chemotherapy is used as an adjuvant to surgery or for palliation. Assess their knowledge of therapy. Teach them about skin care, need for nutrition and fluid intake, and the use of antiemetic drugs. Ensure completion of the designated number of treatments. Care of patients receiving chemotherapy and radiation therapy is discussed in Chapter 16.

When chemotherapy or radiation treatment is continuing after discharge, a referral to home health care may be helpful. The home health nurse can help with recovery and provide support to the patient and caregiver. Provide patients with a list of available community agencies (e.g., American Cancer Society). Encourage them to adhere to the prescribed therapies, keep appointments for chemotherapy or radiation treatments, and notify the HCP of changes in their condition. Cancer recurrence is common. Patients need regular follow-up examinations and imaging assessments. Long-term management of patients with cancer is discussed in Chapter 16.

◆ Evaluation

Expected outcomes for patients with stomach cancer include:

- Have minimal discomfort, pain, or nausea
- Achieve optimal nutrition status
- Maintain a degree of psychologic well-being appropriate to the disease stage

GASTROINTESTINAL STROMAL TUMORS

Gastrointestinal stromal tumors (GISTs) are a rare cancer that originates in cells in the wall of the GI tract. These cells, known as *interstitial cells of Cajal,* help control the movement of food and liquid through the stomach and intestines. About 60% of GISTs are in the stomach; 30% are in the small intestine. The rest are in the esophagus, colon, or peritoneum.[17] Most GISTs occur in people between the ages of 50 and 70. While the exact cause is unknown, genetic mutations likely play a role. A few GISTs occur in people with familial mutations KIT or platelet-derived growth factor receptor a (PDGFRa) or in those with neurofibromatosis type 1.

The manifestations depend on the part of the GI tract affected. Early manifestations are often subtle. They include early satiety, fatigue, bloating, nausea or vomiting, and a change in bowel habits. Because these are like those of many other GI problems, early detection is difficult. Later manifestations may include GI bleeding and obstruction caused by larger tumors.

GISTs are often found during imaging for other problems. Diagnosis is based on histologic examination of biopsied tissue. Endoscopic ultrasound, CT, or MRI are used to determine the extent of disease.

Surgery offers the only permanent cure. GISTs have usually metastasized by the time of diagnosis or often recur. They are unresponsive to conventional chemotherapy. The discovery of genetic mutations led to the development of tyrosine kinase inhibitor drugs (e.g., imatinib mesylate, sunitinib, regorafenib) that are effective against some GISTs.

GASTRITIS

Gastritis is an inflammation of the gastric mucosa. It is a common problem affecting the stomach. Gastritis may be acute or chronic and local or diffuse.

Etiology and Pathophysiology

Gastritis occurs as the result of a breakdown in the normal gastric mucosal barrier. This mucosal barrier normally protects the stomach tissue from the corrosive action of HCl acid and pepsin. When the barrier is broken, HCl acid and pepsin can diffuse back into the mucosa. This back diffusion results in tissue edema, disruption of capillary walls with loss of plasma into the gastric lumen, and possible bleeding.

Risk Factors

Table 46.18 lists risk factors and causes of gastritis. Some risk factors are discussed here.

Helicobacter pylori. *H. pylori* infection causes acute gastritis in most infected persons. Chronic gastritis may develop in some. Prolonged inflammation leads to functional changes in the stomach and may cause stomach cancer. *H. pylori* was discussed earlier in this chapter.

Drug-related gastritis. Drugs contribute to the development of acute and chronic gastritis. NSAIDs and corticosteroids inhibit the synthesis of prostaglandins that protect the gastric mucosa. This makes the mucosa more susceptible to injury. Factors that increase the risk for NSAID-induced gastritis include being female; being over age 60; having a history of ulcer disease; taking anticoagulants, LDA, or corticosteroids; and having a chronic disorder, such as CVD. Some drugs such as digoxin and alendronate have direct irritating effects on the gastric mucosa.

Diet. Diet indiscretions can cause acute gastritis. After binge drinking alcohol, acute damage to the gastric mucosa can range from local injury of superficial epithelial cells to destruction of the mucosa with mucosal congestion, edema, and bleeding. Prolonged damage from repeated alcohol use results in chronic gastritis. Eating large quantities of spicy, irritating foods can cause acute gastritis.

Other risk factors. Although not as common as *H. pylori,* other bacterial, viral, and fungal infections can cause chronic gastritis. Gastritis can occur from reflux of bile salts from the duodenum into the stomach because of anatomic changes after

TABLE 46.18 Causes of Gastritis

Drugs	Microorganisms
• Aspirin • Bisphosphonates • Corticosteroids • Digitalis • Iron supplements • Nonsteroidal antiinflammatory drugs (NSAIDs)	• *H. pylori* • Cytomegalovirus • *Mycobacterium* species • *Salmonella* organisms • *Staphylococcus* organisms • *Treponema pallidum* (syphilis)
Health Problems	**Other Factors**
• Burns • Crohn disease • Large hiatal hernia • Reflux of bile and pancreatic secretions • Renal failure • Sepsis • Shock	• Alcohol use • Endoscopy procedures • Large amounts of spicy, irritating foods • Nasogastric tube • Radiation therapy • Smoking • Stress

surgical procedures (e.g., gastroduodenostomy, gastrojejunostomy). Prolonged vomiting may cause reflux of bile salts. Intense emotional responses and CNS lesions may cause inflammation of the mucosal lining from hypersecretion of HCl acid.

Autoimmune Gastritis

Autoimmune metaplastic atrophic gastritis (or *autoimmune atrophic gastritis*) is an inherited condition in which there is an immune response directed against parietal cells. It most often affects females of northern European descent. Patients often have other autoimmune disorders. The loss of parietal cells leads to low chloride levels, inadequate production of intrinsic factor, cobalamin (vitamin B_{12}) malabsorption, and pernicious anemia. It increases the risk of stomach cancer.

Clinical Manifestations

The symptoms of acute gastritis include anorexia, nausea and vomiting, epigastric tenderness, and a feeling of fullness. GI bleeding is often associated with alcohol use and, at times, is the only symptom. Acute gastritis is self-limiting, lasting from a few hours to a few days. The mucosa should heal completely.

The manifestations of chronic gastritis are like those of acute gastritis. Some patients are asymptomatic. However, when parietal cells are lost because of atrophy, the source of intrinsic factor is also lost. Intrinsic factor is essential for cobalamin absorption. The lack of cobalamin results in pernicious anemia. Cobalamin deficiency anemia is discussed in Chapter 34.

Diagnostic Studies

Acute gastritis is usually diagnosed based on the presence of risk factors. Occasionally, an endoscopic examination with biopsy is needed to make the diagnosis. Breath, urine, serum, stool, and gastric tissue biopsy tests are done to assess for *H. pylori* infection. A CBC may show anemia from blood loss or lack of intrinsic factor. Stools are tested for occult blood. Serum tests for intrinsic factor and antibodies to parietal cells may be done. A tissue biopsy can rule out gastric cancer.

Nursing and Interprofessional Management

Acute Gastritis

Eliminating the cause and preventing or avoiding it in the future are generally all that is needed to treat acute gastritis. The plan of care is supportive and similar to that described for nausea and vomiting. If vomiting is present, rest, NPO status, and IV fluids may be prescribed. Antiemetics are given (Table 46.1). Monitor for dehydration. It can occur rapidly in acute gastritis with vomiting.

In severe cases of acute gastritis, an NG tube may be used to (1) monitor for bleeding, (2) lavage the precipitating agent from the stomach, or (3) keep the stomach empty and free of noxious stimuli. Clear liquids are resumed when symptoms have subsided. Reintroduce solids gradually.

If the patient is at risk for GI bleeding, frequently check vital signs. Test emesis for blood. The management strategies discussed in the section on upper GI bleeding apply to patients with severe gastritis.

Drug therapy focuses on reducing irritation of the gastric mucosa and providing symptomatic relief. H_2 receptor blockers (e.g., cimetidine) or PPIs (e.g., omeprazole) reduce gastric HCl acid secretion (Table 46.10). Teach about the therapeutic effects of PPIs and H_2 receptor blockers.

Chronic Gastritis

The treatment of chronic gastritis focuses on evaluating and eliminating the specific cause. Examples include alcohol cessation or abstaining from drugs. Antibiotic combinations are used to treat *H. pylori* infection (Table 46.14). Patients with pernicious anemia need lifelong cobalamin therapy (see Chapter 34).

Patients may need to adapt to lifestyle changes and strictly adhere to drug therapy. Some patients find a nonirritating diet consisting of 6 small feedings a day helpful. Smoking is contraindicated in gastritis. A team approach in which the HCP, nurse, dietitian, and pharmacist provide consistent information and support will increase the patient's success in making these changes.

UPPER GASTROINTESTINAL BLEEDING

In the United States the incidence of acute upper GI (UGI) bleeding is 80 to 150 cases per 100,000 adults per year. The mortality rate in hospital-admitted patients is 2% to 15%, with 11% succumbing in the ED.[20] Mortality from a UGI bleed increases with age.

Etiology and Pathophysiology

Table 46.19 describes types of UGI bleeding. The severity of bleeding depends on whether the origin is venous, capillary, or arterial. Bleeding from an arterial source is profuse. The blood is

TABLE 46.19 Types of Upper GI Bleeding

Type	Manifestations
Obvious bleeding	
• Hematemesis	Bloody emesis appearing as fresh, bright red blood or "coffee-grounds" appearance (dark, grainy digested blood).
• Melena	Black, tarry stools (often foul smelling) caused by digestion of blood in the GI tract. Black appearance is from the presence of iron.
Occult bleeding	Small amounts of blood in gastric secretions, emesis, or stools not apparent by appearance. Detectable by guaiac test.

bright red because it has not been in contact with gastric HCl acid secretion. Coffee-ground emesis means that the blood has been in the stomach for some time. *Melena* (black, tarry stools) occurs with slow bleeding from an upper GI source. The longer the blood passes through the intestines, the darker the stool color because of the breakdown of hemoglobin and release of iron.

Discovering the cause of the bleeding is not always easy. A variety of areas in the GI tract may be involved. Table 46.20 lists common causes of UGI bleeding.

PUD, due to *H. pylori* infection and NSAID use, is the most common cause of UGI bleeding. About 25% of people on chronic NSAIDs (e.g., ibuprofen) develop PUD. Of these, 2% to 4% will bleed. Even LDA increases risk for GI bleeding. Many OTC preparations contain aspirin.

Bleeding from the esophagus is likely due to chronic esophagitis, Mallory-Weiss tear, or esophageal varices. GERD, smoking, alcohol use, and the use of drugs irritating to the mucosa can cause chronic esophagitis. Esophageal varices most often occur from cirrhosis. Esophageal varices are discussed in Chapter 48.

Stress-related mucosal disease (SRMD), or *physiologic stress ulcers,* describes mucosal damage in the GI tract associated with serious illness. Damage ranges from small single lesions to multiple gastric ulcers and major bleeding. SRMD most often occurs in critically ill patients who have had severe burns, trauma, or major surgery. Patients with coagulopathy, liver disease, continuous-flow left ventricular assist devices, or organ failure and those receiving renal replacement therapy are at highest risk for SRMD.[21]

Diagnostic Studies

Endoscopy is the primary tool for diagnosing the source (e.g., esophageal varices, PUD, gastritis) of UGI bleeding. Angiography is used when endoscopy cannot be done or when bleeding persists after endoscopic therapy. Angiography requires preparation and setup time and may not be appropriate for high-risk, unstable patients. In this procedure, a catheter is inserted into the femoral artery and advanced to the left gastric or superior mesenteric artery until the site of bleeding is found.

Laboratory studies include CBC, blood urea nitrogen (BUN), electrolytes, prothrombin time, partial thromboplastin time, liver enzymes, arterial blood gases (ABGs), and a type and crossmatch for possible blood transfusions. Emesis and stools are tested for gross and occult blood. Hemoglobin and hematocrit values are not of immediate help in estimating the degree of blood loss, but they provide a baseline for guiding further treatment. The initial hematocrit may be normal. It may not reflect the loss until 4 to 6 hours after fluid replacement since initially the loss of plasma and RBCs is equal. With significant bleeding, GI tract bacteria break down proteins, resulting in increased BUN levels. An increased BUN level may also show renal hypoperfusion or renal disease.

TABLE 46.20 Causes of Upper GI Bleeding

Esophagus
- Esophagitis
- Mallory-Weiss tear
- Varices

Stomach and Duodenum
- Drug-induced
  - Corticosteroids
  - NSAIDs
  - Salicylates
- Erosive gastritis
- Peptic ulcer disease
- Polyps
- Stress-related mucosal disease
- Stomach cancer

Systemic Diseases
- Blood dyscrasias (e.g., leukemia, aplastic anemia)
- Kidney failure

Interprofessional Care

The most serious loss of blood from a UGI bleed has a sudden onset. A massive UGI hemorrhage is a loss of more than 1500 mL of blood or 25% of intravascular blood volume. Although 80% to 85% of patients with massive hemorrhage spontaneously stop bleeding, the cause must be identified and treatment started at once.

Endoscopic Therapy

The first-line management of UGI bleeding is endoscopy. Endoscopy within the first 24 hours of bleeding is important for diagnosis, determining the need for surgical intervention, and providing treatment.

The goal of endoscopic hemostasis is to coagulate or thrombose the bleeding vessel. Several techniques are used. These include (1) mechanical therapy with clips or bands, (2) thermal ablation, and (3) injection (e.g., epinephrine). Clips and bands directly compress the bleeding vessel. Thermal ablation cauterizes tissue through applying heat to the bleeding site. Common devices include neodymium:yttrium-aluminum-garnet (YAG) laser, monopolar or bipolar electrocoagulation, heater probes, and argon plasma coagulation (APC).

For variceal bleeding, other strategies include variceal ligation, injection sclerotherapy, and balloon tamponade (see Chapter 48).

Surgical Therapy

Surgical intervention is needed when bleeding continues despite therapy and there is an identified site of bleeding. Surgery may be done if bleeding continues after rapid transfusion of up to 2000 mL of whole blood or shock is still present after 24 hours. The site of the bleeding determines the choice of surgery. Mortality rates increase greatly in older patients.

Drug Therapy

During the acute phase of UGI bleeding, drugs are used to decrease bleeding, decrease HCl acid secretion, and neutralize HCl acid. Empiric PPI therapy with high-dose IV bolus and subsequent infusion to decrease acid secretion is often started before endoscopy (Table 46.10).[20] Efforts are made to reduce acid secretion because the acidic environment can alter platelet function and interfere with clot stabilization. This may decrease the amount of bleeding and need for endoscopic therapy.

After an acute phase of bleeding, antacids may be given hourly, either orally or through the NG tube. If an NG tube is in place, aspirate the stomach contents and test periodically for pH level. If pH is less than 5, intermittent suction may be used or the frequency or dosage of the antacid or antisecretory agent increased.

NURSING MANAGEMENT: UPPER GASTROINTESTINAL BLEEDING

Assessment

Subjective and objective data to obtain from patients or caregivers are outlined in Table 46.21. A complete history of events leading to the bleeding episode is deferred until emergency care has been started. A thorough assessment is essential. Check the abdomen for distention, guarding, and peristalsis. To facilitate early intervention, focus your assessment on identifying signs and symptoms of shock. Vital signs indicate whether shock is present from blood loss and provide a baseline BP and pulse for monitoring a patient's progress. Signs and symptoms of shock include low BP; rapid, weak pulse; prolonged capillary refill; cold, clammy skin; and restlessness. Monitor vital signs every 15 to 30 minutes. Inform the HCP of any significant changes.

Patients may not be able to give specific information about the cause of the bleeding until immediate physical needs are met. Once the immediate interventions have begun, obtain a history. Focus on the presence of any factors that may contribute to bleeding or interfere with treatment. Ask if the patient has a religious preference that prohibits the use of blood or blood products.

TABLE 46.21 NURSING ASSESSMENT

Upper GI Bleeding

Subjective Data

Important Health Information

Health history: Events before bleeding episode, prior bleeding episodes and treatment, PUD, esophageal varices, esophagitis, acute and chronic gastritis, stress-related mucosal disease

Medications: Aspirin, NSAIDs, corticosteroids, anticoagulants

Functional Health Patterns

Health perception—health management: Family history of bleeding, smoking, alcohol use

Nutritional-metabolic: Nausea, vomiting, weight loss, thirst

Elimination: Diarrhea. Black, tarry stools. Decreased urine output. Sweating

Activity-exercise: Weakness, dizziness, fainting

Cognitive-perceptual: Epigastric pain, abdominal cramps

Coping—stress tolerance: Acute or chronic stress

Objective Data

General

Fever

Cardiovascular

Tachycardia, weak pulse, orthostatic hypotension, slow capillary refill

GI

Red or coffee-grounds emesis. Tense, rigid abdomen, ascites. Hypoactive or hyperactive bowel sounds. Black, tarry stools

Neurologic

Agitation, restlessness. Decreasing level of consciousness

Respiratory

Rapid, shallow respirations

Skin

Clammy, cool, pale skin. Pale mucous membranes, nail beds, and conjunctivae. Spider angiomas, jaundice, peripheral edema

Urinary

Decreased urine output, concentrated urine

Possible Diagnostic Findings

↓ Hematocrit and hemoglobin, hematuria. Guaiac-positive stools, emesis, or gastric aspirate. ↓ Levels of clotting factors, ↑ liver enzymes, abnormal endoscopy results

Planning

The overall goals are that patients with UGI bleeding will (1) have no further GI bleeding, (2) have the cause of the bleeding identified and treated, and (3) return to a normal hemodynamic state.

Implementation

Health Promotion

You play a key role in identifying patients at high risk for GI bleeding. Consider patients with a history of chronic gastritis, cirrhosis, or PUD at high risk. Patients who had a UGI bleeding episode are more likely to have another bleed. Patients on LDA and anticoagulants are at risk for UGI bleeding, especially those over 60 years old with a history of PUD.

Teach patients who take regular doses of drugs that cause GI toxicity (PUD, bleeding), such as corticosteroids and NSAIDs, about the risk for GI bleeding. They may need to receive long-term treatment with a PPI, H_2 receptor blocker, or misoprostol. Taking these drugs with meals or snacks lessens irritation.

Teach at-risk patients to avoid known gastric irritants, such as alcohol and smoking, and to take only prescribed medications. OTC drugs can be harmful because they may contain ingredients (e.g., aspirin) that increase the risk for bleeding.

Review how to test emesis or stools for occult blood. Teach them to report positive results promptly to the HCP.

Patients with blood dyscrasias (e.g., aplastic anemia) or liver problems or those who are taking chemotherapy drugs are at risk due to a decrease in clotting factors and platelets. Teach patients about their disease process, drugs, and increased risk for GI bleeding.

Acute Care

Emergency management of acute GI bleeding is outlined in Table 46.22. Place IV lines, preferably 2, with a 16- or 18-gauge needle for fluid and blood replacement. Give fluid or blood replacement as ordered. The type and amount of fluids infused are based on physical and laboratory findings. Generally, we start an isotonic crystalloid solution (e.g., lactated Ringer's solution). Whole blood, packed RBCs, and fresh frozen plasma may be used for volume replacement in massive hemorrhage. When UGI bleeding is less profuse, isotonic saline solution followed by packed RBCs restores the hematocrit more quickly and does not create complications related to fluid volume overload.

An accurate intake and output record is essential so you can assess hydration status. Urine output is one of the best measures of vital organ perfusion. An indwelling urinary catheter is inserted so we can assess hourly output. Hemodynamic monitoring provides an accurate and quick assessment of blood flow and pressure in the cardiovascular system (see Chapter 35). A central venous pressure line can assess fluid volume. If the patient has a history of valvular heart disease, coronary artery disease, or heart failure, a pulmonary artery catheter may be placed. Record readings every 1 to 2 hours.

Apply ECG monitoring. Monitor vital signs closely, especially in patients with CVD, because dysrhythmias may occur. Observe older adults or patients with CVD closely for signs of fluid overload. Volume overload and pulmonary edema are concerns in all patients who are receiving large amounts of IV fluids within a short time. Auscultate breath sounds. Closely observe the respiratory effort. Elevate the head of the bed to provide comfort and prevent aspiration. Give supplemental O_2 to increase blood O_2 saturation.

TABLE 46.22 EMERGENCY MANAGEMENT

Acute GI Bleeding

Assessment Findings	Interventions
Abdominal and GI Findings • Abdominal pain • Abdominal rigidity • Hematemesis • Melena • Nausea **Hypovolemic Shock** • ↓ BP • Cool, clammy skin • ↑ HR • ↓ Level of consciousness • Slow capillary refill • ↓ Urine output (<0.5 mL/kg/h)	**Initial** • If unresponsive, assess circulation, airway, and breathing. • If responsive, monitor airway, breathing, and circulation. • Establish IV access with large-bore catheter and start fluid replacement therapy. Insert a second large-bore catheter if shock present. • Give O_2 via nasal cannula or nonrebreather mask. • Initiate ECG monitoring. • Obtain blood for CBC, clotting studies, and type and cross-match as needed. • Insert NG tube as needed. • Insert indwelling urinary catheter. • Give IV PPI therapy to decrease acid secretion. **Ongoing Monitoring** • Monitor vital signs, level of consciousness, O_2 saturation, ECG, bowel sounds, and intake/output. • Assess amount and character of emesis. • Keep patient NPO. • Provide reassurance and emotional support to patient and caregiver.

CHECK YOUR PRACTICE

You are admitting a 71-year-old male to the unit from the ED. He has a diagnosis of UGI bleeding. He reports heartburn and pain (6 on a scale of 10) in the upper epigastric region. He just had a 250 mL coffee-grounds emesis.

- What assessment data do you need to obtain?
- What are the priority nursing interventions?

When an NG tube is present, keep it in proper position. Check the aspirate for blood. Although some HCPs prescribe gastric lavage (room temperature, cool, iced), its effectiveness as a treatment for UGI bleeding is questionable. With lavage, around 50 to 100 mL of fluid is instilled at a time into the stomach. The lavage fluid may be aspirated from the stomach or drained by gravity. When aspirating, it is important to stop if you feel resistance. The tip of the NG tube may be up against the gastric mucosal lining. When resistance is a factor, use the gravity method. There is a risk for perforation and peritonitis. Do a thorough abdominal assessment. Note the presence of a tense, rigid, board-like abdomen and the presence or absence of bowel sounds.

Provide care in a calm manner to help decrease anxiety level. Use caution when giving sedatives for restlessness. It is a warning sign of shock and may be masked by the drugs.

Assess the stools for blood (black-tarry, bright red). Black, tarry stools usually indicate prolonged bleeding. Determine whether menses is a source of blood in the stool. When emesis contains blood, but the stool contains no gross or occult blood, the hemorrhage is likely of short duration.

When beginning oral intake, observe for symptoms of nausea and vomiting and a recurrence of bleeding. Start with feedings with clear fluids. Give fluids hourly until tolerance is determined. Gradually introduce foods if there are no signs of problems.

When bleeding is the result of chronic alcohol use, closely observe for delirium tremens as alcohol withdrawal takes place. Symptoms indicating the onset of delirium tremens are agitation, uncontrolled shaking, sweating, and hallucinations. Alcohol withdrawal is discussed in Chapter 11.

Discharge teaching focuses on ways to avoid future bleeding episodes. Encourage patients and caregivers to adhere to drug therapy. Emphasize the need to not take any drugs (especially aspirin, NSAIDs) other than those prescribed by the HCP. Support smoking and alcohol cessation. Long-term follow-up care may be needed because of possible recurrence. Teach patients and caregivers what to do if acute bleeding occurs in the future.

◆ Evaluation

Expected outcomes for patients with UGI bleeding include:

- Be free from UGI bleeding
- Maintain normal fluid volume
- Understand potential risk factors and make lifestyle modifications

GASTRIC SURGERY

Gastric surgeries are done to treat stomach cancer, as well as polyps, perforation, chronic gastritis, and PUD. Surgeries include partial gastrectomy, gastrectomy, vagotomy, and pyloroplasty. Partial gastrectomy with removal of the distal two-thirds of the stomach and anastomosis of the gastric stump to the duodenum is a *gastroduodenostomy* or *Billroth I* operation (Fig. 46.16A). If the gastric stump is anastomosed to the jejunum, the surgery is a *gastrojejunostomy* or *Billroth II* operation (Fig. 46.16B). A total gastrectomy involves resecting the lower esophagus, removing the entire stomach, and anastomosis of the esophagus to the jejunum.

Vagotomy, the severing of the vagus nerve, decreases gastric acid secretion. It may be total *(truncal)* or selective *(highly selective vagotomy). Pyloroplasty* is the surgical enlargement of the pyloric sphincter to promote the easy passage of contents from the stomach. It is often done after vagotomy or to enlarge an opening that is constricted from scar tissue.

Postoperative Complications

As with all surgeries, acute postoperative bleeding at the surgical site can occur. Monitoring is similar to that described in the acute upper GI bleeding section. The most common long-term postoperative complications from gastric surgery are (1) dumping syndrome, (2) postprandial hypoglycemia, and (3) bile reflux gastritis.

Dumping Syndrome

Dumping syndrome is the direct result of surgical removal of a large part of the stomach and pyloric sphincter. Normally, gastric chyme enters the small intestine in small amounts. After surgery, the stomach no longer has control over the amount of gastric chyme entering the small intestine. A large bolus of hypertonic fluid enters the intestine, drawing fluid into the bowel lumen. This creates a decrease in plasma volume, distention of the bowel lumen, and rapid intestinal transit.

Symptoms begin within 15 to 30 minutes after eating. Patients usually report weakness, sweating, palpitations, and dizziness. Symptoms are due to the sudden decrease in plasma volume. Patients may have abdominal cramps, *borborygmi* (audible abdominal sounds made by hyperactive intestinal peristalsis), and the urge to defecate. These manifestations usually last less than 1 hour after eating. A short rest period after each meal reduces the chance of dumping syndrome.

Postprandial Hypoglycemia

Postprandial hypoglycemia is a variant of dumping syndrome. It is the result of uncontrolled gastric emptying of a bolus of fluid high in carbohydrate into the small intestine. This causes hyperglycemia and the release of excess amounts of insulin into the circulation. This results in reflex hypoglycemia. Symptoms are like those of any hypoglycemic reaction. They include sweating, weakness, mental confusion, palpitations, tachycardia, and anxiety. Symptoms generally occur 2 hours after eating.

Bile Reflux Gastritis

Gastric surgery that involves reconstruction or removal of the pylorus can result in reflux of bile into the stomach. Prolonged contact with bile causes damage to the gastric mucosa, chronic gastritis, and PUD.

The main symptom is continuous epigastric distress that increases after meals. Vomiting relieves distress, but only temporarily. Although only a small number of patients have bile reflux gastritis, caution patients to notify the HCP of any continuous epigastric distress after meals. Cholestyramine before or with meals can help treat this problem. It binds with the bile salts that are the source of gastric irritation.

❖ NURSING MANAGEMENT: GASTRIC SURGERY

Preoperative Care

Surgery can involve laparoscopic or open surgical techniques. The HCP will provide the necessary information about the procedure and expected outcomes so patients can make an informed decision. Help by answering questions. Teach them what to expect after surgery, including comfort measures, pain relief, coughing and breathing exercises, use of an NG tube, and IV fluid administration. See Chapter 18 for more on preoperative care.

Postoperative Care

Postoperative care focuses on maintaining fluid and electrolyte balance, preventing respiratory complications, maintaining comfort, and preventing infection. Complications include atelectasis, pneumonia, anastomotic leak, deep vein thrombosis, pulmonary embolus, and bleeding. Morbidly obese patients have a higher risk for complications.

After surgery, an NG tube is used for decompression. This decreases pressure on suture lines and allows edema and inflammation resulting from surgical trauma to resolve. Observe the gastric aspirate for color, amount, and odor. Expect small volumes of bloody drainage from the NG tube for the first 2 to 3 hours because bleeding at the anastomotic site is common. Report bright red bleeding that does not decrease after this period or bleeding that becomes excessive (more than 75 mL/h) immediately to the HCP. The NG aspirate should gradually darken within the first 24 hours after surgery. Normally the color changes to yellow-green within 36 to 48 hours. After total gastrectomy, the NG tube does not drain a large quantity of secretions because removing the stomach has eliminated the reservoir capacity.

Observe the NG tube closely because blood easily clots and clogs the tube. Notify the HCP immediately if the tube stops draining or appears obstructed with blood. If the tube becomes clogged, the HCP may order periodic gentle irrigations with normal saline solution. It is essential that the NG suction is working and that the tube stays patent so that accumulated gastric secretions do not put a strain on the anastomosis. This can lead to distention of any remaining part of the stomach and result in (1) rupture of the sutures, (2) leakage of gastric contents into the peritoneal cavity, (3) bleeding, and (4) abscess formation. If the tube must be replaced or repositioned, call the HCP to perform this task because of the danger of perforating the gastric mucosa or disrupting the suture line.

While the NG tube is connected to suction, maintain IV therapy. Before the NG tube is removed, patients begin clear liquids to determine the tolerance level. In a partial gastrectomy, the stomach may be aspirated within 1 or 2 hours to assess the amount remaining and its color and consistency. When patients tolerate fluids, the NG tube is removed. Solids are added gradually with the goal of resuming a normal diet.

Monitor vital signs frequently. Give pain medications as needed. Be aware that pain could be from an anastomosis leak. Closely observe for an anastomotic leak and notify the HCP at once if you suspect one. A leak occurs when there is a breakdown of the suture line in an anastomosis that allows gastric or intestinal contents to enter the abdomen or mediastinum. It requires immediate treatment to prevent sepsis and death. Signs and symptoms include tachycardia, dyspnea, fever, abdominal pain, anxiety, and restlessness.

Since most procedures are done laparoscopically, there is less risk for respiratory complications. In an open surgical approach, the incision is in the epigastrium and respiratory complications may occur. Perform a respiratory assessment. Have patients cough, deep breathe, and use incentive spirometry to expand the lungs. Pain may interfere with deep breathing and coughing. Splint the area with a pillow. Splinting protects the abdominal suture line from rupturing during deep breathing and coughing. Encourage early ambulation and frequent position changes.

Postoperative wound healing may be impaired because of poor nutrition. Abdominal wounds need frequent assessment. Note the amount and type of drainage, wound healing, and signs of infection. Implement measures to control nausea and vomiting. Measure and record the intake and output. Obtain daily weights.

Patients who have had a total gastrectomy and are frail may need skilled care after discharge. For those going home, assist the patient and caregiver with symptom management. Make plans for pain relief, including comfort measures and analgesic use. Teach wound care (if needed) to the primary caregiver. Dressings, special equipment, or special services may be needed. Collaborate with the dietitian to provide teaching about the diet that will optimize nutrition.

Nutrition Therapy

You need to understand the patient's surgery and their resulting anatomy. Long-term, many patients have malnutrition, metabolic bone disease, anemia, and weight loss. Nutrition interventions help minimize the occurrence of expected complications and maximize nutrient intake (Table 46.23). Start nutrition teaching

TABLE 46.23 NUTRITION THERAPY

Postgastrectomy Dumping Syndrome

The amount of time these restrictions should be followed varies. The HCP decides the amount of time to remain on this prescribed diet according to clinical condition and progress.

Purposes

- Slow the rapid passage of food into the intestine.
- Control symptoms of dumping syndrome (dizziness, sense of fullness, diarrhea, tachycardia), which sometimes occurs after a partial or total gastrectomy.

Diet Principles

- Divide meals into 6 small feedings to avoid overloading the stomach and intestine at mealtimes.
- Do not take fluids with meals but at least 30–45 min before or after meals. This helps prevent distention or a feeling of fullness.
- Avoid concentrated sweets (e.g., honey, sugar, jelly, jam, candies, pastries, sweetened fruit). They sometimes cause dizziness, diarrhea, and a sense of fullness.
- Protein intake is unlimited to promote rebuilding of body tissues. Meat and eggs are specific foods to increase in the diet.
- Milk contains lactose, which may be hard to digest. Introduce milk and milk products slowly several weeks after surgery.
- Avoid carbonated beverages and foods that are gas forming to help prevent gastric distention.
- Low-roughage and raw foods are allowed as tolerated a few weeks after surgery.
- Increase complex carbohydrates (e.g., bread, vegetables, rice, potatoes) and fats to meet energy needs.

as soon as the immediate postoperative period has passed. The dietitian usually provides diet instructions. You reinforce them. Following diet measures will decrease symptoms and is essential to long-term adherence.

For those who were malnourished preoperatively, a small bowel feeding tube may be placed during surgery. EN may be started on postoperative day 1 and adjusted depending on how oral intake is tolerated. Some may be discharged with nighttime tube feedings. PN is an option when patients cannot tolerate EN or oral nutrition.

Pernicious anemia is a long-term complication of total gastrectomy and may occur after partial gastrectomy. It is due to the loss of intrinsic factor, which is made by the parietal cells. *Intrinsic factor* is essential for the absorption of cobalamin in the terminal ileum. Cobalamin is essential for RBC growth and maturation. Patients will require cobalamin replacement therapy (see Chapter 34). Patients should take multivitamins with folate, calcium, vitamin D, and iron for life.

Because partial gastrectomy decreases the stomach's reservoir, patients must reduce their meal size accordingly. For the first few weeks after surgery, patients should consume soft, bland foods with low fiber and high complex carbohydrates and protein content. Teach them to eat in small portions and not to drink fluids with meals. They should avoid simple sugars, lactose, and fried foods. Teach patients to avoid extreme temperatures in food and to chew food thoroughly.

TABLE 46.24 Bacterial Food Poisoning

Type and Cause	Sources	Manifestations	Treatment and Prevention
Botulism			
Toxin from *Clostridium botulinum;* ingested toxin absorbed from gut and blocks acetylcholine at neuromuscular junction	Improperly canned or preserved food, home-preserved vegetables (most common), preserved fruits and fish, canned commercial products	*Onset:* 12–36 h *GI:* Nausea, vomiting, abdominal pain, constipation, distention *CNS:* Headache, dizziness, muscular incoordination, weakness, inability to talk or swallow, diplopia, breathing problems, paralysis, delirium, coma	*Treat:* Maintain ventilation, polyvalent antitoxin, guanidine hydrochloric acid (enhances acetylcholine release) *Prevent:* Correct processing of canned foods, boiling of suspected canned foods for 15 min before serving
Clostridial			
Clostridium perfringens	Meat or poultry dishes cooked at low temperature (stew, pot pie), rewarmed meat dishes, gravies, improperly canned vegetables	*Onset:* 8–24 h Diarrhea, nausea, abdominal cramps, midepigastric pain	*Treat:* Symptomatic, fluid replacement *Prevent:* Correct preparation of meat dishes. Serving food immediately after cooking or rapid cooling of food
Escherichia coli			
E. coli 0157:H7	Contaminated beef, pork, milk, cheese, fish, cookie dough	*Onset:* 8 h to 1 week (varies by strain) Bloody stools, hemolytic uremic syndrome, abdominal cramping, profuse diarrhea	*Treat:* Symptomatic, fluid and electrolyte replacement *Prevent:* Correct food preparation
Salmonella			
Salmonella typhimurium (grows in gut)	Improperly cooked poultry, pork, beef, lamb, and eggs	*Onset:* 8 h to several days Nausea and vomiting, diarrhea, abdominal cramps, fever, and chills	*Treat:* Symptomatic, fluid and electrolyte replacement *Prevent:* Correct food preparation
Staphylococcal			
Toxin from *Staphylococcus aureus*	Meat, bakery products, cream fillings, salad dressings, milk Skin and respiratory tract of food handlers	*Onset:* 30 min to 7 h Vomiting, nausea, abdominal cramping, diarrhea	*Treat:* Symptomatic, fluid and electrolyte replacement, antiemetics *Prevent:* Immediate food refrigeration, monitoring food handling

TABLE 46.25 PATIENT & CAREGIVER TEACHING

Preventing Food Poisoning

Include these instructions when teaching patients and caregivers how to prevent food poisoning:

1. Cook all ground beef and hamburger thoroughly.
   - Use a digital instant-read meat thermometer to ensure thorough cooking. Ground beef can turn brown before disease-causing bacteria are killed.
   - Cook ground beef until a thermometer inserted into several parts of the patty, including the thickest part, reads at least 160°F.
   - People who cook ground beef without using a thermometer can decrease their risk for illness by not eating ground beef patties that are still pink in the middle.
2. If you are served an undercooked hamburger or other ground beef product in a restaurant, send it back for further cooking. Ask for a new bun and a clean plate.
3. Avoid spreading harmful bacteria. Keep raw meat separate from ready-to-eat foods. Wash hands, counters, and utensils with hot soapy water after they touch raw meat. Never place cooked hamburgers or ground beef on the unwashed plate that held raw patties. Wash meat thermometers in between tests of patties that need more cooking.
4. Drink pasteurized milk, juice, or cider.
5. Wash fruits and vegetables thoroughly, especially those you are not cooking.
6. Do not eat raw food products that are supposed to be cooked. Follow package directions for cooking at proper temperatures.
7. Avoid eating alfalfa sprouts if you are immunocompromised until you are sure of their safety.

To avoid hypoglycemic episodes, patients should limit the amount of sugar consumed with each meal and eat small, frequent meals with moderate amounts of protein and fat. Immediate intake of sugared fluids or candy relieves hypoglycemic symptoms.

FOODBORNE ILLNESS

Foodborne illness (food poisoning) is a nonspecific term that describes acute GI symptoms such as nausea, vomiting, diarrhea, and abdominal pain caused by the intake of contaminated food or liquids.[22] Each year 1 in 6 Americans, or 48 million people, gets a foodborne illness. Of these, 128,000 are hospitalized and around 3000 die.[22]

Bacteria account for most foodborne illnesses (see Table 47.1). The most common source is raw foods that become contaminated during growing, harvesting, processing, storing, shipping, or final preparation. Bacteria multiply quickly when the temperature of food is between 40°F and 140°F. So, bacteria can multiply if hot food is not kept hot enough or cold food is not cold enough. The most common bacterial food poisonings are described in Table 46.24.

Focus interventions on preventing infection. Teaching includes correct food preparation and cleanliness, adequate cooking, and refrigeration (Table 46.25). For hospitalized patients, emphasize correcting fluid and electrolyte imbalances from diarrhea and vomiting.

CASE STUDY

Peptic Ulcer Disease

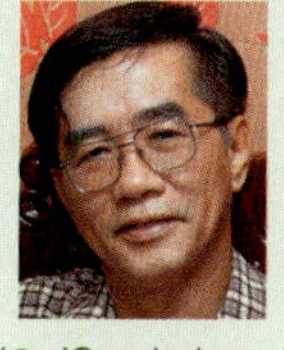

(© iStockphoto/ Thinkstock.)

Patient Profile

F.H., a 40-year-old male immigrant from Vietnam, has a 1-year history of epigastric distress. Increasingly, it is not relieved by over-the-counter omeprazole. He is scheduled for an upper endoscopy this morning.

Subjective Data

- Reports increasing substernal pain, especially 2 to 3 h after eating
- Currently avoids alcohol and is taking an over-the-counter PPI
- Smoking history of 1 pack of cigarettes per day for 20 years
- Has had increasing fatigue with exercise
- Reports occasional black bowel movement

Objective Data

- Height 5 ft, 5 in tall and weight 140 lb

Diagnostic Studies

- Endoscopy reveals a duodenal ulcer
- Hgb 10.2 g/dL; Hct 30%
- Histology of biopsied tissue reveals *H. pylori* infection

Interprofessional Care

- Omeprazole 20 mg twice daily × 10 days
- Clarithromycin 500 mg twice daily × 10 days
- Amoxicillin 1 gram twice daily × 10 days

Discussion Questions

1. ***Recognize:*** What risk factors does F.H. have for PUD?
2. ***Analyze:*** What assessment findings are consistent with PUD?
3. ***Plan:*** How will you consider F.H.'s cultural preferences in planning care?
4. ***Prioritize:*** Based on the data provided, what are the priority clinical problems?
5. ***Prioritize:*** What are the priority nursing interventions?
6. ***Act:*** What lifestyle interventions would you recommend for F.H.?
7. ***Evaluation:*** F.H. asks you if the treatment will work and this will be the end of his problems. How will you respond?

Answers available at http://evolve.elsevier.com/Lewis/medsurg.

BRIDGE TO NCLEX EXAMINATION

The number of the question corresponds to the same-numbered outcome at the beginning of the chapter.

1. M.J. calls the clinic and tells the nurse that her 85-year-old mother has been nauseated all day and has vomited twice. Before calling the HCP, the nurse would tell M.J. to
   - **a.** administer antiemetic drugs and assess her mother's skin turgor.
   - **b.** give her mother sips of water and elevate the head of her bed to prevent aspiration.
   - **c.** offer her mother large quantities of Gatorade to decrease the risk for sodium depletion.
   - **d.** give her mother a high-protein liquid supplement to drink to maintain her nutrition needs.
2. The nurse explains to the patient with Vincent's infection that treatment will include
   - **a.** tetanus vaccinations.
   - **b.** viscous lidocaine rinses.
   - **c.** amphotericin B suspension.
   - **d.** topical application of antibiotics.
3. The nurse teaching young adults about behaviors that put them at risk for oral cancer would include
   - **a.** discouraging chewing gum.
   - **b.** avoiding perfumed lip gloss.
   - **c.** avoiding smokeless tobacco use.
   - **d.** discouraging drinking of carbonated beverages.
4. Which instructions would the nurse include in discharge teaching for a patient with mild gastroesophageal reflux disease (GERD)?
   - **a.** "The best time to take an as-needed antacid is 1 to 3 hours after meals."
   - **b.** "A glass of warm milk at bedtime will decrease your discomfort at night."
   - **c.** "Do not chew gum; the excess saliva will cause you to secrete more acid."
   - **d.** "Limit your intake of foods high in protein because they take longer to digest."
5. A patient who had an esophagectomy for esophageal cancer develops increasing pain, fever, and dyspnea after starting a full-liquid diet. These symptoms are *most* indicative of
   - **a.** an intolerance to the feedings.
   - **b.** extension of the tumor into the aorta.
   - **c.** leakage of fluids into the mediastinum.
   - **d.** esophageal perforation with fistula formation into the lung.
6. The nurse monitors a patient with gastritis for pernicious anemia due to
   - **a.** chronic autoimmune destruction of cobalamin stores in the body.
   - **b.** progressive gastric atrophy from chronic breakage in the mucosal barrier and blood loss.
   - **c.** a lack of intrinsic factor normally produced by acid-secreting cells of the gastric mucosa.
   - **d.** hyperchlorhydria from an increase in acid-secreting parietal cells and degradation of RBCs.
7. The nurse is teaching the patient and family that peptic ulcers are
   - **a.** caused by a stressful lifestyle and other acid-producing factors, such as *H. pylori.*
   - **b.** inherited within families and reinforced by bacterial spread of *Staphylococcus aureus* in childhood.
   - **c.** promoted by factors that cause oversecretion of acid, such as excess diet fats, smoking, and alcohol use.
   - **d.** promoted by a combination of factors that cause erosion of the gastric mucosa, including certain drugs and *H. pylori.*
8. An optimal teaching plan for an outpatient with stomach cancer receiving radiation therapy should include information about
   - **a.** cancer support groups, alopecia, and stomatitis.
   - **b.** nutrition supplements, ostomy care, and support groups.
   - **c.** prosthetic devices, wound and skin care, and grief counseling.
   - **d.** wound and skin care, nutrition, drugs, and community resources.
9. Discharge teaching for patients after an acute episode of upper GI bleeding includes information about the importance of (**Select all that apply.**)
   - **a.** limiting alcohol intake to 1 serving per day.
   - **b.** only taking aspirin with milk or bread products.
   - **c.** avoiding taking aspirin and drugs containing aspirin.
   - **d.** only taking drugs prescribed by the health care provider.
   - **e.** taking all drugs 1 hour before mealtime to prevent further bleeding.
10. Several patients come to the urgent care center with nausea, vomiting, and diarrhea that began 2 hours ago while attending a large family reunion potluck dinner. You ask the patients specifically about foods they ingested containing
    - **a.** beef.
    - **b.** meat and milk.
    - **c.** poultry and eggs.
    - **d.** home-preserved vegetables.

1. b; 2. d; 3. c; 4. a; 5. c; 6. c; 7. d; 8. d; 9. c, d; 10. b.

For rationales to these answers and even more NCLEX review questions, visit http://evolve.elsevier.com/Lewis/medsurg.

REFERENCES

To access the References for this chapter, please scan the QR code with a mobile device.

47

Lower Gastrointestinal Problems

Mariann M. Harding

http://evolve.elsevier.com/Lewis/medsurg/

CONCEPTUAL FOCUS

Cellular Regulation
Elimination
Fluid and Electrolytes
Inflammation
Nutrition
Pain
Stress and Coping

LEARNING OUTCOMES

1. Explain common causes and interprofessional and nursing management of diarrhea, fecal incontinence, and constipation.
2. Describe common causes and the management of patients with acute abdominal pain.
3. Select nursing interventions to manage patient care after abdominal surgery.
4. Describe the interprofessional and nursing management of appendicitis and peritonitis.
5. Compare and contrast ulcerative colitis and Crohn disease, including pathophysiology, clinical manifestations, complications, and interprofessional and nursing management.
6. Discern between small and large bowel obstructions, including causes, clinical manifestations, and interprofessional and nursing management.
7. Describe the clinical manifestations and interprofessional and nursing management of colorectal cancer.
8. Discuss the clinical manifestations and interprofessional and nursing management of patients with diverticulitis.
9. Compare and contrast the types of hernias, including etiology and interprofessional care.
10. Describe the types of malabsorption syndromes and interprofessional care of celiac disease, lactase deficiency, and short bowel syndrome.
11. Describe the types, clinical manifestations, and interprofessional and nursing management of anorectal conditions.

KEY TERMS

anal fistula
appendicitis
bowel obstruction
bowel resection
celiac disease
constipation
Crohn disease
diarrhea
diverticulitis
fecal incontinence
fistula
hemorrhoids
hernia
inflammatory bowel disease (IBD)
irritable bowel syndrome (IBS)
ostomy
paralytic ileus
peritonitis
short bowel syndrome (SBS)
ulcerative colitis (UC)

The wide variety of gastrointestinal (GI) problems discussed in this chapter includes diarrhea, constipation, and fecal incontinence; inflammatory and functional bowel problems; colorectal cancer (CRC); abdominal surgery; and malabsorption problems. Conceptually, patients often have problems with impaired elimination and nutrition. Many have inflammation and pain and are at risk for fluid and electrolyte problems. Promoting optimal bowel habits and nutrition is a common goal.

GENERAL GI AND ABDOMINAL PROBLEMS

DIARRHEA

Diarrhea is the passage of at least 3 loose or liquid stools per day. It may be acute, lasting 14 days or less, or persistent, lasting 2 to 4 weeks. Chronic diarrhea lasts 30 days or longer. Health care–associated diarrhea is acute diarrhea in a hospitalized patient that was not present on admission and starts after 3 days of being hospitalized. It is fairly common, developing in up to one-third of patients.

Etiology and Pathophysiology

Most cases of acute diarrhea are infectious in origin (Table 47.1).[1] Viruses, particularly norovirus, cause most cases in the United States. It is a leading cause of foodborne outbreaks of acute gastroenteritis. Bacterial infection with *Escherichia coli* O157:H7 is a common cause of bloody diarrhea in the United States. It is transmitted by contaminated water or food. Other pathologic *E. coli* strains are endemic in developing countries. They often cause travelers' diarrhea.

Infectious pathogens attack the intestines in different ways. Some (e.g., rotavirus A, norovirus) change the secretion and/or absorption of enterocytes in the small intestine. They do not cause inflammation. Others (e.g., *C. difficile*) impair absorption by destroying cells, causing inflammation in the colon, and producing toxins that cause damage. *Secretory diarrhea* occurs when ingested pathogens survive in the GI tract long enough to absorb into the enterocytes. The resulting chain reaction changes cell permeability and causes the oversecretion of water, sodium, and chloride into the bowel.

Many pathogens enter the body in contaminated food or drinking water. Travelers often get diarrhea, especially if they travel to countries with poorer sanitation than their own. Infection can also spread from person to person via the fecal-oral route. For example, day care workers can transmit infection from one resident to another if they do not wash their hands after changing soiled diapers.

Age, gastric acidity, intestinal microflora, and immune status influence susceptibility to pathogens. Older adults are most likely to have life-threatening diarrhea. Because stomach acid kills ingested pathogens, taking drugs to decrease stomach acid (proton pump inhibitors [PPIs]) increases the chance that pathogens will survive.

Antibiotics kill the normal flora in the colon, making the person more susceptible to common viral, parasitic, and bacterial infections. For example, patients receiving broad-spectrum antibiotics are susceptible to pathogenic strains of *C. difficile.*

People who are immunocompromised because of disease or immunosuppressive drugs are susceptible to GI tract infection. Immunocompromised patients receiving jejunal enteral nutrition (EN) are especially prone to infections. These feedings do not contain the poorly digestible fiber that normal colon bacteria need to survive.

Diarrhea is not always caused by infection. Many drugs, radiation and chemotherapy, and food intolerances can cause diarrhea. Large amounts of undigested carbohydrate, lactose intolerance, and certain laxatives (e.g., lactulose, magnesium citrate) produce osmotic diarrhea. The rapid GI transit prevents fluid and electrolyte absorption. Chronic diarrhea may occur with cancer, cystic fibrosis, and pancreatic problems.[1] Diarrhea from celiac disease and short bowel syndrome (SBS) results from malabsorption in the small intestine.

Clinical Manifestations

Most viral infections are mild and last less than 24 hours. Besides diarrhea, patients may have cramping, abdominal pain, nausea, urgency, tenesmus, or loss of bowel control. Other symptoms, depending on the cause, may include fever, vomiting, and chills (Table 47.1). Infections of the colon and distal small bowel (e.g., *Shigella, Salmonella, C. difficile*) cause frequent bloody diarrhea with a small volume.

Patients may have manifestations of dehydration, electrolyte problems (e.g., hypokalemia), and acid-base imbalances (metabolic acidosis). Weight loss or malnutrition may occur with chronic diarrhea.

Diagnostic Studies

Stool cultures are usually done only in patients who are very ill; have a fever, bloody diarrhea, or diarrhea lasting longer than 3 days; or were exposed during an outbreak. Those with travelers' diarrhea lasting longer than 14 days should be assessed for parasitic infections. Leukocytes, blood, and mucus may be present in the stool, depending on the cause.

Blood cultures should be done in those with signs of sepsis or systemic infection (e.g., high fever) or who are immunocompromised. The white blood cell (WBC) count may be high. People with long-standing diarrhea can develop anemia from iron and folate deficiencies. Increased hematocrit, blood urea nitrogen (BUN), and creatinine levels are signs of fluid deficit.

In patients with chronic diarrhea, measuring stool electrolytes, pH, and osmolality helps determine whether the diarrhea is from decreased fluid absorption or increased fluid secretion. Measuring stool fat and undigested muscle fibers may show fat and protein malabsorption conditions. Some patients with secretory diarrhea have high serum levels of GI hormones, such as vasoactive intestinal polypeptide and gastrin.

Interprofessional Care

Treatment of diarrhea depends on the cause. Acute infectious diarrhea is usually self-limiting. The major concerns are preventing transmission, replacing fluid and electrolytes, and protecting the skin. Most patients tolerate oral fluids. Solutions containing glucose and electrolytes may be enough to replace losses from mild diarrhea. If losses are severe, it will be necessary to give IV fluids, electrolytes, vitamins, and nutrition.

TABLE 47.1 Causes and Manifestations of Acute Infectious Diarrhea

Organism	Manifestations	Source/Susceptibility
Bacterial		
Campylobacter jejuni	• Diarrhea, abdominal cramps, fever. Sometimes nausea, vomiting • Lasts about 7 days	• Undercooked poultry, untreated water, and unpasteurized milk
C. difficile	• Watery diarrhea, fever, anorexia, nausea, abdominal pain • Can progress to severe colitis and intestinal perforation	• Antibiotic, immunosuppressant, and gastric acid–suppressing therapy
Clostridium perfringens	• Diarrhea, abdominal cramps, nausea • Occurs 6–24 h after eating contaminated food and lasts about 24 h	• Meats, gravies • Settings where large groups are served and keeping food at proper temperatures is difficult
Enterohemorrhagic *Escherichia coli* (e.g., *E. coli* O157:H7)	• Severe abdominal cramping, bloody diarrhea, vomiting, fatigue • Lasts 5–7 days • May progress to life-threatening renal failure	• Water or food contaminated with infected feces • Undercooked beef, raw milk • Working with cattle • Not washing hands after using the bathroom
Enterotoxigenic *E. coli*	• Watery or bloody diarrhea, abdominal cramps, nausea, fever • Lasts 5–7 days	• Leading cause of travelers' diarrhea • Water or food contaminated with infected feces
Salmonella	• Diarrhea, fever, abdominal cramps • Lasts 4–7 days	• Touching infected animals, their feces, or their environment, especially turtles, lizards, snakes, chicks, young birds • Undercooked poultry, meat, foods prepared with raw eggs
Shigella	• Diarrhea (sometimes bloody), fever, abdominal pain • Lasts 5–7 days • Postinfection arthritis may occur	• Fecal-oral route or in food or water contaminated with infected feces • Contaminated recreational water, such as pools
Staphylococcus	• Nausea, vomiting, abdominal cramps, diarrhea • Usually mild • Occurs 30 min to 8 h after eating contaminated food and lasts about 24 h	• 25% of people are carriers in mucous membranes, skin, hair • Food contaminated by food workers who are carriers or through contaminated milk and cheese
Parasitic		
Cryptosporidium	• Watery diarrhea, abdominal cramps, nausea, vomiting, fever, dehydration, weight loss • May be fatal in those who are immunocompromised • Lasts 1–2 wk	• Lives in human intestines • Stool of infected human or animal • Outer shell allows it to live for long periods outside of body and makes it resistant to chlorine • Cause of waterborne disease (pools, lakes, drinking water, food contaminated with feces)
Entamoeba histolytica	• Diarrhea, abdominal cramping • May last 2 wk	• Fecal-contaminated food, water, or hands • In the United States, high-risk groups include travelers to or immigrants from tropical places with poor sanitation, men who have sex with men
Giardia lamblia	• Abdominal cramps, nausea, diarrhea, bloating • Lasts 2–6 wk	• Highly contagious • Fecal-oral route • Found in fresh lakes and rivers • Can be transmitted in pools, water parks, hot tubs
Viral		
Norovirus	• Nausea, vomiting, diarrhea, stomach cramping • Rapid onset • Lasts 1–2 days	• Very contagious • Person to person through contaminated food, water, surfaces • Virus present in stool and emesis • Laboratory testing useful when several people simultaneously have gastroenteritis and there is an avenue for virus transmission, such as a shared location or food
Rotavirus	• Fever, vomiting, profuse watery diarrhea, abdominal pain • Lasts 3–8 days	• Highly contagious • Mainly by fecal-oral route; can be through contaminated surfaces, hands

TABLE 47.2 Drug Therapy

Antidiarrheal Drugs

Drug	Mechanism of Action	Nursing Considerations
bismuth subsalicylate (Pepto-Bismol)	Decrease secretions. Weak antibacterial activity. Prevent and treat travelers' diarrhea.	May cause tinnitus and confusion. Do not use with GI bleeding or bleeding problems.
difenoxin with atropine	Decrease peristalsis and intestinal motility.	Limit alcohol use. May cause drowsiness. Take as directed. Overdose may be life-threatening.
diphenoxylate with atropine (Lomotil)	Decrease peristalsis and intestinal motility. Opioid and anticholinergic.	Blurred vision, dry mouth, drowsiness may occur. Take as directed. Overdose may be life-threatening.
loperamide (Imodium)	Decrease peristalsis and intestinal motility. Increase fluid absorption from GI tract.	Limit alcohol use. Do not use with GI bleeding. May cause drowsiness. Use caution with hazardous activities.
octreotide acetate (Sandostatin)	Increase fluid absorption from GI tract. Decrease intestinal motility and serotonin secretion.	Given subcut, IM, IV. May cause gallbladder or liver problems. Limit alcohol use. Use caution with hazardous activities.
paregoric (camphorated tincture of opium)	Opioid. Decrease peristalsis and intestinal motility.	Taken after each stool; up to 6 doses per day. May cause drowsiness. Use caution with hazardous activities.

Antidiarrheal drugs have limited short-term use. They coat and protect mucous membranes, absorb irritating substances, inhibit intestinal transit, decrease intestinal secretions, or decrease central nervous system stimulation of the GI tract (Table 47.2). Antidiarrheal drugs are not used in treating some infectious diarrheas because they potentially prolong exposure to the organism. They are used cautiously in inflammatory bowel disease (IBD) because of the danger of causing *toxic megacolon* (colon dilation greater than 5 cm).

Antibiotics rarely have a role in treating acute diarrhea. They are given only for certain infections or when the infected person is severely ill or immunosuppressed. The 2 antibiotics recommended for adults are a fluoroquinolone, such as ciprofloxacin, and azithromycin.

C. difficile Infection

C. difficile infection (CDI) is the most common cause of health care–associated diarrhea. The risk for contracting CDI is highest in patients receiving antimicrobial, chemotherapy, gastric acid–suppressing, or immunosuppressive drugs.[2] *C. difficile* spores can survive for up to 70 days on objects, including commodes, bedside tables, and floors. Health care workers who do not adhere to strict infection control precautions can transmit *C. difficile* from patient to patient. *Lactobacillus* probiotics may be used to prevent CDI or as an adjunct therapy to help prevent the risk for recurrent CDI.

CDI is treated with oral vancomycin or fidaxomicin. All nonessential antibiotics, stool softeners, laxatives, and antidiarrheal drugs should be stopped. Metronidazole is an option when patients cannot be treated with vancomycin or fidaxomicin. Patients with severe, complicated CDI with shock, hypotension, ileus, or megacolon should receive oral vancomycin with IV metronidazole. Patients with an ileus can receive vancomycin via enema.

Recurrent CDI occurs in about 20% of patients. The risk increases with the use of antibiotics and CDI recurrences. *Fecal microbiota transplantation* (FMT) is an effective treatment for recurrent CDI.[3] With FMT, stool from a healthy donor is transferred into a patient's GI tract to reestablish healthy intestinal flora. The donor stool is placed in the GI tract via an enema, nasoenteral tube, or during colonoscopy. The major concern with FMT is the potential for transmitting infectious agents in the donor stool. Donors go through careful screening to decrease this risk. Most patients have diarrhea right after the procedure.

NURSING MANAGEMENT: ACUTE DIARRHEA

Assessment

Begin your assessment with the history (Table 47.3). Ask patients to describe their stool pattern and symptoms (Fig. 47.1). Focus on the duration, frequency, character, and consistency of stool and the relationship to other symptoms, such as pain and vomiting. Ask about medical problems that may cause diarrhea. Is the person taking drugs that are known to cause diarrhea, decrease stomach acidity, or cause immunosuppression? Ask if other family members are ill. Obtain a food history. Assess food preparation practices, food intolerances, and changes in diet and appetite. Is there a fever or signs of dehydration? Assess the abdomen for distention, pain, and guarding.

Clinical Problems

Clinical problems for patients with acute infectious diarrhea include:

- Impaired bowel elimination
- Fluid imbalance
- Electrolyte imbalance

For more information on clinical problems and interventions for diarrhea, see eNursing Care Plan 47.1 on the website for this chapter.

TABLE 47.3 NURSING ASSESSMENT

Diarrhea

Subjective Data

Important Health Information

Health history: Travel, hospitalization, infections, water exposure, food history. Diverticulitis or malabsorption, metabolic disorders, IBD, irritable bowel syndrome

Medications: Antibiotics, laxatives or enemas, immunosuppressants, acid-blocking drugs, antidiarrheal drugs

Surgery or other treatments: Stomach or bowel surgery, radiation, chemotherapy

Functional Health Patterns

Health perception–health management: Malaise

Nutritional-metabolic: Ingestion of fatty and spicy foods, food intolerances. Anorexia, nausea, vomiting, weight loss. Thirst

Elimination: Increased stool frequency, volume, and looseness. Change in color and character of stools. Steatorrhea, abdominal bloating. Decreased urine output

Cognitive-perceptual: Abdominal tenderness, pain or cramping, tenesmus

Objective Data

General

Lethargy, fever, malnutrition, ↓ BP, ↑ HR

GI

Frequent soft to liquid stools that may alternate with constipation, altered stool color. Abdominal distention, guarding, hyperactive bowel sounds. Pus, blood, mucus, or fat in stools. Fecal impaction

Skin

Pallor, dry mucous membranes, perianal irritation

Urinary

Decreased output, concentrated urine

Possible Diagnostic Findings

Abnormal serum electrolyte levels. Anemia, ↑ WBC, eosinophilia. Positive stool cultures. Ova, parasites, leukocytes, blood, or fat in stool. Abnormal sigmoidoscopy or colonoscopy findings. Abnormal lower GI series

IBD, Inflammatory bowel disease.

Type 1	Separate hard lumps, like nuts (hard to pass)
Type 2	Sausage-shaped but lumpy
Type 3	Like a sausage but with cracks on its surface
Type 4	Like a sausage or snake, smooth and soft
Type 5	Soft blobs with clear-cut edges (passed easily)
Type 6	Fluffy pieces with ragged edges, mushy
Type 7	Watery, no solid pieces, entirely liquid

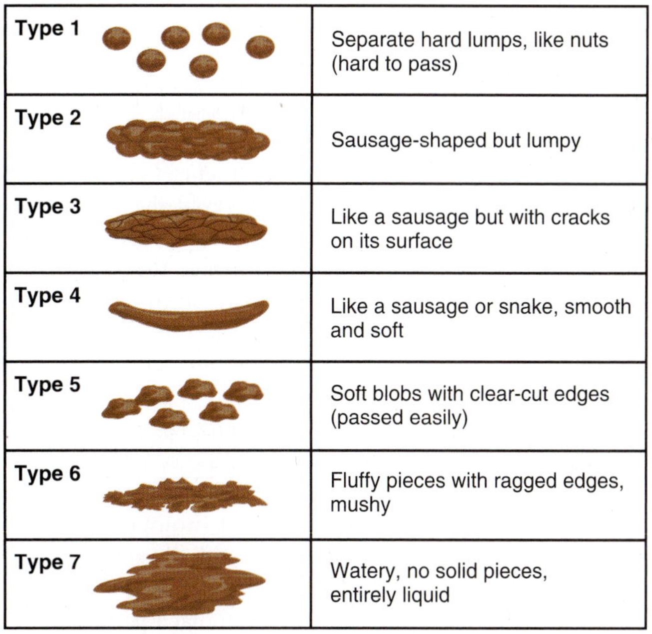

Fig. 47.1 Bristol Stool Scale showing fecal consistency.

TABLE 47.4 NURSING MANAGEMENT

Diarrhea

- Replenish fluid and electrolyte loss:
  - Encourage oral fluids containing glucose and electrolytes.
  - Administer IV fluids and electrolytes as ordered.
- Give antidiarrheal and antibiotic drugs as ordered.
- Implement proper isolation and infection control precautions.
- Monitor for manifestations of fluid and electrolyte balance.
  - Maintain intake and output; weigh daily.
  - Record color, volume, frequency, and consistency of stools.
- Provide perianal care.
  - Assess perianal area for irritation.
  - Apply a moisturizing skin barrier cream as needed.
  - Keep the perineum dry and clean at regular intervals.
- Implement measures to make toileting easier for patients, such as:
  - Call light in reach
  - Easy-to-manage clothing
  - Assistive devices available
- Provide privacy for toileting and use a deodorizer.
- Encourage the patient to consume low-fiber foods.
- Teach the patient good hand washing and the need to avoid foods and fluids known to worsen diarrhea.

◆ Planning

The overall goals are that patients with diarrhea will have (1) normal bowel patterns; (2) fluid, electrolyte, and acid-base balance; and (3) no perianal/perineal skin breakdown.

◆ Implementation

Nursing care of patients with diarrhea is outlined in Table 47.4. Implement measures to maintain hydration status. Encourage oral fluids containing glucose and electrolytes to prevent and treat dehydration. Older adults and chronically ill patients may be unable to consume enough fluids to make up for fluid loss. If dehydration occurs, IV fluid replacement may be needed.

Consider all cases of acute diarrhea as infectious until the cause is known. Infection precautions are needed to prevent the illness from spreading. Use good hand washing. Teach patients the principles of hygiene, infection control, and the potential dangers of an illness that is infectious to themselves and others.

Viruses and *C. difficile* spores are hard to kill. Good hand washing with soap and water is extremely important in limiting the spread of CDI. Alcohol-based hand cleaners are ineffective. Put patients with CDI in contact isolation.

FECAL INCONTINENCE

Etiology and Pathophysiology

Fecal incontinence is the uncontrolled passage of feces for a duration of at least 3 months in a person who previously had control.[4] It occurs when the normal structures that maintain continence are damaged or disrupted. Problems with motor function (contraction of sphincters and rectal floor muscles) and/or sensory function (ability to perceive the presence of stool or have the urge to defecate) can result in fecal incontinence. Other risk factors include altered bowel habits, damage to the nerves that innervate the anorectum, and anal tissue damage (Table 47.5).

For females, obstetric trauma is the most common cause of sphincter injury. Aging and menopause are contributing factors. People with normal functioning defecation can have incontinence if mobility problems prevent prompt access to a toilet or stool is accidentally discharged with diarrhea. Chronic constipation can lead to *fecal impaction,* a collection of hardened feces in the rectum or sigmoid colon that a person cannot expel. Incontinence occurs as liquid stool seeps around the hardened feces. Fecal impaction is common in a person with limited mobility.

TABLE 47.5 Risk Factors for Fecal Incontinence

GI Problems
- Diarrhea
- Celiac disease
- Constipation
- Fecal impaction
- Inflammatory bowel disease
- Irritable bowel syndrome
- Rectal sensation disorders

Injury
- Anorectal surgery for hemorrhoids, fistula, fissures, cancer
- Childbirth-related injury
- Pelvic floor dysfunction, such as fistula, prolapse
- Perineal trauma or pelvic fracture
- Radiation

Medical Problems
- Congenital abnormalities (e.g., spina bifida, myelomeningocele)
- Dementia
- Diabetes
- Multiple sclerosis
- Neuropathy
- Spinal cord injury
- Stroke

Patient-Level Factors
- Long-term care resident
- Multiple chronic illnesses
- Obesity
- Physical or mobility problems

Diagnostic Studies

The diagnosis of fecal incontinence requires a history and physical assessment. A rectal examination can reveal reduced anal canal muscle tone and contraction strength of the external sphincter. We can assess for fissures, prolapse, rectocele, hemorrhoids, masses, and fecal impaction. Other tests, such as anorectal manometry, ultrasound, and defecography, are done depending on the suspected cause.

Interprofessional Care

Treatment depends on the cause. Diet fiber, fiber supplements, and bulk-forming laxatives, like psyllium, improve symptoms. They increase stool bulk, firm the consistency, and promote the sensation of rectal filling. Drugs that decrease motility, such as antidiarrheal drugs, and drugs that increase anal sphincter tone, such as bile acid resins and tricyclic antidepressants, are options. Patients may need to reduce the intake of foods that cause diarrhea and rectal irritation.

Pelvic floor rehabilitation can improve sensation, coordinate internal and external anal sphincters, and increase the strength of external sphincter contraction.[4] Fecal incontinence from fecal impaction usually resolves after manual removal of the hard feces and cleansing enemas.

Sacral nerve stimulation targets communication problems between the brain and nerves that control the pelvic floor muscles and sphincters. Surgery, such as a sphincter repair procedure, is an option when other conservative treatments fail, there is a full-thickness prolapse, or the anal sphincter needs repair. A colostomy is sometimes done.[4] Other treatments include bowel control systems and sphincter augmentation with injectable bulking agents.

NURSING MANAGEMENT: FECAL INCONTINENCE

Assessment

The first step is to identify fecal incontinence by asking about it. It is significantly underreported because of embarrassment. Be sensitive to the patient's feelings when discussing incontinence.

Ask about bowel patterns before the incontinence developed; current bowel habits; stool consistency, volume, and frequency; and symptoms, including pain during defecation and a feeling of incomplete evacuation *(tenesmus)*. The Bristol Stool Scale is helpful to assess stool consistency (Fig. 47.1). Assess whether the patient has a sensation of urgency to evacuate the bowel or sensation of passing flatus and leaking stool.

The unpredictable nature makes it hard to maintain school, work, and physical activities. It hampers social and intimate contact. Ask about daily activities, diet, family and social activities, and the degree to which incontinence interferes with these activities.

Check the perineal area for irritation or breakdown. Patients who have fecal incontinence are at risk for *incontinence-associated dermatitis* (IAD). IAD results from chemical irritants in the feces causing skin damage. Symptoms include redness, skin loss, and rash. IAD usually occurs in the perianal or perineal area, buttocks, or upper thighs. Fungal infection is common and seen as a dark red center surrounded by satellite lesions.

◆ Implementation

Whatever the cause, bowel training is effective for many patients. The best time to schedule elimination is within 30 minutes after breakfast. For hospitalized patients, placement on a bedpan, help to a bedside commode, or walks to the bathroom at a regular time daily help establish regular defecation. Teach patients to pause and perform Kegel exercises when they feel an episode coming on.[4]

If these techniques are not effective in establishing bowel regularity, administer bisacodyl, a glycerin suppository, or a small enema 15 to 30 minutes before the usual evacuation time. These stimulate the anorectal reflex. Because stimulation will not occur unless the suppository or enema touches the rectal wall, first check for stool in the rectum and digitally remove it. Once a regular pattern is established, stop these drugs. Digital stimulation is another way to stimulate the anorectal reflex. It is often part of bowel programs for people with neurogenic bowels (e.g., from spinal cord injury). Irrigating the rectum and colon at regular intervals may achieve continence in patients with neurogenic bowel.

Maintaining perineal skin integrity is a priority. Perform frequent skin assessments. Implement a skin care program. This includes prompt cleansing, moisturizing, and skin protection. Cleanse the skin gently, using a skin cleanser. Options include hydrating cleansing foam, incontinence clean-up cloths, or baby wipes. Avoid products that contain alcohol. They cause drying of the skin and discomfort if the skin is irritated. Pat the skin dry or use a blow dryer on a cool setting. Apply a moisture barrier and, if needed, a skin barrier cream for more protection. For patients unable to care for themselves at home, teach caregivers how to maintain skin integrity. Change briefs or pads promptly after each episode of incontinence.

Feces can contaminate wounds, damage skin, and cause bladder infections. Fecal containment may be needed. One way to contain stool is a stool management system (e.g., Flexi-Seal). A system can remain in place for weeks. Use may decrease the risk for CDI, skin damage from exposure to stool, IAD, and pressure injuries. Do not use a rectal tube or urinary catheter as a stool catheter. They can reduce the responsiveness of the rectal sphincter and ulcerate the rectal mucosa.

Fecal incontinence is associated with significant distress. Teach patients ways to reduce incontinence episodes and better cope with them when they do occur. Help patients identify food triggers that may worsen symptoms. Tell them to try to use bathrooms when they are available. Patients may be more confident when they use discreet, disposable briefs or pads. Have them wear dark-colored clothing that they can quickly remove for toileting. Ready access to a spare set of clothing and cleansing cloths is important.

CONSTIPATION

People with **constipation** have fewer than 3 stools per week, often accompanied by straining, a feeling of incomplete evacuation, a need for digital assistance to evacuate stool, bloating, and hard or lumpy stools. Constipation can be acute, usually lasting less than 1 week, or chronic, lasting over 3 months.

Etiology and Pathophysiology

Risk factors for chronic constipation include a low-fiber diet and decreased physical activity (Table 47.6). Ignoring the urge to defecate for a prolonged period can cause the muscles and mucosa of the rectum to become insensitive to the presence of feces. Prolonged fecal retention results in drying of stool because of water absorption. The harder and drier the feces are, the harder they are to expel. Emotions, including depression and stress, affect the GI tract and can contribute to constipation. Many drugs, especially opioids, cause constipation (Table 47.7).

Some people think they are constipated if they do not have a daily bowel movement. This can result in chronic laxative use and *cathartic colon syndrome*, a condition in which the colon

TABLE 47.6 Common Causes of Constipation

Colon Related
- Cancer
- Diverticular disease
- Inflammatory bowel disease
- Intestinal stenosis
- Intussusception
- Obstructing lesions
- Prolapse
- Rectocele

Systemic
- Amyloidosis
- Diabetes
- Electrolyte imbalance: Hypokalemia, hypercalcemia
- Hypothyroidism
- Kidney problems
- Multiple sclerosis
- Neurofibromatosis
- Parkinson disease
- Scleroderma
- Spinal cord lesions or injury
- Stroke
- Systemic lupus erythematosus
- Systemic sclerosis (scleroderma)

Other
- Diet, particularly low fiber
- Drug side effect (see Table 47.7)
- Emotions, including anxiety, depression, stress
- Inactivity
- Ignoring the urge to or delaying defecation
- Pregnancy

TABLE 47.7 Drugs Associated With Constipation

Cardiovascular	• Antihypertensives (β-adrenergic blockers, calcium channel blockers) • Furosemide • Hypolipidemics (cholestyramine, colestipol, statins)
Central nervous system	• Analgesics (opiates and derivatives) • Antidepressants (tricyclics, selective serotonin reuptake inhibitors) • Antiepileptics (carbamazepine, phenytoin, clonazepam) • Antipsychotics (butyrophenones, phenothiazines, barbiturates) • Benzodiazepines
GI	• Antacids containing aluminum, calcium • Antidiarrheals • Proton pump inhibitors • Supplements (bismuth, calcium, iron)

becomes dilated and atonic (lacking muscle tone). Ultimately, the person cannot defecate without a laxative.

Clinical Manifestations

Constipation varies from mild discomfort to a more severe event mimicking an "acute abdomen." Stools are absent or hard, dry, and difficult to pass. Abdominal distention, bloating, increased flatus, and increased rectal pressure may be present.

Hemorrhoids are a common complication of chronic constipation. They result from venous engorgement caused by repeated *Valsalva maneuvers* (straining) and venous compression from hard, impacted stool. The Valsalva maneuver may have serious outcomes for patients with heart failure, cerebral edema, hypertension, and coronary artery disease. During straining, the patient inspires deeply and holds their breath while contracting abdominal muscles and bearing down. This increases intra-abdominal and intrathoracic pressures and reduces venous return to the heart. The heart rate temporarily decreases along with a decrease in cardiac output. This results in a transient drop in arterial pressure. When the patient relaxes, thoracic pressure falls, resulting in a sudden flow of blood into the heart, increased heart rate, and an immediate rise in arterial pressure. These changes may be fatal for patients who cannot compensate for the sudden increased blood flow returning to the heart.

Rectal mucosal ulcers and fissures may occur from stool stasis or straining. Diverticulosis is another potential complication. It is more common in older patients. In the presence of *obstipation* (absolute constipation with no passage of gas or stool) or fecal impaction from constipation, colon perforation may occur.

Diagnostic Studies

The diagnosis of constipation is often based on the history and physical assessment. The physical should include an abdominal assessment, inspection of the perianal and rectal region, and digital rectal examination (DRE). Concerning signs include a sudden, persistent change in bowel habits (>6 weeks) in those over 50 years, rectal bleeding or bloody stools, iron deficiency anemia, weight loss, significant abdominal pain, family or personal history of CRC, or IBD and a palpable mass. If any of these are present, tests, such as colonoscopy, are done to rule out problems such as CRC. Patients with severe constipation may undergo anorectal manometry, GI tract transit studies, balloon expulsion test, or defecography.

Interprofessional Care

Increased fiber intake, fluid intake, and exercise can treat and prevent many cases of constipation.[5] Laxatives (Table 47.8) and enemas are other treatment options. Patients with severe constipation related to bowel motility or mechanical disorders may need more intense treatment. Biofeedback therapy may help patients who have constipation because of *anismus* (uncoordinated contraction of the anal sphincter during straining). Patients with unrelenting constipation may need a colostomy, ileostomy, or continent fecal diversion. These procedures are discussed later in this chapter.

Nutrition Therapy

Diet is a key factor in preventing and treating constipation. Many patients have improved symptoms when they increase their fiber intake. Fiber adds to the stool bulk directly by attracting water. Fiber is found in fruits, vegetables, and grains (Table 47.9). Adequate fluid intake (2 L/day) is essential. Large, bulky stools move through the colon much more quickly than small stools. However, the recommended fluid intake may be contraindicated in patients with heart disease or renal failure. Tell patients that increasing fiber intake may increase gas production because of fermentation in the colon.[5] This effect decreases over several days.

Drug Therapy

There are many prescription and over-the-counter (OTC) agents. All promote bowel movements, but each class works differently. Which one a patient receives depends on the severity and duration of constipation and the patient's health. Those with low diet fiber intake should take a fiber supplement with psyllium.[5] In patients with chronic constipation who do not respond to diet and lifestyle changes, osmotic laxatives are recommended. Stimulant laxatives are given to patients who do not respond to osmotic laxatives.

Enemas are fast-acting and offer immediate treatment of constipation. They must be used cautiously. Those containing sodium phosphate and magnesium can cause electrolyte imbalances in older adults and patients with heart and kidney problems. Other therapies target specific patient needs. Peripherally acting opioid receptor antagonists, such as methylnaltrexone, decrease constipation from opioid use.

TABLE 47.8 **Drug Therapy**

Constipation

Mechanism of Action	Indications	Drugs	Nursing Considerations
Bulk Forming			
Absorb water. Increase bulk, stimulating peristalsis. *Action:* Usually within 24 h	Acute and chronic constipation, IBS, diverticulosis	methylcellulose (Citrucel) psyllium (Metamucil, Konsyl, Hydrocil, Fiberall)	Do not use in patients with abdominal pain, nausea, vomiting, those suspected of having appendicitis, biliary tract obstruction, or acute hepatitis. Must be taken with fluids (≥8 oz). Best choice for initial treatment of constipation.
Emollients			
Lubricate intestinal tract and soften feces, making hard stools easier to pass. *Action:* Softeners in 72 h, lubricants in 8 h	Acute and chronic constipation, fecal impaction, anorectal conditions	*Softeners:* docusate (Colace) *Lubricants:* mineral oil (Fleet Mineral Oil Enema)	Can block absorption of fat-soluble vitamins, such as vitamin K, which may increase risk for bleeding in patients on anticoagulants.
Prosecretory Drugs			
Increase intestinal fluid secretion through direct action on epithelial cells, speeds colon transit *Action:* Usually within 24 h	Chronic idiopathic constipation, IBS-C (females only)	linaclotide (Linzess) lubiprostone (Amitiza) plecanatide (Trulance)	Do not use in patients with history of mechanical GI obstruction. Can cause nausea and watery diarrhea.
Saline and Osmotic Solutions			
Cause retention of fluid in intestinal lumen, reducing stool consistency and increasing volume *Action:* Within 15 min to 3 h	Chronic constipation, bowel preparation for diagnostic tests and surgery	lactulose magnesium salts (magnesium citrate, Milk of Magnesia) sodium phosphates (Fleet Enema) polyethylene glycol (MiraLAX, GoLYTELY)	May cause abdominal distention, diarrhea. Overuse of magnesium or sodium phosphates in older adults or those with renal failure can lead to fluid and electrolyte imbalances. Least effective agents in this class.
Stimulants			
Increase peristalsis and speed colonic transit by irritating colon wall and stimulating enteric nerves *Action:* Usually within 12 h	Acute constipation, bowel preparation for diagnostic tests and surgery	anthraquinones (cascara sagrada, senna) sennosides (Ex-Lax, Senokot) bisacodyl (Correctol, Dulcolax)	Cause melanosis coli (brown or black pigmentation of colon). Most widely abused laxatives. Should not be used in patients with impaction or obstipation.

NURSING MANAGEMENT: CONSTIPATION

Assessment

Table 47.10 outlines the subjective and objective data to obtain from patients with constipation.

Assess the patient's usual defecation patterns and habits. Ask about the onset and duration of symptoms, the shape and consistency of the stool, and any difficulty with evacuation (Fig. 47.1). Is there a feeling of incomplete evacuation or the need to use fingering to expel the feces? Ask about laxative use and any history that could contribute to problems with defecation.

Implementation

Tailor the nursing management to the patient. Teach patients about the role of diet, adequate fluid intake, and regular exercise in preventing and treating constipation (Table 47.11). Emphasize the importance of a high-fiber diet. Stress using laxatives and enemas as ordered.

Teach patients to establish a regular time to defecate and not to suppress the urge to defecate. Defecation is easiest when the person is sitting on a commode with the knees higher than the hips. The sitting position allows gravity to aid defecation, and flexing the hips straightens the angle between the anal canal and rectum so that stool flows out more easily. Place a footstool in front of the toilet to promote flexion of the hips. It is challenging to defecate while sitting on a bedpan. For patients in bed, raise the head of the bed as high as they can tolerate.

The sights, odors, and sounds of defecation embarrass most people. Provide as much privacy as possible and use an odor eliminator. Encourage patients to maintain abdominal muscle tone. Prompt patients to contract abdominal muscles several times a day. Sit-ups and straight-leg raises can help improve abdominal muscle tone.

For patients whose perceived constipation is related to rigid beliefs about bowel function, start a discussion about these concerns. Provide information on normal bowel function and discuss the adverse consequences of overuse of laxatives and enemas.

CHRONIC ABDOMINAL PAIN

Chronic abdominal pain may originate from abdominal structures or be referred from a site with the same or a similar

TABLE 47.9 NUTRITION THERAPY

High-Fiber Foods

	Fiber/ Serving (g)	Serving Size	Calories/ Serving
Vegetables			
Asparagus	3.5	½ cup	18
Beans			
• Navy	8.4	½ cup	80
• Kidney	9.7	½ cup	94
• Lima	8.3	½ cup	63
• Pinto	8.9	½ cup	78
• String	2.1	½ cup	18
Broccoli	3.5	½ cup	18
Carrots, raw	1.8	½ cup	15
Corn	2.6	½ medium ear	72
Peas, canned	6.7	½ cup	63
Potatoes			
• Baked	1.9	½ medium	72
• Sweet	2.1	½ medium	79
Squash, acorn	7.0	1 cup	82
Tomato, raw	1.5	1 small	18
Fruits			
Apple	2.0	½ large	42
Blackberries	6.7	¾ cup	40
Orange	1.6	1 small	35
Peach	2.3	1 medium	38
Pear	2.0	½ medium	44
Raspberries	9.2	1 cup	42
Strawberries	3.1	1 cup	45
Grain Products			
Bread, whole wheat	1.3	1 slice	59
Cereal			
• All Bran (100%)	8.4	⅓ cup	70
• Corn Flakes	2.6	¾ cup	70
• Shredded Wheat	2.8	1 biscuit	70
Popcorn	3.0	3 cups	62

nerve supply. The pain is often described as dull, aching, or diffuse. Common causes include irritable bowel syndrome (IBS), IBD, peptic ulcer disease, chronic pancreatitis, gastroesophageal reflux, pelvic inflammatory disease, malabsorption, and endometriosis.

Diagnosing the cause begins with a history and detailed pain assessment, including severity, location, duration, and onset. Assess pain frequency and factors that increase or decrease the pain, such as eating, defecation, and activities. Endoscopy, CT scan, MRI, laparoscopy, and barium studies may be done. Treatment for chronic abdominal pain depends on the underlying cause.

ACUTE ABDOMINAL PAIN

Etiology and Pathophysiology

Acute abdominal pain may signal a life-threatening problem, so it requires immediate attention. Causes include damage to organs in the abdomen and pelvis, which leads to inflammation, infection, obstruction, bleeding, and perforation (Fig. 47.2). GI tract perforation results in irritation of the *peritoneum* (serous membrane lining the abdominal cavity) and peritonitis. Hypovolemic shock from bleeding or obstruction and peritonitis can cause large amounts of fluid to move from the vascular space into the abdomen.

TABLE 47.10 NURSING ASSESSMENT

Constipation

Subjective Data

Important Health Information

Health history: Colorectal disease, neurologic problems, bowel obstruction, environment changes, cancer, inflammatory bowel disease, diabetes

Medications: Table 47.7

Functional Health Patterns

Health perception–health management: Chronic laxative, enema use. Rigid beliefs about bowel function. Malaise

Nutritional-metabolic: Change in diet or mealtime. Fiber and fluid intake. Anorexia, nausea, vomiting, weight change

Elimination: Change in usual bowel patterns. Hard, difficult-to-pass stool; decrease in stool frequency and amount. Flatus, abdominal distention, bloating. Straining, tenesmus, rectal pressure. Fecal incontinence (if impacted)

Activity-exercise: Daily activity routine. Immobility. Ability to toilet.

Cognitive-perceptual: Dizziness, headache, anorectal pain. Abdominal pain on defecation

Coping–stress tolerance: Acute or chronic stress

Objective Data

GI

Abdominal distention. Hypoactive or absent bowel sounds. Palpable abdominal mass. Fecal impaction. Small, hard, dry stool. Stool with blood

Skin

Anorectal fissures, hemorrhoids, abscess, perianal skin ulcers

Possible Diagnostic Findings

Guaiac-positive stools. Abdominal x-ray showing stool in lower colon

Clinical Manifestations

Pain is the most common symptom of an acute abdominal problem. There may be nausea, vomiting, diarrhea, constipation, flatulence, fatigue, fever, rebound tenderness, and bloating.

Diagnostic Studies

Diagnosis begins with a history and physical assessment. Description of the pain (frequency, timing, duration, location), accompanying symptoms, and sequence of symptoms (e.g., pain before or after vomiting) provide vital clues. Note the patient's position. The fetal posture is common with peritoneal irritation (e.g., appendicitis). Patients may be supine

TABLE 47.11 PATIENT & CAREGIVER TEACHING

Constipation

Include the following instructions when teaching the patient and caregiver about managing constipation:

1. Eat fiber
   Eat 20 to 30 g of fiber per day. Gradually increase the amount of fiber eaten over 1 to 2 weeks. Fiber softens hard stool and adds bulk to stool, promoting evacuation. Eat prunes or drink prune juice daily. Prunes stimulate defecation. Fiber supplements, such as Metamucil or Fiber-Con, may help.
2. Drink fluids
   Fluid softens hard stools. Drink 2 L/day. Drink water or fruit juices. Avoid caffeinated coffee, tea, and cola. Caffeine stimulates fluid loss through urination.
3. Exercise regularly
   Walk, swim, or bike at least 3 times per week. Contract and relax abdominal muscles when standing or by doing sit-ups to strengthen muscles and prevent straining. Exercise stimulates bowel motility and moves stool through the colon.
4. Establish a regular time to defecate
   First thing in the morning or after the first meal of the day is the best time because people often have the urge to defecate at this time.
5. Do not delay defecation
   Respond to the urge to have a bowel movement as soon as possible. Delaying defecation results in hard stools and a decreased "urge" to defecate. Water is absorbed from stool by the colon over time. The colon becomes less sensitive to the presence of stool in the rectum.
6. Record your bowel elimination pattern
   Develop a habit of recording when you have a bowel movement. Regular monitoring of bowel movements will help you identify a problem early.
7. Use laxatives and enemas as ordered
   Do not overuse laxatives and enemas because they cause dependence. People who overuse them become unable to have a bowel movement without them.

with outstretched legs with visceral pain. Restlessness and inability to find a comfortable position occur with obstructions from kidney stones and gallstones.

Physical assessment includes assessing the abdomen, rectum, and pelvis. A complete blood count (CBC), urinalysis, abdominal x-ray, and ECG are done, along with an ultrasound or CT scan. A negative pregnancy test can rule out ectopic pregnancy.

Interprofessional and Nursing Management

Emergency management of patients with acute abdominal pain is shown in Table 47.12. The goal is to identify and treat the cause and monitor and treat complications, especially shock. General care involves managing fluid and electrolyte imbalances, pain, and anxiety. An immediate surgical consult may be needed.

Take vital signs and assess level of consciousness immediately and then at frequent intervals. Increased pulse and decreasing BP indicate impending shock. A fever suggests an inflammatory or infectious process. Altered mental status occurs with poor cerebral perfusion. Skin color, skin temperature, and peripheral pulse strength give information about perfusion. Intake and output give essential information about the adequacy of vascular volume.

Inspect the abdomen for distention, masses, abnormal pulsation, symmetry, hernias, rashes, scars, and pigmentation changes. Auscultate bowel sounds. Decreased or absent bowel sounds in a quadrant may occur with a bowel obstruction, peritonitis, or paralytic ileus. Perform gentle palpation to help determine the location and level of the pain. Assess for guarding and rigidity, which occur with peritoneal irritation. Note the amount, color, consistency, and odor of any emesis. A nasogastric (NG) tube with low suction may decrease vomiting and relieve discomfort from gastric distention. Ask about usual bowel patterns and habits and any changes.

Assess pain at regular intervals. Ask patients about the onset, location, intensity, duration, frequency, and character of pain. Note whether the pain has spread or moved to new sites (quadrants) and what makes the pain worse or better. Ask if the pain is related to other symptoms, such as nausea, vomiting, changes in bowel and bladder habits, or vaginal discharge in females. Provide medication and other comfort measures.

ABDOMINAL TRAUMA

Etiology and Pathophysiology

Various trauma can cause abdominal injury (Table 47.13). Common abdominal injuries include lacerated liver, ruptured spleen, mesenteric artery tears, diaphragm rupture, urinary bladder rupture, great vessel tears, kidney or pancreas injury, and stomach or intestine rupture.

Blunt trauma often occurs with motor vehicle accidents, direct blows, and falls. It may not be obvious because it does not leave an open wound. Both compression injuries (e.g., direct blow to the abdomen) and shearing injuries (e.g., rapid deceleration in a motor vehicle crash allowing some tissue to move forward while other tissues stay stationary) occur with blunt trauma.[6] Seat belts can produce blunt trauma to abdominal organs by pressing the intestine and pancreas into the spinal column.

Penetrating injuries occur when a gunshot or stabbing produces an obvious, open wound into the abdomen. When solid organs (liver, spleen) are injured, bleeding can be profuse, resulting in hypovolemic shock. When contents from hollow organs (e.g., bladder, stomach, intestines) spill into the peritoneal cavity, the patient is at risk for peritonitis.

Another risk is abdominal compartment syndrome with high pressure in the abdomen. Anything that increases the volume in the abdominal cavity (e.g., edema, bleeding) increases abdominal pressure. This high pressure restricts ventilation, leading to respiratory failure. The high pressure decreases cardiac output, venous return, and arterial perfusion of organs. Decreased renal perfusion can lead to kidney failure.

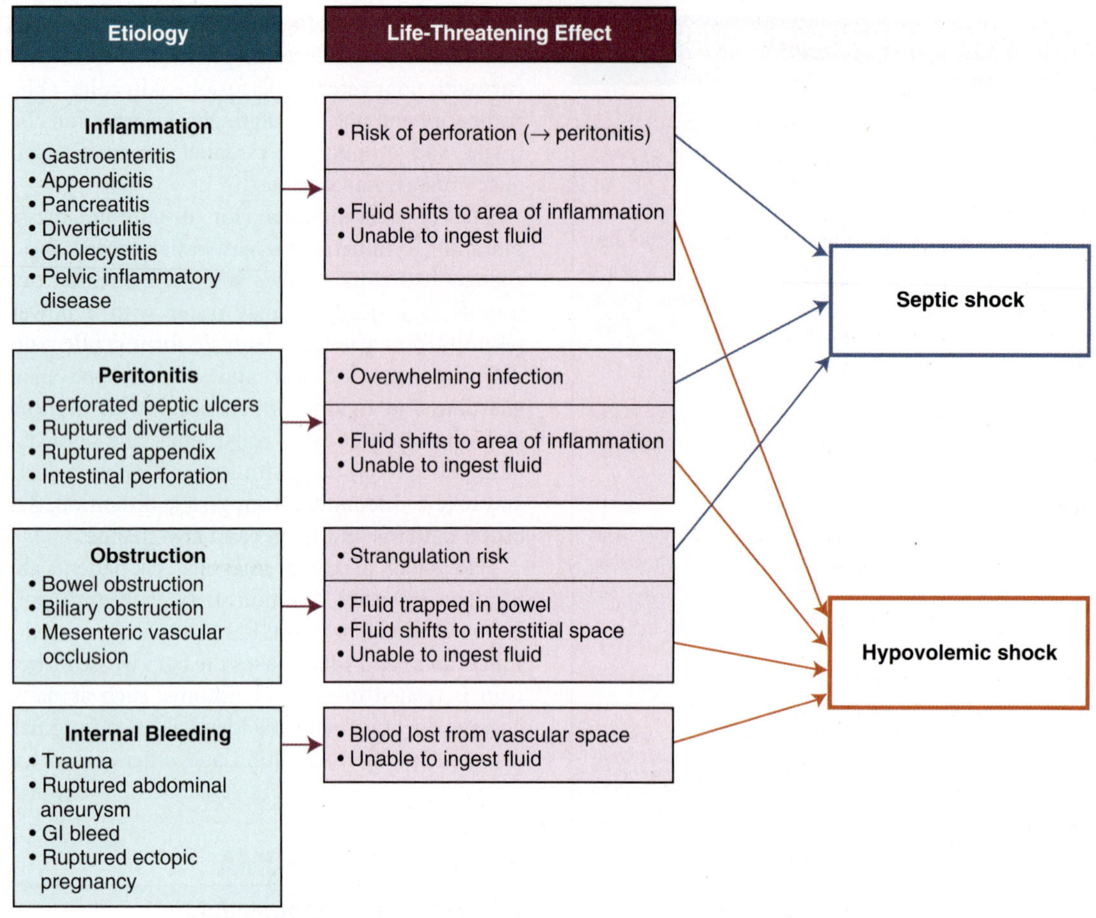

Fig. 47.2 Cause of acute abdominal pain and pathophysiologic sequelae.

TABLE 47.12 EMERGENCY MANAGEMENT

Acute Abdominal Pain

Etiology	Assessment Findings	Interventions
Gynecologic • Ectopic pregnancy • Ovarian cyst, torsion • Pelvic inflammatory disease **Inflammation** • Appendicitis • Cholecystitis • Diverticulitis • Hepatitis • Inflammatory bowel disease • Pancreatitis • Pyelonephritis **Vascular** • Aortic aneurysm • Mesenteric ischemia **Other** • Abdominal organ perforation or obstruction • GI bleeding • GI infection • Kidney stones • Myocardial infarction • Trauma	**GI** • Diffuse, local, dull, burning, sharp abdominal pain or tenderness • Abdominal rigidity • Absent, ↑ or ↓ bowel sounds • Change in bowel habits • Diarrhea • Distention • Guarding • Hematemesis • Melena • Nausea and vomiting • Rebound tenderness **Hypovolemic Shock** • ↓ BP • Cool, clammy skin • Fever • ↓ Level of consciousness • ↑ HR • ↓ Urine output (<0.5 mL/kg/h)	**Initial** • Ensure patent airway. • Apply O_2 via nasal cannula or nonrebreather mask. • Establish IV access with large-bore catheter and infuse IV fluids as ordered. Insert another large-bore catheter if shock present. • Obtain blood for CBC and electrolyte levels. Amylase level, pregnancy tests, clotting studies, and type and crossmatch as appropriate. • Insert indwelling urinary catheter. • Obtain urinalysis. • Insert NG tube as needed. **Ongoing Monitoring** • Monitor vital signs, level of consciousness, O_2 saturation. • Initiate intake/output. • Obtain pain assessment. Administer analgesia as ordered. • Assess amount and character of emesis. Administer antiemetics as ordered. • Anticipate surgical intervention. • Keep patient NPO.

TABLE 47.13 EMERGENCY MANAGEMENT

Abdominal Trauma

Etiology	Assessment Findings	Interventions
Blunt • Assault with a blunt object • Bicycle accident • Crush injury • Falls • Motor vehicle accident • Pedestrian event • Sports injury • Work accident **Penetrating** • Explosions • Gunshot wounds • Impalement • Knife	**Abdominal and GI Findings** • Abdominal pain • Absent or ↓ bowel sounds • Distention • Hematemesis • Hematuria • Nausea and vomiting • Rebound tenderness • Rigidity **Hypovolemic Shock** • ↓ BP • ↑ HR • ↓ Level of consciousness • Tachypnea **Surface Findings** • Abrasions, bruising on abdominal wall, flank, peritoneum • Impaled object • Open wounds: lacerations, eviscerations, puncture wounds, gunshot wounds	**Initial** • If unresponsive, assess circulation, airway, and breathing. • If responsive, monitor airway, breathing, and circulation. • Apply appropriate O_2 therapy. • Control external bleeding with direct pressure or sterile pressure dressing. • Establish IV access with 2 large-bore catheters and infuse IV fluids as ordered. • Obtain blood for type and crossmatch and CBC. • Remove clothing. • Stabilize impaled objects with bulky dressing—*do not remove.* • Cover protruding organs or tissue with sterile saline dressing. • Insert indwelling urinary catheter if there is no blood at the meatus, pelvic fracture, or boggy prostate. • Obtain urine for urinalysis. • Insert NG tube if no evidence of facial trauma. • Anticipate diagnostic peritoneal lavage. **Ongoing Monitoring** • Monitor vital signs, level of consciousness, O_2 saturation, and urine output. • Maintain patient warmth using blankets, warm IV fluids, or warm humidified O_2.

Clinical Manifestations

Classic manifestations of abdominal trauma are (1) guarding and splinting of the abdominal wall (indicating peritonitis); (2) a hard, distended abdomen from intraabdominal bleeding; (3) decreased or absent bowel sounds; (4) abrasions or bruising over the abdomen; (5) abdominal pain; (6) hematemesis or hematuria; and (7) signs of hypovolemic shock (Table 47.13). Bruising around the umbilicus *(Cullen sign)* or flanks *(Grey Turner sign)* may mean retroperitoneal hemorrhage. If the patient was in an automobile accident, a contusion or abrasion across the lower abdomen may indicate internal organ trauma from the seat belt. Loss of bowel sounds occurs with peritonitis. If the diaphragm ruptures, you may hear bowel sounds (if present) in the chest. Assess patients for other injuries. Intraabdominal injuries are often associated with rib fractures, fractured pelvis, spinal injury, and thoracic injury.[6]

Diagnostic Studies

Laboratory tests include a baseline CBC and urinalysis. Even when bleeding, patients will have normal hemoglobin and hematocrit because fluids are lost at the same rate as the red blood cells. Deficiencies are evident after fluid resuscitation begins. Blood in the urine may be a sign of kidney or bladder damage. Other laboratory work includes arterial blood gases (ABGs), prothrombin time, electrolytes, BUN and creatinine, and type and crossmatch (in anticipation of possible blood transfusions). An abdominal CT scan and focused abdominal ultrasound are the most common diagnostic methods, but patients must be stable before going for CT. Peritoneal lavage can detect blood, bile, intestinal contents, and urine in the peritoneal cavity.

Interprofessional and Nursing Management

Emergency management of abdominal trauma is outlined in Table 47.13. Volume expanders or blood is given if the patient is hypotensive. An NG tube with low suction will decompress the stomach and prevent aspiration. Frequent, ongoing assessment is needed to monitor fluid status, detect deterioration in condition, and determine the need for surgery. The decision about whether to do surgery depends on clinical findings, diagnostic test results, and the response to conservative management. Do not remove an impaled object. This can cause further injury and bleeding.

ABDOMINAL SURGERY

LAPAROTOMY AND LAPAROSCOPY

The HCP may perform a laparoscopy or laparotomy to explore the abdomen and diagnose and treat various problems. The HCP can inspect abdominal organs, obtain biopsy specimens, make repairs, and remove organs. A laparotomy, or open abdominal surgery, is done when laparoscopic techniques are inadequate. Either is definitive therapy if the cause of an acute abdomen or other health problem is surgically removed (e.g., inflamed appendix) or repaired (e.g., ruptured abdominal aneurysm).

Preoperative Care

Preoperative care includes the general care of preoperative patients (see Chapter 18). For some patients, include general care of patients with acute abdominal pain (Table 47.12).

Postoperative Care

Postoperative care depends on the type of surgery. See eNursing Care Plan 20.1, a general plan for postoperative patients, on the website for Chapter 20.

Some patients will have an NG tube with low suction to empty the stomach and prevent gastric dilation. If the upper GI tract was entered, drainage from the NG tube may be dark brown to dark red for the first 12 hours. Later it should be light yellowish-brown, or it may have a greenish tinge because of bile. If a dark red color continues or you see bright red blood, notify the HCP because of the risk for hemorrhage. "Coffee-ground" drainage means the blood has been changed by acidic gastric secretions.

Nausea and vomiting are common from the surgery, decreased peristalsis, and pain medications. Antiemetics, such as ondansetron, may be given. Monitor fluid and electrolyte status along with BP, heart rate, and respirations. See Chapter 46 for information about managing nausea and vomiting.

Swallowed air and reduced peristalsis from decreased mobility, manipulation of the abdominal organs during surgery, and anesthesia can result in abdominal distention and gas pains. Early ambulation speeds recovery. It helps restore peristalsis, expel flatus, and reduce gas pain. Gradually, as intestinal activity increases, distention and gas pain disappear. Initially, patients start on clear liquids after surgery and then, if tolerated, progress to a regular diet.

Teach patients and caregivers about any modifications in activity, incision care, diet, and drug therapy. Normal activities are resumed gradually with planned rest periods. Patients often have restrictions not to lift anything heavier than a few pounds. Patients and caregivers should be aware of possible complications. Teach them to notify the HCP at once if fever, vomiting, pain, weight loss, incisional drainage, or changes in bowel function occur.

BOWEL RESECTION AND OSTOMY SURGERY

A **bowel resection** is surgery to remove any part of the bowel. Surgical resection may be done to (1) remove tumors or masses; (2) repair a perforation, fistula, or traumatic injury; (3) relieve an obstruction or stricture; and (4) treat an abscess, inflammatory disease, or hemorrhage (Table 47.14).

TABLE 47.14 Common Intestinal Surgical Procedures

Procedure	Description
Abdominal-perineal resection (APR)	Removal of entire rectum with creation of a permanent colostomy.
Anterior rectosigmoid resection	Removal of part of descending colon, sigmoid colon, and upper rectum with descending colon anastomosed to remaining rectum.
Colectomy	Removal of entire colon with ileum anastomosed to rectum.
Left hemicolectomy	Removal of splenic flexure, descending colon, and sigmoid colon with transverse colon anastomosed to rectum.
Low anterior resection (LAR)	Removal of rectum with anastomosis of colon to anal canal. Temporary ileostomy or colostomy may be done to divert stool and allow time for anastomosis to heal. After 8–12 weeks, ostomy can be "taken down" and ends of colon surgically reconnected.
Proctocolectomy with ileostomy	Removal of colon, rectum, and anus with closure of anal opening. End of terminal ileum brought out through abdominal wall to form a permanent ileostomy.
Proctocolectomy with ileal pouch/anal anastomosis (IPAA)	2 surgeries, 8–12 weeks apart. The first includes colectomy, rectal mucosectomy, ileal pouch (reservoir) construction, ileoanal anastomosis, and temporary ileostomy. Diverting ileostomy is done, and ileal pouch is created and anastomosed directly to anus (Fig. 47.4). Second surgery involves closure of ileostomy to direct stool toward new pouch.
Right hemicolectomy	Removal of ascending colon and hepatic flexure with ileum anastomosed to transverse colon.

Ostomy

An **ostomy** is a surgically created opening on the abdomen that allows the discharge of body waste when the normal elimination route is no longer possible. The outermost part that is visible is a *stoma.* The stoma is the result of the large or small bowel being brought to the outside of the abdomen and sutured in place. When a stoma is created as a fecal diversion, feces will drain through the stoma instead of the anus.

Ostomies are named according to their location (Fig. 47.3). An ostomy in the ileum is an ileostomy. An ostomy in the colon is a colostomy. The ostomy is further described by its anatomic site (ascending, transverse, descending, sigmoid). The more distal the ostomy, the more functioning bowel remains and the more likely that the intestinal contents will resemble the feces that would have been eliminated from an intact colon and rectum. Ileostomy output will be a liquid to thin paste because it did not enter the colon. An ileostomy drains frequently. Patients must wear a pouch to collect the drainage. Sigmoid colostomy output resembles normal formed stool. See Table 47.15 for a comparison of colostomies and ileostomies.

Ostomies may be temporary or permanent. Permanent ostomies may be continent or traditional. *Continent ileostomies* (e.g., Koch pouch) use part of the terminal ileum to fashion an internal pouch and abdominal stoma. The pouch replaces the rectum as a reservoir for stool. It can hold around 500 mL of material. Patients must drain the pouch manually by inserting a catheter. At first, this is done every 1 to 2 hours. As the pouch enlarges, the frequency decreases to 4 times daily and as needed. They must keep the stool consistency relatively fluid by following a low-residue diet.

Traditional ostomies include end, end with mucus fistula, and loop ostomy.[7]

End

An end stoma is made by dividing the bowel and bringing out the proximal end as a single stoma, making a colostomy or ileostomy. The distal part of the GI tract is surgically removed, or the distal segment is oversewn and left in the abdominal cavity with its mesentery intact. If the distal bowel is removed, the stoma is permanent. When the distal bowel is oversewn and not removed, the procedure is called a *Hartmann pouch* (Fig. 47.4). With a Hartmann pouch, the potential exists for the bowel to be reanastomosed and the stoma closed (called a *takedown*).

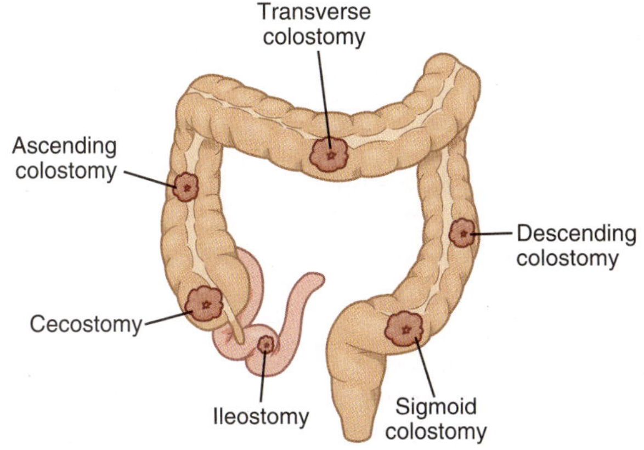

Fig. 47.3 Locations of ostomies.

End With Mucus Fistula

To create a double-barreled stoma, the HCP divides the bowel, and both ends are brought through the abdominal wall as separate stomas (Fig. 47.4). The proximal stoma is the functioning stoma. The distal, nonfunctioning stoma is a *mucus fistula.* A double-barreled stoma is usually temporary.

Loop

A loop stoma is made by bringing a loop of bowel to the abdominal surface and then opening the anterior wall of the bowel to provide fecal diversion. This results in 1 stoma with a proximal opening for feces and a distal opening for mucus drainage from the distal colon. An intact posterior wall separates the 2 openings. A plastic rod holds the loop of bowel in place for 7 to 10 days after surgery to prevent it from slipping back into the abdominal cavity (Fig. 47.4). A loop stoma is usually temporary.

NURSING MANAGEMENT: BOWEL RESECTION AND OSTOMY SURGERY

Preoperative Care

Preoperative care includes the general care of preoperative patients (see Chapter 18). Care that is unique to ostomy surgery includes preparation for the ostomy and selecting the best site for the stoma. If available, a wound, ostomy, and continence nurse (WOCN) should visit with the patient and caregiver.

Psychologic preparation and emotional support are important as the person begins to cope with the changes in body image and elimination. Assess the patient's ability to perform self-care and identify support systems. Patients and caregivers should understand the surgery planned. Provide them with opportunities to share concerns and questions. This will enhance feelings of control and ability to cope.

An experienced provider should choose where the stoma will be and mark the abdomen. The site should be within the rectus muscle, on a flat surface, and in a place that the patient is able to see. A flat site makes it much easier to create a good seal and avoid bag leakage. Being able to see the stoma makes caring

TABLE 47.15 Comparison of Ileostomy and Colostomy

		COLOSTOMY		
Characteristic	**Ileostomy**	**Ascending**	**Transverse**	**Sigmoid**
Stool consistency	Liquid to semiliquid	Semiliquid	Semiliquid to semiformed	Formed
Fluid requirement	↑	↑	Possibly ↑	No change
Bowel regulation	No	No	No	Yes, if there is a history of a regular bowel pattern
Pouch and skin barriers	Yes	Yes	Yes	Dependent on regulation
Indications for surgery	Ulcerative colitis, Crohn disease, diseased or injured colon, familial polyposis, trauma, cancer	Perforating diverticulum in lower colon, trauma, rectovaginal fistula, inoperable tumors of colon, rectum, or pelvis	Same as for ascending	Cancer of the rectum or rectosigmoid area, perforating diverticulum, trauma

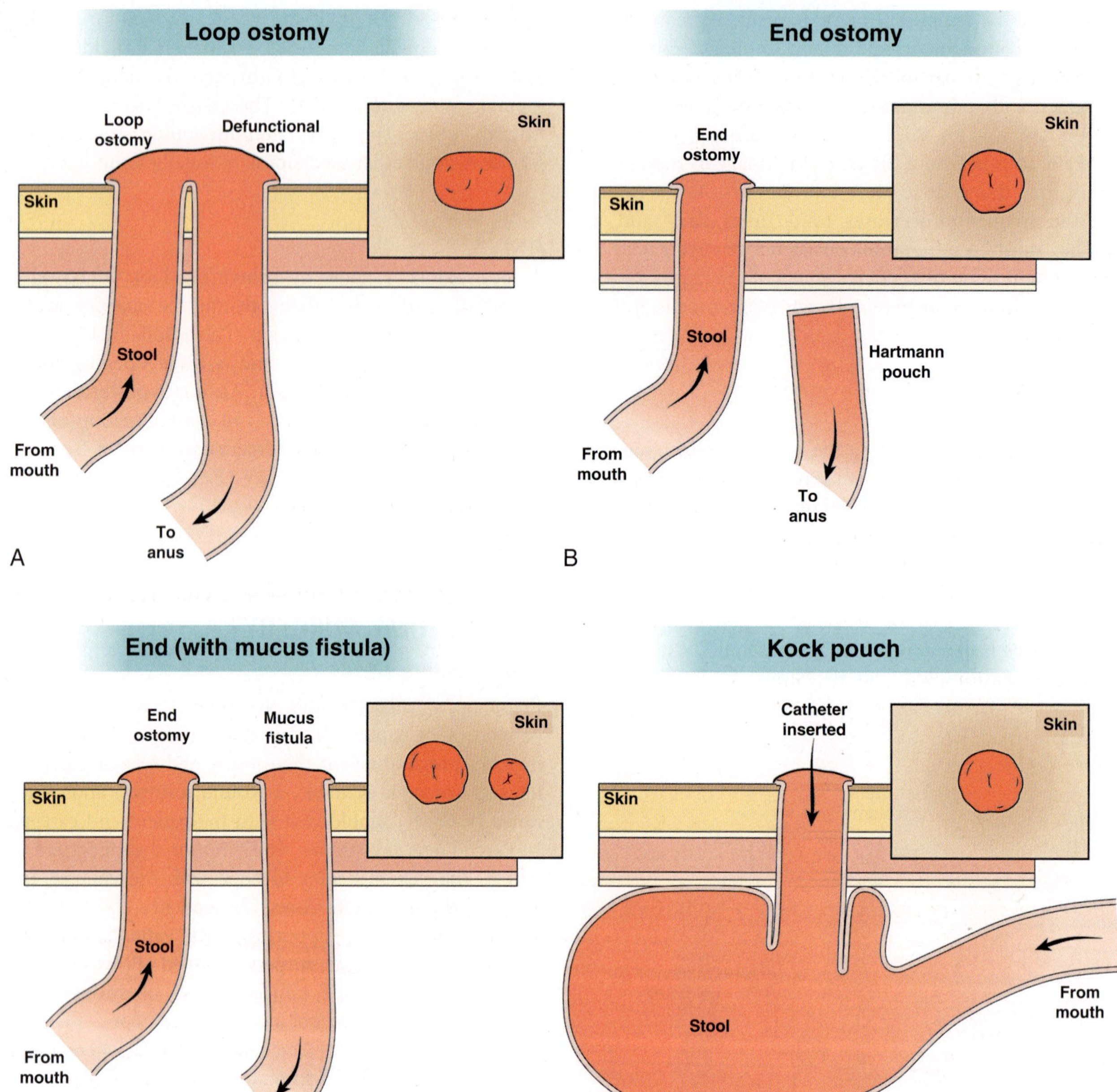

Fig. 47.4 Types of ostomies. (A) Loop ostomy, (B) end ostomy with Hartmann pouch, (C) end ostomy with mucus fistula, and (D) the continent ileostomy (Kock pouch). (From Hedrick TL, Sherman A, Cohen-Mekelburg S, et al: AGA clinical practice update on management of ostomies, *Clin Gastroenterol Hepatol* 21:2473, 2023.)

for it easier. Whenever possible, it should be discreetly hidden under clothing and appropriate for normal activities.

Postoperative Care

Postoperative care depends on the type of surgery. See eNursing Care Plan 20.1, a general plan for postoperative patients, on the website for Chapter 20.

Assess the incision and the area around any drains for signs of infection. Note any edema, redness, and drainage, in addition to a fever and a high WBC count. Monitor for complications, including delayed wound healing, hemorrhage, and fistulas. Keep the area around any drains clean and dry.

Patients who have an open wound with packing need meticulous care. Reinforce dressings and change them often during the first several hours postoperatively when drainage is likely to be profuse. Assess all drainage for amount, color, and consistency. The drainage is usually serosanguineous.

Early ambulation is important.[8] Patients can resume activities of daily living within 6 to 8 weeks but should avoid heavy lifting. Patients can bathe and shower with or without the pouching system in place because water does not harm the stoma.

Ostomy Care

If an ostomy is present, assess the stoma and place a clear pouching system. The stoma should be rosy pink to red and mildly swollen (Table 47.16). Assess stoma color every 4 hours. Ensure there is no excess bleeding. Report any sustained color changes or bleeding to the HCP. Edema will resolve over the first 6 weeks.

The colostomy starts functioning when peristalsis returns. Record the volume, color, and consistency of the drainage. When a colostomy is done on a colon that was not cleaned out before surgery, stool will drain when peristalsis returns. If the bowel was cleansed before surgery, it will not begin producing stool until a few days after the patient is eating again. Excess gas is common during the first 2 weeks. Because this can be distressing to patients, assure them this is temporary.

In the first 24 to 48 hours after surgery, the amount of drainage from an ileostomy may be negligible. When peristalsis returns, ileostomy output may be as high as 1500 to 1800 mL/24 h. Patients are at risk for fluid deficits and electrolyte imbalances, so administer fluids and encourage early oral intake.[8] Maintain intake and output. As the proximal small bowel adapts, fluid absorption will increase. Then, feces will thicken, and the volume will decrease to around 500 mL/day. Patients with an ileostomy must always wear a pouch because they have no control over the drainage. An open-ended, drainable pouch is best so drainage can be easily emptied.

Patients with an ascending or transverse colostomy can use a drainable pouch. A drainable pouch may last up to 4 to 7 days. Patients with a colostomy in the descending or sigmoid colon can use a drainable pouch or a disposable, closed-end pouch. Charcoal filters can deodorize and automatically release flatus. They are available for both types of pouches. Each time the pouch is changed, assess the skin for irritation. If the peristomal skin is irritated and raw, more products may have to be applied. Do not allow feces to remain on the skin, or irritation will quickly develop. Change a pouch that has failed at once.

TABLE 47.16 Stoma Assessment

Characteristic	Description or Cause
Color	
Rose to brick-red	Viable stoma mucosa
Pale	Anemia
Blanching, dark red to dusky blue or purple	Inadequate blood supply to the stoma or bowel
Brown-black	Necrosis
Edema	
Mild to moderate edema	Normal in initial postoperative period, trauma to the stoma
Moderate to severe edema	Obstruction of the stoma, allergic reaction to food, gastroenteritis
Bleeding	
Small amount	Oozing from stoma mucosa when touched is normal because of its high vascularity
Moderate to large amount	Lower GI bleeding, coagulation factor deficiency, stomal varices from portal hypertension

After an ileal pouch/anal anastomosis (IPAA), patients may have 4 to 6 stools or more daily. Adaptation over the next 3 to 6 months will result in fewer bowel movements. Patients can control defecation at the anal sphincter.

After surgical manipulation of the anal canal, transient incontinence of mucus may occur. Have patients start Kegel exercises about 4 weeks after surgery to strengthen the pelvic floor and sphincter muscles (see Table 50.18). Perianal skincare is important. Gently clean the skin with a mild cleanser, rinse well, and dry thoroughly. A moisture barrier ointment and a perineal pad may be used. Some patients have phantom rectal pain or still feel as if they need to have a bowel movement. This is normal and often subsides over time.

Colostomy irrigation is an option when the stoma is in the distal colon. It can stimulate emptying of the colon. Patients may need to wear only a pad or small pouch over the stoma if spillage should occur between irrigations. Irrigation requires manual dexterity and adequate vision. People who irrigate should have ostomy bags in case they develop diarrhea.

Sexual Function

Problems with sexual function depend on the surgery. Pelvic surgery can disrupt nerve and vascular supplies to the genitalia. Unfortunately, any pelvic surgery that removes the rectum has the potential of damaging the parasympathetic nerve plexus. The HCP should discuss the possibility with patients.

For males, the main concern is erection and ejaculation. Erection depends on intact parasympathetic and nonadrenergic noncholinergic nerves and an adequate blood supply. Sympathetic nerve damage in the presacral area can disrupt the ability to ejaculate. This can occur with an abdominal-perineal resection (APR). Sexual problems may be temporary and resolve in 3 to 12 months. Nerve-sparing surgical techniques are used when possible to preserve sexual function.

For females, nerve damage can result in vaginal dryness and decreased sensation in the vagina and clitoris, making arousal and achieving orgasm more challenging. Experimenting with positions and using lubrication may help.

Most patients with an ostomy have sexual concerns. Patients may fear rejection or that others will not find them desirable. Discuss their concerns. Help patients realize that it takes time to adjust before feeling secure with sexual function. Teach patients to empty the pouch before sexual activities. Some may apply a smaller pouch or use a pouch cover or wrap during sexual activity. Wearing a short slip or similar lingerie is an option.

Patient Teaching and Support

Major aspects of nursing care are (1) patient and caregiver teaching and (2) emotional support as patients cope with a change in body image (Table 47.17). With shorter hospital stays, focus teaching on the critical aspects that patients need to master. This includes (1) basic skills about managing the ostomy, (2) diet, and (3) how to get help for problems. Home care and outpatient follow-up may be helpful. Patient and caregiver teaching is outlined in Table 47.18. Nursing care for patients with an ostomy is discussed in eNursing Care Plan 47.3 on the website.

Teach patients about the importance of fluids and a healthy diet. Patients need to increase fluid intake to at least 2 to 3 L/day or more when there are excess fluid losses from heat and sweating. They may need to ingest more sodium. Teach them signs and symptoms of fluid and electrolyte imbalance so that they can take action.

TABLE 47.17 NURSING MANAGEMENT

Ostomy Care

- Assess stoma and peristomal skin appearance.
- Assess the patient with a new ostomy for readiness for ostomy care.
- Assist the patient with managing the psychologic impact of the stoma and its effect on body image and self-esteem.
- Choose appropriate ostomy pouching system for patient.
- Monitor the volume, color, and odor of the ostomy drainage.
- Develop skin care plan for peristomal area.
- Teach ostomy self-care to patient and caregiver (Table 47.18).
- Irrigate new colostomy, if indicated.
- Supervise AP:
  - Empty ostomy bag and measure liquid contents.
  - Place the ostomy pouching system for an established ostomy.
  - Assist stable patient with colostomy irrigation.

TABLE 47.18 PATIENT & CAREGIVER TEACHING

Ostomy Self-Care

Include the following points when teaching the patient and/or caregiver about self-care of an ostomy:

- What an ostomy is and how it functions
- How to perform ostomy care, including skin care and how to apply, empty, clean, and remove the pouch
- How to receive help if needed, including dietitian and ostomy nurse
- How to obtain ostomy supplies
- Diet and fluid management, including:
  - Well-balanced diet and supplements to prevent nutrition problems
  - Foods to avoid to reduce diarrhea or gas (Table 47.19)
  - Fluid intake of least 3000 mL/day to prevent dehydration (unless contraindicated)
  - Increase fluid intake during hot weather, excess perspiration, and diarrhea to replace losses and prevent dehydration
  - Chew food very well to reduce the chance of blockage
- How to recognize problems (fever, diarrhea, skin irritation, fluid and electrolyte imbalance, stomal problems)
- Community resources to assist with adjustment to the ostomy
- Importance of follow-up care
- Managing effects on sexual activity, social life, work, and recreation

The effect of food on stoma output is individual. Most patients with colostomies can eat anything they want. However, some choose to avoid certain foods because of possible increased gas, odor, or stoma output (Table 47.19). An ileostomy is susceptible to obstruction because the lumen is less than 1 inch in diameter. Foods such as nuts, raisins, popcorn, coconut, mushrooms, olives, stringy vegetables, foods with skins, dried fruits, and meats with casings must be chewed very well before swallowing.

The response to a new ostomy is highly individual. Some have little difficulty and view their ostomy positively. It may be curative if their presenting condition was cancer. Other patients may have a grief reaction and be angry or depressed. Concerns about leaking, odor, sounds of flatus, and changes in lifestyle are common.[7] You can help patients learn to live a full life with an ostomy and accept the changes in body image.

Help patients develop confidence and competence in managing the stoma. Their emotional state may limit the ability to take part in teaching and ostomy care. Help patients identify ways of coping. Support from their caregivers is vital. It reassures patients of their value. Encourage patients to share their concerns and ask questions.

Give contact information for support groups. The Wound Ostomy Continence Nurses Society (www.wocn.org), local support groups, and United Ostomy Associations of America (www.ostomy.org) provide practical information about living with an ostomy. Online support groups and visitors programs are available. These give patients and caregivers an opportunity to talk with a person who has adjusted well to an ostomy and had some of the same feelings and concerns they have.

INFLAMMATORY PROBLEMS

APPENDICITIS

Appendicitis is inflammation of the appendix, a narrow blind tube that extends from the inferior part of the cecum (Fig. 47.5). It is the most common reason for emergency abdominal surgery.[9]

TABLE 47.19 NUTRITION THERAPY

Effects of Food on Stoma Output

Odor Producing	Gas Forming	Diarrhea Causing
Alcohol	Beer and alcoholic seltzers	Alcohol
Asparagus	Broccoli	Broccoli
Broccoli	Cabbage	Cabbage
Cabbage	Carbonated beverages	Caffeinated beverages
Eggs	Dairy products	Fruits (raw)
Fish	Onions	Green beans
Garlic	Spicy or fried foods	Spicy foods
Onions		Spinach

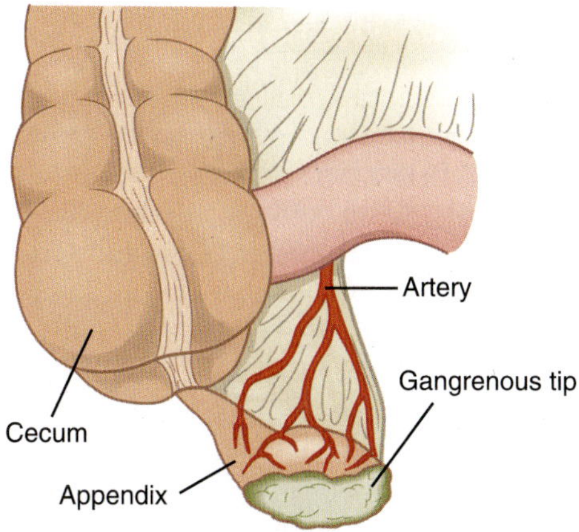

Fig. 47.5 In appendicitis, the blood supply of the appendix is impaired by inflammation and bacterial infection, which may result in gangrene.

Etiology and Pathophysiology

Appendicitis is most common in those 10 to 30 years of age. We think it is caused by luminal obstruction leading to local infection.[9] Subsequent swelling results in distention, venous engorgement, and the accumulation of mucus and bacteria. This can lead to gangrene, perforation, and peritonitis.

Clinical Manifestations

Diagnosis can be difficult because some patients do not have classic symptoms.[9] Appendicitis typically begins with dull periumbilical pain, followed by anorexia, nausea, and vomiting. The pain is persistent and continuous, eventually shifting to the right lower quadrant and localizing at the *McBurney point* (halfway between the umbilicus and right iliac crest). A low-grade fever may develop. Further assessment reveals rigidity, rebound tenderness, and muscle guarding. Positive psoas (pain with extension of right thigh), obturator (pain with passive internal rotation of the flexed thigh), and Rovsing signs (increased right lower quadrant pain occurring with left lower quadrant palpation) lend to the diagnosis. Coughing or sneezing worsens pain. Patients usually prefer to lie still, often with the right leg flexed.

Diagnostic Studies and Interprofessional Care

Diagnosis includes a history, physical assessment, and a differential WBC count. Most patients have a mildly to moderately high WBC count. A urinalysis is done to rule out genitourinary conditions. CT scan is the preferred diagnostic procedure. Ultrasound and MRI are options.

If there is a delay in diagnosis and treatment, the appendix can rupture, and the resulting peritonitis can be fatal. The standard treatment is an immediate *appendectomy* (surgical removal of appendix). Antibiotics and fluid resuscitation are started before surgery. If the appendix has ruptured and there is evidence of peritonitis or an abscess, giving IV fluids and antibiotic therapy for 6 to 8 hours before surgery helps prevent dehydration and sepsis.

NURSING MANAGEMENT: APPENDICITIS

Managing patients who potentially have appendicitis focuses on preventing fluid volume deficit, relieving pain, and preventing complications. To ensure the stomach is empty in case surgery is needed, keep the patient NPO until the HCP evaluates the patient. Monitor vital signs. Perform ongoing assessment to detect any deterioration in condition. Give IV fluids, analgesics, and antiemetics as ordered. Provide comfort measures.

Postoperative care for patients who had an appendectomy is similar to patients after a laparotomy. Patients are usually discharged within 24 hours after an uncomplicated laparoscopic appendectomy. Ambulation begins a few hours after surgery. The diet is advanced as tolerated. Those who had a perforation usually have a longer length of stay and need IV antibiotic therapy. Most patients resume normal activities 2 to 3 weeks after surgery.

CHECK YOUR PRACTICE

A 28-year-old female patient comes to the emergency department with acute abdominal pain.

- What manifestations would make you suspect appendicitis is the cause of the abdominal pain?

PERITONITIS

Etiology and Pathophysiology

Peritonitis, inflammation of the peritoneum, may result from contamination of the peritoneal cavity with bacteria, irritating chemicals, or both. Common causes are listed in Table 47.20. Primary peritonitis occurs when blood-borne organisms enter the peritoneal cavity. It is not related to any other intra-abdominal problem.

Secondary peritonitis is more common. It occurs when abdominal organs perforate or rupture and release their contents (bile, enzymes, bacteria) into the peritoneal cavity.

TABLE 47.20 Common Causes of Peritonitis

Primary
- Blood-borne pathogens
- Cirrhosis with ascites

Secondary
- Appendicitis with rupture
- Blunt or penetrating abdominal trauma
- Diverticulitis with rupture
- Inflammatory bowel disease
- Ischemic bowel disorders
- Pancreatitis
- Pelvic inflammatory disease
- Perforated intestine, uterus, urinary bladder, stomach
- Perforated peptic ulcer
- Postoperative abdominal surgery complication

Common causes include a ruptured appendix, perforated ulcer, and diverticulitis. Peritoneal dialysis–associated peritonitis, which is a distinct subtype, is discussed in Chapter 51.

Intestinal contents and bacteria irritate the normally sterile peritoneum and produce an initial chemical peritonitis. Bacterial peritonitis develops a few hours later. The resulting inflammatory response leads to massive fluid shifts (peritoneal edema) and adhesions as the body tries to wall off the infection.

Clinical Manifestations

Manifestations vary, depending on the severity and acuteness of the underlying condition. A universal sign is tenderness over the involved area. Rebound tenderness, rigidity, and spasm are other signs of peritoneal irritation. Patients may lie still and take only shallow breaths because movement worsens the pain. Abdominal distention, fever, tachycardia, tachypnea, nausea, vomiting, and altered bowel habits may be present. Complications include hypovolemic shock, sepsis, intraabdominal abscess formation, paralytic ileus, and acute respiratory distress syndrome. Peritonitis can be fatal if treatment is delayed.

Diagnostic Studies and Interprofessional Care

A CBC is done to assess for an elevated WBC count and evaluate fluid volume status. Peritoneal aspiration may be done with the fluid analyzed for blood, bile, pus, bacteria, fungus, and amylase content. An abdominal x-ray may show dilated loops of bowel consistent with paralytic ileus, free air if perforation has occurred, or air and fluid levels if an obstruction is present. Ultrasound and CT scans may identify ascites and abscesses. Peritoneoscopy may be helpful in patients without ascites. It allows for direct examination of the peritoneum and the ability to obtain specimens for diagnosis.

Patients with milder cases of peritonitis or those who are poor surgical risks receive conservative care. Treatment consists of antibiotics, NG suction, analgesics, and IV fluid administration. Surgery is done to locate the cause of the inflammation, drain purulent fluid, and repair any damage, such as to perforated organs.

NURSING MANAGEMENT: PERITONITIS

Assessment

Nursing care of patients with peritonitis is outlined in Table 47.21. Obtain a complete pain assessment, including location and quality. Note the presence of bowel sounds. Is there a change in bowel habits? Assess for increasing abdominal distention, guarding, rigidity, nausea, vomiting, and fever. Are there manifestations of hypovolemic shock?

Implementation

Patients with peritonitis are extremely ill and need skilled supportive care (Table 47.21).[10] Plan to give IV fluids to replace fluid lost to the peritoneal cavity and antibiotic therapy. Monitor patients for pain and administer analgesics. You may position patients with knees flexed to increase comfort. Sedatives may relieve anxiety and promote rest.

Monitor intake and output and electrolyte status to determine replacement therapy. Frequently monitor vital signs. Give antiemetics to decrease nausea and vomiting and prevent further fluid and electrolyte losses. Place patients on NPO status. Patients may need an NG tube to decrease gastric distention and further leakage of bowel contents into the peritoneum. Give O_2 therapy as needed.

TABLE 47.21 NURSING MANAGEMENT

Peritonitis

- Assess at regular intervals:
  - Vital signs with O_2 saturation
  - Pain assessment, including location and quality
  - Abdominal assessment, including bowel sounds, distention, rigidity
- Monitor results of CBC, including WBC, differential, and electrolytes, including glucose
- Administer IV fluids, electrolytes, and antibiotic therapy as ordered
- Implement measures to manage nausea/vomiting, including giving antiemetics (see Table 46.1)
- Implement measures to manage fever (see Table 12.5)
- Implement measures to manage pain (see Chapter 9)
- Apply O_2 to maintain O_2 saturation
- NPO status; advance diet as tolerated; obtain diet consult as needed
- NG to low-intermittent suction
- Implement VTE prophylaxis and encourage early ambulation
- Elevate head of bed and maintain a position of comfort
- Implement measures to promote rest and relieve anxiety
- Implement measures to prevent hyperglycemia

INFLAMMATORY BOWEL DISEASE

Crohn disease and ulcerative colitis are **inflammatory bowel disease (IBD)**. With IBD there is chronic inflammation of the GI tract characterized by exacerbations and periods of remission. We classify IBD based on clinical manifestations (Table 47.22). **Ulcerative colitis (UC)** is usually limited to the colon. **Crohn disease** can involve any part of the GI tract. About 1.3 million Americans have IBD. The peak incidence is in the 2nd to 4th decades of life.[11]

Etiology

We do not know the exact cause of the inflammation that leads to the tissue destruction in IBD. It is likely a combination of genetic and environment factors. Some agent or a combination of agents, such as bacteria, viruses, or food, triggers the body's immune system to produce inflammation. It may be an autoimmune disease, where there is an overactive or inappropriate immune response to these triggers in a genetically susceptible person.

The strongest risk factor is family history. Many people with IBD have a family member with the disorder. IBD occurs more often in someone with certain genetic syndromes, such as cystic fibrosis. There is a higher prevalence in those with other inflammatory disorders, such as psoriasis and multiple sclerosis. IBD occurs more often in those of White and Ashkenazic Jewish descent. It is also more common in people who live in urban areas, developed countries, and northern climates.[12]

The high diet intake of refined sugar, total fats, and ultra-processed foods common in developed countries seems to increase IBD risk.[11] Eating more raw fruits and vegetables and fiber decreases risk.[13] Lifestyle factors, such as smoking, obesity, and stress, do not cause IBD but can aggravate it. Nonsteroidal anti-inflammatory drugs (NSAIDs) and antibiotic use increase risk.[12]

Genetic Link

Over 200 genes are associated with IBD. Certain genetic mutations are associated with Crohn disease, others with UC, and many with both. Genetic variation may explain differences in patient responses to drug therapies for IBD. Many of the major genes, including *NOD2,* are involved in immune system function. The proteins made from these genes help the immune system sense and respond to bacteria in the GI tract. Changes in the *NOD2* gene prevent normal immune responses, allowing bacteria to grow unchecked and invade intestinal cells.[12]

TABLE 47.22 Comparison of Ulcerative Colitis and Crohn Disease

Characteristic	Ulcerative Colitis	Crohn Disease
Clinical		
Abdominal pain	Common, severe constant	Common, cramping
Diarrhea	Common	Common
Fever	During acute attacks	Common
Malabsorption and nutrition deficiencies	Minimal incidence	Common
Rectal bleeding	Common	Sometimes
Tenesmus	Common	Rare
Weight loss	Rare	Common, may be severe
Pathologic		
Location	Usually starts in rectum and spreads in a continuous pattern up the colon	Occurs anywhere along GI tract Most common site is distal ileum
Cobblestone mucosa	Rare	Common
Depth of involvement	Mucosa, or inner layer	All layers of bowel wall
Distribution	Continuous areas of inflammation	Healthy tissue interspersed with areas of inflammation (skip lesions)
Pseudopolyps	Common	Rare
Colorectal cancer risk	Higher	Lower
Main complications	Bleeding CDI Perforation with peritonitis Toxic megacolon	Bowel obstruction and strictures CDI Fistulas and fissures Perianal abscess

CDI, C. difficile infection.

Pathophysiology

There are key differences between Crohn disease and UC (Fig. 47.6). Crohn disease can occur anywhere in the GI tract. It most often involves the distal ileum and proximal colon. Segments of normal bowel can occur between diseased portions, called *skip lesions.* The inflammation in Crohn disease involves all layers of the bowel wall. Typically, ulcerations are deep, longitudinal, and penetrate between islands of inflamed edematous mucosa, causing the classic cobblestone appearance. Strictures at the areas of inflammation can cause bowel obstruction. Because the inflammation goes through the entire wall, microscopic leaks can allow bowel contents to enter the peritoneal cavity and cause abscesses or peritonitis. Fistulas are common.

UC is a disease of the colon. Inflammation and ulcerations occur in the mucosal layer, the innermost layer of the bowel wall. Fistulas and abscesses are rare because inflammation does not extend through all bowel wall layers. Because water and electrolytes are not absorbed through inflamed mucosa, diarrhea with large fluid and electrolyte losses occurs. Cell breakdown results in protein loss through the stool. Areas of inflamed mucosa form *pseudopolyps,* finger-like projections into the bowel lumen.

Based on location, there are 3 types of UC. In pancolitis, inflammation involves the entire colon. In ulcerative proctitis,

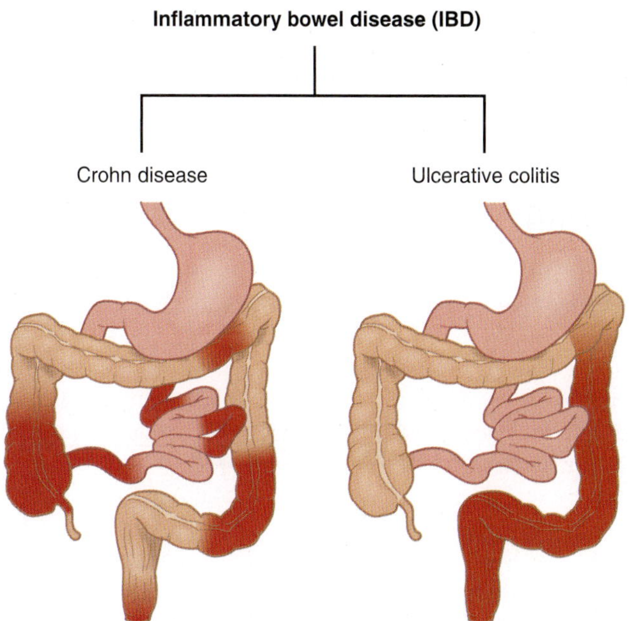

Fig. 47.6 Comparison of distribution patterns of UC and Crohn disease.

inflammation occurs only in the rectum. With left-sided UC, there is inflammation from the rectum to the descending colon.[14]

Clinical Manifestations

IBD is a chronic disorder with acute exacerbations that occur at unpredictable intervals. Although the hallmark symptoms are similar (diarrhea, weight loss, abdominal pain, fever, fatigue), there are differences (Table 47.22). In Crohn disease, diarrhea and cramping abdominal pain are common. Inflammation in the small intestine causes malabsorption and weight loss. Rectal bleeding occurs less often.

In UC, the main problems are bloody diarrhea and abdominal pain. Pain may vary from the mild lower abdominal cramping associated with diarrhea to severe, constant pain from perforations. With *mild disease,* diarrhea may consist of no more than 4 semiformed stools daily that contain small amounts of blood. Patients may have no other manifestations. In *moderate disease,* patients have increased stool output (up to 10 stools/day), increased bleeding, and systemic symptoms (fever, malaise, mild anemia, anorexia). In *severe disease,* diarrhea is bloody, contains mucus, and occurs 10 to 20 times a day. Fever, rapid weight loss, anemia, tachycardia, and dehydration are present.

Complications

Patients with IBD have both GI tract and systemic complications (Fig. 47.7). GI tract complications include hemorrhage,

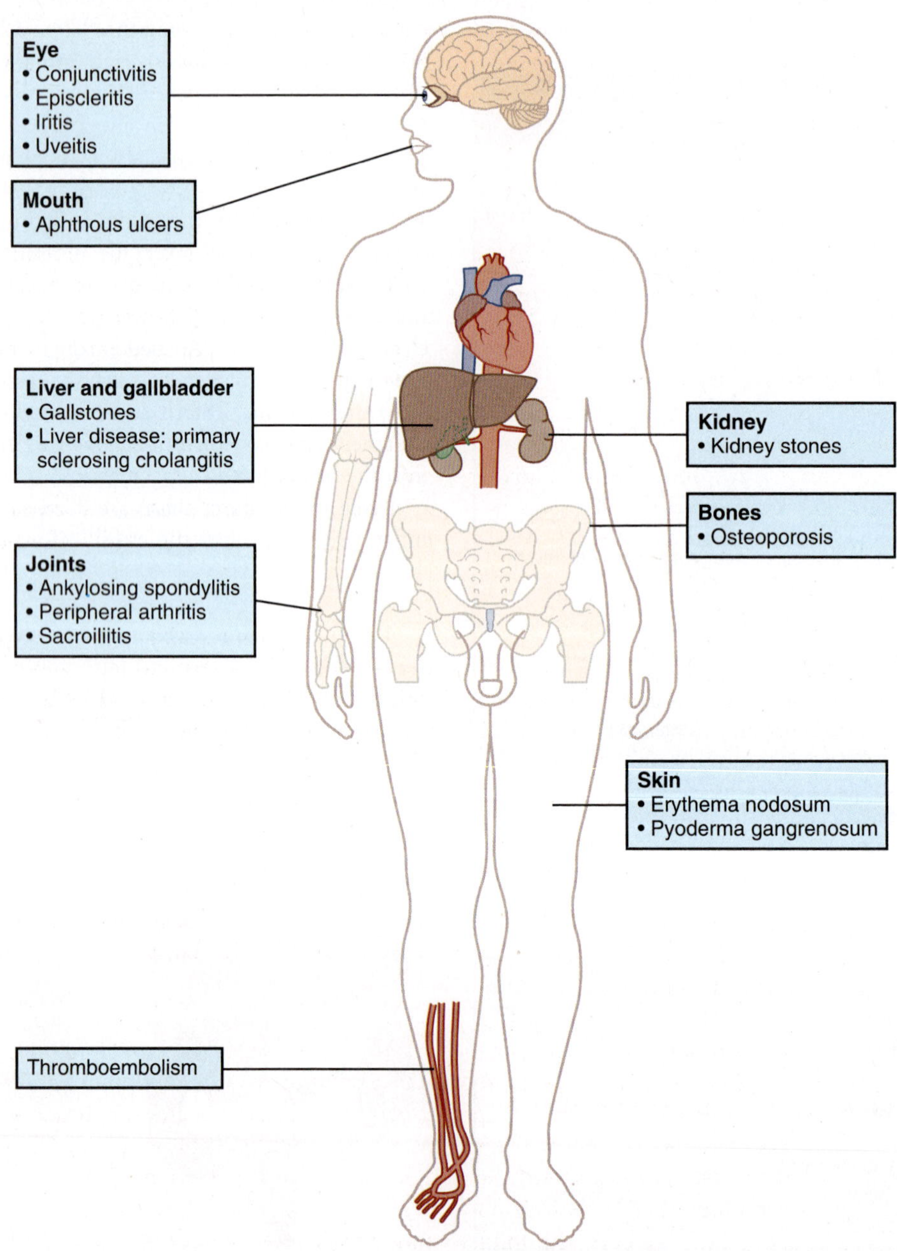

Fig. 47.7 Extraintestinal manifestations of IBD.

strictures, perforation (with possible peritonitis), abscesses, fistulas, and toxic megacolon. Toxic megacolon is more common with UC. Patients with toxic megacolon are at risk for perforation and may need an emergency colectomy. Perineal abscesses and fistulas occur in up to a third of patients with Crohn disease. CDI increases in frequency and severity. There is an increased risk for CRC.

Some systemic complications are related to inflammatory activity in the bowel. They occur with active inflammation and improve when IBD improves. Other complications include malabsorption, primary sclerosing cholangitis, and osteoporosis. Routine liver function tests are important because primary sclerosing cholangitis can lead to liver failure. Patients need a bone density scan at baseline and every 2 years.

Diagnostic Studies

The diagnosis of IBD involves the history and physical assessment, laboratory results, and imaging. The stool is examined for blood, pus, and mucus. Stool cultures determine whether CDI or other infection is present. A CBC typically shows iron deficiency anemia from blood loss. A high WBC count may be a sign of toxic megacolon or perforation. Decreased serum sodium, potassium, chloride, bicarbonate, and magnesium levels occur because of fluid and electrolyte losses from diarrhea and vomiting. Low albumin is present with severe disease because of protein loss. Increased erythrocyte sedimentation rate, C-reactive protein, and WBCs reflect inflammation.

The gold standard for diagnosis is endoscopy. Capsule endoscopy allows the HCP to see mucosal inflammatory changes in the small intestine. Colonoscopy allows for examination of the entire large intestine and sometimes the distal ileum. The HCP can assess the extent of inflammation, ulcerations, pseudopolyps, and strictures and obtain biopsy specimens. Other imaging studies include barium contrast studies, ultrasound, CT, and MRI.

Interprofessional Care

The goals of treatment of IBD are to (1) rest the bowel, (2) control inflammation, (3) correct malnutrition, (4) provide symptom relief, and (5) improve quality of life. There is no cure for IBD. Drug therapy is the main treatment (Table 47.23).

TABLE 47.23 Interprofessional Care

Inflammatory Bowel Disease

Diagnostic Assessment

- History and physical assessment
- Laboratory testing: CBC, erythrocyte sedimentation rate, chemistries
- Testing of stool for occult blood and infection
- Imaging
  - Endoscopy: Capsule endoscopy, colonoscopy
  - Barium contrast
  - Ultrasound studies

Management

- Diet therapy
  - High-calorie, high-vitamin, high-protein diet
  - Enteral nutrition during exacerbations
- Drug therapy (Table 47.24)
- Physical and emotional rest
- Referral for counseling or support group
- Surgical therapy (Table 47.25)

Drug Therapy

The goal of drug treatment is to induce and maintain remission. Several classes of drugs are used (Table 47.24). Drug choice depends on the disease location and severity. Antiinflammatory drugs are given to reduce inflammation with Crohn disease. The recommended treatment to induce and maintain remission in mild to moderate UC is a mesalazine agent.[14] They are available as suppositories, enemas, foams, or oral formulas. Oral mesalazine combined with a mesalazine enema is more effective than either alone.[13] Patients with mild or moderate proctitis should receive rectal mesalazine therapy. Rectal use delivers the drug directly to the affected tissue.

Patients with more severe disease need corticosteroids and biologics for symptom relief. Maintenance therapy relies on immunosuppressants, biologics, and small molecules.

Biologics reduce inflammation by blocking specific proteins that play a role in inflammation. There are 3 main classes: anti–tumor necrosis factor (TNF) agents, alpha 4–integrin inhibitors, and interleukin (IL)-12/23 antagonists (see Table 14.18). The anti-TNF agents are the most effective. They include infliximab (Remicade), adalimumab, and certolizumab pegol. Alpha 4–integrin inhibitors such as vedolizumab (Entyvio) are limited to those who have not had a good response with other therapies.

Oral prednisone is given to patients with mild to moderate disease who did not respond to mesalazine. Those with severe inflammation may need a short course of IV corticosteroids. Corticosteroids are given for the shortest possible time because of the side effects from long-term use. Dosage must be tapered when surgery is planned to reduce complications (e.g., infection, delayed wound healing).

Symptom treatment includes antidiarrheals, antiemetics, and antispasmodics. Patients with an infection or fistula receive antibiotics. Commonly used drugs include ciprofloxacin, vancomycin, and metronidazole.

Surgical Therapy

Indications for surgery are outlined in Table 47.25. Surgery is usually only done for acute complications or those who do not respond to therapy. Because UC affects only the colon, a total colectomy with ileostomy or IPAA is curative. Many patients with Crohn disease eventually need surgery. The most common surgery involves resecting the diseased segments with

TABLE 47.24 Drug Therapy

Inflammatory Bowel Disease

Class	Action	Examples
5-Aminosalicylates (5-ASA)	Decrease inflammation by suppressing proinflammatory cytokines and other inflammatory mediators in the intestine. Maintain remission and prevent flare-ups in mild to moderate UC.	*Systemic:* balsalazide (Colazal), mesalamine (Apriso, Delzicol, Lialda, Pentasa), olsalazine (Dipentum), sulfasalazine (Azulfidine) *Topical:* 5-ASA enema, foam, suppositories
Biologic therapies (see Table 14.18)	*Anti-TNF agents:* Induce and maintain remission.	adalimumab (Humira), certolizumab pegol (Cimzia), golimumab (Simponi), infliximab (Remicade)
	Integrin receptor antagonists: Induce and maintain remission.	natalizumab (Tysabri), vedolizumab (Entyvio)
	IL-12/23 antagonists: Induce and maintain remission.	risankizumab (Skyrizi), ustekinumab (Stelara)
Corticosteroids	Prevent or decrease inflammation of the intestinal mucosa. Mainly induction therapy.	*Systemic:* prednisone, prednisolone, budesonide, methylprednisolone *Topical:* hydrocortisone suppository, foam (Cortifoam), enema (Cortenema)
Immunomodulators	Suppress immune response. Have a delayed onset of action. Not useful for acute flare-ups. Best for maintenance therapy.	azathioprine, cyclosporine, methotrexate, 6-mercaptopurine, tacrolimus
Synthetic small molecule	Decrease inflammation in the gut by targeting parts of the immune system. Cannot be taken with other biologic or immunosuppressive therapies. For moderate to severe UC.	filgotinib (Jyseleca), ozanimod (Zeposia), tofacitinib (Xeljanz), upadacitinib (Rinvoq)

IL, Interleukin; *TNF,* tumor necrosis factor; *UC,* ulcerative colitis.

TABLE 47.25 Indications for Surgery for Inflammatory Bowel Disease

- Abscess
- Bowel obstruction
- Cancer
- Fistula
- GI hemorrhage
- Lack of response to conservative therapy
- Perforation, impending or actual
- Severe anorectal disease
- Strictures

reanastomosis of the remaining intestine. Unfortunately, the disease often recurs at the anastomosis site. Repeated removal of sections of the small intestine can lead to SBS, which is discussed later in this chapter.

The other common surgery for Crohn disease is strictureplasty. This opens narrowed areas obstructing the bowel. Because the intestine stays intact, it reduces the risk of developing SBS and its associated complications. Recurrences at the site are rare.

Nutrition Therapy

The goals of diet management are to (1) correct and prevent malnutrition, (2) replace fluid and electrolyte losses, and (3) prevent weight loss. Many patients with IBD are malnourished. This makes an individualized diet an important part of treating IBD. Patients need a balanced, healthy diet with enough calories, protein, and nutrients. Consult a dietitian about the ideal diet.

The severity of malnutrition is influenced by the activity, duration and extent of disease, and the degree of inflammation.[11] Blood loss and malabsorption lead to iron deficiency anemia (see Chapter 34). Patients may need oral iron supplements. IV iron is an option for those who cannot tolerate oral iron or if anemia is severe.

Disease in the terminal ileum reduces absorption of cobalamin and bile acids. Reduced cobalamin contributes to anemia. Those who develop anemia should receive cobalamin injections. Bile salts are important for fat absorption and contribute to osmotic diarrhea. Cholestyramine, an ion-exchange resin that binds unabsorbed bile salts, helps control diarrhea.

Drug therapy can contribute to nutrition problems. Patients taking sulfasalazine or methotrexate should take folic acid daily to decrease the chance of folate deficiency.[11] Those receiving corticosteroids are prone to osteoporosis and need calcium supplements.

If oral feeding is not tolerable or insufficient, patients should receive EN. EN is preferred over parenteral nutrition (PN) because atrophy of the gut and bacterial overgrowth occur when the GI tract is not used. Patients with SBS, an obstruction, or other complications may need PN. Patients who are malnourished may need EN and/or PN before IBD surgery.

There are no universal food triggers for IBD. Some find that certain foods cause diarrhea. A food diary helps to identify problem foods to avoid. We usually teach patients to avoid or limit foods that cause GI distress or worsen symptoms.

NURSING MANAGEMENT: INFLAMMATORY BOWEL DISEASE

Assessment

Table 47.26 outlines the subjective and objective data to obtain from patients with IBD.

Clinical Problems

Clinical problems for patients with IBD include:

- Impaired bowel elimination
- Nutritionally compromised
- Difficulty coping
- Pain

For more information on clinical problems and interventions for IBD, see eNursing Care Plan 47.2 on the website for this chapter.

TABLE 47.26 NURSING ASSESSMENT

Inflammatory Bowel Disease

Subjective Data

Important Health Information

Health history: Infection, autoimmune disorders

Medications: Antidiarrheal drugs

Functional Health Patterns

Health perception–health management: Family history of IBD. Fatigue, malaise

Nutritional-metabolic: Nausea, vomiting, anorexia. Weight loss

Elimination: Diarrhea. Blood, mucus, pus in stools

Cognitive-perceptual: Pain, cramping, tenesmus

Coping-stress: Impact of symptoms on quality of life, coping with symptoms

Objective Data

General

Intermittent fever, emaciated appearance, fatigue, weight loss

Cardiovascular

↑ HR, ↓ BP

GI

Abdominal distention, hyperactive bowel sounds, abdominal pain, cramping. Diarrhea. Rectal bleeding

Skin

Pale skin with poor turgor, dry mucous membranes. Skin lesions, anorectal irritation, fistulas, skin tags

Possible Diagnostic Findings

Anemia, ↑ WBC, CRP. Electrolyte imbalance, low albumin, vitamin and trace metal deficiencies. Guaiac-positive stool. Abnormal endoscopy and/or barium contrast study findings

CRP, C-reactive protein.

Planning

The overall goals are that patients with IBD will (1) have fewer and less severe exacerbations, (2) maintain fluid and electrolyte balance, (3) be free from discomfort, (4) maintain nutrition balance, and (5) have an improved quality of life.

Implementation

Acute Care

During the acute phase, focus your attention on hemodynamic stability, pain control, fluid and electrolyte balance, and nutrition support (Table 47.27). Give IV fluids, electrolytes, analgesics, and antiinflammatory drugs as prescribed. Monitor serum electrolytes, CBC, and vital signs, being alert for changes related to diarrhea and dehydration. Teach patients with orthostatic hypotension to change position slowly and use safety precautions.

Postoperative care after surgery for IBD is similar to that described in the sections on bowel resection and ostomy surgery and in the general nursing care of postoperative patients (see Chapter 20).

Chronic Care

Assist patients in accepting the chronicity of IBD and learning ways to cope with its recurrent, unpredictable nature (Box 47.1). Teaching includes (1) rest and diet management, (2) perianal care, (3) drug action and side effects, (4) symptoms of recurrence of disease, (5) when to seek medical care, and (6) ways to reduce stress. Excellent teaching resources are available from the Crohn and Colitis Foundation of America (www.crohnscolitisfoundation.org). They also host local and online support groups that can help patients cope.

Patients and caregivers may need your help setting realistic short- and long-term goals. Patients may have severe fatigue, which limits their energy for physical activity. Rest is important. Patients may lose sleep because of frequent episodes of diarrhea and abdominal pain. Nutrition deficiencies and anemia worsen

TABLE 47.27 NURSING MANAGEMENT

Patient With Acute Inflammatory Bowel Disease

- Give IV fluids and electrolyte replacement as ordered
- Monitor for signs of dehydration and electrolyte imbalances
- Implement pain management measures and promote a restful environment
- Maintain intake and output and obtain daily weight
- Implement measures to control diarrhea and reduce perianal irritation
- Assess for blood in stools and emesis
- Evaluate daily calorie intake
- Assess the abdomen, including bowel sounds; note pain, distention
- Consult with a dietitian about diet modifications and the need for nutrition supplements
- Report signs of peritonitis, bowel perforation to HCP
- Provide patient teaching about diet, drug therapy, coping strategies, perianal care, and when to contact the HCP

BOX 47.1 EVIDENCE-BASED PRACTICE

Online Support for Patients With IBD

You are working in an outpatient clinic in a small community hospital. Many patients who come to the clinic live in rural areas and must drive 45 to 90 minutes one way to receive care for IBD. Many express feelings of being unsupported between office visits, leading to increased emotional stress and more frequent exacerbations of IBD.

Making Clinical Decisions

Synthesis of Best Available Evidence

Rural patients with IBD face unique challenges extending beyond disease management, including economic hardship and social isolation. Research findings highlight the need for tailored interventions to bridge health care gaps and improve the quality of life for rural patients.

Clinician Expertise

The clinic nursing staff previously developed a standard education program for patients with IBD. The program's goal is to help patients manage their symptoms so they can have improved quality of life. This program was designed for in-person delivery accompanied by an optional patient support group meeting once a week. Through a coordinated effort, the program was redesigned to give patients online or telephone-based access to education information with a video conference option for the weekly peer support meetings.

Patient Preferences and Values

Nurses contacted all patients with IBD to offer enrollment in the revised program. Within 3 months, there was an overall 30% increase in patient participation in the educational program, with a 45% increase in peer support group participation. Patients shared feeling less isolated and more in control of their IBD symptoms.

Implications for Nursing Practice

1. What questions could you ask program participants to assess for improvement in self-care strategies and lessened feelings of isolation?
2. How could a similar program be implemented for patients with other chronic conditions?

Reference for Evidence

Boscoe V, Mercuri C, Daldo P, et al: The lived experience of adults with inflammatory bowel disease in rural areas: a phenomenological study, *Nurs Health Sci, 27*:e70058, 2025.

fatigue and leave patients feeling weak. Teach them to schedule activities around rest periods.

Given the uncertainty of the frequency and severity of flares, many patients struggle with depression and anxiety. Behavioral therapy may help patients deal with their feelings about the disease and help manage their symptoms. Because of the relationship between emotions and the GI tract, teach patients ways to manage stress (see Chapter 7). Talk with those who smoke who have Crohn disease about quitting because it can cause more severe disease.

Evaluation

The expected outcomes are that patients with IBD will:

- Have a decrease in the number of diarrhea stools
- Maintain body weight within a normal range
- Be free from discomfort
- Use effective coping strategies

Gerontologic Considerations: Inflammatory Bowel Disease

The cause, natural history, and clinical course of IBD are similar to those seen in younger patients, though some differences exist. In older patients, proctitis and left-sided UC are more common. Drug therapy and surgery have an increased risk for adverse events, hospitalization, and mortality. Immunomodulator and biologic therapies have a higher risk for infection and cancer. Anemia and malnutrition are more common. They are more vulnerable to volume depletion from diarrhea.

FUNCTIONAL GI PROBLEMS

IRRITABLE BOWEL SYNDROME

Irritable bowel syndrome (IBS) is a disorder characterized by chronic abdominal pain and altered bowel patterns. Patients may have diarrhea or constipation or a mix of both. IBS more commonly affects females and people under age 50.

IBS has no known cause. The most well-recognized trigger is an episode of acute gastroenteritis. This occurs in around 10% of patients.[15] Genetics, hypersensitivity, GI motility problems, or altered GI microbiota may be involved. Many factors appear to worsen IBS. These include increased stress, anxiety, depression, and Celiac disease.[15] Foods high in fermentable oligo-, di-, and monosaccharides and polyols (FODMAPs) lead to increased GI water secretion and increased fermentation in the gut. This causes distention, bloating, and gas.

IBS is diagnosed solely on symptoms. The Rome IV criteria for diagnosing IBS require the presence of abdominal pain and/or discomfort at least 1 day per week for 3 months that is associated with 2 or more of the following: related to defecation, change in stool frequency, and change in the stool form.[15] Depending on the stool patterns, IBS is categorized as IBS with constipation (IBS-C), IBS with diarrhea (IBS-D), IBS mixed, and IBS unsubtyped. Other common symptoms include abdominal distention, nausea, flatulence, bloating, urgency, mucus in the stool, and sensation of incomplete evacuation. Non-GI symptoms may include fatigue, headache, and sleep problems.

The key to diagnosis is the history and physical assessment. Ask patients to describe symptoms, health history, family history, and drug and diet history. Assess if and how IBS symptoms interfere with school, work, and social activities. Diagnostic tests are used to rule out other disorders, such as CRC, IBD, food allergies, and malabsorption disorders (lactose intolerance, celiac disease).

No single therapy is effective for all patients with IBS. Treatment includes psychologic support, diet and lifestyle changes, and drugs to regulate stool output and reduce discomfort. Patients may benefit from keeping a diary of symptoms, diet, and episodes of stress to help identify any factors that trigger IBS symptoms. Cognitive-behavior therapy and stress management techniques may help patients cope. Regular exercise reduces bloating, constipation, and stress-related symptoms.

Traditional diet teaching focuses on eating regular meals, reducing caffeine and alcohol intake, and maintaining adequate hydration.[15] Fiber intake is increased in patients with constipation and reduced if they have diarrhea. Tell patients with bloating or flatulence to avoid common gas-producing foods, such as legumes. Probiotics can improve symptoms.

If traditional diet approaches are ineffective, patients should consider an exclusion diet. The FODMAP diet (fermentable oligosaccharides, disaccharides, monosaccharides, and polyols) is the most widely used.[16] Restricting the intake of FODMAPs may improve symptoms by changing the GI microbiota.

Drug therapy focuses on the dominant bowel symptom and pain. Patients can benefit from tricyclic antidepressants and antispasmodic agents (hyoscyamine, dicyclomine).[17,18] Antispasmodics decrease GI motility and smooth muscle spasms, reducing pain.

Treatment for IBS-D includes rifaximin, eluxadoline, and alosetron.[17] Eluxadoline decreases colon contractions to reduce diarrhea and pain. Alosetron is only given to females with severe IBS-D that did not respond to other therapy. Because of serious side effects (severe constipation, ischemic colitis), it is available only in a restricted access program. Rifaximin is given as a 2-week course of treatment with up to 2 repeated courses.

Besides laxative therapy, treatment for IBS-C focuses on drugs that increase peristalsis and intestinal fluid volume. These include linaclotide, plecanatide, and tenapanor. Females with IBS-C may receive lubiprostone.[18]

BOWEL OBSTRUCTION

A **bowel obstruction**, or intestinal obstruction, occurs when intestinal contents cannot pass through the GI tract. The obstruction may occur in the small (SBO) or large (LBO) intestine. It can be partial or complete, simple or strangulated. Partial obstructions do not completely occlude the intestinal lumen, allowing for some fluid and gas to pass through. They usually resolve with conservative treatment. A complete obstruction totally occludes the lumen and usually requires surgery. A simple obstruction has an intact blood supply; a strangulated one does not.

Types

Bowel obstructions are mechanical or nonmechanical.

Mechanical

In *mechanical obstruction,* there is a physical obstruction of the intestinal lumen. Most occur in the small intestine. Surgical adhesions are the most common cause of SBO. They can occur within days of surgery or years later (Fig. 47.8). Other causes of SBO are hernia, tumors, and strictures from Crohn disease. The

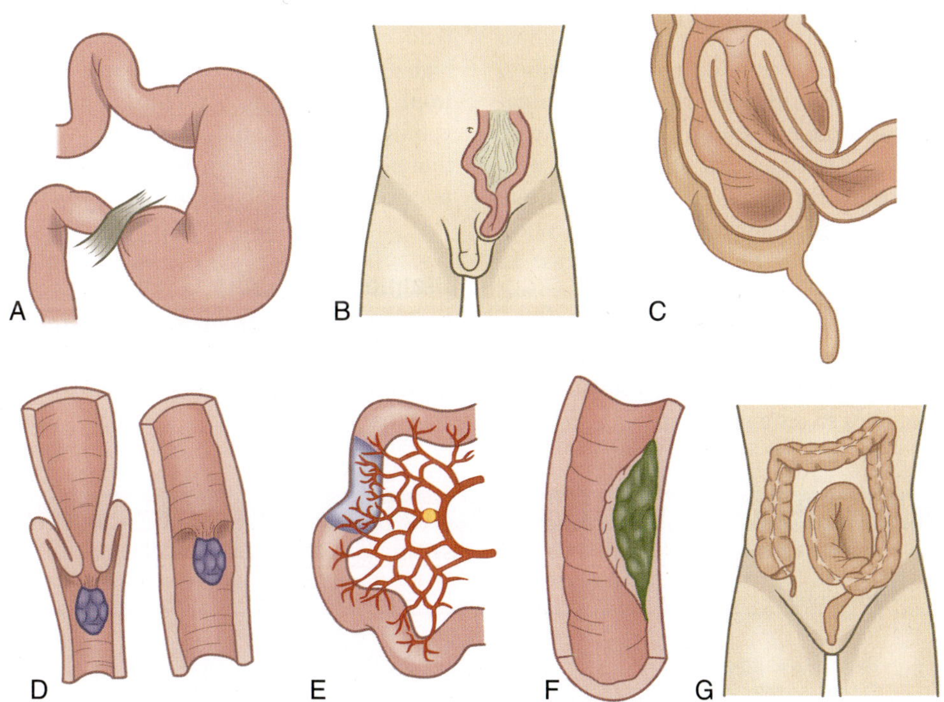

Fig. 47.8 Bowel obstructions. (A) Adhesions. (B) Strangulated inguinal hernia. (C) Ileocecal intussusception. (D) Intussusception from polyps. (E) Mesenteric occlusion. (F) Neoplasm. (G) Volvulus of the sigmoid colon.

most common cause of LBO is CRC, followed by diverticular disease. Other causes include volvulus, hernias, and IBD.[19]

Nonmechanical

A *nonmechanical obstruction* occurs with reduced or absent peristalsis caused by altered neuromuscular transmission of the parasympathetic innervation to the bowel. It may result from a neuromuscular or vascular problem. **Paralytic ileus** (lack of intestinal peristalsis and bowel sounds) is the most common form of nonmechanical obstruction. It occurs to some degree after abdominal surgery. Other causes of paralytic ileus include peritonitis, inflammation (e.g., acute pancreatitis, appendicitis), and electrolyte imbalances (especially hypokalemia).

Pseudoobstruction is a GI motility disorder that mimics a mechanical obstruction. Patients have symptoms of obstruction but without any cause found with imaging. Several conditions are associated with pseudoobstruction. These include neurologic problems, myocardial infarction, kidney disease, and trauma. Patients who use opiates or recently had major orthopedic surgery are at risk.[19]

Vascular obstructions from an interference with the blood supply to a part of the intestines are rare. The most common causes are emboli and atherosclerosis of the mesenteric arteries. Emboli may originate from thrombi in patients who have chronic atrial fibrillation, diseased heart valves, and prosthetic valves. Venous thrombosis may occur in conditions of low blood flow, such as heart failure and shock.

Pathophysiology

When an obstruction occurs, fluid, gas, and intestinal contents accumulate proximal to the obstruction. Distention reduces fluid absorption and initially stimulates intestinal secretions. Distal to the obstruction, the bowel empties and then collapses. As distention increases in the proximal bowel, intraluminal bowel pressure rises. The increased pressure leads to an increase in capillary permeability and extravasation of fluids and electrolytes into the peritoneal cavity. Eventually, the intestinal muscle becomes fatigued, and peristalsis stops. Fluid retention in the intestine and peritoneal cavity leads to a decrease in circulating blood volume. This leads to hypotension and hypovolemic shock.

If blood flow is inadequate, bowel tissue becomes ischemic, then necrotic. The bowel may perforate. In the most dangerous situation, the bowel becomes so distended that the blood flow stops, causing edema, cyanosis, and gangrene of a bowel segment. This is called *intestinal strangulation* or *intestinal infarction.* If not quickly corrected, the bowel will become necrotic and rupture, leading to infection, septic shock, and death.

Clinical Manifestations

The 4 hallmark manifestations of an obstruction are abdominal pain, vomiting, distention, and constipation. The order and degree in which these appear vary by the cause, location, and type of obstruction (Table 47.28). Colicky abdominal pain is usually the first symptom.[19] In SBO, the pain is often of sudden onset and severe. Patients with LBO have persistent, cramping abdominal pain.

With SBO there is a short interval between the onset of pain and vomiting. The nature of the vomit gives a clue to the level of obstruction. In a proximal obstruction, patients rapidly develop vomiting. It may be projectile and contain bile. Vomiting usually gives temporary relief from abdominal pain in higher obstructions. As the site of the obstruction moves more distal, vomiting is more gradual in onset and more fecal and foul smelling. In LBO, vomiting is rare.

The more distal the obstruction, the greater the degree of abdominal distention. Absolute constipation, or the failure to pass stool or flatus, occurs earlier in LBO. Bowel sounds are usually present and become progressively hypoactive. Bowel sounds are usually absent with paralytic ileus.

With both types, abdominal tenderness and rigidity occur. Patients appear acutely ill, with signs of dehydration and sepsis. These include tachycardia, dry mucous membranes, and hypotension. The temperature may rise above 100°F (37.8°C).

The location of the obstruction determines the extent of fluid, electrolyte, and acid-base imbalances. If the obstruction is high (e.g., upper duodenum), metabolic alkalosis may result from the loss of gastric hydrochloric (HCl) acid through vomiting or NG intubation and suction. With SBO, dehydration occurs rapidly. Dehydration and electrolyte imbalances do not occur early in LBO.

Diagnostic Studies

Perform a history and physical assessment. Imaging can identify an obstruction and guide decisions about surgery. Abdominal x-rays and CT scan may be done. Sigmoidoscopy or colonoscopy provides direct visualization of an LBO.

TABLE 47.28 Manifestations of Bowel Obstructions

	SMALL INTESTINE		
Manifestation	**Proximal**	**Distal**	**Large Intestine**
Onset	Rapid	Rapid	Gradual
Vomiting	Frequent and copious	Less frequent	Late or absent
Pain	Colicky, cramping, occurs at frequent intervals	Colicky, occurs more intermittently	Persistent, cramping
Bowel movement	Feces for a short time	Gradual constipation	Obstipation
Abdominal distention	Minimal	↑	↑

Blood tests include a CBC and blood chemistries. A high WBC count may mean strangulation or perforation. Decreased hemoglobin and hematocrit values may mean bleeding from cancer or strangulation with necrosis. Monitor serum electrolytes, BUN, and creatinine to assess for dehydration.

Interprofessional Care

The goal is to regain intestinal patency and resolve the obstruction. Treatment depends on the cause. Surgery may involve simply resecting the obstructed segment of bowel and anastomosing the remaining healthy bowel back together. Partial or total colectomy, colostomy, or ileostomy may be done with an extensive obstruction or necrosis. If a strangulated obstruction or perforation is present, patients will need emergency surgery to relieve the obstruction.

Sometimes an obstruction may resolve without surgery. Colonoscopy offers a means to remove polyps, dilate strictures, and remove tumors. Stents can be placed via endoscopy. They are used for palliative purposes or as "a bridge to surgery," allowing patients to avoid emergency surgery. This gives time to correct fluid volume and other problems, thus improving surgical outcomes.

Patients need fluid and electrolyte replacement. Some may have an NG tube for decompression. Some patients need PN to allow bowel rest and improve nutrition status before surgery. Corticosteroids with antiemetic properties that decrease inflammation may be used.

NURSING MANAGEMENT: BOWEL OBSTRUCTION

An obstruction is potentially life threatening. Major concerns are preventing fluid and electrolyte imbalances and early recognition of deterioration (e.g., hypovolemic shock, sepsis; Table 47.29). Obtain a history and physical assessment. Determine the location, duration, intensity, and frequency of abdominal pain. Implement pain management measures.

Record the onset, frequency, color, odor, and amount of vomitus. Assess bowel function, including the passage of flatus.

TABLE 47.29 NURSING MANAGEMENT

Patient With a Bowel Obstruction

- Give IV fluids and electrolyte replacement as ordered
- Monitor for signs of dehydration and electrolyte imbalances
- Maintain the patient on NPO status
- Implement pain management measures and promote a restful environment
- Maintain intake and output; obtain daily weight
- Insert an indwelling urinary catheter; report if the urine output is less than 0.5 mL/kg/h
- Provide frequent oral care and water-soluble lubricant for the lips
- Implement measures to control nausea and vomiting (see Chapter 46)
- Check the NG tube every 4 hours for patency

Auscultate for bowel sounds. Inspect the abdomen for scars, visible masses, and distention. Assess whether abdominal tenderness or rigidity is present. Measure the abdominal girth. Check for signs of peritoneal irritation (e.g., muscle guarding, rebound pain). If the HCP decides to wait to see if the obstruction resolves on its own, assess the patient regularly. Notify the HCP of changes in vital signs, changes in bowel sounds, decreased urine output, increased abdominal distention, and pain.

Implement measures to promote fluid and electrolyte balance. Maintain a strict intake and output record, including emesis and tube drainage. A urinary catheter allows for hourly monitoring of urine output.[19] Report if the urine output is less than 0.5 mL/kg of body weight per hour. This indicates inadequate vascular volume and the potential for acute kidney injury. Monitor laboratory and ABG values. Rising serum creatinine and BUN levels are other indicators of acute kidney injury. Administer fluids and electrolyte replacement as ordered. If the patient has abdominal surgery, provide care appropriate for the type of surgery.

LARGE INTESTINE POLYPS

Polyps arise from the mucosal surface of the colon and project into the lumen. They may be *sessile* (flat, broad-based, and attached directly to the intestinal wall) or *pedunculated* (attached to the bowel wall by a thin stalk). Polyps tend to be sessile when small and become pedunculated as they enlarge. They may be found anywhere in the large intestine. As patients age, polyps are increasingly present in the proximal colon. Most patients with polyps are asymptomatic. Rectal bleeding and occult blood in the stool are the most common signs.

The most common types of polyps are hyperplastic and adenomatous. *Hyperplastic polyps* are noncancerous. They rarely grow larger than 5 mm and never cause clinical symptoms. Other benign polyps include inflammatory polyps, lipomas, and juvenile polyps.

Adenomatous polyps are neoplastic and closely linked to CRC. There are 3 types: tubular, tubulovillous, and villous. Villous or large adenomatous polyps are more likely to have cancers develop in them. Removing adenomatous polyps decreases the occurrence of CRC.

Genetic Link

Familial adenomatous polyposis (FAP) is the most common polyposis syndrome.[20] It is a genetic disorder characterized by hundreds or sometimes thousands of polyps in the colon. They appear during adolescence and early adulthood. They eventually become cancerous, usually by age 40. Because CRC is inevitable, the colon and rectum are removed, usually by age 25, by proctocolectomy with an IPAA or an ileostomy. Patients with classic FAP are at risk for cancers of the thyroid, stomach, small intestine, liver, and brain, so lifetime cancer surveillance is essential.

Colonoscopy, barium enema, and virtual colonoscopy (CT or MRI colonography) are used to discover polyps. All polyps are considered abnormal. They should be removed *(polypectomy)* during colonoscopy or with surgery. After polypectomy, watch patients for rectal bleeding, fever, severe abdominal pain, and abdominal distention. These may indicate hemorrhage or perforation.

COLORECTAL CANCER

CRC is the second leading cause of cancer-related deaths. Each year about 153,000 people in the United States are diagnosed with CRC and 53,000 people die of CRC.[21]

Although about 85% of new CRC cases are detected in people older than 50, this rate has been slowly decreasing. The number of cases in people aged 20 to 49 years is rising and is expected to continue to do so.[21] We think this is related to diet, physical inactivity, and increasing rates of obesity.

Etiology and Pathophysiology

No single risk factor accounts for most cases of CRC (Table 47.30). It is higher in those with first-degree relatives with CRC and people with IBD. About 30% of cases of CRC occur in patients with a family history of CRC. About 5% of people have inherited gene mutations, including FAP and hereditary nonpolyposis colorectal cancer (HNPCC) syndrome (Box 47.2).[21]

About 30% to 50% of people with CRC have an abnormal *KRAS* gene. The *KRAS* gene, which is involved in regulating cell division, belongs to a class of genes known as *oncogenes.* When mutated, oncogenes have the potential to cause normal cells to become cancerous.

CRC usually starts as a polyp on the inner lining of the colon or rectum that grows over a period of 10 to 20 years. Most polyps are adenomas, which arise from the cells that make mucus. As the tumor grows, the cancer invades and penetrates the wall of the colon or rectum (Fig. 47.9). Eventually, cancer cells gain access to the lymph nodes and vascular system and spread to distant sites. Because venous blood leaving the colon and rectum flows through the portal vein and the inferior rectal vein, the liver is a common site of metastasis. The cancer spreads from the liver to other sites, including the lungs, bones, and brain. CRC can spread directly into adjacent structures.

TABLE 47.30 Risk Factors for Colorectal Cancer

- Age
- Alcohol (≥4 drinks/week)
- Cigarette smoking
- Family history of CRC in first-degree relative
- Family or personal history of familial adenomatous polyposis (FAP)
- Family or personal history of hereditary nonpolyposis colorectal cancer (HNPCC) syndrome
- Inflammatory bowel disease
- Obesity (body mass index ≥30 kg/m^2)
- Red meat (≥7 servings/week)

Clinical Manifestations

CRC develops slowly. Symptoms often do not appear until the disease is advanced. Nonspecific findings in early disease include fatigue and weight loss. As the disease progresses, patients may have abdominal pain and tenderness with a change

BOX 47.2 GENETICS IN CLINICAL PRACTICE

Hereditary Nonpolyposis Colorectal Cancer (HNPCC)

Genetic Basis

- Autosomal dominant disorder
- Mutations in *MSH2, MLH1, MSH6,* or *PMS2* genes
- These genes are involved with the repair of mistakes in DNA replication

Incidence

- Affects 1 in 500 to 2000 people

Clinical Implications

- Accounts for 3% to 5% of all colorectal cancer (CRC) cases
- Depending on the genetic mutation, the risk for developing CRC is from 50% to 80%
- If colon polyps are present, they occur at an earlier age than do polyps in the general population and are more prone to become cancerous
- Have increased risk for stomach, brain, ovary, uterus, skin, urinary tract, small bowel, and bile duct cancers
- Colonoscopy is recommended every 1 to 2 years
- Females with HNPCC should undergo ovarian and endometrial cancer screening

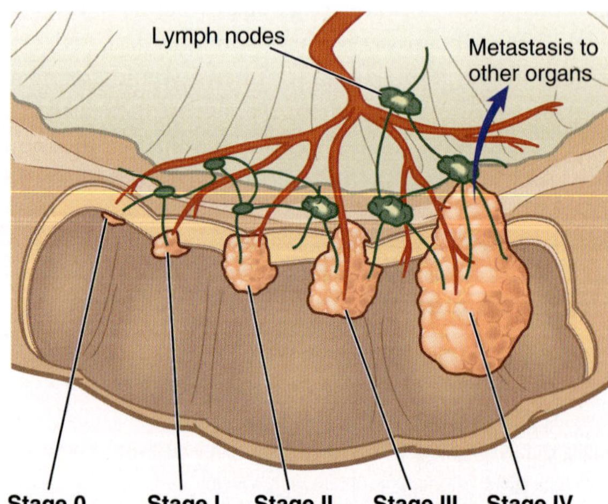

Fig. 47.9 The 5 stages of CRC. Stage 0 cancer has not grown beyond the mucosal layer. Stage I cancer has grown beyond the mucosa into the submucosa, but no lymph nodes are involved. Stage II cancer has grown beyond the submucosa into the muscle, but there is no lymph node involvement or metastasis. Stage III cancer is any tumor with lymph node involvement but no metastasis. Stage IV cancer is any tumor with lymph node involvement and metastasis.

in bowel habits. There may be a palpable abdominal mass, hepatomegaly, or ascites.

Bleeding can occur with both right- and left-sided CRC. Bleeding on the right side is more common than on the left side. It is often unrecognized. An early manifestation is often anemia. Hematochezia (fresh blood in the stool) is more often caused by left-sided CRC than right-sided CRC.

Right-sided cancers are more likely to cause diarrhea. Left-sided cancers are usually detected later and could present with LBO (Fig. 47.10). Other complications include perforation, peritonitis, and fistula formation.

Diagnostic Studies

Obtain a health history with close attention to family history (Table 47.31). Because symptoms of CRC often are not evident until the disease is advanced, there is an increased emphasis on screening. Beginning at age 45 and continuing until age 75, those at average risk for CRC should have a stool-based or visual screening test to detect polyps and cancer:

- Visual tests:
  - Flexible sigmoidoscopy (every 5 years)
  - Colonoscopy (every 10 years)
  - CT colonography (virtual colonoscopy) (every 5 years)
- Stool-based tests:
  - High-sensitivity fecal occult blood test (FOBT) (every year)
  - Fecal immunochemical test (FIT) (every year)
  - Stool DNA test (every 3 years)

Colonoscopy is the gold standard for CRC screening. It allows the entire colon to be examined, biopsies obtained, and polyps removed. People at average risk for CRC should undergo colonoscopy every 10 years beginning at age 45. For persons age 76 to 85, the decision to screen should be based on history, CRC risk, and patient preference. Screening is not recommended after age 85.[22]

Persons at risk (Table 47.30) should begin screening earlier and have screening done more often. Those who have a first-degree relative who developed CRC before age 60 or have 2 first-degree relatives with CRC should have a colonoscopy every 5 years beginning at age 40 or 10 years earlier than when the youngest relative developed cancer. Those who have 1 first-degree relative who had CRC after age 60 should have a colonoscopy every 10 years beginning at age 40.

FOBT and FIT look for blood in the stool. These tests must be done yearly. Tumor bleeding occurs at intervals and may easily be missed if a single test is done. Stool DNA tests (PreGen-Plus, Cologuard) can detect cells with DNA mutations that may occur with CRC in the stool.

Once tissue biopsies confirm the diagnosis of CRC, patients need a CBC to check for anemia and liver function tests. A CT scan, PET scan, or MRI will be done to detect metastases and determine the depth of penetration of the tumor into the bowel wall.

Carcinoembryonic antigen (CEA) is a complex glycoprotein sometimes made by CRC cells. It may be used to detect CRC and monitor for recurrence after surgery or chemotherapy. It is not the best screening tool because of the large number of false-positive findings. CEA levels may be increased in noncolon cancers (e.g., gastric, pancreatic, breast, thyroid cancers) and noncancerous conditions, like IBD, pancreatitis, cirrhosis, and chronic obstructive pulmonary disease.

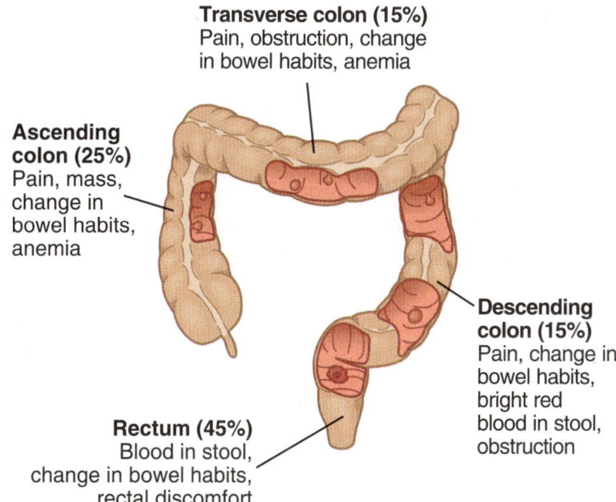

Fig. 47.10 Signs and symptoms of CRC by location of primary tumor.

TABLE 47.31 Interprofessional Care

Colorectal Cancer

Diagnostic Assessment
- History and physical assessment
- Digital rectal examination
- Testing of stool for occult blood
- CBC
- Liver function tests
- Barium enema
- Sigmoidoscopy and/or colonoscopy with biopsy
- Abdominal CT scan, ultrasound, or MRI
- Carcinoembryonic antigen (CEA) test

Management
- Surgical resection
- Chemotherapy
- Targeted therapy
- Radiation therapy

Interprofessional Care

The prognosis and treatment of CRC correlate with the staging. The most common staging system is the tumor, node, metastasis (TNM) staging (Table 47.32). As with other cancers, prognosis worsens with greater size and depth of tumor, lymph node involvement, and metastasis.

Surgical Therapy

The standard treatment for CRC is complete surgical resection of the tumor, surrounding tissues, and nearby lymph nodes.

Other surgical goals include exploring the abdomen to see if the cancer has spread and restoring bowel continuity to promote normal bowel function. Radiation and chemotherapy may be done before surgery to reduce tumor size.

The decision for surgery depends on the staging and location of the cancer and the ability to restore normal bowel function and continence (Table 47.33). If the tumor is in the distal rectum (1 to 2 cm from the anorectal junction) and the sphincters cannot be preserved, the patient will undergo an APR. The entire rectum and tumor will be removed, and the patient will have a permanent colostomy.

If the tumor is in the mid or proximal rectum, it may be possible to preserve the sphincters with a low anterior resection (LAR). An LAR involves removing the rectum and anastomosing the colon to the anal canal. A temporary ostomy may be done to divert stool and allow time for the anastomosis to heal. Another option if the anal sphincters remain is for the HCP to create an alternative reservoir with a J-pouch or coloplasty (Fig. 47.4).

If metastasis is present, removing the cancer and small areas of spread can help patients live longer. A few patients with limited lung or liver metastases can achieve a cure after primary and metastatic tumor resection and chemotherapy. If CRC has spread too much to cure it with surgery, chemotherapy and targeted therapy may control the cancer.

Some patients receive radiation therapy as an adjuvant to surgery and chemotherapy or as a palliative measure with metastatic cancer. As a palliative measure, the primary goal is to reduce tumor size and provide symptomatic relief. Radiation therapy is described in Chapter 15.

TABLE 47.32 Tumor, Node, Metastasis (TNM) Classification of Colorectal Cancer

T	**Primary Tumor**
T_x	Cannot assess primary tumor.
T_{is}	Carcinoma in situ. Cancer is in earliest stage and has not grown beyond mucosa layer.
T_1	Tumor invades the submucosa.
T_2	Tumor invades muscularis propria.
T_3	Tumor invades the pericolorectal tissues.
T_4	Tumor invades the visceral peritoneum or invades or adheres to adjacent organ or structure.
N	**Lymph Node Involvement**
N_x	Cannot assess lymph nodes.
N_0	No regional lymph node involvement is found.
N_1	Cancer is found in 1–3 lymph nodes.
N_2	Cancer is found in 4 or more lymph nodes.
M	**Metastasis**
M_0	No distant metastasis.
M_1	Distant or peritoneal metastasis present.

TABLE 47.33 Classification System Used to Stage Colorectal Cancer

Stage	TNM[a]	Treatment
0	T_{is} N_0 M_0	Surgery
I	T_1 N_0 M_0	Surgery
	T_2 N_0 M_0	Surgery
II	Any T, N_0 M_0	Surgery, chemotherapy
III	Any T, N_{1-2} M_0	Surgery, chemotherapy, radiation
IV	Any T, any N, M_1	Surgery, chemotherapy, targeted therapy, radiation

[a]See Table 47.32.

Chemotherapy and Targeted Therapy

Chemotherapy can be used to shrink the tumor before surgery, as adjuvant therapy after bowel resection, and as palliative treatment for nonresectable cancer (Table 47.33). Current protocols include varying doses of oxaliplatin with fluorouracil (FU)/leucovorin (LV) or capecitabine. Irinotecan can be given with FU/LV or with FU/LV and oxaliplatin. Capecitabine, FU/LV, and irinotecan can be used alone with or without target therapies.[23]

Targeted therapies have a role in treating metastatic CRC as part of chemotherapy regimens.[23] Angiogenesis inhibitors inhibit the blood supply to tumors. These include aflibercept (Zaltrap), bevacizumab (Avastin), and ramucirumab (Cyramza). Cetuximab (Erbitux) and panitumumab (Vectibix) block the epidermal growth factor receptor.

Regorafenib (Stivarga) is a multikinase inhibitor that blocks several enzymes that promote cancer growth. It or trifluridine-tipiracil is given to patients with metastatic CRC who no longer respond to other therapies. Trifluridine impairs DNA function and angiogenesis. Tipiracil prevents the rapid metabolism of trifluridine, thus increasing its bioavailability.

NURSING MANAGEMENT: COLORECTAL CANCER

Assessment

Table 47.34 outlines the subjective and objective data to obtain from patients with CRC.

Implementation

Health Promotion

Encourage all persons over 45 to have regular CRC screening. Help identify those at high risk who need screening at an earlier age. Discuss with patients how taking part in cancer screening helps decrease mortality rates. Realize that barriers exist, including lack of accurate information and fear of diagnosis. Provide teaching about risk factors. Discuss maintaining a healthy weight, being physically active, limiting alcohol use, not smoking, and eating a diet with large amounts of fruits, vegetables, and grains.

Visual procedures can only reveal polyps when the bowel has been properly prepared. Provide teaching about bowel cleansing for outpatient diagnostic procedures and give cleansing preparations to inpatients (see Chapter 43).

Acute Care

Routine postoperative care is appropriate after a bowel resection. If enough healthy bowel remained that the HCP could reconnect the bowel ends, normal bowel function is maintained. Patients with more extensive surgery, such as an APR, may have an open wound and drains (e.g., Jackson-Pratt, Hemovac) and a permanent ostomy. Nursing care includes sterile dressing changes, care of drains, and patient and caregiver teaching about the ostomy.

Chronic Care

Provide psychologic support for patients and caregivers as they deal with a cancer diagnosis. Discuss the patient's feelings about the prognosis. The special needs of cancer patients are discussed in Chapter 16. You may need to address issues surrounding palliative care, end-of-life issues, and hospice (see Chapter 10).

Patients with CRC need to know how to manage changes that result from cancer and cancer treatment. Those who had sphincter-sparing surgery may have diarrhea and incontinence of feces and gas. They may need antidiarrheal drugs or bulking agents to control the diarrhea. A dietitian or WOCN consult may help patients and caregivers understand how to manage food and fluid options. Ostomy rehabilitation, including teaching and ongoing support, should be available for all ostomy patients. Patients with skin changes from incontinence and/or radiation therapy will need help with managing these conditions.

 TABLE 47.34 **NURSING ASSESSMENT**

Colorectal Cancer

Subjective Data

Important Health Information

Health history: Previous cancer, familial polyposis, villous adenoma, adenomatous polyps, inflammatory bowel disease

Medications: Medications affecting bowel function (e.g., laxatives, antidiarrheal drugs)

Functional Health Patterns

Health perception–health management: Family history of colorectal or other cancer; weakness, fatigue

Nutritional-metabolic: High-calorie, high-fat, low-fiber diet. Anorexia, nausea and vomiting, weight loss

Elimination: Change in bowel habits, alternating diarrhea and constipation, defecation urgency. Rectal bleeding, mucoid stools. Black, tarry stools. Flatus, decrease in stool caliber. Feelings of incomplete evacuation.

Cognitive-perceptual: Abdominal and low back pain, tenesmus

Objective Data

General

Pallor, cachexia, lymphadenopathy (later signs)

GI

Palpable abdominal mass, distention, ascites and hepatomegaly (liver metastasis)

Possible Diagnostic Findings

Anemia. Guaiac-positive stools, palpable mass on digital rectal examination. Positive sigmoidoscopy, colonoscopy, barium enema, or CT scan. Positive biopsy

DIVERTICULOSIS AND DIVERTICULITIS

Diverticula are saccular dilations or outpouchings of the mucosa in the colon (Fig. 47.11). Diverticulosis is the presence of multiple noninflamed diverticula. **Diverticulitis** occurs when 1 or more diverticula become inflamed and, in some cases, infected. Diverticula are common, especially in older adults. Most people never develop diverticulitis.

Etiology and Pathophysiology

Diverticula are most common in the left (descending, sigmoid) colon.[24] They seem to occur at weak points in the intestinal wall, such as where the blood vessels pass through the muscle layer. We think the cause includes genetic and environment factors. The main risk factors are diet and lifestyle. The disease is more prevalent in Western, industrial populations, where people tend to consume diets low in fiber and high in red meat and refined carbohydrates. Other risk factors are obesity, constipation, inactivity, smoking, and excess alcohol use. Aspirin, corticosteroids, and NSAID drugs are associated with diverticulitis.

Clinical Manifestations and Complications

Most patients with diverticulosis have no symptoms. Those with symptoms typically have abdominal pain, bloating, flatulence, and changes in bowel habits. In more serious situations, diverticula bleed or diverticulitis develops. Common signs and symptoms of diverticulitis are acute pain in the left lower quadrant, distention, decreased or absent bowel sounds, nausea, vomiting, and systemic symptoms of

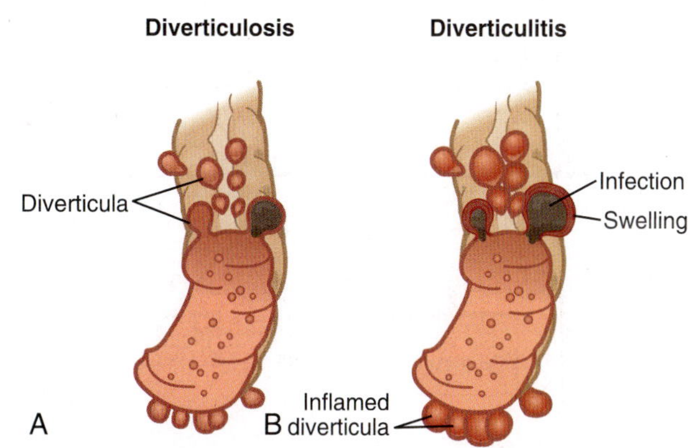

Fig. 47.11 (A) Diverticula are outpouchings of the colon. (B) Diverticulitis occurs when 1 or more diverticula become inflamed and, in some cases, infected.

infection. Older adults with diverticulitis may be afebrile, with a normal WBC count and little, if any, abdominal tenderness. Diverticulitis can cause erosion of the bowel wall and perforation into the peritoneum (Fig. 47.12). A local abscess develops when the body walls off the perforated area. Peritonitis develops if it cannot be contained. Bleeding, a fistula, or LBO may develop.

Diagnostic Studies

Diverticular disease is typically found during routine sigmoidoscopy or colonoscopy. Diagnosis of diverticulitis is based on the physical assessment, CBC, and imaging (Table 47.35). The preferred diagnostic test is a CT scan with or without IV contrast.[24] MRI is an option.

Interprofessional and Nursing Management

In acute diverticulitis, the goal of treatment is to let the colon rest and the inflammation subside (Table 47.36). Some patients can be managed at home with a clear liquid diet and bed rest. They may receive acetaminophen for pain and antispasmodics, such as dicyclomine hydrochloride.

Patients with severe disease are hospitalized for IV antibiotics and fluids. For recurring diverticulitis or complications, such as an abscess or obstruction, surgery may be done. The usual procedure involves resecting the involved colon with a primary anastomosis.[24] If the HCP is not able to anastomose the colon, patients will have a temporary diverting colostomy. After the colon heals, the temporary colostomy can be taken down and the ends of the colon reconnected.

Teach patients about the condition. Those who understand the disease and adhere to the treatment plan are less likely to have an exacerbation. Teach them to follow a high-fiber diet, mainly from fruits and vegetables, with a decreased intake of fat and red meat (Table 47.9). Encourage a fluid intake of at least 2 L/day. They should avoid increased intraabdominal pressure because it may precipitate an attack. Factors that increase intraabdominal pressure are straining at stool, vomiting, bending, heavy lifting, and wearing tight, restrictive clothing. Weight loss (see Chapter 45) is important for the person with obesity. Encourage smoking cessation.

PATHOPHYSIOLOGY MAP

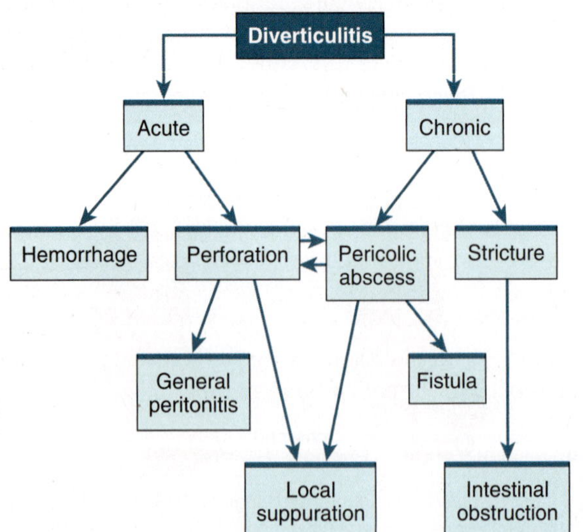

Fig. 47.12 Complications of diverticulitis.

TABLE 47.35 Interprofessional Care

Diverticulosis and Diverticulitis

Diagnostic Assessment
- History and physical assessment
- Testing of stool for occult blood
- CBC
- Urinalysis
- CT scan with oral contrast
- Abdominal and/or chest x-ray
- MRI
- Ultrasound

Management

Conservative Therapy
- High-fiber diet
- Fiber supplements
- Weight loss (if overweight)
- Smoking cessation

Acute Care: Diverticulitis
- Antibiotic therapy
- NPO status
- IV fluids
- Analgesics
- NG suction
- Surgery
  - Possible resection of involved colon
  - Possible temporary colostomy

TABLE 47.36 NURSING MANAGEMENT

Patient With Acute Diverticulitis

- Give IV fluids and electrolyte replacement as ordered.
- Place the patient on NPO status, moving to clear liquids with improvement.
- Administer IV fluids and antibiotics as ordered.
- Observe for signs of abscess, bleeding, and peritonitis.
- Monitor the CBC, noting WBC count.
- Implement pain management measures.
- Keep the patient on bed rest.
- Maintain intake and output; obtain daily weight.
- Provide frequent oral care and water-soluble lubricant for the lips.
- Implement measures to control nausea and vomiting (see Chapter 46).
- Institute NG suctioning and check every 4 hours for patency.
- Monitor for signs of perforation and notify HCP if present.
- Provide patient teaching about diet, drug therapy, and when to contact the HCP.

FISTULAS

A **fistula** is an abnormal tract between 2 hollow organs or a hollow organ and the skin. Fistulas are named by the track that they take from one body part to another. For example, an enterovaginal fistula is between the small intestine and vagina. It would allow stool and gas to drain through the vagina.

Fistulas are classified as simple or complex and by the amount of output. A simple fistula has only one short, direct tract. A complex fistula is associated with an abscess, involves multiple organs, and may open into the base of a wound. High-output fistulas drain more than 500 mL/day, moderate-output fistulas drain 200 to 500 mL/day, and low-output fistulas drain less than 200 mL/day.

A GI fistula occurs between the lumen of the GI tract and another organ. GI fistulas are a serious complication associated with increased morbidity and mortality, extended hospital stays, and increased costs. Most fistulas occur after surgery or trauma. Other times fistulas can form with IBD, cancer, perforation, radiation, diverticulitis, or pancreatitis.

Fever and abdominal pain are early signs of a fistula. Other manifestations depend on the type. With an enterocutaneous fistula, there may be pus or intestinal contents draining through the skin opening. A colocutaneous (colon to skin) fistula may drain stool or pus. Manifestations of a colovesical (colon to urinary tract) fistula include fecaluria (passing stool with urination), urinary tract infections, dysuria, and hematuria.

Interprofessional and Nursing Management

Treatment requires (1) identifying the fistula tract, (2) maintaining fluid and electrolyte balance, (3) controlling infection, (4) protecting the surrounding skin, (5) managing output, and (6) providing nutrition support. Managing a fistula is often a difficult and complex process. It can be disheartening for patients and caregivers. Surgery may be needed if there are complications.

Fluid and electrolyte replacement can be challenging when patients have a high-output fistula. Monitor urine output and the volume of fistula output, as these guide fluid replacement. Assess the drainage. Note the color, consistency, and odor. Monitor laboratory values. Low serum levels of potassium, magnesium, and phosphorus from the loss of GI fluids are common. Give IV fluids and electrolyte replacement as ordered. Measure vital signs frequently and watch for signs of dehydration.

Many patients are NPO, as this reduces intestinal output. They may receive acid suppression with a PPI or histamine H_2-receptor blocker. Antimotility drugs (e.g., loperamide) decrease intestinal fluid loss.

Malnutrition is a problem, especially if patients are NPO or have a small intestinal fistula. Consult a dietitian. High-calorie, high-protein PN or EN is needed to provide enough calories and protein to replace losses and support healing. Many patients need trace elements (e.g., copper, zinc, magnesium) and vitamin supplements.

Maintaining skin integrity and optimizing healing are essential. Consult a WOCN if available. Low-output fistulas may be managed with a simple absorbent dressing. A high-output enterocutaneous fistula often needs advanced techniques, including specialty pouches; barrier creams, powders, and sealants to protect the skin; and negative pressure wound therapy.

CHECK YOUR PRACTICE

A 51-year-old female is 4 days postop after a proctocolectomy for UC. You note 2.5 cm of redness in the center of her incision with heavy, foul-smelling, tan drainage pooling on her skin. Suspecting she is developing an enterocutaneous fistula, you notify the HCP and WOCN.

- What will you do to protect her skin?

HERNIAS

A **hernia** is a protrusion of tissue, such as the intestines, through the tissues in which it is normally contained. A hernia may occur in any part of the body, but it usually occurs within the abdominal cavity. *Reducible* hernias easily return into the abdominal cavity. Reducing can be done manually or may occur spontaneously when the person lies supine. *Irreducible,* or *incarcerated,* hernias cannot be placed back into the abdominal cavity. They have abdominal contents trapped in the opening. Strangulation occurs if the blood supply to the contents trapped in an irreducible hernia becomes compromised. The result is an acute bowel obstruction. Gangrene and necrosis of the hernia contents are possible.

Types

The *inguinal hernia* is the most common type of hernia (Fig. 47.13). It occurs at the point of weakness in the abdominal wall where the spermatic cord (in males) or the round ligament (in females) emerges. An *umbilical hernia* occurs when the rectus muscle is weak (as with obesity) or the umbilical opening does not close after birth. A *femoral hernia* occurs when there is a protrusion through the femoral ring into the femoral canal. It appears as a bulge below the inguinal ligament. Femoral hernias easily strangulate.

Incisional hernias are caused by weakness of the abdominal wall at the site of an incision or stoma. Risk factors include obesity, smoking, older age, chronic steroid use, and diabetes. Surgical factors include having emergency surgery, multiple surgeries in the same area, incision location, and a history of wound infection or poor wound healing.[25]

Clinical Manifestations

Pain is the classic symptom of a hernia. It may worsen with activities that increase intraabdominal pressure, such as lifting,

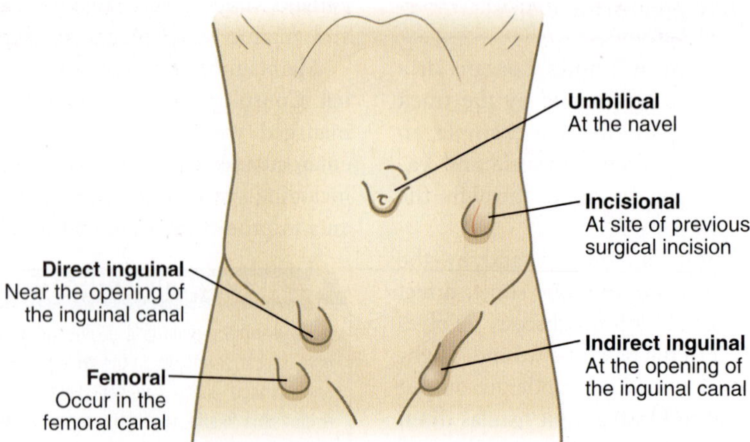

Fig. 47.13 Types of abdominal hernias.

coughing, and straining. A hernia may be readily visible, especially when the person tenses the abdominal muscles. If the hernia becomes strangulated, patients will have severe pain and symptoms of bowel obstruction, such as vomiting, cramping, abdominal pain, and distention.

Interprofessional and Nursing Management

Diagnosis is based on history and physical assessment. Ultrasound, CT, and MRI can help identify a hernia and determine the contents. Laparoscopic surgery is the treatment of choice. The surgical repair of a hernia, or *herniorrhaphy,* is usually an outpatient procedure. Reinforcing the weakened area with wire, fascia, or mesh is known as a *hernioplasty.* Emergency surgery is needed for strangulated hernias or inflamed, irreducible hernias. Surgery for strangulated hernias involves resecting the involved area with possible placement of a temporary colostomy.

After a hernia repair, patients may have problems voiding. Measure intake and output. Observe for a distended bladder. Encourage deep breathing but not coughing. Teach patients to splint the incision and keep their mouths open when coughing or sneezing is unavoidable. Patients may be restricted from heavy lifting (>10 lb) for 6 to 8 weeks. After inguinal hernia repair, there may be scrotal edema. A scrotal support, icing, and elevating the scrotum may help relieve pain and edema.

MALABSORPTION PROBLEMS

MALABSORPTION

Malabsorption results from impaired absorption of fats, carbohydrates, proteins, minerals, and vitamins. The stomach, small intestine, liver, and pancreas regulate normal digestion and absorption. Digestive enzymes ordinarily break down nutrients so that absorption can take place. Malabsorption may occur if this process is interrupted at any point. Several problems can cause malabsorption (Table 47.37). Lactose intolerance is the most common malabsorption disorder, followed by IBD, celiac disease, tropical sprue, and cystic fibrosis.

The most common signs of malabsorption are weight loss and diarrhea. Other signs include fatigue, abdominal pain, and *steatorrhea* (bulky, foul-smelling, yellow-gray, greasy stools with putty-like consistency) (Table 47.38).

A complete history and physical along with testing are needed to make a diagnosis. Laboratory studies include a CBC, prothrombin time (to see if vitamin K absorption is adequate), liver function tests, and serum levels of vitamin A, carotene, electrolytes, iron, and calcium. Stool studies include assessing for fat (e.g., Sudan III stain), doing a microbiologic analysis, and assessing secretory function through elastase or chymotrypsin testing to assess pancreatic function.

Imaging studies include a CT scan and endoscopy. Barium studies can identify structural problems. Capsule endoscopy is useful in assessing the small intestine for changes in mucosal integrity and inflammation. Treatment depends on the cause.

CELIAC DISEASE

Celiac disease is an autoimmune disease that causes damage to the small intestinal mucosa. It is triggered by ingesting gluten, a protein in wheat, barley, and rye. It can occur at any age. *Celiac sprue* and *gluten-sensitive enteropathy* are other names for celiac disease. Untreated celiac disease can lead to other autoimmune diseases, like multiple sclerosis and type 1 diabetes. Those with celiac disease have a higher risk for heart disease and small bowel cancer.[26]

Etiology and Pathophysiology

Many factors are involved in developing celiac disease. These include genetics, gluten ingestion, and an immune response. First-degree relatives of someone with celiac disease have a 10% chance of developing the disorder.[26] About 95% of people with celiac disease have human leukocyte antigen (HLA) allele HLA-DQ2.[27] The other 5% have HLA-DQ8. However, not everyone with these genetic markers develops celiac disease. Some people with celiac disease do not have either of these HLA alleles.

TABLE 47.37 Causes of Malabsorption

Bacterial Proliferation
- Parasitic infection
- Tropical sprue

Biochemical or Enzyme Deficiencies
- Biliary tract obstruction
- Chronic pancreatitis
- Cystic fibrosis
- Lactase deficiency
- Pancreatic insufficiency
- Zollinger-Ellison syndrome

Disturbed Lymphatic and Vascular Circulation
- Heart failure
- Ischemia
- Lymphangiectasia
- Lymphoma

Small Intestinal Mucosal Disruption
- Celiac disease
- Crohn disease
- Whipple disease

Surface Area Loss
- Billroth II gastrectomy
- Distal ileal resection, disease, or bypass
- Short bowel syndrome

The tissue destruction that occurs with celiac disease is the result of chronic inflammation. Gluten contains specific peptides called *prolamins.* Partial digestion of gluten releases prolamin peptides, which are absorbed into the intestinal submucosa. In genetically susceptible persons, the peptides bind to HLA-DQ2 and/or HLA-DQ8 and activate an inflammatory response. Inflammation damages the microvilli and brush border of the small intestine, decreasing the amount of surface area available for nutrient absorption. Damage is most severe in the duodenum, probably because it has more exposure to gluten. The inflammation lasts as long as gluten ingestion continues.

Clinical Manifestations

Classic manifestations include foul-smelling diarrhea, abdominal pain, flatulence, and abdominal distention. Some people have no obvious GI symptoms and instead have atypical signs and symptoms. These include joint pain, liver problems, fatigue, peripheral neuropathy, and reproductive problems.[26] An intensely pruritic, vesicular skin lesion called *dermatitis herpetiformis* is sometimes present. It is a rash on the buttocks, scalp, face, elbows, and knees.

Protein, fat, and carbohydrate absorption are affected. Weight loss, muscle wasting, and other signs of malnutrition may be present. Abnormal serum folate, iron, and cobalamin levels can lead to anemia. Patients may have lactose intolerance and need to refrain from lactose-containing products until the disease is under control. Inadequate calcium intake and vitamin D absorption can lead to decreased bone density and osteoporosis.

TABLE 47.38 Manifestations of Malabsorption

Manifestations	Pathophysiology
Cardiovascular	
Hypotension	Dehydration
Peripheral edema	Protein malabsorption, protein loss in diarrhea
Tachycardia	Hypovolemia, anemia
GI	
Diarrhea	Impaired absorption of water, sodium, fatty acids, bile salts, carbohydrates
Flatulence	Bacterial fermentation of unabsorbed carbohydrates
Glossitis, cheilosis, stomatitis	Deficiency of iron, riboflavin, cobalamin, folic acid, other vitamins
Steatorrhea	Undigested and unabsorbed fat
Weight loss	Malabsorption of fat, carbohydrates, protein leading to loss of calories; decrease in caloric intake or ↑ use of calories
Hematologic	
Anemia	Impaired absorption of iron, cobalamin, folic acid
Hemorrhagic tendency	Vitamin C deficiency; vitamin K deficiency inhibiting production of clotting factors II, VII, IX, and X
Musculoskeletal	
Bone pain	Osteoporosis from impaired calcium absorption; osteomalacia from hypocalcemia, hypophosphatemia, inadequate vitamin D
Muscle wasting	Protein malabsorption
Tetany	Hypocalcemia, hypomagnesemia
Weakness, muscle cramps	Anemia, electrolyte depletion (especially potassium)
Neurologic	
Altered mental status	Dehydration
Night blindness	Thiamine deficiency, vitamin A deficiency
Paresthesias	Cobalamin deficiency
Peripheral neuropathy	Cobalamin deficiency
Skin	
Brittle nails	Iron deficiency
Bruising	Vitamin K deficiency
Dermatitis	Fatty acid deficiency, zinc deficiency, niacin, other vitamin deficiencies
Hair thinning and loss	Protein deficiency

Diagnostic Studies

Celiac disease is diagnosed by the history, physical assessment, and serology testing. Have patients complete diagnostic testing before starting a gluten-free diet because the diet will change the results. The best serologic test is the tissue transglutaminase IgA antibody, plus an IgA antibody.[26] Though not done as often, histologic evidence is the gold standard for confirming the diagnosis. Biopsies show flattened mucosa and noticeable losses of villi. Genetic testing for HLA-DQ2 and/or HLA-DQ8 antigens may be done in susceptible families.

Interprofessional and Nursing Management

A strict gluten-free diet (Table 47.39) is the only treatment for celiac disease.[28] Most patients need to stay on a gluten-free diet for the rest of their lives. Periodic nutrition evaluations and laboratory monitoring are done to check for anemia and malnutrition. Many take daily vitamin and mineral supplements. Patients should have bone density screening every 2 to 3 years.

Refer all patients for a diet consultation.[28] You can work with a dietitian to teach patients how to eat a nutritionally adequate diet while considering food preferences, cultural traditions, and food availability. Teach patients to read medication and food labels. Some medications and many food additives, preservatives, and stabilizers contain gluten. Patients need to know where to buy gluten-free products. Good sources are health food stores, many grocery stores, and Internet sites.

Maintaining a gluten-free diet can be hard, especially when traveling or eating in restaurants. Teach patients to read menus. Talk about how to discuss gluten-free menu options with restaurant staff or when dining in others' homes. Mobile phone users will find apps listing gluten-free menu options at popular restaurants helpful. Many restaurants now indicate which food choices are gluten-free. The Celiac Disease Foundation (www.celiac.org) provides suggestions for maintaining a gluten-free diet and living with celiac disease.

LACTASE DEFICIENCY

Lactase deficiency is a condition in which the lactase enzyme is deficient or absent. Lactase is the enzyme that breaks down lactose into 2 simple sugars: glucose and galactose. Most people with the condition have primary lactase insufficiency. They have normal lactase activity at birth, but the activity will gradually decrease with age to 5% to 10% of the initial level.[28] It is a genetic disorder. The incidence differs among races and regions.

In secondary lactose intolerance, infectious, inflammatory, or other diseases injure the intestinal mucosa resulting in a decrease in lactase activity. Common causes include IBD, celiac disease, and chemotherapy. Lactase activity may be restored to normal after the small intestine recovers. Less common causes include premature birth and congenital lactase deficiency, a rare genetic disorder.

Manifestations include bloating, flatulence, abdominal pain, and diarrhea after ingesting lactose. The undigested lactose ferments in the large intestine by microorganisms, producing a gas. This causes bloating and abdominal pain. Diarrhea results from the undigested lactose and gaseous mixture attracting water, thus decreasing water reabsorption. Decreased calcium absorption can affect growth in children and cause rickets or osteoporosis in adults.[29]

Lactose problems are often diagnosed with lactose tolerance tests, hydrogen breath tests, or genetic testing. Treatment aims to improve symptoms and prevent malnutrition. Limiting the intake of lactose-containing products improves symptoms. Lactase-containing milk products and calcium supplements are recommended. Enzyme supplements contain lactase, which breaks down lactose in milk and milk-containing products. They are available as tablets or drops. Some people have improved symptoms by taking prebiotics or probiotics that produce lactase in the gut.

Teach patients which foods to limit. Hard cheese may be easier to digest. Live culture yogurt has less lactose because the bacteria help digest it. Teach patients to read labels to detect any hidden sources of lactose. Some people tolerate lactose better if taken with meals.

TABLE 47.39 NUTRITION THERAPY

Celiac Disease

Foods that contain or often contain gluten:

- Baked goods, including muffins, cookies, cakes, pies, donuts, rolls
- Barley
- Bread, including wheat bread, white bread, bagels
- Breakfast foods, such as pancakes, French toast
- Crackers
- Dressings, croutons
- Flour
- Flour tortillas
- Gluten stabilizers
- Granola
- Oats
- Pasta, noodles
- Pizza
- Rye
- Wheat

Foods that may contain gluten:

- Candy and candy bars
- Cream-based soups
- Energy bars
- French fries
- Potato chips, tortilla chips
- Processed lunch meat
- Salad dressings, marinades

SHORT BOWEL SYNDROME

Patients with **short bowel syndrome (SBS)** have less than 200 cm of small intestine.[30] There is not enough surface area in the small intestine to absorb enough nutrients to meet energy, fluid, electrolyte, and nutrition needs to stay healthy on a normal diet. Causes of SBS include diseases that damage the intestinal mucosa, surgical removal of small intestine (e.g., with cancer), trauma, and congenital defects.

Functional SBS can be present in patients with more than 200 cm of small intestine if the function of the small intestine present is impaired by factors such as disease (e.g., Crohn disease) or rapid intestinal transit.[30]

The length and area of the small intestine present and the presence of the colon and ileocecal valve affect the outcome. SBS is common in patients with an end jejunostomy. If the terminal ileum, ileocecal valve, and colon are intact, patients will have fewer problems with SBS.[30]

Clinical Manifestations

SBS results in reduced nutrient, fluid, and electrolyte absorption. This leads to dehydration, weight loss, diarrhea, malnutrition, vitamin deficiencies, and electrolyte imbalances. Other manifestations include abdominal pain, flatulence, and steatorrhea. Patients may develop lactase deficiency and bacterial overgrowth. Those who are malnourished may have manifestations from specific deficiencies. For example, patients may have peripheral neuropathy from vitamin B_{12}, vitamin E, copper, or thiamine deficiencies or fatigue caused by anemia from decreased folate or iron.

Interprofessional Care

Treatment goals are that patients will maintain normal nutrition and be free from complications. The main treatment is nutrition support involving PN, EN, medications, and a tailored diet. In the immediate period after a major bowel resection, patients receive PN and IV fluids to replace fluid, electrolyte, and nutrient losses and rest the bowel. They may need PN indefinitely. Continuous EN and an oral diet are resumed to help the remaining intestine to function better. Some can eventually stop PN. PN and EN are discussed in Chapter 44.

The diet should maximize nutrient and fluid absorption and decrease stool output. Refer patients to a dietitian. The ideal diet is high in protein and complex carbohydrates and low in fat and simple sugars. Patients should eat at least 6 small meals per day to increase the time of contact between food and the intestine. Oral vitamin and mineral supplements may be needed. Patients with severe malabsorption may need PN or EN at night.

The mainstay of drug therapy involves antidiarrheal agents (loperamide, diphenoxylate) to reduce fluid losses and slow intestinal motility. Other drug therapy includes somatropin and teduglutide (Gattex). Somatropin improves water, electrolyte, and nutrient absorption in the intestine. Teduglutide increases the surface area of the intestine and improves intestinal absorption of fluids and nutrients. Patients receive a PPI to reduce gastric acid secretion.[31]

ANORECTAL PROBLEMS

HEMORRHOIDS

Hemorrhoids are abnormally dilated hemorrhoidal veins. They may be internal (above the internal sphincter) or external (outside the external sphincter) (Fig. 47.14). Hemorrhoids can appear periodically, depending on the amount of anorectal pressure.

Etiology and Pathophysiology

Hemorrhoids are thought to develop because of increased anal pressure and weakening of the connective tissue that supports the hemorrhoidal veins. Weakened supporting tissue allows for downward displacement of the veins, causing them to dilate. Impaired blood flow may be present. A clot in a vein results in a thrombosed external hemorrhoid. Many factors increase the risk for hemorrhoids. These include pregnancy, constipation with straining, diarrhea, heavy lifting, anal intercourse, obesity, and ascites.[32]

Clinical Manifestations

Internal hemorrhoids most often cause painless, bright red bleeding with stools, on the toilet paper, or dripping into the toilet water. If internal hemorrhoids become constricted, patients will report pain. Internal hemorrhoids can prolapse into the anal canal or externally. Symptoms of prolapse include pressure with defecation, itching, and a protruding mass.

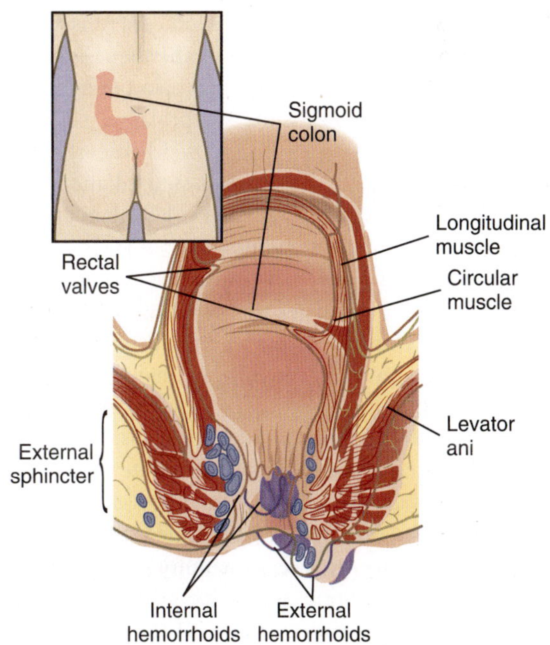

Fig. 47.14 Anatomic structures of the rectum and anus with external and internal hemorrhoids.

External hemorrhoids are reddish-blue and seldom bleed. There may be itching, burning, and edema. They usually do not cause pain unless thrombosis (blood clots) is present. Thrombosed hemorrhoids are a bluish-purple tinge and palpable at the anal orifice. They usually cause pain and inflammation. The clot can erode through the overlying stretched skin, causing bleeding with defecation. Constipation or diarrhea can worsen symptoms.

It is easy to diagnose hemorrhoids with visual inspection and DRE. Sigmoidoscopy or colonoscopy is done to assess for comorbid issues like polyps, cancer, and other anorectal problems.[32]

Interprofessional and Nursing Management

Initial treatment involves diet and lifestyle changes. Teach patients ways to prevent constipation (Table 47.11). A more bulky stool may decrease stool leakage and itching. Stool softeners can keep the stools soft. Warm sitz baths (15 to 20 minutes, 2 or 3 times each day) may reduce discomfort and swelling.

OTC ointments, creams, and suppositories specifically made for hemorrhoid treatment can be used to shrink the mucous membranes and relieve pain. These drugs often contain anesthetics, corticosteroids, protectants, or antiseptics. Corticosteroid use should be limited to 1 week or less to prevent side effects, such as contact dermatitis and mucosal atrophy. NSAIDs can be taken for pain.

Prolapsed or bleeding internal hemorrhoids or thrombosed external hemorrhoids may need medical treatment. Nonsurgical approaches (rubber band ligation, infrared coagulation, sclerotherapy, laser treatment) are options. Rubber band ligation is the most widely used technique. The HCP places a rubber band around the hemorrhoid to constrict circulation. The tissue becomes necrotic, separates, and sloughs off. There is some local discomfort with this procedure, but no anesthetic is needed.

A *hemorrhoidectomy* is the surgical excision of hemorrhoids. Surgery is needed when there is marked prolapse, excess pain or bleeding, or large or multiple thrombosed hemorrhoids. After removing the hemorrhoids, the tissue is sutured and the wound heals by primary intention or the area is left open and healing takes place by secondary intention.

Nursing care focuses on pain control and promoting wound healing (Table 47.40). Be aware that although the procedure is minor, the pain is severe and feared by many. Most patients receive multimodal analgesia. This may involve an opioid and NSAID in conjunction with topical preparations that provide anesthesia or reduce internal sphincter spasms, such as topical lidocaine, 2% diltiazem, and glyceryl trinitrate.

Patients usually dread the first bowel movement and often resist the urge to defecate. Give pain medication before the bowel movement to reduce discomfort. Stool softeners (e.g., docusate) and bulking agents are given to help form a soft, bulky stool that is easier to pass. If the patient does not have a bowel movement within 2 or 3 days, an oil-retention enema is given.

TABLE 47.40 NURSING MANAGEMENT

Care of the Patient After a Hemorrhoidectomy

- Administer analgesics as ordered, especially before bowel movements.
- Administer stool softeners and bulking agents as ordered.
- Encourage the patient to change positions frequently.
- Apply ice to the area several times a day for 10 min at a time.
- Warm sitz baths can help with urination and bowel movements.
- Teach the patient to use a pressure relief cushion, not a ring or "doughnut," when sitting.
- Have the patient use baby wipes or medicated pads instead of toilet paper.
- Assess for rectal bleeding, especially in those taking anticoagulants.
- Provide as much privacy as possible when providing wound care and performing assessments.
- Teach the patient care of the anal area, symptoms of complications (especially bleeding), and ways to avoid constipation and straining.

A warm sitz bath provides comfort and keeps the anal area clean. A sponge ring in the sitz bath helps relieve pressure on the area. Initially, do not leave patients alone because of the possibility of weakness or fainting. Patients may have packing in the rectum to absorb drainage, with a T-binder to hold the dressing in place. Packing is usually removed on the first or second postoperative day.

ANAL FISSURE

An *anal fissure* is a linear skin tear in the anal mucosa. Many times, the inciting event is trauma from passing hard stools. Fissures can occur with trauma (anal intercourse, foreign body insertion, childbirth), local infection (syphilis, gonorrhea, *Chlamydia,* herpes simplex virus, HIV), or inflammation. An anal fissure is acute when it is of recent onset (less than 6 weeks) and chronic if it has been present for a longer period. Chronic fissures have a characteristic appearance that includes perianal skin tags and fibrotic edges.

Anal tissue ulcerates because of ischemia caused by a combination of high pressure in the internal anal sphincter and poor blood supply. The ischemic tissue may ulcerate spontaneously or with trauma, such as with hard stools, which would not normally cause tissue breakdown. Ischemia must be corrected for a fissure to heal.

The hallmark of an anal fissure is severe anal pain. It is worse with defecation and with direct pressure on the site, such as from sitting. Acute fissures tend to bleed slightly. Patients may report red blood on the toilet paper. Constipation results because of fear of pain when having bowel movements.

Anal fissures are easy to diagnose with a physical assessment. Conservative care with fiber supplements, stool softeners, sitz baths, and topical analgesics is successful in most cases, especially with an acute fissure. Topical nitrates or calcium channel blockers relax muscles and increase blood flow. Local injections of botulinum toxin can decrease rectal pressure.[32]

If conservative treatment fails, patients may have an internal sphincterotomy. It carries the risk of fecal incontinence. Postoperative nursing care is the same as the care for patients who have had a hemorrhoidectomy.

ANORECTAL ABSCESS

An *anorectal abscess* is a collection of perianal pus from an infection (Fig. 47.15). It is usually caused by an obstructed anal gland. Risk factors include anal fissures, trauma, pregnancy, sexually transmitted infections, and IBD. The most common organisms are *E. coli,* staphylococci, and streptococci. Manifestations include local severe pain and swelling, foul-smelling drainage, tenderness, and fever. Ultrasound, CT, or MRI is done to evaluate the involved area and surrounding tissues. Fistulas are common.[32]

Anorectal abscesses require surgical drainage. Large abscesses need packing afterward with impregnated gauze or placement of drains. The area then heals by granulation. Patients with diabetes, cellulitis, or are immunocompromised (e.g., chemotherapy) may need antibiotic therapy. Nursing care includes warm, moist heat applications and changing packing daily. Patients are usually more comfortable lying on the abdomen or side. A low-fiber diet is given. Teach patients about wound care and the importance of sitz baths, thorough cleaning after urinating or bowel movements, and follow-up visits with the HCP.

ANAL FISTULA

An **anal fistula** is an abnormal tunnel from the anus or rectum to the surface of the skin around the anus or the vagina. Most are caused by an anorectal abscess or infection. Other causes include Crohn disease, cancer, chronic diarrhea, trauma, or radiation.

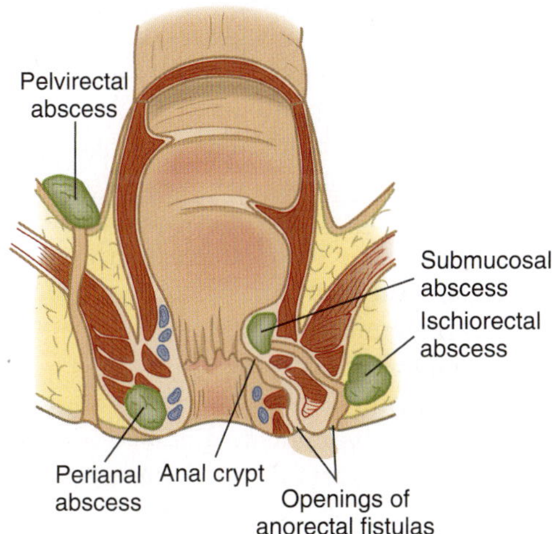

Fig. 47.15 Common sites of anorectal abscesses and fistula formation.

Feces may enter the fistula and cause an infection. There may be persistent, bloody, or purulent discharge or stool leakage from the fistula. Patients may need to wear a pad to avoid staining clothes.

Fistulas are treated surgically. In a fistulotomy, the HCP opens the fistula, and healthy tissue is allowed to granulate in the wound. Care is the same as after a hemorrhoidectomy. Options for complex fistulas include ligation of the fistula tract (LIFT) or the use of rectal flaps, plugs, or fibrin glue to seal the fistula.

ANAL CANCER

Anal cancer is rare, but the incidence is increasing. It is more common in people over 50 years. Human papillomavirus (HPV) is associated with about 90% of the cases. Less common risk factors include HIV, anal warts, immunosuppression, anoreceptive intercourse, and smoking.[32]

Rectal bleeding is the most common presenting sign. Other symptoms include rectal pain, itching, pressure, or a full feeling. There may be a change in bowel frequency or size. Patients may report increased straining or a palpable growth.

We can screen high-risk persons using DRE and anal Pap tests. In an anal Pap test, the anal lining is swabbed and the cells are examined to identify any cell changes (e.g., dysplasia, neoplasia). Anoscopy allows the HCP to assess the mucosa and obtain a biopsy. Disease extent is assessed with ultrasound, CT, or MRI.

Treatment depends on the size and depth of the lesions. The primary treatment is a combination of low-dose radiation and chemotherapy. Chemotherapy regimens include combinations of mitomycin, cisplatin, and FU.[32] Options for precancerous lesions are surgical removal or treatment with topical imiquimod (Aldara) and FU. If the tumor involves the rectum and requires removal of the anal sphincters, the anus is sutured shut and a permanent ostomy created.

PILONIDAL SINUS

A *pilonidal sinus* is a small tract under the skin between the buttocks in the sacrococcygeal area. It is lined with epithelium and hair, hence the name *pilonidal* ("a nest of hair"). Movement of the buttocks causes the short, wiry hair to penetrate the skin. If the irritated skin becomes infected, it forms a pilonidal cyst or abscess. There are no symptoms with a pilonidal sinus unless there is an infection. Then patients may have pain and swelling at the base of the spine.

An abscess requires incision and drainage. The wound may be closed or left open to heal by secondary intention. The wound is packed, and sitz baths are ordered. Nursing care includes warm, moist heat applications when an abscess is present. Patients are usually more comfortable lying on the abdomen or side. Teach patients to avoid contaminating the dressing when urinating or defecating and to avoid straining.

CASE STUDY

Colorectal Cancer

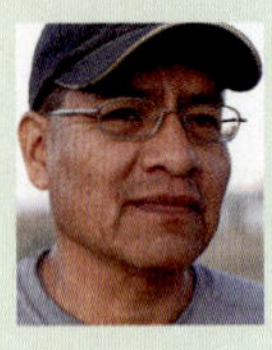
((© iStockphoto/ Thinkstock.))

Patient Profile

L.C., a 58-year-old Native American male, is from a Pueblo tribe in northern New Mexico. L.C.'s wife and family drove 50 miles to take him to the Indian Health Service hospital because of his deteriorating health (see the case study in Chapter 43).

Subjective Data

- See the case study in Chapter 43.
- Currently rates pain as a 7 on a scale of 0 to 10
- States he is not passing flatus

Objective Data

Physical Assessment

- 5 ft 9 in tall, weight 132 lb
- BP 140/72, Heart rate 90, RR 20, temperature 99.4°F (37.4°C), O_2 saturation 97% on room air
- Wound site and staples are intact, dry, without bleeding or signs of infection
- Abdomen slightly distended with hypoactive bowel sounds
- Lungs clear to auscultation, slightly diminished in posterior bases

Laboratory Tests

- CT scan and colonoscopy show 2 medium-sized tumors in the transverse colon
- Hgb of 8.8 g/dL, Hct of 24%.

Interprofessional Care

Surgical Procedure

- Had a transverse hemicolectomy with lymph node biopsies
- Pathology results: Adenocarcinoma has invaded the muscle wall of colon, 2 of 5 lymph nodes are positive for cancer

Postoperative

- Feels like his life has ended and does not want to leave the hospital
- States that there is "no one" to take care of him at his home, and he is far away from the hospital

Follow-Up Treatment

- Scheduled for outpatient chemotherapy

Discussion Questions

1. ***Recognize:*** What signs and symptoms of CRC did L.C. have (see the case study in Chapter 43)?
2. ***Analyze:*** What stage of CRC does L.C. likely have? What treatment is recommended for this stage?
3. ***Plan:*** What is a culturally sensitive way for you to support L.C. and his family in making decisions about his health care?
4. ***Plan:*** What referrals may be indicated at this time?
5. ***Prioritize:*** Based on the assessment data, what are the priority clinical problems?
6. ***Prioritize:*** What are the priority nursing interventions for L.C. at this stage of his illness?
7. ***Act:*** How would you provide emotional support to L.C. and his family?
8. ***Act:*** L.C. is worried that other members of his family may have colon cancer. What can you tell him about the recommendations for CRC screening?
9. ***Evaluate:*** What outcomes would indicate nursing interventions were successful?

Answers available at http://evolve.elsevier.com/Lewis/medsurg.

BRIDGE TO NCLEX EXAMINATION

The number of the question corresponds to the same-numbered outcome at the beginning of the chapter.

1. Nursing care for a patient with acute diarrhea caused by a viral infection would include
   a. initiating NPO status.
   b. administering an antibiotic.
   c. inserting a nasogastric tube.
   d. placing the patient on contact precautions.
2. Priority nursing interventions for a patient admitted to the emergency department with acute abdominal pain would include (**Select all that apply.**)
   a. establishing IV access.
   b. initiating a clear liquid diet.
   c. recording intake and output.
   d. obtaining ordered laboratory work.
   e. monitoring vital signs and pulse oximetry.
3. Assessment findings that suggest a patient has developed peritonitis include (**select all that apply**)
   a. abdominal pain.
   b. rebound tenderness.
   c. a soft, distended abdomen.
   d. shallow respirations with bradypnea.
   e. observing that the patient is lying still.
4. In planning care for the patient with Crohn disease, the nurse recognizes that a major difference between ulcerative colitis and Crohn disease is that Crohn disease
   a. often results in toxic megacolon.
   b. causes fewer nutrition deficiencies than ulcerative colitis.
   c. often recurs after surgery, while ulcerative colitis is curable with a colectomy.
   d. is manifested by rectal bleeding and anemia more often than is ulcerative colitis.
5. The nurse performing an abdominal assessment of a patient with a suspected large bowel obstruction would expect to find (**Select all that apply.**)
   a. persistent abdominal pain.
   b. marked abdominal distention.
   c. diarrhea that is loose or liquid.
   d. colicky, severe, intermittent pain.
   e. profuse vomiting that relieves abdominal pain.

6. Teaching for a patient with stage I colorectal cancer scheduled for surgery would include an explanation that
   a. radiation before surgery will reduce the size of the tumor.
   b. chemotherapy will begin after the patient recovers from the surgery.
   c. both chemotherapy and radiation will be used as palliative treatments.
   d. follow-up colonoscopies will be needed to ensure that the cancer does not recur.
7. The nurse determines a patient undergoing ileostomy surgery understands the procedure when the patient states
   a. "I should only have to change the pouch every 4 to 7 days."
   b. "The drainage in the pouch will look like my normal stools."
   c. "I may not need to wear a drainage pouch if I irrigate it daily."
   d. "Limiting my fluid intake should decrease the amount of output."
8. Discharge teaching for a patient with diverticulitis would include the need to (**Select all that apply.**)
   a. avoid heavy lifting.
   b. increase fluid intake.
   c. avoid nuts and popcorn.
   d. limit the red meat in the diet.
   e. increase intake of fruits and vegetables.
9. A nursing action to decrease pain and edema after an inguinal herniorrhaphy is to
   a. maintain the patient on bed rest.
   b. allow the patient to stand to void.
   c. support the incision during coughing.
   d. apply a scrotal support with an ice bag.
10. The nurse determines that the goals of diet teaching have been met when the patient with celiac disease selects from the menu
   a. scrambled eggs and sausage.
   b. buckwheat pancakes with syrup.
   c. oatmeal, skim milk, and orange juice.
   d. yogurt, strawberries, and rye toast with butter.
11. Which point would be included in discharge teaching after a hemorrhoidectomy?
   a. Take mineral oil before bedtime.
   b. Eat a low-fiber diet to rest the colon.
   c. Use a daily oil-retention enema to empty the colon.
   d. Take prescribed pain medications before a bowel movement.

1. d; 2. a, c, d, e; 3. a, b, e; 4. c; 5. a, b; 6. d;
7. a; 8. a, b, d, e; 9. d; 10. a; 11. d.

For rationales to these answers and even more NCLEX review questions, visit http://evolve.elsevier.com/Lewis/medsurg.

REFERENCES

To access the References for this chapter, please scan the QR code with a mobile device.

48

Liver, Biliary Tract, and Pancreas Problems

Lori Cogan

http://evolve.elsevier.com/Lewis/medsurg/

CONCEPTUAL FOCUS

Health Promotion
Infection
Inflammation
Nutrition
Pain

LEARNING OUTCOMES

1. Distinguish among the types of viral hepatitis.
2. Describe the interprofessional and nursing management of patients with viral hepatitis.
3. Explain the pathophysiology, clinical manifestations, complications, and interprofessional and nursing management of patients with cirrhosis and end-stage liver disease.
4. Describe the clinical manifestations and management of liver cancer.
5. Distinguish between acute and chronic pancreatitis related to pathophysiology, clinical manifestations, complications, and interprofessional and nursing management.
6. Explain the clinical manifestations and interprofessional and nursing management of patients with pancreatic cancer.
7. Describe the pathophysiology, clinical manifestations, and interprofessional care of gallbladder disorders.
8. Describe the nursing management of patients undergoing surgical treatment of cholecystitis and cholelithiasis.

KEY TERMS

acute liver failure
acute pancreatitis
ascites
asterixis
cholecystitis
cholelithiasis
chronic pancreatitis
cirrhosis
esophageal varices
gastric varices
hepatic encephalopathy
hepatitis
jaundice
portal hypertension

This chapter focuses on the care of patients with liver, pancreatic, and gallbladder problems. These organs are closely positioned together anatomically and highly associated with their digestive functions. Liver and pancreas problems can lead to altered nutrient absorption and use, causing malnutrition and impaired elimination. Inflammation may be present, with patients having pain, nausea, and vomiting. Nursing care focuses on helping patients and caregivers manage symptoms and cope with the diagnosis and, sometimes, prognosis. Health promotion focuses on reducing risk through immunizations and avoiding substance use.

LIVER PROBLEMS

HEPATITIS

Hepatitis is inflammation of the liver. The most common cause is viral. Other causes include substances (e.g., alcohol, medications, chemicals), autoimmune diseases, and metabolic problems. The overall mortality rate for acute hepatitis is less than 1%. The mortality rate is higher in older adults and those with underlying debilitating illnesses (including chronic liver disease).

Viral Hepatitis

There are several types of viral hepatitis. We designate each type by a letter (A, B, C, D, E). The different types have similar manifestations. Their modes of transmission and disease course vary (Table 48.1). Some can lead to chronic liver disease. Other less common viruses can also cause liver disease. These include cytomegalovirus (CMV), Epstein-Barr virus (EBV), herpesvirus, coxsackievirus, and rubella virus.

Hepatitis A Virus

Hepatitis A is a self-limiting infection. It can cause a mild flu-like illness and jaundice (Fig. 48.1). In more severe cases, it can cause acute liver failure. Hepatitis A virus (HAV) is a ribonucleic acid (RNA) virus. The virus is in feces. It is transmitted primarily through the fecal-oral route.

Poor hygiene, improper food handling, homelessness, crowded situations, and poor sanitary conditions are risk factors.[1] Transmission occurs between family members, institutionalized persons, and children in daycare centers. Foodborne outbreaks are usually due to food contaminated by an infected food handler. Small outbreaks can occur with fecal contamination of food or drinking water. People at increased risk for infection include drug users (both IV and noninjection drugs), males who have sex with males (MSM), and persons traveling to developing countries.

The greatest risk for transmission occurs before symptoms appear. It can be transmitted up to 2 weeks before the onset of symptoms and at least 1 week after the onset of illness. This means it can be carried and transmitted by persons who have undetectable infection. It is present only briefly in blood, usually less than 3 weeks. Fecal excretion can occur in infants for months.

Antibody to HAV immunoglobulin M (IgM) (HAV IgM) appears during the acute phase. The presence of HAV IgM indicates acute hepatitis. Levels stay high for about 8 weeks. HAV IgG without HAV IgM indicates past infection. IgG antibody provides lifelong immunity (Fig. 48.2). HAV vaccination and thorough hand washing are the best ways to prevent outbreaks. In the United States the incidence of HAV is low among persons who are vaccinated.

TABLE 48.1 Characteristics of Hepatitis Viruses

Incubation Period and Mode of Transmission	Sources of Infection	Infectivity
Hepatitis A Virus (HAV) *Incubation:* 15–50 days (average 28) Fecal-oral (primarily fecal contamination and oral ingestion)	• Contaminated food, milk, water, shellfish • Crowded conditions (e.g., day care, nursing home) • Persons with subclinical infections, infected food handlers, sexual contact, IV drug users • Poor personal hygiene • Poor sanitation	• Most infectious during 2 weeks before onset of symptoms • Infectious until 1–2 weeks after the start of symptoms
Hepatitis B Virus (HBV) *Incubation:* 40–90 days (average 60) Percutaneous (parenteral) or mucosal exposure to blood or blood products Sexual contact Perinatal transmission	• Contaminated needles, syringes, and blood products • HBV-infected mother (perinatal transmission) • Sexual activity with infected partners. Asymptomatic carriers • Tattoos or body piercing with contaminated needles	• Before and after symptoms appear • Infectious for months • Carriers continue to be infectious for life
Hepatitis C Virus (HCV) *Incubation:* 14–180 days (average 56) Percutaneous (parenteral) or mucosal exposure to blood or blood products High-risk sexual contact Perinatal contact	• Blood and blood products • Needles and syringes • Sexual activity with infected partners, low risk	• 1–2 weeks before symptoms appear • Continues during clinical course • 75%–85% develop chronic HCV and remain infectious
Hepatitis D Virus (HDV) *Incubation:* 2–26 weeks HBV must precede HDV Chronic carriers of HBV always at risk	• Same as HBV • Can cause infection only when HBV is present	• Blood infectious at all stages of HDV infection
Hepatitis E Virus (HEV) *Incubation:* 15–64 days (average 26–42 days) Fecal-oral route	• Contaminated water, poor sanitation • Found in Asia, Africa, and Mexico • Not common in United States but is increasing in some areas	• Not known • May be similar to HAV

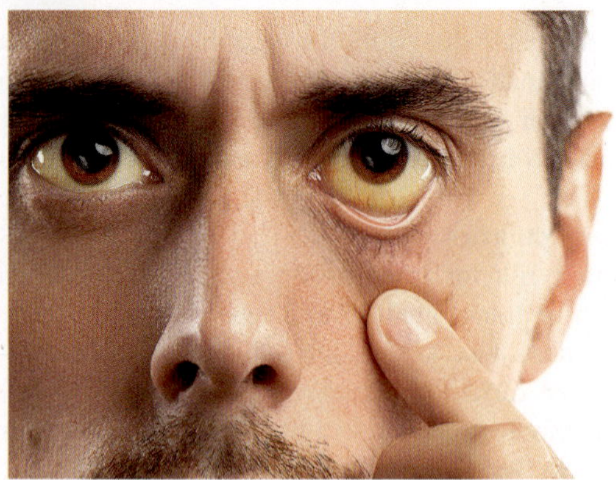

Fig. 48.1 Jaundiced person. (© Jun/iStock.com.)

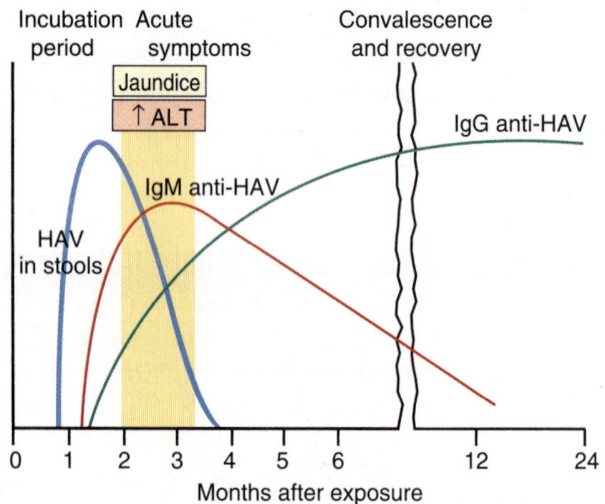

Fig. 48.2 Course of infection with hepatitis A virus *(HAV). ALT,* Alanine aminotransferase. (From McCance KL, Huether SE: *Pathophysiology: the biologic basis for disease in adults and children*, ed 8, St Louis, 2019, Mosby.)

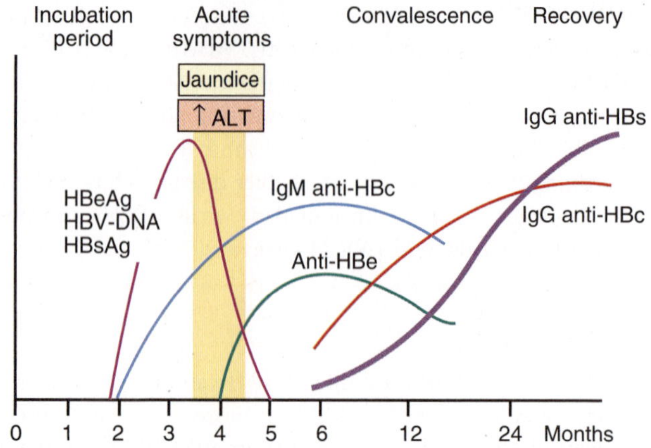

Fig. 48.3 Course of infection with hepatitis B virus *(HBV). ALT,* Alanine aminotransferase; *anti-HBc,* antibody to hepatitis B core antigen; *anti-HBe,* antibody to HBeAg; *anti-HBs,* antibody to HBsAg; *HBeAg,* hepatitis B e antigen; *HBsAg,* hepatitis B surface antigen. (From McCance KL, Huether SE: *Pathophysiology: the biologic basis for disease in adults and children*, ed 8, St Louis, 2019, Mosby.)

Hepatitis B Virus

Hepatitis B virus (HBV) is a blood-borne pathogen that can cause either acute or chronic hepatitis. The global prevalence of HBV is around 3.5% to 5%. The disease burden is largely in Sub-Saharan Africa, Western Pacific Regions, and Southeast Asia. The United States has policies to prevent HBV transmission through immunization of newborns, children, and high-risk populations.[2]

HBV is a deoxyribonucleic acid (DNA) virus. It can be transmitted in several ways: (1) perinatally from mothers infected with HBV to their infants; (2) percutaneously (e.g., IV drug use, accidental needle-stick punctures); or (3) via small cuts on mucosal surfaces and exposure to infectious blood, blood products, or other body fluids (e.g., semen, vaginal secretions, saliva).

Sexual transmission is a common mode of HBV transmission. MSM (especially those practicing unprotected anal intercourse) are at an increased risk. Most believe that casual encounters, like hugging, kissing, and sharing utensils, do not transmit the disease. Other at-risk persons include those who live with chronically HBV-infected persons, patients on hemodialysis, health care personnel, public safety workers, blood product recipients, prisoners, veterans, and persons without stable shelter.

HBV has been detected in almost every body fluid. Infected semen, cervicovaginal secretions, and saliva contain much lower HBV concentrations than blood, but the virus can be transmitted via these secretions. If gastrointestinal (GI) bleeding occurs, virus in the blood can contaminate feces. There is no evidence of fecal-oral transmission. Organ and tissue transplants are another potential source of infection. In some patients with acute HBV, there is no readily identifiable risk factor.

HBV is a complex structure with 3 distinct antigens: surface antigen (HBsAg), core antigen (HBcAg), and e antigen (HBeAg). Each antigen, along with its corresponding antibody, may appear or disappear in blood depending on the phase of infection and immune response.

In most people who acquire HBV infection as an adult, the infection completely resolves without any long-term complications. In those who develop chronic HBV infections, there is an association with liver cancer and severe liver inflammation and scarring (fibrosis). Those who become chronically infected have an increase in comorbidities. These include cardiovascular disease, hypertension, hyperlipidemia, renal disease, and osteoporosis.[3]

Screening for HBV includes identifying those at high risk for infection and testing the blood for the presence of hepatitis B surface antigen (HBsAg), hepatitis B antibody (anti-HBs), and hepatitis B core antibody (anti-HBc). The presence of anti-HBs indicates immunity from the HBV vaccine or from past HBV infection (Fig. 48.3). HBsAg in the blood for 6 months or longer after infection indicates chronic HBV infection.

Hepatitis C Virus

Hepatitis C virus (HCV) is a blood-borne RNA virus that can cause acute illness and chronic infection. It is mainly transmitted percutaneously.[4] Acute HCV can be hard to detect unless a diagnosis is made with laboratory testing. Common modes of HCV transmission are sharing contaminated needles and equipment among persons who inject drugs or having sex with a person with HCV.

Many people infected with HCV develop chronic infection. However, because signs and symptoms of HCV infection are generally mild, most people are not aware of their infection. We think that greater than 50% of people in the United States infected with HCV are undiagnosed. About 20% develop cirrhosis and eventually liver failure and/or liver cancer if left untreated. HCV hepatitis is a common reason for a liver transplant in the United States.[4]

Persons at risk for HCV infection are also at risk for HBV and HIV infections. About 30% to 40% of HIV-infected patients also have HCV. This high rate of coinfection is primarily related to IV drug use. Coinfection with HIV and HCV places patients at greater risk for progression to cirrhosis if HCV is untreated. A positive antibody test for HCV (anti-HCV) is followed by a positive viral load (HCV RNA) test to confirm active infection because anti-HCV can also indicate past infection.

With the use of direct-acting antiviral (DAA) medications, it is possible to cure HCV in most cases. The focus of care in chronic HCV is on preventing transmission, screening, and providing needed health care.[5]

Hepatitis D Virus

Hepatitis D virus (HDV), also called *delta virus,* is uncommon in the United States. HDV is a defective single-stranded RNA virus that cannot survive on its own. It requires HBV surface Ag to serve as its outer shell and to infect the hepatocyte. So, only those who with HBV infection can be infected with HDV. It can be acquired at the same time as HBV or a person with HBV can be infected with HDV later. HDV is transmitted like HBV. It causes more rapid progression of liver disease and mortality than HBV infection alone. There is no vaccine for HDV. However, HBV vaccination reduces the risk for HDV coinfection.[6]

Hepatitis E Virus

Like HAV, the hepatitis E virus (HEV) is an RNA virus transmitted by the fecal-oral route. The usual mode of transmission is through contaminated water. HEV infection epidemics occur in the tropics, but it is widely circulating in the West. It is generally acute and self-resolving. Chronicity in immunosuppressed persons, such as liver transplant recipients and persons with HIV, can occur. Pregnant females may be affected severely. An IgM antibody test is available to test for acute hepatitis E.[7]

Pathophysiology

Liver

In viral hepatitis, hepatocytes become targets of the virus in 1 of 2 ways: through direct action of the virus (as in HCV infection) or through a cell-mediated immune response to the virus (as in HBV and HCV infection).

During acute viral hepatitis, large numbers of infected hepatocytes are destroyed. This destruction leads to a wide range of liver-related dysfunction. Bile production, coagulation, glucose, and protein metabolism can be affected. Detoxification and processing of drugs, hormones, and metabolites (e.g., ammonia from protein catabolism) may be disrupted. The acute phase is the period of maximal infectivity.

After acute infection resolves, liver cells can regenerate. If no complications occur, the liver can resume its normal appearance and function. In some patients, acute hepatitis becomes so severe and irreversible that they develop acute liver failure, which can be fatal.

Chronic viral hepatitis can be insidious and silent, causing persistent and continual destruction of infected hepatocytes. Over time scar tissue can develop, which leads to fibrosis. This can cause cirrhosis, compromised liver function, and liver failure.

Systemic Effects

In the early phases of viral hepatitis, antigen-antibody complexes between the virus and its corresponding antibody may form circulating immune complexes. The circulating immune complexes activate the complement system (see Chapter 12). The manifestations of this activation are rash, angioedema, arthritis, fever, and malaise. *Cryoglobulinemia* (abnormal proteins found in the blood), glomerulonephritis, vasculitis, and involvement of other organs can occur from immune complex activation.

Clinical Manifestations and Complications

We classify the manifestations of viral hepatitis infections into acute hepatitis and chronic hepatitis (Table 48.2).

Acute Hepatitis

Many patients with acute hepatitis have no symptoms. They may not even know they are infected. Others may have anorexia, lethargy, nausea, vomiting, skin rashes, diarrhea or constipation, malaise, fatigue, muscle pain, joint pain, other flu-like symptoms, and right upper quadrant (RUQ) tenderness (caused by liver inflammation).

Although the acute phase of viral hepatitis varies depending on the type of hepatitis, it usually lasts from 1 to 6 months. During this time, patients may have a decreased sense of smell and find food repugnant. Smokers may have distaste for cigarettes. Assessment often reveals hepatomegaly, lymphadenopathy, abdominal tenderness, and sometimes splenomegaly.

Patients in the acute phase of hepatitis may be *icteric* (jaundiced) or anicteric. **Jaundice**, a yellowish discoloration of body tissues, results from a change in normal bilirubin metabolism or disruption of the flow of bile into the hepatic or biliary duct systems. Table 48.3 describes the types of jaundice.

The urine may appear darker due to the kidneys excreting excess bilirubin. If conjugated bilirubin cannot pass into the intestines from the liver because of obstruction or inflammation of the bile ducts, the stools will be clay colored.

Pruritus (intense general itching) sometimes accompanies jaundice. It occurs from the accumulation of bile salts beneath the skin. Itching can be intolerable to patients. Levels of bile salts (bile acid) can be measured in the blood.

As jaundice fades, the convalescent phase begins. The convalescent phase can last for weeks to months, with an average of 2 to 4 months. During this period, patients often have malaise and fatigue. Hepatomegaly remains for several weeks. Splenomegaly (if present) subsides during this period.

Most patients with acute viral hepatitis recover completely. Almost all cases of acute hepatitis A resolve. However, some patients may have a relapse in the first 2 to 3 months after the infection. The disappearance of jaundice does not mean a patient has totally recovered. Some HBV infections and most HCV infections result in chronic hepatitis.

Complications of acute hepatitis include chronic hepatitis, cirrhosis, portal hypertension, and liver cancer. Sometimes, acute liver failure (fulminant hepatic failure) may occur. It is a serious condition with a poor prognosis. Manifestations include encephalopathy, coagulation problems, and jaundice. Multiple complications can develop. A liver transplant may cure these patients.

TABLE 48.2 Manifestations of Hepatitis

Acute Hepatitis	Chronic Hepatitis
• Anorexia • Clay-colored stools • Dark urine • Diarrhea, constipation • Fatigue, lethargy, malaise • Flu-like symptoms (e.g., headache) • Hepatomegaly • Jaundice • Joint and muscle pain • Low-grade fever • Lymphadenopathy • Nausea, vomiting • Pruritus • RUQ tenderness • Splenomegaly • ↓ Taste and smell • Weight loss	• ↑ ALT, AST (may be normal in some people) • Ascites and lower extremity edema • Asterixis ("liver flap") • ↑ Bilirubin • Bleeding problems (thrombocytopenia, easy bruising, prolonged clotting time) • Fatigue, malaise • Hepatic encephalopathy: confusion, problems concentrating, easy agitation • Hepatomegaly • Jaundice • Joint and muscle pain • Palmar erythema • Spider angiomas

Chronic Hepatitis

Table 48.2 shows the manifestations of chronic hepatitis. Chronic HBV is more likely to develop if the person acquired the infection at birth or during childhood. Chronic HBV can remain asymptomatic for years. Complications such as cirrhosis, liver failure, and liver cancer develop in 15% to 40% of people with HBV.[8]

HCV infection is more likely than HBV to become chronic. Many patients with chronic HCV infection develop chronic liver disease, cirrhosis, portal hypertension, and liver cancer if untreated. In some patients, coinfection with HIV may cause complications or require treatment modification.

Skin manifestations may include spider angiomas, palmar erythema, and gynecomastia. Some patients with advanced fibrosis have spleen, liver, or cervical lymph node enlargement.

TABLE 48.3 Classification of Jaundice

	Hemolytic Jaundice	Hepatocellular Jaundice	Obstructive Jaundice
Causes	• Blood transfusion reactions, hemolytic anemia, sickle cell crisis	• Cirrhosis, hepatitis, liver cancer	• Cirrhosis, hepatitis, liver cancer • Common bile duct obstruction from stone(s), biliary strictures, pancreatic cancer, sclerosing cholangitis
Description	• Increased breakdown of RBCs, which increases amount of unconjugated bilirubin in blood • Liver is unable to handle increased load	• Liver's altered ability to take up bilirubin from blood or to conjugate or excrete it • In hepatocellular disease, damaged hepatocytes leak bilirubin	• Decreased or obstructed flow of bile through liver or bile duct system • Obstruction may occur in intrahepatic or extrahepatic bile ducts • Intrahepatic obstructions are due to swelling or fibrosis of the liver's canaliculi and bile ducts
Diagnostic Findings			
Bilirubin			
Unconjugated (indirect)	↑	↑	↑
Conjugated (direct)	Normal	↑ or ↓ (severe disease)	↑
Urine bilirubin	Negative	↑	↑
Urobilinogen			
Stool	↑	Normal, ↓	↓
Urine	↑	Normal, ↑	↓

In patients with decompensated cirrhosis, *hepatic encephalopathy*, a potentially life-threatening spectrum of neurologic, psychiatric, and motor disturbances, can occur. Hepatic encephalopathy results from the liver's inability to remove toxins (especially ammonia) from the blood.

Ascites is the accumulation of excess fluid in the peritoneal cavity. It is a common manifestation of hepatitis (especially from cirrhosis due to chronic hepatitis). Fluid accumulates due to reduced protein levels in the blood, which reduces the plasma oncotic pressure. Stiffness of the liver can prevent natural blood flow, leading to portal hypertension.

Diagnostic Studies

The only definitive way to distinguish among the types of viral hepatitis is by testing the blood for the specific antigen or antibody (Table 48.4). In some types of viral hepatitis, we can test the blood for the viral load (viral level). Many liver function tests show significant abnormalities, as shown in Table 48.5.

Several tests are available to determine the presence of HCV. The screening test for HCV infection is HCV antibody testing. Antibodies can be detected within 4 weeks of infection. If the antibody test is positive, HCV RNA testing assesses for chronic infection and quantifies viral load. A positive result confirms chronic infection. A few patients may have a false-positive HCV antibody result with a negative HCV RNA test. If we suspect recent HCV infection, HCV RNA testing is usually done because it may take several weeks or longer for HCV antibodies to develop.

HCV RNA testing may be used for immunocompromised patients (e.g., persons with HIV). Because of altered or delayed antibody response to HCV, these patients may not have detectable antibody levels even if they are infected with HCV.

Viral genotype testing is done in patients receiving drug therapy for HBV or HCV infection. HBV has at least 10 different genotypes (A to J).[9] In some centers, we do HBV genotyping before starting treatment. HBV genotype may be useful in predicting disease course and treatment outcomes. HBV core Ab (HBVcAb) IgG shows if patients have a history of recovered HBV infection. HBV may reactivate in these patients if they become immunosuppressed.

A liver biopsy is done in acute hepatitis if the diagnosis is in doubt. In chronic hepatitis, a liver biopsy allows for histologic examination of liver cells and determination of the degree of inflammation, fibrosis, or cirrhosis that may be present. Patients with a bleeding disorder may not be able to have a percutaneous liver biopsy because of the risk for bleeding. In these patients, a transjugular biopsy may be done, or patients may receive platelets or fresh frozen plasma immediately before the biopsy.

Noninvasive assessment of liver fibrosis is increasingly replacing the need for liver biopsy. One option is the use of

TABLE 48.4 Diagnostic Studies

Viral Hepatitis

Virus	Tests	Significance
A (HAV)	HAV immunoglobulin M (IgM)	Acute infection
	HAV immunoglobulin G (IgG)	Previous infection or immunization Not routinely done in clinical practice
B (HBV)	HBsAg (hepatitis B surface antigen)	Marker of infectivity Present in acute or chronic infection Positive in chronic carriers
	Anti-HBs (hepatitis B surface antibody)	Previous natural immunity from cleared HBV infection or immunity from immunization
	HBeAg (hepatitis B e antigen)	High infectivity Determine the clinical management of patients with chronic HBV
	Anti-HBe (hepatitis B e antibody)	Less active phase of infection In chronic HBV, indicates a low viral load and low degree of infectivity
	Anti-HBc (antibody to hepatitis B core antigen) IgM	Acute infection Does not appear after vaccination
	Anti-HBc IgG	Previous infection or ongoing infection with HBV Does not appear after vaccination
	HBV DNA quantitation	Active ongoing viral replication Best indicator of viral replication; reflects therapy effectiveness of therapy with chronic HBV
	HBV genotyping	Genotype of HBV
C (HCV)	Anti-HCV (antibody to HCV)	Marker for acute or chronic infection with HCV
	HCV RNA quantitation	Active ongoing viral replication
	HCV genotyping	Genotype of HCV
D (HDV)	Anti-HDV	Present in past or current infection with HDV
	HDV Ag (hepatitis D antigen)	Present within a few days after infection; must have HBV coinfection
E (HEV)	Anti-HEV IgM and IgG	Present 1 week to 2 months after illness onset
	HEV RNA quantitation	Active ongoing viral replication

TABLE 48.5 Diagnostic Findings in Acute Hepatitis

Test	Abnormal Finding	Cause
Alkaline phosphatase	Moderately ↑	Impaired excretory function of liver
γ-Glutamyl transpeptidase (GGT)	↑	Liver cell injury
Aminotransferases		
• Aspartate aminotransferase (AST)	↑ in acute phase Decrease as jaundice disappears	Liver cell injury
• Alanine aminotransferase (ALT)	↑ in acute phase Decrease as jaundice disappears	Liver cell injury
Proteins		
• Albumin	Normal or ↓	Liver cell injury
• γ-Globulin	Normal or ↓	Impaired clearance from liver
Prothrombin time	Prolonged	↓ Prothrombin production by liver
Total bilirubin	↑ to about 8–15 mg/dL (137–257 μmol/L)	Liver cell injury
Urine bilirubin	↑	Conjugated hyperbilirubinemia
Urine urobilinogen	↑ 2–5 days before jaundice	↓ Urobilinogen reabsorption

ultrasound elastography (e.g., FibroScan). It uses an ultrasound transducer to determine the degree of liver stiffness, which is converted to a quantified estimation of fibrosis. Magnetic resonance elastography (MRE) is another noninvasive imaging technique to measure liver fibrosis. FibroSure (FibroTest) is one of several biomarkers that use the results of blood tests to assess the extent of liver fibrosis.[10]

Interprofessional Care

There is no specific treatment for acute viral hepatitis. Most patients are managed at home. Emphasis is on providing adequate nutrition and measures to rest the body and help the liver to regenerate and repair (Table 48.6). Rest reduces the metabolic demands on the liver and promotes liver cell regeneration. In patients with chronic viral hepatitis, care may involve liver specialists, infectious disease specialists, pharmacists, dietitians, and mental health or substance use specialists. The role and extent of involvement of team members is based on the patient's specific needs.

Drug Therapy

Acute hepatitis. There are no drug therapies for treating acute HAV infection. Treatment of acute HBV may be indicated only in patients with severe hepatitis and liver failure. In acute HCV, some patients may choose to be monitored for spontaneous clearance of the infection. Patients who choose treatment may receive a DAA. This class of antiviral drugs is discussed later in the section on chronic hepatitis. Supportive drug therapy may include antihistamines, gallstone dissolution agents, or bile acid binding resins for general itching. Antiemetics are used for nausea.

Chronic hepatitis B. Drug therapy for chronic HBV focuses on decreasing viral load and liver enzymes, and in turn, slowing the rate of disease progression. Long-term goals are preventing the development of cirrhosis, portal hypertension, liver failure, and liver cancer.[11] Current drug therapies do not eradicate the virus. They suppress viral replication and prevent complications. First-line therapies primarily include nucleoside and nucleotide analogs (Table 48.7) and sometimes interferon therapy. Patients who are immunosuppressed, or are undergoing cancer treatment, should be treated for hepatitis B to prevent a flare. Patients with HIV and HBV coinfection must remain on hepatitis B treatment in addition to their HIV treatment regimens. Care must be taken to ensure that changes in HIV regimens do not eliminate hepatitis B treatment unintentionally.

Nucleoside and nucleotide analogs. Nucleoside and nucleotide analogs inhibit viral DNA replication. HBV reproduces by making copies of its viral DNA nucleosides and nucleotides. The nucleoside and nucleotide analog drugs mimic normal building blocks for DNA but are actually faulty viral DNA building blocks. Once they become included in the viral DNA, they halt DNA synthesis.

TABLE 48.6 Interprofessional Care

Viral Hepatitis

Diagnostic Assessment

- History and physical assessment
- Liver testing (Table 48.5)
- Hepatitis testing (Table 48.4)
  - *Hepatitis A (HAV):* HAV IgM, HAV IgG, HAV total antibody
  - *Hepatitis B (HBV):* HBsAg, anti-HBs, HBeAg, anti-HBe, anti-HBc IgM and IgG, HBV DNA quantitation, HBV genotyping
  - *Hepatitis C (HCV):* Anti-HCV, HCV RNA quantitation, HCV genotyping
  - *Hepatitis D (HDV):* Anti-HDV, HDV Ag, HDV RNA
  - *Hepatitis E (HEV):* Anti-HEV IgM, anti-HEV IgG
- Ultrasound elastography (FibroScan)
- Fibrosis biomarkers (FibroSure, FibroTest)

Management

Acute and Chronic

- Well-balanced diet
- Vitamin supplements
- Rest (degree needed varies)
- Avoid alcohol and drugs detoxified by liver
- Protect kidney function
- Monitor for liver failure

Chronic HBV and HCV

- Drug therapy (Table 48.7)
- Screening for liver cancer

TABLE 48.7 **Drug Therapy**

Viral HBV and HCV

Drug Class	Examples	Mechanism of Action	Indication
Immune modulator	pegylated interferon (Pegasys, PegIntron)	Has antiviral, antiproliferative, immune-regulating actions	Chronic HBV
Nucleoside and nucleotide analogs	adefovir[a] entecavir (Baraclude) lamivudine (Epivir HBV) tenofovir (Vemlidy, Viread)	Inhibits HBV DNA polymerase enzyme by competing with natural substrates. Prevents viral replication	Chronic HBV
Direct-acting antivirals for HCV			
NS3/4A protease inhibitors	glecaprevir[b] grazoprevir[c] voxilaprevir[b]	Blocks viral protease enzyme. Prevents viral replication in genotype 1 HCV	Chronic HCV
NS5A inhibitors	elbasvir[b] ledipasvir[c] pibrentasvir[b] velpatasvir[b]	Blocks nonstructural protein 5A (NS5A) at early stage in RNA HCV replication	Chronic HCV
NS5B polymerase inhibitors	sofosbuvir (Sovaldi)	Nucleotide inhibitor and nonnucleoside inhibitor of HCV polymerase. Prevent replication of RNA HCV	Chronic HCV
Combination therapies	elbasvir + grazoprevir (Zepatier) ledipasvir + sofosbuvir (Harvoni) pibrentasvir + glecaprevir (Mavyret) velpatasvir + sofosbuvir (Epclusa) velpatasvir + sofosbuvir + voxilaprevir (Vosevi)	Drugs are combined in 1 tablet. Drugs may be from the same or different classes	Chronic HCV

[a]Not preferred.
[b]Used only in combination therapy.
[c]Used with CYP3A inhibitor to enhance action.

Nucleoside and nucleotide analogs do not prevent all viral reproduction. They can substantially lower viral load or the amount of virus in the body. These drugs include lamivudine (Epivir), adefovir (Hepsera), entecavir (Baraclude), and tenofovir (Viread). They are used to treat chronic HBV when there is evidence of significant active viral replication and liver inflammation. These drugs also decrease liver damage and decrease liver enzyme levels. Most patients with HBV need long-term treatment. When these drugs are stopped, many patients' (except those who have seroconverted) HBV DNA and liver enzyme levels return to pretreatment levels.

Severe exacerbations can develop after ending treatment. If these drugs are stopped for any reason, we monitor patients' liver enzymes for several months.

Interferon. Interferon is a naturally occurring immune protein made by the body during an infection to recognize and respond to pathogens. It has antiviral, antiproliferative, and immune-modulating effects (see Chapter 14). Pegylated interferon (PEG-Intron, Pegasys) is given by subcutaneous injection. The many side effects of therapy, including flu-like symptoms (e.g., fever, malaise, fatigue), make adherence hard for some patients. The availability of better tolerated and more effective oral treatments limits interferon use. However, it is still used to treat some patients with HBV because it can have an increased viral response.

Patients receiving interferon should have a complete blood count (CBC) and liver function tests every 4 to 6 weeks. Thyroid function should also be checked intermittently. Depression is a side effect of therapy. Screen patients for depression and other mood disorders before starting treatment and monitor them frequently while on therapy.

Chronic hepatitis C. Treatment of chronic HCV is patient specific. It is based on the genotype of the HCV, severity of liver disease, and presence of other health problems (e.g., HIV). The goal of drug therapy is eradicating the virus and preventing HCV-related complications.

Treatment for HCV primarily includes the use of DAAs (Table 48.7), which block proteins needed for HCV replication. DAA therapy can take 8 to 12 weeks, depending on the treatment used. Almost all (>95%) of those who complete DAA treatment see a cure of their chronic HCV infection.[5]

Many patients with HIV also have HCV. Patients who have stable HIV and intact immune systems ($CD4^+$ counts greater than 200/μL) receive HCV treatment with the goal of eradicating HCV and reducing the risk for progression to cirrhosis. HCV treatment regimens are equally effective for treating hepatitis C in persons with both HCV and HIV coinfection. Patients with advanced fibrosis or cirrhosis can receive drug therapy if liver decompensation (e.g., ascites, variceal rupture, jaundice, wasting, encephalopathy) is not present.

NURSING MANAGEMENT: VIRAL HEPATITIS

Assessment

Subjective and objective data that you should obtain from a person with hepatitis are outlined in Table 48.8. Assess for jaundice. In persons with light skin, jaundice is usually seen first in the sclera of the eyes and later in the skin. In persons with dark skin, jaundice is seen in the hard palate of the mouth and inner canthus of the eyes. The urine may have a dark-brown or brownish-red color from bilirubin excretion from the kidneys.

Clinical Problems

Clinical problems for patients with viral hepatitis may include:

- Nutritionally compromised
- Activity intolerance
- Risk for bleeding

Additional information on clinical problems and interventions for patients with hepatitis is presented in eNursing Care Plan 48.1 available on the website for this chapter.

Planning

The overall goals are that patients with viral hepatitis will (1) have relief of discomfort, (2) be able to resume normal activities, (3) return to normal liver function without complications, and (4) avoid disease transmission.

Implementation

Health Promotion

Viral hepatitis is a public health problem. Your role is important in the prevention and control of this disease. It is helpful to understand the different types of viral hepatitis when considering control measures. Preventive and control measures for hepatitis A, B, and C are outlined in Table 48.9.

A suggested guideline to prevent you from contracting viral hepatitis from diagnosed and undiagnosed patients and carriers is for you to wear personal protective equipment (PPE) when fecal or blood contamination is likely in handling (1) soiled bedpans, urinals, and catheters and (2) when patients' bed linens are soiled by body excreta or secretions. Preventing needlestick injuries is important.

Hepatitis A. Viral hepatitis outbreaks are usually due to HAV. Preventive measures include personal and environment hygiene and health education to promote good sanitation. Hand washing is the most important precaution. Teach about careful hand washing after bowel movements and before eating. Avoiding raw and undercooked food and tap water in areas where there are high rates of hepatitis A infection and poor sanitation is important.

Isolation is not needed for HAV infection. For patients with HAV infection, use infection control precautions. Place patients who are incontinent of stool or have poor personal hygiene in a private room.

TABLE 48.8 NURSING ASSESSMENT

Hepatitis

Subjective Data

Important Health Information

Health history: Exposure to infected persons, ingestion of contaminated food or water. Exposure to benzene, carbon tetrachloride, or other hepatotoxic agents. Crowded, unsanitary living conditions. Exposure to contaminated needles or sharp objects, including drug implements. Recent travel, organ transplant, cancer, new drug therapy, hemodialysis, hemophilia, blood or blood products transfusion before 1992. HIV status (if known)

Medications: Acetaminophen, new medications or supplements

Functional Health Patterns

Health perception–health management: IV drug and chronic alcohol use. Malaise, distaste for cigarettes (in smokers), high-risk sexual behaviors

Nutritional-metabolic: Weight loss, anorexia, nausea, vomiting. Feeling of RUQ fullness

Elimination: Dark urine, light-colored stools, constipation or diarrhea, skin rashes, hives

Activity-exercise: Fatigue, muscle pain, joint pain

Cognitive-perceptual: RUQ pain, liver tenderness, headache, itching

Role-relationship: Exposure as health care worker, resident in long-term care institution, incarceration, homelessness

Objective Data

General

Low-grade fever, lethargy, lymphadenopathy

GI

Hepatomegaly, splenomegaly

Skin

Rash or other skin changes, jaundice, icteric sclera, injection sites

Possible Diagnostic Findings

↑ Liver enzyme levels. ↑ Total bilirubin, hypoalbuminemia, anemia. Bilirubin in urine and urobilinogen. Prolonged PT time. Positive tests for hepatitis (see Table 48.4). Abnormal liver scan, abnormal liver biopsy results

Vaccination is the best protection against HAV. All children at 1 year of age should receive the vaccine series. Adults at risk should also receive the vaccine. These include travelers to areas with increased rates of hepatitis A, MSM, IV and noninjecting drug users, and homelessness. Others who should receive the vaccine include persons with clotting factor disorders (e.g., hemophilia) and chronic liver disease.

HAV vaccine is inactivated HAV protein. There are 2 forms of HAV vaccine in the United States: Havrix and Vaqta. Primary immunization consists of 1 dose given IM in the deltoid muscle. A booster is recommended 6 to 12 months after the first dose to ensure adequate antibody titers and long-term protection. Primary immunization provides immunity within 30 days after 1 dose in more than 97% to 100% of those vaccinated.[1]

Twinrix, a combined HAV and HBV vaccine, is available for people over 18 years of age. It consists of 3 doses, given on a 0-, 1-, and 6-month schedule (the same schedule as the single HBV

TABLE 48.9 Preventing Viral Hepatitis

Hepatitis A

General Measures

- Hand washing
- Proper personal hygiene
- Food safety
- Control and screening (signs, symptoms) of food handlers
- Serologic screening for those carrying virus
- Active immunization: HAV vaccine series

Use of Immune Globulin

- Early administration (1–2 weeks after exposure) to those exposed
- Prophylaxis for travelers to areas where hepatitis A is common if not vaccinated with HAV vaccine

Hepatitis B and C

Percutaneous Transmission

- Screen donated blood
- Use disposable needles and syringes
- Avoid shared drug paraphernalia
- Avoid unprofessional tattoo placement, maintaining new ink and needles
- Avoid shared piercing implements
- HBV: Screening in endemic areas to prevent vertical transmission

Sexual Transmission

- Acute exposure: HBIG administration to sexual partner of HBsAg-positive person
- Give HBV vaccine series to uninfected sexual partners
- Use condoms for vaginal and anal intercourse

General Measures

- Hand washing
- Avoid sharing toothbrushes and razors
- HBIG administration for one-time exposure (needle stick, contact of mucous membranes with infectious material)
- Active immunization: HBV vaccine series

Special Considerations for Health Care Personnel

- Use infection control precautions
- Reduce contact with blood or blood-containing secretions
- Handle the blood of patients as potentially infective
- Dispose of needles properly
- Use needleless IV access devices when available

vaccine). Twinrix may be given to high-risk persons, including patients with chronic liver disease, persons who inject drugs, patients on hemodialysis, MSM, and people with clotting factor disorders who receive therapeutic blood products. The side effects are mild. They include soreness and redness at the injection site.

Both HAV vaccine and immune globulin (IG) are used to prevent HAV infection after exposure to an infected person *(postexposure prophylaxis)*. The vaccine is used for preexposure prophylaxis. We can give IG either before or after exposure. IG gives temporary (1 to 2 months) passive immunity. It is effective for preventing HAV if given within 2 weeks after exposure. IG is given to persons who do not have HAV antibodies and were exposed by close (household, daycare center) contact with persons who have HAV or foodborne exposure. Because patients with HAV are most infectious just before the onset of symptoms, those exposed through household contact or foodborne outbreaks should receive the HAV vaccine. They may receive IG based on risk factors. Although IG may not prevent infection, it may lessen the illness to a subclinical infection.

Hepatitis B. The best way to reduce HBV infection is to identify those at risk, screen them for HBV, and vaccinate those who are not infected. Teach those at high risk for contracting HBV to reduce risks by following good hygienic practices, including hand washing and using gloves when expecting contact with blood. Patients should not share razors, toothbrushes, and other personal items. Teach patients to use a condom for sexual intercourse. In addition, the partner should be vaccinated.

The HBV vaccine is the best means of prevention. There are different types of HBV vaccines available.[12] One type of HBV vaccine (Recombivax HB, Engerix-B) contains HBsAg. HBsAg promotes the synthesis of specific antibodies directed against HBV. The vaccine is given in a series of 3 IM injections in the deltoid muscle. It is given on a 0-, 1-, and 6-month schedule. The vaccine is 95% effective. Minor reactions include transient fever and soreness at the injection site. The vaccine can be given in pregnancy. Heplisav-B is another type of HBV vaccine that is approved for persons 18 years or older. It is given in 2 doses, spaced 4 weeks apart.

The traditional HBV vaccine of 3 doses is normally given in childhood. The first dose of HBV vaccine should be given at birth. The vaccine series is completed by age 6 to 18 months. Older children and adolescents who did not receive the HBV vaccine should be vaccinated. It is important to vaccinate adults who are in the at-risk groups and are not immune. Household members of patients with HBV should be tested and vaccinated if they are HBsAg and antibody negative. HBV vaccination is recommended for patients with chronic kidney disease before they start dialysis. Patients who receive dialysis should routinely have their antibody titer levels checked to determine the need for revaccination.

For postexposure prophylaxis, the HBV vaccine series and hepatitis B immune globulin (HBIG) are given. HBIG has antibodies to HBV and confers temporary passive immunity. HBIG is prepared from the plasma of donors with a high titer of anti-HBs. HBIG is recommended for postexposure prophylaxis in cases of needle stick, mucous membrane contact, or sexual exposure and for infants born to mothers who are positive for HBsAg. Ideally, we should give HBIG within 24 hours of exposure. Giving antiviral therapy (e.g., tenofovir) to pregnant females in the third trimester with viral levels over 200,000 IU/mL can prevent the small risk for neonatal infection that may occur even with postnatal immunization and vaccination.

The Centers for Disease Control and Prevention (CDC) recommends following standard precautions for patients with HBV (see Table 15.13). This includes using disposable needles and syringes and disposing of them in puncture-resistant units without recapping, bending, or breaking.

Hepatitis C. No vaccine is currently available for HCV. So, it is important to identify those at high risk for contracting HCV and teach them how to reduce their risks. Measures to prevent HCV transmission include (1) screening of blood, organ, and tissue donors; (2) using infection control precautions; and (3) modifying behaviors that increase the risk of transmission.

In the United States many people have undiagnosed HCV. They acquired HCV when they were younger but were never screened or diagnosed. The current U.S. screening guidelines recommend one-time HCV testing for everyone 18 years and older. Annual HCV screening is recommended for persons who inject drugs.

Acute Care

Most patients with viral hepatitis are at home. Assess patients for any complications. These include bleeding tendencies with increasing prothrombin (PT) time values, encephalopathy, bloody or tarry stools, vomiting of blood, or high liver enzymes. Note a sudden increase in weight and abdominal girth, which may indicate fluid retention and/or ascites.

Comfort measures to relieve itching, headache, and joint pain are helpful.

> **CHECK YOUR PRACTICE**
>
> You are caring for a patient with acute hepatitis who was admitted to the hospital for IV hydration and monitoring. The patient says, "My skin feels so itchy, I can't stop scratching. Isn't there something you can do to help me?"
> - How would you handle this situation?
> - What information and teaching will you give him?

Ensure that patients receive adequate nutrition. Anorexia and distaste for food may cause nutrition problems. Emphasize a well-balanced diet that patients can tolerate. Adequate calories are important because patients usually lose weight. If patients do not tolerate fat content because of decreased bile production, it should be reduced. Assess the tolerance of specific foods and eating patterns. Small, frequent meals may be preferable to 3 large ones and may help prevent nausea. Often patients with hepatitis find that anorexia is not as severe in the morning, so it is easier to eat a good breakfast than a large dinner. Include measures to stimulate the appetite, such as mouth care, antiemetics, and attractively served meals in pleasant surroundings. Drinking carbonated beverages and avoiding very hot or cold foods may help ease anorexia. Adequate fluid intake (2500 to 3000 mL/day) is important. Patients may receive vitamin supplements, particularly B-complex and vitamin K. If anorexia, nausea, and vomiting are severe, we may give IV glucose solutions or supplemental enteral nutrition (EN).

The degree of rest depends on the severity of symptoms. Usually, alternating periods of activity and rest are adequate. Assess the response to the rest and activity plan. Modify it as needed based on liver function tests and symptoms. Limited activity may produce anxiety and restlessness in some patients. Diversion activities, such as reading and hobbies, may help patients cope with the plan of care and ensure adequate rest.

Discharge teaching includes how to prevent transmission to other family members and notifying contacts for testing and prophylaxis, if needed. Caution patients about overexertion and the need to follow the HCP's advice about when to return to work. For patients who have fatigue, tell them to plan activities after periods of rest when energy levels are highest.

Patients should have regular follow-ups for at least 1 year after the diagnosis of hepatitis. Because relapses occur with HBV and HCV, teach patients the symptoms of recurrence and the need for follow-up care. All patients with chronic HBV or HCV should avoid alcohol as it can accelerate disease progression. Remind patients who are positive for HBsAg (chronic carrier status) or HCV antibody that they cannot be blood donors. Patients who have chronic hepatitis B infection, with or without cirrhosis, should have regular screening for liver cancer. Patients who have hepatitis C cirrhosis, even if they have cleared the virus, should have regular screening for liver cancer.[5]

◆ Evaluation

Expected outcomes are that patients with hepatitis will
- Maintain food and fluid intake adequate to meet nutrient needs
- Avoid alcohol and other hepatotoxic agents
- Show gradual increase in activity tolerance
- Demonstrate behaviors that prevent disease transmission
- Have regular follow-up with HCP to screen for progression of disease and liver cancer

DRUG- AND CHEMICAL-INDUCED LIVER DISEASES

Alcohol use can cause injury and necrosis of liver tissue. The manifestations can range from a mild elevation in liver enzymes to acute alcoholic hepatitis. Advanced fibrosis and cirrhosis can occur after decades of excess alcohol use. Patients may have serious liver disease caused by another chronic disease (e.g., chronic viral infection or autoimmune liver disease) in combination with alcoholic liver disease, which can compound the problem.

Acute alcoholic hepatitis is a syndrome of hepatomegaly, jaundice, increased liver enzymes (AST, ALT, alkaline phosphatase), and low-grade fever. Ascites and prolonged PT time are possible. These manifestations may improve if alcohol use ceases.

Even at the end-stage of cirrhosis, abstinence can result in significant reversal in some patients. If liver function does not recover after abstaining from alcohol for 6 months or longer, a liver transplant may be an option.[13]

Chemical hepatotoxicity is liver injury caused by exposure to certain compounds (e.g., carbon tetrachloride, gold compounds). Some agents can cause hepatotoxicity, while others may induce cholestasis, necrosis, or liver cancer. Fortunately, because of the decreased use of these agents, the incidence of chemically induced liver toxicity has decreased since the 1980s.

Drug-induced liver injury (DILI) can present similarly to other forms of liver disease, with different degrees of biliary, or immune-mediated injury. The pattern of injury depends on the drug causing the reaction. Many drugs can cause an increase in liver enzymes and in severe cases jaundice and acute liver failure. The main cause of DILI is antimicrobial agents, especially amoxicillin-clavulanate. The most common cause of acute liver failure is acetaminophen. In patients with chemical hepatotoxicity or DILI, all drugs identified as the cause of liver injury should be stopped.[14]

Older adults are particularly vulnerable to DILI. This is due to several factors, including the increased use of multiple prescription and OTC drugs, which can lead to drug interactions and potential drug toxicity. Decreases in liver function result in decreased drug metabolism and a decreased ability to recover from drug-induced injury.

DRUG ALERT

Acetaminophen

- Safe when taken at recommended levels.
- Its prevalence in a variety of pain relievers, fever reducers, and cough medicines may mean that patients do not know they are taking several drugs that all contain acetaminophen. This can cause an overdose.
- Acute liver failure can occur because of overdosing, either intentionally or unintentionally.
- Combining the drug with alcohol increases the risk for liver damage.

AUTOIMMUNE, GENETIC, AND METABOLIC LIVER DISEASES

Autoimmune Hepatitis

Autoimmune hepatitis is a chronic inflammatory liver disorder in which the immune system attacks the liver. The cause is unknown. It is thought to originate from triggers such as the environment, including viral illnesses, drug exposure, and changes to the gut microbiome. It is characterized by the presence of autoantibodies and high levels of immunoglobulins. It often occurs with other autoimmune diseases.

Most patients with autoimmune hepatitis are females. Laboratory tests useful in the diagnosis include antinuclear antibody (ANA), anti–smooth muscle antibody (ASMA), and antimitochondrial antibody (AMA) testing. A liver biopsy can confirm the diagnosis and guide the treatment decision.

Although autoimmune hepatitis can cause acute liver failure, the spectrum of disease is variable. Most patients develop chronic hepatitis. Untreated autoimmune hepatitis can progress to cirrhosis. Prednisone with or without azathioprine (Imuran) is the recommended treatment for active autoimmune hepatitis. Cyclosporine, tacrolimus, budesonide, methotrexate, mercaptopurine, and mycophenolate mofetil are options in those who do not respond to prednisone and azathioprine. Mycophenolate is most often used for those who are intolerant to azathioprine.[15]

Wilson Disease

Wilson disease is an autosomal recessive disorder involving cellular copper metabolism.[16] A defect in biliary excretion leads to copper accumulation in the liver and other tissues. This causes progressive liver injury and cirrhosis.

Once cirrhosis occurs, copper leaks into the plasma, leading to multiple problems, including neurologic, hematologic, and psychiatric symptoms. The hallmark of Wilson disease is corneal Kayser-Fleischer rings. These are brownish-red rings seen in the cornea near the limbus on eye examination. Low ceruloplasmin levels and markedly elevated copper levels from liver biopsy samples are present. Diagnosis is based on clinical findings. First-degree relatives of patients with Wilson disease need to be screened for the disease.

The recommended first treatment of symptomatic patients or those with active disease is chelating agents, such as D-penicillamine or trientine (Syprine). They promote the excretion of urinary copper. Zinc acetate (Galzin), another therapy, interferes with copper absorption. Once we have reduced the amount of copper in the body, treatment focuses on preventing copper from building up again. A liver transplant may be an option with severe liver damage.

Hemochromatosis

Hemochromatosis is a condition in which excess iron accumulates in the body.[17] It is mainly caused by a genetic defect *(hereditary hemochromatosis).* Iron accumulation in the liver can also be caused by liver disease and chronic blood transfusions used to treat thalassemia and sickle cell disease. Hemochromatosis is discussed in Chapter 34.

Primary Biliary Cholangitis

Primary biliary cholangitis (PBC), or primary biliary cirrhosis, is a chronic disease of the small bile ducts of the liver.[18] In PBC, there is a T-cell–mediated attack of the small bile duct cells. This causes a narrowing and loss of bile ducts and blockage of bile flow. Over time, this leads to liver fibrosis and cirrhosis.

Most patients diagnosed with PBC are middle-aged females. The disease is associated with other autoimmune disorders, such as rheumatoid arthritis, Sjögren syndrome, and scleroderma. High alkaline phosphatase, AMA, ANA, and lipid levels are present.

The goals of treatment are suppressing ongoing liver damage, preventing complications, and symptom management. Drugs for PBC include ursodiol, a bile acid, and obeticholic acid (Ocaliva). These drugs decrease bile acids in the liver. Care focuses on preventing or minimizing malabsorption, hyperlipidemia, vitamin deficiencies, anemia, and fatigue. Care is taken to manage skin effects, such as itching and xanthomas (cholesterol deposits in the skin). Cholestyramine is used to treat itching. Patients are monitored for progression to cirrhosis. Liver transplant is an option for end-stage liver disease.

Primary Sclerosing Cholangitis

Primary sclerosing cholangitis (PSC) is characterized by chronic inflammation, fibrosis, and narrowing of the medium and large bile ducts both inside and outside the liver.[19] We do not know the cause. Most patients with PSC also have ulcerative colitis or, less often, Crohn disease. Complications include cholangitis, cholestasis with jaundice, bile duct cancer, and cirrhosis.

Drug therapy has no proven benefit, although many HCPs use ursodiol. Treatment is directed at reducing the incidence of biliary complications and screening for bile duct and colorectal cancer, which is related to the high incidence of ulcerative colitis. Patients with advanced liver disease may need a liver transplant.

Metabolic Dysfunction–Associated Steatotic Liver Disease and Metabolic Dysfunction–Associated Steatohepatitis

Metabolic dysfunction–associated steatotic liver disease (MASLD) refers to a wide spectrum of liver diseases ranging from steatosis (fat deposits in the liver) to metabolic dysfunction–associated steatohepatitis (MASH), to cirrhosis.[20] The fundamental characteristic of liver steatosis is the accumulation of fatty infiltration in the hepatocytes. In MASH, fat accumulation is associated with varying degrees of inflammation and fibrosis of the liver. If MASH is untreated, it can lead to cirrhosis, liver cancer, and liver failure.

Liver steatosis is more prevalent in patients with metabolic disease and obesity. Rates of progression of fibrosis vary based on baseline disease severity, genetic makeup, and environment. Anyone with risk factors, including obesity, diabetes, hyperlipidemia, and hypertension (or *metabolic syndrome*), should be screened for MASH.

Elevated liver function tests (ALT, AST) are often the first sign of MASLD. Ultrasound and CT scans can be used to diagnose MASLD. Definitive diagnosis is by a liver biopsy; however, there are other noninvasive methods (elastography) for identifying fat in the liver and liver stiffness.

There are no currently approved drugs for MASLD. There are studies looking at the benefit of GLP-1 receptor agonists. The goal of therapy is weight loss of at least 10% of body weight, if overweight or obese, and exercise. Bariatric surgery for morbidly obese persons reduces the risk of MASLD. Reducing other risk factors, including hyperlipidemia, hypertension, and diabetes, is important (Box 48.1).

BOX 48.1 EVIDENCE-BASED PRACTICE

MASLD Program

You are caring for a 32-year-old male who was recently diagnosed with MASLD. He arrives today saying he feels tired and concerned that he will end up with liver cancer. He says it is difficult to ask his HCP questions and receive follow-up care.

Making Clinical Decisions

Best Available Evidence

MASLD is often associated with other conditions, including type 2 diabetes and hypertension. This can lead to a complex treatment plan with follow-up care to monitor disease progression and complications. Research shows a novel, nurse-delivered community-based program for people with MASLD achieved increased access to care. Patients reported a decrease in anxiety and stress.

Clinician Expertise

Your clinic partners with another clinic in the community to explore how patients with MASLD could receive follow-up care in a more efficient manner through a nurse-run protocol at the clinic. As the nurse, you believe this patient would benefit from additional education, improved follow-up care, and the ability to talk with other patients diagnosed with MASLD.

Patient Preferences and Values

You approach the patient about the new protocol, and he agrees to enroll. Six months later, he returns to your clinic and states he "feels much better" about his current follow-up appointments and is "less anxious" about getting liver cancer.

Implications for Nursing Practice

1. What information would you anticipate patients receiving at the nurse-run clinic?
2. What follow-up diagnostic studies would be completed to best monitor the patient's disease status?

Reference for Evidence

Allen M, Tulleners R, Brain D, et al: Implementation of nurse-delivered community-based liver screening and assessment program for people with metabolic-dysfunction–associated steatotic liver disease, *BMC Hel Serv Res,* 25:421, 2025.

CIRRHOSIS

Cirrhosis is the end stage of liver disease.[21] It is characterized by extensive degeneration and destruction of the liver cells. This results in the replacement of liver tissue by fibrosis (scar tissue) and regenerative nodules that occur from the liver's attempt to repair itself. Developing cirrhosis usually happens after decades of chronic liver disease.

Etiology and Pathophysiology

Any chronic liver disease can cause cirrhosis. The most common causes in the United States are chronic HCV infection, MASH, and alcohol-induced liver disease. In patients with alcohol-induced liver disease, malnutrition adds to the damage caused by the alcohol. Some cases of nutrition-related cirrhosis have resulted from extreme dieting, malabsorption, and obesity. Environment and genetic predisposition may lead to developing cirrhosis.

Chronic inflammation and cell necrosis from viral hepatitis can result in progressive fibrosis and cirrhosis. Chronic hepatitis combined with alcohol use has a synergistic effect in accelerating liver damage. Biliary causes include PBC and PSC.

Cardiac cirrhosis includes a spectrum of liver problems that result from long-standing, severe, right-sided heart failure. It causes hepatic venous congestion, parenchymal damage, necrosis of liver cells, and fibrosis over time. Treatment is aimed at managing the underlying heart failure.

In cirrhosis, the liver cells try to regenerate, but the regenerative process is disorganized. This results in abnormal blood vessel and bile duct architecture. The overgrowth of new and fibrous connective tissue distorts the liver's normal lobular structure, resulting in lobules of irregular size and shape with impeded blood flow. Eventually, irregular and disorganized liver regeneration, poor cell nutrition, and hypoxia (from inadequate blood flow and scar tissue) result in decreased liver function.

Clinical Manifestations

Early Manifestations

Patients may be unaware of their liver condition because there are few symptoms in early-stage disease. If a person does have symptoms, these may include fatigue or an enlarged liver. Blood tests may show normal liver function (compensated cirrhosis). The diagnosis of cirrhosis is often made later when patients present with symptoms of more advanced liver disease.

Late Manifestations

Late manifestations result from liver failure and portal hypertension (Fig. 48.4). Jaundice, peripheral edema, and ascites develop gradually. Other late manifestations include skin lesions, hematologic problems, endocrine problems, and peripheral neuropathies (Fig. 48.5). In the advanced stages, the liver becomes small and nodular. Liver function is dramatically impaired.

Jaundice. Jaundice results from decreased ability to conjugate and excrete bilirubin into the small intestines (Table 48.3). There is an overgrowth of connective tissue in the liver, which compresses the bile ducts and leads to an obstruction. This results in an increase in the bilirubin in the vascular system,

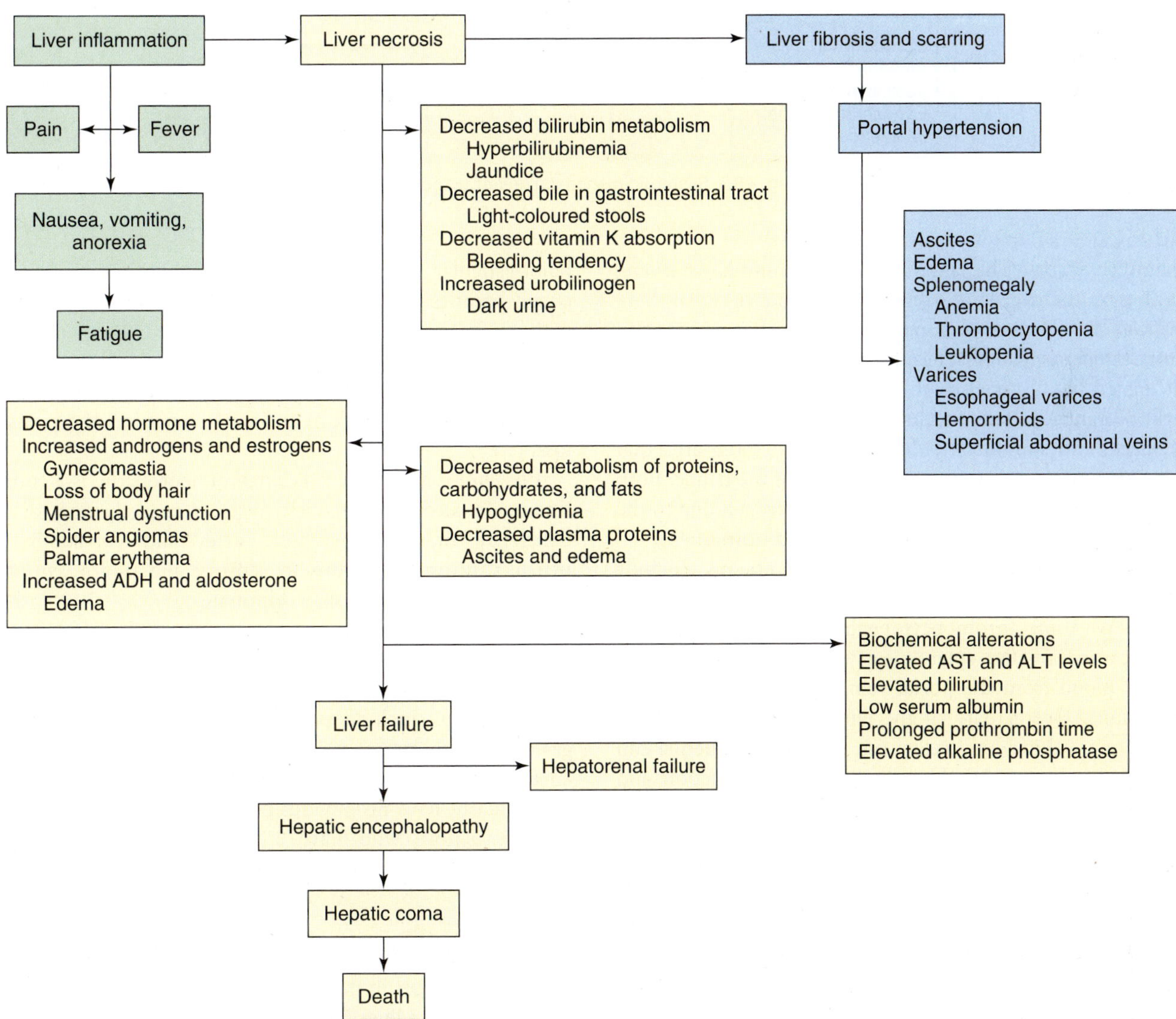

Fig. 48.4 Continuum of liver dysfunction in cirrhosis and resulting manifestations. (Adapted from Huether SE, McCance KL: *Understanding pathophysiology*, ed 2, St Louis, 2023, Mosby.)

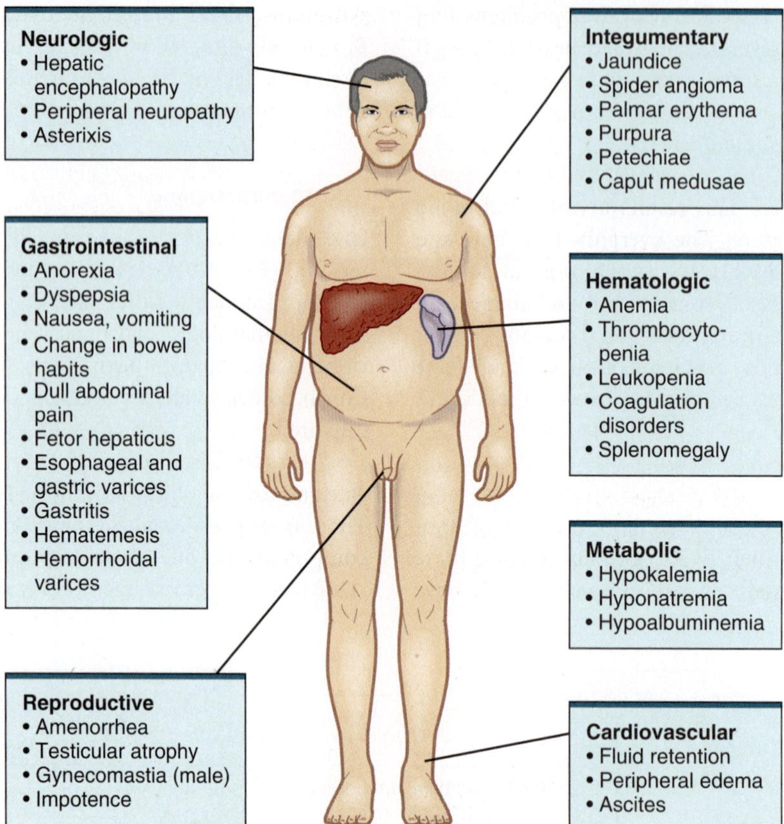

Fig. 48.5 Systemic manifestations of cirrhosis.

and jaundice occurs. The jaundice may be minimal or severe, depending on the degree of liver damage.

Skin lesions. Various skin manifestations often occur with cirrhosis. *Spider angiomas* (telangiectasia or spider nevi) are small, dilated blood vessels with a bright red center point and spiderlike branches. They occur on the nose, cheeks, upper trunk, neck, and shoulders. *Palmar erythema* (a red area that blanches with pressure) occurs on the palms of the hands. Both lesions are due to an increase in circulating estrogen due to the damaged liver's inability to metabolize steroid hormones.

Hematologic problems. Hematologic problems include thrombocytopenia, leukopenia, anemia, and coagulation problems. We think thrombocytopenia, leukopenia, and anemia are caused by the splenomegaly that results from the backup of blood from the portal vein into the spleen (portal hypertension). Overactivity of the enlarged spleen results in increased removal of blood cells from circulation. Anemia can result from inadequate red blood cell (RBC) production and survival, poor diet, poor folic acid absorption, and bleeding from varices.

Coagulation problems result from the liver's inability to make prothrombin and other factors essential for blood clotting. Manifestations include nosebleeds, purpura, petechiae, easy bruising, gingival bleeding, and heavy menses.

Endocrine problems. The liver plays a vital role in the metabolism of hormones, such as estrogen and testosterone. In males with cirrhosis, gynecomastia, loss of axillary and pubic hair, testicular atrophy, and impotence with loss of libido may occur because of increased estrogen levels. Younger females with cirrhosis may develop amenorrhea. Older females may have unexpected vaginal bleeding. If the liver does not metabolize aldosterone properly, it can lead to hyperaldosteronism with sodium and water retention and potassium loss.

Peripheral neuropathy. Peripheral neuropathy is a common finding in alcohol-related cirrhosis. It is likely due to a diet deficiency of thiamine, folic acid, and cobalamin. The neuropathy usually results in sensory and motor symptoms, but sensory symptoms may dominate.

Complications

Complications include portal hypertension, esophageal and gastric varices, peripheral edema, abdominal ascites, hepatic encephalopathy, and hepatorenal syndrome. Patients who are cirrhotic but have no obvious complications have *compensated cirrhosis.* Those who have 1 or more complications have *decompensated cirrhosis.*

Portal Hypertension and Esophageal and Gastric Varices

Structural changes in the liver lead to obstruction of blood flow in and out of the liver. This results in increased pressure within the liver's circulatory system (**portal hypertension**). Portal hypertension is characterized by increased venous pressure in the portal circulation, splenomegaly, large collateral veins, ascites, and gastric and esophageal varices.

To reduce pressure, the body develops alternate circulatory pathways, referred to as *collateral circulation.* The collateral channels often form in the lower esophagus, anterior abdominal wall, parietal peritoneum, and rectum. Varicosities (distended veins) develop in areas where the collateral and systemic circulations communicate, resulting in esophageal and gastric varices, *caput medusae* (ring of varices around the umbilicus), and hemorrhoids.

Esophageal varices are a complex of tortuous, enlarged veins at the lower end of the esophagus. **Gastric varices** are found in the upper part of the stomach. These varices are fragile and do not tolerate high pressure, so they can bleed easily. Large varices are more likely to bleed. Esophageal varices can cause variceal hemorrhages with a 5-year risk of mortality of up to 27%. Patients may present with melena or hematemesis. Ruptured esophageal varices are the most life-threatening complication of cirrhosis and are considered a medical emergency.

Peripheral Edema and Ascites

Peripheral edema occurs in the lower extremities and presacral area. Peripheral edema can occur before, concurrently with, or after ascites development. Edema results from decreased colloidal oncotic pressure from impaired liver synthesis of albumin and increased portacaval pressure from portal hypertension.

Ascites is the accumulation of serous fluid in the peritoneal or abdominal cavity. It is a common manifestation of cirrhosis. Several mechanisms lead to ascites. One mechanism occurs with portal hypertension, which causes proteins to shift from the blood vessels into the lymph space (Fig. 48.6). When the lymphatic system is unable to carry off the excess proteins and water, they leak into the peritoneal cavity. The osmotic pressure of the proteins pulls more fluid into the peritoneal cavity.

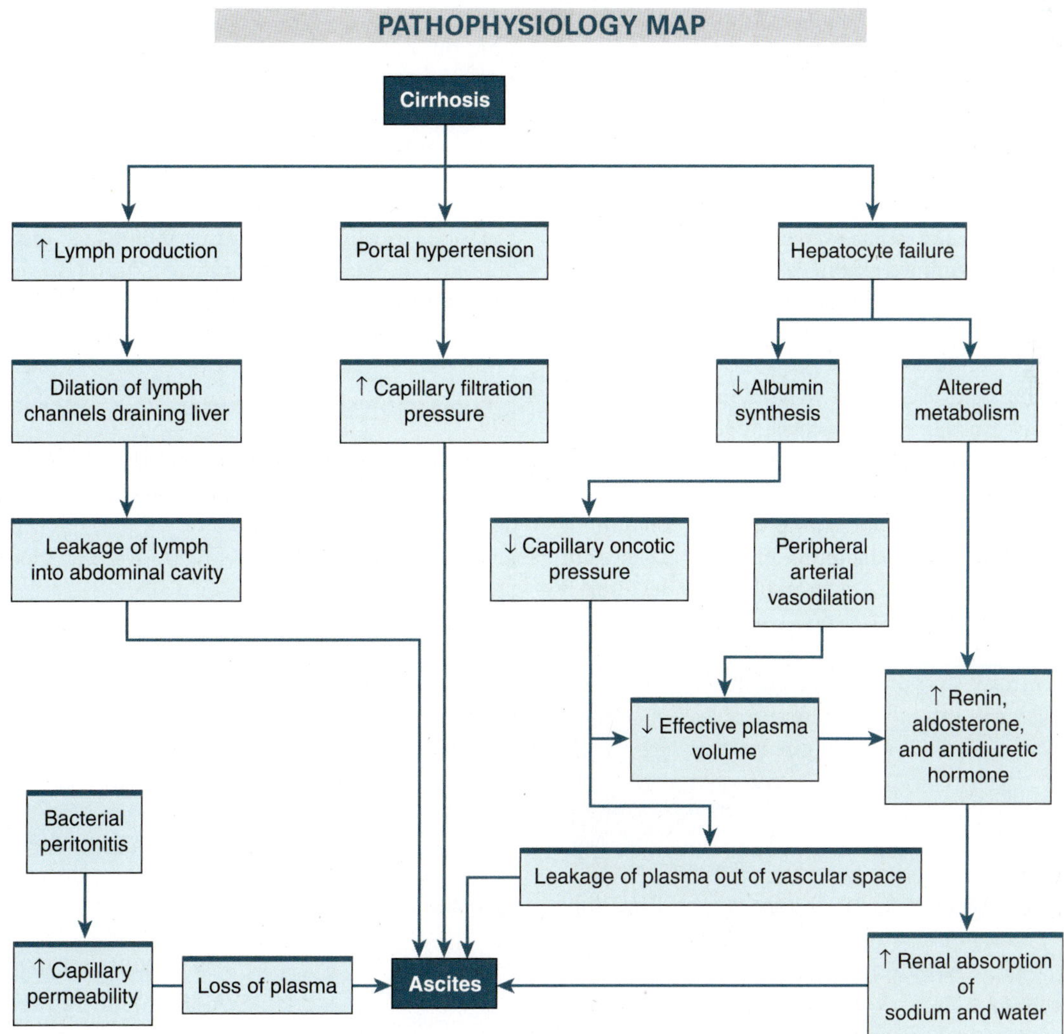

Fig. 48.6 Mechanisms for development of ascites. (Adapted from Huether SE, McCance KL: *Understanding pathophysiology*, ed 5, St Louis, 2012, Mosby.)

A second mechanism of ascites formation is hypoalbuminemia resulting from the liver's decreased ability to synthesize albumin. Hypoalbuminemia results in decreased colloidal oncotic pressure.

A third mechanism of ascites is hyperaldosteronism, which occurs when the damaged hepatocytes metabolize aldosterone. The increased aldosterone level causes increased sodium reabsorption by the renal tubules. Sodium retention, combined with an increase in antidiuretic hormone in blood, leads to further water retention and edema. Edema decreases intravascular volume with decreased renal blood flow and glomerular filtration.

Ascites is manifested by abdominal distention with weight gain (Fig. 48.7). If the ascites is severe, the increase in abdominal pressure from fluid accumulation may cause eversion of the umbilicus (hernia). Abdominal striae with distended abdominal wall veins may be present. Patients may have signs of dehydration and a decrease in urine output. Hypokalemia is common. It is due to excess potassium loss from hyperaldosteronism. Low potassium levels can also result from diuretic therapy used to treat the ascites. Those with severe ascites are at risk for pleural effusion.

Because of decreased immune function with cirrhosis, patients with ascites are at risk for *spontaneous bacterial peritonitis* (SBP). SBP is a bacterial infection of the ascitic fluid. In SBP, bacteria normally found in the intestines move into the peritoneal space. The bacteria most often responsible for the infection are gram-negative enteric pathogens, such as *Escherichia coli.* SBP is a common complication of hospitalized patients with cirrhosis and ascites. Worsening vasodilation contributes to the development of SBP.

Hepatic Encephalopathy

Hepatic encephalopathy is a neuropsychiatric manifestation of liver disease. The cause is multifactorial.[22] It includes the neurotoxic effects of ammonia, abnormal neurotransmission, astrocyte swelling, and inflammatory cytokines. A major source of ammonia is the bacterial and enzymatic deamination of amino acids in the intestines. The ammonia that results from deamination normally goes to the liver via the portal circulation, where it is converted to urea. The kidneys then excrete urea. When blood is shunted past the liver via the collateral vessels or the liver is so damaged that it is unable to convert ammonia to urea, the ammonia levels in the systemic circulation increase. The ammonia crosses the blood-brain barrier and produces neurologic manifestations.

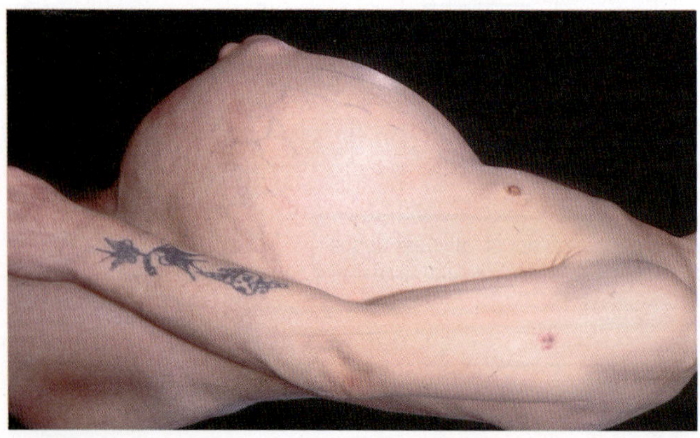

Fig. 48.7 Ascites. (Jarnagin WR: *Blumgart's surgery of the liver, biliary tract and pancreas,* ed 7, St. Louis, 2023, Elsevier.)

Factors that increase ammonia may precipitate hepatic encephalopathy (Table 48.10). Hepatic encephalopathy can occur after placement of a transjugular intrahepatic portosystemic shunt (TIPS). TIPS reduces portal hypertension by diverting blood flow around the liver.

Manifestations include neurologic and mental status changes. These include impaired consciousness and inappropriate behavior, ranging from sleep problems to trouble concentrating to deep coma. Changes may occur suddenly from an increase in ammonia in response to bleeding varices or infection or gradually as ammonia levels slowly rise. We often use a grading system to classify the stage of hepatic encephalopathy (Table 48.11).

A characteristic manifestation is **asterixis** (flapping tremors). This may take several forms, with the most common involving the arms and hands. When asked to hold the arms and hands stretched out, the patients are unable to hold this position and perform a series of rapid flexion and extension movements of the hands.

Writing impairments include difficulty moving the pen or pencil from left to right and *apraxia* (inability to construct simple figures). Other signs include hyperventilation, hypothermia, twitching of the tongue, and grimacing and grasping reflexes. *Fetor hepaticus* (musty, sweet odor of the breath) occurs in some patients. This odor is from the accumulation of digestive by-products that the liver is unable to degrade.

TABLE 48.10 Risk Factors for Hepatic Encephalopathy

Factor	Mechanism
Cerebral depressants (e.g., opioids)	↓ Metabolism by liver, causing ↑ drug levels and cerebral depression
Constipation	↑ Ammonia production from bacterial action on feces
Dehydration	Potentiates ammonia toxicity
GI bleeding	↑ Ammonia in GI tract
Hypokalemia	Potassium needed by brain to metabolize ammonia
Hypovolemia	↑ Ammonia because of hepatic hypoxia Impaired cerebral, liver, and renal function because of ↓ blood flow
Infection	↑ Metabolic rate and cerebral sensitivity to toxins
Metabolic alkalosis	Facilitate transport of ammonia across blood-brain barrier ↑ Renal production of ammonia
↑ Metabolism	↑ Workload of liver
Paracentesis	Loss of sodium and potassium ions ↓ Blood volume
Uremia (renal failure)	Retention of nitrogenous metabolites

TABLE 48.11 Grading Scale for Hepatic Encephalopathy

Grade	Level of Consciousness	Intellectual Function	Neurologic Findings
0	Normal to minimal change	Subtle to no change in personality, behavior, memory, concentration	Asterixis absent. May have abnormal psychometric test
1	Lack of awareness, sleep disturbance	Short attention span, impaired computational skills, personality change, impaired short-term memory, mild confusion, depression	Incoordination, asterixis may be absent
2	Lethargy, drowsiness	Disoriented to time, inappropriate behavior, deficits in executive function	Asterixis, abnormal reflexes
3	Somnolent, arousable	Disoriented to time, loss of meaningful conversation, marked confusion, incomprehensible speech	Asterixis, abnormal reflexes
4	Not arousable, comatose	Absent	Decerebrate May be responsive to painful stimuli

Hepatorenal Syndrome

Hepatorenal syndrome is a type of renal failure with azotemia, oliguria, and intractable ascites. The cause is likely to be portal hypertension along with liver decompensation, resulting in splanchnic and systemic vasodilation and decreased arterial blood volume. As a result, renal vasoconstriction occurs, and renal failure follows. Liver transplants can reverse renal failure. In patients with cirrhosis, hepatorenal syndrome can follow diuretic therapy, GI bleeding, or paracentesis.

Diagnostic Studies

Most liver function tests are abnormal in patients with cirrhosis. Enzyme levels, including alkaline phosphatase, AST, ALT, and γ-glutamyl transpeptidase (GGT), are initially high due to their release from inflamed liver cells. However, in end-stage liver disease, AST and ALT levels may be normal due to the death and loss of hepatocytes. Patients will have low total protein and albumin, increased bilirubin and globulin levels, and prolonged PT time. Low cholesterol levels reflect changes in fat metabolism.

A liver biopsy can identify liver cell changes. It is the gold standard for a definitive diagnosis of cirrhosis. Although a liver ultrasound may be able to detect cirrhosis, it is not a reliable diagnostic test for cirrhosis. Ultrasound elastography (Fibroscan) is a noninvasive test used to quantify the degree of liver fibrosis.

Interprofessional Care

The goal of treatment is to slow the progression of cirrhosis and to prevent and treat any complications. Interprofessional care measures are listed in Table 48.12. Management of specific problems from cirrhosis is described next.

Ascites

Management of ascites focuses on sodium restriction, diuretics, and fluid removal. Patients may need to limit sodium intake to 2 g/day. Very low-sodium intake can result in reduced nutrient intake and malnutrition. Patients are usually not on restricted fluids unless severe ascites develops. Monitor fluid and electrolyte balance. An albumin infusion may help maintain intravascular volume and adequate urine output by increasing plasma colloid oncotic pressure.

TABLE 48.12 Interprofessional Care

Cirrhosis

Diagnostic Assessment
- History and physical assessment
- Liver function tests
- Albumin
- Electrolytes
- PT time
- Complete blood count
- Liver biopsy (percutaneous needle)
- Liver ultrasound (e.g., FibroScan)
- Upper endoscopy (esophagogastroduodenoscopy)
- CT scan, MRI

Management

Conservative Therapy
- Rest
- B-complex vitamins
- Avoiding alcohol
- Minimizing or avoiding aspirin, acetaminophen, and NSAIDs
- Drug therapy (see Table 48.13)

Ascites
- Low-sodium diet
- Diuretics
- Paracentesis (if needed)

Esophageal and Gastric Varices
- Endoscopic band ligation or sclerotherapy
- Balloon tamponade
- TIPS

Diuretic therapy is an important part of management. Often a combination of drugs that work at multiple sites of the nephron is more effective than a single agent. Spironolactone (Aldactone) is an effective diuretic, even in patients with severe ascites. Spironolactone is an aldosterone antagonist and is potassium sparing. A high-potency loop diuretic (e.g., furosemide) is often used with a potassium-sparing drug. Hyponatremia is a common problem in patients on diuretics. It causes an increase in water excretion, resulting in an increase in sodium concentration.

A *paracentesis* is a sterile procedure in which a catheter is used to withdraw fluid from the abdominal cavity. This procedure can diagnose a medical condition or relieve pain, pressure, or problems breathing. In patients with cirrhosis, this procedure is done for patients with impaired respiration or abdominal discomfort caused by severe ascites who do not respond to diuretic therapy. It is only a temporary measure because the fluid tends to reaccumulate rapidly.

TIPS is used to treat ascites that does not respond to diuretics. A peritoneovenous shunt is a surgical procedure that provides continuous reinfusion of ascitic fluid into the venous system. It is rarely used due to the high rate of complications.

Esophageal and Gastric Varices

The main therapeutic goal for esophageal and gastric varices is to prevent bleeding and variceal rupture by reducing portal pressure.[23] Patients with esophageal and/or gastric varices should avoid alcohol, aspirin, and nonsteroidal antiinflammatory drugs (NSAIDs).

All patients with cirrhosis should have an upper endoscopy (esophagogastroduodenoscopy [EGD]) to screen for varices. Patients with varices who are at risk for bleeding often receive a nonselective β-blocker (nadolol, propranolol) to reduce bleeding risk. β-Blockers decrease high portal pressure, which decreases the risk for rupture.

When variceal bleeding occurs, the first step is to stabilize the patient and manage the airway. IV therapy is started and may include giving blood products. Care then moves toward stopping the bleeding, identifying the source, and applying interventions to prevent further bleeding. Management that involves a combination of drug therapy and endoscopic therapy is more successful than either approach alone.

Drug therapy for bleeding varices may include the somatostatin analog octreotide (Sandostatin) or vasopressin. Both produce vasoconstriction of the splanchnic arterial bed, decrease portal blood flow, and decrease portal hypertension. Octreotide is used more often because it has fewer side effects than vasopressin.

At the time of endoscopy, band ligation or sclerotherapy of varices may be used to prevent rebleeding. Endoscopic variceal ligation (EVL, or "banding") is done by placing a small rubber band (elastic O-ring) around the base of the *varix* (enlarged vein). Sclerotherapy involves injecting a sclerosing solution into the swollen veins through a needle placed through the endoscope.

Balloon tamponade is an option when endoscopy does not control acute esophageal or gastric variceal hemorrhage. Balloon tamponade controls massive bleeding by mechanical compression of the varices. Several types of tubes are available. They have multiple lumens, including ones for gastric and esophageal balloons.

! SAFETY ALERT

Balloon Tamponade

- Label each lumen to avoid confusion.
- Secure the tube to prevent movement of the tube that could result in airway occlusion.
- Deflate balloons for 5 minutes every 8 to 12 hours per agency policy to prevent tissue necrosis.

Supportive measures during an acute variceal bleed include giving packed RBCs, vitamin K, and proton pump inhibitors (PPIs; e.g., pantoprazole). Lactulose and rifaximin (Xifaxan) may be given to prevent hepatic encephalopathy from breakdown of blood and the release of ammonia in the intestine. Antibiotics are given to prevent bacterial infection.

Because of the high incidence of recurrent bleeding with each bleeding episode, continued therapy is necessary. Long-term management of patients who have had an episode of bleeding includes nonselective β-blockers, repeated band ligation of the varices, and portosystemic shunts in patients who develop recurrent bleeding.

Shunting. Nonsurgical and surgical methods of shunting blood away from the varices are available. Shunting procedures tend to be done more after a second major bleeding episode than during an initial bleeding episode. TIPS is a nonsurgical procedure in which a tract (shunt) between the systemic and portal venous systems is created to redirect portal blood flow. A catheter is placed in the jugular vein and then threaded through the superior and inferior vena cava to the hepatic vein. The wall of the hepatic vein is punctured, and the catheter is directed to the portal vein. Stents are positioned along the passageway, overlapping in the liver tissue and extending into both veins.

TIPS reduces portal venous pressure and decompresses the varices, thus controlling bleeding. It does not interfere with a future liver transplant. Limitations include the increased risk for hepatic encephalopathy (toxin-containing blood bypasses the liver) and stenosis of the stent. TIPS is contraindicated in patients with severe hepatic encephalopathy, liver cancer, severe hepatorenal syndrome, and portal vein thrombosis.

Various surgical shunting procedures can decrease portal hypertension by diverting some of the portal blood flow while allowing adequate liver perfusion. Currently, the surgical shunts most often used are the portacaval shunt and the distal splenorenal shunt (Fig. 48.8).

Hepatic Encephalopathy

The goal of management of hepatic encephalopathy is to reduce ammonia formation and improve symptoms such as fatigue, memory lapses, and confusion. Lactulose, a drug that traps ammonia in the gut, reduces ammonia formation in the intestines. We can give it orally, as an enema, or through a nasogastric (NG) tube. The drug's laxative effect expels the ammonia from the colon. Antibiotics, such as rifaximin, may be given, especially in patients who do not respond to lactulose.

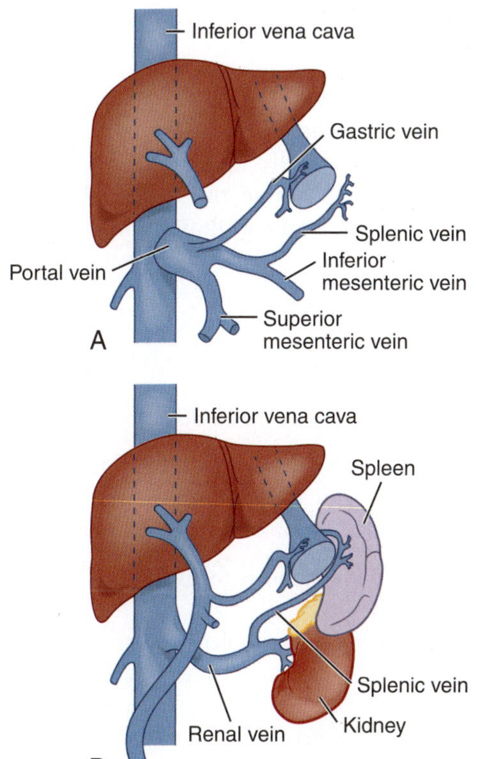

Fig. 48.8 Portosystemic shunts. (A) Portacaval shunt. The portal vein is anastomosed to the inferior vena cava, diverting blood from the portal vein to the systemic circulation. (B) Distal splenorenal shunt. The splenic vein is anastomosed to the renal vein. The portal venous flow stays intact while esophageal varices are selectively decompressed. The short gastric veins are decompressed. The spleen conducts blood from the high pressure of the esophageal and gastric varices to the low-pressure renal vein.

Regular and frequent bowel movements are necessary to minimize ammonia buildup, so use measures to prevent constipation.

Control of hepatic encephalopathy involves treating risk factors (Table 48.10). This includes preventing and controlling GI bleeds and, in the case of a bleed, removing the blood promptly from the GI tract to decrease the protein accumulation in the gut.

Drug Therapy

There is no specific drug therapy for cirrhosis. However, several drugs are used to treat symptoms and complications of advanced liver disease (Table 48.13).

Nutrition Therapy

The diet for patients without complications is high in calories (3000 cal/day). It is high in carbohydrate content with moderate to low levels of fat.

Patients with alcoholic cirrhosis often have protein-calorie malnutrition. Oral supplements containing protein from branched-chain amino acids that are metabolized by the muscles may be needed. These supplements provide protein that the liver can more easily metabolize. Parenteral nutrition (PN) or EN is given for severe malnutrition (see Chapter 44).

Patients with ascites and edema receive a low-sodium diet. The degree of sodium restriction depends on the patient's condition. Teach patients and caregivers about the degree of restriction. Review which foods are high in sodium. Review how to read labels for sodium content (see Fig. 44.4). Offer suggestions about how to make the diet more palatable. Seasonings, like garlic, parsley, onion, lemon juice, and spices, may make food more appetizing. Collaborate with a dietitian about diet strategies.

TABLE 48.13 Drug Therapy

Cirrhosis

Drug	Mechanism of Action
Diuretics	
furosemide	Acts on distal tubule and loop of Henle to ↓ reabsorption of sodium and water
spironolactone	Blocks actions of aldosterone
Other Therapy	
Nonselective β-blocker (e.g., propranolol)	↓ Portal venous pressure and esophageal variceal bleeding
lactulose	Acidifies feces in bowel and traps ammonia, causing its elimination in feces
magnesium sulfate	Corrects low magnesium that may occur with liver dysfunction
neomycin sulfate rifaximin	↓ Bacterial flora, thus reducing ammonia formation
octreotide vasopressin	Hemostasis and control of bleeding in esophageal and gastric varices, constricts splanchnic arterial bed
PPIs (e.g., pantoprazole)	↓ Gastric acidity
Vitamin K	Corrects clotting problems from decreased vitamin K levels

❖ NURSING MANAGEMENT: CIRRHOSIS

◆ Assessment

Subjective and objective data that you should obtain from patients with cirrhosis are outlined in Table 48.14. Assess the patient's physical status. Is jaundice present? Where is it seen—sclera, skin, hard palate? What is the progression of jaundice? Note the color of urine and stools and assess for improvement or normalization of color. When jaundice is present, the urine is often dark brown, and the stool is gray or tan.

◆ Clinical Problems

Clinical problems for patients with cirrhosis may include:

- Nutritionally compromised
- Activity intolerance
- Fluid imbalance

TABLE 48.14 NURSING ASSESSMENT

Cirrhosis

Subjective Data

Important Health Information

Health history: Hepatitis. Alcohol use, metabolic syndrome, chronic biliary obstruction and infection, autoimmune disease, severe right-sided heart failure, family history of liver disease, lung disease (e.g., cystic fibrosis, alpha-1 antitrypsin deficiency).

Medications: Adverse reaction to any medication. Use of anticoagulants, aspirin, NSAIDs, acetaminophen, supplements, herb products.

Functional Health Patterns

Health perception–health management: Chronic alcohol use. Weakness, fatigue

Nutritional-metabolic: Anorexia, weight loss, dyspepsia, nausea and vomiting, gingival bleeding. Dry, yellow skin, bruising

Elimination: Dark urine, decreased urine output, light-colored or black stools, red blood in stool

Cognitive-perceptual: Dull, RUQ or epigastric pain. Memory loss, confusion, somnolence, itching

Sexuality-reproductive: Impotence, amenorrhea, gynecomastia, irregular menses

Objective Data

General

Fever, cachexia, wasting of extremities

GI

Abdominal distention, ascites, distended abdominal wall veins, palpable liver and spleen, foul breath. Hematemesis. Black, tarry stools; rectal bleeding. Hemorrhoids

Neurologic

Altered mentation, asterixis

Reproductive

Loss of libido; gynecomastia, testicular atrophy, and impotence (men); amenorrhea, heavy menses (women)

Respiratory

Shallow, rapid respirations. Nosebleeds

Skin

Icteric sclera, jaundice, petechiae, bruising, spider angiomas, palmar erythema, alopecia, loss of axillary and pubic hair, peripheral edema

Possible Diagnostic Findings

Anemia, thrombocytopenia; leukopenia. ↓ Albumin, potassium. Abnormal liver enzyme studies. ↑ INR, ↓ platelets, ↑ ammonia, ↑ bilirubin levels. Abnormal abdominal ultrasound, CT, or MRI

Additional information on clinical problems and interventions for patients with cirrhosis is presented in eNursing Care Plan 48.2 available on the website for this chapter.

◆ Planning

The overall goals are that patients with cirrhosis will (1) have relief of discomfort, (2) have minimal to no complications, and (3) return to as normal a lifestyle as possible.

◆ Implementation

Health Promotion

Common risk factors include alcohol use, malnutrition, viral hepatitis, biliary obstruction, obesity, and right-sided heart failure. Prevention and early treatment of cirrhosis focus on reducing or eliminating these risk factors. Urge patients to abstain from alcohol. Encourage those with chronic alcohol use to enroll in support programs that help patients maintain sobriety. The treatment of alcohol use is discussed in Chapter 11.

Adequate nutrition, especially for the person who uses alcohol and other people at risk for or with cirrhosis, is essential to promote normal liver regeneration. Identify and treat acute hepatitis early so that it does not progress to chronic hepatitis and cirrhosis.

Acute Care

Care for patients with cirrhosis focuses on conserving strength while maintaining muscle strength and tone. When patients need complete bed rest, implement measures to prevent pneumonia, thromboembolic problems, and pressure injuries. Modify the activity and rest schedule according to signs of improvement (e.g., decreasing jaundice, reduced fluid overload, improved liver function studies).

Anorexia, nausea and vomiting, pressure from ascites, and poor eating habits interfere with adequate nutrient intake. Oral hygiene before meals may improve patients' taste sensation. Make between-meal snacks available so that patients can eat them at times when food is best tolerated. Offer preferred foods whenever possible. Explain the reason for any diet restrictions to patients and caregivers.

If itching accompanies jaundice, use measures to relieve itching. Cholestyramine, hydroxyzine (Atarax), or ursodiol may help. Cholestyramine is a resin that binds bile salts in the intestine, increasing their excretion in the feces. It comes in powder form that you mix with milk or juice. Side effects include nausea, vomiting, diarrhea or constipation, and skin reactions. It may bind with other medications, so check drug-to-drug interactions. Ursodiol helps bile flow and helps with the secretion of bile acids. Other measures to relieve itching include baking soda or moisturizing bath oils (Alpha Keri), lotions containing calamine, antihistamines, soft or old linens, and control of the temperature (not too hot and not too cold). Keep patients' nails short and clean. Teach patients to rub with their knuckles rather than scratch with their nails when they cannot resist scratching.

Edema and ascites require assessment and intervention. Record intake and output and daily weight. Measuring extremities and abdominal girth helps in the ongoing assessment of the location and extent of the edema. Mark the abdomen with a permanent marker so that you measure the girth at the same location each time. Care for patients having a paracentesis is outlined in Table 48.15.

Dyspnea is a frequent problem for patients with severe ascites. A semi-Fowler or Fowler position allows for maximal respiratory efficiency. Use pillows to support the arms and chest to increase patients' comfort and ability to breathe. Monitor the

TABLE 48.15 NURSING MANAGEMENT

Care of the Patient Undergoing Paracentesis

Preprocedure

- Have the patient void or insert an indwelling catheter.
- Insert IV.
- Obtain baseline vital signs and pulse oximetry. Weigh patient. Assess abdomen and measure abdominal girth.
- Assess baseline laboratory values (e.g., platelets, electrolytes, coagulation studies, renal function).
- Give any sedation or analgesia, if ordered.
- Teach patient to remain immobile during the procedure.
- Place the patient in a sitting position with feet on the floor or left lateral recumbent position.

Postprocedure

- Perform assessment and compare with baseline: vital signs, pulse oximetry, abdominal girth, abdominal pain. Watch for signs of intestinal perforation and hypovolemia.
- Help the patient remain in an upright position.
- Label and send the fluid for laboratory analysis.
- Check the dressing for bleeding and/or leakage of ascitic fluid.
- Give IV fluid and/or albumin as ordered.
- Measure any drainage and describe the collected fluid.
- Reweigh the patient and monitor intake and output.
- Maintain bed rest per agency protocol.
- Provide discharge instructions if applicable for showering, and signs of complications.
- Ensure patient has a follow-up visit with their HCP and contact information for changes in clinical status.

O_2 level and vital signs. Implement measures such as coughing and deep breathing to prevent respiratory problems.

CHECK YOUR PRACTICE

A patient with advanced cirrhosis and ascites tells you that he is having difficulty breathing and feels short of breath.

- What is your priority concern?

Good skin care is essential because edematous tissues are prone to break down. Use an alternating air pressure mattress or other special mattress. Adhere to a turning schedule (minimum of every 2 hours). Support the abdomen with pillows. If the abdomen is taut, cleanse it gently. Patients will tend to avoid moving because of abdominal discomfort and dyspnea. Range-of-motion exercises are helpful. The lower extremities may be elevated. If scrotal edema is present, a scrotal support gives some comfort.

When patients are taking diuretics, monitor sodium, calcium, potassium, chloride, and bicarbonate levels. Monitor renal function (blood urea nitrogen [BUN], creatinine) routinely and with any change in the diuretic dosage. Observe for signs of fluid and electrolyte imbalance, especially hypokalemia. Dysrhythmias, hypotension, tachycardia, and muscle weakness may occur with hypokalemia. Muscle cramping, weakness, lethargy, and confusion may be present with hyponatremia from water excess.

Observe for and provide nursing care for any hematologic problems. These include bleeding tendencies, anemia, and increased susceptibility to infection.

Assess the patient's response to altered body image resulting from jaundice, muscle wasting, spider angiomas, palmar erythema, ascites, umbilical hernia, and gynecomastia. Patients may have anxiety and embarrassment about these changes. Explain these phenomena. Be a supportive listener. Provide care to help patients maintain their self-esteem.

Bleeding varices. If patients have esophageal or gastric varices, observe for any signs of bleeding from the varices, such as hematemesis and melena. If hematemesis occurs, assess patients for bleeding and call the HCP. Be ready to transfer patients to the endoscopy suite and/or assist with equipment to control the bleeding. Maintain the airway. Ensure patients have venous access for blood or fluid administration. Patients with bleeding varices are usually admitted to the intensive care unit (ICU).

Balloon tamponade is an option for patients who have bleeding that is unresponsive to band ligation or sclerotherapy. When balloon tamponade is used, explain to the patients and caregivers the use of the tube and how the balloon is inserted. Check the balloons for patency. It is usually the HCP's responsibility to insert the tube by either the nose or mouth. Then the gastric balloon is inflated with 250 mL of air, and the tube is retracted until resistance (lower esophageal sphincter) is felt. The tube is secured by placing a piece of sponge or foam rubber at the nostrils (nasal cuff). For continued bleeding, the esophageal balloon is then inflated. A sphygmomanometer is used to measure and maintain the desired pressure at 20 to 40 mm Hg. An x-ray confirms the balloon's position.

Monitor for complications of rupture or erosion of the esophagus, regurgitation and aspiration of gastric contents, and airway occlusion by the balloon. If the gastric balloon breaks or deflates, the esophageal balloon will slip upward, obstructing the airway and causing asphyxiation. If this happens, cut the tube or deflate the esophageal balloon. Keep scissors at the bedside. Minimize regurgitation by oral and pharyngeal suctioning and keeping patients in a semi-Fowler position.

Patients are unable to swallow saliva because the inflated esophageal balloon occludes the esophagus. Encourage them to expectorate. Provide an emesis basin and tissues. Frequent oral and nasal care offers relief from the taste of blood and irritation from mouth breathing.

Hepatic encephalopathy. Nursing care focuses on maintaining a safe environment, sustaining life, and assisting with measures to reduce the formation of ammonia and other neurotoxins that build up due to liver dysfunction. Plan your care of patients based on the severity of the encephalopathy. Assess neurologic status at least every 2 hours. Include an exact description of the patient's behavior. Patients may be somnolent or confused and at risk for falls or other injuries. Note any sensory and motor problems (e.g., hyperreflexia, asterixis, motor coordination). Institute measures to prevent falls or injuries. Assess for fluid, electrolyte, and acid-base imbalances. Evaluate the response to treatment measures. In patients with altered levels of consciousness or whose airway may become compromised, have emergency equipment readily available.

Control factors known to precipitate encephalopathy as much as possible. Any GI bleeding may worsen encephalopathy. Measures to minimize constipation are important to reduce ammonia production and absorption. Give ordered drugs, laxatives, and enemas. Encourage fluids, if not contraindicated. Assess patients taking lactulose for diarrhea and fluid and electrolyte losses.

Chronic Care

Cirrhosis is a chronic disease. People can live many years with symptoms and complications from cirrhosis. Cirrhosis affects all aspects of a patient's life. Patients and caregivers need to understand the importance of continual health care. Supportive measures include proper diet, rest, avoiding hepatotoxic drugs such as acetaminophen in high doses, and abstaining from alcohol.

Abstinence from alcohol is important and results in improvement in most patients. However, some patients find abstinence difficult and need emotional support. Encourage those with chronic alcohol use to enroll in support programs that help patients maintain sobriety. The treatment of alcohol use is discussed in Chapter 11. Explore your own attitude toward patients whose cirrhosis is from chronic alcohol use (Box 48.2).

Teach patients and caregivers about complications and when to seek medical attention (Table 48.16). Include instructions about adequate rest periods, how to detect early signs of complications, skin care, drug therapy side effects, observation for bleeding, and protection from infection.

Referral to a community or home health nurse may help ensure patient adherence to prescribed therapy. Home care for patients with cirrhosis focuses on helping them with activities of daily living while maintaining the highest level of wellness possible.

◆ Evaluation

Expected outcomes are that patients with cirrhosis will:

- Maintain food and fluid intake adequate to meet nutrient needs
- Maintain skin integrity with relief of edema and itching
- Have normal fluid and electrolyte balance
- Acknowledge and get treatment for a substance use problem

ACUTE LIVER FAILURE

Acute liver failure, or *fulminant hepatic failure,* is a potentially life-threatening clinical syndrome.[22] It is characterized by a rapid onset of severe liver dysfunction in someone with no history of liver disease. It is often accompanied by hepatic encephalopathy, coagulopathy, and jaundice.

The most common cause is drugs, usually acetaminophen. Other drugs that can cause acute liver failure include isoniazid,

BOX 48.2 ETHICAL/LEGAL DILEMMAS

Rationing

Situation

J.R. is a 40-year-old female with cirrhosis, who is frequently admitted to the hospital. She has been told that her continued alcohol use will inevitably lead to her death. She now has GI bleeding and needs blood transfusions. She is a Jehovah's Witness and will not accept a blood transfusion. She commits to abstinence at this time because of how ill she feels. "I will do whatever it takes to live and see my children grow up." She will accept an organ transplant, but the waiting list is long. Her younger brother, who is 30, who also has children, is willing to donate a portion of his liver to her and serve as a living donor. Should you ask for an ethics consult?

Ethical/Legal Points for Consideration

- *Rationing,* or the controlled distribution of scarce resources, is a difficult ethical problem. The needs of an individual patient or group of patients are weighed against the needs of many patients, who may have a greater chance of recovery, and the availability of resources.
- Health interests can supersede the interests or rights of a person. For example, in anticipation of an anthrax attack, the government could confiscate all relevant antibiotics and restrict their use to treat the disease.
- Individual rights that must be considered are the (1) constitutional right to privacy and (2) right to consent to or refuse medical procedures and therapy.
- The competent adult is the only person who may consent to or refuse treatment for their health care problems.
- If J.R. consents to a liver transplant, an intervening party may be allowed to refuse that treatment only given substantial intervening circumstances and not as a threat to compel adherent future behavior.
- If involved parties cannot reach an agreement, legal intervention by way of a court order may become necessary.

Discussion Questions

1. Do you think patients with diseases that have a behavior component, like substance use, deserve aggressive treatment?
2. Would you request an ethics consult in J.R.'s case?
3. Would your opinions change if liver transplant were curative, and the patient agreed to undergo long-term substance overuse counseling and treatment?

TABLE 48.16 PATIENT & CAREGIVER TEACHING

Cirrhosis

When teaching the patient and caregiver about management of cirrhosis, include:

- Cirrhosis is a chronic illness that requires continual health care.
- Symptoms of complications and when to seek medical attention to enable prompt treatment.
- Avoid hepatotoxic over-the-counter drugs because the diseased liver is unable to metabolize them.
- Abstinence from alcohol. Continued use increases the rate of liver disease progression and risk for liver complications.
- Patient with esophageal or gastric varices need to avoid aspirin and NSAIDs.
- Patients with portal hypertension and varices need to avoid straining with defecation, coughing, sneezing, and retching and vomiting that increase risk for variceal hemorrhage.

sulfa-containing drugs, and anticonvulsants. Herb and diet supplements can cause acute liver failure. Drugs can cause hepatocyte damage by disrupting essential intracellular processes or causing an accumulation of toxic metabolic products. Other causes can include autoimmune hepatitis, Wilson disease, and viral hepatitis, especially HBV. HAV is a less common cause.

Clinical Manifestations and Diagnostic Studies

Manifestations include jaundice, coagulation problems, and encephalopathy. Changes in cognitive function are often the first clinical sign. Patients are susceptible to a wide variety of complications. These include cerebral edema, renal failure, hypoglycemia, metabolic acidosis, sepsis, and multiorgan failure.

Bilirubin is high. The PT time is prolonged. Liver enzyme levels (AST, ALT) are often markedly increased. Other laboratory tests include blood chemistries (especially glucose, since hypoglycemia may be present and need correction), CBC, acetaminophen level, screening for other drugs and toxins, viral hepatitis serology (especially HAV and HBV), ceruloplasmin (enzyme made in liver) and α_1-antitrypsin levels, iron levels, ammonia levels, urine copper, and autoantibodies (ANAs and ASMAs).

CT or MRI can provide information about the liver size and contour, presence of ascites or tumors, and patency of the blood vessels.

Interprofessional and Nursing Management

Outcomes depend on the cause. Acute liver failure may progress rapidly, with hour-by-hour changes in consciousness. Patients are usually transferred to the ICU once the diagnosis is made. Planning for transfer to a transplant center should begin in patients with grade 1 or 2 encephalopathy because they may worsen rapidly. Early transfer is important because the risks involved with transport may increase or even prevent transfer if stage 3 or 4 encephalopathy develops (Table 48.11). Liver transplant has a significant survival benefit in patients with a low probability of spontaneous recovery.

Renal failure is a frequent complication. It may be due to dehydration, hepatorenal syndrome, or acute tubular necrosis. The frequency of renal failure is greater with acetaminophen overdose or other toxins with which direct renal toxicity occurs. Although few patients die of renal failure alone, it increases mortality and worsens the prognosis. Protect renal function by maintaining adequate fluid balance, avoiding nephrotoxic agents (e.g., aminoglycosides, NSAIDs), and promptly identifying and treating infection.

Monitoring and management of hemodynamic and renal function, as well as glucose, electrolytes, and acid-base status, are critical. Conduct frequent neurologic evaluations for signs of increased intracranial pressure. Report any changes to the HCP. Avoid giving sedatives due to their effects on mental status. The effects can be confused with worsening encephalopathy. Use only minimal doses of benzodiazepines due to their delayed metabolism by the failing liver. Implement fall and seizure precautions. Position the patient with the head elevated at 30 degrees. Avoid excess patient stimulation. Maneuvers that cause straining or Valsalva-like movements may increase intracranial pressure (ICP). See more about ICP monitoring in Chapter 61.

Monitor intake and output for renal function. Provide good skin and oral care to avoid breakdown and infection. Changes in level of consciousness may compromise oral intake. Many patients receive vitamin supplements. Other factors, such as coagulation problems, may influence whether we start EN. An NG tube may be irritating to the nasal and esophageal mucosa and cause bleeding.

LIVER CANCER

Primary liver cancer starts in the liver. The most common types of liver cancer are hepatocellular carcinoma (HCC) and intrahepatic cholangiocarcinoma (bile duct cancer). Around 40,000 people in the United States are diagnosed with liver cancer every year with about 30,000 deaths.[24] Liver diseases that increase the risk of liver cancer include chronic HBV and HCV infection, cirrhosis, and MASLD. Treatment of chronic alcohol use may lower the risk for liver cancer.

In primary liver cancer, lesions may be singular or numerous and nodular or diffusely spread over the entire liver. Some tumors infiltrate other organs, such as the gallbladder, or move into the peritoneum or the diaphragm. Primary liver cancer often metastasizes to the lung.

Metastatic cancer in the liver is more common than primary liver cancer. The liver is a common site of metastatic growth because of its high rate of blood flow and extensive capillary network. Cancer cells in other parts of the body are often carried to the liver via the portal circulation.

Clinical Manifestations and Diagnostic Studies

The early manifestations of liver cancer can be absent or subtle. They are often a result of an underlying problem rather than the actual liver tumor(s). Patients may present with hepatomegaly, splenomegaly, fatigue, peripheral edema, ascites, and other complications from portal hypertension. The cancer often progresses rapidly, with patients having complications from the advancing cancer and declining liver function. In late stages, patients will often have fever, chills, jaundice, anorexia, weight loss, palpable mass, and RUQ pain. Without treatment, death may occur within 6 to 12 months. Death most often results from hepatic encephalopathy or blood loss from GI bleeding.

Diagnostic tests include ultrasound, CT, and MRI. Recent advances in MRI scanning have allowed for accurate diagnosis and staging of liver cancer without the need for a percutaneous biopsy. Sometimes, a biopsy is only done when diagnostic imaging studies are inconclusive or tissue is needed to guide treatment. Risks of a biopsy include bleeding and potential tumor cell seeding along the needle tract. Ultrasound combined with α-fetoprotein (AFP) levels has a high rate of detection of early-stage HCC. Screening at-risk patients (e.g., those with cirrhosis) usually involves a combination of AFP and CT, MRI, or liver ultrasound.

Interprofessional and Nursing Management

Treatment depends on the stage of cancer: number, size, and location of tumors; blood vessel involvement; patient age and overall health; and extent of underlying liver disease. Liver resection (partial hepatectomy) offers the best chance for a cure. However, only about 15% of people have enough healthy liver tissue for this to be an option. Underlying cirrhosis and portal hypertension often compromise liver function and may cause liver failure after surgery. Many patients are diagnosed at an advanced stage of cancer when surgery is not an option. For those patients who have early-stage liver cancer, liver transplant offers a good prognosis.

Nonsurgical therapies include percutaneous ablation, chemoembolization, radioembolization, and systemic therapies. In ablation, a thin needle is inserted into the core of the tumor. Then various substances can be injected (ethanol, acetic acid) and the temperature of the probe (radiofrequency, microwave, cryotherapy) can be altered to destroy the tumor. This procedure is done percutaneously, laparoscopically, or through an open incision. It is limited by the number, size, and location of liver tumors. It is usually offered to patients with early-stage liver cancer. Complications are uncommon but include infection, bleeding, dysrhythmias, and skin burn.

Embolization is an option in patients with multinodular HCC or intermediate-stage liver cancer. There are 2 common methods: transarterial chemoembolization (TACE) or transarterial radioembolization (TARE). TACE and TARE are minimally invasive procedures done by interventional radiologists. A catheter is placed via the femoral artery or radial artery and advanced to the arterial blood supply of the tumors. Either a chemotherapy drug (TACE) or radioactive beads (TARE) along with embolizing agents are then injected into the arteries of the tumor(s) region. TACE works by shutting off the blood supply to the tumors and exposing the tumor cells to the chemotherapy drug. TARE destroys the tumor(s) by slowly releasing radioactive material directly to the site of the tumor. It can take up to 3 months for complete results.

Systemic therapy options include chemotherapy and immune-based therapy, such as monoclonal antibodies, tyrosine kinase inhibitors, and immune checkpoint inhibitors (see Table 16.12).[25] These drugs have the potential to slow tumor progression and prolong life. Nursing care focuses on keeping patients as comfortable as possible. Since these patients have the same problems as any patient with advanced liver disease, the interventions discussed for cirrhosis apply to these patients.

LIVER TRANSPLANTS

A liver transplant is an option for many people with end-stage liver disease or local HCC. The most common reasons for a liver transplant in adults are chronic liver failure from cirrhosis caused by hepatitis C or chronic alcohol use. Other indications include MASH, chronic hepatitis B, acute liver failure, liver cancer, autoimmune hepatitis, biliary atresia, and inborn errors of metabolism.

Liver transplant candidates go through a rigorous evaluation before being placed on the transplant list. This is done to confirm the diagnosis of end-stage liver disease and assess for other comorbid conditions (e.g., cardiovascular disease, chronic kidney disease) that may affect the outcome. The evaluation includes physical assessment, laboratory tests (CBC, liver function tests), cardiac and pulmonary evaluations, endoscopy, CT scan, and psychologic testing. Potential recipients receive counseling about cigarette smoking and alcohol abstinence. Contraindications include severe extrahepatic disease, advanced HCC or other cancer, ongoing drug or chronic alcohol use, and inability to understand or adhere with posttransplant care.

There is no age cutoff for liver transplants. However, patients over 70 years old have lower survival rates at 1 year and 5 years after transplant. Because older adults tend to have more comorbid conditions, a transplant has more risks for complications. Therefore older adults may not be good candidates for liver transplants.

Liver transplants are done using both deceased (cadaver) and live donor livers. The live donor liver transplant was first developed for children whose parents wanted to serve as donors. Today, some liver transplant centers are performing live liver transplant procedures for adults. In this procedure, the living person donates a part of their liver to another. However, live liver donation poses potential risks to the donor, including biliary problems, hepatic artery thrombosis, wound infection, postoperative ileus, and pneumothorax.

Because of the limited number of donor livers, when a liver becomes available for transplant, it may be divided into 2 parts (split liver transplant) and implanted into 2 recipients. The decision to use a split donor liver is based on the donor's size and health. The recipients of the split liver generally are smaller than the donor. The success rate of split liver transplants is lower than that of whole organ transplant.

Postoperative complications include bleeding, infection, and rejection. However, the liver is subject to a less aggressive immunologic attack than other organs, like the kidneys. Immunosuppressive therapy generally involves a combination of corticosteroids, a calcineurin inhibitor (cyclosporine or tacrolimus), and an antiproliferative agent (e.g., azathioprine). Tacrolimus is superior to cyclosporine in liver transplants. Standard immunosuppressive regimens often change over the course of the recipient's life. Corticosteroid withdrawal is relatively safe to do in liver transplant recipients. Transplants and immunosuppressive therapy are discussed in Chapter 14.

About 80% of patients live more than 5 years after liver transplant. Long-term survival depends on the cause of liver failure (e.g., local HCC, chronic HBV or HCV, biliary disease). Patients who have liver disease from HBV or HCV often have reinfection of the transplanted liver if they do not receive antiretroviral treatment. For patients with HBV, treating HBV after surgery with a nucleoside or nucleotide analog reduces the rate of reinfection of the transplanted liver. Some patients may also receive IV HBIG. For patients with HCV, treatment with a DAA that can cure HCV infection has provided the opportunity to use liver grafts from donors with HCV. Research is ongoing to decide if DAAs should be started before or after transplant.

Patients who have had a liver transplant need highly skilled nursing care, either in an ICU or other special unit. After surgery, we monitor electrolyte levels, neurologic status, and urine output and note signs of bleeding, infection, and rejection. Common respiratory problems are pneumonia, atelectasis, and pleural effusions. To prevent these complications, encourage patients to cough, deep breathe, use incentive spirometry, and frequently reposition. Measure the drainage from the Jackson–Pratt drain, NG tube, and T tube and note the color and consistency of the drainage at regular intervals.

Infections are possible days, weeks, or years after patients receive a transplant. Immunosuppressive therapy makes the risk of infection higher, especially during the first 6 months after surgery. Causes of infection can be viral, fungal, or bacterial. Fever may be the only sign of infection. Some patients may not be able to mount a fever response due to their immunosuppressed state. Adhering to the medication plan can be hard, especially in the beginning. Emotional support and teaching for patients and caregivers are essential to transplant success.

Gerontologic Considerations: Liver Disease

The incidence of liver disease increases with age. The liver's size decreases, and hepatobiliary function changes. The liver has a decreased capacity to respond to injury. This especially applies to regeneration after injury.

Chronic alcohol use and obesity contribute to cirrhosis, fatty liver inflammation (MASH), and liver failure. Because of many older adults' concomitant cardiovascular and lung diseases and possible anticoagulant therapy, variceal bleeding can cause significant morbidity and mortality and needs immediate medical intervention. In older adults with liver disease, we sometimes misdiagnose hepatic encephalopathy as dementia.

PANCREAS PROBLEMS

ACUTE PANCREATITIS

Acute pancreatitis is an acute inflammation of the pancreas. Spillage of pancreatic enzymes into surrounding pancreatic tissue causes autodigestion and severe pain. The degree of inflammation varies from mild edema to severe hemorrhagic necrosis.

Etiology and Pathophysiology

Many factors can cause injury to the pancreas. In the United States the most common cause is gallbladder disease (gallstones). This is more common in females. The second most common cause is chronic alcohol use. This is more common in males. Less common causes include drug reactions, pancreatic cancer, and hypertriglyceridemia (levels over 1000 mg/dL). Biliary sludge and microlithiasis, a mix of cholesterol crystals and calcium salts, can be present in patients with acute pancreatitis.

The most common pathogenic mechanism in acute pancreatitis is autodigestion of the pancreas (Fig. 48.9). The causative factors injure pancreatic cells or activate the pancreatic enzymes in the pancreas rather than in the intestine. This may be due to reflux of bile acids into the pancreatic ducts through an open or distended sphincter of Oddi. This reflux may be caused by blockage created by gallstones. Obstruction of pancreatic ducts results in pancreatic ischemia.

We do not know exactly how chronic alcohol use predisposes a person to pancreatitis. We think that alcohol increases the production of digestive enzymes in the pancreas.

The pathophysiologic involvement of acute pancreatitis is either *mild pancreatitis* (*edematous* or *interstitial pancreatitis*) or *severe pancreatitis* (*necrotizing pancreatitis*) (Fig. 48.10). In

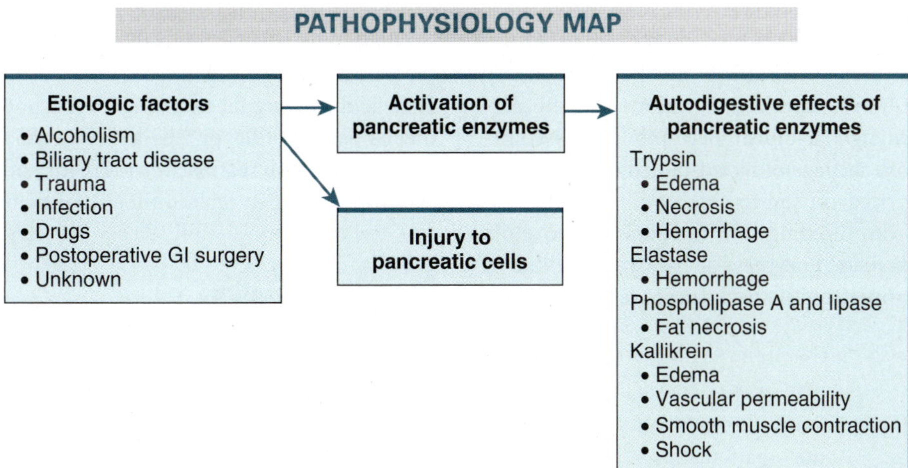

Fig. 48.9 Pathogenic process of acute pancreatitis.

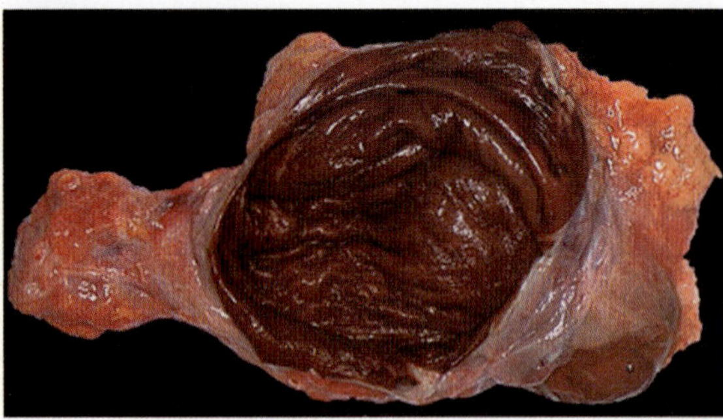

Fig. 48.10 Pancreatitis with large pseudocyst. (From Connolly A, Finkbeiner W, Ursell P, et al: *Atlas of gross autopsy pathology,* ed 3, Philadelphia, 2016, Elsevier.)

severe pancreatitis, about half the patients have permanent decreases in pancreatic endocrine and exocrine function. Patients with severe pancreatitis are at high risk for developing pancreatic necrosis, organ failure, and septic complications. Hospitalization rates for acute pancreatitis are rising, but the overall fatality rate has decreased to about 1%.

Clinical Manifestations

Abdominal pain is the main manifestation. The pain is due to distention of the pancreas, peritoneal irritation, and biliary tract obstruction. It is usually in the left upper quadrant but may be midepigastric. It often radiates to the back due to the retroperitoneal location of the pancreas. The pain has a sudden onset. It is described as severe, deep, piercing, and continuous or steady. Eating worsens the pain. Pain is not relieved by vomiting and may be accompanied by flushing, cyanosis, and dyspnea. It often starts when the patient is recumbent. The patient may assume various positions involving flexion of the spine to try to relieve the severe pain.

Other manifestations include nausea and vomiting, low-grade fever, leukocytosis, hypotension, tachycardia, and jaundice. Abdominal tenderness with muscle guarding is common.

Bowel sounds may be decreased or absent. Paralytic ileus may occur and causes marked abdominal distention. The lungs are often involved with crackles present. Intravascular damage from circulating trypsin (a proteolytic enzyme) may cause areas of cyanosis or greenish to yellow-brown discoloration of the abdominal wall. Other areas of bruising are the flanks (*Grey Turner spots* or *sign,* a bluish flank discoloration) and the periumbilical area (*Cullen sign,* a bluish periumbilical discoloration). These result from seepage of bloodstained exudate from the pancreas and may occur in severe cases.

Shock may occur from bleeding into the pancreas, toxemia from the activated pancreatic enzymes, or hypovolemia due to fluid shift into the retroperitoneal space (massive fluid shifts).

Complications

The severity of acute pancreatitis depends on the extent of pancreatic destruction. Acute pancreatitis can be life threatening. Some patients recover completely. Others have recurring attacks, and some develop chronic pancreatitis.

Two significant local complications are pseudocyst and abscess. A *pancreatic pseudocyst* is an accumulation of fluid, pancreatic enzymes, tissue debris, and inflammatory exudates surrounded by a wall next to the pancreas. Manifestations are abdominal pain, palpable epigastric mass, nausea, vomiting, and anorexia. The amylase level is often high. CT, MRI, and endoscopic ultrasound (EUS) may detect a pseudocyst. The cysts usually resolve spontaneously within a few weeks but may perforate, causing peritonitis or rupture into the stomach or the duodenum.

A *pancreatic abscess* can result when a pseudocyst gets infected. It contains pus and necrotic material. It may rupture or perforate into adjacent organs. Manifestations of an abscess include upper abdominal pain, abdominal mass, high fever, and leukocytosis. Pancreatic abscesses need prompt surgical drainage to prevent sepsis.

The main systemic complications are cardiovascular and pulmonary (pleural effusion, atelectasis, pneumonia, acute respiratory distress syndrome [ARDS]). Pulmonary complications are due to the passage of exudate-containing pancreatic enzymes from the peritoneal cavity through transdiaphragmatic lymph channels. Enzyme-induced inflammation of the diaphragm occurs, with the result being atelectasis caused by reduced diaphragm movement. Trypsin can activate prothrombin and plasminogen, increasing the risk for intravascular thrombi, pulmonary emboli, and DIC. Hypotension can occur from fluid shifts and sepsis.

Tetany, which can be caused by hypocalcemia, is a sign of severe disease. It is due in part to the combining of calcium and fatty acids during fat necrosis. We do not understand the exact mechanisms of how or why hypocalcemia occurs. Patients with severe acute pancreatitis are at risk for abdominal compartment syndrome from intraabdominal hypertension and edema.

TABLE 48.17 Diagnostic Findings

Acute Pancreatitis

Laboratory Test	Abnormal Finding
Serum and urinary amylase	↑
Lipase	↑
Bilirubin	↑
Glucose	↑
Calcium	↓
Liver enzymes	↑
Triglycerides	↑

Diagnostic Studies

The primary diagnostic tests for acute pancreatitis are amylase and lipase (Table 48.17). The amylase level is usually high early and stays high for 24 to 72 hours. Lipase level is high in acute pancreatitis. It is an important test because other disorders (e.g., mumps, cerebral trauma) may increase amylase levels.

TABLE 48.18 Interprofessional Care

Acute Pancreatitis

Diagnostic Assessment

- History and physical assessment
- Amylase and lipase
- Glucose, calcium, glycerides, liver enzymes
- Abdominal ultrasound
- Endoscopic ultrasound (EUS)
- MRCP
- ERCP
- Contrast-enhanced CT of pancreas
- Chest x-ray

Management

- NPO with NG tube to suction
- Albumin (if shock present)
- IV calcium gluconate (10%) (if tetany present)
- Lactated Ringer solution
- Drug therapy (see Table 48.19)

TABLE 48.19 Drug Therapy

Acute and Chronic Pancreatitis

Drug	Mechanism of Action
Acute Pancreatitis	
Antacids	Neutralize gastric hydrochloric (HCl) acid secretion ↓ Production and secretion of pancreatic enzymes and bicarbonate
Antispasmodics (e.g., dicyclomine)	↓ Vagal stimulation, motility, pancreatic outflow (↓ volume and concentration of bicarbonate and enzyme secretion) Contraindicated in paralytic ileus
Carbonic anhydrase inhibitor (acetazolamide)	↓ Volume and bicarbonate concentration of pancreatic secretion
Morphine	Pain relief
PPIs (e.g., omeprazole)	↓ HCl acid secretion (HCl acid stimulates pancreatic activity)
Chronic Pancreatitis	
Insulin	Treat diabetes or hyperglycemia, if needed
Pancreatic enzyme products (pancrelipase [Pancreaze, Creon])	Replacement therapy for pancreatic enzymes

Diagnostic testing is aimed at determining the cause. An abdominal ultrasound, x-ray, or contrast-enhanced CT scan may identify pancreatic problems. CT scan is the best imaging test for pancreatitis and related complications, such as pseudocysts and abscesses. Endoscopic retrograde cholangiopancreatography (ERCP) is an option (although it can cause acute pancreatitis). Other tests include EUS, magnetic resonance cholangiopancreatography (MRCP), and angiography. Chest x-rays may show atelectasis and pleural effusions.

Interprofessional Care

Goals of interprofessional care include (1) pain relief, (2) prevent or alleviate shock, (3) reduce pancreatic secretions, (4) correct fluid and electrolyte imbalances, (5) prevent or treat infection, and (6) remove the precipitating cause, if possible (Table 48.18).[26]

Conservative Therapy

Treatment focuses on supportive care. This includes aggressive hydration, pain management, managing metabolic complications, and minimizing pancreatic stimulation. Treatment and control of pain are very important. Some patients may need IV opioid analgesics. Pain medications may be given with an antispasmodic agent. Atropine and other anticholinergic drugs are avoided when paralytic ileus is present because they can decrease GI mobility, making the problem worse. Other drugs that relax smooth muscles (spasmolytics), such as nitroglycerin or papaverine, may be used.

If shock is present, we give blood volume replacements. Patients may receive plasma or plasma volume expanders, such as dextran or albumin. Lactated Ringer solution or other electrolyte solutions can correct fluid and electrolyte problems. Central venous pressure readings can help determine fluid replacement requirements. Vasoactive drugs, such as dopamine, may be needed to increase systemic vascular resistance in those with hypotension.

It is important to reduce or suppress pancreatic enzymes to decrease stimulation of the pancreas and allow it to rest. We do this in several ways. First, the patient is NPO. Second, NG suction may be used to reduce vomiting and gastric distention and to prevent gastric acidic contents from entering the duodenum. Certain drugs are given to suppress gastric acid secretion (Table 48.19).

The inflamed and necrotic pancreatic tissue is a good medium for bacterial growth. In patients with acute necrotizing pancreatitis, infection is the leading cause of death. Therefore it is important to prevent infections. Because many of the organisms come from the intestine, EN reduces the risk for necrotizing pancreatitis. Monitor patients closely so that antibiotic therapy can be started early if necrosis and infection occur.

Surgical Therapy

When the acute pancreatitis is related to gallstones, an urgent ERCP plus stone removal, stenting, or endoscopic *sphincterotomy* (severing of the muscle layers of the sphincter of Oddi) may be done. Laparoscopic cholecystectomy may follow ERCP to reduce the potential for recurrence. Surgery may be done when the diagnosis is uncertain or if patients do not respond to conservative therapy.

Patients may need drainage of necrotic fluid collections. This is done surgically, under CT guidance, or endoscopically.

Percutaneous drainage of a pseudocyst can be done, and a drainage tube left in place. Some patients will need surgery. Treatment options include surgical drainage, percutaneous catheter placement and drainage, and endoscopic drainage.

Drug Therapy

Several different drugs are used to prevent and treat problems associated with pancreatitis (Table 48.19). Currently, there are no drugs that cure pancreatitis.

Nutrition Therapy

Initially, the patient is NPO to reduce pancreatic secretion. Depending on the severity, we start EN. Because of infection risk, PN is reserved for patients who cannot tolerate EN (see Chapter 44). If patients are receiving IV lipids, monitor triglyceride level.

As pancreatitis resolves, the patient resumes oral intake. When food is allowed, start with small, frequent feedings. The diet is high in carbohydrate content because that is the least stimulating to the exocrine part of the pancreas. Foods with higher fat content are more likely to exacerbate pain. Suspect intolerance to oral foods if a patient reports pain, has increasing abdominal girth, or has increased amylase and lipase levels. Fat-soluble vitamin supplements may be given since patients may not have adequate intake or full absorption of vitamins.

CHECK YOUR PRACTICE

Your patient is admitted for acute pancreatitis. He is upset because his sister is getting married in 3 weeks and he was told he cannot have alcohol. "I don't understand how a little bit of alcohol will be a problem. Why can't I have something to drink?"

- How would you respond?

TABLE 48.20 NURSING ASSESSMENT

Acute Pancreatitis

Subjective Data

Important Health Information

Health history: Biliary tract disease, alcohol use, abdominal trauma, duodenal ulcers, infection, metabolic disorders

Medications: Thiazides, NSAIDs, azathioprine, statins, naproxen, metformin, hormone replacement therapy, proton pump inhibitors

Surgery or other treatments: Surgery on the pancreas, stomach, duodenum, or biliary tract. ERCP, stent placement, cholecystectomy

Functional Health Patterns

Health perception–health management: Chronic alcohol use, fatigue

Nutritional-metabolic: Nausea and vomiting, anorexia

Activity-exercise: Dyspnea

Cognitive-perceptual: Severe midepigastric or left upper quadrant pain that may radiate to the back, worsened by food and alcohol use, not relieved by vomiting

Objective Data

Cardiovascular

Tachycardia, hypotension

GI

Abdominal distention, tenderness, and muscle guarding. Decreased bowel sounds

General

Restlessness, anxiety, low-grade fever

Respiratory

Tachypnea, basilar crackles

Skin

Flushing, diaphoresis, discoloration of abdomen and flanks, cyanosis, jaundice. Decreased skin turgor, dry mucous membranes

Possible Diagnostic Findings

↑ Amylase, lipase, glucose. Leukocytosis, hypocalcemia. Abnormal ultrasound and CT scans of pancreas, abnormal ERCP or MRCP

NURSING MANAGEMENT: ACUTE PANCREATITIS

Assessment

Subjective and objective data that should be obtained from patients with acute pancreatitis are outlined in Table 48.20.

Clinical Problems

Clinical problems for patients with acute pancreatitis may include:

- Pain
- Fluid imbalance
- Electrolyte imbalance
- Nutritionally compromised

Additional information on clinical problems and interventions for patients with acute pancreatitis is presented in eNursing Care Plan 48.3 available on the website for this chapter.

Planning

The overall goals are that patients with acute pancreatitis will have (1) pain relief, (2) normal fluid and electrolyte balance, (3) minimal to no complications, and (4) no recurrent attacks.

Implementation

Health Promotion

Assess for risk factors and encourage measures to address these factors to prevent acute pancreatitis. Encourage patients to cease alcohol intake, especially if they have had pancreatitis before. Recurrent attacks of pancreatitis may become milder or disappear if they stop alcohol use. Encourage early diagnosis and treatment of biliary tract disease, such as gallstones. Smoking cessation is beneficial.

Acute Care

The care of patients with acute pancreatitis is outlined in Table 48.21. During the acute phase, it is important to monitor vital signs. Hypotension, fever, and tachypnea may compromise hemodynamic stability. Monitor the response to IV fluids. Closely assess fluid and electrolyte balance. Frequent vomiting, along with gastric suction, may result in decreased chloride, sodium, and potassium levels.

Respiratory failure may develop in patients with severe acute pancreatitis. Assess respiratory function (e.g., lung sounds, O_2 saturation levels). Apply O_2 to maintain O_2 saturation greater than 95%. In patients with severe pancreatitis, we monitor glucose levels for hyperglycemia. If ARDS develops, patients may need intubation and mechanical ventilation support.

Because hypocalcemia can occur, observe for symptoms of tetany, including jerking, irritability, and muscular twitching. Numbness or tingling around the lips and in the fingers is an early sign of hypocalcemia. Assess for a positive Chvostek sign or Trousseau sign (see Fig. 17.15). Give calcium gluconate as ordered to treat symptomatic hypocalcemia. Monitor magnesium levels since hypomagnesemia may develop.

A major focus of your care is pain relief. Pain and restlessness can increase the metabolic rate and contribute to hemodynamic instability. Opioids may be used for pain relief. Assess and document the duration of pain relief. Comfortable positioning, frequent changes in position, and relief of nausea and vomiting help reduce the restlessness that usually accompanies the pain. Assuming positions that flex the trunk and draw the knees up to the abdomen may decrease pain. A side-lying position with the head elevated 45 degrees decreases tension on the abdomen and may help.

For patients who are NPO or have an NG tube, provide frequent oral and nasal care to relieve the dryness of the mouth and nose. Oral care is essential to prevent parotitis. Patients taking anticholinergics to decrease GI secretions will have a dry mouth. If patients are taking antacids to neutralize gastric acid secretion, they should be sipped slowly or inserted in the NG tube.

Observe for fever and other signs of infection. Respiratory tract infections are common and cause patients to take shallow, guarded abdominal breaths. Measures to prevent respiratory tract infections include turning, coughing, deep breathing, and assuming a semi-Fowler position.

Assess for signs of paralytic ileus, renal failure, and mental changes. Measure glucose levels to assess damage to the β cells of the islets of Langerhans in the pancreas.

Patients who had surgery to drain necrotic fluid or treat a cyst may need special wound care for an anastomotic leak or a fistula. To prevent skin irritation, use skin barriers (e.g., Stomahesive, Karaya Paste), pouching, and drains. Besides protecting the skin, pouching allows a more accurate determination of fluid losses and increases patient comfort. Sterile pouching systems are available. Consult with a clinical specialist or wound, ostomy, and continence nurse (WOCN).

After acute pancreatitis, patients may need home care follow-up. Because of loss of physical and muscle strength, physical therapy may be needed. Continued care to prevent infection and detect any complications is important. Counseling about abstinence from alcohol is important to prevent future attacks of acute pancreatitis and chronic pancreatitis. Because nicotine can stimulate the pancreas, they should avoid smoking.

Provide teaching about the treatment plan, including the importance of taking the required medications and following the recommended diet. Diet teaching should include fat restriction. Fats stimulate cholecystokinin secretion, which then stimulates the pancreas. Encourage carbohydrates as they are less stimulating to the pancreas. Teach patients to avoid crash and binge dieting because they can precipitate attacks.

Teach patients and caregivers to recognize and report symptoms of infection, diabetes, or steatorrhea. These changes indicate ongoing destruction of pancreatic tissue and pancreatic insufficiency. Patients may need exogenous enzyme supplements.

TABLE 48.21 Care of the Patient With Acute Pancreatitis

- Monitor vital signs and pulse oximetry.
- Administer prescribed antibiotic and IV fluid therapy.
- Administer prescribed analgesics and implement pain management strategies.
- Implement measures to manage fever (see Table 12.5).
- Maintain NPO status.
- Monitor laboratory values, including CBC, calcium, glucose, and potassium.
- Implement measures for nausea and give prescribed antiemetics.
- Monitor intake and output and obtain daily weight.
- Keep the head of the bed elevated at least 30 degrees.
- Assess respiratory function and apply supplemental O_2 to maintain saturation over 95%.
- Maintain patency of NG tube. Provide frequent oral and nasal care.
- Provide ordered VTE and GI prophylaxis.
- Assess for hypocalcemia and administer ordered calcium gluconate
- Encourage the patient to cough, deep breathe, and use the incentive spirometer.
- Turn and reposition the patient every 2 h to promote lung expansion and mobilize secretions.

Collaborate With Dietitian

- Assess and monitor nutrition status.
- Recommend optimal diet.

Collaborate With Physical Therapist

- Perform ROM exercises.
- Assist with early and progressive ambulation.

◆ Evaluation

The expected outcomes are that patients with acute pancreatitis will:

- Have adequate pain control
- Maintain adequate fluid and electrolyte balance
- Be knowledgeable about the treatment plan to restore health
- Get help for alcohol use and smoking cessation (if needed)

CHRONIC PANCREATITIS

Chronic pancreatitis is a continuous, prolonged, inflammatory, and fibrosing process of the pancreas. The pancreas is progressively destroyed as it is replaced by fibrotic tissue. Strictures and calcifications may occur in the pancreas.

Etiology and Pathophysiology

The most common cause of nonobstructive pancreatitis (the most common type of chronic pancreatitis) is chronic alcohol use. There is inflammation and sclerosis, mainly in the head of the pancreas and around the pancreatic duct. In some people who drink alcohol, a genetic factor may predispose them to the direct toxic effect of the alcohol on the pancreas.

The most common cause of obstructive pancreatitis is inflammation of the sphincter of Oddi from gallstones. Cancer of the ampulla of Vater, duodenum, or pancreas can also cause obstructive pancreatitis.

Chronic pancreatitis may follow acute pancreatitis. It may occur with systemic diseases (e.g., systemic lupus erythematosus), autoimmune pancreatitis, and cystic fibrosis. Some patients have no identifiable risk factor, or idiopathic pancreatitis.

Clinical Manifestations

A major manifestation of chronic pancreatitis is abdominal pain. The pain is chronic (recurrent attacks at intervals of months or years). There may be episodes of acute pain. The attacks may become more frequent until they are almost constant. Sometimes they decrease as pancreatic fibrosis develops. The pain occurs in the same areas as in acute pancreatitis. It is usually described as a heavy, gnawing feeling or sometimes as burning and cramp-like. Food or antacids do not relieve the pain.

Other manifestations result from pancreatic insufficiency. They include malabsorption with weight loss, constipation, mild jaundice with dark urine, steatorrhea, and diabetes. The steatorrhea may become severe, with voluminous, foul-smelling, fatty stools. Some abdominal tenderness may be present.

Chronic pancreatitis can cause a variety of complications. These include pseudocyst formation, bile duct or duodenal obstruction, pancreatic ascites or pleural effusion, splenic vein thrombosis, pseudoaneurysms, and pancreatic cancer.

Diagnostic Studies

Confirming the diagnosis of chronic pancreatitis can be hard. The diagnosis is based on signs and symptoms, laboratory studies, and imaging. In chronic pancreatitis, amylase and lipase levels may be increased slightly or not at all, depending on the degree of pancreatic fibrosis. Bilirubin and alkaline phosphatase levels may be increased. There is usually mild leukocytosis and a high sedimentation rate.

ERCP can visualize the pancreatic and common bile ducts. Imaging studies, such as CT, MRI, MRCP, endoscopic ultrasound, and abdominal ultrasound, can show a variety of changes, including calcifications, ductal dilation, pseudocysts, and enlargement of the pancreas.

Stool samples are examined for fecal fat content. Deficiencies of fat-soluble vitamins and cobalamin, glucose intolerance, and diabetes may occur. A secretin stimulation test can assess the degree of pancreatic dysfunction.

Interprofessional and Nursing Management

When patients with chronic pancreatitis have an acute attack, the therapy is identical to that for acute pancreatitis. At other times, the focus is on preventing further attacks, pain relief, and controlling pancreatic exocrine and endocrine insufficiency. It sometimes takes frequent doses of analgesics (morphine, fentanyl patch) to relieve the pain if diet measures and enzyme replacement are not effective.

Diet, pancreatic enzyme replacement, and diabetes control are ways to control pancreatic insufficiency. Small, bland, frequent meals that are low in fat decrease pancreatic stimulation. Teach patients not to consume alcohol and caffeinated beverages. If the patient is dependent on alcohol, refer them to other resources as needed (see Chapter 11). Smoking can accelerate progression of chronic pancreatitis.

Pancreatic enzyme products, such as pancrelipase, contain amylase, lipase, and trypsin. They are used to replace the deficient pancreatic enzymes. The enzymes are usually enteric coated to prevent their breakdown or inactivation by gastric acid. They are usually taken with meals and snacks. Teach patients and caregivers to monitor stools for steatorrhea to help determine the effectiveness of the enzymes. Some pancreatic enzyme replacement therapy must be taken with PPIs for optimal efficacy. Bile salts may be given to help with fat-soluble vitamin (A, D, E, and K) absorption and prevent further fat loss.

If diabetes develops, the patient often needs insulin. Provide teaching about testing glucose levels and drug therapy (see Chapter 53). Acid-neutralizing drugs (e.g., antacids) and acid-inhibiting drugs (e.g., H_2-receptor blockers, PPIs) may be given to control gastric acidity. Antidepressants can reduce any neuropathic pain.

Treatment sometimes requires endoscopic therapy or surgery. When biliary disease is present or obstruction or pseudocyst develops, surgery may be needed. Surgical procedures can divert bile flow or relieve ductal obstruction. A choledochojejunostomy diverts bile around the ampulla of Vater, where there may be spasm or hypertrophy of the sphincter. In this procedure, the common bile duct is anastomosed into the jejunum. Another surgical diverting procedure is the Roux-en-Y pancreatojejunostomy. The pancreatic duct is opened, and an anastomosis is made with the jejunum. Pancreatic drainage procedures can relieve ductal obstruction and are often done with ERCP. Some patients may have an

ERCP with sphincterotomy and/or stent placement at the site of obstruction. These patients need follow-up procedures, such as ERCP, to either exchange or remove the stent.

PANCREATIC CANCER

Pancreatic cancer has a low incidence rate of around 1.6%. The median age at diagnosis is around 68 years of age.[27] Most pancreatic tumors are adenocarcinomas that begin in the epithelium of the ductal system. More than half of the tumors occur in the head of the pancreas. As the tumor grows, the common bile duct becomes obstructed and obstructive jaundice develops. Tumors starting in the body or tail often remain silent until their growth is advanced. Most cancers have metastasized at the time of diagnosis. The prognosis of patients with cancer of the pancreas is poor. Most patients die within 5 to 12 months of diagnosis. The 5-year survival rate is only 9%. If diagnosed early when the cancer is local, patients have a 44% relative survival at 5 years.

Etiology and Pathophysiology

The cause of pancreatic cancer is unknown. Two significant risk factors are cigarette smoking and heavy alcohol use. These are thought to cause cell damage, inflammation, and scarring, making the risk higher than in nonusers. Other risks include obesity, diabetes familial pancreatitis, age, and first-degree relatives with inherited genetic mutations associated with cancer syndromes.

Clinical Manifestations

The signs and symptoms are similar to those of chronic pancreatitis. They may not become apparent until the cancer is more advanced. Symptoms include jaundice, itching due to biliary obstruction, weight loss, and pain. In general, pain is common and is related to the cancer's location. The pain is often in the upper abdomen or left hypochondrium and often radiates to the back. Extreme, unrelenting pain is related to extension of the cancer into the retroperitoneal tissues and nerve plexuses. Weight loss is due to poor digestion and absorption caused by a lack of digestive enzymes from the pancreas. Some patients can develop steatorrhea due to obstructions of the main pancreatic duct. Gastric outlet obstruction may cause bloating, discomfort, and vomiting. Venous thrombus formation can occur.

Diagnostic Studies

Abdominal ultrasound or EUS, spiral CT scan, ERCP, MRI, and MRCP are the most often used diagnostic imaging techniques for pancreatic cancer. EUS involves imaging the pancreas with the use of an endoscope positioned in the stomach and duodenum. EUS also allows for fine-needle aspiration of the tumor for biopsy. CT scan is often the first study and gives information on metastasis and vascular involvement of the tumor. ERCP allows us to see the pancreatic duct and biliary system. With ERCP, pancreatic secretions and tissue can be obtained for biopsy and analysis of tumor markers. MRI, PET, PET/CT scans, and MRCP may be done to confirm a cancer diagnosis and determine staging. They can monitor progress and response to therapy.

Tumor markers are used for diagnosing pancreatic cancer and monitoring the response to treatment. Cancer-associated antigen 19-9 (CA 19-9) is increased in pancreatic cancer. It is the most commonly used tumor marker. CA 19-9 also can be increased in gallbladder cancer, bile duct cancers, and benign conditions, such as pancreatitis, hepatitis, and biliary obstruction.

Interprofessional Care

Surgery is the most effective treatment for pancreatic cancer. Only 15% to 20% of patients have resectable tumors at the time of diagnosis. With the use of chemotherapy before surgery, more patients can eventually become surgical candidates. The type of surgery depends on the size and location of the tumor. Pancreatic head tumors require the classic Whipple procedure or pancreaticoduodenectomy (Fig. 48.11). In the Whipple surgery, the proximal pancreas (proximal pancreatectomy), along with duodenum (duodenectomy), distal segment of the common bile duct, and distal part of the stomach (partial gastrectomy), are removed. The pancreatic duct, common bile duct, and stomach are anastomosed to the jejunum. Pancreatic body and/or tail tumors require a distal pancreatectomy procedure. Sometimes, a total pancreatectomy is done. It causes diabetes and patients must receive insulin therapy and pancreatic enzyme supplements for life. If the pancreatic tumor cannot be removed surgically, palliative measures, such as a cholecystojejunostomy, to relieve biliary obstruction and/or endoscopically placed biliary stents, can be done.

Radiation therapy has little effect on survival but may help with pain relief. External radiation is most common, but implanting internal radiation seeds into the tumor has been used. The role of chemotherapy is limited and can have a significant side effect profile. There are various chemotherapy regimens used, including FOLFIRINOX. This is a combination of 5-fluorouracil, leucovorin, irinotecan, and oxiplatin. Other combinations include gemcitabine alone or in combination with agents such as nab-paclitaxel (see Chapter 16).

❖ NURSING MANAGEMENT: PANCREATIC CANCER

Because patients with pancreatic cancer have many of the same problems as patients with pancreatitis, nursing care includes many of the same measures. Provide symptomatic and supportive nursing care. This includes giving medications and providing comfort measures to relieve pain.

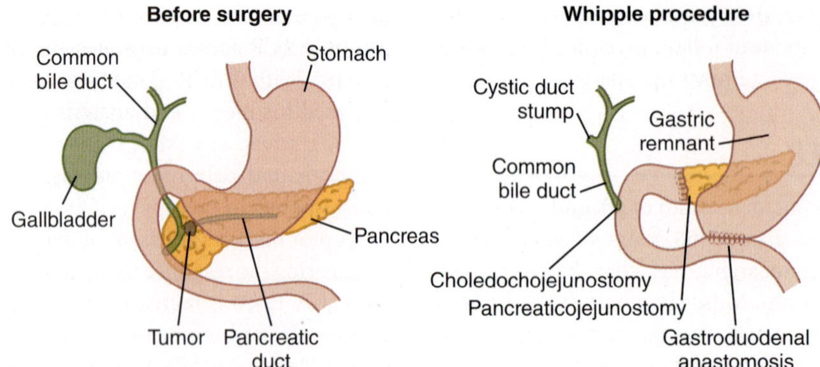

Fig. 48.11 Whipple procedure or radical pancreaticoduodenectomy. This surgery involves resecting the proximal pancreas, adjoining duodenum, distal part of the stomach, and distal part of the common bile duct. An anastomosis of the pancreatic duct, common bile duct, and stomach to the jejunum is done.

Adequate nutrition is important. Frequent and supplemental feedings may be needed. Include measures to stimulate the appetite as much as possible and to manage anorexia, nausea, and vomiting. If the patient is receiving radiation therapy or chemotherapy, observe for adverse reactions, such as anorexia, nausea, vomiting, diarrhea. Assess for skin irritation in those receiving radiation therapy.

The prognosis for patients with pancreatic cancer is poor. Psychologic support to patients and caregivers is essential. Help them cope with the diagnosis and prognosis. Chapter 10 provides information on palliative and end-of-life care.

BILIARY TRACT PROBLEMS

CHOLELITHIASIS AND CHOLECYSTITIS

The most common disorder of the biliary system is **cholelithiasis** (stones in the gallbladder) (Fig. 48.12). The gallstones may lodge in the neck of the gallbladder or in the cystic duct. **Cholecystitis** (inflammation of the gallbladder wall) is usually associated with gallstones. They usually occur together, although a person can have gallstones without cholecystitis. Cholecystitis may be acute or chronic.

Gallbladder disease is a common health problem in the United States. Up to 10% of American adults have cholecystitis caused by gallstones. The actual number is not known because many persons with stones are asymptomatic. *Cholecystectomy* (removal of the gallbladder) is among the most common surgeries done in the United States.

Gallstones are more common in females, especially multiparous females and females over 40 years of age. Postmenopausal females on estrogen replacement therapy and younger females on oral contraceptives are at an increased risk for gallbladder disease. Oral contraceptives affect cholesterol production and increase gallbladder cholesterol saturation. Other factors are a sedentary lifestyle, a familial tendency, and obesity. Obesity causes increased cholesterol secretion in bile. The incidence of gallbladder disease is especially high in the Native American population.

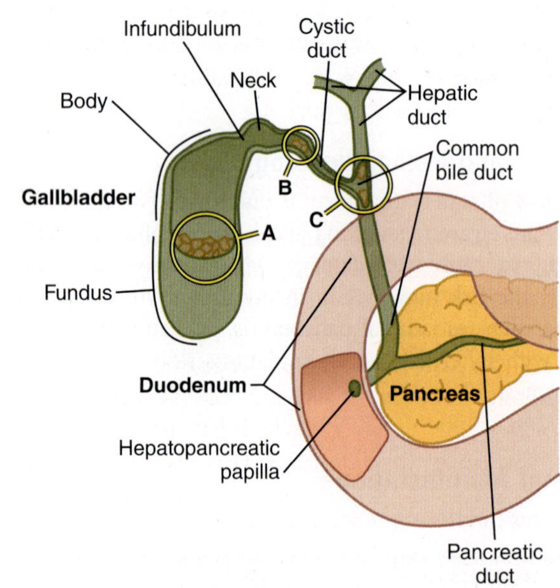

Fig. 48.12 (A) Gallstones. Problems arise if a stone leaves the gallbladder and causes obstruction elsewhere in the biliary system. (B) If a gallstone enters the cystic duct and becomes lodged there, it can lead to cholecystitis. (C) Obstruction of either the hepatic or common bile duct blocks the exit of bile from the liver where it is formed.

Etiology and Pathophysiology

Cholelithiasis

We do not know the cause of gallstones. They develop when the balance that keeps cholesterol, bile salts, and calcium in solution is changed so that these substances precipitate. Mixed cholesterol stones, which are mainly cholesterol, are the most common gallstones. Other components of bile that precipitate into stones are bilirubin and protein.

Conditions that lead to gallstone formation include supersaturation of bile with cholesterol, decreased bile acids that dissolve cholesterol, excess mucus production, and gallbladder dysmotility and stasis. Normally, bile contains enough chemicals to dissolve the cholesterol the liver excretes. If the liver excretes more cholesterol than bile can dissolve, the excess cholesterol may form into crystals and eventually stones. The bile secreted by the liver may be supersaturated with cholesterol (lithogenic bile). The bile in the gallbladder then becomes supersaturated with cholesterol and precipitation of cholesterol. Bile stasis can promote the progression of supersaturation and changes in the chemical composition of the bile (biliary sludge). Immobility, pregnancy, and inflammatory or obstructive lesions in the biliary system decrease bile flow. Hormonal factors during pregnancy may cause delayed emptying of the gallbladder, resulting in bile stasis.

The stones may stay in the gallbladder or migrate to the cystic duct or the common bile duct. They cause pain as they pass through the ducts. Stones can lodge in the ducts and cause an obstruction. Small stones are more likely to move into a duct and cause obstruction. Table 48.22 describes the changes and manifestations that occur when the stones obstruct the common bile duct. If the blockage occurs in the cystic duct, the bile can continue to flow into the duodenum directly from the liver. However, when the bile in the gallbladder cannot escape, bile stasis may lead to cholecystitis.

Cholecystitis

Cholecystitis is most often associated with obstruction caused by gallstones or biliary sludge. Cholecystitis in the absence of obstruction *(acalculous cholecystitis)* occurs most often in older adults and in patients who are critically ill. Acalculous cholecystitis is also associated with prolonged immobility and fasting, prolonged PN, and diabetes. We think the main cause of this illness is bile stasis. Critically ill patients are more predisposed because of increased bile viscosity due to fever and dehydration and because of prolonged absence of oral feeding resulting in a decrease or absence of cholecystokinin-induced gallbladder contraction. Other risk factors include adhesions, cancer, anesthesia, and opioids.

Once acalculous cholecystitis is present, secondary infection with enteric pathogens, including *E. coli, Enterococcus faecalis, Klebsiella, Pseudomonas,* and *Proteus,* is common. Perforation occurs in severe cases.

Inflammation is the major issue. It may be confined to the mucous lining or involve the entire wall of the gallbladder. During an acute attack of cholecystitis, the gallbladder is edematous and hyperemic. It may be distended with bile or pus. The cystic duct is also involved and may become occluded. The wall of the gallbladder becomes scarred after an acute attack. Decreased functioning will occur if large amounts of tissue become fibrotic.

TABLE 48.22 Manifestations of Obstructed Bile Flow

Manifestation	Cause
Bleeding tendencies	Lack of or ↓ vitamin K absorption, resulting in ↓ prothrombin production
Clay-colored stools	No bilirubin reaching small intestine to be converted to urobilinogen
Dark amber to brown urine, which foams when shaken	↑ Water-soluble (conjugated) bilirubin elimination in urine
Fever and chills	Bacterial reflux from biliary tract to systemic circulation
Intolerance for fatty foods	No bile in small intestine for fat digestion
Jaundice	No bile flow into duodenum, bilirubin accumulates in blood
Pruritus	Deposition of bile salts in skin tissues
Steatorrhea	Undigested fatty components of food are eliminated in stool. Occurs because no bile in small intestine, thus preventing emulsion, digestion, and absorption of fat
Urobilinogen absent in urine	No bilirubin reaching small intestine to be converted to urobilinogen

Clinical Manifestations

Gallstones may cause a range of symptoms. The severity depends on whether the stones are stationary or mobile and whether obstruction is present (Fig. 48.12). When a stone is lodged in the ducts or when stones are moving through the ducts, spasms may result in response to the stone. This sometimes causes severe pain, which is termed *biliary colic.* The pain is often steady and severe. The pain may be accompanied by tachycardia, diaphoresis, and prostration. The severe pain may last up to an hour, and when it subsides, there is residual RUQ tenderness. Pain often occurs 3 to 6 hours after a high-fat meal or when the patient lies down.

When total obstruction occurs, symptoms related to bile blockage occur (Table 48.22). If the common bile duct is obstructed, no bilirubin will reach the small intestine to be converted to urobilinogen. Thus the kidneys will excrete bilirubin, causing dark amber to brown urine.

Manifestations of cholecystitis vary from indigestion to moderate to severe pain, fever, chills, and jaundice. Initial symptoms of acute cholecystitis include indigestion and acute pain and RUQ tenderness. Pain may be referred to the right shoulder and scapula. There may be nausea and vomiting, restlessness, and diaphoresis. Inflammation results in leukocytosis and fever. Physical findings include RUQ or epigastrium tenderness and abdominal rigidity. Chronic cholecystitis may present with a history of fat intolerance, dyspepsia, heartburn, and flatulence.

Complications

Complications of gallstones and cholecystitis include gangrenous cholecystitis, subphrenic abscess, pancreatitis, *cholangitis* (inflammation of biliary ducts), biliary cirrhosis, fistulas, and rupture of the gallbladder, which can cause bile peritonitis. In older adults and those with diabetes, gangrenous cholecystitis and bile peritonitis are the most common complications of cholecystitis. *Choledocholithiasis* (stone in the common bile duct) may occur, producing symptoms of obstruction.

Diagnostic Studies

Ultrasound is often used to diagnose gallstones (see Table 43.13). It is especially useful for patients with jaundice and those who are allergic to contrast medium. ERCP allows for visualization of the gallbladder, cystic duct, common hepatic duct, and common bile duct. Bile or bile duct brushings are taken during ERCP and sent for culture to identify possible infecting organisms. Biopsies can be done.

Percutaneous transhepatic cholangiography is the insertion of a needle directly into the gallbladder duct followed by injection of contrast materials. It is generally done after ultrasound shows a bile duct blockage.

Laboratory tests may show an increased WBC count because of inflammation. Liver enzymes (e.g., alkaline phosphatase, ALT, and AST), direct and indirect bilirubin levels, and urine bilirubin levels may be increased if an obstructive process is present (Table 48.22). Amylase is increased if the pancreas is involved.

Interprofessional Care

Once gallstones become symptomatic, a cholecystectomy is usually done (Table 48.23). However, in some cases, conservative therapy may be considered, including medical therapy or interventional procedures including stent and tube placements.

TABLE 48.23 Interprofessional Care

Cholelithiasis and Acute Cholecystitis

Diagnostic Assessment
- History and physical assessment
- Ultrasound
- ERCP
- Percutaneous transhepatic cholangiography
- Liver function tests
- WBC count

Management

Conservative Therapy
- IV fluid
- NPO with NG tube, later progressing to low-fat diet
- Antiemetics
- Analgesics
- Fat-soluble vitamins (A, D, E, and K)
- Anticholinergics (antispasmodics)
- Antibiotics (for secondary infection)
- Transhepatic biliary catheter
- ERCP with sphincterotomy (papillotomy)
- Extracorporeal shock-wave lithotripsy

Dissolution Therapy
- Chenodiol
- Ursodiol

Surgical Therapy
- Laparoscopic cholecystectomy
- Incisional (open) cholecystectomy

Conservative Therapy

Cholelithiasis. The treatment of gallstones depends on the stage.[28] Bile acids (cholesterol solvents), such as ursodiol and chenodiol, are used to dissolve stones. However, the gallstones may recur. We usually do not treat gallstones with drugs because of the high use and success of laparoscopic cholecystectomy.

ERCP with endoscopic sphincterotomy (papillotomy) may be used to remove stones. ERCP allows for visualization of the biliary system, dilation (balloon sphincteroplasty), and placement of stents and sphincterotomy (Fig. 48.13). Special catheters with wire baskets or inflatable balloon tip may be used for stone removal. When a stent is placed, it is generally removed or changed after a few months.

Extracorporeal shock-wave lithotripsy (ESWL) is an alternative treatment used when endoscopic approaches cannot remove stones. In ESWL, a lithotripter uses high-energy shock waves to disintegrate gallstones. It usually takes 1 to 2 hours to disintegrate the stones. The stone fragments pass through the common bile duct and into the small intestine. Usually, ESWL and oral dissolution therapy are used together.

Cholecystitis. During an acute episode of cholecystitis, treatment focuses on pain control, control of infection with antibiotics, and maintaining fluid and electrolyte balance. Treatment is supportive and focused on symptom management. If nausea and vomiting are severe, NG tube insertion and gastric decompression may be used to prevent further gallbladder stimulation. A cholecystostomy may be used to drain purulent material from the obstructed gallbladder. Opioids are given for pain management. Anticholinergics can decrease GI secretions and counteract smooth muscle spasms.

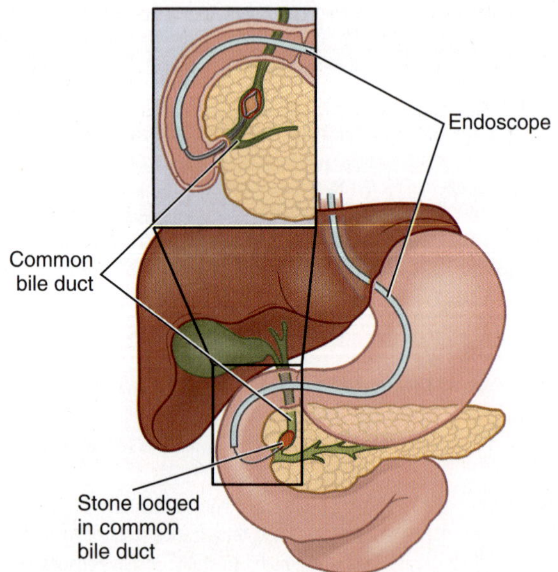

Fig. 48.13 During endoscopic sphincterotomy, an endoscope is advanced through the mouth and stomach until its tip sits in the duodenum opposite the common bile duct. *Inset,* After widening the duct mouth by incising the sphincter muscle, the HCP advances a basket attachment into the duct and snags the stone.

Surgical Therapy

Laparoscopic cholecystectomy is the treatment of choice for symptomatic gallstones. In this procedure, the gallbladder is removed through 1 to 4 small punctures in the abdomen. The HCP makes a small cut below the umbilicus and inserts a needle into the area. CO_2 gas is passed into the abdomen to expand the area. This allows the HCP to see the organs more clearly and gives more room to work. The HCP inserts the laparoscope, which has a camera attached, and grasping forceps into the abdomen through the punctures. Using closed-circuit monitors to view the abdominal cavity, the HCP retracts and dissects the gallbladder and removes it with the forceps. The few contraindications to laparoscopic cholecystectomy include peritonitis, cholangitis, gangrene or perforation of the gallbladder, portal hypertension, and serious bleeding disorders.

This is a safe and routine procedure with minimal morbidity and quick recovery time. Most patients have minimal postoperative pain. They are discharged the day of surgery or the day after. They can usually resume normal activities and return to work within 1 week. The main complications of surgery include injury to the common bile duct and bile leak.

Some patients may need an incisional (open) cholecystectomy. This involves removing the gallbladder through a right subcostal incision. A T tube may be placed in the common bile duct during a common bile duct exploration surgery (Fig. 48.14). It keeps the duct patent until the edema from the trauma of exploring and probing the duct subsides. It allows excess bile to drain while the small intestine is adjusting to receiving a continuous flow of bile.

Transhepatic Biliary Catheter

The transhepatic biliary catheter can be used preoperatively in biliary obstruction and in liver dysfunction from obstructive jaundice. It also can be part of palliative care when inoperable liver, pancreatic, or bile duct cancer obstructs bile flow. The catheter is used when endoscopic drainage has been unsuccessful. The catheter is inserted percutaneously and allows for decompression of obstructed extrahepatic bile ducts so that bile can flow freely. After placement of the catheter into the obstructed duct internally, the external catheter is connected to a drainage bag. Encourage patients to replace fluids lost in the drainage bag with electrolyte-rich drinks. Cleanse the skin around the catheter insertion site daily with an antiseptic. Observe for bile leakage at the insertion site and any signs or symptoms of an occluded or malfunctioning drain. These include sudden abdominal pain, nausea, fever, or chills. It is expected that stool may be lighter in color since bile is being diverted into the bag.

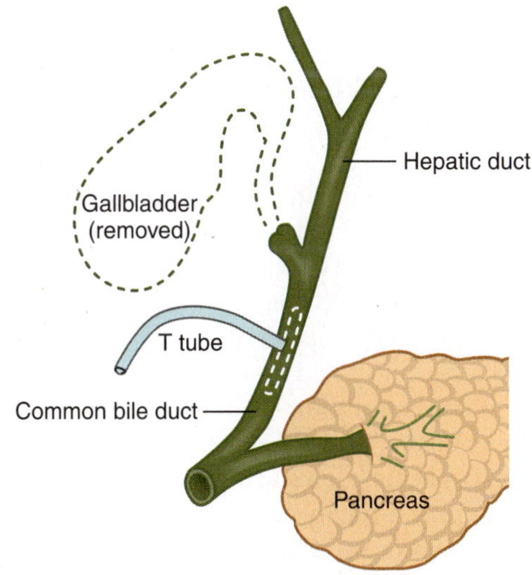

Fig. 48.14 Placement of T tube. *Dotted lines* show parts removed.

Drug Therapy

The most common drugs used in the treatment of gallbladder disease are analgesics, anticholinergics (antispasmodics), fat-soluble vitamins, and bile salts. Morphine may be used initially for pain management. Anticholinergics, such as atropine and other antispasmodics, may be used to relax the smooth muscle and decrease ductal tone.

Patients with chronic gallbladder disease or any biliary tract obstruction may need fat-soluble vitamin (A, D, E, and K) replacement. Bile salts can help with digestion and vitamin absorption. Cholestyramine may provide relief from itching.

Nutrition Therapy

Eating smaller, more frequent meals with some fat at each meal promotes gallbladder emptying. If obesity is a problem, recommend a reduced-calorie diet. The diet should be low in saturated fats (e.g., butter, shortening, lard) and high in fiber and calcium. Avoid rapid weight loss because it can promote gallstone formation.

After a laparoscopic cholecystectomy, teach patients to have liquids for the rest of the day and eat light meals for a few days. After an incisional cholecystectomy, patients will progress from liquids to a regular diet once bowel sounds have returned. The amount of fat in the postoperative diet depends on a patient's tolerance of fat. A low-fat diet may be helpful if the flow of bile is reduced (usually only in the early postoperative period) or if the patient is overweight. Sometimes patients must restrict fats for 4 to 6 weeks. Otherwise, no special diet is needed other than to eat nutritious meals and avoid excess fat intake.

NURSING MANAGEMENT: GALLBLADDER DISEASE

Assessment

Subjective and objective data that you should obtain from patients with gallbladder disease are outlined in Table 48.24.

Planning

The overall goals are that patients with gallbladder disease will have (1) relief of pain and discomfort, (2) no complications, and (3) no recurrent attacks of cholecystitis or gallstones.

TABLE 48.24 NURSING ASSESSMENT

Cholecystitis or Cholelithiasis

Subjective Data

Important Health Information

Health history: Obesity, multiparity, infection, cancer, extensive fasting, pregnancy

Medications: Estrogen or oral contraceptives

Surgery or other treatments: Abdominal surgery

Functional Health Patterns

Health perception–health management: Positive family history, sedentary lifestyle

Nutritional-metabolic: Weight loss, anorexia, indigestion, fat intolerance, nausea and vomiting, dyspepsia, chills

Elimination: Clay-colored stools, steatorrhea, flatulence. Dark urine

Cognitive-perceptual: Moderate to severe RUQ pain that may radiate to the back or scapula. Itching

Objective Data

Cardiovascular

Tachycardia

GI

Abdominal guarding, distention

General

Fever, restlessness

Respiratory

Tachypnea, splinting during respirations

Skin

Jaundice, icteric sclera, diaphoresis

Possible Diagnostic Findings

↑ Liver enzymes, alkaline phosphatase, bilirubin. Absence of urobilinogen in urine, ↑ urinary bilirubin, leukocytosis. Abnormal gallbladder ultrasound

◆ Implementation

Nursing goals for patients receiving conservative therapy include (1) treat pain, (2) relieve nausea and vomiting, (3) provide comfort and emotional support, (4) maintain fluid and electrolyte balance and nutrition, and (5) observe for complications.

With conservative therapy, nursing care depends on symptoms and whether surgery is planned. Provide any diet teaching. The diet is usually low in fat. Patients may need to take fat-soluble vitamin supplements. If needed, review a weight-reduction diet. Review the signs and symptoms of obstruction (e.g., stool and urine changes, jaundice, itching). Explain the importance of continued care follow-up.

Patients with acute cholecystitis or gallstones often have severe pain. Give the drugs ordered to relieve the pain as needed before pain becomes severe. Observe for side effects of the drugs as part of the continued assessment. Provide comfort measures, such as comfortable positioning and oral care.

Some patients have more severe nausea and vomiting than others. For these patients, an NG tube and gastric decompression may be needed. Eliminating intake of food and fluids prevents further stimulation of the gallbladder. Maintain accurate intake and output NG suction. For patients with less severe nausea and vomiting, antiemetics are usually adequate. When the patient is vomiting, provide comfort measures, such as frequent mouth rinses. Remove any vomitus at once from view. Provide oral hygiene and care of nares. If itching occurs with jaundice, use measures to relieve itching. These can include antihistamines or other treatments as previously discussed.

Assess for symptom progression and complications. Observe for signs of obstruction of the ducts by stones. These include jaundice; clay-colored stools; dark, foamy urine; steatorrhea; fever; and increased WBC count.

When an obstruction is present (Table 48.22), bleeding may result from decreased prothrombin production by the liver. Common sites to observe for bleeding are the mucous membranes of the mouth, nose, gingivae, and injection sites. When giving injections, use a small-gauge needle and apply gentle pressure afterward. Know the PT time and use it to guide your assessment.

Assess for infection. Monitor vital signs. A temperature elevation with chills and jaundice may indicate choledocholithiasis.

Care of patients after ERCP with papillotomy includes assessing for complications, such as pancreatitis, perforation, infection, and bleeding. Monitor vital signs. Abdominal pain, fever, and increasing amylase and lipase may indicate acute pancreatitis. Patients should be on bed rest for several hours and NPO until the gag reflex returns. Teach patients the need for follow-up if the stent is to be removed or changed.

Postoperative Care

Postoperative nursing care after a laparoscopic cholecystectomy includes monitoring for complications, such as bleeding, making the patient comfortable, and preparing the patient for discharge. Patients may report referred pain in the shoulder because of the CO_2 that the HCP uses to inflate the abdominal cavity during surgery. It may not be released or absorbed by the body. CO_2 can irritate the phrenic nerve and diaphragm, causing some difficulty breathing. Place patients on their left side with right knee flexed to move the gas pocket away from the diaphragm. Encourage deep breathing along with movement and ambulation. NSAIDs, simethicone, or codeine can usually relieve pain. Patients start clear liquids and can walk to the bathroom to void. Most patients are discharged soon after the surgery, so home care and teaching are important (Table 48.25).

Postoperative nursing care for incisional cholecystectomy focuses on promoting ventilation and preventing respiratory complications. Other nursing care is the same as general postoperative nursing care (see Chapter 20). Tell patients to avoid heavy lifting for 4 to 6 weeks. Most patients tolerate a regular diet with no problems but should avoid excess fats. Sometimes, patients need to remain on a low-fat diet for 4 to 6 weeks.

If the patient has a T tube (Fig. 48.14), maintain the system, and monitor T-tube function and drainage. The T tube is usually connected to a closed gravity drainage system. If the Penrose or Jackson-Pratt drain or the T tube is draining large amounts of

TABLE 48.25 PATIENT & CAREGIVER TEACHING

Postoperative Laparoscopic Cholecystectomy

Postoperative teaching should include:

1. Remove the bandages on the puncture sites the day after surgery and you can shower.
2. Notify your HCP if any of the following signs and symptoms occurs:
   - Redness, swelling, bile-colored drainage or pus from any incision
   - Severe abdominal pain, nausea, vomiting, fever, chills
3. You can gradually resume normal activities.
4. Return to work within 1–2 weeks of surgery.
5. You can resume your usual diet. Many tolerate a low-fat diet better for several weeks after surgery.
6. If you have a T-tube, wash hands well before touching the drainage bag and tube. Use barrier cream to protect the skin around the tube. Do not let the tube get kinked. Empty the bag before it is full, measuring the output each time in milliliters. Call the HCP if the drainage suddenly ceases.

bile, it is helpful to use a sterile pouching system to protect the skin. Encourage oral intake to replace lost fluids and electrolytes.

◆ Evaluation

The overall expected outcomes are that patients with gallbladder disease will:

- Appear comfortable and have pain relief
- Remain free from complications

GALLBLADDER CANCER

Gallbladder cancer has an incidence rate of 1.4 per 100,000 in females and 0.8 per 100,000 in males in the United States.[29] Most gallbladder cancers are adenocarcinomas. Many patients are asymptomatic. The early symptoms are insidious and similar to those of chronic cholecystitis and gallstones. This makes the diagnosis difficult. Most cancers are found incidentally. Many have advanced disease at the time of diagnosis leading to high mortality rates. Later symptoms are usually those of biliary obstruction.

Diagnosis and staging of gallbladder cancer are done using EUS, abdominal ultrasound, CT, MRI, and/or MRCP. When found early, surgery can be curative. Several factors influence successful surgical outcomes. These include the depth of cancer invasion, extent of liver involvement, venous or lymphatic invasion, and lymph node metastasis. Extended cholecystectomy with lymph node dissection has improved outcomes for those with gallbladder cancer.

When surgery is not an option, endoscopic stenting of the biliary tract can reduce obstructive jaundice. Adjuvant therapies, including radiation therapy and chemotherapy, may be used depending on the disease state. Overall, gallbladder cancer has a poor prognosis.

Nursing management involves palliative care with special attention to nutrition, hydration, skin care, and pain relief. Nursing care measures used for patients with cholecystitis and gallstones and for patients with cancer (see Chapter 16) are appropriate.

CASE STUDY

Cirrhosis

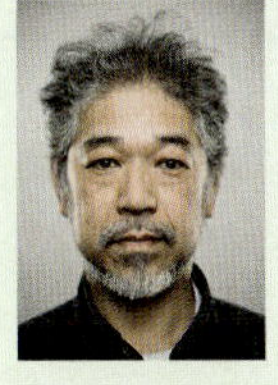

(© SensorSpot/ iStock.com.)

Patient Profile

J.T. arrives in the emergency department via ambulance with reports of having "dizzy spells," feeling "forgetful," and "almost passing out" at home. He has chronic HBV, cirrhosis, depression, and asthma. Upon further questioning, he reports having reddish colored stools for the past 2 days.

Subjective Data

- Close with his 3 adopted children, has a male partner for 15 years.
- Has had cirrhosis for 6 years
- States he drank heavily for 18 years but has been sober for the past 3 years
- Reports anorexia, nausea, abdominal discomfort, and unintentional weight loss over the past 6 months

Objective Data

Physical Assessment

- Moderate ascites
- Jaundice of sclera and skin
- 2+ pitting edema of the lower extremities
- Liver and spleen are palpable, 1 cm below the right costal margin, with a span of 5 cm, and spleen is smooth and palpable near the mid abdomen.

Laboratory Values

- Total bilirubin: 4 mg/dL
- AST: 60 U/L
- ALT: 80 U/L
- Albumin 2.8 g/dL
- Platelets: 29,000/μL
- eGFR: 70 mL/min

Ultrasound shows a nodular shrunken liver, with patent vasculature. There is a 3 cm hepatic lesion suspicious for hepatocellular carcinoma in the left lobe. The gall bladder is decompressed without inflammation. The spleen is enlarged, and there is moderate abdominal ascites. The kidneys are unremarkable.

Discussion Questions

1. ***Recognize:*** Based on the history, what type of cirrhosis does J.T. likely have?
2. ***Analyze:*** Explain the significance of the results of his laboratory values and ultrasound findings.
3. ***Analyze:*** What are possible causes of his GI bleeding and weight loss?
4. ***Plan:*** If J.T. begins to have somnolence, and confusion what would that be called? What would you monitor? What measures would be used to control or decrease encephalopathy?
5. ***Prioritize:*** Based on the assessment data, what are the priority clinical problems?
6. ***Act:*** What interventions do you need to implement in this situation?
7. ***Act:*** J.T. discusses his prognosis with you. He says, "Will my children, my parents, or my partner catch this?" How would you respond to his question?
8. ***Evaluate:*** What would you need to monitor to decide if care was effective?
9. ***Safety:*** Given J.T.'s bleeding history and current ultrasound result, identify areas of concern and priority. What care do you think he will need?
10. Develop a conceptual care map for J.T.

Answers and a corresponding conceptual care map available at evolve.elsevier.com/Lewis/medsurg.

BRIDGE TO NCLEX EXAMINATION

The number of the question corresponds to the same-numbered outcome at the beginning of the chapter.

1. What information would the nurse include when teaching a patient about hepatitis A transmission?
- **a.** Poor sanitary conditions is a risk factor.
- **b.** Injection drug use is the primary mode of transmission.
- **c.** Mothers can pass the virus to their babies during pregnancy.
- **d.** Unprotected vaginal intercourse is one route of transmission.

2. A patient with chronic hepatitis B asks you why the nurse practitioner ordered an ultrasound. You tell him the ultrasound is likely going to be looking for which of the following? **(Select all that apply.)**
- **a.** Ascites
- **b.** Spleen size
- **c.** Liver function
- **d.** Hepatocellular carcinoma
- **e.** Surface texture of the liver

3. High levels of toxins, such as ammonia, in persons with late-stage cirrhosis is referred to as
- **a.** MASLD
- **b.** Portal hypertension
- **c.** Hepatorenal syndrome
- **d.** Hepatic encephalopathy

4. You would plan care for a patient with hepatocellular cancer based on what knowledge?
- **a.** Radiation alone is a curative treatment.
- **b.** There is no cure for hepatocellular cancer.
- **c.** Chemotherapy is the preferred option for cure.
- **d.** A liver transplant is performed to achieve a cure.

5. Which lifestyle changes would you stress with a patient being discharged after acute pancreatitis in order to avoid recurrence? **(Select all that apply.)**
- **a.** Avoid alcohol
- **b.** Eat a low-fat diet
- **c.** Limit fluid intake
- **d.** Avoid smoking tobacco
- **e.** Eat small but frequent meals

6. A patient with pancreatic cancer reports increased yellowing of the sclera over the past 3 weeks. What is the most likely cause?
- **a.** Diabetes
- **b.** Alcohol overuse
- **c.** Nutritional compromise
- **d.** Blockage of the bile duct

7. Which finding can indicate gallstones and gallbladder obstruction?
- **a.** Ascites
- **b.** Pitting edema bilaterally
- **c.** Referred pain to the right shoulder
- **d.** Left lower quadrant tenderness with palpation

8. Discharge teaching for the patient with a transhepatic biliary tube would include which point?
- **a.** Avoid drinks high in electrolytes
- **b.** Keep the tube clamped at all times
- **c.** Remove and replace the tube daily
- **d.** Call the HCP if there is increased abdominal pain

1. a; 2. a, b, d, e; 3. d; 4. d; 5. c; 6. d; 7. c; 8. d.

For rationales to these answers and even more NCLEX review questions, visit https://evolve.elsevier.com/Lewis/medsurg.

REFERENCES

To access the References for this chapter, please scan the QR code with a mobile device.

CASE STUDY

Applying Clinical Judgment With Multiple Patients

The following 4 patients are among the 7 you are assigned to care for today on the medical unit. You have 1 LPN and 1 AP who are assigned to help you.

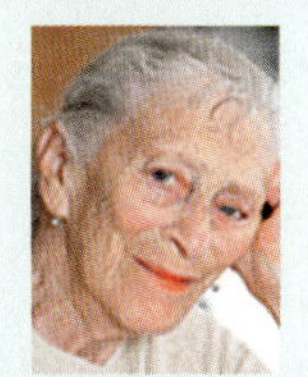 (© iStockphoto/Thinkstock.)	M.S. is a 70-year-old female who was admitted with weakness and malnutrition. She is 5 ft, 4 in tall and weighs 100 lb, with a 30-lb weight loss in past 2 months. Her history includes a recent stroke with hemiparesis and dysphagia. She has been NPO for the past 24 hours and started EN via PEG tube placed yesterday afternoon.
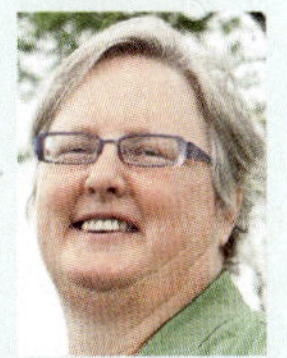 (© Christa Brunt/iStock/ Thinkstock.)	S.R. is a 48-year-old female admitted with chest pain. She has a history of type 2 diabetes, hypertension, and osteoarthritis. She is 5 ft, 6 in tall and weighs 230 lb. The last 2 glucose levels were over 250 mg/dL and she received sliding scale insulin. Cardiac enzymes and ECG are normal. She is scheduled to have a cardiac stress test at 10 AM. Vital signs: 160/110, 102, RR 22, O_2 saturation 94% with O_2 2 L/min via nasal cannula.
(© iStockphoto/Thinkstock.)	F.H., a 40-year-old male, was admitted yesterday with upper GI bleeding. He had just finished treatment with omeprazole, clarithromycin, and amoxicillin for a duodenal ulcer and *H. pylori.* He came to the ED yesterday with severe epigastric pain and melena. He is on a pantoprazole IV infusion and scheduled for a repeat EGD today.
(© SensorSpot/iStock.com.)	J.T. is a 58-year-old male admitted early this morning after reporting dizziness and cognitive problems for 2 days. His history includes chronic HBV, cirrhosis, and asthma. He currently has anorexia, nausea, and abdominal discomfort with severe ascites, jaundice, and 4+ pitting edema. CT scan is suspicious for liver cancer. His liver enzymes are high and platelet count is 29,000/μL. Vital signs: 102/54, 102, RR 22, O_2 saturation 94% with O_2 2 L/min via nasal cannula.

1. Highlight all the findings above that require your immediate attention.
2. After receiving report, which patient should you see first?
3. Which tasks could you delegate to the LPN? **(Select all that apply.)**
   a. Change M.S.'s PEG tube dressing.
   b. Administer a bolus enteral feeding to M.S.
   c. Give a scheduled dose of oral lactulose solution to J.T.
   d. Teach F.H.'s wife about his disease because she speaks English.
   e. Perform bedside glucose reading and administer sliding scale insulin to S.R.
4. Which diagnostic finding would you report to the HCP immediately?
   a. Glucose level 220 mg/dL for S.R.
   b. Hemoglobin 6.9 g/dL and hematocrit 21% for F.H.
   c. Sodium 134 mEq/L and potassium 3.4 mEq/L for M.S.
   d. Total bilirubin 3.2 mg/dL with positive urine bilirubin for J.T.
5. As you are assessing M.B., the LPN tells you that F.H. just vomited a large amount of bright red blood. What initial action would be *most* appropriate?
   a. Have the LPN administer an antiemetic to F.H.
   b. Ask the LPN to notify F.H.'s HCP immediately.
   c. Leave J.T.'s room to perform a focused assessment on F.H.
   d. Ask the AP to obtain a unit of packed RBCs from the blood bank.

Case Study Progression

When you enter F.H.'s room, he tells you that his pain actually feels somewhat relieved since he vomited. However, you note that his skin is cool and clammy, his BP is 90/54 mm Hg, and his heart rate is 116 bpm. You notify his HCP.

6. Which interventions would you expect the HCP to order for F.H.? **(Select all that apply.)**
   a. Stat hemoglobin and hematocrit
   b. Emergent endoscopy with band ligation
   c. Discontinue the pantoprazole IV infusion
   d. Start a second IV and administer a 500 mL normal saline bolus
   e. Contact HCP and notify operating room that patient is unstable and needs surgery
7. You see that you need to complete J.T.'s medication reconciliation for the new HCP orders. Choose the most likely options for the information missing from the table below by selecting from the lists of options provided.

Medication	Dose, Route, Frequency	Drug Class	Indication
Propranolol	1	β-blocker	Decrease portal venous pressure
2	100 mg oral daily	Potassium-sparing diuretic	Excrete fluid with ascites
Lactulose	15 mL oral twice daily	Laxative	3
Vasopressin	10 units subcut 3 times daily	4	Decrease portal blood flow

Options for 1	Options for 2	Options for 3	Options for 4
20 mg IV every 12 hours 320 mg oral twice daily 640 mg oral daily	acetazolamide chlorothiazide spironolactone	Decrease bacterial flora Decrease gastric acidity Fecal elimination of ammonia	Anticoagulant Antihypertensive Hormone analog

8. Which interventions to treat ascites would you expect the HCP to order for J.T.? **(Select all that apply.)**
   a. Thoracentesis
   b. 2 g sodium diet
   c. Diuretic therapy
   d. 1800 mL/day fluid restriction
   e. Shunt insertion from peritoneum to heart

Continued

CASE STUDY—cont'd

Applying Clinical Judgment With Multiple Patients

9. While you are administering M.S.'s bolus feeding of EN, you perform her assessment. For each assessment finding, use an X to indicate whether the interventions were *Effective* (helped meet expected outcomes) or *Ineffective* (did not help meet expected outcomes).

Assessment Finding	Effective	Ineffective
Electrolyte values within normal limits		
Weight gain of 2 lb in 1 week		
Onset of 2+ bilateral pedal edema		
Improved activity intolerance		
Increased muscle strength		
Wound around PEG tube not healing properly		

10 After giving M.S. the bolus feeding, it would be *most* important to
   a. assess for gastric residual.
   b. obtain an abdominal x-ray.
   c. keep head of bed elevated 30 to 45 degrees.
   d. record the total amount of fluid administered.

11. As you enter the nurse's station, you overhear derogatory comments made by the AP to the LPN about S.R.'s weight. Which response would be *most* appropriate?
   a. Report the incident to charge nurse for follow-up.
   b. Talk to the AP to discuss a possible HIPAA violation.
   c. Talk to S.R. about the impact of AP's bias on the patient's self-image.
   d. Set up an in-service to teach staff members to recognize obesity as a disease process.

Answers available at http://evolve.elsevier.com/Lewis/medsurg.

49

Assessment: Urinary System

Amanda Sanders

http://evolve.elsevier.com/Lewis/medsurg/

CONCEPTUAL FOCUS

Elimination | **Fluids and Electrolytes**

LEARNING OUTCOMES

1. Identify the structure and functions of the kidneys, ureters, bladder, and urethra.
2. Explain the physiologic events involved in the formation and passage of urine.
3. Link the age-related changes of the urinary system to differences in assessment findings.
4. Obtain subjective and objective data related to the urinary system.
5. Distinguish normal from abnormal findings of a urinary assessment.
6. Describe the purpose, significance of results, and nursing responsibilities related to diagnostic studies of the urinary system.
7. Evaluate findings of a urinalysis.

KEY TERMS

costovertebral angle (CVA)
creatinine
cystoscopy (Table 49.11)
glomerular filtration rate (GFR)
glomerulus
nephron
renal biopsy (Table 49.11)
urinalysis

The *upper urinary system* consists of 2 kidneys and 2 ureters. The *lower urinary system* consists of the urinary bladder and urethra (Fig. 49.1). Adequate kidney function is essential to health. If a person has kidney failure and treatment is not provided, death is inevitable. This chapter discusses the structures and functions, assessment, and diagnostic studies of the urinary system.

URINARY SYSTEM STRUCTURES AND FUNCTIONS

Kidneys

The kidneys are the principal organs of the urinary system. Their main functions are to (1) regulate the volume and composition of extracellular fluid (ECF) and (2) excrete waste products from the body. Through the formation of urine, the kidneys filter the blood and maintain the body's internal homeostasis. The kidneys also make erythropoietin, activate vitamin D, regulate acid-base balance, and help control BP.

Macrostructure

The kidneys are bean-shaped organs located retroperitoneally (behind the peritoneum) on either side of the vertebral column at about the level of the 12th thoracic (T12) vertebra to the 3rd lumbar (L3) vertebra. Each kidney weighs 4 to 6 oz (113 to 170 g) and is about 5 in (12.5 cm) long. The right kidney, positioned at the level of the 12th rib, is lower than the left. An adrenal gland lies on top of each kidney.

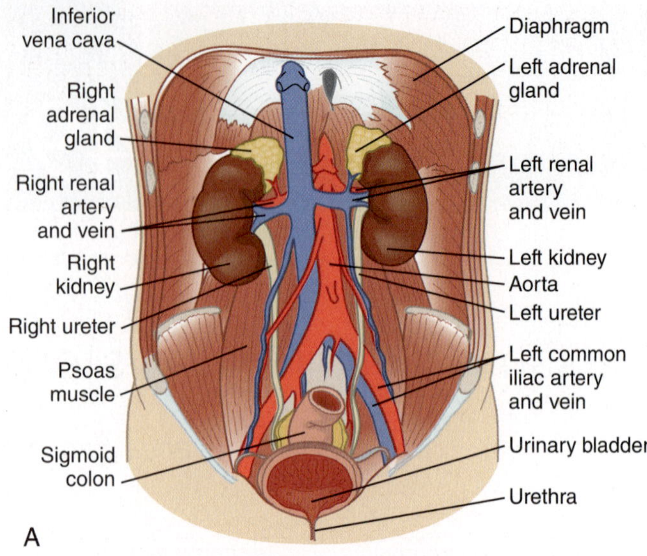

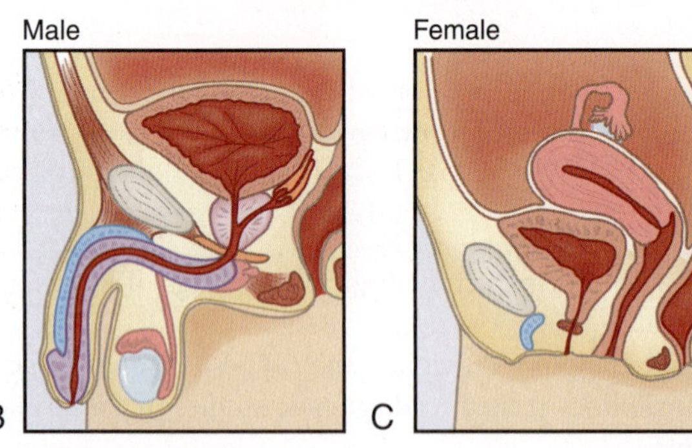

Fig. 49.1 Organs of the urinary system. (A) Upper urinary tract in relation to other anatomic structures. (B) Male urethra in relation to other pelvic structures. (C) Female urethra.

Each kidney is surrounded by a large amount of fat and connective tissue that cushion, support, and help the kidney to maintain its position. A thin, smooth layer of fibrous membrane called the *capsule* covers the surface of each kidney. The capsule protects the kidney and serves as a shock absorber if this area receives a sudden force or strike. The *hilus* on the medial side of the kidney serves as the entry site for the renal artery and nerves and as the exit site for the renal vein and ureter.

The *parenchyma* is the actual tissue of the kidney (Fig. 49.2). The outer layer of the parenchyma is the *cortex*. The inner layer is the *medulla*. The medulla consists of a number of pyramids. The apices (tops) of these pyramids are the *papillae*, through which urine passes to enter the calyces. The minor calyces widen and merge to form major calyces, which form a funnel-shaped sac called the *renal pelvis*. The minor and major calyces transport urine to the renal pelvis, and from there it drains through the ureter to the bladder. The renal pelvis can store a small volume of urine (3 to 5 mL).

Microstructure

The **nephron** is the functional unit of the kidney. Each kidney has around 1 million nephrons. Each nephron is composed of

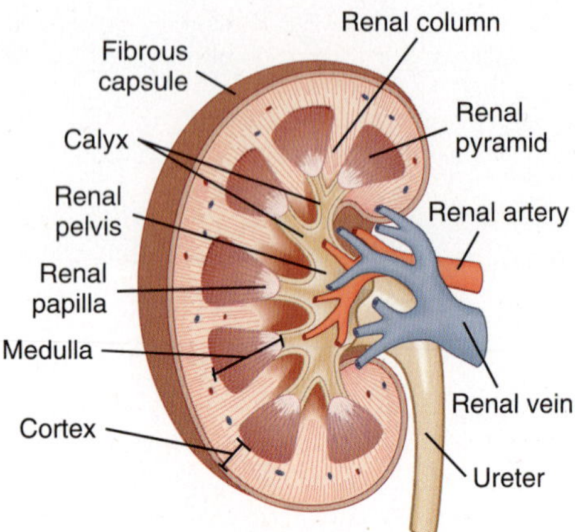

Fig. 49.2 Longitudinal section of the kidney.

the glomerulus, Bowman capsule, and a tubular system. The tubular system consists of the proximal convoluted tubule, loop of Henle, distal convoluted tubule, and collecting tubules (Fig. 49.3). The glomerulus, Bowman capsule, proximal tubule, and distal tubule are in the cortex of the kidney. The loop of Henle and collecting tubules are in the medulla. Several collecting tubules join to form a single collecting duct. The collecting ducts eventually merge into a pyramid that empties through the papilla into a minor calyx.

Blood Supply

Blood flow to the kidneys is around 1200 mL/min. This is 20% to 25% of the cardiac output. Blood reaches the kidneys via the renal artery, which enters the kidney through the hilus. The renal artery divides into secondary branches and then into still smaller branches, each of which forms an afferent arteriole. The afferent arteriole divides into a capillary network, the **glomerulus**, which is a collection of up to 50 capillaries (Fig. 49.3). The capillaries of the glomerulus unite in the efferent arteriole. The efferent arteriole then splits to form a capillary network (peritubular capillaries) that surrounds the tubular system. All peritubular capillaries drain into the venous system. The renal vein empties into the inferior vena cava.

Physiology of Urine Formation

Urine formation is the outcome of a complex, multistep process of filtration, reabsorption, secretion, and excretion of water, electrolytes, and metabolic waste products. Urine is formed in the kidneys. After the glomerulus has filtered the blood, essential constituents are returned to the blood and dispensable substances pass into urine. Urine drains through the ureters to be stored in the bladder and then passes out of the body through the urethra. These processes are discussed in detail next.

Glomerular function. Urine formation begins at the glomerulus, where blood is filtered. The glomerulus is a semipermeable membrane that allows filtration (Fig. 49.3). The hydrostatic pressure of the blood within the glomerular capillaries causes a portion of blood to be filtered across the

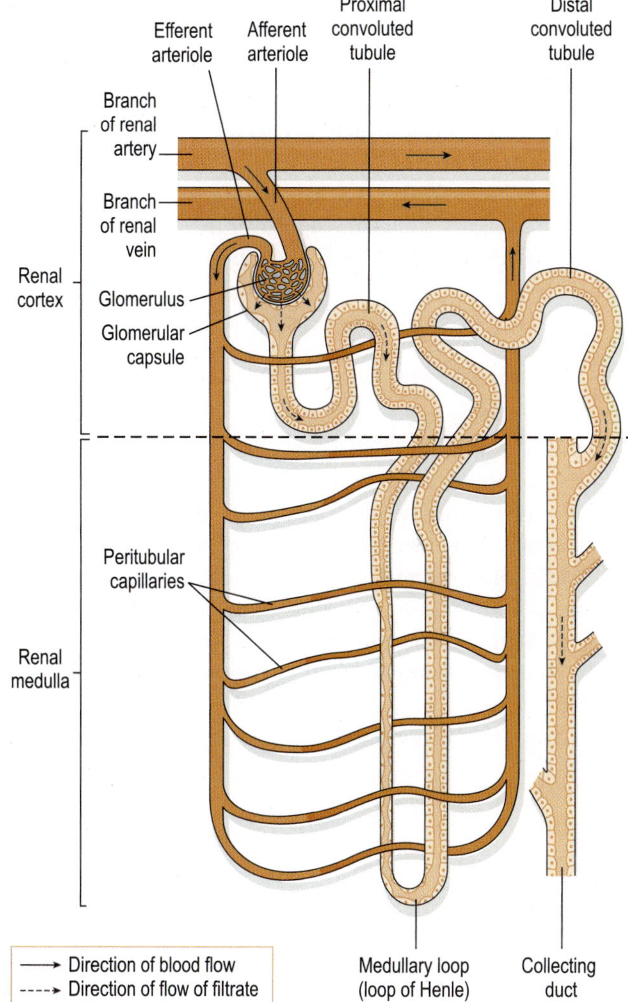

Fig. 49.3 The nephron is the basic functional unit of the kidney. This shows a single nephron unit with the surrounding blood vessels. (From Rankin J: *Physiology in childbearing,* ed 5, St Louis, 2025, Elsevier.)

semipermeable membrane into Bowman capsule. There, the filtered portion of the blood (glomerular filtrate) begins to pass down to the tubule. Filtration is more rapid in the glomerulus than in ordinary tissue capillaries because the glomerular membrane is porous. The glomerular filtrate is similar in composition to blood except that it lacks blood cells, platelets, and large plasma proteins. Under normal conditions, capillary pores are too small to allow the large blood components through. However, in many kidney diseases, capillary permeability increases, which allows plasma proteins and blood cells to pass into the urine.

The amount of blood filtered each minute by the glomeruli is the **glomerular filtration rate (GFR)**. The normal GFR is about 125 mL/min. The peritubular capillary network reabsorbs most of the glomerular filtrate before it reaches the end of the collecting duct. Therefore only 1 mL/min (on average) is excreted as urine.

Tubular function. The tubules and collecting ducts are responsible for reabsorbing essential materials and excreting nonessential ones (Table 49.1). They do this through

TABLE 49.1 Functions of Nephron Segments

Segment	Function
Glomerulus	Selective filtration
Proximal tubule	Reabsorption of 80% of electrolytes and water, glucose, amino acids, HCO_3^-
	Secretion of H^+ and creatinine
Loop of Henle	Concentration of filtrate
	Reabsorption of Na^+ and Cl^- in ascending limb and water in descending loop
Distal tubule	Reabsorption of water (regulated by ADH) and HCO_3^-
	Regulation of Ca^{2+} and PO_4^{2-} by parathyroid hormone
	Regulation of Na^+ and K^+ by aldosterone
	Secretion of K^+, H^+, and ammonia
Collecting duct	Reabsorption of water (requires ADH)

ADH, Antidiuretic hormone.

reabsorption and secretion. *Reabsorption* is the passage of a substance from the lumen of the tubules through the tubule cells and into the capillaries. This process involves both active and passive transport mechanisms. Tubular *secretion* is the passage of a substance from the capillaries through the tubular cells into the lumen of the tubule. Reabsorption and secretion cause many changes in the composition of the glomerular filtrate as it moves through the entire length of the tubule.

In the proximal convoluted tubule, about 80% of the electrolytes are reabsorbed. Normally, this includes all glucose, amino acids, and small proteins. As reabsorption continues in the loop of Henle, water is conserved, which is important for concentrating the filtrate. The descending loop is permeable to water and moderately permeable to sodium, urea, and other solutes. In the ascending limb, chloride ions (Cl^-) are actively reabsorbed, followed by passive reabsorption of sodium ions (Na^+). About 25% of the filtered sodium is reabsorbed in the ascending limb.

Two key functions of the distal convoluted tubules are final regulation of water balance and acid-base balance. Antidiuretic hormone (ADH) is needed for water reabsorption in the kidney. It is important in water balance. ADH makes the distal convoluted tubules and collecting ducts permeable to water. This allows water to be reabsorbed into the peritubular capillaries and eventually returned to the circulation.

Osmoreceptors in the anterior hypothalamus detect decreases in plasma osmolality. These osmoreceptors send neural input to superoptic nuclei cells in the hypothalamus. These cells have neuronal axons that end in the posterior pituitary gland. They inhibit ADH secretion. In the absence of ADH, the tubules are essentially impermeable to water. Thus any water in the tubules leaves the body as urine.

Aldosterone (from the adrenal cortex) acts on the distal tubule to cause reabsorption of Na^+ and water. In exchange for

Na^+, potassium ions (K^+) are excreted. Circulating blood volume and plasma concentrations of Na^+ and K^+ influence aldosterone secretion.

Acid-base regulation involves reabsorbing and conserving most of the bicarbonate (HCO_3^-) and secreting excess hydrogen ions (H^+). The distal tubule has different ways to keep the pH of ECF within a range of 7.35 to 7.45 (see Chapter 17).

Myocyte cells in the right atrium secrete atrial natriuretic peptide (ANP) in response to atrial distention from an increase in plasma volume. ANP acts on the kidneys to increase sodium excretion. ANP inhibits renin, ADH, and the action of angiotensin II on the adrenal glands, thereby suppressing aldosterone secretion. These combined effects of ANP result in a large volume of dilute urine. ANP also relaxes the afferent arteriole, thus increasing the GFR.

The renal tubules are involved in calcium balance. The parathyroid gland releases parathyroid hormone (PTH) when calcium levels are low. PTH maintains calcium levels by increasing tubular reabsorption of calcium (Ca^{2+}) and decreasing tubular reabsorption of phosphate (PO_4^{2-}). In kidney disease, the effects of PTH may have a major effect on bone metabolism.

Vitamin D is a hormone that we obtain in the diet or make by the action of ultraviolet radiation on cholesterol in the skin. These forms of vitamin D are inactive. They go through 2 steps to become metabolically active. The first step occurs in the liver; the second step occurs in the kidneys. Active vitamin D is essential for calcium absorption in the gastrointestinal (GI) tract. Patients with kidney failure *(renal failure)* will have a deficiency of the active metabolite of vitamin D and problems with calcium and phosphate balance (see Chapter 51).

Other Functions of Kidneys

The kidneys have a role in red blood cell (RBC) production and BP regulation. Erythropoietin is a hormone made in the kidneys. It is secreted in response to hypoxia and decreased renal blood flow. Erythropoietin stimulates RBC production in the bone marrow. A deficiency of erythropoietin occurs in kidney failure, leading to anemia.

Renin is important in BP regulation. It is made and secreted by the kidney's juxtaglomerular cells (Fig. 49.4). Renin is released into the bloodstream in response to decreased renal

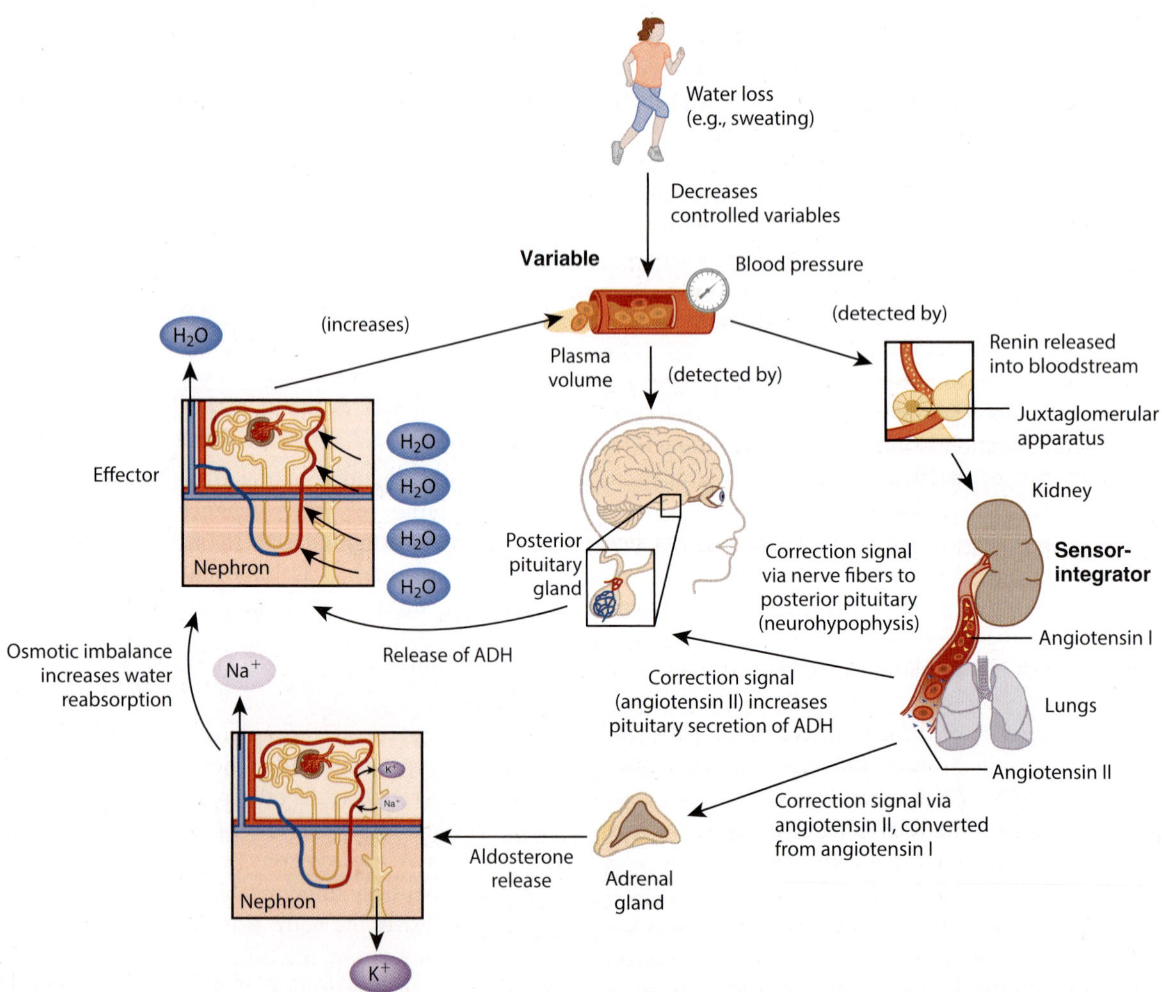

Fig. 49.4 Feedback renin-angiotensin-aldosterone system to fluid loss.

perfusion, decreased arterial BP, decreased ECF, decreased Na^+ concentration, and increased urine Na^+ concentration. The plasma protein angiotensinogen (from the liver) is activated to angiotensin I by renin. Angiotensin I is then converted to angiotensin II by angiotensin-converting enzyme (ACE). ACE is found on the inner surface of all blood vessels, with especially high levels in the vessels of the lungs. Angiotensin II stimulates the release of aldosterone from the adrenal cortex. This causes Na^+ and water retention, leading to increased ECF volume. Angiotensin II also causes increased peripheral vasoconstriction. An elevated BP inhibits renin release. Excess renin production caused by impaired kidney perfusion may be a contributing factor in hypertension (see Chapter 36).

Most body tissues make prostaglandins (PGs) from the precursor arachidonic acid in response to specific stimuli. (See Chapter 12 and Fig. 12.2 for more about PGs.) In the kidney, PG synthesis (mainly PGE_2 and PGI_2) occurs primarily in the medulla. These PGs have a vasodilating action, thus increasing renal blood flow and promoting Na^+ excretion. They counteract the vasoconstrictive effect of substances such as angiotensin. Renal PGs may help lower BP by decreasing systemic vascular resistance. In kidney failure with a loss of functioning tissue, these renal vasodilator factors are lost, which may contribute to hypertension (see Chapter 36).

Ureters

The ureters are tubes that carry urine from the renal pelvis to the bladder (Fig. 49.1). Each ureter is about 10 to 12 inches (25 to 30.5 cm) long and 0.08 to 0.3 inches (0.2 to 0.8 cm) in diameter. Arranged in a meshlike outer layer, circular and longitudinal smooth muscle fibers contract to promote the peristaltic, 1-way flow of urine through the ureters. Distention, neurologic and endocrine influences, and drugs can affect these muscle contractions.

The narrow area where each ureter joins the renal pelvis is the *ureteropelvic junction* (UPJ). The ureters insert into either side of the bladder base at the *ureterovesical junctions* (UVJs). Because the ureteral lumens are narrowest at these junctions, the UPJ and UVJ are often sites of obstruction. The narrow ureteral lumens can be easily obstructed internally (e.g., urinary stones) or externally (e.g., tumors, adhesions, inflammation). Sympathetic and parasympathetic nerves, along with the vascular supply, surround the mucosal lining of the ureters. Stimulation of these nerves during passage of a stone may cause acute, severe pain, termed *renal colic.*

Because the renal pelvis holds only 3 to 5 mL of urine, kidney damage can result from a backflow of more than that amount of urine. The UVJ relies on the ureter's angle of bladder insertion and muscle fiber attachments with the bladder to prevent the backflow *(reflux)* of urine, which predisposes a person to an ascending infection. The distal ureter enters the bladder laterally at its base. It then courses along obliquely through the bladder wall for about 1.5 cm and intermingles with muscle fibers of the bladder base. Circular and longitudinal bladder muscle fibers adjacent to the embedded ureter help secure it. When bladder pressure rises (e.g., during voiding or coughing), muscle fibers that the ureter shares with the bladder base contract first, promoting ureteral lumen closure. Next, the bladder contracts against its base, ensuring UVJ closure and preventing urine reflux through the junction.

Bladder

The urinary bladder is behind the symphysis pubis and anterior to the vagina and rectum (Fig. 49.5). Its functions are to serve as a reservoir for urine and eliminate waste products from the body. The bladder is a stretchable, saclike organ that contracts when it is empty. The *trigone* is the triangular area at the base of the bladder formed by the 2 ureteral openings and bladder neck. The trigone is attached to the pelvis by connective tissue and ligaments. It maintains its shape during bladder filling and emptying.

The bladder muscle *(detrusor)* is composed of intertwined layers of smooth muscle fibers. These fibers are capable of considerable distention during bladder filling and contraction during emptying. The dome and the anterior and lateral aspects of the bladder expand and contract in response to urine volume. The median umbilical ligament anchors the bladder to the anterior abdominal wall. This is why, as the bladder fills, it rises toward the umbilicus.

The bladder has the same mucosal lining as that of the renal pelvises, ureters, and bladder neck. The bladder is lined by transitional cell epithelium referred to as the *urothelium.* Unique to the urinary tract, the urothelium is resistant to absorption of urine. This means that after waste products (made

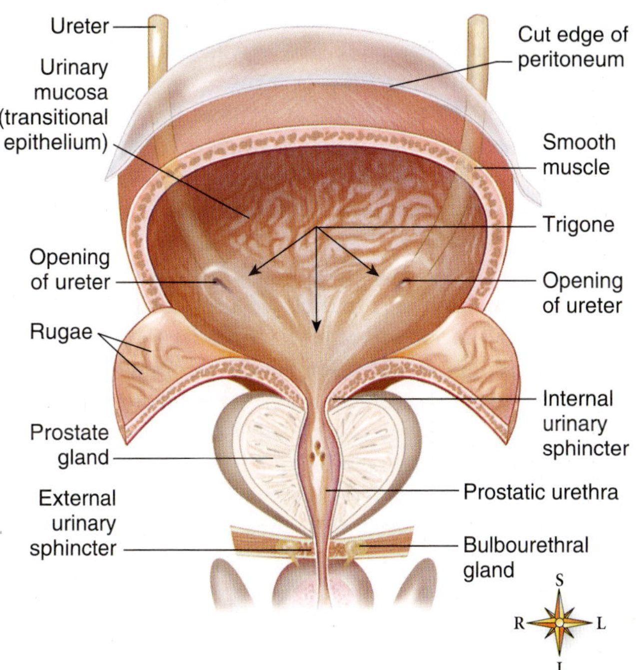

Fig. 49.5 Distended male urinary bladder. (From Patton KT, Thibodeau GA: *The human body in health & disease,* ed 7, St Louis, 2018, Mosby.)

by the kidneys) have left the kidneys, they cannot be reabsorbed in the urinary system. Microscopically, urothelium is only several cells deep. However, as urine enters the bladder, these cells can stretch to accommodate filling. As the bladder empties, the urothelium resumes its multicellular layer formation.

Urethra

The urethra is a small tube that incorporates the smooth muscle of the bladder neck and extends to the striated muscle of the external meatus. The urethra's primary functions are to (1) control voiding and (2) serve as a conduit for urine from the bladder to the outside of the body during voiding.

The female urethra is 1 to 2 in (2.5 to 5 cm) long. It lies behind the symphysis pubis but anterior to the vagina (Fig. 49.1C). The male urethra, which is about 8 to 10 in (20 to 25 cm) long, starts at the bladder neck and extends the length of the penis (Fig. 49.1B).

Urethrovesical Unit

The bladder, urethra, and pelvic floor muscles form the *urethrovesical unit.* Voluntary control of this unit is defined as *continence.* Stimulating and inhibiting impulses are sent from the brain through the thoracolumbar (T11 to L2) and sacral (S2 to S4) areas of the spinal cord to control voiding. Bladder distention stimulates stretch receptors within the bladder wall. Impulses are transmitted to the sacral spinal cord and then to the brain, causing the desire to urinate or void.

Normal adult urine output is around 1500 mL/day, which varies with food and fluid intake. The volume of urine at night is less than half of that formed during the day because of hormonal influences (e.g., ADH). This diurnal pattern of urination is normal. Typically, a person will urinate 5 or 6 times during the day and sometimes at night.

On average, 200 to 250 mL of urine in the bladder causes moderate distention and the urge to urinate. When the quantity of urine reaches 400 to 600 mL, the person feels uncomfortable. Bladder capacity varies with the person, but generally ranges from 600 to 1000 mL.

If you cannot void at a given time, inhibitor impulses in the brain are stimulated and transmitted back through the thoracolumbar and sacral nerves innervating the bladder. In a coordinated fashion, the detrusor muscle accommodates to the pressure (does not contract) while the sphincter and pelvic floor muscles contract to resist bladder pressure.

If you can void, cerebral inhibition is voluntarily suppressed. Impulses are transmitted via the spinal cord for the bladder neck, sphincter, and pelvic floor muscles to relax and for the bladder to contract. The sphincter closes, and the detrusor muscle relaxes when the bladder is empty.

Any disease or trauma that affects the function of the brain, spinal cord, or nerves that directly innervate the bladder, bladder neck, external sphincter, or pelvic floor can affect bladder function. These conditions include diabetes, multiple sclerosis, paraplegia, and quadriplegia. Drugs affecting nerve transmission can affect bladder function.

Gerontologic Considerations: Effects of Aging on the Urinary System

Age-related changes in the urinary system and differences in assessment findings are outlined in Table 49.2. Anatomic changes include a 10% decrease in kidney mass each decade starting at age 30. There is an increase in fat in the kidney. There is a similar decline in glomerular function starting at age 40.[1] Atherosclerosis accelerates the decrease in kidney size with age.

Other changes include decreased renal blood flow, resulting in a decreased GFR. Changes in hormone levels (ADH, aldosterone, ANP) result in decreased urinary concentrating ability and changes in water, sodium, potassium, and acid excretion. Despite these changes, older adults maintain homeostasis unless they have other problems. After abrupt changes in blood volume, acid load, or other insults, the kidney may not be able to function effectively because much of its renal reserve has been lost.

TABLE 49.2 GERONTOLOGIC ASSESSMENT DIFFERENCES

Urinary System

Gerontologic Changes	Differences in Assessment Findings
Kidney	
• ↓ Amount of kidney tissue	• Less palpable
• ↓ Number of nephrons and renal blood vessels. Thickened basement membrane of Bowman capsule and glomeruli	• ↓ Creatinine clearance, ↑ BUN and creatinine
• ↓ Function of loop of Henle and tubules	• Changes in drug excretion, nocturia, loss of normal diurnal urination because of ↓ ability to concentrate urine; less concentrated urine
Ureter, Bladder, and Urethra	
• ↓ Elasticity and muscle tone	• Palpable bladder after urination because of retention
• Weakening of urinary sphincter	• Stress incontinence (especially during Valsalva maneuver), dribbling of urine after urination
• ↓ Bladder capacity and sensory receptors	• Frequency, urgency, nocturia, overflow incontinence
• Estrogen deficiency leading to thin, dry vaginal tissue	• Stress or overactive bladder, dysuria, urinary tract infection (UTI)
• ↑ Prevalence of unstable bladder contractions	• Overactive bladder
• Prostate enlargement	• Hesitancy, frequency, urgency, nocturia, straining to urinate, retention, dribbling

The female urethra, bladder, vagina, and pelvic floor lose elasticity and muscle support. Consequently, older females are more prone to bladder infections and incontinence. As males age, the prostate enlarges, affecting the proximal urethra. This can affect urinary patterns, causing hesitancy, retention, slow stream, and bladder infections.

URINARY SYSTEM ASSESSMENT

Subjective Data

Important Health Information

Health history. Ask about the presence or history of kidney disease or other urologic problems. Note specific urinary problems, such as cancer, infections, benign prostatic hyperplasia (BPH), and stones. Are there other health problems that may affect kidney function? The two most common are hypertension and diabetes.[2]

Medications. Obtain a complete medication history. Drugs affect the urinary tract in several ways. Many drugs can be nephrotoxic (Table 49.3). Some drugs alter the quantity and character of urine output (e.g., diuretics). Others can change the color of urine. Phenazopyridine turns urine orange. Nitrofurantoin turns urine dark yellow to brown. Many antidepressants, calcium channel blockers, antihistamines, and drugs used for neurologic and musculoskeletal problems affect the ability of the bladder or sphincter to contract or relax normally.

Surgery or other treatments. Ask about hospitalizations related to urinary problems. Have they had surgery, especially pelvic surgery, and urinary tract instrumentation (e.g., catheterization)? Ask about any radiation or chemotherapy treatments. Note the duration, severity, and patient's perception of any problem and its treatment.

TABLE 49.3 Potentially Nephrotoxic Agents

Antimicrobials	Other Drugs	Other Agents
• aminoglycosides	• ACE inhibitors	• Gold
• amphotericin B	• captopril	• Heavy metals
• antivirals	• cimetidine	
• cephaloridine	• cisplatin	
• cephalothin	• cocaine	
• polymyxin B	• cyclosporine	
• sulfonamides	• heroin	
• vancomycin	• lithium	
	• methotrexate	
	• nitrosoureas (e.g., carmustine)	
	• NSAIDs (e.g., ibuprofen, indomethacin)	
	• quinine	
	• rifampin	
	• salicylates (large quantities)	
	• statins	

CASE STUDY

Patient Introduction

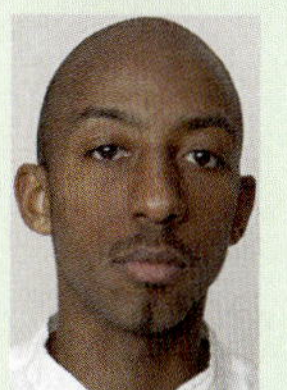
((© iStockphoto/ Thinkstock.))

A.K. is a 28-year-old male who comes to the emergency department (ED) in acute distress with severe abdominal pain. The pain began about 6 hours ago after he finished a 10-mile run as part of his training for a marathon. He says that the pain has steadily increased, and he is nauseous. His urine is a dark, smoky color.

Discussion Questions

1. What are the possible causes of A.K.'s symptoms?
2. What assessment questions will you ask him?

You will learn more about A.K. and his condition as you read this assessment chapter.

Answers available at http://evolve.elsevier.com/Lewis/medsurg.

Functional Health Patterns

Table 49.4 lists key questions to ask patients with problems related to the urinary system.

Health perception–health management. Ask patients about their general health. Abnormal kidney function may be suspected if patients report changes in weight or appetite, excess thirst, fluid retention, headache, pruritus, blurred vision, or "feeling tired all the time." An older adult may report malaise and general abdominal discomfort as the only symptoms of a urinary tract infection (UTI). Obtain a smoking history. Cigarette smoking is a major risk factor for bladder and kidney cancer.[3]

Exposure to certain chemicals can affect the urinary system. Aromatic amines and some organic chemicals increase the risk for bladder cancer. Phenol and ethylene glycol are examples of nephrotoxic chemicals. Obtain an occupational history. Machinists, painters, hairdressers, printers, and truck drivers have an increased risk for bladder cancer.[3] Smokers who work with cancer-causing chemicals have an even higher risk for bladder cancer.

Nutritional-metabolic. The usual quantity and types of fluid a patient drinks are important. Dehydration may contribute to UTIs, stone formation, and kidney failure. Large intake of specific foods, such as dairy products or foods high in proteins, may lead to stone formation. Asparagus may cause the urine to smell musty. Red urine caused by beet ingestion may be mistaken for bloody urine. Caffeine, alcohol, carbonated beverages, some artificial sweeteners, citrus, tomatoes/tomato-based products, or spicy foods often worsen urinary inflammatory diseases. Many teas and caffeine-containing drinks cause diuresis. An unexplained weight gain may be the result of fluid retention from a kidney problem.

Elimination. Questions about urine elimination are the cornerstone of the health history in patients with a lower urinary tract problem. Begin with asking how the patient manages urine elimination. Ask about daytime voiding frequency and the frequency of nocturia. Do they have lower urinary tract symptoms, including urgency, incontinence, or urinary retention? Tables 49.5 and 49.6 list some common manifestations of urinary tract problems.

Changes in the color and appearance of urine are often significant and need to be evaluated. If blood is visible in the

TABLE 49.4 HEALTH HISTORY

Urinary System

Health Perception–Health Management

- Describe your general health.
- How is your energy level compared with 1 year ago?
- Have you ever smoked? If yes, how many packs per day?
- Tell me about the types of jobs you have had.

Nutritional-Metabolic

- How is your appetite?
- Has your weight changed over the past year?[a]
- Do you take vitamins, herbs, or other supplements?[a]
- How much and what kinds of fluids do you drink daily?
- How many dairy products and how much meat do you eat?
- Do you drink coffee? Colas? Tea? Citrus juices?
- Do you spice your food heavily?[a]

Elimination

- Are you able to sit through a 2-h meeting or ride in a car for 2 h without urinating?
- Do you awaken at night to urinate? If so, how many times does this occur during an average night?
- Do you ever have blood in your urine?[a] If so, at what point in the urination does it occur?
- Have you noticed any change in the color or smell of your urine?[a]
- Do you ever pass urine when you do not intend to? When?
- Do you use special devices or supplies for urine elimination or control?[a]
- How often do you move your bowels?
- Do you ever have constipation or diarrhea?[a]
- Do you ever have problems controlling your bowels?[a]

Activity-Exercise

- Tell me about your usual daily activities. Have these changed?[a]
- Do certain activities worsen your urinary problem?[a]
- Has your urinary problem caused you to alter or stop any activity or exercise?[a]
- Do you need help getting to the bathroom?[a]

Sleep-Rest

- Do you awaken at night from an urge to urinate?[a] Does this disturb your sleep?
- Do you awaken at night from pain or other problems and urinate as a matter of routine before returning to sleep?[a]
- Do you have daytime sleepiness and fatigue because of nighttime urination?[a]

Cognitive-Perceptual

- Do you ever have pain when you urinate?[a] If so, where is the pain?

Self-Perception–Self-Concept

- How does your urinary problem or diversion make you feel about yourself?

Role-Relationship

- Does your urinary problem interfere with your relationships with family or friends?[a]
- Has your urinary problem caused a change in your job status or affected your ability to work?[a]

Sexuality-Reproductive

- Has your urinary problem caused any change in your sexual pleasure or performance?
- Do hygiene concerns interfere with sexual activities?

Coping–Stress Tolerance

- What strategies are you using to cope with your urinary problem?

[a]If yes, describe.

TABLE 49.5 Manifestations of Urinary System Problems

	SPECIFIC MANIFESTATIONS RELATED TO THE URINARY SYSTEM				
General	**Edema**	**Pain**	**Urination Patterns**	**Urine Output**	**Urine Composition**
• Anorexia • ↑ BP • Blurred vision • Change in weight • Chills • Cognitive changes • Fatigue • Headaches • Nausea and vomiting • Thirst	• Ankle • Ascites • Facial (periorbital) • General • Sacral	• Dysuria • Flank or costovertebral angle • Groin • Suprapubic	• Change in stream • Dribbling • Frequency • Hesitancy • Incontinence • Nocturia • Retention • Stress incontinence • Urgency	• Anuria • Oliguria • Polyuria	• Color (red, brown, yellowish green) • Concentrated • Dilute • Hematuria • Pyuria

urine, determine whether it occurs at the beginning of, throughout, or at the end of urination. If urinary incontinence is present, ask how the patient is managing the problem.

Assess bowel function. Problems with fecal incontinence may signal neurologic causes for bladder problems because of shared nerve pathways. Constipation and fecal impaction can partially obstruct the urethra, causing inadequate bladder emptying, overflow incontinence, and infection.

Discuss how the patient manages a urinary problem. A patient may already be using a catheter or collection device. Sometimes, they must assume a specific position to urinate or perform maneuvers, such as pressing on the lower abdomen (Credé's method) or straining (Valsalva maneuver), to empty the bladder.

Activity-exercise. Assess the activity level. A sedentary person is more likely to have stasis of urine and thus is predisposed to infection and stones. Bone demineralization in people with limited physical activity can cause increased urine calcium precipitation.

An active person may find that increasing activity worsens the urinary problem. Patients who had prostate surgery or have weakened pelvic floor muscles may leak urine when trying certain activities, such as running or lifting. Some males develop chronic inflammatory prostatitis or epididymitis after long-distance driving from not voiding.

Sleep-rest. Nocturia is a common and bothersome symptom. It often leads to sleep deprivation, daytime sleepiness, and fatigue. Nocturia occurs in multiple problems affecting the lower urinary tract. These include incontinence, urinary retention, and interstitial cystitis. It may be related to polyuria from diabetes, excess fluid intake, or heart failure.

Determine whether the need to urinate causes the person to arise from sleep or if pain or other symptoms interrupt sleep. Ask if they urinate as a matter of habit before returning to bed. Up to 1 episode of nocturia is normal in younger adults, and up to 2 episodes are acceptable in adults aged 65 years or older. If an older adult has more than 2 episodes during the night, assess the amount and timing of fluid intake. This information will help determine whether further assessment is needed.

Cognitive-perceptual. Pain is a frequent symptom of urinary problems. Patients may report dysuria, groin pain, costovertebral pain, or suprapubic pain. Assess pain and note the location, character, and duration. The absence of pain when other urinary symptoms exist is significant. Many urinary tract cancers are painless in the early stages.

Assess the level of mobility, visual acuity, and dexterity. These are important to evaluate, especially when urine retention or incontinence is a problem. Does the patient understand instructions? Can they recall instructions when needed? In older adults with a UTI, family members may report the patient is disoriented, has fallen, or has increased confusion.

Role-relationship. Urinary problems can affect many aspects of a person's life, including the ability to work and relationships with others. These factors have implications for managing the problem.

Urinary system problems may be serious enough to cause problems in job-related and social situations. Chronic dialysis therapy often makes regular employment or management of home and family responsibilities difficult. Concurrent poor health and negative body image can seriously affect existing roles.

Sexuality-reproductive. Assess the effect of urinary problems on sexual satisfaction. Problems related to personal hygiene and fatigue can negatively affect sexual relationships. Incontinence can have a devastating effect on self-esteem and social and intimate relationships. Counseling for the patient and partner may be needed.

TABLE 49.6 FOCUSED ASSESSMENT

Urinary System

Use this checklist to ensure that you complete key assessment steps.

Subjective

Ask about the following and note responses:

Painful urination
Changes in color of urine (blood, cloudy)
Change in characteristics of urination (decreased, excess)
Problems with frequent nighttime urination (nocturia)

Objective: Diagnostic

Check the following laboratory results for critical values:

Blood urea nitrogen
Creatinine
Urinalysis
Urine culture and sensitivity

Objective: Physical Assessment

Inspect

Abdomen
Urinary meatus for inflammation or discharge

Palpate

Abdomen for bladder distention, masses, or tenderness

Percuss

Costovertebral angle for tenderness

CASE STUDY

Subjective Data

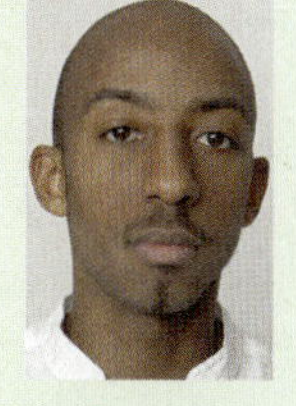

((© iStockphoto/ Thinkstock.))

A focused subjective assessment of A.K. revealed the following:

Medical History: History of 1 isolated incidence of gout 6 years ago. He stopped drinking alcohol with no further occurrence. Appendectomy 12 years ago.

Medications: None.

Health Perception–Health Management: A.K. states that he is usually healthy. He does not smoke or drink alcohol. He has never had this type of pain before. Describes the pain as being sharp and colicky (coming in waves). Rates the pain as 9 on a scale of 0 to 10.

Nutritional-Metabolic: Currently on a high-protein diet as he trains for the marathon. Eats a lot of chicken, beef, and seafood. He drinks milk-based protein shakes and water after exercising but admits that he does not think he drinks enough to replace fluid loss from perspiration. He drinks coffee for energy but avoids sodas.

Elimination: Denies any problems with urination, constipation, or diarrhea. This is the first time he has ever noticed a change of color in his urine.

Activity-Exercise: Prides himself on his ability to exercise and run without difficulty.

Sleep-Rest: Does not awaken at night to urinate.

Cognitive-Perceptual: Denies pain on urination.

Coping–Stress Tolerance: Worried that this pain may interfere with his marathon training.

Discussion Questions

1. Which subjective assessment findings concern you most?
2. What would be your priority assessment of A.K.?
3. What would you include in the physical assessment? What would you be looking for?

You will learn more about the physical assessment of the urinary system in the next section.

Answers available at http://evolve.elsevier.com/Lewis/medsurg.

Objective Data

Physical Assessment

Findings from a general physical assessment can reflect the systemic effects of a urinary tract problem. Direct physical assessment of the urinary system is limited. The assessment focuses on the costovertebral angle, abdomen, rectum, and genitals (see Chapter 55).[4] Table 49.6 describes the approach to assessing the urinary system. Table 49.7 describes specific assessment abnormalities of the urinary system. Assessment findings may vary in the older adult. Table 49.2 outlines age-related differences in assessment findings.

Inspection. Assess for changes in the following:

- *Skin:* Pallor, yellow-gray cast, excoriations, bruises, texture (e.g., rough, dry skin)
- *Mouth:* Stomatitis, ammonia breath odor
- *Abdomen:* Abdominal contour for midline mass in lower abdomen (may indicate bladder distention and urinary retention) or unilateral mass (sometimes seen in adults, indicating kidney enlargement from large tumor or polycystic kidney)
- *Weight:* Weight gain from edema. Weight loss and muscle wasting in kidney failure.
- *General health:* Edema, lethargy, decreased alertness

Palpation. The kidneys are posterior organs protected by the abdominal organs, ribs, and heavy back muscles. A landmark useful in locating the kidneys is the **costovertebral angle (CVA)** formed by the rib cage and the vertebral column. The normal-sized left kidney is rarely palpable because the spleen lies directly on top of it. Sometimes, the lower pole of the right kidney is palpable.

To palpate the right kidney, place your left (anterior) hand behind and support the patient's right side between the rib cage and the iliac crest (Fig. 49.6). Elevate the right flank with the left hand. Use your right hand to palpate deeply for the right

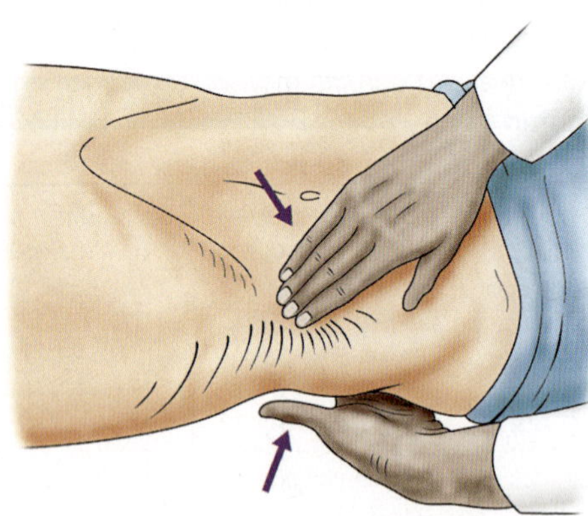

Fig. 49.6 Palpating the right kidney. (From Garden JO, Parks RW, Wigmore S: *Principles and practice of surgery*, ed 8, St Louis, 2023, Elsevier.)

TABLE 49.7 ASSESSMENT ABNORMALITIES

Urinary System

Finding	Description	Possible Cause and Significance
Anuria	Technically no urination (24-h urine output <100 mL)	Acute kidney injury, end-stage renal disease (ESRD), bilateral ureteral obstruction
Burning on urination	Stinging pain in urethral area	Urethral irritation, urinary tract infection (UTI), urethral stone, sexually transmitted infection (STI)
Dysuria	Painful or difficult urination	UTI, interstitial cystitis, urethral stones, STI, wide variety of problems
Enuresis	Involuntary nocturnal urination	Lower urinary tract disorder
Frequency	↑ Incidence of urination	Acutely inflamed bladder, retention with overflow, excess fluid intake, intake of bladder irritants, urethral stones, pelvic organ prolapse
Hematuria	Blood in the urine	Cancer of genitourinary tract, blood dyscrasias, kidney disease, UTI, stones in kidney or ureter, anticoagulants
Hesitancy	Delay or difficulty in initiating urination	Partial urethral obstruction, benign prostatic hyperplasia (BPH)
Incontinence	Inability to voluntarily control discharge of urine	Neurogenic bladder, bladder infection, injury to external sphincter
Nocturia	Frequent urination at night	Kidney disease with impaired concentrating ability, bladder obstruction, heart failure, diabetes, kidney transplant, excess evening and nighttime fluid intake, sleep apnea, alcohol use, liver disease
Oliguria	↓ Amount of urine in a time period (24-h urine output of 100–400 mL)	Severe dehydration, shock, transfusion reaction, kidney disease
Pain	Suprapubic pain (related to bladder), urethral pain (irritation of bladder neck), flank pain, costovertebral angle (CVA) tenderness	Infection, urinary retention, foreign body in urinary tract, urethritis, pyelonephritis, renal colic, stones
Pneumaturia	Passage of urine containing gas	Fistula connections between bowel and bladder, gas-forming UTI
Polyuria	Large volume of urine in a given period	Diabetes, arginine vasopressin (AVP) disorder, chronic kidney disease, diuretics, excess fluid intake, obstructive sleep apnea
Retention	Inability to urinate even though bladder contains excess amount of urine	Pelvic surgery, childbirth, anesthesia; urethral stricture or obstruction; prostate enlargement; neurogenic bladder, constipation, medication side effect
Stress incontinence	Involuntary urination with ↑ pressure (sneezing or coughing)	Poor sphincter control, lack of estrogen, urinary retention

kidney. The lower pole of the right kidney may be felt as a smooth, rounded mass that descends on inspiration. If the kidney is palpable, note its size, contour, and tenderness. Kidney enlargement suggests cancer or other serious problem.

The bladder is normally not palpable unless it is distended with urine. If the bladder is full, it may be felt as a smooth, round, firm organ and is sensitive to palpation.

Percussion. Flank tenderness may be detected by fist percussion *(kidney punch)*. Perform fist percussion by striking the fist of one hand against the dorsal surface of the other hand, which is placed flat along the posterior CVA margin (Fig. 49.7). Normally, this action should not elicit pain. If CVA tenderness and pain are present, it may indicate a kidney infection or polycystic kidney disease.[5]

A bladder does not percuss until it contains at least 150 mL of urine. If the bladder is full, dullness is heard above the symphysis pubis. A distended bladder may be percussed as high as the umbilicus.

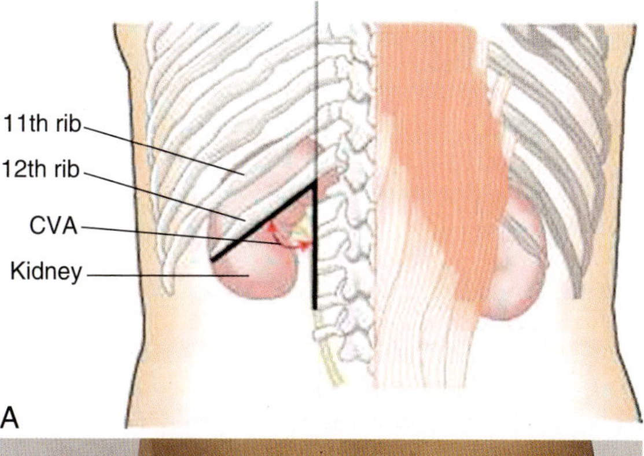

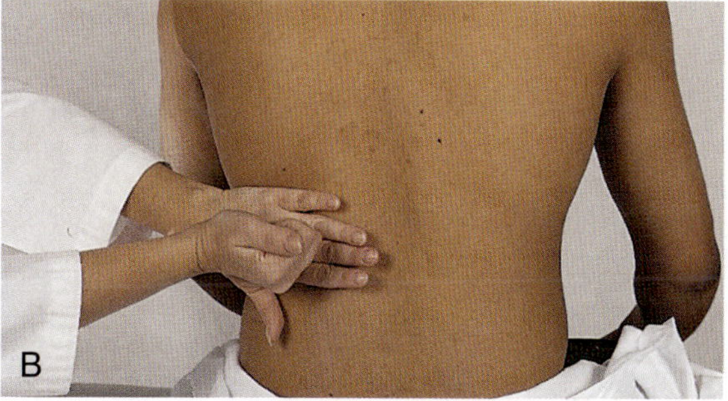

Fig. 49.7 (A) Costovertebral angle. (B) Indirect fist percussion of the costovertebral angle *(CVA)*. To assess the kidney, place one hand over the 12th rib at the CVA on the back. Thump that hand with the ulnar edge of the other fist. (From Jarvis C: *Physical examination and health assessment,* ed 8, St Louis, 2020, Elsevier.)

CASE STUDY

Objective Data: Physical Assessment

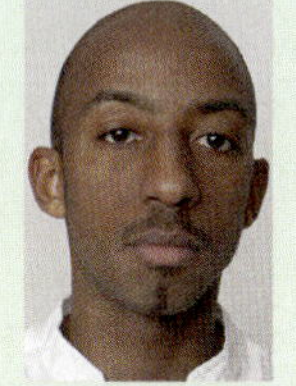

((© iStockphoto/ Thinkstock.))

A focused assessment of A.K. reveals the following: A.K. is lying with his knees bent and drawn to his abdominal area. He appears restless and keeps moving from back to side to reduce his discomfort. Vital signs: BP 156/70, HR 108, respiratory rate 24, temp 37.4°C, SpO_2 96% on room air. Awake, alert, and oriented × 3. Lungs are clear to auscultation. Abdomen nondistended with positive bowel sounds in all 4 quadrants. No rebound tenderness. Positive left costovertebral tenderness. Voiding small amounts of dark, smoky urine.

Discussion Questions

1. Which physical assessment findings concern you most?
2. Based on the results of the subjective and physical assessment findings, what diagnostic studies do you think may be ordered for A.K.?

You will learn more about diagnostic studies related to the urinary system in the next section.

Answers available at http://evolve.elsevier.com/Lewis/medsurg.

DIAGNOSTIC STUDIES OF THE URINARY SYSTEM

Many diagnostic studies are used to assess urinary system problems. Tables 49.8, 49.9, 49.10, and 49.11 describe the most common studies. Select studies are described in more detail here.

Urine Studies

Urinalysis is one of the first studies done to evaluate disorders of the urinary tract (Table 49.8). Results from the urinalysis may show abnormalities, suggest the need for further studies, or show progression in a previously diagnosed problem.

It is best to obtain the first specimen urinated in the morning. This concentrated specimen is more likely to contain abnormal constituents if they are present in the urine. The specimen should be examined within 1 hour of urinating. Otherwise, bacteria multiply rapidly, RBCs hemolyze, *casts* (molds of renal tubules) disintegrate, and the urine becomes alkaline because of urea-splitting bacteria. If it is not possible to send the specimen to the laboratory immediately, refrigerate it. However, for the best results, coordinate specimen collection with routine laboratory hours.

Other studies that we use to test urine are described in Table 49.9. A urine culture is not a routine part of a urinalysis. It is done to definitively diagnose UTI and identify the causative organism.

Creatinine and Creatinine Clearance

Common tests that analyze urinary system problems are creatinine and creatinine clearance. Creatinine is a waste product made by muscle breakdown. Healthy kidneys filter creatinine out of the blood. If the kidneys are not working properly, creatinine levels can rise.

Because almost all creatinine is excreted by the kidneys, creatinine clearance is the most accurate indicator of kidney function. The result of a creatinine clearance test closely approximates the GFR. Normal creatinine clearance values range from 87 to 139 mL/min (Table 49.10). After age 40, the creatinine clearance rate decreases at a rate of about 1 mL/min/year. We should obtain a blood specimen to measure serum creatinine while collecting urine.

TABLE 49.8 Urinalysis

General examination of urine to establish baseline information or provide data to establish a tentative diagnosis and determine whether further studies are needed.

Before: Wash perineal area before collecting specimen.

During: Try to obtain first urinated morning specimen.

After: Ensure specimen is examined within 1 h of urinating.

Test	Normal	Abnormal Finding	Possible Cause and Significance
Bilirubin	None	Present	Liver problems. May appear before jaundice is visible (see Chapter 48)
Casts	None Occasional hyaline	Present	Molds of the renal tubules that may contain protein, WBCs, RBCs, or bacteria. Noncellular casts (hyaline in appearance) sometimes found in normal urine
Color	Amber yellow	Dark, smoky color	Hematuria
		Yellow-brown to olive green	Excess bilirubin
		Orange-red or orange-brown	phenazopyridine (Pyridium), rifampin
		Cloudiness of freshly voided urine	Urinary tract infection (UTI)
		Colorless urine	Excess fluid intake, kidney disease, AVP disorder
Culture for organisms	No organisms in bladder $<10^4$ organisms/mL result of normal urethral flora	Bacteria counts $>10^5$/mL	UTI; most common organisms are *Escherichia coli*, enterococci, *Klebsiella*, *Proteus*, streptococci
Glucose	None	Glycosuria	Diabetes, low kidney threshold for glucose reabsorption (if glucose level is normal). Pituitary problems
Ketones	None	Present	Altered carbohydrate and fat metabolism in diabetes and starvation; dehydration, vomiting, severe diarrhea
Odor	Aromatic	Ammonia-like odor	Urine allowed to stand
		Unpleasant odor	UTI
Osmolality	50–1200 mOsm/kg (50–1200 mmol/kg)	<50 mOsm/kg >1200 mOsm/kg	Tubular dysfunction. Kidney lost ability to concentrate or dilute urine
pH	4.6–8.0 (average, 6.0)	>8.0	UTI. Urine allowed to stand at room temperature (bacteria decompose urea to ammonia)
Protein	Random protein (dipstick): 0–trace	Persistent proteinuria	Characteristic of acute and chronic kidney disease, especially involving glomeruli. Heart failure
	24-h protein (quantitative): 50–80 mg/day		In absence of disease: high-protein diet, strenuous exercise, dehydration, fever, stress, contamination by vaginal secretions
RBCs	0–4/hpf	<4.0	Respiratory or metabolic acidosis
		>4/hpf	Stones, cystitis, cancer, glomerulonephritis, tuberculosis, kidney biopsy, UTI, trauma
Specific gravity	1.005–1.030	Low	Dilute urine, excess diuresis, AVP disorder
	Maximum concentrating ability of kidney in morning urine (1.025–1.030)	High	Dehydration, albuminuria, glycosuria
		Fixed at about 1.010	Kidney inability to concentrate urine; end-stage renal disease
WBCs	0–5/hpf	5/hpf	UTI, inflammation.

AVP, Arginine vasopressin; *hpf*, high-powered field; *RBC*, red blood cell; *WBC*, white blood cell.

TABLE 49.9 Diagnostic Studies

Urine

Study	Description and Purpose	Nursing Responsibility
Composite urine collection	Measures specific components, such as electrolytes, glucose, protein, 17-ketosteroids, catecholamines, creatinine, and minerals. Composite urine specimens collected over a period ranging from 2 to 24 h.	*During:* Have patient urinate and discard this 1st urine specimen. This time is the start of the test. Save all urine from subsequent urinations in a container for a designated period. At end of period, have patient urinate and add this urine to container. Remind patient to save all urine during study period. Specimens may need refrigeration or preservatives added to container used for collecting urine.
Concentration test	Evaluates kidney concentration ability. Measured by specific gravity readings. *Reference interval:* 1.005–1.030.	*Before:* Have patient fast after given time in evening. *During:* Collect 3 urine specimens at hourly intervals in morning.

TABLE 49.9 Diagnostic Studies—cont'd

Urine

Study	Description and Purpose	Nursing Responsibility
Creatinine clearance	Waste product of protein breakdown. Creatinine clearance by kidney approximates glomerular filtration rate (GFR). Measure urine creatinine during 24-h period. Reference interval: *Male:* 107–139 mL/min/1.73 m^2 *Female:* 87–107 mL/min/1.73 m^2 (corrected for body surface area)	*During:* Collect 24-h urine specimen. Discard 1st urination when test is started. Save urine from all subsequent urinations for 24 h. Have patient urinate at end of 24 h and add specimen to collection. Draw blood creatinine level.
Protein determination		
• Dipstick (Albustix, Combistix)	Detects protein (mainly albumin) in urine. *Reference interval:* 0 to trace.	*During:* Dip end of stick in urine and read result by comparing to color chart on label. Grade from 0 to 4+. Interpret with caution. Positive result may not indicate significant proteinuria. Some drugs may give false-positive readings.
• Quantitative protein test	24-h collection gives an accurate indication of amount of protein in urine. Persistent proteinuria usually indicates glomerular kidney disease. *Reference interval:* 50–80 mg/day (mainly albumin).	*During:* Perform 24-h urine collection as noted earlier.
Residual urine	Determines amount of urine left in bladder after urinating. Finding may be abnormal in problems with bladder innervation, sphincter impairment, prostate enlargement, urethral strictures. *Reference interval:* ≤50 mL urine (↑ with age).	*During:* Immediately after patient urinates, catheterize patient or use bladder ultrasound equipment. If a large amount of residual urine is obtained, HCP may leave catheter in bladder.
Urine culture ("clean catch," "midstream")	Confirms urinary tract infection and identifies causative organisms. *Reference interval:* If properly collected, stored, and handled: $<10^3$ organisms/mL usually indicates no infection. 10^3–10^5/mL is usually not diagnostic. Test may need to be repeated. $>10^5$/mL indicates infection.	*During:* Use sterile container to collect urine. Touch only outside of container. *For females:* Wipe the periurethral area from front to back, dry the area thoroughly with sterile swab, separate labia with one hand. *For males:* Retract foreskin (if present), cleanse glans around urethra, replace foreskin after cleaning. After cleaning, have patient start voiding, and collect the specimen 1–2 sec after voiding starts. The initial voided urine flushes out most contaminants in the urethra and perineal area. Catheterization may be needed if patient is unable to perform procedure.
Urine cytologic study	Identifies abnormal cell structures that occur with bladder cancer. Used to follow the progress of bladder cancer after treatment.	*During:* Obtain specimens by voiding, catheterization, or bladder irrigation. Do not use morning's 1st voided specimen because epithelial cells may change in appearance in urine held in bladder overnight. *After:* Specimen should be fresh or brought to laboratory within the hour. Alcohol-based fixative is added to preserve cell structure.

TABLE 49.10 Blood Studies

Urinary System

Test	Reference Interval	Significance
Bicarbonate	22–26 mEq/L (22–26 mmol/L)	Most patients in kidney failure have metabolic acidosis and low HCO_3^- levels.
Blood urea nitrogen (BUN)	10–20 mg/dL (3.6–7.1 mmol/L)	Used to detect kidney problems. BUN regulated by rate at which kidney excretes urea. Nonkidney factors may ↑ BUN (e.g., cell destruction from infections, fever, GI bleeding, trauma, athletic activity, excess muscle breakdown).
BUN/creatinine ratio	12:1–20:1	↑ Ratio may be caused by conditions that ↓ blood flow to kidneys (e.g., heart failure, dehydration, GI bleeding) or by increased protein intake. ↓ Ratio may occur with liver disease (from ↓ urea formation) and malnutrition.
Creatinine	*Male:* 0.6–1.2 mg/dL (53–106 μmol/L) *Female:* 0.5–1.1 mg/dL (49.97 μmol/L)	More reliable than BUN as a determinant of kidney function. Creatinine is a product of muscle and protein metabolism. It is released at a constant rate.
Phosphorus	3.0–4.5 mg/dL (0.97–1.45 mmol/L)	In kidney disease, phosphorus levels are high because the kidney is the main excretory organ.
Potassium	3.5–5.0 mEq/L (3.5–5.0 mmol/L)	Kidneys excrete most of body's potassium. In kidney disease, K^+ is one of the first electrolytes to become abnormal. High K^+ levels >6 mEq/L can lead to muscle weakness and dysrhythmias.
Uric acid	*Male:* 4.0–8.5 mg/dL (0.24–0.51 mmol/L) *Female:* 2.7–7.3 mg/dL (0.16–0.43 mmol/L)	Screening test for disorders of purine metabolism. Can indicate kidney disease. Values depend on kidney function, purine metabolism, and dietary intake of purine-rich foods.

TABLE 49.11 Diagnostic Studies

Urinary System

Study	Description and Purpose	Nursing Responsibility
Endoscopy		
Cystoscopy	Inspects interior of bladder with a tubular lighted scope (cystoscope) (Fig. 49.8). Can be used to insert ureteral catheters, remove stones, obtain biopsy specimens of bladder lesions, treat bleeding lesions. Done under local or general anesthesia, depending on patient need and condition. Complications: Urinary retention, urinary tract hemorrhage, bladder infection, bladder perforation.	*Before:* Give IV fluids if general anesthesia is to be used. Ensure consent form is signed. Explain procedure to patient. Give preoperative medication. *After:* Explain that burning on urination, pink-tinged urine, and urinary frequency are expected. Observe for bright red bleeding, which is not normal. Help with ambulation because orthostatic hypotension may occur. Offer warm sitz baths, heat, mild analgesics to relieve discomfort.
Radiologic Procedures		
CT scan (CT urogram)	Visualizes kidneys, ureters, and bladder. Can detect tumors, abscesses, suprarenal masses (e.g., adrenal tumors), obstructions. Done with or without contrast media.	*Before:* Before contrast medium used, evaluate kidney function. May need to be NPO 4 h before study. *During:* Warn patient that contrast injection may cause a feeling of being warm and flushed. Patient must lie completely still during scan. *After:* Encourage patient to drink fluids to avoid kidney problems with any contrast.
Cystogram	Visualizes bladder and evaluates vesicoureteral reflux. Evaluates neurogenic bladder and recurrent urinary tract infections. Can delineate bladder problems (e.g., diverticula, stones, tumors). Contrast media instilled into bladder via cystoscope or catheter.	*Before:* Explain procedure. *During:* If done via cystoscope, follow nursing care related to cystoscopy.
Intravenous pyelogram (IVP)	Visualizes urinary tract after IV injection of contrast media. Evaluates size and shape of kidneys, ureters, and bladder. Cysts, tumors, and ureteral obstructions distort normal appearance of these structures. Patient with decreased kidney function should not have IVP because contrast media can be nephrotoxic.	*Before:* Cathartic or enema given night before. Assess for iodine sensitivity to avoid anaphylactic reaction. *During:* Warn patient that contrast injection may cause a feeling of being warm and flushed. *After:* Force fluids to avoid kidney problems with contrast.
Kidneys, ureters, bladder (KUB)	X-ray examination of abdomen and pelvis. Delineates size, shape, and position of kidneys, ureter, and bladder. Can see radiopaque stones and foreign bodies.	*Before:* No special preparation needed.
Loopogram	Detects obstructions, anastomotic leaks, stones, and reflux when patient has a urinary pouch or ileal conduit. Because urinary diversions are created with bowel, there is risk for absorption of contrast media.	*Before:* Explain procedure. *During:* Monitor for reactions to the contrast media.
Magnetic resonance angiography	Visualizes renal vasculature. Gadolinium-enhanced studies allow visualization of renal artery.	Same as renal arteriogram. Does not require femoral artery puncture.
MRI	Visualizes kidneys. Not useful for detecting stones or calcified tumors.	*Before:* Oral and/or IV contrast injection may be used. Check for pregnancy, allergies, and kidney function. Have patient remove all metal objects and metallic foil patches. Contraindicated for persons with implanted metallic devices or other metal fragments unless MRI-safe. Ask about staples, plates, dental bridges, or other metal appliances. May need to be fasting. Assess for claustrophobia and need for antianxiety medication. *During:* Must lie completely still during scan.
Nephrostogram (antegrade pyelogram)	Evaluates upper urinary tract when patient has allergy to contrast media, decreased kidney function, or abnormalities that prevent passage of a ureteral catheter. Contrast media may be injected percutaneously into renal pelvis or via a nephrostomy tube that is already in place when determining tube function or ureteral integrity after trauma or surgery.	*Before:* Explain procedure and prepare as for IVP. *During and after:* Watch for complications (e.g., hematuria, infection, hematoma).

TABLE 49.11 Diagnostic Studies—cont'd

Urinary System

Study	Description and Purpose	Nursing Responsibility
Renal arteriogram (angiogram)	Visualizes renal blood vessels. Can aid in diagnosing renal artery stenosis (Fig. 49.9), extra or missing renal blood vessels, and renovascular hypertension. Can aid in distinguishing between a cyst and tumor. Included in workup of potential kidney transplant donor. A catheter is inserted into the femoral artery and passed up the aorta to the level of renal arteries (Fig. 49.10). Contrast media injected to outline renal blood supply.	*Before:* Cathartic or enema may be used the night before. Before injection of contrast material, assess for iodine sensitivity. Tell patients they may feel a transient warm feeling along the course of blood vessel when contrast media is injected. *After:* Place a pressure dressing over femoral artery injection site. Observe site for bleeding and inflammation. Maintain bed rest with affected leg straight. Take peripheral pulses in the involved leg every 30–60 min to detect occlusion of blood flow (from thrombus or emboli).
Renal biopsy	Obtains kidney tissue for examination to determine type of kidney disease or to follow progress of kidney disease. Usually done as a skin (percutaneous) biopsy through needle insertion into lower lobe of kidney under CT or ultrasound guidance. Absolute contraindications: Bleeding disorders, single kidney, uncontrolled hypertension. Relative contraindications: Suspected kidney infection, hydronephrosis, possible vascular lesions.	*Before:* Obtain type and crossmatch. Ensure consent form is signed. Assess coagulation status through history, medication history, CBC, hematocrit, PT/INR. Patient should not be taking aspirin or warfarin. *After:* Apply pressure dressing and keep patient on affected side for 30–60 min. Bed rest for 24 h. Vital signs every 5–10 min, 1st hour. Assess for flank pain, hypotension, decreasing hematocrit, fever, chills, urinary frequency, dysuria, and gross or microscopic hematuria. Inspect biopsy site for bleeding. Teach patient to avoid lifting heavy objects for 5–7 days and to not take anticoagulant drugs until allowed by HCP.
Renal scan	Evaluates anatomic structures, perfusion, and function of kidneys. IV radioactive isotopes are injected. Radiation detector probes are placed over kidney, and scintillation counter monitors radioactive material in kidney. Radioisotope distribution in kidney is scanned and mapped. Shows location, size, and shape of kidney and assesses blood flow, glomerular filtration, tubular function, and urinary excretion. Abscesses, cysts, and tumors may appear as cold spots because of nonfunctioning tissue. Monitors function of transplanted kidney.	*Before:* No diet or activity restriction. Tell patients there should not be any discomfort during test.
Renal ultrasound	Detects kidney masses (tumors, cysts) and obstructions. Small external ultrasound probe is placed on skin. Conductive gel applied to skin. Noninvasive procedure involves passing sound waves into body structures and recording images as they are reflected. Computer interprets tissue density based on sound waves and displays it in picture form.	*Before:* Explain procedure. *During:* Because radiation exposure is avoided, can obtain repeated images over a brief period.
Retrograde pyelogram	X-ray of urinary tract taken after injection of contrast material into kidneys. May be done if an IVP does not visualize the urinary tract or with decreased kidney function. A cystoscope is inserted, and ureteral catheters are inserted through it into the renal pelvis. Contrast media injected through catheters.	*Before:* Prepare patient as for IVP. Tell patients there may be pain from distention of pelvis and discomfort from cystoscope. Anesthesia may be given for procedure. *After:* Complications similar to after cystoscopy.
Urethrogram	Similar to a cystogram. Contrast media injected retrograde into urethra to identify strictures, diverticula, or other urethral pathologic conditions. When urethral trauma is suspected, a urethrogram is done before catheterization.	*Before:* Explain procedure.
Voiding cystourethrogram (VCUG)	Voiding study of bladder opening (bladder neck) and urethra. Bladder filled with contrast media. Fluoroscopic films are taken to visualize bladder and urethra. After urination, another film is taken to assess for residual urine. Detect abnormalities of lower urinary tract, urethral stenosis, bladder neck obstruction, vesicoureteral reflux, and prostate enlargement.	*Before:* Explain procedure.
Urodynamic Studies		
Cystometrogram	Evaluates bladder capacity to contract and expel urine. Involves inserting a catheter and instilling water or saline solution into bladder. Measures pressure exerted against bladder wall. If measuring abdominal pressure, a 2nd tube is inserted into rectum or vagina. This tube is attached to a small fluid-filled balloon to allow pressure recording.	*Before:* Explain procedure. *During:* Ask patient about sensations of bladder filling, usually including the 1st desire (urge) to urinate, a strong desire to urinate, and perception of bladder fullness. *After:* Observe for UTI.

Continued

TABLE 49.11 Diagnostic Studies—cont'd

Urinary System

Study	Description and Purpose	Nursing Responsibility
Radionuclide cystography (RNC)	Detects and grades vesicoureteral reflux. Like VCUG with a small dose of radioisotope tracer instilled into the bladder via urethral catheter. More sensitive than VCUG. Radiation dose is 1/1000 that of the VCUG.	*Before:* Explain procedure to patient as in VCUG.
Sphincter electromyography (EMG)	Recording of electrical activity created when nervous system stimulates muscle tissue. By placing needles, percutaneous wires, or patches near the urethra, pelvic floor muscle activity can be assessed. During test, sphincter EMG is used to identify voluntary pelvic floor muscle contractions and response of these muscles to bladder filling, coughing, and other provocative actions.	*Before:* Explain procedure.
Urine flow study (uroflow)	Measures urine volume in a single voiding expelled in a period. Used to (1) assess the degree of outflow obstruction caused by such conditions as BPH, (2) assess bladder or sphincter dysfunction effects on voiding, and (3) evaluate effects of treatment for lower urinary tract problems. Graphic displays can illustrate straining and intermittent flow patterns or other abnormal voiding disorders. *Normal maximum flow rate:* Males: 20–25 mL/sec; females: 25–30 mL/sec. Volume voided and age can affect the flow rate.	*Before:* Explain procedure. *During:* Have the patient start the test with a comfortably full bladder, urinate into a designated container, and try to empty completely. *After:* Measure residual urine volume immediately after a urinary flow study because this will help identify the degree of chronic urinary retention that often occurs with abnormal flow patterns.
Videourodynamics	Combination of cystometrogram, sphincter EMG, and/or urinary flow study with anatomic imaging of the lower urinary tract, typically via fluoroscopy. Identifies an obstructive lesion and characterizes anatomic changes in bladder and lower urinary tract.	*Before:* Explain procedure.
Voiding pressure flow study	Combines a urinary flow rate, cystometric pressures (intravesical, abdominal, and detrusor pressures), and sphincter EMG for detailed evaluation of micturition. Patient urinates while various pressure tubes and EMG apparatus remain in place.	*Before:* Explain procedure to patient. *During:* Assist the patient to the specialized toileting area.
Whitaker study	Measures pressure differential between renal pelvis and bladder, determines ureteral obstruction. Percutaneous access to renal pelvis obtained by placing a catheter in renal pelvis. A catheter is placed in bladder. Fluid is perfused through the percutaneous tube or needle at a rate of 10 mL/min. Pressure data are then collected. Pressure measurements are combined with fluoroscopic imaging to find the level of obstruction.	*Before:* Explain procedure.

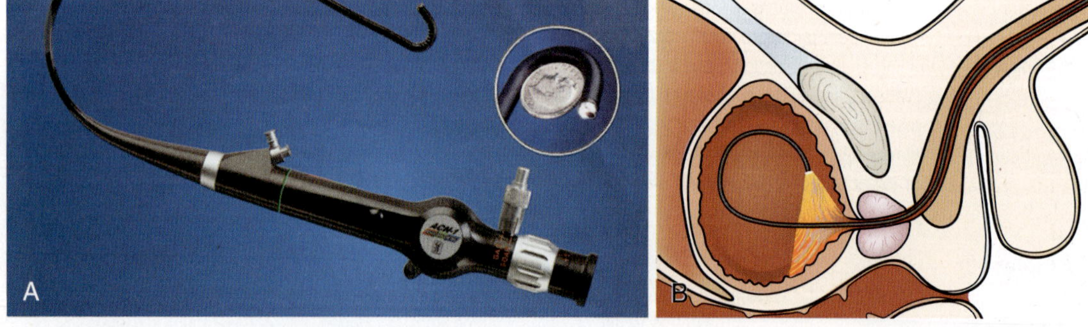

Fig. 49.8 Cystoscopic examination of the bladder in a male. (A) Flexible cystonephroscope. (B) Scope inserted into bladder. (A, Courtesy Circon Corporation, Santa Barbara, CA.)

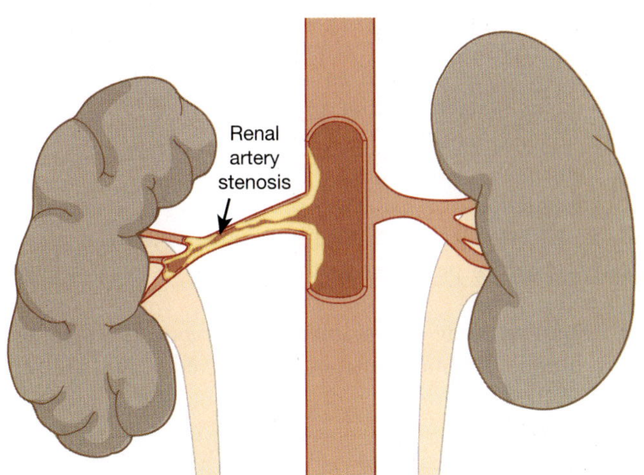

Fig. 49.9 Left renal artery stenosis *(arrow)*.

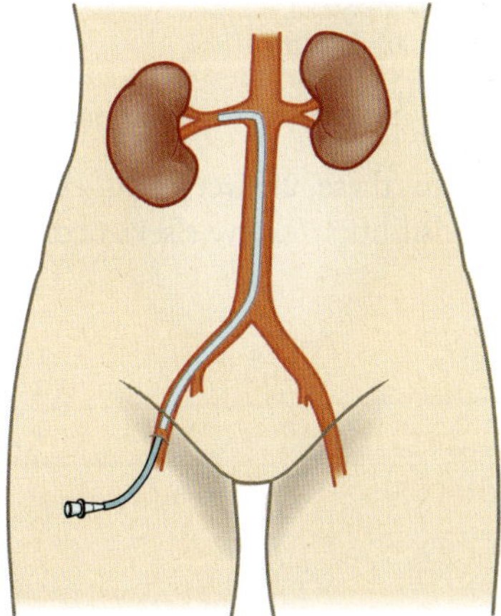

Fig. 49.10 Catheter insertion for a renal arteriogram.

Urodynamic Studies

Urodynamic studies measure urinary tract function. Urodynamic tests study the storage of urine within the bladder and the flow of urine through the urinary tract to the outside of the body. A combination of techniques may be used for a detailed assessment of urinary function (Table 49.11).

Radiologic Studies

Many radiologic studies require a bowel preparation the evening before the study to clear the lower GI tract of feces and flatus. Because the kidneys lie in a retroperitoneal location, colon contents can obstruct visualization of the urinary tract. If the bowel preparation does not adequately clear the lower GI tract, the study may be unsuccessful and need to be rescheduled. Common bowel preparations include enemas, magnesium citrate, and bisacodyl (Dulcolax) tablets or suppositories. Patients with kidney failure should not receive bowel preparations with magnesium or saline laxative enemas because the kidneys cannot excrete the magnesium.

Iodine-based contrast media used in some diagnostic studies may cause contrast-induced kidney injury (CIN) and allergic reactions. Keeping patients hydrated is important. Some patients may need IV fluids started hours before the procedure. N-acetylcysteine—a renal vasodilator and antioxidant—is sometimes given to reduce the incidence of CIN. It can be given by the oral or IV route.

When patients have multiple diagnostic studies, it is important to maintain hydration. Patients are at risk for dehydration when they have had nothing by mouth for consecutive days, extended time in the radiology department, and bowel preparations. Severe dehydration, especially in debilitated or older patients and patients with diabetes, may lead to acute kidney injury. Ensure that patients are hydrated and given adequate nourishment between studies. Check with the HCP about insulin dosage for patients with diabetes who are NPO.

CASE STUDY

Objective Data: Diagnostic Studies

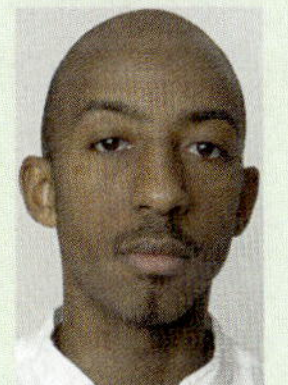

((© iStockphoto/ Thinkstock.))

The HCP orders the following initial diagnostic studies:

- Complete blood count (CBC), basic metabolic panel (electrolytes, blood urea nitrogen [BUN], creatinine)
- Urinalysis and culture if indicated
- Renal ultrasound

A.K.'s CBC and metabolic panel results are within normal limits. His urinalysis shows moderate hematuria. A renal ultrasound shows several stones in the left ureter. There is no hydronephrosis at present. The HCP prescribes IV opioids for pain management and admits A.K. to a medical unit.

Discussion Questions

1. Which diagnostic study results are abnormal?
2. Which diagnostic study result most concerns you?

Answers available at http://evolve.elsevier.com/Lewis/medsurg.

BRIDGE TO NCLEX EXAMINATION

The number of the question corresponds to the same-numbered outcome at the beginning of the chapter.

1. A stone in the pelvis of the kidney will change kidney function by interfering with the
   a. structural support of the kidney.
   b. regulation of the concentration of urine.
   c. entry and exit of blood vessels at the kidney.
   d. collection and drainage of urine from the kidney.
2. A patient with kidney disease has oliguria and a creatinine clearance of 40 mL/min. These findings most directly reflect abnormal function of
   a. tubular secretion.
   b. glomerular filtration.
   c. capillary permeability.
   d. concentration of filtrate.
3. Diminished ability to concentrate urine, associated with aging of the urinary system, is caused by
   a. a decrease in bladder sensory receptors.
   b. a decrease in the number of functioning nephrons.
   c. decreased function of the loop of Henle and tubules.
   d. thickening of the basement membrane of Bowman capsule.
4. The nurse identifies a risk for urinary stones in a patient who relates a health history that includes
   a. dehydration.
   b. hyperaldosteronism.
   c. serotonin deficiency.
   d. adrenal insufficiency.
5. Normal findings expected on assessment of the urinary system include (**Select all that apply.**)
   a. nonpalpable bladder.
   b. nonpalpable left kidney.
   c. auscultation of renal artery bruit.
   d. no CVA tenderness elicited by a kidney punch.
   e. full bladder percusses as dullness above the symphysis pubis.
6. A diagnostic study that evaluates renal blood flow, glomerular filtration, tubular function, and excretion is a(n)
   a. IVP.
   b. VCUG.
   c. renal scan.
   d. loopogram.
7. On reading the urinalysis results of a dehydrated patient, the nurse would expect to find
   a. a pH of 8.4.
   b. RBCs of 4/HPF.
   c. color: yellow, cloudy.
   d. specific gravity of 1.035.

1. d; 2. b; 3. c; 4. a; 5. a, b, d, e; 6. c; 7. d.

For rationales to these answers and even more NCLEX review questions, visit http://evolve.elsevier.com/Lewis/medsurg.

REFERENCES

To access the References for this chapter, please scan the QR code with a mobile device.

50

Renal and Urologic Problems

Hazel A. Dennison

http://evolve.elsevier.com/Lewis/medsurg/

CONCEPTUAL FOCUS

Elimination
Fluids and Electrolytes
Infection
Pain

LEARNING OUTCOMES

1. Discuss the pathophysiology, clinical manifestations, and interprofessional and nursing management of infections in the urinary tract.
2. Distinguish the etiology, clinical manifestations, and interprofessional and nursing management of acute and chronic glomerulonephritis and nephrotic syndrome.
3. Compare and contrast the etiology, clinical manifestations, and interprofessional and nursing management of urinary calculi.
4. Distinguish the common causes and management of renal trauma, renal vascular problems, and hereditary kidney diseases.
5. Describe the clinical manifestations and interprofessional and nursing management of kidney and bladder cancers.
6. Describe the common causes and management of urinary incontinence and urinary retention.
7. Distinguish among types of urinary catheters regarding indications for use and nursing responsibilities.
8. Explain the nursing management of patients undergoing nephrectomy and urinary diversion surgery.

KEY TERMS

cystitis
glomerulonephritis
ileal conduit
interstitial cystitis (IC)
lithotripsy
nephrolithiasis
nephrosclerosis
nephrotic syndrome
polycystic kidney disease (PKD)
pyelonephritis
renal artery stenosis
stricture
urethritis
urinary incontinence (UI)
urinary retention
urinary tract infection (UTI)
urosepsis

A wide range of renal and urologic problems contribute to impaired elimination. This chapter discusses problems of the upper urinary tract (kidneys and ureter) and lower urinary tract (bladder and urethra). Many patients are at risk for fluid, electrolyte, and acid-base imbalances because of the kidneys' vital role in homeostasis. The person may have discomfort, incontinence, disrupted sleep, and impaired skin integrity.

INFECTIOUS AND INFLAMMATORY URINARY PROBLEMS

URINARY TRACT INFECTION

Urinary tract infections (UTIs) are infections of the urinary tract. They are the most common outpatient infection. UTIs can be broadly described as an upper or lower UTI according to the location within the urinary system (Fig. 50.1). We use specific terms to describe the location of a UTI. For example, **urethritis** is an inflammation of the urethra. **Cystitis** is an inflammation of the bladder. **Pyelonephritis** implies inflammation (usually caused by infection) of the renal parenchyma and collecting system. **Urosepsis** is a UTI that has spread systemically. It is a life-threatening condition requiring emergency treatment.

We can classify a UTI as complicated or uncomplicated. *Uncomplicated UTIs* occur in an otherwise normal urinary tract. They usually only involve the bladder. *Complicated UTIs* occur in a person with an underlying disease or with a structural or functional problem in the urinary tract. Examples include obstruction, stones, catheters, acute kidney injury (AKI), chronic kidney disease (CKD), kidney transplant, diabetes, or neurologic disease. They can also occur when a person has developed antibiotic resistance, is immunocompromised, or has pregnancy-induced changes. The person with a complicated infection is at risk for pyelonephritis, urosepsis, and renal damage.

Etiology and Pathophysiology

The urinary tract above the urethra is normally sterile. Several mechanical and physiologic defense mechanisms aid in maintaining sterility and preventing UTIs. These defenses include normal voiding with complete bladder emptying, ureterovesical junction (UVJ) competence, and ureteral peristaltic activity that propels urine toward the bladder. The antibacterial properties of urine are maintained by a slightly acidic pH (6.0 to 7.5) and abundant antimicrobial proteins and peptides that interfere with bacterial growth. A change in any of these defense mechanisms increases the risk for a UTI (Table 50.1).

The organisms that usually cause UTIs originate in the perineum. They are introduced via the ascending route from the urethra. Most infections are caused by gram-negative bacilli normally found in the gastrointestinal (GI) tract (Table 50.2). *Escherichia coli* is the most common pathogen causing a UTI. It causes 75% of cases without urinary tract structural abnormalities or stones and 65% of complicated UTIs.[1] Fungal and

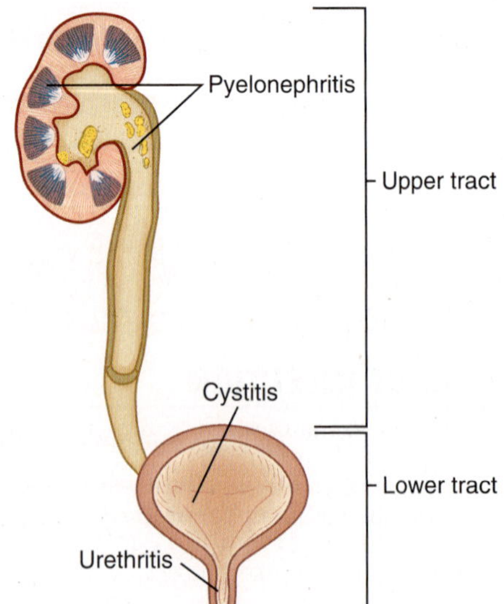

Fig. 50.1 Sites of infections in the upper and lower urinary tracts.

TABLE 50.1 Risk Factors for UTIs

Anatomic Factors
- Congenital defects leading to obstruction or urinary stasis
- Fistula exposing urinary stream to skin, vagina, or fecal stream
- Obesity
- Shorter female urethra and colonization from normal vaginal flora

Compromised Immunity
- Aging
- Cancer
- Diabetes
- HIV infection
- Immunosuppression

Factors Increasing Urinary Stasis
- Extrinsic obstruction (tumor, fibrosis compressing urinary tract)
- Intrinsic obstruction (stone, tumor of urinary tract, urethral stricture, benign prostatic hyperplasia)
- Renal impairment
- Urinary retention (e.g., neurogenic bladder)

Foreign Bodies
- Catheters (indwelling, external condom catheter, ureteral stent, nephrostomy tube, intermittent catheterization)
- Urinary tract instrumentation (cystoscopy)
- Urinary tract stones

Functional Disorders
- Constipation
- Voiding dysfunction with detrusor sphincter muscle incoordination

Other Factors
- Debilitation
- Habitual delay of urination ("nurse's bladder," "teacher's bladder")
- Menopause
- Poor personal hygiene
- Pregnancy
- Sexual activity (female)
- Use of spermicidal agents, contraceptive diaphragm (female), bubble baths, feminine sprays

TABLE 50.2 Common Infectious Causes of UTIs

- *Candida* species
- *Enterobacter*
- *Enterococcus*
- *Escherichia coli*
- *Klebsiella pneumoniae*
- *Proteus mirabilis*
- *Pseudomonas aeruginosa*
- *Serratia*
- *Staphylococcus aureus*
- Streptococci, group B

parasitic infections sometimes cause UTIs. These are more common in patients who are immunosuppressed, have diabetes or kidney problems, or received multiple courses of antibiotic therapy. Residents of long-term care facilities, especially females, may have chronic asymptomatic bacteriuria.

A common factor contributing to ascending infection is urologic instrumentation (e.g., catheterization, cystoscopic examinations). Instrumentation allows bacteria that are normally present at the opening of the urethra to enter the urethra or bladder. Sexual intercourse can cause minor urethral trauma that allows bacteria from the vagina and perineum to enter the urethra, predisposing females to UTIs.

UTIs can result from blood-borne bacteria invading the kidneys, ureters, or bladder from elsewhere in the body. For a kidney infection to occur this way, there must be prior injury to the urinary tract, such as obstruction of the ureter, damage caused by stones, or renal scars.

UTIs are the most common health care–associated infection (HAI). They are mainly the result of having an indwelling catheter. *Catheter-associated urinary tract infections (CAUTIs)* are often caused by *E. coli* and, less often, *Pseudomonas* organisms. CAUTIs lead to extended hospital stays, increased health care costs, and increased mortality.[2]

Clinical Manifestations

Manifestations of UTIs range from painful urination in uncomplicated urethritis or cystitis to severe systemic illness with abdominal or back pain, fever, and sepsis.

Lower urinary tract symptoms (LUTS) include dysuria, frequency (voiding more than every 2 hours), urgency, and suprapubic discomfort or pressure (Table 50.3). The urine may have grossly visible blood (hematuria) or sediment, giving it a cloudy appearance. LUTS are related to bladder storage or bladder emptying. Upper UTIs (involving the renal parenchyma, pelvis, and ureters) typically cause fever, chills, and flank pain. A UTI confined to the lower urinary tract does not usually have systemic manifestations. People with significant bacteriuria may have no symptoms or may have nonspecific symptoms, such as fatigue or anorexia.

The common manifestations of a UTI are often absent in older adults. Older adults tend to have general abdominal discomfort rather than dysuria and suprapubic pain. They may have impaired cognition or overall clinical deterioration. Older adults are less likely to have a fever with a UTI.[3]

Multiple problems may produce LUTS similar to the symptoms of a UTI. For example, patients with bladder tumors or those receiving intravesical chemotherapy or pelvic radiation usually have urinary frequency, urgency, and dysuria. Interstitial cystitis/painful bladder syndrome produces urinary symptoms that are similar to and sometimes confused with a UTI.

A small number of healthy people have some bacteria colonizing the bladder. We call this *asymptomatic bacteriuria.* It does not justify screening or treatment except in pregnant females, those with a recent kidney transplant, or those having a urologic procedure.

TABLE 50.3 Lower Urinary Tract Symptoms (LUTS)

Symptoms	Description
Emptying Symptoms	
Dysuria	• Painful or difficult urination
Hesitancy	• Difficulty starting urine stream • Delay between initiation of urination (because of urethral sphincter relaxation) and beginning of flow of urine • Diminished urinary stream
Intermittency	• Interruption of urinary stream while voiding
Postvoid dribbling	• Urine loss after completing voiding
Urinary retention or incomplete emptying	• Inability to empty urine from bladder • Caused by atonic bladder or obstruction of urethra • Can be acute or chronic
Storage Symptoms	
Incontinence	• Involuntary or accidental urine loss or leakage
Nocturia	• Awakened by urge to void 2 or more times during sleep • May be diurnal or nocturnal depending on sleep schedule
Nocturnal enuresis	• Adult loss of urine during sleep
Urgency	• Sudden, strong, or intense desire to void immediately • Often accompanied by frequency
Urinary frequency	• More than 8 times in 24-h period • Often <200 mL each voiding

Diagnostic Studies

In patients suspected of having a UTI, first obtain a dipstick urinalysis. This test can identify the presence of nitrites (indicating bacteriuria), white blood cells (WBCs), and leukocyte esterase (an enzyme present in WBCs indicating pyuria). Microscopic urinalysis can confirm these findings. Counts as low as 10^2 to 10^3 CFU/mL in a person with signs and symptoms are indicative of UTI. Bacterial counts of 10^5 CFU/mL or higher typically indicate a clinically significant UTI.

After confirmation of bacteriuria and pyuria, we may do a urine culture. A urine culture is needed in persistent bacteriuria, complicated or recurring UTIs (more than 2 or 3 per year), CAUTI, or HAI UTIs. We may culture urine when the infection is not responsive to empiric therapy or the diagnosis is questionable.

A voided midstream technique *(clean-catch urine sample)* is best for obtaining a urine culture in most circumstances (see Table 49.8). When we cannot obtain an adequate clean-catch specimen, we may do catheterization. A specimen from catheterization gives more accurate results than a clean-catch specimen. *Sensitivity testing* determines the bacteria's susceptibility to a variety of antibiotic drugs. The results allow the HCP to prescribe the antibiotic capable of killing the bacteria causing the UTI.

Some patients need imaging studies such as an ultrasound or CT scan of the urinary tract if we suspect an obstruction or UTIs recur.

Interprofessional Care

The interprofessional care and drug therapy of UTIs are outlined in Table 50.4. Once a UTI has been diagnosed, antimicrobial therapy is started. An antibiotic may be chosen based on the HCP's best judgment *(empiric therapy)* or the results of sensitivity testing.

Uncomplicated UTIs are treated with a short-term course of antibiotics, typically for 3 days. Complicated UTIs need a longer period of treatment, lasting 7 to 14 days or more.[4] Asymptomatic bacteriuria is often not treated.

First-choice drugs to treat uncomplicated or initial UTIs are trimethoprim/sulfamethoxazole (TMP/SMX), nitrofurantoin, and fosfomycin.[4] TMP/SMX has the advantage of being inexpensive and taken twice daily. Nitrofurantoin is taken 4 times daily, but a twice-daily formulation is available.

DRUG ALERT

Nitrofurantoin

- Avoid use if the creatinine clearance <30 mL/min.
- Notify the HCP at once if fever, chills, cough, chest pain, dyspnea, rash, or numbness or tingling of fingers or toes develops.

Other antibiotics used in the treatment of uncomplicated UTI include ampicillin, amoxicillin, and cephalosporins. Fluoroquinolones (e.g., levofloxacin, ciprofloxacin) are given to treat complicated UTIs. *E. coli* resistance to TMP/SMX, β-lactams, and ciprofloxacin is an increasing problem in the United States. In patients with UTIs from fungi, fluconazole is the preferred therapy.

A urinary analgesic, such as oral phenazopyridine, may relieve discomfort caused by severe dysuria. Phenazopyridine is an azo dye excreted in urine. It exerts a topical analgesic effect on the urinary tract mucosa. It is taken up to 2 concurrent days. Teach patients that this drug causes the urine to turn orange or red.

Patients who have repeated UTIs may receive prophylactic or suppressive antibiotics. A low dose of TMP/SMX, nitrofurantoin, or another antibiotic taken daily may prevent recurring UTIs. A single dose may be taken after an event likely to provoke a UTI, such as sexual intercourse. Although suppressive therapy is often effective in the short term, use is limited because of the risk for antibiotic resistance, which leads to breakthrough infections with increasingly virulent pathogens.

TABLE 50.4 Interprofessional Care

UTI

Diagnostic Assessment

- History and physical assessment
- Urinalysis (midstream, "clean-catch" voided specimen)
- Urine for culture and sensitivity (if indicated)
- Imaging studies of urinary tract (if indicated): CT scan, ultrasound, cystoscopy

Management

Uncomplicated UTI

- Patient teaching
- Adequate fluid intake (8–9 8-oz glasses/day)

Drug Therapy

- Antibiotics
  - cephalosporins
  - fluconazole (in patients with fungal UTI)
  - fosfomycin (Monurol)
  - nitrofurantoin (Macrodantin, Macrobid)
  - TMP/SMX (Bactrim, Bactrim DS)
  - trimethoprim alone (in patients with sulfa allergy)
- Phenazopyridine

Recurrent or Chronic UTI

- Repeat urinalysis with culture and sensitivity testing
- Adequate fluid intake (8–9 8-oz glasses/day)
- Repeat patient teaching
- Imaging studies of urinary tract

Drug Therapy

- Antibiotic: nitrofurantoin, TMP/SMX
- Sensitivity-guided antibiotic therapy: ampicillin, amoxicillin, 1st- or 2nd-generation phalosporin, fluoroquinolones
- 3- to 6-month trial of suppressive or prophylactic antibiotic therapy
- Postcoital antibiotic prophylaxis: cephalexin, nitrofurantoin, TMP/SMX, fosfomycin, trimethoprim

❖ NURSING MANAGEMENT: URINARY TRACT INFECTION

◆ Assessment

Subjective and objective data that you should obtain from patients with a UTI are shown in Table 50.5.

◆ Clinical Problems

Clinical problems for patients with a UTI may include:

- Impaired urinary elimination
- Infection
- Pain

More information on clinical problems and interventions for patients with a UTI is presented in eNursing Care Plan 50.1 (available on the website for this chapter).

◆ Planning

The overall goals are that patients with a UTI will have (1) symptom relief, (2) no upper urinary tract involvement, and (3) no recurrence.

◆ Implementation

Health Promotion

It is important to recognize people who are at risk for a UTI (Table 50.1). Health promotion measures can help decrease the frequency of UTIs and support early detection of infection. These activities include teaching preventive measures, including (1) emptying the bladder regularly and completely, (2) evacuating the bowel regularly, (3) wiping the perineal area from front to back after voiding and defecation, and (4) drinking an adequate amount of liquid each day.

Routine and thorough perineal hygiene is important for all hospitalized patients, especially after using a bedpan, after a bowel movement, or if fecal incontinence is present. Answer call lights quickly. Offer the bedpan or urinal to bedridden patients at frequent intervals. These measures can prevent incontinence and decrease the number of incontinence episodes.

Prevention of CAUTI. All patients undergoing catheterization of the urinary tract are at risk for developing CAUTI.[5] You play a key role in preventing CAUTI by following evidence-based practices. Avoiding unnecessary catheterization and early removal of indwelling catheters are the most effective means for reducing CAUTI. Always follow aseptic technique during these procedures. Wash your hands before and after contact with each patient. Wear gloves for care of urinary catheters.

TABLE 50.5 NURSING ASSESSMENT

UTI

Subjective Data

Important Health Information

Health history: Previous UTI. Urinary stones, reflux, strictures, or retention. See Table 50.1

Medications: Antibiotics, anticholinergics, antispasmodics

Functional Health Patterns

Cognitive-perceptual: Suprapubic or low back pain, bladder spasms, dysuria, burning on urination

Elimination: Urinary frequency, urgency, hesitancy, dysuria, nocturia

Health perception–health management: Urinary hygiene practices. Lassitude, malaise

Nutritional-metabolic: Nausea, vomiting, anorexia. Chills and fever

Sexuality-reproductive: Sexual activity, use of spermicidal agents or contraceptive diaphragm (females)

Objective Data

General

Fever, chills, dysuria

Atypical presentation in older adults: afebrile, absence of dysuria, loss of appetite, altered mental status

Urinary

Hematuria. Cloudy, foul-smelling urine

Possible Diagnostic Findings

Leukocytosis. Urinalysis positive for bacteria, pyuria, RBCs, WBCs, and nitrites. Positive urine culture. Ultrasound, CT scan, MRI, voiding cystourethrogram (VCUG), cystoscopy showing urinary tract abnormalities

Acute Care

Acute care for patients with a UTI includes ensuring adequate daily fluid intake unless contraindicated. Maintaining adequate fluid intake may be hard because of patient concerns that fluid will increase the pain and urinary frequency. Tell patients that fluids will increase frequency of urination. This will dilute the urine and make the bladder less irritable. Fluids will help flush out bacteria before they have a chance to colonize in the bladder. Teach them to avoid caffeine, alcohol, citrus juices, chocolate, and highly spiced foods or beverages because they are bladder irritants.

Applying heat to the suprapubic area or lower back may relieve discomfort. Have patients apply a heating pad (turned to its lowest setting) against the back or suprapubic area. A warm shower or sitting in a tub of warm water filled above the waist can give temporary relief.

Teach patients and caregivers about the need for ongoing care (Table 50.6). This includes voiding regularly (every 3 to 4 hours) and voiding before and after intercourse. Have patients temporarily stop using a diaphragm. Review the prescribed drug therapy. Stress the importance of taking the full course of antibiotics. Often patients stop antibiotic therapy once symptoms disappear. This can lead to inadequate treatment, recurrent infection, or bacterial resistance to antibiotics.

Sometimes a second drug or a reduced dosage of drug is given after the first course to suppress bacterial growth in patients susceptible to recurrent UTI. Teach patients to monitor for signs of improvement (e.g., cloudy urine becomes clear) with a decrease in or cessation of symptoms. Tell them to report to the HCP any (1) persistence of LUTS beyond the antibiotic treatment course, (2) onset of flank pain, or (3) fever.

If treatment is complete and the symptoms are still present, the patient requires follow-up care. Recurrent symptoms typically occur within 1 to 2 weeks after completing therapy. If the patient has followed the treatment plan, a relapse indicates the need for further evaluation.

TABLE 50.6 PATIENT & CAREGIVER TEACHING

UTI

When teaching a patient and caregiver measures to prevent a recurrence of a UTI, include:

1. Take all antibiotics as prescribed. Symptoms may improve after 1–2 days of therapy, but organisms may still be present.
2. Practice good hygiene, including:
   - Carefully clean the perineal region by separating the labia in females, or in males pulling back the foreskin if present when cleansing.
   - Wipe from front to back after urinating.
   - Cleanse with warm, soapy water after each bowel movement.
3. Empty the bladder before and after sexual intercourse.
4. Void regularly, about every 3–4 hours during the day.
5. Maintain adequate fluid intake.
6. Avoid vaginal douches and harsh soaps, bubble baths, powders, and sprays in the perineal area.
7. Report to the HCP symptoms or signs of recurrent UTI (e.g., fever, cloudy urine, pain on urination, urgency, frequency).

Evaluation

The expected outcomes are that patients with a UTI will:

- Have normal urinary elimination patterns
- Report relief of symptoms
- State knowledge of the treatment plan

ACUTE PYELONEPHRITIS

Etiology and Pathophysiology

Pyelonephritis is an inflammation of the renal parenchyma and collecting system, including the renal pelvis (Fig. 50.2). The most common cause is bacterial infection. Fungi, protozoa, or viruses can also infect the kidney.[6]

Urosepsis is a systemic infection arising from a urologic source. Its prompt diagnosis and effective treatment are critical because it can lead to septic shock and death unless promptly treated. Septic shock is discussed in Chapter 42.

Pyelonephritis usually begins with colonization and infection of the lower urinary tract via the ascending urethral route. Bacteria normally found in the GI tract, including *E. coli* or *Proteus, Klebsiella,* or *Enterobacter* species, often cause pyelonephritis. A preexisting factor can be present, like *vesicoureteral reflux* (retrograde [backward] movement of urine from lower to upper urinary tract) or dysfunction of the lower urinary tract (e.g., obstruction from benign prostatic hyperplasia [BPH], stricture, stones).

Acute pyelonephritis often starts in the renal medulla and spreads to the adjacent cortex. Pregnancy-induced physiologic changes in the urinary system are an important risk factor for acute pyelonephritis. Recurring episodes of pyelonephritis, especially in patients with an obstructive problem, can lead to chronic pyelonephritis.

Clinical Manifestations and Diagnostic Studies

The classic manifestations include (1) fever/chills, (2) nausea/vomiting, (3) malaise, and (4) flank pain. There may be LUTS, such as dysuria, urgency, and frequency. *Costovertebral angle tenderness* to percussion (costovertebral angle [CVA] pain) is typically present on the affected side. Some patients develop renal scarring and decreased kidney function. Potentially life-threatening urosepsis can occur.

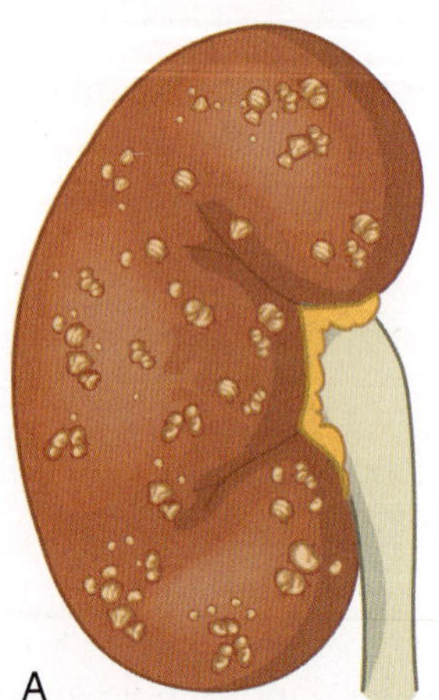

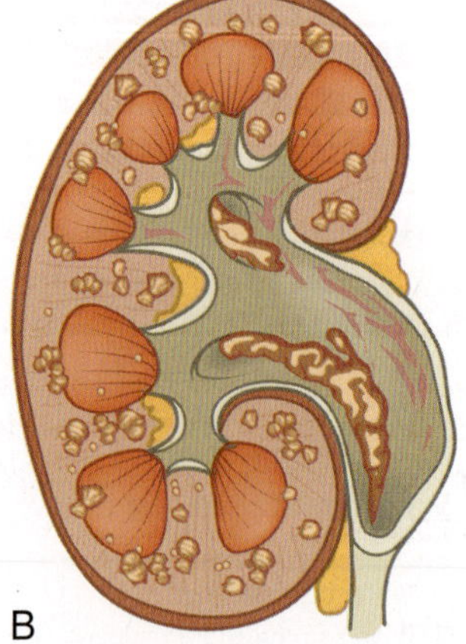

Fig. 50.2 Acute pyelonephritis with (A) multiple small abscesses on the surface and (B) in cortex.

Urinalysis results may show pyuria, bacteriuria, and varying degrees of hematuria. WBC casts in the urine may indicate renal parenchyma involvement. Urine cultures with sensitivities are done when pyelonephritis is suspected. Blood cultures may be done on hospitalized patients with more severe illness.

Ultrasound can identify anatomic abnormalities, hydronephrosis, renal abscesses, or an obstructing stone. CT scans are the preferred imaging studies. They can assess for signs of infection in the kidney and complications of pyelonephritis, such as impaired renal function, scarring, chronic pyelonephritis, or abscesses.

Interprofessional Care

The diagnostic tests and interprofessional care of acute pyelonephritis are outlined in Table 50.7. Patients with severe infections or complicating factors, such as nausea and vomiting with dehydration, need to be hospitalized.

Patients with mild symptoms may be treated as an outpatient with antibiotics for 5 to 14 days (Table 50.7). IV antibiotics are often given initially in the hospital to rapidly establish high serum and urinary drug levels.[6] Symptoms and signs typically improve or resolve within 48 to 72 hours after starting therapy. Patients are discharged when initial treatment resolves acute symptoms and they tolerate oral fluids and drugs. Oral antibiotics continue for 14 more days. Relapses may be treated with a different course of antibiotics. Antibiotic prophylaxis also may be used for recurrent infections.

Urosepsis is characterized by bacteriuria and bacteremia (bacteria in blood). Close observation and vital sign monitoring are essential. Prompt recognition and treatment of septic shock may prevent irreversible damage or death.

NURSING MANAGEMENT: ACUTE PYELONEPHRITIS

Assessment

Subjective and objective data that you should obtain from patients with pyelonephritis are similar to those for patients with a UTI (Table 50.5).

Implementation

Interventions vary depending on the severity of symptoms. Teach patients about the disease. Stress (1) taking antibiotic therapy as prescribed, (2) having a follow-up urine culture, and (3) recognizing signs of recurrence or relapse (Table 50.6). Encourage patients to drink at least 8 glasses of fluid every day, even after the infection has been treated. Rest will increase patient comfort. Patients who have frequent relapses or reinfections may receive long-term, low-dose antibiotics. Making

TABLE 50.7 Interprofessional Care
Acute Pyelonephritis

Diagnostic Assessment
- History and physical assessment
- Urinalysis with culture and sensitivity
- Imaging studies: ultrasound (initially), CT scan, MRI, cystoscopy, voiding cystourethrogram (VCUG)
- CBC count with WBC differential
- Blood culture (if bacteremia is suspected)
- Percussion for flank (CVA) pain

Management
Mild Symptoms
- Outpatient management or short hospitalization
- Adequate fluid intake
- NSAIDs or antipyretic drugs
- Follow-up urine culture and imaging studies

Drug Therapy
- Empirically selected broad-spectrum antibiotics: fluoroquinolones (ciprofloxacin, levofloxacin), cephalosporins preferred. TMP/SMX or an oral β-lactam can be used if infection expected to be susceptible
- Short course of IV antibiotics, such as an extended-spectrum cephalosporin or penicillin, fluoroquinolone (e.g., ciprofloxacin, levofloxacin), or an aminoglycoside without or with amoxicillin
- Switch to sensitivity-guided therapy when urine and blood culture results available

Severe Symptoms
- Hospitalization
- Adequate fluid intake (IV initially; switch to oral fluids as nausea, vomiting, and dehydration subside)
- NSAIDs or antipyretic drugs to reverse fever and relieve discomfort
- Follow-up urine culture and imaging studies

Drug Therapy
- IV antibiotics
  - Empirically selected broad-spectrum antibiotics: carbapenem (e.g., imipenem, meropenem), vancomycin, daptomycin, linezolid
  - Switch to sensitivity-guided antibiotic therapy when results of urine and blood culture are available
- Oral antibiotics when patient tolerates oral intake

certain patients understand the reason for therapy is important to increase adherence.

CHRONIC PYELONEPHRITIS

In *chronic pyelonephritis,* the kidneys are continually infected. This leads to inflammation and fibrosis (scarring). There may be a loss of renal function and renal atrophy (shrinkage). Chronic pyelonephritis is usually the result of significant anatomic abnormalities, such as vesicoureteral reflux or recurring infections involving the upper urinary tract. It can occur because of a substantial inflammatory response from an infection.

Radiologic imaging studies can confirm the diagnosis of chronic pyelonephritis and possible contributing factors. A renal biopsy can show the loss of functioning nephrons, infiltration of the parenchyma with inflammatory cells, and fibrosis.

Kidney function in chronic pyelonephritis depends on whether 1 or both kidneys are affected, the extent of scarring, and the presence of coexisting infection. Chronic pyelonephritis can progress to end-stage renal disease (ESRD). Monitoring and treating infections and correcting any underlying contributing factors are important. Care of patients with CKD is discussed in Chapter 51.

URETHRITIS

Urethritis is inflammation of the urethra. Causes include a bacterial or viral infection (e.g., herpes simplex virus), *Trichomonas,* monilial infection (especially in females), chlamydial infection, *Mycoplasma,* and gonorrhea.

In males, the causes of urethritis are usually sexually transmitted. Purulent discharge can indicate gonococcal urethritis. A clear or mucoid discharge typically signifies a nongonococcal urethritis. Sexually transmitted infections (STIs) are discussed in Chapter 57. Urethritis can cause LUTS, including dysuria, urgency, and frequency, similar to those seen with cystitis. Males may have penile burning.

In females, urethritis can be hard to diagnose. It should be considered when WBCs are present on urinalysis but there are no bacteria. It often produces LUTS, but urethral discharge may not be present.

Treatment of urethritis is based on identifying and treating the cause and providing symptom relief. Drugs used for bacterial infections include TMP/SMX, doxycycline (Vibramycin), ceftriaxone, and nitrofurantoin. Metronidazole (Flagyl) and tinidazole (Tindamax) are options for treating *Trichomonas* infection. Drugs used to treat monilial infections include nystatin, clotrimazole, or fluconazole. In chlamydial infections, doxycycline or azithromycin are options. Females with negative urine cultures and no pyuria usually do not respond to antibiotics.

Warm sitz baths may temporarily relieve bothersome symptoms. Teach patients to (1) avoid using vaginal deodorant sprays and contraceptive gels, (2) cleanse the perineal area after bowel movements and voiding, and (3) avoid sexual intercourse for at least 7 days. Tell patients with sexually transmitted urethritis to refer their sex partners for evaluation and testing if they had sexual contact in the 60 days before the onset of the symptoms or diagnosis.

URETHRAL DIVERTICULA

Urethral diverticula are local outpouchings of the urethra. Females have a much higher incidence than males. The rare cases in males usually are associated with congenital lower urinary tract anomalies or surgical trauma.

Risk factors include obstructed periurethral glands or infection. The periurethral glands are found along the distal two-thirds of the urethra. Other risk factors include urethral trauma, vaginal delivery, urethral instrumentation, and urethral dilation.

Classic symptoms include dysuria, postvoid dribbling, and dyspareunia (painful intercourse). Other symptoms include frequency (voiding more often than every 2 hours), urgency, suprapubic discomfort or pressure, pelvis or urethral pain, and a feeling of incomplete bladder emptying. Urinary incontinence (UI) is often present. Females can be asymptomatic.

The urine may have gross blood (hematuria) or sediment, which gives it a red or cloudy appearance. The diverticula can protrude into the anterior vaginal wall, causing an anterior wall mass. The mass may be felt on assessment. When palpated, the mass is often quite tender and can express urine and/or purulent discharge through the urethra.

Radiographic studies, such as ultrasound and MRI, are helpful in determining the size of the diverticulum in relation to the urethral lumen. A urethroscopy may be of benefit. It is done as an adjunct to radiologic studies.

Surgical options include transvaginal diverticulectomy, marsupialization (creation of a permanent opening) of the diverticular sac into the vagina *(Spence procedure)*, and urethroscopic surgical excision. Stress UI, infection, bleeding, and urethral-vaginal fistula are potential complications of the surgery.

INTERSTITIAL CYSTITIS/PAINFUL BLADDER SYNDROME

Interstitial cystitis (IC) is a chronic, painful disease of the bladder characterized by urgency, frequency, and pain in the bladder and/or pelvis. IC is also called *bladder pain syndrome* or *painful bladder syndrome* (PBS). The term *IC/PBS* refers to cases of urinary pain that we cannot attribute to other causes, such as UTI or urinary stones. IC/PBS is more common in females. It affects about 3 to 8 million females and 1 to 4 million males each year.[7]

The cause of IC/PBS is unknown. It is likely multifactorial. Possible causes include neurogenic hypersensitivity of the lower urinary tract, changes in mast cells in the muscle and/or mucosal layers of the bladder, bladder attacked by the immune system, or production of a toxic substance in the urine.

Clinical Manifestations and Diagnostic Studies

The 2 primary manifestations are pain and LUTS (e.g., frequency, urgency). People with severe cases may void as often as 60 times daily, including nighttime urination. The pain is usually in the suprapubic area, but may involve the vagina, labia, or entire perineal region, including the rectum and anus. The pain varies from mild to severe. The pain may get worse with bladder filling, postponed urination, physical exertion, pressure against the suprapubic area, certain foods, exercise, or prolonged sitting. Voiding temporarily relieves pain. LUTS are similar to a UTI. The condition may be misdiagnosed as a recurring or chronic UTI or, in males, chronic prostatitis.

There may be periods of remission and exacerbation. Females often report pain that occurs before menstruation. Sexual intercourse or emotional stress can worsen pain. Some patients have symptoms that disappear altogether after a period of weeks to months. Others have persistent symptoms over months to years.

IC/PBS is a diagnosis of exclusion. A history and physical assessment can rule out other problems that have similar symptoms, such as cancer, infection, or pelvic abnormalities. Cystoscopy may reveal a small bladder capacity, Hunner lesions (distinct inflammatory areas on the bladder wall), and glomerulations (superficial ulcerations with pinpoint bleeding). These findings are not always present.

Interprofessional Care

No single treatment consistently reverses or relieves symptoms. Various therapies have been effective, including nutrition and drug therapy. The tricyclic antidepressants amitriptyline (preferred) and nortriptyline may reduce burning and urinary frequency. Pentosan polysulfate sodium (Elmiron) is the only oral agent approved for treating IC symptoms. It enhances the protective effects of the glycosaminoglycan layer of the bladder and relieves pain by reducing the irritative effects of urine on the bladder wall. This drug provides relief over time (weeks to months). It does not give immediate relief for acute symptoms. Because of reports of macular eye changes, this medication has an FDA-approved warning label regarding eye toxicity.

Pelvic physical therapy and bladder hydrodistention therapy may be useful. Dimethyl sulfoxide (DMSO) can be directly instilled into the bladder through a small catheter. DMSO decreases inflammation and desensitizes pain receptors in the bladder wall. Heparin, lidocaine, or sodium bicarbonate can also be instilled into the bladder to relieve acute symptoms. Intradetrusor botulinum toxin and cyclosporine A may be of some help.

A UTI may occur during IC/PBS management because of diagnostic instrumentation and frequent bladder instillations. A UTI is likely to cause an acute exacerbation of LUTS, dysuria (not typically present with IC/PBS), odorous urine, and hematuria.

Surgery is an option to improve severe, debilitating pain. Sacral neuromodulation or fulguration (using high-frequency energy to destroy a lesion) and resection of Hunner lesions are options. Urinary diversion, such as an ileal conduit, without or with removal of the bladder, is an option when other measures fail. Unfortunately, some patients have pain within the urinary diversion, which means that some factor in the urine may contribute to IC/PBS in some cases.

❖ NURSING MANAGEMENT: IC/PBS

Assess the characteristics of the pain. Ask about specific diet or lifestyle factors that relieve pain or make it worse. Teach patients to keep a bladder log or voiding diary over a period of at least 3 days to determine voiding frequency and patterns of nocturia. Keeping a pain record at the same time may be useful.

Eliminating foods and beverages that are likely to irritate the bladder may give some symptom relief. Common bladder irritants include coffee and tea (caffeinated and decaffeinated); alcohol; citrus products; carbonated drinks; chocolate; foods containing vinegar, curries, or hot peppers; and foods or beverages likely to lower urinary pH, including fruits such as cranberries. Calcium glycerophosphate (Prelief) or 1 tablespoon of baking soda mixed with water alkalinizes the urine. It may provide relief from the irritating effects of some foods. Discuss proper nutrition, especially considering the broad diet restrictions. Tell patients to take a multivitamin containing no more than the recommended daily allowance for essential vitamins. They should avoid high-potency vitamins because they may irritate the bladder.

Because stress can worsen symptoms or cause flare-ups, stress management techniques such as relaxation breathing and imagery (see Chapter 7) may be helpful. Using lubrication or changing positions may decrease pain from sexual intercourse. Patients should avoid clothing that creates suprapubic pressure, such as pants with tight belts or waistlines.

Information about coping with the need for frequent urination and the emotional burden of IC/PBS is available from the Interstitial Cystitis Association (www.ichelp.org). They also have recipes and menus for a well-balanced diet that avoids bladder-irritating foods and beverages. Reassurance that IC/PBS is a real condition experienced by others and that it can be treated may relieve the anxiety, anger, guilt, and frustration related to having chronic pain and voiding dysfunction in the absence of a clear-cut diagnosis and treatment strategy.

GENITOURINARY TUBERCULOSIS

Genitourinary tuberculosis (GUTB) is the 3rd most common type of extrapulmonary tuberculosis (TB). Between 2% and 20% of patients with pulmonary TB develop GUTB. Onset can occur 1 to 33 years after the primary lung infection.[8,9] When the kidney is first infected with bacilli, patients are often asymptomatic. They may have incidental microscopic hematuria and/or pyuria. The progression of the infection involves the bladder. Symptoms of urgency, frequency, dysuria, and/or nocturia develop in about 50% of patients. A third of patients have back pain and gross hematuria.

A diagnosis of GUTB is based on finding *Mycobacterium tuberculosis* bacilli in the urine. A CT scan with contrast and ultrasound can help determine the extent and severity of the disease. A TB test should be done.

Long-term complications depend on the duration of the disease. Scarring of the renal parenchyma, calcifications, hydronephrosis, and ureteral strictures can occur. The earlier treatment is started, the less likely renal failure will develop. Patients may need long-term urologic follow-up. Care of patients with TB is discussed in Chapter 30.

GLOMERULAR DISEASES

GLOMERULONEPHRITIS

Glomerulonephritis (inflammation of the glomeruli) affects both kidneys equally. It is the 3rd leading cause of ESRD in the United States. Although the glomerulus is the primary site of inflammation, tubular and interstitial changes with vascular scarring and hardening *(glomerulosclerosis)* in the kidney can occur.[10]

A variety of conditions are associated with glomerulonephritis. These range from kidney infections, drugs toxic to the kidneys, problems with the immune system, and systemic diseases (Table 50.8). Glomerulonephritis can be acute or chronic. With *acute glomerulonephritis,* symptoms come on suddenly. They may be temporary or reversible. An example of this is acute poststreptococcal glomerulonephritis (APSGN). *Chronic glomerulonephritis* typically progresses slowly and can lead to irreversible renal failure.

Diagnostic studies and the history, including any recent infection, such as a sore throat or upper respiratory tract infection, or a diagnosis of diabetes, aid in identifying the type of glomerulonephritis present.

Acute Poststreptococcal Glomerulonephritis

Acute poststreptococcal glomerulonephritis is the most common type of acute glomerulonephritis worldwide. It is most common in children aged 5 to 7 years old and adults older than 60 years. APSGN develops about 1 to 6 weeks after an infection of the tonsils, pharynx, or skin (e.g., streptococcal sore throat, impetigo) by nephrotoxic strains of group A β-hemolytic streptococci.[11] The person makes antibodies to the streptococcal antigen. Although the exact mechanism is not known, tissue injury occurs as the antigen-antibody complexes are deposited in the glomeruli, complement is activated (see Chapter 12), and inflammation results.

Manifestations vary. They include general edema, hypertension, oliguria, hematuria, and proteinuria. Fluid retention occurs because of decreased glomerular filtration. At first, edema appears in low-pressure tissues, such as those around the eyes *(periorbital edema).* Later it progresses to involve the whole body. Red to brown urine occurs with bleeding in the upper urinary tract. The degree of proteinuria varies with the severity. Hypertension results from increased fluid volume. Patients may have abdominal or flank pain. Sometimes they may be asymptomatic. The problem is found on routine urinalysis.

The diagnosis of APSGN is based on the history and physical assessment. An immune response to streptococci is often shown by the Streptozyme test. It measures 5 different streptococcal antibodies, including antistreptolysin-O (ASO). The finding of decreased complement components (especially C3 and CH50) indicates an immune-mediated response. A renal biopsy can confirm the disease.

TABLE 50.8 Causes and Risk Factors for Glomerulonephritis (GN)

Cause or Risk Factor	Description
Conditions Causing Scarring of Glomeruli	
Diabetic nephropathy	• Primary cause of end-stage renal disease in the United States (see Chapter 51) • Microvascular changes of diffuse glomerulosclerosis involving thickening of glomerular basement membrane (GBM)
Focal segmental glomerulosclerosis	• Scattered scarring of glomeruli • May result from another disease or occur for unknown reasons
Hypertension	• Nephrosclerosis is a complication of hypertension • GN can cause hypertension
Immune Disease	
Anti-GBM disease	• Autoimmune disorder that causes lung and kidney disease • Causes bleeding into lungs and GN
Immunoglobulin A (IgA) nephropathy	• Results from deposits of IgA in the glomeruli • Recurrent episodes of hematuria
Scleroderma	• Causes widespread changes in connective tissue and vascular lesions in many organs (see Chapter 69) • In the kidney, vascular lesions are associated with fibrosis • Severity of renal involvement varies
Systemic lupus erythematosus (SLE)	• Autoimmune disorder characterized by the involvement of several tissues and organs, especially joints, skin, and kidneys (see Chapter 69) • GN often occurs in SLE and has a poor prognosis
Infections	
Infective endocarditis	• Bacteria can cause an infection of 1 or more of the heart valves (see Chapter 40) • People at risk include those with a heart defect, such as a damaged or artificial heart valve • GN may be caused by glomerular membrane deposits of complement and immunoglobulin
Poststreptococcal glomerulonephritis	• GN may develop 1–3 weeks after a streptococcal throat infection or 3–6 weeks after a skin infection • Antibodies (Ab) to strep antigen (Ag) develop, and the Ag-Ab deposit in the glomeruli, causing inflammation
Viral infections	• Viral infections can trigger GN • Common viruses include HIV, hepatitis B, and hepatitis C viruses
Vasculitis	
Granulomatosis with polyangiitis	• Form of vasculitis affecting small and medium blood vessels • Most often affects kidneys, lungs, and upper respiratory tract
Polyarteritis nodosa	• Rare disease, possibly autoimmune, that affects small and medium blood vessels • Can affect any organ but common in heart, kidneys, and intestines
Other Causes	
Amyloidosis	• Caused by infiltration of tissues with amyloid (hyaline substance) • Hyaline bodies consist largely of protein • Kidney involvement is common • Proteinuria is often the first clinical manifestation
Illegal drug use	• People who use these drugs are at increased risk for GN

Dipstick urinalysis and urine sediment microscopy can show significant numbers of red blood cells (RBCs) with or without casts. Proteinuria may range from mild to severe. Blood tests include blood urea nitrogen (BUN) and serum creatinine to assess the extent of renal impairment.

Interprofessional and Nursing Management

More than 90% of patients with APSGN recover completely or improve rapidly with supportive management. Accurate recognition and assessment are critical. Chronic glomerulonephritis can develop if the patient is not treated appropriately.

Management focuses on symptom relief. Rest is recommended until the signs of glomerular inflammation (proteinuria, hematuria) and hypertension subside. Restricting sodium and fluid intake and giving diuretics can reduce edema. Severe hypertension is treated with antihypertensive drugs. We may restrict protein intake if there is evidence of an increase in nitrogenous wastes (e.g., increased BUN). The protein restriction varies with the degree of proteinuria. Low-protein, low-sodium, fluid-restricted diets are discussed in Chapter 51. Antibiotics are given if the streptococcal infection is still present.

One of the most important ways to prevent APSGN is to encourage early diagnosis and treatment of sore throats and skin lesions. If a culture is positive for streptococci, antibiotic therapy is essential. Teach patients to take the full course of antibiotics to ensure that the bacteria are completely gone. Good personal hygiene is a key factor in preventing the spread of cutaneous streptococcal infections.

In most cases, recovery from the acute glomerulonephritis is complete. However, in rare cases, hypertension, proteinuria, and/or renal insufficiency can occur.

Chronic Glomerulonephritis

Chronic glomerulonephritis is a syndrome of permanent and progressive renal fibrosis involving the glomeruli. It can progress to ESRD. Most types of glomerulonephritis and nephrotic syndrome can eventually lead to chronic glomerulonephritis. Some people who develop chronic glomerulonephritis have no history of kidney disease. We may not find the cause of chronic glomerulonephritis. An inherited disorder (e.g., Alport syndrome) or an autoimmune disorder may be the cause.

With chronic glomerulonephritis, symptoms develop slowly over time. Patients are often unaware that progressive kidney impairment is occurring, even if it is severe, until they have a diagnostic evaluation. Chronic glomerulonephritis is often discovered by finding an abnormality on a urinalysis, high BP, or increased serum creatinine. Patients slowly develop uremia and ESRD (see Chapter 51) because of decreasing renal function.

Manifestations include varying degrees of hematuria (ranging from microscopic to gross), proteinuria, and urinary excretion of various formed elements, including RBCs, WBCs, and casts. Increased BUN and serum creatinine levels are common. Ultrasound and CT scans are the preferred radiologic studies. A renal biopsy may be done to determine the cause.

The history provides vital information. Assess exposure to drugs (e.g., nonsteroidal antiinflammatory drugs [NSAIDs]) and infections (e.g., hepatitis). Evaluate patients for other immune disorders, such as systemic lupus erythematosus (SLE). Is there a history of renal problems?

Treatment depends on the cause. It includes supportive and symptomatic care. Management of CKD is discussed in Chapter 51.

ANTIGLOMERULAR BASEMENT MEMBRANE DISEASE

Antiglomerular basement membrane (anti-GBM) disease (formerly called Goodpasture syndrome) is an autoimmune disease characterized by antibodies that attack the glomerular and alveolar basement membranes. Damage to the kidneys and lungs results when binding of the antibody causes an inflammatory reaction mediated by complement activation (see Chapter 12).

Anti-GBM is a rare disease that occurs mainly in older children and adults, especially those in their 30s and into their 60s. The manifestations can include weakness, pallor, and pulmonary symptoms, such as cough, mild shortness of breath, hemoptysis, crackles, and pulmonary insufficiency. Renal involvement includes hematuria, proteinuria, and anemia. It can proceed quickly to renal failure. Pulmonary involvement can occur before or at the same time as glomerular abnormalities.

Current management includes glucocorticoids, immunosuppressive drugs (e.g., cyclophosphamide, rituximab), plasmapheresis (see Chapter 14), and, if needed, dialysis. Plasmapheresis removes the circulating anti-GBM antibodies. Immunosuppressive therapy inhibits further antibody production. Those with ESRD may be a candidate for a kidney transplant. Anti-GBM disease rarely occurs in the transplanted kidney. Patients receive care appropriate for critically ill patients who have AKI (see Chapter 51) and respiratory distress (see Chapter 32). Death may occur from bleeding in the lungs and respiratory failure.

RAPIDLY PROGRESSIVE GLOMERULONEPHRITIS

Rapidly progressive glomerulonephritis (RPGN) is a type of glomerular disease with glomerular crescent formations. With RPGN, there is rapid, progressive loss of renal function over days to months.

There are 3 types of RPGN: (1) anti-GBM disease, (2) as a result of immune complex disease (e.g., SLE, postinfectious), (3) or pauci-immune disease where no or few immune deposits are seen on electron or immunofluorescence microscopy.

Manifestations of renal insufficiency (hypertension, edema, hematuria, and reduced urine output) often occur. Treatment aims include correcting fluid overload, hypertension, and uremia and reducing inflammatory injury to the kidney. Treatment often includes corticosteroids and cyclophosphamide. Plasmapheresis may be an option. Dialysis or a kidney transplant may be an option if the patient has progressed to ESRD. After a kidney transplant, RPGN may recur.

NEPHROTIC SYNDROME

Nephrotic syndrome results when the glomerulus is overly permeable to plasma protein, causing proteinuria that leads to low plasma albumin and edema.

Etiology and Clinical Manifestations

Common causes of nephrotic syndrome are listed in Table 50.9. Minimal change disease is the most common cause in children. For adults, 30% of nephrotic syndrome cases are caused by systemic diseases such as diabetes, SLE, or amyloidosis.[12]

The common manifestations are peripheral edema, massive proteinuria, hyperlipidemia, hypoalbuminemia, and foamy urine. The increased glomerular membrane permeability is responsible for the massive excretion of protein in the urine. This results in decreased total serum protein and subsequent edema formation. Ascites and *anasarca* (massive, general edema) develop if there is severe hypoalbuminemia. Decreased plasma oncotic pressure from decreased serum proteins stimulates lipoprotein synthesis. Significant increases in the lipid profile (e.g., cholesterol, low-density lipoprotein (LDL) triglycerides) can occur. Fat bodies (fatty casts) often appear in the urine, causing foamy urine.

Immune responses are impaired. As a result, there is an increased risk of infection. Calcium and skeletal abnormalities may occur, including hypocalcemia, blunted calcium response to parathyroid hormone, hyperparathyroidism, and osteomalacia.

Hypercoagulability is a serious issue. It increases the risk for arterial and venous thromboembolism, including pulmonary embolism and deep vein or renal thrombus.

Interprofessional and Nursing Management

Specific treatment of nephrotic syndrome depends on the cause. The goals are to cure or control the primary disease and relieve the symptoms. Corticosteroids and cyclophosphamide may be used. Prednisone has been effective to varying degrees for some causes of nephrotic syndrome (e.g., membranous glomerulonephritis, lupus nephritis). Managing diabetes is important when nephrotic syndrome is related to diabetes.

Angiotensin-converting enzyme inhibitors or angiotensin receptor blocker drugs may reduce urine protein losses. Diuretics (typically loop diuretics) can improve edema. The treatment of hyperlipidemia includes lipid-lowering agents (see Table 37.6). Anticoagulant therapy may be given if thrombosis is present.

TABLE 50.9 Causes of Nephrotic Syndrome

Primary Glomerular Disease
- Focal-segmental glomerulosclerosis
- Membranous glomerulopathy
- Minimal-change disease

Secondary Causes

Cancers
- Hodgkin lymphoma
- Leukemias
- Solid tumors of lungs, colon, stomach, breast, renal, prostate

Drugs
- Captopril
- Heroin
- Lithium
- NSAIDs
- Penicillamine

Infections
- Bacterial (streptococcal, syphilis)
- Protozoal (malaria)
- Viral (hepatitis, HIV, mononucleosis)

Multisystem Disease
- Amyloidosis
- Diabetes
- Systemic lupus erythematosus

Patients are placed on a low-sodium (less than 2 g/day), low-moderate protein (1 g/kg/day) diet. If urine protein losses are high (more than 10 g/day), more protein may be needed. Patients are usually anorexic. They can become malnourished from the excess loss of protein in the urine. Serve small, frequent meals to encourage intake.

A major nursing focus is on managing edema. Assess edema by (1) weighing patients daily, (2) recording intake and output, and (3) measuring abdominal girth or extremity size. Compare this information daily to assess the effectiveness of treatment. Clean edematous skin carefully. Avoid trauma to the skin.

Because patients are susceptible to infection, teach them to avoid exposure to persons with known infections. Provide patients support, especially in coping with an altered body image. They may feel embarrassment and shame because of their edematous appearance.

OBSTRUCTIVE PROBLEMS

Urinary obstruction refers to any anatomic or functional condition that blocks or impedes the flow of urine (Fig. 50.3). It may be congenital or acquired. Damaging effects from an obstruction affect the urinary system above the level of the obstruction. The severity of these effects depends on the location, duration of obstruction, amount of pressure or dilation, and presence of urinary stasis or infection. Infection increases the risk for irreversible damage.[13]

When obstruction occurs at the level of the bladder neck or prostate, significant bladder changes can occur. Detrusor muscle fibers *hypertrophy* (increase in size) to contract harder to push urine out a narrower pathway. Over a long period, the detrusor loses its ability to compensate for this resistance, eventually leading to a large residual urine volume in the bladder.

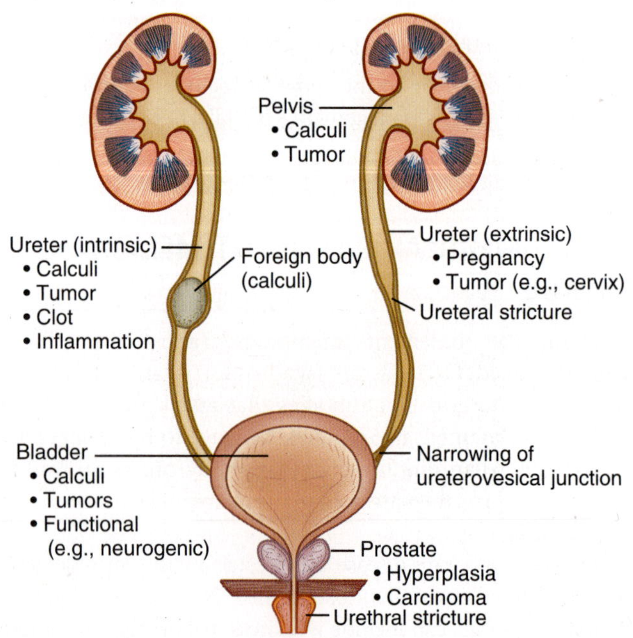

Fig. 50.3 Sites and causes of upper and lower urinary tract obstruction.

When *bladder outlet obstruction* is present, pressure increases during bladder filling or storage. This pressure can be transmitted to the ureters. Pressure can lead to *reflux* (backflow, or backward movement, of urine), *hydroureter* (ureteral dilation and distention), vesicoureteral reflux (backflow of urine from the lower to upper urinary tract), and *hydronephrosis* (dilation or enlargement of the renal pelvises and calyces; Fig. 50.4). Chronic pyelonephritis and renal atrophy may develop. If only 1 kidney is obstructed, the other kidney may try to compensate by enlarging.

Partial obstruction may occur in the ureter or at the ureteropelvic junction (UPJ), where the renal pelvis narrows into the ureter. If the pressure stays low or moderate, the kidney may continue to dilate with no noticeable loss of function. Urinary stasis and reflux increase the risk for pyelonephritis. If only 1 kidney is involved and the other kidney is functioning, patients may be asymptomatic.

If both kidneys are involved or if the patient has only 1 kidney, changes in renal function (e.g., increased BUN and serum creatinine levels) occur. Progressive obstruction can lead to renal failure. Treatment involves finding and relieving the blockage. This can include insertion of a tube (e.g., urethral, ureteral), surgical correction, or diverting the urinary stream above the level of blockage.

URINARY TRACT CALCULI

In their lifetime, 11% of males and 7% of females in the United States will have **nephrolithiasis** (kidney stone disease, renal calculi). The term *calculus* refers to the stone, and *lithiasis* refers to stone formation.

Most patients are middle-aged adults. The risk for developing kidney stones increases with age.[14] Stone formation occurs more often in White and Asian persons. The incidence is higher in those with a family history of stone formation. Stones recur in up to 50% of patients. In the United States the incidence of stone disease is highest in the South and Southwest. Stone formation occurs more often in the summer months, supporting the possible contributing factors of a hot climate and dehydration.

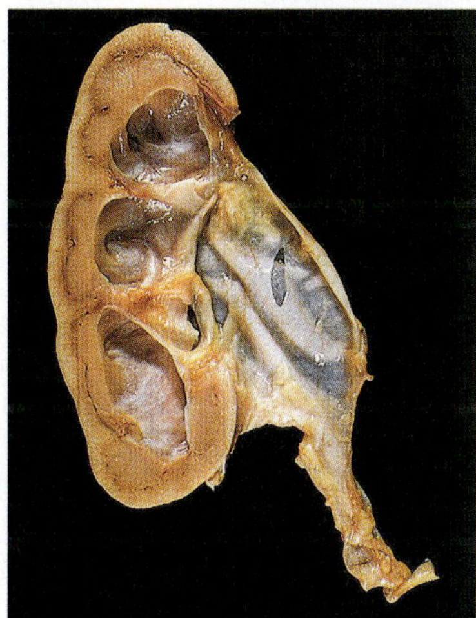

Fig. 50.4 Hydronephrosis. Note the marked dilation of the pelvis and calyces and thinning of the renal parenchyma. (From Kumar V, Abbas AK, Aster JC, et al: *Robbins and Cotran pathologic basis of disease,* ed 10, St Louis, 2021, Elsevier.)

Etiology and Pathophysiology

Many factors are involved in the incidence and type of stones. These factors include climate, diet, genetic, metabolic, and lifestyle (Table 50.10). No single theory accounts for stone formation in all cases. We think kidney stones form when certain crystal-forming substances are not diluted by the kidney and/or the kidney's ability to keep crystals from sticking together is reduced. Crystals, when in a supersaturated concentration, can precipitate and unite to form a stone. Urinary pH, solute load, and inhibitors in the urine affect stone formation. When a substance is not very soluble in fluid, it is more likely to precipitate. The higher the pH (alkaline), the less soluble elements are calcium and phosphate. The lower the pH (acidic), the less soluble elements are uric acid and cystine.

Other key factors in stone formation include obstruction with associated urinary stasis and UTI with urea-splitting bacteria (e.g., *Proteus, Klebsiella, Pseudomonas,* some species of staphylococci). These bacteria cause the urine to become alkaline and contribute to the formation of struvite stones. Infected stones, trapped in the kidney (Fig. 50.5), may assume a staghorn configuration as the stone branches to occupy a larger part of the collecting system. These stones can lead to a renal infection, hydronephrosis, and loss of kidney function.

TABLE 50.10 Risk Factors for Urinary Tract Stones

Age

Climate

- Warm climates that cause increased fluid loss, low urine volume, and increased urine solute concentration

Diet

- Excess amounts of tea or fruit juices that increase urinary oxalate level
- Large intake of diet proteins that increases uric acid excretion
- Large intake of salt, low calcium intake
- Low fluid intake that increases urine concentration

Genetic factors

- Family history of stone formation, cystinuria, gout, renal acidosis

Lifestyle

- Immobility
- Obesity
- Sedentary occupation

Metabolic

- Abnormalities that result in increased urine pH, calcium, oxalate, or uric acid levels, or low citrate

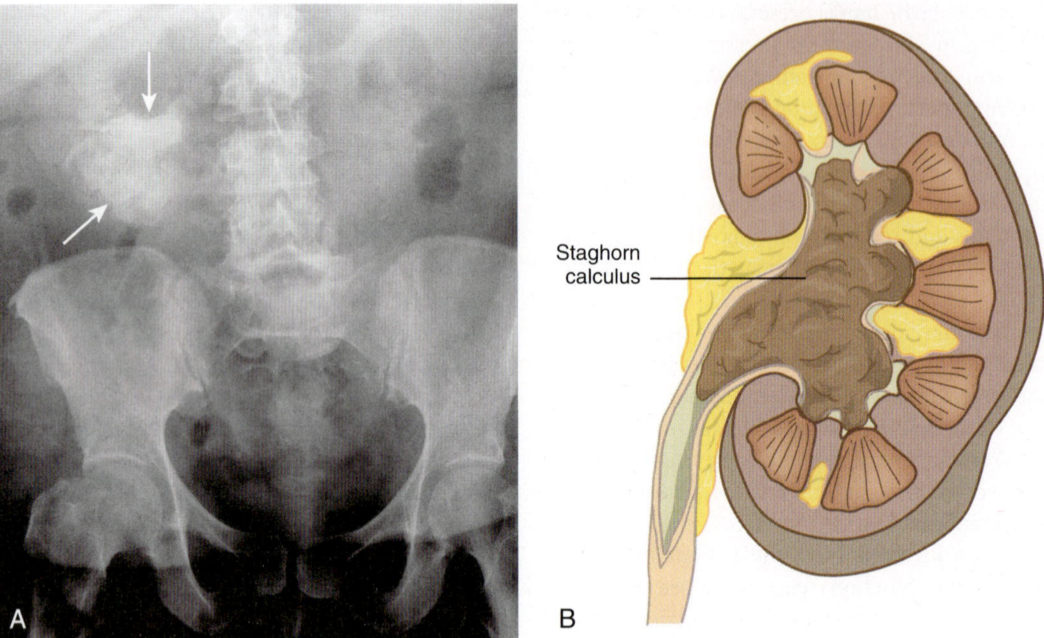

Fig. 50.5 (A) Bilateral staghorn stones *(arrows)* shown on x-ray. (B) Staghorn stone. The renal pelvis is filled with a large stone that is shaped to its contours, resembling the horns of a stag. (A, From Torigian DA, Ramchandani P: *Radiology secrets plus,* ed 4, Philadelphia, 2017, Elsevier.)

Genetic factors may contribute to stone formation. Cystinuria, an autosomal recessive disorder, causes a large increase in the urinary excretion of cystine.

Types of Urinary Stones

The 5 main types of stones are (1) calcium oxalate, (2) calcium phosphate, (3) cystine, (4) struvite (magnesium ammonium phosphate), and (5) uric acid (Table 50.11). Calcium stones are the most common. Stone composition may be mixed. For example, calcium stones can be calcium oxalate, calcium phosphate, or a mix of both. Stones occur in various sites in the urinary tract (Figs. 50.3 and 50.5).

Clinical Manifestations

The first symptom of a kidney stone is usually severe pain that begins suddenly. Typically, a person feels a sharp, severe pain in the flank area, back, or lower abdomen. People describe the pain as the most excruciating that a person can endure. We call this *renal colic.* It results from the stretching, dilation, and spasm of the ureter in response to the obstructing stone. Nausea and vomiting may occur because of severe pain. Patients with renal colic have a hard time being still. They go from walking to sitting to lying down, and then they repeat the process. Some people refer to this as the "kidney stone dance."

Urinary stones cause manifestations when they obstruct urinary flow. Common sites of obstruction are at the UPJ and UVJ. Pain can vary depending on the location of the stone. If the obstruction is in a calyx or at the UPJ, patients may have costovertebral flank pain or renal colic. Pain resulting from the passage of a stone down the ureter can be intense, colicky, and radiate into the genital region. If the stone is nonobstructing, pain may be absent.

Patients may be in mild shock with cool, moist skin. As a stone nears the UVJ, pain moves around toward the abdomen and down toward the lower quadrant. Males may have testicular pain, while females may have labial pain. Both can have groin pain and manifestations of a UTI with dysuria, fever, and chills.

Diagnostic Studies

We can easily diagnose stones with a CT scan or ultrasound. A urinalysis helps confirm the diagnosis of a urinary stone by assessing for hematuria and crystalluria. Measuring urine pH is useful in the diagnosis of struvite stones (tendency to alkaline or high pH) and uric acid or cystine stones (tendency to acidic or low pH).

Retrieval and analysis of the stone(s) are important in diagnosing an underlying problem contributing to stone formation. We measure serum calcium, phosphorus, sodium, potassium, bicarbonate, uric acid, BUN, and creatinine levels. Patients who have recurrent stone formation have a 24-hour urinary measurement of calcium, phosphorus, magnesium, sodium, oxalate, citrate, cysteine, sulfate, potassium, uric acid, and total urine volume.

Interprofessional Care

Care of patients with stones consists of 2 concurrent approaches. The first approach is aimed at managing the acute attack by treating the pain, infection, and/or obstruction.

TABLE 50.11 Types of Urinary Tract Stones

Characteristics	Predisposing Factors	Treatment
Calcium Oxalate		
Most common type of stone. More frequent in males. *Incidence:* 70%–80%	Idiopathic hypercalciuria, hyperoxaluria, independent of urinary pH, family history	• Increase hydration. • Reduce oxalate, animal protein, sodium intake. • Increase calcium, fruit, vegetable intake. • Thiazide diuretics. • Potassium citrate to maintain alkaline urine. • Avoid vitamin C and calcium supplements.
Calcium Phosphate		
Mixed stones (typically), with struvite or oxalate stones. *Incidence:* 15%	Alkaline urine, primary hyperparathyroidism	• Increase hydration. • Treat underlying causes and other stones. • Reduce sodium and animal protein intake. • Increase calcium intake.
Cystine		
Genetic autosomal recessive defect. Defective absorption of cystine in GI tract and kidney, excess concentrations causing stone formation. *Incidence:* 1%–2%	Acidic urine	• Increase hydration. • Captopril, α-penicillamine, tiopronin to prevent cystine crystallization. • Potassium citrate to keep urine alkaline.
Struvite (Magnesium Ammonium Phosphate)		
More common in females. Associated with UTIs. Large staghorn type (usually) (Fig. 50.5). *Incidence:* 1%	UTIs (urease-producing bacteria, usually *Proteus*)	• Antimicrobial agents. • Acetohydroxamic acid. • Typically need surgery to remove stone. • Measures to acidify urine.
Uric Acid		
Predominant in males. *Incidence:* 5%–8%	Gout, acidic urine, high urinary uric acid	• Increase hydration. • Reduce urinary concentration of uric acid. • Alkalinize urine with potassium citrate. • Consider allopurinol. • Reduce purine intake (Table 50.12).

Opioids and/or NSAIDs can relieve renal colic pain. Most stones are 4 mm or less in size and pass spontaneously. However, it may take weeks for a stone to pass. α-Adrenergic blockers, such as tamsulosin or terazosin, which relax the smooth muscle in the ureter, can help stone passage. These drugs also relax the muscle tissue in the prostate in males with BPH.

The second approach is determining the cause of the stone formation and preventing further stone development. Treatment to prevent or minimize stone formation requires a comprehensive approach. Adequate hydration, sodium restrictions, dietary changes, and drugs are used (Table 50.11). Depending on the specific problem underlying the stone formation, various drugs are prescribed. These drugs prevent stone formation in several ways. These include altering urine pH, preventing excess urinary excretion of a substance, or correcting a primary disease (e.g., hyperparathyroidism).

Treatment of struvite stones typically requires surgical intervention (e.g., percutaneous nephrolithotomy). Chronic antibiotic therapy may be given to patients unable to tolerate surgery. It may also be given after surgically removing a stone. Acetohydroxamic acid may be used in those with a retained stone or with recurrent struvite stones. Acetohydroxamic acid inhibits urease produced by bacteria.

Endourology, lithotripsy, or open surgical stone removal may be used if (1) stones are too large for spontaneous passage (usually greater than 5 mm); (2) stones with bacteriuria or symptomatic infection are present; (3) stones are causing impaired renal function; (4) stones are causing persistent pain, nausea, or paralytic ileus; (5) the patient is unable to be treated medically; and (6) the patient has only 1 kidney.[15]

Endourologic Procedures

If the stone is in the bladder, a cystoscopy is done to remove small stones. For larger stones (Fig. 50.6), a *transurethral or percutaneous suprapubic cystolitholapaxy* is done. In this procedure, ultrasonic or laser energy or an instrument called a *lithotrite* (stone crusher) is used to break up the stone. The bladder is then irrigated, and the crushed stones washed out. A *cystoscopic lithotripsy* uses ultrasonic waves to break up stones. Sometimes, we may need to remove the stone with an open suprapubic cystotomy. Complications of these procedures include hemorrhage, retained stone fragments, and infection.

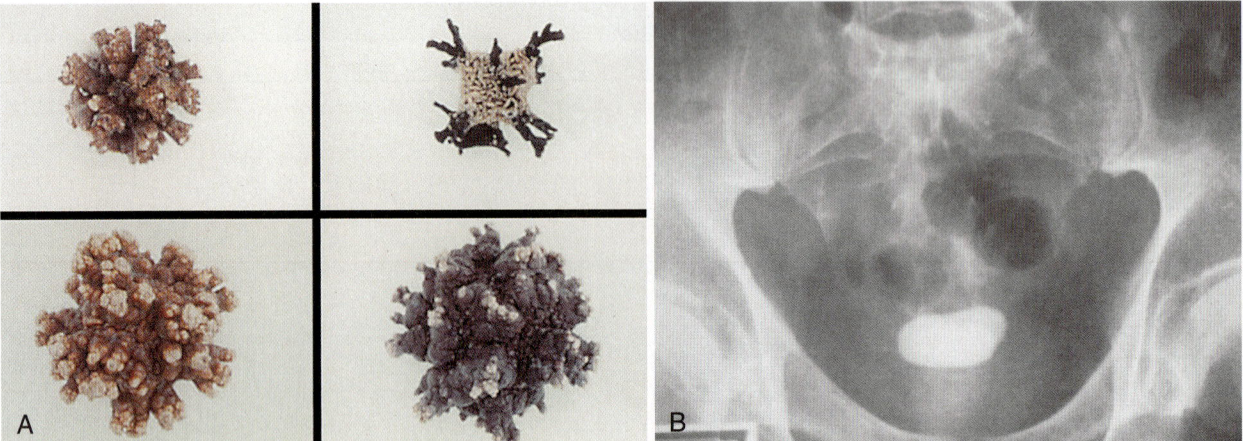

Fig. 50.6 (A) Calcium oxalate stones. (B) Abdominal x-ray showing large bladder stone. (From Bullock N, Doble A, Turner W, et al: *Urology: an illustrated colour text,* London, 2008, Churchill Livingstone.)

Flexible or rigid *ureteroscopes* can remove stones from the renal pelvis and upper urinary tract. Ultrasonic, laser, or electrohydraulic lithotripsy may be used in conjunction with ureteroscopy to break up the stone.

In *percutaneous nephrolithotomy,* a nephroscope is inserted into the kidney pelvis through a tract (using a sheath) in the skin of the patient's back. The kidney stones can be fragmented using ultrasound, electrohydraulic, or laser lithotripsy. The stone fragments are removed, and the renal pelvis is then irrigated. A percutaneous nephrostomy tube can be left in place to make sure that the ureter stays unobstructed. Complications include bleeding, injury to adjacent structures, and infection.

Lithotripsy

Lithotripsy is a procedure used to break up stones, thus allowing them to pass from the urinary tract. Lithotripsy techniques include (1) laser lithotripsy, (2) extracorporeal shockwave lithotripsy, (3) ultrasonic lithotripsy, and (4) electrohydraulic lithotripsy. *Laser lithotripsy* is used to shatter ureteral and large bladder stones. To access ureteral stones, a ureteroscope is used to get close to the stone. A small fiber is inserted up the scope so that the tip (which emits the laser energy) can come in contact with the stone. A holmium laser in direct contact with the stone is often used. The intense energy breaks the stone into small pieces. The pieces are then extracted or flushed out. This minimally invasive treatment usually requires general anesthesia.

In *extracorporeal shockwave lithotripsy (ESWL),* patients receive general or spinal anesthesia to ensure they stay in the same position during the procedure. The HCP uses fluoroscopy or ultrasound to focus the lithotripter over the stone. Then, a high-voltage spark generator produces high-energy acoustic shockwaves that shatter the stone. The small pieces of stone are then excreted in the urine. Complications of ESWL include incomplete breakup of the stone, which can lead to possible obstruction, kidney damage, decreased renal function, and elevated BP.

In *ultrasonic lithotripsy,* high-frequency sound waves are used to break the stone into sandlike particles, and patients receive general or spinal anesthesia. In *electrohydraulic lithotripsy,* electrical shockwaves are used to break the stone into small fragments, and patients need general anesthesia.

Complications of lithotripsy are rare. They include hemorrhage, infection, and obstruction. Hematuria is common and can last a few days to a few weeks. The first few times that the patient voids, the urine is often bright red. As the bleeding subsides, the urine can become dark red or a smoky color. Antibiotics are given to reduce the risk for infection.

Afterward, patients usually have mild to moderate pain. Severe colicky pain can occur as the pieces of stone pass. Most patients can return to their normal activities in a day or so. For those with a large stone, a self-retaining ureteral stent may be placed to aid in passing the shattered stone. This helps prevent obstruction. The stent is typically removed within 2 weeks after lithotripsy. Encourage fluids to help dilute the urine and reduce the pain from passing stone fragments.

Surgical Therapy

A small group of patients needs open surgery. The primary indications for surgery include pain, infection, and obstruction. The type of surgery depends on the location of the stone. A *nephrolithotomy* is an incision into the kidney to remove a stone. A *pyelolithotomy* is an incision into the renal pelvis for stone removal. If the stone is in the ureter, a *ureterolithotomy* is done. A *cystotomy* may be indicated for bladder stones. For open surgery on the kidney or ureter, there is usually a flank incision directly below the diaphragm and across the side. The most common complications after surgery for stone removal are bleeding and infection.

Nutrition Therapy

To manage an obstructing stone, patients should drink adequate fluids to avoid dehydration. Do not force excess fluids because it does not promote the passage of stones in the urine. Forcing fluids may increase the pain or precipitate renal colic.

After an episode of urolithiasis, encourage a high fluid intake (around 3 L/day) to produce a urine output of at least 2.5 L/day unless contraindicated. High urine output prevents supersaturation of minerals (i.e., dilutes the urine) and promotes excretion of minerals in the urine, thus preventing stone formation. A low-sodium diet is best. High-sodium intake increases calcium excretion in the urine. Table 50.12 shows foods high in calcium, oxalate, and purines.

NURSING MANAGEMENT: URINARY TRACT CALCULI

Assessment

Subjective and objective data you should obtain from patients with urinary tract stones are outlined in Table 50.13. Is there a history of prolonged illness with immobilization, dehydration, or disease or surgery involving the GI or GU tract? Is there a personal or family history of stone formation? What is their geographic residence? Obtain a nutrition assessment, including fluid intake and the intake of vitamins C and D. Review their activity pattern (active or sedentary). Obtain a medication history.

Clinical Problems

Clinical problems for patients with urinary tract stones include:

- Impaired urinary elimination
- Pain

More information on clinical problems and interventions for patients with urinary tract stones is presented in eNursing Care Plan 50.2 (on the website for this chapter).

TABLE 50.12 NUTRITION THERAPY

Urinary Tract Stones

Depending on the type of stone, modifying the diet can be helpful in preventing recurrence.

Calcium

High: Milk, cheese, ice cream, yogurt, sauces containing milk; all beans (except green beans), lentils; fish with fine bones (e.g., sardines, kippers, herring, salmon); dried fruits, nuts; Ovaltine, chocolate, cocoa

Oxalate

High: Dark roughage, spinach, rhubarb, asparagus, cabbage, tomatoes, beets, nuts, celery, parsley, runner beans; grapefruit, orange, raspberries; chocolate, cocoa, instant coffee, Ovaltine, tea; Worcestershire sauce

Purine

High: Sardines, anchovies, herring, mussels, scallops, organ meats, kidney, goose

Moderate: Chicken, salmon, crab, veal, mutton, bacon, pork, beef, ham

Planning

The overall goals are that patients with urinary tract stones will have (1) pain relief, (2) no urinary tract obstruction, and (3) knowledge of ways to prevent stone recurrence.

Implementation

Pain management is a key nursing responsibility when patients have an obstructing stone and renal colic. To retrieve any spontaneously passed stones, strain all urine with a gauze or a urine strainer. Encourage ambulation to promote movement of the stone from the upper to the lower urinary tract. To ensure

TABLE 50.13 NURSING ASSESSMENT

Urinary Tract Stones

Subjective Data

Important Health Information

Health history: Recent or chronic UTI. Immobilization. Previous urinary tract stones, obstruction, or kidney disease with urinary stasis. Gout, benign prostatic hyperplasia, hyperparathyroidism, chronic diarrhea

Medications: Drug therapy to prevent or treat UTI, allopurinol, analgesics, loop diuretics, thiazide diuretics

Surgery or other treatments: External urinary diversion, long-term indwelling urinary catheter

Functional Health Patterns

Health perception–health management: Family history of urinary tract stones, sedentary lifestyle

Nutritional-metabolic: Nausea, vomiting. Intake of purines, calcium, salt, oxalates, phosphates, and supplements. Low fluid intake. Chills

Elimination: Decreased urine output, urinary urgency, frequency, feeling of bladder fullness

Cognitive-perceptual: Acute, severe, colicky pain in flank, back, abdomen, groin, or genitalia. Burning on urination, dysuria. Anxiety

Objective Data

General

Guarding, back pain, fever, dehydration

GI

Abdominal distention, absence of bowel sounds

Skin

Warm, flushed skin or pallor with cool, moist skin (mild shock)

Urinary

Oliguria, hematuria, tenderness on palpation of renal areas, passage of stone or stones

Possible Diagnostic Findings

↑ BUN and serum creatinine levels. Urinalysis showing RBCs, WBCs, pyuria, crystals, casts, minerals, bacteria. ↑ Uric acid, calcium, phosphorus, oxalate, or cystine values on 24-h urine sample. Stones or anatomic changes on x-ray, CT scan, or renal/bladder ultrasound. Visualization of obstruction on cystourethroscopy

safety, tell patients with acute renal colic to ask for help when ambulating, especially if they are receiving opioid analgesics.

Most people who had urinary stones can lower their risk for recurrence by changing their lifestyle and diet habits. Adequate fluid intake is important to produce a urine output of around 2.5 L/day. Consult with the HCP about specific recommendations for fluid intake. The moderately active, ambulatory person should drink around 3 to 4 L/day. Water is the preferred fluid. Limit colas, coffee, and tea intake because they increase the risk for recurring urinary stones.

Increasing fluid intake is important for patients at risk for dehydration, including those who (1) are active in sports, (2) live in a dry climate, (3) perform physical exercise, (4) have a family history of stone formation, or (5) work outside or in an occupation that requires a great deal of physical activity.

Additional measures for patients who are on bed rest or immobile for a prolonged time include turning patients every few hours and helping patients sit or stand, if possible, to maximize urinary flow. Other preventive measures focus on reducing metabolic or secondary risk factors. For example, restricting purine intake may help those at risk for uric acid stones. Review the dosage, scheduling, and potential side effects of drugs used to reduce the risk for stone formation (Table 50.11). You may teach some patients to monitor urinary pH or urine output.

◆ Evaluation

The expected outcomes are that patients with urinary tract stones will:

- Maintain free flow of urine with minimal hematuria
- Report satisfactory pain relief
- State understanding of the disease and ways to prevent recurrence

STRICTURES

A ureteral or urethral **stricture** is a narrowing of the lumen of the ureter or urethra.

Ureteral Strictures

Ureteral strictures can affect the entire length of the ureter, from the UPJ to UVJ. Although these can be congenital, they are usually from adhesions or scar formation after surgery or radiation. They may be caused by extrinsic factors, such as large tumors in the peritoneal cavity. Depending on its severity, ureteral obstruction can threaten kidney function.

Manifestations include mild to moderate colic, flank pain, and CVA tenderness. This pain may be moderate to severe in intensity, especially if patients drink a large volume of fluids, such as alcohol, over a brief period. Infection is unusual unless a stone or foreign object, such as a stent or nephrostomy tube, is present.

The obstruction of a ureteral stricture may be temporarily bypassed by placing a stent using endoscopy or by diverting urine flow through a nephrostomy tube placed in the renal pelvis of the affected kidney. Definitive correction requires surgery. Ureteral strictures under 1 cm can be treated using an endoscopic procedure *(endoureterotomy)*. In some patients, open surgery may be done to excise the stenotic area and reanastomose the ureter to the contralateral ureter *(ureteroureterostomy)* or to the renal pelvis. Alternatively, distal ureteral strictures may be treated by a *ureteroneocystostomy* (reimplantation of the ureter into the bladder wall).

Urethral Strictures

A *urethral stricture* is caused by fibrosis or inflammation of the urethral lumen. Causes include urethral trauma, STIs (especially gonorrhea), surgery (especially prostate or urethral), repeated catheterizations, or a congenital defect. A history of UTI is common, especially if the stricture involves the distal urethra. However, many cases are idiopathic and lack a clear cause.

Once the process of inflammation and fibrosis begins, the lumen of the urethra narrows and its compliance (ability to close or open in response to bladder filling or voiding) is compromised. Meatal stenosis, a narrowing of the urethral opening at the tip of the penis, develops because of irritation in this region.

Manifestations include a diminished force of the urinary stream, straining to void, sprayed stream, postvoid dribbling, or a split urine stream. Patients may report feelings of incomplete bladder emptying with urinary frequency and nocturia. Moderate to severe obstruction of the bladder outlet may lead to acute urinary retention. Retrograde urethrography (RUG), ultrasound urethrography, voiding cystourethrogram, and cystourethroscopy are used to identify stricture length, location, and caliber.

Initial management can include dilation. Dilation places a metal instrument (urethral sound) or a series of progressively larger stents (followers) into the urethra to expand the lumen. Alternatively, patients may have an endoscopic urethrotomy, a closed procedure involving an incision of the urethra. An open surgical procedure *(urethroplasty)* may be done for an obstructive urethral stricture. Shorter strictures may be treated by resecting the fibrotic area followed by reanastomosis of the urethra. Longer strictures may require the use of a skin flap as a substitute urethral segment.

RENAL TRAUMA

Renal trauma is especially likely with an injury to the abdomen, flank, or back. Around 10% of patients with abdominal trauma have renal trauma. Renal trauma can be blunt or penetrating. *Blunt trauma* is the most common cause. Injury to the kidney can occur with sports injuries, motor vehicle accidents, and falls. *Penetrating injuries* may result from violent encounters (e.g., gunshot, stabbing incidents).

The severity of renal trauma depends on the extent of the injury. Obtain a history of trauma to the area of the kidneys. Gross or microscopic hematuria may be present. Diagnostic studies include contrast-enhanced CT and CT pyelography.

Both the injured kidney and the uninvolved kidney need evaluation. Patients with renal trauma are often admitted for observation. Up to 60% to 70% need surgery.[16]

Nursing care depends on the type of trauma and the extent of any associated injuries. Your priority interventions are to (1) evaluate the patient and vital signs frequently; (2) monitor for shock, especially in a penetrating injury; (3) monitor intake and output; (4) provide for pain relief; and (5) assess for hematuria and myoglobinuria.

RENAL VASCULAR PROBLEMS

Vascular problems involving the kidney include (1) nephrosclerosis, (2) renal artery stenosis, and (3) renal vein thrombosis.

NEPHROSCLEROSIS

Nephrosclerosis is sclerosis of the small arteries and arterioles of the kidney. The decreased blood flow results in ischemia, interstitial fibrosis, and necrosis of parts of the kidney. *Benign nephrosclerosis* usually occurs in adults over 60 years old. It is caused by vascular changes from hypertension and narrowing of blood vessels. Vascular changes account for most of the loss of renal function from aging. The degree of nephrosclerosis is related to the severity of hypertension. Benign nephrosclerosis generally does not progress to significant loss of renal function or ESRD.

With accelerated nephrosclerosis (acute hypertensive or malignant nephrosclerosis), we see a significantly high BP (systolic BP ≥180 and/or diastolic BP ≥120 mm Hg) with concurrent acute impairment of 1 of more organ systems. It can begin suddenly and is a medical emergency. With renal involvement, damage to the kidney can progress rapidly.

The availability and use of antihypertensive drugs have improved the prognosis for patients with nephrosclerosis. Treatment for benign nephrosclerosis is the same as that for essential hypertension (see Chapter 36). Malignant nephrosclerosis is treated with antihypertensive therapy. We generally lower the BP over a 24-hour period. The prognosis for patients with untreated or refractive malignant hypertension is poor. These conditions can lead to death.

RENAL ARTERY STENOSIS

Renal artery stenosis is a partial occlusion of 1 or both renal arteries and their major branches. It can be the result of atherosclerotic narrowing or fibromuscular hyperplasia. Renal artery stenosis can be a cause of secondary hypertension. When hypertension develops suddenly or is difficult to treat, renal artery stenosis should be considered.

Diagnostic tests used to assess for renal artery stenosis include a renal duplex Doppler ultrasonography, CT or MRI angiography, and renal arteriography.

The goals of therapy are to control BP and restore perfusion to the kidney. Percutaneous transluminal renal angioplasty, with or without stenting, for unilateral renal artery stenosis can be done but only if there is a high chance of success.

Surgical revascularization of the kidney is an option in complex cases. Revascularization may result in the BP becoming normotensive. Surgery usually involves anastomosis between the kidney and another major artery, usually the splenic artery or aorta. In some cases of unilateral renal involvement, unilateral nephrectomy may be done.

RENAL VEIN THROMBOSIS

Renal vein thrombosis may occur unilaterally or bilaterally. It can develop acutely or chronically. Causes include trauma, extrinsic compression (e.g., tumor, aortic aneurysm), kidney cancer, pregnancy, contraceptive use, and nephrotic syndrome.

Patients can be asymptomatic or have acute flank pain/tenderness, hematuria, fever, worsening renal function, and/or worsening proteinuria. Anticoagulation is used to prevent progression and the development of an embolus. Patients may undergo percutaneous thrombectomy. Other options include thrombolysis and placement of suprarenal inferior vena cava (IVC) filters. Surgical thrombectomy is rarely needed.

HEREDITARY KIDNEY DISEASE

POLYCYSTIC KIDNEY DISEASE

Polycystic kidney disease (PKD) is a common genetic disorder. In PKD, cysts form in the kidneys that can cause them to change shape and enlarge over time. PKD affects 500,000 people in the United States. The disease usually progresses from loss of kidney function to ESRD by age 65 in 85% of patients.[17] It is the 4th leading cause of ESRD, affecting 5% of those with ESRD. A nongenetic PKD (acquired cystic kidney disease [ACKD]) can occur in those with severe kidney scarring and damage who typically receive dialysis. After 8 years on dialysis, 90% of patients will have ACKD.[17]

PKD has 2 hereditary forms: one usually diagnosed in early childhood and one in adulthood. The childhood form of PKD is a rare autosomal recessive disorder that is often rapidly progressive (Box 50.1). The adult form is an autosomal dominant disorder (ADPKD). If 1 parent has the disease, there is a 50% chance that the disease will pass to the child.

ADPKD involves both kidneys. Large, thin-walled cysts that are several millimeters to several centimeters in diameter fill the cortex and medulla (Fig. 50.7). The cysts enlarge and destroy surrounding tissue by compression. They are filled with fluid and may contain blood or pus. ADPKD kidneys can become enlarged and look like they are filled with golf balls.

The condition can be symptomless for many years. Signs and symptoms usually develop between 30 and 50 years of age.[17] Symptoms can appear when the renal cysts begin to enlarge. Often the first manifestations are hypertension, hematuria, proteinuria, loss of kidney function, and/or a feeling of pain or heaviness in the back, side, or abdomen.

Acute and chronic pain is a common problem. Acute pain can develop from kidney stone formation, UTIs, or cyst hemorrhage. The pain can be constant and severe in those with

BOX 50.1 GENETICS IN CLINICAL PRACTICE

Polycystic Kidney Disease

	Adult	Child
Genetic basis	• Autosomal dominant	• Autosomal recessive
Incidence	• 90% of cases	• 10% of cases
Gene location	• *PKD1* gene on chromosome 16 or *PKD2* gene on chromosome 4 • Genes code for polycystins (proteins that promote normal kidney development and function) • Mutations in genes lead to formation of thousands of cysts that disrupt the normal function of kidneys and other organs	• Polycystic kidney and hepatic disease *(PKHD1)* gene on chromosome 6p21, DZIP1L gene may be affected • *PKHD1* gene codes for fibrocystin • Mutations in gene lead to cyst formation
Age of onset	• Kidney function usually starts worsening in the 40s, but symptoms can start earlier	• Infancy or childhood
Clinical implications	• Multisystem involvement • Systemic hypertension is common, occurs in 60% of patients before kidney function worsens • Increased risk for cerebral aneurysms	• Up to 30% of affected newborns die within 1 wk after birth • If infant survives the newborn period, chances of survival are good • Often need dialysis or transplant by adulthood

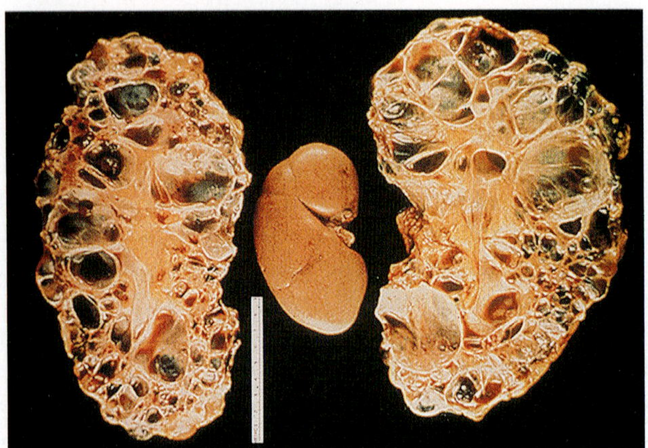

Fig. 50.7 Comparison of polycystic kidney with normal kidney. (From Johnson RJ, Tonelli M, Floege J: *Comprehensive clinical nephrology,* ed 7, St Louis, 2024, Elsevier.)

enlarged kidneys. Bilateral enlarged kidneys are often palpable. Those with ADPKD can have no symptoms, which can delay diagnosis.

ADPKD can affect the liver (liver cysts), pancreas, heart (abnormal heart valves), blood vessels (aneurysms), and intestines (diverticulosis). The most serious complication is a cerebral aneurysm, which can rupture.

Diagnosis is based on manifestations, family history, ultrasound (best screening measure), or CT scan (provides more precise images).

Interprofessional and Nursing Management

There is no cure for PKD. Tolvaptan is an approved treatment for rapidly progressive ADPKD. It works to slow growth of renal cysts, helping to preserve kidney function. Other treatment aims include preventing or treating UTIs. Nephrectomy may be done if pain, bleeding, or infection becomes a chronic, serious problem. Dialysis and kidney transplant may be needed to treat ESRD (see Chapter 51).

When patients begin to have progressive renal failure, the interventions depend on the remaining renal function. Measures are the same as those for managing ESRD. They include diet changes, fluid restriction, and drugs (e.g., antihypertensives). Help patients and caregivers cope with having a chronic disease. Patients with ADPKD often have children by the time the disease is diagnosed. Those children should receive genetic counseling. Patients need counseling about plans for having more children. You can find more resources at the PKD Foundation website (www.pkdcure.org).

CHECK YOUR PRACTICE

You are doing a rotation in the dialysis unit. You have been doing vital sign checks on a 45-year-old male who receives dialysis 3 times a week. When you ask him why he is on dialysis, he tells you that he has ADPKD. After further discussion, he tells you that he has 1 son who is now 23 years old, but they do not speak. He does not want to tell him about his medical problems or why he is on dialysis.

- How would you respond to this patient?

MEDULLARY CYSTIC KIDNEY DISEASE

In *medullary cystic kidney disease,* cysts form in the medulla, or center, of the kidneys. It is a rare, autosomal dominant disorder. Patients have loss of renal function often starting in their teens. Most progress to ESRD by the time they are age 65. The kidneys are typically normal or small in size with significant tubular-interstitial fibrosis. Defects in the kidneys' concentrating ability result in polyuria, which is a hallmark of the disease. Hyperuricemia is common. Genetic counseling may help with family planning. Treatment measures are those related to ESRD (see Chapter 51). A similar disease, familial juvenile nephronophthisis, is found in young children. It is autosomal recessive and leads to 15% of pediatric ESRD cases.

ALPORT SYNDROME

Alport syndrome, or *chronic hereditary nephritis,* is an inherited disease that affects the glomeruli. The basic defect is a mutation in a gene for collagen that results in altered synthesis of the GBM.[18]

There are 3 genetic types of Alport syndrome: X-linked, autosomal recessive, and autosomal dominant. In X-linked, the most common type, the earliest manifestation is chronic asymptomatic microscopic hematuria. These patients can have progressive hearing loss and deformities of the lens of the eye. Ocular changes and sensorineural hearing loss occur with the autosomal recessive type but are rare in the autosomal dominant type.

Alport syndrome can cause progressive kidney damage, leading to ESRD. Those with X-linked and autosomal recessive types generally progress to ESRD between ages 16 and 35. People with autosomal dominant Alport syndrome usually develop ESRD around ages 45 to 60.

There is no specific treatment. Care is supportive. A kidney transplant is usually successful. The disease itself does not recur after a kidney transplant, but there is small risk of developing anti-GBM antibody disease.

URINARY TRACT TUMORS

KIDNEY CANCER

Tumors that arise from the cortex, pelvis, or calyces may be benign or cancerous. Most cases of kidney cancer are renal cell carcinomas (renal adenocarcinoma). It occurs twice as often in males. The average age at diagnosis is 64 years.[19] It is rare in those under 45 years old. Smoking and obesity are significant risk factors. An increased incidence occurs in first-degree relatives of people who have or had renal cell cancer. Other risk factors include hypertension and exposure to certain chemicals such as trichloroethylene and cadmium.

Clinical Manifestations and Diagnostic Studies

Early stage kidney cancer usually has no symptoms, so many patients go undiagnosed until the disease has significantly progressed. Many are diagnosed as incidental findings on imaging studies used to evaluate symptoms for unrelated conditions.

Kidney tumors cause symptoms by compressing, stretching, or invading structures near or within the kidney. The most common presenting symptoms are hematuria and flank pain. Other manifestations include weight loss, fever, anemia, fatigue, hypercalcemia, and/or a palpable mass in the flank or abdomen.

About 33% of patients have metastasis at the time of diagnosis. Local extension of kidney cancer into the renal vein and vena cava is common. The most common sites of metastases include lungs, lymph nodes, bone, and liver.

CT scan is often used in the diagnosis and can detect small kidney tumors. Ultrasound has improved the ability to distinguish between a solid mass tumor and a cyst. This is significant because most masses detected on imaging are cysts. Partial nephrectomy or total nephrectomy is typically done at the time of biopsy.

Interprofessional and Nursing Management

Preventive measures include quitting smoking, maintaining a healthy weight, controlling BP, and reducing exposure to toxins. Patients in high-risk groups should be aware of their increased risk. Teach them about early manifestations (e.g., hematuria, flank pain). A cure for kidney cancer may be possible if it is found and treated early.

Table 50.14 outlines the interprofessional care of patients with kidney cancer. Staging provides a basis for determining treatment options. The following is a simple description of staging of kidney cancer based on the primary tumor:

Stage I: The tumor can be up to 7 cm in diameter and is confined to the kidney.

Stage II: The tumor is larger than a stage I tumor but still confined to the kidney.

Stage III: The tumor extends beyond the kidney to the surrounding tissue. It has not spread to the adrenal gland or to Gerota fascia.

Stage IV: Cancer spreads outside the kidney beyond Gerota fascia. It can involve multiple lymph nodes or spread to distant parts of the body, such as bones, brain, liver, or lung.

The treatment of choice for some kidney cancers is a partial nephrectomy (for smaller tumors), simple total nephrectomy, or a radical nephrectomy (for larger tumors). Radical nephrectomy involves removal of the kidney, adrenal gland, surrounding fascia, and draining lymph nodes. Nephrectomy can be done by a conventional (open) approach or laparoscopically. Other treatment options include cryoablation (freezing

TABLE 50.14 Interprofessional Care

Kidney Cancer

Diagnostic Assessment	Management

• History and physical assessment
• Urinalysis
• Ultrasound
• Abdominal CT scan
• MRI
• Renal biopsy
• Renal scan
	• Surgical therapy
	  • Partial nephrectomy
	  • Radical nephrectomy
	• Ablation
	  • Cryoablation
	  • Radiofrequency ablation
	• Immunotherapy
	• Targeted therapy

technique) and radiofrequency ablation (destroying the tumor by using radiofrequency heat). These procedures can be used when surgery is not an option (e.g., patient has comorbid conditions) and for small renal tumors.

Kidney cancer is relatively resistant to most chemotherapy drugs. Although kidney cancer can be resistant to radiation therapy, such therapy may be useful in certain situations, such as metastasis to bone, brain, or lungs.

Immunotherapy, including α-interferon and interleukin-2 (IL-2), is a treatment option in metastatic disease (see Chapter 16). Another drug used as immunotherapy is nivolumab (Opdivo) without or with ipilimumab (anti–CTLA-4 antibody). Nivolumab targets PD-1, a protein on T cells that normally helps keep these cells from attacking other cells in the body. By blocking PD-1, this drug boosts the immune response against cancer cells. This can shrink some tumors or slow their growth.

Targeted therapy is another treatment option for metastatic kidney cancer. Kinase inhibitors, a class of targeted therapies, block certain proteins (kinases) that play a role in tumor growth and cancer progression. Bevacizumab (Avastin) inhibits the formation of new blood vessel growth to the tumor. Temsirolimus (Torisel) and everolimus (Afinitor) inhibit a specific protein known as the *mechanistic target of rapamycin* (mTOR).[20] These drugs are discussed in Table 16.12. The mechanisms of action are shown in Fig. 16.16.

The diagnosis of kidney cancer is devastating. Often the cancer has already metastasized by the time a person is diagnosed. See more about the care of patients with cancer in Chapter 16.

BLADDER CANCER

Bladder cancer is the most common cancer of the urinary system.[21] About 83,730 new cases are diagnosed each year. About 17,240 deaths occur every year. Ninety percent of cases occur in those over the age of 55. It is far more common in males and in White persons.[22] Some bladder tumors are benign growths.

Urothelial cancer, or transitional cell cancer (TCC), is by far the most common type of bladder cancer. TCC can easily spread to other urinary tract areas given that the mucosal lining throughout the urinary tract is the same. Cancer recurrence within the bladder is common.

About half of bladder cancers are related to cigarette smoking.[21] Other risk factors include exposure to certain chemicals, treatment with pelvic radiation for cancer, having received cyclophosphamide or aristolochic acid, and having an indwelling catheter for long periods. People with chronic, recurrent urinary tract stones, often in the bladder, and chronic lower UTIs have an increased risk for nonurethral bladder cancer such as squamous cell carcinoma.

Clinical Manifestations and Diagnostic Studies

Microscopic or gross, painless hematuria (chronic or intermittent) is the most common manifestation. Bladder irritability with dysuria, frequency, and urgency are other early symptoms.

When cancer is suspected, the patient has a urologic workup. This includes obtaining urine specimens to identify any cancer cells. Exfoliated cells from the bladder's epithelial surface are often found in voided specimens. Urine cytology and testing for bladder tumor antigens can be done. CT without and with contrast is the recommended study of choice. Alternatively, IV pyelogram and MRI are options. Cancer is confirmed by cystoscopy and biopsy.[23]

Interprofessional and Nursing Management

Most bladder cancers are diagnosed at an early stage when the disease is treatable. Before starting treatment, bladder cancers are graded based on the cell type and staged based on the extent and invasiveness of the cancer. We use a grading system to classify the cancerous potential of tumor cells, using a scale from well differentiated (closely resembling the normal tissue) to undifferentiated (poorly differentiated).

Clinical staging is based on the depth of invasion of the bladder wall and surrounding tissue (Fig. 50.8). The following is a simple description of staging of bladder cancer:

Stage I: Cancer is in the inner lining of the bladder but has not invaded the bladder muscle wall.

Stage II: Cancer has invaded the bladder wall but is still confined to the bladder.

Stage III: Cancer has spread through the bladder wall to surrounding tissue.

Stage IV: Cancer has spread to the bowels, prostate, vagina, and/or uterus.

Interprofessional care of bladder cancer includes surgery, radiation, chemotherapy, targeted therapy, immunotherapy, and intravesical therapy (Table 50.15).

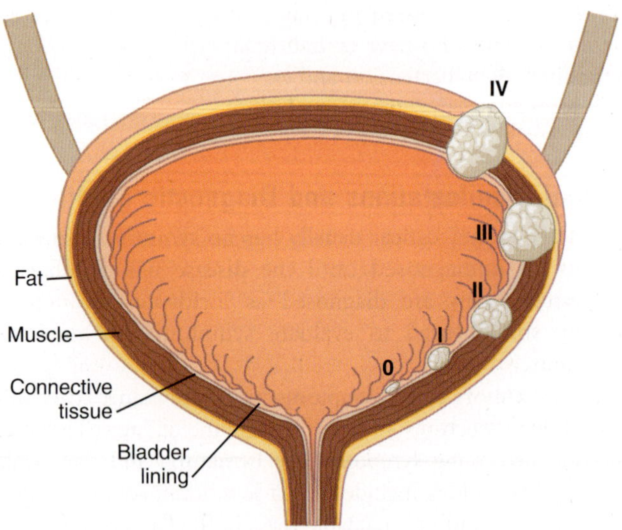

Stages of Bladder Cancer

IV
III
II
I
0
Fat
Muscle
Connective tissue
Bladder lining

Fig. 50.8 Stages of bladder cancer.

TABLE 50.15 Interprofessional Care

Bladder Cancer

Diagnostic Assessment
- History and physical assessment
- Urinalysis
- Urine cytology studies
- Cystoscopy with biopsy
- CT scan

Management
- Surgical therapy
  - Transurethral resection of bladder tumor
  - Partial cystectomy
  - Radical cystectomy
- Radiation therapy
- Immunotherapy
- Targeted drug therapy
- Intravesical immunotherapy
  - Bacille Calmette-Guérin (BCG)
  - α-interferon (Intron A)
- Intravesical chemotherapy
  - epirubicin
  - gemcitabine
  - mitomycin
  - valrubicin
- Systemic chemotherapy and immunotherapy

Surgical Therapy

Surgical therapy includes a variety of procedures. *Transurethral resection of the bladder tumor* (TURBT) is used for superficial lesions of the bladder's inner lining. The HCP uses a wire loop inserted through the cystoscope or a resectoscope with an attached loop to remove the tumor and tissue, which are sent for pathologic evaluation. After the tumor is removed, the tissue in the area where the tumor was may be burned. This is called *fulguration*. Cells can also be destroyed with a high-energy laser. Those with a low- or intermediate-risk tumor may get a one-time dose of intravesical chemotherapy in the immediate postoperative period. Repeat TURBT is often done 6 weeks later for those with higher-grade tumors. The primary disadvantages of TURBT include the chance of incomplete removal of the tumor, bleeding, and bladder perforation.[24]

A *segmental cystectomy (partial cystectomy)* is used to treat larger tumors or those that involve only 1 area of the bladder. The part of the bladder wall containing the tumor is removed along with a margin of normal tissue.

When the tumor is invasive and involves muscle, a radical cystectomy with urinary diversion is the treatment of choice. A *radical cystectomy* involves removal of the bladder, prostate, and seminal vesicles in males and the bladder, uterus, cervix, anterior vagina, and ovaries in females. After a radical cystectomy, a new way for urine to leave the body, or urinary diversion, must be created.

Postoperative instructions for these procedures include drinking a large volume of fluid for the first week afterward. Teach patients to monitor the color and consistency of the urine. Hematuria is common, but the blood in the urine should not contain clots and/or appear thick.

Give analgesics and stool softeners for a brief period after the procedure. Help patients and caregivers cope with fears about cancer, surgery, and sexuality. Discuss the importance of regular follow-up care. Follow-up cystoscopies are done on a regular basis after surgery for bladder cancer.

Radiation Therapy, Chemotherapy, Targeted Therapy, and Immunotherapy

Radiation therapy can be used in combination with cystectomy or as the primary therapy when the cancer is inoperable or the patient refuses surgery. Chemotherapy is often used in combination with radiation. Targeted therapy includes fibroblast growth factor receptor (FGFR) inhibitors (e.g., erdafitinib) that affect proteins that help the cancer cells grow. Immunotherapy can be used to treat bladder cancer. Options include immune checkpoint inhibitors, PD-1 and PD-L1 inhibitors, and intravesical Bacillus Calmette-Guérin (BCG).

Intravesical Therapy

In intravesical therapy, chemotherapy or immunotherapy is placed directly into the bladder by a urethral catheter. The drug is then retained for 1 to 2 hours. During that time, patients may need to change position every 15 minutes so the solution washes over the entire bladder. The bladder must be empty before instillation. Intravesical therapy is usually given once per week for 6 to 12 weeks. Maintenance therapy after the initial induction regimen may be given.

BCG, a weakened strain of *Mycobacterium bovis,* is the treatment of choice for high-risk bladder tumors. It can also treat intermediate-risk tumors. BCG stimulates the immune system to attack the cancer cells. Interferon-alpha therapy may be given with BCG. Other intravesical chemotherapy options include mitomycin, epirubicin, gemcitabine, and valrubicin.

Most patients have irritative voiding symptoms and hematuria after intravesical therapy. BCG may cause flulike symptoms, increased urinary frequency, hematuria, and, rarely, systemic infection. Other side effects of chemotherapy (e.g., nausea, vomiting, hair loss) do not occur with intravesical chemotherapy.

Encourage patients to increase their daily fluid intake and quit smoking. Assess for a secondary UTI. Stress the need for routine urologic follow-up. Patients may have fears or concerns about sexual activity or bladder function that we must address. Because of the high rate of disease recurrence and progression in bladder cancer, follow-up is important.

BLADDER DYSFUNCTION

URINARY INCONTINENCE

Urinary incontinence (UI) is an involuntary leakage of urine. Although UI is more prevalent among older adults, it is not a natural consequence of aging. UI has a major effect on quality of life and contributes to emotional, social, and potential serious health problems, especially in older adults.

Etiology and Pathophysiology

UI occurs when bladder pressure exceeds urethral closure pressure. Anything that interferes with internal and/or external urethral sphincter control can result in UI. There are many risk factors for UI. These include obesity, BPH, smoking, recurrent UTIs, GU surgeries, vaginal delivery, impaired functional status, certain drugs, certain neurologic problems, and a family history of UI. Patients may have more than 1 type of UI (Table 50.16). The combination of stress and urge incontinence is called *mixed incontinence.*

Diagnostic Studies

The basic evaluation includes a focused history, physical assessment, and urinalysis. Obtain information about the onset of UI, factors that provoke urine leakage, any associated systemic symptoms, use of caffeine and alcohol, medications taken, and associated conditions. Pay special attention to factors known to produce transient UI, especially when the onset of urine loss is sudden. It may be useful to have patients keep a bladder log or voiding diary. Have them record the timing of urinations, episodes of urinary leakage, and frequency of nocturia for a minimum period of 3 to 7 days if possible. Nursing staff can keep this record if the person is in an inpatient or long-term care facility.

Begin the assessment by looking at general health and functional issues related to urination, including mobility, dexterity, and cognitive function. A pelvic examination may be done. Carefully inspect the perineal skin for signs of erosion or rashes related to UI. Is there any pelvic organ prolapse? Assess local innervation and pelvic floor muscle strength. Perform a digital examination of the pelvic floor muscle to assess for weakness or tension.

A urinalysis can identify factors contributing to transient UI (e.g., UTI, diabetes). A bladder stress test can be useful when we suspect stress incontinence. Measuring postvoid residual (PVR) urine may be of use. PVR volume is obtained by asking the patient to void, followed by catheterization or the use of a bladder ultrasound (preferably within 10 to 20 minutes).

Some patients have urodynamic testing. Imaging studies of the upper and lower urinary tract (e.g., ultrasound) and cystoscopy may also be done.

Interprofessional Care

Many cases of UI can be cured or significantly improved. Transient, reversible factors are first corrected, followed by management of the type of UI (Table 50.16). In general, we try less invasive treatments before more invasive ones (e.g., surgery). The choice of the initial treatment is patient specific, based on patient preference, the type and severity of UI, and associated anatomic defects.

Several behavior therapies may improve UI (Table 50.17). Pelvic floor muscle training (Kegel exercises) is used to treat UI, especially stress UI (Table 50.18).[25] Biofeedback can help patients identify, isolate, contract, and relax the pelvic muscles. Bladder training may help.

Drug Therapy

Drug therapy varies according to the UI type (Table 50.19). No drugs are approved to treat stress UI. In urge and reflex UI, however, drugs play a key role.

Anticholinergic drugs (muscarinic receptor blockers) block the action of acetylcholine at muscarinic receptors. They relax the bladder muscle and inhibit overactive detrusor contractions (Table 50.19). Side effects include dry mouth and eyes, constipation, blurred vision, and sleepiness.

OnabotulinumtoxinA (Botox) can be used to treat UI from detrusor overactivity. Botox is injected into the bladder. It results in bladder relaxation, an increase in its storage capacity, and a decrease in UI.

DRUG ALERT

Antimuscarinic Agents

- Overdosage can result in severe anticholinergic effects.
- These effects include constipation, decreased sweating, eye pain, blurred vision, and difficulty starting urination and/or completely emptying the bladder.

Surgical Therapy

Surgical techniques vary depending on the type of UI. Surgical correction of stress UI is aimed at making the urinary structures more receptive to intraabdominal pressure and augmenting the urethral resistance of the internal sphincter. It may involve repositioning the urethra and/or creating a backboard of support to stabilize the urethra and bladder neck and make them more receptive to changes in intraabdominal pressure.

Another technique for stress UI augments the urethral resistance of the intrinsic sphincter with a sling or periurethral injectable. Placing a suburethral sling, typically midurethral, using the person's own fascia or a synthetic material, can correct stress UI in females. Complications include vascular and bowel injury, urinary retention, mesh or sling erosion, infection, urgency, and bladder perforation. Suburethral slings have better success rates compared with conservative therapy.

TABLE 50.16 Types of Urinary Incontinence

Description	Causes	Treatment
Functional Incontinence		
• Loss of urine resulting from cognitive, functional, environmental factors	• Neurologic and/or muscular limitations (e.g., severe arthritis) • Cognitive problems (e.g., dementia) • Psychologic issues • Environment barriers	• Modify environment or care plan to promote regular, easy access to toilet and patient safety • Includes better lighting, ambulatory assistance, adaptive clothing, timed voiding, toileting equipment
Incontinence After Trauma or Surgery		
• In females, vesicovaginal or urethrovaginal fistula may occur • In males, inadequate urethral sphincter function, can lead to stress, urge, overflow, or mixed urinary incontinence	• Fistulas may occur as a complication of pregnancy and delivery of baby, after hysterectomy or invasive cancer of cervix, or after radiation therapy • Postoperative complication of radical prostatectomy, and rarely transurethral resection of the prostate	• External condom catheter • External female catheter • Penile clamp • Sling surgery (male) • Surgery to correct fistula • Periurethral balloons
Overflow Incontinence		
• Pressure of urine in overfull bladder overcomes sphincter control and/or detrusor underactivity • Leakage of small amounts of urine is frequent or continual throughout day and night • Concurrent incomplete bladder emptying • Bladder can stay distended and is usually palpable	• Bladder or urethral outlet obstruction (bladder neck obstruction, urethral stricture, pelvic organ prolapse) or by underactive detrusor muscle caused by myogenic or neurogenic factors (e.g., herniated disc, diabetic neuropathy) • May occur after pelvic floor surgery • Neurogenic bladder (flaccid type)	• Urinary catheterization to decompress bladder • α-Adrenergic blockers (Table 50.20) • 5α-Reductase inhibitors (Table 50.20) to decrease outlet resistance • Bethanechol to enhance bladder contractions • Intermittent catheterization • Intravaginal device, such as a pessary, to support prolapse • Surgery to correct underlying problem
Reflex Incontinence		
• Occurs with no warning, periodic involuntary urination • Urination can be frequent, large in volume • Occurs equally during day and night	• CNS problems, including multiple sclerosis, brain tumor, stroke, Parkinson disease, spinal cord injury	• Treat underlying cause • Intermittent self-catheterization • Behavior therapy including bladder training, pelvic floor muscle exercises • Drug therapy includes anticholinergics, β3-adrenergic agonist, tricyclic antidepressants, topical estrogen (females)
Stress Incontinence		
• Sudden increase in intraabdominal pressure causes involuntary passage of urine • Can occur during coughing, laughing, sneezing, or physical activities, such as heavy lifting, exercising • Leakage usually is in small amounts and may not be daily	• Most common in female with relaxed pelvic floor musculature (from delivery, use of instrumentation during vaginal delivery, multiple pregnancies) • Structures of female urethra atrophy when estrogen decreases • After benign prostatic hyperplasia or prostate cancer surgery	• Pelvic floor muscle exercises (e.g., Kegel exercises), weight loss if obese, topical estrogen products, transurethral bulking agents, surgery • Continence pessary • Duloxetine
Urge Incontinence		
• Overactive bladder • Occurs randomly when urgency precedes involuntary urination • Leakage is periodic but can be frequent and varies in amount • Nocturnal frequency and incontinence common	• Uncontrolled contraction or overactive detrusor muscle • Bladder escapes central inhibition and contracts reflexively • Conditions include: • CNS problems (e.g., stroke, Alzheimer disease, brain tumor, Parkinson disease) • Bladder disorders (e.g., cancer, radiation effects, interstitial cystitis) • Interference with spinal inhibitory pathways (e.g., cancer in spinal cord, spondylosis) • Bladder outlet obstruction	• Treat underlying cause • Biobehavior interventions (bladder retraining with urge suppression, decrease in diet irritants, bowel regularity, pelvic floor muscle exercises) • Anticholinergic drugs (Table 50.20) • mirabegron (Myrbetriq) • Vaginal estrogen creams • Containment devices (e.g., external condom catheters or external female catheters) • Absorbent products

TABLE 50.17 Interventions for Urinary Incontinence

Intervention	Description
Lifestyle changes	• Self-management to reduce or eliminate risk factors, including: • Smoking cessation • Weight reduction • Bowel regimen • Reduce intake of bladder irritants (e.g., caffeine, aspartame artificial sweetener, citrus juices) • Fluid modifications for urge incontinence
Scheduled Voiding Regimens	
Bladder retraining and urge-suppression strategies	• Scheduled toileting with progressive voiding intervals. • Teach urge control using relaxation and distraction techniques, self-monitoring, reinforcement techniques, other strategies, such as conscious contraction of pelvic floor muscles.
Habit retraining	• Scheduled toileting with adjustments of voiding intervals (longer or shorter) based on the person's voiding pattern.
Prompted voiding	• Scheduled toileting that requires prompts to void from a caregiver (typically every 3 h). • Used with operant conditioning to reward people for maintaining continence and toileting.
Timed voiding	• Toileting on a fixed schedule; typically every 2–3 h during waking hours.
Pelvic Floor Muscle Rehabilitation	
Biofeedback	• Feedback from vaginal pressure sensor about pelvic floor contractions.
Electrical stimulation	• Application of low-voltage electric current to sacral and pudendal afferent fibers through vaginal, anal, or surface electrodes. • Used to inhibit bladder overactivity and improve awareness, contractility, and efficiency of pelvic muscle contraction.
Pelvic floor muscle (Kegel) exercises or training	• See Table 50.18.
Vaginal weight training	• Active retention of vaginal weights (devices designed and shaped to exercise and strengthen pelvic floor muscles) at least twice a day. • Typically used with pelvic floor muscle exercises.
Antiincontinence Devices	
Incontinence clamps (penile compression devices)	• Mechanical fixed compression applied to the penis to prevent any flow or leakage via the urethra. • Must be released to void.
Intraurethral occlusive device (urethral plug)	• Device worn in the urethra to provide mechanical obstruction to prevent urine leakage. • Removed for voiding and after several hours of wearing.
Intraurethral valve pump	• Replaceable urinary prosthesis in females who have impaired detrusor contractility (cannot contract muscles to push urine out of the bladder). • Draws urine out to empty bladder and blocks urine flow when continence is desired.
Intravaginal support devices (pessaries)	• Devices support bladder neck, relieve minor pelvic organ prolapse, and change pressure transmission to the urethra.
Containment Devices	
Absorbent products	• Variety of reusable and disposable pads and undergarment systems.
External collection devices	• Male external catheter (condom) systems (e.g., penile sheaths) direct urine into a drainage bag. • Female external catheters: Soft, flexible wick is seated between the labia and uses suction to direct urine into a collecting device.

A bulking agent can be injected underneath the mucosa of the urethra to correct stress UI. Bulking agents include glutaraldehyde cross-linked bovine collagen (GAX collagen), autologous fat, carbon beads, carbon hydroxylapatite, and polydimethylsiloxane injections. Although treatment with bulking agents avoids the risk from open surgery, reinjection is typically needed after several years.

In artificial urethral sphincter surgery, the bladder sphincter that no longer works is replaced with an artificial one. An inflatable cuff is placed around the urethra internally. Patients inflate it to stop the flow and deflate it when the need to empty occurs. Patients must be able to work the internal pump. It is usually done in males. This procedure is done only as a last resort.[26]

❖ NURSING MANAGEMENT: URINARY INCONTINENCE

It is important to recognize the physical and emotional problems from UI. Maintain and enhance the patient's dignity, privacy, and feelings of self-worth. This involves a 2-step

TABLE 50.18 PATIENT & CAREGIVER TEACHING

Pelvic Floor Muscle (Kegel) Exercises

Include the following instructions when teaching the patient to perform Kegel exercises:

What Are the Pelvic Floor Muscles?

- Your pelvic floor muscles provide support for your bladder and rectum and, in females, the vagina and uterus.
- If the muscles weaken or are damaged, they cannot support these organs and their position can change.
- This causes problems with the normal bladder and rectal function.
- If you have weak pelvic floor muscles, you may want to do special exercises to make the muscles stronger, prevent unwanted urine leakage, and lessen urinary urgency.

Finding the Pelvic Floor Muscles

- Without tensing the muscles of your leg, buttocks, or abdomen, imagine that you are trying to control the passing of gas or pinching off a stool.
- Imagine you are in an elevator full of people and feel the urge to pass gas. What do you do?
- You tighten or pull in the ring of muscle around your rectum.
- You should feel a lifting sensation in the area around the vagina or a pulling in of your rectum.

How to Do the Exercises

1. Squeeze the pelvic floor muscles.
2. Hold the muscle contraction for 3–5 seconds, building up over time to longer and harder contractions.
3. Relax the pelvic floor muscles for 3–5 seconds.

Do these exercises 10 times at 3 different times of the day each day.

When to Do These Exercises

- You can do these exercises anytime and anywhere.
- You can do these exercises in any position, but sitting or lying down may be the easiest.

How Long Does It Take Before I Notice a Change?

- After a few weeks or months of doing these exercises, you should start to see less urine leakage and urinary urgency.

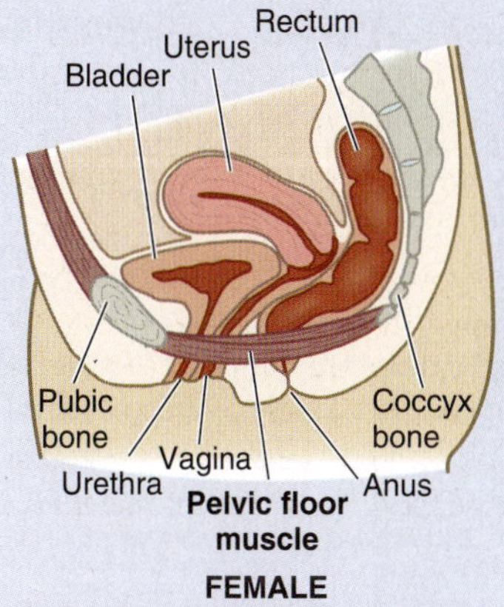

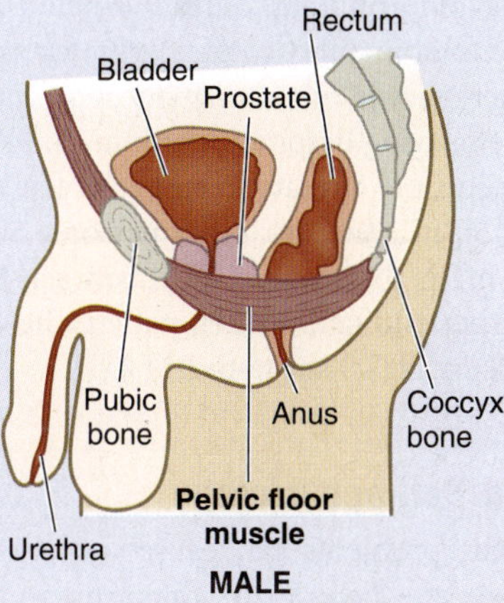

(Courtesy Diane Newman.)

approach with (1) containment devices to manage existing urinary leakage and (2) a plan to reduce or resolve the factors leading to UI.

CHECK YOUR PRACTICE

You are doing BP and glucose screening at the community senior center. While you are checking the BP on a 78-year-old female, she starts to sob quietly. You tell her that her BP is 134/84 and gently place your hand on her arm. You ask her what is wrong. She tells you, "I have to pee all the time. I soak the bed, and my husband won't sleep with me anymore. I am washing sheets and my clothes all the time. Our whole house smells like urine."

- How would you respond to her?

Management options are shown in Tables 50.17 and 50.18. Behavior treatments include scheduled voiding regimens (timed voiding, habit training, prompted voiding), bladder retraining, and pelvic floor muscle training. Have patients maintain a regular, flexible schedule of urination, usually every 3 to 4 hours while awake. In inpatient or long-term care facilities, maximize toilet access. This may take the form of offering the urinal or bedpan or helping patients to the bathroom every 3 to 4 hours or at scheduled times. Ensure that toilets are accessible to patients and provide privacy to allow effective urine elimination.

Assess how the patient contains urine and offer alternatives if needed (Table 50.20). Many females use feminine hygiene pads. Some use household products, such as rags, paper towels, or folded toilet tissue. Unfortunately, none of these products wicks urine away from the skin, prevents soiling of clothing, and eliminates odor. Provide information on products specifically designed to contain urine. For example,

TABLE 50.19 Drug Therapy

Voiding Dysfunction

Class and Mechanism of Action	Drug
α-Adrenergic Blockers	
Reduce urethral sphincter resistance to urinary outflow	alfuzosin (Uroxatral) doxazosin (Cardura) phenoxybenzamine (Dibenzyline) prazosin (Minipress) silodosin (Rapaflo) tamsulosin (Flomax) terazosin (Hytrin)
5α-Reductase Inhibitors	
Suppress androgen resulting in epithelial atrophy and decrease in prostate size	dutasteride (Avodart) finasteride (Proscar)
β_3-Adrenergic Agonist	
Improve bladder storage capacity by relaxing bladder muscle during filling	mirabegron (Myrbetriq)
Anticholinergics (Muscarinic Receptor Blockers)	
Reduce overactive bladder contractions in urge incontinence	darifenacin (Enablex) fesoterodine (Toviaz)
Relax bladder muscle during filling and improve the storage capacity of bladder	oxybutynin (Ditropan, Oxytrol Transdermal System) solifenacin (Vesicare) tolterodine (Detrol, Detrol LA) trospium (Sanctura)
Hormone Therapy	
Local application reduces urethral irritation and increases host defenses against UTI	estrogen cream (Premarin) estrogen vaginal ring (Estring)
Serotonin-Norepinephrine Reuptake Inhibitor	
Unclear mechanism, decreases urinary incontinence in some patients	duloxetine (Cymbalta)
Tricyclic Antidepressants	
Reduce sensory urgency and burning pain of interstitial cystitis Reduce overactive bladder contractions	amitriptyline (Elavil) imipramine (Tofranil)

patients with mild to moderate UI often benefit from incontinent pads containing superabsorbent material, designed to absorb many times their weight in water. Patients with higher-volume urine loss or those with urinary and fecal incontinence may need disposable or reusable incontinence-protective underwear, briefs, or pad/pant systems. External catheters may be a consideration for continued incontinence care.

Provide teaching about lifestyle interventions. Tell patients to consume an adequate volume of fluids and reduce or eliminate bladder irritants, especially caffeine and alcohol, from the diet. Advise patients to quit smoking because it increases the risk for stress UI. Teach patients about the relationships among constipation, UI, and urinary retention. Management of constipation is recommended. Begin with ensuring adequate fluid intake, increasing fiber, lightly exercising, and judiciously using stool softeners (see Chapter 47).

TABLE 50.20 NURSING MANAGEMENT

Caring for the Patient With Incontinence

- Assess for risk factors for UI or urinary retention.
- Determine type of UI that patient has.
- Develop plan of care to decrease UI (Table 50.17).
- Teach patients ways to decrease UI, such as pelvic floor muscle (Kegel) exercises (Table 50.18).
- Assist patients in choosing products to contain urine.
- Use bladder scanner to estimate the postvoid residual volume (PVR).
- Catheterize patients and measure PVR.
- Give medications to decrease UI or urinary retention.
- Supervise AP:
  - Help patients with toileting at regular intervals.
  - Clean patient and provide skin care.
  - Notify RN about new-onset UI in a previously continent patient.

URINARY RETENTION

Urinary retention is the inability to empty the bladder when a person voids or the accumulation of urine in the bladder because of an inability to void. In some cases, there is urinary leakage or postvoid dribbling, called *overflow UI. Acute urinary retention* is the total inability to pass urine via micturition. It is a medical emergency. *Chronic urinary retention* is an incomplete bladder emptying despite urination. The PVR volumes in patients with chronic urinary retention vary widely. Normal PVR is under 50 mL and, for older persons, 50 to 100 mL. A PVR over 200 mL is abnormal. A PVR between 100 and 200 mL can justify further evaluation when patients have issues such as recurring UTIs or LUTS suggestive of UTI.

Etiology and Pathophysiology

Several different problems can cause urinary retention. The most common are neurologic impairment, bladder outlet obstruction, and deficient detrusor (bladder muscle) contraction strength. *Bladder outlet obstruction* leads to urinary retention when the blockage is so severe that the bladder can no longer evacuate its contents despite a detrusor contraction. A common cause of obstruction in males is an enlarged prostate.

Deficient detrusor contraction strength leads to urinary retention when the muscle is no longer able to contract with enough force or for enough time to completely empty the bladder. Common causes include neurologic impairment, diabetic neuropathy, overdistention, chronic alcohol use, and drugs (e.g., anticholinergic drugs).

Diagnostic Studies

Diagnostic studies for urinary retention are similar to the ones used for UI. Other studies include PVR measurement, ultrasound, urodynamic evaluation, video urodynamic evaluation, cystourethroscopy, and electromyography.

Interprofessional Care

Behavior therapies for UI may be used in managing urinary retention. Scheduled toileting and double voiding may be effective in chronic urinary retention with moderate PVR volumes. *Double voiding* is an attempt to maximize bladder evacuation. The patient is asked to void, sit on the toilet for 3 to 4 minutes, and void again before exiting the bathroom.

Catheterization may be needed. Intermittent catheterization allows patients to remain free of an indwelling catheter with its associated risk of CAUTI and urethral irritation. In some situations, an indwelling catheter is preferred (e.g., if a patient is unwilling or unable to perform intermittent catheterization). An indwelling catheter is used when urethral obstruction makes intermittent catheterization uncomfortable or infeasible.

Drug Therapy

Several drugs may be given to promote bladder evacuation. For patients with dysfunctional voiding, an α-adrenergic blocker may be prescribed. These drugs relax the smooth muscle of the bladder neck and prostatic urethra and may decrease urethral resistance. Examples of α-adrenergic blockers are listed in Table 50.20. They are given to patients with BPH and may help with bladder neck or detrusor sphincter dyssynergia (muscle incoordination).

Surgical Therapy

Surgical interventions are used to manage retention from an obstruction. Transurethral or open surgical techniques are used to treat benign or cancerous prostatic enlargement, bladder neck contracture, urethral strictures, or dyssynergia of the bladder neck. Pelvic reconstruction using an abdominal or transvaginal approach can correct bladder outlet obstruction in females with severe pelvic organ prolapse.

Although surgery has had a minimal role in managing urinary retention caused by deficient detrusor contraction strength, there are procedures that may help. Sacral neuromodulation involves a stimulator device and placement of a lead wire into the S3 foramen. Placement of an intraurethral valve pump, which empties the bladder on command, may be another option.

❖ NURSING MANAGEMENT: URINARY RETENTION

Acute urinary retention is a medical emergency that requires prompt recognition and bladder drainage. Insert a catheter as ordered. Use a catheter with a retention balloon in anticipation of the need for an indwelling catheter.

Teach patients with acute urinary retention and patients predisposed to these episodes ways to minimize risk. Have them pay attention to when they need to urinate and to void when they feel the need to do so. Take medications as prescribed. Pelvic floor muscle exercises may help. Teach patients to drink small amounts throughout the day and avoid the intake of large volumes of fluid over a brief period. Tell patients (if chilled) to warm up before trying to void. They should avoid excess alcohol use because it leads to polyuria and a diminished awareness of the need to void until the bladder is distended. Tell patients that sitting in a tub of warm water or taking a warm shower may help them void. If these measures do not lead to successful urination, have patients seek immediate care.

Chronic urinary retention may be managed by behavior methods, indwelling or intermittent catheterization, surgery, or drugs. Scheduled toileting and double voiding are the main behavior interventions used for chronic retention. Scheduled toileting can reduce, rather than expand, bladder capacity. In this case have patients void every 3 to 4 hours regardless of the desire to void. This is especially useful in patients with chronic overdistention, diabetes, or chronic alcohol use with a large bladder capacity and diminished or delayed sensations of bladder filling and urgency.

CATHETERIZATION

INDICATIONS FOR AND COMPLICATIONS OF CATHETERIZATION

Urinary catheterization can be used in managing hospitalized patients. Indications for short-term urinary catheterization are listed in Table 50.21. Catheterization for sterile urine specimens

TABLE 50.21 Indications for Urinary Catheterization

Indwelling Catheter
- Relieve urinary retention caused by lower urinary tract obstruction, paralysis, or inability to void
- Bladder decompression preoperatively and operatively for lower abdominal or pelvic surgery
- Facilitate surgical repair of urethra and surrounding structures
- Splinting of ureters or urethra to promote healing after surgery or other trauma in area
- Accurate measurement of urine output
- Contamination of stage 3 or 4 pressure injuries with urine that has impeded healing, despite personal care for the incontinence
- Terminal illness or severe impairment, which makes positioning or clothing changes uncomfortable or which is associated with intractable pain

Intermittent (Straight, In-and-Out) Catheter
- Relieve urinary retention caused by lower urinary tract obstruction, paralysis, or inability to void
- Study of anatomic structures of urinary system
- Urodynamic testing
- Collect sterile urine sample in certain situations
- Instill medications into bladder
- Measure residual urine after voiding (postvoid residual [PVR]) if portable ultrasound not available

may be needed if patients have a history of complicated UTI. The risk for CAUTI is too high to perform catheterization for (1) routine acquisition of a urine specimen for laboratory analysis or (2) the convenience of the health care team or caregivers. A catheter should be the last resort to provide a dry environment to prevent skin breakdown and protect dressings or skin lesions.

Having a catheter is not without serious complications. Complications that are seen with long-term use (more than 28 days) of indwelling catheters include CAUTI, bladder spasms, periurethral abscess, chronic pyelonephritis, urosepsis, urethral trauma or erosion, fistula or stricture formation, and stones. CAUTIs are the most common HAI (Box 50.2).

Aseptic technique is mandatory when inserting a urinary catheter (Table 50.22). After insertion, maintaining the closed drainage system and preventing infection are major nursing responsibilities. Do not routinely irrigate the catheter. Only irrigate if ordered. While the catheter is in place, manage fluid intake and provide for patient comfort. Address the psychologic implications of urinary drainage. Patient concerns can include embarrassment, an altered body image, and fear that care of the catheter will result in increased dependency.

CATHETER CONSTRUCTION

Catheters vary in construction materials, size of the lumen, and tip shape (Fig. 50.9). Catheter materials include polyvinyl chloride, red rubber, silicone, and latex. Some are DEHP-free. Catheters coated with antimicrobial agents may prevent CAUTIs.

A coudé tip catheter is often used in males. We size catheters using the French scale. Each French unit (Fr) equals 0.33 mm of diameter. The diameter listed is the external diameter of the

BOX 50.2 EVIDENCE-BASED PRACTICE

Nurse-Driven Protocol for Catheter Removal

You are caring for M.B., a 42-year-old patient who had a total vaginal hysterectomy for dysfunctional uterine bleeding. She had an indwelling urinary catheter placed before surgery. On the 1st postoperative day, M.B. asks you when the catheter will be removed.

Making Clinical Decisions

Synthesis of Best Available Evidence

Catheter-associated urinary tract infections (CAUTI) lead to extended hospital stays, increased health care costs, and increased mortality. All patients undergoing catheterization of the urinary tract are at risk for developing CAUTI. Avoiding unnecessary catheterization and early removal of indwelling catheters are the most effective means for reducing CAUTI. Nurse-driven protocols for directed assessment of catheter need and decision for removal may be a way to decrease catheter days and CAUTI occurrence.

Clinician Expertise

As part of the unit's efforts to decrease occurrence of CAUTI, you receive education on daily assessment of specific indications for continued catheterization. In your agency, use of an indwelling catheter typically does not exceed 24 hours after a hysterectomy. You assess M.B. based on identified criteria and find the time appropriate for catheter removal. You explain the process to M.B. and remove the indwelling urinary catheter.

Patient Preferences

M.B. expresses concern about getting a UTI related to catheterization.

Implications for Nursing Practice

1. How would you explain the catheter removal protocol and its rationale to M.B.?
2. How can you demonstrate engagement with and ownership of this unit practice?

Reference for Evidence

Jones AE, Nagle C, Ahern T, et al: Evidence for a nurse-led protocol for removing urinary catheters: a scoping review, *Collegian* 30:190, 2023.

TABLE 50.22 NURSING MANAGEMENT

Care of the Patient With a Urethral Catheter

The following measures can be used to manage patients with a urethral catheter and prevent a catheter-associated urinary tract infection (CAUTI):

- Determine need for catheterization, but HCP must order.
- Choose catheter type and size.
- Implement measures to reduce the risk for CAUTI:
  - Insert catheter using sterile technique.
  - Maintain a sterile, closed drainage system.
  - Do not disconnect the distal urinary catheter and proximal drainage tube.
  - Use sterile technique whenever the collecting system is open. If frequent irrigations are needed in short-term catheterization to maintain catheter patency, a triple-lumen catheter may be preferable, permitting continuous irrigations within a closed system.
  - Remove the catheter as early as possible.
- Consider alternatives to indwelling catheterization, including intermittent catheterization and external catheters.
- Teach catheter care to the patient, especially one who is ambulatory.
- A routine catheter change is not needed if the patient is catheterized for less than 2 weeks. For long-term use of an indwelling catheter, replace the catheter based on patient assessment and not on a routine changing schedule.
- When ordered, aspirate small volumes of urine for culture from the catheter sampling port using a sterile syringe and needle. Prepare the puncture site with an antiseptic solution.
- With long-term use of a catheter, a leg bag may be used. If the collection bag is reused, wash it in soap and water and rinse thoroughly. When it is not reused immediately, fill it with ½ cup of vinegar and drain. Vinegar is effective against *Pseudomonas* and other organisms and eliminates odors.
- Ensure that AP:
  - Maintain unobstructed downhill flow of urine.
  - Empty the collecting bag regularly and accurately record the urine output.
  - Provide perineal care (once or twice a day and when needed), cleaning the meatus-catheter junction with soap and water.
  - Do not use lotion or powder near the catheter.
  - Apply a securement device. Anchor catheter to upper thigh in females and lower abdomen in males to prevent catheter movement and urethral tension.

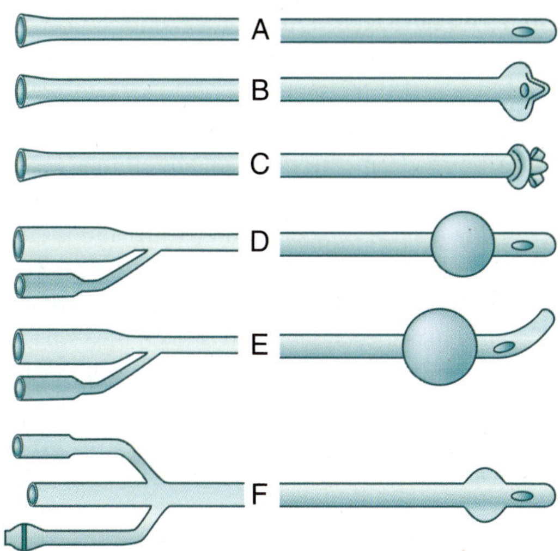

Fig. 50.9 Types of urinary catheters. (A) Simple urethral catheter. (B) Mushroom-tip de Pezzer catheter (can be for suprapubic catheterization). (C) Wing-tip Malecot catheter (wings hold catheter in place for temporary drainage). (D) Indwelling urethral catheter with inflated balloon. (E) Indwelling Tiemann catheter with coudé tip (slightly curved tip allows for passage past obstruction). (F) Three-way indwelling catheter (third lumen can be used for irrigation).

catheter. The size used varies with the patient's size and the purpose of catheterization. In females, urethral catheter sizes 10Fr to 12Fr are the most common. In males, the most common sizes are 14Fr to 16Fr. Balloon sizes are 5 or 30 mL. The primary problem from using too large a catheter is tissue erosion from excessive pressure on the meatus or urethra.

TYPES OF CATHETERS

Four routes are used for urinary tract catheterization: urethral, ureteral, suprapubic, and via a nephrostomy tube.

Urethral Catheterization

Urethral catheterization is the most common route of catheterization. It involves the insertion of a catheter through the external meatus into the urethra, past the internal sphincter, and into the bladder.

Ureteral Catheters

A *ureteral catheter* is often called a *ureteral stent*. It is placed through the ureters into the renal pelvis. The catheter is inserted by (1) being threaded up the urethra and bladder to the ureters under cystoscopic observation or (2) surgical insertion through the abdominal wall into the ureters. The ureteral catheter is used during surgery with removal immediately afterward or after surgery to splint the ureters and prevent them from being obstructed by edema.

A self-retaining ureteral catheter is often inserted after a lithotripsy procedure or when ureteral obstruction from adjacent tumors or fibrosis threatens renal function. They can be placed short- or long-term. When used long-term, we replace the catheter every 3 to 6 months. A double-J ureteral catheter is often used. It allows patients to ambulate. One end coils up in the kidney pelvis, and the other coils in the bladder.

Care of these catheters is similar to that of urethral catheters. Avoid situations that could cause catheter dislodgement or displacement. If the output is decreased, notify the HCP immediately.

Suprapubic Catheters

Suprapubic catheterization requires surgical placement. It is the oldest method of urinary diversion. The 2 ways to insert a suprapubic catheter are (1) through an open approach with a small incision made in the abdominal wall or (2) through a percutaneous approach. The catheter is placed under general anesthesia for another procedure or at the bedside with a local anesthetic. The catheter may be sutured into place. Tape the catheter to prevent dislodgment. Teaching includes the need to stay well hydrated and how to monitor for infection, catheter obstruction or kinking, and urinary leakage around the catheter.

Suprapubic catheters can be used short- or long-term. Common situations where a suprapubic catheter may be placed include acute urinary retention, urethra trauma, need for long-term urinary diversion, and to aid in treating a complicated UTI. The catheter should be changed at least monthly.

A suprapubic catheter is prone to poor drainage because of mechanical obstruction of the catheter tip by the bladder wall, sediment, and clots. To ensure patency of the tube, (1) prevent tube kinking by coiling the excess tubing and maintaining gravity drainage, (2) have the patient turn from side to side, and (3) milk the tube. If these measures are not effective, obtain an order from the HCP to irrigate the catheter using sterile technique.

If patients have bladder spasms that are hard to control, urinary leakage may result. Oxybutynin or solifenacin can decrease bladder spasms.

Nephrostomy Tubes

The *nephrostomy tube* (catheter) is typically inserted on a temporary basis but can be placed long-term to preserve renal function. Nephrostomy tubes are placed most often for urinary obstruction. The tube is inserted through a small flank incision directly into the pelvis of the kidney and attached to connecting tubing for closed drainage. The principle is the same as with other catheters—that is, the catheter should never be kinked, twisted, or tugged on. If patients have excess pain in the area or if there is excess drainage around the tube, check catheter patency. Use aseptic technique when performing irrigation. Gently instill no more than 5 mL of sterile saline solution at one time to prevent overdistention of the kidney pelvis and renal damage. Good wound care is critical. Infection, including pyelonephritis, is a common complication.

Intermittent Catheterization

An alternative approach to a long-term indwelling catheter is *intermittent catheterization,* often referred to as "straight" or "in-and-out" catheterization. The main goal of intermittent catheterization is to prevent urinary retention, stasis, and compromised blood supply to the bladder caused by prolonged pressure.[27]

It can be used short- or long-term and for conditions such as neurogenic bladder dysfunction (e.g., spinal cord injuries, chronic neurologic diseases). Barriers to intermittent catheterization include obesity, patient unwillingness, discomfort from the catheterization, urinary obstruction, and limited upper extremity strength and/or movement.

The technique consists of inserting a urethral catheter into the bladder every 4 to 6 hours, including first thing upon awakening and before going to bed. Some patients perform intermittent catheterization only once or twice a day to measure residual urine and ensure an empty bladder.

The techniques for intermittent catheterization vary. Catheters can be sterile (single use) or clean (multiple use). Research shows no evidence that any technique (sterile or clean), catheter type (coated or uncoated), method (single-use or multiple-use), person (self or other), or strategy is better than any other.

We often use sterile technique in the hospital or long-term care facility. Depending on agency policy, you may see clean technique used. Clean intermittent catheterization done correctly at home does not seem to increase the risk for UTIs and is more cost-effective. For home care, clean technique includes good hand washing with soap and water. Teach patients to wash and rinse the catheter before and after catheterization.

Using a lubricant makes catheterization more comfortable and minimizes trauma. Catheters come coated (prelubricated) or uncoated. Patients may prefer one type of catheter for use at home and another type while at work or during travel. Patients, caregivers, or HCPs may insert the catheter.

Teach patients to observe for signs of UTI so it can be treated early. Some patients receive prophylactic antibiotics. Complications include urethritis, urethral sphincter damage (especially if there is a forceful catheterization against a closed sphincter), urethral stricture, and creation of a false passage. Urethral damage from intermittent catheterization in males is similar to problems seen with indwelling catheterization.

URINARY TRACT SURGERY

RENAL AND URETERAL SURGERY

The most common indications for nephrectomy are a renal tumor, polycystic kidneys that are bleeding or severely infected, massive traumatic injury to the kidney, and the elective removal of a kidney for transplant into a person with ESRD. Surgery involving the ureters and kidneys can be done to remove stones that become obstructive, correct congenital anomalies, and divert urine when necessary. It is important that patients having a nephrectomy have 1 working kidney to maintain normal renal function.

Surgical Procedure

Nephrectomy can be done by a conventional (open) approach or laparoscopically. In the open approach, an incision of about 8 to 12 inches is made through several layers of muscle. The incision can be made in the flank or abdominal area. With a laparoscopic nephrectomy, there are 3 to 5 puncture sites. When removing a kidney for donation, 1 incision is enlarged to 6 to 9 cm so the kidney can be removed in 1 piece. The kidney can also be removed through morcellation. Once dissected, the kidney is placed in a special sac, then broken into smaller pieces before being removed. The laparoscopic approach is less painful, involves a shorter hospital stay, and has a faster recovery.

Nursing Care

The basic needs of patients having renal and ureteral surgery are similar to those of any patient who has surgery (see Chapters 18 and 20). Specific postoperative needs of patients are related to urine output, respiratory status, and abdominal distention.

Urine Output

In the immediate postoperative period, measure and record the urine output at least every 1 or 2 hours. Measure drainage from the various catheters and record it separately. Do not clamp or irrigate the catheter or tube without a specific order. The total urine output should be at least 0.5 mL/kg/h. It is important to assess for urine drainage on the dressing and to estimate this amount. Observe and monitor the color and consistency of urine. Urine with increased amounts of mucus, blood, or sediment may occlude the drainage tubing or catheter.

Obtain a daily weight. A significant change in daily weight can indicate fluid retention, which increases the risk for heart failure. Fluid retention can increase the work required of the remaining kidney to perform its functions.

Respiratory Status

A nephrectomy can be done through a flank incision just below the diaphragm. It is important to ensure adequate ventilation. Patients are often reluctant to turn, cough, and breathe deeply because of the incisional pain. Give adequate pain medication to ensure comfort and the ability to perform coughing and deep-breathing exercises. Have patients use an incentive spirometer every 2 hours while awake. Early and frequent ambulation helps maintain respiratory function.

Abdominal Distention

Abdominal distention is present to some degree in most patients who have had surgery on their kidneys or ureters. It is often the result of paralytic ileus caused by manipulation and compression of the bowel during surgery. We restrict oral intake until bowel sounds are present (usually 24 to 48 hours after surgery). Give IV fluids as ordered until oral intake resumes. Progression to a regular diet follows.

URINARY DIVERSION

Urinary diversion procedures are done when urine needs to be redirected from the bladder. Common reasons include bladder cancer, neurogenic bladder, congenital anomalies, strictures, bladder trauma, and chronic bladder inflammation. Numerous urinary diversion techniques and bladder substitutes are possible. These include an incontinent urinary diversion, a continent urinary diversion catheterized by the patient, or an orthotopic neobladder so that the patient voids urethrally.[28] Surgical procedures for urinary diversion are described in Table 50.23 and Fig. 50.10. Urinary diversion may be done with or without cystectomy.

TABLE 50.23 Urinary Diversion Surgery

Description	Advantages	Disadvantages	Special Considerations
Cutaneous Ureterostomy			
Ureters excised from bladder and brought through abdominal wall, and stoma is created. Ureteral stomas may be created from both ureters, or ureters may be brought together, and 1 stoma created.	No need for major surgery.	External pouch needed because of continuous urine drainage. Possible stricture or stenosis of small stoma.	Periodic catheterizations may be needed to dilate stomas to maintain patency.
Ileal Conduit			
Ureters implanted into part of ileum or colon that has been resected from GI tract. Abdominal stoma is created.	Relatively good urine flow with few physiologic alterations.	External pouch needed to continually collect urine.	Surgery is complex. Increased risk for complications. Metabolic complications include electrolyte imbalances. Meticulous attention necessary to care for stoma and collecting device.
Nephrostomy			
Catheter inserted into pelvis of kidney. May be done to 1 or both kidneys. May be temporary or permanent. Most often done in advanced disease as palliative procedure.	No need for major surgery.	High risk for renal infection.	May have to change nephrostomy tube every 10–12 wk. Never clamp the catheter.

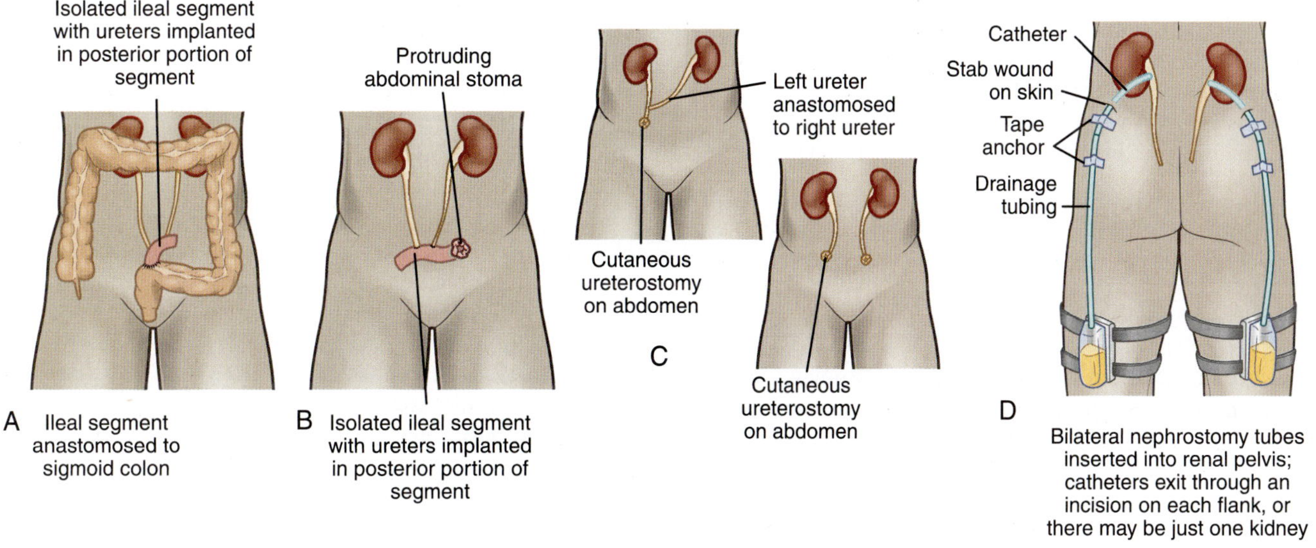

Fig. 50.10 Methods of urinary diversion. (A) Ureteroileosigmoidostomy. (B) Ileal loop (ileal conduit). (C) Ureterostomy (transcutaneous ureterostomy and bilateral cutaneous ureterostomies). (D) Nephrostomy.

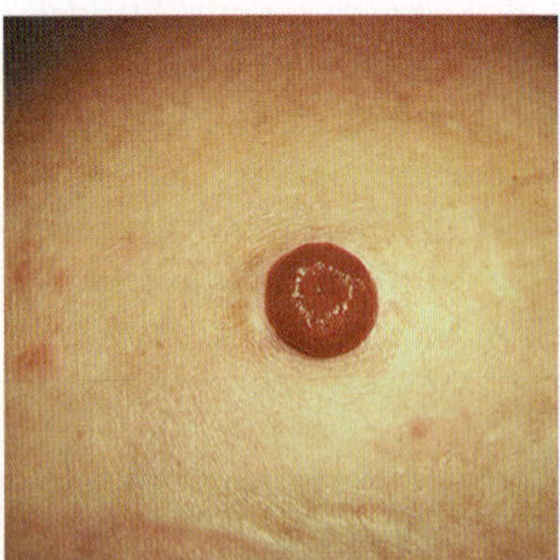

Fig. 50.11 Urinary stoma. Symmetric, no skin breakdown, protrudes about 1.5 cm. Mucosa is healthy red. This configuration is flat when the patient is upright or supine. (Courtesy Lynda Brubacher, Virginia Mason Hospital, Seattle, WA.)

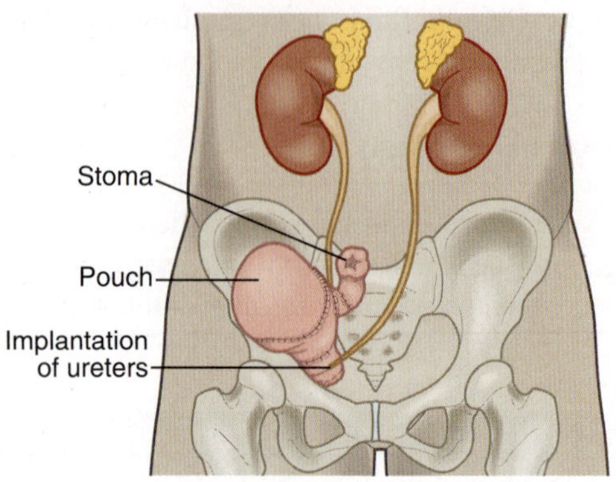

Fig. 50.12 Creation of a Kock pouch with implantation of ureters into one intussuscepted part of the pouch and creation of a stoma with the other intussuscepted part.

Incontinent Urinary Diversion

Incontinent urinary diversion is diversion to the skin, requiring a pouch. The simplest form is the cutaneous ureterostomy. However, complications (e.g., scarring, ureteral strictures) have led to the more frequent use of ileal or colonic conduits. The most common diversion procedure is the **ileal conduit** (ileal loop). In this procedure a 4- to 6-in (10- to 15-cm) segment of the ileum is converted into a conduit for urinary drainage. The colon (colon conduit) can also be used. The ureters are anastomosed into one end of the conduit. The other end of the bowel is brought out through the abdominal wall to form a stoma (Fig. 50.11). The bowel is anastomosed and continues to function normally.

Because there is no valve and no voluntary control over the stoma, drops of urine flow from the stoma every few seconds, requiring a permanent external collecting device. The visible stoma and need for external collection devices are disadvantages. The lifelong need to care for and deal with the stoma and collection devices may be difficult. These problems have led to the increasing use of continent diversions and neobladder substitutes.

Continent Urinary Diversions

A *continent urinary diversion* is an intraabdominal urinary reservoir that can be catheterized. Continent diversions are internal pouches created similarly to the ileal conduit. Reservoirs are constructed from the ileum, ileocecal segment, or ascending colon. Large segments of bowel are altered to prevent peristaltic action. A surgically created valve and the large, low-pressure reservoir help prevent involuntarily leakage. Patients with a continent reservoir need to self-catheterize every 4 to 6 hours but do not need to wear external attachments. Patients may wear a small bandage on the stoma to collect any mucous drainage or excess drainage. Examples of continent diversions are the Kock (Fig. 50.12), Indiana (most often used), and Miami pouches. The main difference among the diversions is the bowel segment used. For example, the Indiana pouch uses part of the ilium, cecum, and ascending colon as the reservoir.

Orthotopic Bladder Reconstruction

Orthotopic bladder reconstruction, or orthotopic neobladder, is the construction of a new bladder in the bladder's normal anatomic position, with discharge of urine through the urethra. The neobladder is surgically shaped from intestinal segments to make a low-pressure reservoir. An isolated segment of the terminal ileum is often used. The ureters and urethra are sutured into the neobladder. There are multiple procedure types based on the type of intestine and the construction technique used.

Orthotopic bladder reconstruction has become a more viable option if cancer does not involve the bladder neck or prostate apex. Ideal patients have normal renal and liver function, longer than 1- to 2-year life expectancy, adequate motor skills, and no history of inflammatory bowel disease or colon cancer. The advantage of an orthotopic bladder is that it allows for natural micturition. Incontinence is a possible problem. Intermittent catheterization may be needed.

❖ NURSING MANAGEMENT: URINARY DIVERSION

Preoperative Care

Teaching is important for patients and caregivers awaiting cystectomy and urinary diversion surgery. Assess their ability and readiness to learn before starting a teaching program. Anxiety and fear may be decreased by providing information. Discuss the psychosocial aspects of living with a stoma. This may calm some fears. Additional interventions are discussed in eNursing Care Plan 50.3 for patients with an ileal conduit (on the website for this chapter).

Postoperative Care

Plan interventions during the postoperative period to prevent surgical complications, such as atelectasis (see Chapter 20). After pelvic surgery, there is an increased incidence of thrombophlebitis and UTI. Removing part of the bowel increases the

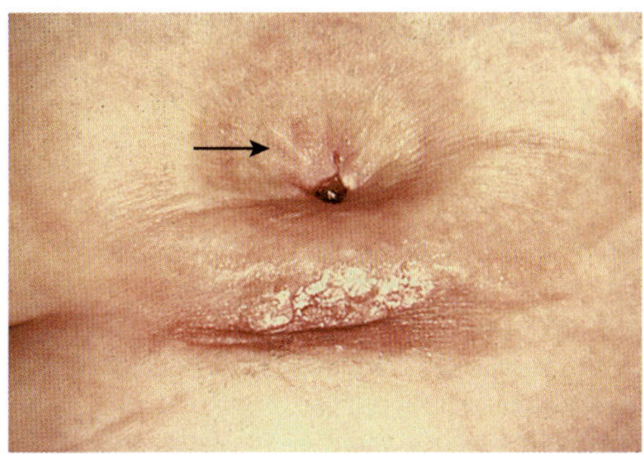

Fig. 50.13 Retracted urinary stoma with pressure injury from faceplate above stoma *(arrow)*. (Courtesy Lynda Brubacher, Virginia Mason Hospital, Seattle, WA.)

risk of paralytic ileus and small bowel obstruction. Patients are NPO. They may need a nasogastric tube for a few days.

Prevent injury to the stoma and maintain urine output. Mucus in the urine is normal. The mucus is secreted by the mucosa of the intestine (used to create the ileal conduit) in response to the irritating effect of urine. Encourage a high fluid intake to "flush" the ileal conduit or continent diversion and prevent obstruction.

Provide meticulous care for the skin around the stoma. Alkaline encrustations with dermatitis may occur when alkaline urine comes in contact with exposed skin. The urine is often kept slightly acidic to prevent alkaline encrustations. Other common peristomal skin problems include yeast infections, product allergies, and shearing-effect excoriations.

Patients are fitted for a pouching system to collect urine passed out of the stoma. It may be refitted later, depending on the degree of stoma healing and shrinkage. There are 2 types of pouching systems. There is a 1-piece pouch that has an attached skin barrier. The other type is a 2-piece system composed of a skin barrier with a detachable pouch. A properly fitting pouch helps prevent skin problems (Fig. 50.13). The pouch should be more than $\frac{1}{8}$ inch (3 mm) larger than the stoma. It is normal for the stoma to shrink within the first few weeks after surgery. Table 50.24 describes how to change the pouch.

Teach patients with a continent diversion (e.g., Indiana pouch) to catheterize at first every few hours. Over time this can be extended to every 4 to 6 hours. Irrigation of the pouch with normal saline or sterile water is often needed.

Patients with a neobladder may have postoperative urinary retention and need catheterization. They may have problems with incontinence, especially nocturnal. It may take up to 6 months to gain bladder control. Patients empty their neobladders by relaxing their outlet sphincter muscles and bearing down with their abdominal muscles. Because there is no longer neurologic feedback between the reservoir and the brain, patients should not expect a normal desire to void. To avoid bladder overdistention, patients should void at least every 2 to 3 hours, sit during voiding, and practice pelvic floor muscle relaxation to aid voiding.

Discharge teaching includes teaching about symptoms of obstruction and infection and care of the ostomy. Follow-up with an HCP is important to monitor recovery, detect complications, and assess renal function. Acceptance of the surgery and changes in body image ensures the best adjustment to a urinary diversion. Concerns include fear that the stoma will be offensive to others and will interfere with sexual, personal, professional, and recreational activities. Teach patients that few activities will be restricted because of the urinary diversion.

Discuss the psychosocial aspects of living with a stoma. Include clothing options, exercise, and odor control. Discuss concerns about sexual activity, and let them know that counseling is available. Tell patients and caregivers about where to buy supplies, emergency telephone numbers, and follow-up visits with a wound, ostomy, and continence nurse (WOCN). A visit from or meeting and sharing feelings with similar patients in a support group can help.

TABLE 50.24 PATIENT & CAREGIVER TEACHING

Ileal Conduit Appliances

Include the following instructions when teaching a patient or a caregiver how to change an ileal conduit appliance:

Temporary

1. Cut hole in pouch to fit over stoma (pouch 0.1 in [0.2 cm] larger than stoma).
2. Remove old pouch.
3. Clean area gently and remove old adhesive.
4. Wash area with warm water.
5. Place wick (rolled-up 4 × 4–in pad) over stoma to keep area dry during rest of procedure.
6. Dry skin around stoma.
7. Unless recommended by ostomy nurse or HCP, avoid using creams or powders on the skin around the stoma.
8. Apply pouch by first smoothing its edges toward side and lower part of body.
9. Remove wick and complete application of pouch.
   - If patient is usually in bed, apply pouch so that it lies toward side of body.
   - If patient is ambulatory, apply pouch so that it lies vertically.
10. Connect drainage tubing to pouch.
11. Keep drainage pouch on same side of bed as stoma.

Permanent

1. Keep pouch in place for 3–4 days. May need to be changed more or less often as needed.
2. Change pouch when fluid intake has been restricted for several hours.
3. Sit or stand in front of mirror.
4. Can moisten edge of faceplate with warm water or adhesive solvent and gently remove.
5. Use warm water and a washcloth to clear the skin around the stoma. Use soap to remove any adhesive solvent.
6. Dry skin and inspect.
7. Place wick (rolled-up 4 × 4–inch pad) over stoma to keep skin free of urine.
8. Place pouch over stoma.

CASE STUDY

Painful Bladder and Frequent Urination

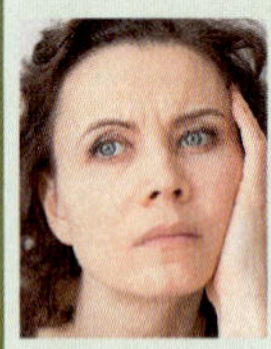
(© marilook/ iStock/ Thinkstock.)

Patient Profile

L.T., a 38-year-old female, comes to the HCP's office today for the 8th time in the past year for a history of pelvic pain with urinary frequency during the day, nocturia, and urgency to void. All previous urine cultures were negative for bacteria. A recent evaluation by her gynecologist was negative for endometriosis.

Subjective Data

- Has a history of suprapubic and vaginal pain, urinary frequency, and urgency
- Reports bladder pain that increases with bladder filling
- States this is her 3rd attack of suprapubic pain and painful urination in 2 months
- Constant pain and discomfort that are physically and emotionally exhausting
- Worried that she has cancer and no one cares
- Had 4 pregnancies with uneventful vaginal deliveries
- Normal menstrual cycles
- Her husband and she rarely have sexual intercourse because she has pain with intercourse
- Has a bowel movement every day; denies constipation and/or diarrhea
- Recalls having many UTIs as a child

Objective Data

Physical Assessment

- Lungs clear. Temp 36.6°C (97.9°F). BP 132/86. Heart rate 86/min. Respiratory rate 18/min. Abdomen soft, tender in suprapubic region.

Diagnostic Studies

- Urinalysis today: normal
- Previous urine cytology ordered to rule out cancer: normal
- Recent referral to urologist for cystoscopy, which was done 2 weeks ago

Interprofessional Care

- Cystoscopy results show glomerulations and Hunner lesions
- Urologist diagnosed interstitial cystitis
- Urologist prescribed pentosan, which she has not started yet
- Follow-up in 4 weeks with the urologist

Discussion Questions

1. ***Recognize:*** After taking L.T.'s history, would you consider a UTI as a cause of her symptoms? Why or why not?
2. ***Analyze:*** What further testing and assessment would be helpful?
3. ***Analyze:*** What is the significance of the cystoscopy findings?
4. ***Analyze:*** What is the reason for giving pentosan?
5. ***Prioritize:*** What are the priority clinical problems?
6. ***Plan:*** How would you involve the dietitian in L.T.'s care?
7. ***Act:*** How can you help L.T. deal with her diagnosis and treatment plan?
8. ***Act:*** L.T. asks you how she can control her interstitial cystitis. How would you respond?

Answers available at http://evolve.elsevier.com/Lewis/medsurg.

BRIDGE TO NCLEX EXAMINATION

The number of the question corresponds to the same-numbered outcome at the beginning of the chapter.

1. The nurse teaches the female patient who has frequent UTIs to
 a. take tub baths with bubble bath.
 b. void before and after sexual intercourse.
 c. take prophylactic sulfonamides for the rest of her life.
 d. restrict fluid intake to prevent the need for frequent voiding.

2. One of the *most* important nursing roles in relation to acute poststreptococcal glomerulonephritis (APSGN) is to
 a. promote early diagnosis and treatment of sore throats and skin lesions.
 b. encourage patients to obtain antibiotic therapy for upper respiratory tract infections.
 c. teach patients that long-term prophylactic antibiotic therapy is needed to prevent recurrence.
 d. monitor for respiratory symptoms that indicate the disease is affecting the alveolar basement membrane.

3. The nurse's *first priority* in managing the patient with severe renal colic is to
 a. administer opioids as prescribed.
 b. obtain supplies for straining all urine.
 c. encourage fluid intake of 3 to 4 L/day.
 d. keep the patient NPO in preparation for surgery.

4. The nurse recommends genetic counseling for the children of a patient with
 a. nephrotic syndrome.
 b. chronic pyelonephritis.
 c. malignant nephrosclerosis.
 d. adult-onset polycystic kidney disease.

5. Which factor from the health history is a risk factor for kidney and bladder cancer?
 a. Aspirin use
 b. Tobacco use
 c. Chronic alcohol use
 d. Use of artificial sweeteners

6. Nursing interventions to increase bladder control in patients with urinary incontinence include? **(Select all that apply.)**
 a. Teaching the patient to use Kegel exercises
 b. Clamping and releasing a catheter to increase bladder tone
 c. Teaching biofeedback mechanisms to train pelvic floor muscles
 d. Counseling the patient about choosing incontinence containment devices
 e. Developing a fluid modification plan, focusing on decreasing intake before bedtime

7. A patient with a ureterolithotomy returns from surgery with a nephrostomy tube in place. Postoperative nursing care includes
   a. clamping the tube for 10 minutes every hour to decrease spasms.
   b. encouraging fluids of at least 2 to 3 L/day after nausea has subsided.
   c. notifying the provider if nephrostomy tube drainage is more than 30 mL/h.
   d. irrigating the nephrostomy tube with 10 mL of normal saline solution as needed.

8. Four days after surgery, the nurse notes mucous shreds in the pouch of a patient who had a cystectomy and ileal conduit diversion. The nurse would
   a. notify the provider.
   b. notify the charge nurse.
   c. irrigate the drainage tube.
   d. document it as a normal observation.

1. b; 2. a; 3. a; 4. d; 5. b; 6. a, c; 7. b; 8. d.

For rationales to these answers and even more NCLEX review questions, visit http://evolve.elsevier.com/Lewis/medsurg.

REFERENCES

To access the References for this chapter, please scan the QR code with a mobile device.

51

Acute Kidney Injury and Chronic Kidney Disease

Lillian A. Pryor

http://evolve.elsevier.com/Lewis/medsurg/

CONCEPTUAL FOCUS

Acid-Base Balance
Adherence
Coping
Elimination
Fluids and Electrolytes
Nutrition

LEARNING OUTCOMES

1. Outline criteria used to classify acute kidney injury (AKI) using the acronym RIFLE.
2. Relate the clinical course of AKI.
3. Explain the interprofessional and nursing management of patients with AKI.
4. Define chronic kidney disease (CKD) and delineate its 5 stages based on glomerular filtration rate.
5. Identify risk factors for CKD.
6. Explain the conservative interprofessional care and related nursing management of patients with CKD.
7. Distinguish among renal replacement therapy options for patients with end-stage renal disease.
8. Discuss nursing care for patients receiving renal replacement therapy.
9. Discuss the role of nurses in managing patients who receive a kidney transplant.

KEY TERMS

acute kidney injury (AKI)
acute tubular necrosis (ATN)
arteriovenous fistula (AVF)
arteriovenous grafts (AVGs)
automated peritoneal dialysis (APD)
azotemia
chronic kidney disease (CKD)
CKD mineral and bone disorder (CKD-MBD)
continuous renal replacement therapy (CRRT)
dialysis
end-stage renal disease (ESRD)
hemodialysis (HD)
peritoneal dialysis (PD)
renal replacement therapy (RRT)
uremia

Kidney failure, also called *renal failure,* is the partial or complete impairment of kidney function. It results in the inability to excrete metabolic waste products and water. Kidney failure contributes to problems with all body systems. Persons with kidney failure have problems with fluid, electrolyte, and acid-base imbalance. Adhering to diet therapy and the treatment plan can be challenging. The person must deal with changes in lifestyle, occupation, relationships, and self-image that can lead to withdrawal and depression. The person grieves the loss of kidney function and independence.

We classify kidney failure as acute or chronic (Table 51.1). Acute kidney injury (AKI) has a rapid onset. It can develop over hours or days. Chronic kidney disease (CKD) is gradual with a progressive decline in kidney function.

KIDNEY FAILURE

ACUTE KIDNEY INJURY

Acute kidney injury (AKI) is the term used to encompass the entire scope of the syndrome, ranging from a slight deterioration in kidney function to severe impairment. AKI is characterized by a rapid loss of kidney function with or without decreased urine output. This loss is accompanied by progressive increases in blood urea nitrogen (BUN), creatinine, and potassium. **Azotemia**, an accumulation of nitrogenous waste products (urea nitrogen, creatinine) in the blood, can develop.

AKI usually affects people with other life-threatening problems (Table 51.2).[1] It often follows severe, prolonged hypotension, hypovolemia, or exposure to a nephrotoxic agent.

Hospitalized patients develop AKI at a high rate and have a high mortality rate. When AKI develops in intensive care unit (ICU) patients, the mortality rate can be as high as 80%.[1] The most common cause of death in AKI is infection. A high number of patients with COVID-19 develop AKI. We do not know the exact cause of AKI in COVID-19. It may be from direct damage to the kidney or linked to lung and heart failure.[2]

Etiology and Pathophysiology

The causes of AKI are multiple and complex. We categorize them as prerenal, intrarenal (or intrinsic), and postrenal causes (Table 51.2 and Fig. 51.1).

Prerenal

Prerenal causes are factors that reduce systemic circulation, causing decreased renal blood flow. There is no damage to the kidney tissue (parenchyma). The oliguria is caused by a decrease in circulating blood volume (e.g., severe dehydration, heart failure [HF]), leading to decreased glomerular perfusion and filtration of the kidneys. Prerenal azotemia results in decreased sodium excretion (less than 20 mEq/L), increased sodium and water retention, and decreased urine output.

Prerenal oliguria is readily reversible with proper treatment.[3] Prerenal problems can contribute to intrarenal AKI. If decreased perfusion persists for an extended time, the kidneys

TABLE 51.1 Comparison of AKI and CKD

	AKI	CKD
Onset	Sudden	Gradual, often over many years
Most common cause	Acute tubular necrosis	Diabetic nephropathy
Diagnostic criteria	Acute reduction in urine output *AND/OR* ↑ Creatinine	GFR <60 mL/min/1.73 m² for >3 months *AND/OR* Kidney damage >3 months
Reversibility	Potentially	Progressive and irreversible
Main cause of death	Infection	CVD

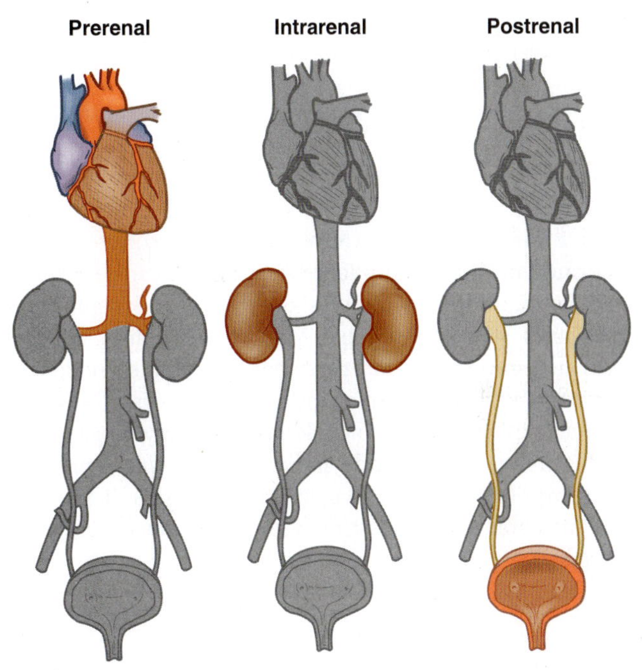

Fig. 51.1 Prerenal, intrarenal, and postrenal causes of AKI.

TABLE 51.2 Common Causes of AKI

Prerenal	Intrarenal	Postrenal
Decreased Cardiac Output • Cardiogenic shock • Dysrhythmias • HF • MI **Decreased Peripheral Vascular Resistance** • Anaphylaxis • Neurologic injury • Septic shock **Decreased Renal Blood Flow** • Bilateral renal vein thrombosis • Embolism • Hepatorenal syndrome • Renal artery thrombosis **Hypovolemia** • Burns • Dehydration • Diuresis • GI losses (diarrhea, vomiting) • Hemorrhage • Hypoalbuminemia	**Interstitial Nephritis** • Allergies: antibiotics (sulfonamides, rifampin), NSAIDs, ACE inhibitors • Infections: bacterial (acute pyelonephritis), viral (Epstein-Barr), fungal (candidiasis) **Nephrotoxic Injury** • Chemical exposure: ethylene glycol, lead, arsenic, carbon tetrachloride • Contrast media • Drugs: aminoglycosides (gentamicin), amphotericin B • Hemolytic blood transfusion reaction • Severe crush injury **Other** • Acute glomerulonephritis • Malignant hypertension • Prolonged prerenal ischemia • Systemic lupus erythematosus • Thrombotic disorders • Toxemia of pregnancy	• BPH • Bladder cancer • Calculi formation • Neuromuscular disorders • Prostate cancer • Spinal cord disease • Strictures • Trauma (back, pelvis, perineum)

lose their ability to compensate and damage to kidney tissue occurs (intrarenal damage).

Intrarenal

Intrarenal causes of AKI (Table 51.2) cause direct damage to the kidney tissue, resulting in impaired nephron function. Damage can result from prolonged ischemia or nephrotoxins (e.g., aminoglycosides, contrast media). Hemoglobin from hemolyzed red blood cells (RBCs) or myoglobin from necrotic muscle cells can block the tubules and cause renal vasoconstriction. Kidney diseases, such as acute glomerulonephritis and systemic lupus erythematosus (SLE), may cause AKI.

Nephrotoxins can cause obstruction of intrarenal structures by crystallizing or causing damage to the epithelial cells of the tubules. The necrotic tubular epithelial cells slough off and plug the tubules.

Acute tubular necrosis (ATN) is the most common intrarenal cause of AKI in hospitalized patients. It can result from ischemia, nephrotoxins, or sepsis. Ischemic and nephrotoxic ATN causes 90% of intrarenal AKI.[3] Severe kidney ischemia causes a disruption in the basement membrane and patchy destruction of the tubular epithelium. Other risk factors for ATN while in the hospital include major surgery, shock, blood transfusion reaction, muscle injury from trauma, and prolonged hypotension. ATN is potentially reversible if the basement membrane is not destroyed and the tubular epithelium regenerates.

Postrenal

Postrenal causes of AKI involve mechanical obstruction in the outflow of urine. With the flow of urine obstructed, urine refluxes into the renal pelvis, impairing kidney function. The most common postrenal causes are benign prostatic hyperplasia (BPH), prostate cancer, stones, trauma, and extrarenal tumors. Bilateral ureteral obstruction leads to *hydronephrosis* (kidney dilation), increase in hydrostatic pressure, and tubular blockage, resulting in a progressive decline in kidney function. If bilateral obstruction is relieved within 48 hours of onset, complete recovery is likely. Prolonged obstruction can lead to tubular atrophy and irreversible kidney fibrosis. Postrenal causes of AKI account for less than 10% of AKI cases.[3]

Clinical Manifestations

Prerenal and postrenal AKI that has not caused intrarenal damage usually resolves quickly with treatment. When tissue damage occurs from prerenal or postrenal causes, or when damage occurs directly as with intrarenal causes, AKI has a prolonged course. Clinically, AKI may progress through phases: oliguric, diuretic, and recovery. When a patient does not recover from AKI, CKD may develop.

The RIFLE classification describes the stages of AKI (Table 51.3). *R*isk, the first stage of AKI, is followed by *I*njury, the second stage. Then AKI increases in severity to the last, or third, stage, *F*ailure. The 2 outcome variables are *L*oss and *E*nd-stage renal disease.[3]

Oliguric Phase

Urinary changes. The most common initial manifestation of AKI is *oliguria*, a reduction in urine output to less than 400 mL/day. It usually occurs within 1 to 7 days of the injury to the kidneys. If the cause is ischemia, oliguria often occurs within 24 hours. When nephrotoxic drugs are involved, the onset may be

TABLE 51.3 Diagnostic Criteria

RIFLE Classification for Acute Kidney Injury

Stage	GFR Criteria	Urine Output Criteria	Clinical Example
Risk	Creatinine increased × 1.5 *OR* GFR decreased by 25%	Urine output <0.5 mL/kg/h for 6 h	68-year-old patient with type 2 diabetes, hypertension, CAD, CKD. Scheduled for emergency coronary artery bypass graft. Creatinine is 1.8 mg/dL (increased), weight 60 kg. Calculated GFR is 35 mL/min/1.73 m^2. Has stage 3b CKD
Injury	Creatinine increased × 2 *OR* GFR decreased by 50%	Urine output <0.5 mL/kg/h for 12 h	During surgery, hypotensive for a sustained period. Diagnosed with acute tubular necrosis. After surgery: creatinine 3.6 mg/dL, urine output 28 mL/h
Failure	Creatinine increased × 3 *OR* GFR decreased by 75% *OR* Creatinine >4 mg/dL with acute rise ≥0.5 mg/dL	Urine output <0.3 mL/kg/h for 24 h (oliguria) *OR* Anuria for 12 h	72 h after surgery, develops ventilator-associated pneumonia and sepsis while in ICU. Creatinine rises to 5.2 mg/dL, urine output drops to 10 mL/h. BP remains low despite dopamine therapy
Loss	Persistent acute kidney failure. Complete loss of kidney function >4 weeks	—	Starts on continuous venovenous HD. After 3 weeks of therapy has a cardiac arrest and does not survive
End-stage renal disease	Complete loss of kidney function >3 months	—	—

delayed for as long as 1 week. This phase lasts on average 10 to 14 days. It can last months in some cases. The longer the oliguric phase lasts, the poorer the prognosis for complete recovery of kidney function.

Nonoliguric AKI has a urine output greater than 400 mL/day. About 50% of patients will be nonoliguric. This makes their initial diagnosis more difficult.[1] Nonoliguric AKI occurs with acute interstitial nephritis and ATN.[1]

While changes in urine output often do not correspond to changes in glomerular filtration rate (GFR), they can help us determine the cause of AKI. For example, *anuria* (no urine output) is usually seen with urinary tract obstruction. Oliguria often occurs with prerenal causes.

Urinalysis may show casts, RBCs, and white blood cells (WBCs). Casts form from mucoprotein impressions of the necrotic renal tubular epithelial cells, which slough into the tubules. The specific gravity may be fixed at around 1.010, with urine osmolality at about 300 mOsm/kg (300 mmol/kg). This is the same specific gravity and osmolality as plasma, thus reflecting tubular damage and the loss of concentrating ability by the kidney. Proteinuria may be present if AKI is related to glomerular membrane dysfunction.

Fluid volume. Hypovolemia can worsen all forms of AKI. When urine output decreases, fluid retention occurs. The severity of the manifestations depends on the extent of the fluid overload. In the case of reduced urine output (anuria, oliguria), the neck veins may become distended with a bounding pulse. Edema and hypertension may develop. Fluid overload can eventually lead to HF, pulmonary edema, and pericardial and pleural effusions.

Metabolic acidosis. Impaired kidneys cannot excrete hydrogen ions or the acid products of metabolism. Bicarbonate (HCO_3^-) production decreases from defective reabsorption and regeneration of HCO_3^- ions. HCO_3^- is depleted through buffering of acidic hydrogen ions and metabolic end products. Patients with severe acidosis may develop rapid, deep respirations to try to compensate by increasing CO_2 exhalation.

Sodium balance. Damaged tubules cannot conserve sodium. Urine sodium excretion may increase, resulting in normal or below-normal sodium levels. Excess sodium intake is avoided because it can lead to volume expansion, hypertension, and HF. Uncontrolled hyponatremia or water excess can lead to cerebral edema.

Potassium excess. Hyperkalemia is one of the most serious complications in AKI because it can cause life-threatening dysrhythmias. The kidneys normally excrete 80% to 90% of the body's potassium. In AKI the potassium level increases because the kidney's ability to excrete potassium is impaired. The risk for hyperkalemia increases if AKI is caused by massive tissue trauma because the damaged cells release potassium into the extracellular fluid (ECF). Bleeding and blood transfusions may cause cell destruction, releasing more potassium into the ECF. Metabolic acidosis worsens hyperkalemia as hydrogen ions enter the cells, and potassium is driven out of the cells into the ECF.

While patients with hyperkalemia are often asymptomatic, some may have weakness with severe hyperkalemia. Acute or rapid development of hyperkalemia may result in ECG changes (see Fig. 17.14).[4] Emergency treatment may be needed.

Waste product accumulation. The kidneys are the main excretory organs for urea (a product of protein metabolism) and creatinine (product of endogenous muscle metabolism). BUN and creatinine levels are increased in kidney disease. An increased BUN level also can be caused by dehydration, corticosteroids, or catabolism resulting from infections, fever, severe injury, or GI bleeding. The best serum indicator of AKI is creatinine because it is not affected by other factors.

Neurologic problems. Neurologic changes can occur as nitrogenous waste products accumulate in the brain and other nervous tissue. The manifestations can be as mild as fatigue and difficulty concentrating and escalate to seizures, stupor, and coma.

Diuretic Phase

During the diuretic phase of AKI, daily urine output is usually around 1 to 3 L. It may reach 5 L or more. The nephrons are still not fully functional even as urine output increases. The high urine volume is caused by osmotic diuresis from the high urea concentration in the glomerular filtrate and the inability of the tubules to concentrate the urine. Hypovolemia and hypotension can occur from massive fluid losses. The kidneys, though, have recovered their ability to excrete waste.

Patients who had an oliguric phase will have greater diuresis as kidney function returns. Large losses of fluid and electrolytes require us to monitor for hyponatremia, hypokalemia, and dehydration. The diuretic phase may last 1 to 3 weeks. Near the end of this phase, acid-base, electrolyte, and waste product (BUN, creatinine) values stabilize.

Recovery Phase

The recovery phase begins when the GFR increases, allowing the BUN and creatinine levels to decrease. Major improvements occur in the first 1 to 2 weeks of this phase. It may take 12 months for kidney function to stabilize. Patients' overall health, severity of kidney injury, and number and type of complications influence their outcome. Some patients do not recover and progress to end-stage renal disease (ESRD). The older adult is less likely to have a complete recovery of kidney function. Patients who recover may achieve clinically normal kidney function but remain in an early stage of CKD.

Diagnostic Studies

The history is essential for diagnosing the cause of AKI. Consider prerenal causes when there is a history of dehydration, hypotension, or blood loss. Suspect intrarenal causes if the patient was exposed to nephrotoxic drugs or contrast media. A history of changes in the urinary stream, stones, BPH, or bladder or prostate cancer suggests postrenal causes.

Although changes in urine output and creatinine occur late in the course of AKI, they are diagnostic indicators. An increase in creatinine may not be present until there is a loss of more than 50% of kidney function. The rate of increase in creatinine is important in determining the severity of injury.

Urinalysis is an important diagnostic test. Urine sediment containing abundant cells, casts, or proteins suggests intrarenal disorders. The urine osmolality, sodium content, and specific gravity help distinguish the causes of AKI. Urine sediment may be normal in prerenal and postrenal AKI. In intrarenal problems, hematuria, pyuria, and crystals may be seen. Other testing may be done (Table 51.4). A kidney ultrasound is often the first test done. It provides imaging without exposure to nephrotoxic contrast agents. It can evaluate kidney disease and urinary tract obstruction. A renal scan can assess abnormalities in kidney blood flow, tubular function, and the collecting system. A CT scan can show lesions, masses, obstructions, and vascular anomalies. A renal biopsy is the best way to confirm intrarenal causes of AKI.

Having an MRI or magnetic resonance angiography (MRA) study with the contrast media gadolinium is not advised in patients with kidney failure. Giving gadolinium can be potentially fatal.

Interprofessional Care

Because AKI is potentially reversible, the main goals of treatment are to eliminate the cause, manage the signs and symptoms, and prevent complications while the kidneys recover (Table 51.4). The first step is to determine whether there is adequate intravascular volume and cardiac output to ensure adequate kidney perfusion.[4] Fluid replacement is often enough to treat many forms of AKI, especially prerenal causes. Loop diuretics (e.g., furosemide, bumetanide) or an osmotic diuretic (e.g., mannitol) may be given. If AKI is established, forcing fluids and diuretics will not be effective and may be harmful. Closely monitor fluid intake during the oliguric phase.

The general rule for calculating the fluid restriction is to add all losses for the previous 24 hours (e.g., urine, diarrhea, emesis, blood) plus 600 mL for insensible losses (e.g., respiration, diaphoresis). For example, if a patient excreted 300 mL of urine on Tuesday with no other losses, the fluid allocation on Wednesday would be 900 mL.

Therapies used to treat high potassium levels are listed in Table 51.5. Insulin and sodium bicarbonate promote a transient shift of potassium into the cells. Potassium will eventually diffuse back into the bloodstream. Calcium gluconate raises the threshold at which dysrhythmias occur, temporarily stabilizing the myocardium. Dialysis removes potassium rapidly from the body.

TABLE 51.4 Interprofessional Care

Acute Kidney Injury

Diagnostic Assessment

- History and physical assessment
- Identify cause
- Electrolytes, creatinine, BUN levels
- Urinalysis
- Renal ultrasound
- Renal scan
- CT scan

Management

- Treat cause
- Fluid restriction (600 mL plus previous 24-h fluid loss)
- Nutrition therapy
  - Adequate protein intake (0.8–1.0 g/kg/day) depending on degree of catabolism
  - Enteral nutrition
  - PN
  - Diet restrictions (potassium, phosphate, sodium)
- Measures to lower potassium (if high) (Table 51.5)
- Calcium supplements or phosphate-binding agents
- RRT

TABLE 51.5 Therapies for High Potassium Levels

Regular Insulin IV

- Potassium moves into cells when insulin is given
- IV glucose given concurrently to prevent hypoglycemia
- When effects of insulin decrease, potassium shifts back out of cells

Sodium Bicarbonate

- May be given to correct acidosis and cause a shift of potassium into cells

Calcium Gluconate IV

- Generally used in advanced cardiac toxicity (hyperkalemic ECG changes)
- Lowers the threshold for excitation, treating dysrhythmias

Sodium Polystyrene Sulfonate (Kayexalate)

- Given by mouth or retention enema
- When resin is in the bowel, potassium is exchanged for sodium
- Produces osmotic diarrhea, allowing for evacuation of potassium-rich stool
- Removes 1 mEq of potassium per 1 g of drug
- Do not give to a patient with a paralytic ileus as bowel necrosis can occur

Patiromer (Veltassa) and Sodium Zirconium Cyclosilicate (SZC)

- Oral suspension that binds potassium in GI tract
- Used to treat patients with CKD
- Has a delayed onset of action
- Do not give to a patient with a paralytic ileus as bowel necrosis can occur

Hemodialysis

- Most effective therapy to remove potassium
- Works within a short time

Diet Restriction

- Potassium intake is limited to 40 mEq/day
- Used to prevent recurrent elevation, not for acute elevation

Conservative therapy may be all that is necessary until kidney function improves. If conservative therapy is not effective in treating AKI, then *renal replacement therapy* (RRT) is used. Controversy exists about the timing of RRT in AKI.[5] The most common indications for RRT in AKI are (1) volume overload, resulting in compromised cardiac and/or pulmonary status; (2) high potassium level; (3) metabolic acidosis (HCO_3^- level less than 15 mEq/L [15 mmol/L]); (4) BUN level greater than 120 mg/dL (43 mmol/L); (5) significant change in mental status; and (6) pericarditis, pericardial effusion, or cardiac tamponade.[6] Although laboratory values provide rough parameters, the best guideline is the patient's clinical status.

There is no consensus about the best approach for RRT.[6] Even though peritoneal dialysis (PD) is a viable option for RRT, it is not often used. Intermittent hemodialysis (HD) and continuous renal replacement therapy (CRRT) have both been used effectively.

Nutrition Therapy

The goal of nutrition therapy in AKI is to provide adequate calories to prevent catabolism despite restrictions that prevent electrolyte and fluid problems and azotemia. Intake must provide adequate calories (30 to 35 kcal/kg and 0.8 to 1.0 g of protein/kg of desired body weight) to prevent the breakdown of body protein.

Adequate energy should mainly come from carbohydrate and fat sources to prevent ketosis from endogenous fat breakdown and gluconeogenesis from muscle protein breakdown. Essential amino acids may be supplemented. Potassium and sodium are regulated per plasma levels. Sodium is restricted as needed to prevent edema, hypertension, and HF.[7] Fat intake is increased so that the patient receives at least 30% to 40% of total calories from fat. IV fat emulsion infusions are a good source of nonprotein calories. If a patient cannot maintain adequate oral intake, enteral nutrition is preferred for nutrition support (see Chapter 44). When the GI tract is not functional, parenteral nutrition (PN) can provide adequate nutrition. Patients treated with PN may need daily HD or CRRT to remove the excess fluid. Concentrated PN formulas minimize fluid volume.

NURSING MANAGEMENT: ACUTE KIDNEY INJURY

Assessment

Several assessments are essential for developing the plan of care. Daily weights, strict intake and output, and vital signs are key. Daily monitoring of urine output has prognostic value. It is crucial for determining therapy and daily fluid volume replacement. Assess the urine for color, specific gravity, glucose, protein, blood, and sediment. Note the general appearance, including skin color. Is there any edema, neck vein distention, or bruises? If a patient is receiving dialysis, check the access site for inflammation and exudate. Assess mental status and level of consciousness. Check the oral mucosa for dryness and inflammation. Auscultate the lungs for crackles, wheezes, or decreased breath sounds. Monitor the heart for an S_3 gallop, murmurs, or a pericardial friction rub. Assess ECG readings for dysrhythmias. Review all laboratory values and diagnostic test results.

Clinical Problems

Clinical problems for patients with AKI include:

- Electrolyte imbalance
- Fluid imbalance
- Risk for infection

Planning

The overall goals are that patients with AKI will (1) completely recover without any loss of kidney function, (2) maintain normal fluid and electrolyte balance, (3) have decreased anxiety, and (4) adhere to and understand the need for careful follow-up care.

Implementation

Health Promotion

Prevention and early recognition of AKI are the most important aspects of care. Prevention is directed toward identifying and monitoring high-risk populations, controlling exposure to nephrotoxic drugs and chemicals, and preventing prolonged episodes of hypotension and hypovolemia. In the hospital, factors that increase the risk for AKI are CKD, older age, massive trauma, major surgery, extensive burns, HF, sepsis, and obstetric complications.[8] Dehydration is a predisposing factor. It can occur from polypharmacy (diuretics, laxatives, drugs that suppress consciousness), acute febrile illness, and immobility.

Monitor weight, intake and output, and fluid and electrolyte balance. Prompt replacement of fluid losses helps prevent ischemic tubular damage from trauma, burns, and extensive surgery. Intake and output and weight are valuable indicators of fluid volume status. Aggressive diuretic therapy for patients with fluid overload can decrease renal blood flow.

Contrast-induced nephropathy (CIN) can occur when contrast media for diagnostic studies causes nephrotoxic injury. In patients with diabetes receiving metformin, the drug should be held for 48 hours before and after the use of contrast media to decrease the risk for lactic acidosis. The best way to avoid CIN is to avoid exposure to contrast media by using other diagnostic tests, such as ultrasound.[9]

! SAFETY ALERT

- When you give contrast media to high-risk patients, ensure adequate fluid intake.
- Administer the lowest possible dose or a lower osmolality contrast agent.

Monitor kidney function in persons who are taking drugs that are potentially nephrotoxic (see Table 49.3). These drugs should be used sparingly in high-risk patients. When they must be used, they should be given in the smallest effective doses for the shortest possible periods. Caution patients about over-the-counter (OTC) analgesics (especially nonsteroidal antiinflammatory drugs [NSAIDs]). They may worsen kidney function in patients with mild CKD.

Angiotensin-converting enzyme (ACE) inhibitors can decrease perfusion pressure and cause hyperkalemia. If other measures, such as diet changes and diuretics, cannot control hyperkalemia, ACE inhibitors may have to be reduced or stopped. However, ACE inhibitors are often used to prevent proteinuria and progression of kidney disease, especially in patients with diabetes.

Acute Care

Patients with AKI are critically ill. They may have other problems (e.g., diabetes, cardiovascular disease [CVD]) in addition to AKI. Focus on patients holistically since they will have many physical and emotional needs. Usually, the changes caused by AKI arise suddenly. Patients may need help understanding how kidney disease affects the entire body.

You have a key role in managing fluid and electrolyte balance during the oliguric and diuretic phases. Observe and record intake and output. Take daily weights with the same scale at the same time each day to detect excess fluid gains or losses. Assess for signs and symptoms of hypervolemia (in the oliguric phase) or hypovolemia (in the diuretic phase), potassium and sodium problems, and other electrolyte imbalances that may occur in AKI (see Chapter 17).

Because infection is the leading cause of death in AKI, meticulous aseptic technique is critical. Protect patients from those with infectious diseases. Be alert for local manifestations of infection (e.g., swelling, redness, pain) as well as systemic manifestations (e.g., fever, malaise, leukocytosis).

If patients with renal failure have an infection, be aware that they may not have a fever. Patients with AKI have a blunted febrile response to infection (e.g., pneumonia). If antibiotics are given to treat infection, we carefully consider the type, frequency, and dosage because the kidneys are the main route of excretion for many antibiotics. Dosages may be decreased depending on the kidney function if the drug is eliminated by the kidneys. Nephrotoxic drugs (see Table 49.3) are given with caution.

Perform good skin care. Take measures to prevent pressure injuries if mobility is impaired. Mouth care is important to prevent stomatitis, which develops when ammonia (made by bacterial breakdown of urea) in saliva irritates the mucous membranes.

Chronic Care

Recovery from AKI is highly variable. It depends on whether other body systems fail, patients' general health and age, the length of the oliguric phase, and the severity of nephron damage. Protein and potassium intake are dictated by kidney function. Regular evaluation of kidney function is necessary. Teach patients the signs and symptoms of recurrent kidney disease. Emphasize measures to prevent the recurrence of AKI.

The long-term convalescence of 3 to 12 months may cause psychosocial and financial hardships for patients and caregivers. Make appropriate referrals for counseling. If the kidneys do not recover, the patient will need to transition to life on RRT or a possible transplant.

◆ Evaluation

The expected outcomes are that patients with AKI will:

- Regain and maintain normal fluid and electrolyte balance
- Adhere to the treatment regimen
- Have no complications
- Have a complete recovery

Gerontologic Considerations: Acute Kidney Injury

Older adults are at an increased risk for AKI. The GFR declines with age. The aging kidney is less able to compensate for changes in fluid volume, solute load, and cardiac output. Common causes of AKI in the older adult include hypotension, diuretic therapy, aminoglycoside therapy, obstructive disorders (e.g., BPH), surgery, infection, and contrast media. Patients over 65 years of age are less likely to recover from AKI.

CHRONIC KIDNEY DISEASE

Chronic kidney disease (CKD) involves progressive, irreversible loss of kidney function. More than 37 million American adults, or 1 out of every 7, have CKD. CKD is much more common than AKI (Table 51.1). Because the kidneys are highly adaptive, CKD is often not recognized until there has been considerable loss of nephrons. Patients with CKD are often asymptomatic. We think more than 85% of people with CKD are unaware that they have the disease.[10]

CKD has many different causes. The leading ones are diabetes (about 50%) and hypertension (about 25%) (Table 51.6).[11,12] We partially attribute the prevalence of CKD

TABLE 51.6 Risk Factors for CKD

Risk Factors	Prevention and Management
Age >60 years	Prevent insult or injury to kidneys
Cardiovascular disease	Institute risk factor reduction measures
Diabetes	Achieve optimal glycemic control
Ethnic minority (e.g., Black, Native American)	Teach about risk and assist with screening (BP measurement, urinalysis)
Exposure to nephrotoxic drugs	Limit exposure and give sodium bicarbonate as treatment
Family history of CKD	Teach about risk and assist with screening
Hypertension	Maintain BP in normal range with ACE inhibitors or ARBs

to increased risk factors, including an aging population, and increased rates of obesity, diabetes, and hypertension. Less common causes include glomerulonephritis, cystic diseases, and urologic diseases.

Kidney Disease Improving Global Outcomes (KDIGO) Clinical Practice Guidelines define CKD as the presence of kidney damage or a decreased GFR less than 60 mL/min/1.73 m^2 for longer than 3 months.[11] Table 51.7 shows the stages of CKD. The last stage of kidney disease, **end-stage renal disease (ESRD)**, occurs when the GFR is less than 15 mL/min. At this point, RRT (dialysis, transplant) is needed to maintain life.[11] Patients with ESRD have a high mortality rate. Mortality rates are as high as 19% to 24% for patients with ESRD on dialysis.[13]

The prognosis and course of CKD are highly variable. They depend on the cause, patients' health and age, and adequacy of health care follow-up. Some people live normal, active lives with kidney disease, while others may rapidly progress to ESRD (stage 5).

Clinical Manifestations

As kidney function deteriorates, all body systems become affected. The manifestations result from retained urea, creatinine, phenols, hormones, electrolytes, and water. **Uremia** is a syndrome in which kidney function declines to the point that symptoms may develop in multiple body systems (Fig. 51.2). It often occurs when the GFR is 15 mL/min or less. The manifestations of uremia vary depending on the cause, comorbid problems, age, and degree of adherence to the treatment plan. Many patients are tolerant of the changes caused by declining kidney function because they occur gradually.[10]

TABLE 51.7 Diagnostic Criteria

Stages of CKD

Description	GFR (mL/min/1.73 m^2)	Clinical Action Plan
Stage 1 Kidney damage with normal or ↑ GFR	≥90	Diagnosis and treatment CVD risk reduction Slow progression
Stage 2 Kidney damage with mild ↓ GFR	60–89	Estimate progression
Stage 3a Moderate ↓ GFR	45–59	Evaluate and treat complications
Stage 3b Moderate ↓ GFR	30–44	More aggressive treatment of complications
Stage 4 Severe ↓ GFR	15–29	Preparation for RRT (dialysis, kidney transplant)
Stage 5 Kidney failure	<15 (or dialysis)	RRT (if uremia present and patient desires treatment)

Urinary System

In the early stages of CKD, patients usually do not report any change in urine output. Since diabetes is the main cause of CKD, polyuria may be present, but not necessarily from kidney disease. As CKD progresses, patients have increasing difficulty with fluid retention and need diuretic therapy. After a period on dialysis, patients may develop anuria.

Metabolic Disturbances

Waste product accumulation. As the GFR decreases, BUN and creatinine levels increase. The BUN increase is not only from kidney disease but also protein intake, fever, corticosteroids, and catabolism. For this reason, creatinine clearance determinations (calculated GFR) are more accurate indicators of kidney function than BUN or creatinine (Table 51.8). Significant increases in BUN contribute to nausea, vomiting, lethargy, fatigue, impaired cognition, and headaches.

Altered carbohydrate metabolism. Impaired glucose metabolism, from cell insensitivity to the normal action of insulin, causes defective carbohydrate metabolism. Mild to moderate hyperglycemia and hyperinsulinemia may occur.

Insulin and glucose metabolism may improve (but not to normal values) after starting dialysis. Patients with diabetes who use insulin before starting dialysis may need less insulin therapy when they start dialysis, and their kidney disease progresses. Patients with diabetes who develop uremia may need less insulin than before the onset of CKD. Insulin, which depends on the kidneys for excretion, stays in the circulation longer. Insulin dosing is patient specific. We monitor glucose levels carefully.

CHECK YOUR PRACTICE

You are working in a community-based HD unit. One of your patients is a 56-year-old female who has been on HD for 3 weeks. You are reviewing her medications with her. She is surprised that her dose of glargine insulin has been decreased. She tells you, "I have been a diabetic for 10 years. This is the first time ever that my dose of insulin has been decreased."

- How would you respond?

Elevated triglycerides. High insulin levels stimulate the liver to produce triglycerides. Many patients develop dyslipidemia, with increased very-low-density lipoproteins (VLDLs), increased low-density lipoproteins (LDLs), and decreased high-density lipoproteins (HDLs). The altered lipid metabolism is related to decreased lipase levels, an enzyme that is important in the breakdown of lipoproteins. Most patients with CKD die of CVD.[12]

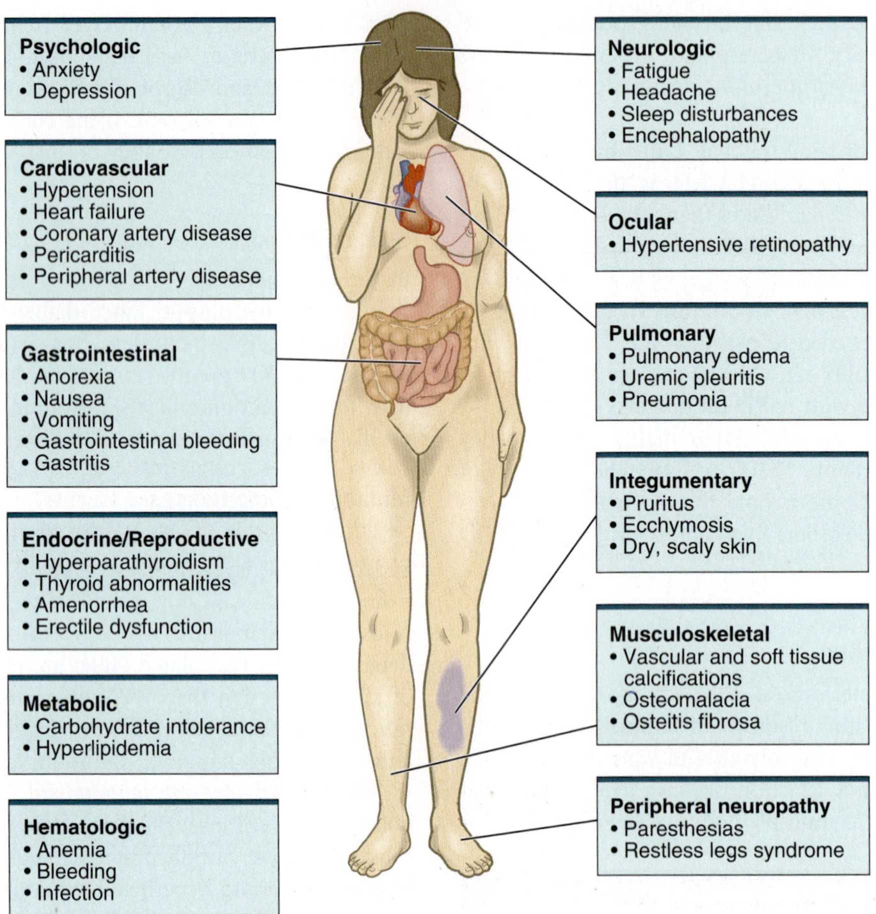

Fig. 51.2 Possible manifestations of CKD.

TABLE 51.8 Interprofessional Care

CKD

Diagnostic Assessment

- History and physical assessment
- Renal ultrasound, renal scan, CT scan
- Renal biopsy
- BUN, creatinine, creatinine clearance, electrolyte levels
- Lipid profile
- Urinalysis
- Protein-to-creatinine ratio in 1st morning voided specimen
- Hematocrit and hemoglobin levels

Management

- Correct fluid volume overload or deficit
- RRT (dialysis, kidney transplant)
- Nutrition therapy (Table 51.10 and Table 17.7)
- Measures to lower potassium (Table 51.5)

Drug Therapy

- Calcium supplementation, phosphate binders, or both
- Antihypertensive therapy
- ACE inhibitors or ARBs
- Erythropoietin therapy
- Lipid-lowering drugs
- Adjust drug dosages to degree of renal function

Electrolyte and Acid-Base Imbalances

Potassium. Hyperkalemia results from the kidneys excreting less potassium, the breakdown of cell protein, and metabolic acidosis. Fatal dysrhythmias can occur when the potassium level reaches 7 to 8 mEq/L (7 to 8 mmol/L). Potassium may come from foods, diet supplements, drugs, and IV infusions.

Sodium. Sodium may be high, normal, or low in kidney disease. Because of impaired sodium excretion, sodium is retained with water. If large quantities of water are retained, dilutional hyponatremia occurs. Sodium retention can contribute to edema, hypertension, and HF.

Metabolic acidosis. Metabolic acidosis results from the kidneys' impaired ability to excrete excess acid and from defective reabsorption and regeneration of HCO_3^-. The average adult makes 80 to 90 mEq of acid per day. This acid is normally buffered by HCO_3^-. In kidney disease, plasma HCO_3^-, which is an indirect measure of acidosis, usually falls to a new steady state at around 16 to 20 mEq/L (16 to 20 mmol/L). The decreased plasma HCO_3^- reflects its use in buffering metabolic acids. The HCO_3^- level often does not progress below this level because H^+ production is balanced by buffering from bone demineralization.

Hematologic System

Anemia. Normocytic, normochromic anemia is associated with CKD. Anemia in CKD is due to decreased erythropoietin production. Other factors contributing to anemia are nutrition deficiencies, decreased RBC life span, increased RBC hemolysis, frequent blood sampling, and GI bleeding. For patients receiving maintenance HD, blood loss in the dialyzer contributes to anemia. Increased parathyroid hormone (PTH) can inhibit erythropoiesis, shorten RBC survival, and cause bone marrow fibrosis, which can result in decreased numbers of hematopoietic cells.

Sufficient iron stores are needed for erythropoiesis. Many patients with kidney disease are iron deficient and need iron supplementation. Oral iron supplements may not be effective for the person with CKD. Medications, such as proton pump inhibitors or phosphate binders, decrease absorption. Patients on dialysis may need IV iron to restore iron levels. Folic acid, needed for RBC maturation, is dialyzable because it is water soluble. Many patients receive folic acid supplements (1 mg/day).[14]

Bleeding. The most common cause of bleeding is a defect in platelet function. This is caused by impaired platelet aggregation and impaired release of platelet factor III. Changes in the coagulation system occur due to increased concentrations of factor VIII and fibrinogen. Altered platelet function, bleeding tendencies, and GI bleeding susceptibility can usually be corrected with regular HD or PD.

Infection. Patients with advanced CKD have an increased risk of infection. This is due to changes in WBC function and altered immune response and function. Cellular and humoral immune responses are suppressed. Other factors contributing to the increased risk for infection include hyperglycemia and external trauma (e.g., catheters, needle insertions into vascular access sites).

Cardiovascular System

The most common cause of death in patients with CKD is CVD. Causes of death include myocardial infarction (MI), peripheral arterial disease, HF, cardiomyopathy, and stroke.[15] CVD and CKD are so closely linked that if patients develop cardiac events (e.g., MI, HF), kidney function is evaluated.

CVD may be related to vascular calcification and arterial stiffness. Calcium deposits in the vascular medial layer can cause stiffening of the blood vessels. The mechanisms involved are multifactorial. They include (1) vascular smooth muscle cells changing into chondrocytes or osteoblast-like cells, (2) high total body amount of calcium and phosphate resulting from abnormal bone metabolism, (3) impaired renal excretion, and (4) drug therapies to treat the bone disease (e.g., calcium-phosphate binders).[16]

Hypertension, which is prevalent in patients with CKD, is both a cause and a consequence of CKD. Hypertension is worsened by sodium retention and increased ECF volume.[15] In some people, increased renin production contributes to hypertension. Hypertension and diabetes are contributing risk factors for vascular complications. Long-standing hypertension, volume overload, and anemia contribute to left ventricular hypertrophy that may eventually lead to cardiomyopathy and HF. Because of the many effects of hypertension, BP control is one of the most important goals in CKD management.[15]

Patients with CKD are susceptible to dysrhythmias from hyperkalemia and decreased coronary artery perfusion. Uremic pericarditis can develop and sometimes progresses to pericardial effusion and cardiac tamponade.

Respiratory System

With severe acidosis, the respiratory system may try to compensate with Kussmaul breathing, which increases CO_2 removal by exhalation (see Chapter 17). Dyspnea may occur because of fluid overload, pulmonary edema, uremic pleuritis, pleural effusion, and respiratory infections (e.g., pneumonia).

GI System

Stomatitis with exudates and ulcerations, a metallic taste in the mouth, periodontal disease, and *uremic fetor* (a urinous odor of the breath) often occur in CKD. Anorexia, nausea, and vomiting may develop if CKD progresses to ESRD and is not treated with dialysis. Weight loss and malnutrition may occur. Diabetic *gastroparesis* (delayed gastric emptying) can compound the effects of malnutrition for patients with diabetes. GI bleeding is a risk because of mucosal irritation and platelet defects.

Constipation may be due to ingesting iron salts or calcium-containing phosphate binders. Limits on fluid intake and physical inactivity increase the risk for constipation.

Neurologic System

Neurologic changes are expected as kidney disease progresses. They are the result of increased nitrogenous waste products, electrolyte imbalances, metabolic acidosis, and atrophy and demyelination of nerve fibers. The central nervous system (CNS) becomes depressed, resulting in lethargy, apathy, decreased ability to concentrate, fatigue, irritability, and altered mental ability. Seizures and coma may result from a rapidly increasing BUN and hypertensive encephalopathy.

Peripheral neuropathy initially manifests as a slowing of nerve conduction to the extremities. Patients may describe paresthesia in the feet and legs as a burning sensation. Eventually, motor involvement may lead to bilateral foot drop, muscular weakness and atrophy, and loss of deep tendon reflexes. Muscle twitching, jerking, *asterixis* (hand-flapping tremor), and nighttime leg cramps may occur. In patients with diabetic neuropathy, uremic neuropathy can compound symptoms. Those with advanced stage 5 CKD may develop restless legs syndrome.

Dialysis should improve general CNS problems and may slow or halt the progression of neuropathies. Motor neuropathy may not be reversible. The treatment for neurologic problems is dialysis or a transplant. Altered mental status, a late manifestation of CKD stage 5, rarely occurs unless a patient has chosen not to have RRT.

Musculoskeletal System

CKD mineral and bone disorder (CKD-MBD) is a systemic disorder of mineral and bone metabolism caused by progressive deterioration in kidney function (Fig. 51.3). It is a common complication of CKD.

Activated vitamin D is necessary to optimize absorption of calcium from the GI tract. As kidney function declines, less vitamin D is converted to its active form. Low levels of active vitamin D result in decreased serum calcium levels.[17] Low calcium levels stimulate the parathyroid gland to secrete PTH, which stimulates bone demineralization, releasing calcium from the bones. Phosphate is also released, leading to high phosphate levels. Hyperphosphatemia also results from decreased phosphate excretion by the kidneys. High phosphate levels inhibit a renal enzyme needed to activate vitamin D, thus further decreasing serum calcium levels.

CKD-MBD results in skeletal, vascular, and soft tissue (extraskeletal) complications. Skeletal complications include (1) *osteomalacia* from demineralization from slow bone turnover and defective mineralization of newly formed bone and (2) *osteitis fibrosa*, decalcification of the bone and replacement of bone tissue with fibrous tissue. The weakened bone matrix increases the risk for fractures.

Soft tissue complications result from vascular calcifications. Vascular calcifications are a significant contributing factor to CVD. Irritation from calcium deposits in the eye can cause "uremic red eye." Cardiac calcifications can disrupt the conduction system and cause cardiac arrest.

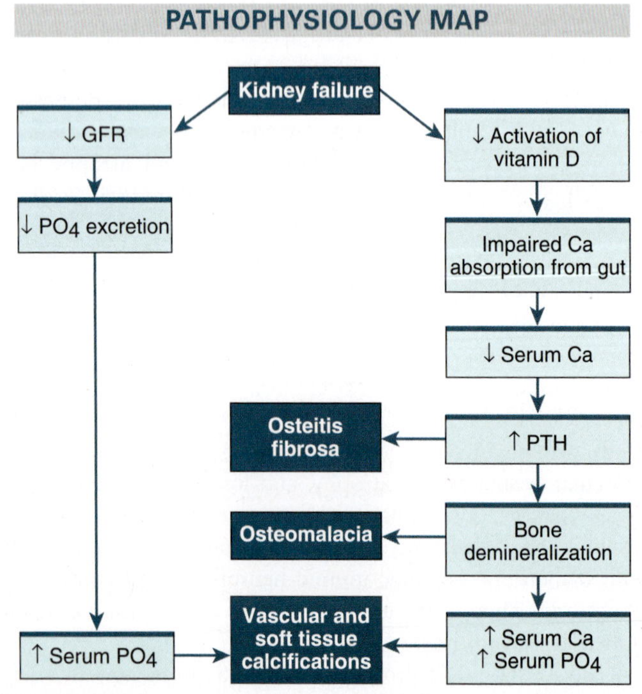

Fig. 51.3 Mechanisms of CKD-MBD. *GFR*, Glomerular filtration rate; *PTH*, parathyroid hormone.

Skin

A small number of patients develop refractory itching that can have a devastating impact on their well-being and quality of life. Itching has multiple causes, including dry skin, calcium-phosphate deposition in the skin, and sensory neuropathy. It is more common in patients receiving dialysis. The itching may be so intense that it can lead to bleeding or infection from scratching. Uremic frost is a rare condition in which urea crystallizes on the skin. It is usually seen only when BUN levels are very high (e.g., over 200 mg/dL).

Reproductive System

Patients can have infertility and a decreased libido. Females usually have low levels of estrogen, progesterone, and luteinizing hormone, causing anovulation and menstrual changes (usually amenorrhea). Menses and ovulation may return after starting dialysis. Males have loss of testicular consistency, decreased testosterone levels, and low sperm counts.

Peripheral neuropathy can cause impotence in males and anorgasmia in females. Other factors that may cause changes in sexual function are psychologic problems (e.g., anxiety, depression), anemia, stress, and drug side effects. Sexual function may improve with maintenance dialysis and become normal after a transplant.

Patients who become pregnant while receiving dialysis have been able to carry a fetus to term, but there is significant risk to the mother and infant. Pregnancy in patients with a kidney transplant is more common, but there is still considerable risk to the mother and fetus.

Psychologic Changes

Personality and behavior changes, emotional lability, withdrawal, and depression often occur in patients with CKD. Fatigue and lethargy contribute to the feeling of illness. Changes in body image occur with edema, skin changes, and access devices (e.g., fistulas, catheters). Decreased ability to concentrate and slowed mental activity can give the appearance of dullness and disinterest in the environment. Patients must deal with significant changes in lifestyle, occupation, family responsibilities, and financial status. Long-term survival depends on medications, diet restrictions, dialysis, and possibly a transplant. Patients grieve the loss of kidney function and independence.

Diagnostic Studies

Persistent proteinuria is usually the first sign of kidney damage.[17] Screening for CKD involves a dipstick evaluation of the urine for protein and albumin. The urine of patients with diabetes must be checked for albuminuria if no protein is present on routine urinalysis. A person with persistent proteinuria (1+ protein on standard dipstick testing 2 or more times over a 3-month period) should have further assessment of risk factors and a diagnostic workup with blood and urine tests to evaluate for CKD.

Urinalysis can detect RBCs, WBCs, protein, casts, and glucose. A renal ultrasound can detect any obstructions and determine the size of the kidneys. Other diagnostic studies (Table 51.9) help establish the diagnosis and cause of CKD. A kidney biopsy may be needed to provide a definitive diagnosis. The standard for diagnosing CKD-MBD is a bone biopsy.

Creatinine alone poorly reflects kidney function. GFR is the preferred way to determine kidney function. There are several GFR calculators. The equations used most often are the Cockcroft-Gault formula and Modification of Diet in Renal Disease (MDRD) Study equation. MDRD is the preferred method of calculation.[18]

Interprofessional Care

The overall goals of CKD therapy are to preserve existing kidney function, reduce the risk for CVD, prevent complications, and provide comfort. Early recognition, diagnosis, and treatment can prevent the progression of kidney disease. Patients with CKD need a referral to a nephrologist. Every effort is made to detect and treat potentially reversible causes of kidney failure (e.g., HF, dehydration, infections, nephrotoxins, urinary tract obstruction, glomerulonephritis, renal artery stenosis).

Patients with CKD have a high incidence of CVD. More patients die of CVD than live to need dialysis. When a patient has CKD, therapy is aimed at treating CVD plus slowing the progression of kidney disease (Table 51.8).

A focus during stages 1 through 4 (Table 51.7) before the need for dialysis (stage 5) includes controlling blood pressure, hyperparathyroidism, CKD-MBD, anemia, and dyslipidemia. The next section focuses on the drug and nutrition aspects of care.

Drug Therapy

Hyperkalemia. We use several strategies to manage hyperkalemia (Table 51.5). These include restricting high-potassium foods and drugs. Acute hyperkalemia may need treatment with IV glucose and insulin or IV 10% calcium gluconate.

Sodium polystyrene sulfonate, a cation-exchange resin, is often given to lower potassium levels in stage 4 CKD. Sodium polystyrene sulfonate has an osmotic laxative action and ensures potassium evacuation from the bowel. Tell patients to expect some diarrhea. Since this drug exchanges sodium ions for potassium ions, observe for sodium and water retention. If ECG changes appear, HD may be done to remove excess potassium.

Patiromer (Veltassa) is an oral suspension that binds potassium in the GI tract. It should not be used in emergency situations to treat hyperkalemia because of its delayed onset of action. Because patiromer binds other oral medications, it must be taken at least 6 hours before or after other oral medications. Sodium zirconium cyclosilicate (SZC) is another long-term drug for hyperkalemia. It is an oral solution that should be given at least 2 hours apart from other medications.[19]

Hypertension. For some, the progression of CKD can be delayed by controlling hypertension.[15] Treatment of hypertension includes (1) weight loss (if needed), (2) lifestyle changes (e.g., exercise, avoid alcohol use, smoking cessation), (3) diet recommendations (DASH Diet), and (4) antihypertensive drugs. Drug therapy depends on whether a patient has diabetes. ACE inhibitors and ARBs are given to patients with diabetes and those with nondiabetic proteinuria.[11] They decrease proteinuria and may delay the progression of CKD. They must be used with caution as they can further decrease the GFR and increase potassium levels. The treatment of hypertension is discussed in Chapter 36.

CKD-MBD. Interventions for CKD-MBD include limiting phosphorus intake, giving phosphate binders, supplementing vitamin D, and controlling hyperparathyroidism.[16] Phosphate intake is not usually restricted until the patient needs RRT. At

TABLE 51.9 NUTRITION THERAPY

CKD

	Pre-ESRD	Hemodialysis	Peritoneal Dialysis
Calcium	About 1000–1500 mg/day	Patient specific	Patient specific
Calories	30–35 kcal/kg/day	30–35 kcal/kg/day	25–35 kcal/kg/day (includes calories from dialysate glucose absorption)
Fluid allowance	As desired or depends on urine output	Urine output plus 600–1000 mL	Unrestricted if weight and BP controlled and residual renal function
Iron	Supplement recommended if receiving erythropoietin	Supplement recommended if receiving erythropoietin	Supplement recommended if receiving erythropoietin
Phosphate	Patient specific or 1.0–1.8 g/day	Patient specific or about 0.6–1.2 g/day	Patient specific or about 0.6–1.2 g/day
Potassium	Based on laboratory values	Patient specific or about 2–4 g/day	Usually not restricted
Protein	Patient specific or 0.6–1.0 g/kg/day (low protein)	1.2 g/kg/day	1.2–1.3 g/kg/day
Sodium	Patient specific or 1–3 g/day	Patient specific or 2–3 g/day	Patient specific or 2–4 g/day

that time, phosphate is usually limited to about 1 g/day, but diet control alone is usually not enough.

Phosphate binders include calcium carbonate and calcium-based binders such as calcium acetate. They bind phosphate in the bowel and then excrete it in the stool. Giving calcium increases the calcium load, which increases the risk for vascular calcifications. When calcium levels are increased or there are signs of existing vascular or soft tissue calcifications, non—calcium-based phosphate binders are used. These include lanthanum carbonate (Fosrenol), sevelamer carbonate (Renvela), and iron-based, calcium-free phosphate binders, such as sucroferric oxyhydroxide (Velphoro) and ferric citrate (Auryxia). To be most effective, give phosphate binders with each meal. Constipation is a frequent side effect. Stool softeners may be needed.

Because bone disease is associated with excess aluminum, aluminum preparations should be used with caution in patients with kidney disease. Do not use magnesium-containing antacids (e.g., Maalox, Mylanta) because magnesium depends on the kidneys for excretion.

Hypocalcemia is a problem in the later stages of CKD due to the inability of the GI tract to absorb calcium in the absence of active vitamin D. If hypocalcemia persists even if the phosphate levels are normal, calcium and vitamin D supplements may be given. Assess vitamin D levels to determine the need for a supplement. If the levels are low, vitamin D is given in the form of cholecalciferol.

Treatment of secondary hyperparathyroidism in ESRD patients requires the activated form of vitamin D because the kidneys cannot activate vitamin D. Active vitamin D is available as oral or IV calcitriol (Rocaltrol), IV paricalcitol (Zemplar), or oral or IV doxercalciferol (Hectorol). Their use can reduce high PTH levels. Cinacalcet (Sensipar), a calcimimetic agent, can control secondary hyperparathyroidism. Calcimimetics mimic calcium and increase the sensitivity of the calcium receptors in the parathyroid glands. As a result, the parathyroid glands detect calcium at lower serum levels and decrease PTH secretion.

If parathyroid disease becomes severe, a subtotal or total parathyroidectomy may be done to decrease the synthesis and secretion of PTH. In most cases, a total parathyroidectomy is done and parathyroid tissue transplanted into the forearm. The transplanted cells make PTH as needed. If PTH production becomes excessive, some cells can be removed from the forearm.

Hypercalcemia may occur with calcium and vitamin D supplements. If hypercalcemia occurs, vitamin D may be withheld, and calcium-based phosphate binders replaced with non—calcium-based phosphate binders.

Anemia. Treatment of CKD-related anemia is patient specific with the goal being to reduce the need for blood transfusions. We often give exogenous erythropoietin (EPO). One option is epoetin alfa (Epogen, Procrit). It can be given IV or subcutaneously, usually 2 or 3 times per week. Darbepoetin alfa (Aranesp) is longer acting and can be given weekly or biweekly.

Hemoglobin and hematocrit levels may take 2 to 3 weeks to increase. There is no target hemoglobin or widely accepted EPO dosing strategy. Teach people who are prescribed EPO about the risks and benefits and allow them to decide about their treatment plan.

Higher doses of EPO increase the risk of thromboembolic events and death from CV events (MI, HF, stroke). The recommendation is to use the lowest possible dose of EPO. EPO can increase BP. It is contraindicated in uncontrolled hypertension.

EPO therapy may lead to iron deficiency from the increased demand for iron to support erythropoiesis. Iron supplements are recommended if the ferritin concentrations fall below 100 ng/mL. Most patients with CKD receive an iron supplement. Iron can be given by mouth or IV. Oral use is limited due to GI side effects. Oral iron should not be taken at the same time as phosphate binders because calcium binds the iron, preventing its absorption. Most patients receiving HD are prescribed IV iron sucrose (Venofer) or sodium ferric gluconate complex. Folic acid supplements are usually given because it is needed for RBC formation and is removed by dialysis.

Blood transfusions are avoided unless patients have acute blood loss or symptomatic anemia (i.e., dyspnea, excess fatigue, tachycardia, palpitations, chest pain). Transfusions increase the development of antibodies. This makes it harder to find a compatible donor for a kidney transplant. Multiple blood transfusions may lead to iron overload since each unit of blood has about 250 mg of iron.

Dyslipidemia. Dyslipidemia, a risk factor for CVD, is a common problem in CKD. Statins (HMG-CoA reductase inhibitors), such as atorvastatin, can lower LDL cholesterol levels (see Table 37.6). Statins should be used in patients with CKD, especially those with diabetes, not yet on dialysis.[15]

Fibrates (fibric acid derivatives), such as gemfibrozil (Lopid), are used to lower triglyceride levels and can increase HDLs. Specific drugs used in these classes depend on the patient response and HCP recommendation.

Complications of drug therapy. The kidneys partially or totally excrete many drugs. CKD causes decreased elimination that leads to an accumulation of drugs and the potential for drug toxicity. Drug doses and frequency are adjusted based on the severity of the kidney disease. Increased sensitivity may result as drug levels increase in the blood and tissues. Drugs of particular concern include digoxin, diabetic agents (metformin, glyburide), antibiotics (e.g., vancomycin, gentamicin), and opioid drugs.

Nutrition Therapy

Protein restriction. The current diet for the person with CKD is designed to maintain good nutrition (Table 51.9). Calorie-protein malnutrition is a potential, serious problem that results from altered metabolism, anemia, dental problems, anorexia, and nausea. Other factors leading to malnutrition include depression and complex diets that restrict protein, phosphorus, potassium, and sodium. Frequent monitoring of laboratory tests and anthropometric measurements are needed to evaluate nutrition status. All patients with CKD should be referred to a dietitian for nutrition teaching.

For CKD stages 1 through 4, many HCPs encourage a diet with normal protein intake. For patients on HD, protein is not routinely restricted. Patients should avoid high-protein diets and supplements because they may overburden the diseased kidneys.[20]

Protein guidelines for PD differ from those for HD because of protein loss through the peritoneal membrane. During PD, protein intake must be high enough to compensate for the losses so that the nitrogen balance is maintained. The recommended protein intake is at least 1.2 g/kg of ideal body weight (IBW) per day. This can be increased depending on the patient's needs.

For patients with malnutrition or inadequate caloric or protein intake, commercially prepared products that are high in protein but low in sodium and potassium are available (e.g., Nepro, Amin-Aid). As an alternative, patients may drink liquid or powder breakfast drinks.

Fluid restriction. Water and any other fluids are not routinely restricted in patients with CKD stages 1 to 5 who are not receiving HD. To reduce fluid retention, diuretics are often used. Patients on HD have a more restricted fluid intake than patients on PD. For those on HD, as their urine output decreases, fluids are restricted. Recommended fluid intake depends on the daily urine output. Generally, 600 mL (from insensible loss) plus an amount equal to the previous day's urine output is allowed for patients on HD.

Foods that are liquid at room temperature (e.g., gelatin, ice) are counted as fluid intake. Space fluid allotment throughout the day so that patients do not become thirsty. Teach patients to limit fluid intake so that weight gains are no more than 1 to 3 kg between dialyses (interdialytic weight gain).

Sodium and potassium restriction. Teach patients with CKD to restrict sodium. Sodium-restricted diets may vary from 2 to 4 g/day. Teach patients to avoid high-sodium foods. Potassium restriction depends on the kidneys' ability to excrete potassium. Restrictions range from 2000 to 3000 mg (39 mg = 1 mEq). Teach patients receiving HD to avoid foods that are high in potassium (see Table 17.7). Patients using PD do not usually need potassium restrictions. They may need oral potassium supplements because of the loss of potassium with dialysis exchanges.

Phosphate restriction. As kidney function declines, phosphate elimination by the kidneys is decreased. Patients develop high phosphorus levels. By the time patients reach ESRD, they need to limit phosphate to around 1 g/day. Foods that are high in phosphate include meat and dairy products. Many foods that are high in phosphate are also high in protein. When patients eat a diet containing protein, phosphate binders are given to control the phosphate level.

NURSING MANAGEMENT: CHRONIC KIDNEY DISEASE

Assessment

Obtain a complete history of any existing kidney disease or family history of kidney disease. Some kidney disorders, including Alport syndrome and polycystic kidney disease, have a genetic component. Other problems that can lead to CKD are diabetes, hypertension, and SLE.

Because many drugs are potentially nephrotoxic, obtain a medication history. Decongestants and antihistamines that contain pseudoephedrine and phenylephrine cause vasoconstriction and can lead to an increase in BP. Magnesium and aluminum from antacids can accumulate in the body because they cannot be excreted. Some antacids have high salt levels. This also contributes to hypertension.

NSAIDs (aspirin, ibuprofen, naproxen) can contribute to the progression of CKD, especially when taken in higher doses than recommended. If taken as prescribed, these analgesics are usually considered safe.[21]

Assess diet habits and discuss any problems with intake. Measure height and weight. Evaluate any recent weight changes. Assess for respiratory difficulty, edema, and signs of fluid overload.

CKD and its long-term treatment affect virtually every area of a person's life, including family relationships, social and work activities, self-image, and emotional state. Assess support systems. The choice of treatment may be related to the support systems available.

Clinical Problems

Clinical problems for patients with CKD include:

- Fluid imbalance
- Electrolyte imbalance
- Impaired cardiac function
- Difficulty coping

More information on clinical problems and interventions for patients with CKD is presented in eNursing Care Plan 51.1, available on the website for this chapter.

Planning

The overall goals are that patients with CKD will (1) be engaged in and adhere to the treatment plan, (2) have effective coping strategies, and (3) continue with activities of daily living within their limitations.

Implementation

Health Promotion

Identify those at risk for CKD (Table 51.6). At-risk persons include those diagnosed with diabetes or hypertension and people with a personal or family history of kidney disease or repeated urinary tract infections (UTIs). They should have regular checkups that include a routine urinalysis and calculation of the estimated GFR. Monitor kidney function in patients receiving nephrotoxic drugs.

People with diabetes need to have their urine checked for albuminuria if routine urinalysis is negative for protein. Teach patients with diabetes to report any changes in urine appearance (color, odor), frequency, or volume to the HCP. Those at risk must take measures to prevent or delay the progression of CKD. Most important are measures to reduce the risk or progression of CVD. These include glycemic control for patients with diabetes (see Chapter 53), BP control (see Chapter 36), and lifestyle changes, including smoking cessation.

Chronic Care

Most of the care of patients with CKD occurs on an outpatient basis. In-hospital care is needed for management of complications and kidney transplants. Teach patients and caregivers about the diet, drugs, and follow-up care (Table 51.10). Patients need to understand the drugs and common side effects. The dietitian should meet with patients and caregivers on a regular basis for diet planning. A diet history and consideration of cultural variations help with diet planning and adherence.

Most patients need PD or HD. Most patients use HD. Explain what is involved in PD or HD. Offer information about all treatment options so that patients can be involved in the decision-making process, giving a sense of control over life-altering decisions. Tell them that even while on dialysis, transplant is still an option. Let them know that if a transplanted organ fails, they can return to dialysis.

Patients can complete an evaluation for a kidney transplant before the need to start dialysis. Patients may receive a transplant before ever having to start dialysis. Even though a transplant offers the best outcome for many ESRD patients, the critical shortage of donor organs limits this option for many patients.

Discuss palliative care as needed. Patients themselves often start the conversation about palliative care. Focus the discussion on moving from the curative approach to promotion of comfort care and consideration of hospice care. Listen to patients and caregivers. Pay attention to their hopes and fears. Palliative and end-of-life care is discussed in Chapter 10.

TABLE 51.10 PATIENT & CAREGIVER TEACHING

CKD

Include the following information in the teaching plan for patients and caregivers:

1. Diet (sodium, potassium, phosphate) and fluid restrictions.
2. Common problems patients will encounter in modifying diet and fluid intake.
3. Signs and symptoms of electrolyte imbalance, especially high potassium.
4. Alternative ways of reducing thirst, such as sucking on ice cubes, lemon, or hard candy.
5. Reasons for prescribed drugs and common side effects. *Examples:*
    - Phosphate binders (including calcium supplements used as phosphate barriers) should be taken with meals.
    - Take calcium supplements prescribed to treat hypocalcemia on an empty stomach, but not at the same time as iron supplements.
    - Iron supplements should be taken between meals.
6. The need to avoid OTC drugs such as NSAIDs and aluminum- and magnesium-based laxatives and antacids.
7. How to take BP; importance of daily BP measurements.
8. The importance of reporting any weight gain >4 lb (2 kg), increasing BP, shortness of breath, edema, increasing fatigue or weakness, or confusion or lethargy.
9. Need for support and encouragement. Share concerns about lifestyle changes, living with a chronic illness, and decisions about type of dialysis or transplantation.

◆ Evaluation

The expected outcomes are that patients with CKD will maintain:

- Fluid and electrolyte levels within normal ranges
- An acceptable weight

RENAL REPLACEMENT THERAPY

GENERAL PRINCIPLES OF RENAL REPLACEMENT THERAPY

Renal replacement therapy (RRT) replaces the nonendocrine kidney function in patients with renal failure. It also can be used to treat drug overdoses and poisoning. Techniques include **peritoneal dialysis (PD)**, **hemodialysis (HD)**, and continuous renal replacement therapy (CRRT). All techniques exchange solute and remove fluid from the blood using dialysis and filtration.[22] They do not correct endocrine problems, including decreased erythropoietin. RRT can ease many of the symptoms of CKD and, if started early, prevent certain complications.

Since 1972, the United States has covered most of the costs of dialysis through Medicare benefits. Under Title XVIII of the Social Security Act, ESRD was recognized as a disability. Medicare pays for 80% of eligible charges. The state, private insurance, or patient covers the rest.[23]

Dialysis is started when uremia can no longer be adequately treated with conservative medical management. Generally, this is when the GFR is less than 15 mL/min/1.73 m^2.[24] This criterion can vary widely in different clinical situations. The nephrologist discusses with the patient when to start dialysis based on clinical status. Certain uremic complications, such as encephalopathy, neuropathies, hyperkalemia, pericarditis, and accelerated hypertension, indicate a need for immediate dialysis.

Most patients with ESRD are treated with dialysis because (1) there is a lack of donated organs, (2) some patients are physically or mentally unsuitable for a transplant, or (3) some patients do not want transplants. An increasing number of people, including older adults and those with complex medical problems, are receiving maintenance dialysis. Age is not a factor in determining candidacy for dialysis.[23]

The yearly death rate of patients receiving maintenance HD is around 19% to 24%. CVD (stroke, MI) causes most deaths. Mortality rates are similar between in-center HD patients and PD patients for the first few years. After about 2 years, mortality rates for patients receiving PD increase, especially for the older person with diabetes and patients with a prior history of CVD.[22] Infectious complications are the second leading cause of death.

Clinically, **dialysis** is a technique in which substances move from the blood through a semipermeable membrane and into a dialysis solution *(dialysate)*. In PD the peritoneal membrane acts as the semipermeable membrane (Table 51.11). In HD a semipermeable artificial membrane (usually made of cellulose-based or synthetic materials) is used and in contact with the blood.[24]

Solutes and water move across the semipermeable membrane from the blood to the dialysate or from the dialysate to the blood per concentration gradients. Diffusion, osmosis, and ultrafiltration are involved in dialysis (Fig. 51.4). *Diffusion* is the movement of solutes from an area of greater concentration to an area of lesser concentration. In kidney failure, urea, creatinine, uric acid, and electrolytes (potassium, phosphate) move from the blood to the dialysate with the net effect of lowering their concentration in the blood. RBCs, WBCs, and plasma proteins are too large to diffuse through the pores of the membrane. Small-molecular-weight substances can pass from the dialysate into the blood, so we must monitor and control the water purity used for dialysis.

Osmosis is the movement of fluid from an area of lesser concentration to an area of greater concentration of solutes. Glucose in the dialysate creates an osmotic gradient across the membrane, pulling excess fluid from the blood.

Ultrafiltration (water and fluid removal) results when there is an osmotic gradient or pressure gradient across the membrane. In PD, excess fluid is removed by increasing the osmolality of the dialysate (osmotic gradient) with glucose. In HD, the gradient is created by increasing pressure in the blood compartment (positive pressure) or decreasing pressure in the dialysate compartment (negative pressure). ECF moves into the dialysate because of the pressure gradient. The excess fluid is removed by creating a pressure differential between the blood and the dialysate solution with a combination of positive pressure in the blood compartment and negative pressure in the dialysate compartment.

PERITONEAL DIALYSIS

Catheter Placement

Peritoneal access is obtained by inserting a catheter through the anterior abdominal wall (Fig. 51.5). The catheter is about 24 in

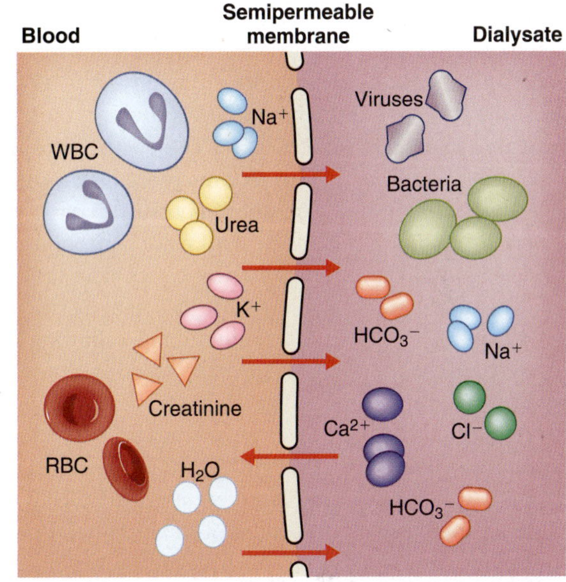

Fig. 51.4 Osmosis and diffusion across a semipermeable membrane.

TABLE 51.11 Comparison of Peritoneal Dialysis and Hemodialysis

	Peritoneal Dialysis (PD)	Hemodialysis
Advantages	• Immediate initiation in almost any hospital • Less complicated • Portable system with CAPD • Fewer diet restrictions • Short training time • Usable in patient with vascular access problems • Less cardiovascular stress • Home based • Preferable for patient with diabetes	• Rapid fluid removal • Rapid removal of urea and creatinine • Effective potassium removal • Less protein loss • Lowers triglycerides • Home dialysis possible • Can place temporary access at bedside
Disadvantages	• Bacterial or chemical peritonitis • Protein loss into dialysate • Exit site and tunnel infections • Hyperglycemia • Surgery for catheter placement • Contraindicated in patient with multiple abdominal surgeries, trauma, unrepaired hernia • Requires completion of education program • Catheter can migrate • Best instituted with willing partner	• Vascular access problems • Diet and fluid restrictions • Heparinization may be necessary • Extensive equipment necessary • Hypotension during dialysis • Added blood loss that contributes to anemia • Specially trained personnel necessary • Surgery for permanent access placement

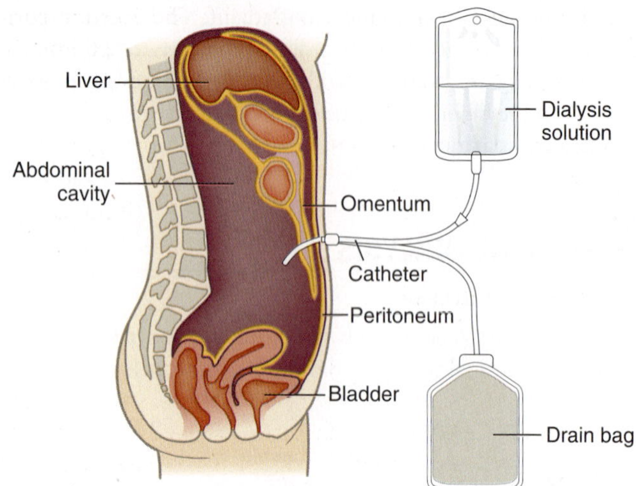

Fig. 51.5 PD showing peritoneal catheter inserted into peritoneal cavity.

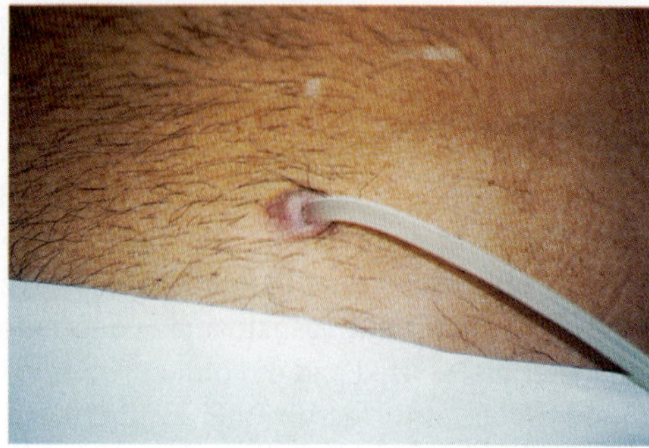

Fig. 51.6 Peritoneal catheter exit site. (Courtesy Mary Jo Holechek, Baltimore, MD.)

(60 cm) long and has 1 or 2 Dacron cuffs. The cuffs act as anchors and prevent the migration of microorganisms into the peritoneum. Within a few weeks, fibrous tissue grows into the Dacron cuff, holding the catheter in place and preventing bacterial penetration into the peritoneal cavity. The tip of the catheter rests in the peritoneal cavity. It has many perforations spaced along the distal end of the tubing, allowing fluid movement through the catheter.

The technique for catheter placement varies. It is usually placed surgically so that the catheter can be seen directly, minimizing potential complications. After placement, PD may be started at once with low-volume exchanges or delayed for 2 weeks pending healing and sealing of the exit site. Once the catheter incision site is healed, patients may shower and then pat the catheter and exit site dry.[22] Daily catheter care varies. Some patients just wash with soap and water and go without a dressing (Fig. 51.6). Others need daily dressing changes. Showering is preferred to bathing.

In PD it is critical to maintain aseptic technique to avoid peritonitis. Several tubing connections and devices are available to help maintain an aseptic system. Teach all patients to check their catheter site for signs of infection.

Dialysis Solutions and Cycles

PD is done by putting dialysis solution into the peritoneal space. The 3 phases of the PD cycle are inflow (fill), dwell (equilibration), and drain. Together, the 3 phases are an *exchange*. For manual PD, it takes about 30 to 50 minutes to complete an exchange. During *inflow*, a prescribed amount of solution, usually 2 L, is infused through an established catheter over about 10 minutes. The flow rate may be decreased if the patient has pain. After infusing the solution, the inflow clamp is closed.

The next part of the cycle is the *dwell* phase, or equilibration. This is when diffusion and osmosis occur between the blood and peritoneal cavity. The duration of the dwell time is usually between 4 and 6 hours. *Drain* time takes 15 to 30 minutes. It may be facilitated by gently massaging the abdomen or changing position. The cycle starts again with the infusion of another 2 L of solution.

PD solutions vary. The exchange volume is mainly determined by the size of the peritoneal cavity. An average-size person typically uses a 2-L exchange. A larger person may need a 3-L exchange volume. Smaller exchange volumes are used for patients with a smaller body, pulmonary compromise (the added pressure of the large volume may cause respiratory problems), or inguinal hernias.

Ultrafiltration (fluid removal) during PD depends on osmotic forces. Dextrose is the most often used osmotic agent in PD solutions. It is safe and inexpensive. It is associated with high rates of peritoneal glucose absorption. This can lead to problems with high triglycerides, hyperglycemia, and long-term peritoneal membrane dysfunction.

Alternatives to dextrose PD solution include icodextrin and amino acid solutions. Icodextrin is an isoosmolar preparation. It induces ultrafiltration by its oncotic effect. It is relatively slow compared with dextrose solution. Amino acid PD solutions are an option for patients who need added nutrition.

Peritoneal Dialysis Systems

Automated Peritoneal Dialysis

Automated peritoneal dialysis (APD) is the most popular form of PD because it allows patients to do dialysis while they sleep. An automated device called a *cycler* delivers the dialysate for APD (Fig. 51.7). The automated cycler times and controls the fill, dwell, and drain phases. The machine cycles 4 or more exchanges per night with 1 to 2 hours per exchange. Alarms and monitors built into the system make it safe for patients to sleep while dialyzing. Patients disconnect from the machine in the morning. They usually leave fluid in the abdomen during the day. It is hard to achieve the required solute and fluid clearance solely with nighttime APD. One or 2 daytime manual exchanges may be needed to ensure adequate dialysis.

Continuous Ambulatory Peritoneal Dialysis

Continuous ambulatory peritoneal dialysis (CAPD) is done every few hours during the day. Patients may perform an exchange of

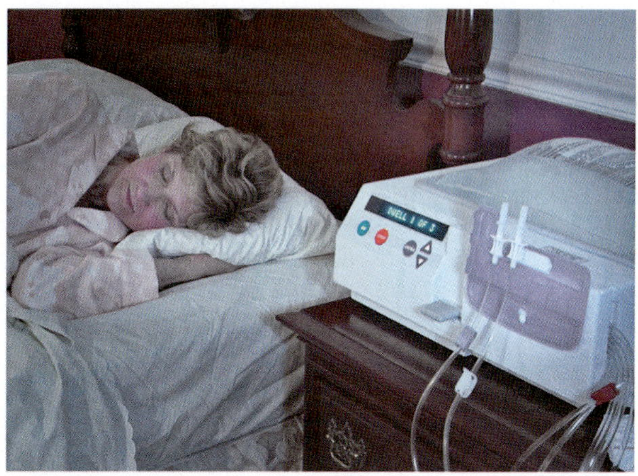
Fig. 51.7 Automated PD can be used while patients are sleeping.

2 L of peritoneal dialysate 4 times daily, with dwell times averaging 4 hours. A common schedule includes exchanges at 7 AM, 12 noon, 5 PM, and 10 PM.

In CAPD, the person instills 2 to 3 L of dialysate from a plastic bag into the peritoneal cavity through a disposable administration line. The bag and line are then disconnected. After the equilibration period, the line is reconnected to the catheter, the dialysate (effluent) is drained from the peritoneal cavity, and a new 2- to 3-L bag of dialysate solution is infused.

Complications of Peritoneal Dialysis

Exit Site Infection

Infection of the peritoneal catheter exit site is most often caused by *Staphylococcus aureus* or *Staphylococcus epidermidis* (from skin flora). Manifestations include redness at the site, tenderness, and drainage. Superficial exit site infections caused by these organisms generally resolve with antibiotic therapy. If not treated quickly, subcutaneous tunnel infections may progress and cause peritonitis, requiring catheter removal.

Peritonitis

Peritonitis results from contact contamination or an exit site or tunnel infection. Most often it occurs because of improper technique when connections for exchanges are contaminated. Peritonitis is usually caused by *S. aureus* or *S. epidermidis.* It rarely results from bacteria in the intestine crossing into the peritoneal cavity.

The main manifestations are abdominal pain, rebound tenderness, and cloudy peritoneal effluent with a WBC count greater than 100 cells/μL (more than 50% neutrophils) or bacteria in the peritoneal effluent shown by Gram stain or culture. GI manifestations may include diarrhea, vomiting, abdominal distention, and hyperactive bowel sounds. Fever may be present. To determine whether the peritoneal effluent is cloudy, drain the effluent and place the drained bag on reading material, such as a newspaper. If you cannot read the print through the effluent, it is cloudy.

Cultures, Gram stain, and a WBC differential of the peritoneal effluent are used to confirm the diagnosis of peritonitis. Antibiotics can be given orally, IV, or intraperitoneally. In most cases, patients are treated on an outpatient basis.

Adhesions in the peritoneum can result from repeated infections. They can interfere with the peritoneal membrane's ability to act as a dialyzing surface. Repeated infections may require the removal of the peritoneal catheter and a temporary or permanent change of modality to HD.

Hernias

Increased intraabdominal pressure from the dialysate volume can cause hernias to develop in predisposed persons, such as multiparous females and older males. After hernia repair, PD often can be resumed after several days using small dialysate volumes and keeping the patient supine.

Lower Back Problems

Increased intraabdominal pressure can cause or worsen lower back pain. The lumbosacral curvature is increased by intraperitoneal infusion of dialysate. Orthopedic binders and a regular exercise program for strengthening the back muscles are helpful for some patients.

Bleeding

After peritoneal catheter placement, it is common for the PD effluent drained after the first few exchanges to be pink or slightly bloody from trauma after catheter insertion. Bloody effluent over several days or the new appearance of blood in the effluent can indicate active intraperitoneal bleeding. If this occurs, check the BP and hematocrit. Blood may be present in the effluent of females who are menstruating or ovulating. This requires no intervention.

Pulmonary Complications

Atelectasis, pneumonia, and bronchitis may occur from repeated upward displacement of the diaphragm, resulting in decreased lung expansion. Longer dwell times increase the risk for pulmonary problems. Frequent repositioning and deep-breathing exercises can help. When patients are lying in bed, elevate the head of the bed to prevent these problems.

Protein Loss

The peritoneal membrane is permeable to plasma proteins, amino acids, and polypeptides. These substances are lost in the dialysate fluid. The amount of loss is usually about 0.5 g/L of dialysate drainage, but it can be as high as 10 to 20 g/day. This loss may increase to as much as 40 g/day with peritonitis as the peritoneal membrane becomes more permeable. Unresolved peritonitis can cause protein loss that can result in malnutrition. PD may need to stop temporarily or sometimes permanently.

HEMODIALYSIS

Vascular Access Sites

HD requires a very rapid blood flow and access to a large blood vessel. Obtaining vascular access is one of the biggest issues with HD. Enough time is needed to determine the best access for HD. The types of vascular access include AV fistulas (AVFs), AV grafts (AVGs), and temporary vascular access.[25]

Arteriovenous Fistulas and Grafts

A subcutaneous **arteriovenous fistula (AVF)** is usually created in the forearm or upper arm with an anastomosis between an artery and a vein (usually cephalic or basilic) (Figs. 51.8A and 51.9). The fistula allows arterial blood to flow through the vein.

The vein becomes "arterialized," increasing in size and developing thicker walls. The arterial blood flow is essential to supply the rapid blood flow needed for HD. As the fistula matures, it is more amenable to repeated venipunctures. Maturation may take 6 weeks to months. AVF should be placed at least 3 months before starting HD.

Normally, a *thrill* (buzzing sensation) can be felt by palpating the fistula, and a *bruit* (rushing sound) can be heard with a stethoscope. The thrill and bruit are created by arterial blood moving at a high velocity through the vein.

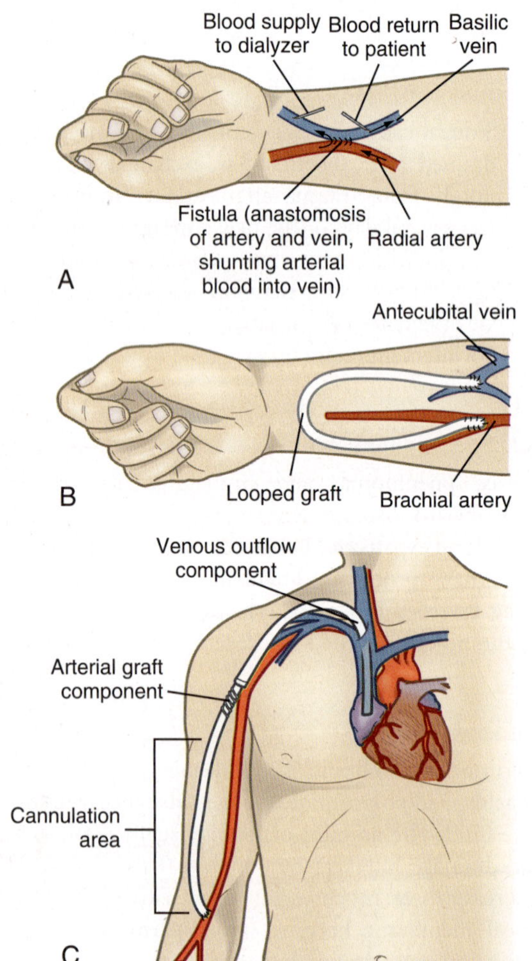

Fig. 51.8 Vascular access for hemodialysis. (A) AVF. (B) AVG. (C) HeRO graft.

CHECK YOUR PRACTICE

It is your first time working with an HD patient on your unit. You are helping an HD tech "hook up" a 56-year-old male to HD. He has been on HD for 5 years due to polycystic kidney disease. You take his vital signs, palpate his AV fistula, and then use your stethoscope to auscultate the AV fistula. You are concerned because you feel a super-strong pulse and hear a very loud "whoosh" sound. The patient turns to you and just smirks, "I bet you have never had a thrill like that."

- You are very flustered and not sure how to respond. What should you say to him?

AVFs are harder to create in patients with a history of severe peripheral vascular disease (e.g., people with diabetes), those with prolonged IV drug use, and obese females. These people may need a synthetic graft.

Arteriovenous grafts (AVGs) are made of synthetic materials (polytetrafluoroethylene [PTFE, Teflon]). They form a "bridge" between the arterial and venous blood supplies. Grafts are placed under the skin and surgically anastomosed between an artery (usually brachial) and a vein (usually antecubital) (Fig. 51.8B). An interval of 2 to 4 weeks is usually needed to allow the graft to heal, but it may be used earlier. Because grafts are made of artificial materials, they are more likely than AVFs to become infected and tend to form clots. When AVG infections occur, they may need to be surgically removed, since it is hard to resolve infection from the synthetic material.

A common problem is central venous stenosis (CVS) or occlusion. CVS is serious because the central veins are the final pathway for blood flow to the heart. As CVS progresses, vascular access for HD is often lost.

A special bridge graft can be used in patients when other access options are exhausted. The Hemodialysis Reliable Outflow (HeRO) consists of 2 pieces: a reinforced tube to bypass blockages in veins and a graft anastomosed to an artery for HD access (Fig. 51.8C). It is placed under the skin, like a fistula and standard graft. It bypasses the venous system and provides blood flow directly from a target artery to the heart. You may find it harder to auscultate the bruit or feel the thrill because of the absence of a venous anastomosis.

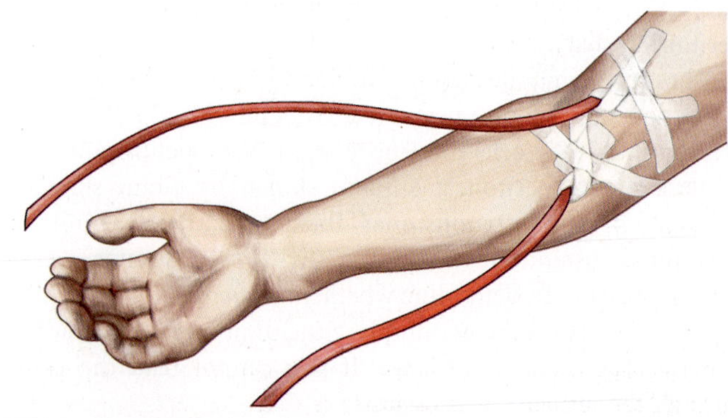

Fig. 51.9 AVF with cannulation needles for HD access.

Surgical creation of AV access for HD has several risks. These include distal ischemia *(steal syndrome)* and pain because too much arterial blood is being shunted or "stolen" from the distal extremity. Manifestations of steal syndrome are pain distal to the access site, numbness or tingling of fingers that may worsen during HD, and poor capillary refill. Aneurysms can develop in the AV access and can rupture if left untreated.

! SAFETY ALERT

AV Fistulas and Grafts

- Never perform BP measurements, IV insertion, or venipuncture in an extremity with AV access.
- These precautions are taken to prevent infection and clotting of the vascular access.
- Place signs in patient's room and label the arm with a band that says, "No BP, blood draws, or IV in this arm."

Temporary Vascular Access

When immediate vascular access is needed, catheterization of the internal jugular or femoral vein is done (Fig. 51.10). The catheters usually have a double external lumen with an internal septum separating the 2 internal segments. One lumen is used for blood removal and the other for blood return (Fig. 51.11A and B). Temporary catheters have high rates of infection, dislodgment, and malfunction. Patients should not be discharged from the hospital with a temporary catheter in place.

Long-term cuffed HD catheters are often used for temporary vascular access. These catheters give temporary access while patients are waiting for fistula placement or as long-term access when other forms of access have failed. They exit on the upper chest wall and are tunneled subcutaneously to the internal or external jugular vein (Fig. 51.11C). The catheter tip rests in the right atrium. It has 1 or 2 subcutaneous Dacron cuffs that prevent infection from tracking along the catheter and anchor the catheter, eliminating the need for sutures.

Dialyzers

The HD dialyzer is a plastic cartridge that has thousands of parallel hollow tubes or fibers. The fibers are semipermeable

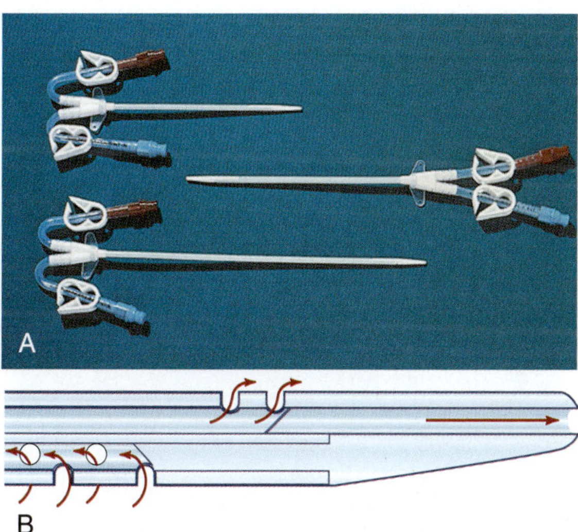

Fig. 51.10 Temporary double-lumen vascular access catheter for acute hemodialysis. (A) Soft, flexible double-lumen tube is attached to a Y hub. (B) The distance between the arterial intake lumen and the venous return lumen typically provides recirculation rates of 5% or less. (A, Courtesy Quinton Instrument Co., Seattle, WA.)

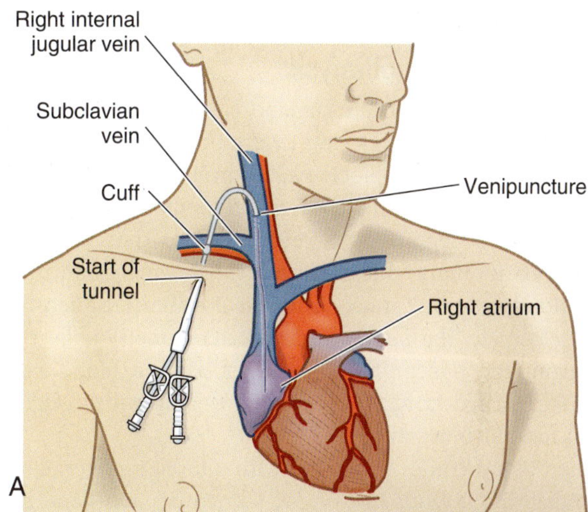

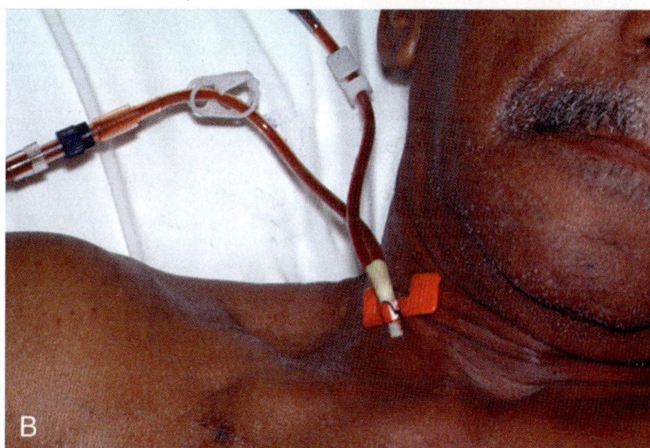

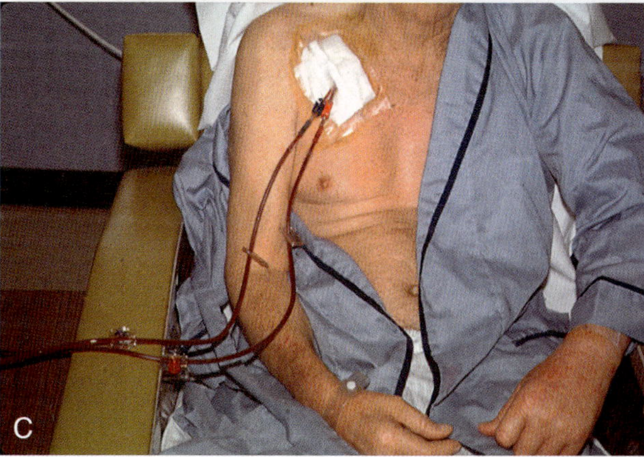

Fig. 51.11 (A) Right internal jugular placement for a tunneled, cuffed semipermanent catheter. (B) Temporary hemodialysis catheter in place. (C) Long-term cuffed hemodialysis catheter. (B and C, Courtesy Dr. Stephen Van Voorst, MD.)

membranes made of cellulose-based or other synthetic materials. The blood is pumped into the top of the cartridge and dispersed into all the fibers. Dialysis fluid *(dialysate)* is pumped into the bottom of the cartridge and bathes the outside of the fibers. Ultrafiltration, diffusion, and osmosis occur across the pores of this semipermeable membrane. When the dialyzed blood reaches the end of the thousands of semipermeable fibers, it converges into a single tube that returns it to the patient. Dialyzers differ in surface area, membrane composition and thickness, clearance of waste products, and removal of fluid.

Procedure for Hemodialysis

The needles used for HD are large bore, usually 15 or 16 gauge. They are inserted into the fistula or graft to obtain access to the blood. One needle pulls blood away from the circulation to the HD machine (arterial line). The other needle returns the dialyzed blood to the patient (venous line). The needles are attached via tubing to dialysis lines. If a patient has a catheter, the 2 blood lines are attached to the 2 catheter lumens. The needle closer to the fistula (red catheter lumen) pulls blood away from the patient to the dialyzer using a blood pump. Blood is returned from the dialyzer to the patient through the second needle (blue catheter lumen).[24]

When blood comes in contact with a foreign material, such as the dialyzer, it tends to clot. We sometimes add heparin via the system to prevent clotting.

In addition to the dialyzer, we use a dialysate delivery and monitoring system (Fig. 51.12). This system pumps the dialysate through the dialyzer, countercurrent to the blood flow. To end the treatment, saline solution returns the blood in the extracorporeal circuit back to the patient through the vascular access. The needles are removed from the patient. Firm pressure is applied to the venipuncture sites until the bleeding stops.

Before beginning treatment, assess fluid status (weight, peripheral edema, lung and heart sounds), condition of vascular access using the "One Minute Check," and vital signs. The difference between the last postdialysis weight and the present predialysis weight determines the ultrafiltration or the amount of weight (from fluid) to be removed. While patients are on HD, take vital signs at least every 30 minutes because rapid BP changes may occur.

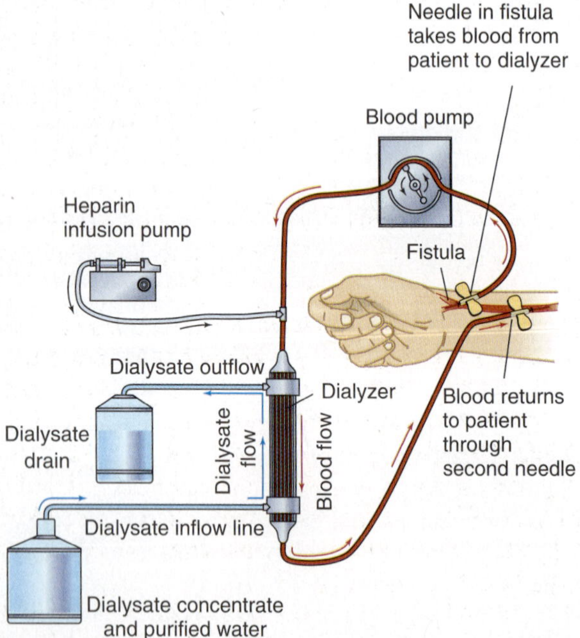

Fig. 51.12 Parts of a hemodialysis system. Blood is removed via a needle inserted in a fistula or via catheter lumen. A pump moves the blood to the dialyzer. Heparin is infused as a predialysis bolus or through a heparin pump to prevent clotting. Dialysate flows in the opposite direction of the blood. The dialyzed blood is returned to the patient through a second needle or catheter lumen. Dialysate with waste products and ultrafiltrate are drained and discarded.

Settings and Schedules for Hemodialysis

Most HD patients are treated in a community-based center. They dialyze for 3 to 4 hours 3 days/week. Other schedule options are short daily HD and long nighttime HD. Patients receiving long nighttime HD have the advantage of sleeping while dialyzing. Each nighttime treatment lasts 6 to 8 hours. Patients dialyze up to 6 times per week.

Home HD may be an option (Fig. 51.13). The use of home HD often depends on a person's choice, as well as caregiver support. One of the main advantages of home HD is that it allows greater freedom in choosing dialysis times. In short daily HD, patients dialyze for 2½ to 3 hours per session 5 to 6 days/week. Short daily HD is usually done at home.

Patients who choose daily or nighttime dialysis may have fewer uremic symptoms, tend to need fewer medications, and have fewer HD-related side effects (e.g., hypotension, cramps). Although daily home HD offers the potential of significant health benefits, the number of people that dialyze at home is low. However, the number has increased from around 6% in 2010 to 13% in 2020.[24]

The wearable artificial kidney is a miniature dialysis machine that can be worn on the body. The carrier resembles a tool belt. The device connects to a patient via a catheter. Like conventional dialysis machines, it filters the blood of ESRD patients.

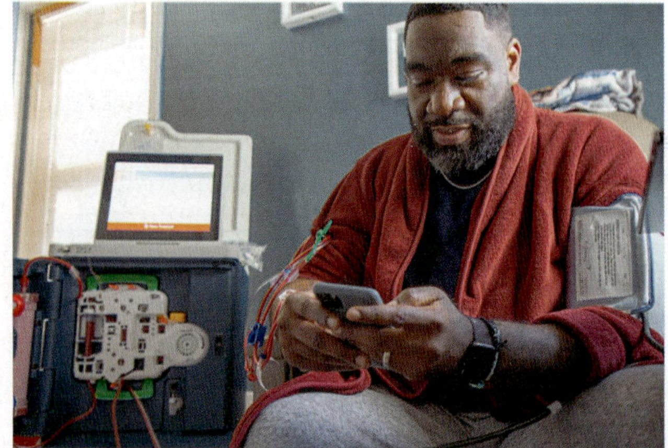

Fig. 51.13 Home hemodialysis is growing in popularity, and machines are more compact. (Courtesy Outset Medical, Inc.)

Unlike current portable or stationary dialysis machines, it can run continuously on batteries. The present version weighs about 10 lb. The wearable artificial kidney has improved the quality of life for some ESRD patients.

Complications of Hemodialysis

Hypotension

Hypotension during HD often results from rapid removal of vascular volume (hypovolemia), decreased cardiac output, and decreased systemic vascular resistance. The drop in BP may cause lightheadedness, nausea, vomiting, seizures, vision changes, and chest pain from cardiac ischemia. The usual treatment includes decreasing the volume of fluid removed and infusing 0.9% saline solution.

Muscle Cramps

We do not completely understand the cause of muscle cramps in HD. They are associated with hypotension, hypovolemia, high ultrafiltration rate (UFR), and low-sodium dialysis solution. Treatment includes reducing the UFR and giving fluids (saline, mannitol).

Loss of Blood

Blood loss may result from blood not being completely rinsed from the dialyzer, accidental separation of blood tubing, dialysis membrane rupture, or bleeding after removing the needles at the end of HD. If a patient has received too much heparin or has clotting problems, postdialysis bleeding can occur. It is essential to rinse back all blood, avoid excess anticoagulation, and hold firm but nonocclusive pressure on access sites until the risk for bleeding has passed.

Hepatitis

Hepatitis B used to have a high prevalence in HD patients, but the incidence today is low. Outbreaks still occur, likely from breaks in infection control practices. To prevent transmission, all patients and personnel in dialysis units receive hepatitis B vaccine. Hepatitis C virus (HCV) causes most cases of hepatitis in HD patients (see Chapter 48). About 10% of patients receiving dialysis in the United States are positive for anti-HCV, which indicates a previous infection. Infection control precautions are mandated in caring for patients with hepatitis C (see Chapter 15).

NURSING MANAGEMENT: HEMODIALYSIS

Nursing care for patients receiving HD is outlined in Table 51.12. Key nursing goals are to (1) help patients maintain a healthy self-image and (2) return patients to the highest level of function possible, including returning to work. Adaptation to maintenance HD varies considerably. At first, many patients feel positive about the dialysis because it makes them feel better and keeps them alive, but it has adverse physical and psychologic complications. Dependence on a machine is a reality. Several problems, such as fatigue, depression, and sleep problems, play a role in reducing the quality of life of HD patients (Box 51.1).

TABLE 51.12 NURSING MANAGEMENT

Care of the Patient Receiving HD

- Monitor blood chemistries (e.g., creatinine, BUN, sodium, potassium) before and after treatment and note manifestations of electrolyte imbalances
- Record baseline vital signs and lung sounds; monitor during treatment and after per agency protocol
- Obtain daily weight, preprocedure weight, and postprocedure weight
- Maintain intake and output records
- Monitor for cardiac manifestations of hyperkalemia and initiate ECG monitoring as needed
- Implement measures to reduce hypervolemia between treatments, include fluid restrictions
- Administer prescribed drug therapy, including calcium, vitamin D
- Plan medication administration to regulate fluid and electrolyte shifts between treatments and accommodate treatment schedule
- Provide a safe environment if neuromuscular manifestations occur
- Monitor for manifestations of electrolyte imbalance
- Monitor and maintain patency of the vascular access graft
- Monitor for dialysis complications, including bleeding, infection
- Identify sources of community support
- Implement measures to promote positive coping
- Provide patient and caregiver education about HD and CKD (Table 51.10)

Collaborate

Dialysis Technician

- Institute and discontinue dialysis according to agency protocol
- Provide HD treatment and adjust filtration pressure, length of dialysis

Dietitian

- Assess nutrition status and monitor trends in weight
- Provide nutrition teaching regarding the optimal diet (Table 51.9)
- Encourage adherence to diet plan

CONTINUOUS RENAL REPLACEMENT THERAPY

Continuous renal replacement therapy (CRRT) is a method for treating AKI. It provides a means by which uremic toxins and fluids are removed while acid-base status and electrolytes are adjusted slowly and continuously in hemodynamically unstable patients. The principle of CRRT is to dialyze patients in a more physiologic way (over 24 hours), just like the kidneys. CRRT is contraindicated if patients have life-threatening manifestations of uremia (hyperkalemia, pericarditis) that need rapid treatment. CRRT can be used with HD.

Several types of CRRT are available (Table 51.13). CRRT often uses a venovenous approach. Examples include continuous venovenous hemofiltration (CVVH), continuous venovenous hemodialysis (CVVHD), and continuous venovenous hemodiafiltration (CVVHDF).

Vascular access for CRRT is achieved with a double-lumen catheter as used in HD (Figs. 51.10 and 51.11) placed in the

BOX 51.1 EVIDENCE-BASED PRACTICE

Sleep Hygiene for Hemodialysis Patients

You are a working in a dialysis clinic. One morning you overhear 2 patients talking about how they are each having difficulty falling and staying asleep many nights. They say they feel "tired and listless" and take several naps throughout the day.

Making Clinical Decisions

Synthesis of Best Available Evidence

More than half of patients receiving hemodialysis report sleep problems, including insomnia. The resulting daytime fatigue can lead to irritability and depression, which can interfere with work and social functioning. Improving sleep quality through sleep hygiene can decrease these negative effects.

Clinician Expertise

You ask the patients about their sleep habits and bedtime routine and determine that both may have insomnia. In addition to reviewing sleep hygiene habits, you consider suggesting that they add relaxation breathing to their bedtime routine. Performing relaxation breathing 15 to 20 minutes before going to sleep has been found to decrease time to falling asleep and to increase length of sleep.

Patient Preferences and Values

You review sleep hygiene with the patients and teach them relaxation breathing. They agree to try the exercises for 1 month and keep a sleep log. After 1 month, both reported taking less time falling asleep and sleeping 30 to 60 minutes longer per night on average.

Implications for Nursing Practice

1. What other nonpharmacologic interventions could you recommend to the patients to improve sleep quality?
2. How could patients monitor their own sleep patterns when implementing new interventions to improve sleep?

Reference for Evidence

Ebrahimi F, Sokhtseraei S, Navidian A: The effect of sleep hygiene education on sleep quality, depression, and fatigue of hemodialysis patients, *Med Surg Nurs J* 12:1 2023.

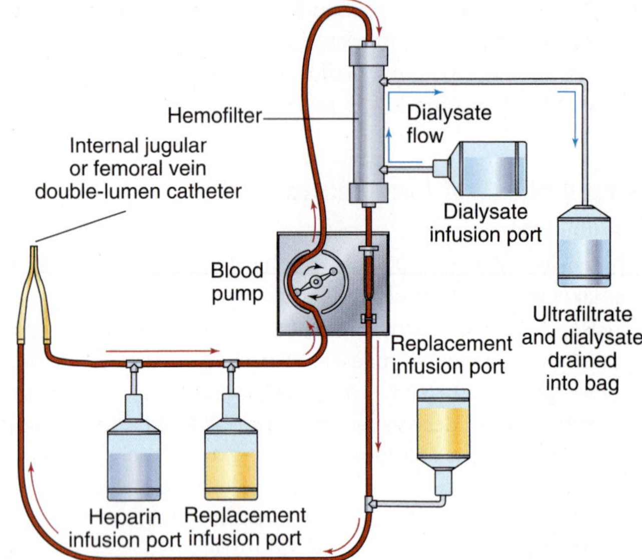

Fig. 51.14 Basic schematic of continuous venovenous therapies. A blood pump is needed to pump blood through the circuit. Replacement ports are used for instilling replacement fluids and can be given prefilter or postfilter. Dialysate port is used for infusing dialysis solution. Ultrafiltrate is drained via the ultrafiltration drain port.

TABLE 51.13 Continuous Renal Replacement Therapies

Therapy	Abbreviation	Purpose
Continuous venovenous hemofiltration	CVVH	Removes fluid and solutes Requires replacement fluid
Slow continuous ultrafiltration	SCUF	Simplified version of CVVH Removes fluid No fluid replacement required
Continuous venovenous hemodialysis	CVVHD	Removes fluids and solutes Requires dialysate and replacement fluid
Continuous venovenous hemodiafiltration	CVVHDF	Removes fluids and solutes Requires dialysate and replacement fluid

jugular or femoral vein. A blood pump propels the blood through the circuit. A highly permeable, hollow-fiber hemofilter removes plasma water and nonprotein solutes, which are collectively termed *ultrafiltrate.* The UFR may range from 0 to 500 mL/h. Under the influence of hydrostatic pressure and osmotic pressure, water and nonprotein solutes pass out of the filter into the extracapillary space and drain through the ultrafiltrate port into a collection device (drainage bag) (Fig. 51.14). The remaining fluid continues through the filter and returns to the patient via the return port of the double-lumen catheter.

As ultrafiltrate drains out of the hemofilter, fluid and electrolyte replacements can be infused through a port found before or after the filter as the blood returns to the patient. Replacement fluid is designed to replace volume and solutes, such as sodium, chloride, HCO_3^-, and glucose. The infusion rate of replacement fluid is determined by the degree of fluid and electrolyte imbalance. Replacement fluid infused into the infusion port before the hemofilter allows for greater clearance of urea and can decrease filter clotting. An infusion port after the filter dilutes intravascular fluid and decreases the concentration of unwanted solutes, such as BUN, creatinine, and potassium. Anticoagulants are given to prevent blood clotting. They may be infused as a bolus at the start of CRRT or through an infusion port before the hemofilter.

The type of CRRT is determined by patient needs. Some types involve giving replacement fluids. CVVHD and CVVHDF use dialysate. Dialysis fluid is attached to the distal end of the hemofilter, and the fluid is pumped countercurrent to the blood flow (Fig. 51.14). As in HD, diffusion of solutes and ultrafiltration via hydrostatic pressure and osmosis occur. This is an ideal treatment for patients who need fluid and solute control but cannot tolerate the rapid fluid shifts associated with HD.

Several features of CRRT differ from HD:

- The blood pump in CRRT runs at a slower (150 mL/min average) rate. This may improve hemodynamic stability.
- Continuous. Fluid volume can be removed over days (24 hours to more than 2 weeks) versus hours (3 to 4 hours).
- Solute removal can occur by *convection* (no dialysate needed) in addition to osmosis and diffusion.
- Causes less hemodynamic instability (e.g., hypotension)
- Does not need constant monitoring by a specialized HD nurse but does require a trained ICU nurse
- Does not require complicated HD equipment

CRRT can be continued for as long as 30 to 40 days. Change the hemofilter every 24 to 48 hours because of loss of filtration efficiency or potential for clotting. The ultrafiltrate should be clear yellow. Specimens may be obtained for chemistries. If the ultrafiltrate becomes bloody or blood tinged, suspect a rupture in the filter membrane. Stop treatment to prevent blood loss.

Specific nursing care includes obtaining weights and monitoring laboratory values daily to ensure adequate fluid and electrolyte balance. Assess hourly intake and output, vital signs, and hemodynamic status. Although we expect central venous pressure and pulmonary artery pressure to decrease, there should be little change in mean arterial pressure or cardiac output. Assess and maintain the patency of the CRRT system. Provide care for vascular access sites to prevent infection. Once AKI is resolved or there is a decision to withdraw treatment, CRRT is stopped and the needle(s) removed.

KIDNEY TRANSPLANTS

A kidney transplant is the best treatment option for patients with ESRD. Kidney transplants are very successful. One-year graft survival rates are over 90% for deceased donor transplants and 95% for live donor transplants.[26] General information about organ transplants is in Chapter 14.

An advantage of a kidney transplant compared with dialysis is that it reverses many of the pathophysiologic changes associated with renal disease. It eliminates the dependence on dialysis and accompanying diet and lifestyle restrictions. A transplant is less expensive than dialysis after the first year.

Every year thousands are waiting for kidney transplants (more than 120,000 are currently on the list), yet only about 24,000 transplants take place every year. Most die while waiting. This is due to the large disparity between the supply and demand for kidneys. There is usually a long wait for a transplant from a deceased (cadaveric) donor. Average wait times in the United States for a deceased kidney usually range from 2 to 5 years.[26]

Recipient Selection

Appropriate recipient selection is important for a successful outcome. Candidacy is determined by several medical and psychosocial factors (Box 51.2). These factors vary among transplant centers. Some programs exclude patients who are morbidly obese or continue to smoke despite smoking cessation interventions. A careful evaluation is done to identify and minimize potential complications after the transplant. Certain patients, particularly those with CVD and diabetes, are considered high risk. They must be carefully evaluated and then monitored closely after the transplant.

For a small number of patients who are approaching ESRD, a *preemptive transplant* (before dialysis is needed) is possible if they have a living donor. This approach is best for patients with diabetes because they have a higher mortality rate on dialysis.

Contraindications to a transplant include advanced cancer, refractory or untreated heart disease, chronic respiratory failure, extensive vascular disease, chronic infection, and unresolved psychosocial disorders (e.g., nonadherence to treatment plan, alcohol use, drug use).

BOX 51.2 ETHICAL/LEGAL DILEMMAS

Allocation of Resources

Situation

T.H., a transplant nurse coordinator, is considering her feelings about 2 patients who are being evaluated for placement on the deceased kidney transplant waiting list. One patient is a 40-year-old schoolteacher. She is married and has 2 children. The other patient is a 22-year-old unemployed male. He misses 3 or 4 dialysis treatments per month and does not take his antihypertensive drugs consistently.

Ethical/Legal Points for Consideration

- Ethical principles that are important in the allocation of human organs include utility and justice.
- Allocation policies based on utility require we use standardized outcome measures to give a rough estimate about which allocation would produce the greatest good. Factors considered include patient survival, quality of life, availability of alternative treatments, and age.
- We must give equal respect and concern to each patient. Allocation based on social characteristics (e.g., socioeconomic class, education) conflicts with the principle of justice and violates constitutional law. ANA recognizes impartiality begins with the individual nurse and should occur within every health care organization. All nurses must recognize the potential impact of unconscious bias and practices contributing to discrimination, and actively seek opportunities to promote inclusion of all people in the provision of quality health care while eradicating disparities. ANA supports policy initiatives directed toward abolishing all forms of discrimination (https://doi.org/10.3912/OJIN.Vol24No03PoSCol01).
- Constitutional laws prohibit discrimination based on race, gender, religion, and ethnic background. It is possible that definitions of unhealthy behavior, such as substance use, alcohol use, smoking, and obesity, may be used to screen out candidates.
- Nurses are concerned about social justice because of their health advocacy role. Today the situation is immensely more complex because of the cost and availability of care.

Discussion Questions

1. What does the ANA Code of Ethics say about how you as a nurse should view patients?
2. What are your thoughts about which patient should receive the next available kidney transplant?

Patients may need other surgeries before having a transplant. Coronary artery bypass or angioplasty may be needed for advanced coronary artery disease. Cholecystectomy may be necessary for patients with a history of gallstones, biliary obstruction, or cholecystitis. On rare occasions, bilateral nephrectomies are done for patients with refractory hypertension, recurrent UTIs, or grossly enlarged kidneys from polycystic kidney disease. In general, the recipient's own kidneys are not removed before receiving a kidney transplant.

Donor Sources

Kidneys for transplants are obtained from compatible blood-type deceased donors, blood relatives, emotionally related (close and distant) living donors (e.g., spouses, distant cousins), and altruistic living donors who are known (friends) or unknown to the recipient. Living donation accounts for around 27% of all kidney transplants in the United States. Most transplant centers regard them as the preferred donation modality.[26]

Live Donors

Advantages of a live donor kidney include (1) better patient and graft survival rates, (2) immediate organ availability, (3) immediate function due to minimal *cold time* (kidney out of body and not getting blood supply), and (4) the opportunity to have the recipient in the best possible health since the surgery is elective.

Live donors undergo an extensive evaluation to ensure that they are in good health and have no history of disease that would place them at risk for developing kidney disease or operative complications. They see a nephrologist for a history and physical assessment and laboratory and diagnostic studies. Histocompatibility studies, including human leukocyte antigen (HLA) testing and crossmatching, are done (see Chapter 14). Laboratory studies include a 24-hour urine study for creatinine clearance and total protein, complete blood count, and chemistry and electrolyte profiles. Hepatitis B and C, HIV, and cytomegalovirus (CMV) testing is done to assess for transmitted diseases. An ECG and chest x-ray are done. A renal ultrasound and renal arteriogram or 3-dimensional CT scan are done to ensure that the blood vessels supplying each kidney are adequate and that no anomalies exist and to see which kidney will be used in the transplant.

A transplant psychologist or social worker determines whether the person is emotionally stable and able to deal with the issues related to organ donation. All donors must be informed about the risks and benefits of donation, potential complications, and what to expect during the hospitalization and recovery phases. Kidney donation is considered safe without any long-term health consequences. Although the recipient's insurance covers the costs of the evaluation and surgery, no compensation is available for lost wages during the posthospitalization recovery period. This period can last 6 weeks or longer.

When there is ABO incompatibility between a donor and recipient, paired donor exchange is a viable alternative. *Paired organ donation* occurs when one donor/recipient pair who are incompatible or poorly matched with each other find another donor/recipient pair with whom they can exchange kidneys. For example, a spouse (person A) who wants to donate a kidney to his wife (person B) but is incompatible is paired with another donor/recipient pair involving a son with ESRD (person C) and his mother (person D). In this example, person A would donate his kidney to person C, and person D would donate her kidney to person B. Paired organ donation is the practice of matching incompatible donor/recipient pairs to permit a transplant to both candidates.

Another option for ABO incompatibility or a positive crossmatch between the donor and recipient is to use plasmapheresis to remove antibodies from the recipient. This allows transplant candidates to receive kidneys from live donors with blood types that we have traditionally considered incompatible. After the transplant, patients have more plasmapheresis treatments.

Deceased Donors

Deceased (cadaver) kidney donors are fairly healthy persons who have an irreversible brain injury and are declared brain dead. The brain-dead donor must have effective CV function and be supported on a ventilator to preserve the organs.

In deceased kidney donation, the kidneys are removed and preserved. They can be preserved for up to 72 hours. Most transplant surgeons prefer to transplant kidneys before the cold time (time outside of the body when being transported from the deceased donor to the recipient) reaches 24 hours. Prolonged cold time increases the chance that the kidney will not function immediately. ATN may develop.

The United Network for Organ Sharing (UNOS) distributes deceased donor kidneys using an objective computer point system. The kidney allocation system (KAS) provides all donor kidneys with a kidney donor profile index (KDPI). The KDPI includes 10 donor factors that evaluate the risk for a kidney transplant failure. The KDPI can help predict how long a kidney may function. Each kidney transplant candidate gets an Estimated Post-Transplant Survival (EPTS) score. This score ranges from 0% to 100%. The score is related to how long a candidate will need a functioning kidney transplant compared with other candidates. For example, a person with an EPTS score of 20% is likely to need a kidney longer than 80% of other candidates. The EPTS score is based on age, length of time on dialysis, previous transplants, and having diabetes. Emergency transplants receive priority because the patient is facing imminent death if not transplanted.

When a donor becomes available, the donor's key information is compared with the data of all patients awaiting a transplant locally and nationwide. When a kidney arrives at the recipient's transplant center, a final crossmatch is done. It must be negative for the deceased donor transplant to proceed.

The only exception is if a patient needs an emergency transplant or if a donor and recipient match on all 6 HLA antigens (zero antigen mismatch). Patients meeting either of these criteria go to the top of the list. If a zero-antigen mismatch patient is found nationally, since statistically these grafts have better survival rates, 1 of the donor kidneys must be sent to that recipient's transplant center regardless of location.

Surgical Procedure

Live Donor

A transplant surgeon performs the live donor nephrectomy. The donor's surgery begins 1 to 2 hours before the recipient's surgery. The recipient is surgically prepared for the kidney transplant in a nearby operating room.

Laparoscopic donor nephrectomy is the most common technique for removing a kidney in a living donor. Laparoscopic nephrectomy is discussed in Chapter 50. After the kidney is removed, it is flushed with a chilled, sterile electrolyte solution and prepared for immediate transplant into the recipient. The use of this procedure is minimally invasive, with fewer risks and shorter recovery time. It decreases hospital stay, pain, operative blood loss, debilitation, and length of time off work. This has increased the number of people willing to donate a kidney significantly.

Kidney Transplant Recipient

The transplanted kidney is usually placed extraperitoneally in the iliac fossa (Fig. 51.15). The right iliac fossa is preferred to facilitate anastomoses of the blood vessels and ureter and minimize paralytic ileus.

Rapid revascularization is critical to prevent ischemic injury to the kidney. The donor artery is anastomosed to the recipient's internal iliac (hypogastric) or external iliac artery. The donor vein is anastomosed to the recipient's external iliac vein. The clamps are released, and blood flow to the kidney is reestablished. The kidney should become firm and pink. Urine may begin to flow from the ureter at once. The donor ureter is then tunneled through the bladder submucosa before entering the bladder cavity and being sutured in place. This approach is called *ureteroneocystostomy.* This allows the bladder wall to compress the ureter as it contracts for micturition, thereby preventing reflux of urine up the ureter into the transplanted kidney. A urinary catheter is placed into the bladder, and an antibiotic solution is instilled to distend the bladder and decrease the risk for infection. Transplant surgery takes about 3 to 4 hours.

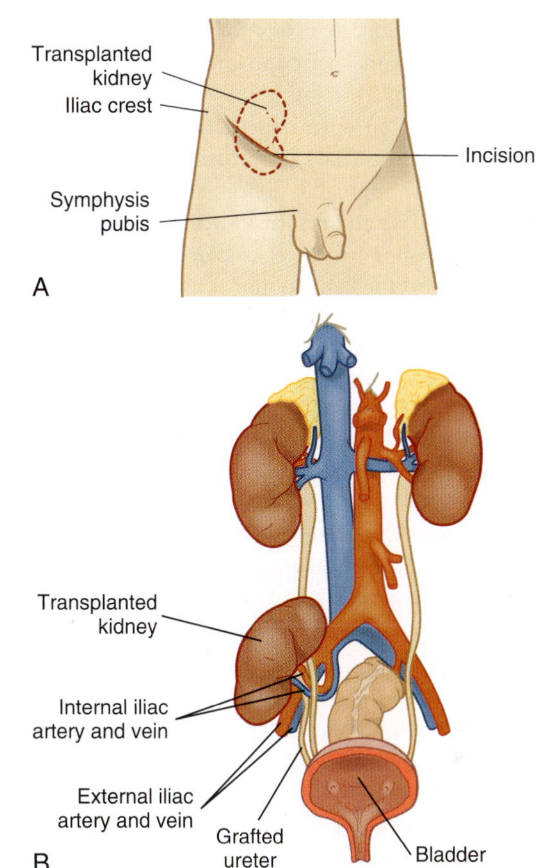

Fig. 51.15 (A) Surgical incision for a renal transplant. (B) Surgical placement of transplanted kidney.

❖ NURSING MANAGEMENT: KIDNEY TRANSPLANT RECIPIENT

Preoperative Care

Nursing care includes emotional and physical preparation for surgery. Because patients and caregivers may have been waiting years for the kidney transplant, a review of the operative procedure and what can be expected in the immediate postoperative recovery period is necessary. Stress that there is a chance the kidney may not function at once, and dialysis may be needed for days to weeks. Review the need for immunosuppressive drugs and measures to prevent infection.

To ensure patients are in the best health for surgery, an ECG, chest x-ray, and laboratory studies are done. Crossmatches are repeated about a week before a live donor transplant to ensure that no antibodies to the donor are present or that the antibody titer is below the allowed level. Dialysis may be needed before surgery for fluid overload or hyperkalemia. Because dialysis may be needed after the transplant, we must maintain patency of the vascular access. Label the vascular access extremity "dialysis access, no procedures" to prevent use of that extremity for BP measurement, blood drawing, or IV infusions. Patients on PD must empty the peritoneal cavity of all dialysate solution before going to surgery and have the PD catheter capped.

Postoperative Care

Live Donor

Postoperative care for the donor is similar to that after open (conventional) or laparoscopic nephrectomy (Chapter 50).

Monitor renal function to assess for impairment. Assess for bleeding. Monitor pain levels and provide pain management strategies.

Donors who had an open approach are usually discharged from the hospital in 4 or 5 days and return to work in 6 to 8 weeks. With a laparoscopic approach, donors are discharged from the hospital in 2 to 4 days and return to work in 4 to 6 weeks. The surgeon sees the donor 1 to 2 weeks after discharge.

Nurses caring for the living donor must acknowledge the gift that this person has given. The donor has taken physical, emotional, and financial risks to help the recipient. It is vital that the donor is not forgotten after surgery. The donor will need support if the donated organ does not work at once or for some reason fails.

Kidney Transplant Recipient

The priority during the postoperative period is maintaining fluid and electrolyte balance. Kidney transplant recipients require close monitoring and spend the first 12 to 24 hours in the ICU. Large volumes of urine may be made soon after the blood supply to the transplanted kidney is reestablished. This diuresis is due to the (1) new kidney's ability to filter BUN, which acts as an osmotic diuretic; (2) fluids given during the surgery; and (3) initial renal tubular dysfunction, which inhibits the kidney from concentrating urine normally. Urine output during this phase may be as high as 1 L/h. It gradually decreases as the BUN and creatinine levels return toward normal. Urine output is replaced with fluids milliliter for milliliter hourly for the first 12 to 24 hours.

Central venous pressure readings are essential for monitoring fluid status. Dehydration is avoided to prevent renal hypoperfusion and renal tubular damage. Assess for hyponatremia and hypokalemia. They can occur with rapid diuresis. Treatment with potassium supplements or infusion of 0.9% normal saline may be needed. IV sodium bicarbonate may be given if develops metabolic acidosis from a delay in the return of kidney function.

ATN in the transplanted kidney can occur because of prolonged cold times causing ischemic damage or the use of marginal cadaveric donors (those who are medically suboptimal). While patients are in ATN, dialysis is needed to maintain fluid and electrolyte balance. Some patients have high-output ATN with the ability to excrete fluid but not metabolic wastes or electrolytes. Other patients have oliguric or anuric ATN. These patients are at risk for fluid overload in the immediate postoperative period. Assess closely for the need for dialysis. ATN can last from days to weeks, with gradually improving kidney function. Most patients with ATN are discharged from the hospital on dialysis. This is discouraging for patients, who need reassurance that renal function usually improves. Dialysis is stopped when urine output increases and creatinine and BUN begin to normalize.

A sudden decrease in urine output in the early postoperative period is a cause for concern. It may be due to dehydration, rejection, a urine leak, or obstruction. A common cause of early obstruction is a blood clot in the urinary catheter. Maintain catheter patency since the catheter stays in the bladder for 3 to 5 days to allow the ureter-bladder anastomosis to heal. If you suspect blood clots, gentle catheter irrigation (if ordered) can reestablish patency.

Identify and address discharge planning and teaching needs early. Patient teaching ensures a smooth transition from the hospital to home. Include how to recognize signs of rejection, infection, and any complications of surgery. Frequent blood tests and clinic visits help detect rejection early.

Immunosuppressive Therapy

The goal of immunosuppression is to adequately suppress the immune response to prevent rejection of the transplanted kidney while maintaining sufficient immunity to prevent overwhelming infection. Immunosuppressive therapy is discussed in Chapter 14.

Complications of Transplants

Complications of PD, HD, and kidney transplants are compared in Table 51.14.

Rejection

Rejection is a major problem after a kidney transplant. Rejection can be hyperacute, acute, or chronic. The types of rejection

TABLE 51.14 Complications of Dialysis and Transplants

Peritoneal Dialysis (PD)	Hemodialysis (HD)	Transplant

• Abdominal pain
• Carbohydrate abnormalities
• Catheter outflow
• CVD
• Encapsulating sclerosing peritonitis
• Exit site infection
• Hernias
• Lipid abnormalities
• Lower back pain
• Peritonitis
• Protein loss
• Pulmonary problems
  • Atelectasis
  • Pneumonia
  • Bronchitis
	• CVD
	• Disequilibrium syndrome
	• Exsanguination
	• Hepatitis
	• Hypotension
	• Infection
	• Muscle cramps
		• Cancer
		• Corticosteroid-related complications
		• CVD
		• Recurrent kidney disease
		• Susceptible to infection
		• Transplant rejection
		  • Hyperacute
		  • Acute
		  • Chronic

are discussed in Chapter 14. Patients with chronic rejection may be placed on the transplant list to be retransplanted before they need dialysis.

Infection

Infection is a significant cause of mortality after a transplant. The transplant recipient is at risk for infection because of suppression of the body's normal defense mechanisms by surgery, immunosuppressive drugs, and the effects of ESRD. Underlying systemic illness, such as diabetes or SLE, malnutrition, and older age, can further compound the negative effects on the immune response. The signs and symptoms of infection can be subtle. You must be astute in your assessment of the recipient. Prompt diagnosis and treatment of infection improves patient outcomes.

The common infections seen in the first month after a transplant are like those of any postoperative patient. These include pneumonia, wound infections, UTIs, and IV line and drain infections. Fungal and viral infections are common due to immunosuppression. Fungal infections include *Candida, Cryptococcus,* and *Aspergillus* organisms and *Pneumocystis jirovecii.* Fungal infections are hard to treat, require prolonged treatment periods, and often involve the administration of nephrotoxic drugs. Transplant recipients usually receive prophylactic antifungal drugs to prevent these infections, such as clotrimazole, fluconazole, and trimethoprim/sulfamethoxazole.

Viral infections, including CMV, Epstein-Barr virus, herpes simplex virus (HSV), and varicella-zoster virus, can be primary infections or reactivations of existing disease. Primary infections occur as new infections from an exogenous source such as the donated organ or a blood transfusion. Reactivation occurs when a virus exists in a patient and becomes reactivated because of immunosuppression.

CMV is one of the most common viral infections. If a recipient has never had CMV and receives an organ from a donor with a history of CMV, antiviral prophylaxis will be needed (e.g., ganciclovir, valganciclovir). To prevent HSV infections, patients receive oral acyclovir for several months after the transplant.

Cardiovascular Disease

CVD is the leading cause of death after a kidney transplant.[26] Transplant recipients have an increased incidence of CVD. Hypertension, dyslipidemia, diabetes, smoking, rejection, infections, and increased homocysteine levels can contribute to CVD. Immunosuppressants can worsen hypertension and dyslipidemia.

Teach patients to control risk factors, such as high cholesterol, triglycerides, glucose, and weight gain. Adherence to the prescribed antihypertensive regimen is essential to prevent CV events and damage to the new kidney.

Cancers

The overall incidence of cancer in kidney transplant recipients is greater than in the general population, mainly because of immunosuppressive therapy. Immunosuppressants suppress the ability to fight the production of abnormal cells, including cancer cells. The most common types of cancer after transplant are (1) skin cancers—basal and squamous cell cancers and melanoma—and (2) posttransplant lymphoproliferative disorder (PTLD). Most PTLDs are of B-cell origin, related to Epstein-Barr virus (EBV). They cause aggressive lymphomas (Hodgkin and non-Hodgkin lymphoma). Most cases of PTLD occur within the first year of transplant.

Patients are at risk for cancers of the colorectum, breast, cervix, liver, stomach, oropharynx, anus, vulva, and penis. Regular screening for cancer is an important part of the transplant recipient's preventive care.

Recurrence of Original Kidney Disease

Recurrence of the original disease that destroyed the native kidneys occurs in some kidney transplant recipients. It is most common with certain types of glomerulonephritis, immunoglobulin A (IgA) nephropathy, diabetic nephropathy, and focal segmental sclerosis. Disease recurrence can result in the loss of a functioning kidney transplant. We must advise patients before the transplant if they have a disease known to recur.

Corticosteroid-Related Complications

Many transplant programs have corticosteroid-free drug regimens because of the problems of long-term corticosteroid use. Other centers withdraw patients from corticosteroids after the transplant. For patients who stay on corticosteroids, vigilant monitoring for side effects and prompt treatment are essential. Corticosteroid therapy as immunosuppression is discussed in Chapter 14.

Gerontologic Considerations: Chronic Kidney Disease

The care of older patients is particularly challenging because of the normal changes of aging and the increased presence of disabilities, chronic diseases, and comorbid problems. When conservative therapy for CKD is no longer effective, older patients need to consider the best treatment modality based on physical and emotional health, personal preferences, and availability of support. Rationing dialysis based on age alone is not a reasonable decision for health care professionals to make. Older adults have successfully used dialysis, especially PD. Many choose treatment with in-center HD due to a lack of help in the home and reluctance to manage the technology of home HD or PD. Establishing vascular access for HD may be difficult because of atherosclerotic changes.

Although a transplant is an option, older adults are carefully screened to ensure that the benefits outweigh the risks. Although a living donor is preferable, this may not be an option for many older patients.

The most common cause of death in older ESRD patients is CVD (MI, stroke), followed by withdrawal from dialysis. If a competent patient decides to withdraw from dialysis, it is essential to support the patient and family. Ethical issues (Box 51.3) include patient competency, benefit versus burden of treatment, and futility of treatment. Withdrawal from treatment is not a failure if the patient is well informed and comfortable with the decision.

BOX 51.3 ETHICAL/LEGAL DILEMMAS

Withdrawing Treatment

Situation

L.R., a 70-year-old patient with diabetes and ESRD, has been on dialysis for 10 years. He tells you that he wants to stop his dialysis. His quality of life has declined during the past 2 years since his wife died. He is not a transplant candidate.

Ethical/Legal Points for Consideration

- Informed consent includes the legal right to refuse treatment. The right to refuse may be difficult if (1) it is contrary to the wishes of family and friends, (2) the treatment is still effective, and (3) the treatment has been in place for some time.
- Quality-of-life decisions often outweigh the benefit against the burden of treatment. When a treatment becomes too burdensome, the patient, if competent, may request to withdraw the treatment.
- It must be determined whether some other treatable problem, such as depression, may be clouding the patient's judgment.
- Although there is no ethical or legal difference between withdrawing treatment and withholding treatment, withdrawing treatment feels different because it requires an action.
- Some health care professionals become conflicted when asked to withdraw treatment, since they may think they are contributing to the patient's premature death.
- If a decision is made to withdraw treatment, the interprofessional care team, patient, and family should develop a follow-up plan that includes palliative care and hospice support.

Discussion Questions

1. How should you respond to L.R.'s request?
2. What is the ANA's position on withdrawing or withholding treatment that no longer benefits the patient or causes suffering?

CASE STUDY

Chronic Kidney Disease

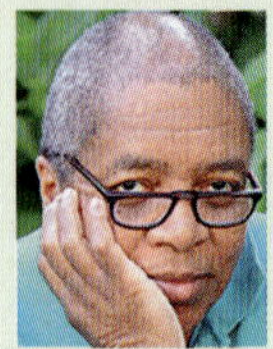

(© iStockphoto/ Thinkstock.)

Patient Profile

M.B. is a 56-year-old college professor. He is having a well visit with his primary HCP. He has not seen an HCP in a little over a year. M.B. reports malaise, frequent urination, and "increasing thirst." His history includes borderline hypertension and dyslipidemia. He smokes 1 pack of cigarettes per day. His efforts to quit have been unsuccessful.

Subjective Data

- Family history: father died of an MI at age 62, brother had coronary artery bypass graft at age 50, mother died from complications of diabetes
- Becomes "winded" when walking from his car to his office at the university
- Wakes up at night to urinate and has more frequent urination
- Increasing thirst

Objective Data

Laboratory Data

- Calculated creatinine clearance using the MDRD equation: 42 mL/min/1.73 m^2
- Creatinine 6.5 mg/dL; BUN 85 mg/dL
- Glucose 264 mg/dL
- Hgb 13 g/dL
- Cholesterol 236 mg/dL

Physical Assessment

- Weight 220 lb, height 5 ft, 11 in
- BP 168/104 mm Hg

Discussion Questions

1. ***Recognize:*** What may have caused M.B.'s kidney disease?
2. ***Analyze:*** What stage of chronic kidney disease does he have?
3. ***Analyze:*** Identify the abnormal diagnostic study results and why each would occur.
4. ***Plan:*** How can the interprofessional team work together with M.B. to plan the best form of renal replacement therapy?
5. ***Prioritize:*** Based on the assessment data provided, what are the priority clinical problems?
6. ***Plan:*** What are the measures that the interprofessional team can plan to provide for M.B.?
7. ***Act:*** What interventions would help promote M.B.'s self-management of his disease?
8. ***Act:*** M.B. tells you that he has not been taking his BP medications regularly. When he asks you how important they are, what will you tell him?

Answers available at http://evolve.elsevier.com/Lewis/medsurg.

BRIDGE TO NCLEX EXAMINATION

The number of the question corresponds to the same-numbered outcome at the beginning of the chapter.

1. The nurse using RIFLE to determine the early stage of AKI evaluates the
   a. blood pressure and urine osmolality.
   b. fractional excretion of urine sodium.
   c. creatinine or urine output from baseline.
   d. estimate of GFR with the MDRD equation.

2. During the oliguric phase of AKI, the nurse monitors for (**Select all that apply.**)
   a. hypotension.
   b. ECG changes.
   c. hypernatremia.
   d. pulmonary edema.
   e. urine with high specific gravity.

3. The nurse must monitor for which electrolyte imbalances when a patient is in the diuretic phase of AKI?
   a. Hyperkalemia and hyponatremia
   b. Hyperkalemia and hypernatremia
   c. Hypokalemia and hyponatremia
   d. Hypokalemia and hypernatremia
4. The nurse assesses patients with chronic kidney disease with the understanding that this condition is characterized by
   a. progressive irreversible destruction of the kidneys.
   b. a rapid decrease in urine output with an elevated BUN.
   c. an increasing creatinine clearance with a decrease in urine output.
   d. prostration, somnolence, and confusion with coma and imminent death.
5. Nurses can screen patients at risk for developing chronic kidney disease. Those considered to be at increased risk include (**Select all that apply.**)
   a. patients with an STI.
   b. patients more than 60 years old.
   c. those with a history of pancreatitis.
   d. those with a history of hypertension.
   e. those with a history of type 2 diabetes.
6. Which points must the nurse consider when planning nutrition support for patients with chronic kidney disease? (**Select all that apply.**)
   a. Sodium may be restricted in someone with advanced CKD.
   b. Fluid is not usually restricted for patients on peritoneal dialysis.
   c. Decreased fluid intake and a low-potassium diet are needed for a patient on hemodialysis.
   d. Decreased fluid intake and a low-potassium diet are needed for a patient on peritoneal dialysis.
   e. Decreased fluid intake and a diet of protein-rich foods are part of a diet for a patient on hemodialysis.
7. An ESRD patient receiving hemodialysis is considering asking a relative to donate a kidney for a transplant. In helping the patient decide about treatment, the nurse informs the patient that
   a. successful transplant usually provides better quality of life than that offered by dialysis.
   b. if rejection of the transplanted kidney occurs, no further treatment for the renal failure is available.
   c. hemodialysis replaces normal kidney functions, and they do not have to live with the continual fear of rejection.
   d. immunosuppressive therapy after a transplant makes the person ineligible to receive other treatments if the kidney fails.
8. To assess the patency of a newly placed arteriovenous graft, the nurse should (**Select all that apply.**)
   a. monitor the BP in the affected arm.
   b. irrigate the graft daily with low-dose heparin.
   c. palpate the area of the graft to feel a normal thrill.
   d. listen with a stethoscope over the graft to detect a bruit.
   e. assess the pulses and neurovascular status distal to the graft.
9. A kidney transplant recipient has had fever, chills, and dysuria over the past 2 days. What is the *first* action that the nurse should take?
   a. Assess temperature and start workup to rule out infection.
   b. Reassure the patient that this is common after a transplant.
   c. Provide warm covers to the patient and give 1 gram oral acetaminophen.
   d. Notify the nephrologist that the patient has manifestations of acute rejection.

1. c; 2. b, d; 3. c; 4. a;
5. b, d, e; 6. a, b, c; 7. a; 8. c, d, e; 9. a.

For rationales to these answers and even more NCLEX review questions, visit http://evolve.elsevier.com/Lewis/medsurg.

REFERENCES

To access the References for this chapter, please scan the QR code with a mobile device.

CASE STUDY

Applying Clinical Judgment With Multiple Patients

You are working on the medical-surgical unit and have been assigned to care for the following 4 patients. You are also assigned to receive the next admission. You have 1 AP on your team to help you.

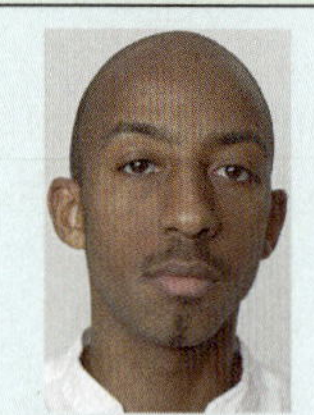 (© iStockphoto/Thinkstock.)	A.K., a 28-year-old male, was admitted with several kidney stones in the left ureter. He is receiving IV morphine sulfate for pain. His current pain level is 4 (1—10 scale). He is voiding dark, smoky-colored urine. He has positive costovertebral tenderness. Vital signs: 156/70, 94, RR 24.
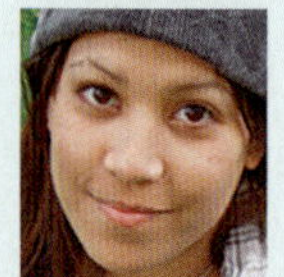 (© iStockphoto/Thinkstock.)	S.U., a 29-year-old female with type 1 diabetes, was admitted with acute pyelonephritis from a recent UTI. She has bilateral flank pain and abdominal tenderness. UA shows pyuria and hematuria. Blood culture results are pending. The next dose of IV antibiotics is due at 0900. Laboratory results: WBC 14,800/μL, glucose 215 mg/dL. Vital signs: 126/74, 94, RR 20, temp 101.5°F (38.6°C).
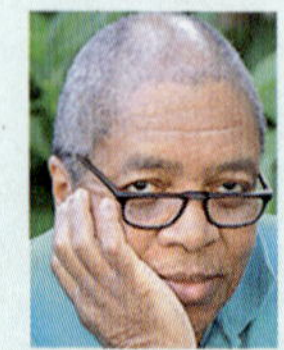 (© iStockphoto/Thinkstock.)	M.B., a 56-year-old male, was admitted with uncontrolled hypertension and CKD. He smokes 1 pack of cigarettes per day and is having some nicotine withdrawal symptoms. BP on admission was 224/102. He is receiving IV metoprolol 5 mg q4h prn for SBP >180 mm Hg. Laboratory results: BUN 85 mg/dL, creatinine 6.5 mg/dL, glucose 264 mg/dL. Vital signs: 178/86, 88, RR 18.
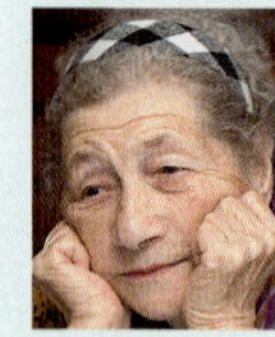 (© iStockphoto/Thinkstock.)	D.M., an 82-year-old female, was admitted with dehydration, heart failure, and AKI. She is confused. Her potassium is 6.3 mEq/L. Urine output for the past 8 hours was 90 mL. Vital signs: 142/86, 98, RR 22.

1. Highlight all the findings above that require your follow-up.
2. After receiving report, which patient should you see first? Second?
3. Which tasks could you delegate to the AP? **(Select all that apply.)**
   a. Obtain vital signs on M.B.
   b. Strain A.K.'s voided urine.
   c. Report D.M.'s potassium level to the HCP.
   d. Measure D.M.'s urine output and report the results to the RN.
   e. Assess S.U. for manifestations of sepsis and diabetic ketoacidosis.
4. As you are assessing D.M., the AP tells you that M.B.'s BP is 190/106. He is asymptomatic. Then the charge nurse calls and tells you that you will receive a patient with heart failure from the ED in 20 min. Which action would be *most* appropriate?
   a. Ask the charge nurse to assign the new admission to someone else.
   b. Have the AP admit the new patient while you administer M.B.'s IV metoprolol.
   c. Call the ED and have them hold the new admission until after you have assessed all your patients.
   d. Ask the charge nurse to give M.B.'s IV metoprolol while you complete your assessment of D.M. and S.U.

Case Study Progression

As you complete your assessment of D.M., you note she has 1+ pitting edema in her lower extremities. Her BP is 160/90 mm Hg, heart rate 108 beats/min, and respiratory rate 32/min. Auscultation reveals crackles in the lung bases and O_2 saturation is 88% on room air. The skin is cool, and she is reporting dyspnea.

5. Based on these assessment findings, you suspect D.M. is experiencing _____1_____. You notify the HCP, expecting orders for _____2_____, _____2_____, and _____2_____.

Options for 1	Options for 2
Pulmonary edema	12-lead ECG and continuous ECG monitoring
Pulmonary embolism	furosemide
Unstable angina	heparin
	nitroglycerin
	O_2 therapy

6. A.K. is reporting pain rated as 8 (1—10 scale) and requests IV morphine. What would you do first to safely administer the medication?
   a. Assess the patency of A.K.'s IV site.
   b. Prepare the dose using sterile technique.
   c. Determine the last time A.K. received IV morphine.
   d. Scan A.K.'s ID band and the medication according to agency policy.
7. You begin S.U.'s scheduled infusion of IV ceftriaxone and perform her assessment. Use an X for the nursing actions listed below that are *Indicated* (appropriate or necessary) or *Contraindicated* (could be harmful) for S.U. at this time.

Nursing Action	Indicated	Contraindicated
Monitor BUN and creatinine levels.		
Maintain intake and output.		
Medicate with ibuprofen every 6 h as needed for pain.		
Initiate a fluid restriction.		
Encourage her to void every 3–4 h while awake.		
Insert an indwelling urinary catheter.		

8. Which statement would be *most* appropriate when teaching S.U. about her kidney infection?
   a. "The damage to your kidneys will likely require dialysis."
   b. "You will need to be in the hospital for a 2-week course of IV antibiotics."
   c. "It is very important that you maintain adequate hydration to flush your kidneys."
   d. "You will not need further antibiotics once you are discharged from the hospital."

Continued

CASE STUDY—cont'd

9. As the AP prepares the room for the patient being admitted from the ED, you overhear her telling a coworker that she does all your work for you. What is your *best* initial action?
   a. Report the incident to the charge nurse for follow-up.
   b. Ask the AP to discuss her concerns with you in private.
   c. Tell the AP how much you appreciate and value her input on your team.
   d. Immediately clarify the situation by telling the AP all the tasks you are completing.
10. You are reviewing S.U.'s latest assessment findings. For each assessment finding, use an X to indicate whether the interventions were *Effective* (helped meet expected outcomes) or *Ineffective* (did not help meet expected outcomes).

Assessment Finding	Effective	Ineffective
BUN 55 mg/dL, creatinine 3.5 mg/dL		
Reports wiping front to back after voiding		
No flank pain or dysuria		
Clear, yellow urine		
Voiding 5–6 times per day		
UA shows hematuria		

Answers available at http://evolve.elsevier.com/Lewis/medsurg.

52

Assessment: Endocrine System

Julia A. Hitch

http://evolve.elsevier.com/Lewis/medsurg/

CONCEPTUAL FOCUS

Homeostasis
Hormonal Regulation
Reproduction

LEARNING OUTCOMES

1. Describe the common characteristics and functions of hormones.
2. Identify the locations of the endocrine glands.
3. Describe the functions of hormones secreted by the pancreas and pituitary, thyroid, parathyroid, and adrenal glands.
4. Link age-related changes in the endocrine system to differences in assessment findings.
5. Obtain subjective and objective assessment data related to the endocrine system.
6. Perform a physical assessment of the endocrine system.
7. Distinguish normal from common abnormal findings of an endocrine physical assessment.
8. Describe the purpose, significance of results, and nursing responsibilities related to diagnostic studies of the endocrine system.

KEY TERMS

aldosterone
antidiuretic hormone (ADH)
catecholamines
circadian rhythm
corticosteroid
cortisol
hormones
insulin
negative feedback
positive feedback
thyroxine (T_4)
triiodothyronine (T_3)
tropic hormones

ENDOCRINE SYSTEM STRUCTURE AND FUNCTION

Hormones

The endocrine system has 5 general functions: (1) maintaining homeostasis, (2) responding to emergency demands, (3) a role in reproductive and central nervous system (CNS) development in the fetus, (4) stimulating growth and development during childhood and adolescence, and (5) sexual reproduction.

Hormones are chemical substances made by endocrine glands that control and regulate the activity of certain target cells or organs (Fig. 52.1). Many are made in one part of the body and control and regulate the activity of certain cells or organs in another part of the body. The thyroid gland makes the hormone thyroxine, which affects many body tissues when released directly into the circulation. Other hormones act locally on cells where they are released and never enter the bloodstream. We call this local effect *paracrine action.* The action of sex steroids on the ovary is an example of paracrine action.

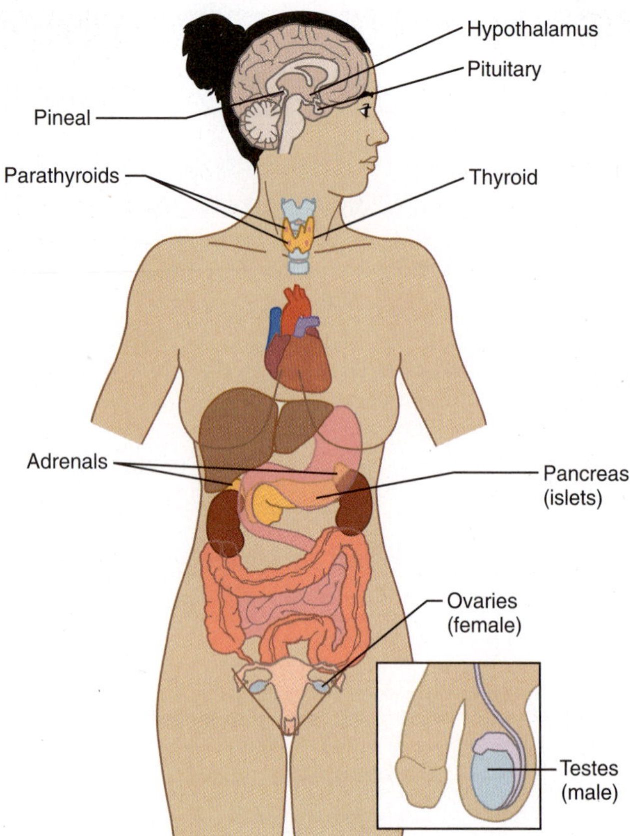

Fig. 52.1 Location of the major endocrine glands.

Most hormones have common characteristics. They are (1) secreted in small amounts at variable but predictable rates, (2) regulated by feedback systems, and (3) able to bind to specific target cell receptors. Table 52.1 reviews the main hormones, the glands or tissues that make the hormones, their target organs or tissues, and their functions. Hormones exert their effects by attaching to receptor sites in their target tissues in a "lock-and-key" type of mechanism. This is why a hormone only acts on cells with a receptor specific to that hormone (Fig. 52.2).

Organs can act as endocrine glands by secreting hormones. For example, the kidneys secrete erythropoietin. It stimulates red blood cell production. The heart secretes atrial natriuretic peptide (ANP). The gastrointestinal (GI) tract secretes many peptide hormones (e.g., gastrin) that aid in digestion. These hormones are discussed in their respective assessment chapters.

We classify hormones by their chemical structure as lipid or water soluble. Solubility is important in understanding how the hormone interacts with the target cell (Fig. 52.3). Lipid-soluble hormones (steroids, thyroid) are bound to plasma proteins as they travel to target cells. They cross the cell membrane by simple diffusion. Water-soluble hormones (insulin, growth hormone [GH]) circulate freely in the blood and act directly on target tissues.

Hormone Regulation

Specific mechanisms control endocrine activity by either stimulating or inhibiting hormone synthesis and secretion. These include positive and negative feedback, nervous system control, and physiologic rhythms.

Feedback. **Negative feedback** relies on the blood level of a hormone or other chemical compound regulated by the hormone (e.g., glucose). It is the most common type of endocrine feedback system. It results in the gland increasing or decreasing the release of a hormone. An example of negative feedback is calcium and parathyroid hormone (PTH) regulation. Low levels of calcium stimulate the parathyroid gland to release PTH. PTH acts on the bone, intestine, and kidneys to increase calcium levels. The increased calcium level then inhibits PTH release.

With **positive feedback**, increasing hormone levels cause another gland to release a hormone that stimulates further release of the first hormone. Something must stop the release of the first hormone (e.g., follicle death), or its release will continue. The ovarian hormone estradiol works by this type of feedback. Increased estradiol levels made by the follicle during the menstrual cycle result in the production and release of follicle-stimulating hormone (FSH) by the anterior pituitary. FSH causes further increases in estradiol until the death of the follicle. This results in a drop in FSH levels.

Nervous system control. Nervous system activity directly affects some endocrine glands. Pain, fear, sexual excitement, and other stressors can stimulate the nervous system to control hormone secretion. For example, when the CNS senses or perceives stress, the sympathetic nervous system (SNS) secretes catecholamines (e.g., epinephrine), which maximize heart and lung function and vision to deal with the stress more effectively. Chronic exposure to some stressors can increase heart rate and BP and cause changes in the endocrine system. This puts patients at risk for chronic disease, such as hypertension.

Rhythms. A common physiologic rhythm is the **circadian rhythm**. It is a 24-hour rhythm that is driven by sleep-wake or dark-light 24-hour (diurnal) cycles. Hormone levels and the responsiveness of target tissues fluctuate predictably during these cycles. Cortisol, made by the adrenal cortex, rises early in the day, declines toward evening, and rises again toward the end of sleep to peak by morning (Fig. 52.4). GH, thyroid-stimulating hormone (TSH), and prolactin levels peak during sleep. Reproductive cycles are often longer than 24 hours *(ultradian)*. An example is the menstrual cycle. We must consider these rhythms when interpreting laboratory results for hormone levels.

Glands

Hypothalamus

The hypothalamus releases substances that either stimulate or inhibit the production and release of hormones from the pituitary gland (Table 52.2). Examples of these hormones include corticotropin-releasing hormone (CRH) and thyrotropin-releasing hormone (TRH). Somatostatin inhibits GH release. Neurons in the hypothalamus receive input from the CNS, including the brainstem, limbic system, and cerebral cortex. These neurons create a circuit that helps coordinate the endocrine system and autonomic nervous system (ANS). The hypothalamus also coordinates the expression of complex behavioral responses, such as anger, fear, and pleasure.

TABLE 52.1 Endocrine Glands and Hormones

Hormones	Target Tissue	Functions
Anterior Pituitary		
Adrenocorticotropic hormone (ACTH)	Adrenal cortex	Foster growth of adrenal cortex Stimulate corticosteroid secretion
Gonadotropic hormones • Follicle-stimulating hormone (FSH) • Luteinizing hormone (LH)	Reproductive organs	Stimulate sex hormone secretion, reproductive organ growth, reproductive processes
Growth hormone (GH), or somatotropin	All body cells	Promote protein anabolism (growth, tissue repair) and lipid mobilization and catabolism
Melanocyte-stimulating hormone (MSH)	Melanocytes in skin	↑ Melanin production in melanocytes
Prolactin	Ovary and mammary glands in females Testes in males	Stimulate milk production in lactating females. ↑ Follicles response to LH and FSH Stimulate testicular function in men
Thyroid-stimulating hormone (TSH), or thyrotropin	Thyroid gland	Stimulate synthesis and release of thyroid hormones, growth and function of thyroid gland
Posterior Pituitary		
Antidiuretic hormone (ADH)	Renal tubules, vascular smooth muscle	Promote reabsorption of water from the renal tubules, vasoconstriction
Oxytocin	Uterus, mammary glands	Stimulate milk secretion, uterine contractility
Thyroid		
Calcitonin	Bone tissue	Regulate calcium and phosphorus levels. ↓ Calcium levels
Thyroxine (T_4)	All body tissues	Precursor to T_3
Triiodothyronine (T_3)	All body tissues	Regulate metabolic rate of all cells and cell growth and tissue differentiation
Parathyroids		
Parathyroid hormone (PTH) or parathormone	Bone, intestine, kidneys	Regulate calcium and phosphorus levels. Promote bone demineralization and intestinal calcium absorption to ↑ calcium levels
Adrenal Medulla		
Epinephrine (adrenaline)	Catecholamine	↑ In response to stress. Enhance and prolong effects of sympathetic nervous system
Norepinephrine (noradrenaline)	Catecholamine	↑ In response to stress. Enhance and prolong effects of sympathetic nervous system
Adrenal Cortex		
Androgens (e.g., dehydroepiandrosterone [DHEA], androsterone) and estradiol	Reproductive organs	Promote growth spurt in adolescence, secondary sex characteristics, and libido
Corticosteroids (e.g., cortisol, hydrocortisone)	All body tissues	Promote metabolism. ↑ In response to stress. Antiinflammatory
Mineralocorticoids (e.g., aldosterone)	Kidney	Regulate sodium and potassium balance and thus water balance
Pancreas (Islets of Langerhans)		
Amylin (from β cells)	Liver, stomach	↓ Gastric motility, glucagon secretion, and endogenous glucose release from liver. ↑ Satiety
Glucagon (from α cells)	General	Stimulate glycogenolysis and gluconeogenesis
Insulin (from β cells)	General	Promote glucose transport from the blood into the cell
Pancreatic polypeptide	General	Influence regulation of pancreatic exocrine function and metabolism of absorbed nutrients
Somatostatin	Pancreas	Inhibit insulin and glucagon secretion
Gonads		
Females: Ovaries		
Estrogen	Reproductive system, breasts	Stimulate development of secondary sex characteristics, preparation of uterus for fertilization, and fetal development. Stimulates bone growth
Progesterone	Reproductive system	Maintain lining of uterus needed for successful pregnancy
Males: Testes		
Testosterone	Reproductive system	Stimulate development of secondary sex characteristics, spermatogenesis

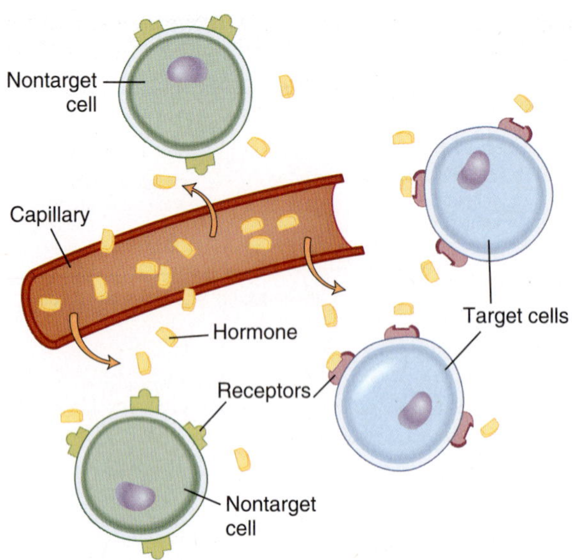

Fig. 52.2 The target cell concept. Hormones act only on cells with receptors specific to that hormone since the receptor's shape determines which hormone can react with it. This is an example of the lock-and-key model of biochemical reactions.

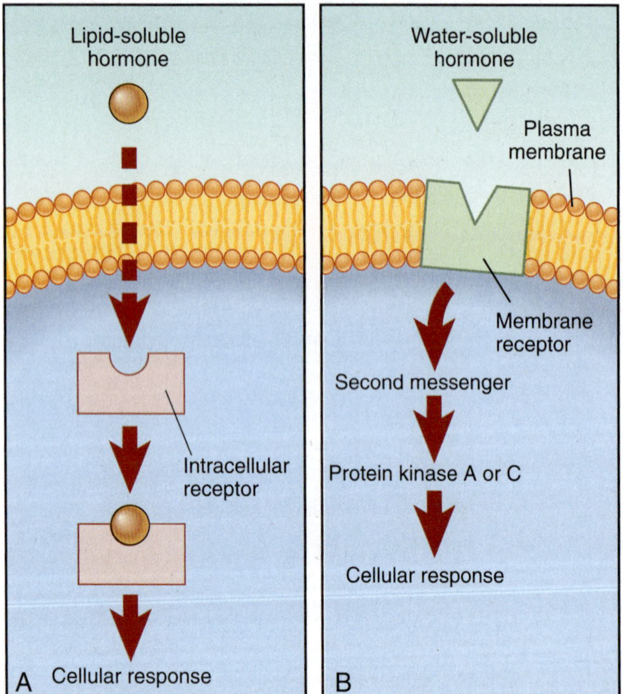

Fig. 52.3 (A) Lipid-soluble hormones (e.g., steroid hormones) penetrate the cell membrane and interact with intracellular receptors. (B) Water-soluble hormones (e.g., protein hormones) bind to receptors in the cell membrane. The hormone-receptor interaction stimulates various cell responses. (Modified from McCance KL, Huether SE: *Pathophysiology: the biologic basis for disease in adults and children,* ed 6, St Louis, 2010, Mosby.)

Pituitary

The pituitary gland *(hypophysis)* is in the sella turcica under the hypothalamus at the base of the brain above the sphenoid bone (Fig. 52.1). The infundibular *(hypophyseal)* stalk connects the pituitary and hypothalamus. The stalk relays information between the hypothalamus and pituitary, creating a strong neuroendocrine connection. The pituitary consists of 2 main parts, the anterior lobe *(adenohypophysis)* and posterior lobe *(neurohypophysis).* A smaller intermediate lobe makes melanocyte-stimulating hormone (MSH).

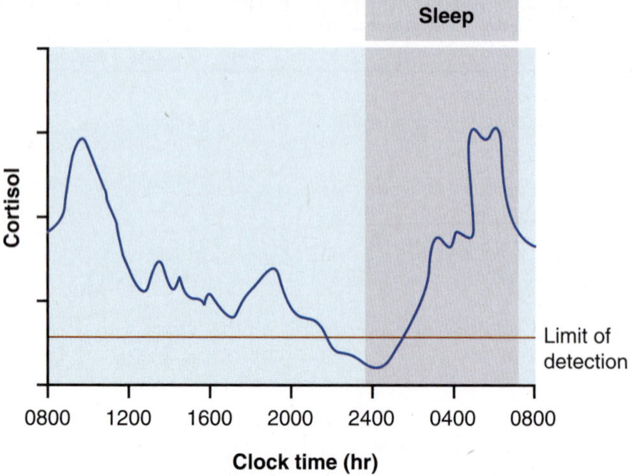

Fig. 52.4 Circadian rhythm of cortisol secretion.

TABLE 52.2 Hormones of the Hypothalamus

The following hormones from the hypothalamus target the anterior pituitary:

Releasing Hormones

- Corticotropin-releasing hormone (CRH)
- Thyrotropin-releasing hormone (TRH)
- Growth hormone—releasing hormone (GHRH)
- Gonadotropin-releasing hormone (GnRH)
- Prolactin-releasing factor

Inhibiting Hormones

- Somatostatin
- Prolactin-inhibiting factor

Anterior Pituitary

The anterior lobe accounts for 80% of the gland by weight. The hypothalamus regulates the anterior lobe through releasing and inhibiting hormones. These hypothalamic hormones reach the anterior pituitary through a network of capillaries known as the *hypothalamus-hypophyseal portal system.* These releasing and inhibiting hormones, in turn, affect the secretion of 6 hormones from the anterior pituitary.

We refer to several hormones secreted by the anterior pituitary as **tropic hormones**. Tropic hormones control the secretion of hormones by other glands. TSH stimulates the thyroid gland to secrete thyroid hormones. Adrenocorticotropic hormone (ACTH) stimulates the adrenal cortex to secrete corticosteroids. FSH stimulates secretion of estrogen and the development of ova in females and sperm in males. Luteinizing hormone (LH) stimulates ovulation in females and secretion of sex hormones in males and females.

GH affects the growth and development of all body tissues. It has many biologic actions, including a role in protein, fat, and carbohydrate metabolism. Prolactin, or lactogenic hormone, stimulates the breast development needed for lactation after childbirth.

Posterior Pituitary

The posterior pituitary is composed of nerve tissue and is essentially an extension of the hypothalamus. Communication between the hypothalamus and posterior pituitary occurs through nerve tracts. The hormones secreted by the posterior pituitary, **antidiuretic hormone (ADH)** and oxytocin, are made in the hypothalamus. These hormones travel down the nerve tracts from the hypothalamus to the posterior pituitary and are stored there until stimuli trigger their release.

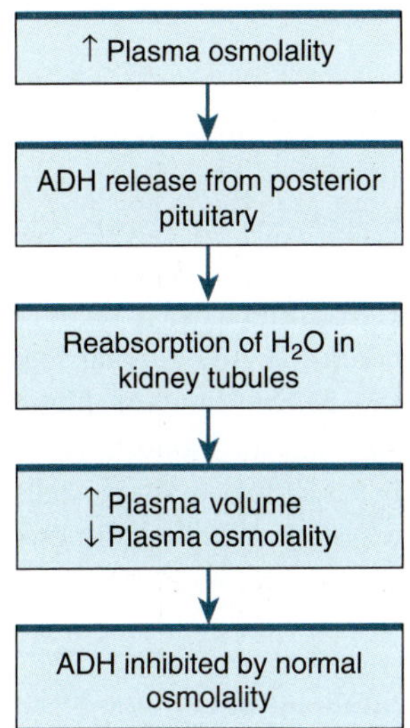

Fig. 52.5 Relationship of serum osmolality to ADH release and action.

The main physiologic role of ADH *(arginine vasopressin)* is to regulate fluid volume. It causes the renal tubules to reabsorb water, making the urine more concentrated. A rise in serum osmolality or hypovolemia causes specialized neurons in the hypothalamus, called *osmoreceptors,* to stimulate ADH release from the posterior pituitary (Fig. 52.5). When ADH release is inhibited, renal tubules do not reabsorb water, resulting in more dilute urine. Volume receptors in large veins, heart atria, and carotid arteries that sense pressure changes (from hypovolemia) also contribute to ADH control. ADH is also a potent vasoconstrictor.

Pineal Gland

The pineal gland is in the brain. It is composed of photoreceptive cells. The gland helps to regulate circadian rhythms and the reproductive system at the onset of puberty.

Its primary function is the secretion of the hormone *melatonin.* Melatonin secretion increases in response to exposure to the dark and decreases in response to light exposure.

Thyroid Gland

The thyroid gland is in the anterior part of the neck in front of the trachea. It consists of 2 encapsulated lateral lobes connected by a narrow isthmus (Fig. 52.6). The thyroid gland is highly vascular. Its size is related to TSH secretion by the anterior

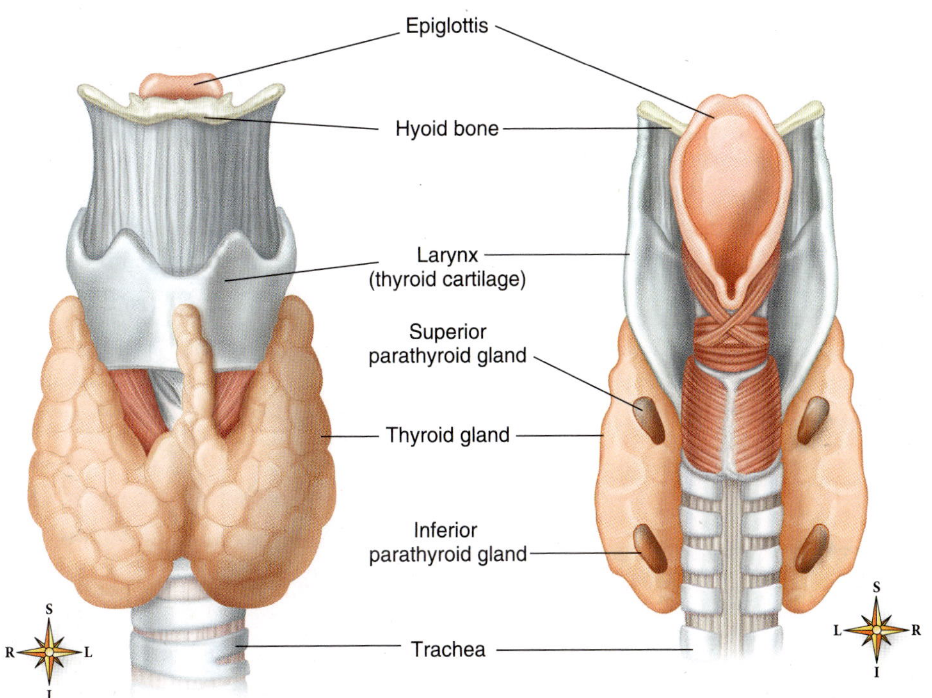

Fig. 52.6 Thyroid and parathyroid glands. Note the surrounding structures. (From Patton KT, Thompson T, Bell FB, et al: *Structure and function of the body,* ed 17, St. Louis, 2025, Elsevier.)

pituitary. The 3 hormones made and secreted by the thyroid gland are thyroxine (T_4), triiodothyronine (T_3), and calcitonin.

Thyroxine (T_4) accounts for 90% of thyroid hormone made by the thyroid gland. **Triiodothyronine (T_3)** is much more potent and has greater metabolic effects. The thyroid gland directly secretes about 20% of circulating T_3. The rest comes from the conversion of T_4 after its release into the bloodstream. Iodine is needed to produce T_3 and T_4. Both hormones affect metabolic rate, caloric requirements, O_2 consumption, carbohydrate and lipid metabolism, growth and development, brain function, and other nervous system activities. More than 99% of thyroid hormones are bound to plasma proteins, especially thyroxine-binding globulin made by the liver. Only the unbound "free" hormones are biologically active.

TSH from the anterior pituitary gland stimulates thyroid hormone production and release (Fig. 52.7). When circulating levels of thyroid hormone are low, the hypothalamus releases TRH. TRH causes the anterior pituitary to release TSH. High circulating thyroid hormone levels inhibit the secretion of TRH from the hypothalamus and TSH from the anterior pituitary gland.

Calcitonin is made by C cells (parafollicular cells) of the thyroid gland in response to high circulating calcium levels. Calcitonin lowers calcium levels by (1) inhibiting the transfer of calcium from the bone to blood, (2) increasing calcium storage in bone, and (3) increasing renal excretion of calcium and phosphorus. Calcitonin and PTH regulate calcium balance.

Parathyroid Glands

There are usually 2 pairs of parathyroid glands lying behind each thyroid lobe (Fig. 52.6). Although there are usually 4 glands, their number may range from 2 to 6.

The parathyroid glands secrete PTH, or *parathormone.* PTH's major role is to regulate calcium levels. It increases calcium levels by acting on bone, the kidneys, and indirectly on the GI tract. PTH stimulates the transfer of calcium from the bone into the blood. In the kidney, PTH promotes calcium reabsorption and phosphate excretion. PTH stimulates the renal conversion of vitamin D to its most active form (1,25-dihydroxyvitamin D_3). This form of vitamin D promotes calcium and phosphorus absorption in the GI tract. PTH secretion is regulated by a negative feedback system. When calcium or magnesium levels are low, PTH secretion increases. When calcium or active vitamin D levels are high, PTH secretion falls.

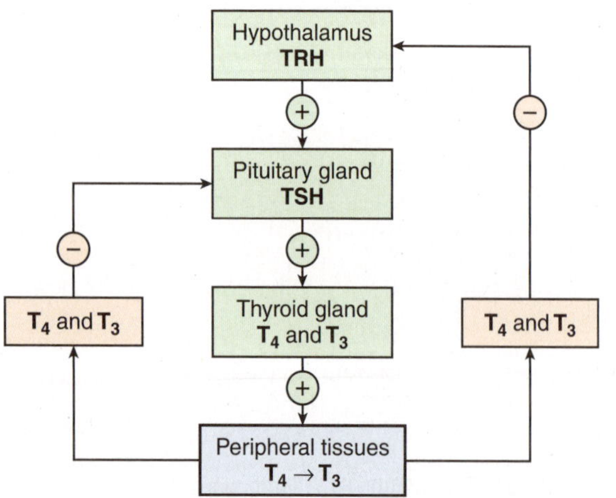

Fig. 52.7 Regulation of thyroid hormone secretion.

Adrenal Glands

The adrenal glands are small, paired, highly vascular glands located on the upper part of each kidney. Each gland consists of 2 parts: medulla and cortex (Fig. 52.8). Each part has distinct functions and acts independently from the other.

Adrenal Medulla

The adrenal medulla is the inner part of the adrenal gland. It consists of sympathetic postganglionic neurons. The medulla secretes the **catecholamines** *epinephrine* (adrenaline), *norepinephrine* (noradrenaline), and *dopamine.* We consider catecholamines neurotransmitters when secreted by neurons and hormones when secreted by the adrenal medulla. They are an essential part of the SNS's "fight or flight" response. Catecholamines travel through the bloodstream and affect multiple organ systems. When secreted by nerve cells in the brain and peripheral nervous system, catecholamines act as neurotransmitters, sending impulses across nerve synapses.

Adrenal Cortex

The adrenal cortex is the outer part of the adrenal gland. It secretes several steroid hormones, including *glucocorticoids, mineralocorticoids,* and *androgens.* Cholesterol is the precursor for steroid hormone synthesis. Glucocorticoids (e.g., cortisol) are named for their effects on glucose metabolism. They inhibit the inflammatory response and are considered anti-inflammatory. Mineralocorticoids (e.g., aldosterone) are essential for maintaining fluid and electrolyte balance. The term **corticosteroid** refers to glucocorticoids and mineralocorticoids.

Cortisol, the most abundant and potent glucocorticoid, is necessary to maintain life and protect the body from stress. It is

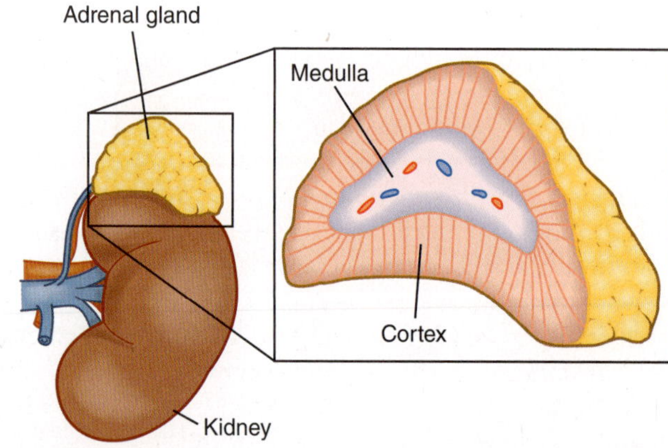

Fig. 52.8 The adrenal gland is composed of the cortex and medulla.

secreted in a diurnal pattern (Fig. 52.4). A negative feedback mechanism controls cortisol secretion. The release of CRH from the hypothalamus stimulates the anterior pituitary to secrete ACTH.

A key function of cortisol is regulating glucose levels by stimulating hepatic glucose formation *(gluconeogenesis)*. Cortisol inhibits peripheral glucose use in the fasting state, inhibits protein synthesis, and stimulates the mobilization of glycerol and free fatty acids. It helps maintain vascular integrity and fluid volume through its action on mineralocorticoid receptors. Cortisol decreases the inflammatory response by stabilizing the membranes of cellular lysosomes and preventing increased capillary permeability. Stress, burns, infection, fever, acute anxiety, and hypoglycemia increase cortisol levels.

Aldosterone is a potent mineralocorticoid that maintains extracellular fluid volume. It acts on the renal tubule to promote renal reabsorption of sodium and excretion of potassium and hydrogen ions. Hyponatremia, hyperkalemia, and angiotensin II stimulate aldosterone synthesis and secretion. ANP and hypokalemia inhibit aldosterone synthesis and release.

The adrenal cortex secretes small amounts of androgens. They are converted to sex steroids in peripheral tissues: testosterone in males and estrogen in females. The most common adrenal androgens are dehydroepiandrosterone (DHEA) and androstenedione. Because they are precursors to other sex steroids, their actions are like those of testosterone and estrogen. In postmenopausal females, the main source of estrogen is the peripheral conversion of adrenal androgens to estrogen.

Pancreas

The pancreas is a long, tapered, lobular, soft gland located behind the stomach and anterior to the first and second lumbar vertebrae. The pancreas has exocrine and endocrine functions. The hormone-secreting part of the pancreas is the *islets of Langerhans*. The islets account for less than 2% of the gland. They consist of 4 types of hormone-secreting cells: α, β, delta, and F cells. The α cells make and secrete the hormone glucagon. The β cells make and secrete insulin and amylin. Delta cells make and secrete somatostatin. F (or PP) cells secrete pancreatic polypeptide.

Pancreatic α cells release *glucagon* in response to low glucose levels, protein ingestion, and exercise. Glucagon increases glucose, providing fuel for energy by stimulating glycogenolysis (breakdown of glycogen into glucose), gluconeogenesis (formation of glucose from noncarbohydrate molecules), and ketogenesis. Glucagon and insulin function in a reciprocal manner to maintain normal glucose levels.

Insulin is the main regulator of metabolism and storage of ingested carbohydrates, fats, and proteins. Insulin facilitates glucose transport into cells, transport of amino acids across muscle membranes, and the synthesis of amino acids into protein in the peripheral tissues. After a meal, insulin is responsible for how we use and store nutrients *(anabolism)*. An increased glucose level is the major stimulus for insulin synthesis and secretion. Low glucose levels, glucagon, somatostatin, hypokalemia, and catecholamines usually inhibit insulin secretion.

Gerontologic Considerations: Effects of Aging on the Endocrine System

Normal aging has many effects on the endocrine system (Table 52.3). These include (1) decreased hormone production and secretion, (2) altered hormone metabolism and biologic activity, (3) decreased responsiveness of target tissues to hormones, and (4) changes in circadian rhythms.

Assessing the effects of aging on the endocrine system may be difficult. The subtle changes of aging may mimic manifestations of endocrine problems. Endocrine problems may manifest differently in an older adult. Older adults may have multiple comorbidities and take medications that change the body's usual response to endocrine function. Symptoms of endocrine problems, such as fatigue, constipation, or mental impairment, may be attributed to aging, resulting in delayed treatment.

TABLE 52.3 GERONTOLOGIC ASSESSMENT DIFFERENCES

Endocrine System

Changes	Clinical Significance
Thyroid	
Atrophy of thyroid gland	↑ Incidence of hypothyroidism
↑ T_3, T_4, TSH secretion	Most maintain adequate thyroid function
↑ Nodules	Lower dosage of thyroid hormone replacement
Parathyroid	
↑ PTH secretion	↑ Calcium resorption from bone
↑ Basal level of PTH	Hypercalcemia, hypercalciuria (may reflect defective renal mechanism)
Adrenal Cortex	
Becomes more fibrotic, slightly smaller	↓ Metabolic clearance rate for glucocorticoids
↓ Cortisol metabolism	
↓ Adrenal androgens and aldosterone levels	
Adrenal Medulla	
↑ Secretion and basal level of norepinephrine	↓ Responsiveness to β-adrenergic agonists and receptor blockers
↓ β-Adrenergic receptor response to norepinephrine	May partly explain ↑ incidence of hypertension with aging
Pancreas	
↑ Fibrosis and fatty deposits in pancreas	May partly contribute to ↑ incidence of diabetes with advanced aging
↑ Glucose intolerance with ↓ sensitivity to insulin	
Gonads	
Females: ↓ Estrogen secretion	Menopausal symptoms Risk for arteriosclerosis, osteoporosis
Males: ↓ Testosterone secretion	May or may not have symptoms

CASE STUDY

Patient Introduction

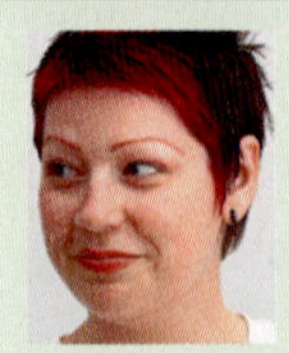

(© iStockphoto/ Thinkstock.)

L.M. is a 35-year-old female who comes to the clinic saying she is "just not feeling well." Her husband, H.M., is with her. L.M. states that she has gained a lot of weight despite trying to watch her diet and just seems to be getting more tired. H.M. voices concerns about the changes in his wife's energy level.

Discussion Questions

1. What are the possible causes of L.M.'s weight gain, fatigue, and irritability?
2. What would be your priority assessment of L.M.?
3. What questions would you ask L.M.?

You will learn more about L.M. and her condition as you read this assessment chapter.

Answers available at http://evolve.elsevier.com/Lewis/medsurg.

ENDOCRINE SYSTEM ASSESSMENT

Subjective Data

Important Health Information

Health history. Patients with endocrine problems often present with nonspecific complaints. The onset of symptoms is often gradual. They may report not just one but a group of symptoms. The most common presenting problems include fatigue, weakness, menstrual problems, and weight changes. It is important to determine whether the onset of symptoms has been gradual or sudden and what the patient has done about them.

Endocrine problems generally result from too much or too little of a specific hormone. Be alert for these specific signs of problems. Some of the more general signs are the easiest to overlook. Evaluate any reported or observed changes in weight, appetite, skin, libido, mental acuity, emotional stability, or energy levels.

Medications. Obtain a complete medication history. Ask about the reason for taking the drug, the dosage, and the length of time the drug has been taken. Are they using hormone replacements, such as insulin, thyroid hormone, or corticosteroids (e.g., prednisone)? This will alert you to potential adverse drug events. For example, corticosteroids may increase glucose levels and cause bone loss with long-term use. Thyroid agents may cause tachycardia or dysrhythmias. Drug-to-drug interactions and adverse effects of nonhormone medications can contribute to endocrine problems.

Surgery or other treatments. Ask about medical, surgical, and obstetric history. Include the number of pregnancies and live births. Assess growth patterns and stages of physical and emotional development. For example, knowing about radiation therapy to the head and neck is important when you suspect thyroid or pituitary problems.

Functional Health Patterns

Key questions to ask patients with an endocrine problem are outlined in Table 52.4.

Health perception–health management. Heredity plays a key role in the development of endocrine problems. Ask about first-degree relatives with diabetes, thyroid disease, multiple endocrine neoplasia, and endocrine cancers.[1] A genetic assessment of family members may be needed.

Nutritional-metabolic. Changes in appetite and weight can indicate an endocrine problem. Ask about a history of weight distribution and changes. Weight loss with increased appetite may occur with hyperthyroidism or diabetes. Weight gain may occur with hypothyroidism or hypercortisolism. Patients who are obese are more likely to develop type 2 diabetes (T2DM).

Ask if there are problems with nausea, vomiting, or diarrhea. An enlarged thyroid gland can cause problems swallowing or a change in neck size. Increased SNS activity, including nervousness, palpitations, sweating, and tremors, may occur with thyroid problems or a rare tumor of the adrenal medulla *(pheochromocytoma)*. Heat or cold intolerance occurs with hyperthyroidism or hypothyroidism, respectively.

Ask about changes in the patient's skin, especially on the face, neck, hands, or body creases. Changes in skin texture and skin that seems thicker or drier may suggest an endocrine problem. Patients with hypothyroidism or excess GH may have skin that feels coarse or leathery. Ask if the patient has noticed any change in the distribution of hair anywhere on the body.

Elimination. Because maintaining fluid balance is a key role of the endocrine system, questions related to fluid intake and elimination patterns may uncover endocrine problems. For example, increased thirst and urination can indicate diabetes (pancreas problem) or arginine vasopressin (AVP) disorder (pituitary problem). Ask about the frequency and consistency of bowel movements. Diarrhea can occur with hyperthyroidism or thyroid cancer. Constipation occurs with hypothyroidism, hypoparathyroidism, and hypopituitarism.

Activity-exercise. Determine whether there are any acute or gradual changes in energy level or persistent fatigue. Patients with chronic fatigue from hypothyroidism, hypocortisolism, or diabetes may report changes in activity level.

Cognitive-perceptual. Memory deficits may occur with hypothyroidism and changes in sodium levels. Syndrome of inappropriate diuresis (SIAD) or pituitary tumors can cause hyponatremia. These issues can occur gradually. Gathering information from the patient and family about memory, cognitive abilities, and balance can increase the chances of an earlier diagnosis.

Self-perception–self-concept. Many endocrine problems may affect patients' self-esteem because of associated changes in physical appearance. For example, weight gain from hypothyroidism or exophthalmos and goiter from hyperthyroidism can cause body image concerns.

Role-relationship. Questions related to roles and relationships can highlight depression, chronic fatigue, and sleep problems. With chronic fatigue, depression, and anxiety, patients and their families will have stressed relationships. Ask about patients' home life and their ability to fulfill their roles.

TABLE 52.4 HEALTH HISTORY

Endocrine System

Health Perception–Health Management

- What is your usual day like?
- Have you noticed any changes in your ability to perform your usual activities compared with last year? 5 years ago?[a]

Nutritional-Metabolic

- What are your weight and height?
- Have there been any changes in your appetite or weight?[a]
- Have you noticed any changes in the distribution of the hair anywhere on your body?[a]
- Have you noticed any changes in the color of your skin, especially on your face, neck, hands, or body creases?[a]
- Has the texture of your skin changed? For example, does it seem thicker and drier than it used to?[a]
- Have you noticed any problems swallowing, throat pain, or hoarseness? Is the top button on your shirt or blouse hard to button?[a]
- Do you feel more nervous than you used to? Do you notice your heart pounding or that you sweat when you do not think you should be sweating?
- Is it hard to hold things because of shakiness of your hands?[a]
- Do you feel that most rooms are too hot or too cold? Do you often have to put on a sweater, or feel hot or cold when others seem comfortable?[a]
- Do you have, or have you had, any wounds that were slow to heal?[a]

Elimination

- Do you have to get up at night to urinate? If so, how many times? Do you keep water by your bed at night?
- Have you ever had a kidney stone?[a]
- Describe your usual bowel pattern. Have you noted any bowel changes?[a]

Activity-Exercise

- Describe your activity during a typical day.
- Do you feel you are able to do what you think you can do? If not, why not?
- Do you have a planned exercise program? If yes, what is it and have you had to make any changes in this routine lately? If so, why, and what kinds of changes?
- Do you have fatigue with or without activity?[a]

Sleep-Rest

- How many hours do you sleep at night? Do you feel rested on awakening?
- Are you ever awakened by sweating during the night?[a]
- Do you have nightmares?[a]

Cognitive-Perceptual

- How is your memory? Have you noticed any changes?[a]
- Have you had any blurring or double vision?[a]
- When was your last eye examination?

Self-Perception–Self-Concept

- Have you noticed any changes in your physical appearance or size?[a]
- Does your health problem affect how you feel about yourself?[a]

Role-Relationship

- Do you have a support system or partner? Are you married? Do you have any children? Do you think you are able to take care of your family and home? If not, why not?
- Where do you work? What kind of work do you do? Are you able to do what is expected of you and what you expect of yourself?
- Are you retired? What type of work did you do before you retired? How do you spend your time now that you have retired?

Sexuality-Reproductive

- Are you trying to have children but cannot?[a]

Females

- When did you start to menstruate? Was this earlier or later than other females in your family?
- When was your last menstrual period? Describe your menstrual flow.
- How many children have you had? How much did they weigh at birth? Were you told you had diabetes during any pregnancy?[a]
- Are you menopausal? If so, for how long?

Males

- Have you noticed any changes in your ability to get and maintain an erection?[a]

Coping–Stress Tolerance

- What types of stressors do you have?
- How do you deal with stress or problems?
- What is your support system? To whom do you turn when you have a problem?

Value-Belief

- Do any of your prescribed therapies cause any conflict in your values or beliefs?[a]

[a]If yes, describe.

Sexuality-reproductive. Menstrual problems, hirsutism, infertility, decreased libido, and growth problems can result from endocrine problems.[2] Obtain a detailed history of menstruation and pregnancy. A history of large-birth-weight babies or gestational diabetes increases the risk of T2DM. Some females develop hypothyroidism during or after menopause. Other patients develop T2DM during middle age when sex hormones are changing. Assess for abnormal secondary sex characteristics, such as facial hair *(hirsutism)* in females. Male sexual problems may include impotence, infertility, or the lack of development of secondary sex characteristics. Retrograde ejaculation can occur in diabetes.

Coping–stress tolerance. Because stress worsens some endocrine conditions, ask patients about their stress level and usual coping patterns. Patients with adrenal insufficiency have difficulty dealing with stress. These patients are at risk for developing hypotension and fluid and electrolyte imbalance.

CASE STUDY

Subjective Data

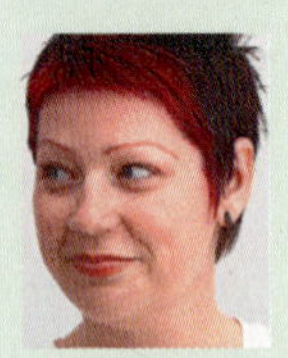

(© iStockphoto/ Thinkstock.)

A focused subjective assessment of L.M. revealed the following information:

- ***Medical History:*** Denies any medical or surgical history. Has not seen an HCP for 8 years.
- ***Medications:*** None.
- ***Health Perception–Health Management:*** L.M. works as a receptionist for a law firm. She says it is all she can do to make it through the workday. She often goes to bed and wakes up with a headache, describing it as a dull, throbbing ache between her eyes. She rates the pain as a 4 on a scale of 0 to 10. Ibuprofen does not ease the pain. The pain is typically worse on arising in the morning. It slowly decreases during the day. She does not have the energy she had 6 months ago. She used to enjoy gardening and going out with friends but now can barely manage work and coming home.
- ***Nutritional-Metabolic:*** L.M. reports a steady weight gain over the past 6 months, mainly in her abdominal area. She feels as if she looks pregnant but knows that is not possible. Her appetite has decreased, but she is not able to lose any weight. She says she feels "bloated." She has new facial hair and notices she is bruising easily. L.M. denies problems with swallowing, hoarseness, palpitations, or tremors.
- ***Elimination:*** Denies any changes or problems with urination or bowel movements.
- ***Activity-Exercise:*** L.M. states that she has no ambition to exercise. She is just too tired at the end of the workday and has no energy on the weekends either. She reports leg cramps with walking.
- ***Sleep-Rest:*** Sleeps 10+ h at night but does not feel rested on awakening.
- ***Cognitive-Perceptual:*** L.M. finds herself easily angered and irritable, often snapping at coworkers and her husband. She says this is not her usual self. At first, she thought it was because she was dealing with the headache. Lately, she has noticed that her vision is blurry, making work and life more stressful.
- ***Self-Perception–Self-Concept:*** L.M. says that she cannot believe what she sees when she looks in the mirror. She feels as if she has aged 10 years over the past 6 months. She has gained weight in her face, neck, and trunk. Her scalp hair is thinning, and she is growing a beard. She tells you she feels "old and ugly."
- ***Coping–Stress Tolerance:*** L.M. states that she is finding it harder to cope with the stresses of her job, her relationship with her husband, and life in general. She believes her emotions are very "raw and labile," so different from the easy-going, smiling person she had once prided herself in being.

Discussion Questions

1. Which subjective assessment findings concern you most?
2. Based on the subjective assessment findings, what should you include in the physical assessment? What would you be looking for?

You will learn more about the physical assessment of the endocrine system in the next section.

Answers available at http://evolve.elsevier.com/Lewis/medsurg

Objective Data

Except for the thyroid and testes, most endocrine glands are inaccessible to direct assessment. We may assess the function of a gland by monitoring the target tissue. Assessment abnormalities related to the endocrine system are outlined in Table 52.5. Specific clinical findings for the various endocrine problems are discussed in Chapters 53 and 54. A focused assessment of the endocrine system is shown in Box 52.1.

Physical Assessment

Endocrine problems may cause changes in mental and emotional status. Throughout the assessment, note the patient's orientation, alertness, memory, cognitive abilities, affect, personality, and appropriateness of their behavior.

Take a full set of vital signs. Variations in temperature, heart rate, and BP can occur with endocrine problems. Obtain height and weight. Calculate body mass index (BMI) to assess nutrition status.

Integument. Assess the color, moisture, and texture of the skin and nails. Decreased skin pigment can occur in hypopituitarism, hypothyroidism, and hypoparathyroidism. Hyperpigmentation, or "bronzing" of the skin, especially on knuckles, elbows, knees, genitalia, and palmar creases, is a classic finding with Addison disease. Is there bruising and delayed wound healing? Assess hair distribution on the head, face, trunk, genitalia, and extremities. Note the hair's appearance and texture. Hair loss, excess hair growth, or dull, brittle hair may suggest endocrine problems. Changes in genital hair distribution can occur with hormone problems.

Head. Inspect the size and contour of the head. Hyperreflexia and facial muscle contraction upon percussion of the facial nerve *(Chvostek sign)* may occur in hypoparathyroidism. Inspect the eyes for position, symmetry, and shape. Large and protruding eyes (exophthalmos) can occur with hyperthyroidism. Assess visual acuity. Visual field loss may occur with a pituitary tumor. In the mouth, inspect the buccal mucosa, condition of teeth, and tongue size. Vision and hearing loss are common in acromegaly from excess GH.[3]

Neck. The thyroid gland is not usually visible during inspection. A feature that distinguishes the thyroid from other masses in the neck is its upward movement on swallowing. Inspect the neck while the patient swallows a sip of water. The neck should appear symmetric without lumps or bulging.

Palpate the thyroid for size, shape, symmetry, tenderness, and any nodules. In a normal person, the thyroid is often not palpable. If palpable, it usually feels smooth with a firm consistency. It is not tender with gentle pressure.[4] If nodules, enlargement, asymmetry, or hardness is present, refer patients for further evaluation. Auscultate the lateral lobes of an enlarged thyroid gland with the stethoscope bell to hear a *bruit.* A bruit can occur with a goiter or hyperthyroidism.

Goiter, an enlarged thyroid gland, can occur with thyroid problems. Do not press too hard or massage an enlarged thyroid gland. This can cause a sudden release of thyroid hormone into an already overloaded system. An experienced clinician should perform palpation in patients with hyperthyroidism.

Perform palpation using a posterior or anterior approach. For *anterior palpation,* stand in front of the patient with the patient's neck flexed. Place your thumb horizontally with the

TABLE 52.5 ASSESSMENT ABNORMALITIES

Endocrine System

Finding	Description	Possible Etiology and Significance
Cardiovascular		
Chest pain	Angina caused by increased metabolic demands, effusions	Thyroid problems
Dysrhythmias	Tachycardia, atrial fibrillation	Thyroid problems hypoparathyroidism, hyperparathyroidism, pheochromocytoma
Fluid overload, signs of heart failure	Crackles in the lungs, edema, shortness of breath	SIAD, hypothyroidism, myxedema
Hypertension	High BP caused by ↑ metabolic demands and catecholamines	Hyperthyroidism, pheochromocytoma, Cushing syndrome
GI		
Constipation	Passage of infrequent hard stools	Hypothyroidism, hyperparathyroidism
Head and Neck		
Exophthalmos	Eyeball protrusion from orbits	Hyperthyroidism because of fluid accumulation in eye and retroorbital tissue
Goiter	Enlargement of thyroid gland	Thyroid problems, iodine deficiency
Moon face	Periorbital edema and facial fullness	Cushing syndrome because of ↑ cortisol secretion
Myxedema	Puffiness, periorbital edema, masklike affect	Mucopolysaccharides accumulate in dermis with hypothyroidism
Thyroid nodule(s)	Local enlargement of thyroid gland	May be benign or malignant
Vision changes	↓ Visual acuity and/or ↓ peripheral vision	Pituitary gland enlargement or tumor pressing on optic nerve
Integument		
Bruises easily	Bruising over body	Cushing syndrome
Changes in hair distribution	Hair loss	Thyroid problems, ↓ pituitary secretion
	↓ Axillary and pubic hair	Cortisol deficiency
	Hirsutism	Cushing syndrome, prolactinoma (a pituitary tumor)
Changes in skin texture	Thick, cold, dry skin	Hypothyroidism
	Thick, leathery, oily skin	GH excess (acromegaly)
	Warm, smooth, moist skin	Hyperthyroidism
Depigmentation (vitiligo)	Patchy areas of light skin	May be a marker of autoimmune endocrine problems
Edema	General edema	Mucopolysaccharide accumulation in tissue in hypothyroidism
Hyperpigmentation	Darkening of the skin, especially in skinfolds and creases	↑ Secretion of MSH from Addison disease, acanthosis nigricans
Skin ulcers	Areas of ulcerated skin, most often found on legs and feet	Peripheral neuropathy and peripheral vascular disease, which contribute to diabetic foot ulcers
Striae	Purplish red marks below the skin surface. Usually seen on abdomen, breasts, and buttocks	Cushing syndrome
Musculoskeletal		
Changes in muscular strength or muscle mass	General weakness and/or fatigue	Pituitary, thyroid, parathyroid, and adrenal problems
		Diabetes, AVP disorder
	↓ Muscle mass	Protein wasting with GH deficiency, Cushing syndrome
Enlargement of bones and cartilage	Coarsening of facial features. ↑ Size of hands and feet over several years	GH excess in adults. Acromegaly due to pituitary dysfunction
Neurologic		
↑ Deep tendon reflexes	Hyperreflexia	Hyperthyroidism, hypoparathyroidism
Lethargy	Mental sluggishness or somnolence	Hypothyroidism
Seizure	Sudden involuntary contraction of muscles	Pituitary tumor
		Hypervolemia and hyponatremia with SIAD
		Complication of diabetes, severe hypothyroidism
Tetany	Intermittent involuntary muscle spasms usually involving the extremities	Severe hypocalcemia that can occur with hypoparathyroidism
Nutrition		
Changes in weight	Weight loss	Hyperthyroidism caused by ↑ in metabolism, type 1 diabetes
	Weight gain	Hypothyroidism, Cushing syndrome, type 2 diabetes
Glucose levels altered	↑ Glucose	Diabetes, Cushing syndrome, GH excess

Continued

TABLE 52.5 ASSESSMENT ABNORMALITIES—cont'd

Endocrine System

Finding	Description	Possible Etiology and Significance
Reproductive		
Changes in reproductive function	Menstrual irregularities, ↓ libido, ↓ fertility, impotence	Pituitary hypofunction, GH excess, thyroid problems, adrenocortical problems
Other		
↓ Urine output	↓ Water reabsorption from kidney tubules	SIAD
Polydipsia	Excess thirst	Extreme water losses in diabetes (with severe hyperglycemia), AVP disorder, dehydration
Polyuria	Excess urine output	Diabetes, AVP disorder (due to ↓ ADH)
Thermoregulation	Cold insensitivity	Hypothyroidism with slowing of metabolic processes
	Heat intolerance	Hyperthyroidism with excess metabolism

BOX 52.1 FOCUSED ASSESSMENT

Endocrine System

Use this checklist to ensure you complete key assessment steps.

Subjective

Ask the patient about any of the following and note responses:

- Excess or increased thirst
- Excess or decreased urination
- Excess hunger
- Heat or cold intolerance
- Excess sweating
- Recent weight gain or loss

Objective: Diagnostic

Check the following laboratory results for critical values:

- Potassium
- Glucose
- Sodium
- Glycosylated hemoglobin (A1C)
- Thyroid studies: TSH, T_3, T_4
- Serum osmolality

Objective: Physical Assessment

Inspect/Measure

- Temperature
- Height and weight
- Alertness and emotional state
- Skin for changes in color and texture
- Hair for changes in color, texture, and distribution

Auscultate

- Heart rate, BP

Palpate

- Extremities for edema
- Skin for texture and temperature
- Neck for thyroid size, shape

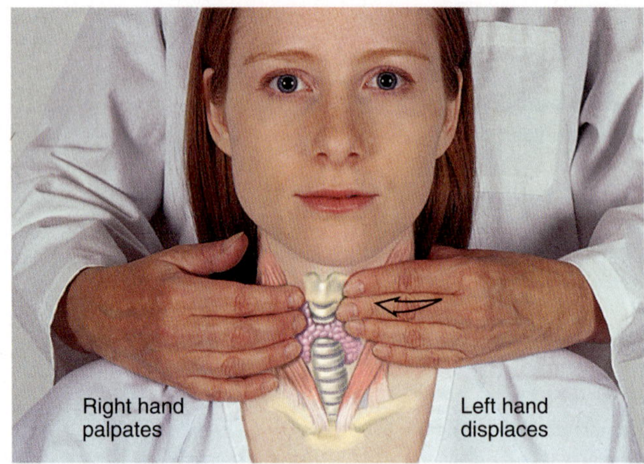

Fig. 52.9 Posterior palpation of the thyroid gland. (From Jarvis C: *Physical examination and health assessment,* ed 6, St Louis, 2012, Saunders.)

upper edge along the lower border of the cricoid cartilage. Then move your thumb over the isthmus as the patient swallows water. Place your fingers laterally to the anterior border of the sternocleidomastoid muscle and palpate each lateral lobe before and while the patient swallows water.

For *posterior palpation,* stand behind the patient (Fig. 52.9). With the thumbs of both hands resting on the nape of the patient's neck, use your index and middle fingers of both hands to feel for the thyroid isthmus and the anterior surfaces of the lateral lobes. Ask the patient to flex the neck slightly forward and to the right to relax the neck muscles. Displace the thyroid cartilage to the right with your left hand and fingers. Palpate with your right hand after placing the thumb deep and behind the sternocleidomastoid muscle with the index and middle fingers in front of it. Ask the patient to swallow water and feel for the thyroid to move up.

Thorax. Inspect the thorax. Note the presence of breast gynecomastia in males. Auscultate lung sounds and heart sounds. Note any adventitious lung sounds (wheezing, decreased sounds) or extra heart sounds. Signs of fluid overload or heart failure may be present in patients with SIAD or hypothyroidism.

Abdomen. Inspect the contour of the abdomen. Note the symmetry and color. Cushing syndrome (hypercortisolism) causes the skin to be fragile, resulting in purple-blue striae across the abdomen. Note general obesity or truncal obesity. Auscultate bowel sounds.

Extremities. Assess the size, shape, symmetry, and general proportion of hands and feet. Patients with acromegaly from pituitary tumors may have large hands and feet.[3] Assess for lesions and edema. Test muscle strength and deep tendon reflexes. Are there any tremors? Test for Trousseau sign, which may be present with hypoparathyroidism.

CASE STUDY

Objective Data: Physical Assessment

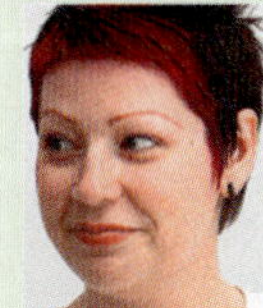
(© iStockphoto/ Thinkstock.)

A focused assessment of L.M. reveals the following: L.M. appears anxious. Her BP is 190/80, heart rate 84, respiratory rate 20, temp 98.6°F (37°C). Her weight is 160 lb. She is 5 ft 4 in tall. L.M.'s face is reddened and puffy. She has a lump on the back of her neck and shoulders. There is some acne on her face and some hair growth on her upper lip and chin area. Her abdomen is protruding, but her arms and legs are thin. She has +1 edema in her ankles bilaterally. There are several bruises on her upper and lower extremities, and purple stretch marks on her abdomen.

Discussion Questions

1. Which physical assessment findings concern you most?
2. What diagnostic studies would you expect to be ordered?

You will learn more about diagnostic studies related to the endocrine system in the next section.

Answers available at http://evolve.elsevier.com/Lewis/medsurg.

DIAGNOSTIC STUDIES OF THE ENDOCRINE SYSTEM

Findings from the history and physical assessment guide the selection of diagnostic studies. Tests used to evaluate glucose metabolism are important in the diagnosis and management of diabetes. See Chapter 53 for information about diagnostic studies for diabetes. Diagnostic studies of the endocrine system are shown in Tables 52.6 and 52.7.

Imaging studies can identify pituitary tumors, thyroid nodules, or adrenal tumors. Laboratory studies may include direct measures of hormone levels or an indirect measure of gland function by evaluating blood or urine components affected by the hormone, such as glucose or electrolytes. We can measure releasing and stimulating hormones. For example, we can evaluate thyroid function by measuring TSH.

We can assess hormones with constant basal levels, such as T_4, with a single measurement. Note the time of the sample collection on the laboratory slip. Information about night shift work is important for hormones with circadian or sleep-related secretion (e.g., cortisol). Evaluating other hormones may require multiple blood samplings. Examples include suppression tests (e.g., dexamethasone) and stimulation tests (e.g., glucose tolerance). In these situations, it is often necessary to obtain IV access to give the testing medication and fluids and draw multiple blood samples.

Pituitary gland problems can manifest in a wide variety of ways because of the number of hormones produced. Many diagnostic studies evaluate these hormones either directly or indirectly.

Several tests are available to evaluate thyroid function. The most sensitive and accurate laboratory test is a TSH level. It is often the first test performed to evaluate thyroid function. Follow-up tests ordered when the TSH level is abnormal include total T_4, free T_4, and total T_3. Free T_4 is the unbound thyroxine. It more accurately reflects thyroid function than total T_4.[5]

The only hormone secreted by the parathyroid glands is PTH. Because PTH regulates calcium and phosphate levels, these levels reflect problems with PTH secretion. For this reason, parathyroid gland testing typically includes PTH, calcium, and phosphate levels.

Tests assessing adrenal cortex function focus on measuring blood and urine levels of the 3 types of hormones secreted: glucocorticoids, mineralocorticoids, and androgens. Urine studies often require a 24-hour urine collection to eliminate the impact of fluctuations in blood hormone levels.

CASE STUDY

Objective Data: Diagnostic Studies

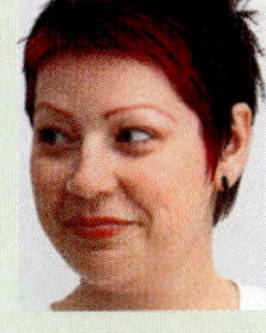
(© iStockphoto/ Thinkstock.)

The HCP orders the following initial diagnostic studies to be drawn in the morning after an 8-h fast:

- CBC, basic metabolic panel (electrolytes, BUN, creatinine)
- Fasting glucose
- TSH, free T_4
- Cortisol and ACTH levels

CBC results reveal a WBC of 12,200/µL and a decreased lymphocyte count at 800 cells/µL. The rest of the CBC is within normal limits (WNL). The FBG is 130 mg/dL. The blood cortisol and ACTH levels are high. Thyroid studies are WNL.

Discussion Questions

1. Which diagnostic study results are of most concern to you?
2. Do you expect the HCP to order any other diagnostic studies for L.M.?

Answers available at http://evolve.elsevier.com/Lewis/medsurg.

TABLE 52.6 Serology and Urine Studies

Endocrine System

Study	Reference Interval	Purpose and Description	Nursing Responsibility
Adrenal Studies			
Blood Studies			
Adrenal steroid precursors • Androstenedione (AD) • Dehydroepiandrosterone (DHEA) • Dehydroepiandrosterone sulfate (DHEA S) • 11-Deoxycortisol	AD • *Female:* 0.05–2.05 ng/mL • *Male:* 0.04–1.06 ng/mL DHEA • *Female:* 0.14–7.88 ng/mL • *Male:* 0.11–6.73 ng/mL DHEA S • *Female:* 7–488 mcg/dL • *Male:* 7–371 mcg/dL 11-Deoxycortisol • *Adults:* 10–79 ng/dL	Assess for congenital adrenal hyperplasia, sex hormone changes, adrenal or gonadal tumors.	*Before:* Grade Tanner stages I–V of physical development. Determine date of last menstrual period (LMP). Should be done 1 week before or after menstrual cycle. *After:* Note date of LMP on laboratory slip.
Adrenocorticotropic hormone (ACTH, corticotropin)	*Female:* 6–58 pg/mL *Male:* 7–69 pg/mL	Measures amount of ACTH made by the anterior pituitary gland. Determines whether there is an overproduction or underproduction of cortisol and whether cause is an adrenal or pituitary gland problem.	*Before:* NPO after midnight. Do morning blood draw between 6 and 8 AM. *During:* Use prechilled blood tube and place on ice.
ACTH stimulation test with cosyntropin (cortisol stimulation test)	*Rapid test:* Cortisol levels increase more than 7 mcg/dL from baseline *24-h test:* Cortisol levels >40 mcg/dL *3-day test:* Cortisol levels greater than 40 mcg/dL	Evaluate cause of adrenal insufficiency. If cortisol levels increase after cosyntropin injection, the cause of adrenal insufficiency is the pituitary gland. If there is no or little rise in cortisol levels, the cause of adrenal insufficiency is the adrenal gland.	*Before:* Obtain baseline cortisol level at beginning of cosyntropin infusion. *During:* Inject bolus of IV cosyntropin with a plastic syringe. Draw cortisol samples 30 and 60 min after bolus. Monitor site and rate of IV infusion. Ensure sample collection at correct times.
Aldosterone	*Supine:* 3–10 ng/dL (0.08–0.30 nmol/L) *Upright:* • *Female:* 5–30 ng/dL (0.14–0.08 nmol/L) • *Male:* 6–22 ng/dL (0.17–0.61 nmol/L)	Identify hyperaldosteronism. Helps distinguish primary aldosteronism from adrenal disease versus secondary aldosteronism from extraadrenal disease.	*Before:* Morning blood sample is best. Tell patient that the required position (supine/sitting/standing) must be maintained for 2 h before specimen is drawn.
Cortisol (hydrocortisone, cortisol)	*8 AM:* 5–23 mcg/dL (138–635 nmol/L) *4 PM:* 3–13 mcg/dL (83–359 nmol/L)	Measures cortisol level to evaluate adrenal activity. Cortisol levels are normally highest in the morning, slowly drop during the day, and are lowest around midnight.	*Before:* Morning blood sample is best. Note if patient works night shift. Mark time of blood draw on laboratory slip. Stress and excess physical activity produce elevated results.
Dexamethasone suppression (DST, prolonged/rapid DST, cortisol suppression test, ACTH suppression test)	Prolonged method: • *Low dose:* >50% reduction of cortisol and 17-hydroxycorticosteroid (17-OCHS) • *High dose:* >50% reduction of cortisol and 17-OCHS Rapid (overnight) method: • Cortisol levels suppressed to <2 mcg/dL	Helps to identify and determine cause of adrenal hyperactivity (e.g., Cushing syndrome).	*Before:* NPO 8–10 h prior. Do not test acutely ill patients or those under stress. Stress-stimulated ACTH may override suppression. Screen for drugs, such as estrogen and corticosteroids, which may give false-positive results. *Overnight method:* Dexamethasone 1 mg (low dose) or 4 mg (high dose) is given at 2300 to suppress secretion of corticotropin-releasing hormone. Plasma cortisol sample is drawn at 0800.

TABLE 52.6 Serology and Urine Studies—cont'd

Endocrine System

Study	Reference Interval	Purpose and Description	Nursing Responsibility
Metanephrine, free (fractionated metanephrine)	*Normetanephrine:* <0.5 nmol/L or 18–111 pg/mL by HPLC *Metanephrine:* <0.9 nmol/L or 12–60 pg/mL by HPLC	Identify pheochromocytoma.	*Before:* Ask about recent history of vigorous exercise, high stress levels, or starvation (may artificially ↑ levels). Assess for drugs (e.g., caffeine, alcohol, levodopa, nitroglycerin, acetaminophen, and those containing epinephrine or norepinephrine) that can alter results.
Urine Studies			
Cortisol (hydrocortisone, urine cortisol, free cortisol)	*24-h specimen:* <100 mcg/24 h (<276 nmol/day)	Measures urine cortisol level to evaluate adrenal activity.	*Before:* Explain 24-h urine collection and need to avoid stressful situations and excess physical exercise. Assess for drug use (e.g., reserpine, diuretics, phenothiazines, insulin, amphetamines) that may alter results.
17-Hydroxycorticosteroids (17-OCHS)	*24-h specimen:* Adults: • *Male:* 3–10 mg/24 h (8.3–27.6 μmol/day) • *Female:* 2–8 mg/24 h (5.2–22.1 μmol/day)	Measures 17-OCHS, a cortisol metabolite, to evaluate adrenocortical function. Older adults may have slightly lower values.	*Before:* Explain 24-h urine collection and need to avoid stressful situations and excess physical exercise. Assess for drug use (e.g., erythromycin, spironolactone) that may alter results.
17-Ketosteroids (17-KS)	24-h specimen: • *Male:* 6–20 mg/24 h (20–70 μmol/day) • *Female:* 6–17 mg/24 h (20–60 μmol/day)	Evaluates adrenocortical and gonadal functions by measuring urine androgen metabolites. Older adults may have slightly lower values.	*Before:* Explain 24-h urine collection.
Vanillylmandelic acid (VMA)	*24-h specimen:* <6.8 mg/24 h (<35 μmol/24 h)	Measures the excretion of catecholamine metabolite. Used to identify catecholamine-producing tumors, such as pheochromocytoma.	*Before:* Explain 24-h urine collection. Must follow VMA-restricted diet 2–3 days before and during the urine collection. *During:* Keep 24-h urine collection at pH <3.0 with HCl acid as preservative. Keep on ice.
Pancreatic Studies			
Blood Studies			
C-peptide (connecting peptide insulin, insulin C-peptide, proinsulin C-peptide)	*Fasting:* 0.78–1.89 ng/mL (0.26–0.62 nmol/L) *1 h after glucose load:* 5–12 ng/mL	Measures amount of C-peptide, which is released with insulin. Distinguishes between type 1 (low levels) and type 2 diabetes (normal or high levels).	*Before:* NPO 8–12 h prior. Water intake allowed.
Glucagon	50–100 pg/mL (50–100 ng/L)	Assess for glucagonoma (α islet cell tumor). Evaluates pancreatic function, especially in people with diabetes with hypoglycemia.	*Before:* NPO 8–12 h prior. Water intake allowed.
Glucose (blood sugar, fasting blood glucose [FBG])	*Fasting* (no caloric intake for at least 8 h): 74–106 mg/dL (4.1–5.9 mmol/L) *Casual* (any time of day): ≤200 mg/dL (<11.1 mmol/L)	Aids in the diagnosis of diabetes.	*Before:* NPO 8–12 h prior. Water intake allowed. Assess for medications that may influence results.

Continued

TABLE 52.6 Serology and Urine Studies—cont'd

Endocrine System

Study	Reference Interval	Purpose and Description	Nursing Responsibility
Glucose, postprandial (2-hour postprandial glucose [2-h PPG])	*0–50 years:* <140 mg/dL (<7.8 mmol/L) *50–60 years:* <150 mg/dL *60 years and older:* <160 mg/dL	Aids in diagnosing diabetes.	*Before:* NPO 8–12 h, then eat a meal of at least 75 g of carbohydrate. Patient NPO after eating the meal until blood is drawn. No exercise during test.
Glucose tolerance test (GTT, oral glucose tolerance test [OGTT])	Nonpregnancy: • *Fasting:* <110 mg/dL (<6.1 mmol/L) • *1 h:* <180 mg/dL (<11.1 mmol/L) • *2 h:* <140 mg/dL (<7.8 mmol/L)	Assess glucose levels in people with symptoms of hypoglycemia. Aids in diagnosing diabetes.	*Before:* NPO 8–12 h prior. Many drugs may influence results, including caffeine and smoking. The diet 3 days before test should include 150–300 g of carbohydrate with at least 1500 cal/day.
Glycosylated hemoglobin (GHb, GHB, glycohemoglobin, hemoglobin A1c [HbA1c], diabetic control index, glycated protein)	*Nondiabetic adult/child:* 4%–5.6%	Measure of average glucose for past 90 days. Used to diagnose and screen diabetes treatment plans.	Explain the test to the patient.
Insulin assay	6–26 μU/mL (43–186 pmol/L)	Assess insulin levels in people with symptoms of hypoglycemia. Assess for insulinomas and carbohydrate and lipid absorption abnormalities.	*Before:* NPO 8–12 h prior. Water intake allowed.
Urine Studies			
Glucose	*Random specimen:* negative *24-h specimen:* 50–300 mg/day (0.3–1.7 mmol/day)	Measure amount of glucose in urine. Assess diabetes management.	*Before:* Use freshly voided urine. Many drugs alter glucose readings. Follow directions exactly to avoid errors.
Ketones	None or negative	Measure amount of ketones in urine. Assess for diabetic ketoacidosis.	*Before:* Use freshly voided urine specimen. Often obtain blood glucose at same time. Follow directions. Certain drugs can produce false-positive or false-negative results.
Parathyroid Studies			
Blood Studies			
Calcium (total)	9.0–10.5 mg/dL (2.25–2.62 mmol/L)	Assess function of parathyroid gland and calcium absorption.	*Before:* NPO 8–12 h prior. Assess for drug use (e.g., albuterol, heparin, diuretics) that may alter results. *After:* Keep sample on ice.
Calcium (ionized)	4.5–5.6 mg/dL (1.05–1.3 mmol/L)	Free form of total calcium. Unchanged by inconsistent albumin levels that occur in certain populations, such as critically ill patients.	*Before:* NPO 8–12 h prior. *After:* Keep sample on ice.
Parathyroid hormone (PTH, parathormone)	*Intact (whole):* 10–65 pg/mL (10–65 ng/L) *N terminal:* 8–24 pg/mL *C terminal:* 50–330 pg/mL	Determine cause of changes in calcium levels from parathyroid or nonparathyroid problems. Monitored in patients with chronic kidney disease, especially those on dialysis.	*Before:* NPO 8–12 h prior. Obtain sample in the morning. *During:* Obtain calcium level at same time.
Phosphate (PO_4), phosphorus (P)	3.0–4.5 mg/dL (0.97–1.45 mmol/L)	Measure amount of inorganic phosphate in blood. Assess for problems related to calcium and phosphorus.	*Before:* NPO 8–12 h prior. If possible, hold IV fluids containing glucose for 8 h prior.

TABLE 52.6 Serology and Urine Studies—cont'd

Endocrine System

Study	Reference Interval	Purpose and Description	Nursing Responsibility
Pituitary Studies			
Blood Studies			
Antidiuretic hormone (ADH, vasopressin, Arginine vasopressin [AVP])	1–5 pg/mL	Assess for AVP disorder, SIAD.	*Before:* NPO 8–12 h prior.
Gonadotropins • Follicle-stimulating hormone (FSH) assay • Luteinizing hormone (LH assay, Lutropin)	FSH (adult) • *Male:* 1.42–15.4 IU/L • *Female:* *Follicular phase:* 1.37–9.9 IU/L *Ovulatory phase:* 6.17–17.2 IU/L *Luteal phase:* 1.09–9.2 IU/L *Postmenopause:* 19.3–100.6 IU/L LH (adult) • *Male:* 1.24–7.8 IU/L • *Female:* *Follicular phase:* 1.68–15 IU/L *Ovulatory phase:* 21.9–56.6 IU/L *Luteal phase:* 0.61–16.3 IU/L *Postmenopause:* 14.2–52.3 IU/L	Assess pituitary and infertility problems. Evaluate puberty and menopause.	*During:* Note on the laboratory slip time of LMP or if female is menopausal.
Growth hormone (GH, somatotropin hormone [SH])	*Male:* <5 ng/mL *Female:* <10 ng/mL	Evaluates GH secretion and pituitary gland function.	*Before:* NPO 8–12 h prior. Stress may alter results. Note NPO status and recent activity level on the laboratory slip.
GH stimulation (GH provocation, insulin tolerance test [ITT], arginine test)	GH levels >10 mg/mL	Identify GH deficiency and problems due to decreased pituitary hormone production.	*Before:* NPO 10–12 h prior. Water allowed on morning of test. Establish IV access for medication administration and blood sampling. *During:* Assess for hypoglycemia and hypotension. Keep 50% dextrose and 5% dextrose IV solution at the bedside in case severe hypoglycemia occurs.
Insulin-like growth factor (IGF-1, somatomedin C, insulin-like growth factor binding proteins [IGF BP])	42–110 ng/mL	Evaluate GH and pituitary gland function. Accurate reflection of mean GH concentration because it is not subject to circadian rhythm and fluctuations.	*Before:* NPO 8–12 h prior.
Urine Studies			
Water deprivation (ADH stimulation)	*Arginine vasopressin (AVP) disorder:* >9% rise in urine osmolality *AVP-R:* <9% rise in urine osmolality *Psychogenic polydipsia:* <9% rise in urine osmolality	Distinguishes among types of AVP disorder.	*Before:* Obtain baseline weight and urine and serum osmolality. Should be done only if sodium is normal and urine osmolality is <300 mOsm/kg. *During:* May need to be NPO. Severe dehydration may occur. Assess urine hourly for volume and specific gravity. Send hourly urine samples to laboratory for osmolality determination. Send blood samples for sodium and osmolality every 2 h. Stop test and rehydrate if weight drops >2 kg at any time. *After:* Rehydrate with oral fluids. Check orthostatic BP and pulse to ensure adequate fluid volume.

Continued

TABLE 52.6 Serology and Urine Studies—cont'd

Endocrine System

Study	Reference Interval	Purpose and Description	Nursing Responsibility
Thyroid Studies			
Blood Studies			
Antithyroglobulin antibody (thyroid autoantibody, thyroid antithyroglobulin antibody, thyroglobulin antibody, thyroid peroxidase antibody [TPO])	<116 IU/mL	Measures thyroid antibody levels. Diagnoses autoimmune thyroid disease and separates it from other forms of thyroiditis. One or more antibody tests may be ordered depending on symptoms.	Explain the procedure to the patient.
Thyroglobulin (Tg, thyrogen-stimulated thyroglobulin)	*Male:* 0.5–53 ng/mL *Female:* 0.5–43.0 ng/mL	Identifies functioning thyroid tissue and thyroid cancer cells. Tumor marker for patients being treated for thyroid cancer.	Same as above.
Thyroid-stimulating hormone (TSH, thyrotropin)	2–10 μU/mL	Most sensitive test for evaluating thyroid function. Helps distinguish primary (thyroid), secondary (pituitary), and tertiary (hypothalamus) hypothyroidism.	Same as above.
Thyroxine-binding globulin (TBG, thyroid-binding globulin)	*10–19 years:* • *Male:* 1.4–2.6 mg/dL • *Female:* 1.4–3.0 mg/dL *20 years:* 1.7–3.6 mg/dL *Oral contraceptives:* 1.5–5.5 mg/dL	Measures TBG, the main thyroid hormone protein carrier. Assess thyroid function when T_4 and T_3 levels are abnormal.	Same as above.
Thyroxine, total and free (T_4, thyroxine screen, FT_4)	*Free T_4:* 0.8–2.8 ng/dL (10–36 pmol/L) *Total T_4:* • *Male:* 4–12 mcg/dL (51–154 nmol/L) • *Female:* 5–12 mcg/dL (64–154 nmol/L) • *>60 years:* 5–11 mcg/dL (64–142 nmol/L)	Evaluate thyroid function and monitor thyroid replacement or suppressive therapy. Free T_4 levels not affected by protein levels like total T_4 is, so it is thought to be more precise marker of thyroid function.	Same as above.
Triiodothyronine (total T_3 radioimmunoassay [T_3 by RIA], free T_3)	*16–20 years:* 80–210 ng/dL *20–50 years:* 70–205 ng/dL (1.2–3.4 nmol/L) *>50 years:* 40–180 ng/dL (0.6–2.8 nmol/L)	Evaluate thyroid function. Free T_3 measures the active component of total T_3. Diagnose hyperthyroidism if TSH is abnormal and T_4 levels are normal. May be used to monitor drug therapy.	Same as above.
T_3 uptake (thyroid hormone–binding ratio [THBR], T_3 resin uptake)	24%–39%	Used with T_4 to assess thyroid function. Indirectly measures binding capacity of thyroid-binding globulin.	Same as above.

TABLE 52.7 Radiologic Studies

Endocrine System

Study	Description and Purpose	Nursing Responsibility
Adrenal arteriography (adrenal angiography)	Assess for arterial obstructive conditions and/or tumors of the adrenal glands.	*Before:* Assess for allergies, especially to contrast dye. NPO 6–12 h prior. Give sedative and other drugs, as ordered. *During:* Patient will feel flushed when dye is injected. *After:* Check pressure dressing site after procedure. Monitor BP, pulse, and circulation distal to injection site. Place compression device over site. Maintain IV and/or oral fluid intake.
CT scan	*Abdominal:* Detect adrenal hyperplasia and tumors or pancreatic problems, such as pancreatitis, tumors, or cysts. *Brain:* Detect a pituitary tumor and its size. *Neck:* Locate thyroid nodules and assess for thyroid cancer.	*Before:* If contrast medium used, assess renal function. Check for shellfish allergy since contrast is iodine based. May need to be NPO 4 h before study. If taking metformin, hold the day of test to prevent hypoglycemia or acidosis. *During:* Warn patient that contrast injection may cause a feeling of being warm and flushed. Must lie completely still during scan. *After:* Encourage patient to drink fluids to avoid renal problems with any contrast.
Magnetic resonance cholangiopancreatography (MRCP)	Assess for the source of pancreatitis and detect pancreatobiliary tumors.	*Before:* May need to be NPO. Oral and/or IV contrast injection may be used. Check for pregnancy, allergies, and renal function. *During:* Must lie completely still during scan.
MRI	*Abdominal:* Can distinguish benign tumors from adrenal cancers. *Brain:* Study of choice for radiologic evaluation of the pituitary gland and hypothalamus. Used to identify tumors in these glands.	*Before:* Oral and/or IV contrast injection may be used. Check for pregnancy, allergies, and renal function before test. Have patient remove all metal objects. Ask about any history of surgical insertion of staples, plates, dental bridges, or other metal appliances. Remove metallic foil patches. May need to be NPO. Assess for claustrophobia and need for antianxiety medication. *During:* Must lie completely still during scan.
Parathyroid scan (parathyroid scintigraphy)	Obtains image of parathyroid glands and any abnormally active areas. Radioactive isotopes are taken up by cells in parathyroid glands.	*Before:* Check for iodine allergy. Some foods and medications are restricted a few weeks before the scan.
Radioactive iodine uptake (RAIU)	Direct measure of thyroid activity and evaluates function of thyroid nodules. • *For 2–4 h:* 3%–19%. • *For 24 h:* 11%–30%.	*Before:* Radioactive iodine given orally or IV. Check for allergies. *During:* Uptake by thyroid gland is measured with a scanner at several time intervals, such as 2–4 h and at 24 h. *After:* Encourage increased fluid intake as radionuclide takes 6–24 h to be eliminated from body.
Thyroid scan	Evaluate thyroid nodules. Benign nodules appear as warm spots because they take up radionuclide. Cancer appears as cold spots because they tend not to take up radionuclide.	*Before:* Radioactive isotopes given orally or IV. Check for allergies. *After:* Encourage increased fluid intake as radionuclide takes 6–24 h to be eliminated from body.
Thyroid ultrasound	Evaluate thyroid nodules to determine size and characteristics (cystic or solid). Management and surveillance of nodules and unaffected portions of the gland.	*Before:* Explain that gel and a transducer will be used over the neck.

BRIDGE TO NCLEX EXAMINATION

The number of the question corresponds to the same-numbered outcome at the beginning of the chapter.

1. A characteristic common to all hormones is that they
   a. circulate in the blood bound to plasma proteins.
   b. influence cellular activity of specific target tissues.
   c. accelerate the metabolic processes of all body cells.
   d. enter a cell and change the cell's metabolism or gene expression.
2. The nurse monitors the patient receiving radiation therapy for renal cancer for signs and symptoms of damage to the
   a. pancreas.
   b. thyroid gland.
   c. adrenal glands.
   d. posterior pituitary gland.
3. The normal hormone response in a patient with a sodium level of 152 mEq/L (152 mmol/L) is
   a. release of ADH.
   b. release of ACTH.
   c. secretion of aldosterone.
   d. secretion of corticotropin-releasing hormone.
4. Endocrine problems often go unrecognized in the older adult because
   a. symptoms are often attributed to aging.
   b. older adults rarely have identifiable symptoms.
   c. endocrine problems are uncommon in an older adult.
   d. older adults usually have endocrine problems with lesser symptoms.
5. When obtaining subjective data during an endocrine assessment, the nurse asks specifically about
   a. energy level.
   b. intake of vitamin C.
   c. employment history.
   d. frequency of intercourse.
6. An appropriate technique to use during physical assessment of the thyroid gland is
   a. asking the patient to hyperextend the neck during palpation.
   b. percussing the neck for dullness to define the size of the thyroid.
   c. having the patient swallow water during inspection and palpation of the gland.
   d. using deep palpation to determine the extent of a visibly enlarged thyroid gland.
7. Abnormal findings during an endocrine assessment include **(Select all that apply.)**
   a. excess facial hair on a female.
   b. blood pressure of 100/70 mm Hg.
   c. soft, formed stool every other day.
   d. 3-lb weight gain over last 6 months.
   e. hyperpigmented coloration in lower legs.
8. A patient has a total calcium level of 3 mg/dL (1.5 mEq/L). If this finding reflects hypoparathyroidism, the nurse expects further diagnostic testing to reveal
   a. decreased PTH.
   b. increased ACTH.
   c. increased glucose.
   d. decreased cortisol levels.

1. b; 2. c; 3. a; 4. a; 5. a; 6. c; 7. a, e; 8. a.

For rationales to these answers and even more NCLEX review questions, visit http://evolve.elsevier.com/Lewis/medsurg.

REFERENCES

To access the References for this chapter, please scan the QR code with a mobile device.

Diabetes

Jane K. Dickinson

http://evolve.elsevier.com/Lewis/medsurg/

CONCEPTUAL FOCUS

Glucose Regulation
Infection
Nutrition
Self-Management
Sensory Perception

LEARNING OUTCOMES

1. Describe the pathophysiology of type 1 and type 2 diabetes.
2. Outline the clinical manifestations of diabetes.
3. Describe the interprofessional care of patients with diabetes.
4. Describe the role of nutrition and exercise in managing diabetes.
5. Discuss the nursing management of patients with diabetes with an acute health problem.
6. Outline the nursing management of a person with diabetes.
7. Relate the pathophysiology and interprofessional care of patients experiencing an acute complication of diabetes.
8. Explain the interprofessional care and nursing management of patients with chronic complications of diabetes.

KEY TERMS

basal-bolus plan
dawn phenomenon
diabetes mellitus (DM)
diabetes-related ketoacidosis (DKA)
diabetes-related nephropathy
diabetes-related neuropathy
diabetes-related retinopathy
hyperglycemia
hyperosmolar hyperglycemia syndrome (HHS)
hypoglycemia
insulin resistance
prediabetes
Somogyi effect

PATHOGENESIS

Diabetes mellitus (DM), or diabetes, is marked by high blood glucose levels (hyperglycemia) resulting from an absent or insufficient insulin supply and/or ineffective use of the body's available insulin, or both. DM is a prevalent and growing health problem throughout the world. In the United States an estimated 38.4 million people, or 11.6% of the population, have DM. Prediabetes affects 97.6 million adults.[1] About 8.7 million people with DM have not been diagnosed and are unaware that they have the disease. DM is the 8th leading cause of death in the United States.[2]

The American Diabetes Association (ADA) recognizes 4 different classes of DM. The 2 most common classes are type 1 (T1D) and type 2 DM (T2DM) (Table 53.1). The 2 other classes are gestational DM and DM due to specific causes.

ETIOLOGY AND PATHOPHYSIOLOGY

Normal Glucose and Insulin Metabolism

Insulin is a hormone made by the β cells in the islets of Langerhans of the pancreas. Under normal conditions, the pancreas continuously releases insulin into the bloodstream in small amounts. Release increases when we ingest food (Fig. 53.1). Insulin lowers glucose and facilitates a stable glucose range of about 74 to 106 mg/dL (4.1 to 5.9 mmol/L).

TABLE 53.1 **Comparison of T1D and T2DM**

Factor	Type 1 DM	T2DM
Age at onset	More common in young people but can occur at any age	More common in adults but can occur at any age. Incidence increasing in children
Type of onset	Signs and symptoms usually abrupt, although disease process may be present for several years	Gradual, may go undiagnosed for years
Prevalence	5%–10% of DM	90%–95% of DM
Endogenous insulin	Absent	Initially increased in response to insulin resistance. Secretion decreases over time
Environment factors	Virus, toxins	Genetics, higher weight, lack of exercise
Islet cell antibodies	Often present at onset	Absent
Primary defect	Absent or minimal insulin production	Insulin resistance, decreased insulin production over time, and changes in adipokine production
Symptoms	Polydipsia, polyuria, polyphagia, fatigue, weight loss without trying	Often none. Fatigue, recurrent infections. May also have polyuria, polydipsia, and polyphagia, blurred vision
Ketosis	Present at onset or during insulin deficiency	Usually not present; can occur during infection or high stress
Insulin therapy	Required for all	Required for some. Progressive. Insulin may need to be added to treatment plan
Body type	Any body type	Often higher weight with visceral adiposity ("apple shape")

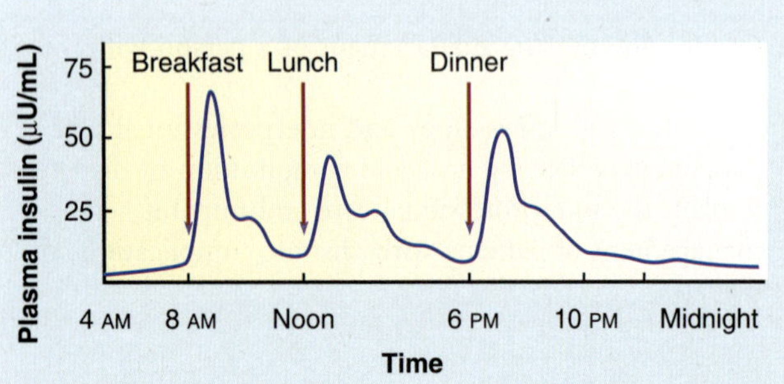

Fig. 53.1 Normal endogenous insulin secretion. After meals, insulin concentrations rise rapidly in blood and peak at about 1 hour. Then insulin concentrations promptly decline toward preprandial values as carbohydrate absorption from the GI tract declines. After carbohydrate absorption from the GI tract is complete and during the night, insulin concentrations are low and fairly constant, with a slight increase at dawn.

The amount of insulin secreted daily by an adult is about 40 to 50 U, or 0.6 U/kg of body weight.

Insulin promotes glucose transport from the bloodstream across the cell membrane to the cytoplasm of the cell (Fig. 53.2). Cells break down glucose to make energy. Liver and muscle cells store excess glucose as glycogen. The rise in plasma insulin after a meal inhibits gluconeogenesis, enhances fat deposition of adipose tissue, and increases protein synthesis. For this reason, insulin is an *anabolic*, or storage, hormone. The fall in insulin level during normal overnight fasting promotes the release of stored glucose from the liver, protein from muscle, and fat from adipose tissue.

Skeletal muscle and adipose tissue have specific receptors for insulin. They are considered insulin-dependent tissues. Insulin is required to "unlock" these receptor sites, allowing the transport of glucose into the cells to be used for energy. Other tissues (e.g., brain, liver, blood cells) do not directly depend on insulin for glucose transport but do require an adequate glucose supply for normal function. Although liver cells are not insulin

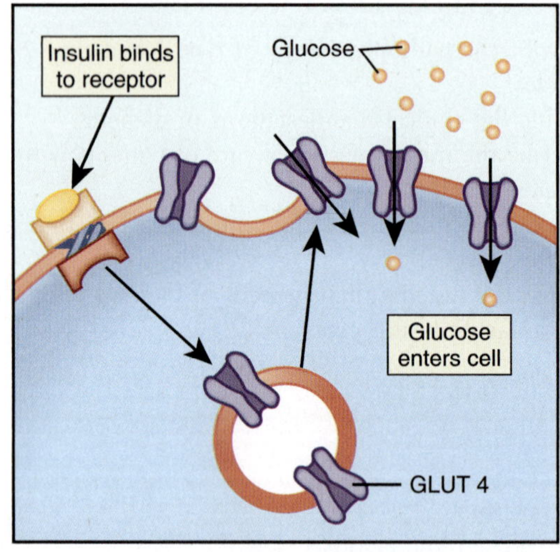

Fig. 53.2 Normal glucose metabolism. Insulin binds to receptors along the cell walls of muscle, adipose, and liver cells. Glucose transport proteins *(GLUT 4s)* then attach to the cell wall and allow glucose to enter the cell. There it is stored or used to make energy.

dependent, insulin receptor sites on the liver facilitate uptake of glucose and its conversion to glycogen.

Other hormones (glucagon, epinephrine, growth hormone [GH], cortisol) work against the effects of insulin. These *counterregulatory* hormones increase glucose levels by (1) stimulating glucose production and release by the liver and (2) decreasing the movement of glucose into cells. The counterregulatory hormones and insulin work together to maintain glucose levels within the normal range by regulating the release of glucose for energy during food intake and periods of fasting.

Insulin is synthesized from its precursor, proinsulin. Enzymes split proinsulin to form insulin and C-peptide. The 2 substances are released in equal amounts. Therefore measuring C-peptide in blood and urine is an indicator of pancreatic β-cell function and insulin levels.

Type 1 Diabetes

T1D accounts for about 5% to 10% of all people with DM. T1D generally affects people under 40 years of age, although it can occur at any age.[3]

Etiology and Pathophysiology

T1D is an autoimmune disorder in which the body develops antibodies against insulin and/or the pancreatic β cells that make insulin. This eventually results in not enough insulin for a person to survive. A genetic predisposition and exposure to a virus are factors that may contribute to developing T1D (Box 53.1).

Predisposition to T1D is related to human leukocyte antigens (HLAs) (see Chapter 14). In theory, when a person with certain HLA types is exposed to a viral infection, the β cells of the pancreas are destroyed, either directly or through an autoimmune process.

Idiopathic type 1 diabetes is a form of ketosis-prone diabetes that is not related to autoimmunity. It only occurs in a small number of people with T1D.[4] *Latent autoimmune diabetes in adults* (LADA) is a slowly progressing autoimmune form of T1D. It occurs in adults and is often mistaken for T2DM.

Onset

In T1D, the islet cell autoantibodies responsible for β-cell destruction are present for months to years before the onset of symptoms. Manifestations develop when the pancreas can no longer make enough insulin to maintain normal glucose levels. Once this occurs, the onset of symptoms is usually rapid. Patients often present with impending or actual ketoacidosis. There is usually a history of recent and sudden weight loss and the classic symptoms of *polydipsia* (excess thirst), *polyuria* (frequent urination), and *polyphagia* (excess hunger).

Persons with T1D require insulin from an outside source *(exogenous insulin)* to sustain life. Without insulin, they will develop diabetes-related ketoacidosis (DKA), a life-threatening condition causing metabolic acidosis. Newly diagnosed patients may have a remission, or "honeymoon" period, for 3 to 12 months after starting treatment. During this time, patients need little injected insulin because β-cell insulin production is still sufficient for healthy glucose levels. Eventually, as more β cells are destroyed and glucose levels increase, the honeymoon period ends. Patients then require insulin on a permanent basis.

Type 2 Diabetes

T2DM accounts for about 90% to 95% of people with DM.[5] Many risk factors contribute to developing T2DM. These include having a family history of T2DM, having higher weight, and being older. The incidence is rising in children because of the increasing prevalence of childhood obesity. T2DM is more prevalent in some ethnic populations. This increase is related to genetic predisposition, environment factors, and diet choices.

Etiology and Pathophysiology

T2DM is characterized by a combination of inadequate insulin secretion and insulin resistance. The pancreas usually makes some *endogenous* (self-made) insulin. However, the body does not make enough insulin, does not use it effectively, or both. Although we do not fully understand the genetics of T2DM, it is likely that multiple genes are involved (Box 53.1). We have found genetic mutations that lead to insulin resistance and a higher risk for obesity in many people with T2DM.

BOX 53.1 GENETICS IN CLINICAL PRACTICE

Diabetes

Type 1 DM	Type 2 DM	Maturity-Onset Diabetes of the Young (MODY)
Genetic Basis		
• Increased susceptibility (40%–50%) when a person has specific human leukocyte antigens (HLA-DR3, HLA-DR4; HLA-DR7; HLA-DR9) • Polygenic (>40 genes influence susceptibility)	• Polygenic (>25 genes influence susceptibility) • Persons with a first-degree relative with the disease are 10 times more likely to develop T2DM	• Autosomal dominant • Monogenic (single gene) • Caused by mutations in any of 6 MODY genes (types 1–6) • Gene mutations lead to β-cell dysfunction
Risk to Offspring		
• Risk to offspring of mothers with DM is 1%–4% • Risk to offspring of fathers with DM is 5%–6% • When 1 identical twin has type 1 DM, the other gets DM about 30%–40% of the time	• Risk to offspring is 40%–70% • When 1 identical twin has type 2 DM, the other gets DM about 60%–75% of the time	• If 1 parent has MODY, a child has a 50% chance of developing MODY • If 1 parent has MODY, a child has a 50% chance of being a carrier
Clinical Implications		
• Result of interaction of genetic, autoimmune, and environment factors	• Result of genetic interactions and other metabolic factors • Environment factors, such as body weight and exercise, can modify metabolic factors	• Accounts for 1%–5% of people with DM • Young age of onset (often before age 25) • Not related to obesity or hypertension • Treatment depends on the genetic mutation that caused MODY

Metabolic problems have a role in developing T2DM (Fig. 53.3). The first factor is *insulin resistance.* This is a condition in which body tissues do not respond to the action of insulin because insulin receptors are unresponsive, insufficient in number, or both. Most insulin receptors are located on skeletal muscle, fat, and liver cells. When insulin is not properly used, the entry of glucose into the cell is impeded, causing hyperglycemia. In the early stages of insulin resistance, the pancreas responds to high glucose levels by producing more insulin (if β-cell function is normal). This temporary state of hyperinsulinemia coexists with hyperglycemia.

A second factor is a marked decrease in the ability of the pancreas to make insulin. The β cells become fatigued from the compensatory overproduction of insulin or when β-cell mass is lost. We do not know the reason the β cells fail to adapt. It may be the result of the adverse effects of chronic hyperglycemia or high circulating free fatty acids. In addition, the α cells of the pancreas increase glucagon production.

A third factor is inappropriate glucose production by the liver. Instead of properly regulating the release of glucose in response to blood levels, the liver does so in a haphazard way that does not correspond to the body's needs at the time.

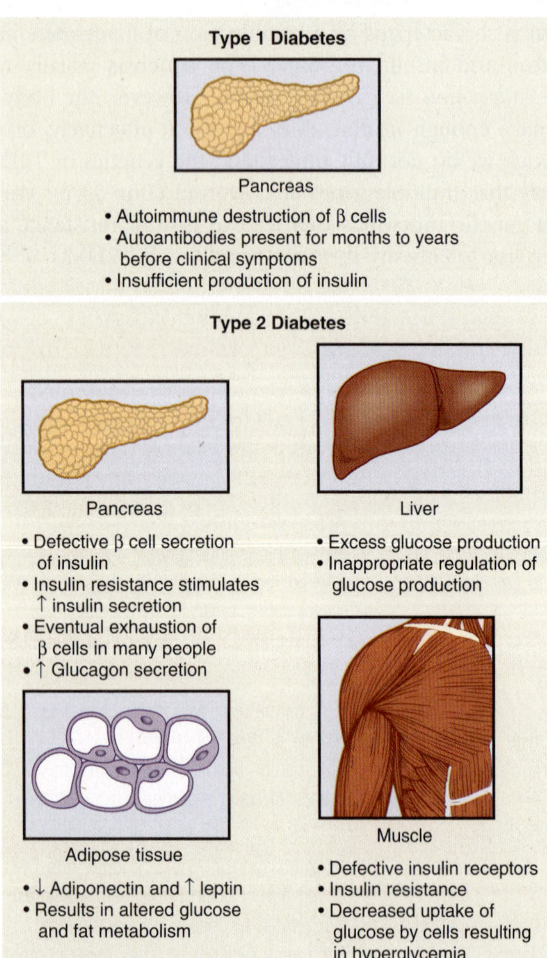

Fig. 53.3 Altered mechanisms in T1D and T2DM.

The last factor is the complex role of hormones and cytokines. Adipokines secreted by adipose tissue appear to play a role in glucose and fat metabolism. They are likely to contribute to developing T2DM.[6] We think adipokines cause chronic inflammation, a factor involved in insulin resistance, T2DM, and cardiovascular disease (CVD). The 2 main adipokines thought to affect insulin sensitivity are adiponectin and leptin. Finally, the brain, kidneys, and gut have roles in developing T2DM.

People with *metabolic syndrome* have an increased risk of developing T2DM. Metabolic syndrome has 5 components: increased glucose levels, abdominal obesity, high BP, high triglyceride levels, and decreased high-density lipoprotein (HDL) levels (see Table 45.12). A person with 3 of the 5 components is considered to have metabolic syndrome.[7] Persons with higher weight and metabolic syndrome can reduce their risk for DM through food choices and regular physical activity.

Onset

The disease onset is usually gradual. The person may go for many years with undetected hyperglycemia and few, if any, symptoms. Many people are diagnosed on routine laboratory testing or when they undergo treatment for other problems, and they have high glucose or glycosylated hemoglobin (A1C) levels. The signs and symptoms of hyperglycemia develop when about 50% to 80% of β cells are no longer secreting insulin. At the time of diagnosis, the average person has had T2DM for 6½ years.

Prediabetes

Persons with prediabetes are at increased risk for developing T2DM. **Prediabetes** is defined as *impaired glucose tolerance* (IGT), *impaired fasting glucose* (IFG), or both. It is an intermediate stage between normal glucose homeostasis and DM. Glucose levels are high but not high enough to meet the diagnostic criteria for DM. A diagnosis of IGT is made if the 2-hour oral glucose tolerance test (OGTT) values are 140 to 199 mg/dL (7.8 to 11.0 mmol/L). IFG is diagnosed when fasting glucose levels are 100 to 125 mg/dL (5.56 to 6.9 mmol/L).

Persons with prediabetes usually do not have symptoms. However, long-term damage to the body, especially the heart and blood vessels, may be occurring. It is important for people to undergo screening and understand risk factors for DM. Encourage those with prediabetes to have their glucose level and A1C checked regularly and monitor for symptoms of DM, such as fatigue or frequent infections. People with prediabetes can take action to prevent or delay developing T2DM. This includes maintaining a healthy weight, exercising regularly, and making healthy food choices.

Gestational Diabetes

Gestational diabetes develops during pregnancy. It occurs in about 2% to 10% of pregnancies in the United States.[8] Females with gestational DM have a higher risk for cesarean delivery. Their babies are at increased risk for perinatal death, birth injury, and neonatal complications. Females who are at high risk for gestational DM are screened at the first prenatal visit. Those at high risk include females who are obese, are of advanced maternal age, or have a family history of DM. We screen patients with an average risk for gestational DM using an OGTT at 24 to 28 weeks of gestation. Most females with gestational DM have normal glucose levels within 6 weeks postpartum. Those who had gestational DM have up to a 63% chance of developing T2DM within 16 years. Gestational DM and managing pregnant patients with DM are not covered in detail here. Consult an obstetric text for more information.

Specific Types of Diabetes

DM sometimes occurs because of another medical condition or treatment of a medical condition that causes abnormal glucose levels. Conditions that may cause DM can result from injury to, interference with, or destruction of the β-cell function in the pancreas. These include Cushing syndrome, hyperthyroidism, pancreatitis, cystic fibrosis, hemochromatosis, and parenteral nutrition. Common drugs that can induce DM include corticosteroids, thiazides, phenytoin (Dilantin), and atypical antipsychotics (e.g., clozapine). DM caused by medical conditions or drugs can resolve when the underlying condition is treated or the drug is discontinued. Maturity-onset diabetes of the young (MODY) is a rare inherited form of DM.

CLINICAL MANIFESTATIONS

Type 1 Diabetes

Because the onset of T1D is rapid, the first manifestations are usually acute. The classic symptoms are *polyuria, polydipsia,* and *polyphagia.* The osmotic effect of excess glucose in the bloodstream causes polydipsia and polyuria. Polyphagia is a result of cell malnourishment when insulin deficiency prevents cells from using glucose for energy. Weight loss may occur because the body cannot get glucose and instead breaks down fat and protein to try to make energy. Weakness and fatigue may result because cells lack needed energy from glucose. DKA, a common complication in those with untreated T1D, has additional manifestations.

Type 2 Diabetes

The manifestations of T2DM are often nonspecific. Some common manifestations are fatigue, recurrent infections, recurrent vaginal yeast or *Candida* infections, prolonged wound healing, and vision problems. Although not common, it is possible for a person with T2DM to have classic symptoms associated with T1D, including polyuria, polydipsia, and polyphagia.

DIAGNOSTIC STUDIES

The diagnosis is made using 1 of 4 methods (Table 53.2). If a patient has a hyperglycemic crisis or clear symptoms of hyperglycemia (polyuria, polydipsia, polyphagia) with a random plasma glucose level of 200 mg/dL or greater, repeat testing is not needed. Otherwise, criteria 1 through 3 require confirmation by repeat testing. The repeat test should be the same test used initially. For example, if a random high glucose was the initial measurement, that same measure should be used to confirm a diagnosis.

The accuracy of laboratory results depends on patient preparation and attention to the many factors that influence the results. Factors that can falsely increase values include recent severe restrictions of carbohydrate intake, acute illness, drugs (e.g., contraceptives, corticosteroids), and restricted activity, such as bed rest. Patients with impaired gastrointestinal (GI) absorption or who have recently taken acetaminophen may have false-negative results.

A1C measures the amount of glycosylated hemoglobin (Hgb) as a percentage of total Hgb. For example, an A1C of 6.5% means that 6.5% of the total Hgb has glucose attached to it. The amount of glycosylated Hgb depends on the glucose level. When glucose levels are high over time, the amount of glucose attached to Hgb increases. This glucose stays attached to the red blood cell (RBC) for the life of the cell (about 120 days). Therefore A1C provides an average measure of glucose levels over the previous 2 to 3 months. Increases in the A1C reflect higher average glucose levels. A1C does not, however, consider fluctuations in glucose. It does not give a good indicator of how often someone has high or low glucose levels. An advantage of the A1C includes greater convenience because fasting is not needed. Diseases affecting RBCs (e.g., iron deficiency anemia, sickle cell anemia) can influence the A1C and should be considered when interpreting results.

Teach patients with DM and prediabetes to have their A1C regularly monitored to determine whether they are meeting their glycemic goals. The ADA identifies an A1C goal of less than 7.0% for people with DM. When the A1C is maintained at near-normal levels, the risk for developing microvascular and macrovascular complications is greatly reduced. For people with prediabetes, monitoring the A1C can detect overt DM and provide feedback on efforts to prevent it.

More people with DM are using continuous glucose monitoring (CGM). CGM reports include "time in range." It is a more accurate way to look at daily glucose levels and fluctuations than A1C. Until CGM is more widely used, A1C remains a good tool for monitoring glucose over time.

TABLE 53.2 Diagnostic Criteria

DM

The diagnosis of DM is made using 1 of 4 methods:

1. A1C of 6.5% or higher
2. Fasting plasma glucose (FPG) level of 126 mg/dL (7.0 mmol/L) or greater. *Fasting* is defined as no caloric intake for at least 8 hours
3. A 2-hour plasma glucose level of 200 mg/dL (11.1 mmol/L) or greater during an oral glucose tolerance test, using a glucose load of 75 g
4. In a person with classic symptoms of hyperglycemia (polyuria, polydipsia, unexplained weight loss) or hyperglycemic crisis, a random plasma glucose level of 200 mg/dL (11.1 mmol/L) or greater

Fructosamine is formed by a chemical reaction of glucose with plasma protein. Fructosamine levels may show a change in glucose levels before A1C does. It reflects glycemia in the previous 1 to 3 weeks. It is used for people with abnormal hemoglobin or short-term measurement of glucose levels, for instance, after a change in medication or during pregnancy.

Islet cell autoantibody testing can help distinguish between autoimmune T1D and DM from other causes. Autoantibodies can develop into 1 or several autoantigens, including GAD65, IA-2, or insulin.

INTERPROFESSIONAL AND NURSING MANAGEMENT

The goals of DM management are to reduce symptoms, promote well-being, prevent acute complications related to hyperglycemia and hypoglycemia, and prevent or delay the onset and progression of chronic complications. These goals are most likely to be met when patients maintain glucose levels as near to normal as possible. Meeting goals for what we refer to as the "ABCs of diabetes" can help persons manage DM and lower their risk for CVD. The ABCs refer to (1) A1C, (2) BP, (3) cholesterol, and (4) stop smoking. Patient teaching, which enables patients to self-manage their own care, is essential to achieve glycemic goals. Nutrition therapy, drug therapy, exercise, and glucose monitoring are the tools used in managing DM (Table 53.3).

TABLE 53.3 Interprofessional Care

DM

Diagnostic Assessment

- History and physical assessment
- Blood tests, including glucose levels (Table 53.2), A1C, fructosamine, lipid profile, BUN and creatinine, electrolytes, islet cell autoantibodies
- Urine for complete urinalysis, albuminuria, and acetone (if indicated)
- BP
- ECG (if indicated)
- Dilated eye examination
- Dental examination
- Neurologic examination, including monofilament test for sensation to lower extremities
- Ankle-brachial index (ABI) (if indicated)
- Foot (podiatric) examination
- Monitoring of weight

Management

- Patient and caregiver teaching and evaluation (Tables 53.15 and 53.16)
- Nutrition therapy (Table 53.9)
- Exercise therapy (Table 53.10)
- Glucose monitoring (Table 53.11)

Drug Therapy

- Insulin (Fig. 53.3 and Tables 53.4 and 53.5)
- Oral agents (OAs) and noninsulin injectable agents (Tables 53.7 and 53.8)
- Antiplatelet therapy (see Table 41.10)
- BP medications (see Table 36.6)
  - Angiotensin-converting enzyme (ACE) inhibitors
  - Angiotensin II receptor blockers (ARBs)
  - Statin therapy (see Table 37.6)

DRUG THERAPY

The 3 major types of glucose-lowering agents (GLAs) used in DM treatment are insulin, oral agents (OAs), and noninsulin injectable agents.[9]

Insulin

Exogenous (injected) insulin is needed when someone has inadequate insulin to meet specific metabolic needs. People with T1D require exogenous insulin to survive. They often use multiple daily injections of insulin (often 4 or more) or continuous insulin infusion via an insulin pump to adequately manage glucose levels. People with T2DM may need exogenous insulin during periods of severe stress, such as illness or surgery. Because T2DM is progressive, over time, the combination of nutrition, exercise, OAs, and noninsulin injectable agents may no longer adequately manage glucose levels. At that point, we add exogenous insulin to their management plan. People with T2DM may also need up to 4 injections per day or a continuous infusion to maintain healthy glucose levels.

Insulin Types and Plans

Genetically engineered human insulin is made in laboratories. Types of insulin differ by their onset, peak action, and duration (Fig. 53.4). They are categorized as rapid-acting, short-acting, intermediate-acting, and long-acting insulin (Table 53.4).

Table 53.5 shows examples of insulin plans. The insulin approach that most closely mimics endogenous insulin production is the **basal-bolus plan** (often called *intensive* or *physiologic insulin therapy*). It consists of multiple daily insulin injections or an insulin pump together with frequent glucose monitoring or CGM. Injections include rapid- or short-acting (bolus) insulin before meals and intermediate- or long-acting (basal) background insulin once or twice a day. The goal is to achieve a glucose level as close to normal as possible, as much of the time as possible. We refer to this as "time in range."

Other, less intense plans can promote healthy glucose levels for some people. Ideally, patients and HCPs work together to choose a plan. Selection is based on the desired and feasible glucose levels and the patient's lifestyle, food choices, and activity. If a less intense plan is not giving optimal results, the HCP may encourage a more intense approach.

Mealtime insulin (bolus). To manage postprandial glucose levels, the timing of rapid- and short-acting insulin in relation to meals is crucial. Rapid-acting insulin most closely mimics natural insulin secretion in response to a meal. It should be injected within 15 minutes of eating. Older agents (aspart

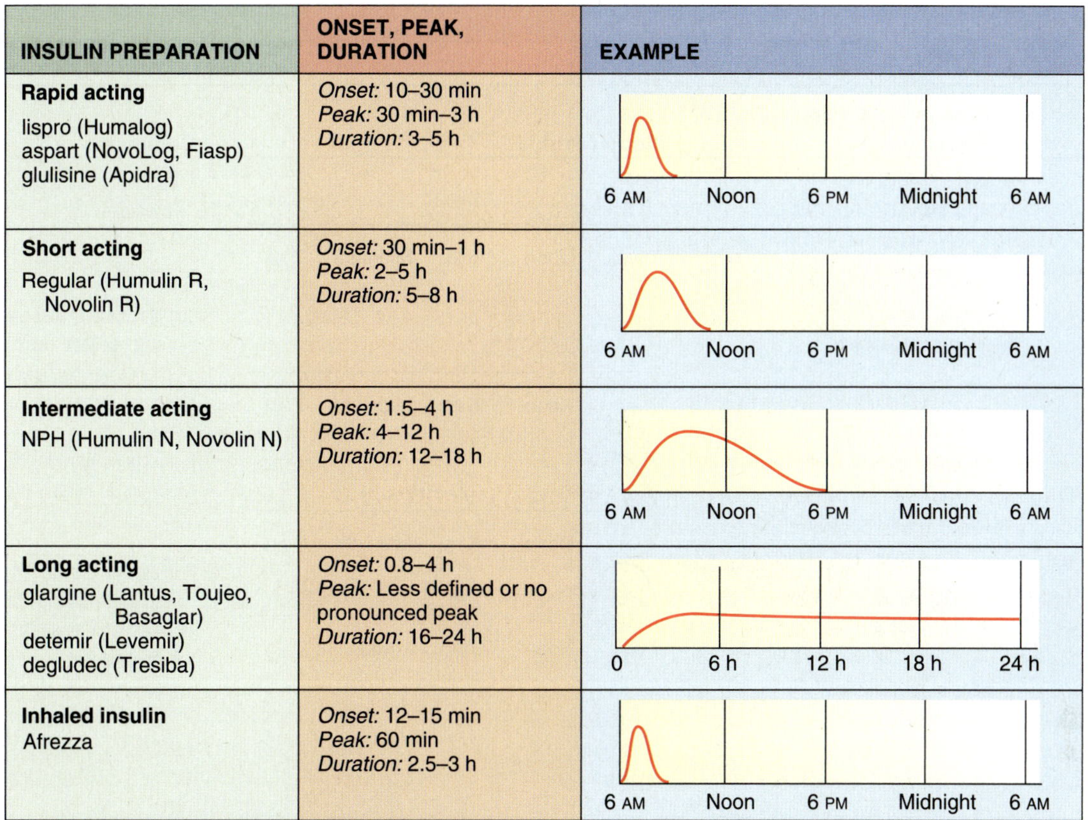

INSULIN PREPARATION	ONSET, PEAK, DURATION	EXAMPLE
Rapid acting lispro (Humalog) aspart (NovoLog, Fiasp) glulisine (Apidra)	*Onset:* 10–30 min *Peak:* 30 min–3 h *Duration:* 3–5 h	6 AM Noon 6 PM Midnight 6 AM
Short acting Regular (Humulin R, Novolin R)	*Onset:* 30 min–1 h *Peak:* 2–5 h *Duration:* 5–8 h	6 AM Noon 6 PM Midnight 6 AM
Intermediate acting NPH (Humulin N, Novolin N)	*Onset:* 1.5–4 h *Peak:* 4–12 h *Duration:* 12–18 h	6 AM Noon 6 PM Midnight 6 AM
Long acting glargine (Lantus, Toujeo, Basaglar) detemir (Levemir) degludec (Tresiba)	*Onset:* 0.8–4 h *Peak:* Less defined or no pronounced peak *Duration:* 16–24 h	0 6 h 12 h 18 h 24 h
Inhaled insulin Afrezza	*Onset:* 12–15 min *Peak:* 60 min *Duration:* 2.5–3 h	6 AM Noon 6 PM Midnight 6 AM

Fig. 53.4 Available insulin preparations showing onset, peak, and duration of action. Patient responses to each type of insulin are different and affected by many factors.

TABLE 53.4 Drug Therapy

Types of Insulin

Classification	Examples
Rapid-acting	aspart (NovoLog, Fiasp) glulisine (Apidra) lispro (Humalog, Lyumjev)
Short-acting (regular)	regular (Humulin R, Novolin R)
Intermediate-acting	NPH (Humulin N, Novolin N)
Long-acting	degludec (Tresiba) detemir (Levemir) glargine (Basaglar, Lantus, Semglee, Toujeo)
Combination (premixed)	aspart protamine/aspart 70/30[a] (NovoLog Mix 70/30) degludec/aspart 70/30 (Ryzodeg) lispro protamine/lispro 75/25[a] (Humalog Mix 75/25) lispro protamine/lispro 50/50[a] (Humalog Mix 50/50) NPH/regular 70/30[a] (Humulin 70/30, Novolin 70/30) NPH/regular 50/50[a] (Humulin 50/50)
Concentrated	Humulin R U-500 Toujeo U-300 (insulin glargine) Humalog U-200 (insulin lispro)
Inhaled	Afrezza

[a]These numbers refer to percentages of each type of insulin.

[NovoLog], lispro [Humalog]) have an onset of action of about 15 minutes. Newer agents (aspart [Fiasp], lispro [Lyumjev]) start working faster.

Short-acting regular insulin has an onset of action of 30 to 60 minutes. It is injected 30 to 45 minutes before a meal to ensure that the insulin is working at the same time as meal absorption. Because timing an injection 30 to 45 minutes before a meal is hard for some people to do with their lifestyles, those taking insulin with their meals often prefer the flexibility of rapid-acting insulins. Short-acting insulin is more likely to cause hypoglycemia because of its longer duration of action.

Basal (background) insulin. People with T1D use a long- or intermediate-acting basal (background) insulin to maintain glucose levels in between meals and overnight. Without 24-hour background insulin, people with T1D are more prone to developing DKA. Many people with T2DM who use OAs need basal insulin to maintain healthy glucose levels. If OAs and long-acting insulin are not adequate to achieve glycemic goals, people with T2DM may need to add mealtime insulin.

The long-acting insulins include degludec (Tresiba), detemir (Levemir), and glargine (Lantus, Toujeo). Long-acting insulin is released steadily and continuously. For many people, it does not have a peak of action. The action time for long-acting insulin varies (Fig. 53.4). Although they can be given once daily, detemir is often given twice daily. Because they lack peak action time, their risk for hypoglycemia is greatly reduced. Glargine

TABLE 53.5 Drug Therapy

Insulin Plans

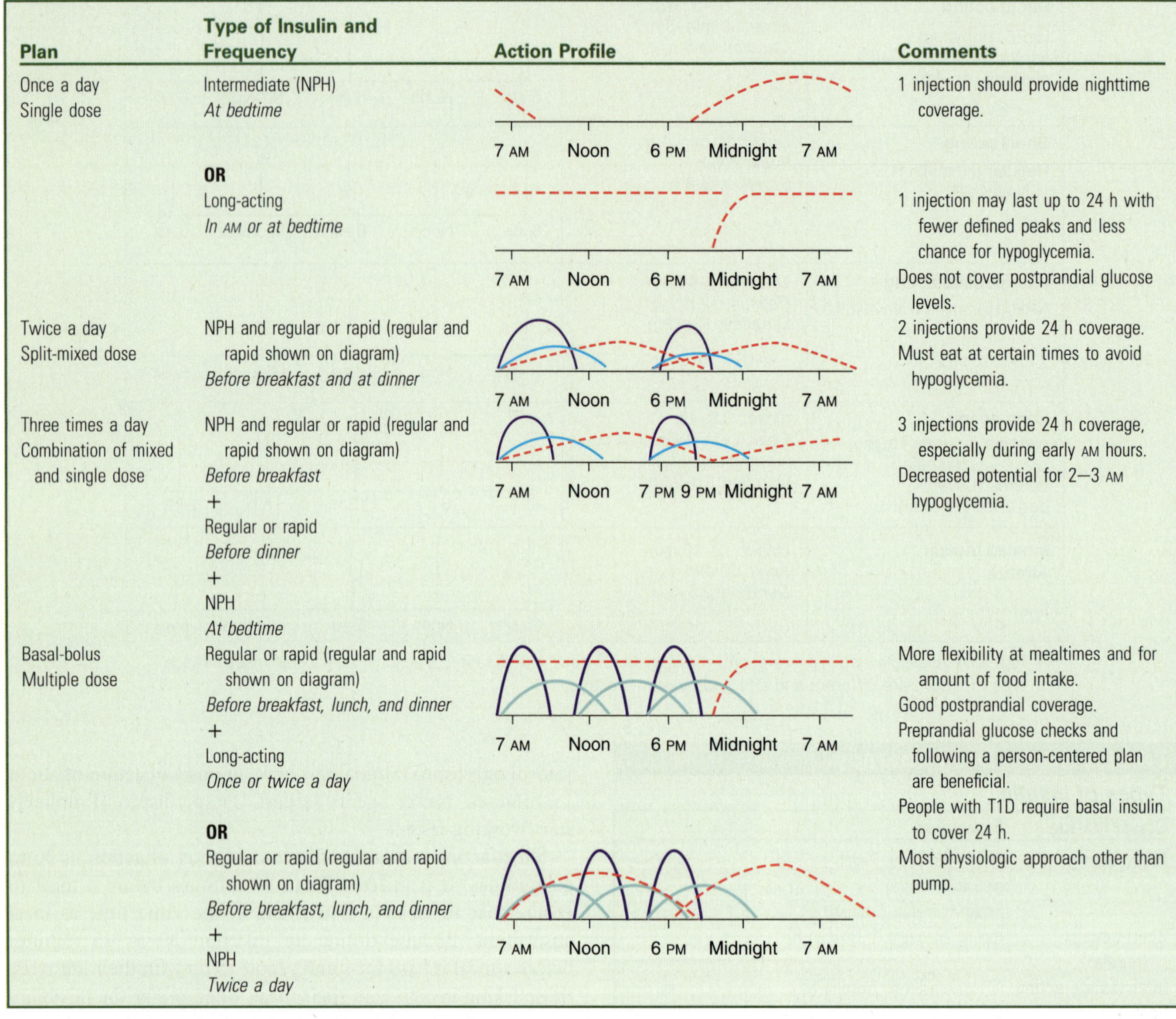

Plan	Type of Insulin and Frequency	Action Profile	Comments
Once a day Single dose	Intermediate (NPH) *At bedtime*	7 AM Noon 6 PM Midnight 7 AM	1 injection should provide nighttime coverage.
	OR Long-acting *In AM or at bedtime*	7 AM Noon 6 PM Midnight 7 AM	1 injection may last up to 24 h with fewer defined peaks and less chance for hypoglycemia. Does not cover postprandial glucose levels.
Twice a day Split-mixed dose	NPH and regular or rapid (regular and rapid shown on diagram) *Before breakfast and at dinner*	7 AM Noon 6 PM Midnight 7 AM	2 injections provide 24 h coverage. Must eat at certain times to avoid hypoglycemia.
Three times a day Combination of mixed and single dose	NPH and regular or rapid (regular and rapid shown on diagram) *Before breakfast* + Regular or rapid *Before dinner* + NPH *At bedtime*	7 AM Noon 7 PM 9 PM Midnight 7 AM	3 injections provide 24 h coverage, especially during early AM hours. Decreased potential for 2–3 AM hypoglycemia.
Basal-bolus Multiple dose	Regular or rapid (regular and rapid shown on diagram) *Before breakfast, lunch, and dinner* + Long-acting *Once or twice a day*	7 AM Noon 6 PM Midnight 7 AM	More flexibility at mealtimes and for amount of food intake. Good postprandial coverage. Preprandial glucose checks and following a person-centered plan are beneficial. People with T1D require basal insulin to cover 24 h. Most physiologic approach other than pump.
	OR Regular or rapid (regular and rapid shown on diagram) *Before breakfast, lunch, and dinner* + NPH *Twice a day*	7 AM Noon 6 PM Midnight 7 AM	

Rapid-acting (lispro, aspart, glulisine) insulin.
Short-acting (regular) insulin.
Intermediate-acting (NPH) or long-acting (glargine, detemir, degludec) insulin.

and detemir must not be diluted or mixed with any other insulin or solution in the same syringe.

Intermediate-acting insulin (NPH) can be used as basal insulin. It has a duration of 12 to 18 hours. The disadvantage of NPH is that its action peaks 4 to 12 hours after injection, which can result in hypoglycemia. NPH can be mixed with short- and rapid-acting insulins. It is never given IV.

CHECK YOUR PRACTICE

You are preparing a patient's NPH insulin injection. When you look at the vial, you notice that it is cloudy. You think that you should throw away the vial because it has become contaminated.

- Before you take this action, what should you do?

All insulins are clear solutions except NPH, lispro protamine, and aspart protamine. They are cloudy because they contain a protein called *protamine,* which makes them work longer. These insulins must be gently agitated before administration.

Combination insulin therapy. For those who want to use only 1 or 2 injections per day, a short- or rapid-acting insulin is mixed with intermediate-acting insulin in the same syringe. This allows the person to have mealtime and basal coverage without having to give 2 separate injections. Although this may be more appealing, most people achieve target glucose levels with basal-bolus therapy. Patients may mix the 2 types of insulin themselves or use a commercially premixed formula or pen (Table 53.4). Premixed formulas offer convenience, as people do not have to draw up and mix insulin from 2 different vials. This is helpful to those who lack the visual, manual, or cognitive skills to mix insulin themselves. However, it is harder to achieve target glucose levels because there is less opportunity for flexible dosing based on need.

Insulin Storage

As a protein, insulin has special storage considerations. Extreme temperatures alter insulin and can make it less effective. Insulin vials and pens in use may be left at room temperature for up to 4 weeks. The room temperature cannot be higher than 86°F (30°C) or below freezing (<32°F [0°C]). Teach patients to avoid exposing their insulin to direct sunlight. A person who is traveling in hot climates may store insulin in a thermos or cooler to keep it cool (not frozen). Store unopened insulin vials and pens in the refrigerator.

People who are traveling or caregivers of patients with impaired vision or who cannot fill their own syringes may prefill insulin syringes. Prefilled syringes with 2 different insulins are stable for up to 1 week when stored in the refrigerator. Syringes with only 1 type of insulin are stable for up to 30 days.

Teach patients to store syringes in a vertical position with the needle pointed up to avoid clumping of suspended insulin in the needle. Before injection, gently roll prefilled syringes between the palms 10 to 20 times to warm the insulin and resuspend the particles. Some insulin combinations cannot be prefilled and stored because the mixture can alter the onset, action, and/or peak times of either insulin. Consult a reference as needed when mixing and prefilling different types of insulin.

Insulin Administration

Routine doses of insulin are given by subcutaneous injection. Regular insulin can be given IV when immediate onset of action is desired. Insulin is not taken orally because it is inactivated by gastric fluids. Teach patients to avoid injecting insulin IM because rapid and unpredictable absorption could result in hypoglycemia.

The steps in giving a subcutaneous insulin injection are outlined in Table 53.6. Teach this technique to new insulin users and review it periodically with long-term users. Never assume that because a patient already uses insulin, they know and practice the correct insulin injection technique. They may not have understood prior instructions, or changes in eyesight may result in incorrect preparation. Patients may not see air bubbles in the syringe or may improperly read the scale on the syringe. Those receiving mixed insulins in the same syringe need to learn the right technique for combining them if they are not using commercially prepared premixed insulin.

The speed with which peak blood concentrations are reached varies with the injection site. The fastest subcutaneous absorption is from the abdomen, followed by the arm, thigh, and buttock. Although the abdomen is often the preferred injection site, other sites work well (Fig. 53.5). Caution patients about injecting into a site that will be exercised. For example, injecting into the thigh and then going jogging could increase body heat and circulation. This could increase the rate of insulin absorption and speed the onset of action, causing hypoglycemia.

TABLE 53.6 PATIENT & CAREGIVER TEACHING

Preparing an Insulin Injection

Include the following instructions when teaching patients and caregivers about insulin therapy:

1. Wash hands thoroughly.
2. Always inspect insulin bottle or pen before using it. Make sure that it is the right type and concentration, the expiration date has not passed, and the top of the bottle is in perfect condition. Insulin solutions (except for NPH, lispro protamine, and aspart protamine) should look clear and colorless. Discard if it appears discolored or you see particles in the solution.
3. For intermediate-acting insulin (which is normally cloudy), gently roll the insulin bottle between the palms of the hands to mix the insulin. Do not agitate clear insulin. Do not shake insulin to decrease air bubbles.
4. Choose the right injection site (Fig. 53.5).
5. Ensure that the site is clean and dry.
6. Push the needle straight into the skin (90-degree angle). If you are very thin, muscular, or using an 8- or 12-mm needle, you may need to pinch the skin and/or use a 45-degree angle. Most people benefit from a short or very short insulin needle. Pen needles need to be changed frequently to avoid insulin crystallizing and causing the pen to malfunction.
7. Push the plunger all the way down, leave needle in place for 5 sec to ensure that all insulin is injected, and then remove needle.
8. Destroy and dispose of single-use syringe safely.

Teach patients to rotate the injection within and between sites. This allows for better insulin absorption. It may be helpful to think of the abdomen as a checkerboard, with each ½-in square representing an injection site. Injections are rotated systematically across the board, with each injection site at least ½ to 1 inch away from the previous injection site. It can be helpful to inject fast-acting insulin into faster-absorbing sites and slow-acting insulin into slower absorbing sites.

In the United States most commercial insulin is available as U100. This means that 1 mL contains 100 U of insulin. U100 insulin must be used with a U100-marked syringe. Disposable plastic insulin syringes are available in a variety of sizes, including 1.0, 0.5, and 0.3 mL. The 0.5-mL size is for doses of 50 U or less. The 0.3-mL syringe is for doses of 30 U or less. The 0.5- and 0.3-mL syringes are in 1-unit increments. This provides more accurate delivery when the dose is an odd number. The 1.0-mL syringe is necessary for patients who inject more than 50 U of insulin. The 1.0-mL syringe is in 2-unit increments. When patients change from a 0.3- or a 0.5-mL to a 1.0-mL syringe, tell them of the dose increment difference.

Insulin syringe needles come in 3 lengths: 5 mm 3⁄16 in, 8 mm (5⁄16 in), and 12.7 mm (½ in).[10] Needle gauges vary among syringes. The needle gauges available are 28, 29, 30, and 31. The higher the gauge number, the smaller the diameter. This results in a more comfortable injection. Only the person using the syringe should recap the needle. Patients performing

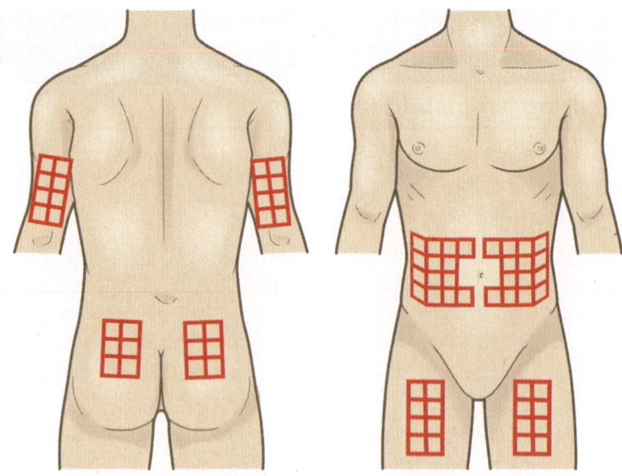

Fig. 53.5 Insulin injection sites.

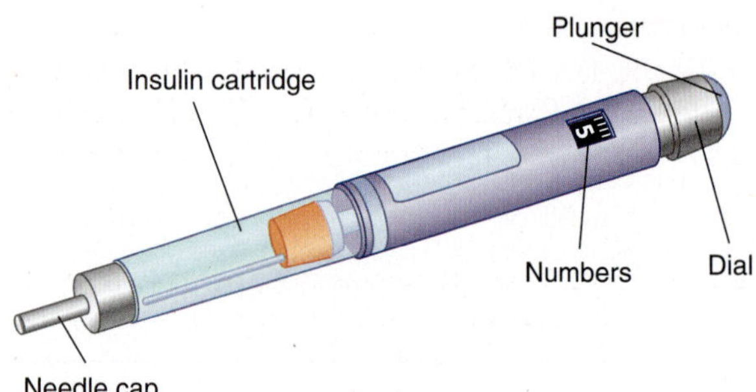

Fig. 53.6 Parts of insulin pen.

self-injection can prepare the site with routine hygiene, such as washing with soap and rinsing with water.

! SAFETY ALERT

- Never recap a needle used for a patient.
- When injecting a patient, prepare the site with alcohol to prevent health care–associated infection.

Insulin is typically injected at a 90-degree angle. For very thin or muscular patients in the hospital, perform injections at a 45-degree angle. At home, patients inject at a 90-degree angle using the shortest needle desired. We no longer pinch up the skin to avoid IM injection because of the use of short needles.

An insulin pen is a compact device loaded with an insulin cartridge that serves the same function as a needle and syringe (Fig. 53.6). Pen needles are available in lengths of 4 mm (5⁄32 in), 5 mm (3⁄16 in), 8 mm (5⁄16 in), and 12.7 mm (½ in) and in 3 gauges: 29, 31, and 32. Insulin pens offer convenience and flexibility. They provide consistent and accurate dosing. For patients with poor vision, the pen is a better option. They can hear the pen click as they dial the dose. Insulin pens come packaged with printed instructions, including pictures of the steps to take when using the pen. These instructions are helpful when teaching new pen users and reviewing technique with current users. Smart pens connect with a phone app that provides many reminders and helps people calculate doses.

Insulin pump. An *insulin pump* delivers a continuous subcutaneous insulin infusion through a small device worn on the belt, in a pocket, or under clothing.[11] Insulin pumps use rapid-acting insulin. Insulin is loaded into a reservoir or cartridge and connected via plastic tubing to a catheter inserted into the subcutaneous tissue. Insulet Corporation has an insulin pump that is a tubing-free system (Fig. 53.7). All insulin pumps are programmed to deliver a continuous infusion of rapid-acting insulin 24 hours a day, known as the *basal rate.* Pump users need different basal rates at different times of the day. Basal insulin can be temporarily increased or decreased based on carbohydrate intake, activity, or illness.

A major advantage of the insulin pump is the potential for keeping glucose levels in a tighter range with the goal of eliminating high and low glucose. With careful programming and constant monitoring, this is possible because insulin delivery is similar to the normal physiologic pattern. Insulin pump users check their glucose level at least 4 times per day and/or use a CGM system. Monitoring 8 times or more per day is common. This offers more flexibility with meals and activities. At mealtime, the person programs the pump to deliver a bolus infusion of insulin appropriate to the amount of carbohydrate ingested and an additional amount, if needed, to bring down, or "correct," high preprandial glucose.

Potential challenges of pump therapy include infection at the insertion site, an increased risk for DKA if the infusion is disrupted, the cost of the pump and supplies, and being attached to a device. Infusion sets are changed every 2 to 3 days and placed in a new site to avoid infection and promote good insulin absorption.

Hybrid closed-loop insulin pumps deliver insulin automatically by adjusting basal doses constantly throughout the day. The person must program bolus doses, which is why they are called "hybrid."

Problems With Insulin Therapy

Problems associated with insulin therapy include hypoglycemia, allergic reactions, lipodystrophy, and the Somogyi effect. Hypoglycemia is discussed later in this chapter.

Allergic reactions. Local inflammatory reactions to insulin may occur. These include itching, redness, and burning around the injection site. Local reactions may be self-limiting within 1 to 3 months or may improve with a low dose of antihistamine. A true insulin allergy is rare. It is manifested by a systemic response with urticaria and possibly anaphylactic shock. Preservatives in the insulin and the latex or rubber stoppers on the vials have caused allergic reactions.

Lipodystrophy. *Lipodystrophy* (changes in subcutaneous fatty tissue) may occur if the same injection sites are used frequently. *Atrophy,* which is uncommon, is the wasting of subcutaneous tissue. It presents as indentations in injection sites. *Hypertrophy* happens more often and is a thickening of the subcutaneous tissue. It eventually regresses if the person does not use the site for at least 6 months. Injecting into a hypertrophied site may cause erratic insulin absorption.

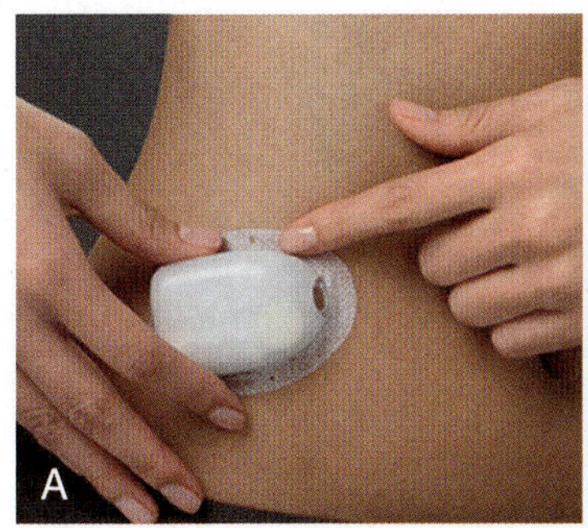
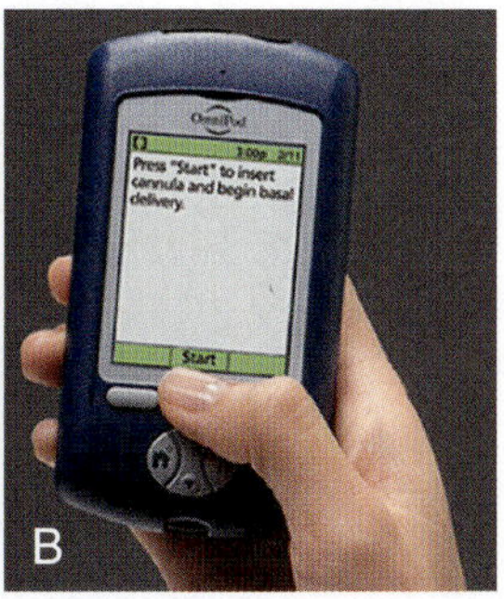

Fig. 53.7 (A) OmniPod Insulin Management System. The Pod holds and delivers insulin. (B) The Personal Diabetes Manager (PDM) wirelessly programs insulin delivery via the Pod. The PDM has a built-in glucose meter. (Courtesy Insulet Corporation.)

Somogyi effect and dawn phenomenon. Hyperglycemia in the morning may be caused by the **Somogyi effect.** A high dose of insulin causes a decline in glucose levels during the night. As a result, counterregulatory hormones (e.g., glucagon, epinephrine, GH, cortisol) are released. They stimulate lipolysis, gluconeogenesis, and glycogenolysis, which in turn cause rebound hyperglycemia. The danger of this effect is that when glucose levels are measured in the morning, hyperglycemia is present, and the patient or the HCP may increase the insulin dose. The patient may report headaches on awakening and recall having night sweats or nightmares.

The **dawn phenomenon** is also characterized by hyperglycemia that is present on awakening. Two counterregulatory hormones (GH and cortisol), which are excreted in increased amounts in the early morning hours, may be the cause. The dawn phenomenon affects many people with DM. It tends to be most severe when GH is at its peak in adolescence and young adulthood.

Careful assessment is needed to diagnose the Somogyi effect or dawn phenomenon because the treatment for each differs. The treatment for Somogyi effect is a bedtime snack, reducing the dose of insulin, or both. The treatment for dawn phenomenon is an increase in insulin or an adjustment in administration time. Your assessment must include insulin dose, injection sites, and variability in the time of meals or insulin administration.

Have patients measure bedtime, nighttime (between 2:00 and 4:00 AM), and morning fasting glucose levels on several occasions. If the glucose levels between 2:00 and 4:00 AM are less than 60 mg/dL (3.3 mmol/L) and signs and symptoms of hypoglycemia are present, it is the Somogyi effect. The insulin dose should be reduced. If the 2:00 to 4:00 AM glucose is high, suspect dawn phenomenon. The insulin dose should be increased. Discuss appropriate bedtime snacks.

Inhaled Insulin

Afrezza is a rapid-acting inhaled insulin. It is given at the beginning of each meal or within 20 minutes after starting a meal. Afrezza must be used in combination with long-acting insulin in those with T1D. It should not be used to treat DKA. People with chronic lung disease, such as asthma or chronic obstructive pulmonary disease (COPD), or who smoke should not use Afrezza because bronchospasm can occur. Other side effects include hypoglycemia, cough, and throat pain or irritation.

Oral and Noninsulin Injectable Agents

OAs and noninsulin injectable agents work to improve the mechanisms by which the body makes and uses insulin and glucose. These drugs primarily work on 3 defects of T2DM: (1) insulin resistance, (2) decreased insulin production, and (3) increased liver glucose production (Fig. 53.8). They may be used in combination with drugs from other classes or with insulin to achieve glucose goals. Table 53.7 lists OAs and noninsulin injectable agents. Table 53.8 lists combination OAs.

Biguanides

The most widely used OA is metformin. It is the only drug in the biguanide class available in the United States. Metformin is the most effective first-line treatment for T2DM. It is available as an immediate-release and an extended-release oral medication. The primary action of metformin is to reduce glucose production by the liver. It enhances insulin sensitivity at the tissue level and improves glucose transport into the cells. It has beneficial effects on lipid levels.

Because it may cause moderate weight loss, metformin may be useful for people with T2DM or prediabetes and overweight or obesity. It may prevent or delay T2DM in those with prediabetes who are younger than age 60 and have risk factors, such as hypertension or a history of gestational DM.

Patients who are having surgery or radiologic procedures that involve the use of a contrast medium need to temporarily discontinue metformin before surgery or the procedure. This reduces the risk of contrast-induced kidney injury (CIN) (see Chapter 49). They should not resume the metformin until 48 hours afterward once their creatinine has been checked and is normal.

DRUG ALERT

Metformin

- Do not use in patients with kidney disease, liver disease, or heart failure. Lactic acidosis is a rare complication of metformin accumulation.
- IV contrast media that contain iodine pose a risk for CIN, which could worsen metformin-induced lactic acidosis.
- To reduce risk for CIN, discontinue metformin 2 days before the procedure.
- May be resumed 48 hours after the procedure, assuming kidney function is normal.
- Do not use in people who drink excess amounts of alcohol.

Sulfonylureas

Sulfonylureas include glimepiride (Amaryl), glipizide (Glucotrol XL), and glyburide (DiaBeta, Glynase). Their primary action is to increase insulin production by the pancreas. This makes hypoglycemia the major side effect.

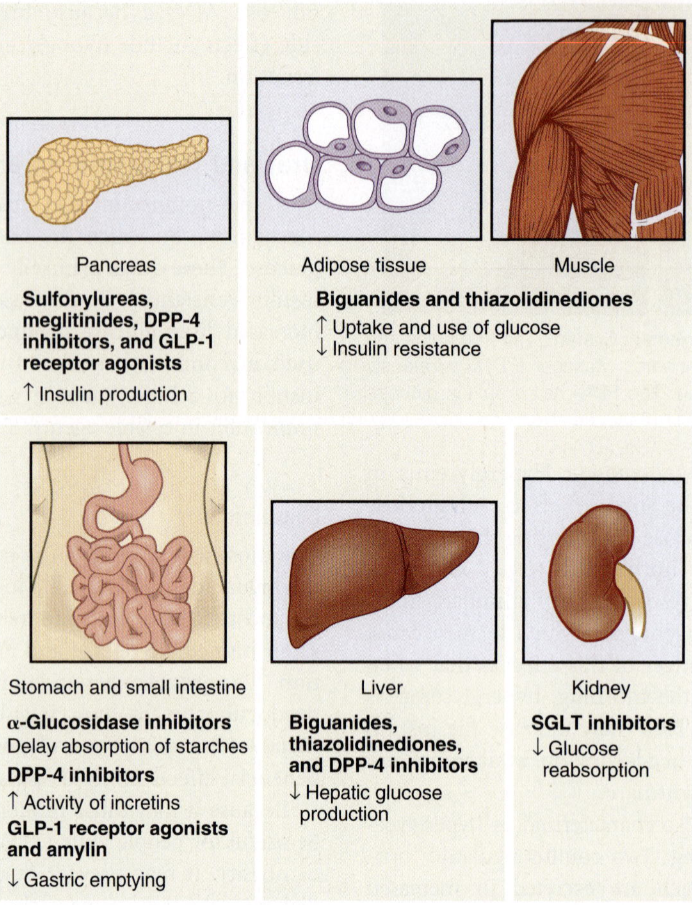

Fig. 53.8 Sites and mechanisms of action of T2DM drugs. *DDP-4,* Dipeptidyl peptidase; *GLP-1,* glucagon-like peptide-1; *SGLT,* sodium-glucose cotransporter.

Meglitinides

Meglitinides (nateglinide, repaglinide) increase insulin production by the pancreas. Because they are rapidly absorbed and eliminated, they are less likely to cause hypoglycemia. When taken just before meals, pancreatic insulin production increases during and after the meal, mimicking the normal response to eating.

α-Glucosidase Inhibitors

These drugs, also known as "starch blockers," work by slowing down carbohydrate absorption in the small intestine. Acarbose and miglitol (Glyset) are the available drugs in this class. They are most effective in lowering postprandial glucose. Their effectiveness is measured by checking 2-hour postprandial glucose levels.

Thiazolidinediones

Thiazolidinediones, sometimes called "insulin sensitizers," include pioglitazone (Actos) and rosiglitazone. They are most effective for people who have insulin resistance. These drugs improve insulin sensitivity, transport, and use at target tissues. Because they do not increase insulin production, they do not cause hypoglycemia. These drugs are rarely used because of their adverse effects. Rosiglitazone can cause cardiovascular events (e.g., myocardial infarction [MI]). It can be obtained only through restricted access programs.

Dipeptidyl Peptidase-4 Inhibitors

Normally, the intestines release incretin hormones throughout the day. When glucose levels are normal or high, incretins increase insulin synthesis and release from the pancreas and decrease liver glucose production. Incretin levels increase after a meal. The 2 main incretin hormones are gastric inhibitory peptide (GIP) and glucagon-like peptide-1 (GLP-1). They are quickly inactivated by the enzyme dipeptidyl peptidase-4 (DPP-4).

DPP-4 inhibitors (or *gliptins*) block the action of DPP-4, which inactivates incretin hormones. The result is an increase in insulin release, a decrease in glucagon secretion, and a decrease in liver glucose production. Because DPP-4 inhibitors are glucose dependent, they have a lower potential for hypoglycemia. Their main benefits over other drugs with similar effects are their pill forms and the absence of weight gain as a side effect.

TABLE 53.7 Drug Therapy

Oral Agents and Noninsulin Injectable Agents

Type	Mechanism of Action	Side Effects	Considerations
Oral Agents			
α-Glucosidase Inhibitors			
acarbose miglitol (Glyset)	Delays absorption of complex carbohydrates (starches) from GI tract.	Gas, abdominal pain, diarrhea	Take with the first bite of each main meal.
Biguanides			
metformin (Fortamet, Glumetza)	↓ Liver glucose production. ↑ Insulin sensitivity. Improves glucose uptake by tissues, especially muscles.	Diarrhea, lactic acidosis	Must be held 1–2 days before IV contrast media given and for 48 h after. Take with food to decrease GI side effects.
Dipeptidyl Peptidase-4 (DPP-4) Inhibitors			
alogliptin (Nesina) linagliptin (Tradjenta) saxagliptin sitagliptin (Januvia, Zituvio)	↑ Activity of incretins. ↑ Insulin release from pancreatic β-cells. ↓ Liver glucose production.	Pancreatitis, allergic reactions	Take with or without food.
Dopamine Receptor Agonists			
bromocriptine (Cycloset)	Activates dopamine receptors in central nervous system. Unknown how it improves glucose levels.	Orthostatic hypotension, nausea, headache, fatigue	Take with food at the same time each day. Change positions slowly.
Meglitinides			
nateglinide repaglinide	Stimulates a rapid and short-lived release of insulin from the pancreas.	Weight gain, hypoglycemia	Take any time from 30 min before each meal right up to the time of the meal. Should not be taken if a meal is skipped.
Sodium-Glucose Cotransporter 2 (SGLT2) Inhibitors			
bexagliflozin (Brenzavvy) canagliflozin (Invokana) dapagliflozin (Farxiga) empagliflozin (Jardiance) ertugliflozin (Steglatro) sotagliflozin (Inpefa)	↓ Renal glucose reabsorption. ↑ Urine glucose excretion.	Increased risk of genital and urinary tract infections. Hypoglycemia	Take in the morning before the first meal of the day. Drink 1–2 glasses of water each day above their normal intake.
Sulfonylureas			
glimepiride (Amaryl) glipizide glyburide (DiaBeta, Glynase)	↑ Insulin release from pancreatic islets. ↓ Glycogenolysis and gluconeogenesis. Enhances cellular sensitivity to insulin.	Weight gain, hypoglycemia	Take 30 min before meals. Avoid alcohol use.
Thiazolidinediones			
pioglitazone (Actos) rosiglitazone	↑ Glucose uptake in muscle. ↓ Endogenous glucose production.	Weight gain, edema *Pioglitazone:* ↑ Risk for bladder cancer, worsen heart failure *Rosiglitazone:* ↑ Risk for cardiovascular events (e.g., myocardial infarction, stroke)	Taken with or without food.
Noninsulin Injectable Agents			
Amylin Analogs			
pramlintide (Symlin)	Slows gastric emptying. ↓ Glucagon secretion and endogenous glucose output from liver. ↑ Satiety.	Hypoglycemia, nausea, vomiting, decreased appetite, headache	Inject subcutaneous into the thigh or abdomen before meals. Do not inject into the arm because absorption is too variable. Can give concurrently with insulin. Do not mix in syringe with insulin.
Glucagon-Like Peptide-1 (GLP-1) Receptor Agonists			
dulaglutide (Trulicity) exenatide (Byetta) exenatide extended release (Bydureon) liraglutide (Victoza) semaglutide (Ozempic) tirzepatide (Mounjaro, Zepbound)	↑ Insulin release. ↓ Glucagon secretion and slow gastric emptying. ↑ Satiety.	Nausea, vomiting, hypoglycemia, diarrhea, headache	Delayed gastric emptying may affect absorption of other oral drugs. Take fast-acting oral agents at least 1 h before injecting a GLP-1 agonist drug. May cause pancreatitis.

TABLE 53.8 Combination Oral GLAs

Components	Drug
Actoplus Met, Actoplus Met XR	Metformin and pioglitazone
Duetact	Pioglitazone and glimepiride
Glyxambi	Empagliflozin and linagliptin
Invokamet, Invokamet XR	Canagliflozin and metformin
Janumet, Janumet XR	Metformin and sitagliptin
Jentadueto, Jentadueto XR	Linagliptin and metformin
Kazano	Alogliptin and metformin
Kombiglyze	Saxagliptin and metformin
Oseni	Alogliptin and pioglitazone
Qtern	Dapagliflozin and saxagliptin
Qternmet XR	Dapagliflozin, saxagliptin, and metformin XR
Segluromet	Metformin and ertugliflozin
Steglujan	Sitagliptin and ertugliflozin
Synjardy, Synjardy XR	Metformin and empagliflozin
Trijardy	Empagliflozin, linagliptin, and metformin XR
Xigduo	Dapagliflozin and metformin

Glucagon-Like Peptide-1 Receptor Agonists

GLP-1 receptor agonists stimulate GLP-1, an incretin hormone that is decreased in people with T2DM. These drugs increase insulin synthesis and release from the pancreas, inhibit glucagon secretion, slow gastric emptying, and reduce food intake by increasing satiety. They may be used alone or with another T2DM treatment when OAs have not achieved optimal glucose levels.

Except for the oral form of semaglutide, all are given using a subcutaneous injection. Exenatide is given twice daily. Liraglutide is given once daily. Dulaglutide, exenatide extended release, and tirzepatide are given weekly.

DRUG ALERT

GLP-1 Receptor Agonists

- Do not use in patients with a personal or family history of medullary thyroid cancer.
- Acute pancreatitis may occur.

Sodium-Glucose Cotransporter 2 Inhibitors

Sodium-glucose cotransporter 2 (SGLT2) is responsible for the kidneys reabsorbing about 90% of glucose back into the bloodstream. SGLT2 inhibitors work by blocking glucose reabsorption, thus increasing urine glucose excretion. Drugs in this class include canagliflozin, dapagliflozin, and empagliflozin.

Dopamine Receptor Agonist

Bromocriptine is a dopamine receptor agonist that improves glucose levels. The mechanism of action is unknown. We think people with T2DM have low dopamine levels in the morning. These low dopamine levels may interfere with the body's ability to control glucose. Bromocriptine increases dopamine receptor activity. It can be used alone or with another T2DM treatment.

Amylin Analogs

Pramlintide is the only amylin analog. Amylin is a hormone secreted by the pancreatic β cells in response to food intake. It slows gastric emptying, reduces glucagon secretion, and increases satiety. People with high glucose levels on insulin therapy take pramlintide with their mealtime insulin.

Concurrent use of pramlintide and insulin increases the risk for severe hypoglycemia during the 3 hours after injection, especially in those with T1D. Teach patients to eat a meal with at least 250 calories and fast-acting glucose on hand in case hypoglycemia develops. When using pramlintide, the bolus insulin dose should be reduced.

NUTRITION THERAPY

Nutrition therapy is a cornerstone of care for people with DM and prediabetes. Achieving nutrition goals requires a coordinated team effort that considers the person's behavior, cognitive, socioeconomic, cultural, and religious backgrounds and preferences. Changing eating habits can be challenging for many people.[12] Because of these complexities, a dietitian with expertise in DM management should work with the person with DM. The dietitian starts with a nutrition assessment and develops a person-centered food plan. Other team members may include nurses, certified diabetes care and education specialists (CDCESs), clinical nurse specialists, social workers, and other HCPs. Monitoring glucose levels, A1C, lipids, and BP gives feedback on how well the goals of nutrition management are being met.

ADA guidelines state that, within the context of an overall healthy eating plan, a person with DM can eat the same foods as a person without DM. This means that the same principles of healthy nutrition that apply to the general population apply to the person with DM. Table 53.9 describes nutrition guidelines for people with DM. The overall goal of nutrition therapy is to help people with DM make healthy food choices that will lead to achieving and/or maintaining safe and healthy glucose levels. Additional goals include:

- Maintain glucose levels as close to normal as safely possible to prevent or reduce the risk for DM complications.
- Achieve lipid profiles and BP levels that reduce the risk for CVD.
- Prevent or slow the development of chronic complications by modifying diet and lifestyle.
- Maintain the pleasure of eating by encouraging a variety of healthy food choices.

Type 1 Diabetes

People with T1D base their meal planning on usual food intake and preferences balanced with insulin and exercise patterns.[13] Patients coordinate insulin dosing with eating habits and

TABLE 53.9 NUTRITION THERAPY

DM

Component	Recommendations
Meal plan in general	• A personal meal plan should address nutrient quality, calories, and metabolic goals
Carbohydrate	• Carbohydrates should come from nutrient-rich sources, such as vegetables (especially non-starchy), whole grains, fruits, legumes, and dairy products • Monitor intake by counting carbohydrates, using exchange lists, or using proportion sizes • Limit processed foods with added fat, sugar, and sodium • Fiber intake at least 14 g/1000 kcal/day • Replace sugar-sweetened beverages with water
Salt	• Aim for no more than 2300 mg of sodium per day
Fat	• Eat heart-healthy fish at least twice a week; avoid fried fish • Consume fats from plant products • Limit intake of saturated fat and trans fat
Alcohol	• Limit to moderate amount (1 drink per day for females, 2 drinks per day for males) • Consume alcohol with food to reduce risk for hypoglycemia in those using insulin or drugs that promote insulin secretion • Some effects of alcohol (e.g., drowsiness) resemble hypoglycemia, so it can be difficult to recognize a true diabetic emergency

activity in mind. Day-to-day consistency in timing and amount of food eaten makes it much easier to manage glucose levels, especially for those using conventional, fixed insulin plans. Those using rapid-acting insulin can adjust the dose before each meal based on the current glucose level and the carbohydrate content of the meal. Intensified insulin therapy, such as multiple daily injections or the use of an insulin pump, allows considerable flexibility in food selection and can be adjusted for changes from usual eating and exercise habits. This does not diminish or replace the need for healthy food choices and a well-balanced diet.

Type 2 Diabetes

Nutrition therapy in T2DM emphasizes achieving glucose, lipid, and BP goals. Modest weight loss may improve insulin sensitivity. Therefore weight loss is recommended for all persons with DM who are overweight or obese. A weight loss of 5% to 7% of body weight often improves glucose levels, even if desirable weight is not achieved.

There is no one proven strategy for weight loss. Weight loss is best achieved by a moderate decrease in calories and regular exercise. A nutritionally adequate meal plan with appropriate serving sizes, a reduction of saturated and *trans* fats, and lower carbohydrates can decrease calorie consumption. Spacing meals is another strategy that spreads nutrient intake throughout the day.

Food Composition

A healthy balance of nutrients is essential to maintain glucose levels and overall health. Energy from food intake can be balanced with energy output. Teach patients to outline their meal plan with their lifestyle and health goals in mind. There is no special eating plan for people with DM. The person can work with their HCP to determine which plan works best for them, keeping in mind portions and effects on glucose, lipids, and BP.

The ADA recommends individualizing protein and carbohydrate intake. Carbohydrates are an important source of energy, fiber, vitamins, and minerals. They are needed by all people, including those with DM. Lean meats and foods containing carbohydrates from whole grains, fruits, vegetables, and low-fat dairy are part of a healthy meal plan. The amount of daily protein for people with DM and normal kidney function is the same as the general population. People with DM should consume a minimum of 14 g of diet fiber per 1000 kcal. At least half of the grain intake should come from whole intact grains.

Nutritive and nonnutritive sweeteners may be included in a healthy meal plan in moderation. Nonnutritive sweeteners include the sugar substitutes saccharine, aspartame, sucralose, stevia, neotame, and acesulfame-K.

Fat provides energy, transports fat-soluble vitamins, and provides essential fatty acids. The ADA recommends 20% to 35% of total calorie intake from fat. People with DM benefit from eating fewer combination foods that contain carbohydrates and high total fat. Healthy fats are those that come from plants, such as olives, nuts, and avocados.

Alcohol

Alcohol inhibits gluconeogenesis by the liver. This can cause severe hypoglycemia in people who take insulin or OAs that increase insulin secretion. Alcohol use can make DM harder to manage. Create a trusting environment in which patients feel comfortable talking openly about their alcohol use.

Moderate alcohol use can be safely included in the meal plan if the person monitors glucose levels and is not at risk for other alcohol-related problems. Moderate use is defined as 1 drink per day for females and 2 drinks per day for males. A person can reduce the risk for alcohol-induced hypoglycemia by eating carbohydrates when drinking alcohol. Mixed drinks often contain sweetened mixers and can increase glucose levels. To decrease the carbohydrate content, recommend using sugar-free mixes and drinking dry, light wines.

Patient Teaching Related to Nutrition Therapy

Most often, the dietitian initially teaches the principles of nutrition management. Whenever possible, work with dietitians as part of the DM care team. Some patients who have limited insurance coverage or live in remote areas do not have access to a dietitian. In these cases, you may need to assume responsibility for teaching basic nutrition principles to patients with DM.

Whenever possible, include family members and caregivers in nutrition education and counseling, especially the person who cooks for the household. However, the responsibility for maintaining a healthy eating plan still belongs to the person with DM. Reliance on someone else to make health decisions interferes with the person's ability to develop self-care skills, which are essential in managing DM.

Discuss traditional and favorite foods with patients. Explore the influences of culture on food choices and meal planning with that person. Individualize food choices considering patient preferences. Ask about cultural food preferences. Access nutrition resources designed for members of different cultural groups from the ADA.

Carbohydrate counting is a meal planning technique used to keep track of the amount of carbohydrate eaten at each meal and per day. Teach patients to keep carbohydrate intake within a healthy range. The amount of total carbohydrate per day depends on glucose levels, age, weight, activity level, patient preference, and drug therapy. A serving size of carbohydrate is 15 g. A typical adult might start with 45 to 60 g of carbohydrate per meal. Some people tailor insulin doses to the amount of carbohydrate foods that they will consume at the meal, with a set number of units of insulin given per gram of carbohydrate (e.g., 1 U/15 g carbohydrate, 2 U/25 g carbohydrate). Teach patients about foods that contain carbohydrates, how to read food labels, and appropriate serving sizes.

Diabetes exchange lists are another method for meal planning. The person selects a specific number of servings from a list of exchanges for each meal and snack. The exchanges are starches, fruits, milk, meats, vegetables, fats, and free foods. The person chooses foods from the various exchanges based on the prescribed meal plan. This method may be easier for some people than carbohydrate counting. Another advantage is that this approach helps the person limit portion sizes and overall food intake, an important part of weight management.

EXERCISE

Regular, consistent exercise is an essential part of DM and prediabetes management (Table 53.10). Exercise decreases insulin resistance and can have a direct effect on lowering glucose levels. It contributes to weight loss, which further decreases insulin resistance. The therapeutic benefits of regular activity may result in a decreased need for GLAs to reach target glucose goals in people with T2DM. Regular exercise may help reduce triglyceride and low-density lipoprotein (LDL) cholesterol levels, increase HDL, reduce BP, and improve circulation.

The ADA recommends that people with DM engage in at least 150 minutes/week (30 minutes, 5 days/week) of a moderate-intensity aerobic activity. They encourage people with DM to perform resistance training 2 to 3 times a week unless contraindicated. Teach patients how to work exercise safely into their day. Encourage them to be active every day. Medical clearance may be needed for new, intensive exercise programs. Teach patients to start slowly and gradually progress toward the desired goal. Encourage them to interrupt prolonged sitting with activity every 30 minutes. Patients who use insulin, sulfonylureas, or meglitinides are at increased risk for hypoglycemia when they increase physical activity, especially if they exercise at the time of peak drug action or eat too little to maintain adequate glucose levels. This can also occur if normally sedentary patients with DM have an unusually active day.

The glucose-lowering effects of exercise can last up to 48 hours after the activity, so it is possible for hypoglycemia to occur long after the activity. People who use drugs that can cause hypoglycemia should exercise about 1 hour after a meal or have a 10- to 15-g carbohydrate snack and check their glucose before exercising. It is preferable not to increase caloric intake for exercise. If needed, they can eat small carbohydrate snacks every 30 minutes during exercise to prevent hypoglycemia. Patients using drugs that place them at risk for hypoglycemia should always carry a fast-acting source of carbohydrate, such as glucose tablets or hard candies, when exercising. If they have frequent lows from exercise, the dose may need to be lowered.

The body can perceive strenuous activity as stress, causing a release of counterregulatory hormones and a temporary increase in glucose. In a person with T1D who has hyperglycemia

TABLE 53.10 PATIENT & CAREGIVER TEACHING

Exercise for Patients With DM

Include the following information in the exercise teaching plan for patients and caregivers:

1. Exercise does not have to be vigorous to be effective. The glucose-reducing effects of exercise can be reached with activities such as brisk walking.
2. Choose activities that are enjoyable to foster regularity.
3. Use properly fitting footwear to avoid rubbing or injury.
4. The exercise session includes a warm-up period and a cool-down period. Start the exercise program gradually and increase slowly.
5. Exercise is best done after meals when the glucose level is rising.
6. Exercise plans are patient-specific and monitored by the HCP.
7. Monitor glucose levels before, during, and after exercise to determine the effect exercise has on glucose levels at specific times of the day.
8. Before exercise, if glucose $\leq$100 mg/dL, eat a 15-g carbohydrate snack. After 15–30 min, recheck glucose levels. Delay exercise if $<$100 mg/dL. Talk to HCP about lowering drug dose(s) if hypoglycemia occurs consistently.
9. Before exercise, if glucose $\geq$250 mg/dL in a person with T1D and ketones are present, delay vigorous activity until ketones are gone. Drink fluids.
10. Exercise-induced hypoglycemia may occur several hours after completing exercise.
11. With extensive planned or spontaneous activity, monitor glucose levels and adjust the insulin dose (if taken) and food intake.

and ketones, exercise can worsen these conditions. Teach patients to delay activity if the glucose level is over 250 mg/dL *and* ketones are present in the urine. If hyperglycemia is present without ketosis, it is not necessary to postpone exercise.

GLUCOSE MONITORING

Glucose monitoring is an essential part of DM management. It provides patients with a tool for achieving and maintaining glycemic goals. With current glucose readings, people make decisions about food intake, activity patterns, and drug dosages. They can see daily glucose fluctuations and trends and monitor for changes in glucose related to drugs, food, and exercise. They are alerted to acute episodes of hyperglycemia and hypoglycemia. It is recommended for all people who use insulin to manage their DM.

Many people use portable meters to perform blood glucose monitoring (BGM). A wide variety of meters are available (Fig. 53.9). Disposable lancets are used to get a small drop of capillary blood (usually from a finger stick) that is placed in a reagent strip. After a specified time, the meter displays a reading of the capillary glucose value. Technology is rapidly changing. More convenient systems are introduced on an ongoing basis.

Monitoring frequency depends on several factors: glycemic goals, type of DM, drug plan, patients' ability to check glucose independently, access to supplies and equipment, and patients' willingness and ability to do so. The recommendation for people who use multiple insulin injections or insulin pumps is to monitor their glucose 4 to 8 times each day (upon waking, before and after meals, when feeling symptoms of hypoglycemia, and before and during exercise). Those using less frequent insulin injections, noninsulin therapy, or nutrition management may monitor as often as needed to achieve their glycemic goals.

CGM systems are another route for monitoring glucose (Fig. 53.10).[14] Using a sensor inserted subcutaneously, the CGM systems display new glucose values every 1 to 5 minutes. CGM assesses interstitial glucose, which lags behind blood glucose by 5 to 10 minutes. The person inserts the sensor using an automatic insertion device. Data are sent from the sensor to a transmitter, which displays the glucose value on an insulin pump, a pager-like receiver, or a smartphone. The CGM can be used with or without an insulin pump. CGMs can also "share" data with friends and family via smartphone. Insurance coverage and cost are the most common limiting factors.

CGMs help patients and HCPs identify trends and patterns in glucose levels. The goal is to increase "time in range" (70 to 180 mg/dL) and have fewer highs and lows. They alert the person to episodes of hypoglycemia and hyperglycemia. This allows them to take corrective action quickly.

Glucose meters are reliable when used consistently and correctly. It is not necessary to compare their readings with laboratory readings. If the A1C result does not correspond to the glucose readings on the home meter, troubleshoot any problems with the meter, technique, strips, and hand washing.

Because errors in technique can cause errors in management strategies, patient teaching is essential. Follow the initial instruction with regular reassessment. Review the instructions that come with each product. If a product has a control solution, teach patients to use and interpret control solutions. A control should be done when first using a meter or when there is a reason to believe that the readings are not correct. Table 53.11 lists the steps to include when teaching patients how to perform glucose monitoring.

People with T1D often check their glucose before meals. This is because many people use insulin pumps or multiple daily injections and base the insulin dose on the amount of carbohydrate in a meal or the preprandial glucose value. Checking glucose 2 hours after the first bite of food helps a person determine whether the bolus insulin dose was adequate for that meal.

Teach patients to check glucose whenever they suspect hypoglycemia and then take immediate action. During times of illness, check glucose levels at 4-hour intervals (or more often) to determine the effects of the illness on glucose levels. Teach patients to check glucose before and after exercise to determine the effects of exercise on glucose levels. This is especially important for the person with T1D.

Patients with impaired vision, cognitive impairment, or limited dexterity need careful assessment to see if they can monitor glucose independently. We may need to identify caregivers who can assume this responsibility. Adaptive devices are available to help patients with certain limitations. These

Fig. 53.9 Blood glucose meters are used to measure glucose levels. (© iStock.com/kolesnikovserg.)

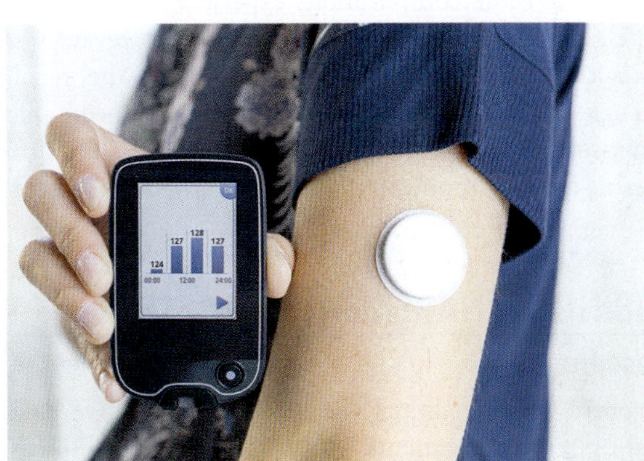

Fig. 53.10 Continuous glucose meter showing a reading after scanning the sensor of the glucose monitoring system placed on the arm. (©Click_and_Photo/iStock.com.)

TABLE 53.11 PATIENT & CAREGIVER TEACHING

Blood Glucose Monitoring (BGM)

Include the following instructions when teaching patients and caregivers about BGM:

1. Wash and dry hands completely. It is not necessary to clean the site with alcohol, and it may interfere with results.
2. If it is hard to get an adequate drop of blood for monitoring, warm the hands in warm water or let the arms hang dependently for a few minutes before making the finger puncture.
3. A lancing device is often used. Place the lancet in the device, following the instructions that come with it. If the puncture is made on the finger, use the side of the finger pad rather than near the center. There are fewer nerve endings along the side of the finger pad.
4. Set the lancing device to make a puncture just deep enough to get a sufficiently large drop of blood. Unnecessarily deep punctures may cause pain and bruising. Current meters need very small amounts of blood.
5. Follow instructions on meter for checking the glucose level.
6. Record results. Compare with personal glucose goals.

include talking monitors and other equipment for the visually impaired.

PANCREAS TRANSPLANT

Pancreas transplant is an option for select persons with T1D. Candidates include patients who have end-stage renal disease (ESRD) and have had or plan to have a kidney transplant. Kidney and pancreas transplants are often done together, or a pancreas may be transplanted after a kidney transplant. If renal failure is not present, the ADA recommends that a pancreas transplant be considered only for people who meet 3 criteria: (1) a history of frequent, acute, and severe metabolic complications (e.g., hypoglycemia, hyperglycemia, DKA) requiring medical attention; (2) clinical and emotional problems with the use of insulin therapy that are so severe as to be incapacitating; and (3) consistent failure of insulin-based management to prevent acute complications.

A successful transplant can improve quality of life by eliminating the need for insulin therapy and glucose monitoring. It can eliminate acute complications experienced by people with T1D (e.g., hypoglycemia, hyperglycemia). However, a transplant is only partially successful in reversing the renal and neurologic complications of DM. Patients need lifelong immunosuppression to prevent organ rejection. Complications can result from immunosuppressive therapy (see Chapter 14).

NURSING MANAGEMENT: DIABETES

Assessment

Table 53.12 provides initial subjective and objective data you should obtain from patients with DM. After the initial assessment, perform periodic assessments on a regular basis.

Clinical Problems

Clinical problems for patients with DM may include:

- Altered glucose level
- Deficient knowledge
- Risk for injury
- Impaired endocrine function
- Neurologic problem

Additional information on clinical problems and interventions for patients with DM is presented in eNursing Care Plan 53.1, available on the website.

Planning

The overall goals are patients with DM will (1) engage in self-care behaviors to actively manage DM, (2) have few or no hyperglycemia or hypoglycemia emergencies, (3) maintain safe and healthy glucose levels, (4) reduce the risk for chronic complications, and (5) adjust health behaviors to accommodate the DM plan with minimal stress. The goal is for patients with DM to safely and effectively fit DM into life rather than living life around DM.

Implementation

Health Promotion

Your role in health promotion is to identify, monitor, and teach people at risk for DM. Obesity is a key risk factor. The ADA recommends routine screening for T2DM for all adults who are overweight or obese (BMI 25 kg/m^2 or greater) or have 1 or more risk factors. A risk test is available at www.diabetes.org/risk-test. The risk test determines whether the person is at risk for prediabetes or DM based on the number of risk factors present. For those who do not have risk factors for DM, begin screening at age 35. Table 53.13 provides criteria to screen for prediabetes and DM. If results are normal, repeat screening at 3-year intervals.

Primary prevention is a cost-effective approach (Box 53.2). Current recommendations for primary prevention include health behavior modifications for at-risk people. A modest weight loss of 5% to 7% of body weight and 150 minutes of physical activity a week lower the risk for developing T2DM by 34% to 58%.

Acute Care

Acute situations involving patients with DM include hypoglycemia, DKA, and hyperosmolar hyperglycemic syndrome (HHS). Management for these situations is discussed in more detail later in this chapter. A key nursing responsibility is managing patients when they are undergoing surgery or are acutely ill with another health problem (Table 53.14).

Acute illness, injury, stress, and surgery may evoke a counterregulatory hormone response, causing hyperglycemia. Even common illnesses, such as an upper respiratory tract infection or the flu, can cause this response. Patients may require more intense treatment, such as extra insulin and more frequent

TABLE 53.12 NURSING ASSESSMENT

DM

Subjective Data

Important Health Information

Health history: Mumps, rubella, coxsackievirus, or other viral infections. Recent trauma, infection, or stress. Pregnancy, gave birth to infant >9 lb. Pancreatitis, Cushing syndrome, acromegaly, family history of T1D or T2DM.

Medications: Use of glucose-lowering agents, corticosteroids, diuretics, phenytoin.

Surgery or other treatments: Any recent surgery.

Functional Health Patterns

Health perception—health management: Positive family history, malaise.

Nutrition-metabolic: Obesity, weight loss (type 1), weight gain (type 2). Thirst, hunger, nausea, and vomiting. Poor healing (especially involving the feet), eating habits.

Elimination: Constipation or diarrhea, frequent urination, frequent bladder infections, nocturia, urinary incontinence.

Activity-exercise: Muscle weakness, fatigue.

Cognitive-perceptual: Abdominal pain, headache, blurred vision, numbness or tingling of extremities, pruritus.

Sexuality-reproductive: Erectile dysfunction, frequent vaginal infections, vaginal dryness, or pain, ↓ libido.

Adaptation: Depression, irritability, apathy.

Value-belief: Health beliefs, commitment to lifestyle changes involving food, medication, and activity patterns.

Objective Data

Cardiovascular

Hypotension.[a] Weak, rapid pulse.[a]

Eyes

Soft, sunken eyeballs.[a] History of vitreal hemorrhages, cataracts.

GI

Dry mouth, vomiting.[a] Fruity breath.[a]

Musculoskeletal

Muscle wasting.[a]

Neurologic.

Altered reflexes, restlessness, confusion, stupor, coma.[a]

Respiratory

Rapid, deep respirations (Kussmaul respirations).[a]

Skin

Dry, warm, inelastic skin. Pigmented lesions (on legs), ulcers (especially on feet), loss of hair on toes, acanthosis nigricans.

Possible Findings

Abnormal electrolytes. Fasting glucose level ≥126 mg/dL. OGTT >200 mg/dL, random glucose ≥200 mg/dL. Leukocytosis. ↑ BUN, creatinine, triglycerides, cholesterol, LDL, VLDL. ↓ HDL. A1C >6.0% (A1C >7.0% in those with diagnosed DM), glycosuria, ketonuria, albuminuria. Acidosis.

[a]Indicates manifestations of DKA.

HDL, High-density lipoprotein; *LDL,* low-density lipoprotein; *OGTT,* oral glucose tolerance test; *VLDL,* very low-density lipoprotein.

TABLE 53.13 Screening for DM in Asymptomatic, Undiagnosed Persons

Who to Screen

1. Consider screening adults with overweight or obesity (BMI ≥25 kg/m^2 or ≥23 kg/m^2 in Asian persons) who have 1 or more risk factors:
   - First-degree relative with DM
   - High-risk race and ethnicity (e.g., African American, Latino, Native American, Asian American)
   - Cardiovascular disease
   - Hypertension (≥130/80 mm Hg or on therapy for hypertension)
   - HDL cholesterol level <35 mg/dL (<0.9 mmol/L) and/or a triglyceride level >250 mg/dL (>2.8 mmol/L)
   - Polycystic ovary syndrome
   - Physical inactivity
2. People with prediabetes (A1C ≥5.7% [≥39 mmol/mol], impaired glucose tolerance, impaired fasting glucose) should be screened yearly.
3. Females who had gestational diabetes should have lifelong screening at least every 3 years.
4. For people without risk factors, screening should begin at age 35 years.

Screening Tests

To screen for DM or to assess risk of future DM, A1C, fasting plasma glucose (FPG), or 2-h OGTT is appropriate (Table 53.2).

If results are normal, repeat screening at least every 3 years, with more frequent screening depending on initial results and risk status.

HDL, High-density lipoprotein.

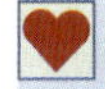

BOX 53.2 PROMOTING POPULATION HEALTH

Preventing DM

- Be physically active with 150 min of moderate activity each week.
- Maintain a healthy weight.
- Eat a balanced, nutritional diet. Limit the intake of processed foods. Choose healthy fats and increase the intake of whole grains, fruits, and vegetables.
- Follow DM screening recommendations.
- Avoid cigarette smoking and tobacco products.
- Limit alcohol use to moderate levels.
- Follow the prescribed treatment plan for hypertension.

glucose monitoring, to maintain glycemic goals and avoid hyperglycemia.

Patients with T1D may need an increase in insulin to prevent DKA. High glucose levels can lead to poor healing and infection. Patients with T2DM may need insulin therapy to prevent or treat hyperglycemia symptoms and avoid an acute hyperglycemia emergency. In critically ill patients, insulin therapy may be started if the glucose is persistently greater than 180 mg/dL. These patients have a higher target glucose level, which is usually 140 to 180 mg/dL.

TABLE 53.14 NURSING MANAGEMENT

Caring for Patients With DM and Acute Health Problems

- Implement measures to avoid hypoglycemia or hyperglycemia:
- Perform glucose monitoring before meals for patients who are eating and every 4–6 hours for patients who are not eating.
- Time administration of GLAs to patient condition and meals.
- Determine acid-base status by evaluating arterial blood gases (ABGs) and trends in pH, $Paco_2$, and HCO_3^-.
- Review laboratory results to evaluate glucose levels, electrolyte values, and kidney function.
- Assess for acute complications and implement actions for hypoglycemia, DKA, and HHS if they occur.
- Provide a safe environment for the patient with neuromuscular manifestations by initiating fall and seizure precautions.
- Give prescribed IV fluids and encourage appropriate oral fluid intake.
- Provide education to patients and caregivers about DM management, including glucose monitoring, drug therapy, nutrition, activity, and preventing and managing acute and chronic complications.

Collaborate With Other Team Members

Dietitian

- Determine needed diet.
- Work with patients and caregivers to create a person-centered meal plan.
- Provide meal plan instructions as needed.

Physical Therapist

- Assess current fitness level.
- Develop an activity plan with the patient.

Occupational Therapist

- Teach patients with impaired vision how to use devices to draw up and measure insulin.
- Provide teaching on how to use adaptive glucose meters.
- Develop protective techniques for activities that involve exposure to heat, cold, and sharp objects.

Social Worker

- Aid patients in finding resources to meet health and financial needs.
- Help with coping with DM, including managing problems within the family or workplace.

During the intraoperative period, we often adjust the DM plan to ensure safe and healthy glucose levels. We administer IV fluids and insulin (if needed) just before, during, and after surgery when there is no oral intake. Explain to patients with T2DM who have been taking OAs that this is a temporary measure, not a sign of worsening DM.

When caring for unconscious surgical patients receiving insulin, be alert for signs of hypoglycemia, such as sweating, tachycardia, and tremors. Frequent glucose monitoring can prevent episodes of hypoglycemia.

If patients are outside of the acute care setting, encourage them to check their glucose at least every 4 hours. Teach patients with T1D and glucose greater than 240 mg/dL (13.3 mmol/L) to check urine for ketones every 3 to 4 hours. They should contact the HCP when glucose levels are over 300 mg/dL twice in a row or urine ketone levels are moderate to high.

Food intake is important during times of stress and illness when the body needs extra energy. If patients can eat normally, they can continue with their regular meal plan while increasing the intake of noncaloric fluids, such as water, sugar-free gelatin, and other decaffeinated beverages, and continue taking GLAs as prescribed. When illness causes patients to eat less than normal, they can continue to take GLAs while supplementing food intake with carbohydrate-containing fluids. Examples include low-sodium soups, juices, and regular, sugar-sweetened decaffeinated soft drinks. Teach patients to contact an HCP if they are unable to keep down food or fluid.

Chronic Care

Effective DM management involves ongoing interaction among patients, caregivers, and the health care team. Because DM is a complex chronic disease, a great deal of patient contact takes place in outpatient and home settings. The major goal of patient care in these settings is to enable patients (with the help of a caregiver as needed) to reach an optimal level of independence in self-management. You play a vital role in promoting DM self-management through providing comprehensive patient and caregiver education (Table 53.15). Patients who actively manage their DM care have better outcomes. Advocate for an education approach that facilitates informed decision-making (Box 53.3).

Having DM affects each person in many ways. DM self-management is demanding. It requires making daily decisions about foods to eat, glucose monitoring, medication, and activities. The requirements of scheduled meals, glucose monitoring, and taking GLAs may interfere with patients' other responsibilities. Any change in the daily routine can be hard. Consider patients' financial and social situation and the effect of multiple drugs, eating habits, and quality-of-life issues.

Assess the patient's knowledge of DM and health behaviors when planning teaching. What does it mean to the person to have DM? Assess knowledge frequently so that you can help with gaps in knowledge or correct misinformation. Many people face challenges that can affect self-management. DM increases the risk for chronic complications. These include impaired vision, lower extremity problems that affect mobility, and other functional limitations related to a stroke. Other barriers may include feelings of inadequacy about their abilities, unwillingness to make behavior changes, ineffective coping strategies, and cognitive problems.

Identify the patient's support system. Include them in planning, teaching, and counseling. When we include family members and other persons close to the patient, they can support the patient's self-management. They can provide care if self-care is not possible. Encourage the family and caregivers to provide emotional support and encouragement as the patient deals with the reality of living with a chronic disease.

Patient education issues include those related to altered vision, mobility, cognitive status, and functional ability. Plan

BOX 53.3 EVIDENCE-BASED PRACTICE

Digital Self-Management Interventions in DM

You are a nurse working in a clinic with J.H., a patient who has had T2DM for 2 years. His A1C results have risen from 6.9% (at diagnosis) to 9.4% today. J.H. tells you he wants to be more involved in his DM care and make diet and exercise changes. You see that he is motivated to better manage his DM.

Making Clinical Decisions

Best Available Evidence

Digital innovations have become a way to provide patient education based on individual needs and learning capacity. Including digital technology in the patient's education plan has proven to strengthen knowledge, improve self-efficacy levels, and expand self-care—all components of effective DM self-management.

Clinician Expertise

Interactive self-management strategies are effective in helping patients manage their care. You believe that J.H. would benefit from using a smartphone application that includes diet, medication, and activity tracking.

Patient Preferences and Values

J.H. and you discuss DM self-management. He agrees that using an application may be helpful. You review available options and together select one that seems suited to his needs and learning capacity.

Implications for Nursing Practice

1. Why is it important to measure J.H.'s knowledge and skills?
2. What outcomes would you assess to determine the impact of application use?

Reference for Evidence

Shaban MM, Sharaa H, Amer F, et al: Effect of digital based nursing intervention on knowledge of self-care behaviors and self-efficacy of adult clients with diabetes, *BMC Nurs* 23:130, 2024.

patient teaching based on patient needs. Use a slower pace with simple printed or audio materials in patients with cognitive and functional limitations. If patients or caregivers with cognitive, physical, and other barriers cannot make decisions related to DM management, consider a referral to a CDCES, social worker, or other resources in the community. A CDCES has the special knowledge and skills to teach and support self-care behaviors.

Tables 53.16 and 53.17 present guidelines to use for patient and caregiver teaching. The ADA website (www.diabetes.org) has extensive information for the public and health care professionals. They offer resources for patients in the form of pamphlets, booklets, books, and their website. The ADA publishes materials and sponsors conferences for health care professionals concerned with DM care, education, and research. Most drug companies that make DM-related products have free education materials for patients and HCPs.

Insulin therapy. Nursing management of patients taking insulin includes proper administration, assessing the response

TABLE 53.15 PATIENT & CAREGIVER TEACHING

DM Management

Include the following instructions when teaching patients and caregivers how to manage DM:

Component	What to Teach
Disease process	• How insulin is made • Relationship between insulin and glucose • The type of DM the patient has
Drug therapy	• The drug plan and need to take GLAs as prescribed • Side effects and safety issues • Need to keep an adequate supply of GLAs on hand
Exercise (Table 53.10)	• Effect of exercise on managing glucose and improving cardiovascular function and health • How exercise affects glucose levels • When to eat and monitor glucose in relation to exercise
Meal planning	• Importance of a well-balanced diet as part of a DM management plan (Table 53.9) • Impact of food choices on glucose levels • Need to eat regular meals at regular times • Limit the amount of alcohol, as use may lead to low-glucose events
Monitoring glucose	• How to monitor glucose (Table 53.10) • When to check glucose levels, how to record them, and how to adjust insulin levels, if necessary • Obtain A1C blood test every 3–6 months as an indicator of long-term glucose levels
Risk reduction	• Signs and symptoms and how to respond to hypoglycemia and hyperglycemia (Table 53.18) • Need to carry a form of rapid-acting glucose to treat hypoglycemia quickly • Teach family members how and when to use glucagon if the patient is unresponsive because of hypoglycemia • Proper foot care (Table 53.17) • What to do when sick, such as with influenza • Have an annual eye examination by an ophthalmologist • Obtain annual urine monitoring for protein • Always carry identification that says you have DM • Have other medical problems treated, especially high BP and high cholesterol • Have a yearly influenza vaccination • Smoking cessation • Effect stress can have on glucose
Psychosocial	• Available resources to help with the adjustment and answer questions about living with DM • Feelings about living with and managing DM • Encourage patients to meet other people with DM through support groups and social media

TABLE 53.16 **Evaluating Patients Receiving Glucose-Lowering Agents**

Category	Assessment
Patients With Newly Diagnosed DM or Reevaluation of Drug Plan	
Affective	• What emotions and attitudes are patient and caregiver displaying concerning DM diagnosis and insulin or other treatment?
Cognitive	• Is patient or caregiver able to understand why insulin or other drugs are part of DM management? • Is patient or caregiver able to understand concepts of asepsis, combining insulins, and drug side effects? • Is patient able to remember to take >1 dose/day? • Does patient take medications at right times in relation to meals?
Psychomotor	• Is patient or caregiver physically able to prepare and give accurate drug doses?
Patient Follow-up	
Effectiveness of therapy	• Is patient having symptoms of hyperglycemia? • What patterns does the glucose record show for glucose levels in or out of the target range? • Is A1C in a safe range and consistent with glucose records, and do patient and caregiver understand what A1C is?
Self-management behaviors	• If patient is having hyperglycemia or hypoglycemia, how do they manage the episodes? • Can patient determine reason for hyperglycemia or hypoglycemia? • How much insulin or other drug is patient taking and at what time of day? Does patient understand how to adjust insulin dose? Under what circumstances and by how much? • Has the exercise pattern changed? • Is patient making healthy food choices? Are meals taken at times corresponding to peak insulin action?
Side effects of therapy	• Is atrophy or hypertrophy present at injection sites? • How often does patient experience hypoglycemia? What time of day? What were their symptoms of hypoglycemia? • Are there reports of nightmares, night sweats, or early morning headaches? • Has patient had a skin rash or GI upset since taking DM drugs? • Has patient gained or lost weight?

to insulin therapy, and teaching about administration, storage, and side effects of insulin.

Assess new patients using insulin for their ability to safely manage therapy. This includes the ability to understand the interaction of insulin, food, and activity and to recognize and treat the symptoms of hypoglycemia. If a patient does not have the cognitive skills to do these things, identify and teach a responsible person. Patients or caregivers must have the cognitive and manual skills needed to prepare and inject insulin. Otherwise, additional resources are needed. Assistive devices for self-administration of insulin include syringe magnifiers, vial stabilizers, and dosing aids for the visually impaired.

Assess patients' beliefs and concerns about starting insulin. Many people are fearful when they first begin using insulin. Some find it hard to self-inject because they are afraid of needles or the pain associated with an injection. Others may think that they do not need insulin or that they will have hypoglycemia after an injection. Often people think that being prescribed insulin means they have failed. Dispel this myth and support patients who need insulin.

Follow-up assessment of patients using insulin therapy includes inspecting injection sites for signs of lipodystrophy and other reactions, reviewing insulin preparation and injection technique, taking a history of the occurrence of hypoglycemia, and assessing how they managed hypoglycemia. Review glucose readings to assess how patients are doing and make any adjustments.

Oral and noninsulin injectable agents. Your responsibilities for patients taking OAs and noninsulin injectable agents are

TABLE 53.17 **PATIENT & CAREGIVER TEACHING**

Foot Care

Include the following instructions when teaching patients and caregivers about foot care:

1. Wash feet daily with mild soap and warm water. First, test water temperature with elbow.
2. Pat feet dry gently, especially between toes.
3. Examine feet daily for cuts, blisters, swelling, and red, tender areas. Do not depend on feeling sores. If eyesight is poor, have others inspect feet.
4. Use lanolin on feet to prevent skin from drying and cracking. Do not apply between toes.
5. Use mild foot powder on sweaty feet.
6. Do not use commercial remedies to remove calluses or corns.
7. Cleanse cuts with warm water and mild soap, covering with clean dressing. Do not use iodine, rubbing alcohol, or strong adhesives.
8. Report skin infections or nonhealing sores to HCP at once.
9. Cut toenails evenly with rounded contour of toes. Do not cut down corners. The best time to trim nails is after a shower or bath.
10. Separate overlapping toes with cotton or lamb's wool.
11. Avoid open-toe, open-heel, and high-heel shoes. Leather shoes are preferred to plastic ones. Wear slippers with soles. Do not go barefoot. Inspect feet, socks, and shoes for foreign objects before putting on.
12. Wear clean, absorbent (cotton or wool) socks or stockings that have not been mended. Colored socks must be colorfast.
13. Do not wear clothing that leaves impressions, hindering circulation.
14. Do not use hot water bottles or heating pads to warm feet. Wear socks for warmth.
15. Guard against frostbite.
16. Exercise feet daily by walking or by flexing and extending feet in suspended position. Avoid prolonged sitting, standing, and crossing of legs.

similar to those for patients taking insulin (Table 53.16). Proper storage and administration, assessing the patient's use of and response to these drugs, and teaching are essential nursing actions.

Your assessment is valuable in determining the most appropriate drug for patients. Factors such as mental status, eating habits, home environment, learning ability, resources, attitude toward DM, and medication history all play a significant role in determining the most appropriate drug. For example, frail older adults who live alone are at high risk for severe hypoglycemia because low glucose is often undetected or untreated. This is especially true for patients with cognitive impairment. In these cases, an OA that does not cause hypoglycemia or a shorter-acting OA would be most appropriate.

Patient teaching is essential. Some patients may assume that their DM is not a serious condition if they are only taking a pill to treat it. Teach patients that OAs help manage glucose and prevent serious long- and short-term complications. Discuss how OAs and noninsulin injectable agents are part of the DM plan with food choices and activity. Stress the importance of following their meal and activity plans. Teach patients not to take extra pills if they have overeaten. If patients use sulfonylureas and metformin, teach them how to prevent, recognize, and manage hypoglycemia.

Personal hygiene. The risk for infection requires diligent skin and dental hygiene practices. Because of the susceptibility to periodontal disease, encourage daily brushing and flossing and regular dental visits. When having dental work done, teach patients to tell the dentist they have DM.

Routine care includes regular bathing, with an emphasis on foot care.[15] Teach patients to inspect their feet daily, avoid going barefoot, and wear shoes that are supportive and comfortable (Table 53.17). If cuts, scrapes, or burns occur, treat them promptly and monitor them carefully. Wash the area and apply a nonabrasive or nonirritating antiseptic ointment. Cover the area with a dry, sterile pad. Teach patients to notify the HCP at once if the injury does not begin to heal within 24 hours or if signs of infection develop.

Medical identification and travel. Teach patients to carry medical identification indicating that they have DM. Police, paramedics, and many people know to look for this identification when working with a sick or unconscious person. An identification card (Fig. 53.11) can supply valuable information, such as the name of the HCP, the type of DM, and the type and dose of GLAs.

Travel for a person with DM requires planning. Being sedentary for long periods may raise the glucose level. Encourage patients to get up and walk at least every 2 hours to lower the risk for deep vein thrombosis and prevent high glucose levels. Teach patients to have a full set of DM care supplies in their carry-on luggage. This includes glucose monitoring equipment, medications, syringes, insulin pens, and pen needles.

Best practices for traveling with DM supplies change frequently. Encourage patients to check current guidelines before traveling at https://www.diabetes.org/resources/know-your-rights/what-can-i-bring-with-me. Notify security screeners if an insulin pump is used so that they can inspect it while it is on the body, rather than removing it.

Teach patients taking insulin or OAs that can cause hypoglycemia to keep snack items and a quick-acting carbohydrate source for treating hypoglycemia in their carry-on luggage. Keep extra insulin available in case a bottle breaks or is lost. For longer trips, carry a full day's supply of food in case of canceled flights, delayed meals, or closed restaurants. If a patient is planning a trip out of the country, it is wise to have a letter from the HCP explaining that the person has DM and requires all the materials, especially syringes, for ongoing health care.

When travel involves time zone changes, patients should plan an insulin schedule with the HCP. During travel, most people find it helpful to keep watches set to the time of the city of origin until they reach their destination. The key to travel when taking insulin is to know the type of insulin being taken, its onset of action, the anticipated peak time, and mealtimes. Pump and CGM clocks can be set to the local time when the person arrives at their destination.

I have DIABETES

If unconscious or behaving abnormally, I may be having a reaction associated with diabetes or its treatment.

If I can swallow, give me a sweet drink, orange juice, LifeSavers, or low-fat milk.

If I do not recover promptly, call a physician or send me to the hospital.

If I am unconscious or cannot swallow, do not attempt to give me anything by mouth, but call 911 or send me to the hospital immediately.

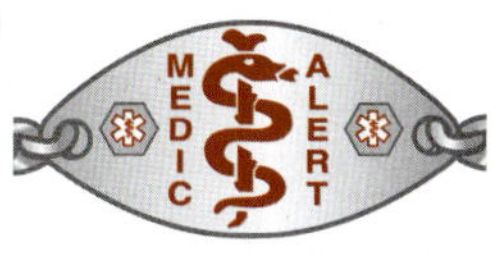

Fig. 53.11 Medical alerts. A patient with DM should carry a card and wear a bracelet or necklace that indicates DM. If the patient with DM is unconscious, these measures will ensure prompt attention.

Evaluation

The expected outcomes are that patients with DM will:

- State key elements of the treatment plan
- Describe measures that may prevent or slow progression of chronic complications
- Maintain a balance of nutrition, activity, and insulin availability that results in stable, safe, and healthy glucose levels
- Have no injury from decreased sensation in the feet

ACUTE COMPLICATIONS

Acute complications associated with DM are hyperglycemia and hypoglycemia. Hyperglycemia (high glucose) occurs when there is not enough insulin working. Hypoglycemia (low glucose) occurs when there is too much insulin working. Many signs and symptoms overlap. It is important to distinguish between them because hypoglycemia worsens rapidly and is a serious threat if action is not immediately taken. Table 53.18 compares the manifestations, causes, management, and prevention of hyperglycemia and hypoglycemia.

TABLE 53.18 Comparison of Hyperglycemia and Hypoglycemia

Hyperglycemia	Hypoglycemia
Manifestations	
• High glucose • ↑ Urination • ↑ Appetite followed by anorexia • Weakness, fatigue • Blurred vision • Headache • Glycosuria • Nausea and vomiting • Abdominal cramps • Progression to DKA or HHS • Mood swings	• Glucose <70 mg/dL (3.9 mmol/L) • Cold, clammy skin • Numbness of fingers, toes, mouth • Tachycardia • Emotional changes • Headache • Nervousness, tremors • Faintness, dizziness • Unsteady gait, slurred speech • Hunger • Changes in vision • Seizures, coma
Causes	
• Illness, infection • Corticosteroids • Too much food • Too little or no DM medication • Inactivity • Emotional, physical stress • Poor absorption of insulin	• Alcohol intake without food • Too little food—delayed, omitted, inadequate intake • Too much DM medication • Too much exercise without adequate food intake • DM medication or food taken at wrong time • Loss of weight without change in medication • Use of β-adrenergic blockers interfering with recognition of symptoms
Clinical Course	
• More gradual onset • Definition of high glucose varies by person, based on personal glucose targets	• More rapid onset • Pattern of manifestations changes over time
Treatment	
• Get medical care • Continue DM medication as prescribed • Check glucose frequently and check urine for ketones; record results • Drink fluids at least on an hourly basis • Contact HCP about ketonuria	• Follow the Rule of 15 • See Table 53.21 for emergency treatment of hypoglycemia
Prevention	
• Take prescribed dose of medication at proper time • Accurately give insulin, noninsulin injectables, OA • Make thoughtful food choices • Follow sick-day rules when ill • Check glucose routinely • Wear or carry DM identification	• Take prescribed dose of medication at proper time • Accurately give insulin, noninsulin injectables, OA • Coordinate eating with medications • Eat adequate food intake needed for calories for exercise • Be able to recognize symptoms and treat them immediately • Carry simple carbohydrates • Teach family and caregiver about symptoms and treatment • Check glucose routinely • Wear or carry DM identification

DIABETES-RELATED KETOACIDOSIS

Etiology and Pathophysiology

Diabetes-related ketoacidosis (DKA) is caused by a profound deficiency of insulin. It is characterized by hyperglycemia, ketosis, acidosis, and dehydration. It is most likely to occur in people with T1D. DKA may occur in people with T2DM if there is severe illness or stress and the pancreas cannot meet the extra demand for insulin. Precipitating factors include illness; infection; inadequate insulin dose; undiagnosed T1D; lack of education, understanding, or resources; and neglect.

When the circulating supply of insulin is insufficient, glucose cannot be properly used for energy. The body compensates by breaking down fat stores as a secondary source of fuel (Fig. 53.12). Ketones are acidic by-products of fat metabolism. When there are too many ketones in the blood, they change the pH, causing metabolic acidosis. Ketonuria occurs because ketones are excreted in the urine. During this process, the kidney excretes cation electrolytes with the anionic ketones to try to maintain balance.

Insulin deficiency impairs protein synthesis and causes protein degradation. This results in nitrogen losses from the tissues. Insulin deficiency stimulates glucose production from amino acids (from proteins) in the liver and leads to further hyperglycemia. Because of insulin deficiency, the body cannot use the extra glucose, and the glucose level rises further. This adds to the osmotic diuresis.

If not treated, patients will develop severe depletion of sodium, potassium, chloride, magnesium, and phosphate. Vomiting caused by acidosis results in more fluid and electrolyte losses. Eventually, hypovolemia, followed by shock, will ensue. Renal failure, which may eventually occur from hypovolemic shock, causes the retention of ketones and glucose. The acidosis progresses. Untreated, patients become comatose from dehydration, electrolyte imbalance, and acidosis. If they are not treated, death is inevitable.

Clinical Manifestations

Dehydration occurs in DKA with dry mucous membranes, tachycardia, and orthostatic hypotension. Early symptoms may include lethargy and weakness. Abdominal pain may be present and accompanied by anorexia, nausea, and vomiting. Acetone is noted on the breath as a sweet, fruity odor.

Kussmaul respirations (rapid, deep breathing associated with dyspnea) are the body's attempt to reverse metabolic acidosis through exhaling excess CO_2. See Chapter 17 for a discussion of respiratory compensation of metabolic acidosis. Laboratory findings include a glucose level of 250 mg/dL (13.9 mmol/L) or greater, arterial blood pH less than 7.30, and bicarbonate level less than 16 mEq/L (16 mmol/L). Moderate to large ketones are present in the urine or blood.

Interprofessional Care

DKA is a serious condition that proceeds rapidly and must be treated promptly. Hospitalization may not be needed to treat patients with DKA. If fluid and electrolyte imbalances are not

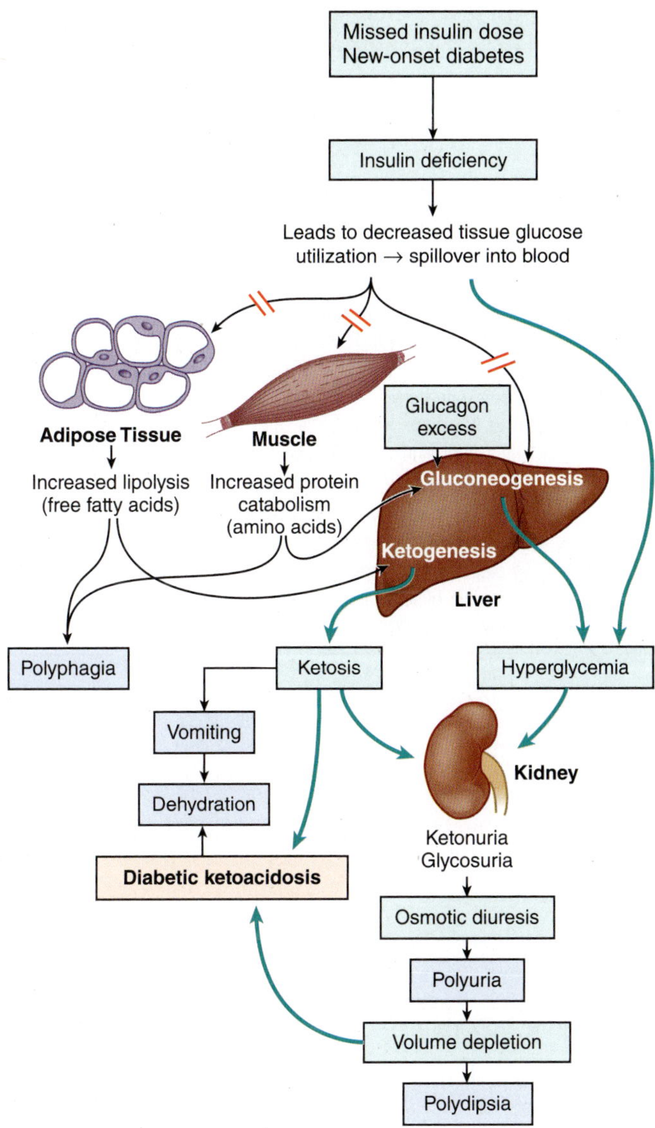

Fig. 53.12 Metabolic events leading to DKA.

severe and glucose levels can be safely monitored at home, DKA can be managed on an outpatient basis (Table 53.19). Other factors to consider when deciding where we manage patients include the presence of fever, nausea, vomiting, and diarrhea; altered mental status; the cause of the DKA; and availability of communication with the HCP (every few hours). Patients with DKA who have an illness such as pneumonia or a urinary tract infection (UTI) usually need admission to the hospital.

Table 53.20 describes the emergency management of patients with DKA. Because fluid imbalance is potentially life-threatening, the first goal of therapy is to establish IV access and begin fluid and electrolyte replacement. The aim of fluid and electrolyte therapy is to replace extracellular and intracellular water and to correct deficits of sodium, chloride, bicarbonate, potassium, phosphate, and magnesium.

The initial fluid therapy often involves an IV infusion of 0.45% or 0.9% NaCl at a rate to raise BP and restore urine output to 30 to 60 mL/h. When glucose levels approach 250 mg/dL (13.9 mmol/L), 5% to 10% dextrose is added to prevent hypoglycemia and a sudden drop in glucose that can cause cerebral edema. Rapid rehydration, especially with hypotonic IV solutions, can cause cerebral edema.

IV insulin therapy is given to correct hyperglycemia and hyperketonemia. It is important to prevent rapid drops in glucose to avoid cerebral edema. A glucose reduction of 36 to 54 mg/dL/h (2 to 3 mmol/L/h) will avoid complications. Insulin allows water and potassium to enter the cell along with glucose and can lead to a depletion of vascular volume and hypokalemia.

Obtain a potassium level before starting insulin. If patients are hypokalemic, giving insulin will further decrease potassium levels, making early potassium replacement essential. Although initial potassium may be normal or high, levels can rapidly decrease once therapy starts as insulin drives potassium into the cells, leading to life-threatening hypokalemia.

TABLE 53.19 Interprofessional Care

DKA and HHS

Diagnostic Assessment

- History and physical assessment
- Blood studies, including glucose, CBC, pH, ketones, electrolytes, BUN, arterial or venous blood gases
- Urinalysis, including specific gravity, glucose, acetone

Management

- IV fluid administration
- IV administration of short-acting insulin
- Electrolyte replacement
- Assess mental status
- Record of intake and output
- Central venous pressure monitoring (if indicated)
- Monitor glucose levels
- Assess blood and urine for ketones
- ECG monitoring
- Assess cardiovascular and respiratory status

HYPEROSMOLAR HYPERGLYCEMIA SYNDROME

Hyperosmolar hyperglycemia syndrome (HHS) is a life-threatening syndrome that can occur in people with DM who are able to make enough insulin to prevent DKA but not enough to prevent severe hyperglycemia, osmotic diuresis, and extracellular fluid depletion (Fig. 53.13). HHS is less common than DKA (Table 53.19). It often occurs in patients over 60 years of age with T2DM.

Common causes include UTIs, pneumonia, sepsis, an acute illness, and newly diagnosed T2DM. HHS is often related to impaired thirst sensation and/or a functional inability to replace fluids. There is usually a history of inadequate fluid intake, mental depression or impaired cognition, and polyuria.

TABLE 53.20 EMERGENCY MANAGEMENT

DKA

Etiology	Assessment Findings	Interventions
• Undiagnosed DM • Inadequate treatment of existing DM • Insulin not taken as prescribed • Illness, infection • Drastic change in eating, insulin, or exercise plan • Malfunction of insulin pump/non-delivery of insulin • Insulin has gone bad (outdated, exposed to extreme temperatures)	• Abdominal pain • Breath odor of ketones (fruity) • Dry mouth • Eyes appearing sunken • Fever • Flushed, dry skin • Glucosuria and ketonuria • Increasing restlessness, confusion, lethargy • Labored breathing (Kussmaul respirations) • Nausea and vomiting • Rapid, weak pulse • Glucose >250 mg/dL (13.9 mmol/L) • Thirst • Urinary frequency	**Initial** • Ensure patent airway. • Give O_2 via nasal cannula or nonrebreather mask. • Establish IV access with large-bore catheter. • Begin fluid resuscitation with 0.9% NaCl solution 1 L/h until BP stabilized and urine output 30–60 mL/h. • Begin continuous regular insulin drip 0.1 U/kg/h. • Identify history of DM, time of last food, and time and amount of last insulin dose. **Ongoing Monitoring** • Monitor vital signs, level of consciousness, ECG, O_2 saturation, and urine output. • Assess breath sounds for fluid overload. • Monitor glucose and potassium. • Give potassium to correct hypokalemia. • Give sodium bicarbonate if severe acidosis (pH <7.0). • Add dextrose to IV fluid for glucose <250 mg/dL.

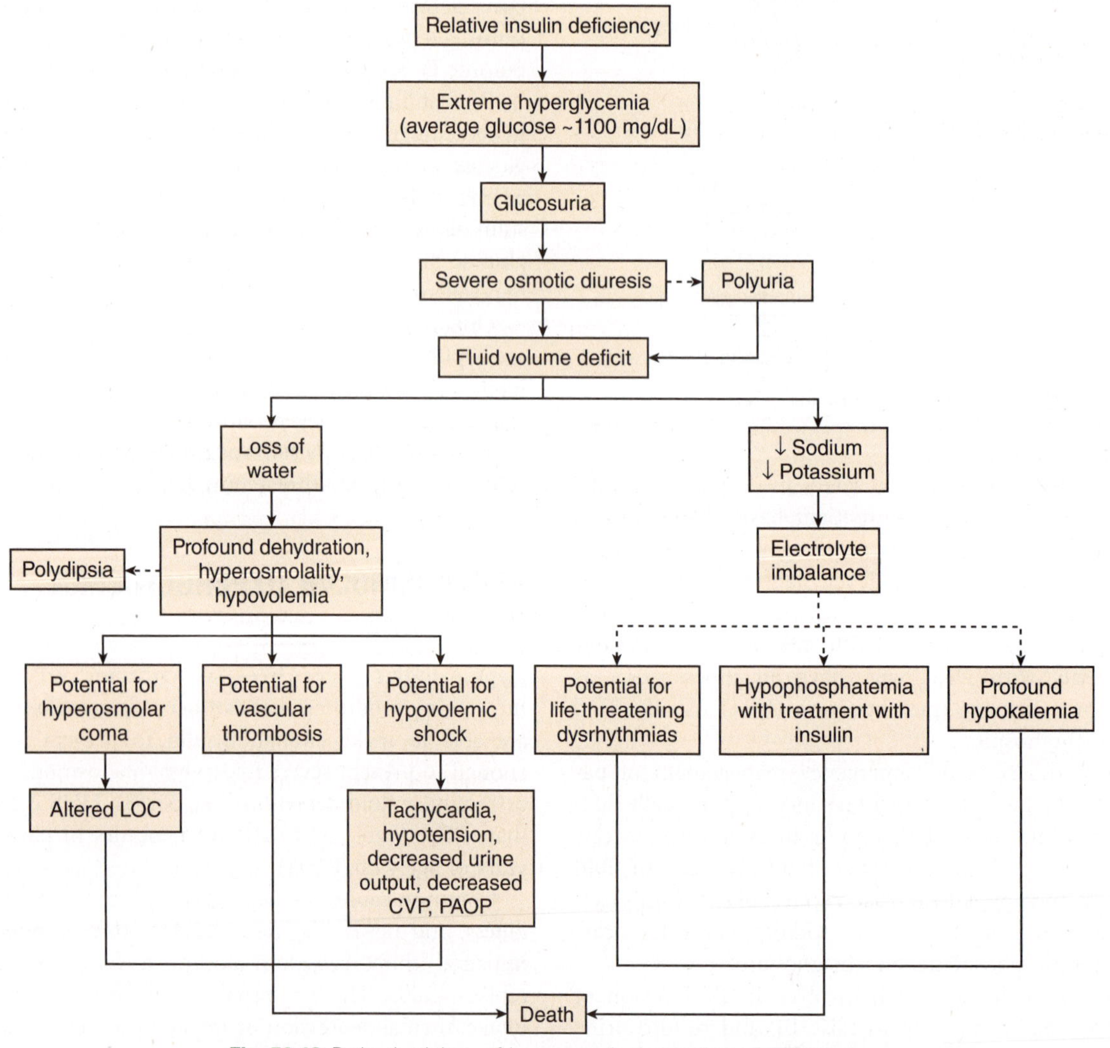

Fig. 53.13 Pathophysiology of hyperosmolar hyperglycemic syndrome.

The main difference between HHS and DKA is that patients with HHS usually have enough circulating insulin so that ketoacidosis does not occur. Because HHS has fewer symptoms in the earlier stages, glucose levels can climb quite high before the problem is recognized. The higher glucose levels increase osmolality and cause more severe neurologic manifestations, such as somnolence, coma, seizures, hemiparesis, and aphasia. Because these manifestations resemble a stroke, immediate determination of the glucose level is critical for correct diagnosis and treatment. Laboratory values in HHS include a glucose level greater than 600 mg/dL (33.33 mmol/L) and a marked increase in osmolality. Ketone bodies are absent or minimal in blood and urine.

Interprofessional Care

HHS is a medical emergency. It has a high mortality rate. The management of HHS is similar to DKA. It includes immediate IV administration of insulin and 0.9% or 0.45% NaCl. HHS usually requires large volumes of fluid replacement. This should be done slowly and carefully. When glucose levels fall to about 250 mg/dL (13.9 mmol/L), IV fluids containing dextrose are given to prevent hypoglycemia.

NURSING MANAGEMENT: DKA AND HHS

Monitor hospitalized patients with blood and urine tests. Evaluate glucose and urine for output and ketones, and use laboratory data to guide patient care. Monitor IV fluid administration to correct dehydration and insulin therapy to reduce glucose and ketone levels. Assess vital signs, intake and output, neurologic status, and laboratory values to check the efficacy of fluid and electrolyte replacement. Monitor osmolality. Frequently assess cardiac and renal status. Patients with heart or kidney problems may require hemodynamic monitoring to avoid fluid overload during fluid replacement.

Electrolytes are monitored and replaced as needed. Assess for signs of potassium imbalance resulting from low levels of insulin and osmotic diuresis (see Chapter 17). When insulin treatment is started, potassium levels may rapidly decrease as potassium moves into the cells once insulin is available. This movement of potassium into and out of extracellular fluid influences cardiac function. ECG monitoring is useful in detecting changes in potassium levels (see Fig. 17.14). Watch for fever, hypovolemic shock, tachycardia, and Kussmaul respirations.

CHECK YOUR PRACTICE

A patient with DKA has a glucose level of 554 mg/dL. You are trying to regulate the IV rate. You know that giving IV fluids too rapidly and quickly lowering glucose can lead to cerebral edema and other complications. Before starting IV insulin, you review the laboratory tests and note that the potassium is 3.2 mEq/L

- What are you concerned about, and what would you do next?

HYPOGLYCEMIA

Hypoglycemia, or low glucose, occurs when there is too much insulin in proportion to available glucose in the blood. This causes the glucose level to drop to less than 70 mg/dL (3.9 mmol/L). When glucose drops below 70 mg/dL, the body releases counterregulatory hormones and activates the autonomic nervous system. Suppressing insulin secretion and producing glucagon and epinephrine provide a defense against hypoglycemia. Epinephrine release causes manifestations that include shakiness, palpitations, nervousness, diaphoresis, anxiety, hunger, and pallor. Because the brain needs a constant supply of glucose in sufficient quantities to function properly, hypoglycemia can affect mental functioning. These "neuroglycopenia" manifestations are difficulty speaking, visual changes, stupor, confusion, and coma. Manifestations of hypoglycemia can mimic alcohol intoxication. Untreated hypoglycemia can progress to loss of consciousness, seizures, coma, and death.

Causes are often related to a mismatch in the timing of food intake and the peak action of insulin or OAs that increase insulin secretion or circulation. Common causes include receiving too much insulin or medication, ingesting too little food, delaying the time of eating, and performing unusual or unexpected exercise. Hypoglycemia can occur at any time. It most often occurs when the OA or insulin is at its peak of action or when patients' daily routine is disrupted without adequate adjustments in diet, drugs, and activity. Hypoglycemia is most common with insulin therapy. It can occur with non-insulin injectable agents and OAs and may persist for an extended time because of the longer duration of action of these drugs.

Hypoglycemia unawareness is a condition in which a person does not have the warning signs and symptoms of hypoglycemia until the glucose level reaches a critical point. Then the person may become incoherent and combative or lose consciousness. This is often a result of DM autonomic neuropathy that interferes with the secretion of counterregulatory hormones that cause these symptoms. Patients at risk for hypoglycemia unawareness include those who have had repeated episodes of hypoglycemia, older adults, and patients who use β-adrenergic blockers. Using intensive treatment to lower glucose levels in patients who have or are at risk for hypoglycemia unawareness may not be an appropriate goal. These patients usually keep glucose levels higher than those who can detect and manage the onset of hypoglycemia.

Symptoms of hypoglycemia may occur when a very high glucose level falls too rapidly (e.g., a glucose level of 300 mg/dL [16.7 mmol/L] falling quickly to 150 mg/dL [10 mmol/L]). The sudden metabolic shift can cause hypoglycemia symptoms. Aggressively managing glucose levels, lowering high glucose levels for the first time, or lowering glucose with insulin after a long period of hyperglycemia can cause this situation.

NURSING MANAGEMENT: HYPOGLYCEMIA

Hypoglycemia can usually be quickly reversed with effective treatment. At the first sign of hypoglycemia, check the glucose, if possible. If it is less than 70 mg/dL (3.9 mmol/L), immediately begin treatment for hypoglycemia. If the glucose is greater than 70 mg/dL, look for other possible causes of the signs and symptoms. If patients have manifestations of hypoglycemia and monitoring equipment is not available or they have a history of fluctuating glucose levels, assume hypoglycemia and start treatment.

Follow the "Rule of 15" to treat hypoglycemia (Table 53.21). A glucose value less than 70 mg/dL is treated by ingesting 15 to 20 g of a simple (fast-acting) carbohydrate, such as 4 to 6 oz of fruit juice or a regular soft drink. Encourage patients to carry or have available glucose tablets, gels, and powders for use in such situations. Recheck the glucose 15 minutes later. If the value is still less than 70 mg/dL, ingest 15 to 20 g more of carbohydrate and recheck the glucose in 15 minutes. If no significant improvement occurs after 2 or 3 doses, contact the HCP. After an acute episode of hypoglycemia, patients may need a snack with carbohydrate and protein if the next meal is more than an hour away or if they are being active.

Avoid treatment with carbohydrates that contain fat, such as candy bars, cookies, whole milk, and ice cream. The fat in those foods will slow glucose absorption and delay the response to treatment. Do not overtreat with large quantities of quick-acting carbohydrates because a rapid fluctuation to hyperglycemia can occur.

In an acute care setting, patients with hypoglycemia may receive 20 to 50 mL of 50% dextrose IV. If patients are not alert enough to swallow and no IV access is available, another option is to give 1 mg of glucagon by IM or subcutaneous injection. An IM injection in a site such as the deltoid muscle will result in a quicker response. Glucagon stimulates the liver to convert glycogen to glucose and makes glucose rapidly available. Nausea is a common reaction after glucagon injection. To prevent aspiration if vomiting occurs, turn the patient on the side until they are alert. Patients with minimal glycogen stores will not respond to glucagon. This includes patients with alcohol-related liver disease, starvation, and adrenal insufficiency. Teach family members and others likely to be present if severe hypoglycemia occurs when and how to inject glucagon.

Once the episode is resolved, explore the reasons why the situation developed. This assessment may indicate the need for further patient teaching to avoid future episodes of hypoglycemia.

CHRONIC COMPLICATIONS

ANGIOPATHY

Chronic complications associated with DM are primarily those of end-organ disease from damage to blood vessels *(angiopathy)* from chronic hyperglycemia (Fig. 53.14). Angiopathy is a leading cause of diabetes-related deaths.[16] These chronic blood vessel dysfunctions are divided into 2 categories: macrovascular and microvascular complications.

Several theories exist as to how and why chronic hyperglycemia damages cells and tissues. Possible causes include (1) the accumulation of damaging by-products of glucose metabolism, such as sorbitol, which damage nerve cells; (2) the formation of abnormal glucose molecules in the basement membrane of small blood vessels, such as those that circulate to the eyes and

TABLE 53.21 EMERGENCY MANAGEMENT

Hypoglycemia

Etiology	Assessment	Interventions
• Too little food—delayed, omitted, inadequate intake • Too much DM medication • Too much exercise without adequate food intake • DM medication or food taken at wrong time • Alcohol use without food intake	• Glucose <70 mg/dL (3.9 mmol/L) • Cold, clammy skin • Numbness of fingers, toes, mouth • Tachycardia • Emotional changes • Headache • Nervousness, tremors • Faintness, dizziness • Unsteady gait, slurred speech • Hunger • Changes in vision • Unresponsiveness, seizures, coma	**Initial** • Check glucose. • Determine cause of hypoglycemia (after correcting condition). **Management** ***Conscious Patient*** • Have patient eat or drink 15–20 g of quick-acting carbohydrate (4–6 oz of regular soda, 5–8 LifeSavers, 1 Tbsp syrup or honey, 4 tsp jelly, 4–6 oz orange juice, commercial dextrose products [per label instructions]). • Wait 15 min. Check glucose level. • If glucose is still <70 mg/dL, have patient eat or drink another 15–20 g of carbohydrate. • Once the glucose level is stable, give patient additional food of carbohydrate plus protein or fat (e.g., crackers with peanut butter or cheese) if the next meal is more than 1 h away or patient is engaged in physical activity. • Immediately notify HCP or emergency service (if patient outside hospital) if symptoms do not subside after 2 or 3 doses of quick-acting carbohydrate. ***Worsening Symptoms or Unconscious Patient*** • Give 1 mg glucagon subcutaneous or IM or 20–50 mL of 50% glucose IV. • Turn the patient on the side to prevent aspiration.

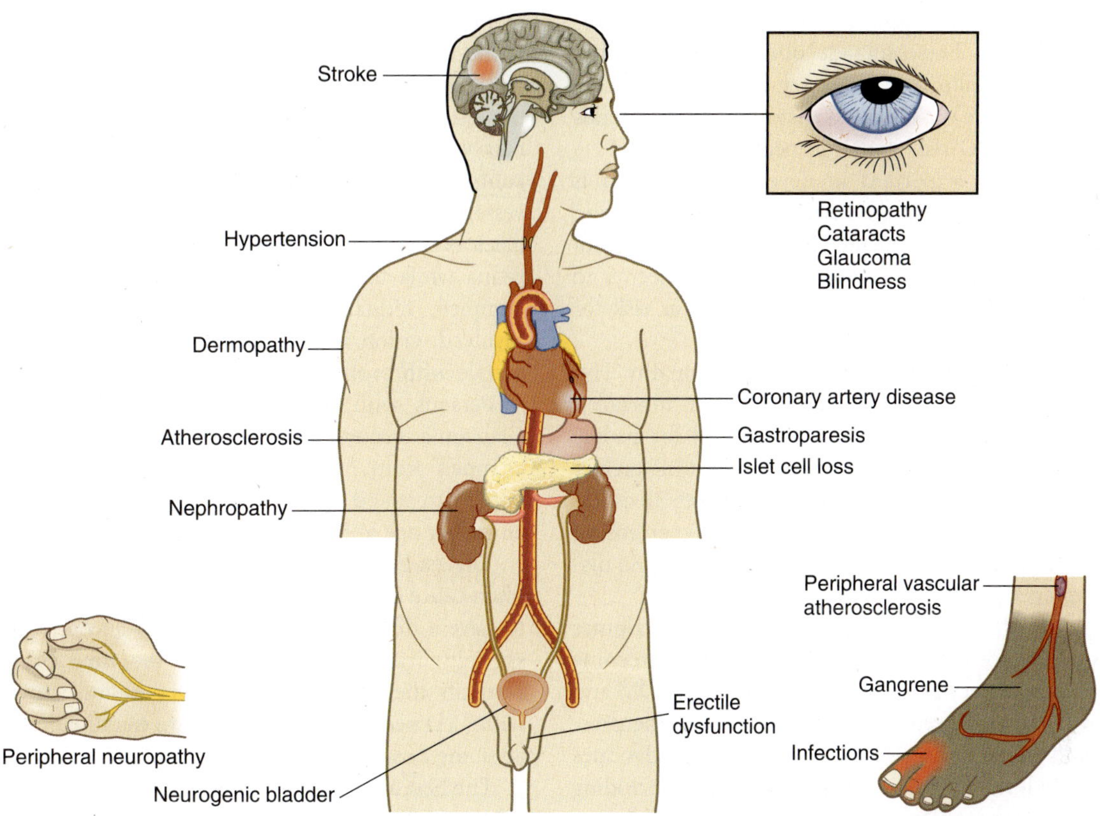

Fig. 53.14 Chronic complications of DM.

kidneys; and (3) a problem with RBC function that leads to a decrease in tissue oxygenation.

The risk for microvascular complications is reduced by keeping glucose levels as near to normal as possible for as much of the time as possible *(tight or intensive therapy)*.[17] Those who maintained tight glucose levels reduced their risk for developing eye and kidney problems, common microvascular complications. Specific targets for each patient must consider their risk for severe or undetected hypoglycemia as a side effect of tight management.

Because of the devastating effects of chronic complications, people with DM need scheduled and ongoing monitoring for the detection and prevention of chronic complications. Recommendations for evaluation are shown in Table 53.22. It is essential that patients understand the importance of regular follow-up visits.

Macrovascular Complications

Macrovascular complications are diseases of the large- and medium-size blood vessels that occur with greater frequency and with an earlier onset in people with DM. Macrovascular diseases include cerebrovascular, cardiovascular, and peripheral vascular disease. Females with DM have a 4 to 6 times increased risk for CVD. Males with DM have a 2 to 3 times increased risk for CVD compared with those without DM.

TABLE 53.22 Monitoring for Chronic Complications Related to DM

Complication	Type of Examination	Frequency
Retinopathy	• Retinal examination • Fundus photography	• Annually
Nephropathy	• Urine albumin level • Creatinine	• Annually
Neuropathy (foot and lower extremities)	• Visual examination of foot	• Daily by patient
	• Foot examination (e.g., integrity, toenails, callous formation) • Vibration or pinprick sensation; monofilament exam	• Annually • Foot examination at every visit if patients have a history of foot ulcers, loss of sensation in their feet, or other foot problems
Cardiovascular disease	• BP measurement	• Every visit
	• Risk factor assessment • Screen for PAD (e.g., pulses temperature)	• At least annually
	• Routine ECG	• Every 3–5 yr
	• Exercise stress testing, CT angiography	• As needed, based on risk factors

Several modifiable risk factors are associated with macrovascular complications. These include obesity, smoking, hypertension, high fat intake, and sedentary lifestyle. The ADA recognizes that DM alone is a CVD risk factor and recommends yearly screening for CVD risk factors in people with DM.[16]

Insulin resistance is important in developing CVD. It is implicated in the pathogenesis of essential hypertension and dyslipidemia. We do not completely understand the role of insulin resistance in the pathogenesis of CVD. It seems to combine with dyslipidemia in contributing to greater risk for CVD in people with DM.

Optimizing BP is significant in decreasing angiopathy. Hypertension in people with DM causes an increase in mortality. The ADA recommends BP screening at every visit for people with DM. They recommend health counseling for BP greater than 120/80 mm Hg and treatment to achieve a target BP of less than 130/80 mm Hg for most patients with DM. Hypertension is discussed in Chapter 36, and coronary artery disease is discussed in Chapter 37.

People with DM have an increase in lipids that contributes to the increased risk for CVD. The ADA recommends screening all adults for dyslipidemia when they are diagnosed with DM and starting statin therapy as needed. Dosing is based on the presence of age and other CVD risk factors. The ADA advocates treating high lipid levels with health behavior changes, including nutrition, exercise, weight loss, and smoking cessation.

Smoking is especially dangerous for people with DM. It significantly increases the risk for blood vessel and CVD, stroke, and lower extremity amputation.

Microvascular Complications

Microvascular complications result from thickening of the vessel membranes in the capillaries and arterioles (small vessels) in response to chronic hyperglycemia. Although microangiopathy can be found throughout the body, the areas most noticeably affected are the eyes (retinopathy), kidneys (nephropathy), and nerves (neuropathy). Microvascular changes are present in some people with T2DM at the time of diagnosis.

RETINOPATHY

Etiology and Pathophysiology

Diabetes-related retinopathy refers to the microvascular damage to the retina from chronic hyperglycemia, nephropathy, and hypertension in people with DM. DM retinopathy is the leading cause of new cases of adult blindness.

We classify retinopathy as nonproliferative or proliferative. In *nonproliferative retinopathy,* the most common form, partial occlusion of the small blood vessels in the retina causes microaneurysms to develop in the capillary walls. The walls of these microaneurysms are so weak that capillary fluid leaks out, causing retinal edema and eventually hard exudates or intraretinal hemorrhages. This may cause mild to severe vision loss, depending on which parts of the retina are affected. If the center of the retina (macula) is affected, vision loss can be severe.

Proliferative retinopathy, the most severe form, involves the retina and vitreous. When retinal capillaries become occluded, the body compensates by forming new blood vessels to supply the retina with blood, a process called *neovascularization.* These new vessels are very fragile and bleed easily, causing vitreous contraction. Eventually, light cannot reach the retina as the vessels break and bleed into the vitreous cavity. Patients see black or red spots or lines. If these new blood vessels pull the retina while the vitreous contracts, causing a tear, partial or complete retinal detachment will occur. If the macula is involved, vision is lost. Without treatment, more than half of people with proliferative retinopathy will be blind.

Persons with DM are prone to other visual problems. Glaucoma occurs because of the occlusion of the outflow channels from neovascularization. This type of glaucoma is hard to treat and often results in blindness. Cataracts develop at an earlier age and progress more rapidly in people with DM.

The earliest and most treatable stages of DM retinopathy often cause no changes in the vision. Teach patients with T2DM to have a dilated eye examination by an ophthalmologist or a specially trained optometrist at the time of diagnosis and annually thereafter for early detection and treatment.[18] Those with T1D need to have a dilated eye examination within 5 years after the onset of DM and then annually.

The best approach to managing DM eye disease is to prevent it by maintaining safe glucose levels and managing hypertension. Laser photocoagulation therapy can reduce the risk for vision loss in people with proliferative retinopathy or macular edema and, sometimes, nonproliferative retinopathy. Laser photocoagulation destroys the ischemic areas of the retina that make growth factors that encourage neovascularization. Patients who develop vitreous hemorrhage and retinal detachment may need to undergo vitrectomy (see Chapter 22). Another treatment involves an intravitreal implant that releases the corticosteroid fluocinolone acetonide for 36 months.

Vascular endothelial growth factor (VEGF) plays a key role in developing DM retinopathy. We are currently studying drugs injected into the eye that block the action of VEGF and reduce inflammation for their effectiveness in treating retinopathy.

NEPHROPATHY

Diabetes-related nephropathy is associated with damage to the small blood vessels that supply the glomeruli of the kidney. It is the leading cause of ESRD in the United States and is seen in 20% to 40% of people with DM. Risk factors include hypertension, genetic predisposition, smoking, and chronic hyperglycemia. Keeping glucose levels in a healthy range is critical in preventing DM nephropathy.

Patients are screened for nephropathy annually with a random spot urine collection to assess for albuminuria and measure the albumin-to-creatinine ratio. Creatinine is measured to give an estimate of the glomerular filtration rate and the degree of kidney function.

Patients with albuminuria take angiotensin-converting enzyme (ACE) inhibitor drugs (e.g., lisinopril) or angiotensin

II receptor blockers (e.g., losartan). These drugs are used to treat hypertension and delay the progression of nephropathy in patients with DM. Hypertension significantly accelerates the progression of nephropathy. Aggressive BP management is indicated for people with DM and hypertension. Patients with DM and hypertension need aggressive BP management (see Chapter 36). See Chapter 51 for a discussion of renal failure.

NEUROPATHY

Diabetes-related neuropathy is nerve damage that occurs from the metabolic imbalances associated with DM. About 60% to 70% of patients with DM have some degree of neuropathy. The most common type affecting persons with DM is sensory neuropathy. This can lead to the loss of sensation in the lower extremities. Coupled with other factors, it significantly increases the risk for complications that result in lower limb amputation. More than 60% of nontraumatic amputations in the United States occur in people with DM. Neuropathy can precede, accompany, or follow the diagnosis of DM. Screening for neuropathy begins at the time of diagnosis in patients with T2DM and 5 years after diagnosis in patients with T1D.[19]

Etiology and Pathophysiology

We do not completely understand the pathophysiology of DM neuropathy. Theories include metabolic, vascular, and autoimmune factors. The prevailing theory is that persistent hyperglycemia leads to sorbitol and fructose accumulating in the nerves that causes damage. How they cause damage is unknown. The result is reduced nerve conduction and demyelination. Ischemic damage by chronic hyperglycemia in blood vessels that supply the peripheral nerves is implicated in developing DM neuropathy.

Classification

The 2 major categories of DM neuropathy are *sensory neuropathy,* which affects the peripheral nervous system, and *autonomic neuropathy.* Each type has several forms.

Sensory Neuropathy

The most common form of sensory neuropathy is distal symmetric polyneuropathy. It affects the hands and/or feet bilaterally. We sometimes call this *stocking-glove neuropathy.* Characteristics include loss of sensation, abnormal sensations, pain, and paresthesias. Patients describe the pain as burning, cramping, crushing, or tearing. It is usually worse at night and may occur only at that time. The paresthesias may be associated with tingling, burning, and itching sensations. They may report a feeling of walking on pillows or numb feet. The skin can become so sensitive (hyperesthesia) that patients cannot tolerate even light pressure from bed sheets. Complete or partial loss of sensitivity to touch and temperature is common. Foot injury and ulcerations can occur without ever having pain (Fig. 53.15). Neuropathy can cause atrophy of the small muscles of the hands and feet, causing deformity and limiting fine movement.

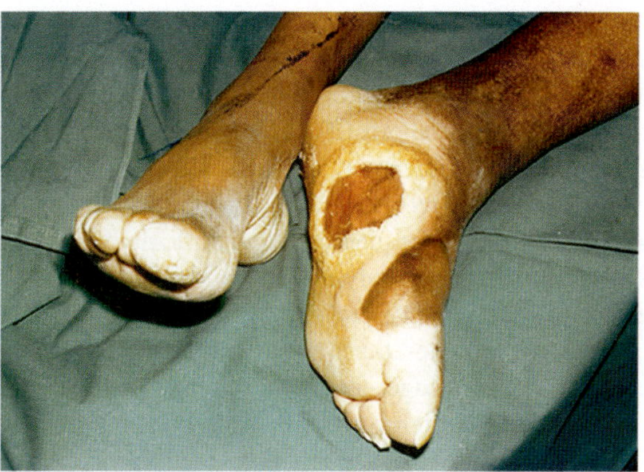

Fig. 53.15 Neuropathy: Neurotrophic ulceration.

Managing glucose is the only treatment for DM neuropathy. It is effective in many, but not all, cases. Drug therapy may be used to treat neuropathic symptoms, especially pain. At the start of therapy, symptoms usually increase, followed by relief of pain in 2 to 3 weeks.

Common drugs used include topical creams (e.g., capsaicin), tricyclic antidepressants (e.g., amitriptyline), selective serotonin and norepinephrine reuptake inhibitors (e.g., duloxetine), and antiseizure drugs (e.g., gabapentin). Capsaicin is a moderately effective topical cream made from chili peppers. It depletes the accumulation of pain-mediating chemicals in the peripheral sensory neurons. The cream is applied 3 or 4 times a day.

Tricyclic antidepressants are moderately effective in treating DM neuropathy. They inhibit the reuptake of norepinephrine and serotonin, which are neurotransmitters thought to play a role in pain transmission. We think duloxetine relieves pain by increasing the levels of serotonin and norepinephrine, which improves the body's ability to regulate pain. Antiseizure drugs decrease the release of neurotransmitters that transmit pain.

Autonomic Neuropathy

Autonomic neuropathy can affect nearly all body systems and lead to hypoglycemia unawareness, bowel incontinence and diarrhea, and urine retention. *Gastroparesis* (delayed gastric emptying) is a complication of autonomic neuropathy that can cause anorexia, nausea, vomiting, gastroesophageal reflux, and persistent feelings of fullness. Gastroparesis can trigger hypoglycemia by delaying food absorption. Cardiovascular problems from autonomic neuropathy include postural hypotension, resting tachycardia, and painless myocardial infarction (MI). Assess for postural hypotension to determine whether there is a risk for falls. Teach patients with postural hypotension to change from a lying or sitting position slowly.

DM can affect sexual function. Erectile dysfunction (ED) in males with DM is common. It is often the first manifestation of autonomic neuropathy. ED is associated with other factors, including vascular disease, high glucose levels, endocrine problems, psychogenic factors, and other drugs. Decreased libido is a problem for some females with DM. Candida and nonspecific vaginitis are common. ED and sexual problems require sensitive counseling for patients and their partners. See Chapter 59 for more about ED.

A neurogenic bladder may develop as the sensation in the inner bladder wall decreases, causing urine retention. Patients with retention have infrequent voiding, difficulty voiding, and a weak stream of urine. Emptying the bladder every 3 hours in a sitting position helps prevent stasis and infection. Tightening the abdominal muscles during voiding and using the Credé maneuver (mild massage downward over the lower abdomen and bladder) may help with complete bladder emptying. Cholinergic agonist drugs, such as bethanechol, may be used. Patients may need to learn self-catheterization.

COMPLICATIONS OF FEET AND LOWER EXTREMITIES

People with DM are at high risk for foot ulcerations, serious infection, and lower extremity amputations. DM-related foot complications can be the result of a combination of microvascular and macrovascular diseases. Sensory neuropathy and peripheral artery disease (PAD) are risk factors for foot complications. Clotting problems, impaired immune function, and autonomic neuropathy have a role. Smoking has a negative effect on lower extremity blood vessels and increases the risk for amputation.

Sensory neuropathy is a major risk factor for lower extremity amputation in people with DM. *Loss of protective sensation* (LOPS) can prevent patients from being aware that a foot injury has occurred. Improper footwear and injury from stepping on foreign objects while barefoot are common causes of undetected foot injury in the person with LOPS. Because the primary risk factor for lower extremity amputation is LOPS, annual screening with monofilament testing is important (Fig. 53.16).

PAD increases the risk for amputation by reducing blood flow to the lower extremities. With decreased blood flow, oxygen, white blood cells (WBCs), and vital nutrients are not available to the tissues. Wounds take longer to heal, and the risk for infection increases. Signs of PAD include intermittent claudication, pain at rest, cold feet, loss of hair, delayed capillary refill, and dependent rubor. PAD is diagnosed by history, ankle-brachial index (ABI), and angiography. Management includes reducing risk factors, especially smoking, and managing cholesterol and hypertension. Bypass or graft surgery is needed in some patients. PAD is discussed in Chapter 41.

If the patient has LOPS or PAD, aggressive measures must be taken to teach them how to prevent foot ulcers. Guidelines for patient teaching are listed in Table 53.17. Proper care of a foot ulcer is critical for wound healing. Several treatments can be used. Casting can redistribute the weight on the plantar surface of the foot. Wound care for the ulcer can include debridement, dressings, advanced wound healing products, vacuum-assisted closure, ultrasound, hyperbaric O_2, and skin grafting.

Neuropathic arthropathy, or *Charcot foot,* results in ankle and foot changes that lead to joint problems and footdrop. These changes occur gradually. They promote an abnormal distribution of weight over the foot. This increases the chances of developing a foot ulcer as new pressure points appear. Foot deformity should be recognized early and proper footwear fitted before ulceration occurs.

SKIN COMPLICATIONS

Up to two-thirds of persons with DM develop skin problems. DM-related dermopathy, the most common skin lesion, is characterized by reddish-brown, round or oval patches. They

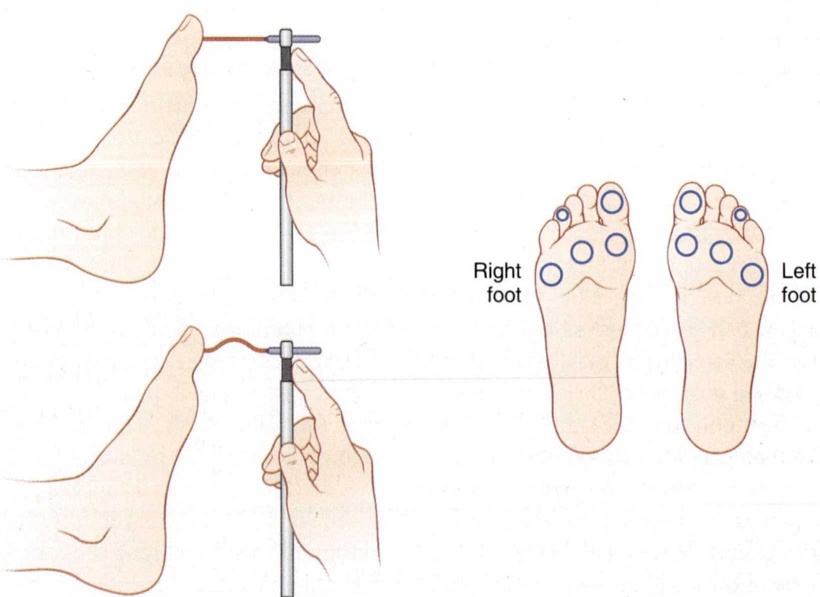

Fig. 53.16 Monofilament testing. Press the monofilament lightly until it bows in each area of the foot that is being tested. Record the presence of sensation in that area. (From Dehn R: *Essential clinical procedures,* St. Louis, 2021, Elsevier.)

initially are scaly, then they flatten out and become indented. The lesions appear most often on the shins but can occur on the front of the thighs, forearm, side of the foot, scalp, and trunk.

Acanthosis nigricans is a manifestation of insulin resistance. It can appear as a velvety light brown to black skin thickening, mainly on flexures, axillae, and the neck (Fig. 53.17). *Necrobiosis lipoidica diabeticorum* usually appears as red-yellow lesions, with atrophic skin that becomes shiny and transparent, revealing tiny blood vessels under the surface. This condition is uncommon. It occurs more often in young females. It may appear before other signs and symptoms of DM. Because the thin skin is prone to injury, special care must be taken to protect affected areas from injury and ulceration.

INFECTION

A person with DM is more susceptible to infections because of a defect in the mobilization of WBCs and impaired phagocytosis by neutrophils and monocytes. Recurring or persistent infections, such as *Candida albicans,* boils, and furuncles in undiagnosed patients, often lead the HCP to suspect DM. Loss of sensation (neuropathy) may delay the detection of an infection.

Persistent glycosuria predisposes people to bladder infections, especially those with a neurogenic bladder. Decreased circulation resulting from angiopathy can prevent or delay the immune response. Treatment of infections must be prompt and vigorous. Teach patients to prevent infection by practicing good hand hygiene, avoiding exposure to persons who have a communicable illness, and getting an annual influenza vaccine and pneumococcal vaccine.

PSYCHOLOGIC CONSIDERATIONS

People with DM have high rates of distress, anxiety, and eating disorders. Depression and distress contribute to diminished DM self-care, feelings of helplessness related to managing a chronic disease, and poor outcomes. DM distress encompasses the stress, fear, and burden of living with and managing a demanding chronic disease. Assess patients for manifestations of depression and/or DM distress. Open communication helps identify these behaviors early.

Disordered eating behaviors (DEBs) can occur. DEBs include anorexia, bulimia, binge eating, extreme calorie restriction, and intense exercise. Adolescent females with DM are more than twice as likely to develop DEB.[20] Patients may intentionally decrease their dose of insulin or omit the dose. This is called "diabulimia." It leads to weight loss, hyperglycemia, and glycosuria because the food ingested cannot be used for energy without adequate insulin. Insulin omission and DEBs can have serious consequences, including retinopathy, neuropathy, abnormal lipids, DKA, and death. Refer patients with DEB to a mental health professional with expertise in DEB and an understanding of DM management.

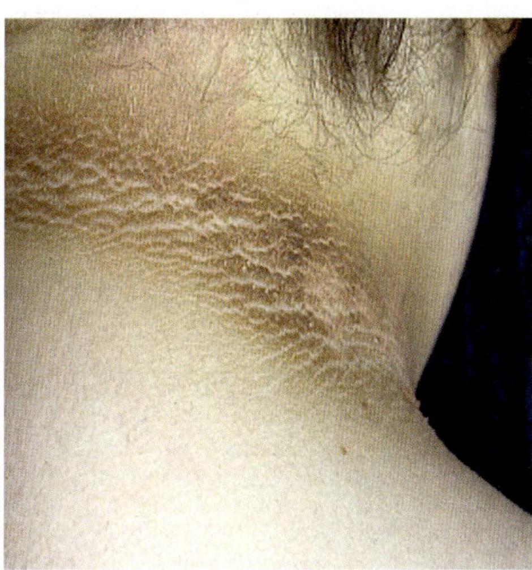

Fig. 53.17 Acanthosis nigricans of the neck. (From Strauss J: *Yen and Jaffe's reproductive endocrinology*, St Louis, 2019, Elsevier.)

GERONTOLOGIC CONSIDERATIONS: DM

DM is present in more than 25% of people over 65 years of age. This age group is the fastest-growing segment of the population developing it. Older people with DM have higher rates of premature death, functional disability, and coexisting illnesses, such as hypertension and stroke. The prevalence of DM increases with age. A major reason for this is that the aging process is associated with a reduction in β-cell function, decreased insulin sensitivity, and altered carbohydrate metabolism. Aging is associated with conditions that are more likely to be treated with drugs that impair insulin action (e.g., corticosteroids, antihypertensives, phenothiazines). Undiagnosed and untreated DM is more common in older adults. This in part occurs because manifestations of DM, such as low energy levels, dizziness, confusion, and chronic UTIs, are wrongly attributed to normal age-related changes.

Several factors affect setting glycemic goals for an older adult. One is that hypoglycemia unawareness is more common in older adults, making them more likely to have adverse consequences from glucose-lowering therapy. They may have problems that could interfere with the ability to treat hypoglycemia. Other factors include patients' desire for treatment and coexisting medical problems, such as cognitive impairment. Compounding the challenge, DM can increase the rate of cognitive decline. Although treatment is needed to prevent complications, intensive DM management may be hard and dangerous to achieve, especially in older adults.

Meal planning and exercise are recommended therapies for older adults with DM. Consider functional limitations that may interfere with physical activity and the ability to prepare meals. Because of the physiologic changes that occur with aging, the therapeutic outcome for the older adult who takes OAs may be altered. Assess renal function and creatinine clearance in those over 80 years of age taking metformin. Monitor those taking sulfonylurea drugs (e.g., glipizide) for hypoglycemia and kidney and liver problems. Insulin therapy may be started if OAs are not effective. However, older adults are more likely to have limitations in the dexterity and visual acuity needed for accurate insulin administration. Insulin pens may be a safer alternative.

CASE STUDY
HHS

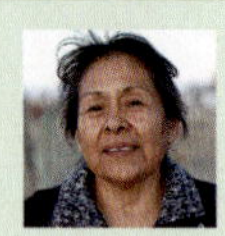
(©eyecrave productions/ iStock.com.)

Patient Profile

T.K. is a 78-year-old female with T2DM and hypertension who is being admitted for hyperosmolar hyperglycemia syndrome. Before admission, she was diagnosed with community-acquired pneumonia the preceding week at an urgent care center and had been recovering at home. She was brought to the emergency room earlier today after her son noted that she was becoming confused and was sleeping more than usual.

Subjective Data (Provided by Son)

- Diagnosed with T2DM 10 years ago
- Takes metformin twice daily and semaglutide once weekly
- Treated for pneumonia last week with oral antibiotics
- Stopped taking her GLAs because of fatigue and malaise. Has not been eating or drinking much because of recent illness

Objective Data

Physical Assessment

- Dry mucous membranes
- Skin flushed and dry
- Heart rate 118 beats/min; BP 98/60 mm Hg, O_2 sat 93%
- Difficult to arouse with decreased level of consciousness

Diagnostic Studies

- Glucose level 730 mg/dL (40.5 mmol/L)
- Blood pH 7.32
- Ketones negative

Discussion Questions

1. ***Recognize:*** Briefly explain the pathophysiology behind T.K.'s hyperosmolar hyperglycemia syndrome (HHS).
2. ***Recognize:*** What factors precipitated T.K. developing HHS?
3. ***Analyze:*** What clinical manifestations of HHS does T.K. have?
4. ***Analyze:*** What distinguishes this case history from one of DKA?
5. ***Prioritize:*** Based on the assessment data presented, what are the priority clinical problems?
6. ***Prioritize:*** What are the priority nursing interventions for T.K.?
7. ***Act:*** What teaching do you need to provide for T.K. and her family?
8. ***Act:*** How can the health care team work together in caring for T.K.?
9. ***Evaluate:*** What outcomes would indicate that interprofessional care was effective?
10. Develop a conceptual care map for T.K.

Answers and a corresponding concept map are available at http://evolve.elsevier.com/Lewis/medsurg.

BRIDGE TO NCLEX EXAMINATION

The number of the question corresponds to the same-numbered outcome at the beginning of the chapter.

1. Patient education about the function of insulin would include that it
- **a.** Increases glucose levels
- **b.** Decreases after consuming a meal
- **c.** Is produced by β cells in the islets of Langerhans
- **d.** Promotes transport of glucose from cells into the bloodstream

2. Which point would the nurse include when teaching a patient with newly diagnosed with type 1 diabetes about their condition?
- **a.** "You will require lifelong treatment with insulin."
- **b.** "Losing weight may prevent or reverse your condition."
- **c.** "Oral treatment with metformin is considered the best option for you."
- **d.** "You are still able to make insulin, your body just does not use it effectively."

3. Goals of managing patients with diabetes include (**Select all that apply.**)
- **a.** keeping the target A1C at 8% or higher.
- **b.** preventing injuries by limiting exercise.
- **c.** teaching self-monitoring of glucose levels.
- **d.** preventing complications of hypoglycemia.
- **e.** maintaining the LDL cholesterol greater than 100 mg/dL (2.6 mmol/L).

4. The nurse is teaching a patient with diabetes about exercise. Which patient statement indicates that further teaching is needed?
- **a.** "I cannot exercise if I am taking insulin and metformin."
- **b.** "Exercise can help improve my cholesterol and blood pressure."
- **c.** "Exercise decreases insulin resistance, so I may need to adjust my medication."
- **d.** "I should try to get about 150 minutes of moderate-intensity aerobic activity weekly."

5. The nurse is caring for a patient who has just returned from having a CT scan with IV contrast for abdominal pain. The patient usually takes metformin orally twice daily and is due for their second dose now. Which nursing action is a priority?
- **a.** Hold the metformin for at least 48 hours after the dose of IV contrast
- **b.** Notify the HCP to change the order from oral metformin to IV push
- **c.** Check the patient's glucose level and hold metformin if it is <120 mg/dL
- **d.** Administer metformin now and provide orange juice to avoid hypoglycemia

6. During a home visit, a patient with type 2 diabetes tells the nurse about a leg wound that they have had for the past 2 weeks that is red and tender. What is the **priority** nursing action?
   a. Check the patient's glucose level.
   b. Administer acetaminophen for the pain.
   c. Assess the wound and notify the HCP of the findings.
   d. Reassure the patient that wounds heal slower in persons with diabetes.
7. Emergency management of patients in acute diabetes-related ketoacidosis includes
   a. Fluid resuscitation.
   b. Giving oral metformin.
   c. Withholding oral fluids.
   d. Administering naloxone.
8. Strategies to reduce the risk of diabetes-related nephropathy include (**Select all that apply.**)
   a. avoiding diet protein sources.
   b. maintaining normal glucose levels.
   c. smoking cessation for persons who smoke.
   d. keeping the blood pressure in a normal range.
   e. taking an ACE inhibitor or angiotensin II receptor blocker if albuminuria is present.

1. c; 2. a; 3. c, d; 4. a; 5. a; 6. c; 7. a, 8. b, c, d, e.

For rationales to these answers and even more NCLEX review questions, visit http://evolve.elsevier.com/Lewis/medsurg.

REFERENCES

To access the References for this chapter, please scan the QR code with a mobile device.

54

Endocrine Problems

Ann H. Crawford

http://evolve.elsevier.com/Lewis/medsurg/

CONCEPTUAL FOCUS

Coping
Fluids and Electrolytes
Hormonal Regulation
Nutrition
Perfusion
Reproduction
Thermoregulation
Tissue Integrity

LEARNING OUTCOMES

1. Explain the pathophysiology, clinical manifestations, and interprofessional and nursing management of patients with anterior pituitary gland problems.
2. Describe the pathophysiology, clinical manifestations, and interprofessional and nursing management of patients with posterior pituitary gland problems.
3. Explain the pathophysiology, clinical manifestations, and interprofessional and nursing management of patients with thyroid problems.
4. Describe the pathophysiology, clinical manifestations, and interprofessional and nursing management of patients with parathyroid problems.
5. Identify the pathophysiology, clinical manifestations, and interprofessional and nursing management of patients with adrenal cortex problems.
6. Outline the nursing management of patients receiving corticosteroid therapy.
7. Describe the pathophysiology, clinical manifestations, and interprofessional and nursing management of patients with pheochromocytoma.

KEY TERMS

acromegaly
Addison disease
arginine vasopressin (AVP) disorder
Cushing syndrome
goiter
Graves disease
hyperaldosteronism
hyperparathyroidism
hyperthyroidism
hypoparathyroidism
hypopituitarism
hypothyroidism
myxedema
pheochromocytoma
syndrome of inappropriate antidiuresis (SIAD)
thyroiditis
thyrotoxicosis

Endocrine problems may cause many homeostatic changes because of the wide range of hormonal actions. Regulating fluid and electrolyte balance and temperature may be difficult. There may be adverse effects on perfusion, metabolism, skin integrity, and nutrition. Patients may have problems with growth and reproductive processes because these are hormone dependent. There may be a wide range of psychologic responses, including anxiety and depression.

ANTERIOR PITUITARY GLAND PROBLEMS

The anterior pituitary gland secretes growth hormone (GH), prolactin, and 4 tropic hormones—adrenocorticotropic hormone (ACTH), thyroid-stimulating hormone (TSH), follicle-stimulating hormone (FSH), and luteinizing hormone (LH). These hormones affect growth, sexual maturation, reproduction, metabolism, stress response, and fluid balance. As a result, pituitary gland disorders manifest in a variety of ways.

Pituitary gland tumors account for 5% to 20% of primary intracranial tumors.[1] The most common, a pituitary adenoma, is a slow-growing, benign tumor. It often occurs in adults between 40 and 60 years of age. Hypersecretory pituitary adenomas secrete an excess of a specific hormone causing manifestations related to the action of that hormone. The most common are prolactinomas and GH- and ACTH-secreting adenomas.[1]

ACROMEGALY

Acromegaly is a rare condition characterized by an overproduction of GH. Acromegaly most often occurs because of a benign GH-secreting pituitary adenoma. The excess GH results in an overgrowth of soft tissues and bones in the hands, feet, and face. Around 3 cases per 1 million people in the United States are diagnosed each year.[2] The mean age at the time of diagnosis is 40 to 45 years old.

Clinical Manifestations

The changes resulting from excess GH in adults can occur slowly, over many years. They may go unnoticed by the person, family, and friends. Thickening and enlargement of the bony and soft tissues on the face, feet, and head occur (Fig. 54.1). Because the problem develops after epiphyseal closure, the bones of the arms and legs do not grow longer. Patients may have proximal muscle weakness, carpal tunnel syndrome, and peripheral neuropathy. Joint pain can range from mild to crippling. Carpal tunnel syndrome and peripheral neuropathy may be present.

Tongue enlargement causes dental and speech problems. The voice deepens because of hypertrophy of the vocal cords. Sleep apnea may occur because of upper airway narrowing and obstruction from increased amounts of pharyngeal soft tissues. The skin becomes thick, leathery, and oily with acne outbreaks.

Vision changes may occur from pressure on the optic nerve from a pituitary adenoma. Headaches are common. Since GH antagonizes the action of insulin, glucose intolerance and manifestations of diabetes may occur, including increased thirst and polyuria.

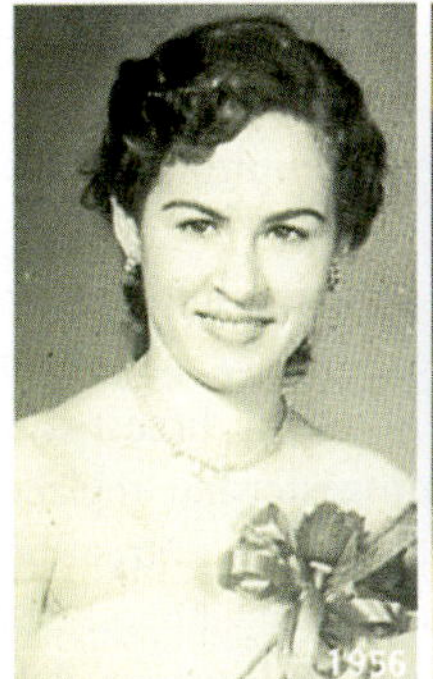
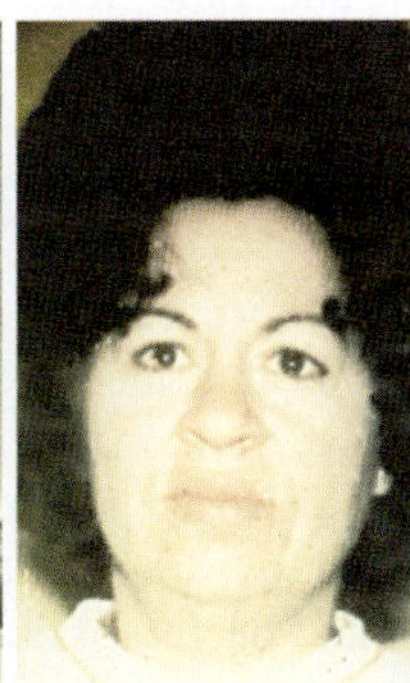
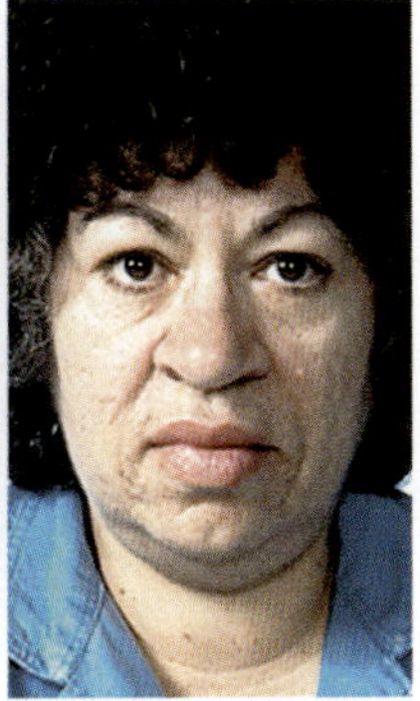

Fig. 54.1 Progressive development of facial changes from acromegaly. (Courtesy Linda Haas, Seattle, WA.)

Diagnostic Studies

In addition to the history and physical assessment, a diagnosis requires measuring insulin-like growth factor-1 (IGF-1) levels and GH response to an oral glucose tolerance test (OGTT). IGF-1 mediates the peripheral actions of GH. As GH levels rise, so do IGF-1 levels. Since GH is released in a pulsatile fashion, we need several samples to obtain an accurate assessment. Serum IGF-1 levels are more constant, giving a reliable diagnostic measure of acromegaly. During an OGTT, GH concentration falls because glucose inhibits GH secretion. In acromegaly, GH levels do not fall and in some cases GH levels rise.

MRI or high-resolution CT scan with contrast can detect pituitary adenomas. A complete eye examination, including visual fields, is done because a tumor may cause pressure on the optic chiasm or optic nerves.

Interprofessional and Nursing Management

The overall goal is to return GH levels to normal. The prognosis depends on the age at onset, age when treatment started, and tumor size. Treatment can stop bone growth and reverse tissue hypertrophy. Life expectancy is reduced by 5 to 10 years. Patients are prone to cardiovascular disease (CVD), diabetes, and colorectal cancer.[3] Even if patients are cured or the disease is well controlled, manifestations such as joint pain and deformities often remain.

Treatment consists of surgery, radiation therapy, drug therapy, or a combination of these. Surgery (hypophysectomy) is the treatment of choice. It offers the best chance for a cure and optimal symptom management, especially for smaller tumors.[4] Surgery results in an immediate reduction in GH levels. IGF-1 levels fall within a few weeks. Patients with larger tumors or those with GH levels greater than 45 ng/mL may need radiation or drug therapy. Surgery and radiation therapy for pituitary tumors are discussed later in this chapter.

Drug therapy is an option for patients whose surgery did not result in a cure and/or in combination with radiation therapy. The main drug used is octreotide (Sandostatin), a somatostatin analog. It reduces GH levels to normal in many patients. Octreotide is given by subcutaneous injection 3 times a week. Long-acting somatostatin analogs, octreotide (Sandostatin LAR), pasireotide (Signifor), and lanreotide SR (Somatuline Depot), are available as IM injections given every 4 weeks. GH levels are measured every 2 weeks to guide drug dosing and then every 6 months until the desired response is achieved.

Dopamine agonists (e.g., bromocriptine, cabergoline) may be given alone or with somatostatin analogs if surgery does not result in a complete remission. These drugs reduce GH secretion from the tumor.

GH antagonists (e.g., pegvisomant [Somavert]) reduce the effect of GH by blocking liver production of IGF-1. Most patients taking this drug achieve normal IGF-1 levels with symptom improvement.

Serial photographs showing improvement in appearance may be helpful to patients' recovery. Psychosocial effects of acromegaly include body image problems, sexual problems, and depression. Fatigue and sleep problems may persist after surgery. Patients will need strategies for dealing with these symptoms. Referral to a support group may be helpful.

EXCESSES OF OTHER TROPIC HORMONES

Excess prolactin or tropic hormone (e.g., ACTH, TSH) secretion by the anterior pituitary gland will cause other endocrine glands to overproduce certain hormones. An excess of these hormones (discussed later in the chapter) can cause significant problems in metabolism and general health.

A prolactin-secreting adenoma is a *prolactinoma.* They account for about 40% of pituitary tumors.[5] Females with prolactinomas may have galactorrhea, anovulation, infertility, infrequent or absent menses, decreased libido, and hirsutism. In males, impotence, decreased sperm density, and decreased libido may result. Compression of the optic chiasm can cause vision changes and signs of increased intracranial pressure, including headache, nausea, and vomiting.

Because prolactinomas do not typically grow, drug therapy is usually the first-line treatment. The dopamine agonists cabergoline and bromocriptine are given to block prolactin release. Surgery may be an option, depending on the extent and size of the tumor. Radiation therapy can reduce the risk for tumor recurrence for patients with large tumors.

PITUITARY GLAND HYPOFUNCTION

Hypopituitarism is a rare disorder that involves a decrease in 1 or more of the pituitary hormones. A deficiency of only 1 pituitary hormone is called *selective hypopituitarism.* Total failure of the pituitary gland results in deficiency of all pituitary hormones—a condition called *panhypopituitarism.* The most common hormone deficiencies from hypopituitarism involve GH and gonadotropins (e.g., LH, FSH).

Etiology and Pathophysiology

The usual cause is a pituitary tumor. Other causes include autoimmune disorders, infections, pituitary infarction (Sheehan syndrome), or destruction of the pituitary gland (from trauma, radiation, surgery). Anterior pituitary hormone deficiencies can lead to end organ failure. TSH and ACTH deficiencies are life threatening. ACTH deficiency can lead to acute adrenal insufficiency and hypovolemic shock from sodium and water depletion.

Clinical Manifestations and Diagnostic Studies

The manifestations vary with the type and degree of dysfunction. Early manifestations of a tumor include headaches, vision changes (decreased visual acuity, decreased peripheral vision), loss of smell, nausea and vomiting, and seizures. Manifestations associated with hyposecretion of the target glands vary widely (Table 54.1).

TABLE 54.1 Manifestations of Hypopituitarism

Hormone Deficiency	Manifestations
Adrenocorticotropic hormone (ACTH)	Cortisol deficiency: weakness, fatigue, headache, dry and pale skin, ↓ axillary and pubic hair, ↓ resistance to infection, fasting hypoglycemia
Follicle-stimulating hormone (FSH) and luteinizing hormone (LH)	*Females:* Menstrual irregularities, loss of libido, changes in secondary sex characteristics (e.g., ↓ breast size) *Males:* Testicular atrophy, ↓ spermatogenesis, loss of libido, impotence, ↓ facial hair and muscle mass
Growth hormone (GH)	Subtle, nonspecific findings: truncal obesity, osteoporosis, ↓ muscle mass and strength, weakness, fatigue, depression, or flat affect
Thyroid-stimulating hormone (TSH)	Hypothyroidism: Table 54.6

In addition to a history and physical assessment, diagnostic studies such as MRI and CT can identify a pituitary tumor. Laboratory tests involve the direct measurement of pituitary hormones (e.g., TSH) or an indirect determination of the target organ hormones (e.g., triiodothyronine [T_3], thyroxine [T_4]). See Chapter 52 for more information about diagnostic studies.

Interprofessional and Nursing Management

Treatment often consists of surgery or radiation therapy followed by lifelong hormone therapy. Surgery and radiation therapy for pituitary tumors are discussed in the next section. Appropriate hormone therapy is given (e.g., corticosteroids, thyroid hormone). Hormone therapies are discussed later in this chapter.

Somatropin (Genotropin, Humatrope, Omnitrope) is recombinant human GH. It is used for long-term hormone therapy in adults with GH deficiency. Patients often respond well to GH replacement. They have increased energy, increased lean body mass, a feeling of well-being, and improved body image. Side effects include fluid retention with peripheral edema, muscle and joint pain, and headache. GH is given daily as a subcutaneous injection, preferably in the evening. The dosing is variable and adjusted based on symptoms, IGF-1 levels, and side effects.

Hormone therapy will improve sexual function and general well-being. It is contraindicated in those with certain health problems, such as phlebitis, pulmonary embolism, breast cancer, and prostate cancer. Estrogen and progesterone replacement therapy may be given to hypogonadal females to treat hot flashes, vaginal dryness, and decreased libido (see Chapter 58). Testosterone is used to treat males with gonadotropin deficiency. The benefits of testosterone therapy include a return of male secondary sex characteristics, improved libido, and increased muscle mass, bone mass, and bone density. Hormone therapy for males is discussed in Chapter 59.

PITUITARY SURGERY

A *hypophysectomy* is the surgical removal of the pituitary gland. It is the treatment of choice for tumors in the pituitary area, especially smaller pituitary adenomas. Most surgeries are done by an endoscopic *transsphenoidal* approach (Fig. 54.2). When the entire pituitary gland is removed, there is permanent loss of all pituitary hormones. Patients will need lifelong replacement therapy with thyroid hormone, sex hormones, and corticosteriods.[6]

Radiation therapy can reduce the tumor size before surgery. It is also used when surgery does not produce a cure or when patients are not surgical candidates. The full effects may take months to years. Radiation therapy may lead to hypopituitarism, which then requires lifelong hormone replacement therapy. Stereotactic radiosurgery (Gamma Knife surgery, proton beam, linear accelerator) is an option for small, surgically inaccessible pituitary tumors or in place of conventional radiation.

Cerebrospinal fluid (CSF) leaks and nosebleeds are other common complications after surgery. The HCP may place a petroleum jelly–coated ribbon of gauze or a balloon-tipped catheter (like an indwelling urinary catheter) in the sphenoid sinus. It is usually removed after 24 hours. It can be left in for 2 to 3 days if there is concern for bleeding or CSF leak.

Monitor the "moustache" dressing regularly for any drainage. Check any clear drainage with a urine dipstick for glucose and protein. If present, notify the HCP of a possible CSF leak. A sample can be sent to the laboratory. A glucose level greater than 30 mg/dL (1.67 mmol/L) indicates CSF leakage from an open connection with the brain. If this happens, patients are at increased risk for meningitis. A persistent and severe general or supraorbital headache may indicate CSF leakage into the sinuses. A CSF leak usually resolves within 72 hours when treated with head elevation and bed rest. If the leak persists, daily spinal taps can reduce pressure to below-normal levels.

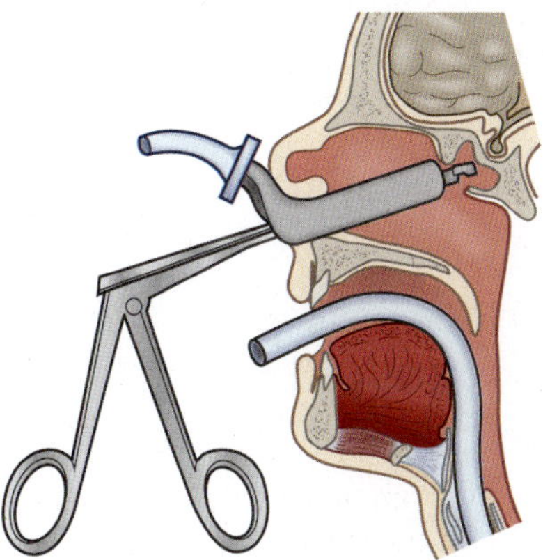

Fig. 54.2 Surgery on the pituitary gland is most often done by a transsphenoidal approach. An incision is made in the inner aspect of the upper lip and gingiva. The sella turcica is entered through the floor of the nose and sphenoid sinuses.

After surgery, you need to assess for a hematoma compressing the optic nerve or optic chiasma. Monitor peripheral vision, visual acuity, extraocular movements, and pupil response. Report changes at once. Prompt intervention may prevent vision changes from becoming permanent (Table 54.2).

Keep the head of the bed elevated at a 30-degree angle. This avoids pressure on the sella turcica and decreases headaches. Monitor pupil response, speech patterns, and extremity strength to detect neurologic complications. Gentle mouth care every 4 hours keeps the surgical site clean and free of debris. Have patients avoid brushing their teeth for at least 10 days to protect the suture line.

CHECK YOUR PRACTICE

You are caring for a 52-year-old patient who had a hypophysectomy for a pituitary adenoma. As you are preparing to give oral pain medication, the patient reports increasing headache. The patient also reports difficulty focusing and has difficulty seeing.

- How do you respond?
- What complication do you suspect could be occurring?
- What assessments do you need to make?
- Describe the actions needed if this complication is occurring.

Fluid and electrolyte problems can occur if the body's ability to produce or use antidiuretic hormone (ADH) is affected. Transient arginine vasopressin (AVP) disorder, previously known as diabetes insipidus, may occur because of the loss of ADH, which is stored in the posterior lobe of the pituitary gland, or cerebral edema from manipulation of the pituitary during surgery. AVP disorder may be permanent

TABLE 54.2 NURSING MANAGEMENT

Care of Patients After Pituitary Surgery

- Monitor vital signs. Assess peripheral pulses and watch for orthostatic hypotension.
- Monitor neurologic and cognitive status (e.g., level of consciousness, orientation, speech) hourly for the first 24 h and then every 4 h.
- Assess extremity strength and reflexes.
- Monitor field of vision, visual acuity, extraocular movements, and pupil response. Notify HCP of any changes.
- Assess dressing for type and amount of drainage. Notify HCP for excess bleeding or CSF drainage.
- Maintain intake and output and monitor fluid balance. Assess for AVP disorder or SIAD.
- Keep head of bed elevated at least 30 degrees.
- Encourage deep-breathing exercises and incentive spirometer use.
- Monitor pain and give prescribed analgesics.
- Encourage high-fiber diet to decrease risk for constipation.
- Patients must not blow their nose for 48 h.
- Perform oral care every 4 h.
- Teach patients to:
  - Avoid vigorous coughing and sneezing
  - Avoid bending over at the waist or straining at stool
  - Avoid using a toothbrush until incision heals
  - Follow replacement hormone therapy plan

after surgery. To assess for AVP disorder, monitor urine output and measure specific gravity. Report a urine output of more than 200 mL/h for more than 3 consecutive hours or a specific gravity level of less than 1.005. Patients with AVP disorder will have a high sodium level and extreme thirst. We treat AVP disorder by giving desmopressin acetate (DDAVP). Fluid replacement may be needed to avoid hypovolemia from high urine output.

Syndrome of inappropriate antidiuresis (SIAD) can occur after surgery. SIAD typically occurs later than AVP disorder, usually around the 4th postoperative day. It may be due to manipulation of the pituitary causing release of ADH. The fluid retention caused by circulating ADH leads to dilutional hyponatremia. AVP disorder and SIAD are discussed in the next section.

After a hypophysectomy, patients need lifelong ADH, cortisol, and thyroid hormone replacement. Surgery may result in permanent loss or deficiencies in FSH and LH. This can lead to decreased fertility. Assist patients in working through the grieving process associated with these losses.

POSTERIOR PITUITARY GLAND PROBLEMS

SYNDROME OF INAPPROPRIATE ANTIDIURESIS

Etiology and Pathophysiology

Syndrome of inappropriate antidiuresis (SIAD) results from an overproduction of ADH or the release of ADH despite normal or low osmolarity (Fig. 54.3). ADH increases the permeability of the renal distal tubule and collecting duct, which leads to the reabsorption of water into the circulation. Extracellular fluid volume expands, osmolality declines, glomerular filtration rate increases, and sodium levels decline (dilutional hyponatremia). Thus features of SIAD are fluid retention, serum hypoosmolality, dilutional hyponatremia, hypochloremia, and concentrated urine in the presence of normal or increased intravascular volume.

PATHOPHYSIOLOGY MAP

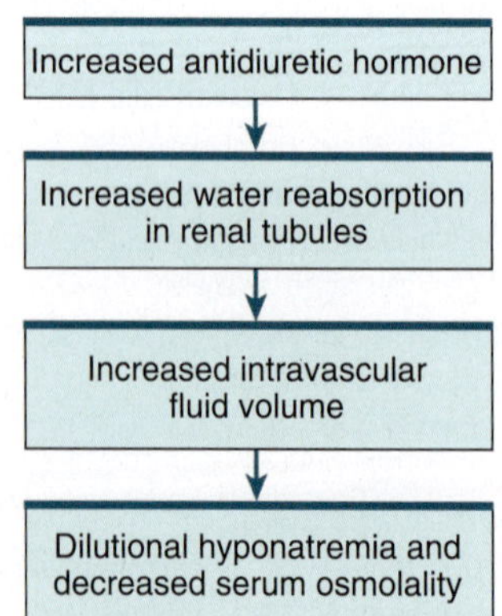

Fig. 54.3 Pathophysiology of SIAD.

SIAD occurs more often in older adults. The most common cause is cancer, especially small cell lung cancer (Table 54.3). SIAD tends to be self-limiting when caused by head trauma or drugs. It can occur after any intracranial surgery. It can be chronic when caused by tumors or metabolic diseases.

Clinical Manifestations and Diagnostic Studies

Patients with SIAD have low urine output and increased body weight. At first, patients have thirst, dyspnea on exertion, and fatigue. Mild hyponatremia causes muscle cramping, irritability, and headache. As sodium levels fall (usually below 120 mEq/L [120 mmol/L]), manifestations become more severe. They include vomiting, decreased level of consciousness, and muscle twitching. As osmolality and sodium levels continue to decline, cerebral edema may occur, leading to confusion, seizures, and coma.

The diagnosis is made by simultaneous measurements of urine and serum osmolality. Dilutional hyponatremia is indicated by a sodium level less than 135 mEq/L, osmolality less than 280 mOsm/kg (280 mmol/kg), and urine specific gravity

TABLE 54.3 Causes of SIAD

Cancer
- Colorectal cancer
- Lymphoid cancers (Hodgkin lymphoma, non-Hodgkin lymphoma, lymphocytic leukemia)
- Pancreatic cancer
- Prostate cancer
- Small cell lung cancer
- Thymus cancer

CNS Problems
- Brain tumors
- Guillain-Barré syndrome
- Head injury (skull fracture, subdural hematoma, subarachnoid hemorrhage)
- Infection (encephalitis, meningitis)
- Stroke
- Systemic lupus erythematosus

Drug Therapy
- Carbamazepine
- Chemotherapy agents (vincristine, vinblastine, cyclophosphamide)
- General anesthesia agents
- Opioids
- Oxytocin
- Thiazide diuretics
- Selective serotonin reuptake inhibitor (SSRI) antidepressants
- Tricyclic antidepressants

Miscellaneous
- Adrenal insufficiency
- COPD
- HIV
- Hypothyroidism
- Lung infection (pneumonia, tuberculosis, lung abscess)
- Positive pressure mechanical ventilation

greater than 1.030. An osmolality much lower than the urine osmolality shows the body is inappropriately excreting concentrated urine in the presence of dilute serum.

Interprofessional and Nursing Management

When assessing patients at risk and those who have confirmed SIAD, be alert for low urine output with a high specific gravity, a sudden weight gain without edema, or a decreased sodium level. Monitor intake and output, vital signs, and heart and lung sounds. Obtain daily weights. Observe for signs of hyponatremia, including seizures, headache, vomiting, and decreased neurologic function.

Treatment is directed at the underlying cause.[7] Medications that stimulate ADH release should be avoided or discontinued (Table 54.3). If symptoms are mild and the sodium level is greater than 125 mEq/L (125 mmol/L), the only treatment may be a fluid restriction of 800 to 1000 mL/day. This restriction should result in weight loss and a gradual rise in sodium level and osmolality and an improvement in symptoms. Provide frequent oral care and distractions to decrease discomfort related to thirst from the fluid restriction.

A loop diuretic, such as furosemide, may be used to promote diuresis. Since loop diuretics cause sodium loss, sodium levels must be at least 125 mEq/L (125 mmol/L). Because furosemide increases potassium, calcium, and magnesium loss, patients may need supplements. Demeclocycline also may be given. It blocks the effect of ADH on the renal tubules, resulting in more dilute urine.

Initiate seizure and fall precautions if patients have an altered sensorium or are having seizures. Keep the head of the bed flat or elevated no more than 10 degrees. This promotes venous return to the heart and increases left atrial filling pressure, thus reducing ADH release. Frequent turning, positioning, and range-of-motion exercises are important to maintain skin integrity and joint mobility.

In cases of severe hyponatremia (less than 120 mEq/L), especially with neurologic manifestations, such as seizures, small amounts of IV hypertonic saline solution (3% sodium chloride) may be given. We must correct hyponatremia slowly. The level should not increase by more than 8 to 12 mEq/L in the first 24 hours. Quickly increasing levels can cause osmotic demyelination syndrome with permanent damage to nerve cells in the brain. A fluid restriction of 500 mL/day may be needed for those with severe hyponatremia.

Vasopressor receptor antagonists block the activity of ADH. They are used to treat euvolemic hyponatremia in hospitalized patients. Two drugs are approved for use in the United States: conivaptan (Vaprisol) and tolvaptan (Samsca). Conivaptan is given IV; tolvaptan is given orally. Neither should be given to patients with liver disease because they worsen liver function.

Help patients with chronic SIAD to self-manage their treatment. In chronic SIAD, a fluid restriction of 800 to 1000 mL/day is recommended. Ice chips or sugarless chewing gum help decrease thirst. Teach them to supplement the diet with sodium and potassium, especially if taking loop diuretics. Have patients obtain a daily weight to monitor changes in fluid balance. Teach patients the symptoms of fluid and electrolyte imbalances, especially those involving sodium and potassium (see Chapter 17).

ARGININE VASOPRESSIN (AVP) DISORDER

Etiology and Pathophysiology

Arginine vasopressin (AVP) disorder (or diabetes insipidus) is caused by deficient production or secretion of ADH or a decreased renal response to ADH.[8] The decrease in ADH results in fluid and electrolyte imbalances caused by increased urine output and increased osmolality (Fig. 54.4). Depending on the cause, AVP disorder may be transient or a chronic, lifelong condition. There are two types of AVP disorder (Table 54.4). *AVP-deficiency (AVP-D)* is the most common.

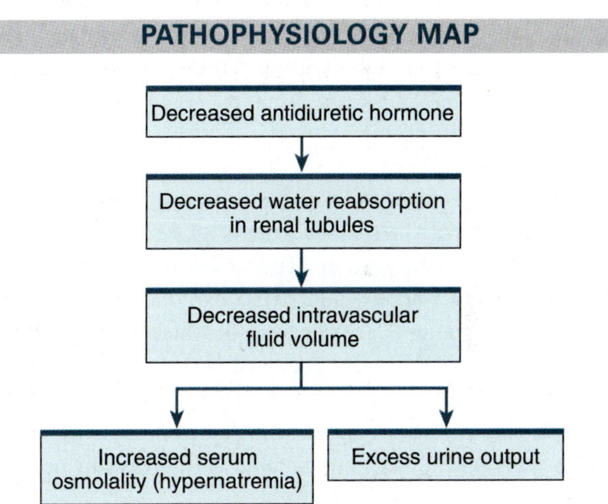

Fig. 54.4 Pathophysiology of arginine vasopressin (AVP) disorder.

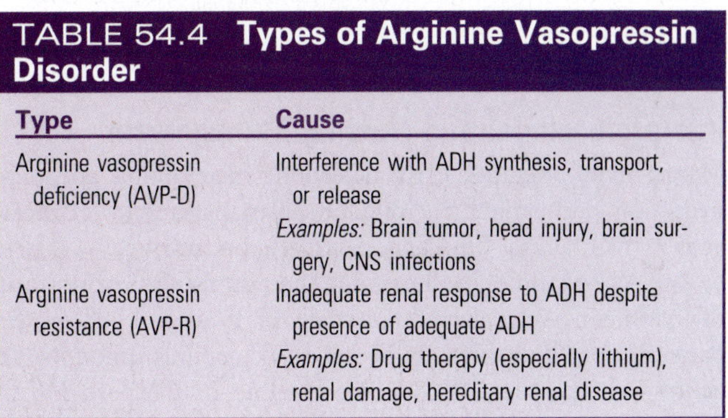

TABLE 54.4 Types of Arginine Vasopressin Disorder

Type	Cause
Arginine vasopressin deficiency (AVP-D)	Interference with ADH synthesis, transport, or release *Examples:* Brain tumor, head injury, brain surgery, CNS infections
Arginine vasopressin resistance (AVP-R)	Inadequate renal response to ADH despite presence of adequate ADH *Examples:* Drug therapy (especially lithium), renal damage, hereditary renal disease

Clinical Manifestations

Key features of AVP disorder are polydipsia and polyuria. Patients excrete large quantities of urine (2 to 20 L/day) with a very low specific gravity (less than 1.005) and urine osmolality of less than 100 mOsm/kg (100 mmol/kg). Serum osmolality is increased (usually greater than 295 mOsm/kg [295 mmol/kg]) because of hypernatremia (sodium level greater than 145 mg/dL) from pure water loss in the kidneys. Most patients compensate for fluid loss by drinking large amounts of water so that serum osmolality stays normal or is somewhat increased. They may be tired from nocturia and have weakness. Uncorrected hypernatremia can cause brain shrinkage and intracranial bleeding.

The onset of AVP-D is usually acute and accompanied by excess fluid loss. After intracranial surgery, AVP-D has a triphasic pattern: (1) an acute phase with an abrupt onset of polyuria, (2) an interphase in which urine volume normalizes, and (3) a third phase in which AVP-D may become permanent. The third phase occurs 10 to 14 days after surgery. AVP-D from head trauma is often self-limiting. It improves with treatment of the underlying problem. Although the manifestations of arginine vasopressin resistance (AVP-R) are like those of AVP-D, the onset and amount of fluid loss are less dramatic.

Severe dehydration can result if oral intake cannot keep up with urinary losses. Patients will have hypotension, tachycardia, and hypovolemic shock. Increasing osmolality and hypernatremia can cause central nervous system (CNS) manifestations, ranging from irritability and mental dullness to coma.

Diagnostic Studies

Patients with AVP disorder excrete dilute urine at a rate greater than 200 mL/h with a specific gravity of less than 1.005. We diagnose AVP-D with a water deprivation test. Before the test, we measure body weight, and urine osmolality, volume, and specific gravity. Patients are deprived of water for 8 to 12 hours and then given DDAVP subcutaneously or nasally. Patients with AVP-D have a dramatic increase in urine osmolality (from 100 to 600 mOsm/kg) and a significant decrease in urine volume. Patients with AVP-R will not be able to increase urine osmolality to greater than 300 mOsm/kg.

We can distinguish AVP-D from APV-R by measuring ADH levels after giving an ADH analog (e.g., desmopressin). If the cause is AVP-D, the kidneys will respond to the hormone by concentrating urine. If the kidneys do not respond, the cause is nephrogenic.

Interprofessional and Nursing Management

Management includes early detection, maintaining adequate hydration, and patient teaching for self-management. A clinical goal is maintaining fluid and electrolyte balance.

For AVP-D, fluid and hormone therapy are the cornerstone of treatment. We replace fluids orally or IV, depending on the patient's condition and ability to drink copious amounts. In acute AVP disorder, IV hypotonic saline or dextrose 5% in water (D_5W) is given and titrated to replace urine output. If IV glucose solutions are used, monitor glucose levels. Hyperglycemia and glycosuria can lead to osmotic diuresis, which increases the fluid volume deficit. Monitor BP, heart rate, urine output, level of consciousness, and specific gravity. They may be done hourly in acutely ill patients. Assess for signs of acute dehydration. Evaluate intake and output and daily weights to assess fluid volume. Adjustments in fluid replacement should be made accordingly.

DDAVP, an analog of ADH, is the hormone replacement of choice for AVP-D. DDAVP can be given orally, IV, subcutaneously, or as a nasal spray. Assess the response to DDAVP by monitoring pulse, BP, level of consciousness, intake and output, and specific gravity. Another ADH replacement drug is aqueous vasopressin. Medications such as carbamazepine (Tegretol) can help decrease thirst associated with AVP-D.

Because the kidney is unable to respond to ADH in AVP-R, hormone therapy has little effect. Instead, the treatment includes a low-sodium diet and thiazide diuretics (e.g., chlorothiazide), which may reduce flow to the ADH-sensitive nephrons. Limiting sodium intake to no more than 3 g/day often helps decrease urine output. If a low-sodium diet and thiazide drugs are not effective, indomethacin may be prescribed. It is a nonsteroidal antiinflammatory drug (NSAID) that helps increase renal responsiveness to ADH.

THYROID PROBLEMS

Thyroid problems are among the most common endocrine problems. Thyroid gland problems include goiter, benign and malignant nodules, inflammatory conditions leading to hyperthyroidism, and hypothyroidism (Fig. 54.5).

GOITER

A **goiter** is an enlarged thyroid gland. The person may have an overactive thyroid (hyperthyroidism) or an underactive thyroid (hypothyroidism). The most common cause of goiter worldwide is a lack of diet iodine. In the United States where most people use iodized salt, goiter is more often due to the overproduction or underproduction of thyroid hormones or to nodules in the thyroid gland. *Goitrogens* (foods or drugs that contain thyroid-inhibiting substances) can cause a goiter (Table 54.5).

A nontoxic goiter is a diffuse enlargement of the thyroid gland that does not result from cancer or inflammation. The thyroid hormone levels are normal. *Nodular goiters* are thyroid hormone–secreting nodules. They function independently of TSH stimulation. There may be multiple nodules (multinodular goiter) or a single nodule (solitary autonomous nodule). The nodules are usually benign follicular adenomas. If these nodules cause hyperthyroidism, they are called *toxic*

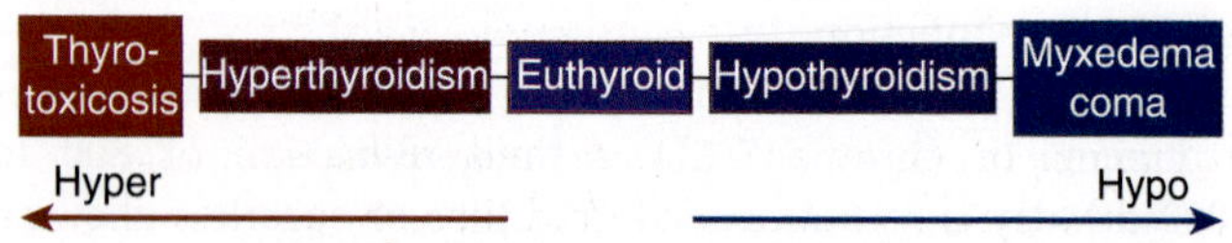

Fig. 54.5 Continuum of thyroid dysfunction.

TABLE 54.5 Goitrogens

Thyroid Inhibitors	Select Foods
• Iodine in large doses • Methimazole • Propylthiouracil (PTU)	• Broccoli • Brussels sprouts • Cabbage • Cauliflower • Kale • Mustard • Peanuts • Strawberries • Turnips
Other Drugs • Amiodarone • Lithium • p-Aminosalicylic acid • Salicylates • Sulfonamides	

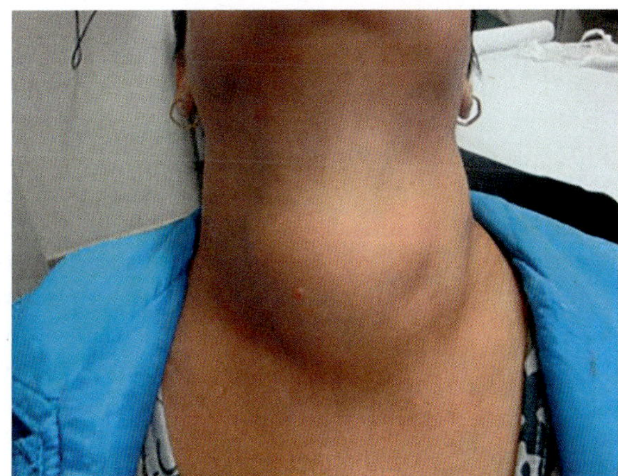

Fig. 54.6 Goiter. (From Iyomasa RM, Tagliarini JV, Rodrigues SA, et al: Laryngeal and vocal alterations after thyroidectomy, *Braz J Otorhinolaryngol* 85:3, 2019.)

nodular goiters.[9] This type of goiter is often found in patients with Graves disease (Fig. 54.6). They most often occur in people over 40 years of age.

We measure TSH and T_4 levels to determine whether a goiter is associated with normal thyroid function, hyperthyroidism, or hypothyroidism. Thyroid antibodies may show the presence of thyroiditis. Treatment with thyroid hormone may prevent further thyroid enlargement. Surgery can remove large goiters. Goiter as a manifestation of thyroid problems is discussed in the next sections.

THYROIDITIS

Thyroiditis, an inflammation of the thyroid gland, encompasses several clinical problems. It is a frequent cause of goiter. We think that *subacute granulomatous thyroiditis* is caused by a viral infection. *Acute thyroiditis* is due to bacterial or fungal infection. Subacute and acute forms of thyroiditis have an abrupt onset. Patients report pain in the thyroid area or radiating to the throat, ears, or jaw. Systemic manifestations include fever, chills, sweats, and fatigue.

Hashimoto thyroiditis (chronic autoimmune thyroiditis) is caused by the destruction of thyroid tissue by antibodies.[10] It is the most common cause of hypothyroid goiters in the United States. Risk factors include female gender, a family history, older age, and White ethnicity. The goiter may develop gradually or rapidly. If it enlarges rapidly, it may compress structures in the neck (e.g., trachea, laryngeal nerves), changing the voice and affecting breathing. As antibodies destroy thyroid tissue, there may be a transient phase of hyperthyroidism due to leaking thyroid hormone from the damaged tissues.

Silent, painless thyroiditis, which may be early Hashimoto thyroiditis, can occur in postpartum females. This condition is usually seen in the first 6 months after delivery. It may be due to an autoimmune reaction to fetal cells in the mother's thyroid gland.

At first, T_4 and T_3 levels increase in subacute, acute, and silent thyroiditis. They decrease with time. Suppressed radioactive iodine uptake (RAIU) occurs in subacute and silent thyroiditis. In Hashimoto thyroiditis, T_4 and T_3 levels are usually low and the TSH level is high. Antithyroid antibodies are present in Hashimoto thyroiditis.

Recovery from acute or subacute thyroiditis may be complete in weeks or months without any treatment. NSAIDs (e.g., aspirin, naproxen) can relieve symptoms. With more severe pain, corticosteroids (e.g., prednisone up to 40 mg/day) can relieve discomfort. Propranolol or atenolol may relieve cardiovascular symptoms related to a hyperthyroid state. Patients who are hypothyroid need thyroid hormone therapy.

Nursing care includes patient teaching about the disease process and treatment. Teach patients not to stop medications abruptly. Tell them to remain under close health care supervision so that progress can be monitored. Review changes in symptoms to report to the HCP, such as trouble breathing or swallowing, swelling to face and extremities, or rapid weight gain or loss. Those receiving thyroid hormone need to know the expected side effects and ways to manage them.

Patients with Hashimoto thyroiditis are at risk for other autoimmune diseases, such as Addison disease, pernicious anemia, or Graves disease. Teach patients the signs and symptoms of these problems.

HYPERTHYROIDISM

Hyperthyroidism is hyperactivity of the thyroid gland with sustained increase in synthesis and release of thyroid hormones.[11] It occurs in females, with the highest frequency in persons 20 to 40 years old. The most common cause is Graves disease (Fig. 54.7). Other causes include toxic nodular goiter, thyroiditis, excess iodine intake, pituitary tumors, and thyroid cancer. Since hyperthyroidism may be caused by iodinated contrast media used in CT scans and other radiologic studies, monitor those at risk after iodinated contrast media exposure.

Thyrotoxicosis refers to the physiologic effects or clinical syndrome of hypermetabolism resulting from excess circulating levels of T_4, T_3, or both. Hyperthyroidism and thyrotoxicosis

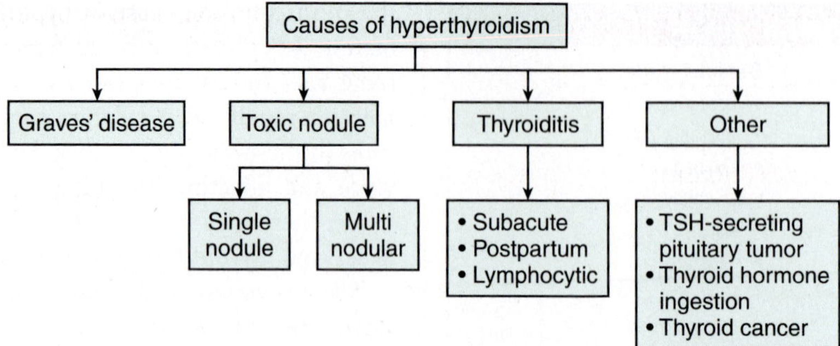

Fig. 54.7 Causes of hyperthyroidism.

usually occur together. Subclinical hyperthyroidism occurs when the TSH level is below 0.4 mU/L with normal T_4 and T_3 levels. Overt hyperthyroidism is defined by low or undetectable TSH and increased T_4 and T_3 levels. Patients may or may not have symptoms of hyperthyroidism.

Etiology and Pathophysiology

Graves disease is an autoimmune disease characterized by thyroid enlargement and excess thyroid hormone secretion. It accounts for 75% of the cases of hyperthyroidism. We do not know the exact cause. Risk factors, such as a lack of iodine, smoking, infection, and stress, may interact with genetic factors to cause Graves disease.

In Graves disease, patients develop antibodies to TSH receptors. These antibodies attach to the receptors and stimulate the thyroid gland to release T_3, T_4, or both. Excess thyroid hormones lead to the manifestations of thyrotoxicosis. Remissions and exacerbations occur, with or without treatment. It may progress to destruction of the thyroid tissue, causing hypothyroidism. Patients may have another autoimmune problem, such as rheumatoid arthritis, pernicious anemia, systemic lupus erythematosus, Addison disease, celiac disease, or vitiligo.

Clinical Manifestations

The manifestations are related to the effect of excess circulating thyroid hormones (Table 54.6). They directly increase metabolism and tissue sensitivity to sympathetic nervous system stimulation. Patients in the early stages may only have weight loss and increased nervousness. Manifestations in older adults and younger adults are compared in Table 54.7.

Palpation of the thyroid gland may reveal a goiter. When the thyroid gland is excessively large, you may be able to see a goiter (Fig. 54.6). Auscultating the thyroid gland may reveal bruits from the increased blood supply. A classic finding in Graves disease is *exophthalmos,* a protrusion of the eyeballs from the orbits (see Fig. 22.9). Exophthalmos results from increased fat deposits and fluid (edema) in the orbital tissues and ocular muscles. The increased pressure forces the eyeballs outward. The upper lids are usually retracted and elevated, with the sclera visible above the iris. When the eyelids do not close completely, the exposed corneal surfaces become dry and irritated. Corneal ulcers and loss of vision can occur. Changes in the ocular muscles result in muscle weakness, causing diplopia.

Complications

Acute thyrotoxicosis (thyrotoxic crisis or *thyroid storm)* is an acute, severe, rare condition that occurs when excess amounts of thyroid hormones are released into the circulation. Although considered a life-threatening emergency, death is rare when treatment is started early. We think that it results from stressors (e.g., infection, trauma, surgery) in patients with preexisting hyperthyroidism. Patients having a thyroidectomy are at risk because manipulation of the hyperactive thyroid gland results in the increased release of hormones.

In acute thyrotoxicosis, all the symptoms of hyperthyroidism are prominent and severe. Manifestations include severe tachycardia, heart failure, shock, fever, agitation, delirium, seizures, abdominal pain, vomiting, and diarrhea.

Diagnostic Studies

The primary laboratory findings used to confirm the diagnosis of hyperthyroidism are low or undetectable TSH levels ($<$0.4 mU/L) and increased free T_4 levels (Table 54.8). Total T_3 and T_4 levels may be assessed, but they are not as definitive. Total T_3 and T_4 determine free and bound (to protein) hormone levels. The free hormone is the only biologically active form of these hormones.

The RAIU test can distinguish Graves disease from other forms of thyroiditis. Patients with Graves disease have a diffuse, homogeneous uptake of 35% to 95%. Patients with thyroiditis show an uptake of less than 2%. Patients with a nodular goiter have an uptake in the high normal range.

Interprofessional Care

The goals of care are to block the adverse effects of excess thyroid hormone, suppress thyroid hormone secretion, and prevent complications. There are several treatment options. They include antithyroid medications, radioactive iodine (RAI) therapy, and surgery (Table 54.9). Supportive therapy is aimed at managing respiratory distress, reducing fever, replacing fluid,

TABLE 54.6 Manifestations of Thyroid Problems

Hyperfunction	Hypofunction
Cardiovascular	
• ↑ BP	• ↑ Capillary fragility
• ↑ Rate and force of cardiac contractions	• ↓ Rate and force of contractions
• Bounding, rapid pulse	• Varied changes in BP
• ↑ Cardiac output	• Cardiac hypertrophy
• Systolic murmurs	• Distant heart sounds
• Dysrhythmias	• Anemia
• Palpitations	• Heart failure
• Angina	• Angina
GI	
• ↑ Appetite, thirst	• ↓ Appetite
• Weight loss	• Weight gain
• ↑ Peristalsis	• Nausea and vomiting
• Diarrhea, frequent defecation	• Constipation
• ↑ Bowel sounds	• Distended abdomen
• Splenomegaly	• Enlarged, scaly tongue
• Hepatomegaly	
Musculoskeletal	
• Fatigue	• Fatigue
• Weakness	• Weakness
• Proximal muscle wasting	• Muscular aches and pains
• Dependent edema	• Slow movements
• Osteoporosis	• Arthralgia
Nervous	
• Hyperactive deep-tendon reflexes	• Prolonged relaxation of deep tendon reflexes
• Depression	• Anxiety, depression
• Lack of ability to concentrate	• Slowed mental processes
• Rapid speech	• Slow, slurred speech
• Insomnia	• Sleepiness
• Difficulty focusing eyes	• Apathy
• Nervousness	• Lethargy
• Fine tremor of fingers and tongue	• Forgetfulness
• Lability of mood, delirium	• Hoarseness
• Restlessness	• Stupor, coma
• Personality changes of irritability, agitation	• Paresthesias
• Stupor, coma	
Reproductive	
• Menstrual irregularities	• Prolonged menstrual periods or amenorrhea
• Amenorrhea	• ↓ Libido
• ↓ Libido	• Infertility
• ↓ Fertility	
• Impotence and gynecomastia in males	
Respiratory	
• Dyspnea on mild exertion	• Dyspnea
• ↑ Respiratory rate	
Skin	
• Warm, smooth, moist skin	• Dry, thick, inelastic, cold skin
• Thin, brittle nails detached from nail bed	• Thick, brittle nails
• Hair loss (may be patchy)	• Dry, sparse, coarse hair
• Clubbing of fingers (thyroid acropachy)	• Poor turgor
• Palmar erythema	• General edema
• Fine, silky hair	• Puffy face
• Premature graying	• ↓ Sweating
• Diaphoresis	• Pallor
• Vitiligo	
• Pretibial myxedema	
Other	
• Goiter (Fig. 54.6)	• Goiter
• Intolerance to heat	• Hearing problems
• Lid lag	• Intolerance to cold
• Eyelid retraction	• ↑ Risk for infection
• Exophthalmos	• ↑ Sensitivity to opioids, barbiturates, anesthesia
• ↑ Temperature	

and eliminating or managing the initiating stressor(s). The choice of treatment depends on patients' age and preferences, coexisting health problems, and pregnancy status.

Drug Therapy

Drugs used to treat hyperthyroidism include antithyroid drugs, iodine, and β-adrenergic blockers. These drugs are useful in treating thyrotoxic states but are not curative. Radiation therapy or surgery may be needed.

Antithyroid drugs. The first-line antithyroid drugs are propylthiouracil and methimazole. These drugs inhibit thyroid hormone synthesis. Reasons for use include Graves disease in young patients, hyperthyroidism during pregnancy, and the need to achieve a euthyroid state before surgery or radiation therapy. Propylthiouracil is generally used for patients who are in the first trimester of pregnancy, have had an adverse reaction to methimazole, or need a rapid reduction in symptoms. It is the first-line therapy in thyrotoxicosis since it blocks the peripheral conversion of T_4 to T_3. An advantage of propylthiouracil is that it achieves the goal of being euthyroid more quickly. However, it must be taken 3 times per day. Methimazole is given in a single daily dose.

Improvement usually begins 1 to 2 weeks after the start of drug therapy. We usually see results within 4 to 8 weeks. Therapy is usually continued for 6 to 15 months to allow for spontaneous remission, which occurs in 20% to 40% of patients. Teach patients the importance of adhering to the drug plan. Abruptly stopping drug therapy can result in a return of hyperthyroidism.

TABLE 54.7 Comparison of Hyperthyroidism in Younger and Older Adults

	Younger Adult	Older Adult
Common causes	Graves disease in >90% of cases	Graves disease, toxic nodular goiter
Common symptoms	Nervousness, irritability, weight loss, heat intolerance, warm moist skin	Anorexia, weight loss, apathy, lassitude, depression, confusion
Goiter	Present in >90% of cases	Present in ~50% of cases
Ophthalmopathy	Exophthalmos (Fig. 54.6) present in 20%–40% of cases	Exophthalmos less common
Cardiac features	↑ HR and palpitations common but without heart failure	Angina, dysrhythmia (especially atrial fibrillation with rapid ventricular response), heart failure may occur

TABLE 54.8 Laboratory Results for Hyperthyroid and Hypothyroid Patients

		HYPOTHYROID	
Test	**Hyperthyroid**	**Primary**	**Secondary**
Thyroid-stimulating hormone (TSH)	↓	↑	↓
T_4 (thyroxine)	↑	↓	↓
Total cholesterol	N	↑	↑
Low-density lipoproteins (LDLs)	↓	↑	↑
Triglycerides	N	↑	↑
Creatine kinase (CK)	N	↑	↑
Basal metabolic rate (BMR)	↑	↓	↓
Thyroid peroxidase (TPO) antibody	N	+ (in autoimmune hypothyroidism)	N

N, Normal; +, positive.

Iodine. Iodine is available as saturated solution of potassium iodine (SSKI) and Lugol solution. Iodine is used with other antithyroid drugs to prepare patients for thyroidectomy or treat thyrotoxicosis. Quickly giving large doses of iodine inhibits T_3 and T_4 synthesis and blocks their release into circulation. It decreases the vascularity of the thyroid gland, making surgery safer and easier. The maximal effect usually occurs within 1 to 2 weeks. Long-term iodine therapy is not an effective treatment because the therapeutic effect declines.

Iodine is mixed with water or juice and given after meals. Sipping it through a straw decreases the chance of it staining the teeth. Assess for signs of iodine toxicity. These include swelling of the buccal mucosa and other mucous membranes, excess salivation, nausea and vomiting, and skin reactions. If toxicity occurs, hold the iodine and notify the HCP.

TABLE 54.9 Interprofessional Care

Hyperthyroidism

Diagnostic Assessment

- History and physical assessment
- Ophthalmologic examination
- ECG
- Laboratory tests (Table 54.8)
  - TSH levels, free and total T_4, total T_3
  - Thyroid antibodies (e.g., thyroid peroxidase [TPO] antibody)
- Radioactive iodine uptake (RAIU)

Management

Drug Therapy

- Antithyroid drugs
  - Methimazole
  - Propylthiouracil
- Iodine (SSKI)
- β-Adrenergic blockers

Radiation Therapy

- Radioactive iodine

Surgical Therapy

- Subtotal thyroidectomy

Nutrition Therapy

- High-calorie, high-protein diet
- Frequent meals

β-Adrenergic blockers. β-Adrenergic blockers are used to relieve symptoms of thyrotoxicosis. They block the effects of sympathetic nervous stimulation, thereby decreasing tachycardia, nervousness, irritability, and tremors. Propranolol is usually given with antithyroid agents. Atenolol is the preferred β-adrenergic blocker in patients with asthma or heart disease.

Radioactive Iodine Therapy

RAI therapy is the treatment of choice for most nonpregnant adults. RAI damages or destroys thyroid tissue, thus limiting thyroid hormone secretion. RAI has a delayed response. The maximum effect may not be seen for up to 3 months. For this reason, patients are usually treated with antithyroid drugs and propranolol before and for 3 months after starting RAI until the effects of radiation become apparent. After treatment, 80% of patients are hypothyroid and need lifelong thyroid hormone therapy. Teach patients the symptoms of hypothyroidism and to seek medical help if these symptoms occur.

RAI therapy is usually given on an outpatient basis. A pregnancy test is done before starting therapy for all females who have menstrual cycles. Tell patients that radiation thyroiditis and parotitis are possible and may cause dryness and irritation of the mouth and throat. Relief may be obtained with frequent sips of water, ice chips, or a salt and soda gargle 3 or 4 times per day. Make this gargle by dissolving 1 tsp of salt and 1 tsp of baking soda in 2 cups of warm water. The discomfort should subside in 3 to 4 days. A mixture of antacid (Mylanta, Maalox), diphenhydramine, and viscous lidocaine can be used to swish and spit, increasing patient comfort when eating.

To limit radiation exposure to others, teach patients receiving RAI home precautions. These include (1) using private toilet facilities, if possible; (2) flushing 2 or 3 times after each use; (3) separately laundering towels, bed linens, and clothes daily at home; and (4) not preparing food for others that needs prolonged handling with bare hands. They should avoid being close to pregnant females and children for 7 days after therapy.

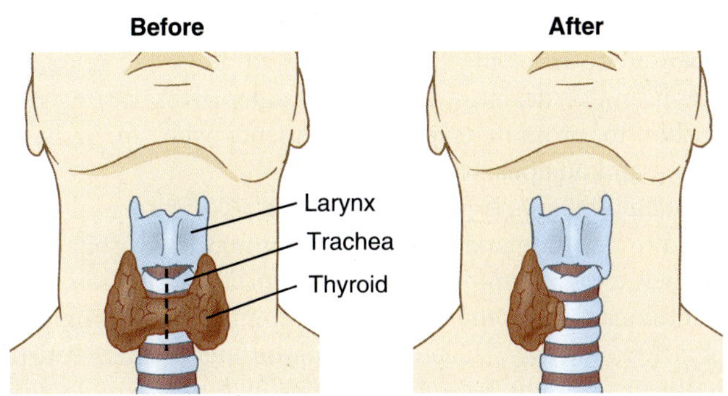

Fig. 54.8 Subtotal thyroidectomy. Part of the thyroid gland is removed.

Surgical Therapy

A thyroidectomy is done for those who have (1) a large goiter causing tracheal compression, (2) a lack of response to antithyroid therapy, or (3) thyroid cancer (Fig. 54.8). Surgery may be done when a person is not a candidate for RAI. One advantage that thyroidectomy has over RAI is a more rapid reduction in T_3 and T_4 levels. A *subtotal thyroidectomy* is the preferred surgical procedure. It involves removing a large portion (90%) of the thyroid gland.

Some patients may have minimally invasive endoscopic or robotic thyroidectomy. Endoscopic thyroidectomy is appropriate for patients with small nodules (less than 3 cm) and no evidence of cancer. Robotic surgery is best for those who are not overweight and have small nodules on only 1 side of the gland. Advantages of these procedures include less scarring, less pain, and a faster return to normal activity.

Nutrition Therapy

With the increased metabolic rate in hyperthyroid patients, there is a high risk for nutrition problems. A high-calorie diet (4000 to 5000 cal/day) may be needed to satisfy hunger, prevent tissue breakdown, and decrease weight loss. Patients may need 6 full meals a day and snacks high in protein, carbohydrates, minerals, and vitamins. The protein content should be 1 to 2 g/kg of ideal body weight. Increase carbohydrate intake to compensate for increased metabolism. Carbohydrates provide energy and decrease the use of body-stored protein. Teach patients to avoid highly seasoned and high-fiber foods because they can further stimulate the already hyperactive GI tract. Have them avoid caffeine-containing liquids, such as coffee, tea, and cola, to decrease the restlessness and sleep problems. Refer patients to a dietitian for help in meeting their nutrient needs.

❖ NURSING MANAGEMENT: HYPERTHYROIDISM

◆ Assessment

Subjective and objective data you should obtain from patients with hyperthyroidism are outlined in Table 54.10.

TABLE 54.10 NURSING ASSESSMENT

Hyperthyroidism

Subjective Data

Important Health Information

Health history: Preexisting goiter. Recent infection or trauma, immigration from iodine-deficient area, autoimmune disease

Medications: Thyroid hormones, drug therapies that may contain thyroid hormone

Functional Health Patterns

Health perception–health management: Positive family history of thyroid or autoimmune disorders

Nutritional-metabolic: Iodine intake, weight loss, ↑ appetite, thirst, nausea, vomiting

Elimination: Diarrhea, polyuria, sweating

Activity-exercise: Dyspnea on exertion, palpitations, muscle weakness, fatigue

Sleep-rest: Insomnia

Cognitive-perceptual: Chest pain, nervousness, heat intolerance, pruritus

Sexuality-reproductive: ↓ Libido, impotence and gynecomastia (males), amenorrhea (females)

Coping–stress tolerance: Emotional lability, irritability, restlessness, personality changes, delirium

Objective Data

Cardiovascular

↑ HR, bounding pulse, systolic murmurs, dysrhythmias, ↑ BP, bruit over the thyroid gland

Eyes

Exophthalmos, eyelid retraction, infrequent blinking

General

Agitation, rapid speech and body movements, anxiety, restlessness, fever, enlarged or nodular thyroid gland

GI

↑ Bowel sounds. ↑ Appetite, diarrhea, weight loss, liver and/or spleen enlargement

Neurologic

Hyperreflexia; diplopia. Fine tremors of hands, tongue, eyelids

Musculoskeletal

Muscle wasting

Reproductive

Menstrual irregularities, infertility, impotence, gynecomastia in males

Respiratory

Tachypnea, dyspnea on exertion

Skin

Warm, diaphoretic, velvety skin. Thin, loose nails. Fine, silky hair and hair loss. Palmar erythema, clubbing, white pigmentation of skin (vitiligo), pedal edema

Possible Diagnostic Findings

↑ T_3, ↑ T_4, ↑ T_3 *resin* uptake, ↓ or undetectable TSH. Chest x-ray showing enlarged heart. ECG findings of tachycardia, atrial fibrillation

◆ Clinical Problems

Clinical problems for patients with hyperthyroidism include:

- Impaired endocrine function
- Activity intolerance

Additional information on clinical problems and interventions is presented in eNursing Care Plan 54.1 for patients with hyperthyroidism (available on the website for this chapter).

◆ Planning

The overall goals are that patients with hyperthyroidism will (1) have relief of symptoms, (2) have no serious complications related to the disease or treatment, (3) maintain balanced nutrition, and (4) cooperate with the therapeutic plan.

◆ Implementation

Acute Care

Patients with hyperthyroidism are usually treated in an outpatient setting. However, those who develop acute thyrotoxicosis or undergo thyroidectomy need hospitalization and acute care.

Acute thyrotoxicosis. Acute thyrotoxicosis requires aggressive treatment, often in an intensive care unit (ICU).[12] Give medications that block thyroid hormone production and sympathetic nervous system effects. Provide supportive therapy, including monitoring for dysrhythmias and decompensation and ensuring adequate oxygenation. Give IV fluids to replace fluid and electrolyte losses. This is important in patients who have fluid losses from vomiting and diarrhea (Table 54.11).

Ensuring adequate rest may be a challenge because of irritability and restlessness. Use light bed coverings and change the linen often if the patient is diaphoretic. Encourage and assist with exercise involving large muscles to allow the release of tension and restlessness. Establish a supportive, trusting relationship to promote coping by patients who are irritable, restless, and anxious.

If exophthalmos is present, there is a risk for corneal injury related to irritation and dryness. Patients may have orbital pain. To relieve eye discomfort and prevent corneal ulceration, apply artificial tears to soothe and moisten conjunctival membranes. Restricting salt may help reduce periorbital edema. Patients should sit upright as much as possible to promote fluid drainage from the periorbital area.

Dark glasses reduce glare and prevent irritation from smoke, air currents, dust, and dirt. If the eyelids cannot be closed, lightly tape them shut for sleep. To maintain flexibility, teach patients to exercise the intraocular muscles several times a day by turning the eyes in the complete range of motion. Good grooming can help promote self-esteem from an altered body image. If the exophthalmos is severe, treatment options include corticosteroids, radiation of retroorbital tissues, orbital decompression, or corrective lid or muscle surgery.

Thyroid surgery. When a subtotal thyroidectomy is planned, patients must be adequately prepared to avoid complications. Before surgery, antithyroid drugs, iodine, and β-adrenergic blockers may be given to achieve a euthyroid state. Iodine decreases the vascularization of the thyroid gland, reducing the risk for bleeding.

Teach patients about routine postoperative care (see Chapter 18). Show them how to support the head manually while turning in bed, since this minimizes stress on the suture line after surgery. Have patients practice neck range-of-motion exercises. Tell patients that talking is likely to be difficult for a short time after surgery.

TABLE 54.11 EMERGENCY MANAGEMENT

Acute Thyrotoxicosis

Cause	Assessment Findings	Interventions

• Infection, surgery, trauma in a patient with hyperthyroidism
• Thyroidectomy
	• Abdominal pain
	• Agitation
	• Delirium
	• Diarrhea
	• Fever (up to 106°F [41.1°C])
	• Heart failure
	• Seizures
	• Severe tachycardia
	• Shock
	• Vomiting
		• IV fluid replacement with isotonic saline infusions containing dextrose.
		• Monitor airway, breathing, and circulation.
		• Monitor vital signs at least every 30 min.
		• Apply continuous O_2 saturation and ECG monitoring.
		• Monitor electrolytes, glucose, ABGs, calcium levels.
		• Monitor urine output hourly.
		• Apply ice packs and cooling blankets to reduce fever. Acetaminophen as needed.
		• Provide pulmonary hygiene.
		• Assess for manifestations of heart failure or pulmonary edema (e.g., extra heart sounds, adventitious lung sounds).
		• Provide calm, quiet environment.
		• Restrict visitors, if needed.
		• Give prescribed drugs and monitor effects:
		  • β-Adrenergic blockers
		  • Antithyroid agents
		  • Iodine compounds
		  • Glucocorticoids

TABLE 54.12 NURSING MANAGEMENT

Care of Patients After Thyroid Surgery

- Assess vital signs every 15 min until stable and then every 30 min for the first 24 h after surgery.
- Monitor airway and respiratory status (patency, rate, rhythm, depth, and effort).
- Assess every 2 h for 24 h for signs of hemorrhage or tracheal compression (e.g., irregular breathing, neck swelling, frequent swallowing, choking, blood on the dressings, sensations of fullness at the incision site).
- Assist the patient with coughing and deep breathing.
- Apply O_2 therapy with humidification as ordered.
- Have suction equipment and a tracheostomy kit available for immediate use.
- Assess the ability to speak aloud, noting voice quality, tone, and any problems speaking. Notify the HCP of any permanent hoarseness or loss of vocal volume.
- Monitor calcium levels. Assess for signs of tetany and hypocalcemia (e.g., tingling in toes, fingers, around the mouth; muscular twitching; apprehension) and any trouble with speaking or hoarseness. Check Trousseau sign and Chvostek sign (see Fig. 17.15).
- Keep IV calcium (calcium gluconate, calcium chloride) available for immediate use.
- Assess surgical site and dressing. Monitor the area under the neck and shoulders for drainage.
- Keep the patient in a semi-Fowler position. Support the head and neck with pillows. Avoid neck flexion to prevent tension on the suture line.
- Provide comfort measures and give prescribed analgesics.
- Give oral fluids as soon as tolerated. Start a soft diet the day after surgery.

Postoperative complications include hypothyroidism, damage to or inadvertent removal of parathyroid glands (causing hypoparathyroidism and hypocalcemia), bleeding, injury to the recurrent or superior laryngeal nerve, thyrotoxicosis, and infection. Recurrent laryngeal nerve damage leads to vocal cord paralysis. If both cords are paralyzed, spastic airway obstruction will occur, requiring an immediate tracheostomy.

SAFETY ALERT

Airway Obstruction

- Airway obstruction after thyroid surgery is an emergency.
- Keep O_2, suction equipment, and a tracheostomy tray available in the room.

Respiration may become difficult because of excess swelling of the neck tissues, bleeding, and hematoma formation. *Laryngeal stridor* (harsh, vibratory sound) may occur because of laryngeal nerve edema. It may be related to tetany from hypocalcemia, which occurs if the parathyroid glands were removed or damaged during surgery. To treat tetany, have IV calcium salts (e.g., calcium gluconate) available (Table 54.12).

Rebreathing may partially relieve the acute neuromuscular symptoms from hypocalcemia, including muscle cramps and mild tetany. Have patients breathe in and out of a paper bag or breathing mask. This reduces CO_2 excretion from the lungs, increases carbonic acid levels in the blood, and lowers the pH. A lower pH (acidic environment) enhances calcium ionization. This causes more total body calcium to be available in the active form.

Because of the surgical site location and the risk for hypocalcemia perform frequent assessments. Monitor vital signs. Assess for airway obstruction, bleeding, and tetany. Expect some hoarseness for 3 or 4 days after surgery because of edema. If recovery is uneventful, patients ambulate within hours after surgery.

DRUG ALERT

IV Calcium

- Give IV calcium slowly.
- Use ECG monitoring when giving calcium since high calcium levels can cause hypotension, dysrhythmias, or cardiac arrest.
- Assess IV patency as venous irritation and inflammation can occur.
- Extravasation may cause cellulitis, necrosis, and tissue sloughing.

The appearance of the incision may be distressing to patients. Reassure them that the scar will fade in color and eventually look like a normal neck wrinkle. A scarf, jewelry, a high collar, or other covering can effectively camouflage the scar.

Chronic Care

Teach patients and caregivers that thyroid hormone balance will be monitored periodically. Most patients have a period of relative hypothyroidism soon after surgery because of the substantial reduction in the size of the thyroid. The remaining tissue usually hypertrophies over time and recovers the ability to make hormones. We usually do not give thyroid hormone because the exogenous hormone inhibits pituitary production of TSH and delays or prevents the restoration of normal gland function and tissue regeneration.

To prevent weight gain, caloric intake must be greatly reduced to less than the amount that was needed before surgery. Adequate iodine is needed to promote thyroid function, but excesses can inhibit the thyroid gland. Seafood once or twice a week or normal use of iodized salt should provide enough iodine intake. Encourage regular exercise to stimulate the thyroid gland. Teach patients to avoid high environment temperatures because they inhibit thyroid regeneration.

Regular follow-up care is needed. Patients should see the HCP biweekly for a month and then at least semiannually to assess thyroid function. Tell patients who had a complete thyroidectomy about the need for lifelong thyroid hormone replacement. Teach them the signs and symptoms of thyroid failure and to seek medical care promptly if these develop.

◆ Evaluation

The expected outcomes are patients with hyperthyroidism will:

- Have relief of symptoms
- Have no serious complications related to the disease or treatment
- Cooperate with the therapeutic plan
- Maintain balanced nutrition

HYPOTHYROIDISM

Hypothyroidism is a deficiency of thyroid hormone that causes a general slowing of the metabolic rate. About 4% of the U.S. population has mild hypothyroidism, with about 0.3% having more severe disease. Hypothyroidism is more common in females. Subclinical hypothyroidism occurs when the TSH is greater than 4.5 mU/L, but the T_4 levels are normal. Up to 10% of females older than 60 years have subclinical hypothyroidism. Patients with overt hypothyroidism have increased TSH and decreased T_4 levels. Critically ill patients may present with nonthyroidal illness syndrome (NTIS).[13] Those with NTIS have low T_3, T_4, and TSH levels.

Etiology and Pathophysiology

We classify hypothyroidism as primary or secondary. *Primary hypothyroidism* is caused by destruction of thyroid tissue or defective hormone synthesis. *Secondary hypothyroidism* is caused by pituitary disease with decreased TSH secretion or hypothalamic dysfunction with decreased thyrotropin-releasing hormone (TRH) secretion. Hypothyroidism can be brief and related to thyroiditis or stopping thyroid hormone therapy.

Iodine deficiency is the most common cause of hypothyroidism worldwide. In the United States the most common cause of primary hypothyroidism is atrophy of the thyroid gland. Atrophy is the result of Hashimoto thyroiditis or Graves disease. These autoimmune diseases destroy the thyroid gland. Hypothyroidism can develop after treatment for hyperthyroidism, specifically thyroidectomy or RAI therapy, or radiation therapy in the head and neck area. Drugs such as amiodarone, which contains iodine, and lithium, which blocks hormone production, can cause hypothyroidism. Other risk factors include age, type 1 diabetes, Down syndrome, and a family history of thyroid disease.[14]

Hypothyroidism that develops in infancy *(cretinism)* results from thyroid hormone deficiencies during fetal or early neonatal life. In the United States we screen all infants for decreased thyroid function at birth.

Clinical Manifestations

With hypothyroidism we see a slowing of body processes (Table 54.6). Manifestations vary depending on the severity and the duration of thyroid deficiency and age at onset. Symptoms may develop over months to years, unless hypothyroidism occurs after a thyroidectomy, after thyroid ablation, or during treatment with antithyroid drugs.

Patients are often tired and lethargic. There may be personality and mental changes, including impaired memory, slowed speech, decreased initiative, and somnolence. Many appear depressed. Weight gain is a result of a decreased metabolic rate.

Hypothyroidism may cause significant cardiovascular problems, especially in a person with a history of CVD. It can cause decreased cardiac contractility and decreased cardiac output. Patients may have low exercise tolerance and shortness of breath on exertion. High cholesterol and triglyceride levels and the accumulation of mucopolysaccharides in the intima of small blood vessels can result in coronary atherosclerosis. Anemia is common.

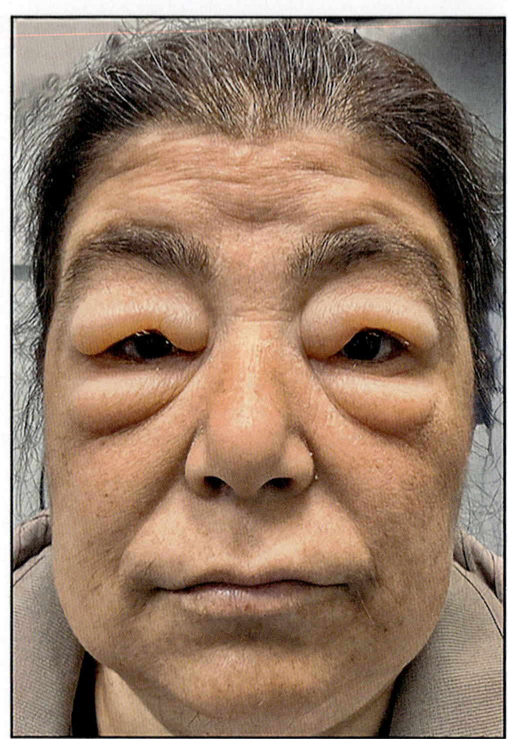

Fig. 54.9 Facial appearance of hypothyroidism. The patient has periorbital edema and coarse, sparse hair. (From Levinkron O, Ah-kye L, Vahdani K: Rapid resolution of periorbital myxedema after hypothyroidism treatment, *Ophthalmology*, 2024.)

Patients with severe, long-standing hypothyroidism may have **myxedema**. Myxedema results from the accumulation of hydrophilic mucopolysaccharides in the dermis and other tissues (Fig. 54.9). It alters the physical appearance of the skin and subcutaneous tissues with puffiness, facial and periorbital edema, and a mask-like affect. Patients may have an altered self-image related to their altered appearance.

In the older adult, we may attribute manifestations of hypothyroidism (fatigue, cold and dry skin, hair loss, constipation, cold intolerance) to normal aging. For this reason, symptoms may not raise suspicion of an underlying condition. Older adults who have confusion, lethargy, and depression should be screened for thyroid disease.

Complications

Hypothyroidism may progress suddenly to a notable impairment of consciousness or coma. This situation, termed *myxedema coma,* is a medical emergency. Cause of myxedema coma include infection, drugs (especially opioids, tranquilizers, and barbiturates), exposure to cold, and trauma. Manifestations include low temperature, hypotension, and hypoventilation. Cardiovascular collapse can result from hypoventilation, hyponatremia, hypoglycemia, and lactic acidosis. For patients to survive myxedema coma, we must support vital functions and give IV thyroid hormone replacement.

Diagnostic Studies

TSH and free T_4 values, correlated with findings from the history and physical assessment, confirm the diagnosis of hypothyroidism (Table 54.8).[14] TSH levels help determine the cause. TSH is high when the defect is in the thyroid and low when it is in the pituitary or the hypothalamus. The presence of thyroid antibodies suggests an autoimmune origin. Other abnormal laboratory findings are high cholesterol and triglycerides, anemia, and increased creatine kinase.

Interprofessional Care

The treatment goal is to restore a euthyroid state as safely and quickly as possible with hormone therapy (Table 54.13). Levothyroxine (Synthroid) is the drug of choice to treat hypothyroidism. In young and otherwise healthy patients, the maintenance replacement dosage is based on their clinical response and laboratory findings. When beginning thyroid hormone therapy, the first dosages are low to avoid increases in resting heart rate and BP. In patients with compromised cardiac status, monitoring is needed when starting and adjusting the dosage because the usual dose may increase myocardial O_2 demand. This may cause angina and dysrhythmias.

DRUG ALERT

Levothyroxine

- Monitor patients with CVD who take this drug.
- Assess heart rate and report pulse greater than 100 beats/min or an irregular heartbeat.
- Promptly report chest pain, weight loss, nervousness, tremors, or insomnia.

TABLE 54.13 Interprofessional Care

Hypothyroidism

Diagnostic Assessment
- History and physical assessment
- TSH, total and free T_4, total T_3
- Thyroid peroxidase (TPO) antibodies

Management
- Thyroid hormone replacement (e.g., levothyroxine)
- Monitor thyroid hormone levels and adjust dosage as needed
- Nutrition therapy to promote weight loss
- Patient and caregiver teaching (Table 54.14)

In patients without side effects, the dose is increased at 4- to 6-week intervals as needed based on the TSH levels. It may take 8 weeks to see the full effect of hormone therapy. Levothyroxine has a peak of action of 1 to 3 weeks. Patients must regularly take replacement medication. Lifelong thyroid therapy is usually needed.

NURSING MANAGEMENT: HYPOTHYROIDISM

Assessment

Assessment may reveal early and subtle changes in patients suspected of having hypothyroidism. Note any history of hyperthyroidism and treatment with antithyroid medications, RAI, or surgery. Ask patients about using iodine-containing medications (Table 54.5). Note any changes in appetite, weight, activity level, speech, memory, and skin (e.g., increased dryness or thickening). Assess for cold intolerance, constipation, and signs of depression. Further assessment should focus on heart rate, tenderness over the thyroid gland, and edema in the extremities and face.

Clinical Problems

Clinical problems for patients with hypothyroidism may include:

- Impaired endocrine function
- Activity intolerance
- Constipation

Additional information on clinical problems and interventions is presented in the eNursing Care Plan 54.2 for patients with hypothyroidism (available on the website for this chapter).

Planning

The overall goals are that patients with hypothyroidism will (1) have relief of symptoms, (2) maintain a euthyroid state, (3) maintain a positive self-image, and (4) adhere with lifelong thyroid therapy.

Implementation

Acute Care

Most people with hypothyroidism are treated on an outpatient basis. The person who develops myxedema coma needs acute nursing care, often in the ICU. They often need mechanical respiratory support and cardiac monitoring.

Give thyroid hormone therapy and all other medications IV because severe gastric hypomotility may prevent the absorption of oral agents. Monitor the core temperature for hypothermia that often occurs in myxedema coma. Use gentle soap. Moisturize often to prevent skin breakdown. Frequent position changes and a low-pressure mattress help maintain skin integrity.

Monitor patients' progress by assessing vital signs, weight, intake and output, and edema. Cardiac assessment is important because the cardiovascular response to hormone therapy determines the medication regimen. Note energy level and mental alertness. They should improve within 2 to 14 days and continue a steady progression to normal levels. Neurologic status and TSH levels are used to determine continuing treatment.

Chronic Care

Provide patient teaching about medication management and complications (Table 54.14). Hypothyroidism can significantly impair quality of life due to the symptoms associated with the condition. Even with treatment, many persons continue to have fatigue and other issues that affect their well-being (Box 54.1).

Stress the need to follow lifelong drug therapy as prescribed. Some patients notice weight loss and are tempted to increase dosing to achieve a desired weight. Review the side effects, including the signs and symptoms of hypothyroidism and hyperthyroidism (Table 54.6). The manifestations of overdose are the same as hyperthyroidism. Tell patients to contact the HCP at once if symptoms are present.

Patients with diabetes should check glucose levels at least daily because the return to the euthyroid state often increases insulin requirements. Thyroid drugs increase the effects of anticoagulants. Stress the need to remain under close medical observation until stable.

TABLE 54.14 PATIENT & CAREGIVER TEACHING

Hypothyroidism

Include the following instructions when teaching patients and caregivers about managing hypothyroidism:

1. Discuss thyroid hormone therapy:
   - Need for lifelong therapy
   - Taking thyroid hormone in the morning before food
   - Need for regular follow-up care and monitoring of thyroid hormone levels
   - Avoid abruptly stopping drugs
   - Do not double up on doses for any reason
   - Side effects, including hypothyroidism and hyperthyroidism
   - When to contact the HCP
2. Caution patients not to switch brands of the hormone since the bioavailability of thyroid hormones may differ.
3. Teach ways to prevent skin breakdown. Use soap sparingly. Apply lotion to skin.
4. Caution patients, especially older adults, to avoid sedatives. If they must be used, suggest that the lowest dose be used. Caregivers should closely monitor mental status, level of consciousness, and respirations.
5. Discuss ways to minimize constipation, including:
   - Gradual increase in activity and exercise
   - Increased fiber in diet
   - Use of stool softeners
   - Regular bowel elimination time
   - Avoid using enemas. They cause vagal stimulation, which can be hazardous if heart disease is present

With treatment, striking transformations occur in appearance and mental function. Most adults return to a normal state. Cardiovascular conditions may persist after correcting the hormone imbalance. Relapses occur if treatment is interrupted.

◆ Evaluation

The expected outcomes are that patients with hypothyroidism will:

- Have relief from symptoms
- Maintain an euthyroid state with normal thyroid hormone and TSH levels
- Avoid complications of therapy
- Adhere to lifelong therapy

BOX 54.1 EVIDENCE-BASED PRACTICE

Quality of Life in Patients With Hypothyroidism

You are working in the clinic when B.F., a 53-year-old patient, checks in for an appointment. B.F. was diagnosed with hypothyroidism about 9 months ago. Despite treatment, B.F.'s TSH levels continue to fluctuate. Her husband is with her today. While B.F. is having blood drawn for laboratory testing, he tells you she seems depressed and continues to have memory problems. He adds, "She is not interested in much lately."

Making Clinical Decisions

Synthesis of Best Available Evidence

Living with hypothyroidism can significantly impair quality of life and a sense of well-being. In addition to traditional therapy, research suggests a holistic approach incorporating alternative therapies such as yoga and gentle exercise helps improve quality of life and stabilize thyroid hormone levels.

Clinician Expertise

When B.F. returns, you take her vital signs and begin the usual intake questions. You ask, "How have you been sleeping? Do you have enough energy for regular activity?" She looks at her husband but initially says nothing. You continue, "We know that people with hypothyroidism often feel fatigued and may even become depressed." B.F. responds, "Some days I don't really feel like doing much. I know I need to get active again to try to lose weight." You encourage B.F. by responding, "Let's talk about the things you like to do that will help you become more active again. Would you consider attending a new program where we focus on holistic care, including meditation and other relaxation techniques, to help patients cope with their illness?"

Patient Preferences and Values

B.F. returns to the clinic for follow-up 4 months after starting the program. She states she feels much better, is finally enjoying life again, and does not feel so exhausted. Serum TSH levels are stable and no further medication adjustments have been needed in the past 8 weeks.

Implications for Nursing Practice

1. What aspects of health-related quality of life may be affected by hypothyroidism?
2. How can we best address these issues with our patients?

Reference for Evidence

Salina S, Leena KC: Effect of nurse led multi-intervention program on quality of life, subjective well-being, and level of thyroid hormones among patients with hypothyroidism: a quasi-experimental double arm study, *J Clin Diag Res*, 17:18, 2023.

THYROID NODULES AND CANCER

A *thyroid nodule* (growth in the thyroid gland) may be benign or malignant (thyroid cancer). More than 95% of thyroid gland nodules are benign. The risk of developing a thyroid nodule increases with age. Benign nodules are usually not dangerous. They can cause tracheal compression if they become too large.

Thyroid cancer is the most common type of endocrine cancer. Around 62,450 new cases of thyroid cancer are diagnosed each year. The incidence of thyroid cancer has increased significantly in the past 25 years. Thyroid cancer affects more females. The incidence is higher in White persons and Asian Americans. Adults at risk include those who had head and neck radiation therapy during childhood, were exposed to radioactive fallout, or have a personal or family history of goiter.[15]

Types of Thyroid Cancer

The 4 main types of thyroid cancer are papillary, follicular, medullary, and anaplastic. *Papillary* thyroid cancer is the most common type. It accounts for about 70% to 80% of thyroid cancers.[9] Papillary cancer tends to grow slowly. It initially spreads to lymph nodes in the neck.

Follicular thyroid cancer makes up about 15% of thyroid cancers. It tends to occur in older patients. Follicular cancer first metastasizes into the cervical lymph nodes and then spreads to the neck, lungs, and bones.

Medullary thyroid cancer accounts for only 10% of thyroid cancers. It is more likely to occur in families and be associated with other endocrine problems. It is diagnosed by genetic testing for a proto-oncogene called *RET.* Medullary thyroid cancer is a type of multiple endocrine neoplasia (MEN).[16] It is associated with early metastasis.

Anaplastic thyroid cancer occurs in less than 2% of patients with thyroid cancer. It is the most advanced and aggressive thyroid cancer, and patients are least likely to respond to treatment and have a poor prognosis.

Clinical Manifestations and Diagnostic Studies

The primary manifestation of thyroid cancer is a painless, palpable nodule or nodules in an enlarged thyroid gland. Most nodules are found during routine palpation of the neck. Firm, palpable, cervical masses suggest lymph node metastasis. Some patients may have trouble swallowing or breathing if tumor growth invades the trachea or esophagus. Hemoptysis and airway obstruction may occur if the trachea is involved. Patients generally are euthyroid.

Any nodular enlargement or palpation of a thyroid mass requires further evaluation. Ultrasound is often the first test used.[14] Follow-up testing may involve CT, MRI, and ultrasound-guided fine-needle aspiration (FNA). An FNA is done when a tissue sample for pathologic examination is needed. A thyroid scan may be done. The scan shows whether nodules on the thyroid are "hot" or "cold." "Hot" tumors take up RAI. They are almost always benign. If the nodule does not take up the RAI, it appears "cold." There is a higher risk for cancer.

Increased calcitonin is associated with medullary thyroid cancer. In papillary and follicular cancers, thyroglobulin is high. In families with a history of medullary thyroid cancer, we encourage genetic testing and thyroid screening on a regular basis.

Interprofessional and Nursing Management

Surgical removal of the tumor is the main treatment for thyroid cancer. Procedures range from unilateral total lobectomy to near-total thyroidectomy with bilateral lobectomy. Lymph nodes in the neck may be removed to determine whether the cancer has spread. Some patients may receive RAI after surgery to destroy any remaining cancer cells. RAI therapy improves survival rates in patients with papillary and follicular thyroid cancer. External beam radiation is a palliative treatment for metastatic thyroid cancer.

Many thyroid cancers are TSH dependent. Thyroid hormone therapy in high doses is often prescribed to inhibit TSH secretion. Chemotherapy, including doxorubicin, may be used for advanced disease. Targeted therapies for metastatic cancer include vandetanib (Caprelsa), lenvatinib (Lenvima), sorafenib tosylate (Nexavar), and cabozantinib (Cometriq). These drugs inhibit tyrosine kinases, enzymes that promote cancer cell growth. Nursing care for patients with thyroid cancer is similar to that of patients undergoing thyroidectomy (Table 54.12).

MULTIPLE ENDOCRINE NEOPLASIA

Multiple endocrine neoplasia (MEN) is an inherited condition characterized by hormone-secreting tumors.[16] It is caused by the mutation of 1 of 2 genes, *MEN1* or *RET,* that normally control cell growth. Tumors may develop in childhood or later in life.

The 2 major types are type 1 and type 2. Both are often inherited as autosomal dominant disorders. Persons with type 1 often have hyperparathyroidism. Other signs may include hyperactivity of the pituitary gland (prolactinoma) and pancreas (gastrinoma). In most cases, the tumors are initially benign. Some tumors later become malignant. Persons with type 2 neoplasia often have medullary thyroid carcinoma. They may develop pheochromocytoma (tumor of the adrenal glands).

Treatment includes conservative management (watchful waiting), drugs to block the effects of excess hormone, and surgical removal of the gland and/or tumor. Patients must have regular screening visits with the HCP so that new tumors may be detected early and existing tumors carefully monitored.

PARATHYROID GLAND PROBLEMS

HYPERPARATHYROIDISM

Etiology and Pathophysiology

Hyperparathyroidism is a condition involving an increased parathyroid hormone (PTH) secretion. PTH helps regulate calcium and phosphate levels by stimulating bone resorption of calcium, renal tubular reabsorption of calcium, and vitamin D activation. Thus PTH oversecretion causes increased calcium levels.

There are primary, secondary, and tertiary forms. *Primary hyperparathyroidism* is due to an increased PTH secretion.[17] It affects 25 of 100,000 persons per year. The peak incidence is in the 40s and 50s. It affects twice as many females. The most common cause is a benign tumor (adenoma) in the parathyroid gland. Patients who have had head and neck radiation have an increased risk for developing a parathyroid adenoma. Long-term lithium therapy is a risk factor.

Secondary hyperparathyroidism is a compensatory response to conditions that induce or cause hypocalcemia, the main stimulus of PTH secretion. These include vitamin D deficiencies, malabsorption, chronic kidney disease, and high phosphorus levels.

Tertiary hyperparathyroidism occurs when there is excess growth of the parathyroid glands and a loss of negative feedback from circulating calcium levels. Thus there is autonomous PTH secretion even with normal calcium levels. This may happen in patients who have a kidney transplant after a long period of dialysis treatment for chronic kidney disease (see Chapter 51).

Clinical Manifestations

High PTH levels usually lead to hypercalcemia and hypophosphatemia. Multiple body systems are affected (Table 54.15). Loss of appetite, constipation, fatigue, emotional problems, shortened attention span, and muscle weakness, especially in the proximal muscles of the lower extremities, often occur. Decreased bone density can occur because of PTH's effect on bone resorption and bone formation activity. Patients may have osteoporosis and long bone, rib, and vertebral fractures. The kidneys cannot reabsorb the excess calcium. This leads to high urine calcium levels (hypercalciuria). This excess calcium, along

TABLE 54.15 Manifestations of Parathyroid Problems

Hyperfunction	Hypofunction
Cardiovascular	
• ↑ BP	• ↓ BP
• Angina	• Edema
• Dysrhythmias	• Dysrhythmias
• Shortened ST segment	• Elongation of ST segment
• Shortened QT interval	• Prolonged QT interval
• ↑ Digitalis effect	• ↓ Cardiac output
Gastrointestinal	
• Vague abdominal pain	• Abdominal cramps
• Anorexia	• Fecal incontinence (in older adult)
• Nausea and vomiting	• Malabsorption
• Constipation	
• Pancreatitis	
• Peptic ulcer disease	
• Cholelithiasis	
• Weight loss	
Laboratory Findings	
• ↑ Calcium	• ↓ Calcium
• ↓ Phosphorus	• ↑ Phosphorus
Musculoskeletal	
• Weakness, fatigue	• Weakness, fatigue
• Skeletal pain	• Painful muscle cramps
• Backache	• Skeletal x-ray changes, osteosclerosis
• Pain on weight bearing	• Soft tissue calcification
• Osteoporosis	• Problems walking
• Pathologic fractures of long bones	
• Compression fractures of spine; kyphosis	
• ↓ Muscle tone, muscle atrophy	
Neurologic	
• Lethargy, weakness, fatigue	• Weakness, fatigue
• Psychosis, depression	• Depression
• Depressed reflexes	• Hyperreflexia, muscle cramps
• Personality changes	• Personality changes
• Irritability	• Irritability
• Impaired memory	• Impaired memory
• Delirium, confusion, coma	• Disorientation, confusion (in older adult)
• Headache	• Headache, ↑ intracranial pressure
• Poor coordination	• Tetany, seizures
• Gait abnormalities	• Positive Chvostek and Trousseau signs
• Psychomotor retardation	• Tremor
• Paresthesias	• Paresthesias of lips, hands, feet
Renal/Urinary	
• Hypercalciuria	• Urinary frequency
• Kidney stones	• Urinary incontinence
• Urinary tract infections	
• Polyuria	
Skin	
• Skin necrosis	• Dry, scaly skin
• Moist skin	• Hair loss on scalp and body
	• Brittle nails, transverse ridging
	• Lack of tooth enamel
Visual	
• Impaired vision	• Eye changes, including lenticular opacities, cataracts, papilledema
• Corneal calcification	

with a large amount of urine phosphate, can lead to stone formation and kidney failure.

Diagnostic Studies

Patients with hyperparathyroidism have increased PTH levels. Calcium levels usually exceed 10 mg/dL (2.50 mmol/L). Because of its inverse relation with calcium, the phosphorus level is usually less than 3 mg/dL (0.1 mmol/L). Asymptomatic hypercalcemia is often found through a routine chemistry panel. Bone density measurements may be used to detect bone loss. Conversely, those with bone loss on a screening dual energy x-ray absorptiometry (DEXA) scan should be screened for high calcium levels. MRI, CT, and/or ultrasound can detect an adenoma.

Interprofessional Care

The goal of treatment is to relieve symptoms and prevent complications caused by excess PTH. The choice of therapy depends on patients' condition, calcium levels, and underlying cause.

Surgical Therapy

The most effective treatment of primary and secondary disease is surgery. Surgery involves partial or complete removal of the parathyroid glands. The most common procedure involves outpatient endoscopy. Criteria for surgery include increased calcium levels, hypercalciuria (greater than 400 mg/day), markedly reduced bone mineral density, overt symptoms (e.g., neuromuscular effects, kidney stones), or age under 50 years. Parathyroidectomy leads to a rapid reduction of high calcium levels.

Patients who have multiple parathyroid glands removed may undergo autotransplantation of normal parathyroid tissue in the forearm or near the sternocleidomastoid muscle. This allows PTH secretion to continue with normal calcium levels. If autotransplantation is not possible or if it fails, patients will need to take calcium supplements for life.

Nonsurgical Therapy

A conservative approach is often used in patients who are asymptomatic or have mild symptoms. Ongoing care includes regular measurement of PTH, calcium, phosphorus, alkaline phosphatase, creatinine and blood urea nitrogen (BUN) (to assess renal function), and urine calcium excretion. Annual x-rays and DEXA scans assess for metabolic bone loss. Continued ambulation and avoiding immobility are important. Diet measures include high fluid and moderate calcium intake.

Severe hypercalcemia is managed with IV sodium chloride and loop diuretics, such as furosemide, to increase urine calcium excretion. Several drugs help lower calcium levels. Bisphosphonates (e.g., alendronate) inhibit osteoclastic bone resorption, normalizing calcium levels and improving bone mineral density. IV bisphosphonates (e.g., pamidronate) can quickly lower calcium in patients with dangerously high levels. Phosphates are given if patients have normal renal function and low phosphate levels.

Calcimimetic agents (e.g., cinacalcet [Sensipar]) increase the sensitivity of calcium receptors on the parathyroid gland, resulting in decreased PTH secretion and calcium levels. They are useful in treating secondary hyperparathyroidism in patients with parathyroid cancer or chronic kidney disease on dialysis.

❖ NURSING MANAGEMENT: HYPERPARATHYROIDISM

Nursing care for patients after a parathyroidectomy is similar to that for patients after thyroidectomy (Table 54.12). The major complications are bleeding and fluid and electrolyte problems. *Tetany* from a sudden decrease in calcium levels is a concern. It is usually apparent early in the postoperative period but may develop over several days. Mild tetany, characterized by unpleasant tingling of the hands and around the mouth, may be present. It should decrease over time. If tetany becomes more severe (e.g., muscular spasms, laryngospasms), IV calcium may be given. Keep IV calcium gluconate available in case acute tetany occurs.

Monitor intake and output to evaluate fluid status. Assess calcium, potassium, phosphate, and magnesium levels frequently. Monitor Chvostek and Trousseau signs (see Fig. 17.15). Encourage mobility to promote bone calcification.

If surgery is not done, treatment to relieve symptoms and prevent complications is started. Help patients adapt the meal plan to their lifestyle. A referral to a dietitian may be helpful. Because immobility can worsen bone loss, stress the importance of an exercise program. Encourage patients to keep their follow-up appointments. Teach patients the symptoms of high and low calcium levels and to report them if they occur. Calcium imbalances are discussed in Chapter 17.

HYPOPARATHYROIDISM

Hypoparathyroidism is an uncommon condition associated with inadequate circulating PTH. Hypocalcemia occurs due to a lack of PTH to maintain calcium levels. The most common cause is iatrogenic. This may include accidental removal of the parathyroid glands or damage to the vascular supply of the glands during neck surgery (e.g., thyroidectomy).

Idiopathic hypoparathyroidism from the absence, fatty replacement, or atrophy of the glands is rare. It usually occurs early in life and may be associated with other endocrine problems. Affected patients may have antiparathyroid antibodies. Severe hypomagnesemia (e.g., malnutrition, alcohol use, kidney failure) can suppress PTH secretion. Other causes include tumors and heavy metal poisoning. PTH resistance at the cell level may occur *(pseudohypoparathyroidism)*. This is caused by a genetic defect resulting in hypocalcemia despite normal or high PTH levels. It is often associated with hypothyroidism and hypogonadism.

The features of acute hypoparathyroidism are due to hypocalcemia (Table 54.15). Sudden decreases in calcium levels cause tetany, characterized by tingling of the lips and stiffness in the extremities. Painful tonic spasms of smooth and skeletal muscles can cause dysphagia and laryngospasms, which compromise breathing. Lethargy, anxiety, and personality changes may occur. Laboratory findings include decreased calcium and PTH and increased phosphate levels.

Interprofessional and Nursing Management

Treatment goals are to treat acute complications, such as tetany, maintain normal calcium levels, and prevent long-term complications. Emergency treatment of tetany after thyroid or parathyroid surgery requires IV calcium administration (Table 54.12). Teach patients how to manage long-term drug and nutrition therapy. Most receive oral calcium and magnesium supplements and vitamin D. Vitamin D enhances intestinal calcium absorption. A high-calcium meal plan includes foods, such as dark green vegetables, soybeans, and tofu. Tell patients to avoid foods containing oxalic acid (e.g., spinach, rhubarb) because they inhibit calcium absorption. Teach patients about the need for follow-up care, including monitoring of calcium levels 3 or 4 times a year.

ADRENAL CORTEX PROBLEMS

CUSHING SYNDROME

Etiology and Pathophysiology

Cushing syndrome is a clinical condition that results from chronic exposure to excess glucocorticoids (cortisol).[18] Several conditions can cause Cushing syndrome. The most common is iatrogenic administration of exogenous corticosteroids (e.g., prednisone). About 85% of the cases of endogenous Cushing syndrome are due to an ACTH-secreting pituitary adenoma (Cushing disease). Less common causes include adrenal tumors and ectopic ACTH production by tumors (usually of the lung or pancreas) outside of the hypothalamic-pituitary-adrenal axis. Cushing disease and primary adrenal tumors are more common in females 20 to 40 years old. Ectopic ACTH production is more common in males.

Clinical Manifestations

Manifestations occur in most body systems. Most are related to excess cortisol levels (Table 54.16). Patients have pronounced

TABLE 54.16 Manifestations of Adrenocortical Problems

System	Cushing Syndrome	Addison Disease
Glucocorticoids		
General appearance	Truncal obesity, thin extremities, rounding of face (moon face), fat deposits on back of neck and shoulders (buffalo hump) (Fig. 54.11A)	Weight loss, emaciation
Cardiovascular	↑ BP, hypervolemia, edema of lower extremities	↓ BP, tendency to develop refractory shock, vasodilation
GI	↑ Secretion of pepsin and HCl acid, risk for peptic ulcer disease, anorexia	Anorexia, nausea and vomiting, cramping abdominal pain, diarrhea
Immune	Inhibition of immune response, suppression of allergic response	Tendency for coexisting autoimmune diseases
Metabolic	Hyperglycemia, negative nitrogen balance, dyslipidemia	↓ Sodium, insulin sensitivity, fever
Musculoskeletal	Muscle wasting in extremities, fatigue, osteoporosis, awkward gait, back pain, weakness, compression fractures	Fatigue
Psychologic	Euphoria, irritability, depression, insomnia, anxiety	Depression, exhaustion or irritability, confusion, delusions
Renal/urinary	Glycosuria, hypercalciuria, risk for kidney stones	
Skin	Thin, fragile skin, purplish red striae (Fig. 54.11A). Petechial hemorrhages, bruises. Florid cheeks (plethora), acne, poor wound healing	Bronzed or smoky hyperpigmentation of face, neck, hands (especially creases), buccal membranes, nipples, genitalia, and scars (if pituitary function normal). Vitiligo, alopecia
Mineralocorticoids		
Cardiovascular	↑ BP, hypervolemia	Hypovolemia, tendency toward shock, decreased cardiac output
Fluid and electrolytes	Marked sodium and water retention, edema, marked ↓ potassium, alkalosis	Sodium loss, ↓ volume of extracellular fluid, ↑ potassium, salt craving
Androgens		
Musculoskeletal	Muscle wasting and weakness	↓ Muscle size and tone
Reproductive	*Females:* Menstrual irregularities and enlargement of clitoris *Males:* Gynecomastia and testicular atrophy	*Females:* ↓ Libido *Males:* No effect
Skin	Hirsutism, acne, hyperpigmentation	↓ Axillary and pubic hair (in females)

changes in their physical appearance. Weight gain is the most common. It results from the accumulation of adipose tissue in the trunk (centripetal obesity), face ("moon face"), and cervical areas ("buffalo hump") (Fig. 54.10). Glucose levels are high because of cortisol-induced insulin resistance and increased gluconeogenesis by the liver. Muscle wasting causes weakness, especially in the extremities. A loss of bone matrix leads to osteoporosis and back pain. The loss of collagen makes the skin weaker, thinner, and more easily bruised. Purplish red striae (usually depressed below the skin surface) appear on the abdomen, breast, or buttocks (Fig. 54.11). Catabolic processes lead to a delay in wound healing.

Mineralocorticoid excess may cause hypokalemia from potassium excretion and hypertension from fluid retention. Adrenal androgen excess may cause severe acne, the development of male characteristics in females, and feminization in males. Menstrual problems and hirsutism in females and gynecomastia and impotence in males occur more often with adrenal cancer.

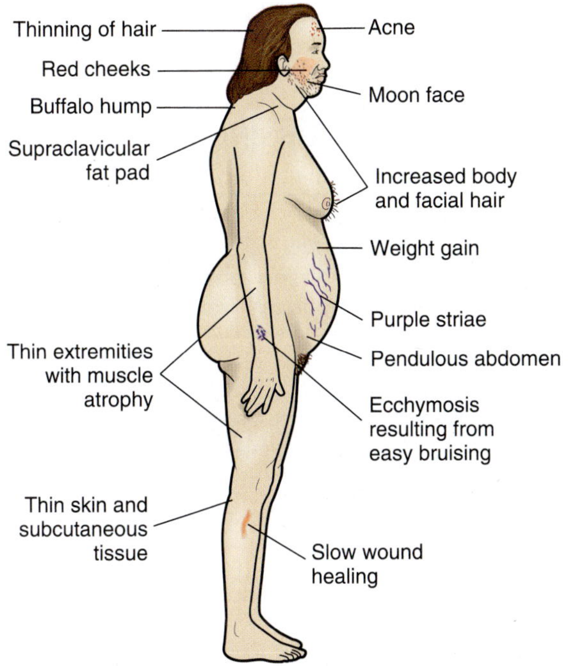

Fig. 54.10 Manifestations of Cushing syndrome.

Diagnostic Studies

Diagnosing Cushing syndrome begins with confirming increased cortisol levels. We use 3 tests: (1) midnight or late-night salivary cortisol, (2) low-dose dexamethasone suppression test, and (3) 24-hour urine cortisol. Urine cortisol levels higher than 100 mcg/24 h indicate Cushing syndrome. Urine levels of 17-ketosteroids may be high. A CT scan or MRI of the pituitary and adrenal glands can detect a tumor.

ACTH levels may be low, normal, or high, depending on the underlying cause. High or normal ACTH levels indicate Cushing disease. Low or undetectable levels indicate an adrenal or medication cause. Other findings that may be present but are not diagnostic of Cushing syndrome include leukocytosis, lymphopenia, eosinopenia, hyperglycemia, glycosuria, hypercalciuria, and osteoporosis. Hypokalemia and alkalosis occur with ectopic ACTH syndrome and adrenal cancer.

Interprofessional Care

The primary goal of treatment is to normalize hormone secretion. The treatment depends on the underlying cause

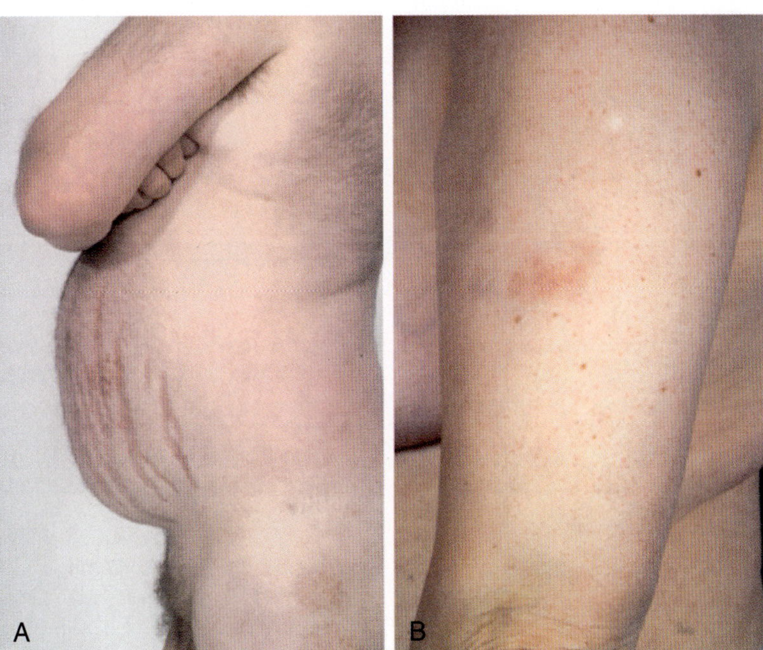

Fig. 54.11 Cushing syndrome. (A) Truncal obesity with broad, purple striae. (B) Typical bruising with thin skin. (From Auchus RJ, Melmed S, Kopp PA, et al: *Williams textbook of endocrinology,* ed 15, St. Louis, 2025, Elsevier.)

(Table 54.17). If the cause is a pituitary adenoma, the standard treatment is surgical removal of the pituitary tumor using the transsphenoidal approach. Radiation therapy is an option for patients who are not surgical candidates.

An adrenalectomy is done if Cushing syndrome is caused by adrenal tumors or hyperplasia. Sometimes, bilateral adrenalectomy is needed. A laparoscopic approach is used unless adrenal cancer is suspected. Then an open surgical adrenalectomy is usually done.

Patients with ectopic ACTH-secreting tumors are best managed by removing the tumor (usually lung or pancreas). This is usually possible when the tumor is benign. If a cancerous tumor has already metastasized, surgical removal may not be possible or successful.

When a patient is a poor candidate for surgery or prior surgery has failed, we can try drug therapy. The goal of drug therapy is to suppress the synthesis and secretion of cortisol from the adrenal gland. Drugs used include ketoconazole and mitotane.[18] These are used cautiously because they are often toxic at the dosages needed to reduce cortisol secretion. Hydrocortisone or prednisone may be needed to avoid adrenal insufficiency. Mifepristone (Korlym) can help control glucose levels in patients with endogenous Cushing syndrome who have type 2 diabetes.

If Cushing syndrome developed because of prolonged use of corticosteroids (e.g., prednisone), we may try several options. We can gradually discontinue corticosteroid therapy, reduce the dosage, or convert to alternate-day dosing. Gradual tapering of the corticosteroids is necessary to avoid potentially life-threatening adrenal insufficiency. In alternate-day dosing, twice the daily dosage of a shorter-acting corticosteroid is given every other morning to minimize hypothalamic-pituitary-adrenal suppression, growth suppression, and altered appearance. This plan is not an option if the corticosteroids are given as hormone therapy.

TABLE 54.17 Interprofessional Care
Cushing Syndrome

Diagnostic Assessment
- History and physical assessment
- Dexamethasone suppression test
- 24-h urine for free cortisol and 17-ketosteroids
- Plasma and salivary cortisol levels
- ACTH levels
- CBC with WBC differential
- Electrolytes (sodium, potassium), glucose
- CT scan, MRI

Management

Pituitary Adenoma
- Transsphenoidal resection
- Radiation therapy

Adrenocortical Adenoma, Cancer, or Hyperplasia
- Adrenalectomy (open or laparoscopic)
- Drug therapy (e.g., ketoconazole, mitotane, mifepristone)

Ectopic ACTH-Secreting Tumor
- Treatment of the tumor (surgical removal or radiation)

Exogenous Corticosteroid Therapy
- Discontinue or change dose of exogenous corticosteroids

NURSING MANAGEMENT: CUSHING SYNDROME

Assessment

Subjective and objective data that should be obtained from patients with Cushing syndrome are outlined in Table 54.18.

TABLE 54.18 NURSING ASSESSMENT
Cushing Syndrome

Subjective Data

Important Health Information

Health history: Pituitary tumor (Cushing disease). Adrenal, pancreatic, or pulmonary cancer. GI bleeding, frequent infections

Medications: Corticosteroids

Functional Health Patterns

Health perception–health management: Malaise

Nutritional-metabolic: Weight gain, anorexia. Prolonged wound healing, easy bruising

Elimination: Polyuria

Activity-exercise: Weakness, fatigue

Sleep: Insomnia, poor sleep quality

Cognitive-perceptual: Headache. Back, joint, bone, and rib pain. Poor concentration and memory

Self-perception–self-concept: Negative feelings about changes in personal appearance

Sexuality-reproductive: Amenorrhea, impotence, ↓ libido

Coping–stress tolerance: Anxiety, mood changes, emotional lability, psychosis

Objective Data

Cardiovascular

↑ BP

General

Truncal obesity, supraclavicular fat pads, buffalo hump, moon face

Musculoskeletal

Muscle wasting, thin extremities, awkward gait

Reproductive

Gynecomastia, testicular atrophy (in males), enlarged clitoris (in females)

Skin

Hirsutism, thinning of head hair. Thin, friable skin. Acne, petechiae, purpura, hyperpigmentation. Purplish red striae on breasts, buttocks, and abdomen. Edema of lower extremities

Possible Diagnostic Findings

↑ Glucose, ↓ potassium, dyslipidemia, polycythemia, lymphocytopenia, eosinopenia. ↑ Cortisol, ↑ salivary cortisol. High, low, or normal ACTH levels. Abnormal dexamethasone suppression test. ↑ Urine free cortisol, 17-ketosteroids. Glycosuria, hypercalciuria. Osteoporosis

◆ Clinical Problems

Clinical problems for patients with Cushing syndrome may include:

- Impaired endocrine function
- Risk for infection
- Disturbed body image
- Impaired tissue integrity

Additional information on clinical problems and interventions is presented in eNursing Care Plan 54.3 for patients with Cushing syndrome (available on the website for this chapter).

◆ Planning

The overall goals are that patients with Cushing syndrome will (1) have relief of symptoms, (2) avoid serious complications, (3) maintain a positive self-image, and (4) actively take part in the therapeutic plan.

◆ Implementation

Health Promotion

Health promotion focuses on identifying patients at risk for Cushing syndrome. Patients receiving long-term, exogenous corticosteroids are at risk. Teaching related to medications and side effects is an important preventive measure.

Acute Care

Patients with Cushing syndrome are seriously ill. Because the therapy has many side effects, assessment focuses on signs and symptoms of hormone and drug toxicity and complicating conditions (e.g., CVD, diabetes, infection). Monitor vital signs, weight, and glucose. Assess for infection. Because signs and symptoms of inflammation (e.g., fever, redness) may be minimal or absent, assess for pain, loss of function, and purulent drainage. Monitor for thromboembolic events (venous thromboembolism [VTE]).

Another important focus of care is emotional support. Changes in appearance, such as truncal obesity, multiple bruises, hirsutism in females, and gynecomastia in males, can be distressing. Patients may feel unattractive, repulsive, or unwanted. Be sensitive to their feelings and offer unconditional acceptance. Reassure them that the physical changes and much of the emotional lability will resolve when hormone levels return to normal.

Adrenalectomy. Before surgery, patients should be in optimal physical condition. High BP and glucose levels must be under control. Hypokalemia must be corrected with diet and potassium supplements. A high-protein diet helps correct protein depletion. Provide teaching about the expected care after surgery.

Surgery on the adrenal glands poses great risks. Because the adrenal glands are vascular, there is an increased risk for bleeding. After laparoscopic and open adrenalectomy, patients may have a nasogastric tube, a urinary catheter, IV therapy, and central venous pressure monitoring. Initiate VTE prophylaxis.

Manipulating glandular tissue during surgery may release large amounts of hormones into the circulation. This can produce marked fluctuations in the metabolic processes affected by these hormones. After surgery, BP, fluid balance, and electrolyte levels may be unstable due to these hormone fluctuations.

High doses of corticosteroids (e.g., hydrocortisone) are given IV during surgery and for several days afterward to ensure adequate responses to the stress of the procedure. If large amounts of endogenous hormones were released into the systemic circulation during surgery, patients are likely to have hypertension, increasing the risk for bleeding. High corticosteroid levels cause problems with glucose control, increase risk for infection, and delay wound healing.

The critical period for circulatory instability is 24 to 48 hours after surgery. During this time, you must be alert for signs of corticosteroid imbalance. Report any rapid or significant changes in BP, respirations, or heart rate. Monitor intake and output and assess for imbalances. Give prescribed IV corticosteroids. The dosage is adjusted depending on the manifestations and fluid and electrolyte balance. Oral doses are given as tolerated. After IV corticosteroids are withdrawn, keep the IV line open for quick administration of corticosteroids or vasopressors. Obtain morning urine samples at the same time each morning for cortisol measurement to evaluate the surgery's effectiveness.

If corticosteroid dosage is tapered too quickly after surgery, acute adrenal insufficiency may develop. Vomiting, weakness, dehydration, and hypotension are signs of hypocortisolism. Patients may have painful joints, itching, or peeling skin and severe emotional problems. Report these signs and symptoms so that drug doses can be adjusted as needed.

Patients are usually kept on bed rest until the BP stabilizes. Implement measures to prevent infection. Be alert for subtle signs of infection because the usual inflammatory responses are suppressed.

Chronic Care

Discharge teaching is based on patients' lack of endogenous corticosteroids and resulting inability to react physiologically to stressors. Consider a home health nurse referral, especially for older adults, because of the need for ongoing evaluation and teaching. Teach patients to always wear a Medic Alert bracelet and carry medical identification and instructions in a wallet or purse. They need to avoid exposure to extreme temperatures, infections, and emotional situations. Stress may cause acute adrenal insufficiency because the remaining adrenal tissue cannot meet an increased hormone demand. Many patients need lifetime replacement therapy. It may take several months to adjust the hormone dose satisfactorily. Teach patients to adjust their corticosteroid replacement therapy by their stress levels. Consult with the HCP to determine the parameters for dosage changes if this plan is feasible. If patients cannot adjust their own medication or if weakness, fainting, fever, or nausea and vomiting occur, they should contact the HCP for a possible adjustment in corticosteroid dosage.

◆ Evaluation

The expected outcomes are that patients with Cushing syndrome will:

- Have no signs or symptoms of infection
- Maintain weight appropriate for height
- State acceptance of appearance and treatment plan
- Show healing of skin and maintaining intact skin

ADRENOCORTICAL INSUFFICIENCY

Etiology and Pathophysiology

Adrenocortical insufficiency (hypofunction of the adrenal cortex) may be from a primary cause (**Addison disease**) or a secondary cause (lack of pituitary ACTH secretion). In Addison disease, glucocorticoids (cortisol), mineralocorticoids, and adrenal androgens are reduced or lost. In secondary adrenocortical insufficiency, glucocorticoids and androgens are deficient but, rarely, mineralocorticoids. ACTH deficiency may be caused by pituitary disease or suppression of the hypothalamic-pituitary axis because of the use of exogenous corticosteroids.

Up to 80% of Addison disease cases in the United States are caused by an autoimmune response.[19] Autoimmune adrenalitis causes the adrenal cortex to be destroyed by antibodies. These patients often have other autoimmune disorders, such as type 1 diabetes, autoimmune thyroid disease, pernicious anemia, and celiac disease. Other endocrine problems may be present. This is known as *autoimmune polyglandular syndrome.* It is most common in White females.

Although tuberculosis causes Addison disease worldwide, it is now an uncommon cause in the United States. Other causes include amyloidosis, fungal infections (e.g., histoplasmosis), AIDS, and metastatic cancer. Iatrogenic Addison disease may be due to adrenal hemorrhage, often related to anticoagulant therapy, chemotherapy, or bilateral adrenalectomy.

Clinical Manifestations

Because manifestations do not tend to become evident until 90% of the adrenal cortex is destroyed, the disease is often advanced before it is diagnosed. Manifestations often have a slow onset. They include anorexia, nausea, weakness, fatigue, and weight loss (Fig. 54.12). Increased ACTH causes the striking bronze-colored skin hyperpigmentation. It is seen mainly in sun-exposed areas of the body, at pressure points, over joints, and in the creases, especially palmar creases. Skin changes are likely due to increased secretion of β-lipotropin (which contains melanocyte-stimulating hormone [MSH]).

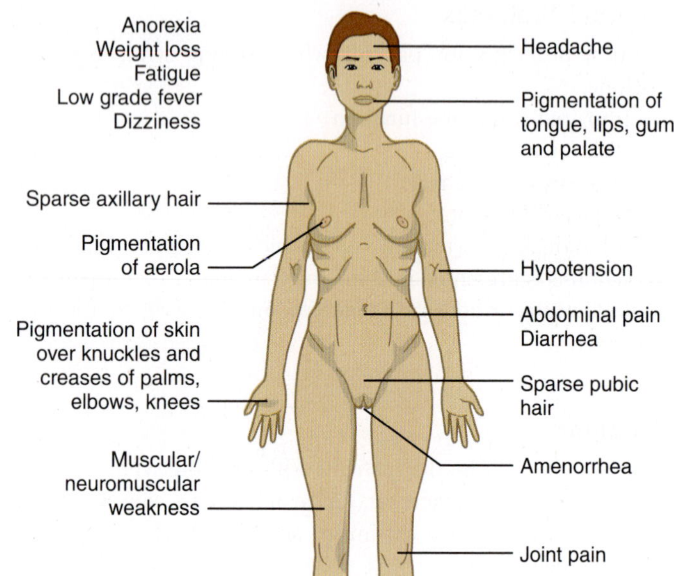

Fig. 54.12 Manifestations of Addison disease.

Patients may crave salt. Irritability and depression may occur in primary adrenal hypofunction.

Patients with secondary adrenocortical hypofunction may have many signs and symptoms similar to those of patients with Addison disease. However, they usually do not have hyperpigmented skin because ACTH levels are low.

Acute Adrenal Insufficiency

Patients with adrenocortical insufficiency are at risk for acute adrenal insufficiency *(addisonian crisis).*[20] It is a life-threatening emergency caused by insufficient adrenocortical hormones or a sudden sharp decrease in these hormones (Fig. 54.13). Triggers of addisonian crisis include (1) stress (e.g., infection, surgery), (2) sudden withdrawal of corticosteroid hormone therapy, (3) adrenal surgery, or (4) sudden pituitary gland destruction.

During acute adrenal insufficiency, patients have severe manifestations of cortisol and mineralocorticoid deficiencies. These include hypotension, tachycardia, dehydration, fever, weakness, and confusion. Hypotension may lead to shock. Shock from adrenal insufficiency is often unresponsive to the usual treatment (vasopressors and fluid replacement). GI manifestations include severe vomiting, diarrhea, and pain in the abdomen. Pain may occur in the lower back and legs.

Diagnostic Studies

The ACTH stimulation test is a common test to diagnose adrenal insufficiency. Baseline cortisol and ACTH levels are measured, and patients are given an IV injection of synthetic ACTH (cosyntropin). Cortisol and ACTH levels are rechecked after 30 and 60 minutes. The normal response is a rise in cortisol levels. People with Addison disease have little or no

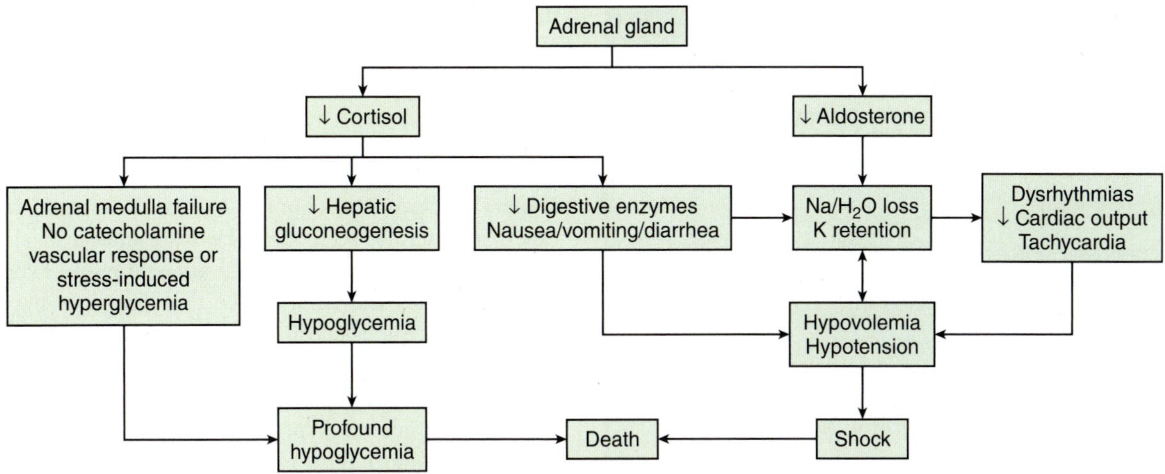

Fig. 54.13 Acute adrenal insufficiency.

increase in cortisol levels. Those with primary adrenal insufficiency have a high ACTH level.

When the response to the ACTH test is abnormal, a corticotropin-releasing hormone (CRH) stimulation test may be done. Patients are given an IV injection of synthetic CRH, and blood is taken after 30 and 60 minutes. Those with Addison disease have high ACTH levels but no cortisol. People with secondary adrenal insufficiency from pituitary or hypothalamus problems do not make ACTH or have a delayed response.

Other abnormal laboratory findings may include hyperkalemia, hyponatremia, hypoglycemia, anemia, and increased BUN levels. An ECG may show changes from hyperkalemia (see Fig. 17.14). CT scans and MRI can identify other causes, including tumors, fungal infections, tuberculosis, or adrenal calcification.

Interprofessional and Nursing Management

Treatment focuses on managing the underlying cause when possible. The mainstay is often lifelong hormone therapy with corticosteroids and mineralocorticoids (Table 54.19). Overall, patients who take their medications consistently can expect a normal life expectancy. Hydrocortisone, the most common form of hormone therapy, has corticosteroid and mineralocorticoid properties. Mineralocorticoids are replaced with fludrocortisone. Females need androgen replacement with dehydroepiandrosterone (DHEA) as their only source of androgen production is the adrenal glands.

Acute Care

When patients with Addison disease are hospitalized, nursing care focuses on monitoring patients while correcting fluid and electrolyte balance. Assess vital signs and neurologic status. Monitor for signs of fluid volume deficit and electrolyte imbalance. Obtain a daily weight. Keep an intake and output record. Take a medication history to see if there are drugs that can interact with corticosteroids. These drugs include oral hypoglycemics, cardiac glycosides, oral contraceptives, anticoagulants, and NSAIDs.

Note changes in BP, weight gain, weakness, and other manifestations of Cushing syndrome. Guard patients against exposure to infection and help with daily hygiene. Protects patients from noise, light, and temperature extremes. Patients cannot cope with these stresses because of the inability to make corticosteroids.

Addisonian crisis is a life-threatening emergency requiring aggressive management. Treatment is directed toward shock management and high-dose hydrocortisone replacement. Large volumes of IV fluid are given to reverse hypotension and electrolyte imbalances until BP returns to normal.

TABLE 54.19 Interprofessional Care

Addison Disease

Diagnostic Assessment
- History and physical assessment
- ACTH stimulation test
- Cortisol and ACTH
- Urine cortisol and aldosterone
- CRH suppression test
- Electrolytes
- CT scan, MRI

Management
- Daily glucocorticoid (e.g., prednisone, hydrocortisone) replacement (two-thirds on awakening in morning, one-third in late afternoon)
- Daily mineralocorticoid (fludrocortisone) in morning
- ↑ Salt in the diet
- Androgen replacement with dehydroepiandrosterone (DHEA) for females
- Salt supplement for excess heat or humidity
- ↑ Doses of glucocorticoid for stress situations (e.g., surgery, hospitalization)

TABLE 54.20 PATIENT & CAREGIVER TEACHING

Addison Disease

Include the following information in the teaching plan for patients with Addison disease and caregivers:

1. Names, dosages, and actions of drugs
2. Symptoms of overdosage and underdosage
3. Conditions requiring increased dosage (e.g., trauma, infection, surgery, emotional crisis)
4. Action to take related to changes in medication
   - Increased dose of corticosteroid
   - Self-administration of large dose of corticosteroid IM
   - Consult with HCP
5. Preventing infection and need for prompt and vigorous treatment of existing infections
6. Need for lifelong replacement therapy
7. Need for lifelong medical supervision
8. Need to carry medical identification
9. How to give an IM injection
10. Fall prevention
11. Adverse effects of corticosteroid therapy and prevention techniques
12. Special instruction for patients with diabetes and management of glucose when taking corticosteroids

Chronic Care

As a nurse, you have a key role in the long-term management of Addison disease. The serious nature of the disease and the need for lifelong hormone therapy necessitate a comprehensive teaching plan. Table 54.20 outlines the major areas to include in a teaching plan.

Corticosteroids are usually given in divided doses, two-thirds in the morning and one-third in the afternoon. Mineralocorticoids are given once daily, preferably in the morning. This schedule reflects normal circadian rhythm in endogenous hormone secretion and decreases the side effects of therapy. Teach patients taking mineralocorticoid therapy how to take their BP, increase salt intake, and report any significant changes to the HCP.

Patients with Addison disease need an increased dosage of corticosteroids in stressful situations to prevent addisonian crisis. Examples include fever, illness, surgery, and rigorous physical activity, such as playing sports on a hot day or distance running. If vomiting or diarrhea occurs, as may happen with gastroenteritis, patients should notify the HCP at once. They may need electrolyte replacement and IV cortisol administration.

Teach patients the signs and symptoms of corticosteroid deficiency and excess (Cushing syndrome) and to report these signs to the HCP so that the drug dose can be adjusted. They should wear an identification bracelet and carry a wallet card saying they have Addison disease so that therapy can be started in an emergency. Patients should carry an emergency kit with 100 mg of IM hydrocortisone and syringes. Teach patients and caregivers how to give an IM injection.

HYPERALDOSTERONISM

Hyperaldosteronism (Conn syndrome) is characterized by excess aldosterone secretion. The main effects of aldosterone are (1) sodium retention and (2) potassium and hydrogen ion excretion. Thus the hallmark of this disease is hypertension with hypokalemic alkalosis. *Primary hyperaldosteronism* (PA) is most often caused by a single, small adrenocortical adenoma. Sometimes, multiple lesions are involved and are associated with bilateral adrenal hyperplasia.

PA affects more females. It usually occurs between 30 and 50 years of age. A genetic link has been found in some patients. PA causes up to 2% of all cases of hypertension. *Secondary hyperaldosteronism* occurs in response to a nonadrenal cause of increased aldosterone levels, such as renal artery stenosis, renin-secreting tumors, and chronic kidney disease.

Increased aldosterone levels cause sodium retention and potassium excretion. Sodium retention leads to hypernatremia, hypertension, and headache. Edema does not usually occur because the rate of sodium excretion increases, preventing more severe sodium retention. Potassium wasting leads to hypokalemia, which causes muscle weakness, fatigue, dysrhythmias, glucose intolerance, and metabolic alkalosis that may lead to tetany.

Hyperaldosteronism should be suspected in hypertensive patients with hypokalemia who are not being treated with diuretics. PA causes increased sodium and aldosterone levels, decreased potassium levels, and decreased renin activity. A CT scan or MRI can detect an adenoma. If a tumor is not found, we measure 18-hydroxycorticosterone after overnight bed rest. A level greater than 50 ng/dL indicates an adenoma.

Interprofessional and Nursing Management

The preferred treatment for PA is surgical removal of the adenoma (adrenalectomy).[21] A laparoscopic approach is most often used. Before surgery, patients should receive potassium-sparing diuretics (e.g., spironolactone) and antihypertensive agents to normalize potassium levels and BP. Spironolactone and eplerenone block the binding of aldosterone to the mineralocorticoid receptor in the terminal distal tubules and collecting ducts of the kidney, thus increasing sodium and water excretion and potassium retention. Oral potassium supplements and sodium restrictions may be needed. However, potassium supplements and potassium-sparing diuretics should not be started simultaneously because of the risk for hyperkalemia.

Patients with bilateral adrenal hyperplasia are treated with a potassium-sparing diuretic. Calcium channel blockers may be used to control BP. Dexamethasone may be used to decrease overgrowth of the adrenal glands.

Nursing care includes assessment of fluid and electrolyte balance (especially potassium) and cardiovascular status. Monitor BP frequently before and after surgery. Unilateral adrenalectomy is successful in controlling hypertension in only 80% of patients. Teach patients receiving spironolactone about the possible side effects of gynecomastia, impotence, and menstrual problems, as well as the signs and symptoms of hypokalemia and hyperkalemia. Review how to monitor their BP and the need for frequent monitoring. Stress the need for continued health care.

CORTICOSTEROID THERAPY

Corticosteroids are effective in treating many problems (Table 54.21). However, long-term corticosteroid therapy at therapeutic doses often leads to serious complications and side effects (Table 54.22). For this reason, corticosteroid therapy is not recommended for minor chronic conditions. Therapy should be reserved for problems that have a risk for death, permanent loss of function, or for which short-term therapy is likely to produce remission or recovery. We must weigh the potential benefits of treatment against the risks.

TABLE 54.21 Drug Therapy
Problems Treated With Corticosteroids

Allergic Reactions
- Anaphylaxis
- Bee stings
- Contact dermatitis
- Drug reactions
- Serum sickness
- Urticaria

Connective Tissue Problems
- Mixed connective tissue disorders
- Polymyositis
- Polyarteritis nodosa
- Rheumatoid arthritis
- Systemic lupus erythematosus

Endocrine Problems
- Adrenal insufficiency
- Hypercalcemia
- Hashimoto thyroiditis
- Thyrotoxicosis

GI Problems
- Inflammatory bowel disease
- Celiac disease

Liver Problems
- Alcoholic hepatitis
- Autoimmune hepatitis

Neurologic Problems
- Cerebral edema and increased intracranial pressure
- Head trauma

Pulmonary Diseases
- Aspiration pneumonia
- Asthma
- Chronic obstructive pulmonary disease

Other Problems
- Skin diseases
- Cancer, leukemia, lymphoma
- Immunosuppression
- Inflammation
- Nephrotic syndrome

CHECK YOUR PRACTICE

You are working in the outpatient clinic. Your 30-year-old female patient has Cushing syndrome from high doses of prednisone use for autoimmune hepatitis. At her office visit today, she tells you, "I haven't been taking my prednisone because I'm gaining weight and I'm not happy with the way I look."

- How would you respond to her?

A beneficial effect of corticosteroids in one situation may be a harmful one in another. For example, decreasing inflammation in arthritis is an important therapeutic effect, but increasing the risk for infection is a harmful effect. Suppressing inflammation and the immune response may help save lives in persons with anaphylaxis and in those receiving an organ transplant, but it can activate latent tuberculosis and increase the risk for cancer. The vasopressive effect of corticosteroids is critical in allowing a person to function in stressful situations but can cause hypertension when used for drug therapy.

DRUG ALERT
Corticosteroids

- Teach patients not to abruptly stop therapy.
- Monitor for signs of infection.
- Have patients with diabetes closely monitor glucose.

Provide detailed teaching to ensure patient adherence. Corticosteroids given as nonreplacement therapy are taken once daily or once every other day. They should be taken early in the morning with food to decrease GI irritation. Because exogenous corticosteroid use may suppress endogenous ACTH and cortisol (suppression is time and dose dependent), emphasize the danger of abruptly stopping corticosteroid

TABLE 54.22 Drug Therapy
Side Effects of Corticosteroids

- Delayed wound healing with ↑ risk for wound dehiscence
- Fat from extremities redistributed to trunk and face
- Glucose intolerance
- Hypertension with ↑ risk for heart failure
- Hypocalcemia related to anti–vitamin D effect
- Hypokalemia
- ↑ Risk for infection
- Infection develops more rapidly and spreads more widely
- Mood and behavior changes
- Pathologic fractures, especially compression fractures of the vertebrae (osteoporosis)
- Peptic ulcer disease
- Pituitary ACTH synthesis suppressed
- Skeletal muscle atrophy and weakness
- Suppressed inflammatory response

TABLE 54.23 PATIENT & CAREGIVER TEACHING

Corticosteroid Therapy

Include the following instructions when teaching patients and caregivers to manage corticosteroid therapy:

1. Follow a diet high in protein, calcium (at least 1500 mg/day), and potassium and low in fat and concentrated simple carbohydrates, such as sugar, syrups, and candy.
2. Ensure adequate rest and sleep, such as daily naps and avoiding caffeine late in the day.
3. Take part in an exercise program to help maintain bone integrity.
4. Recognize edema and ways to restrict sodium intake to <2000 mg/day if edema occurs.
5. Monitor glucose levels and recognize symptoms of hyperglycemia (e.g., polydipsia, polyuria, blurred vision). Report hyperglycemic symptoms or glucose levels >120 mg/dL (10 mmol/L).
6. Notify HCP if heartburn after meals or epigastric pain that is not relieved by antacids occurs.
7. See an eye specialist yearly to assess for cataracts.
8. Use safety measures, such as getting up slowly from bed or a chair and good lighting, to avoid accidental injury.
9. Maintain hygiene practices.
10. Avoid contact with persons with colds or other contagious illnesses to prevent infection.
11. Inform all HCPs about long-term corticosteroid use.
12. Recognize need for higher doses of corticosteroids in times of physical and emotional stress.
13. Never abruptly stop the corticosteroids because this could lead to addisonian crisis and death.

therapy to patients and caregivers. Corticosteroids taken for longer than 1 week will suppress adrenal production, and oral corticosteroids must be tapered. Ensure that higher doses of corticosteroids are prescribed in situations of physical or emotional stress.

Corticosteroid-induced osteoporosis is an important concern for patients who receive corticosteroid treatment for long periods (longer than 3 months).[22] Therapies to reduce bone resorption include increased calcium intake, vitamin D supplements, bisphosphonates (e.g., alendronate), and a low-impact exercise program. Measures to minimize the side effects and complications of corticosteroid therapy are outlined in Table 54.23.

ADRENAL MEDULLA PROBLEMS

PHEOCHROMOCYTOMA

Pheochromocytoma is a rare condition caused by a tumor in the adrenal medulla. It affects the chromaffin cells, resulting in excess production of catecholamines (epinephrine, norepinephrine). The most dangerous immediate effect is severe hypertension. If untreated, it may lead to encephalopathy, diabetes, cardiomyopathy, multiple organ failure, and death. It most often occurs in young to middle-aged adults. Pheochromocytoma may be inherited in persons with MEN.

The most striking findings are severe, episodic hypertension accompanied by a classic trio of symptoms: severe, pounding headache; tachycardia with palpitations; and profuse sweating. Some patients have abdominal or chest pain. Attacks can be induced by direct trauma, mechanical pressure to the tumor, stress (e.g., surgery, exercise, defecation, sexual intercourse, alcohol use, smoking), or many drugs, including antihypertensives, opioids, radiologic contrast media, and tricyclic antidepressants. Attacks can last from a few minutes to several hours.

The most reliable diagnostic test is measurement of urinary fractionated metanephrines (catecholamine metabolites) and fractionated catecholamines and creatinine, usually done as a 24-hour urine collection.[23] Values are increased in most persons with pheochromocytoma. Serum catecholamines may be increased during an "attack." CT scans and MRI can detect tumors. Do not palpate the abdomen of a patient with suspected pheochromocytoma. It may cause the sudden release of catecholamines and severe hypertension.

Interprofessional and Nursing Management

The main treatment is surgical removal of the tumor. Treatment with α- and β-adrenergic receptor blockers is needed before surgery to control BP and prevent an intraoperative hypertensive crisis. Therapy begins with an α-adrenergic receptor blocker (e.g., doxazosin, prazosin, phenoxybenzamine) 10 to 14 days before surgery to reduce BP. After adequate α-adrenergic blockade, β-adrenergic receptor blockers (e.g., propranolol) are used to decrease tachycardia and dysrhythmias. If β-blockers are started too early, unopposed α-adrenergic stimulation can cause a hypertensive crisis. Therapy can cause orthostatic hypotension. Teach patients to change positions slowly. Monitor the BP often, especially if a patient is having an "attack." Keep patients as comfortable as possible. Monitor glucose levels to assess for diabetes. Patients need rest, proper nutrition, and emotional support during this period.

Surgery is usually done using a laparoscopic approach. Removing the adrenal tumor often cures the hypertension. Monitor BP after surgery because hypertension persists in 10% to 30% of patients. If surgery is not an option, metyrosine (Demser) can decrease catecholamine production by the tumor.

Surgical care is similar to that for any patient undergoing adrenalectomy. Note that BP fluctuations from catecholamine excesses tend to be severe and must be monitored. Emphasize the importance of follow-up and routine BP monitoring because of persistent hypertension.

CASE STUDY

Graves Disease

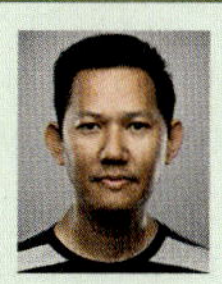

(© SensorSpot/ iStock.com.)

Patient Profile

J.G., a 34-year-old male, was admitted with palpitations and anxiety. Based on his history, assessment, and laboratory findings, the HCP diagnosed J.G. with Graves disease.

Subjective Data

- Reports recent unintentional weight loss, insomnia, and erectile dysfunction
- Symptoms include irritability, heat intolerance, vision changes, fatigue, muscle weakness, and diarrhea
- Reports no significant medical history but states family history of thyroid disorders

Objective Data

- Fever of 103°F (39.4°C)
- BP of 148/86 mm Hg, pulse of 134 beats/min, and respiratory rate of 26 breaths/min
- Hot, moist skin, with thickened and reddened shins
- Fine tremors of the fingers
- 4+ deep tendon reflexes and muscle strength of 1 to 2 out of 5
- Swelling to the anterior neck with audible bruit
- Tearing of the eyes with periorbital edema

Interprofessional Care

- Subtotal thyroidectomy planned for 2 months later
- Started on methimazole and propranolol

Discussion Questions

1. ***Recognize:*** Explain the cause of J.G.'s symptoms.
2. ***Analyze:*** What diagnostic studies were probably ordered? What would the results have been to establish the diagnosis of Graves disease?
3. ***Analyze:*** Why was surgery delayed?
4. ***Prioritize:*** What is the interprofessional team's top priority at this time for J.G.?
5. ***Prioritize:*** Based on the assessment data, what are the priority clinical problems?
6. ***Plan:*** What are his teaching needs at this time?
7. ***Act:*** What teaching will you provide after surgery so that J.G. can successfully self-manage his care?
8. ***Evaluate:*** What is the expected outcome of drug therapy?
9. ***Safety:*** Why is J.G. counseled to give up his long-standing cigarette smoking habit?

Answers available at http://evolve.elsevier.com/Lewis/medsurg.

BRIDGE TO NCLEX EXAMINATION

The number of the question corresponds to the same-numbered outcome at the beginning of the chapter.

1. Which interventions would be in the plan of care for a patient who had a transsphenoidal excision of the pituitary gland? (**Select all that apply.**)
   - **a.** Position the patient flat on their back
   - **b.** Allow the patient to brush teeth vigorously
   - **c.** Perform frequent neurologic assessments
   - **d.** Encourage vigorous coughing to clear airways
   - **e.** Monitor for signs of cerebrospinal fluid (CSF) leakage
   - **f.** Monitor for signs of arginine vasopressin (AVP) disorder
2. Which laboratory results would support the diagnosis of arginine vasopressin (AVP) disorder? (**Select all that apply.**)
   - **a.** Decreased urine output
   - **b.** Increased sodium level
   - **c.** Increased urine osmolality
   - **d.** Increased plasma osmolality
   - **e.** Decreased antidiuretic hormone
3. Which manifestations would lead you to believe a patient has developed Hashimoto's thyroiditis?
   - **a.** Weight gain, fatigue
   - **b.** Hyperactivity, tremors
   - **c.** Heat intolerance, diarrhea
   - **d.** Muscle weakness, tachycardia
4. After thyroid surgery, a patient reports headache, fatigue, numbness in the hands and feet, and muscle spasms. Which electrolyte problem is most likely causing these manifestations?
   - **a.** Low calcium
   - **b.** High sodium
   - **c.** High potassium
   - **d.** Low magnesium
5. The nurse is teaching a patient about Cushing disease. Which patient statement would indicate to the nurse that further education is required?
   - **a.** "I should monitor my blood sugar levels regularly."
   - **b.** "I need to avoid consuming any foods that contain calcium."
   - **c.** "I should wear a medical alert bracelet indicating my diagnosis."
   - **d.** "I should inform my provider if taking new medications or supplements."

6. The nurse teaches patients with Addison disease who are prescribed corticosteroid therapy to:
   a. Monitor glucose levels regularly
   b. Limit fluid intake to prevent fluid retention
   c. Skip doses if experiencing gastrointestinal upset
   d. Take medication on an empty stomach for better absorption

7. What is a priority nursing intervention for patients with a pheochromocytoma?
   a. Monitor blood pressure frequently
   b. Initiate aggressive diuresis to reduce fluid volume
   c. Encourage patients to consume caffeine to improve alertness
   d. Administer high-dose corticosteroids to suppress adrenal function

1. c, e, f; 2. b, d, e; 3. a; 4. a; 5. b; 6. a; 7. a.

For rationales to these answers and even more NCLEX review questions, visit http://evolve.elsevier.com/Lewis/medsurg.

REFERENCES

To access the References for this chapter, please scan the QR code with a mobile device.

55

Assessment: Reproductive System

Anthony Richard Lutz and Robyn Schafer

http://evolve.elsevier.com/Lewis/medsurg/

CONCEPTUAL FOCUS

Hormonal Regulation
Reproduction
Sexuality

LEARNING OUTCOMES

1. Describe the structures and functions of the male and female reproductive systems.
2. Outline the functions of the major hormones essential for the function and neuroendocrine regulation of the reproductive system.
3. Explain physiologic stages of the menstrual cycle and sexual response.
4. Link age-related changes of the reproductive system to differences in assessment findings.
5. Obtain significant subjective and objective assessment data related to sexual and reproductive health.
6. Perform a reproductive system physical assessment.
7. Distinguish normal from common abnormal findings from the reproductive system assessment.
8. Describe the purpose, significance of results, and nursing responsibilities related to diagnostic studies of the reproductive system.

KEY TERMS

epididymis
estrogen
follicle-stimulating hormone (FSH)
gonads
luteinizing hormone (LH)
menarche
menopause
menstrual cycle
progesterone
spermatogenesis
testes
testosterone
uterus
vulva

Understanding sexual and reproductive health is essential nursing knowledge. This chapter presents foundational information about anatomy, physiology, assessment, and diagnostic studies related to the human reproductive system. We use the terms "female" and "male" throughout this chapter to reflect reproductive anatomy from birth. Although binary terms are used, some people are born with anatomy or sex characteristics that are a combination of male and female traits (known as intersex).[1] It is important to recognize that a person's reproductive anatomy and sex assigned at birth may not match their gender identity. People who identify as transgender or gender nonconforming may have had gender-affirming hormone therapies or surgery. Care for these persons is outside the scope of this chapter. Nurses should use terms to accurately identify a person's reproductive anatomy and represent their gender identity.

STRUCTURES AND FUNCTIONS OF THE REPRODUCTIVE SYSTEM

The female and male reproductive systems consist of primary and secondary organs. In both males and females, the **gonads** are the primary reproductive organs. These are ovaries in females and testes in males. Gonads secrete hormones and produce sex cells called gametes. These are ova (eggs) in females and sperm in males. During fertilization, gametes unite to form a new cell called a *zygote*. In pregnancy, the zygote divides and multiplies to form an embryo, which develops into a fetus.

In addition to the gonads, the reproductive system includes organs, ducts, and glands. These are all considered secondary (or accessory) reproductive organs. Secondary organs begin their maturity at puberty under the influence of sex hormones. They are responsible for transporting and nourishing the ovum (egg) and sperm and preserving and protecting the fertilized ovum. Female breasts are also considered secondary reproductive organs because they produce milk to nurture an infant.

Female Reproductive System

The main roles of the female reproductive system are to (1) produce ova, (2) secrete hormones, and (3) facilitate sexual activity and pregnancy. The primary female organs are the ovaries. Secondary organs include the fallopian tubes (ducts), uterus, vagina, external genitalia (vulva), and sex glands.

Pelvic Organs

Ovaries. The ovaries are found on either side of the uterus, just behind and below the fallopian tubes (Fig. 55.1). The almond-shaped ovaries are around 0.6 inches (1.5 cm) wide and 1.2 inches (3 cm) long. The ovaries produce ova. They also secrete hormones estrogen and progesterone.

The outer zone of the ovary has follicles with germ cells called *oocytes.* Each follicle contains a primordial (immature) oocyte surrounded by granulosa and theca cells. These 2 layers protect and nourish the oocyte until the follicle reaches maturity and ovulation occurs. Not all follicles reach maturity. In a process termed *atresia,* most of the immature follicles become smaller and are reabsorbed by the body. Over time, the number of follicles declines from around 1 million at birth to around 400,000 at menarche (first menstruation).[2] This is the lifetime supply of sex cells. The number and quality of oocytes decline with age across the reproductive life span.

Fallopian tubes. The fallopian tubes (oviducts or ovarian tubes) transport the ovum from the ovary to the uterus. The tubes are uterine appendages that end by curling around the ovary. Fallopian tubes average 4.8 inches (12 cm) in length, extending from the fimbriae to the superior lateral borders of the uterus. The distal ends of the tubes are open into the abdominal cavity. During ovulation, the fimbriae sweep the ovum from the ruptured ovarian follicle into the tube.

Normally, each month during the reproductive years, one follicle reaches maturity. The ovary expels the ovum through the stimulus of the gonadotropic hormones follicle-stimulating hormone (FSH) and luteinizing hormone (LH). The ovum then travels through a fallopian tube, where fertilization by sperm may occur if sperm are present. Fertilization usually takes place within the outer one-third of the fallopian tubes within 24 hours after release of the ovum.

Uterus. The **uterus** is a pear-shaped, hollow, muscular organ found between the bladder and rectum (Fig. 55.1). In a *nulliparous* female (one who has never been pregnant), the uterus is about 2.4 to 3.2 inches (6 to 8 cm) long and 1.6 inches (4 cm) wide. The uterus consists of the body (or corpus) and cervix. The body makes up about 80% of the uterus. The uterine body walls consist of an outer serosal layer, the *perimetrium;* a middle muscular layer, the *myometrium;* and an inner mucosal layer, the *endometrium.* The dome-shaped top of the uterine body is known as the *fundus.* The lower portion of the uterus is called the isthmus. At the bottom of the uterus, the body connects with the cervix. The cervix projects into the anterior wall of the vaginal canal. It makes up about 15% to 20% of the uterus in the nulliparous female. The cervical canal is 0.8 to 1.6 inches (2 to 4 cm) long. The cervix consists of the ectocervix, the outer part that protrudes into the vagina, and the inner canal known as the endocervix. The part of the cervix that opens into the vagina is the external *cervical os.*

The ectocervix is covered with squamous epithelial cells. It appears smooth and pink. The endocervix is lined with columnar epithelial cells, which give it a rough, reddened appearance. The junction at which the 2 types of epithelial cells (squamous and columnar) meet is the *squamocolumnar junction* (Fig. 55.2). Cells from the squamocolumnar junction are

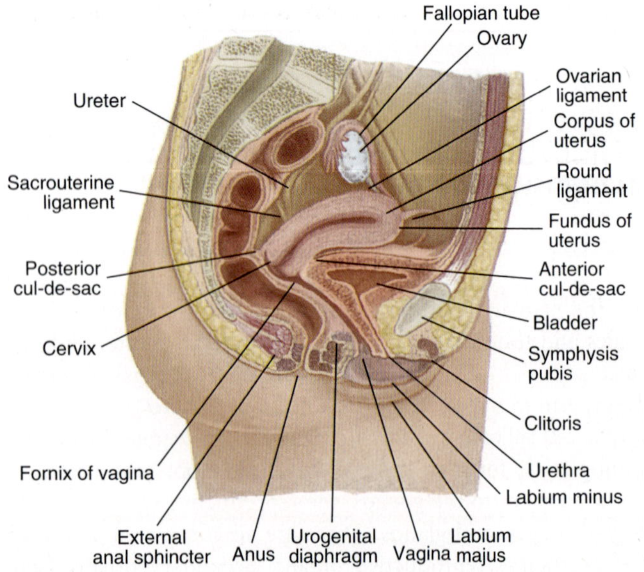

Fallopian tube
Ovary
Ureter
Ovarian ligament
Corpus of uterus
Sacrouterine ligament
Round ligament
Fundus of uterus
Posterior cul-de-sac
Anterior cul-de-sac
Bladder
Cervix
Symphysis pubis
Clitoris
Fornix of vagina
Urethra
Labium minus
External anal sphincter
Anus
Urogenital diaphragm
Vagina
Labium majus

Fig. 55.1 Female reproductive tract. (Modified from Ball JW, Dains JE, Flynn JA, et al: *Seidel's guide to physical examination,* ed 9, St. Louis, 2019, Elsevier.)

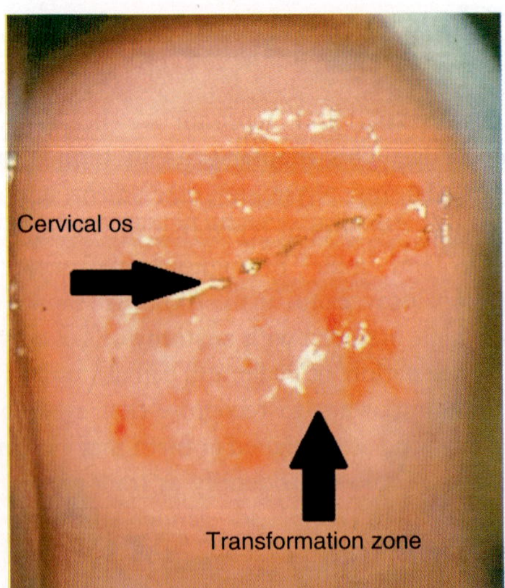

Fig. 55.2 Cervical os and squamocolumnar junction (transformation zone). (Courtesy Candy Tedschi, NP, Great Neck, NY.)

sampled for cervical cancer screening through a Papanicolaou test or "Pap smear."[3]

The external cervical os is relatively tightly closed. It is open slightly to allow menstrual blood to be expelled and sperm to enter the uterus. Mucus made by the cervix under the influence of estrogen and progesterone regulates the entrance of sperm into the uterus. During ovulation, cervical mucus is watery, stretchy, and abundant. Postovulatory cervical mucus is thick and inhibits sperm passage. During pregnancy and birth, the cervix undergoes dramatic transformation in response to hormone changes.

Vagina. The vagina is a tubular structure 3 to 4 inches (7.6 to 10 cm) long. The anterior vaginal wall lies along the urethra and bladder. The posterior vaginal wall is next to the rectum. It is lined with squamous epithelium. In reproductive-age females, the vagina has multiple transverse folds, or *rugae.* The muscular and erectile tissue of the vaginal walls allows enough dilation and contraction to accommodate penetration during sex and the passage of the fetus during childbirth. Vaginal secretions consist of cervical mucus, desquamated epithelium, and, during sexual stimulation, a watery secretion. The vagina has a delicate balance of microorganisms (yeast and bacteria) called the vaginal *microbiome.* Disruption of the microbiome can cause infection and abnormal vaginal discharge.

External Genitalia

The external part of the female reproductive system is the vulva (Fig. 55.3). The vulva consists of the mons pubis, labia majora, labia minora, clitoris, vestibule, urethral meatus, and vaginal introitus (opening). Although not externally visible, paraurethral and vestibular glands are also part of the female reproductive system.

The *mons pubis* is a fatty layer lying over the pubic bone. It is covered with coarse hair in a triangular pattern. The labia are folds of tissue. The labia majora form the outer borders of the vulva. The labia minora form the borders of the vaginal orifice and extend anteriorly to enclose the clitoris. The clitoris is a highly sensitive, erectile sex organ. Only a small part of the clitoris is visible externally. It extends under the tissue of the vulva. The clitoral glans and hood are visible where the labia minora meet at the top of the vestibule. The *vestibule* is the space between the labia minora that contains openings to the urethra (the urethral meatus) and vagina (the introitus). The vestibule extends from the clitoris to the *posterior fourchette,* a mucous membrane band that forms the posterior ends of the labia minora. At birth, the vaginal introitus is surrounded by thin membranous tissue called the *hymen* or *hymenal ring.* In reproductive-age females, the hymen usually appears as folds or tags. The *perineum* is the area between the introitus and the anus.

Paraurethral glands (Skene's glands) lie alongside the urinary meatus. They are similar to the prostate gland in males. These glands secrete mucus, which provides lubrication during sexual arousal and may lubricate the urethral meatus. Vestibular glands (Bartholin's glands) are located at the posterior and lateral aspects of the vaginal orifice. They secrete a mucus that lubricates the vagina and vulva during sexual arousal.

Breasts

Female breasts undergo significant development during puberty, pregnancy, and lactation in response to hormone changes. Adult breasts extend from the 2nd to the 6th ribs. There is wide variation in breast size. Breast tissue includes adipose (fatty) tissue, connective tissue, and glandular tissue (or lobules) that produce milk during lactation. The extension of breast tissue into the upper-outer quadrant into the axilla is an area referred to as the *tail of Spence* (Fig. 55.4). The breast has many blood and lymph vessels. The fully mature breast is dome shape. The pigmented center is the *areola.* At the center of the areola is the nipple. In lactation, milk (or mammary) ducts carry the milk from the lobules to the nipple. The nipple has 5 to 9 ductal openings and many sensory nerve endings. The

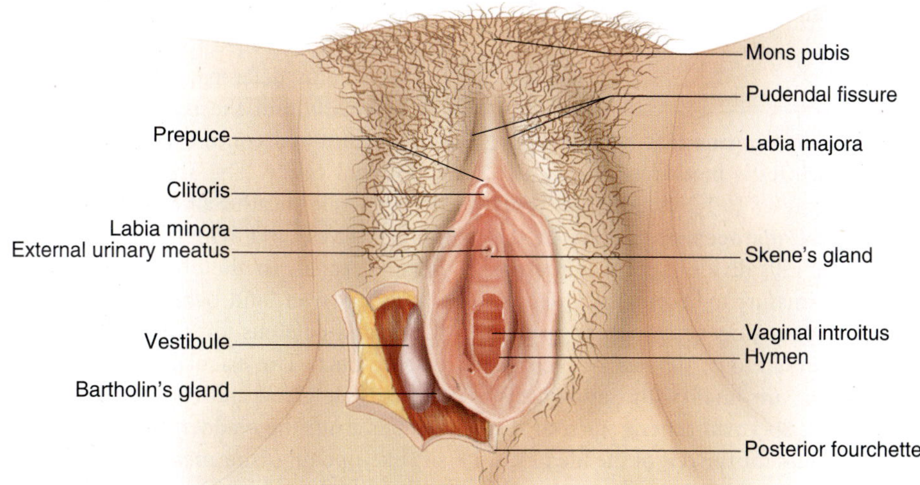

Fig. 55.3 External female genitalia. (Modified from Patton KT, Thibodeau GA: *Anatomy and physiology,* ed 8, St Louis, 2013, Mosby.)

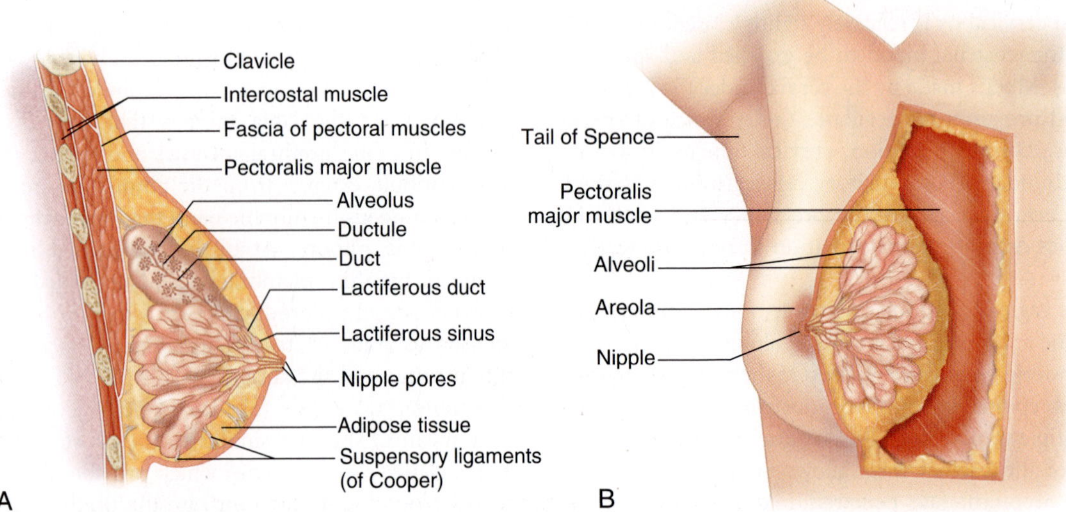

Fig. 55.4 The lactating female breast. (A) Glandular structures are anchored to the overlying skin and the pectoralis muscle by suspensory ligaments of Cooper. Each lobule of glandular tissue is drained by a lactiferous duct that eventually opens through the nipple. (B) Anterior view of a lactating breast. In nonlactating breasts, glandular tissue is less evident, with adipose tissue making up most of the breast. (Modified from Patton KT, Thibodeau GA: *Anatomy and physiology,* ed 8, St Louis, 2013, Mosby.)

nipple and areola have several sebaceous and sweat glands, including areolar glands (or Montgomery tubercles), which secrete lubrication for the nipple. Occasionally, people have supernumerary (accessory) nipples located in other areas of the body.

Male Reproductive System

The main roles of the male reproductive system are to (1) produce and transport sperm, (2) release sperm to facilitate sexual activity and fertilization, and (3) secrete hormones. The primary male organs are the testes. Secondary organs include ducts (epididymis, ductus deferens, ejaculatory duct, urethra), sex glands (prostate gland, Cowper glands, seminal vesicles), and the external genitalia (scrotum, penis) (Fig. 55.5).

Testes

The **testes** are ovoid, smooth, firm organs that lie within the scrotum, typically as a pair. Each testis measures about 1.4 to 2.2 inches (3.5 to 5.6 cm) long and 0.8 to 1.2 inches (2 to 3 cm) wide. Sperm production, or **spermatogenesis**, occurs in the testes. In spermatogenesis, germ cells divide to form immature *spermatogonia,* which ultimately mature to become *spermatozoa* (sperm). Within the testes, spermatogenesis occurs in the seminiferous tubules. The seminiferous tubules are coiled structures within the testes that are lined with Sertoli cells, which facilitate spermatogenesis. Spermatogenesis starts at the beginning of puberty and continues for the rest of the life of the male. Leydig cells lie between the seminiferous tubules. Leydig cells make and release the sex hormone testosterone. Both males and females have testosterone. In males, testosterone is the primary sex hormone.

Ducts

Sperm formed in the seminiferous tubules move through a series of ducts. These ducts transport sperm from the testes to the outside of the body. As sperm leave the testes, they pass through the epididymis, ductus deferens, ejaculatory duct, and urethra. Fig. 55.6 shows a cross section of the internal anatomy of the testis, epididymis, and ductus deferens. The **epididymis** is a comma-shaped structure attached to the back and top of each testis within the scrotum. It is a tightly coiled ridge-like structure. Sperm mature and develop motility as they travel through the epididymis. Sperm exit the epididymis through a long, thick tube called the *ductus deferens.*

The ductus deferens *(vas deferens)* is continuous with the epididymis within the scrotal sac. It travels upward through the scrotum and continues through the inguinal ring into the abdominal cavity. The *spermatic cord* is composed of a connective tissue sheath that encloses the ductus deferens, arteries, veins, nerves, and lymph vessels as it ascends through the inguinal canal. In the abdominal cavity, the ductus deferens travels up, over, and behind the bladder. Behind the bladder, the ductus deferens joins the seminal vesicle to form the ejaculatory duct. The ejaculatory duct passes downward through the prostate gland and connects with the urethra. The urethra extends from the bladder, through the prostate, and ends in a slit-like opening (the meatus) on the ventral side of the *glans* (the tip of the penis). During ejaculation, sperm travel through the urethra and out of the penis.

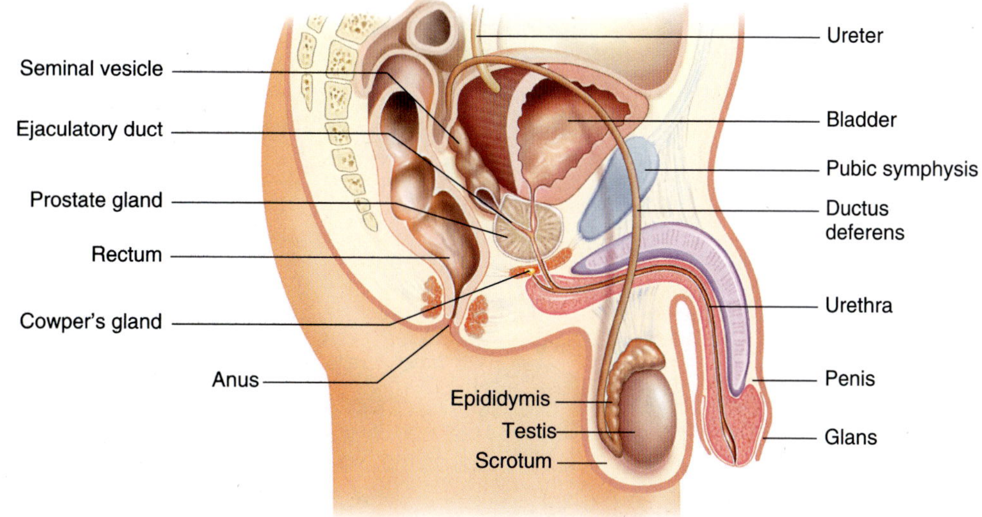

Fig. 55.5 Male reproductive tract. (Modified from Patton KT, Thibodeau GA: *Anatomy and physiology,* ed 8, St Louis, 2013, Mosby.)

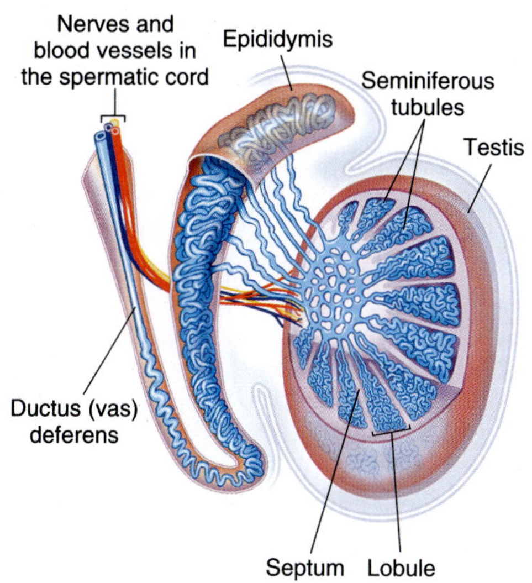

Fig. 55.6 Seminiferous tubules, testis, epididymis, and ductus (vas) deferens in the male. (Modified from Patton KT, Thibodeau GA: *Anatomy and physiology,* ed 8, St Louis, 2013, Mosby.)

Glands

The seminal vesicles, prostate gland, and Cowper (bulbourethral) glands are accessory glands. These glands make and secrete seminal fluid *(semen),* which surrounds the sperm and forms the *ejaculate.* Seminal fluid serves as a medium for the transport of sperm. It creates an alkaline, nutritious environment that promotes sperm motility and survival.

The seminal vesicles lie behind the bladder, between the bladder and rectum. The ducts of the seminal vesicles fuse with the ductus deferens to form the ejaculatory ducts. They enter the prostate gland, which lies beneath the bladder. Its posterior surface is in contact with the rectal wall. The prostate normally measures 0.8 inches (2 cm) wide and 1.2 inches (3 cm) long. It is divided into 5 lobes: right lateral, left lateral, median, anterior, and posterior. Cowper glands lie on each side of the urethra and slightly behind it, just below the prostate. The ducts of these glands enter directly into the urethra.

External Genitalia

The male external genitalia are the penis and scrotum. The penis consists of the shaft and tip *(glans).* The glans is covered by a fold of skin, the prepuce (or foreskin), that forms at the junction of the glans and shaft of the penis. In circumcised males, the prepuce has been removed. The components of the penile shaft include the corpus cavernosum (erectile tissue), the corpus spongiosum (which surrounds the urethra), and the urethra. The skin covering the penis is thin and loose. The *scrotum* is a loose protective sac below the penis that is composed of a thin outer layer of skin over a tough connective tissue layer. The scrotum holds and protects the testes.

Neuroendocrine Regulation of the Reproductive System

The hypothalamus, pituitary gland, and gonads secrete several hormones (see Chapter 52). These hormones regulate ovulation, sperm formation, fertilization, and secondary sex characteristics. The hypothalamus secretes gonadotropin-releasing hormone (GnRH). GnRH stimulates the anterior pituitary gland to secrete its hormones, including **follicle-stimulating hormone (FSH)** and **luteinizing hormone (LH)**. These hormones stimulate the gonads (ovaries, testes) to secrete hormones we call gonadotropins. The gonadal hormones are estrogen, progesterone, and testosterone. They regulate ovarian and testicular function and are essential for reproductive system function.

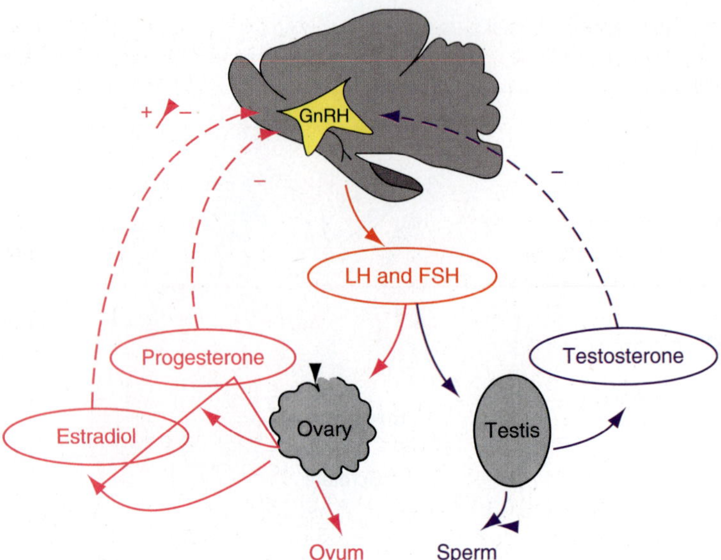

Fig. 55.7 Hypothalamic-pituitary-gonadal axis. Only the major pituitary hormone actions are depicted. *FSH,* Follicle-stimulating hormone; *GnRH,* gonadotropin-releasing hormone; *ICSH,* interstitial cell–stimulating hormone; *LH,* luteinizing hormone. (Brown BB, Prinstein MJ: *Encyclopedia of adolescence,* Cambridge, Mass, 2011, Academic Press.)

The hypothalamus, anterior pituitary, and gonads are all connected through a feedback loop. This loop is called the hypothalamic-pituitary-ovarian (HPO) axis in females or the hypothalamic-pituitary-gonadal (HPG) axis in males (Fig. 55.7). Receptors within the hypothalamus and pituitary are sensitive to the circulating blood levels of the hormones. Increased hormone levels stimulate a hypothalamic response to decrease the high circulating levels. Low circulating levels provoke a hypothalamic response that increases the low circulating levels. We refer to this as a *negative feedback loop.* For example, low testosterone levels stimulate the hypothalamus to secrete GnRH. This triggers the anterior pituitary to secrete greater amounts of FSH and LH, which then increase testosterone production. The high testosterone level signals a decrease in GnRH production, and thus FSH and LH.[4]

In males, **testosterone** is the major gonadal hormone. Testosterone in males is responsible for the development and maintenance of secondary sex characteristics and adequate spermatogenesis. Testosterone plays an important role in libido, muscle mass, bone health, and mood. FSH stimulates the Sertoli cells to promote sperm production in the seminiferous tubules of the testes. LH stimulates the Leydig cells to promote testosterone production in the testes.

In females, FSH and LH stimulate the ovaries to secrete **progesterone** and **estrogen**. Together, these hormones regulate the menstrual cycle (Fig. 55.7). They also affect pregnancy and breast development. These hormones are connected through both negative and positive feedback loops. Negative feedback occurs when estrogen and progesterone levels rise, triggering the hypothalamus to decrease secretion of GnRH. Positive feedback occurs in ovulation, when high levels of estrogen trigger the hypothalamus to increase GnRH secretion. This causes a surge of FSH and LH, which stimulates release of the ovum (ovulation).

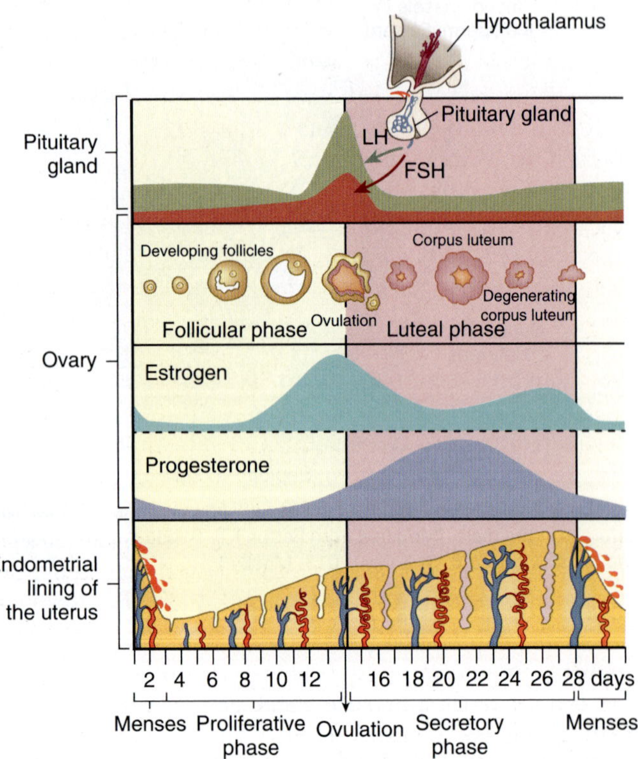

Fig. 55.8 Events of the menstrual cycle. The *lines* depict the changes in blood hormone levels, the development of the follicles, and the changes in the endometrium during the cycle. (Modified from Patton KT, Thibodeau GA: *Anatomy and physiology,* ed 8, St Louis, 2013, Mosby.)

Menstrual Cycle

The major functions of the ovaries are ovulation and the secretion of hormones. These functions are accomplished during the normal **menstrual cycle**, a monthly process mediated by the hormone activity of the hypothalamus, pituitary gland, and ovaries (Fig. 55.8). Menstruation occurs during each month in which an ovum is not fertilized. The length of the menstrual cycle ranges from 21 to 35 days, with an average of 28 days. The onset of menstruation is called **menarche**. Menarche usually occurs around age 12 but can occur normally between 10 and 16 years of age. Menstrual cycles are often irregular for the first 1 to 2 years after menarche with *anovulatory cycles* (cycles without ovulation). Most reproductive age females have regular menstrual cycles. Irregular cycles may occur and can be due to a variety of factors, such as hormone fluctuations, medications, or conditions, such as uterine fibroids. Table 55.1 describes characteristics of the menstrual cycle.

The menstrual cycle is divided into distinct phases based on changes in the ovaries and uterus. The ovarian phases are follicular, ovulation, and luteal. The uterine phases are the proliferative, secretory, and menstrual phases. The menstrual cycle begins on the 1st day of menstrual bleeding. Bleeding typically lasts 3 to 6 days. This is known as the menstrual phase. During this phase, estrogen and progesterone levels are low. FSH and LH stimulate the growth and development of ovarian follicles (the follicular phase). The follicles develop FSH and LH receptors. They also produce estrogen. As estrogen increases, FSH decreases in response. The follicle with the most FSH receptors emerges as dominant and will continue to grow and produce estrogen. The other follicles will atrophy. Estrogen also affects the uterine lining (the endometrium). Estrogen stimulates the growth of the uterine lining (the proliferative phase).

A peak in estrogen levels stimulates a surge of LH. LH triggers the release of the ovum (ovulation) about 24 to 36 hours later. The LH surge is the best indicator of ovulation and is the basis of at-home ovulation predictor tests. After ovulation, the ovaries enter the luteal phase. This phase lasts about 14 days. During this time, the ruptured follicle transforms into a temporary functional cyst we call the corpus luteum. The corpus luteum produces progesterone. Progesterone affects the endometrium, changing it from the proliferative phase to secretory phase in preparation for implantation of a fertilized ovum. Progesterone results in a decrease in FSH and LH through a negative feedback loop. If no pregnancy occurs, the corpus luteum will degenerate, and progesterone levels will decline. This triggers a shift in hormones and the onset of the next menstrual cycle. The blood vessels contract, and tissue begins to slough (fall away). This sloughing results in menses and the start of the menstrual phase, beginning a new cycle.

TABLE 55.1 Characteristics of the Menstrual Cycle

Normal Characteristics	Implications
Menarche	
• Occurs between ages 10 and 16 years • Average age at onset is 12–13 years	• Delayed onset of menarche may indicate endocrine or development problems
Interval	
• Normally 21–35 days • Regular cycles as short as 17 days or as long as 45 days are considered normal if pattern is consistent for the person	• Irregular menstrual cycles may occur with endocrine problems or hormone changes • Some drugs and stressful life events can result in irregular bleeding patterns • Bleeding between menses can be caused by cervical or uterine problems
Duration	
• Menstrual flow generally lasts 2–8 days	• Bleeding longer than 8 days should be assessed for underlying endocrine or hematologic complications • Anatomic changes and cancer can cause prolonged menses
Amount	
• Menstrual flow varies from 20–80 mL per menses • Amount varies for different people and same person at different times • It is usually heaviest first 2 days	• Heavy menstrual bleeding can interfere with quality of life • Heavy menstrual bleeding may indicate uterine problems • Hormone, hematologic, or pregnancy-related complications can present with heavy menses
Composition	
• Menstrual discharge is a mixture of endometrium, blood, mucus, and vaginal cells • Dark red, less viscous than blood, and usually does not clot	• Clots indicate heavy flow or vaginal pooling of blood

Sexual Response

Human sexual response is a complex physiologic process. Healthy sexual activity and expression can take many different forms and include a wide range of behaviors. Historically, sexual response was understood as a linear process with 4 physiologic phases: excitement, plateau, orgasm, and resolution.[5] In this model, sexual stimulation leads to vasoconstriction (excitement), then pelvic floor muscle elevation (plateau), followed by a climax of muscle contraction (orgasm) and a subsequent return to baseline preexcitation (resolution). This 4-stage model provides a general framework for male sexual response: Sexual stimulation leads to penile erection during the *excitement phase.* The erection is maintained in the *plateau phase,* with a slight increase in vasocongestion. In the *orgasm phase,* vasocongestion is released, and rhythmic contractions of the penile and urethral musculature release and propel sperm and seminal fluid outward by *ejaculation.* Then in the *resolution phase,* the penis returns to a flaccid state.[6]

In females, physiologic response to sexual stimulation similarly includes vasocongestion of the clitoris, secretion of vaginal lubrication, and contraction of pelvic muscles. Sexual response in females is often nonlinear. Response phases may overlap, repeat, or be absent from female sexual experiences.

This nonlinearity is one of several reasons why we now know that this 4-stage model is inadequate to describe human sexual response.[7] Recent research shows that sexual response is influenced by emotional, situation, and psychologic factors. Environment, stress, culture, emotional intimacy, satisfaction in interpersonal relationships, and pleasure affect sexual response. We also now know that sexual stimulus affects more than just reproductive organs. Circulatory, nervous, and musculoskeletal systems are involved in sexual response.

Gerontologic Considerations: Effects of Aging on Reproductive Systems

With advancing age, changes occur in the reproductive systems (Table 55.2). Many of these changes are related to decreased hormone production. In females, these changes are related to **menopause**, which is the physiologic cessation of menses from declining ovarian function. Menopause is discussed in Chapter 58. Estrogen, progesterone, and testosterone all decrease with menopause. Decreased hormone levels can result in urogenital atrophy, reduced bone mass, atherosclerosis, vaginal dryness, and sexual dysfunction. After menopause, the vaginal pH becomes more acidic. Breast density and size often decrease.

With aging, males experience a decrease in testosterone. Testosterone levels gradually decrease by an average of 1.6% per year starting in the mid-30s to early 40s age ranges.[8] Age-related gradual decreases in testosterone can lead to physiologic changes, sexual dysfunction, and psychologic manifestations. Physiologic changes include prostate enlargement, decreased bone mineral density and muscle mass, cardiovascular disease, and loss of body/facial hair. Sexual changes can include decreased libido, erectile dysfunction, decreased sperm production and ejaculate volume, and reduction in testicular size and firmness. Psychologic changes can include fatigue, depression, and mood changes. Prostate-specific antigen (PSA) commonly increases with age.

Many factors affect sexuality in later life. The cumulative effects of these changes, as well as the negative social attitude toward sexuality in older adults, can affect the sexual practices of older adults. Illness, disability, medicines, and surgeries can affect the ability to take part in sexual activities. Nurses play a vital role in providing accurate and unbiased information about sexuality and age. Emphasize the normalcy of sexual activity in older adults and refer them to resources that address such issues.

CASE STUDY

Patient Introduction

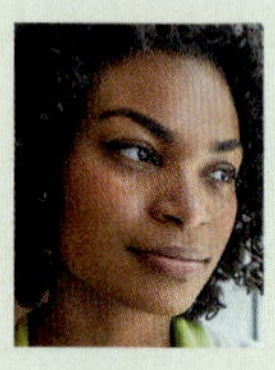

(© Benjamin A. Peterson/Mother Image/mother image/Fuse/Thinkstock.)

C.W. is a 23-year-old cisgender female who is being seen for pelvic pain and irregular menstrual bleeding for the past several months. She takes oral contraceptive pills (OCPs) but occasionally forgets to take them. C.W. takes naproxen as needed for pain with menses.

Discussion Questions

1. What are the possible causes for C.W.'s irregular menstrual bleeding?
2. What assessment questions would you ask C.W.?
3. How would you individualize the assessment based on her age and condition?

You will learn more about C.W. and her condition as you read this assessment chapter.

Answers available at http://evolve.elsevier.com/Lewis/medsurg.

REPRODUCTIVE SYSTEM ASSESSMENT

Subjective Data

Important Health Information

Many people consider reproduction and sexual issues personal and private. The extent and depth of the interview about sexuality and reproductive health depend on the presenting concern, your expertise, and patients' willingness to discuss the topic.

A professional demeanor is important when taking a sexual history. Develop trust with patients. Work to increase your comfort in discussing aspects of sexual health. Conduct interviews in an environment that provides privacy and confidentiality. Do not make any assumptions about gender, sexual orientation, or sexual activity. Have a nonjudgmental attitude. Be sensitive. Use gender-neutral terms when asking about partners. Maintain an awareness of a patient's culture and beliefs. Begin with the least sensitive information (e.g., general health history) before asking questions about more sensitive issues, such as sexual practices. It also requires a nonjudgmental attitude. Acknowledge there is wide variation in sexual activities and sexual responses that can be normal and healthy.

Health history. The health history should include information about major illnesses, hospitalizations, immunizations, and surgeries. Ask about current health status and any acute or chronic health problems. Chronic illnesses, such as cardiovascular disease, respiratory problems, anemia, cancer, and kidney and urinary tract problems, may affect the reproductive system and sexual function. For females, ask about specific medical conditions that affect eligibility for hormone contraceptives. These include history of venous thromboembolism, stroke, breast cancer, and migraine headaches with aura. Ask about pregnancy and lactation status.

In males, ask about prior cardiovascular history and metabolic conditions. Diabetes may lead to erectile dysfunction (ED) and retrograde ejaculation. Stroke or a myocardial

TABLE 55.2 GERONTOLOGIC ASSESSMENT DIFFERENCES

Reproductive Systems

Structure	Changes	Assessment Findings
Female		
Breasts	↓ Subcutaneous fat, increased fibrous tissue	Less resilient, looser, more pendulous tissue ↓ Size
Ovaries	↓ Ovarian function	Nonpalpable ovaries are normal postmenopause
Urethra	↓ Muscle tone, mucosal thinning	Possible UTIs, painful urination (dysuria), urgency, frequency, incontinence
Uterus	↓ Thickness of myometrium	Uterine prolapse
Vagina	Tissue atrophy, ↓ muscle tone, alkaline pH	Mucosa becomes pale, dry, smooth, thin Vagina narrows and shortens
Vulva		Atrophy ↓ Amount of pubic hair
Sexual function	↑ Vaginal dryness ↓ Size of clitoris and labia	Pain with intercourse ↓ Arousal and orgasm ↓ Libido and interest in sex
Male		
Breasts	Enlargement	Gynecomastia (abnormal enlargement)
Penis	↓ Subcutaneous fat	Easily retractable foreskin (if uncircumcised) ↓ Size and rigidity ↓ Ability to attain or sustain erection ↑ Stimulation necessary for erection
Prostate	Benign hyperplasia	Enlargement, urinary obstruction, incontinence
Testes	↓ Testosterone production	↓ Size, firmness ↓ Libido and interest in sex

infarction (MI) may cause physiologic or psychologic ED. Post-MI medication, such as β-blockers, may also worsen ED.

Ask about mental health. Has the patient had treatment for mental health conditions? Ask questions relating to possible endocrine problems, including diabetes, hypothyroidism, and hyperthyroidism. In females, these conditions can affect menstruation, sexual health, and pregnancy.

Take an immunization history. Is there a history of any childhood or adult infections? Infections such as mumps and rubella can affect reproductive function in males. This history also identifies risk for infection in pregnancy and the need for immunizations in preconception care in females.

Note any allergies. Is the patient allergic to latex or drugs, including sulfonamides, macrolides, cephalosporins, tetracyclines, or penicillin? These drugs are often used to treat reproductive and genitourinary (GU) problems, such as STIs and urinary tract infections (UTIs). Silicone and latex are often used in diaphragms and condoms. An allergy to these substances precludes their use as contraception.

Obtain a surgical history. Common surgeries involving the female reproductive system are listed in Table 58.7. Common surgeries involving the male reproductive system are detailed in Chapter 59.

Sexual history. Tell the patient you would like to ask them about their sexual health. An accurate and detailed sexual history is important to guide risk-based screening, counseling, and interventions. A detailed sexual history includes sexual partners, practices, protection from STIs, history of STIs, and pregnancy intention.[9] Table 55.3 outlines the CDC's *5 "P"s of Taking a Sexual History* approach for taking a sexual health history. Do they have any concerns related to their sexual health they would like to discuss? Screen for intimate partner violence and history of sexual trauma.

Menstrual and reproductive history. For females, complete a menstrual and reproductive history. The menstrual history includes the first day of the last menstrual period (LMP), age of menarche, and qualities of menstruation such as the timing, duration, and characteristics of menses. Has the patient had any bleeding or spotting since their last menstrual period? Menstrual history data are used to detect pregnancy, infertility, and many gynecologic problems. Terminology that describes abnormal uterine bleeding patterns is discussed in Chapter 58. For females beyond the reproductive years, ask about perimenopausal symptoms or age of menopause. Ask about prior cervical cancer screening tests or related procedures. Discuss contraceptive history and desire for pregnancy.

Reproductive history is typically recorded using the GTPAL system (Table 55.4). GTPAL includes the total number of pregnancies, term and preterm births, pregnancy losses including spontaneous abortions (or "miscarriages") and pregnancy terminations, and the number of living children. In some cases, we may use a shortened version of the pregnancy

TABLE 55.3 The CDC's Five "P"s of Taking a Sexual History

The 5 *Ps*	Questions
1. Partners	• Are you currently having sex of any kind with anyone? If no, have ever had sex of any kind with another person? • What is/are the gender(s) of your sexual partner(s)? • In recent months, how many sexual partners have you had? • Do you or your partner(s) have other sex partners?
2. Practices	• To understand your risk for STIs, I need to understand the kinds of sex you have had recently. Would that be okay? • Genital (penis in vagina) • Anal (penis in anus) • Oral (mouth on penis, vagina, or anus) • Have you or any of your partners used drugs? • Have you exchanged sex for your needs (money, housing, drugs)?
3. Protection from STIs	• Do you and your partner(s) discuss STI prevention? If you use prevention tools, what methods do you use? • How often do you use these methods? • Have you received HPV, hepatitis A, and/or hepatitis B shots? • Are you aware of PrEP?
4. History of STIs	• Have you ever been tested for STIs and HIV? Would you like to be tested? • Have you been diagnosed with an STI in the past? When? Did you get treatment? • Have you had any symptoms that keep coming back? • Has your current or former partner been diagnosed or treated for an STI?
5. Pregnancy intention	• Do you think you would like to have (more) children at some point? When do you think that might be? • How important is it to you to prevent pregnancy (until then)? • Are you or your partner using contraception or any form of birth control?

Note: Modify this guide as needed to be culturally appropriate, based on culture or gender dynamics.
Adapted from https://www.cdc.gov/std/treatment/sexualhistory.htm#five-ps.

history that includes gravidity and parity. *Gravidity* is the total number of pregnancies, regardless of the pregnancy outcome. *Parity* is the number of pregnancies that reached 20 weeks and 0 days gestation or beyond, regardless of the number of fetuses or pregnancy outcomes. Record the course of each pregnancy. Include the duration of each pregnancy, date of each birth, weight of the infant, any problems that occurred, and the need for any treatment.

Medications. Obtain a complete medication history. Include the reason for use, dosage, and length of time that the drug has been taken. Ask about the use of complementary or alternative therapies such as herbal or nutrition supplements. Many medications can interfere with sexual function.[10]

In females, note the use of hormone agents including contraceptives, selective estrogen receptor modulators (such as tamoxifen, raloxifene), and hormone therapy (HT). Long-term use of combined HT can increase risk for complications such as stroke, breast cancer, deep vein thrombosis, and gallbladder disease.[11] Ask about the use of any vaginal products such as spermicides, douches, gels, or creams. Do they have a contraceptive intrauterine device (IUD) or implant? Some hormone contraceptives are taken for menstrual regulation, not just pregnancy prevention. Ask about the reason for contraceptive use.

In males, it is important to note cardiovascular medication history, as medications like nitrates that are used for angina are contraindicated with oral medications for ED due to risk for hypotension. Antihypertensives, such as amlodipine, propranolol, and clonidine, may cause ED. Antidepressants and other psychotropic medications can also cause or worsen ED. Hormone medications to treat prostate cancer (such as leuprolide) can worsen ED.[12] Ask about chronic opioid or corticosteroid use, as these medications can cause testosterone deficiency.

Family history. An accurate family history is vital. Ask about a history of cancer, especially of the reproductive organs. Note a family history of any chronic conditions such as diabetes, hypothyroidism, hyperthyroidism, hypertension, stroke, angina, MI, endocrine problems, or anemia. Ask about any genetic conditions, congenital abnormalities, or intellectual or developmental disabilities in the family.

Social and environment history. Social and environment factors can have significant impacts on sexual function. Alcohol, marijuana, and other illegal or misused substances can affect sexual and reproductive health. Ask about tobacco use. Tobacco increases risk of complications with hormone agents and worsens ED. Assess for exposure to chemicals or teratogens that could affect sexual function and fertility, including chemotherapies and radiation. Diet and exercise affect sexual and reproductive health. Ask about diet, any past or current eating disorders, and type and frequency of exercise. Screen for any current or historic intimate partner violence or sexual trauma.

Functional Health Patterns

Key questions to ask patients with a reproductive problem are outlined in Table 55.5.

Health perception–health management. Discuss the patient's perception of their own health and measures that they take to maintain health. Ask about self-examination practices and screenings. Breast and cervical cancer screenings are important for females. Males are at risk for testicular and

TABLE 55.4 Reproductive (Pregnancy) History: GTPAL

Abbreviation	Aspect of History	Definition
G	Gravidity	Total number of pregnancies, regardless of outcome (including current one if pregnant)
T	Term births	Number of pregnancies that reached 37 weeks' gestation
P	Preterm births	Number of pregnancies that reached 20 weeks' gestation and did not exceed $36\frac{6}{7}$ weeks' gestation (regardless of pregnancy outcome)
A	Abortion	Number of spontaneous or induced abortions (prior to 20 weeks' gestation)
L	Living children	Number of living children (which usually equals total of term and preterm numbers but may be greater if patient had multiple gestations or less if any children have died)

TABLE 55.5 Reproductive Health History

Health Perception–Health Management

- How would you describe your overall health?
- Describe the health of your family members. Any history of breast, uterine, ovarian, or prostate cancer?[a]

Females

- Are you currently pregnant or lactating?
- Have you noticed any changes in your breasts?
- When was your last Pap test?[a]
- Have you ever had an abnormal Pap test; if so, what did it find?
- When was your last mammogram?[a]
- Have you ever had an abnormal mammogram; if so, what did it find?

Males

- Do you perform testicular self-examination? Any concerns?

Nutritional-Metabolic

- Describe what you usually eat and drink.
- Have you had any changes in weight?[a]
- How do you feel about your current weight?
- Do you take any nutrition supplements, such as calcium or vitamins?[a]
- Do you have any diet restrictions?[a]

Elimination

- Do you have problems with urination (e.g., pain, burning, dribbling, incontinence, frequency)?[a]
- Have you had bladder infections? If so, when? How often?
- Do you have problems with bowel movements?[a]
- Do you have any constipation, loose stools, or blood with stools?[a]
- Do you use laxatives?[a]

Activity-Exercise

- What activities do you typically do each day?
- Do you have enough energy for your desired activities?

Sleep-Rest

- How many hours do you typically sleep each night?
- Do you feel rested after sleep?
- Do you have any problems sleeping?[a]

Cognitive-Perceptual

- Do you have pain? If yes, where?
- Do you have pain during sexual activity?[a]

Self-Perception–Self-Concept

- How would you describe yourself?
- Have there been any recent changes that have made you feel differently about yourself?[a]
- Are you having any problems that are affecting your sexuality?[a]

Role-Relationship

- Describe your living arrangements. With whom do you live?
- Do you have a significant other? If yes, is this relationship satisfying?
- Are you having any role-related problems in your family?[a] At work?[a]
- What are the relationships among your family members?

Sexuality-Reproductive

- Are you sexually active? If so, how many partners do you have?
- What kind of sex do you engage in (oral, vaginal, anal)?
- How do you protect yourself against sexually transmitted infections and unwanted pregnancy?
- Are you satisfied with your present means of sexual expression? If not, explain.
- Have you had any recent changes in your sexual practices?[a]

Females

- Menstrual history: How old were you when you had your first menstrual period? What was the first day of your last menstrual period? Describe your period. How many days does it last? How often does it come (e.g., every 28 days)? Do you have any problems with your periods?
- Menopause history: How old were you when you went through menopause? Have you had any postmenopausal bleeding or spotting?[a]
- Pregnancy history (Table 55.4): How many times have you been pregnant? How many living children do you have? Have you ever had any miscarriages or abortions? Did they need medical intervention?

Males

- Do you have any problem obtaining or sustaining an erection?
- Do you have any problems with ejaculation?

Coping–Stress Tolerance

- Have there been any major changes in your life within the past couple of years?[a]
- What is stressful in your life right now?
- How do you handle health problems when they occur?
- Do you feel safe in your home? Work? Has anyone ever tried to hurt or harm you?

Value-Belief

- Do you use any complementary or alternative therapies or home remedies?[a]
- Do you have any religious or personal beliefs that affect your sexual or reproductive health?[a]

[a]If yes, describe.

prostate cancer. However, controversy exists about the benefits of routine screening for these cancers.[13] All patients should discuss the benefits and risks of screening with their HCP.

Nutritional-metabolic. Anemia is a common problem in females in their reproductive years, especially during pregnancy and the postpartum period. Evaluate their diet with this in mind. Folic acid deficiency in pregnancy can result in spina bifida and other fetal neural tube defects. Iron deficiency anemia is the most common cause of anemia in menstruating females. Take a thorough nutrition and psychologic history to assess for an eating disorder. Anorexia nervosa can cause amenorrhea (loss of menses). Obesity can be related to polycystic ovary syndrome. Adequate calcium and vitamin D intake help prevent osteoporosis.

Nutrition can affect sperm quality. For males, the Mediterranean diet may benefit semen quality. Encourage adequate fiber and antioxidant intake in the diet. Discourage diets high in processed foods, excess animal proteins, trans fats, and saturated fats, as these can negatively affect semen quality.[14]

Elimination. Genitourinary problems can be caused by changes in the reproductive system. For example, as females age, they experience relaxation of the pelvic musculature, which can lead to pelvic organ prolapse and urinary incontinence. Similarly, benign prostatic hyperplasia (BPH) is common in older males. It can cause urinary retention or difficulty in starting the urinary stream.

Sexual health conditions can lead to GU problems. Urinary tract infections can result from spermicide use, diaphragms, and sexual activity. Males may have urethritis, an inflammation of the urethra, which may be caused by an STI. Urethritis can cause painful urination.

Activity-exercise. Record the amount, type, and intensity of activity and exercise. In females, excess exercise can cause amenorrhea. Lack of weight-bearing exercise is important in the developing osteoporosis after menopause. Anemia can result in fatigue and activity intolerance and interfere with performing activities of daily living.

In males, a sedentary lifestyle and lack of exercise can lead to increased adipose tissue, especially abdominal fat, which can worsen sexual function. Increased estradiol levels in central adipose tissue can negatively affect natural testosterone production. Some research shows that adequate physical exercise may have similar sexual health benefits for some males as ED medications.[15]

Sleep-rest. Many aspects of sexual and reproductive health can negatively affect sleep. In females, hormone changes of menstruation can cause insomnia.[16] Physiologic changes of pregnancy alter sleep needs and can cause fatigue. Perimenopausal hot flashes and night sweats often disrupt sleep. In males, frequent urination at night can disturb sleep. Nocturia could be related to prostate enlargement or hormone therapy for prostate cancer.

Cognitive-perceptual. In females, pelvic pain can occur with various gynecologic problems, such as pelvic inflammatory disease, ovarian cysts, and endometriosis. Sexual pain worsens self-esteem and relationships. These conditions can negatively affect quality of life. Complications of menstrual, reproductive, or sexual health can lead to anxiety or depression. Hormone shifts and physiologic changes in pregnancy and menopause may affect cognitive function. In males, chronic pelvic pain, urethritis, and chronic testicular pain can have similar negative effects.

Self-perception—self-concept. Gender identity and sexual orientation strongly affect self-perception. Changes associated with sexuality and advancing age lead to alterations in self-concept. For example, females may struggle with urinary incontinence and vaginal dryness. In males, a decrease in penis size may lead to distress. Sexual dysfunction can cause a negative view of self.

Role-relationship. Obtain information about the family structure and occupation. Ask about recent changes in work-related relationships or family conflict. Assess the patient's role in the family as a starting point to determine family dynamics. Changes within the family, such as marriage, divorce, or birth of a child, affect roles and relationships. Sexual health and function are important to many people and affect intimate relationships.

Sexuality-reproductive. Sexual health, safety, and satisfaction are essential to overall health and well-being. Ask about satisfaction with sexuality. Explore any unexplained changes in sexual practices or performance. Discuss desire for pregnancy. Ask about family planning needs and preferences.

Coping—stress tolerance. In females, gynecologic, sexual, and reproductive complications are often stressful. Normal changes associated with pregnancy or menopause can strain coping mechanisms. In males, changes in erectile function over time can cause significant personal and relationship stress. Side effects from treatments for prostate cancer, including ED and urinary incontinence, can strain coping mechanisms in males.

Determine the support people and systems in the patient's life. Explore ways to manage stress. Encourage patients to share their concerns. Help them identify and develop strategies to reduce stress and improve coping related to sexual and reproductive health.

Value-belief. Sexual and reproductive function is often closely related to cultural, religious, moral, and ethical values. Recognize and sensitively react to personal beliefs associated with issues around reproductive and sexual health.

Objective Data

Approach to Intimate Physical Assessment

Assessing the reproductive system including genitals, rectum, and breasts is considered intimate or sensitive. Ensure patient safety, comfort, and privacy during these exams. Patients may experience embarrassment, fear, and vulnerability. They can also trigger prior trauma. Not all patients who experienced prior trauma will disclose this information. A trauma-informed approach to care is essential for all patients. Ensure patients are informed and consent to the assessment. Explain what will happen. Take measures to protect privacy and modesty. This may include a private space for undressing and gowns or drapes. Provide emotional support. Continue to reassess

CASE STUDY

Subjective Data

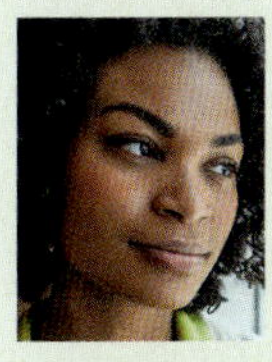

(© Benjamin A. Peterson/ Mother Image/ mother image/ Fuse/ Thinkstock.)

A focused assessment of C.W. revealed the following information:

Health Perception–Health Management: In good health. Pap smear 2 years ago was normal. Has not had any surgeries

Nutritional-Metabolic: 5 ft 2 in, 130 lb (BMI 23.7 kg/m^2). Does not take any vitamins or supplements, follows a "normal" diet. Eats out 2x week otherwise cooks own meals at home with friends

Elimination: Denies any changes with urination or bowel movements

Activity-Exercise: Exercises at gym, 45 min 2 times a week

Sleep-Rest: Sleeps 6 to 7 hours per night

Cognitive-Perceptual: Denies dyspareunia

Self-Perception–Self Concept: Cisgender female, identifies as "bisexual," has positive view of self and body image

Role-Relationship: Full-time graduate school student, single and lives with 2 other young females in off-campus housing, feels socially connected and safe in relationships

Sexuality-Reproductive: Menarche at age 12. Last menstrual period 2 weeks ago. Menses is usually every 28 days, lasting 4 days, but has noted periods are longer and more painful over past few months, with occasional "spotting" between periods. Sexually active with males and females, for past 2 years in a mutually monogamous relationship with cisgender male partner. Practices vaginal and oral sex. Does not desire pregnancy and is using oral contraceptive pills (OCPs).

Coping–Stress Tolerance: Reports "moderate" levels of stress with school, exercises and socializes for stress relief

Value-Belief: Raised Catholic, not actively involved with a religious/spiritual community

Discussion Questions

1. Which subjective assessment findings concern you most?
2. What would you include in the physical assessment?

You will learn more about physical assessment of the reproductive system in the next section.

Answers available at http://evolve.elsevier.com/Lewis/medsurg.

consent and comfort throughout the examination. Patients may defer, decline, or revoke consent for an exam at any time, and if so, it should be recorded in the medical record.

Nurses may serve as a chaperone for HCPs during these exams. Chaperones should be trained on expectations for the normal procedure and any variations or deviations from norms. Chaperones should be aware of the specific policies to report any concerns or questionable practices they observe.

Table 55.6 gives an example of documentation for normal physical assessment findings. A focused assessment is used to evaluate the status of identified reproductive problems and monitor for signs of new problems. A focused assessment of the reproductive system is shown in Box 55.1.

Physical assessment: female. Physical assessment often begins with inspection and palpation of the breasts and axillae, then proceeds to the abdomen and, when appropriate, genital and pelvic examination. Abdominal exam is discussed in Chapter 43. It provides an opportunity to detect pain or any masses that may involve the GU system.

Breasts. To perform a breast examination, first examine the breasts by visual inspection. With the patient seated, inspect the breasts for symmetry, size, shape, color, vascular patterns. Note any skin changes such as dimpling, scars, or lesions (Table 55.7). Inspect the nipple shape and presence of any discharge. Ask them to put the arms at the sides, arms overhead, lean forward, and press hands on hips. Observe for changes during these maneuvers. After washing hands, palpate the axillae and clavicle areas for enlarged lymph nodes. Ask the patient to recline into a supine position with their arm above the head. This position flattens breast tissue to improve palpation of abnormal tissue. Palpate the lymph nodes and breast in a systematic, linear fashion (see Fig. 56.4). Use flat surface of the finger pads of the index, middle, and ring fingers for palpation. Include the axillary tail of Spence. This area of the breast lies adjacent to the upper outer quadrant. It is where most breast cancer develops. Palpate the area around the areolae for masses.

TABLE 55.6 Normal Physical Assessment of Breasts and External Genitalia

Female	Male
Breasts	
Symmetric without dimpling. Nipples soft. No drainage, retraction, or lesions noted. No masses or tenderness. No lymphadenopathy.	Nipples soft. No lumps, nodules, swelling, or enlarged tissue noted. No masses or tenderness.
External Genitalia	
Triangular hair distribution. Genitalia dark pink, no lesions, redness, swelling, or inflammation in perineal region. No tenderness with palpation of paraurethral or vestibular glands.	Diamond-shaped hair distribution. No penile lesions or discharge noted. Scrotum symmetric, no masses, descended testes. No inguinal hernia.
Anus	
No hemorrhoids, fissures, or lesions noted.	No hemorrhoids, fissures, or lesions.

Pelvic examination. Pelvic exams are typically only done when indicated by the history or symptoms. For asymptomatic, nonpregnant females, shared decision making that considers patients' preferences for routine pelvic examination is appropriate. When performed, comprehensive genital and pelvic assessment of the female reproductive system has 3 parts:

BOX 55.1 FOCUSED ASSESSMENT

Reproductive System

Use this checklist to ensure the key assessment steps have been done.

Subjective

Ask the patient about any of the following and note responses:

Breasts: changes in shape or size, masses, nipple discharge
Vagina or vulva: discharge, lesions, itching, unusual bleeding, odor
Penis or testes: lesions, masses, irritation, penile discharge
Anus: lesions, hemorrhoids, inflammation
Pain or tenderness: breasts, pelvis, or genitalia
Medications: antihypertensives, psychotropics, hormones, contraceptives

Objective: Diagnostic

Check the following for results and critical values:

Serology studies: CBC, TSH, PSA, hCG, hormone studies (e.g., testosterone, progesterone, estrogen, FSH, LH, prolactin)
STIs: *Chlamydia,* gonorrhea, *Trichomonas,* HIV, syphilis, HPV
In-office testing: urine hCG, wet mount (microscopy), pH assessment
Mammography
Cytology (Pap smear) or colposcopy
Semen analysis
Ultrasound or MRI: breast, pelvic, transvaginal, penile, testicular, rectal

Objective: Physical Assessment

Inspect

Breasts and nipples for size and symmetry, dimpling, retraction, discharge, redness, scars, lesions
External genitalia for hair distribution, redness, swelling, discharge, lesions
Anus for lesions, fissures, hemorrhoids

Palpate

Breasts and axillae for masses or tenderness
External genitalia for masses or tenderness

FSH, Follicle-stimulating hormone; *hCG,* human chorionic gonadotropin; *LH,* luteinizing hormone; *NAAT,* nucleic acid amplification test; *PSA,* prostate-specific antigen; *STI,* sexually transmitted infection; *TSH,* thyroid-stimulating hormone.

external, speculum, and internal bimanual. Not all 3 components may be necessary based on the presenting concern.

Before beginning, it is essential to ensure informed consent. Have patients use the bathroom beforehand. Wash hands and wear gloves. Supplemental lighting is often needed for optimal visualization. Drapes and gowns should be provided to ensure modesty. A variety of positions may be used to ensure comfort. Commonly, the knees are bent and the feet are placed on the exam table or specialized footrests, with the knees out to sides.

External pelvic examination. External examination starts with inspection of the mons pubis, vulva, and anus. Assess for hair distribution, presence of body lice, lesions, redness, edema, or discharge (Table 55.8). Many females remove hair from the genital region via shaving, waxing, or laser hair removal. Hair removal may result in folliculitis (infection of the hair follicle).

Talk to the patient throughout. Explain what you are going to do. If palpation is required, reestablish consent before proceeding. You may need to separate the labia to fully inspect the clitoris, urethral meatus, vaginal orifice, and paraurethral and vestibular glands. Spread the buttocks apart to inspect the anus for fissures, lesions, and hemorrhoids. Be attentive for any signs of discomfort and pause until the patient is ready to continue.

Internal pelvic examination. HCPs or nurses with special training usually do this part of the examination. A vaginal speculum is inserted to inspect the walls of the vagina and cervix for inflammation, discharge, or other problems. Specimens for cervical cytology (Pap test), microscopy, or nucleic acid amplification tests (NAATs) for STIs may be obtained. Internal bimanual examination may be done to assess the size, shape, consistency, and sensitivity of the internal reproductive organs or musculature.

Physical assessment: male. Assessment of the external male genitalia includes inspection and palpation of the pubis, penis, and scrotum. The patient may be supine or standing. A standing position is preferred. Sit in front of the standing patient. Wash hands and wear gloves when assessing the male genitalia. Explain what you are going to do for the examination and why. Reconfirm consent prior to proceeding with palpation.

If breast cancer is suspected or there is a strong family history of breast cancer in a male patient, a clinical breast examination is done in the same pattern for male patients as for a female breast examination.

Pubis. Assess hair distribution. Normally, the hair is in a diamond-shaped pattern and coarser than scalp hair (Table 55.9). The absence of hair is not normal unless patients are shaving or waxing the pubic hair. Assess the skin for irritation and inflammation.

Penis and scrotum. Inspect the penis for any lesions, bleeding, or swelling. Note the location of the urethral meatus and the presence or absence of foreskin. If present, retract the foreskin and note any redness, discharge, irritation, lesions, or swelling from the meatus. Replace the foreskin over the glans after observation. Inspect the scrotum by lifting each testis to inspect all sides of the scrotal sac. Palpate the testes for tenderness or masses. The left testis usually hangs lower than the right. An undescended testis *(cryptorchidism)* is a major risk factor for testicular cancer and a potential cause of male infertility.

Anus. Note if the buttocks have any lesions, swelling, or inflammation. Spread the buttocks apart with both hands to expose the anus. Inspect the anal sphincter and perineal regions for fissures, lesions, masses, and hemorrhoids. The anus should be free from inflammation or skin changes.

Prostate. Digital rectal examination (DRE) to examine the prostate is typically done by HCPs with advanced or special training. Informed consent is obtained before a DRE. Patients may be positioned standing and instructed to bend forward at the waist or may be positioned on their side with knees pulled up to the abdomen. Wearing gloves, the HCP inserts a lubricated finger into the rectum. They gently palpate the posterior lobe of the prostate to evaluate for any firm nodules or masses that could represent prostate cancer then remove their finger. If the prostate feels boggy or tender to palpation, that could

TABLE 55.7 ASSESSMENT ABNORMALITIES

Breast

Finding	Description	Possible Cause and Significance
Dimpling	Unilateral, recent onset, no pain	Cancer
Nipple inversion or retraction	Recent onset, redness, pain, unilateral	Abscess, inflammation, cancer
Nipple scaling or irritation	Unilateral or bilateral, crusting, possible ulcer	Eczema, infection, cancer
Nipple discharge		
• Galactorrhea (female)	Milky, no relationship to lactation, unilateral or bilateral, intermittent or consistent	Side effect of certain medications, endocrine dysfunction, hypothalamus or pituitary tumor
• Galactorrhea (male)	Milky, bilateral	Chorioepithelioma of testes, pituitary tumor
• Multicolored or dark green discharge	Thick, sticky, often bilateral	Ductal ectasia
• Purulent	Gray-green or yellow color. Often unilateral. May have pain, redness, induration, nipple inversion	Puerperal (after birth) mastitis or abscess, infected sebaceous cyst
• Serosanguineous or bloody drainage	Unilateral	Papillomatosis (widespread development of nipple-like growths), intraductal papilloma, cancer (male and female)
• Serous discharge	Clear appearance, unilateral or bilateral, intermittent or consistent	Intraductal papilloma
Nodules, lumps, or masses	Multiple, bilateral, well-delineated, soft or firm, mobile cysts. Pain. Premenstrual occurrence	Fibrocystic or cyclical changes
	Rubbery consistency, fluid-filled interior, pain	Ductal ectasia
	Soft, mobile, well-delineated cyst, painless	Lipoma, fibroadenoma
	Redness, tenderness, induration	Infected sebaceous cysts, abscesses
	Usually singular, hard, irregularly shaped, poorly delineated, nonmobile	Cancer

TABLE 55.8 ASSESSMENT ABNORMALITIES

Female Reproductive System

Finding and Description	Possible Cause and Significance
Vaginal Discharge	
Thin gray or white, malodorous/fishy	Bacterial vaginosis
White, thick, curdy, itchy	Candidiasis (*Candida* or yeast infection)
Mucopurulent, bloody	*Chlamydia trachomatis* or *Neisseria gonorrhoeae* infection, menstruation, trauma, cancer
Frothy, green or yellow, malodorous	Trichomoniasis
Vulvar Growths	
Soft, fleshy growth, nontender	Condyloma acuminatum (genital warts)
Flat and warty appearance, nontender	Condyloma latum
Same as either of above, possible pain	Cancer
Red base, vesicles, and small erosions; pain	Lymphogranuloma venereum, genital herpes, chancroid
Indurated, firm ulcers, no pain	Chancre (syphilis), granuloma inguinale
Vulvar Appearance	
Bright or beefy red color, itching	*Candida albicans,* allergy, chemical vaginitis
Red base, painful vesicles or ulcers	Genital herpes
Macules or papules, itching	Chancroid, contact dermatitis, scabies, pediculosis
Abdominal Pain, Tenderness, or Pelvic Masses	
Intermittent or consistent tenderness in right or left lower quadrant	Salpingitis, ectopic pregnancy, ruptured ovarian cyst, pelvic inflammatory disease, tubal or ovarian abscess
Periumbilical location, consistent occurrence	Cystitis, endometritis, ectopic pregnancy
Abdominal or pelvic pain, especially with menses, radiates to back, rectum, or vagina	Endometriosis
Pelvic masses	Fibroids, ovarian cysts, cancer

TABLE 55.9 ASSESSMENT ABNORMALITIES
Male Reproductive System

Finding and Description	Possible Cause and Significance
Inguinal Masses	
Bulging unilateral mass during straining	Inguinal hernia
1–3 cm nodules	Lymphadenopathy
Penile Discharge	
Clear to purulent color, minimal to copious flow	Urethritis or gonorrhea, *Chlamydia trachomatis* infection, trauma
Penile Growths or Masses	
Indurated, smooth, disk-like appearance. Painless, single lesion	Chancre (syphilis)
Papular to irregularly shaped ulcer with pus, no induration	Chancroid
Ulcer with induration and nodularity	Cancer
Flat, wartlike nodule	Condyloma latum
Raised, fleshy, moist, elongated projections with single or multiple projections	Condyloma acuminatum (genital warts)
Local swelling with retracted, tight foreskin	Paraphimosis (inability to replace foreskin to its normal position after retraction), trauma
Scrotal Masses	
Local swelling with tenderness, unilateral or bilateral	Epididymitis, testicular torsion, orchitis (mumps)
Swelling, tenderness	Incarcerated hernia
Swelling without pain. Unilateral or bilateral. Translucent, cordlike, or wormlike appearance	Hydrocele, spermatocele, varicocele, hematocele
Firm, nodular testes or epididymis. Often unilateral	Tuberculosis, cancer
Vesicles, Erosions, or Ulcers	
Macules and papules	Scabies, pediculosis
Painful, reddened base. Vesicular or small erosions	Genital herpes, balanitis, chancroid
Painless, singular, small erosion with eventual lymphadenopathy	Lymphogranuloma venereum, cancer

represent prostatitis. It is possible to palpate internal hemorrhoids. The utility and frequency of DREs is a topic of debate among primary care and specialty HCPs.

CASE STUDY
Objective Data: Physical Assessment

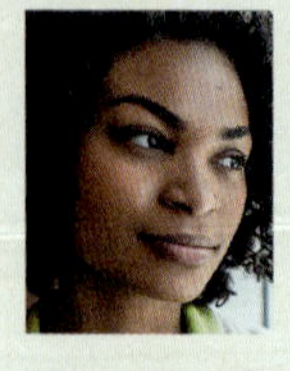

(© Benjamin A. Peterson/Mother Image/mother image/Fuse/Thinkstock.)

Focused assessment of C.W. reveals the following: BP is 108/72 mm Hg; her pulse is 78 beats/min and regular. Temp 97.8°F. Urine hCG is negative. Skin is warm and dry without lesions. She has facial acne. Thyroid is slightly enlarged. Abdomen is soft, nontender, nondistended. External genitalia are normal. Bimanual examination by the HCP is negative for cervical motion tenderness or uterine anomalies. She has left-sided tenderness with palpation of the left adnexa. No masses are palpated.

Discussion Questions

1. Based on the subjective and objective assessment findings, what diagnostic tests would you anticipate being ordered for C.W.?

You will learn more about diagnostic studies related to the reproductive system in the next section.

Answers available at http://evolve.elsevier.com/Lewis/medsurg.

DIAGNOSTIC STUDIES OF THE REPRODUCTIVE SYSTEM

The most common diagnostic studies used to assess the reproductive systems are described in Tables 55.10 through 55.14. Diagnostic studies of the endocrine system may also be done in a person with a reproductive system problem (see Tables 52.6 and 52.7).

Nursing Responsibility for Diagnostic Procedures

Before a procedure, teach patients about the procedure and ensure informed consent. Explain steps for any advance preparation such as taking pain medication or abstaining from food or drink. During procedures, nurses can assist HCPs as appropriate, provide ongoing assessment, and ensure patients' comfort. After the procedure, assess for complications such as pain. Provide information about pain medication as prescribed by the HCP. Explain how to follow up to obtain test results.

For vaginal procedures, assess for bleeding and pain. Teach about common symptoms such as mild cramping or light vaginal bleeding. Provide information about warning signs of complications as prolonged or excess vaginal bleeding (soaking through more than one menstrual pad an hour), foul-smelling vaginal discharge, worsening or severe pain, or fever/chills.

TABLE 55.10 Serology Studies

Study	Reference Interval	Commonly Associated Conditions
Female		
Estradiol (estrogen)	Follicular phase: 20–350 pg/mL Luteal phase: 30–450 pg/mL Postmenopause: ≤20 pg/mL	Abnormal uterine bleeding Infertility Menopausal status Ovarian tumor Precocious puberty Response to hormone replacement therapy
Follicle-stimulating hormone (FSH)	Follicular phase: 1.37–9.9 IU/mL Ovulatory phase: 6.17–17.2 IU/mL Luteal phase: 1.09–9.2 IU/mL Postmenopause: 19.3–100.6 IU/mL	Infertility Pituitary problems Precocious puberty Menopause status Menstrual irregularities
Human chorionic gonadotropin (hCG)	Negative: <5 mIU/mL Indeterminate: 5–25 IU/L Positive: >25 IU/L	Pregnancy Hydatidiform mole Choriocarcinoma
Luteinizing hormone (LH)	Follicular phase: 1.68–15 IU/mL Ovulatory phase: 21.9–56.6 IU/mL Luteal phase: 0.61–16.3 IU/mL Postmenopause: 14.2–52.3 IU/mL	Infertility Ovulation Pituitary problems Precocious puberty Menopausal status Menstrual problems
Progesterone	Follicular phase: <50 ng/dL Luteal phase: 300–2500 ng/dL Postmenopause: <40 ng/dL First trimester pregnancy: 725–4400 ng/dL	Adrenal hyperplasia or tumor Amenorrhea Choriocarcinoma Hydatidiform mole Luteal ovarian cysts Ovulation Pregnancy viability
Prolactin	Nonpregnant: 3–27 ng/mL	Galactorrhea Pituitary tumor Menstrual irregularities
Male		
Estradiol	*Male:* 10–50 pg/mL (37–184 pmol/L)	Erectile dysfunction Infertility Testosterone deficiency Testicular tumor
Follicle-stimulating hormone (FSH)	*Male:* 1.42–15.4 mU/mL	Infertility Pituitary problems Testosterone deficiency
Human chorionic gonadotropin (hCG)	Qualitative: Negative Quantitative: <5 mIU/mL (<5 IU/L) (males and nonpregnant females)	Infertility Testosterone deficiency Testicular tumor
Luteinizing hormone (LH)	*Male:* 1.8–8.6 IU/L	Erectile dysfunction Infertility Pituitary problems Testosterone deficiency
Prolactin	*Male:* 3.0–14.7 ng/mL (3.0–14.7 mg/L)	Infertility Pituitary problems Prolactinoma Testosterone deficiency
Prostate-specific antigen (PSA)	*Male:* <2.5 ng/mL (<2.5 mcg/L)	Benign prostate conditions Prostate cancer, screening, follow-up
Testosterone	In 24-h urine samples: • *Male:* 40–135 mcg/24 h (139–469 nmol/24 h) In blood: • *Male:* 280–1100 ng/dL (10.4–38.17 nmol/L)	Decreased libido Erectile dysfunction Infertility Pituitary problems Response to hormone treatment for prostate cancer Testosterone deficiency

From Pagana KD, Pagana TJ, Pagana TN: *Mosby's diagnostic and laboratory test reference,* St. Louis, 2023, Elsevier.

Caution against inserting anything into the vagina until bleeding is resolved and the site is healed.

Teach male patients about expected side effects and warning signs specific to the location of the procedure. For testicular procedures, discuss the potential for mild testicular or scrotal swelling and discomfort after the procedure. Teach patients to contact the HCP if they develop severe pain or swelling, penile discharge, dysuria, fever, or chills. For prostate procedures, discuss the potential for mild temporary blood in the urine, stool, and semen. Review complications including persistent bleeding per rectum with lightheadedness or dizziness, an inability to urinate, fevers, or chills. Caution against bicycle riding for several weeks after a prostate procedure, as repetitive trauma to the perineal area could worsen prostate bleeding or pain.

TABLE 55.11 Radiologic Studies

Study	Description and Purpose
CT scan	Detect masses or tumors in pelvis.
Mammography	X-ray image used to assess breast tissue and detect masses. See Chapter 56 for mammography screening guidelines.
MRI	In females, may detect abnormalities in internal reproductive organs. Breast MRI with mammography can detect breast cancer. In males, pelvic/prostate MRI may detect prostate tumors.
Ultrasound	
Breast	Detect masses or cysts in breasts. Used with mammography for dense breast tissue.
Pelvic	May be transabdominal or transvaginal. Used to detect pelvic problems, such as ectopic pregnancy, ovarian cysts, fibroids, cancer. Reproductive and pregnancy-related assessment.
Testicular	Detect testicular masses and testicular torsion.
Rectal	Detect prostate tumors.

CASE STUDY

Objective Data: Diagnostic Studies

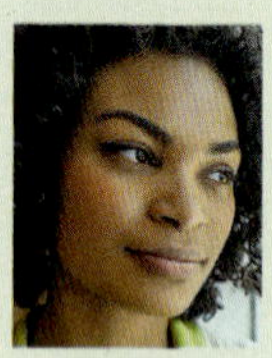

(© Benjamin A. Peterson/Mother Image/mother image/Fuse/Thinkstock.)

The following laboratory and diagnostic tests are ordered for C.W.: hCG, complete blood count (CBC), thyroid-stimulating hormone (TSH), FSH, LH, prolactin, testosterone, STI panel (HIV, syphilis, gonorrhea, chlamydia), and pelvic and transvaginal ultrasound. The results are:

- *hCG:* <5 mIU/mL
- *CBC:* Hemoglobin 14.1 g/dL, hematocrit 36.5%, WBC 11.5
- *TSH:* 0.3 IU/L
- *Hormone testing (FSH, LH, prolactin, testosterone):* Within normal ranges
- *HIV antigen/antibody:* Nonreactive (negative)
- *Syphilis:* Nonreactive (negative)
- *Gonorrhea and chlamydia tests:* Negative

The pelvic and transvaginal ultrasound revealed a normal uterus and ovaries except for a round, 4-cm, simple ovarian cyst with good blood flow in the left ovary.

Discussion Questions

1. Which diagnostic and laboratory test results are of concern to you?
2. What teaching can you provide C.W. based on her diagnostic test results?

Answers available at http://evolve.elsevier.com/Lewis/medsurg.

TABLE 55.12 Intervention Studies

Study	Description	Commonly Associated Conditions
Female		
Colposcopy	Visualize cervix with macroscope, allows magnification of cervix, study of cell abnormalities, and identification of lesions for cervical biopsy	Abnormal cervical cancer screening tests (i.e., Pap smear)
Conization (cervical cone biopsy or loop electrosurgical excision procedure [LEEP])	Remove cone-shaped sample of cervical tissue. Done with a scalpel (called cold-knife conization) or electrosurgical loop (loop electrosurgical excision procedure [LEEP])	Abnormal cervical cytology or colonoscopy results
Dilation and curettage (D&C) with or without suction (uterine aspiration)	Remove endometrial tissue following dilation of cervix and insertion of instruments. May be done with a curette or suction or vacuum pump	Abnormal uterine bleeding Pregnancy termination or loss
Endometrial biopsy	Remove small sample of tissue from uterine lining (endometrium) to assess for cell changes or cancer	Abnormal uterine bleeding Endometrial cancer Postmenopausal bleeding
Hysterosalpingogram (HSG)	Evaluate uterine cavity and tubes using x-ray with contrast media injected through cervix	Infertility Suspected uterine anomalies

Continued

TABLE 55.12 Intervention Studies—cont'd

Study	Description	Commonly Associated Conditions
Hysteroscopy	Visualize uterine lining through insertion of scope through cervix	Abnormal uterine bleeding Infertility
Laparoscopy	Visualize pelvic structures via fiberoptic scopes inserted through small abdominal incisions	Infertility Gynecologic surgery Pelvic pain
Saline-infused sonohysterography	Visualize uterine cavity using fluid injected through cervix with transvaginal ultrasound	Abnormal uterine bleeding Infertility
Male		
Microdissection TESE (microTESE)	Examine sperm and extraction of sperm from seminiferous tubules via a very small incision in testis	Infertility
Penile Doppler ultrasound	Evaluate penile blood flow with ultrasound, with or without intracavernosal injection of medications to cause erection	Erectile dysfunction
Testicular sperm extraction (TESE)	Examine for sperm and, if possible, extraction of sperm from seminiferous tubules via a small incision in testis	Infertility
Transrectal ultrasound	Evaluate prostate size and assessment for any prostate masses that might need further evaluation for possible prostate cancer, with an ultrasound probe inserted into rectum	Benign prostatic hypertrophy (BPH) Abnormal digital rectal exam (DRE) Prostate cancer
Transrectal ultrasound-guided prostate biopsy	Remove small samples of prostate tissue under ultrasound guidance to evaluate for prostate cancer or other cell changes. Use a thin needle that passes along an ultrasound probe inserted into rectum	Abnormal digital rectal exam (DRE) Elevated PSA Prostate cancer

TABLE 55.13 Cytology and Microbiologic Studies

Study	Description and Purpose
Cultures	Specimens from urine to assess for gonorrhea, chlamydia, or UTIs. Rectal and throat cultures may be taken depending on sexual history.
Gram stain	Rapid detection of gonorrhea. Gram-negative intracellular diplococci generally need treatment. Alternative chlamydia test.
Nucleic acid amplification test (NAAT)	Nonculture test used to identify small amounts of DNA or RNA in test samples. Sensitivity similar to culture tests. Uses ligase or polymerase chain reaction that amplifies signal of nucleic acids in sample so they are easier to identify. Preferred method to test for gonorrhea, chlamydia, trichomoniasis. Done on a wide variety of samples, including vaginal, endocervical, urethral, urine, rectal, pharyngeal.
Papanicolaou (Pap) test	Microscopic study of exfoliated cervical cells to detect abnormal cells. *Conventional cytology* entails fixing cells directly to a slide at the time of collection and sending the slide to the laboratory for interpretation. In *liquid-based cytology* the specimen is sent in a liquid solution that preserves it and is processed for microscopic evaluation at the laboratory. HPV testing can be done on specimen obtained for liquid-based Pap test.
Wet mount (microscopy)	Direct microscopic examination of vaginal discharge specimen. Assessment of vaginal infections such as candidiasis (yeast), bacterial vaginosis, trichomoniasis.

TABLE 55.14 Fertility Studies

Study	Description and Purpose
Female	
Basal body temperature assessment	Indirectly indicates whether ovulation has occurred. Temperature rises at ovulation and stays high during secretory phase of normal menstrual cycle.
Serum anti-Müllerian hormone, estradiol, FSH, progesterone	Same as serology studies. See Table 55.10.
Urinary LH	"Ovulation predictor kit." Identifies midcycle LH surge that precedes ovulation by 1–2 days.
Male	
Semen analysis	Assesses semen for volume (2–5 mL), viscosity, sperm count (>20 million/mL), sperm motility (60% motile), percent of abnormal sperm (60% with normal structure).

BRIDGE TO NCLEX EXAMINATION

The number of the question corresponds to the same-numbered outcome at the beginning of the chapter.

1. The nurse would anticipate which change in reproductive function in a patient who had an orchiectomy?
   a. Increase in PSA
   b. Decrease in PSA
   c. Increase in testosterone
   d. Decrease in testosterone
2. A spike in which hormone is the best indicator of ovulation?
   a. Estrogen
   b. Progesterone
   c. Luteinizing hormone (LH)
   d. Follicle-stimulating hormone (FSH)
3. Ejaculation occurs in which phase of the male sexual response?
   a. Plateau phase
   b. Orgasm phase
   c. Resolution phase
   d. Excitement phase
4. A normal age-related finding when assessing an older male's reproductive system is:
   a. Increased libido
   b. Increased skin turgor
   c. Increased muscle tone
   d. Increased prostate size
5. The 5 "P"s of sexual history taking include asking questions about (**Select all that apply.**):
   a. Last menstrual period
   b. Libido and erectile function
   c. The gender(s) of sexual partner(s)
   d. Anatomic sites involved in sexual activity
   e. Frequency of using methods of STI prevention
   f. Past medical history, including diabetes and hypertension
6. What position is optimal for palpating breast tissue?
   a. Sitting, hands on hips
   b. Sitting, leaning forward
   c. Supine, arm above the head
   d. Supine, hands on the abdomen or thighs
7. Which condition would the nurse suspect in a patient with thick, white vaginal discharge and vulvar itching?
   a. Candidiasis
   b. Genital herpes
   c. Trichomoniasis
   d. Condyloma acuminatum
8. A patient's Pap smear results came back with abnormal cell changes. What follow-up testing is the HCP most likely to recommend?
   a. Colposcopy
   b. Mammogram
   c. Endometrial biopsy
   d. Transvaginal ultrasound

1. d; 2. c; 3. b; 4. d; 5. c, d, e; 6. c; 7. a; 8. a.

For rationales to these answers and even more NCLEX review questions, visit http://evolve.elsevier.com/Lewis/medsurg.

REFERENCES

To access the References for this chapter, please scan the QR code with a mobile device.

Breast Problems

Maura Abbott

http://evolve.elsevier.com/Lewis/medsurg/

CONCEPTUAL FOCUS

Cellular Regulation
Coping
Infection
Pain
Sexuality

LEARNING OUTCOMES

1. State screening guidelines for the early detection of breast cancer.
2. Explain the types, causes, clinical manifestations, and interprofessional and nursing management of common benign breast problems.
3. State the risk factors for breast cancer.
4. Describe the pathophysiology and clinical manifestations of breast cancer.
5. Describe the interprofessional and nursing management of breast cancer.
6. Specify the physical and psychologic aspects of nursing management for patients undergoing breast cancer surgery.
7. Explain the indications for, types and complications of, and nursing management after reconstructive breast surgery.

KEY TERMS

ductal ectasia
fibroadenoma
fibrocystic changes
galactorrhea
gynecomastia
intraductal papilloma
lumpectomy
lymphedema
mammoplasty
mastalgia
mastitis
Paget disease

Breast problems are a significant health concern. Whether the actual diagnosis is a benign condition or cancer, the initial discovery of a lump or change in the breast often triggers anxiety and fear. The potential loss of a breast, or part of a breast, may be devastating because of the associated significant psychologic, social, sexual, and body image implications.

The most common breast problems are fibrocystic changes, fibroadenoma, intraductal papilloma, ductal ectasia, and breast cancer. In a female's lifetime, there is a 1 in 8 (12%) chance that she will be diagnosed with breast cancer.[1] Although rare, breast cancer does occur in males. Being aware of personal risk, including genetic factors, and taking part in recommended screening are important health promotion activities.

ASSESSMENT OF BREAST PROBLEMS

Breast Cancer Screening Guidelines

Screening guidelines for the early detection of breast cancer vary depending on a patient's age and risk (Table 56.1).[2] Females at increased risk for breast cancer (family history, genetic link, prior breast cancer, history of thoracic radiation therapy, or certain atypical findings on a prior breast biopsy) should talk with their HCP about the benefits and limitations of starting screening earlier with 3D mammography and breast MRI and having more frequent clinical breast encounters. A clinical encounter includes an assessment of risk factors, instruction in ways to reduce the risk factors, and a clinical breast examination (CBE).[3]

Consistent breast self-examination (BSE) may be a useful way to increase self-awareness of how one's breasts normally look and feel. Research shows that BSE has no effect on reducing deaths from breast cancer. However, you still need to teach patients the importance of knowing how their breasts look and feel and to report breast changes (e.g., nipple discharge, a lump) to their HCP.[3]

If someone wants to learn about BSE, include information about the potential benefits and limitations. Allow time for questions and a return demonstration. Teach the method described at www.breastcancer.org/symptoms/testing/types/self_exam/.

Diagnostic Studies

Radiologic Studies

We use several techniques to screen for breast problems or help diagnose a suspicious physical finding. *Mammography* is used to view the breast's internal structure using x-rays (Fig. 56.1). It can detect suspicious lumps that cannot be felt. Mammography has significantly improved the early and accurate detection of breast cancer. Improved imaging technology has reduced the radiation dose from mammography.

TABLE 56.1 Breast Cancer Screening Guidelines

The American Cancer Society (ACS) recommends the following guidelines for screening females at average risk for breast cancer:

- Females should undergo regular screening mammography starting at age 45 years
- Females should be offered the chance to begin annual screening between the ages of 40 and 44
- Females aged 45–54 years should be screened annually
- Females 55 years and older can switch to every-other-year screening or can continue screening annually
- Females should continue screening if their overall health is good and they have a life expectancy of 10 years or longer

A comparison of current and prior mammograms may show early tissue changes. Early detection by mammography allows for earlier treatment and the prevention of metastasis. In younger females, mammography is less sensitive because of the greater density of breast tissue, resulting in more false-negative results. Having dense breasts makes mammographic detection of cancer more difficult.

With *digital mammography* x-ray images are digitally coded and stored in a computer (Fig. 56.1). It is more accurate than traditional film mammography in younger females with dense breasts. The availability and associated costs of digital mammography are issues.

3D mammography, or tomosynthesis mammography, produces a 3D image of the breast. It gives a clearer view of overlapping breast tissue structures. It can increase the number of cancers detected and decrease the number of false-positive results (a result stating a cancer is present when it is not).

Calcifications are the most easily recognized mammogram abnormality (Fig. 56.1). They are deposits of calcium crystals that form in the breast. Causes include inflammation, trauma, and aging. Although most calcifications are benign, they may occur with breast cancer.

About 10% to 15% of all breast cancers may not be seen on mammography. They may be detected by palpation or other breast imaging studies, such as ultrasound and MRI. If the clinical findings are suspicious and the mammogram is normal, an ultrasound or MRI may be done. Based on these findings, a biopsy may be done.

Ultrasound is used in conjunction with mammography to discern a solid mass from a cystic mass, to evaluate a mass in a

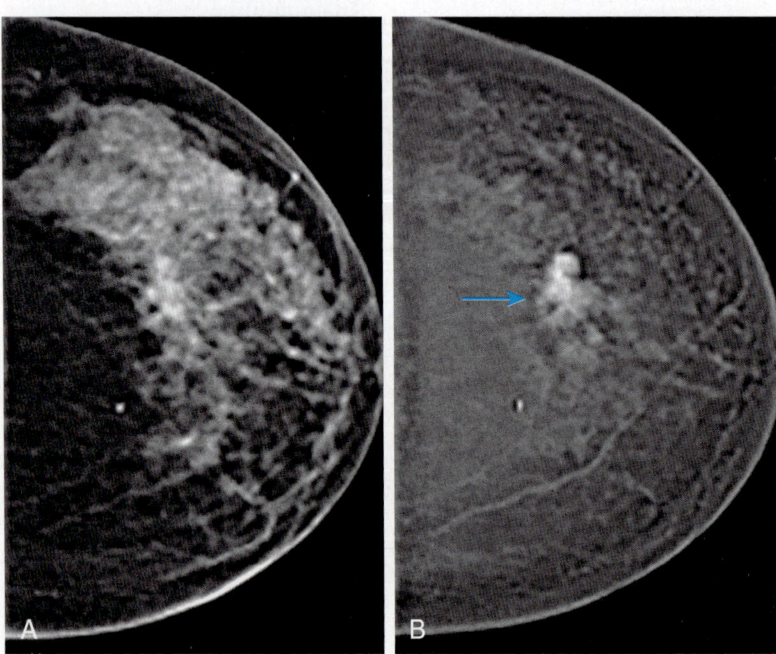

Fig. 56.1 Screening mammogram showing dense breast tissue and benign, scattered microcalcifications. (A) Using conventional x-rays. (B) Using digital x-rays. (From Patel B, Lobbes M, Lewin J: Contrast enhanced spectral mammography: a review, *Semin Ultrasound CT MR* 39[1]:70, 2018.)

pregnant or lactating female, and to locate and biopsy a suspicious lesion. MRI is recommended as a screening tool in addition to mammography for females who are at high risk for breast cancer (e.g., first-degree relative with a *BRCA* mutation).

Biopsies

A definitive diagnosis of a suspicious area is made by analyzing biopsied tissue. Biopsy techniques include *fine-needle aspiration* (FNA), core (core needle), vacuum-assisted, and excisional biopsies.

FNA biopsy is done by inserting a needle into a lesion to sample fluid from a breast lesion, remove cells from intercellular spaces, or sample cells from a solid mass. Before the procedure, the breast area is first locally anesthetized. Then, the needle is placed into the breast, and fluid and cells are aspirated into a syringe. Usually, 3 or 4 passes are made. If the results are negative with a suspicious lesion, another biopsy may be necessary.

A *core (core needle) biopsy* involves removing small samples of breast tissue using a hollow "core" needle. For palpable lesions, this is done by fixing the lesion with one hand and performing a needle biopsy with the other. In the case of nonpalpable lesions, *stereotactic mammography*, ultrasound, or MRI image guidance is used. Stereotactic mammography uses computers to pinpoint the exact location of a breast mass based on mammograms. With ultrasound, the HCP watches the needle on the ultrasound monitor to help guide it to the area of concern. A core biopsy is more accurate because it removes more tissue than an FNA.

Vacuum-assisted biopsy is a newer version of core biopsy that uses a vacuum technique to help collect tissue samples. In core biopsy, several separate needle insertions are used to obtain multiple samples. During vacuum-assisted biopsy, the needle is inserted only once into the breast, and the needle can be rotated, allowing for multiple samples through a single needle insertion.

Minimally invasive breast biopsies have become the standard of care for diagnosing abnormalities found either on imaging studies or through CBE. In some cases, an *excisional biopsy*, which is when the entire suspicious tumor and some surrounding tissue are removed, is recommended. An excisional biopsy is done in an operating room.

BENIGN BREAST PROBLEMS

MASTALGIA

Mastalgia, or breast pain, is the most common breast-related symptom reported in females. The most common form is *cyclic mastalgia*, which coincides with the menstrual cycle.[4] Females describe it as diffuse bilateral breast tenderness or heaviness. Breast pain may last 2 or 3 days or most of the month. It is related to hormone sensitivity. Symptoms often decrease with menopause.

Noncyclic mastalgia has no relationship to the menstrual cycle. It can continue into menopause. Pain may be constant or intermittent throughout the month and last for several years. Symptoms include a burning, aching, or soreness in the breast. It usually affects only 1 breast. The pain may be from trauma, fat necrosis, ductal ectasia, costochondritis, or arthritic pain in the chest or neck radiating to the breast.

For patients with breast pain, mammography and targeted ultrasound are often done to exclude cancer and provide information on the cause of the pain. Reassure patients that mastalgia is not a usual sign of breast cancer.[4]

There is no specific treatment for breast pain. Some relief for cyclic pain may occur by reducing intake of caffeine and fat; taking vitamin E or gamma-linolenic acid (evening primrose oil); and continually wearing a supportive bra. Compresses, ice, analgesics, and antiinflammatory drugs may help. Tamoxifen may provide relief in 70% to 90% of females with cyclic mastalgia and 50% to 60% of females with noncyclic mastalgia with few side effects. Bromocriptine, a prolactin inhibitor, may provide some with relief. It causes GI upset and lightheadedness. Danazol is an FDA-approved treatment. The androgenic side effects (acne, edema, hirsutism) make this therapy unacceptable for many females.

BREAST INFECTIONS

Mastitis

Mastitis is an inflammatory breast condition.[5] It occurs most often in lactating females (Table 56.2). *Lactational mastitis* presents as a local area that is red, painful, and tender to palpation. Fever is often present. The infection develops when pathogens (usually staphylococci) gain access to the breast through a cracked nipple. In its early stages, mastitis can be cured with antibiotics. Breastfeeding should continue unless an abscess is forming or there is purulent drainage. The mother may wish to use a nipple shield or to hand-express milk from the involved breast until the pain subsides. The female should see her HCP promptly to begin antibiotic therapy. Any breast that stays red, tender, and not responsive to antibiotics requires follow-up care and evaluation for inflammatory breast cancer.

Mastitis sometimes develops in females who are not lactating. This is called *periductal mastitis*. It occurs most often in regular smokers aged late 20s to early 30s. Treatment is the same as for lactating mastitis.

Lactational Breast Abscess

If lactational mastitis persists after several days of antibiotic therapy, a lactational breast abscess may be present. In this condition, the skin may become red and edematous over the involved breast, often with a corresponding palpable mass. Patients may have a fever. Antibiotics alone are insufficient treatment for a breast abscess. Ultrasound-guided drainage of the abscess or surgical incision and drainage are done. The drainage is cultured, and sensitivities are obtained. Antibiotic therapy is started. Breastfeeding can continue in most cases with ongoing treatment.

TABLE 56.2 Common Benign Breast Problems

Disorder	Risk Factors	Clinical Manifestations
Lactational mastitis	Occurs in up to 33% of postpartum lactating mothers (both primipara and multipara). Usually within first 3 months after birth.	• Warm to touch, indurated, painful, often unilateral • Most often caused by *Staphylococcus aureus*
Fibrocystic changes	Most common between ages 30 and 50.	• Not usually discrete masses—nodularity instead • Usually accompanied by cyclic pain and tenderness • Mass(es) often cyclic in occurrence (movable, soft)
Cysts	Most common over age 35. Incidence decreases after menopause. Develop in over half of females in North America.	• Palpable fluid-filled mass (movable, soft, tender) • Multiple cysts can occur and recur • Rarely associated with breast cancer
Fibroadenoma	Often occurs in teens and those in their 20s.	• Palpable mass (firm, movable), usually 1–3 cm in size • Rarely associated with breast cancer
Fat necrosis	History of trauma to breast.	• Usually a hard, tender, mobile, indurated mass with irregular borders
Ductal ectasia	Most common in females over 60 years old. Considered a normal part of aging. May be caused by duct obstruction or mastitis.	• Nipple fixation, usually accompanied by nipple discharge of thick gray material • Breast pain often present

FIBROCYSTIC CHANGES

Fibrocystic changes are benign conditions characterized by changes in breast tissue (Fig. 56.2).[6] They are the most common breast disorder, occurring in 30% to 60% of females of reproductive age. Many patients report premenstrual problems, early menarche or late menopause, or a history of spontaneous abortion. Others at risk include nulliparous females and nonusers of oral contraceptives.

Fibrocystic changes include excess fibrous tissue, hyperplasia of the epithelial lining of the mammary ducts, proliferation of mammary ducts, and cysts. We think these changes are caused by a heightened responsiveness of breast tissue to circulating estrogen and progesterone. They may cause pain from chronic inflammation, edema, nerve irritation, and fibrosis. Pain and nodularity often increase over time. They tend to subside after menopause unless the female is taking high doses of estrogen replacement. Symptoms often worsen in the premenstrual phase and subside after menstruation.

Manifestations of fibrocystic breast changes include 1 or more palpable lumps that are often round, well delineated, and freely movable within the breast (Table 56.2). Discomfort ranging from tenderness to pain may occur. The lump usually increases in size and tenderness before menstruation. Cysts may enlarge or shrink rapidly. Nipple discharge from fibrocystic breasts is often green or dark brown, not bloody.

Alone, fibrocystic changes do not increase breast cancer risk. Masses or nodules can appear in both breasts. They often occur in the upper outer quadrants and usually bilaterally.

Mammography may be helpful in distinguishing fibrocystic changes from breast cancer. In some females, the breast tissue is so dense that it is hard to obtain a mammogram. In these situations, ultrasound can better distinguish a fluid-filled cyst from a solid mass.

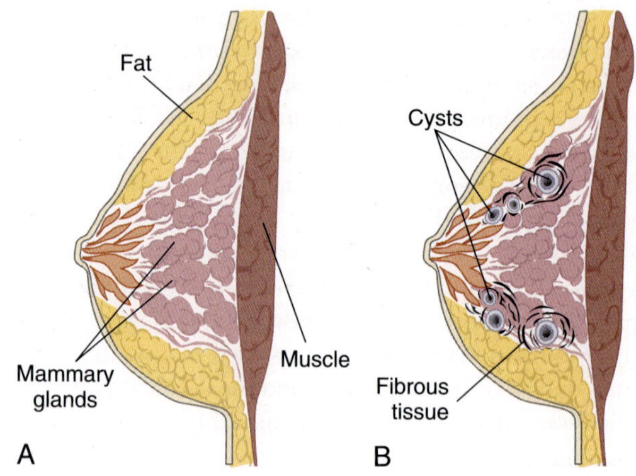

Fig. 56.2 (A) Normal breast tissue. (B) Fibrocystic breast tissue.

Interprofessional and Nursing Management

With the discovery of a discrete mass in the breast by a female or the HCP, aspiration or biopsy may be done. If the nodularity is recurrent, we may wait 7 to 10 days to see if any changes are related to the menstrual cycle. With large or frequent cysts, an excisional biopsy may be done if (1) no fluid is found on aspiration, (2) the fluid is hemorrhagic, or (3) a residual mass remains after fluid aspiration.

Severe fibrocystic changes may make palpating the breast more difficult. Teach patients with cystic changes to maintain regular follow-up care with the HCP. Encourage breast self-awareness and to report any changes found so they can be evaluated.

Treatment for a fibrocystic condition is similar to that described earlier for mastalgia. Teach patients with fibrocystic breasts that cysts may recur in 1 or both breasts until menopause and that the cysts may enlarge or become painful just before menstruation. Reassure her that the cysts do not "turn into" cancer. Tell her that the HCP should examine any new lump that does not respond in a cyclic manner over 1 to 2 weeks.

FIBROADENOMA

Fibroadenoma is the most common cause of discrete benign breast lumps in young females. It generally occurs in females in their teens and 20s. They occur most often in Black females.

The possible cause may be increased estrogen sensitivity in a local area of the breast. Fibroadenomas are usually small (but can be large [2 to 3 cm]), painless, round, well delineated, and mobile. They are usually solid, firm, and rubbery in consistency. The fibroadenoma may appear as a single unilateral mass, although multiple bilateral fibroadenomas may occur. Growth is slow and often ceases when the size reaches 2 to 3 cm. Menstruation does not affect size. Pregnancy can stimulate dramatic growth.

Fibroadenomas are easily detected by physical assessment. They may be visible on mammography and ultrasound. Definitive diagnosis requires a biopsy and tissue examination to exclude cancer. Treatment can include observation with regular monitoring if cancer is not present, there are no symptoms, and the mass stays less than 3 cm. A fibroadenoma that increases in size and/or is symptomatic should be removed by surgical resection or, in some cases, cryotherapy. All new lesions should be evaluated by breast ultrasound and possible biopsy.

NIPPLE DISCHARGE

Nipple discharge may occur spontaneously or because of nipple manipulation. Secretions can be clear, serous, bloody, or brown to green. A milky secretion is the result of inappropriate lactation, or **galactorrhea.**

Nipple discharge can occur with benign breast conditions, such as fibrocystic changes, intraductal papilloma, or ductal ectasia. It may be a result of certain medicines or endocrine or neurologic problems. Sometimes there is no known cause. In most cases, nipple discharge is not caused by cancer. Spontaneous, unilateral discharge that can be reproduced on examination warrants further evaluation. A cytology slide of the secretion can help determine the specific cause and recommended treatment.

ATYPICAL HYPERPLASIA

Atypical hyperplasia is usually found after a biopsy is done to evaluate a suspicious area found on a mammogram or during a CBE. It can be in either the ducts (atypical ductal hyperplasia) or in the lobules (atypical lobular hyperplasia). Both increase the risk for breast cancer. To follow up on a diagnosis of atypical hyperplasia, an excisional biopsy or lumpectomy may be done to remove all the affected tissue.

INTRADUCTAL PAPILLOMA

An **intraductal papilloma** is a benign, soft or hard, wartlike growth found in the mammary ducts. It is usually unilateral. Typically, the nipple has a bloody discharge that can be intermittent or spontaneous. Most intraductal papillomas are beneath the areola. They may be hard to palpate. They usually occur in females 35 to 55 years of age. A single duct or several ducts may be involved. Papillomas have a slightly increased risk for developing breast cancer, so a core biopsy is recommended. If there are any abnormal cells, surgical excision of the papilloma and the involved duct or duct system is done.[7]

DUCTAL ECTASIA

Ductal ectasia (duct dilation) is a benign breast disease of perimenopausal and postmenopausal females involving the ducts in the subareolar area. It usually involves several bilateral ducts. Nipple discharge is the main symptom. Ductal ectasia is initially painless but may progress to burning, itching, pain around the nipple, and swelling in the areolar area. Inflammatory signs are often present. The nipple may retract. The discharge may become bloody in more advanced disease. It is not associated with cancer. If an abscess develops, warm compresses and antibiotics are usually effective treatments. Therapy consists of close follow-up examinations or surgical excision of the involved ducts.

MALE GYNECOMASTIA

Gynecomastia is a transient, noninflammatory enlargement of 1 or both breasts. It is the most common breast problem in males. The condition is usually temporary and benign. Gynecomastia itself is not a risk factor for breast cancer. The most common cause is a change in the normal ratio of active androgen to estrogen in plasma or within the breast itself.[8]

Gynecomastia can occur in puberty. During puberty, there is often a transient relative imbalance between estrogen and testosterone, leading to gynecomastia. It usually resolves by age 20 years when the person reaches adult androgen-to-estrogen ratios. Reassure the parent and teenager about the benign nature of the condition.

Gynecomastia can also be a sign of other problems. It may occur with testicular tumors, adrenal cancer, pituitary adenomas, hyperthyroidism, and liver disease. It can be a side effect of drug therapy, especially estrogen, androgen, digitalis, isoniazid, ranitidine, and spironolactone. Marijuana use can cause gynecomastia.

Senescent Gynecomastia

Senescent gynecomastia occurs in many older males. The likely cause is high plasma estrogen levels with the increased conversion of androgens to estrogens in peripheral circulation. Although initially unilateral, the tender, firm, centrally located enlargement may become bilateral. A discrete, circumscribed mass with gynecomastia must be biopsied to determine whether it is the rare breast cancer in males. Senescent hyperplasia needs no treatment. It usually regresses within 6 to 12 months.

GERONTOLOGIC CONSIDERATIONS: AGE-RELATED BREAST CHANGES

The loss of subcutaneous fat and structural support and the atrophy of mammary glands often result in pendulous breasts in the postmenopausal female. Encourage older females to wear a well-fitting bra. Adequate support can improve physical appearance and reduce pain in the back, shoulders, and neck. It can also prevent *intertrigo,* dermatitis caused by friction between opposing surfaces of skin.

The decrease in glandular tissue makes a breast mass easier to palpate. This decreased density likely results from age-related decreases in estrogen. Rib margins may be palpable in a thin female and can be confused with a mass. That is why it is so important that females become familiar with their own breasts and what is normal for them. Because the incidence of breast cancer increases with age, encourage breast awareness in older females. Encourage them to have an annual mammogram and CBE and have any breast-related concern evaluated by their HCP.

BREAST CANCER

Breast cancer is the most common cancer in American females except for skin cancer. It is second only to lung cancer as the leading cause of death from cancer in females. In the United States around 13% of females will develop breast cancer in their lifetime. About half of all U.S. females who develop breast cancer are diagnosed at age 62 or younger. Males account for almost 3000 cases of breast cancer diagnosis each year.

The incidence of breast cancer is slowly increasing (0.6%), with a slight decrease in the number of deaths. This decline may be a result of the decreased use of hormone therapy after menopause, earlier detection, and treatment advances. The 5-year survival rate of cancer that is detected early is 99%.[9] Breast cancer survivors are the largest group of all cancer survivors.

ETIOLOGY AND RISK FACTORS

We do not completely understand the cause of breast cancer. We know there are several risk factors (Table 56.3). Risk factors appear to be cumulative and interacting. So, the presence of multiple risk factors may greatly increase the overall risk, especially for females with a positive family history.

Female Risk Factors

The strongest risk factors include female gender and advancing age.[10] Ninety-nine percent of breast cancers occur in females. Modifiable risk factors include excess weight gain during adulthood, sedentary lifestyle, smoking, fat intake, obesity, nightshift work, and alcohol use. Environment factors, such as radiation exposure and using hair dyes and straighteners, may play a role.

TABLE 56.3 Risk Factors for Breast Cancer

Risk Factor	Comments
Age ≥55 years	Majority found in postmenopausal females Incidence ↑ after age 60
Alcohol use	Drinking ≥1 alcoholic beverage per day
Benign breast disease with atypical epithelial hyperplasia, lobular carcinoma in situ	Atypical changes in breast biopsy
Chemicals in environment, cosmetics (parabens, phthalates), food	Emerging risk, may be hormone disruptors
Early menarche (before age 12), late menopause (after age 55)	A long menstrual history
Exposure to ionizing radiation	Radiation damages DNA (e.g., prior treatment for Hodgkin lymphoma)
Family history	Breast cancer, ovarian, pancreatic, and high-grade prostate cancer in a first-degree relative, particularly when premenopausal or bilateral
Female	Females account for 99% of breast cancer cases
First full-term pregnancy after age 30, nulliparity, no breastfeeding	Prolonged exposure to unopposed estrogen
Genetic factors (BRCA1, BRCA2, P53, PTEN, PALB2, ATM, CHEK2, NBM)	Gene mutations play a role in up to 10% of breast cancer cases
Hair chemicals in permanent dyes and hair straightening products	Emerging risk, especially in Black females
Height, being taller	May be caused by factors related to early growth
Hormone use	Use of estrogen and/or progesterone as hormone therapy, especially in postmenopausal females
Light exposure at night	Emerging risk, seen in night shift workers
Long-term heavy smoking	May ↑ risk, especially in females who begin smoking before first pregnancy
Obesity, weight gain after menopause	Fat cells store estrogen
Personal history of breast, colon, endometrial, or ovarian cancer	Personal history significantly ↑ risk for breast cancer, risk for cancer in other breast, and recurrence
Physical inactivity	Risk ↑ most after menopause
Race and ethnicity	White and Black females have the highest incidence Black females have lower survival rates, even when diagnosed at an early stage Hispanic and Black females more likely to have triple-negative cancer and be diagnosed at a later stage

Hormone regulation of the breast is related to cancer development, but we do not understand exactly how. The hormones estrogen and progesterone may act as tumor promoters to stimulate breast cancer growth if cancer changes in the cells have already occurred. Combined hormone therapy (estrogen plus progesterone) (1) increases the risk for breast cancer after as little as 2 years of use and (2) increases the risk for having a larger, more advanced breast cancer at diagnosis. This risk decreases within 5 years of stopping hormone therapy. Some studies show that using estrogen therapy alone for longer than 15 years (for females with a prior hysterectomy) increases long-term risk. A link also exists between oral contraceptive use and increased risk for breast cancer. This risk decreases when use stops and is gone after 10 years.

Male Risk Factors

Risk factors for breast cancer in males include estrogen use, hyperestrogenism, a family history of breast cancer, and radiation exposure. Examining the male breast should be a routine part of a physical assessment. Males in *BRCA*-positive families should consider genetic testing. Teach patients who test positive for a *BRCA* gene mutation to be aware of how their breasts look and feel and to report any changes to their HCP. They should have a CBE every year starting at age 35.[11] We do not recommend screening mammography, as research shows this to be of no benefit. Males with a history of breast cancer treated with lumpectomy should have an ipsilateral annual mammogram. Those with a history of breast cancer and a genetic mutation with an increased risk of breast cancer should have a contralateral mammogram. These patients should begin prostate screening at age 35, as they have an increased risk for prostate cancer.

Genetic Link

Family history of breast cancer is an important risk factor, especially if the family member also had ovarian cancer, was premenopausal, or had bilateral breast cancer. Having any first-degree relative (mother, father, sister, brother, daughter) with breast cancer doubles a female's risk for breast cancer, especially if the relative was diagnosed at a young age. A breast cancer risk assessment tool for HCPs is available (www.cancer.gov/bcrisktool). Genetic counseling must be considered for those at high risk for breast cancer.

Up to 10% of all breast cancers are hereditary. This means that the patient inherited specific genetic abnormalities that contribute to breast cancer (Box 56.1). Most inherited breast cancer cases are related to mutations in 2 genes: *BRCA1* and *BRCA2*. *BRCA* stands for *BR*east *CA*ncer. Everyone has *BRCA* genes. The *BRCA1* gene, found on chromosome 17, is a tumor suppressor gene that inhibits tumor development when functioning normally. The *BRCA2* gene, found on chromosome 11, is another tumor suppressor gene. Females with a mutation of this gene have a similar risk for breast cancer.[12]

BOX 56.1 GENETICS IN CLINICAL PRACTICE

Breast Cancer

Genetic Basis

- Mutations occur in *BRCA1* and/or *BRCA2* genes.
- Normally, these genes are tumor suppressor genes involved in DNA repair.
- Transmission is autosomal dominant.
- Other genes may increase the risk for breast cancer.

Incidence

- Up to 10% of breast cancers are related to *BRCA1* and *BRCA2* gene mutations.
- As many as 1 in 300 to 800 females in the United States have *BRCA1* and *BRCA2* gene mutations.[11]
- Females with *BRCA1* and *BRCA2* gene mutations have a 41% to 90% lifetime risk for developing breast cancer.
- Mutations in *BRCA* genes may cause as many as 90% of all inherited breast cancers.
- *BRCA1* and *BRCA2* gene mutations are associated with early-onset breast cancer that is more likely to involve both breasts.
- Males with mutations in *BRCA1* and *BRCA2* have an increased risk for breast cancer and prostate cancer.
- Family history of both breast and ovarian cancer increases the risk for having a *BRCA* mutation.

Genetic Testing

- DNA testing is available for *BRCA1* and *BRCA2* gene mutations.

Clinical Implications

- Bilateral oophorectomy and/or bilateral mastectomy reduces the risk for breast cancer and ovarian cancer in females with *BRCA1* and *BRCA2* mutations.
- Females with *BRCA* mutations have a higher risk for developing ovarian, colon, pancreatic, and uterine cancers.[11]

Genetic counseling and testing for *BRCA* mutations should be offered to patients whose personal or family history puts them at high risk for a genetic predisposition to breast cancer.

In addition to *BRCA* gene mutations, we have found many other abnormal genes that increase the risk of breast cancer. These include genes that normally suppress tumor growth, including *PALB2* (which partners with *BRCA* to suppress tumor growth), *TP53*, *CHEK2*, and *PTEN*. Other genes that may be abnormal include *ATM* and *NBM* (help repair damaged DNA), *CDH1* (makes a protein to bind cells together), and *STK11* (provides instructions to make a tumor suppressor enzyme).

Most people (90%) who develop breast cancer do not have an abnormal breast cancer gene or a family history of breast cancer. Their cancer is associated with genetic changes that occurred after they were born (somatic mutations). There is no risk for passing on the mutated gene to children.

PATHOPHYSIOLOGY

The main components of the breast are lobules (milk-producing glands) and ducts (milk passages that connect the lobules and the nipple). In general, breast cancer arises from the epithelial lining of the ducts *(ductal carcinoma)* or from the epithelium of the lobules *(lobular carcinoma)*. Breast cancers may be in situ (within the duct) or invasive (invading through the duct wall).

Metastatic breast cancer is breast cancer that has spread to other organs. The most common sites are the bone, liver, lung, and brain. Cancer growth rates can range from slow to rapid. Factors that affect cancer prognosis are tumor size, axillary node involvement (the more nodes involved, the worse the prognosis), tumor differentiation, estrogen and progesterone receptor (PR) status, and *human epidermal growth factor receptor 2* (HER-2) status. HER-2 is a protein that helps regulate cell growth.[13]

TYPES OF BREAST CANCER

Breast cancer can be classified as (1) ductal, lobular, or other or (2) noninvasive or invasive (Table 56.4). We can also classify it based on hormone status and genetic subtypes. Each type is characterized by different pathologic findings and clinical behaviors.

TABLE 56.4 Classification of Breast Cancer

Based on Tissue Type
- Ductal carcinoma (affects milk ducts)
  - Medullary
  - Tubular
  - Colloid (mucinous)
- Lobular carcinoma (affects milk-producing glands)
- Other
  - Inflammatory
  - Paget disease
  - Phyllodes tumor

Based on Invasiveness
Noninvasive (In Situ)
- Ductal carcinoma in situ (DCIS)
- Pure Paget disease

Invasive (Spreading to Other Locations)
- Invasive ductal carcinoma
- Invasive lobular carcinoma

Based on Hormone Receptor and Genetic Status
Estrogen and Progesterone Receptor Status
- Estrogen receptor positive
- Estrogen receptor negative
- Progesterone receptor positive
- Progesterone receptor negative

HER-2 Genetic Status
- HER-2 positive
- HER-2 negative

Noninvasive Breast Cancer

Around 20% of breast cancers are noninvasive. Noninvasive cancer stays within the milk ducts or lobules. It does not grow into or invade normal tissues within or beyond the breast. This cancer is sometimes called *carcinoma in situ* ("in the same place") or precancer. It includes *ductal carcinoma in situ* (DCIS) and pure Paget disease.

DCIS tends to be unilateral. It may progress to invasive breast cancer if left untreated. Treatment options include breast-conserving treatment (lumpectomy) with or without radiation therapy, total mastectomy with or without sentinel lymph node biopsy (SLNB), and/or hormone therapy (e.g., tamoxifen) to prevent recurrences.[14]

Lobular carcinoma in situ (LCIS) is a benign condition that is a risk factor for developing breast cancer. No surgical or radiation treatment is indicated for LCIS. Hormone therapy may be used as a preventive measure to reduce breast cancer risk for some patients.

Invasive Ductal Carcinoma

Invasive (infiltrating) ductal carcinoma is the most common type of breast cancer. It accounts for about 80% of all invasive breast cancers. It starts in the milk ducts and then breaks through the walls of the duct, invading the surrounding tissue. From there, it may metastasize to other parts of the body. Subtypes of invasive ductal carcinoma include medullary, tubular, colloid (mucinous), papillary, and metaplastic.

Invasive Lobular Carcinoma

Invasive (infiltrating) lobular carcinoma begins in the lobules of the breast. It accounts for about 10% to 15% of invasive breast cancers. The cancer cells can break out of the lobule and metastasize to other areas of the body. Invasive lobular carcinoma usually presents as a subtle thickening in the upper outer quadrant of the breast. It is often not detected by mammography.

Other Types of Breast Cancer

Inflammatory Breast Cancer

Inflammatory breast cancer is an aggressive and fast-growing cancer with a high risk for metastasis. It accounts for about 1% to 3% of all breast cancers. In the early stages, it is often mistaken for mastitis. However, the inflammatory changes do not improve with antibiotics. Cancer cells block the lymph channels in the skin of the breast. Because of skin involvement, the breast looks red, feels warm, and has a thickened appearance that is often described as looking like an orange peel *(peau d'orange)*. Sometimes, the breast develops ridges and small bumps that look like hives. A breast mass may not be present. Changes may not show up on mammograms, making diagnosis difficult. Inflammatory breast cancer has a worse prognosis compared with invasive ductal and lobular breast cancers.[15]

Paget Disease

Paget disease is a rare breast cancer that starts in the breast ducts and spreads to the nipple and areola. It causes about 1% of all breast cancers. It is different from Paget disease of the bone (see Chapter 68). Most females with Paget disease have underlying ductal carcinoma. Only in rare cases is the cancer confined to the nipple (in situ) and not invasive.

Itching, burning, bloody nipple discharge with superficial skin erosion, and ulceration may be present. Nipple changes are often diagnosed as an infection or dermatitis, which can lead to treatment delays.

The treatment is surgical removal of the involved tissue by either central lumpectomy or mastectomy with or without SLN biopsy. Radiation therapy may be used after surgery. The prognosis is good when the cancer is confined to the nipple.

Phyllodes Tumor

A phyllodes tumor is a rare tumor that develops in the connective tissue (stroma) of the breast. The tumors tend to grow quickly, within a period of weeks or months, to a size of 2 to 3 cm or sometimes larger. Although most are benign, some are cancerous. Treatment is usually excision with a wide margin. Axillary surgery is not necessary.

Triple-Negative Breast Cancer

Patients whose breast cancer tests negative for all 3 receptors (estrogen, progesterone, HER-2) have *triple-negative breast cancer.*[16] The incidence of triple-negative breast cancer is higher in females who are Black, Hispanic, premenopausal, and/or have a *BRCA1* mutation. Patients tend to have more aggressive tumors with a poorer prognosis. These cancers do not respond to hormone therapy or therapy for HER-2. Chemotherapy is more successful in treating triple-negative breast cancer.

CLINICAL MANIFESTATIONS

Breast cancer is usually detected as a lump or thickening in the breast or mammography abnormality. It occurs most often in the upper outer quadrant of the breast, which is the location of most of the glandular tissue (Fig. 56.3). Breast cancers vary in their growth rate. If palpable, breast cancer is characteristically hard and may be irregularly shaped, poorly delineated, nonmobile, and nontender.

A small number of breast cancers cause nipple discharge. The discharge is usually unilateral. It may be clear or bloody.

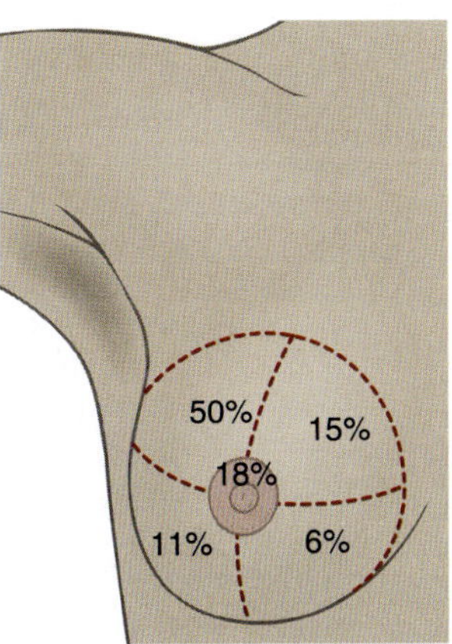

Fig. 56.3 Distribution of where breast cancer occurs.

Nipple retraction may be present. Peau d'orange may occur because of plugging of the dermal lymphatics. In large cancers, infiltration, induration, and dimpling (pulling in) of the overlying skin may occur.

COMPLICATIONS

The main complication of breast cancer is recurrence (Table 56.5). Recurrence may be *local* or *regional* (skin or soft tissue near the mastectomy site, axillary or internal mammary lymph nodes) or distant. Widely disseminated or metastatic disease involves the growth of cancerous breast cells in parts of the body distant from the breast. Most often involved are the bone, lung, brain, and liver. Metastases primarily occur through the lymphatics, usually those of the axilla (Fig. 56.4). However, metastatic disease can occur anywhere.

DIAGNOSTIC STUDIES

In addition to radiologic and biopsy studies used to diagnose breast cancer, we use other tests to predict the risk for local or systemic recurrence. These tests include axillary lymph node

TABLE 56.5 Sites of Breast Cancer Recurrence and Metastasis

Site	Manifestations
Local Recurrence	
Skin, chest wall	Firm, discrete nodules. Sometimes pruritic, usually painless, often in or near a scar.
Regional Recurrence	
Lymph nodes	Enlarged nodes in axilla or supraclavicular area, usually nontender.
Distant Metastasis	
Bone marrow	Anemia, infection, ↑ bleeding, bruising, petechiae. Weakness, fatigue, mild confusion, lightheadedness, dyspnea.
Brain	Headache, unilateral sensory loss, focal muscular weakness, hemiparesis, incoordination (ataxia), nausea and vomiting not related to medication, cognitive changes.
Liver	Abdominal distention. Right lower quadrant abdominal pain sometimes radiating to scapular area. Nausea and vomiting, anorexia, weight loss. Weakness and fatigue. Hepatomegaly, ascites, jaundice. Peripheral edema. High liver enzymes.
Lung (including lung nodules and pleural effusions)	Shortness of breath, tachypnea, nonproductive cough.
Skeletal	Local pain of gradually increasing intensity, percussion tenderness at involved sites, pathologic fracture caused by involvement of bone cortex.
Spinal cord	Progressive back pain, local and radiating. Change in bladder or bowel function. Loss of sensation in lower extremities.

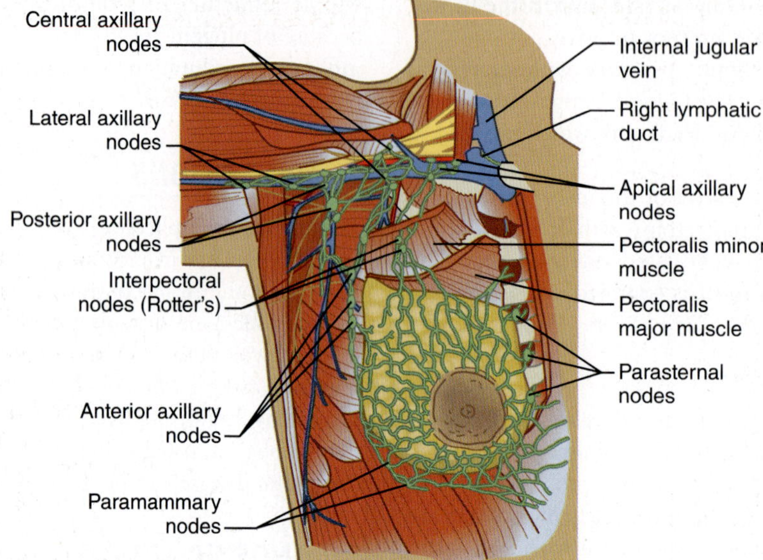

Fig. 56.4 Lymph nodes and drainage in the axilla. A complete axillary dissection would remove all nodes.

analysis, tumor size, estrogen and PR status, cell-proliferative indices (number of cells that are dividing), and genomic assays.

Axillary Lymph Node Analysis

Axillary lymph node involvement is an important prognostic factor in breast cancer. *Axillary lymph nodes* are often examined to see if cancer has spread to the axilla on the same side of the breast as the cancer (Fig. 56.4). The more nodes involved, the greater the risk for recurrence.

A *sentinel lymph node biopsy* helps to identify the lymph node(s) that drain first from the tumor site. Those nodes are *sentinel node(s)*. In SLNB, a radioisotope and/or blue dye, which will travel the same route as the cancer, is injected into the affected breast. Then, in surgery, the HCP determines whether the radioisotope (using a radioactive detector) or dye (visually see blue nodes) is found in any SLNs. A local incision is made in the axilla, and the HCP dissects the blue-stained and/or radioactive SLNs. Generally, with SLNB, 1 to 4 axillary lymph nodes are removed. The nodes are sent for pathologic analysis. If the SLNs are negative, no further axillary surgery is needed.

If the SLNs are positive or the SLN cannot be identified, patients may have a complete *axillary lymph node dissection* (ALND). In an ALND, the HCP will typically remove 12 to 20 lymph nodes. SLNB is less invasive and has a lower mortality rate than ALND.

Tumor Size

Tumor size is a prognostic variable. In general, the larger the tumor, the poorer the prognosis. The wide variety of biologic types of breast cancer explains the variability of disease behavior. In general, the more well differentiated (like the original cell type) the tumor, the less aggressive it is. The cells of poorly differentiated (unlike the original cell type) tumors appear morphologically disorganized, and they are more aggressive.

Estrogen and Progesterone Receptor Status

Estrogen receptor (ER) and progesterone receptor (PR) status is another diagnostic test useful for decisions about treatment and prognosis. Hormone receptor testing is done with any newly diagnosed primary or metastatic breast cancer and on DCIS. Receptor-positive tumors (1) often show histologic evidence of being well differentiated, (2) have a lower chance for recurrence, (3) often have a *diploid* (more normal) DNA content and low proliferative indices, and (4) are often hormone dependent and responsive to hormone therapy. Receptor-negative tumors (1) are often poorly differentiated histologically, (2) often recur, (3) have a high incidence of *aneuploidy* (abnormally high or low DNA content) and higher proliferative indices, and (4) are usually unresponsive to hormone therapy. Ploidy status (number of chromosomes in a cell) correlates with tumor aggressiveness. Diploid tumors have a much lower risk for recurrence than aneuploid tumors.

Genomic Assay

An important *genomic assay* is to determine HER-2, which is a prognostic indicator. Overexpression of HER-2 is associated with unusually aggressive tumor growth, a greater risk for recurrence, and a poorer prognosis. It is overexpressed in 10% to 20% of patients with breast cancer. The presence of HER-2 helps in the selection and sequence of drug therapy and predicts response to treatment. HER-2 testing is done with any newly diagnosed primary or metastatic breast cancer.

A *gene expression assay* test uses a sample of the breast cancer tissue to analyze the activity of a group of genes that can affect how a cancer is likely to behave and respond to treatment. Knowing whether certain genes are present or absent, or overly active or not active enough, can provide information about the risk for recurrence and the expected benefit of chemotherapy or hormone therapy. The 21-gene recurrence (OncotypeDX) test is the most often used genomic test.[17] Other genomic tests are MammaPrint, PAM50 (Prosigna), EndoPredict, and the Breast Cancer Index.

Cell-Proliferative Indices

Cell-proliferative indices indirectly measure the rate of tumor cell proliferation. The number of tumor cells in the synthesis (S) phase of the cell cycle is another important prognostic indicator. Patients with cells that have high S-phase fractions have a higher risk for recurrence and earlier cancer death.

Breast Cancer Staging

The most widely accepted staging method for breast cancer is the TNM system. This system uses anatomic factors of tumor size (T), nodal involvement (N), and presence of metastasis (M) to determine the stage of disease (Table 56.6). The stages range from 0 to IV, with stage 0 being in situ cancer with no lymph node involvement and no metastasis. Stage IV indicates metastatic spread, regardless of tumor size or lymph node involvement. This system is used worldwide to communicate the size of a breast cancer and the extent to which it has spread. It provides an accurate prediction of the outcome of a group of patients.

The latest cancer staging guidelines now include biologic factors to help more accurately determine the stage, predict outcomes, and guide treatment decisions. These factors include tumor grade, hormone receptor expression, HER-2 overexpression and/or amplification, and genomic panels.

For example, some larger tumors may be classified as stage I rather than stage II based on favorable biologic features. Specifically, patients with hormone receptor–positive, HER2-negative, node-negative tumors and a low-risk genomic recurrence score can be downstaged to the same prognostic group as T1a or T1b tumors. Patients with triple-negative breast cancers are staged higher due to their poorer prognosis, even when the anatomic stage is lower.

TABLE 56.6 Breast Cancer Staging

Stage	Tumor Size	Lymph Node Involvement	Metastasis
0	TIS (tumor in situ)	No	No
I			
A	<2 cm	No	No
B	<2 cm	<2 mm	No
II			
A	No evidence of tumor ranging to 5 cm	No, or 1–3 axillary nodes and/or internal mammary nodes	No
B	Ranging from ≤2 to >5 cm	No, or 1–3 axillary nodes and/or internal mammary nodes	No
III			
A	Ranging ≤2 to >5 cm	Yes, 1–9 axillary nodes and/or internal mammary nodes	No
B	Any size with extension to chest wall or skin	No, or 1–9 axillary nodes and/or internal mammary nodes	No
C	Any size	Yes, ≥10 axillary nodes, internal mammary nodes, or infraclavicular nodes	No
IV	Any size	Any type of nodal involvement	Yes

INTERPROFESSIONAL CARE

A wide range of treatment options is available (Table 56.7). The treatment plan is often determined by prognostic factors, the clinical stage, and biology of the cancer.

Surgical Therapy

Surgery is the main treatment for breast cancer. Table 56.8 describes the most common procedures used. The most common options for operable breast cancer are (1) breast conservation surgery (lumpectomy [segmental mastectomy]) and (2) mastectomy with or without reconstruction. Most females diagnosed with early-stage breast cancer (tumors smaller than 5 cm) are candidates for either surgery. The overall survival rate with lumpectomy and radiation is the same as with mastectomy.

Breast reconstruction is an option for any female having surgery for breast cancer. Females having a mastectomy can have breast reconstruction at the time of the surgery or months or even years later. Some females choose to not have reconstruction and use a breast prosthesis instead.

Breast-Conserving Surgery

Breast-conserving surgery, or **lumpectomy,** involves removing the entire tumor along with a margin of normal surrounding tissue (Fig. 56.5A). In some cases, it may take 2 or 3 more surgeries to remove all the cancer from the margins. After surgery, radiation therapy is usually delivered to the entire breast, ending with a boost to the tumor bed. If the risk for recurrence is high, patients may receive chemotherapy before starting radiation.

TABLE 56.7 Interprofessional Care

Breast Cancer

Diagnostic Assessment

Prediagnosis

- Health history, including risk factors
- Physical assessment, including breast and lymph nodes
- Mammography
- Ultrasound (if indicated)
- Breast MRI (if indicated)
- Biopsy

Postdiagnosis

- Lymph node analysis
- Estrogen and progesterone receptor status
- Cell-proliferative indices
- HER-2 marker
- Genetic assays (e.g., MammaPrint, Oncotype DX)

Staging

- Complete blood count
- Liver function tests
- Chest x-ray (if indicated)
- CT scan of chest, abdomen, pelvis (if indicated)
- PET/CT, MRI, bone scans (if indicated)

Management

Surgical Therapy

- Breast-conserving surgery (lumpectomy) with sentinel lymph node biopsy (SLNB) and/or axillary lymph node dissection
- Simple (total) mastectomy with SLNB and/or axillary lymph node dissection
- Modified radical mastectomy
- Reconstructive surgery

Radiation Therapy

- External radiation
- Brachytherapy
- Palliative radiation therapy

Drug Therapy (Table 56.9)

- Chemotherapy
- Hormone therapy
- Immunotherapy
- Targeted therapy

Not everyone is a candidate for breast conservation surgery. Contraindications include breast size too small in relation to the tumor size to yield an acceptable cosmetic result, multifocal masses and calcifications, multicentric masses (in more than 1 quadrant), diffuse calcifications in more than 1 quadrant, or prior radiation therapy. Because of the time commitment (5 to 7 weeks of daily radiation therapy treatments) and travel distances to access radiation therapy treatment centers, some patients may choose mastectomy over breast conservation surgery.

Mastectomy

A *total* or *simple mastectomy* removes the entire breast. A *modified radical mastectomy* includes removal of the breast and axillary lymph nodes. It preserves the pectoralis major muscle (Fig. 56.5B). For females desiring breast reconstruction, a skin-sparing mastectomy provides the best cosmetic result and does not increase the chance of the cancer recurring. In a *nipple-sparing mastectomy,* the nipple and/or areola are left in place and the breast tissue under them is removed. Females who have a small, low-grade cancer near the outer part of the breast, with no signs of cancer in the skin or near the nipple, may be able to have nipple-sparing surgery.

For females who have a mastectomy, breast reconstruction either can be done with the mastectomy or it can be delayed. Some females choose not to have reconstruction. There are 2 main types of breast reconstruction procedures: implant reconstruction or procedures that use autologous tissue transplantation (pedicled or microsurgical flaps from the abdomen, back, buttocks or thigh, and/or fat grafting) (Table 56.8).

Prophylactic Oophorectomy and Mastectomy

In females with *BRCA1* or *BRCA2* mutations, prophylactic bilateral oophorectomy can decrease the risk for breast and ovarian cancers. Removing the ovaries lowers the risk for breast cancer because the ovaries are the main source of estrogen in a premenopausal female. Removing the ovaries does not reduce the risk for breast cancer in postmenopausal females because the ovaries are not the main producers of estrogen in these patients. Females with *BRCA* mutations have a higher risk for developing breast cancer in the unaffected (contralateral) breast. They may choose, as might any female who has a high risk for developing breast cancer, in consultation with their HCP and genetic counselor, to undergo prophylactic bilateral mastectomy.

In deciding whether and when to undergo this surgery, females should receive counseling about the risks and benefits of prophylactic oophorectomy, including fertility issues. Patients need to consider the options and make decisions with which they feel comfortable. There is a small risk that cancer can develop in the areas where the breasts used to be. Close follow-up is necessary even after prophylactic surgery.

CHECK YOUR PRACTICE

You are doing a preoperative assessment on a female who is scheduled to have an elective bilateral mastectomy based on her *BRCA* testing, which revealed that she is high risk. You note that she appears tearful and anxious. She asks you, "I saw what happened to my mother, who died of breast cancer, but I am concerned that I'm being too aggressive. What do you think?"

- How would you respond to her?

Radiation Therapy

Radiation therapy may be used to (1) prevent local breast cancer recurrences after breast-conserving surgery; (2) prevent local and lymph node recurrences after mastectomy; or (3) relieve pain caused by local, regional, or distant cancer spread.

TABLE 56.8 Surgical Procedures for Breast Cancer

Procedure	Side Effects	Complications	Patient Issues
Breast-Conserving Surgery (Lumpectomy) With Radiation Therapy			
Excision of tumor with no tumor at margins, sentinel lymph node biopsy (SLNB) and/or axillary lymph node dissection (ALND) Radiation therapy	Arm swelling Breast edema Breast soreness Sensory changes in breast and arm Skin reactions	*Short-term:* moist desquamation[a] hematoma, seroma, infection *Long-term:* fibrosis,[a] lymphedema,[b] myositis, pneumonitis,[a] rib fractures[a]	Impaired arm mobility[b] Prolonged treatment[a] Texture and sensitivity changes in breast
Mastectomy			
Simple Mastectomy			
Removal of breast, preservation of pectoralis muscle, SLNB may be done at same time ***Modified Radical Mastectomy*** Removal of breast with ALND, pectoralis muscle is spared	Chest wall tightness, scar Impaired range of motion Lymphedema Phantom breast sensations Sensory changes	*Short-term:* skin flap necrosis, seroma, hematoma, infection *Long-term:* sensory loss, muscle weakness, lymphedema	Body image Impaired arm mobility Incision Loss of breast Need for prosthesis
Breast Implants and Tissue Expansion			
Expander used to slowly stretch tissue. Saline gradually injected into reservoir over weeks to months Insertion of implant under musculofascial layer of chest wall Fat grafting can sometimes replace implant	Chest wall tightness Pain	*Short-term:* skin flap necrosis, wound separation, seroma, hematoma, infection *Long-term:* capsular contractions, displacement of implant	Body image HCP visits to expand implants Potential added surgeries for nipple construction, symmetry
Breast Reconstruction Tissue Flap Procedures[c]			
Transverse Rectus Abdominis Musculocutaneous (TRAM) Flap			
Musculocutaneous flap (muscle, skin, fat, blood supply) is transposed from abdomen to the mastectomy site May be done concurrently with mastectomy	Pain related to 2 surgical sites and extensive surgery	*Short-term:* delayed wound healing, infection, skin flap necrosis, abdominal hernia, hematoma	Longer postoperative recovery
Deep Inferior Epigastric Artery Perforator (DIEP) Flap			
Free flap that transfers skin and fat from the abdomen to the chest. Differs from TRAM flap because no muscle is moved	More time in surgery than pedicle TRAM flap Pain related to 2 surgical sites	Needs close monitoring first 24–48 h after surgery; if flap fails, patient needs surgery	Less pain and impaired movement than with a pedicle TRAM flap

[a]Specific to radiation therapy.
[b]If ALND (less likely with SLNB).
[c]This list is not inclusive; other breast reconstruction options are available.

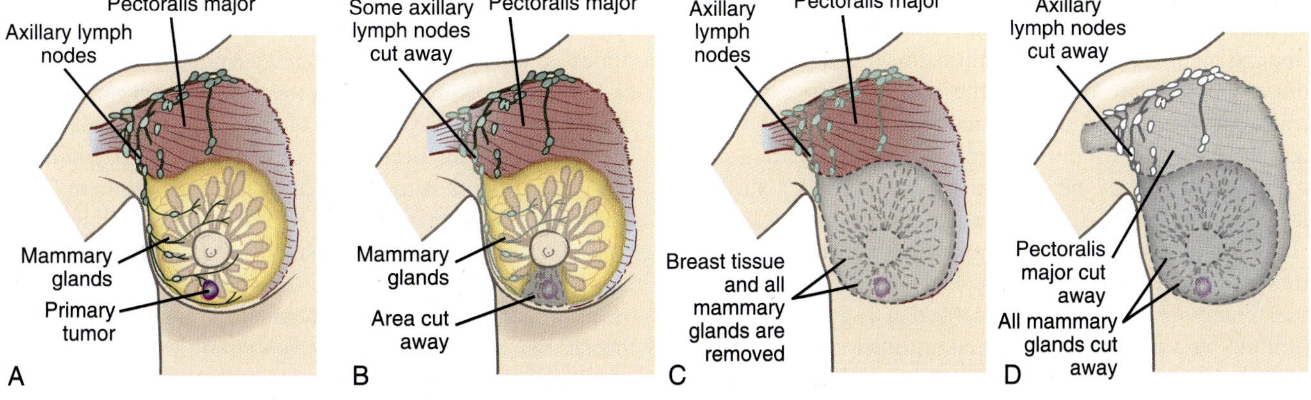

Fig. 56.5 Breast cancer surgery. (A) Preoperative. (B) Lumpectomy. (C) Simple mastectomy. (D) Modified radical mastectomy.

External Radiation Therapy

When radiation therapy is a primary treatment, it is usually done after surgery. The decision to use radiation after mastectomy is based on the chance that local residual cancer cells are present. Radiation of the axilla and/or supraclavicular nodes may be done when lymph nodes are involved to decrease the risk for axillary recurrence. Radiating a local area does not prevent distant metastasis.

With traditional whole breast and, in some cases, regional lymph node treatment, the area is radiated 5 days per week over the course of about 5 to 7 weeks. External beam of radiation delivers daily fractions of usually 1.8 to 2 Gy per day to a total dose of 46 to 50 Gy. Patients who have had breast-conserving surgery may receive a "boost" dose of radiation to the area where the original tumor was located. It is given by external beam and adds 4 to 8 more treatments to the total number given.

Newer and preferred regimens use a type of accelerated external beam radiation called *hypofractionation*. This type of radiation shortens the schedule to daily for 3 to 4 weeks, with the daily treatment delivering a higher dose. The total dose is 40 to 42.5 Gy.

Fatigue, skin changes, and breast edema are temporary side effects of external radiation therapy. Nursing care of patients receiving radiation therapy is discussed in Chapter 16.

Brachytherapy

Brachytherapy (internal radiation) is used for partial-breast radiation. It is an alternative to traditional external radiation treatment for some patients with early-stage breast cancer. This method has the same chance for local recurrence as whole breast radiation. However, the cosmetic results may not be as good.

Brachytherapy is minimally invasive. The radiation is delivered directly into the cavity left after a tumor is surgically removed by a lumpectomy. Because the radiation is concentrated and focused on the area with the highest risk for tumor recurrence, it only requires 5 treatments. Therapy is delivered using a multicatheter method or balloon-catheter system.

In the *multicatheter method* (e.g., strut-adjusted volume implant [SAVI]), many small catheters are placed in the breast at the site of the tumor. The SAVI is inserted through a small incision, and the catheter bundle expands uniformly. The ends of the catheters stick out through little holes in the skin. Small radioactive seeds are placed in the catheters. The seeds are left in place just long enough to deliver the radiation dose (e.g., 5 to 10 minutes) and then removed. The radiation does not stay in the body between treatments or after the last treatment is over.

In the *balloon-catheter system,* a balloon is placed where the tumor was located. The balloon is filled with fluid to keep it in place, then radioactive seeds are inserted (Fig. 56.6). Radiation is emitted by a tiny radioactive seed attached by a wire to an afterloader, a computer-controlled machine. The seed travels through the MammoSite applicator into the inflated balloon. As with the multicatheter system, the radiation does not stay in the body between treatments or after the last treatment is over. After the last session, the balloon is deflated and the system is removed.

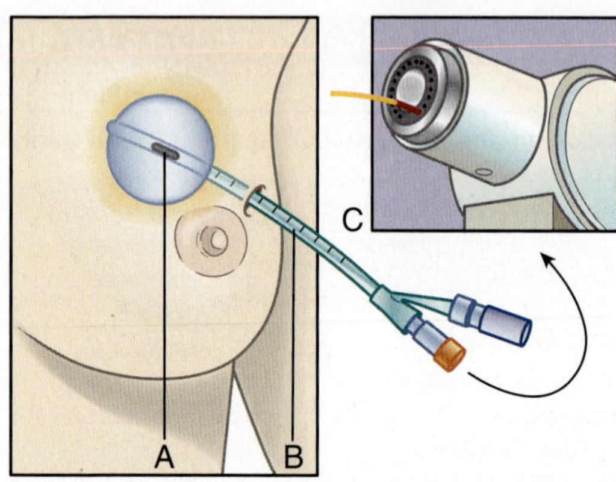

Fig. 56.6 High-dose brachytherapy for breast cancer. The MammoSite system involves the insertion of a single small balloon catheter (B) at the time of the lumpectomy or shortly thereafter into the tumor resection cavity (the space that is left after the HCP removes the tumor). A tiny radioactive seed (A) is inserted into the balloon, connected to an afterloader (C), and delivers the radiation therapy.

Palliative Radiation Therapy

Reducing the primary tumor mass with radiation often results in a decrease in pain. Radiation is a treatment option for symptomatic metastatic lesions in such sites as bone, soft tissue organs, brain, and chest. It often relieves pain and is successful in controlling recurrent or metastatic disease.

Drug Therapy

Drug therapy includes chemotherapy, hormone therapy, immunotherapy, and targeted therapy. When drug therapy is given before surgery, we call it *neoadjuvant therapy.* Neoadjuvant therapy is given to shrink the size of the tumor enough to make surgical removal possible or allow for breast-conserving surgery in females who would have been recommended to have a mastectomy. It also allows time for genetic testing to occur (if appropriate) so patients can make more informed treatment decisions. It provides evidence whether the tumor is responsive to the selected agent(s).

Drug therapy after surgery is called *adjuvant therapy.* Drug therapy can decrease the rate of recurrence and increase the length of survival. Because of the risk for recurrent disease, nearly all patients with evidence of node involvement, particularly those who are hormone receptor negative, will have some type of drug therapy. Some patients, especially those with a more aggressive tumor, have a higher risk for recurrent or metastatic disease. They may receive drug therapy even when there is no evidence of node involvement. Weighing the risks and benefits of drug therapy is a complex process.

Chemotherapy

Chemotherapy is the use of cytotoxic drugs to destroy cancer cells. A combination of drugs is usually better than using a single drug. Combination treatment is best because the drugs have different mechanisms of action and work at different phases of the cell cycle. When used in the neoadjuvant and adjuvant setting, chemotherapy is usually given for 3 to 6 months. Patients with metastasis may receive chemotherapy for the rest of their lives.

Common combination-therapy protocols in the adjuvant and neoadjuvant setting are (1) CMF: cyclophosphamide, methotrexate, and fluorouracil; (2) AC: doxorubicin and cyclophosphamide, with or without a taxane, such as paclitaxel or docetaxel (Taxotere); or (3) CEF or CAF: cyclophosphamide, epirubicin (Ellence) or doxorubicin, and fluorouracil.

Because chemotherapy affects healthy cells, many side effects accompany chemotherapy. The incidence and severity of common side effects are related to specific drug combinations, drug schedule, and dosage. Nursing care of patients receiving chemotherapy is discussed in Chapter 16.

DRUG ALERT

Doxorubicin

- Monitor for cardiotoxicity and heart failure (e.g., shortness of breath, pedal edema, decreased activity tolerance, dysrhythmias, ECG changes).
- Tell patients not to have immunizations without the HCP's approval.

Hormone Therapy

Estrogen can promote the growth of breast cancer cells if the cells are ER positive. Hormone therapy promotes tumor regression by either (1) blocking ERs or (2) suppressing estrogen synthesis by inhibiting aromatase, an enzyme needed for estrogen synthesis (Table 56.9).

ER and PR status assays can identify females whose breast cancers are likely to respond to hormone therapy. These assays predict whether hormone therapy is a treatment option. Chances of tumor regression are much higher in females whose tumors have ERs and PRs. The 21-gene recurrence score (OncotypeDX) can identify which females with hormone-positive breast cancer can be treated with hormone therapy alone and do not need chemotherapy.

Premenopausal females with ER-positive breast cancers may benefit from the removal or suppression of their ovaries. Ovarian ablation can be done surgically or by using luteinizing hormone–releasing hormone (LHRH) analogs, such as goserelin (Zoladex) or leuprolide (Lupron).

Estrogen Receptor Blockers

ER blockers include tamoxifen, toremifene (Fareston), and fulvestrant (Faslodex). Tamoxifen has been the hormone therapy of choice in ER-positive females at all stages of breast cancer for the past 30 years. It also may be used in high-risk females to prevent breast cancer. Common side effects include hot flashes, mood swings, vaginal discharge and dryness, and other effects associated with decreased estrogen. It increases the risk for blood clots, cataracts, stroke, and endometrial cancer in postmenopausal females.

DRUG ALERT

Tamoxifen

- Irregular vaginal bleeding or spotting may occur.
- Decreased visual acuity, corneal opacity, and retinopathy can occur in females receiving high doses (240–320 mg/day for >17 months). These problems may not be reversible.
- Teach patients to report any vision changes.
- Monitor for signs of venous thromboembolism (VTE) and stroke.

Aromatase inhibitors. Aromatase inhibitors lower estrogen levels by stopping aromatase, an enzyme in fat tissue, from changing other hormones into estrogen. These drugs include anastrozole, letrozole, and exemestane. They do not stop the ovaries from making estrogen. Thus they are of little benefit and may be harmful in premenopausal females. They are used to treat breast cancer in postmenopausal females.

Because they block estrogen production in postmenopausal females, osteoporosis and bone fractures may occur. Side effects include night sweats, nausea, and joint and muscle pain.

Estrogen receptor modulators. Raloxifene is a selective ER modulator that has both estrogen-agonistic effects on bone and estrogen-antagonistic effects on breast tissue (see Chapter 68).

Targeted Therapy

As we learn more about genetic changes in breast cancer, we have developed drugs that specifically target cells that have altered gene expression. One of these genetic changes is the overexpression of HER-2. Tumors that overexpress the HER-2 protein tend to be more aggressive and are more likely to recur.

HER-2 inhibitors work by attaching to the HER-2 receptors on the surface of the breast cancer cells and blocking them from receiving signals that tell them to proliferate. Trastuzumab is one HER-2 inhibitor. It can be used alone or in combination with chemotherapy agents. The most common side effects are flulike symptoms (fever, chills, myalgia), nausea and vomiting, diarrhea, and infusion reactions. A possible, but more serious, side effect is heart damage. Trastuzumab-qyyp and trastuzumab-pkrb are biosimilars of trastuzumab.

DRUG ALERT

Trastuzumab

- Use with caution in females with preexisting heart disease.
- Monitor for heart failure.

Other drugs that target HER-2 include pertuzumab, adotrastuzumab emtansine, and lapatinib. Neratinib is an option for extended adjuvant therapy for some high-risk females. Using 2 of these agents together for neoadjuvant therapy can

TABLE 56.9 Drug Therapy

Breast Cancer

Drug Class	Mechanism of Action	Indications
Hormone Therapy		
Aromatase Inhibitors		
anastrozole (Arimidex) exemestane (Aromasin) letrozole (Femara)	Prevents estrogen production by inhibiting aromatase	ER-positive breast cancer in postmenopausal females only
Estrogen Receptor (ER) Blockers		
fulvestrant (Faslodex)	Blocks ERs and increases their degradation	ER-positive breast cancer in postmenopausal females only
tamoxifen	Selectively blocks ERs	ER-positive breast cancer in premenopausal and postmenopausal females Used as a preventive measure in high-risk premenopausal and postmenopausal females
toremifene (Fareston)	Blocks ERs	ER-positive breast cancer in postmenopausal females only
Estrogen Receptor Modulator		
raloxifene (Evista)	In breast, blocks the effect of estrogen. In bone, promotes effect of estrogen and prevents bone loss	Postmenopausal females
Targeted Therapy		
HER-2 Inhibitors		
lapatinib (Tykerb)	Blocks the function of HER-2 related kinases inside the cell	HER-2–positive breast cancer
margetuximab-cmkb (Margenza) pertuzumab (Perjeta) trastuzumab (Herceptin) trastuzumab-pkrb (Herzuma) trastuzumab-qyyp (Trazimera)	Blocks HER-2 receptor	HER-2–positive breast cancer
ado-trastuzumab emtansine (Kadcyla)	Trastuzumab with a chemotherapy drug called DM1	HER-2–positive breast cancer
fam-trastuzumab deruxtecan-nxki (Enhertu)	HER-2–directed antibody and a topoisomerase inhibitor	Advanced or metastatic HER-2–positive breast cancer after 2 other HER-2 therapies
Kinase Inhibitors		
abemaciclib (Verzenio) palbociclib (Ibrance) ribociclib (Kisqali)	CDK4/6 kinase inhibitors	ER-positive, HER-2–negative breast cancer in postmenopausal females
neratinib (Nerlynx) tucatinib (Tukysa)	Tyrosine kinase inhibitor	Advanced or metastatic HER-2–positive breast cancer after 1 other HER-2 therapy, includes patients with brain metastasis
alpelisib (Piqray)	P13 kinase inhibitor	*PIK3CA*-mutated, HER-2–negative advanced breast cancer
everolimus (Afinitor)	mTOR inhibitor suppressing T-cell activation and proliferation	ER-positive, HER-2–negative breast cancer in postmenopausal females
olaparib (Lynparza) talazoparib (Talzenna)	PARP inhibitors	Patients with metastatic breast cancer positive for *BRCA* mutations
entrectinib (Rozlytrek) larotrectinib (Vitrakvi)	NTRK inhibitors	In NTRK-positive breast cancers (very rare) when no other options exist
Immunomodulators		
atezolizumab (Tecentriq)	PD-1 inhibitor	PD-L1–positive triple-negative advanced or metastatic breast cancer
pembrolizumab (Keytruda)	PD-1 inhibitor	Any MSI-H breast cancer when no other options exist
sacituzumab govitecan-hziy (Trodelvy)	Monoclonal antibody that targets Trop-2 protein and a topoisomerase 1 inhibitor	Metastatic triple-negative disease after 2 other therapies

increase the number of tumors that become undetectable. Survival improves when used for adjuvant therapy.

Kinase inhibitors prevent cells from dividing, thus slowing cancer growth. Drugs in this class include palbociclib, ribociclib, and abemaciclib. They are used for ER-positive, HER-2–negative cancer in postmenopausal females.

Other targeted drugs include everolimus. It works by blocking mammalian target of rapamycin (mTOR), a protein that normally promotes cell growth and division. The PARP inhibitors olaparib and talazoparib are used in patients with metastatic breast cancer positive for *BRCA* mutations. Alpelisib, a PI3K inhibitor, is used for patients with advanced or metastatic disease with a *PIK3CA* mutation. For the rare breast cancers that test positive for *NTRK* fusion genes, the NTRK inhibitors larotrectinib and entrectinib may be tried after other treatments are exhausted. Immunotherapy and targeted therapy are discussed in Chapter 16.

Immunotherapy

Atezolizumab, an immune checkpoint inhibitor, was the first FDA-approved immunotherapy agent. It is used with chemotherapy to treat locally advanced triple-negative breast cancer in patients with a PD-L1 (programmed death ligand 1)–positive biomarker.

Adding pembrolizumab to chemotherapy as part of neoadjuvant therapy for triple-negative breast cancer increased the chance of a complete response. Pembrolizumab is an option with advanced breast cancer that tests microsatellite instability-high (MSI-H) when no other therapies are available.

NURSING MANAGEMENT: BREAST CANCER

Assessment

You must consider many factors when assessing patients with a breast problem. The history helps establish a diagnosis. Investigate the presence of nipple discharge, pain, rate of growth of the lump, breast asymmetry, and correlation with the menstrual cycle. Record the size and location of the lump(s). Assess the lesion, including consistency, mobility, and shape. If nipple discharge is present, note the color and consistency. Does it occur from 1 or both breasts?

Subjective and objective data to obtain from a person suspected of having or diagnosed with breast cancer are outlined in Table 56.10.

Clinical Problems

Clinical problems for patients diagnosed with breast cancer vary. After diagnosis and before a treatment plan has been selected, the following would apply:

- Difficulty coping
- Deficient knowledge

If surgery is planned, the nursing diagnoses and interventions may include those in eNursing Care Plan 56.1 (available on the website for this chapter).

Planning

The overall goals are that patients with breast cancer will (1) take part in decision-making related to treatment, (2) adhere to the therapeutic plan, (3) communicate about and manage the side effects of therapy, (4) be supported by significant others and the health care team, and (5) adhere to recommended follow-up and surveillance after treatment.

TABLE 56.10 NURSING ASSESSMENT

Breast Cancer

Subjective Data

Important Health Information

Health history: Benign breast disease with atypical changes. Previous unilateral breast cancer. Menstrual history (early menarche with late menopause), pregnancy history (nulliparity or first full-term pregnancy after age 30). Endometrial, ovarian, or colon cancer. Hyperestrogenism and testicular atrophy (males)

Medicines: Hormones, especially as postmenopausal hormone therapy and in oral contraceptives. Infertility treatments

Surgery or other treatments: Exposure to therapeutic radiation (e.g., Hodgkin lymphoma or thyroid radiation)

Functional Health Patterns

Health perception–health management: Family history of breast cancer (young age at diagnosis). History of abnormal mammogram or atypical prior biopsy. Palpable change found on BSE. Known *BRCA* mutation carrier, first-degree relative of *BRCA* carrier (but untested)

Nutritional-metabolic: Obesity; unexplained severe weight loss (may indicate metastasis)

Activity-exercise: Level of usual activity

Cognitive-perceptual: Changes in cognition, headache, bone pain (may indicate metastasis)

Sexuality-reproductive: Unilateral nipple discharge (clear, milky, bloody). Change in breast contour, size, or symmetry

Coping–stress tolerance: Psychologic stress

Self-perception–self-concept: Anxiety about threat to self-esteem

Objective Data

General

Axillary and supraclavicular lymphadenopathy

GI

Hepatomegaly, jaundice, ascites (may indicate liver metastasis)

Respiratory

Pleural effusions (may indicate metastasis)

Skin

Hard, irregular, nonmobile breast lump, most often in upper outer sector, possibly fixated to fascia or chest wall. Thickening of breast. Nipple inversion or retraction, erosion. Edema (*peau d'orange*), redness, induration, infiltration, or dimpling (in later stages). Firm, discrete nodules at mastectomy site (may indicate local recurrence). Peripheral edema (may indicate metastasis)

Possible Diagnostic Findings

Finding of mass or change in tissue on breast examination. Abnormal mammogram, ultrasound, or breast MRI. Positive results of fine-needle aspiration or surgical biopsy; similar results with a needle biopsy

◆ Implementation

Health Promotion

Review the risk factors in Table 56.3. Maintaining a healthy weight, exercising regularly, limiting alcohol, eating nutritious food, and never smoking (or quitting if currently smoking) are ways to reduce risk.

Encourage females to adhere to the breast cancer screening guidelines shown in Table 56.1. Those at high risk need a personal plan with the HCP. Early detection can decrease mortality from breast cancer. Discuss genetic testing for *BRCA* and other gene mutations in those at risk. If testing was done in the past and was negative, a conversation about repeat testing with a genetic counselor is worthwhile, as newer tests examine a much wider range of genes. People with a personal history of breast cancer, especially those diagnosed at age 45 or earlier; those older with unknown family history; those with a second breast cancer at any age; those of Ashkenazi Jewish ancestry; males of any age, and anyone with 1 or more close relatives with breast, ovarian, pancreatic, or high-grade prostate cancers should be tested.

Prophylactic surgery decisions require a great deal of thought, patience, and discussion with the HCP, genetic counselor, and family. In females with an abnormal *BRCA1* or *BRCA2* gene, prophylactic oophorectomy may reduce their risk of developing breast and ovarian cancer. In deciding whether and when to undergo this surgery, females should receive counseling about the risks and benefits of prophylactic oophorectomy, including fertility issues.

Patients need to consider the options and make decisions with which they feel comfortable. Removing both breasts and ovaries does not eliminate the risk for breast cancer. A small risk exists that cancer can develop in the areas where the breasts used to be. Close follow-up is necessary even after prophylactic surgery.

Acute Care

The times of waiting for the initial biopsy results and the HCP to make treatment recommendations are difficult for patients and their families. Even after the HCP has discussed treatment options, patients often rely on you to clarify and expand on these options. During this stressful time, patients may not be coping effectively. Provide support as they make decisions.

Provide patients with enough information to ensure informed consent. Some seek extensive, detailed information to maintain a sense of control. Others avoid information to decrease anxiety and fear. Be sensitive to the patient's need for and preferred type of information. These include (1) instructions on pain control and what to expect after surgery (e.g., dressing and drain care, turning, coughing, deep breathing), (2) a review of mobility restrictions and postoperative exercises, and (3) an explanation of the recovery period.

The female who has breast-conserving surgery usually has an uncomplicated postoperative course with variable pain intensity. Pain depends primarily on the extent of the lymph node sampling procedure. If an ALND has been done or if the patient had a mastectomy, drains are often left in place and patients are discharged home with them. Provide teaching about how to manage the drains at home.

Most patients are discharged from the hospital 24 to 48 hours after a mastectomy, depending on if reconstructive surgery was done. Restoring arm function on the affected side after breast cancer surgery is a key nursing goal. Arm and shoulder exercises, which are started gradually, may begin before discharge (Fig. 56.7). These exercises aim to prevent contractures and muscle shortening, maintain muscle tone, and improve lymph and blood circulation. The difficulty and pain encountered in performing what used to be simple tasks may cause frustration and depression. The goal of all exercise is a gradual return to full range of motion.

Minimize discomfort by giving analgesics regularly when patients are in pain and about 30 minutes before starting exercises. When patients can shower, the warm water on the involved shoulder often relaxes the muscle and reduces joint stiffness.

Explain the specific follow-up plan. Stress the importance of ongoing monitoring and self-care. Teach patients to report symptoms, such as fever, inflammation at the surgical site, redness, and unusual swelling. Other changes to report are new

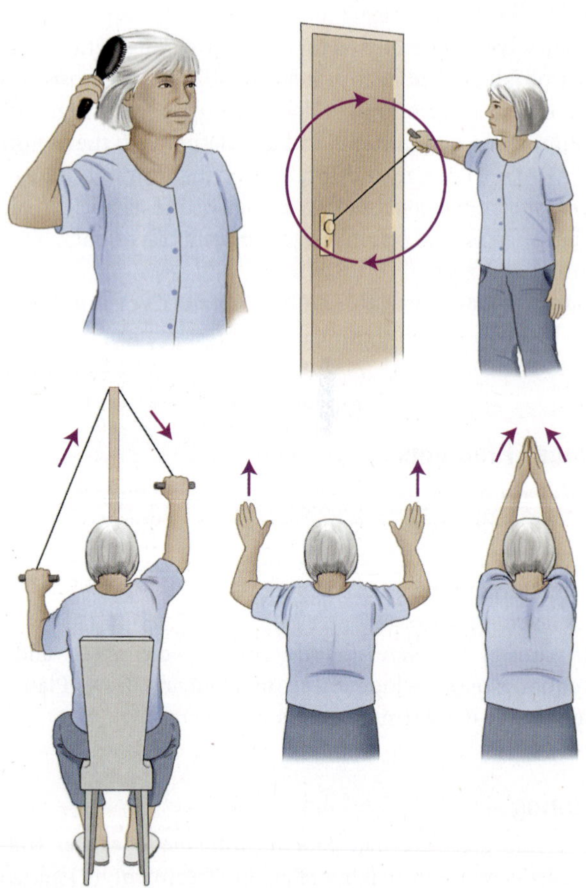

Fig. 56.7 Postoperative exercises for patients after a mastectomy or lumpectomy with axillary lymph node sampling and/or dissection.

back pain, weakness, shortness of breath, and change in mental status, including confusion.

For females who have had a mastectomy without breast reconstruction, a variety of products are available. Your role is to present the choices and resources. Options include garments such as camisoles with soft breast prosthetic inserts or a fitted prosthesis with a bra. Should the female choose a breast prosthesis, a certified fitter can help her choose a comfortable, more permanent weighted prosthesis and bra. This is done 4 to 8 weeks after surgery.

Lymphedema. Lymphedema is an accumulation of lymph in soft tissue. It can occur because of the lymph node sampling procedure or radiation therapy (Fig. 56.8). When the axillary nodes cannot return lymph fluid to the central circulation, the fluid accumulates in the arm, hand, or breast, causing obstructive pressure on the veins and venous return. Patients may have heaviness, impaired motor function in the arm, and numbness and paresthesia of the fingers. Cellulitis and progressive fibrosis of the skin can result from untreated lymphedema.

Upper extremity lymphedema can occur at any point after treatment for breast cancer. Teach patients ways to prevent and reduce lymphedema. These include no BP readings, venipunctures, or injections on the affected arm, if possible. The affected arm should not be dependent for long periods. Caution should be used to prevent infection, burns, or compromised circulation on the affected side. Encourage exercise and maintaining a normal weight.

If trauma to the arm occurs, teach patients to thoroughly wash the area with soap and water and observe. A topical antibiotic ointment and a bandage or other sterile dressing may be needed.

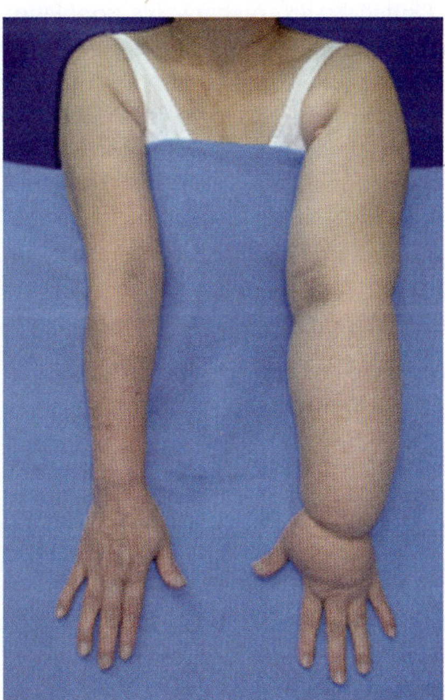

Fig. 56.8 Lymphedema. Accumulation of fluid in the tissue after excision of lymph nodes. (From Pappalardo M, Cheng M: *Principles and practice of lymphedema surgery,* St Louis, 2022, Elsevier.)

With acute lymphedema, we usually start complete decongestive therapy. Specially trained professionals perform this therapy. It consists of a massage-like technique to mobilize the subcutaneous accumulation of fluid. This may be followed by compression bandaging with use of an intermittent pneumatic compression sleeve. The sleeve applies mechanical massage to the arm and helps move lymph drainage up toward the heart. Elevating the arm so that it is level with the heart and performing isometric exercises reduce the fluid in the arm. To maintain maximum volume reduction, patients may need to wear a fitted compression sleeve during waking hours and preventively during air travel.

Post–breast therapy pain syndrome. *Post–breast therapy pain syndrome* (PBTPS) occurs in some people who had procedures for breast cancer. It is often caused by injury to nerves during surgery. Other causes include chemotherapy and radiation therapy. The most common theory is that PBTPS results from injury to intercostobrachial nerves. These are sensory nerves that exit the chest wall muscles and provide sensation to the shoulder and upper arm.

PBTPS symptoms range from mild to debilitating. Common symptoms include chest and upper arm pain, tingling down the arm, continuous aching and burning, numbness, shooting or pricking pain, and unbearable itching that persists beyond the normal 3-month healing time. Edema may be present.

Treatment includes nonsteroidal antiinflammatory drugs (NSAIDs), low-dose antidepressants, topical anesthetics (e.g., EMLA [lidocaine and prilocaine]), and antiseizure drugs (e.g., gabapentin). Other treatments include biofeedback, physical therapy to prevent "frozen shoulder" syndrome from inadequate movement, guided imagery, and psychologic counseling with a therapist trained in the management of chronic pain syndromes.

Phantom breast pain. *Phantom breast pain* is feeling pain in the breast after it was removed with mastectomy. It occurs for the same reasons that phantom limb sensation occurs after limb amputations. The brain continues to send signals to nerves in the breast area that were cut during surgery, even though the breast is no longer physically there.

CHECK YOUR PRACTICE

You are reviewing discharge instructions with a 56-year-old female who had a right radical mastectomy. Although you are speaking to her, she appears distracted and keeps staring down at the floor. You ask her if she has any questions, and she says, "I feel like no one will find my body attractive anymore."

- How would you respond?

Psychosocial support. Throughout history, the female breast has been a symbol of beauty, femininity, sexuality, and motherhood. The potential loss of a breast, or part of a breast, may be devastating for many females because of the significant psychologic, social, sexual, and body image implications associated with it. In some cases, psychosocial concerns may increase the physical effects of cancer, such as pain, fatigue, sleep problems, fear of recurrence, and cognitive changes. Males diagnosed with breast cancer may feel isolation and embarrassment related to the diagnosis. You must be aware of resources for these patients (https://mbcglobalalliance.org/).

Screening all cancer patients for psychosocial distress is a Commission on Cancer accreditation requirement.[18] From the time of diagnosis through treatment, survivorship, or metastatic disease, patients may have distress or tension (e.g., tachycardia, muscle tension, sleep problems, restlessness, changes in appetite or mood). Assess patients' body language and affect during periods of high stress so that you can begin appropriate interventions.

Be sensitive to the psychologic impact that a cancer diagnosis and breast surgery can have on patients and their families (Box 56.2). Cultural values and meanings associated with body image, sexuality, and motherhood influence how patients respond to and cope with breast cancer and treatment.

With an accepting attitude and the offer of resources, you can help patients cope with feelings of fear, anger, anxiety, and depression (Table 56.11). Refer patients to support resources, such as Breastcancer.org (www.Breastcancer.org), American Cancer Society (www.cancer.org), Living Beyond Breast Cancer (www.lbbc.org), Susan G. Komen for the Cure (www.komen.org), the Cancer Support Community, or local breast cancer organizations. The National Cancer Institute (www.nccn.org) provides materials to help you meet the special needs of patients with breast cancer. In addition to in-person and online support programs, free smartphone applications are available through national cancer organizations that provide reliable and current information.

If you are comfortable, begin a discussion of sexuality by inviting questions about relationships or intimacy concerns. Often, the partner and/or family members need help dealing with their emotional reactions to the diagnosis and surgery before they can provide effective support for the patient. There are no physical reasons why a mastectomy would prevent sexual satisfaction. A female taking hormone therapy may have a decreased sexual drive or vaginal dryness. She may need to use lubrication to prevent pain during intercourse. If difficulty adjusting or other problems develop, single or couples counseling may be useful to deal with distress.

Depression and anxiety may occur with the continued stress and uncertainty of a cancer diagnosis. A patient's self-esteem and identity may be threatened. The support of family and friends and taking part in a cancer support group and/or counseling are important aspects of care that may improve quality of life.

Survivorship. Almost 3 million breast cancer survivors are alive in the United States, making this population the largest group of cancer survivors. We expect this number to grow because of an aging population and improved methods for early detection and treatment. After treatment for breast cancer, patients will have ongoing survivorship care.[19]

BOX 56.2 EVIDENCE-BASED PRACTICE

Caregiver Burden With Breast Cancer Patients

In the oncology clinic where you work, many patients are receiving chemotherapy to treat breast cancer. You are finding that more of their partners are expressing anxiety and concern about the treatments. Several state concerns about childcare and financial burdens due to missing work. This leads you to consider how they may be better supported.

Making Clinical Decisions

Best Available Evidence

Research shows that education, social support, and relaxation techniques such as exercise, meditation, deep breathing, and imagery can have beneficial effects on caregivers' well-being. These benefits include reduced distress and caregiver burden, as well as improved coping and self-efficacy. The content and mode of these interventions can vary depending on the methods used.

Clinician Expertise

As a nurse, you know that the taxing nature of cancer treatment often demands the active involvement of family or close friends in a caregiving role. These caregivers devote time and energy to supporting the patient, often at the expense of their own physical and emotional well-being. Before they can provide effective support, many caregivers need help processing their own stress and emotional responses.

Patient Preferences and Values

The nursing staff, in collaboration with the instruction technology and medical teams, enhance the support program for caregivers. The program now includes an application with words of encouragement, spiritual messages, and video and audio vignettes with relaxation techniques. There is a forum for questions and answers and links to both virtual and online weekly caregiver support groups. Each caregiver can choose what resources they need.

Implications for Nursing Practice

1. Identify tools you could use to assess caregiver burden.
2. How would you assess if the support program was effective in decreasing caregiver burden?

Reference for Evidence

Zhang Y, Tang R, Wang D, et al: Family-centered online positive psychological intervention for breast cancer patients and family caregivers: a single-arm pre-post study of feasibility and preliminary effects, *BMC Psychol* 13:1, 2025.

TABLE 56.11 NURSING MANAGEMENT

Managing Distress in Breast Cancer

- Screen all patients for distress.
- Provide a safe environment for expressing feelings.
- Identify sources of support and strength, such as the partner, family, and spiritual or religious practices.
- Encourage patients to identify and learn personal coping strengths.
- Promote communication among the patient, family, and friends.
- Assess the willingness, availability, and resilience of family and friends to serve as supportive caregivers.
- Provide teaching and answer questions about the disease, treatment options, and reproductive, fertility, or lactation issues.
- Make resources available for mental health counseling.
- Offer information about local and national community resources.

A history and physical assessment is recommended 1 to 4 times per year as clinically appropriate for 5 years, then annually thereafter. Teach breast cancer survivors to perform monthly BSE and chest wall self-examination and report any changes to their HCP. Local recurrence of breast cancer is usually at the surgical site. Breast cancer survivors should have an annual mammogram. Other breast imaging studies, such as a breast ultrasound or breast MRI, are an adjunct to mammography and are not used for routine surveillance. Cancer survivorship is discussed in Chapter 16.

◆ Evaluation

Expected outcomes are that patients after breast cancer surgery will:

- Identify activities that can reduce postoperative edema and improve mobility
- Show effective use of coping strategies
- Discuss feelings about and the meaning of changes in physical appearance
- Identify community and online resources, counseling, and support groups

Gerontologic Considerations: Breast Cancer

A major risk for breast cancer is increasing age. More than half of all breast cancers occur in females who are age 55 or older. Screening and treatment decisions should be based on overall health rather than biologic age because health status has a greater influence on tolerance to treatment and long-term prognosis. In addition to comorbidities and life expectancy, treatment decisions for the older female with breast cancer should be based on nutrition and functional status; vision, gait, and balance; and the presence of dementia or depression.

Breast cancer treatment is similar for older patients, including the use of surgery, radiation therapy, and drug therapy. For healthy older females, breast cancer survival rates are similar to those of younger females when matched by cancer stage.

MAMMOPLASTY

Mammoplasty is the surgical change in the size or shape of the breast. It may be done electively for cosmetic purposes to either enlarge or reduce the size of the breasts. Mammoplasty reconstructs the breast after a mastectomy.

A professional attitude and clear information about surgical options are useful for females engaged in decision-making about mammoplasty. The desire to change the appearance of the breasts has special significance for each female as she attempts to change or recreate her body image. Be aware of the cultural value that the female places on the breast. Help patients set realistic expectations about what mammoplasty can achieve and possible complications (e.g., hematoma formation, hemorrhage, infection). If an implant is involved, capsular contracture and loss of the implant are possible.

BREAST RECONSTRUCTION

Breast reconstructive surgery is a type of surgery for females who have had all or part of a breast removed. It can achieve symmetry and restore or preserve body image. It may be done simultaneously with a mastectomy or some time afterward. The timing of reconstructive surgery is based on physical and psychologic needs.[20]

Indications

The main indications for breast reconstruction are to improve self-image, regain a sense of normalcy, and assist in coping with the loss of the breast. It restores the contour of the breast without the use of an external prosthesis. Although the breast will not fully resemble its premastectomy appearance, the reconstructed appearance usually is an improvement over the mastectomy scar (Fig. 56.9). Reconstruction cannot restore lactation, nipple sensation, or erectility.

Types of Reconstruction

Breast Implants and Tissue Expansion

Implants have a silicone shell filled with either silicone gel or saline. Some newer types use a cohesive gel, which is a thicker silicone gel. Implant surgery can be done in 1 or 2 stages. In the 1-stage procedure, the implant is placed at the same time as the mastectomy. The implant is usually placed under the pectoralis muscle.

In the 2-stage procedure, a tissue expander is inserted after the mastectomy. The expander stretches the skin and muscle at the mastectomy site before inserting permanent implants (Fig. 56.10). It is placed in a pocket under the pectoralis muscle, which protects the implant and provides soft tissue coverage. The expander is minimally inflated, then gradually filled by weekly injections of sterile saline solution. This procedure stretches the skin and muscle and can be painful. A small magnet embedded in most expanders helps locate the port where the fluid is injected. Patients should not have an MRI with a magnet in place.

The expander can be (1) surgically removed and a permanent implant is inserted or (2) remain in place to become the implant, thus eliminating the need for a second surgery. Tissue expansion does not work well in those with extensive scar tissue from surgery or radiation therapy.

The body's natural response to the presence of a foreign substance is the formation of a fibrous capsule around the implant. If excessive capsular formation occurs because of infection, hematoma, trauma, or reaction to a foreign body, a contracture can develop, resulting in deformity. Although HCPs differ in their approaches to the prevention of contracture formation, gentle manual massage around the implant is

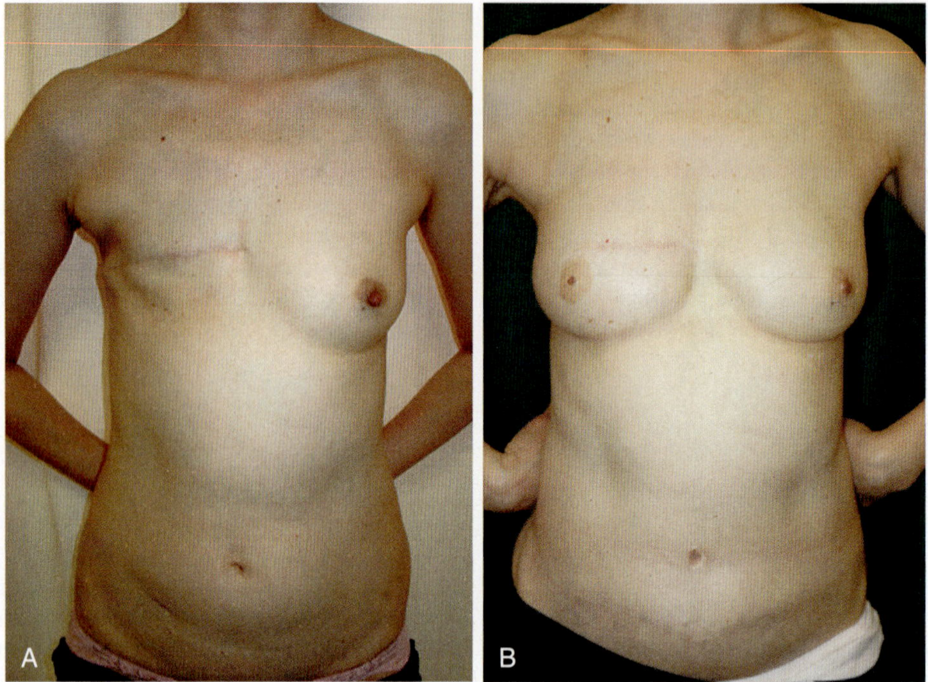

Fig. 56.9 (A) Appearance of the chest after right modified mastectomy. (B) Breast reconstruction after nipple-areolar reconstruction. (From Satake T, Muto M, Kou S, et al: Contralateral unaffected breast augmentation using zone IV as a SIEA flap during unilateral DIEP flap breast reconstruction, *J Plast Reconstr Aesthet Surg* 72:1537, 2019.)

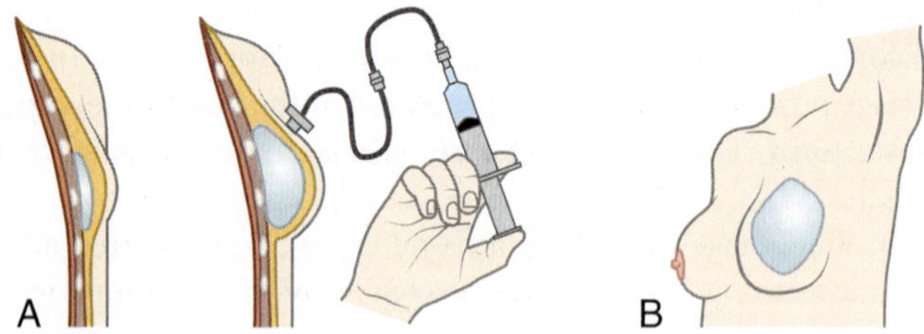

Fig. 56.10 (A) Tissue expander with gradual expansion. (B) Tissue expander in place after mastectomy.

routine. Other adverse outcomes include wrinkling, scarring, asymmetry, pain, and infection at the incision site. There is a small chance of anaplastic large cell lymphoma. This has mostly occurred with textured implants.

Tissue Flap Procedures

We can use autologous (the person's own) tissue to re-create a breast mound. In autologous reconstruction, tissue from the abdomen, back, thighs, or buttocks is used to create a reconstructed breast. The most common types of tissue flap procedures are *transverse rectus abdominis musculocutaneous (TRAM) flap, deep inferior epigastric artery perforator (DIEP) flap,* and *latissimus dorsi flap.*

The TRAM flap is a common flap surgery. The rectus abdominis muscles are paired flat muscles running from the rib cage down to the pubic bone. Arteries running inside the muscles provide branches at many levels, and these branches supply the fat and skin across a large expanse of the abdomen.

There are 2 different types of TRAM flaps: pedicle and free. In a pedicle flap, the tissue stays attached to the rectus muscle and is tunneled under the skin to the chest (Fig. 56.11). In a free flap, the tissue is completely separated from the muscle and its blood supply and moved to the new place on the chest. The tissue is molded and fashioned to form a breast. The abdominal incision is closed, yielding a result that is similar to having an abdominoplasty ("tummy tuck"). The procedure can last 6 to 8 hours with recovery taking 6 to 8 weeks. Some patients report pain and fatigue for up to 3 months. Complications include bleeding, hernia, infection, and low back pain.

Perforator flaps are a type of free flap (a perforator artery connects a superficial artery with a deep one) that does not use muscle tissue. A *DIEP flap* is the type done most often. With the DIEP flap, only the skin and fat are taken from the same lower abdominal area as the TRAM flap. Patients may have less pain and impaired movement with this procedure. The *superficial inferior epigastric artery perforator (SIEAP)* is another option using the abdominal area.

The *latissimus dorsi flap* is a pedicle flap. In this type of flap, a block of skin and muscle from the back replaces tissue removed during mastectomy. A small implant may be needed under the flap to gain reasonable breast shape and size. A disadvantage is a scar on the back.

Less often, flaps are taken from the buttocks, hips, or thighs. The transverse upper gracilis flap, or inner thigh flap, is one type of free flap. Tissue, including the gracilis muscle, is taken from the bottom fold of the buttock extending into the inner

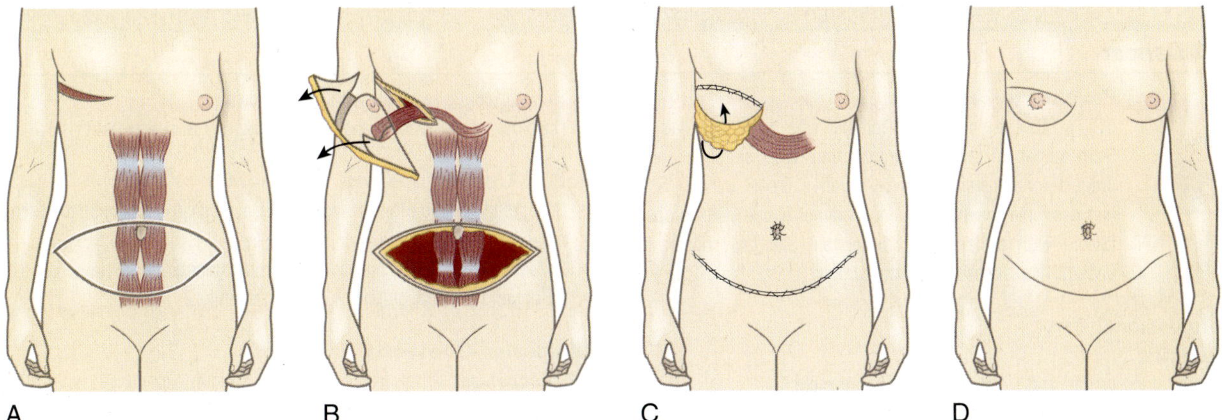

Fig. 56.11 Transverse rectus abdominis musculocutaneous (TRAM) flap. (A) TRAM flap is planned. (B) The abdominal tissue, while attached to the rectus muscle, nerve, and blood supply, is tunneled through the abdomen to the chest. (C) The flap is trimmed to shape the breast. The lower abdominal incision is closed. (D) Nipple and areola are reconstructed after the breast is healed.

thigh. The inferior or superior gluteal artery perforators are used for flaps taken from the buttocks.

Nipple-Areolar Reconstruction

Many patients having breast reconstruction also have nipple-areolar reconstruction. Nipple reconstruction gives the reconstructed breast a much more natural appearance (Fig. 56.9B). Nipple-areolar reconstruction is usually done a few months after breast reconstruction. Tissue to construct a nipple may be taken from the opposite breast or from a small flap of tissue on the reconstructed breast mound. Most often, the areola is tattooed with a permanent pigmented dye. Improved techniques allow skilled tattoo artists to create a complete 3D nipple-areola complex. Polyurethane removable nipples are also available.

BREAST AUGMENTATION

In *augmentation mammoplasty* (a procedure to enlarge the breasts), an implant is placed in a surgically created pocket between the capsule of the breast and pectoral fascia or ideally under the pectoralis muscle.

BREAST REDUCTION

For some females, large breasts can be a source of physical and psychologic discomfort. They can interfere with normal daily activities, such as walking, using a computer, and driving a car. The weight of large breasts can lead to back, shoulder, and neck problems, including degenerative nerve changes. Overly large breasts can interfere with self-esteem, self-image, and comfort in wearing some clothing. Reducing breast size can have positive effects on psychologic and physical health.

Reduction mammoplasty is done by resecting wedges of tissue from the upper and lower quadrants of the breast. The excess skin is removed. The areola and nipple are relocated on the breast. Lactation usually can still occur if massive amounts of tissue are not removed and the nipples are left connected during surgery.

BREAST LIFT

A breast lift, or mastopexy, is a surgical procedure that changes the shape of the breasts. During a breast lift, excess skin is removed and the tissue reshaped to raise the breast. Most females who have this procedure do so to lift sagging breasts. A breast lift does not change the size of the breast. It is often done with breast augmentation or reduction.

❖ NURSING MANAGEMENT: BREAST AUGMENTATION AND REDUCTION

Breast augmentation and breast reduction may be done in the outpatient surgical area or involve overnight hospitalization. General anesthesia is used. Drains are often placed in the surgical site to prevent hematoma formation and then removed when drainage is under 20 to 30 mL/day. Assess drainage for color and odor to detect infection or hemorrhage. Monitor the temperature. Change dressings as needed using sterile technique.

After surgery, assure the female that the breast's appearance will improve when healing is complete. Depending on HCP preference, patients may wear a bra that provides good support continuously for 2 or 3 days after breast reduction or augmentation. Depending on the extent of the surgery, most females resume normal activities within 2 to 3 weeks. They must avoid strenuous exercise for several weeks.

CASE STUDY

Breast Cancer

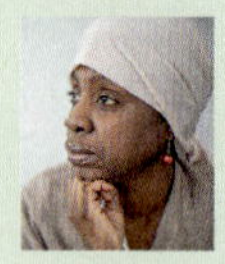

(© FatCamera/ iStock.com)

Patient Profile

L.S., a 60-year-old divorced female, was diagnosed with a 3-cm tumor of the left breast that was estrogen- and progesterone-positive, HER-2—negative breast cancer. She had a simple mastectomy and sentinel lymph node biopsy (SLNB) with axillary node dissection. She has chosen to undergo breast reconstruction surgery.

Interprofessional Care

Preoperative

- "I cannot sleep or eat, and I just pace the floor at night."
- "My mother died of breast cancer when she was 61, and my younger sister got it when she was 42 and still has to be monitored."
- Expresses concern that her 2 daughters (34 and 32) and their daughters are going to get "this horrible disease."
- Appointment made with genetic counselor.

Operative Procedure

- Simple mastectomy and SLNB; 4 lymph nodes removed; breast implant expander inserted
- Tumor was removed with clear margins
- No cancer cells in the sentinel lymph nodes
- Tissue specimen sent for a 21-gene recurrence score genomic test

Postoperative

- Does not want to leave hospital and refuses to get out of bed or eat
- Swelling and restricted range of motion in left arm
- Pain not controlled well with pain medication
- Oncology social worker and physical therapy to see patient

Follow-Up Findings and Treatment

- Scheduled for radiation oncology and a medical oncologist to discuss hormone and need for radiation therapy
- 21-Gene recurrence score is 11, low risk; genetic panel negative
- L.S. joined support group for cancer patients

Discussion Questions

1. ***Recognize:*** What in L.S.'s breast cancer experience with her family members may influence her coping response?
2. ***Analyze:*** What complication did she develop after surgery?
3. ***Plan:*** Which exercises will L.S. need to perform after surgery?
4. ***Prioritize:*** What is the most important information you would provide L.S. about radiation treatment and hormone therapy?
5. ***Act:*** What information would you provide L.S. about her surgery and why the 21-gene recurrence test was done and how it may affect her treatment?
6. ***Act:*** What information would you provide L.S. and her daughters? What early detection measures are important for them to know?
7. ***Act:*** What types of referrals may be indicated for L.S.?
8. ***Act:*** What information would you provide for L.S. about how long her postoperative complications may last and long-term complications?
9. ***Evaluate:*** What outcomes would indicate nursing interventions were successful for L.S.?
10. Develop a conceptual care map for L.S.

Answers and a corresponding conceptual care map available at http://evolve.elsevier.com/Lewis/medsurg.

BRIDGE TO NCLEX EXAMINATION

The number of the question corresponds to the same-numbered outcome at the beginning of the chapter.

1. A 38-year-old female with no family history or other risk factors for breast cancer asks the nurse when is the optimal time to begin breast cancer screening. An appropriate response would be
- **a.** "Screening begins at age 50."
- **b.** "Screening is recommended starting now."
- **c.** "If you had a clinical breast examination, that is all you need."
- **d.** "You can speak with your HCP about starting screening at age 40."

2. A 28-year-old female noted a 2-cm, painless, mobile lump in her left breast. What information should the nurse include when teaching the patient about next steps?
- **a.** Counsel her on the need for a mastectomy.
- **b.** Inform her that she will likely need an ultrasound.
- **c.** Tell the patient that she will need antibiotic therapy.
- **d.** The patient should avoid getting her blood pressure taken in her left arm.

3. Which are considered risk factors for breast cancer in females? **(Select all that apply.)**
- **a.** Menarche at age 11
- **b.** Having a BMI of 22 kg/m^2
- **c.** Having a mother with breast cancer
- **d.** Smoking 1 pack per day × 15 years
- **e.** Having twins and breastfeeding at age 28

4. A nurse is teaching a female newly diagnosed with invasive ductal carcinoma about her disease. Which statement demonstrates an understanding of the pathophysiology of breast cancer?
- **a.** "The nipples and areola are the primary sites of invasion."
- **b.** "Most cancers arise from the lining of the ducts in the breast."
- **c.** "Cancer cells arise first in the lymph nodes, then migrate to the breast."
- **d.** "Persistent mastitis and inflammation are the main cause of cancer development."
- **e.** "I will have a low-risk genetic score on 21-gene testing."

5. The nurse teaches a patient starting hormone therapy for breast cancer that is ER positive that this treatment works by
   a. blocking HER-2 receptors.
   b. decreasing estrogen production.
   c. increasing the number of macrophages.
   d. preventing the production of aromatase.
6. Priorities in providing care for a patient who underwent mastectomy include (**Select all that apply.**)
   a. teaching the patient to shower with cool water.
   b. promoting exercises to restore arm function on the affected side.
   c. not measuring blood pressure or having blood drawn in the affected arm.
   d. screening for psychologic distress, such as fear, anger, anxiety, and depression.
   e. administering analgesics only when the patient reports a pain score of 5 or higher.
7. A patient with breast cancer who underwent mastectomy is asking about reconstructive surgery. Which information would the nurse provide? (**Select all that apply.**)
   a. Breast implants are not advised.
   b. Some people use the rectus abdominis muscle for a breast mound.
   c. Most people will require surgical drains after reconstructive surgery.
   d. Patients must wait 3 months after mastectomy before reconstruction can begin.
   e. Although a breast mound can be created, it will never have a nipple or areola.

1. d; 2. b; 3. a, c, d; 4. b; 5. b; 6. b, c, d; 7. b, c.

For the rationales to these answers and even more NCLEX review questions, visit http://evolve.elsevier.com/Lewis/medsurg.

REFERENCES

To access the References for this chapter, please scan the QR code with a mobile device.

57

Sexually Transmitted Infections

Daniel P. Worrall

http://evolve.elsevier.com/Lewis/medsurg/

CONCEPTUAL FOCUS

Infection
Pain
Reproduction
Sexuality

LEARNING OUTCOMES

1. Identify current trends in sexually transmitted infections (STIs) in the United States.
2. Describe the etiology, clinical manifestations, and interprofessional care for STIs with discharge, cervicitis, or urethritis.
3. Explain the etiology, clinical manifestations, and interprofessional care for STIs with genital lesions or ulcers.
4. Discuss the nursing assessment for patients who have an STI.
5. Summarize the nursing role in prevention of STIs.
6. Describe the nursing management of patients with STIs.

KEY TERMS

chlamydial infections
genital herpes
genital warts
gonorrhea
sexually transmitted infections (STIs)
syphilis
trichomoniasis

EPIDEMIOLOGY

Sexually transmitted infections (STIs) are infectious diseases that spread through sexual contact with the penis, vagina, anus, mouth, or sexual fluids of an infected person. Mucosal tissues in the genitals (urethra in males, vagina in females), rectum, and mouth are susceptible to the bacteria and viruses that cause STIs. A list of common STIs is shown in Table 57.1. Some STIs, such as human papillomavirus (HPV), can spread from direct skin-to-skin contact with an infected person. Other STIs, such as HIV, may be contracted via blood products, semen, or vaginal secretions or be transmitted from mother to baby during pregnancy or labor and delivery. Some STIs can spread through *autoinoculation* (spread of infection by touching or scratching an infected area and transferring it to another part of the body).

The incidence of STIs continues to rise. Reports suggest that any decrease in the number of infections during the pandemic was caused by a lack of testing and treatment at the time.[1] These numbers are again on the rise. In the United States, all cases of gonorrhea, chlamydia, and syphilis must be reported to public health authorities for surveillance purposes for federally funded control programs and partner notification. Surveillance and partner notification are a major part of the effort to prevent and control the spread of STIs. Nurses and other HCPs play a vital role. They are mandated to report STIs to public health authorities. Despite this requirement, only a small number of infections are reported. This means that the cases of gonorrhea, chlamydia, and syphilis reported in the United States annually do not represent the actual number of infections.

Many factors contribute to the high rate of STIs. Earlier reproductive maturity and increased longevity make for a longer sexual life span. Other factors include greater sexual freedom, individual sexual behaviors, the media's emphasis on sexuality without mentioning safer sex, and sexual network characteristics. Alcohol and substance use can contribute to unsafe sexual practices by impairing judgment. Risk factors for STIs are outlined in Table 57.2. Rates are rising in older adults.[2] They are less likely to use condoms and may have a hard time discussing sexual health issues.

TABLE 57.1 Causes of STIs

STI	Cause
Bacterial Infections	
Chlamydial	*Chlamydia trachomatis*
Gonorrhea	*Neisseria gonorrhoeae*
Syphilis	*Treponema pallidum*
Viral Infections	
Genital herpes	Herpes simplex virus (HSV 1 or 2)
Genital warts (condylomata acuminata)	Human papillomavirus (HPV)
HIV	HIV (see Chapter 15)
Hepatitis B and C	Hepatitis B and C viruses (see Chapter 48)
Molluscum	*Molluscum contagiosum*
Parasitic/Protozoan Infection	
Trichomoniasis	*Trichomonas vaginalis*

TABLE 57.2 Risk Factors for STIs

High-Risk Behaviors
- Alcohol or substance use (inhibits judgment)
- Having new sexual partners
- Having more than 1 sexual partner
- Having sexual partners who have/have had multiple partners
- Inconsistent or incorrect use of condoms or other barrier methods
- Exchanging sex for money, shelter, or other needs

High-Risk Medical History
- Having 1 STI is a risk factor for getting another
- Not being vaccinated for STIs or other infections that may be transmitted through some forms of sexual activity (HPV, hepatitis A and B)
- Receiving multiple courses of nonoccupational postexposure prophylaxis to prevent HIV infection

High-Risk Populations
- Adolescents and young adults (under age 25)
- Ethnicity/race (e.g., Black, American Indian/Alaskan Native, Hispanic)
- Men who have sex with men (MSM)
- Persons in correctional facilities
- Transgender women
- Victims of sexual assault
- Females

All STIs have an *incubation period.* It is the time from initial infection to the time when symptoms first appear or screening tests for the infection are positive. This can lead to the transmission of disease from an asymptomatic (but infected) person to another person, even before any signs or symptoms begin.

STIs affect certain groups of people disproportionately (Box 57.1). This includes youth and young adults under age 25, men who have sex with other men (MSM), transgender women, and those who are socially and economically disadvantaged.[1] Many minority groups have rates of STIs greater than that of non-Hispanic White persons. These include Black/African American persons, Hispanic ethnicity groups, Native American Indian/Alaskan Native, and those with multiracial backgrounds.[3] Socioeconomic factors and access to quality sexual health care contribute.[1]

Trends in methods of contraceptive use affect the rate of STIs. The male condom is one of the best forms of protection (other than abstinence) against STIs. Although condom use has increased in the United States, many people do not use them. Most females use hormone (e.g., oral contraceptive pills, patch, injectables) or long-acting reversible contraceptives (e.g., intrauterine devices). These do not provide barrier protection against STIs.

BOX 57.1 Incidence of STIs

- Depending on their age and gender, non-Hispanic Black/African American persons:
  - Have 32.4% of all cases of chlamydia, gonorrhea, and syphilis cases in the United States (32.4%) despite being only 12.6% of the population
  - Have 29.5% of congenital syphilis cases (n = 1146) despite being 14.1% of live births
- Hispanic persons:
  - Are infected with both chlamydia and gonorrhea at a rate higher than that of non-Hispanic White persons
  - Have 21% of all primary and secondary syphilis cases in the United States
  - Account for 1172 congenital syphilis cases in the United States
- Men who have sex with men (MSM):
  - Have the highest proportion of all primary and secondary syphilis cases in the United States (32.7%) and an even higher proportion of cases when the gender of sexual partners is known (57.5%)
  - Have the highest proportion of gonorrhea cases in the United States (21.8%)
  - Have an increased risk for HIV, hepatitis C, and HSV-2
- Despite their small proportion of overall cases, non-Hispanic American Indian/Alaska Native persons:
  - Have seen the greatest increase in reportable STIs in recent years
  - Have the highest rates of primary and secondary syphilis infection in the United States (63.6 per 100,000)
  - Have the second highest infection rates of gonorrhea and chlamydia in the United States
  - Have the highest rates of congenital syphilis in the United States (680.8 per 100,000), followed by non-Hispanic Native Hawaiian or Pacific Islander persons (295.6 per 100,000)

Factors Influencing Disparities
- Social and economic disadvantages can make it hard for people to care for their overall health, including their sexual health.
- People who cannot afford basic necessities may have trouble accessing and affording sexual health services.
- Fear and distrust of HCPs and institutions can negatively affect racial and ethnic minorities from seeking health care.
- In communities with a higher prevalence of STIs, it may be hard to reduce infection rates because a person has a higher chance of having an infected partner.

This chapter covers the most common STIs. HIV infection is covered in Chapter 15. Anyone who contracts an STI may be at risk for HIV infection. HIV preexposure prophylaxis (PrEP) or nonoccupational postexposure prophylaxis (nPEP) may be appropriate. See Chapter 15 for more about PrEP and nPEP.

STIS WITH DISCHARGE, CERVITIS, OR URETHRITIS

CHLAMYDIAL INFECTIONS

Chlamydia is the most common reportable STI in the United States. More than 1.6 million cases are reported annually.[1] Because many infections are asymptomatic, we believe the actual number of cases is higher.

Etiology and Pathophysiology

Chlamydial infections are caused by *Chlamydia trachomatis,* a gram-negative bacterium and intracellular pathogen. *Chlamydia* is transmitted through vaginal, anal, or oral sex. Ejaculation does not have to occur for transmission. The incubation period for chlamydia is 1 to 3 weeks. Prior infection with *Chlamydia* does not provide protection from reinfection. This means that people who were treated for chlamydia can be reinfected.

The most common site for infection in males is the urethra. Infection in the male urethra is called *urethritis.* The most common site for infection for females is the cervix. Infection of the female cervix is called *cervicitis.* Males and females can get chlamydia of the rectum from receptive anal sex or the oropharynx from giving oral sex. Because the vagina acts as a natural reservoir for infectious secretions, STI transmission is more efficient from males to females than it is from females to males.

There are many serotypes of *C. trachomatis.* The more common are the cause of nongonococcal urethritis (NGU) in males or cervicitis in females. A small subset of serotypes can cause another STI, lymphogranuloma venereum (LGV), when spread to the rectum. Although rare, this is more common in MSM.

Clinical Manifestations

Patients with chlamydia often have no symptoms. If symptoms develop in males, they may have pain with urination (dysuria) or urethral discharge. Rarely, males have testicular pain or swelling caused by infection of the epididymis (Fig. 57.1). In females, symptoms include mucopurulent vaginal discharge (mucus with pus), abnormal vaginal bleeding, dysuria, and pain with intercourse. Symptoms of rectal chlamydia include anorectal pain, discharge or bleeding, anal pruritus, tenesmus, mucus-coated stools, or painful bowel movements. Most patients with chlamydia in the throat will have no symptoms. A few may have a sore throat.

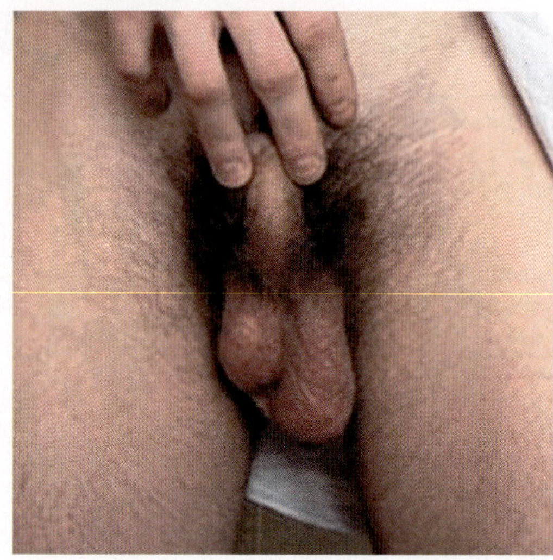

Fig. 57.1 Unilateral testicular swelling from chlamydial epididymitis. (From Jordan S, Geisler W: *Infectious diseases,* St. Louis, 2017, Elsevier.)

Complications

Complications often develop from poorly managed, inaccurately diagnosed, or undiagnosed chlamydia. Although males rarely have long-term complications from infection, epididymitis can result in male infertility. More often, chlamydia can affect a female's reproductive tract, resulting in *pelvic inflammatory disease* (PID). PID can damage fallopian tubes and increase the risk for an ectopic pregnancy, infertility, and chronic pelvic pain.[4] The risk for developing PID increases with repeated infection. The more episodes of PID, the more likely a female will experience infertility. Although rare, patients can develop reactive arthritis, an autoimmune response to infection with *C. trachomatis.*

Diagnostic Studies

Diagnosis requires an accurate sexual history, physical assessment, and laboratory tests. The preferred method for diagnosing chlamydia is a nucleic acid amplification test (NAAT) (Table 57.3). NAAT is used to identify small amounts of DNA

TABLE 57.3 Interprofessional Care

Chlamydial Infections

Diagnostic Assessment
- History and physical assessment
- Nucleic acid amplification test (NAAT)
- Testing for other STIs (gonorrhea, HIV, syphilis)

Management
- Doxycycline
- Alternative regimen: azithromycin or levofloxacin
- Teach to abstain from sexual contact for 7 days after completing treatment
- Treat all sexual partners, who must also wait 7 days before resuming sexual contact

or RNA in test samples. It can be done on urine, rectal, and oropharyngeal swabs from males and females; endocervical or vaginal swabs from females; and urethral swabs from males.

Interprofessional Care

The preferred treatment is doxycycline (Vibramycin) twice a day for 7 days (Table 57.3).[5] All sexual contacts within 60 days should be tested and treated to prevent reinfection and further transmission. Teach patients to abstain from sexual contact for 7 days after treatment or until all partners have been treated and have also abstained from sexual contact for 7 days. Review ways to reduce risk of reinfection or infection with another STI in the future. Anyone diagnosed and treated for chlamydia should return for repeat testing 3 months after treatment to ensure cure or detect reinfection. Tell patients to return sooner if symptoms persist or recur.

DRUG ALERT

Doxycycline

- Take doses on an empty stomach either 1 h before eating or 2 h after eating.
- Avoid taking with antacids, iron products, or dairy products.
- Remain upright for at least 30 min after taking a dose.
- Avoid prolonged or excessive exposure to sunlight.
- Pregnant females should not take doxycycline.

Unfortunately, there is a high rate of recurrence. This often occurs when the sexual partners of people with an STI are not treated. This "ping-pong" effect (treatment, reexposure, reinfection) can end only when all partners are treated appropriately. Because of this issue, we recommend *expedited partner therapy* (EPT).[6] With EPT, HCPs give drugs or prescriptions to patients with STIs to give to their partners without the HCP having to examine their partners. EPT varies from state to state, but few states prohibit it. EPT is often not recommended for partners of MSM because of a higher risk for coexisting infections, especially undiagnosed syphilis or HIV. It is not recommended for female partners who are symptomatic because of the risk for PID.

GONOCOCCAL INFECTIONS

Gonorrhea remains the second most common reportable STI in the United States, with over 600,000 cases reported each year.[1] As with chlamydia, we think the actual number of cases is higher.

Etiology and Pathophysiology

Gonorrhea is caused by *Neisseria gonorrhoeae*, a gram-negative, diplococcus bacterium. Gonorrhea can be transmitted by exposure to sexual fluids during vaginal, anal, or oral sex. Ejaculation does not have to occur for it to be transmitted. The incubation period ranges from 1 to 14 days. Prior infection does not provide protection from reinfection. The most common site for infection for males is the urethra and for females, the cervix.

Clinical Manifestations

Most males will be symptomatic within a few days of infection. The most common symptoms of gonococcal urethritis are dysuria, purulent urethral discharge (Fig. 57.2), or epididymitis. Most females are asymptomatic or have minor symptoms that they often overlook. In females, common symptoms are increased vaginal discharge, dysuria, frequency, or bleeding after sex. Often, redness and swelling occur at the cervix or urethra along with a purulent exudate (Fig. 57.3).

Anyone can contract rectal gonorrhea during anal intercourse or oropharyngeal gonorrhea during oral sex. Symptoms of rectal infection include mucopurulent rectal discharge or bleeding, anorectal pain, anal pruritus, tenesmus, mucus-coated stools, or painful bowel movements. Most patients with gonorrhea in the throat have no symptoms. A few may have a sore throat.

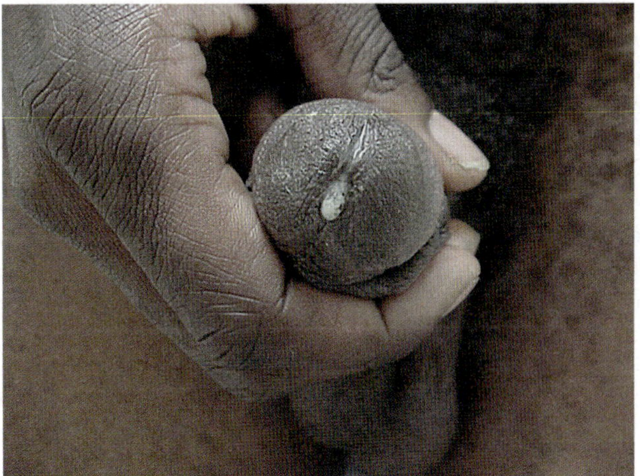

Fig. 57.2 Profuse, purulent drainage in a patient with gonorrhea. (From CDC: *Sexually transmitted infections.* Retrieved from https://www.cdc.gov/sti/php/training/picture-cards.html.)

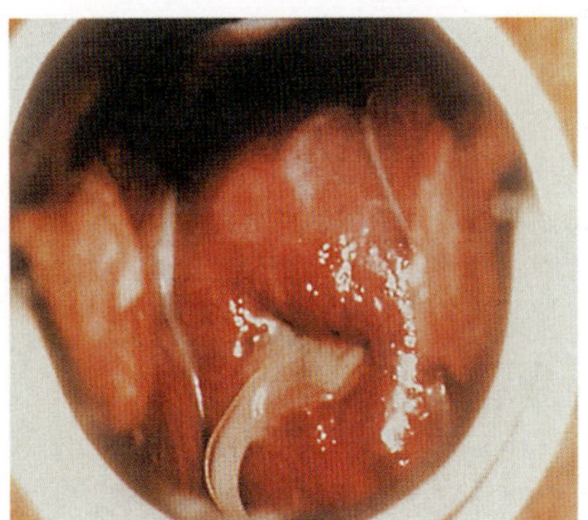

Fig. 57.3 Endocervical gonorrhea. Cervical redness and edema with discharge. (From Morse S, Moreland A, Holmes K: *Atlas of sexually transmitted diseases and AIDS,* London, 1996, Mosby-Wolfe.)

CHECK YOUR PRACTICE

You are caring for a 23-year-old male who is being treated for gonorrhea. He said he has only been with 1 partner in the past month. They just had oral sex. His partner denies any symptoms. "I think my partner must be lying to me about being with other people."

- How would you respond?

Complications

Because males are more often symptomatic and seek treatment earlier, they are less likely to develop serious complications. Those who do can develop epididymitis, a progression of the infection to the testes. It can cause infertility.

Because females are more likely to be asymptomatic and therefore seldom seek early treatment, serious complications are more common. Untreated gonorrhea can cause an infection in the Bartholin glands or Skene glands or result in PID. PID increases the risk for ectopic pregnancy, infertility, and chronic pelvic pain.

Although rare, patients can develop disseminated gonococcal infection (DGI). DGI can cause skin lesions, fever, arthralgia, arthritis, and/or endocarditis (Fig. 57.4).

Neonates can develop gonococcal conjunctivitis *(ophthalmia neonatorum)* from exposure to an infected mother during delivery that can result in permanent blindness. Almost all states have laws or health department regulations requiring the use of prophylactic eye treatment of all newborns to prevent such infections. Because of improved prenatal screening for gonorrhea and prophylactic treatment plans, *ophthalmia neonatorum* is rare.

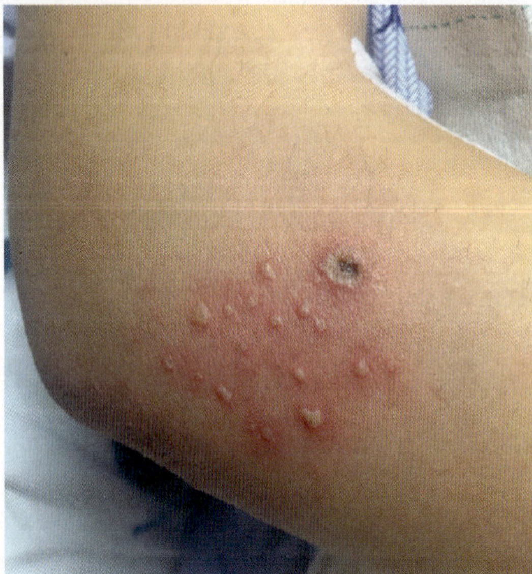

Fig. 57.4 Red, pustular rash with skin lesion from disseminated gonococcal infection. (From Earle M, Nelson D: A teen with rash and arthralgia, *Vis J Emerg Med* 22:100914, 2020.)

Diagnostic Studies

For males, the diagnosis of gonorrhea can be made if there is a history of sexual contact with a new or infected partner followed within a few days by the development of urethral discharge. For females, making a diagnosis based on symptoms is difficult. Most females are asymptomatic or have symptoms that may be confused with other conditions, such as a urinary tract infection.

The preferred method for diagnosing gonorrhea is through NAAT (Table 57.4). This can be done on endocervical or vaginal swabs from females, urethral swabs from males, and urine, rectal, and oropharyngeal swabs from males or females. A culture may be used to diagnose infection. Gram stains of urethral secretions can be used, but the sensitivity is not as good as other methods.

Interprofessional Care

Over the years, *N. gonorrhoeae* has developed resistance to many classes of antibiotics, including fluoroquinolones (e.g., ciprofloxacin, levofloxacin), tetracyclines (e.g., doxycycline), and macrolides (e.g., azithromycin). First-line treatment is currently high-dose IM ceftriaxone (Table 57.4).[5] Patients who persistently test positive after treatment should have culture of the infected site with antibiotic sensitivity testing to check for resistance.

All sexual contacts within 60 days before diagnosis should be tested and treated to prevent reinfection and further transmission. Teach patients to abstain from sexual contact for 7 days after treatment or until all partners have been treated and have also abstained from sexual contact for 7 days. Anyone diagnosed and treated for gonorrhea should return for repeat testing 3 months after treatment to ensure cure or detect reinfection.

TABLE 57.4 Interprofessional Care

Gonococcal Infections

Diagnostic Assessment

- History and physical assessment
- Gram-stained smears of urethral or endocervical exudate
- Culture for *Neisseria gonorrhoeae* with antibiotic sensitivity testing if available
- Nucleic acid amplification test (NAAT) to detect *N. gonorrhoeae*
- Testing for other STIs (syphilis, HIV, chlamydial infection)

Management

- Uncomplicated gonorrhea: high-dose ceftriaxone IM
- Gonorrhea with chlamydia coinfection: high-dose ceftriaxone IM plus doxycycline
- Testing and treatment of sexual contacts
- Teach to abstain from sexual contact for 7 days after treatment
- Treat all sexual partners, who must also wait 7 days before resuming sexual contact
- Reexamination if symptoms persist or recur after treatment

TRICHOMONIASIS

Trichomoniasis ("trich") is an STI caused by the protozoan parasite *Trichomonas vaginalis.* It is another common STI in the United States. It is much more common among females than males, especially among females with HIV.

Etiology and Pathophysiology

Trichomonas can be transmitted by exposure to sexual fluids during vaginal, anal, or oral sex, even if ejaculation does not occur. The incubation period is usually 1 week to 1 month but can be much longer. Prior infection does not provide protection from reinfection.

The most common site for infection in males is the urethra and in females is the cervix. It is uncommon for *Trichomonas* to infect the rectum. It is not known to infect the oropharynx. Routine screening should be considered for females in high-risk populations, those receiving care in high-risk settings, and females seeking care for vaginal discharge.[5]

Clinical Manifestations

Most people do not have symptoms. Males may have burning with urination, ejaculation, or urethral discharge. Females may have painful urination, vaginal itching, painful intercourse, bleeding after sex, or a yellow-green discharge with a foul odor. The cervix can have a "strawberry" appearance.

Complications

The main complications of untreated infection are related to the inflammation and irritation that it causes in the genital tract. Inflammation makes an infected person more likely to contract or transmit another STI, particularly HIV. Trichomoniasis is associated with PID in females with HIV.

Diagnostic Studies

The preferred method of diagnosing trichomoniasis is by NAAT of vaginal or endocervical secretions or urine. Other methods include culture, point-of-care testing, or direct visualization of trichomonads under the microscope. Identifying motile trichomonads in vaginal secretions confirms infection. Tests can be done on liquid-based cervical Pap samples. In males, NAAT is recommended.[5]

Interprofessional Care

Patients and their partners should be treated with either metronidazole (Flagyl) or tinidazole (Tindamax). Teach patients to abstain from sexual contact for 7 days after treatment or until all sexual partners have completed a full course of treatment and abstained from sexual contact for 7 days. Tell patients to return if symptoms persist or recur. Any sexual partner within the preceding 60 days should be treated. Teach patients to use condoms or other barrier methods with every sexual contact. Because of a high rate of recurrence, recommend repeat testing 3 months after treatment.

STIs WITH GENITAL LESIONS OR ULCERS

GENITAL HERPES INFECTIONS

Genital herpes is a common, lifelong, incurable but treatable infection. There are 2 strains of herpes: herpes simplex virus type 1 (HSV-1) and herpes simplex virus type 2 (HSV-2). More than 50% of the population has HSV-1 and 12% have HSV-2. Most new infections are transmitted by someone who does not know they are infected.[7]

Etiology and Pathophysiology

The herpes virus enters through the mucous membranes or breaks in the skin during contact with an infected person. The virus reproduces inside the cell and spreads to the surrounding cells. The virus then enters the peripheral or autonomic nerve endings and ascends to the sensory or autonomic nerve ganglion near the infection site. There, it often becomes dormant. Viral reactivation (recurrence or "outbreak") occurs when the virus descends to that initial site of infection, either the mucous membranes or skin.

When a person is infected with HSV-1 or HSV-2, the virus persists within the person for life. Transmission of either strain of HSV to others occurs easiest through direct contact with skin or mucous membranes when an infected person is symptomatic. However, both can be transmitted without any apparent symptoms, called *asymptomatic viral shedding.* It is impossible to predict when asymptomatic shedding will occur or for how long. HSV-2 is more likely to shed than HSV-1.

HSV-1 or HSV-2 can cause genital, anal, or orolabial infections. In most cases, HSV-1 infections involve the gingivae, dermis, upper respiratory tract and, rarely, the central nervous system (CNS). HSV-1 is often associated with oral lesions, known as "cold sores" or "fever blisters" (Fig. 57.5). An

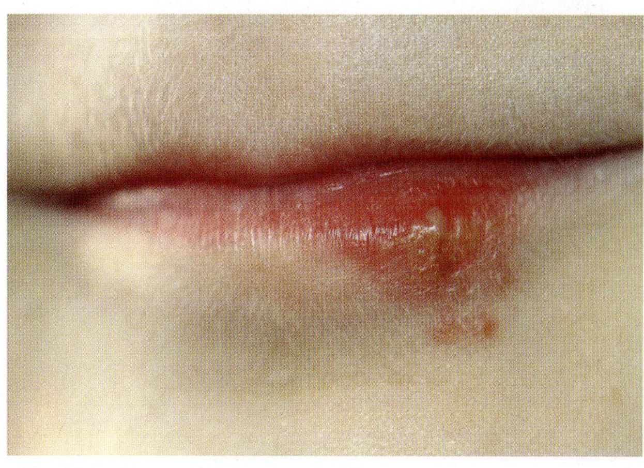

Fig. 57.5 Herpes simplex virus (HSV). (© Gulay Erun/iStock.com.)

increasing proportion of new anogenital HSV-1 infections affect young females and MSM.[8] HSV-2 almost always infects sites "below the waist," or the genital tract, perineum, or anus. It is rare to have HSV-2 infection of the mouth. Having HSV-2 infection protects against getting HSV-1.

Clinical Manifestations

Primary Episode

A *primary (initial) episode* of genital herpes has an incubation period of 2 to 12 days. Most people do not have any symptoms of primary HSV genital infection. If symptoms do occur, they follow a series of stages. During the *prodromal stage,* the period before lesions appear, patients may have burning, itching, or tingling at the site of inoculation. In the *vesicular stage,* few to multiple small, often painful vesicles (blisters) may appear on the buttock, inner thigh, penis, scrotum, vulva, perineum, perianal region, vagina, or cervix. The vesicles have large quantities of infectious viral particles (Fig. 57.6). Next, in the *ulcerative stage,* the lesions rupture and form shallow, moist ulcerations. In the *final stage,* spontaneous crusting and epithelialization of the erosions occur.

Regional (inguinal node) lymphadenopathy and systemic flulike symptoms, including fever, headache, malaise, and myalgia, may occur with the primary episode. Urination may be painful from the urine touching active lesions. The whole process from prodrome to healing varies. It may take up to 3 weeks. Autoinoculation can occur if active lesions are touched or scratched, causing additional and potentially recurrent infection at extragenital sites.

Recurrent Episodes

Recurrent genital herpes occurs in many people during the year after the primary episode. The symptoms of recurrent episodes are less severe. The lesions usually heal more quickly. HSV-1 genital infections recur less often than HSV-2 genital infections. Over time, both decrease in frequency.

Common triggers of recurrence include stress, fatigue, sunburn, general illness, immunosuppression, menses, or local trauma at the site of infection. Many patients can predict a recurrence by noticing the prodromal symptoms of tingling, burning, and itching at the site where the lesions will recur. The greatest risk for transmitting infection exists when active lesions are present. However, it is possible to transmit the virus when no visible lesions or symptoms are present. Most HSV transmission occurs during these asymptomatic periods.[7]

Complications

Both HSV-1 and HSV-2 can cause rare but serious complications, including blindness, encephalitis, and aseptic meningitis. Autoinoculation can result in extragenital lesions in the buttocks, groin, thighs, fingers, and eyes. Genital ulcers increase the risk for contracting HIV. HSV lesions can be more severe and more persistent in HIV-infected patients.

Pregnant females with HSV can transmit the virus to the baby, especially if the virus is shed while the infant passes through the birth canal. Females with a primary episode of HSV near the time of delivery have the highest risk for transmitting genital herpes to the neonate.[8] The virus can infect the neonate's skin, eyes, mouth, or the CNS or become widespread and cause significant mortality. An active genital lesion at the time of delivery is an indication for cesarean delivery.

One of the most profound consequences for people with genital herpes is the overall impact it can have on their psychologic well-being, relationships, and sexual lives. Teach patients how to talk to sexual partners about HSV. Refer patients who need counseling. Teach patients with herpes that it is a common, manageable, non–life-threatening condition. Help them understand their treatment options.

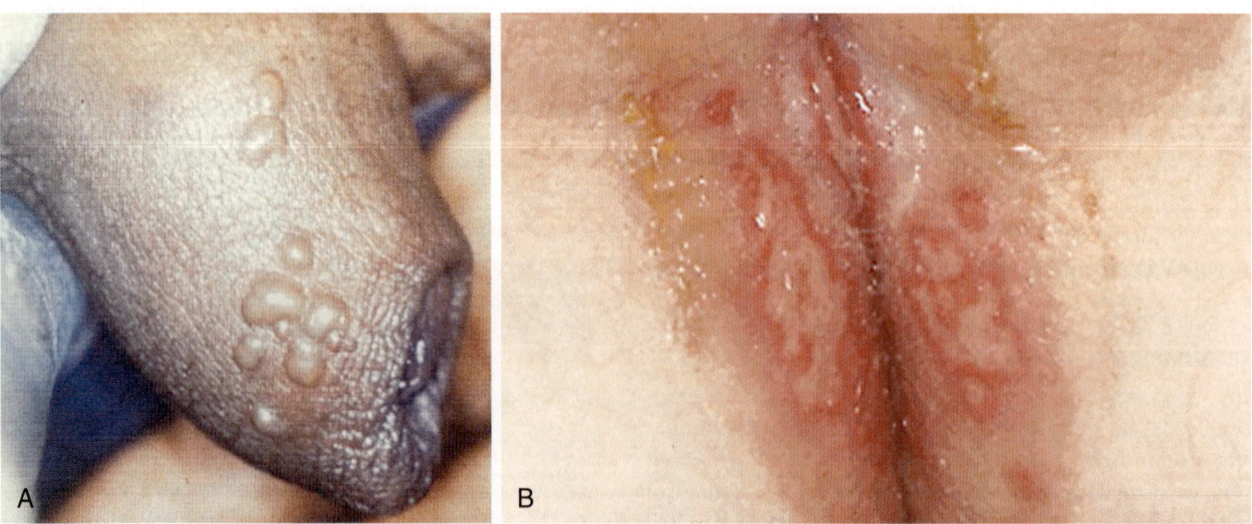

Fig. 57.6 Herpes simplex virus type 2. (A) Vesicular stage. Clear, grouped vesicles on the penis. (B) Ulcerative stage. Vesicles and ulceration of vulvar area. (From *Elsevier Point of Care,* St. Louis, 2020, Elsevier.)

Diagnostic Studies

Diagnosis is often based on the symptoms, then confirmed by visual examination. Viral culture or polymerase chain reaction (PCR) from open skin eruptions can be used to diagnose HSV and distinguish between HSV-1 and HSV-2. Highly accurate blood tests for antibodies are available for HSV-1 and HSV-2. Antibodies usually appear by 12 weeks after exposure. These tests do not show the location of the infection.

Interprofessional Care

There is no cure for HSV infection. Antiviral drugs can shorten the duration of HSV viral shedding, shorten the healing time of eruptions, and reduce the frequency of outbreaks by up to 80%.[8] Treatment of HSV should start before diagnostic results are available because early treatment reduces the duration of the ulcers and risk for transmission (Table 57.5).

Three antiviral agents are available for treating HSV: acyclovir (Zovirax), famciclovir (Famvir), and valaciclovir (Valtrex).[5] These drugs inhibit herpetic viral replication (see Table 15.10). They are prescribed for both primary and recurrent infections. Taken daily at a lower dose, they can be used as suppressive therapy to decrease frequency and severity of anogenital recurrences. They reduce, but do not eliminate, the risk of transmission to others. IV acyclovir is reserved for severe or life-threatening infections in which hospitalization is needed to treat eye or widespread infections, CNS infections (e.g., meningitis), or pneumonitis.

Teach patients with active outbreaks to maintain good hygiene, wear loose-fitting cotton undergarments, and avoid sexual contact until the outbreak has completely healed. Patients with oral lesions should avoid kissing or performing oral sex until fully healed.

The main goal is to keep eruptions clean and dry. Ways to reduce pain with urination include pouring water onto the perineal area while voiding to dilute the urine or voiding in the shower. Patients may need a local anesthetic, such as lidocaine gel, or analgesics, such as ibuprofen, acetaminophen, or acetaminophen with codeine. Ice packs to the affected area may give some relief.

TABLE 57.5 Interprofessional Care

Genital Herpes

Diagnostic Assessment
- History and physical assessment
- Antibody assay for HSV type
- Viral isolation by culture, polymerase chain reaction (PCR) testing

Management
- Identify triggering factors
- Abstain from sexual contact while lesions are present and until fully healed
- Symptomatic care
- Confidential counseling and testing for HIV

Primary (Initial) Infection (see Table 15.10)
- Acyclovir, valacyclovir, or famciclovir

Recurrent Episodic Infection
- Acyclovir, valacyclovir, or famciclovir for shorter duration

Suppressive Therapy
- Acyclovir, valacyclovir, or famciclovir daily at a lower dose

Severe Infection
- IV acyclovir until clinical improvement, followed by oral antiviral therapy

GENITAL WARTS

Genital warts *(condylomata acuminata)* are caused by HPV. More than 200 strains of HPV can infect different areas of the body. At least 40 of these are sexually transmitted.[9] "Low-risk" strains of the virus can cause warts on the skin. "High-risk" strains can lead to cancers of the genital tract, anus, or oropharynx. HPV types 6 and 11 cause about 90% of genital and anal warts. HPV types 16 and 18 cause about 70% of cervical cancer, most anal cancers, and some throat cancers.[10] Many sexually active people will be infected with some type of HPV at some point in their lives. In most states, HPV is not a reportable infection. Cervical HPV infection is discussed in Chapter 58.

Etiology and Pathophysiology

HPV is transmitted by skin-to-skin contact, most often during vaginal or anal sex. It can also be transmitted during non-penetrating sexual activity. The basal epithelial cells infected with HPV undergo transformation and proliferation to form a warty growth (Fig. 57.7). The incubation period can range from weeks to months to years. Infection with 1 type of HPV does not prevent infection with another type.

In most people, HPV is transient (virus is "cleared" or resolves spontaneously after 1 to 2 years). For others, it persists even when the warts themselves are not visible after treatment. We do not know whether removing visible warts helps a person to clear the virus, cures the virus, or reduces their ability to transmit the virus.[9]

Clinical Manifestations

Most people with HPV do not know that they are infected because they have no symptoms. Genital or anal warts are discrete single or multiple papillary growths. They may grow and coalesce to form large, cauliflower-like masses, although most patients will have few lesions. Growths may be pink, pink-flesh colored, or hyperpigmented depending on the skin type.

In males, warts occur on the penis and scrotum, in or around the anus, or in the urethra. In females, warts occur on the inner thighs, vulva, vagina, or cervix; perineum; or internal or external anus (Fig. 57.7). Itching may occur with anogenital warts. Bleeding on defecation may occur with anal warts. Usually there are no other signs or symptoms.

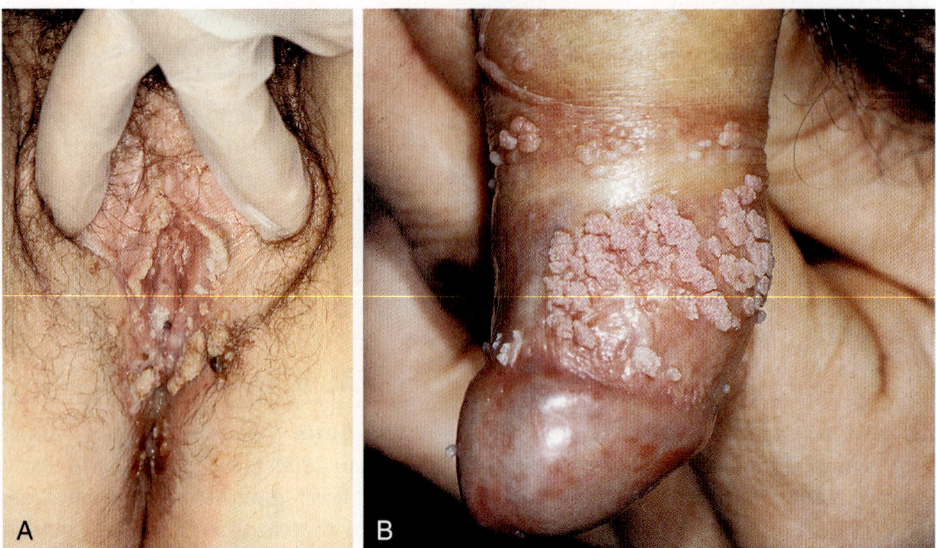

Fig. 57.7 Genital warts. (A) Vulvar warts. (B) Multiple warts on the penis. (From Habif TP: *Clinical dermatology,* ed 6, St Louis, 2015, Mosby.)

Diagnostic Studies

Most early lesions caused by HPV are undetectable by visual examination. A diagnosis of genital warts can be made based on the characteristic appearance of the lesions (Fig. 57.7). Warts may be confused with *condylomata lata* of secondary syphilis, cancer, or benign growths. Testing should be done to rule out other conditions. At present, the only definitive diagnostic procedure is biopsy of any questionable growth. Testing for cervical HPV is discussed in Chapter 58.

Complications

Genital and anal warts have few long-term complications. The HPV strains that cause warts do not cause cancer. For some people, the lesions can cause psychosocial burden because of stigma, the cosmetic appearance of lesions, or the need for long courses of HPV-related treatment. During pregnancy, warts tend to grow rapidly and increase in size. Persistent infection with "high-risk" strains of HPV (especially types 16 and 18) can lead to cancers of the cervix, vagina, vulva, penis, anus, and oropharynx.[9]

Interprofessional Care

HPV Vaccine

It may be possible to eradicate some HPV types over the next few decades, especially if all youth are vaccinated. A 9-valent vaccine (Gardasil 9) is the only vaccine available in the United States. It protects against HPV types 6, 11, 16, 18, and 5 other high-risk HPV types.[10] The vaccine is given in 2 or 3 IM doses over a 6-month period. There are few side effects. The Centers for Disease Control and Prevention (CDC) recommends that all children, male and female, be vaccinated at age 11 to 12. Vaccination can be started as early as age 9. Routine vaccination is recommended up to age 26. Gardasil 9 is also approved for use in those ages 27 through 45 who may be at risk.[11]

The HPV vaccine offers protection against strains causing 90% of anogenital warts and cervical cancers. This protection extends to other HPV-related cancers, including penile, anal, and throat cancers. Remember that the vaccine does not treat active HPV infection. Ideally persons should receive the vaccine before the start of sexual activity or before the potential for infection.

Drug Therapy

Treatment of genital or anal warts is hampered by the high proportion of asymptomatic and undiagnosed infections and lack of curative treatment. The primary goal of treatment is the removal of symptomatic warts.

In-office treatment consists of chemical or ablative (removal with laser or electrocautery) methods. A common treatment is the use of trichloroacetic acid (TCA) or bichloroacetic acid (BCA) applied directly to the wart surface. Petroleum jelly applied with a cotton swab to the surrounding normal skin can minimize irritation. A sharp, stinging pain is often felt with initial acid contact, but this quickly subsides.

Patient-applied treatments are available. Podofilox liquid and gel are available by prescription (Condylox, Condylox Gel). Patients apply the solution or gel for 3 successive days, then stop for 4 days in cycles. Treatment can be repeated for up to 4 weeks or until resolution of the lesions. Imiquimod cream is an immune response modifier applied at bedtime for up to 16 weeks. Sinecatechin ointment (Veregen) is a green tea derivative that has antioxidant properties. It is applied 3 times daily for up to 16 weeks.

Treatment of warts may not decrease infectivity because the virus causing warts may still be present. Anogenital warts are hard to treat and often need more than 1 treatment or modality. Therapy should be modified if a patient has not improved or cannot tolerate the side effects of certain treatments.

If the warts do not resolve with topical therapies, treatments such as cryotherapy with liquid nitrogen, electrocautery, laser therapy, local α-interferon injections, or surgical excision may be done. Teach patients that because treatment does not destroy the virus (merely the infected tissue), recurrence and reinfection are possible. Long-term follow-up is needed.

SYPHILIS

Syphilis is a sexually transmitted bacterial infection that can cause serious long-term complications if not identified and treated. Infections in the United States continue to increase. Over 200,000 cases were reported in 2023.[1] As with other infections, we think this number is higher. Recent increases in cases staged as unknown duration or late syphilis may reflect the delayed diagnosis of infections occurring during the COVID-19 pandemic, when STI prevention and care services were disrupted.

Etiology and Pathophysiology

Syphilis is caused by *Treponema pallidum,* a bacterial spirochete. It is transmitted by direct contact with a syphilitic ulcer *(chancre)* or through the mucosal membranes of an infected person. A chancre can occur externally on the genitals, anus, or lips or internally in the vagina, rectum, or mouth or tongue (Fig. 57.8). Transmission can occur during vaginal, anal, or oral sex. The incubation period can range from 10 to 90 days (average 21 days). Having the infection does not provide protection from reinfection, even after successful treatment. An infected pregnant female can transmit syphilis to her fetus during her pregnancy. There is a high risk for stillbirth or having babies who develop complications after birth, including seizures and death. Unfortunately, the incidence of congenital syphilis in the United States continues to increase.[1]

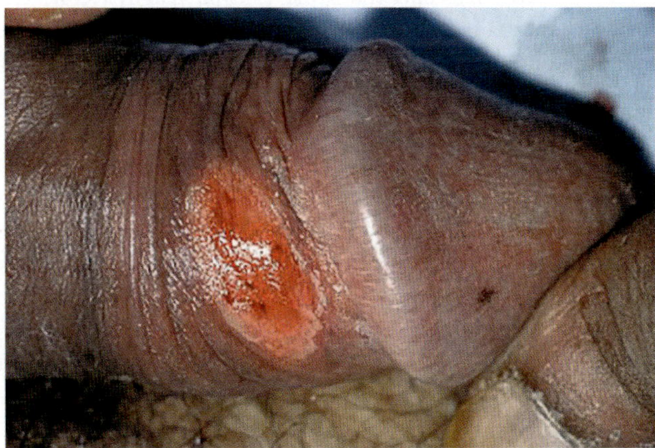

Fig. 57.8 Primary syphilis chancre. (From Elston DM, Treat JR, James WD, Rosenbach MA: *Andrews' diseases of the skin,* ed 14, St. Louis, 2026, Elsevier.)

Clinical Manifestations

Syphilis is called *the great imitator* because it can present with a variety of signs and symptoms that mimic other diseases. Compared with other STIs, syphilis is harder to recognize, which can delay treatment. If it is not diagnosed and treated, specific clinical stages occur with the progression of the disease (Table 57.6).

The primary stage is the development of a chancre at the site of transmission (Fig. 57.9). This can appear days to months after infection. In most patients, it occurs by 3 weeks. Chancres can be found on the genitals but often go unnoticed when inside the mouth, vagina, or anus. As the chancre begins to heal or shortly after, patients will progress to the secondary stage of infection if untreated. This stage is usually characterized by a maculopapular rash. The classic rash appears as round, reddish "spots" on the palms of the hands or soles of the feet. It may involve the trunk or extremities (Fig. 57.10). Without

TABLE 57.6 Stages of Syphilis

Primary
- *Infectivity:* Highly infectious
- *Duration of stage:* 3–6 wk
- Single or multiple chancres (painless indurated lesions) of penis, vulva, lips, mouth, vagina, and rectum; Fig. 57.8); occurs 10–90 days after inoculation
- Regional lymphadenopathy (microorganisms drain into the lymph nodes)
- Exudate and blood from chancre are highly infectious

Secondary
- *Infectivity:* Highly infectious
- *Duration of stage:* Occurs a few weeks after primary chancre heals, lasts 1–2 yr
- Flulike symptoms: malaise, fever, sore throat, headaches, fatigue, arthralgia, general adenopathy
- Mucous patches in mouth (Fig. 57.9), tongue, or cervix
- Symmetric, nonpruritic rash bilaterally that appears on trunk, palms, and/or soles (Fig. 57.10)
- Condylomata lata (moist, weeping warts) in the anogenital area
- Weight loss, alopecia

Latent
- *Infectivity:* Early (<1 yr)—infectious; late (≥1 yr)—noninfectious
- *Duration of stage:* Throughout life or progression to late stage
- No signs or symptoms
- Diagnosis based on positive treponemal antibody test with normal cerebrospinal fluid and absence of clinical manifestations

Late
- Infectivity: Noninfectious
- Duration of stage: Chronic (without treatment), occurs 1–20 yr after initial infection
- Gummas (chronic, destructive lesions affecting any organ of body, especially skin, bone, liver, mucous membranes; Fig. 57.11)
- Cardiovascular: Aneurysms, heart valve insufficiency, heart failure, aortitis
- Neurosyphilis: Can occur at any stage of syphilis
- General paresis: Personality changes from minor to psychotic, tremors, physical and mental deterioration
- Tabes dorsalis (ataxia, areflexia, paresthesias, lightning pains, damaged joints)

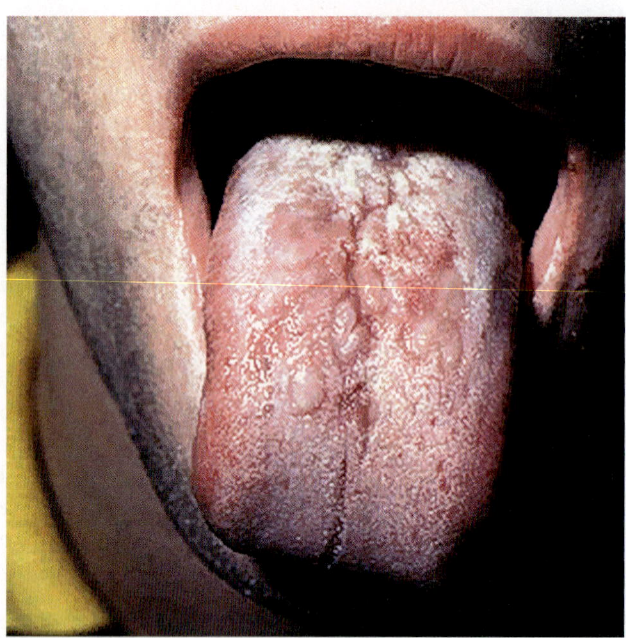

Fig. 57.9 Secondary syphilis. Mucous patches in the mouth. (From CDC: *Sexually transmitted infections*. Retrieved from https://www.cdc.gov/sti/php/training/picture-cards.html.)

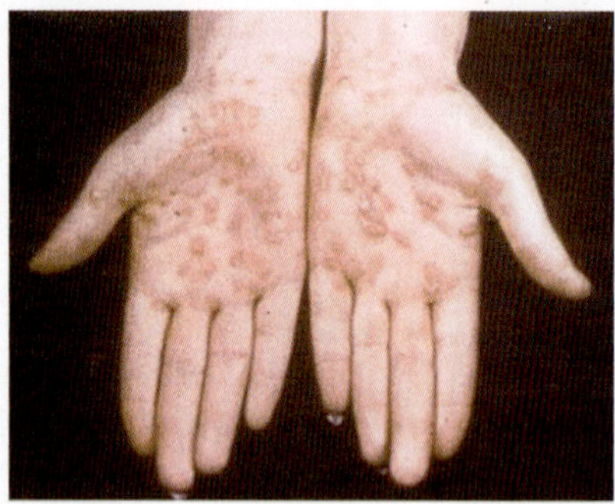

Fig. 57.10 Secondary syphilis. Palmar rash. (From Centers for Disease Control and Prevention Public Health Image Library. Courtesy Robert Sumpter.)

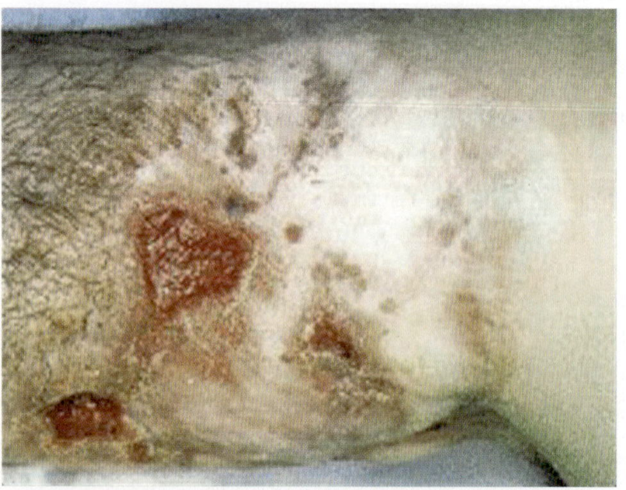

Fig. 57.11 Destructive skin gummas from tertiary syphilis. (From Gawkrodger D, Ardern-Jones M: *Dermatology*, ed 6, St Louis, 2016, Mosby.)

treatment, the rash will resolve, but the patient still has syphilis and is infectious for some time. There may be other systemic symptoms at this stage.

Tertiary, or late syphilis, is the final stage. Patients will not have obvious symptoms. During this stage, the organism is silently causing organ damage over many years. The formation of *gummas,* an inflammatory tumor-like response to syphilis, can lead to serious complications (Fig. 57.11).

Complications

Gummas may cause irreparable damage to skin, bone, or liver. In cardiovascular syphilis, the resulting aneurysm may press on structures such as the intercostal nerves, causing pain. The risk for rupture exists as the aneurysm increases in size. Scarring of the aortic valve can cause aortic valve insufficiency and heart failure.

Neurosyphilis occurs when *T. pallidum* invades the CNS. It can occur at any stage of syphilis. Impaired vision, *tabes dorsalis* (progressive locomotor ataxia), and dementia are rare, extreme manifestations.

Chancres on or inside the genitalia or anus enhance HIV transmission. Patients with HIV and syphilis are at greatest risk for significant CNS involvement. They may need more intensive treatment than other patients with syphilis.

Diagnostic Studies

Blood tests can diagnose syphilis. We classify tests for syphilis as those done for screening and those done that help stage the infection and ensure an infected person was effectively treated. The fluorescent treponemal antibody absorption (FTA-Abs) test, *T. pallidum* particle agglutination (TP-PA) test, and syphilis qualitative enzyme-linked immunoassay (EIA) treponemal tests detect antibodies to *T. pallidum.* They are positive if a patient has ever been infected with syphilis. They remain positive even after treatment, so another test is used to ensure cure and determine when someone has been reinfected.

Nontreponemal tests detect antibodies that are not specific for syphilis. These include the Venereal Disease Research Laboratory (VDRL) test and the rapid plasma reagin (RPR) test. These tests usually become positive 10 to 14 days after the appearance of a chancre. When positive, or "reactive," the test will read as a titer and will increase exponentially (e.g., 1:1, 1:2, 1:4, 1:8). This titer will continue to climb, reaching levels of up to 1:2048 during the primary and secondary stages of infection. After treatment, this titer will fall back to "nonreactive" or negative. It will take time for this to happen, usually several months. If the titer does not return to nonreactive or continues to elevate, this could indicate treatment failure or reinfection.

False-negative and false-positive test results can occur with the nontreponemal tests (VDRL, RPR). A false-negative result may occur with primary syphilis if the test is done before the person has had time to make these nonspecific antibodies. A false-positive may occur in patients who have other diseases or inflammatory conditions that produce these nonspecific

TABLE 57.7 Interprofessional Care
Syphilis

Diagnostic Assessment
- History and physical assessment
- Treponemal and/or nontreponemal serologic testing
- Testing for other STIs (HIV, gonorrhea, chlamydial infection)

Management
- Antibiotic therapy:
  - Penicillin G benzathine
  - Doxycycline or tetracycline (if penicillin contraindicated)
- Confidential counseling and testing for HIV infection
- Surveillance
- Repeat of nontreponemal tests at 6 and 12 mo
- Cerebrospinal fluid examination at 1 yr if treatment involves alternative antibiotics or treatment failure has occurred

antibodies. If treatment with antibiotics is started early in suspected cases of syphilis, the serologic nontreponemal test may not react or elevate.

Interprofessional Care

Because of the serious complications of untreated syphilis, screening programs for high-risk groups are important for reducing morbidity and mortality. The evaluation of all patients with syphilis should include HIV testing. Patients with HIV should have annual syphilis testing (Table 57.7).[5]

Drug Therapy

Management is aimed at starting treatment early. Penicillin G benzathine is the recommended treatment for all stages (Table 57.7).[5] When penicillin is contraindicated, doxycycline or tetracycline may be used with close follow-up. Aqueous procaine penicillin G is the treatment of choice for neurosyphilis. Treatment cannot reverse damage that is already present in the later stages of the disease. All sexual contacts from the preceding 90 days should be treated. Reexamination and follow-up testing are recommended every 6 months for up to 2 years to ensure cure. Repeat HIV testing should be done on all HIV-negative patients diagnosed with primary or secondary syphilis given the higher risk for HIV transmission during these stages.

Doxycycline Postexposure Prophylaxis (Doxy PEP)

Doxycycline postexposure prophylaxis (doxy PEP) is recommended as a preventative measure against bacterial STIs, especially chlamydia, gonorrhea, and syphilis.[12] It is advised for MSM and TGW who have had one of these bacterial STIs in the last 12 months. Patients take a single 200-mg dose of doxycycline within 72 hours after unprotected oral, anal, or vaginal sex. It is important that they understand doxy PEP may reduce, but will not eliminate, chlamydia, gonorrhea, and syphilis and that it does not provide protection against HIV or other STIs.

NURSING MANAGEMENT: STIs

Assessment

Subjective and objective data that you should obtain from patients with an STI are outlined in Table 57.8. Screen patients based on risk history and sexual behaviors. Assess the risk for contracting an STI. Questions to ask include the number of sexual partners (in the last month, year), gender of partners, type of birth control used (if applicable), use of condoms or other barrier methods, and history of an STI. Do they use social media or other networking apps to meet partners? Do they use drugs and alcohol or exchange sex for drugs or money? Are there violence and personal safety concerns?[13] Plan teaching based on patients' responses.

Interpersonal skills needed for this interview include respect, compassion, and a nonjudgmental attitude. Tailor counseling to the patient, and protect their privacy. Sexual practices are deeply personal. Interview patients alone, without parents or partners present whom they may not want to disclose all activities in front of. Provide a safe space to encourage honest discussion. Start by asking how they define themselves, including their gender identity and sexual preferences. Finally, do not assume that older people are not at risk. Sex and sexuality are dynamic across the life cycle. Sexually active older adults can be at risk for STIs.[13]

CHECK YOUR PRACTICE

You are working on the medicine unit caring for a 71-year-old female admitted for IV penicillin for neurosyphilis. The nurse whom you are working with says, "I can't believe that patient got syphilis—she is as old as my grandparents."
- How would you respond?
- What should you discuss with your colleague?

Clinical Problems

Clinical problems for patients with an STI include:
- Impaired sexual functioning
- Infection
- Deficient knowledge

Planning

The overall goals are that patients with an STI will (1) understand the mode of transmission and the risks related to STIs, (2) complete treatment and return for follow-up and testing, (3) notify or assist in notifying sexual contacts about their need for testing and treatment, (4) abstain from sexual contact until the infection is resolved and all partners have been treated, and (5) show knowledge of safer sex practices.

TABLE 57.8 NURSING ASSESSMENT

Sexually Transmitted Infections

Subjective Data

Important Health Information

Sexual health history: Sexual activity, history of STIs, number of sexual partners, unsafe sexual practices, alcohol and substance use, social media apps.

Medications: Allergy to antibiotics.

Functional Health Patterns

Health perception–health management: Unsafe sexual practices, drug and/or alcohol use.

Nutritional-metabolic: Nausea, vomiting, anorexia. Pharyngitis, oral lesions, chills. Alopecia.

Elimination: Dysuria, urinary frequency, urethral discharge, pain with bowel movements.

Cognitive-perceptual: Arthralgia, headache, painful, burning lesions, itching or irritation at infected site.

Sexuality-reproductive: Dyspareunia, vaginal or penile discharge, bleeding with sex, genital or perianal lesions.

Objective Data

General

Fever, lymphadenopathy (general or inguinal).

GI

Rectal discharge, rectal lesions.

Reproductive

Cervical mucopurulent discharge, cervical erythema, cervical bleeding; penile purulent discharge, epididymitis, proctitis, genital lesions.

Skin

Syphilis:

Primary: Painless, indurated genital, oral, or perianal lesions.

Secondary: Bilateral, symmetric rash on palms, soles, or entire body. Mucous patches on mouth or tongue; alopecia; condylomata lata.

Genital herpes: Painful genital or anal vesicular lesions.

Genital warts: Single or multiple flesh-colored, hyperpigmented, genital or anal warts.

Urinary

Urethral discharge, erythema.

Possible Diagnostic Findings

Chlamydia: Positive NAAT cervical, urethral, anal, oropharyngeal, or urine samples.

Gonorrhea: Positive cultures or NAAT from cervical, urethral, anal, oropharyngeal, or urine samples.

Genital herpes: Positive HSV-1 or HSV-2 serum antibody test. Positive viral culture or PCR from an active lesion indicating HSV-1 or HSV-2.

Syphilis: Positive findings on fluorescent treponemal antibody absorption (FTA-Abs) test, *T. pallidum* particle agglutination (TP-PA) test, or syphilis qualitative enzyme-linked immunoassay (EIA) test and/or a reactive VDRL or RPR test with elevated titer.

Trichomoniasis: ↑ pH and positive motile protozoa on wet preparation of discharge. Positive FDA-approved rapid test or liquid-based Pap positive for trichomoniasis.

NAAT, Nucleic acid amplification test; *PCR,* polymerase chain reaction; *RPR,* rapid plasma reagin; *VDRL,* Venereal Disease Research Laboratory.

◆ Implementation

Health Promotion

Many approaches to stopping the spread of STIs have had varying degrees of success (Box 57.2). Be prepared to discuss "safer" sex practices and harm reduction with all patients, not only those you perceive to be at risk. These practices include abstinence, monogamy, avoiding high-risk sexual behaviors, and correctly using condoms and other barriers with every sexual act. Sexual abstinence is the only certain method of avoiding all STIs, but few people consider this option. Limiting sexual contacts to an established, monogamous relationship in which both partners have been tested for STIs can reduce the risk. Addressing issues related to drug and alcohol use is important for promoting healthy sexual behavior.

Be prepared to teach special populations about their risks, including people of different racial and ethnic backgrounds, MSM, and transgender persons (Table 57.9). Encourage routine testing in people who are at higher risk so STIs can be identified early. This will help decrease the potential for complications and reduce transmission to others. A teaching guide for patients with an STI is shown in Table 57.10.

Measures to prevent infection. Help patients to be aware of specific signs and symptoms of infection. Encourage patients to take notice of a sexual partner's genitalia before sex. They should note any discharge, sores, blisters, lesions, or rashes. This can help them to make good decisions about whether to continue sexual activity with safer-sex modifications or to choose not to have sexual contact at all. Remind patients that most STIs may have no symptoms but can still be transmitted. Many are transmitted through oral sex. Emphasize that when they have sex, they are exposed to the infections of everyone with whom their partner has ever had sex.

Proper condom use is a highly effective mechanical barrier to infections that may be transmitted by or to a penis. Partners should openly discuss any objections to condom use, such as interference with spontaneity and the presence of a barrier. Information about the mechanics of sexual arousal and incorporating a condom into sex can help overcome resistance to its use. Refusing sexual activity with

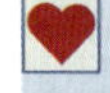

BOX 57.2 PROMOTING POPULATION HEALTH

Preventing STIs

- Follow "safer" sex practices every time you have sexual contact, and be responsible for your own protection.
- Have sexual activity only in an established, monogamous relationship, and limit the number of sexual partners otherwise.
- Obtain vaccinations to help prevent some types of HPV.
- Know your sex partners. Be comfortable saying "no" to sexual activity.
- Limit alcohol use to moderate levels, and avoid substance use.
- If you are sexually active and at risk, obtain testing regularly and encourage partners to do the same.

TABLE 57.9 Working With Special Populations

When working with the following populations at risk for STIs, consider cultural, behavior, social networking, and other factors that may place them at increased risk.

Racial and Ethnic Minorities

- When approaching patients of different backgrounds, be sensitive to their culture, religion, and social norms.
- Remember that there may be limited access to care, varying education levels, and lower health literacy among certain populations.
- Use an interpreter when communicating with non–English-speaking patients.
- Acknowledge that some communities may not be open to talking about sex or sexual practices for religious or cultural reasons.
- Be aware that some males in the Black, Hispanic, or Middle Eastern communities may not be comfortable disclosing that they are having sex with other males. They may be in a relationship with a female partner because of cultural or community pressures.

Men Who Have Sex With Men

- Assess risk for STIs. Be comfortable asking questions about sexual identity and practices, including insertive and receptive anal sex. Do not assume all MSM engage in the same sexual activities.
- Ask about social media and networking apps used to connect with other men for casual dating and sex. These have been traced to outbreaks of STIs.
- Counsel MSM without HIV who acquire another STI about options for HIV prevention, including preexposure prophylaxis (PrEP) and nonoccupational postexposure prophylaxis (nPEP) (see Chapter 15). Review the potential benefits of doxycycline postexposure prophylaxis (doxy PEP) in reducing some STIs.

Transgender Persons

- *Transgender man* is a term used to describe a person assigned female at birth but who identifies as male. *Transgender woman* is a term used to describe a person assigned male at birth but who identifies as female.
- Not all transgender persons have had gender reassignment surgery and may still have the anatomy present at birth. Screen these persons for STIs based on both risk history and site of exposure. For example, a transgender man may still have a vagina and cervix, requiring a vaginal examination and testing for trichomoniasis. Assess if transgender women are appropriate for doxy PEP.

any partner who will not use a condom is a safe and legitimate option.

The *female condom,* a lubricated polyurethane sheath designed for vaginal use, is an option for some females. Teach patients to avoid the spermicide nonoxynol 9 (N-9), which can be used alone to prevent pregnancy or as a condom lubricant. N-9 is one of the least effective methods of birth control when used alone. It can be irritating to the vagina and rectum, increasing the risk for acquiring an STI.

Screening programs. Screening programs are a way to identify, treat, prevent, and control the spread of STIs. At present, there are CDC-recommended screening programs for certain populations, including young people, MSM, pregnant females, and anyone at increased risk for exposure to an STI (e.g., new partners, multiple relationships, not using condoms).[5]

TABLE 57.10 PATIENT & CAREGIVER TEACHING

STIs

When teaching patients with an STI:

1. Explain precautions to take, such as:
    - Using condoms and other barrier methods with every sexual encounter
    - When being monogamous, defining what monogamy means with your partner
    - Limiting the number of sexual partners
    - Asking potential partners about their sexual history
    - Asking potential partners if they have been tested for STIs
    - Avoiding sex with partners who have visible oral, inguinal, genital, perineal, or anal lesions or those who use IV drugs
    - Voiding and washing genitalia and surrounding area after sex to flush out/wash away organisms to reduce potential for transmitting infection
2. Explain the importance of taking all antibiotics or antiviral agents as prescribed. Symptoms will improve after 1–2 days of treatment, but organisms may still be present.
3. Teach patients diagnosed with gonorrhea, chlamydia, syphilis, or trichomoniasis that all sexual partners need treatment to prevent transmission and reinfection.
4. Teach patients to abstain from sexual contact during and for 7 days after treatment. Review the use of condoms or other barrier methods when sexual activity is resumed to prevent spread of infection and reinfection.
5. Explain the importance of follow-up examination and retesting at least once after treatment (if needed) to confirm a cure.
6. Allow patients and partners to voice their concerns and clarify areas that need explanation.
7. Teach patients about the signs and symptoms of complications and need to report problems to their HCP to ensure proper follow-up and early treatment of reinfection.
8. Tell patients of the infectious nature of these conditions to avoid a false sense of security, which may result in careless sexual practices or poor personal hygiene.
9. Tell patients about health department requirements for anonymously reporting certain STIs.

Case finding. Interviewing and case finding are other methods used to control the spread of STIs. These activities are directed toward finding and examining all sexual contacts of patients with reportable STIs so that they receive treatment. Public health professionals, often nurses, are aware of the social implications of STIs and the need for discretion in finding partners. Sexual contacts are not told about the origin of the information naming them as a contact or the timing of exposure to ensure patient privacy mandates.

Partner notification and treatment impose a heavy burden on public health departments. As a result, notification often becomes the responsibility of the infected partner. The infected partner may choose not to tell sexual partners, and the partners may choose not to seek treatment. Unfortunately, this perpetuates the disease.

Education programs. Encourage your community to provide education about STIs. High-risk populations (e.g., MSM, people of color, young people under age 25) should be a target.

Knowledge and understanding can decrease the incidence of STIs. Encourage the HPV vaccine before the start of sexual activity. Accurate and current information may help reduce parental fears related to the vaccine. Consider stressing cancer prevention as a reason for the vaccine. This may be more productive and less controversial, thus making the parent and adolescent more receptive.

Acute Care

Patient education, counseling, and referrals are essential nursing roles for promoting health and optimal sexual well-being. If you work in public health facilities, clinics, or other outpatient settings, you are more likely to care for patients with an STI than if you work in a hospital setting. Patient education, counseling, and referrals are essential nursing roles for promoting health and optimal sexual well-being (Table 57.10).

Because many STIs are cured with a single dose or short course of antibiotic therapy, many patients are casual about the outcome. The consequences of this attitude can include treatment delays, nonadherence, treatment failure, reinfection, and complications. Single-dose treatment for gonorrhea and syphilis helps prevent problems from nonadherence with drug therapy. Stress to patients receiving multiple-dose therapy the need to complete the prescribed treatment. Teach them about problems resulting from nonadherence.

All patients should return to the treatment center for repeat testing of the infected sites or for serologic testing at designated times to determine the effectiveness of the treatment. Explaining that they may not be cured with the first treatment can reinforce the need for a follow-up visit.

Tell patients to inform sexual partners of the need for testing and treatment as a contact, regardless of whether they are free of or have symptoms (Box 57.3). Because young people ages 15 to 24 represent about 50% of new STIs annually, almost every state and the District of Columbia have laws that allow minors to consent to STI services without parental involvement. However, the minimum age does vary by state.

Patients with infection-related complications may need prolonged treatment and surgery. Major surgery, such as an aneurysm resection or aortic valve replacement, may be needed to treat cardiovascular problems caused by syphilis. Pelvic surgery and procedures to correct fertility problems from an STI may be needed. If not successful, patients may need assisted reproductive technologies to achieve a pregnancy.

Hygiene measures. Emphasize the importance of certain hygiene measures, such as frequent hand washing. Tell patients not to scratch infection sites to avoid autoinoculation of STIs that can be spread to other parts of the body. Washing with soap and water and voiding after sex may have some benefit in decreasing the exposure to STIs but does not give adequate protection against transmission. Teach patients not to douche after sex. It can push bacteria higher into the reproductive tract or undermine local immune responses.

Sexual activity. Sexual abstinence is needed during the communicable phase of any STI. Long-term precautions must be taken with those STIs that are chronic or recurrent. Emphasize that even single-dose treatments can take up to 1 week to clear the infection. Thus patients are infectious during this period and should avoid all sexual contact. Remind patients that all partners must be treated as contacts to prevent reinfection. Emphasize the importance of using condoms or other barrier methods to help prevent the spread of infection and reinfection after all have been treated.

BOX 57.3 ETHICAL/LEGAL DILEMMAS

Confidentiality and HIPAA

Situation

O.P. is a 22-year-old female who recently tested positive for gonorrhea. You tell her she must tell her sexual partners of the infection so they may be treated. She refuses to tell her boyfriend because he will then know that she had sex with someone else. You later learn that the patient's boyfriend works at the hospital laboratory and the patient is worried that he will find out.

Ethical/Legal Points for Consideration

- Each state has requirements for reporting communicable diseases and other health-related data. Inform patients of the reporting requirements for communicable diseases.
- Nurses and other HCPs have both a legal and an ethical obligation to maintain confidentiality of patient information. The Health Insurance Portability and Accountability Act (HIPAA) ensures the privacy of personal health information.
- The duty to maintain confidentiality is not absolute and may be limited, as needed, to protect the patient or other parties, or by law or regulation, such as mandated reporting for safety or public health reasons.
- Your main obligation is to the patient seeking care. Teaching is a way to establish a partnership with this patient. Share information about the effects of the disease, the consequences of reinfection, and the effect of the disease on others who may not know that they are infected. Then encourage the patient to tell partners of the diagnosis and discuss the option of expedited partner treatment (EPT) where applicable.

Discussion Questions

1. What are your state's requirements for reportable conditions?
2. In your opinion, what is the best way to balance the needs of a patient with those of the public?
3. What are the risks to agencies for the breach of confidentiality and HIPAA?

Reference

Code of Ethics for Nurses. Retrieved from https://www.nursingworld.org/practice-policy/nursing-excellence/ethics/code-of-ethics-for-nurses/.

Remind patients that complications can follow if sexual activity occurs before treatment completion or if all partners are not treated as needed. Patients need to discuss retreatment or continued treatment with an HCP. During treatment, patients can choose to relate to a partner in an intimate way that avoids penetrative, oral-genital contact, or skin-to-skin contact.

Psychologic support. The diagnosis of an STI may be met with a variety of emotions, such as embarrassment, shame, guilt, anger, or even a desire for vengeance. Having an STI can affect a person's well-being, their relationships, and their sexual lives. Encourage patients to voice their feelings. Couples in marital or committed relationships have an added problem when an STI is diagnosed, as this suggests sexual activity outside the relationship. The STI raises other concerns about their relationship and may serve as an incentive for further problem-solving. A referral for professional counseling to explore the impact of the STI on their relationship may be needed.

Patients with genital herpes are faced with the fact that future outbreaks are likely to occur and that no cure is available. This can be frustrating and disruptive to their physical, emotional, social, and sexual life. Help them identify and avoid any factors that may precipitate outbreaks, such as stress, local trauma, or sun exposure. Tell patients that the frequency and severity of recurrences will decrease over time. Stress that herpes is a common, manageable condition and does not pose a risk to their overall health.

Genital or anal warts often involve a prolonged course of treatment. Clearing the virus takes time and is not always possible. Patients can become frustrated and fatigued from frequent office visits, associated costs, treatment side effects, and effects the infection has on future health and sexual relationships. Support and a willingness to listen are needed. Local or online support groups are available for most STIs. Help patients to connect with support groups.

◆ Evaluation

Expected outcomes for patients with an STI are that patients will:

- Understand the course, modes of transmission, and treatment options for the STI
- Relate the potential long-term complications of untreated infection
- Adhere to the treatment plan and follow-up protocol
- Understand the importance of partner notification and treatment
- Practice STI risk-reducing behaviors

CASE STUDY

Syphilis Infection

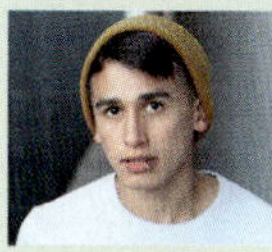

(© ajr_images/ iStock.com.)

Patient Profile

S.M. is a 32-year-old bisexual male who presents to the outpatient clinic with a rash. He noticed "red spots" on his chest when getting out of the shower a few days ago. These have since spread to his back, abdomen, and hands. They do not itch, and he has no other symptoms. S.M. reports having had unprotected receptive anal sex with a new male partner 4 weeks ago. He reports he is currently seeing a new female partner. They have not had any intimate or sexual contact yet. S.M. has a history of gonorrhea treated 6 months ago.

Subjective Data

- Recent unprotected receptive anal sex
- History of gonorrhea 6 months ago
- Appears anxious

Objective Data

- Skin: Maculopapular rash on the chest, back, trunk, and palms of the hands
- No cervical, axillary, epitrochlear, or inguinal lymphadenopathy
- No penile or anorectal discharge, no lesions or ulcers on the penis or anus
- Serologies are positive for treponemal antibodies and a rapid plasma reagin (RPR) of 1:256; last RPR 6 months ago was nonreactive
- HIV test is nonreactive

Interprofessional Care

- Penicillin G benzathine 2.4 million units IM now

Discussion Questions

1. ***Recognize:*** What are S.M.'s risk factors for acquiring syphilis?
2. ***Analyze:*** What complications could occur if S.M.'s infection is not treated?
3. ***Plan:*** What impact could the diagnosis have on S.M.'s relationship with his new female partner?
4. ***Prioritize:*** What is the priority of care for S.M.?
5. ***Act:*** S.M. mentions he is on preexposure prophylaxis (PrEP) for protection against HIV but has heard about doxy PEP. How would you advise him on using this for STI prevention?
6. ***Act:*** What instructions should S.M. receive to ensure successful treatment? To prevent reinfection? To prevent further transmission?
7. ***Safety:*** S.M. tells you he still has contact information for the partner with whom he had sex 4 weeks ago but is too embarrassed to notify him of the infection. What assistance in notifying this partner should you consider?

Answers available at http://evolve.elsevier.com/Lewis/medsurg.

BRIDGE TO NCLEX EXAMINATION

The number of the question corresponds to the same-numbered outcome at the beginning of the chapter.

1. Which groups are at high risk for sexually transmitted infections in the United States? (**Select all that apply.**)
   a. Transgender women
   b. Adults 35 to 45 years of age
   c. Youth and young adults 25 and under
   d. Men who have sex with men (MSM)
   e. People at social or economic disadvantage
2. The nurse is reviewing treatment orders for a patient diagnosed with syphilis. What is *most* important to consider?
   a. Congenital syphilis is rising.
   b. Repeat testing is needed after treatment to ensure cure.
   c. Symptoms of syphilis are often confused with other medical problems.
   d. Penicillin G should not be used if patients report an allergy to amoxicillin.
3. What would the nurse include in a teaching plan for a patient with newly diagnosed genital herpes? (**Select all that apply.**)
   a. Herpes is best treated with doxycycline.
   b. Acyclovir only works for oral herpes infection.
   c. Avoid sexual contact until the lesions have fully healed.
   d. Antivirals can reduce the duration and severity of outbreaks.
   e. Applying a heating pad to the lesions can help reduce the pain.
4. What symptoms may be present in a male patient with gonococcal urethritis? (**Select all that apply.**)
   a. Sore throat
   b. Testicular pain
   c. Pain with urination
   d. Purulent urethral discharge
   e. Flesh-colored lesions at the base or tip of the penis
5. Which statement about reducing STI transmission would the nurse include when teaching a patient with PID caused by chlamydia and gonorrhea infections?
   a. "Condoms are the only way to reduce the risk of STIs."
   b. "All STIs can be treated, so don't worry if you get it again."
   c. "It is recommended that you get repeat STI screening in 3 months."
   d. "Only partners with symptoms should be encouraged to get tested."
6. A patient asks the nurse how chlamydia is transmitted. The best response would be
   a. From an open sore.
   b. Through skin-to-skin contact.
   c. Through oral, vaginal, and anal sex.
   d. From touching an object, such as a toilet seat.

1. a, c, d, e; 2. b; 3. c, d; 4. a, b, c, d; 5. c; 6. c.

For rationales to these answers and even more NCLEX review questions, visit http://evolve.elsevier.com/Lewis/medsurg.

REFERENCES

To access the References for this chapter, please scan the QR code with a mobile device.

58

Female Reproductive Problems

Robyn Schafer

http://evolve.elsevier.com/Lewis/medsurg/

CONCEPTUAL FOCUS

Cellular Regulation
Hormonal Regulation
Infection
Inflammation
Pain
Reproduction
Sexuality

LEARNING OUTCOMES

1. Outline strategies for the diagnosis and treatment of female infertility.
2. Identify risk factors and nursing and interprofessional management of early pregnancy loss and ectopic pregnancy.
3. Describe the etiology and clinical manifestations of menstrual problems and abnormal uterine bleeding.
4. Describe physiologic changes related to menopause and management of perimenopausal symptoms.
5. Outline the etiology and clinical manifestations of genital tract infections.
6. Identify the pathophysiology and interprofessional and nursing care for benign gynecologic problems.
7. Explain the clinical manifestations, diagnostic studies, and treatment of gynecologic cancers.
8. Discuss the interprofessional and nursing care for survivors of sexual assault.

KEY TERMS

abnormal uterine bleeding (AUB)
dysmenorrhea
early pregnancy loss
ectopic pregnancy
endometriosis
infertility
menopause
pelvic inflammatory disease (PID)
pelvic organ prolapse
perimenopause
polycystic ovary syndrome (PCOS)
premenstrual syndrome (PMS)
sexual assault
sexual dysfunction
spontaneous abortion
uterine aspiration

Gynecologic, sexual, and reproductive health are important aspects of well-being across the life span. Problems with gynecologic and sexual health profoundly affect health and well-being. This chapter discusses common female reproductive system problems. Care often includes screening and prevention, health teaching and promotion, and assessment and treatment of complications.

While we refer to these as female reproductive system problems, the terms "female" and "woman" may not reflect the gender identity of patients with these problems. These problems may be present in transgender, gender-nonconforming, and gender-diverse persons assigned female sex at birth. Use of gendered terms here is not meant to exclude any person who has these problems.

OBSTETRIC PROBLEMS

INFERTILITY

Infertility is the inability to achieve a successful pregnancy. Infertility is diagnosed after at least 1 year of vaginal-penile intercourse without contraception in females under 35 years of age or after 6 months in those 35 years of age or older.[1] Around 15% of heterosexual couples experience infertility. It is more common with advancing age.

Etiology and Pathophysiology

Infertility affects both males and females. It is caused by male, female, and combined (male and female) factors. As many as 30% of infertility cases are unexplained, with no identifiable cause. Male factor infertility is discussed in Chapter 59. We discuss female factor infertility here. The most common identifiable causes are hormone imbalances and structure problems.

Diagnostic Studies

Formal evaluation of infertility is usually done after 12 months of regular, unprotected intercourse (Table 58.1). Earlier evaluation is appropriate in females over the age of 35 or if there are known medical or physical problems. Evaluation starts with a history and physical assessment (Table 58.2). Based on the findings, laboratory tests and diagnostic imaging may be done. These explore common causes of infertility, including diminished ovarian reserve, ovulatory dysfunction, and structure problems of the fallopian tubes and uterus.[2] Diagnostic studies for male factors, such as semen analysis, are also done.

Interprofessional and Nursing Management

There are multiple treatment options for infertility. These include lifestyle changes, drug therapy, and surgery. The approach is tailored to the underlying cause. A patient-centered approach is essential in treating infertility. The process of assessing and managing infertility is often expensive, stressful, and emotionally difficult for patients and their partners. Teaching about fertility, ovulation, and intercourse is important. This information often improves conception rates. Involve patients in determining the plan of care and weighing the efficacy, safety, and advantages and disadvantages of treatment options. Discuss concerns about ethical issues related to infertility technology and procedures.

Lifestyle changes include weight loss, smoking cessation, and reduced alcohol and caffeine intake. Intercourse should be timed around ovulation. Medical treatment for female infertility focuses on stimulating the ovaries (known as *ovulation induction*). Table 58.3 reviews common drugs used in fertility treatment. Surgery may address blockages in the ovarian tubes or uterine problems. *Assisted reproductive technology* (ART) procedures include insemination through intracervical insemination (ICI), intrauterine insemination (IUI), or in vitro fertilization (IVF). The National Infertility Association (RESOLVE) is a useful resource to support patients in exploring treatment options.[3]

TABLE 58.1 Diagnostic Criteria

Infertility

Infertility is diagnosed after a person has not been able to conceive after regular (frequent) intercourse without contraception for:

- 12 months in females less than 35 years of age; OR
- 6 months in females 35 years of age and older.

TABLE 58.2 Interprofessional Care

Infertility

Diagnostic Assessment

- History and physical assessment of both partners
  - Detailed menstrual, sexual, reproductive, and gynecologic history
  - Height, weight, and body mass index
  - Pelvic examination
- Laboratory tests
  - CBC
  - Thyroid-stimulating hormone (TSH)
  - STI screening
  - Hormone levels (FSH, LH, antimüllerian hormone, progesterone, prolactin)
- Imaging
  - Transvaginal ultrasound
  - Hysterosalpingogram

Management

- Lifestyle changes
- Drug therapy (Table 58.3)
- Surgery
- Assisted reproductive technologies (ARTs)

PREGNANCY LOSS

Pregnancy loss is the term used to describe the loss of a nonviable pregnancy up to 20 weeks gestation. **Early pregnancy loss** occurs in the first trimester (the first 13 weeks of pregnancy). It is the most common type of pregnancy loss. *Abortion* is another term used to describe spontaneous

TABLE 58.3 Drug Therapy

Infertility

Class	Drugs	Mechanism of Action
Aromatase inhibitor	letrozole (Femara)	↓ Estrogen by preventing the conversion of androgens to estrogens in the ovaries
Biguanide	metformin	↓ Hyperinsulinemia. May lead to enhanced spontaneous ovulation with PCOS
Dopamine agonist	bromocriptine (Parlodel) cabergoline	↓ Prolactin to restore normal ovulation. Reduces risk of ovarian hyperstimulation
Gonadotropin	follicle-stimulating hormone (Gonal-f) human chorionic gonadotropin (hCG) human menopausal gonadotropin (Menopur)	Stimulates follicle growth and maturation by mimicking the body's natural hormones
Selective estrogen receptor modulator (SERM)	clomiphene citrate	Stimulates ovulation by binding estrogen receptors in the hypothalamus. Leads to ↑ gonadotropin-releasing hormone (GnRH) production and ↑ LH and FSH secretion in the pituitary

pregnancy loss and induced termination of pregnancy at any gestation. Pregnancy loss can lead to grief and psychologic distress.

Spontaneous Abortion

Spontaneous abortion (or "miscarriage") is the natural loss of pregnancy before 20 weeks of gestation. Around 20% of pregnancies result in spontaneous abortion. Most occur in the first trimester. Table 58.4 lists risk factors for spontaneous abortions. Patients experiencing a spontaneous abortion often present with vaginal bleeding and cramping. Following a history and physical assessment, blood work is done to assess human chorionic gonadotropin levels (hCG, β-hCG) and blood type. A transvaginal ultrasound may be done.

> **CHECK YOUR PRACTICE**
>
> You are working in the ED. Your patient is a 36-year-old female who is 10 weeks' gestation. She presents with cramping and scant vaginal bleeding. The HCP suspects spontaneous abortion. The patient is crying, "This is the second time this has happened to me. I can't go through this again. I'm never going to be able to have children."
>
> - As her nurse, what are your priorities?
> - How would you respond to her?

There are 3 treatment approaches of spontaneous abortion: (1) expectant management, (2) medication abortion, and (3) procedural abortion (uterine aspiration).[4] We use a patient-centered approach to determine the plan of care based on patients' preferences and values. Patients with signs of acute complications such as hemorrhage or infection need emergency care.

Expectant management involves waiting for the pregnancy tissue (*products of conception [POC]*) to pass on its own. When criteria are met, this approach is about 75% effective in the 1st trimester. This option is the least invasive. However, it is not as predictable or effective as other approaches. Provide teaching about warning signs. We need to monitor for complications and have a clear plan for follow-up.

Medication abortion involves taking misoprostol (Cytotec) and mifepristone (Mifeprex) to induce passage of the POC from the uterus. This approach offers more predictable timing than expectant management. It is also less invasive than uterine procedures. The combination of both agents is 95% effective. However, mifepristone is not available in all settings.[5] Misoprostol alone is an alternative for medication management. With medication abortion, patients will likely pass the POC at home. Teaching about side effects and anticipatory guidance is essential to safety in this approach.

Procedural abortion involves using medical instruments to empty the uterus. The most common type of procedural abortion is **uterine aspiration** (suction). Uterine aspiration can be either manual vacuum aspiration (MVA) or electric vacuum aspiration (EVA) (Fig. 58.1). This procedure can be done in an office, clinic, or ambulatory care setting. Local anesthesia or sedation may be offered. Some patients may choose a dilation and curettage (D&C) procedure. This is done at a health care facility under general anesthesia. Procedural abortion is the most effective and invasive option for managing a spontaneous abortion. It offers predictable timing and rapid resolution of pregnancy loss. Complications such as infection, hemorrhage, uterine perforation, or incomplete abortion are rare.

Teach patients to call the HCP for heavy vaginal bleeding, fever, foul-smelling vaginal discharge, or severe pain. Discuss the use of pain medications, such as ibuprofen. Patients who are RhD-negative blood type should receive Rho(D) immune globulin (Rhogam) for alloimmunization prevention. Give resources or referrals for psychologic support and grief counseling to reduce mental health complications such as depression and anxiety. Review contraceptive options or planning for a subsequent pregnancy. Ovulation can resume within days or weeks after a pregnancy loss. Patients can try to become pregnant again as soon as they feel ready. They do not need to wait.

TABLE 58.4 Risk Factors for Spontaneous Abortion

- Advanced maternal age (>35 years)
- Chronic stress
- Endocrine problems
- Embryonic chromosomal abnormalities
- Exposure to certain medications, environment toxins
- Infection
- Obesity
- Prior pregnancy loss
- Obesity
- Substance use

Pregnancy Termination

The term *abortion* is also used to describe *pregnancy termination* (sometimes called an "induced abortion"). In the United States pregnancy termination is regulated by state and federal laws and statutes. The most common methods of pregnancy termination are medical abortion and procedural abortion (Table 58.5). The approach used depends on the gestational

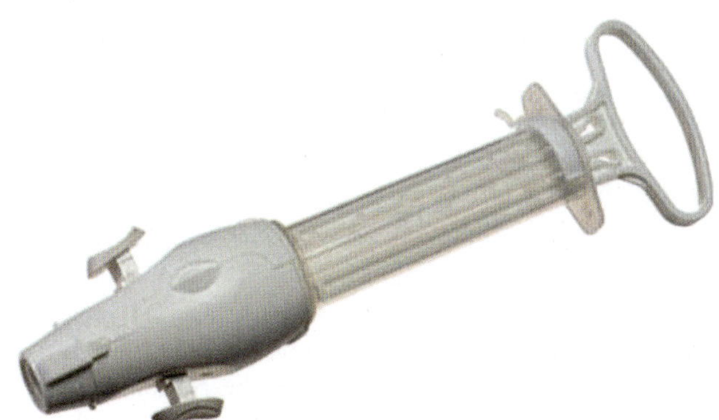

Fig. 58.1 Manual vacuum uterine aspiration device for management of early pregnancy failure. (Ipas, Chapel Hill, NC, USA.)

TABLE 58.5 Common Ways to Induce Abortions

Method	Medication Abortion	Procedural Abortion
Description	Combination of oral or buccal drugs (most often mifepristone and misoprostol) to soften and dilate the cervix and expel the pregnancy tissue	Products of conception are removed through medical instruments that are introduced through the cervix and attached to manual or electric vacuum aspirator
Timing	Up to 10–11 weeks' gestation	Up to 14 weeks' gestation (uterine aspiration) More advanced gestational age (dilation and evacuation or "D&E")
Success rate	High (98%–99%)	High (99%)
Setting	Telehealth Clinic or office	Clinic or office Health care facility or hospital
Common side effects	GI distress, abdominal cramping, vaginal bleeding	Abdominal cramping, vaginal bleeding

length of the pregnancy, patient preference, and availability of care. Considering all relevant laws and regulations, engage patients in decision making about the risks, benefits, and alternatives. Where appropriate, provide resources and referrals to ensure safe abortion care. Educate that pregnancy termination does not negatively affect future pregnancies. Nursing care for pregnancy termination is similar to care for spontaneous abortion, discussed above.

ECTOPIC PREGNANCY

An **ectopic pregnancy** is the implantation of a fertilized ovum outside the uterus. Almost all ectopic pregnancies occur within the fallopian tube (Fig. 58.2). When this happens, there is a risk that the pregnancy could rupture the fallopian tube. This can lead to excess intraabdominal blood loss. It is a life-threatening emergency. Early detection of ectopic pregnancy is essential.

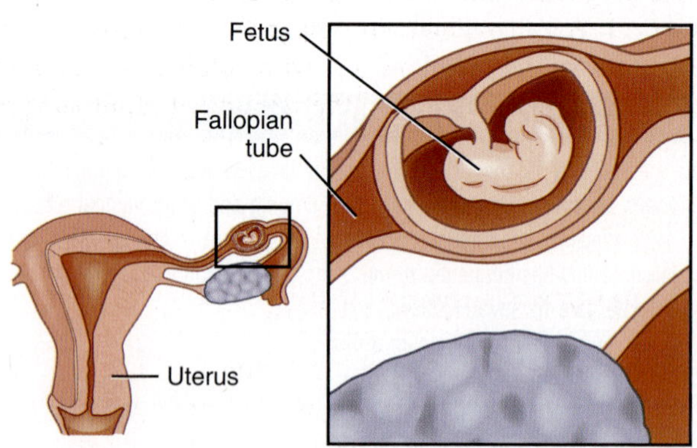

Fig. 58.2 Ectopic pregnancy in the fallopian tube.

Etiology and Pathophysiology

Tubal complications or blockages from infection, surgery, or deformity increase the chance that implantation will occur in the fallopian tube. Rarely, ectopic pregnancies can occur in other sites such as the cervix, ovaries, scar tissue, or abdomen. Embryos that implant outside of the uterus are not able to develop normally. As the embryo grows, it can cause organ rupture leading to severe internal bleeding and, if untreated, death.

Risk factors for ectopic pregnancy include a history of prior ectopic pregnancy, tubal surgery, or pelvic infection or inflammatory disease. When a pregnancy occurs with an IUD present, it has increased risk of being ectopic.

Clinical Manifestations

Ectopic pregnancies often cause abdominal or pelvic pain and unexplained vaginal bleeding. These symptoms should trigger immediate evaluation when a female has a positive pregnancy test. Pregnancy testing should be done in someone who presents with these symptoms and might be pregnant. Ectopic pregnancy symptoms typically present about 6 to 8 weeks after the last menstrual period. Pain is typically caused by distention of the fallopian tube. Some patients do not have any pain. When present, vaginal bleeding can vary in quantity and color from scant, brown spotting to bright red, heavy bleeding. In severe cases, patients have severe, sharp, unilateral pelvic or abdominal pain and sudden onset of vaginal bleeding. Secondary symptoms include those of early pregnancy, such as absent or late menses, nausea, frequent urination, and breast tenderness. Any patients who present with severe hemorrhage or symptoms of shock, such as hypotension or feeling dizzy or faint, should be treated as a medical emergency.

Diagnostic Studies

Physical assessment, diagnostic imaging, and laboratory studies are used to diagnose an ectopic pregnancy. Tenderness of the cervix or adnexa on palpation or visualization of an adnexal mass on ultrasound may be present. Serial transvaginal ultrasound and measurement of β-hCG may be done to guide management decisions.

Interprofessional and Nursing Management

Ectopic pregnancy can be treated with medication or surgery. Both options are equally effective. When diagnosed early in stable patients, ectopic pregnancy can be managed with medication. Methotrexate stops the growth of rapidly dividing cells, including fetal and early placenta cells, by inhibiting DNA synthesis and disrupting cell multiplication. It is given as an IM injection. The most common side effect is cramping or abdominal pain, which usually occurs during the first 2 to 3 days after treatment. When therapy is ineffective or a patient has severe symptoms or high risk of rupture, surgery is needed. Surgical options include a *salpingectomy* (removal of the fallopian tube) or *salpingostomy* (surgically opening the tube and removing the pregnancy tissue). Surgery may be done laparoscopically. For a small number of very low-risk patients, expectant management with close monitoring may be an option.

Nursing care includes closely monitoring symptoms and vital signs. Assess for signs of shock. Teach patients about ectopic pregnancy and treatment options. Provide emotional support. Prepare patients for diagnostic procedures, drug therapy, or surgery. Follow up with additional laboratory tests or imaging based on the treatment approach and symptoms.

MENSTRUAL PROBLEMS

PREMENSTRUAL DISORDERS

Most females have physical and emotional symptoms during specific phases of the menstrual cycle. For example, many have mild bloating, breast tenderness, or mood swings in the premenstrual phase. While often referred to as PMS, these mild symptoms do not meet the criteria for PMS. Clinically, we use the term **premenstrual syndrome (PMS)** in situations in which 1 or more recurrent physical and behavior symptoms cause severe distress or interfere with daily functioning. PMS can affect health, relationships, work performance, or academic performance. *Premenstrual dysphoric disorder* (PMDD) is a severe form of PMS that often includes behavior and affective symptoms.

Etiology and Pathophysiology

We do not know the exact cause of premenstrual disorders. Most likely, they are the result of a combination of hormone and psychosocial factors. Genetics, nutrition, drug therapy, and underlying medical or mental health problems may be contributing factors.

Clinical Manifestations

PMS presents with a wide variety of recurrent, cyclical symptoms. Symptoms may be physical, emotional, behavioral, or cognitive. Onset of symptoms occurs in the luteal phase of the menstrual cycle. Resolution of symptoms occurs within days of onset of menses. Common physical symptoms are breast discomfort, bloating and swelling, headache, and cramping. Emotional symptoms include mood swings, irritability, and feeling anxious or depressed. Changes in behavior such as food cravings or increased appetite are common. Some patients have cognitive symptoms like difficulty concentrating. With PMDD, patients often have irritability, anger, fatigue, anxiety, and depressed mood. PMDD may be superimposed on other psychiatric conditions.

Diagnostic Studies

To diagnose premenstrual disorders, we rule out problems that may present with similar symptoms. Obtain a history, including detailed menstrual and psychiatric histories. Physical and laboratory assessments may be helpful. Evaluation for mood or anxiety disorders, thyroid problems, or perimenopausal symptoms may be appropriate. Use of a symptom diary or calendar can aid the diagnosis.

Interprofessional and Nursing Management

Care focuses on symptom management. A holistic approach includes lifestyle and behavior interventions, complementary and alternative therapies such as acupuncture, and consideration of drug options.[6] Health promotion should include guidance and support for improved nutrition, exercise, sleep, and stress management. Behavior interventions such as relaxation techniques may be helpful. Cognitive behavior therapy is an option to manage moderate to severe symptoms. Drug treatment options include selective serotonin reuptake inhibitors (SSRIs) and/or combined hormone contraceptives such as an oral contraceptive pill (OCP). Calcium supplements and other vitamins or herbs may help manage symptoms. NSAIDs can be taken for pain.

Nursing care includes teaching about the condition and ways to manage symptoms (Table 58.6). Acknowledging the diagnosis can be therapeutic and validating. Helping patients monitor their symptoms and set realistic goals can improve functioning and quality of life. Patients with PMDD are at increased for suicide. Provide counseling and resources for suicide prevention.

TABLE 58.6 Interprofessional Care

Premenstrual Disorders

Diagnostic Assessment

- Health history including medication, menstrual, psychiatric history
- Symptom diary
- Physical assessment
- Laboratory studies as indicated

Management

- Health promotion (diet, sleep, exercise)
- Stress reduction and relaxation
- Cognitive behavior therapy
- Complementary and alternative therapy (acupuncture, calcium supplements)
- Medications (SSRIs, hormonal contraceptives)

DYSMENORRHEA

Etiology and Pathophysiology

Dysmenorrhea is painful menstruation. It is one of the most common gynecologic problems. Although most females have some discomfort during menses, dysmenorrhea is cyclic pain that interferes with activities of daily living.

Dysmenorrhea can be primary or secondary. In *primary dysmenorrhea,* no underlying problem or disease process is causing the symptoms. We think it is caused by excess production of prostaglandin, a hormone secreted by the *endometrium* (uterine lining) during menstruation. Prostaglandin stimulates the uterus to contract. Uterine contractions and constriction of small endometrial blood vessels lead to tissue ischemia and increased sensitization of pain receptors. This results in painful menstrual cramps. As menstruation continues, prostaglandin levels decrease, and menstrual cramping improves. Primary dysmenorrhea is most common in adolescents around the time of menarche.

In *secondary dysmenorrhea,* the symptoms are due to an underlying pathology. The most common causes are endometriosis, adenomyosis, or uterine fibroids. There may be an association between dysmenorrhea and chronic pain conditions.

Clinical Manifestations

Both forms of dysmenorrhea present with similar symptoms. Patients have pain with the start of menses or a day or two before. Most commonly, it is felt in the lower abdomen. Symptoms often resolve spontaneously within 2 or 3 days after onset. There may be back pain, nausea and vomiting, and symptoms of premenstrual disorders. Dysmenorrhea can impair functioning and quality of life. Severe dysmenorrhea can lead to absenteeism and decreased productivity at work or school. Depending on the cause, secondary dysmenorrhea may be associated with *dyspareunia* (painful intercourse), heavy or irregular vaginal bleeding, or infertility.

Diagnostic Studies

Evaluation begins with the history. Obtain detailed menstrual and sexual histories. Use of a symptom diary may help aid diagnosis. Diagnosis is based on the presentation of symptoms in the absence of other suspected causes of pain. Testing may be done to screening for chlamydia and gonorrhea in sexually active patients. Screening for urinary tract infection may be appropriate. Pelvic examination may not be necessary for adolescents who present with classic symptoms of primary dysmenorrhea. Assessment for secondary dysmenorrhea includes pelvic examination and transvaginal or pelvic ultrasound imaging.

Interprofessional Care

Treatment for primary dysmenorrhea includes drug and nonpharmacologic therapies. First-line drug therapy includes nonsteroidal antiinflammatory drugs (NSAIDs). NSAIDs inhibit prostaglandins and decrease pain. Acetaminophen and hormone therapies such as oral conceptive pills may be used. Nonpharmacologic options include heat, exercise, and transcutaneous electrical nerve stimulation (TENS).

Treatment of secondary dysmenorrhea depends on the cause. Some symptoms are improved by the same approaches used to treat primary dysmenorrhea. However, management of the underlying problem may be needed to relieve symptoms. Common surgical treatments for dysmenorrhea include *endometrial ablation* (surgical destruction of the uterine lining) and *hysterectomy* (removal of the uterus) (Table 58.7).

Nursing care includes teaching about the cause, symptoms, and treatment options. Validate patients' pain and experience. Provide psychosocial support. Teach patients about lifestyle changes. Regular exercise and good nutrition to improve symptoms. Provide teaching about drug therapy and nonpharmacologic options. Follow up on test results as appropriate.

ABNORMAL UTERINE BLEEDING

Abnormal uterine bleeding (AUB) is any uterine bleeding that is abnormal in quantity, duration, or timing. AUB can have

TABLE 58.7 Common Gynecologic Surgeries

Type of Surgical Procedure	Description
Dilation and curettage (D&C)	Opening (dilation) of cervix and removal (scraping) of endometrial tissue
Endometrial ablation	Destroys endometrial lining using heat, cold, or electrical energy
Hysterectomy	Removal of the uterus Several types: • Vaginal: uterus removed through an incision in the vagina • Abdominal: uterus removed through an incision in the abdomen • Laparoscopic: laparoscope and instrument inserted through abdominal incisions • Robotic-assisted laparoscopy: surgical robot manipulates surgical instruments
Hysteroscopy	Examine uterine cavity using a hysteroscope (lighted, flexible viewing instrument), inserted through the cervix
Myomectomy	Removal of fibroids from the uterus, leaving the uterus in place
Oophorectomy	Removal of the ovary, can be unilateral or bilateral
Salpingectomy	Removal of the fallopian tube, can be unilateral or bilateral
Uterine artery embolization	Minimally invasive surgery to inject embolic agents into uterine arteries to block blood supply to uterine fibroids
Vaginectomy	Removal of vagina, may be partial or total
Vulvectomy	Removal of part or all the vulva

significant negative effects on quality of life. AUB is defined as acute or chronic. *Acute AUB* is an episode of uterine bleeding (in a nonpregnant female of reproductive age) that requires immediate treatment. *Chronic AUB* is abnormal uterine bleeding that has been present for most of the past 6 months. The most common forms of AUB are heavy menstrual bleeding, intermenstrual bleeding (between periods), and irregular bleeding (frequent or infrequent periods). Other terms we have used to describe AUB include dysfunctional uterine bleeding (DUB), menorrhagia, and metrorrhagia. Though we no longer recommended their use, you may still hear them used in some settings.

The absence of menses *(amenorrhea)* is a common menstrual abnormality. *Primary amenorrhea* refers to the failure of menstrual cycles to begin by 15 years of age. *Secondary amenorrhea* occurs when menstrual cycles stop for more than 3 months after previously regular menstrual cycles or more than 6 months in those with irregular menses.

Etiology and Pathophysiology

There are many different problems that cause AUB. The most common causes are outlined in the PALM-COEIN classification system for AUB (Fig. 58.3). PALM stands for common structural causes of bleeding: polyps, adenomyosis, leiomyoma, and malignancy or hyperplasia. The COEIN acronym represents common nonstructural causes. Those are coagulopathy, ovulatory dysfunction (including hypothalamic-pituitary-ovarian axis disorders and polycystic ovary syndrome), endometrial, iatrogenic, and not otherwise classified. AUB may also be related to medication use such as hormone contraception.

Clinical Manifestations

AUB is defined in contrast to normal menstruation (see Chapter 55). Bleeding that is outside the norms of frequency, duration, volume, and timing is classified as abnormal. For example, normal menstruation occurs every 21 to 35 days, lasts no more than 7 days, and has a blood loss that does not interfere with quality of life.

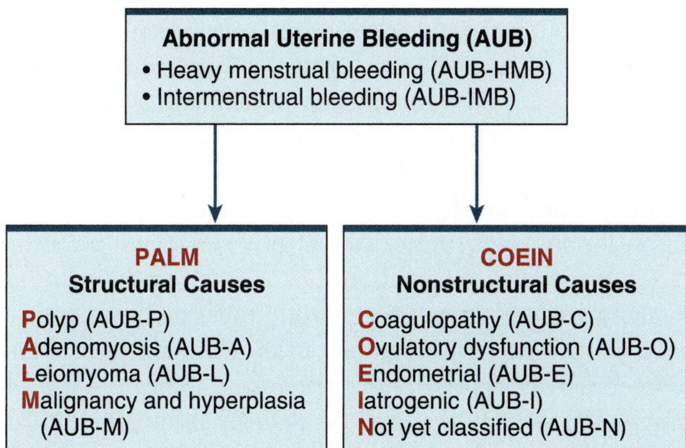

Fig. 58.3 PALM-COIEN classification system for abnormal uterine bleeding. (Used with permission from Munro MG, Critchley HO, Broder MS, et al: FIGO classification system [PALM–OEIN] for causes of AUB in nongravid females of reproductive age, *Int J Gynecol Obstet* 11:3, 2011.)

Diagnostic Studies

Evaluation of AUB begins with the history, including detailed menstrual, sexual, gynecologic, and obstetric histories. Physical assessment should determine rule out other (nonuterine) potential sources of bleeding. Pelvic examination is useful to assess for any masses or structural problems. Laboratory tests may be done to assess for pregnancy, sexually transmitted infections, hormone imbalances, coagulation problems, or endocrine disorders. Additional tests may include cervical cancer screening (Pap test), pelvic or transvaginal ultrasound, endometrial biopsy, and hysteroscopy or saline infusion sonohysterography (SIS).

Interprofessional Care

The treatment depends on the cause (Table 58.8).[7] Treatment goals may be to improve quality of life or prevent further complications such as cancer and severe anemia. Future fertility goals are important in guiding the treatment plan. Care for *heavy menstrual bleeding (HMB)* focuses on medical or surgical treatments. Drug therapy for HMB includes hormone therapy such as OCPs, NSAIDs, and tranexamic acid (Lysteda). IUDs are another option for HMB. Surgical therapy for HMB includes D&C, endometrial ablation, uterine artery embolization, or hysterectomy (Table 58.7). Medical and surgical treatment options include hormone therapy, antibiotics for suspected infections, and polyp removal (polypectomy).

Nursing care focuses on patient teaching. Teach about the menstrual cycle and characteristics of normal bleeding to help patients identify variations (see Table 55.1). Encourage patients to report excessively heavy bleeding, passing of clots, or bleeding of extended duration. Nutrition teaching is appropriate, especially for adolescents and those at risk for anemia. Ensure that patients understand the cause of their bleeding and the various treatment options. Follow up to assess treatment effectiveness and improvement in symptoms and quality of life.

MENOPAUSE

Menopause is the cessation of menstruation. *Natural menopause* is the permanent cessation of menstrual periods. It is diagnosed retrospectively after 12 months of amenorrhea without any other suspected cause. The median age for menopause is 51 years, but it can occur normally between 40 and 58 years of age. The menopausal transition is known as **perimenopause**. Perimenopause often begins about 4 years before the *final menstrual period (FMP)*. Menopause and perimenopausal symptoms are a major health focus for females during midlife. These include menstrual cycle and endocrine changes as well as mood symptoms and hot flashes. The Stages of Reproductive Aging Workshop (STRAW) +10 System

TABLE 58.8 Interprofessional Care

Abnormal Uterine Bleeding

Diagnostic Assessment

- History
  - Detailed menstrual history
  - Bleeding patterns, perceived severity of bleeding (clots, soaking through clothing)
- Physical assessment
  - Inspection of the source of bleeding
  - Pelvic examination
  - Evaluation for obesity/hirsutism (suggestive of PCOS)
- Laboratory tests (as indicated)
  - Pregnancy test
  - CBC
  - Thyroid-stimulating hormone (TSH)
  - STI screening
  - Screening for bleeding disorders
  - Hormone levels (e.g., FSH, LH, prolactin, testosterone)
  - Liver and renal function tests
- Imaging studies and tissue sampling
  - Endometrial biopsy
  - Hysteroscopy
  - Transvaginal/pelvic ultrasound
  - Saline infusion sonohysterography

Management

Based on the cause, may include:

- Hormone therapy
- NSAIDs
- Tranexamic acid (Lysteda)
- Antibiotics
- Surgery
  - D&C
  - Endometrial ablation
  - Uterine artery embolization
  - Hysterectomy

describes reproductive aging in females (Fig. 58.4). Table 58.9 lists common menopause terms.

Etiology and Pathophysiology

Natural menopause occurs in response to normal physiologic changes of aging in the hypothalamic-pituitary-ovarian axis. Fluctuations in hormone levels cause perimenopausal symptoms. Menopause can be induced. *Induced menopause* occurs after surgery to remove the ovaries or due to side effects of chemotherapy, radiation therapy, or other drugs. *Primary ovarian insufficiency* is permanent or temporary menopause that occurs at less than 40 years of age. Causes include drugs, chromosome abnormalities, or health problems such as endocrine or autoimmune disorders.

Clinical Manifestations

Perimenopause is characterized by erratic hormone fluctuations and irregular menstrual cycles. Common symptoms are outlined in Table 58.10. The experience of perimenopause varies widely. Many females have vasomotor changes such as hot flashes, experienced as an intense heat sensation. Sleep disruptions, mood changes, and decreased sexual function are common. Some find perimenopausal symptoms disrupt their quality of life and well-being, while others may report no bothersome symptoms. In postmenopause, estrogen and progesterone deficiency increases the risk for cardiovascular disease, urogenital atrophy, bone mineral density loss, and dementia.

Diagnostic Studies

Menopause is a retrospective diagnosis after 12 consecutive months of amenorrhea. A diagnosis of perimenopause is based on clinical symptoms. A detailed history, including menstrual and sexual histories, and physical assessment guide diagnosis. A symptom diary may be useful. Laboratory tests are not needed in females over age 45 with typical perimenopausal symptoms. Some HCPs measure follicle-stimulating hormone (FSH). However, FSH varies widely throughout the menstrual cycle and is not a reliable indicator of perimenopause. HCPs should assess for other potential causes of clinical manifestations such as pregnancy or thyroid disease. Further assessment is needed in females under 40 years of age or those with atypical symptoms. This may include laboratory assessment of hormone levels or diagnostic imaging such as pelvic ultrasound.

CHECK YOUR PRACTICE

In an outpatient clinic, your 58-year-old patient is reporting symptoms of menopause. She tells you, "I keep getting hot flashes and am so fatigued. I just can't function like this anymore."

- How would you respond?
- What can she do to improve her symptoms?

Interprofessional Care

Treatment options include options to target specific symptoms and systemic effects. The Menopause Society has patient information, tools, and a mobile app to help patients and HCPs engage in patient-centered care around treatment decisions.[8] Hormone therapy is an option. Estrogen comes in many forms including pills, patches, vaginal preparations, and topical creams, lotions, and sprays. Patient preference and symptoms often inform which preparation they use. In females who have not had a hysterectomy, progesterone must be given with estrogen to prevent endometrial cancer from estrogen-related endometrial hyperplasia. Progesterone comes in several different forms including oral or vaginal administrations and an IUD. Estrogen and progesterone may be given as a combination oral or transdermal therapy.

A patient-centered approach is important. We need to address patients' needs and preferences against the potential risks from hormone therapy. Hormone therapy can reduce

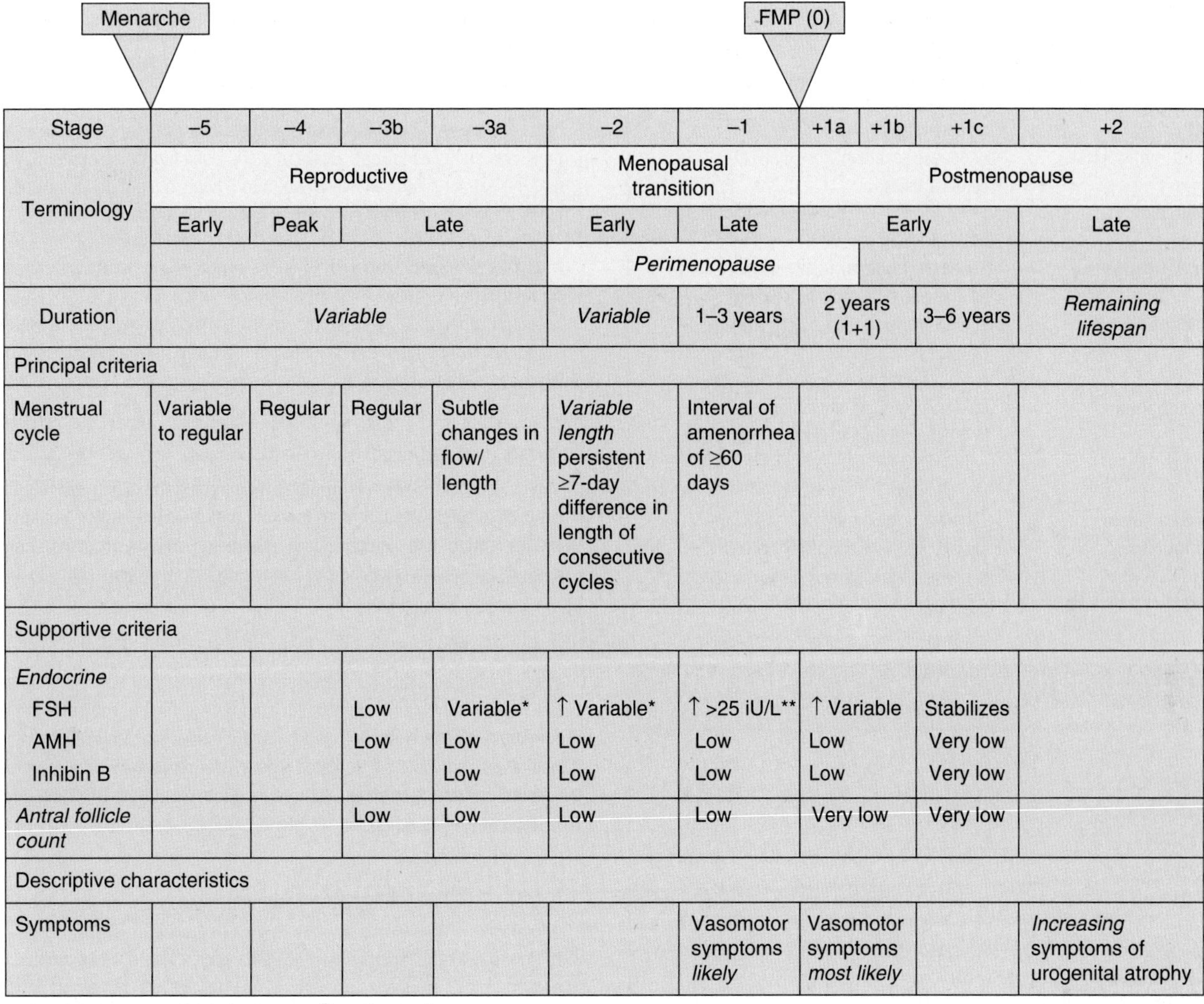

Stage	−5	−4	−3b	−3a	−2	−1	+1a	+1b	+1c	+2
Terminology	Reproductive				Menopausal transition		Postmenopause			
	Early	Peak	Late		Early	Late	Early			Late
					Perimenopause					
Duration	*Variable*				*Variable*	1–3 years	2 years (1+1)		3–6 years	*Remaining lifespan*
Principal criteria										
Menstrual cycle	Variable to regular	Regular	Regular	Subtle changes in flow/length	*Variable length* persistent $\geq$7-day difference in length of consecutive cycles	Interval of amenorrhea of $\geq$60 days				
Supportive criteria										
Endocrine										
FSH			Low	Variable*	$\uparrow$ Variable*	$\uparrow$ >25 iU/L**	$\uparrow$ Variable		Stabilizes	
AMH			Low	Low	Low	Low	Low		Very low	
Inhibin B				Low	Low	Low	Low		Very low	
Antral follicle count			Low	Low	Low	Low	Very low		Very low	
Descriptive characteristics										
Symptoms						Vasomotor symptoms *likely*	Vasomotor symptoms *most likely*			*Increasing* symptoms of urogenital atrophy

* Blood draw on cycle days 2–5. $\uparrow$ = elevated.
** Approximate expected level based on assays using current international pituitary standard.

Fig. 58.4 Stages of Reproductive Aging Workshop + 10 staging system for reproductive aging in females. (From Harlow SD, Gass M, Hall JE, et al: Executive summary of the Stages of Reproductive Aging Workshop + 10: addressing the unfinished agenda of staging reproductive aging, *J Clin Endocrinol Metab* 2012. © 2012, The Endocrine Society.)

symptoms and improve quality of life. However, there is an increased risk of breast and endometrial cancer and cardiovascular disease. Assess for contraindications to hormone therapy such as a history of breast cancer, coronary heart disease, stroke, thromboembolic disorders, or liver disease. Females who are not candidates for hormone therapy or want alternatives may try nonhormone drug treatment options. These include antidepressants (SSRIs or SNRIs), gabapentin, and fezolinetant (Veozah). There is no evidence to support the safety and efficacy of herb, compounded, or complementary and alternative therapies for perimenopausal symptoms.

❖ NURSING MANAGEMENT: MENOPAUSE

Menopause is a time of great physical and psychologic transition. Many females have symptoms for years during the perimenopausal period, while others transition without any difficulty. Menopause may be occurring simultaneously with role changes in personal and professional life. Many females will not seek treatment for common menopausal symptoms such as hot flashes, sleep disturbances, or mood changes. Asking about midlife health issues, including menopausal symptoms, during routine health encounters can help identify concerns.

Provide teaching about menopause and common symptoms (Box 58.1). Provide support for physical, psychologic, and emotional effects of menopause. Discuss lifestyle changes that can improve symptoms and quality of life. Encourage smoking cessation. Suggest wearing breathable or moisture-wicking fabrics and layered clothing to improve comfort during hot flashes. Support stress management and reduction strategies. Cognitive behavior therapy may be helpful.

TABLE 58.9 Menopause Terminology

Term	Definition
Final menstrual period (FMP)	Last menstrual period; the point of menopause
Induced menopause	Menopause resulting from medical or surgical therapy
Menopause	A point in time 12 consecutive months after the FMP
Natural menopause	Menopause resulting from normal, spontaneous, physiologic changes
Perimenopause	Period of transition before menopause. Often lasts around 4 years. Associated with fluctuations in hormone levels
Postmenopause	Period of time after menopause. Characterized by symptoms associated with decreased estrogen and progesterone
Primary ovarian insufficiency	Temporary or permanent menopause at <40 years of age. May be called premature menopause

TABLE 58.10 Symptoms Associated With Perimenopause

- Changes in menstrual bleeding patterns
- Depression
- Headache
- Joint pain
- Libido
- Memory loss
- Poor concentration
- Sexual dysfunction
- Sleep problems
- Urinary frequency/urgency
- Vaginal dryness
- Vasomotor symptoms (e.g., hot flashes)

BOX 58.1 EVIDENCE-BASED PRACTICE

Sleep and Quality of Life in Menopause

You are caring for a 57-year-old female who presents to the clinic seeking help for fatigue. She states that she feels like she wants to "sleep all the time" and struggles to keep awake at work. Upon further assessment, you find that the patient sleeps an average of 5 to 6 hours a night and awakens 2 to 3 times a night due to feeling warm or getting up to urinate.

Making Clinical Decisions

Synthesis of Best Available Evidence

Research shows that sleep problems are common during menopause due to decreases in estrogen and magnesium. Patients may experience insomnia, increased daytime sleepiness, multiple awakenings, and strange movements. The poor quality of sleep can negatively influence quality of life.

Clinician Expertise

Nurses can play a key role in understanding and managing the relationship between menopause and sleep quality. Asking about midlife health issues during routine health encounters can help identify concerns. Providing teaching about sleep hygiene and lifestyle recommendations can help improve sleep quality and menopause symptoms.

Patient Preferences and Values

After further discussion, you recommend that the patient begin a sleep journal and keep a consistent schedule for sleep/wake times. You refer her to an evening menopause support group where relaxation techniques, including meditation and yoga, are featured. Lastly, you recommend she avoid screen time an hour before bedtime. You communicate this to the HCP, and a follow-up appointment is scheduled for 8 weeks.

Implications for Nursing Practice

1. What nonpharmacological interventions can you recommend for the patient?
2. How would you assess sleep quality?

Reference for Evidence

Hadiabad SFN, Abdollahi M, Sadrzadeh SM, et al: The relationship between sleep quality and quality of life among postmenopausal women, *JCCNC* 9:47, 2023.

Review the risks, benefits, and alternatives of various treatment options. Ensure patients are getting adequate intake or supplements of calcium and vitamin D to reduce risk of bone fractures (see Table 68.16). Encourage health promotion measures such as depression screening, bone density screening, mammography, and ways to reduce risk of cardiovascular disease.

GENITAL TRACT INFECTIONS

LOWER GENITAL TRACT INFECTIONS

Lower genital tract infections include infections resulting from a disruption in the vaginal microbiome and STIs. The *vaginal microbiome* contains microorganisms like yeast and healthy bacteria that protect against infection by maintaining an acidic environment. Inflammation of the vagina, known as *vaginitis,* can occur from a disruption of the vaginal flora. Vaginal infections associated with vaginitis are shown in Table 58.11. STIs are discussed in Chapter 57. If not treated, lower genital tract infections can lead to long-term health problems.

Etiology and Pathophysiology

Common problems associated with vaginitis are bacterial vaginosis, vulvovaginal candidiasis, and STIs such as trichomoniasis. Exposure to irritating substances and foreign bodies (such as tampons or condoms) left in the vagina can disrupt the vaginal microbiome and cause lower genital infections.

Bacterial vaginosis (commonly called "BV") is the most common infection. It is characterized by a disruption in the microbiota shifting away from healthy *Lactobacillus* species toward other organisms such as anaerobic bacteria, leading to a rise in vaginal pH. Bacteria causing BV can be transmitted by

TABLE 58.11 Vaginal Infections Associated With Vaginitis

Infection	Manifestations	Common Treatment Options
Bacterial vaginosis (bacterial infection)	"Fishy" odor Gray or white vaginal discharge	Oral or vaginal antibiotics • clindamycin (Cleocin) • metronidazole (Flagyl) • tinidazole (Tindamax)
Trichomonas vaginalis (protozoan infection)	Genital itching and inflammation Dysuria Frothy, thin, yellowish-greenish vaginal discharge Deep red or pink cervix and vagina ("strawberry cervix")	Oral and vaginal agents • metronidazole (Flagyl) • tinidazole (Tindamax) • secnidazole (Solosec) Treat partner(s)
Vulvovaginal candidiasis (yeast infection)	Vaginal itching Red, swollen vulva Thick, white, curdy vaginal discharge	Oral or vaginal antifungals • butoconazole (Gynazole) • clotrimazole • fluconazole (Diflucan) • miconazole (Monistat)

sexual activity, especially receptive oral sex. Vaginal douching, smoking, and having an STI are risk factors for BV.

The second most common cause of vaginitis symptoms is vulvovaginal candidiasis. *Vulvovaginal candidiasis* is caused by an overgrowth of *Candida,* a naturally occurring part of the vaginal flora. The cause of the disruption of normal vaginal flora is not always known. Certain drugs (e.g., broad-spectrum antibiotics), behaviors (e.g., vaginal douching), and chronic problems (e.g., diabetes) increase the risk of vulvovaginal candidiasis.

STIs such as *trichomoniasis,* a protozoan infection, can cause vaginitis. STIs are passed from person to person through sexual contact. They are transmitted through body fluids such as blood, semen, and vaginal fluids. High-risk sexual behaviors, such as having multiple sex partners, increase the risk for STIs. Common STIs are listed in Table 58.12 and discussed in Chapter 57.

TABLE 58.12 Common STIs

- Bacterial vaginosis
- Chlamydia
- Gonorrhea
- Hepatitis
- Herpes simplex virus
- HIV
- Human papillomavirus (HPV)
- Pelvic inflammatory disease (PID)
- Pubic lice or crabs
- Scabies
- Syphilis
- Trichomoniasis
- Zika virus

Clinical Manifestations

The manifestations depend on the type of infection. Many patients are asymptomatic. Vaginal discharge that is abnormal in color, quantity, odor, or consistency is a common symptom. For example, a "fishy" odor is a common symptom of bacterial vaginosis. Discharge that is thick, white, and curdy is characteristic of vulvovaginal candidiasis. Many patients have itching, burning, or irritation. Pain during intercourse or urination is common.

Interprofessional and Nursing Management

Assessment starts with the history, including a sexual history. Routine screening for vaginitis infections is not recommended in asymptomatic people. For patients with lower genital tract infection symptoms, assessment should include speculum examination. Evaluating vaginal secretions by pH testing, microscopic examination, culture, and/or other laboratory tests aids in diagnosis. Treatment options depend on the type of infection. Screening and treatment for STIs are discussed in Chapter 57. A follow-up visit is often recommended to evaluate treatment effectiveness and teach sexual health and contraception.

Teach patients about behavior and lifestyle measures to reduce the risk for infection. This includes keeping the vulvar area dry and avoiding products like harsh laundry detergents, scented menstrual products, or spermicides that can cause irritation. Discuss how to clean the vulva and vagina to reduce infections and avoiding douching. Provide education about any recommended treatments, such as how to insert vaginal applicators for topical therapies. Review sexual practices to prevent infections, such as condom use.

PELVIC INFLAMMATORY DISEASE

Pelvic inflammatory disease (PID) is a clinical syndrome that includes a spectrum of infectious and inflammatory diseases of the upper genital tract. Ascending organisms cause inflammation in the endometrium, fallopian tubes, ovaries, and pelvic peritoneum (Fig. 58.5). There are about 1 million cases of PID each year in the United States. PID is most common among sexually active young females.

Etiology and Pathophysiology

PID is caused by an infectious organism ascending from the vagina or upper urogenital tract. Untreated sexually transmitted *Neisseria gonorrhoeae* and *Chlamydia trachomatis* are common causes, as are microbes associated with bacterial vaginosis. Organisms can ascend past the endocervical barrier through normal processes like menstruation or gynecologic procedures (e.g., IUD insertion). Other risk factors include high-risk sexual behaviors, young age, vaginal douching, recent cervical manipulation, and history of PID.

Clinical Manifestations

The classic presentation of acute PID is pelvic or lower abdominal pain with tenderness in the cervix, uterus, or adnexa. Pain varies from mild to severe. The pain often occurs with intercourse and urination. Movement, such as walking, can increase the pain. Spotting after intercourse and purulent cervical or vaginal discharge may occur. Fever and chills may be present.

Complications

If not diagnosed and treated promptly, PID can cause serious complications. These include infertility, ectopic pregnancy, chronic pelvic pain, or tubo-ovarian abscess (TOA). These complications result from scarring, adhesions, or obstruction of the fallopian tubes. TOA or perihepatitis (Fitz-Hugh-Curtis Syndrome) are potential immediate and serious risks of untreated PID.

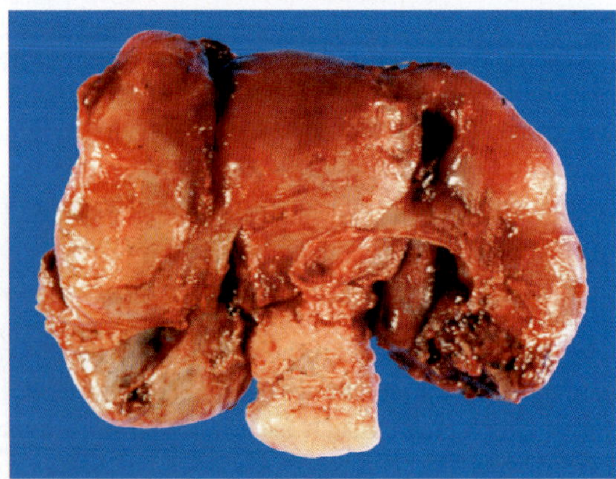

Fig. 58.5 Pelvic inflammatory disease (PID). (From Kumar V, Abbas AK, Aster JC, et al: *Robbins & Cotran pathologic basis of disease,* ed 8, Philadelphia, 2010, Saunders.)

Diagnostic Studies

A health and sexual history and physical assessment are important to explore the presenting symptoms and rule out other causes of abdominal or pelvic pain. Physical assessment will include abdominal, pelvic, and speculum examinations. No laboratory tests are needed to begin treatment. Microscopic examination of vaginal discharge and testing for gonorrhea and chlamydia can support the diagnosis. Testing for other STIs such as HIV is recommended. A pregnancy test is done to rule out a possible ectopic pregnancy. Ultrasound, endometrial biopsy, or laparoscopy may be useful to rule out other potential complications. Some HCPs may order blood tests, such as a complete blood count (CBC), erythrocyte sedimentation rate, or C-reactive protein.

Interprofessional and Nursing Management

Treatment is started promptly, based on the symptoms and history. PID is usually treated on an outpatient basis with a combination of broad-spectrum antibiotics (see Table 15.8). Antibiotic regimens recommended by the Centers for Disease Control and Prevention (CDC) are outlined in Chapter 57. Symptoms should improve within 72 hours of starting treatment. Hospitalization may be needed for patients with suspected PID who do not respond within 48 to 72 hours, are pregnant, or have severe symptoms such as high fever. In those instances, IV antibiotics, further tests, or surgery may be needed. Recent sexual partners should be treated presumptively for gonorrhea and chlamydia.

Prevention, early recognition, and prompt treatment can prevent PID and associated complications. Data that you should obtain from patients with PID are outlined in Table 58.13. For hospitalized patients, you have a key role in implementing drug therapy and monitoring health status. Record vital signs. Note the character, amount, color, and odor of any vaginal discharge. Assess pain and provide analgesics and supportive measures to decrease pain.

Teaching about PID is important. Provide anticipatory guidance about symptom improvement. Stress the importance of completing the prescribed therapy. Advise them to abstain from sexual intercourse until treatment is completed and sexual partners have been treated. Provide teaching about sexual practices and health screening to reduce transmission of STIs in the future.

BENIGN GYNECOLOGIC PROBLEMS

Many benign problems affect the female reproductive organs. While they are benign in that they are not life-threatening or cancerous, they can still significantly affect quality of life. Problems that affect the skin, such as vulvar dermatoses, are discussed in Chapter 55. This section focuses on those benign conditions affecting the cervix, uterus, or adnexa.

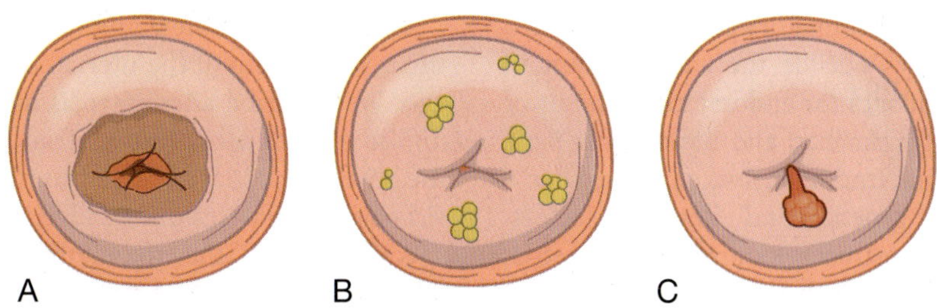

Fig. 58.6 Benign cervical lesions. (A) Cervical ectropion. (B) Nabothian cyst. (C) Cervical polyp.

TABLE 58.13 NURSING ASSESSMENT

PID

Subjective Data

Important Health Information

Health history: Previous STIs or PID. Recent IUD insertion, termination of pregnancy, or gynecologic procedure

Sexual history: Age of first sexual encounter. Number and sex of sexual partners. Exposure to partner with STIs. Types of sexual activities. Use of condoms and other preventive measures for STIs

Medications: Hormone agents, including contraception

Allergies: Allergies to antibiotics or other drugs

Functional Health Patterns

Health perception–health management: Malaise

Nutritional-metabolic: Nausea, vomiting; chills, fever

Elimination: Urinary frequency, urgency

Cognitive-perceptual: Lower abdominal pain, pelvic pain, low back pain, onset of pain just after a menstrual cycle; dyspareunia, dysuria, vulvar pruritus

Sexuality-reproductive: Abnormal vaginal discharge, unscheduled vaginal bleeding

Objective Data

Reproductive

Mucopurulent cervicitis, vulvar maceration, vaginal discharge (heavy and purulent to thin and mucoid), cervical motion tenderness, uterine or adnexal tenderness. Inflammatory masses on palpation

Possible Diagnostic Findings

White blood cells on wet mount (saline microscopy of vaginal fluid), ↑ erythrocyte sedimentation rate, laboratory confirmation of gonorrheal or chlamydial infection, abscess or inflammation on ultrasonography

CERVICAL PROBLEMS

The cervix may have benign growth or lesions such as cervical ectropion, cysts, or polyps. These may be seen with a speculum examination (Fig. 58.6). *Cervical ectropion* occurs when the cervix becomes slightly everted, exposing underlying cells that may be more sensitive or prone to bleeding. This condition is not due to underlying pathology. It is common in adolescents and pregnancy.

Nabothian cysts (mucus or epithelial inclusion cysts) are a common finding on speculum examination. They are caused by mucus-producing cells being covered by epithelial cellular growth. Nabothian cysts do not usually cause symptoms or require treatment. They may resolve spontaneously.

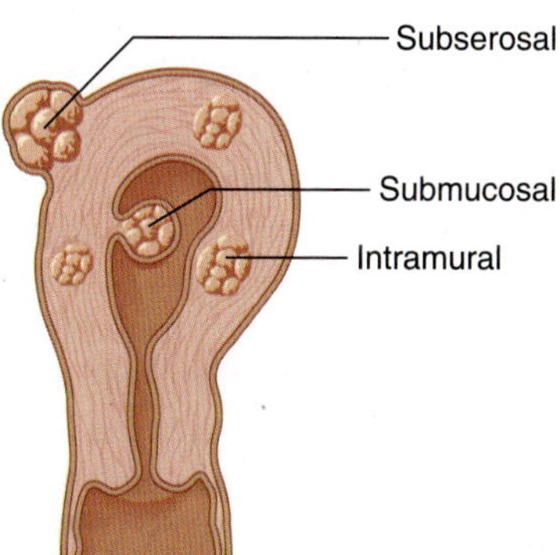

Fig. 58.7 Uterine fibroids. (From McCance KL, Huether SE: *Pathophysiology: the biologic basis for disease in adults and children*, ed 6, St. Louis, 2010, Mosby.)

Cervical polyps are benign growths that may be found during routine speculum examination. Polyps are usually red or purple and small, measuring less than 3 cm in length. Their cause is not known but hormone factors may play a role. Polyps may be removed if they are large or cause complications, such as bleeding after intercourse. Other cervical problems include cervicitis (inflammation), trauma (lacerations), condylomas (HPV infection), and cervical cancer.

UTERINE PROBLEMS

The most common benign uterine problems are uterine fibroids, endometriosis, and adenomyosis. Uterine fibroids (or leiomyomas, myomas) are noncancerous smooth-muscle tumors.[9] They appear most often in females of reproductive age. We think they are caused by hormone and genetic factors. Fibroids are classified as either subserosal, intermural, or submucosal based on their location (Fig. 58.7).

Many patients with fibroids have no symptoms. Others will have pelvic pain, AUB, or infertility. On physical assessment, the uterus may be enlarged or irregularly shaped. Pelvic imaging is used to confirm the diagnosis. The approach to treatment depends on a patient's age, severity of symptoms, and desire for pregnancy. Expectant management may be appropriate since most fibroids reduce in size after menopause. Drug therapy, such as hormone contraception or gonadotropin-releasing hormone (GnRH) agonists, can reduce bleeding and pain. Surgery such as removal of uterine fibroids (myomectomy), hysterectomy, or uterine artery embolization may be used for severe symptoms affecting quality of life or fertility.

Endometriosis is a benign inflammatory condition in which endometrial tissue accumulates outside the endometrium of the uterus. The most frequent sites for endometriosis are in or near the ovaries, uterosacral ligaments, and uterovesical peritoneum (Fig. 58.8). We think endometriosis is caused by a combination of hormone, genetic, and immune factors. Retrograde menstruation (menstrual blood and endometrial tissue flow backward into the pelvis during menses) may be a factor.

Endometriosis may be suspected based on manifestations of infertility, vaginal bleeding, and pain. Pain may be chronic or occur during menses, intercourse, urination, or defecation. Tenderness or nodules in the pelvic region may be noted on physical assessment. Some patients may not have any symptoms but are diagnosed with endometriosis during fertility treatment or gynecologic surgery. Laparoscopy with biopsy is needed for a definitive diagnosis. Imaging such as ultrasound and MRI may be used to aid in the diagnosis.

Management includes both medical and surgical approaches. The treatment depends on a patient's age, desire for pregnancy, severity of symptoms, and extent and location of the disease. Drug therapy is used to relieve pain, reduce inflammation, and suppress endometrial tissue growth. Common agents include NSAIDs, hormone contraceptives, aromatase inhibitors, and GnRH analogs (e.g., leuprolide).

The only cure for endometriosis is surgical removal of all endometrial tissue and adhesions. For females with infertility who desire pregnancy, efforts are made to restore pelvic anatomy to allow the ovaries and fallopian tubes to work better. Therapy may involve removing implants blocking the fallopian tube. Adhesions are removed from the tubes, ovaries, and pelvic structures.

DRUG ALERT

Leuprolide

- Assess for pregnancy before starting therapy.
- Monitor for dysrhythmias and palpitations.
- Teach patient to use nonhormone contraceptive measures during therapy.

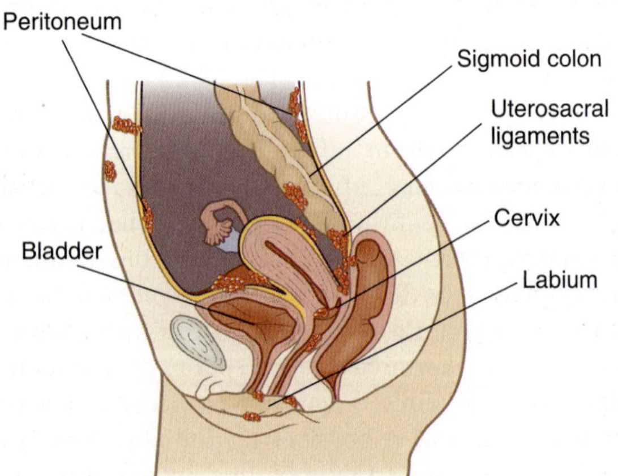

Fig. 58.8 Common sites of endometriosis.

Adenomyosis is the benign growth of endometrial tissue in the myometrium of the uterus. It is most common in middle age. We describe adenomyosis as either diffuse or focal. In *diffuse adenomyosis,* endometrial tissue is found throughout the myometrial layer of the uterus. *Focal adenomyosis* consists of nodular lesions (called adenomyomas) confined to specific areas of the myometrium. The growth of endometrial tissue causes uterine enlargement and can lead to painful and heavy menstruation, pain during intercourse, or chronic pelvic pain. Diagnosis is made through pelvic ultrasound or MRI. Adenomyosis is often treated with hysterectomy. Uterine artery embolization or ablation can improve symptoms in some patients. Hormone contraceptives and GnRH agonists are options for those who prefer nonsurgical approaches.

POLYCYSTIC OVARY SYNDROME

Polycystic ovary syndrome (PCOS) is an endocrine disorder that affects menstruation and fertility. This syndrome is characterized by menstrual irregularity, ovulatory dysfunction, and hyperandrogenism. It is the most common cause of infertility. The cause of PCOS is not known. The underlying pathophysiology includes excess androgen production in the ovaries, often accompanied by insulin resistance. There are many long-term health consequences associated with PCOS. Patients with PCOS are at increased risk for diabetes, cardiovascular disease, mood disorders, and endometrial cancer.

Clinical Manifestations

Manifestations include signs of hyperandrogenism such as hirsutism and acne, irregular menstrual cycles, and obesity. Amenorrhea or oligomenorrhea and anovulation are common. Signs of insulin resistance, such as metabolic syndrome, may be present.

Diagnostic Studies

PCOS should be considered in a female of reproductive age based on the presence of classical manifestations of irregular menstrual cycles, such as infrequent menstruation or anovulation, with signs of hyperandrogenism. Laboratory tests and pelvic imaging are not needed to make a diagnosis. Testing may be useful to identify high androgen levels in the absence of symptoms. These diagnostic studies can also rule out other potential causes of symptoms such as pregnancy or nonclassic congenital adrenal hyperplasia. Polycystic ovaries may be visible on ultrasound, although this is not required for diagnosis (Fig. 58.9).

Interprofessional Care

The approach to treating PCOS depends on the symptoms and desire for pregnancy. For overweight patients, weight loss is recommended and improves ovulatory dysfunction. Hormone

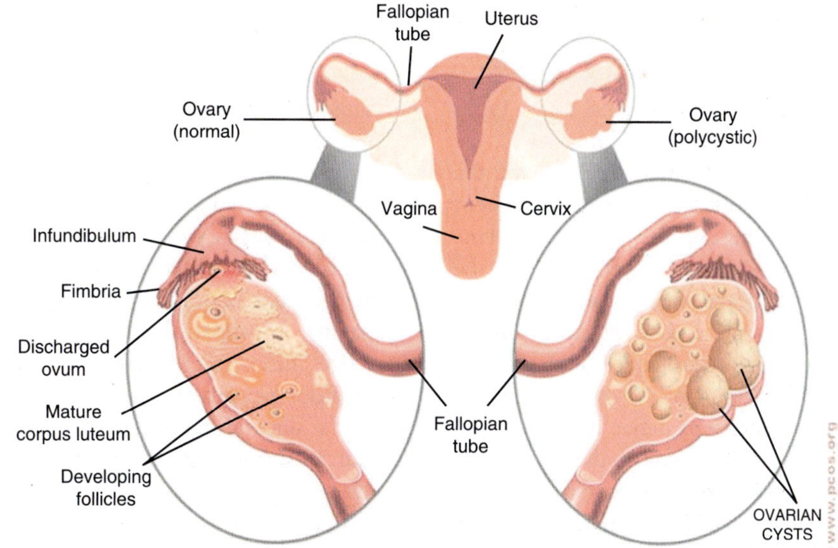

Fig. 58.9 PCOS. (From Thakur D, Singh SS, Tripathi M: Effect of yoga on polycystic ovarian syndrome: a systematic review, *J Bodyw Mov Ther* 27:281, 2021.)

contraceptives are often used in patients not pursuing pregnancy. Medications such as spironolactone (Aldactone), letrozole (Femara), eflornithine hydrochloride, or metformin may be prescribed to manage associated symptoms. Resources such as the National PCOS Association's PCOS Challenge may be helpful to provide support and resources to patients with PCOS.[10]

DRUG ALERT

Spironolactone

- Check for drug interactions.
- Monitor for hypotension and electrolyte imbalances.
- Discuss the importance of a low-potassium diet.

Uterus

Ovarian cyst

Fig. 58.10 Large ovarian cyst. (McPherson MBA: *Colour atlas of obstetrics and gynecology*, London, 1994, Mosby.)

ADNEXAL MASSES

Adnexal masses are those found in the ovary, fallopian tube, or connective tissue. There are many different causes of adnexal masses. HCPs need to consider and assess for serious conditions such as ectopic pregnancy, TOA, or cancer. The most common benign adnexal masses are ovarian cysts and benign tumors.

Follicular or *corpus luteal cysts* are associated with normal, physiologic ovarian function (see Chapter 55). Occasionally, these cysts may become enlarged or painful (Fig. 58.10). Diagnosis is made by ultrasound or MRI. Cysts usually resolve spontaneously. In rare instances, complications such as rupture or hemorrhage may cause pain and bleeding requiring surgical treatment.

Adnexal masses can also be caused by benign tumors, such as dermoid cysts or endometriomas. A dermoid cyst (teratoma) is an ovarian germ cell tumor. Patients with teratomas are often asymptomatic. The cysts may be identified incidentally on pelvic examination or imaging. Surgical removal of the cyst (cystectomy) is recommended since they may become cancerous. Endometriomas are a type of benign mass resulting from growth of endometrial tissue in the adnexal region. They are a form of endometriosis.

An acute condition associated with an adnexal mass is ovarian or adnexal torsion. This happens when an ovary or fallopian tube becomes abnormally rotated and partially or completely cut off from its blood supply. Torsion can cause pelvic pain, flank pain, and nausea and vomiting. Ovarian mass is often present on pelvic ultrasound. However, false-positive diagnosis based on ultrasound is common. Definitive diagnosis is made through visualization of the rotated ovary or tube during surgery. Treatment for ovarian or fallopian tube torsion is surgery. HCPs may remove or drain the cyst, manually rotate the ovary or tube (detorsion), or remove the ovary or tube (salpingectomy or oophorectomy).

PELVIC ORGAN PROLAPSE

Pelvic organ prolapse is a common, benign condition in which the pelvic organs herniate to or beyond the vaginal walls. Types of prolapse include *cystocele* or urethrocele (prolapse of the bladder) (Fig. 58.11), *rectocele* or enterocele (bulging of the rectum in the vagina) (Fig. 58.12), and *uterine prolapse* (descent of the uterus into the vaginal canal). We describe uterine prolapse by degrees (Fig. 58.13). In first-degree prolapse, the cervix rests in the lower part of the vagina. Second-degree prolapse means the cervix is at the vaginal opening. Third-degree prolapse means the uterus protrudes through the introitus.

The cause of pelvic organ prolapse is pelvic floor dysfunction from weak pelvic floor muscles or connective tissue. Patients may have physiologic pelvic organ prolapse as they age. Other risk factors include having multiple pregnancies, history of vaginal births, obesity, connective tissue disorders, and chronic constipation.

Some patients with pelvic organ prolapse have no symptoms. For others, this condition can be uncomfortable and limit their quality of life and daily functioning. Pelvic pressure or bulging is a common concern. Other manifestations are difficulty with urination and defecation, decreased sexual function, and backache.

Evaluation starts with the history and physical assessment, including abdominal and pelvic examination. The assessment includes evaluation of pelvic floor function. The Pelvic Organ Prolapse Quantification (POP-Q) tool from the American Urogynecologic Society is used to assess and grade the stage of prolapse.[11]

A patient-centered approach is important to identify the severity and impact of symptoms and goals for treatment. Treatment is often unnecessary in the absence of bothersome symptoms such as pelvic pain/pressure, sexual dysfunction, or bowel or bladder dysfunction. In those cases, provide patient teaching and reassurance. Lifestyle changes such as weight loss, managing constipation, and eliminating heavy lifting can improve minor symptoms. Nonsurgical treatments include pelvic floor physical therapy (see Table 50.18) or vaginal pessaries (a silicone supportive device inserted into the vagina, similar to a diaphragm). When these interventions are ineffective or symptoms are severe, surgery may be needed. Surgical options include hysterectomy, suspension of prolapsed organs, and repair of vaginal walls.

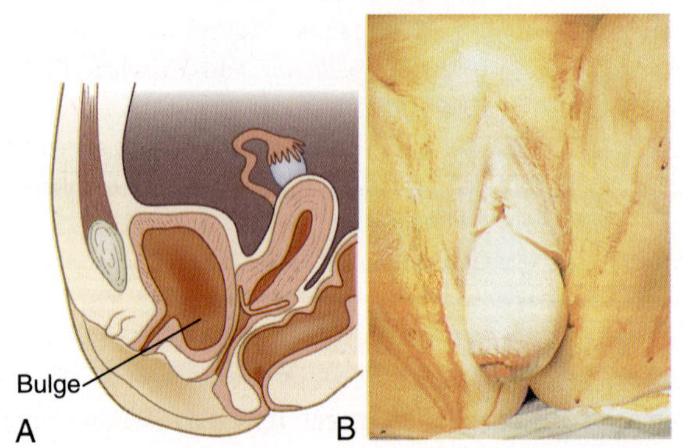

Fig. 58.11 (A) Cystocele. (B) Bladder has prolapsed into the vagina.

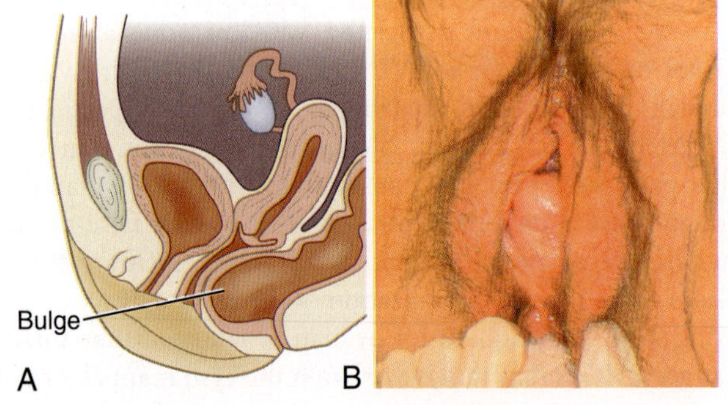

Fig. 58.12 (A) Rectocele. (B) Rectum has prolapsed into the vagina. (B, From Townsend CM: *Sabiston textbook of surgery*, ed 18, St. Louis, 2009, Mosby.)

VAGINAL FISTULA

A *vaginal fistula* is an abnormal opening between the vagina and another organ, such as the bladder or rectum. Fistulas can be caused by gynecologic surgery, cancer, radiation, inflammation, or obstetric trauma through childbirth. When *vesicovaginal* fistulas (between the vagina and bladder) develop, some urine leaks into the vagina. With *rectovaginal or anovaginal* fistulas (between the vagina and rectum or anus), flatus and feces escape into the vagina. Both can cause pain and irritation. Offensive odors may develop, causing embarrassment and limiting socialization.

Interprofessional and Nursing Management

HCPs may use a variety of tests to evaluate fistulas. These include a dye test or imaging (such as ultrasound, MRI, or CT

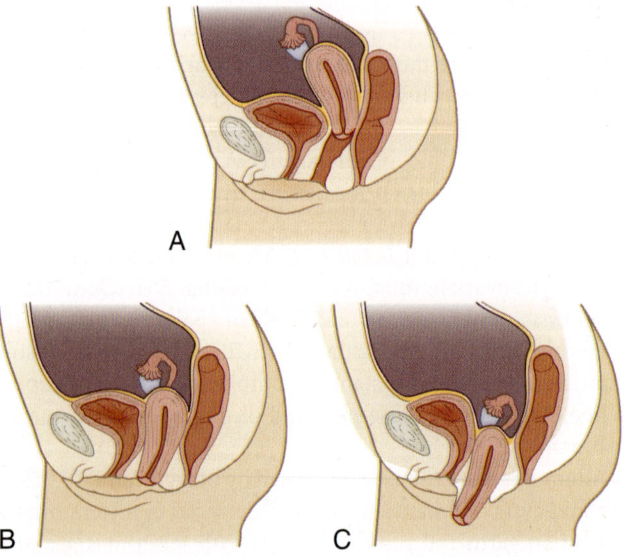

Fig. 58.13 Uterine prolapse. (A) First-degree. (B) Second-degree. (C) Third-degree.

scan). They may also perform a colonoscopy or cystourethroscopy to determine the location.

Because small fistulas may heal spontaneously within a matter of months, treatment may not be needed. If the fistula does not heal, surgery is often recommended. Multiple surgeries may be required. Fistulectomy (removal of the fistula) may result in patients having an ileal conduit or temporary colostomy. Surgical repair is not always effective, even in the best conditions.

Preoperative care includes a liquid diet, mechanical bowel cleansing, and prophylactic antibiotics. After surgery, emphasize ways to avoid stress on the repaired areas and prevent infection. Change perineal pads often. Give stool softeners or mild laxatives as ordered. A special, low-residue diet is often recommended. Enemas should be avoided. Urinary retention is common. Bladder catheters and drains may be needed for up to 2 weeks.

FEMALE REPRODUCTIVE CANCERS

There are 5 main types of gynecologic cancer: cervical, ovarian, uterine, vaginal, and vulvar.[12] Combined, these cancers affect around 100,000 patients each year in the United States. Signs and symptoms of gynecologic cancers are shown in Table 58.14. When cancer is present, patients are referred to gynecologic oncologists. Depending on the extent of the cancer, treatment options include surgery, chemotherapy, or radiation (see Chapter 16).

CERVICAL CANCER

Historically, cervical cancer was a common cause of cancer-related death. However, as cervical cancer screening and prevention measures have become widespread, the mortality rate from cervical cancer has significantly declined. One of the key measures in preventing cervical cancer is vaccination for high-risk strains of HPV, the leading cause of cervical cancer (see Chapter 57).

Cervical cancer is the only gynecologic cancer with a reliable screening approach.[13] A *Pap test* (also called Papanicolaou test or Pap smear) screens for cell changes to the cervix such as precancerous or cancerous cervical lesions. The Pap test obtains a sample through speculum examination and use of endocervical sampler (e.g., spatula, brush). This test can be used alone or in combination with testing for the virus that causes most cervical cancer (HPV).

There are different screening recommendations for cervical cancer in the United States. The recommendations include cytology (Pap test) alone, primary HPV testing, or cotesting (both Pap and HPV testing). Screening typically starts at age 21 and ends at age 65. In females under the age of 21, abnormalities including HPV infection most often go away on their own. Over the age of 65, females who have a history of normal testing are unlikely to develop high risk complications. Based on age and risk factors, testing repeats every 3 to 5 years. Patients with abnormal findings may require more frequent testing. Those at increased risk for cervical cancer due to immunosuppression, HIV infection, or in utero exposure to diethylstilbestrol (DES) may be screened more often. The goal of screening is to detect cancer early without leading to overdiagnosis and unnecessary treatment. Some early cancer conditions can resolve on their own. Gynecologic procedures following abnormal cervical cancer screening results can permanently change the cervix and cause problems with infertility or pregnancy.

Early cervical cancer often has no symptoms. Some females have vaginal bleeding after sex, after menopause, or between menstrual periods. Pelvic pain or painful sexual intercourse may be present. Abnormal vaginal discharge that is watery, bloody, or foul-smelling can occur. Pain, weight loss, anemia, and muscle wasting are late symptoms.

Management of abnormal screening results should follow the American Society of Colposcopy and Cervical Pathology (ASCCP) guidelines.[14] The ASCCP has both an online and mobile app to guide HCPs in screening and management recommendations. The primary diagnostic method is colposcopy. *Colposcopy* is an outpatient procedure where the HCP examines the cervix using a magnification device (colposcope) after applying an acetic acid solution (Fig. 58.14). When abnormalities are seen on colposcopy, a biopsy may be done. Cryotherapy, loop electrosurgical excision procedure (LEEP), laser therapy, or cone biopsy can remove abnormal cells and prevent progression to cervical cancer. Treatment depends on the stage of the cancer and if fertility is a concern. The main treatment

TABLE 58.14 Symptoms of Gynecologic Cancers

Symptom	Cervical Cancer	Ovarian Cancer	Uterine Cancer	Vaginal Cancer	Vulvar Cancer
Abdominal or back pain		X			
Abnormal vaginal bleeding or discharge	X	X	X	X	
Bloating		X			
Changes in vulva color or skin, such as a rash, sores, or warts					X
Feeling full too quickly or difficulty eating		X			
Pelvic pain or pressure		X	X		
Urgent or frequent need to urinate and/or constipation		X		X	
Vulvar pain, itching, burning, tenderness of the vulva					X

Adapted from CDC Common Symptoms of Gynecological Cancers.

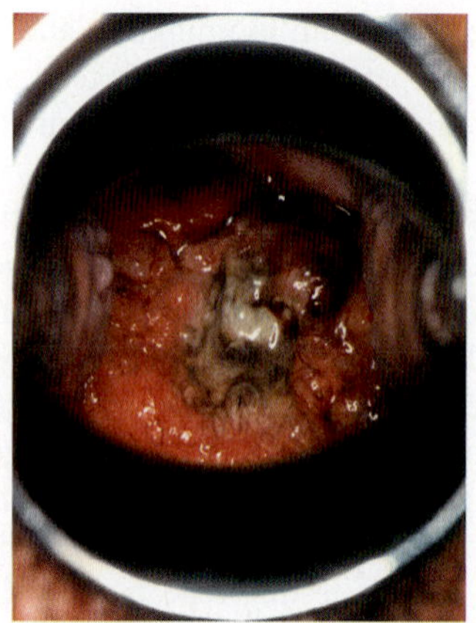

Fig. 58.14 Cervical cancer. (From Drake RL et al: *Gray's anatomy for students,* ed 2, Edinburgh, 2010, Churchill Livingstone.)

for early cancer is surgery or radiation therapy (Table 58.7). Care for more advanced cancer can include a combination of surgery, chemotherapy, and radiation.

OVARIAN CANCER

Ovarian cancer is the most common cause of death related to gynecologic cancers. Ovarian cancer often affects postmenopausal females. Risk factors include a personal or family history of cancer, genetic predisposition (Box 58.2), family history of Lynch syndrome (hereditary nonpolyposis colorectal cancer [HNPCC]), endometriosis, nulliparity (never having given birth), and infertility. Females who have given birth, breastfed, or used hormone contraceptive pills for 5 or more years have a reduced risk of ovarian cancer. These factors may have a protective effect because they reduce the number of ovulatory cycles over the lifetime.

There are 3 major types of ovarian cancer. About 90% of ovarian cancers are epithelial cancers that arise from surface epithelial cells. Germ cell tumors account for another 3%, and sex cord stromal, 2%. Histologic grading is important to determine the prognosis. Intraperitoneal dissemination is common in ovarian cancer. It metastasizes to the uterus, bladder, bowel, and omentum. In advanced disease, it can spread to the stomach, colon, liver, and other parts of the body.

Ovarian cancer is often found at a late stage. Early ovarian cancer usually has no obvious symptoms. There may be nonspecific symptoms such as pelvic or abdominal pain, bloating, urinary urgency or frequency, and difficulty eating or feeling full quickly. In later stages, abdominal enlargement with ascites (fluid in the abdominal cavity), unexplained weight loss or gain, nausea, and abnormal vaginal discharge or bleeding may occur. Adnexal mass or lymphadenopathy may be present on physical exam. A mass may be identified on pelvic imaging such as ultrasound or MRI.

No accurate screening test exists for early detection of ovarian cancer. For those at increased risk, screening may include tumor marker CA-125 and pelvic ultrasound. The CA-125 test is positive in 80% of females with advanced ovarian cancer. CA-125 is used to monitor the course of the disease and response to treatment. The problem is that CA-125 levels can be high with other cancers (e.g., pancreatic cancer) or with benign gynecologic problems, including fibroids and endometriosis.

Options for high-risk females based on family and health history include prophylactic removal of the ovaries and fallopian tubes and the use of OCPs. While salpingo-oophorectomy significantly reduces the risk for ovarian cancer, it does not completely eliminate the risk for cancer in the peritoneum.

The initial treatment for all stages of ovarian cancer is a total abdominal hysterectomy and bilateral salpingo-oophorectomy (TAH-BSO) with removal of as much of the tumor as possible (e.g., tumor debulking). Depending on the grade and stage of cancer, treatment options include intraperitoneal and systemic chemotherapy, intraperitoneal instillation of radioisotopes, and external abdominal and pelvic radiation therapy. Combination chemotherapy and radiation therapy is preferred over single-modality treatment.

The most used chemotherapy agents are taxanes (paclitaxel, docetaxel) and platinums (carboplatin, cisplatin). Among the targeted therapies used to treat advanced ovarian cancer are bevacizumab (Avastin), rucaparib (Rubraca), and olaparib (Lynparza). Rucaparib and olaparib are PARP inhibitors. They block enzymes involved in repairing damaged DNA. They are used for females with cancer associated with defective *BRCA* genes.

BOX 58.2 GENETICS IN CLINICAL PRACTICE

Ovarian Cancer and* BRCA *Genetic Mutations

Genetic Basis
- Normally these are tumor suppressor genes involved in DNA repair.
- Transmission is autosomal dominant.
- Mutations are passed down from either mother or father.

Incidence
- About 15% of cases of ovarian cancer are related to *BRCA1* and *BRCA2* mutations.
- Females with *BRCA1* mutations have a 40% lifetime risk for developing ovarian cancer.
- Females with *BRCA2* mutations have a 15% lifetime risk for developing ovarian cancer.
- Family history of both breast and ovarian cancer increases the risk of having a *BRCA* mutation.

Genetic Testing
- DNA testing is available for *BRCA1/2* genetic mutations.
- All patients with ovarian cancer should be offered testing for *BRCA1/2* mutations.

Clinical Implications
- Genetic counseling and testing for *BRCA* mutations should be offered to those with a personal or family history that puts them at increased risk for ovarian cancer.
- Bilateral salpingectomy-oophorectomy reduces the risk for ovarian cancer in females with *BRCA1/2* mutations.

UTERINE CANCER

Uterine cancer is the most common gynecologic cancer in high-income countries. Cancer of the endometrium (lining of the uterus) is the most common site and type of uterine cancer. Other types of uterine cancer are rare, such as gestational trophoblastic tumors (hydatidiform mole) and uterine sarcoma.

Endometrial cancer mainly affects females over 50. The major risk factor is exposure to estrogen, especially unopposed estrogen therapy (without progesterone). Obesity is a risk factor because of increased estrogen in adipose tissue. Other risk factors include family history of cancer or Lynch syndrome, infertility, and use of tamoxifen. Protective factors include taking OCPs, breastfeeding, increased number of pregnancies, and physical activity.

AUB (especially postmenopause) is the classic sign of endometrial cancer. Other exam findings are often normal. Late symptoms can include dysuria, dyspareunia, unintentional weight loss, and pelvic pain. A thickened endometrium may be seen on ultrasound.

There is no routine screening test for uterine cancer. Diagnosis of endometrial cancer is based on tissue sampling, usually obtained by endometrial biopsy. Alternatively, HCPs may obtain a specimen using curettage or following hysterectomy. Most patients with endometrial cancer have a good prognosis due to early diagnosis. Surgery (total hysterectomy and bilateral salpingo-oophorectomy) is the main treatment for uterine cancer (Table 58.7). It is often curative (Fig. 58.15). For complex cases, chemotherapy, radiation, or hormone therapy are part of the treatment plan.

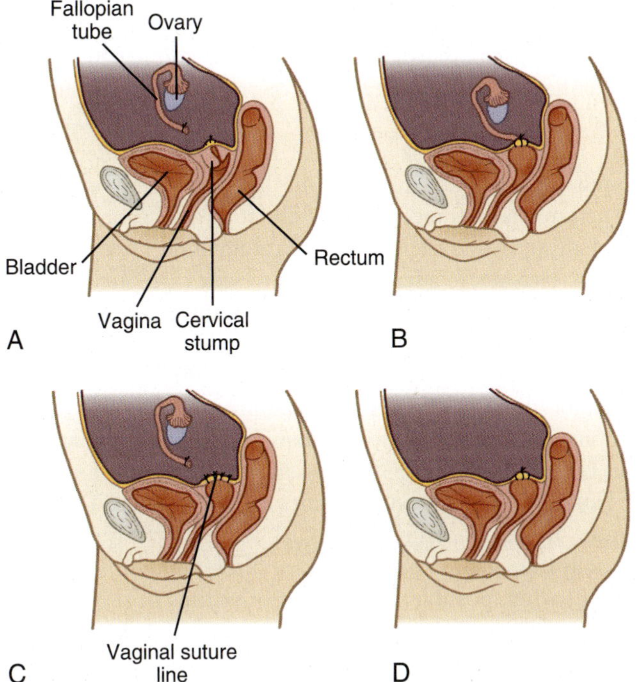

Fig. 58.15 Hysterectomies. (A) Subtotal hysterectomy. Cervical stump, fallopian tubes, and ovaries remain. (B) Total hysterectomy. Fallopian tubes and ovaries remain. (C) Vaginal hysterectomy. Fallopian tubes and ovaries remain. (D) Total hysterectomy, salpingectomy, and oophorectomy. Uterus, fallopian tubes, and ovaries are removed.

CHECK YOUR PRACTICE

You are working in the surgical unit. Your patient is a 55-year-old single mother of 2 children who underwent a TAH-BSO for uterine cancer. When you ask her how she is doing, she tells you that she is worried because she is afraid about her future and her teenage daughters.

- How would you approach this situation?
- What information would you provide?

VAGINAL AND VULVAR CANCER

Cancers of the vagina and vulva account for 6% to 7% of all gynecologic cancers in the United States. Both are associated with HPV infection. Most are squamous cell cancers. Melanoma, sarcoma, basal cell, and adenocarcinoma are less common. Primary vaginal cancer is rare. More often, vaginal cancer results from metastasis from another gynecologic cancer.

These cancers often affect postmenopausal females. Risk factors include smoking, multiple sex partners, immunodeficiency (e.g., HIV), chronic vulvar itching/burning, and having other gynecologic cancers. Having vulvar lichen sclerosus increases risk.

Manifestations include abnormal vaginal discharge or bleeding, frequent urination, hematuria, feeling constipated, change in bowel habits, and pelvic pain. Assessment includes bimanual, speculum, and rectovaginal examinations. A vaginal mass and enlarged inguinal lymph nodes may be present. Vulvar cancer presents with vulvar skin changes such as redness and lesions. Vulvar itching or burning, dysuria, dyspareunia, and pelvic pain may be present. Diagnostic evaluation often includes cytology, colposcopy, and biopsy. Treatment depends on the location, size, and stage of the cancer. Options include surgery, radiation, and/or chemotherapy.

NURSING MANAGEMENT: FEMALE REPRODUCTIVE SYSTEM CANCERS

The overall goals of nursing care are that patients will (1) take part in treatment decisions, (2) achieve satisfactory pain and symptom management, (3) recognize and report complications, (4) maintain quality of life, and (5) practice cancer detection. Key concerns with gynecologic cancer include pain, disturbed body image, and impaired sexual functioning.

Health promotion is an important aspect of nursing care. Teach patients about the importance of HPV vaccination and cervical cancer screening. HPV vaccination can reduce the risk of vaginal and vulvar cancers. Teach about risk factors for cancers of the reproductive system. When high-risk behaviors are identified, help patients change their lifestyles to decrease risk.

Acute Intervention Related to Surgery

Common types of gynecologic surgery are described in Table 58.7. Many patients feel anxious about surgical procedures. They may have concerns about its effect on their body and sexual functions. Be willing to listen to patients' feelings and concerns.

Standard preoperative care includes perineal or abdominal preparation and urinary catheter insertion (see Chapter 18).

After surgery, pain management, bowel and bladder care, and encouraging ambulation and exercise are important. Initiate venous thromboembolism (VTE) prophylaxis. Teach patients about postoperative care and expectations for recovery. Radiation therapy is discussed in Chapter 16.

SEXUAL DYSFUNCTION

Female sexual response is a complex process affected by multiple biologic, psychologic, cultural, and environment factors. **Sexual dysfunction** is a complication of sexual desire, arousal, orgasm, or pain that causes personal distress. Out of every 8 females, 1 reports sexual dysfunction. It can strongly affect quality of life. Common types of sexual dysfunction include sexual interest/arousal disorder, orgasmic disorder, genitopelvic pain/penetration disorder, and medication-induced sexual dysfunction.

There are many potential causes of sexual dysfunction. They include psychologic issues (e.g., anxiety, relationship stress), medication or substance use (e.g., SSRIs, hormone agents), medical problems (e.g., diabetes, hypertension, thyroid disease), structural problems (e.g., female genital mutilation, gynecologic surgery), gynecologic problems (e.g., endometriosis, uterine fibroids), and physiologic changes (e.g., breastfeeding, menopause).[15] Sexual dysfunction may also be caused by a combination of personal or relationship factors.

Females with sexual dysfunction may present with concerns of low libido or sexual arousal, difficulty in achieving orgasm, genital or pelvic pain, pain with penetration, medication- or substance-induced changes in sexual response, or other distress with sexual activities.

Given the complexity and sensitivity of sexual dysfunction, it may be appropriate to provide a referral to an HCP with experience in female sexual medicine for assessment, diagnosis, and treatment. Assessment begins with the history, including gynecologic, obstetric, sexual, menstrual, and psychiatric histories. Symptom diaries and symptom checklists can help define the extent and type of dysfunction. Physical assessment may include speculum and pelvic examination. In the absence of underlying medical conditions, laboratory tests are not part of diagnosing sexual dysfunction.

The management is patient-centered and specific to the condition. Care may include counseling, sex education and sexual skills training, physical therapy, and gynecologic care. Stress reduction, cognitive behavior therapy, and relationship counseling are often important aspects of treatment. Teaching anatomy, sexual response, and methods to achieve sexual health goals can improve sexual functioning. Pelvic floor physical therapy can reduce pain.

Management includes both drugs and nonpharmacologic treatment options. If the patient takes drugs associated with sexual dysfunction, such as certain antidepressants or antipsychotics, they may be discontinued. Hormone therapy or use of ospemifene (Osphena), a selective estrogen receptor modulator [SERM]), may help with sexual dysfunction due to menopause or estrogen deficiency. Transdermal testosterone, flibanserin (Addyi), a serotonin receptor agonist/antagonist, or bremelanotide (Vyleesi), a melanocortin receptor agonist, may be used to treat sexual interest and arousal disorders. Bupropion, an antidepressant, may be appropriate for dysfunction associated with psychologic conditions. Estrogen may be used for menopausal patients. Vaginal lubricants and moisturizers, topical anesthesia, and vaginal dilators can improve pain symptoms.

Nursing care starts with an understanding of normal female sexual response. Approach patients with a nonjudgmental, sex-positive attitude to support patients in discussing their concerns. Provide teaching about sexual health and functioning. Suggest books or other resources for more information. Review safe sex practices and measures to prevent unintended pregnancy. Teach patients about lifestyle changes to support sexual health and well-being. Help create a plan to reduce stress. Provide sexual medicine specialists, sex or couples therapists, or pelvic floor physical therapy referrals. Follow up to assess the effectiveness of treatment and next steps to promote sexual health.

SEXUAL ASSAULT

Sexual violence is any sexual activity in which consent was not freely given. It is a serious public health problem that affects millions of people each year. Nearly 1 in 3 females will experience some form of sexual violence in their lifetime. Sexual violence may take many forms, such as unwanted sexual contact, sexual coercion, or rape.[16] Persons of all ages, races, genders, sexual orientations, and socioeconomic statuses experience sexual violence. It has long-lasting consequences on physical and mental health. Nurses play a key role in caring for survivors of sexual violence in both the short and long term. This section focuses on gynecologic nursing care for females who have been recent victims of sexual assault.

Sexual assault is nonconsensual sexual contact, such as penetration of the survivor's body. The terms sexual assault and rape are often used interchangeably. Rape is completed or attempted nonconsensual vaginal, anal, or oral penetration, no matter how slight, with any object or part of the body (such as a finger or penis). There are many complex factors associated with an increased risk of sexual assault. Most often, sexual assault is committed by someone known to the victim. The perpetrator is a stranger in only about 20% of cases.

Many survivors will not seek medical attention. Others may wait days or even weeks after the assault to seek care. Survivors may present with physical trauma or injury on any area of the body, in addition to psychologic trauma. A medical forensic exam may be needed to collect evidence. You should be familiar with the legal definition of sexual crimes and rape in your state.[17] A forensic examination is not mandatory. It requires informed consent. HCPs may be asked to testify if sexual assault charges are filed.

Nursing care for a sexual assault victim is complex. Due to the unique needs of caring for sexual assault victims, involve a specially trained provider such as a sexual assault nurse examiner (SANE) when possible. Assessment of victims of sexual assault includes (1) treatment of acute traumatic injuries including anogenital injuries, (2) evaluation for STIs, (3) pregnancy screening and prevention, (4) assessment and support for psychologic health, and (5) forensic examination (Table 58.15).

First, we must establish consent for care and ensure patients' physical and psychologic safety. Caring for any acute traumatic injuries or urgent medical problems is the priority. Once the patient is stable, contact appropriate services such as a social worker, psychiatric HCP, rape advocate, medical forensic examiner, or SANE. Explain that you are not offering to clean the patient until evidence has been collected. Collaborate with the health care team to obtain a history, perform a physical assessment, and collect forensic evidence. Monitor vital signs. Provide emotional support. Perform baseline screening for HIV and STIs. Teach patients that it is often not possible to assess for STIs after a recent sexual assault and stress the importance of seeking follow-up care for this screening. Discuss pregnancy prevention measures such as emergency contraception. Provide referrals for counseling services and follow-up care.

TABLE 58.15 Assessment of Victims of Sexual Assault

Assessment

1. Medicolegal
   - Informed consent for assessment and care
   - Informed consent for forensic examination and collection of evidence
   - Appropriate "chain of evidence" documentation
2. History
   - Details of the assault (who, what, when, where)
   - Activities since assault that may affect evidence collection (e.g., changed clothes, showered, douched)
   - Review of symptoms, including any loss of consciousness or memory loss
   - Alcohol or drug intake
   - Health history including menstrual, gynecologic, contraceptive, sexual, and immunization history
3. Physical assessment
   - Vital signs and general appearance
   - Psychologic assessment
   - Extragenital and/or anogenital trauma (e.g., bruising, lacerations, abrasions, edema, redness)
   - Pelvic and speculum examination
4. Laboratory tests and diagnostic imaging
   - STI testing (e.g., HIV, hepatitis B, syphilis, chlamydia, gonorrhea, trichomonas)
   - Microscopic analysis of vaginal fluids
   - Pregnancy test
   - Toxicology for victims who may have been drugged
   - Radiology for trauma assessment
5. Forensic samples
   - Clothing
   - Anogenital and/or oral swabs
   - Combed specimens from scalp or pubic hair
   - Fingernail scrapings or clippings
   - Blood, urine, saliva, and hair samples

Treatment Considerations

- Care of any traumatic injuries and pain management
- Empiric treatment for STIs (e.g., gonorrhea, chlamydia)
- Postexposure prophylaxis treatment for HIV
- Tetanus and hepatitis B boosters
- Emergency contraception
- HPV vaccination
- Psychologic support and referrals for mental health services
- Protection of legal rights and compliance with mandatory reporting based on local requirements
- Recommendation of continued follow-up and services of rape crisis center

CASE STUDY

PID

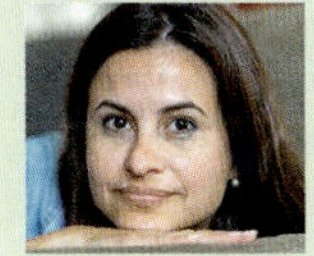

(© Juanmonino/ iStock.com.)

Patient Profile

C.C., a 26-year-old female, was admitted with lower abdominal pain, fever, and vaginal discharge for the past week. She started on oral antibiotics for PID by her primary care provider, but she continued to have ongoing abdominal pain and low-grade fevers. She has never been pregnant and has no history of STIs. She reports menarche at age 14, irregular menses, and no periods in the past 2 months. She states she hoped she might be pregnant but has had multiple negative urine pregnancy tests. She has been feeling depressed and has not been sleeping well for the past year. She is not currently taking any drugs and reports no allergies.

Subjective Data

- History of asthma
- Reports lower pelvic pain, vaginal discharge, nausea, low-grade fever
- No pain with urination, no vaginal bleeding

Objective Data

- BP 118/870 mm Hg, pulse 100 beats/min, respirations 14 breaths/min, temperature 101.2°F
- Height 5 ft, 6 in; weight 187 lb; BMI 30 kg/m^2
- Abdomen is soft, with mild tenderness in bilateral lower quadrants
- Pelvic and speculum examination reveal + mucopurulent discharge with cervical motion tenderness and adnexal tenderness

Diagnostic Studies

- Pregnancy test negative
- Depression screen negative
- Gonorrhea: positive
- Chlamydia: negative
- HIV: nonreactive
- Syphilis: nonreactive

Plan of Care

- IV antibiotics and fluids
- Referral for counseling

Discussion Questions

1. ***Recognize:*** What would you include when assessing a patient with PID?
2. ***Analyze:*** What is the relationship between PID and infertility?
3. ***Plan:*** C.C. expresses concern because she wants to get pregnant but is worried about how PID may affect her chances to conceive. What other team members would you involve?
4. ***Prioritize:*** Based on the assessment data, what are the priority clinical problems?
5. ***Act:*** What teaching will you provide C.C. so she can successfully self-manage her care?
6. ***Safety:*** What measures can C.C. take to avoid long-term health complications associated with PID?

Answers available at http://evolve.elsevier.com/Lewis/medsurg.

BRIDGE TO NCLEX EXAMINATION

The number of the question corresponds to the same-numbered outcome at the beginning of the chapter.

1. A 37-year-old female patient is receiving fertility treatments due to difficulty conceiving. What information would the nurse include as part of patient teaching to help optimize the patient's health? (**Select all that apply.**)
   - **a.** Limiting exercise
   - **b.** Smoking cessation
   - **c.** Maintaining a healthy weight
   - **d.** Reducing alcohol consumption
   - **e.** Getting no more than 7 hours of sleep
2. What tests will likely be ordered for a female who presents to the emergency department with severe right-sided abdominal pain and heavy vaginal bleeding? (**Select all that apply.**)
   - **a.** β-hCG
   - **b.** FSH and LH
   - **c.** Endometrial biopsy
   - **d.** Transvaginal ultrasound
   - **e.** Estradiol and progesterone
3. A patient with abnormal uterine bleeding from endometriosis is likely to present with what other clinical finding?
   - **a.** Acne
   - **b.** Facial hair
   - **c.** Pelvic pain
   - **d.** Urinary tract infection
4. The nurse teaching a perimenopausal female about hormone therapy states that progesterone is usually prescribed to
   - **a.** preserve fertility.
   - **b.** improve sexual functioning.
   - **c.** decrease the risk of depression.
   - **d.** reduce the risk of endometrial cancer.
5. The nurse suspects that the patient with white, curd-like vaginal discharge that sticks to the vaginal wall most likely has
   - **a.** syphilis.
   - **b.** gonorrhea.
   - **c.** bacterial vaginosis.
   - **d.** vulvovaginal candidiasis.
6. In caring for a patient with endometriosis, the nurse teaches that although some interventions can improve symptoms, the only cure is through
   - **a.** radiation therapy.
   - **b.** insertion of a hormonal intrauterine device (IUD).
   - **c.** surgical removal of endometrial tissue and adhesions.
   - **d.** consistent use of nonsteroidal antiinflammatory drugs (NSAIDs).
7. Current national recommendations are that screening for cervical cancer for low-risk patients should begin
   - **a.** at age 21.
   - **b.** with menarche.
   - **c.** after the first pregnancy.
   - **d.** at the onset of sexual activity.
8. When caring for a patient who presents for care after a sexual assault, it is important to (**Select all that apply.**)
   - **a.** empirically treat for STIs.
   - **b.** document emotional status.
   - **c.** provide referrals for counseling.
   - **d.** stabilize acute traumatic injuries.
   - **e.** prioritize washing off blood or other body fluids.

1. b, c, d; 2. a, d; 3. c; 4. d; 5. d; 6. c; 7. a; 8. a, b, c, d.

For rationales to these answers and even more NCLEX review questions, visit http://evolve.elsevier.com/Lewis/medsurg.

REFERENCES

To access the References for this chapter, please scan the QR code with a mobile device.

59

Male Reproductive Problems

Anthony Lutz

http://evolve.elsevier.com/Lewis/medsurg/

CONCEPTUAL FOCUS

Cellular Regulation
Infection
Pain
Reproduction
Sexuality

LEARNING OUTCOMES

1. Describe the pathophysiology, clinical manifestations, interprofessional care, and nursing management of benign prostatic hyperplasia.
2. Describe the pathophysiology, clinical manifestations, and interprofessional care of prostate cancer.
3. Explain the nursing management of prostate cancer.
4. Describe the pathophysiology, clinical manifestations, and interprofessional care of prostatitis and problems of the penis.
5. Explain the clinical manifestations and interprofessional care of scrotal and testicular cancer.
6. Describe the pathophysiology, clinical manifestations, and interprofessional care of problems related to male sexual and reproductive function.

KEY TERMS

benign prostatic hyperplasia (BPH)
epididymitis
erectile dysfunction (ED)
orchitis
paraphimosis
phimosis
prostate cancer
prostatitis
radical prostatectomy
testicular cancer
testicular torsion
transurethral resection of the prostate (TURP)
vasectomy

This chapter discusses male reproductive system problems. While we refer to these as male reproductive system problems, the terms "male" and "men" may not reflect the patient's gender identity. These conditions may be present in transgender, gender-nonconforming, and gender-diverse persons who were assigned male sex at birth. Use of gendered terms here is not meant to exclude any person who has these problems. The male reproductive system involves a variety of structures, including the prostate, penis, urethra, testes, epididymis, and rectum. Many of these problems can profoundly affect sexuality and reproduction. Sexual dysfunction from prostate problems or erectile dysfunction (ED) can cause psychologic and body image problems. Patients may be anxious because of a perceived loss of their sex role, self-esteem, or quality of sexual interaction with their partner. Patient teaching and counseling are essential to promote health and optimal sexual well-being.

PROSTATE GLAND PROBLEMS

BENIGN PROSTATIC HYPERPLASIA

Benign prostatic hyperplasia (BPH) is a condition in which the prostate gland increases in size, disrupting the outflow of urine from the bladder through the urethra. Over half of males will have some signs of BPH by the age of 60. That number increases to more than 80% for males 80 years old.[1]

Etiology and Pathophysiology

There are several factors that may play a role in the development and progression of BPH. We think that hormone changes associated with aging are a contributing factor. Dihydroxytestosterone (DHT), one of several sex hormones, stimulates prostate cell growth. Excess DHT can cause overgrowth of prostate tissue. As males age, they continue to make and accumulate high levels of DHT. This increases prostate size.

Another possible cause of BPH is an increased proportion of estrogen compared with testosterone. Throughout their lives, males make testosterone and small amounts of estrogen. As males age, the amount of testosterone they make decreases. This leaves a higher proportion of estrogen. A higher amount of estrogen within the prostate gland increases the activity of substances (including DHT) that promote prostate cell growth.

BPH usually develops in the inner part of the prostate, called the transition zone. As the transition zone of the prostate enlarges, it gradually compresses the urethra, leading to partial or complete obstruction (Fig. 59.1). This compression of the urethra leads to the development of clinical manifestations. There is no direct relationship between prostate size and the severity of manifestations or degree of obstruction.[2] The location of the enlargement is most significant in the development of obstructive symptoms (Fig. 59.2). For example, it is possible for mild prostate enlargement to cause severe obstructive symptoms or for extreme prostate enlargement to cause few obstructive symptoms.

Risk factors for BPH include aging, obesity (especially increased waist circumference), lack of physical activity, a high intake of red meat and animal fat, alcohol use, ED, smoking, and diabetes.[3] A family history of BPH in a first-degree relative also may be a risk factor.

Clinical Manifestations

Manifestations occur gradually. They may go unnoticed until prostate enlargement has been present for some time. Early symptoms may not cause many problems because the bladder can compensate for a small amount of resistance to urine flow. As the severity of urethral obstruction increases, symptoms gradually worsen.

We place symptoms into 2 groups: irritative and obstructive. *Irritative symptoms* include nocturia, frequency, urgency, dysuria, bladder pain, and incontinence. These symptoms are related to inflammation or infection. Nocturia is often the first symptom that patients notice. *Obstructive symptoms,* caused by prostate enlargement, include a decrease in the caliber and force of the urine stream, difficulty in starting a stream, intermittency (stopping and starting stream several times while voiding), and dribbling at the end of urination. These symptoms are due to the increased effort of the bladder as it tries to empty through the decreased diameter of the urethra. As a group, both irritative and obstructive symptoms are considered lower urinary tract symptoms (LUTS).

The American Urological Association (AUA) symptom index (AUA-SI) for BPH (Table 59.1) is a widely used tool to assess voiding symptoms from obstruction.[4] This tool is not diagnostic. It helps determine the extent of symptoms and guide treatment. Higher scores on this tool mean greater symptom severity.

Complications

Some males may have acute urine retention. They will have the sudden and painful inability to urinate. Treatment involves inserting a catheter to drain the bladder. Surgery may be needed in severe situations. Bladder damage can occur if treatment is delayed. Renal failure can occur due to *hydronephrosis* (distention of the renal pelvis and calyces by urine that cannot flow through the ureter to the bladder).

Urinary tract infection (UTI) can be a complication. Since the bladder is unable to empty completely, bacteria can grow in the residual urine that remains in the bladder and cause infection. In more severe cases, infection can progress into the kidney and cause pyelonephritis. In severe cases, infection can spread into the bloodstream and sepsis can develop. Bladder calculi (stones) may develop because of the alkalinization of the residual urine. So, the finding of bladder stones often indicates obstruction from BPH.

Bladder
Enlarged prostate gland
Compressed urethra
Rectum

Fig. 59.1 BPH. The enlarged prostate compresses the urethra.

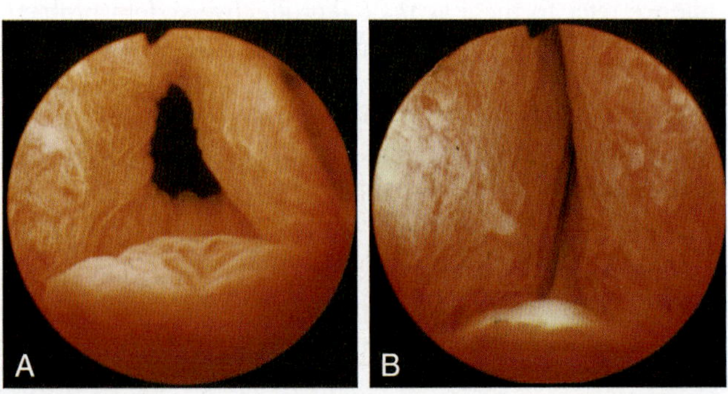

Fig. 59.2 Views of the prostate by cystoscopy. (A) Normal appearance. (B) Moderate BPH with urethral obstruction. (From Townsend CM, Beauchamp RD, Evers BM, et al: *Sabiston textbook of surgery,* ed 19, Philadelphia, 2012, Saunders.)

TABLE 59.1 AUA Symptom Index to Determine Severity of Prostatic Problems

Questions	AUA SYMPTOM SCORE (CIRCLE 1 NUMBER ON EACH LINE)					
	Not At All	Less Than 1 Time in 5	Less Than Half the Time	About Half the Time	More Than Half the Time	Almost Always
Over the Past Month						
1. How often do you have the sensation that your bladder is not completely empty after you finish urinating?	0	1	2	3	4	5
2. How often do you have to urinate again, less than 2 h after you finish urinating?	0	1	2	3	4	5
3. How often do you stop and start again several times when you urinate?	0	1	2	3	4	5
4. How often do you find it difficult to postpone urination?	0	1	2	3	4	5
5. How often do you have a weak urine stream?	0	1	2	3	4	5
6. How often do you have to push or strain to begin urination?	0	1	2	3	4	5
7. Do you usually get up to urinate from the time you go to bed at night until the time you get up in the morning?	0 (none)	1 (1 time)	2 (2 times)	3 (3 times)	4 (4 times)	5 (5 times or more)
Sum of circled numbers (AUA Symptom Score): ____						
Score is interpreted as follows: 0–7, mild; 8–19, moderate; 20–35, severe.						

From Barry MJ, Fowler FJ, O'Leary MP, et al: The AUA symptom index for benign prostatic hyperplasia, *J Urol* 148:1549, 1992. Used with permission.

Diagnostic Studies

The history and physical assessment are important. Diagnostic studies are outlined in Table 59.2. A digital rectal examination (DRE) is done to estimate the prostate size, symmetry, and consistency. In BPH, the prostate is symmetrically enlarged, firm, and smooth.

A urinalysis (UA) and culture with sensitivity can detect bacteria, nitrites, leukocyte esterase, white blood cells (WBCs), or microscopic hematuria (RBCs), which could indicate infection or inflammation.

A prostate-specific antigen (PSA) blood test can screen for prostate cancer. Patients with BPH may have slightly increased PSA levels. PSA is released into the bloodstream by benign and malignant prostate cells. Creatinine levels can evaluate renal insufficiency. If creatinine levels are high, a renal ultrasound may show hydronephrosis if the cause is obstruction. Because symptoms of BPH and neurogenic bladder are similar, a neurologic assessment may be done.

In patients with an abnormal DRE and high PSA, testing options include a transrectal ultrasound (TRUS), pelvic MRI, or TRUS-guided prostate biopsy. If abnormal areas are seen on MRI, these areas can be targeted on a TRUS prostate biopsy (MRI-fusion targeted biopsy). Assessments with MRI prior to biopsy and MRI-targeted biopsy are more accurate than a TRUS biopsy in males at risk for prostate cancer.[5]

Uroflowmetry (measures the volume of urine expelled from the bladder) helps determine the extent of urethral blockage and the treatment needed. Postvoid residual urine volume can determine the degree of urine flow obstruction. Cystoscopy is done if the diagnosis is unclear or to see the degree of prostatic enlargement. If the diagnostic picture is unclear, urodynamic/pressure flow studies can help evaluate bladder function and assess for obstruction.

Interprofessional Care

The goals of care are to (1) restore bladder drainage, (2) relieve symptoms, and (3) prevent or treat the complications of BPH. Treatment is based on the degree to which the symptoms bother patients or the presence of complications rather than the size of the prostate. Alternatives to surgery include surveillance, drug therapy, and minimally invasive procedures. The most conservative treatment is called *active surveillance,* or watchful waiting. When patients have mild symptoms (AUA symptom scores of 0 to 7), we usually take a wait-and-see approach. If patients begin to have signs or symptoms that indicate an increase in obstruction, further treatment is needed.

Drug Therapy

The 2 main classes of drugs to treat BPH include 5α-reductase inhibitors and α-adrenergic receptor blockers. Combination therapy with both types of drugs may be more effective in reducing symptoms than using 1 drug. An erectogenic drug can also help treat BPH.

5α-Reductase inhibitors. 5α-Reductase inhibitors reduce the size of the prostate gland. They block the 5α-reductase type 1 and 2 isoenzymes, which are necessary for the conversion of testosterone to DHT. Prostate size is directly related to the

TABLE 59.2 Interprofessional Care

BPH

Diagnostic Assessment

- History and physical assessment with DRE
- UA and urine culture and sensitivities
- PSA
- Creatinine
- Postvoid residual (by ultrasound)
- Renal ultrasound (if increased creatinine, assess for hydronephrosis)
- TRUS
- Uroflowmetry
- Cystoscopy
- Urodynamic/pressure flow studies

Management

Active Surveillance

- Annual PSA and DRE
- Repeat AUA symptom score and postvoid residual if any symptoms change

Drug Therapy

- 5α-Reductase inhibitors (e.g., dutasteride, finasteride)
- α-Adrenergic receptor blockers (e.g., alfuzosin, doxazosin, tamsulosin)
- Combination 5α-reductase inhibitor and α-adrenergic receptor blocker (e.g., dutasteride plus tamsulosin [Jalyn])
- Erectogenic drugs (e.g., tadalafil)

Minimally Invasive Therapy (Table 59.3)

- Laser enucleation of the prostate (HoLEP or ThuLEP)
- Photoselective vaporization of the prostate (PVP)
- Prostatic urethral lift (PUL)
- Water vapor thermal therapy

Surgical Therapy (Table 59.3)

- Transurethral incision of the prostate (TUIP)
- Transurethral resection of the prostate (TURP)
- Simple prostatectomy (open, laparoscopic, robotic assisted)

amount of DHT. By blocking DHT, overly enlarged prostates can decrease in size. These agents are more effective for males with larger prostates who have bothersome symptoms.

Finasteride inhibits only the type 2 isoenzyme. It is a treatment for males with a moderate to severe symptom score on the AUA-SI (Table 59.1). Although most males who are treated with the drug have symptom improvement, it can take 6 months to be effective. It must be taken on a regular basis to have an effect. Because it blocks the enzyme needed for conversion of testosterone to DHT, decreased libido is a common side effect.

PSA levels may appear decreased by 50% when taking finasteride. Therefore to "correct" for the apparent decrease caused by finasteride, the HCP should double the PSA value for patients who have been taking a 5α-reductase inhibitor for at least 6 months. This allows for a more accurate comparison to premedication PSA levels. Dutasteride (Avodart) has the same effect on prostatic tissue as finasteride. It is a dual inhibitor of 5α-reductase types 1 and 2 isoenzymes.

These drugs may lower the risk for some prostate cancers. However, using them to prevent prostate cancer is not recommended, and research is ongoing. Patients who develop a high PSA level while taking these drugs should have further evaluation. Encourage patients to discuss prostate cancer screening with the HCP.

DRUG ALERT

Finasteride

- Females who may be or are pregnant should not touch tablets due to potential risk to male fetus (anomaly).

α-Adrenergic receptor blockers. α-Adrenergic receptor blockers are another drug treatment option for BPH. These drugs selectively block α_1-adrenergic receptors, which are abundant in the prostate and increased in hyperplastic prostate tissue. They relax the smooth muscle of the prostate that surrounds the urethra, thus promoting urine flow through the urethra. These agents do not decrease the size of the prostate.

α-Adrenergic blockers include alfuzosin (Uroxatral), doxazosin (Cardura), prazosin (Minipress), tamsulosin (Flomax), and silodosin (Rapaflo). Symptom improvement can often be seen within days to weeks of starting therapy. Because they relax the smooth muscle of the prostatic urethra, a common side effect is retrograde ejaculation. The combination of a 5α-reductase inhibitor (dutasteride) and an α-adrenergic receptor blocker (tamsulosin) is available in a single oral medication (Jalyn).

Erectogenic drugs. Tadalafil (Cialis) can be used in males who have symptoms of BPH alone or in combination with ED. It can be effective in reducing symptoms for both conditions.

Herb therapy. Some patients take plant extracts, such as saw palmetto. Research shows that saw palmetto has no benefit over a placebo.[6] Advise patients to discuss these therapies with their HCP.

Minimally Invasive Therapy

Minimally invasive therapies are becoming more common as an alternative to watchful waiting and surgery (Table 59.3). A benefit of these procedures is a decreased length of stay in the hospital. They are associated with fewer adverse events. Many minimally invasive therapies have outcomes comparable to surgery.

Photoselective vaporization. *Photoselective vaporization of the prostate* (PVP) uses a high-power green laser light to vaporize prostate tissue. Laser therapy through visual or ultrasound guidance is an effective alternative to transurethral resection of the prostate (TURP). The laser beam is delivered through a fiber instrument inserted into the meatus and through the urethra. It can cut, coagulate, and vaporize prostatic tissue. Improvements in urine flow and symptoms are almost immediate. PVP works well for larger prostate glands. Irritative voiding symptoms may persist for several weeks. Urine retention can be a complication. Patients often go home with an indwelling urinary catheter for 2 to 7 days to maintain urine flow and promote the passing of small

TABLE 59.3 Treatment for BPH

Description	Advantages	Disadvantages
Minimally Invasive		
Laser Enucleation of the Prostate		
Laser beams rapidly vaporize and coagulate prostate tissue. Laser does not penetrate deep tissue. 2 types of lasers: holmium laser enucleation of the prostate (HoLEP), thulium laser enucleation of the prostate (ThuLEP).	• Outpatient procedure • Better coagulative properties in tissue compared with TURP • Comparable results to TURP and PVP • Minimal bleeding • Fast recovery time	• Catheter needed after for 24–48 h • Irritative voiding symptoms, urine incontinence • Hematuria • Retrograde ejaculation • May be more difficult to perform compared with PVP
Photoselective Vaporization of the Prostate (PVP)		
Uses a laser beam to cut or destroy part of the prostate. May be more effective for small to moderate-sized prostates.	• Short procedure • Comparable results to TURP • Minimal bleeding • Fast recovery time • Rapid symptom improvement • Very effective	• Catheter needed up to 7 days after due to edema and urine retention • Delayed sloughing of tissue • Takes several weeks to reach optimal effect • Retrograde ejaculation
Prostatic Urethral Lift (PUL)		
Permanent transprostatic implants/tension sutures placed transurethrally via cystoscope. Mechanically open the prostatic urethra by compressing the prostate tissue/parenchyma.	• Outpatient procedure • ED, urine incontinence, retrograde ejaculation are minimal • No change in PSA since no prostate tissue ablated	• Lack of long-term durability/results • Treatment response rates slightly lower compared with TURP • If unsuccessful, may need repeat PUL or TURP in the future
Transurethral Vaporization of Prostate (TUVP)		
Electrosurgical modification of the standard TURP. Vaporization and desiccation used to destroy prostatic tissue. Can use a variety of energy delivery mediums (e.g., button, rollerball, vaportrode).	• Minimal risks • Minimal bleeding and sloughing	• Retrograde ejaculation • Intermittent hematuria
Water Vapor Thermal Therapy		
Heated water vapor/steam used to destroy obstructive prostate tissue. Delivered transurethrally via hand-held device with a retractable needle that releases the water vapor in 9-second doses.	• Outpatient procedure • Can be done in an outpatient office setting • ED, urine incontinence, retrograde ejaculation are rare • Precise delivery of steam to desired area • Little pain	• Relatively new so lacks long-term results • Irritative voiding symptoms and UTI • Hematuria
Surgical Therapy		
Transurethral Incision of the Prostate (TUIP)		
Involves transurethral incisions into prostatic tissue to relieve obstruction. Effective for small to moderate prostates.	• Outpatient procedure • Minimal complications • Low occurrence of ED or retrograde ejaculation • Outcomes similar to TURP	• Urinary catheter needed after
Transurethral Resection of the Prostate (TURP)		
Excision and cauterization to remove prostate tissue via cystoscope. Standard for treatment of BPH.	• ED unlikely	• Bleeding, clot retention • Retrograde ejaculation • Catheter needed after
Simple Prostatectomy (Open, Laparoscopic, or Robotic Assisted)		
Surgery of choice for males with large prostates (often >100 g), bladder damage, or other complicating factors. If open, involves an external incision with retropubic or perineal approach (Fig. 59.6). If laparoscopic and/or robotic assisted, involves several small abdominal incisions and 1 slightly larger incision near the umbilicus.	• Complete visualization of the prostate and surrounding tissue	• ED • Bleeding • Pain • Risk for infection

clots or necrotic tissue. Antibiotics, pain medication, and bladder antispasmodics can be used to treat and prevent postprocedure problems.

Laser enucleation. Laser enucleation involves delivering a laser beam transurethrally through a fiber instrument. It is used for rapid coagulation and vaporization of prostatic tissue. There are 2 types of lasers in this class: holmium laser enucleation of the prostate (HoLEP) and thulium laser enucleation of the prostate (ThuLEP). Neither penetrates deep tissue, which decreases side effects.

Prostatic urethral lift. *Prostatic urethral lift* (PUL) involves permanent transprostatic implants or tension sutures delivered transurethrally via cystoscope. They mechanically open the prostatic urethra by compressing the prostate tissue. This alters prostate anatomy without ablating any tissue. PUL is typically considered for prostates less than 80 grams in size and without an obstructive median lobe.[2] There is a lack of long-term data on the durability of PUL over time and the rates of needing repeat treatment or progression to TURP.

CHECK YOUR PRACTICE

You are caring for a patient who is scheduled for PVP for BPH. He appears anxious. He tells you he is worried about not being able to urinate normally after the procedure.

- What type of information and teaching would you provide?

Transurethral vaporization of the prostate. *Transurethral vaporization of the prostate* (TUVP) is an electrosurgical modification of the standard TURP. Vaporization and desiccation are used together to destroy obstructive prostatic tissue. There are a variety of energy delivery mediums that can be used to deliver the energy (e.g., button, rollerball, vaportrode). This is why many call it a "button TURP." The results, side effects, and long-term outcomes are equal to TURP. Because TUVP uses a bipolar energy delivery surface, an energy current is not passed through the body to a grounding pad. This allows the HCP to use saline irrigation during the procedure, which decreases the risk for TUR syndrome.

Water vapor thermal therapy. *Water vapor thermal therapy* uses heated water vapor/steam to destroy obstructive prostate tissue. The steam is delivered transurethrally directly into the prostate by a hand-held device with a retractable needle. It releases the heated water vapor in 9-second doses. It is potentially a good option for patients who are looking to minimize the risk for postprocedure ED. This treatment is typically recommended for prostates less than 80 grams in size. It lacks long-term durability data.

Surgical Therapy

Invasive treatment of symptomatic BPH involves surgery. The approach used depends on the size and location of the prostatic enlargement and patient factors, such as age and surgical risk. Table 59.3 describes common surgeries.

Surgery is indicated when a decrease in urine flow causes pain, persistent residual urine, acute urine retention because of obstruction with no reversible precipitating cause, or hydronephrosis. Intermittent catheterization or insertion of an indwelling catheter can temporarily reduce symptoms and bypass the obstruction. We avoid long-term catheter use because of the increased infection risk.

Transurethral incision of the prostate. Transurethral incision of the prostate (TUIP) is a surgical procedure done under local anesthesia for males with moderate to severe symptoms. Several small incisions are made into the prostate gland to expand the urethra, which relieves pressure on the urethra and improves urine flow. TUIP is an option for patients with a small or moderately enlarged prostate gland.

Transurethral resection of the prostate. **Transurethral resection of the prostate (TURP)** involves the removal of prostate tissue using a resectoscope inserted through the urethra. TURP is the gold standard for surgical treatment of obstructing BPH. Most patients have marked improvements in symptoms and urine flow rates.

In a TURP there is no external incision. A resectoscope is inserted through the urethra to excise and cauterize obstructing prostatic tissue (Fig. 59.3). A large 3-way indwelling catheter with a 30-mL balloon is inserted into the bladder after the procedure to provide hemostasis and to promote urine drainage. If there is a large amount of hematuria with clots after surgery, then the bladder can be irrigated, continuously or intermittently, for the first 24 hours to prevent obstruction from blood clots.

TURP has relatively low risk. We do have to assess for transurethral resection syndrome (TUR or TURP syndrome). Signs and symptoms include nausea, vomiting, confusion, bradycardia, and hypertension. TUR syndrome is due to hyponatremia from long operative times and prolonged intraoperative bladder irrigation with hypotonic fluid. If the HCP uses saline irrigation during the procedure, the risk for TUR syndrome dramatically decreases.

Other complications include bleeding and clot retention. Patients taking aspirin, warfarin, or other anticoagulants must stop taking these several days before surgery. BPH medications are stopped after the procedure.

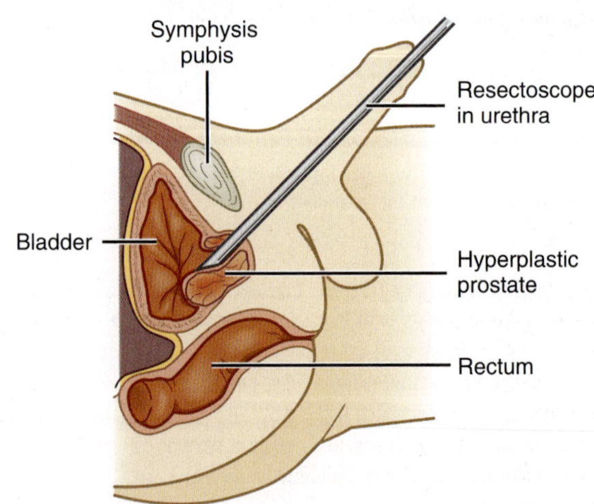

Fig. 59.3 Transurethral resection of the prostate.

NURSING MANAGEMENT: BPH

Because you may care for patients with BPH having surgery, the focus of this section is on perioperative nursing care.

Assessment

Subjective and objective data that you should obtain from patients with BPH are outlined in Table 59.4.

Clinical Problems

Clinical problems for patients with BPH before surgery may include:

- Pain
- Risk for infection
- Impaired urinary elimination

Clinical problems and interventions for patients with BPH who have surgery are presented in eNursing Care Plan 59.1 (available on the website for this chapter).

Planning

The overall preoperative goals for patients having surgery are to (1) restore urine drainage; (2) resolve any UTI; and (3) understand the procedure, implications for sexual function, and urine control. The overall postoperative goals are to have (1) no complications, (2) restoration of urine control, (3) complete bladder emptying, and (4) satisfying sexual expression.

Implementation

Health Promotion

Teaching patients to make lifestyle changes can help relieve early or mild symptoms (Box 59.1). Some males find that consuming alcohol, caffeine, or other bladder irritants tends to increase prostatic voiding symptoms because the diuretic effect increases bladder distention and overactivity. Compounds found in common cough and cold remedies, such as pseudoephedrine (e.g., Sudafed) and phenylephrine, often worsen the symptoms of BPH. These drugs are α-adrenergic agonists

TABLE 59.4 NURSING ASSESSMENT

BPH

Subjective Data

Important Health Information

Medications: Testosterone supplementation

Surgery or other treatments: Previous BPH treatment

Functional Health Patterns

Health perception—health management: Knowledge of the condition

Nutritional-metabolic: Voluntary fluid restriction

Elimination: Urgency, diminution in caliber and force of urinary stream. Hesitancy in starting voiding. Postvoid dribbling, urine retention, urine incontinence

Sleep-rest: Nocturia

Cognitive-perceptual: Dysuria, sensation of incomplete voiding, bladder discomfort

Sexuality-reproductive: Anxiety about sexual dysfunction

Objective Data

General

Older adult male

Urinary

Distended bladder on palpation. Smooth, firm, elastic enlargement of prostate on rectal examination

Possible Diagnostic Findings

Enlarged prostate on ultrasonography, bladder neck obstruction on cystoscopy, residual urine with postvoiding ultrasound or catheterization. WBCs, bacteria, or microscopic hematuria with bladder infection. ↑ Creatinine levels with renal involvement

BOX 59.1 EVIDENCE-BASED PRACTICE

BPH and Quality of Life

J.H., a 60-year-old patient, comes to the clinic seeking help with urinary symptoms. He states that he was told he has an "enlarged prostate." J.H. now states that the symptoms are worse, causing "daily living to be difficult," including "relations" with his wife. Your assessment reveals frequent nocturia, lower abdominal discomfort, dysuria, and occasional dribbling.

Making Clinical Decisions

Synthesis of Best Available Evidence

Nurse-directed education focusing on lifestyle modifications among BPH patients can result in substantial improvement in BPH symptom severity and reported quality of life. Teaching should include self-management strategies (fluid management, avoiding caffeine and alcohol), specific behavior changes (bladder retraining, pelvic floor exercises, double voiding, voiding urge suppression), and avoiding constipation with diet changes.

Clinician Expertise

You know that lower urinary tract symptoms in men with BPH can negatively affect their quality of life. This can lead to challenges in self-care, activity restrictions, and feelings of discomfort, anxiety, and/or depression. Sexual dysfunction can cause psychologic and body image problems because of a perceived loss of sex role or low-quality sexual interactions.

Patient Preferences and Values

J.H. had several questions about ways to improve his symptoms. You recommend J.H. decrease his fluid intake 3 hours before going to bed and limit caffeine and alcohol use. You discuss his eating a well-balanced diet that contains adequate fiber and beginning walking 3 to 4 times a week.

Implications for Nursing Practice

1. What feedback would support that J.H. is experiencing an improved quality of life?
2. What are the next treatments at this point in time?

Reference for Evidence

Choudhary D, Kalal N, Kumar A, et al: The feasibility trial of nurse-directed education programme among benign prostatic hyperplasia patients. *Int J Urol Nurs*, 18:e12378, 2024.

that cause smooth muscle contraction. If this occurs, patients should avoid these drugs.

A timed voiding schedule (bladder retraining) may reduce symptoms and eliminate the need for further treatment. Teach patients with obstructive symptoms to urinate every 2 to 3 hours and when they first feel the urge. This will minimize urine stasis and acute retention. Teach patients to maintain a normal level of fluid so that they do not become dehydrated. Patients may think that if they restrict fluid intake, symptoms will be less severe. This actually increases the risk of infection while concentrating the urine.

Acute Care

The following discussion focuses on perioperative care for patients undergoing a TURP.

Preoperative care. Antibiotics are usually given before any invasive genitourinary (GU) procedure. UTI must be treated before surgery. Restoring urine drainage and encouraging a high fluid intake (2 to 3 L/day unless contraindicated) are helpful in managing infection.

Prostatic obstruction may result in acute retention or inability to void. A urinary catheter may be needed to restore bladder drainage. In many health care settings, 2% lidocaine gel is inserted into the urethra before catheter placement. The lidocaine gel acts as a lubricant, provides local anesthesia, and helps open the urethral lumen. If a sizable obstruction of the urethra exists, the HCP may need to use a special catheter or dilation tools to pass through the obstruction. Aseptic technique is important to avoid introducing bacteria into the bladder.

Patients may be concerned about the impact of the surgery on sexual function. Provide an opportunity for patients and partners to express their concerns. Tell them that ejaculate volume may be decreased or absent afterward. Most prostatic surgeries result in some degree of *retrograde ejaculation.* This is a condition in which some semen travels back into the bladder during orgasm instead of traveling out of the penis. This may decrease orgasmic sensations felt during ejaculation. Retrograde ejaculation is not harmful. The semen is voided with the next urination.

Postoperative care. The main complications after surgery are bleeding, bladder spasms, urine incontinence, and infection. Adjust the plan of care to the type of surgery, reasons for surgery, and the patient's response to surgery.

After surgery, patients will have a standard 2-way or 3-way urinary catheter. Bladder irrigation is typically done to remove clotted blood from the bladder and ensure drainage of urine (Fig. 59.4). The bladder is irrigated manually on an intermittent basis or more often, as continuous bladder irrigation (CBI) with sterile normal saline solution or another prescribed solution. If the bladder is manually irrigated, instill 50 mL of irrigation solution. Then withdraw with a syringe to remove clots that may be in the bladder and catheter. Painful bladder spasms often occur with manual irrigation.

With CBI, irrigation solution is continuously infused and drained from the bladder. The rate of infusion is based on the color of drainage. The urine drainage should be light pink without clots. Monitor the inflow and outflow of the irrigant (Table 59.5). If outflow is less than inflow, assess the catheter patency for kinks or clots. If the outflow is blocked and you cannot reestablish patency by manual irrigation, stop the CBI and notify the HCP.

Blood clots are expected after prostate surgery for the first 24 to 36 hours. However, large amounts of bright red blood in the urine can indicate bleeding. Bleeding may occur from catheter displacement, dislodgment of a large clot, or increased abdominal pressure.

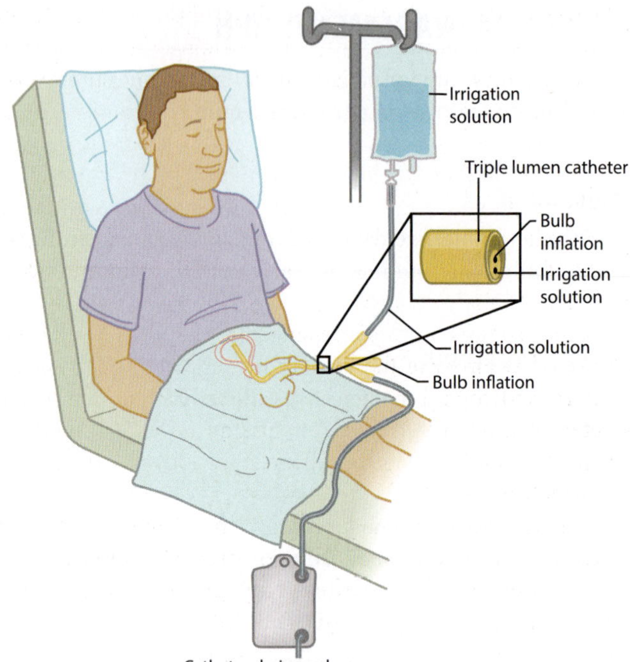

Fig. 59.4 Bladder irrigation with a triple lumen urinary catheter.

TABLE 59.5 NURSING MANAGEMENT

Patient Receiving Bladder Irrigation

- Monitor the inflow and outflow of the irrigant.
- Assess for bleeding and the presence of bladder spasms.
- Assess catheter patency for kinks or clots.
- Manually irrigate catheter if bladder spasms or decreased outflow occurs.
- Use careful aseptic technique because you can easily introduce bacteria into the urinary tract.
- Maintain a closed drainage system.
- Give prescribed antispasmodics and analgesics.
- Monitor catheter drainage for increased blood or clots.
- Do not disconnect the system unless it is being removed, changed, or irrigated.
- Discontinue CBI and notify HCP if obstruction occurs.
- Secure the catheter to the leg with tape or a catheter strap to prevent urethral irritation and minimize the risk for infection.
- Teach patient Kegel exercises after catheter removal.
- Provide care instructions for patient discharged with indwelling catheter.

Release or displacement of the catheter dislodges the balloon that provides counterpressure on the operative site. Traction on the catheter may be applied to provide counterpressure on the bleeding site in the prostate to decrease bleeding. This traction can result in local necrosis if pressure is applied for too long. Pressure should be relieved on a scheduled basis by qualified personnel.

Patients should avoid activities that increase abdominal pressure in the recovery period. These include sitting or walking for prolonged periods and straining to have a bowel movement (Valsalva maneuver).

Bladder spasms are a distressing complication. They occur because of irritation of the bladder mucosa from the insertion of the resectoscope, presence of a catheter, or clots leading to catheter obstruction. If bladder spasms develop, check the catheter for clots. If present, remove the clots by irrigation so that urine can flow freely. Tell patients not to urinate around the catheter because this increases the chance of spasm. Belladonna and opium suppositories, diazepam suppositories, or other antispasmodics (e.g., oxybutynin), along with relaxation techniques, can relieve pain and decrease spasm.

We often remove the catheter 2 to 4 days after surgery. Patients should have a voiding trial after catheter removal. If they cannot urinate, they will have a catheter reinserted for a few days or perform clean intermittent self-catheterization.

Poor sphincter tone right after catheter removal may cause urine incontinence or dribbling. This is often distressing. Performing Kegel exercises (pelvic floor muscle technique) 10 to 20 times per hour while awake (see Table 50.18) can strengthen sphincter tone. Encourage patients to practice starting and stopping the stream several times during urination. This helps patients to target the correct pelvic floor muscles when doing Kegel exercises.

It can take several weeks to achieve continence. Sometimes, control of urine is not fully regained. Continence can improve for up to 12 months. If continence has not been achieved by that time, patients may be referred to a continence clinic. A variety of methods, including biofeedback, have been used to achieve results.

Teach patients how to use a penile clamp, a condom catheter, or incontinence pads or briefs to avoid embarrassment from dribbling. In severe cases, an occlusive cuff that serves as an artificial sphincter can be surgically implanted to restore continence. Help patients find ways to manage the problem that allow them to continue socializing and interacting with others. Urine incontinence is discussed in Chapter 50.

Observe for infection. If an external wound is present (e.g., from an open, laparoscopic, or robotic-assisted prostatectomy), assess the area for redness, heat, swelling, and purulent drainage. Take special care if a perineal incision is present because of the proximity of the anus. Avoid rectal procedures, such as enemas. The insertion of well-lubricated suppositories is acceptable.

Diet intervention and stool softeners are important to prevent straining with bowel movements. Straining increases intraabdominal pressure, which can lead to bleeding at the operative site. A high-fiber diet promotes the passage of stool.

Chronic Care

Discharge planning is important after prostate surgery. Teaching, especially about the procedure and the possible complications, directly affects quality of life. Teaching includes (1) caring for a urinary catheter (if present), (2) managing urine incontinence, (3) maintaining fluid intake, (4) observing for signs and symptoms of infection, (5) preventing constipation, (6) avoiding heavy lifting, and (7) refraining from driving or intercourse after surgery as directed by the HCP.

Patients may have a change in sexual function after surgery. Recovery depends on the type of surgery done and the interval of time between when symptoms first appeared and the date of surgery. For example, it may take 2 years for maximal sexual function recovery after nerve-sparing prostatectomy. Many males have retrograde ejaculation because of trauma to the internal urethral sphincter. ED may occur if the nerves are cut or damaged during surgery. Patients may be anxious over the change because of a perceived loss of sex role, self-esteem, or quality of sexual interaction with their partner. Discuss these changes with patients and their partners. Allow them to ask questions and express their concerns. Sexual counseling and treatment options may be needed if ED becomes a chronic issue.

The bladder may take 2 to 3 months to return to its normal capacity. Teach patients to drink at least 2 to 3 L of fluid per day and urinate every 2 to 3 hours to flush the urinary tract. Have them avoid or limit the amounts of bladder irritants, such as caffeine products, carbonated drinks, citrus juices, and alcohol. Because patients may have incontinence or dribbling, they may incorrectly believe that decreasing fluid intake will relieve this problem.

Urethral strictures may result from instrumentation or catheterization. Treatment may include intermittent clean self-catheterization or having a urethral dilation.

Teach patients to discuss the need for a yearly DRE with their HCP if they had any procedure other than complete removal of the prostate. Hyperplasia or cancer can occur in the remaining prostatic tissue.

◆ Evaluation

The expected outcomes are that patients with BPH who have surgery will report:

- Acceptable pain control
- Improved urinary function with no pain or incontinence

PROSTATE CANCER

Prostate cancer is a tumor of the prostate gland. Prostate cancer is the most common cancer among males, excluding skin cancer. It is the second leading cause of cancer death in males, exceeded only by lung cancer. A male has a 1 in 8 risk for developing prostate cancer in his lifetime. More than 3.3 million males in the United States are prostate cancer survivors.[7]

Etiology and Pathophysiology

Prostate cancer is a slow-growing, androgen-dependent cancer. It is most likely to develop in the outer part of the prostate, called the peripheral zone. It can spread by 3 routes: by direct extension, through the lymph system, or through the bloodstream. Spread by direct extension involves the seminal vesicles, urethral mucosa, bladder wall, and external sphincter. The cancer later spreads through the lymphatic system to the regional lymph nodes. The bloodstream is the mode of spread to the axial skeleton (e.g., pelvic bones, head of the femur, lower lumbar spine), liver, and lungs.

Age, ethnicity, and family history are known risk factors for prostate cancer. The incidence of prostate cancer rises markedly after age 50. The median age at diagnosis is 66 years old. However, many cases occur in younger males. They sometimes have a more aggressive type of cancer. Black males are diagnosed with prostate cancer at an earlier age, have more advanced disease at the time of diagnosis, and have a high mortality rate.

Diet factors and obesity may be related to prostate cancer. A diet high in red and processed meat and high-fat dairy products along with a low intake of vegetables and fruits may increase the risk of prostate cancer. Environment may play a role. There is an increased prevalence of prostate cancer in farmers and commercial pesticide applicators. This might be due to chemicals found in pesticides. It is not clear if smoking is a risk factor.

Genetic Link

Currently no known single gene causes prostate cancer. Some genes or gene mutations are more common in males with prostate cancer. From a genetics viewpoint, we classify prostate cancer into 3 categories.

Most prostate cancers (about 75%) are *sporadic,* which means that damage to the genes occurs by chance after a person is born. Prostate cancer that runs in a family, called *familial prostate cancer,* is less common (about 20%). It occurs because of a combination of genes and environment or lifestyle factors. Familial prostate cancer is when 2 or more first-degree relatives (father, brother, son) have prostate cancer.

Hereditary (inherited) prostate cancer is rare (5% to 10%). It occurs when gene mutations are passed down in a family from one generation to the next. In hereditary prostate cancer, a family has any of the following characteristics: (1) 3 or more first-degree relatives with prostate cancer, (2) prostate cancer in 3 generations on the same side of the family, and (3) 2 or more close relatives (father, brother, son, grandfather, uncle, nephew) on the same side of the family diagnosed with prostate cancer before age 55.

Having a family history does not mean that a male will develop prostate cancer. It means that they have an increased risk. Males with a family history of prostate cancer should talk with their HCP about their concerns. It is important for the HCP to obtain a detailed family history. Depending on the findings, a referral to a genetic counselor may be appropriate.

Hereditary breast and ovarian cancer (HBOC) syndrome is associated with mutations in the *BRCA1* and/or *BRCA2* genes (*BRCA* stands for *BR*east *CA*ncer). Males with HBOC have an increased risk for breast cancer and prostate cancer. Mutations in *BRCA1* and *BRCA2* cause only a small number of familial prostate cancers. Genetic testing may be appropriate for families with prostate cancer that have HBOC.

Clinical Manifestations and Complications

Prostate cancer typically has no symptoms in the early stages. Eventually, patients may have LUTS similar to those of BPH. Pain in the lumbosacral area that radiates down to the hips or the legs, when combined with urine symptoms, may indicate metastasis.

The tumor can spread to pelvic lymph nodes, bones, bladder, lungs, and liver. Once the tumor has spread to distant sites, the major problem becomes pain. As the cancer spreads to the bones (common site of metastasis), pain can become severe, especially in the back and legs because of spinal cord compression and bone destruction.

Diagnostic Studies

Most males in the United States with prostate cancer are diagnosed by PSA screening. As prostate cancer screening has become more widespread, smaller cancers are being found in older males. In most cases, slow-growing cancers do not need to be treated. Many males live and die *with* prostate cancer, but most will not die *of* it.

Males can make an informed decision with their HCP about whether to be screened for prostate cancer. Males should be told about the potential risks (e.g., subsequent evaluation and treatment that may not be needed) and benefits (early detection of prostate cancer) of PSA screening before being tested. After this discussion, males who want to be screened may have an annual PSA test and DRE. On DRE, an abnormal prostate may feel hard, nodular, and asymmetric.

The AUA states that males ages 55 to 69 have the greatest potential benefit from PSA screening. They recommend shared decision making and potential screening every 2 years. Males at higher risk (Black males, males with a first-degree relative with prostate cancer) should have a more personalized screening schedule.

The ACS recommends males decide about screening after they discuss information about the risks and benefits with their HCP.[8] This discussion should take place at:

- Age 50 for males who are at average risk for prostate cancer and expected to live at least 10 more years.
- Age 45 for males at high risk for developing prostate cancer. This includes Black males and males with a first-degree relative (father, brother, son) diagnosed with prostate cancer at an early age (younger than age 65).
- Age 40 for males at even higher risk (those with more than 1 first-degree relative who had prostate cancer at an early age).

High PSA levels do not always indicate prostate cancer. Mild PSA increases may occur with aging, BPH, recent ejaculation, constipation, prostatitis, or after long bike rides. Cystoscopy, indwelling urinary catheters, and prostate biopsies may cause transient increases in PSA levels.

If PSA levels are continually high or if the DRE is abnormal, a prostate biopsy is usually done. Biopsy can confirm the diagnosis of prostate cancer. The biopsy is typically done using a transrectal approach. In a TRUS procedure, an ultrasound probe allows the HCP to see abnormalities in the prostate. When a suspicious area is found, biopsy needles are inserted through the wall of the rectum into the prostate to obtain tissue samples. A pathologic exam of the specimen is done to assess for cancer. For patients at a high risk for infection with a transrectal biopsy or a history of prior postbiopsy sepsis, a transperineal approach is another option if it is available. There can be a lower risk for infection with the transperineal approach as the biopsy needles do not pierce the rectal wall. It is typically done in the operating room.

Another approach for biopsies is to use an MRI/ultrasound fusion biopsy. In this approach, pelvic MRI 3-dimensional images are fused with real-time, TRUS images. This technique is more accurate than the traditional approach. Typically, males who undergo this procedure have a history of a previous negative ultrasound-guided biopsy and increasing PSA. This approach may be used for males who are on active surveillance. Recent studies show risk assessment with MRI before biopsy and MRI-targeted biopsy are better than standard TRUS biopsy in males at risk for prostate cancer who have not had a prostate biopsy before.[5]

The regular measurement of PSA levels after treatment is used to monitor treatment and possible recurrence of prostate cancer.[8] When treatment has been successful, with prostatectomy or hormone therapy, PSA levels should decrease to undetectable levels. With successful radiation therapy, the PSA level should decrease to a very low number and remain stable.

With advanced prostate cancer, alkaline phosphatase can be increased because of bone metastases. Other tests used to determine the location and extent of the spread of the cancer may include a nuclear medicine whole body bone scan, CT scan of the abdomen and pelvis, and MRI of the pelvis with special attention to the prostate.

Interprofessional Care

Chemoprevention of prostate cancer is an active area of research. Finasteride and dutasteride, used to treat BPH, may reduce the chance of getting prostate cancer. Males who are concerned about prostate cancer should discuss with their HCP the risks and benefits of taking finasteride or dutasteride.

Early recognition and treatment are important to control tumor growth, prevent metastasis, and preserve quality of life. Most patients with prostate cancer are diagnosed when the cancer is at a local or regional stage.[8] The 5-year survival rate with a diagnosis at this stage is almost 100%.

The most common classification system for staging prostate cancer is the tumor, node, and metastasis (TNM) system (Table 59.6). The tumor is graded based on tumor histology using 2 different grading systems: the Gleason score and the Grade Group. The Gleason score grades the tumor from 3 to 5 based on the degree of glandular differentiation. Grade 3 is the most well-differentiated or lowest grade (most like the original cells). Grade 5 is the most poorly differentiated (unlike the original cells) or highest grade. The 2 most commonly occurring patterns of cells are graded, and we add the 2 scores to create a Gleason score. Gleason score ranges from 6 to 10. Currently the lowest risk Gleason score is Gleason 6 (3 + 3).

The Grade Group system grades the cells based on their differentiation. The Grade Group assigns the tumor a number on a scale from 1 to 5. Grade Group 1 is the lowest risk, and Grade Group 5 is the highest risk. Currently, we use the Gleason score and the Grade Group system together. A low-risk, well-differentiated prostate cancer may be graded as Grade Group 1, Gleason 6 (3 + 3) prostate cancer. The trend is moving toward Grade Group scoring only.

The PSA level at diagnosis and the Gleason score and Grade Group are used with the TNM system to determine the stage of the tumor, which helps guide treatment options.

The care of patients with prostate cancer depends on the stage of the cancer, Gleason score, PSA, and patients' overall health (Table 59.7). None of the diagnostic options can predict the progression of prostate cancer. The decision of which treatment to pursue should be made jointly by patients, their partners, and the health care team.[8]

Active Surveillance

Low-grade prostate cancer is slow growing. Therefore a conservative approach is active surveillance, or "watchful waiting." This strategy is appropriate when patients have (1) a life expectancy of less than 10 years (low risk for dying of the disease); (2) a low-grade, low-stage tumor; and (3) serious coexisting medical conditions. With active surveillance, patients are

TABLE 59.6 Staging of Prostate Cancer

Stage	Tumor Size	Lymph Node Involvement	Metastasis	PSA Level	Gleason Score
I	Not felt on DRE. Not seen by visual imaging.	No	No	<10	≤6
II	Felt on DRE. Seen by imaging. Tumor confined to prostate.	No	No	10–20	6–7
III	Cancer outside prostate. Possible spread to seminal vesicles.	No	No	Any level	Any score
IV	Any size.	Any nodal involvement	Yes	Any level	Any score

Adapted from ACS: *How is prostate cancer staged?* Retrieved from https://www.cancer.org/Cancer/ProstateCancer/DetailedGuide/prostate-cancer-staging.

TABLE 59.7 Interprofessional Care

Prostate Cancer

Diagnostic Assessment

- History and physical assessment
- Digital rectal examination (DRE)
- Prostate-specific antigen (PSA)
- Transrectal ultrasound (TRUS) or pelvic MRI
- Prostate biopsy
- Whole-body bone scan to assess for bone metastases
- CT abdomen and pelvis with contrast to assess for metastatic disease

Management

Active Surveillance

- Closely monitor PSA and DRE (annually, at minimum)
- Repeat/surveillance prostate biopsies
- Repeat imaging
- Genomic testing on biopsy tissue

Surgery

- Radical prostatectomy
- Cryotherapy

Radiation Therapy

- External beam for primary, adjuvant, and recurrent disease
- Brachytherapy

Drug Therapy

- Androgen deprivation therapy (Table 59.8)
- Chemotherapy for metastatic disease

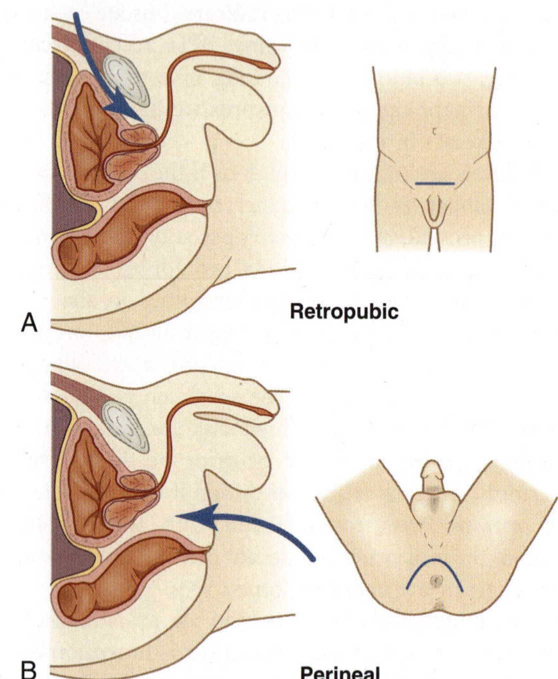

Fig. 59.5 Common approaches used to perform a prostatectomy. (A) Retropubic approach involves a midline abdominal incision. (B) Perineal approach involves an incision between the scrotum and the anus.

typically followed with frequent PSA levels and DRE to monitor the progress of the disease. Significant changes in PSA level, DRE, or the development of symptoms warrant a reevaluation of treatment options.

Surgical Therapy

Radical prostatectomy. With radical prostatectomy, the entire prostate gland, seminal vesicles, and part of the bladder neck (ampulla) are removed. The entire prostate is removed because the cancer tends to be in many different places within the gland. A pelvic lymph node dissection is typically done to assess for nodal metastases in the local pelvic area. Typically, a higher number of lymph nodes are removed if the prostate cancer is higher grade/higher risk on biopsy. Surgery is usually not an option for advanced-stage disease except to relieve symptoms from obstruction.

Traditional surgical approaches for an open radical prostatectomy include retropubic and perineal approaches (Fig. 59.5). With the *retropubic* approach, a low midline abdominal incision is made to access the prostate gland and dissect pelvic lymph nodes. With the *perineal* resection, the incision is between the scrotum and anus.

With a robotic-assisted (e.g., da Vinci system) prostatectomy, the HCP sits at a computer console while controlling high-resolution cameras and microsurgical instruments. Robotics is being used more often since it allows for increased precision, visualization, and dexterity by the HCP when removing the prostate gland. It results in less bleeding, less pain, and a faster recovery compared with other approaches.[9]

Two major adverse outcomes after a radical prostatectomy are ED and urine incontinence. The incidence of ED depends on patients' age, preoperative sexual function, whether nerve-sparing surgery was done, and the HCP's ability. Sexual function tends to return gradually over at least 24 months or more. Phosphodiesterase type 5 (PDE5) inhibitor drugs may help improve sexual function.

Problems with urine control may occur for the first few months after surgery because the bladder must be reattached to the urethra after the prostate is removed. Over time, the bladder adjusts, and most males regain urine continence. Kegel exercises strengthen the pelvic floor muscles and the urinary sphincter. They may help improve continence (see Table 50.18). Other complications of surgery include bleeding, lymphocele, urinary retention, infection, wound dehiscence, and VTE.

Nerve-sparing procedure. Near the prostate gland are neurovascular bundles that maintain erectile function. The preservation of these bundles during a prostatectomy is possible while still removing all the cancer. Nerve-sparing prostatectomy is not indicated for patients with cancer outside of the prostate gland. Although the risk for ED is reduced with this procedure, there is no guarantee that potency will be maintained.

Cryotherapy. *Cryotherapy* (cryoablation) is a surgical technique that destroys cancer cells by freezing the tissue. It is an initial treatment or a second-line treatment after radiation therapy has failed. A TRUS probe is inserted to see the prostate gland. Probes containing liquid nitrogen are then inserted into the prostate. Liquid nitrogen delivers freezing temperatures, thus destroying the tissue. The treatment takes about 2 hours under general or spinal anesthesia. It does not involve an abdominal incision.

Complications include damage to the urethra and, in rare cases, a urethrorectal fistula (an opening between the urethra and rectum) or a urethrocutaneous fistula (an opening between the urethra and skin). Tissue sloughing, ED, urinary incontinence, prostatitis, and bleeding can occur.

Radiation Therapy

Radiation therapy is another common treatment. Radiation therapy may be the only treatment, or it may be used with surgery or with hormone therapy. Salvage radiation therapy given for prostate cancer recurrence after a radical prostatectomy may improve survival in some males.

External beam radiation. External beam radiation is the most widely used method of delivering radiation treatments for prostate cancer. This therapy can be used to treat cancer confined to the prostate and/or surrounding tissue. Patients are usually treated on an outpatient basis 5 days a week for 4 to 8 weeks. Each treatment lasts less than 1 hour.

Side effects from radiation can be acute (occurring during treatment or within 90 days that follow) or delayed (occurring months or years after treatment). The most common side effects involve changes to the skin (dryness, redness, irritation, pain), gastrointestinal tract (diarrhea, abdominal cramping, bleeding, radiation proctitis), urinary tract (dysuria, hematuria, frequency, hesitancy, urgency, nocturia, radiation cystitis), and sexual function.[10] Fatigue may occur. There is a rare risk for secondary cancers after radiation to the pelvic area (e.g., bladder cancer, rectal cancer). In patients with local prostate cancer, cure rates with external beam radiation are comparable with those with radical prostatectomy.

Brachytherapy. *Brachytherapy* involves placing radioactive seed implants into the prostate gland. This delivers high doses of radiation directly to the tissue while sparing the surrounding tissue (rectum and bladder). The radioactive seeds are placed in the prostate gland with a needle through a grid template guided by TRUS (Fig. 59.6) to ensure correct placement of the seeds.

Because brachytherapy is a 1-time outpatient procedure, many patients find this more convenient than external beam radiation treatment. Brachytherapy is best suited for patients with early-stage disease. The most common side effect is the development of urinary irritative or obstructive problems. Some males may have ED. The AUA-SI (Table 59.1) can measure urine function for patients undergoing brachytherapy and can be part of nursing management. For those with more advanced tumors, brachytherapy may be used with external beam radiation treatment. Brachytherapy is discussed in Chapter 16.

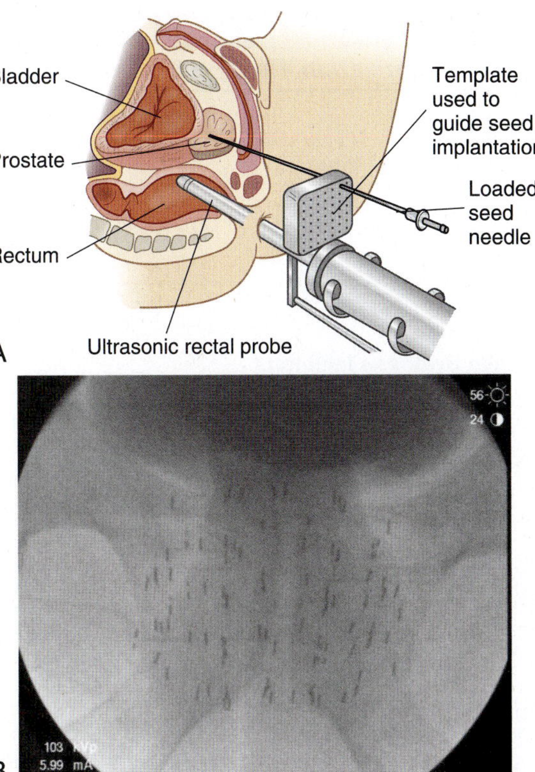

Fig. 59.6 (A) Prostate brachytherapy. Implantation of radioactive seeds with a needle guided by ultrasound and a template grid. (B) Radioactive seeds. (B, From Calvert AD, Dyer AW, Montgomery VA: Embolization of prostatic brachytherapy seeds to pulmonary arteries, *Radiol Case Rep* 12:34, 2017.)

Drug Therapy

Drug therapy for the treatment of advanced or metastatic prostate cancer includes androgen deprivation (hormone) therapy, chemotherapy, or a combination.

Androgen deprivation therapy. Prostate cancer growth is largely dependent on the presence of androgens. *Androgen deprivation therapy* (ADT) reduces the levels of circulating androgens to reduce the tumor growth. Androgen deprivation can be produced by inhibiting androgen production or blocking androgen receptors (Table 59.8).

One of the biggest challenges with ADT is that almost all tumors treated become resistant to this therapy *(hormone refractory)* within a few years. A high PSA level is often the first sign that this therapy is no longer effective. Patients taking ADT have an increased risk for cardiovascular side effects, including high cholesterol and triglyceride levels and coronary artery disease.[11]

Osteoporosis and fractures may occur in those receiving ADT. Drugs recommended to reduce bone mineral loss include zoledronic acid (Reclast) and raloxifene (Evista). Zoledronic acid is a bisphosphonate therapy given IV. A rare complication of therapy is osteonecrosis of the jaw. Denosumab (Prolia, Xgeva), a drug that slows the breakdown of bone, may be used to increase bone mass in males with nonmetastatic prostate cancer.

TABLE 59.8 Drug Therapy

Androgen Deprivation Therapy for Prostate Cancer

Therapy	Mechanism of Action	Side Effects
Androgen Receptor Blockers		
apalutamide (Erleada) bicalutamide (Casodex) darolutamide (Nubeqa) enzalutamide (Xtandi) nilutamide (Nilandron)	• Block action of testosterone by competing with receptor sites	• Loss of libido, ED • Hot flashes • Breast pain, gynecomastia
Androgen Synthesis Inhibitors ***CYP17 Enzyme Inhibitor***		
abiraterone (Zytiga)	• Inhibit *CYP17,* an enzyme needed to produce testosterone • Inhibit testosterone synthesis from testes, adrenal glands, and prostate cancer cells	• Joint swelling, fluid retention • Muscle aches • Hot flashes • Diarrhea
LHRH Agonists		
goserelin (Zoladex) leuprolide (Eligard, Lupron Depot) triptorelin (Trelstar)	• ↓ LH and FSH secretion • ↓ Testosterone production	• Hot flashes, gynecomastia, ↓ libido, ED • Depression, mood changes
LHRH Antagonist		
degarelix (Firmagon)	• Block LH receptors • Immediate testosterone suppression	• Pain, redness, swelling at injection site • ↑ Liver enzymes

Androgen synthesis inhibitors. The hypothalamus produces luteinizing hormone–releasing hormone (LHRH), which stimulates the anterior pituitary to produce luteinizing hormone (LH) and follicle-stimulating hormone (FSH). LH stimulates the testicular Leydig cells to make testosterone. *LHRH agonists* superstimulate the pituitary, downregulating the LHRH receptors and leading to a condition in which the anterior pituitary is unresponsive to LHRH. This produces a chemical castration similar to the effects of an orchiectomy. These drugs cause an initial transient increase in LH and FSH; testosterone abruptly rises resulting in a *flare.* Symptoms may worsen during this time. With continued administration, LH and testosterone levels will decrease. They are given by subcutaneous or IM injections.

Degarelix is an LHRH antagonist. It lowers testosterone levels to castration levels. Degarelix does not cause a testosterone flare because it acts directly to block LH and FSH receptors. It is given as a subcutaneous injection. Results are seen in 3 days.

Abiraterone (Zytiga) inhibits the enzyme CYP17, which is needed to produce testosterone. This drug is given orally to males with castration-resistant prostate cancer, usually in combination with prednisone. It improves overall survival by 4 to 5 months.

Androgen receptor blockers. Androgen receptor blockers are another class of antiandrogen drugs that compete with circulating androgens at the receptor sites. They are taken orally each day. They be used in combination with an LHRH agonist (e.g., goserelin). Combining an androgen receptor blocker with an LHRH agonist results in combined androgen blockade.

Chemotherapy. Chemotherapy is limited to treatment for those with hormone-refractory prostate cancer (HRPC) in late-stage disease. In HRPC the cancer is progressing despite treatment. This occurs in patients who have taken an antiandrogen for a certain period. The goal of chemotherapy is mainly palliative. Common chemotherapy drugs include cabazitaxel (Jevtana), cyclophosphamide, docetaxel (Taxotere), mitoxantrone, paclitaxel (Abraxane), and vinblastine.

Males with advanced prostate cancer who have HRPC may receive a vaccine (sipuleucel-T [Provenge]). We do not know exactly how, but the vaccine stimulates the immune system against the cancer. Use prolongs survival by about 4 months. It is individually prepared for each male by a process that combines his own WBCs with granulocyte-macrophage colony-stimulating factor (GM-CSF), which then attacks the prostate tumor cells.

Radiotherapy. Radium-223 dichloride (Xofigo) can be used in treating patients with castration-resistant prostate cancer, symptomatic bone metastases, and no known visceral metastatic disease. It is an alpha particle–emitting radiotherapy drug that mimics calcium and forms complexes with hydroxyapatite at areas of increased bone turnover, such as bone metastases.

Orchiectomy. A bilateral orchiectomy may be done alone or after prostatectomy. It is the gold standard for androgen deprivation. For advanced stages of prostate cancer, an orchiectomy is an option for cancer control, with rapid relief of bone pain associated with advanced tumors. Orchiectomy may shrink the prostate, thus relieving urine obstruction in the later stages of disease when surgery is not an option. After an orchiectomy, weight gain and loss of muscle mass can change a man's physical appearance. These physical changes can affect self-esteem, leading to grief and depression. Because this procedure is permanent, many males prefer drug therapy over an orchiectomy.

NURSING MANAGEMENT: PROSTATE CANCER

Assessment

Subjective and objective data that you should obtain from patients with prostate cancer are outlined in Table 59.9.

Clinical Problems

Clinical problems for patients with prostate cancer depend on the stage of the cancer. These may include:

- Pain
- Impaired urinary elimination
- Impaired sexual function
- Difficulty coping

Planning

The overall goals are that patients with prostate cancer will (1) be an active participant in the treatment plan, (2) have acceptable pain control, (3) follow the treatment plan, (4) understand the effect of the treatment plan on sexual function, and (5) find an acceptable way to manage bladder and bowel function.

Implementation

Health Promotion

A key role in relation to prostate cancer is to encourage patients, in consultation with their HCPs, to have annual prostate screening (PSA, DRE). Because of their increased risk for prostate cancer, Black males and other males at high risk, such as those with a family history of prostate cancer, should discuss the need for annual PSA and DRE beginning at age 45.[12]

Acute Care

Care of patients after a radical prostatectomy is similar to surgical procedures for BPH. After surgery, patients have a large urinary catheter with a 10- or 30-mL balloon placed in the bladder via the urethra. A drain placed in the surgical site helps remove drainage from the area. This drain is typically removed after a few days. Because the perineal approach has a higher risk for infection (location of the incision related to the anus), careful dressing changes and perineal care after each bowel movement are important for comfort and to prevent infection. Depending on the type of surgery, the hospital stay is from 1 to 3 days.

Care of patients receiving radiation therapy and chemotherapy is discussed in Chapter 16. Another consideration is the psychologic response to the cancer diagnosis. Provide sensitive, caring support for patients and their families to help them cope with the diagnosis. Prostate cancer support groups are available for males and their families to encourage them to be active, informed participants in their own care.

Teach catheter care if patients are discharged with a urinary catheter in place. Teach patients to clean the urethral meatus with soap and water once a day; always keep the collection bag lower than the bladder; and keep the catheter securely anchored to the inner thigh or abdomen. Tell them to report any signs of bladder infection, such as bladder spasms, fever, or hematuria. They should maintain a high fluid intake.

If urine incontinence is a problem, encourage patients to practice pelvic floor muscle exercises (Kegel exercises) at every urination and throughout the day. Continuous practice during the 4- to 6-week healing process improves the success rate. Products used for incontinence specifically designed for males are available through home care product catalogs and retail stores. Urinary incontinence is discussed in Chapter 50.

TABLE 59.9 NURSING ASSESSMENT

Prostate Cancer

Subjective Data

Important Health Information

Medications: Testosterone supplements. Use of drugs affecting urinary tract such as morphine, anticholinergics, monoamine oxidase inhibitors, tricyclic antidepressants

Functional Health Patterns

Health perception—health management: Positive family history. ↑ Fatigue and malaise

Nutritional-metabolic: High-fat diet. Anorexia, weight loss (may indicate metastasis)

Elimination: Hesitancy or straining to start stream, urgency, frequency, retention with dribbling, weak stream, hematuria

Sleep-rest: Nocturia

Cognitive-perceptual: Dysuria. Low back pain radiating to legs or pelvis, bone pain (may indicate metastasis). Pain level

Self-perception—self-concept: Anxiety about self-concept

Objective Data

General

Older adult male. Pelvic lymphadenopathy (late sign)

Urinary

Distended bladder on palpation. Unilaterally hard, enlarged, fixed prostate on rectal examination

Possible Diagnostic Findings

PSA. Alkaline phosphatase. Nodular and irregular prostate on ultrasonography, positive biopsy results. Anemia

Chronic Care

Palliative and end-of-life care are often appropriate and beneficial to patients with advanced disease and their families (see Chapter 10). Common problems with advanced prostate cancer include fatigue, bladder outlet obstruction and ureteral obstruction (caused by compression of the urethra and/or ureters from tumor mass or lymph node metastasis), severe bone pain and fractures (from bone metastasis), spinal cord compression (from spinal metastasis), and leg edema (from lymphedema, VTE). Nursing care must focus on managing these problems.

Pain management is important. Pain control involves pain assessment, prescribed analgesics, and nonpharmacologic methods of pain relief (e.g., relaxation breathing). Pain management is discussed in Chapter 9.

◆ Evaluation

The outcomes are that patients with prostate cancer will:

- Be an active participant in the treatment plan
- Have acceptable pain control
- Follow the treatment plan
- Understand the effect of the treatment on sexual function
- Find an acceptable way to manage bladder or bowel function

PROSTATITIS

Etiology and Pathophysiology

Prostatitis is a broad term that describes a group of inflammatory and noninflammatory conditions affecting the prostate gland. Prostatitis is one of the most common urologic disorders. We believe that 10% of all males in the United States will have prostatitis in their lifetime.[13] Almost 2 million males are treated for prostatitis every year.

The 4 categories of prostatitis syndromes are (1) acute bacterial prostatitis, (2) chronic bacterial prostatitis, (3) chronic prostatitis/chronic pelvic pain syndrome, and (4) asymptomatic inflammatory prostatitis.

Acute and chronic bacterial prostatitis generally result from organisms reaching the prostate gland by ascending from the urethra, descending from the bladder, or invading via the bloodstream or the lymphatic channels. Common causative organisms are *Escherichia coli* (most common), *Klebsiella, Pseudomonas, Enterobacter, Proteus, Chlamydia trachomatis, Neisseria gonorrhoeae,* and group D streptococci.

Chronic bacterial prostatitis differs from acute prostatitis in that it involves recurrent episodes of infection. It is the most common reason for recurrent UTIs in adult males.

Chronic prostatitis/chronic pelvic pain syndrome describes a syndrome of prostate and urinary pain in the absence of an obvious infectious process. The cause of this syndrome is not known. It may occur after a viral illness, or with a sexually transmitted infection (STI), especially in younger adults. A culture reveals no causative organisms. WBCs may be found in prostatic secretions.

Asymptomatic inflammatory prostatitis is usually diagnosed in those who have no symptoms but have an inflammatory process in the prostate. These patients are usually diagnosed during the evaluation of other GU tract problems. WBCs are present in the seminal fluid from the prostate. We do not know the cause.

Clinical Manifestations and Complications

Common manifestations of acute prostatitis include fever, chills, back pain, and perineal pain. Acute urinary symptoms such as dysuria, frequency, urgency, and cloudy urine may occur. Patients may progress to acute urine retention caused by prostatic swelling if untreated. With DRE, the prostate is extremely swollen, extremely tender, and boggy. The clinical features of prostatitis can mimic those of a UTI. However, remember that acute cystitis is not common in males.

Manifestations of chronic prostatitis are similar but generally milder than those of acute bacterial prostatitis. They include irritative voiding symptoms (frequency, urgency, dysuria), backache, perineal and pelvic pain, and ejaculatory pain. Obstructive symptoms are rare unless there is coexisting BPH. With DRE, the prostate feels enlarged and soft or boggy. It may be slightly tender with palpation. Chronic prostatitis can predispose patients to recurrent UTIs.

Complications include epididymitis and cystitis. Sexual function may be affected. Manifestations include post-ejaculation pain, libido problems, and ED. Prostatic abscess is a potential but rare complication.

Diagnostic Studies

Because patients with prostatitis have urinary symptoms, a UA and urine culture and sensitivities are needed. Often WBCs and bacteria are present. Patients with a fever need blood cultures and a complete blood count (CBC) to check the WBC count. The PSA test may be done to rule out prostate cancer. PSA levels are often increased with prostatic inflammation or infection. Thus, when inflammation or infection is present, the PSA may not be diagnostic.

Microscopic evaluation and culture of expressed prostate secretion can potentially be useful in the diagnosis of prostatitis. Expressed prostate secretion is obtained using a premassage and postmassage test. Patients are asked to void into a specimen cup just before and just after a vigorous prostate massage. Prostatic massage (for expressed prostate secretion) is becoming less common unless all other diagnostic options are exhausted. It should not be done if acute bacterial prostatitis is suspected. Compression is extremely painful and can increase the risk for bacterial spread. TRUS is not useful in the diagnosis of prostatitis. TRUS or MRI can rule out an abscess in the prostate.

Interprofessional and Nursing Management

Common antibiotics used for acute and chronic bacterial prostatitis include fluoroquinolones (e.g., ciprofloxacin, levofloxacin, ofloxacin), clindamycin, cephalexin, doxycycline, trimethoprim/sulfamethoxazole (Bactrim), or tetracycline. Antibiotics are usually given orally for up to 4 weeks for acute bacterial prostatitis. If patients have a high fever or other signs of sepsis, they need to be hospitalized and receive IV antibiotics.

Chronic bacterial prostatitis may be treated with oral antibiotic therapy for 8 to 12 weeks. Antibiotics may be given for a lifetime if patients are immunocompromised. A short course of oral antibiotics is usually prescribed for those with chronic prostatitis in case of bacterial infection. Antibiotic therapy is often not effective for patients whose prostatitis is not due to bacteria.

Patients with bacterial prostatitis tend to have a great amount of pain. The pain resolves as the infection resolves. Many patients have residual pain for several weeks because it takes time for the prostate to return to normal. Managing pain for patients with chronic prostatitis is difficult because the pain persists for weeks to months. No single approach provides relief for everyone. Antiinflammatory agents (e.g., ibuprofen, naproxen) may help provide some relief.

Warm sitz baths may help relieve pain. α-Adrenergic blockers (e.g., tamsulosin, alfuzosin) relax muscle tissue in the prostate. They are effective in reducing pain for some males.

Acute urinary retention can develop in acute prostatitis, requiring insertion of a urinary catheter. However, passage of a urethral catheter is often contraindicated due to the risk of increasing inflammation or causing trauma. Such patients may need a suprapubic catheter. Prostatic massage may be recommended as an adjunct therapy. It can relieve congestion in the prostate by squeezing out excess prostatic secretions, providing pain relief. Prostatic massage is contraindicated in acute bacterial infection due to the risk of sepsis. Like massage, measures to stimulate ejaculation (masturbation, intercourse) may help drain the prostate and provide some relief.

Encourage patients to drink plenty of fluids. They have increased fluid needs from fever and infection. Managing fever is important (see Table 12.5).

PROBLEMS OF THE PENIS

We describe problems of the penis as congenital, problems of the prepuce, problems with the erectile mechanism, and cancer. Penis problems are rare once we exclude STIs (see Chapter 57).

CONGENITAL PROBLEMS

Hypospadias is a urologic problem in which the urethral meatus is on the ventral surface of the penis. This can be anywhere from the corona to the perineum. Causes include hormone influences in utero, environment factors, and genetic factors. Surgical repair of hypospadias, especially those that are close to the scrotum or perineum, is usually done while the boy is young. Surgery may be done if it is associated with *chordee* (a painful downward curvature of the penis during erection) or if it prevents intercourse or normal urination. Surgery may be considered for cosmetic reasons or emotional well-being in older boys and adult males.

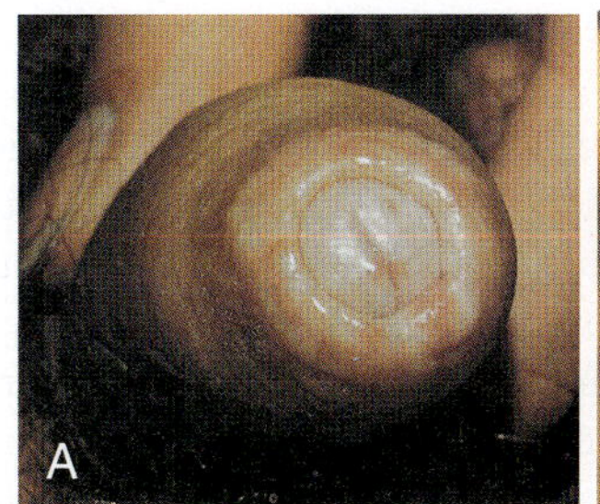

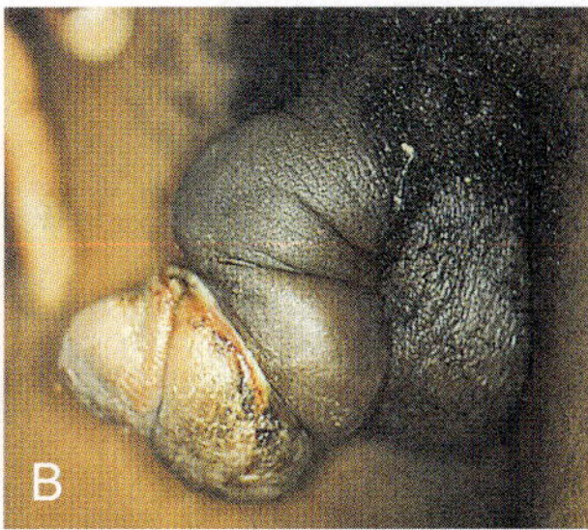

Fig. 59.7 (A) Phimosis: inability to retract the foreskin due to secondary lesions on the prepuce (foreskin). (B) Paraphimosis: ulcer with edema from foreskin remaining contracted over the prepuce (foreskin).

PROBLEMS OF PREPUCE

Problems of the prepuce (foreskin) are not as common in the United States as in most other countries because circumcision is a routine procedure for many male infants. When these conditions do occur, they can be very painful and potentially an emergency.

Phimosis is a tightness or constriction of the foreskin around the head of the penis, making retraction difficult (Fig. 59.7A). It is caused by chronic inflammation of the foreskin. It is usually related to poor hygiene techniques that allow bacterial and yeast organisms to become trapped under the foreskin. Topical corticosteroid cream, with or without an antifungal, applied 2 or 3 times daily to the exterior and interior of the tip of the foreskin may be effective in treating inflammation. Definitive treatment is circumcision or a dorsal slit surgery.

Paraphimosis is tightness of the foreskin resulting in the inability to pull it forward from a retracted position, thus preventing normal return over the glans. It is a urologic emergency. A tightly retracted phimotic ring can decrease arterial flow to the glans. An ulcer can develop if the foreskin stays contracted (Fig. 59.7B). Paraphimosis can occur when the foreskin is pulled back during bathing, use of urinary catheters, or intercourse and is not placed back in the forward position. Replacing the foreskin after careful cleaning helps prevent this condition. The goal of treatment is to return the foreskin to its natural position over the glans penis through manual reduction. One strategy involves pushing the glans back through the prepuce by applying constant thumb pressure while the index fingers pull the prepuce over the glans. Ice and/or hand compression on the foreskin, glans, and penis may be applied before to reduce edema. Treatment may include antibiotics or warm soaks. Definitive treatment is circumcision or a dorsal slit.

PROBLEMS OF ERECTILE MECHANISM

Priapism is a painful erection lasting longer than 4 hours. It is caused by complex vascular and neurologic factors that result in an obstruction of venous outflow in the penis. Conditions that may be associated with priapism include sickle cell disease, diabetes, trauma to the spinal cord, degenerative lesions of the spine, and drugs (e.g., cocaine, trazodone). Vasoactive drugs (e.g., alprostadil) injected into the corpora cavernosa for ED can cause priapism. Complications include penile tissue necrosis caused by lack of blood flow or hydronephrosis from bladder distention. Without immediate medical treatment, the risk for permanent ED is high.

Treatment varies depending on the cause. Patients with sickle cell disease may need a blood exchange transfusion. Other patients may receive sedatives, an injection of a smooth muscle relaxant directly into the penis, or aspiration and irrigation of the corpora cavernosa with a large-bore needle.

Peyronie disease is caused by plaque formation in the corpora cavernosa of the penis that results in inelasticity during erection. The palpable, nontender, hard plaque formation may occur spontaneously or result from trauma to the penile shaft. The plaque prevents adequate blood flow into the spongy tissue, which results in a curvature during erection. The condition is not dangerous but can result in painful erections, ED, or embarrassment. Patients may improve slightly over time, stabilize, or need surgery. Collagenase clostridium histolyticum (Xiaflex) and intralesional verapamil (ILV) are other options. Each is given as a series of injections into the plaque. The goal of therapy is to reduce the curvature and avoid surgery.

CANCER OF PENIS

Cancer of the penis is rare in the United States. More than 95% are squamous cell cancer. It occurs more often in males who have human papillomavirus (HPV) infection and phimosis or uncircumcised males.[14] The tumor may appear as a superficial ulceration or a pimple-like nodule. Pain is rare. This contributes to a delay in seeking treatment. The nontender warty lesion may be mistaken for a genital wart. Treatment in the early stages is laser removal. A radical resection of the penis may be needed if the cancer has spread. Surgery, radiation, or chemotherapy are options, depending on the extent of the disease, lymph node involvement, and metastasis.

PROBLEMS OF THE SCROTUM AND TESTES

INFLAMMATORY AND INFECTIOUS PROBLEMS

Skin Problems

The skin of the scrotum is susceptible to several common skin problems. The most common are fungal infections, dermatitis (neurodermatitis, contact dermatitis, seborrheic dermatitis), and parasitic infections (scabies, lice). These conditions involve discomfort but cause few severe complications (see Chapter 25).

Epididymitis

Epididymitis is an acute, painful inflammatory process of the epididymis (Fig. 59.8). It is often due to an infectious process, trauma, or urine reflux down the ductus (vas) deferens. It is usually unilateral. Swelling may progress to the point that the epididymis and testis are indistinguishable. In males younger than 35 years of age, the most common cause is gonorrhea or chlamydial infection. In males older than 35, the most common cause is *E. coli* infection. BPH and prostatitis are common contributors in older males.

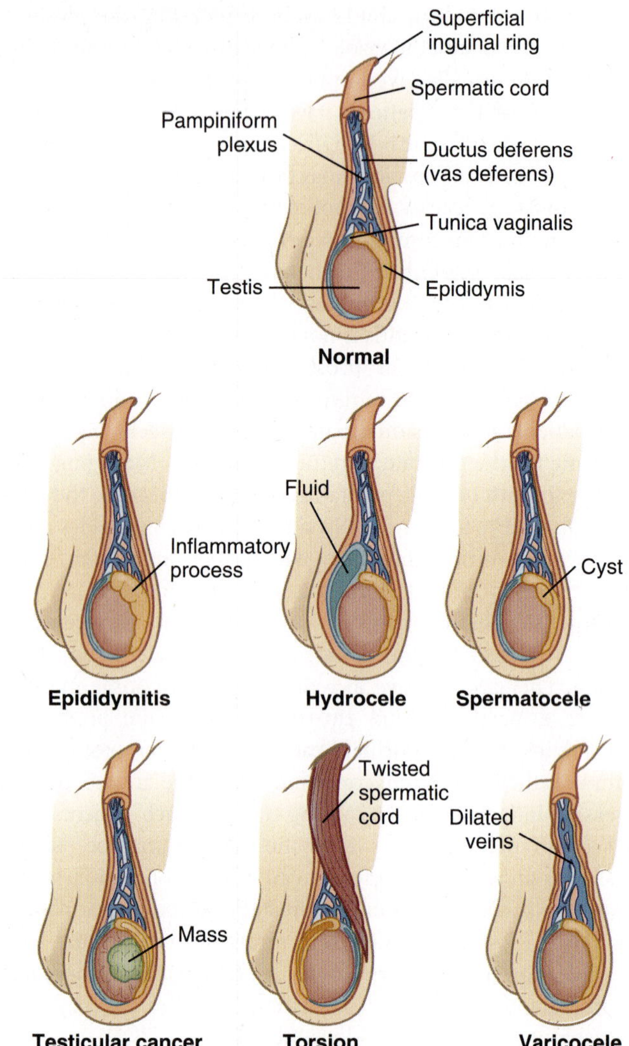

Fig. 59.8 Scrotal masses.

Antibiotic treatment is important. We treat both partners if the transmission is through sexual contact. Encourage patients to refrain from sexual intercourse until treatment is complete. They should use a condom if they do engage in intercourse. Conservative treatment consists of elevating the scrotum, ice packs, and analgesics. Ambulation places the scrotum in a dependent position and increases pain. Acute tenderness subsides within 1 week, although some pain and swelling may last for weeks or months.

Orchitis

Orchitis is an acute inflammation of the testis. In orchitis, the testis is painful, tender, and swollen. It often occurs after an episode of bacterial or viral infection, such as mumps, pneumonia, tuberculosis, or syphilis. It can be a side effect of epididymitis, trauma, infectious mononucleosis, influenza, catheterization, or complicated UTI. Mumps orchitis can cause infertility. It can be avoided by childhood vaccination against mumps. Treatment is similar to that for epididymitis.

CONGENITAL PROBLEMS

Cryptorchidism (undescended testes) is failure of the testes to descend into the scrotal sac before birth. It is the most common congenital testicular condition. The condition may occur bilaterally or unilaterally. It is more common on the right. We believe it is a contributing factor to male infertility if corrective surgery is not done by age 2. The incidence of testicular cancer is higher if the condition is not corrected before puberty. Surgery is done to locate and suture the testis or testes to the scrotum.

ACQUIRED PROBLEMS

Hydrocele

A *hydrocele* is a nontender, fluid-filled mass that results from interference with lymphatic drainage of the scrotum and swelling of the tunica vaginalis that surrounds the testis (Figs. 59.8 and 59.9). Diagnosis is aided by shining a flashlight through the scrotum (transillumination). No treatment is needed unless the swelling becomes large and uncomfortable, then surgical repair is needed. Hydrocele repair is avoided in males who have not started their family or seek to add to their family as repair can contribute to subfertility or infertility.

Spermatocele

A *spermatocele* is a firm, sperm-containing cyst of the epididymis. It may be visible with transillumination (Fig. 59.8). The cause is unknown. They can become large, tense, and painful. Their size can wax and wane with time. Spermatocele repair is avoided in males who have not started their family or seek to add to their family as repair can contribute to subfertility or infertility.

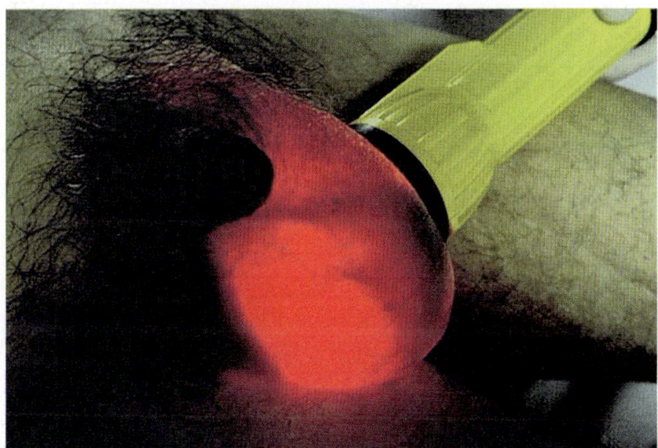

Fig. 59.9 Hydrocele. (From Klatt EC: *Robbins and Cotran atlas of pathology,* ed 4, St. Louis, 2021, Elsevier.)

Varicocele

A *varicocele* is a dilation of the veins that drain the testes (Fig. 59.8). The scrotum can feel worm-like when palpated if the venous dilation is significant. We do not know the cause of the problem. A varicocele is usually on the left side of the scrotum because of retrograde blood flow from the left renal vein.

Varicoceles are associated with 40% to 50% of cases of infertility. We think that the varicocele damages the sperm. Surgery is considered if fertility is a concern. Repair options include injecting a sclerosing agent or surgical ligation of the spermatic vein.

Testicular Torsion

Testicular torsion involves a twisting of the spermatic cord that supplies blood to the testes and epididymis (Fig. 59.8). It is a surgical emergency. It most often occurs in males younger than age 20. It can occur spontaneously or because of trauma or an anatomic abnormality.

Patients have severe, sudden onset of scrotal pain, tenderness, swelling, nausea, and vomiting. The pain does not usually subside with rest or elevating the scrotum. The cremasteric reflex is absent on the side of the swelling. Normal anatomic landmarks are lost due to tissue edema.

A Doppler ultrasound is done to assess blood flow within the testicle. Decreased or absent blood flow confirms the diagnosis. Torsion is an emergency! If the blood supply to the affected testicle is not restored within 4 to 6 hours, ischemia to the testis will occur, leading to necrosis. Unless the torsion resolves spontaneously, surgery to untwist the cord and restore the blood supply must be done emergently.

TESTICULAR CANCER

Etiology and Pathophysiology

Testicular cancer is relatively rare. It accounts for less than 1% of all cancers in males. In the United States about 9760 new cases occur annually.[15] It is the most common cancer in young males between 15 and 34 years of age.

Testicular tumors are more common in males who had undescended testes (cryptorchidism) or a family history of testicular cancer or anomalies. Other predisposing factors include orchitis, HIV infection, maternal exposure to exogenous estrogen, and testicular cancer in the other testis.

Most testicular cancers develop from 2 types of embryonic germ cells: seminomas and nonseminomas. Seminoma germ cell cancers are the most common but are the least aggressive. Nonseminoma testicular germ cell tumors are rare but very aggressive. Non–germ cell tumors arise from other testicular tissue. These include Leydig cell and Sertoli cell tumors. They cause less than 10% of testicular cancers.

Clinical Manifestations

Testicular cancer may have a slow or rapid onset depending on the type of tumor (Fig. 59.8). There may be a painless, firm lump in the scrotum and scrotal swelling. Some patients report a dull ache or heavy sensation in the lower abdomen, perianal area, or scrotum. Acute pain is the first symptom in about 10% of patients. Manifestations of advanced disease vary. They include lower back or chest pain, cough, and dyspnea.

Diagnostic Studies

Palpation of the scrotal contents is the first step in diagnosing testicular cancer. A cancerous mass is firm and does not transilluminate. Ultrasound is done if testicular cancer is suspected (e.g., palpable mass) or when persistent or painful testicular swelling is present. Tumor markers include α-fetoprotein (AFP), lactate dehydrogenase (LDH), and human chorionic gonadotropin (hCG) levels.

Chest x-ray, CBC, basic metabolic panel, and liver function tests may be done. Anemia may be present. Liver function levels may be increased in metastatic disease. If cancer is confirmed by pathology, then a CT scan of the abdomen and pelvis (and possibly the chest) is done to further stage and assess for metastases.

Interprofessional and Nursing Management

Testicular cancer is one of the most curable cancers. Treatment generally involves a radical inguinal orchiectomy (removal of the affected testis, spermatic cord, and regional lymph nodes). Some patients with early-stage disease do not need further treatment after an orchiectomy. Retroperitoneal lymph node dissection and removal also may be done in early-stage disease. These nodes are the primary route for metastasis.

Postorchiectomy treatment may involve radiation therapy or chemotherapy depending on the stage of the cancer. Radiation therapy is mainly used for patients with seminoma, which is very sensitive to radiation. Radiation does not work well for nonseminomas.

Testicular germ cell tumors are more sensitive to systemic chemotherapy than any other adult solid tumor. Chemotherapy protocols use a combination of agents, including bleomycin, cisplatin, etoposide, and ifosfamide (Ifex). Retroperitoneal lymph node dissection may be done after chemotherapy in patients with advanced testicular cancer.

The prognosis for males with testicular cancer has greatly improved; 95% obtain complete remission if the disease is found in the early stages. Because of treatment successes, many males with testicular cancer are long-term survivors. All patients with testicular cancer need surveillance and regular physical assessments, chest x-rays, CT scans, and tumor markers (hCG, AFP, LDH). The goal is to detect relapse when the tumor burden is minimal.

Some drugs used to treat testicular cancer can cause serious long-term side effects. These include lung problems, kidney damage, nerve damage (which can cause numbness and tingling), and hearing loss (from nerve damage). Secondary cancers can occur after chemotherapy (see Chapter 16).

Pretreatment subfertility or impaired fertility is identified at diagnosis. Chemotherapy with cisplatin and/or pelvic radiation often damages the testicular germ cells. Spermatogenesis can return in some patients. Because of the high risk for infertility, the cryopreservation of sperm in a sperm bank before treatment begins should be discussed and recommended. Ejaculatory dysfunction may result from retroperitoneal lymph node dissection. These issues may be hard to discuss with newly diagnosed patients. Males may feel the disease is a threat to their masculinity and self-worth.

CHECK YOUR PRACTICE

You are working on the urologic oncology unit caring for a 35-year-old male who recently had an orchiectomy for testicular cancer. His wife is at the bedside. The patient appears quiet and nonengaged when you assess him. His wife tells you that the patient has been worried that he will never have a normal sex life and will never enjoy sex again.

- How would you respond? What kind of support and information would you provide?

SEXUAL AND REPRODUCTIVE FUNCTION

VASECTOMY

Vasectomy is the bilateral surgical ligation or resection of the ductus deferens done for the purpose of sterilization (Fig. 59.10). The procedure takes only 15 to 30 minutes. It is usually done under local anesthesia on an outpatient basis. Although we consider vasectomy a permanent form of sterilization, successful vasectomy reversals *(vasovasostomy, vasoepididymostomy)* are common.

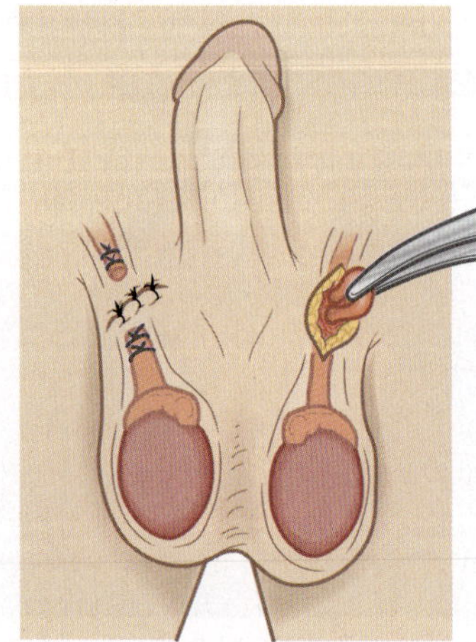

Fig. 59.10 Vasectomy procedure. The ductus deferens is ligated or resected for sterilization.

After vasectomy, patients should not notice any difference in the look or feel of the ejaculate because its major components are seminal and prostatic fluid. They must use a different form of contraception until semen examination reveals no sperm. Sperm cells continue to be made by the testes but are stored in the epididymis and reabsorbed by the body rather than being passed through the ductus deferens. Vasectomy does not affect the hormone production, ability to ejaculate, or physiologic mechanisms related to erection or orgasm. Psychologic adjustment may be a problem after surgery. It may be hard for patients to separate vasectomy from castration at a subconscious level. Some males develop psychogenic ED or feel the need to be more sexually active than they were to prove their masculinity.

ERECTILE DYSFUNCTION

Erectile dysfunction (ED) is the inability to attain or maintain an erection that allows satisfactory sexual activity. ED is significant because of its prevalence. More than 10 million males in the United States have ED. The incidence increases with age. We believe that 50% of males between ages 40 and 70 have at least some degree of ED. In younger males, we attribute an increase in ED to substance use (e.g., recreational drugs, alcohol), stress, and anxiety.

Etiology and Pathophysiology

ED can be due to many factors (Table 59.10). Common causes include diabetes, vascular disease, drug side effects, surgery (e.g., prostatectomy), trauma, chronic illness, stress, difficulty in a relationship, or depression. Since ED results from reduced blood flow to the penis, there is a potential association with cardiovascular disease because the risk factors are the same.

Normal physiologic age-related changes are associated with changes in erectile function. They may be an underlying cause of ED for some males. Table 55.2 lists age-related changes in sexual function. Review age-related changes (if necessary) to reassure an anxious older male about normal changes in his sexual abilities.

Clinical Manifestations and Complications

The typical symptom is a patient's self-report of problems with erectile activity, describing an inability to attain or maintain an erection. The symptoms may occur only occasionally, may be continual with a gradual onset, or may have a sudden onset. A gradual onset of symptoms is usually due to physiologic factors. A sudden or rapid onset of symptoms may be related to psychologic issues. It is common for younger males with ED to have diabetes, hypertension, depression, or high cholesterol levels.

A man's inability to perform sexually can cause great distress in his interpersonal relationships and interfere with his concept of himself as a male. It can affect the relationship between the male and his partner. ED can lead to personal issues, including anger, anxiety, and depression.

Diagnostic Studies

The first step in the diagnosis of ED is a sexual, health, and psychosocial history. Self-administered questionnaires may be used as primary screening tools. For example, the International Index of Erectile Function (IIEF) assesses a man's response to 5 key areas of male sexual function: erectile function, orgasmic function, sexual desire, intercourse satisfaction, and overall satisfaction.

The physical assessment should focus on secondary sexual characteristics. Note if secondary sexual characteristics reflect the person's chronologic age (Tanner stage). A DRE is done to assess prostate size, consistency, and presence of nodules. Assess BP and peripheral pulses. Auscultate the femoral arteries.

Further testing is typically based on findings from the history and physical assessment. A lipid profile, glucose, and hemoglobin A1C (HbA1c) are recommended to rule out diabetes. Hormone levels for testosterone, prolactin, LH, and thyroid hormones may show endocrine-related problems. PSA level and CBC may help identify other diseases.

Other diagnostic tests may be done to diagnose ED. Nocturnal penile tumescence and rigidity testing is a

TABLE 59.10 Common Risk Factors for ED

Drug Induced
- Alcohol
- Antiandrogens
- Antihypertensives
- Antilipidemic agents
- Major tranquilizers (diazepam, alprazolam)
- Marijuana, cocaine
- Nicotine
- Tricyclic antidepressants (e.g., amitriptyline)

Endocrine
- Diabetes
- Hypogonadism
- Obesity

Genitourinary
- Radical prostatectomy
- Renal failure

Neurologic
- Cerebrovascular disease
- Parkinson disease
- Trauma to the spinal cord
- Tumors or transection of spinal cord

Psychologic
- Anxiety
- Depression
- Stress

Vascular
- Atherosclerosis
- Hypertension
- Peripheral vascular disease

Other
- Aging

noninvasive method that involves the continuous measurement of penile circumference and axial rigidity during sleep. These tests distinguish between physiologic and psychogenic causes of ED. Vascular studies, including penile arteriography, penile blood flow study, and duplex Doppler ultrasound studies, can assess penile blood inflow and outflow. These tests help identify vascular problems interfering with erection.

Interprofessional and Nursing Management

The goal of therapy is for the patient and partner to achieve a satisfactory sexual relationship. The treatment for ED can be based on the underlying cause. In general, males are moved directly into treatment without a costly workup. A variety of treatment options are available (Table 59.11). Tell patients that no option will restore ejaculation or tactile sensations if they were absent before treatment.

It is important to determine whether ED is reversible before treatment is started. For example, if ED is a side effect of prescribed drugs, other treatments can be explored. With an established diagnosis of testicular failure (hypogonadism), androgen replacement therapy may be part of the prescribed treatment. For ED that is psychologic in nature, counseling (with or without his partner) is recommended. This counseling should be with a qualified sex therapist.

Erectogenic Drugs

PDE5 inhibitors cause smooth muscle relaxation and increased blood flow into the corpus cavernosum, promoting penile erection. Most are taken orally before sexual activity. These drugs are generally safe and effective for the treatment of most types of ED. They are ineffective in the absence of arousal.

Side effects include headaches, leg/back pain, dyspepsia, flushing, and nasal congestion. Rare side effects are blurred or blue-green vision problems, sudden hearing loss, and an erection lasting more than 4 hours (priapism). Teach patients to seek immediate medical attention if any of these reactions occur. Because these drugs may potentiate the hypotensive effect of nitrates, they are contraindicated for those taking nitrates (e.g., nitroglycerin).

DRUG ALERT

Phosphodiesterase Type 5 (PDE5) Inhibitors

- Should not be used with nitrates (nitroglycerin) in any form.
- Can potentiate hypotensive effects of nitrates.

TABLE 59.11 Interprofessional Care

ED

Diagnostic Assessment
- History and physical assessment
- Sexual history
- Glucose and lipid profile
- Testosterone, prolactin, and thyroid hormone levels
- Nocturnal penile tumescence and rigidity testing
- Vascular studies

Management
- PDE5 inhibitors: avanafil (Stendra), sildenafil (Viagra), tadalafil (Cialis), vardenafil
- Modify reversible causes
- Sexual counseling

Devices and Implants
- Intraurethral medication pellet
- Intracavernosal self-injection
- Penile implants
- Vacuum erection device (VED)

Vacuum Erection Devices

Vacuum erection devices (VEDs) are suction devices that are applied to a flaccid penis. They produce an erection by pulling blood up into the corporeal bodies. A penile ring or constrictive band is placed around the base of the penis to retain venous blood, preventing the erection from subsiding.

Intraurethral Devices and Intracavernosal Injections

Intraurethral devices include the use of vasoactive drugs applied as a topical gel or a medication pellet inserted into the urethra using a medicated urethral system for erection (MUSE) device. Intracavernosal self-injections may be combined with medication injected directly into the corpus cavernosum.

Alprostadil (Caverject, Edex) is a vasoactive drug that enhances blood flow into penile arteries. It can be given by injection or as a transurethral pellet (suppository). When given as a suppository, the drug is placed into the opening at the tip of the penis. When injected, a needle and syringe are used to inject the drug directly into the corpus cavernosum. Trimix (a combination product) includes alprostadil, papaverine, and phentolamine.

Penile Implants

Penile implants are placed into the corporeal bodies to provide an erection firm enough for penetration. The inflatable implant consists of cylinders in the penis, a small pump in the scrotum, and a reservoir in the lower abdomen. The main complications of penile prostheses are infection, erosion, and, rarely, mechanical failure. Implantation requires surgery. It can sometimes be done in an outpatient setting.

Sexual Counseling

The male with ED needs a great deal of emotional support for him and his partner. Males often do not feel comfortable discussing their problems because of their perception of society's expectations of a man's sexual abilities. Many males delay seeking medical care or expect immediate solutions to ED. The health care team should provide a support system and accurate information.

Sexual counseling can be recommended at any point during treatment for ED. It may be most effective in cases with a component of psychogenic ED. Counseling should address psychologic or interpersonal factors that may enhance sexual expression, as well as other factors that are of concern. It can include their partner, especially if patients are in a long-term relationship.

HYPOGONADISM

Hypogonadism is a gradual decline in androgen secretion that occurs in most males as they age. Thus we also call it *late-onset hypogonadism* or *hypogonadism of old age.* It can begin as early as age 40. The primary male androgen that is reduced is testosterone (Fig. 59.11). It is unclear what causes the decline in testosterone. Obesity is a contributing factor.

Manifestations of low testosterone include decreased libido, fatigue, ED, depression and mood swings, and sleep problems. Since many of these manifestations can be associated with aging, some patients may not mention this to their HCP, or the HCP may not recognize these manifestations as signs of low testosterone. Long-term effects of low testosterone include loss of muscle mass and strength, which may contribute to an increased risk for falls and fractures.

Hypogonadism is diagnosed with a blood test and physical assessment. Replacement testosterone therapy is considered if total testosterone levels are less than 300 ng/dL on 2 separate early morning measurements/occasions and there are manifestations of low testosterone.[16] Therapy may be started earlier depending on severity of symptoms. Testosterone replacement therapy (TRT) should not be started until patients, in consultation with their HCP, consider the risks and benefits of therapy. Rare effects include lower levels of high-density lipoprotein (HDL) cholesterol, increased hematocrit, and worsening sleep apnea. Since TRT may cause increased growth of prostate tissue, TRT is contraindicated in patients with unmanaged BPH or prostate cancer. Before starting treatment, a DRE and PSA are done. Once TRT begins, we closely monitor patients.

Replacement therapy is available in different forms, including injection, transdermal, topical, buccal, or intranasal preparations. IM injections, such as testosterone cypionate (Depo-Testosterone) and testosterone enanthate, are available in varying doses. These drugs create a cyclic rise and fall in testosterone levels. The highest levels occur 2 to 3 days after the injection. Testosterone levels slowly decrease until the next injection. One side effect of IM TRT is mood swings with the hormone fluctuations.

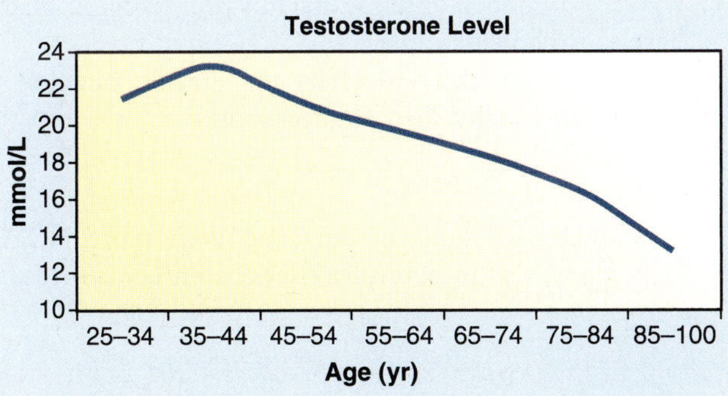

Fig. 59.11 Changes in testosterone levels as males age.

Transdermal preparations, including patches and gels (e.g., Testim), are often prescribed. They are applied to the skin at product-specific sites, including the back, arm, and abdomen. Skin irritation is a common side effect.

Stress the importance of hand washing with soap and water after applying testosterone preparations to the skin. Have patients cover the area with clothing until the preparation has dried. Females of childbearing age and children should not touch testosterone products. Testosterone may cause early signs of puberty in young children and changes (virilization) in the external genitalia of a female fetus.

INFERTILITY

Infertility in a couple is the inability to conceive after 1 year of frequent unprotected intercourse. Infertility is a problem with the couple, not of a person. For this reason, both partners must be involved in evaluating infertility. Some estimate up to 50% of infertility cases are related to male factors.[17]

We consider the physical causes of infertility in 3 categories: pretesticular, testicular, and posttesticular. The remaining 40% are *idiopathic,* or of unknown causes. The *pretesticular* or endocrine causes occur in only about 3% of the cases. They can generally be treated with medication or surgery.

Testicular problems make up 50% of the cases. The most common cause of male infertility is a varicocele. Other factors that influence the testes include infection (e.g., mumps virus, STIs, bacterial infections), congenital anomalies, drugs, radiation, substance use (alcohol, nicotine, drugs), and environment hazards. *Posttesticular* causes account for 5% to 7% of the cases. Obstruction, infection, and the result of a surgical procedure are the primary causes.

The history is a starting point for determining cause and treatment. The history should include age; occupation; past injury, surgery, or infections of the genital tract; lifestyle issues (e.g., hot tubs, weight training, wearing tight undergarments); sexual practices; frequency of intercourse; and emotional factors, such as stress level. Have they fathered a child? Record the use of drugs, such as chemotherapeutic agents, anabolic steroids or testosterone, sulfasalazine, cimetidine, and recreational drugs. These drugs can reduce the sperm count. The assessment may identify a varicocele, Peyronie disease, or other physical findings.

The first test in the male infertility evaluation is a semen analysis to evaluate sperm concentration, motility, and morphology. Hormone studies, including testosterone, LH, and FSH levels, are helpful. Be tactful in dealing with male patients undergoing infertility studies. Many cultures equate fertility and masculinity. Male and female partners should undergo evaluation simultaneously to avoid potential treatment delays.

Treatment options for the male include drugs, conservative lifestyle changes (e.g., avoiding scrotal heat, substance use, high stress), in vitro fertilization techniques, and corrective surgery. Infertility can seriously strain a relationship. The couple may need counseling and discussion of alternatives if they do not achieve conception. Female infertility is discussed in Chapter 58.

CASE STUDY

Benign Prostatic Hyperplasia With Acute Urinary Retention

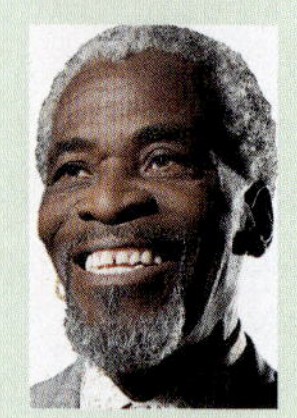

(© IPGGutenberg UKLtd/iStock/ Thinkstock.)

Patient Profile

B.G. is a 60-year-old Black male with hypertension, COPD, and coronary artery disease, who had a green light laser photovaporization of the prostate (PVP) 2 days ago. He was discharged that evening with a urinary catheter, with plans to remove the catheter with his local urologist in 2 days. He presents to the emergency department the next day because of increasing pressure and pain in his bladder. He tells the nurse that the catheter has not been draining for the past 8 hours. There is urine leaking around the catheter at the meatus.

Subjective Data

- Reports the urge to void, and pain in the lower abdomen
- Reports gradually worsening gross hematuria for the past 24 hours
- Appears restless, anxious, and agitated

Objective Data

- Tender and palpable bladder above the umbilicus
- Urinalysis (from catheter): >50 WBC, >50 RBC, positive bacteria and nitrites
- PSA test: 8 ng/mL

Interprofessional Care

- Attempted to irrigate indwelling urinary catheter at the bedside, without success. The catheter balloon was deflated, and the catheter was removed intact. The nurse inserted a new 22-French 3-way catheter.
- Once the new catheter was placed, 900 mL of cloudy urine with gross hematuria drained from the bladder with relief of symptoms.
- Admitted for observation.

Discussion Questions

1. ***Recognize:*** What risk factors are present for prostate problems?
2. ***Analyze:*** Interpret B.G.'s high PSA level.
3. ***Analyze:*** Based on the assessment, what problem does B.G. have?
4. ***Plan:*** What treatment options are possible?
5. ***Prioritize:*** What is the most important problem to manage right now?
6. ***Act:*** What teaching will you provide so B.G. can successfully self-manage care?
7. ***Evaluate:*** What do you need to continually monitor?
8. ***Safety:*** What risk factors does B.G. have for VTE? Infection?

Answers available at http://evolve.elsevier.com/Lewis/medsurg.

BRIDGE TO NCLEX EXAMINATION

The number of the question corresponds to the same-numbered outcome at the beginning of the chapter.

1. A patient who had a transurethral resection of the prostate (TURP) has continuous bladder irrigation (CBI) running via a 3-way urinary catheter with a 30 mL balloon. On assessment, CBI outflow is light pink. The patient reports intermittent bladder spasms. The nurse would
   a. inflate the balloon to 40 mL to decrease bulk in the bladder.
   b. stop the irrigation and immediately notify the HCP of possible obstruction.
   c. deflate and then reinflate the balloon to ensure that the balloon is functioning.
   d. tell him spasms are expected so he should not try to force urine around the catheter.
2. Which factors increase the risk for prostate cancer? **(Select all that apply.)**
   a. Black ethnicity
   b. Asian ethnicity
   c. Cigarette smoking
   d. Working as a farmer
   e. Age between 40 and 50 years old
   f. Working spreading commercial pesticides
3. A patient who is recovering from a radical prostatectomy for prostate cancer expresses concern that he will have erectile dysfunction. In responding to the patient, the nurse knows that
   a. ejaculation will be spared if a nerve-sparing prostatectomy was done.
   b. PDE5 inhibitors are contraindicated in patients who had a prostatectomy.
   c. erectile dysfunction can occur even if a nerve-sparing prostatectomy was done.
   d. testosterone replacement therapy is prescribed after prostatectomy to improve erectile dysfunction.
4. The nurse explains to the patient with chronic bacterial prostatitis that **(Select all that apply.)**
   a. all patients require hospitalization for 2 to 4 weeks.
   b. antibiotic treatment duration is generally 8 to 12 weeks.
   c. warm sitz baths should be avoided, as they will worsen pain.
   d. long-term antibiotic therapy may be needed in immunocompromised patients.
   e. if the condition is not treated appropriately, they are at increased risk for prostate cancer.
5. The most common assessment finding in a patient with testicular cancer is
   a. painful ejaculation with visible blood.
   b. painless firm lump on one of the testes.
   c. significant testicular swelling that transilluminates.
   d. rapid onset of dysuria with scrotal swelling and fever.
6. When discussing the emotional impact of sexual dysfunction with a male patient, the nurse knows that
   a. sexual counseling must include the patient and their partner to be successful.
   b. vasectomy alters hormone levels, which causes physiologic erectile dysfunction.
   c. with ED of sudden onset, sexual function symptoms likely have a psychologic cause.
   d. stress is more likely to affect the erectile function of middle-aged males than younger males.

1. d; 2. a, d, f; 3. c; 4. b, d; 5. b; 6. c.

For rationales to these answers and even more NCLEX review questions, visit http://evolve.elsevier.com/Lewis/medsurg.

REFERENCES

To access the References for this chapter, please scan the QR code with a mobile device.

CASE STUDY

Applying Clinical Judgment With Multiple Patients

You are working on the medical-surgical unit. The following are 4 of the 6 patients you have been assigned to care for this shift. An LPN and an AP assist another RN and you.

Chapter 52 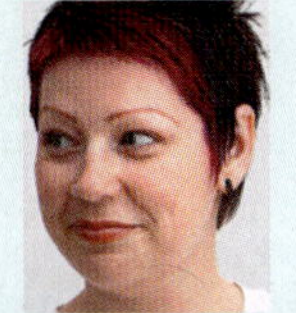 (© iStockphoto/Thinkstock.)	L.M. is a 35-year-old female admitted for hypertension caused by newly diagnosed Cushing syndrome. She has been depressed and crying because of her appearance. Vital signs: 194/94, 84, RR 18.
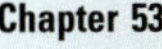 **Chapter 53** 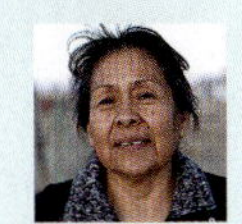 (© eyecrave productions/ iStock.com.)	T.K. is a 78-year-old female with T2DM and hypertension, who was admitted yesterday for hyperosmolar hyperglycemia syndrome. Remains difficult to arouse. Heart rate 118 beats/min; BP 98/ 60 mm Hg, O_2 sat 93%. Last glucose 396 mg/dL.
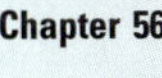 **Chapter 56** 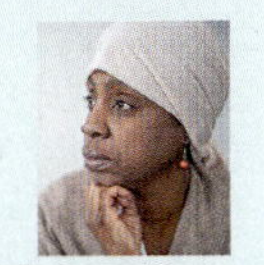 (© FatCamera/iStock.com.)	L.S. is a 60-year-old female with cancer of her left breast. She had a mastectomy and axillary node dissection yesterday. She has a Jackson-Pratt drain in her left chest. Her last pain medication was given 1 hour ago, at which time she rated her pain as a 7 (0 −10 scale).
Chapter 54 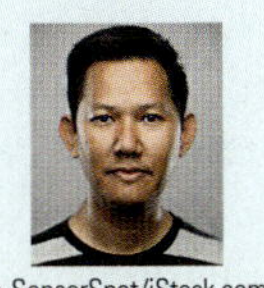 (© SensorSpot/iStock.com.)	J.G., a 52-year-old male with Graves disease, had a subtotal thyroidectomy yesterday. Is to start a soft diet and ambulate in the hall this morning. In report it was noted that his voice has become slightly "hoarse" in the last hour.

1. Highlight all the findings above that require your follow-up.
2. After receiving report, which patient should you see first? Second?
3. Which tasks could you delegate to AP? **(Select all that apply.)**
   a. Assist L.M. to ambulate in the hallway.
   b. Obtain daily weights for L.S. and T.K.
   c. Take J.G.'s vital signs and report the results to you.
   d. Assess L.S.'s mastectomy incision for signs of infection.
   e. Listen to L.M. talk about her feelings while helping her with AM care.
4. While you are assessing J.G., the LPN tells you that L.S.'s chest dressing is totally saturated with bloody drainage. Which *initial* action would be most appropriate?
   a. Ask the LPN to call the laboratory for a stat hemoglobin (Hgb) and hematocrit (Hct) on L.S.
   b. Tell the LPN to reinforce the dressing with sterile 4 × 4 gauze pads.
   c. Have the LPN stay with J.G. while you assess L.S.'s Jackson-Pratt drain.
   d. Ask the LPN to stay with L.S., have the AP monitor J.G. while you call L.S.'s HCP.

Case Study Progression

L.S.'s Jackson-Pratt drain was not functioning properly. You get it working and change the chest dressing. The incision is well approximated without signs of infection. When you leave the room, the Jackson-Pratt has a small amount of serosanguineous drainage in it. As you enter J.G.'s room, you notice he is having a carpal spasm on the same arm on which the LPN is taking his BP. You obtain a focused assessment and notify the health care provider.

5. Which assessment findings would be *most* important to include in a discussion with the health care provider about J.G.? **(Select all that apply.)**
   a. Patient is anxious
   b. Hoarseness of voice
   c. Most recent Hgb and Hct
   d. BP of 138/76 and heart rate of 78
   e. Carpal spasm upon inflation of BP cuff
6. Based on J.G.'s assessment findings, the priority need will be prevention of _____1_____. To reduce this risk, the most important intervention is to _____2_____.

Options for 1	Options for 2
bleeding	administer IV calcium gluconate
respiratory distress	increase IV fluids and apply a pressure dressing
thyrotoxicosis	start O_2 therapy

7. Which intervention would be of *highest* priority in caring for L.M.?
   a. Assess her for fall risk.
   b. Assess her for signs and symptoms of hypoglycemia.
   c. Teach her the need for a high-carbohydrate, low-protein diet.
   d. Reassure her that her physical appearance will improve with treatment.
8. You are concerned that T.K.'s glucose is still increased and she continues to be dehydrated. For each assessment finding, use an X to indicate whether it is *Expected* (no follow-up is required) or *Requires Follow-up* (potentially requires intervention) at this time.

Assessment Finding	Expected	Requires Follow-up
Urine output 60 mL/h		
Lungs sounds clear bilaterally		
Somnolence		
Slightly labored respirations		
Reports of dizziness when ambulating		
Skin pink, warm, and dry		

Continued

CASE STUDY—cont'd

9. You see that you need to review T.K.'s medication record for new HCP orders. Choose the most likely options for the information missing from the table by selecting from the lists of options provided.

Medication	Dose, Route, Frequency	Drug Class	Indication
Insulin glargine	1	Long-acting insulin	Decrease glucose levels
2	20 mEq IV in 250 mL 0.9% over 2 h	Electrolyte replacement	Reverse low potassium levels
enoxaparin sodium	40 units subcut daily	Anticoagulant	3
Ondansetron	4 mg IV q8h as needed	4	Reduce feelings of nausea and vomiting

Options for 1	Options for 2	Options for 3	Options for 4
20 units IV daily 22 units subcut daily 100 units subcut daily	Magnesium, potassium, sodium sulfates Penicillin G potassium Potassium chloride	Decrease insulin resistance Reduce risk of atrial fibrillation VTE prophylaxis	Antiemetic Antihyperglycemic Hormone analog

10. The LPN is assigned to give medications to T.K., including her sliding scale Novolog insulin with lunch. The AP, who is also a senior nursing student, tells you that the LPN gave T.K.'s insulin at least 30 minutes after the patient ate his lunch. What is your *best* initial action?
    a. Report the incident to the charge nurse for follow-up.
    b. Talk to the LPN about the importance of timely medication administration.
    c. Ask the LPN what time the insulin was given and when the patient ate breakfast.
    d. Ask the AP to first discuss the concern with the LPN to follow lines of communication.

Answers available at http://evolve.elsevier.com/Lewis/medsurg

60

Assessment: Nervous System

Kristen J. Keller

http://evolve.elsevier.com/Lewis/medsurg/

CONCEPTUAL FOCUS

Cognition
Functional Ability
Intracranial Regulation
Sensory Perception

LEARNING OUTCOMES

1. Compare the functions of neurons and glial cells.
2. Explain the anatomic location and functions of the cerebrum, brainstem, cerebellum, spinal cord, peripheral nerves, and cerebrospinal fluid.
3. Identify the major arteries supplying the brain.
4. Describe the functions of the 12 cranial nerves.
5. Compare the functions of the 2 divisions of the autonomic nervous system.
6. Link the age-related changes in the neurologic system to the differences in assessment findings.
7. Obtain significant subjective and objective data related to the nervous system.
8. Perform a physical assessment of the nervous system.
9. Discern normal from common abnormal findings of a nervous system assessment.
10. Describe the purpose, significance of results, and nursing responsibilities related to diagnostic studies of the nervous system.

KEY TERMS

autonomic nervous system (ANS)
blood-brain barrier
central nervous system (CNS)
cerebrospinal fluid (CSF)
cranial nerves (CNs)
dermatome
meninges
neurons
neurotransmitters
peripheral nervous system (PNS)
reflex
synapse

The nervous system is one of the most complex systems in the human body, controlling all the body's activities. Having a good understanding of the nervous system is critical to being able to examine and interpret clinical findings. This chapter reviews the structures and functions, assessment, and diagnostic studies of the nervous system.

STRUCTURES AND FUNCTIONS OF THE NERVOUS SYSTEM

The nervous system is responsible for the control and integration of the body's many activities. It is divided into the central nervous system and peripheral nervous system. The central nervous system (CNS) includes the cerebrum (cerebral hemispheres), cerebellum, brainstem, and spinal cord. The peripheral nervous system (PNS) includes all the neuronal structures that lie outside the CNS. It consists of the spinal and cranial nerves, their associated ganglia (groupings of cell bodies), and parts of the autonomic nervous system.

Nervous System Cells

The nervous system is made up of 2 types of cells: neurons and supportive glial cells.

Neurons

Neurons are the main functional unit of the nervous system. Neurons come in many shapes and sizes. They share 3 characteristics: (1) excitability, or the ability to generate a nerve impulse; (2) conductivity, or the ability to transmit an impulse; and (3) the ability to influence other neurons, muscle cells, or glandular cells.

A typical neuron consists of a cell body, multiple dendrites, and an axon (Fig. 60.1). The cell body contains the nucleus and cytoplasm. It is the metabolic center of the neuron. Dendrites are short processes extending from the cell body. They receive impulses or signals from other neurons and conduct them toward the cell body.

The axon projects varying distances from the cell body. It carries nerve impulses to other neurons or to end organs, such as smooth and striated muscles and glands. Many axons in the CNS and PNS are myelinated, or covered by a *myelin sheath.* It is a white, lipid protein substance that acts as an insulator for impulse conduction.

Glial Cells

Glial cells (glia, neuroglia) provide support, nourishment, and protection to neurons. Glial cells make up about half of the brain and spinal cord mass. They are divided into microglia and macroglia. *Microglia* are specialized macrophages capable of phagocytosis. They protect the neurons. These cells are mobile within the brain and multiply when the brain is damaged.

Macroglial cells include astrocytes, oligodendrocytes, and ependymal cells. *Astrocytes* are found mainly in gray matter. They provide structural support to neurons. Their delicate processes form the *blood-brain barrier* with the endothelium of the blood vessels. They play a role in *synaptic transmission* (impulse conduction between neurons). When the brain is injured, astrocytes act as phagocytes for cleaning up neuronal

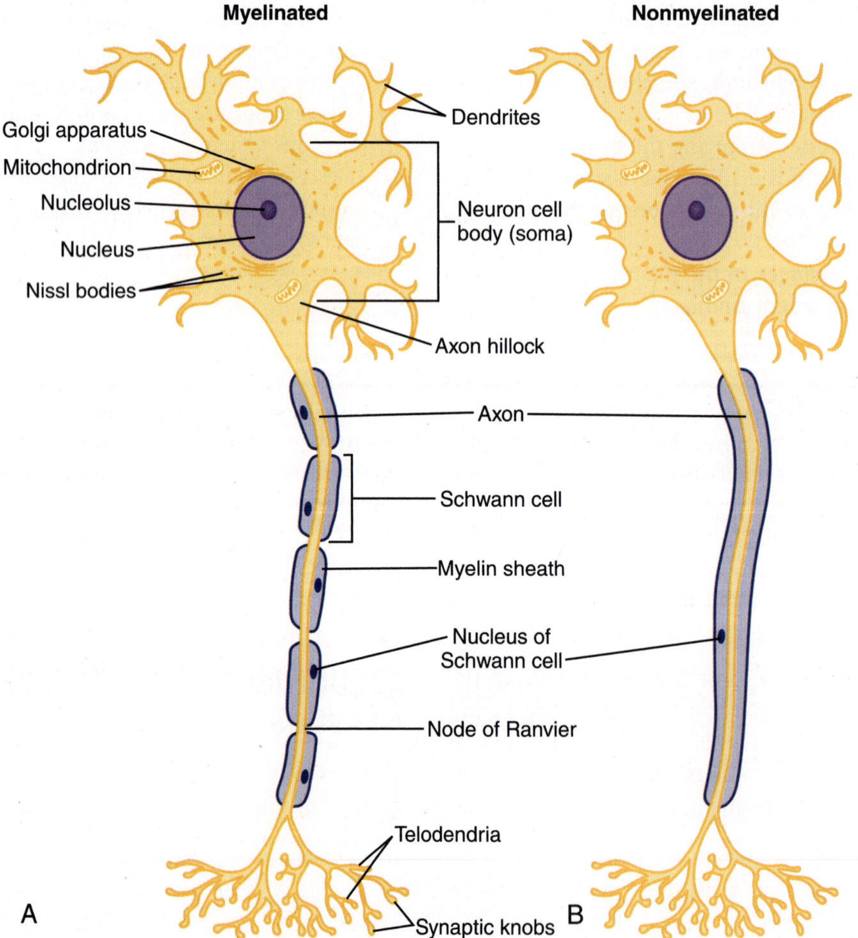

Fig. 60.1 Structure of neurons: dendrites, cell body, and axons in an (A) unmyelinated neuron and (B) myelinated neuron.

debris. They help restore the neurochemical milieu and provide support for repair. Proliferation of astrocytes contributes to the formation of scar tissue *(gliosis)* in the CNS.

Oligodendrocytes produce the myelin sheath of nerve fibers in the CNS. They are found mainly in the white matter of the CNS. *Ependymal cells* line the brain ventricles. They aid in cerebrospinal fluid (CSF) secretion.

Nerve Regeneration

If the axon of the nerve cell is damaged, the cell tries to repair itself. Damaged nerve cells try to grow back to their original destinations by sprouting many branches from the damaged ends of their axons. Axons in the CNS are generally less successful than peripheral axons in regeneration.[1]

Schwann cells myelinate the nerve fibers in the PNS. Injured nerve fibers in the PNS can regenerate by growing within the protective myelin sheath of the Schwann cells if the cell body is intact and the environment is optimal.[2] The final result of nerve regeneration depends on the number of axon sprouts that join with Schwann cell columns and reinnervate end organs.

Neurons have long been thought to be nonmitotic. That is, after being damaged, neurons could not be replaced. Recent research shows a subset of astrocytes proliferates after some CNS injuries, and neurogenesis may occur from stem cells.[3] These findings support the potential for patients to have a certain amount of recovery after neuronal injury.

Nerve Impulse

The purpose of a neuron is to initiate, receive, and process messages about events both within and outside the body. The initiation of a neuronal message *(nerve impulse)* involves the generation of an action potential. A series of action potentials travels along the axon. When the impulse reaches the end of the nerve fiber, a chemical interaction involving neurotransmitters transfers the impulse across a synapse. A synapse is the structural and functional junction between 2 neurons (Fig. 60.2). The chemical interaction generates another set of action potentials in the next neuron. These events continue until the nerve impulse reaches its destination. Nerve impulses also can be transmitted from neurons to glands or muscles.

Because of its insulating quality, myelination of axons speeds the conduction of an action potential. Many peripheral nerve axons have *nodes of Ranvier* (gaps in the myelin sheath) that allow an action potential to travel much faster by jumping from node to node. We call this *saltatory* (hopping) *conduction.* In an unmyelinated fiber, conduction is slower. The wave of depolarization travels the entire length of the axon, with each part of the membrane becoming depolarized in turn.

Neurotransmitters

Neurotransmitters are chemicals that affect the transmission of impulses across a synapse. *Excitatory neurotransmitters* (e.g., epinephrine, norepinephrine, glutamate) activate postsynaptic receptors that increase the chance that an action potential will be generated. *Inhibitory neurotransmitters* (e.g., serotonin, γ-aminobutyric acid [GABA], dopamine) activate postsynaptic receptors to decrease the chance that an action potential will be generated. For example, endorphins block pain transmission, while substance P (a neuropeptide) makes nerves more sensitive to pain.

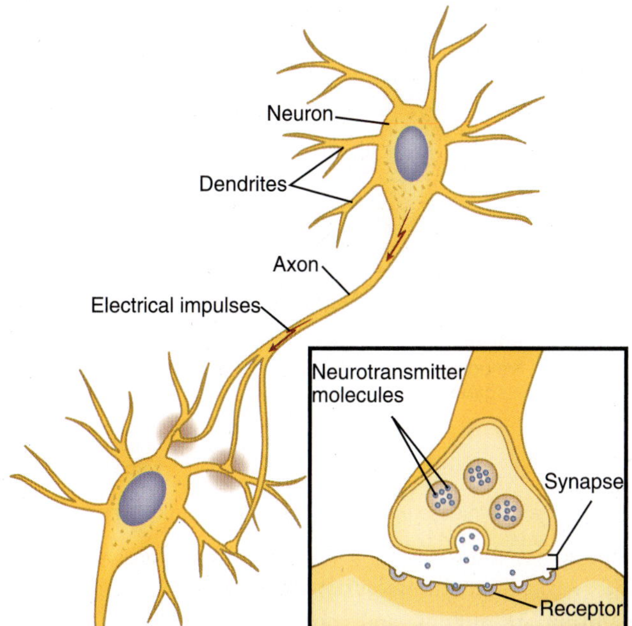

Fig. 60.2 Impulse generation between neurons. Synapse shown with neurotransmitters and receptors.

In general, the total effect (excitatory or inhibitory) depends on the number of presynaptic neurons releasing neurotransmitters on the postsynaptic cell. A presynaptic cell that releases an excitatory neurotransmitter does not always cause the postsynaptic cell to depolarize enough to generate an action potential.

When many presynaptic cells release excitatory neurotransmitters on a single neuron, the sum of their input is enough to generate an action potential. Neurotransmitters continue to combine with the receptor sites at the postsynaptic membrane until they are inactivated by enzymes, taken up by the presynaptic endings, or diffuse away from the synaptic region. Drugs and toxins can affect neurotransmitters by changing their function or blocking their attachment to receptor sites on the postsynaptic membrane. Cerebral microdialysis can measure neurotransmitter levels in the cerebral cortex.

Central Nervous System

Brain

The brain has 3 major intracranial components: cerebrum, cerebellum, and brainstem.

Cerebrum. The *cerebrum* is composed of the right and left cerebral hemispheres. It is divided into 4 lobes: frontal, temporal, parietal, and occipital (Fig. 60.3). The functions of the

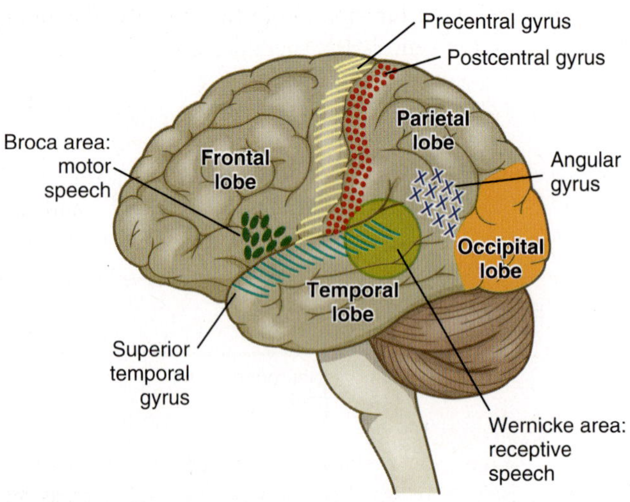

Fig. 60.3 Left hemisphere of cerebrum, lateral surface, showing major lobes and areas of the brain.

cerebrum are multiple and complex (Table 60.1). The *frontal lobe* controls higher cognitive function, memory retention, voluntary eye and motor movements, and motor functions involved in speech production *(Broca area)*. The *temporal lobe* integrates somatic, visual, and auditory data. It contains the *Wernicke receptive speech area.* The *parietal lobe* interprets spatial information. It contains the sensory cortex. Processing of sight takes place in the *occipital lobe.*

The neocortex (gray matter) makes up the outer layer of the cerebral hemispheres. Neurons in specific parts of the neocortex are essential for various complex and sophisticated functions. These include language, memory, and interpreting visual-spatial relationships.

The basal ganglia, thalamus, hypothalamus, and limbic system are specific groups of neuron clusters in the cerebrum. The *basal ganglia* are found centrally in the cerebrum and midbrain. Most of them are on both sides of the thalamus. The function of the basal ganglia includes the initiation, execution, and completion of voluntary movements; learning; emotional response; and automatic movements associated with skeletal muscle activity (e.g., swallowing saliva, blinking, swinging the arms while walking).

The *thalamus* lies directly above the brainstem (Fig. 60.4). It is the major relay center for sensory input from the body, face, retina, and cochlear and taste receptors. Motor relay nuclei in the thalamus connect the cerebellum and basal ganglia to the frontal cortex.

The *hypothalamus* is just below the thalamus and slightly in front of the midbrain. It has a direct influence on release of hormones from the anterior pituitary gland. It has a rich capillary connection to the pituitary gland to aid in the transport of hormones. These hormones include thyroid-stimulating hormone, growth hormone, luteinizing hormone, and prolactin-releasing hormone (see Chapter 52). In contrast, the supraoptic and paraventricular neurons travel directly through the pituitary stalk to the posterior pituitary. There, they release vasopressin and oxytocin. The hypothalamus contains the satiety center that regulates appetite. With input from the limbic system, it regulates body temperature, water balance (through vasopressin secretion), circadian rhythm, and expression of emotion. The *limbic system* is found near the inner surfaces of the cerebral hemispheres. It is concerned with emotion, aggression, feeding behavior, and sexual response.

TABLE 60.1 Function of Cerebrum

Part	Location	Function
Cortical Areas		
Motor		
Primary	Precentral gyrus	Motor control and movement on opposite side of body
Supplemental	Anterior to precentral gyrus	Facilitates proximal muscle activity, including activity for stance and gait, and spontaneous movement and coordination
Sensory		
Association areas	Parietal lobe	Integrates somatic and sensory input
	Posterior temporal lobe	Integrates visual and auditory input for language comprehension
	Anterior temporal lobe	Integrates past experiences
	Anterior frontal lobe	Controls higher-order processes (e.g., judgment, reasoning)
Auditory	Superior temporal gyrus	Registers auditory input
Somatic	Postcentral gyrus	Sensory response from opposite side of body
Visual	Occipital lobe	Registers visual images
Language		
Comprehension	Wernicke area in dominant posterior temporal lobe	Integrates auditory language (understanding of spoken words)
Expression	Broca area in dominant frontal lobe	Regulates motor speech
Basal Ganglia	Near lateral ventricles of both cerebral hemispheres	Controls and refines learned and automatic movements
Thalamus	Below and slightly posterior to basal ganglia	Relays sensory and motor input to and from cerebrum
Hypothalamus	Below and anterior to thalamus	Regulates endocrine and autonomic functions
Limbic System	Lateral to hypothalamus	Influences emotional behavior and basic drives, such as feeding and sexual behavior

Cerebellum. The *cerebellum* is in the posterior cranial fossa below the occipital lobe. It coordinates voluntary movement and maintains trunk stability and equilibrium. The cerebellum

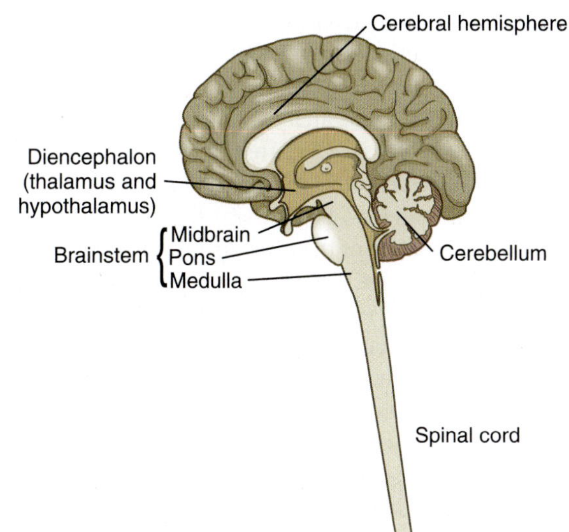

Fig. 60.4 Major divisions of the CNS.

receives information from the cerebral cortex, muscles, joints, and inner ear. It influences motor activity through axonal connections to the thalamus, motor cortex, and brainstem nuclei and their descending pathways.

Ventricles and cerebrospinal fluid. The ventricles are 4 interconnected fluid-filled cavities. The lower part of the 4th ventricle becomes the central canal in the lower part of the brainstem. The spinal canal extends centrally through the full length of the spinal cord.

Cerebrospinal fluid (CSF) is made largely in the choroid plexuses of the brain within the ventricles. It circulates within the subarachnoid space that surrounds the brain, brainstem, and spinal cord and flows from the cranial cavity to the spinal cavity. CSF cushions the brain and spinal cord and carries nutrients through passive diffusion and active transport. We make about 500 mL/day of CSF. The ventricles and central canal are filled with an average of 150 mL at any given time. Changes in CSF production or absorption can occur. This leads to a change in the volume within the ventricles and central canal. Too much CSF results in *hydrocephalus.*

CSF circulates throughout the ventricles and flows into the subarachnoid space surrounding the brain and spinal cord. It is absorbed mainly through the *arachnoid villi* (tiny projections into the subarachnoid space) into the intradural venous sinuses and eventually into the venous system.

Analyzing CSF composition provides useful diagnostic information related to certain nervous system diseases. We often measure CSF pressure in patients with actual or suspected intracranial injury. Increased intracranial pressure, indicated by increased CSF pressure, can force downward (central) herniation of the brain and brainstem. The signs indicating this development are part of herniation syndrome (see Chapter 61).

Brainstem. The *brainstem* includes the midbrain, pons, and medulla (Fig. 60.4). Ascending and descending fibers to and from the cerebrum and cerebellum pass through the brainstem. The nuclei of cranial nerves (CNs) III through XII are in the brainstem. The vital centers concerned with respiratory, vasomotor, and heart function are in the medulla. The brainstem contains the centers for sneezing, coughing, vomiting, sucking, and swallowing.

The *reticular formation* is a diffusely arranged group of neurons and their axons that extends from the medulla to the thalamus and hypothalamus. It relays sensory information, influences excitatory and inhibitory control of spinal motor neurons, and controls vasomotor and respiratory activity. The *reticular activating system* (RAS) is a complex system that requires communication among the brainstem, reticular formation, and cerebral cortex. The RAS regulates arousal and sleep-wake transitions.

Spinal Cord

The *spinal cord* is continuous with the brainstem. It exits from the cranial cavity through the foramen magnum. A cross section of the spinal cord reveals gray matter that is centrally located in an H shape and surrounded by white matter. Gray matter contains the cell bodies of voluntary motor neurons, preganglionic autonomic motor neurons, and association neurons (interneurons). White matter contains the axons of the ascending sensory and descending motor fibers. The myelin surrounding these fibers gives them their white appearance. The spinal pathways or tracts are named for the point of origin and the point of destination (e.g., spinocerebellar tract [ascending], corticospinal tract [descending]).

Ascending tracts. In general, the ascending tracts carry specific sensory information to higher levels of the CNS. This information comes from special sensory receptors in the skin, muscles and joints, viscera, and blood vessels. It enters the spinal cord by way of the dorsal roots of the spinal nerves. The ascending tracts are organized by sensory modality and anatomy. The fasciculus gracilis and the fasciculus cuneatus (*dorsal* or *posterior columns*) carry information about touch, deep pressure, vibration, position sense, and kinesthesia (appreciation of movement, weight, and body parts). The *spinocerebellar tracts* carry information about muscle tension and body position to the cerebellum for coordination of movement. The *spinothalamic tracts* carry pain and temperature sensations.

Other ascending tracts may also carry sensory information. The signs and symptoms of various neurologic problems suggest there are other pathways for touch, position sense, and vibration.

Descending tracts. Descending tracts carry impulses that are responsible for muscle movement. Important descending tracts are the corticobulbar and corticospinal tracts, collectively termed the *pyramidal tract.* These tracts carry voluntary impulses from the cerebral cortex to the cranial and peripheral nerves. Another group of descending motor tracts carries impulses from the extrapyramidal system (all motor tracts except the pyramidal) concerned with voluntary movement. It includes pathways originating in the brainstem, basal ganglia, and cerebellum. The motor output exits the spinal cord through the ventral roots of the spinal nerves.

Reflex arc. A reflex is an involuntary response to stimuli. In the spinal cord, reflex arcs play a key role in maintaining muscle tone, posture, and stability. The components of a monosynaptic reflex arc (Fig. 60.5) are a receptor organ, afferent neuron, effector neuron, and effector organ (e.g., skeletal muscle). The afferent neuron synapses with the efferent neurons in the gray matter of the spinal cord, producing an involuntary response to a perceived stimulation. This initiates a signal that does not require processing by the brain to prevent injury or harm from the perceived sensory stimulation.

Lower and upper motor neurons. *Upper motor neurons (UMNs)* originate in the cerebral cortex and project downward. The corticobulbar tract ends in the brainstem, and the corticospinal tract descends into the spinal cord. These neurons influence skeletal muscle movement. UMN lesions generally cause weakness or paralysis, disuse atrophy, hyperreflexia, and increased muscle tone (spasticity).

Lower motor neurons (LMNs) are the final common pathway through which descending motor tracts influence skeletal muscle. The cell bodies of LMNs, which send axons to innervate the skeletal muscles of the arms, trunk, and legs, are found in the anterior horn of the corresponding segments of the spinal cord (e.g., cervical segments contain LMNs for the arms). LMNs for skeletal muscles of the eyes, face, mouth, and throat are found in the corresponding segments of the brainstem. These cell bodies and their axons make up the somatic motor components of the CNs. LMN lesions generally cause weakness or paralysis, denervation atrophy, hyporeflexia or areflexia, and decreased muscle tone (flaccidity).

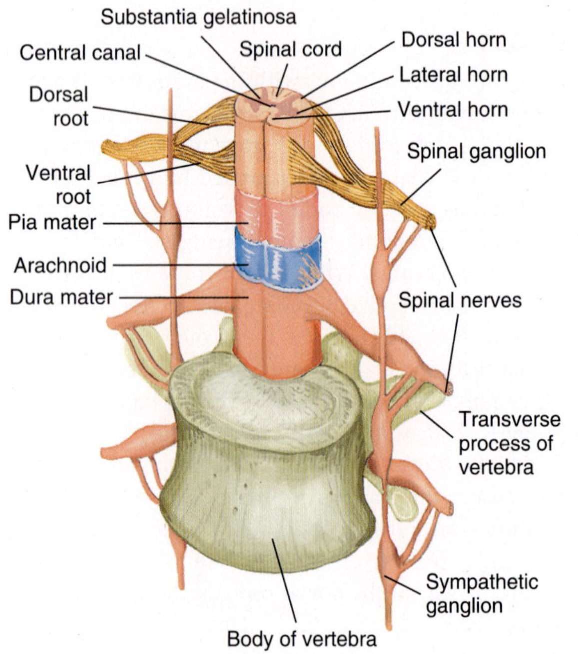

Fig. 60.5 Cross section of spinal cord showing attachments of spinal nerves and coverings of the spinal cord.

Peripheral Nervous System

Spinal Nerves

The spinal cord can be seen as a series of spinal segments, each on top of another with no visible boundaries. In addition to the cell bodies, each segment has a pair of dorsal (afferent) sensory nerve fibers or roots and ventral (efferent) motor fibers or roots. They innervate a specific region of the body. This combined motor-sensory nerve is called a *spinal nerve* (Fig. 60.6). The cell bodies of the voluntary motor system are in the anterior horn of the spinal cord gray matter. The cell bodies of the autonomic (involuntary) motor system are in the anterolateral part of the spinal cord gray matter. The cell bodies of sensory fibers are in the dorsal root ganglia just outside the spinal cord. On exiting the spinal column, each spinal nerve divides into ventral and dorsal rami, a collection of motor and sensory fibers that eventually goes to peripheral structures (e.g., skin, muscles, viscera).

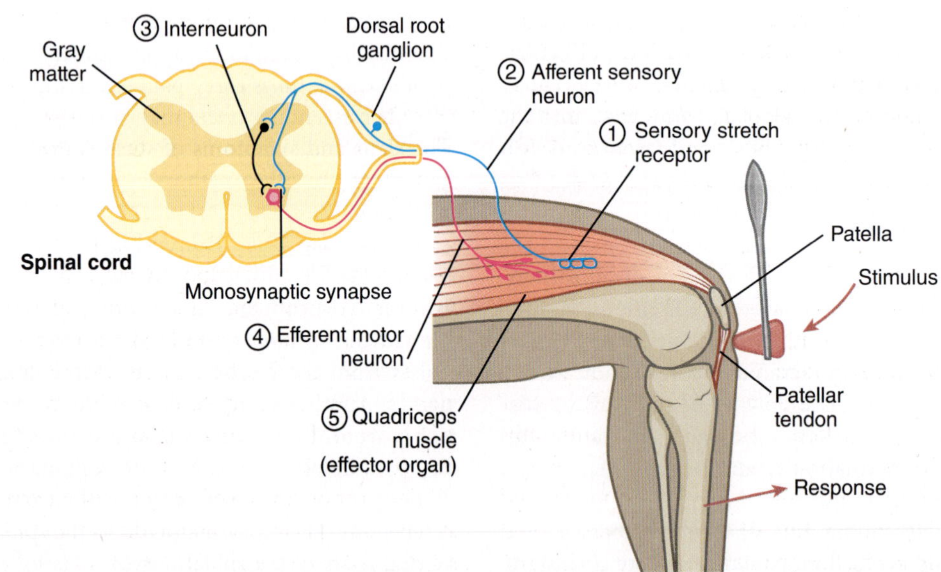

Fig. 60.6 An illustration of the knee-jerk reflex with the spinal cord and the knee. Basic diagram of the patellar "knee jerk" reflex arc, including the *(1)* sensory stretch receptor, *(2)* afferent sensory neuron, *(3)* interneuron, *(4)* efferent motor neuron, and *(5)* quadriceps muscle (effector organ).

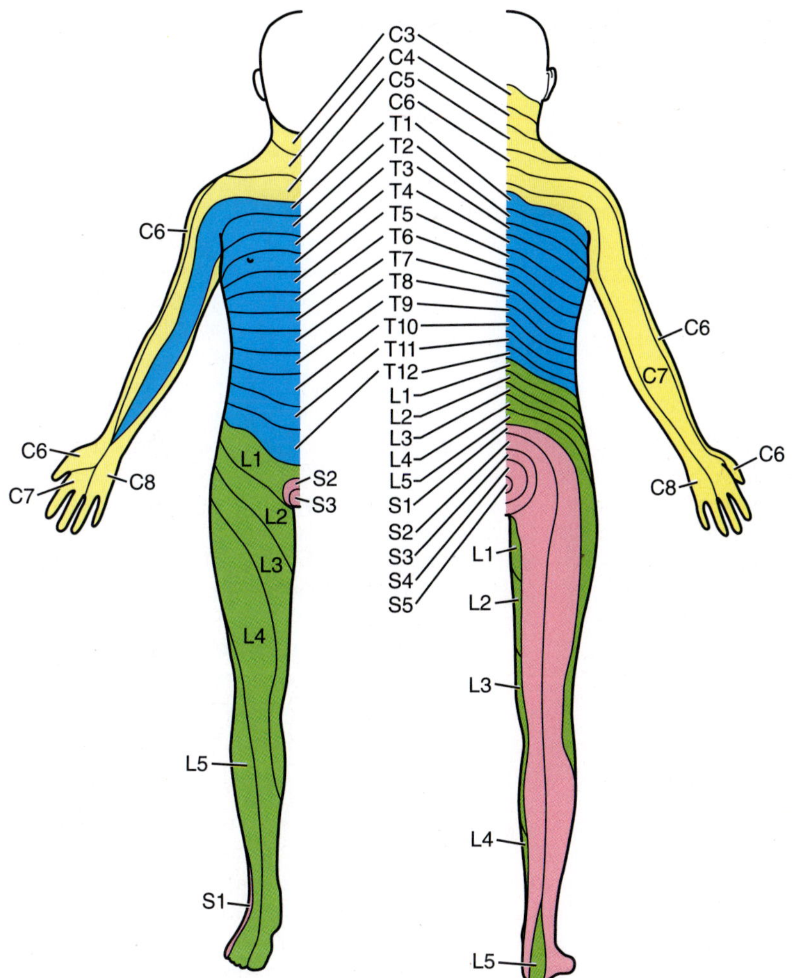

Fig. 60.7 Dermatomes of the body.

A **dermatome** is the area of skin innervated by the sensory fibers of a single dorsal root of a spinal nerve (Fig. 60.7). The dermatomes give a general picture of somatic sensory innervation by spinal segments. A *myotome* is a muscle group innervated by the primary motor neurons of a single ventral root. The dermatomes and myotomes of a given spinal segment overlap with those of adjacent segments because of the development of ascending and descending collateral branches of nerve fibers.

Cranial Nerves

The **cranial nerves (CNs)** are the 12 paired nerves composed of cell bodies with fibers that exit from the cranial cavity. Unlike the spinal nerves, which always have both afferent sensory and efferent motor fibers, some CNs are only sensory, some only motor, and some both.

Table 60.2 outlines the motor and sensory components of the CNs. Fig. 60.8 shows the position of the CNs in relation to the brain and spinal cord. Just as the cell bodies of the spinal nerves are in specific segments of the spinal cord, cell bodies (nuclei) of the CNs are in specific segments of the brainstem. Exceptions are the nuclei of the olfactory and optic nerves. The primary cell bodies of the olfactory nerve are in the nasal epithelium. The cell bodies of the optic nerve are in the retina.

Autonomic Nervous System

The **autonomic nervous system (ANS)** is divided into the sympathetic and parasympathetic systems. The ANS governs involuntary functions of heart muscle, smooth muscle, and glands through both efferent and afferent pathways. The 2 systems function together to maintain a relatively balanced internal environment. The preganglionic cell bodies of the *sympathetic nervous system* (SNS) are found in spinal segments T1 through L2. The neurotransmitter released by the preganglionic fibers is acetylcholine. The major neurotransmitter released by the postganglionic fibers of the SNS is norepinephrine.

The preganglionic cell bodies of the *parasympathetic nervous system* (PSNS) are found in the brainstem and sacral spinal segments (S2 through S4). Acetylcholine is the neurotransmitter released at both preganglionic and postganglionic nerve endings.

TABLE 60.2 Cranial Nerves

Function and Assessment

Nerve	Function	Assessment
I Olfactory	*Sensory:* from olfactory (smell)	Ask patient to close 1 nostril at a time and identify easily recognized odors (e.g., coffee). Any asymmetry in sense of smell is important.
II Optic	*Sensory:* from retina of eyes (vision)	Examine each eye separately. *Visual fields:* Position yourself opposite the patient. Ask them to look at the bridge of your nose and indicate when an object (finger, pencil tip) presented from the periphery of each of the visual fields is seen (Fig. 60.15). *Visual acuity:* Ask patient to read a Snellen chart. Record the number on the lowest line the patient can read with 50% accuracy. Patients who wear glasses should wear them during testing unless they are used only for close reading. If a Snellen chart is not available, ask the patient to read newsprint for gross assessment of acuity. Record the distance from patient to newsprint needed for accurate reading.
III Oculomotor	*Motor:* 4 eye movement muscles and levator palpebrae muscle *Parasympathetic:* smooth muscle in eyeball	Ask the person to hold the head steady and to follow the movement of your finger, pen, or penlight only with the eyes. Hold the target back about 12 inches so that the person can focus on it comfortably. Move the target to each of the 6 positions (right and up, right, right and down, left and up, left, left and down), hold it momentarily, and then move back to center. Progress clockwise. A normal response is parallel tracking of the object with both eyes. Check for pupil constriction and *accommodation* (pupils constricting with near vision). To test pupil constriction, shine a light into the pupil of 1 eye; look for ipsilateral constriction of the same pupil and contralateral (consensual) constriction of the opposite eye. Note the size and shape of the pupils. The optic nerve must be intact for this reflex to occur.
IV Trochlear	*Motor:* 1 eye movement muscle, the superior oblique muscle	See testing for CN III. Because the oculomotor (CN III), trochlear (CN IV), and abducens (CN VI) nerves help move the eye, they are tested together.
V Trigeminal		
• Ophthalmic branch	*Sensory:* from forehead, eye, superior nasal cavity	*Sensory:* Have patient close eyes and identify light touch (cotton wisp) and pinprick in each of the 3 divisions (ophthalmic, maxillary, and mandibular) of nerve on both sides of face.
• Maxillary branch	*Sensory:* from inferior nasal cavity, face, upper teeth, mucosa of superior mouth	*Motor:* Ask patient to clench teeth and then palpate masseter muscles just above the mandibular angle. Muscles should feel equally strong on both sides.
• Mandibular branch	*Sensory:* from surfaces of jaw, lower teeth, mucosa of lower mouth, and anterior tongue *Motor:* to muscles of mastication	*Corneal (blink) reflex:* Assesses CN V and CN VII simultaneously. Sensory component (corneal sensation) is innervated by the ophthalmic division of CN V. The motor component (eye blink) is innervated by the facial nerve (CN VII). Have patient look up and away. Then from the other side, lightly touch the cornea with cotton wisp. Look for normal blink reaction of both eyes. Repeat on other side.
VI Abducens	*Motor:* to the lateral rectus muscle of the eye (1 eye movement)	See testing for CN III. Because CN III, CN IV, and CN VI nerves help move the eye, they are tested together.
VII Facial	*Motor:* to facial muscles of expression and cheek muscle *Sensory:* taste from anterior two-thirds of tongue	Ask patient to raise eyebrows, close eyes tightly, purse lips, draw back the corners of mouth in an exaggerated smile, and frown. Note any asymmetry in the facial movements because this can indicate damage to nerve.
VIII Vestibulocochlear		
• Vestibular branch	*Sensory:* from equilibrium sensory organ (vestibular apparatus)	Not routinely tested unless the patient has dizziness, vertigo, unsteadiness, or auditory problems.
• Cochlear branch	*Sensory:* from auditory sensory organ (cochlea), hearing	Have patient close eyes and indicate when they hear the rustling of your fingertips. For more precise assessment of hearing, perform the Weber and Rinne tests or use an audiometer (see Table 23.6).
IX Glossopharyngeal	*Sensory:* from pharynx and posterior tongue, including taste *Motor:* to superior pharyngeal muscles	Glossopharyngeal and vagus nerves (CN IX and CN X) are tested together because both innervate the pharynx. To test the gag reflex, touch the sides of the posterior pharynx or soft palate with a tongue blade. If the reflex is weak or absent, the patient is in danger of aspirating food or secretions. For the awake, cooperative patient, ask the patient to say "ah." Note the bilateral symmetry of elevation of the soft palate. If a patient has an endotracheal tube, the cough reflex (elicited when the suction catheter contacts the *carina* of the respiratory tree) is a method of assessing the vagus nerve.

TABLE 60.2 **Cranial Nerves—cont'd**

Nerve	Function	Assessment
X Vagus	*Sensory:* from much of viscera of thorax and abdomen *Motor:* to larynx and middle and inferior pharyngeal muscles *Parasympathetic:* to heart, lungs, most of digestive system	See testing for CN IX. Glossopharyngeal and vagus nerves (CN IX and CN X) are tested together because both innervate the pharynx.
XI Accessory	*Motor:* to sternocleidomastoid and trapezius muscles	Ask patient to shrug the shoulders and to turn head to either side against resistance. Sternocleidomastoid and trapezius muscles should contract smoothly. Note symmetry, atrophy, or fasciculation of muscle.
XII Hypoglossal	*Motor:* to muscles of tongue	Ask patient to protrude tongue. It should protrude in midline. Next ask the patient to move the tongue up and down and side to side. Finally, the patient should be able to push the tongue to either side against the resistance of a tongue blade. Note any asymmetry, atrophy, or fasciculation.

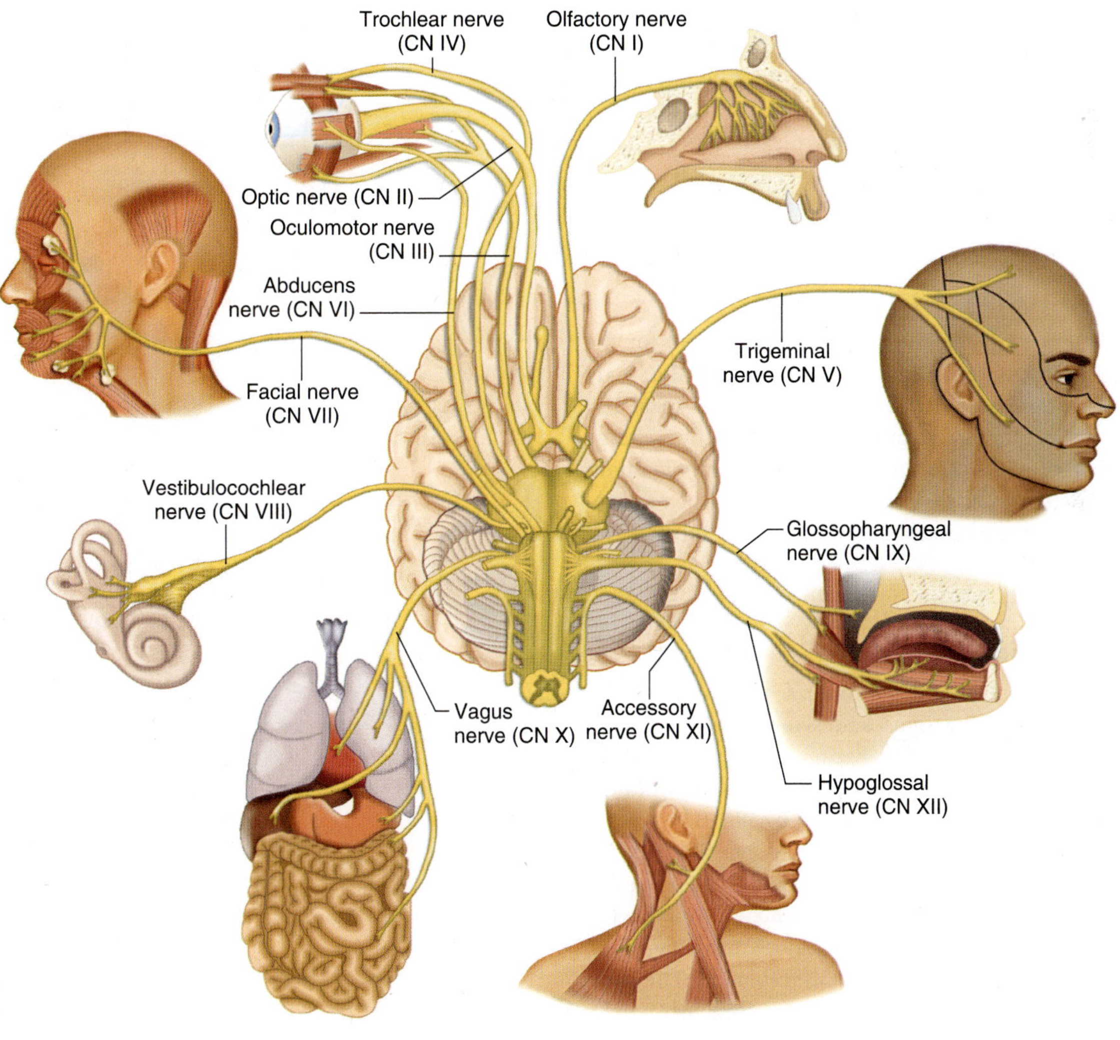

Fig. 60.8 The cranial nerves and their functions. The cranial nerves are numbered by the order in which they leave the brain. (From Williamson P, Thompson T, Bell F, et al: *Human body in health and disease,* ed 8, St Louis, 2024, Mosby.)

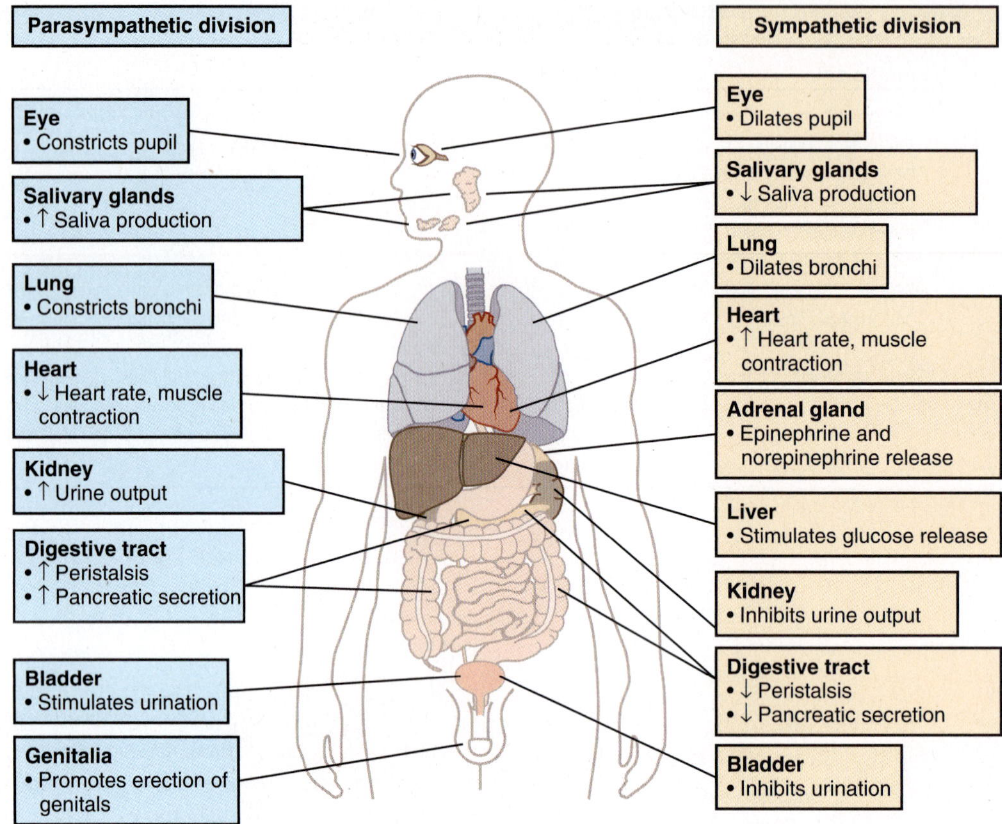

Fig. 60.9 Effects of the sympathetic and parasympathetic systems.

SNS stimulation activates the mechanisms required for the "fight-or-flight" response that occurs throughout the body (Fig. 60.9). In contrast, the PSNS is geared to act in local and discrete regions. It conserves and restores the body's energy stores. The ANS provides dual and often reciprocal innervation to many structures. For example, the SNS increases the rate and force of heart contraction, and the PSNS decreases the rate and force.

Cerebral Circulation

Knowing the distribution of the brain's major arteries is essential for evaluating the signs and symptoms of cerebrovascular disease and trauma. The brain's blood supply arises from the internal carotid arteries (anterior circulation) and the vertebral arteries (posterior circulation) (Fig. 60.10).

The internal carotid arteries provide blood flow to the anterior and middle portions of the cerebrum. The vertebral arteries join to form the basilar artery. It branches to supply the middle and lower parts of the temporal lobes, occipital lobes, cerebellum, brainstem, and part of the diencephalon. The main branch of the basilar artery is the posterior cerebral artery. The *circle of Willis* is formed by communicating arteries that join the basilar and internal carotid arteries (Fig. 60.11). It plays a key role in cerebral blood flow. Interestingly, research shows the formation of the circle of Willis varies greatly. Imaging shows that many people have an incomplete formation.[4]

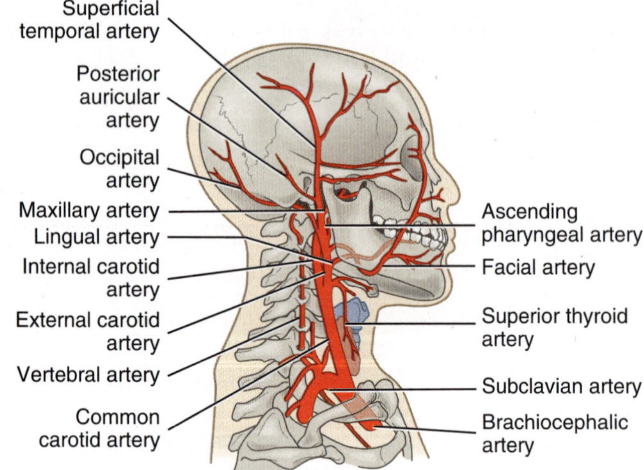

Fig. 60.10 Arteries of the head and neck. Brachiocephalic artery, right common carotid artery, right subclavian artery, and their branches. The major arteries to the head are the common carotid and vertebral arteries. (Modified from Thibodeau GA, Patton KT: *Anatomy and physiology,* ed 8, St Louis, 2013, Mosby.)

Arising from the circle of Willis, 3 pairs of arteries supply blood to the left and right hemispheres. The anterior cerebral artery feeds the medial and anterior portions of the frontal lobes. The middle cerebral artery feeds the outer portions of the frontal, parietal, and superior temporal lobes. The posterior cerebral artery feeds the medial portions of the occipital and

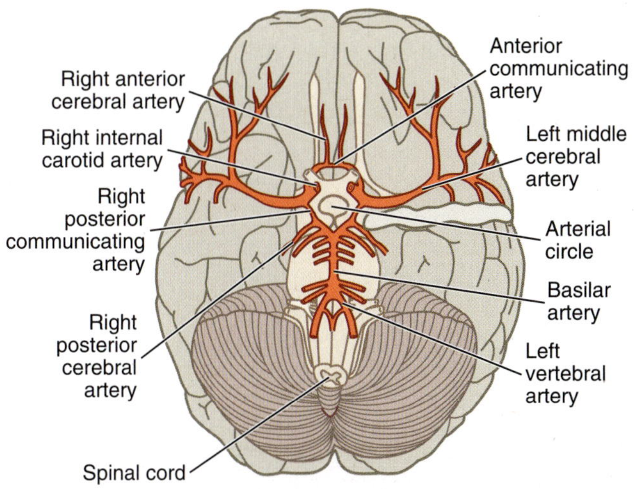

Fig. 60.11 Arteries at the base of the brain. The arteries that compose the circle of Willis are the 2 anterior cerebral arteries joined to each other by the anterior communicating cerebral artery and to the posterior cerebral arteries by the posterior communicating arteries. (Modified from Thibodeau GA, Patton KT: *Anatomy and physiology*, ed 8, St Louis, 2013, Mosby.)

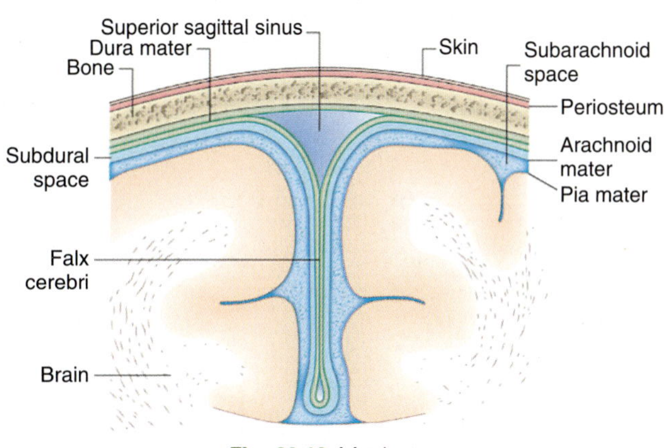

Fig. 60.12 Meninges.

inferior temporal lobes. Venous blood drains from the brain through the dural sinuses, which form channels that drain into the jugular veins.

Blood-Brain Barrier

The **blood-brain barrier** is a physiologic barrier between blood capillaries and brain tissue. This barrier protects the brain from harmful agents, while allowing nutrients and gases to enter. The structure of brain capillaries differs from that of other capillaries. Substances that normally pass into most tissues are prevented from entering brain tissue. Lipid-soluble compounds enter the brain easily. Water-soluble and ionized drugs enter the brain and the spinal cord slowly. Thus the blood-brain barrier affects drug penetration. Only some drugs can enter the CNS from the bloodstream.

Protective Structures

Meninges

The **meninges** consist of 3 protective membranes that surround the brain and spinal cord: the dura mater, arachnoid, and pia mater (Fig. 60.12). The thick *dura mater* forms the outermost layer. The *falx cerebri* is a fold of the dura that separates the 2 cerebral hemispheres. It slows expansion of brain tissue in conditions such as a rapidly growing tumor or acute hemorrhage. The *tentorium cerebelli* is a fold of dura that separates the cerebral hemispheres from the posterior fossa (which contains the brainstem and cerebellum).

The *arachnoid* layer is a fragile, weblike membrane that lies between the dura mater and *pia mater* (the vascular innermost layer of the meninges). The area between the arachnoid layer and pia mater *(subarachnoid space)* is filled with CSF. Structures such as arteries, veins, and CNs passing to and from the brain and skull must pass through the subarachnoid space. A larger subarachnoid space in the region of the 3rd and 4th lumbar vertebrae is the area used to obtain CSF during a lumbar puncture (LP).

Skull

The *skull* protects the brain from external trauma. It is composed of 8 cranial bones and 14 facial bones. The top and sides of the inside of the skull are fairly smooth. The bottom surface is uneven. It has many ridges, prominences, and foramina (holes through which blood vessels and nerves enter the intracranial vault). The largest hole is the *foramen magnum*, through which the brainstem extends to the spinal cord. The foramen magnum is the only major space for the expansion of brain contents when increased intracranial pressure occurs.

Vertebral Column

The *vertebral column* protects the spinal cord, supports the head, and provides flexibility. The vertebral column is made up of 33 individual vertebrae: 7 cervical, 12 thoracic, 5 lumbar, 5 sacral (fused into 1), and 4 coccygeal (fused into 1). Each vertebra has a central opening through which the spinal cord passes. A series of ligaments holds the vertebrae together. Intervertebral discs occupy the spaces between vertebrae, allowing cushion and movement of the column. Fig. 60.13 shows the natural curves of the spinal column and its relation to the trunk.

Gerontologic Considerations: Effects of Aging on the Nervous System

Changes in assessment findings result from age-related changes in the nervous system (Table 60.3). In the CNS, the gradual loss of neurons in certain areas of the brainstem, cerebellum, and cerebral cortex begins in early adulthood. With loss of neurons, the ventricles widen or enlarge, brain weight decreases, and cerebral blood flow decreases. CSF production declines.

In the PNS, degenerative changes in myelin cause a decrease in nerve conduction. Coordinated neuromuscular activity, such

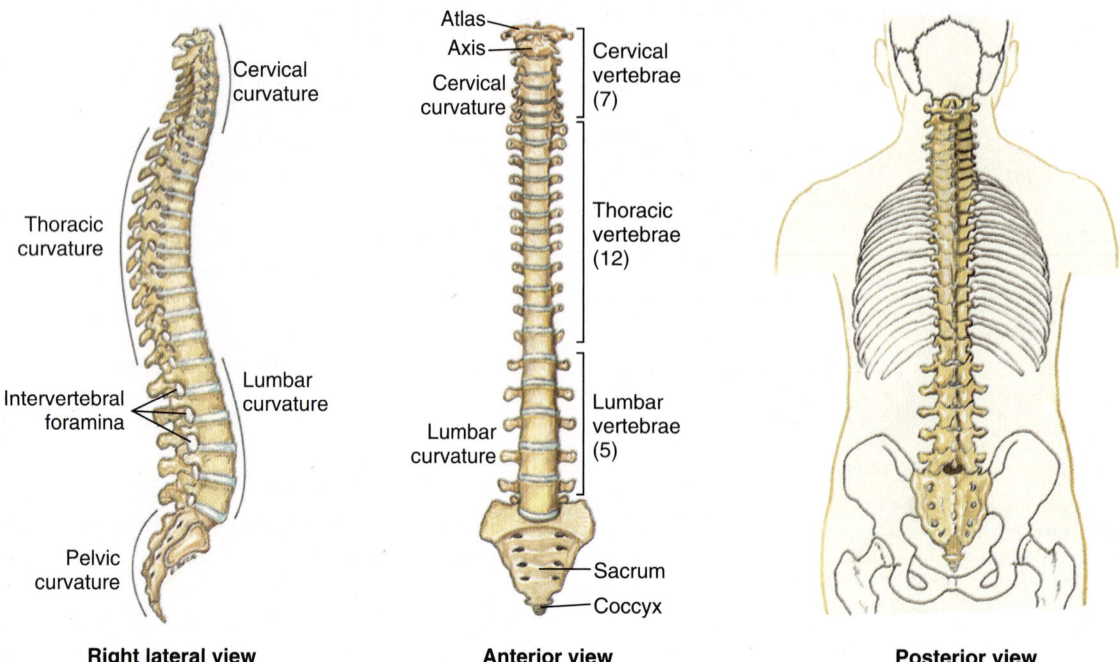

Fig. 60.13 The vertebral column (3 views). (Modified from Thibodeau GA, Patton KT: *Anatomy and physiology,* ed 8, St Louis, 2013, Mosby.)

TABLE 60.3 GERONTOLOGIC ASSESSMENT DIFFERENCES

Nervous System

Component	Changes	Differences in Assessment Findings
Central Nervous System		
Brain	↓ Cerebral blood flow and metabolism Cerebral tissue atrophy and ↑ size of ventricles ↓ Efficiency of temperature-regulating mechanism ↓ Neurotransmitters, loss of neurons ↓ O_2 supply	• Altered balance, vertigo, syncope, ↑ postural hypotension • Changes in gait and ambulation • Changes in mental functioning • ↓ Kinesthetic sense • ↓ Ability to adapt to environment temperature • ↓ Proprioception, ↓ sensory input • Slowed conduction of nerve impulses, with slowed response time
Peripheral Nervous System		
Cranial and Spinal Nerves	Cell degeneration, death of neurons Loss of myelin and ↓ conduction time	• ↓ Reaction time in specific nerves • ↓ Speed and intensity of neuronal reflexes
Functional Divisions		
Motor	↓ Muscle bulk	• ↓ Strength, tone, agility
Sensory	Atrophy of taste buds Degeneration and loss of fibers in olfactory bulb Degenerative changes in nerve cells in inner ear, cerebellum, and proprioceptive pathways ↓ Electrical activity ↓ Sensory receptors	• ↓ Sense of touch, pain, and temperature • Slowing of or change in sensory reception • Malnutrition, weight loss • ↓ Sense of smell • Poor ability to maintain balance, widened gait
Reflexes	↓ Deep tendon reflexes ↓ Sensory conduction velocity	• Below-average reflex score • Sluggish reflexes, slowed reaction time
Reticular Formation		
Reticular activating system	Modification of hypothalamic function ↓ Stage IV sleep	• Changes in sleep patterns
Autonomic Nervous System		
Sympathetic nervous system and parasympathetic nervous system	Morphologic features of ganglia Slowed autonomic nervous system responses	• Orthostatic hypotension, systolic hypertension

as maintaining BP in response to changing from a lying to a standing position, is altered. As a result, older adults are more likely to have orthostatic hypotension. Coordination of neuromuscular activity to maintain body temperature becomes less efficient. Thus older adults are less able to adapt to extremes in ambient temperature. They are more vulnerable to hypothermia and hyperthermia.

Other changes include decreases in memory, vision (see Table 22.1), hearing (see Table 23.1), vibration, position sense, muscle strength, and reaction time. Decreases in taste and smell may result in decreased intake in the older adult. Reduced hearing and vision can result in perceptual confusion.[5] Problems with balance and coordination can put the older adult at risk for falls.[6]

CASE STUDY

Patient Introduction

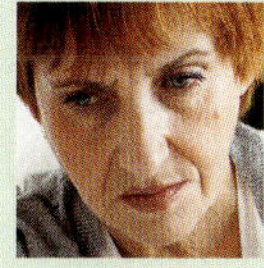

(© TatyanaGl/iStock/Thinkstock.)

J.K., a 57-year-old female, went to see her HCP for severe, persistent headaches that she has had for a few weeks. She lives alone and has a stressful job as an office manager in an engineering office. When her HCP did a neurologic assessment, he noted that she had a visual field deficit, especially in the upper left quadrant of her visual field. During the visit, J.K. had a seizure in his office. Staff called 911. She was admitted to the hospital, and the on-call neurologist was notified.

Discussion Questions

1. What are the possible causes of J.K.'s headaches and seizure?
2. Is her condition stable or an emergency?
3. What assessment questions do you need to ask her?

You will learn more about J.K. and her condition as you read this assessment chapter.

Answers available at http://evolve.elsevier.com/Lewis/medsurg.

NERVOUS SYSTEM ASSESSMENT

Subjective Data

Important Health Information

Health history. When performing a neurologic assessment, first determine whether an emergency exists. For example, is the level of consciousness decreasing? Is the patient a reliable historian and able to give detailed information? Patients with a neurologic problem may not be aware of it or may be a poor historian. If not, interview someone with firsthand knowledge of the history and current problem. They may have noticed any mental or physical changes in the patient.

Second, the mode of onset and course of the illness are important aspects of the history. Often these facts alone can reveal the nature of a nervous system problem. Obtain all pertinent data in the history of the present illness, especially the characteristics and progression of the symptoms. In some cases, the history may include birth injury (e.g., cerebral palsy from hypoxia) and/or other neurologic insults, such as a traumatic brain injury, stroke, or degenerative disease.

Growth and developmental history can be important in determining whether a nervous system problem was present at an early age. Ask about major developmental tasks, such as walking and talking. Obtain a family history.

Medications. Obtain a medication history. Include the use of sedatives, opioids, tranquilizers, and mood-elevating drugs. Many drugs have neurologic side effects. Ask patients to describe their treatment plan to determine adherence to prescribed therapies.

Surgery or other treatments. Ask about any surgery involving any part of the nervous system, such as the head, spine, or sensory organs. If patients have had surgery, determine the date, procedure, recovery, and current status. Note any history of eye surgery to determine the relevance of abnormal pupil assessment.

Functional Health Patterns

Key questions to ask patients with a neurologic problem are outlined in Table 60.4.

Health perception–health management. Ask about health practices that affect the nervous system. Include substance use, smoking, adequate nutrition, BP management, safe participation in exercise and recreation activities, and use of seat belts or helmets. Ask about hospitalizations for neurologic problems. If patients have an existing neurologic problem, assess how it affects daily living and the ability to perform self-care.

Nutritional-metabolic. Neurologic problems can result in poor nutrition. Problems related to chewing, swallowing, facial nerve paralysis, and muscle coordination could make it difficult to ingest adequate nutrients. Certain vitamins, such as thiamine (B_1), niacin, and pyridoxine (B_6), are essential for the health of the CNS. Deficiencies in any of these can result in nonspecific problems, such as depression, apathy, neuritis, weakness, confusion, and irritability. Cobalamin (vitamin B_{12}) deficiency can occur in older adults. They may have problems with vitamin absorption from supplements in addition to natural food sources, such as meat, fish, and poultry. Untreated, cobalamin deficiency can cause mental function decline.

Elimination. Bowel and bladder problems often occur with neurologic problems, such as stroke, head injury, spinal cord injury, MS, and dementia. Determine whether the bowel or bladder problem was present before or after the current neurologic event. Retention and incontinence of urine and feces are common problems. For example, nerve root compression (as occurs in cauda equina conditions) leads to a sudden onset of incontinence. Note key details, such as number of episodes, accompanying sensations or lack of sensations, and measures to control the problem.

Activity-exercise. Many neurologic disorders can cause problems with mobility, strength, and coordination. These problems can affect activity and exercise and increase fall risk.[6] Assess the person's activities of daily living. Neurologic problems can affect the ability to perform motor tasks, which increases the risk for injury.

Sleep-rest. Sleep pattern changes can be both a cause of and a response to neurologic problems. Pain and reduced ability to change position because of muscle weakness and paralysis

TABLE 60.4 HEALTH HISTORY

Nervous System

Health Perception–Health Management
- What are your usual daily activities?
- Do you use alcohol, tobacco, or recreational drugs?[a]
- What safety practices do you follow in a car? On a motorcycle? On a bicycle?
- Do you have hypertension? If so, how is it managed?
- Have you ever been hospitalized for a neurologic problem?[a]
- Do you take any medication to manage neurologic problems? If so, what?

Nutritional-Metabolic
- Are you able to feed yourself?
- Do you have any problems getting adequate nutrition because of chewing or swallowing problems, facial nerve paralysis, or poor muscle coordination?[a]
- Ask for a 24-h diet recall.

Elimination
- Do you have bowel or bladder incontinence?[a]
- Do you ever have problems with urinary hesitancy, urgency, or retention?[a]
- Do you postpone your bowel movements?[a]

Activity-Exercise
- Describe any problems you have with usual activities and exercise because of a neurologic problem.
- Do you have weakness or lack of coordination?[a]
- Are you able to perform your personal hygiene needs alone?[a]

Sleep-Rest
- Describe your sleep pattern.
- When you have trouble sleeping, what do you do?

Cognitive-Perceptual
- Have you noticed any changes in your memory?[a]
- Do you have dizziness, heat or cold sensitivity, numbness, or tingling?[a]
- Do you have chronic pain?[a]
- Do you have any problem with verbal or written communication?[a]
- Have you noticed any changes in vision or hearing?[a]

Self-Perception–Self-Concept
- How do you feel about yourself, about who you are?
- Describe your general emotional pattern.

Role-Relationship
- Have you had changes in roles such as spouse, parent, or primary wage earner?[a]

Sexuality-Reproductive
- Are you satisfied with your sexual function?[a]
- Are problems related to your sexual function causing tension in an important relationship?[a]
- Do you feel the need for professional counseling related to your sexual function?[a]

Coping–Stress Tolerance
- Describe your usual coping pattern.
- Do you think your present coping pattern is adequate to meet the stressors of your life?[a]
- What needs are unmet by your current support system?

Value-Belief
- Describe any culturally specific beliefs and attitudes that may influence your care.

[a]If yes, describe.

could interfere with sleep quality. Hallucinations from dementia or drugs can interrupt sleep. Assess sleep pattern and bedtime routines.

Cognitive-perceptual. Because the nervous system controls cognition and sensory integration, many neurologic problems affect these functions. Consider culture, age, and education when assessing communication because they play a role in our interaction with others. Assess memory, language, calculation ability, problem-solving ability, insight, and judgment. Ask hypothetical questions, such as "What is a reasonable price for a cup of coffee?" or "What would you do if you saw a car crash outside your house?" Do their plans and goals match their physical and mental capabilities? Note factors affecting intellectual capacity, such as impaired cognition, hallucinations, delusions, and dementia.

Assess a person's ability to use and understand language. Appropriateness of responses is a useful indicator of cognitive and perceptual ability. Determine their understanding and ability to carry out needed treatments. Neurologic-related cognitive changes can interfere with understanding of the disease and adherence to treatment.

Pain is common with many neurologic problems. It is often the reason patients seek care. Carefully assess pain. Pain assessment is discussed in Chapter 9.

Self-perception–self-concept. Neurologic problems can drastically change patients' control over life and create dependency on others for meeting daily needs. Physical appearance and emotional control can be affected. Sensitively ask patients about their evaluation of self-worth, perception of abilities, body image, and general emotional pattern.

Role-relationship. Physical impairments, such as weakness and paralysis, can alter or limit participation in usual roles and activities. Cognitive changes can permanently alter a person's ability to maintain previous roles. These changes can dramatically affect patients and caregivers. Ask them if a role change has occurred (e.g., spouse or breadwinner) because of neurologic problems and determine how long it has lasted. Caregivers should take part in decision making when neurologic problems affect the ability to make decisions.

Sexuality-reproductive. Assess the ability to take part in sexual activity. Many neurologic problems can affect sexual response. Cerebral lesions may inhibit the desire phase or the reflex responses of the excitement phase. The hypothalamus stimulates the pituitary gland to release hormones that influence sexual desire. Brainstem and spinal cord lesions may partially or completely interrupt the desire or ability to have intercourse. Neuropathies and spinal cord lesions may prevent reflex activities of the sexual response or affect sensation and decrease desire.

Coping–stress tolerance. The physical sequelae of a neurologic problem can strain patients' coping ability. Often the problem is chronic, and patients must learn new coping skills. Assess if the coping skills are adequate to deal with the stress of this problem. Evaluate patients' support system.

CASE STUDY

Subjective Data

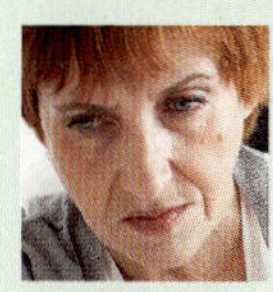

(© TatyanaGl/iStock/Thinkstock.)

After her admission to the hospital, a subjective assessment of J.K. revealed the following information:

Medical History: No history of seizures, migraine, or other headache before the current headaches and seizure.

Medications: Lisinopril 10 mg orally daily.

Health Perception–Health Management: Never smoked. Occasional social alcohol use. Reports good health other than mild hypertension.

Nutritional-Metabolic: J.K. is 5 ft 5 in tall; weight 145 lb.

Activity-Exercise: Moderate activity. No formal exercise or participation in sports.

Cognitive-Perceptual: Says her headaches led her to get her eyes tested. Has had only minor decrease in visual acuity.

Coping–Stress Tolerance: Is depressed and fearful. She is worried that something serious is wrong. Denies dizziness, change in hearing, or memory deficits.

Discussion Questions

1. Which subjective assessment findings concern you the most?
2. Based on these subjective assessment findings, what would be included in the physical assessment?

You will learn more about the physical assessment of the neurologic system in the next section.

Answers available at http://evolve.elsevier.com/Lewis/medsurg.

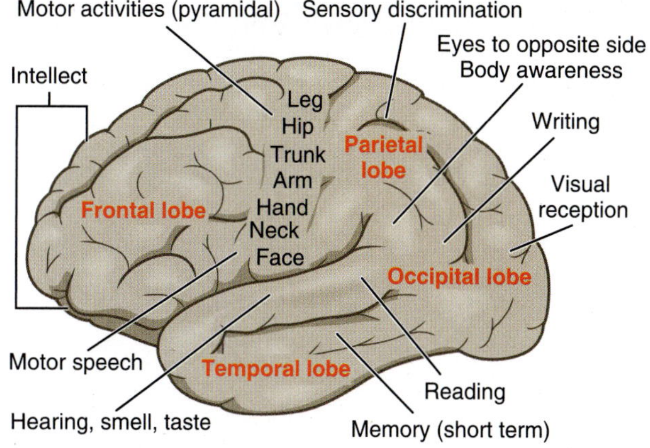

Fig. 60.14 Each area of the brain controls a particular activity.

TABLE 60.5 Normal Physical Assessment of the Nervous System

Parameter	Findings
Mental status	• Alert and oriented, orderly thought processes. • Appropriate mood and affect.
Cranial nerves May be recorded as "CN I to XII intact"	• Smell intact to soap or coffee. • Visual fields full to confrontation. • Intact extraocular movements. • No nystagmus. PERRLA. • Intact facial sensation to light touch and pinprick. • Full facial movements. • Hearing intact bilaterally. • Intact gag and swallow reflexes. Symmetric smile. Midline protrusion of tongue. • Full strength with head turning and shoulder shrugging.
Motor system	• Normal gait and station. Normal tandem walk. Negative Romberg test. • Normal and symmetric muscle bulk, tone, strength. • Smooth performance of finger-nose, heel-shin movements.
Sensory system	• Intact sensation to light touch, position sense, pinprick, heat, and cold.
Reflexes	• Biceps, triceps, brachioradialis, patellar, and Achilles tendon reflexes 2/5 bilaterally. • Toes pointed down with plantar stimulation.

Objective Data

Physical Assessment

The standard neurologic assessment helps determine the presence, location, and nature of nervous system disease (Fig. 60.14). The assessment looks at 6 categories of function: mental status, CN function, motor function, sensory function, cerebellar function, and reflexes.[7] Table 60.5 is an example of a normal neurologic physical assessment. Abnormal assessment findings of the neurologic system are shown in Table 60.6. A *focused assessment* is used to assess the status of previously identified neurologic problems and to monitor for signs of new problems. A focused assessment of the neurologic system is shown in Box 60.1.

Mental status. Assessing mental status gives a general impression of how the patient is functioning. It involves determining complex and high-level cerebral functions governed by many areas of the cerebral cortex. Begin your assessment when you first see a patient and continue throughout your interaction. For example, assess language and memory when asking for details of the illness and past events. Consider age, cultural background, and level of education when evaluating mental status.

The components of the mental status assessment include:

- *General appearance and behavior:* Assess level of consciousness (awake, asleep, comatose), motor activity, body posture, dress and hygiene, facial expression, and speech pattern. Patients with deficits in self-care as shown by poor grooming are more likely to have other cognitive problems.

TABLE 60.6 ASSESSMENT ABNORMALITIES

Nervous System

Finding	Description	Possible Cause and Significance
Cranial Nerves		
Dysphagia	Difficulty swallowing	Lesions involving motor pathways of CN IX and CN X (including lower brainstem)
Ophthalmoplegia	Paralysis of eye muscles	Lesions in brainstem
Eyes		
Anisocoria	Inequality of pupil size	Oculomotor nerve injury Sympathetic pathway injury
Diplopia	Double vision	Lesions affecting nerves of extraocular muscles, cerebellar damage
Homonymous hemianopsia	Loss of vision in 1 side of visual field	Lesions in the contralateral occipital lobe
Papilledema	"Choked disc," swelling of optic nerve head	Increased intracranial pressure
Mental Status		
Altered consciousness	Stuporous, mute, ↓ response to verbal cues or pain	Intracranial lesions, metabolic problem, psychiatric disorders
Anosognosia	Inability to recognize bodily defect or disease	Lesions in right parietal cortex
Motor System		
Apraxia	Inability to perform learned movements despite having desire and physical ability to perform them	Cerebral cortex lesion
Ataxia	Lack of coordination of movement	Lesions of sensory or motor pathways, cerebellum Antiseizure drugs, sedatives, hypnotic drug toxicity (including alcohol)
Dyskinesia	Impaired voluntary movement, resulting in fragmentary or incomplete movements	Disorders of basal ganglia, idiosyncratic reaction to psychotropic drugs
Hemiplegia	Paralysis on 1 side	Stroke and other lesions involving contralateral motor cortex
Nystagmus	Jerking or bobbing of eyes as they track moving object	Lesions in cerebellum, brainstem, vestibular system Antiseizure drugs, sedatives, hypnotic toxicity (including alcohol)
Reflexes		
Deep tendon reflexes	↓ or absent motor response	Lower motor neuron lesions
Extensor plantar response	Toes pointing up with plantar stimulation	Suprasegmental or upper motor neuron lesion
Sensory System		
Analgesia	Loss of pain sensation	Lesion in spinothalamic tract or thalamus Analgesic drugs
Anesthesia	Absence of sensation	Lesions in spinal cord, thalamus, sensory cortex, or peripheral sensory nerve Anesthesia drugs
Astereognosis	Inability to recognize form of object by touch	Lesions in parietal cortex
Paresthesia	Abnormal sensation, such as numbness or tingling	Lesions in the posterior column or sensory cortex
Speech		
Aphasia, dysphasia	Loss of or impaired language faculty (comprehension, expression, or both)	Left cerebral cortex lesion
Dysarthria	Lack of coordination in articulating speech	Cerebellar or CN lesion Antiseizure drugs, sedatives, hypnotic drug toxicity (including alcohol)
Spinal Cord		
Bladder dysfunction		
• Atonic (autonomous)	Absence of muscle tone and contractility, enlargement of capacity, no discomfort, overflow with large residual, inability to voluntarily empty	Early stage of spinal cord injury
• Hypertonic	↑ Muscle tone, ↓ capacity, reflex emptying, dribbling, incontinence	Lesions in pyramidal tracts (efferent pathways)
• Hypotonic	More ability than atonic bladder but less than normal	Interruption of afferent pathways from bladder
Paraplegia	Paralysis of lower extremities	Spinal cord transection or mass lesion (thoracolumbar region)
Tetraplegia (quadriplegia)	Paralysis of all extremities	Spinal cord transection or mass lesion (cervical region)

BOX 60.1 FOCUSED ASSESSMENT

Nervous System

Use this checklist to make sure the key assessment steps have been done.

Subjective

Ask about any of the following and note responses:

Blackouts/loss of memory

Weakness, numbness, tingling in arms or legs

Headaches, especially new onset

Loss of balance/coordination

Orientation to person, place, time, and situation

Objective: Diagnostic

Check the following diagnostic results for critical values:

Lumbar puncture

CT or MRI of brain

EEG

Objective: Physical Assessment

Inspect/Observe

General level of consciousness/orientation

Oropharynx for gag reflex and soft palate movement

Peripheral sensation of light touch and pinprick (face, hands, feet)

Smell with coffee or soap

Eyes for extraocular movements, PERRLA, peripheral vision, nystagmus

Gait for smoothness and coordination

Palpate

Strength of neck, shoulders, arms, and legs for fullness and symmetry

Percuss

Reflexes

- *Cognition:* Note orientation to time, place, person, and situation. Note memory, general knowledge, insight, judgment, problem-solving, and calculation. Common questions are "Who were the last 3 presidents?" "What do people use to cut paper?" "Can you count backward from 100 by 7s?" We often use a structured mental status questionnaire to assess these functions and provide baseline data for evaluating changes over time. Common tools include the Mini-Mental State Examination (MMSE) (see Table 64.9) and Montreal Cognitive Assessment (MoCA).[8] Delirium is an acute and transient disorder of cognition that can occur at any time during illness. As discussed in Chapter 64, delirium is often an early indicator of various illnesses (see Table 64.17). The Confusion Assessment Method tool is used to assess for delirium (see Table 64.19).
- *Mood and affect:* Note any agitation, anger, depression, or euphoria and the appropriateness of these states. Use suitable questions to reveal a patient's feelings.

Cranial nerves. Testing each CN is an essential part of the neurologic assessment (Table 60.2).

Olfactory nerve. Chronic rhinitis, sinusitis, and heavy smoking may decrease the sense of smell. Problems with smell may occur with a tumor involving the olfactory bulb or a basilar skull fracture that has damaged the olfactory fibers. *Anosmia*

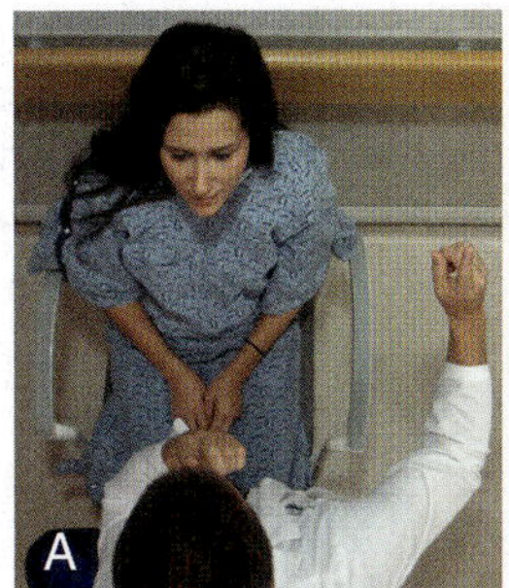

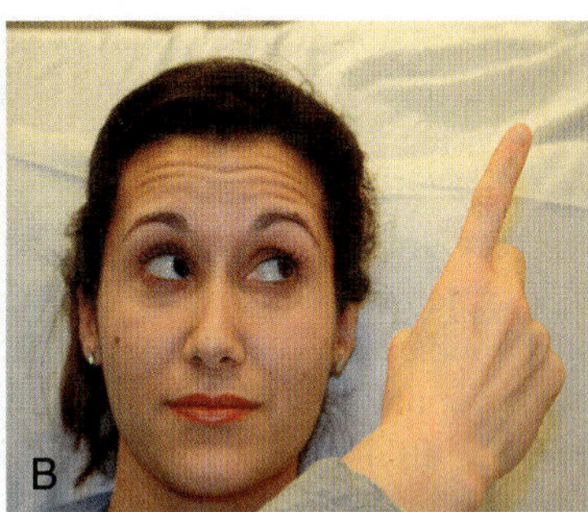

Fig. 60.15 (A) Nurse checking visual fields. (B) Nurse checking extraocular movement (EOM). (Courtesy DaiWai Olson, RN, PhD, CCRN, Dallas, TX.)

(loss of sense of smell) and *hyposmia* (reduced sense of smell) are early signs in Parkinson disease and Alzheimer disease.[9]

Optic nerve. Visual field deficits may arise from lesions of the optic nerve, optic chiasm, or tracts that extend through the temporal, parietal, or occipital lobes. Visual field changes resulting from brain lesions include *hemianopsia* (half of the visual field is affected), *quadrantanopia* (25% of the visual field is affected), *bitemporal hemianopsia* (bilateral peripheral vision is affected), or monocular vision.

Oculomotor, trochlear, and abducens nerves. Because the oculomotor (CN III), trochlear (CN IV), and abducens (CN VI) nerves help move the eye, we test them together (Table 60.2). With weakness or paralysis of an eye muscle, the eyes do not move together and the patient has a *disconjugate gaze.* Note the presence and direction of *nystagmus* (fine, rapid jerking movements of the eyes). This condition most often indicates vestibulocerebellar problems (Fig. 60.15).

Because the oculomotor nerve exits at the top of the brainstem at the tentorial notch, it can be compressed easily by expanding mass lesions. When this occurs, sympathetic input to the pupil is unopposed; the pupil changes shape and becomes dilated. The lack of pupil constriction is an early sign of central herniation (see Chapter 61).

Two abbreviations we often use to record the reaction of the pupils are *PERRL* (*P*upils are *E*qual [in size], *R*ound, and *R*eactive to *L*ight) and *PERRLA* (*P*upils are *E*qual, *R*ound, and *R*eactive to *L*ight and *A*ccommodation). The *PERRL* abbreviation is appropriate when accommodation cannot be assessed, as in unconscious patients. Test convergence and accommodation by having the patient focus on your finger as it moves toward their nose.

Another function of the oculomotor nerve is to keep the eyelid open. Damage to the nerve can cause *ptosis* (drooping eyelid), pupil abnormalities, and eye muscle weakness.

Motor system. The motor system assessment includes strength, tone, coordination, and symmetry of the major muscle groups. Test muscle strength by asking the patient to push and pull against the resistance of your arm as it opposes flexion and extension of the muscle. Test all 4 extremities and note any asymmetry in strength or movement. Ask the patient to offer resistance at the shoulders, elbows, wrists, hips, knees, and ankles. Mild arm weakness is demonstrated by downward drifting of the arm or pronation of the palm *(pronator drift).*

The pronator drift test is an excellent measure of strength in the upper extremities. It is especially sensitive with vasospasm or increasing edema in 1 cerebral hemisphere. Have the patient close their eyes and hold the arms out with palms facing up (like they are holding a large pizza). The patient should hold this position for 30 seconds. Downward drift with palm pronation indicates a problem in the opposite motor cortex. Asking the patient to raise the foot from the bed or to bend the knees up in bed is a good assessment of lower extremity strength.

Test muscle tone by passively moving the limbs through their range of motion. You should identify a slight resistance to these movements. Abnormal tone is described as *hypotonia* (flaccidity) or *hypertonia* (spasticity). Note any involuntary movements, such as tics, tremor, *myoclonus* (spasm of muscles), *athetosis* (slow, writhing, involuntary movements of extremities), *chorea* (involuntary, purposeless, rapid motions), and *dystonia* (impaired muscle tone).

Test cerebellar function by assessing balance and coordination. A good screening test for both balance and muscle strength is to observe stature (posture while standing) and gait. Note the pace and rhythm of the gait. Observe for normal symmetric and oppositional arm swing. The ability to ambulate helps to determine the level of nursing care needed and the risk for falling.

The finger-to-nose test (having a patient alternately touch the nose, then touch the examiner's finger) and the heel-to-shin test (having a patient stroke the heel of 1 foot up and down the shin of the opposite leg) assess coordination and cerebellar function. Reposition your finger while the patient is touching the nose so that the patient must adjust to a new distance each time your finger is touched. These movements should be smooth and accurate. Other tests include asking the patient to pronate and supinate both hands rapidly and to do a shallow knee bend, first on 1 leg and then on the other. Note any dysarthria or slurred speech because it is a sign the speech muscles lack coordination.

Sensory system. We evaluate several modalities in the somatic sensory assessment. Each modality is carried by a specific ascending pathway in the spinal cord before it reaches the sensory cortex. As a rule, perform the assessment with the patient's eyes closed to avoid providing the patient with clues. Ask "How does this feel?" rather than "Is this sharp?" In the routine assessment, sensory testing of the anterior torso, posterior torso, and all extremities is sufficient. However, if you identify a problem in sensory function, delineate the boundaries of that dysfunction carefully along the dermatome.

Touch, pain, and temperature. Light touch is usually tested first using a cotton wisp or light pinprick. Gently touch each extremity. Ask patients to indicate when they feel the stimulus. Test pain by alternately touching the skin with the sharp and dull ends of a pin. Tell patients to respond "sharp" or "dull." Assess each limb separately.

Extinction is assessed by simultaneously touching both sides of the body symmetrically. Normally, the simultaneous stimuli are both perceived (sensed). An abnormal response occurs when the patient perceives the stimulus on only 1 side. The other stimulus is *extinguished.*

Test temperature sensation by applying tubes of warm and cold water to the skin and asking the patient to identify the stimuli with the eyes closed. If pain sensation is intact, you do not have to assess temperature sensation because the same ascending pathways carry both sensations.

Vibration sense. Assess vibration sense by applying a vibrating tuning fork to the fingernails and bony prominences of the hands, legs, and feet. Ask the patient if the vibration or "buzz" is felt. Then ask them to indicate when the vibration stops.

Position sense. Assess position sense *(proprioception)* by placing your thumb and forefinger on either side of a patient's forefinger or great toe and gently moving their digit up or down. Ask the patient to close the eyes and state the direction in which the digit is moved.

Another test of proprioception is the Romberg test. Ask the patient to stand with feet together and then close their eyes. If the patient can maintain balance with the eyes open but sways or falls with the eyes closed (i.e., a positive Romberg test), vestibulocochlear problems in the posterior columns of the spinal cord may be present. Be aware of patient safety during this test.

Cortical sensory functions. Several tests assess cortical integration of sensory perceptions (which occurs in the parietal lobes). Explain these tests beforehand, while their eyes are still open. Assess *2-point discrimination* by placing the 2 points of a calibrated compass on the tips of the fingers and toes. The minimum recognizable separation is 4 to 5 mm in the fingertips and a greater degree of separation elsewhere. This test is important in diagnosing diseases of the sensory cortex and PNS.

Test *graphesthesia* (ability to feel writing on skin) by having the patient identify numbers traced on the palms of the hands. Test *stereognosis* (ability to perceive the form and nature of objects) by having the patient close the eyes and identify the size and shape of easily recognized objects (e.g., coins, keys, safety pin) placed in the hands.

Reflexes. Tendons have receptors that are sensitive to stretch. A reflex contraction of the skeletal muscle occurs when the tendon is stretched. In general, we test the biceps, triceps, brachioradialis, patellar, and Achilles tendon reflexes. Initiate a simple muscle stretch reflex by briskly tapping the tendon of a stretched muscle, usually with a reflex hammer (Fig. 60.16). Measure the response (muscle contraction of the corresponding muscle) on a 0 to 5 scale as follows: 0 = absent reflex; 1 = weak response, seen only with reinforcement; 2 = normal response; 3 = brisk response; 4 = hyperreflexia with no sustained clonus; and 5 = hyperreflexia with sustained clonus. *Clonus,* an abnormal response, is a continued rhythmic contraction of the muscle with continuous application of the stimulus.

Elicit the *biceps reflex,* with the patient's arm partially flexed and palm up, by placing your thumb over the biceps tendon in the antecubital space and striking the thumb with a hammer. The normal response is flexion of the arm at the elbow or contraction of the biceps muscle that you can feel with your thumb.

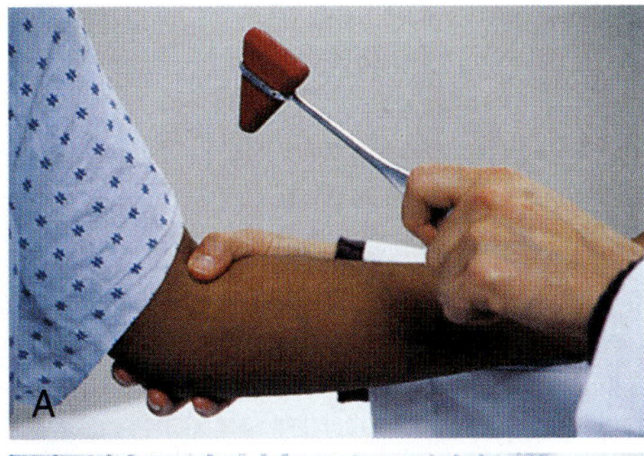

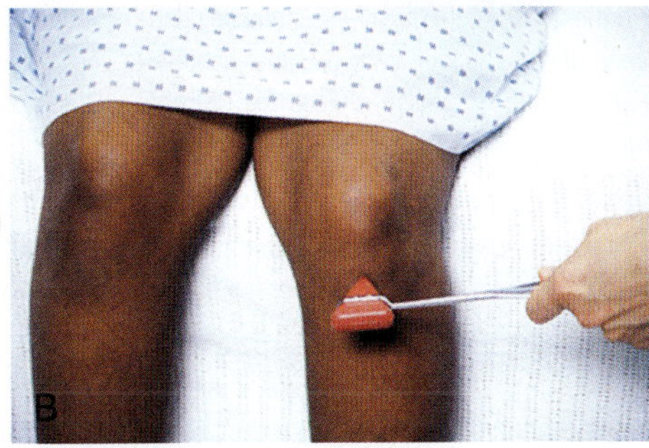

Fig. 60.16 The examiner strikes a swift blow over a stretched tendon to elicit a stretch reflex. (A) Biceps reflex. (B) Patellar reflex.

Elicit the *triceps reflex* by striking the triceps tendon above the elbow while the patient's arm is flexed. The normal response is extension of the arm or visible contraction of the triceps.

Elicit the *brachioradialis reflex* by striking the radius 3 to 5 cm above the wrist while the patient's arm is relaxed. The normal response is flexion and supination at the elbow or visible contraction of the brachioradialis muscle.

Elicit the *patellar reflex* by striking the patellar tendon just below the patella. The patient can be sitting or lying, as long as the leg being tested hangs freely. The normal response is extension of the leg with contraction of the quadriceps.

Gently dorsiflex the patient's foot at the ankle. Elicit the *Achilles tendon reflex* by striking the Achilles tendon while the patient's leg is flexed at the knee. The normal response is plantar flexion at the ankle.

CASE STUDY

Objective Data: Physical Assessment

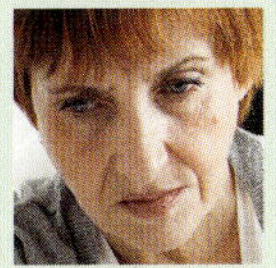
(© TatyanaGl/ iStock/ Thinkstock.)

A physical assessment of J.K. reveals the following:

- BP 145/80, HR 78, RR 20, T 98.6°F (37°C)
- Alert, oriented, and appropriate, but anxious
- Strength 5/5 on all extremities
- Visual field deficits in upper left quadrant of visual field

Discussion Questions

1. Which physical assessment findings concern you most?
2. Based on the results of the subjective and physical assessment, what diagnostic studies do you think may be ordered for J.K.?

You will learn more about diagnostic studies related to the neurologic system in the next section.

Answers available at http://evolve.elsevier.com/Lewis/medsurg.

DIAGNOSTIC STUDIES OF THE NERVOUS SYSTEM

Many diagnostic studies are available to assess the nervous system. CSF analysis provides information about a variety of CNS diseases. Normal CSF is clear, colorless, odorless, and free of red blood cells. It contains little protein. Normal CSF values are listed in Table 60.7. CSF may be obtained through LP or, on occasion, ventriculostomy.

During LP, the HCP aspirates CSF through a needle inserted into the L3—L4 or L4—L5 interspace. A manometer attached to the needle is used to obtain CSF pressure. CSF is withdrawn in a series of tubes and sent for analysis. LP is contraindicated in the presence of increased intracranial pressure because of the risk for downward herniation from CSF removal or if there is infection present at the intended puncture site. Nursing care of patients undergoing LP is outlined in Table 60.8.

Tables 60.9 and 60.10 describe a number of other studies. Nerve, muscle, brain, and arterial tissue biopsies are useful in diagnosing several disorders (e.g., tumors, infectious disease, degenerative diseases). A brain biopsy is usually done using a stereotactic procedure.

TABLE 60.7 Cerebrospinal Fluid Analysis

Parameter	Normal Value
Specific gravity	1.007
pH	7.35
Appearance	Clear, colorless
RBCs	None
WBCs	0–5 cells/μL (0–5 × 10^6 cells/L)
Protein	
• Lumbar	15–45 mg/dL (0.15–0.45 g/L)
• Cisternal	15–25 mg/dL (0.15–0.25 g/L)
• Ventricular	5–15 mg/dL (0.05–0.15 g/L)
Glucose	40–70 mg/dL (2.2–3.9 mmol/L)
Microorganisms	None
Pressure	60–150 mm H_2O

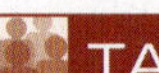

TABLE 60.8 NURSING MANAGEMENT

Care of the Patient Undergoing Lumbar Puncture

Preprocedure

- Obtain vital signs and a baseline neurologic assessment. Notify HCP of signs of increased intracranial pressure (see Chapter 61).
- Assess coagulation studies to reduce the risk for epidural hematoma.
- Provide teaching about procedure. Tell the patient they may feel temporary, sharp pain or tingling radiating down the leg as a sterile needle is passed between 2 lumbar vertebrae.
- Give sedative and analgesia as ordered.
- Have patient void.
- Place patient in a side-lying or sitting position (Fig. 60.17).

Postprocedure

- Monitor neurologic signs and vital signs.
- Monitor for headache intensity and drainage from the puncture site.
- Apply pressure and a pressure dressing to the puncture site.
- Keep the patient in a reclining position for 1 hour or up to several hours to decrease the risk for spinal headache. They may turn from side to side if the head is not raised.
- Properly label CSF specimens and send to laboratory.
- Teach the patient to report numbness, tingling, and movement of the extremities; pain at the injection site; and the inability to void.
- Encourage fluids with a straw to replace the CSF that was removed.
- Give ordered analgesia, as needed.

TABLE 60.9 Radiologic Studies

Nervous System

Study	Description and Purpose	Nursing Responsibility
Cerebral angiography	Serial x-rays of intracranial and extracranial blood vessels done to detect vascular lesions (aneurysms, hematomas, arteriovenous malformations) and brain tumors. Catheter is inserted into the femoral (sometimes brachial) artery and passed through the aortic arch into the base of a carotid or a vertebral artery for injection of contrast medium. Timed-sequence radiographic images obtained as contrast flows through arteries, smaller vessels, and veins.	*Before:* Assess for stroke risk because thrombi may be dislodged during procedure. May need to be NPO. *During:* Warn that contrast injection may cause a feeling of being warm and flushed. Must lie completely still during scan. *After:* Monitor neurologic signs and VS every 15–30 min for first 2 h, every hour for next 6 h, then every 2 h for 24 h. Maintain bed rest for 6 h (1 h if a closure device is used). Assess for bleeding. Report any neurologic status changes.
CT scan	Rapid way to obtain radiographic images of the brain. Computer-assisted x-ray of multiple cross sections of body parts to detect problems such as hemorrhage, tumor, cyst, edema, infarction, brain atrophy, and other abnormalities. Contrast medium may be used to enhance visualization of brain structures.	*Before:* Note renal function before contrast medium used. Assess for allergy to shellfish because the contrast is iodine based. If taking metformin, hold it the day of the test to prevent kidney damage. *During:* Warn that contrast injection may cause a feeling of being warm and flushed. Must lie completely still during scan. *After:* Encourage patient to drink fluids to avoid renal problems with any contrast.
• CT angiography (CTA)	Noninvasive imaging of vascular system (e.g., aneurysms). Evaluates blood volume, flow, and mean transit time as a measure of perfusion. Fewer complications than cerebral angiography; less expensive.	Similar to CT (see earlier).
MRI	Imaging of brain, spinal cord, and spinal canal by means of magnetic energy. Can detect strokes, multiple sclerosis, tumors, trauma, herniation, and seizures. Provides greater detail than CT. Takes a longer time to complete and may not be appropriate in life-threatening emergencies. Contrast medium can enhance visualization. The contrast agent *gadolinium* has a lower incidence of allergy than iodine used in CT.	*Before:* Oral and/or IV contrast injection may be used. Check for pregnancy, allergies, and renal function. Have patient remove all metal objects. Ask about a history of surgical insertion of staples, plates, dental bridges, or other metal appliances. Remove metallic foil patches. May need to be fasting. Assess for claustrophobia and need for antianxiety medication. *During:* Must lie completely still.
• Magnetic resonance angiography (MRA)	Uses differential signal characteristics of flowing blood to assess extracranial and intracranial blood vessels. Provides both anatomic and hemodynamic information. Can be done with contrast medium.	Similar to MRI (see earlier).
• Functional MRI (fMRI)	MRI technique that provides time-related images that evaluate how the brain responds to various stimuli. Makes it possible to detect the brain areas involved in a task, process, or an emotion.	Similar to MRI (see earlier).
• MR spectroscopy (MRS)	Noninvasive. Measures biochemical changes in the brain, especially the presence of tumors. Compares chemical composition of normal brain tissue with abnormal tumor tissue. Can detect tissue changes in stroke and epilepsy.	Similar to MRI (see earlier).

TABLE 60.9 **Radiologic Studies—cont'd**

Study	Description and Purpose	Nursing Responsibility
Myelogram	X-ray of spinal cord and vertebral column after injection of contrast medium into subarachnoid space. Detects spinal lesions (e.g., herniated or ruptured disc, spinal tumor).	*Before:* Give sedative as ordered. Have patient empty bladder. Tell patient that test is done with patient on tilting table that is moved during test. *After:* Should lie flat for 1–2 h to prevent spinal headache. Encourage fluids. Monitor neurologic signs and VS. Headache, nausea, and vomiting may occur.
Positron emission tomography (PET)	Measures metabolic activity of brain to assess cell death or damage. Uses radioactive material that shows up as a bright spot on the image. Can diagnose stroke, Alzheimer disease, seizure disorders, Parkinson disease, tumors.	*Before:* Explain procedure. Tell patient not to take sedatives or tranquilizers. Have patient empty bladder. Insert 2 IV lines. *During:* May be asked to perform different activities during test.
Single-photon emission computed tomography (SPECT)	Method of scanning similar to PET but uses more stable substances and different detectors. Radiolabeled compounds are injected, and their photon emissions can be detected. Resulting images are accumulation of labeled compound. Assesses blood flow and O_2 and glucose metabolism in the brain. Can diagnose strokes, brain tumors, seizure disorders.	Similar to PET (see earlier).
Skull and spine x-rays	Simple x-ray of skull and spinal column. Can detect fractures, bone erosion, calcifications, abnormal vascularity.	*Before:* Remove any radiopaque objects that can interfere with results. Explain procedure.
Ultrasound		
Carotid artery duplex scan	Noninvasive. Assess degree of stenosis of carotid and vertebral arteries. Combines ultrasound and Doppler technology. Probe is placed over the carotid artery and slowly moved along the course of the common carotid artery. Frequency of reflected ultrasound signal corresponds to blood velocity. Increased blood flow velocity can indicate stenosis of a vessel.	*Before:* Explain procedure.
Transcranial Doppler	Same technology as carotid duplex but evaluates blood flow velocities of intracranial blood vessels. Probe placed on skin at various "windows" in the skull (areas in the skull that have only a thin bony covering) to record velocities of the blood vessels.	*Before:* Explain procedure.

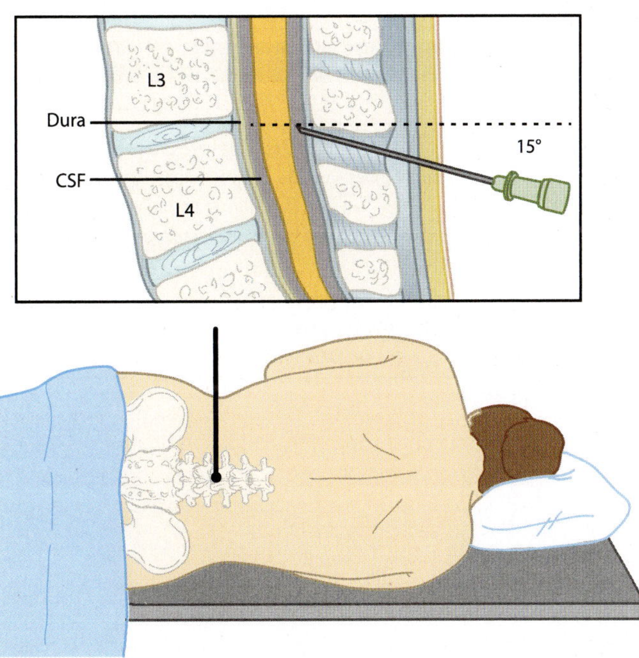

Fig. 60.17 The lateral position for an LP. The hips, knees, and neck are flexed with the knees bent up toward the chest.

TABLE 60.10 Electrographic Studies

Nervous System

Study	Description and Purpose	Nursing Responsibility
Electroencephalography (EEG)	Electrical activity of brain recorded using scalp electrodes. Evaluates seizure disorders, cerebral disease, CNS effects of systemic diseases, brain injury, brain death. Specific tests may be done to assess brain's electrical response to lights and loud noises.	*Before:* Tell patient procedure is noninvasive and without danger of electric shock. Determine whether any medications (e.g., tranquilizers, antiseizure drugs) should be withheld. *After:* Resume medications. Wash electrode paste out of hair.
Electromyography (EMG)	Recording of electrical activity associated with skeletal muscle contraction. Needle electrodes are inserted into the muscle to record specific motor units. Normal muscle at rest shows no electrical activity. Activity may be altered in muscle diseases (e.g., myopathic conditions), disorders of muscle innervation (e.g., segmental or LMN lesions, peripheral neuropathic conditions).	*Before:* Explain procedure. Include that pain and discomfort are common with insertion of needles. HCPs may restrict stimulants (e.g., caffeine) 2–3 h prior. *After:* Assess needle sites for hematoma or inflammation. Give as-needed analgesics.
Electroneurography (nerve conduction studies)	Measures nerve conduction velocity of peripheral nerves. Involves applying a brief electrical stimulus to a distal portion of a sensory nerve and recording resulting wave of depolarization at a point proximal to the stimulation. Time between stimulus onset and first wave of depolarization at the recording electrode is measured. Damaged nerves have slower conduction velocities.	*Before:* Explain procedure.
Evoked potentials	Electrical activity associated with nerve conduction along sensory pathways is recorded by electrodes placed on skin and scalp. A stimulus generates the impulse. Increase in normal time from stimulus onset to a given peak (latency) indicates slowed nerve conduction or nerve damage. Can diagnose disease (e.g., multiple sclerosis), locate nerve damage, monitor function during surgery. Can diagnose visual or auditory system problems because it shows if a sensory impulse is reaching the right part of brain.	*Before:* Explain procedure. Shampoo hair before test.
Magnetoencephalography (MEG)	Uses a biomagnetometer to detect magnetic fields generated by neural activity. Can accurately pinpoint the part of the brain involved in a stroke, seizure, or other disorder or injury. Measures extracranial magnetic fields and scalp electric field (EEG).	*Before:* Explain procedure. MEG, a passive sensor, does not make physical contact with patient.

LMN, Lower motor neuron.

CASE STUDY

Objective Data: Diagnostic Studies

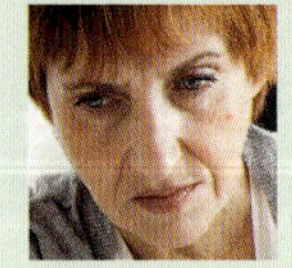

(© TatyanaGl/ iStock/ Thinkstock.)

MRI/MRA results show a temporal-parietal glioblastoma that has extended into the margins of the occipital lobes.

Discussion Questions

1. Did you expect this diagnostic study to be ordered?
2. What is the implication of the diagnostic study result?

This case study is continued in Chapter 62.

Answers available at http://evolve.elsevier.com/Lewis/medsurg.

BRIDGE TO NCLEX EXAMINATION

The number of the question corresponds to the same-numbered outcome at the beginning of the chapter.

1. In a patient with a disease that affects the myelin sheath of nerves, such as multiple sclerosis, the glial cells affected are the
   a. microglia.
   b. astrocytes.
   c. ependymal cells.
   d. oligodendrocytes.
2. A patient taking a drug that impairs function of the extrapyramidal system may have loss of
   a. sensations of pain and temperature.
   b. regulation of the autonomic nervous system.
   c. integration of somatic and special sensory inputs.
   d. automatic movements associated with skeletal muscle activity.
3. During the neurologic assessment, the nurse finds the patient has speech problems with weakness of the right arm and lower face. The nurse would expect a CT scan to show pathology in the distribution of the
   a. basilar artery.
   b. left middle cerebral artery.
   c. right anterior cerebral artery.
   d. left posterior communicating artery.
4. A patient is seen in the emergency department after diving into the pool and hitting the bottom with a blow to the face that hyperextended the neck and scraped the skin off the nose. The patient reports double vision when looking down. During the neurologic assessment, the nurse finds the patient is unable to abduct their left eye. The nurse recognizes this finding is related to
   a. a basal skull fracture.
   b. an injury to CN VI.
   c. a stiff neck from the hyperextension injury.
   d. facial swelling from the scrape on the bottom of the pool.
5. Stimulation of the parasympathetic nervous system results in **(Select all that apply.)**
   a. constriction of the bronchi.
   b. dilation of skin blood vessels.
   c. increased secretion of insulin.
   d. increased blood glucose levels.
   e. relaxation of the urinary sphincters.
6. When assessing the muscle strength of an older adult, the nurse cannot compare the findings with those of a younger adult because
   a. nutrition status is better in young adults.
   b. muscle tone and strength decrease in older adults.
   c. muscle strength should be the same for all adults.
   d. most young adults exercise more than older adults.
7. A patient is admitted with a headache, fever, and general malaise. The HCP has asked that the patient be prepared for a lumbar puncture. What is a *priority* nursing action to avoid complications?
   a. Review laboratory results for changes in the white cell count.
   b. Give acetaminophen for the headache and fever before the procedure.
   c. Notify the provider if signs of increased intracranial pressure are present.
   d. Administer antibiotics before the procedure to treat the potential meningitis.
8. During neurologic testing, the patient can perceive pain elicited by pinprick. Based on this finding, the nurse may omit testing for
   a. position sense.
   b. patellar reflexes.
   c. temperature perception.
   d. heel-to-shin movements.
9. A patient's eyes jerk while the patient looks to the left. The nurse records this finding as
   a. nystagmus.
   b. papilledema.
   c. CN VI palsy.
   d. oculocephalic response.
10. The nurse caring for a patient with peripheral neuropathy who is scheduled for electromyography (EMG) studies should
    a. ensure the patient has an empty bladder.
    b. teach the patient about the risk for electric shock.
    c. ensure the patient has no metallic jewelry or metal fragments.
    d. teach the patient that pain may be experienced during the study.

1. d; 2. d; 3. b;
4. b; 5. a, b, c, e; 6. b; 7. c; 8. c; 9. a; 10. d.

For rationales to these answers and even more NCLEX review questions, visit http://evolve.elsevier.com/Lewis/medsurg.

REFERENCES

To access the References for this chapter, please scan the QR code with a mobile device.

61

Acute Intracranial Problems

Kristen J. Keller

http://evolve.elsevier.com/Lewis/medsurg/

CONCEPTUAL FOCUS

Cognition
Functional Ability
Intracranial Regulation
Mobility
Safety
Sensory Perception

LEARNING OUTCOMES

1. Explain the mechanisms that maintain normal intracranial pressure.
2. Describe the common etiologies, clinical manifestations, and interprofessional care of patients with increased intracranial pressure.
3. Describe the nursing management of patients with increased intracranial pressure.
4. Compare types of head injury by mechanism of injury and clinical manifestations.
5. Describe the interprofessional and nursing management of patients with a head injury.
6. Compare the types, clinical manifestations, and interprofessional care of patients with brain tumors.
7. Discuss the nursing management of patients with a brain tumor.
8. Describe the nursing management of patients undergoing cranial surgery.
9. Distinguish among the primary causes and interprofessional and nursing management of brain abscess, meningitis, and encephalitis.

KEY TERMS

cerebral edema
concussion
diffuse axonal injury (DAI)
encephalitis
epidural hematoma
Glasgow Coma Scale (GCS)
head injury
intracerebral hematoma
intracranial pressure (ICP)
meningitis
nuchal rigidity
subdural hematoma
unconsciousness

The body has various mechanisms by which it regulates the intracranial space to promote optimal brain function. Acute intracranial problems can disrupt these processes, leading to increased intracranial pressure (ICP), reduced blood flow to the brain, and brain tissue damage. This chapter discusses the mechanisms that maintain normal ICP and problems that lead to increased ICP (IICP).

INTRACRANIAL REGULATION

Normal Compensatory Adaptations

The skull is an enclosed space with 3 essential volume components: brain tissue, blood, and cerebrospinal fluid (CSF) (Fig. 61.1). Brain tissue makes up about 78% of this volume. Blood in the arterial, venous, and capillary network makes up 12% of the volume. The remaining 10% is CSF. A variation in any of these components may lead to neurologic symptoms and IICP.

The Monro-Kellie doctrine states that the 3 components must stay at a relatively constant volume within the closed skull. If the volume of any 1 of the 3 components increases within the skull and the volume from another component is displaced, the total intracranial volume will not change. This hypothesis is applicable only when the skull is closed. The hypothesis does not apply in persons with displaced skull fractures or craniectomy (removal of part of the skull).

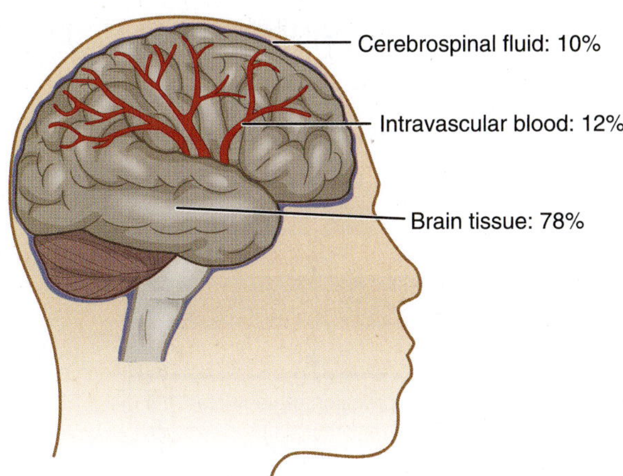

Fig. 61.1 Components of the brain.

Intracranial pressure (ICP) is the hydrostatic force measured in the brain CSF compartment. Normal ICP ranges from 5 to 15 mm Hg.[1] Under normal conditions in which intracranial volume is relatively constant, the balance among the 3 components (brain tissue, blood, CSF) maintains normal ICP. Factors that influence ICP under normal conditions are changes in (1) arterial pressure, (2) venous pressure, (3) intraabdominal and intrathoracic pressure, (4) posture, (5) temperature, and (6) blood gases, especially CO_2 levels. The degree to which these factors increase or decrease ICP depends on the brain's ability to adapt to changes.

In applying the Monro-Kellie doctrine, the body can adapt to volume changes within the skull in 3 different ways to maintain a normal ICP. The first compensatory mechanisms can include changes in CSF volume. CSF volume can be changed by altering CSF absorption or production and by displacing CSF into the spinal subarachnoid space. Second, changes in intracranial blood volume can occur through the collapse of cerebral veins and dural sinuses, regional cerebral vasoconstriction or dilation, and changes in venous outflow. Third, brain tissue volume compensates through distention of the dura or compression of brain tissue.

Initially an increase in volume does not increase ICP because of these compensatory mechanisms. However, there is a limited ability to compensate for changes in volume. As the volume increase continues, ICP rises and decompensation occurs. This results in compression, ischemia, and resulting neurologic compromise.

Cerebral Blood Flow

Cerebral blood flow (CBF) is the amount of blood in milliliters passing through 100 g of brain tissue in 1 minute. CBF is about 50 mL/min/100 g of brain tissue. Maintaining blood flow to the brain is critical because the brain requires a constant supply of O_2 and glucose. The brain uses 20% of the body's O_2 and 25% of its glucose.[2]

The brain regulates its own blood flow in response to its metabolic needs despite wide fluctuations in systemic arterial pressure. *Cerebral autoregulation* is the automatic adjustment in the diameter of the cerebral blood vessels by the brain to maintain a constant blood flow with changes in arterial BP. This ensures a consistent CBF to provide for the metabolic needs of brain tissue and maintain cerebral perfusion pressure (CPP) within normal limits.

TABLE 61.1 Calculating Cerebral Perfusion Pressure

$$CPP = MAP - ICP$$
$$MAP = DBP + 1/3\ (SBP - DBP)$$
OR
$$MAP = \frac{SBP + 2\ (DBP)}{3}$$

Example: Systemic BP = 122/84 mm Hg
MAP = 97 mm Hg
ICP = 12 mm Hg
CPP = 85 mm Hg

The lower limit of systemic arterial pressure at which autoregulation is effective is a mean arterial pressure (MAP) of 70 mm Hg. Below this, CBF decreases, and symptoms of cerebral ischemia, such as syncope and blurred vision, occur. The upper limit of systemic arterial pressure at which autoregulation is effective is a MAP of 150 mm Hg. When this pressure is exceeded, the vessels are maximally constricted and further vasoconstrictor response is lost.

Cerebral perfusion pressure is the pressure needed to ensure blood flow to the brain. CPP is equal to the MAP minus the ICP (CPP = MAP − ICP). See the example in Table 61.1. Normal CPP is 60 to 100 mm Hg. As CPP decreases, autoregulation fails and CBF decreases. A CPP of less than 50 mm Hg is associated with ischemia and neuron death. A CPP of less than 30 mm Hg results in ischemia and, if sustained, is incompatible with life. This is why it is important to maintain MAP when ICP is increased.

Although CPP is clinically used, it does not consider the effect of cerebrovascular resistance. Cerebrovascular resistance is generated by the arterioles within the cranium. It links CPP and blood flow as follows:

$$CPP = Flow \times Resistance$$

When cerebrovascular resistance is high, blood flow to brain tissue is impaired. Normally, autoregulation maintains an adequate CBF and CPP by adjusting the diameter of cerebral blood vessels and metabolic factors that affect ICP.

CPP may not reflect perfusion pressure in all parts of the brain. There may be local areas of swelling and compression that limit perfusion pressure. Thus these patients may need a higher CPP to prevent local tissue damage. For example, patients with an acute stroke may need a higher BP, increasing MAP and CPP, to increase perfusion to the brain and prevent further tissue damage.

Factors Affecting Cerebral Blood Flow

CO_2, O_2, and hydrogen ion concentration affect cerebral blood vessel tone. An increase in the partial pressure of CO_2 in arterial blood ($Paco_2$) relaxes smooth muscle, dilates cerebral vessels, decreases cerebrovascular resistance, and increases CBF. A decrease in $Paco_2$ constricts cerebral vessels, increases cerebrovascular resistance, and decreases CBF.

Cerebral O_2 tension of less than 50 mm Hg results in cerebrovascular dilation. Dilation decreases cerebrovascular resistance, increases CBF, and increases O_2 tension. However, if O_2 tension is not increased, anaerobic metabolism begins, resulting in a buildup of lactic acid. As lactic acid increases and hydrogen ions accumulate, the environment becomes more acidic. Within this acidic environment, further vasodilation occurs in a continued attempt to increase blood flow. The combination of a severely low partial pressure of O_2 in arterial blood (Pao_2) and increased hydrogen ion concentration (acidosis), which are potent cerebral vasodilators, may produce a state in which autoregulation is lost and compensatory mechanisms do not meet tissue metabolic demands.

CBF can be affected by cardiac or respiratory arrest, systemic bleeding, and other pathophysiologic states (e.g., infections, toxicities). Regional CBF can be affected by trauma, tumors, cerebral bleeding, or stroke. When regional or global autoregulation is lost, CBF is no longer maintained at a constant level, but is directly influenced by changes in systemic BP, hypoxia, or catecholamines.

INCREASED INTRACRANIAL PRESSURE

Mechanisms of Increased Intracranial Pressure

IICP is a potentially life-threatening situation that results from an increase in any or all of the 3 components (brain tissue, blood, CSF) within the skull. IICP is clinically significant because it decreases CPP and increases risks for brain ischemia and infarction. It has a poor prognosis. Common causes include a mass (e.g., hematoma, contusion, abscess, tumor) and cerebral edema (e.g., brain tumors, hydrocephalus, head injury, brain inflammation).

Cerebral insults increase the formation and spread of cerebral edema. This may result in hypercapnia, cerebral acidosis, impaired autoregulation, and systemic hypertension. Edema distorts brain tissue, further increasing ICP, and leads to even more tissue hypoxia and acidosis. Fig. 61.2 shows the progression of IICP.

One of the most common causes of IICP is traumatic brain injury. We categorize brain injury in 2 phases: primary and secondary injury. *Primary injury* occurs at the initial time of an injury (e.g., impact of car accident, blunt-force trauma). It results in displacement, bruising, or damage to any cranial component (brain tissue, blood, CSF).

Secondary injury is the resulting hypoxia, ischemia, hypotension, edema, or IICP that follows the primary injury. Secondary injury can occur several hours to days after the initial injury. It is a modifiable concern when managing brain injury. Managing patients with an acute intracranial problem must include managing secondary injury and preventing IICP.

PATHOPHYSIOLOGY MAP

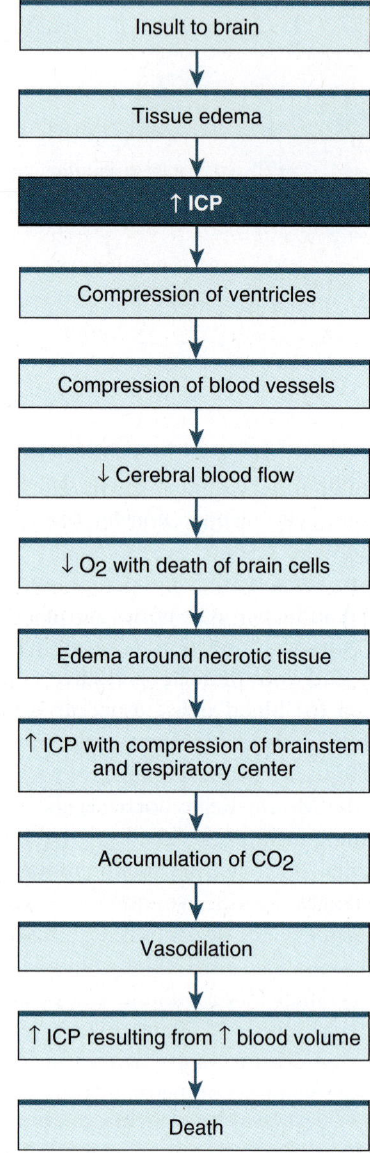

Fig. 61.2 Progression of increased ICP.

We must maintain CBF to preserve tissue and minimize secondary injury. Sustained increases in ICP result in brainstem compression and brain herniation. *Herniation* occurs as the brain tissue is forcibly shifted from a compartment of greater pressure to a compartment of less pressure.

Displacement and herniation of brain tissue can cause a potentially reversible process to become irreversible. Ischemia and edema are further increased, compounding the preexisting problem. Compression of the brainstem and cranial nerves (CNs) may be fatal. Fig. 61.3 shows types of herniation. Central herniation forces the cerebellum and brainstem downward through the foramen magnum. If brainstem compression is not relieved, respiratory arrest will occur from compression of the respiratory control center in the medulla.

In this situation, intense pressure is placed on the brainstem and decreases CBF. If herniation continues, brainstem death is imminent.

Cerebral Edema

There are a variety of causes of **cerebral edema** (increased accumulation of fluid in the extravascular spaces of brain tissue) (Table 61.2). Cerebral edema results in an increase in tissue volume that can increase ICP. The extent and severity of the original insult are factors that determine the degree of cerebral edema. There are 3 types of cerebral edema: vasogenic, cytotoxic, and interstitial. A patient may have more than 1 type.

Vasogenic Cerebral Edema

Vasogenic cerebral edema is the most common type of cerebral edema. It occurs mainly in the white matter and results from disruption of the blood-brain barrier. This allows large molecules (protein, blood products) to enter brain tissue. This exposes brain cells to toxic products from the blood and results in an osmotic gradient that causes fluid to flow from the intravascular to extravascular space. The result is an increase in the extracellular fluid volume. Systemic BP, site of the brain injury, and extent of the blood-brain barrier defect influence the extent of the spread of edema.

Edema may produce a continuum of symptoms. These range from headache to a decrease in consciousness, including coma and focal (specific to a certain area of the brain) neurologic deficits. In cases of cerebral edema, a headache can quickly progress to coma and death. So, you must be vigilant in your assessment.

TABLE 61.2 Causes of Cerebral Edema

Cerebral Infections • Encephalitis • Meningitis	**Lesions** • Brain abscess • Brain tumor (primary, metastatic) • Hematoma (intracerebral, subdural, epidural) • Hemorrhage (intracerebral, cerebellar, brainstem)
Encephalopathies • Hepatic encephalopathy • Lead or arsenic intoxication • Uremia	**Vascular Insult** • Anoxic and ischemic episodes • Cerebral infarction (thrombotic, embolic) • Venous sinus thrombosis
Head Injuries and Brain Surgery • Contusion • Hemorrhage • Posttraumatic brain swelling	

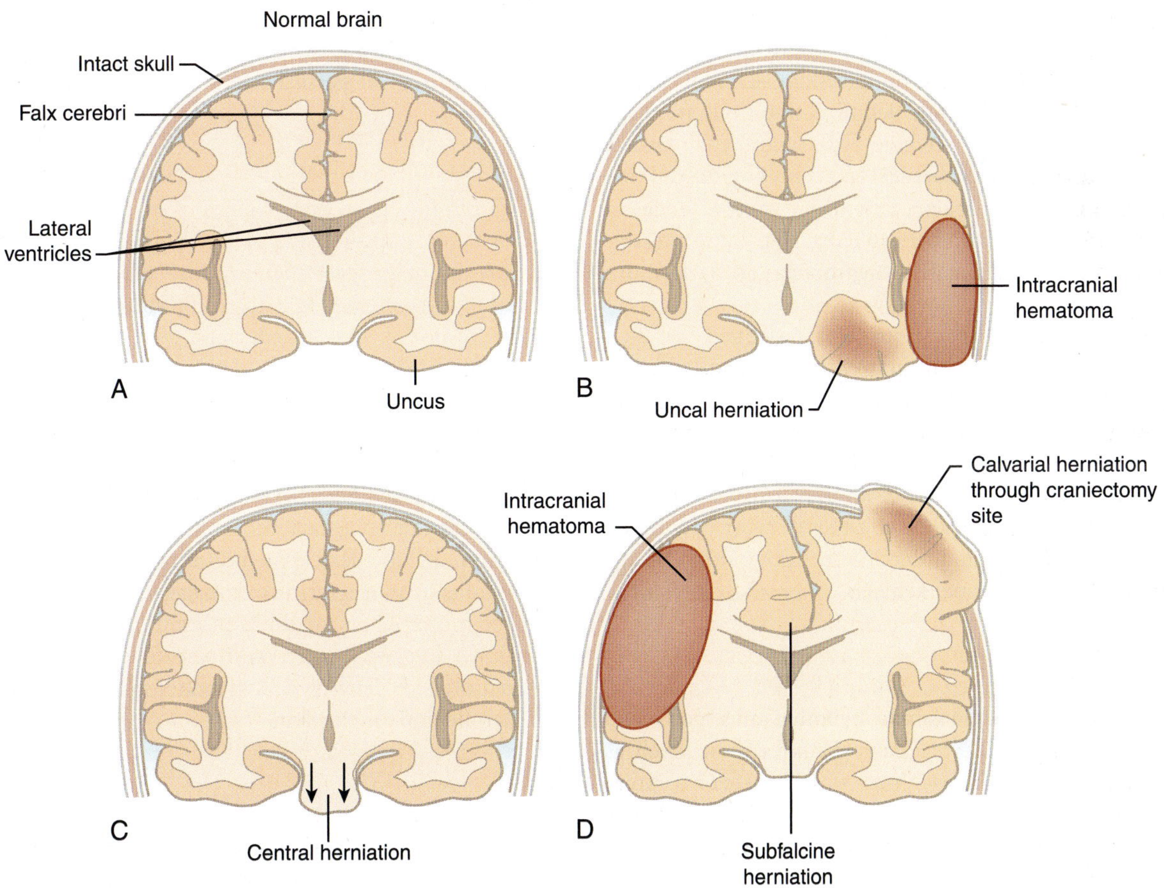

Fig. 61.3 Herniation. (A) Normal relationship of intracranial structures. (B, C, and D) Shifts of intracranial structures.

Cytotoxic Cerebral Edema

Cytotoxic cerebral edema results from disruption of the integrity of the cell membranes. It develops from destructive lesions or trauma to brain tissue, resulting in cerebral hypoxia or anoxia and syndrome of inappropriate antidiuresis (SIAD). In this type of edema, the blood-brain barrier stays intact. Cerebral edema occurs from fluid and protein shifts from the extracellular space directly into the cells, with subsequent swelling and loss of cell function.

Interstitial Cerebral Edema

Interstitial cerebral edema is usually a result of hydrocephalus. *Hydrocephalus* is a buildup of fluid in the brain. It is manifested by ventricular enlargement. It can be due to excess CSF production, obstructed CSF flow, or an inability to reabsorb the CSF.

Clinical Manifestations

The manifestations of IICP can take many forms, depending on the cause, location, and rate of increase in ICP. Any patient who becomes unconscious acutely, regardless of the cause, should be suspected of having IICP.

Change in Level of Consciousness

Level of consciousness (LOC) is the most sensitive and reliable indicator of neurologic status. Changes in LOC are a result of impaired CBF, which causes O_2 deprivation to the cells of the cerebral cortex and reticular activating system (RAS). The RAS is found in the brainstem, with neural connections to many parts of the nervous system. An intact RAS can maintain a state of wakefulness even in the absence of a functioning cerebral cortex. Interruptions of impulses from the RAS or changes in functioning of the cerebral hemispheres can cause **unconsciousness,** an abnormal state of complete or partial unawareness of self or environment.

The patient's state of consciousness is defined by their clinical responses and pattern of brain activity (recorded by an electroencephalogram [EEG]). A change in consciousness may be dramatic (as in coma) or subtle (e.g., flattening of affect, change in orientation). In the deepest state of unconsciousness, patients do not respond to painful stimuli. Corneal and pupillary reflexes are absent. They cannot swallow or cough and are incontinent of urine and feces. The EEG pattern shows suppressed or absent neuronal activity.

Changes in Vital Signs

Increasing pressure on the thalamus, hypothalamus, pons, and medulla causes changes in vital signs. Manifestations such as *Cushing triad* (systolic hypertension with a widening pulse pressure, bradycardia with a full and bounding pulse, irregular respirations) may be present. However, they often do not appear until ICP has been increased for some time or is suddenly and markedly increased (e.g., head trauma). Cushing triad is a medical emergency. It is a sign of brainstem compression and impending death. A change in body temperature may occur because IICP affects the hypothalamus.

> **CHECK YOUR PRACTICE**
>
> You are monitoring vital signs of an 82-year-old female who has a head injury. She fell while walking on the sidewalk, hitting her head on a fire hydrant. She was confused on admission with stable vital signs: BP 150/86, pulse 84, respirations 14/min; 2 h after admission, her vital signs are BP 166/74, pulse 54, respirations 10 to 16/min.
>
> - What is your interpretation of her vital signs?

Ocular Signs

Compression of CN III, the oculomotor nerve, results in pupil dilation on the same side *(ipsilateral)* as the mass lesion. There may be sluggish or no pupil response to light, inability to move the eye upward and adduct, and ptosis of the eyelid. These signs result from the brain shifting from midline, compressing the trunk of CN III, and paralyzing the muscles controlling pupillary size and shape. In this situation, a fixed, unilateral, dilated pupil is a neurologic emergency that indicates brain herniation.

Other CNs may be affected, including the optic (CN II), trochlear (CN IV), and abducens (CN VI) nerves. Signs of problems with these CNs include blurred vision, diplopia, and changes in extraocular eye movements. *Central herniation* may initially manifest as sluggish but equal pupil response. *Uncal herniation* may cause a dilated unilateral pupil. *Papilledema* (an edematous optic disc seen on retinal examination) is a nonspecific sign of persistent increases in ICP.

Decrease in Motor Function

As ICP continues to rise, we see changes in motor ability. A *contralateral* (opposite side of the mass lesion) hemiparesis or hemiplegia may develop depending on the location of the source of the increased ICP. If painful stimuli are used to elicit a motor response, the patient may localize to the stimuli or withdraw from them.

Noxious stimuli may elicit *decorticate* (flexor) or *decerebrate* (extensor) posturing (Fig. 61.4). Decorticate posture consists of internal rotation and adduction of the arms with flexion of the elbows, wrists, and fingers. It is a result of interruption of voluntary motor tracts in the cerebral cortex. Extension of the legs may be seen. A decerebrate posture may indicate more serious damage. It results from disruption of motor fibers in the midbrain and brainstem. In this position, the arms are stiffly extended, adducted, and hyperpronated. There is hyperextension of the legs with plantar flexion of the feet.

Headache

Although the brain itself is insensitive to pain, compression of other intracranial structures, such as arteries, veins, and CNs, can cause a headache. A nocturnal headache and/or a headache

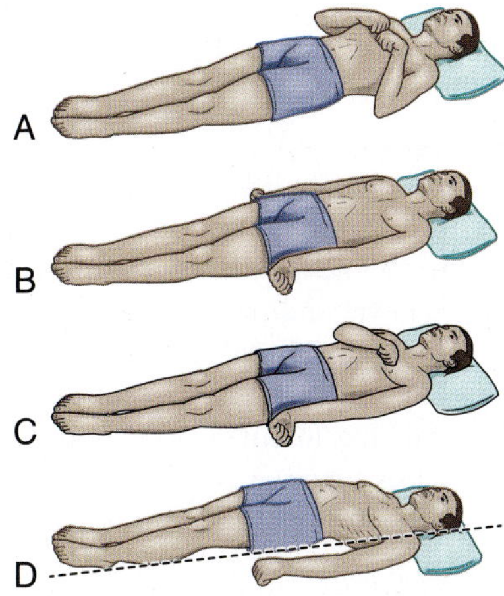

Fig. 61.4 Decorticate and decerebrate posturing. (A) Decorticate response. Flexion of arms, wrists, and fingers with adduction in upper extremities. Extension, internal rotation, and plantar flexion in lower extremities. (B) Decerebrate response. All 4 extremities in rigid extension, with hyperpronation of forearms and plantar flexion of feet. (C) Decorticate response on right side of body and decerebrate response on left side of body. (D) Opisthotonic posturing.

TABLE 61.3 Interprofessional Care

Increased Intracranial Pressure

Diagnostic Assessment

- History and physical assessment
- Vital signs, neurologic assessments, ICP measurements
- Skull, chest, and spinal x-ray studies
- CT scan, MRI, cerebral angiography, EEG, PET
- Transcranial Doppler studies
- Infrascanner
- ECG
- Evoked potential studies
- Lumbar puncture (not done if there is a risk for herniation)
- Laboratory studies, including CBC, coagulation profile, electrolytes, serum creatinine, ABGs, ammonia level, drug and toxicology screen
- CSF analysis (protein, WBC, glucose)

Management

- Mechanical ventilation
- ICP monitoring
- Cerebral oxygenation monitoring ($PbtO_2$, $SjvO_2$)
- Maintain fluid balance
- Maintain systolic BP between 100 and 160 mm Hg
- Maintain cerebral perfusion pressure (CPP) >60 mm Hg
- Reduction of cerebral metabolism (e.g., high-dose barbiturates)

Drug Therapy

- Osmotic diuretic (mannitol)
- Hypertonic saline
- Antiseizure drugs (e.g., phenytoin)
- Corticosteroids for brain tumors, bacterial meningitis
- Proton pump inhibitor (e.g., pantoprazole) to prevent GI ulcers

in the morning is cause for concern. It may indicate a tumor or other space-occupying lesion that is causing IICP. Straining, agitation, or movement may worsen the pain.

Vomiting

Vomiting not preceded by nausea is called *unexpected vomiting.* It is often a nonspecific sign of increasing ICP that is related to pressure changes within the skull. Projectile vomiting may occur.

Complications

The major complications of uncontrolled IICP are inadequate cerebral perfusion and cerebral herniation (Fig. 61.3). To help you understand cerebral herniation, we are going to describe 2 important structures in the brain. The *falx cerebri* is a thin wall of dura that folds down between the cortex, separating the 2 cerebral hemispheres. The *tentorium cerebelli* is a rigid fold of dura that separates the cerebral hemispheres from the cerebellum (Fig. 61.3). It is called the *tentorium* (meaning tent) because it forms a tentlike cover over the cerebellum.

Tentorial herniation (central herniation) occurs when a mass lesion in the cerebrum forces the brain to herniate downward through the opening created by the brainstem (the foramen magnum). Uncal herniation occurs when there is lateral and downward herniation. Cingulate herniation occurs when there is lateral displacement of brain tissue beneath the falx cerebri.

Diagnostic Studies

Diagnostic studies can be used to identify the cause of IICP (Table 61.3). CT and MRI can discover many conditions and assess the effect of treatment.

Other tests include EEG, cerebral angiography, ICP monitoring, brain tissue oxygenation measurement, positron emission tomography (PET), transcranial Doppler studies, and evoked potential studies. In general, a lumbar puncture (LP) is contraindicated when we suspect increased ICP. The reason is that cerebral herniation could occur from the sudden release of the pressure in the skull from the area above the LP.

In some agencies, a handheld near-infrared scanner (Infrascanner) is used to detect life-threatening intracranial bleeding. The scanner directs a wavelength of light that can penetrate tissue and bone. Blood from intracranial hematomas absorbs the light differently from other areas of the brain. Transcranial Doppler can monitor changes in cerebrovascular resistance.

Monitoring ICP and Cerebral Oxygenation

Indications for ICP Monitoring

ICP monitoring is used to guide care when patients are at risk for or have IICP. It may be used in patients with a variety of neurologic problems, including stroke, hemorrhage, tumor, infection, or traumatic brain injury (TBI). ICP should be monitored in patients admitted with a *Glasgow Coma Scale* (GCS) score of 8 or less and an abnormal CT scan or MRI. These results could show bleeding, contusion, edema, or other problems, putting them at risk for IICP.

Methods of Measuring ICP

Patients with conditions known to increase ICP, except those with irreversible problems or advanced neurologic disease, usually undergo ICP monitoring in an intensive care unit (ICU). Multiple methods and devices are available to monitor ICP (Fig. 61.5).

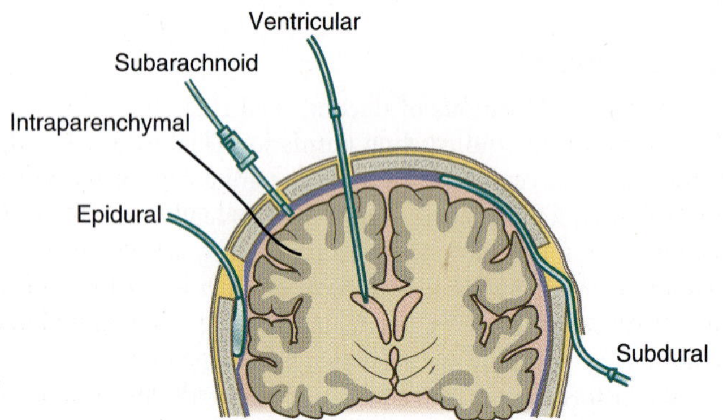

Fig. 61.5 Coronal section of brain showing potential sites for placement of ICP monitoring devices.

The gold standard for monitoring ICP is the *ventriculostomy,* in which a special catheter is inserted into the lateral ventricle and coupled to an external transducer (Figs. 61.6 and 61.7). This technique directly measures the pressure within the ventricles, facilitates removal and/or sampling of CSF, and allows for intraventricular drug administration. The transducer is external. We must ensure that the transducer is at the right height and level with the foramen of Monro (Fig. 61.8A). A reference point for this foramen is the tragus of the ear. Every time a patient is repositioned, assess the system to ensure it is level.

The *fiberoptic catheter,* an alternative technology, uses a sensor transducer found within the catheter tip. The sensor tip is placed within the ventricle or the brain tissue and gives a direct measurement of brain pressure. *Air pouch/pneumatic technology* uses an air-filled pouch to measure ICP. Pressure changes within the skull are transmitted through the changes exerted on this pouch to the monitor.

ICP is represented on the monitor as a mean pressure in millimeters of mercury (mm Hg). If a CSF drainage device is in

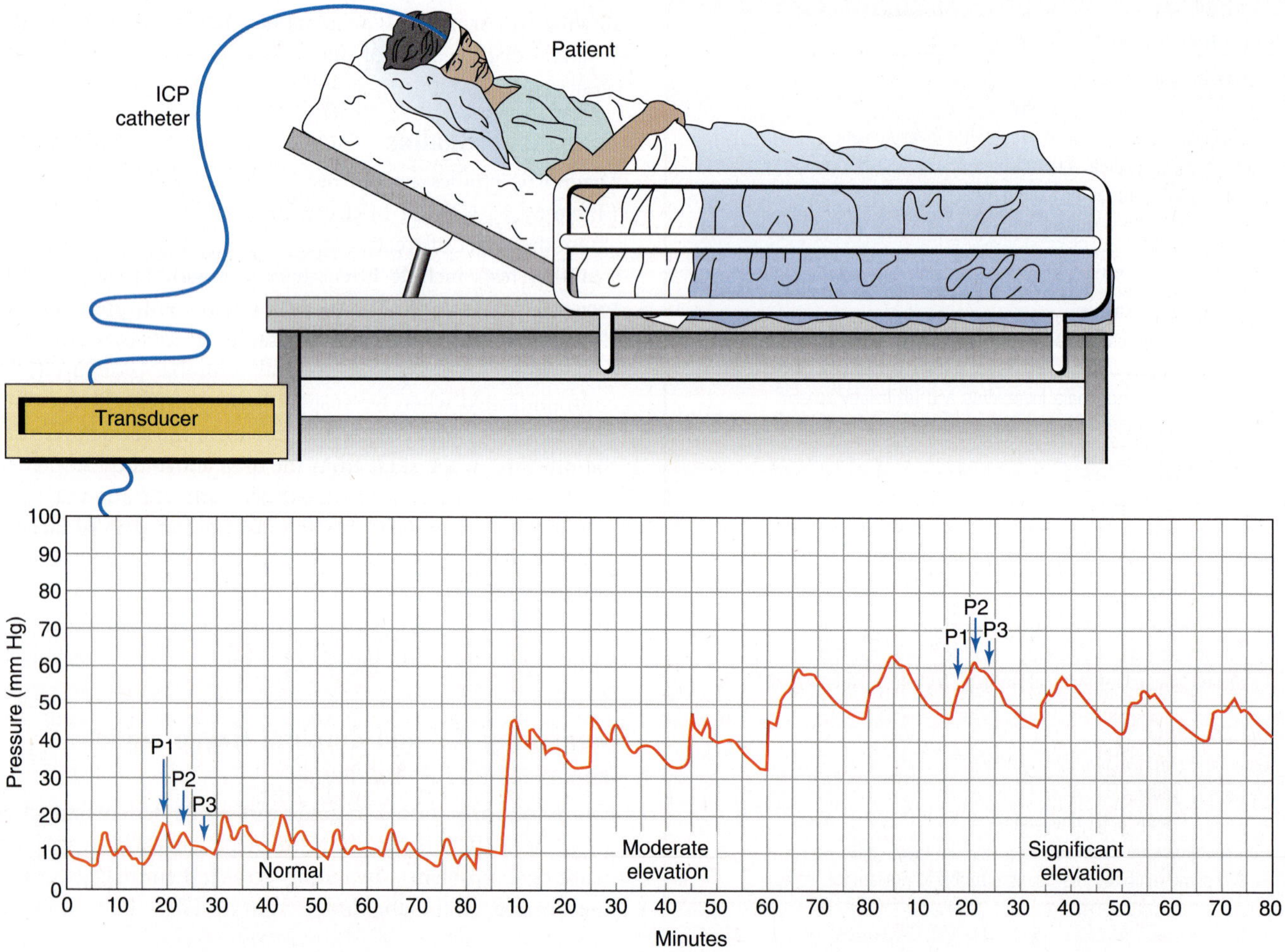

Fig. 61.6 ICP monitoring can continuously measure ICP. The ICP tracing shows normal, elevated, and plateau waves. At high ICP, the P2 peak is higher than the P1 peak, and the peaks become less distinct and plateau. (From Copstead-Kirkhorn LC, Banasik JL: *Pathophysiology,* ed 6, St Louis, 2019, Mosby.)

place, the drain must be closed for at least 6 minutes to ensure an accurate reading. Record the waveform strip along with other pressure monitoring waveforms. The normal ICP waveform has 3 phases (Fig. 61.6 and Table 61.4). It is important to monitor the ICP waveform and the mean CPP. When ICP is normal, P1, P2, and P3 resemble a staircase. As ICP increases, P2 rises above P1. This indicates poor ventricular compliance (Fig. 61.6). Consider the rate at which changes occur and the patient's condition. Neurologic deterioration may not occur until the ICP increase is pronounced and sustained. Immediately report to the HCP any increase in ICP or abnormal waveforms.

Causes of inaccurate ICP readings include CSF leaks around the monitoring device, obstruction of the intraventricular catheter (from tissue or blood clot), a difference between the height of the catheter and the transducer, kinks in the tubing, and incorrect height of the drainage system relative to the reference point. Bubbles or air in the tubing can dampen the waveform.

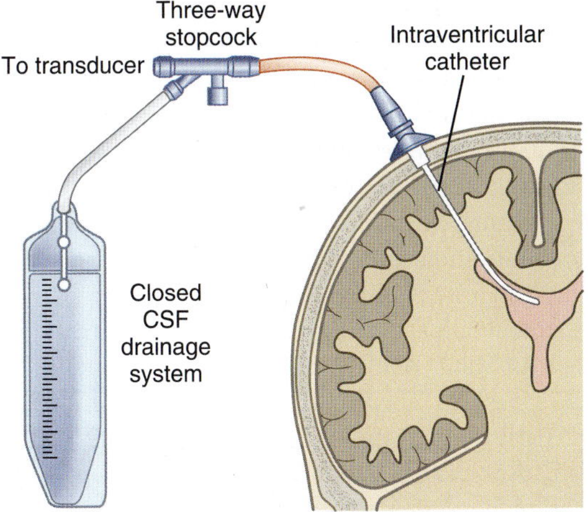

Fig. 61.7 Ventriculostomy in place. Cerebrospinal fluid *(CSF)* can be drained via a ventriculostomy when ICP exceeds the upper pressure parameter set by the HCP. Intermittent drainage involves opening the 3-way stopcock to allow CSF to flow into the drainage bag for brief periods (30 to 120 seconds) until the pressure is less than the upper pressure parameters.

Infection is a serious complication with ICP monitoring. Factors that contribute to infection include ICP monitoring for more than 5 days, use of a ventriculostomy, a CSF leak, and a concurrent systemic infection. Assess the insertion site and use aseptic technique. Monitor the CSF for a change in drainage color or clarity.

Cerebrospinal Fluid Drainage

With a ventricular catheter, it is possible to control ICP by removing CSF (Fig. 61.7). Draining CSF relieves pressure inside the skull (Fig. 61.8B). There are no universal guidelines for CSF removal. Guidelines are typically based on agency or HCP preference.[3] The HCP typically orders a specific level at which to start drainage (e.g., if ICP is greater than 20 mm Hg) and the frequency of drainage (intermittent or continuous).

The 2 options for CSF drainage are intermittent or continuous. With intermittent drainage, you open the system at the

TABLE 61.4 Normal Intracranial Pressure Waveforms

Waveform (Fig. 61.6)	Meaning
P1 Percussion wave	Represents arterial pulsations Normally the highest of the 3 waveforms
P2 Rebound wave or tidal wave	Reflects intracranial compliance or relative brain volume When P2 is higher than P1, intracranial compliance is compromised
P3 Dicrotic wave	Follows dicrotic notch Represents venous pulsations Normally the lowest waveform

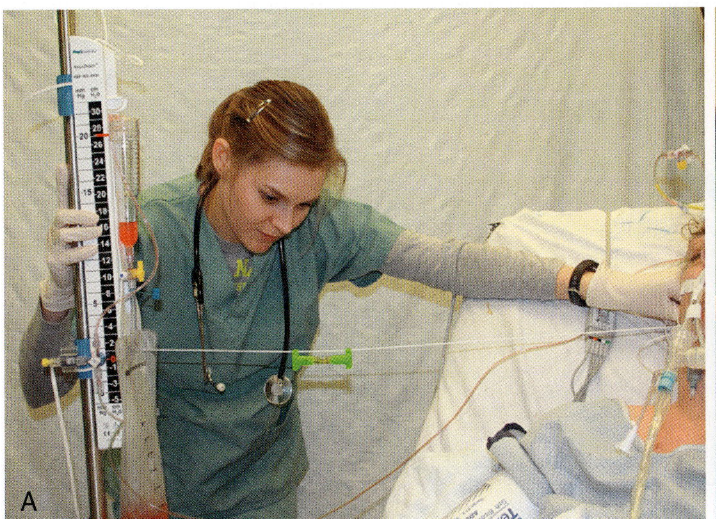

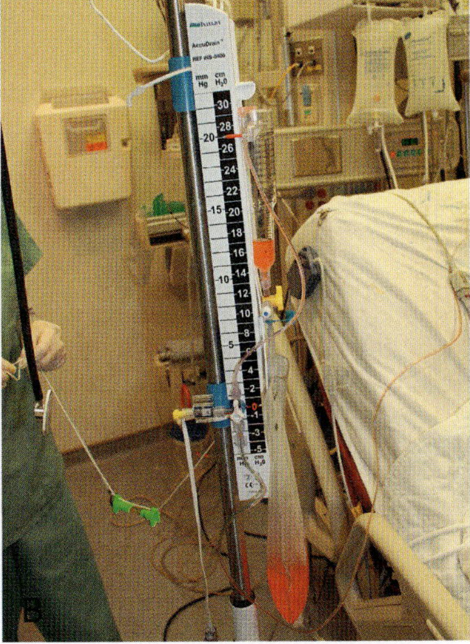

Fig. 61.8 (A) Leveling a ventriculostomy. (B) Cerebrospinal fluid is drained into a drainage system. (Courtesy Meg Zomorodi, RN, PhD, CNL, Raleigh, NC.)

indicated ICP and allow CSF to drain for 2 to 3 minutes. Then close the stopcock to return the ventriculostomy to a closed system. With continuous ICP drainage, carefully monitor the amount of CSF drained. Normal CSF production is about 20 to 30 mL/h. There is a total CSF volume of about 150 mL. Implement measures to prevent the removal of too much CSF, which can cause serious complications. Close the system when repositioning or transporting patients. Post a sign above the bed to notify anyone who turns, moves, or suctions the patient.

Complications include ventricular collapse, infection, and herniation or subdural hematoma formation from rapid decompression. Use strict aseptic technique during dressing changes or sampling of CSF to prevent infection. Keep the system intact to ensure that the ICP readings are accurate because treatment is based on the pressures.

Cerebral Oxygenation Monitoring

Technology is available to measure cerebral oxygenation and assess perfusion. Three intracranial devices used in ICU settings are the Licox catheter, Neurovent catheter, and jugular venous bulb catheter.

The Licox and Neurovent catheters are placed in healthy white matter (Fig. 61.9). They provide continuous monitoring of the O_2 pressure in brain tissue ($PbtO_2$). Normal $PbtO_2$ is 20 to 40 mm Hg. A low $PbtO_2$ level indicates ischemia or regional tissue hypoxia.[4] These catheters can also measure brain temperature. A cooler brain temperature (96.8°F [36°C]) may produce better outcomes.

Jugular venous bulb oximetry measures jugular venous O_2 saturation ($SjvO_2$), which indicates total venous brain tissue extraction of O_2. This is a measure of cerebral O_2 supply and demand. The normal $SjvO_2$ range is 60% to 75%. Values less than 50% indicate impaired cerebral oxygenation.

Interprofessional Care

The goals of interprofessional care (Table 61.3) are to (1) identify and treat the cause of IICP and (2) support brain function. The earlier IICP is recognized and treated, the better the outcome.

For patients with IICP, it is important to maintain adequate oxygenation to support brain function and prevent secondary injury. Patients may need mechanical ventilation to ensure adequate oxygenation. Arterial blood gas (ABG) analysis guides the O_2 therapy. The goal is to maintain the Pao_2 at 100 mm Hg or greater and to keep $Paco_2$ in normal range at 35 to 45 mm Hg.

If IICP is caused by a mass (e.g., tumor, hematoma), surgical removal of the mass is the best treatment. In aggressive situations, a craniectomy (removal of part of the skull) may be done to reduce ICP and prevent herniation.

Drug Therapy

Drug therapy plays an important part in managing IICP. Mannitol (Osmitrol) (25%) is an osmotic diuretic given IV. Its immediate plasma-expanding effect reduces the hematocrit and blood viscosity. This increases CBF and cerebral O_2 delivery. Mannitol creates a vascular osmotic gradient. The decrease in the total brain fluid content causes fluid to move from the tissues into the blood vessels, reducing ICP. Monitor fluid and electrolyte status when osmotic diuretics are used. Mannitol may be contraindicated with renal disease and increased osmolality.

Hypertonic saline solution is another option. It produces movement of water out of edematous swollen brain cells and into blood vessels. This movement can reduce swelling and improve CBF. During an infusion, monitor BP and sodium levels because intravascular fluid volume excess can occur. Hypertonic saline infusion is just as effective as mannitol when treating IICP. They are often used concurrently when caring for patients with a severe brain injury.

Corticosteroids (e.g., dexamethasone) are used to treat vasogenic edema around tumors and abscesses. These drugs are not recommended for TBI. Corticosteroids stabilize the cell membrane and inhibit prostaglandin synthesis (see Fig. 12.2), preventing the formation of proinflammatory mediators.

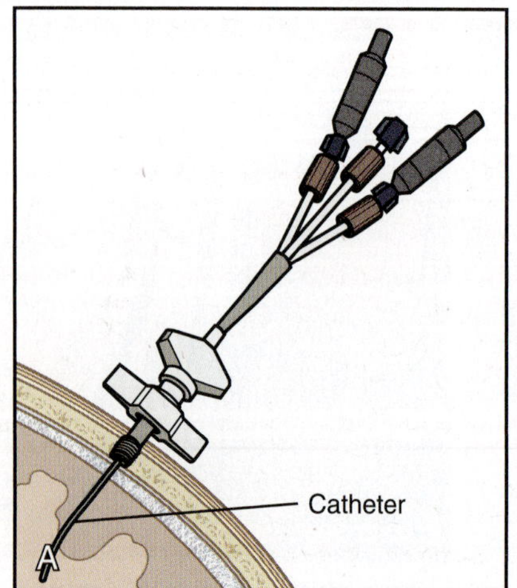

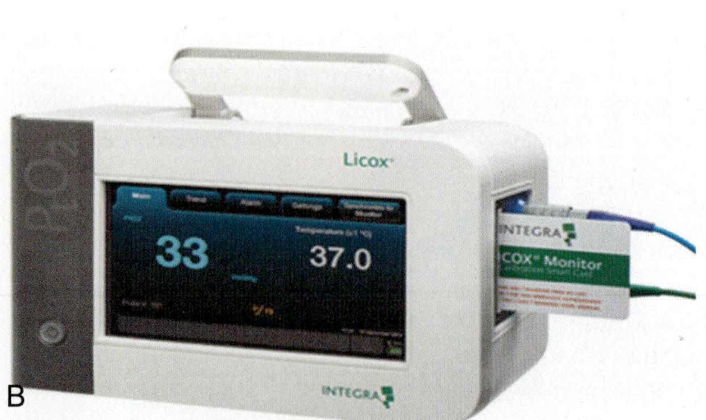

Fig. 61.9 (A) The Licox brain tissue O_2 system involves insertion of a catheter. (B) The system measures O_2 in the brain ($PbtO_2$), brain tissue temperature, and ICP. (B, Courtesy Integra LifeSciences Corporation, Plainsboro, NJ.)

Corticosteroids also improve neuronal function by improving CBF and restoring autoregulation.

Complications of corticosteroids include hyperglycemia, infections, and gastrointestinal (GI) bleeding. Monitor fluid intake, electrolyte, and glucose levels. Perform glucose monitoring at least every 6 hours. Patients receiving corticosteroids should receive a histamine (H_2)-receptor blocker or proton pump inhibitor (e.g., pantoprazole) to prevent GI ulcers and bleeding.

IV 0.9% sodium chloride is the preferred solution for giving secondary medications. If 5% dextrose in water or 0.45% sodium chloride is used, serum osmolality decreases and an increase in cerebral edema may occur.

Drug therapy to reduce cerebral metabolism may be an effective way to control ICP. Reducing the metabolic rate decreases CBF and therefore ICP. High doses of barbiturates (e.g., pentobarbital, thiopental) are used in patients with IICP refractory to other treatments. Barbiturates decrease cerebral metabolism, decreasing ICP and cerebral edema. With this treatment, monitor ICP, blood flow, and EEG. Barbiturate dosing is typically based on analysis of the bedside EEG tracing and the ICP. The HCP orders the barbiturate infusion at a rate that achieves a desired level of brain wave suppression to control ICP. *Total burst suppression,* recognized by the absence of spikes showing brain activity on the EEG monitor, shows that maximal therapeutic effect has been achieved.

Nutrition Therapy

Because malnutrition promotes continued cerebral edema, maintaining optimal nutrition is important. Patients with IICP are in a hypermetabolic and hypercatabolic state that increases the need for glucose as fuel for metabolism of the injured brain. If a patient cannot maintain an adequate oral intake, we should start other means of meeting nutrition needs, such as enteral feedings or parenteral nutrition.

Early feeding after brain injury may improve patient outcome. Nutrition replacement should meet caloric needs by at least day 5 after injury.[3] Fluid and electrolyte status and metabolic needs should guide feedings or supplements. We often keep patients euvolemic. Continuously evaluate clinical factors such as urine output, electrolytes, and serum and urine osmolality.

NURSING MANAGEMENT: INCREASED INTRACRANIAL PRESSURE

Assessment

You can obtain subjective data from patients or from caregivers or family members who are familiar with them. Assess LOC and body functions. Describe LOC by noting the specific behaviors seen. Record vital signs, including BP, pulse, respiratory rate, and temperature. Be aware of Cushing triad, which indicates severe IICP. Note the respiratory pattern. Specific respiratory patterns are associated with severe IICP (Fig. 61.10).

Glasgow Coma Scale

The Glasgow Coma Scale (GCS) is a quick, practical, and standard system for assessing LOC. The 3 areas assessed in the GCS are patients' ability to (1) open the eyes when a verbal or painful stimulus is applied, (2) speak, and (3) obey commands. Specific assessments evaluate the response to varying degrees of stimulus. Three indicators of response are evaluated: (1) opening of the eyes, (2) best verbal response, and (3) best motor response (Table 61.5).

Specific behaviors observed as responses to the testing stimulus are given a numeric value. Your responsibility is to elicit the best response on each of the scales. The subscale scores are especially important if patients are untestable in an area. For example, severe periorbital edema may make eye opening impossible.

The total GCS score is the sum of the numeric values assigned to each of the 3 areas. The higher the scores, the higher the level of brain functioning. The highest GCS score is 15 for a fully alert person. The lowest possible score is 3. A GCS score of 8 or less generally indicates coma. Plot GCS scores on a graph. Use the data to determine whether a patient is stable, improving, or deteriorating.

The GCS offers several advantages in the assessment of unconscious patients. It allows different health care professionals to arrive at the same conclusion about a patient's status. It can be used to distinguish between different or changing states.

We sometimes use other scales, such as the *Full Outline of Unresponsiveness (FOUR) scale.*[4] In cases of stroke or hemorrhage with IICP, use the National Institutes of Health (NIH)

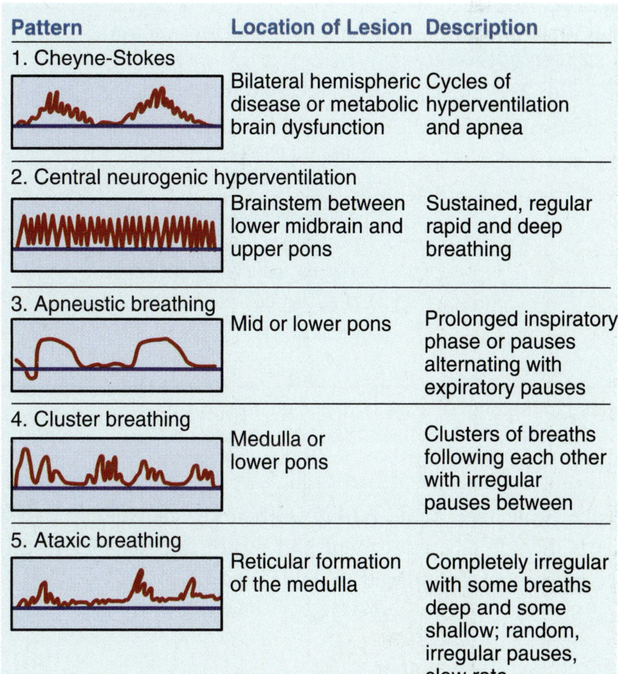

Fig. 61.10 Common abnormal respiratory patterns associated with coma.

TABLE 61.5 Glasgow Coma Scale

Appropriate Stimulus	Response	Score
Eyes Open		
• Approach to bedside • Verbal command • Pain	Spontaneous response	4
	Opening of eyes to name or command	3
	Lack of opening of eyes to previous stimuli but opening to pain	2
	Lack of opening of eyes to any stimulus	1
	Untestable[a]	U
Best Verbal Response		
• Verbal questioning with maximum arousal	Appropriate orientation, conversant. Correct identification of self, place, year, and month	5
	Confusion. Conversant, but disorientation in 1 or more spheres	4
	Inappropriate or disorganized use of words (e.g., cursing), lack of sustained conversation	3
	Incomprehensible words, sounds (e.g., moaning)	2
	Lack of sound, even with painful stimuli	1
	Untestable[a]	U
Best Motor Response		
• Verbal command (e.g., "raise your arm, hold up 2 fingers") • Pain (pressure on proximal nail bed)	Obeys commands	6
	Localize pain, lack of obedience but attempts to remove offending stimulus	5
	Flexion withdrawal,[a] flexion of arm in response to pain without abnormal flexion posture	4
	Abnormal flexion, flexing of arm at elbow and pronation, making a fist	3
	Abnormal extension, extension of arm at elbow, usually with adduction and internal rotation of arm at shoulder	2
	Lack of response	1
	Untestable[a]	U

[a]Added to the original scale by some centers.

Stroke Scale (see Table 62.12). Other key neurologic assessments include CN assessment and motor and sensory testing. CN assessment is outlined in Table 60.4.

Neurologic Assessment

Compare the pupils for size, shape, movement, and reactivity (Fig. 61.11). If the oculomotor nerve (CN III) is compressed,

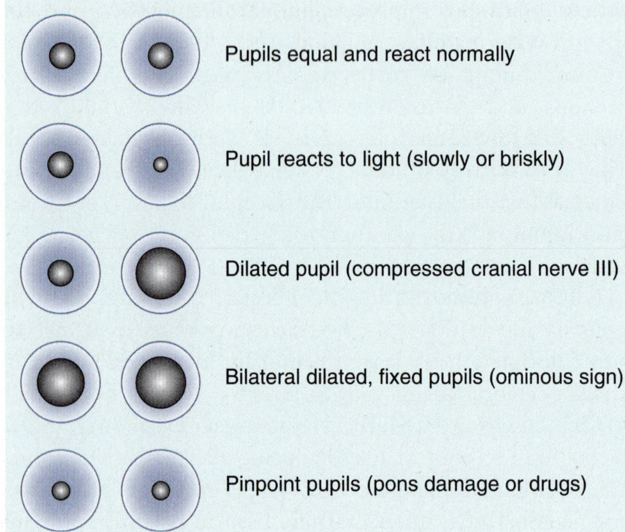

Fig. 61.11 Pupillary check for size and response.

the pupil on the affected side *(ipsilateral)* becomes larger until it fully dilates. If ICP continues to increase, both pupils dilate.

Test pupillary reaction with a penlight. The normal reaction is brisk constriction when the light is shone directly into the eye. Note a consensual response (slight constriction in the opposite pupil) at the same time. A sluggish reaction can indicate early pressure on CN III. A fixed pupil unresponsive to light stimulus usually indicates IICP. However, there are other causes of a fixed pupil. These include direct injury to CN III, previous eye surgery, atropine administration, and mydriatic eye drops.

In some agencies, we are using a handheld device *(pupillometer)* to measure the pupil reactivity and size. The device removes any subjectivity from the pupil evaluation.

Assess eye movements controlled by CN III, CN IV, and CN VI in patients who are awake and able to follow commands. This can assess brainstem function. Testing the corneal reflex gives information about CN V and CN VII. If this reflex is absent, start routine eye care to prevent corneal abrasion (see Chapter 22).

We can assess uncooperative or unconscious patients by testing the oculocephalic and oculovestibular reflexes. Both tests are done in the evaluation of brain death.

To test the oculocephalic reflex (doll's eye), turn the patient's head briskly to the left or right while holding the eyelids open. A normal response is movement of the eyes across the midline in the direction opposite that of the turning. Next, quickly flex and then extend the neck. Eye movement should be opposite to the direction of head movement—up when the neck is flexed and down when it is extended. Abnormal responses can help locate an intracranial lesion.

To test the oculovestibular reflex (cold caloric), position the patient with the head of the bed elevated. Instill a syringe of ice-cold water into the external auditory ear canal. Then, assess the eyes for a total of 1 minute. The absence of eye movement or response indicates severe neurologic demise. This test requires patent external auditory ear canals and tympanic membranes.

◆ Clinical Problems

Clinical problems for patients with IICP include:

- Increased intracranial pressure
- Inadequate tissue perfusion
- Risk for injury

Additional information on clinical problems and interventions for patients with IICP is presented in eNursing Care Plan 61.1 (available on the website for this chapter).

◆ Planning

The overall goals for patients with IICP are to (1) maintain a patent airway; (2) have ICP within normal limits; (3) have normal fluid, electrolyte, and nutrition balance; and (4) prevent complications from immobility and decreased LOC.

◆ Implementation

Nursing management of patients with IICP is outlined in Table 61.6.

Respiratory Function

Maintaining a patent airway is critical. It is a major nursing responsibility. As the LOC decreases, there is an increased risk for airway obstruction from the tongue dropping back and occluding the airway or from accumulation of secretions. An oral airway facilitates breathing and provides an easier suctioning route in comatose patients. In general, any patient with a GCS of 8 or less or an altered LOC who is unable to maintain a patent airway or effective ventilation needs intubation and mechanical ventilation.

! SAFETY ALERT

Altered Breathing

- Be alert to altered breathing in patients with IICP.
- Snoring sounds indicate obstruction and require immediate intervention.

TABLE 61.6 NURSING MANAGEMENT

Care of Patients With IICP

- Monitor patients diligently:
  - Vital signs and neurologic assessment
  - Electrolytes, especially glucose, sodium, potassium, magnesium, osmolality
  - Calculate cerebral perfusion pressure (CPP) and maintain >60 mm Hg
  - Amount, rate, and characteristics of cerebrospinal fluid (CSF) drainage
  - Cerebral oxygenation monitoring ($PbtO_2$, $SjvO_2$)
  - Intake and output with daily weight
- Maintain systolic BP between 100 and 160 mm Hg
- Analyze ICP waveforms and maintain ICP monitoring systems
- Provide appropriate ventilatory support, including mechanical ventilation
  - Only suction patients as needed; limit suctioning passes to less than 10 sec
  - Evaluate arterial blood gas (ABG) values
  - Evaluate tissue O_2 delivery (e.g., Sao_2, cardiac output), if used
- Give prescribed IV fluids, diuretics, corticosteroids, and antiseizure drugs
- Maintain systolic BP between 100 and 160 mm Hg, and administer prescribed inotropic or vasoconstrictive agents
- Maintain nasogastric (NG) tube suctioning
- Provide ordered sedation and analgesia and implement measures to control pain
- Keep a quiet, calm environment with minimal noise and interruption
  - Coordinate with team members to minimize procedures that may cause agitation
  - Monitor ICP and neurologic response to activity
  - Allow ICP to return to baseline between activities
- Elevate head of bed to 30 degrees with head in a neutral position
- Provide measures to minimize complications of immobility, including atelectasis, VTE, and contractures
- Implement seizure and fall risk precautions
- Maintain normothermia and implement measures to manage any fever
- Assist with needs related to nutrition, elimination, hydration, and personal hygiene

Frequently monitor and evaluate ABG values. Take measures to maintain levels within prescribed or acceptable parameters. Ventilatory support can be ordered based on Pao_2 and $Paco_2$ values.

Prevent hypoxia and hypercapnia to minimize secondary injury. Suctioning and coughing cause transient decreases in Pao_2 and increase ICP. Keep suctioning to a minimum and less than 10 seconds in duration. Give 100% O_2 before and after to prevent decreases in the Pao_2. To avoid cumulative increases in the ICP with suctioning, limit suctioning to 2 passes per suction procedure, if possible. Patients with IICP are at risk for lower CPP during suctioning.

Try to prevent abdominal distention, because it can interfere with respiratory function. Inserting a nasogastric (NG) tube to aspirate the stomach contents can prevent distention, vomiting, and aspiration. In patients with facial and skull fractures, an NG tube is contraindicated because of the risk for inadvertent intracranial placement. Oral insertion of a gastric tube is preferred.

Sedation

Pain, anxiety, and fear related to the primary injury, therapeutic procedures, or noxious stimuli can increase ICP and BP. The appropriate choice or combination of sedatives, paralytics, and analgesics for symptom management is a challenge. Giving these agents may alter the neurologic state, thus masking true neurologic changes. We may need to temporarily stop drug therapy to assess neurologic status. The choice, dose, and combination of agents may vary depending on the history, neurologic state, and clinical presentation.

Opioids, such as morphine sulfate and fentanyl, are rapid-onset analgesics with minimal effect on CBF or O_2

metabolism. The IV sedative propofol (Diprivan) is used to manage anxiety and agitation in the ICU because of its rapid onset and short half-life. We can do an accurate neurologic assessment soon after stopping an infusion of propofol.

Dexmedetomidine (Precedex), an α_2-adrenergic agonist, is used for continuous IV sedation of mechanically ventilated patients in the ICU setting for up to 24 hours. When using continuous IV sedatives, be aware of the side effects of these drugs, especially hypotension. Hypotension can lower CPP.

Nondepolarizing neuromuscular blocking agents (e.g., vecuronium) are useful for achieving complete ventilatory control in the treatment of refractory intracranial hypertension. Because these agents paralyze muscles without blocking pain or noxious stimuli, they must be used in combination with sedatives, analgesics, or benzodiazepines. Ensure patients are adequately sedated before giving a paralytic agent.

Benzodiazepines, although useful for sedation, are usually avoided when managing IICP because of the hypotensive effect and long half-life. If used, they are usually given as an adjunct to neuromuscular blocking agents.

Keep a quiet, calm environment with minimal noise and interruptions. Use a calm, reassuring approach. Touch and talk to the patient, even one who is in a coma. Observe for signs of agitation, irritation, or frustration. Teach the caregiver and family about decreasing stimulation. Coordinate with team members to minimize procedures that may cause agitation.

Fluid and Electrolyte Balance

Fluid and electrolyte problems can have an adverse effect on ICP. Closely monitor IV fluids with the use of an accurate IV infusion control device or pump. Intake and output, accounting for insensible losses, and daily weights are important in assessing fluid balance. Monitor electrolytes, especially glucose, sodium, potassium, magnesium, and osmolality. Discuss abnormal values with the HCP.

Monitor urine output to detect problems related to arginine vasopressin (AVP) disorder and SIAD. AVP disorder is caused by a decrease in antidiuretic hormone (ADH). It results in increased urine output and hypernatremia. The usual treatment is fluid replacement, vasopressin, or desmopressin acetate (see Chapter 54). If it is not quickly identified and treated, severe dehydration will occur.

SIAD is caused by excess secretion of ADH. SIAD results in decreased urine output and dilutional hyponatremia. It may result in cerebral edema, changes in LOC, seizures, and coma. SIAD is described in Chapter 54.

Monitoring ICP

ICP monitoring is used with other parameters to guide patient care and assess the response to treatment. Suctioning, hypoxemia, and arousal from sleep are factors that can increase ICP. Be alert to these factors and try to minimize them. Increased intrathoracic pressure can increase ICP by impeding the venous return. So, patients should avoid coughing, straining, sneezing, and the Valsalva maneuver.

Metabolic demands, such as fever (greater than 100.4°F [38°C]), agitation, shivering, pain, and seizures, can increase ICP. Implement measures to reduce these metabolic demands to lower ICP in at-risk patients. Monitor patients for seizure activity. They may need prophylactic antiseizure medication. Maintain the temperature at 96.8°F to 98.6°F (36°C to 37°C) by using antipyretics (e.g., acetaminophen), cool baths, cooling blankets, ice packs, or intravascular cooling devices as needed. Do not let patients shiver. This increases the metabolic workload on the brain. If this occurs, you may give sedatives or apply a different cooling method.

Body Position

Proper head positioning is important. Maintain a head-up position. Keep the head in a midline position, avoiding extreme neck flexion. Flexion can cause venous obstruction and increase ICP. Adjust the body position to decrease the ICP and improve the CPP. Elevating the head of the bed promotes drainage from the head and decreases the vascular congestion that can produce cerebral edema. However, raising the head of the bed more than 30 degrees can decrease the CPP by lowering systemic BP. Carefully evaluate the effects of elevating the head of the bed on ICP and CPP. Position the bed so that it lowers the ICP while optimizing the CPP and other indices of cerebral oxygenation.

Turn patients with slow, gentle movements. Rapid changes in position may increase ICP. Prevent discomfort when turning and positioning because pain or agitation increases pressure. Avoid extreme hip flexion to decrease the risk for raising the intraabdominal pressure, which increases ICP. Decorticate or decerebrate posturing is a reflex response in some patients with IICP. Turning, skin care, and even passive range of motion can elicit posturing.

Provide care to minimize complications of immobility, such as atelectasis and contractures. Turn patients at least every 2 hours.

Protection From Injury

Patients with IICP and decreased LOC need protection from injury. Confusion, agitation, and the possibility of seizures increase the risk for injury. Use restraints carefully in agitated patients. If restraints are necessary to keep patients from removing tubes or falling out of bed, they should be secure enough to be effective. Observe the skin area under the restraints regularly for irritation. Agitation may increase with the use of restraints, which indicates the need for other measures to protect patients from injury. Light sedation with sedative agents may be needed. Having a family member stay with the patient may have a calming effect.

Place patients with or at risk for seizures on seizure precautions. These include padded side rails, an Ambu bag at the bedside, readily available suction, accurate and timely administration of antiseizure drugs, and close observation.

Antiseizure prophylaxis against early seizures (within the first 7 to 10 days) is recommended in severe brain injury. This practice is controversial for mild to moderate brain injury.[5]

Psychologic Considerations

Be aware of the psychologic well-being of patients and their families. There is a need for support and teaching of patients and families. Anxiety over the diagnosis and prognosis can be distressing to patients and family. Your competent and assured manner in performing care is reassuring. Short, simple explanations are appropriate. Provide patients and family with the amount of information they desire. Assess family members' desires to help with providing patient care and allow for their participation as appropriate. Encourage interprofessional management (e.g., social work, chaplain) involving patients and their families as much as possible.

◆ Evaluation

The expected outcomes are that patients with IICP will:

- Maintain ICP and cerebral perfusion within normal parameters
- Have no sustained increases in ICP during or after care activities
- Have no complications of immobility

HEAD INJURY

Head injury includes any injury or trauma to the scalp, skull, or brain. A serious form of head injury is *traumatic brain injury* (TBI). Around 214,000 TBI-related hospitalizations occur each year with 69,500 deaths.[6] People age 75 years and older had the highest numbers and rates of TBI-related hospitalizations and deaths. At least 5.3 million Americans (2% of the U.S. population) currently live with disabilities from TBI.

The most common causes of head injury are falls and motor vehicle accidents. Other causes include firearms, assaults, sports-related trauma, recreational injuries, and war-related injuries. Males are twice as likely to sustain a TBI.

Head trauma has a high potential for a poor outcome (Box 61.1). Deaths from head trauma occur at 3 points after injury: immediately after the injury, within 2 hours after injury, and about 3 weeks after injury. Most deaths occur immediately after the injury, from direct head trauma or massive bleeding and shock. Deaths within a few hours of the trauma are caused by progressive worsening of the brain injury or bleeding.[7]

Deaths occurring 3 weeks or more after the injury result from multisystem failure. Expert nursing care in the weeks after the injury is crucial in decreasing mortality and optimizing outcomes.[8]

BOX 61.1 ETHICAL/LEGAL DILEMMAS

Brain Death

Situation

The emergency nurse receives a call from emergency response system (ERS) personnel, who are en route with R.G., a young man involved in a motorcycle crash. He was not wearing a helmet and has a large open skull fracture. Transport from the accident scene was delayed by 45 min because of a severe thunderstorm and the location. R.G. has fixed, dilated pupils and is in cardiac arrest. Estimated arrival at the hospital is still another 30 min because of the weather. ERS personnel request permission to stop resuscitation efforts.

Ethical/Legal Points for Consideration

- Criteria for brain death include coma or unresponsiveness, absence of brainstem reflexes, and apnea (see Chapter 10).
- In a situation in which the professional responsible for determining death is in remote contact with the patient but the monitoring devices available provide virtual contact, a remote diagnosis of death may be legally acceptable.
- Cardiopulmonary resuscitation (CPR) is not appropriate when survival is not expected or the patient is expected to survive without the ability to communicate. Quantitative futility implies that survival is not expected after CPR under given circumstances. In the absence of mitigating factors, prolonged resuscitative efforts are unlikely to be successful and can be stopped if there is no return of spontaneous circulation at any time during 30 minutes of cumulative advanced life support.
- It is ethical for ED personnel to stop treatment started by ERS personnel in the prehospital setting if there is valid, after-the-fact evidence that these interventions are now inappropriate.

Discussion Questions

1. What are your feelings about cessation of brain function versus cessation of heart and lung function as the criteria for death?
2. What are your state's laws or practices about stopping CPR efforts by ERS personnel in the field?

Types of Head Injuries

Scalp Lacerations

Scalp lacerations are an easily recognized type of external head trauma. Because the scalp contains many blood vessels with poor constrictive abilities, profuse bleeding occurs with most scalp lacerations. Even relatively small wounds can bleed significantly. The major complications are blood loss and infection.

Skull Fractures

Skull fractures often occur with head trauma and are described in several ways: (1) linear or depressed; (2) simple, comminuted, or compound; and (3) closed or open (Table 61.7). Fractures may be closed or open, depending on the presence of a scalp laceration or extension of the fracture into the air sinuses or dura. The type and severity of a skull fracture depend on the velocity, momentum, direction, and shape (blunt or sharp) of the injuring object and site of impact. Skull fractures are associated with intracranial infection, hematoma, and meningeal and brain tissue damage.

The location of the fracture determines the manifestations (Table 61.8). For example, a basilar skull fracture is a special type of linear fracture involving the base of the skull. Manifestations can evolve over the course of several hours. They vary with the location and severity of fracture. These may include CN deficits, Battle sign (postauricular bruising), and periorbital bruising

TABLE 61.7 Types of Skull Fractures

Type	Description	Cause
Comminuted	Multiple linear fractures with fragmentation of bone into many pieces	Direct, high-momentum impact
Compound	Depressed skull fracture and scalp laceration with communicating pathway to intracranial cavity	Severe head injury
Depressed	Inward indentation of skull	Powerful blow
Linear	Break in continuity of bone without change of relationship of parts	Low-velocity injuries
Simple	Linear or depressed skull fracture without fragmentation or communicating lacerations	Low to moderate impact

TABLE 61.8 Manifestations of Skull Fractures

Fracture Location	Manifestations
Basilar	CSF or brain otorrhea, bulging of tympanic membrane caused by blood or CSF, Battle sign, tinnitus or hearing difficulty, rhinorrhea, facial paralysis, conjugate deviation of gaze, vertigo
Frontal	Exposure of brain to contaminants through frontal air sinus, possible association with air in forehead tissue, CSF rhinorrhea, pneumocranium (air between cranium and dura mater)
Orbital	Periorbital bruising (raccoon eyes), optic nerve injury
Parietal	Deafness, CSF or brain otorrhea, bulging of tympanic membrane caused by blood or CSF, facial paralysis, loss of taste, Battle sign
Posterior fossa	Occipital bruising resulting in cortical blindness, visual field defects, rare appearance of ataxia or other cerebellar signs
Temporal	Boggy temporal muscle because of extravasation of blood, oval-shaped bruise behind ear in mastoid region (Battle sign), CSF otorrhea, middle meningeal artery disruption, epidural hematoma

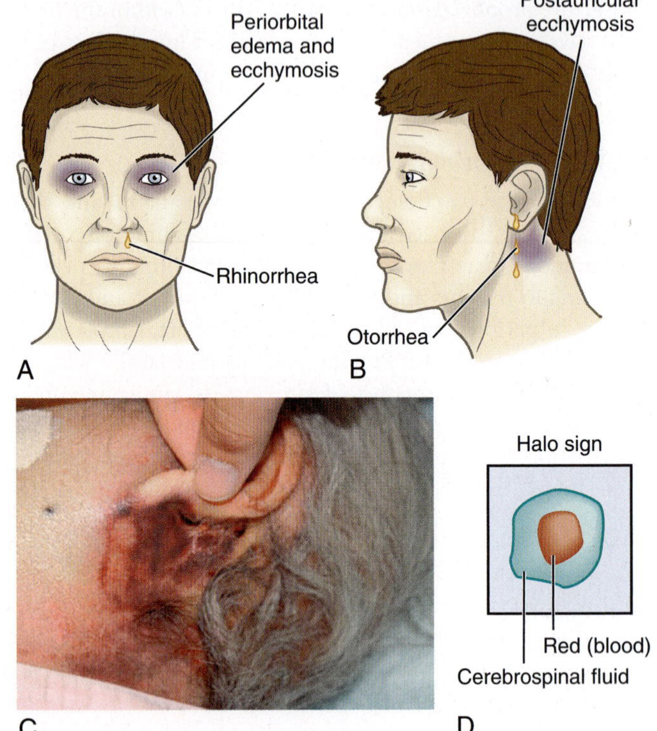

Fig. 61.12 (A) Raccoon eyes and rhinorrhea. (B) Battle sign (postauricular bruising) with otorrhea. (C) Battle sign. (D) Halo or ring sign. (C, From Takahashi C, Okudera H, Kobayashi K, et al: An extensive retropharyngeal hematoma associated with pyramidal fracture, *Inj Extra* 40:162, 2009.)

(raccoon eyes) (Fig. 61.12). This fracture is often associated with a tear in the dura and subsequent leakage of CSF.

Rhinorrhea (CSF leakage from the nose) or *otorrhea* (CSF leakage from the ear) can confirm that a fracture has traversed the dura (Fig. 61.12). Rhinorrhea may also manifest as postnasal sinus drainage. It may be overlooked unless we assess for this finding. The risk for meningitis is high with a CSF leak. Antibiotics should be given as a preventive measure.

We use 2 ways to test whether fluid leaking from the nose or ear is CSF. One method is to test the leaking fluid with a Dextrostix or Tes-Tape strip to see if glucose is present. CSF gives a positive reading for glucose. If blood is present in the fluid, testing for glucose is unreliable because blood contains glucose. In this case look for the *halo* or *ring* sign (Fig. 61.12D). Allow the leaking fluid to drip onto a white gauze pad (4 × 4) or towel and then observe the drainage. Within a few minutes, the blood coalesces into the center, and a yellowish ring encircles the blood if CSF is present. Note the color, appearance, and amount of leaking fluid because both tests can give false-positive results.

Head Trauma

We categorize brain injuries as diffuse (general) or focal (local). In a *diffuse* injury (e.g., concussion, diffuse axonal injury), damage to the brain is not in a specific area. In a *focal injury* (e.g., contusion, hematoma), the damage is to a specific area of the brain. We also classify brain injury as *minor* (GCS 13 to 15), *moderate* (GCS 9 to 12), or *severe* (GCS 3 to 8).

Diffuse injury. A **concussion** is a sudden transient mechanical head injury with disruption of neural activity and a change in the LOC. It is a minor diffuse head injury. Typical signs include a brief disruption in LOC, amnesia about the event (retrograde amnesia), and headache. Patients may or may not lose consciousness. The manifestations are often of short duration. It usually resolves spontaneously.

For some, the signs and symptoms may be the beginning of a more serious, progressive problem, especially in patients with a history of a concussion or head injury. If the patient has not lost consciousness or if the loss of consciousness lasts less than 5 minutes, they are usually discharged with instructions to notify the HCP if symptoms persist or if behavior changes occur. Give patients and caregivers instructions for observation and accurate reporting of symptoms or changes in neurologic status.

Postconcussion syndrome may develop in some patients, usually from 2 weeks to 2 months after the injury. Manifestations include persistent headache, lethargy, personality and behavior changes, shortened attention span, decreased short-term memory, and changes in intellectual ability. This syndrome can significantly affect the ability to perform activities of daily living.

Diffuse axonal injury. Diffuse axonal injury (DAI) is widespread axonal damage occurring after a mild, moderate, or severe TBI. The damage occurs primarily around axons in the subcortical white matter of the cerebral hemispheres, basal ganglia, thalamus, and brainstem.[9] This injury typically occurs with rapid acceleration-deceleration forces. Initial shear trauma sets off a cascade of events causing changes in membrane permeability, hypoxia, free radical formation, and inflammation.

DAI is graded in severity depending on its extent of injury deep into the brain. The clinical signs vary. They may include a decreased LOC, IICP, decortication or decerebration, and cerebral edema. Patients with DAI who survive the initial event are admitted to the ICU. There, they will be vigilantly watched for signs of IICP and treated accordingly. Patients with severe injury have a poor functional prognosis.[10]

Focal injury. Focal injury can be minor to severe and local to an area of injury. Focal injury consists of lacerations, contusions, hematomas, and CN injuries.

Lacerations involve actual tearing of the brain tissue. They often occur in depressed and open fractures and penetrating injuries. Tissue damage is severe. Surgical repair of the laceration is impossible because of the nature of brain tissue. Management consists of antibiotics (until meningitis is ruled out) and preventing secondary injury from IICP. If bleeding is deep into the brain tissue, focal and general signs develop.

With major head trauma, many delayed responses can occur. These include bleeding, hematoma formation, seizures, and cerebral edema. Intracerebral hemorrhage is generally caused by a cerebral laceration. This bleeding manifests as a space-occupying lesion accompanied by unconsciousness, hemiplegia on the contralateral side, and a dilated pupil on the ipsilateral side. As the hematoma expands, signs of IICP become more severe. Subarachnoid hemorrhage and intraventricular hemorrhage can occur from head trauma.

Intracerebral hematoma occurs from bleeding within the brain tissue. It usually happens in the frontal and temporal lobes, possibly from rupture of intracerebral vessels at the time of injury. The size and location of the hematoma are key in determining the outcome. These injuries can be caused by trauma or nontraumatic insults, such as extreme hypertension.

A *contusion* is bruising of the brain tissue within a focal area. It is usually associated with a closed head injury and trauma. A contusion often worsens over time. There may be areas of bleeding, infarction, necrosis, and edema.

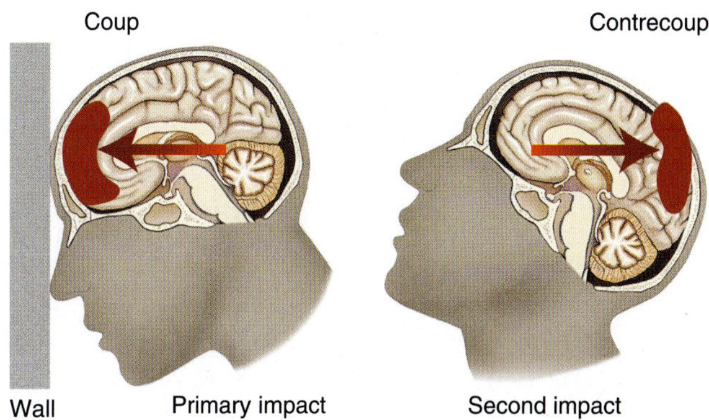

Fig. 61.13 Coup-contrecoup injury. After the head strikes the wall, a coup injury occurs as the brain strikes the skull (primary impact). The contrecoup injury (the second impact) occurs when the brain strikes the skull surface opposite the site of the original impact.

With contusion, the phenomenon of *coup-contrecoup injury* may occur (Fig. 61.13). Injuries can range from minor to severe. Damage from coup-contrecoup injury occurs when the brain moves inside the skull because of high-energy or high-impact injury mechanisms. Contusions or lacerations occur at the site of the direct impact of the brain on the skull *(coup)* and at a second area of damage on the opposite side away from injury *(contrecoup)*, leading to multiple contused areas. *Contrecoup* injuries tend to be more severe. The overall prognosis depends on the amount of bleeding around the contusion site.

Contusions may continue to bleed or rebleed and appear to "blossom" on subsequent CT scans. Bleeding worsens the neurologic outcome. Neurologic assessment may show focal and general manifestation, depending on the contusion's size and location. Seizures can occur, especially when the injury involves the frontal or temporal lobes. Anticoagulant, antiplatelet use, and coagulopathy are associated with increased bleeding, more severe head injury, and an increased mortality rate.[11] This is especially important with older adults who are taking anticoagulants. If they fall, their contusion is likely to be more severe because of anticoagulant use.

Complications

Epidural Hematoma

An epidural hematoma results from bleeding between the dura and inner surface of the skull (Fig. 61.14). An epidural hematoma is a neurologic emergency. It is usually the result of a linear fracture crossing a major artery in the dura, causing a tear. It can have a venous or arterial origin. Venous epidural hematomas are caused by a tear of the dural venous sinus and develop slowly. With arterial hematomas, the middle meningeal artery lying under the temporal bone is often torn. Bleeding occurs into the epidural space, which lies between the dura and inner surface of the skull (Fig. 61.14). Because this is arterial bleeding, the hematoma develops rapidly.

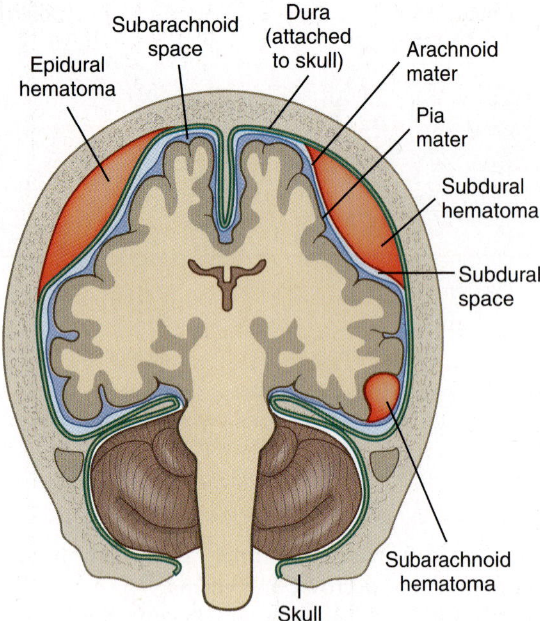

Fig. 61.14 Locations of epidural, subdural, and subarachnoid hematomas. (From Copstead-Kirkhorn LC, Banasik JL: *Pathophysiology,* ed 4, St Louis, 2010, Mosby.)

Classic signs include an initial period of unconsciousness, with a brief lucid interval followed by a decrease in LOC. Other manifestations may be a headache, nausea and vomiting, or focal findings. Rapid surgical treatment to evacuate the hematoma and prevent cerebral herniation, along with medical management for increasing ICP, dramatically improves outcomes.

Subdural Hematoma

A **subdural hematoma** occurs from bleeding between the dura mater and arachnoid layer of the meninges (Fig. 61.14). It usually results from injury to the brain tissue and its blood vessels. The veins that drain from the surface of the brain into the sagittal sinus are the source of most subdural hematomas. Because it is usually venous in origin, a subdural hematoma may be slower to develop. Arterial bleeds that cause a subdural hematoma often develop more rapidly.

Subdural hematomas may be acute, subacute, or chronic (Table 61.9). An *acute subdural hematoma* manifests within hours of the injury.[12] The signs and symptoms are similar to those of brain tissue compression in IICP. They include decreasing LOC and headache. The size of the hematoma determines the presentation and prognosis. Patients' appearance may range from drowsy and confused to unconscious. The ipsilateral pupil dilates and becomes fixed if ICP is significantly increased. Blunt-force injuries that produce acute subdural hematomas may cause significant underlying brain injury, resulting in cerebral edema. The resulting increase in ICP from the cerebral edema can increase mortality despite surgery to evacuate the hematoma.

A *subacute subdural hematoma* usually occurs within 2 to 14 days of the injury. After the initial bleeding, this hematoma may appear to enlarge over time as the breakdown products of the blood draw fluid into the subdural space.

TABLE 61.9 Types of Subdural Hematomas

Occurrence After Injury	Symptom Progression	Treatment
Acute		
24–48 h after severe trauma	Immediate deterioration	Craniotomy, evacuation, and decompression
Subacute		
48 h–2 wk after severe trauma	Decline in mental status as hematoma develops Progression dependent on size and location of hematoma	Evacuation and decompression
Chronic		
Weeks or months, usually >20 days after injury Often injury seemed trivial or was forgotten by patient	Nonspecific, nonlocalizing progression Progressive change in LOC	Evacuation and decompression, membranectomy

A *chronic subdural hematoma* develops over weeks or months after a seemingly minor head injury.[12] They are more common in older adults because of a potentially larger subdural space from brain atrophy. With atrophy, the brain stays attached to the supportive structures and tension is increased. This makes it subject to tearing. Because the subdural space is larger, the presenting problem is focal symptoms rather than IICP.[12] Patients with a history of alcohol use are prone to subdural hematomas because of an increased incidence of falls.

There may be a delay in diagnosing a subdural hematoma in the older adult because symptoms mimic other health problems in this age group, such as confusion, lethargy, and memory loss. Manifestations of a subdural hematoma are often attributed to vascular disease (stroke, transient ischemic attack [TIA]) or dementia.

CHECK YOUR PRACTICE

You are doing BP screenings in the senior center when you meet a 76-year-old man and his wife. As you perform their BP screening, the wife tells you that her husband has been getting severe headaches, is dizzy, and sometimes has difficulty talking. Based on your advice, they go to an urgent care center, where a CT scan is done. The results show he has a chronic subdural hematoma. When you find out the diagnosis, you are puzzled because you thought he was having a stroke and cannot understand how he got a subdural hematoma.

- What could you have done differently when screening this patient?

Diagnostic Studies

In general, the diagnostic studies for head trauma are similar to those used for patients with IICP (Table 61.3). CT scan allows for rapid diagnosis and intervention in the acute care setting.

TABLE 61.10 EMERGENCY MANAGEMENT

Head Injury

Etiology	Assessment Findings	Interventions
Blunt • Assault • Fall • Motor vehicle collision • Sports injury **Penetrating** • Arrow • Gunshot • Knife	**Neurologic** • Asymmetric facial movements • Combativeness • Confusion • CSF leaking from ears or nose • Decerebrate or decorticate posturing • Depressed or hyperactive reflexes • Dilated or unequal pupils, photophobia • Flaccidity • Garbled speech, abusive speech • GCS score <12 • Incontinence • Involuntary movements • ↓ LOC • Seizures **Respiratory** • Hyperventilation • Cheyne-Stokes respirations • ↓ O_2 saturation • Pulmonary edema **Surface Findings** • Bruises or contusions on face, Battle sign • Fracture or depressions in skull • Raccoon eyes • Scalp lacerations	**Initial** • If unresponsive, assess circulation, airway, and breathing. • If responsive, monitor airway, breathing, and circulation. • Assume neck injury with head injury. • Stabilize cervical spine. • Apply O_2 via nonrebreather mask. • Establish IV access with 2 large-bore catheters to infuse normal saline or lactated Ringer solution. • Intubate if Glasgow Coma Scale score <8. • Control external bleeding with sterile pressure dressing. • Remove patient's clothing. **Ongoing Monitoring** • Maintain normothermia using blankets, warm IV fluids, as needed. • Monitor vital signs, LOC, O_2 saturation, cardiac rhythm, GCS score, pupil size and reactivity. • Expect intubation if gag reflex is impaired or absent. • Assess for rhinorrhea, otorrhea, scalp wounds. • Give fluids cautiously to prevent fluid overload and increasing ICP.

MRI, PET, and evoked potential studies may be used to diagnose head injuries. An MRI scan is more sensitive than a CT scan in detecting small lesions. Transcranial Doppler studies can measure CBF velocity. A cervical spine x-ray series, CT scan, or MRI of the spine may be done because cervical spine trauma often occurs at the same time as a head injury.

Interprofessional Care

Emergency management of patients with a head injury is outlined in Table 61.10. The key treatment of head injuries is prompt diagnosis and surgery (if needed). We also institute measures to prevent secondary injury by treating cerebral edema and managing IICP. For patients with concussion and contusion, observation and management of IICP are the main management strategies.

The treatment of skull fractures is usually conservative. For depressed fractures and fractures with loose fragments, a craniotomy is done to elevate the depressed bone and remove the free fragments. If large amounts of bone are destroyed, the bone may be removed (craniectomy). A cranioplasty will be needed later.

In cases of large acute subdural and epidural hematomas or those that have significant neurologic impairment, the blood must be removed through surgical evacuation. A craniotomy is usually done to see and allow control of the bleeding vessels. Burr-hole openings may be used in an extreme emergency for a more rapid decompression, followed by a craniotomy. A drain may be placed after surgery for several days to prevent blood from reaccumulating. When extreme swelling is expected (e.g., DAI, bleeding), a craniectomy may be done. This involves removing a piece of skull to reduce the pressure inside the skull and reduce the risk for central herniation.

NURSING MANAGEMENT: HEAD INJURY

Assessment

Patients with a head injury always have the potential to develop IICP, which has higher mortality rates and poorer functional outcomes. Objective data are obtained by applying the GCS (Table 61.5), assessing and monitoring neurologic status, and determining whether a CSF leak has occurred. Nursing assessment related to IICP was discussed earlier in this chapter. Assessment of patients with a head injury is outlined in Table 61.11.

Clinical Problems

Clinical problems for patients with a head injury may include:

- Increased intracranial pressure
- Inadequate tissue perfusion
- Altered temperature

TABLE 61.11 NURSING ASSESSMENT

Head Injury

Subjective Data

Important Health Information

Health history: Mechanism of injury: motor vehicle collision, sports injury, industrial incident, assault, falls.

Medications: Anticoagulant drugs.

Functional Health Patterns

Health perception—health management: Alcohol or recreational drugs. Risk-taking behaviors.

Cognitive-perceptual: Headache, mood or behavior change, mentation changes, aphasia, dysphasia, impaired judgment.

Coping—stress tolerance: Fear, denial, anger, aggression, depression.

Objective Data

Cardiovascular

Impending herniation: Cushing triad (systolic hypertension with widening pulse pressure, bradycardia with full and bounding pulse, irregular respirations).

GI

Vomiting, projectile vomiting, bowel incontinence.

Musculoskeletal

Motor deficit/impairment, weakness, palmar drift, paralysis, spasticity, decorticate or decerebrate posturing, muscular rigidity or increased tone, flaccidity, ataxia.

Neurologic

Altered LOC, altered mental status, seizure activity, pupil dysfunction, cranial nerve deficit(s).

Respiratory

Rhinorrhea, impaired gag reflex, inability to maintain a patent airway. Impending herniation: altered/irregular respiratory rate and pattern.

Skin

Lacerations, contusions, abrasions, hematoma, Battle sign, periorbital edema and bruising, otorrhea, exposed brain matter.

Urinary

Bladder incontinence.

Possible Diagnostic Findings

Location and type of hematoma, edema, skull fracture, and/or foreign body on CT scan and/or MRI; abnormal EEG; positive toxicology screen or alcohol level, ↓ or ↑ glucose level; ↑ ICP.

◆ Planning

The overall goals are that patients with an acute head injury will (1) maintain adequate cerebral oxygenation and perfusion, (2) stay afebrile, (3) be free of discomfort, (4) be free from infection, (5) have adequate nutrition, and (6) attain maximal cognitive, motor, and sensory function.

◆ Implementation

Health Promotion

One of the best ways to prevent head injuries is to prevent car and motorcycle accidents. Be active in campaigns that promote driving safety (Box 61.2). Speak about the dangers of distracted driving and driving after drinking alcohol or using drugs. Helmets for motorcycle riders are the most effective way to increase survival after crashes.

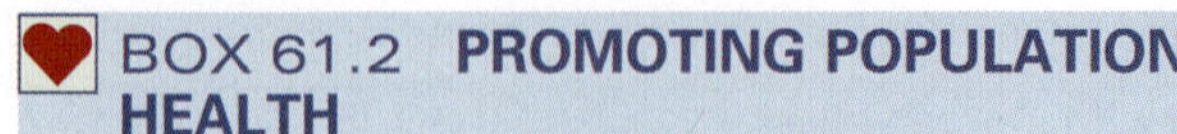

BOX 61.2 PROMOTING POPULATION HEALTH

Reducing the Risk for Head Injuries

- Always wear car seat belts in motor vehicles.
- Do not drive after using drugs or alcohol.
- Do not text and drive or drive distracted.
- Wear helmets while bicycling, skating, skateboarding, skiing, and playing contact sports.
- Athletes should follow safe playing techniques and the rules of the game.
- Assess home safety and implement any corrective measures needed.
- Older adults should continue to exercise regularly to improve strength and balance.
- Follow workplace safety precautions, including wearing helmets and protective gear.

Acute Care

Management at the scene can have a significant impact on the outcome of a head injury. Emergency management of head injury is outlined in Table 61.10. The general goal of nursing management of patients with head injury is to maintain cerebral oxygenation and perfusion.

The major focus of nursing care for patients with a brain injury relates to IICP (Table 61.6). Monitoring for changes in neurologic status is important. Patients may deteriorate rapidly, requiring emergency surgery. Appropriate nursing interventions are started if surgery is anticipated. Because of the close association between hemodynamic status and cerebral perfusion, be aware of any coexisting injuries or conditions.

Perform neurologic assessments at intervals based on the patient's condition. The GCS is useful in assessing the LOC (Table 61.5). Report any signs of a deteriorating neurologic state, no matter how subtle, such as a decreasing LOC or motor strength, to the HCP.

Explain the need for frequent neurologic assessments to patients and caregivers. Behavior manifestations can result in frightened, disoriented patients who are combative and resist help. Your approach should be calm and gentle. A family member may be available to stay with the patient to decrease their anxiety and fear. An important need of the caregivers and family members in the acute injury phase is information about a patient's diagnosis, treatment plan, and reason for the interventions. Other teaching points are described in Table 61.12.

Eye problems may include loss of the corneal reflex, periorbital bruising and edema, and diplopia. Loss of the corneal reflex may require lubricating eye drops or taping the eyes shut to prevent abrasion. Periorbital bruising and edema decrease with time. Cold and, later, warm compresses provide comfort and hasten healing. Wearing an eye patch can relieve diplopia. Consider a consult with an ophthalmologist.

TABLE 61.12 PATIENT & CAREGIVER TEACHING

Head Injury

Include the following instructions when teaching patients and caregivers about care during the first 2 or 3 days after a head injury:

1. Notify your HCP immediately if you have signs and symptoms that may indicate complications. These include:
   - Increased drowsiness (e.g., difficulty arousing, confusion)
   - Nausea or vomiting
   - Worsening headache or stiff neck
   - Seizures
   - Vision changes (e.g., blurring) or sensitivity to light (photophobia)
   - Behavior changes (e.g., irritability, anger)
   - Motor problems (e.g., clumsiness, difficulty walking, slurred speech, weakness in arms or legs)
   - Sensory problems (e.g., numbness)
   - Heart rate <60 beats/min
2. Have someone stay with you.
3. Abstain from alcohol.
4. Check with your HCP before taking drugs that may increase drowsiness, including muscle relaxants, tranquilizers, and opioid analgesia.
5. Avoid driving, using heavy machinery, playing contact sports, and taking hot baths.

Fever may occur from injury to or inflammation of the hypothalamus. Fever can increase CBF, cerebral blood volume, and ICP. Increased metabolism from fever increases metabolic waste. This causes further cerebral vasodilation. Avoid fever, with a goal of a temperature of 96.8°F to 98.6°F (36°C to 37°C). Use interventions to reduce fever and prevent shivering (see Table 12.5).

If CSF rhinorrhea or otorrhea occurs, inform the HCP at once. The head of the bed may be raised to decrease the CSF pressure so that a tear can seal. A loose collection pad may be placed under the nose or over the ear. Do not place a dressing in the nasal or ear cavities. Record the amount of drainage each shift. Teach patients not to sneeze or blow the nose. Do not use NG tubes. Do not perform nasotracheal suctioning because of the high risk for meningitis.

Implement measures specific to the care of immobilized patients, such as those related to bladder and bowel function, skin care, and infection. Nausea and vomiting may be a problem. Administer antiemetic drugs as ordered. Acetaminophen or small doses of codeine can help control headaches.

Patients who deteriorate may need intracranial surgery. They may need a burr-hole opening or craniotomy, depending on the underlying injury. The emergency nature of the surgery may hasten the usual preoperative preparation. Consult with the HCP to determine specific preoperative nursing measures.

Patients are often unconscious before surgery, making it necessary for a family member to sign the consent form for surgery. This is a difficult and frightening time for the caregivers and family and requires sensitive nursing management. The suddenness of the situation makes it especially hard for the family to cope. Use a team approach, including social workers, to help patients and family throughout the hospitalization and recovery time.

Chronic Care

Once their condition has stabilized, patients are usually transferred for acute rehabilitation management. There may be chronic problems related to motor and sensory deficits, communication, memory, and intellectual functioning. Conditions we may need to manage include nutrition problems, bowel and bladder problems, spasticity, dysphagia, and hydrocephalus. Many of the principles for managing patients after a stroke are appropriate (see Chapter 62).

Seizure disorders may occur in patients with nonpenetrating head injury. They may develop during the first week after the head injury or not until years later. Antiseizure drugs may be used prophylactically to manage posttraumatic seizure activity. However, this practice is controversial.

The mental and emotional sequelae are often the most incapacitating problems. One of the consequences of TBI is that the person may not realize that a brain injury has occurred. Many patients with head injuries who were comatose for more than 6 hours may have some personality change. They may have loss of concentration and memory and defective memory processing. Personal drive may decrease. Apathy may increase. Euphoria and mood swings, along with a seeming lack of awareness of the seriousness of the injury, may occur. There may be a loss of social restraint, judgment, tact, and emotional control.

Progressive recovery may continue for years. Specific nursing management in the posttraumatic phase depends on specific residual deficits. Being able to return to work and maintaining employment are challenges during the recovery period.[13] Patients' outward physical appearance does not necessarily reflect what has happened in the brain. It is not a good indicator of how well they will ultimately function in the home or work environment.

Give the family special consideration. They need to understand what is happening. The family often has unrealistic expectations of the patient as the coma begins to recede. They may expect a full return to pretrauma status. In reality, the patient usually has a reduced awareness and ability to interpret environment stimuli. Prepare the family for the patient's emergence from coma. Explain that the process of awakening often takes several weeks. Help the patient and family to remain hopeful. Arrange for social work and chaplain consults for the family.

When it is time for discharge planning, patients and family may benefit from specific instructions to avoid family-patient friction. Special "no" policies may include no alcohol use, no driving, no use of firearms, no working with hazardous implements and machinery, and no unsupervised smoking. Help the family involve the patient in family activities whenever possible. Family members, especially spouses, go through role transition as the role changes from that of spouse to that of caregiver. Provide guidance and referrals for financial aid, childcare, and other personal needs.

◆ Evaluation

The expected outcomes are that patients with a head injury will:

- Maintain normal CPP
- Achieve maximal cognitive, motor, and sensory function
- Have no infection or fever

BRAIN TUMORS

Around 23,400 people are diagnosed each year with brain tumors in the United States. Brain tumors most often occur in middle-aged persons, but they may be seen at any age.

Types

Brain tumors can occur in any part of the brain or spinal cord. They may be *primary*, arising from tissues within the brain, or *secondary*, resulting from a metastasis of cancer from elsewhere in the body.[14] Metastatic brain tumors are the most common brain tumor. The brain is a frequent site for metastasis.[14] Cancers that most often metastasize to the brain are lung and breast.

We usually classify primary brain tumors according to the tissue from which they arise (Table 61.13). Meningiomas are the most common primary brain tumor. Other common brain tumors are gliomas (e.g., astrocytoma, glioblastoma [most common form of glioma]).

More than half of brain tumors are malignant. They infiltrate the brain tissue and are not amenable to complete surgical removal. Other tumors may be histologically benign but are located such that complete removal is not possible.

Brain tumors rarely metastasize outside the central nervous system (CNS) because they are contained by structural (meninges) and physiologic (blood-brain) barriers. Table 61.13 compares the most common brain tumors. Sites of common tumors are shown in Fig. 61.15.

Clinical Manifestations and Complications

The manifestations depend mainly on their location and size (Table 61.14). A wide range of manifestations is possible. Headaches are common. Tumor-related headaches tend to be worse at night and may awaken patients. The headaches are usually dull and constant but sometimes throbbing. Seizures are common in gliomas and brain metastases. Brain tumors can cause nausea and vomiting from IICP. Impaired cognition, including memory problems and mood or personality changes, is common, especially in patients with brain metastases. Muscle weakness, sensory losses, aphasia, and visual-spatial dysfunction may occur.

If the tumor obstructs the ventricles or occludes the outlet, ventricular enlargement (hydrocephalus) can occur. As the tumor expands, it may produce IICP, cerebral edema, or obstruction of the CSF pathways. Unless treated, all brain tumors eventually cause death from increasing tumor size leading to IICP.

Diagnostic Studies

A history and neurologic examination are done in the workup and may provide data with respect to location. New onset of

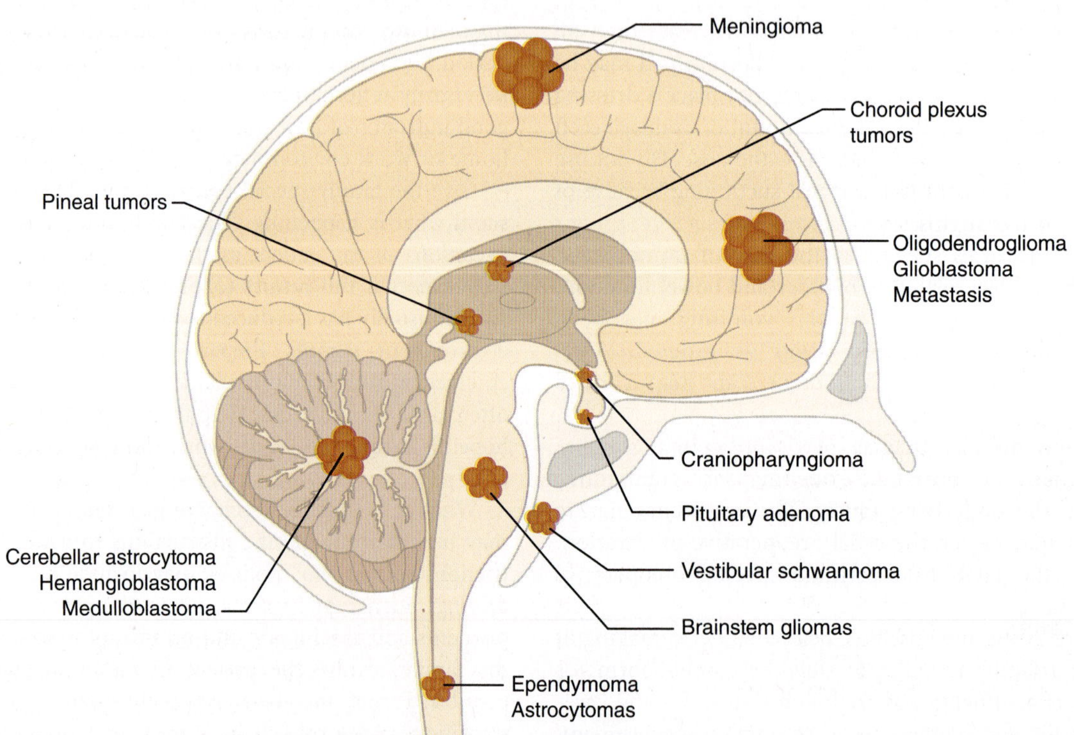

Fig. 61.15 Common sites of occurrence for CNS tumors.

TABLE 61.13 Types of Brain Tumors

Type	Tissue of Origin	Characteristics
Acoustic neuroma (schwannoma)	Cells that form myelin sheath around nerves. Often affects cranial nerve VIII.	Many grow on both sides of the brain. Usually benign or low grade.
Gliomas		
• Astrocytoma	Supportive tissue, glial cells, and astrocytes	Can range from low grade to moderate grade.
• Ependymoma	Ependymal epithelium	Range from benign to highly malignant. Most are benign and encapsulated.
• Glioblastoma	Primitive stem cell (glioblast)	Highly malignant and invasive. Among the most devastating of primary brain tumors.
• Medulloblastoma	Primitive neuroectodermal cell	Highly malignant and invasive. Metastatic to spinal cord and remote areas of brain.
• Oligodendroglioma	Oligodendrocytes	Benign (encapsulation and calcification).
Hemangioblastoma	Blood vessels of brain	Rare and benign. Surgery is curative.
Meningioma	Meninges	Can be benign or malignant. Most are benign.
Metastatic tumors	Lungs and breast (most common)	Malignant.
Pituitary adenoma	Pituitary gland	Usually benign.
Primary central nervous system lymphoma	Lymphocytes	↑ Incidence in transplant recipients and patients with AIDS.

TABLE 61.14 Manifestations of Brain Tumors

Tumor Location	Manifestations
Brainstem tumors	Headache on awakening, drowsiness, vomiting, ataxic gait, facial muscle weakness, hearing loss, dysphagia, dysarthria, "crossed eyes" or other vision changes, hemiparesis
Cerebellopontine tumors	Tinnitus and vertigo, deafness
Cerebral hemisphere	
• Frontal lobe (unilateral)	Unilateral hemiplegia, seizures, memory deficit, personality and judgment changes, vision changes
• Frontal lobe (bilateral)	Symptoms of unilateral frontal lobe tumors. Ataxic gait
• Parietal lobe	Speech problems (if tumor is in the dominant hemisphere), inability to write, spatial disorders, unilateral neglect
• Occipital lobe	Vision changes, seizures
• Temporal lobe	Few symptoms. Seizures, dysphagia, hallucinations, auras
Fourth ventricle and cerebellar tumors	Headache, nausea, papilledema (occur from ↑ ICP). Ataxic gait, changes in coordination
Meningeal tumors	Symptoms of compression of the brain and depend on tumor location
Metastatic tumors	Headache, nausea, or vomiting (occur from ↑ ICP). Other symptoms depend on tumor location
Subcortical	Hemiplegia: other symptoms may depend on area of infiltration
Thalamus and sellar tumors	Headache, nausea, vision changes, papilledema, nystagmus (from ↑ ICP). Arginine vasopressin (AVP) disorder may occur

seizures or adult-onset migraines may indicate a brain tumor and should be assessed. Diagnostic studies are similar to those used for patients with IICP (Table 61.3).

CT with contrast and MRI are used to identify the lesion location. The sensitivity of MRI and PET scans allows for detection of small tumors and may provide better diagnostic information than a CT scan. Other tests include magnetic resonance spectroscopy, functional MRI (fMRI), and single-photon emission computed tomography (SPECT). An EEG can rule out seizures but is of less importance. Cerebral angiography can assess blood flow to the tumor and further localize the tumor. Other studies are done to rule out a primary lesion elsewhere in the body. Endocrine studies are done if a pituitary adenoma is suspected (see Chapter 54).

The diagnosis of a brain tumor can be made by obtaining tissue for histologic study. In most patients, tissue is obtained at the time of surgery. Computer-guided stereotactic biopsy is also an option. A smear or frozen section can be done in the operating room for a preliminary interpretation of the histologic type. With this information, the HCP can make a better decision about the extent of surgery.

Interprofessional Care

Treatment goals are aimed at (1) identifying the tumor type and location, (2) removing or decreasing tumor mass, and (3) preventing or managing IICP.

Surgical Therapy

Surgical removal is the preferred treatment for brain tumors. The outcome of surgery depends on the tumor type, size, and location. Complete removal of the tumor is not always possible because the tumor is not always accessible or may involve vital parts of the brain. Surgery can reduce tumor mass, which decreases ICP, provides relief of symptoms, and extends survival time.

Meningiomas and oligodendrogliomas can usually be completely removed. The more invasive gliomas and medulloblastomas may be only partially removed. Stereotactic surgery is used to perform a biopsy and remove small brain tumors. Computer-guided stereotactic biopsy, ultrasound, MRI, and cortical mapping can localize brain tumors during surgery.

Ventricular Shunts

Hydrocephalus caused by a tumor obstructing the CSF flow can be treated by placing a ventricular shunt. A catheter with 1-way valves is placed in the lateral ventricle and then tunneled under the skin to drain CSF into the peritoneal cavity. Rapid decompression of ICP can cause total body collapse and weakness. Headache may be prevented by gradually introducing patients to the upright position.

Manifestations of shunt malfunction, which are related to IICP, include decreasing LOC, restlessness, headache, blurred vision, or vomiting. This may require shunt revision or replacement. Infection may occur, with high fever, headache, and stiff neck. Antibiotics are used to treat the infection. In some situations, the shunt is replaced. CSF drainage is managed with an extraventricular drainage system while the infection is treated.

Radiation Therapy and Stereotactic Radiosurgery

Radiation therapy may be used as a follow-up measure after surgery. Radiation seeds can be implanted into the brain. Cerebral edema and rapidly increasing ICP may be complications of radiation therapy. These problems can usually be managed with high doses of corticosteroids. Radiation therapy is discussed in Chapter 16.

Stereotactic radiosurgery delivers a highly concentrated dose of radiation to a precise location within the brain. It may be used when conventional surgery has failed or is not an option because of the tumor location.

Chemotherapy and Targeted Therapy

The effectiveness of chemotherapy is limited by the difficulty with getting drugs across the blood-brain barrier, tumor cell heterogeneity, and tumor cell drug resistance. Chemotherapy drugs called *nitrosoureas* (e.g., carmustine, lomustine) are used to treat brain tumors. Normally the blood-brain barrier prohibits the entry of most drugs into the brain. Cancer tumors can cause a breakdown of the blood-brain barrier in the area of the tumor, thus allowing chemotherapy to be used to treat the cancer. Chemotherapy-laden biodegradable wafers (e.g., Gliadel wafer [polifeprosan with carmustine implant]) implanted at the time of surgery can deliver chemotherapy directly to the tumor site. Other drugs being used include methotrexate and procarbazine (Matulane). Another way to deliver chemotherapy directly to the CNS is intrathecal administration via an Ommaya reservoir.

Temozolomide (Temodar) is an oral chemotherapy agent that can cross the blood-brain barrier. In contrast with many chemotherapy drugs, which require metabolic activation to exert their effects, temozolomide can convert spontaneously to a reactive agent that directly interferes with tumor growth. It does not interact with other common drugs taken by patients with brain tumors, such as antiseizure drugs, corticosteroids, and antiemetics.

DRUG ALERT

Temozolomide

- Causes myelosuppression. Before using, the absolute neutrophil count should be $\geq$1500/μL and platelet count should be $\geq$100,000/μL.
- To reduce nausea and vomiting, take on an empty stomach or at bedtime.

Bevacizumab (Avastin) is used to treat patients with glioblastoma that continues to progress after standard therapy. It is a targeted therapy that inhibits the action of vascular endothelial growth factor, which helps form new blood vessels. These vessels can feed a tumor, helping it to grow, and provide a pathway for cancer cells to circulate in the body.

Other Therapies

The Optune System is used to treat glioblastoma that recurs or progresses after receiving chemotherapy and radiation therapy. With this system, electrodes are placed on the surface of the scalp to deliver low-intensity, changing electrical fields called *tumor treatment fields* (TTFs) to the tumor site.

NURSING MANAGEMENT: BRAIN TUMORS

Assessment

Ask about the medical history, intellectual abilities and education, and history of nervous system infections and trauma. Is there a history of dementia? Loss of emotional control, confusion, disorientation, memory loss, impulsivity, and depression may be signs of a frontal lobe lesion. Patients often do not perceive these changes. Having patients or caregivers explain the problem can be helpful to determine limitations and obtain information about their insight. Use this information to design a realistic patient-specific care plan. Record initial data to provide a baseline for comparison to determine whether a patient is improving or deteriorating.

Structure the initial assessment to provide baseline data of patients' neurologic status. Assess LOC, motor abilities, sensory perception, integrated function (including bowel and bladder function), balance, and proprioception. Determine the presence of seizures, syncope, nausea, vomiting, and headaches or other pain. Assess the coping abilities of patients and family members. Watching patients perform activities of daily living and listening to their conversation can be part of the neurologic assessment.

◆ Clinical Problems

Clinical problems for patients with a brain tumor may include:

- Inadequate tissue perfusion
- Pain
- Anxiety
- Neurologic problem

◆ Planning

The overall goals are that patients with a brain tumor will (1) maintain normal ICP, (2) maximize neurologic functioning, (3) achieve control of pain and discomfort, and (4) be aware of the long-term implications with respect to prognosis and cognitive and physical functioning.

◆ Implementation

Help the caregiver and family understand what is happening and provide support. A frontal lobe tumor can cause behavior and personality changes. These changes can be disturbing and frightening to caregivers and family members. They can also cause distancing to occur between patients and family.

Confused patients with behavior instability can be a challenge. Protecting patients from self-harm is an important part of nursing care. Essential interventions include close supervision of activity, use of side rails, judicious use of restraints, appropriate sedation, padding of the rails and the area around the bed, and a calm, reassuring approach.

Temporal lobe tumors can cause hallucinations. Perceptual problems from frontal and parietal lobe tumors contribute to disorientation and confusion. Minimize environment stimuli, create a routine, and use reality orientation for confused patients.

Seizures, which often occur with brain tumors, are managed with antiseizure drugs. Use seizure precautions for safety. Some behavior changes are a result of seizure disorders and can improve with adequate seizure control. Patients at risk for seizures may be unable to drive. Be aware of the extra resources needed and collaborate with the social worker and family. Seizure disorders are discussed in Chapter 63.

Motor and sensory problems interfere with activities of daily living. Encourage patients to provide as much self-care as physically possible. Self-image often depends on patients' ability to take part in care within the limitations of physical deficits.

Language deficits may be present. Motor (expressive) or sensory (receptive) dysphasia may occur. The problem with communication can be frustrating for patients and may interfere with your ability to meet their needs. Try to establish a communication system that patients and staff can use.

Nutrition intake may be decreased because of patients' inability to eat, loss of appetite, or loss of desire to eat. Assess nutrition status and ensure adequate nutrition intake. Encourage patients to eat. Some patients may need enteral or parenteral nutrition (see Chapter 44).

Provide help and support during the adjustment phase and in long-range planning. Social work and home health nurses may help the caregiver with discharge planning. They can help the family adjust to role changes and psychosocial and socioeconomic factors. Issues related to palliative and end-of-life care must be discussed with patients and family (see Chapter 10).

◆ Evaluation

The expected outcomes are that patients with a brain tumor will:

- Achieve control of pain, vomiting, and other discomforts
- Maintain ICP within normal limits
- Have maximal neurologic function given the location and extent of the tumor
- Maintain optimal nutrition status
- Accept the long-term consequences of the tumor and its treatment

CRANIAL SURGERY

Indications for cranial surgery include brain tumors, CNS infection (e.g., abscess), vascular abnormalities, craniocerebral trauma, seizure disorder, or intractable pain (Table 61.15).

Types

Various cranial surgeries are outlined in Table 61.16.

Craniotomy

Depending on the location of the pathologic condition, a *craniotomy* may be frontal, parietal, occipital, temporal, suboccipital, or a combination of any of these. The HCP drills a set of burr holes and uses a saw to connect the holes to remove the bone flap (Fig. 61.16). Sometimes operating microscopes are used to magnify the site. After surgery, the bone flap is secured with small plates or wired shut. Sometimes drains are placed to remove fluid and blood. Patients usually receive care in the ICU until stable.

Stereotactic Radiosurgery

Stereotactic procedures use a precision apparatus (often computer guided) to help the HCP precisely target an area of the brain. This reduces the damage to surrounding tissue. Stereotactic biopsy can be done to obtain tissue samples for histologic examination. CT scanning and MRI image the targeted tissue. With the patient under general or local anesthesia, the HCP drills a burr hole or creates a bone flap for an entry site and then introduces a probe and biopsy needle. Stereotactic procedures are used for removal of small brain tumors and abscesses, drainage of hematomas, ablative procedures for extrapyramidal diseases (e.g., Parkinson disease), and repair of arteriovenous malformations.

Stereotactic radiosurgery is not a form of surgery in the traditional sense. Instead, radiosurgery uses high-dose radiation to destroy precisely targeted tumor cells and other abnormal growths. Computers create 3-dimensional images of the brain.

TABLE 61.15 Indications for Cranial Surgery

Indication	Cause	Surgical Procedure
Aneurysm repair	Dilation of weak area in arterial wall (usually near anterior portion of circle of Willis)	Dissection and clipping or coiling of aneurysm
Arteriovenous (AV) malformation	Congenital tangle of arteries and veins (often in middle cerebral artery)	Excision of malformation
Brain abscess	Bacteria that caused intracranial infection	Excision or drainage of abscess
Brain tumors	Benign or malignant cell growth	Excision or partial resection of tumor
Hydrocephalus	Overproduction of CSF, obstruction to flow, defective reabsorption	Placement of ventriculoperitoneal or (rarely) ventriculoatrial shunt
Intracranial bleeding	Rupture of cerebral vessels because of trauma or stroke	Surgical evacuation through burr holes or craniotomy
Skull fractures	Trauma to skull	Debridement of fragments and necrotic tissue, elevation and realignment of bone fragments

TABLE 61.16 Types of Cranial Surgery

Type	Description
Burr hole	Opening into the cranium with a drill. Used to remove local fluid and blood beneath the dura.
Craniectomy	Excision into the cranium to cut away bone flap.
Cranioplasty	Repair of cranial defect resulting from trauma, malformation, or previous surgery. Artificial material used to replace damaged or lost bone.
Craniotomy	Opening into cranium with removal of bone flap and opening the dura to remove a lesion, repair a damaged area, drain blood, or relieve ↑ ICP.
Shunt procedures	Alternative pathway to redirect cerebrospinal fluid from one area to another using a tube or implanted device. Examples include ventricular shunt and Ommaya reservoir.
Stereotactic procedure	Precise localization of a specific area of the brain using a frame or frameless system based on 3-dimensional coordinates. Used for biopsy, radiosurgery, or dissection.

These images are used to guide the focused radiation while the patient's head is held still in a stereotactic frame. The ionizing radiation can be generated by a linear accelerator, Gamma Knife, or CyberKnife. The dose of radiation is delivered in a single treatment lasting a few hours or in multiple sessions. Side effects include fatigue, headache, and nausea.

In combination with stereotactic procedures to identify and localize tumor sites, lasers can be used to destroy tumors. They work by creating thermal energy, which destroys the tissue on which it is focused. Laser therapy provides the benefit of reducing damage to surrounding tissue.

NURSING MANAGEMENT: CRANIAL SURGERY

The general nursing care for patients undergoing cranial surgery is similar to that of patients with IICP. Patients (if conscious and coherent), caregivers, and family members will be concerned about the potential physical and emotional problems that can result from surgery. The uncertainty about the prognosis and outcome requires compassionate nursing care in the preoperative period. Preoperative teaching is important in allaying their fears and in preparing them for the postoperative period. Provide general information about the type of surgery and what they can expect. Explain that some hair may be shaved to allow for better exposure and to prevent contamination. The hair is usually removed in the operating room after induction of anesthesia. Tell them that the patient will be in an ICU or special care unit after surgery.

The main goal of care after cranial surgery is preventing IICP. Frequent neurologic assessment is essential during the first 48 hours. Monitor fluid and electrolyte levels and serum osmolality to detect changes in sodium regulation, the onset of AVP disorder, or severe hypovolemia. Manage problems associated with IICP.

Monitor for pain and nausea. Nausea and vomiting are common after surgery. Administer antiemetic drugs as ordered. Although the brain itself does not have pain receptors, patients often report headache caused by edema or pain at the incision site. Control pain with short-acting opioids.

The dressing is usually in place for a few days. When the incision over the skull is in the anterior or middle fossa, elevate the head of the bed at least 30 degrees. If the surgical approach is in the posterior fossa or they have a burr hole, keep the patient flat or at a slight elevation (10 to 15 degrees).

Turning and positioning patients will depend on the site of the operation. If a bone flap was removed (craniectomy), do not place the patient on the operative side. Place a sign at the head of the bed, alerting everyone to the craniectomy site and position of the surgical site. Observe the dressing for color, odor, and amount of drainage. Notify the HCP immediately of any excess bleeding or clear drainage. Check drains for placement. Assess the area around the dressing. Scalp care should include meticulous care of the incision to prevent wound infection. Cleanse the area and treat it following agency protocol or the HCP's orders. Once the dressing is removed, use an antiseptic soap for washing the scalp. The psychologic impact of hair removal can be lessened by using a wig, turban, scarves, or caps. Teach patients receiving radiation to use sunblock and head covering if any sun exposure is expected.

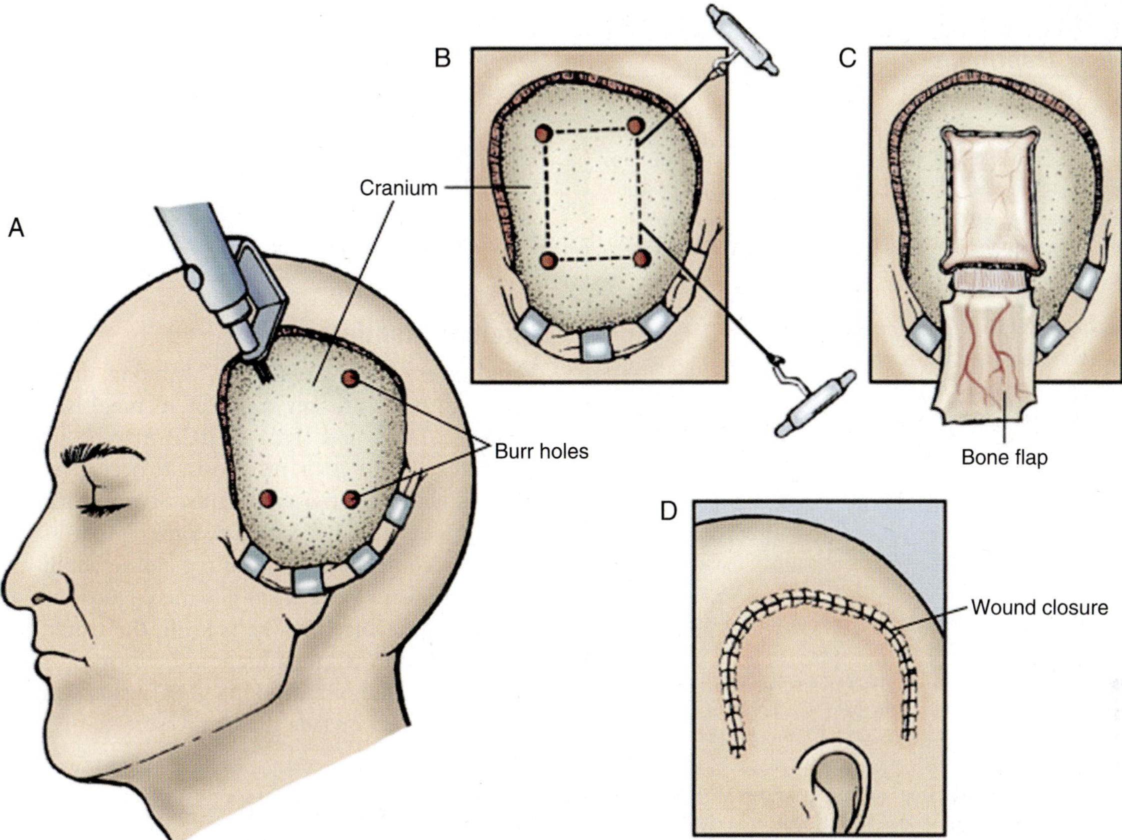

Fig. 61.16 Craniotomy. (A) Burr holes are drill into skull. (B) Skull is cut between burr holes with a surgical saw. (C) Bone flap is turned back to expose cranial contents. (D) Bone flap is replaced and wound closed. (From Monahan F, Sands J, Neighbors M, et al: *Phipps' medical-surgical nursing: health and illness perspectives,* ed 9, St Louis, 2007, Mosby.)

The rehabilitative potential depends on the reason for the surgery, postoperative course, and their general state of health. Base your care on a realistic appraisal of these factors. Specific rehabilitation potential cannot be determined until cerebral edema and IICP subside postoperatively (Box 61.3). An overall goal is to foster independence for as long as possible and to the highest degree possible.

Take care to maintain as much function as possible through measures such as careful positioning, meticulous skin and mouth care, regular range-of-motion exercises, bowel and bladder care, and adequate nutrition. Address the needs and problems of each patient individually because many variables affect the plan.

Collaborate with other specialists. The physical therapist may provide an exercise plan to regain functional deficits. A speech therapist will help patients with communication and swallowing skills. The patient's mental and physical deterioration, including seizures, personality disorganization, apathy, and wasting, is difficult for families and health care professionals. Cognitive and emotional residual deficits are often harder to accept than are motor and sensory losses. Social workers can help patients and family members adapt to changes in their home life, work, and financial circumstances.

INFLAMMATORY BRAIN CONDITIONS

Brain abscesses, meningitis, and encephalitis are the most common inflammatory conditions of the brain and spinal cord (Table 61.17). Inflammation can be caused by bacteria, viruses, fungi, and chemicals (e.g., contrast media used in diagnostic tests, blood in the subarachnoid space). CNS infections may occur via the bloodstream, by extension from a primary site, or along cranial and spinal nerves.

The mortality rate for inflammatory conditions of the brain is about 10% to 15%. Rates are higher in older and immunosuppressed patients. Some who recover have long-term neurologic deficits, including hearing loss.[15]

BACTERIAL MENINGITIS

Meningitis is an acute inflammation of the meningeal tissues surrounding the brain and spinal cord. It usually occurs in fall, winter, or early spring and is often related to a viral respiratory disease. Older adults and persons who are debilitated are affected more often. College students living in dormitories and people living in institutions (e.g., prisoners) have a high risk for

BOX 61.3 ETHICAL/LEGAL DILEMMAS

Withholding Treatment

Situation

C.J., a 26-year-old patient in a permanent vegetative state after a craniotomy for brain trauma, is diagnosed with her 15th bladder infection. As the home care nurse, you must determine whether to seek antibiotics for this infection. The family members have expressed that no heroic measures be used to extend her life. However, they do not want to stop enteral nutrition. Should antibiotics be withheld?

Ethical/Legal Points for Consideration

- Patients in a persistent vegetative state do not recover.
- The main legal issue here is who has the legal right to refuse or consent to treatment for this incapacitated patient. You need to know if a guardian has been appointed by the court or if her parents retain a form of guardianship to make health care decisions for her.
- You need to know when the vegetative state began. Did the patient ever have the right to consent, having reached the age of majority as a competent adult, or did the vegetative state begin while she was a minor? If the patient did become a competent adult before the vegetative state, did she ever express any preference for quality-of-life and end-of-life decision making?
- The courts have widespread legal precedents for accepting the decision of the patient's guardian or parents or the patient's clearly expressed preferences for quality-of-life decision making.
- Life-sustaining treatment is any treatment that serves to prolong life without reversing the underlying medical condition. Common life-sustaining treatments include mechanical ventilation, dialysis, chemotherapy, antibiotics, and artificial nutrition and hydration.
- There is no ethical distinction between withdrawing and withholding life-sustaining treatment. If there is not adequate evidence of the incompetent patient's preferences and values, the decision should be based on the best interests of the patient (i.e., what outcome will promote the patient's well-being).

Discussion Questions

1. How would you approach C.J.'s family?
2. What are your feelings about providing nutrition, hydration, and treatments that will prolong life in a patient for whom there is no hope of recovery?
3. What options are available to the family for the care of their daughter once a decision is made about withholding antibiotics?

meningitis. Untreated bacterial meningitis has a high mortality rate.[16]

Etiology and Pathophysiology

Streptococcus pneumoniae and *Neisseria meningitidis* are the leading causes of bacterial meningitis. *N. meningitides* has at least 13 different subtypes (serogroups), with 5 of them (A, B, C, Y, W) causing most cases. *Haemophilus influenzae* vaccination has significantly decreased meningitis from this organism.

Organisms usually gain entry to the CNS through the upper respiratory tract or bloodstream. Less often, they may enter by direct extension from penetrating skull wounds or through fractured sinuses in basilar skull fractures.

The inflammatory response to the infection increases CSF production with a moderate increase in ICP. In bacterial meningitis, the purulent secretions quickly spread to other areas of the brain through the CSF and cover the CNs and other intracranial structures. If this process extends into the brain parenchyma or if concurrent encephalitis is present, cerebral edema and IICP become more of a problem. ICP can increase from swelling around the dura and increased CSF volume.

Clinical Manifestations

Fever, severe headache, nausea, vomiting, and **nuchal rigidity** (neck stiffness) are key signs of meningitis. Photophobia, a decreased LOC, and signs of IICP may be present. Coma is associated with a poor prognosis. It occurs in 5% to 10% of patients with bacterial meningitis. Seizures occur in one-third of all cases. The headache becomes progressively worse. It may be accompanied by vomiting and irritability.

If the infecting organism is a meningococcus, a skin rash is common. Petechiae may be seen on the trunk, lower extremities, and mucous membranes. Perform a *tumbler test* by pressing the base of a drinking glass against the rash. The rash does not blanch or fade under pressure.

Complications

The most common acute complication of bacterial meningitis is IICP, and most patients have it. IICP is the major cause of an altered mental status.

Another complication is residual neurologic problems. It often involves many CNs. CN irritation can have serious sequelae. The optic nerve (CN II) is compressed by IICP. Papilledema is often present. Blindness may occur. When CN III, CN IV, and CN VI are irritated, ocular movements are affected. Ptosis, unequal pupils, and diplopia are common. CN V irritation results in sensory losses and loss of the corneal reflex. Irritation of CN VII results in facial paresis. Irritation of CN VIII causes tinnitus, vertigo, and deafness. The dysfunction usually disappears within a few weeks. For a few, hearing loss is permanent.

Hemiparesis, dysphasia, and hemianopsia may occur. These signs usually resolve over time. If they do not, suspect a cerebral abscess, subdural empyema, subdural effusion, or persistent meningitis. Acute cerebral edema may cause seizures, CN III palsy, bradycardia, hypertensive coma, and death.

Headaches may occur for months until the irritation and inflammation have completely resolved. It is important to implement pain management for chronic headaches.

A noncommunicating hydrocephalus may occur if the exudate causes adhesions that prevent the normal flow of CSF from the ventricles. CSF reabsorption by the arachnoid villi may be obstructed by the exudate. In this situation, surgical implantation of a shunt is the only treatment.

Waterhouse-Friderichsen syndrome is a complication of meningococcal meningitis. The syndrome is manifested by

TABLE 61.17 Cerebral Inflammatory Conditions

	Meningitis	Encephalitis	Brain Abscess
Cause	Bacteria (*Streptococcus pneumoniae, Neisseria meningitidis,* group B streptococci, viruses, fungi)	Bacteria, fungi, parasites, herpes simplex virus (HSV), other viruses (e.g., West Nile virus)	Streptococci, staphylococci through bloodstream
Cerebrospinal Fluid (Reference Interval)			
Pressure (<20 mm H_2O)	Bacterial: 200–500 Viral: ≤250	Normal to slight ↑	↑
WBC count (0–5 cells/μL)	Bacterial: >1000/μL (mainly neutrophils) Viral: 25–500/μL (mainly lymphocytes)	500/μL, neutrophils (early), lymphocytes (later)	25–300/μL (neutrophils)
Protein (15–45 mg/dL [0.15–0.45 g/L])	Bacterial: >500 mg/dL Viral: 50–500 mg/dL	Slight ↑	Normal
Glucose (50–77 mg/dL [2.2–3.9 mmol/L])	Bacterial: 5–40 Viral: Normal or low >40	Normal	↓ or absent
Appearance	Bacterial: Turbid, cloudy Viral: Clear or cloudy	Clear	Clear
Diagnostic Studies	CT scan, Gram stain, smear, culture, PCR	CT scan, EEG, MRI, PET, PCR, IgM antibodies to virus in serum or CSF	CT scan
Treatment	Antibiotics, dexamethasone, supportive care, prevent ↑ ICP	Supportive care, prevent ↑ ICP, acyclovir (Zovirax) for HSV	Antibiotics, incision and drainage Supportive care

petechiae, disseminated intravascular coagulation (DIC), adrenal hemorrhage, and circulatory collapse. DIC and shock, which are some of the most serious complications of meningitis, are associated with meningococcemia. DIC is discussed in detail in Chapter 34.

Diagnostic Studies

A blood culture and CT scan should be done for patients with manifestations that suggest bacterial meningitis. Diagnosis is usually verified by doing an LP with CSF analysis (Table 61.17). An LP should be done only after the CT scan has ruled out an obstruction in the foramen magnum to prevent a fluid shift resulting in herniation.

CSF, sputum, and nasopharyngeal secretions are taken for culture before the start of antibiotic therapy to identify the causative organism. A Gram stain can detect bacteria. Neutrophils are the main white blood cell type in the CSF with bacterial meningitis.

Skull x-rays may show infected sinuses. CT scans and MRI may be normal in uncomplicated meningitis. In other cases, CT scans may show signs of IICP or hydrocephalus.

Interprofessional Care

Bacterial meningitis is a medical emergency. Rapid diagnosis based on history and physical assessment is crucial because patients are usually in a critical state when health care is sought. When meningitis is suspected, antibiotic therapy is begun after collecting cultures, even before the diagnosis is confirmed (Table 61.18).

Ampicillin, penicillin, vancomycin, cefuroxime, ceftriaxone, and ceftazidime are the main drugs given to treat bacterial meningitis. Dexamethasone may be given before or with the first dose of antibiotics. Collaborate with the HCP to manage the headache, fever, and nuchal rigidity from meningitis.

NURSING MANAGEMENT: BACTERIAL MENINGITIS

Assessment

Initial assessment should include vital signs, neurologic assessment, fluid intake and output, and evaluation of the lungs and skin.

Clinical Problems

Clinical problems for patients with bacterial meningitis may include:

- Increased ICP
- Inadequate tissue perfusion
- Altered body temperature
- Pain

Additional information on clinical problems and interventions for patients with bacterial meningitis is presented in eNursing Care Plan 61.2 (available on the website for this chapter).

TABLE 61.18 Interprofessional Care

Bacterial Meningitis

Diagnostic Assessment
- History and physical assessment
- Analysis of CSF (for protein, WBC, glucose), Gram stain, and culture
- CBC, coagulation profile, electrolyte levels, glucose, platelet count
- Blood culture
- CT scan, MRI, PET scan
- Skull x-ray studies

Management
- Rest
- IV fluid
- Hypothermia

Drug Therapy
- IV antibiotics
  - ampicillin, penicillin
  - cephalosporin (e.g., ceftriaxone)
- codeine for headache
- dexamethasone
- acetaminophen or aspirin for temperature >100.4°F (38°C)
- IV phenytoin
- IV mannitol (Osmitrol) for diuresis

◆ Planning

The overall goals for patients with bacterial meningitis are to (1) return to maximal neurologic functioning, (2) resolve the infection, and (3) control pain and discomfort.

◆ Implementation

Health Promotion

Prevention of respiratory tract infections through vaccination programs for pneumococcal pneumonia and influenza is important. Meningococcal vaccines are available that protect against the serogroups that occur most often in the United States. However, they will not prevent all cases. Two types of meningococcal vaccines are available in the United States:

- Meningococcal conjugate vaccines (MCV4) (Menactra, Menveo)
- Serogroup B meningococcal vaccines (Bexsero, Trumenba)

Early treatment of respiratory tract and ear infections is important. Persons who have close contact with anyone who has bacterial meningitis should receive prophylactic antibiotics.

Acute Care

Patients with bacterial meningitis are usually acutely ill. Changes in mental status and LOC depend on the degree of IICP. Assess vital signs, neurologic status, intake and output, skin, and lung sounds at regular intervals based on patients' condition. Implement measures to manage IICP. Administer antibiotics as scheduled to maintain therapeutic blood levels.

Head pain is often severe. Neck and head pain with movement requires attention. Codeine provides some pain relief without undue sedation for most patients. Assist patients to a position of comfort, often curled up with the head slightly extended. Elevate the head of the bed slightly.

All patients have some degree of mental distortion and hypersensitivity. They may be frightened and misinterpret the environment. Make every attempt to minimize environment stimuli and prevent injury. For patients with delirium, low lighting may decrease hallucinations. A darkened room and a cool cloth over the eyes relieve photophobia. A familiar person at the bedside may have a calming effect. Be efficient with care while conveying an attitude of caring and unhurried gentleness. The use of touch and a soothing voice to give simple explanations of activities is helpful.

Irritation of the cerebral cortex may cause seizures. If seizures occur, assess the patient and take protective measures. Give antiseizure drugs, such as phenytoin or levetiracetam, as ordered.

The fever is high. Fever is vigorously treated because it increases cerebral edema and the risk for seizures. Neurologic damage may result from a high fever over a prolonged time. Acetaminophen or aspirin may be given. If the fever is resistant to aspirin or acetaminophen, more vigorous means are needed (e.g., cooling blanket). Do not reduce the temperature too rapidly because shivering may result, causing a rebound effect and increasing the temperature and ICP. Wrap the extremities in soft towels or a blanket covered with a sheet to reduce shivering. If a cooling blanket is not available or desirable, tepid sponge baths with water may be effective in lowering the temperature. Protect the skin from excessive drying and injury and prevent breaks in the skin.

Because high fever increases the metabolic rate and insensible fluid loss, assess for dehydration and adequacy of fluid intake. Calculate replacement fluids as 800 mL/day for respiratory losses and 100 mL for each degree of temperature greater than 100.4°F (38°C). Supplemental feeding (e.g., enteral nutrition) may be needed to maintain adequate nutrition.

Meningococcal meningitis is highly contagious. Maintain respiratory isolation until the cultures are negative. Other causes of meningitis may pose minimal to no infection risk with patient contact. They do not need isolation.

After the acute period has passed, patients need several weeks of recovery before resuming normal activities. In this period, stress the importance of adequate nutrition. Encourage a high-protein, high-calorie diet in small, frequent feedings.

Muscle rigidity may persist in the neck and back of the legs. Progressive range-of-motion exercises and warm baths are useful. Have patients gradually increase activity as tolerated, but encourage adequate rest and sleep.

Residual effects can result in sequelae such as dementia, seizures, deafness, hemiplegia, and hydrocephalus. Assess vision, hearing, cognitive skills, and motor and sensory abilities after recovery. Provide patients with needed referrals. Throughout the acute and recovery periods, be aware of the anxiety and stress felt by the caregiver and other family members.

◆ Evaluation

The expected outcomes are that patients with bacterial meningitis will:

- Maintain baseline cognitive function
- Maintain body temperature within normal range
- Report satisfaction with pain control

VIRAL MENINGITIS

The most common causes of viral meningitis are enteroviruses, arboviruses, HIV, and herpes simplex virus (HSV). Enteroviruses most often spread through direct contact with respiratory secretions. Viral meningitis usually presents as a headache, fever, photophobia, and stiff neck.[16] The fever may be moderate or high.

Many laboratories perform molecular testing through polymerase chain reaction (PCR) techniques. This allows faster results than previous viral-only testing and produces results for bacterial, viral, and fungal pathogens. Results are available within hours of symptom onset.[16]

Antibiotics should be given after the LP while awaiting the results of the CSF analysis. We can discontinue them if the meningitis is found to be viral.

Viral meningitis is managed symptomatically because the disease is self-limiting. A full recovery is expected. Rare sequelae include persistent headaches, mild mental impairment, and incoordination.

BRAIN ABSCESS

Brain abscess is an accumulation of pus within the brain tissue from a local or systemic infection. Direct extension from an ear, tooth, mastoid, or sinus infection is the main cause. Other causes include spread from a distant site (e.g., pulmonary infection, bacterial endocarditis), skull fracture, and prior brain trauma or surgery. Streptococci and *Staphylococcus aureus* are the most common infective organisms.

Manifestations are similar to meningitis and encephalitis. They include headache, fever, and nausea and vomiting. Signs of IICP may include drowsiness, confusion, and seizures. Focal symptoms may reflect the local area of the abscess. For example, visual field defects and seizures are common with a temporal lobe abscess. Vision problems and hallucinations may accompany an occipital abscess. CT and MRI are used to diagnose a brain abscess.

Antimicrobial therapy is the main treatment. Other manifestations are treated symptomatically. If drug therapy is not effective, the abscess may have to be drained or removed if it is encapsulated.

Nursing care is similar to those for patients with meningitis and IICP. The nursing care for patients with surgical drainage or removal is similar to that for patients having cranial surgery.

ENCEPHALITIS

Encephalitis is an acute inflammation of the brain. It is a serious and sometimes fatal disease. Several thousand cases occur in the United States each year. It is usually caused by a virus. Many different viruses can cause encephalitis. Some are associated with certain seasons of the year or endemic to certain geographic areas.

Ticks and mosquitoes transmit epidemic encephalitis, such as La Crosse and West Nile.[16] Nonepidemic encephalitis may occur as a complication of measles, chickenpox, or mumps. HSV encephalitis is the most common cause of acute nonepidemic viral encephalitis. Cytomegalovirus encephalitis occurs in patients with AIDS.

Clinical Manifestations and Diagnostic Studies

Encephalitis can be acute or subacute. The onset is typically nonspecific, with fever, headache, nausea, and vomiting. CNS signs appear on day 2 or 3. They vary from minimal changes in mental status to coma. Virtually any CNS problem can occur, including hemiparesis, tremors, seizures, CN palsies, personality changes, impaired memory, amnesia, and dysphasia.

Early diagnosis and treatment are essential for favorable outcomes. Diagnostic findings are shown in Table 61.17. Brain imaging techniques include CT, MRI, and PET. PCR tests allow for early detection of HSV and West Nile encephalitis. West Nile virus should be strongly considered in adults over 50 years old who develop encephalitis or meningitis in summer or early fall. The best diagnostic test for West Nile virus is a blood test that detects viral RNA. This test is also used to screen donated blood, organs, cells, and tissues.

Interprofessional and Nursing Management

Encephalitis prevention focuses on mosquito control. Measures include cleaning rain gutters, removing old tires, draining bird baths, and removing water where mosquitoes can breed. Insect repellent should be used during mosquito season.

Management is symptomatic and supportive. In the initial stages of encephalitis, many patients need intensive care. We treat seizure disorders with antiseizure drugs. Prophylactic treatment with antiseizure drugs may be used in severe cases of encephalitis.

Acyclovir (Zovirax) is used to treat encephalitis caused by HSV infection. Its use reduces mortality rates, although neurologic complications may still occur. For maximal benefit, it should start before the onset of coma. Treatment of cytomegalovirus encephalitis in patients with AIDS is discussed in Chapter 15.

CASE STUDY

Traumatic Brain Injury

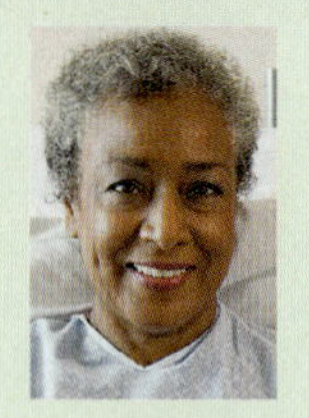

(© monkeybusiness images/iStock.com.)

Patient Profile

C.G. is a 74-year-old female who presents to the emergency room today after sustaining a fall. She tripped over a rock while walking her dog, falling forward and striking the right side of her face. The incident occurred 1 week ago. She was able to get up and walk the rest of the way home. She lives alone. She takes a "blood thinner" but cannot recall which one.

Subjective Data

- Reports a progressive headache since the fall and feels her left arm is weak
- Rates her headache 7/10 in severity with some associated nausea, but not vomiting

Objective Data

- Awake and alert, oriented × 4
- Left arm is slightly weaker than her right arm
- No facial asymmetry noted
- Right eye periorbital hematoma, appears subacute
- CN II–XII intact
- Vital signs: Afebrile, HR 87 to 120 irregular, BP 178/90, RR 18, SpO_2 94% on RA
- Right pupil, 3 mm sluggishly reactive; left pupil, 3 mm briskly reactive

An ECG strip is shown here:

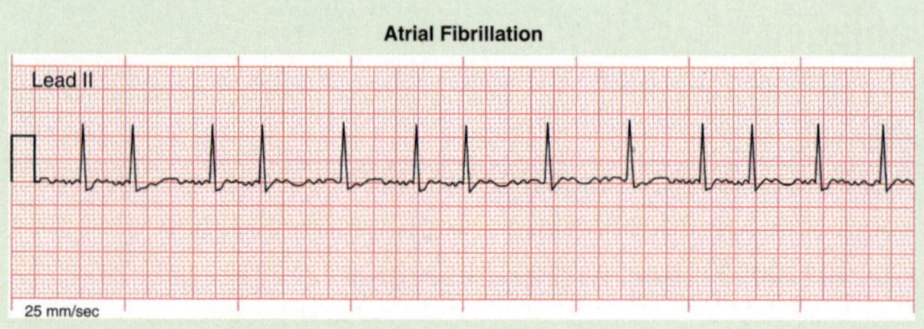

(© alfa md/iStock.com.)

Diagnostic Studies

- CT scan of the head shows a subacute subdural hematoma with a 2-mm midline shift; negative for skull fractures
- CT scan of neck negative for fractures or dislocations

Discussion Questions

1. ***Recognize***: What risk factors do you identify that led to C.G.'s condition?
2. ***Analyze***: Based on the assessment data presented, what are the priority clinical problems?
3. ***Prioritize***: What are the care priorities for C.G. right now?
4. ***Plan***: How can the interprofessional team work together to meet her needs?
5. ***Act***: What priority interventions would you include in the plan of care?
6. ***Safety***: What measures would you implement to promote C.G.'s safety?
7. ***Evaluate***: What do you need to monitor?

Answers available at http://evolve.elsevier.com/Lewis/medsurg.

BRIDGE TO NCLEX EXAMINATION

The number of the question corresponds to the same-numbered outcome at the beginning of the chapter.

1. Vasogenic cerebral edema increases intracranial pressure by
- **a.** shifting fluid in the gray matter.
- **b.** disrupting the blood-brain barrier.
- **c.** leaking molecules from the intracellular fluid to the capillaries.
- **d.** altering the osmotic gradient flow into the intravascular component.

2. A patient with intracranial pressure monitoring has a pressure of 12 mm Hg. The nurse understands that this pressure reflects
- **a.** a severe decrease in cerebral perfusion pressure.
- **b.** an alteration in the production of cerebrospinal fluid.
- **c.** the loss of autoregulatory control of intracranial pressure.
- **d.** a normal balance among brain tissue, blood, and cerebrospinal fluid.

3. The *best* way to position patients with increased intracranial pressure is to
- **a.** keep the head of the bed flat.
- **b.** elevate the head of the bed to 30 degrees.
- **c.** maintain patients on the left side with the head supported on a pillow.
- **d.** use a continuous-rotation bed to continuously change patient position.

4. The nurse would monitor for a possible acute subdural hematoma in the patient who
- **a.** has a linear skull fracture crossing a major artery.
- **b.** has focal symptoms of brain damage with no recollection of a head injury.
- **c.** develops decreased level of consciousness and a headache within 48 hours of a head injury.
- **d.** has an immediate loss of consciousness with a brief lucid interval followed by decreasing level of consciousness.

5. During admission of a patient with a severe head injury to the emergency department, the nurse places the *highest* priority on assessment of
- **a.** airway patency.
- **b.** presence of a neck injury.
- **c.** neurologic status with the Glasgow Coma Scale.
- **d.** cerebrospinal fluid leakage from the ears or nose.

6. A patient suspected of having a brain tumor has memory deficits, vision changes, right upper and lower extremity weakness, and personality changes. The nurse determines that the tumor is likely located in the
- **a.** frontal lobe.
- **b.** parietal lobe.
- **c.** occipital lobe.
- **d.** temporal lobe.

7. Management of patients with a brain tumor includes (**Select all that apply.**)
   a. discussing with patients methods to control inappropriate behavior.
   b. using diversion techniques to keep patients stimulated and motivated.
   c. assisting and supporting the family in understanding any behavior changes.
   d. limiting self-care activities until patients regain maximum physical functioning.
   e. planning for seizure precautions and teaching patients and caregivers about antiseizure drugs.
8. The nurse on the clinical unit is assigned to 4 patients. Which patient would be assessed *first*?
   a. Patient with a skull fracture whose nose is bleeding
   b. A patient with an acute stroke who is confused and whose daughter is present
   c. Patient with meningitis who is suddenly agitated and reporting a headache of 10 on a 0 to 10 scale
   d. Patient 2 days postoperative after a craniotomy for a brain tumor who has had continued vomiting
9. A nursing measure that can reduce the potential for seizures and increased intracranial pressure in patients with bacterial meningitis is
   a. administering codeine for relief of head and neck pain.
   b. controlling fever with prescribed drugs and cooling techniques.
   c. maintaining strict bed rest with the head of the bed slightly elevated.
   d. keeping the room dark and quiet to minimize environment stimulation.

1. b; 2. d; 3. b; 4. c; 5. a; 6. a; 7. c, e; 8. c; 9. b.

For rationales to these answers and even more NCLEX review questions, visit http://evolve.elsevier.com/Lewis/medsurg.

REFERENCES

To access the References for this chapter, please scan the QR code with a mobile device.

62

Stroke

Rebekah O. Filson

http://evolve.elsevier.com/Lewis/medsurg/

CONCEPTUAL FOCUS

Family Dynamics
Functional Ability
Intracranial Regulation
Mobility
Safety
Sensory Perception

LEARNING OUTCOMES

1. Describe risk factors for stroke.
2. Compare and contrast the etiology and pathophysiology of ischemic and hemorrhagic strokes.
3. Correlate the clinical manifestations of stroke with the underlying pathophysiology.
4. Identify diagnostic studies done for patients with strokes.
5. Distinguish the interprofessional care for patients with ischemic strokes and hemorrhagic strokes.
6. Describe the acute nursing management of patients with a stroke.
7. Describe the rehabilitative care of patients with a stroke.

KEY TERMS

aneurysm
aphasia
cerebrovascular accident (CVA)
dysarthria
dysphasia
embolic stroke
hemorrhagic strokes
intracerebral hemorrhage
ischemic stroke
stroke
subarachnoid hemorrhage (SAH)
thrombotic stroke
transient ischemic attack (TIA)

Stroke, or **cerebrovascular accident (CVA)**, occurs when there is (1) *ischemia* (inadequate blood flow) to a part of the brain or (2) *hemorrhage* (bleeding) into the brain that results in the death of brain cells. In a stroke, functions such as movement, sensation, thinking, talking, or emotions that were controlled by the affected area of the brain are lost or impaired. The severity of the loss of function varies based on the location and extent of the brain damage.

Stroke is a major public health concern. About 800,000 people have a stroke each year with more than 160,000 deaths.[1] An estimated 7.8 million adults in the United States have had a stroke. With an aging population, we can expect these numbers to increase. A stroke can occur at any age. About 38% of strokes occur in people younger than 65 years old.[1]

A stroke is a lifelong change for the stroke survivor and family. Stroke is the leading cause of long-term disability. Up to 30% of survivors have a permanent disability. Common long-term disabilities include *hemiparesis* (partial paralysis on 1 side), inability to walk, complete or partial dependence for activities of daily living (ADLs), *aphasia* (dysfunction in communication), and depression.

RISK FACTORS

The most effective way to decrease the burden of stroke is prevention and teaching, especially about risk factors. We divide risk factors into nonmodifiable and modifiable (Table 62.1). Stroke risk increases with multiple risk factors. Modifiable risk factors are those that can potentially be altered through lifestyle changes and medical treatment, thus reducing stroke risk. Thus primary prevention focuses on reducing modifiable risk factors.

TABLE 62.1 Risk Factors for Stroke

- Age
- Alcohol use
- Atrial fibrillation
- Blood clotting disorders (e.g., factor V Leiden mutation)
- Cardiomyopathy
- Diabetes
- Diet and nutrition
- Dyslipidemia
- Early-onset menopause
- Endometriosis
- Estrogen therapy for gender affirmation
- Ethnicity/race
- Family history
- Gender
- Heart valve disease and prosthetic heart valves
- Hypertension
- Illicit drug use, especially cocaine
- Inflammatory conditions (e.g., rheumatoid arthritis)
- Migraines with aura
- Myocardial infarction
- Physical inactivity
- Obesity
- Obstructive sleep apnea
- Sickle cell disease
- Smoking

Nonmodifiable

Nonmodifiable risk factors include age, gender, ethnicity or race, and family history. Stroke risk increases with age, doubling each decade after 55 years of age. Two-thirds of all strokes occur in persons older than 65 years. Strokes are more common in males, but more females die of stroke. Because females tend to live longer, they have more opportunity to have a stroke.[2]

Black people have twice the incidence of stroke and a higher death rate from stroke compared with any other ethnic group.[1] This may be related in part to higher rates of hypertension, obesity, and diabetes.

A person with a family history of stroke has an increased risk of having a stroke.[3] We think that genes encoding products involved in lipid metabolism, thrombosis, and inflammation are genetic factors for stroke. People who have at least 2 first-degree relatives with a history of subarachnoid hemorrhage (SAH) or aneurysm should be screened to rule out anomalies in their cerebral blood vessels.

Modifiable

Hypertension is the single most important modifiable risk factor.[4] Increases in systolic BP (SBP) and diastolic BP (DBP) independently increase stroke risk. Treating hypertension reduces stroke risk up to 50%. Guidelines include a goal of SBP less than 130 mm Hg.[5]

Heart disease, including atrial fibrillation, myocardial infarction (MI), cardiomyopathy, cardiac valve abnormalities, and congenital heart defects, is a risk factor for stroke. Atrial fibrillation causes about 25% of strokes after age 80. People with atrial fibrillation are 5 times more likely to have a stroke than people with a regular heart rhythm. Anticoagulants (e.g., warfarin, dabigatran) and adherence to their therapy play a key role in stroke prevention.

Diabetes is a significant risk factor for stroke. High glucose levels cause destructive changes in the blood vessels in the brain. If glucose levels are high at the time of a stroke, then brain damage is usually more severe.[4]

The effect of alcohol on stroke risk depends on the amount consumed. Females who drink more than 1 alcoholic drink per day and males who drink more than 2 alcoholic drinks per day are at higher risk for hypertension, which increases their chance of stroke. Increased alcohol consumption may be related to a higher risk of hemorrhagic stroke.

Physical inactivity and obesity are associated with hypertension, diabetes, and heart disease, which all increase stroke risk. A waist circumference to hip circumference ratio equal to or above the midvalue for the population increases the risk for ischemic stroke 3-fold.[4] Benefits of physical activity can occur with even light to moderate regular activity. The American Heart Association (AHA) recommends 150 minutes of moderate-intensity exercise or 75 minutes of vigorous-intensity exercise per week.[5] A diet high in fat and low in fruits and vegetables may increase stroke risk.

Use of hormone contraceptive in those with specific risk factors (age >35 years, tobacco use, hypertension, migraine with aura) increases stroke risk. The AHA recommends smoking cessation and alternatives to estrogen oral contraceptives for those females to reduce their risk of stroke.[5] Hormones used for gender transition can place patients in a higher risk category.

Transient Ischemic Attack

Another risk factor associated with stroke is a history of a **transient ischemic attack (TIA)**. A TIA is a transient episode of neurologic dysfunction caused by focal brain, spinal cord, or retinal ischemia, but without acute brain infarction. Symptoms typically last less than 1 hour.

TIAs may be due to microemboli that temporarily block the blood flow. TIAs are a warning sign of progressive cerebrovascular disease. There is no way to predict if a TIA will resolve or if it will progress to a stroke. In general, about 20% of people who have a TIA will progress to a stroke, with almost half occurring within 2 days.[6] The ABCD^2 score is a tool used to predict stroke risk after a TIA (Table 62.2).[7]

The signs and symptoms of a TIA depend on the blood vessel that is involved and the area of the brain that is ischemic. If the carotid system is involved, patients may have a temporary loss of vision in 1 eye *(amaurosis fugax),* transient hemiparesis, numbness or loss of sensation, or a sudden inability to speak.

Signs of a TIA involving the vertebrobasilar system may include tinnitus, vertigo, darkened or blurred vision, diplopia, ptosis, dysarthria, dysphagia, ataxia, and unilateral or bilateral numbness or weakness.

TABLE 62.2 ABCD² Score

The ABCD² score is a risk assessment tool. It is designed to predict stroke risk 2 days after a transient ischemic attack (TIA). Calculate the score by adding up points for 5 factors.

Risk Factor	Points
Age ≥60 years	1
Systolic BP ≥140 mm Hg *OR* diastolic BP ≥90 mm Hg	1
Clinical features of TIA (choose 1)	
• Unilateral weakness with or without impaired speech *OR*	2
• Impaired speech without unilateral weakness	1
Duration	
• TIA duration ≥60 min *OR*	2
• TIA duration 10–59 min	1
Diabetes	1
Total ABCD² score	0–7

ABCD² Score	2-Day Stroke Risk (%)	Care Needed
0–3	1.0	Hospitalization not needed unless there is another indication (e.g., new atrial fibrillation)
4–5	4.1	Hospitalization in most situations
6–7	8.1	Hospitalization

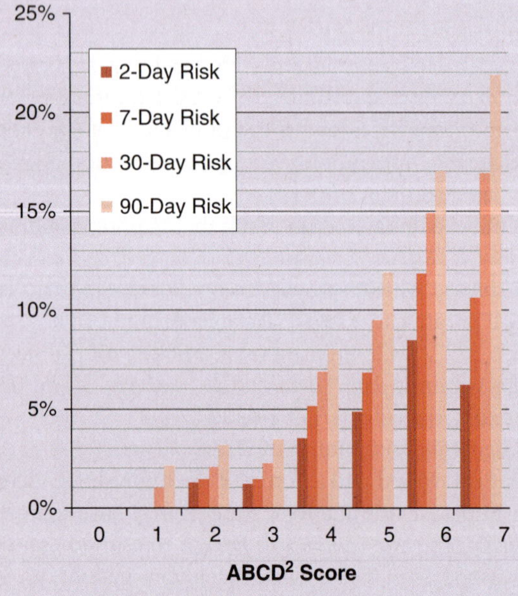

25%
20%
15%
10%
5%
0%
2-Day Risk
7-Day Risk
30-Day Risk
90-Day Risk
0 1 2 3 4 5 6 7
ABCD² Score

Permission obtained from National Stroke Association. Retrieved from https://www.stroke.org.

A TIA is considered a medical emergency since it can lead to an ischemic stroke. Teach people at risk for TIAs to seek medical attention at once with any stroke-like symptoms and to identify the time of onset of symptoms.

CHECK YOUR PRACTICE

You are talking with your uncle at your family reunion. He knows that you are a nurse and seems very eager to talk with you. He tells you that earlier this morning, he was having problems talking, got dizzy, and then "blanked" out for a while. He found himself just lying on the floor in his room. He says, "I think it is just all the excitement of the reunion."

- How would you respond?

TYPES OF STROKES

We classify strokes as ischemic or hemorrhagic based on the cause and underlying pathophysiologic findings (Fig. 62.1 and Table 62.3).

Ischemic Stroke

An **ischemic stroke** results from inadequate blood flow to the brain from partial or complete occlusion of an artery. About 87% of strokes are ischemic.[1] We classify ischemic strokes as thrombotic or embolic strokes.

Thrombotic Stroke

A **thrombotic stroke** occurs from injury to a blood vessel wall and formation of a blood clot (Fig. 62.1A). The lumen of the blood vessel becomes narrowed, and, if it becomes occluded, infarction occurs. Thrombosis develops readily where atherosclerotic plaques have already narrowed blood vessels. Thrombotic stroke is the most common cause of stroke. They are more common in older adults, especially those with high cholesterol, atherosclerosis, or diabetes. Most thrombotic strokes are associated with hypertension or diabetes, both of which accelerate atherosclerosis. Many times, a TIA precedes thrombotic strokes.

The extent of the stroke depends on rapidity of onset, size of the damaged area, and presence of collateral circulation. Most patients with ischemic stroke do not have a decreased level of consciousness (LOC) in the first 24 hours, unless it is due to a brainstem stroke or other condition, such as seizure, increased ICP, or hemorrhage. Manifestations of ischemic stroke may progress in the first 72 hours as infarction and cerebral edema increase.

Embolic Stroke

Embolic stroke occurs when an embolus lodges in and occludes a cerebral artery, resulting in infarction and edema of the area supplied by the involved vessel (Fig. 62.1B). Embolism is the second most common cause of stroke. Embolic strokes

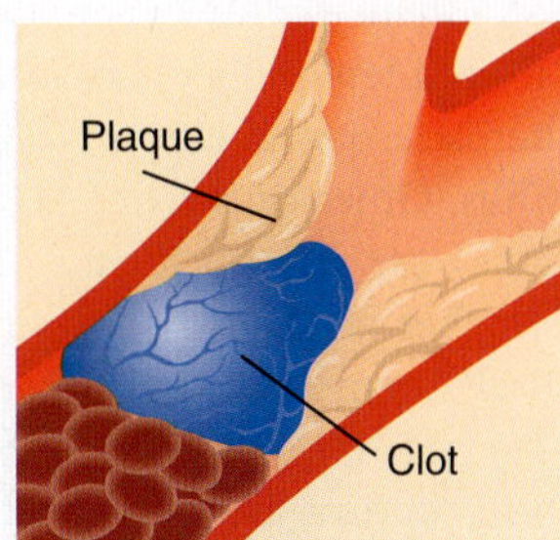

Thrombotic stroke. The process of clot formation (thrombosis) results in a narrowing of the lumen, which blocks the passage of the blood through the artery.

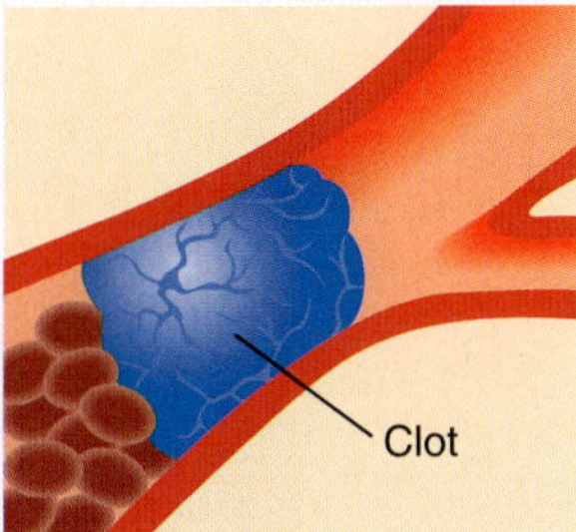

Embolic stroke. An embolus is a blood clot or other debris circulating in the blood. When it reaches an artery in the brain that is too narrow to pass through, it lodges there and blocks the flow of blood.

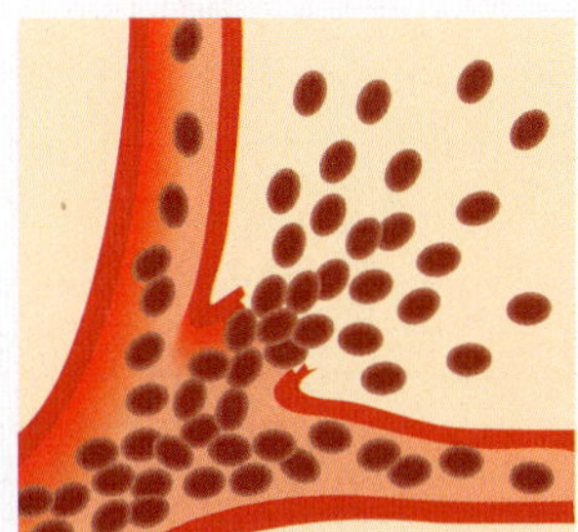

Hemorrhagic stroke. A burst blood vessel may allow blood to seep into and damage brain tissues until clotting shuts off the leak.

Fig. 62.1 Major types of strokes.

TABLE 62.3 Types of Strokes

Warning and Onset	Prognosis
Ischemic	
Embolic	
Warning: TIA (uncommon) *Onset:* Sudden onset, most likely to occur during activity	Single event. Signs and symptoms develop quickly, usually some improvement. Recurrence common without aggressive treatment of underlying disease.
Thrombotic	
Warning: TIA (30%–50% of cases) *Onset:* Often during or after sleep	Stepwise progression. Signs and symptoms develop slowly, usually some improvement. Recurrence in 20%–25% of survivors.
Hemorrhagic	
Intracerebral	
Warning: Headache (25% of cases) *Onset:* Activity (often)	Progression over 24 h. Poor prognosis, fatality more likely with presence of coma.
Subarachnoid	
Warning: Headache (common) *Onset:* Activity (often), sudden onset, most often related to head trauma	Usually single sudden event. Fatality more likely with presence of coma.

often occur rapidly, giving little time to accommodate an obstructed blood vessel by developing collateral circulation.

Most emboli originate in the endocardial (inside) layer of the heart when a plaque breaks off from the endocardium and enters the circulation. The embolus travels upward to the cerebral circulation and lodges where a vessel narrows or bifurcates (splits). Heart conditions, including atrial fibrillation, MI, infective endocarditis, heart valve disease and prostheses, and patent foramen ovale, cause most embolic ischemic strokes. Less common causes of emboli include air and fat from long bone (e.g., femur) fractures. Rheumatic heart disease is a cause of embolic stroke in young to middle-aged adults. An embolus from an atherosclerotic plaque is more common in older adults.

Patients with an embolic stroke often have a sudden onset of neurologic deficits that reach maximal intensity within minutes and then gradually improve. Patients may have a decline in mental status or change in level of consciousness. They may have a headache. The effects can be temporary if the clot breaks up and allows blood to flow. Smaller emboli then continue to obstruct smaller vessels, which in turn involve smaller portions of the brain with fewer deficits noted.

The prognosis is related to the amount of brain tissue deprived of its blood supply. Recurrence of embolic stroke is common unless the underlying cause is treated.

Hemorrhagic Stroke

Hemorrhagic strokes result from bleeding into the brain tissue itself (intracerebral or intraparenchymal hemorrhage) or into the subarachnoid space or ventricles (SAH or intraventricular hemorrhage).

Intracerebral Hemorrhage

Intracerebral hemorrhage is bleeding within the brain caused by a rupture of a vessel (usually in the basal ganglia) (Fig. 62.1C). The prognosis of patients with intracerebral hemorrhage is poor. The 30-day mortality rate is 40%.[8] Half of the survivors die in the first 2 years after the initial hemorrhage.

Hypertension is the most common cause (Fig. 62.2). Other causes include vascular malformations, coagulation disorders, anticoagulant and thrombolytic drugs, trauma, brain tumors, and ruptured aneurysms. Hemorrhage often occurs during periods of activity. Most often, there is a sudden onset of symptoms, with progression over minutes to hours because of ongoing bleeding. The extent of the symptoms varies depending on the amount, location, and duration of the

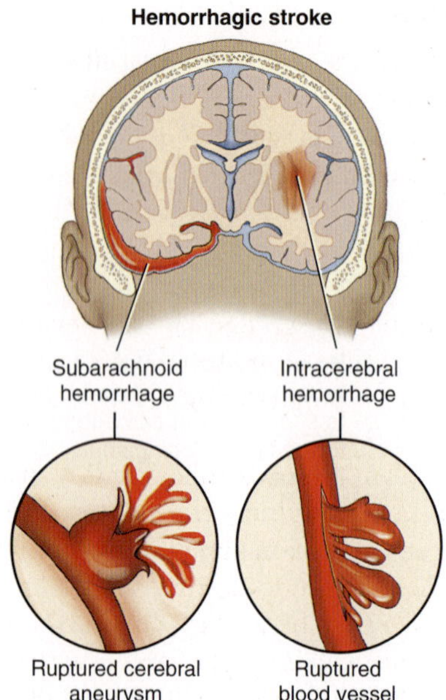

Fig. 62.2 Hemorrhagic strokes. (From Lafleur Brooks D, Brooks ML, Levinsky DM: *Basic medical language with flash cards,* ed 7, 2023, Elsevier.)

bleeding. A blood clot within the closed skull can result in a mass that causes pressure on brain tissue, displaces brain tissue, and decreases cerebral blood flow (CBF), leading to ischemia and infarction.

Most intracerebral hemorrhages occur in the cerebral lobes, cerebellum, pons, thalamus, subcortical white matter, internal capsule, or a part of the basal ganglia called the putamen. At first, patients have a severe headache with nausea and vomiting. Manifestations of putamen and internal capsule bleeding include weakness of 1 side (including the face, arm, and leg), slurred speech, and deviation of the eyes. Progression of symptoms related to a severe hemorrhage includes hemiplegia, fixed and dilated pupils, abnormal body posturing, and coma. Thalamic hemorrhage results in hemiplegia with more sensory than motor loss. Bleeding into the subthalamic areas of the brain leads to problems with vision and eye movement. Cerebellar hemorrhages are characterized by severe headache, vomiting, loss of ability to walk, dysphagia, dysarthria, and eye movement changes.

Hemorrhage in the pons is the most serious because basic life functions (e.g., respiration) are rapidly affected. Hemorrhage in the pons can be characterized by hemiplegia leading to complete paralysis, coma, abnormal body posturing, fixed pupils, hyperthermia, and death.

Subarachnoid Hemorrhage

Subarachnoid hemorrhage (SAH) occurs when there is intracranial bleeding into the cerebrospinal fluid (CSF)–filled space between the arachnoid and pia mater membranes on the surface of the brain. SAH is often caused by rupture of a cerebral **aneurysm** (congenital or acquired weakness and ballooning of vessels). Aneurysms may be saccular or berry aneurysms, ranging from a few millimeters to 20 to 30 mm in size, or fusiform atherosclerotic aneurysms. Most aneurysms are in the circle of Willis. Other causes of SAH include trauma and illicit drug (cocaine) use. The incidence of SAH increases with age. The rate is higher in females.

In general, cerebral aneurysms are viewed as a "silent killer" since people do not have warning signs or symptoms of an aneurysm until rupture has occurred. Patients may have warning signs and symptoms if the ballooning artery applies pressure to brain tissue. Minor warning symptoms may result from leaking of an aneurysm before major rupture.

CHECK YOUR PRACTICE

You are watching your husband's soccer game. He leaves the game and is kneeling on the ground. When you try to assess what is going on, he says, "I have a terrible headache. It just started." Knowing that he sometimes gets headaches when he is stressed, you ask him if he is feeling stressed. He almost screams back at you, "NO! This is the worst headache of my life!"

- What are 3 priority interventions?

LOC may range from alert to comatose, depending on the severity of the bleed. Other manifestations include focal neurologic deficits (including cranial nerve deficits), nausea, vomiting, seizures, and stiff neck.

Complications of aneurysmal SAH include rebleeding before surgery or other therapy is started and cerebral vasospasm (narrowing of the blood vessels), which can result in cerebral infarction. Cerebral vasospasm is likely due to an interaction between blood metabolites and the vascular smooth muscle. This occurs when the subarachnoid blood clots break down or dissolve, releasing metabolites that can cause endothelial damage and vasoconstriction. The release of endothelin (a potent vasoconstrictor) may play a key role in inducing cerebral vasospasm after SAH. Patients with SAH who are at risk for vasospasm are often in the intensive care unit (ICU) until the threat of vasospasm is reduced. Peak time for vasospasm is 6 to 10 days after the initial bleed.

Despite improvements in surgical techniques and management, many patients with SAH die. Some die almost immediately when a rupture occurs. Others die of subsequent bleeding. Survivors can have significant deficits, including cognitive problems.

CLINICAL MANIFESTATIONS

Neurologic manifestations do not significantly differ between ischemic and hemorrhagic stroke. This is because neural tissue destruction is the basis for neurologic dysfunction caused by both types of strokes. The manifestations are related to the location of the stroke. Specific manifestations related to the type of stroke were discussed in the previous section. General manifestations of ischemic and hemorrhagic stroke are discussed together here.

A stroke can affect many body functions, including motor activity, bladder and bowel function, intellect, spatial perception, personality, emotions, affect, sensation, swallowing, and communication. The functions affected are directly related to the artery involved and area of the brain that it supplies (Table 62.4). Manifestations related to right- and left-brain damage differ somewhat. These are shown in Fig. 62.3.

TABLE 62.4 Stroke Manifestations Related to Involved Artery

Artery	Manifestations
Anterior cerebral	Motor and/or sensory deficit (contralateral), sucking or rooting reflex, rigidity, gait problems, loss of proprioception and fine touch
Middle cerebral	*Dominant side:* Aphasia, motor and sensory deficit, hemianopsia *Nondominant side:* Neglect, motor and sensory deficit, hemianopsia
Posterior cerebral	Hemianopsia, visual hallucination, spontaneous pain, motor deficit
Vertebral	Cranial nerve deficits, diplopia, dizziness, nausea, vomiting, dysarthria, dysphagia, and/or coma

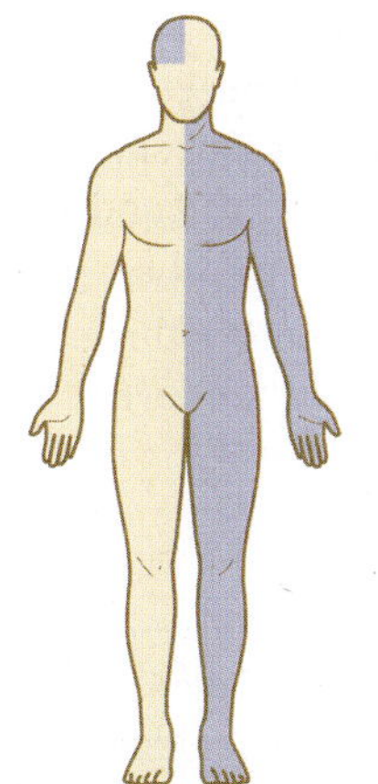

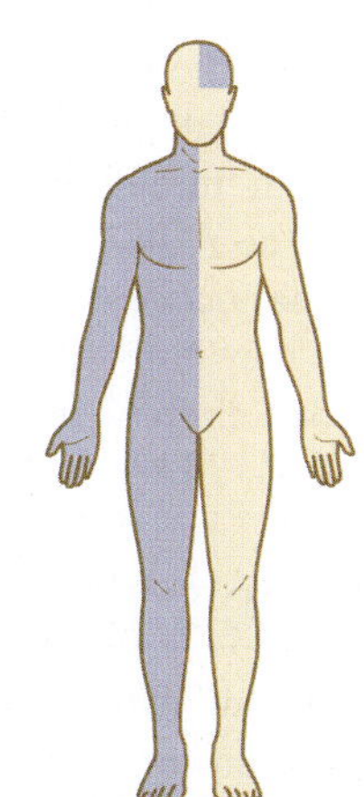

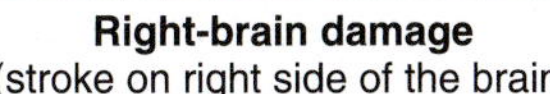

Right-brain damage
(stroke on right side of the brain)

- Paralyzed left side: hemiplegia
- Left-sided neglect
- Spatial-perceptual deficits
- Tends to deny or minimize problems
- Rapid performance, short attention span
- Impulsive, safety problems
- Impaired judgment
- Impaired time concepts

Left-brain damage
(stroke on left side of the brain)

- Paralyzed right side: hemiplegia
- Impaired speech/language aphasias
- Impaired right/left discrimination
- Slow performance, cautious
- Aware of deficits: depression, anxiety
- Impaired comprehension related to language, math

Fig. 62.3 Manifestations of right-brain and left-brain stroke.

Motor Function

Motor deficits are the most obvious effect. Motor deficits include impaired (1) mobility, (2) respiratory function, (3) swallowing and speech, (4) gag reflex, and (5) self-care abilities. Symptoms are caused by the destruction of motor neurons in the pyramidal pathway (nerve fibers from the brain that pass through the spinal cord to the motor cells). Characteristic motor deficits include loss of skilled voluntary movement *(akinesia),* impaired integration of movements, changes in muscle tone, and altered reflexes. The initial *hyporeflexia* (depressed reflexes) progresses to *hyperreflexia* (hyperactive reflexes) for most patients.

Motor deficits after a stroke follow certain specific patterns. Because the pyramidal pathway crosses at the level of the medulla, a lesion on 1 side of the brain affects motor function on the opposite side of the body (contralateral). The arms and legs of the affected side may be weakened or paralyzed to different degrees depending on which part of and to what extent cerebral circulation was compromised. A stroke affecting the middle cerebral artery leads to greater weakness in the upper extremity than the lower extremity. The affected shoulder tends to rotate internally, and the hip rotates externally. The affected foot is plantar flexed and inverted. An initial period of flaccidity may last from days to several weeks. It is related to nerve damage. Muscle spasticity follows the flaccid stage. It is related to interruption of upper motor neuron influence.

Communication

The left hemisphere is dominant for language skills in right-handed people and in most left-handed persons. Language disorders involve expression and comprehension of written and spoken words. Patients may have **aphasia**. Types of aphasia include *receptive aphasia* (loss of comprehension), *expressive aphasia* (inability to produce language), or *global aphasia* (total inability to communicate). Aphasia occurs when a stroke damages the dominant hemisphere of the brain.

Dysphasia refers to impaired ability to communicate. In most settings, the terms *aphasia* and *dysphasia* are used interchangeably. Aphasia is the more common term. Patterns of aphasia may differ since a stroke affects different portions of the brain. We describe aphasia as *nonfluent* (minimal speech activity with slow speech that requires obvious effort) or *fluent* (speech is present but has little meaningful communication) (Table 62.5). Most types of aphasia are mixed, with both impaired expression and understanding. A massive stroke may result in global aphasia.

Many patients have **dysarthria**, a problem with the muscle control and mechanics of speech. Impairment may involve pronunciation, articulation, and phonation. Dysarthria does not affect the meaning of communication or language comprehension. Some patients have a combination of aphasia and dysarthria.

Affect

Patients who had a stroke may have a hard time controlling their emotions. Emotional responses may be exaggerated or

TABLE 62.5 Types of Aphasia

Type	Characteristics
Broca	• Type of nonfluent aphasia • Damage to frontal lobe of brain • Often speak in short phrases that make sense but take great effort • Often omit small words (e.g., is, and, the) • May say, "Walk dog," meaning, "I will take the dog for a walk," or "Book 2 table," for "There are 2 books on the table" • Typically understands others' speech • Often aware of their difficulties and can become easily frustrated
Global	• Type of nonfluent aphasia • Results from damage to extensive portions of language areas of brain • Have severe communication difficulties • May be limited in ability to speak or understand language
Wernicke	• Type of fluent aphasia • Damage occurs in left temporal lobe, although it can result from damage to right lobe • May speak in long sentences that have no meaning, add unnecessary words, and even create made-up words • May say, "You know that smoodle pinkered and that I want to get him round and take care of him like you want before" • Usually have great difficulty understanding speech • Often unaware of their mistakes • Often difficult to follow what person is trying to say
Other	• From damage to different language areas in brain • Some may have trouble repeating words and sentences, even though they can speak and understand the meaning of the word or sentence • May have trouble naming objects, even though they know what the object is and what its use is

unpredictable. Depression and feelings due to changes in body image and loss of function can make this worse. Mobility and communication problems increase frustration.

Intellectual Function

A stroke may impair memory and judgment. These impairments can occur with strokes affecting either side of the brain. Patients may find it hard to make generalizations, interfering with their ability to learn.

A left-brain stroke is more likely to result in memory problems related to language. Patients with a right-brain stroke tend to be impulsive and move quickly. An example is that they try to rise quickly from a wheelchair without locking the wheels or raising the footrests. Patients with a left-brain stroke often are cautious in making judgments. They would move slowly and cautiously from the wheelchair.

Spatial-Perceptual Problems

Those who had a stroke on the right side of the brain are more likely to have problems with spatial-perceptual orientation. However, this can occur in people with left-brain stroke. Patients may or may not be aware of their spatial-perceptual problems. You need to assess for these problems as they will affect rehabilitation and recovery.

Spatial-perceptual problems fall within 4 categories:

- An incorrect perception of self and illness. Patients may deny their illnesses or not recognize their own body parts. This results from parietal lobe damage.
- Spatial neglect. This occurs when patients neglect all input from the affected side (erroneous perception of self in space). This may be worsened by *homonymous hemianopsia,* in which blindness occurs in the same half of the visual fields of both eyes. Patients have trouble with spatial orientation, such as judging distances.
- *Agnosia.* The inability to recognize an object by sight, touch, or hearing.
- *Apraxia.* The inability to carry out learned, sequential movements on command.

Elimination

Most urinary and bowel elimination problems are temporary. When a stroke affects 1 hemisphere of the brain, the prognosis for normal bladder function is excellent. At least partial sensation for bladder filling remains, and voluntary urination is present. At first, patients may have frequency, urgency, and incontinence. Although motor control of the bowel is usually not a problem, patients are often constipated. Constipation is associated with immobility, weak abdominal muscles, dehydration, and decreased response to the defecation reflex. Incontinence may occur if patients are not able to say they need to eliminate or they have difficulty managing clothing. Scheduled toileting and clothes that are easily removed encourage independence.

DIAGNOSTIC STUDIES

When manifestations of a stroke occur, diagnostic studies are done to (1) confirm that it is a stroke and (2) identify the likely cause of the stroke. Diagnostic study results guide decisions about therapy (Table 62.6). A key assessment is to determine the time of the onset of symptoms. This is especially important for ischemic strokes, since time can affect treatment decisions.

When a person suspected of TIA or stroke arrives in the emergency department or mobile stroke unit, it is important for them to rapidly undergo a noncontrast head CT or MRI. These tests can rapidly distinguish between ischemic and hemorrhagic stroke. They help determine the size and location of the stroke and treatment options. MRI is more effective in identifying ischemic stroke than CT scans. However, a CT scan is a rapid diagnostic tool to rule out hemorrhage. Serial scans can assess the effectiveness of treatment and evaluate recovery.

TABLE 62.6 Diagnostic Studies

Stroke

Diagnosis of Stroke (Including Extent of Involvement)
- CT scan
- CT angiography (CTA)
- CT/MRI perfusion and diffusion imaging
- MRI
- Magnetic resonance angiography (MRA)

Cerebral Blood Flow
- Carotid angiography
- Carotid duplex scanning
- Cerebral angiography
- Digital subtraction angiography
- Transcranial Doppler ultrasonography

Cardiac Assessment
- Cardiac markers (troponin, creatine kinase-MB)
- Chest x-ray
- Echocardiography (transthoracic, transesophageal)
- ECG

Additional Studies
- Coagulation studies: prothrombin time, activated partial thromboplastin time
- CBC (including platelets)
- Electrolyte panel with glucose
- Lipid profile
- Renal and hepatic studies

CT angiography (CTA) provides visualization of cerebral blood vessels. It can be done after or at the same time as the noncontrast CT scan. CTA can give an estimate of perfusion and detect filling defects in the cerebral arteries. Magnetic resonance angiography (MRA) can detect vascular lesions and blockages, similar to CTA. CT/MRI perfusion and diffusion imaging are other options.

If we suspect the cause of the stroke includes emboli from the heart, diagnostic cardiac tests are done. Cardiac imaging is recommended because many strokes are caused by blood clots from the heart. Blood tests can help identify conditions contributing to stroke and guide treatment (Table 62.1).

Angiography can identify cervical and cerebrovascular occlusion, atherosclerotic plaques, and malformation of vessels. Cerebral angiography can find the source of SAH. Risks of angiography include dislodging an embolus, causing vasospasm, inducing further hemorrhage, and provoking an allergic reaction to contrast media.

Intraarterial digital subtraction angiography (DSA) involves injecting a contrast agent to visualize blood vessels in the neck and the large vessels of the circle of Willis. It reduces the dose of contrast material, uses smaller catheters, and shortens the length of the procedure compared with conventional angiography. It is considered safer because there is less vascular manipulation.

Transcranial Doppler (TCD) ultrasonography is a noninvasive study that measures blood flow in the major cerebral arteries. TCD is effective in detecting microemboli and vasospasm. It is ideal for patients suspected of having an SAH. Carotid duplex scanning is used to detect the cause of the stroke and stratify patients for either medical management or carotid intervention if they have carotid stenosis.

An LP can determine whether red blood cells are present in the CSF if we suspect SAH and the CT does not show hemorrhage. An LP is avoided if we suspect an obstruction in the foramen magnum or other signs of increased ICP because of the danger of brain herniation. This could lead to pressure on cardiac and respiratory centers in the brainstem and potentially death.

The LICOX system may be used as a diagnostic tool to evaluate stroke progression. It measures brain oxygenation and temperature.

INTERPROFESSIONAL CARE

Preventive Therapy

Primary prevention is a priority for decreasing stroke. The goals of stroke prevention include adopting a healthy lifestyle and managing modifiable risk factors. Health promotion focuses on (1) healthy diet, (2) weight control, (3) regular exercise, (4) no smoking, (5) glucose control, (6) cholesterol control, and (7) BP management. Patients with known risk factors (e.g., diabetes, hypertension, obesity, high lipids, heart disease) need close management.

Preventive Drug Therapy

We use measures to prevent the development of a thrombus or embolus in patients with TIAs since they are at high risk for stroke. Antiplatelet drugs are a first-line treatment to prevent stroke in patients who had a TIA. Aspirin, at a dose of 81 mg/day, is the most often used antiplatelet agent. Some additional agents include ticlopidine, clopidogrel (Plavix), dipyridamole, and combined dipyridamole and aspirin (Aggrenox). Statins (e.g., atorvastatin) are effective for those with high cholesterol levels who had a TIA.

DRUG ALERT

Ticlopidine and Clopidogrel (Plavix)

- Inform all HCPs and dentists that the drug is being taken before surgery or major dental procedures.
- Therapy may be stopped 10 to 14 days before surgery if the antiplatelet effect is not desired.
- Monitor patients to determine whether there are any symptoms of a stroke.

For patients with atrial fibrillation, oral anticoagulation can include warfarin (Coumadin) and direct factor Xa inhibitors: rivaroxaban (Xarelto), dabigatran (Pradaxa), and apixaban (Eliquis). Other medications continue to be trialed and show a promising future. The advantage of direct factor Xa inhibitors compared with warfarin is that they do not need close monitoring or dosage adjustments.

Left Atrial Appendage Occlusion

The left atrial appendage (LAA) is a pouch that extends off the left atrium. We think the LAA is the source of many stroke-causing emboli in patients with atrial fibrillation. Removing or occluding the LAA decreases the risk of strokes. LAA occlusion can help prevent blood clot formation in patients with atrial fibrillation. It is an alternative for patients who cannot use oral anticoagulants, such as warfarin. After LAA occlusion, patients may be able to stop taking anticoagulants.

Patent Foramen Ovale

Patients with a patent foramen ovale have a hole between the left and right atriums. Blood clots can pass through this opening and go to the brain, leading to ischemia. An occlusion device implanted in the opening can prevent clot dislodgment and reduce the risk of stroke.[9]

Surgical/Endovascular Therapy for TIA and Stroke Prevention

Surgical interventions for patients with TIAs due to carotid disease include carotid endarterectomy (CEA), transluminal angioplasty, and stenting. In a *carotid endarterectomy,* the atheromatous lesion is removed from the carotid artery to improve blood flow.

Transluminal angioplasty involves inserting a balloon to open a stenosed artery in the brain and improve blood flow. The balloon is threaded up to the carotid artery through a catheter inserted in the femoral artery.

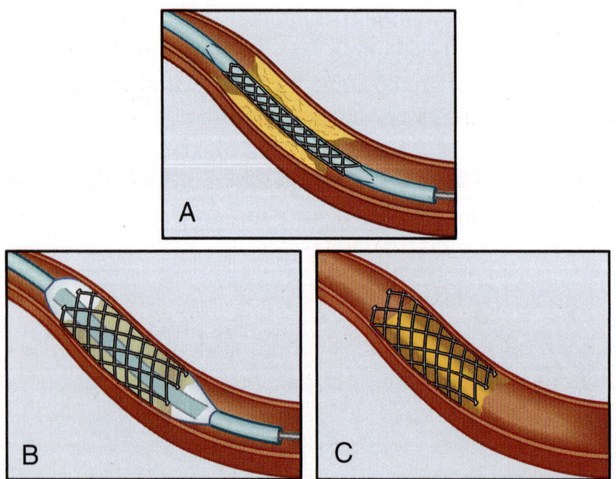

Fig. 62.4 Brain stent used to treat blockages in cerebral blood flow. (A) A balloon catheter is used to implant the stent into an artery of the brain. (B) The balloon catheter is moved to the blocked area of the artery and then inflated. The stent expands due to inflation of the balloon. (C) The balloon is deflated and withdrawn, leaving the stent permanently in place, holding the artery open, and improving the flow of blood.

Stenting involves the intravascular placement of a stent to try to maintain patency of the artery (Fig. 62.4). The stent can be inserted during angioplasty. Once in place, the system can be used with a tiny filter that opens like an umbrella. The filter catches and removes the debris that is stirred up during the stenting procedure before it floats to the brain, where it can trigger a stroke.

Care after stenting or angioplasty includes neurovascular assessment and BP management. Monitor vital signs. Assess for complications, including stent occlusion and bleeding. Minimize the risk for bleeding at the insertion site by keeping the leg straight for the prescribed time.

Acute Care for Ischemic Stroke

Care goals during the acute phase are preserving life, preventing further brain damage, and reducing disability (Table 62.7). For emergency care, patients should be transported to the closest certified stroke center. If one is not available, they should be sent to the closest place offering special emergency stroke care.[10] Some places have a mobile stroke unit that offers onsite emergency CT and point-of-care testing. Meeting 60-minute door-to-treatment time initiatives promotes better patient outcomes (Table 62.8).[11] The stroke (STK) core measures (Table 62.9) are proven standards of care that reduce complications and lead to better outcomes.

Table 62.10 outlines the emergency management of patients with a stroke. During initial evaluation, the single most important point in the history is the time of onset of symptoms. In the unresponsive person, acute care begins with assessing circulation, airway, and breathing. Patients may have difficulty keeping an open and clear airway because of a decreased LOC or decreased or absent gag and swallowing reflexes. Maintaining adequate oxygenation is important. O_2 administration, artificial airway insertion, and mechanical ventilation may be needed. Perform a baseline neurologic assessment.

Elevated BP is common right after a stroke. It may be a protective response to maintain cerebral perfusion. However, it can be detrimental. In patients with an ischemic stroke who do not receive thrombolytic therapy, the use of drugs to lower BP is recommended if BP is markedly increased (SBP greater than 220 mm Hg or DBP greater than 120 mm Hg). In patients who are receiving thrombolytic therapy, the BP must be less than 185/110 mm Hg and then maintained at or below 180/105 mm Hg for at least 24 hours after ending therapy. In an acute stroke, IV antihypertensives, such as labetalol and nicardipine, are preferred.

Although low BP right after a stroke is uncommon, we correct hypotension and hypovolemia if present. The goal is to keep patients adequately hydrated to promote perfusion and decrease further brain injury. We take care to control fluid and electrolyte balance. Overhydration may compromise perfusion by increasing ICP and cerebral edema.

Monitor urine output. If secretion of antidiuretic hormone (ADH) increases in response to the stroke, urine output

TABLE 62.7 Interprofessional Care

Acute Stroke

Diagnostic Assessment
- History and physical assessment
- Diagnostic studies (Table 62.5)

Management

Drug Therapy
- Platelet inhibitors (e.g., aspirin)
- Anticoagulation therapy for patients with atrial fibrillation

Surgical Therapy
- Carotid endarterectomy
- Stenting of carotid artery
- Transluminal angioplasty
- Surgical interventions for aneurysms at risk for bleeding

Acute Care
- Maintain airway
- Fluid therapy
- Treat cerebral edema
- Prevent secondary injury

Ischemic Stroke
- Tissue plasminogen activator (tPA) IV or intraarterial
- Endovascular therapy

Hemorrhagic Stroke
- Surgical decompression if indicated
- Clipping or coiling of aneurysm

Role of Interprofessional Team Members

Speech Therapy
- Assess swallowing reflex
- Evaluate for communication defects (e.g., aphasia)

Occupational Therapy
- Evaluate ability to perform self-care
- Teach to perform activities of daily living and adapting tasks

Physical Therapy
- Recommend functional position
- Assess function and, together with patient, plan a rehabilitation program

TABLE 62.8 Example of 60-Minute Stroke Time Interval Goals

Action	Time
Door to provider	≤5 min
Door to stroke team	≤10 min
Door to CT/MRI	≤25 min
Door to CT/MRI results	≤45 min
Door to IV thrombolytics	≤60 min

decreases, and fluid is retained. Low sodium (hyponatremia) may occur. We avoid hypotonic IV solutions because they may further increase cerebral edema and ICP. Glycemic control should be maintained. In general, decisions about fluid and

TABLE 62.9 Stroke (STK) Core Measure Set

Measure	Topic
STK-1	Venous thromboembolism (VTE) prophylaxis
STK-2	Discharged on antithrombotic therapy
STK-3	Anticoagulation therapy for atrial fibrillation/flutter
STK-4	Thrombolytic therapy
STK-5	Antithrombotic therapy by end of hospital day 2
STK-6	Discharged on statin medication
STK-8	Stroke education
STK-10	Assessed for rehabilitation

From The Joint Commission: *Stroke core measures.* Retrieved from https://www.jointcommission.org/stroke.

electrolyte replacement therapy are based on the extent of intracranial edema, manifestations of increased ICP, central venous pressure, electrolyte levels, and intake and output.

Drug Therapy for Ischemic Stroke

IV thrombolytics can reestablish blood flow through a blocked artery and prevent cell death in patients with the acute onset of ischemic stroke. Thrombolytics must be given within 4.5 hours of the onset of signs of ischemic stroke.[12] We must screen patients carefully before they receive thrombolytics. Screening includes a noncontrast CT scan or MRI to rule out hemorrhagic stroke and blood tests for coagulation disorders. Contraindications include recent history of stroke, spinal or intracranial surgery, or head trauma within the past 3 months; brain tumor; or active bleeding.[12] Thrombolytic therapy is discussed in Chapter 37.

During and after a thrombolytic administration, monitor vital signs and neurologic status to assess for improvement or for potential deterioration related to intracerebral hemorrhage. Control of BP (SBP less than 185 mm Hg) is critical during treatment and for 24 hours following.

Anticoagulant (e.g., heparin) use in the emergency phase after an ischemic stroke is not recommended because of the risk for intracranial hemorrhage. Aspirin at a higher dose may be started within 24 to 48 hours after the onset of an ischemic stroke. Complications of high-dose aspirin include GI bleeding. Aspirin should be given cautiously if there is a history of peptic ulcer disease.

To prevent further clot formation, patients with strokes caused by thrombi and emboli may be treated with anticoagulants and platelet inhibitors. For patients with atrial fibrillation, oral anticoagulant options include warfarin and direct factor Xa inhibitors (e.g., rivaroxaban, dabigatran, apixaban). Platelet inhibitors include aspirin, ticlopidine, clopidogrel, and dipyridamole. The use of statins is effective after an ischemic stroke.

Endovascular Therapy for Ischemic Stroke

Stent retrievers are an option for some patients. They are a way of opening blocked arteries in the brain by using a removable

TABLE 62.10 EMERGENCY MANAGEMENT
Stroke

Etiology	Assessment Findings	Interventions
• Aneurysm • Arteriovenous malformation • Embolism • Hemorrhage • Sudden vascular compromise causing disruption of blood flow to brain • Thrombosis • Trauma	• Altered level of consciousness • Bladder or bowel incontinence • ↑ BP • Difficulty swallowing • Facial drooping on affected side • Heart rate ↑ or ↓ • Numbness, weakness, or paralysis of part of body • Respiratory distress • Seizures • Severe headache • Speech or vision changes • Unequal pupils • Vertigo	• If unresponsive, assess circulation, airway, and breathing. • If responsive, monitor airway, breathing, and circulation. • Call stroke code or stroke team. • Remove dentures. • Perform pulse oximetry. • Maintain adequate oxygenation (Sa_{O_2} >95%) with supplemental O_2, if needed. • Establish IV access with normal saline. • Maintain BP according to guidelines. • Remove clothing. • Obtain CT scan or MRI. • Perform baseline laboratory tests (including glucose) immediately and treat if hypoglycemic. • Position head in midline. • Elevate head of bed 30 degrees if no symptoms of shock or injury. • Institute seizure precautions. • Anticipate thrombolytic therapy for ischemic stroke. • Keep patient NPO until swallow reflex evaluated. • Emotional support for patient and family.

stent system.[13] During the procedure, a catheter is used to guide the small stent from the femoral or radial artery into the part of the artery where a blood clot has formed. The stent expands the interior walls of the artery and allows blood to get to the brain immediately to prevent as much brain damage as possible. The clot seeps into the mesh of the stent. Then, after a few minutes, the stent and clot are removed together.

Acute Care for Hemorrhagic Stroke
Drug Therapy for Hemorrhagic Stroke

Drug therapy for patients with hemorrhagic stroke involves managing hypertension. Oral and IV agents may be used to maintain BP within a normal to high-normal range (SBP less than 160 mm Hg). Seizure prophylaxis is patient specific.[14] Anticoagulants and platelet inhibitors are contraindicated in patients with hemorrhagic strokes.

Surgical Therapy for Hemorrhagic Stroke

Surgery for hemorrhagic stroke includes immediate evacuation of aneurysm-induced hematomas or cerebellar hematomas larger than 3 cm. Those who have an arteriovenous malformation (AVM) may have a hemorrhagic stroke if the AVM ruptures. The treatment of AVM is surgical resection and/or radiosurgery. Catheter embolization of affected vessels can block the blood supply to the AVM.

SAH is usually caused by a ruptured aneurysm. Patients may have multiple aneurysms. Treatment of an aneurysm often involves clipping or coiling the aneurysm to prevent rebleeding (Figs. 62.5 and 62.6). In clipping the aneurysm, the HCP places a metallic clip on the neck of the aneurysm to block blood flow and prevent rupture. The clip stays in place for life.

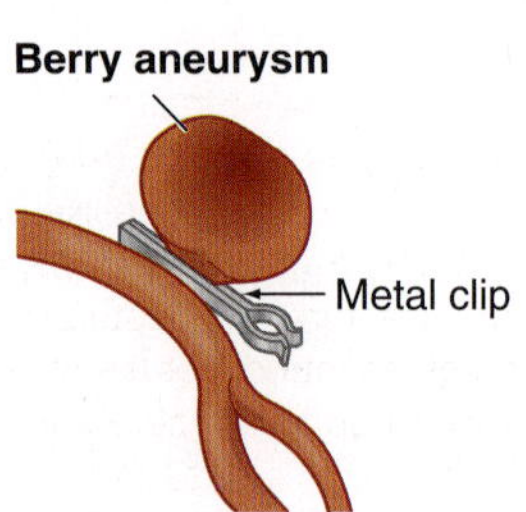

Fig. 62.5 Clipping of aneurysms.

Interventional radiology procedures include coiling and flow diversion. With coiling, a hydrogel-coated platinum coil is inserted into the lumen of the aneurysm (Fig. 62.6). Coils protect against hemorrhage by reducing the blood pulsations within the aneurysm. Eventually, a thrombus forms within the aneurysm. The aneurysm becomes sealed off from the parent vessel by the formation of an endothelialized layer of connective tissue. Flow diverters placed in the parent blood vessel divert blood flow away from an aneurysm.

After clipping or coiling, hyperdynamic therapy (induced hypertension using vasoconstricting agents, such as phenylephrine or dopamine, and hypervolemia) may be started to increase the mean arterial pressure and cerebral perfusion. Volume expansion is achieved with crystalloid or colloid solutions.

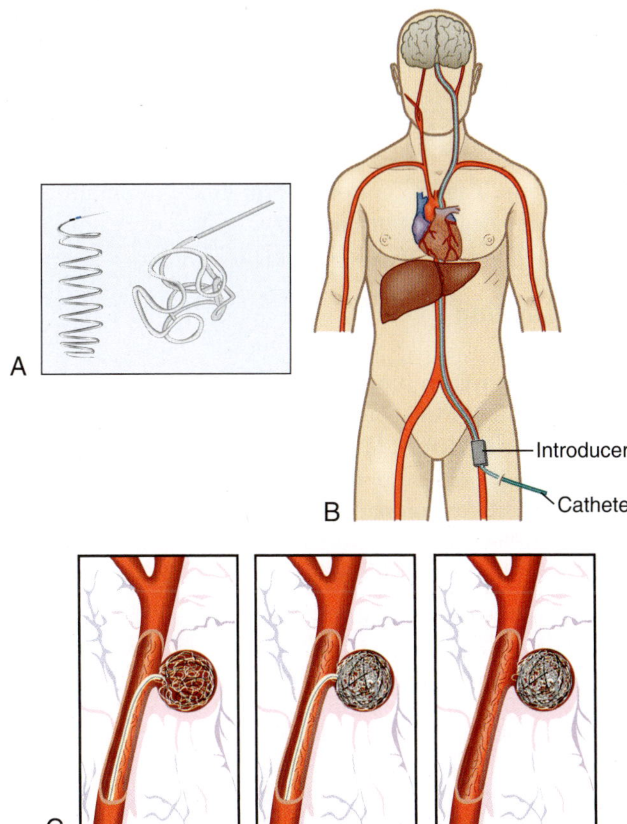

Fig. 62.6 Guglielmi detachable coil (GDC). (A) A coil is used to occlude an aneurysm. Coils are made of soft, spring-like platinum. The softness of the platinum allows the coil to assume the shape of irregularly shaped aneurysms while posing little threat of rupture of the aneurysm. (B) A catheter is inserted through an introducer (small tube) in an artery in the leg. The catheter is threaded up to the cerebral blood vessels. (C) Platinum coils attached to a thin wire are inserted into the catheter and then placed in the aneurysm until the aneurysm is filled with coils. Packing the aneurysm with coils prevents the blood from circulating through the aneurysm, reducing the risk for rupture.

With SAH, bleeding from a damaged vessel causes blood to accumulate between the brain and skull. The leaked blood can irritate, damage, or destroy the surrounding brain cells. When blood enters the subarachnoid space, it mixes with the CSF. This can block CSF circulation, thus increasing pressure on the brain. The open spaces in the brain (ventricles) may enlarge, causing hydrocephalus. This further increases ICP (due to the large accumulation of blood) and can result in further brain injury. Inserting a ventriculostomy for CSF drainage can improve outcomes by reducing ICP. Goals for managing ICP are the same for patients with SAH as they are for patients dealing with acute stroke. The management of ICP is discussed in Chapter 61.

Patients may receive the calcium channel blocker nimodipine to treat cerebral vasospasms and minimize cerebral damage. We think it dilates narrowed blood vessels around the area of the bleeding, so blood flows more easily. This minimizes cerebral damage.

DRUG ALERT

Nimodipine

- Assess BP and pulse before administration.
- If pulse is ≤60 beats/min or SBP is <90 mm Hg, hold the medication and contact the HCP.

Rehabilitation Care

After patients have been stable for 12 to 24 hours, care goals shift from preserving life to lessening disability and reaching optimal function. Many of the interventions started in the acute phase are continued. Patients may be evaluated by a physiatrist (physician who specializes in physical medicine and rehabilitation). Some aspects of rehabilitation begin in the acute care phase as soon as patients are stable. Specific rehabilitation measures are discussed under Chronic Care later in this chapter.

NURSING MANAGEMENT: STROKE

Assessment

Subjective and objective data that you should obtain from patients who had a stroke are detailed in Table 62.11. The key assessments focus on neurologic, cardiac, and respiratory status. Obtain a history from the patient, if stable, and family. Include (1) description of the current illness with attention to initial symptoms, including symptom onset and duration, nature (intermittent or continuous), and changes; (2) history and having had similar symptoms before; (3) current medications; (4) risk factors and other illnesses, such as hypertension; and (5) family history of stroke, aneurysm, and cardiovascular disease.

The primary assessment tool to evaluate and document neurologic status in patients with acute stroke is the NIHSS (Table 62.12).[15] The NIHSS, which measures stroke severity, is a predictor of short- and long-term outcomes. It serves as a data collection tool for planning patient care and exchanging information among HCPs. Other assessment data includes (1) LOC; (2) cognition; (3) motor abilities; (4) cranial nerve function; (5) sensation; (6) proprioception; (7) cerebellar function; and (8) deep tendon reflexes. Documentation of initial and ongoing neurologic assessment is essential to note changes in status.

Clinical Problems

Clinical problems for patients with a stroke may include:

- Neurologic problems
- Increased intracranial pressure
- Impaired communication
- Difficulty coping
- Risk for aspiration
- Musculoskeletal problems
- Risk for injury

TABLE 62.11 NURSING ASSESSMENT

Stroke

Subjective Data

Important Health Information

Health history: Hypertension, previous stroke, TIA, aneurysm, cardiac disease (including recent myocardial infarction, dysrhythmias, heart failure, valvular heart disease, infective endocarditis), hyperlipidemia, polycythemia, blood clotting disorders, diabetes, gout

Family history: Neurologic disorders, aneurysms, stroke, TIA, diabetes, hypertension, coronary artery disease

Medications: Oral contraceptives; use of and adherence with antihypertensive and anticoagulant therapy; illicit substance use

Functional Health Patterns

Health perception–health management: Alcohol use, smoking, drug use

Nutritional-metabolic: Anorexia, nausea, vomiting. Dysphagia, altered sense of taste and smell

Elimination: Change in bowel and bladder patterns

Activity-exercise: Loss of movement and sensation. Syncope, weakness on one side, general weakness, easy fatigability

Cognitive-perceptual: Numbness, tingling of one side of the body, loss of memory. Change in speech, language, problem-solving ability. Pain, headache (possibly sudden and severe) (hemorrhage). Vision changes. Denial of illness

Objective Data

Cardiovascular

↑ BP, ↑ HR, carotid bruit

General

Emotional lability, lethargy, apathy or combativeness, fever

Gastrointestinal

Loss of gag reflex, bowel incontinence, decreased or absent bowel sounds, constipation

Neurologic

Contralateral motor and sensory deficits, including weakness, paresis, paralysis, anesthesia. Unequal pupils, hand grasps. Akinesia, aphasia (expressive, receptive, global), dysarthria (slurred speech), agnosia, apraxia, vision deficits, perceptual or spatial problems, altered level of consciousness (drowsiness to deep coma), and Babinski sign, ↓ followed by ↑ deep tendon reflexes, flaccidity followed by spasticity, amnesia, ataxia, personality change, nuchal rigidity, seizures

Respiratory

Loss of cough reflex, labored or irregular respirations, tachypnea, wheezes (aspiration), airway occlusion (tongue), apnea, coughing when eating, or delayed coughing

Urinary

Frequency, urgency, incontinence

Possible Diagnostic Findings

Positive CT, CT angiography, MRI, magnetic resonance angiography, or other neuroimaging scans showing size, location, and type of lesion. Positive Doppler ultrasonography and angiography showing stenosis

More information on clinical problems and interventions is presented in eNursing Care Plan 62.1 (available on the website for this chapter).

◆ Planning

Establish the goals of nursing care with patients and family. Typical goals are that patients will (1) maintain a stable or improved LOC, (2) attain maximum physical functioning, (3) attain optimal self-care abilities, (4) maintain stable body functions (e.g., bladder control), (5) maximize communication, (6) maintain adequate nutrition, (7) avoid complications, and (8) maintain effective personal and family coping.

◆ Implementation

Health Promotion

You have a key role in promoting a healthy lifestyle (Box 62.1). Teaching should focus on stroke prevention, especially for persons with risk factors. Most strokes are caused by modifiable risk factors. Measures to reduce risk factors for stroke are similar to those for coronary artery disease (see Chapter 37).

Uncontrolled or undiagnosed hypertension is the primary cause of stroke. Therefore be involved in BP screening and ensuring that patients adhere to their antihypertensive therapy. If a person has diabetes, it is important that it is well controlled. If a person has atrial fibrillation, anticoagulant therapy reduces stroke risk. Because smoking is a major risk factor for stroke, help patients to stop smoking (see Chapter 11).

An important aspect is teaching patients and families about early symptoms of stroke or TIA and the need to treat them as a medical emergency. Table 62.13 presents information on when to seek health care for these symptoms. After the onset of a stroke, immediate medical attention is crucial to decrease disability and the risk of death.

Acute Care

Respiratory system. During the acute phase after a stroke, managing the respiratory system is a priority. Patients are vulnerable to respiratory problems. Advancing age and immobility increase the risk for atelectasis and pneumonia.

Interventions to support adequate respiratory function are tailored to meet patients' specific needs (Table 62.14). Some patients, especially those with brainstem or hemorrhagic stroke, may need endotracheal intubation and mechanical ventilation. An oropharyngeal airway in comatose patients may prevent the tongue from falling back and obstructing the airway and provide access for suctioning. Alternatively, a nasopharyngeal airway may be used to provide airway protection and access. When an artificial airway is needed for a prolonged time, a tracheostomy may be done.

Frequently assess airway patency and function. Provide O_2 therapy as ordered. Suction patients as needed and encourage deep breathing. Implement measures to reduce the risk of ventilator-assisted pneumonia in patients who are on mechanical ventilation (see Table 28.10).

Position patients to prevent aspiration. Risk for aspiration pneumonia is high because of impaired consciousness or dysphagia. Dysphagia after stroke is common. Airway obstruction can occur because of problems with chewing and swallowing, food pocketing (food remaining in the buccal cavity of the mouth), and the tongue falling back. Enteral

TABLE 62.12 National Institutes of Health Stroke Scale

Description

NIH Stroke Scale (NIHSS) is a 15-item neurologic examination used to evaluate the effect of an acute stroke. Total scores on the NIHSS range from 0 to 42. Higher values reflect more severity.

Procedure for Use

A trained observer rates the patient's ability to answer questions and perform activities. Ratings for each item are scored, and there is an allowance for untestable (UN) items. If an item is untested, a detailed explanation must be clearly written on the form. Free training is available at www.nihstrokescale.org.

Item	Scale Definition
Level of consciousness	0 = Alert 1 = Not alert, but arousable by minor stimulation 2 = Not alert, requires repeated stimulation to get attention 3 = Responds only with reflex motor or autonomic effects or unresponsive, flaccid, areflexic
Level of consciousness questions	0 = Answers both questions correctly 1 = Answers 1 question correctly 2 = Answers neither question correctly
Level of consciousness commands	0 = Performs both tasks correctly 1 = Performs 1 task correctly 2 = Performs neither task correctly
Best gaze	0 = Normal 1 = Partial gaze palsy 2 = Forced deviation, or total gaze paresis
Visual	0 = No vision loss 1 = Partial hemianopsia 2 = Complete hemianopsia 3 = Bilateral hemianopsia or blind
Facial palsy	0 = Normal symmetric movement 1 = Minor paralysis 2 = Partial paralysis 3 = Complete paralysis of 1 or both sides
Motor and drift (for each extremity)	0 = No drift 1 = Drift 2 = Some effort against gravity 3 = No effort against gravity, limb falls 4 = No movement UN = Amputation
Limb ataxia	0 = Absent 1 = Present in 1 limb 2 = Present in 2 limbs
Sensory	0 = Normal 1 = Mild to moderate sensory loss 2 = Severe to total sensory loss
Best language	0 = No aphasia, normal 1 = Mild to moderate aphasia 2 = Severe aphasia 3 = Mute, no usable speech or auditory comprehension
Dysarthria	0 = Normal 1 = Mild to moderate 2 = Severe UN = Intubated or other physical barrier
Extinction or inattention	0 = No abnormality 1 = Inattention or extinction to bilateral stimulation 2 = Does not recognize own hand
Distal motor function	0 = Normal (no flexion after 5 sec) 1 = At least some extension but not fully extended 2 = No voluntary extension after 5 sec

From National Institutes of Health: *NIH Stroke Scale*. Retrieved from https://www.stroke.nih.gov/resources/scale.htm.

nutrition (EN) increases the risk for aspiration pneumonia. Assess patients for their ability to swallow. Keep them NPO until dysphagia is ruled out.

Neurologic. Perform ongoing neurologic assessments, including the NIHSS, mental status, pupil response, and extremity movement and strength. Note signs of increasing neurologic deficit. A decreasing LOC may indicate increasing ICP. Monitor ICP and cerebral perfusion pressure for patients in the ICU. Record your assessment promptly to communicate neurologic status to the stroke team.

Increased ICP is more likely to occur with hemorrhagic strokes but can occur with ischemic strokes. Increased ICP from cerebral edema usually peaks in 72 hours and may cause brain herniation. Management of increased ICP includes practices that improve venous drainage. These include elevating the head of the bed, keeping the head and neck in alignment, and avoiding hip flexion. Other measures for reducing ICP include managing fever, pain management, and preventing constipation. CSF drainage is an option in some patients to reduce ICP. The management of increased ICP is discussed in Chapter 61 and Table 61.6.

Cardiovascular. Nursing goals for cardiovascular care are aimed at maintaining homeostasis. Many patients with stroke have decreased cardiac reserves from cardiac disease. Fluid retention, overhydration, dehydration, or BP changes may further compromise cardiac efficiency. Central venous pressure, pulmonary artery pressure, or hemodynamic monitoring may be used to assess fluid balance and cardiac function in the ICU.

Monitor vital signs and maintain ECG monitoring. Hypertension sometimes occurs after a stroke as the body tries to increase CBF. It is important to assess for orthostatic hypotension before ambulating patients for the first time. Neurologic changes can occur with a sudden decrease in BP.

Calculate intake and output, noting imbalances. Regulate IV infusions and adjust fluid intake to meet patient needs. Monitor lung sounds for crackles and wheezes, which may indicate pulmonary congestion.

Patients are at risk for venous thromboembolism (VTE), especially in the weak or paralyzed lower extremity. VTE is related to immobility, loss of venous tone, and decreased muscle pumping activity in the leg. The most effective prevention is to keep patients moving. Teach active range-of-motion (ROM) exercises if patients have voluntary movement in the affected extremity. For patients with hemiplegia, perform passive ROM exercises several times a day. Other measures to prevent VTE include positioning to minimize the effects of dependent edema and using intermittent pneumatic compression.[16] VTE prophylaxis may include low-molecular-weight heparin (e.g., enoxaparin). Observe for swelling of the lower extremities, note unusual warmth of the leg, and ask patients about pain in the calf.

Musculoskeletal. The nursing goal for the musculoskeletal system is to maintain optimal function by preventing joint contractures and muscular atrophy. In the acute phase, ROM exercises and positioning are important nursing interventions. Passive ROM exercise begins on the first day of hospitalization. Muscle atrophy from lack of innervation and activity can develop after a stroke, so exercise is an important intervention for rehabilitation and recovery.

The paralyzed or weak side needs special attention when patients are positioned. Position each joint higher than the joint proximal to it to prevent dependent edema. Specific deformities on the weak or paralyzed side that may be present include internal rotation of the shoulder; flexion contractures of the hand, wrist, and elbow; external rotation of the hip; and plantar flexion of the foot. Subluxation of the shoulder on the affected side is common. Careful positioning and moving of the affected arm may prevent the development of a painful shoulder condition. Immobilization of the affected upper extremity may precipitate a painful shoulder-hand syndrome.

Interventions to promote musculoskeletal function include (1) trochanter roll at the hip to prevent external rotation; (2) hand cones (not rolled washcloths) to prevent hand

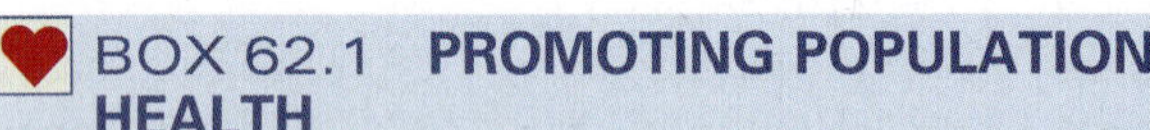

BOX 62.1 PROMOTING POPULATION HEALTH

Stroke Prevention

- Reduce salt and sodium intake.
- Maintain a normal body weight.
- Follow a diet low in saturated fat and high in fruits and vegetables.
- Limit alcohol use to moderate levels.
- Maintain a systolic BP less than 140 mm Hg.
- Avoid cigarette smoking and tobacco products.
- Maintain a normal glucose level and control diabetes.
- Follow the prescribed treatment plan for diagnosed heart problems.
- Moderate exercise for 150 min/week or vigorous exercise for 75 min/week.

TABLE 62.13 PATIENT & CAREGIVER TEACHING

FAST Warning Signs of Stroke

FAST is an easy way to remember the signs of stroke. Include the following information in the teaching plan for patients at risk for stroke and caregivers:

F: Face drooping	Ask the person to smile. Does one side of the face droop, or is it numb? Is the smile uneven?
A: Arm weakness	Ask the person to raise both arms. Does one arm drift downward? Is one arm weak?
S: Speech difficulties	Ask the person to repeat a simple phrase such as, "The sun is yellow." Is speech slurred? Is the person unable to speak or hard to understand? Is the sentence repeated correctly?
T: Time	Time is CRITICAL! If someone shows any of these signs (even if they go away), call 911. Note the time when the signs first appeared.

In addition, report the sudden onset of the following:

- Confusion, trouble speaking
- Numbness or weakness, especially in 1 side of the body
- Severe headache with no known cause
- Trouble seeing in one or both eyes
- Trouble walking, dizziness, loss of balance or coordination

From Centers for Disease Control and Prevention: *Signs and symptoms of stroke.* Retrieved from https://www.cdc.gov/stroke/signs-symptoms/index.html.

TABLE 62.14 NURSING MANAGEMENT

Caring for Patients With an Acute Stroke

- Assess manifestations of stroke and determine onset and duration.
- Screen patient for contraindications for thrombolytic therapy.
- Infuse thrombolytic therapy for patients with ischemic stroke who meet criteria.
- Assess respiratory status and start needed actions, such as O_2, oropharyngeal or nasopharyngeal airways, suctioning.
- Position patient to prevent aspiration and atelectasis.
- Assess neurologic status, including intracranial pressure (ICP), if needed.
- Monitor cardiovascular status, including hemodynamic monitoring, if needed.
- Calculate intake and output, noting imbalances.
- Regulate IV infusions and adjust fluid intake to patient needs.
- Assess swallowing ability in conjunction with the speech therapist.
- Give ordered anticoagulant and antiplatelet drugs.
- Implement measures to prevent venous thromboembolism and pressure injuries.
- Delegate to AP:
  - Obtain vital signs and report these to RN.
  - Measure and record urine output.
  - Help with positioning and turning patient at least every 2 h.
  - Perform passive and active range-of-motion exercises.

contractures; (3) arm supports with slings and lap boards to prevent shoulder displacement; (4) avoiding pulling patients by the arm to avoid shoulder displacement; and (5) posterior leg splints or high-top tennis shoes to prevent footdrop.

Using a footboard for patients with spasticity is controversial. Rather than preventing plantar flexion (footdrop), the sensory stimulation of a footboard against the bottom of the foot increases plantar flexion. Likewise, experts disagree on whether hand splints decrease spasticity. The decision about using footboards or hand splints is made on an individual patient basis.

Skin. The skin is susceptible to breakdown related to loss of sensation, decreased circulation, and immobility. Advanced age, poor nutrition, dehydration, edema, and incontinence compound the risk.

Measures to prevent skin breakdown include (1) pressure relief by position changes, special mattresses, or wheelchair cushions; (2) good skin hygiene; (3) emollients applied to dry skin; (4) early mobility; and (5) nutrition. Position patients on the weak or paralyzed side for only 30 minutes. Controlling pressure is key in preventing and treating skin breakdown. Use pillows under lower extremities to reduce pressure on the heels. See more information on preventing pressure injuries in Chapter 12.

Gastrointestinal. The most common bowel problem after stroke is constipation. Fluid and fiber intake goals are determined with the stroke team based on nutrition and fluid status. Patients may be placed on stool softeners and/or fiber (e.g., psyllium). Laxatives, suppositories, or additional stool softeners may be ordered if there is no response to increased fluid and fiber. Enemas are used only if suppositories and digital stimulation are ineffective because they cause vagal stimulation and increase ICP. Physical activity promotes bowel function. If a patient has liquid stools, check for stool impaction.

Bowel retraining may be needed and continued into the rehabilitation phase. A bowel management program consists of placing patients on the bedpan or bedside commode or taking them to the bathroom at a regular time daily to reestablish bowel regularity. A good time for a bowel movement is 30 minutes after breakfast because eating stimulates the gastrocolic reflex and peristalsis. The timing may need to be adjusted as bowel habits vary.

Urinary. In the acute stage of stroke, the primary urinary problem is poor bladder control, resulting in incontinence. Take steps to promote normal bladder function and avoid the use of indwelling catheters. If an indwelling catheter is used initially, remove it as soon as patients are medically and neurologically stable. Long-term use of an indwelling catheter is associated with urinary tract infections and delayed bladder retraining.

Avoid bladder overdistention. An intermittent catheterization program may be used for patients with urinary retention to lower the risk of urinary infections. An alternative to intermittent catheterization for male patients is an external catheter. External catheters do not address problems with urine retention.

Often patients have functional incontinence, which is associated with communication, mobility, and dressing problems. A bladder retraining program consists of (1) adequate fluid intake, with most of it given between 7:00 AM and 7:00 PM; (2) scheduled toileting every 2 hours using bedpan, commode, or bathroom; (3) usual position for urinating (standing or sitting); (4) observing for signs of restlessness, which may indicate the need for urination; and (5) assessing for bladder distention. Encourage patients to wear pants without drawstrings, buttons, or zippers. These can be hard to manage if motor or sensory deficits exist.

We often assess postvoid residual volume using bladder ultrasound. The ultrasound measures how much urine is in the bladder after voiding. If urine stays in the bladder, incomplete emptying is a problem and may cause urinary tract infections. A coordinated program by the entire nursing staff is needed to achieve urinary continence.

Nutrition. Patients should have their nutrition needs addressed in the first 24 hours of admission because nutrition is important for recovery and healing. Those with severe impairment may need EN or parenteral nutrition.

Many patients have dysphagia after a stroke. Keep patients NPO until a speech therapist performs a swallowing evaluation. This should be done in the first 24 hours after the stroke. You or another health care team member may perform the screen if a speech therapist cannot perform the formal evaluation. Follow agency guidelines.

! SAFETY ALERT

Oral Feeding After Stroke

- Dysphagia is common after stroke.
- Keep patients on NPO status until a speech therapist does a swallowing evaluation.

Before starting feeding, assess the gag reflex. If the gag reflex is absent, defer the feeding and begin exercises to stimulate swallowing. The speech therapist or occupational therapist is usually responsible for designing this program. You may be involved in helping to develop the program in some settings.

The speech therapist may recommend specific foods. Refer to the speech therapist's recommendations and guidelines. If you do not have recommendations, then consider the following: Foods should be easy to swallow and provide enough texture, temperature (warm or cold), and flavor to stimulate a swallow reflex. Crushed ice can be used as a stimulant. Pureed foods are not usually the best choice because they are often bland or too smooth. Thin liquids are often hard to swallow and may promote coughing. We can thicken thin liquids with a commercially available thickening agent.

Mouth care before feeding helps stimulate sensory awareness and salivation and can help swallowing. Keep patients in the high-Fowler position, preferably in a chair, for the feeding and 30 minutes afterward. While feeding, keep the head flexed forward. Place food in the unaffected side of the mouth. Teach patients to swallow and then swallow again. Follow feedings with good oral hygiene because food may collect in the affected side of the mouth.

A dietitian can help determine the daily caloric intake based on patients' size, weight, and activity level. If patients are unable to take in an adequate oral diet and dysphagia persists, a percutaneous endoscopic gastrostomy (PEG) tube may be used for EN. EN is described in Chapter 44.

The inability to self-feed can be frustrating and may result in malnutrition and dehydration. Interventions to promote self-feeding include using the unaffected upper extremity to eat; employing assistive devices, such as rocker knives, plate guards, and nonslip pads for dishes; and removing unnecessary items from the tray or table, which can reduce spills. Provide a calm environment (e.g., turn off the television) to decrease sensory overload and distraction. Introduce these interventions in the acute care setting so that maximum rehabilitation can occur after discharge. We evaluate the effectiveness of the diet program in terms of weight, adequate hydration, and patient satisfaction.

Communication. Speech, comprehension, and language deficits are the most difficult problems for patients and family. Assess the ability to speak and understand. Their response to simple questions can guide you in structuring explanations and instructions. Collaborate with the speech therapist to assess and develop a plan of care to enhance communication.

Interventions that support communication include communicating often and meaningfully, using visual cues. Allow time for patients to comprehend and answer. Use simple, short sentences and structure the conversation so that it allows simple answers. If patients cannot understand words, use gestures to support verbal cues.

Alert patients are usually anxious because of what has happened and problems with communication or the inability to communicate. Verbal stimuli can easily overwhelm patients with aphasia. Give them extra time to understand and respond to communication. Guidelines for communicating with patients with aphasia are outlined in Table 62.15. A picture board may be helpful. The speech therapist often does further evaluation and treatment of language and communication deficits once patients have stabilized. It is important to teach the family these communication strategies.

Sensory-perceptual problems. Patients often have perceptual deficits. Patients with a stroke on the right side of the brain usually have difficulty judging position, distance, and rate of movement. These patients are often impulsive and impatient. They tend to deny problems related to strokes. They may not correlate spatial-perceptual problems with the inability to perform activities, such as guiding a wheelchair through the doorway. They best understand directions given verbally. Break down the task into simple steps for ease of understanding. Patients with a right-brain stroke and left hemiplegia are at higher risk for injury because of mobility problems. Environment control (e.g., removing clutter, using good lighting) aids in concentration and safer mobility. Provide nonslip socks at all times. One-sided neglect is common for patients with right-brain stroke. You may need to help or remind patients to dress the weak or paralyzed side or shave the forgotten side of the face.

Patients with a left-brain stroke (right hemiplegia) often are slower in organizing and performing tasks. They tend to have impaired spatial discrimination. These patients usually admit to deficits and have a fearful, anxious response to a stroke. Their behaviors are slow and cautious. Nonverbal cues and instructions are helpful.

Homonymous hemianopsia (blindness in the same half of each visual field) is common after a stroke. Persistent disregard of objects in part of the visual field should alert you to this possibility. At first, help patients compensate by arranging the environment within their perceptual field, such as arranging the food tray so that all foods are on one side to accommodate for the field of vision (Fig. 62.7). Later, they learn to compensate for the vision defect by consciously attending to or by scanning the neglected side. They should check weak or paralyzed extremities for adequacy of dressing, hygiene, and trauma.

It is often hard to tell between a visual field cut and a neglect syndrome. Both problems may occur with strokes affecting the right or left side of the brain. A person may have homonymous hemianopsia and a neglect syndrome, which increases the inattention to the weak or paralyzed side. Neglect syndrome results in decreased safety awareness and places patients at high risk for injury. Immediately after the stroke, anticipate safety

TABLE 62.15 Communicating With Patients With Aphasia

The following are guidelines for communicating with patients with aphasia:

1. Decrease stimuli that may be distracting and disrupting to communication efforts.
2. Speak with normal volume and tone.
3. Present a single thought or idea at a time.
4. Keep questions simple or ask questions that can be answered with "yes" or "no."
5. Let patients speak. Do not interrupt. Allow time for them to complete thoughts.
6. Make use of gestures as an alternative form of communication. Encourage this by saying, "Show me" or "Point to what you want."
7. Do not pretend to understand if you do not. Calmly say you do not understand. Encourage the use of nonverbal communication or ask patients to write out what they want.
8. Give patients time to process information and generate a response before repeating a question or statement.
9. Allow body contact (e.g., clasp of a hand, touching) as much as possible. Realize that touching may be the only way patients can express feelings.
10. Organize the day by preparing and following a schedule (the more familiar the routine, the easier it will be).
11. Do not push communication if patients are tired or upset. Aphasia worsens with fatigue and anxiety.
12. Teach communication techniques to caregivers and family members.

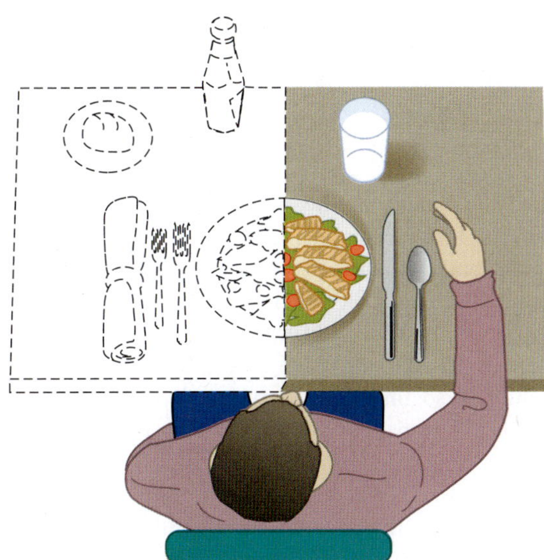

Fig. 62.7 Spatial and perceptual deficits in stroke. Perception of a patient with homonymous hemianopsia shows that food on the left side is not seen and thus is ignored.

hazards and provide protection from injury. Safety measures include closely observing patients, elevating side rails, lowering the height of the bed, and using video monitors.

Other visual problems may include *diplopia* (double vision), loss of the corneal reflex, and *ptosis* (drooping eyelid), especially if the stroke is in the vertebrobasilar distribution. Diplopia is often treated with an eye patch. If the corneal reflex is absent, there is a risk for corneal abrasion. Prevent corneal abrasions with artificial tears or gel to keep the eyes moist and an eye shield (especially at night). We usually only treat ptosis if it inhibits vision.

Coping. During the acute stage of stroke, your role in meeting patients' psychologic needs is primarily supportive. A stroke is usually a sudden, very stressful event. Stroke is often a family disease, affecting the family emotionally, socially, and financially. Roles and responsibilities change within the family. Patients and their families may perceive the stroke as a threat to life and their accustomed lifestyle. Reactions to this threat vary considerably. They may involve fear, apprehension, denial of the severity of the stroke, depression, anger, and sorrow. Nursing interventions that promote coping involve teaching and providing emotional support.

Give clear, understandable explanations about what has happened and diagnostic and therapeutic procedures. Reinforce as needed. Decision making and upholding patients' wishes during this challenging time are important (Box 62.2). Advance directives should be honored. Update the family daily. Hold family meetings about feeding tube placement or tracheostomy.

Give family a careful, detailed explanation of what has happened. If they are anxious and upset during the acute phase, you may have to repeat explanations later. Because family usually have not had time to prepare for the illness, they may need help in arranging care for family members or pets and for transportation and finances. A social services referral is often helpful.

BOX 62.2 ETHICAL/LEGAL DILEMMAS

Competence

Situation

M.T., a 60-year-old male in the ICU with an LVAD, had a stroke that left him paralyzed on his right side. He is only able to answer yes/no questions by shaking his head. M.T. has needed mechanical ventilation since his stroke. For the past 2 weeks, he has needed hemodialysis because of renal failure. Recently, when you suction him, he turns his head away from you and bites down on the endotracheal tube. His wife and daughter tell you that, on many occasions before these events, he expressed that he would not want to live if he lost his independence. They are asking to have the mechanical ventilator withdrawn.

Ethical/Legal Points for Consideration

- Decisional capacity for informed consent related to treatment decisions involves 4 elements: (1) information provided about possible treatment options must be understood by patients, (2) patients must have the capacity to deliberate about the treatment choices and their consequences, (3) patients' treatment decisions must be freely chosen and made without coercion, and (4) patients must be able to communicate their decisions.
- Review how your state defines legal competence. The ability to respond to questions by signaling a yes or no may be enough to prove understanding of the questions, ability to discriminate between choices, and ability to communicate choices, providing that the answers make sense and are appropriate.
- Next of kin are the legal decision makers in the absence of advance directives if the patient is unable to make decisions for himself. Decisional capacity should be tested without assuming it is absent.
- Some courts have accepted past assertions of preferences, past behavior, and assertions of their parties as evidence to support end-of-life preferences in the absence of advance directives.
- Know your agency's policies and local laws and regulations about informed consent and end-of-life decision making.

Discussion Questions

1. What would you do next given M.T.'s behavior and the information from his wife?
2. What are your feelings and concerns about caring for a patient for whom withdrawal of treatment will result in death?

CHECK YOUR PRACTICE

You are working in the outpatient stroke clinic, counseling the family of one of your favorite patients. He is a well-respected 65-year-old business owner who has returned home after a stroke. His family tells you that during meals, he becomes frustrated and begins to cry because of the difficulty getting food into his mouth and chewing. His family cannot understand why a previously very competent male is so emotional.

- What measures can you take to support the family?

Chronic Care

Care transitions. Patients are usually discharged from the acute care setting to home, an intermediate- or long-term care facility, or a rehabilitation facility. Ideally, discharge planning starts early in the hospitalization and promotes a smooth transition between care settings. The stroke team provides guidance for the care needed after discharge. Factors we consider include patients' medical needs and independence in performing ADLs, caregiver's ability to provide care, and community setting. If patients need a short- or long-term health care facility, the team can make referrals that allow time to select and arrange for care.

If patients are returning home, the team can make referrals for needed equipment and services. You can prepare patients and caregivers through teaching. Evaluate the transition plan for any barriers. Follow-up care is planned to allow continued nursing care; physical, occupational, and speech therapy; and medical care. Identify community resources to provide recreation activities, group support, spiritual assistance, respite care, adult day care, and home assistance based on patients' needs.

Rehabilitation. After patients have stabilized for 12 to 24 hours, care goals shift from preserving life to lessening disability and reaching optimal function. The goals of rehabilitation are to prevent deformity and maintain and improve function. Many interventions started in the acute phase of care continue throughout rehabilitation. Ongoing rehabilitation is essential to maximize abilities. Most patients recover in the first 6 months after a stroke, with a maximum benefit 1 year after a stroke.[1]

Rehabilitation requires an interprofessional team approach so that patients and caregivers can benefit from the team's combined, expert care. The team must communicate and coordinate care to achieve patients' goals. As a nurse, you can facilitate this process and are often the key to successful rehabilitation. The team is composed of many other members. These include physicians; psychiatrists or psychologists; physical, occupational, speech, vocational, recreation, and respiratory therapists; registered dietitians; social workers; pharmacists; and chaplains.

Physical therapy focuses on mobility, progressive ambulation, transfer techniques, and equipment needed for mobility. Occupational therapy emphasizes retraining for skills of daily living, including eating, dressing, hygiene, and cooking. Occupational therapists are skilled in cognitive and perceptual evaluation and training. Speech therapy focuses on speech, communication, cognition, and eating abilities.

The rehabilitation nurse assesses patients, caregivers, and family with attention to (1) rehabilitation potential, (2) physical status, (3) complications caused by the stroke or other chronic conditions, (4) cognitive status, (5) family resources and support, and (6) expectations related to the rehabilitation program.

Musculoskeletal function. The initial assessment consists of determining the stage of recovery of muscle function. If the muscles are still flaccid several weeks after the stroke, the prognosis for regaining function is poor, and care focuses on preventing further loss.

Most patients begin to show signs of spasticity with exaggerated reflexes within 48 hours after the stroke. Spasticity at this phase denotes progress toward recovery. As improvement continues, small voluntary movements of the hip or shoulder may be accompanied by involuntary movements in the rest of the extremity. The last stage of recovery occurs when there is voluntary control of isolated muscle groups.

Interventions advance in a manner of progressive activity. Balance training is the first step. It begins with the patient sitting up in bed or dangling the legs over the edge of the bed. Assess tolerance by noting dizziness or syncope caused by vasomotor instability. Loss of postural stability is common after stroke. When the nondominant hemisphere is involved, walking apraxia and loss of postural control are usually apparent. The patient may be unable to sit upright and tends to fall sideways. Provide support with pillows or cushions.

Assess if patients autocorrect their posture when sitting on the edge of the bed. If a patient can straighten their posture instead of leaning to the weaker side, they may be ready for the next step of transferring from bed to chair. Place the chair beside the bed so that the patient can lead with the stronger arm and leg. The patient sits on the side of the bed, stands, places the strong hand on the far wheelchair arm, and sits down. You may either supervise the transfer or provide minimal aid by guiding the patient's strong hand to the wheelchair arm, standing in front of the patient while blocking their knees with your knees to prevent knee buckling, and guiding the patient into a sitting position.

Supportive or assistive equipment, such as canes, walkers, and leg braces, may be needed on a short- or long-term basis for mobility. The physical therapist usually selects the right supportive device(s) to meet specific needs and teaches patients about use. Include physical therapy activities in patients' daily routine for added practice and repetition of rehabilitation efforts (Fig. 62.8).

In some rehabilitation units, the Bobath method is used as an approach to mobility. The Bobath method helps patients gain control over spasticity by inhibiting abnormal reflex patterns. Therapists and nurses use the Bobath approach to encourage normal muscle tone, normal movement, and bilateral function of the body. An example is to have the patient transfer into the wheelchair using the weak or paralyzed side and the stronger side to facilitate more bilateral functioning.

Another approach is *constraint-induced movement therapy* (CIMT) (Fig. 62.9). CIMT encourages patients to use the weakened extremity by restricting movement of the normal extremity.[17] This approach can be challenging. It is used only under the supervision of physical or occupational therapy. Movement training, skill acquisition, stretching, and exercise are other therapies used.

Survivorship and coping. Patients may have many losses, including sensory, intellectual, communicative, functional, role behavior, emotional, social, and vocational. Patients and family often go through the process of grief and mourning associated with the losses. Some develop long-term depression, with symptoms including anxiety, weight loss, fatigue, poor appetite, and sleep problems. The time and energy needed to perform previously simple tasks can result in anger and frustration.

The magnitude of disability and changes in total function can leave patients wondering if they can ever return to their "old self." Loss of independence may be a major concern. The ability to perform ADLs may require many adaptive changes because of residual deficits. Patients may become fearful and depressed because they think they may have another stroke or die. The fear can become immobilizing and interfere with effective rehabilitation.

Patients and family need help coping with the losses from the stroke. Provide assistance by (1) supporting communication; (2) discussing lifestyle changes resulting from stroke deficits; (3) discussing changing roles and responsibilities within the family; and (4) allowing the expression of fear, frustration, and anxiety. Include patients and family in short- and long-term goal planning and patient care and support family conferences.

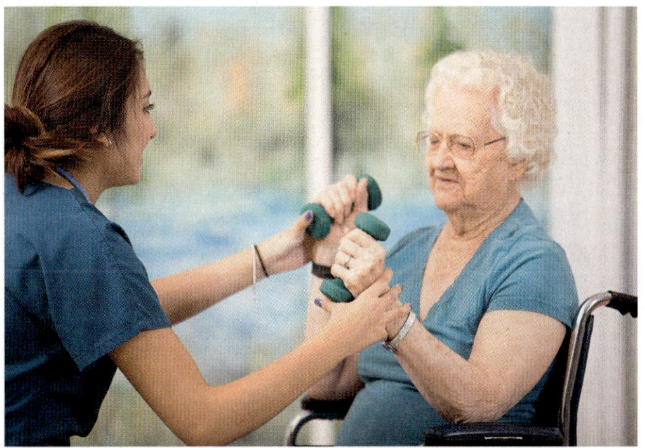

Fig. 62.8 A patient who had a stroke works with a physical therapist to improve arm strength. (© Thinkstock 78783452.)

Changes may occur in the patient-partner relationship. The dependency resulting from a stroke may threaten the relationship. The partner may be older or have chronic health problems that affect their ability to care for the stroke survivor. Patients may not want anyone other than their partner to provide care, thus putting a significant burden on the partner. There may be limited family members, including adult children, living nearby to provide help.

Patients who had a stroke may appear apathetic, depressed, fearful, anxious, weepy, frustrated, and angry. Some patients, especially those with a stroke on the left side of the brain (right hemiplegia), have exaggerated mood swings. They may be unable to control emotions and suddenly burst into tears or laughter. This behavior is out of context and often unrelated to the patient's underlying emotional state. Interventions for atypical emotional response are to (1) distract patients who suddenly become emotional, (2) explain to patients and family that emotional outbursts may occur after a stroke, (3) maintain a calm environment, and (4) avoid shaming or scolding patients during outbursts.

Maladjusted dependence with inadequate coping occurs when patients do not maintain optimal functioning for self-care, family responsibilities, decision making, or socialization. This situation can cause resentment with a negative cycle of interpersonal dependency and control. Family therapy is often helpful. Caregivers and family must cope with 3 aspects of

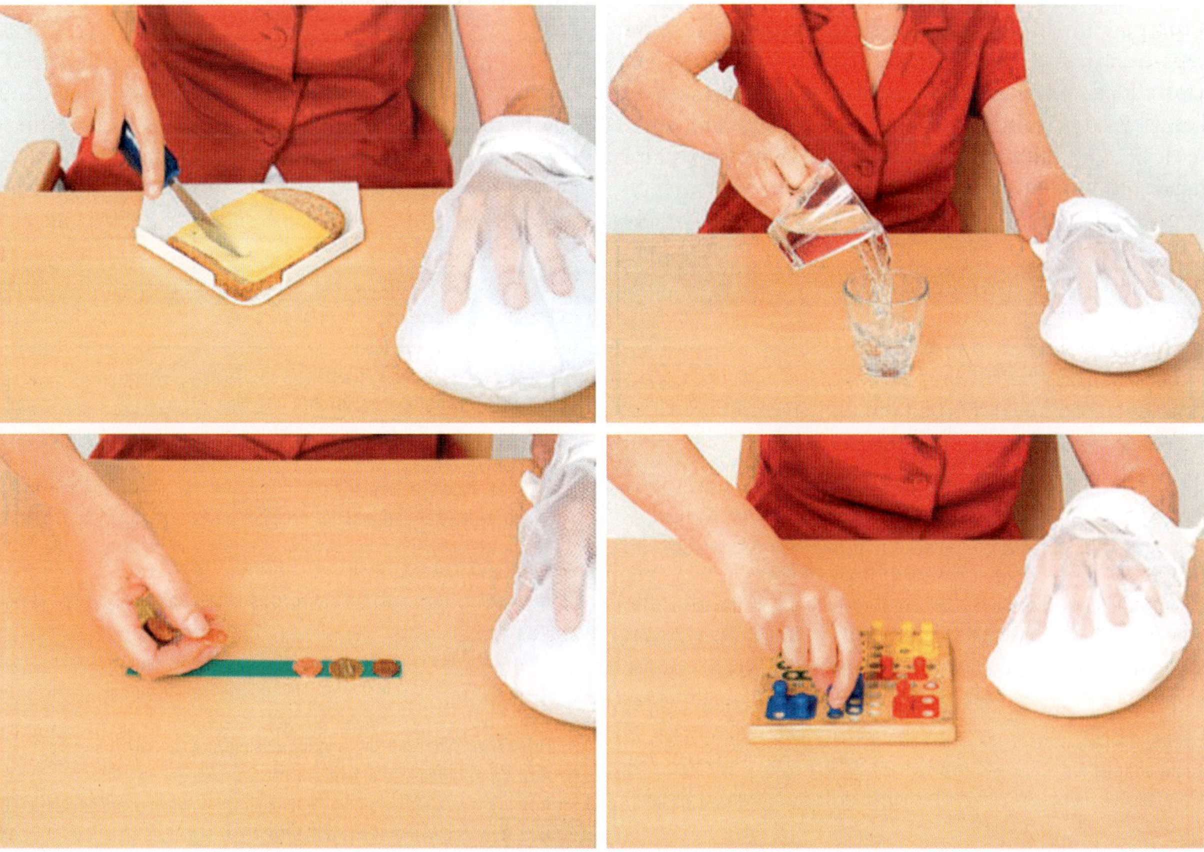

Fig. 62.9 Constraint-induced movement therapy after stroke. (From Kwakkel G, Veerbeek JM, van Wegen EE, et al: Constraint-induced movement therapy after stroke, *Lancet Neurol* 14:224, 2015. Reprinted with permission from Elsevier.)

patient behavior: (1) recognition of behavior changes resulting from neurologic deficits that are not changeable, (2) responses to multiple losses by patients and family, and (3) behaviors that may have been reinforced during the early stages of stroke as a continued dependency.

Sexual function. Patients may be concerned about the loss of sexual function. Many patients are comfortable talking about their anxieties and fears about sexual function if you are comfortable and open to the topic. You can start a discussion about the topic with patients and their partners. Common concerns include impotence and the chance of another stroke occurring during sex. Interventions include teaching about (1) optional positioning of partners, (2) timing for peak energy periods, and (3) patient and partner counseling.

Community integration. Successful community integration after stroke may be hard for patients because of persistent problems with cognition, coping, physical deficits, and emotional changes that interfere with functioning. Older adults who had a stroke often have more severe deficits and multiple health problems. Failure to continue rehabilitation at home may result in deterioration and further complications.

Community resources can be an asset to patients and their families (Box 62.3). Stroke support groups help survivors and their caregivers cope with the physical and emotional challenges of post-stroke recovery and offer a sense of community, education, and resources. The National Stroke Association provides information, resources, referral services, and quarterly newsletters on stroke. The American Stroke Association (ASA) has information about stroke, hypertension, diet, exercise, and assistive devices. They sponsor self-help groups in many areas. Easter Seals may supply wheelchairs and other assistive devices. Local groups can offer help with meals and transportation.

BOX 62.3 EVIDENCE-BASED PRACTICE

Rehabilitation in Patients With Strokes

You are working on a stroke rehabilitation unit. The director has communicated to the nursing staff that postdischarge attendance at physical therapy, nutrition classes, and the family-patient stroke support group is declining.

Making Clinical Decisions

Synthesis of Best Available Evidence

Recent studies have raised the importance of patients taking part in a rehabilitation program as soon as they are discharged to prevent further deterioration of physical abilities and to help maintain their ability to live independently in the community. Support groups play a vital role in providing education, support, and resources to both survivors and their caregivers.

Clinician Expertise

The nursing staff follows a structured stroke education program and collaborates with physical therapy to review rehabilitative exercises. The nurse who facilitates the support group offers expert knowledge on stroke recovery and management and connects participants with community resources. The HCAHPS reports reveal that some patients are not participating in the program due to mobility limitations and the time and cost of traveling.

Patient Preferences and Values

Your peers and you decide to offer support group meetings and nutrition classes in both face-to-face and virtual formats. Patients and families are encouraged to choose what format works best for them. A nurse calls each patient weekly to discuss concerns and answer questions about their recovery. After 3 months, there is a 28% increase in participation in the rehabilitation activities.

Implications for Nursing Practice

1. What information would be important to include in the classes?
2. How can you make the information interactive?
3. How could you overcome any technology literacy problems?

Reference for Evidence

Wong AK, Kwok VW, Wong FK, et al: Improving post-acute stroke follow-up care by adopting telecare consultations in a nurse-led clinic. *J Adv Nurs* 80:1222, 2024.

CASE STUDY

Stroke

Patient Profile

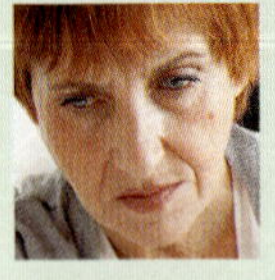

(© iStockphoto/ Thinkstock.)

J.K. is a 57-year-old female who was diagnosed with a temporal-parietal glioblastoma that extends into the occipital lobes (see the Case Study in Chapter 60). She was diagnosed after presenting with persistent headaches, a seizure in her HCP's office, and left-side upper visual field loss and neglect. J.K. lives alone and holds a management position. She was concerned about her ability to return to work after her surgery.

J.K. returned to the neurosurgery unit after surgery to debulk the tumor. She was drowsy but followed commands. Her pupils were equal and responded to light. During the night, J.K. developed left-sided weakness in both arm and leg. She is now having difficulty answering questions.

Subjective Data

- Left arm and leg are weak and feel numb
- Trying to answer questions but looks confused and cannot follow commands

Objective Data

- BP 150/90 mm Hg
- Right gaze preference
- Left homonymous hemianopsia
- Left arm weakness (3/5) greater than leg weakness (4/5)
- Decreased sensation on left arm and leg
- Has speech but not clear. Difficulty with word finding and following commands
- CT scan shows a hemorrhagic stroke into the site of the tumor bed, and temporal-parietal and anterior occipital areas extending into the thalamus

Discussion Questions

1. ***Recognize:*** How did J.K.'s diagnosis of glioblastoma put her at risk for a stroke?
2. ***Analyze:*** What potential complications is J.K. at highest risk for developing?
3. ***Plan:*** How would you involve other interprofessional team members in J.K.'s care?
4. ***Prioritize:*** What are the priority nursing interventions for J.K.?
5. ***Act:*** What nursing interventions can you delegate to AP?
6. ***Act:*** What strategies can you implement to improve communication for J.K.?
7. ***Act:*** How can you address J.K.'s concerns about her finances and self-care?
8. ***Safety:*** How can you ensure safety for J.K. in light of her homonymous hemianopsia and left-sided neglect?
9. Develop a conceptual care map for J.K.

Answers available at http://evolve.elsevier.com/Lewis/medsurg.

BRIDGE TO NCLEX EXAMINATION

The number of the question corresponds to the same-numbered outcome at the beginning of the chapter.

1. Which patient has the *highest* risk for having a stroke?
   a. 65-year-old Black male with hypertension
   b. 50-year-old Native American with obesity
   c. 40-year-old Asian American female who smokes
   d. 35-year-old White female taking oral contraceptives
2. Patient information that would help distinguish a hemorrhagic stroke from a thrombotic stroke includes
   a. sensory changes.
   b. a history of hypertension.
   c. presence of motor weakness.
   d. sudden onset of severe headache.
3. A patient after a stroke has difficulty finding words and weakness in his right arm. What area of the brain is *most* likely involved?
   a. Brainstem
   b. Vertebral artery
   c. Left middle cerebral artery
   d. Right middle cerebral artery
4. Which test would provide the best initial diagnostic information for a patient who presents to the emergency department with a potential stroke?
   a. Noncontrast head CT
   b. Cerebral angiography
   c. Transcranial Doppler ultrasonography
   d. Intraarterial digital subtraction angiography
5. A patient having TIAs is scheduled for a carotid endarterectomy. The nurse explains that the purpose of this procedure is to
   a. decrease cerebral edema.
   b. reduce the brain damage that occurs during a stroke in evolution.
   c. prevent a stroke by removing atherosclerotic plaques blocking cerebral blood flow.
   d. provide a circulatory bypass around thrombotic plaques obstructing cranial circulation.
6. The *most* important piece of information that the nurse would obtain from a patient who is suspected of having a stroke is
   a. time of the patient's last meal.
   b. time at which stroke symptoms first appeared.
   c. patient's hypertension history and management.
   d. family history of stroke and other cardiovascular diseases.
7. A patient who recently had a stroke is home after 1 month of rehabilitation. The home care nurse is concerned when the patient says **(Select all that apply.)**
   a. "I just don't want to do anything anymore."
   b. "My daughter visits twice a day and helps me."
   c. "I just cannot sleep at night. I wake up every hour."
   d. "I understand that my atrial fibrillation caused my stroke."
   e. "I have no problem going up the stairs. Why is everyone so worried?"

1. a; 2. d; 3. c; 4. a; 5. c; 6. b; 7. a, c, e.

For rationales to these answers and even more NCLEX review questions, visit http://evolve.elsevier.com/Lewis/medsurg.

REFERENCES

To access the References for this chapter, please scan the QR code with a mobile device.

63

Chronic Neurologic Problems

Cynthia Bernat Amerson

http://evolve.elsevier.com/Lewis/medsurg/

CONCEPTUAL FOCUS

Cognition
Coping
Functional Ability
Inflammation
Intracranial Regulation
Mobility
Safety

LEARNING OUTCOMES

1. Compare the etiology, clinical manifestations, and interprofessional and nursing management for primary headaches.
2. Describe the clinical manifestations, diagnostic studies, and interprofessional and nursing management of seizure disorder and restless legs syndrome.
3. Discern the clinical manifestations and nursing and interprofessional management of multiple sclerosis, Parkinson disease, and myasthenia gravis.
4. Outline the nursing care for patients with a degenerative neurologic disease.

KEY TERMS

absence seizure
amyotrophic lateral sclerosis (ALS)
aura
cluster headache
focal-onset seizures
generalized-onset seizures
Huntington disease (HD)
migraine headache
multiple sclerosis (MS)
myasthenia gravis (MG)
myasthenic crisis
Parkinson disease (PD)
restless legs syndrome (RLS)
seizure
seizure disorder
status epilepticus
tension-type headache (TTH)
tonic-clonic seizure
trigeminal autonomic cephalgia (TAC)

This chapter discusses headaches, chronic neurologic disorders, and degenerative neurologic disorders. Patients with these diseases have many similar concerns and problems. Treatment seeks to reduce symptoms and help patients maintain optimal function. Patients must deal with the disease and its impact on quality of life. Many have concerns about safety, nutrition, mobility, self-care, and coping. Patients and caregivers need psychosocial support, especially as the disease progresses and disability worsens.

HEADACHES

Headache is one of the most common types of pain. Most people have functional headaches, such as migraine or tension-type headaches. Other headaches are organic, caused by intracranial or extracranial disease.

Pain-sensitive structures in the head include venous sinuses, dura, cranial blood vessels, and cervical nerves. Pain occurs when these structures experience pull, displacement, inflammation, or swelling. Signals are sent to the trigeminal nerve (cranial nerve [CN] V), facial nerve (CN VII), and glossopharyngeal nerve (CN IX). These nerves have motor and sensory functions, so pain intensity can increase when a person moves.

We classify headaches as primary or secondary based on the International Headache Society (IHS) classification.[1] *Primary headaches* include tension-type, migraine, and trigeminal autonomic cephalgia (TAC) (Table 63.1). They are not caused by a disease or medical problem. These classifications have further subtypes. *Secondary headaches* are caused by another disease or problem, such as sinus infection, neck injury, or brain tumor. Patients may have more than 1 type of headache.

TENSION-TYPE HEADACHE

Tension-type headache (TTH), or *stress headache,* is a very common type of headache.[2] TTH is usually of mild or moderate intensity. It lasts minutes to days. TTHs are divided into 3 categories by frequency: infrequent, frequent, or chronic.

TABLE 63.1 Interprofessional Care

Comparison of Headaches

Tension-Type Headaches	Migraine Headache	Trigeminal Autonomic Cephalgia
Location		
Bilateral, bandlike pressure at base of skull	Unilateral in 60%, may switch sides; often anterior location	Unilateral, radiating up or down from 1 eye
Quality		
Constant, squeezing, tightness	Throbbing, synchronous with pulse	Severe, bone crushing
Frequency		
Cycles for many years	Periodic, cycles of several months and years	Up to 8/day. May have months or years between attacks. Occurs in clusters over 2–12 wk
Duration		
30 min–7 days	4–72 h	5 min–3 h
Time and Mode of Onset		
Not related to time	May be preceded by prodromal symptoms or aura Onset after awakening Improves with sleep	Nocturnal, often awakens person from sleep
Associated Symptoms		
Palpable neck and shoulder muscle tension Stiff neck Tenderness	Aura: visual, sensory, aphasic Irritability, sweating Nausea, vomiting Photophobia Phonophobia Prodromal sensory, motor, or psychic phenomena	Facial flushing or pallor Unilateral lacrimation, ptosis, rhinitis
Treatment: Abortive and Symptomatic Drugs		
Nonopioid analgesics: aspirin, acetaminophen, NSAIDs Analgesic combinations • butalbital/acetaminophen/caffeine • butalbital/aspirin/caffeine (Fiorinal) Muscle relaxants	α-Adrenergic blockers • ergotamine • dihydroergotamine NSAIDs Serotonin receptor agonists • almotriptan • eletriptan (Relpax) • frovatriptan (Frova) • lasmiditan (Reyvow) • naratriptan (Amerge) • rizatriptan (Maxalt) • sumatriptan (Imitrex) • zolmitriptan (Zomig) • acetaminophen/caffeine/aspirin • sumatriptan/naproxen (Treximet) CGRP antagonists Nasal lidocaine	α-Adrenergic blockers • ergotamine • dihydroergotamine Serotonin receptor agonists • almotriptan • eletriptan • frovatriptan • naratriptan • rizatriptan • sumatriptan • zolmitriptan High-flow 100% O_2

Continued

TABLE 63.1 Interprofessional Care—cont'd

Comparison of Headaches

Tension-Type Headaches	Migraine Headache	Trigeminal Autonomic Cephalgia
Treatment: Preventive		
Antiseizure drugs • topiramate (Topamax) • divalproex (Depakote) β-Adrenergic blockers Botulinum toxin A mirtazapine (Remeron) Muscle relaxation training Selective serotonin reuptake inhibitors • fluoxetine (Prozac) • paroxetine (Paxil) Tricyclic antidepressants • amitriptyline • doxepin • nortriptyline	Antiseizure drugs β-Adrenergic blockers Botulinum toxin A CGRP antagonists Tricyclic antidepressants Monoclonal antibodies	α-Adrenergic blockers • ergotamine tartrate Antiseizure drugs • gabapentin • topiramate Corticosteroids CGRP antagonists Lithium verapamil

CGRP, Calcitonin gene-related peptide.

Chronic TTH occurs more than 15 days per month for at least 3 months. They can lead to decreased quality of life and severe disability.[1]

Etiology and Pathophysiology

We do not know the cause of TTH. Triggers include inadequate sleep, stress, anxiety, or depression. They may develop after exposure to caffeine or smoking. Many patients have tight cervical muscles and general pain in the back, hips, and knees. Episodic headaches can evolve into chronic headaches. Headaches may occur intermittently for weeks, months, or years. TTH may occur more frequently in those with an increased sensitivity to pain.

Clinical Manifestations

TTH manifests with a bilateral frontal-occipital headache (Fig. 63.1). The pain is a constant, dull pressure or a tight band. Increased cervical and neck muscle tone with neck pain is common. Patients may be sensitive to light *(photophobia)* or sound *(phonophobia)*. Activity increases the pain. TTH has no *prodromal symptoms* (symptoms of impending headache). Patients can have a combination of migraine headache and TTH.

Diagnostic Studies

The history is the most useful tool for diagnosing TTH (Table 63.2). If a TTH is present during assessment, increased resistance to passive movement of the head and tenderness in the head and neck may be present. Electromyography (EMG) may show sustained contraction of neck, scalp, or facial muscles. Imaging is done when symptoms reveal a possible organic cause.

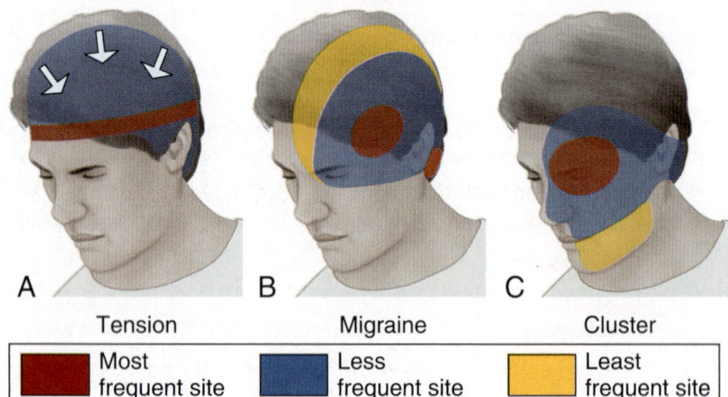

Fig. 63.1 Location of pain for common headache syndromes. (A) Tension headache is often described as feeling of a weight in or on the head or a band squeezing the head. (B) Migraine headache is usually unilateral, in the temple on 1 side of the head. The pain can be bilateral. (C) Cluster headache pain is focused in and around 1 eye.

MIGRAINE HEADACHE

Migraine headache is a recurring headache characterized by unilateral throbbing pain. Migraines are most common between the ages of 25 and 55. Over 10% of Americans are diagnosed with migraine.[2] Migraines are a leading cause of disability in females aged 15 to 50.[3] The IHS divides migraines into 3 categories: migraine without aura, migraine with aura, and chronic migraine.[1]

Etiology and Pathophysiology

We do not know the exact cause of migraines. The trigeminal vascular system is activated causing release of proinflammatory

TABLE 63.2 Interprofessional Care

Headaches

Diagnostic Assessment

- History and physical assessment
  - Neurologic assessment
  - Inspect for local infection
  - Palpate head for tenderness, bony swellings
  - Auscultate for bruits over major arteries, especially neck
- Laboratory studies
  - CBC
  - Electrolytes
  - Urinalysis
- Diagnostic studies
  - Angiography
  - CT scan, MRA, MRI
  - EEG
  - Lumbar puncture

Management

- Drug therapy (Table 63.1)
- Biofeedback
- Cognitive behavior therapy
- Relaxation therapy
- Sleep modification therapy

mediators. Serotonin deficiency may play a role. Calcitonin gene-related polypeptide, a potent vasodilator promoting pain and inflammation, binds to the trigeminal nerve fibers spreading inflammation to the meninges and vessels in the pia mater. The input spreads across the brain. The aura is thought to come from a prolonged wave of neural depolarization (cortical spreading).[4] Patients with migraines have neuron hyperexcitability in the cerebral cortex, especially in the occipital cortex.

There is 3 times greater risk of migraine if a first-degree relative has migraines.[4] Other risk factors include female gender, obesity, and stressful life events. Patients with migraines have increased risk of seizure disorder, ischemic stroke, asthma, depression, anxiety, sleep disorders, and hypertension.[5]

For some patients, specific factors, or triggers, may initiate a migraine. Triggers include hormone fluctuations, bright lights, loud noises, barometric pressure changes, skipping meals, odors, alcohol, lack of sleep, and stress. Some patients have food triggers. Common food triggers include caffeine, monosodium glutamate, and high-tyramine foods. Some foods once thought to be triggers (e.g., chocolate) are now believed to be prodromal food cravings.[6]

Clinical Manifestations

Migraine has 4 stages: prodrome, aura, headache, and postdrome. Prodromal symptoms occur hours or days before the onset of the headache or aura. Prodromal symptoms include a change in activity level, depression, fatigue, food cravings, yawning, or difficulty concentrating.

An **aura** is a group of neurologic symptoms that occur before a headache begins but may continue into the headache. Aura occurs in about 20% of patients. Symptoms of an aura are completely reversible. There are 4 main types of aura: visual, sensory, aphasic, and motor. Visual symptoms include flashes of bright lights, blind spots, or zigzag lines. They are the most common aura. Sensory auras may start as tingling or numbness in the fingers or in the mouth, hearing nonexistent voices, or smelling unusual odors. Aphasic and motor auras are rare.

The headache stage lasts 4 to 72 hours. Patients describe the pain as steady, pounding, or throbbing. It is synchronous with the pulse and worsens with movement. The pain is unilateral (Fig. 63.1). Patients may try to avoid noise, light, odors, and stress. Postdrome can leave patients tired and unable to concentrate.

Diagnostic Studies

The history is the key to diagnosis. Diagnostic testing is done to rule out organic causes (Table 63.2). No specific laboratory or radiologic test can diagnose migraine headache. Neuroimaging techniques (e.g., CT scan, MRI) are not part of the evaluation unless the neurologic assessment is abnormal.

TRIGEMINAL AUTONOMIC CEPHALGIA

Trigeminal autonomic cephalgia (TAC) is the most severe form of primary headache. Age at onset is often between 20 and 40. Symptoms often decline after age 65.[7] Males have TAC 3 times more often.

The most common headache in this class is the **cluster headache**. It is considered the most painful type of headache. Headaches happen in clusters of 1 to 8 headaches a day.[8] A cluster typically lasts 4 to 12 weeks. There may be months to years between clusters. Because cluster periods often occur seasonally, headaches may be mistaken for allergy symptoms. About 20% of patients do not have pain-free intervals between clusters.[8]

Etiology and Pathophysiology

We do not know the cause of cluster headaches. Genetic influence is likely. A sudden release of histamine or serotonin at the trigeminal nerve may initiate symptoms. Imaging studies show the hypothalamus and trigeminal vascular complex are activated when the headache begins. Alcohol, caffeine, and food high in tyramine can be triggers. Pain may start within 1 hour of drinking alcohol. Strong odors (e.g., gasoline, paint fumes) or becoming overheated are other triggers. Cluster headaches may occur at high altitudes when less oxygen is available in the air.

Clinical Manifestations

TAC causes severe, intense pain lasting 15 minutes to 3 hours. The pain is described as sharp, stabbing, or excruciating. Pain is unilateral, focused around the eye, radiating to the temple, forehead, cheek, nose, or jaw along the CN V pathway (Fig. 63.1). Headaches usually occur at the same time each day. Attacks often occur at night, waking the person with severe pain after falling asleep. Parasympathetic autonomic symptoms include swelling around the eye, lacrimation (tearing), facial sweating, nasal congestion or rhinorrhea, ptosis, and miosis. Patients may be agitated and restless.

Diagnostic Studies

The diagnosis is based on the history. Timing, duration, location, and associated symptoms help determine the type and cause of headaches. Laboratory tests can identify physical causes of headache. CT scan, MRI, or magnetic resonance angiography (MRA) may rule out an aneurysm, infection, or intracranial masses. A lumbar puncture (LP) may rule out bleeding, infection, or other problems.

OTHER TYPES OF HEADACHES

Other types of headaches may be related to external or internal causes. A headache may be the first symptom of more serious illness or from head trauma. Headache can occur with intracranial hemorrhage, tumors, allergies, systemic illness (e.g., infection), substance withdrawal, and eye, nose, or dental problems. Because of the varied causes of headache, assessment is critical. Management is based on the cause.

Medication Overuse Headaches

Patients with frequent headaches may overuse drugs for headache treatment. *Medication overuse headache* (MOH) is a term used to describe new headache or worsening of a preexisting headache associated with frequent treatment. Drugs known to cause MOH are acetaminophen, aspirin, nonsteroidal antiinflammatory drugs (NSAIDs), NSAIDs with caffeine, triptans, barbiturates, and ergotamine. Patients who take these agents for more than 15 days a month for longer than 3 months are at risk. MOH often occurs daily and is present on wakening. Patients may also have nausea, restlessness, lack of energy, decreased memory, difficulty concentrating, and irritability. Treatment involves stopping the offending drug and using alternative agents, such as amitriptyline.

INTERPROFESSIONAL CARE: HEADACHES

The type of headache guides therapy (Table 63.1). Cognitive behavior therapy, sleep modification therapy, and progressive relaxation therapy may produce up to a 60% reduction in frequency and severity of headache.[9] Biofeedback helps some patients reduce headache frequency. It uses physiologic monitoring equipment to monitor the body's stress responses. Positive reinforcement occurs when patients reduce physiologic signs of stress. Acupuncture, acupressure, and hypnosis help some patients. Actions to decrease headache pain include resting in a dark, quiet area, placing cool cloths on the head, drinking fluids, and consuming small amounts of caffeine (Table 63.2).

Drug Therapy

Tension-Type Headache

Drug therapy for TTH usually involves aspirin, acetaminophen, or NSAIDs (see Table 9.8). They may be used alone or in combination with caffeine, sedatives, or muscle relaxants. Analgesics are often only partly effective, even at maximum dose. Stronger analgesics provide no added benefit. Tricyclic antidepressants, antiseizure medications, or muscle relaxants may be used as preventive therapy.

Migraine Headache

The aim of drug therapy during acute migraine is stopping or decreasing symptoms. Many people with mild migraine headache can get relief with NSAIDs or aspirin, alone or with caffeine. Analgesia with caffeine provides increased efficacy compared with analgesia alone for migraine and TTH.[3] For moderate to severe migraine pain, triptans are the first line of therapy (Table 63.1).[2]

Triptans (e.g., sumatriptan) increase cerebral serotonin. This reduces neurogenic inflammation and vasoconstricts cerebral blood vessels. Triptans are most effective when taken at the start of a migraine or during the aura. Sumatriptan is available in several forms and delivery systems (oral, subcutaneous, nasal spray, transdermal). It is the only ultrafast-acting triptan. A combination of oral sumatriptan and naproxen sodium (Treximet) is highly effective for symptom relief. Triptans are contraindicated for people with cardiovascular disease due to vasoconstriction.

When triptans are contraindicated or ineffective, other drugs are prescribed. The serotonin (5-HT) receptor agonist lasmiditan (Reyvow) increases serotonin, reduces inflammation, and relieves pain during a migraine. It is safe for patients with cardiovascular disease because it does not cause vasoconstriction.[3] Other agents used to treat acute migraine include dihydroergotamine (DHE 45) and other ergot-based agents. Patients with cardiovascular disease or those taking other vasoconstrictors should use ergot agents with caution.

DRUG ALERT

Sumatriptan

- Should not be used by patients with a history of angina, stroke, myocardial infarction, or hypertension.
- Excess dosage may cause tremors and decrease respirations.
- Limit use to 10 days per month.

Calcitonin gene-related peptide (CGRP) increases in migraine causing inflammation and vasodilation. CGRP receptor antagonists block this effect. Patients take these injectable drugs (erenumab [Aimovig], fremanezumab [Ajovy], galcanezumab [Emgality]) at the onset of an attack. Other forms include ubrogepant (Ubrelvy), given orally, and zavegepant (Zavzpret), a rapidly acting nasal spray.

Preventive treatment is an important part of migraine management. The decision to start preventive treatment is based on frequency, severity, and disability related to headaches. Patients having migraines more than 3 days a week often take preventive medication. Antiseizure drugs (e.g., topiramate, divalproex, valproate) may be taken daily for migraine prevention. They take 2 to 3 months to reach full effectiveness. Antiseizure drugs should never be abruptly stopped because seizures may develop. Provide teaching to promote safe use. Extended-release medication promotes adherence, with fewer cognitive effects.[3]

Other medications include β-adrenergic blockers such as propranolol (Inderal) or atenolol (Tenormin). They should be used cautiously in patients with asthma and diabetes. Tricyclic antidepressants like amitriptyline are options.

Botulinum toxin A (Botox) may be an effective prophylactic treatment for adults who have chronic migraines at least 15 days each month or migraines unresponsive to other medications. Botox is given by multiple injections around the head and neck into the pain fibers. Injections are given every 3 months. Maximum benefit may not be seen for 6 months. During this time, patients should continue their regular medications. The most common reactions are neck pain and headache. A slight risk exists for the toxin to migrate to the face and neck, causing difficulty swallowing and breathing. Patients should seek immediate medical attention if this occurs.

CGRP antagonists, atogepant (Qulipta) and rimegepant (Nurtec ODT), are approved for migraine prevention. Eptinezumab (Vyepti) and galcanezumab are monoclonal antibody (mAb) treatments that can reduce the frequency and severity of chronic migraines by acting on CGRP pathways.

Other prophylactic treatments for migraine include supraorbital transcutaneous electrical stimulation, vagal nerve stimulation (VNS), and single pulse transcranial magnetic stimulation. These treatments use energy stimulation to prevent headache. Complementary approaches for migraine prophylaxis include riboflavin, coenzyme Q10, magnesium, and butterbur.[9]

Cluster Headache

Triptans (e.g., sumatriptan, zolmitriptan) given by injection or nasally are the standard treatment for occasional cluster headache. Intranasal dihydroergotamine or 4% lidocaine are other effective options for pain relief. The lidocaine may be repeated in 15 minutes if needed.

Nondrug options for patients with refractory cluster headaches include invasive nerve blocks, deep brain stimulation (DBS), vagal or trigeminal stimulators, and ablative neurosurgical procedures (e.g., percutaneous radiofrequency).[9] Alternatively, 7 to 12 L/min of 100% O_2 by nonrebreather mask for 20 minutes is well-tolerated, safe, and effective treatment for TAC. O_2 causes vasoconstriction and reduces inflammation in the brain. Treatment may be repeated after a 5-minute rest.

Those with chronic cluster headaches often seek preventive treatment. High-dose verapamil is the first-choice drug to prevent cluster headache. We monitor patients carefully during treatment. An ECG should be done every 6 months and with dose changes. Galcanezumab and topiramate are used for preventive treatment of TAC. Prednisone may be used for a short time until the preventive medications reach a therapeutic level.

NURSING MANAGEMENT: HEADACHES

Assessment

The history and neurologic assessment are key to defining the type of headache. The assessment is often normal with primary headaches. The history is focused on specific characteristics of the headaches (Table 63.3). Include location and type of pain, onset, frequency, duration, relation to events (emotional, psychologic, physical), and time of day of the occurrence. What are the effects on daily activities? Has the character, intensity, or location of the headache changed? Obtain a medication history.

Encourage patients to keep a diary of headaches with specific details. This helps monitor frequency, precipitating events, and treatment effectiveness. Avoiding diet triggers is helpful for many patients with cluster and migraine headache.

Clinical Problems

Clinical problems for patients with headaches may include:

- Pain
- Deficient knowledge

Additional information on clinical problems and interventions is presented in eNursing Care Plan 63.1 for patients with headaches (available on the website for this chapter).

Planning

The overall goals are that patients with headaches will (1) have reduced or no pain, (2) understand triggers and treatments, (3) use positive coping strategies, and (4) have increased quality of life.

Implementation

Table 63.4 addresses teaching for patients with headaches. Patients benefit from engaging in stress reduction techniques. An inability to cope with daily stressors can cause headaches. Help patients examine their daily routine, recognize stressful situations, and develop coping strategies. Help them identify precipitating factors and develop ways to avoid or minimize them. Encourage daily exercise, relaxation periods, and socialization as ways to decrease headaches. Suggest meditation, yoga, and other ways to reduce stress. Encourage a consistent daily routine with adequate sleep and regular, well-balanced meals.

TABLE 63.3 NURSING ASSESSMENT

Headaches

Subjective Data

Important Health Information

Health history: Seizures, cancer, recent fall or other trauma, cranial infection, stroke. Asthma or allergies. Relationship of headache to overwork, stress, menstruation, exercise, food, sexual activity, travel, bright lights, or noxious environment stimuli

Medications: Hydralazine, bromides, nitroglycerin, ergotamine (withdrawal), NSAIDs (in high daily doses), estrogen preparations, oral contraceptives, OTC medications

Surgery: Craniotomy, sinus surgery, facial surgery

Functional Health Pattern

Health perception—health management: Positive family history. Malaise

Nutritional-metabolic: Ingesting alcohol, caffeine, cheese, chocolate, monosodium glutamate, aspartame, lunch meats (nitrites in cured meats), sausage, hot dogs, onions, avocados. Anorexia, nausea, vomiting; unilateral lacrimation (cluster)

Activity-exercise: Vertigo, fatigue, weakness, paralysis, fainting

Sleep-rest: Insomnia

Cognitive-perceptual:

- *Tension type:* Bilateral, bandlike, dull and persistent, base-of-skull headache, neck tenderness
- *Migraine:* Aura. Unilateral, severe, throbbing headache (possible switching of side). Vision changes, photophobia, phonophobia, dizziness, tingling or burning sensations
- *Cluster:* Unilateral and severe, nocturnal headache. Nasal stuffiness

Self-perception—self-concept: Depression

Coping—stress tolerance: Stress, anxiety, irritability, withdrawal

Objective Data

General

Anxiety, apprehension

Musculoskeletal

Resistance of head and neck movement, nuchal rigidity (meningeal, tension type), palpable neck and shoulder muscle tension (tension type)

Neurologic

Restlessness (cluster), hemiparesis (migraine)

Skin

Migraine: Edema, pallor, diaphoresis

Cluster: Forehead diaphoresis, pallor, unilateral facial flushing with cheek/eye edema, conjunctivitis

Possible Diagnostic Findings

Disease, deformity, or infection on brain imaging (CT, MRI, MRA), cerebral angiogram, lumbar puncture, EEG, EMG

Teach patients about drugs prescribed for preventive and symptomatic treatment. Encourage patients with acute migraine to seek a quiet, dimly lit environment and take medication as soon as the headache or aura begins. Massage and cool or hot packs to the neck and head can help. If headaches are triggered by food, plan ways to eliminate those foods. Active challenge testing (designed specifically to provoke symptoms) with suspect foods helps determine causative agents.

TABLE 63.4 PATIENT & CAREGIVER TEACHING

Headaches

Include the following instructions when teaching patients with headaches and caregivers:

- Keep a diary of headaches, symptoms, and possible precipitating events.
- Avoid possible headache triggers:
  - Alcohol (especially red wine)
  - Drugs: ergot-containing preparations (ergotamine tartrate) and monoamine oxidase inhibitors
  - Fatigue
  - Foods: aged cheese, ice cream, onions, oranges, vinegar
  - Aspartame
  - Caffeine
  - Fermented or marinated foods
  - Monosodium glutamate
  - Nitrites (processed lunch meats, hot dogs)
  - Nicotine
- Learn the purpose, action, dosage, and side effects of drugs taken.
- Self-administer sumatriptan nasally or subcutaneously, if prescribed.
- Use stress management techniques (see Chapter 7).
- Take part in regular exercise.
- Avoid smoking and exposure to environment triggers, such as strong perfumes.
- Contact HCP if any of the following occur:
  - Symptoms become more severe, last longer than usual, or are resistant to medication
  - Nausea and vomiting (if severe or not typical), change in vision, or fever occurs with the headache
  - Problems occur with any drug

◆ Evaluation

Expected outcomes are that patients with headaches will:

- Report satisfaction with pain management
- Use measures to manage pain
- Report optimal quality of life

CHRONIC NEUROLOGIC PROBLEMS

SEIZURE DISORDER

A **seizure** is a sudden, abnormal, excess electrical discharge of neurons in the brain. During a seizure, multiple neurons fire at a rate much faster than normal, causing involuntary movements, sensory phenomena, emotional expression, and unusual behaviors.[10] **Seizure disorder**, or *epilepsy*, is a group of neurologic diseases marked by recurring seizures. Patients with 2 or more seizures, more than 24 hours apart, without an underlying problem that caused the seizure, may have seizure disorder.[10] Seizures from systemic or metabolic problems that stop when the underlying problem is corrected are not seizure disorder. About 1.2% of Americans have seizure disorder.[11]

Etiology and Pathophysiology

Seizure disorder is characterized by a group of abnormal neurons that fire without a clear cause. This may be due to the release of excitatory neurotransmitters or by an absence of neuroinhibitory activity. Both lead to excess electric activity. Any stimulus that causes the neuron's cell membrane to depolarize can cause this firing, which spreads through physiologic pathways.

For most people, the cause of seizure disorder is unknown. This is known as *idiopathic generalized epilepsy (IGE).* Some patients may have seizures due to medical problems. Known causes of seizure disorder include stroke, brain tumors, cerebral infection, traumatic brain injury, hypoxic birth injury, neurodevelopment disorders (e.g., autism spectrum disorders), and neurodegenerative disease. Other common causes include low or very high glucose levels, abnormal electrolyte levels (sodium, magnesium, calcium), eclampsia, lack of sleep, and alcohol withdrawal. Children may have seizures with high fever. Patients with autoimmune disease, like systemic lupus erythematosus (SLE) or autoimmune encephalitis, have cerebral inflammation that increases seizure risk.

Genetic Link

Interaction between genetics and the environment may cause seizure disorder. Environment exposures may cause genetic changes. Some genetic diseases cause brain malformations that lead to a seizure disorder. Gene mutations that cause a low seizure threshold, change in nutrient metabolism, altered neural signaling, or altered neural migration in brain development can lead to seizure disorder. Patients with chromosomal disorders (e.g., Down syndrome) often have seizure disorder.

Clinical Manifestations

Specific manifestations of a seizure are determined by the site of the electrical disturbance. The International League Against Epilepsy classification system divides seizures into 3 major classes based on where the seizure activity begins: *generalized onset, focal onset,* and unknown onset.[12] Focal onset accounts for about 60% of seizures (Table 63.5). Seizures within each classification are also characterized as *motor* or *nonmotor* and by level of awareness. These descriptors address what occurs during the seizure.

A seizure occurs in 4 phases: (1) *prodromal phase,* sensations or behavior changes that precede a seizure by hours or days; (2) *aural phase,* part of the seizure, a sensory warning that is similar each time a seizure occurs; (3) *ictal phase,* the first symptoms to the end of seizure activity; and (4) *postictal phase,* the recovery period after the seizure. Not all patients have every phase.

TABLE 63.5 Classification of Seizures

Generalized-Onset Seizure (Involves Both Hemispheres of Brain)

- Motor seizure
  - Atonic
  - Clonic
  - Epileptic spasms
  - Myoclonic
  - Myoclonic-atonic
  - Myoclonic-tonic-clonic
  - Tonic
  - Tonic-clonic
- Nonmotor (absence) seizure
  - Typical
  - Atypical
  - Myoclonic
  - Eyelid myoclonia

Focal-Onset Seizure (Limited to 1 Hemisphere of Brain)

- Aware (no impairment of awareness/consciousness)
- Impaired awareness (impairment of awareness/consciousness)
- Motor onset
  - Automatisms
  - Atonic
  - Clonic
  - Epileptic spasms
  - Hyperkinetic
  - Myoclonic
  - Tonic
- Nonmotor onset
  - Autonomic
  - Behavior arrest
  - Cognitive
  - Emotional
  - Sensory

Unknown Onset Seizure

Due to inadequate information or inability to assign to other categories above

Adapted from Fisher RS, Cross JH, D'Souza C, et al: Instruction manual for the ILAE 2017 operational classification of seizure types, *Epilepsia* 58:4, 2017.

Generalized-Onset Seizures

Generalized-onset seizures start over wide areas of both sides of the brain. They are characterized by bilateral, synchronous neural discharges. Patients usually have impaired consciousness for a few seconds to several minutes. Generalized seizures are motor or nonmotor. Motor movements are bilateral.

Generalized-onset motor seizures. Tonic-clonic seizure is the most common generalized-onset motor seizure. During a tonic-clonic seizure, patients lose consciousness and fall to the ground. The body stiffens (tonic phase) for 10 to 20 seconds and then the extremities jerk (clonic phase) for 30 seconds to several minutes. Cyanosis, excess salivation, tongue or cheek biting, and incontinence may occur during the seizure. In the postictal phase, patients usually have muscle soreness, feel tired, and may sleep for several hours. Some patients do not feel normal for several hours or days after a seizure. They have no memory of the seizure.

Other types include tonic and clonic. Tonic seizures involve a sudden onset of increased tone in the extensor muscles, contributing to sudden stiff movements. Tonic seizures most often occur in sleep and affect both sides of the body. Tonic seizures usually last less than 20 seconds. Patients usually stay aware. Clonic seizures begin with loss of awareness and sudden loss of muscle tone, followed by rhythmic limb jerking that may or may not be symmetric.

An *atonic seizure* (or *drop attack*) involves a brief, sudden loss of muscle tone. It may affect just the head and neck or result in the person falling to the ground. Seizures typically last a few seconds. A brief loss of consciousness is followed with brief postictal confusion. Patients with atonic seizure are at great risk for head injury. They may need protective helmets.

Generalized-onset nonmotor seizures. **Absence seizure** most often occurs in females between ages 4 and 14. They rarely occur beyond adolescence. They may stop altogether or evolve into another type of seizure as the child matures. A typical absence seizure is marked by a sudden onset brief staring spell that resembles daydreaming with sudden recovery. Eye fluttering and an upward gaze may occur. It often goes unnoticed because it lasts less than 10 to 20 seconds. Usually, patients are unresponsive when spoken to during the seizure.[13]

In *atypical absence seizure,* the staring spell is accompanied by additional signs, such as rapid eye blinking, jerking movements of the lips, or repetitive movements (automatisms). This type of seizure lasts 20 seconds or more and has a gradual beginning and end. Seizure activity may be hard to identify if patients have a coexisting cognitive disorder. Atypical absence seizures can continue into adulthood.

Focal-Onset Seizures

Focal-onset seizures (formerly called *partial* or *partial focal seizures*) are the second major class of seizures (Table 63.5). Focal seizures begin in 1 hemisphere of the brain in a local region of the cortex. They cause sensory, motor, cognitive, or emotion manifestations based on the function of the involved area of the brain. For example, if the discharging focus is in the medial aspect of the postcentral gyrus, patients may have paresthesia in the leg on the side opposite the focus.

Focal seizures are motor or nonmotor. Motor activities are atonic (loss of muscle tone, relaxed muscles), tonic (sustained stiffening), clonic (rhythmic jerking), or myoclonic (very rapid, irregular, brief jerking).[13] Some people show strange behavior, such as lip smacking, picking at clothes, or other repetitive, purposeless actions (automatisms).

We further describe focal-onset seizure as aware or impaired awareness. In *focal awareness seizures,* patients are conscious and alert but have unusual feelings or sensations. They may have sudden and unexplainable feelings of joy, anger, sadness, or nausea. They may hear, smell, taste, see, or feel things that are not real. Some have local twitching. In a *focal impaired awareness seizure,* patients have a loss of consciousness or a change in awareness producing a dreamlike state. Their eyes are open. Their movements may seem purposeful, but they cannot interact with others. During a seizure, people may do things that can be dangerous or embarrassing, such as walking into traffic or removing clothes. They may continue an activity started before the seizure, such as counting coins or choosing items from a grocery shelf. After the seizure they do not remember the activity performed during the seizure. Seizures last 1 to 2 minutes. Patients are tired or confused after the seizure and do not return to normal activity for hours. *Subclinical seizures* are a form of seizure in which sedated patients seize but there are no external physical movements because of the sedative use.

Psychogenic Nonepileptic Seizures

Psychogenic nonepileptic seizures (PNES) imitate seizures but are not due to neuron activity. They are triggered by emotional events. Because of the close resemblance, PNES may be misdiagnosed as seizure disorder. Proper diagnosis requires video-EEG monitoring during the attack. A history of emotional or physical abuse or a traumatic event often exists. Treatment includes cognitive behavior therapy and serotonin reuptake inhibitors.

Complications

People with seizure disorder have higher mortality rates. Injury or death can result from trauma suffered during a seizure. Patients who lose consciousness during a seizure are at greatest risk. Other deaths are due to accidents during seizures, underlying diseases, sudden unexpected death in epilepsy (SUDEP), or status epilepticus.

Status epilepticus (SE) is defined as seizures lasting longer than 5 minutes or occurring so close together that patients cannot recover between them.[14] They do not return to consciousness between seizures. The longer a seizure lasts, the less likely it is to stop without drug therapy.

SE is a neurologic emergency. SE can occur with any type of seizure. The highest incidence occurs in children and older adults. Common causes in adults include stroke, metabolic disease, or low levels of seizure medications. Many patients who have SE do not have a history of seizure disorder.[14]

During repeated seizures, the brain uses more energy than the body can supply. As neurons become exhausted and cease to function, permanent damage may result. *Convulsive status epilepticus* (CSE) is the most common form. It occurs with prolonged, repeated tonic-clonic or other motor seizures. The goal of therapy is to rapidly end clinical and electrical seizure activity before neuronal damage occurs. Without prompt treatment, CSE can lead to respiratory insufficiency, hypoxemia, dysrhythmias, hyperthermia, and systemic acidosis. The prognosis is related to the cause, length of the seizures, age, and time to treatment. *Nonconvulsive status epilepticus* is a long or recurrent focal impaired awareness seizure. Symptoms may be subtle, making it hard to tell recovery from seizure symptoms.

Refractory status epilepticus (RSE) is continuous seizure activity despite administration of first- and second-line therapy.

TABLE 63.6 Interprofessional Care

Seizure Disorder

Diagnostic Assessment

History and Physical Assessment

- Health history
  - Birth and development
  - Significant illnesses and injuries
  - Family history
- Febrile seizures
- Neurologic assessment
- Seizure history
- Precipitating factors
- Seizure description (aura, onset, duration, frequency, postictal state, movements, awareness)

Diagnostic Studies

- CBC, metabolic panel
- Urinalysis
- Lumbar puncture for CSF analysis
- Imaging scans: CT, MRI, MRA, MRS, PET
- EEG

Management

- Antiseizure drugs (Table 63.7)
- Surgery
- Vagal nerve stimulation
- Deep brain stimulation
- Responsive neurostimulation
- Counseling
- Physical therapy

RSE has a high risk for mortality and neurologic damage. Treatment should be rapidly escalated to avoid progression. *Superrefractory SE* is the presence of medically refractory seizures that continue 24 hours or more after starting anesthesia or when seizure activity persists after 7 days of continuous general anesthesia.

SUDEP affects about 1in 1000 persons with uncontrolled seizures each year.[14] The cause is unknown. It occurs most often with tonic-clonic seizures. SUDEP is more common at night, in those taking multiple antiseizure drugs, and in patients with poorly managed seizures. Having seizure disorder from a young age increases risk. Seizures may interfere with vital functions in the brainstem. Ictal and postictal apnea and hypoxia may play a role. Seizures may cause dysrhythmias. Specific teaching about drug therapy and controlling seizures is critical to reduce SUDEP risk.

Diagnostic Studies

An accurate, comprehensive description of seizures and the health history is essential to diagnosis (Table 63.6). Once diagnosed with seizure disorder, the seizure type must be identified to determine the correct treatment. An electroencephalogram (EEG) can help determine the type of seizure and pinpoint the seizure focus. An EEG should be done within 24 hours of a suspected seizure. Only a small number of patients have abnormal EEG findings the first time they have an EEG. Repeated EEGs, continuous EEG monitoring, or video-EEG may be needed to detect abnormalities. Many patients with seizure disorder have normal EEG results between seizures. Magnetoencephalography (MEG) may be done with the EEG. MEG has greater sensitivity in detecting small fields of neuron activity.

A CT scan or MRI should be done with any new-onset seizure to rule out a structural lesion. If an MRI shows a lesion but EEG results differ, MEG can determine whether the abnormal brain waves are coming from the lesion. Other imaging tests or angiography may be done. A complete blood count (CBC), chemistries, and liver and kidney function tests assess for metabolic problems.

Interprofessional Care

Drug Therapy

The main treatment for seizure disorder is antiseizure medication (Table 63.7). Because a cure is not possible, the goal of therapy is to prevent seizures with minimal drug side effects. Many drugs are effective for multiple seizure types. Most drugs stabilize nerve cell membranes by blocking sodium or calcium channels or increasing GABA to prevent spread of epileptic discharges.[15] Therapy should begin with a single drug based on the patients' age, weight, and type, frequency, and cause of the seizure. Dosage should be increased until seizures are under control or toxic side effects occur. Antiseizure drugs successfully control seizures for about 70% of patients. About 30% of patients have *medically refractory epilepsy* (drug-resistant epilepsy).

If seizure control is not achieved with a single drug, we change the dose or timing or add a second drug. Many patients need combination therapy for control. Therapy should provide the best control with the least amount of medication. Each drug has a therapeutic range. Above that range, most patients have toxic side effects. Below that range, most continue to have seizures. Therapeutic drug ranges are guides for therapy. Drug levels are monitored if seizures continue to occur, frequency increases, or drug adherence is questioned. Many newer drugs do not require drug-level monitoring.

The main drugs to manage generalized-onset motor and focal-onset seizures are levetiracetam (Keppra), carbamazepine (Tegretol), lamotrigine (Lamictal), divalproex (Depakote), gabapentin (Neurontin), and topiramate (Topamax). The drugs used most often to treat generalized-onset nonmotor and myoclonic seizures include ethosuximide (Zarontin) and clonazepam (Klonopin).

Rapid-acting benzodiazepines are used to treat SE. Options include midazolam IM autoinjector (Seizalam) or intranasal/buccal midazolam (Nayzilam).[16] IV lorazepam may be used if an IV is present. Because these drugs are short-acting, long-acting antiseizure drugs are added. If seizures do not stop, continuous IV antiseizure and anesthetic drugs are given.

Long-acting antiseizure drugs (e.g., phenytoin, phenobarbital, lamotrigine, topiramate) increase adherence because the drug does not have to be taken at work or school. Many seizure drugs are teratogenic (divalproex, phenytoin, carbamazepine). Education and family planning are recommended.

Side effects of antiseizure drugs include vision changes, drowsiness, ataxia, and mental slowness. Neurologic assessment for dose-related toxicity involves testing for nystagmus, hand and gait coordination, cognitive function, and alertness.

TABLE 63.7 Drug Therapy

Select Antiseizure Agents

Drug	Route	Side Effects	Considerations
GABA Analogs			
gabapentin (Neurontin)	Oral	Ataxia Dizziness Drowsiness Vision changes Weight gain	Monitor weight. Avoid pregnancy. Use safety measures if CNS effects occur. Avoid alcohol.
pregabalin (Lyrica)	Oral	Dizziness Drowsiness Edema Vision problems Weight gain	Avoid pregnancy. Use safety measures if CNS effects occur. Avoid alcohol. Monitor weight.
vigabatrin (Sabril)	Oral	Dizziness Drowsiness Impaired memory Vision changes	Stop if vision changes occur. Avoid pregnancy. Use safety measures if CNS effects occur. Avoid alcohol.
Hydantoins			
phenytoin (Dilantin) fosphenytoin (Cerebyx, Sesquient)	IV, oral IM, IV	Ataxia Drowsiness GI distress Gingival hyperplasia Liver toxicity Nystagmus Rash	Avoid alcohol, direct sunlight. Monitor drug levels. Monitor site when giving IV. Monitor CBC and liver function tests. May change urine color to pink or red-brown. Maintain good oral hygiene.
Iminostilbenes			
carbamazepine (Tegretol) oxcarbazepine (Trileptal)	Oral Oral	Bleeding Dizziness Gait changes GI distress Headache Rash Vision problems	Take with meals; avoid grapefruit juice. Avoid direct sunlight. Monitor drug levels, CBC, and liver function tests. Avoid pregnancy. Use safety measures if CNS effects occur. Avoid alcohol.
Miscellaneous			
brivaracetam (Briviact)	IV, oral	Dizziness GI distress Suicidal thoughts	Avoid alcohol. Monitor for depression.
cenobamate (Xcopri)	Oral	Dizziness Drowsiness Suicidal thoughts Vision problems	Use safety measures if CNS effects occur. Monitor for depression. Avoid alcohol.
clonazepam (Klonopin)	Oral	Confusion Dizziness Drowsiness	Do not stop suddenly. Use safety measures if CNS effects occur. Can develop tolerance. Monitor liver function tests.
divalproex (Depakote)	Oral	Bleeding Drowsiness GI distress Liver toxicity Suicidal thoughts Vision changes Weight gain	Use safety measures if CNS effects occur. Monitor for depression. Monitor CBC, liver function tests. Monitor weight.

TABLE 63.7 **Drug Therapy—cont'd**

Select Antiseizure Agents

eslicarbazepine (Aptiom)	Oral	Depression Drowsiness GI distress Rash Speech problems Vision changes	Monitor for depression. Avoid alcohol. Use safety measures if CNS effects occur. Avoid pregnancy. Monitor liver function tests.
ethosuximide (Zarontin)	Oral	Drowsiness GI distress Liver toxicity Rash	Monitor liver function tests. Use safety measures if CNS effects occur. Avoid alcohol. Avoid pregnancy. Stop if rash occurs.
felbamate (Felbatol)	Oral	Decreased appetite with weight loss Liver toxicity Vision changes	Monitor CBC, liver function tests. Monitor weight.
lacosamide (Vimpat)	IV, oral	Dizziness Drowsiness Dysrhythmias GI distress	Use safety measures if CNS effects occur. Avoid alcohol. Avoid pregnancy.
lamotrigine (Lamictal)	Oral	Dizziness Drowsiness GI distress Rash Vision changes	Use safety measures if CNS effects occur. Monitor liver function tests. Stop if rash occurs.
levetiracetam (Keppra)	Oral	Dizziness GI distress Suicidal thoughts	Avoid alcohol. Monitor for depression.
perampanel (Fycompa)	Oral	Anxiety Dizziness GI distress Suicidal thoughts	Give at bedtime. Monitor for depression. Avoid alcohol. Use safety measures if CNS effects occur. Avoid pregnancy.
tiagabine (Gabitril)	Oral	Agitation Dizziness GI distress Rash Suicidal thoughts	Monitor for depression. Avoid in pregnancy. Avoid alcohol. Use safety measures if CNS effects occur.
topiramate (Topamax)	Oral	Ataxia Drowsiness GI distress Vision changes	Stop if vision changes occur. Use safety measures if CNS effects occur. Avoid alcohol. Avoid pregnancy.
valproic acid (Depakene)	Oral	Bleeding Drowsiness GI distress Weight gain	Avoid use in pregnancy. Take with food; avoid carbonated beverages. Monitor bleeding times, CBC, drug levels, liver function tests. Use safety measures if CNS effects occur.
zonisamide (Zonegran)	Oral	Confusion Drowsiness Gait changes GI distress Kidney stones	Use safety measures if CNS effects occur. Encourage fluids.

DRUG ALERT
Antiseizure Drugs

- Abrupt withdrawal after long-term use may cause seizures.
- Patients must be seizure free for a prolonged period (e.g., 2 to 5 years) and have a normal neurologic assessment and EEG for weaning to be initiated.

Gerontologic Considerations: Seizure Disorder and Drug Therapy

Older adults' symptoms of seizure are often confused with other health issues. Repetitive movements of a seizure may be mistaken as a tremor. A patient found on the ground may be presumed to have fallen. Older adults are more likely to have SE than other age groups. Older adults are more responsive to antiseizure drugs than younger adults, but they are more likely to have side effects at lower drug levels. Older adults have prolonged postictal states and increased incidence of postictal confusion.[17]

Because the liver metabolizes phenytoin, it should not be used in older patients with liver dysfunction. The potential effects on cognitive function and bone demineralization make carbamazepine less desirable for older adults. Newer agents like gabapentin, lamotrigine, and levetiracetam may have fewer cognitive effects and fewer drug interactions.

Surgical Therapy

Over 30% of patients with seizures are drug resistant. People with a defined site of seizure origin (epileptogenic zone) can benefit from lesionectomy, focal resection, laser ablation, or radiosurgery. For severe cases, hemispherectomy or corpus callosotomy can be done. Patients should stay on seizure control medication for 2 years after surgery. About 80% of patients are seizure free and have improved quality of life after surgery.[18]

Extensive preoperative evaluation is important. Continuous EEG monitoring, MEG, and other tests to ensure precise localization of the focal point. Localizing the seizure focus (the place where the seizure originates) is critical to the success of surgical treatment. Surgical treatment destroys or removes brain tissue, so it is best for seizures that do not arise from critical areas.

Other Therapies

Several neurostimulation devices are used for drug-resistant epilepsy. These treatments involve surgically implanting an electrode that can deliver a stimulation to reduce or stop seizures. In vagal nerve stimulation (VNS), a surgically implanted electrode in the neck is programmed to deliver electrical impulses to CN X at specific intervals or when the pulse elevates. Elevated pulse occurs with seizures. Contraindications include a history of dysrhythmias or sleep apnea.

Responsive neurostimulation (RNS) continually monitors the EEG to detect abnormalities, record seizure activity, and respond to seizure activity. RNS delivers electrical stimulation to a precise location, which stops the seizure. RNS is the only device that will respond to seizure activity immediately.

Deep brain stimulation (DBS) consists of electrodes placed in the brain at defined sites. The electrodes are connected to a neurostimulator placed under the skin in the chest. The neurostimulator delivers electrical stimulation to stop the signals that trigger seizures.

A ketogenic diet is a high-fat, low-carbohydrate diet that helps control seizures in some people. A person on this diet makes more ketones that pass into the brain, where they replace glucose as an energy source. Meals are carefully planned to restrict the amount of protein and carbohydrate intake. Modified Atkins diets and low glycemic index diets have been shown to control seizures as well. Most people on these diets must continue their antiseizure medications but often take lower doses. Seizures worsen if the diet is stopped abruptly. Long-term effects of ketogenic diets are not clear. Kidney function and lipids are monitored while on these diets.[19]

NURSING MANAGEMENT: SEIZURE DISORDER

Assessment

Subjective and objective data to obtain from patients with seizure disorder are outlined in Table 63.8. Obtain data related to a specific seizure episode from a witness.

Clinical Problems

Clinical problems for patients with seizure disorder may include:

- Impaired respiratory function
- Difficulty coping
- Risk for injury

Additional information on clinical problems and interventions for patients with seizure disorder is presented in eNursing Care Plan 63.2 (available on the website for this chapter).

Planning

The overall goals are that patients with seizure disorder will (1) be free from injury during a seizure, (2) have optimal functioning while taking antiseizure drugs, and (3) have acceptable psychosocial function.

Implementation

Acute Care

Most seizures are self-limiting and do not require emergency medical care. However, if injury occurs, or if the event is a first-time seizure, medical care should be sought immediately.

TABLE 63.8 NURSING ASSESSMENT

Seizure Disorder

Subjective Data

Important Health Information

Health history: Seizures, birth defects or injuries, anoxic episodes. CNS trauma, tumors, or infections. Stroke, metabolic disorders, alcohol use, exposure to metals or carbon monoxide, hepatic or renal failure, fever, pregnancy, systemic lupus erythematosus

Medications: Adherence to antiseizure medication plan. Barbiturate or alcohol withdrawal. Use or overdose of cocaine, amphetamines, lidocaine, theophylline, penicillin, lithium, phenothiazines, tricyclic antidepressants, benzodiazepines

Functional Health Patterns

Health perception–health management: Family history

Cognitive-perceptual: Headaches, aura, mood, or behavioral changes before seizure. Mentation changes, abdominal pain, muscle pain (postictal)

Self-perception–self-concept: Anxiety, depression. Loss of self-esteem, social isolation

Sexuality-reproductive: Decreased sexual drive, erectile dysfunction. Increased sexual drive (postictal)

Objective Data

Cardiovascular

Hypertension, tachycardia, or bradycardia (ictal)

General

Precipitating factors, including severe metabolic acidosis or alkalosis, hyperkalemia, hypoglycemia, dehydration, water intoxication

GI

Bowel incontinence, excess salivation

Musculoskeletal

Weakness, paralysis, ataxia (postictal)

Neurologic

Generalized Onset

Tonic-clonic: Loss of consciousness, muscle tightening, then jerking. Dilated pupils. Hyperventilation, then apnea. Postictal somnolence

Absence: Altered consciousness (5–30 sec), minor facial motor activity

Focal Onset

Aware: Aura. Focal sensory, motor, cognitive, or emotional phenomena (focal motor)

Impaired awareness: Altered consciousness with inappropriate behaviors, automatisms, amnesia of event

Respiratory

Abnormal respiratory rate, rhythm, or depth. Apnea (ictal). Absent or abnormal breath sounds, possible airway occlusion

Skin

Bitten tongue, soft tissue damage, cyanosis, diaphoresis (postictal)

Urinary

Incontinence

Possible Diagnostic Findings

Positive toxicology screen or blood alcohol level. Altered electrolytes, acidosis or alkalosis, low blood glucose, ↑ blood urea nitrogen or creatinine, abnormal liver function tests, ammonia; abnormal CT scan or MRI of head, abnormal findings from LP. Abnormal discharges on EEG

TABLE 63.9 NURSING MANAGEMENT

Care of Patients With Seizure Disorder

- Initiate safety precautions for the patient at risk for seizures.
  - Place suction equipment, bag-valve-mask, and O_2 at the bedside.
  - Remove potentially harmful objects from the bedside and pad side rails.
- Assess and record details of seizure events, including events preceding the seizure; length of each phase of the seizure; course and nature of seizure activity; and level of consciousness, vital signs, and activity during the postictal period.
- Provide emergency care for patients experiencing a seizure (Table 63.10).
- Give prescribed antiseizure medications as scheduled.
- Make referrals to community agencies to help patients manage finances, work training, employment, and living arrangements.
- Provide patient and caregiver teaching (Table 63.11).
- Evaluate patient self-management of medication therapy.
- Assess the impact of disorder and encourage discussion of feelings.
- Assist patient to identify positive strategies to deal with limitations and manage needed lifestyle or role changes.
- Supervise AP:
  - Immediately report any seizure activity to the RN.
  - Provide no food or fluid until awake
  - Obtain vital signs during the postictal period.

Collaborate With Other Team Members

Respiratory Therapist

- Assess airway patency and suction as needed.
- Provide needed respiratory support.

Social Worker

- Help patient identify and obtain needed resources.
- Offer counseling to develop positive coping skills.

Nursing care for hospitalized patients with seizure disorder or patients who have had seizures due to other factors involves observation and acute treatment of the seizure, patient and caregiver teaching, and psychosocial intervention (Table 63.9).

CHECK YOUR PRACTICE

You are making your morning rounds and check a patient who was admitted the night before with increased seizure activity. When you go to the room, a visitor is yelling, "Help, help!" You find the patient is on the floor jerking and stiffening and not responding to you.

- What would you do?

Nurses monitor seizure activity and ensure patient safety. Table 63.10 outlines care of patients having a tonic-clonic seizure and status epilepticus. When a seizure occurs, carefully observe and record details of the event. The diagnosis and subsequent treatment often rest on the seizure description. What events preceded the seizure? When did the seizure occur? How long did each phase last? What occurred during each phase?

TABLE 63.10 EMERGENCY MANAGEMENT

Tonic-Clonic Seizures and Status Epilepticus

Etiology	Assessment Findings	Interventions
Drug-Related • Ingestion, inhalation • Overdose • Withdrawal of alcohol, opioids, antiseizure drugs **Head Trauma** • Cerebral contusion • Epidural hematoma • Intracranial hematoma • Subdural hematoma • Traumatic birth injury **Idiopathic Infection** • Encephalitis • Meningitis • Sepsis **Intracranial** • Brain tumor • Hypertensive crisis • Increased ICP • Stroke • Subarachnoid hemorrhage **Medical Problems** • Heart, liver, lung, or kidney disease • Systemic lupus erythematosus **Metabolic Problems** • Fluid and electrolyte imbalance • Hypoglycemia **Other** • Cardiac arrest • High fever • Psychiatric problems	**Aural Phase** • Bowel and bladder incontinence • Diaphoresis • Loss of consciousness • Pallor, flushing, or cyanosis • Peculiar sensations that precede seizure • Tachycardia • Warm skin **Tonic Phase** • Continuous muscle contractions • Extreme muscular rigidity lasting 5–15 sec **Clonic Phase** • Rigidity and relaxation alternating in rapid succession **Postictal Phase** • Altered level of consciousness, lethargy • Confusion and headache	**Initial** • Note time of onset, duration, behavior in each stage, and awareness. • Ensure patent airway. • Protect patient from injury during seizure. Do not restrain. Pad side rails. • Remove sharp objects and glasses. • Remove or loosen tight clothing. • Establish IV access. • Stay with patient until seizure has passed. • Anticipate benzodiazepines (e.g., diazepam, midazolam, lorazepam) to stop seizures. May repeat after 5 minutes. • Administer fosphenytoin, phenytoin, levetiracetam, or valproic acid **Ongoing** • Provide supplemental O_2 and respiratory support. • Suction as needed. • Monitor vital signs, level of consciousness, O_2 saturation, pupil size and reactivity. • Reassure and orient patients after seizure. • Give IV dextrose for hypoglycemia. • Maintain NPO until awake with gag reflex. • If seizures persist, begin continuous infusion of midazolam, pentobarbital, or thiopental. • With prolonged seizure activity, anesthesia agents may be given.

Note (1) the description of aura (if any); (2) the exact time of onset ; (3) the course and nature of the seizure activity (awareness, motor movements, automatisms); (4) body parts involved, their sequence of involvement; (5) autonomic signs (dilated pupils, excess salivation, altered breathing, cyanosis, flushing, diaphoresis, or incontinence); and (6) postictal activity. Assessment during the postictal period includes level of consciousness, vital signs, pupil size and position of the eyes, memory loss, muscle soreness, speech disorders (aphasia, dysarthria), weakness or paralysis, and sleep period.

After the seizure, the patient may need suctioning, O_2, or repositioning to open and maintain the airway. A seizure can be frightening for the patient and others who witnessed it. Assess their level of understanding and provide information about how and why the event occurred. This is an opportunity to discuss misconceptions about seizures.

Chronic Care

Preventing recurring seizures is a major goal. We have a vital role in teaching patients and caregivers (Table 63.11). Encourage patients to maintain a seizure diary monitoring frequency, triggers, and associated symptoms. This can aid in ongoing management. Help patients identify events or situations that trigger seizures. Review how patients can handle these situations.

Encourage patients to keep regular appointments with the HCP. Help patients understand drugs must be taken consistently for treatment to be effective. Review the treatment plan and what to do if a medication dose is missed. Usually, the dose is made up if the omission is remembered within 24 hours. Caution patients not to adjust drug dosages without HCP guidance because this can increase seizure frequency and cause SE.

TABLE 63.11 PATIENT & CAREGIVER TEACHING

Seizure Disorder

Include the following information in the teaching plan for the patient with seizure disorder:

1. Take antiseizure medications as prescribed. Report all drug side effects to the HCP.
2. When needed, blood is drawn to ensure therapeutic drug levels. Schedule regular visits with the HCP to discuss treatment options.
3. Do not add any supplements without HCP approval.
4. Use nondrug techniques, such as relaxation therapy and diet modification, to try to reduce the number of seizures.
5. Be aware of community and online resources for education and help with tracking and explaining seizure activity.
6. Wear a medical alert bracelet or necklace and carry an identification card.
7. Avoid excess alcohol use, fatigue, and loss of sleep.
8. Eat regular meals and snacks in between if feeling shaky, faint, or hungry.
9. Be knowledgeable as a female of childbearing age about antiseizure medications and contraceptive use.

Caregivers should receive the following information:

Focal-Onset Seizures

1. Stay calm. Guide patient to safety to prevent injury but do not restrain.
2. Observe for asymmetry of activity and focus on specific actions, such as lip smacking and abnormal movements.
3. Assess patient's level of consciousness and ability to converse and respond appropriately.
4. Note the time the seizure started and stopped. Take note of the time of return to baseline.
5. Provide respect and explanation of occurrence.

Generalized-Onset Tonic-Clonic Seizures

1. When seizure occurs outside the hospital setting, activate EMS if (1) the duration is greater than 5 min; (2) events recur without the patient recovering to baseline; (3) the patient is unable to establish a normal breathing pattern, is injured, or is pregnant; or (4) you do not know if this is a first-time seizure event.
2. Maintain patient safety. Lower the patient to the floor or bed, remove glasses if worn, and loosen restrictive clothing.
3. Do not place anything in the patient's mouth. Patient's teeth/dentures may be damaged. Caregiver may be bitten.
4. Position patient on side (if possible) to improve the patient's ability to drain oral secretions.
5. Note the time the seizure started and stopped. Take note of the time of return to baseline.
6. Assess for any injury and lingering motor weakness.

Teach patients about drug side effects. Review side effects patients need to report. Common side effects of phenytoin are gingival hyperplasia (excess growth of gingival tissue) and hirsutism, especially in young adults. Good dental hygiene can decrease gingival hyperplasia. If gingival hyperplasia is extensive, phenytoin may be replaced with another drug.

Teach caregivers to manage seizures. Remind them they do not need to call an ambulance or send a person to the hospital after a single seizure unless the seizure is prolonged (longer than 5 minutes), another seizure immediately follows, or injury has occurred.

Patients may have concerns or fears related to recurrent seizures, incontinence, or loss of self-control. Support patients through teaching and by helping them use effective coping strategies. Perhaps the greatest challenge is adjusting to any limits imposed by the illness. Discrimination in employment is a serious problem facing the person with seizure disorder. For issues relating to job discrimination, refer patients to the state department of vocational rehabilitation or the U.S. Equal Employment Opportunity Commission (EEOC).

Perhaps the most common complication is the effect on a patient's lifestyle. Patients who have seizures that are difficult to control have an increased incidence of anxiety and depression. Screen patients for symptoms and help them to pursue treatment options. A small number of patients have ictal or postictal psychosis, a loss of contact with reality during the ictal or postictal period. This is different from psychosis unrelated to seizures.[18]

Many agencies that offer services to patients with seizure disorder offer teaching aids and support. Help patients find community resources. Support groups and varied services may be identified through the Epilepsy Foundation (EF; www.epilepsy.com). Refer patients who need counseling to a community mental health center.

Social workers and government programs can help with financial implications and living arrangements. State agencies specializing in vocational rehabilitation can provide vocational assessment, counseling, and funding for training. They can help with job placement for patients whose seizures are not well controlled. Financial assistance for transportation and medical costs may be available.

Driving laws for patients who have had a seizure vary from state to state. They may require up to a year seizure free before reissuing a driver's license. The EF provides current information on driving laws for each state.

Medical alert bracelets, necklaces, and identification cards are available through the EF, local pharmacies, or companies specializing in identification devices (e.g., Medic Alert). Using medical identification is optional.

◆ Evaluation

Expected outcomes are that patients with seizure disorder will:

- Have no seizure-related injury
- Perform optimal self-management
- Maintain positive mood

RESTLESS LEGS SYNDROME

Etiology and Pathophysiology

Restless legs syndrome (RLS) *(Willis-Ekbom disease)* is a movement disorder with unpleasant sensory (paresthesia) and motor abnormalities of 1 or both legs. It is a fairly common sleep problem. Up to 8% of the U.S. population has RLS.

There are 2 types of RLS: primary (idiopathic) and secondary. Most people have primary RLS. Common causes of secondary RLS include iron deficiency, renal disease, hemodialysis, or chronic neuropathy. Many pregnant females develop RLS in the final trimester.[20] Patients who develop RLS before age 40 likely have a genetic predisposition.

We do not know the exact cause of primary RLS. There may be impaired dopamine (DA) transmission in the brain's basal ganglia.[21] DA helps with smooth and purposeful movements. Disruption in these pathways can cause involuntary movement. Iron deficiency during pregnancy, infancy, and childhood increases the risk of RLS later in life.[20]

Clinical Manifestations

The sensory symptoms range from infrequent minor discomfort to severe pain. A few people have symptoms that affect their quality of life. Patients describe numb, tingling, itching, "creepy-crawling," or throbbing sensations in their calf muscle, accompanied by an irresistible urge to move. Symptoms are worsened by sleep deprivation, sleep apnea, stress, sedentary lifestyle, obesity, alcohol, nicotine, caffeine, diabetes, and some medications (antihistamines, antiemetics, lithium, and many antipsychotics).

Symptoms typically begin when patients are inactive or lying still, most commonly at night. Some have symptoms after sitting for long periods. Discomfort may occur in the arms too. RLS worsens over time. Symptoms become more frequent and last longer.

Pain at night disrupts sleep. Physical activity, such as walking, stretching, rocking, or kicking, temporarily relieves the discomfort. In severe cases, patients sleep only a few hours at night. This causes daytime fatigue and disrupts the daily routine. Motor problems include restlessness and periodic, involuntary movements. Fatigue worsens symptoms.

Diagnostic Studies

RLS is diagnosed based on history or the report of the bed partner about nighttime activity. The HCP may ask patients to keep a sleep diary to aid in diagnosis and treatment. Diagnosis is made when patients meets 5 specific criteria: (1) overwhelming urge to move the legs, often with uncomfortable or unpleasant sensations in the legs; (2) urge to move the legs worsens during rest or inactivity; (3) urge to move the legs is partially or totally relieved by movement, as long as the activity continues; (4) urge to move the legs becomes worse in the evening or night; and (5) these features are not due to another medical problem.[20]

Patients may have polysomnography studies during sleep to discern RLS from other problems that disturb sleep. Periodic leg movements are not exclusive to RLS. Blood tests, such as a CBC, ferritin, glucose, and renal function tests, may help identify secondary causes of RLS.

Interprofessional Care

There is no cure. The goals of care are to reduce discomfort and improve sleep quality. In secondary RLS treatment is focused on the underlying medical conditions. Lifestyle changes may help persons with mild to moderate RLS. Decreasing the use of caffeine, alcohol, or tobacco; maintaining regular sleep habits; relaxation techniques; and massaging or stretching the legs daily may help. Regular daily exercise improves symptoms. Warm baths prior to bed provide some relief. Patients should avoid antihistamine-containing medications. Devices used to decrease symptoms include foot wraps, vibration pads, and noninvasive peripheral nerve stimulation.[20]

No medication effectively manages RLS for all patients. Antiseizure drugs affecting calcium channels (gabapentin enacarbil, pregabalin) are first-line drugs for RLS. They decrease the sensory symptoms and nerve pain. Patients with low ferritin levels receive iron supplements with vitamin C.[20] Other supplements that may help include magnesium, zinc, and vitamin D.[21]

Other medications for RLS increase the amount of DA in the brain. DA agonists like ropinirole (Requip) and rotigotine (Neupro) treat pain and provide more restful sleep. DA agonists can lead to a worsening of RLS symptoms after extended use. Caution patients because DA agonists can cause impulse disorders like gambling or shopping. Some patients benefit from carbidopa/levodopa as needed.

Other drugs treat specific symptoms of RLS. Very low doses of opioids may help patients with severe symptoms unresponsive to other therapies. Patients may need to use concurrent stool softeners due to the side effects of constipation. Short-acting benzodiazepines (e.g., lorazepam) may help patients obtain more restful sleep. They should only be used for a short time if other treatments do not work.

DEGENERATIVE NEUROLOGIC PROBLEMS

MULTIPLE SCLEROSIS

Multiple sclerosis (MS) is a chronic, unpredictable, progressive, degenerative disorder of the CNS. It is characterized by disseminated demyelination of nerve fibers in the brain and spinal cord. The onset of MS is usually between ages 20 and 40 years. People diagnosed at 50 years of age or older often have more progressive disease. Almost a million people are living with MS in the United States.

Etiology and Pathophysiology

Females account for 75% of MS patients.[22] MS becomes more prevalent further away from the equator. MS is most common in the Northeast and the Midwest regions of the United States.[22] MS is most prevalent in people of Northern European ancestry. Other risk factors include low vitamin D levels, smoking, and having a direct relative with MS.[23]

The exact cause of MS is unknown. MS is not inherited, but there are over 200 genetic variables that play a part in MS risk. It is believed a genetically susceptible person experiences an environment exposure, such as a viral infection, which triggers the autoimmune process. No specific virus has been implicated, but Epstein-Barr is most consistently linked to MS.[22] Some viral proteins are structurally similar to myelin. The antigen activates T cells in the lymphatic system. Blood vessels bring the activated T cells to the brain where they begin the inflammatory process, which damages myelin. Killer T cells directly attack myelin cells with specific antigens. B cells create antibodies to these proteins. T-regulatory cells (Tregs) should limit excess inflammatory response preventing an attack on self-antigens. In patients with MS, the Tregs fail to stop inflammation.

Successive antigen-antibody reactions within the CNS lead to further demyelination and destruction.

MS is marked by chronic inflammation, demyelination, and gliosis in the CNS. The immune system attack on the myelin proteins damages the myelin sheath (Fig. 63.2A–C). Transmission of nerve impulses slows. Patients may have impaired function (e.g., weakness, numbness). Inflammation ceases and recovery can occur. Symptoms all or partially disappear. At that point, the patient is in remission.

As inflammation recurs, nearby oligodendrocytes are affected, and myelin loses the ability to regenerate. Damage eventually occurs to the axon, which disrupts impulse transmission. Nerve function can be permanently lost (Fig. 63.2D). Glial scar tissue replaces damaged myelin. Hard, rigid plaques form (Fig. 63.3) throughout the white matter of the CNS. With disease progression the dendrites are damaged as well. In late disease cerebral cortex atrophy occurs. MS can reduce life expectancy. Infection or complications of immobility are the usual causes of death.

Clinical Manifestations

The onset of MS is usually gradual. Vague symptoms occur periodically over months or years. Patients may not seek medical attention over these nonspecific symptoms. MS may not be diagnosed until long after the first symptom.

Because damage from MS has a spotty distribution in the CNS, symptoms vary based on the area involved. Some have severe symptoms early in the disease. Others have minimal symptoms for several years. Some have rapid, progressive deterioration leading to disability. Most patients have remissions and exacerbations. With repeated exacerbations, the overall trend is progressive deterioration in neurologic function. MS occurs in 1 of 4 primary patterns based on the clinical course (Table 63.12). A 5th classification, radiologically isolated syndrome, is not considered a form of MS. It is used to describe patients with spinal cord lesions like MS, but with no neurologic symptoms.

Vision changes like double vision or scotoma occur (Fig. 63.4). Patients describe muscle weakness and difficulty with coordination and balance. Partial or complete paralysis happens in the worst cases. Most have numbness and tingling in affected areas. *Lhermitte's sign* is a temporary sensory symptom described as an electric shock sensation going down the spine with neck flexion. Some patients report pain from muscle spasm especially around the low thoracic and abdominal regions. This "MS hug" is from muscle spasm in intercostal and abdominal muscles. Other frequent problems include speech problems, hearing loss, tremors, and dizziness. Cerebellar signs include nystagmus, ataxia, dysarthria, and dysphagia. Many patients have severe, even disabling fatigue. Heat, humidity, deconditioning, and medication side effects worsen fatigue.

Rigid plaques in areas of the CNS that control elimination alter bowel and bladder function. Many patients have constipation. Urinary problems vary. Spastic bladder causing unchecked bladder contractions is common. Urinary urgency and frequency with dribbling or incontinence results. A flaccid (hypotonic) bladder causes urinary retention because there is no sensation, no pressure or desire to void. Urodynamic studies diagnose urinary dysfunction. Some patients have remission during pregnancy.

Sexual problems may occur. Males have erectile dysfunction from spinal demyelination. Females may have decreased libido, difficulty with orgasm, painful intercourse, and decreased sensation preventing a normal sexual response. The emotional impact of chronic illness and the loss of self-esteem contribute to loss of sexual response.

About half of people with MS develop cognitive problems. These include difficulty with multitasking, concentration, short-term memory, speed of processing, and word finding. Intellect is preserved. Emotional changes include anger, depression, or euphoria.

Diagnostic Studies

No diagnostic test specific for MS exists. The history and manifestations are important diagnostic cues. Lab work is done

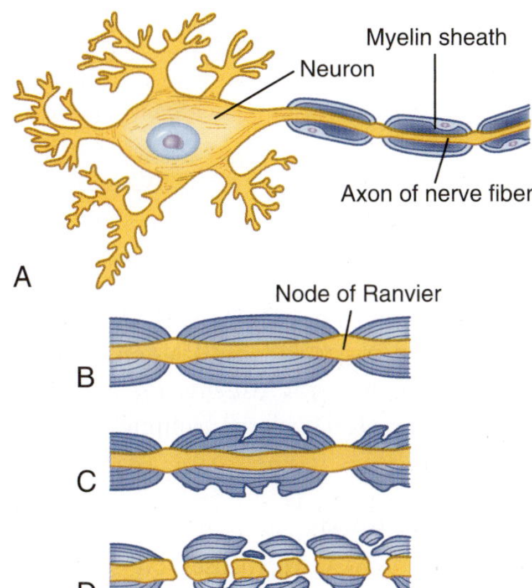

Fig. 63.2 Pathogenesis of multiple sclerosis. (A) Normal nerve cell with myelin sheath. (B) Normal axon. (C) Myelin breakdown. (D) Myelin totally disrupted; axon not functioning.

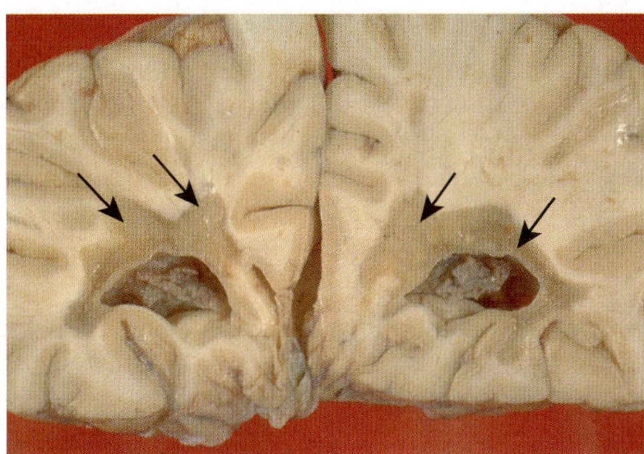

Fig. 63.3 Plaque lesions *(arrows)* from multiple sclerosis. (From Vanderah TW: *Nolte's the human brain in photographs and diagrams,* ed 5, St. Louis, 2020, Elsevier.)

TABLE 63.12 Patterns of Multiple Sclerosis

Category	Characteristics
Clinically isolated syndrome	• Single attack followed by complete or near complete recovery. Silent damage may be present on MRI. No further attacks.
Relapsing-remitting	• Clearly defined attacks of worsening neurologic function *(relapses)* with partial or complete recovery *(remission)* between attacks. • 85% of people first diagnosed with this type.
Primary-progressive	• Steadily worsening neurologic function from the beginning with periodic minor improvements but no distinct relapses or remissions. • 10% of people first diagnosed with this type.
Secondary-progressive	• A relapsing-remitting initial course, followed by progression with or without occasional relapses, minor remissions, and plateaus. • New treatments may slow progression. • Most people initially diagnosed with relapsing-remitting MS eventually transition to this type.

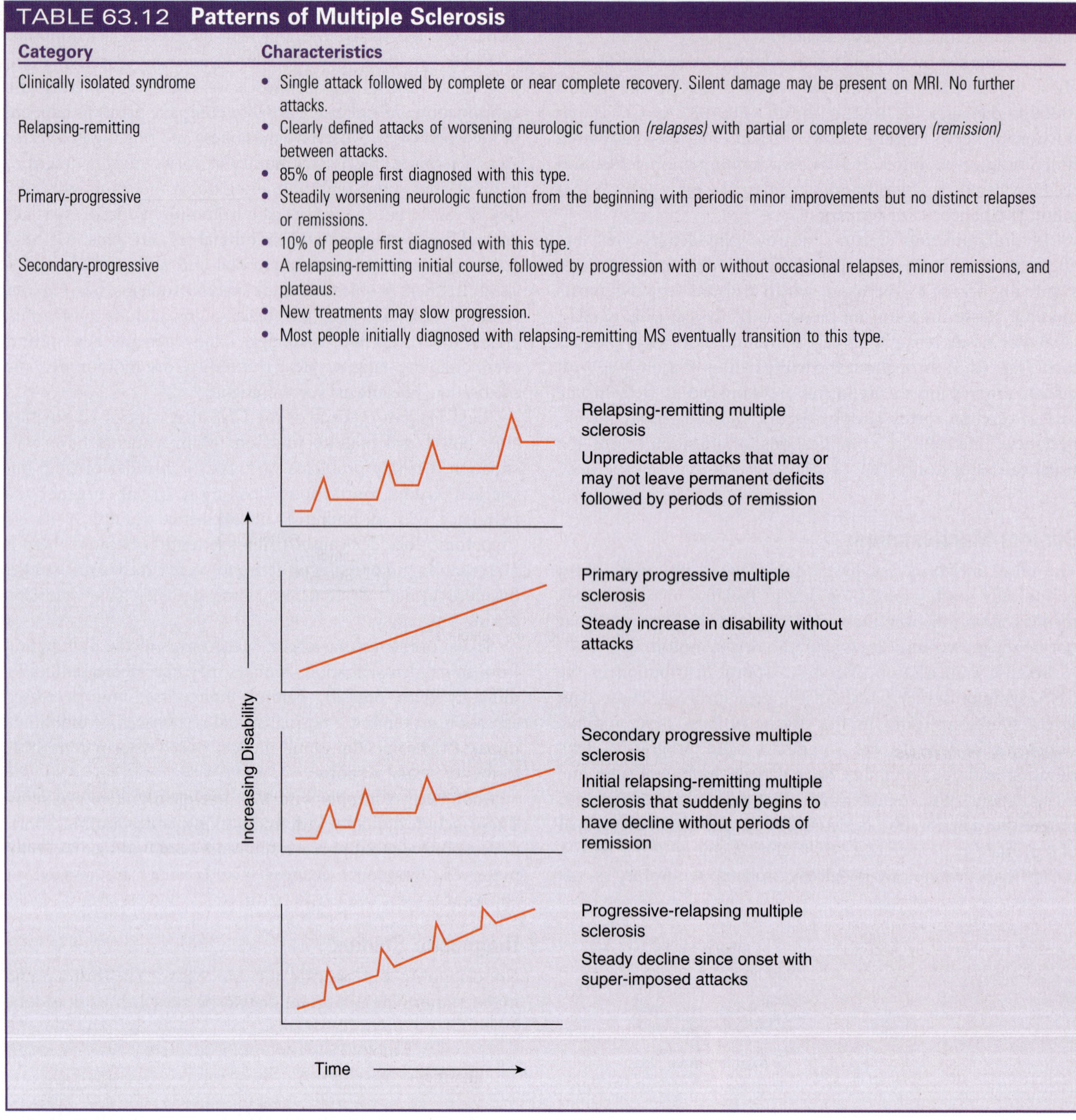

to rule out diseases with similar manifestations, such as Lyme disease or neurosyphilis. An MRI with contrast of the brain and spinal cord may show plaques, inflammation, atrophy, and tissue destruction. Cerebrospinal fluid (CSF) analysis reveals increased immunoglobulin G and the presence of oligoclonal banding indicating inflammation. Visual evoked potential testing may reveal delayed nerve conduction from the eye to the brain.[24]

Diagnostic criteria for MS specify that patients must have (1) evidence of at least 2 inflammatory demyelinating lesions in at least 2 locations within the CNS, (2) 2 or more attacks occurring 1 month or more apart, and (3) other diagnoses ruled out. If evidence exists for only 1 lesion or only 1 clinical attack the HCP will monitor patients for another attack or confirm the presence of oligoclonal banding in the CSF.[24]

Interprofessional Care

No cure exists for MS. Care focuses on reducing relapses, slowing neurologic degeneration, and providing symptomatic relief (Table 63.13). Since no cases of MS are alike, the disease pattern and symptoms guide therapy.

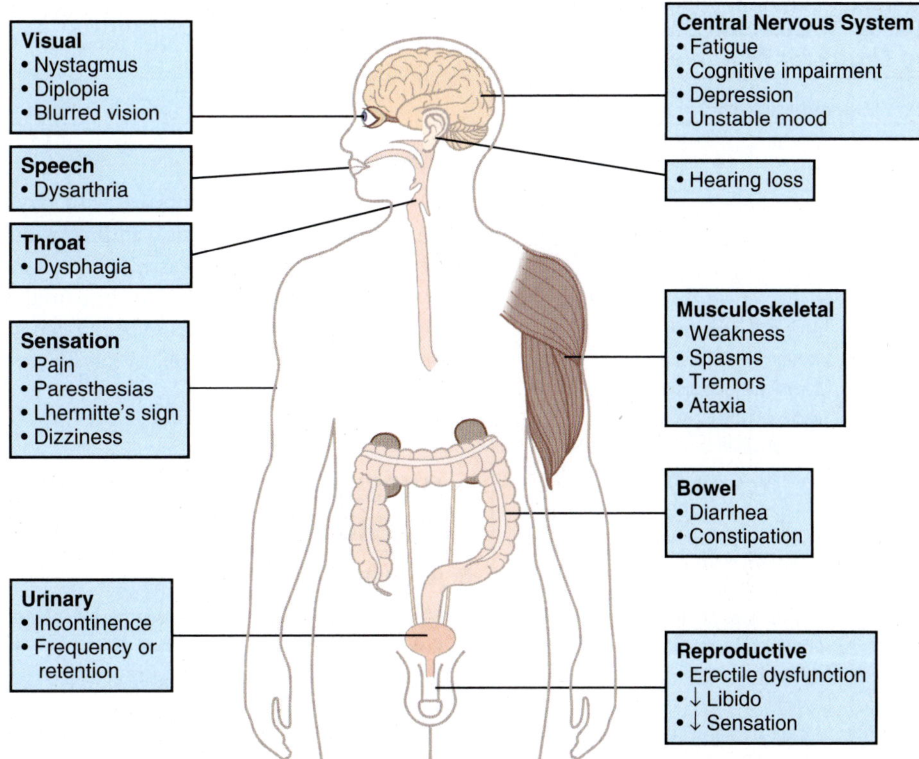

Fig. 63.4 Manifestations of multiple sclerosis.

TABLE 63.13 Interprofessional Care

Multiple Sclerosis

Diagnostic Assessment

- History and physical assessment
- CSF analysis
- CT scan
- MRI, MRS (magnetic resonance spectroscopy)
- Evoked potential testing
- Somatosensory evoked potential (SSEP)
- Auditory evoked potential (AEP)
- Visual evoked potential (VEP)

Management

- Drug therapy
  - Disease-modifying drugs (Table 63.14)
  - Corticosteroids
  - Symptom-specific drugs (Table 63.15)
- Surgical therapy
- Thalamotomy (unmanageable tremor)
- Neurectomy, rhizotomy, cordotomy (unmanageable spasticity)
- Physical therapy
- Occupational therapy

Drug Therapy

Primary treatment includes disease-modifying therapies that limit inflammation, slow disease progression, and prevent relapse (Table 63.14). Treatment is more effective when started early in the course of MS. Delays in treatment are linked to poor outcomes. Medications include interferons, monoclonal antibodies, and biologic and biosimilar agents. The patient and provider select therapy considering medication dose, schedule, route, action, efficacy, adverse effects, and patient preference.

Common medications for initial treatment are given orally or by subcutaneous self-injection. These include glatiramer acetate, dimethyl fumarate (Tecfidera), fingolimide (Gilenya), and teriflunomide (Aubagio).[23] Adverse effects include life-threatening liver toxicity, immunosuppression, diarrhea, and cancer. Some MS treatments cause *progressive multifocal leukoencephalopathy* (PML), a fatal viral infection.

For more active forms of MS, IV monoclonal antibodies suppress immunologic activity. These include natalizumab, alemtuzumab, and ocrelizumab. These are recommended for those who had an inadequate response to other treatments. These medications slow disease progression and improve symptoms, but increase the risk for PML, infection, and cancer.[23] Antihistamines and antipyretics given before infusion decrease transfusion reactions.

Autologous human stem cell therapy (aHST) can improve symptoms and slow attacks. Stem cell therapy may be done once in the course of MS. Human stem cells are pharmacologically stimulated in the patient. The cells are gathered 15 days later. The patient receives immunosuppressive therapy, and the stem cells are returned to the patient by IV. Close monitoring is required.[25]

TABLE 63.14 Drug Therapy

Disease-Modifying Drugs for Multiple Sclerosis

Drug	Considerations
Injectable	
β-1a interferon (Rebif, Plegridy, Avonex) β-1b interferon (Betaseron, Extavia)	• Teach self-injection techniques. • Rotate injection sites. • Treat flu-like symptoms with an NSAID or acetaminophen. • Monitor for depression.
glatiramer acetate (Copaxone, Glatopa)	• Teach self-injection techniques. • Monitor liver function tests.
ofatumumab (Kesimpta)	• Monoclonal antibody. • Teach self-injection techniques. • Avoid pregnancy. • Monitor liver function tests.
Oral Agents	
cladribine (Mavenclad)	• Avoid pregnancy. • No contact with large crowds and people who have an infection. • Follow cancer screening guidelines. • Monitor liver tests.
dimethyl fumarate (Tecfidera)	• Manage GI side effects.
fingolimod (Gilenya)	• Monitor for infection. • Monitor BP and heart rate regularly. • Avoid pregnancy.
monomethyl fumarate (Bafiertam)	• Report side effects. • Avoid pregnancy.
ponesimod (Ponvory)	• Monitor for bradyarrhythmia. • Monitor for infection. • Avoid pregnancy.
siponimod (Mayzent)	• Report side effects. • Monitor BP and heart rate regularly. • Avoid pregnancy.
teriflunomide (Aubagio)	• Report side effects. • Avoid pregnancy. • Limit contact with large crowds or people with infection. • Monitor liver function tests.
IV Infusions	
alemtuzumab (Lemtrada) natalizumab (Tysabri) ocrelizumab (Ocrevus) ublituximab-xiiy (Briumvi)	• Report side effects. • Avoid pregnancy. • Monitor for infusion-related reactions. • Follow cancer screening guidelines. • No live virus vaccines for 4 weeks prior to the infusion. • Provide antihistamine and antipyretic prior to the infusion.

IV corticosteroids are used to treat acute MS exacerbations. They speed recovery by reducing edema and acute inflammation at the site of demyelination. Corticosteroids do not affect residual neurologic symptoms.[26] Therapeutic plasma exchange (plasmapheresis), Acthar Gel, and IV immunoglobulin G may be considered during exacerbation when treatment with corticosteroids alone does not improve symptoms. Many other drugs and treatments are used to treat MS symptoms (Table 63.15).

Other Therapies

Neurologic symptoms improve with physical therapy. Exercise during periods of remission improves daily function. Exercise decreases spasticity, increases coordination, and retrains unaffected muscles to substitute for impaired ones. Water exercise is especially beneficial (Fig. 63.5). Water gives buoyancy to the body and allows patients to perform activities that would otherwise be too hard.

NURSING MANAGEMENT: MULTIPLE SCLEROSIS

Assessment

MS symptoms are widespread and affect many facets of life. Subjective and objective data that are obtained from patients with MS are outlined in Table 63.16.

Clinical Problems

Clinical problems for patients with MS include:

- Musculoskeletal problems
- Fatigue
- Difficulty coping
- Impaired urinary elimination

Additional information on clinical problems and interventions for patients with MS is presented in the eNursing Care Plan 63.3 (available on the website for this chapter).

Planning

The overall goals are that patients with MS will (1) maximize neuromuscular function, (2) maintain independence in activities of daily living (ADLs), (3) manage fatigue, (4) optimize psychosocial well-being, and (5) reduce factors that trigger exacerbations.

Implementation

During the diagnostic phase, reassure patients that multiple tests are done to rule out other disorders, even if a tentative diagnosis of MS has been made. Help them deal with stress caused by the diagnosis of a disabling illness. Patients newly diagnosed with MS may need support with grieving.

During an acute exacerbation, patients may be immobile and confined to bed. The focus of nursing care at this phase is to prevent complications of immobility including respiratory complications, UTIs, and pressure injuries. Discuss ways to prevent illness including avoiding fatigue, stress, and exposure to infection. Treat infection early when it occurs.

TABLE 63.15 Symptom Management of Multiple Sclerosis

Symptom	Interventions
Anxiety,depression, grief	• Counseling • Antidepressants to elevate or stabilize mood • Stay in touch with navigator or HCP • Exercise daily • Reduce stress • Relaxation exercises or meditation • Maintain a social support group, join an MS community • Acknowledge your feelings • Journaling to express stressors and emotions • Avoid alcohol or addictive substances
Bladder incontinence, urgency, dribbling	• Drink fluids during the day • Stop drinking fluids 3 hours before bedtime • Scheduled voiding • Frequent breaks when traveling • Keep bladder protection pads available • Wear easily manageable clothing • Keep a change of clothes, underwear, catheters, and wipes available • Anticholinergic medication
Constipation	• High-fiber diet choices • Drink >48 oz. of fluid daily • Exercise daily • Stool softeners, bulk-forming supplements, enemas, suppositories, manual stimulation
Cognitive changes	• Maintain cognitive reserve (reading, working, active leisure, puzzles, learning new activities) • Maintain a regular sleep and activity schedule • MIND diet: leafy vegetables, berries, nuts, fish; less fried foods, butter, cheese, red and processed meats, sweets • Visualize items when having difficulty with recall of words • Do 1 activity at a time • Organize, simplify, consolidate living and workspaces • Set reminders, calendars, use technology
Dizziness	• Dimenhydrinate, cyclizine, meclizine • Short-term corticosteroids
Double vision, opticneuritis	• Patching one eye • Special glasses • Corticosteroids • Plan for support when driving is unsafe • Audio books if reading is difficult
Dysesthesia	• Exercise • Loose clothing • Medications: antiseizure, muscle relaxants, topical lidocaine • Relaxation techniques • Warm compresses
Fatigue, weakness	• Occupational therapy to simplify tasks and conserve energy • Physical therapy for energy-saving ways of walking and performing tasks • Sleep schedule • Stress management • Cognitive behavior therapy • Avoid overheating • Stimulants (modafinil)
Gait difficulty	• Physical therapy • Walkers • Canes • Medications for spasticity • Dalfampridine
Neuropathic pain, paresthesia	• Acupuncture • Hypnosis • Medications: antidepressant, antiseizure, muscle relaxants, NSAIDs • Mindfulness and meditation • Physical therapy with massage, stretching • Water therapy
Numbness and tingling	• Corticosteroids • Vitamin B_{12}
Sexual dysfunction	Males: • Erectile dysfunction medications • Penile vacuum pumps Females: • Clitoral pumps • Vibrators • Water-soluble personal lubricant
Spasticity	• Baclofen oral or via intrathecal pump • Botulinum toxin A • Dorsal-column electrical stimulation • Muscle relaxants • Physical therapy • Stretching • Surgery (e.g., neurectomy, rhizotomy, cordotomy) • Yoga
Tremor	• Assistive devices for ADLs • Deep brain stimulation • Thalamotomy

Patients should know their treatment plan, how to manage drug side effects, and avoid drug interactions. Teach them to notify the HCP at the first signs of relapse. Help patients manage symptoms that affect many facets of life. Patients with MS should be aware of triggers that worsen the disease. These include infection, trauma, sleep deficit, and stress. Help them develop plans to avoid triggers or decrease their effects. Becoming overheated worsens symptoms of MS. If patients live in a warm climate, cooling vests may help maintain function. Avoiding the midday heat will help manage symptoms in the

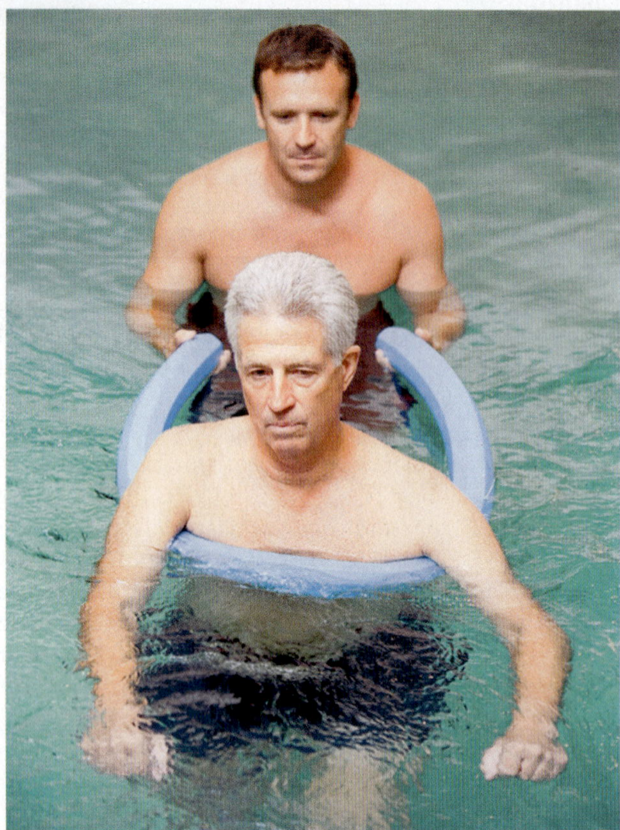

Fig. 63.5 Water therapy provides exercise and recreation for the patient with a chronic neurologic disease. (© Photos.com/AbleStock.com/Thinkstock.)

summer. Teach patients to balance exercise and rest. Eating a healthy diet, encouraging antioxidant-rich fruits and vegetables, and minimizing caffeine intake helps maintain immune health.

Patients and caregivers must adjust to the disease unpredictability, necessity for lifestyle changes, and challenge of avoiding precipitating factors. The uncertainty of disease progression, fatigue, and decreased abilities can cause anxiety and depression. Help patients identify resources to meet needs. Many assistance programs are available to help with costly medication and supplies. The National Multiple Sclerosis Society offers a variety of services to meet the needs of patients with MS.

◆ Evaluation

The expected outcomes are that patients with MS will:

- Maintain or improve muscle strength and mobility
- Maintain urinary continence
- Make decisions about health and lifestyle modifications to manage MS
- Maintain independence in ADLs

PARKINSON DISEASE

Parkinson disease (PD) is a chronic, progressive neurodegenerative movement disorder characterized by slowed initiation and execution of movement *(bradykinesia)*, increased muscle tone *(rigidity)*, tremor at rest, and postural instability.[27] It is the most common form of *parkinsonism*, a syndrome of several disorders with similar symptoms.

Almost 1 million Americans are living with PD in the United States. Incidence of PD increases with age. The average age of onset is around 65 years. Males are 1.5 times more likely to have PD.[27]

TABLE 63.16 NURSING ASSESSMENT
Multiple Sclerosis

Subjective Data

Important Health Information

Health history: Recent or past viral infections or vaccinations, other recent infections, residence in cold or temperate climates, physical or emotional stress, pregnancy, exposure to extremes of heat and cold

Medications: Adherence to treatment plan (corticosteroids, immunomodulators, immunosuppressants, cholinergics, anticholinergics, antispasmodics)

Functional Health Patterns

Health perception—health management: Positive family history; malaise

Nutritional-metabolic: Weight loss; difficulty in chewing, dysphagia

Elimination: Urinary frequency, urgency, dribbling or incontinence, retention; constipation

Activity-exercise: Muscle weakness, muscle fatigue; tingling and numbness; ataxia (clumsiness)

Cognitive-perceptual: Eye, back, leg, joint pain; painful muscle spasms; vertigo; blurred or lost vision; diplopia; tinnitus

Sexuality-reproductive: Impotence, decreased libido

Coping—stress tolerance: Anger, depression, euphoria, social isolation

Objective Data

General

Apathy, inattentiveness

Musculoskeletal

Muscle weakness, paresis, paralysis, spasms, foot dragging, dysarthria

Neurologic

Nystagmus, ataxia, tremor, spasticity, hyperreflexia, decreased hearing

Possible Diagnostic Findings

↓ T suppressor cells, demyelinating lesions on MRI or MRS scans, ↑ IgG or oligoclonal banding in CSF, delayed evoked potential responses

MRS, Magnetic resonance spectroscopy.

Etiology and Pathophysiology

PD is likely caused by an interplay of genetic and environment risk factors. Traumatic brain injury has been shown to increase the risk of PD. Exposure to industrial manganese, pesticides, herbicides (paraquat), industrial solvents, and chemicals (polychlorinated biphenyl) increases risk.[28]

Genetic factors influence the development of PD. Genetic mutations in some ethnic groups, such as Ashkenazi Jews and North African Berbers, lead to increased incidence of PD. Genetic factors cause 10% to 15% of PD. Onset of PD before age 50 is linked to genetic mutations *PRKN* and *PINK1*. *SNCA* mutation is associated with alpha-synuclein changes.

Changes in PD occur throughout the brain. Degeneration of the DA-producing neurons in the substantia nigra of the midbrain (Figs. 63.6 to 63.8) occurs. This disrupts the balance between DA and acetylcholine (ACh) in the basal ganglia. DA is essential for normal function of the extrapyramidal motor system, including control of posture and involuntary movement. Initial symptoms of PD do not occur until 60% to 80% of DA-producing neurons are lost. Signals to the corpus striatum that provide smooth, purposeful movement are impaired. Imbalance of monoamine neurotransmitters (norepinephrine, epinephrine) is present.[27]

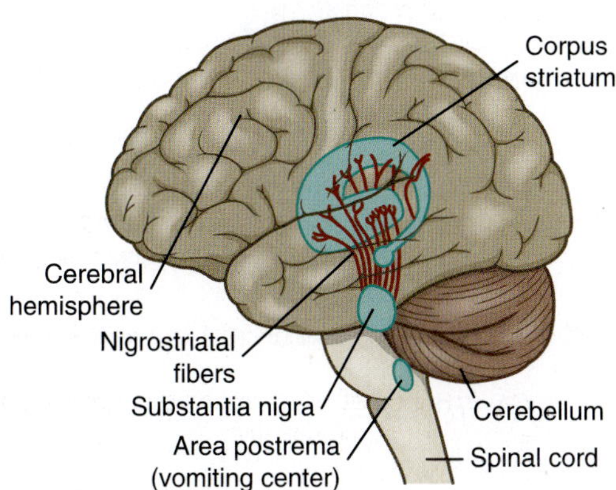

Fig. 63.6 Nigrostriatal disorders produce parkinsonism. Left-sided view of the human brain showing the substantia nigra and the corpus striatum *(shaded area)* lying deep within the cerebral hemisphere. Nerve fibers extend upward from the substantia nigra, divide into many branches, and carry dopamine to all regions of the corpus striatum.

Unusual clumps of protein called Lewy bodies are found in the brains of patients with PD. We believe these contribute to neuronal death. Their presence indicates abnormal brain function. Lewy body dementia is discussed in Chapter 64. Alpha synuclein is a presynaptic protein that assists with regulation of DA release. Abnormal alpha synuclein is linked to PD and other Lewy body diseases.[27]

Because of their similarity, PD and parkinsonism can be confused. Parkinsonism is a syndrome made up of disorders that mimic PD. Many forms of secondary *(atypical)* parkinsonism exist. Parkinsonism has occurred after exposure to a variety of chemicals and metals. Drug-induced parkinsonism can occur with use of metoclopramide, methyldopa, lithium, and many first-generation antipsychotic agents like chlorpromazine. Parkinsonism has occurred after methamphetamine use. After removing the cause, symptoms of parkinsonism often disappear.

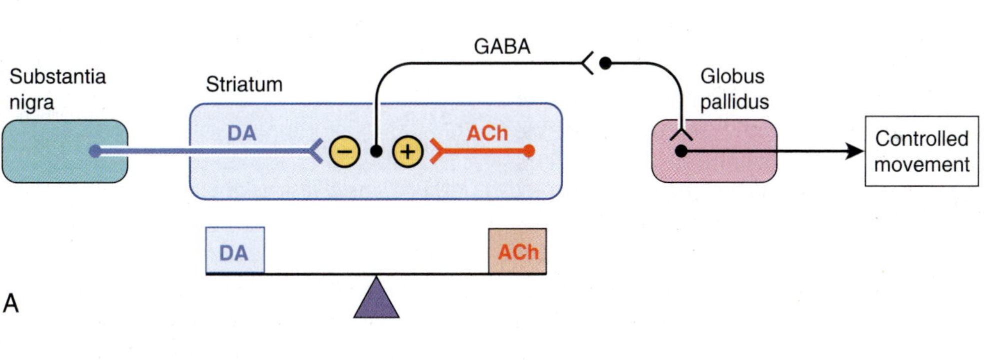

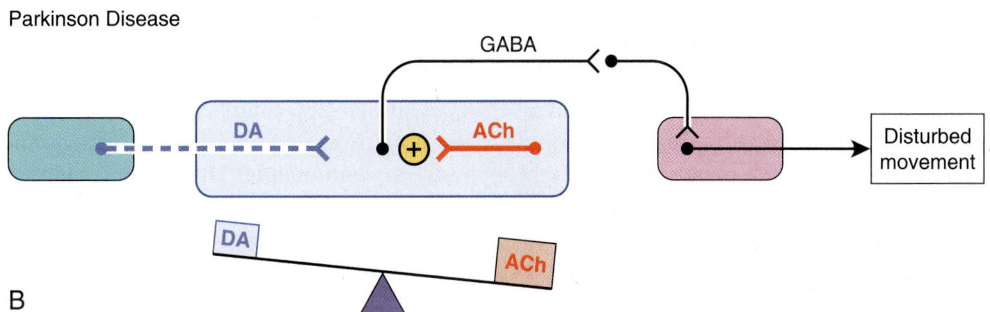

Fig. 63.7 A deficit in dopamine *(DA)* exists in PD. This deficit creates an imbalance between DA and the excitatory neurotransmitter acetylcholine *(ACh)*. (A) In a healthy person, DA released from neurons in the substantia nigra inhibits the firing of neurons in the striatum that release γ-aminobutyric acid *(GABA)*. Conversely, neurons in the striatum, which release ACh, excite the GABAergic neurons. Under normal conditions, inhibitory actions of DA are balanced by excitatory actions of ACh, and controlled movement results. (B) In PD, neurons in the substantia nigra that supply DA to the striatum degenerate. When a deficit of DA occurs, excitatory effects of ACh go unopposed and disturbed movements (tremor, rigidity) result. (From Lehne RA: *Pharmacology for nursing care,* ed 12, St Louis, 2025, Elsevier.)

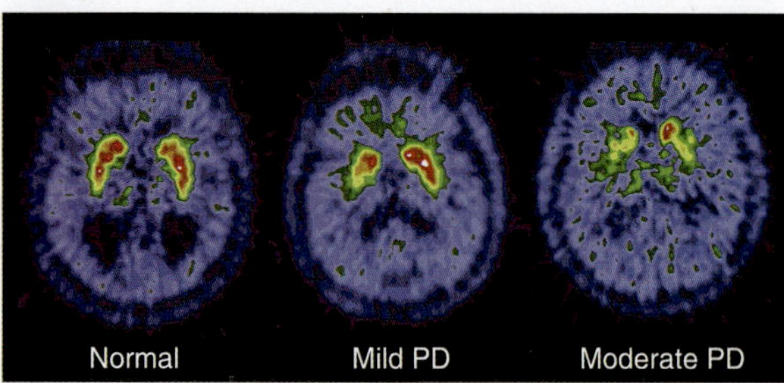

Fig. 63.8 In PD, PET scan showing reduced fluorodopa uptake in the basal ganglia *(right)* compared with a normal control *(left)*. (From Winn HR: *Youmans and Winn neurological surgery*, ed 8, St. Louis, 2023, Elsevier.)

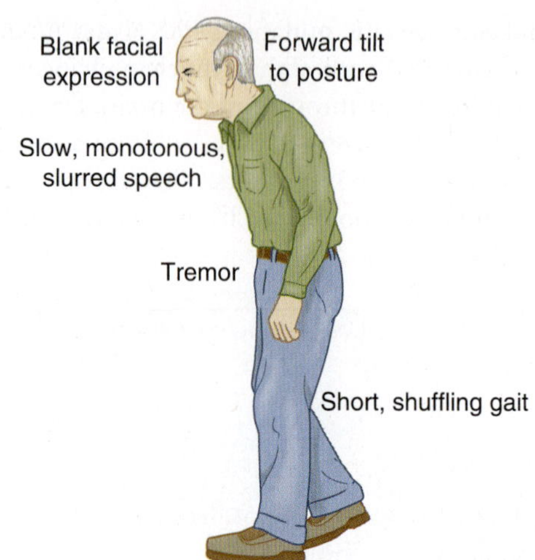

Fig. 63.9 Characteristic appearance of a patient with PD.

Clinical Manifestations

The onset of PD is gradual with ongoing progression. It begins in only 1 side of the body or 1 limb. Primary manifestations of PD are tremors, rigidity, bradykinesia (slowed movement), and postural instability. Early in the disease mild tremor, flat affect, slowing of ADLs (dressing, feeding), or decreased arm swing are present. Shoulder rigidity may be mistaken for arthritis. With disease progression, patients develop a propulsive gait (stiff stooped posture, forward bending of the neck, rapid short steps).

Nonmotor symptoms like apathy, fatigue, pain, urine incontinence, constipation, and erectile dysfunction disturb daily activities. PD impairs executive functioning. Patients have an inability to make plans, problem solve, or limit risky behavior. Neuropsychiatric problems include depression, PD psychosis with hallucinations, and dementia.

Problems with eating include early satiety, loss of taste, and difficulty swallowing. *Hypokinetic dysarthria* occurs, causing monotone, quiet, and poorly articulated speech. Patients have trouble communicating.[29] Sleep problems include difficulty staying asleep at night, restless sleep, and excess daytime sleepiness. About one-third of patients develop rapid eye movement (REM) sleep behavior disorder. This causes violent dreams and potentially dangerous motor activity during REM sleep.

Tremor

Tremor appears early in PD. It occurs at rest and lessens with purposeful movement *(nonintention tremor)*. Tremor increases with stress, caffeine, and fatigue. The hand tremor is described as "pill rolling" because the thumb and forefinger appear to move in a rotary fashion as if rolling a pill. Tremor contributes to increasingly smaller and cramped handwriting. Tremor can involve the diaphragm, tongue, lips, and jaw. Nonintention tremor should not be confused with benign *essential tremor.* Essential tremor occurs during voluntary movement and is not a symptom of PD.

Rigidity

Rigidity is the increased resistance to movement or stiffness. Parkinsonian rigidity is jerky *(cogwheel rigidity)*, as if there were occasional catches in the movement of a joint. The alternating contraction and relaxation in opposing muscle groups (e.g., biceps and triceps) is inhibited. Muscles do not relax. Sustained muscle contraction causes stiffness, muscle soreness, aching, and fatigue. Pain may occur in the upper body, spine, or legs. Rigidity enhances bradykinesia.

Bradykinesia

Bradykinesia is present in spontaneous and automatic movements. Decreased impulses from the basal ganglia cause slowed response and difficulty initiating movement. This leads to the masked face (deadpan expression), slowed blinking, drooling of saliva, and shuffling gait (Fig. 63.9). Tasks that were once easy are now frustratingly slow.

Postural Instability

Postural instability is the inability to sustain a stable upright posture. Patients describe being unable to stop themselves from going forward *(propulsion)* or backward *(retropulsion)*. This increases the risk of falling. Assessment of postural instability includes the "pull test." The examiner stands behind the patient and gives a tug backward on the shoulder. Patients with PD will lose their balance and are unable to take a corrective step backward.

Complications

As PD progresses, complications increase. Swallowing difficulty can lead to aspiration or malnutrition. Increasing weakness leads to immobility. Dyskinesia (spontaneous involuntary movements) may develop. Orthostatic hypotension is common. A loss of postural reflexes, weakness, and orthostatic changes increase fall risk. Patients with PD are at increased risk for melanoma.[29] Skin assessment should be done annually.

Diagnostic Studies

Diagnosis is based on the history and assessment. The presence of 2 of the 4 primary manifestations (tremor, rigidity, bradykinesia, and postural instability) with an asymmetric onset is required for diagnosis of PD. Confirmation occurs with a positive response to an antiparkinsonian drug trial with levodopa or a DA agonist. The Unified Parkinson's Disease Rating Scale is used to assess and document findings. This scale establishes a baseline, monitors treatment effectiveness, and tracks disease progression.[30] MRI and CT imaging studies are usually normal but may help rule out other diagnoses. DaTscan imaging may be done to detect a loss of DA producing neurons and distinguish PD from similar diseases.

Interprofessional Care

Because PD has no cure, interprofessional care focuses on symptom management (Table 63.17).

TABLE 63.17 Interprofessional Care

Parkinson Disease

Diagnostic Assessment

- History and physical assessment
- Positive response to antiparkinsonian drugs
- MRI

Management

- Antiparkinsonian drugs (Table 63.18)
- Surgical therapy
- Deep brain stimulation
- Ablation
- Physical therapy
- Occupational therapy
- Speech therapy
- Dietitian consult for nutrition therapy

Drug Therapy

Drug therapy is aimed at correcting the imbalance of neurotransmitters within the CNS (Table 63.18). Antiparkinsonian drugs enhance the release of DA, increase supply of DA (dopaminergic), or block the effects of overactive cholinergic neurons (anticholinergic) (Fig. 63.7).

Drug doses are carefully adjusted. Excess amounts of dopaminergic drugs can cause *paradoxic intoxication,* worsening rather than improving symptoms. Treatment with only 1 drug is preferable because fewer side effects occur and dose adjustments are easier. However, as PD progresses, combination therapy is often necessary.

Levodopa with carbidopa is the primary treatment for symptomatic patients. Levodopa is a chemical precursor of DA. DA cannot cross the blood-brain barrier, but levodopa can. Levodopa is converted to DA in the basal ganglia. Carbidopa inhibits the enzyme dopa-decarboxylase, which breaks down levodopa before it reaches the brain. The net result is that more levodopa reaches the brain. Carbidopa/levodopa reduces symptoms but does not stop PD progression.[31]

PD is unpredictable. Symptoms improve or worsen during the day. The periods of worsening are called "off" time. Off episodes occur toward the end of a dosing interval with medications (end-of-dose wearing off) or at unpredictable times (spontaneous "on/off"). Prolonged use of levodopa often results in dyskinesias and "off/on" periods when the drug will unpredictably stop or start working.

DRUG ALERT

Carbidopa/Levodopa

- Levodopa has many drug and food interactions and side effects.
- Monitor for signs of dyskinesia and report uncontrolled movement of the face, eyelids, mouth, tongue, arms, hands, or legs.
- Stress that effects may be delayed for several weeks to months.
- Teach patients to report mental changes, palpitations, high fever, and excess sweating.

HCPs may prefer to start therapy with a DA receptor agonist that directly stimulates DA receptors. Ropinirole (Requip) and pramipexole (Mirapex) may be used alone or in combination with carbidopa/levodopa. Many drugs are available in extended-release forms that improve the ability to adhere to treatment. Rotigotine, a DA receptor agonist, is a transdermal patch applied once daily. The DA receptor agonist apomorphine (Apokyn) can improve movement in "off" episodes. Patients must take it with an antiemetic drug because it causes severe nausea and vomiting when taken alone. It cannot be taken with serotonin (5-HT3) receptor antagonists (e.g., ondansetron) because the combination causes very low BP and loss of consciousness.[27] Amantadine, an antiviral, may increase the activity of DA, but its effectiveness decreases after several months of use.

DRUG ALERT

Apomorphine

- May be taken up to 5 times per day.
- Take BP and pulse before and after administration.
- May cause falls, dizziness, and spontaneous sleepiness.
- Take with an antiemetic (not $5HT_3$ antagonist).

Anticholinergic drugs, such as trihexyphenidyl and benztropine, decrease the activity of ACh. Providing balance between cholinergic and dopaminergic actions can help with tremors and rigidity. Monoamine oxidase type B (MAO-B) inhibitors like selegiline and rasagiline may be given with carbidopa/levodopa. Inhibiting MAO-B, the enzyme that degrades DA, increases DA levels. MAO-B inhibitors are less effective at treating motor symptoms than DA receptor agonists.

Table 63.18 discusses drugs used to treat off time and other PD symptoms. Entacapone (Comtan) and opicapone (Ongentys) block the enzyme catechol *O*-methyltransferase (COMT), which breaks down levodopa in the peripheral circulation. This prolongs the effect of carbidopa/levodopa. They are used as adjuncts to therapy when patients experience "wearing off" at the end of the dosing interval. Istradefylline (Nourianz) is an adenosine blocker used to

TABLE 63.18 Drug Therapy

Parkinson Disease

Drug	Mechanism of Action	Side Effects	Considerations
Dopaminergics			
Dopamine Precursors			
levodopa (L-dopa) levodopa/carbidopa (Sinemet) levodopa/carbidopa enteral suspension (Duopa) levodopa inhalation (Inbrija)	Converted to dopamine (DA) in basal ganglia	Dry mouth GI distress	Do not take with meals. Limit vitamin B_6 intake. Teach ways to decrease dry mouth. Used if having 3 or more "off" hours a day. May use up to 5 times a day to reduce "off" periods.
Dopamine Receptor Agonists			
pramipexole (Mirapex) ropinirole (Requip, Requip XL) rotigotine (Neupro [transdermal patch])	Stimulate DA receptors	Dizziness GI distress Hallucinations Insomnia Orthostatic BP	Monitor orthostatic BP. Change positions slowly. Use safety measures if CNS effects occur. Rotate patch sites.
Dopamine Agonists			
amantadine amantadine ER capsules (Gocorvi)	Blocks NMDA-type glutamate receptors, increases DA release, and blocks DA reuptake	Dizziness Insomnia	Do not stop abruptly. Use safety measures if CNS effects occur. Take extended-release capsules at bedtime.
apomorphine (Apokyn)	Stimulates postsynaptic DA receptors	Chest pain Drowsiness GI distress Liver toxicity Sweating	Monitor liver function. Rotate injection sites. Give in abdomen, thigh, upper arm. Sublingual dosing for reduction in "off time."
Anticholinergics			
benztropine (Cogentin) trihexyphenidyl (Artane)	Block cholinergic receptors, helping to balance cholinergic and dopaminergic activity	Dizziness Dry mouth Urinary retention Vision changes	Stop if swallowing problems occur. Avoid alcohol, hot weather. Use safety measures if CNS effects occur.
Antihistamine			
diphenhydramine	Anticholinergic effect	Drowsiness Dry mouth Urinary retention Vision changes	Avoid alcohol. Use safety measures if CNS effects occur. Do not take with MAO inhibitors.
Monoamine Oxidase Type B Inhibitors			
rasagiline (Azilect) safinamide (Xadago) selegiline (Elepryl)	Block breakdown of DA	Dizziness Dry mouth Headache Orthostatic BP	Use safety measures if CNS effects occur. Avoid tyramine-containing foods. Many drug interactions. Avoid direct sunlight. Change positions slowly.
Catechol O-Methyltransferase (COMT) Inhibitors			
entacapone (Comtan) opicapone (Ongentys)	Block COMT and slow the breakdown of levodopa, prolonging the action of levodopa	Confusion Dizziness GI distress Hypotension	Only give with levodopa. Avoid pregnancy. Use safety measures if CNS effects occur.
Adenosine A2 Antagonist			
istradefylline (Nourianz)	Blocks adenosine receptors next to dopamine receptors in basal ganglia	Hallucination Strong urges (gambling, spending, binge eating)	Used with levodopa and carbidopa. Avoid pregnancy. Do not stop abruptly.

TABLE 63.18 **Drug Therapy—cont'd**

Parkinson Disease

Other			
droxidopa (Northera)	Temporarily increases epinephrine to improve dizziness	Confusion Dysrhythmias Supine hypertension, Hyperpyrexia	Take at least 3 h before bedtime. Avoid pregnancy. Do not stop abruptly.
incobotulintoxinA (Xeomin)	Neuromuscular blocking agent to reduce drooling	Dysphagia Dyspnea Ptosis	Facial injection every 3–4 months. Report new onset of problems breathing, swallowing.
pimavanserin (Nuplazid)	Serotonin antagonist/inverse agonist used for PD psychosis	Confusion Edema Nausea Prolonged QT interval	Avoid use in patients with dysrhythmias. Do not stop abruptly.

reduce "off" symptoms in patients taking levodopa/carbidopa.[31]

Surgical Therapy

Patients with severe motor complications or dyskinesia may find relief with surgical intervention. Surgical procedures include deep brain stimulation (DBS) and ablation. The most common surgical treatment is DBS. An electrode is placed in the targeted areas that control movement and connected to a generator placed subcutaneously in the upper chest (Fig. 63.10). The device delivers electrical stimulation to the targeted cells. Some providers prefer DBS to ablation because it is reversible.[32]

Ablation surgery involves finding, targeting, and destroying an area of the brain affected by PD. The goal is to destroy tissue that produces abnormal chemical or electrical impulses leading to PD symptoms. Typical targets of ablation are the thalamus *(thalamotomy)* and globus pallidus *(pallidotomy)*. Gamma knife surgery uses multiple radiation beams to destroy the target tissue. Unilateral focused ultrasound (FUS) uses MRI-guided high-intensity ultrasound to destroy target tissue causing PD symptoms.

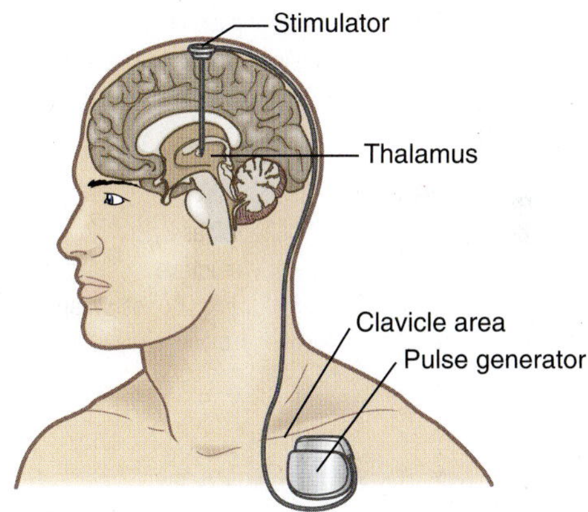

Fig. 63.10 DBS can be used to treat tremors and uncontrolled movements of PD. Electrodes are surgically placed in the brain and connected to a neurostimulator (pacemaker device) in the chest.

Additional information on clinical problems and interventions for patients with PD is presented in eNursing Care Plan 63.4 (available on the website for this chapter).

NURSING MANAGEMENT: PARKINSON DISEASE

Assessment

Table 63.19 lists subjective and objective data that should be assessed in patients with PD.

Clinical Problems

Clinical problems for patients with PD may include:

- Neurologic problem
- Nutritionally compromised
- Risk for injury
- Impaired communication
- Difficulty coping

Planning

The overall goals are that patients with PD will (1) maximize neurologic function, (2) maintain independence in ADLs as long as possible, (3) prevent injury, and (4) optimize well-being.

Implementation

Because PD is a chronic progressive degenerative disorder, teaching and nursing care are directed toward maintaining good health, encouraging independence, and avoiding complications, such as aspiration and falls. The American Parkinson Disease Association (www.apdaparkinson.org) can connect patients and families with support groups and education materials that can be used by caregivers and health care professionals.

Promoting physical exercise is a major nursing concern. Exercise will not stop disease progress, but it will enhance functional ability. Exercise limits the effects of decreased

TABLE 63.19 NURSING ASSESSMENT

Parkinson Disease

Subjective Data

Important Health Information

Health history: CNS trauma, cerebrovascular disorders, exposure to metals and carbon monoxide, encephalitis or other infections

Medications: Major tranquilizers, especially haloperidol, phenothiazines, reserpine, methyldopa, amphetamines

Functional Health Patterns

Health perception–health management: Fatigue

Nutritional-metabolic: Excess salivation, dysphagia, weight loss, satiety

Elimination: Constipation, incontinence, excess sweating

Activity-exercise: Difficulty in initiating movements, frequent falls, loss of dexterity, slowing of movements, micrographia (handwriting deterioration)

Sleep-rest: Insomnia, nightmares, daytime sleepiness

Cognitive-perceptual: Diffuse pain in head, shoulders, neck, back, legs, and hips. Muscle soreness and cramping, impulse control

Role-relationship: Decreased libido, impotence

Self-perception–self-concept: Depression, mood swings, hallucinations

Objective Data

Cardiovascular

Postural hypotension

General

Blank (masked) facial expression, slow and monotonous speech, infrequent blinking

GI

Drooling, difficulty swallowing, rigid tongue and jaw

Musculoskeletal

Cogwheel rigidity, dysarthria, bradykinesia, contractures, stooped posture, shuffling gait, dysphonia

Neurologic

Tremor at rest, first in hands (pill rolling), later in legs, arms, face, and tongue. Aggravation of tremor with anxiety, absence in sleep. Poor coordination, cognitive impairment and dementia, impaired postural reflexes

Skin

Seborrhea, dandruff; ankle edema, moles

Possible Diagnostic Findings

No specific tests. Diagnosis based on history and physical findings and ruling out other diseases. Improvement with levodopa confirms diagnosis.

mobility, such as muscle atrophy, weakness, or constipation. A physical therapist can design a personal exercise program to strengthen and stretch specific muscles.

Patients should work with a speech pathologist early in the disease process to perform exercises that strengthen and support swallowing and speech function. Special voice amplifiers can be used for soft vocal tones. An occupational therapist can help patients with ADLs.

CHECK YOUR PRACTICE

You are working at a rehabilitation facility with a 78-year-old male with PD. He was at your facility briefly 6 months ago with a fractured hip after falling in his yard. The family has asked to talk with you about their fear of taking him for a walk in the hallways because he is so unstable.

- How would you advise them?

Work with caregivers to promote independence and self-care. Patients can get out of a chair more easily by using an upright chair with arms and placing the back legs of the chair on small (2-inch) blocks. Encourage environment changes to improve safety. These include removing rugs and excess furniture to avoid stumbling and using an elevated toilet seat to help patients get on and off the toilet. Elevating the legs can decrease dependent ankle edema. Dressing can be simplified by using slip-on shoes and Velcro, hook-and-loop fasteners, or zippers instead of buttons. Allow extra time for all ADLs.

A well-balanced diet is important. Malnutrition can result from dysphagia, bradykinesia, fatigue, and difficulty chewing. Patients need appetizing foods that are easy to chew and swallow. The diet should have adequate fiber to reduce constipation. Eating 6 small meals a day may be less fatiguing than 3 large meals a day. Plan adequate time for eating to avoid frustration. Cut food into bite-sized pieces. Protein ingestion can impair the absorption of levodopa. Limiting protein intake to the evening meal can decrease this problem. Vitamin B_6 found in a multivitamin or fortified cereal can inhibit levodopa, but this does not occur when taking carbidopa with levodopa.

Effective management of sleep problems can improve quality of life. Some patients find satin nightwear or satin sheets helpful. Sleep hygiene is discussed in Chapter 8.

In the early stages of PD, patients often have depression and anxiety. Patients need to adjust their lifestyle, including work and home responsibilities. Help patients by listening, providing teaching, gently correcting distorted thoughts, and encouraging social interaction. Counseling may be necessary.

Family members care for most patients with PD. Their burden increases as the disease progresses and their mental health declines. PD causes subtle changes in cognitive function that can progress to PD psychosis or dementia. This may lead to long-term care placement. Information on care of patients with dementia is discussed in Chapter 64. Help caregivers find resources for the distressing delusions, hallucinations, or memory loss.

◆ Evaluation

The expected outcomes are that patients with PD will:

- Maintain optimal muscle function
- Use needed assistive devices
- Maintain adequate nutrition
- Have unimpaired swallowing
- Use communication methods that allow interaction with others

MYASTHENIA GRAVIS

Myasthenia gravis (MG) is an autoimmune disease of the neuromuscular junction marked by skeletal muscle weakness that worsens with activity. MG occurs in all ages and races. Around 87,000 people in the United States have MG.[33] In females, MG often starts before age 40. Males usually develop MG after age 60.[34]

Etiology and Pathophysiology

In MG, autoantibodies attack and destroy acetylcholine (ACh) receptors at the neuromuscular junction. This results in fewer ACh receptor (AChR) sites. ACh molecules cannot stimulate muscle contraction because they cannot bind to the receptors. For many patients with MG, the thymus gland fails to shrink after puberty. The thymus remains active and may develop a thymoma. The thymus may give incorrect instructions to developing lymphocytes, causing them to make AChR antibodies (ab).[33] AChRab are in the serum of most patients with MG. The autoantibodies muscle-specific tyrosine kinase (MuSK) and low-density lipoprotein receptor–related protein 4 (LRP4) are present. Some patients have no autoantibodies.

Clinical Manifestations and Complications

The key feature of MG is skeletal muscle weakness that gets worse with activity and improves with rest. Many muscles are affected, but muscles engaged in repetitive movements are affected the most. This includes muscles that control blinking, chewing, swallowing, speaking, and breathing. Muscles are strongest in the morning. They become exhausted with continued activity and weakness is prominent by the end of the day. A period of rest usually restores strength.

For about half of patients with MG, the first muscles involved are the ocular muscles, causing ptosis (drooping of the eyelids) in 1 or both eyes and double vision (Fig. 63.11).[35] MG is limited to the ocular muscles in some patients. In others, facial muscles are affected. Facial mobility and expression are impaired. Patients may have difficulty with chewing and swallowing. Speech may slur and the voice fade after long conversations. The muscles of the trunk and limbs easily fatigue especially proximal muscles of the neck, shoulders, and hips. Neonates can acquire autoantibodies from their mother and have symptoms for 2 to 3 months after birth.[34]

The course of MG is highly variable. Patients may have fluctuations from day to day, have short-term remissions, or have severe progressive disease. Fatigue, pregnancy, illness, trauma, temperature extremes, stress, and hypokalemia can exacerbate MG. Prescribed β-adrenergic blockers, calcium channel blockers, lithium, quinidine, statins, and aminoglycoside antibiotics worsen MG symptoms.[36]

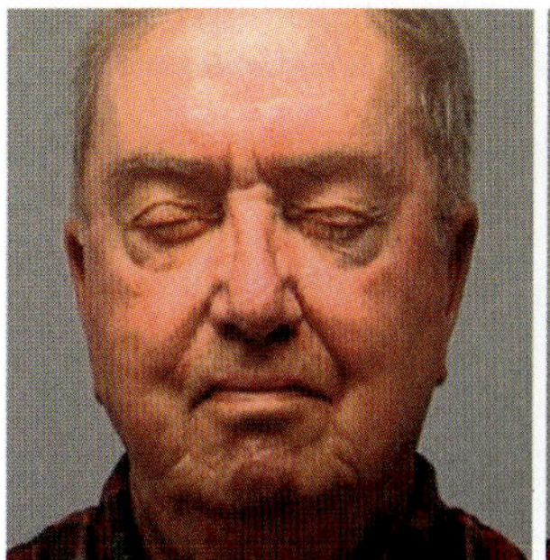
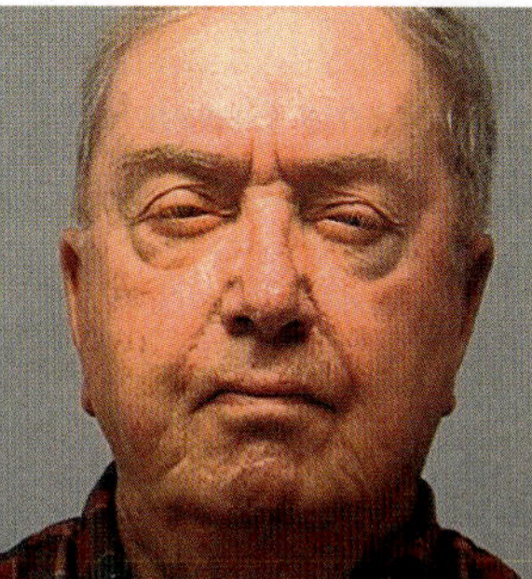

Fig. 63.11 "Peek" sign in myasthenia gravis. During sustained forced eyelid closure, he is unable to bury his eyelashes *(left)*. After 30 seconds, he cannot keep the lids fully closed *(right)*. (From Sanders DB, Massey JM: Clinical features of myasthenia gravis. In AG Engel, editor: *Neuromuscular junction disorders: handbook of clinical neurology*, New York, 2008, Elsevier.)

Myasthenic crisis is acute worsening of muscle weakness. Stressors and inadequate treatment are triggers. During myasthenic crisis, weakness occurs in muscles that affect swallowing and breathing. This requires urgent intervention. Aspiration or respiratory insufficiency can occur. Patients may need a ventilator or noninvasive respiratory support (BiPAP).

Diagnostic Studies

The history and physical assessment are the foundation of diagnosis. Single-fiber EMG showing impaired nerve-muscle transmission helps confirm MG.[34] Repetitive nerve stimulation testing examines the response of muscles to stimulus. Serology testing may show increased levels of AChRab or anti-MuSK antibodies. In patients who are antibody negative, diagnosis may be confirmed by administering medications used to treat MG and observing for symptom improvement. A chest CT scan may be done to evaluate the thymus.

Interprofessional Care

Drug Therapy

Drug therapy for MG includes anticholinesterase drugs, corticosteroids, immunosuppressants, FcRN inhibitors, and complement inhibitors (Table 63.20). Anticholinesterase drugs inhibit acetylcholinesterase, prolong the action of ACh, and improve impulse transmission at the neuromuscular junction. For long-term treatment of MG, pyridostigmine (Mestinon) is the preferred drug.[34] Tailoring the dose to avoid a myasthenic or a cholinergic crisis presents a challenge. Inadequate dosing can cause myasthenic crisis. Excess dosing will cause a cholinergic crisis from too much cholinesterase inhibition. Table 63.21 distinguishes these complications.

TABLE 63.20 Interprofessional Care

Myasthenia Gravis

Diagnostic Assessment
- History and physical assessment
  - Fatigability with prolonged upward gaze (2–3 min)
  - Muscle weakness
- EMG
- Edrophonium test
- Acetylcholine receptor antibodies
- Chest x-ray

Management
- Drug therapy
  - Anticholinesterase agents
  - Corticosteroids
  - Immunosuppressive agents
  - FcRn inhibitors
  - Complement inhibitors
- Surgery (thymectomy)
- Plasmapheresis
- IV immunoglobulin G

TABLE 63.21 Comparison of Myasthenic and Cholinergic Crises

Myasthenic Crisis	Cholinergic Crisis
Causes	
Exacerbation of myasthenia after precipitating factors, failure to take drug as prescribed, or drug dose too low	Overdose of anticholinesterase drugs resulting in ↑ ACh at the receptor sites, remission (spontaneous or after thymectomy)
Differential Diagnosis	
Improved strength after IV administration of anticholinesterase drugs	Weakness within 1 h after ingestion of anticholinesterase drugs
↑ Weakness of skeletal muscles: Ptosis, bulbar signs (e.g., difficulty swallowing, difficulty articulating words), dyspnea	↑ Weakness of skeletal muscles: ptosis, bulbar signs, dyspnea Effects on smooth muscle include pupillary miosis, salivation, diarrhea, nausea or vomiting, abdominal cramps, ↑ bronchial secretions, sweating, lacrimation

Several monoclonal antibodies are available to treat patients who are seropositive for AChRab. Efgartigimod alfa-fcab (Vygart) inhibits FcRn causing AChRab to be removed from the body. Ravulizumab-cwvz (Ultomiris) and eculizumab (Soliris) decrease autoimmune activity by AChRab. Corticosteroids and immunosuppressants (prednisone, azathioprine, mycophenolate) reduce ACh antibody production.

Surgical Therapy

The thymus gland enhances the production of AChR antibodies in MG. Removing the thymus gland improves symptoms in most patients. Up to 50% of patients can attain long-lasting remission.[34] It can take 2 years to attain results after surgery. Thymectomy is recommended for MG patients under 50 years old who meet criteria.

Other Therapies

Plasmapheresis and IV immunoglobulin G can yield short-term improvement in symptoms. These are indicated for patients in myasthenic crisis or before surgery. Plasmapheresis directly removes circulating AChR antibodies from the plasma, leading to a decrease in symptoms. IV immunoglobulin G reduces autoantibody activity.

NURSING MANAGEMENT: MYASTHENIA GRAVIS

Assessment

Assess the severity of MG by asking about fatigue. Some patients become so fatigued they cannot work or even walk. What muscles are affected? How severe is their weakness? Assess coping abilities and understanding of MG. Obtain a thorough medication history. Many drugs are contraindicated or must be used with caution in patients with MG.

Objective data include respiratory rate and depth, O_2 saturation, arterial blood gas analyses, and pulmonary function tests. Assess for respiratory distress in patients with acute myasthenic crisis. Assess muscle strength of all face and limb muscles. Evaluate swallowing, speech (volume and clarity), and cough and gag reflexes.

Clinical Problems

Clinical problems for patients with MG may include:
- Impaired respiratory function
- Activity intolerance
- Risk for injury

Planning

The overall goals are that patients with MG will (1) have a return of normal muscle strength, (2) manage fatigue, (3) avoid complications, and (4) maintain quality of life.

Implementation

Hospital admission for patients with MG is usually due to respiratory tract infection or acute myasthenic crisis. The focus of nursing care is maintaining adequate ventilation, continuing drug therapy, and monitoring for side effects of therapy. Nurses must be able to tell a cholinergic from myasthenic crisis. Both cause muscle weakness, but their causes and treatment differ greatly.

BOX 63.1 EVIDENCE-BASED PRACTICE

Exercise in Patients With Myasthenia Gravis

Your patient today is M.S., a 51-year-old who was diagnosed with myasthenia gravis (MG) 6 months ago. During your assessment, you note that M.S. appears withdrawn and is not speaking with you except to answer your questions. M.S. says, "I used to be so active, and now I do nothing. I miss hiking and riding my bike with my family. I feel like such a burden."

Making Clinical Decisions

Synthesis of Best Available Evidence

Patients with MG tend to live a less active lifestyle due to increased muscle weakness with activity. Recent evidence shows that exercise can increase muscle strength, improve daily functioning, and enhance respiratory muscle function.

Clinician Expertise

You know that the type and intensity of exercise should be adapted to patients' needs and capabilities, taking into account the severity of their MG and other factors. While exercise can be beneficial, you must be mindful of fatigue and avoid overexertion, as MG can cause significant fatigue. You believe a walking program would be the best option for M.S. at this time.

Patient Preferences and Values

Following discussion with the HCP, M.S. agrees to attend a walking program and follow up weekly with you to discuss questions or concerns about exercising. After 4 months, M.S. states he is "enjoying the program" despite some days being "more challenging." He adds that he is happy that someone in his family goes with him at least once a week.

Implications for Nursing Practice

1. What barriers might be present when recommending exercise for a patient with MG?
2. What outcomes would indicate a positive effect of an exercise program?

Reference for Evidence

Alsop T, Cassimatis M, Williams K, et al: Perspectives of people with myasthenia gravis on physical activity advice from health professionals in the Australian context: a qualitative study, *Disability and Rehab* 47:1, 2025.

As with other chronic illnesses, focus care on the neurologic deficits and their impact on daily living. Teach patients about a balanced diet that can easily be chewed and swallowed. Semisolid foods may be easier to eat. Scheduling doses of drugs to reach peak action at mealtime may make eating easier. Arrange activities that match the patient's interests and abilities (Box 63.1). Plan ADLs and rest to avoid fatigue.

Discuss the treatment plan, adverse drug reactions, and preventing complications. Teach patients to be prepared for an MG crisis. Have a bag packed in case emergency hospitalization is needed. Have an emergency wallet card or medical ID so EMS and health care workers can be aware of treatment requirements. Explore community resources such as the Myasthenia Gravis Foundation of America and MG support groups.

◆ Evaluation

The expected outcomes are that patients with MG will:

- Maintain optimal muscle function
- Be free from side effects of drugs
- Have no complications
- Maintain a quality of life appropriate to the disease course

AMYOTROPHIC LATERAL SCLEROSIS

Amyotrophic lateral sclerosis (ALS) is a rare progressive degenerative neuromuscular disorder marked by loss of motor neurons. ALS usually leads to death 3 to 5 years after diagnosis. A few patients may survive longer. Those diagnosed in early adulthood have an increased likelihood of longer survival. Many call ALS *Lou Gehrig's disease* after the famous baseball player who died from ALS. The well-known physicist Stephen Hawking lived with ALS for 50 years. About 30,000 Americans have ALS.[37] The median age of onset is 55 years. ALS is more common in White persons, males, and military veterans. Genetics causes about 10% of cases. The most common gene mutations are in *C9ORF72* and *SOD1*.[38] Factors that affect ALS include smoking, metals, solvents, radiation, electromagnetic fields, pesticides, and viruses.

In ALS, upper and lower motor neurons in the brainstem and spinal cord degenerate. We do not know the cause. Early in the disease mitochondrial changes lead to excess glutamate. Excess glutamate activates neuron damaging enzymes. Destroyed motor neurons cannot produce or transport signals to muscles. Consequently, electrical and chemical messages originating in the brain do not reach the muscles to activate them.

Progressive muscle weakness and atrophy are the classic signs of ALS. Some initially have symptoms only in arms or legs. The person may have trouble with tasks requiring fine motor skills (e.g., writing, typing) or notice they are tripping or dropping things. Those who first develop problems with slurred speech or swallowing have "bulbar onset" ALS.

Muscle wasting, involuntary contractions, and twitching result from denervation of the muscles. Other symptoms include pain, spasticity, hyperreflexia, drooling, emotional lability, and constipation. Eventually patients will not be able to communicate. As the ability to move decreases, impaired swallowing leads to aspiration. Sleep problems from respiratory muscle weakness and muscle spasm occur. Death often results from compromised respiratory function due to muscle weakness and paralysis.

No cure exists for ALS. Medication may slow the decline for a few months or a year. Riluzole (Rilutek) reduces damage to motor neurons by decreasing glutamate release. Edaravone

(Radicava) is a free radical scavenger that slows ALS progression. It is given orally, by feeding tube, or IV. Toferson (Qalsody) is given intrathecally to lower the SOD1 protein in CSF. Given early, it is believed to slow the rate of disease progression.[38]

The course of ALS is devastating because patients are cognitively intact while wasting away. They may have some difficulty with decision making and memory. Common problems are grief and impaired role performance. Care focuses on (1) facilitating communication, (2) reducing aspiration risk, (3) early identification of respiratory problems, (4) decreasing pain, (5) decreasing risk for fall-related injury, (6) providing diversional activities, such as reading and companionship, and (7) providing compassionate end-of-life care.

Moderate-intensity, endurance-type exercises for the trunk and limbs reduce spasticity. Communication can be helped with the use of computer-based speech synthesizers. Mobility can be improved with the use of brain-computer interface systems that allow control of equipment with brain activity. As the respiratory muscles begin to decline, the use of noninvasive ventilation may be used.

Provide patients and caregivers support. Include grieving related to the loss of motor function and impending death. Discuss advance directives and artificial ventilation with patients and caregivers. Provide the caregiver with resources to combat fatigue and stress.

HUNTINGTON DISEASE

Huntington disease (HD) is a progressive, degenerative brain disorder causing deterioration of physical, emotional, and cognitive abilities. It is a genetically transmitted, autosomal dominant disorder. There are about 41,000 affected people in the United States.[39] The onset of HD is usually between ages 30 and 50 years. Diagnosis is often made after the affected person has had children. Patients live 15 to 25 years after diagnosis.[39]

The diagnosis begins with a review of the family history and clinical symptoms. Genetic testing confirms excess cytosine-adenine-guanine (CAG) nucleotide protein repeats in the *HTT* (huntingtin) gene. People with a family history of HD who are asymptomatic must decide if they want genetic testing. If the test is positive, the person will develop HD but will not know when. If HD is present in a family, genetic testing is recommended to aid in family planning. Refer those wishing to have a child without the gene to a fertility specialist.

HD involves a deficiency of the neurotransmitters ACh and γ-aminobutyric acid (GABA). This leads to excess DA in the basal ganglia and extrapyramidal motor system.

Manifestations include movement, cognitive, and psychologic symptoms. Early in the disease patients are "fidgety." They have difficulty staying on task, planning, or remembering. Movement symptoms are marked by abnormal and excess involuntary movements *(chorea)*. These are writhing, twisting movements of the face, limbs, tongue, and body. The chorea gets worse as the disease progresses. Movements are uncoordinated. Patients have difficulty with movement sequences (getting out of bed, pouring a cup of tea). Inability to sustain intentional movement occurs and they may not be able to hold a glass, make a bed, or perform other tasks. Facial movements involving speech, chewing, and swallowing are affected. Aspiration is likely. The excess movement causes unintentional weight loss. The gait deteriorates, and patients have difficulty balancing. They will lose the ability to drive and work. Eventually all psychomotor processes are impaired.

Psychologic symptoms are present in HD, even before the onset of motor symptoms. Depression is common. Other mental health concerns include anxiety, agitation, impulsivity, apathy, withdrawal, and mood swings. Personality change often occurs. Cognitive deterioration leads to forgetfulness and slowed mental processing and will progress to dementia. Patients have difficulty thinking through a problem and putting tasks in order. Perception and learning deficits are present. At the end of the disease, patients are nonverbal, bedridden, and require help with all ADLs. The most common cause of death is pneumonia, followed by suicide.

HD has no cure; treatment is palliative. Drugs are available to control movement and cognitive changes. Tetrabenazine (Xenazine) and deutetrabenazine (Austedo) treat involuntary movements by decreasing DA at the nerve synapse. Antipsychotics such as risperidone treat chorea with psychiatric symptoms if tetrabenazine is not effective. Cognitive disorders are treated with nondrug therapies (e.g., counseling, memory books). Selective serotonin reuptake inhibitors, such as sertraline (Zoloft), help treat depression.

The goals of nursing management are to provide the most comfortable environment possible for patients and caregivers, maintain physical safety, treat symptoms, and provide emotional support.

Because of the chorea, caloric requirements are high. Patients may need as many as 4000 to 5000 kcal/day to maintain body weight. As HD progresses, meeting calorie needs becomes a greater challenge because patients have difficulty swallowing and cannot hold their head still. Depression and cognitive decline compromise nutrition intake. Enteral or parenteral nutrition may be needed.

Discuss end-of-life issues with patients and caregivers. Include care in home or a long-term care facility, artificial methods of feeding, advance directives, and guardianship. Address these topics throughout the course of the disease as patients and caregivers adapt to increasing disability.

CASE STUDY

Seizure Disorder With Headache

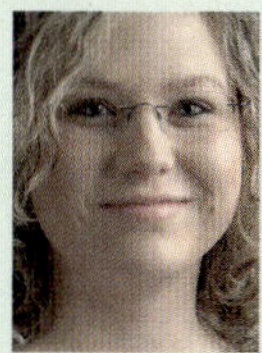

(© Purestock/ Thinkstock.)

Patient Profile

M.A. is a 28-year-old female diagnosed with seizure disorder at age 17. At that time, a heat-related injury and electrolyte imbalance causing a tonic-clonic seizure occurred. A second seizure occurred 2 months later, and divalproex was prescribed. No further seizures occurred until 6 months ago. In the past 6 months, M.A. has had 2 generalized-onset seizures with throbbing headaches after both. M.A. now has headaches several days a week. M.A. says she is planning her wedding and has taken on more responsibilities at work. M.A. expresses fear the headaches and seizures will cause her to lose her job and interfere with the wedding.

Subjective Data

- Describes throbbing headache pain on the right side of her forehead
- Has vomited during headaches
- Describes vision changes, including blurring and flashing lights before the start of a headache
- Headache occurs several times a week and lasts several hours
- Headaches have not improved with ibuprofen or acetaminophen

Objective Data

- Neurologic assessment is normal
- Divalproex levels are within therapeutic range
- EEG and CT of head are unremarkable
- CBC and metabolic panel are within normal limits

Discussion Questions

1. ***Recognize:*** What assessment findings are significant?
2. ***Analyze:*** What type of headache is M.A. describing?
3. ***Plan:*** What therapy do you expect for her headaches and seizures?
4. ***Prioritize:*** Based on the assessment data, what are the priority clinical problems?
5. ***Act:*** What teaching will you provide so M.A. can manage her care?
6. ***Act:*** What lifestyle changes would you recommend?
7. ***Evaluate:*** What outcomes would indicate M.A.'s care has been successful?
8. ***Safety:*** To ensure M.A.'s safety, what nursing interventions are needed?

Answers available at http://evolve.elsevier.com/Lewis/medsurg.

BRIDGE TO NCLEX EXAMINATION

The number of the question corresponds to the same-numbered outcome at the beginning of the chapter.

1. A patient in the clinic describes a recent increase in frequency of migraine headaches. They report a headache most mornings, treated with a combination acetaminophen, aspirin, and caffeine medication. To assist with determining the cause of this change, what assessment data would the nurse collect?
   - **a.** When the increased frequency started
   - **b.** If the headaches cause photosensitivity
   - **c.** Are the headaches causing difficulty with ADLs
   - **d.** Have they recently begun using a vagal nerve stimulator
2. The rapid response team is called to the cafeteria. They find a 22-year-old with a known seizure disorder having a tonic-clonic seizure. What actions will be taken during the seizure? **(Select all that apply.)**
   - **a.** Establish IV access.
   - **b.** Insert an oral airway.
   - **c.** Gently hold the arms to prevent injury.
   - **d.** Administer prescribed intranasal midazolam.
   - **e.** Turn the person to their side and pad their head.
3. A patient with multiple sclerosis receives natalizumab every 6 months and modafinil and dalfampridine daily. What assessment findings would indicate that the treatment plan was successful? **(Select all that apply.)**
   - **a.** Blurred vision
   - **b.** Improved walking
   - **c.** Decreased fatigue
   - **d.** No change in spasticity
   - **e.** Reduced exacerbation frequency
4. A 28-year-old patient whose mother has Huntington disease is discussing family planning with the nurse. The patient says she wants to have a child but is concerned. What statement will the nurse make?
   - **a.** "Only about 1 in 10 people who have the gene pass it to their children."
   - **b.** "Both parents must have the gene for your child to inherit this disease."
   - **c.** "If you have the Huntington mutation, you will not be able to have children."
   - **d.** "Genetic testing can be done to determine whether you can pass this trait to a child."

1. a; 2. a, d, e; 3. b, c, e; 4. d.

For rationales to these answers and even more NCLEX review questions, visit http://evolve.elsevier.com/Lewis/medsurg.

REFERENCES

To access the References for this chapter, please scan the QR code with a mobile device.

64

Dementia and Delirium

Janice Smolowitz

http://evolve.elsevier.com/Lewis/medsurg/

CONCEPTUAL FOCUS

Caregiving
Cognition
Family Dynamics
Functional Ability
Safety

LEARNING OUTCOMES

1. Define dementia and delirium.
2. Explain the etiology, pathophysiology, clinical manifestations, diagnostic studies, and nursing and interprofessional care for patients with dementia.
3. Explain the pathophysiology of AD.
4. Discuss the clinical manifestations of AD.
5. Describe the diagnostic studies and interprofessional care for patients with AD.
6. Discuss the nursing management for patients with Alzheimer disease.
7. Explain the etiology, pathophysiology, clinical manifestations, diagnostic studies, and nursing and interprofessional care for patients with delirium.

KEY TERMS

Alzheimer disease (AD)
delirium
dementia
dementia with Lewy bodies (DLB), Table 64.2
frontotemporal lobar degeneration (FTLD), Table 64.2
mild cognitive impairment (MCI)
mixed dementia
retrogenesis
sundowning

This chapter discusses dementia and delirium, with a focus on the care of patients with Alzheimer disease (AD). *Cognitive impairment* refers to any deficit in intellectual function, including problems with memory, orientation, attention, and concentration.[1] The term *dementia* describes a group of symptoms that adversely affect a person's ability to function and fulfill responsibilities. Symptoms include problems with short-term memory, language, problem-solving, and other thinking skills. In most cases, these problems are caused by changes in the brain that occur over a long period.

DEMENTIA

Dementia is a disorder characterized by cognitive decline from the previous level of function in 1 or more domains: complex attention, executive function, language, learning and memory, perceptual-motor, and social cognition.[2] This decline interferes with the ability to perform daily activities. The function most often lost is the ability to recall events specific to a time and place. This decline does not occur with the onset of acute confusion, such as delirium, or the onset of another major mental health problem, such as depression.

The number of patients with dementia is increasing. Globally, we estimate that 50 million people have dementia. AD is the most common form of dementia. It accounts for 60% to 80% of all cases (Fig. 64.1).

Etiology and Pathophysiology

Dementia is caused by treatable and untreatable conditions. The most common cause is aging. We estimate that 10% of people over the age of 70 years have memory loss that can be identified on clinical examination. This increases to 20% to 40% among persons over age 85 years.[3]

Table 64.1 describes types of dementia and their underlying causes. Treatable causes may initially be reversible. However,

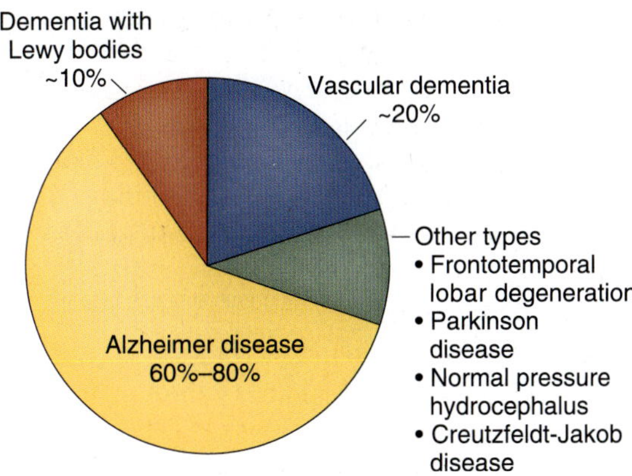

Fig. 64.1 Causes of dementia.

irreversible changes can occur with prolonged exposure or disease. The most common causes are neurodegenerative conditions that cannot be reversed (Table 64.2). Most of these are the result of AD.[4] Other causes include dementia with Lewy bodies (DLB), frontotemporal dementia (FTD), and Parkinson disease with dementia (PDD).

Vascular or multiinfarct dementia (VaD) is a loss of cognitive function caused by vascular disease. It may be caused by a single infarct (stroke) or multiple strokes.[5] It is more common among males. Subcortical dementia is the most common type of VaD. It occurs when small vessels deep in the brain develop thick walls and become stiff. This reduces blood flow, which damages the nerve fibers because of a lack of oxygen.

Mixed dementia occurs when 2 or more types of dementia are present at the same time. It is usually characterized by the hallmark abnormalities of AD and another type of dementia. More than 50% of people with AD may have mixed dementia.[1] Mixed dementia is usually found among persons aged 85 years and or older.

Normal-pressure hydrocephalus is a rare problem where an obstruction in cerebrospinal fluid (CSF) flow causes a buildup of CSF in the brain. Manifestations include dementia, urinary incontinence, and difficulty walking. If diagnosed early, it is treatable by surgery in which a shunt is inserted to divert the fluid away from the brain.

Clinical Manifestations

Although the cause of dementia cannot be determined based only on the history of symptom progression, patterns can guide your thinking. The onset of manifestations varies depending on the cause. Manifestations of neurologic degeneration usually occur gradually and progress over time. Symptoms of VaD may appear abruptly or progress in a stepwise pattern. An acute change that occurs over days to weeks or a subacute change that occurs over weeks to months may indicate an infectious or metabolic cause of dementia, such as encephalitis, meningitis, hypothyroidism, or drug-related dementia. Other manifestations are discussed in the section on clinical manifestations of AD.

TABLE 64.1 Causes of Dementia

Type of Dementia	Cause
Neurodegenerative disorders	• AD • Amyotrophic lateral sclerosis (ALS) • Dementia with Lewy bodies (DLB) • Down syndrome • Frontotemporal lobar degeneration (FTLD) • Huntington disease • Parkinson disease
Vascular diseases	• Chronic subdural hematoma[a] • Subarachnoid hemorrhage[a] • Vascular (multiinfarct) dementia
Immunologic diseases or infections	• AIDS • Encephalitis[a] • Infections (e.g., Creutzfeldt-Jakob disease) • Meningitis[a] • Multiple sclerosis • Neurosyphilis[a] • Systemic exertion intolerance disease • Systemic lupus erythematosus[a]
Medications[b]	• Anticholinergics • Antiparkinsonian drugs • Cardiac drugs: digoxin, methyldopa • Cocaine • Heroin • Hypnotics • Opioids • Phenytoin (Dilantin) • Tranquilizers
Metabolic or nutrition problems	• Alcohol use disorder • Cobalamin (vitamin B_{12}) deficiency[a] • Folate deficiency[a] • Hyperthyroidism[a] • Hypothyroidism[a] • Thiamine (vitamin B_1) deficiency[a]
Systemic diseases	• Dialysis dementia[a] • Hepatic encephalopathy[a] • Uremic encephalopathy[a] • Wilson disease
Trauma	• Head injury[a]
Tumors	• Brain tumors (primary)[a] • Metastatic tumors[a]
Ventricular disorders	• Hydrocephalus[a]

[a]Potentially reversible.
[b]Examples of drugs that may cause cognitive impairment that is potentially reversible.

Persons with dementia and delirium may have symptoms of depression. Depression and dementia are often mistaken for one another, especially among older adults. Manifestations of depression may include sadness, difficulty concentrating, fatigue, apathy, feelings of despair, and inactivity. When depression is severe, poor concentration and inattention may result, causing memory and functional impairment. When dementia and depression occur together, there can be marked intellectual decline.[1] Table 64.3 compares key features of dementia, delirium, and depression.

TABLE 64.2 Neurodegenerative Causes of Dementia

Neurodegenerative Disorder	Characteristics	Management
Dementia With Lewy Bodies (DLB)		
• Characterized by presence of Lewy bodies (abnormal deposits of protein α-synuclein) in brainstem and cortex • Has features of AD and Parkinson disease	• Diagnosis based on manifestations • Typically have manifestations of parkinsonism, hallucinations, short-term memory loss, unpredictable cognitive shifts, sleep problems • Pneumonia is a common complication	• Drug therapy: levodopa/carbidopa, acetylcholinesterase inhibitors • Manage dementia, dysphagia, and immobility • Swallowing problems can lead to impaired nutrition • At risk for falls from impaired mobility and balance
Frontotemporal Lobar Degeneration (FTLD)		
• Caused by atrophy of frontal and temporal lobes of brain • In Pick disease, a type of FTLD, brain may have abnormal microscopic deposits called Pick bodies • Often misdiagnosed as a psychiatric problem because of strange behaviors	• Changes in behavior, sleep, eventually memory • Progresses relentlessly • May lead to language impairment, erratic behavior, dementia • Tends to occur at a younger age than does AD, typically about age 60	• No specific treatment • Antidepressants and antipsychotics to treat behavior manifestations
Vascular (Multiinfarct) Dementia		
• Caused by a single infarct (stroke) or multiple strokes • Prognosis is poor • Symptoms may begin suddenly, with decline after each small stroke	• More common in males • Typically begins between ages 60 and 75 • Symptoms are similar to AD • Often occurs with AD	• See Chapter 62 • No treatment • Focus on preventing future strokes by controlling problems that increase stroke risk

TABLE 64.3 Comparison of Dementia, Delirium, and Depression

Feature	Dementia	Delirium	Depression
Onset	Subtle, gradual.	Abrupt, although initially can be subtle.	Often coincides with life changes. Often abrupt.
Progression	Slow.	Abrupt. Can fluctuate from day to day.	Variable, rapid to slow but may be uneven.
Duration	Years (average of 8, can be longer).	Hours to days to weeks. Can be prolonged.	Can be several months to years, especially if not treated.
Thinking	Difficulty with abstract thinking, impaired judgment, words difficult to find.	Disorganized, distorted. Slow or accelerated incoherent speech.	Intact but with apathy and fatigue. May be indecisive. Feels a sense of hopelessness. May not want to live.
Perception	Misperceptions often present. Delusions and hallucinations.	Distorted. Delusions and hallucinations.	May deny or be unaware of depression. May have feelings of guilt.
Psychomotor behavior	May pace or be hyperactive. As disease progresses, may not be able to perform tasks or movements when asked.	Variable. Can be hyperactive or hypoactive, or mixed.	Often withdrawn and hypoactive.
Sleep-wake cycle	Sleeps during the day. Frequent awakenings at night. Fragmented sleep.	Disturbed sleep. Reversed sleep-wake cycle.	Disturbed, often with early morning awakening.

Diagnostic Studies

The diagnosis is focused on determining the cause. An important first step is a thorough medical, neurologic, and psychologic history.[6] During the history, give attention to the cognitive and behavior changes that have occurred. Family members and significant others can give important information. Obtain information about (1) problems with judgment; (2) reduced interest in hobbies/activities; (3) repeating questions, stories, or statements; (4) trouble learning how to use a tool or appliance; (5) forgetting the month or year; (6) problems handling financial affairs; (7) difficulty remembering appointments; and (8) consistent problems with thinking and/or memory.

Obtain information about diet and nutrition, alcohol and drug use, and medications. Ask about drugs that can impair cognition, such as analgesics, anticholinergics, psychotropics, and sedative-hypnotics.

The physical assessment is done to assess for other medical problems. For example, slow movement, rigidity, asymmetric tremor of an extremity, and shuffling gait suggest parkinsonism. Dementia, urinary incontinence, and ataxic gait suggest normal-pressure hydrocephalus.[7] The neurologic assessment includes a mental status screening test. Agreement among assessment findings, screening tests, and history helps confirm the presence of dementia.

Based on the history and physical assessment, diagnostic studies are ordered to confirm the most likely cause and exclude other possible conditions. Routine screening tests include electrolyte panel, liver function tests, vitamin B_{12} level, complete blood count (CBC), and thyroid function tests. Special laboratory tests, such as red blood cell folate in patients with alcohol use disorder or ionized calcium in patients with multiple myeloma, are ordered based on history. Head CT or MRI may show strokes, tumors, and other changes. Positron emission tomography (PET) can examine brain activity. In some instances, genetic testing may be considered based on family history.

Interprofessional and Nursing Management

If there is an identifiable cause, care is aimed at treating that cause. Other management measures are similar to the care of patients with AD. Preventive measures for VaD include treating risk factors, such as hypertension, diabetes, tobacco use, atrial fibrillation, and cardiovascular disease (CVD). Stroke is discussed in Chapter 62. Drugs given to patients with AD are useful for patients with VaD.

ALZHEIMER DISEASE

Alzheimer disease is a chronic, progressive, irreversible neurodegenerative brain disease. More than 6.9 million people are living with AD in the United States.[1] It most often affects persons age 65 and older. As the population ages, the prevalence is expected to increase. A small number of people younger than 60 years of age develop AD. When AD develops in someone younger than 60 years, it is called *early-onset AD*. It is the 5th leading cause of death among persons age 65 and older. The average clinical duration after diagnosis is 4 to 8 years, although this is variable.[8]

Etiology

AD is caused by a combination of factors. The 3 most important risk factors are aging, family history, and genetics. These risk factors cannot be modified. There are other risk factors that can be modified.

Aging

The greatest risk factor for AD is age. Most people with the condition are diagnosed at age 65 or older, which is called *late-onset AD*. Although age is the greatest risk factor, AD is not a normal part of aging, and age alone does not cause AD.[1]

Family History

Family history of AD is an important risk factor. Persons with a first-degree relative (parent or sibling) with dementia are more likely to develop AD. Those who have more than 1 first-degree relative with dementia are at even higher risk for developing it.[1]

 Genetic Link

Many genes have been identified that increase and decrease the risk of AD. The presence of ApoE-4 increases the risk of developing late-onset AD (Box 64.1). *ApoE* contains the instructions to make a protein that helps to carry cholesterol and other types of fat in the bloodstream.[1]

BOX 64.1 GENETICS IN CLINICAL PRACTICE

AD

Genetic Basis

Early Onset (Familial) (<60 Years Old at Onset)

- Autosomal dominant disorder
- Various mutations in the following genes:
  - Amyloid precursor protein *(APP)* gene on chromosome 21
  - Presenilin-1 *(PSEN1)* gene on chromosome 14
  - Presenilin-2 *(PSEN2)* gene on chromosome 1

Late Onset (Sporadic) (>60 Years Old at Onset)

- There are 3 forms of the apolipoprotein (ApoE) gene: e-2, e-3, and e-4.
- One form is inherited from each parent.
- Having the *ApoE-4* allele on chromosome 19 increases risk for developing AD.
- Having the *ApoE-2* allele is associated with a lower risk for AD.

Incidence

Early Onset

- Rare form of AD, accounts for <5% of cases
- 50% risk for disease for children of affected parents
- May occur in people as young as 30 years

Late Onset

- *ApoE-4* is present in 40% to 65% of people with late-onset AD.
- Many *ApoE-4*—positive people do not develop AD.

Genetic Testing

Early Onset

- Genetic screening is available for mutations on chromosomes 1, 14, and 21.

Late Onset

- Blood tests can identify the *ApoE* allele but cannot predict who will develop disease.
- In a patient who meets the clinical criteria for AD, finding *ApoE-4* increases the reliability of the diagnosis.

Clinical Implications

- Genetic testing for family members of patients with early-onset AD may be appropriate.
- Testing should be done with genetic counseling, especially when asymptomatic family members are involved.
- If a person tests positive for *ApoE-4,* it does not mean they will develop AD.

Among persons who develop AD before age 65, 3 key genes, presenilin-1 *(PSEN1)*, presenilin-2 *(PSEN2)*, and amyloid precursor protein *(APP)*, have been identified as causative factors.[1] When these genes mutate, they cause brain cells to overproduce β-amyloid. People with Down syndrome have 3 copies of chromosome 21 (trisomy 21). They are at increased risk for developing AD as they age. Chromosome 21 has the gene that encodes for APP production. Among people with AD, APP is cut into β-amyloid fragments that accumulate, forming plaques in the brain. The extra copy of chromosome 21 may increase β-amyloid fragment production.

Cardiovascular Factors

Brain health is linked to heart and blood vessel health. Brain function depends on a good blood supply and nutrients delivered to it by that blood supply.

Many factors increase CVD risk. These include diabetes, hypertension, obesity, hypercholesterolemia, and smoking. Diabetes increases the risk of AD and other types of dementia. Diabetes can contribute to dementia in several ways. Chronic high levels of insulin and glucose may be directly toxic to brain cells. Insulin resistance, which can lead to type 2 diabetes, may interfere with the body's ability to break down amyloid, a protein that forms brain plaques in AD. High glucose and cholesterol have a role in atherosclerosis, which contributes to VaD.

Diabetes may contribute to poor memory and decreased mental function in other ways. Diabetes causes microangiopathy, which damages small blood vessels throughout the body. Ongoing damage to blood vessels in the brain may be one reason people with diabetes are at a higher risk for cognitive problems as they age. People with diabetes may lose brain volume, especially gray matter, as diabetes progresses. Factors that decrease CVD risk can decrease the risk of dementia. These include being physically active, following a heart-healthy diet, and managing cholesterol levels.[9]

Head Trauma

Head trauma is a risk factor for dementia. People with a history of moderate to severe traumatic brain injury (TBI) have a 2- to 4-fold increased risk of developing dementia. Professional football players and military veterans who had a TBI have an increased risk for AD and other types of dementia.[1]

Pathophysiology

Changes in the brain's structure and function with AD include (1) amyloid plaques, (2) neurofibrillary tangles, (3) loss of connections between neurons, and (4) neuron death. Fig. 64.2 shows the pathologic changes in AD.

As a part of aging, people develop some plaques in their brain tissue. In AD, more plaques appear in certain parts of the brain affecting memory. Other plaques develop in areas of the brain used for memory and cognitive function, including the hippocampus. The hippocampus is important in forming and storing short-term memories. Eventually, AD attacks the cerebral cortex, especially the areas responsible for language and reasoning.

Plaques are clusters of insoluble deposits of a protein called β-amyloid, other proteins, remnants of neurons, nonnerve cells such as microglia (cells that surround and digest damaged cells or foreign substances), and other cells, such as astrocytes. β-Amyloid is cleaved from APP, which is associated with the cell membrane (Fig. 64.3). Genetic factors may play a critical role in how the brain processes the β-amyloid protein. Overproduction of β-amyloid is an important risk factor for AD. Abnormally high levels of β-amyloid cause cell damage either directly or by eliciting an inflammatory response and ultimately neuron death.

Neurofibrillary tangles are abnormal collections of twisted protein threads inside nerve cells. The main component of these structures is a protein called *tau*. Tau proteins in the central nervous system (CNS) provide support for intracellular structure through their support of microtubules. Tau proteins hold the microtubules together like railroad ties. In AD, tau protein is altered. As a result, the microtubules twist together in a helical fashion (Fig. 64.3). This forms the neurofibrillary tangles found in the neurons of people with AD.

Plaques and neurofibrillary tangles are not unique to patients with AD or dementia. They are found in the brains of people without cognitive impairment. However, they are more abundant in the brains of those with AD.

The other feature of AD is the loss of connections between neurons and neuron death. These processes result in structural damage. Affected parts of the brain begin to shrink in a process called *brain atrophy*. By the final stage of AD, brain tissue has shrunk significantly (Fig. 64.4).

Clinical Manifestations and Diagnostic Criteria

AD is considered on a spectrum. The main stages are preclinical AD, mild cognitive impairment, and dementia due to AD: mild, moderate, and severe (Table 64.4). Dementia is the last stage. Symptoms do not always directly relate to abnormal changes in the brain caused by AD. The rate of progression from mild to severe is highly variable and may be affected by factors including age and genetics.[1]

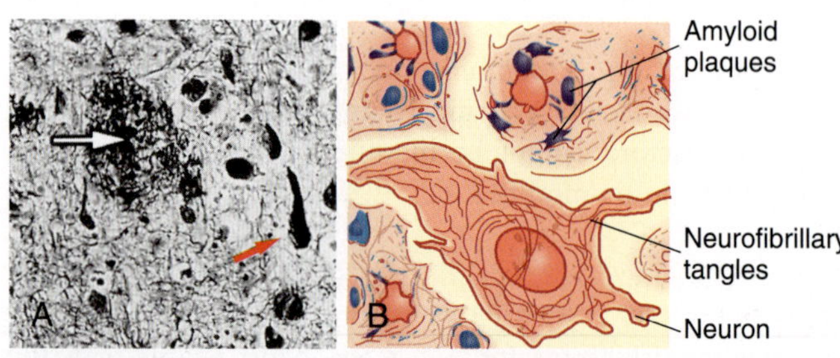

Fig. 64.2 Pathologic changes in AD. (A) Plaque with central amyloid core *(white arrow)* next to a neurofibrillary tangle *(red arrow)* on the histologic specimen from a brain autopsy. (B) Schematic representation of amyloid plaque and neurofibrillary tangle.

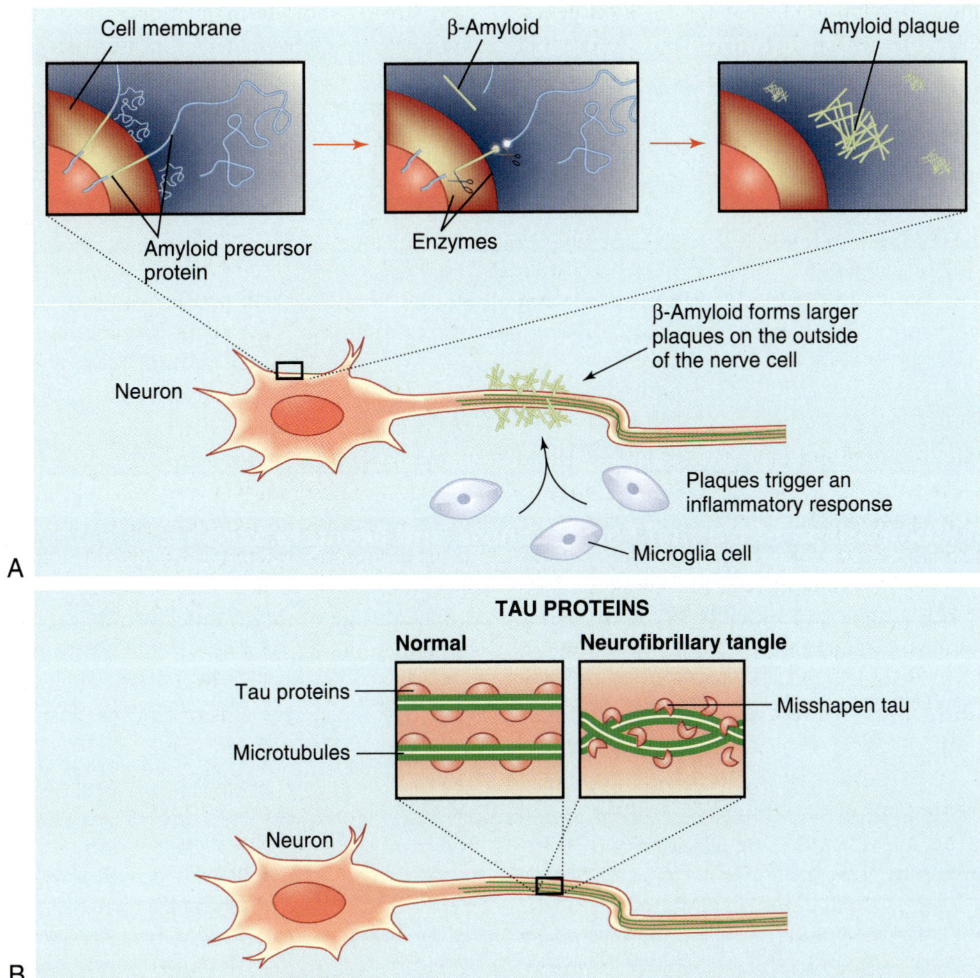

Fig. 64.3 Current theories about the development of AD. (A) Abnormal amounts of β-amyloid are cleaved from the amyloid precursor protein (APP) and released into the circulation. The β-amyloid fragments come together in clumps to form plaques that attach to the neuron. Microglia react to the plaque. This results in an inflammatory response. (B) Tau proteins provide structural support for the neuron microtubules. Chemical changes in the neuron cause structural changes in tau proteins. This results in twisting and tangling (neurofibrillary tangles).

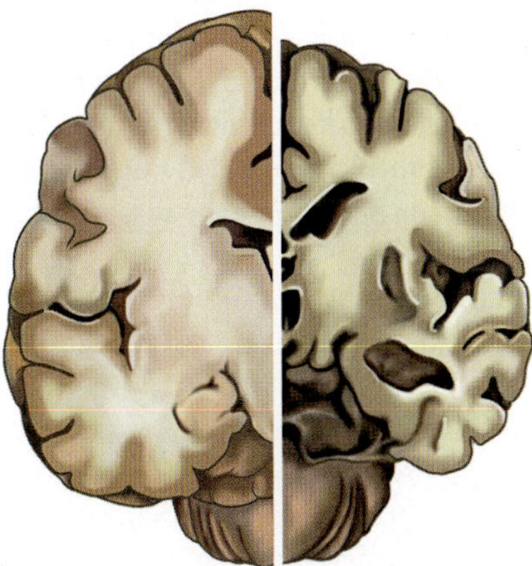

Fig. 64.4 Effects of AD on the brain. This figure compares a normal brain *(left)* with a brain affected by AD *(right)*.

Preclinical Stage

Research suggests AD causes pathologic changes in the brain at least 20 years before manifestations appear.[1] A long lag exists between pathologic changes in the brain and manifestations of AD. The future goal would be to modify the disease process before it becomes symptomatic. Once plaques and tangles have formed in sufficient quantity, it may be too late to intervene to prevent the disease or its progression.

Mild Cognitive Impairment

Mild cognitive impairment (MCI) is the second stage in the AD spectrum. The person with MCI may have problems with memory, language, and thinking.[10] The memory and language problems are severe enough to be noticed by the person having them. People who are close to the person may see changes in abilities and behaviors (Table 64.5). If the person is working, job performance declines.

We classify MCI based on the cognitive skills affected. MCI that primarily affects memory is called *amnestic MCI.* With amnestic MCI, a person may forget important information that they would have recalled easily, such as appointments. MCI that

TABLE 64.4 Stages of Dementia Due to AD

Mild	Moderate	Severe
• Forgetfulness beyond what is seen in a normal person • Short-term memory impairment, especially for new learning • Loss of initiative and interests • May forget recent events or the names of people or things • Impatient • May no longer be able to solve simple math problems • Slowly loses the ability to plan and organize	• Memory loss and confusion become more obvious • Has more trouble organizing, planning, and following directions • May need help getting dressed • May start having incontinence • Trouble recognizing family members and friends • Agitation, restlessness • May lack judgment and begin to wander, gets lost • Sleep problems • Delusions, hallucinations, paranoia • Behavior problems	• Severe impairment of all cognitive functions • Little memory, unable to process new information • Unable to perform self-care activities • Often needs help with daily needs • May not be able to talk • Cannot understand words • May have problems eating, swallowing • May not be able to walk or sit up without help • Immobility • Incontinence

TABLE 64.5 Comparison of Normal Forgetfulness and Memory Loss

Normal Forgetfulness	Memory Loss in Mild Cognitive Impairment	Memory Loss in AD
• Sometimes misplaces keys, eyeglasses, or other items	• Often misplaces items	• Forgets what an item is used for or puts it in an inappropriate place
• Momentarily forgets an acquaintance's name	• Often forgets people's names and is slow to recall them	• May not remember knowing a person
• Sometimes searches for a word	• Has increasing difficulty finding desired words	• Begins to lose language skills and may withdraw from social interaction
• Sometimes forgets to run an errand	• Begins to forget important events and appointments	• Loses sense of time, does not know what day it is
• May forget an event from the distant past	• May forget recent events or newly learned information	• Seriously impaired recent memory. Problems learning and remembering new information.
• When driving, may momentarily forget where to turn, but quickly orients self	• Becomes temporarily lost more often. Trouble understanding and following a map	• Becomes easily disoriented or lost in familiar places, sometimes for hours
• Jokes about memory loss	• Worries about memory loss. Family and friends notice lapses	• May have little or no awareness of cognitive problems

Adapted from Rabins P: Memory. In *The Johns Hopkins white papers,* Baltimore, 2007, Johns Hopkins University.

affects other cognitive skills is *nonamnestic MCI.* Skills that may be affected include the ability to make sound decisions or complete a complex task. Some people with MCI show no progression and do not go on to develop AD. Assessing for changes in memory and thinking skills that indicate a worsening of symptoms or a progression to AD or another dementia is critical.

Dementia Due to AD

With mild dementia, symptoms of memory loss are obvious. Most people can function independently in most activities. Although they may not have difficulty driving, working, or taking part in favorite activities, they may have difficulty with complex activities such as managing finances. They may not be able to act in a socially appropriate manner or remember major events like holidays or birthdays.[1]

In the moderate stage, the person can no longer manage on their own and needs assistance with maintaining adequate nutrition and housing. Memory and language are increasingly impaired. They may no longer recognize people who were well known to them. Bathing and dressing are difficult. They may have incontinence. Behavior changes such as suspicion and agitation may occur.

In the severe stage, continued damage to the brain results in decreased communication, swallowing issues, and mobility issues. The person is wheelchair or bed bound. Round-the-clock care may be required. Because of the loss of function, patients in this stage are at risk for skin breakdown, skin infections, and aspiration pneumonia.

Retrogenesis

Retrogenesis is the process in which the decline in AD mirrors, in reverse order, brain development that occurs from birth.[11] Thus, it compares the development stages of childhood with the deterioration of patients with AD. As seen in Fig. 64.5, a relationship exists between development stage and deterioration of function. For example, a patient in the moderate stage may enjoy putting together puzzles that belong to his 3-year-old grandson. In fact, they may play well together on the same task or project.

Stage	Alzheimer Disease	Reisberg Stage*	Developmental Age	Diversion/Distraction Activities
Mild	No difficulty at all.	1		
	Some memory trouble begins to affect job/home. Forgets familiar names.	2		
	Much difficulty maintaining job performance. Withdrawal from difficult situations.	3	12+ yr	Can function with understanding. Enjoy things previously enjoyed—watch TV, play and listen to music, play games.
	Can no longer hold a job, plan and prepare meals, handle personal finances, etc. Driving becomes difficult, although can drive to familiar places.	4	8–12 yr	Can still enjoy simple games, watch TV and videos. Enjoys family photos and memories.
Moderate	Can no longer select proper clothing for occasion or season. Needs help to remain safe in home. Forgets to bathe.	5	5–7 yr	Needs age-appropriate toys and games.
	Requires assistance with dressing.	6a	4–5 yr	Enjoy many of the same activities as preschoolers.
	Requires assistance with bathing.	6b	4–5 yr	
	Can no longer use toilet without assistance.	6c	4 yr	
	Urinary incontinence.	6d	3–4.5 yr	
	Fecal incontinence.	6e	2–3 yr	
Severe	Speech now limited to about 6 words per day.	7a	15 mo	Enjoys infant toys, mobiles, dangling ribbons.
	Speech now limited to 1 word per day.	7b	1 yr	
	Can no longer walk without assistance.	7c	1 yr	
	Can no longer sit up without assistance.	7d	6–10 mo	
	Can no longer smile.	7e	2–4 mo	
	Can no longer hold up head.	7f	1–3 mo	

Fig. 64.5 Retrogenesis (back to birth) in AD. *Based on Functional Assessment Staging. (From Reisberg B: Functional Assessment Staging [FAST], *Psychopharmacol Bull* 24:653, 1988.)

Diagnostic Studies

No single test can determine if a person has AD. We use a combination of the health history, neurologic exams, cognitive and functional assessments, brain imaging, and CSF and blood tests to make a diagnosis (Tables 64.6 and 64.7).[12] Neuropsychologic testing is important for diagnosis and to establish a baseline for monitoring changes. These tests are repeated at regular intervals to assess changes in cognitive status. Brief screening tools, such as the Mini-Cog (Table 64.8), are useful for routine screening, especially when time is limited. The clock drawing test can be used as part of the Mini-Cog or by itself to assess cognitive function (Fig. 64.6). More detailed screening tests, such as the Mini-Mental State Examination (MMSE) (Table 64.9) and Montreal Cognitive Assessment (MoCA), can detect MCI.

The 2 main CSF biomarkers for diagnosing AD are β-amyloid and tau proteins. Elevated tau and or reduced β-amyloid suggest the presence of AD pathology.[12] Brain imaging, preferably MRI, helps detect structural changes and may help monitor treatment.[12] In AD, atrophy occurs in several brain regions, and decreased brain volume correlates with neurodegeneration. PET scanning can help discern AD from other forms of dementia (Fig. 64.7). PET assesses brain metabolism using glucose tracers and can detect amyloid.

Interprofessional Care

There is no cure for AD. Treatment does not stop the deterioration of brain cells. Care is aimed at controlling undesirable behavior manifestations and providing support for family caregivers (Table 64.7).

TABLE 64.6 Diagnostic Criteria

AD

Stage	Description	Recommendations for Biomarkers
Preclinical AD	• Brain changes, including amyloid buildup and other early neuron changes, may already be in process • Significant symptoms are not evident • In some people, PET scans and CSF analysis can detect amyloid buildup	• Use of imaging and biomarker tests at this stage is only for research • Biomarkers are still being developed, not used by clinicians in general practice
Mild cognitive impairment (MCI) due to AD	• Symptoms of memory problems, enough to be noticed and measured, but not compromising a patient's independence • May or may not progress to AD	• Used mainly by researchers • May be used in clinical settings to supplement standard tests to help determine possible causes of MCI • May help confirm that impairment is related to AD
Dementia due to AD	• Memory, thinking, and behavior symptoms that impair ability to function in daily life • Dementia marks the terminal stage of AD • Encompasses all stages shown in Table 64.4	• Can increase level of certainty about a diagnosis of AD • May be used to discern AD from other dementias

CSF, Cerebrospinal fluid; *PET,* positron emission scanning.

From National Institute on Aging: *Diagnostic criteria for Alzheimer's disease.* Retrieved from https://www.nia.nih.gov/health/alzheimers-disease-diagnostic-guidelines.

TABLE 64.7 Interprofessional Care

AD

Diagnostic Assessment

- History and physical assessment
  - Psychologic evaluation, including depression screening
  - Neuropsychologic testing, including Mini-Cog (Table 64.8) and Mini-Mental State Examination (Table 64.9)
- Brain imaging tests: MRI, PET
- CSF fluid analysis: β-amyloid and tau proteins
- CBC
- ECG
- Glucose, creatinine, BUN
- Vitamin B_1, B_6, B_{12} levels
- Thyroid function tests
- Liver function tests

Management

- Drug therapy for cognitive problems (Table 64.10)
- Behavior modification
- Moderate exercise
- Assistance with functional independence
- Assistance and support for caregivers

Drug Therapy

AD medications do not cure or reverse the progression of the disease (Table 64.10). They help many people for a time by leading to a modest decrease in the rate of decline of cognitive function.[13]

Cholinesterase inhibitors block the normal breakdown of acetylcholine (ACh) into acetate and choline. This increases the level and duration of action of acetylcholine (Fig. 64.8). These drugs include donepezil (Aricept), rivastigmine (Exelon), and galantamine (Razadyne).[13]

Memantine blocks the N-methyl-D-aspartate (NMDA) subtype of glutamate receptors, which prevents overactivation

TABLE 64.8 The Mini-Cog

The Mini-Cog is used as a brief assessment tool for cognitive impairment. It can be quickly administered and can guide the need for further evaluation.

Administration

- Tell the patient to listen carefully to and remember 3 unrelated words and then to repeat the words. *Example:* apple, table, penny. (This initial step is not scored.) The same 3 words may be repeated to the patient up to 3 times to register all 3 words.
- Tell the patient to draw the face of a clock, either on a blank sheet of paper or on a sheet with the clock circle already drawn on the page. After the patient puts the numbers on the clock face, ask them to draw the hands of the clock to read a specific time (11:10). The test is considered normal if all numbers are present in the correct sequence and position and the hands readably display the requested time.
- Ask the patient to repeat the 3 previously stated words.

Scoring (Out of 5 Total Points)

- Give 1 point for each recalled word after the clock drawing test.
  - Patients recalling none of the 3 words are classified as cognitively impaired (score = 0).
  - Patients recalling all 3 words are classified as not cognitively impaired (score = 3).
  - Patients with intermediate word recall of 1 or 2 words are classified on the clock drawing test.
- The clock drawing test is scored 2 if normal and 0 if abnormal.

Interpretation of Results

0–2: Positive screen for dementia
3–5: Negative screen for dementia

From Borson S, Scanlan J, Brush M, et al: The Mini-Cog: a cognitive "vital signs" measure for dementia screening in multi-lingual elderly, *Intern J Geriatr Psychiatry* 15:1021, 2000.

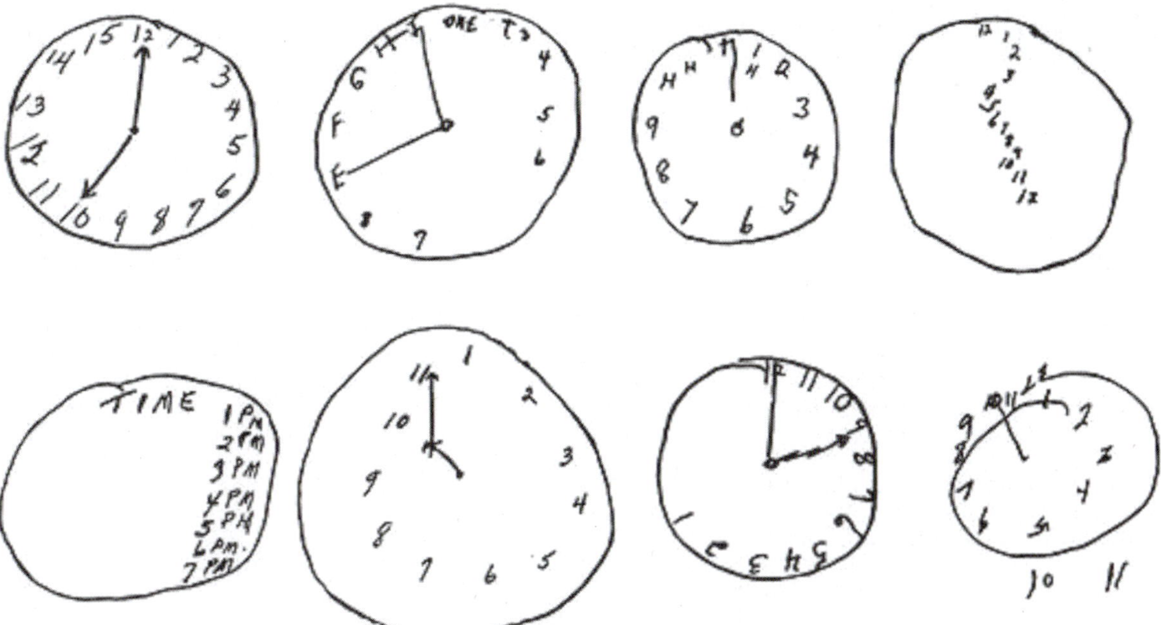

Fig. 64.6 Clock drawing is a simple test that can be used to assess for dementia. The patient is asked to draw a clock, put in all the numbers, and set the hands at 11:10. Clocks drawn by people with AD. (From Mendez M: *Mental status examination handbook,* St. Louis, 2022, Elsevier.)

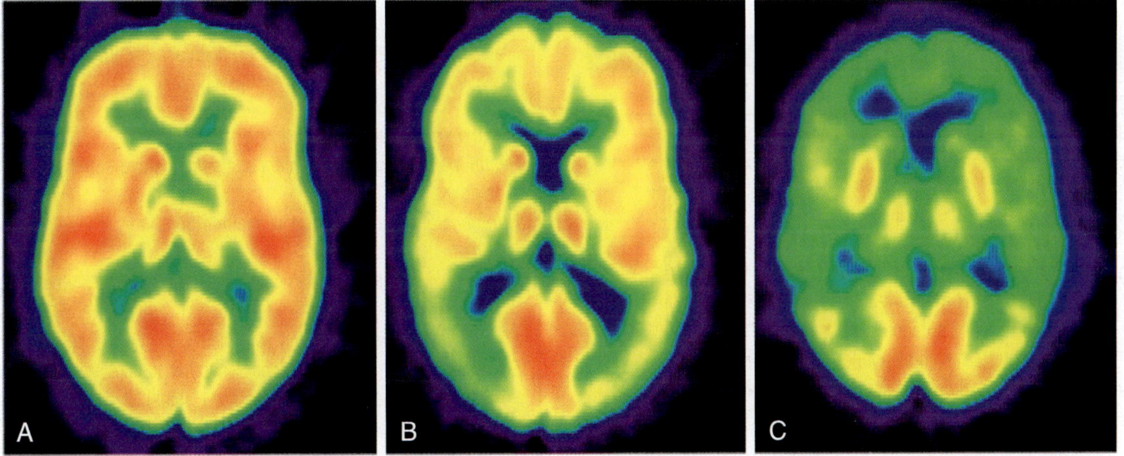

Fig. 64.7 PET scans assist in diagnosing AD. Radioactive fluorine is applied to glucose (fluorodeoxyglucose), and the *yellow areas* show metabolically active cells. (A) A normal brain. (B) Early AD. (C) Advanced AD, with hypometabolism in many areas of the brain. (From Rice L, Bisdas S: The diagnostic value of FDG and amyloid PET in Alzheimer's disease, *Eur J Radiol* 94:16, 2017.)

of glutamate and facilitates normal activity. The medication counteracts excess glutaminergic activity in the CNS, which contributes to the neurotoxicity in AD.[14]

Treating depression with selective serotonin reuptake inhibitors may improve cognitive function. These include fluoxetine, sertraline, and citalopram. The antidepressant trazodone may help with sleep problems.

Antipsychotic drugs can be used to manage agitation and aggressive behavior, which occurs in some patients. These drugs can increase the risk for death and cognitive decline. They should be used only when symptoms of agitation and psychosis are severe, dangerous, and/or cause significant distress.

NURSING MANAGEMENT: ALZHEIMER DISEASE

Assessment

Subjective and objective data that you should obtain from patients with AD are outlined in Table 64.11. Gather information about changes in cognition, activities of daily living, mood, neuropsychiatric symptoms, and sensory and motor function. Useful questions are, "When did you first notice the memory loss?" and "How has the memory loss progressed since then?"[1]

TABLE 64.9 Mini-Mental State Examination (MMSE)

Sample Items

Orientation to Time
"What is the date?"

Registration
"Listen carefully. I am going to say 3 words. You say them back after I stop. Ready? Here they are HOUSE (pause), CAR (pause), LAKE (pause). Now repeat those words back to me." (Repeat up to 5 times but score only the first trial.)

Naming
"What is this?" (Point to a pencil or pen.)

Reading
"Please read this and do what it says." (Show examinee the words CLOSE YOUR EYES on the stimulus form.)

TABLE 64.10 Drug Therapy

AD

Problem	Drugs
Decreased memory and cognition	Cholinesterase inhibitors • donepezil (Aricept) • galantamine (Razadyne) • rivastigmine (Exelon) N-methyl-d-aspartate (NMDA) receptor antagonist • memantine (Namenda)
Depression	Selective serotonin reuptake inhibitors (SSRIs) • citalopram (Celexa) • fluoxetine (Prozac) • sertraline (Zoloft) • fluvoxamine (Luvox) Atypical antidepressants • mirtazapine (Remeron) • trazodone
Behavior problems (e.g., agitation, physical aggression, disinhibition)	Antipsychotics • aripiprazole (Abilify) • haloperidol (Haldol) • olanzapine (Zyprexa) • quetiapine (Seroquel) • risperidone (Risperdal) Benzodiazepines • clonazepam (Klonopin) • lorazepam (Ativan)
Sleep problems	Sedative-hypnotics • zolpidem (Ambien)

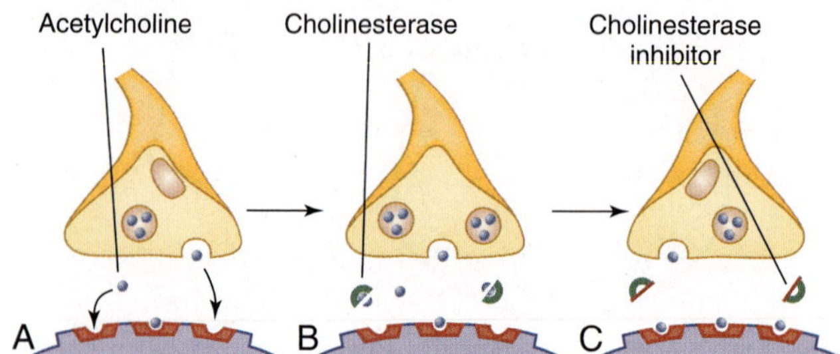

Fig. 64.8 Mechanism of action of cholinesterase inhibitors. (A) Acetylcholine is released from the nerve synapses and carries a message across the synapse. (B) Cholinesterase breaks down acetylcholine. (C) Cholinesterase inhibitors block cholinesterase, thus giving acetylcholine more time to transmit the message.

TABLE 64.11 NURSING ASSESSMENT

AD

Subjective Data

Important Health Information

Health history: Repeated head trauma, stroke, CNS infection, family history of dementia.

Medications: Use of any drug to decrease symptoms (e.g., tranquilizers, hypnotics, antidepressants, antipsychotics).

Functional Health Patterns

Health perception–health management: Positive family history. Emotional lability.

Nutritional-metabolic: Anorexia, malnutrition, weight loss.

Elimination: Incontinence.

Activity-exercise: Poor personal hygiene, gait instability, weakness, inability to perform ADLs.

Sleep-rest: Frequent nighttime awakening, daytime napping.

Cognitive-perceptual: Forgetfulness, inability to cope with complex situations, difficulty with problem solving (early signs), depression, withdrawal, suicidal ideation (early).

Objective Data

General

Disheveled appearance, agitation.

Neurologic

Mild: Loss of recent memory, disorientation to date and time, flat affect, lack of spontaneity. Impaired abstraction, cognition, and judgment.

Moderate: Agitation, impaired ability to recognize close family and friends, loss of remote memory, confusion, apraxia, agnosia, alexia (inability to understand written language); aphasia, inability to do simple tasks.

Severe: Inability to do self-care, incontinence, immobility, limb rigidity, flexor posturing.

Possible Diagnostic Findings

Diagnosis by exclusion, cerebral cortical atrophy on CT scan, poor scores on mental status tests, hippocampal atrophy on MRI scan, abnormal changes on PET.

Clinical Problems

Clinical problems for patients with AD may include:

- Impaired cognition
- Risk for injury
- Impaired role performance

Additional information on clinical problems and interventions for patients with AD is presented in eNursing Care Plan 64.1 (available on the website for this chapter).

Planning

The overall goals for patients with AD are to (1) maintain functional ability for as long as possible, (2) be in a safe environment, (3) have personal care needs met, and (4) have dignity maintained. The overall goals for caregivers of patients with AD are to (1) reduce caregiver stress; (2) maintain personal, emotional, and physical health; and (3) cope with the long-term effects of caregiving.

Implementation

Health Promotion

Can AD be prevented? Although there is no known definitive way to prevent AD, there are several things that we can do to keep our brain healthy and lower the risk of developing dementia (Table 64.12). Early recognition and treatment of AD are important. Review early signs of AD with patients and families (Table 64.13).[10] In the early stages, patients are often aware that their memory is faulty and do things to mask the problem.

Chronic Care

Nursing management of patients with AD is outlined in Table 64.14. The diagnosis is traumatic for patients and families. It is not unusual for patients to have depression, denial, worry, fear, and feelings of loss and dread. Family members may be in denial and not seek medical attention early in AD. Assess their ability to accept and cope with the diagnosis.

Ongoing monitoring of patients and caregivers is important. Patients need to be aware that the progression of AD is variable. The health care team works with caregivers and patients to manage symptoms, which change over time. The care patients need changes as AD progresses, which emphasizes the need for regular assessment and support. The severity of the problems and amount of care needed increase over time. The specific manifestations depend on the area of the brain involved. Nursing care focuses on decreasing manifestations, preventing harm, and supporting patients and family. Effective management may slow symptom progression and decrease the burden on patients and families (Box 64.2).

Decisions related to care should be made with the patient, family members, and health care team early. You have a role in advising patients and caregivers to initiate health care decisions, including advance directives, while the patient has the capacity to do so. This can ease the burden for the caregiver as AD progresses.

TABLE 64.12 PROMOTING POPULATION HEALTH

Decreasing Risk for Cognitive Decline

The following are tips to reduce the risk for cognitive decline and dementia:

1. Avoid harmful substances.
   Excess drinking and drug use can damage brain cells. Stop smoking because it increases the risk for cognitive decline.
2. Challenge your mind.
   Read often, do crossword puzzles. Play games. Keep mentally active. Learn new skills. Go back to school. This strengthens the brain connections and promotes new ones.
3. Exercise regularly.
   Even low- to moderate-level activity, such as walking or gardening 3 to 5 times per week, can make you feel better. Daily physical activity, even in older adults, can decrease the risk for cognitive decline.
4. Stay socially active.
   Pursue social activities that have meaning to you. Family, friends, church, and a sense of community may all contribute to better brain health.
5. Avoid trauma to the brain.
   Because traumatic brain injury may be a risk factor for developing AD, promote safety in physical activities and driving. Use the car seat belt. Wear a helmet when playing contact sports or riding a bike. Fall-proof your home.
6. Take care of your mental health.
   Recognize and treat depression early. Depression may cause or worsen memory loss and other cognitive problems.
7. Treat diabetes.
   Better glucose control can help prevent the cognitive decline from diabetes.
8. Take care of your heart.
   Risk factors for cardiovascular disease and stroke (hypertension, obesity) negatively affect your cognitive health. Heart health is linked to brain health.
9. Get enough sleep.
   Not getting enough sleep may result in problems with memory and thinking.
10. Get the right fuel.
   A healthy and balanced diet low in fats and sugary foods and high in vegetables and fruits helps to reduce the risk for cognitive decline.

Adapted from Alzheimer's Association: *10 ways to love your brain.* Retrieved from https://www.alz.org/help-support/brain_health/10_ways_to_love_your_brain.

Patients with AD may have other acute and chronic illnesses that require hospitalization or surgery. Hospitalization can be traumatic for patients with AD. It can precipitate a worsening of dementia or the development of delirium.

SAFETY ALERT

Patients With AD in Acute Care

- Observe patients with AD more closely because of safety concerns.
- Provide frequent reassurance and orient to place and time.
- Reduce anxiety or disruptive behavior by using consistent nursing staff.
- When a patient resists or pulls tubes or dressings, cover these items with stretch tube gauze or remove them from the visual field.

TABLE 64.13 PATIENT & CAREGIVER TEACHING

Early Warning Signs of AD

1. Memory loss that affects job skills
   - Frequent forgetfulness or unexplainable confusion at home or in the workplace may signal that something is wrong.
   - This type of memory loss goes beyond forgetting an assignment, colleague's name, deadline, or phone number.
2. Problems with abstract thinking
   - For the patient with AD, this goes beyond challenges, such as balancing a checkbook.
   - The patient with AD may not be able to recognize numbers or do basic calculations.
3. Difficulty doing familiar tasks
   - It is normal for most people to become distracted and to forget something (e.g., leave something on the stove too long).
   - People with AD may cook a meal, then forget not only to serve it but also that they made it.
4. Poor or decreased judgment
   - Many people from time to time may choose not to dress appropriately for the weather (e.g., not bringing a coat or sweater on a cold evening).
   - The patient with AD may dress inappropriately in more noticeable ways, such as wearing a bathrobe to the store or a sweater on a hot day.
5. Problems with language
   - Most people have trouble finding the "right" word from time to time.
   - People with AD may forget simple words or substitute incorrect words, making their speech hard to understand.
6. Misplacing things
   - For many people, temporarily misplacing keys, purses, or wallets is a normal, albeit frustrating, event.
   - The patient with AD may put items in inappropriate places (e.g., eating utensils in clothing drawers) but have no memory of how they got there.
7. Changes in mood
   - Most people have mood changes.
   - Patients with AD tend to have more rapid mood swings for no apparent reason.
8. Changes in personality
   - As most people age, they may have some change in personality (e.g., become less tolerant).
   - Patients with AD can change dramatically, either suddenly or over time (e.,g., someone who is easygoing may become angry, suspicious, or fearful).
9. Loss of initiative
   - Patients with AD may become and remain uninterested and uninvolved in many or all of their usual pursuits.

Adapted from Alzheimer's Association: *10 early signs and symptoms of Alzheimer's*. Retrieved from https://www.alz.org/alzheimers_disease_know_the_10_signs.asp.

Currently, family members and friends care for many people with AD in their homes. Adult day care is an available option. They can provide respite for the family and a protective environment. Programs vary in size, structure, physical environment, and staff experience. Other patients with AD live in various types of facilities, including long-term care and assisted living. A facility that is good for one patient may not be good for another. What is helpful for a patient at one point in the disease process may be completely different from what is best when AD progresses.

TABLE 64.14 NURSING MANAGEMENT

Caring for Patients With AD

Assess patients on an ongoing basis, including:
- Memory and level of function
- Presence of any coexisting problems
- Ability to perform ADLs
- Diet and fluid intake and develop a plan to ensure adequate intake
- Ability to meet self-care needs related to elimination and hygiene
- Safety concerns

Determine possible precipitating factors for behavior changes and develop strategies to address difficult behavior.

Assess family caregivers' stress level and coping strategies.

Implement a plan to meet areas of identified need for elimination, nutrition, hydration, and hygiene.

Provide for patient needs:
- Communicate with patients in a therapeutic manner (Table 64.15).
- Use memory aids and reorient to time, place, and person often.
- Use distraction to manage agitated behavior.
- Provide measures to manage pain, fever, nausea, and other symptoms.
- Maintain a consistent daily routine.
- Encourage continued mobility if appropriate.
- Present changes in the patient's routine gradually, if possible.
- If patients use eyeglasses or a hearing aid, have them available.

Provide a safe, optimal environment:
- Implement measures to decrease fall risk and address wandering.
- Reduce noise and provide adequate nonglare lighting.
- Provide a soothing atmosphere.
- Assign consistent nursing staff.

Implement measures to promote sleep (see Chapter 8).

Provide caregiver support:
- Make referrals for community services, such as adult day care and respite care.
- In long-term care, encourage visitation by significant others and include them in planning, providing, and evaluating care to the extent desired.
- Teach patients and caregivers about measures to manage AD (Table 64.16).

Delegate to LPN/VN:
- Monitor for behavior changes that may indicate physiologic problems.
- Check the environment for safety hazards.
- Give ordered enteral feedings.
- Give ordered medications.

Supervise AP:
- Help patients to use the toilet, commode, or bedpan at frequent intervals.
- Provide personal hygiene, skin care, and oral care.
- Help patients with eating.
- Aid patients with daily activities.
- Use bed alarms and surveillance to decrease risk for falls.

Collaborate With Other Team Members

Dietitian
- Assess nutrition status and provide prescribed nutrition support.
- Offer practical suggestions to enhance diet intake.

Occupational Therapist
- Suggest ways to help patients retain self-care ability as long as possible.

Social Worker
- Help caregivers identify and obtain needed resources.
- Provide support and counseling to caregivers.

BOX 64.2 EVIDENCE-BASED PRACTICE

Activities in Patients With AD

You care for patients in a locked memory care unit in a long-term care facility. Despite scheduled interactive activities, including storytelling, art, and yoga provided by the memory care team, you note that patients are experiencing cognitive decline within 6 weeks of admission.

Making Clinical Decisions

Synthesis of Best Available Evidence

Evidence supports that engaging patients with moderate AD in fine movement, life, sensory, language, and math activities may slow the progression of cognitive decline. Although these activities do not cure AD, they can contribute to an improved quality of life and reduce caregiver stress.

Clinician Expertise

Patients with AD can benefit from stimulating activities that encourage independence and decision making in a protective environment. You question whether offering a wider variety of scheduled activities could increase cognition, thereby improving independence and quality of life.

Patient Preferences and Values

Following consultation with the memory care team and family members, new activities including sorting buttons, making themed collages, completing simple jigsaw puzzles, and participating in sing-along exercises were incorporated into each patient's routine for 15-minute intervals. After 3 months, you note that patients are more engaged with family members and have less agitation.

Implications for Nursing Practice

1. What other activities could be successful in slowing cognitive decline in the patient with AD?
2. What other behavior or cognitive observations would indicate a positive outcome?

Reference for Evidence

Wang W, Said F: Research on the application of Montessori education method in cognitive training of patients with Alzheimer's disease, *J Clin Nurs Res* 8:5, 2024.

TABLE 64.15 NURSING MANAGEMENT

Promoting Communication With Patients With AD

Do

- Treat patients with respect and dignity, even when behavior is childlike.
- Use gentle touch and direct eye contact.
- Remain flexible, calm, and understanding.
- Expect challenging behaviors because AD affects the ability to think logically.
- Give directions using gestures or pictures.
- Simplify tasks. Focus on one thing at a time.
- Avoid questions/topics that require extensive thought, memory, or words.
- Be flexible. If one approach does not work, try another.
- Use distraction, changing the subject, redirecting to another activity.
- Provide reassurance. Praise sincerely for success.

Do Not

- Criticize, correct, or argue.
- Rush or hurry patients.
- Force participation in activities or events.
- Talk about patients as if they are not there.
- Take challenging behaviors personally. These behaviors are caused by the disease.
- Use condescending terms, such as "honey" or "sweetie."
- Use threatening gestures.
- Overreact.
- Try to explain "why" or rationalize.

In the early stages of AD, memory aids, such as calendars, may be helpful. Patients often become depressed during this phase. Depression may be related to the diagnosis of an incurable disorder and the impact on activities of daily living (ADLs), including driving, socializing, and taking part in recreation activities. Antidepressant drugs and counseling may be needed. Teach caregivers to perform tasks needed to maximize quality of life and patient safety.

During the early and moderate stages of AD, patients can still benefit from stimulating activities that encourage independence and decision making in a protective environment. Patients return home tired, content, less frustrated, and ready to be with the family. The respite from the demands of care allows the caregiver to be more responsive to the patient's needs.

As AD progresses, the demands on the caregiver eventually exceed the resources. The patient may need to be placed in a long-term care facility. Special dementia or memory care units are common. The dementia unit is designed with an emphasis on safety. Many have designated areas that allow patients to walk freely in the unit. The unit is secured so patients cannot wander outside.

At the late stage, the patient is severely impaired. They have difficulty with basic functions, including walking and talking. Total care is needed. Specific problems relate to the care of patients in all phases of AD. These problems are described next.

Behavior problems. Behavior problems occur in about 90% of patients with AD. These problems include asking the same question repeatedly, delusions, hallucinations, agitation, aggression, sleep problems, wandering, hoarding, and resisting care. Many times, these behaviors are unpredictable and may challenge caregivers. Caregivers must be aware that these behaviors are not intentional and are often difficult to control. Behavior problems are often the reason that patients are placed in a facility.[15]

These behaviors are often the patient's way of responding to pain, frustration, temperature extremes, or anxiety. When these behaviors become problematic, you must plan interventions carefully. Assess physical status. Check for changes in vital signs, urinary and bowel patterns, and pain that could account for behavior problems. Are factors in the environment triggering the behavior? Extremes in temperature or excess noise may lead to behavior changes. When environment conditions are agitating the patient, move the patient or remove the stimulus.

Nursing strategies that address difficult behavior include redirection, distraction, and reassurance. Table 64.15 lists tips for promoting communication. When a patient is restless or agitated, use redirection. Change the patient's focus by having them perform activities, such as sweeping, raking, or dusting. Providing snacks, taking a car ride, sitting on a porch swing or rocker, listening to favorite music, watching videotapes, looking at family photographs, or walking may distract agitated patients. Reassure patients that you are present to keep them safe. Repetitive activities, including songs, poems, music, massage, aromas, or a favorite object can be soothing. Animal-assisted therapy helps some persons.

Do not threaten to restrain an agitated patient. Ask a calming family member to stay with them. Monitor the patient frequently. As verbal skills decline, you and the caregiver must rely more on the patient's body language to communicate care needs. Positive nursing actions can reduce the use of chemical (drug therapy) restraints.

Antipsychotic drugs may be used to treat disruptive behaviors (Table 64.10). However, they have adverse effects. We should exhaust all other ways of treating behavior issues before starting drug treatment.

CHECK YOUR PRACTICE

You are working in a secure Alzheimer's unit. While making rounds at 1600, you see Dan, one of the APs, screaming at an 84-year-old male resident. When you approach Dan and the resident, you ask what is going on. Dan responds, "Every day about this time he gets so agitated and starts yelling at me, so I yell back."

- How would you manage the situation? What teaching does Dan need?

A specific type of agitation, **sundowning,** is when patients become more confused and agitated in the late afternoon or evening. Behaviors related to sundowning include agitation, aggressiveness, wandering, resistance to redirection, and increased verbal activity, such as yelling. The cause of sundowning is unclear. It may be caused by a disruption of circadian rhythms. Other causes include pain, hunger, unfamiliar environment and noise, medications, reduced lighting, and fragmented sleep.[16]

Managing sundowning can be challenging for you, the patient, and the family. When patients have sundowning, remain calm and avoid confrontation. Assess for possible causes. Interventions to use include (1) create a quiet, calm environment; (2) maximize exposure to daylight by opening blinds and turning on lights during the day; (3) evaluate medications to determine whether any cause sleep problems; (4) limit naps and caffeine; and (5) consult with the HCP about drug therapy.

Safety. Patients are at risk for problems related to personal safety. Hazards include falling, ingesting dangerous substances, wandering, injuring others and self with sharp objects, being burned, and being unable to respond to crisis situations. These concerns require careful attention in the home environment to minimize risk. Supervision is needed. As cognitive function declines over time, they may have problems navigating physical spaces and interpreting environment cues. Help the caregiver assess the home environment for safety risks.

Wandering is a major concern.[17] It may be related to loss of memory or to medication side effects. Wandering also may be an expression of a physical or emotional need, restlessness, curiosity, or stimuli that trigger memories of earlier routines. As with other behaviors, observe for factors or events that may precipitate wandering. For example, patients can be sensitive to stress and tension in the environment. In such cases, wandering may reflect an attempt to leave.

Pain management. Because of difficulties with oral and written language, patients may have a hard time expressing physical problems, including pain. You need to rely on other clues, such as their behavior. Pain can result in behavior changes, including increased vocalization, agitation, withdrawal, and changes in function. Pain should be recognized and treated promptly and the response monitored.

Eating and swallowing problems. Undernutrition is a problem in the moderate and severe stages of AD. Loss of interest in food, decreased ability to self-feed, and comorbid conditions can result in significant nutrition problems. In long-term care facilities, inadequate help with feeding may add to the problem.

Use pureed foods, thickened liquids, and nutrition supplements when chewing and swallowing become problematic. Patients may need reminders to chew their food and to swallow. A quiet and unhurried environment without distractions (e.g., television) at mealtimes can help. Low lighting, music, and simulated nature sounds may improve eating behaviors. Easy-grip eating utensils and finger foods may allow patients to self-feed. Offer liquids frequently.

When oral feeding is not possible, explore alternative routes. Nasogastric (NG) feeding may be used for short periods. However, an NG tube is uncomfortable and may add to the agitation. A percutaneous endoscopic gastrostomy (PEG) tube is another option. PEG tubes can be problematic because patients with AD are vulnerable to aspiration of feeding formula and tube dislodgment. The potential positive outcomes from nutrition therapies must be considered in light of overall goals and potential adverse effects of the specific therapy. Nutrition therapy is described in Chapter 44.

Oral care. In the late stages, patients are unable to perform oral self-care. With decreased tooth brushing and flossing, dental problems are likely to occur. Because of swallowing problems, patients may retain food in the mouth, adding to the risk for tooth decay. Dental caries and tooth abscess can cause discomfort and increase agitation. Inspect the mouth regularly. Provide mouth care to those who cannot perform self-care.

Infection prevention. Urinary tract infection and pneumonia are the most common infections in patients with AD. Such infections are a common cause of death. Because of feeding and swallowing problems, patients are at risk for aspiration pneumonia. Immobility can also predispose patients to pneumonia.

Reduced fluid intake, prostate enlargement, poor hygiene, and urinary drainage devices can predispose patients to bladder infection. Any manifestations of infection, such as a change in behavior, fever, cough, or pain on urination, require prompt evaluation and treatment.

Skin care. Monitor the skin over time. Note and treat rashes, areas of redness, and skin breakdown. In the late stages, incontinence along with immobility and undernutrition can place patients at risk for skin breakdown. Keep the skin clean and dry. Change the patient's position regularly to avoid areas of pressure over bony prominences.

Elimination problems. During the moderate and severe stages of AD, urinary and fecal incontinence lead to an increased need for nursing care. Scheduled toileting may help decrease incontinence. Constipation is a common problem. Causes include immobility, reduced fiber intake, and decreased fluid intake. Treatment includes increased diet fiber, fiber supplements, and stool softeners. Ways to manage constipation are discussed in Chapter 47.

Caregiver support. The burden of caring for patients with AD is well documented.[1] Caregiving tasks include performing household chores, shopping, preparing meals, driving, managing appointments and finances, administering or reminding the person to take medications, assisting with ADLs, and managing symptoms.

More than 11 million Americans provide unpaid care for people with AD or other dementias.[1] Most of these are family members providing care in the home (Fig. 64.9). Almost two-thirds of informal caregivers are females. Commonly, daughters care for aging parents. Wives are more likely to be caregivers for their husbands.

Caregivers for people with AD describe it as very stressful. It is often important to them to keep people with AD at home. They describe a sense of duty and love in this role. However, they often have adverse consequences to their own health. The chronic and often severe stress of caregiving increases the risk for dementia in spouse caregivers. It could be that the effects of chronic stress from caregiving affect the area of the brain responsible for memory.

As AD progresses, the relationship between the caregiver and patient changes. Family roles may be altered or reversed. A child may care for a parent. Decisions must be made. When do patients have to stop driving or doing activities that may have become dangerous? When do families need help? When should patients be placed in adult day care or a long-term care facility?

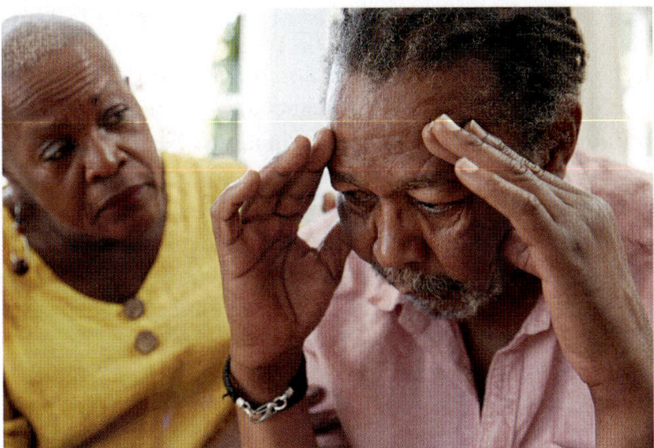

Fig. 64.9 Caregivers of patients with dementia face incredible challenges. (© monkeybusinessimages/iStock.com.)

With early-onset AD, patients are affected during their most productive years in terms of career and family. The consequences can be devastating to patients and families.

AD seriously affects sexual relationships. As AD progresses, sexual interest may decline for the patient and partner. Reasons for this include fatigue, memory impairment, and incontinence. Some patients become sexually driven and uninhibited.[18]

Work with caregivers to assess stressors and identify coping strategies to reduce caregiving burden. Ask which behaviors are most disruptive to family life at a given time. This is likely to change as AD progresses. Determining what is most disruptive or distressful to the caregiver can help establish priorities.

Patient safety is a high priority. Assess what the caregiver's expectations are about the patient's behavior. Are the expectations reasonable given the stage? A family and caregiver teaching guide based on the stages is shown in Table 64.16. A

TABLE 64.16 **PATIENT & CAREGIVER TEACHING**

AD

Include the following instructions when teaching families and caregivers the management of patients with AD:

Mild Stage

- Many treatable (and potentially reversible) conditions can mimic dementia (Table 64.2). Try to establish a diagnosis.
- Get the patient to stop driving. Confusion and poor judgment can impair driving skills and potentially put others at risk.
- Encourage activities such as visiting with friends and family, listening to music, enjoying hobbies, and exercising.
- Provide cues in the home, establish a routine, and determine a specific location where essential items (e.g., glasses) must be kept.
- Do not correct misstatements or faulty memory.
- Register with MedicAlert + Alzheimer's Association Safe Return, a program established by the MedicAlert Foundation and the Alzheimer's Association to locate those who wander from their homes.
- Make plans in terms of advance directives, care options, financial concerns, and personal preference for care.

Moderate Stage

- Install door locks for patient safety.
- Provide protective wear for incontinence.
- Ensure that the home has good lighting, install handrails in stairways and bathrooms, and remove area rugs.
- Label drawers and faucets (hot and cold) to ensure safety.
- Develop ways, such as distraction and diversion, to cope with behavior problems. Identify and reduce potential triggers (e.g., reduce stress, extremes in temperature) for disruptive behavior.
- Provide memory triggers, such as pictures of family and friends.

Severe Stage

- Follow a regular schedule for toileting to reduce incontinence.
- Provide care to meet needs, including oral care and skin care.
- Monitor diet and fluid intake to ensure their adequacy.
- Continue communication through talking and touching.
- Consider placement in a long-term care facility when providing total care becomes too difficult.

nursing care plan for the family caregiver (eNursing Care Plan 64.2) is available on the website for this chapter.

Support groups for caregivers and family members (Fig. 64.10) can provide an atmosphere of understanding and give current information about AD and related topics, such as safety, legal, ethical, and financial issues. The Alzheimer's Association has many education and support systems available to help family caregivers (www.alz.org).[1]

◆ Evaluation

Expected outcomes are that patients with AD will:

- Function at the highest level of cognitive ability
- Perform basic personal care ADLs, by self or with assistance, as needed
- Be injury free

DELIRIUM

Delirium is a state of confusion that develops over hours to days.[2] Attention and awareness are disturbed. Memory, orientation, language, or visual perceptual ability can be affected. The symptoms cannot be explained by dementia and do not occur in the context of a severely impaired level of consciousness.

Delirium most often occurs among hospitalized older adults. Around half of people aged 65 and older who are hospitalized experience delirium. It is related to longer hospital stays and higher mortality rates. Delirium has been reported in 48% of persons in skilled nursing facilities and up to 83% of people at the end of life.

Etiology and Pathophysiology

We do not know the exact cause of delirium. Most often delirium occurs when acute stress is placed on a vulnerable brain. Structural lesions; vascular lesions; and neuroinflammatory, neurodegenerative, and aging changes in the brain increase vulnerability. Multiple neurotransmitter abnormalities are involved. There is cholinergic deficiency, excess release of dopamine, and changes in serotonin activity. In response to a severe illness, the sympathetic and immune systems are activated. There is increased hypothalamic-pituitary-adrenal axis activity with hypercortisolism and release of cerebral cytokines, which alter neurotransmitter systems.

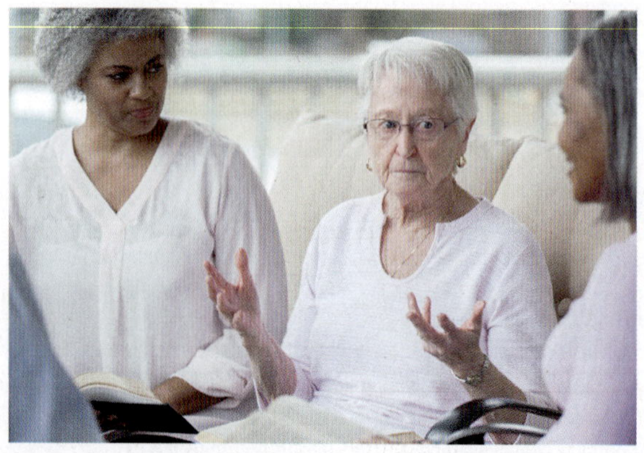

Fig. 64.10 Support groups are an effective way to help caregivers cope. (© SDI Productions/iStock.com.)

Delirium is rarely caused by a single factor. Common factors that can lead to delirium are listed in Tables 64.17 and 64.18. Major risk factors include increased age, preexisting dementia, hypertension, alcohol use, and severe illness on admission to an acute care facility. Dementia is a leading risk factor for delirium. Likewise, delirium is a risk factor for developing dementia. Delirium may cause permanent neuronal damage and lead to dementia.

Environment factors that can contribute to delirium include sleep deprivation, stress, sensory overload, and immobilization. Certain drugs (e.g., sedatives [benzodiazepines], opioids) are linked with delirium, especially in older or vulnerable patients. It may occur in persons with life-threatening illnesses such as pneumonia or urosepsis.

Delirium can occur after a relatively minor insult in vulnerable patients. For example, patients with underlying health problems, such as heart failure (HF), cancer, cognitive impairment, or sensory limitations, may develop delirium in response to a minor change, such as using a sleeping medication. In other less vulnerable patients, it may take a combination of factors, such as anesthesia, major surgery, mechanical ventilation, infection, and prolonged sleep deprivation, to precipitate delirium. Pain and depression contribute to delirium, especially among older adults.

Clinical Manifestations

Delirium can have a variety of manifestations, ranging from hypoactivity and lethargy to hyperactivity, agitation, and hallucinations.[19] Patients can have mixed delirium, with hypoactive and hyperactive symptoms. Delirium usually develops over a 2- to 3-day period. It can last from 1 to 7 days. However, delirium may persist for months or years. Some patients do not fully recover.

During a delirious state, patients often have a reduced ability to focus, sustain, and shift attention. Memory, judgment, and orientation are impaired. Speech is rapid, rambling, and/or incoherent. Other manifestations include disorganized thinking, irritability, insomnia, loss of appetite, and restlessness. Later manifestations may include agitation, misperception, misinterpretation, and hallucinations.

The manifestations are sometimes confused with those of dementia. A key distinction between them is that patients who have sudden cognitive impairment, disorientation, or clouded sensorium are more likely to have delirium rather than dementia. Table 64.3 compares delirium and dementia.

Diagnostic Studies

Diagnosing delirium is complicated because many critically ill patients cannot communicate their needs. A careful history and

TABLE 64.17 Risk Factors for Delirium

Demographic
- Age 65 years or older
- Male

Cognitive Status
- Cognitive impairment
- Dementia
- Depression
- History of delirium

Decreased Oral Intake
- Dehydration
- Malnutrition

Drugs
- Alcohol or drug use or withdrawal
- Aminoglycosides
- Anticholinergics
- Opioids
- Sedative-hypnotics
- Treatment with multiple drugs
- Vasopressors

Environment
- Admission to ICU
- Pain (especially untreated)
- Use of restraints
- Sleep deprivation
- Stress

Functional Status
- Functional dependence
- History of falls
- Immobility

Medical Problems
- Acute infection, sepsis, fever
- Chronic kidney or liver disease
- Electrolyte imbalances
- Fracture or trauma
- Hemodynamic instability
- History of stroke
- Hypertension
- Hypoxia
- Neurologic disease
- Severe acute illness
- Terminal illness

Sensory
- Impaired vision or hearing
- Sensory deprivation
- Sensory overload

Surgery
- Cardiac surgery
- Orthopedic surgery
- Prolonged cardiopulmonary bypass

physical assessment are the first steps in diagnosing delirium and its underlying cause. This includes careful attention to medications. The Confusion Assessment Method (CAM) is a reliable tool for assessing delirium (Table 64.19). The version of the CAM may vary depending on the clinical setting. Determine whether delirium is related to underlying dementia.

Once delirium has been diagnosed, explore potential causes. Review the health history and medication record. Laboratory tests include CBC, serum electrolytes, blood urea nitrogen (BUN), and creatinine levels; ECG; urinalysis; liver and thyroid function tests; and O_2 saturation. Drug and alcohol levels may be obtained. If unexplained fever or nuchal rigidity is present and meningitis or encephalitis is suspected, a lumbar puncture may be done. CSF is examined for glucose, protein, and bacteria. If the history includes head injury, x-rays or scans may be ordered. In general, brain imaging studies, such as CT and MRI, are used only when head injury is known or suspected.

Interprofessional and Nursing Management

Treatment is important, as many cases of delirium are potentially reversible.[19] In caring for patients with delirium, you are responsible for prevention, early recognition, and treatment

TABLE 64.18 Mnemonic for Causes of Delirium

Dementia, dehydration
Electrolyte imbalances, emotional stress
Lung, liver, heart, kidney, brain
Infection, intensive care unit
Rx drugs
Injury, immobility
Untreated pain, unfamiliar environment
Metabolic disorders

TABLE 64.19 Confusion Assessment Method

Delirium is diagnosed with the presence of features 1 and 2 and either 3 or 4.

Feature 1
Acute Onset and Fluctuating Course
Data usually obtained from a family member or nurse.
Positive responses to the following questions:
- Is there evidence of an acute change in mental status from baseline?
- Did the abnormal behavior fluctuate during the day (i.e., tend to come and go or increase and decrease in severity)?

Feature 2
Inattention
Positive response to the following question:
- Did the patient have problem focusing attention (e.g., being easily distractible or having problem keeping track of what was being said)?

Feature 3
Disorganized Thinking
Positive response to the following question:
- Is the patient's thinking disorganized or incoherent, such as rambling or irrelevant conversation, unclear or illogical flow of ideas, or unpredictable switching from subject to subject?

Feature 4
Altered Level of Consciousness
Any answer other than "alert" to the following question:
- Overall, how would you rate the patient's level of consciousness: alert, vigilant [hyperalert], lethargic, stupor [hard to arouse], or coma?

Adapted from Inouye S, van Dyck C, Alessi C, et al: Clarifying confusion: the confusion assessment method, *Ann Intern Med* 113:941, 1990.

(Table 64.20). Prevention involves recognition of patients at high risk, including those with neurologic disorders, such as dementia or stroke. Table 64.17 lists common risk factors.

Care focuses on eliminating precipitating factors. If it is drug induced, medications are discontinued. Keep in mind that delirium can accompany drug and alcohol withdrawal. Depending on the history, drug screening may be done. Fluid and electrolyte imbalances and nutrition deficiencies (e.g., thiamine) are corrected. Antibiotic therapy may be started if an infection is present. Similarly, if delirium is the result of

TABLE 64.20 NURSING MANAGEMENT

Caring for Patients With Delirium

Determine potential cause for delirium and initiate measures to address it

Assess for delirium

- Administer screening tools, such as the Confusion Assessment Method (CAM) (Table 64.19)
- Screen for any coexisting problems
- Review diagnostic test results

Determine ability to meet self-care needs related to nutrition, elimination, hydration, and hygiene and implement a plan to meet any areas of identified need

Provide for patient needs:

- Provide the patient with reassurance
- Talk to the patient and reorient to time, place, and person often
- Use distraction to manage agitated behavior
- Institute measures to manage pain, fever, nausea, and other symptoms
- Encourage early mobility if appropriate
- If patients use eyeglasses or a hearing aid, have them available

Provide a safe, optimal environment:

- Reduce noise and provide adequate nonglare lighting
- Provide a soothing atmosphere
- Plan for consistent nursing staff

Implement measures to promote sleep (see Chapter 8)

Teach patients and caregivers about causes and manifestations of delirium

chronic illness, such as chronic kidney disease or HF, treatment focuses on these conditions.

If the problem is related to an overstimulating environment, then changes should be made. Reduce environment stimuli, including noise and light levels. Limit noise levels by muting phones. Set alarms based on the patient's condition and reduce unnecessary alarms. Limit overhead paging and all unnecessary noise in patient care areas.

Conversation is a stressful noise, especially when it concerns the patient and is held in the presence of, but without participation from, the patient. Find suitable places for patient-related discussions. Whenever possible, include the patient and caregiver in the discussion.

CHECK YOUR PRACTICE

You are working in the medical ICU. Your patient is an 82-year-old male who had a hip replacement 3 days ago. He was doing well after surgery and then developed bilateral pneumonia. He was transferred to the ICU yesterday. When you walk into his room, you notice his daughter is staring out the window and does not respond to your greeting. When you approach her, you notice she is very upset. When you ask her what is wrong, she bursts out crying, "How can this be? My dad is a brilliant man. Now look at him. He talks to himself. He screams at me. He thinks I am his wife. Mom died 5 years ago. What happened to him?"

- How would you assess the situation?
- What can you do to help the daughter?

Implement measures to protect patients from harm. Give priority to creating a calm and safe environment. The presence of a caregiver may help. Provide familiar objects and family photos, transfer the patient to a private room or one closer to the nurses' station, and plan for consistent nursing staff if possible. Use reorientation and behavior interventions. Provide patients with reassurance and reorienting information as to place, time, and procedures. Clocks, calendars, and lists of scheduled activities are helpful. Removing lines no longer needed and early mobility are effective.

Reorient patients who are confused during assessments to provide comfort and direction. Personal contact through touch and verbal communication can be an important reorienting strategy. If patients use eyeglasses or a hearing aid, they should be available because sensory deprivation can precipitate delirium. Other interventions, including relaxation techniques, music therapy, and massage, may be appropriate for some patients.

You may need to address polypharmacy, pain, nutrition, and potential for incontinence. Patients with delirium are at risk for the adverse consequences of immobility, including skin breakdown. Give attention to increasing physical activity or providing range-of-motion exercises, when appropriate, and maintaining skin integrity.

Focus on supporting the family and caregivers during episodes of delirium. Family members need to understand factors that may have precipitated the delirium, in addition to the potential outcomes. Patient education materials are available at www.ICUdelirium.org.

Drug Therapy

Drug therapy is reserved for patients with severe agitation, especially when it interferes with medical care. Agitation can put patients at risk for falls and injury. Drug therapy is used cautiously because many of the drugs used to manage agitation have psychoactive properties. Drugs should be used only when nonpharmacologic interventions have failed.

The use of low-dose antipsychotics (e.g., haloperidol, risperidone), though common practice, is controversial. Their use does not change the duration of delirium or the length of hospitalization. Haloperidol can produce sedation. Other side effects include hypotension; extrapyramidal side effects, including *tardive dyskinesia* (involuntary muscle movements of face, trunk, and arms) and *athetosis* (involuntary writhing movements of the limbs); muscle tone changes; and anticholinergic effects. Monitor older patients receiving antipsychotic agents.

Short-acting benzodiazepines (e.g., lorazepam) can be used to treat delirium from sedative and alcohol withdrawal or in conjunction with antipsychotics to reduce extrapyramidal side effects. However, these drugs may worsen delirium caused by other factors and must be used cautiously.

CASE STUDY

Alzheimer Disease

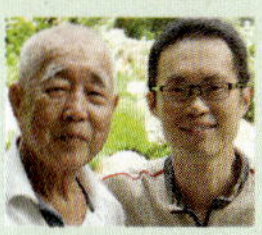

(© iStock/ Thinkstock.)

Patient Profile

T.Y., a 78-year-old male, was diagnosed with AD 3 years ago, shortly after his wife died. Today, his 45-year-old son brings him to the emergency department because he wandered from his son's home, fell, and injured his left hip.

Subjective Data

- Can say his name, confused as to place and time
- Denies memory of wandering or falling
- Agitated, trying to get up
- Denies pain

Objective Data

Physical Assessment

- Left leg shorter than the right leg
- Tense and anxious

Diagnostic Studies

- X-ray of left hip indicates a fracture
- Mini-Cog testing indicates cognitive impairment

Discussion Questions

1. ***Recognize:*** What is the pathogenesis of AD?
2. ***Analyze:*** What factors may have resulted in T.Y.'s fall?
3. ***Plan:*** Surgery is planned to repair the hip fracture. Why is he at risk for delirium?
4. ***Prioritize:*** What is the priority nursing intervention for T.Y.?
5. ***Act:*** What nursing activities can you delegate to AP?
6. ***Act:*** What teaching plan should you develop for T.Y. and his son?
7. ***Safety:*** What safety precautions need to be taken when caring for T.Y.?

Answers available at *http://evolve.elsevier.com/Lewis/medsurg.*

BRIDGE TO NCLEX EXAMINATION

The number of the question corresponds to the same-numbered outcome at the beginning of the chapter.

1. Dementia is defined as a
- **a.** syndrome that results only in memory loss.
- **b.** disease associated with abrupt behavior changes.
- **c.** disease that is always caused by reduced blood flow to the brain.
- **d.** syndrome characterized by cognitive dysfunction and loss of memory.

2. Vascular dementia is associated with
- **a.** transient ischemic attacks.
- **b.** viral infection of nerve tissue.
- **c.** cognitive changes from cerebral ischemia.
- **d.** abrupt changes in cognitive function that are irreversible.

3. Which factor from the health history places the patient at the *highest* risk for Alzheimer disease?
- **a.** Diabetes
- **b.** Cardiovascular disease
- **c.** Family history of early-onset Alzheimer disease
- **d.** Parkinsonian symptoms, including muscle rigidity

4. Which statements describe patients with mild cognitive impairment? **(Select all that apply.)**
- **a.** Patients will pass standard screening tests.
- **b.** Patients may appear normal to the casual observer.
- **c.** Family members may see changes in the patient's abilities.
- **d.** Problems patients experience interfere with their daily activities.
- **e.** Patients are usually aware that there is a problem with their memory.

5. A patient with cognitive impairment would receive a diagnosis of Alzheimer disease based on
- **a.** CT or MRI.
- **b.** brain biopsy.
- **c.** electroencephalogram.
- **d.** history and cognitive assessment.

6. A priority nursing goal for patients with Alzheimer disease is to
- **a.** maintain patient safety.
- **b.** maintain or increase body weight.
- **c.** return to a higher level of self-care.
- **d.** enhance functional ability over time.

7. Which patient is at the highest risk for developing delirium?
- **a.** A 35-year-old female with cholecystitis
- **b.** A 39-year-old male with a fractured femur
- **c.** A 42-year-old female having a total hysterectomy for ovarian cancer
- **d.** A 78-year-old male admitted to the medical unit with complications of heart failure

1. d; 2. c; 3. c; 4. b, c, e; 5. d; 6. a; 7. d.

For rationales to these answers and even more NCLEX review questions, visit http://evolve.elsevier.com/Lewis/medsurg.

REFERENCES

To access the References for this chapter, please scan the QR code with a mobile device.

65

Spinal Cord and Nerve Problems

Kristen J. Keller

http://evolve.elsevier.com/Lewis/medsurg/

CONCEPTUAL FOCUS

Family Dynamics
Functional Ability
Mobility
Pain
Sensory Perception

LEARNING OUTCOMES

1. Outline the classification of spinal cord injuries (SCIs) and associated clinical manifestations.
2. Describe the acute interprofessional management of patients with SCI.
3. Describe the acute nursing management of patients with SCI.
4. Discuss rehabilitation care and the relationship to the level of disruption in SCI.
5. Explain the types, clinical manifestations, and interprofessional and nursing management of spinal cord tumors.
6. Explain the etiology, clinical manifestations, and interprofessional and nursing management of trigeminal neuralgia and Bell palsy.
7. Describe the etiology, clinical manifestations, and interprofessional and nursing management of Guillain-Barré syndrome and inflammatory demyelinating polyneuropathy.

KEY TERMS

autonomic dysreflexia (AD)
Bell palsy
Guillain-Barré syndrome (GBS)
neurogenic bladder
neurogenic (vasogenic) shock
paraplegia
spinal cord injury (SCI)
spinal shock
tetanus
tetraplegia
trigeminal neuralgia (TN)

This chapter discusses spinal cord and nerve problems, including spinal cord injuries (SCIs), spinal cord tumors, cranial nerve problems, and polyneuropathies. We focus on the nursing management of the problems encountered by patients with SCI. The potential for disruption of family dynamics, economic loss from unemployment, and the high cost of rehabilitation and long-term health care make SCI a major problem. Although many people with SCI can care for themselves independently, those with the highest level of injury need around-the-clock care. The nurse's role in providing holistic care significantly affects patients' general health and well-being.

SPINAL CORD PROBLEMS

SPINAL CORD INJURY

Spinal cord injury (SCI) is caused by trauma or damage to the spinal cord. It can result in temporary or permanent alteration in spinal cord function. About 17,000 Americans have SCIs each year. Around 282,000 persons in the United States are living with SCI. The average life expectancy for persons with SCI is shortened and has not improved since the 1980s. In the first year after injury, mortality rates are high. There is a 30% chance of rehospitalization.[1]

Etiology and Pathophysiology

SCI is usually a result of trauma. The 4 most common causes are motor vehicle collisions (37.5%), falls (31.7%), violence (15.4%), and sports injuries (8%).[1]

Types of Injury

Neurologic damage from SCI occurs in 2 phases: *primary injury* (initial physical disruption of the spinal cord) and *secondary injury* (from processes such as ischemia, hypoxia, hemorrhage, and edema).

Primary injury. *Primary injury* results from direct physical trauma to the spinal cord due to blunt or penetrating trauma. Trauma can cause spinal cord compression by bone displacement, interruption of blood supply, or distraction from pulling. Penetrating trauma, such as gunshot and stab wounds, can cause tearing and transection.

Secondary injury. *Secondary injury* refers to the ongoing, progressive damage that occurs after the primary injury. Secondary injury causes further permanent damage. It begins a few minutes after injury and lasts for months. The cascade of events results in edema, ischemia, and inflammation. This causes cell death, disruption of the blood-brain barrier, and demyelination. This can extend the level of deficit and worsen long-term outcomes.

The edema from the inflammatory response is especially harmful because of limited space for tissue expansion. Thus compression of the spinal cord occurs. Edema extends above and below the injury, increasing ischemic damage. Within 24 hours, permanent damage may occur from edema.

Apoptosis (programmed cell death) continues for weeks and contributes to postinjury demyelination. The inflammatory response at the site of the initial injury focuses on clearing up the initial cellular debris without damaging normal tissue. This results in a central nonneural core of connective tissue that we refer to as a *glial scar* (Fig. 65.1). The glial scar creates a physical barrier. It restricts the cells in the spinal cord from migration and regeneration. This leads to irreversible nerve damage and permanent neurologic deficit.

Classification of SCI

We classify SCI by the (1) mechanism of injury, (2) level of injury, and (3) degree of injury.

Mechanisms of injury. The major mechanisms of injury include flexion, flexion-rotation, hyperextension, vertical compression, extension-rotation, and lateral flexion (Fig. 65.2). Flexion-rotation injury is often the most unstable because ligaments that stabilize the spine are torn. This injury most often contributes to severe neurologic deficits.

Level of injury. *Skeletal level* of injury is the vertebral level with the most damage to vertebra and related ligaments. *Neurologic level* is the lowest segment of the spinal cord with normal sensory and motor function on both sides of the body. The level of injury may be cervical, thoracic, lumbar, or sacral. Cervical and lumbar injuries are most common because those areas of the spine are associated with the greatest flexibility and movement.

Fig. 65.3 shows affected structures and functions at different levels of cord injury. Injury from C1 to T1 can cause paralysis of all 4 extremities, resulting in **tetraplegia** (formerly called *quadriplegia*). The degree of impairment in the arms after cervical injury depends on the level of injury. The lower the level, the more function is retained in the arms. **Paraplegia** (paralysis and loss of sensation in the legs) can occur in SCI below the level of T2.[2]

Degree of injury. The degree of spinal cord involvement may be complete or incomplete (partial). *Complete cord involvement* results in total loss of sensory and motor function below the level of injury. *Incomplete cord involvement* results in a mixed loss of voluntary motor activity and sensation and leaves some tracts intact. The degree of sensory and motor loss depends on the level of injury and reflects specific damaged nerve tracts.

Five major syndromes are associated with incomplete injuries: central cord syndrome, anterior cord syndrome, Brown-Séquard syndrome, cauda equina syndrome, and conus medullaris syndrome (Table 65.1).

Clinical Manifestations

The manifestations are the result of trauma that causes cord compression, ischemia, edema, and possible cord transection. They are related to the level and degree of injury. Patients with an incomplete injury may have a mix of manifestations.

Motor and Sensory Effects

The American Spinal Injury Association (ASIA) Impairment Scale is used to classify the severity of impairment from SCI and identify rehabilitation potential. It combines motor and sensory

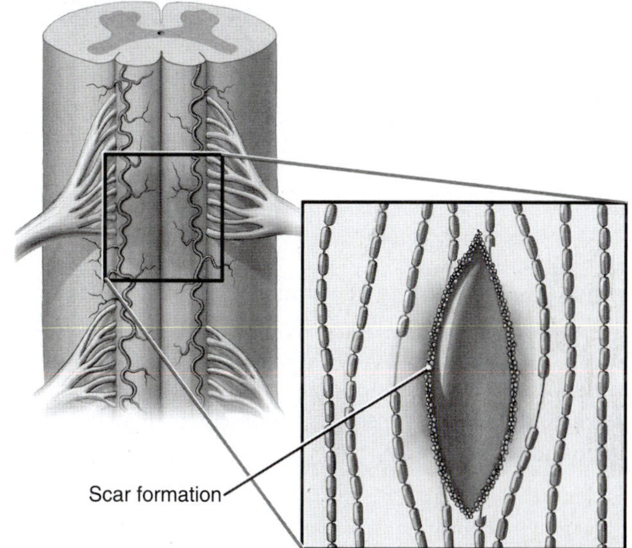

Fig. 65.1 One to 2 days after the injury, astrocytes proliferate and surround the edges of the fibrotic scar. This confines inflammation to the area of injury and protects neighboring neural tissue from further damage. This process may take 7 to 10 days. (Used with permission from Barrow Neurological Institute, Phoenix, AZ.)

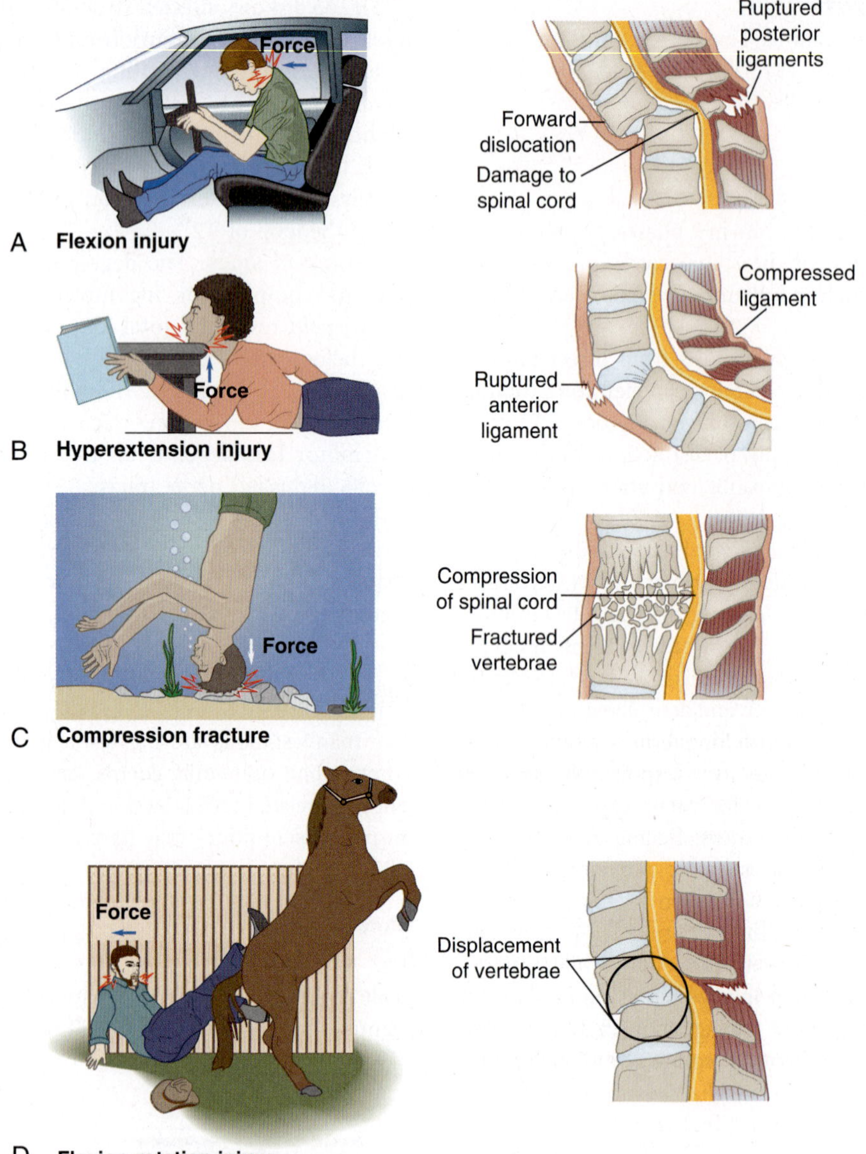

Fig. 65.2 Examples of mechanisms of spinal cord injury. (A) Flexion injury of the cervical spine ruptures the posterior ligaments. (B) Hyperextension injury of the cervical spine ruptures the anterior ligaments. (C) Compression fractures crush the vertebrae and force bony fragments into the spinal canal. (D) Flexion-rotation injury of the cervical spine often results in tearing of ligamentous structures that normally stabilize the spine. (A–C, From Copstead-Kirkhorn LC, Banasik JL: *Pathophysiology,* ed 5, St Louis, 2014, Mosby.)

function assessments to determine neurologic level and completeness of injury (Fig. 65.4).[3] We can use it to record changes in neurologic status. Movement and rehabilitation potential related to specific locations of SCI are described in Table 65.2. In general, sensory function closely matches motor function at all levels.

Respiratory

Respiratory complications closely correspond to the level of injury. Cervical injuries above C3 present special problems because of the total loss of respiratory muscle function. These patients have respiratory arrest within minutes of injury if not intubated. Patients with high cervical injury (C3–C5) have respiratory insufficiency due to loss of phrenic nerve innervation to the diaphragm and decreased chest and abdominal wall strength.[4] Patients with complete SCI above C5 should be intubated at once. Patients with incomplete SCI injury will have variability in their respiratory function.

Cervical and thoracic injuries cause paralysis of abdominal muscles and often the intercostal muscles. Patients cannot cough effectively enough to remove secretions. This increases the risk for aspiration, atelectasis, and pneumonia. Hypoventilation and impairment of the intercostal muscles lead to decreased vital capacity and tidal volume.

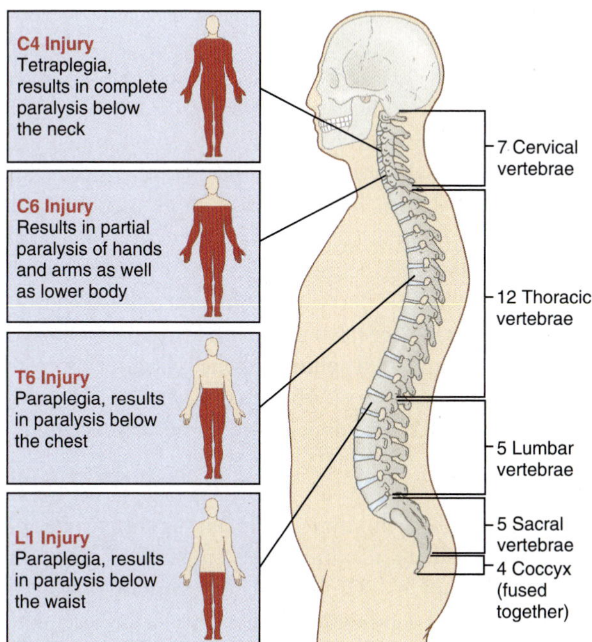

Fig. 65.3 Symptoms, degree of paralysis, and potential for rehabilitation depend on level of spinal injury.

Associated traumatic injuries, such as lung contusions, can further compromise lung function. Fluid overload can cause pulmonary edema. Neurogenic pulmonary edema may occur because of a dramatic increase in sympathetic nervous system (SNS) activity at the time of injury.

Maintaining an arterial saturation above 92% reduces hypoxemia, which can lead to bradycardia and worsen secondary injury. We assess patients for respiratory distress, including dyspnea, decreased vital capacity, and P_{CO_2} greater than 20 mm Hg above baseline, and their ability to manage their secretions. Patients in distress may need mechanical ventilation.

Cardiovascular

Any cord injury above T6 leads to SNS dysfunction. The result may be bradycardia, peripheral vasodilation, and hypotension (neurogenic shock). Peripheral vasodilation causes relative hypovolemia because of the increase in the capacity of the dilated veins. It reduces venous return of blood to the heart. Cardiac output then decreases, leading to hypotension. Other injuries can cause hemorrhagic shock and further reduce BP. It is essential to identify all causes of hypotension in the person with SCI.

Venous thromboembolism (VTE) is a common problem caused by hypercoagulability, venous stasis, and venous endothelial injury.[5] Immobilization promotes venous stasis and thrombi of the lower extremities. It may be hard to detect a deep venous thrombosis (DVT) because usual signs and symptoms, such as pain and tenderness, are not present.

TABLE 65.1 Incomplete Spinal Cord Injury Syndromes

Description	Manifestations
Anterior Cord Syndrome	
• Damage to anterior spinal artery • Results in compromised blood flow to anterior spinal cord • Results from acute compression of anterior part of the spinal cord • Common with flexion injury	• Motor paralysis and loss of pain and temperature sensation below level of injury • Because posterior cord tracts are not injured, sensations of touch, position, vibration, and motion are intact
Brown-Séquard Syndrome	
• Damage to half of the spinal cord • Often results from penetrating injury to spinal cord	• *Contralateral* (opposite side of injury): Loss of pain and temperature sensation below level of injury • *Ipsilateral* (same side as injury): Loss of motor function, light touch, pressure, position, and vibratory sense
Cauda Equina Syndrome	
• Damage to cauda equina (lumbar and sacral nerve roots)	• Asymmetric distal weakness, patchy sensation in lower extremities • May cause flaccid paralysis of lower extremities • Complete loss of sensation between legs and over buttocks, inner thighs, and backs of legs (*saddle area*) • Areflexic (flaccid) bladder and bowel • Severe, radicular, asymmetric pain
Central Cord Syndrome	
• Damage to central spinal cord • Occurs most often in cervical cord region • More common in older adults • Caused by hyperextension injury in people with degenerative disease	• Motor weakness and altered sensation present in upper extremities • Lower extremities not usually affected • Burning pain in upper extremities
Conus Medullaris Syndrome	
• Damage to conus medullaris (lowest part of spinal cord)	• Motor function in legs may be preserved, weak, or flaccid • Decrease in or loss of sensation in perianal area • Areflexic bowel and bladder • Impotence

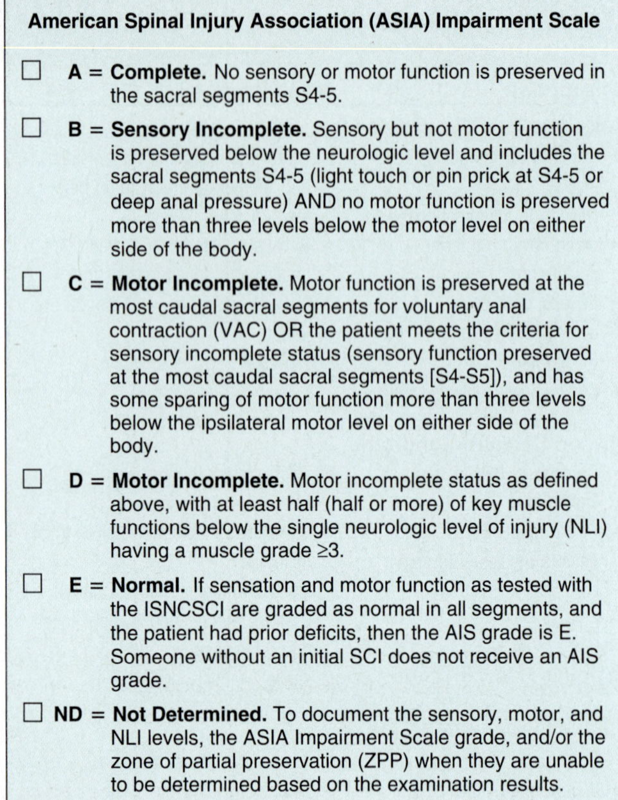

American Spinal Injury Association (ASIA) Impairment Scale

- ☐ **A = Complete.** No sensory or motor function is preserved in the sacral segments S4-5.
- ☐ **B = Sensory Incomplete.** Sensory but not motor function is preserved below the neurologic level and includes the sacral segments S4-5 (light touch or pin prick at S4-5 or deep anal pressure) AND no motor function is preserved more than three levels below the motor level on either side of the body.
- ☐ **C = Motor Incomplete.** Motor function is preserved at the most caudal sacral segments for voluntary anal contraction (VAC) OR the patient meets the criteria for sensory incomplete status (sensory function preserved at the most caudal sacral segments [S4-S5]), and has some sparing of motor function more than three levels below the ipsilateral motor level on either side of the body.
- ☐ **D = Motor Incomplete.** Motor incomplete status as defined above, with at least half (half or more) of key muscle functions below the single neurologic level of injury (NLI) having a muscle grade ≥3.
- ☐ **E = Normal.** If sensation and motor function as tested with the ISNCSCI are graded as normal in all segments, and the patient had prior deficits, then the AIS grade is E. Someone without an initial SCI does not receive an AIS grade.
- ☐ **ND = Not Determined.** To document the sensory, motor, and NLI levels, the ASIA Impairment Scale grade, and/or the zone of partial preservation (ZPP) when they are unable to be determined based on the examination results.

Fig. 65.4 The ASIA Impairment Scale. (From American Spinal Injury Association.)

Urinary

Urinary dysfunction occurs in most patients after SCI. Neurogenic bladder describes any type of bladder dysfunction related to abnormal or absent bladder innervation. After SCI, the ability of the bladder muscles and the micturition center in the brain to transmit information is impaired. Both the detrusor muscle (bladder wall) and sphincter muscle may be overactive because of the lack of brain control. This may cause high bladder pressures and urinary retention. Incontinence results from reflex emptying and failure to store urine.

Depending on the injury, a neurogenic bladder may (1) have no reflex detrusor contractions *(flaccid, hypotonic)*, which can result in bladder stretching from overdistention; (2) have hyperactive reflex detrusor contractions *(spastic)*, seen in SCI above T12, leading to incontinence; or (3) lack coordination between detrusor contraction and urethral relaxation *(dyssynergia)*, resulting in reflux of urine into the kidneys. Reflux into the kidneys can lead to stone formation, hydronephrosis, pyelonephritis, and renal failure.[6]

Gastrointestinal

Decreased gastrointestinal (GI) motor activity contributes to gastric distention and paralytic ileus. Gastric emptying may be delayed, especially in patients with higher-level SCI. Excess hydrochloric acid (HCl) release in the stomach may cause stress ulcers. Dysphagia may be present in patients who need mechanical ventilation, tracheostomy, or anterior spine surgery.

Intraabdominal bleeding may be hard to diagnose because the person with SCI may not have pain or tenderness. Continued hypotension and decreases in hemoglobin and hematocrit may be the only signs of bleeding.

Loss of voluntary control of the bowel results in neurogenic bowel. SCI above the level of the conus medullaris results in a *hyperreflexic* bowel with increased rectal and sigmoid compliance. Combined with increased anal sphincter tone and the inability to sense a full rectum, this causes stool retention and constipation.[7] SCI at or below the conus medullaris causes the bowel to be *areflexic.* Peristalsis is impaired. The defecation reflex may be damaged and anal sphincter tone relaxed. This leads to constipation, increased risk for incontinence, and possible impaction, ileus, or megacolon. Hemorrhoids can occur.

Thermoregulation

Poikilothermia is the inability to maintain a constant core temperature, with patients assuming the temperature of the environment. It occurs in SCI because interruption of the SNS prevents peripheral temperature sensations from reaching the hypothalamus. There is a decreased ability to sweat or shiver below the level of injury, which affects the ability to regulate body temperature. The degree of poikilothermia depends on the level of injury. Cervical injuries are associated with a greater loss of ability to regulate temperature than are thoracic or lumbar injuries.

Metabolic Needs

The person with SCI has increased nutrition needs because of increased metabolism and more protein breakdown. Lean body mass decreases and muscles atrophy, leading to weight loss. In the acute injury phase, stress on the body from hemodynamic instability and medical interventions, such as surgery, can worsen stress. Adequate nutrition helps prevent skin breakdown, reduces infection, and decreases muscle atrophy.

Pain

Pain differs in type and severity. Patients' physical functioning and emotions influence pain. Pain can be nociceptive or neuropathic. Nociceptive pain can result from musculoskeletal, visceral, and/or other types of injury (e.g., skin ulceration, headache). Patients often describe musculoskeletal pain as dull or aching. It starts or worsens with movement. Visceral pain is in the thorax, abdomen, and/or pelvis. It may be dull, tender, or cramping.

Neuropathic pain occurs from damage to the spinal cord or nerve roots. The pain can be at or below the level of injury. Patients often describe the pain as hot, burning, tingling, pins and needles, cold, and/or shooting. They may be very sensitive to stimuli. Even light touch can cause significant pain. Pain is discussed in Chapter 9.

Spinal and Neurogenic Shock

Spinal shock may occur shortly after acute SCI. It is characterized by a temporary loss of deep tendon and sphincter

TABLE 65.2 Level of SCI and Rehabilitation Potential

Movement Remaining	Rehabilitation Potential
Tetraplegia	
C1–C3	
• Often fatal • Movement in neck and above, loss of innervation to diaphragm, absence of independent respiratory function	• Able to drive electric wheelchair equipped with portable ventilator by using chin control or mouth stick, headrest to stabilize head • Computer use with mouth stick, head wand, or noise control • Care 24 h/day, able to instruct others
C4	
• Sensation and movement in neck and above • May be able to breathe without ventilator	• Same as C1–C3
C5	
• Full neck, partial shoulder, back, biceps • Gross elbow, inability to roll over or use hands • ↓ Respiratory reserve	• Able to drive electric wheelchair with hand supports • Indoor mobility in manual wheelchair • Able to feed self with setup and adaptive equipment • Care 10 h/day
C6	
• Shoulder and upper back abduction and rotation at shoulder • Full biceps to elbow flexion, wrist extension, weak grasp of thumb • ↓ Respiratory reserve	• Able to help with transfer and perform some self-care • Feed self with hand devices • Push wheelchair on smooth, flat surface • Drive adapted van from wheelchair • Independent computer use with adaptive equipment • Care 6 h/day
C7–C8	
• All triceps to elbow extension, finger extensors, and flexors • Good grasp with some decreased strength • ↓ Respiratory reserve	• Able to transfer self to wheelchair • Roll over and sit up in bed • Push self on most surfaces • Perform most self-care • Independent use of wheelchair • Able to drive car with powered hand controls (in some patients) • Care 0–6 h/day
Paraplegia	
T1–T6	
• Full innervation of upper extremities • Back, essential intrinsic muscles of hand • Full strength and dexterity of grasp • ↓ Trunk stability, decreased respiratory reserve	• Full independence in self-care and in wheelchair • Able to drive car with hand controls (in most patients) • Independent standing in standing frame
T6–T12	
• Full, stable thoracic muscles and upper back • Functional intercostal muscles, resulting in ↑ respiratory reserve	• Full independent use of wheelchair • Able to stand erect with full leg brace, ambulate on crutches with swing (although gait difficult) • Unable to climb stairs
L1–L2	
• Varying control of legs and pelvis • Instability of lower back	• Good sitting balance • Full use of wheelchair • Ambulation with long leg braces
L3–L4	
• Quadriceps and hip flexors • Absence of hamstring function, flail ankles	• Completely independent ambulation with short leg braces and canes • Unable to stand for long periods

reflexes, loss of sensation, and flaccid paralysis below the level of injury. This syndrome lasts days to weeks. It often masks postinjury neurologic function.[8]

Neurogenic (vasogenic) shock can occur in cervical or high thoracic injury (T6 or higher). It occurs from unopposed parasympathetic response because of loss of SNS innervation. It causes peripheral vasodilation, venous pooling, and decreased cardiac output. Manifestations include significant hypotension (<90 mm Hg), bradycardia, and temperature dysregulation. Neurogenic shock may persist for as long as 5 weeks after injury.[9] Hypotension can result in poor perfusion and oxygenation to the spinal cord and worsen spinal cord ischemia.

Diagnostic Studies

CT scan is the preferred imaging study to diagnose the location and degree of injury and the degree of spinal canal compromise. Cervical x-rays are done when a CT scan is not readily available. However, it is hard to see C7 and T1 on a cervical x-ray, decreasing the ability to fully evaluate a cervical spine injury. MRI can assess soft tissue injury, neurologic changes, unexplained neurologic deficits, or worsening neurologic conditions.

We perform a comprehensive neurologic examination and assess for other injuries or trauma. Patients with cervical injuries who have altered mental status may need a CT angiogram of the neck to rule out vascular injuries.

Interprofessional Care

Prehospital

Goals immediately after injury include maintaining a patent *airway*, adequate ventilation/*breathing*, and adequate *circulating* blood volume (ABCs) and preventing extension of spinal cord damage (secondary injury). Table 65.3 outlines emergency management of patients with SCI. Spinal motion should be restricted with a combination of a rigid cervical collar and a supportive backboard with straps. Most patients are kept

TABLE 65.3 EMERGENCY MANAGEMENT

SCI

Etiology	Assessment Findings	Interventions
Blunt Trauma • Compression, flexion, extension, or rotation injuries to spinal column • Diving • Falls • Motor vehicle crash • Pedestrian accidents • Sports injuries **Penetrating Trauma** • Gunshot wounds • Stab wounds • Stretched, torn, crushed, or lacerated spinal cord	• Bowel and bladder incontinence • Changes in sensation • ↓ Rectal sphincter tone • Muscle weakness, paralysis, or flaccidity • Neurogenic shock: hypotension, bradycardia, cool or warm dry skin • Numbness, paresthesia • Pain, tenderness, deformities, or muscle spasms adjacent to vertebral column • Priapism • Spinal shock • Respiratory distress/difficulty breathing • Urinary retention • Wounds, cuts; bruises; on head, face, neck, or back	**Initial** • Ensure patent airway and adequate breathing. • Maintain Sa_{O_2} >90%. Apply O_2 via nasal cannula, nonrebreather mask, or endotracheal tube. • Maintain SBP >90 mm Hg. • Establish IV access with 2 large-bore catheters to infuse normal saline or lactated Ringer's solution. • Immobilize and stabilize cervical spine. • Assess for other injuries. • Control external bleeding. • Obtain appropriate imaging. **Ongoing Monitoring** • Monitor vital signs, level of consciousness, motor and sensory function, O_2 saturation, cardiac rhythm, urine output. • Anticipate need for intubation if in respiratory distress or gag reflex absent. • Maintain normal temperature.

supine. Some may be placed in reverse Trendelenburg position. Sedation may be given to keep combative patients safe from further injury.

Intubation to secure the airway is done as soon as possible for patients with respiratory distress. End-tidal CO_2 monitoring can help determine the need for rapid-sequence intubation (RSI). Patients with stable airways in the field may need intubation at the medical facility. After cervical injury, all body systems must be maintained until we evaluate the full extent of the damage. After stabilization at the injury scene, the person should be transferred to the nearest medical facility. The preferred facility is one that specializes in acute SCI care. A thorough assessment determines the degree of deficit and the level and severity of injury.

Acute Care

Interprofessional care during the acute phase for patients with a cervical injury is described in Table 65.4. Compared with cervical injury, patients with SCI of the thoracic and lumbar vertebrae need less intense support. Respiratory compromise is not as severe at this level of injury. Other problems are treated symptomatically.

Obtain a history. How did the incident occur? Assess the extent of injury perceived by the patient or the emergency response system (ERS) personnel right after the event. Initial assessment occurs in the emergency department (ED). It includes managing the ABCs and vital signs. Ensure a secure airway. Maintain oxygenation saturation (Sa_{O_2}) greater than 92% and mean arterial pressure (MAP) greater than 85 mm Hg. Avoid systolic BP (SBP) less than 90 mm Hg. Neurogenic shock is treated with IV fluids and vasopressors to maintain SBP greater than 90 mm Hg after other causes of hypotension, including bleeding, are ruled out. Medical interventions and diagnostics are implemented to ensure hemodynamic stability.

Perform a complete neurologic assessment using the ASIA tool (Fig. 65.5). Muscle groups are tested with and against gravity, alone and against resistance, on both sides of the body. Record strength, symmetry, and spontaneous movement. Complete a sensory assessment, including touch and pain, as tested by pinprick. Start at the toes and work upward toward the head. If time and conditions permit, assess position sense and vibration. Assess rectal tone. Note the presence of *priapism.* Voluntary anal contractions indicate incomplete SCI.

Mechanisms of injury that cause spinal cord trauma, especially involving the cervical cord, may result in brain injury and/or vertebral artery injury. Is there a history of unconsciousness? Note signs of concussion and increased intracranial pressure (see Chapter 61). Assess for musculoskeletal injuries and trauma to internal organs. Because there may be altered or no muscle, bone, or visceral sensations below the level of injury, the only clue to internal trauma with bleeding may be a rapidly decreasing BP and increasing pulse. Imaging and diagnostic tests are done to evaluate injuries.

Move the patient in alignment as a unit *(logroll)* during transfers and when repositioning to prevent further injury. Monitor respiratory, cardiac, urinary, and GI functions. Some

TABLE 65.4 Interprofessional Care

Cervical Cord Injury

Diagnostic Assessment
- History and physical assessment, including complete neurologic examination
- ABGs
- Electrolytes, serum glucose, coagulation profile, hemoglobin, hematocrit
- Urinalysis
- CT scan, MRI, EMG (measure evoked potentials)
- Spinal x-rays
- Serial bedside pulmonary function tests (PFTs)

Management

Acute Care
- Immobilization and stabilization of vertebral column
- ABCs (airway, breathing, circulation)
  - O_2 by high-humidity mask (Pa_{O_2} >60 mm Hg)
  - Intubation (if indicated by ABGs and PFTs)
  - Maintain heart rate (e.g., atropine) and BP (e.g., dopamine) (SBP >90 mm Hg, MAP >85)
  - Administer IV fluids
- Insert NG tube and attach to suction
- Assessment and management of nutrition
- Maintain normal body temperature
- Indwelling urinary catheter
- Pain management
- VTE prophylaxis
- Pressure injury prevention
- Stress ulcer prophylaxis
- Bowel and bladder care and training
- Mobilization once spine stabilized
- Physical, occupational, speech therapy and physiatrist consults

Rehabilitation
- Physical therapy (ROM, mobility, strength, equipment)
- Occupational therapy (splints, ADLs training)
- Speech therapy (swallow and cognition)
- Pain management
- Spasticity management
- Bowel and bladder training
- Autonomic dysreflexia prevention
- Pressure injury prevention
- Recreational therapy
- Patient and caregiver teaching

EMG, Electromyography; *MAP,* mean arterial pressure.

patients go directly to surgery after the initial evaluation or to the intensive care unit (ICU) for monitoring and management.

Nonoperative stabilization. Nonoperative treatments involve stabilizing the injured spinal segment and decompression, either through traction or realignment. Stabilization eliminates damaging motion at the injury site. It is meant to prevent secondary spinal cord damage caused by narrowing of the spinal canal or continued contusion or compression of the spinal cord at the level of the injury. Early realignment of an unstable fracture-dislocation injury by closed reduction through craniocervical traction is effective and safe.

Surgical stabilization. Surgical treatment after acute SCI is used to manage instability and decompress the spinal cord. It may reduce secondary injury and improve outcomes. Early surgery (within 24 hours after the injury) is recommended for persons with central cord syndrome and for adults with acute SCI at any level.[10] The type of surgery depends on the severity and level of the injury, mechanism of injury, and location and degree of compression.

Surgery to stabilize the spine can be done from the back of the spine *(posterior approach)* or from the front of the spine *(anterior approach)*. In some cases, both approaches are needed. Fixation involves attaching metal screws, plates, or other devices to the bones of the spine to help keep them aligned. This procedure is usually done when 2 or more vertebrae are injured. Small pieces of bone may be attached to the injured bones to help them fuse into 1 solid piece. The bone is obtained from the patient's spinal bone harvested during surgery, from another bone in the patient's body, or from donor bone.

Drug Therapy

Evidence for using methylprednisolone is mixed. Guidelines for managing SCIs by both the American Association of Neurological Surgeons and Congress of Neurological Surgeons do not recommend its use for treating acute SCI.[11] The AOSPine 2017 Guidelines suggest a 24-hour infusion of high-dose methylprednisolone within 8 hours of acute SCI.[11] So, some HCPs may give an infusion.

VTE prophylaxis with low-molecular-weight heparin (LMWH) (e.g., enoxaparin) or fixed, low-dose heparin should start within 72 hours after injury unless contraindicated. For those with abnormal kidney function, heparin is best, as LMWH is mainly excreted by the kidneys.

Vasopressors (e.g., phenylephrine, norepinephrine) are used in the acute phase of injury as adjuvant treatment. They maintain MAP to improve perfusion to the spinal cord. Vasopressors have significant risk for complications. These include ventricular tachycardia, troponin elevation, metabolic acidosis, and atrial fibrillation. Dopamine has more complications than phenylephrine in SCI. Considerations for vasopressor selection include level of injury, patient age, and comorbidities (e.g., heart problems).

NURSING MANAGEMENT: SCI

Assessment

Subjective and objective data you should obtain from patients with SCI are outlined in Table 65.5.

Clinical Problems

Clinical problems for patients with SCI depend on the severity of the injury and level of dysfunction. Clinical problems may include:

- Impaired respiratory function
- Neurologic problems

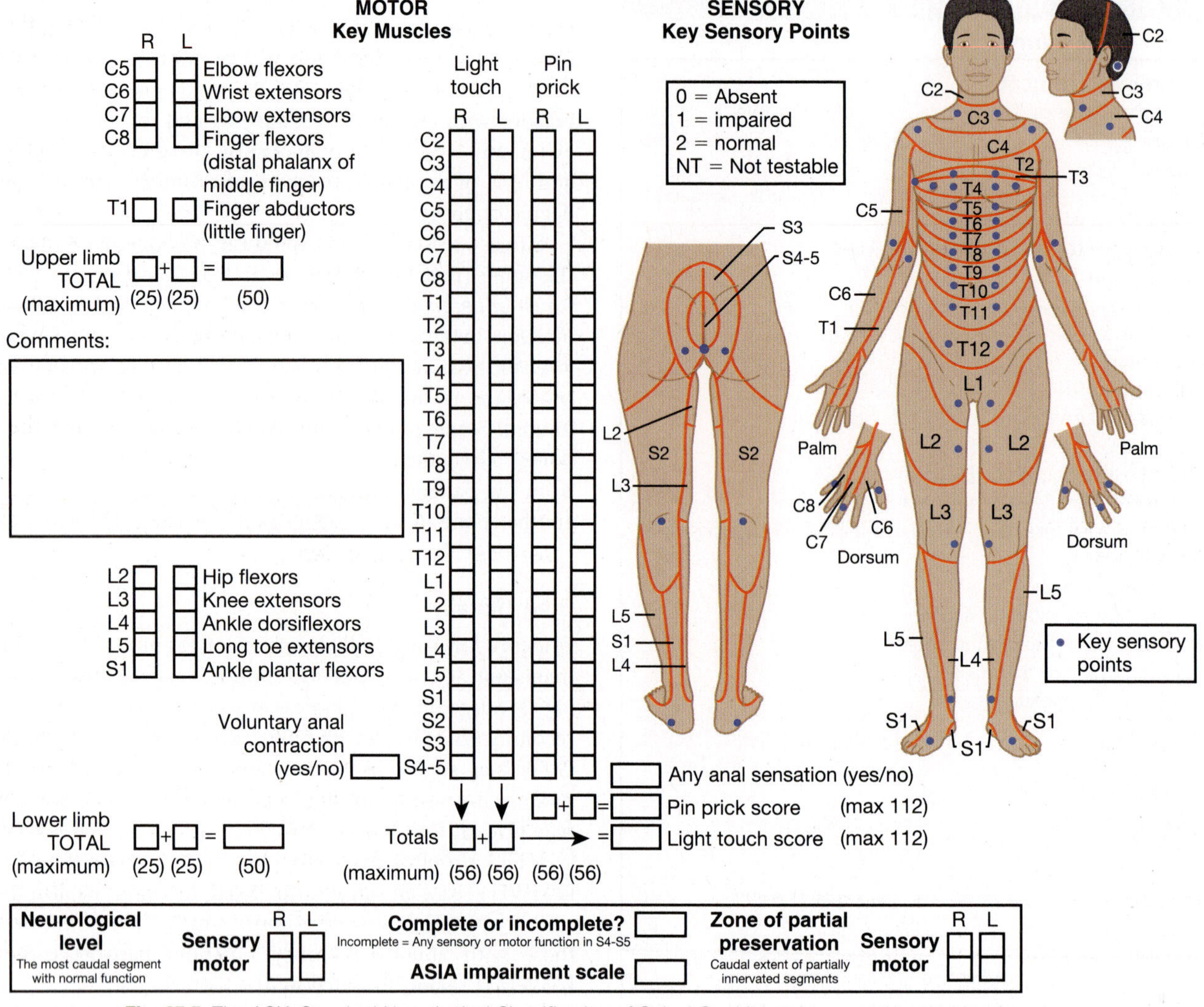

Fig. 65.5 The ASIA Standard Neurological Classification of Spinal Cord Injury is an assessment used to score the motor and sensory impairment and severity of an SCI.

- Nutritionally compromised
- Inadequate tissue perfusion
- Impaired tissue integrity
- Impaired urinary elimination
- Difficulty coping

Additional information on clinical problems and interventions for patients with complete cervical SCI is presented in eNursing Care Plan 65.1 (available on the website for this chapter).

◆ Planning

Overall goals are that patients with SCI will (1) maintain an optimal level of neurologic functioning; (2) have minimal or no complications of immobility; (3) be able to care for self or direct others to do so; and (4) return home at an optimal level of functioning.

◆ Implementation

Health Promotion

Nursing interventions for preventing SCI include identifying high-risk persons and providing teaching. Support measures to combat distracted and impaired driving. Teach people to use child safety seats and helmets for motorcyclists and bicyclists. Promote programs for reducing accidents, deaths, and injuries (e.g., ThinkFirst).[12]

Emphasize the importance of health promotion and screening behaviors after SCI. Health-promoting behaviors after SCI can have a significant impact on overall health and well-being. Provide teaching and counseling. Refer patients as needed to smoking cessation or alcohol treatment programs. Explore available recreation programs. They should continue to receive routine care for nonneurologic problems. Make sure facilities are accessible to and accommodate people with SCI. Schedule wheelchair-accessible examination rooms and allow extra time, if needed, for appointments.

TABLE 65.5 NURSING ASSESSMENT

SCI

Subjective Data

Important Health Information

Health history: Motor vehicle crash, sports injury, industrial incident, gunshot or stabbing injury, falls

Functional Health Patterns

Health perception–health management: Use of alcohol or recreational drugs. Risk-taking behaviors.

Activity-exercise: Loss of strength, movement, and sensation below level of injury. Dyspnea, inability to breathe adequately ("air hunger").

Cognitive-perceptual: Tenderness, pain at or above level of injury. Numbness, tingling, burning, twitching of extremities.

Coping–stress tolerance: Fear, denial, anger, depression.

Objective Data

Cardiovascular

Injury above T6: Bradycardia, hypotension, postural hypotension, absence of vasomotor tone

General

Poikilothermia (unable to regulate body heat)

GI

↓ Or absent bowel sounds (paralytic ileus in injuries above T5), abdominal distention, constipation, fecal incontinence, fecal impaction

Musculoskeletal

Muscle atony (in flaccid state), contractures (in spastic state)

Neurologic

Complete: Areflexic, flaccid paralysis and anesthesia below level of injury resulting in tetraplegia (injuries above C8) or paraplegia (injuries below C8), hyperactive deep tendon reflexes and bilaterally positive Babinski test (after resolution of spinal shock)

Incomplete: Mixed loss of voluntary motor activity and sensation

Pain

Neuropathic, musculoskeletal, and/or visceral

Reproductive

Priapism, altered sexual function

Respiratory

Injury at C1–C3: Apnea, inability to cough

Injury at C4: Poor cough, diaphragmatic breathing, hypoventilation

Injury at C5–T6: ↓ Respiratory reserve

Skin

Warm, dry skin below level of injury (neurogenic shock)

Urinary

Retention (for injuries at T1–L2), flaccid bladder (acute stages), spasticity with reflex bladder emptying (later stages)

Possible Diagnostic Findings

Location of level and type of bony involvement on spinal x-ray. Injury, edema, compression on CT scan and MRI; positive finding on myelogram.

Acute Care

High cervical cord injury caused by flexion-rotation is the most complex SCI. It is the focus of this section. Interventions for this type of injury can be modified for patients with less severe injuries.

Immobilization. To restrict spinal motion, maintain the neck in a neutral position. For cervical injuries, closed reduction with skeletal traction is used for early realignment *(reduction)*. Crutchfield (Fig. 65.6) or Gardner-Wells tongs or halo (halo ring) can provide this type of traction. A rope extends from the center of the device over a pulley to weights attached at the end. Traction must be always maintained. Possible displacement of the skull pins is a disadvantage of tongs. If pin displacement occurs, hold the patient's head in a neutral position and get help. Immobilize the head while the HCP reinserts the tongs.

! SAFETY ALERT

Cervical Spine Injuries

- Always keep the body in correct alignment.
- Turn the patient as a unit (e.g., logrolling) to prevent movement of the spine.

No specific guidelines address the maximum weight for traction. The HCP may start with 10 lb and add 5 lb for each level to the injury. The goal is spinal reduction. Awake patients are monitored with x-ray and neurologic and pain assessment. Comatose patients need serial x-rays to evaluate the effects of traction. The need for surgery is determined after the spine is reduced. After cervical fusion or other stabilization surgery, patients may have a hard cervical collar or sternal-occipital-mandibular immobilizer brace (Fig. 65.7).

Some patients with spinal fractures with or without acute SCI may not be able to have surgery but still need immobilization for their cervical fracture. In these patients, the halo frame can be attached to a special vest (halo vest) (Fig. 65.8). This allows patients to move and ambulate while cervical bones fuse. Surgery is used instead of the halo if there is ligament instability from the injury, severe cervical deformity, or if the patient is morbidly obese, older, cachectic, or noncompliant.

Infection at the tongs or pin insertion sites is a potential problem. Preventive care is based on agency protocol. A common protocol involves cleansing sites twice a day with chlorhexidine. Antibiotic ointment is then applied to act as a mechanical barrier to the entrance of bacteria. Patient and caregiver teaching for a patient with a halo vest is outlined in Table 65.6.

Patients with stable thoracic or lumbar spine injuries may be immobilized with a custom thoracolumbar sacral orthosis (TLSO, body jacket). TLSO limits spinal flexion, extension, and rotation. A Jewett brace may be used instead to restrict forward flexion. Unstable injuries may require surgical decompression and fusion in addition to the TLSO or lumbosacral orthotic (LSO).

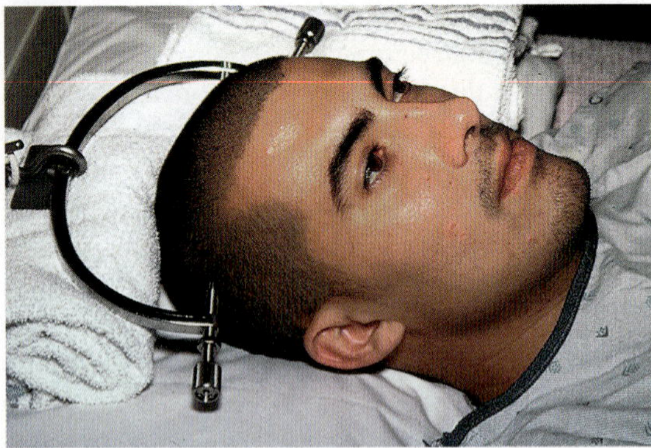

Fig. 65.6 Cervical traction is attached to tongs inserted in the skull. A U-shaped cervical traction is attached to tongs and inserted into the skull of a patient. The tongs cover the upper portion of the head. (Courtesy Michael S. Clement, MD, Mesa, AZ.)

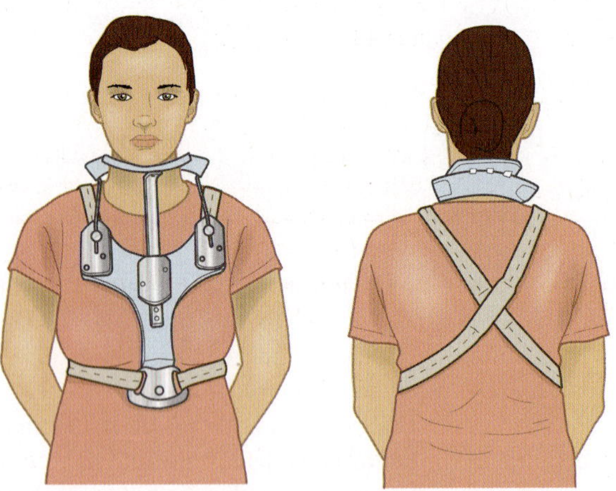

Fig. 65.7 Sternal-occipital-mandibular immobilizer brace.

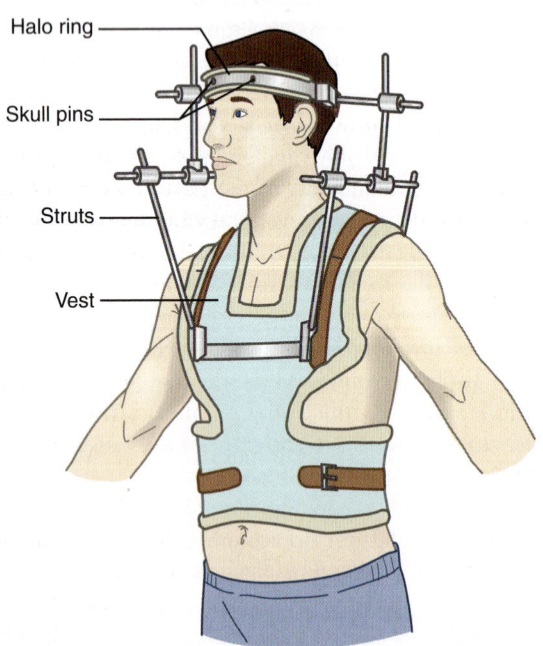

Fig. 65.8 Halo vest. The halo traction brace immobilizes the cervical spine, which allows patients to ambulate and take part in self-care.

TABLE 65.6 PATIENT & CAREGIVER TEACHING

Halo Vest Care

Include the following instructions when teaching patients and caregivers management of a halo vest:

1. Inspect the pins on the halo traction ring. Report to HCP if pins are loose or signs of infection are present, including redness, tenderness, swelling, or drainage at insertion sites.
2. Clean around pin sites carefully with chlorhexidine, water, or half-strength peroxide on a cotton swab as directed.
3. Apply antibiotic ointment as prescribed.
4. For skin care, have patient lie down with the head resting on a pillow to reduce pressure on the brace. Loosen 1 side of the vest. Gently wash the skin under the vest with soap and water, rinse area, and then dry it thoroughly. At the same time, check the skin for pressure points, redness, swelling, bruising, or chafing. Close the open side and repeat the procedure on the other side.
5. If the vest becomes wet or damp, carefully dry it with a blow dryer.
6. Encourage patient to use assistive device (e.g., cane, walker) to improve balance; encourage use of flat shoes.
7. Teach patient to turn the entire body, not just the head and neck, when trying to look sideways.
8. Keep a set of wrenches close to the halo vest in case they are needed for an emergency.
9. Mark the vest strap to maintain consistent buckling and fit.
10. Avoid grabbing bars or vest to help the patient.
11. Keep sheepskin pad under vest. Change and wash pad at least weekly.
12. If perspiration or itching is a problem, encourage patient to wear a cotton T-shirt under the sheepskin. The T-shirt can be modified with a Velcro seam closure on one side.

Skin care is vital because decreased sensation and circulation increase the risk for skin breakdown. Remove the backboard as soon as possible. Replace it with other forms of immobilization to prevent skin breakdown in the coccygeal and occipital areas. Fit cervical collars properly. Assess areas under any device used for immobilization.

Respiratory care. Respiratory complications are the leading cause of mortality.[4] Respiratory dysfunction is present in up to 65% of patients with cervical SCI. During the first 48 hours after injury, spinal cord edema may increase the level of dysfunction, and respiratory distress may occur. Injury at or above C4 affects the phrenic nerve. This leads to the diaphragm, and breathing can stop.

Monitor for respiratory compromise. Be prepared for quick action if arrest occurs. Regularly assess (1) breath sounds, (2) arterial blood gases (ABGs), (3) tidal volume, (4) vital capacity, (5) skin color, (6) breathing patterns (especially use of accessory muscles), (7) subjective comments about the ability to breathe, and (8) amount and color of sputum. A Pao_2 greater than 60 mm Hg and a $Paco_2$ less than 45 mm Hg are acceptable values in patients with uncomplicated tetraplegia. Patients who are unable to count to 20 aloud without taking a breath need immediate attention.

Provide measures to maintain ventilation. Apply O_2 and provide appropriate ventilatory support until ABGs stabilize. If exhaustion from labored breathing occurs or ABGs show inadequate oxygenation, endotracheal intubation or tracheostomy and mechanical ventilation are needed. Patients with chest trauma or difficulty weaning from the ventilator may need a tracheostomy for long-term airway management.

Clearing secretions reduces the risk for lung complications and respiratory failure.[4] Perform tracheal suctioning if crackles or coarse breath sounds are present. Chest physiotherapy and assisted (augmented) coughing can help. Perform assisted coughing either manually or mechanically with an insufflation-exsufflation device. Encourage the use of incentive spirometry.

The older adult has more difficulty responding to hypoxia and hypercapnia. Chest physiotherapy, adequate oxygenation, and proper pain management are needed to maximize respiratory function and gas exchange.

Cardiovascular care. Heart rate is slowed, often to less than 60 beats/min, because of unopposed vagal response. Any increase in vagal stimulation, as occurs with turning or suctioning, can cause cardiac arrest. Loss of SNS tone in peripheral vessels results in chronic low BP with potential orthostatic hypotension. The lack of muscle tone to aid venous return can cause sluggish blood flow and predispose patients to VTE. Dysrhythmias may occur.

Frequently assess vital signs. If bradycardia is symptomatic, give an anticholinergic drug, such as atropine. Some patients need a temporary or permanent pacemaker. Maintain SBP greater than 90 mm Hg and keep MAP between 85 and 90 mm Hg for the first 7 days after SCI.[9] Manage hypotension with fluid replacement and a vasopressor agent, such as phenylephrine or norepinephrine.

Maintain a normal blood volume. If blood loss has occurred from other injuries, monitor hemoglobin and hematocrit and give blood according to protocol. Assess for hypovolemic shock from hemorrhage.

Orthostatic hypotension is likely to occur in patients with injury at T6 and above. Patients may have lightheadedness, dizziness, and nausea. Assess orthostatic BP when mobilizing patients. Some lose consciousness when moved from the bed to a chair. For symptomatic patients, use an abdominal binder and graduated compression stockings to promote venous return. Drugs used to increase intravascular volume include salt tablets and fludrocortisone. Midodrine may be given to promote blood vessel contraction and increase venous return.

Use LMWH or low-dose heparin in combination with intermittent pneumatic compression devices or graduated compression stockings to promote venous return and reduce the risk for VTE. Remove stockings every 8 hours for skin care. Assess thighs and calves every shift for signs of VTE. Regularly perform range-of-motion (ROM) exercises and stretching. Continue VTE prophylaxis for 3 months after injury.

Fluid and nutrition management. During the first 48 to 72 hours after the injury, the GI tract may stop functioning *(paralytic ileus)*. We may insert a nasogastric (NG) tube if severe ileus occurs. Because the patient cannot have oral intake, monitor fluid and electrolyte status.

We estimate that 52% of patients entering rehabilitation facilities are malnourished. This makes nutrition support early in the acute phase of injury imperative.[13] Nutrition should be started within the first 72 hours after injury. Specific solutions and additives are determined by individual requirements. Because of severe catabolism, a high-protein, high-calorie diet is needed for energy and tissue repair. Patients who cannot be fed through the GI system, either orally or with enteral nutrition (EN), may receive parenteral nutrition (PN).

Once bowel sounds are present or flatus is passed and the patient is off mechanical ventilation, they have a formal swallow evaluation. If no risk for aspiration is identified, gradually introduce oral food and fluids. If the patient fails the swallow evaluation or is unable to eat because of an endotracheal tube or tracheostomy, a feeding tube may be placed in the stomach or jejunum (see Chapter 44).

CHECK YOUR PRACTICE

You are working in the spinal cord unit. Your 28-year-old male patient with SCI at T6 weighs 168 lb. When he was admitted 3 weeks ago, he weighed 196 lb. He asks you, "Well, what is my weight? Are you going to make me eat now? You know you can't do that."

- What assessment data do you need to obtain?
- What interventions would help him avoid further weight loss and regain lean body mass?

Patients may have anorexia due to depression, boredom with agency food, or discomfort at being fed (often by a hurried person). Some patients have a normally small appetite. Sometimes refusal to eat is a way of asserting control. If a patient is not eating adequately, assess the cause.

Based on assessment findings, make a contract with patients with mutual goal setting for the diet. This contract gives patients increased control and often results in improved intake. General measures may be effective. For example, provide a pleasant eating environment and allow adequate time to eat (including any self-feeding the patient can achieve). Encourage the family to bring in special foods. Plan social rewards for eating.

Consult a dietitian to ensure evaluation of laboratory markers and develop the treatment plan. Keep a calorie count. Record daily weight to evaluate progress. If possible, have patients take part in recording calorie intake. Diet supplements may be needed to meet nutrition goals. Increase diet fiber to promote bowel function.

Bladder and bowel management. Immediately after the injury, urine retention occurs because of the loss of autonomic and reflex control of the bladder and sphincter *(neurogenic bladder)*. Because there is no sensation of fullness, overdistention of the bladder can result in reflux into the kidney and cause renal failure. Bladder overdistention may even result in rupture of the bladder. An indwelling catheter may be inserted soon after injury. Maintain catheter patency. Prevent kinking and ensure free flow of urine. While the catheter is in place, encourage a large fluid intake.

Catheter-acquired urinary tract infection (CAUTI) is a common problem. Use strict aseptic technique for catheter care to prevent infection. The best way to prevent CAUTI is regular and complete bladder drainage. Once the patient is stabilized, assess the best means of managing long-term urinary function. Clean intermittent catheterization (CIC) is the preferred method for emptying the bladder. CAUTI and CIC are discussed in Chapter 50.

CIC should be done 4 to 6 times daily to prevent bacterial overgrowth from urinary stasis. Keep urine residuals under 500 mL to prevent bladder distention. If the urine is cloudy or has a strong odor or if patients develop symptoms of a urinary tract infection (UTI) (e.g., chills, fever, malaise), send a specimen for culture.

Consider age-related changes in renal function. The older adult is more likely to develop renal stones. Older males may have benign prostatic hyperplasia, which may interfere with urinary flow and complicate management of urinary problems. It can affect the ability to complete CIC.

Start a bowel program to combat constipation from neurogenic bowel. This involves inserting a rectal stimulant (suppository or small-volume enema) daily at a regular time, followed by gentle digital stimulation or manual evacuation until evacuation is complete. At first, the program may be done in bed with the patient in the side-lying position. As soon as the patient has resumed sitting, they should be in the upright position on a padded bedside commode chair. These programs typically take 30 to 60 minutes to complete. Measures to reduce constipation include adequate fluid intake, a diet high in fiber and vegetables, and increased activity and exercise as able.

Temperature control. Monitor the environment to maintain an appropriate temperature. Assess temperature. Do not use excess covers or unduly expose a patient (e.g., during bathing). If an infection with fever develops, implement measures to control temperature (see Table 12.5).

Stress ulcers. Stress ulcers can occur because of the physiologic response to severe trauma and psychologic stress. Peak incidence of stress ulcers is 6 to 14 days after injury. Monitor the hematocrit for a slow drop. Prophylactic histamine (H_2)-receptor blockers or proton pump inhibitors (e.g., pantoprazole) decrease HCl secretion and prevent ulcers.

Sensory deprivation. To prevent sensory deprivation, compensate for absent sensations by stimulating patients above the level of injury. Conversation, music, and interesting foods can be a part of the care plan. If the head of the bed must stay flat, provide prism glasses to help patients read and watch television.

Help patients avoid withdrawing from the environment. Promote adequate rest and sleep. Assess for changes in mood. Depression is common.

Pain management. Musculoskeletal nociceptive pain can develop from injuries to bones, muscles, and ligaments. The pain is worse with movement or palpation. Antiinflammatory drugs, such as ibuprofen, may help with pain. Opioids may be used to manage nociceptive pain.

Visceral nociceptive pain is a dull, tender, or cramping pain in the thorax, abdomen, or pelvis. It may originate in the bladder or bowel. Assess bowel and bladder function to avoid bladder distention or constipation. Other causes of nociceptive pain include UTI and renal stones. Notify the HCP if a patient has persistent pain despite treatment. Diagnostic testing may be needed to determine the cause.

Neuropathic pain in the initial phase is usually at the level of SCI. It may occur on one or both sides of the body within the affected dermatome and up to 3 levels below. Patients will describe hot, burning, tingling, shooting, electric pain. Pregabalin (Lyrica) and gabapentin (Neurontin) may reduce symptoms.

Neuropathic pain can occur months or years after SCI, become chronic, and negatively affect sleep. Mood, sudden noise, constipation, and infection can affect the pain. Teach patients and caregivers about possible pain triggers and offer relaxation therapy. Treatments may include tricyclic antidepressants, intrathecal drugs, epidural stimulation, and destructive surgical intervention.

Skin care. The most common long-term complication in SCI is a pressure injury (PI). PIs can occur quickly and lead to infection and sepsis. Constant pressure in 1 position can compress blood vessels and limit blood supply, causing cell death and PI. Factors that increase risk for PI include duration of SCI, higher level of injury, smoking, being underweight, and comorbid medical conditions.[14]

Preventing PI requires diligent nursing care. Perform a risk assessment with a daily skin assessment. Areas most vulnerable to breakdown include the sacrum, ischia, trochanters, and heels. Assess surgical incisions for healing and skin integrity under collars and braces. Regularly assess nutrition status. Both weight loss and gain can contribute to skin breakdown. Teach patients and caregivers PI prevention.[14]

A consult with the wound, ostomy, and continence nurse (WOCN) can assist with prevention and management strategies (e.g., surface overlays).[14] Monitor incontinence. Implement neurogenic bowel and bladder management. Apply skin barrier creams.

Carefully position and reposition the patient at least every 2 hours. Gradually increase the times between turns if no redness over bony prominences is seen when turning. While the patient is supine in bed, float the heels to reduce pressure. Consider prophylactic dressings to prevent sacral and heel injury. Move patients carefully during turns and transfers to avoid stretching and shear.

We often place patients on special beds (Fig. 65.9). Kinetic therapy involves continuous side-to-side rotation to 40 degrees or more to help prevent lung complications. This lateral rotation redistributes pressure, helping to prevent PIs. We may use specialty mattresses.[14] When patients are moved to a chair or wheelchair, use pressure-relieving cushions. Schedule pressure relief every 15 to 20 minutes when patients are in a chair. It should last 30 to 60 seconds each time.

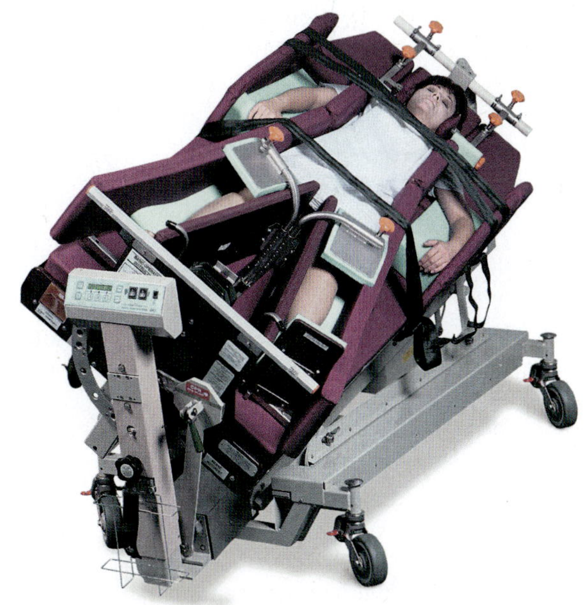

Fig. 65.9 RotoRest Therapy System helps prevent and treat lung complications for immobile patients, including those with unstable cervical, thoracic, and lumbar fractures. Kinetic therapy, the continual side-to-side bilateral rotation, redistributes pulmonary blood flow and mobilizes secretions to improve ventilation and perfusion matching. The therapy system helps to prevent pressure injuries. (Courtesy Arjo Huntleigh, Addison, IL.)

Reflexes. Once spinal cord shock is resolved, return of reflexes may complicate rehabilitation. Lacking control from the higher brain centers, reflexes are often hyperactive and have exaggerated responses. Penile erection can occur from a variety of stimuli, causing embarrassment and discomfort. Spasms ranging from mild twitches to convulsive movements below the level of injury may occur. Patients or caregivers may interpret this reflex activity as a return of function. Tactfully explain the reason for the activity. Teach patients the positive use of these reflexes in sexual, bowel, and bladder retraining. Antispasmodic drugs, such as baclofen (Lioresal), dantrolene (Dantrium), and tizanidine (Zanaflex), may help control spasms. Botulism toxin injections may be given to treat severe spasticity.

Autonomic dysreflexia. The return of reflexes after the resolution of spinal shock means patients with injury at T6 or higher may develop autonomic dysreflexia. **Autonomic dysreflexia (AD)** is a massive, uncompensated cardiovascular reaction mediated by the SNS. It involves stimulation of sensory receptors below the level of the SCI. The intact SNS below the level of injury responds to the stimulation with a reflex arteriolar vasoconstriction that increases BP. The parasympathetic nervous system cannot directly counteract these responses via the injured spinal cord. Baroreceptors in the carotid sinus and aorta sense the hypertension and stimulate the parasympathetic system. This causes a decrease in heart rate. Visceral and peripheral vessels do not dilate because efferent impulses cannot pass through the injured spinal cord. The higher the level of the SCI, the greater the risk of developing AD.[15]

The most common precipitating cause is a distended bladder or rectum. However, any sensory stimulation, including contraction of the bladder or rectum, skin stimulation, or stimulation of pain receptors, can cause AD. AD is a life-threatening condition that requires immediate resolution. Proper identification and elimination of the inciting stimulus for AD can resolve the event. If uncorrected, it can lead to status epilepticus, stroke, myocardial infarction, and even death.

Manifestations include hypertension, throbbing headache, marked diaphoresis above the level of injury, bradycardia (30 to 40 beats/min), piloerection from pilomotor spasm, flushing of the skin above the level of injury, blurred vision or spots, nasal congestion, anxiety, and nausea. Measure BP when a patient with SCI reports a headache. Suspect AD with SBP elevation of 20 to 40 mm Hg above baseline.[15]

Immediate interventions include elevating the head of the bed 45 degrees or sitting the patient upright (to lower the BP) and determining the cause (bowel impaction, urinary retention, UTI, PI, tight clothing). Notify the HCP. The most common cause is bladder irritation. Immediate catheterization to relieve bladder distention may be done. Instill lidocaine jelly in the urethra before catheterization. If a catheter is already in place, check it for kinks or folds. If it is plugged, perform small-volume irrigation slowly and gently to open the catheter or insert a new catheter.

Stool impaction can cause AD. Apply an anesthetic ointment to avoid increasing symptoms, and then perform a digital rectal examination (if trained). Remove all skin stimuli, such as constrictive clothing and tight shoes. Monitor BP often during the episode. If symptoms persist after the source has been relieved, the HCP may order a rapid-onset and short-duration agent, such as nitroglycerin, nitroprusside, or hydralazine. Continue careful monitoring until vital signs stabilize.

Teach patients and caregivers to recognize causes and symptoms of AD (Table 65.7). They must understand the life-threatening nature of AD, know how to relieve the cause, and activate the ERS, if needed.

Chronic Care

Rehabilitation of patients with SCI is complex. With physical and psychologic care and intensive and specialized rehabilitation, patients can learn to function at the highest level of wellness. All patients with a new SCI should receive comprehensive inpatient care in a unit or center that specializes in SCI rehabilitation.[16] Rehabilitation is an interprofessional team effort. Team members include rehabilitation nurses, HCPs, physical therapists, occupational therapists, speech therapists, vocational counselors, psychologists, therapeutic recreation specialists, prosthetists, orthotists, case managers, social workers, and dietitians.

Many problems that begin in the acute period become chronic and continue throughout life. Rehabilitation focuses on retraining physiologic processes and extensive patient and

TABLE 65.7 PATIENT & CAREGIVER TEACHING

Autonomic Dysreflexia

For patients at risk for autonomic dysreflexia, include the following information in the teaching plan:

1. Signs and symptoms
    - Sudden onset of acute headache
    - Elevation in BP and/or reduction in pulse rate
    - Flushed face and upper chest (above level of injury) and pale extremities (below level of injury)
    - Sweating above level of injury
    - Nasal congestion
    - Feeling of apprehension
2. Immediate interventions
    - Raise the person to a sitting position.
    - Remove the noxious stimulus (fecal impaction, kinked urinary catheter, tight clothing).
    - Call the HCP if these actions do not relieve the signs and symptoms.
3. Measures to decrease the incidence of autonomic dysreflexia
    - Maintain regular bowel function.
    - If manual rectal stimulation is used to promote bowel function, use a local anesthetic to prevent autonomic dysreflexia.
    - Monitor urine output.
    - Teach patients to wear a Medic Alert bracelet indicating a history of risk for autonomic dysreflexia.

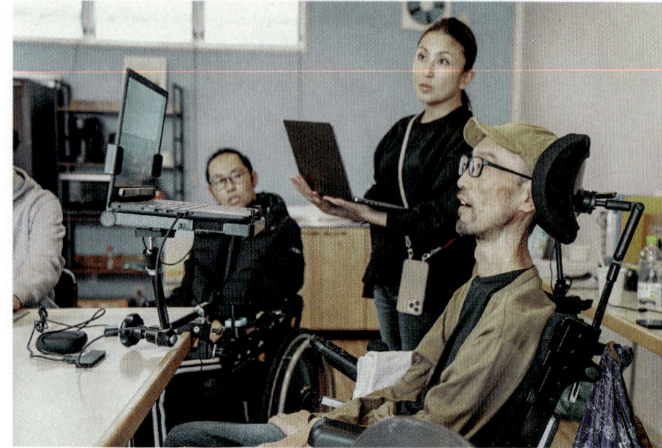

Fig. 65.10 SCI rehabilitation is a complex, team effort. (© tdub303/iStock.com.)

caregiver teaching about how to manage the physiologic and life changes resulting from the injury (Fig. 65.10).

Rehabilitation care depends on patients' goals and needs. Patients are expected to be involved in therapies and learn self-care for several hours each day. Such intensive work at a time when patients are dealing with the sudden change in health and function can be stressful. Progress may be slow. The rehabilitation nurse has a key role in providing encouragement, specialized nursing care, and patient and caregiver teaching and in helping to coordinate efforts of the rehabilitation team.

Respiratory rehabilitation. Patients with mechanical ventilation will need around-the-clock caregivers to provide respiratory hygiene and tracheostomy care. The rehabilitation nurse and respiratory therapist should teach patients and caregivers about home ventilator and tracheostomy care. Patients may need chest percussion or postural drainage to manage secretions to lower the risk for atelectasis and pneumonia. Refer to community agencies as needed.

Some patients with high cervical SCI have improved respiratory function with phrenic nerve stimulators or electronic diaphragmatic pacemakers.[4] These devices are not appropriate for all ventilator-dependent patients. But they are safe and effective for those with an intact phrenic nerve. Some ventilators are portable, allowing ventilator-dependent patients with tetraplegia to be mobile and less dependent.

If a patient was weaned from the ventilator during hospitalization, downsizing (gradual decrease in size) and removing the tracheostomy would be done during rehabilitation. Stress regular assisted coughing, incentive spirometry, and breathing exercises to patients who are not ventilator dependent. They should limit exposure to persons with fever, cold, and cough. Adhering to swallowing precautions (e.g., proper positioning of head and neck) and diet recommendations can prevent aspiration.

Neurogenic bladder. Types of neurogenic bladder are described in Table 65.8. The type of bladder dysfunction determines management options. After the patient's overall condition is stable and assessment shows return of neurologic reflexes, urodynamic testing (see Table 49.11) and a urine culture may be done. Diagnostic and interprofessional care of neurogenic bladder is described in Table 65.9.

Patients with a neurogenic bladder need a comprehensive program to manage bladder function. The goal is to improve quality of life and safety through preserving renal function, minimizing UTI and bladder stones, and developing a plan for urinary continence. Many factors are considered when selecting a bladder management strategy. These include patient preference, upper extremity function, and caregiver availability. For the selected strategy, teach patients and caregivers successful self-management. Review management techniques, how to obtain supplies, care of supplies and equipment, and when to seek health care.

Anticholinergic drugs (e.g., oxybutynin, tolterodine) may be used to suppress bladder contraction. α-Adrenergic blockers (e.g., terazosin, doxazosin) can relax the urethral sphincter. Antispasmodic drugs (e.g., baclofen) may decrease spasticity of pelvic floor muscles. *Botulinum toxin* is an effective alternative in patients with neurogenic detrusor overactivity who cannot tolerate or have an inadequate response to anticholinergic drugs.[17]

Numerous drainage methods are possible. These include bladder reflex retraining (if partial voiding control remains), indwelling catheter, CIC, and external catheter (condom catheter). Evaluate long-term use of an indwelling catheter because of the associated high incidence of CAUTI, fistula formation, and diverticula. However, this is the best option for

TABLE 65.8 **Types of Neurogenic Bladder**

Type	Characteristics	Causes	Manifestations
Uninhibited bladder (spastic, overactive)	• No inhibitions influence time and place of voiding • Bladder empties in response to stretching of bladder wall	• Lesions above the pons • Seen in stroke, brain tumor, brain trauma	• Incontinence, frequency, urgency • Voiding is unpredictable and incomplete

Upper motor neuron bladder (flaccid, spastic/overactive)	• Mixed A type (most common):
	  • Bladder is flaccid and external sphincter is spastic, leading to urinary retention.
	• Mixed B type:
	  • Bladder is spastic with flaccid external sphincter leading to urinary incontinence.
		• Lesions between pons and sacral spinal cord
		• Seen in SCI or multiple sclerosis involving the cervicothoracic spinal cord
			• Detrusor-sphincter dyssynergia
			• Can lead to high bladder pressures and kidney damage from urinary reflex
			• Sensory function impaired

Lower motor neuron bladder (flaccid, underactive, areflexic)	• Bladder acts as if all motor functions were paralyzed • Bladder fills without emptying	• Lower motor neuron injury caused by trauma involving S2–S4 or below • Lesions of cauda equina, pelvic nerves	• If sensory function intact, patient feels bladder distention and hesitancy • No control of micturition, resulting in urinary retention, overdistention of bladder, overflow incontinence, and UTI

TABLE 65.9 **Interprofessional Care**

Neurogenic Bladder

Diagnostic Assessment
- History and physical assessment, including neurologic and pelvic examinations
- Laboratory: Urinalysis, urine culture and sensitivity, blood urea nitrogen, serum creatinine, creatinine clearance
- Urodynamic testing (postvoid residual, cystometric testing, EMG, urethral pressure profile)

Management
- Patient teaching
- Voiding diary
- Bladder retraining: time voiding, manual expression, intermittent catheterization
- Fluid schedule: intake of 1800–2000 mL/day
- Indwelling urinary catheter

Drug Therapy
- Tricyclic antidepressants
- Anticholinergic drugs
- α-Adrenergic blockers
- Antispasmodics
- Botulinum toxin injection into bladder wall

Bladder and/or Urethral Surgical Therapy
- Bladder augmentation
- Sphincter resection or removal *(sphincterotomy)*
- Electrode placement for electrical stimulation
- Urinary diversion
- Urethral stents and balloon dilation
- Artificial urinary sphincter

some patients. Patients with indwelling catheters need to have adequate fluid intake (at least 3 to 4 L/day). Regularly check catheter patency. Frequency of routine catheter changes ranges widely depending on the type of catheter used and agency policy.

CIC is the first-line option for bladder management (see Chapter 50). Assessment is essential in selecting the time interval between catheterizations. At first, catheterization is done every 4 hours. Measure bladder volume before catheterization using bladder ultrasound. If less than 200 mL of urine is present, the time interval until catheterization may be extended. If more than 500 mL of urine is present, the time interval is shortened. CIC is usually done 4 to 6 times daily.

Suprapubic catheters are a safe option in select patients. Because of personal preference or the inability to catheterize as a result of neurologic dysfunction, 30% of patients with SCI use indwelling urethral or suprapubic catheters. The incidence of bacteriuria after catheter introduction is 5% to 10% per day.

Traditional bladder management options include *urinary diversion surgery* for patients with recurrent UTI with renal involvement or recurring stones. Surgical treatment includes bladder neck revision (sphincterotomy), bladder augmentation (augmentation cystoplasty), perineal ureterostomy, cystotomy, vesicostomy, and anterior urethral transplantation. Placement of a sacral cord stimulator, penile prosthesis, or artificial sphincter is possible. Urinary diversion procedures are discussed in Chapter 50.

Neurogenic bowel. Management of bowel evacuation is necessary for patients with SCI because voluntary control may be lost. Usual measures for preventing constipation include a high-fiber diet and adequate fluid intake (see Table 47.9).

Patient and caregiver teaching is needed to promote successful independent bowel management. Guidelines related to bowel management are outlined in Table 65.10.

These measures may not be adequate to stimulate evacuation. Suppositories (e.g., bisacodyl) or small-volume enemas and digital stimulation (done 20 to 30 minutes after suppository insertion) by the nurse or patient may be needed. In patients with an upper motor neuron injury, digital stimulation can relax the external sphincter to promote defecation. A stool softener can help regulate stool consistency. Oral stimulant laxatives should be used only if necessary and not on a regular basis.

Valsalva maneuver and manual stimulation are useful in patients with lower motor neuron injuries. Because the Valsalva maneuver requires intact abdominal muscles, it is used in patients with injuries below T12. In general, a bowel movement every other day is adequate. However, consider preinjury bowel patterns. Fecal incontinence can result from too much stool softener or a fecal impaction.

Timing of defecation is important. Planning bowel evacuation for 30 to 60 minutes after the first meal of the day may enhance success by taking advantage of the gastrocolic reflex induced by eating. This reflex may also be stimulated by drinking a warm beverage right after the meal. Discuss timing of the bowel program so there are no interruptions when the patient is doing therapy (e.g., swimming pool therapy). Record all bowel movements, including amount, time, and consistency.

Spasticity. Spasticity can be both beneficial and undesirable. It aids with mobility, especially for patients with incomplete SCI. Spasticity improves circulation by promoting venous return, decreasing orthostatic hypotension and the risk for VTE. Unfortunately, patients with marked spasticity and tone may have difficulty with positioning and mobility from spasms. Spasms can cause significant pain and make activities of daily living (ADLs) difficult.

You can use the Ashworth and Modified Ashworth Scales to evaluate spasticity. Treatment includes ROM exercises to prevent muscle and joint tightness and reduce the risk for contracture. Antispasmodic drugs, such as baclofen or tizanidine, may be given. Botulinum toxin injection is useful for specific muscle involvement.

Skin care. Prevention of PI is part of the lifelong treatment plan. Nurses are responsible for teaching patients and caregivers about daily skin care. PI may not be noticed until severe damage has occurred. Include information on the importance of adequate nutrition to skin condition. Provide anticipatory guidance about potential risks. Patient and caregiver teaching about skin care is outlined in Table 65.11.

Pain management. Acute pain from the initial injury may persist during the first few weeks of rehabilitation. Chronic pain can result from overuse of muscles in the shoulders and arms for movement and repositioning. Pain often disrupts sleep. Assess, evaluate, and treat pain routinely. Use analgesics and interventions, such as massage and repositioning, to help patients during therapy. Patients may benefit from referral to a pain management specialist.

TABLE 65.10 PATIENT & CAREGIVER TEACHING

Bowel Management After SCI

For a patient with SCI, include the following information about bowel management in the teaching plan:

1. Optimal nutrition intake includes:
   - 3 well-balanced meals each day
   - 2 servings from the milk group
   - 2 or more servings from the meat group, including beef, pork, poultry, eggs, fish
   - 4 or more servings from the vegetable and fruit groups
   - 4 or more servings from the bread and cereal group
2. Fiber intake should be about 20–30 g/day. Increase the amount of fiber eaten gradually over 1–2 wk.
3. Consume at least 2–3 L of fluid per day unless contraindicated. Drink water or fruit juices (fluid softens hard stools). Limit caffeinated beverages, such as coffee, tea, and cola (caffeine stimulates fluid loss through urination).
4. Avoid foods that produce gas (e.g., beans) or upper GI upset (e.g., spicy foods).
5. Timing: Follow a regular schedule for bowel elimination. A good time is 30 min after the first meal of the day.
6. Position: If possible, an upright position with feet flat on the floor or on a step stool enhances bowel evacuation. Staying on the toilet, commode, or bedpan for longer than 20–30 min may cause skin breakdown. Based on stability, someone may need to stay with the patient.
7. Activity: Exercise is important for bowel function. In addition to improving muscle tone, it increases appetite and GI transit time. Exercise muscles, including stretching, ROM, position changing, and functional movement.
8. Drug treatment: Suppositories may be needed to stimulate a bowel movement. Manual stimulation of the rectum may be helpful in starting defecation. Use stool softeners as needed to regulate stool consistency. Use oral laxatives only if necessary.

Sexuality. Sexuality is an important issue regardless of age or gender. Open discussion about sexual rehabilitation is essential. A nurse or other rehabilitation professional trained in sexual counseling should provide support for the patient and the partner. Alternative methods of obtaining sexual satisfaction, such as oral-genital sex, may be options. Explicit films may help, such as a film showing sexual activities of a patient with paraplegia and a nondisabled partner. Use graphics cautiously because they may focus too much on the mechanics of sex rather than on the relationship.

We need to know the level and completeness of injury to understand a male patient's potential for orgasm, erection, fertility, and capacity for sexual satisfaction. Males normally have 2 types of erections: psychogenic and reflex. The process of *psychogenic erection* begins in the brain with sexual thoughts. Signals from the brain are sent through the nerves of the spinal cord to the T10–L2 levels. The signals are then relayed to the penis and trigger an erection. Males with low-level incomplete injuries are more likely to have psychogenic erection than those with higher-level incomplete injuries. Males with complete injuries are less likely to have psychogenic erection.[18]

TABLE 65.11 PATIENT & CAREGIVER TEACHING

Skin Care After SCI

To prevent skin breakdown in patients with SCI, include the following instructions when teaching patients and caregivers:

Change Position Frequently
- If in a wheelchair, lift self and shift weight every 15–30 min.
- If in bed, change position with a regular turning schedule (at least every 2 h) that includes sides, back, and abdomen.
- Use pressure-reducing mattresses and wheelchair cushions (not eggcrate).
- Use pillows to protect bony prominences when in bed.

Monitor Skin Condition
- Inspect skin often for areas of redness, swelling, and breakdown.
- If a wound develops, follow standard wound care procedures.

Protect Skin
- Do not sit too close to fires, space heaters, or other sources of heat.
- Use sunscreen liberally when outdoors.
- Keep fingernails trimmed to avoid scratches and abrasions.
- Do not wear clothes that are too tight or too loose.
- Dress warmly in cold weather to prevent frostbite.
- Do not put hot food in your lap without protection.

A *reflex erection* occurs with direct physical contact to the penis or other erotic areas. This short-lived, uncontrolled erection is involuntary. It does not require sexually stimulating thoughts. Most males with SCI can have a reflex erection with physical stimulation if the S2–S4 nerve pathways are not damaged.

Treatment for erectile dysfunction includes drugs, vacuum devices, and surgery. Phosphodiesterase inhibitors (e.g., sildenafil) are the first-line treatment in males with SCI between T6 and L5. Sexual stimulation is needed to get an erection after taking the medication. Penile injection of vasoactive substances (papaverine, alprostadil, or a combination) is another treatment. Risks include scarring, bruising, and infection. Use may lead to priapism. Vacuum suction devices use negative pressure to encourage blood flow into the penis. A constriction band placed at the base of the penis maintains the erection. The main surgical option is implantation of a penile prosthesis.[18] Erectile dysfunction is discussed in Chapter 59.

SCI affects male fertility, causing poor sperm motility and ejaculatory dysfunction. Sperm retrieval methods include penile vibratory stimulation and rectal probe electroejaculation. Surgical removal of sperm is a last resort for sperm retrieval. Once retrieved, sperm can be directly injected into an egg via intracytoplasmic sperm injection (ICSI). These techniques have changed the prognosis for males with SCI to father children from unlikely to a reasonable chance of successful outcomes.[18]

The effect of SCI on female sexual response is less clear. A female of childbearing age with SCI usually stays fertile. The injury does not affect the ability to become pregnant or deliver normally through the birth canal. Menses may cease for as long as 6 months after injury. If sexual activity is resumed, discuss protection against unplanned pregnancy. Pregnancy increases the risk for diabetes and UTI and higher rates of AD, PI, increased spasticity, and catheter-related issues. Labor and delivery have high rates of complications.[19]

Care must be taken not to dislodge an indwelling catheter during sexual activity. Patients with an external catheter should refrain from fluids and remove the catheter before sexual activity. Teach patients about the risk for AD. The bowel program should include evacuation on the morning of sexual activity. Encourage the patient to tell the partner that incontinence is always possible. The female may need a water-soluble lubricant to supplement decreased vaginal secretions and ease vaginal penetration. Females with some residual pelvic innervation can achieve orgasm.[20]

Grief and depression. Patients with SCI may feel an overwhelming sense of loss. They may temporarily lose control over everyday activities as they depend on others for ADLs and for life-sustaining measures. Patients may feel they are useless and burdens to their families. At a life stage when independence is of great importance, they may be totally dependent on others.

Working through grief is a hard, lifelong process for which patients need support and encouragement. Table 65.12 outlines the grief response to SCI and nursing interventions. Your role in grief work is to provide support and to allow mourning as part of the rehabilitation process. Maintaining hope is important during the grieving process. It should not be viewed as denial. With recent advances in rehabilitation, patients are often independent physically and discharged from the rehabilitation center before completing the grief process.

The goal of recovery is related more to adjustment than to acceptance. *Adjustment* implies the ability to go on with living with certain limitations. Problem-based strategies are effective in supporting positive adjustment. When the patient accepts the current new normal, levels of coping and adjustment are improved. Nonacceptance is more predictive of psychologic distress, disengagement, denial, fantasy, and drug and alcohol use.

Include and encourage patients to participate in care planning. A primary nurse relationship is helpful. To adjust, patients need continual support throughout the rehabilitation process in the form of acceptance, affection, and caring. Be attentive when a patient needs to talk and sensitive to needs at various stages of the grief process.

Depression after SCI is common and disabling. Some patients become clinically depressed and need treatment for depression. Evaluation by a psychiatric nurse or psychiatrist is recommended. Treatment may include drugs and therapy. Treatment is maximized when the patient's personal preferences are identified and care is tailored to patient needs (Box 65.1).

Caregivers need counseling to avoid promoting dependency in the patient through guilt or misplaced sympathy. A support group of family members and friends of patients with SCI can help them increase their participation and knowledge of the grieving process, physical problems, rehabilitation plan, and meaning of the disability.

TABLE 65.12 Grief Response in SCI

Patient Behavior	Nursing Intervention
Shock and Denial	
Struggle for survival, complete dependence, excess sleep, withdrawal, fantasies, unrealistic expectations	• Provide honest information. • Use simple diagrams to explain injury. • Encourage patient to begin road to recovery. • Establish agreement to use and improve all current abilities while not denying the possibility of future improvement.
Anger	
Refusal to discuss paralysis, ↓ self-esteem, manipulation, hostile and abusive language	• Coordinate care with patient and encourage self-care. • Support family members. • Use humor appropriately. • Allow patient outbursts of emotions. • Do not allow fixation on injury.
Depression	
Sadness, pessimism, anorexia, nightmares, insomnia, agitation, "blues," suicidal preoccupation, refusal to take part in any self-care activities	• Encourage family involvement and use of community resources. • Plan graded steps in rehabilitation to give success with minimal opportunity for frustration. • Give cheerful and willing assistance with ADLs. • Avoid sympathy. • Use firm kindness.
Adjustment and Acceptance	
Planning for future, actively taking part in therapy, finding personal meaning in experience and continuation of growth, returning to premorbid personality	• Remember patients have unique personalities. • Balance support systems to encourage independence. • Set goals with patient input. • Emphasize potential.

BOX 65.1 ETHICAL/LEGAL DILEMMAS

Right to Refuse Treatment

Situation

R.D., a 25-year-old male, had an SCI to C7–C8 after a motorcycle accident. He was diagnosed with anterior cord syndrome and has motor paralysis. He has become very depressed and no longer wishes to live. Because of his emotional state, R.D. is now refusing to eat. Can we force him to receive enteral nutrition (EN)?

Ethical/Legal Points for Consideration

- Withholding treatment in a newly injured but otherwise healthy young adult may present an ethical dilemma for some nurses. They may consider it assisted suicide and believe that it violates the ethical principles of beneficence and nonmaleficence.
- A competent adult has the right to consent to or refuse medical treatment under the right to privacy, the Fourteenth Amendment of the Constitution, and case law (*Cruzan v. Director, Missouri Department of Health,* 497 U.S. 261, 1990. Retrieved from www.supreme.justia.com/cases/federal/us/497/261). Case law has supported the concept that forced treatment is battery (unlawful use of force on somebody). A mentally competent, physically incapacitated adult can refuse EN. The health agency must follow the patient's wishes (*Bouvia v. Superior Court,* 1986. Retrieved from http://law.justia.com/cases/california/calapp3d/179/1127.html).
- To be competent to take part in informed consent or refusal, an adult must be able to understand the information provided about the procedure or treatment, consider choices among available alternatives, and make a choice based on values and preferences. Depression may not be a factor in determining competency to make informed treatment choices.
- If, after adequate evaluation and treatment for pain, depression, or other medical conditions, the patient persists in their refusal, their wishes must be respected.
- Refusal to eat or drink has never been upheld as illegal, and the alternative—forced eating and drinking—is clearly a violation of patient rights and the criminal act of battery.

Discussion Questions

1. What are your feelings about requests to withhold treatment in a young person with a newly acquired disability?
2. What resources are available to help R.D., his family, and nursing staff deal with this emotionally charged and ethically complex situation?

◆ Evaluation

Expected outcomes are that patients with SCI will:

- Maintain adequate ventilation and have no signs of respiratory distress
- Maintain adequate circulation and BP
- Maintain intact skin over bony prominences
- Maintain adequate nutrition
- Establish a bowel and bladder management program
- Have no episodes of AD

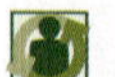 Gerontologic Considerations: SCI

Falls are the leading cause of SCI for people aged 65 and older. Older adults with traumatic injuries have more complications, are hospitalized longer, and have higher mortality rates. Rehabilitation may take longer because of preexisting conditions and poorer health status at the time of initial injury. Chronic illnesses can have a serious impact on older adults living with SCI. As patients with SCI age, both aging changes and length of time since injury can affect functional ability. For example, bowel and bladder dysfunction can increase with the duration and severity of SCI.

Health promotion and screening are important for older patients with SCI. Daily skin inspections and UTI prevention measures are critical. Regular breast examinations for females and prostate cancer screening for males are recommended. Heart disease is the most common cause of mortality among older adults with SCI. The lack of sensation, including chest pain, in persons with high-level injuries may mask acute myocardial ischemia. Altered autonomic nervous system function and decreases in physical activity can place patients at risk for heart problems, including hypertension.

SPINAL CORD TUMORS

Spinal cord tumors can have a devastating impact due to spinal compression and neurologic dysfunction. We classify tumors as *primary* (arising from some part of the spinal cord, dura, nerves, or vessels) or *secondary* (from primary growths in other places in the body that have metastasized to the spinal cord).

Etiology and Pathophysiology

Spinal cord tumors are either *extradural* (outside the dura), *intradural-extramedullary* (between the spinal cord and dura), or *intramedullary* (within the substance of the spinal cord itself; Fig. 65.11 and Table 65.13).

Extradural tumors include metastatic cancer and benign schwannomas. Many patients with cancer will have metastasis to the spine. Metastatic lesions can invade into the dura and compress the spinal cord. Tumors that often metastasize to the spinal epidural space are those that spread to bone, such as prostate, breast, lung, and kidney cancer. Intradural-extramedullary lesions include meningiomas that develop in the arachnoid membrane, schwannomas and neurofibromas that extend from the nerve root, and ependymomas found at the end of the spinal cord. Intramedullary tumors arise from glial or ependymal cells found throughout the entire spinal cord. The most common lesions are astrocytes and ependymomas.[21]

Many spinal cord tumors are slow growing. Their symptoms are caused by the mechanical effects of slow compression and irritation of nerve roots, spinal cord displacement, or gradual obstruction of the blood supply. The slowness of growth does not cause secondary injury as in traumatic SCI. Thus complete functional restoration may be possible when the tumor is removed.

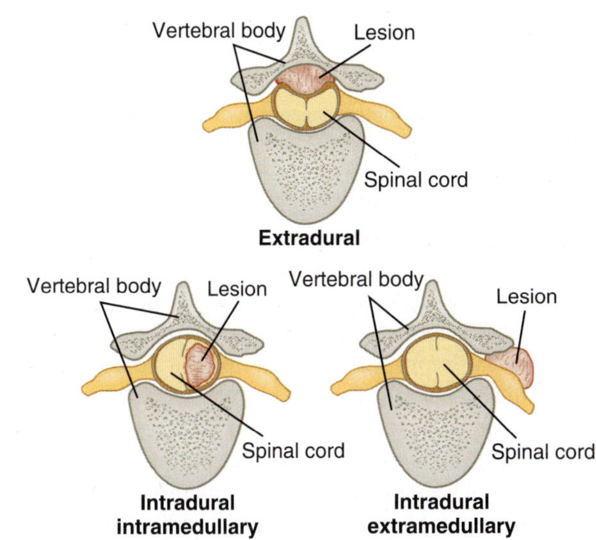

Fig. 65.11 Types of spinal cord tumors.

Clinical Manifestations

Sensory and motor problems may result. The location and extent of the tumor determine the severity and extent of the problem. The most common early symptom of a spinal cord tumor is back pain or pain radiating along the compressed nerve route.[21] Location of the pain depends on the level of compression. Pain may worsen with activity, coughing, straining, and/or lying down. There may be slowly increasing clumsiness, weakness, and spasticity. Paralysis can develop. Sensory disruption occurs as coldness, numbness, and tingling in 1 or more extremities. Neurogenic bowel and bladder are marked by incontinence, constipation, and urgency with difficulty in starting the flow, progressing to retention with overflow incontinence.

Interprofessional and Nursing Management

Extradural tumors can be seen on routine spinal x-rays. Intradural extramedullary and intramedullary tumors require MRI, CT scan, or CT myelogram for detection. Cerebrospinal fluid (CSF) analysis may reveal tumor cells. Patients with tumors suspicious for metastatic disease need an oncology referral and further diagnostic testing to identify the primary cancer.[22]

Spinal cord compression is an emergency. The goal of care is to relieve ischemia related to compression. Indications for surgery depend on the type of tumor and neurologic deficit. Emergency surgery may be needed to decompress the spinal cord, obtain tissue for biopsy, and help determine treatment.[22] Primary spinal tumors may be removed with the goal of cure. In patients with metastatic tumors, treatment is mainly palliative. The goal is to restore or preserve neurologic function, stabilize the spine, and alleviate pain.

Radiation and/or chemotherapy are other treatment options. Surgery and radiation therapy may cause more inflammation. Corticosteroids (e.g., dexamethasone) may be used to relieve tumor-related edema.[22]

Other care goals include relieving pain and maximizing neurologic function. Assess neurologic status before and after treatment. Giving analgesia as needed is an important nursing responsibility. Depending on the amount of neurologic dysfunction, patient care may be similar to that of patients after SCI.

CRANIAL NERVE PROBLEMS

Cranial nerve problems usually involve the motor and/or sensory branches of a single nerve *(mononeuropathies)*. Causes include tumors, trauma, infection, inflammatory processes, and idiopathic (unknown) causes. The 2 cranial nerve problems discussed here are trigeminal neuralgia (TN) and Bell palsy.

TRIGEMINAL NEURALGIA

Trigeminal neuralgia (TN) *(tic douloureux)* is characterized by sudden, usually unilateral, severe, brief, stabbing, recurrent

TABLE 65.13 Classification of Spinal Cord Tumors

Type	Incidence	Treatment	Prognosis
Extradural			
Outside spinal cord in extradural space	Metastatic lesions Benign schwannomas	Relief of cord pressure by surgical laminectomy, radiation, chemotherapy, or combination approach	*Benign:* Excellent with resection *Metastatic:* Poor, treatment usually palliative
Intradural Extramedullary			
Within dura mater but outside spinal cord	Mostly benign Meningiomas, neurofibromas, schwannomas	Complete surgical removal of tumor (if possible) Partial removal followed by radiation	Usually very good if no damage to cord from compression
Intramedullary			
Within spinal cord	Mostly benign Astrocytomas, ependymomas	Complete surgical removal of tumor (if possible) Partial removal followed by radiation	Usually very good if no damage to cord from compression Complete surgical resection of astrocytomas difficult

episodes of pain in the distribution of the trigeminal nerve. It occurs in about 12 per 100,000 Americans each year. TN is more common in females and in people over age 50. We classify TN as *classic* (TN 1) or *atypical* (TN 2). Patients may have both types.

Etiology and Pathophysiology

The trigeminal nerve, the 5th cranial nerve (CN V), has both motor and sensory branches. TN most often affects the sensory (afferent) branches of the second and third divisions (maxillary and mandibular branches) of CN V (Fig. 65.12).

Most cases result from vascular compression of the trigeminal nerve root by an abnormal loop of the superior cerebellar artery. This artery compresses the nerve as it exits the brainstem. Constant compression appears to lead to chronic injury, causing flattening and atrophy of the nerve and damage to the myelin sheath.[23] In some cases, TN may be related to underlying pathology, such as multiple sclerosis (MS), shingles, or masses in the cerebellum or brainstem.

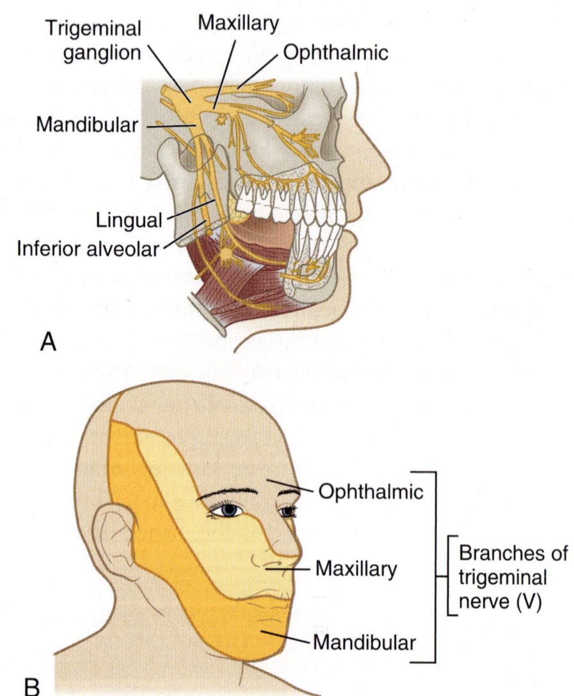

Fig. 65.12 (A) Trigeminal (fifth cranial) nerve and its 3 main divisions: ophthalmic, maxillary, and mandibular nerves. (B) Cutaneous innervation of the head. (Modified from Patton KT, Thibodeau GA: *Anatomy and physiology,* ed 8, St Louis, 2013, Mosby.)

Clinical Manifestations

The pain intensity and lifestyle disruption that accompany TN can cause marked physical and psychologic dysfunction. The first episode of TN is sudden, with a memorable onset. In TN 1, patients have an abrupt onset of waves of excruciating pain. It is described as a burning, knifelike, or lightning-like shock in the lips, upper or lower gums, cheek, forehead, or side of the nose.[23] Facial twitching, grimacing, and frequent blinking and tearing of the eye can occur during the acute attack (giving rise to the term *tic douloureux*). Some patients may have facial sensory loss. Attacks are usually brief, lasting only seconds to 2 or 3 minutes. They may become longer and more intense over time.[23]

Pain episodes are usually started by a triggering mechanism of light touch at a specific point *(trigger zone)* along the distribution of the nerve branches. Precipitating stimuli include chewing, brushing the teeth, feeling a hot or cold blast of air on the face, washing the face, yawning, or even talking. As a result, patients may eat improperly, neglect hygienic practices, wear a cloth over the face, and withdraw from interaction with others. Patients may sleep to cope with pain.

TN 2 manifests as constant aching, burning, crushing, or stabbing pain. The pain has a lower intensity and does not subside completely.[24] The distinct attacks of TN 1 do not occur in TN 2.

Diagnostic Studies

Diagnosis is based almost entirely on history and results from physical and neurologic assessments. Other disorders that cause facial pain are ruled out before TN is diagnosed. MRI can rule out sinusitis, cancer, MS, or masses in the cerebellopontine angle. 3D reconstruction and angiography MRI are helpful with seeing the specific brain anatomy, nerve roots, and vasculature involved. Other specialists, such as neuroradiology, neurosurgery, dentistry, maxillofacial surgery, and pain management, may be involved.

Interprofessional Care

The goal is to relieve pain (Tables 65.14 and 65.15). Electrical nerve stimulation and nerve blocks with local anesthetics or botulinum toxin are options.

Antiseizure drugs may reduce pain by stabilizing the neuronal membrane and blocking nerve firing. These drugs are usually effective in treating TN 1. They are less effective in TN 2. First-line drugs include carbamazepine (Tegretol) and oxcarbazepine (Trileptal). Topiramate (Topamax), clonazepam (Klonopin), phenytoin, lamotrigine (Lamictal), gabapentin, and valproic acid are other options.[24]

Tricyclic antidepressants, such as amitriptyline or nortriptyline, can help treat the constant burning or aching pain. Analgesics or opioids are usually not effective in controlling pain in TN 1.

If a conservative approach is ineffective or patients cannot tolerate drug therapy, surgical therapy is available (Table 65.15 and Fig. 65.13). In percutaneous procedures, affected nerve fibers are damaged to eliminate pain. The different surgical techniques have varying degrees of efficacy and recurrent pain rates.[25]

NURSING MANAGEMENT: TRIGEMINAL NEURALGIA

Patients usually receive outpatient treatment. Assess the attacks in detail, including triggering factors, characteristics, frequency, and pain management techniques. This information helps you to plan care. Evaluate the degree of pain and its effects on lifestyle, drug use, emotional state, and suicidal tendencies. Note behavior, including withdrawal.

Monitor the response to drug therapy. Note any side effects. Discuss complementary pain management measures, such as acupuncture, biofeedback, and yoga. Environment assessment is essential during an acute period to decrease triggering stimuli. The room should be kept at an even, moderate

TABLE 65.14 Interprofessional Care

Trigeminal Neuralgia

Diagnostic Assessment

- History and physical assessment, including neurologic examination
- MRI

Management

- Drug therapy
  - Antiseizure drugs (e.g., carbamazepine, oxcarbazepine, gabapentin)
  - Tricyclic antidepressants (e.g., amitriptyline)
- Local nerve block
- Surgical therapy (Table 65.15)

TABLE 65.15 Therapies for Trigeminal Neuralgia

Procedure	Description
Percutaneous Procedures	
Balloon compression	• Cannula is inserted through cheek and guided to a natural opening in the base of skull. • Soft catheter with a balloon tip is threaded through cannula. • Balloon is inflated and mechanical compression damages trigeminal nerve.
Glycerol rhizotomy (injection into 1 or more branches of trigeminal nerve; Fig. 65.14)	• Thin needle inserted through puncture in cheek and guided through natural opening in base of skull. • Glycerol is injected into trigeminal ganglion. • Procedure can be repeated multiple times.
Radiofrequency thermal lesioning	• Needle passed through cheek through a natural opening in base of skull. • Patient is awakened, and then a small electric current is passed through the needle, causing tingling. • When the needle is positioned so the tingling occurs in the same area of pain, patient is sedated again, then radiofrequency current is used to destroy part of the nerve. • Can result in facial numbness (although some degree of sensation may be retained), corneal anesthesia, trigeminal motor weakness.
Surgical Procedures	
Microvascular decompression, with or without neurectomy	• Small craniotomy done behind the ear (suboccipital craniotomy). • Blood vessels that appear to be compressing the nerve at the root entry zone where it exits the pons are then displaced and repositioned. • If there is no compression, cutting of the nerve (neurectomy) may be done.
Stereotactic radiosurgery (Gamma Knife, CyberKnife)	• Uses stereotactic localization to focus high doses of radiation to area where trigeminal nerve exits the brainstem. • Radiation causes slow formation of a lesion on nerve and disrupts transmission of pain signals to brain. • Pain relief may take several months.

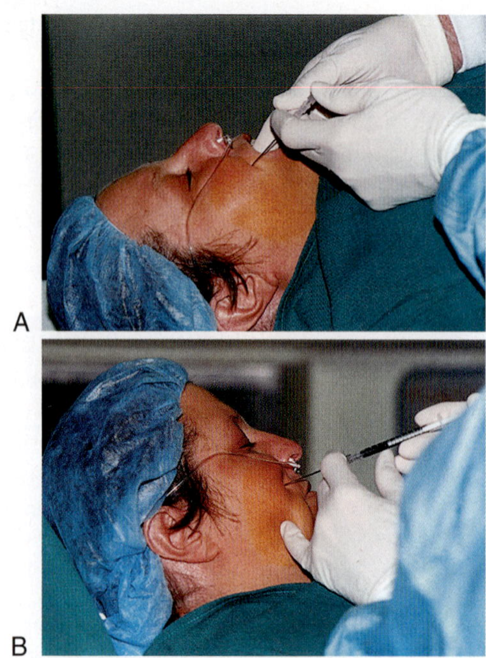

Fig. 65.13 Glycerol rhizotomy for the treatment of trigeminal neuralgia. (A) Patient with trigeminal neuralgia having needle placed. (B) HCP injecting glycerol. (Courtesy Joe Rothrock, Media, PA.)

temperature and free of drafts. Patients may prefer to complete all self-care activities, fearing someone else will inadvertently cause injury.

Assess nutrition status and hygiene, especially oral. Teach patients the importance of nutrition, hygiene, and oral care. Convey understanding if oral neglect is apparent. A small, soft-bristled toothbrush or a warm mouthwash helps promote oral care. Hygiene activities are best done when analgesia is at its peak.

Encourage food that is high in protein and calories and easy to chew. Serve food lukewarm. Encourage small, frequent meals. If oral intake is sharply reduced and patients are nutritionally compromised, an NG tube can be inserted on the unaffected side for EN.

The teaching related to surgery depends on the procedure planned. Patients need to know they will be awake during local procedures to cooperate when corneal and ciliary reflexes and facial sensations are checked. After the procedure, compare pain with the preoperative intensity. Evaluate the corneal reflex, extraocular muscles, hearing, sensation, and facial nerve function (see Chapter 60). If the corneal reflex is impaired, take care to protect the eyes. This includes using artificial tears or eye shields.

After a percutaneous radiofrequency procedure, apply an ice pack to the jaw on the operative side for 3 to 5 hours. To avoid injuring the mouth, patients should not chew on the operative side until sensation has returned. If intracranial surgery was done, general postoperative nursing care after a craniotomy is appropriate. Nursing care related to craniotomy is discussed in Chapter 61.

Plan for regular follow-up care. Teach patients about drug therapy. Encourage patients to keep environment stimuli to a moderate level and use stress management techniques. Long-term management after surgery depends on residual effects of the procedure. If anesthesia is present or the corneal reflex is altered, teach patients to (1) chew on the unaffected side; (2) avoid hot foods or beverages, which can burn the mucous membranes; (3) check the oral cavity after meals to remove food particles; (4) practice good oral hygiene and continue with semiannual dental visits; (5) protect the face against temperature extremes; (6) use an electric razor; (7) wear a protective eye shield and avoid rubbing eyes; and (8) examine eyes regularly for symptoms of infection or irritation.

BELL PALSY

Bell palsy is an acute, usually temporary, facial paresis (or palsy) resulting from damage or trauma of the facial nerve (CN VII). It usually affects only 1 side of the face, but both sides can be affected.

Bell palsy is the most common facial nerve disorder.[26] It occurs equally between males and females. The peak incidence is between ages 15 and 60 years. There is a high incidence during pregnancy and in persons with upper respiratory tract conditions (e.g., flu, colds). Risk factors include obesity, diabetes, and hypertension.[26]

Etiology and Pathophysiology

We do not know the exact cause. Several theories exist. Some think it is a reactivation of herpes simplex virus isoform (HSV-1) and/or herpes zoster virus (HZV). The viral infection causes inflammation, leading to nerve compression and the subsequent clinical features (Fig. 65.14). Another cause may be acute demyelination, similar to what happens in Guillain-Barré syndrome.

The prognosis is often good. The extent of nerve damage determines the extent of recovery. Most begin to get better within 2 weeks after the onset and recover some or all facial function within 6 months. There may be residual effects in some cases, including facial asymmetry or abnormal facial movements.

Clinical Manifestations

CN VII is a mixed cranial nerve with motor, sensory, and autonomic function, which accounts for the manifestations. The key feature is the acute onset of unilateral lower motor facial weakness. Fifty to sixty percent have pain around and behind the ear and neck. Other manifestations include drooping of the eyelid and corner of the mouth, drooling, facial twitching, dryness of the eye or mouth, facial numbness, altered taste, hearing loss, and excess tearing in 1 eye.[26] Most often, these symptoms begin suddenly. They reach their peak within 48 to 72 hours.

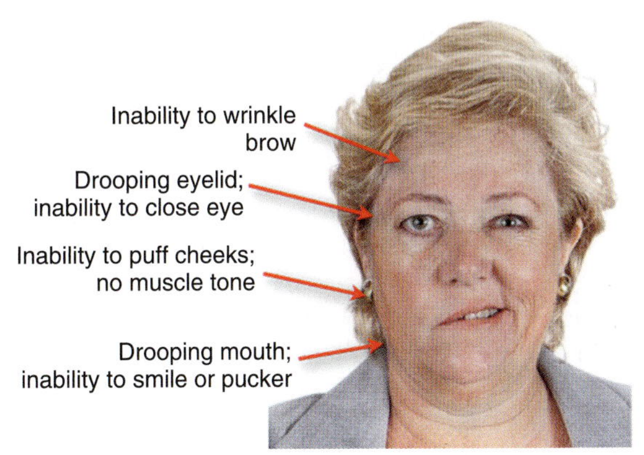

Fig. 65.14 Facial characteristics of a person with Bell palsy. (© Jo Ann Snover/123RF Stock Photo/123rf.com.)

Quality of life is often decreased due to eating, swallowing, speech, and taste problems. Patients may have psychologic withdrawal because of changes in appearance, muscle stretching, and facial spasms and contractures. They may have malnutrition, dehydration, mucous membrane trauma, or corneal abrasions.

Diagnostic Studies

Bell palsy is a clinical diagnosis. No definitive diagnostic test exists. The assessment and typical pattern of onset guide the diagnosis and prognosis. Patients should be referred to a neurologist or otolaryngologist as soon as possible to exclude other neurologic conditions. If indicated, MRI and CT can eliminate other causes for facial paralysis. Blood tests can diagnose infections or other diseases. Electromyography (EMG) can confirm the presence of nerve damage.

Interprofessional Care

Care focuses on relieving symptoms, preventing complications, and protecting the eye on the affected side. Early treatment improves the chance of a complete recovery. Oral corticosteroid therapy to reduce inflammation and swelling should be started within 72 hours of onset.[26] Some patients should also receive an antiviral agent, such as acyclovir. Surgical decompression of the facial nerve is controversial but an option in refractory cases.

NURSING MANAGEMENT: BELL PALSY

Mild analgesics can relieve pain. Moist heat can reduce discomfort and aid circulation. Electrical stimulation of the nerve, facial massage, and physical therapy help maintain muscle tone and ease pain. When function begins to return, active facial muscle exercises are done several times a day. Tell patients to protect the face from cold and drafts because trigeminal *hyperesthesia* (extreme sensitivity to pain or touch) may occur.

> **CHECK YOUR PRACTICE**
>
> You are working in the outpatient neurology clinic. Your patient is a 68-year-old female with Bell palsy. Her main problem today is dry eyes. When you are doing an assessment, she tells you, "I hate the way I look. I cannot go anywhere, and I am afraid to leave the house. I am so ugly."
>
> - How can you help her cope?
> - What can you suggest to increase moisture in the affected eye?

Eye protection is important. Patients may wear dark glasses for protective and cosmetic reasons. Frequent use of artificial tears during the day can prevent drying of the cornea. Ointment and an impermeable eye shield can be used at night to retain moisture. Some patients may need to tape the lids closed at night. Teach patients to report eye pain, drainage, or discharge.

Maintaining good nutrition is important. Teach patients to chew on the unaffected side of the mouth to avoid trapping food and enjoy the taste of food. After each meal, thorough oral hygiene helps prevent parotitis, caries, and periodontal disease from accumulated residual food.

The change in physical appearance can be devastating. Reassure patients that chances for a full recovery are good. Enlisting support from family and friends is important. Tell patients most people recover within 3 to 6 months after onset of symptoms.

POLYNEUROPATHIES

GUILLAIN-BARRÉ SYNDROME

Guillain-Barré syndrome (GBS) is an autoimmune process that occurs a few days or weeks after a viral or bacterial infection. It is rare, affecting about 1 to 2 persons in every 100,000.[27] The most common type is *acute inflammatory demyelinating polyneuropathy* (AIDP). Other types include acute motor axonal neuropathy (AMAN) and acute motor-sensory axonal neuropathy (AMSAN). AMAN is more common in children.

Etiology and Pathophysiology

The cause is unknown. Both cellular and humoral immune responses likely play a role in AIDP. Humoral responses appear to cause AMAN.[28] After an infection, immune responses cause injury to either the myelin sheath (AIDP) or the nerve axon itself (AMAN). Edema and inflammation of affected nerves are present. The result is segmental loss of the myelin sheath with exposed nerve membranes in nerve terminals and the nodes of Ranvier. Transmission of nerve impulses is stopped or slowed. This leads to flaccid paralysis with muscle denervation and atrophy. In the recovery phase, remyelination occurs slowly. Neurologic function returns in a proximal-to-distal pattern.

Most GBS cases follow a viral or bacterial infection of the GI or upper respiratory tract. Cytomegalovirus is the most common viral cause. *Campylobacter jejuni* gastroenteritis is the most common bacterial cause, especially for AMAN. Other related infections include Epstein-Barr virus, *Mycoplasma pneumoniae, Haemophilus influenza,* hepatitis (A, B, E), COVID-19, and Zika virus.[27] Surgery and trauma may trigger GBS.

Clinical Manifestations and Complications

The main features include acute, ascending, rapidly progressive, symmetric weakness of the limbs. The first symptoms are weakness, *paresthesia* (numbness and tingling), and *hypotonia* (reduced muscle tone) of the limbs. Reflexes in the affected limbs are weak or absent. Maximal weakness is reached in 4 weeks.

Autonomic nervous system dysfunction occurs with AIDP and AMAN, causing orthostatic hypotension, hypertension, and abnormal vagal responses (bradycardia, heart block, asystole). Other autonomic dysfunction effects include bowel and bladder dysfunction, facial flushing, and diaphoresis. CN involvement manifests as facial weakness and paresthesia, extraocular eye movement problems, and dysphagia.

Pain is common. It can include paresthesia, muscular aches and cramps, and hyperesthesia. It is often worse at night. Pain may contribute to decreased appetite and interfere with sleep.

The most serious complication is respiratory failure. It occurs if the paralysis progresses to nerves that innervate the thoracic area. Assess the respiratory system by checking respiratory rate and depth to determine the need for immediate intervention, including intubation and mechanical ventilation. Respiratory infection or UTI may occur. Immobility from paralysis can cause paralytic ileus, muscle atrophy, VTE, PIs, orthostatic hypotension, and nutrition deficiencies.[27]

Diagnostic Studies

Diagnosis is based mainly on history and assessment. Clinical features required for diagnosis include progressive weakness of more than 1 limb and decreased or absent reflexes. Electrolyte levels, liver function tests, creatinine phosphokinase, and erythrocyte sedimentation rates are evaluated. CSF analysis helps exclude other causes. In GBS, the CSF has more protein than normal.[27] EMG and nerve conduction studies (NCSs) are used after 2 weeks to confirm the diagnosis and aid in selecting treatment. NCSs allow the HCP to diagnose the subtype. NCSs in AIDP show demyelination.

Interprofessional and Nursing Management

The management of GBS is supportive. Ventilatory support is critical during the acute phase. Patients may be in the ICU for hemodynamic monitoring. Immunomodulating treatments, such as plasma exchange (PE) *(plasmapheresis)* or high-dose IV immunoglobulin (IVIG), are most effective if used within the first 2 weeks of symptom onset. They are equally effective. PE removes antibodies and other immune factors. It is used 5 times, either daily or every other day, in the first 2 weeks (see Chapter 14). IVIG interferes with antigen presentation. It is given over 5 days. It is readily available and is the preferred treatment in many centers.[28] After 4 weeks past disease onset, PE and IVIG therapies have little value.

Assessment is important during the acute phase. During the neurologic assessment, evaluate motor and sensory function. Report changes in motor function (e.g., ascending paralysis), reflexes, CN function (gag, cornea, swallow), and level of consciousness.

Monitor respiratory and cardiac function. Assess ABGs and vital capacity. Monitor BP and cardiac rate and rhythm during the acute phase because dysrhythmias, orthostatic hypotension, and increased or decreased BP and heart rate may occur. Vasopressor agents and volume expanders may be needed to treat the low BP. If fever develops, obtain sputum and blood cultures to identify the pathogen. Appropriate antibiotic therapy is then started.

Nutrition needs must be met despite possible delayed gastric emptying, paralytic ileus, and potential for aspiration if the gag reflex is lost. In addition to testing for the gag reflex, note drooling and other problems with secretions that may indicate an inadequate gag reflex. EN or PN may be used to ensure adequate caloric intake.

Throughout the course of the illness, provide support and encouragement to patients and caregivers. Coordinate early referrals for physical, occupational, and speech therapy. Counseling may help patients adjust to the sudden disabling syndrome and dependence on others.

Most patients will start to recover spontaneously at about 28 days. Eighty percent of patients walk independently at 6 months, with 60% making a full recovery in 1 year. Patients who have a GI infection, are older in age, have poor upper extremity motor strength, or need mechanical ventilation have a poorer prognosis.[27]

CHRONIC INFLAMMATORY DEMYELINATING POLYNEUROPATHY

Chronic inflammatory demyelinating polyneuropathy (CIDP) is a motor and sensory neuropathy. It is a rare autoimmune disorder, affecting 1 to 2 persons per 100,000. CIDP is more common in males and those in their 50s and 60s.

There are different types of CIDP. It differs from GBS in that symptoms gradually occur over 8 weeks. There is no acute onset. CIDP is not self-limiting (with an end to the acute phase). Early recognition and treatment can help patients avoid significant disability.

Etiology and Pathophysiology

We do not know the exact cause of CIDP. Research supports an autoimmune basis. CIDP seems to be associated with infection,

HIV, hepatitis C, Sjögren syndrome, inflammatory bowel disease, melanoma, lymphoma, and diabetes.

Clinical Manifestations and Diagnostic Studies

The classic presentation of CIPD includes progressive symptoms lasting over 2 months, more weakness than sensory deficits, symmetric weakness in the arms and legs, impaired sensation (from distal to proximal), paresthesia and dysesthesia, and absent or decreased reflexes in all extremities. Tremors, facial weakness, and papilledema may be present. There may be sensory ataxia and impaired vibration and pinprick sensation.

CIDP diagnostic tests are similar to those for GBS. CSF shows high protein levels. MRI may show changes. Key identifying features include nerve conduction block and slowed conduction velocity, possibly because of demyelination. Nerve biopsy is done when other studies do not confirm a diagnosis.

Interprofessional and Nursing Management

Early recognition and diagnosis are key to reducing permanent disability. The goal of treatment is to halt the immune response and stop nerve inflammation and demyelination. IVIG, high-dose corticosteroids, and PE are all effective treatments.

Patients continue therapy until maximum clinical improvement is achieved or until they reach a plateau. Patients need maintenance therapy to prevent relapse or progression. Coordinate needed referrals to rehabilitation to promote maximum recovery. Therapy may improve muscle strength, function, and mobility while minimizing muscle atrophy and joint distortion.

TETANUS

Tetanus (lockjaw) is a severe nervous system infection affecting spinal and cranial nerves. In the United States because of widespread immunization and careful wound care, there are fewer than 50 cases per year.[29]

Tetanus results from the effects of a potent neurotoxin (tetanospasmin) released by the anaerobic bacillus *Clostridium tetani.* The spores of the bacillus are present in soil, garden mold, and manure. Tetanospasmin binds to motor nerves and enters the axons. From there, it can travel to the brain and spinal cord and stop the release of inhibitory neurotransmitters. This causes sustained muscle contraction. Many different muscles can be affected if the toxin reaches the blood or lymph system.

C. tetani enters the body through a wound that provides an appropriate low-O_2 environment for the organisms to mature and make toxin. Examples of such wounds include IV drug use injection sites, human and animal bites, puncture wounds from stepping on a nail, gardening injuries, burns, frostbite, open fractures, and gunshot wounds. The incubation period is typically 4 to 14 days. The shorter the period, the more severe the symptoms.

The hallmark feature of tetanus is muscle rigidity and spasms. Patients may have muscle soreness, cramping, or difficulty swallowing. Facial muscles are affected first with stiffness in the jaw *(trismus).* They may have a sardonic smile *(risus sardonicus)* from facial muscle contractions. The neck muscles, back, abdomen, and extremities become increasingly rigid as the disease progresses. In severe forms, continuous tonic seizures may occur with *opisthotonos* (extreme arching of the back and retraction of the head). Laryngeal and respiratory spasms cause apnea and anoxia. The slightest noise, jarring motion, or bright light can set off a painful seizure.

Tetanus prevention and immunizations are the key factors influencing incidence. Adults should receive a tetanus and diphtheria toxoid booster every 10 years. Teach patients that immediate, thorough cleansing of all wounds with soap and water is important to prevent tetanus. If an open wound occurs and the patient has not been immunized within 5 years, contact the HCP so they can get a tetanus booster.

Tetanus is a medical emergency that requires hospitalization. Patients receive tetanus immune globulin (TIG). It provides temporary immunity by directly providing antitoxin. Drugs to control spasms are essential. Diazepam or barbiturates are given to promote sedation and skeletal muscle relaxation. In severe cases, neuromuscular blocking agents (e.g., vecuronium) are given to paralyze skeletal muscles. Opioid analgesics are used for pain management. A 10- to 14-day course of penicillin, metronidazole, tetracycline, or doxycycline inhibits further growth of *C. tetani.*

Because of laryngospasm and the potential need for neuromuscular blocking drugs, patients are placed on mechanical ventilation. IV fluids are needed for proper hydration due to sustained muscle contraction. Any wound should be debrided or abscess drained. Antibiotics may be given to prevent secondary infections.

CASE STUDY

SCI

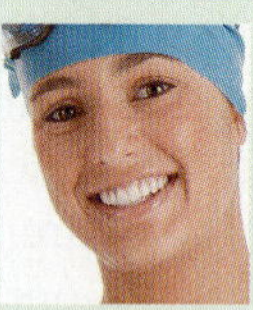

(© Comstock Images/ Stockbyte/ Thinkstock.)

Patient Profile

Acute Phase

S.W., an 18-year-old woman, is admitted to the ED with a cervical SCI. S.W. was swimming at a neighbor's backyard pool. She dove into the shallow end, striking her head on the bottom of the pool. Her friends noticed she did not resurface. They rescued her and brought her to the side of the pool. They maintained neck immobilization until emergency personnel arrived.

Subjective Data

- Awake and alert
- Reporting neck pain
- Anxious and asking why she cannot move her legs
- Asking to see her family

Objective Data

- Weak elbow flexion (biceps) movement bilaterally
- No triceps movement bilaterally
- Gross shoulder movement present bilaterally
- No movement in bilateral lower extremities
- Decreased sensation from the shoulders down
- No bladder or bowel control
- BP 85/50 mm Hg; pulse 56 beats/min; respirations 32 breaths/min and labored

Diagnostic Studies

- CT C-spine shows C5 subluxation and compression fracture
- MRI C-spine shows severe spinal cord compression at C5–C6

Interprofessional Care

- Intubated and started on mechanical ventilation
- Placed in tongs and traction on arrival to ICU

Discussion Questions

1. ***Recognize:*** What are the priorities in her initial emergency management? What signs and symptoms would indicate respiratory distress?
2. ***Analyze:*** What physiologic problems are causing S.W. to have hypotension and bradycardia?
3. ***Plan:*** What would be the initial treatment for S.W.'s hypotension and bradycardia?
4. ***Prioritize:*** What nursing activities would be a priority on S.W.'s arrival in the ICU?
5. ***Act:*** What interventions can decrease S.W.'s anxiety?

Patient Profile

Rehabilitation Phase

S.W. is now 1-month post injury and has been transferred to a local inpatient SCI rehabilitation center. She is extubated and using a wheelchair to mobilize. She eats 3 meals a day with help and is on a strict bowel and bladder program.

Subjective Data

- Awake and alert but anxious
- Reporting a severe headache, blurred vision, and nausea

Objective Data

- Flushed and diaphoretic above the level of injury
- No bowel movement for 2 days
- BP 235/106 mm Hg, pulse 32 beats/min, respirations 30 breaths/min and labored

Discussion Questions

1. ***Analyze:*** What physiologic problem is causing S.W.'s hypertension and bradycardia?
2. ***Prioritize:*** What initial priority nursing interventions would be appropriate?
3. ***Plan:*** Once you notify the HCP, what other interventions would be appropriate?
4. ***Act:*** Patient and caregiver involvement in rehabilitation is vital. What teaching will you provide about bowel management?
5. ***Act:*** S.W. and her family are concerned about autonomic dysreflexia. What effective strategies to prevent autonomic dysreflexia would you discuss with them?
6. ***Evaluation:*** What outcomes would indicate that nursing interventions were successful?

Answers available at http://evolve.elsevier.com/Lewis/medsurg.

BRIDGE TO NCLEX EXAMINATION

The number of the question corresponds to the same-numbered outcome at the beginning of the chapter.

1. A patient with spinal cord injury has severe neurologic deficits. What was the *most* likely mechanism of injury?
   a. Compression
   b. Hyperextension
   c. Flexion-rotation
   d. Extension-rotation

2. What treatment would the nurse anticipate for a patient with a T4 spinal cord injury and neurogenic shock?
   a. Giving low-dose heparin
   b. Administering IV fluids
   c. Maintaining mechanical ventilation
   d. Inserting an indwelling urinary catheter

3. A patient with a C7 spinal cord injury tells the nurse he must have the flu because he has a bad headache and nausea. The nurse's *first priority* is to
   a. call a code blue.
   b. check the temperature.
   c. measure the blood pressure.
   d. elevate the head of the bed to 90 degrees.

4. During rehabilitation, a patient with spinal cord injury begins to ambulate with long leg braces. Which level of injury does the nurse associate with this degree of recovery?
   a. L1–L2
   b. T6–T7
   c. T1–T2
   d. C7–C8

5. The most common early symptom of a spinal cord tumor is
   a. urinary incontinence.
   b. back pain that worsens with activity.
   c. paralysis below the level of involvement.
   d. impaired sensation of pain, temperature, and light touch.
6. When assessing patients with trigeminal neuralgia, the nurse would (**Select all that apply.**)
   a. inspect all aspects of the mouth and teeth.
   b. assess the gag reflex and respiratory rate and depth.
   c. lightly palpate the affected side of the face for edema.
   d. test for temperature and sensation perception on the face.
   e. ask the patient to describe factors that initiate an episode.
7. During routine assessment of a patient with Guillain-Barré syndrome, the nurse finds the patient is short of breath. The respiratory distress is caused by
   a. elevated protein levels in the CSF.
   b. immobility resulting from ascending paralysis.
   c. degeneration of motor neurons in the brainstem and spinal cord.
   d. paralysis ascending to the nerves that stimulate the thoracic area.

1. c; 2. b; 3. c; 4. a; 5. b; 6. a, d, e; 7. d.

For rationales to these answers and even more NCLEX review questions, visit http://evolve.elsevier.com/Lewis/medsurg.

REFERENCES

To access the References for this chapter, please scan the QR code with a mobile device.

66

Assessment: Musculoskeletal System

Mariann M. Harding

http://evolve.elsevier.com/Lewis/medsurg/

CONCEPTUAL FOCUS

Functional Ability
Mobility
Safety

LEARNING OUTCOMES

1. Describe the gross and microscopic anatomy of bone.
2. Explain the classification system for joints and movements at synovial joints.
3. Describe the functions of cartilage, muscles, ligaments, tendons, fascia, and bursae.
4. Link age-related changes in the musculoskeletal system to differences in assessment findings.
5. Obtain subjective and objective assessment data related to the musculoskeletal system.
6. Perform a physical assessment of the musculoskeletal system.
7. Distinguish normal from common abnormal findings of the musculoskeletal system assessment.
8. Describe the purpose, significance of results, and nursing responsibilities related to diagnostic studies of the musculoskeletal system.

KEY TERMS

arthrocentesis, Table 66.9
arthroscopy, Table 66.9
atrophy, Table 66.4
contracture, Table 66.4
crepitus, Table 66.4
isometric contractions
i1sotonic contractions
kyphosis, Table 66.4
range of motion (ROM)
scoliosis
x-ray

The musculoskeletal system is composed of the bones and joints, skeletal muscles, and the ligaments, tendons, and parts that connect these tissues. These provide support and stability for the body and allow coordinated movement. *Mobility* refers to purposeful physical movement. Large muscle, fine motor, and coordinated movements depend on the synchronized efforts of the musculoskeletal and nervous systems. Being mobile requires energy, muscle strength, skeletal stability, joint function, and neuromuscular coordination. This chapter reviews the structure and function of the musculoskeletal system to enable nursing assessment and evaluation of assessment findings.

STRUCTURES AND FUNCTIONS OF THE MUSCULOSKELETAL SYSTEM

Bone

The main functions of bone are support, protection of body organs, voluntary movement, and blood cell production. They serve as a storage site for inorganic minerals, including calcium and phosphorus.[1] Bones provide the supporting framework that keeps the body from collapsing. They allow the body to bear weight. Bones protect underlying vital organs and tissues. For example, the skull encloses the brain and vertebrae surround the spinal cord. The rib cage protects the lungs and heart.

Bones serve as a point of attachment for muscles and ligaments. Muscles are connected to bones by tendons. Bones act as a lever for muscles. Movement occurs because of muscle contractions applied to these levers.

Bone is a dynamic tissue that continuously changes form and composition. It contains organic material (collagen) and inorganic material (calcium, phosphate). The internal and external growth and remodeling of bone are ongoing processes that vary throughout the life span.

Microscopic Structure

We classify bone according to structure as *cortical* (compact and dense) or *cancellous* (spongy). In *cortical bone,* cylindrical structural units called *osteons (Haversian systems)* fit closely together to create a dense bone structure (Fig. 66.1A). Within the systems, the Haversian canals run parallel to the bone's long axis. They contain the blood vessels that travel to the bone's interior from the periosteum. Surrounding each osteon are concentric rings called *lamellae,* which indicate mature bone. Smaller canals *(canaliculi)* extend from the Haversian canals to the *lacunae,* where mature bone cells are embedded.

Cancellous bone has a different structure. The lamellae occur along the lines of maximum stress placed on the bone. Cancellous bone is filled with red or yellow marrow. Bone marrow contains the tissues responsible for making red and white blood cells. Blood reaches the bone cells by passing through spaces in the marrow.

The 3 types of bone cells are osteocytes, osteoblasts, and osteoclasts. Osteocytes are mature bone cells. Osteoblasts are the basic bone-forming cells. The inner layer of bone is made mostly of osteoblasts with a few osteoclasts. Osteoclasts help break down old bone tissue (resorption).[2] Normal adult bone undergoes constant turnover in a balanced process of bone resorption by osteoclasts and bone production by osteoblasts. This process, called *bone remodeling,* maintains bone strength by continuously replacing old, damaged bone with new bone.

Gross Structure

The anatomic structure of bone is best represented by a typical long bone, such as the tibia (Fig. 66.1B). Each long bone consists of the epiphysis, diaphysis, and metaphysis. The *epiphysis,* the widened area at each end of a long bone, is made mostly of cancellous bone. The wide epiphysis allows greater weight distribution and provides stability for the joint. The epiphysis is a main location for muscle attachment. Articular cartilage covers the ends of the epiphysis. It provides a smooth, low-friction surface for joint movement.

The *diaphysis* is the main shaft of the long bone. It provides structural support and is composed of cortical bone. Its tubular structure allows it to withstand bending and twisting forces more easily. The *metaphysis* is the flared area between the epiphysis and diaphysis. It is composed of cancellous bone.

The *epiphyseal plate* (physis or growth plate) is the cartilaginous area between the epiphysis and metaphysis. In skeletally immature children who still have open growth plates, the epiphyseal plate actively makes chondrocytes that become mature bone. Chondrocyte division causes longitudinal bone growth in children. Injury to the epiphyseal plate in a growing child can cause the formation of new bone to stop at the growth plate. This leads to a shorter extremity and may contribute to major functional problems. In the adult, the metaphysis and epiphysis become joined when chondrocyte formation at the growth plate stops and bone formation is complete.

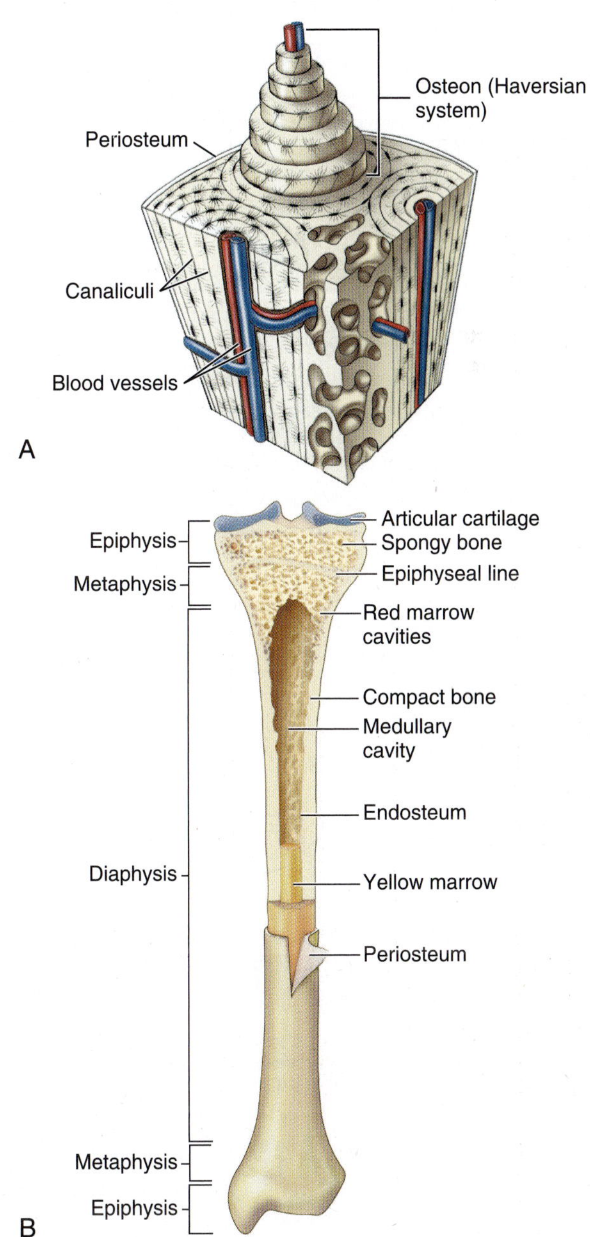

Fig. 66.1 Bone structure. (A) Cortical bone showing numerous structural units called osteons. (B) Anatomy of a long bone (tibia) showing cancellous and compact bone. (A, From Patton KT, Thibodeau GA: *Anatomy and physiology,* ed 9, St Louis, 2016, Mosby. B, From Patton KT, Thibodeau GA: *The human body in health and disease,* ed 7, St Louis, 2018, Mosby.)

The *periosteum* is composed of fibrous connective tissue that covers the bone. Tiny blood vessels penetrate the periosteum to bring nutrition to underlying bone. Musculotendinous fibers attach to the outer layer of the periosteum. Collagen bundles attach the inner layer of the periosteum to the bone. There is no periosteum on the articular surfaces of long bones. These bone ends are covered by articular cartilage.

The medullary *(marrow)* cavity in the center of the diaphysis contains red or yellow bone marrow. In adults, red marrow is found mainly in the flat bones, such as the pelvis, sternum, and scapula, and cancellous bone at the epiphyseal ends of long bones, such as the femur and humerus. Red bone marrow is involved in blood cell production (hematopoiesis). In an adult, the medullary cavity of long bones contains yellow bone marrow (mainly adipose tissue). It serves as a storage site for triglycerides. Yellow marrow is involved in hematopoiesis in times of great blood cell need.

Types

The skeleton consists of 206 bones. We classify bones by shape as long, short, flat, irregular, or sesamoid. Long bones have a central shaft (diaphysis) and 2 widened ends (epiphyses) (Fig. 66.1B). Examples include the femur, humerus, and tibia. Short bones are composed of cancellous bone covered by a thin layer of compact bone. Examples include the carpals in the hand and tarsals in the foot.

Flat bones have 2 layers of compact bone separated by a layer of cancellous bone. The spaces in the cancellous bone contain bone marrow. Flat bones include the pelvis, skull, sternum, ribs, vertebrae, and scapula. Irregular bones appear in a variety of shapes and sizes. Examples include the sacrum, mandible, and ear ossicles. *Sesamoid bones* are round or oval bones (such as the patella), which develop in tendons.

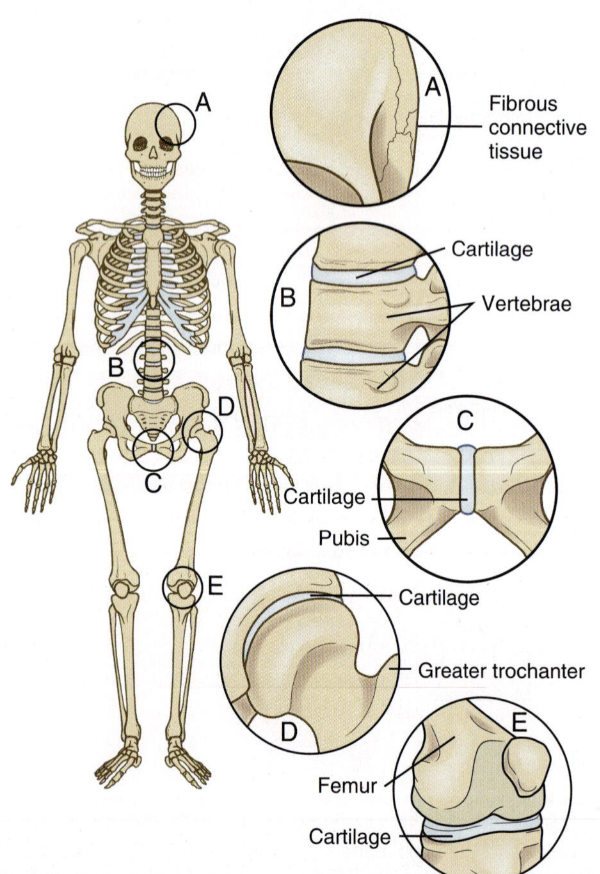

Fig. 66.2 Classification of joints. (A–C) Synarthrotic (immovable) and amphiarthrotic (slightly movable) joints. (D and E) Diarthrodial (freely movable) joints.

Joints

A *joint* (articulation) is a place where the ends of 2 bones are close and move in relation to each other. Joints are classified by the degree of movement that they allow (Fig. 66.2).

The most common joint is the freely movable *diarthrodial* (synovial) type. This joint is enclosed in a capsule of fibrous connective tissue, which joins the 2 bones together to form a cavity (Fig. 66.3). The capsule is lined by a synovial membrane, which secretes thick synovial fluid. This fluid lubricates the joint, reduces friction, and allows opposing surfaces to slide smoothly over each other. It supplies oxygen and nutrients to and removes carbon dioxide and metabolic wastes from the chondrocytes within articular cartilage. The end of each bone is covered with articular (hyaline) cartilage. Supporting structures (e.g., ligaments, tendons) reinforce the joint capsule. They provide limits and stability to joint movement. Types of diarthrodial joints are shown in Fig. 66.4.

Cartilage

The 3 types of *cartilage* are hyaline, elastic, and fibrous. *Hyaline cartilage* is the most common. It has a moderate amount of

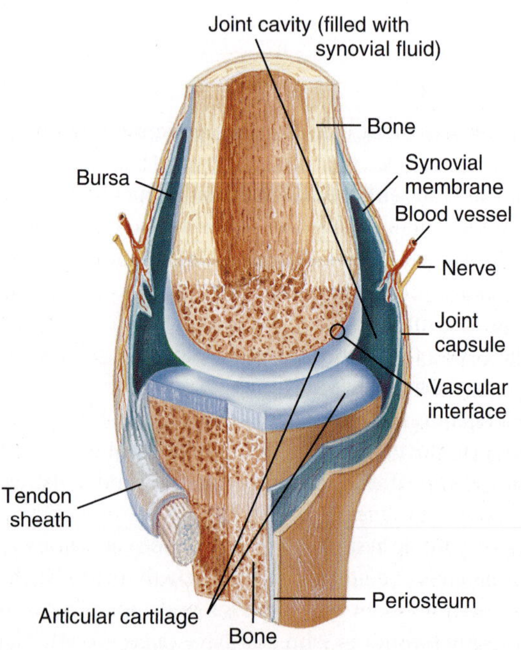

Fig. 66.3 Structure of diarthrodial (synovial) joint.

Joint	Movement	Examples	Illustration
Hinge joint	Flexion, extension	Elbow joint (shown), interphalangeal joints, knee joint	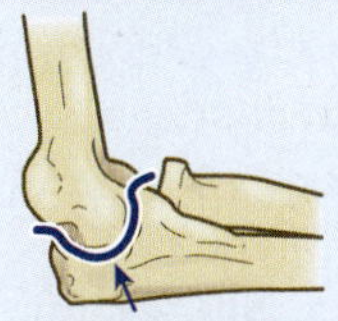
Ball and socket (spheroidal)	Flexion, extension; adduction, abduction; circumduction	Shoulder (shown), hip	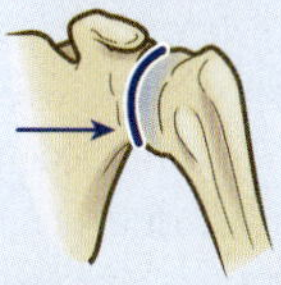
Pivot (rotary)	Rotation	Atlas-axis, proximal radioulnar joint (shown)	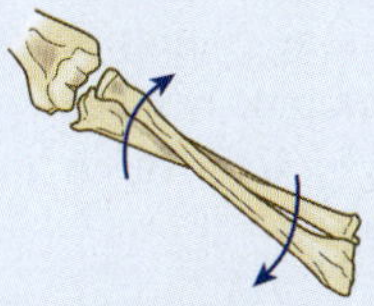
Condyloid	Flexion, extension; abduction, adduction; circumduction	Wrist joint (between radial and carpals) (shown)	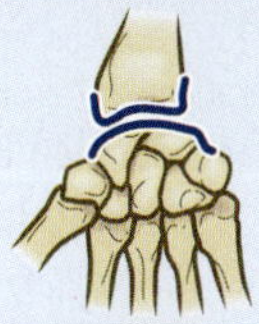
Saddle	Flexion, extension; abduction, adduction; circumduction, thumb-finger opposition	Carpometacarpal joint of thumb (shown)	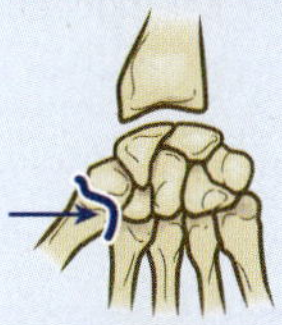
Gliding	One surface moves over another surface	Between tarsal bones, sacroiliac joint, between articular processes of vertebrae, between carpal bones (shown)	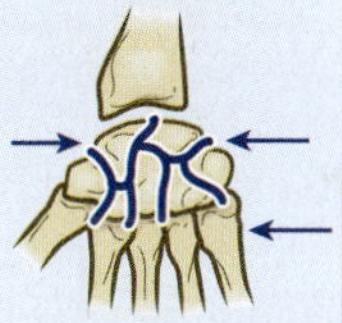

Fig. 66.4 Types of diarthrodial (synovial) joints.

collagen fibers. It is found in the trachea, bronchi, nose, epiphyseal plate, and articular surfaces of bones.

Elastic cartilage, which has both collagen and elastic fibers, is more flexible than hyaline cartilage. It is found in the ear, epiglottis, and larynx. Fibrous cartilage consists mostly of collagen fibers. It is a tough tissue that often functions as a shock absorber. Fibrous cartilage is found between the vertebral discs. It forms a protective cushion between the bones of the pelvic girdle, knee, and shoulder.

Cartilage in synovial joints serves as a support for soft tissue and provides the articular surface for joint movement. It protects underlying tissues. Because articular cartilage is avascular, it must receive nourishment by the diffusion of material from the synovial fluid. The lack of a direct blood supply explains why healing and repair of cartilage tissue occur slowly. The cartilage in the epiphyseal plate is involved in the growth of long bones before we reach physical maturity.[3]

Muscle

The 3 types of muscle tissue are cardiac (striated, involuntary), smooth (nonstriated, involuntary), and skeletal (striated, voluntary) muscle. *Cardiac muscle* is found only in the heart. Its contractions are spontaneous. *Smooth muscle* is found in the walls of hollow structures, such as airways, arteries, gastrointestinal (GI) tract, bladder, and uterus. Smooth muscle contraction is controlled by neuronal and hormonal influences. *Skeletal muscle* requires neuronal stimulation for contraction. It accounts for about half of a human's body weight.

Skeletal Muscle

Skeletal muscle fibers are bound together by connective tissue called perimysium into bundles called fascicles. Fascicles are bound into larger bundles, which collectively form the muscle. A connective tissue layer called the *endomysium* surrounds each

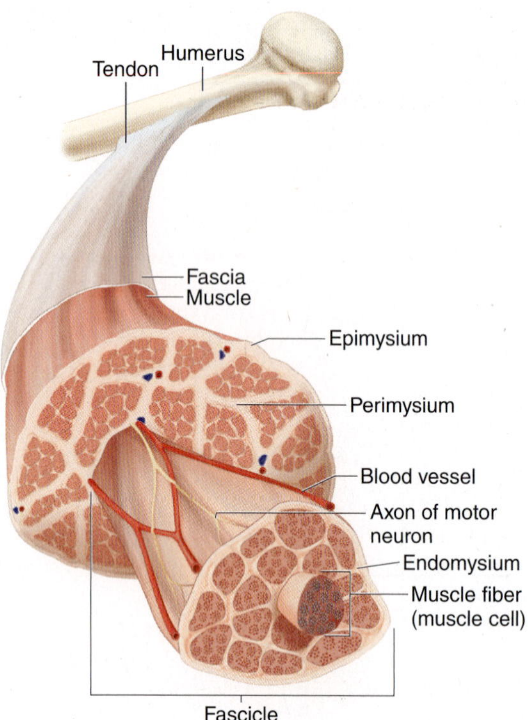

Fig. 66.5 Myofibrils of a skeletal muscle fiber and overall organization of skeletal muscle.

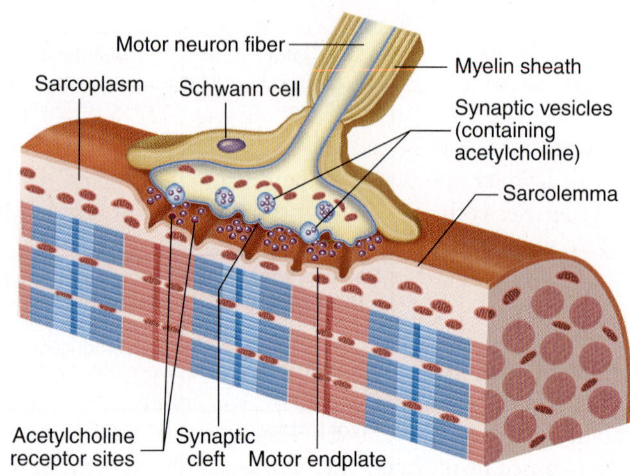

Fig. 66.6 Motor units of a muscle. (From McCance KL, Huether SE. *Pathophysiology: the biological basis for disease in adults and children*, ed 8, St. Louis, 2019, Elsevier.)

fiber (Fig. 66.5). The entire muscle is covered by the *epimysium.* The epimysium helps muscles slide over nearby structures. It is continuous with the tendon and connective tissue around the fascicles.

The structural unit of skeletal muscle is the muscle cell or muscle fiber. It is highly specialized for contraction. Skeletal muscle fibers are long, multinucleated strands. They contain protein called myofibrils, which are made up of sarcomeres. A *sarcomere* is the contractile unit of a myofibril. Myofibrils have striations or bands. The dark (thick) bands are made of the protein myosin. Light (thin) bands contain the protein actin. Muscle contraction occurs as thick and thin filaments slide past each other, causing the sarcomeres to shorten.

Muscle contractions allow posture maintenance, body movement, and facial expressions. Most skeletal muscles work in groups. **Isometric contractions** increase the tension within a muscle but do not produce movement. **Isotonic contractions** shorten a muscle to produce movement. Most contractions are a combination of tension *(isometric)* and shortening *(isotonic).* Repeated isometric and/or isotonic contractions provide stress to stimulate muscle growth. Muscular *atrophy* (decrease in size) occurs with the absence of contractions. Increased muscular activity leads to *hypertrophy* (increase in size).

Skeletal muscle fibers are divided into 2 groups based on the type of activity they show. *Slow-twitch muscle fibers* support prolonged muscle activity, such as marathon running. Because they support the body against gravity, they help maintain posture. *Fast-twitch muscle fibers* are used for rapid muscle contraction needed for activities such as blinking the eye, jumping, or sprinting. Fast-twitch fibers tire more quickly than slow-twitch fibers.

Skeletal muscle has many mitochondria to support its high metabolic activity. The direct energy source for muscle contractions is adenosine triphosphate (ATP). ATP is synthesized through cellular oxidative metabolism in the mitochondria. It is rapidly depleted through conversion to adenosine diphosphate (ADP) and must be rephosphorylated. Phosphocreatine provides a rapid source for the resynthesis of ATP, but it is, in turn, converted to creatine. Glycolysis can serve as a source of ATP when the O_2 supply is inadequate for metabolic needs of the muscle tissue.

Neuromuscular Junction

Skeletal muscle fibers require a nerve impulse to contract. A nerve fiber and the skeletal muscle fibers it stimulates are called a *motor endplate.* The junction between the axon of the nerve cell and the adjacent muscle cell is called the *myoneural* or *neuromuscular junction* (Fig. 66.6).

Presynaptic neurons release acetylcholine. It diffuses across the neuromuscular junction to bind with receptors on the motor endplate of the muscle. In response to this stimulation, the sarcoplasmic reticulum releases calcium into the cytoplasm.[4] The presence of calcium triggers contraction in the myofibrils. When calcium is low, *tetany* (involuntary skeletal muscle contractions) can occur.

Ligaments and Tendons

Ligaments and tendons are composed of dense, fibrous connective tissue with bundles of closely packed collagen fibers arranged in the same plane for more strength. *Tendons* attach muscles to bones. They are an extension of the muscle sheath that adheres to the periosteum. *Ligaments* connect bones to bones (e.g., tibia to femur at knee joint). They have a higher elastic content than tendons. Ligaments provide stability at joints while allowing controlled movement.

Ligaments and tendons have a poor blood supply. This can make their repair after injury a slow process. For example, the stretching or tearing of ligaments that occurs with a sprain may require a long time to mend.

Fascia

Fascia are layers of connective tissue with intermeshed fibers that can withstand limited stretching. Superficial fascia lies right under the skin. Deep fascia is a dense, fibrous tissue that surrounds muscle bundles, nerves, and blood vessels. It encloses individual muscles, allowing them to act independently and glide over each other during contraction. Fascia provides strength to muscle tissues.

Bursae

Bursae are small sacs of connective tissue lined with synovial membrane that contain viscous synovial fluid. They act as padding between structures to relieve pressure and decrease friction caused by moving parts.[5] Bursae are found between the (1) patella and skin (prepatellar bursae), (2) olecranon process of the elbow and skin (olecranon bursae), (3) head of the humerus and acromion process of the scapula (subacromial bursae), and (4) greater trochanter of the proximal femur and skin (trochanteric bursae).

Gerontologic Considerations: Effects of Aging on Musculoskeletal System

Many functional problems in an older adult are related to changes in the musculoskeletal system. These may affect the older adult's ability to complete self-care tasks and pursue usual activities. Effects of musculoskeletal changes may range from mild discomfort and decreased ability to perform activities of daily living (ADLs) to severe, chronic pain and immobility. Assess the impact of age-related changes on functional status. Ask about changes in self-care habits and ability to be independent in the home environment. Functional limitations that are accepted by the older adult as a normal part of aging can often be addressed with preventive strategies.

Joints are often affected by degenerative problems. Cartilage softens and thins. Joint surfaces become rough. There may be joint space narrowing with bone spur growth. Osteoarthritis is more likely to affect joints in the older adult (see Chapter 69).

The bone remodeling process changes as we age. Increased bone resorption and decreased bone formation cause a loss of bone density. This contributes to osteoporosis (see Chapter 68). Muscle mass and strength decrease. Almost 30% of muscle mass is lost by age 70. Motor neuron loss can cause problems with skeletal muscle movement. Tendons and ligaments become less flexible, making movement more rigid.

Fall risk increases due in part to loss of strength.[6] Aging can change balance, making a person unsteady. *Proprioception* (awareness of self in relation to the environment) may be altered. Identify any musculoskeletal changes that increase fall risk.

Carefully distinguish between expected changes and signs of problems. Table 66.1 outlines age-related changes in the musculoskeletal system and differences in assessment findings.

TABLE 66.1 GERONTOLOGIC ASSESSMENT DIFFERENCES

Musculoskeletal System

Changes	Differences in Assessment Findings
Bone	
• ↓ Bone density and strength • Slowed remodeling process	• Loss of height and deformity, such as kyphosis, from vertebral compression and degeneration • Back pain, stiffness • ↑ Risk for osteoporosis and fractures
Joints	
• ↑ Risk for cartilage erosion that leads to direct contact between bone ends and overgrowth of bone around joint margins	• Joint stiffness, ↓ mobility, limited ROM, possible crepitation on movement • Pain with motion and/or weight bearing
• Loss of water from discs between vertebrae, ↓ height of intervertebral spaces	• Loss of height and shortening of trunk from disc compression. Posture change
Muscles	
• ↓ Number and diameter of muscle cells • Replacement of muscle cells by fibrous connective tissue • ↓ Elasticity and deterioration of cartilage • ↓ Ability to store glycogen. ↓ Ability to release glycogen as energy during stress • ↓ Conduction of nerve impulses along motor units • ↓ Mitochondria function	• ↓ Muscle strength and mass • Abdominal protrusion • ↑ Rigidity in neck, shoulders, back, hips, and knees • ↓ Fine motor dexterity, ↓ agility • Slowed reaction times and reflexes • Earlier fatigue with activity

CASE STUDY

Patient Introduction

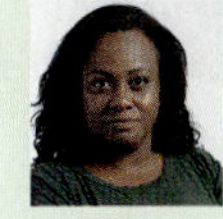

(© Studio CJ/ iStock.com.)

G.A. is a 58-year-old female whose husband brought her to the emergency department (ED) this morning after she awoke with a sudden onset of excruciating pain in her left great toe. She denies any injury to her foot. She says she has never had this type of pain before.

Discussion Questions

1. What are the possible causes for G.A.'s acute pain in her great toe?
2. What type of assessment would be most appropriate: comprehensive, focused, or emergency? What is the basis for your decision?
3. What assessment questions will you ask G.A.?

You will learn more about how to assess G.A.'s condition as you read this chapter.

Answers available at http://evolve.elsevier.com/Lewis/medsurg.

MUSCULOSKELETAL SYSTEM ASSESSMENT

Subjective Data

Important Health Information

Pain is the most common symptom reported by someone with a musculoskeletal problem. Other manifestations are weakness, swelling, limited movement, stiffness, and joint crepitation. Ask patients about changes in sensation, such as numbness. Determine weight-bearing status.

Ask if there is a history of a chronic musculoskeletal problem. Focus questions on symptoms of arthritic and connective tissue diseases (e.g., gout, arthritis, systemic lupus erythematosus [SLE]). Is there an underlying neurologic problem?

Trauma is a common reason for seeking health care. Patients who are good historians can recount minor and major injuries. Have they had a broken bone, strain, or other injury to a muscle, joint, tendon, or ligament? Record information and include:

- Mechanism and circumstances of the injury (e.g., twist, crush, stretch)
- Treatment received
- Current ability and progress related to the injury
- Need for assistive devices and ability to perform ADLs

Certain illnesses affect the musculoskeletal system directly or indirectly. Ask patients about problems such as tuberculosis, polio, diabetes, parathyroid problems, hemophilia, and rickets. Ask about sources of a secondary bacterial infection, such as ears, tonsils, teeth, sinuses, lungs, or genitourinary tract. These infections can enter the bones via the blood, causing osteomyelitis or joint destruction. Get a detailed account of the course and treatment of any problem.

Is there a family history of problems such as rheumatoid arthritis, SLE, osteoarthritis, gout, osteoporosis, and scoliosis (Box 66.1)? Patients may have a genetic predisposition to these or other musculoskeletal problems.

Medications. Obtain a complete medication history. Ask about the use of skeletal muscle relaxants, opioids, nonsteroidal antiinflammatory drugs, corticosteroids, and calcium and vitamin D supplements. Ask patients about tetanus, pertussis, and polio immunizations. Review the use of drugs that can have negative effects on the musculoskeletal system. These include antiseizure drugs (osteomalacia), corticosteroids (avascular necrosis, decreased bone and muscle mass), and potassium-depleting diuretics (muscle cramps and weakness). Ask postmenopausal females about the use of hormone therapy.

Surgery and treatments. Ask about any surgeries or hospitalizations due to a musculoskeletal problem. Note the reason; the date and duration; and the treatment. Have they had fracture repair or knee or hip replacements? With prolonged immobilization, consider the possibility of disuse osteoporosis and muscle atrophy.

BOX 66.1 GENETICS IN CLINICAL PRACTICE

- Many autoimmune diseases of the musculoskeletal system have a genetic basis involving human leukocyte antigens (HLAs). These diseases include ankylosing spondylitis, rheumatoid arthritis, and systemic lupus erythematosus.
- Genetic factors contribute to osteoporosis by influencing bone mineral density and bone size, quality, and turnover.
- A genetic predisposition is a contributing risk factor in gout, scoliosis, and osteoarthritis.
- The most common types of muscular dystrophy are X-linked recessive disorders.

Functional Health Patterns

Musculoskeletal problems can affect overall health. Table 66.2 outlines specific questions to ask using functional health patterns.

Health perception–health management. Ask patients if there has been a perceived change in health status within the last several days, months, or years. With many musculoskeletal problems, declines occur slowly over many years. Ask about health practices related to the musculoskeletal system. This includes maintaining avoiding excess stress on muscles and joints and using proper body mechanics when lifting objects. Safety practices can affect the predisposition for certain injuries and illnesses. Ask about work, home, and recreation safety practices. For example, if a patient works with computers, do they use ergonomic adaptations that decrease the risk for carpal tunnel syndrome? Identifying problems in this area will direct your patient teaching.

Occupational activity can affect the musculoskeletal system. For example, a desk job can negatively affect muscle flexibility and strength. Jobs that require heavy lifting or pushing can lead to damage of joints and supporting structures. Ask about work-related musculoskeletal injuries.

Nutritional-metabolic. A patient's description of a typical day's diet can reveal areas of nutrition concern that can affect the musculoskeletal system. Adequate intake of vitamins C and D, calcium, and protein is essential for a healthy musculoskeletal system. Nutrition problems can contribute to osteoporosis. Maintaining normal weight is an important goal. Obesity places added stress on weight-bearing joints, such as the knees, hips, and spine.

Elimination. Questions about mobility may reveal problems with ambulating to the toilet. Bowel or bladder incontinence may occur when ambulation is a problem. Ask patients if an assistive device, such as an elevated toilet seat or a grab bar, is needed to manage toileting. Decreased mobility can lead to constipation.

Activity-exercise. Get a detailed account of the type, duration, and frequency of exercise and recreational activities. What

TABLE 66.2 HEALTH HISTORY

Musculoskeletal System

Health Perception–Health Management
- Has there been a change in your health within the last several days, months, or years?
- Describe your daily routine. Do you need help in completing your usual daily activities because of a musculoskeletal problem?[a]
- Do you have to lift heavy objects? Does your work or exercise involve repetitive motion or joint stress? Describe any special equipment you use or wear when you work or exercise that helps protect you from injury.
- Have you had a work-related musculoskeletal injury?[a]
- Do you take any drugs to manage your musculoskeletal problem? If so, what and what are the expected effects?
- Have you ever used tobacco? If yes, in what form, how much, and for how long?
- How often and how much alcohol do you drink?

Nutritional-Metabolic
- Describe your usual daily intake of food and snacks.
- Do you have problems preparing your food?
- What diet supplements do you take? Do you take calcium or vitamin D supplements?
- What is your weight? Describe any recent weight loss or gain.

Elimination
- Does your musculoskeletal problem make it hard for you to reach the toilet in time?[a]
- Do you need any assistive devices or equipment to manage toileting?[a]
- Do you have constipation related to decreased mobility or drugs taken for your musculoskeletal problem?[a]

Activity-Exercise
- Describe your usual exercise. Do you have musculoskeletal symptoms before, during, or after exercising?[a]
- Are you able to move all your joints comfortably through full range of motion?
- Do you use any prosthetic or orthotic devices?[a]

Sleep-Rest
- Do you have any problems sleeping because of a musculoskeletal problem?[a]
- Do you need frequent position changes at night?[a]
- Do you wake up at night because of musculoskeletal pain?[a]
- Describe any practices you use to help you sleep at night.[a]

Cognitive-Perceptual
- Describe any musculoskeletal pain you have. How do you manage your pain?

Self-Perception–Self-Concept
- Have changes in your musculoskeletal system (posture, walking, muscle strength) and decreased ability to do certain things affected how you feel about yourself?[a]
- Have these changes affected your lifestyle?[a]

Role-Relationship
- Who do you live with?
- Describe how family, friends, or others help you with your musculoskeletal problem.
- Describe the effect of your musculoskeletal problem on your work and your social relationships. Describe what you do if you have trouble dressing, preparing meals, feeding yourself, performing hygiene, writing, using the phone, or maintaining your home.

Sexuality-Reproductive
- Describe any sexual concerns related to your musculoskeletal problem.

Coping–Stress Tolerance
- Describe how you deal with problems such as pain, weakness, or immobility that have resulted from your musculoskeletal problem.

Value-Belief
- Describe any cultural practices or religious beliefs that may influence the treatment of your musculoskeletal problem.

[a]If yes, describe.

are their warm-up activities? Compare daily, weekend, and seasonal patterns because occasional exercise can be a problem. Ask about limitations in movement, pain, weakness, or any change in bones or joints that interferes with daily activities. Obtain a fall risk assessment.

Note the use of a prosthetic or assistive device such as a cane. Is the fit correct? Does the patient know the safe and correct technique for using the device? Ask patients if they use the device regularly. If not, assess for reasons for inconsistent use.

Sleep-rest. Discomfort from a musculoskeletal problem can interfere with sleep and lead to fatigue. Ask about sleep problems. If patients describe poor sleep because of a musculoskeletal problem, ask about the type of bedding and pillows used, bedtime routine, sleeping partner, and sleeping positions.

Cognitive-perceptual. Discuss any reports of pain reported from a musculoskeletal problem. Ask patients to describe the intensity and measures used to manage pain.

Self-perception–self-concept. Many chronic musculoskeletal problems lead to deformities and a reduction in activities. This can have a serious negative impact on body image and sense of worth. Assess patients' feelings about these changes and any effect on interactions with family and friends.

Role-relationship. Ask about role performance and relationships. Impaired mobility and chronic pain can negatively affect the ability to perform in roles of spouse, parent, and/or employee. The ability to maintain meaningful social and personal relationships can be adversely affected. Ask who the patient lives with. Assess how much help is available from family, friends, and other caregivers. It may be hard for patients who live alone to continue to do so. Find out if other resources are needed, such as physical therapy and home health care.

Coping–stress tolerance. Mobility limitations and pain are serious potential stressors that challenge patients' coping resources. Explore if a musculoskeletal problem is causing difficulties for patients, families, or significant others.

CASE STUDY

Subjective Data

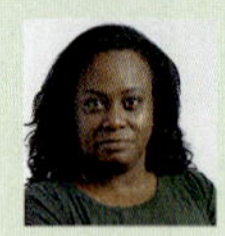

(© Studio CJ/ iStock.com.)

A focused subjective assessment of G.A. revealed:

Medical History: Hypertension for 6 years. Type 2 diabetes for 11 years.

Medications: Metformin 500 mg orally bid; hydrochlorothiazide 50 mg orally bid.

Health Perception–Health Management: Drinks alcohol at night.

Nutritional-Metabolic: 5 ft, 2 in tall and weighs 160 lb (BMI 29.3 kg/m^2). Does not take any nutrition supplements. Avoids milk and other dairy products because they make her "gassy."

Activity-Exercise: Minimally active; does not exercise. Able to perform ADLs without assistance. Denies any history of musculoskeletal problems.

Cognitive-Perceptual: Rates toe pain at 8 on a scale of 0 to 10. Describes sharp, burning pain that increases in intensity with any movement. Denies any numbness.

Coping–Stress Tolerance: Is asking for pain medicine "as strong as you can give me."

Discussion Questions

1. What subjective assessment findings concern you most?
2. Is this an appropriate time to talk with G.A. about her weight?
3. Based on these subjective findings, what should be included in the physical assessment?

You will learn more about the physical assessment of the musculoskeletal system in the next section.

Answers available at http://evolve.elsevier.com/Lewis/medsurg.

Objective Data

Physical Assessment

The basic musculoskeletal physical assessment involves observation, inspection, palpation, neurovascular assessment, and range of motion, strength, and reflex testing. There are some special tests we use to assess for specific conditions. Assessment of reflexes is discussed in Chapter 60. Table 66.3 shows an example of how to record a normal musculoskeletal system assessment. Abnormal musculoskeletal system assessment findings are described in Table 66.4. A *focused assessment* is used to evaluate previously identified musculoskeletal problems and to monitor for signs of new problems (Box 66.2).

Compare sides simultaneously. Expect symmetry of structure and function of the corresponding areas. Note any subtle variations in muscle strength when comparing patients' dominant and nondominant sides. Use the opposite body part for comparison when you suspect a problem.

TABLE 66.3 Normal Physical Assessment of the Musculoskeletal System

- Ordinary spinal curvatures
- No muscle atrophy or asymmetry
- No joint swelling, deformity, or crepitation
- No tenderness on palpation of spine, joints, or muscles
- Full ROM of all joints without pain or laxity
- Muscle strength of 5/5

Ideally, begin your assessment before the patient is aware of being observed.

Note the degree of disability, level of function, posture, and gait. Pay attention to cues about pain or discomfort patients report that they are experiencing. Observe them sitting and rising to a standing position. Combined with gait, you will have information about weight bearing and strength of push-off.

Inspection. Perform a systematic inspection. Start at the head and neck then move to the upper extremities, lower extremities, and trunk. Inspect the skin for color, scars, and signs of previous injury or surgery. Is there redness, bruising, or abrasions? Note posture and body build, muscle size and symmetry, and symmetry and contour of joints. Observe for swelling, deformity, and nodules. Is there a difference in limb length or muscle size?

If patients can move independently, assess posture and gait by watching them walk, stand, and sit. Note any lordosis, kyphosis, or scoliosis. If you find unequal limb length or problems, measure limb length and circumferential muscle mass.[7] Measure muscle mass circumference at the largest area of the muscle. Record the exact location at which the measurements were obtained (e.g., left quadriceps muscle measured 15 cm above the patella). This tells the next examiner the exact area to measure and ensures consistency with reassessment.

Scoliosis is a lateral S-shaped curvature of the thoracic and lumbar spine. We usually see unequal shoulder and scapula height when we observe patients from the back (Fig. 66.7). Have them stand up straight with arms at their sides. Have them bend forward at a 90-degree angle with their arms hanging down as if they are trying to touch their toes. Note the straightness of the spine. Assess for unevenness of the shoulders, ribs, and hips.

Palpation. Examine the neck, shoulders, elbows, wrists, hands, back, hips, knees, ankles, and feet. Warm your hands to prevent muscle spasm, which can interfere with identifying essential landmarks or soft tissue structures. Carefully palpate any specific areas of concern because of a subjective report or abnormal appearance on inspection.

TABLE 66.4 ASSESSMENT ABNORMALITIES

Musculoskeletal System

Finding	Description	Possible Cause
Achilles' tendonitis	Pain in ankle and posterior calf, initially when running or walking. Can progress to pain at rest.	Stress on Achilles tendon over time causing inflammation.
Ankylosis	Stiffness and fixation of a joint.	Chronic joint inflammation and destruction (e.g., rheumatoid arthritis).
Ataxic gait	Staggering, uncoordinated gait often with sway.	Neurogenic problems (e.g., spinal cord lesion).
Atrophy	↓ Size and strength of muscle leading to ↓ function and tone.	Muscle denervation, contracture, prolonged disuse from immobilization.
Boutonnière deformity	Finger abnormality, flexion of proximal interphalangeal (PIP) joint and hyperextension of the distal interphalangeal (DIP) joint of the fingers (see Fig. 69.4B).	Rheumatoid and psoriatic arthritis. Caused by disruption of extensor tendons over the fingers.
Contracture	Resistance of movement of muscle or joint due to fibrosis of supporting soft tissues.	Shortening of muscle or ligaments, tightness of soft tissue, incorrect positioning of immobilized extremity.
Crepitus	Frequent, audible crackling sound with palpable grating that accompanies movement.	Fracture, dislocation, temporomandibular joint dysfunction, osteoarthritis.
Dislocation	Separation of 2 bones from their normal position within a joint.	Trauma, surrounding soft tissue problem.
Festinating gait	While walking, neck, trunk, and knees flex and the body is rigid. Delayed start with short, quick, shuffling steps. Speed may ↑ as if patient is unable to stop (festination).	Neuromuscular problems, such as Parkinson disease.
Ganglion cyst	Small fluid-filled mass over a tendon sheath or joint, usually on dorsal surface of wrist or foot.	Inflammation of tissues around a joint, which can increase in size or disappear.
Hypertonicity	Abnormally ↑ muscle tension.	Parkinson disease, cerebral palsy, trauma, stroke, multiple sclerosis.
Kyphosis	Exaggerated thoracic curvature.	Poor posture, tuberculosis, arthritis, osteoporosis, growth disturbance of vertebral epiphyses, vertebral fractures.
Lateral epicondylitis (tennis elbow)	Dull ache along outer aspect of elbow, worsens with twisting and grasping motions.	Injury, inflammation, and/or partial tearing of tendon at its insertion on epicondyle.
Limited range of motion (ROM)	Joint does not achieve expected degrees of motion.	Injury, inflammation, contracture.
Lordosis (swayback)	Exaggerated lumbar curvature.	Other spinal deformities, muscular dystrophy, obesity, flexion contracture of hip, congenital dislocation of hip.
Muscle spasticity	↑ Muscle tone with sustained muscle contractions (spasms) that increase with movement; stiffness or tightness may interfere with gait, movement, speech.	Neuromuscular problems, such as multiple sclerosis, cerebral palsy.
Myalgia	General muscle tenderness and pain.	Chronic pain syndromes (e.g., fibromyalgia). Overuse, injury, or strain. Statin therapy.
Paresthesia	Numbness and tingling, often described as a "pins and needles" sensation.	Compromised sensory nerves, often due to edema in a closed space (e.g., cast, bulky dressing). Spinal stenosis.
Pes planus (flatfoot)	Abnormal flatness of the sole and arch of the foot.	Hereditary, muscle paralysis, mild cerebral palsy, muscular dystrophy, posterior tibial tendon injury.
Plantar fasciitis	Burning, sharp pain on heel and sole of foot. Worse in the morning with first step out of bed.	Chronic degenerative/reparative cycle resulting in inflammation.
Scoliosis	Asymmetric elevation of shoulders, scapulae, and iliac crests with lateral spine curvature (Fig. 66.8).	Idiopathic, congenital, or neuromuscular condition, fracture or dislocation, osteomalacia.
Short-leg gait	A limp, unless corrective footwear used.	Leg length discrepancy of 1 inch or more, often structural (e.g., arthritis, fracture).
Spastic gait	Short steps with dragging of foot. Jerky, uncoordinated, cross-knee (scissor) movement.	Neurogenic problems (e.g., cerebral palsy, hemiplegia).
Steppage gait	↑ Hip and knee flexion to clear the foot from the floor. Footdrop is present, foot slaps down and along walking surface.	Neurogenic problems (e.g., peroneal nerve injury, paralyzed dorsiflexor muscles).
Subluxation	Partial dislocation of joint.	Instability of joint capsule and supporting ligaments (e.g., trauma, arthritis).
Swan neck deformity	Hyperextension of the PIP joint with flexion of the metacarpophalangeal (MCP) and DIP joints of the fingers (see Fig. 69.4D).	Typical deformity of rheumatoid and psoriatic arthritis. Caused by contracture of muscles and tendons.

TABLE 66.4 ASSESSMENT ABNORMALITIES—cont'd

Musculoskeletal System

Finding	Description	Possible Cause
Swelling	Enlargement, often of a joint due to fluid collection. Usually leads to pain, stiffness.	Trauma, inflammation.
Tenosynovitis	Superficial swelling, pain, and tenderness along a tendon sheath.	Inflammation that often occurs with infection, injury, or overuse.
Torticollis (wryneck)	Neck is rotated and laterally bent in unusual position to one side.	Prolonged contraction of neck muscles.
Tremor	Involuntary muscle quivering.	Neuromuscular problems, such as multiple sclerosis, Parkinson disease, dystonia. Muscle fatigue.
Ulnar deviation (ulnar drift)	Fingers drift to ulnar side of forearm (see Fig. 69.4A).	Typical deformity of rheumatoid arthritis due to tendon contracture.
Valgum deformity (knock-knees)	When knees are together and there is <1 in (2.5 cm) between the medial malleoli.	Poliomyelitis, congenital deformity, arthritis.
Varum deformity (bowlegs)	When knees are apart and the medial malleoli are together, a space of >1 in (2.5 cm) exists.	Arthritis, congenital deformity.

BOX 66.2 FOCUSED ASSESSMENT

Musculoskeletal System

Use this checklist to be sure key assessment steps have been done.

Subjective

Ask the patient about the following and note responses:

Joint pain or stiffness

Muscle weakness

Swelling, redness

Objective: Diagnostic

Check the results of the following diagnostic studies:

X-ray

MRI or CT scan

Bone scan

Ultrasound

Objective: Physical Assessment

Inspect and Palpate

Spine and extremities for alignment, contour, symmetry, size, gross deformities

Joints for ROM, tenderness or pain, warmth, crepitus, swelling, deformity

Muscles for size, symmetry, tone, tenderness, or pain

Posture and gait for stride, balance

Both superficial and deep palpation are usually done consecutively. Consider the underlying anatomy structures and landmarks you are palpating. Palpate muscles and joints to assess temperature, tenderness, swelling, and crepitation. Look at the general contour. Note the specific anatomic location of any abnormal findings.

Motion. Assess joint mobility by evaluating active and passive **range of motion (ROM)**. ROM is the full movement potential of a joint. Common movements that occur at the synovial joints, including *abduction, adduction, flexion,* and *extension,* are described in Table 66.5. Measurements should

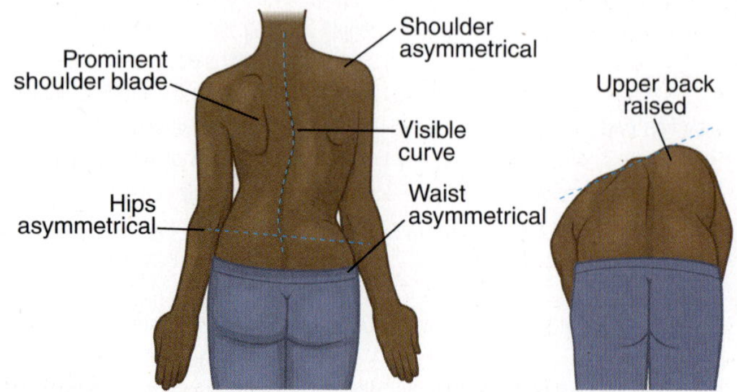

Fig. 66.7 Scoliosis assessment. (A) Standing. (B) Forward bending.

TABLE 66.5 Synovial Joint Movements

Movement	Description
Abduction	Movement of part away from midline of body
Adduction	Movement of part toward midline of body
Circumduction	Circular motion of a body part from a combination of flexion, abduction, extension, and adduction
Dorsiflexion	Flexion of the ankle and toes toward the shin
Eversion	Turning of sole outward away from midline of body
Extension	Straightening of joint that ↑ angle between 2 bones
External rotation	Movement along longitudinal axis away from midline of body
Flexion	Bending of joint from muscle contraction that causes ↓ angle between 2 bones
Hyperextension	Extension in which angle exceeds 180 degrees
Internal rotation	Movement along longitudinal axis toward midline of body
Inversion	Turning of sole inward toward midline of body
Opposition	Moving the first and fifth metacarpals anteriorly from a flattened palm ("cupping position"); makes it possible to hold objects between the thumb and fingers
Plantar flexion	Flexion of the ankle and toes toward the plantar surface of the foot ("toes pointed")
Pronation	Turning of palm downward
Supination	Turning of palm upward

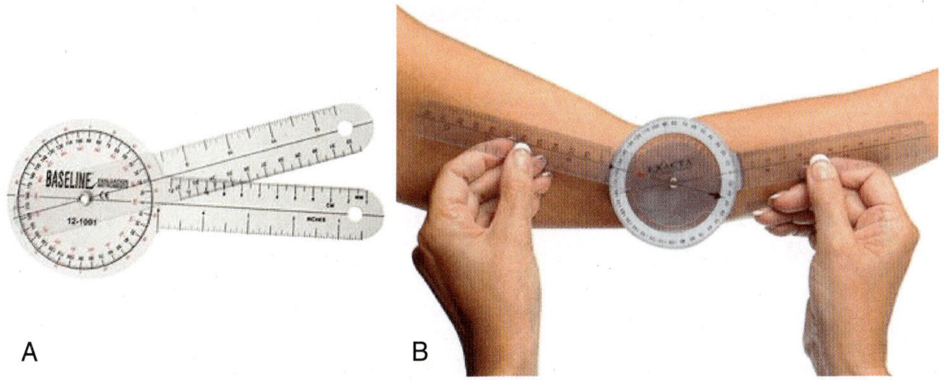

Fig. 66.8 (A) Goniometer. (B) Measurement of joint ROM using a goniometer. (From LaSala TT, Run-Kowzun T, Figueroa M: The effect of a Hatha yoga practice on hamstring flexibility, *J Bodyw Move Ther* 28:439–449, 2021.)

TABLE 66.6 Muscle Strength Scale

0/5	No detection of muscular contraction
1/5	Barely detectable flicker or trace of contraction with observation or palpation
2/5	Active movement of body part with elimination of gravity
3/5	Active movement against gravity only and not against resistance
4/5	Active movement against gravity and some resistance
5/5	Active movement against full resistance without fatigue (normal muscle strength)

be similar for active and passive maneuvers. Be careful in performing passive ROM because of the risk for injury to underlying structures. If pain or resistance occurs, stop at once.

If you note deficits in active or passive ROM, assess function. Are joint changes affecting the ability to perform ADLs? Ask patients if activities, such as eating, grooming, dressing, and bathing, require help or cannot be done at all.

Use a goniometer to accurately assess ROM and measure joint angles (Fig. 66.8). We do not usually measure specific degrees of ROM of all joints. If a specific musculoskeletal problem has been identified, measure ROM of the affected joint.

Perform the *straight-leg-raising test* on patients with sciatica or leg pain. With the patient supine, passively raise the leg 60 degrees or less. The test is positive if the patient reports pain along the distribution of the sciatic nerve. A positive test shows nerve root irritation from intervertebral disc prolapse and herniation, especially at level L4–5 or L5–S1.

Muscle strength. Assess the strength of individual muscles or groups of muscles using a 5-point scale (Table 66.6). Grade normal muscle strength with full resistance to opposition as a 5/5 bilaterally. To test resistance to opposition, have the patient apply resistance as you exert a force. For example, have the patient extend the elbow while you flex it. Assess dorsi and plantar flexion and knee and hip flexion. Assess hand grip strength.

Neurovascular assessment. Perform a neurovascular assessment to assess sensory function and peripheral circulation. In addition to motor function, assess the color and temperature of the extremities. Note peripheral pulse quality and measure capillary refill. Test for any areas of numbness and problems with sensation.

MUSCULOSKELETAL SYSTEM DIAGNOSTIC STUDIES

Many diagnostic studies are used to help determine a diagnosis and treatment plan. Tables 66.7 and 66.8 present the most common studies.

The x-ray is the most common diagnostic study.[7] Dense areas, like bone, show as white on the standard x-ray. X-rays provide information about bone deformity, joint congruity, bone density, and soft tissue calcifications. X-rays are used for diagnosing fractures. MRI is best for evaluating soft tissue injuries.[8]

CASE STUDY

Objective Data: Physical Assessment

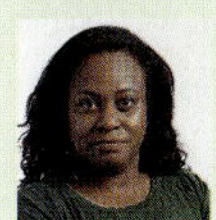
(© Studio CJ/ iStock.com.)

A focused assessment of G.A. reveals: BP 128/94, heart rate 88, respiratory rate 26, temp 96.8°F, O_2 saturation 98%. Alert and oriented ×3. Left great toe is red and swollen. No open wounds. Tremendous pain on palpation and with any movement of the left great toe. +1 Pedal pulses bilaterally. No edema or changes in sensation.

Discussion Questions

1. What physical assessment findings concern you most?
2. Based on the subjective and physical assessment findings, what diagnostic studies might you expect to be ordered for G.A.?

You will learn more about diagnostic studies related to the musculoskeletal system in the next section.

Answers available at http://evolve.elsevier.com/Lewis/medsurg.

TABLE 66.7 Serology Studies

Musculoskeletal System

Test	Reference Intervals	Description and Purpose
Aldolase	22–59 mU/L	Enzyme involved in glycolysis. ↑ in muscular dystrophy, crush injuries.
Alkaline phosphatase	30–120 U/L (0.5–2.0 μkat/L)	Enzyme made by osteoblasts, needed for mineralization of organic bone matrix. ↑ in healing fractures, bone cancer, osteoporosis, osteomalacia, Paget disease.
Anticyclic citrullinated peptide antibody (anti-CCP)	<20.0 U	Presence of CCP antibodies indicates high likelihood of rheumatoid arthritis.
Anti-DNA antibody	<5 IU/mL	Detects serum antibodies that react with DNA. Most specific test for systemic lupus erythematosus (SLE).
Antinuclear antibody (ANA)	Negative at 1:40 dilution	Assess presence of antibodies capable of destroying nucleus of tissue cells. Positive in 95% of patients with SLE. May be positive with scleroderma, rheumatoid arthritis, small number of normal persons.
Calcium (total)	9.0–10.5 mg/dL (2.25–2.62 mmol/L)	Bone is main site for calcium storage. ↓ in osteomalacia, fat embolism, vitamin D deficiency. ↑ in Paget disease, bone metastases.
C-reactive protein (CRP)	<1.0 mg/dL	Made by liver. Present in large amounts in serum 18–24 h after onset of tissue damage. Used to diagnose inflammatory diseases, infections, active widespread cancer.
Creatine kinase (CK)	20–200 U/L	Highest concentration in skeletal muscle. ↑ in muscular dystrophy, polymyositis, traumatic injuries.
Human leukocyte antigen (HLA)–B27	Negative	Often present in autoimmune disorders, such as ankylosing spondylitis, rheumatoid arthritis.
Phosphorus	3.0–4.5 mg/dL (0.97–1.45 mmol/L)	Indirectly related to calcium. ↓ in osteomalacia. ↑ in rhabdomyolysis, crush injuries, bone metastases.
Rheumatoid factor (RF)	Negative or titer <1:17	Presence of the autoantibody rheumatoid factor. Not specific for rheumatoid arthritis. Seen in other connective tissue diseases and small number of normal persons.

TABLE 66.8 Diagnostic Studies

Musculoskeletal System

Study	Description and Purpose	Nursing Responsibilities
Basic x-ray	Evaluates structural or functional changes of bones and joints. Gives general impression of bone density. In anteroposterior view, x-ray beam passes from front to back, allowing 1-dimensional view. Lateral position provides 2-dimensional view.	*Before:* Remove any radiopaque objects that can interfere with results. *During:* Avoid excess exposure of patient and self.
Bone scan	Inject radioisotope (usually technetium [Tc]-99 m) that is taken up by bone. Uniform uptake of isotope is normal. ↑ Uptake with osteomyelitis, arthritis, bone cancer, certain fractures. ↓ Uptake in areas of avascular necrosis.	*Before:* Explain that radioisotope is given 2 h before procedure. Have patient void before scan. Tell patient that no harm will result from isotopes. *During:* Patient must lie completely still during scan. *After:* Increase fluids after scan.
CT	X-ray beam used with a computer to provide a 3D picture. Used to identify soft tissue and bone abnormalities and musculoskeletal trauma.	*Before:* Assess renal function before contrast medium used. Patient may be NPO 4 h prior to study. If the patient is taking metformin, hold it the day of the test to prevent hypoglycemia or lactic acidosis. *During:* Warn patient that contrast injection may cause a feeling of being warm and flushed. Patient must lie completely still during scan. *After:* Encourage patient to drink fluids to avoid renal problems with any contrast.
Discogram	X-ray of cervical or lumbar intervertebral disc done after injecting contrast media into nucleus pulposus. Assesses for intervertebral disc abnormalities.	*Before:* Assess patient for allergy to contrast medium. Explain procedure. *After:* May have mild back pain for 1–2 days. Use as-needed analgesics.
Dual energy x-ray absorptiometry (DEXA)	Measures bone mineral density of spine, femur, forearm, total body. Assesses bone density with minimal radiation exposure. Used to diagnose metabolic bone disease (e.g., osteoporosis), monitor changes in bone density with treatment.	*Before:* Remove any radiopaque objects that can interfere with results.

Continued

TABLE 66.8 **Diagnostic Studies— cont'd**

Study	Description and Purpose	Nursing Responsibilities
Electromyogram (EMG)	Evaluates electrical potential of skeletal muscle contraction. Small-gauge needles are inserted into certain muscles. Needles are attached to leads that send information to EMG machine. Recordings of muscle electrical activity are traced on audio transmitter, oscilloscope, and recording paper. Provides information about lower motor neuron problems and primary muscle disease.	*Before:* Tell patient needle insertion will cause discomfort. Some HCPs restrict stimulants (e.g., caffeine) 2–3 h prior. *After:* Assess needle sites for hematoma or inflammation. Use as-needed analgesics.
MRI	Radio waves and magnetic field used to view soft tissue. Used to diagnose avascular necrosis, disc disease, tumors, osteomyelitis, ligament or cartilage tears. IV contrast may be given to enhance visualization of structures.	*Before:* Check for pregnancy, allergies, and renal function before test. Have patient remove all metal objects. Ask about any surgical insertion of staples, plates, dental bridges, or other metal appliances. Remove metallic foil patches. Patient may need to be fasting. Assess for claustrophobia and the need for antianxiety medication. *During:* Patient must lie completely still during test. *After:* Increase fluids if contrast given.
Myelogram with or without CT	Injection of a radiographic contrast medium into sac around nerve roots. CT scan may follow to show how bone is affecting the nerve roots. Sensitive test for nerve impingement, can detect subtle lesions and injuries.	*Before:* Give sedative as ordered. Have patient empty bladder. Tell patient that test is done with patient on tilting table that is moved during test. *After:* Keep patient flat for 1–2 h after to prevent spinal headache. Encourage fluids. Monitor neurologic signs and VS. Headache, nausea, and vomiting may occur after.
Somatosensory evoked potential (SSEP)	Evaluates evoked potential of muscle contractions. Electrodes are placed on skin that provide recordings of electrical activity of muscle. Used to identify lower motor neuron dysfunction and primary muscle disease. Measures nerve conduction along pathways not accessible by EMG. Transcutaneous or percutaneous electrodes applied to the skin help identify neuropathy and myopathy. Used during spinal surgery for scoliosis to detect neurologic compromise when patient is under anesthesia.	*Before:* Tell patient that procedure is like an EMG but does not involve needles. Electrodes are applied to the skin.
Thermography	Uses infrared detector to measure degree of heat radiating from skin surface. Assess inflamed joint and determine response to drug therapy. Can evaluate skin temperature.	*Before:* Tell patient that procedure is painless and noninvasive.
Ultrasound	Assesses tendon and ligament injuries, bursa, nerve and vascular injuries, infections, and soft tissue masses.	*Before:* Tell patient that procedure is painless and noninvasive.

TABLE 66.9 **Interventional Studies**

Musculoskeletal System

Study	Description and Purpose	Nursing Responsibilities
Arthrocentesis	Incision or puncture of joint capsule to obtain samples of synovial fluid or to remove excess fluid. Local anesthesia and aseptic preparation are used before needle is inserted into joint and fluid aspirated. Used to diagnose joint inflammation, infection, meniscal tears, and subtle fractures.	*Before:* HCP may have patient be NPO prior. Usually done at bedside or in examination room. *After:* Send synovial fluid sample to laboratory. Apply compression dressing and ice to decrease pain and swelling. Observe for blood or fluid on dressing. Assess the joint for any pain, fever, or swelling. Review activity restrictions.
Arthroscopy	Insertion of arthroscope into joint to see interior of joint cavity. Can be used for surgery (removal of loose bodies, biopsy); repair of joint structures; diagnosis of problems with meniscus, articular cartilage, ligaments, joint capsule. Structures that can be seen through an arthroscope include knee, shoulder, elbow, wrist, jaw, hip, ankle (Fig. 66.9).	*Before:* Can be done in outpatient setting. Local or general anesthesia may be used. HCP may have patient be NPO prior. *After:* Cover wound with sterile dressing. Apply ice to decrease pain and swelling. Observe for bleeding. Assess the joint for any pain, weakness, or swelling. Review activity restrictions.

Synovial fluid can be obtained for analysis through arthrocentesis (Table 66.9). The fluid is assessed for volume, color, clarity, viscosity, and mucin clot formation. Normal synovial fluid is transparent, thin, and colorless or straw colored. Fluid from an infected joint may be purulent and thick or gray and thin. In gout, the fluid may be whitish yellow and contain urate crystals. Blood may be aspirated if there is hemarthrosis due to injury or a bleeding disorder. Floating fat globules indicate bone injury. The mucin clot test gives information about the protein in synovial fluid. Normally a white, ropelike mucin clot is formed. With inflammation, the clot fragments easily. A Gram stain and culture may be done to assess for infection.

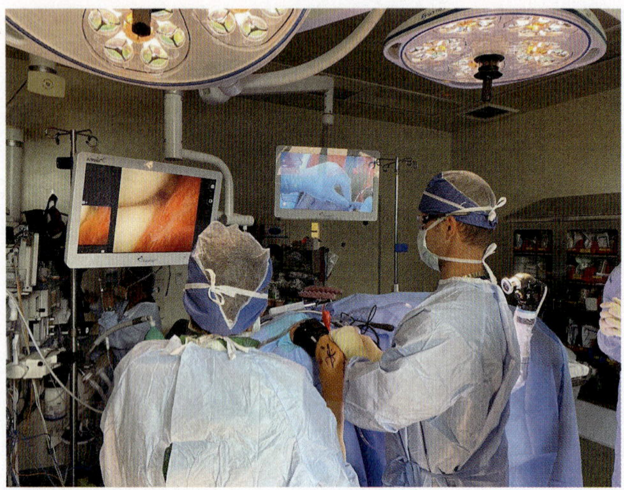

Fig. 66.9 Elbow arthroscopy in progress. Patient is positioned so monitor is clearly visible. (From Fournier M, Corning E, Witt A, et al: Arthroscopically assisted fixation of terrible triad variant injuries of the elbow with small-bore needle arthroscopy, *Arthrosc Tech* 10:e1469–e1474, 2021.)

CASE STUDY

Objective Data: Diagnostic Studies

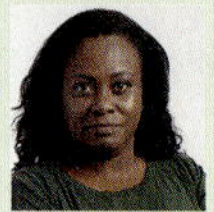

(© Studio CJ/ iStock.com.)

The HCP orders the following diagnostic studies:

- X-ray of left foot
- CBC, electrolytes
- Aspiration of the great toe

The foot x-ray shows minor soft tissue swelling but no signs of fracture. Very mild arthritis is noted at the interphalangeal joint of the great toe. CBC and electrolytes are within normal limits. Aspiration of the interphalangeal joint shows clear synovial fluid. Protein and glucose are within normal limits. Synovial fluid analysis shows urate crystals.

Discussion Questions

1. Which diagnostic results are abnormal?
2. What diagnostic study results concern you most?

Answers available at http://evolve.elsevier.com/Lewis/medsurg.

BRIDGE TO NCLEX EXAMINATION

The number of the question corresponds to the same-numbered outcome at the beginning of the chapter.

1. The bone cells that function in the formation of new bone tissue after a patient sustains a fracture are called
   a. osteoids
   b. osteocytes.
   c. osteoclasts.
   d. osteoblasts.
2. When performing active range of motion with a patient, the nurse puts the knee joint through the movements of
   a. flexion and extension.
   b. pronation and supination.
   c. abduction and adduction.
   d. rotation and circumduction.
3. A patient with a torn shoulder ligament asks what the ligament does. The nurse would respond that ligaments
   a. connect bone to bone.
   b. provide strength to muscle.
   c. lubricate joints with synovial fluid.
   d. relieve friction between moving parts.
4. The increased risk for falls in the older adult is likely due to **(Select all that apply.)**
   a. changes in balance.
   b. decrease in bone mass.
   c. loss of ligament elasticity.
   d. decrease in reaction time.
   e. decrease in muscle mass and strength.
5. The nurse obtained a health history of a patient with a fracture. Which problem, if reported by the patient, would most concern the nurse?
   a. Diabetes
   b. Hypertension
   c. Chronic bronchitis
   d. Nephrotic syndrome
6. When grading muscle strength, the nurse records a score of 3/5. This indicates
   a. no detection of muscular contraction.
   b. a barely detectable flicker of contraction.
   c. active movement against full resistance without fatigue.
   d. active movement against gravity but not against resistance.

7. An abnormal finding during a musculoskeletal assessment is
   a. equal leg length bilaterally.
   b. ulnar deviation and subluxation.
   c. full range of motion in all joints.
   d. muscle strength of 5/5 in all muscles.

8. A patient is scheduled for a bone scan. The nurse explains that this test involves
   a. incision or puncture of the joint capsule.
   b. insertion of small needles into certain muscles.
   c. administration of a radioisotope before the procedure.
   d. placement of skin electrodes to record muscle activity.

1. d; 2. a; 3. a; 4. a, b, c, e; 5. a; 6. d; 7. b; 8. c.

For rationales to these answers and even more NCLEX review questions, visit http://evolve.elsevier.com/Lewis/medsurg.

REFERENCES

To access the References for this chapter, please scan the QR code with a mobile device.

67

Musculoskeletal Trauma and Orthopedic Surgery

Rebekah O. Filson

http://evolve.elsevier.com/Lewis/medsurg/

CONCEPTUAL FOCUS

Functional Ability
Infection
Mobility
Pain
Perfusion
Safety

LEARNING OUTCOMES

1. Discuss the etiology, pathophysiology, manifestations, and interprofessional and nursing management of soft tissue injuries.
2. Relate the sequence of events involved in fracture healing.
3. Compare closed reduction, casting, open reduction, and traction in terms of purpose, complications, and nursing management.
4. Assess the neurovascular condition of an injured extremity.
5. Explain common complications of a fracture and fracture healing.
6. Describe the interprofessional and nursing management of patients with various kinds of fractures.
7. Describe indications for and interprofessional and nursing management of patients with an amputation.
8. Describe types of joint replacement surgery.
9. Prioritize care of patients having joint replacement surgery.

KEY TERMS

amputation
arthrodesis
arthroplasty
bursitis
carpal tunnel syndrome (CTS)
compartment syndrome
dislocation
fat embolism syndrome (FES)
fracture
osteotomy
phantom limb sensation
repetitive strain injury (RSI)
sprain
strain
traction

This chapter discusses musculoskeletal problems resulting from trauma and common orthopedic surgeries. The most common cause of musculoskeletal injury is a traumatic event resulting in fracture and/or soft tissue injury. Most of these injuries are not fatal. However, accidents are 1 of the top 3 causes of death for persons ages 1 to 64 years.[1] The costs in terms of pain, disability, and expense are enormous. After trauma or surgery, the injured area is often immobilized while healing occurs. Nurses have a key role in preventing complications (e.g., pressure injuries, constipation, infection, venous thromboembolism [VTE]) and promoting functional ability.

Nurses play a key role in teaching the public about basic principles of safety and accident prevention. Teach people to take safety precautions while at home or work, driving, or taking part in sports (Box 67.1). Accidents can be reduced if people are aware of hazards, use safety equipment, and apply safety and traffic rules. In the work setting, teach employees and employers to use safety equipment and decrease workplace hazards. Falls cause many injuries. Provide preventive teaching to high-risk persons (e.g., people with gait instability, impaired vision) (Table 67.1).

SOFT TISSUE INJURIES

Soft tissue injuries include sprains, strains, dislocations, and subluxations. They usually result from trauma. As more people have become involved in fitness programs or sports, the incidence of soft tissue injuries has increased. Table 67.2 describes common sports-related injuries. Sports injuries that often result in a visit to the emergency department (ED) for younger patients include sprains and strains, growth plate injuries, and repetitive motion injuries.[2]

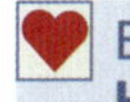

BOX 67.1 PROMOTING POPULATION HEALTH

Reducing the Risk for Musculoskeletal Injuries

- Use proper lifting techniques.
- Use safety equipment at work.
- Warm up and stretch before exercise.
- Use protective athletic equipment (helmets and knee, wrist, and elbow pads).
- Avoid awkward postures by adjusting work heights and minimizing reach distances.
- Follow traffic rules—wear seatbelts, drive within the speed limit, and avoid distracted driving.

TABLE 67.1 PATIENT & CAREGIVER TEACHING

Reducing Risk for Falls

To reduce the risk for falls, include the following instructions when teaching patients and caregivers:

1. Use shoes with good support for safety and comfort.
2. Use caution on wet or slippery surfaces.
3. Remove throw rugs and ensure adequate lighting in the home.
4. Maintain clear paths to the bathroom for nighttime use.
5. Get regular and frequent exercise. Include exercises that focus on balance and strength training.
6. Stress the importance of adequate calcium and vitamin D intake for bone health.
7. Avoid sudden change in position. Rise slowly to a standing position to prevent dizziness, falls, and fractures.
8. Do not walk on uneven surfaces and wet floors. Use ramps in buildings and at street corners instead of steps.

SPRAINS AND STRAINS

Sprains and strains often result from abnormal stretching or twisting forces during vigorous activities. These injuries tend to occur around joints and in the spinal muscles.

A **sprain** is an injury to the ligaments surrounding a joint. Sprains are usually caused by a wrenching or twisting motion. Most occur in the ankle, wrist, and knee joints. We classify sprains according to the degree of ligament damage. A *first-degree (mild) sprain* involves tears in only a few fibers, with mild tenderness and minimal swelling. A *second-degree (moderate) sprain* results in partial disruption of the involved tissue with more swelling and tenderness. A *third-degree (severe) sprain* is a complete tear of the ligament with moderate to severe swelling.[3]

A **strain** is an excess stretching of a muscle and its fascial sheath, often involving the tendon. Most strains occur in the large muscle groups, including the lower back, calf, and hamstrings. We classify strains as first degree (mild or slightly pulled muscle), second degree (moderately torn muscle), or third degree (severely torn or ruptured muscle).[3] The muscle defect may be apparent or palpated through the skin if the muscle is torn. Because areas around joints are rich in nerve endings, strains can be very painful.

Manifestations of sprains and strains are similar. They include pain, edema, decreased function, and bruising. Continued use of the joint, tendon, or ligament makes pain worse. Edema develops in the injured area from the local inflammatory response.

TABLE 67.2 Soft Tissue Injuries

Injury	Description	Treatment
Anterior cruciate ligament tear	Tearing of ligament by deceleration forces with pivoting or odd positions of the knee or leg	PT with rehabilitation, knee brace. If knee instability or further injury, reconstructive surgery may be done.
Impingement syndrome	Entrapment of soft tissues and nerves under coracoacromial arch of shoulder	NSAIDs. Rest until symptoms ↓, then begin gradual ROM and strength exercises.
Ligament injury	Tearing or stretching of ligament. Usually occurs from inversion, eversion, shearing, or torque applied to a joint. Sudden pain, swelling, and instability	Rest, ice, elevation of extremity if possible, NSAIDs. Protect affected extremity with a brace. If symptoms persist, surgical repair may be needed.
Meniscus injury	Injury to fibrocartilage discs in knee. Popping, clicking, tearing sensation, effusion, and/or swelling	Rest, ice, elevation of extremity if possible, NSAIDs. Gradual return to regular activities. If symptoms persist, MRI to assess meniscus injury. Possible arthroscopic surgery.
Rotator cuff tear	Tear within muscle, tendons, or ligaments around shoulder	*If minor tear:* rest, NSAIDs, and gradual mobilization with ROM and strength exercises. *If major tear:* surgical repair.
Shin splints	Inflammation of periosteal bone *(periostitis)* along anterior calf. Caused by improper shoes, overuse, or running on hard pavement	Rest, ice, NSAIDs, proper shoes. Gradual ↑ in activity. If pain persists, x-ray to rule out tibial stress fracture.
Tendonitis	Inflammation of tendon due to overuse or incorrect use	Rest, ice, NSAIDs. Gradual return to sport activity. Protective brace *(orthosis)* may be needed if symptoms recur.

Mild sprains and strains are usually self-limiting. Full function generally returns within 3 to 6 weeks. X-rays may be done to rule out a fracture. A severe sprain can cause an *avulsion fracture,* in which the ligament pulls loose a fragment of bone. The joint structure may become unstable, causing subluxation or dislocation. At the time of injury, *hemarthrosis* (bleeding into a joint space or cavity) or disruption of the synovial lining may occur. Severe strains may need surgical repair of the muscle, tendon, or surrounding fascia.

NURSING MANAGEMENT: SPRAINS AND STRAINS

Implementation

Health Promotion

Warming up muscles before exercising and vigorous activity, followed by stretching, may significantly reduce the risk for soft tissue injury. Balance and endurance exercises are important (Box 67.2). Strength exercises that involve working against resistance build muscle strength and bone density. Balance exercises, which may overlap with some strength exercises, help prevent falls. Exercise should start at a low level of effort and progress gradually.

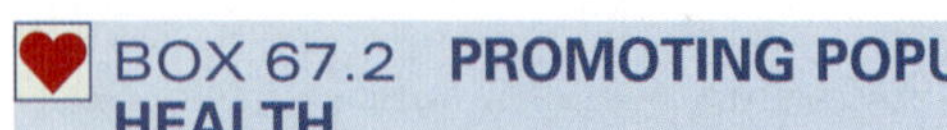

Health Impact of Physical Activity

- Helps with weight management
- Increases lean muscle and decreases body fat
- Helps maintain and improve bone mass
- Increases muscle strength, flexibility, and endurance
- Helps prevent high BP
- Reduces the risk for heart disease, diabetes, and colon cancer
- Enhances sense of well-being and reduces risk for depression

Acute Care

Most strains and sprains are treated in an outpatient setting. Immediate care focuses on (1) limiting movement to the injured part, (2) applying ice packs to the injured area, (3) compressing the involved area, (4) elevating the extremity, and (5) providing analgesia as needed (Table 67.3).

PRICE (*P*rotection, *R*est, *I*ce, *C*ompression, *E*levation) limits swelling and pain and improves healing for most musculoskeletal injuries.[3] Movement should be restricted with the extremity rested as soon as pain is felt. Unless the injury is severe, prolonged rest is usually not needed.

There are several forms of cold therapy. Cold causes vasoconstriction in the soft tissue and reduces the transmission and perception of nerve pain impulses. These changes reduce muscle spasms, inflammation, and edema. Cold is most useful when applied immediately after an injury has occurred and used for 24 to 28 hours. Apply ice for 20 to 30 minutes at a time. Do not apply ice directly to the skin.

Compression helps decrease edema and pain. We often use an elastic compression bandage. It can be wrapped around the injured part. To prevent edema and encourage fluid return, wrap the bandage starting distally (at the point farthest from the trunk of the body) and progress proximally (toward the trunk of the body). The bandage is too tight if there is numbness or tingling below the area of compression or pain or

TABLE 67.3 EMERGENCY MANAGEMENT

Acute Soft Tissue Injury

Cause	Assessment Findings	Interventions
• Crush injury • Direct blows • Falls • Motor vehicle crashes • Sports injuries	• Bruising • ↓ Movement with limited function or inability to bear weight (lower extremity) • ↓ HR, coolness, capillary refill >2 sec • ↓↓ Sensation • Edema • Muscle spasms • Pain, tenderness • Pallor • Shortening or rotation of extremity	**Initial** • Ensure airway, breathing, and circulation. • Perform neurovascular assessment of involved limb. • Elevate involved limb. • Apply compression bandage unless dislocation present. • Apply ice packs to affected area. • Immobilize affected extremity in the position found. Do *not* try to realign or reinsert protruding bones. • Anticipate x-rays of injured extremity. • Give analgesia as needed. • Give antibiotic prophylaxis for open fracture, large tissue defects, mangled extremity injury. • Give tetanus prophylaxis if there is a break in skin. **Ongoing Monitoring** • Monitor for changes in neurovascular status. • Implement weight-bearing restrictions for lower extremity involvement. • Monitor for compartment syndrome.

more swelling occurs beyond the edge of the bandage. Use of an elastic wrap may provide extra support during training, athletic, and work activities.

Elevate the injured part above heart level, even during sleep, for 24 to 48 hours to help mobilize excess fluid from the area and prevent further edema. Mild analgesics and nonsteroidal antiinflammatory drugs (NSAIDs) may be used for discomfort.

After the acute phase (usually 24 to 48 hours), apply warm, moist heat to the affected part to reduce swelling and provide comfort. Heat applications should not exceed 20 to 30 minutes. Allow a "cool-down" time between applications. Encourage patients to use the limb if the joint is protected by a cast, brace, splint, or taping. Joint movement maintains nutrition to the cartilage. Movement helps prevent *contracture* (stiffening) of tendons and ligaments. Muscle contraction improves circulation and helps resolve bruising and swelling.

Emphasize the importance of strength and conditioning exercises to prevent reinjury. The physical therapist may help with pain relief by using ultrasound or other interventions. They can teach patients exercises to improve flexibility and strength.

DISLOCATIONS

Dislocation is the complete displacement or separation of the articular surfaces of the joint. *Subluxation* is a partial or incomplete displacement of the joint surface. Symptoms of subluxation are similar to a dislocation but are less severe. Many structures contribute to joint stability. Injury to, or excess laxity of, ligaments is a major factor in dislocations or subluxations. Weak or atrophied muscles can cause chronic joint instability. Fibrocartilage structures, such as the labrum around hip and shoulder sockets and the meniscus at the knee, play a key role in joint stability. Even small tears to these structures can result in recurrent, chronic dislocations or subluxations.

Dislocations typically result from forces on the joint that disrupt the surrounding soft tissue support structures. The joints most often dislocated in the upper extremity include the thumb, elbow, and shoulder. The shoulder most often dislocates anteriorly. Posterior shoulder dislocation typically only happens after electrocution or seizure. In the lower extremity, the hip is vulnerable to dislocation from severe trauma, often from motor vehicle crashes (Fig. 67.1). The kneecap *(patella)* may dislocate after a sharp, direct blow or sudden twisting inward motion while the planted foot is pointed outward.

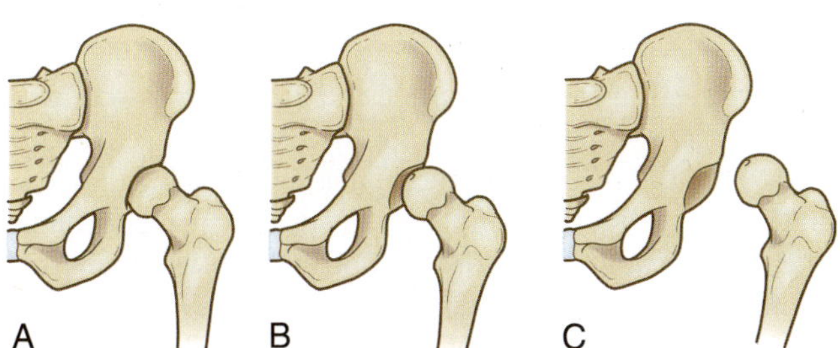

Fig. 67.1 Soft tissue injury of the hip. (A) Normal. (B) Subluxation (partial dislocation). (C) Dislocation.

The most obvious sign of a dislocation is deformity. Other manifestations include local pain, tenderness, loss of function, and swelling of soft tissues near the joint. Major complications include open joint injuries, *intraarticular* fractures (within the joint), *avascular necrosis* (bone cell death from blood supply), and damage to adjacent nerves and blood vessels.

X-rays can determine the extent of displacement. The joint may be aspirated to assess for hemarthrosis or fat cells. Fat cells in the aspirate indicate a probable intraarticular fracture.

Interprofessional and Nursing Management

A dislocation requires prompt attention. It is often considered an emergency because it can cause significant vascular injury. The longer the joint is dislocated, the greater the risk for avascular necrosis and compartment syndrome. The femoral head of the hip joint is especially susceptible to avascular necrosis. Compartment syndrome is due to vascular injury and resulting ischemia. Neurovascular assessment is critical.

The first goal is to realign the dislocated part of the joint to its original anatomic position. Closed reduction (no incision) may be done under local or general anesthesia or IV moderate to deep sedation. Anesthesia is often needed to relax the muscle so that the bones can be manipulated. Sometimes, open reduction (joint visualized through surgery) may be needed. After reduction, the extremity is immobilized by a brace, splint, or sling, or by taping, to allow torn ligaments and surrounding tissue to heal.

Nursing care includes pain management and support and protection of the injured joint. After the joint has been reduced and immobilized, motion is usually restricted. A monitored exercise program can prevent further instability and joint problems. Gentle range-of-motion (ROM) exercises may be done if the joint is stable and well supported. Exercise slowly restores the joint to its original ROM without causing another dislocation. Patients should gradually return to normal activities.

Patients who have dislocated a joint may be at greater risk for repeated dislocations due to damage or laxity to the supporting structures. Activity restrictions may be imposed on the affected joint to decrease the risk for repeated dislocations.

REPETITIVE STRAIN INJURY

Repetitive strain injury (RSI) and *cumulative trauma disorder* are terms used to describe injuries resulting from prolonged force or repetitive movements and awkward postures. Repeated movements strain the tendons, ligaments, and muscles, causing tiny tears that become inflamed. We do not know the exact cause of RSI. No specific diagnostic tests exist, and diagnosis is often difficult.

Persons at risk for RSI include musicians, dancers, butchers, grocery clerks, vibratory tool workers, and those who use a computer mouse and keyboard. Competitive athletes and poorly trained athletes may develop RSI. Swimming, overhead throwing (e.g., baseball), weightlifting, gymnastics, tennis, skiing, and kicking sports (e.g., soccer) require repetitive motion. Overtraining compounds the effects of RSI.

Other risk factors include poor posture and positioning, poor workspace ergonomics, badly designed workplace equipment (e.g., computer keyboard), and repetitive lifting of heavy objects without sufficient muscle rest. Inflammation, swelling, and pain in the muscles, tendons, and nerves of the neck, spine, shoulder, forearm, and hand may result. Symptoms of RSI include pain, weakness, numbness, or impaired motor function.

RSI can be prevented through education and *ergonomics* (the science that promotes efficiency and safety in the interaction of humans and their work environment). For example, ergonomic considerations for those who work at a desk and use a computer include keeping the hips and knees flexed to 90 degrees with the feet flat, keeping the wrist straight to type, having the top of the computer monitor even with the forehead, and taking at least hourly stretch breaks.

Treatment is supportive. Pain management includes heat or cold therapy, NSAIDs, and rest. Physical therapy (PT) focuses on strength and conditioning exercises. Teach patients about lifestyle changes and ways to modify equipment and/or activity.

CARPAL TUNNEL SYNDROME

Carpal tunnel syndrome (CTS) is caused by median nerve compression. The median nerve enters the hand at the wrist through the narrow carpal tunnel (Fig. 67.2). The carpal tunnel is formed by ligaments and bones. CTS is the most common compression neuropathy in the upper extremity. It is associated with hobbies or work that require continuous wrist movement (e.g., musicians, carpenters, computer operators).

CTS is often caused by pressure from trauma or edema (from inflammation of a tendon *[tenosynovitis]*), cancer, rheumatoid arthritis (RA), or soft tissue masses, such as ganglia. Hormones may be involved because CTS often occurs during the premenstrual period, pregnancy, and menopause. Persons with diabetes, peripheral vascular disease (PVD), and RA have a higher incidence due to swelling that changes blood flow to the nerve and narrows the carpal tunnel.[4] Females are more likely to develop CTS, possibly from a smaller carpal tunnel.

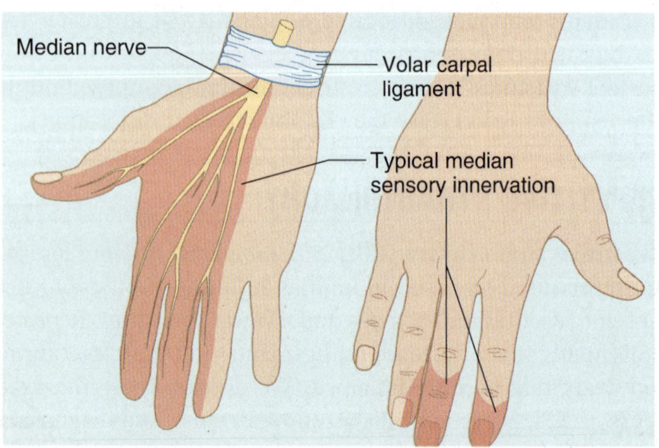

Fig. 67.2 Wrist structures involved in carpal tunnel syndrome. Median nerve distribution. *Shaded areas* show the locations of pain in carpal tunnel syndrome. (From Buttaravoli P: *Minor emergencies,* ed 3, Philadelphia, 2012, Saunders.)

Manifestations include impaired sensation, pain, numbness, or weakness in the distribution of the median nerve (Fig. 67.2). Numbness and tingling may awaken patients at night. Shaking the hands often relieves these symptoms. Clumsiness in performing fine hand movements is common.

Patients may have a positive Tinel sign and Phalen sign. Elicit *Tinel sign* by tapping over the median nerve as it passes through the carpal tunnel in the wrist. A positive response is a sensation of tingling in the distribution of the median nerve over the hand. Test for *Phalen sign* by allowing the wrists to fall freely into maximum flexion and maintain the position for longer than 60 seconds. A positive response is a sensation of tingling in the distribution of the median nerve over the hand. In late stages, atrophy of the muscles around the base of the thumb results in recurrent pain and eventual dysfunction of the hand.

Interprofessional and Nursing Management

To prevent CTS, teach patients to identify risk factors. Adaptive devices, such as wrist splints, may be worn to hold the wrist in a slight extension and relieve pressure on the median nerve. Special keyboard pads and computer mice can help prevent repetitive pressure on the median nerve. Other ergonomic changes include workstation changes, change in body positions, and frequent breaks from work activities.

Care is directed toward relieving the underlying cause of the nerve compression. Early symptoms can usually be relieved by stopping the aggravating movement and by resting the hand and wrist by immobilization in a hand splint. Splints worn at night help keep the wrist in a neutral position. This may reduce night pain and numbness. PT with hand and wrist exercises may lessen symptom severity. A corticosteroid injection directly into the carpal tunnel may give short-term relief.

Carpal tunnel release is generally done if symptoms last more than 6 months or if there is significant impairment to conduction on electromyography (EMG). Surgery involves severing the band of tissue around the wrist to reduce pressure on the median nerve (Fig. 67.2). Surgery is done in the outpatient setting using local anesthesia. The types of carpal tunnel release surgery include open release and endoscopic surgery. In *open release surgery,* an incision is made in the wrist and then the carpal ligament is cut to enlarge the carpal tunnel. *Endoscopic carpal tunnel release* is done through 1 or more small puncture incisions in the wrist and palm. A camera is attached to a tube, and the carpal ligament is cut. The endoscopic approach may allow a faster recovery and cause less discomfort than traditional open release surgery.

Although symptoms may be relieved right after surgery, full recovery may take months. After surgery, assess the hand's neurovascular status. Teach patients about wound care and assessments to perform at home.

ROTATOR CUFF INJURY

The rotator cuff is made up of 4 muscles in the shoulder: the supraspinatus, infraspinatus, teres minor, and subscapularis muscles. These muscles stabilize the humeral head in the glenoid fossa and assist with ROM of the shoulder and rotation of the humerus.

A tear in the rotator cuff may occur as a gradual, degenerative process due to aging, repetitive stress (especially overhead arm motions), or injury to the shoulder. In sports, repetitive overhead motions, such as in swimming, weightlifting, and swinging a racquet (tennis, pickleball), often cause injury. The rotator cuff can tear because of sudden adduction forces applied to the cuff while the arm is held in abduction. Other causes include (1) falling onto an outstretched arm and hand, (2) a blow to the upper arm, (3) heavy lifting, or (4) repetitive work motions.[5]

Manifestations include shoulder weakness, pain, and decreased ROM. Patients usually have severe pain when the arm is abducted between 60 and 120 degrees (the painful arc). A positive *drop arm test* is a sign of rotator cuff injury. In this test, the arm is abducted 90 degrees. The patient is asked to slowly lower the arm to the side. If the arm falls suddenly, rotator cuff injury is suspected. MRI can usually confirm a tear.

Patients with a partial tear or cuff inflammation may be treated with rest, ice, and heat, NSAIDs, corticosteroid injections into the subacromial space, ultrasound, and PT. If there is no response to conservative treatment or if a complete tear is present, surgical repair may be done. Most repairs are arthroscopic procedures done as an outpatient (Fig. 67.3). If the tear is extensive, part of the acromion may be surgically removed *(acromioplasty)* to relieve compression of the rotator cuff during movement. A shoulder immobilizer with an abduction pillow is typically used for 6 weeks after surgery to limit shoulder movement. However, the shoulder should not be immobilized for too long because "frozen" shoulder *(arthrofibrosis)* may occur. Pendulum exercises and other passive exercises typically begin the first postoperative day. Active PT starts after 6 weeks of immobilization. Weight restrictions for lifting are usually given. Full recovery may take 6 to 12 months.

MENISCUS INJURY

The menisci are crescent-shaped pieces of fibrocartilage in the knee. Menisci are also found in other joints, including the acromioclavicular (AC), sternoclavicular, and temporomandibular joints. Meniscus injuries are associated with ligament sprains common among athletes in sports such as basketball, football, soccer, and hockey. These activities produce rotational stress when the knee is in varying degrees of flexion and the foot is planted or fixed. A blow to the knee can cause tearing of the meniscus between the femoral condyles and tibial plateau. Older adults and people who have jobs that require squatting or kneeling are at risk for degenerative tears.

Meniscus injuries alone do not usually cause significant edema because most cartilage is avascular. An acutely torn meniscus may present with local tenderness, pain, and effusion (Fig. 67.4). Pain occurs with flexion, internal rotation, and then extension of the knee *(McMurray's test)*. Patients may feel that the knee is unstable. They often report that the knee "clicks," "pops," "locks," or "gives way." Quadriceps atrophy is usually present if the injury has been present for some time. Traumatic arthritis may occur from repeated meniscus injury and chronic inflammation.

Acromion
Torn supraspinatus muscle
Arthroscope
Biceps tendon
Humerus
Subscapularis muscle (located behind the rib cage)

Fig. 67.3 A torn rotator cuff is repaired using arthroscopic surgery.

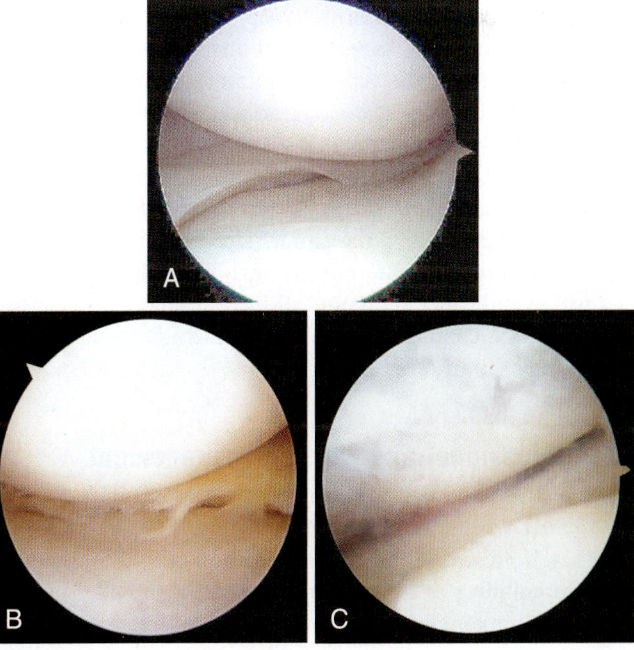

Fig. 67.4 Arthroscopic views of the meniscus. (A) Normal meniscus. (B) Torn meniscus. (C) Surgically repaired meniscus. (A, From David Lintner, MD, Houston, TX, www.drlintner.com. B and C, Courtesy Peter Bonner, Placitas, NM.)

MRI can confirm the diagnosis before arthroscopy. Age, occupation, sport activities, degree of pain, and dysfunction may affect the decision whether to have surgery.

Interprofessional and Nursing Management

Most meniscus injuries are treated in an outpatient setting. The acutely injured knee should be examined within 24 hours of injury. Initial care involves ice, immobilization, and use of crutches with weight bearing as tolerated. A knee brace or immobilizer during the first few days after the injury protects the knee and offers some pain relief.

After acute pain has decreased, PT can help patients regain knee flexion and muscle strength to aid in returning to full function. Teach athletes to do warm-up exercises to reduce the risk for sports-related injuries. In older adults with degenerative meniscus tears, progressive exercise therapy may improve neuromuscular function and muscle strength.

Surgical repair or excision of part of the meniscus *(meniscectomy)* may be needed (Fig. 67.4). Meniscal surgery is done by arthroscopy. Pain relief may include NSAIDs or other analgesics. Rehabilitation starts soon after surgery. PT includes quadriceps and hamstring strength exercises and ROM. When patients' strength is back to its preinjury level, they can resume normal activities.

ANTERIOR CRUCIATE LIGAMENT INJURY

Knee injuries account for more than 50% of all sports injuries. The most injured knee ligament is the anterior cruciate ligament (ACL). ACL injuries are usually noncontact injuries that occur when a person pivots, lands from a jump, or stops abruptly when running. Patients often report coming down on the knee, twisting, and hearing a pop, followed by acute knee pain and swelling. The knee may feel unstable. Athletes usually cannot continue playing. ACL injury can result in a partial tear, a complete tear, or an *avulsion* (tearing away) from the bones that form the knee (Fig. 67.5).

A positive *Lachman's test* suggests an ACL tear. This test is done by flexing the knee 15 to 30 degrees and pulling the tibia forward while stabilizing the femur. The test is positive for an ACL tear if forward motion of the tibia occurs with the feeling of a soft or indistinct endpoint. MRI can diagnose an ACL tear and coexisting conditions, including a fracture, meniscus tear, and ligament injuries.

Interprofessional and Nursing Management

Conservative treatment for an intact ACL injury includes rest, ice, NSAIDs, elevation, and ambulation as tolerated with crutches. If present, a tight, painful effusion may be aspirated. A knee immobilizer or hinged knee brace may provide support. PT can help maintain knee joint motion and muscle tone.

Reconstructive surgery is usually recommended for physically active patients who have sustained severe injury to the ACL and meniscus. In reconstruction, the torn ACL tissue is removed and replaced with graft tissue. ROM is encouraged soon after surgery. The knee is placed in a brace or immobilizer. Rehabilitation with PT is critical. Progressive weight bearing is determined by the type of surgery. A safe return to the prior level of function may take 6 to 8 months.

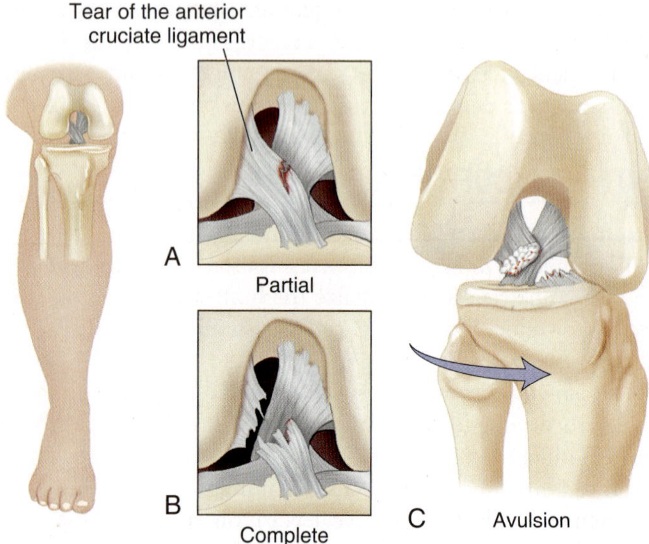

Fig. 67.5 ACL injury. (A) Partial tear. (B) Complete tear. (C) Avulsion.

BURSITIS

Bursae are closed sacs that are lined with synovial membrane and contain a small amount of synovial fluid. They are found at sites of friction, such as between tendons and bones and near the joints. **Bursitis** (inflammation of the bursa) results from repeated or excess trauma or friction, gout, RA, or infection.

Symptoms include warmth, pain, swelling, and limited ROM in the affected part. Common sites are the hands, elbows, shoulders, knees, and greater trochanters of the hip. Improper body mechanics, repetitive kneeling (e.g., carpet layers, coal miners, gardeners), jogging in worn-out shoes, and prolonged sitting with crossed legs are common precipitating activities.

Try to determine and correct the cause of the bursitis. Rest is often the only treatment needed. The affected part may be immobilized in a compression dressing or splint. Ice and NSAIDs can reduce pain and inflammation. Aspiration of the bursal fluid and intraarticular corticosteroid injection may be needed. If the bursal wall has become thickened and continues to interfere with normal joint function, surgical excision *(bursectomy)* may be done. Septic bursae may be treated with oral antibiotics. Patients may need surgical incision and drainage.

FRACTURES

Classification

A **fracture** is a disruption or break in the continuity of bone. Traumatic injuries cause most fractures. Other fractures are due to a disease process, such as cancer or osteoporosis *(pathologic fracture).*

We classify fractures in several ways. Fractures are described as *open* or *closed* based on communication with the external environment (Fig. 67.6). In an *open fracture,* the skin is broken and bone is exposed, causing soft tissue injury. An open fracture usually results from severe external forces. In a *closed fracture,* the skin is intact over the site.

We also describe fractures as complete or incomplete. A fracture is *complete* if the break goes completely through the bone. An *incomplete* fracture occurs partly across a bone shaft, but the bone is still intact. An incomplete fracture is often the result of bending or crushing forces applied to a bone. Fractures are identified by the direction of the fracture line. Types include linear, oblique, transverse, longitudinal, and spiral fractures (Fig. 67.7).

Finally, we describe fractures as displaced or nondisplaced. In a *displaced* fracture, the 2 ends of the broken bone are separated from each other and out of their normal positions. Displaced fractures are often *comminuted* (more than 2 fragments) or *oblique* (Fig. 67.7). In a *nondisplaced* fracture, the bone fragments stay in alignment. Nondisplaced fractures are usually transverse, spiral, or greenstick (Fig. 67.7).

Manifestations

Manifestations include immediate pain, decreased function, and inability to bear weight or use the affected part (Table 67.4). The patient guards and protects the extremity against movement. Obvious deformity may be present.

Fracture Healing

Bone goes through a complex multistage healing process, or union (Fig. 67.8). Healing occurs in 6 stages:

1. *Fracture hematoma:* When a fracture occurs, bleeding creates a hematoma that surrounds the ends of the bone fragments. The hematoma is composed of extravasated blood that changes from a liquid to a semisolid clot in the first 72 hours after injury.
2. *Granulation tissue:* Active phagocytosis absorbs the products of local necrosis. The hematoma converts to granulation tissue. Granulation tissue (consisting of new blood vessels, fibroblasts, and osteoblasts) forms the basis for new bone substance *(osteoid)* during days 3 to 14 after injury.
3. *Callus formation:* As minerals (calcium, phosphorus, and magnesium) and new bone matrix are deposited in the osteoid, an unorganized network of bone is formed and woven about the fracture parts. *Callus* is mainly composed of cartilage, osteoblasts, calcium, and phosphorus. It usually appears by the end of the second week after injury. An x-ray can show evidence of callus formation.
4. *Ossification:* Callus ossification occurs from 3 weeks to 6 months after the fracture and continues until the fracture has healed. Ossification is sufficient to prevent movement at the fracture site when the bones are gently stressed. The fracture is still evident on x-ray. During this stage of clinical union, patients may be allowed limited mobility or we may remove the cast.
5. *Consolidation:* As callus continues to develop, the distance between bone fragments decreases and eventually closes. Ossification continues and can be equated with *radiologic union,* which occurs when an x-ray shows complete bony union. This phase can occur up to 1 year after injury.
6. *Remodeling:* Excess bone tissue is resorbed, and union is complete. Gradual return of the injured bone to its

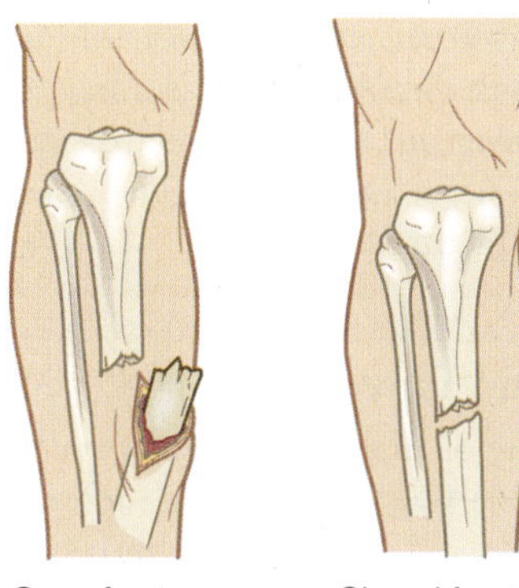

Fig. 67.6 Fracture classification by communication with the external environment.

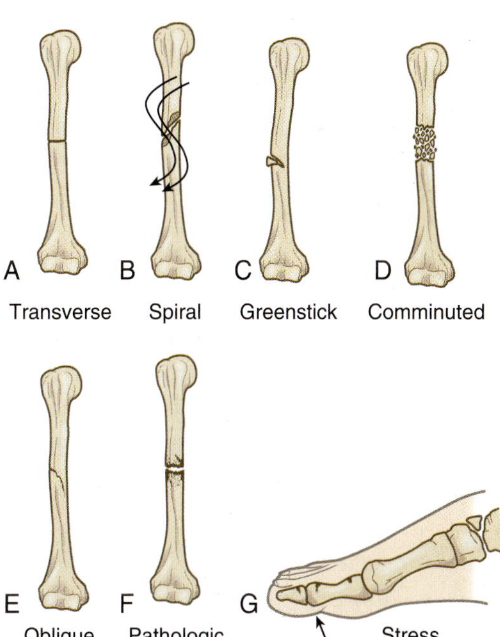

Fig. 67.7 Types of fractures. (A) Transverse fracture: the line of the fracture extends across the bone shaft at a right angle to the longitudinal axis. (B) Spiral fracture: the line of the fracture extends in a spiral direction along the bone shaft. (C) Greenstick fracture: an incomplete fracture with 1 side splintered and the other side bent. (D) Comminuted fracture: a fracture with more than 2 fragments. The smaller fragments appear to be floating. (E) Oblique fracture: the line of the fracture extends across and down the bone. (F) Pathologic fracture: a spontaneous fracture at the site of a diseased bone. (G) Stress fracture: occurs in bone that is subject to repeated stress, such as from jogging or running.

TABLE 67.4 Manifestations of Fracture

Manifestation	Significance
Bruising	
Discoloration of skin from extravasation of blood in subcutaneous tissues.	May appear immediately after injury and distal to injury. Reassure patient that process is normal, and discoloration will resolve.
Crepitation	
Grating or crunching of bony fragments, causing palpable or audible crunching or popping sensation.	May ↑ chance for nonunion if bone ends are allowed to move excessively. Micromovement of fragments (postfracture) helps in osteogenesis (new bone growth).
Deformity	
Abnormal position of extremity, protrusion of bone through skin. Seen as a loss of normal bony contours.	Classic sign of fracture. If uncorrected, it may cause problems with bony union and restoration of function of injured part.
Edema and Swelling	
Disruption or penetration of skin or soft tissues by bone fragments, or bleeding into surrounding tissues.	Unchecked bleeding and swelling in closed space can occlude blood vessels and damage nerves (e.g., ↑ risk for compartment syndrome).
Loss of Function	
Disruption of bone or joint, preventing functional use of limb or part.	Fracture must be managed properly to ensure restoration of function to limb or part.
Muscle Spasm	
Irritation of tissues and protective response to injury and fracture.	May displace nondisplaced fracture or prevent it from reducing spontaneously.
Pain and Tenderness	
Muscle spasm due to involuntary reflex action of muscle, direct tissue trauma, ↑ pressure on nerves, movement of fracture fragments.	Prompt the patient to splint muscle around fracture and reduce motion of injured area.

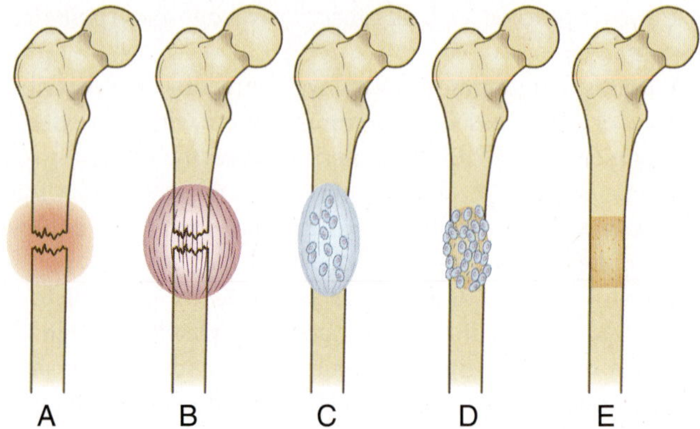

Fig. 67.8 Bone healing (schematic representation). (A) Bleeding at fractured ends of the bone with hematoma formation. (B) Organization of hematoma into fibrous network. (C) Invasion of osteoblasts, lengthening of collagen strands, and deposition of calcium. (D) Callus formation: new bone is built up as osteoclasts destroy dead bone. (E) Remodeling is accomplished as excess callus is resorbed and trabecular bone is laid down.

TABLE 67.5 Complications of Fracture Healing

Complication	Description
Angulation	Fracture heals in abnormal position in relation to midline of structure (type of malunion).
Delayed union	Fracture healing progresses more slowly than expected. Healing eventually occurs.
Malunion	Fracture heals in expected time but in unsatisfactory position. May cause deformity or dysfunction.
Myositis ossificans	Deposition of calcium in muscle tissue at site of significant blunt muscle trauma or repeated muscle injury.
Nonunion	Fracture does not heal despite treatment. No x-ray evidence of callus formation.
Pseudoarthrosis	Type of nonunion occurring at fracture site in which a false joint is formed with abnormal movement at site.
Refracture	New fracture occurs at original fracture site.

preinjury structural strength and shape occurs. Bone remodels in response to physical loading stress. Initially, stress is provided through exercise. Weight bearing is gradually introduced. New bone is deposited in sites subjected to stress and resorbed at areas of little stress.

Many factors influence the time needed for complete fracture healing. They include displacement and site of the fracture, blood supply, other local tissue injury, immobilization, and use of internal fixation devices (e.g., screws, pins). Ossification may be slowed or even stopped by inadequate immobilization, excess movement of fracture fragments, infection, poor nutrition, and systemic disease (e.g., diabetes).[6] Healing time for fractures increases with age. For example, an uncomplicated midshaft femur fracture heals in 3 weeks in an infant and in 20 weeks in an adult. Smoking increases fracture healing time. Fracture healing may not occur in the expected time *(delayed union)* or may not occur at all *(nonunion)*. Table 67.5 describes complications of fracture healing.

Interprofessional Care

The overall goals of fracture treatment are (1) anatomic realignment of bone fragments through reduction, (2) immobilization to maintain realignment, and (3) restoration of normal or near-normal function of the injured part. Table 67.6 outlines the management of fractures.

TABLE 67.6 Interprofessional Care

Fractures

Diagnostic Assessment
- History and physical assessment
- X-ray
- CT scan, MRI

Management

Fracture Reduction
- Manual traction
- Closed reduction
- Skeletal traction
- Open reduction

Fracture Immobilization
- Casting or splinting
- Skeletal traction
- External fixation
- Internal fixation

Open Fractures
- Surgical debridement and irrigation
- Tetanus and diphtheria immunization
- Prophylactic antibiotic therapy

Fracture Reduction

Closed reduction. *Closed reduction* is the nonsurgical, manual realignment of bone fragments to their anatomic position. Traction and countertraction are manually applied to the bone fragments to restore position, length, and alignment. Closed reduction is usually done under local or general anesthesia. Traction, casting, splints, or orthoses (braces) may be used after reduction to maintain alignment and immobilize the injured part until healing occurs.

Open reduction. *Open reduction* is the correction of bone alignment through surgery. It usually includes internal fixation of the fracture with wires, screws, pins, plates, intramedullary rods, or nails. The type and location of the fracture, patient age, and concurrent disease influence the decision to use open reduction with internal fixation (ORIF).

Traction. Traction is the application of a pulling force to an injured or diseased body part or extremity. Traction is used to (1) prevent or reduce pain and muscle spasm (e.g., whiplash, unrepaired hip fracture), (2) immobilize a joint or part of the body, (3) reduce a fracture or dislocation, and (4) treat a pathologic joint condition (e.g., tumor, infection). Traction can also (1) provide immobilization to prevent soft tissue damage, (2) expand a joint space during arthroscopic procedures, and (3) expand a joint space before joint reconstruction.

Traction devices apply a pulling force on a fractured extremity to attain realignment. Realignment depends on the correct positioning and alignment of the patient while the traction forces stay constant. For extremity traction to be effective, forces must be pulling in the opposite direction *(countertraction)*. Countertraction is supplied by the patient's body weight or by weights pulling in the opposite direction.

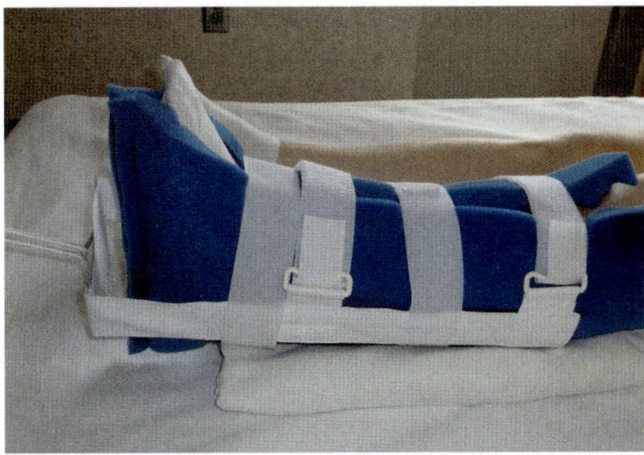

Fig. 67.9 Buck's traction is most often used for fractures of the hip and femur. (Courtesy Mary Wollan, RN, BAN, ONC, Spring Park, MN.)

The most common types of traction are skin traction and skeletal traction. *Skin traction* is generally used for short-term treatment (48 to 72 hours) until skeletal traction or surgery is possible. Tape, boots, or splints are applied directly to the skin. They help decrease muscle spasms in the injured extremity. Traction weights are usually 5 to 10 lb (2.3 to 4.5 kg). *Buck's traction* is a type of skin traction sometimes used for patients with a hip, knee, or femur fracture (Fig. 67.9). Pelvic or cervical skin traction may require heavier weights applied intermittently. In skin traction, regular skin assessment is a priority because pressure points and skin breakdown may develop quickly. Assess key pressure points every 2 to 4 hours.

Skeletal traction is used to align injured bones and joints or to treat joint contractures and congenital hip dysplasia. It provides a long-term pull that keeps the injured bones and joints aligned. To apply skeletal traction, the HCP inserts a pin or wire into the bone, and weights are attached to align and immobilize the injured body part. Weight for skeletal traction ranges from 5 to 45 lb (2.3 to 20.4 kg). Too much weight can result in delayed union or nonunion. The major complications of skeletal traction are infection at the pin insertion site and the effects of prolonged immobility. A common type of skeletal traction is balanced suspension traction (Fig. 67.10). You must keep the weights off the floor and moving freely through the pulleys.

Fracture Immobilization

Fracture immobilization is achieved with immobilizers (e.g., casts, braces, splints) and external and internal fixation devices.

Immobilizers. A *cast* is a temporary immobilization device often applied after closed reduction. A cast usually immobilizes the joints above and below a fracture. This restricts tendon and ligament movement, thus assisting with joint stabilization while the fracture heals. A cast often allows patients to perform many normal activities of daily living (ADLs) while providing stability. Braces and splints are similar in that they immobilize the joint. An advantage is they are made of more flexible material and can be taken on and off.

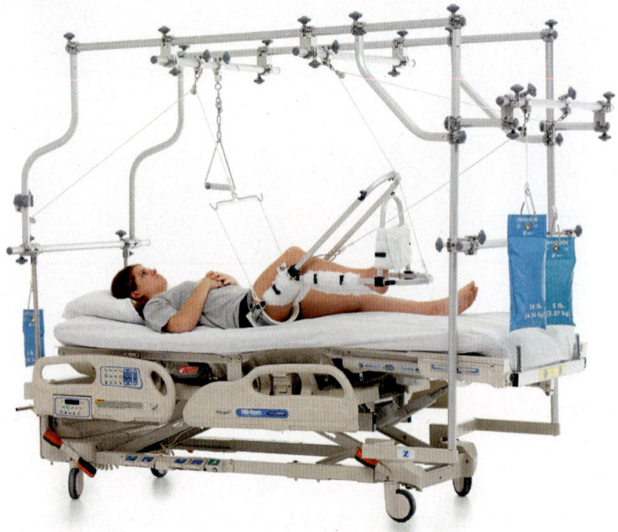

Fig. 67.10 Balanced suspension skeletal traction. Most often used for fractures of the femur, hip, and lower leg. (Courtesy Zimmer, Inc.)

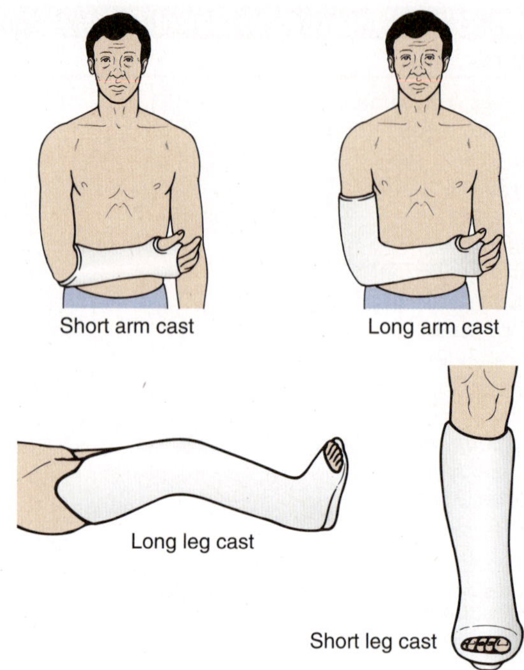

Fig. 67.11 Common types of casts.

The 2 most common cast materials are plaster and fiberglass. We use fiberglass casts most often because they are lighter, relatively waterproof, and longer wearing than plaster. They also allow early weight bearing. Casts made of fiberglass or other synthetic materials (thermolabile plastic, thermoplastic resins, polyurethane) are activated by submersion in cool or tepid water. Then they are molded to fit the torso or extremity.

Plaster is used mainly for contact casting for treating diabetic foot ulcers.[7] Plaster sets within 15 minutes. It is not strong enough for weight bearing until about 36 to 72 hours after application. The decision about weight bearing is made by the HCP. Leave a fresh plaster cast uncovered to allow air circulation. Covering the cast allows heat to build up in the cast. This may cause a burn and delay drying. Avoid direct pressure on the cast during the drying period. Handle the cast gently with an open palm to avoid denting the cast. Once the cast is thoroughly dry, the rough edges may be *petaled* to minimize skin irritation. Petaling also prevents plaster debris from falling into the cast and causing irritation or pressure necrosis. Place several strips (petals) of tape over the rough areas to ensure a smooth cast edge.

Upper extremity injuries. An acute fracture or soft tissue injury of the upper extremity can be immobilized by using a (1) sugar-tong splint, (2) posterior splint, (3) short arm cast, or (4) long arm cast (Fig. 67.11). The *sugar-tong splint* is applied for acute wrist injuries or injuries that may result in significant swelling. Splints are placed over a well-padded forearm, beginning at the phalangeal joints of the hand, extending up the dorsal aspect of the forearm around the distal humerus, and then down the volar aspect of the forearm to the distal palmar crease. The splinting material is wrapped with either elastic bandage or bias stockinette. The sugar-tong posterior splint adjusts for early swelling in the fractured extremity.

The *short arm cast* is often used to treat stable wrist or metacarpal fractures. An aluminum finger splint can be placed in a short arm cast to treat finger injuries. The short arm cast is a circular cast extending from the distal palmar crease to the proximal forearm. This cast immobilizes the wrist and allows unrestricted elbow motion.

The *long arm cast* is often used for stable forearm, elbow, or unstable wrist fractures. It is similar to the short arm cast but extends to the proximal humerus, restricting motion at the wrist and elbow. Support the extremity and reduce edema by elevating the extremity with a sling. When a hanging arm cast is used for a proximal humerus fracture, avoid elevation or use of a supportive sling. The hanging provides traction and maintains fracture alignment.

When a sling is used, ensure the axillary area is well padded to prevent skin breakdown from direct skin-to-skin contact. Apply the sling carefully to avoid putting excess pressure on the neck. Encourage movement of the fingers. This decreases edema by enhancing the pumping action of blood vessels. Teach patients to actively move joints of the upper extremity if not immobilized to prevent stiffness and contractures.

Vertebral injuries. The *body jacket brace* is used for immobilization and support for stable spine injuries of the thoracic or lumbar spine. The brace goes around the chest and abdomen, extending from above the nipple line to the pubis. After applying a brace, assess for superior mesenteric artery syndrome *(cast syndrome)*. This condition occurs if the brace is too tight, compressing the superior mesenteric artery against the duodenum. Patients may have abdominal pain, abdominal pressure, nausea, and vomiting. Assess the abdomen for decreased bowel sounds (there may be a window in the brace over the umbilicus). Treatment of cast syndrome includes gastric decompression with a nasogastric (NG) tube and suction. Assess respiratory status and bowel and bladder function.

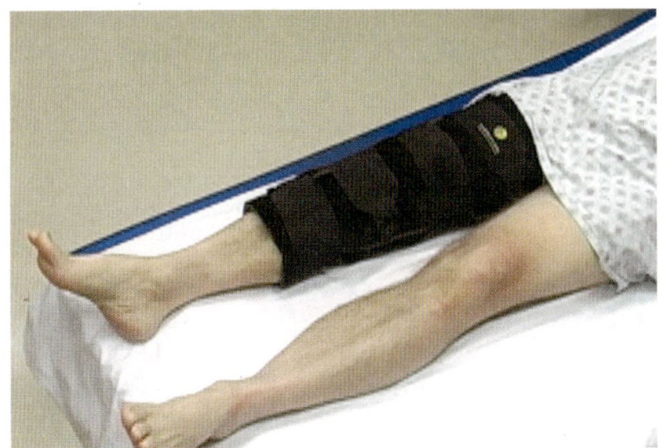

Fig. 67.12 Knee immobilizer. (From Naples RM, Ufberg JW: *Roberts and Hedges' clinical procedures in emergency medicine and acute care*, Philadelphia, 2020, Elsevier.)

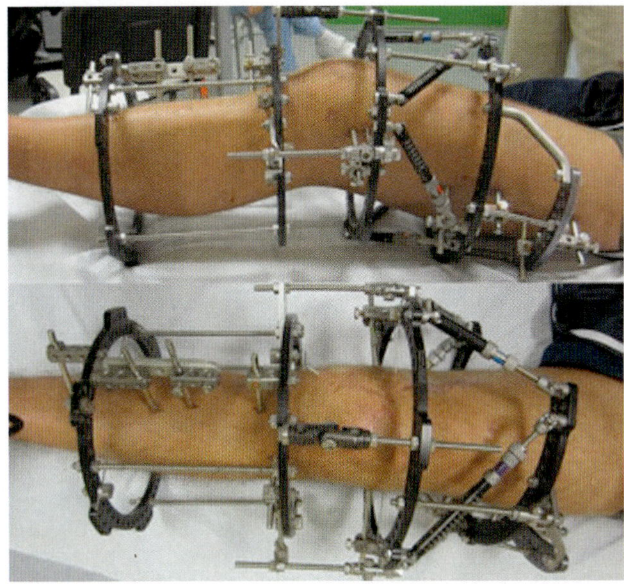

Fig. 67.13 External fixation of tibial fracture. (From Krettke C, Hawi N: *Skeletal trauma: basic science, management, and reconstruction*, ed 6, Philadelphia, 2020, Elsevier.)

Check areas of pressure over the bony prominences, especially the iliac crest. The brace may have to be adjusted or removed if complications occur.

Lower extremity injuries. Lower extremity injuries can be immobilized with a long leg cast, short leg cast, cylinder cast, or prefabricated splint or immobilizer. The usual indications for a long leg cast are an unstable ankle fracture, soft tissue injuries, a fractured tibia, and knee injuries. The cast usually extends from the base of the toes to the groin and gluteal crease. The short leg cast is used for stable ankle and foot injuries. A cylinder cast is used for knee injuries or fractures. It extends from the groin to the malleoli of the ankle. A Robert Jones dressing may be used temporarily to limit mobility of a joint. It is composed of soft padding materials (absorption dressing and cotton sheet wadding), splints, and an elastic wrap or bias-cut stockinette.

With a lower extremity cast or dressing, elevate the extremity above the heart on pillows for the first 24 hours. A casted extremity should not be placed in a dependent position, as this may increase edema. Observe for signs of compartment syndrome. Note increased pressure, especially in the heel, anterior tibia, head of the fibula, and malleoli. Increased pressure presents as pain or a burning feeling in these areas.

Prefabricated knee and ankle splints and immobilizers are used in many settings. This type of immobilization is easy to apply and remove. This allows us to observe the affected joint for swelling and skin breakdown (Fig. 67.12). Depending on the injury, removing the splint or immobilizer promotes ROM of the affected joint and faster return to function.

The *hip spica cast* is mainly used for femur fractures in children to immobilize the affected extremity and trunk. It extends from above the nipple line to the base of the foot (single spica) and may include the opposite extremity up to an area above the knee (spica and a half) or both extremities (double spica). Assess patients with a hip spica cast for the same problems associated with the body jacket brace.

External fixation. An *external fixator* is composed of metal pins and wires that are inserted into the bone and attached to external rods to stabilize the fracture while it heals (Fig. 67.13). It can be used to apply traction or to compress fracture fragments and immobilize reduced fragments when the use of a cast or traction is not appropriate. The external device holds fracture fragments in place similar to a surgically implanted internal device. External fixation is mainly used for complex fractures with extensive soft tissue damage, correcting congenital bony defects, nonunion or malunion, and limb lengthening.

External fixation is often used to try to salvage extremities that otherwise may need amputation. Perform ongoing assessment for pin loosening and infection. Infection may require removing the device. Teach patients and caregivers about how to perform pin care.

Internal fixation. Internal fixation devices (pins, plates, intramedullary rods, metal and bioabsorbable screws) are surgically inserted to realign and maintain position of bony fragments (Fig. 67.14). These metal devices are made from stainless steel, vitallium, or titanium. Proper alignment and bone healing are evaluated regularly by x-rays.

Electrical Bone Growth Stimulation

Electrical bone growth stimulation can promote healing, especially with fracture nonunion or delayed union. It stimulates new bone, cartilage, and blood vessel formation.[8] There are noninvasive, semiinvasive, and invasive methods of electrical bone growth stimulation. Noninvasive stimulators use direct current or pulsed electromagnetic fields (PEMFs) to generate a weak electrical current. Electrodes are typically in a band applied over the skin or cast and worn 10 to 12 hours each day, usually while the patient is sleeping. Semiinvasive or percutaneous bone growth stimulators use an external power supply and electrodes that are inserted through the skin and

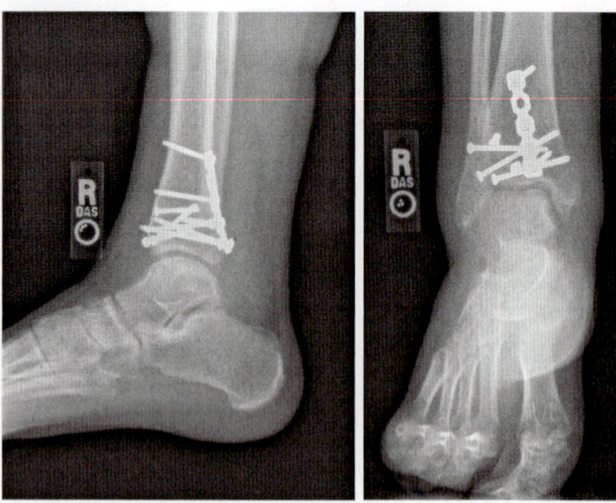

Fig. 67.14 Views of internal fixation devices to stabilize a fractured tibia and fibula. (From Jeremy Lewis, MD, Albuquerque, NM.)

into the bone. Invasive stimulators require surgical implantation of a current generator in an IM or subcutaneous space. An electrode is implanted in the bone fragments.

Drug Therapy

Patients with fractures have varying degrees of pain. Muscle relaxants may be given to manage pain from muscle spasms. We give tetanus and diphtheria toxoid or tetanus immunoglobulin to patients with an open fracture when their immunization status cannot be confirmed. Bone-penetrating antibiotics, such as a cephalosporin, are given prophylactically before surgery.

Nutrition Therapy

Proper nutrition helps ensure optimal soft tissue and bone healing. An adequate energy source promotes muscle strength and tone, builds endurance, and provides energy for ambulation and gait-training skills. The diet must include adequate protein (e.g., 1 g/kg of body weight), vitamins (especially B, C, and D), calcium, potassium, phosphorus, and magnesium. Low serum protein and vitamin C deficiencies interfere with tissue healing. Immobility and bone healing increase calcium needs.

A fluid intake of 2000 to 3000 mL/day promotes optimal bladder and bowel function. Adequate fluid and a high-fiber diet with fruits and vegetables prevent constipation. If immobilized in bed with skeletal traction or in a body jacket brace, patients should eat 6 small meals. This helps avoid overeating that can cause abdominal pressure and cramping.

NURSING MANAGEMENT: FRACTURES

Assessment

Obtain a brief history of the traumatic episode, mechanism of injury, and position in which the patient was found from the patient or witnesses. As soon as possible, the patient should be transported to an ED. There we do a thorough assessment and start treatment (Table 67.7). Subjective and objective data that you should obtain from a person with a fracture are outlined in Table 67.8.

TABLE 67.7 EMERGENCY MANAGEMENT

Fractured Extremity

Cause	Interventions
Blunt Trauma • Direct blow • Fall • Forced flexion or hyperextension • Motor vehicle crash • Pedestrian event • Twisting force **Penetrating Trauma** • Blast • Gunshot **Other** • Pathologic condition • Violent muscle contraction (seizures) • Crush injury	**Initial** • Treat life-threatening injuries first. • If unresponsive, assess circulation, airway, and breathing. • If responsive, monitor airway, breathing, and circulation. • Control external bleeding with direct pressure or sterile pressure dressing and elevation of the extremity. • Assess neurovascular condition distal to injury before and after splinting. • Elevate injured limb if possible. • Do not try to straighten fractured or dislocated joints. • Do not manipulate protruding bone ends. • Apply ice packs to affected area. • Obtain x-rays of affected limb. • Give tetanus prophylaxis if there is a break in skin. • Mark location of pulses to aid repeat assessment. • Splint fracture site, including joints above and below fracture site. **Ongoing Monitoring** • Assess vital signs, level of consciousness, O_2 saturation, neurovascular condition, pain. • Assess for compartment syndrome (excess pain, pain with passive stretch of affected extremity muscles, pallor, paresthesia, with late signs of paralysis and pulselessness). • Assess for fat embolism syndrome (dyspnea, chest pain, temperature elevation).

If a fracture is suspected, immobilize the extremity in the position in which it is found. Unnecessary movement increases the risk for damage to adjacent nerves and blood vessels. It may also convert a closed fracture to an open fracture.

Neurovascular Assessment

Perform a thorough neurovascular assessment of the affected extremity, distal to the fracture site. Musculoskeletal injuries may cause changes in the neurovascular status of an injured extremity. Poor positioning, physiologic responses to the traumatic injury, and application of a cast or constrictive dressing can cause nerve or vascular damage, usually distal to the injury. Record clinical findings before fracture treatment. This way, if a problem occurs later, it will help determine

TABLE 67.8 NURSING ASSESSMENT

Fracture

Subjective Data

Important Health Information

Health history: Traumatic injury, long-term repetitive forces (stress fracture), bone or systemic diseases, prolonged immobility, osteopenia, osteoporosis

Medications: Corticosteroids (osteoporotic fractures); analgesics

Surgery or other treatments: First aid treatment of fracture, musculoskeletal surgeries

Functional Health Patterns

Health perception—health management: Calcium and vitamin D supplementation

Activity-exercise: Loss of motion or weakness of affected part, muscle spasms

Cognitive-perceptual: Sudden and severe pain in affected area; numbness, tingling, loss of sensation distal to injury; ongoing pain that increases with activity (stress fracture)

Objective Data

Cardiovascular

Reduced or absent pulse distal to injury, ↓ skin temperature, delayed capillary refill

General

Apprehension, guarding of injured site

Musculoskeletal

Restricted or lost function of affected part; local bony deformities, unnatural position; shortening, rotation, or crepitation of affected part; muscle spasms and weakness

Neurovascular

Paresthesia (numbness, tingling), absent or ↓ sensation, hypersensation

Skin

Wound over site, exposed bone, pallor and cool skin or bluish and warm skin distal to injury; bruising, edema at fracture site

Possible Diagnostic Findings

Identification and extent of fracture on x-ray, bone scan, CT scan, or MRI

whether it was missed during the original assessment or a result of treatment.

The neurovascular assessment consists of *peripheral vascular assessment* (color, temperature, capillary refill, peripheral pulses, edema) and *peripheral neurologic assessment* (sensation, motor function, pain). Throughout the neurovascular assessment, compare both extremities to obtain an accurate assessment.

Assess an extremity's color (pink, pale, cyanotic) and temperature (hot, warm, cool, cold) around the injury. Pallor or a cool-to-cold extremity below the injury could indicate arterial insufficiency. A warm, cyanotic extremity could indicate poor venous return. Next, assess capillary refill. A delay in returning to its original color (greater than 3 seconds) can occur with arterial insufficiency.

Compare pulses on the unaffected and injured extremities to identify differences in rate or quality. A decreased or absent pulse distal to the injury can indicate vascular problems and insufficiency. Assess peripheral edema. Pitting edema may be present with severe injury.

Assess ulnar, median, and radial nerve function to evaluate sensation and motor innervation in the upper extremity. Assess motor function by asking patients to (1) abduct the fingers (ulnar nerve), (2) oppose the thumb and small finger (median nerve), and (3) flex and extend the wrist (or the fingers, if in a cast) (radial nerve). In the lower extremity, assess the ability to perform dorsiflexion (peroneal nerve) and plantar flexion (tibial nerve). Evaluate sensory function of the peroneal nerve by touching the web space between the big and second toes. Stroke the plantar surface (sole) of the foot to assess sensory function of the tibial nerve.

Patients may report *paresthesia* (abnormal sensation [e.g., numbness, tingling]) and hypersensation or hyperesthesia. Partial or full loss of sensation (paresis or paralysis) may be a late sign of neurovascular damage. Teach patients to immediately report any changes in sensation or the ability to move the digits in the affected extremity.

◆ Clinical Problems

Clinical problems for patients with a fracture may include:

- Musculoskeletal problem
- Risk for infection
- Pain

Additional information on clinical problems and interventions for patients with a fracture is presented in eNursing Care Plan 67.1 (on the website for this chapter).

◆ Planning

The overall goals are that patients with a fracture will (1) have healing with no associated complications, (2) have acceptable pain relief, and (3) achieve maximal rehabilitation potential.

◆ Implementation

Patients with fractures may be treated in an ED or an HCP's office and released to home care. They may need hospitalization for varying amounts of time. Specific nursing measures depend on the setting and type of treatment.

Perioperative Care

If surgery is needed to treat a fracture, patients must be prepared. In addition to the usual preoperative nursing care (see Chapter 18), teach patients about the type of immobilization and expected activity limitations after surgery. In general, nursing care after surgery involves monitoring vital signs and applying general principles of postoperative nursing care (see Chapter 20). Other nursing actions depend on the type of immobilization used.

Perform frequent neurovascular assessment of the affected extremity to detect early and subtle changes. Follow any limitations related to turning, positioning, and extremity support. Minimize pain and discomfort through proper alignment and positioning. Frequently observe for any signs of bleeding or drainage. Report an increase in size of the drainage area to the HCP. If a wound drainage system is in place, regularly measure the volume of drainage and assess its character (e.g., bloody, purulent). Report increased or purulent drainage at once to the HCP. Maintain the patency of any drainage systems, using aseptic technique to avoid contamination.

A blood salvage and reinfusion system may be used to allow recovery and reinfusion of the patient's own blood. The blood is retrieved from a joint space or cavity; then the patient receives this blood in the form of an autotransfusion. Autotransfusion is discussed in Chapter 34.

Immobility

Patients often have reduced mobility. Plan care to decrease risk for possible complications of immobility. Prevent constipation by increasing patient activity. Maintain high fluid intake (more than 2500 mL/day unless contraindicated) and a diet high in bulk and roughage (fresh fruits and vegetables). If these measures are not effective in continuing the normal bowel elimination pattern, give stool softeners, laxatives, or suppositories. Maintain a regular time for elimination to promote bowel regularity (Table 67.9).

Hypercalcemia and kidney stones can develop from bone demineralization due to reduced mobility. Unless contraindicated, maintain a fluid intake of 2500 mL/day to decrease the risk for stone formation. Renal stones are discussed in Chapter 50.

Rapid deconditioning of the cardiopulmonary system can occur from prolonged bed rest, resulting in orthostatic hypotension and decreased lung capacity. Unless contraindicated, decrease these effects by having patients sit on the side of the bed, allowing their lower limbs to dangle over the bedside. Have patients perform standing transfers. When patients are allowed to increase activity, assess for orthostatic hypotension. Assess patients for signs of VTE (see Chapter 41).

Traction

When slings are used with traction, regularly inspect exposed skin areas. Pressure over a bony prominence created by wrinkled sheets or blankets may cause pressure necrosis. Persistent skin pressure may impair blood flow and cause injury to peripheral nerves and blood vessels. Assess skeletal traction or external fixation pin sites for signs of infection. Pin site care may vary. It often includes routine cleansing with chlorhexidine, rinsing with sterile saline, and drying the area with sterile gauze.

If skin traction is ordered before surgery, apply traction without trying to reposition or realign the extremity. Movement of fracture fragments can occur during repositioning, causing increased pain and possible nerve impingement. Keep patients in the center of the bed in a supine position to provide adequate countertraction.

If allowed, encourage participation in a simple exercise program based on activity restrictions. Have patients perform frequent position changes, ROM exercises of unaffected joints, deep-breathing exercises, and isometric exercises. These activities should be done several times each day. Teach patients to use the trapeze bar (if permitted) to raise the body off the bed for linen changes and placement of the bedpan. Encourage and help hospitalized patients to stay connected with friends and family by telephone or through social media resources.

Cast Care

Most uncomplicated fractures are treated in an outpatient setting. Whatever the type of cast material, a cast can interfere

TABLE 67.9 NURSING MANAGEMENT

Caring for Patients With a Cast or Traction

- Perform neurovascular assessment on the affected extremity.
- Assess pain. Give prescribed analgesics and muscle relaxants.
- Determine correct body alignment to enhance traction.
- Monitor skin integrity around cast and at traction pin sites.
- Monitor cast during drying for denting or flattening.
- Teach patients and caregivers about cast care or traction and measures to prevent complications (e.g., ROM exercises).
- Assess for complications of immobility (e.g., constipation, venous thromboembolism, kidney stones, atelectasis) and develop a plan to minimize those complications.
- Supervise AP:
  - Position casted extremity above heart level as directed by RN.
  - Apply ice to cast as directed by RN.
  - Maintain body position and integrity of traction (if trained in this procedure).
  - Help with passive and active ROM exercises.
  - Notify RN about reports of pain, tingling, or decreased sensation in the affected extremity.

Collaborate With Physical Therapist

- Assess current mobility and need for assistance.
- Teach safe ambulation with assistive device based on weight-bearing restrictions.
- Establish exercise plan and teach patient to perform exercises safely.
- Coordinate PT with RN so that patient can receive timely analgesia.
- Discuss home environment with patient and identify modifications to promote safety (e.g., stair training).

Collaborate With Occupational Therapist

- Assess ability to perform ADLs.
- Teach use of assistive devices (e.g., long-handled reacher, shoe donner) to promote self-care while maintaining activity restrictions.

with circulation and nerve function if it is applied too tightly or excess edema occurs after application. Frequent neurovascular assessment of the immobilized extremity is critical. Teach patients to recognize and promptly report tightness of the cast and areas of pressure or discomfort. Explain the importance of elevating the extremity above heart level to promote venous return and applying ice to control or prevent edema during the initial phase. However, if you suspect compartment syndrome, do not elevate the extremity above the heart.

Patient and caregiver teaching is important to prevent complications. Table 67.10 describes patient and caregiver instructions for cast care. Teach patients to exercise joints above and below the cast. Tell them not to scratch or place anything inside the cast because this may cause skin injury and infection. For itching, direct a hair dryer on a cool setting under the cast. Confirm patients and caregivers understanding of these instructions before discharge. A follow-up phone call is appropriate. Home care nursing visits may be needed, especially for patients in a body jacket brace.

The cast is typically removed in the outpatient setting. Patients often fear being cut by the oscillating blade of the cast saw. Reassure them that damage to the skin is unlikely. Prepare patients for possible changes in the appearance of the extremity beneath the cast (e.g., dry, wrinkled skin; atrophied muscle; foul odor). Some patients are scared to use the injured extremity after cast removal.

TABLE 67.10 PATIENT & CAREGIVER TEACHING

Cast Care

After a cast is applied, include the following instructions when teaching the patient and the caregiver:

Do

1. Apply ice directly over fracture site for first 24 h (avoid getting cast wet by keeping ice in plastic bag and protecting cast with cloth).
2. Check with HCP before getting fiberglass cast wet.
3. Dry cast thoroughly if inadvertently exposed to water.
   - Blot dry with towel.
   - Use hair dryer on low setting until cast is thoroughly dry.
4. Elevate extremity above heart level for first 48 h.
5. Regularly move joints above and below cast.
6. Use hair dryer on cool setting for itching inside the cast.
7. Contact HCP for signs of possible problems:
   - Pain that is more than expected or does not improve with elevation, ice, analgesia
   - Swelling with pain and discoloration of toes or fingers
   - New onset of numbness or burning
   - Sores or foul odor under cast
8. Keep appointment to have fracture and cast checked.

Do Not

1. Get cast wet.
2. Remove any padding.
3. Insert any objects inside cast.
4. Bear weight on new cast for 48 h (not all casts are made for weight bearing; check with HCP when unsure).
5. Cover cast with plastic for prolonged periods.

Ambulation

Know the overall goals of PT in relation to patients' abilities, needs, and tolerance. The physical therapist is responsible for mobility training and teaching about the use of assistive aids (cane, crutches, walker). Reinforce these instructions. Patients with lower extremity fractures usually start mobility training when they can sit in bed and dangle their feet over the side. Work with the physical therapist to give analgesia before a PT session.

When patients begin to ambulate, know their weight-bearing status and the correct technique for using any assistive devices. Ambulation occurs in different degrees of weight bearing: (1) non—weight-bearing ambulation (no weight on the involved extremity); (2) touch-down/toe-touch weight-bearing ambulation (contact with floor for balance but no weight borne); (3) partial—weight-bearing ambulation (25% to 50% of weight borne); (4) weight bearing as tolerated (based on pain and tolerance); and (5) full—weight-bearing ambulation (no limitations).

Assistive Devices

Assistive devices range from a cane (can relieve up to 40% of the weight normally borne by a lower limb) to a walker or crutches (may allow for complete non—weight-bearing ambulation). The HCP decides which device is best, balancing the need for maximum stability and safety with the need for maneuverability in small spaces, such as bathrooms. Discuss lifestyle requirements and help patients select a device that helps them feel secure and independent. The technique for using assistive ambulation devices varies. The involved limb is usually advanced at the same time or immediately after advance of the device. The uninvolved limb is advanced last. Canes are held in the hand opposite the involved extremity.

Place a transfer belt (gait belt) around the patient's waist to provide stability while teaching how to use an assistive device. Discourage patients from reaching for furniture or relying on another person for support. Patients with inadequate upper limb strength or poorly fitted crutches bear weight at the axilla rather than at the hands. This can damage the neurovascular bundle that passes across the axilla. If verbal coaching does not correct the problem, teach patients another form of ambulation (e.g., walker) until strength is adequate.

Patients who must ambulate without weight bearing need enough upper limb strength to lift their own weight at each step. Because the muscles of the shoulder girdle and upper arm may not be accustomed to this work, patients require focused training for this task. Push-ups, pull-ups using the overhead trapeze bar, and weightlifting develop the triceps and biceps muscles. Straight-leg raises and quadriceps-setting exercises strengthen the quadriceps muscles.

Psychosocial Concerns

Short-term goals address the transition from dependence to independence in performing simple ADLs. They are directed at preserving or increasing strength and endurance. Long-term rehabilitative goals are aimed at preventing problems from musculoskeletal injury (Table 67.11). During the rehabilitative phase, help patients adjust to any problems caused by the injury (e.g., separation from family, financial impact, loss of income from inability to work, potential for disability). Assess for posttraumatic stress disorder. This is especially important if significant injury to others or fatalities occurred with the incident.

The caregiver may have a key role in providing long-term care. Teach the caregiver how to help with strength and endurance exercises, mobility, and promoting activities that enhance the quality of daily living. Offer support and encouragement while actively listening to patients' and caregivers' concerns.

◆ Evaluation

The expected outcomes are that patients with a fracture will:

- Report satisfactory pain management
- Show proper care of cast or immobilizer
- Have uncomplicated bone healing

FRACTURE COMPLICATIONS

Most fractures heal without complications. Complications may be direct or indirect. *Direct complications* include infection, problems with bone union, and avascular necrosis. *Indirect complications* include compartment syndrome, VTE, fat embolism syndrome (FES), breakdown of skeletal muscle *(rhabdomyolysis)*, and hypovolemic shock. Most musculoskeletal injuries are not life threatening. Death after a fracture is usually due to damage to underlying organs and vascular structures or complications of the fracture or immobility. Open fractures, fractures with severe blood loss, and fractures that damage vital organs (e.g., lung, heart) are medical emergencies requiring immediate attention.

Infection

Open fractures and soft tissue injuries have a high rate of infection. Communication of the fracture site with the outside environment can contaminate the site with microorganisms or foreign bodies. Damage to the surrounding soft tissue and blood vessels impairs the ability of defense mechanisms to respond to microorganisms. Dying or contaminated tissue is an ideal medium for many common pathogens, including anaerobic bacilli, such as *Clostridium tetani.* Measures to prevent infection and osteomyelitis are important.

Open fractures require surgical debridement. The wound is cleaned by saline lavage in the operating room. Gross contaminants are irrigated and mechanically removed. Contused, contaminated, and devitalized tissue (muscle, subcutaneous fat, skin, and bone fragments) is surgically excised *(debridement).* The wound may be irrigated with antibiotic solution. Antibiotic-impregnated beads can be placed in the surgical site. Patients usually receive IV antibiotics for at least 3 days.[9] Surgical management and antibiotics have reduced the occurrence of

TABLE 67.11 Problems Associated With Musculoskeletal Injuries

Problem	Description	Nursing Considerations
Atrophy	• ↓ Muscle mass occurs from disuse after prolonged immobilization. • Loss of nerve function can cause muscle atrophy.	• Isometric strength exercises as able with immobilization device help reduce amount of atrophy. • Muscle atrophy interferes with and prolongs rehabilitation process.
Contracture	• Abnormal condition of joint characterized by flexion and fixation. • Caused by atrophy and shortening of muscle fibers and ligaments or by loss of normal elasticity of skin over joint.	• Can be prevented by frequent position change, correct body alignment, active-passive ROM exercises several times a day. • Intervention requires gradual progressive stretching of muscles or ligaments in region of joint.
Footdrop	• Plantar-flexed position of the foot occurs when Achilles' tendon in ankle shortens because it has been allowed to assume an unsupported position. • Peroneal nerve palsy (a compression neuropathy) can cause footdrop and spinal nerve compression.	• For patient with long-term injuries, support foot in neutral position to ↓ risk for footdrop. • Once footdrop has developed, can significantly hinder ambulation and gait training. • May need splint to keep feet in neutral position. • High-top athletic shoes may help. Apply at scheduled times to keep feet in neutral position.
Muscle spasms	• Caused by involuntary muscle contraction after fracture, muscle strain, or nerve injury. • May last several weeks. • Pain from muscle spasms is often intense and can last from several seconds to several minutes.	• Measures to ↓ intensity of muscle spasms are similar to actions for pain management. • Do not massage muscle spasms. Massage may stimulate muscle tissue contraction that ↑ spasm and pain. • Heat may reduce muscle spasm.
Pain	• Common with fractures, edema, muscle spasm. • May be mild to severe and described as aching, dull, burning, throbbing, sharp, or deep.	• Causes include incorrect positioning and alignment of extremity, incorrect support of extremity, sudden movement of extremity, immobilization device that is applied too tightly or incorrectly, constrictive dressings, motion at fracture site. • Determine causes of pain so that corrective action can be taken.

infection. The amount of soft tissue damage determines whether the wound is closed at the time of surgery or if it needs repeat debridement, closed suction drainage, and/or skin grafting.

Compartment Syndrome

Compartment syndrome is a condition in which swelling causes increased pressure within a limited space (muscle compartment). There are 38 compartments in the upper and lower extremities. A decreased compartment size can result from restrictive dressings, splints, casts, excess traction, or premature closure of fascia. Increased compartment contents can occur with bleeding, inflammation, edema, or IV infiltration. Compartment syndrome may occur initially from the body's physiologic response to the injury, or it may be delayed for several days after the original insult or injury.

Because the fascia surrounding the muscle has limited ability to stretch, swelling can cause pressure that compromises the function of blood vessels and nerves in the compartment. Edema can create enough pressure to obstruct circulation and cause venous occlusion, which further increases edema. Arterial flow is eventually compromised, causing ischemia in the extremity. As ischemia continues, muscle and nerve cells are destroyed. Ischemia can occur within 4 to 8 hours after the onset of compartment syndrome. Delays in diagnosis and treatment may lead to irreversible muscle and nerve ischemia. The extremity may become functionally useless or severely impaired.

Compartment syndrome often involves the leg but can occur in any muscle group. It is usually due to fractures (especially of long bones), extensive soft tissue damage, and crush injury. Distal humerus and proximal tibial fractures are the most common ones associated with compartment syndrome. Compartment injury can occur after knee or leg surgery. Prolonged pressure on a muscle compartment may result when someone is trapped under a heavy object or a person's limb is trapped beneath the body.

Interprofessional Care

Prompt diagnosis of compartment syndrome is critical. Perform regular neurovascular assessment on patients with fractures, especially those with injury of the extremities or soft tissue in these areas. Early recognition and effective treatment are essential to avoid permanent damage to muscles and nerves.

One or more of the "6 *P*s" are specific to compartment syndrome: (1) *pain* out of proportion to the injury that is not managed by opioid analgesics, and *pain* on passive stretch of muscle in the compartment; (2) increasing *pressure* in the compartment; (3) *paresthesia* (numbness and tingling); (4) *pallor,* coolness, and loss of normal color of the extremity; (5) *paralysis* or loss of function; and (6) *pulselessness* (decreased or absent peripheral pulses). Pulselessness and paralysis are late signs of compartment syndrome.

Carefully assess the location, quality, and intensity of pain. Pain unrelieved by drugs and out of proportion to the level of injury is one of the *first* signs of compartment syndrome.

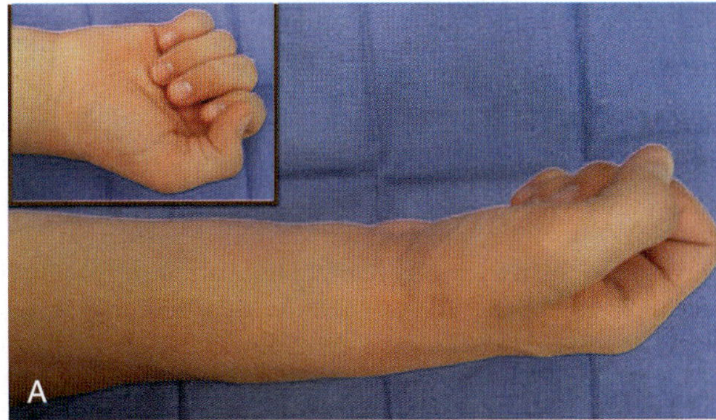

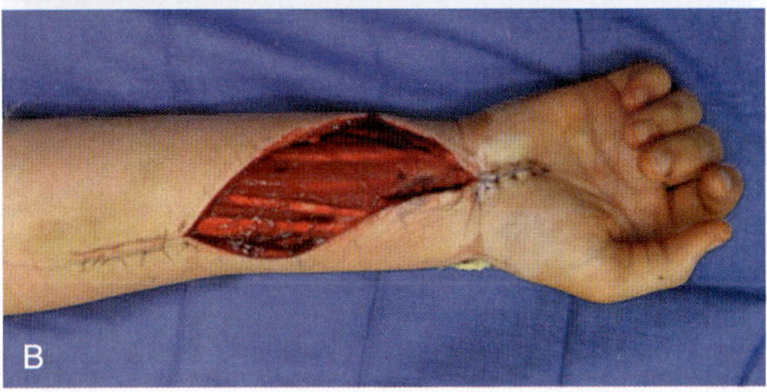

Fig. 67.15 (A) Fracture of the distal radius with distal forearm compartment syndrome. (B) Fasciotomy used to treat compartment syndrome. (From Stevanovic MV, Sharpe F: *Green's operative hand surgery,* ed 7, Philadelphia, 2017, Elsevier.)

Paresthesia is also an early sign. Notify the HCP immediately of these changes. Do not elevate the extremity above the heart or apply cold compresses. Cold causes vasoconstriction and worsens compartment syndrome.

Relieving the source of pressure (e.g., cast is cut [bivalved] or dressing loosened by order of the HCP) typically decreases pain and paresthesia and can avoid compartment syndrome. Reducing traction weight may decrease external pressures on the extremity. Surgical decompression (e.g., fasciotomy) of the involved compartment may be needed (Fig. 67.15). The fasciotomy site is left open for several days to allow adequate soft tissue decompression. Infection resulting from delayed wound closure is a potential problem after fasciotomy. In severe cases of compartment syndrome, amputation is done.

CHECK YOUR PRACTICE

Your 22-year-old male patient had a fall while rock climbing. He returned from surgery 8 hours ago with a long leg cast placed for open fractures of the femur and tibia. He continually reports pain that IV morphine does not seem to help.

- How will you assess his neurovascular status?
- What signs and symptoms suggest compartment syndrome?

Venous Thromboembolism

Veins of the lower extremities and pelvis are at great risk for VTE after total hip or total knee replacement surgery or a fracture, especially a hip fracture. In patients with limited mobility, inactivity of muscles that normally help pump venous blood from the extremities to the heart worsens venous stasis.

Patients should receive prophylactic anticoagulant drugs for at least 10 to 14 days. The choice of drug depends on the surgery and patient. First-line options include low-molecular-weight heparins (LMWHs; e.g., enoxaparin), direct oral anticoagulants (DOAs) (e.g., rivaroxaban, apixaban), and aspirin. Second-line options are unfractionated heparin, fondaparinux, or warfarin. For most patients having knee or hip arthroplasty, the initial agents given in the early perioperative period are LMWHs (e.g., enoxaparin) or DOAs.[10] Have patients dorsiflex and plantar flex the ankle of an affected lower extremity against resistance and perform ROM exercises on the unaffected leg. For upper extremity injuries, have patients flex and extend the wrist if not immobilized by a cast or splint and perform ROM exercises on the unaffected arm. They may wear compression gradient stockings (antiembolism hose) or use intermittent pneumatic compression devices. VTE is discussed in Chapter 41.

! SAFETY ALERT

Anticoagulant Therapy

- Monitor for signs of bleeding (e.g., nosebleeds, hematuria).
- Teach patient signs of bleeding and what to do if bleeding occurs.
- Teach patient safe self-injection if taking an injectable anticoagulant after discharge.
- Encourage patients to keep appointments for laboratory testing to monitor effects of warfarin (if prescribed).

Fat Embolism Syndrome

Fat embolism syndrome (FES) is characterized by fat globules entering the circulatory system from fractures. They collect in areas with abundant blood vessels, especially the lungs and brain. FES contributes to mortality from fractures. The fractures most often associated with FES are those of the femur, humerus, tibia/fibula, and pelvis.[11] FES can occur after joint replacement, burns, pancreatitis, liposuction, crush injuries, and bone marrow transplantation.

Two theories about FES exist. According to the mechanical theory, fat emboli originate from fat released from the marrow of injured bone. The fat enters systemic circulation, where it travels to other organs. As fat droplets become stuck in small blood vessels, local ischemia and inflammation occur. The biochemical theory suggests hormonal changes caused by trauma or sepsis stimulate systemic release of free fatty acids (e.g., chylomicrons) that form the fat emboli.

Clinical Manifestations

Most patients have symptoms within 24 to 72 hours after injury. Severe forms have occurred within hours of injury. The clinical course of FES may be rapid and acute. Fat emboli in the lungs cause hemorrhagic interstitial pneumonitis with signs and symptoms of acute respiratory distress syndrome (ARDS). These include chest pain, tachypnea, dyspnea, apprehension, tachycardia, and hypoxemia. In a short time, skin color can change from pallor to cyanosis. These symptoms are caused by poor O_2 exchange. Changes in mental status due to hypoxemia are common. Petechiae on the neck, anterior chest wall, axilla, and head may help discern FES from other problems.[11] They may appear due to intravascular thromboses caused by decreased oxygenation. However, not all patients have petechiae. They may fade before they are noticed.

No specific laboratory tests aid in the diagnosis. However, certain abnormalities may be present. These include fat cells in blood, urine, or sputum; a decrease of Pao_2 to less than 60 mm Hg; decreased platelet count and hematocrit; and high erythrocyte sedimentation rate (ESR). The ECG may show ST segment and T-wave changes. A chest x-ray may show bilateral pulmonary infiltrates.

Interprofessional Care

Management of FES is supportive and related to managing symptoms. Provide needed respiratory support (see Chapter 28). Administer O_2 to treat hypoxia. ECMO or mechanical ventilation may be an option if a satisfactory Pao_2 cannot be obtained. Some develop pulmonary edema and/or ARDS, leading to increased mortality. Cardiovascular problems are often managed with IV fluids, pulmonary vasodilators, peripheral vasoconstrictors, and inotropic drugs.

Preventing FES is important. Careful immobilization and handling of a long bone fracture are the most important factors in preventing FES. Reposition patients as little as possible before fracture immobilization or stabilization to decrease the risk of dislodging fat droplets into the general circulation.

CHECK YOUR PRACTICE

You are caring for a 24-year-old male patient who had a femur fracture in a motorcycle accident last night. He is scheduled for ORIF later today. While doing your assessment, you notice that he seems very restless. You note some axillary petechiae.

- What complication would you suspect is occurring?
- Why is this patient at risk for this complication?

Rhabdomyolysis

Rhabdomyolysis is a syndrome caused by the breakdown of damaged skeletal muscle cells. This breakdown causes the release of myoglobin into the bloodstream. Myoglobin precipitates and causes obstruction in renal tubules. This results in acute tubular necrosis and acute kidney injury (AKI). Because of possible muscle damage, assess urine output. Common signs are dark reddish-brown urine and symptoms of AKI (see Chapter 51).

CARE OF SPECIFIC FRACTURES

WRIST FRACTURES

Colles and Smith fractures are fractures of the distal radius (Fig. 67.16). The styloid process of the ulna may be involved as well. These usually occur when patients fall on an outstretched

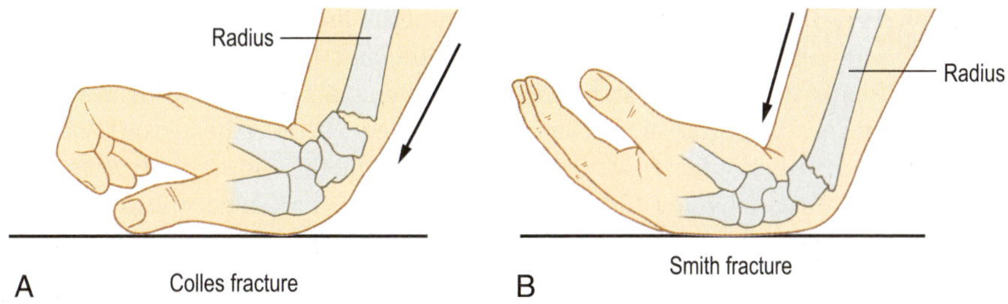

Fig. 67.16 Wrist fractures. (A) Colles and (B) Smith fractures from falling on an outstretched hand. (From Soames RW: *Anatomy and physiology for paramedical practice*, St. Louis, 2024, Elsevier.)

arm and hand. Colles fractures are one of the most common types of fractures in adults. It most often occurs in patients over 50 years old whose bones are osteoporotic (fragility fracture).

Symptoms include pain in the immediate area of injury, pronounced swelling, limited mobility, and distal forearm deformity. Numbness suggests nerve involvement. The major complication is vascular insufficiency from edema. CTS can be a later complication.

Patients are usually managed with closed reduction of the fracture and applying a splint or cast. If displaced, patients may need open reduction and internal or external fixation. Nursing care includes frequent neurovascular assessment and measures to reduce edema. Provide support and protect the extremity. Encourage active movement of the thumb and fingers to reduce edema and increase venous return.

HUMERAL SHAFT FRACTURE

Fractures involving the humeral shaft are common among young and middle-aged adults. The most common symptoms are obvious displacement of the humeral shaft, shortened extremity, abnormal mobility, and pain. Complications include radial nerve injury and injury to the brachial artery due to laceration, transection, or muscle spasm.

Treatment depends on the specific fracture location and displacement. Nonoperative treatment may include a hanging arm cast, shoulder immobilizer, sling and swathe (a type of immobilizer that prevents shoulder movement), or humeral cuff brace (Fig. 67.17). The humeral cuff brace is typically used to stabilize midshaft humerus fractures. Two pieces of molded plastic are fitted together in a clam-shell configuration and held together with Velcro straps. The humeral cuff brace is a good option for nonoperative fracture management if patients are at increased risk for complications.

When these devices are used, elevate the head of the bed to assist gravity in reducing the fracture. Allow the arm to hang freely when patients are sitting or standing. Provide measures to protect the axilla and prevent skin breakdown. Carefully place absorbable composite dressing pads (e.g., ABD pads) in the axilla. Change them twice daily or as needed. Skin or skeletal traction may be used for reduction and immobilization.

During the rehabilitative phase, an exercise program to improve strength and motion of the injured extremity is important. Exercises should include assisted motion of the hand and fingers. The shoulder can be exercised if the fracture is stable. This helps prevent stiffness from frozen shoulder or fibrosis of the shoulder capsule.

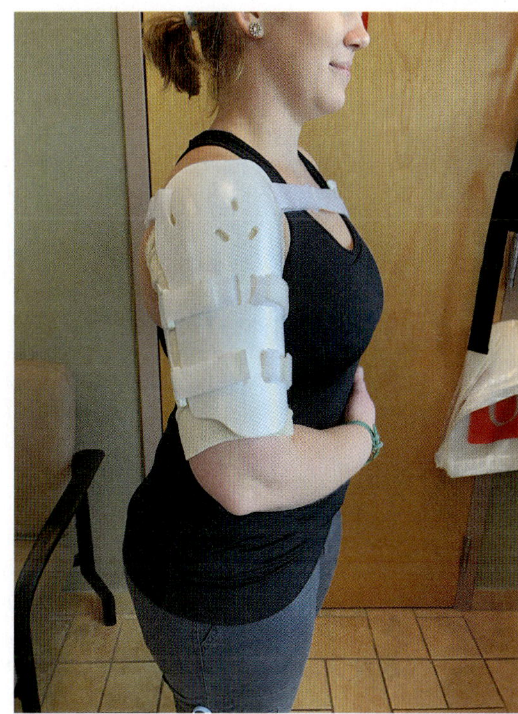

Fig. 67.17 Humeral cuff brace. (Courtesy Matthew C. Price, MS, RN, CNP, ONP-C, RNFA, Columbus, OH.)

CLAVICULAR FRACTURE

The clavicle is a frequently broken bone in children and young adults. Midshaft fractures account for 85% of all clavicle fractures. Injury is usually the result of a fall. Less often it happens from direct trauma to the bone. Common manifestations include pain at the fracture site, with or without obvious deformity, and limited shoulder range of motion. Patients often support the affected side with the other hand and tilt the head toward the side of the fracture.

Most patients do not need surgery. Surgery is usually done only if the fracture is open. Treatment is aimed at maintaining comfort with splinting, ice, and analgesics. PT includes early ROM and strength exercises. Most clavicle fractures heal without complications. Contact sports should be avoided for 8 to 10 weeks.

STABLE VERTEBRAL FRACTURE

In a stable vertebral fracture, the fracture fragments are unlikely to move or cause spinal cord damage. Vertebral bodies are usually protected from displacement by intact spinal ligaments. This injury is often confined to the vertebral body (anterior part of the spinal column) in the lumbar region. Sometimes it involves the cervical and thoracic regions. Stable vertebral fractures are usually caused by motor vehicle crashes, falls, diving, or sports injuries. Patients with osteoporosis have more than 700,000 vertebral compression fractures annually, many of which are stable.

Most patients with stable fractures have only brief periods of disability. If spinal ligaments are significantly disrupted, dislocation of the vertebrae may occur. Instability and injury to the spinal cord may result (unstable fracture). These injuries often require surgery. The most serious complication of vertebral fractures is fracture displacement, which can cause damage to the spinal cord (see Chapter 65). Although stable vertebral fractures are not associated with abnormal spinal cord pathology, all spinal injuries should be considered unstable and potentially serious until diagnostic tests determine the fracture to be stable.

Patients usually have pain and tenderness in the affected region of the spine. There may be a kyphotic deformity (flexion angulation of thoracic vertebrae). We can easily identify this deformity during the physical assessment (see Fig. 68.9). *Lordosis* and cervical spine involvement are possible. Sudden loss of function below the fracture indicates spinal cord impingement and paraplegia. Bowel and bladder problems may occur if there is interruption of the autonomic nervous system nerves or injury to the spinal cord.

The overall goal is to keep the spine in good alignment until union is achieved. Assess for spinal cord trauma (see Chapter 65). Regularly monitor vital signs and bowel and bladder function. Monitor the motor and sensory function of peripheral nerves distal to the injured region. Report any decline in neurovascular condition.

Treatment includes pain medication followed by early mobilization and bracing. The mattress should be firm to support the spinal column, relax muscles, decrease edema, and prevent potential compression on nerve roots. Teach patients to keep the spine straight when turning by moving the shoulders and pelvis together. Patients will need to learn to logroll. Several days after the initial injury, the HCP may apply a specially constructed orthotic device (e.g., thoracolumbar sacral orthosis [TLSO]), a jacket cast, or a removable corset if there is no neurologic deficit. The device gives extra support during healing. It is used for a short period of time.

Lightweight bracing may be used for patients with stable vertebral compression fractures due to osteoporosis. Patients with osteoporosis may undergo balloon kyphoplasty or vertebroplasty. *Balloon kyphoplasty* involves inserting a balloon into the vertebral body and then inflating it. This creates a cavity that is filled with bone cement under low pressure to restore the height of the vertebral body. It is the surgery of choice for compression fractures. This is due to the decreased incidence of bone cement leakage into nearby structures (e.g., colon, lung) compared with vertebroplasty. *Vertebroplasty* uses radioimaging to guide the injection of bone cement into a fractured vertebral body. When hardened, the cement stabilizes the vertebra and prevents further compression. Patients have decreased pain almost at once with these procedures. Later compression fractures of adjacent vertebrae are a risk.

If the fracture is in the cervical spine, patients may wear a hard cervical collar. Some cervical fractures are immobilized with a halo vest (see Fig. 65.8). This consists of a plastic jacket or cast fitted about the chest and attached to a halo held in place by skeletal pins inserted into the cranium. These devices immobilize the spine in the fracture area while allowing patients to ambulate.

Patients with a stable vertebral fracture are discharged after (1) showing safe ambulation, (2) learning care of the cast or orthotic device, and (3) stating ways to address safety and security concerns related to the injury and treatment.

PELVIC FRACTURE

Pelvic fractures range from relatively minor to life threatening, depending on the mechanism of injury and associated vascular damage. They account for only 3% of adult fractures. Pelvic fractures have a high mortality rate. They may cause serious intraabdominal injury, including laceration and hemorrhage of the urethra, bladder, or colon. They can cause acute pelvic compartment syndrome and paralytic ileus. Patients may survive the pelvic injury, only to die of sepsis, FES, or VTE.

Abdominal assessment may show local swelling, tenderness, deformity, unusual pelvic movement, and bruising. Assess the neurovascular condition of the lower extremities and determine associated injuries. Pelvic fractures are diagnosed by x-ray and CT scan.

Treatment depends on the severity of the injury. Stable, nondisplaced fractures require little intervention. Ambulation with weight bearing as tolerated is typically encouraged. Complex or displaced fractures (e.g., open book fracture) need external fixation alone or combined with ORIF (e.g., screws), often done emergently. Use extreme care in handling or moving patients to prevent further injury. Because a pelvic fracture can damage other organs, assess bowel and urinary elimination. Regularly perform distal neurovascular assessment. Provide back care with adequate help or while patients are raised from the bed by independent use of a trapeze (Box 67.3).

FEMORAL SHAFT FRACTURE

Because the femur can bend slightly to absorb stress, femoral shaft fracture occurs from a severe direct force. The force exerted to cause the fracture (e.g., from a motor vehicle crash or gunshot wound) often also damages the adjacent soft tissue.

BOX 67.3 ETHICAL/LEGAL DILEMMAS

Entitlement to Treatment

Situation

D.C., a 35-year-old Spanish tourist, was in a hang-gliding accident while touring the United States. She was taken to the regional trauma center for treatment of internal injuries, blood loss, and severe pelvic fractures. She has become septic, is now in renal failure, and has ARDS. She has no health insurance. Despite a poor chance of survival, her husband and parents want all measures to be taken.

Ethical/Legal Points for Consideration

- Federal law requires hospitals receiving federal funds through Medicare and Medicaid to provide emergency evaluation and treatment to stabilize patients. Once the patient is stabilized, they are under no obligation to continue treatment and may transfer the patient to another facility.
- Discuss with the family treatment goals (e.g., recovery, survival, continued biologic existence) and what they mean by wanting "everything done." There is no legal or ethical obligation to continue medical treatment when treatment goals cannot be met.
- Contact with the Spanish consulate may result in collaboration to stabilize the patient and transport her to Spain.
- Neither HCPs nor hospitals are required to provide medically futile care (care that provides no benefit to the patient).
- Although her home country offers universal health care, D.C. assumed the risk when engaging in a potentially dangerous activity and did not obtain international health insurance coverage for her visit to a foreign country.

Discussion Questions

1. How can the nurse promote discussions with the family about treatment goals for D.C.?
2. Are family members able to state D.C.'s wishes for her own care in such a situation?

These injuries may be more serious than the bone injury. Young adults have a high incidence of this type of fracture. The most common types of femoral shaft fracture include transverse, spiral, comminuted, oblique, and open (Figs. 67.6 and 67.7).

A femoral shaft fracture is marked by pain, notable deformity and angulation, shortening of the extremity, and inability to move the hip or knee. Displacement of fracture fragments often causes increased soft tissue damage. Considerable blood loss (1 to 1.5 L) can occur. Complications include FES; nerve and vascular injury; and problems with bone union, open fracture, and soft tissue damage.

Initial management involves patient stabilization and fracture immobilization. Traction may be used as a temporary measure before surgery or in patients unable to have surgery. Internal fixation with an *intramedullary rod* is the most common surgical treatment for femoral shaft fracture. The metal rod is placed into the marrow canal of the femur. The rod passes across the fracture to keep fragments in position. Plates and screws may be used. Internal fixation reduces the hospital stay and complications of prolonged bed rest. External fixation may be used for an open fracture.

After surgery, gluteal and quadriceps isometric exercises promote and maintain strength in the affected extremity. Encourage patients to perform ROM and strength exercises for all uninvolved extremities to prepare for ambulation. Patients may be allowed to start non–weight-bearing activities with an assistive device (e.g., walker, crutches). Full weight bearing is usually restricted until x-rays show union of fracture fragments. Teach patients to follow the HCP's instructions for weight bearing.

TIBIAL FRACTURE

Strong force is needed to cause a tibial fracture. As a result, soft tissue damage, devascularization, and open fracture are common. The tibia is a common site for stress fracture. Complications include compartment syndrome, FES, delayed union or nonunion, and possible infection with an open fracture.

Treatment for closed tibial fractures is closed reduction followed by immobilization in a long leg cast. ORIF with intramedullary rods, plate fixation, or external fixation is needed for complex fractures and those with extensive soft tissue damage.

Assess the neurovascular condition of the affected extremity at least every 2 hours during the first 48 hours. Have patients perform active ROM exercises with the uninvolved leg and the upper extremities to build the strength needed for crutch walking. When the HCP has determined a patient is ready for gait training, review principles of crutch walking introduced by the physical therapist. Patients may be non–weight bearing for 6 to 12 weeks, depending on healing. Home nursing visits may be needed to monitor progress if a patient is homebound.

HIP FRACTURE

More than 320,000 patients are admitted to hospitals each year with hip fractures. About 88% of hip fractures result from a fall.[12] Hip fractures are common in older adults. Rates are highest among older adults living in rural areas and among those over age 85 years.

Older adults may have low bone density *(osteopenia)* or osteoporosis, which increases their risk for fragility fractures. Factors that increase the risk for a hip fracture from falling in older adults include (1) an altered center of gravity and inability to correct a postural imbalance, (2) decreased fat and muscle to act as local tissue shock absorbers, and (3) reduced skeletal strength. Other factors that increase the older adult's risk for falling include (1) gait and balance problems, (2) vision and hearing problems, (3) slow reflexes, (4) orthostatic hypotension, and (5) medication use.

Hip fracture refers to a fracture of the proximal (upper) third of the femur, which extends 5 cm below the lesser trochanter (Fig. 67.18). Fractures within the hip joint capsule are *intracapsular fractures.* Intracapsular fractures are further identified by their specific locations: (1) *capital* (fracture of the head of the femur), (2) *subcapital* (fracture just below the head of the femur), and (3) *transcervical* (fracture of the femoral neck). These fractures, which are often associated with osteoporosis and minor trauma, are *fragility fractures.*

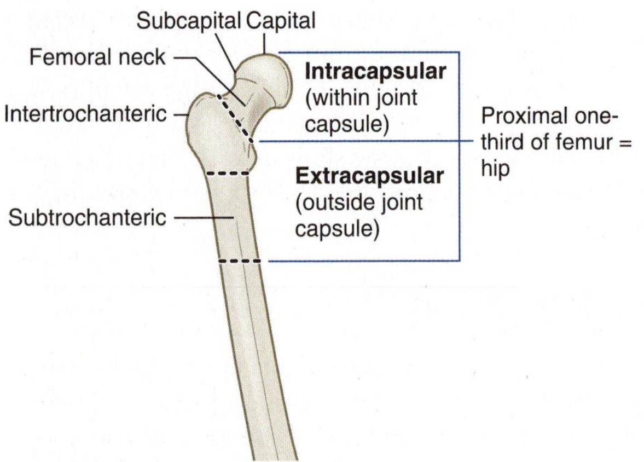

Fig. 67.18 Femur with location of various types of fractures.

Extracapsular fractures occur outside the joint capsule. They are either (1) *intertrochanteric* (in a region between the greater and lesser trochanter) or (2) *subtrochanteric* (below the lesser trochanter). Most are caused by severe direct trauma or a fall.

Clinical Manifestations

Manifestations include external rotation, muscle spasm, shortening of the affected extremity, and severe pain and tenderness around the fracture site. Displaced femoral neck fractures may disrupt blood supply to the femoral head, resulting in avascular necrosis of the femoral head.

Interprofessional Care

Immediate surgery is the standard of care. We may have to delay surgery briefly until the patient's general health is stable. If so, we may immobilize the affected extremity with Buck's traction (Fig. 67.9) until they can have surgery. Buck's traction may be used for 24 to 48 hours to relieve painful muscle spasms.

The type of surgery depends on the location and severity of the fracture and the person's age. Options include (1) closed reduction with percutaneous pinning (CRPP) (minimally invasive surgery to stabilize the femoral neck and head with screws), (2) repair with internal fixation devices (e.g., hip compression screw, intramedullary devices), (3) replacement of the femoral head with a prosthesis (partial hip replacement or *hemi arthroplasty,* often used for fracture of the femoral neck) (Fig. 67.19), and (4) total hip replacement (involves the femur and acetabulum) (Fig. 67.20).

NURSING MANAGEMENT: HIP FRACTURE

Implementation

Preoperative Care

Provide usual preoperative nursing care (see Chapter 18). Most patients do not have an extended preoperative period in which to receive instructions. Many are older adults. Consider the presence of any chronic health problems (e.g., diabetes, heart disease). Begin to consider discharge plans because the length of stay after surgery will be no more than a few days. Many older adults develop disabilities that require long-term care. Before surgery, severe muscle spasms can increase pain. Analgesics or muscle relaxants, comfortable positioning, and skin traction can help manage the spasms.

Postoperative Care

Similar principles of patient care apply to any surgical procedure for hip fractures. See eNursing Care Plan 67.2 for orthopedic surgical patients (available on the website for this chapter). In the initial postoperative period, assess vital signs and intake and output. Monitor respiratory function and encourage deep breathing and coughing. Assess pain and give pain medication. Observe the dressing and incision for signs of bleeding. Provide VTE prophylaxis. An LMWH is preferred.[10]

Neurovascular impairment is possible. Assess the extremity for (1) color, (2) temperature, (3) capillary refill, (4) distal pulses, (5) edema, (6) sensation, (7) motor function, and (8) pain. Decrease edema by elevating the leg when patients are in bed or in a chair. Pain in the affected extremity can be reduced by maintaining limb alignment with pillows between the knees when turning patients to the nonoperative side.

Encourage patients to use the overhead trapeze bar and the opposite side rail to help in position changes. Avoid turning patients to the affected side unless approved by the HCP. Have patients exercise the unaffected leg and both arms.

Weight bearing on the involved extremity varies. Limited weight bearing is typically the only restriction for patients who had ORIF of the hip fracture. The restriction continues until x-rays show adequate healing, usually 6 to 12 weeks. Teach patients and caregivers about weight-bearing status after surgery.

If hemiarthroplasty or total joint replacement was done by a posterior approach, the HCP may prescribe measures to prevent dislocation (Table 67.12). Tell patients and caregivers about positions and activities that increase the risk for dislocation (more than 90 degrees of flexion, adduction across the midline [crossing of legs and ankles], internal rotation of hip). Many daily activities reproduce these positions. These include (1) putting on shoes and socks, (2) crossing the legs or feet while seated, (3) assuming the side-lying position incorrectly, (4) standing up or sitting down while the hip is flexed more than 90 degrees relative to the chair, and (5) sitting on low seats, especially low toilet seats. Teach patients to avoid these activities until the soft tissue capsule around the hip has healed enough to stabilize the prosthesis (usually at least 6 weeks).

Elevated toilet seats and chair alterations (e.g., raising the seat with a folded blanket, keeping a straight back) are needed. Avoid placing a soft pillow in a seat because sitting on it can cause internal rotation. If a foam abduction wedge is ordered to prevent joint dislocation, place it between the legs (Fig. 67.21). Apply the top straps above the knee to avoid putting pressure on the peroneal nerve at the lateral tibial tubercle. Some HCPs want patients to keep the abductor wedge in place except when bathing or walking.

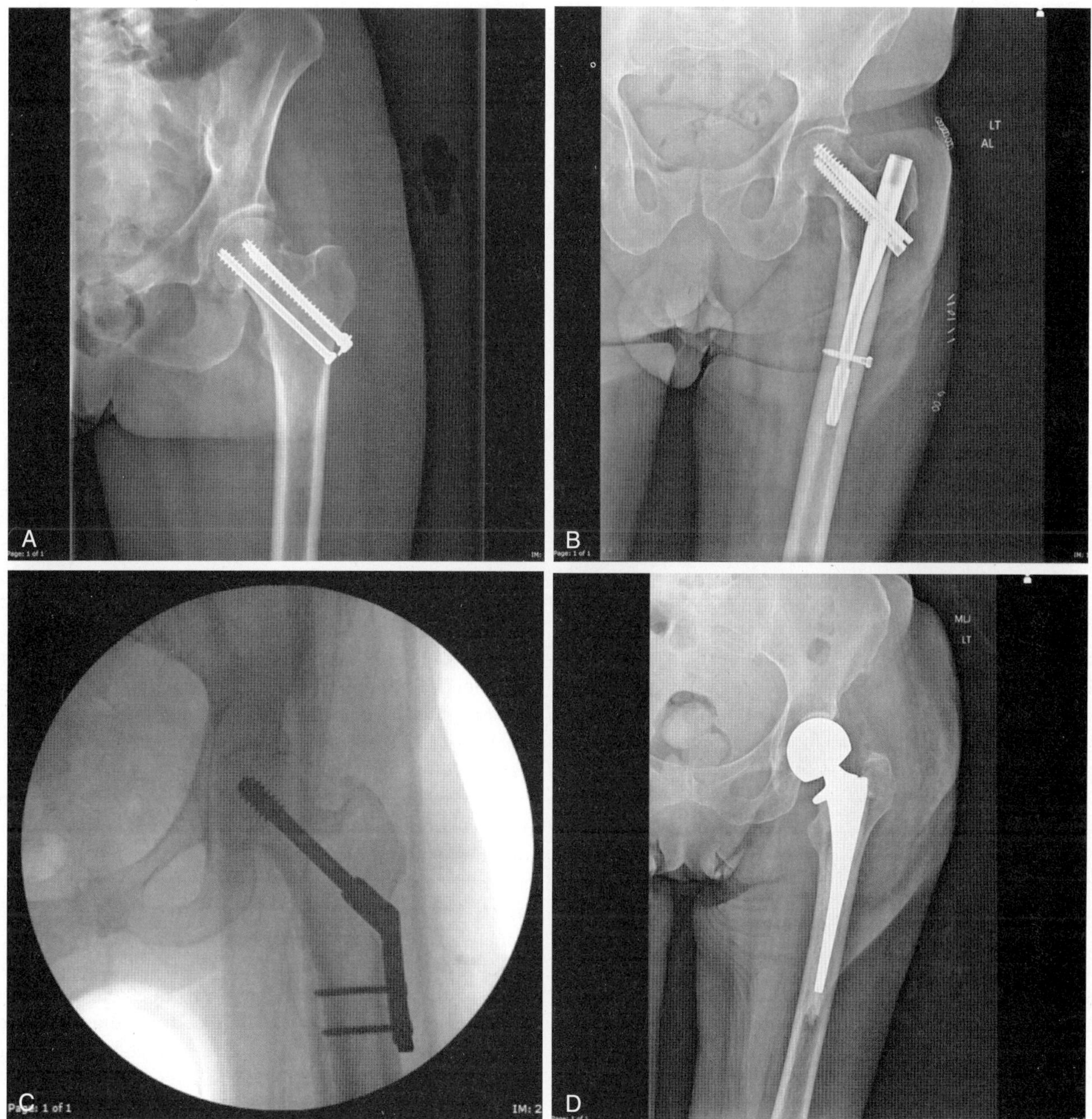

Fig. 67.19 Types of surgical repair for a hip fracture. (A) Closed reduction with percutaneous pinning. (B) Intramedullary nail. (C) Sliding hip screw. (D) Hemiarthroplasty. (Courtesy Matthew C. Price, MS, RN, CNP, ONP-C, RNFA, Columbus, OH.)

If hemiarthroplasty or total joint replacement was done by an *anterior approach* (incision is made in the front of the hip with patient lying on the back), the hip muscles are left intact. This approach provides a more stable hip in the postoperative period with a lower rate of complications. Precautions related to motion and weight bearing are few. They typically include instructions to avoid hyperextension.

Complications of femoral neck fracture include nonunion, avascular necrosis, dislocation, and osteoarthritis (OA). The affected leg may be shorter if the patient had an intertrochanteric fracture. A cane or shoe lift may be needed for safe ambulation.

Sudden severe pain, a lump in the buttock, limb shortening, and external rotation indicate prosthesis dislocation. This requires closed reduction with moderate to deep sedation or open reduction under general anesthesia to realign the femoral head in the acetabulum. If any of these signs occur, keep the patient NPO in anticipation of surgical intervention.

Physical therapists usually supervise exercises for the affected extremity and ambulation when the HCP allows it. They can teach patients how to transfer out of the bed to a chair. Patients are usually out of bed the first postoperative day. Monitor for the proper use of crutches or a walker. To be discharged home, patients must show proper use of crutches or

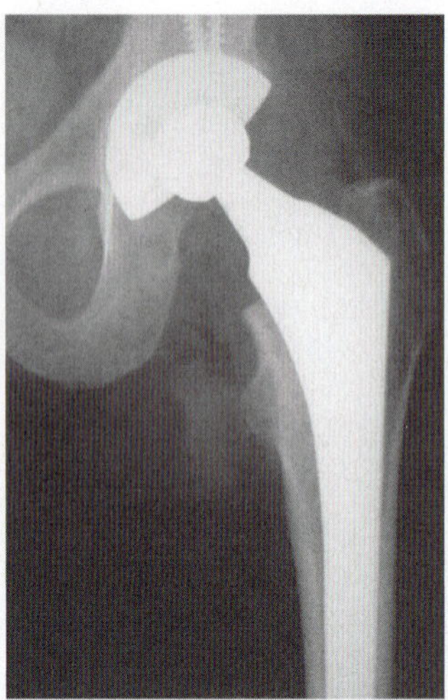

Fig. 67.20 Total hip replacement (arthroplasty) with cementless femoral prosthesis of metal alloy with plastic acetabular socket.

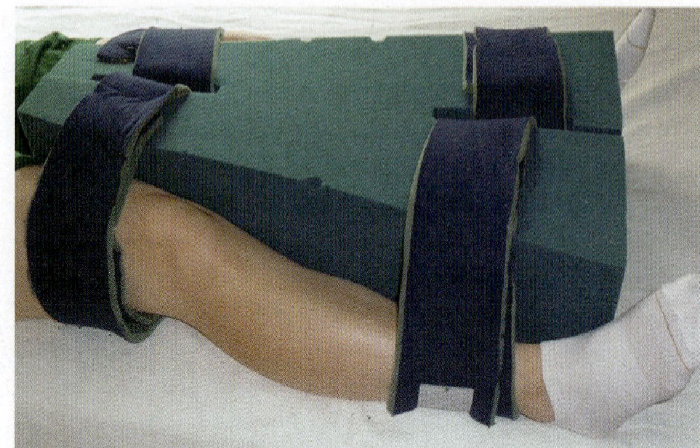

Fig. 67.21 Maintaining abduction after total hip replacement. (Courtesy Mary Wollan, RN, BAN, ONC, Spring Park, MN.)

TABLE 67.12 PATIENT & CAREGIVER TEACHING

Posterior Hip Replacement

After a hip replacement by posterior surgical approach, include the following instructions when teaching a patient and caregiver:

Do

- Use an elevated toilet seat.
- Place chair inside shower or tub and remain seated while washing.
- Use pillow between legs for first 6 weeks when lying on nonoperative side or when supine.
- Keep hip in neutral, straight position when sitting, walking, or lying.
- Notify HCP at once if severe pain, deformity, or loss of function occurs.
- Discuss personal risk factors for prosthetic joint infection with HCP and dentist before dental work.

Do Not

- Flex hip greater than 90 degrees (e.g., sitting in low chairs or toilet seats).
- Adduct hip (e.g., bring legs together at knees).
- Internally rotate hip (e.g., turn toward planted foot on affected side).
- Cross legs at knees or ankles.
- Put on own shoes or stockings without adaptive device (e.g., long-handled shoehorn or stocking-helper) for 4–6 weeks.
- Sit on chairs without arms. The arms of chairs will help the patient rise to a standing position.

a walker over a functional distance (about 150 ft). They must be able to transfer to and from a chair and bed and to go up and down stairs.

Exercises to restore strength and tone in the quadriceps and muscles around the hip are essential to improve function and ROM. These include quadriceps setting (e.g., pressing the kneecap down), gluteal muscle setting (e.g., tightening the buttocks), leg raises in supine and prone positions, and abduction exercises from the supine and standing positions (e.g., swinging the leg out but never crossing midline). Patients continue these exercises for many months after discharge. Teach the exercise program to the caregiver who will be encouraging the patient at home. Patients gradually increase the number of exercise repetitions and may add ankle weights. Swimming and stationary cycling may tone quadriceps and improve cardiovascular fitness. Teach patients to avoid high-impact exercises and sports, such as jogging and tennis, because they may loosen the implant.

Help patients and caregivers adjust to restrictions and dependence. A physical therapist or home care nurse may perform a home assessment to identify hazards that may cause another fall. Provide teaching about ways to decrease falls (Table 67.1).

Patients may not take a tub bath or drive until cleared by the HCP. An occupational therapist (OT) can teach how to use assistive devices, such as long-handled shoehorns, sock assists, and reachers or grabbers, to avoid bending over to pick up something on the floor. The knees must be kept apart. Teach patients to never cross the legs or twist to reach behind.

Calcium and vitamin D supplementation are given to patients with osteopenia or osteoporosis. A bisphosphonate drug (e.g., alendronate) may be prescribed to decrease bone loss or increase bone density. This reduces the chance of fracture. Osteoporosis is discussed in Chapter 68.

CHECK YOUR PRACTICE

You are taking care of an 83-year-old patient who fell down the steps outside her house while getting her mail. She was diagnosed with a femoral neck fracture and Colles fracture. She is returning to the clinical unit after surgery. She had a hemiarthroplasty for the femoral neck fracture and closed reduction of the Colles fracture.

- Based on these injuries, what are some possible complications?
- How will you mobilize a patient with these injuries?
- What are your discharge concerns?

Discharge Care

Hospitalization averages 3 or 4 days. Older adults or patients who live alone may require care in a subacute rehabilitation unit, at a skilled nursing facility, or in an acute rehabilitation facility for a few weeks before returning home. If patients have skilled nursing needs or are homebound for PT after discharge from postacute care, the HCP may order follow-up home health care. Tell patients and caregivers about community services that can help with rehabilitation after hospital discharge.

Home care considerations include pain management, monitoring for infection, and VTE prevention. If incision is closed with metal staples, they will be removed at the HCP's office. Teach patients who are receiving an anticoagulant to report signs of bleeding to the HCP (see Chapter 41). Review how to administer an injectable anticoagulant (if needed).

◆ Evaluation

The expected outcomes are that patients with a hip fracture will:

- Report satisfactory pain management
- Have uncomplicated bone healing
- Take part in exercise therapy

FACIAL FRACTURE

A person can fracture any bone of the face. Trauma, such as a motor vehicle crash, assault, or fall, is a common cause. After facial injury it is important to establish and maintain a patent airway and provide adequate ventilation. Suctioning may be needed to remove foreign material and blood. A surgically created airway *(tracheostomy)* may be needed if a patent airway cannot be maintained.

Facial fractures and cervical spine injuries often occur together. All patients with facial injuries should be treated as if they have a cervical injury until proven otherwise by assessment and CT scan or x-ray. Table 67.13 describes clinical manifestations of common facial fractures.

Related soft tissue injury often makes assessment of facial injury difficult. Perform oral and facial assessments after we have treated life-threatening situations. Assess eye muscles and cranial nerves III, IV, and VI. X-rays help determine the extent of the injury. CT scanning helps discern between bone and soft tissue injury.

Suspect injury to the eye when facial injury occurs, especially if the injury is near the orbit. If an eye-globe rupture is suspected, stop and place a protective shield over the eye. Signs of rupture include vitreous humor forced out of the eye. Brown tissue (iris or ciliary body) may be seen on the surface of the globe or penetrating through a laceration, with an off-center or teardrop-shaped pupil.

Specific treatment depends on the site and extent of the facial fracture and associated soft tissue injury. Immobilization or surgical stabilization may be needed. Maintain a patent airway and adequate nutrition throughout the recovery period.

Be sensitive about changes in appearance that may occur after facial fracture. These changes may be drastic. Edema and discoloration subside with time, but soft tissue injuries can cause permanent scarring.

TABLE 67.13 Manifestations of Facial Fractures

Fracture	Manifestation
Frontal bone	Rapid edema that may mask underlying fractures
Mandible	Tooth fractures, bleeding, limited motion of mandible
Maxilla	Segmental motion (instability) of maxilla and tooth fracture at socket
Nasal bone	Displacement of nasal bones, nosebleed (epistaxis)
Periorbital bone	Possible frontal sinus involvement, entrapment of ocular muscles
Zygomatic arch	Depression of cheek bone (zygomatic arch) and entrapment of ocular muscles

MANDIBULAR FRACTURE

Mandibular fracture may result from trauma to the face or jaw. The fracture may be simple, with no bone displacement, or may involve loss of tissue and bone. Mandibular fracture may need immediate treatment to ensure survival. Long-term treatment is sometimes needed to restore satisfactory appearance and function.

Mandibular fractures may be done therapeutically to correct an underlying alignment problem *(malocclusion)* that cannot be adjusted by orthodontics alone. The mandible is resected during surgery and manipulated forward or backward to correct the occlusion problem.

Surgery includes immobilization, usually by wiring the jaws *(intermaxillary fixation)*. Internal fixation may be done with screws and plates. In a simple fracture with no loss of teeth, the lower jaw is wired to the upper jaw. Wires are placed around the teeth, and then crosswires or rubber bands are used to hold the lower jaw tight against the upper jaw (Fig. 67.22). Arch bars may be placed on the maxillary and mandibular arches of the teeth. Vertical wires placed between the arch bars hold the jaws together. If teeth are missing or bone is displaced, other forms

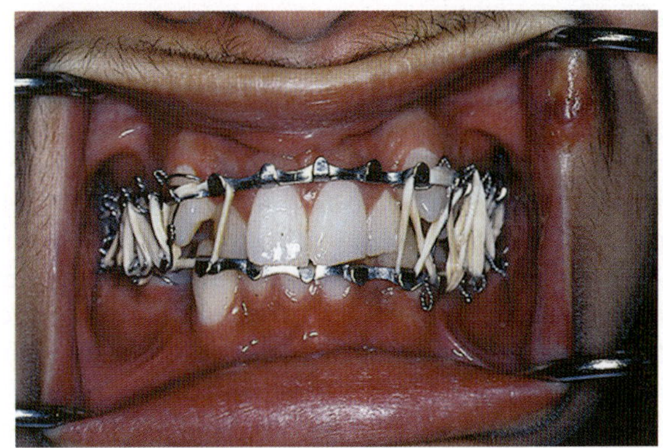

Fig. 67.22 Intermaxillary fixation. (Courtesy R.A. Weinstein, Denver, CO.)

of fixation may be needed (e.g., metal arch bars in the mouth or insertion of a pin in the bone). Bone grafting may be done. Immobilization is usually needed for only 4 to 6 weeks because the fractures often heal rapidly.

❖ NURSING MANAGEMENT: MANDIBULAR FRACTURE

Teach patients before surgery about what is involved in the surgery, how their face will look afterward, and changes caused by the surgery. Reassure them about the ability to breathe normally, speak, and swallow liquids. Hospitalization for respiratory monitoring is brief unless there are other injuries or problems.

Postoperative care focuses on a patent airway, oral hygiene, communication, pain management, and adequate nutrition. Two potential problems in the immediate postoperative period are airway obstruction and aspiration. Because patients cannot open the jaws, an airway must be maintained. Observe for signs of respiratory distress (e.g., dyspnea; changes in rate, quality, and depth of respirations). Place patients on their side with the head slightly elevated.

Tape a wire cutter or scissors (for rubber bands) to the head of the bed. Send it with the patient when they are away from the bedside. The wire cutter or scissors may be used to cut the wires or elastic bands in case of an emergency requiring access to the pharynx or lungs (e.g., cardiac arrest or respiratory distress). Keep a picture nearby showing the appropriate wires to cut in an emergency. In some cases, cutting the wires may cause the entire facial and upper jaw structure to shift or collapse and worsen the problem. Have a tracheostomy or endotracheal tray available.

If the patient begins to vomit or choke, try to clear the mouth and airway. Suction via the nasopharyngeal or oral route, depending on the extent of injury and type of repair. An NG tube can remove fluids and gas from the stomach to help prevent vomiting and aspiration. The NG tube can later be used as a feeding tube. Antiemetics may be given. Teach patients to clear secretions and vomitus.

Oral hygiene is important. Teach patients to remove food debris by rinsing the mouth often, especially after meals and snacks. Warm normal saline solution, water, or alkaline mouthwashes may be used. A syringe and soft irrigation catheter or a Water Pik may be effective for thorough oral cleansing. Inspect the mouth several times a day to see that it is clean. Use a tongue depressor to retract the cheeks. Keep the lips, corners of the mouth, and buccal mucosa moist. Cover any sharp edges of the wires with dental wax to prevent irritation of the buccal mucosa.

Communication may be a problem, especially in the early postoperative period. Establish an effective way of communicating before surgery (e.g., dry erase board, texting). Patients can usually speak well enough to be understood within a few days after surgery.

Adequate nutrition may be a challenge because of the liquid diet. Work with dietitians and patients to plan a diet with adequate calories and protein. Liquid protein supplements may improve nutrition. The low-bulk, high-carbohydrate diet and intake of air through the straw contribute to constipation and gas. Ambulation, prune juice, and bulk-forming laxatives may help relieve these problems.

Patients are usually discharged with the wires in place. Encourage them to share feelings about the changes in appearance. Discharge teaching should include oral care, diet, how to handle secretions, how and when to use wire cutters or scissors, and when to notify the HCP.

AMPUTATION

An **amputation** is the removal of a body extremity by trauma or surgery. About 2 million Americans live with limb loss.[13] About 185,000 amputations occur each year in the United States. Just over half are due to PVD and diabetes. These patients often have peripheral neuropathy that progresses to deep ulcers and gangrene. Trauma is the other major cause. Injuries have affected over 1700 military veterans since 2003, with several losing more than 1 limb (Fig. 67.23).[14] Other reasons for amputation include thermal injuries, tumors, osteomyelitis, and congenital limb disorders.

Diagnostic Studies

Diagnostic studies depend on the underlying reason for the amputation (Table 67.14). An increased white blood cell (WBC) count with abnormal differential may show infection. Vascular tests such as arteriography, Doppler studies, and venography give information about peripheral circulation.

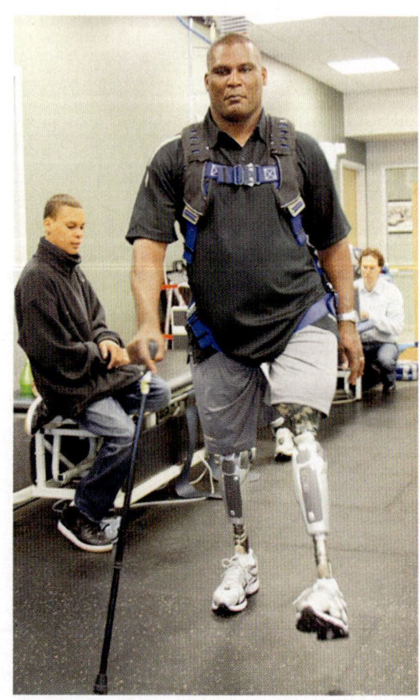

Fig. 67.23 A double amputee fitted with prostheses. (Photo courtesy U.S. Army.)

Interprofessional Care

Chronic illnesses and infection must be managed before an amputation is done. The goal of surgery is to preserve the greatest extremity length and function while removing all infected, pathologic, or ischemic tissue. Fig. 67.24 shows levels of amputation of upper and lower extremities. The type of amputation depends on the reason for the surgery. A closed amputation creates a weight-bearing *residual limb* (or stump). An anterior skin flap with dissected soft tissue padding covers the bony part of the residual limb. The skin flap is sutured posteriorly so that the suture line will not be in a weight-bearing area. Take care to prevent drainage accumulation, which can cause pressure and harbor bacteria that may cause infection.

Disarticulation is an amputation done through a joint. A *Syme's amputation* is a form of disarticulation at the ankle. After an open amputation *(guillotine amputation)*, the surface of the residual limb is left uncovered with skin. This type of surgery is generally done to control actual or potential infection. The wound is usually closed later by a second surgery or closed by skin traction surrounding the residual limb.

TABLE 67.14 Interprofessional Care

Amputation

Diagnostic Assessment
- History and physical assessment
  - Physical appearance of soft tissues
  - Skin temperature
  - Sensory function
  - Quality of peripheral pulses
- Arteriography
- Venography
- Plethysmography (measures blood flow in the arms or legs)
- Transcutaneous ultrasonic Doppler recordings

Management

Medical
- Management of underlying disease
- Stabilize trauma victim

Surgical
- Residual limb management
- Prosthesis fitting

Rehabilitation
- Coordination of prosthesis-fitting and gait-training activities
- Coordination of muscle-strength and PT programs

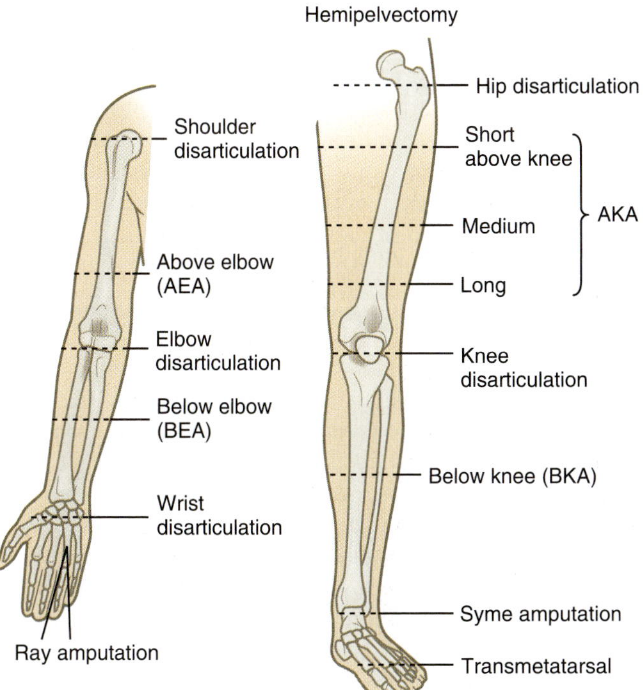

Fig. 67.24 Location and description of amputation sites of the upper and lower extremities. *AKA,* Above-the-knee amputation.

NURSING MANAGEMENT: AMPUTATION

Assessment

Assess for any preexisting illnesses. If amputation is planned or elective, as for patients with PVD, assess general health. Because most amputations are done for vascular problems, vascular and neurologic assessments are important (see Chapters 35 and 60).

Clinical Problems

Clinical problems for patients with an amputation may include:
- Impaired tissue integrity
- Musculoskeletal problem
- Impaired role performance
- Negative self-esteem

Planning

The overall goals are that patients with an amputation will (1) reach maximum rehabilitation potential (with the use of a prosthesis, if indicated), (2) cope with the body image changes, and (3) make satisfying lifestyle adjustments.

Implementation

Health Promotion

Control of illnesses, such as PVD and diabetes, can eliminate or delay the need for amputation. Teach patients with these problems to carefully examine their lower extremities daily for signs of infection or skin breakdown. If a patient cannot do this, the caregiver should help. Teach patients and caregivers to report changes to the HCP. These include decreased or absent sensation, tingling, burning pain, cuts, or abrasions, and changes in skin color or temperature.

Review safety precautions for people taking part in recreational activities and potentially hazardous work. This role is important for the occupational health nurse.

Acute Care

Preoperative care. Reinforce information about reasons for the amputation, proposed prosthesis, and mobility-training program. Help patients and caregivers understand the need for the amputation. Assure them that rehabilitation can help with quality of life. If the amputation is done emergently after trauma, patient management is physically and emotionally more complicated.

Know the level of amputation, type of dressings to be applied, and type of prosthesis to be used. Teach patients to perform upper extremity exercises, such as push-ups in bed or the wheelchair, to promote arm strength for crutch walking and gait training. Discuss general postoperative nursing care. Review positioning, support, and residual limb care. If a compression bandage will be used after surgery, teach patients about its purpose and how it will be applied. If immediate prosthesis use is planned, discuss general ambulation expectations.

Postoperative care. General care for patients who had an amputation depends on their age, general state of health, and reason for the amputation. Monitor patients who had an amputation due to a traumatic injury for posttraumatic stress disorder because they may have had no time to prepare or even take part in the decision to have a limb amputated.

Prevention and detection of complications are important. Monitor vital signs. Assess dressings for hemorrhage. Use sterile technique during dressing changes to reduce the risk for wound infection. If an immediate postoperative prosthesis has been applied, carefully observe the surgical site. If excess bleeding occurs, notify the HCP at once. Keep a tourniquet available for emergency use.

Proper bandaging ensures the residual limb is shaped and molded for eventual prosthesis fitting (Fig. 67.25). The HCP usually orders a compression bandage to be applied right after surgery to support soft tissues, reduce edema, hasten healing, and minimize pain. Compression also promotes residual limb shrinkage and maturation. This bandage may be an elastic roll applied to the residual limb or a residual limb shrinker, which is an elastic stocking that fits tightly over the residual limb.

At first, patients always wear the compression bandage except during PT and bathing. Remove and reapply the bandage several times daily. Take care to apply it snugly but not so tight as to interfere with circulation. Wash and change shrinker bandages daily. After the residual limb is healed, bandage it only when the patient is not wearing the prosthesis. Teach patients to avoid dangling the residual limb over the bedside to decrease edema.

We start active ROM exercises for all joints as soon as possible after surgery. As patients improve, the HCP and physical therapist start and supervise an exercise program. To prepare for mobility, patients should increase triceps and shoulder strength for lower limb support. They will need to learn to balance the altered body. The lost weight of an amputated limb requires adaptation of proprioception and coordination to prevent falls and injury.

Flexion contractures may delay rehabilitation. The most common and debilitating contracture is hip flexion. To prevent flexion contractures, have patients avoid sitting in a chair for more than 1 hour with hips flexed or having pillows under the surgical extremity. Unless contraindicated, patients should lie on their abdomen for 30 minutes 3 or 4 times each day and position the hip in extension while prone.

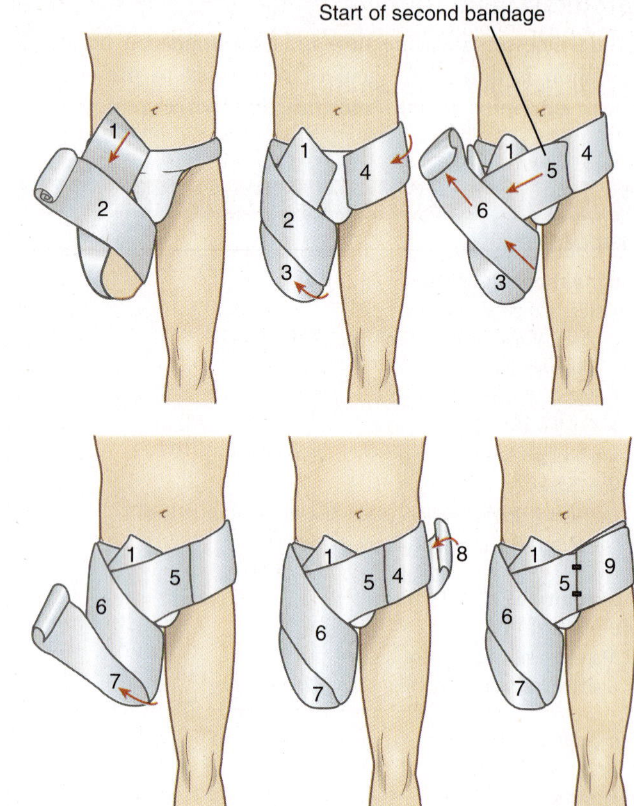

Fig. 67.25 Bandaging for the above-the-knee amputation residual limb. Figure-8 style covers progressive areas of the residual limb; 2 elastic wraps are used.

Crutch walking starts as soon as patients are physically able. Follow orders for weight bearing carefully to avoid injury to the skin flap and delay of tissue healing. Before discharge, teach patients and caregivers about residual limb care, ambulation, contracture prevention, recognition of complications, exercise, and follow-up care (Table 67.15).

Chronic Care

Success of rehabilitation depends on patients' physical and emotional health. Rehabilitation potential depends on a person's age, diagnosis, occupation, personality, resources, and support system. Chronic illness and deconditioning can complicate rehabilitation. A patient's previous ability to ambulate may affect the extent of recovery. Physical and occupational therapy are a key part of the plan of care.

Be aware of the psychologic and social implications of amputation. Body image problems related to amputation often cause patients to go through a grieving process. Use therapeutic communication to help them through this process and develop a realistic attitude about the future. Artificial limbs become an integral part of patients' changed body image.

TABLE 67.15 PATIENT & CAREGIVER TEACHING

Lower Extremity Amputation

After lower extremity amputation, include the following instructions when teaching the patient and caregiver:

1. Inspect the residual limb daily for signs of skin irritation, especially redness, abrasion, and odor. Especially evaluate areas prone to pressure.
2. Stop using the prosthesis if irritation develops. Have the area checked before resuming use of the prosthesis.
3. Wash the residual limb thoroughly each night with warm water and bacteriostatic soap. Rinse thoroughly and dry gently. Expose the residual limb to air for 20 min.
4. Do not use lotions, alcohol, powders, or oil on residual limb unless prescribed by the HCP.
5. Wear only a residual limb sock in good condition and supplied by the prosthetist.
6. Change residual limb sock daily. Launder in mild soap, squeeze, lay flat to dry.
7. Use prescribed pain management techniques.
8. Perform ROM to all joints daily. Perform general strength exercises (including for upper extremities) daily.
9. Do not elevate residual limb on a pillow.
10. Lay prone with hip in extension for 30 min, 3 or 4 times daily.

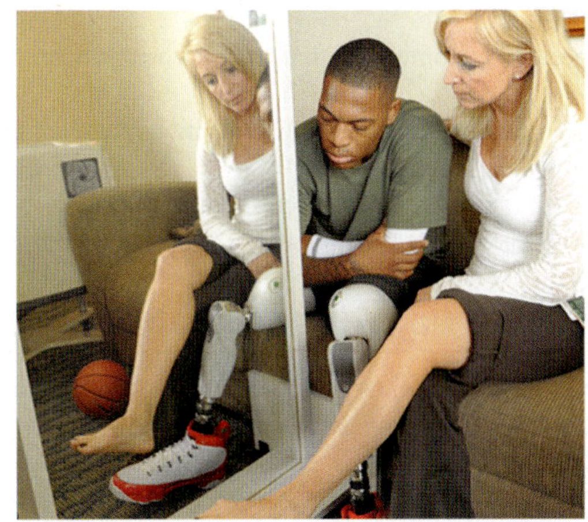

Fig. 67.26 Mirror therapy, a type of treatment that may reduce phantom limb sensation and pain. (U.S. Navy photo courtesy Mass Communication Specialist Seaman Joseph A. Boomhower.)

Prostheses

Timing for the use of a prosthesis depends on satisfactory healing of the residual limb and a patient's general condition. Delayed prosthetic fitting may be the best choice for older adults, patients with infection, or patients who had amputations above the knee or below the elbow. A temporary prosthesis may be used for partial weight bearing after sutures are removed. If there are no problems, patients can bear full weight on a permanent prosthesis about 3 months after amputation.

Not all patients are candidates for prostheses. Using a prosthesis requires significant strength and energy for ambulation. For example, walking with a below-the-knee prosthesis requires 40% more energy than walking on 2 legs. An above-the-knee prosthesis requires 60% more. Seriously ill or debilitated patients may not have the upper body strength and energy needed to use a lower extremity prosthesis. Mobility with a wheelchair may be the most realistic goal for these patients.

When healing has occurred satisfactorily, and the residual limb is well molded, patients are ready for prosthesis fitting. A prosthetist makes a mold of the residual limb and measures landmarks for creation of the prosthesis. The molded limb socket allows the residual limb to fit snugly into the prosthesis. The residual limb is covered with a stocking to ensure good fit and prevent skin breakdown. If the limb continues to shrink, causing a loose fit, a new socket must be made. Patients may need to have the prosthesis adjusted to prevent rubbing and friction between the residual limb and socket. Excess movement of a loose prosthesis can cause severe skin irritation, breakdown, and gait problems.

Teach patients to clean the prosthesis socket daily with mild soap and rinse thoroughly to remove irritants. Leather and metal parts of the prosthesis should not get wet. Encourage patients to have regular maintenance on the prosthesis. Consider the condition of their shoes. A badly worn shoe alters the gait and can damage the prosthesis.

Phantom Limb Syndrome

The amputated limb may feel like it is still present, with patients perceiving pain in the missing part of the limb. This phenomenon, termed **phantom limb sensation**, occurs in many amputees. As recovery and ambulation progress, phantom limb sensations usually subside. For some the pain becomes chronic. Patients may have shooting, burning, or crushing pain as well as feelings of coldness, heaviness, and cramping.

There is no one therapy for phantom limb sensation. Mirror therapy and virtual reality treatment reduce symptoms in some patients (Fig. 67.26). We think these therapies give visual information to the brain, replacing sensory feedback expected from the missing limb.[15]

Upper Limb Amputation

An upper limb amputation is often devastating. Despite technologic advances, we cannot replicate the movements and functional capacity of our hands with upper extremity prostheses. The enforced dependency due to being 1-handed may be depressing and frustrating. Because most upper extremity amputations result from trauma, patients likely have had little time to adjust or be a part of the decision-making process.

Immediate and delayed prosthetic fittings are possible for the below-the-elbow amputee. Prosthetic fitting is delayed for the above-the-elbow amputee. The usual functional prosthesis is the arm and hook. A cosmetic hand is available but has limited functional value. As with the lower limb prosthesis, patient motivation and perseverance are major factors contributing to a satisfactory outcome.

◆ Evaluation

The expected outcomes are that patients with an amputation will:

- Accept changed body image and integrate changes into lifestyle
- Have no evidence of skin breakdown
- Become mobile within limitations imposed by amputation

COMMON JOINT SURGERIES

Surgery plays a vital role in the treatment and rehabilitation of patients with various joint problems. The goals of surgery are to relieve chronic pain, improve joint motion, correct deformity and misalignment, and remove diseased cartilage. If the joint problem is not corrected, contraction with permanent limitation of motion may occur. There will be limited joint motion on physical assessment. Joint-space narrowing can be seen on x-rays.

TYPES OF JOINT SURGERIES

Synovectomy

Synovectomy (removal of synovial membrane) is done to remove inflamed tissue that is causing unacceptable pain or limiting ROM in RA. A synovectomy is best done early in the disease process when there is minimal bone or cartilage destruction. Removing the thickened synovium does not cure RA. It may relieve symptoms temporarily. Common sites include the elbow, wrist, and fingers.

Osteotomy

An **osteotomy** involves removing a wedge or slice of bone to restore alignment (joint and vertebral) and to shift weight bearing, thus relieving pain. Cervical osteotomy may be used to correct kyphosis in patients with ankylosing spondylitis. Halo vests and body jacket braces are worn until fusion occurs (3 to 4 months). Femoral osteotomy may provide some pain relief and improve motion in select patients with hip OA. Tibial osteotomy provides pain relief in some patients with knee instability or OA.

Care of patients who had an osteotomy is similar to that of patients with ORIF of a fracture at a comparable site. Internal wires, screws and plates, bone grafts, or an external fixator usually fixes the bone in place.

Debridement

Debridement is the removal of debris, such as pieces of bone or cartilage *(loose bodies)* or osteophytes, from a joint using a fiberoptic arthroscope. This procedure is usually done on an outpatient basis on the knee or shoulder. A compression dressing is applied after surgery. Weight bearing is permitted after knee arthroscopy. Patient teaching includes monitoring for signs of infection, managing pain, and restricting activity for 24 to 48 hours.

Arthroplasty

Arthroplasty is the reconstruction or replacement of a joint to relieve pain, improve or maintain ROM, and correct deformity. Arthroplasty is most often done on patients with OA, RA, avascular necrosis, congenital deformities or dislocations, and other systemic problems. Types of arthroplasty include surgical reshaping of the bones of the joints, replacement of part of a joint (hemiarthroplasty), and total joint replacement. Over 1 million Americans have knee and hip replacement surgery annually.[16] Arthroplasty is also available for elbows, shoulders, fingers, wrists, ankles, and feet.

Total Hip Arthroplasty

Total hip arthroplasty (THA), or a total hip replacement, provides significant relief of pain and improved function for patients with joint deterioration from OA, RA, and other conditions. THA is also used to treat hip fractures.

In THA, the prosthesis (implant) replaces the ball-and-socket joint formed by the upper shaft of the femur and pelvis (Fig. 67.27). The ball-and-socket components can be cemented in place with polymethyl methacrylate, which bonds to the bone. They may be inserted without cement (cementless). Cementless THA may provide longer stability by enabling growth of new bone tissue into the porous surface coating of the prosthesis. Cementless devices are better for younger, more active patients and patients with good bone quality as there is better bone growth into the components. The nursing care for patients who had a THA is discussed in the section on nursing management of patients with a hip fracture.

Hip Resurfacing Arthroplasty

An alternative to THA is hip resurfacing arthroplasty. It preserves and reshapes the femoral head (ball) rather than replacing it. The resurfaced femoral head is then capped by a metal prosthesis. Hip resurfacing may be an option for patients younger than age 60 with larger frames. A small number of patients have a femoral neck fracture after hip resurfacing.

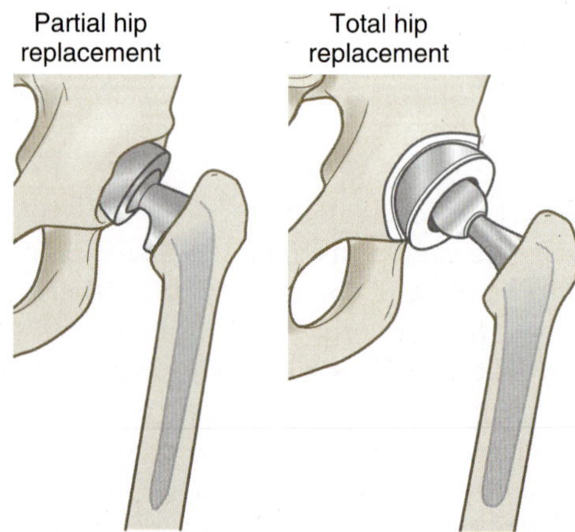

Fig. 67.27 Types of hip replacements.

Metal ions may be released into the bloodstream from the prosthesis. Patients may develop sensitivity or allergy to these ions.[17] Patients receiving a smaller femoral head (including many women) have a higher failure rate with a resurfaced implant compared with patients receiving THA.

Knee Arthroplasty

Unrelieved pain and instability due to severe deterioration of the knee joint are the main reasons for total knee arthroplasty (TKA) or a total knee replacement (Fig. 67.28). Partial arthroplasty can be done on patients with OA limited to 1 part (compartment) of the knee.

Right after surgery a compression dressing may be used to immobilize the knee in extension. This dressing is removed before discharge. If patients are unable to perform a straight leg raise, a knee immobilizer or posterior plastic shell to maintain extension may be used during ambulation and at rest for about 4 weeks.

After surgery, emphasis is on pain management and PT. Managing pain is a primary nursing goal. Doing so decreases the risk for complications and speeds the return to function. Adequate analgesia should be prescribed at discharge to allow patients to continue with the exercise program. Effective pain management is key to achieving positive rehabilitation outcomes.

PT begins early with isometric quadriceps setting. Therapy progresses to straight-leg raises and gentle ROM to increase muscle strength and obtain 90-degree knee flexion. Ambulation starts early with walking short distances, progressing to full weight bearing. An active home exercise program involves progressive ROM with muscle strength and flexibility exercises. After TKA, many patients with OA show significant improvement in mobility, motor function tests, and ability to complete daily tasks.

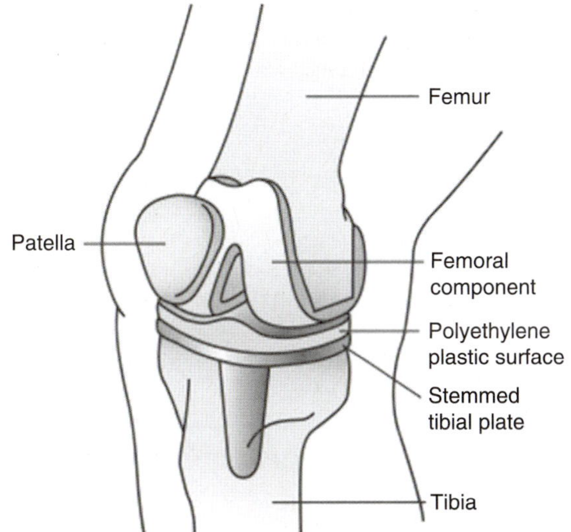

Fig. 67.28 Knee arthroplasty components. Up to 3 bone surfaces can be replaced in a total knee replacement. (Modified from Odom-Forren J: *Drain's perianesthesia nursing,* ed 7, St Louis, 2018, Elsevier.)

Finger Joint Arthroplasty

The main goal of hand surgery is to restore function related to grasp, pinch, stability, and strength rather than to correct cosmetic deformity. A silicone rubber arthroplastic device can restore function in the fingers of patients with RA. Before surgery, teach patients hand exercises, including flexion, extension, abduction, and adduction of the fingers.

After surgery, patients will have a bulk dressing. Keep the hand elevated. Perform regular neurovascular assessment. Monitor for signs of infection. Success of the surgery depends largely on the postoperative treatment plan. An OT plays a key role. After the dressing is removed, a guided splinting program is started. Patients wear splints while sleeping and do hand exercises at least 3 or 4 times a day for 10 to 12 weeks. Teach patients to avoid lifting heavy objects.

Elbow and Shoulder Arthroplasty

Elbow and shoulder replacements are not as common as other arthroplasties. Shoulder replacements are done in patients with severe pain from RA, OA, avascular necrosis, or trauma. A special type of shoulder replacement, called a reverse total shoulder arthroplasty, may be done for pain and dysfunction caused by massive, irreparable rotator cuff tears. Shoulder replacement is usually considered if patients have adequate surrounding muscle strength and bone density.

Rehabilitation is longer and more difficult than with other joint surgeries. If someone needs elbow and shoulder joint replacements, the elbow is usually done first because elbow pain interferes with shoulder rehabilitation. Most patients have no pain at rest or minimal pain with activity after elbow and shoulder arthroplasty. Functional improvements contribute to increased ability to perform ADLs.

Ankle Arthroplasty

Total ankle arthroplasty (TAA) is indicated for RA, OA, trauma, and avascular necrosis. TAA is an alternative to fusion for treatment of severe ankle arthritis in certain patients. Available devices include several fixed-bearing devices and a mobile-bearing cementless prosthesis. This device more closely imitates natural ankle function.

Ankle fusion is preferred over arthroplasty because the result is more durable. However, fusion leaves patients with a stiff foot and the inability to change heel height. TAA achieves a more normal gait pattern. After surgery, patients may not bear weight for 6 weeks. They need to elevate the extremity to reduce edema and maintain immobilization as directed by the HCP.

Arthrodesis

Arthrodesis is the surgical fusion of a joint. This procedure is done only if articular surfaces are too severely damaged or infected to allow joint replacement or if reconstructive surgery fails. Arthrodesis relieves pain and provides a stable but immobile joint. The fusion is usually done by removing the articular hyaline cartilage and adding bone grafts across the joint surface. The affected joint must be immobilized until bone healing has occurred. Common areas fused are wrist, ankle, cervical spine, lumbar spine, and metatarsophalangeal (MTP) joint of the big toe.

NURSING MANAGEMENT: JOINT SURGERY

Preoperative Care

The primary goal of preoperative assessment is to identify risk factors for postoperative complications so we can implement measures to promote optimal outcomes. A careful history includes (1) medical diagnoses and complications, such as diabetes; (2) pain tolerance and management preferences; (3) current functional level and expectations after surgery; (4) current social support; and (5) home care needs after discharge. Patients should be free from infection, breaks in skin integrity, and acute joint inflammation.

Provide preoperative teaching about the expected hospital course and postoperative management at home. Explain postoperative care, including early mobility, the need to maintain hydration, and VTE prophylaxis. A preoperative PT visit allows practice of postoperative exercises and measurement for crutches or other assistive devices. Provide opportunities for practice with assistive devices.

If lower extremity surgery is planned, assess upper extremity muscle strength and joint function to determine the type of assistive devices needed for ambulation and ADL performance. Discuss ways to maximize the usefulness and longevity of the prosthesis. Patients need to realize that recovery does not occur rapidly. Talking with other people who have had joint arthroplasty may help patients better understand their rehabilitation.

Begin discharge planning. Review the duration of the hospital stay and expected postoperative events so that patients and caregivers can prepare. Advanced planning helps to allow for a discharge home. Assess the support system. Identify their care partner. Who is going to help the patient at home? Do they need homemaker or meal services? It is preferable for patients to go home after a total joint arthroplasty. Assess the safety and accessibility of the home environment (e.g., throw rugs, cords). Are the bathroom and bedroom on the first floor? Are door frames wide enough to accommodate a walker? Discharge to a subacute or extended care facility should be planned beforehand. Patients may need to go to a facility for a few weeks to regain independent living skills if there is no social support available.

Postoperative Management

Nursing care of patients having orthopedic surgery is outlined in Table 67.16. Other nursing interventions are presented in eNursing Care Plan 67.2 (available on the website for this chapter). The hospital stay after arthroplasty can be a few hours after surgery to 2 days depending on preoperative planning, postoperative course, and need for PT after surgery. Many hip and knee replacement surgeries are done at ambulatory surgical centers. Same-day surgery is common.

Regularly perform neurovascular assessment. Assess pain often and give prescribed analgesics. Monitor for postoperative complications. Infection is a serious complication of joint surgery. The most common causative organisms are streptococci and staphylococci. Give prescribed antibiotics. Teach patients to report complications. Review signs of infection (e.g., fever, increased pain, drainage) and dislocation of the prosthesis (e.g., pain, loss of function, shortening or malalignment of an extremity).

Assess ROM at regular intervals to promote functional performance. In general, the affected joint is exercised, and we encourage ambulation as early as possible. PT and ambulation enhance mobility, build muscle strength, and reduce the risk for VTE. Specific protocols vary depending on the patient, type of prosthesis, and HCP preference.

VTE is a serious complication, especially after surgery involving the lower extremities. Provide prophylactic measures, such as anticoagulant drugs, use of intermittent pneumatic compression devices, and early ambulation. Most prophylactic anticoagulant drugs are given for at least 10 to 14 days.[10] Some patients need therapy for up to 35 days. If a patient is taking warfarin, therapy starts on the day of surgery, and the INR and prothrombin times are measured daily. Therapy with LMWH (e.g., enoxaparin), apixaban, or rivaroxaban usually starts the morning after surgery. Assess patients for signs of VTE. VTE is discussed in Chapter 41.

TABLE 67.16 NURSING MANAGEMENT

Caring for Patients After Joint Surgery

- Perform neurovascular assessment on the affected extremity.
- Monitor pain intensity and give prescribed analgesics.
- Maintain correct body alignment.
- Provide wound care, including dressing changes.
- Assess for complications of immobility (e.g., constipation, venous thromboembolism) and develop a plan to minimize those complications.
- Assist with initial ambulation then help as needed.
- Assist patient, caregiver(s), and family in planning for discharge care.
- Supervise AP:
  - Record oral intake and output.
  - Obtain vital signs and pulse oximetry.
  - Help patient with nutrition, elimination, and hygiene needs.
  - Maintain body position and assist with ambulation.
  - Help with passive and active ROM exercises.
  - Notify RN about reports of pain, tingling, or decreased sensation in the affected extremity.

Collaborate With Physical Therapist

- Assess current mobility and need for assistance.
- Teach safe ambulation with assistive device based on weight-bearing restrictions.
- Establish exercise plan and teach patient to perform exercises safely.
- Coordinate PT with RN so that patient can receive timely analgesia.
- Discuss home environment with patient and identify modifications to promote safety.

CASE STUDY

Hip Fracture and Revision Arthroplasty

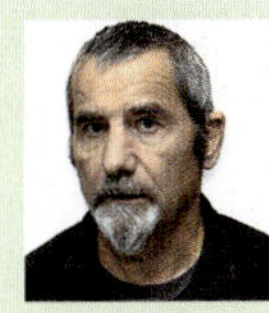

(© aronaze/ iStock.com.)

Patient Profile

M.C. is a 64-year-old male who had both hips replaced (left 6 years ago, right 2 years ago). He has a history of hypothyroidism. He was admitted to the ED after tripping over a short retaining wall in his backyard while gardening. He landed on his right side.

Subjective Data

- Acute, severe pain in right hip, unable to bear weight on right leg.
- Takes cholecalciferol (vitamin D_3) 1000 IU every day without calcium supplement. States calcium upsets his stomach.
- Reports loss of about 30 lb in the last year through diet and exercise. Exercises 3 times a week.
- Lives in a 2-story house with his wife. Bedrooms are on the second level.
- Has smoked ½ pack of cigarettes a day for 30 years.
- Describes himself as "a very light social drinker."

Objective Data

- 5 ft, 9 in tall, 175 lb

Diagnostic Studies

- X-rays show periprosthetic right proximal femur fracture at the greater trochanter with loss of fixation in the femoral part of the THA
- Normal CBC, chest x-ray
- Serum calcium 8.1 mg/dL

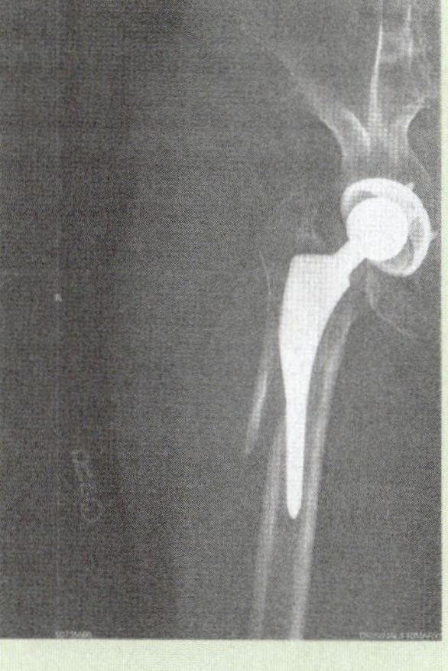

Interprofessional Care

- Revision of femoral part of his right total hip replacement with open reduction of the femoral fracture and fixation with 3 wires
- Medications:
  - IV morphine sulfate 2 mg IV every 3 h as needed
  - Cefazolin 1 gram IV every 8 h for 24 h
  - Enoxaparin 40 mg subcutaneous daily for 4 weeks
  - Calcium citrate 600 mg plus 800 IU vitamin D orally daily
  - Levothyroxine 125 mcg orally daily
- PT for transfers, gait, and stair training
- Occupational therapy for ADLs training
- Discharge planning based on mobility limitations and need for continued PT and OT

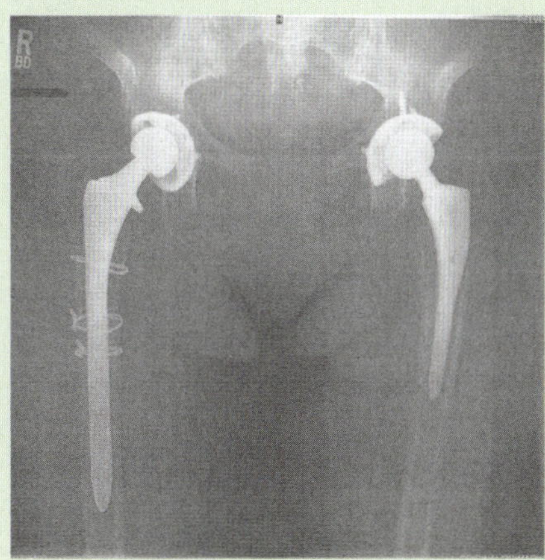

Discussion Questions

1. ***Recognize:*** How do M.C.'s previous total joint surgeries affect his recovery after this surgery?
2. ***Analyze:*** What are the most likely postoperative complications M.C. could develop?
3. ***Plan:*** As you plan care for M.C., what are the priority nursing interventions?
4. ***Prioritize:*** What is the interprofessional team's top priority at this time?
5. ***Act:*** What do you need to assess to determine his readiness for discharge?
6. ***Safety:*** What safety precautions should we implement for M.C.?
7. ***Evaluate:*** Why is satisfactory pain management an important postoperative nursing goal for M.C.?
8. ***Evaluate:*** What outcomes would indicate nursing care was effective?

Answers available at http://evolve.elsevier.com/Lewis/medsurg.

BRIDGE TO NCLEX EXAMINATION

The number of the question corresponds to the same-numbered outcome at the beginning of the chapter.

1. The nurse in urgent care suspects an ankle sprain when a patient describes
   a. being hit by another soccer player during a game.
   b. having ankle pain after sprinting around the track.
   c. dropping a 10-lb weight on his lower leg at the health club.
   d. twisting his ankle while running bases during a baseball game.
2. A patient with a humeral fracture is returning for a 4-week checkup. The nurse explains that initial evidence of healing on x-ray is indicated by
   a. formation of callus.
   b. complete bony union.
   c. hematoma at the fracture site.
   d. presence of granulation tissue.

3. A patient with a comminuted fracture of the tibia is to have an open reduction with internal fixation (ORIF) of the fracture. The nurse explains that ORIF is indicated when
   a. patients cannot tolerate prolonged immobilization.
   b. patients cannot tolerate the surgery for a closed reduction.
   c. other nonsurgical methods cannot achieve adequate alignment.
   d. a temporary cast would be too unstable to provide normal mobility.
4. The nurse suspects a neurovascular problem based on assessment of
   a. exaggerated strength with movement.
   b. increased redness and heat below the injury.
   c. decreased sensation distal to the fracture site.
   d. purulent drainage at the site of an open fracture.
5. A patient with a stable, closed humeral fracture has a temporary splint with bulky padding applied with an elastic bandage. The nurse suspects early compartment syndrome when the patient has
   a. increasing edema of the limb.
   b. muscle spasms of the lower arm.
   c. bounding pulse at the fracture site.
   d. pain when passively extending the fingers.
6. The nurse would monitor a patient with a pelvic fracture for
   a. changes in urine output.
   b. petechiae on the abdomen.
   c. a palpable lump in the buttock.
   d. sudden increase in blood pressure.
7. The nurse teaches the patient with an above-the-knee amputation that the residual limb should not be routinely elevated because this position promotes
   a. hip flexion contracture.
   b. clot formation at the incision.
   c. skin irritation and breakdown.
   d. increased risk for wound dehiscence.
8. The nurse teaches a patient with osteoarthritis who is undergoing total hip arthroplasty that the purpose of the procedure is to (**Select all that apply.**)
   a. fuse the joint.
   b. replace the joint.
   c. prevent further damage.
   d. improve or maintain ROM.
   e. decrease the amount of destruction in the joint.
9. The nurse teaches the patient who had a total ankle replacement surgery that they should avoid
   a. lifting heavy objects.
   b. sleeping on the back.
   c. abduction exercises of the affected ankle.
   d. bearing weight on the affected leg for 6 weeks.

1. d; 2. a; 3. c; 4. c; 5. d; 6. a; 7. a; 8. b, d; 9. d.

For rationales to these answers and even more NCLEX review questions, visit http://evolve.elsevier.com/Lewis/medsurg.

REFERENCES

To access the References for this chapter, please scan the QR code with a mobile device.

68

Musculoskeletal Problems

Rebekah O. Filson

http://evolve.elsevier.com/Lewis/medsurg/

CONCEPTUAL FOCUS

Functional Ability
Mobility
Pain
Safety

LEARNING OUTCOMES

1. Describe the pathophysiology, clinical manifestations, and interprofessional and nursing management of osteomyelitis.
2. Discern among the types, clinical manifestations, and interprofessional management of bone cancer.
3. Discuss the genetic basis and clinical course of muscular dystrophy.
4. Discern between the causes and characteristics of acute and chronic low back pain.
5. Describe the postoperative nursing management of patients who have had spine surgery.
6. Discuss the etiology and nursing management of common neck and foot problems.
7. Describe the etiology, pathophysiology, clinical manifestations, and nursing and interprofessional management of osteomalacia, osteoporosis, and Paget disease.

KEY TERMS

degenerative disc disease (DDD)
hallux valgus
herniated disc
low back pain (LBP)
muscular dystrophy (MD)
osteochondroma
osteomalacia
osteomyelitis
osteoporosis
osteosarcoma
Paget disease
sarcoma

We were made to move! This chapter reviews a variety of acute and chronic musculoskeletal problems unrelated to trauma that affect the musculoskeletal system. These include osteomyelitis, bone cancer, foot problems, back pain, and metabolic bone disease. These problems are a common source of pain and physical limitations that restrict the ability to take part in activities of daily living (ADLs), leading to disability. You play a key role in assessing pain and functional ability and initiating interventions to prevent injury and maintain mobility.

OSTEOMYELITIS

Etiology and Pathophysiology

Osteomyelitis is a severe infection of the bone, bone marrow, and surrounding soft tissue. A number of pathogens can cause osteomyelitis (Table 68.1). *Staphylococcus aureus* is the most common cause.

Infecting microorganisms can invade by indirect or direct entry. *Indirect entry* (hematogenous) occurs when bacteria or fungi invade the bone through the bloodstream. This most often affects children younger than 17 years. Risk factors in adults are older age, being male, immunosuppression, endocarditis, sickle cell disease, and IV drug use. Adults are more likely to have infection in the lumbar, thoracic, or cervical areas.[1]

Direct entry (contiguous) osteomyelitis accounts for 80% of cases. It most often affects adults.[2] It can occur when an open wound (e.g., penetrating wounds, fractures, surgery) allows microorganisms to enter the body. Osteomyelitis can be related to a foreign body, such as an implant or an orthopedic prosthetic device (e.g., plate, total joint prosthesis). This may happen in the feet of patients with diabetes or vascular

TABLE 68.1 Organisms Causing Osteomyelitis

Organism	Predisposing Problem
Escherichia coli	Urinary tract infection
Fungi, mycobacteria	Immunocompromised host
Mycobacterium tuberculosis	Tuberculosis
Neisseria gonorrhoeae	Gonorrhea
Pseudomonas	Puncture wounds, IV drug use
Salmonella	Sickle cell disease
Staphylococcus aureus	Pressure injury, penetrating wound, open fracture, orthopedic surgery, vascular insufficiency (e.g., diabetes, atherosclerosis)
Staphylococcus epidermidis	Indwelling prosthetic devices (e.g., joint replacements, fracture fixation devices)
Streptococcus viridans	Abscessed tooth, gingival disease

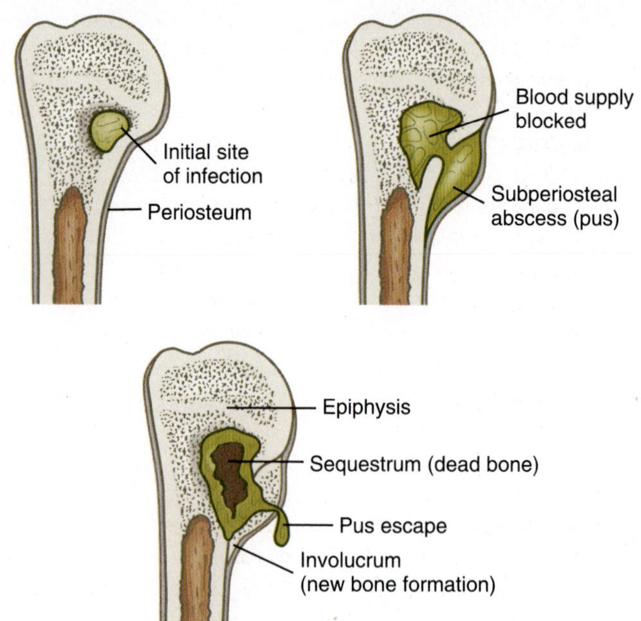

Fig. 68.1 Development of osteomyelitis infection with involucrum and sequestrum.

disease—related ulcers or in the hips or sacrum near a pressure injury. Many cases occur in adults from a nonhealing wound.[2]

After entering the blood, microorganisms grow. Pressure increases because of the nonexpanding nature of most bone. This increased pressure leads to ischemia and vascular compromise of the periosteum. The infection spreads through the bone cortex and marrow cavity, obstructing blood flow and causing necrosis.

Bone death occurs because of ischemia. The area of dead bone eventually separates from the surrounding living bone, forming *sequestra* (Fig. 68.1). Antibiotics or white blood cells (WBCs) have difficulty reaching the sequestrum through the blood. Thus sequestrum may become a reservoir for microorganisms that spread to other sites, including the lungs and brain. If the sequestrum does not resolve or is not debrided surgically, a sinus tract may develop. Chronic, purulent drainage from the tract results.

Clinical Manifestations and Complications

Acute osteomyelitis refers to the initial infection or an infection of less than 1 month in duration. Local manifestations include constant bone pain with swelling, tenderness, and warmth at the site and restricted movement of the affected part. Pain worsens with activity and is unrelieved by rest. Systemic manifestations include fever, night sweats, chills, weight loss, nausea, and fatigue. Later signs include drainage from skin sinus tracts or the fracture site.

Chronic osteomyelitis is a bone infection that lasts longer than 1 month or does not respond to initial antibiotic treatment. It may be a continuous, persistent problem or recurrent, with exacerbations and remissions (Fig. 68.2). Systemic manifestations are lessened. Local signs of infection become more common, including constant bone pain with swelling and

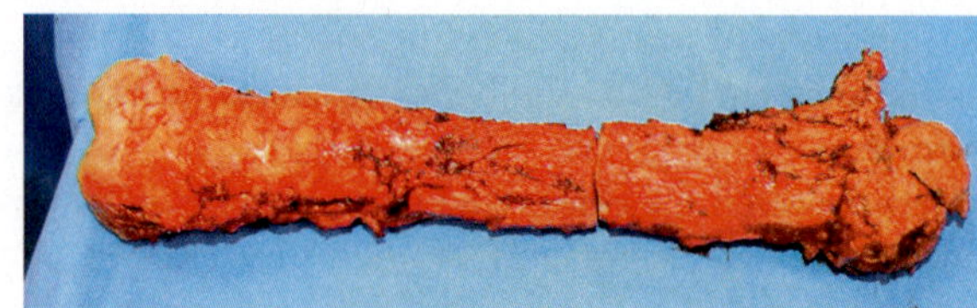

Fig. 68.2 Left femur with severe bone damage caused by osteomyelitis. (From Trung DT, Dinh HN, Le NT, et al: Total femur replacement in a patient with chronic persistence osteomyelitis, *Int J Surg Case Rep* 84:106067, 2021.)

warmth at the infection site. Over time, granulation tissue turns to scar tissue. Avascular scar tissue is an ideal site for continued microorganism growth because it cannot be penetrated by antibiotics.

Long-term, and mostly rare, complications of osteomyelitis include septicemia, septic arthritis, pathologic fractures, and amyloidosis.

Diagnostic Studies

Bone or soft tissue biopsy is the definitive way to identify the causative agent. Blood and wound cultures are often positive. Increased WBC count and erythrocyte sedimentation rate (ESR) may occur. High C-reactive protein (CRP) may occur with acute infection. Signs of osteomyelitis usually do not appear on x-rays until 2 to 4 weeks after the initial symptoms. By this time, the disease will have progressed. CT scan, WBC scan (indium-111—labeled cells), and radionuclide bone scans (technetium-99m) can assess the extent of infection. In the acute phase, MRI may be better than CT in detecting bone marrow edema, an early sign of osteomyelitis.

Interprofessional Care

Prolonged antibiotic therapy is the treatment of choice for acute osteomyelitis if bone ischemia has not yet occurred. Cultures or a bone biopsy should be done, if possible, before starting drug therapy. Any related soft tissue abscess or ulceration often needs surgical debridement or drainage.

Most patients start on IV antibiotics and then switch to oral therapy. Some patients may only receive oral agents. The antibiotic used depends on culture results and the infection itself (e.g., complexity, cause). IV antibiotic therapy may need to continue at home for 4 to 6 weeks. A few patients need therapy for 3 to 6 months. Patients may be discharged to home care or a skilled nursing facility, with antibiotics given through a central venous access device (CVAD).

Treatment of chronic osteomyelitis includes surgical removal of the poorly perfused tissue and dead bone and extended antibiotic therapy. In adults, oral therapy with a fluoroquinolone (e.g., ciprofloxacin) for 6 to 8 weeks may be an option. Oral antibiotics may be given for 4 to 8 weeks after completing IV therapy to ensure the infection is resolved. We monitor the response to drug therapy through bone scans and ESR testing.

Acrylic bead chains containing antibiotics may be implanted to help treat the infection. After debriding the dead, infected tissue, a suction irrigation system may be inserted and the wound closed. Intermittent or constant irrigation of the area with antibiotics may be used. Another option for wound management is negative pressure wound therapy (discussed in Chapter 12).

Hyperbaric O_2 is an adjunct therapy option in refractory cases of chronic osteomyelitis. It stimulates new blood growth and healing in the infected tissue.

If an orthopedic prosthetic device is the source of chronic infection, it must be removed. Muscle flaps or skin grafts provide wound coverage over the dead space in the bone. Bone grafts may help restore blood flow. However, flaps or grafts should never be placed when there is an active or suspected infection.

Amputation may be needed if bone destruction is extensive. Amputation should improve quality of life and may save the patient's life if systemic complications are developing.

NURSING MANAGEMENT: OSTEOMYELITIS

Assessment

Subjective and objective data that you should obtain from patients with osteomyelitis are outlined in Table 68.2.

TABLE 68.2 NURSING ASSESSMENT

Osteomyelitis

Subjective Data

Important Health Information

Health history: Bone trauma, open fracture, open or puncture wounds, other infections (e.g., streptococcal sore throat, endocarditis, pneumonia, sinusitis, skin or tooth infection, urinary tract infection), immunosuppression, diabetes, vascular disease

Medications: Analgesics or antibiotics

Surgery or other treatments: Bone surgery

Functional Health Patterns

Health perception–health management: IV drug and alcohol use. Fatigue.

Nutritional-metabolic: Anorexia, weight loss. Chills, nausea.

Activity-exercise: Weakness, paralysis, muscle spasms around affected area

Cognitive-perceptual: Local tenderness over affected area, ↑ pain with movement of affected area

Coping–stress tolerance: Irritability, withdrawal, dependency, anger

Objective Data

General

Restlessness. High, spiking fever. Night sweats

Musculoskeletal

Restricted movement; wound drainage. Spontaneous fracture

Skin

Diaphoresis. Redness, warmth, edema at site of infection

Possible Diagnostic Findings

Positive blood and/or wound cultures, ↑ ESR, ↑ WBC. Presence of sequestrum and involucrum on x-rays, radionuclide bone scans, CT, and MRI

ESR, Erythrocyte sedimentation rate.

Clinical Problems

Clinical problems for patients with osteomyelitis may include:

- Pain
- Musculoskeletal problems
- Infection

Additional information on nursing diagnoses and interventions for patients with osteomyelitis can be found in eNursing Care Plan 68.1 (available on the website for this chapter).

Planning

The overall goals are that patients with osteomyelitis will (1) have satisfactory pain and fever management, (2) be free from complications, and (3) adhere to the treatment plan.

Implementation

Acute Care

Nursing care of patients with osteomyelitis is outlined in Table 68.3. Some immobilization of the affected limb (e.g., splint, traction) is usually needed to decrease pain and reduce risk for further injury. Casts or braces can protect the limb or the surgical site. Carefully handle the limb. Avoid undue manipulation. This may increase pain and cause a pathologic fracture. Assess for pain. Muscle spasms may cause minor to severe pain. Nonsteroidal antiinflammatory drugs (NSAIDs), opioid analgesics, and muscle relaxants may be given.

Dressings are used to absorb drainage from wounds and debride dead tissue from the wound bed. These include dry, sterile dressings; dressings saturated in saline or antibiotic solution; wet-to-dry dressings; and dressings applied with negative-pressure wound therapy. Handle soiled dressings carefully to prevent transfer of bacteria to other areas of the

TABLE 68.3 NURSING MANAGEMENT

Caring for Patients With Osteomyelitis

- Give IV antibiotics as ordered.
- Assess wound for signs of worsening infection.
- Teach patient and caregiver about antibiotic side effects and length of treatment, signs and symptoms of worsening infection, and use of hyperbaric O_2 if ordered.
- Assess for muscle spasms and give prescribed muscle relaxants.
- Assess pain, and give analgesics as ordered. Assess response.
- Handle affected limb carefully and avoid undue manipulation.
- Assess neurovascular condition of affected limb, and immediately inform HCP of significant changes.
- Encourage nondrug approaches to managing pain (e.g., guided imagery, relaxation breathing; see Chapter 7).
- Change dressing as ordered using sterile technique.
- Implement contact precautions as needed.
- Supervise AP:
  - Handle affected limb carefully based on RN instruction.
  - Help patient with passive ROM of adjacent joints and active ROM exercises of unaffected limb.
  - Notify RN about reports of pain, tingling, or decreased sensation in the affected extremity.

Collaborate With Physical Therapist

- Assess current mobility and need for aid.
- Teach safe ambulation with assistive device based on weight-bearing restrictions.
- Establish exercise plan and teach patient to perform exercises safely.
- Coordinate PT so that patient can receive timely analgesia.
- Discuss home environment with patient and identify modifications needed (e.g., stair training, bed placement on first level).

Collaborate With Occupational Therapist

- Assess impact of condition on ability to perform ADLs.
- Teach use of assistive devices (e.g., long-handled reacher, shoe donner) to promote self-care while maintaining activity restrictions.

wound. Discard dressings appropriately to prevent spread of infection.

Patients are often placed on bed rest in the early stages of acute infection. Good body alignment and frequent position changes promote comfort and prevent complications related to immobility. Flexion contracture of the affected lower extremity is common. Patients often position the leg in a flexed position to promote comfort. Footdrop can develop quickly because of Achilles tendon contracture if the foot is not supported in a neutral position by a splint or boot.

CHECK YOUR PRACTICE

Your patient on the orthopedic unit is a 22-year-old male who was in an all-terrain vehicle accident in a remote area 4 days ago. He is slowly recovering from his head injury and surgical repair of an open fracture of the femur. Yesterday, he was diagnosed with acute osteomyelitis. At times he is angry and disoriented. When you try to assess his leg, he yells at you, "It hurts. Leave it alone!"

- What are your priorities of care?
- What signs and symptoms would suggest the patient's condition is worsening?

Chronic Care

Provide teaching about prolonged high-dose antibiotic therapy (see Table 15.8). Review side effects, including hearing problems, impaired renal function, and neurotoxicity. Assess *Candida albicans* and *C. difficile* genitourinary (GU) and gastrointestinal (GI) tract infections, especially in immunosuppressed and older adult patients. Teach patients to report any changes in the oral cavity (e.g., whitish yellow, curdlike lesions) or the GU tract (e.g., perianal itching, discharge). Stress the importance of continuing to take the full course of antibiotics prescribed, even after symptoms have improved. Reinforce the need for follow-up laboratory testing. Monitor peak and trough blood levels of most antibiotics.

Teach patients and caregivers how to manage the CVAD if receiving IV antibiotics at home. Review how to administer the antibiotic. Dressing changes are often needed if there is an open wound. Patients and caregivers may need supplies and instruction for completing the dressing change.

Patients and caregivers may be anxious and discouraged because of the serious nature of osteomyelitis, the uncertainty of the outcome, and the long, costly treatment. Continued emotional support is a key part of nursing management.

◆ Evaluation

The expected outcomes are that patients with osteomyelitis will:

- Have satisfactory pain management
- Adhere to the recommended treatment plan
- Show a consistent increase in mobility and range of motion (ROM)

BONE TUMORS

Primary bone tumors, both benign and malignant, are rare in adults. They account for only 1% of all tumors. Benign bone tumors are more common than primary malignant tumors. Metastatic bone cancer, in which cancer has spread from another site, is more common.

BENIGN BONE TUMORS

The main types of benign bone tumors are osteochondroma, osteoclastoma, and enchondroma (Table 68.4). **Osteochondroma** is the most common benign bone tumor. It is characterized by an overgrowth of cartilage and bone near the end of the bone at the growth plate. Manifestations include a painless, hard, immobile mass; shorter-than-normal height for age; soreness of muscles close to the tumor; 1 leg or arm longer than the other; and pressure or irritation with exercise. Some may be asymptomatic. Diagnosis is confirmed using x-ray, CT scan, and MRI.

No treatment is needed for asymptomatic osteochondroma. Patients should have regular screenings to detect progression to cancer. If the tumor is causing pain or neurologic manifestations because of compression, surgical removal is usually done.

TABLE 68.4 Types of Primary Bone Tumors

Types	Description
Benign	
Enchondroma	• Intramedullary cartilage tumor usually found in cavity of a single hand or foot bone • Rarely transforms to cancer • If tumor becomes painful, surgical resection is done • Peak incidence in people ages 10–20 yr
Osteochondroma	• Most common benign bone tumor • Often found in pelvis, scapula, or metaphyseal part of long bones • Occurs most often in people ages 10–25 yr • May transform to cancer (chondrosarcoma)
Osteoclastoma (giant cell tumor)	• Arises in cancellous ends of arm and leg bones • Around 10% are locally aggressive and may spread to lungs • High rate of local recurrence after surgery and chemotherapy
Malignant	
Chondrosarcoma	• Most often occurs in cartilage in arm, leg, and pelvic bones of adults ages 50–70 yr • Can arise from benign bone tumors (osteochondromas) • Wide surgical resection is typically done, as tumor rarely responds to radiation and chemotherapy • Survival rate depends on stage, size, and grade of tumor
Ewing sarcoma	• Develops in medullary cavity of pelvis and long bones, especially femur, humerus, and tibia • Usually occurs in children and teenagers • Use of wide surgical resection, radiation, and chemotherapy has improved 5-yr survival rate to 60%
Osteosarcoma	• Most common primary bone cancer • Occurs mostly in males ages 10–25 • Most often in pelvis or bones of arms, legs (Fig. 68.3)

MALIGNANT BONE TUMORS

A **sarcoma** is a malignant tumor that develops in bone, muscle, fat, nerve, or cartilage. The most common types of sarcomas are osteosarcoma, chondrosarcoma, and Ewing sarcoma (Table 68.4). Primary tumors occur most often during childhood and young adulthood. They cause bone destruction and have rapid metastasis.

Osteosarcoma

Osteosarcoma is a highly aggressive bone cancer. It rapidly spreads to distant sites. It often starts in the pelvis or metaphyseal region of the long bones of extremities, especially in the distal femur, proximal tibia, and proximal humerus (Fig. 68.3).

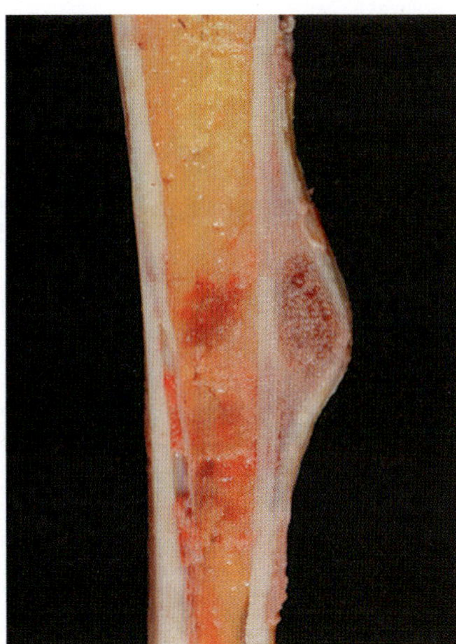

Fig. 68.3 Osteosarcoma. (From Czerniak B: *Dorfman and Czerniak's bone tumors,* ed 2, Philadelphia, 2016, Elsevier.)

Osteosarcoma is the most common bone cancer affecting children and young adults. It can occur in older adults, but not as often. It is most often associated with Paget disease and prior radiation.[3]

The gradual onset of pain and swelling in the affected bone is the most common manifestation. The pain may be worse at night and increase with activity. Metastasis is present in 10% to 20% of people at the time of diagnosis. Diagnosis is confirmed from tissue biopsy, increased alkaline phosphatase and calcium, x-ray, CT or PET scans, and MRI.

Chemotherapy given before surgery can decrease tumor size. Limb salvage procedures are usually considered if a clear 6- to 7-cm margin surrounds the lesion. Limb salvage is usually not possible if patients have major nerve or blood vessel involvement, pathologic fracture, infection, or extensive muscle involvement.

Chemotherapy after amputation or limb salvage has increased the 5-year survival rate to 75% in people without metastasis. Chemotherapy includes combinations of methotrexate, doxorubicin, cisplatin, ifosfamide, cyclophosphamide, gemcitabine, and etoposide.[3]

Metastatic Bone Cancer

The most common type of cancerous bone tumor occurs because of spread (metastasis) from a primary tumor at another site. Common primary sites include breast, colon, prostate, lungs, kidney, and thyroid.[4] Metastatic cancer cells travel from the primary tumor to the bone via the lymph and blood supply. Metastatic bone lesions often occur in the spine, ribs, or pelvis.[4] Pathologic fractures at the site of metastasis are common because the bone is weak. High calcium occurs as damaged bones release calcium.

Once a primary lesion is found, bone scans are often done to detect metastatic lesions. Metastatic bone lesions may occur at any time after diagnosis and treatment of the primary tumor. Bone metastasis should be suspected in patients with local bone pain and a history of cancer. Surgical stabilization of the bone may be indicated for fracture or to prevent fracture in high-risk patients. Prognosis depends on the primary type of cancer and any other sites of metastasis. Possible palliative treatment consists of radiation and pain management (see Chapter 16).

NURSING MANAGEMENT: BONE CANCER

Nursing care of patients with bone cancer does not differ significantly from the general care of patients with cancer (see Chapter 16). Monitor the tumor site for swelling, changes in circulation, and decreased movement, sensation, or joint function.

Use care to prevent pathologic fractures and reduce their complications. Prevent fractures by careful handling and support of the affected extremity and logrolling patients. Note weakness caused by anemia and decreased mobility.

Treatment for hypercalcemia may be started if bone decalcification occurs. Patients may find it hard to take part in activities because of weakness from the disease and treatment, fear of falling and fracturing a bone, and fear of pain. Provide rest periods between activities.

Assess for the location and severity of pain. The pain can be severe. It is often caused by the tumor pressing against nerves and other organs near the bone. New-onset pain or changes in pain severity may indicate pathologic fracture. Provide adequate pain medication. Sometimes radiation therapy is used as a palliative treatment to shrink the tumor and decrease pain.

Assist patients and caregivers in coping with the diagnosis. Assist with managing pain and disability, side effects of chemotherapy, and postoperative care (e.g., after spinal cord decompression or amputation). Stress the importance of follow-up care.

MUSCULAR DYSTROPHY

Muscular dystrophy (MD) is a group of genetic diseases characterized by progressive symmetric wasting of skeletal muscles without neurologic involvement. The types of MD differ in the groups of muscles affected, age of onset, rate of progression, and mode of genetic inheritance (Table 68.5). A gradual loss of strength with increasing disability and deformity occurs with all forms of MD. Duchenne MD is the most common type. Duchenne and Becker MDs are X-linked recessive disorders mainly affecting males (Box 68.1).[5]

Diagnostic studies include genetic testing, muscle enzymes (especially creatine kinase), electromyogram (EMG) testing, and muscle fiber biopsy. Classic findings on muscle biopsy include fat and connective tissue deposits, muscle fiber degeneration and necrosis, and a deficiency of dystrophin. ECG changes may suggest cardiomyopathy.

TABLE 68.5 Select Types of MD

	Genetic Basis	Manifestations
Becker	• X-linked • Mutation of dystrophin gene	• Similar but less severe than Duchenne MD • Onset ages 5–15 • Slower course of pelvic and shoulder muscle wasting than Duchenne • Cardiomyopathy • Respiratory failure • May survive into 50s
Duchenne	• X-linked • Mutation of dystrophin gene	• Most common form of MD • Primarily affects boys • Onset before age 5 • Progressive weakness of pelvic and shoulder muscles • Unable to walk by age 12 • Cardiomyopathy • Respiratory failure in 20s • Mental impairment
Facioscapulohumeral	• Autosomal dominant • Deletion of chromosome *4q35*	• Onset before age 20 • Slowly progressive weakness of face, shoulder muscles, upper arms, and lower legs • Can affect vision and hearing
Limb-girdle	• Autosomal recessive or autosomal dominant • Mutation in any of at least 15 genes affecting proteins needed for muscle function	• Group of disorders affecting voluntary muscles, especially those of hips and shoulders • Onset ranges from early childhood to early adulthood or later • Slow progressive weakness of hip and shoulder muscles

There is no cure. Corticosteroids may slow disease progression for up to 2 years and improve survival.[5] Deflazacort (Emflaza) is the first corticosteroid approved to treat Duchenne MD. Eteplirsen (Exondys 51), viltolarsen (Viltepso), and golodirsen (Vyondys 53) are disease-modifying drugs used to treat patients with Duchenne MD who have specific gene mutations.[5]

The main treatment goals are to preserve mobility and independence through exercise, physical therapy, and use of assistive devices. Progressive muscle weakening around the trunk can cause spinal collapse. Patients may be fitted early with an orthotic jacket to give stability and prevent further deformity or injury.

Cardiomyopathy often occurs and causes heart failure. Gradual decreases in lung function often lead to the need for continuous positive airway pressure (CPAP). Eventually tracheostomy and mechanical ventilation are needed to support respiratory function.

BOX 68.1 GENETICS IN CLINICAL PRACTICE

Duchenne and Becker Muscular Dystrophy

Genetic Basis

- Caused by various mutations in the dystrophin *(DMD)* gene
- Gene provides instructions for making dystrophin, a protein that helps keep muscle fibers intact
- Dystrophin is found mainly in skeletal and cardiac muscle
- Abnormal dystrophin can cause defects in the muscle fiber and muscle fiber degeneration
- Inherited in an X-linked recessive pattern
- Females in affected families have a 50% chance of inheriting and passing the defective gene to their children

Incidence

- Between 400 and 600 young males are born with muscular dystrophy (MD) each year in the United States
- Together they affect 1 in 3500 to 5000 newborn males worldwide

Genetic Testing

- DNA testing can detect mutations in dystrophin gene
- Genetic testing and counseling should be considered for those with a family history of MD

Clinical Implications

- Because there are many types of MD with different genetic bases, knowing the type of MD is important to direct treatment and genetic counseling recommendations

Encourage communication between patients and caregivers to cope with the emotional and physical demands of MD. Teach them range-of-motion (ROM) exercises, principles of good nutrition, and signs of disease progression.

Focus care on keeping patients active as long as possible. Prolonged bed rest should be avoided because immobility can cause more muscle wasting. As the disease progresses, have patients limit sedentary periods to prevent skin breakdown and respiratory complications. Ongoing medical and nursing care is needed.

The Muscular Dystrophy Association (www.mda.org) is an important resource with information about support services for patients and caregivers. The website gives updates about the latest clinical trials and treatment advances.

LOW BACK PAIN

Low back pain (LBP) is most often caused by a musculoskeletal problem. It affects about 80% of adults in the United States at least once during their lives. LBP is second to headache as the most common pain problem. It is the leading cause of job-related disability and a major contributor to missed work.

LBP may be local or diffuse. With local pain, patients feel soreness or discomfort when a specific area of the lower back is palpated or pressed. Diffuse pain occurs over a larger area and comes from deep tissue.

LBP may be radicular or referred. *Radicular pain* is caused by irritation of a nerve root and is not isolated to a single location. Instead, it radiates or moves along a nerve distribution. Sciatica is an example of radicular pain. *Referred pain* is felt in the lower back, but the source of the pain is another location (e.g., kidneys, lower abdomen).

LBP is common because the lumbar region (1) bears most of the weight of the body, (2) is the most flexible region of the spinal column, (3) has nerve roots that are at risk for injury or disease, and (4) has a naturally poor biomechanical structure. Risk factors include lack of muscle tone, obesity, trauma, poor posture, older age, smoking, pregnancy, prior compression fracture of the spine, spinal problems since birth, and a family history of back pain. Jobs that require repetitive heavy lifting, vibration (e.g., a jackhammer operator), and extended periods of sitting are associated with LBP.

Causes of LBP of musculoskeletal origin include (1) acute lumbosacral strain, (2) instability of the lumbosacral bony mechanism, (3) osteoarthritis (OA) of the lumbosacral vertebrae, (4) degenerative disc disease, and (5) herniation of an intervertebral disc.

ACUTE LOW BACK PAIN

Acute low back pain lasts 4 weeks or less.[6] Most acute LBP is caused by trauma or an activity that causes undue stress (often hyperflexion) on the lower back. Examples of trauma or activities that cause acute back pain are heavy lifting; overuse of back muscles during yard work; a sports injury; or a sudden jolt, as in a motor vehicle crash.

Often symptoms do not appear at the time of injury. They develop later (usually within 24 hours) because of a gradual increase in pressure on the nerve from an intervertebral disc and/or associated edema. Symptoms may range from muscle ache to shooting or stabbing pain, limited flexibility or ROM, or an inability to stand upright.

There are few definitive diagnostic changes with nerve irritation and muscle strain. One test is the straight-leg-raising test (see Chapter 66). MRI and CT scans are not done unless trauma or systemic disease (e.g., cancer, spinal infection) is suspected. MRI findings may be limited in the acute phase of an injury because of increased edema near the injury.

NURSING MANAGEMENT: ACUTE LOW BACK PAIN

Assessment

Subjective and objective data that you should obtain from patients with LBP are outlined in Table 68.6.

Implementation

Nursing interventions for patients with LBP are detailed in eNursing Care Plan 68.2 (available on the website for this chapter). If acute muscle spasms and accompanying pain are not severe and unbearable, patients are treated as an outpatient with NSAIDs and muscle relaxants (e.g., cyclobenzaprine).

TABLE 68.6 NURSING ASSESSMENT

Low Back Pain

Subjective Data

Important Health Information

Health history: Acute or chronic lumbosacral strain/trauma, osteoarthritis, degenerative disc disease, obesity

Medications: Opioid analgesics and NSAIDs, muscle relaxants, corticosteroids, over-the-counter remedies (e.g., topical ointments, patches)

Surgery or other treatments: Back surgery, epidural corticosteroid injections

Functional Health Patterns

Health perception–health management: Smoking, lack of exercise

Nutritional-metabolic: Obesity

Activity-exercise: Poor posture, muscle spasms, activity intolerance

Elimination: Constipation

Sleep-rest: Interrupted sleep

Cognitive-perceptual: Pain in back, buttocks, or leg associated with walking, turning, straining, coughing, leg raising. Numbness or tingling of legs, feet, toes

Role-relationship: Occupations requiring heavy lifting, vibrations, or extended driving. Change in role within family structure because of inability to work and provide income

Objective Data

General

Guarded movement

Musculoskeletal

Tense, tight paravertebral muscles on palpation, ↓ range of motion in spine

Neurologic

Depressed or absent Achilles tendon reflex or patellar tendon reflex. Positive straight-leg-raising test, positive crossover straight-leg-raising test, positive Trendelenburg test

Possible Diagnostic Findings

Localization of site of lesion or disorder on myelogram, CT scan, or MRI. Determination of nerve root impingement on electromyography (EMG)

TABLE 68.7 PATIENT & CAREGIVER TEACHING

Low Back Problems

Include the following instructions when teaching patients and caregivers how to manage low back problems:

Do

- Maintain healthy body weight.
- Maintain a neutral pelvic position if standing. Place 1 foot on a low stool if standing for long periods.
- Choose a seat with good lower back support, armrests, and a swivel base. Place a pillow at the lumbar spine to maintain normal curvature. Keep knees and hips level.
- Sleep in a side-lying position with knees and hips bent and a pillow between the knees for support.
- Use a firm mattress.
- Sleep on back with a lift under knees and legs or on back with 10-in-high pillow under knees to flex hips and knees.
- Use proper body mechanics when lifting heavy objects. Bend at the knees, not at the waist, and stand up slowly while holding object close to your body.
- Take part in strength and flexibility training and low-impact aerobic exercise.
- Use local heat and cold application to relieve muscle tension.

Do Not

- Lean forward without bending knees.
- Lift anything above level of elbows.
- Stand unmoving for prolonged time.
- Sleep on abdomen or on back or side with legs out straight.
- Exceed prescribed amount and type of exercises without consulting HCP.
- Smoke or use tobacco products.

Massage, back manipulation, acupuncture, and cold and hot compresses may help some patients. Severe pain may need a brief course of corticosteroids or opioid analgesics.

Some people may need a brief period (1 to 2 days) of rest. They should avoid prolonged bed rest. Most patients do better if they continue their normal activities. Patients should refrain from activities that increase the pain, including lifting, bending, twisting, and prolonged sitting. Symptoms of acute LBP usually improve within 2 weeks. They often resolve without treatment.

If the lumbosacral area is unstable or there is persistent use of poor body mechanics, repeated episodes are likely. The goal is to make an episode of acute LBP an isolated incident. Teach patients about the cause of the pain and ways to prevent further episodes (Table 68.7). Offer advice when patients do activities that could cause LBP. Some HCPs refer patients to a formal program called "Back School." Patients learn ways to minimize back pain and avoid repeat episodes of pain. Teaching is provided by an HCP, nurse, or physical therapist. If the strain is work related, occupational counseling may be needed.

Exercise is aimed at strengthening the supporting muscles. Muscle stretching may be part of the management plan. Referral to a physical therapist or personal trainer to address posture and core and abdomen strength may be needed. Reinforce the type and frequency of prescribed exercise and the reason for the program.

Recommend flat shoes or shoes with low heels and shock-absorbing shoe inserts for females. Stress the importance of smoking cessation. Tobacco use impairs circulation to the intervertebral discs and contributes to LBP. Advise patients to maintain a healthy body weight. Excess body weight places more stress on the lower back and weakens abdominal muscles that support the lower back. Sleeping position is important. Teach patients to avoid sleeping in a prone position. It causes excess lumbar lordosis, placing stress on the lower back. Sleeping in a supine or side-lying position with knees and hips flexed prevents pressure on support muscles, ligaments, and lumbosacral joints. Recommend use of a firm mattress. LBP can cause frustration, pain, and disability. Provide emotional support.

Special Needs of Health Care Personnel

Health care personnel who perform direct patient care activities are at high risk for developing LBP.[7] Lifting and moving patients, excess bending or leaning forward, and frequent twisting can result in LBP. This causes lost productivity and disability. Safe patient handling devices to lift, transfer, and reposition patients are recommended for nurse and patient safety. Serve as a role model by always using proper body mechanics. This includes raising the bed height, bending at the knees, and asking for help in lifting and moving patients.

CHRONIC LOW BACK PAIN

Chronic low back pain lasts more than 3 months or involves repeated incapacitating episodes.[6] It is often progressive. Common causes include (1) degenerative conditions, such as arthritis or disc disease; (2) osteoporosis or other metabolic bone diseases; (3) weakness from the scar tissue of prior injury; (4) chronic strain on lower back muscles from obesity, pregnancy, or stressful postures on the job; and (5) congenital spine problems.

Spinal Stenosis

Spinal stenosis is a narrowing of the spinal canal, which holds the spinal cord. Stenosis in the lumbar spine is a common cause of chronic LBP. Spinal stenosis can be acquired or inherited (e.g., congenital spinal stenosis, scoliosis). A common acquired cause is OA. Arthritic changes (bone spurs, calcification of spinal ligaments, disc degeneration) narrow the space around the spinal canal and nerve roots, eventually leading to compression. Inflammation caused by the compression results in pain, weakness, and numbness. Other acquired conditions that may cause spinal stenosis include rheumatoid arthritis, spinal tumors, Paget disease, and trauma damage to the vertebral column.

The pain from lumbar spinal stenosis often starts in the lower back and then radiates to the buttock and leg. It is worse with walking or prolonged standing. Numbness, tingling, weakness, and heaviness in the legs and buttocks may be present. History of decreased pain when the patient bends forward or sits is often a sign of spinal stenosis. Cold, damp weather may worsen the pain. In most cases, stenosis slowly progresses.

Interprofessional and Nursing Management

The management and treatment of chronic LBP is similar to acute LBP. Manage pain and stiffness with mild analgesics, such as NSAIDs, for daily comfort. Antidepressants (e.g., duloxetine) may help with pain and sleep problems. The antiseizure drug gabapentin may improve walking and relieve leg symptoms.

Weight reduction, rest periods, and exercise and activity throughout the day help keep the muscles and joints mobilized. Physical therapy can reduce pain and improve body posture. Rest and local heat application can decrease pain. Complementary therapies, such as biofeedback, acupuncture, and yoga, may help reduce pain.

Minimally invasive treatments, such as epidural corticosteroid injections and implanted devices that deliver pain medication, are options for those who do not respond to the usual therapies. Surgery may be done in patients with severe pain who received no benefit from conservative care and/or have continued neurologic deficits.

INTERVERTEBRAL DISC DISEASE

Intervertebral discs separate the vertebrae and help absorb shock for the spine. *Intervertebral disc disease* involves deterioration, herniation, or other problem with the intervertebral discs. Disc problems can affect the cervical, thoracic, and lumbar spine.

Etiology and Pathophysiology

Degenerative disc disease (DDD) results from loss of fluid in the intervertebral discs with aging. The discs lose their elasticity, flexibility, and shock-absorbing abilities. Unless it is accompanied by pain, DDD is a normal process. The discs become thinner as the *nucleus pulposus* (gelatinous center of the disc) starts to dry out and shrink. This change limits the disc's ability to distribute pressure between vertebrae. The pressure is then transferred to the *annulus fibrosus* (strong outside part of the disc), causing progressive destruction. When the disc is damaged, the nucleus pulposus may seep through a torn or stretched annulus. This is called a **herniated disc** *(slipped disc)*. The spinal disc bulges outward between the vertebrae (Fig. 68.4).

A herniated disc can result from degeneration with age or repeated stress and trauma to the spine. The most common

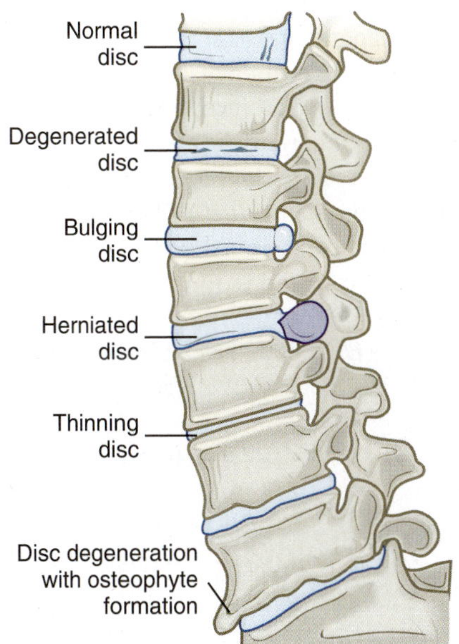

Fig. 68.4 Common causes of degenerative disc damage.

sites of herniation are the lumbosacral discs, specifically L4–L5 and L5–S1. Disc herniation at C5–C6 and C6–C7 may be the result of spinal stenosis. There is a narrowing of the spinal canal that forces the intervertebral disc to bulge.

The spinal nerves emerge from the spinal column through an opening *(intervertebral foramen)* between adjacent vertebrae. Herniated discs can press against these nerves ("pinched nerve"), causing *radiculopathy* (radiating pain, numbness, tingling, decreased strength and/or ROM).

OA of the spine is associated with DDD and the stresses placed on the vertebrae. As the poorly lubricated joints rub against each other, the protective cartilage is damaged and painful bone spurs occur.

Clinical Manifestations

In *lumbar disc disease,* the most common manifestation is LBP. Radicular pain that radiates down the buttock and below the knee, along the distribution of the sciatic nerve, generally indicates disc herniation. Manifestations of lumbar disc herniation are outlined in Table 68.8. A positive straight-leg-raising test may indicate nerve root irritation (see Chapter 66). Back or leg pain may be reproduced by raising the leg.

LBP from other causes may not be accompanied by leg pain. Reflexes may be depressed or absent, depending on the spinal nerve root involved. Numbness and tingling *(paresthesia)* or muscle weakness in the legs, feet, or toes may occur.

Multiple lumbar nerve root compressions *(cauda equina syndrome)* may occur from a herniated disc, tumor, or epidural abscess. Manifestations include severe LBP, progressive weakness, increased pain, and bowel and bladder incontinence or retention. Saddle anesthesia (loss of or altered sensation of the perineum, buttocks, inner thighs, and back of the legs [saddle area]) may be present. Symptoms of cauda equina syndrome may develop suddenly or evolve slowly over time. They may vary in intensity. Cauda equina is a medical emergency. It requires surgical decompression to reduce pressure on the nerves and prevent permanent paralysis.[8]

In *cervical disc disease,* pain radiates into the arms and hands, following the pattern of the involved nerve. Like lumbar disc disease, reflexes may or may not be present. The handgrip is often weak. Because manifestations of cervical disc disease may include shoulder pain and problems, the HCP must rule out shoulder problems as part of the diagnosis.

Diagnostic Studies

X-rays are done to detect any structural defects. A myelogram, MRI, or CT scan is helpful in localizing the damaged site. An epidural venogram or diskogram may be needed if other diagnostic studies are inconclusive. An EMG can determine the severity of nerve irritation or rule out other conditions, such as peripheral neuropathy.

Interprofessional Care

Patients with suspected disc damage are usually managed with conservative therapy (Table 68.9). This includes limiting extremes of spinal movement (e.g., brace, corset, belt), local heat or ice, ultrasound and massage, traction, and transcutaneous electrical nerve stimulation (TENS). Drug therapy to manage pain includes acetaminophen, ibuprofen, naproxen, muscle relaxants, or neuropathic agents (e.g., gabapentin, pregabalin, duloxetine, venlafaxine).[9] Opioids may be used short-term. Epidural corticosteroid injections may reduce inflammation and relieve acute pain. However, pain tends to recur if the underlying cause remains.

When symptoms subside, patients should begin back-strengthening exercises twice a day and continue for life. Teach patients the principles of good body mechanics. Discourage extreme flexion and torsion. Most patients heal after 6 months with a conservative treatment plan.

Surgical Therapy

If conservative treatment is unsuccessful, radiculopathy becomes worse, or loss of bowel or bladder control occurs, surgery may be considered. Surgery for a damaged disc is generally done if patients are in constant pain and/or have a persistent neurologic deficit.

Image-guided procedures are considered minimally invasive treatments. Overall, they have good results and fewer complications than surgery. Heating (e.g., radiofrequency, microwave, laser) or injecting chemicals into the intervertebral disc may alter the internal mechanics of the disc and relieve pain by recreating the intervertebral disc's structure.[10] Examples include intradiscal electrothermoplasty (IDET) and radiofrequency discal nucleoplasty (coablation nucleoplasty). Several drugs can be injected to reduce compression and inflammation, with minimal damage to the surrounding tissues. Steroids and methylene blue can reduce

TABLE 68.8 Manifestations of Lumbar Disc Herniation

Intervertebral Level	Pain	Affected Reflex	Motor Function	Sensation
L3–L4	Back to buttocks to posterior thigh to inner calf	Patellar	Quadriceps, anterior tibialis	Inner aspect of lower leg, anterior part of thigh
L4–L5	Back to buttocks to dorsum of foot and big toe	None	Anterior tibialis, extensor hallucis longus, gluteus medius	Dorsum of foot and big toe
L5–S1	Back to buttocks to sole of foot and heel	Achilles	Gastrocnemius, hamstring, gluteus maximus	Heel and lateral foot

TABLE 68.9 Interprofessional Care

Intervertebral Disc Disease

Diagnostic Assessment
- History and physical assessment
- X-ray
- CT scan
- MRI
- Myelogram
- Diskogram
- Electromyography (EMG)

Management

Conservative Therapy
- Restricted activity for several days, limited total bed rest
- Local ice or heat
- Physical therapy
- Drug therapy
  - Analgesics
  - Muscle relaxants (e.g., cyclobenzaprine)
  - Antiseizure drugs (e.g., gabapentin)
  - Antidepressants
- Epidural corticosteroid injections

Surgical Therapy
- Artificial disc replacement
- Discectomy
- Intradiscal electrothermoplasty (IDET)
- Interspinous device implants
- Laminectomy with or without spinal fusion
- Radiofrequency discal nucleoplasty
- Spinal fusion without or with instrumentation (e.g., plates, screws)

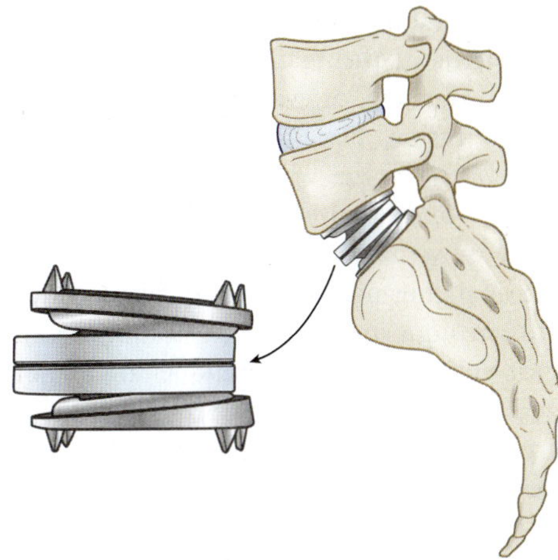

Fig. 68.5 The Charité artificial disc, used to replace a damaged intervertebral disc in degenerative disc disease of the lumbar spine. A movable high-density plastic core is placed between 2 cobalt-chromium alloy end plates. The disc's design helps realign the spine and preserve movement.

inflammation. Inserting biomaterials such as platelet-rich plasma (PRP), stem cells, and hydrogel may regenerate the disk.

Another third minimally invasive procedure involves implanting a device made from titanium, elastomeric compounds, or other materials to decompress and/or stabilize the affected spinal segment. *Interspinous devices* (ISDs) are implanted between the spinous processes to lift vertebrae off the pinched nerve. Newer ISDs include *interspinous dynamic stabilizers* (ISDSs) and *interspinous stabilizers* (ISSs). *ISSs* reduce the degree of extension of the vertebrae with no effect on spinal stability. *ISDSs* stabilize the spinal segment and provide some spacer properties.[10]

Laminotomy with discectomy (or lumbar discectomy) is the most common surgery. The HCP makes a small incision on the back over the involved disc. A small portion of the lamina is removed to expose the nerve root. Next, the herniated portion of the disc that is causing nerve root compression is removed. The goal is to relieve leg pain. It may or may not relieve back pain. Patients may need a short hospital stay.

Minimally invasive procedures to decompress the nerve root are *microdiscectomy* and *endoscopic microdiscectomy.* In the first procedure, the HCP uses a microscope to see the disc and disc space to remove the herniated portion. *Percutaneous discectomy* uses instruments with a tiny camera with fluoroscopy guidance, then uses a laser on the damaged part of the disc.

The goals of artificial disc replacement surgery are to restore movement and eliminate pain. The Charité disc is used in patients with lumbar disc damage from DDD (Fig. 68.5). The surgeon removes the damaged disc and places the device in the spine. The disc restores movement at the level of the implant. The ProDisc-L and activL are 2 other types of artificial lumbar discs. Options for treating DDD of the cervical spine include the Prestige cervical disc, Mobi-C disc, Secure-C, Simplify, and M6-C artificial cervical disc.

A *spinal fusion* stabilizes the spine by creating *ankylosis* (fusion) of adjacent vertebrae with a bone graft. Grafts are from the fibula or iliac crest *(autograft)* or from donated cadaver bone *(allograft).* Metal fixation with rods, plates, or screws can give more stability and decrease vertebral motion. Surgical procedures include posterior lumbar interbody fusion (PLIF), anterior lumbar interbody fusion (ALIF), transforaminal lumbar interbody fusion (TLIF), and extreme lateral interbody fusion (XLIF).[11]

Bone morphogenetic protein (BMP), a genetically engineered protein, may be placed to stimulate bone growth of the graft in spinal fusions. A dissolvable sponge soaked with BMP is implanted into the spine. BMP on the sponge stimulates the body's cells to become active and produce bone, promoting fusion. The body absorbs the sponge, leaving living bone behind.

NURSING MANAGEMENT: SPINE SURGERY

Nursing care after spine surgery is outlined in Table 68.10. A key nursing focus is maintaining proper spinal alignment until it has healed. Depending on the type and extent of surgery and the HCP's preference, patients may be able to dangle the legs at the side of the bed, stand, or even ambulate the day of surgery.

After lumbar fusion, place pillows under the thighs when supine and between the legs when in the side-lying position to provide comfort and ensure alignment. Patients often fear turning or any movement that may increase pain. Have them logroll when changing position in bed. Have enough staff to move patients without undue pain or strain. Reassure patients that you are using proper technique to maintain body alignment.

After surgery, most patients receive IV analgesia for 24 to 48 hours. Once patients receive oral fluids, they can transition to oral drugs. Diazepam may be prescribed for muscle relaxation.

Because the spinal canal may be entered during surgery, cerebrospinal fluid (CSF) leakage is possible. Immediately report leakage of CSF on the dressing or if patients report a severe headache. CSF appears as clear or slightly yellow drainage on the dressing. It has a high glucose concentration and tests positive for glucose with a dipstick. If suspected, place the patient flat.

Assess peripheral neurologic condition and compare with the preoperative assessment. Movement of the arms and legs and assessment of sensation should at least equal the preoperative status. Repeat these assessments every 2 to 4 hours during the first 48 hours after surgery. Paresthesia may not be relieved right after surgery. Report any new muscle weakness or paresthesia at once. Assess extremity circulation using skin temperature, capillary refill, and pulses.

Paralytic ileus and interference with bowel function may occur for several days. Opioids can slow bowel elimination. Assess if patients are passing gas and have bowel sounds. Stool softeners (e.g., docusate) and laxatives may prevent and relieve constipation.

Emptying the bladder may be hard because of activity restrictions, opioids, or anesthesia. Encourage males to dangle the legs over the side of the bed or stand to urinate if allowed by the HCP. Urge patients to use a bedside commode or ambulate to the bathroom when allowed to promote bladder emptying. Patients with problems urinating may need intermittent catheterization or an indwelling urinary catheter. Loss of sphincter tone or bladder tone may indicate nerve damage. Monitor for incontinence or problems with bowel or bladder elimination. Immediately report problems to the HCP.

With cervical spine surgery, be alert for signs of spinal cord edema, such as respiratory distress and a worsening neurologic condition of the upper extremities. After surgery, the neck may be immobilized in a soft or hard cervical collar.

If the patient also had a spinal fusion, a bone graft is usually involved. Healing time will be prolonged compared with a laminectomy. Activity limitations may be needed for an extended time. A rigid orthosis (thoracolumbar sacral orthosis [TLSO] or chairback brace) is often used during this period. Some HCPs want patients to learn to apply and remove the brace by logrolling in bed. Others allow their patients to apply the brace in a sitting or standing position. Verify the preferred method before starting this activity.

Assess the bone graft donor site. The posterior iliac crest is the most often used donor site. The donor site usually causes greater pain than the spinal fusion area. The donor site is bandaged with a pressure dressing to prevent excess bleeding. If the donor site is the fibula, perform frequent neurovascular assessment of the extremity.

After spinal fusion, patients may have some immobility of the spine at the fusion site. Teach them to use proper body mechanics and avoid sitting or standing for prolonged periods. Encourage activities such as walking and shifting weight from 1 foot to the other when standing. Review any lifting restrictions. Encourage patients to think through an activity before starting a potentially injurious task, such as bending or stooping. Any twisting movement of the spine is contraindicated. Teach patients to use the thighs and knees, rather than the back, to absorb the shock of activity and movement. A firm mattress or bed board is essential.

TABLE 68.10 NURSING MANAGEMENT

Care of the Patient After Spine Surgery

- Perform frequent peripheral neurologic and cardiovascular assessments.
- Monitor vital signs, intake and output.
- Maintain proper spinal alignment:
  - Advance activity as ordered
  - Help patent with changing positions
  - Apply any immobilizers, braces, orthotics as ordered
- Assess for the presence of CSF leakage. If suspected, place the patient flat.
- Assess pain and give analgesics as ordered. Assess response.
- Administer IV fluids and antibiotics as prescribed.
- Provide wound care as ordered and assess for signs of infection.
- Assess for constipation and paralytic ileus. Give stool softeners or laxatives as ordered.
- Implement measures to promote elimination. Perform intermittent catheterization as needed.
- Implement prevention measure for VTE and CAUTI (if the patient has an indwelling catheter).
- Immediately report to the HCP:
  - Severe headache
  - Hypotension, tachycardia, fever
  - Suspected CSF leakage
  - Any new muscle weakness or paresthesia
  - Onset of bowel or bladder problems
  - Pain not responsive to analgesics
  - Signs of wound infection

Collaborate With Physical Therapist

- Assess patient's mobility and need for aid.
- Teach safe ambulation with assistive device based on patient's restrictions.
- Establish exercise plan and teach patient to perform exercises safely.
- Coordinate PT so that patient can receive timely analgesia.

CAUTI, Catheter-associated urinary tract infection; *CSF*, cerebrospinal fluid; *VTE*, venous thromboembolism.

TABLE 68.11 Causes of Neck Pain

- Degenerative disc disease, including herniation
- Meningitis
- Osteomyelitis
- Osteoporosis
- Poor posture
- Rheumatoid arthritis
- Spondylosis
- Strain or sprain
- Trauma (e.g., fractures, subluxation)
- Tumor

NECK PAIN

Neck pain can result from various cervical spine problems. It may be caused by disc degeneration, narrowing of the spinal canal, muscle inflammation, strain, or trauma (Table 68.11). In rare cases, it may be a sign of cancer or meningitis. Age, injury, poor posture, or arthritis can lead to degeneration of the bones or joints of the cervical spine, causing disc herniation or bone spurs. Sudden severe injury to the neck may cause disc herniation, whiplash, and vertebral injury.[12]

Patients have stiffness and neck pain with possible radicular pain into the arm and hand. Pain may radiate to the head, anterior chest, thoracic spine region, and shoulders. Weakness or paresthesia of the arm and hand suggests cervical nerve root compression from stenosis, DDD, or herniation.

The history, assessment, x-ray, MRI, CT scan, and myelogram can help diagnose the cause of the pain. An EMG of the upper extremities may show cervical radiculopathy.

The treatment depends on the cause. Most causes of neck pain resolve with time and conservative treatment. Conservative treatment for acute neck pain in patients without serious pathologies includes physical therapy followed by home exercise, gentle traction, and cautious manipulation to prevent possible worsening of symptoms. TENS and acupuncture may be helpful for short-term pain relief. Drug therapy includes analgesics and muscle relaxants. Opioids should be used only for intractable pain in the short term with close supervision by HCPs.[12]

Patient teaching should emphasize self-management and the importance of an active lifestyle. Preventing neck pain that occurs with everyday activities, such as prolonged sitting at a computer or television, sleeping in nonaligned spinal positions, or making jarring movements during exercise, is important. Cognitive-behavioral therapy may assist with psychosocial risk factors.

FOOT PROBLEMS

The foot is the platform that supports the weight of the body and absorbs shock when the person ambulates. It is a complicated structure composed of bony structures, muscles, tendons, and ligaments. The foot can be affected by congenital conditions, structural weakness, and injuries. Many people are prone to foot problems because of poor circulation, atherosclerosis, and decreased sensation in the lower extremities. This is especially true for those with diabetes. Patients may develop an open wound but not feel it because of altered sensation from peripheral vascular disease or diabetic neuropathy. Table 68.12 outlines common foot problems.

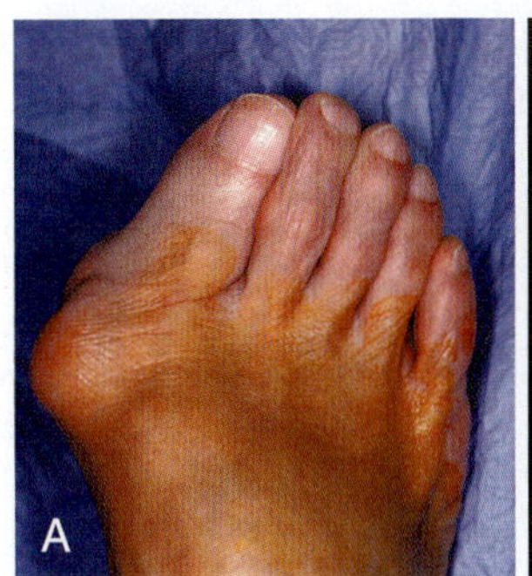

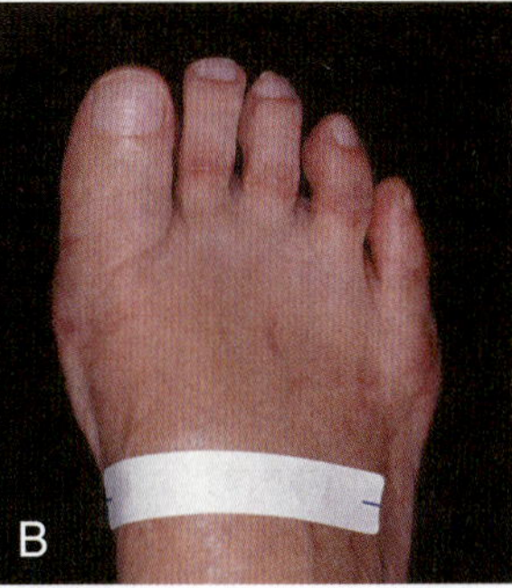

Fig. 68.6 (A) Severe hallux valgus with bursa formation. (B) Postoperative correction. (From Canale ST, Beaty JH: *Campbell's operative orthopaedics,* ed 12, Philadelphia, 2013, Mosby.)

Ill-fitting shoes that are not the right size or shape for your foot are associated with many foot problems. These include plantar fasciitis, bunions, blisters, corns, calluses, and inflammation of the ball of the foot. Small shoes inhibit normal movement of foot muscles. Crowding and angulation of the toes can force the great toe into a position of **hallux valgus** (Fig. 68.6). Prolonged use of improper footwear can cause a *Morton neuroma.* The neuroma compresses an intermetatarsal plantar nerve, resulting in paresthesia and burning.

NURSING MANAGEMENT: FOOT PROBLEMS

Implementation

Health Promotion

Teach patients to inspect their feet daily and report any open wounds or breaks in the skin to their HCP. Stockings should be long enough to avoid wrinkling and causing pressure areas. Trimming toenails straight across helps prevent ingrown toenails and reduces the risk for infection. Teach patients with impaired circulation or diabetes to prevent serious complications from blisters, pressure areas, and infection. Teach patients to perform daily foot care and wear clean stockings.

Well-made and properly fitted shoes are essential for healthy, pain-free feet.[13] Footwear should provide support, stability, protection, and shock absorption. Footwear provides a foundation for orthotics and can treat some foot problems. Women's footwear is often influenced by current styles instead of comfort and support. Stress the importance of having a shoe that conforms to the foot rather than to fashion trends. At the metatarsal head, the shoe should be wide enough to allow foot muscles to move freely and toes to bend. The shank (narrow part of sole under the instep) of the shoe should be rigid enough to give good support. The height

TABLE 68.12 Common Foot Problems

Problem	Description	Treatment
Forefoot		
Hallux rigidus	Painful stiffness of first MTP joint caused by osteoarthritis or local trauma.	• Intraarticular corticosteroids, passive manual stretching of first MTP joint. • Shoe with a stiff sole decreases pain in the joint during walking. • Surgical treatment: Joint fusion or arthroplasty with silicone rubber implant.
Hallux valgus (bunion)	Painful deformity of great toe with lateral angulation of great toe toward second toe, bony enlargement of medial side of first metatarsal head, swelling of bursa, and formation of callus over bony enlargement (Fig. 68.6).	• Wearing shoes with wide forefoot or "bunion pocket" and use of bunion pads to relieve pressure on bursal sac. • Surgical treatment: Removing bursal sac and bony enlargement and correction of lateral angulation of great toe. • May include temporary or permanent internal fixation.
Hammer and claw toes	Hammer toe is a deformity of PIP joint on 2nd to 5th toes causing toe to be permanently bent, resembling a hammer. Mallet toe is a similar condition affecting DIP joint. Claw toe is a similar deformity with dorsiflexion of proximal phalanx on MTP joint combined with flexion of both PIP and DIP joints. Symptoms include burning on bottom of foot and pain and difficulty walking when wearing shoes.	• Passive manual stretching of PIP joint, use of metatarsal arch support. • Surgical treatment: Resecting base of middle phalanx and head of proximal phalanx, bringing raw bone ends together. • Kirschner wire maintains straight position.
Morton neuroma (plantar neuroma)	Neuroma in web space between third and fourth metatarsal heads, causing sharp, sudden attacks of pain and burning sensations. May describe feeling as if a sock is rolled up under their toes.	• Surgical excision.
Midfoot		
Pes cavus	Elevation of longitudinal arch of foot resulting from contracture of plantar fascia or bony deformity of arch.	• Surgical correction needed if condition interferes with ambulation.
Pes planus (flatfoot)	Loss of metatarsal arch causing pain in foot or leg.	• Use of resilient longitudinal arch supports. • Surgical treatment: Triple arthrodesis or fusion of subtalar joint.
Hindfoot		
Calcaneus stress fracture	Heel pain after moderate walking. Common causes are overtraining, running on hard surfaces, osteoporosis.	• Rest, ice, shoe heel pad, NSAIDs. • See HCP to assess for osteoporosis.
Heel pain	Heel pain with weight bearing. Common causes are plantar bursitis, plantar fasciitis, bone spur.	• Corticosteroids injected locally into inflamed bursa. • Sponge-rubber heel cup. • Surgical excision of bursa or spur. • Stretching exercises, ice, shoe heel cup, shockwave therapy, NSAIDs, corticosteroids for plantar fasciitis.
Other Problems		
Callus	Local thickening of skin. Covers wide area and usually found on weight-bearing part of foot.	• Softened with warm water or preparations containing salicylic acid and trimmed with razor blade or scalpel. • Pressure on bony prominences caused by shoes is relieved.
Corn	Local thickening of skin. Caused by continual pressure over bony prominences, especially metatarsal head, often causing local pain.	• Same as with callus.
Plantar wart	Painful papillomatous growth caused by virus that may occur on any part of skin on sole of foot. Warts tend to cluster on pressure points.	• Remedies containing salicylic acid (e.g., Compound W), excision with electrocoagulation, or surgical removal. • Laser treatments. • May disappear without treatment.
Soft corn	Painful lesion caused by bony prominence of a toe pressing against adjacent toe. Usual location is web space between toes. Softness caused by secretions keeping web space relatively moist.	• Pain relieved by placing cotton or spacers between toes to separate them. • Excision of projecting bone spur (if present).

DIP, Distal interphalangeal; *MTP,* metatarsophalangeal; *PIP,* proximal interphalangeal.

of the heel should be realistic in relation to the shoe's purpose. Ideally, the heel of the shoe should not rise more than 1 inch higher than the forefoot support. Wearing higher-heeled shoes with a narrow toe box will cause hammertoes and corns over time.

Acute Care

Many foot problems require referral to a podiatrist. Depending on the problem, conservative therapies are tried first (Table 68.12). These include NSAIDs, ice, physical therapy, footwear changes, stretching, warm soaks, orthotics, ultrasound, and corticosteroid injections. If these methods do not help, surgery may be needed.

> **CHECK YOUR PRACTICE**
>
> A 53-year-old female patient is scheduled for surgical correction of a bunion after a diagnosis of hallux valgus. You are doing her preoperative assessment. She says, "I love shoes and have a whole closet full of fancy ones. Now I have to wear this big ugly shoe. I hope I can wear my nice shoes after surgery."
> - How will you respond?
> - What are the priority learning needs related to her self-care after surgery?

Depending on the type of surgery, pins or wires may extend through the toes, or a protective splint may be placed over the end of the foot. The foot is usually immobilized by a bulky dressing (Fig. 68.7), short leg cast, slipper (plaster) cast, or a platform shoe that fits over the dressing and has a rigid sole (*bunion shoe*).

Elevate the foot with the heel off the bed to reduce discomfort and prevent edema. Assess neurovascular condition during the immediate postoperative period. Inserted devices may interfere with assessment for movement. Evaluating sensation may be hard because patients may be unable to distinguish surgical pain from pain caused by nerve pressure or circulatory impairment.

The type and extent of surgery determine the orders for ambulation. Crutches, a walker, or a cane may be needed. Patients may have pain or a throbbing sensation when lowering the affected leg. Reinforce instructions from the physical therapist. Review the importance of walking with an erect posture with proper weight distribution. Report gait problems or continued pain to the HCP. Encourage frequent rest periods with the foot elevated.

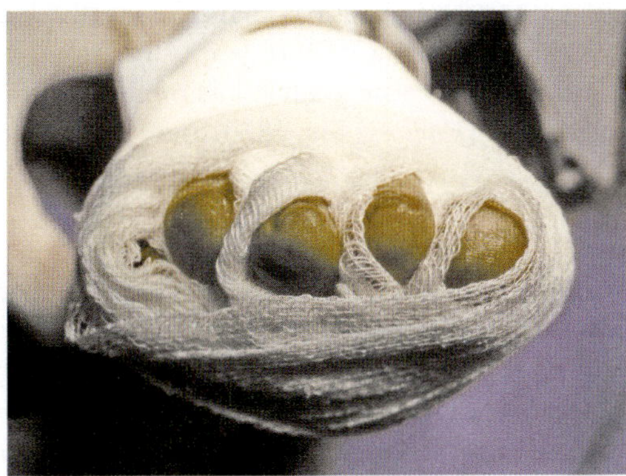

Fig. 68.7 Postoperative supportive dressing for treatment of moderate forefoot deformity. (From Canale ST, Beaty JH: *Campbell's operative orthopaedics,* ed 12, Philadelphia, 2013, Mosby.)

METABOLIC BONE DISEASE

OSTEOMALACIA

Osteomalacia is characterized by inadequate mineralization of bone tissue. It usually results from prolonged vitamin D deficiency that causes weakening and softening bones. Vitamin D is required for calcium absorption from the intestine. Thus insufficient vitamin D can interfere with normal bone mineralization.

Common causes include decreased vitamin D production from limited sun exposure or obesity and decreased GI absorption (GI tract surgery, inflammatory bowel disease, celiac disease). Altered vitamin D metabolism can occur with pregnancy or chronic liver and kidney disease. Drug therapy with antiseizure agents (e.g., phenytoin), antifungals, or corticosteroids can negatively influence vitamin D metabolism.[14]

Common manifestations are bone pain and muscle weakness. The pain is often worse at night and affects the lower back, pelvis, hips, legs, and ribs. Muscle weakness and progressive deformity of weight-bearing bones (e.g., spine, extremities) can lead to problems walking and a waddling gait. Fractures are common and indicate delayed bone healing.

Laboratory findings include decreased calcium and phosphorus, decreased 25-hydroxyvitamin D, and increased alkaline phosphatase.[14] X-rays may show effects of bone demineralization, especially loss of calcium in the bones of the pelvis and associated bone deformity. *Looser transformation zones* (ribbons of decalcification in bone) found on x-ray are diagnostic of osteomalacia.

Treatment is directed toward reversing the underlying cause and correcting vitamin D and other nutrition deficiencies. Patients receive vitamin D_3 (cholecalciferol) or vitamin D_2 (ergocalciferol) supplements. Most should also take at least 1000 mg of calcium per day. Encourage a diet rich in eggs, meat, and oily fish (e.g., salmon, tuna).[14] Milk, yogurt, cheese, orange juice, and bread fortified with calcium and vitamin D should be part of the diet. Exposure to sunlight and weight-bearing exercise are encouraged.

OSTEOPOROSIS

Osteoporosis is a chronic, progressive metabolic bone disease marked by low bone mass and deterioration of bone tissue, leading to increased bone fragility (Fig. 68.8). Bones eventually become so fragile that they cannot withstand normal mechanical stress. More than 54 million persons in the United States have osteoporosis.[15]

Etiology and Pathophysiology

Risk factors for osteoporosis are listed in Table 68.13. Osteoporosis is more common in females. There are several reasons

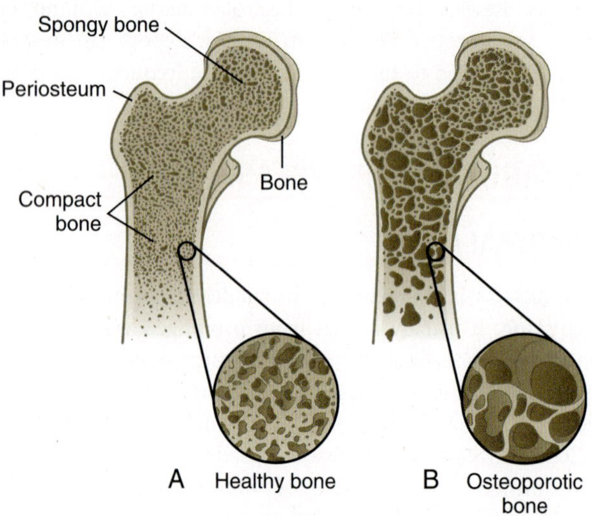

Fig. 68.8 (A) Normal bone. (B) Osteoporotic bone.

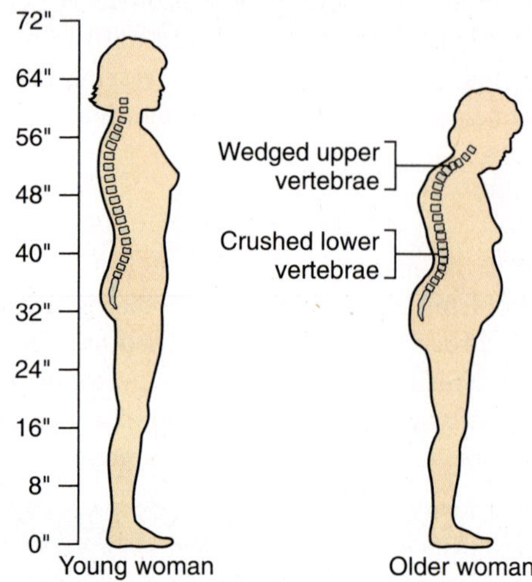

Fig. 68.9 The effects of osteoporosis. Comparison of young female with an older female. (A, From Phillips N: *Berry & Kohn's operating room technique,* ed 12, St Louis, 2013, Mosby.)

TABLE 68.13 Risk Factors for Osteoporosis

- Advancing age (>65 yr)
- Asian or White ethnicity
- Chronic illness: cirrhosis, diabetes, hyperthyroidism, kidney disease, liver disease, rheumatoid arthritis
- Diet low in calcium or vitamin D deficiency
- Estrogen deficiency in females (surgical or age-related menopause)
- Excess use of alcohol (>2 drinks/day)
- Family history of osteoporosis
- Female gender
- Low body weight
- Low testosterone in males
- Medications: corticosteroids, thyroid replacement, heparin, long-acting sedatives, antiseizure drugs, chemotherapy
- Sedentary lifestyle
- Smoking

why. Females have less bone mass because of their smaller frames. Bone loss from midlife (ages 35 to 40 years) onward is inevitable, but the rate of loss varies. At menopause, females have rapid bone loss when the decline in estrogen production is the greatest. The rate of loss then slows and eventually matches the rate of bone lost by males ages 65 to 70 years. Pregnancy and breastfeeding deplete skeletal reserve unless calcium intake is adequate. Females' longevity increases the risk for osteoporosis.

Diseases associated with osteoporosis include inflammatory bowel disease, intestinal malabsorption, hypogonadism, and diabetes. Many drugs can interfere with bone metabolism. Long-term corticosteroid use is a major contributor to osteoporosis. Others include antiseizure drugs (e.g., divalproex sodium, phenytoin), aluminum-containing antacids, and some chemotherapy drugs. When prescribed one of these drugs, teach patients about this possible side effect.

Peak bone mass (maximum bone tissue) is typically achieved before age 20. It is largely determined by 4 factors: heredity, nutrition, exercise, and hormone function. Heredity may be responsible for up to 70% of a person's peak bone mass. Genetic factors influence bone size, quality, and turnover. Low testosterone is a major risk factor in males. Weight-bearing exercise and adequate intake of fluoride, calcium, and vitamin D decrease risk.

Bone is continuously being deposited by osteoblasts and resorbed by osteoclasts, a process called *remodeling.* Rates of bone deposition and resorption are normally equal, so total bone mass stays constant. In osteoporosis, bone resorption exceeds bone deposition.

Clinical Manifestations

Osteoporosis occurs most often in bones of the spine, hips, and wrists. Early manifestations include back pain and spontaneous fractures. The loss of bone mass causes the bone to become mechanically weaker and prone to spontaneous fractures or fractures from minimal trauma. A person who has a vertebral fracture related to osteoporosis has an increased risk for having a second vertebral fracture within 1 year. Over time, vertebral fractures and wedging cause gradual loss of height and a humped thoracic spine (*kyphosis*; Fig. 68.9).

Diagnostic Studies

Bone mineral density (BMD) serves as the basis for diagnosing osteoporosis. It may be measured by quantitative ultrasound (QUS) and dual-energy x-ray absorptiometry (DEXA). QUS uses sound waves to measure bone density in the heel, kneecap, or shin. DEXA measures bone density in the spine and hips. These are the most common sites of fragility fractures from osteoporosis. Most guidelines use DEXA to diagnose osteoporosis and guide the decision on when to start drug therapy

TABLE 68.14 Diagnostic Criteria

Osteoporosis

A diagnosis of osteoporosis is made when patients meet any of the following criteria:

1. Fragility fracture
2. T-score ≤−2.5 at the lumbar spine, femoral neck, total hip or distal one-third radius on dual-energy x-ray absorptiometry (DEXA) examination
3. T-score between −1.0 and −2.5 with elevated fracture risk as determined by the Fracture Risk Assessment Tool (FRAX). In the United States, the cutoffs for 10-year fracture risk estimates are ≥20% risk of major osteoporotic fracture and ≥3% risk of hip fracture.

T-Score	Classification
+1 and −1	Normal
−1 and −2.5	Osteopenia
−2.5 or lower	Osteoporosis
−2.5 or lower with a fracture	Severe osteoporosis

TABLE 68.15 Interprofessional Care

Osteoporosis

Diagnostic Assessment

- History and physical assessment
- Calcium, phosphorus, alkaline phosphatase, vitamin D
- Bone mineral densitometry
- Dual energy x-ray absorptiometry (DEXA) (Table 68.14)

Management

- Adequate diet calcium
- Calcium supplements
- Sun exposure or vitamin D supplements
- Exercise program
- Drug therapy (Table 68.16)
  - Bisphosphonates (recommended)
  - Monoclonal antibodies
  - Recombinant parathyroid hormone
- Minimally invasive procedures
  - Vertebroplasty
  - Kyphoplasty

(Table 68.14).[16] DEXA studies evaluate changes in bone density over time and assess treatment effectiveness.

BMD test results are compared with the ideal or peak BMD of a healthy 30-year-old adult and reported as T-scores. A T-score of 0 means the BMD is equal to the norm for a healthy young adult. Differences are measured in units called *standard deviations (SDs)*. The greater the negative number, the lower the BMD and the higher the risk for fracture. We can calculate a patient's risk for fracture from osteoporosis with the Fracture Risk Assessment (FRAX) tool. The FRAX considers BMD and other clinical factors when assessing fracture risk.

Current guidelines recommend an initial bone density test in all females older than age 65 years.[17] If results are normal and there is a low risk for osteoporosis, another test is not needed for 15 years. Females who are younger than 65 and at high risk (e.g., low body weight, smoker, prior fractures) or have had an adulthood fracture should have a bone density test earlier.

Osteoporosis cannot be detected by conventional x-ray until 25% to 40% of calcium in the bone is lost. Calcium, phosphorus, and alkaline phosphatase levels usually are normal. Alkaline phosphatase may be increased after a fracture.

Interprofessional and Nursing Management

The National Osteoporosis Foundation recommends treatment for osteoporosis for postmenopausal females with (1) a T-score of less than −2.5, (2) a T-score between −1 and −2.5 with other risk factors (Table 68.13), or (3) prior history of a hip or vertebral fracture. Management focuses on proper nutrition, calcium and vitamin D supplements, exercise, prevention of falls and fractures, and drugs (Table 68.15).

The recommended calcium intake is 1000 mg/day for females ages 19 to 50 years and males ages 19 to 70 years and 1200 mg/day in females age 51 years or older and males age 71 years or older. If dietary intake of calcium is inadequate, calcium supplements may be given.

It is hard to absorb calcium in single doses greater than 500 mg. Teach patients to take calcium supplements as divided doses to increase absorption. The amount of elemental calcium varies in calcium preparations. Calcium carbonate has 40% elemental calcium. It should be taken with meals because stomach acid is needed to dissolve and absorb this supplement. Calcium citrate has around 20% elemental calcium but is less dependent on stomach acid for absorption. It is better absorbed by patients taking a proton pump inhibitor (e.g., esomeprazole) or histamine receptor blocker (e.g., cimetidine) for acid reflux. Calcium lactate and calcium gluconate are not recommended because they have small amounts of elemental calcium.

Vitamin D is important in calcium absorption and function and may have a role in bone formation. Most people get enough vitamin D from their diet or naturally through synthesis in the skin from exposure to sunlight. Being in the sun for 20 minutes a day is generally enough. Vitamin D (800 IU) supplements are recommended for postmenopausal females, older males, persons who are homebound or in long-term care settings, and those in northern climates because of decreased sun exposure.

Physical activity is important to build and maintain bone mass. Exercise increases muscle strength, coordination, and balance. The best exercises are weight-bearing exercises that force a person to work against gravity. These include walking, hiking, weight training, stair climbing, tennis, and dancing. Walking is preferred to high-impact aerobics or running. Both may put too much stress on the bones and cause stress fractures. Encourage patients to walk 30 minutes 3 times a week. Teach patients to quit smoking and decrease alcohol use to lessen negative effects on bone mass.[17]

Encourage patients to remain ambulatory to prevent further loss of bone density caused by immobility. Treatment may involve the use of a gait aid to walk safely and protect areas of potential pathologic fractures. For example, a TLSO can maintain the spine in proper alignment after fracture or treatment of a vertebral fracture.

Vertebroplasty and *kyphoplasty* are minimally invasive procedures used to treat osteoporotic vertebral fractures (see Chapter 62). In vertebroplasty, bone cement is injected into the collapsed vertebra to stabilize the spine and improve pain. This procedure does not restore vertebral height or correct deformity. In kyphoplasty, a small balloon is inserted into the collapsed vertebra and inflated to restore vertebral body height before injection of bone cement. Kyphoplasty is the preferred surgical treatment for vertebral compression fractures.

Drug Therapy

Drug therapies for preventing and treating osteoporosis include agents to decrease bone resorption, such as bisphosphonates, denosumab, and the selective estrogen-receptor modulator (SERM) raloxifene (Table 68.16).[18] Bisphosphonates inhibit osteoclast-mediated bone resorption and slow the cycle of bone remodeling. Although a modest increase in BMD is common, bone remodeling may be suppressed to the extent that normal bone formation is impaired and fracture risk increases. A rare but serious side effect of bisphosphonates is *osteonecrosis* (bone death) of the jaw. Its cause is unknown. Those with dental disease, cancer, Paget disease, or renal disease are most at risk for this complication.

DRUG ALERT

Bisphosphonates

Teach patient to:
- Take with full glass of water.
- Take 30 min before food or other drugs.
- Stay upright for at least 30 min after taking.

Females no longer routinely use estrogen replacement therapy or estrogen with progesterone after menopause to

TABLE 68.16 Drug Therapy

Osteoporosis

Drug	Action	Side Effects	Considerations
Bisphosphonates			
alendronate (Fosamax) ibandronate (Boniva) pamidronate (Aredia) risedronate (Actonel, Atelvia) zoledronic acid (Reclast, Zometa)	Inhibit osteoclast-mediated bone resorption and slows cycle of bone remodeling. Increases bone density.	Bone, joint, muscle pain Esophageal irritation Gastritis Osteonecrosis	When taking orally: Take with full glass of water. Take 30 min before food or other drugs. Stay upright for at least 30 min after. Zoledronic acid is once-yearly or every-other-year IV infusion. Monitor calcium and kidney function tests. Patients should see a dentist before beginning treatment and then annually.
Monoclonal Antibodies			
denosumab (Prolia, Xgeva)	Binds to a protein (RANKL) involved in osteoclast function.	Back and extremity pain Dizziness Hypocalcemia Rash	Subcutaneous injection every 6 mo. Give with calcium and vitamin D supplements. Monitor electrolytes.
romosozumab (Evenity)	Inhibits action of sclerostin, a regulatory factor in bone metabolism. Increases bone formation and, to a lesser extent, decreases bone resorption.	Femoral fractures Headache Hypocalcemia Muscle pain Osteonecrosis of jaw	Subcutaneous injection every month for a total of 12 doses. Give with calcium and vitamin D supplements. Monitor electrolytes.
Recombinant Parathyroid Hormone			
abaloparatide (Tymlos) teriparatide (Forteo)	Increases action of osteoblasts and stimulates new bone formation.	Dizziness GI distress Hypercalcemia Muscle cramps ↑ Uric acid levels	Self-administered daily by subcutaneous injection from preloaded pen. Monitor electrolytes and parathyroid hormone levels. Use for up to 2 yr.
Selective Estrogen Receptor Modulator (SERM)			
raloxifene (Evista)	Mimics the effect of estrogen on bone by reducing bone resorption.	Flulike symptoms Leg cramps Venous thromboembolism, including stroke, pulmonary embolism Weight gain	Reduces risk for vertebral, but not hip, fractures. Discontinue if immobilized; resume only after fully ambulatory. Avoid smoking. Teach symptoms to report to HCP.

prevent osteoporosis because of the increased risk for heart disease and breast and uterine cancer. A female who takes short-term estrogen therapy to treat menopause symptoms, such as hot flashes, may receive some protection against bone loss and hip and vertebrae fractures. Estrogen may inhibit osteoclast activity, leading to decreased bone resorption.

Patients receiving corticosteroids should receive the lowest effective dose for the shortest possible time. Ensure an adequate intake of calcium and vitamin D, including supplements, when osteoporosis drugs are prescribed. If osteopenia is present in people who are taking corticosteroids, we may start a bisphosphonate.

PAGET DISEASE

Paget disease *(osteitis deformans)* is a chronic skeletal bone disorder in which excess bone resorption is followed by replacement of normal marrow by vascular, fibrous connective tissue. The new bone is larger, disorganized, and weaker. Areas often affected include the pelvis, long bones, spine, ribs, sternum, and skull. Typically, it develops in people in their 50s, particularly males.[19]

We do not know what causes Paget disease. The cause may be viral or genetic. Up to 50% of all patients with the disease have at least 1 relative with the disorder.[19]

In milder forms of Paget disease, patients do not have any symptoms. The disease may be found incidentally through x-ray or laboratory findings of high alkaline phosphatase. Bone pain may develop gradually and progress to severe intractable pain. Other early manifestations include fatigue and progressive development of a waddling gait. Patients report becoming shorter or their heads are becoming larger (Fig. 68.10). Headaches, dementia, vision problems, and hearing loss can result from an enlarged, thick skull. Increased bone volume in the spine can cause spinal cord or nerve root compression.

Pathologic fracture is the most common complication and may be the first sign of Paget disease. Other complications include osteosarcoma, fibrosarcoma, and osteoclastoma (giant cell) tumors.

Alkaline phosphatase is very high in advanced disease, showing high bone turnover. X-rays may show curvature of an affected bone. The bone cortex becomes thicker and irregular, especially in weight-bearing bones and the cranium. Bone scans using a radiolabeled bisphosphonate show increased uptake in the affected skeletal areas.

Treatment is usually limited to symptomatic and supportive care, with correction of secondary deformities by surgical intervention or braces. Bisphosphonate drugs (Table 68.16) are used to slow bone resorption. Zoledronic acid is the therapy of choice. It is given specifically to build bone. Calcium and vitamin D can decrease hypocalcemia, a common side effect of drug therapy. Monitor drug effectiveness by assessing alkaline phosphatase.

Calcitonin is an option for patients who cannot tolerate bisphosphonates. Its use is limited in duration, as the body's response to this drug quickly decreases. Human calcitonin inhibits osteoclastic activity, prevents bone resorption, relieves acute symptoms, and lowers serum alkaline phosphatase.

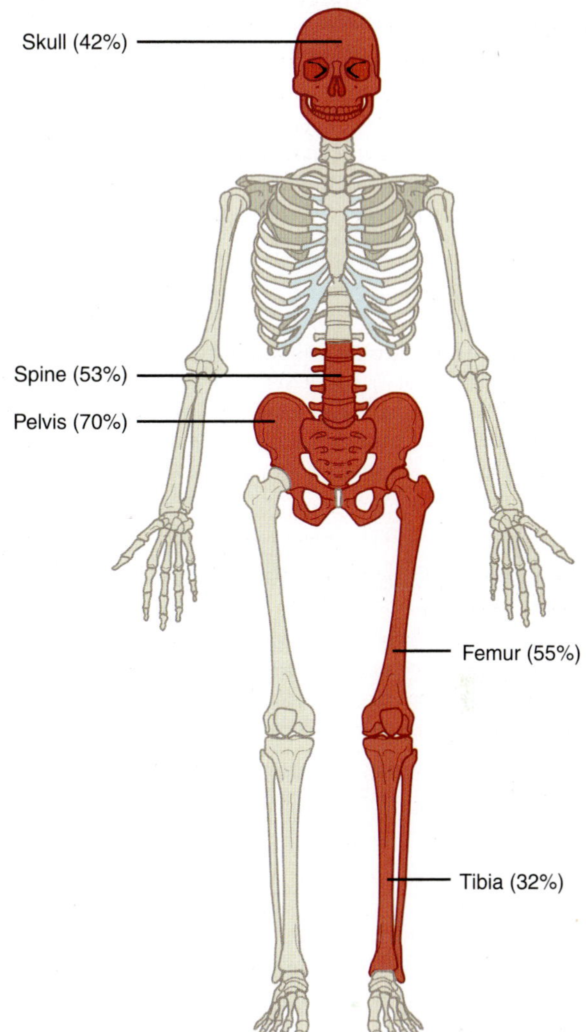

Fig. 68.10 Areas of the skeleton affected by Paget disease.

Pain is usually managed with NSAIDs. Orthopedic surgery for fractures, hip and knee replacement, and knee realignment may be needed.

A firm mattress can provide back support and relieve pain. Patients may need to wear a corset or light brace to relieve back pain and give support when upright. Teach them to correctly apply the device and examine the skin for friction damage. Discourage lifting and twisting. Good body mechanics are essential. Physical therapy may increase muscle strength. A well-balanced diet is important. Vitamin D, calcium, and protein ensure components are available for bone formation. To decrease risk for falls and related fractures, teach patients to use an assistive device and make environmental changes (e.g., do not use throw rugs).

CASE STUDY

Osteoporosis/Hip Fracture

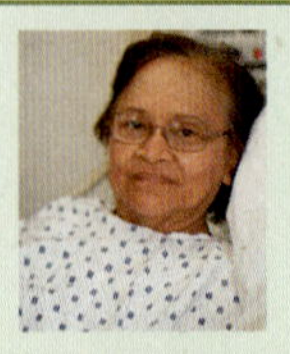
(© azndc/iStock.com.)

Patient Profile

M.K. is a thin 70-year-old Asian female admitted to the emergency department after falling in her driveway. X-ray shows a left femoral neck fracture. She has a history of hypertension and chronic obstructive pulmonary disease (COPD).

Subjective Data

- Denies hitting her head or loss of consciousness
- Reports significant left hip pain, 9 on the 0 to 10 pain scale
- States she has never had a bone density test
- Former 2 pack a day smoker who quit 4 years ago
- Takes atenolol every morning and fluticasone propionate/salmeterol (Advair Diskus) inhaler twice a day

Objective Data

- Left lower extremity slightly shorter and externally rotated compared with right lower extremity
- Unable to bear weight on lower extremities
- Moderate edema with bruising on left hip
- 2+ dorsalis pedis and posterior tibialis pulses bilaterally
- Gross motor/sensation intact in affected extremity

Diagnostic Studies

- Normal CBC, metabolic panel, protime/INR, urinalysis
- Chest x-ray shows hyperinflated lung fields
- 12-lead ECG shows normal sinus rhythm

Interprofessional Care

- Hip arthroplasty for fracture
- Multimodal postoperative pain management
- Physical therapy evaluation and treatment
- Early postoperative mobilization
- Removal of urinary catheter (if applicable) early in postoperative period
- Ambulation using standard walker

Discussion Questions

1. ***Recognize:*** Why did a relatively low-energy injury cause M.K.'s fracture?
2. ***Analyze:*** What postoperative complications is M.K. at risk for developing?
3. ***Plan:*** What are M.K.'s learning needs?
4. ***Prioritize:*** What is the interprofessional team's top priority at this time for M.K.?
5. ***Act:*** What therapy do you expect M.K. to receive?
6. ***Act:*** Describe specific actions you would take to promote patient safety.
7. ***Evaluation:*** What outcomes would indicate that care was effective?

Answers available at http://evolve.elsevier.com/Lewis/medsurg.

BRIDGE TO NCLEX EXAMINATION

The number of the question corresponds to the same-numbered outcome at the beginning of the chapter.

1. What would the nurse include in the teaching plan for a patient with acute osteomyelitis who is being discharged on antibiotic therapy? **(Select all that apply.)**
   - **a.** You will need to have weekly bone scans and cultures.
   - **b.** It is important to finish all the antibiotics even after you feel better.
   - **c.** If the infection comes back, you will need to undergo surgery.
   - **d.** Signs such as fever and fatigue may be present but are usually not severe.
   - **e.** Contact the HCP if signs of infection such as pain and swelling at the site occur.
2. A patient with a history of colon cancer is diagnosed with rib fractures, and the HCP orders a bone scan. The nurse determines the patient understands teaching about the purpose of the procedure when they state
   - **a.** "The bone scan will cure my rib fractures."
   - **b.** "The bone scan will see if my colon cancer may have spread."
   - **c.** "My colon cancer was cured so I really don't think this is necessary."
   - **d.** "The results of the bone scan will only just confirm that I have a rib fracture."
3. The nurse provides counseling to a family of a patient with Duchenne muscular dystrophy with the knowledge that
   - **a.** patients are usually female.
   - **b.** all daughters of a carrier will be carriers.
   - **c.** genetic testing can help determine treatment.
   - **d.** only males can pass the gene to their offspring.
4. Which persons are at high risk for chronic low back pain? **(Select all that apply.)**
   - **a.** A 63-year-old male who is a long-distance truck driver
   - **b.** A 30-year-old nurse who works on an orthopedic unit and smokes
   - **c.** A 55-year-old construction worker who is 6 ft, 2 in and weighs 250 lb
   - **d.** A 44-year-old female chef with prior compression fracture of the spine
   - **e.** A 28-year-old female yoga instructor who is 5 ft, 6 in and weighs 130 lb
5. When caring for a patient after lumbar spinal surgery, the nurse would report which finding to the HCP?
   - **a.** The patient reports mild low back pain.
   - **b.** The patient has a single episode of emesis.
   - **c.** The patient is nauseated and has not voided in 4 hours.
   - **d.** The patient has loss of sensation to the perineum, buttocks, and inner thighs.

6. A patient who ran his first marathon had heel pain that would not resolve and was diagnosed with a calcaneus stress fracture. The nurse will teach the patient to **(Select all that apply.)**
   a. resume running in 1 week.
   b. rest and refrain from running.
   c. wear a shoe heel pad when ambulating.
   d. walk barefoot to decrease pressure on the heel.
   e. apply ice to the heel and take NSAIDs as directed by the HCP.

7. A patient with osteoporosis shows they understand self-care when they state
   a. "I should remove trip hazards such as throw rugs in my house to make it safer."
   b. "I am not using the cane my HCP recommended. I don't want to look that old!"
   c "I can continue to go downhill skiing as long as I'm careful and don't ever fall."
   d. "I need to start running to help strengthen my bones. Walking is just not enough."

1. b, d, e; 2. b; 3. c; 4. a, b, c, d; 5. d; 6. b, c, e; 7. a.

For rationales to these answers and even more NCLEX review questions, visit http://evolve.elsevier.com/Lewis/medsurg.

REFERENCES

To access the References for this chapter, please scan the QR code with a mobile device.

69

Arthritis and Connective Tissue Diseases

Cynthia Bernat Amerson

http://evolve.elsevier.com/Lewis/medsurg/

CONCEPTUAL FOCUS

Coping
Fatigue
Functional Ability
Inflammation
Mobility
Pain
Self-Management

LEARNING OUTCOMES

1. Outline the sequence of events leading to joint destruction in osteoarthritis and rheumatoid arthritis.
2. Detail the clinical manifestations and interprofessional and nursing management of osteoarthritis and rheumatoid arthritis.
3. Describe the pathophysiology, clinical manifestations, and interprofessional care of gout, Lyme disease, and septic arthritis.
4. Discuss the pathophysiology, clinical manifestations, and interprofessional and nursing management of patients with a spondyloarthropathy.
5. Describe the pathophysiology, clinical manifestations, and interprofessional and nursing management of systemic lupus erythematosus, scleroderma, autoimmune myositis, and Sjögren syndrome.
6. Relate possible etiologies, clinical manifestations, and interprofessional and nursing management of fibromyalgia and myalgic encephalomyelitis.

KEY TERMS

arthritis
axial spondylitis (axSpA)
fibromyalgia (FMS)
gout
Lyme disease
Myalgic encephalomyelitis (ME)
osteoarthritis (OA)
psoriatic arthritis (PsA)
Raynaud phenomenon
rheumatoid arthritis (RA)
scleroderma
septic arthritis
Sjögren syndrome
systemic lupus erythematosus (SLE)

This chapter discusses connective tissue diseases, which affect joints, tendons, ligaments, muscles, and bones. These diseases are marked by inflammation, pain, and loss of function in 1 or more of the body's connecting or supporting structures. Patients may have limited function and disability. Fatigue and altered body image challenge their ability to cope. More than 100 kinds of arthritic-related diseases exist.

ARTHRITIS

Arthritis involves inflammation of 1 or more joints. Arthritis affects all ages, races, and genders. It is most common in females and older adults.[1] Osteoarthritis is the most common type. Other types include autoimmune inflammatory arthritis (rheumatoid arthritis, psoriatic arthritis), infectious arthritis (septic arthritis), and gout.[2]

OSTEOARTHRITIS

Osteoarthritis (OA) is a slowly progressive degenerative disorder of the diarthrodial *(synovial)* joints. All areas of the joint are affected. As damage to the joint progresses, pain, muscle weakness, and decreased motion occur.[3]

Etiology and Pathophysiology

OA most often occurs in people over age 40.[4] About 80% of people over 65 have radiographic evidence of OA.[5] Decreased estrogen at menopause may contribute to the increased incidence of OA in aging females. No single cause can be identified. OA may be caused by events or conditions that directly damage cartilage. Obesity, joint injury, and joint instability increase risk (Table 69.1). Genetic traits contribute to developing cartilage defects.[1]

OA involves the gradual destruction of articular cartilage and the development of osteophytes (bone spurs), bone remodeling, and synovial inflammation (Fig. 69.1). Genetic, metabolic, and local factors initiate local inflammation and cytokine release. Collagen protease enzymes degrade the cartilage matrix. Cartilage erodes and thins. Cartilage repair cannot match destruction. The chondrocytes proliferate and become hypertrophic. Remodeling and ossification form bone spurs. Pain occurs when articular cartilage is lost and bony joint surfaces rub each other.

TABLE 69.1 Causes of OA

Cause	Effects on Joint Cartilage
Drugs	Long-term use of some drugs (NSAIDs, corticosteroids) may cause proteoglycan loss and increased cartilage destruction.
Endocrine problems	Estrogen loss may promote joint damage through loss of hormone protection. Metabolic syndrome causes systemic inflammation contributing to joint damage.
Hematologic problems	Chronic hemarthrosis (e.g., from hemophilia) contributes to cartilage deterioration and synovial fluid damage.
Inflammation	Injury and infection begin the inflammatory process. Protease and other enzymes that break down cartilage are released. Exposure to inflammatory mediators degrades cartilage. CD4 and CD8 lymphocytes in synovium contribute to joint breakdown.
Joint instability	Damage to supporting structures (muscle, tendons, bones) or misalignment places uneven stress on joint cartilage.
Mechanical stress	Repetitive physical activities (e.g., sports) can cause cartilage destruction. Obesity increases stress on joints.
Neurologic problems	Pain, loss of reflexes, altered sensation, and altered gait from neurologic disorders can cause injury, stress, and inflammation, contributing to cartilage deterioration.
Skeletal deformities	Congenital or acquired conditions (e.g., dislocated hip) contribute to cartilage deterioration. Uneven stress on joints may occur.
Trauma	Dislocations or fractures may lead to avascular necrosis, stimulate inflammation, and place uneven stress on cartilage. Rapid stops, pivoting, and repetitive movements common to sports can cause injury to knees and ankles.
Age	Oxidative stress over time causes proteoglycan damage. Loss of collagen causes cartilage to be stiff and brittle.
Genetics	Gene expression can cause release of cartilage-destroying enzymes. Females are more likely to have OA.

Clinical Manifestations

Joints

Manifestations range from mild discomfort to significant disability. Joint pain is the main symptom. Patients describe aching pain that worsens with activity. In early stages of OA, rest relieves the joint pain. With advanced OA, pain may be present at rest. Patients may have trouble sleeping because of increased pain. Pain may worsen when the barometric pressure falls before the onset of severe weather.

As OA progresses, continuous pain contributes to disability and loss of function.[5] Pain may be referred to the groin, buttock, outer thigh, or knee. It can be hard to sit down or get up from a chair when the hips are lower than the knees. With OA in the intervertebral *(apophyseal)* joints of the spine, back pain and stiffness are common.

Joint stiffness occurs after periods of rest or immobility *(gelling phenomenon)*. Morning stiffness generally resolves within 30 minutes. Excess activity can cause a mild swelling that temporarily increases stiffness. Crepitus is common. Joint instability and muscle weakness may cause joints to "buckle" or "give way."[5]

OA affects joints on 1 side of the body *(asymmetric)* rather than in pairs. For example, the left knee is affected and the right knee unchanged. Weight-bearing joints (hips, knees), the metatarsophalangeal (MTP) joint of the foot, cervical vertebrae, and lumbar vertebrae are most often involved (Fig. 69.2). Other affected joints include the distal interphalangeal (DIP), proximal interphalangeal (PIP) joints of the fingers, and the metacarpophalangeal (MCP) joint of the thumb.

Deformity

Deformity or instability from OA is specific to the involved joint. For example, *Heberden nodes* and *Bouchard nodes* can occur on the DIP and PIP joints, respectively. They are caused by osteophyte formation and loss of joint space. Heberden and Bouchard nodes are red, swollen, and tender. They do not cause significant loss of function, but the deformity may bother patients.

Knee OA often leads to deformity because of cartilage loss in 1 joint compartment. Patients may become bowlegged *(varus deformity)* from medial joint arthritis. Lateral joint arthritis causes a knock-kneed appearance *(valgus deformity)*. In advanced hip OA, 1 leg may become shorter as the joint space narrows.

Diagnostic Studies

Symptoms and progression of OA vary widely. Assessment reveals pain worsening with activity and resolving with rest, morning stiffness lasting less than 30 minutes, bony joint

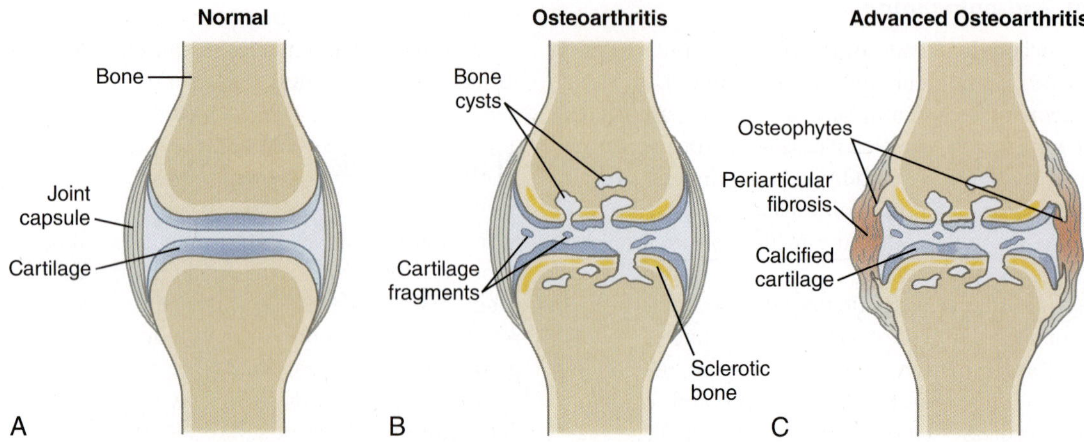

Fig. 69.1 Pathologic changes in OA. (A) Normal synovial joint. (B) Early change in OA is destruction of articular cartilage and narrowing of the joint space. Inflammation and thickening of the joint capsule and synovium are present. (C) With time, thickening of subarticular bone occurs, caused by constant friction of the 2 bone surfaces. Osteophytes form around the periphery of the joint by irregular overgrowths of bone.

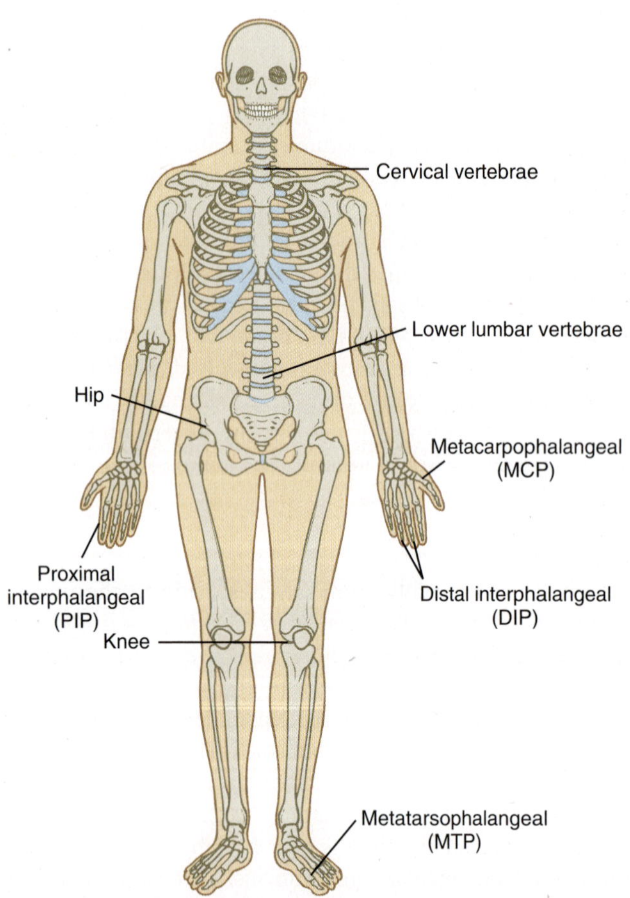

Fig. 69.2 Joints most often involved in OA.

enlargement, and limited range of motion. X-rays help confirm disease and stage of joint damage. As OA progresses, x-rays show joint space narrowing from degradation of cartilage. Osteophytes may be visible. These changes do not always reflect the degree of pain that patients experience. Despite strong x-ray evidence, one patient may have few symptoms, while another has severe pain

TABLE 69.2 Interprofessional Care

OA

Diagnostic Assessment

- History and physical assessment
- Radiologic studies of involved joints (e.g., x-ray, CT scan, MRI, bone scan)
- Synovial fluid analysis

Management

- Nutrition and weight management counseling
- Rest and joint protection, use of assistive devices
- Therapeutic exercise
- Heat and cold applications
- Transcutaneous electrical nerve stimulation (TENS)
- Reconstructive joint surgery
- Relaxation exercises

Drug Therapy (Table 69.3)

- NSAIDs: topical and oral
- Intraarticular corticosteroids
- Capsaicin cream

with only slight x-ray changes. A bone scan, CT scan, or MRI can detect cartilage destruction and early joint changes.[1]

Synovial fluid analysis helps distinguish OA from other types of arthritis. In OA, the fluid is clear yellow with little sign of inflammation. No laboratory tests or biomarkers can diagnose OA. The erythrocyte sedimentation rate (ESR) is normal except during acute inflammation.

Interprofessional Care

OA has no cure. Treatment is aimed at managing pain and inflammation, preventing disability, and maintaining joint function (Table 69.2). Care focuses on self-management, medication, education, therapeutic exercise, weight loss as needed, and adjuvant therapies.

Drug Therapy

Drug therapy is based on the joints affected and symptom severity (Table 69.3). Drug therapy includes topical, oral, and intraarticular agents.[6] Drugs thought to slow OA progression or support joint healing are known as *disease-modifying osteoarthritis drugs (DMOADs).* No DMOAD drugs are approved to modify OA progression.[7]

Nonsteroidal antiinflammatory drugs (NSAIDs) are the first-line treatment for OA. NSAIDs inhibit production of cyclooxygenase (COX). Most NSAIDs are nonspecific, affecting COX-1 and COX-2.[6] These enzymes convert arachidonic acid into prostaglandins (see Fig. 9.5). COX-2 promotes inflammation.

TABLE 69.3 Drug Therapy

OA

Drug	Mechanism of Action	Nursing Considerations
Corticosteroids		
Intraarticular Injections		
methylprednisolone acetate (Depo-Medrol) triamcinolone (Aristospan)	Analgesic Antiinflammatory Inhibit synthesis and/or release of inflammatory mediators	Use aseptic technique for corticosteroid injection. Tell patient that joint may temporarily feel worse right after injection. Teach patient to rest the affected joint right after injection. Improvement lasts weeks to months after injection. Report if no improvement occurs after 4 injections.
Systemic		
dexamethasone hydrocortisone (Solu-Cortef) methylprednisolone (Solu-Medrol) prednisone triamcinolone	Analgesic Antiinflammatory Inhibit synthesis and/or release of inflammatory mediators	Use only in life-threatening exacerbation or when symptoms persist after treatment with less potent antiinflammatory drugs. Give for short time only, taper dose slowly. Abrupt withdrawal of drug worsens symptoms. Monitor BP, weight, CBC, potassium. Limit sodium intake. Report signs of infection. Provide H_2 antagonist or proton-pump inhibitor (PPI).
Nonsteroidal Antiinflammatory Drugs (NSAIDs)		
celecoxib clofenac ibuprofen (Advil) indomethacin (Indocin) ketoprofen (Orudis) meclofenamate (Meclomen) meloxicam (Mobic) nabumetone (Relafen) naproxen (Aleve) oxaprozin (Daypro) piroxicam (Feldene) sulindac (Clinoril)	Antiinflammatory Analgesic Antiinflammatory Inhibit prostaglandin synthesis	Give drug with food, milk, or antacids (as prescribed). Report signs of bleeding, edema, skin rashes, persistent headaches, visual problems. Monitor BP for increases from fluid retention. Use regularly for maximum effect. Monitor for kidney toxicity in older adults. Educate about myocardial and stroke risk, recognition, and prevention. Avoid alcohol.
Salicylate		
aspirin, salicylate	Analgesic Antiinflammatory Inhibit prostaglandin synthesis	Give with food, milk, antacids (as prescribed), or full glass of water. May use enteric-coated aspirin. Report signs of bleeding. Monitor for confusion, ulcer, dizziness, loss of hearing if taking high doses.
Topical Analgesics		
capsaicin cream	Deplete substance P from nerve endings, interrupting pain signals to the brain	Used at regular intervals for maximal effect. Aloe vera cream may decrease burning sensation. Do not use with external heat source (heating pad) because of burn risk. Available in OTC and prescription strengths.
diclofenac sodium gel	Analgesic Antiinflammatory	Avoid sun and ultraviolet (UV) light exposure. Do not use with oral NSAIDs or aspirin because of risk for increased side effects.
Menthol Camphor	Analgesic Vasodilator	Monitor for rash, hives, redness

COX-1 helps protect the stomach lining. Inhibiting COX-1 causes some of the negative effects of oral NSAIDs, including GI distress.

Topical NSAIDS (e.g., diclofenac) are the preferred treatment. Oral NSAID therapy is started in low-dose over-the-counter (OTC) strengths (e.g., ibuprofen 200 mg up to 4 times daily). If GI side effects are a concern, adding a protective agent, such as misoprostol (Cytotec), to NSAID therapy may be needed. Acetaminophen is not effective on OA pain. It is only given if NSAIDs should not be taken.[8]

Patients taking an anticoagulant and an oral NSAID are at high risk for bleeding. Long-term NSAID treatment may negatively affect cartilage metabolism, especially in older patients. COX-2–selective inhibitors like celecoxib (Celebrex) may have fewer negative effects of NSAIDS. Some patients prefer aspirin, but it is not recommended. It should be used cautiously with NSAIDs because both inhibit platelet function and prolong bleeding time.

Topical agents such as capsaicin cream block pain by locally interfering with substance P and the transmission of pain impulses. Capsaicin creams of lower concentration are available OTC. Concentrated capsaicin is available by prescription. OTC products that contain camphor, eucalyptus oil, and menthol (e.g., Bengay, Arthricare) may provide temporary pain relief through heat and vasodilation. Some patients use topical salicylates (e.g., Aspercreme).

Intraarticular corticosteroid injections can help those with local inflammation and swelling in the knees and hips. If a patient has 4 or more injections without relief, alternative interventions should be used. After injections, the patient should rest and use ice on the injection site. Systemic corticosteroids are not used, as they may hasten disease progression. Duloxetine (Cymbalta) is recommended for patients with depression and chronic pain in OA.[6] Hyaluronic acid injection is a controversial treatment for knee OA. Some believe it improves disability, but studies show little benefit. Current guidelines do not recommend hyaluronates.

Surgical Therapy

Symptoms are often managed conservatively for many years. Hand braces, splinting, hand orthoses, and shock-absorbing footwear can support joints and protect them from instability.[2] Loss of joint function, unmanaged pain, and increased dependence for activities of daily living (ADLs) may lead to considering surgery. Reconstructive surgeries (e.g., hip and knee replacements) are discussed in Chapter 67.

Complementary and Alternative Therapies

Complementary and alternative therapies are popular with patients who have not found relief through traditional options. Teach patients to research alternative therapies and avoid replacing conventional treatments with unproven approaches. Acupuncture and subcutaneous needling may reduce pain and improve joint mobility. Relaxation therapy can calm anxiety and relax muscles. Some nutrition supplements may have antiinflammatory effects (e.g., ginger, SAM-e). Despite their popularity, studies on glucosamine and chondroitin are mixed. Their use is not recommended.[6] Patients should discuss any supplement use with their HCP to identify drug interactions.

NURSING MANAGEMENT: OSTEOARTHRITIS

Assessment

Assess the type, location, severity, frequency, and duration of joint pain and stiffness. Explore what makes the pain better or worse. How do symptoms affect the ability to perform ADLs? Review pain management practices. Ask about success of treatments. Assess tenderness, swelling, limitation of movement, joint stability, and crepitation of affected joints. Compare an involved joint with the opposite joint.

Health assessment questionnaires can pinpoint areas of decreased function. They are regularly completed to record disease and treatment progression. Data from the questionnaires can help us develop treatment goals and specific interventions.

Clinical Problems

Clinical problems for patients with OA may include:

- Pain
- Musculoskeletal problems
- Impaired role performance

Planning

Overall goals are that patients with OA will (1) maintain or improve joint function through a balance of rest and activity, (2) use joint protection measures to improve activity tolerance, (3) achieve independence in self-care and maintain optimal role function, and (4) use drug and nondrug strategies to manage pain satisfactorily.

Implementation

Health Promotion

Prevention of OA is possible in some cases. Focus education on modifiable risk factors (Box 69.1). For example, encourage patients to lose weight and reduce occupation or recreation hazards. Athletic instruction and physical fitness programs should include safety measures that protect and reduce trauma to joints.

Chronic Care

OA is a lifelong problem. The interprofessional team may include a family HCP, rheumatologist, nurse, occupational therapist, and physical therapist. Patient and caregiver teaching is important. Provide information about the course and treatment of OA, pain management, body mechanics, use of

BOX 69.1 PROMOTING POPULATION HEALTH

Preventing OA

- Avoid smoking.
- Promptly treat any joint injury.
- Maintain healthy weight and eat a balanced diet.
- Use safety measures to protect and decrease risk for joint injury.
- Exercise regularly, including strength and endurance training.
- Stretch before exercise.
- Avoid repetitive joint motions like knee bending.

assistive devices (e.g., cane, walker), principles of joint protection and energy conservation (Table 69.4), and an exercise program. If patients are overweight, weight reduction is included in the treatment plan. Chapter 45 discusses ways to help patients attain and maintain a healthy body weight.

Assure patients that OA is a local disease and severe deforming arthritis is not usual. Patients may gain support and knowledge through community and online resources.

CHECK YOUR PRACTICE

A 54-year-old female has OA of the left knee. She received an intraarticular corticosteroid injection in the left knee and a prescription for meloxicam 7.5 mg once daily. She has a prescription for physical therapy.

- What self-care information will you reinforce immediately after the injection?
- What information will you provide about meloxicam to ensure safe, effective use?

Heat and Cold Applications

Use of heat or cold is based on symptoms. Heat therapy is useful for stiffness. It relaxes muscles, increases flexibility, and improves blood flow to the area. Treatments include hot packs, whirlpool baths, ultrasound, and paraffin wax baths. Ice is not used as often as heat in OA treatment, but it can help reduce swelling with acute inflammation.

Exercise

Aerobic conditioning, range-of-motion (ROM) exercises, and programs to strengthen muscles around the affected joint help many patients. A physical therapist can help plan an exercise program. Stress the importance of warming up before any exercise to decrease risk for injury. Balance exercises improve the ability to control and stabilize body position. Encourage exercise like tai chi, which focuses on strength and balance.

Rest and Joint Protection

Teach patients to balance rest and activity, maintain functional positioning, use splints and braces to support joints, and modify activities to decrease joint stress. Joint protection is discussed in Table 69.4. Work with the physical therapist regarding the safe use of assistive devices.

TABLE 69.4 PATIENT & CAREGIVER TEACHING

Joint Protection and Energy Conservation

Include the following instructions when teaching patients with arthritis to protect joints and conserve energy:

- Maintain healthy weight.
- Use assistive devices, if needed (e.g., walkers, canes, zipper pulls, buttoning aids, grippers, grab bars, modified handles, Velcro fasteners).
- Avoid forceful repetitive joint movements.
- Maintain neutral positions to reduce stress on joint.
- Use good posture and body mechanics.
- Seek help with needed tasks that cause pain.
- Organize routine tasks and pace yourself to decrease fatigue and joint pain.
- Modify home and work environment to perform tasks in less stressful ways.
- Stop smoking.
- Wear low-heeled or flat shoes.
- Change positions often; alternate between sitting and standing.
- Avoid kneeling and squatting for extended times.
- Engage in simple stretching daily.
- Use splints and braces to support and rest joints.
- Use the strongest joint for tasks (use palms to push from a chair, carry items with arms, not fingers.
- Distribute weight evenly.
- Hold heavy items close to body.
- Do not grasp and hold items with fingers for extended time: steering wheel, pencils, knives when chopping, holding a clutch purse or a book.
- Eat high-calcium green vegetables (romaine lettuce, kale, broccoli, parsley).

Role Performance

Adjust home management goals to meet patients' needs. Include the caregiver, family members, and significant others in goal setting and teaching. Discuss home and work environment modification for patient safety and accessibility. Reduced mobility and self-care can cause safety concerns. Provide teaching about fall prevention. Assistive devices (e.g., canes, walkers, elevated toilet seats) reduce the load on affected joints and promote safety.

Sexual counseling may help patients and their significant other enjoy physical closeness by introducing alternative positions and timing for sexual activity. Encourage patients to take analgesics or a warm bath to decrease joint stiffness before sexual activity.

◆ Evaluation

The expected outcomes are that patients with OA will:

- Have adequate rest and activity
- Achieve acceptable pain management
- Maintain joint flexibility and muscle strength

RHEUMATOID ARTHRITIS

Rheumatoid arthritis (RA) is a chronic, systemic, autoimmune inflammatory disease characterized by inflammation in the diarthrodial (synovial) joints. It is considered one of the most disabling forms of arthritis. Table 69.5 compares RA with OA.

RA affects around 1.5 million adult Americans. It most often begins in females between ages 30 and 60 years. Almost 3 times as many females have RA.[9]

Etiology and Pathophysiology

The cause of RA is unknown. It likely begins when a genetically susceptible person has an initial immune response to an antigen (virus, bacteria) or environment trigger (cigarette smoke). Some risk factors are modifiable. Smoking increases the risk for RA, and patients who smoke are less likely to have disease remission. Obesity is a known risk factor for RA. Weight loss and a diet high in omega-3 fatty acids can reduce the risk. Altered gut and mouth microbiome plays a role in RA and autoimmune response. Presence of the HLA-DRB1 antigen is linked to genetic susceptibility in RA.[10] Human leukocyte antigen (HLA) antigens are discussed in Chapter 14.

The trigger causes formation of an abnormal protein, which leads to the production of autoantibodies rheumatoid factor (RF) and anticyclic citrullinated peptide (anti-CCP). RF and anti-CCP bind with the new protein antigens and form immune complexes in the tissues. The immune complexes deposit on synovial membranes and articular cartilage, leading to inflammation.

Neutrophils are attracted to this inflammation. They release proteolytic enzymes that damage articular cartilage and thicken the synovial lining (Fig. 69.3). Other inflammatory cells include T-helper (CD4) cells, which cause monocytes, macrophages, and synovial fibroblasts to secrete proinflammatory interleukin-1 (IL-1), IL-6, and tumor necrosis factor (TNF). This process leads to osteoclast formation and bone erosion.[10]

Clinical Manifestations

RA is marked by periods of remission and exacerbation. Table 69.6 lists the stages of RA. Symptoms and outcomes vary greatly.

Joints

The onset of RA is subtle. Nonspecific manifestations, such as fatigue, anorexia, weight loss, occasional fever, and general stiffness, may precede the onset of joint symptoms. Stiffness becomes localized in the following weeks to months.

Joint involvement is marked by pain, stiffness, limited motion, and signs of inflammation (e.g., warmth, swelling, pain). Joint symptoms occur symmetrically and often begin in the small joints of the hands (PIP, MCP) and feet (MTP) followed by the larger peripheral joints (e.g., wrists, elbows, shoulders, knees, hips, ankles, jaw). The cervical spine may be affected. Cervical spine instability at C1 or C2 may require urgent intervention.

TABLE 69.5 Comparison of RA and OA

Parameter	RA	OA
Age at onset	Young to middle age	Usually older than 40 yr
Gender	Female-to-male ratio is 3:1. Less difference after age 60	Females 2:1 after age 60; except for traumatic arthritis. Males less affected until age 70 or 80.
Weight	Lost or maintained weight	Often overweight
Disease	Systemic disease with exacerbations and remissions	Localized disease with variable, progressive course
Affected joints	Small joints typically affected first (PIPs, MCPs, MTPs), wrists, elbows, shoulders, knees. Usually bilateral, symmetric involvement	Weight-bearing joints of knees and hips, small joints (MCPs, DIPs, PIPs), cervical and lumbar spine. Asymmetric
Pain characteristics	Stiffness lasts 1 h to all day and may ↓ with joint use. Pain is variable, may disrupt sleep	Stiffness occurs on arising but usually subsides after 30 min. Pain gradually worsens with joint use and disease progression, relieved with joint rest but may disrupt sleep
Effusions	Common	Uncommon
Nodules	Present, especially on extensor surfaces	Heberden (DIPs) and Bouchard (PIPs) nodes
Synovial fluid	WBC count 1500–25,000/mL^3 with mostly neutrophils; ↓ viscosity. Inflammatory cells present	WBC count <2000/mL^3 (mild leukocytosis); normal viscosity. CD4 and CD8 present
X-rays	Joint space narrowing and erosion with bony overgrowths, subluxation with advanced disease. Osteoporosis related to decreased activity, corticosteroid use	Joint space narrowing, osteophytes, subchondral cysts, sclerosis
Laboratory findings	Rheumatoid factor positive in 80% of patients ↑ Antinuclear antibodies (ANAs) titer likely Positive anti-CCP (anti-citrullinated peptide) in 60%–70% ↑ ESR, CRP indicative of active inflammation, used to test disease activity. Not specific to RA	Rheumatoid factor negative ANA negative Anti-CCP negative Transient elevation in ESR related to synovitis

CRP, C-reactive protein; *DIP,* distal interphalangeal joint; *ESR,* erythrocyte sedimentation rate; *MCP,* metacarpophalangeal joint; *MTP,* metatarsophalangeal joint; *PIP,* proximal interphalangeal joint.

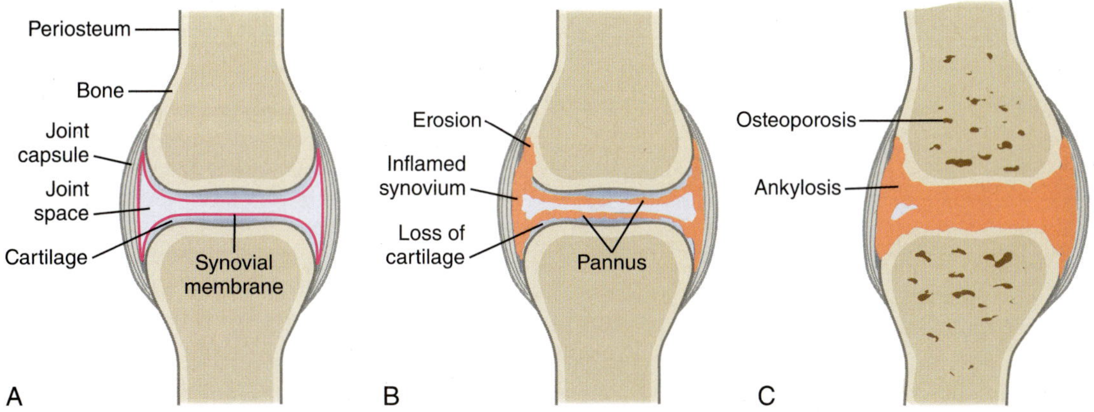

Fig. 69.3 RA. (A) Early pathologic change is rheumatoid synovitis. Synovium becomes inflamed. Lymphocytes and plasma cells increase. (B) Over time, articular cartilage destruction occurs, and vascular granulation tissue grows across the cartilage surface (pannus) from the edges of the joint. Joint surface shows loss of cartilage beneath the extending pannus, most marked at joint margins. (C) Inflammatory pannus causes focal destruction of bone. Osteolytic destruction of bone occurs at joint edges, causing erosions seen on x-rays. This phase is associated with joint deformity.

TABLE 69.6 Stages of RA

Stage	Characteristics
I	• No destructive change on x-ray • X-ray evidence of osteoporosis possible • Joint pain, fatigue • Slight swelling of joints
II	• Persistent joint pain • X-ray evidence of osteoporosis at joint, with or without slight subchondral bone destruction • Cartilage destruction possible • Joint mobility is limited, but no joint deformities noted • Muscle atrophy near joints • Increased joint swelling • Joint stiffness
III	• X-ray evidence of cartilage and bone destruction, osteoporosis at joint • Joint deformity without joint fusion • Extensive muscle atrophy near joints • Soft tissue lesions (nodules) near joints (elbows and hands) • Carpal tunnel possible from wrist inflammation
IV	• Criteria from stage III, plus • Extreme deformity • Extreme pain and swelling • Chronic fatigue • Fibrous or bony joint fusion • Decreased ROM to the point of disability

Joint stiffness occurs after periods of inactivity. Morning stiffness may last from 60 minutes to several hours depending on disease activity. MCP and PIP joints are typically swollen. In early disease, the fingers may become spindle shaped from synovial hypertrophy and thickening of the joint capsule. Joints are tender, painful, and warm to the touch. Joint pain increases with movement. Pain may not be related to the degree of inflammation. Tenosynovitis may affect the tendons around the wrists, causing carpal tunnel symptoms. This makes it hard for patients to grasp objects. Thick, inflamed synovium extends farther into the joint, destroying cartilage and bone. The joint capsule stretches. Changes in the joint cause deformity and disability. Irreversible joint changes can occur within the first year.

Muscle atrophy, weakness, and destruction of ligaments and tendons cause joint surfaces to slip past each other (subluxation). Metatarsal dislocation and subluxation may cause pain and walking disability. Ulnar drift ("zig-zag deformity"), swan neck, and boutonnière deformities are common in the hands (Fig. 69.4).

Extraarticular Manifestations

RA affects nearly every body system (Fig. 69.5). Extraarticular manifestations are more likely to occur in patients with high levels of RF and anti-CCP.

Rheumatoid nodules are the most common extraarticular sign.[10] The nodules are firm, nontender masses under the skin. They may be found on bony areas exposed to pressure, such as the fingers, elbows, and knees. Treatment is usually not needed. Rheumatoid nodules may form in the lungs but are harmless.[11]

Atherosclerosis results from chronic inflammation damaging endothelial cells within the blood vessels. Cholesterol plaques form. When plaques break loose, they can lead to heart attack or stroke. Risk of heart attack is 60% higher in patients with RA.[10] Pericarditis can lead to chest pain and palpitations.[12]

Patients may develop *Sjögren syndrome.* Inflammation in RA can damage the tear-producing (lacrimal) glands, making the eyes feel dry and gritty.[11] Sjögren syndrome is covered later in this chapter.

Felty syndrome is rare but can occur in patients with long-standing RA. It is characterized by an enlarged spleen and low white blood cell (WBC) count. Patients with Felty syndrome are at increased risk for infection and lymphoma.[11]

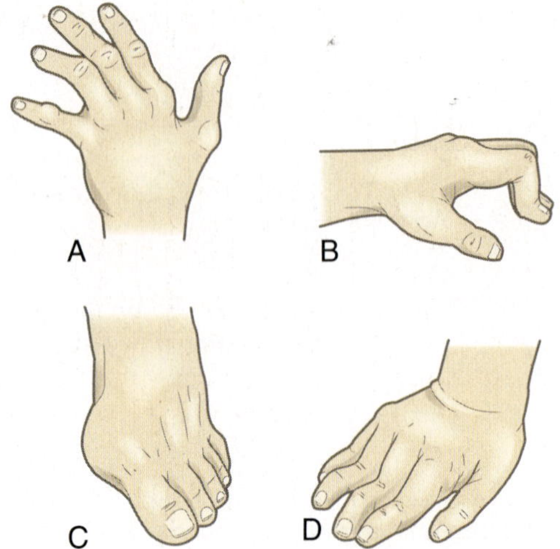

Fig. 69.4 Typical deformities of RA. (A) Ulnar drift. (B) Boutonnière deformity. (C) Hallux valgus. (D) Swan neck deformity.

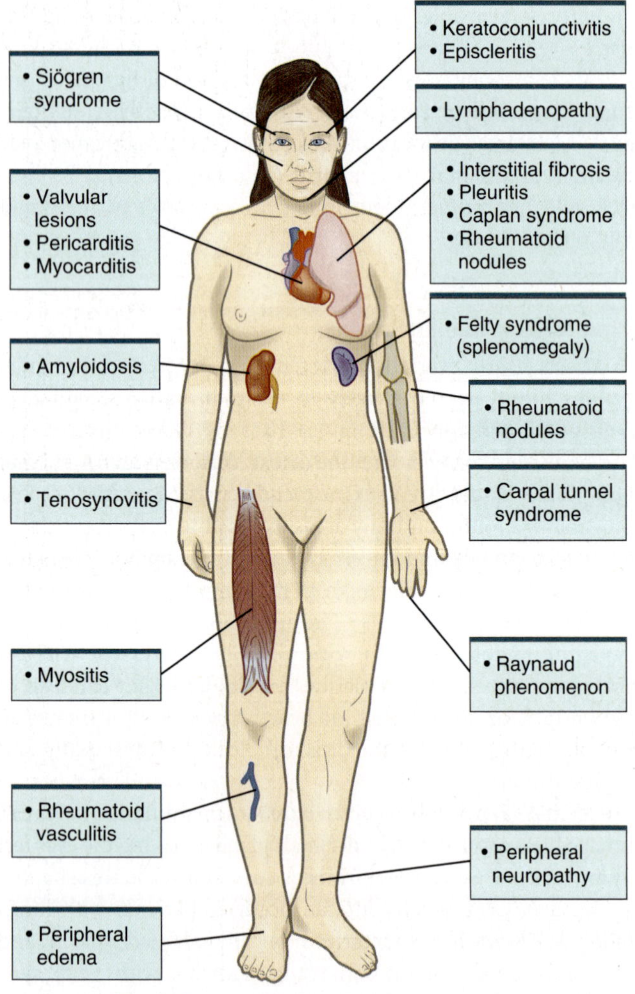

Fig. 69.5 Extraarticular manifestations of RA.

TABLE 69.7 Diagnostic Criteria

Patients With RA

The 2010 American College of Rheumatology and the European League Against Rheumatism (ACR/EULAR) diagnostic criteria for RA.

Screen patients for RA who initially present with:

- At least 1 joint with definite clinical synovitis (swelling)
- Synovitis not better explained by another disease

Classification criteria for RA is a score-based algorithm. Scores for categories A–D are added. A score ≥6 (highest possible total 10) is needed to classify a patient as having RA.

	Score
Joint Involvement	
• 1 large joint (shoulders, elbows, hips, knees, and ankles)	0 points
• 2–10 large joints	1 point
• 1–3 small joints (with or without large joint involvement)	2 points
• 4–10 small joints (with or without large joint involvement)	3 points
• >10 joints (at least 1 small joint)	5 points
Serologic Testing: At least 1 test result needed for classification	
• Negative RF *and* negative anti-CCP	0 points
• Low-positive RF *or* low-positive anti-CCP	2 points
• High-positive RF *or* high-positive anti-CCP	3 points
Acute-Phase Reactants	
• Normal CRP *and* normal ESR	0 points
• Abnormal CRP *or* abnormal ESR	1 point
Duration of Symptoms	
• <6 wk	0 points
• ≥6 wk	1 point

CCP, Citrullinated peptide; *CRP,* C-reactive protein; *ESR,* erythrocyte sedimentation rate; *RF,* rheumatoid factor

Flexion contractures and hand deformities cause decreased grasp strength and affect the ability to perform self-care. Depression may occur. It is unclear if the depression is caused by chronic pain and disability or part of the autoimmune disease process. Depression is associated with poorer outcomes for people with RA.

Other systemic effects from the chronic inflammation in RA include pulmonary fibrosis, causing shortness of breath and dyspnea, and vasculitis, leading to petechiae, purpura, and ulcers.[12] Decreased bone density can cause osteoporosis. Anemia causes fatigue and weakness.

Diagnostic Studies

Criteria for diagnosis of RA are shown in Table 69.7. Positive RF occurs in 80% to 90% of adults with the condition. Titers may rise during flares. Anti-CCP is present in about 70% to 80% of patients with RA. If symptoms are consistent with RA, the presence of anti-CCP and RF helps confirm the diagnosis. Antinuclear antibody (ANA) titers may be present with autoimmune activity. ESR and C-reactive protein (CRP) elevation indicate active inflammation. Periodic laboratory testing is used to monitor RA activity and response to treatment.

Synovial fluid analysis in early disease shows slightly cloudy, straw-colored fluid with fibrin flecks, increased WBCs, and the enzyme MMP-3. MMP-3 is a marker of cartilage breakdown.

Bone scans are useful in detecting early joint changes and confirming the diagnosis. X-rays may show soft tissue swelling and bone demineralization in early disease. A narrowed joint space, articular cartilage destruction, erosion, subluxation, and deformity are seen in later disease. Joint fusion may be seen in advanced disease. X-rays are used to monitor disease progression.

Interprofessional Care

A patient-specific treatment plan considers disease activity, joint function, age, gender, societal roles, and response to previous treatment (Table 69.8). Providing information on patients' options and encouraging shared decision making promote autonomy and self-worth. The progression of joint damage and disease activity can be reduced with aggressive, early treatment.[13] A trusting, long-term relationship with the health care team promotes positive coping.

Drug Therapy

Disease-modifying antirheumatic drugs. Drug therapy is the cornerstone of RA treatment (Table 69.9). Disease-modifying antirheumatic drugs (DMARDs) are started early. These drugs can slow disease progression and decrease risk for joint erosion and deformity. The choice of drug is based on disease activity, a patient's functional ability, and lifestyle considerations. Patients and providers should identify a goal and adjust treatment until the goal is reached. Remission may not be possible for everyone. Minimal disease activity, tight control of inflammation, and maintaining quality of life are ideal.[14]

Methotrexate monotherapy is preferred for early treatment.[14] Serious side effects include bone marrow suppression and liver toxicity. Therapy requires frequent monitoring of complete blood count (CBC) and blood chemistry. Therapeutic effects are seen in 4 to 6 weeks. Oral pills are preferred over infusions.

If patients cannot take methotrexate, alternative DMARDs may be given. Sulfasalazine (Azulfidine) and the antimalarial drug hydroxychloroquine are effective for patients with low disease activity. Leflunomide (Arava) blocks immune cell overproduction. Its efficacy and side effects are similar to sulfasalazine. JAK inhibitors (e.g., baricitinib) interfere with enzymes involved in joint inflammation. Many RA drugs are teratogenic. Pregnancy must be excluded before starting therapy.

Biologic response modifiers. *Biologic response modifiers* (BRMs) are used to slow disease progression. They can be used alone or in combination therapy with a DMARD. BRMs are used to treat patients with moderate to severe RA who have not responded to DMARDs alone.

TNF inhibitors (e.g., adalimumab, etanercept) are BRMs that bind to TNF in circulation before it can bind to the cell surface receptors. TNF inhibitors are recommended concurrently with methotrexate if needed. Other BRMs used in RA include IL receptor antagonists (e.g., tocilizumab), which block the action of the cytokine IL-6. Abatacept (Orencia) blocks T-cell activation. Rituximab (Rituxan) is a monoclonal antibody that targets the CD-20 antigen on B lymphocytes. BRMs are discussed in Chapter 14.

Other drug therapy. Immunosuppressants (azathioprine) and gold salts are rarely used because they are weak treatments compared with DMARDs and BRMs. The effectiveness of CBD in pain management has not been validated. It is currently not recommended.[15]

Corticosteroid therapy can be used to manage symptoms during disease flares. Intraarticular injections may temporarily reduce acute pain and inflammation. Low-dose oral corticosteroids may be used for a limited time to decrease disease activity until the effects from DMARDs or BRMs are evident. Corticosteroids do not stop disease progression. They are not recommended for ongoing treatment of RA.[14]

Patients use various NSAIDs and salicylates to treat pain and inflammation. They do not alter the course of RA. Aspirin may be used in dosages of 3 to 4 g/day in divided doses. Monitor salicylate levels if patients take more than 3600 mg daily.[14] NSAIDs have antiinflammatory and analgesic effects. Some relief may be seen within days of starting treatment with NSAIDs. Full effect may take 2 to 3 weeks (Table 69.3). Selective COX-2 inhibitors are effective in RA.

TABLE 69.8 Interprofessional Care

Rheumatoid Arthritis

Diagnostic Assessment
- History and physical assessment
- CBC
- Erythrocyte sedimentation rate (ESR)
- C-reactive protein (CRP)
- Rheumatoid factor (RF)
- Antibodies to citrullinated peptide (anti-CCP)
- Antinuclear antibody (ANA)
- X-rays of involved joints
- Synovial fluid analysis, synovial biopsy

Management
- Nutrition and weight management counseling
- Therapeutic exercise
- Psychologic support
- Rest and joint protection, use of assistive devices
- Heat and cold applications
- Reconstructive surgery

Drug Therapy
- Disease-modifying antirheumatic drugs (DMARDs) (Table 69.9)
- Biologic response modifiers (BRMs) (Table 69.9)
- NSAIDs
- Intraarticular or systemic corticosteroids (Table 69.3)
- Antidepressants

TABLE 69.9 Drug Therapy

RA

Drug	Mechanism of Action	Nursing Considerations
Disease-Modifying Antirheumatic Drugs (DMARDs)		
leflunomide	Antiinflammatory Immunomodulatory Inhibits proliferation of lymphocytes	Monitor liver function. Avoid pregnancy.
methotrexate (Trexall)	Antimetabolite Inhibits DNA, RNA, protein synthesis	Monitor CBC, liver and renal function. Teach patient to report signs of anemia (fatigue, weakness). Keep patient well hydrated. Avoid pregnancy.
sulfasalazine	Sulfonamide Antiinflammatory Blocks prostaglandin synthesis	Monitor CBC. Tell patient drug may cause orange-yellow discoloration of urine or skin. Space doses evenly around the clock. Take drug after food with 8 oz water. Treatment may be continued even after symptoms are relieved. Encourage oral fluid intake. Wear sunscreen with sun exposure.
hydroxychloroquine	Exact mechanism of action unknown May reduce autoantigen presentation	Monitor CBC, liver function. Response may not occur for up to 6 mo. Teach patient to report vision changes, muscle weakness, ↓ hearing, tinnitus. Have a baseline eye examination with follow-up every 6–12 mo because of risk for vision loss. Avoid pregnancy.
Biologic Response Modifiers (see Table 14.18)		
B-Cell–Depleting Agent		
rituximab	Monoclonal antibody Binds to CD20, an antigen on B cells, destroying B cells and suppressing immune response	Monitor for infection and bleeding. No live virus vaccines during treatment. Monitor for low BP if taking BP medication. Fatigue is common.
Interleukin-1 (IL-1) Receptor Antagonist		
anakinra (Kineret) canakinumab (Ilaris)	Blocks the action of IL-1, ↓ inflammatory response	Do not use with TNF inhibitors. Injection site reaction generally occurs in first month of treatment and decreases with continued therapy. Monitor renal function. Monitor for infection.
IL-6 Receptor Antagonist		
sarilumab tocilizumab (Actemra)	Blocks action of IL-6, thus ↓ inflammatory response	Given to patients for whom other therapies have failed. Monitor BP and for infection. Tell patient of GI effects (e.g., perforation). Monitor liver function, LDL.
JAK (Janus Kinase) Inhibitors		
baricitinib tofacitinib (Xeljanz) upadacitinib (Rinvoq)	Inhibits action of JAK enzymes, signaling pathways inside the cell	Avoid use in patient with severe liver disease. Monitor CBC and liver function. Monitor for infection. Avoid pregnancy. Monitor for heart attack, stroke, venous thromboembolism.
T-Cell Activation Inhibitor		
abatacept	Inhibits T-cell activation, thus suppressing immune response	Do not use with TNF inhibitors. Monitor for infusion reaction if given IV. Assess injection site for reaction. Monitor for infection.
Tumor Necrosis Factor (TNF) Inhibitors		
adalimumab certolizumab (Cimzia) etanercept golimumab (Simponi) infliximab (Remicade)	Bind to TNF, blocks TNF interaction with cell surface receptors. Decreases inflammatory and immune responses.	Monitor CBC, liver function. ↑ Risk for tuberculosis. Monitor for infection, cancers. No live virus vaccines during treatment. For infliximab: Monitor for infusion reaction. Other TNF inhibitors: Teach SC injection. Site reaction generally occurs in first month of treatment and ↓ with continued therapy.

TABLE 69.10 **NURSING ASSESSMENT**

RA

Subjective Data	Objective Data
Important Health Information	***Cardiovascular***
Health history: Recent infections. Precipitating factors, such as emotional upset, infections, overwork, childbirth, surgery. Pattern of remissions and exacerbations	Symmetric pallor and cyanosis of fingers (Raynaud phenomenon). Distant heart sounds, murmurs, dysrhythmias.
Medications: NSAIDs, corticosteroids, DMARDs, BRMs	***General***
Surgery or other treatments: Any joint surgery	Lymphadenopathy, fever
Functional Health Patterns	***GI***
Health perception—health management: Positive family history for RA or other autoimmune disorders. Malaise, ability to take part in treatment plan. Impact of disease on functional ability	Splenomegaly (Felty syndrome)
Nutritional-metabolic: Anorexia, weight loss, dry mucous membranes	***Musculoskeletal***
Activity-exercise: Stiffness and joint swelling, muscle weakness, difficulty walking, fatigue	Symmetric joint involvement with swelling, redness, warmth, tenderness. Deformities. Enlargement of PIP and MCP joints. Limitation of joint movement, decreased ROM, muscle contractures, muscle atrophy, joint instability.
Cognitive-perceptual: Paresthesia of hands and feet, loss of sensation; symmetric joint pain and aching that ↑ with motion or stress on joint, interferes with rest	***Respiratory***
	Bronchiectasis, pleural effusion, respiratory excursion, lung sounds
	Skin
	Scleritis, uveitis, Sjögren syndrome. Subcutaneous rheumatoid nodules on forearms, elbows. Skin ulcers. Shiny, taut skin over involved joints. Peripheral edema, pallor (anemia).
	Possible Diagnostic Findings
	Positive rheumatoid factor (RF), antinuclear antibody (ANA), anti-CCP. ↑ ESR; anemia. ↑ WBCs in synovial fluid. On x-ray evidence of joint space narrowing, bony erosion, deformity, possible osteoporosis.

BRB, Biologic response modifier; *CCP,* citrullinated peptide; *DMARD,* disease-modifying antirheumatic drug; *ESR,* erythrocyte sedimentation rate; *MCP,* metacarpophalangeal; *PIP,* proximal interphalangeal.

Surgical Therapy

Surgery may be needed to relieve severe pain and improve the function of severely deformed joints. Removal of the joint lining *(synovectomy)* and total joint replacement *(arthroplasty)* are common surgeries. Joint surgery is discussed in Chapter 67. Stem cell therapy to control inflammation and improve tissue regeneration is effective for some patients.

NURSING MANAGEMENT: RHEUMATOID ARTHRITIS

Assessment

Subjective and objective data you should obtain from patients with RA are outlined in Table 69.10. Begin with the history and physical assessment (e.g., joint pain, swelling, ROM, health status). Assess psychosocial needs (e.g., family support, sexual satisfaction, emotional stress, career limitations). Are there environment concerns (e.g., transportation, home, or work modifications)? After identifying the problems, plan a program for rehabilitation and education with the interprofessional care team (Table 69.11).

Clinical Problems

Clinical problems for patients with RA may include:

- Impaired musculoskeletal function
- Pain
- Impaired role performance
- Depressed mood

Additional information on clinical problems and interventions for patients with RA is provided in eNursing Care Plan 69.1 (available on the website for this chapter).

Planning

The overall goals are that patients with RA will (1) have acceptable pain management, (2) have minimal loss of function of affected joints, (3) take part in planning and implementing the treatment plan, (4) maintain a positive self-image, and (5) perform self-care to the maximum amount possible.

TABLE 69.11 NURSING MANAGEMENT

Caring for Patients With RA

- Give drug therapy as ordered.
- Teach patient and caregiver about drug therapy, including increased risk for infection with DMARDs and BRMs.
- Assess disease impact on quality of life and joint function.
- Assess pain intensity and give analgesics as ordered. Assess response.
- Develop program for rehabilitation and education with the interprofessional team.
- Teach patient about need for balance of rest and activity, with use of joint protective strategies (Table 69.4).
- Assist with heat and cold therapy.
- Teach energy conservation techniques.
- Supervise AP:
  - Aid with passive ROM of affected joints.
  - Help with self-care needs.

Collaborate With Interprofessional Team Members

Physical Therapist

- Assess current mobility and need for help (e.g., walker).
- Develop exercise plan and teach patient to perform exercises safely.
- Coordinate PT with RN so that patient can receive timely analgesia.
- Recommend and apply thermal therapies.

Occupational Therapist

- Assess impact of condition on ability to perform.
- Teach use of assistive devices (e.g., long-handled reacher, long-handled shoehorn, splints) to improve self-care ability without increasing stress on joints.
- Identify modifications to improve role performance (e.g., kitchen modifications for meal preparation).

Social Worker

- Help with obtaining durable medical equipment (e.g., walker).
- Assess psychosocial and financial impact of disease. Arrange vocational retraining if needed.

BRM, Biologic response modifier; *DMARD,* disease-modifying antirheumatic drug.

◆ Implementation

Care of patients with RA includes a program of drug therapy, self-management strategies, exercise, and teaching. Nondrug management may include the use of therapeutic heat and cold, rest, relaxation techniques, joint protection (Table 69.4), biofeedback, and transcutaneous electrical nerve stimulation (see Chapter 9). Allow patients and caregivers to choose therapies that promote optimal comfort and fit their lifestyle. Connect patients with reliable online resources that provide publications, teaching, and support.

Patients are treated on an outpatient basis. Those with systemic complications or who need surgery may be hospitalized. Work closely with the health care team to help patients regain function and adjust to chronic illness.

Teach patients and caregivers about the disease process and treatment plan. Inflammation may be managed with NSAIDs, DMARDs, and BRMs. Careful timing of drug administration is critical to maintain a therapeutic drug level and reduce inflammation and stiffness. Teach the action and side effects of each drug and any needed laboratory monitoring. Patients take several different drugs. Make the drug plan as understandable as possible. Encourage patients to develop ways to remember to take their medications (e.g., alarms, pill containers).

Rest

Energy conservation requires planning. Alternating scheduled rest periods with activity throughout the day (pacing) helps relieve fatigue and pain. The amount of rest needed varies based on disease severity and the patient's limitations. Patients should rest before becoming exhausted. Total bed rest is avoided to prevent stiffness and other effects of immobility. Patients with mild disease may need daytime rest plus 8 to 10 hours of sleep at night. Help patients alter daily activities to avoid overexertion and fatigue. For example, patients may be able to prepare meals more easily while sitting on a high stool rather than standing.

Teach patients to maintain good body alignment during rest through use of a firm mattress or bed board. Encourage positions of extension and avoid flexion. To decrease the risk for joint contracture, do not place pillows under the knees. Use a small, flat pillow under the head and shoulders if needed.

Joint Protection

Protecting joints from stress is important. Help patients find ways to simplify work and alter routine tasks to put less stress on joints (Table 69.4). Organize activities to avoid going up and down stairs repeatedly. Use carts to carry supplies. Store frequently used items in a convenient, easy-to-reach area. Use joint-protective methods (e.g., smart house technology, electric can opener) whenever possible. Teach patients to delegate tasks to others.

An occupational therapist (OT) helps patients maintain fine motor movement. OT facilitates the use of splints or other assistive devices for joint protection. Lightweight splints can rest an inflamed joint and prevent deformity. Remove the splints regularly to assess skin and perform ROM exercises. After assessment and care, reapply splints as prescribed.

OT may increase independence with assistive devices (e.g., built-up utensils, zipper pulls, modified drawer handles). Encourage patients to make dressing easier by wearing shoes with Velcro fasteners and clothing with closures in the front instead of the back. Use a cane or a walker for support and decreased pain when walking. Avoid activities requiring a fist or contraction of the fingers for extended periods.

Cold and Heat Therapy

Cold and heat applications can help relieve stiffness, pain, and muscle spasm. They can be used several times a day as needed. Ice is especially helpful during periods of increased disease activity and inflammation. Cold application should not exceed 10 to 15 minutes at a time. Plastic bags of small frozen vegetables can easily mold around the joints for an effective home ice pack. Ice cubes or small paper cups of frozen water can be used to massage a painful joint.

Moist heat offers better relief for chronic stiffness. Moist hot packs, paraffin baths, warm baths, and sitting or standing in a warm shower can relieve stiffness and allow patients to take part in therapeutic exercise or perform ADLs more comfortably. Heat application should not exceed 20 minutes at a time. Patients should avoid using a heat-producing cream (e.g., capsaicin) with an external heat device. Heat should be avoided during a flare.[16]

Exercise

Exercise is an important part of the treatment plan. A physical therapist will develop a therapeutic exercise program to improve flexibility, strengthen affected joints, and increase endurance. Encourage participation and reinforce correct performance of the exercises. Progressive joint immobility and muscle weakness can occur if the patient does not move the joints. Overaggressive exercise can increase pain, inflammation, and joint damage. Stress that taking part in recreation activities or doing usual daily activities does not take the place of therapeutic exercise.

Gentle ROM exercises daily can help keep joints functional. Exercising in warm water (78°F to 86°F [25°C to 30°C]) allows easier joint movement because of the buoyancy and warmth of the water. Although movement seems easier, water provides 2-way resistance that makes muscles work harder while supporting the entire joint. During acute inflammation, limit exercise to 1 or 2 repetitions.

Nutrition

Balanced nutrition is important. Fatigue, pain, and depression may cause a loss of appetite. Limited endurance and mobility make it hard to shop for and prepare food. Weight loss may result. The occupational therapist can help patients modify the home environment and use assistive devices for easier food preparation. A plant-based diet with adequate fiber and healthy fats can support gut health and reduce inflammation.

Corticosteroid therapy and decreased mobility may cause unwanted weight gain. Corticosteroids increase the appetite, leading to higher caloric intake. If overweight, a sensible weight loss program reduces stress on affected joints. Teach patients to manage side effects of steroids (see Chapter 54).

Psychologic Support

For effective self-management, help patients understand the course and consequences of RA and the goals of therapy. Discuss changes in sexuality. Consider the patient's value system and perception of the disease.

Evaluate the support system. Financial planning may be needed. Consider community resources, such as home care, homemaker services, and vocational rehabilitation. Some patients benefit from therapeutic groups.

Chronic pain or loss of function may make patients vulnerable to false advertising about unproven or dangerous remedies. Help them recognize psychologic strain faced by those with chronic illness. Living with chronic pain may lead to depression. To decrease depressive symptoms, suggest activities such as listening to music, reading, exercising, and counseling. Hypnosis and biofeedback may be useful. Antidepressants, if needed, can help with mood and have benefits related to pain reduction.[12]

Gerontologic Considerations: Arthritis

The prevalence of arthritis in older adults is high. The disease is accompanied by problems unique to this age group. Areas of concern include:

- The high incidence of OA may keep the HCP from considering other types of arthritis.
- Drugs and comorbid conditions can affect laboratory values.
- Musculoskeletal pain syndromes and weakness may have no physical cause. They may be related to depression and inactivity.
- Physical and metabolic changes of aging may alter sensitivity to therapeutic and toxic effects of drugs.
- Side effects from NSAIDs are more common in the older adult.
- Polypharmacy is a concern.
- Support systems for the older adult are critical to the ability to follow a treatment plan.

The drug plan should be as simple as possible to increase adherence and reduce chances of drug interaction. Osteopenia from corticosteroid use can worsen the problem of decreased bone density from aging and inactivity. The risk for pathologic fractures is increased, especially vertebral compression fractures.

GOUT

Gout is a type of metabolic inflammatory arthritis characterized by elevation of uric acid *(hyperuricemia)* and the deposit of uric acid crystals in 1 or more joints. Sodium urate crystals may be found in articular, periarticular, and subcutaneous tissues. Gout is marked by painful flares lasting days to weeks followed by long periods without symptoms.

In the United States 250,000 people a year are diagnosed with gout.[17] Gout usually develops between ages 30 and 50. Black persons have a higher incidence than other ethnicities.

Males are 3 times more likely to acquire gout. Females rarely develop gout before menopause because estrogen promotes renal excretion of uric acid.[17]

Etiology and Pathophysiology

Uric acid is the end product of purine catabolism. It is excreted by the kidneys. Gout occurs when either the kidneys cannot excrete enough uric acid or there is too much being made for the kidneys to handle.

We classify hyperuricemia as primary or secondary. *Primary hyperuricemia* is genetic. Genetic predisposition causes decreased uric acid excretion. *Secondary hyperuricemia* is caused by conditions that increase uric acid production, decrease uric acid excretion, or drugs that inhibit uric acid excretion.[18] A high rate of nucleic acid metabolism leads to increased uric acid production. Table 69.12 lists causes of hyperuricemia.

Not everyone with high uric acid levels develops gout. Crystallization and inflammation are essential for a person to develop it. Urate levels increase and saturate the synovial fluid or soft tissues. Excess urate crystallizes. These crystals trigger inflammation. Monocytes and macrophages try to remove the crystals through phagocytosis. This causes the release of inflammatory mediators causing more inflammation, pain, and tissue damage.

Gout is likely caused by the interaction of several factors. Metabolic syndrome (obesity, insulin resistance, hypertension, hyperlipidemia) is a significant risk factor. Other risk factors include renal insufficiency and heart failure. Increased intake of foods containing purines (e.g., red and organ meat, shellfish, anchovies, trout, tuna, food and drinks with fructose, asparagus, dried beans, mushrooms) can trigger gout. Thirty percent of uric acid production is related to diet intake.[19] High uric acid may result from prolonged fasting or excess beer and hard liquor intake. These increase the production of keto acids, which inhibit uric acid excretion.

TABLE 69.12 Causes of High Uric Acid Levels

- Acidosis or ketosis
- Alcohol use, especially beer and red wine
- Cancer
- Chemotherapy drugs
- Diabetes
- Drug-induced renal impairment
- Hyperlipidemia
- Hypertension
- Lead exposure
- Medications: aspirin, ACE inhibitors, β-blockers, loop or thiazide diuretics, niacin
- Metabolic syndrome
- Myeloproliferative disorders
- Obesity
- Renal insufficiency
- Sickle cell anemia
- Starvation

Clinical Manifestations and Complications

Acute gout occurs in 1 to 4 joints. Inflammation of the great toe *(podagra)* is the most common initial problem. Other affected joints may include wrists, knees, ankles, elbows, and the midfoot. Affected joints may appear red, dusky, or cyanotic. The joints are very tender. Acute gout can be triggered by events such as trauma, surgery, or systemic infection. Symptom onset typically occurs at night with sudden swelling and severe pain peaking within several hours. The painful area is highly sensitive to light touch. Low-grade fever is common. An attack usually resolves in 2 to 10 days with or without treatment. The affected joint returns to normal. Patients have no symptoms between attacks.

Chronic gout is defined by having 2 or more attacks a year. Multiple joints are often involved. Visible deposits of sodium urate crystals called *tophi* are present in chronic disease. Tophi are hard white nodules. They are found in subcutaneous tissue, synovial membranes, tendons, and other tissues such as the sclera in the eye or renal pyramids (Fig. 69.6). Tophi occur many years after the onset of disease.[20]

The severity of gout arthritis varies. The clinical course may involve infrequent mild attacks or multiple severe episodes marked by gradual disability. In general, patients have more frequent, severe episodes of gout if serum uric acid is high. Chronic inflammation destroys joint tissue, causing joint deformity. Cartilage destruction may lead to secondary OA. Large urate crystal deposits may pierce overlying skin.

Uric acid is filtered through the kidneys. Excess uric acid excretion may lead to stone formation in the kidneys or urinary tract. Over time the crystals can cause damage and scarring, leading to pyelonephritis and obstruction. NSAIDs, which are commonly taken for gout pain, can contribute to kidney disease.[21]

Diagnostic Studies

Normal uric acid levels range from 3.5 to 7.2 mg/dL.[22] The higher the value, the greater the risk for uric acid deposits in joints and future gout attacks. Uric acid levels should be kept below 6 mg/dL for females and below 7 mg/dL for males. Hyperuricemia is not specifically diagnostic of gout because serum values may be normal during an acute gout attack. A 24-hour urine uric acid test can determine whether gout is caused by decreased renal excretion or overproduction of uric acid. The most reliable test for gout is synovial fluid aspiration. Aspiration is done under local anesthesia. Positive findings show monosodium urate crystals in the fluid. This test is the best way to differentiate gout from reactive arthritis or *pseudogout* (calcium phosphate crystals).[22] Aspiration may decrease pain by relieving pressure in a swollen joint capsule.

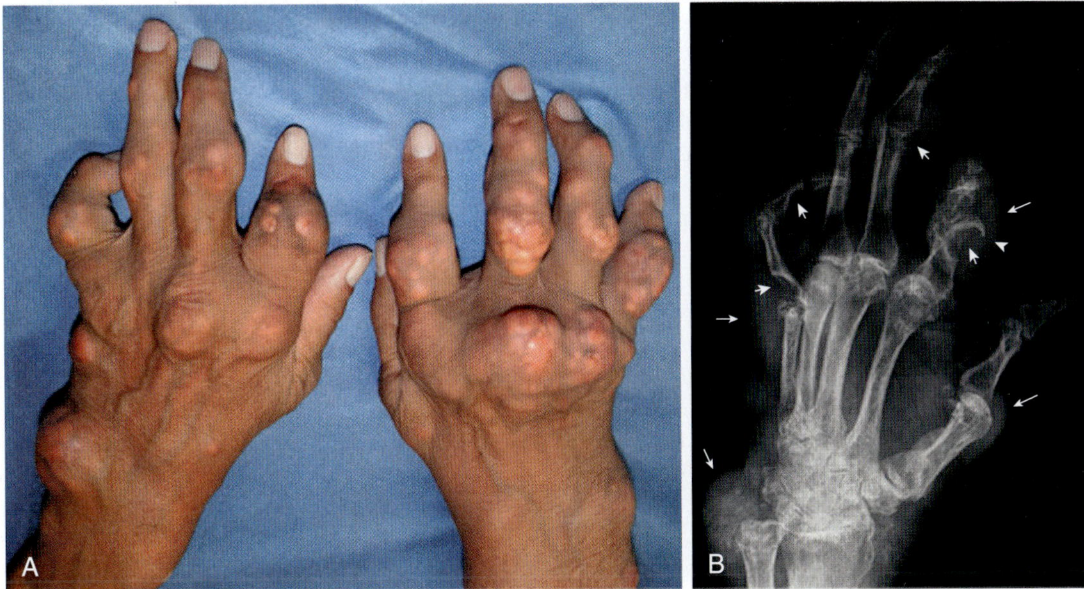

Fig. 69.6 Tophi from chronic gout. (A) The fingers of a patient with chronic gout. Small to large painless nodules are spread across the fingers of the patient filled with uric acid crystals. (B) A radiograph for chronic gout shows swollen nodules on several portions of the fingers indicated by *arrows*. (From Barajas-Ochoa A, Castaneda-Sanchez JJ, Ramos-Remus C: Is gout an easy-to-treat disease?, *Rheumatol Clin* 14:59, 2018.)

X-rays appear normal in the early stages of gout. Ultrasound may show crystals or tophi in joints. Dual-energy CT scan (DECT) can find tophi and crystals that other tests are unable to identify.[22]

Interprofessional and Nursing Management

The goal of care for patients with an acute gout attack is to end the attack with an antiinflammatory agent. Table 69.13 lists interprofessional care for gout. Drug therapy is the primary way to treat acute and chronic gout. Ingesting cherries and vitamin C–rich foods can help decrease uric acid levels during a gout flare.[20] Nursing interventions for patients with acute gout include supportive care of the inflamed joints. Handle inflamed joints carefully to avoid causing pain. Assess motion limitations and degree of pain.

Drug Therapy

Medication is used to treat acute attacks, prevent future attacks, and decrease complications. Acute gout flares are treated with oral colchicine (Colcrys, Mitigare) and NSAIDs. Colchicine works by stopping the process that causes swelling in gout. Colchicine is not an analgesic, so NSAIDs are added for pain management. Colchicine can result in relief when given within 12 hours of an attack. This aids in diagnosis because good response to colchicine is further evidence of gout.

Corticosteroids (intraarticular injection or orally) can be helpful in treating an acute attack. Systemic corticosteroids should be used only if routine therapies are contraindicated or

TABLE 69.13 Interprofessional Care

Gout

Diagnostic Assessment

- History and physical assessment
- Family history of gout or other inflammatory arthritis
- Sodium urate crystals in synovial fluid
- ↑ Uric acid
- ↑ Uric acid excretion in 24-h urine
- X-ray or dual-energy CT scan (DECT) of affected joints

Management

- Joint immobilization
- Local application of cold
- Joint aspiration
- Avoid food and fluids with high purine content (e.g., anchovies, liver, wine, beer)
- Drink at least 2 L/day of water
- Protect tender joints (bed cradle, careful handling)

Drug Therapy

- Colchicine
- NSAIDs (e.g., naproxen)
- Xanthine oxidase inhibitors: allopurinol, febuxostat
- Uricosurics: probenecid
- Pegloticase
- Corticosteroids (e.g., prednisone)
- Intraarticular corticosteroids (methylprednisolone)
- Adrenocorticotropic hormone (ACTH)

ineffective. Adrenocorticotropic hormone (ACTH) is an option for acute treatment of patients for whom NSAIDs, colchicine, or steroids are problematic.

Uric acid–lowering medication is recommended for patients who have more than 1 attack in a year.[23] Patients take a maintenance dose of a xanthine oxidase inhibitor to decrease uric acid production. Allopurinol is the drug used most often. It can be used for patients with uric acid kidney stones or renal impairment. Febuxostat is approved to lower uric acid production. Use of febuxostat is limited to those who cannot take allopurinol because of adverse effects. Pegloticase (Krystexxa) lowers uric acid by metabolizing it to a harmless chemical excreted in the urine. Pegloticase must be given IV every 2 weeks for 6 months.[23] Life-threatening infusion reactions can occur.

DRUG ALERT

Febuxostat

- May cause heart-related death and liver failure.
- Encourage patients with cardiovascular disease to take low-dose aspirin.
- Monitor liver function tests before starting and during treatment.
- Teach patient to notify HCP if symptoms of liver or heart problems occur.

A uricosuric agent, which increases uric acid excretion in the urine, may be added if uric acid levels do not decrease. Probenecid is the most common agent. Salicylates inactivate its effect. Thus OTC medications with salicylates (e.g., aspirin) must be avoided during treatment. Uricosurics can cause renal impairment. They are ineffective when creatinine clearance is reduced. Monitor renal function and drug effectiveness in patients over age 60 years or with renal impairment. They should be taken in the morning with food and water. Teach patients to stay well hydrated and to drink about 2 L of liquid a day when taking uricosurics.

The angiotensin II receptor antagonist losartan (Cozaar) may be effective for treating older patients with gout and hypertension. Losartan promotes urate excretion and may help normalize urate levels.

Patient Education

Hyperuricemia and related inflammation are chronic problems that can be controlled with teaching and adherence to a treatment plan. Explain the importance of drug therapy and the need for regular assessment of uric acid. We check uric acid levels regularly to monitor treatment effectiveness.

Avoiding purine-rich foods helps prevent future gout flares. Limiting alcohol and foods high in purine helps decrease uric acid production. Adequate urine volume and normal renal function (2 to 3 L/day) must be maintained to prevent uric acid precipitation in the renal tubules. Teach patients with obesity about weight reduction (see Chapter 45). Teach patients about other factors that may cause an attack.

CHECK YOUR PRACTICE

A patient comes to the primary care office with acute gout. The right great toe is swollen, red, and painful. He is prescribed colchicine.

- What interventions will you teach the patient to protect the foot and decrease pain?
- What will you discuss with the patient about diet changes to decrease risk for future attacks?

LYME DISEASE

Lyme disease is an infection caused by the spirochete *Borrelia burgdorferi.* It is transmitted by the bite of an infected black-legged tick (deer tick). The tick typically feeds on mice, dogs, cats, cows, horses, deer, and humans. Person-to-person transmission does not occur. Lyme disease is most common in the Northeast, Mid-Atlantic, and upper Midwest regions of the United States. Highest incidence is in children 5 to 15 years and adults over 50 years. Risk of infection is greatest in late spring and summer.[24] Over 63,000 people in the United States test positive for Lyme disease annually.[24]

Symptoms mimic many other diseases, such as mononucleosis and meningitis. The most characteristic symptom of early disease is *erythema migrans* (EM). This "bull's-eye rash" occurs in about 80% of infected persons.[25] It appears at the site of the tick bite within 1 month after exposure (Fig. 69.7). It may occur elsewhere on the body as the disease progresses. The EM lesion begins as a central red macule or papule that slowly expands to include a red outer ring of up to 12 inches. It may be warm to palpation but does not itch or hurt. Other symptoms include low-grade fever, headache, stiff neck, fatigue, lymphadenopathy, and arthralgia. Symptoms usually resolve over weeks or months, even if untreated. With treatment, 5% to 10% of people develop chronic symptoms with lingering pain and fatigue.

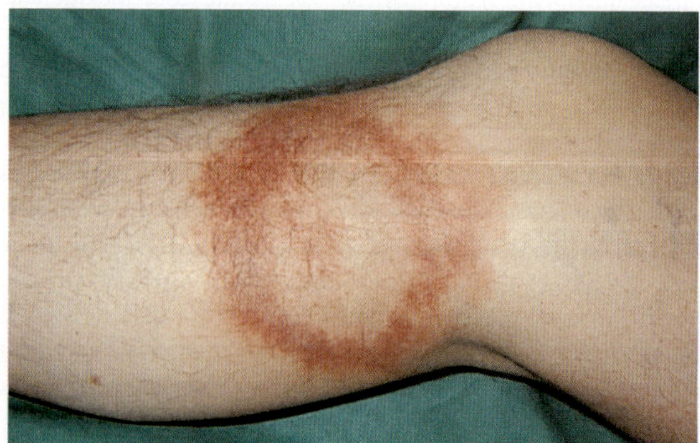

Fig. 69.7 Erythema migrans. Typical skin lesion of Lyme disease occurs at the site of tick bite. (From Silvestri AE, Silvestri LA: *Saunders comprehensive review for the NCLEX-RN© examination,* ed 9, St. Louis, 2023, Elsevier.)

If not treated, days to months after the bite, the spirochete can spread to the heart, joints, and central nervous system (CNS). People with untreated infection may develop chronic arthritic pain and swelling in the large joints, most commonly the knee.[26] Cardiac symptoms, from inflammation and AV heart block *(Lyme carditis)*, may require hospitalization. Death from Lyme disease is rare but increases if carditis develops.[24] Facial palsy is the most common neurologic effect. Months to years later, memory problems and paresthesia in the feet may occur.[26]

Diagnosis is often based on the manifestations, especially EM, and a history of exposure in an at-risk area. A two-step laboratory testing process can confirm the diagnosis.[27] The first step is the enzyme immunoassay (EIA), an antibody test. It will be positive for most people with Lyme disease. If the EIA is positive or inconclusive, a Western blot test is done. Both tests must be positive for a diagnosis of Lyme disease. It takes a few weeks before antibody levels are sufficient to test. False-negative results can happen if the test is done too soon.[27]

Active lesions are treated with oral antibiotics. Ten to fourteen days of doxycycline, cefuroxime, or amoxicillin effectively treat early-stage infection and prevent later stages of the disease.[27] In areas where Lyme disease is endemic, a single dose of doxycycline taken within 72 hours of tick removal is effective in reducing risk of disease. Antibiotic treatment is extended up to 4 weeks for prolonged symptoms.

Reducing exposure to ticks through pesticide use and skin treatment before going to high-risk areas is the best way to prevent Lyme disease. Teaching on avoiding tick bites is outlined in Table 69.14.

SEPTIC ARTHRITIS

Septic arthritis (infectious arthritis) is caused by microorganisms invading the joint cavity. These organisms travel through the bloodstream from another site of active infection and colonize the joint. The joint is highly vascular and may already be damaged from trauma or disease. Organisms can be introduced directly through trauma or surgical incision.

Any infectious agent can cause septic arthritis, especially in immunocompromised patients. *Staphylococcus aureus* is the most common cause.[28] Factors that increase infection risk include (1) decreased host resistance (e.g., RA, systemic lupus erythematosus [SLE]), (2) treatment with corticosteroids or immunosuppressive drugs, (3) debilitating chronic illness (e.g., diabetes), (4) joint trauma or an artificial joint, (5) skin conditions (e.g., psoriasis, eczema), and (6) IV drug use.[28]

Large joints, such as the knee and hip, are most often affected. Local inflammation of the joint cavity causes severe pain, warmth, redness, and swelling. Patients may refuse to move the joint. Septic arthritis of the hip may cause *avascular necrosis.* Fever, chills, and tachycardia are often present.

Diagnosis may be made by joint aspiration *(arthrocentesis)* and synovial fluid culture and Gram stain.[28] WBCs may be elevated with a shift to the left (increased neutrophils and elevated bands). WBC count may be low early in the infectious process, especially in those who are immunosuppressed. Blood

TABLE 69.14 PATIENT & CAREGIVER TEACHING

Prevent Tick Bites

Include the following instructions when teaching patients how to prevent Lyme disease:

- Expect ticks in grassy, brushy, or wooded areas or on animals.
- Treat clothing and gear with products containing 0.5% permethrin.
- Use insect repellents containing DEET, picaridin, IR3535, oil of lemon eucalyptus (OLE), para-menthane-diol (PMD), or 2-undecanone.
- Walk in the center of trails, not on brushy and grassy borders.
- Remove leaf litter from yards.
- Clear tall grasses and brush around homes and at the edge of lawns.
- Place a 3-ft-wide barrier of wood chips or gravel between lawns and wooded areas.
- Mow the lawn frequently.
- Stack wood neatly and in a dry area.
- Keep playground equipment, decks, and patios away from yard edges and trees.
- Fence yards to discourage unwelcome animals (such as deer, raccoons, and stray dogs) from entering your yard.
- Remove old furniture, mattresses, or trash from the yard that may give ticks a place to hide.
- Do not walk in tall grasses and brush or sit on logs.
- Mow grass frequently. Remove brush around paths, buildings, and campsites to create tick-safe zones.
- Move woodpiles and bird feeders away from your house. Discourage deer (main source of food for adult ticks) from being in the area.
- Keep playground equipment and decks away from yard edges and in a sunny location if possible.
- Wear long pants or nylon tights of tightly woven, light-colored fabric so that you can easily see ticks.
- Tuck pants into boots or long socks, wear long-sleeved shirts tucked into pants, and wear closed-toed shoes when hiking.
- Check often for ticks crawling from pant legs to open skin.
- Thoroughly inspect and wash clothes with hot water. Cold and tepid water will not kill ticks. Placing clothing in dryer on high heat kills ticks.
- Examine gear and pets.
- Shower soon after being outdoors. Showering within 2 hours of coming indoors has been shown to reduce your risk of getting Lyme disease.
- Do a full body check for ticks after being outdoors. Check behind ears, under arms, back of knees, around hair line, between legs, and around the waist.
- Have pets wear tick collars and inspect them often. Do not allow pets on furniture or beds.

Include the following instructions when teaching patients and caregivers living in endemic areas:

- Use clean, fine-tipped tweezers to grasp the tick as close to the skin's surface as possible.
- Pull upward with steady, even pressure. Do not twist or jerk the tick; this can cause the mouth parts to break off and remain in the skin. If this happens, remove the mouth parts with tweezers. If you cannot remove the mouth easily with tweezers, leave it alone and let the skin heal.
- After removing the tick, thoroughly clean the bite area and your hands with rubbing alcohol or soap and water.
- If you develop a rash or fever within several days to weeks after removing a tick, see your doctor.
- Never crush a tick with your fingers. Dispose of a live tick by putting it in alcohol, placing it in a sealed bag/container, wrapping it tightly in tape, or flushing it down the toilet.

Data from CDC: *Ticks: preventing tick bites.* Retrieved from https://www.cdc.gov/ticks/prevention/index.html and CDC: *Ticks: what to do after a tick bite.* Retrieved from https://www.cdc.gov/ticks/after-a-tick-bite/index.html.

cultures for aerobic and anaerobic organisms should be obtained. Imaging studies can assess joint effusion, joint damage, or damage to a prosthesis.

Emergent synovial fluid aspiration or surgical drainage by arthroscopy or needle aspirations is a cornerstone of treatment. Permanent joint damage can occur without rapid intervention. Broad-spectrum IV antibiotics are often started before culture results are available. Once the organism is known, more specific antibiotics can be prescribed. IV antibiotics are followed with oral antibiotics. Antibiotic treatment lasts 2 to 6 weeks. If an artificial joint is infected, treatment may involve debridement or removing the joint and replacing it temporarily with a joint spacer. The spacer is made with antibiotic cement. If the artificial joint cannot be removed, several months of oral antibiotics are prescribed to avoid recurrence of infection. If no improvement is seen after 6 days of an antibiotic, Lyme disease should be ruled out.[28]

Assess and monitor joint inflammation, pain, and fever. To manage pain, use resting splints to immobilize affected joints. Typically, immobilization is not required after 3 days. Local hot therapy can decrease pain. Gentle ROM exercises are started as soon as tolerated to prevent muscle atrophy and joint contractures. Explain the need for antibiotic compliance and treatment duration. Use strict aseptic technique when assisting with joint aspiration. Despite antibiotic treatment, mortality occurs in up to 15% of hospitalized patients.

SPONDYLOARTHROPATHIES

The *spondyloarthropathies* are a group of multisystem inflammatory disorders that affect the spine, peripheral joints, and periarticular structures. These disorders include axial (ankylosing spondylitis) and peripheral spondyloarthritis (psoriatic arthritis, reactive arthritis). All spondyloarthropathies are *seronegative arthropathies* (negative for RF). Over 3.2 million adults in the United States have a form of spondyloarthritis.[29]

Pain in the lower back and hips in the morning or after periods of inactivity is the primary symptom of spondyloarthropathies. This may make it hard to discern among them in early disease. Other related conditions may include peripheral joint involvement (mainly of the lower extremities), pain and redness of the eyes (uveitis), intestinal inflammation, and psoriasis. Genetic and environment factors play a role in the development. Inheriting HLA-B27 is strongly associated with these diseases.[30] HLAs and their relationship to autoimmune diseases are discussed in Chapter 14.

AXIAL SPONDYLITIS

Axial spondylitis (axSpA) is a chronic inflammatory disease that mainly affects the axial skeleton, sacroiliac joints, intervertebral disc spaces, and costovertebral articulations. There are 2 types: radiographic axSpA (r-axSpA) and nonradiographic axSpA (nr-axSpA). Males are more likely to develop r-axSpA with spine damage that we can see on x-ray. With nr-axSpA, changes show on MRI rather than x-ray. White, Asian, and Hispanic are at increased risk. AxSpA most often begins between age 30 and 40 but can start in adolescence.[29]

Etiology and Pathophysiology

We do not know the cause of axSpA. The HLA-B27 antigen is found in about 90% of patients with axSpA, but only 8% of the general population. The presence of this antigen makes patients more susceptible to axSpA.[30]

Inflammation where tendons and ligaments attach to bone (*enthesitis*) leads to release of additional proinflammatory cytokines and the formation of granulation tissue. This stimulates new bone growth, forming spurs, fibrous scars, and bone fusion (ankylosis). Inflammation can affect extraarticular tissues, including eyes, lungs, heart, kidneys, and peripheral nervous system.

Clinical Manifestations and Complications

Symmetric sacroiliitis and progressive inflammatory arthritis of the axial skeleton are characteristic of axSpA. Patients may have dull, aching low back pain; stiffness; and limited motion that is worse during the night and in the morning but improves with mild activity. In females, early symptoms may include pain and stiffness in the neck rather than the lower back. Many patients develop uveitis, which can lead to permanent vision damage. This may occur before back and hip pain. Patients with axSpA may have chest pain and sternocostal tenderness, which can be confused with angina.

Most people with axSpA remain fully independent. In advanced disease, disability can occur from postural changes (Fig. 69.8). Impaired spinal ROM and fusion, along with vision

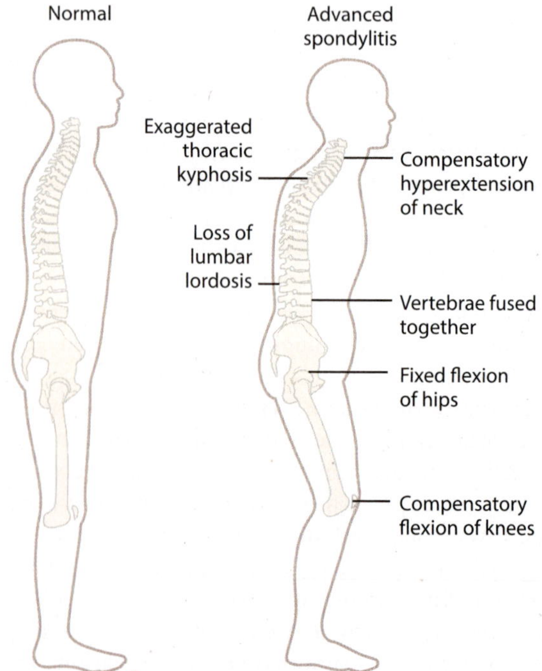

Fig. 69.8 Posture changes in patient with axial spondylitis.

problems, raise concerns about safe ambulation. Osteoporosis from inflammation and immobility increases the risk for fracture. Serious complications include aortic insufficiency, cardiac conduction changes, cardiomyopathy, and pulmonary fibrosis. Compression of nerves at the end of the spinal cord (cauda equina syndrome) can occur. This results in lower extremity weakness, sciatica, sexual dysfunction, urinary retention or incontinence, and bowel incontinence.[31]

Diagnostic Studies

MRI and CT scans are useful in assessing early cartilage changes. X-rays are important in monitoring of axSpA. They are limited in detecting early vertebral changes, but in later disease can detect the appearance of calcifications *(syndesmophytes)* that bridge from one vertebra to another causing spinal fusion (bamboo spine). An increased ESR and mild anemia from chronic inflammation may be seen. HLA-B27 testing may help confirm the diagnosis.

Interprofessional and Nursing Management

Care goals are aimed at maintaining maximal skeletal mobility while decreasing pain and inflammation. Heat applications help relieve stiffness and tight muscles. NSAIDs and salicylates are prescribed for pain and inflammation. If active disease persists, TNF inhibitors like etanercept are recommended. TNF inhibitors reduce active inflammation and improve spinal mobility. Monoclonal antibodies that block cytokine IL-17A are an option.[32] Local corticosteroid injections may help relieve symptoms.

Once pain and stiffness are managed, exercise is essential to increase balance, flexibility, endurance, and bone density. Good posture is important to minimize spinal deformity. PT includes gentle, graded stretching; strengthening the spine; and maintaining ROM. The exercise plan should include back, neck, and chest stretches. Hydrotherapy (e.g., sauna, steam bath) can decrease pain and promote spinal extension. Patients do not usually need surgery, but may choose surgery (spinal osteotomy, joint replacement) to reduce pain and improve mobility (see Chapter 67). Assess chest expansion as part of baseline ROM assessment.

Teach patients about the disease and principles of therapy. The home management program should include regular exercise, attention to posture, local moist heat applications, and drug therapy. Smoking cessation can reduce the risk of lung complications in persons with reduced chest expansion.

Discourage physical exertion during periods of increased disease activity. Proper positioning is essential during exacerbation. Encourage patients to use a firm mattress and sleep on their back with a flat pillow. Stress the need to avoid spinal flexion (e.g., leaning over a desk); heavy lifting; and prolonged walking, standing, or sitting. Encourage sports that involve natural stretching, such as swimming and racquet games. Family counseling and vocational rehabilitation may be needed.

Encourage a plant-based or Mediterranean diet, rich in omega-3 fatty acids, antioxidants, and fiber. Avoid processed foods and sugary snacks. Turmeric, curcumin, and ginger may be used to reduce inflammation. Meditation, hypnosis, relaxation therapy, and music therapy can all relax muscle tension and related pain.[32]

PERIPHERAL SPONDYLOARTHRITIS

Peripheral spondyloarthritis is a group of disorders whose primary symptoms are caused by inflammatory arthritis in the peripheral joints and tendons, rather than the spine and hips.

PSORIATIC ARTHRITIS

Psoriatic arthritis (PsA) is an autoimmune peripheral spondyloarthritis that affects about one-third of people with psoriasis.[33] *Psoriasis* is a common inflammatory skin disorder characterized by red, irritated, and scaly patches on elbows, knees, and scalp. We do not know the exact cause of PsA. A combination of immune, genetic, and environment factors is likely. HLA-B27 antigens make a person more susceptible to PsA. Onset can be at any age. It is generally between 30 and 50. Psoriasis occurs before arthritis symptoms by many years.

PsA occurs in different forms. Asymmetric oligoarticular arthritis involves 1 to 4 different joints on each side of the body. Symmetric polyarthritis affects 5 or more joints on both sides of the body at the same time, like RA. PsA causes inflammation and pain in the distal joints at the end of the fingers. Wrists, knees, and ankles may be involved. Throbbing pain, reduced movement, and fatigue are present. Fingernails and toenails may get small pits and yellow/brown discoloration.[33] *Arthritis mutilans* affects less than 5% of people with PsA. It is the most severe form of the disease, causing complete destruction of small joints. A "pencil in cup" deformity occurs with arthritis mutilans. One end of the metacarpal or phalange is thinned and narrowed to a point, and the bone on the other end of the joint is eroded out like a cup. The bones continue to grind against each other, destroying more bone.

There is no definitive diagnostic test for PsA. Diagnosis is made through history, physical examination, and x-rays. On x-ray, the cartilage loss and erosion are similar to RA. Advanced disease often shows widened joint spaces. Patients may have increased ESR and uric acid levels with mild anemia. Gout and RA must be excluded because of similar presentation. PsA treatment includes splinting, protecting painful inflamed joints, and PT. Starting NSAIDs early in the course of the disease helps with inflammation. Local corticosteroids, DMARDs (methotrexate, tofacitinib), BRMs (etanercept, adalimumab, infliximab), and immunosuppressants (apremilast) are used for joint and skin symptoms.

REACTIVE ARTHRITIS

Reactive arthritis is a peripheral spondyloarthritis associated with a triad of symptoms: urethritis, conjunctivitis, and arthritis. We believe the cause is an autoimmune response to an infection. Some known pathogens causing ReA include *Chlamydia trachomatis, Neisseria gonorrhea, Salmonella enteritidis, Shigella flexneri,* and *Campylobacter jejuni.* Genetic predisposition is present for those positive for HLA-B27. ReA occurs more often in males under 40 years old.

When specific pathogens transmitted by sexual contact or contaminated food enter circulation, they activate cytotoxic T cells, which then attack the synovium and other self-antigens. Unlike septic arthritis, infection is not present in the joints.[34] Urethritis or cervicitis develops within 1 to 2 weeks after exposure to sexually transmitted pathogens. Low-grade fever, conjunctivitis, and asymmetric arthritis may occur over the next several weeks. Arthritis is usually the last symptom to appear. Toes and the large joints of the lower extremities are most often involved. No more than 6 joints are involved at any time. Lower back pain may occur with severe ReA. Lesions involving the skin and mucous membranes occur as small, painless, superficial red bumps or ulcerations on the tongue, oral mucosa, foot, or glans penis. Achilles tendinitis or plantar fasciitis may occur.

Assessment reveals swollen fingers or toes, heel pain, genital ulcerations, or diarrhea within 4 weeks before the onset of arthritis symptoms. Stool, urine, and cervical cultures are examined for causative bacteria. ESR and CRP may be increased. No specific diagnostic test for ReA exists. Synovial fluid aspiration is analyzed. Patients with untreated HIV often have ReA; thus patients diagnosed with ReA should be tested for HIV.

Most patients recover with return of full joint function within 3 to 5 months of initial symptoms. Antibiotics are only used with an active infection. Antibiotics have no effect on arthritis or other symptoms of ReA. Treatment is based on symptoms. NSAIDs are given to treat inflammation and pain. DMARDs (sulfasalazine) may be used if joint symptoms do not resolve with NSAIDs. TNF inhibitors are only used if other treatments fail. Topical ophthalmic corticosteroids are helpful for uveitis. Intraarticular corticosteroids are used to decrease joint inflammation. PT and strengthening exercises may help muscles and joints during recovery. Around 30% develop mild, chronic arthritis.[34]

OTHER AUTOIMMUNE PROBLEMS

SYSTEMIC LUPUS ERYTHEMATOSUS

Systemic lupus erythematosus (SLE) is a multisystem inflammatory autoimmune disease. It affects the skin, joints, and serous membranes (pleura, pericardium). Complications occur in renal, hematologic, cardiac, pulmonary, and neurologic systems. SLE has an unpredictable course with alternating periods of remission and exacerbation (flares).[35]

Over 200,000 people in the United States have SLE.[36] The incidence and severity are highest in Black, Asian American, Hispanic, Native American, and Pacific Islander persons.[36] Black patients are likely to die 10 years earlier than White patients with SLE.[36] Females have 10 times the risk of developing SLE. It usually develops between ages 15 and 44 years.

Etiology and Pathophysiology

SLE originates from complex interactions among genetic, hormonal, environment, and immune factors. We do not know the cause of the autoimmune response in SLE. Genetic influence is suspected based on the high prevalence of SLE among family members. Over 100 contributing gene mutations have been identified. The most common mutations are HLA related.[37] Infections, like Epstein Barr, may stimulate autoimmunity.

Hormones play a role in SLE. Estrogen and prolactin promote autoimmunity. Flares commonly occur around menses, when taking oral contraceptives, or when using estrogen hormone replacement therapy after menopause.

Environment factors like exposure to sun, ultraviolet light, and chemicals contribute to SLE. Exposure to silica dust in agricultural or industrial settings can be a factor. Drug triggers include those that make a person more sensitive to the sun (e.g., sulfa drugs, diuretics, tetracycline). Drug-induced SLE generally occurs after long-term continuous therapy with a causative drug. Procainamide and hydralazine are the most common medications contributing to SLE.

The body makes autoantibodies against nucleic acids (DNA), erythrocytes, coagulation proteins, lymphocytes, platelets, and many other self-proteins. B cells and T cells become overactive. Circulating immune complexes with autoantibodies against DNA are deposited in the basement membranes of capillaries in the joints and other body tissues. These complexes activate the complement system, triggering inflammation and causing tissue destruction and the symptoms of SLE.[37] Specific disease symptoms depend on the involved cell types or organs. SLE is a type III hypersensitivity response (see Chapter 14).

Clinical Manifestations and Complications

The severity of SLE varies widely. It ranges from a mild cutaneous response to a rapidly progressive multiorgan disease (Fig. 69.9). No characteristic pattern occurs in the progression of SLE. The circulating immune complexes can affect any organ. General problems, such as fever, weight loss, joint pain, malaise, and fatigue, may precede a flare. Other commonly reported symptoms include swelling of hands, feet, and periorbital tissue; headaches; low-grade fever; sensitivity to sunlight and fluorescent light; and chest pain with deep breathing.[37]

Skin Problems

Vascular skin lesions can appear anywhere. Lesions are most likely to develop on sun-exposed areas. Severe skin reactions can occur in people who are sensitive to sunlight *(photosensitivity).*

Some forms of SLE are limited to the skin. People with *chronic cutaneous lupus erythematosus* (CCLE) have photosensitive discoid (round, coin-shaped) papules or plaque-type

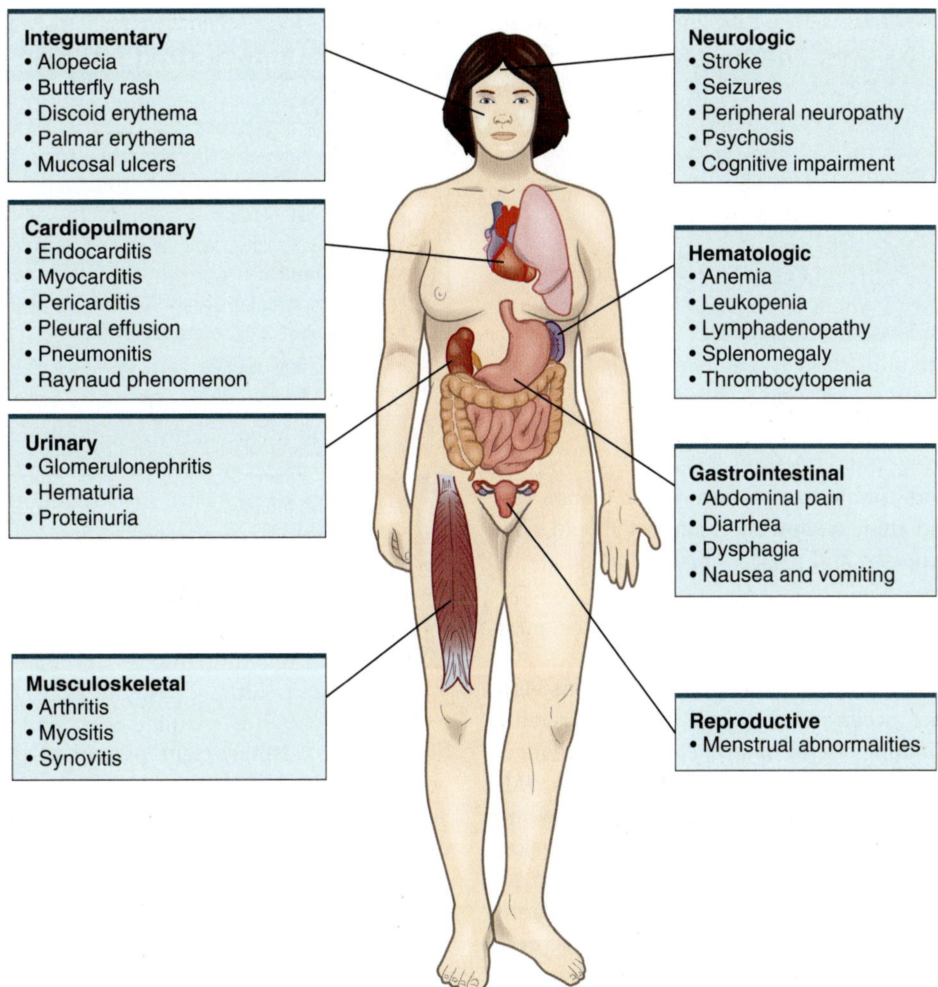

Fig. 69.9 Multisystem involvement in SLE.

lesions on the scalp and face. Some lesions may scar. Some patients with CCLE later develop lupus in other organ systems. *Subacute cutaneous lupus erythematosus* (SCLE) is marked by widespread areas of red, ring-shaped lesions. The lesion of *acute cutaneous lupus* is the flat, red, classic butterfly rash over the cheeks and bridge of the nose *(malar rash)* that looks like a sunburn (Fig. 69.10). It may be a raised, red, and itchy rash on the cheeks and nasal bridge.[36] Alopecia is common. Hair loss may be caused by a dry, scaly, and atrophied scalp. Alopecia can occur in discoid lesions. Hair may grow back during remission. Painless oral or nasopharyngeal ulcers are frequently present.

Musculoskeletal Problems

Arthritis occurs in up to 90% of patients with SLE. Pain and morning stiffness occur in multiple symmetric joints *(polyarthralgia)*. Small joints of the hands, wrist, and knees are commonly affected. Lupus arthritis is nonerosive. Inflammation of the tendons and ligaments can cause joint looseness, bone movement, and deformity (e.g., swan neck deformity of the fingers [Fig. 69.4D], ulnar deviation, and subluxation). Patients have increased risk for bone loss and fracture.

Cardiopulmonary Problems

SLE can cause pleurisy and interstitial pneumonia. Tachypnea and cough are cues to the presence of lung disease. Cardiac involvement may include dysrhythmias resulting from fibrosis of the SA and AV nodes. Inflammation of any layer of the heart may occur, but pericarditis is the most common. This is the leading cause of death among patients with SLE. Cardiac valves develop inflammatory growths and tissue thickening. SLE often causes inflamed coronary arteries and atherosclerosis.[37] People with SLE can get *antiphospholipid syndrome* (APS). Antiphospholipid antibodies attack fat molecules, making the blood more likely to clot in arteries and veins. This increases risk for stroke, gangrene, deep venous thrombosis (DVT), and heart attack.

Renal Problems

About half of patients with SLE develop kidney disease. Renal involvement occurs early in the process. Manifestations vary from mild proteinuria to rapidly progressive glomerulonephritis. Scarring and permanent damage can lead to end-stage renal disease (ESRD). Patients may have hypertension, foamy

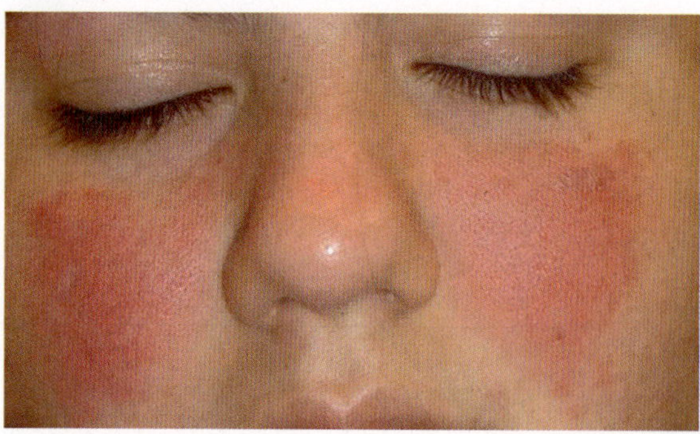

Fig. 69.10 Butterfly rash of SLE. (From Yale Dermatology Residents' Slide Collection. In Bolognia JL, Schaffer JV, Duncan KO, et al: *Dermatology essentials,* Philadelphia, 2014, Elsevier.)

urine, hematuria, and elevated creatinine. Renal biopsy can confirm diagnosis and guide treatment. Treatment should slow progression of nephropathy and preserve renal function.

Nervous System Problems

Central and peripheral nervous system manifestations and psychiatric symptoms occur. These range from intractable headaches to demyelinating disease or stroke. Seizure activity is associated with increased disease activity. Neuropsychiatric SLE (NPSLE) occurs in 1 of 2 ways. *Focal NPSLE* may be caused by clots. This leads to headaches, especially during a flare. Strokes or aseptic meningitis may occur. *Diffuse NPSLE* is caused by inflammation. Cognitive symptoms of memory loss, confusion, difficulty expressing themselves, psychosis, anxiety, or depression can occur.[37]

Hematologic Problems

Antibodies against blood cells lead to chronic anemia, leukopenia, thrombocytopenia, and coagulation problems. Nontender lymphadenopathy is often present. People with SLE are likely to be resistant to the blood-thinning effects of aspirin.

Infection

Patients have increased susceptibility to infection. This may be caused by leukopenia, autoantibodies that attack the immune system, and immunosuppressive effects of medication. The respiratory and urinary tracts are the most common sites for infection. Increased susceptibility to COVID-19, shingles, and candidiasis is present. Vaccinations are safe for patients with SLE. Patients receiving corticosteroids or cytotoxic drugs must avoid live virus vaccines. Sulfa antibiotics are used with caution because they can cause increased sensitivity to light.

Diagnostic Studies

There is no specific diagnostic test for SLE. Differentiating SLE from other autoimmune diseases is necessary. History, physical, and 11 specific criteria are used to establish the diagnosis (Table 69.15). Ninety-eight percent of persons with SLE are positive for ANA.[38]

TABLE 69.15 Diagnostic Criteria for Systemic Lupus Erythematosus

A person is recognized as having SLE if 4 or more of the criteria are present, serially or simultaneously, during any interval of observation:

- Antinuclear antibody (ANA): abnormal titer
- Discoid rash: raised patches with keratotic scaling, follicular plugging; scarring in older lesions
- Hematologic disorder: hemolytic anemia, leukopenia, lymphopenia, or thrombocytopenia
- Immunologic disorder: anti-dsDNA antibody, antibody to Sm (Smith) nuclear antigen, antiphospholipid antibodies
- Malar rash: fixed redness, flat or raised (butterfly rash)
- Oral ulcers: usually painless
- Neurologic disorder: seizures or psychosis (in the absence of causative drugs or known metabolic disorders)
- Nonerosive arthritis: 2 or more peripheral joints with tenderness, swelling, and effusion
- Serositis: pleuritis or pericarditis
- Photosensitivity: worsening symptoms after UV exposure
- Renal disorder: hematuria, persistent proteinuria, casts in urine, reduced kidney function

Testing for anti–double-stranded DNA antibodies (anti-dsDNA), anti-Smith (Sm) antibodies, and antiphospholipid antibodies (anticardiolipin, lupus anticoagulant) is highly specific for SLE. Increased ESR and CRP indicate nonspecific inflammation.

Interprofessional Care

There is no cure for SLE. Treatment goals include preventing organ damage and attaining remission of active disease. Age, sex, social health determinants, comorbidities, and severity influence survival. A major challenge is managing active disease while preventing complications of treatment. SLE has a good prognosis for most people. Early detection and treatment adherence improve outcomes. Prognosis can be improved with ongoing assessment, prompt recognition of organ involvement, and effective treatment plans (Table 69.16). Serial anti-DNA titers and serum complement help monitor disease activity and medication effectiveness.

Drug Therapy

NSAIDs are an important intervention, especially for patients with mild joint pain. Patients may need to try several different NSAIDs to find the most effective one. Monitor those on long-term NSAID therapy for GI, cardiac, and renal effects.

Antimalarial agents, such as hydroxychloroquine (HCQ), are the foundation of treatment for skin and joint manifestations. HCQ has antiinflammatory properties, delays UV light absorption, and reduces flares. It helps prevent pleurisy and pericarditis. HCQ has antithrombotic properties that decrease

TABLE 69.16 Interprofessional Care

SLE

Diagnostic Assessment
- History and physical assessment
- Antibodies (ANA, anti-dsDNA, anti-Sm, antiphospholipid)
- CBC
- Serum complement (C3, C4)
- Urinalysis: renal involvement
- X-ray of affected joints
- Chest x-ray: pleural involvement
- ECG: cardiac involvement

Management

Drug Therapy
- NSAIDs or acetaminophen for mild disease
- DMARD (e.g., methotrexate)
- Antimalarials (e.g., hydroxychloroquine)
- Corticosteroids for flares and severe disease
- Immunosuppressive drugs (e.g., tacrolimus)
- BRMs (belimumab, rituximab)
- Anticoagulants (low-molecular-weight heparin, warfarin)
- Renin-angiotensin blockers

Other Interventions
- Turmeric
- Omega-3
- Acupuncture
- Sleep hygiene
- Stress management
- Sun protection

ANA, Antinuclear antibody; *BRM,* biologic response modifier; *DMARD,* disease-modifying antirheumatic drug.

the risk of clots.[37] Remind patients to tell the provider about other prescription or OTC drugs because of many unsafe drug interactions.

DRUG ALERT

Hydroxychloroquine

- Report an irregular heart rate or chest pain because of the risk of life-threatening dysrhythmia.
- Patients should have an eye examination at the beginning of treatment and every year to monitor for retinopathy.
- Monitor for hypoglycemia.

If a patient cannot tolerate an antimalarial agent, methotrexate may be used. Topical immunomodulators can treat serious skin lesions. Tacrolimus (Protopic, Prograf) and pimecrolimus suppress immune activity in the skin, including malar rash and discoid lesions. Systemic corticosteroids are used for pleurisy and pericarditis. They can rapidly reduce inflammation during a flare. Corticosteroids should be limited to the lowest dose for the shortest possible time. Taper the steroid dose slowly rather than stopping therapy abruptly.

Immunosuppressive drugs, such as azathioprine and cyclophosphamide, reduce end-organ damage. Monitor for toxicity and side effects (glucose control, renal function). Because antiphospholipid antibodies induce life-threatening blood clots, lifelong anticoagulants, such as low-molecular-weight heparin, may be prescribed.

Treatment of lupus nephritis includes renin angiotensin–blocking medications to protect kidney function. The human monoclonal antibody belimumab (Benlysta) may reduce B-cell activity and control autoimmune activity. Immunosuppressive agents (e.g., cyclosporin, tacrolimus) are used if proteinuria is present. Immunosuppressant treatment should be maintained for at least 3 years.[37] IV steroids are used during the initial treatment period for severe nephritis or when cytotoxic agents have not yet taken effect. Kidney failure may require renal replacement therapy, dialysis, or kidney transplant.

NURSING MANAGEMENT: SLE

Assessment

Subjective and objective data you should obtain from patients with SLE are outlined in Table 69.17. During a disease flare, patients may quickly become very ill. Assess the effect of pain and fatigue on ability to perform ADLs. Assess fever, joint inflammation, and limited motion. Monitor weight, intake and output, and cardiac and pulmonary status. Collect 24-hour urine samples for protein and creatinine clearance as ordered. Observe for signs of bleeding resulting from drug therapy (e.g., bruising, tarry stools).

Assess neurologic function. Observe for vision problems, headaches, personality changes, seizures, and memory loss. Psychosis may result from NPSLE or be an effect of corticosteroid therapy. Nerve irritation of the extremities *(peripheral neuropathy)* may cause numbness, tingling, and weakness of the hands and feet.

Clinical Problems

Clinical problems for patients with SLE may include:
- Musculoskeletal problems
- Impaired role performance
- Impaired tissue integrity

Additional information on clinical problems and interventions for patients with SLE is presented in eNursing Care Plan 69.2 (available on the website for this chapter).

Planning

Overall goals are that patients with SLE will (1) have acceptable pain management, (2) show awareness of and avoid activities that increase disease activity, and (3) maintain optimal role function and positive self-image.

Implementation

The unpredictable nature of SLE presents many challenges for patients and caregivers. Physical, psychologic, and sociocultural problems linked to long-term management require varied

TABLE 69.17 NURSING ASSESSMENT

SLE

Subjective Data	Objective Data
Important Health Information	**Cardiovascular**
Health history: Exposure to ultraviolet light or sun, drugs, chemicals, viral infections. Physical or psychologic stress. States of ↑ estrogen activity, pregnancy, postpartum period. Pattern of remissions and flares	Vasculitis, pericardial friction rub, hypertension, edema, dysrhythmias, murmurs. Bilateral, symmetric pallor and cyanosis of fingers, blood clots.
Medications: Oral contraceptives, procainamide, hydralazine, antiseizure drugs, corticosteroids, NSAIDs	**General** Fever, lymphadenopathy, periorbital edema
Functional Health Patterns	**GI** Oral and pharyngeal ulcers; splenomegaly
Health perception–health management: Family history of autoimmune disorders, frequent infections, malaise, impact of disease on functional ability	**Musculoskeletal** Myopathy, myositis, arthritis
Nutritional-metabolic: Weight loss, oral and nasal ulcers, nausea and vomiting, dry mouth *(xerostomia)*, dysphagia, photosensitivity with rash, frequent infections	**Neurologic** Facial weakness, peripheral neuropathies, papilledema, dysarthria, confusion, hallucination, disorientation, psychosis, seizures, aphasia
Elimination: Urine output, bowel activity	**Respiratory** Pleural friction rub, ↓ breath sounds, cough
Activity-exercise: Morning stiffness, joint swelling and deformity, shortness of breath *(dyspnea)*, excessive fatigue, ADLs	**Skin** Alopecia. Dry, scaly scalp. Keratoconjunctivitis, malar rash, discoid lesions, redness at fingernails or toenails, purpura, petechiae.
Sleep-rest: Insomnia	**Possible Diagnostic Findings** Presence of anti-dsDNA, anti-Sm, or antinuclear antibodies. Anemia, leukopenia, thrombocytopenia. ↑ ESR, ↑ creatinine. Microscopic hematuria, proteinuria, casts in urine. Pericarditis or pleural effusion on chest x-ray or ultrasound.
Cognitive-perceptual: Vision problems, vertigo, headache, arthralgia, chest pain (pericardial, pleuritic), abdominal pain. Pain, aching, cold fingers with numbness and tingling	
Sexuality-reproductive: Amenorrhea, irregular menstrual periods	
Coping–stress tolerance: Depression, withdrawal, support system	

ESR, Erythrocyte sedimentation rate.

approaches and skills. Referrals to multiple specialists are likely during the course of the disease. Patient teaching for SLE is covered in Table 69.18.

Patient involvement in treatment decisions is necessary for self-management. Help them understand that adherence to the treatment plan is no guarantee against flares. Encourage patients to keep a journal recording treatments, medications, side effects, and triggers. Discuss these with the treatment team. Help patients and caregivers eliminate or reduce exposure to things that trigger flares. During a flare, patients should rest, reduce stress, eat a balanced diet, and activate their support system.

Explain the nature of SLE, treatments, and all diagnostic procedures. Teach patients about their drug therapy. Include indications, proper administration, and managing side effects. Help patients understand that abruptly stopping a drug may worsen disease activity.

Role Performance

Patients with SLE face many psychosocial issues. Supportive therapies may be as important as medical treatment in helping patients cope with the disease. Provide emotional support for patients and caregivers, especially during a disease flare. Help them find assistance with role responsibilities during flares if necessary.

Stress the need to plan recreational and work activities. Teach patients ways to avoid UV light. Vitamin D supplements may be given. Young adults may find sun restrictions and physical limitations hard to follow. Help patients develop reasonable goals for improving or maintaining mobility, energy, and self-esteem. Connect patients who are worried how SLE may affect marriage and career with counseling. Discuss how to approach employers, teachers, and coworkers about the impact of SLE.

SLE and Pregnancy

Because SLE is most common in females of childbearing age, family planning and contraception are necessary. Pregnancy should be planned when disease has minimal activity. Couples may worry about hereditary aspects and if their children will have SLE.

Many SLE drugs are teratogenic. Drugs like methotrexate should be stopped several months before pregnancy. Infertility may result from organ damage or medication. Immune complexes and inflammation on the placenta and blood vessels increase risk for spontaneous abortion, stillbirth, and

TABLE 69.18 PATIENT & CAREGIVER TEACHING

SLE

Include the following information in the teaching plan for patients with SLE and the caregiver:

- Disease process
- Names of drugs, actions, side effects, dosage, administration
- Pain management strategies
- Energy conservation and pacing techniques
- Therapeutic exercise, heat therapy for arthralgia
- Relaxation therapy: stress management
- Avoid exposure to people with infection
- Plant-based, antiinflammatory diet; avoid high-fat foods
- Encourage vitamin D_3 intake
- Avoid drying soaps, powders, household chemicals
- Use sunscreen protection (at least SPF 15), sunglasses, hats, and protective clothing; avoid sun exposure from 11:00 AM to 3:00 PM
- Need for regular medical and laboratory follow-up
- Marital and pregnancy counseling as needed
- Signs of cardiac, pleural, or renal involvement
- Community resources and health care agencies
- Promote healthy sleep hygiene

intrauterine growth restriction. Hypertension and renal damage also increase the risk of complications. Increased clot formation further endangers the pregnancy. Flares are common during the postpartum period. Patients who show effects in renal, lung, CNS, or cardiovascular systems should discuss if pregnancy is safe with their HCP.

◆ Evaluation

Expected outcomes are that patients with SLE will:

- Use energy-conservation techniques
- Adapt lifestyle to current abilities
- Maintain skin integrity with use of topical treatments and sun protection
- Prevent disease flares

SCLERODERMA

Scleroderma is an autoimmune disorder characterized by fibrotic, degenerative, and inflammatory changes in skin and internal organs. The usual age at onset is between 25 and 55 years. About 300,000 Americans have the disease. Around 80% are female.[39]

Localized scleroderma mainly affects the skin. Children are more frequently affected. Autoantibodies for local scleroderma are more common in Japanese Americans. *Systemic scleroderma (systemic sclerosis [SSc])* affects people of all ethnic groups. Black persons have an increased prevalence and severity.[39] SSc affects skin, blood vessels, synovium, skeletal muscle, and internal organs.

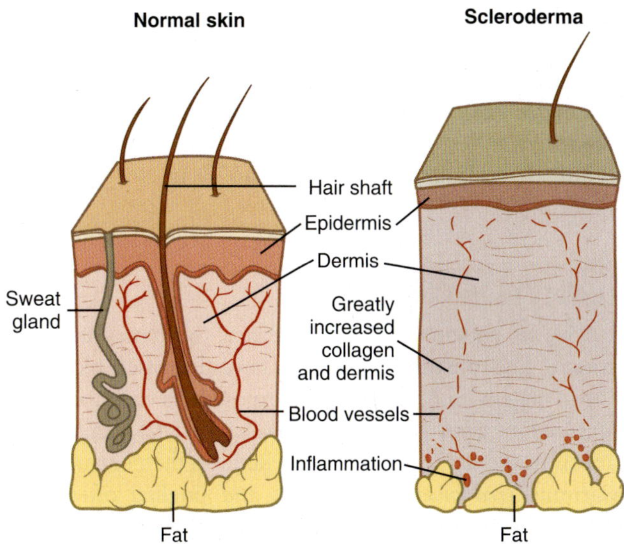

Fig. 69.11 Skin changes in scleroderma.

Etiology and Pathophysiology

We do not know the cause of scleroderma. We think an environment event in a genetically susceptible person causes autoantibodies to attack the body's own proteins. Silica, radiation, plastics, and solvents are known environment triggers. Eleven autoantibodies have been associated with scleroderma. The most common are antitopoisomerase, anticentromere, RNA polymerase III, and antinuclear antibody.[40] Autoimmune activity activates fibroblasts and stimulates excessive production of collagen and other proteins (Fig. 69.11). The excess collagen leads to skin tightening, thickening, and fibrosis. Collagen overproduction alters function in the lungs, heart, and gastrointestinal (GI) tract. Fibrosis and occlusion of small arteries and arterioles are usually present.

Clinical Manifestations

Local scleroderma causes thick patches or streaks that feel waxy. It is usually limited to a few patchy areas on the skin or fibrous thickening on extremities. It usually spreads above the knees or elbows. Local disease may improve without treatment.

SSc is divided into 2 subtypes: limited and diffuse.[41] *Diffuse scleroderma* involves progressive and widespread thickening and hardening of tissue and organs. This occurs in the hands, arms, thighs, chest, abdomen, and face. Organs involved are the blood vessels, heart, joints, muscles, and digestive system. Both types can cause lung problems. *Limited scleroderma,* or CREST syndrome, affects the face, fingers, hands, and lower arms and legs. It has a slow onset. Symptoms include

- **C**alcinosis: painful deposits of calcium in the skin of fingers, forearms, and pressure points
- **R**aynaud phenomenon: intermittent vasospasm of fingertips in response to cold or stress

- **E**sophageal dysfunction: difficulty swallowing because of decreased motility and internal scarring
- **S**clerodactyly: tightening of skin on fingers and toes
- **T**elangiectasia: red spots on skin from capillary dilation and spider veins

Limited and diffuse disease can lead to pulmonary complications.

Raynaud Phenomenon

For 95% of patients with scleroderma, the first symptom is Raynaud phenomenon.[41] Patients have decreased blood flow to the fingers and toes when exposed to cold or stress *(blanching or white phase)*. This vasoconstriction then causes cyanosis in the tissues *(blue phase)*. Redness then occurs during rewarming *(red phase)*. Numbness and tingling often occur. Raynaud phenomenon is discussed in Chapter 41.

Skin and Joint Changes

In diffuse disease, the skin loses elasticity and becomes taut and shiny. This causes the typical expressionless face with tightly pursed lips. Skin changes in the face may contribute to reduced ROM in the temporomandibular joint and chewing difficulty. Reduced ROM in the hands causes the fingers to stay in a semiflexed position *(sclerodactyly)*, with tightened skin to the wrist (Fig. 69.12). Skin may develop areas of hypo- and hyperpigmentation.

Internal Organ Involvement

Lung problems include pleural thickening, pulmonary fibrosis, and abnormal pulmonary function. Patients develop a cough and dyspnea. Pulmonary arterial hypertension and interstitial lung disease can occur. Lung disease is the main cause of death in SSc.

Cardiovascular effects include pericarditis, pericardial effusion, and dysrhythmias. Heart failure from myocardial fibrosis occurs. Inflammation and fibrosis in coronary arteries lead to heart attack. Treatment includes diltiazem, β-blockers, pacemakers, implantable cardiac defibrillators (ICDs), and heart transplant.

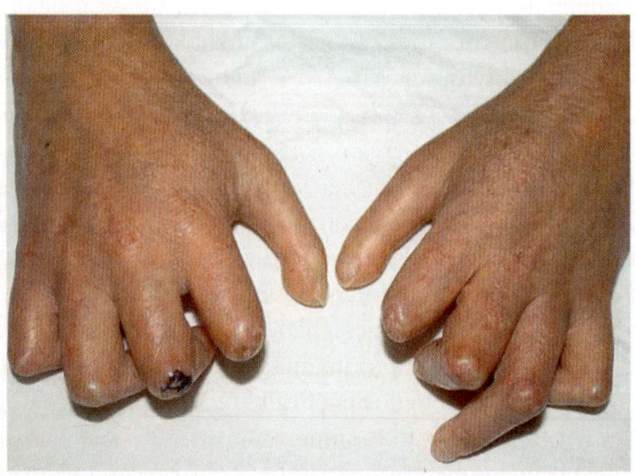

Fig. 69.12 Sclerodactyly in the hands of a patient with scleroderma. (From Bolognia JL, Schaffer JV, Duncan KO, et al: *Dermatology essentials,* ed 2, Philadelphia, 2021, Elsevier.)

Many patients take angiotensin-converting enzyme (ACE) inhibitors (e.g., lisinopril) to help control hypertension and provide renal protection. Occlusion of renal vessels causes rapidly progressive renal insufficiency and malignant hypertension. Malignant hypertension may cause headache, stroke, and seizure. Early recognition of renal involvement and initiating therapy are critical. Patients with SSc should monitor their BP at home. Dialysis and kidney transplant offer hope to patients with renal failure.

Over 20% of people with SSc develop secondary Sjögren syndrome, a condition associated with dry eyes and dry mouth. Sjögren syndrome is discussed later in this chapter.

Diagnostic Studies

No single test can diagnose scleroderma. Diagnosis is based on the manifestations found in the history and physical examination. We can measure and score skin thickness using the Modified Rodnan Skin Score.[40] If scleroderma is suspected, further antibody testing will be done. ANA is present in most patients with scleroderma. Nine other autoantibodies can be tested to determine the type. Nailfold capillary testing can be done to assess abnormal capillary beds at the edge of the cuticle. Pulmonary function tests will be done to identify pulmonary fibrosis, vital capacity, and lung compliance. Pulmonary hypertension will be assessed through ECG and right-sided heart catheterization.

Upper GI testing through endoscopy, gastric emptying studies, and esophageal pressure measurements helps identify GI complications. Serum muscle enzymes and ESR may be monitored. CBC may show mild hemolytic anemia from RBC damage. If renal involvement is present, the creatinine may be increased, and urinalysis may show proteinuria, microscopic hematuria, and casts. Kidney biopsy may be done.

Interprofessional Care

There is no specific treatment and no cure for scleroderma.[42] Supportive care is directed toward preventing or treating complications of involved organs (Table 69.19). PT helps maintain joint mobility and preserve muscle strength. OT assists with maintaining functional abilities.

Drug Therapy

Drug therapy is symptom specific. Vasoactive agents are often prescribed in early disease. Calcium channel blockers (e.g., nifedipine), angiotensin II blockers (losartan, amlodipine), and PDE-5 inhibitors (sildenafil) are common treatments for Raynaud phenomenon. Topical nitroglycerine and botulinum toxin injections may be used.

Immunosuppressants (mycophenolate, cyclophosphamide) treat fibrosis in the skin. BRMs approved to treat and delay

TABLE 69.19 Interprofessional Care
Scleroderma

Diagnostic Assessment
- History and physical assessment
- Autoantibodies to topoisomerase-1
- Anticentromere antibody
- RNA polymerase III
- Antinuclear antibody
- Nail bed capillary microscopy
- Chest x-ray
- Skin or organ biopsy
- Urinalysis (proteinuria, hematuria, casts)
- Pulmonary function tests
- ECG

Management
- Physical therapy
- Occupational therapy

Drug Therapy
- Vasoactive agents: reserpine, bosentan, epoprostenol, β-blockers
- Calcium channel blockers: diltiazem, nifedipine
- ACE inhibitors: lisinopril (Prinivil)
- PDE5 inhibitors: sildenafil, tadalafil
- Immunosuppressive drugs: cyclophosphamide, mycophenolate mofetil

pulmonary fibrosis are nintedanib (Ofev) and tocilizumab. Bosentan (Tracleer) and epoprostenol (Flolan) improve pulmonary blood flow and treat pulmonary hypertension.[42]

NSAIDs and topical agents (capsaicin) may give some relief from joint pain. Short-term oral steroids are sometimes needed. Other therapies prescribed to treat specific systemic problems include (1) loperamide for diarrhea, (2) psyllium husks for constipation, (3) H_2 receptor blockers or proton pump inhibitors for reflux, and (4) antihypertensive agents (e.g., captopril, propranolol) for hypertension. Autologous stem cell transplant and lung transplant may be used for interstitial lung disease in severe disease.[42]

NURSING MANAGEMENT: SCLERODERMA

Assess vital signs, weight, intake and output, respiratory status, bowel function, and joint ROM regularly to plan care and track changes. Avoid finger-stick blood testing because of compromised circulation and poor healing. Protect skin, as injuries will heal slowly.

Teaching is important for self-care. Encourage patients to avoid smoking because of its vasoconstricting effect. Avoid harsh soaps or contact with strong chemicals. Report signs of infection promptly. Use alcohol-free lotions to improve skin dryness and cracking. Rub lotions in for a long time to help absorption through thick skin.

Patients should regularly take part in therapeutic exercises at home to prevent skin retraction and promote vascularization. Mouth excursion (yawning with an open mouth) exercises can help with temporomandibular joint function. Isometric exercises are useful with arthropathy because no joint movement occurs. Promote low-impact exercise that supports circulation and muscle strength. Encourage the use of moist heat applications or paraffin baths to promote skin flexibility in the hands and feet. Teach patients to use assistive devices as needed. Organize activities to preserve strength.

Patients can reduce dysphagia by eating small, frequent meals; taking small bites; chewing carefully; and drinking fluids. Consultation with a dietitian is helpful. Sitting upright for 2 hours after eating decreases the risk for gastroesophageal reflux disease (GERD). Use extra pillows or raise the head of the bed on blocks to reduce reflux at night.

Job adaptations are often needed because of problems with fine motor movement. Patients may be socially withdrawn as skin tightening changes the appearance of the face and hands. Dining out may become socially embarrassing for patients because of their small mouth, swallowing difficulty, and reflux. Some persons with scleroderma wear gloves to protect fingertips and provide extra warmth. Stress daily oral hygiene to avoid dental problems. Help patients find a dentist familiar with scleroderma and limited jaw and mouth movement.[42]

Teach patients to avoid stress and cold temperatures, as these may aggravate Raynaud phenomenon. Refer patients to educational groups. Psychologic support, biofeedback training, and relaxation can reduce stress and improve sleeping habits. Sexual problems from body changes, pain, weakness, limited mobility, decreased self-esteem, erectile dysfunction, and decreased vaginal secretions may require sensitive counseling. Support patients in dealing with chronic uncurable illness and related depression and loss.

CHECK YOUR PRACTICE

A 34-year-old female patient hospitalized for aspiration pneumonia has a 5-year history of scleroderma.
- How could scleroderma have contributed to the aspiration pneumonia?
- What strategies will you suggest to decrease the risk for pneumonia recurrence?

AUTOIMMUNE MYOSITIS

Autoimmune myositis is a rare group of autoimmune disorders causing inflammation of the muscles. The 3 most common types are polymyositis, dermatomyositis, and inclusion body myositis. ***Polymyositis (PM)*** is diffuse, inflammatory myopathy of striated muscle. Bilateral weakness in the muscle groups closest to the center of the body (hips, thighs, upper arms, and neck) is the primary symptom. PM affects people 5 to 15 years and 40 to 65 years old. Inflammatory myopathy accompanied by a patchy purple or red rash is called ***dermatomyositis (DM).*** DM occurs more often in adults aged 31 to 60 and twice as often in females. It is more common in Black persons. Patients with PM tend to have more severe disease than those with DM.

Inclusion body myositis (IBM) is the most common type of myositis. IBM has an insidious onset. It occurs in males and people over age 50.[43] It may cause disability over time.

Etiology and Pathophysiology

We do not know the cause of myositis. Most patients have HLA antibody genes. Several myositis autoantibodies have been identified. Autoantibodies infiltrate the muscles and cause inflammation. Activities that cause muscle swelling (infection, strenuous exercise, injury, cocaine use) may trigger myositis in a genetically susceptible person.

Clinical Manifestations and Complications

Muscular

Patients with autoimmune myositis have gradual muscle weakness, pain, and fatigue. Myositis has flares when symptoms are exacerbated. Patients may have difficulty lifting arms, performing ADLs, rising from sitting to standing, climbing stairs, or combing hair. Repetitive movements worsen symptoms. Muscles are unable to move against resistance. Weak pharyngeal muscles can cause nasal or hoarse voice, weak cough, difficulty swallowing, and increased risk for aspiration. Patients may have contractures and dysgraphia. Weakness, fatigue, and muscle atrophy increase the risk for falls. Patients with PM may get interstitial lung disease causing fibrosis and dyspnea. Myocarditis may occur.[43]

Skin changes of DM include a classic red or purple symmetric rash *(heliotrope)* on the face, chest, back, and elbows, with edema around the eyelids. *Gottron sign* (symmetric red, scaly rash on the backs of hands or knees) or Gottron papules (red, scaly bumps) may be present in DM (Fig. 69.13). During flares patients may have Raynaud phenomenon. Dilated capillaries on the skin around the nail bed are common. Patients with DM may get painful calcium nodules (calcinosis) throughout the muscles and skin. Joint redness, pain, and inflammation occur with limited ROM of joints.

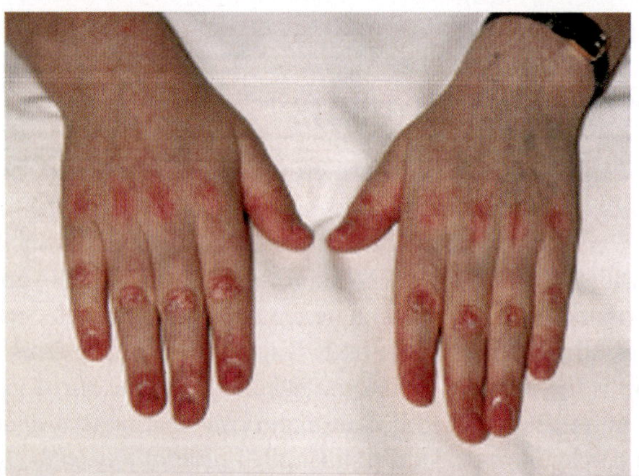

Fig. 69.13 Dermatomyositis skin changes indicating Gottron papules. (From Firestein GS, Budd RC, Gabriel SE, et al: *Kelley's textbook of rheumatology*, ed 9, Philadelphia, 2012, Saunders.)

Diagnostic Studies

Muscle biopsy is the standard for diagnosis. Muscles show degeneration and fibrosis with distinct pathologic findings for myositis. The biopsy should be taken from a muscle with weakness and edema found on MRI or electromyography (EMG). EMG measures electrical activity in the muscles. Myositis-associated autoantibodies are tested. Skin biopsy is done when characteristic lesions of DM are present. Increased muscle enzymes (e.g., aldolase, creatine kinase [CK], myoglobin, lactate dehydrogenase [LDH]) reflect muscle damage. Increased ESR or CRP occurs with active disease.

Interprofessional and Nursing Management

There is no cure. IBM does not respond to any treatment. PM and DM are treated initially with high-dose oral or IV corticosteroids. Steroids can effectively control inflammation and ease pain. Taper the dose as quickly as possible based on patient response. Most patients respond well. Long-term oral corticosteroid therapy may be needed. Serial muscle enzyme values guide treatment.

Immunosuppressive drugs (azathioprine, tacrolimus) may be used if there is no response to steroids. IV immunoglobulin (IVIG) may be used in patients resistant to other treatments.[44]

DRUG ALERT

IV Immunoglobulin

- Give slowly to decrease risk for thromboembolic complications.
- Hydrate patient well to decrease risk for thrombosis and renal failure.
- Treat transient adverse effects, such as headache.
- Premedicate with acetaminophen or diphenhydramine to prevent fever, headache, and backache.

Synthetic ACTH injections may help with muscle strength and skin rash. Exercise can strengthen muscles, reduce inflammation, and improve stamina.[44] During a flare, limit exercise to walking and achieving ADLs. Muscle strengthening is started when disease activity is low.

Teach patients about the disease, therapies, diagnostic tests, and need for regular medical care. Help them understand that the benefits of therapy are often delayed. Encourage a Mediterranean diet, with whole grain and less saturated fats. Stress avoiding processed foods with high fructose corn syrup. Decreased calories may be needed when taking corticosteroids. Calcium, vitamin D, and folic acid supplements may be necessary because of drug interactions. To prevent aspiration, encourage patients to rest before meals, maintain an upright position when eating, and choose easily swallowed foods.

Help patients use pacing to conserve energy. Encourage daily ROM exercises to prevent contractures. Bed rest may be needed during acute exacerbations because of profound muscle weakness. Use assistive devices to decrease risk for falls.

All patients should have routine chest x-rays and pulmonary function tests. Patients with DM should protect their skin from sun. Patients have an increased risk for cancer and should have appropriate screenings.

MIXED CONNECTIVE TISSUE DISEASE

Patients with a combination of clinical features from several rheumatic diseases but no definitive features of a specific disease are described as having *mixed connective tissue disease.* The term describes a disorder with features primarily of SLE, scleroderma, and PM. This disease occurs most often in females in their 20s and 30s. People with one connective tissue disease may develop another related disease over time *(overlap syndrome).* Corticosteroids and immunosuppressants are the cornerstone of medical treatment.

SJÖGREN SYNDROME

Sjögren syndrome is an autoimmune disease caused by lymphocytes attacking moisture-producing exocrine glands. This leads to *xerostomia* (dry mouth) and *keratoconjunctivitis sicca* (corneal and conjunctival inflammation and dry eyes).[45] The eyes, nose, throat, airways, and skin become dry. Other glands may be involved, including those in the stomach, pancreas, lungs, and intestines. This increases the risk for non-Hodgkin lymphoma. The disease is usually diagnosed in people over 40. Between 1 and 4 million people in the United States have Sjögren syndrome, and 90% are female.[45]

People with primary Sjögren syndrome do not have another rheumatic disease. The secondary form occurs in combination with another rheumatic disease (e.g., RA, SLE, scleroderma).[45] People with Sjögren syndrome are more likely to have autoimmune thyroid disorders. Sjögren syndrome appears to have genetic and environment origins. Genes can predispose patients to the disease. An environment trigger like a viral or bacterial infection adversely stimulates the immune system, and leukocytes attack the moisture-producing glands.

Decreased tearing causes dry eyes, which leads to a gritty sensation in the eyes, burning, blurred vision, and photosensitivity. Dry mouth causes buccal membrane fissures, changes in taste, dysphagia, and dental decay. Hoarse voice, difficulty chewing, and dry cough may result. Dry nasal passages may decrease smell and cause nosebleeds. Dry skin, rash, and joint pain may be present. Other exocrine glands can be affected. Vaginal dryness may lead to painful intercourse. As symptoms progress, lymph nodes, bone marrow, and visceral organs become involved.

Autoantibodies anti-SSA and anti-SSB are the most specific laboratory tests for Sjögren syndrome. Eye examination, including Schirmer test for tear production, assessment of salivary gland function, and biopsy of minor salivary glands, aids in diagnosis. Treatment is symptomatic. Instilling preservative-free artificial tears or antiinflammatory eye drops (e.g., cyclosporine) provides adequate hydration and lubrication. Immunosuppressant medication may be prescribed if severe disease affects organs.

Encourage increased fluids with meals. Pilocarpine (Salagen) and cevimeline (Evoxac) can ease dry mouth and decrease risk of dental caries. Toothpaste specifically for dry mouth may be used. Lotion may help dry cracked skin. Increased humidity at home may reduce respiratory infections and soothe mucous membranes. Saline nasal spray helps dry nasal membranes. Vaginal lubrication with a water-soluble product may increase comfort during intercourse.

! SAFETY ALERT

Sjögren Syndrome

To help with chewing and swallowing:

- Moisten food with mayonnaise, sauces, gravy, or yogurt.
- Thin foods with skim milk or broth.
- Finely chop or liquefy foods.
- Try soft, creamy foods (e.g., mashed potatoes, macaroni and cheese).
- Drink high-calorie cold liquids (e.g., breakfast drinks).
- Avoid salty, acidic, and spicy foods.

CHRONIC MUSCLE PAIN SYNDROMES

MYOFASCIAL PAIN SYNDROME

Myofascial pain syndrome is a chronic form of muscle pain and tenderness confined to one area in the chest, neck, shoulders, hips, or lower back. Myofascial pain syndrome is common in those 27 to 60 years old. Symptoms include aching pain, muscle stiffness, stinging or burning pain, fatigue, malaise, poor sleep, tension headaches, and postural changes (e.g., hunching, shoulder rounding, forward head posture). The regions of pain are within the *fascia* that covers skeletal muscles. Injury, overuse, stress, and anxiety form areas of tight muscle fibers called *trigger points.* Pressure on trigger points activates a characteristic pattern of pain that worsens with activity or stress. Pain is unrelenting and does not resolve with rest or massage.[46]

Diagnosis is largely by eliminating other conditions through imaging and tests. The HCP applies gentle pressure to identify tight muscle bands that trigger pain or muscle twitches.

Most treatments focus on trigger points. Interventions include cold laser (low-level light therapy), ultrasound, dry needling, transcutaneous electronic nerve stimulation (TENS), and extracorporeal shockwave therapy. Drug therapy includes NSAIDs, lidocaine patches, muscle relaxants (clonazepam, benzodiazepines), corticosteroid injections, botulinum toxin A (Botox) injections, and antidepressants.[46] Physical therapy, behavior modification, heat, massage, stretching, and acupuncture are helpful. Patients should eat a well-balanced diet, get adequate sleep, and participate in relaxation activities.

FIBROMYALGIA

Fibromyalgia (FMS) is a chronic central pain syndrome marked by widespread, nonarticular, musculoskeletal pain and fatigue with multiple tender points. FMS appears between ages 30 to 55 and affects about 5 million Americans. It is the most common cause of musculoskeletal pain in females.[47] FMS and myalgic encephalomyelitis (ME) share many features (Table 69.20).

Etiology and Pathophysiology

FMS involves abnormal processing of nociceptive pain in the CNS. PET scans of the brains of people with FMS show widespread neuroinflammation. Spinal fluid contains increased substance P. Increased neurotransmitters for pain are present in the brain. Pain is "louder" at the brain and spinal cord, and the pain threshold is lowered. Pain inhibitory pathways do not work effectively. Growth hormone, prolactin, serotonin, and tryptophan levels are low. Familial tendency in FMS points to a genetic link. FMS is not an autoimmune condition, but people with other autoimmune diseases are at greater risk. Viral infection, physical or mental illness, or trauma frequently precede FMS.[47]

Clinical Manifestations and Complications

Patients report widespread pain that fluctuates throughout the course of the day. It is difficult for them to determine whether muscles, joints, or soft tissues are the source of the pain. The pain can accompany temporomandibular joint dysfunction.

TABLE 69.20 Common Features of FMS and ME

Occurrence
Previously healthy young and middle-aged females
Etiology (Theories)
Infection, dysfunction in HPA axis, central nervous system problem
Clinical Manifestations
General musculoskeletal pain, malaise and fatigue, cognitive problems, headaches, sleep problems, depression, anxiety, fever
Disease Course
Variable intensity of symptoms, fluctuates over time
Diagnosis
No definitive laboratory tests or joint and muscle assessments
Diagnosis of exclusion
Management
Symptomatic treatment may include antidepressant drugs, such as amitriptyline and fluoxetine (Prozac)
Nondrug measures include heat, massage, regular stretching, biofeedback, stress management, and relaxation training

HPA, Hypothalamic-pituitary-adrenal.

Assessment shows pain above and below the waist and on both sides of the body. Pain is accompanied by sleep problems, fatigue, cognitive changes, and GI problems.[47] Patients with FMS have pain at 18 tender points (9 pairs) throughout the body (Fig. 69.14). Patients may have pain in response to a stimulus that does not typically cause pain *(allodynia)*. Pain varies from day to day.

Cognitive effects include difficulty concentrating, memory lapses ("fibro fog"), slowed speech, impaired judgment, and a sense of being overwhelmed when dealing with multiple tasks. Patients are less able to manage stress. Many patients have migraine headaches. Depression and anxiety often occur. Stiffness, nonrefreshing sleep, and fatigue are present. Restless legs syndrome is common.

Irritable bowel syndrome with constipation and/or diarrhea, abdominal pain, and bloating is common. Patients may have difficulty swallowing if pain sensitivity in esophageal smooth muscle is involved. Neurotransmitter changes can cause urinary frequency and urgency. Females may have menstrual pain, irregularity, and worsening symptoms of FMS during menstruation.

Diagnostic Studies

A definitive diagnosis of FMS is based on meeting established diagnostic criteria. All criteria must be met. We calculate scores on the Widespread Pain Index (WPI) and Symptom Severity Index (SSI). The WPI considers pain in 19 areas of the body over the previous week. The pain must have been present in 4 of the 5 regions of the WPI, and pain must be present for longer than 3 months. The SSI is based on ranking cognitive symptoms, fatigue, unrefreshed sleep, and other specific symptoms. To be diagnosed with FMS, patients must have a WPI score of 7 or more and an SSI score of 5 or more, or a WPI score between 3 and 6 and an SSI score of 9 or more.[47]

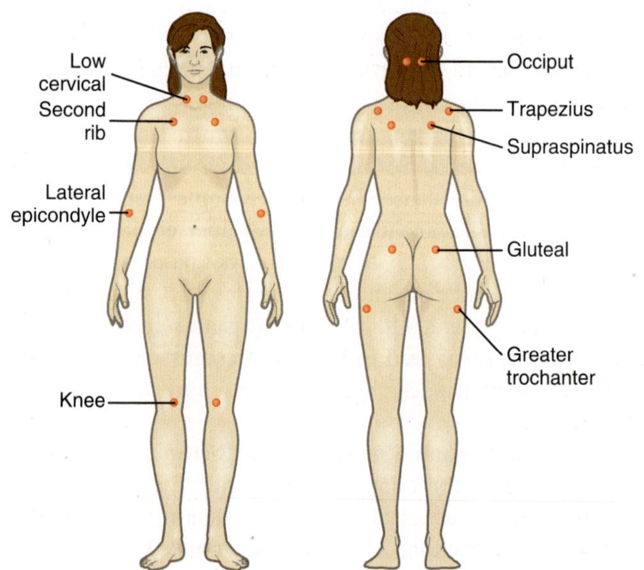

Fig. 69.14 Tender points in fibromyalgia.

Interprofessional and Nursing Management

Treatment is symptomatic. Because of the chronic nature of FMS, patients need consistent support from the health care team. A wide variety of practitioners will be involved. The treatment plan will include diet, medication, exercise, and relaxation. Encourage patients to be an active participant in treatment.

Drug therapy for the chronic widespread neurologic pain includes pregabalin (Lyrica), duloxetine, and milnacipran (Savella). Sometimes pain can be managed with acetaminophen or NSAIDs. Opioid agonists like tramadol (Ultram) may be used if other therapies are not successful. Low-dose tricyclic antidepressants and selective serotonin reuptake inhibitors (SSRIs) may be used for pain or depression. Benzodiazepines (e.g., diazepam) may help with sleep.[48] If pain is local, lidocaine injections are prescribed.

Rest can help the pain and tenderness. Sleep management is addressed in Chapter 8. Short-term use of sleep medication may be used, especially for patients with restless leg syndrome.[48]

Regular, gentle exercise and stretching (e.g., yoga, tai chi) can help maintain muscle tone and decrease pain. Low-impact aerobic exercise, such as walking, can help prevent muscle atrophy. Massage is often combined with ultrasound or alternating heat and cold packs to soothe muscles and increase circulation. Patients may have less pain and stiffness with water therapy, chiropractic treatment, or biofeedback.[48]

Plant-based and Mediterranean diets, rich in antioxidants, can be antiinflammatory. Vitamin and mineral supplements may help correct deficiencies and support immune health. Review weight loss with patients who are obese (see Chapter 45).

Chronic pain and the related symptoms of FMS can be disabling. Patients may not cope well with stress. Mental health support is critical. Psychologic counseling and support groups may be helpful. Patients need initial training for biofeedback, meditation, and cognitive-behavioral interventions, but can practice these in their own homes. Establishing a set schedule and pacing activity every day, even when symptoms are minimal, can help avoid flareups. Stress management is discussed in Chapter 7.

MYALGIC ENCEPHALOMYELITIS

Myalgic encephalomyelitis (ME), also called *chronic fatigue syndrome* or systemic exertion intolerance disease, is a long-term multisystem illness in which physical, emotional, or cognitive exertion is impaired and accompanied by profound fatigue not improved with rest. ME is poorly understood. It can have a devastating impact on the lives of patients and their families.

Over 830,000 people in the United States have ME. The condition is most common in 40- to 60-year-old adults. ME is 3 times more common in females. Black, Latino, and socioeconomically disadvantaged persons are affected more often.

Etiology and Pathophysiology

We do not know the cause or pathology of ME. Possible causes include infection, stress, altered energy production, and genetics.[49] Infectious agents implicated include Epstein-Barr virus (EBV), Ross River virus, *Coxiella burnetii,* and long COVID. ME may also be caused by an altered immune response.

Diagnostic Studies

Diagnosis is made by identifying specific core symptoms and ruling out other possible causes. No laboratory test can diagnose ME or measure its severity. Baseline laboratory work is done to rule out other causes of the symptoms. Patients may become angry and frustrated with HCPs who cannot diagnose a problem. Table 69.21 lists diagnostic criteria for ME.

Clinical Manifestations

ME has 5 major symptoms (Table 69.21). Fatigue is the most common symptom. Patients have postexertional malaise (PEM). They may need a nap or bed rest after any exertion. These symptoms after activity are called a "crash." It may take a week or more to rebound from a crash. Symptoms vary in intensity and may get better or worse in cycles. ME can arise suddenly in a previously active, healthy person. People with ME are not able to do their usual activities and may be confined to bed. Difficulty concentrating and thinking, pain, and dizziness may be present.[49]

Interprofessional and Nursing Management

No definitive treatment exists for ME. Supportive care is essential. NSAIDs can be used to treat headaches, muscle and joint aches, and fever (see Table 12.5). Antianxiety agents may be used if needed. Tricyclic antidepressants (e.g., doxepin, amitriptyline) and SSRIs (e.g., fluoxetine,

TABLE 69.21 Diagnostic Criteria *ME*

Diagnosis of ME requires that the patient have the following 3 symptoms:

1. Fatigue: Impaired ability to engage in preillness level of social, educational, occupational, or other activities. This lasts more than 6 months with fatigue that is not relieved by rest.
2. Malaise after exertion: Patients have worsening symptoms/exhaustion after even minor physical or cognitive exertion, a "crash."
3. Unrefreshing sleep: Patients are tired after a full night's sleep.

At least 1 of the following is required:

1. Cognitive impairment ("brain fog," confusion): problem solving and thinking worsen with exertion or stress.
2. Orthostatic intolerance (lightheadedness, dizziness, imbalance, fainting): symptoms worsen when the patient assumes an upright position.

paroxetine) can be used if depression occurs. They may improve mood and sleep. Clonazepam is an option for sleep difficulty. Stimulants such as methylphenidate may help memory and concentration.

Patients should avoid total bed rest because of self-image and the complications of immobility, but exertion increases exhaustion. Patients should stay within their identified energy limits and pace themselves throughout the day. Daily activities like brushing teeth, bathing, or meal preparation can trigger an episode of PEM. Keeping an activity journal can help identify personal limits. Patients should take part in a planned exercise program. Encourage a well-balanced diet, including fiber and antioxidant-rich fresh fruits and vegetables. Behavior therapy may promote a positive mood and improve fatigue.

Patients may need help with ADLs. Many patients face loss of employment and economic security. Loss of a job often leads to loss of medical insurance. The challenges in receiving a definitive diagnosis can make obtaining disability benefits difficult. Patients with ME may have severe psychosocial losses, including social pressure and isolation from an inability to participate or being labeled as lazy.

ME does not progress. Most patients show improvement and recovery over 6 months to a year. Some do not have any improvement.

CASE STUDY

Axial Spondylitis

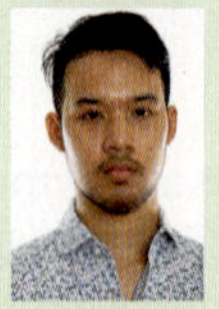

(© Ranta Images/ iStock.com.)

Patient Profile

R.B., a 34-year-old male, comes to the rheumatology clinic with low back pain. He states he has had early morning stiffness that started in the lower back 6 months ago. He says it is interfering with his work, as he "can't move like he used to." He reports aching pain at 6 out of 10 most days.

Subjective Data

- Taking acetaminophen, with minimal relief
- Father diagnosed with psoriatic arthritis 15 years ago
- Expresses concern about continued employment because of increasing pain

Objective Data

Physical Assessment

- Severely limited spinal flexion
- Moderate pain over sacroiliac joints
- Mild sternal tenderness

Diagnostic Studies

- Positive ESR, HLA-B27
- Left sacroiliac sclerosis on MRI

Interprofessional Care

- Diagnosed with axial spondylitis
- Started on etanercept subcutaneously once per week and meloxicam once daily

Discussion Questions

1. ***Recognize:*** How will you explain the pathophysiology of AS to R.B.?
2. ***Analyze:*** R.B. asks you how he could get this disorder. What findings are present in his history, physical, and diagnostic testing that indicate increased susceptibility?
3. ***Plan:*** What referrals may R.B. need?
4. ***Prioritize:*** Based on the assessment data presented, what are the priority clinical problems?
5. ***Act:*** What are some home and work modifications you can suggest to R.B. to promote self-care?
6. ***Act:*** He asks if he should exercise or rest when he is in pain. Why is an exercise program important in the treatment plan for R.B.?
7. ***Evaluate:*** What outcomes would indicate interprofessional care was effective?
8. ***Safety:*** What safety concerns does R.B. have because of his treatment plan?

Answers available at http://evolve.elsevier.com/Lewis/medsurg.

BRIDGE TO NCLEX EXAMINATION

The number of the question corresponds to the same-numbered outcome at the beginning of the chapter.

1. What comment shows a patient understands teaching about how RA causes the joint changes in the hands?
   - **a.** "Enzymes created by my body cause the cartilage to break down and erode into the bone. New bone growth causes bone spurs."
   - **b.** "Anti-dsDNA and anticoagulant antibodies attack the cells in my joints and other tissues, leading to joint and organ dysfunction."
   - **c.** "My kidneys cannot excrete uric acid, so this builds up in the blood and tissue. The uric acid makes crystals that cause swelling, redness, and pain."
   - **d.** "I have autoantibodies attacking my tissues. This causes inflammation that can destroy cartilage and bone and give me deformity in my joints."
2. What health promotion activities will the nurse teach a patient with newly diagnosed osteoarthritis? (**Select all that apply.**)
   - **a.** Weight management
   - **b.** Avoiding joint injury
   - **c.** Regular moderate exercise
   - **d.** Managing fever and autoimmune fatigue
   - **e.** Proper body mechanics and joint alignment
3. A patient with an inflamed great toe on the right foot is in the clinic for an acute gout flare. What medication will the nurse expect to administer?
   - **a.** Allopurinol
   - **b.** Prednisone
   - **c.** Colchicine
   - **d.** Febuxostat

4. A patient with psoriasis is in the rheumatology clinic with throbbing pain and reduced movement of the distal phalangeal joints of the right hand. The HCP diagnosed psoriatic arthritis and ordered infliximab. What is the priority concern when planning care?
   a. Fatigue
   b. Pain at injection site
   c. Electrolyte imbalance
   d. Immune suppression
5. Which assessment findings would support the diagnosis of systemic lupus erythematosus? **(Select all that apply.)**
   a. Fatigue
   b. Jaundice
   c. Pain on respiration
   d. Intractable headaches
   e. Red rash across bridge of nose and cheeks
6. Which patient statement would require further clarification after teaching a patient newly diagnosed with fibromyalgia?
   a. I will walk for a mile daily and do tai chi twice a week.
   b. Taking pregabalin regularly should help control my pain.
   c. Drinking 3 or 4 cups of coffee a day will lessen the fatigue.
   d. Amitriptyline will help with the depression I am experiencing.

1. d; 2. a, b, c, e; 3. c; 4. d; 5. a, c, d, e; 6. c.

For rationales to these answers and even more NCLEX review questions, visit http://evolve.elsevier.com/Lewis/medsurg.

REFERENCES

To access the References for this chapter, please scan the QR code with a mobile device.

CASE STUDY

Applying Clinical Judgment With Multiple Patients

You are working on the medical-surgical unit and have been assigned to care for the following 4 patients. You have an AP who is helping another nurse and you.

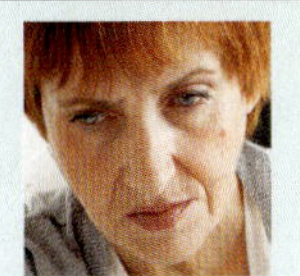	J.K. is a 57-year-old female who had debulking surgery for a temporal-parietal glioblastoma. Four days ago, she had a hemorrhagic stroke into the site of the tumor bed extending into the thalamus. Has left homonymous hemianopsia. Left arm weakness (3/5) greater than leg weakness (4/5). Vital signs: 150/90, 68, RR 20.
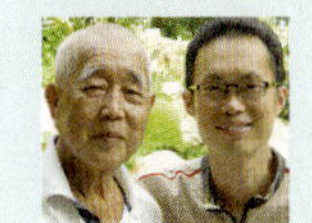	T.Y., a 78-year-old male, had an open reduction and internal fixation (ORIF) 2 days ago for a fractured left hip. He has a 3-year history of Alzheimer disease and is confused to place and time. He has been slightly agitated. He has a personal alarm and bed alarm on for safety. His hip dressing is dry and intact, and the drainage in the Hemovac drain is minimal.
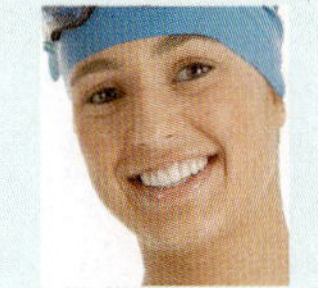	S.W. is an 18-year-old female with a C5 spinal cord injury. After spending 1 week in an inpatient rehabilitation facility, she was admitted this morning with severe headaches. She is reporting periodic blurred vision and nausea. Vital signs: 164/94, 84, RR 18.
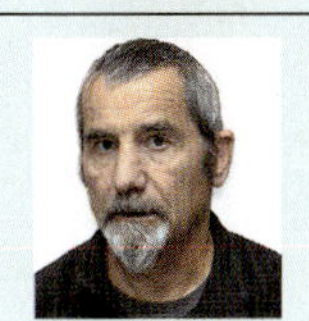	M.C. is a 64-year-old male who had a right proximal femur fracture at the greater trochanter with loss of fixation in the femoral part of a total hip arthroplasty (THA) he had previously. He had surgery 3 days ago, and discharge is planned today.

1. Highlight all the findings that require your follow-up.
2. After receiving report, which patient should you see first? Why?
3. Which tasks could you delegate to the AP? **(Select all that apply.)**
   a. Explain discharge instructions to M.C.
   b. Change the dressing on T.Y.'s left hip.
   c. Obtain vital signs on M.C. before discharge.
   d. Assist S.W. with hygienic care and repositioning.
   e. Assess J.K.'s ability to swallow before feeding her breakfast.
4. When you enter the room to assess S.W., you find her diaphoretic with a flushed face and pale extremities. Her BP is 200/102 mm Hg.

Use an X for the nursing actions listed that are indicated (appropriate or necessary), contraindicated (could be harmful), or nonessential (makes no difference or not necessary) at this time.

Nursing Action	Indicated	Contraindicated
Assess for the presence of any noxious stimuli.		
Direct the AP to stay with S.W. while you contact the HCP.		
Obtain a STAT bladder scan.		
Administer as-needed oral hypertensive medication.		
Place the head of the bed flat.		
Obtain repeat BP measurements.		

CASE STUDY—cont'd

Applying Clinical Judgment With Multiple Patients

Case Study Progression

S.W.'s bladder scan showed 700 mL of urine. Her symptoms subside after you catheterize her. You take this time to teach S.W. about autonomic dysreflexia. You discuss bladder training strategies and how to avoid bladder distention. S.W. is grateful for the information and your caring attitude. As you are finishing, the AP tells you that T.Y. has pulled out his Hemovac drain.

5. What should be your *initial* intervention for T.Y.?
   a. Reinsert the Hemovac drain.
   b. Assess the incision site for a hematoma.
   c. Notify T.Y.'s HCP that the drain was removed.
   d. Apply pressure to the site where the drain was placed.
6. You receive T.Y.'s morning laboratory results and compare them with the day prior.

Laboratory Results

	Postop Day 1	Postop Day 2
RBC	$4.8 \times 10^6/\mu L$	$4.9 \times 10^6/\mu L$
WBC	5000	11,800
Platelets	180,000 µ/L	170,000 µ/L
Hemoglobin	Hgb 10.9 g/dL	Hgb 10.4 g/dL
Hematocrit	Hct 41.2%	Hct 38.2%
Glucose	132 mg/dL	142 mg/dL
INR	1.3	1.4

Choose the most *likely* option for the information missing from statement that follows by selecting from the lists of options provided.

Based on the laboratory results, you determine T.Y. may be experiencing the priority problem of ______**1**______. To manage this problem, you expect that the HCP will order _____**2**_____.

Options for 1	Options for 2
Anemia with hypovolemia	Antibiotic therapy
Hyperglycemia	Blood transfusion
Infection	Insulin

7. As you are preparing J.K.'s medications, the electronic health record (EHR) system alerts you that patient teaching has yet to be documented for some of her medications. For each medication, select the most likely option for drug classification and patient teaching.

Medication	Drug Classification	Patient Teaching
Furosemide	Loop diuretic	Take this medication at bedtime
	Potassium-sparing diuretic	Limit oral fluid intake to 1000 mL/day
	Thiazide diuretic	Include foods high in potassium in the diet
Nimodipine	Calcium-channel blocker	Report a night cough or slowed pulse to the HCP
	ACE inhibitor	This drug may lower blood glucose levels
	Angiotensin receptor blocker	Take on an empty stomach
Phenytoin	Serotonin receptor agonist	Maintain good oral hygiene.
	Antiseizure agent	Report the new onset of signs of depression.
	Antineoplastic	Avoid persons who have an infection.

8. Which intervention would be *most* appropriate in caring for J.K.?
   a. Place her left arm in a sling for support.
   b. Arrange the food tray so that all foods are on the right side.
   c. Position her left leg so that the ankle is lower than the knee.
   d. Call the provider to get an order of warfarin to prevent VTE.
9. As you enter M.C.'s room to discuss his discharge plans, you find him all packed up and ready to go. He tells you the AP already told him what he needed to do. What is your *best* initial action?
   a. Ask M.C. if he has any further questions.
   b. Call the AP to M.C.'s room to find out what she told him.
   c. Review discharge instructions with M.C. to ascertain correct understanding.
   d. Give M.C. a telephone number to call in case he has any concerns when he gets home.

Answers and rationales available at http://evolve.elsevier.com/Lewis/medsurg.

INDEX

Disorder names and key terms are in **boldface**. Page numbers in **boldface** indicate main discussions. Page numbers followed by *b*, *f*, or *t* indicate boxes, figures, or tables, respectively.

B

C

F

O

Q

R

S

U

X

Y

Z